Intensive Care Medicine

Intensive Care

Medicine

*Third Edition
Volume II*

Edited by

James M. Rippe, M.D.
Associate Professor of Medicine, Tufts University School of Medicine, Boston; Director, The Center for Clinical and Lifestyle Research, Shrewsbury, Massachusetts

Richard S. Irwin, M.D.
Professor of Medicine, University of Massachusetts Medical School; Director, Division of Pulmonary, Allergy, and Critical Care Medicine, University of Massachusetts Medical Center, Worcester, Massachusetts

Mitchell P. Fink, M.D.
Johnson & Johnson Professor of Surgery, Harvard Medical School; Surgeon-in-Chief, Beth Israel Hospital, Boston

Frank B. Cerra, M.D.
Dean of the Medical School and Professor of Surgery and Clinical Pharmacy, University of Minnesota Medical School—Minneapolis

Little, Brown and Company
Boston / New York / Toronto / London

Library of Congress Cataloging-in-Publication Data

Intensive care medicine / edited by James M. Rippe . . . [et al.] — 3rd ed.
    p.   cm.
  Includes bibliographical references and index.
  ISBN 0-316-74732-7 (vol. 1). — ISBN 0-316-74731-9 (vol. 2). — ISBN 0-316-74728-9 (set)
  1. Critical care medicine.   I. Rippe, James M.
    [DNLM: 1. Critical Care.   2. Intensive Care Units.   WX 218 I60424 1996]
  RC86.7.I555   1996
  616′.028—dc20
  DNLM/DLC
  for Library of Congress   95-33188
                                                                        CIP

Volume I ISBN 0-316-74732-7
Volume II ISBN: 0-316-74731-9
Set ISBN: 0-316-74728-9

Printed in the United States of America
MV-NY

Editorial: Nancy E. Chorpenning, Robert J. Stuart
Development Editor: Julie M. Jewell
Production Services: Ruttle, Shaw & Wetherill, Inc.
Copyeditors: Jane Grochowski, Julie Gillman, Peg Markow, Tina Rebane, Dana Singer
Cover Designer: Louis C. Bruno, Jr.

To our families
Stephanie, Diane, Rachel, Sara, Jamie, Rebecca,
Jan, Emily, Matthew, Kathie, Nicole, Christa, and Josh

Contents

VIII. Endocrine Problems in the Intensive Care Unit

IX. Hematologic Problems in the Intensive Care Unit

Volume II
X. Overdoses and Poisonings

XI. Surgical Problems in the Intensive Care Unit

XII. Shock and Trauma

XIII. Neurologic Problems in the Intensive Care Unit

XIV. Transplantation

XV. Metabolism and Nutrition

XVI. Pharmacokinetics and Pharmacodynamics

XVII. Dermatologic, Rheumatologic, and Immunologic Problems in the Intensive Care Unit

XVIII. Psychiatric Issues in Intensive Care

XIX. Moral, Ethical, Legal, and Public Policy Issues in the Intensive Care Unit

Notice

The indications and dosages of all drugs in this book have been recommended in the medical literature and conform to the practices of the general medical community. The medications described do not necessarily have specific approval by the Food and Drug Administration for use in the diseases and dosages for which they are recommended. The package insert for each drug should be consulted for use and dosage as approved by the FDA. Because standards for usage change, it is advisable to keep abreast of revised recommendations, particularly those concerning new drugs.

X. Overdoses and Poisonings

Section Editors
Christopher H. Linden and Cynthia K. Aaron

128. General Considerations in the Evaluation and Treatment of Poisoning

Christopher H. Linden

Introduction and Terminology

A poison is a chemical that is capable of producing harmful or toxic effects on a biologic system. The term *toxin* was originally restricted to poisons of animal or plant origin. In common usage, poisons are chemicals or chemical products that are distinctly harmful to humans. Their presence in or on the human body, even in small amounts, is typically associated with undesirable effects. Chemicals generally recognized as unfit for human consumption include cleaning agents, industrial chemicals, herbicides, pesticides, nonedible plants, petroleum distillates, and venoms. In contrast, other chemicals are generally regarded as nontoxic and some are essential for the maintenance or restoration of normal body function. Chemicals usually considered safe for external or internal human consumption include cosmetics, drugs, foods, vitamins, and toiletries. In reality, all chemicals, even those essential for life, such as oxygen and water, are potentially harmful, and the presence or absence of adverse effects depends more on the conditions of exposure than the identity of the chemical. By limiting the dose, chemicals usually thought of as poisons can be rendered harmless. Conversely, the use of ordinarily safe chemicals in excessive amounts or by an inappropriate route can result in harmful effects.

Precise terminology should be used to describe chemically related events. *Poisoning* implies that potentially harmful effects have resulted from a chemical exposure: it is a particular form of adverse chemical reaction in which *adverse* effects are concentration- or dose-related. Such effects may be generalized (i.e., systemic) or limited to exposed body surfaces (i.e., local). They can be objective (e.g., behavioral, biochemical, cognitive, or physiologic abnormalities detected) or subjective (i.e., symptoms only). *Adverse chemical reactions* also include predictable but unwanted *side effects, secondary effects,* and *chemical interactions* and unpredictable *allergic, intolerance,* and *"idiosyncratic"* (i.e., undefined and presumably pharmacogenetic) reactions. In the absence of signs or symptoms, external or internal body contact with a potentially harmful amount of a chemical is merely an *exposure*. An *overdose* is an excessive exposure to a chemical that in specified (e.g., therapeutic) amounts is normally intended for human use. It most commonly denotes excessive drug ingestion. An exposure is not necessarily an overdose; it may simply be an unwanted event. Similarly, an overdose may or may not result in poisoning.

Poisonings, exposures, and overdoses may be characterized by the route, duration, and intent of exposure. Ingestion, dermal or ophthalmic contact, inhalation, and parenteral injection (including bites and stings) are the most common routes but rectal, urethral, vaginal, bladder, peritoneal, intraocular, and intrathecal exposures can also occur. Events that occur once or during a short period of time are considered acute, whereas those that occur repeatedly or over a prolonged time interval are said to be chronic. Intentions can vary with respect to exposure and outcome, and the designation of a particular occurrence as accidental or deliberate sometimes involves value judgments. Events due to unforeseeable circumstances (e.g.,

chemical spills, industrial accidents, environmental contamination), normal childhood behavior (e.g., environmental exploration by tasting), and mistaken chemical identification (e.g., product label missing, not read, or misread) are clearly accidental. In contrast, exposures due to chemical abuse (i.e., for psychotropic effects), addiction, and failure to appreciate the consequences of exposure (e.g., uninformed vocational or avocational use of chemicals; self-medication) are intentional but the induction of harmful effects is not. Hence, if poisoning ensues, it is generally considered accidental. Overdoses and poisonings due to "therapeutic misadventures" (e.g., dosing errors, failure to monitor routinely for adverse reactions or excessive drug concentrations) are usually considered accidental, whereas those due to excessive exposure for the purpose of self-harm (e.g., Münchausen's syndrome, attempted suicide) or for achieving a greater or more rapid therapeutic effect (i.e., misuse) are generally regarded as intentional. Events resulting from chemically induced abortion, attempted murder, child abuse, or product tampering can be considered accidental or intentional depending on whether the perspective is that of the victim or the perpetrator.

Epidemiology

Although comprehensive data regarding the true extent of potentially harmful or unwanted chemical exposure are not available [1], it is clearly a significant medical problem [2–8]. Excluding ethanol and smoke inhalation, an estimated 5 to 10 million such exposures occur in the United States each year. These events are responsible for an average of 5 percent of all emergency department visits, ambulance transportations, and adult medical intensive care unit (ICU) admissions and 2 to 5 percent of pediatric hospital admissions. In addition, 25 percent of routine medical admissions involve some form of drug-related adverse patient event (an adverse drug reaction or noncompliance) and up to 30 percent of acute psychiatric admissions are prompted by attempted self-harm via chemical exposure. Although the incidence of poisoning in children has decreased since introduction of the Poison Prevention Packaging Act in 1970 [9], the overall incidence of poisoning is increasing, particularly that due to suicide attempts in teens, middle-aged adults, and the elderly.

Of exposures reported to poison centers, most are acute (99%), occur in the patient's home (92%), are accidental (87%), cause minor or no harmful effects (83%), result from ingestion (76%), and involve children younger than 6 years of age (60%) [10]. Pharmaceutical preparations are involved in 40 percent of these exposures. The chemicals most frequently involved are cleaning agents, analgesics, cosmetics, plants, and cough and cold preparations. Those most often responsible for fatal poisoning are analgesics, antidepressants, sedative-hypnotics, stimulants and street drugs, cardiovascular medications, alcohols and glycols, gases and fumes, asthma therapies, inorganic chemicals, hydrocarbons, cleaning agents, and pesticides.

Poisoning is second only to firearms as the leading cause of suicide [11,12]. It is estimated that 30,000 people commit suicide by this method in the United States each year and that drugs or alcohol are involved in two-thirds of all suicides. Eighty percent of poisoning fatalities are "coroner's cases." Since the victims are clearly dead when discovered, they are not admitted to the hospital nor included in poison center statistics. Carbon monoxide is the most common cause of poisoning reported by medical examiners. Poisoned patients admitted to ICUs are typically adolescents or young adults with intentional ingestions of more than one chemical. The mortality rate for hospitalized patients is 1 to 2 percent.

Pharmacologic Concepts

Familiarity with mechanisms of chemical action, chemical disposition (pharmacokinetics), and concentration-effect and dose-response relationships (pharmacodynamics) is essential to predict the effect of a particular chemical exposure and hence determine the appropriate treatment and disposition. Only a brief overview of these concepts is presented here. The reader is referred to Chapter 205 and to other sources [3–20] for additional information.

MECHANISMS OF CHEMICAL ACTION. The ability of a particular chemical to cause local poisoning, systemic poisoning, or both depends on its chemical reactivity, physical characteristics, and ability to interact with components of cells or cell membranes. Chemicals that are highly reactive or corrosive (e.g., strong acids and alkali, desiccants, fixatives, oxidizing and reducing agents, potent organic solvents) are nonselective and can disrupt the integrity and function of all cells. Because of their high reactivity, however, they act primarily at surface sites and undergo little if any absorption. In contrast, most chemicals (or their metabolites) that cause systemic poisoning are absorbed and act by binding to and disrupting the function of specific enzymes, proteins, membrane lipids, or neurohumoral receptors. Their effects may be generalized or limited to a specific organ or tissue, depending on the distribution and location of target sites. Systemic poisoning can sometimes occur, however, in the absence of significant chemical absorption (e.g., anoxia due to asphyxia or pulmonary injury, acidosis and shock secondary to localized but severe tissue necrosis).

CHEMICAL ABSORPTION. The absorption of chemicals into the bloodstream involves their translocation across the membranes of cells that make up mucosal surfaces, pulmonary epithelium, and skin, all of which function as biologic barriers to chemical movement. Translocation occurs by filtration or passive diffusion through gaps or pores in membranes (e.g., small molecules), by dissolving in and diffusing through the membrane itself (e.g., lipid-soluble chemicals), or by attaching to "carrier" molecules in the membrane, which actively or passively facilitate diffusion (e.g., water-soluble chemicals). In general, only chemicals that are small (i.e., <4 nm in diameter), have low molecular weight (i.e., <50 d), and are soluble in both water and lipids at the pH of body fluids (in either neutral or ionized states) can readily cross membranes.

The rate and extent of absorption depend on the route of exposure as well as chemical factors. Absorption following intravenous (IV) injection is complete and almost instantaneous. Peak arterial and venous blood concentrations occur within 30 to 90 seconds. The absorption of chemicals by other routes tends to follow *first-order kinetics*: the amount of chemical absorbed per unit of time is directly proportional to its external or extravascular concentration. **Threshold tissue concentrations, and hence the *onset* of effects, are usually noted *sooner* after an overdose than after a therapeutic dose.** The rate of pulmonary absorption of gases and vapors increases as their partial pressure increases and is inversely related to their molecular weight (Fick's law). Pulmonary absorption is rapid but incomplete. Blood concentrations peak (i.e., reach an equilibrium with alveolar concentrations) within seconds to minutes. The absorption of chemicals following intramuscular (IM) or subcutaneous (SC) injection is slower but complete. Peak blood levels generally occur within an hour of administration. Both the rate and extent of absorption following ingestion are variable. Peak blood levels are typically noted within 0.5 to 2 hours of a therapeutic dose. The absorbed dose is proportional but not necessarily equal to the one administered (see Chap. 205 for a discussion of bioavailability). The rate and extent of absorption following contact with other mucosal surfaces (e.g., oral, nasal, ophthalmic, rectal) is similar, but skin absorption, if it occurs at all, is usually considerably slower.

The dissolution of particulate material is generally the rate-limiting step in gastrointestinal (GI) absorption. Hence, chemicals in pill, solid, and suppository forms are generally absorbed more slowly than liquids, powders, or suspensions. Slow dissolution also accounts for the delayed and prolonged absorption of enteric-coated tablets (e.g., aspirin, potassium), sustained-release preparations (e.g., cardiovascular drugs, lithium, phenytoin, theophylline), and drugs that tend to form concretions (e.g., ethchlorvynol, glutethimide, iron, lithium, meprobamate, and salicylates). It is also responsible for the long duration of action of intramuscular "depot" formulations (e.g., neuroleptics). Poor water solubility accounts for the slow absorption of some agents (e.g., carbamazepine and digoxin). **Since the time required for dissolution and solvation increases as the amount and concentration of ingested chemical increase, absorption takes longer and *peak* effects tend to occur *later* following an overdose than they do after a therapeutic dose.**

Ingested chemicals are predominantly absorbed from the small intestine rather than the stomach, since it has a larger surface area. Hence, absorption can also be delayed or prolonged as a result of decreased gastric emptying or bowel activity caused by the presence of food, disease, or the effects of previously absorbed chemicals (e.g., anticholinergics, opioids, sedative-hypnotics, salicylates). Food or other chemicals may also decrease chemical absorption by binding the chemical within the gut lumen or competitively inhibiting its dissolution and translocation. In addition, absorption may be decreased if intestinal motility is excessive.

CHEMICAL DISTRIBUTION. Chemicals are first distributed within the blood. They are subsequently delivered to and taken up by other body parts at a rate determined by the blood flow of individual organs and tissues and their ease of movement across internal membranes. During distribution, chemicals may encounter and become bound to (i.e., inactivated by) endogenous nontarget molecules (e.g., serum proteins). The final distribution of chemical is uneven and reflects its affinity for active and inactive binding sites and the locations of such sites. It is also influenced by biologic variables such as age, sex, weight, and disease states as they relate to body composition (e.g., water, fat, muscle content) and serum protein concentrations. Since distribution is also a translocation process, it is influenced by the same chemical characteristics as absorption and hence follows first-order kinetics. Distribution generally occurs much faster than absorption, as evidenced by the occurrence of peak effects within minutes following IV injection of most chemicals. For some agents (e.g., digitalis, heavy metals, lithium, and salicylates), however, distribution is slow, requiring a number of hours. The extent of distribution of a chemical is reflected by its apparent volume of distribution (V_d), measured in liters per kilogram of body weight, and calculated most simply by dividing the amount of chemical in the body (i.e., the absorbed bioavailable dose) by its plasma concentration (see Chap. 205).

TOXICODYNAMICS. The severity of poisoning reflects the concentration of a chemical at its site(s) of action and is proportional to the dose. For external body surface and inhalational exposures, the duration of exposure also must be considered. Since plasma concentrations of systemically absorbed chemicals are also proportional to the dose, they are sometimes used to assess the severity of poisoning. However, the ability to measure chemical concentrations is often limited and plasma and target site chemical concentrations are not always in steady-state equilibrium. When distribution and redistribution occur more slowly than absorption (e.g., after IV administration, inhalational exposure, and with ingested agents with slow distribution) or more slowly than elimination (e.g., after extracorporeal removal), plasma chemical levels may be relatively higher or lower, respectively, than those in tissue, and they may not accurately correlate with the severity of poisoning. In addition, age, genetic influences, tolerance, underlying disease, and the presence or absence of other chemicals may have synergistic or antagonistic effects and also influence the response to a given level of chemical exposure.

Since overdose studies cannot ethically be performed in humans and animal data may not be available or applicable to humans, relationships between dose or plasma concentration of a chemical and the magnitude of chemical effect are well characterized only for therapeutic doses of a small number of pharmaceutical agents. Prediction of severity following an overdose must therefore be based on toxicodynamic data extrapolated from previously published reports of human poisonings. Unfortunately, such data are often incomplete or altogether unavailable and are always limited by the accuracy of the overdose history.

CHEMICAL ELIMINATION. Elimination of chemicals from the body (detoxification) can be accomplished by urinary, pulmonary, GI, and glandular (e.g., bile, milk, tears, saliva, sweat) excretion or metabolic inactivation. Hepatic metabolism and renal excretion are the major routes of elimination for most chemicals. Pulmonary excretion also plays a major role in the elimination of gases and volatile chemicals.

Elimination generally follows first-order kinetics and can be described by half-life. For some chemicals, however, hepatic metabolism has a finite capacity (i.e., becomes "saturated") and proceeds at a constant rate. This usually occurs only when plasma chemical concentrations are high (Michaelis-Menton kinetics) but can sometimes occur when they are low (zero-order kinetics). When metabolism is saturable and also the primary route of elimination, a small increase in the dose of a chemical can result in a large increase in its plasma and target site concentrations and potential poisoning. Examples of chemicals with saturable metabolism are alcohols, phenytoin, salicylate, and theophylline. Renal excretion is also accomplished by translocation processes (e.g., glomerular filtration, tubular secretion, and reabsorption) and is therefore influenced by the same factors as absorption and distribution. Any condition that impairs hepatic or renal blood flow or function can decrease

chemical elimination (see Chaps. 205 and 206). Metabolic enzymes are also subject to genetic influences and to induction or inhibition resulting from past or current chemical exposures.

Chemical elimination half-lives range from minutes to days but are most often 2 to 24 hours. The duration of effects of a chemical is usually directly proportional to its half-life. Regardless of the mechanism and kinetics of elimination, however, the time for chemical elimination increases as the plasma concentration increases. **Hence, the *duration* of effects tends to be *longer* following an overdose than following a therapeutic dose.**

Many chemicals have metabolites that remain active and contribute to their toxicity following overdosage. Some chemicals undergo metabolic activation, resulting in the production of compounds that are more toxic than the parent one. Examples of chemicals whose metabolites are primarily responsible for poisoning are acetaminophen, ethylene glycol, chlorinated hydrocarbons, meperidine, methanol, paraquat, and some organophosphate insecticides.

OTHER CONSIDERATIONS. Details regarding the disposition and effects of specific chemicals can be found in other chapters and references [4,18,21–26]. Since pharmacokinetic parameters and pharmacodynamic relationships depend on biologic variables, they are distributed (with respect to dose) according to a normal (gaussian) curve within the human population. Numeric values reported in the literature generally refer to population means following the administration of therapeutic doses to healthy subjects. In a particular individual, especially after an overdose, the disposition of and response to a chemical dose may deviate significantly from the norm. Hence, although knowledge of a chemical's pharmacology is important, there will always be some degree of uncertainty when attempting to predict the consequences of exposure in an individual patient.

Poisoning is usually reversible on elimination of the offending chemical. However, if normal activity of the target site is essential for cell viability, chemical exposure may result in irreversible cell or tissue destruction. Although organ systems usually have an excess or reserve functional capacity, if enough cells are affected their function may be permanently impaired. If the damaged organ system is essential for life and its function cannot be artificially maintained, death may ensue. Commonly encountered chemicals that can cause permanent or fatal tissue damage include acetaminophen, carbon monoxide, corrosives, ethylene glycol, heavy metals, methanol, and neurotoxic hydrocarbons.

Clinical Considerations

MANAGEMENT GOALS AND PRIORITIES. The principal objectives in the diagnosis and evaluation of the patient exposed to a chemical are (1) recognition of poisoning, (2) identification of the offending chemical or chemicals, (3) prediction of potential toxicity, and (4) assessment of severity of poisoning. Treatment objectives include (1) provision of supportive care, (2) prevention of chemical absorption, (3) prevention or reversal of poisoning by the use of antidotes, (4) enhancement of chemical elimination, (5) safe disposition, and (6) prevention of subsequent exposures. Accurate diagnostic evaluation is a prerequisite for optimal management.

The priority of assessment and treatment objectives depends on the phase of poisoning [27,28,29]. During the *induction* or *preclinical phase* (i.e., the time between exposure and the onset of clinical or laboratory evidence of toxicity), the priorities are chemical identification, prediction of toxicity, and prevention of absorption (i.e., decontamination). The sooner decontamination is accomplished, the greater its efficacy. Hence, the history, physical examination, and gathering of ancillary test data should initially be brief. Assessment should be directed at determining whether decontamination is indicated (i.e., whether poisoning is likely to ensue).

During the *toxic phase* (i.e., the time between the onset of toxicity and its peak), assessment of the severity of poisoning, provision of supportive care, administration of antidotes, prevention of further chemical absorption, and enhancement of chemical elimination are the primary objectives. If marked vital sign, cardiac rhythm, or mental status abnormalities are present, physical examination should be limited to a general survey and the history and diagnostic evaluation deferred or conducted concurrently with treatment. As always, resuscitation and stabilization of vital signs are the highest priority.

During the *detoxification* or *resolution phase* (i.e., the time between peak toxicity and full recovery), continued supportive care, antidotal therapy, enhancement of elimination, and reassessment of severity (i.e., evaluation of the response to treatment) are the highest priorities. Measures to prevent subsequent reexposure should also be initiated before discharge.

The recognition of poisoning and chemical identification are detailed in Chapter 129. Other management objectives are discussed in the following sections.

PREDICTION OF POTENTIAL TOXICITY.

The prediction of toxicity requires knowledge of the dose and time of exposure as well as the identity of the chemical. For commercial products, the amount and concentration of every ingredient should be identified. Products deemed hazardous by the U.S. Consumer Product Safety Committee are required by law (the Federal Hazardous Substance Act of 1980) to bear a label containing a signal word, the nature of potential toxicity, first aid measures, and a "keep out of reach of children" statement, as well as a list of ingredients. The signal words *caution, warning,* and *danger* identify the product or its constituent chemical(s) as a weak irritant (i.e., may damage mucosal surfaces), strong irritant (i.e., can damage skin as well as mucosa), or corrosive (i.e., can cause permanent tissue damage or death) following topical exposure or moderately toxic, highly toxic, or extremely toxic (oral LD_{50} 50–500 mg/kg, 1–50 mg/kg, or <1 mg/kg, respectively) after ingestion and can be used to predict potential toxicity. However, since labeling is frequently inaccurate or incomplete [28–32], its information should always be confirmed by consulting a reliable toxicology text or current product information source, such as Poisindex [25].

The dose of drug in a pill or tablet can be determined from the sources cited in Chapter 129. For liquids and powders, the dose can be estimated or measured using the container itself or the weights and volumes listed on the label. It may also be reported in teaspoons (3–7 ml for standard flatware), tablespoons (7–14 ml for noncalibrated ones) [33], or swallows. The volume of a swallow varies with the patient's age, height, weight, and sex, the orifice size of the container, and the viscosity of the ingested liquid [34,35]. It ranges from 1 to 5 ml in infants to 4 to 40 ml in adults.

The accuracy and reliability of the history must be evaluated when assessing potential toxicity. The amount and time of ingestion are frequently erroneous when reported by patients with intentional self-poisoning. It is best always to assume a worst-case scenario: the maximum possible dose (i.e., the entire amount available or not clearly accounted for) should be cal-

culated and presumed to have been recently ingested. The potential toxicity can then be predicted from previously reported toxicodynamic data. Again, it should be assumed that the maximum toxicity previously reported following exposure to the estimated dose (or a lower one) will develop and should be treated accordingly.

The time of exposure is important because it allows for prediction of the time of onset of toxicity and the time of peak toxicity based on known pharmacokinetic and pharmacodynamic data. Only when the time between exposure and evaluation has clearly exceeded the longest known or predicted interval between exposure and peak toxicity can the possibility of subsequent poisoning be excluded. For most chemicals, maximal systemic effects are usually noted within 4 to 6 hours of an oral overdose. Important exceptions to this generalization are the "toxic time bombs"—chemicals that characteristically cause delayed or slowly progressive poisoning (Table 128-1). For some of these chemicals (e.g., acetaminophen, ethylene glycol, methanol, paraquat), the serum concentration measured soon after exposure can be used to predict subsequent toxicity. Peak (local) toxicity may also be delayed until 12 to 24 hours after irritant gas inhalation, pulmonary aspiration (e.g., hydrocarbon pneumonitis), and topical or ingestion exposure to corrosives.

ASSESSMENT OF SEVERITY.

The severity of poisoning is primarily determined by findings on physical examination. Since poisoning is far more dynamic than most diseases and illnesses, frequent reevaluations are required to determine the ultimate severity. Poisoned patients can rapidly deteriorate, with few or no warning signs.

A complete physical examination should be performed in all patients. It should initially be directed toward assessment of cardiovascular stability, respiratory function, and neurologic status. Accurate and timely measurement of all vital signs is essential. The respiratory rate should be measured for a full

Table 128-1. "Toxic Time Bombs"

Chemicals with slow GI absorption	Chemicals that undergo metabolic activation
Carbamazepine	Acetaminophen
Digitalis preparations	Chloramphenicol
Dilantin Kapseals	Chlorinated hydrocarbons
Enteric-coated pills	Ethylene glycol
Lomotil (atropine and diphenoxylate)	Methanol
Salicylates	Paraquat
Sustained-release formulations	Some methemoglobin inducers
Chemicals that form gastric concretions	Chemicals that inhibit nucleic acid synthesis
Barbiturates	*Amanita phalloides* and related mushrooms
Ethchlorvynol	Cancer chemotherapeutic agents
Glutethimide	Immunosuppressive agents
Heavy metals (e.g., iron)	Podophylline
Lithium	Viral antimicrobials
Meprobamate	
Salicylates	
Chemicals with slow distribution	Chemicals that inhibit metabolic pathways
Digitalis derivatives	Disulfiram
Heavy metals	Monoamine oxidase inhibitors
Lithium	Salicylates
Salicylates	Thyroid hormone synthesis inhibitors

minute. A core or rectal temperature should be obtained to detect severe or occult abnormalities. It is the sickest patients who are most likely to have significant temperature abnormalities; preoccupation with cardiovascular and respiratory therapy all too often leads to delayed detection of extremes of temperature requiring intervention. In contrast, an abbreviated mental status examination is usually sufficient [36]. The degree of physiologic dysfunction should be objectively described. Scales for the grading of stimulant and depressant poisoning, adapted from now classic publications [37,38], are useful for following the clinical course (Table 128-2).

The number and type of ancillary tests required for metabolic or organ function assessment are determined primarily by clinical severity and secondarily by the history. Asymptomatic but potentially poisoned patients with reliable histories and accidental exposures should have blood and urine samples obtained on presentation. Samples should be saved and sent for later (baseline) analysis in the event of subsequent deterioration. Patients who are symptomatic or suicidal should have serum electrolytes, blood urea nitrogen (BUN), creatinine, and glucose measurements, urinalysis, and 12-lead electrocardiogram (ECG). Arterial blood gas, serum osmolality, and ketone and methemoglobin analyses may also be indicated (see Chap. 129). Anion, osmolal, and oxygen saturation gaps should be calculated whenever their determinants are measured. Assessment of patients with respiratory complaints or grade 2 or greater stimulant or depressant poisoning (see Table 128-2) should include a chest radiograph. A complete blood count, coagulation studies, serum amylase, calcium, magnesium, creatine phosphokinase, and hepatic enzyme levels should also be determined in any patient with grade 2 or greater physiologic dysfunction. Additional testing (e.g., biopsies, invasive monitoring, neurodiagnostic studies, radiologic examinations) should be individualized and based on the findings of physical examination, the history, and the results of routine ancillary studies.

The measurement of chemical concentrations in serum, whole blood, or urine can sometimes help in assessing the severity of poisoning. In contrast to screening tests (see Chap. 129), quantitative analyses generally cost only $25 to $50 (per chemical) and can usually be performed in less than an hour. **Agents for which quantitative measurements are necessary or desirable for optimal patient management include acetaminophen, acetone, alcohols, antiarrhythmics, antiepileptics, barbiturates, carbon monoxide, digoxin, electrolytes (including calcium and magnesium), ethylene glycol, heavy metals, lithium, salicylate, theophylline [27,39–43].** The use of expensive, invasive, potentially hazardous, or poison-specific therapies is difficult to justify without laboratory documentation of toxic levels of these chemicals. Quantitative or qualitative assays for other chemicals are not generally helpful since they serve only to confirm the clinical impression and do not affect treatment (which is either supportive or must be initiated long before laboratory results are available to be effective).

PROVISION OF SUPPORTIVE CARE. Meticulous supportive care is necessary to maintain physiologic and biochemical homeostasis and to prevent secondary complications (e.g., anoxia, aspiration, bedsores, shock-induced organ injury, sepsis) until detoxification can be accomplished by normal mechanisms or therapeutic interventions. As obvious as it seems today, it was not until the late 1960s that the provision of such care, originally called the "Scandinavian method" [44], was shown to be effective in reducing mortality. Despite the development of antidotes and advances in absorption prevention and elimination technology, supportive care remains the most effective therapy for the majority of poisoned patients. Supportive therapy (e.g., treatment of vital sign abnormalities, organ dysfunction, seizures) is discussed in detail in other chapters. Only those considerations of special relevance to the poisoned patient are noted here.

Monitoring. Unless toxicity is minimal and predicted with a high degree of certainty to remain so, venous access should be established and continuous cardiac monitoring initiated. Since fluid resuscitation may become necessary, normal saline is the preferred IV solution. Pulse oximetry should be checked on presentation and monitored frequently if abnormal or if significant (grade 2 or greater) physiologic dysfunction (see Table 128-2) is present. Urine output should also be monitored (via Foley catheter) in such patients. Until the ultimate severity of poisoning is known, frequent or continuous visual observation is also necessary. Patients with intentional self-poisoning also need close behavioral observation until the possibility of a repeat suicide attempt has been evaluated in detail and assessed to be unlikely.

Respiratory Care. Pulmonary aspiration of gastric contents is a relatively common complication of poisoning and its treatment (e.g., GI decontamination procedures) [45,46,47]. Patients with CNS depression or seizures are at risk for aspiration as well as anatomic (i.e., tongue-related) airway obstruction. Although spontaneously breathing patients who can be aroused with painful stimulation can sometimes be successfully managed by "aspiration-preventative positioning" (e.g., left lateral decubitus and Trendelenburg position) and close observation, prophylactic endotracheal intubation is recommended for those who cannot respond to and by voice or who are unable to sit upright and drink fluids without assistance. Reliance on the gag reflex as an indication of the need for intubation should be abandoned. Many normal individuals have an absent gag reflex and many comatose patients will gag if sufficiently stimulated and yet be unable to protect their airways [48]. In addition, attempting to elicit a gag reflex may itself induce vomiting and cause aspiration in a patient with an altered mental state. Prophylactic or therapeutic intubation may also be required for patients with extreme behavioral or physiologic stimulation who require aggressive pharmacologic therapy with sedative,

Table 128-2. Physiologic Grading of the Severity of Poisoning

Severity	Signs and symptoms	
	Stimulant poisoning	Depressant poisoning
Grade 1	Agitation, anxiety, diaphoresis, hyperreflexia, mydriasis, tremors	Ataxia, confusion, lethargy, weakness, verbal, able to follow commands
Grade 2	Confusion, fever, hyperactivity, hypertension, tachycardia, tachypnea	Mild coma (nonverbal but responsive to pain); brainstem and deep tendon reflexes intact
Grade 3	Delirium, hallucinations, hyperpyrexia, tachyarrhythmias	Moderate coma (respiratory depression, unresponsive to pain); some but not all reflexes absent
Grade 4	Coma, cardiovascular collapse, seizures	Deep coma (apnea, cardiovascular depression); all reflexes absent

antipsychotic, anticonvulsant, or paralyzing agents. An endotracheal tube with a low-pressure, high-volume cuff is recommended to prevent aspiration [49], but it is by no means completely effective [50]. In one study, charcoal was recovered from the airway of 25 percent of patients who were given it by nasogastric tube despite prior endotracheal intubation [47]. In intubated patients who can tolerate it, elevation of the upper half of the body (45 degree semi-recumbent positioning) may decrease the incidence of aspiration [51].

As with airway protection, the need for supplemental oxygen or mechanical ventilation, although clinically obvious in patients with high-grade poisoning, may go unrecognized in those with less severe clinical toxicity. Hypoxia may mimic poisoning itself, auscultatory and radiographic evidence of aspiration or acute respiratory distress syndrome may be subtle or delayed in appearance, and clinical assessment of the adequacy of ventilation is not very reliable [52]. Hence, arterial blood gas analysis (or at least oxygen saturation measurement by pulse oximetry) is recommended in all patients except those who are awake and alert and have no respiratory complaints, to determine the need for oxygen and assisted ventilation.

Extracorporeal membrane oxygenation, cardiopulmonary bypass, and hyperbaric oxygen therapy should be considered in patients with reversible poisoning who cannot be adequately oxygenated with 100% endotracheal oxygen administration. Analeptics (i.e., centrally acting respiratory stimulants) such as amphetamines, caffeine, coramine, doxapram, ethamivan, pentylenetetrazole, and picrotoxin are contraindicated for the treatment of respiratory depression due to poisoning. They are ineffective [53], and their use is associated with increased morbidity (i.e., seizures) and mortality [44].

Cardiovascular Therapy. Maintenance or restoration of a normal blood pressure, pulse, and sinus rhythm is the goal of cardiovascular therapy. However, since adverse drug interactions may worsen, rather than alleviate, cardiovascular toxicity, the severity and trend of abnormalities and potential complications of treatment should be considered before instituting pharmacologic therapy. In addition, since the causes of cardiovascular toxicity are varied and multiple mechanisms may be concurrently operative in poisoned patients, invasive hemodynamic (e.g., arterial, central venous, pulmonary artery pressure) and electrophysiologic (e.g., esophageal or intracardiac electrodes) monitoring may sometimes be necessary for accurate diagnosis and optimal treatment. Finally, since poisoning is usually reversible, advanced supportive measures, such as external or internal electrical cardiac pacing, intraaortic balloon pump counterpulsation or cardiopulmonary bypass (partial or full) circulatory assistance, and extracorporeal membrane oxygenation, should be considered in patients unresponsive to routine therapeutic measures.

In the absence of an extremely fast or slow heart rate, *hypotension* due to poisoning is most often caused by loss of peripheral vascular tone rather than pump failure [54,55]. Hence, therapy should generally begin with several liters of normal saline. Fluid input and output and respiratory function should be carefully monitored during volume resuscitation. It is not uncommon for 5 or even 10 liters of fluid to be given without recognizing the volume until the patient develops iatrogenic pulmonary edema. Since many poisons deplete catecholamines, block their receptors, or directly cause myocardial depression, a direct-acting vasopressor with positive inotropic activity, such as norepinephrine or high-dose dopamine, should be used to treat hypotension if there is an incomplete response to fluid administration or evidence of volume overload.

Hypertension is most often caused by sympathomimetics, hallucinogens, or drug withdrawal (see Table 129-1) but is usu-

ally not severe. It often requires only observation or nonspecific treatment with a sedative (see Treatment of Neuromuscular Hyperactivity). If hypertension is extreme or associated with chest pain, ECG evidence of ischemia, headache, or focal neurologic findings, specific therapy is indicated. Since beta blockade may result in unopposed alpha-stimulation with a paradoxical increase in blood pressure and vasodilation may reflexively increase tachycardia, treatment with a nonselective sympatholytic (e.g., labetelol) or the combination of a beta blocker and a vasodilator (e.g., esmolol or propranolol with nitroprusside) is preferred for patients with sympathomimetic poisoning. A vasodilator alone or a selective alpha-blocker (e.g., phentolamine) can be used if hypertension occurs in association with a normal heart rate or reflex bradycardia. Physostigmine, although rarely necessary, is the treatment of choice for severe hypertension secondary to anticholinergic poisoning. Mannitol and diuretics may be useful if hypertension is due to increased intracranial pressure.

As with hypertension, *sinus tachycardia* caused by sympathomimetics, hallucinogens, or drug withdrawal (see Table 129-1) is usually not severe and can be managed by observation or nonspecific sedation. If it is associated with signs or symptoms of myocardial ischemia, a beta-blocker (with or without a vasodilator, depending on the presence or absence of coexisting hypertension) or a calcium channel blocker (e.g., verapamil) should be used for patients with sympathomimetic poisoning. When anticholinergic poisoning is the etiology, physostigmine is the preferred therapy. Tachycardia associated with hypotension is usually a reflex response of vascular tone or volume depletion and should be treated by fluid administration.

Since the general and poison-specific treatment of *ventricular tachyarrhythmias* is discussed in other chapters, only a brief summary is given here. As always, underlying electrolyte and metabolic abnormalities must be corrected. Lidocaine and phenytoin are generally safe for ventricular tachyarrhythmias of any etiology. Sodium bicarbonate, sodium lactate, or hypertonic saline may be effective in treating wide-complex tachycardias due to antiarrhythmics, cyclic antidepressants, and possibly other membrane-active agents (see Chap. 129). Magnesium and overdrive pacing with electricity or isoproterenol should be considered for patients with prolonged QT intervals and *Torsades de pointes* (polymorphous) ventricular tachycardia. Antibodies should be used to treat serious arrhythmias caused by digitalis. Magnesium has also been used with success in patients with digitalis poisoning. Beta-blockers should be reserved for the treatment of tachyarrhythmias that are clearly due to sympathetic hyperactivity. Procainamide and other class IA antiarrhythmics should not be used in patients with arrhythmias caused by membrane-active agents or in those with prolonged QRS or Q–T intervals because of the potential for worsening rhythm disturbances and conduction abnormalities (see Chap. 131). Similarly, physostigmine should not be used for wide-complex tachycardias due to cyclic antidepressants, since these arrhythmias are not anticholinergic in etiology and physostigmine can precipitate asystole in this setting (see Chaps. 133 and 140).

Bradycardias require active intervention only if they are associated with hemodynamic compromise (i.e., hypotension with evidence of organ ischemia). In most cases, atropine and isoproterenol are the agents of choice. Calcium and glucagon are effective for the treatment of bradycardia and hypotension due to calcium channel blocker and beta-blocker poisoning (see Chaps. 135 and 136).

Treatment of Neuromuscular Hyperactivity. *Behavioral* and *muscular hyperactivity* due to sympathomimetic or hallucinogen poisoning and drug withdrawal should initially be treated with nonspecific sedation. In general, benzodiazepines (e.g., diazepam, lorazepam, midazolam) are preferred to neuroleptics (e.g., chlorpromazine, haloperidol), since the latter are more likely to cause hypotension and can lower the seizure threshold. In phencyclidine poisoning, however, haloperidol, a central dopaminergic antagonist, may be more effective than a benzodiazepine, since phencyclidine has central dopaminergic activity. Similarly, chlorpromazine seems to be the most effective agent for sedating patients poisoned by other hallucinogens (see Chap. 152). The combined use of benzodiazepines and neuroleptics is sometimes the most effective therapy; doses and side effects can often be minimized using this approach. For severe hyperactivity due to anticholinergic poisoning, physostigmine is the drug of choice. A bolus of glucose should always be given if the etiology of mental status abnormalities (particularly seizures) is unclear and the glucose level is not known.

Seizures due to the stimulation of central catecholamine receptors by sympathomimetics, hallucinogens, and drug withdrawal and those due to the inhibition of central gamma-aminobutyric acid (GABA) and glycine inhibitory neuroreceptors (e.g., poisoning by isoniazid and strychnine, respectively) appear to be most effectively treated with GABA agonists (e.g., benzodiazepines and barbiturates) [56,57]. Administration of pyridoxine, a precursor of the cofactor pyridoxal phosphate required for GABA synthesis, is usually also necessary to stop seizures caused by isoniazid, since isoniazid also inhibits GABA synthesis and GABA agonists act partly by enhancing the release of this neurotransmitter from presynaptic nerve endings. In contrast, phenytoin, a membrane-active anticonvulsant, is likely to be most useful for seizures caused by agents with membrane-destabilizing effects (as suggested by the presence of prolonged QRS and Q–T intervals on the ECG). Therapy with both a GABA agonist and phenytoin may sometimes be successful when single agent therapy is not. Specific antidotes may be necessary for the treatment of seizures due to certain chemicals (e.g., cyanide).

Severe agitation or prolonged convulsions can cause acidosis, rhabdomyolysis, and hyperthermia. Since each of these complications can result in additional organ dysfunction, paralyzing (neuromuscular blocking) agents should be given to patients who fail to respond to sedatives and anticonvulsants. During paralytic therapy, electroencephalographic monitoring and continued seizure treatment are required to prevent permanent neurologic damage. Nondepolarizing agents (e.g., pancuronium, vecuronium) are preferable to succinylcholine for inducing paralysis, since the latter agent may be hazardous in patients with rhabdomyolysis [58].

Temperature Regulation. Hyperthermia and hypothermia should be treated by routine cooling and warming techniques, respectively. In addition to physical measures, patients with hyperthermia may require anticonvulsants, sedatives, or paralyzing agents if neuromuscular hyperactivity is present. Antipyretics are generally ineffective for drug-induced hyperthermia. They are potentially dangerous in patients who may have unrecognized acetaminophen or salicylate poisoning.

PREVENTION OF CHEMICAL ABSORPTION. Early and effective decontamination (i.e., dose reduction) can limit the surface exposure and systemic absorption of chemicals and prevent subsequent toxicity or reduce its severity and duration. Hence, decontamination is recommended in all patients unless the exposure is clearly nontoxic (Table 128-3). Methods of decontamination are discussed according to the route of chemical exposure.

Table 128-3. Criteria for a Nontoxic Exposure

1. Patient is asymptomatic by both history and physical examination
2. Amount and identity of all chemicals and time of exposure are known with high degree of certainty
3. Exposure dose is less than the smallest dose known or predicted to cause toxicity
4. Time elapsed since exposure is greater than the longest known or predicted interval between exposure and peak toxicity

Body Cavity Exposure. The removal of liquid and powdered chemicals from body cavities (e.g., bladder, external auditory canal, nose, rectum, vagina) is best accomplished by aspiration and irrigation using normal saline. Accessible particulate matter (e.g., pills, suppositories, drug packages) should be manually removed, preferably under direct visualization. The evacuation of drug packages from the GI tract is discussed under Ingestion.

Eye and Skin Exposure. Methods of decontamination following topical exposure include manual removal of particulate material, irrigation of exposed surfaces, and a scrub for skin exposure to noncorrosive chemicals [59]. Since "time is damage," particularly with corrosives, tap water or any other readily available liquid that is clear and drinkable can be used in the prehospital setting. If exposure involves an unknown chemical, its pH should be measured to determine whether it is highly acidic (pH ≤ 2) or alkaline (pH ≥ 12) and hence highly corrosive. Searching for pH paper (e.g., pHydron, usually available in the emergency department or the labor and delivery area), however, should never delay treatment. Irrigation should initially be performed for a minimum of 20 minutes. Prolonged irrigation (up to 24 hours) may be beneficial for corrosive exposures, especially those involving strong alkali.

With eye exposures, blepharospasm secondary to pain can prevent effective irrigation unless treatment is preceded by the instillation of a topical anesthetic (e.g., proparacaine, tetracaine) [60,61]. Particulate material should be removed with a moist cotton-tipped swab or eye spud. Normal saline and lactated Ringer's solution are the traditional irrigation fluids for inhospital use. Although commercially available pH-balanced saline solutions and normal saline adjusted to a pH of 7.4 with sodium bicarbonate are less irritating than normal saline or lactated Ringer's solution [62], they need not be used if an anesthetic is used. The irrigating solutions can be administered via an IV infusion setup, directly through the tubing, or via an irrigating (Morgan) lens attachment. A low-pressure squeeze bottle also may be used. One or 2 liters is usually sufficient. For acid or alkali exposures, the tear pH (normally 7.3–7.7) should be determined after as well as before irrigation; irrigation should continue until the pH is between 5 and 8. To be sure the pH of tears, not that of the irrigation fluid (the pH of normal saline is approximately 5.5 and that of lactated Ringer's solution is 6.5) is tested, the tear pH should be checked several minutes after irrigating.

For skin exposures, treatment should begin with the removal of contaminated clothing. Gloves should be worn to prevent contamination of care-givers. Particulate matter (e.g., dusts, powders) should be removed from the skin using a soft brush, forceps, or hand-held vacuum cleaner before irrigation. Washing the skin with soap and water or isopropyl (rubbing) alcohol more effectively prevents pesticide absorption than simply rinsing with water [63]. For some chemicals, a triple wash (irrigation and washing with soap before and after an alcohol scrub) may provide better decontamination than irrigation alone [64]. Because it contains 30 percent alcohol, tincture of green soap has been recommended as a skin detergent [25].

Inhalational Exposure. The patient should be removed from the contaminated atmosphere and supplemental oxygen (preferably humidified) administered as soon as possible. Under no circumstances should a rescuer enter a hazardous dust, fume, gas, or vapor environment without adequate eye, skin, and respiratory protection. Should assisted ventilation be necessary, bagging methods are preferred, since the mouth-to-mouth technique may result in contamination of the rescuer [65].

Ingestion. Gastrointestinal decontamination can be accomplished by activated charcoal administration, gastric lavage, emesis induction with syrup of ipecac, whole bowel irrigation, and endoscopic or surgical removal of the ingested chemical [27,66–72]. Diluents and cathartics, although often used in conjunction with other treatments, are generally not effective methods of decontamination when used alone. Details regarding the pharmacology, clinical use, contraindications, and complications of each of these therapies and general recommendations for GI decontamination based on current information are presented below.

ACTIVATED CHARCOAL. Activated charcoal can prevent absorption of ingested chemicals by binding them with the gut lumen. Since activated charcoal is neither absorbed nor metabolized, the chemical bound to it is normally eliminated with stool [68,69,70]. The activated charcoal-complex can also be removed from the stomach by inducing emesis or by gastric lavage [73,74].

Activated charcoal is a fine black powder produced by the activation (i.e., pyrolysis, oxidation, and purification) of carbon-containing materials such as bone, coal, peat, petroleum, and wood. It is odorless, tasteless, and insoluble in liquids. The activation process yields particles that have an extensive internal network of minute, branching, irregular, interconnecting channels (i.e., pores) that range in size from about 10 to 100 nm in diameter and account for the extremely large surface area of activated charcoal. The surface area of standard (i.e., USP) charcoal is 950 m^2 per gram, that of the Actidose and Darco brands is 1500 m^2 per gram, that of Norit Supra is 2000 m^2 per gram, and that of SuperChar ("superactivated charcoal") is 3150 m^2 per gram.

The absorption or adherence of chemical molecules to the external and internal surfaces of activated charcoal is rapid (within minutes of contact). It is due to relatively weak van der Waals forces and can be described by the reversible equilibrium: Activated charcoal + Chemical ↔ Activated charcoal-Chemical complex [68]. Hence, as the amount of activated charcoal is increased, the amount or fraction of unbound or free chemical decreases (i.e., the equilibrium shifts to the right according to the law of mass action). At an activated charcoal to chemical ratio of 10:1 or greater, 90 percent or more of most chemicals is adsorbed to the charcoal in vitro [68–71,75,76,77].

Activated charcoal can adsorb most chemicals, but its absorptive capacity (i.e., the amount of chemical that can be absorbed by 1 g in vitro) ranges from a few milligrams to more than 1 gram and depends on the physical characteristics of the chemical, the formulation of activated charcoal, and other factors (Table 128-4) [68–71,75,78]. Small, highly ionized molecules of inorganic compounds, such as acids, alkali, electrolytes (e.g., potassium), and the readily dissociable salts of arsenic, bromide, cyanide, fluoride, iron, and lithium, are not significantly adsorbed by activated charcoal [68,69,70,75,76].

In in vivo studies using toxic as well as therapeutic doses of chemicals administered to animals and therapeutic or slightly greater doses (i.e., "simulated overdoses") in humans, activated charcoal is effective in preventing GI absorption of a wide variety of chemicals (Table 128-5). In agreement with in vitro studies, as the dose of activated charcoal relative to that of a

Table 128-4. Factors Influencing the Adsorptive Capacity of Activated Charcoal

Factor	Effect
Ratio of AC to chemical	Increasing ratio increases percentage and amount of toxin absorbed
Surface area of AC	Adsorptive capacity increases with increasing surface area
Size of AC pores	Adsorption of high-molecular-weight compounds increases with increasing pore size
Size of chemical molecule	Adsorption increases with increasing molecular size until pore size is exceeded
Structure of chemical molecule	Aromatic and branched chain compounds adsorbed better than aliphatic or straight chain compounds of similar molecular size
Dissolution/solubility of chemical	Molecules must be dispersed in gaseous, liquid, or solution state to be adsorbed by AC; compounds with high lipid solubility are adsorbed better than those with low lipid solubility
pKa of chemical/pH of solution	Nonionized compounds are adsorbed better than ionized ones
Presence of competing solutes	Food and other chemicals may decrease the adsorptive capacity of AC

AC = activated charcoal

chemical increases, its efficacy increases; with simultaneous dosing of activated charcoal and chemical at a ratio of 10:1 or greater, charcoal prevents the absorption of most chemicals by more than 90 percent [77–80]. Superactivated charcoal is up to three times more effective than other charcoals in preventing chemical absorption [81–84], and multiple doses of activated charcoal are more effective than a single dose [85,86,87]. The efficacy of multiple-dose charcoal may be partly due to enhanced chemical elimination (see Multiple-Dose Activated Charcoal, following). At a constant charcoal to chemical ratio, the efficacy of activated charcoal in preventing chemical absorption increases as the absolute amount of both agents increases [88], suggesting that the efficacy of activated charcoal may be greater in overdose (provided a high activated charcoal to chemical ratio can be achieved). Diluting a dose of activated charcoal and administering it as aliquots by gastric lavage is less effective than administering the same dose as a single, concentrated bolus [89]. However, administering a dose before as well as after gastric lavage with saline is more effective in preventing chemical absorption than the usual practice of giving only a single dose after lavage [74].

The time between administration of a chemical and administration of activated charcoal also has a significant effect on the in vivo efficacy of charcoal. As this interval (i.e., the time for uninhibited absorption) increases, the ability of activated charcoal to prevent chemical absorption decreases [88,90–96]. In controlled studies using doses of activated charcoal several to many times greater than those of coadministered chemicals,

Table 128-5. Chemicals Whose Gastrointestinal Absorption Is Reduced by Activated Charcoal

Acetaminophen	Diethylaniline	Nicotine
Aconitine	Digitoxin	Nortriptyline
Amiodarone	Digoxin	Paraquat
Aminophylline	Diphenhydramine	Paroxetine
Amitriptyline	Diphenoxylate	Phencyclidine
Ampicillin	Disopyramide	Pheniramine
Amphetamine	Doxepin	Phenylbutazone
Aspirin	Doxycycline	Phenylpropanolamine
Atenolol	Estriol	Phenytoin
Atropine	Ethchlorvynol	Pindolol
Barbiturates	Ethylene dichloride	Piroxicam
Benzene	Ethylene glycol	Promazine
Carbamazepine	Flecainide	Propantheline
Carbaryl	Furosemide	Propoxyphene
Carbon disulfide	Glutethimide	Pyridine
Carbon tetrachloride	Hexachlorophene	Quinine
Chlordane	Imipramine	Quinidine
Chlordecone	Indomethacin	Salicylamide
Chloroquine	Isoniazid	Sotalol
Chlorpheniramine	Kerosine	Strychnine
Chlorpromazine	Malathion	Sulfanilamide
Chlorpropamide	Mefenamic acid	Tetrachlorethane
Cimetidine	Meprobamate	Tetracycline
Cocaine	Mercuric chloride	Tilidine
Dapsone	Methotrexate	Theophylline
Desipramine	Mexiletine	Tolbutamide
Diazepam	N-acetylcysteine	Tolfenamic acid
Diazinon	Nadolol	Trimethoprim
Dichloroethane	Nefopam	Valproic acid
Diethylene dioxide	Neguvon	Yohimbine

chemical absorption is decreased an average of 73 percent (range 12–99%) if charcoal is given within 5 minutes of chemical dosing [76,79,80,82,83,88,91–114], 51 percent (range 17–75%) if it is given 30 minutes after the chemical [74,85,90,94,115–121], and 36 percent (range 6–62%) if it is given after an interval of 60 minutes [81,83,84,85,87,89,90,92,93,118,119,120,122–126]. As expected, lesser effects are noted when activated charcoal is administered more than 1 hour after the chemical [88,89,91,121,127,128]. Activated charcoal can effectively prevent the absorption of chemicals from slow-release preparations when given after an interval of 4 hours [129] and probably longer. However, the ability of a single dose of activated charcoal to prevent the absorption of chemicals from such formulations appears to be less than it is for immediate-release chemicals [69].

The presence of food in the stomach appears to enhance the in vivo efficacy of activated charcoal in preventing chemical absorption, possibly by slowing gastric emptying [78,96]. Coingested cathartics, chocolate, ethanol, and excipients have variable but relatively minor effects on the efficacy of activated charcoal [69,97,109,114,125,126,130–135]. The concomitant administration of antacids does not significantly alter the efficacy of charcoal [78,109,110]. Delayed absorption of aspirin secondary to its desorption from activated charcoal may occur [136], presumably as a result of increased ionization of this drug as the activated charcoal-drug complex moves from the stomach to the more alkaline environment of small intestine.

The ability of activated charcoal to prevent the in vivo absorption of a chemical generally correlates well with its ability to adsorb that chemical in vitro [68,69,76, 80,81,101,109,110,133,137]. However, some chemicals (e.g., cyanide, malathion, tolbutamide) are poorly adsorbed by activated charcoal in vitro [68,75], yet their absorption is significantly reduced by activated charcoal in vivo [98,105,138].

Conversely, some chemicals (e.g., ethanol, ipecac, N-acetylcysteine) are moderately well adsorbed by activated charcoal in vitro [70,139–142] but their in vivo absorption does not appear to be significantly inhibited by charcoal [73,143–148].

Activated charcoal is administered as an aqueous suspension; a minimum of 8 ml of water should be added to each gram of powdered charcoal if a premixed formulation is not available. Some commercial preparations contain lubricants (e.g., propylene glycol or carboxymethyl-cellulose) or a cathartic (i.e., sorbitol). Flavoring agents (e.g., cherry, chocolate, or Coke syrup) can be added to suspensions to increase their palatability. Premixed product containers must be thoroughly agitated to resuspend sedimented charcoal prior to use [149].

Activated charcoal can be given orally to awake patients or by gastric tube to comatose or uncooperative patients. A nippled bottle can be used for infants. Putting the suspension in an opaque container and having the patient sip it through a straw may enhance its acceptability in adults. The recommended dose is at least 10 times the weight of the ingested chemical or as much as possible if the chemical dose is unknown. Due to volume constraints, the maximum single dose is generally limited to 1 to 2 gm per kilogram of body weight. For chemicals that are ingested in large amounts (e.g., ≥5 gm) or that are not well adsorbed by activated charcoal, it may be advantageous to use a high-surface-area charcoal.

Compared with other methods of GI decontamination, the advantages of activated charcoal are ease of administration, rapidity of action, extensively documented and relatively greater efficacy and safety, and lack of absolute contraindications. An additional advantage is its ability to enhance chemical elimination (see Multiple-Dose Activated Charcoal, following). The main disadvantages of activated charcoal are its color (black), gritty taste, and ability to stain clothing (which can limit its acceptance by staff as well as patients) and its low or reversible binding of some chemicals. It can also interfere with management by preventing enteral absorption and enhancing elimination of drugs administered for therapeutic purposes.

Controlled experimental studies have shown that activated charcoal is equal or superior to gastric lavage and emesis in preventing drug absorption [94,99,108,116,122–125]. In fact, prior administration of ipecac negates the superior efficacy of charcoal [122]. Activated charcoal alone has been found to be equal or superior to syrup of ipecac followed by charcoal in awake overdose patients [150–154]. Activated charcoal alone is equally or more effective than gastric lavage followed by charcoal in obtunded patients [152], particularly those who present more than 1 hour after overdose [150] and in awake patients with acetaminophen overdose [153]. Activated charcoal may not, however, be as effective as whole bowel irrigation for preventing the absorption of chemicals from sustained-released pharmaceuticals [129].

Activated charcoal is nonreactive and nonabsorbable and has little or no intrinsic toxicity. No changes in serum chemistry or hematologic parameters are detected following a single 30-gm dose (with sorbitol) [155]. Mice have been fed activated charcoal for up to 18 months and uremic patients have been treated with daily doses of 20 to 50 gm for up to 20 months without adverse effects [156,157]. Chronic inhalation of activated charcoal powder results in carbon deposition in the lungs but little or no inflammation or fibrosis [158]. Adverse effects associated with activated charcoal therapy include nausea, vomiting, abdominal cramps, diarrhea, and constipation. Many of these effects are related to excessive volumes or rapid administration [159], concomitant cathartic therapy [160], prior treatment with syrup of ipecac [122,151,152,154], or the ingested chemical, since they are rarely observed in volunteers given only activated charcoal [68,69,84,160,161,162]. Intestinal obstruction, pseudoobstruction, and nonocclusive intestinal infarction have been reported in patients with decreased bowel motility treated with multiple doses of activated charcoal [163–166]. Aspiration of activated charcoal along with gastric contents can result in large and small airway obstruction as well as pneumonitis [167–170]. Aspiration of an aqueous suspension of activated charcoal can also cause significant increases in airway resistance and pulmonary shunt fraction and decreases in vital capacity [169,170]. If AC accidentally gets into the eyes (e.g., in a comatose patient who regurgitates it), it can cause corneal abrasions.

There are no absolute contraindications to the use of activated charcoal. It is not recommended, however, for patients who have ingested only nonabsorbable corrosives (i.e., most acids and alkali) or hydrocarbons with poor GI absorption and low systemic toxicity (i.e., low-viscosity petroleum distillates and turpentine) [66–69,171]. In the former situation, it is ineffective and obscures endoscopic assessment of the extent of injury; in the latter, it may promote vomiting and increase the risk of pulmonary aspiration. In either case, however, if the history is equivocal and suggests the coingestion of chemicals that can cause systemic poisoning, the benefits of charcoal may outweigh its disadvantages. Current data indicate that previous admonitions against the use of activated charcoal in acetaminophen poisoning are unfounded (see Chap. 130).

GASTRIC LAVAGE. Gastric lavage can directly remove any ingested chemical from the stomach and thereby prevent its absorption [66,67]. As with activated charcoal, the efficacy of gastric lavage appears to decrease as time between ingestion and treatment increases [172]. In controlled experiments using therapeutic and toxic doses of chemicals in animals and therapeutic or slightly greater doses in humans, gastric lavage decreases chemical absorption an average of 52 percent (range 37–90%) if performed within 5 minutes of chemical administration [172,173,174], 26 percent (range 13–38%) if performed 30 minutes after chemical dosing [172,175], and 16 percent (range 8–32%) if performed at 60 minutes [123,124,172]. The efficacy of gastric lavage is enhanced if it is preceded as well as followed by a dose of activated charcoal [74].

Gastric lavage is performed by first aspirating stomach contents and then repetitively instilling and aspirating or siphoning off fluid through a nasogastric or orogastric tube [176–179]. It appears to be most effective if the patient is placed in a left lateral decubitus position with Trendelenburg or a left side-down Sims position. The left lateral decubitus position has also been shown to delay spontaneous drug absorption [180]. An unknown fraction of gastric contents may enter the duodenum during gastric lavage [156]. Although theoretically reasonable and commonly stated as fact, there is no direct evidence that a large-bore tube (i.e., 28–40 Fr.) is more effective than a small-bore (i.e., 16–18 Fr.) tube. On the contrary, no difference in the recovery of either solid (i.e., pill) or liquid formulations with respect to tube size has been found in experimental [173] or clinical [181] studies. Most intact pills will not fit through the lumen of even the largest tube [182], and since most pills are designed to disintegrate rapidly [183], unless lavage is accomplished very soon after ingestion the size of the tube is probably irrelevant.

Due to the risk of complications (see following section), if a large-bore tube is used it should be inserted by the physician and should be inserted orally to avoid unnecessary trauma to nasal passages. Once the tube is in place, lavage can be performed by an assistant. Although automated irrigation devices and lavage sets (e.g., large bags connected to the lavage tube by a Y connector) are commercially available [184], it is far simpler, quicker, and less expensive to use a funnel connected to the lavage tube, raising it 2 to 3 feet above the level of the stomach when administering fluid and lowering it 2 to 3 feet below the stomach to allow for drainage.

The lavage fluid of choice is tap water for patients older than 2 years. Because of the potential for inducing fluid and electrolyte disturbances, normal saline is recommended for younger patients [184,185]. Using warm fluids may increase pill dissolution and inhibit gastric emptying, and massaging the epigastrium may promote the mixing and suspension of gastric contents and enhance the efficacy of gastric lavage [178]. The optimal volume of fluid for each lavage cycle is unclear. Recommended amounts range from 60 to 800 ml for adults and up to 10 ml per kilogram of body weight for children [176–179,181]. Experimental studies suggest that larger aliquots are superior to smaller ones [173]. Hence, an aliquot volume of 5 to 10 ml per kilogram body weight would seem reasonable. Most chemical is recovered with the initial aspiration and first few lavage cycles [181,186,187]. Although inspection of the lavage effluent and estimation of drug recovery on the basis of the visualized pill fragments are unreliable [181] (most of what is seen consists of insoluble excipients and bears little relation to the amount of drug present), gastric lavage should be continued until the return is relatively clear. It is rarely necessary to use more than 5 liters of fluid. Injection of air into the stomach may prevent or reverse mucosal collapse around the large tube orifices and obstruction of drainage. If gastric lavage is properly performed, the amount of fluid recovered should be 90 percent or more of that instilled.

Endotracheal intubation is neither necessary nor sufficient to prevent aspiration during gastric lavage. On the contrary, gastric lavage can safely be performed on awake patients without endotracheal intubation [150,176,186,188], and the presence of an endotracheal tube does not preclude aspiration [47]. In both situations, strict adherence to proper positioning is essential. This is particularly true for elderly patients, because of their lesser ability to protect their airways [189]. In uncooperative awake patients, it is safer to use a small-bore tube than a large one. The practice of physically, sometimes brutally, restraining a combative patient and forcibly inserting a large-bore tube increases the risk of mechanical complications (see following) and should be abandoned. If a large-bore tube is thought to be necessary (e.g., a witnessed ingestion of a clearly lethal quantity of chemical), therapeutic sedation with or without paralysis, along with endotracheal intubation, is recommended. Short-acting agents (e.g., midazolam with or without vecuronium) should be used. The patient can be extubated upon awakening following gastric lavage.

Compared with other methods of GI decontamination, the advantage of gastric lavage is that it can be used in comatose patients. Although rapidity of action is often said to be an advantage, reported times from the initiation to completion of gastric lavage (neglecting set-up time) range from 20 to 35 minutes in relatively asymptomatic children [190] to a mean of 1.3 hours in adults with serious poisoning [181]. The disadvantages are that gastric lavage is a skilled and labor-intensive procedure, it is distinctly unpleasant [191], and it is associated with a relatively high risk of potentially serious or even fatal complications (see following section). In addition, with few exceptions, it is no more effective than other decontamination measures.

In controlled experimental studies, gastric lavage is not as effective as activated charcoal [122,123]. Compared with syrup of ipecac, it is more [174,192,193], less [122,172], or equally [123] effective; there is probably no significant difference. In children with salicylate ingestions treated sequentially with gastric lavage and ipecac, lavage was less effective than ipecac, regardless of whether it preceded or followed ipecac [194]; however, the mean recovery of salicylate was only 50 mg with lavage and 150 mg with ipecac, suggesting that neither treatment was very effective. In adult overdose patients, gastric lavage followed by activated charcoal may be more effective in preventing clinical deterioration than charcoal alone, but only in comatose patients who present within 1 hour of ingestion [150]. In a similar study, however, no difference in these two treatments with respect to clinical outcome was observed [152].

Gastric lavage can remove large amounts of chemicals from some overdose patients. As much as 5.6 gm of barbiturate [186], 20.3 gm of salicylate [188], 2950 mg of tricyclic antidepressant [186], 1118 mg of glutethimide [188], and 165 mg of diazepam [195] has been recovered. However, significant quantities of drug are recovered in only a small fraction of patients undergoing gastric lavage. More than 200 mg of drug was recovered in only 17 percent of 148 patients with barbiturate overdoses and more than 1 gm of drug was recovered in only 25 percent of 25 patients with salicylate ingestions [186]. In 127 patients with a variety of CNS depressant overdoses, more than 2 therapeutic doses were recovered in only 16 percent of patients and more than 10 therapeutic doses in only 7 percent; in 21 percent of patients blood drug levels continued to rise following lavage [195]. In 14 patients with cyclic antidepressant ingestions, more than 100 mg was recovered in only 36 percent [187]. Mean drug recovery was only 110 mg in another series of 13 patients with cyclic antidepressant poisoning, and the maximal amount recovered was only 342 mg [181]. Gastric aspiration removed significant amounts of ethanol (i.e., an amount that could increase the blood alcohol level by more than 40 mg/dl) in only 18 percent of acutely inebriated patients [196]. Examination of intragastric residue by flexible endoscopy following gastric lavage revealed residual solid in the stomach of 88 percent of overdose patients [197].

In agreement with experimental studies, the clinical efficacy of gastric lavage decreases as the time between overdose and initiation of treatment increases. In patients with barbiturate poisoning, more than 200 mg of drug was recovered in 37 percent of those who had lavage within 4 hours of ingestion but in only 15 percent of those treated more than 4 hours following ingestion [186]. Similar findings were noted in a study of patients poisoned by a variety of CNS depressants [195]. In patients with salicylate poisoning, however, large amounts of drug were recovered by gastric lavage up to 9 hours after ingestion [186], probably due to this drug's ability to inhibit gastric emptying and to form concentrations. The efficacy of gastric lavage in patients with barbiturate poisoning increased as the magnitude of the overdose and the severity of coma increased [186], a finding also consistent with drug-induced decreased gut motility.

Gastric lavage can result in significant morbidity and mortality. In one series it contributed to death in 8 of 22 (36%) patients who died following this procedure [198]. Aspiration has been reported in 25 percent of patients with cyclic antidepressant poisoning given activated charcoal by nasogastric tube despite prior endotracheal intubation [47]. Inadvertent placement of the lavage tube in the trachea has resulted in pneumothorax, pneumonia, and death [199,200,201]. Malpositioning of the tube, primarily in the esophagus, has been reported in 50 percent of pediatric patients undergoing gastric lavage [202]. Basing tube insertion length on the child's height or length and radiographic imaging have been suggested as ways to improve and document tube placement. The lavage tube can become kinked and impacted in the esophagus [203,204,205]. Since forceful removal can lead to esophageal perforation [204], inserting a flexible pediatric esophagoscope into the lumen of the tube under fluoroscopy and advancing the kinked area into the stomach

where the tube can be straightened has been recommended as treatment for this complication [205]. Esophageal perforation can occur during tube insertion [150,206]. Laryngospasm [201], hypoxia, ECG changes and dysrhythmias [207], and cardiac arrest [181] have also been reported. Other complications include hematemesis, gastric rupture, charcoal empyema, and pneumoperitoneum [179,203,208]. On endoscopy, esophageal and gastric erosions are noted in almost all patients treated by gastric lavage using a large-bore tube [209].

As with activated charcoal, there are no absolute contraindications to gastric lavage. However, in patients with corrosive and hydrocarbon ingestions, its use is controversial and should be selective [66,67,210–213]. With corrosives, insertion of a tube may increase the risk of perforation (particularly of the esophagus) at sites of transmucosal or transmural injury. Although there are no reports of this actually occurring, it is recommended that gastric lavage be reserved for patients who have ingested large amounts (i.e., more than a swallow) of liquid acid or alkali and who present for treatment within 1 or 2 hours of exposure and for those who have ingested corrosives that can cause systemic toxicity (e.g., heavy metals, hydrazine). Since gastric lavage may increase the risk of pulmonary aspiration following hydrocarbon ingestion [214], it should be reserved for patients with large ingestions of agents that can cause systemic poisoning (i.e., camphor, halogenated and aromatic hydrocarbons, and those containing heavy metals or pesticides).

SYRUP OF IPECAC. Syrup of ipecac can remove ingested chemicals from the stomach and proximal small intestine by inducing emesis [66,67,179,215,216,217]. Ipecac contains the alkaloids cephaeline and emetine, which stimulate the chemoreceptor trigger zone in the medulla and cause direct irritation of gastric mucosa. Systemic absorption of the alkaloids does not appear to be required for the induction of vomiting [218]. Other methods of inducing emesis (e.g., apomorphine, copper sulfate, liquid detergents, mechanical gagging, mustard) either are less effective or are associated with more complications and are not recommended [66,67,179,219,220,221].

The dose of syrup of ipecac is 15 to 30 ml for adults and children 12 years of age or older, 15 ml for children 1 to 11 years old, and 5 to 10 ml for children 6 to 12 months of age [222]. Vomiting occurs in about 20 minutes in 81 to 98 percent of patients [190,223,224,225]. Patients typically have three or four episodes of emesis during the following hour. If vomiting fails to occur within 30 minutes, a second dose is almost certain to be effective [225]. The success rate for patients who have ingested antiemetics is the same as that for patients who have ingested other agents [224,225]. A dose of 30 ml may induce vomiting faster than 15 ml in pediatric patients [226]. Although it is common to administer large volumes of fluid with syrup of ipecac, the time and incidence of vomiting are not affected by the volume [227,228,229], type (e.g., water, milk, carbonated beverage) [230,231], or temperature [232] of the fluid given. Physical activity (e.g., having the child run about) is often recommended, but has no effect on the time of onset of emesis [233].

Syrup of ipecac is significantly less effective in preventing chemical absorption than it is in inducing emesis. As with activated charcoal and gastric lavage, the efficacy of syrup of ipecac decreases as time between ingestion and treatment increases [94,172,225,234]. In controlled experimental studies similar to those described for charcoal and lavage, syrup of ipecac decreases chemical absorption an average of 60 percent (range 28–83%) when given within 5 minutes of chemical ingestion [94,108,172,174,235,236], 32 percent (range 2–59%) when given after an interval of 30 minutes [94,172,175], and

30 percent (range 8–44%) when given at 60 minutes [122,123,124,172,235]. Horizontal positioning does not improve the efficacy of ipecac [237]. Although children given syrup of ipecac within 1 hour of acetaminophen overdose had lower ratios of measured to predicted plasma drug concentrations than those treated later [234], only one study has documented drug recovery in the vomitus of actual overdose patients [194], and the maximal amount recovered was only 791 mg of salicylate. Examination of intragastric residue by flexible fiberoptic endoscopy following ipecac-induced emesis revealed residual solid in the stomach of 38 percent of overdose patients [196].

Compared with other methods of GI decontamination, the advantages of syrup of ipecac are that it is safe, simple to use, and widely available for home administration. As with gastric lavage, ipecac-induced vomiting does not result in clinically important changes in serum electrolytes [185]. The disadvantages of syrup of ipecac are that its action is delayed, vomiting is noxious [191], and it has relatively more contraindications and comparatively less efficacy than lavage or charcoal. In addition, chemical absorption continues during the time between ipecac administration and the onset of emesis, and vomiting may preclude the administration of activated charcoal and oral antidotes (e.g., N-acetylcysteine) [27,122].

In controlled experiments, syrup of ipecac is less effective than activated charcoal [94,108,122,123,124] and more [123,172], less [175,192,193], or equal [124] in efficacy to gastric lavage in preventing chemical absorption. In clinical studies, ipecac alone or followed by charcoal is no more effective [150,152,154] or less effective [151,153] than charcoal alone, and its use is associated with a longer stay in the emergency department and more treatment-related complications [151,154].

Due to the risk of aspiration, syrup of ipecac is contraindicated in patients with CNS depression or seizures and those who have ingested substances that can rapidly cause these events (e.g., cocaine, cyanide, cyclic antidepressants, isoniazid, propoxyphene, strychnine) [66,67,179]. In addition, vomiting may precipitate seizures in patients with stimulant ingestions [179]. As with activated charcoal and gastric lavage, syrup of ipecac is contraindicated in patients with pure ingestions of corrosives and those hydrocarbons with low systemic toxicity but high aspiration potential [66,67,179]. In the former instance, emesis may further expose the relatively thinner wall of the esophagus to gastric contents and increase the risk of esophageal as well as gastric perforation. In the latter, it may increase the risk of pulmonary aspiration.

Complications of syrup of ipecac can be divided into those related to vomiting and those due to direct toxicity. Aspiration can occur if the awake patient becomes obtunded or has a seizure and then vomits [66,67,151,179]. Ipecac-induced vomiting has resulted in esophageal tears [238], death from gastric rupture [239] and gastric herniation into the chest [240], pneumomediastinum and retropneumoperitoneum [241], and fatal intracranial hemorrhage [242]. Adverse side effects of therapeutic doses of syrup of ipecac occur in 10 to 20 percent of children and include protracted emesis (i.e., >4 hours duration), atypical lethargy, and diarrhea [243]. Acute or chronic overdosing of ipecac (e.g., in abused children or by patients with anorexia nervosa and bulimia) may result in myopathy, congestive heart failure, cardiac conduction disturbances, electrolyte abnormalities, intestinal pseudoobstruction, and sudden death [244–255]. Similar complications were reported when the formerly available fluid extract of ipecac, which is 14 times more concentrated than syrup of ipecac, was mistakenly administered as an emetic [215,216].

WHOLE BOWEL IRRIGATION. Whole bowel irrigation (WBI) refers to the enteral administration of large volumes of an electrolyte solution. It is commonly used to cleanse the GI tract before colonoscopy, barium enema radiography, and bowel surgery [256,257]. It can prevent the absorption of ingested chemicals by promoting rectal evacuation [72,258,259,260]. Although less well studied than other methods of GI decontamination for poisoning, in controlled experiments it decreased drug absorption 24 percent when performed 5 minutes after a therapeutic dose of aspirin [261], 67 percent when performed 1 hour after a simulated overdose of ampicillin and sustained-release lithium carbonate [262,263], and 73 percent when initiated 4 hours after ingestion of a supratherapeutic dose of enteric-coated aspirin [129]. Whole bowel irrigation can also be considered a form of "GI dialysis": it has been used in the treatment of uremia [264] and, like multiple-dose activated charcoal, can enhance elimination of previously absorbed chemicals [265].

Whole bowel irrigation is performed by administering a solution that contains electrolytes and polyethylene glycol (e.g., Colyte, Golightly) at a rate of 0.5 liters per hour in children and 2 liters per hour in adults until the rectal effluent is clear. The solution can be swallowed or given by gastric tube. The patient should be maintained in a sitting position during treatment.

Whole bowel irrigation appears to be more effective than gastric lavage or syrup of ipecac in preventing chemical absorption [123,260]. It is more [123,129,262] or less [261] effective than activated charcoal. The combination of charcoal followed by WBI was more effective than WBI alone [261,266] but equally [267] or less [261] effective than charcoal alone. Although clinical experience is limited, WBI appears to be safe [72,256–269]. Fluid and electrolyte abnormalities have not been noted. Whole bowel irrigation may be particularly useful in patients who have ingested enteric-coated or sustained-release pharmaceuticals (e.g., aspirin, theophylline) [129,263,270], potentially toxic foreign bodies (e.g., bezoars, button batteries, drug packets) [259,271,272], and agents that are poorly adsorbed by activated charcoal (e.g., heavy metals) [260,273,274]. It may also be of benefit in patients with extremely large ingestions or those with delayed presentations [72]. The disadvantages of WBI are that it is unpleasant, labor-intensive, and time-consuming; typically 2 to 4 hours is required for completion, and patients must be carefully monitored for potential complications of therapy (e.g., regurgitation, aspiration, abdominal distension).

ENDOSCOPY AND SURGERY. Gastric endoscopy, using baskets or snares to grasp or break up particulate chemicals, can be used with or without gastric lavage to remove potentially toxic foreign bodies (e.g., button batteries that break apart or fail to pass beyond the pylorus), gastric pill bezoars, or concretions (Table 128-1) [275,276,277]. Since it requires specialized equipment and operator expertise and has additional expense and risks, it should be reserved for patients with severe or potentially lethal poisoning, such as those with large amounts of heavy metal visible in the stomach on radiograph, and those who continue to deteriorate and have rising drug levels despite attempts at GI decontamination by other methods. Endoscopy should not be used for the removal of drug packets, since it may cause their rupture [278].

Immediate surgery is indicated for patients who develop toxicity following the ingestion of packets containing cocaine [278]. Surgery (i.e., gastrotomy, enterotomy) should also be considered in those situations when endoscopy is unsuccessful or impossible due to the location of the chemical or foreign body [279,280,281].

CATHARTICS. Cathartics are osmotically active saccharides (e.g., mannitol, sorbitol) or salts (e.g., magnesium citrate, magnesium sulfate, disodium phosphate) that promote rectal evacuation of ingested chemicals. They act by causing retention of fluids within the gut and thereby stimulating GI motility. When used alone or with activated charcoal, gastric lavage, or syrup of ipecac, they have little if any documented efficacy in decreasing absorption of ingested chemicals [66,67,217,282,283,284]. Cathartics are primarily used as an adjunct to charcoal to prevent constipation and enhance elimination of the charcoal-chemical complex. They may be of some benefit in preventing the absorption of chemicals from delayed or sustained-release formulations [268].

Cathartics can be given orally or by gastric tube. The dose for sorbitol and mannitol is 0.5 to 2 gm per kilogram and that for the saline cathartics is 250 mg per kilogram. Sorbitol is more effective than other agents in decreasing the transit time of GI contents [285,286] and appears to be safer. When sorbitol and activated charcoal are administered together, the mean time until a charcoal stool is noted is 1 hour in healthy volunteers [285] and 14 to 16 hours in overdose patients [287,288].

Adverse effects of all cathartics are dose-related and include nausea, vomiting, abdominal cramps, and excessive diarrhea [66,67,282–285,287]. Colonic perforation has also been reported [289]. Magnesium and phosphate can be absorbed, resulting in increased serum magnesium levels and increased serum phosphorus and decreased serum calcium levels, respectively [290–293]. Single doses are unlikely to result in fluid and electrolyte disturbances [155]. When given in repeated doses (e.g., during multiple-dose activated charcoal therapy), however, all cathartics can cause severe and sometimes fatal hypernatremic dehydration [294–298]. Multiple doses of magnesium salts can cause also hypermagnesemia, resulting in lethargy, weakness, loss of reflexes, and even coma [299–302].

Cathartics are contraindicated in patients with corrosive ingestions [282,283]. They are unnecessary in those who have or develop diarrhea and should be used with extreme caution in patients with congestive heart failure and renal dysfunction. Repeated doses of cathartics should not be given to patients with absent bowel sounds. Serum electrolytes, fluid balance, and, depending on the agent used, serum magnesium, phosphorus, and calcium levels should be monitored if multiple doses are administered.

DILUTION. The administration of water, milk, or other drinkable liquids is now recommended as a primary treatment only for corrosive ingestions [303]. In this setting, it may lower the concentration of chemical and limit its toxicity. To be effective, dilution should be accomplished as soon as possible. The volume of fluid should not exceed 5 ml per kilogram, since larger amounts may induce vomiting and cause further esophageal exposure. Dilution is no longer recommended to prevent chemical absorption. On the contrary, it may facilitate the dissolution of solid chemicals, increase the amount of chemical in solution, and stimulate gastric emptying, thereby enhancing chemical absorption [303].

SUMMARY AND GENERAL RECOMMENDATIONS. Despite extensive experimental data documenting the efficacy of GI decontamination measures in preventing chemical absorption, the clinical efficacy of such interventions (e.g., improved outcome) remains inconclusive. Indeed, because of undocumented clinical benefit and potential complications, GI decontamination measures (with the exception of gastric aspiration in awake patients who presented within 1 hour of overdose) were not part of the Scandinavian method (i.e., intensive supportive care) of treating poisoned patients, which was originally described in 1961, and clearly decreased mortality [44]. Given the more sophisticated monitoring and supportive techniques available today, it is very likely that most patients would recover fully without any decontamination therapy. A recent study found no difference in the outcome of asymptomatic overdose patients treated without

GI decontamination when compared to those treated with activated charcoal [152]. There are ample data to suggest, however, that decontamination prevents chemical absorption and is therefore likely to shorten the duration of toxicity and hence the duration of observation and treatment in some patients.

For several reasons it is difficult to document and predict the clinical efficacy of decontamination measures. Since overdose histories are frequently unreliable and the amount of chemical reportedly ingested is often inconsistent with observed toxicity or quantitative chemical analyses, it is difficult to assess the effects of treatment. In addition, patients often present for treatment at a time when the efficacy of GI decontamination remains to be established (the mean time between ingestion and arrival at a hospital is more than 1 hour in children and more than 3 hours in adults) [150–154,223]. Given the poor reliability of the overdose history (see Chap. 129), it impossible to identify with any degree of certainty which patients will benefit from decontamination. However, since some patients may indeed benefit, it is difficult to justify the use of control groups (i.e., patients not treated with decontamination) to prove or disprove the efficacy of these procedures.

Despite these uncertainties, it is recommended that all patients with intentional ingestions and those with accidental ingestions of unknown or potentially toxic amounts of chemicals be treated by decontamination unless they are asymptomatic and it is certain that more than 4 hours has elapsed since the time of ingestion. The choice of decontamination procedure(s) should be based on the actual and predicted severity of poisoning and the relative efficacy, availability, risks, and contraindications of the procedure. As noted in previous sections, activated charcoal appears to have equal or greater efficacy, fewer contraindications, and less frequent and less serious complications than other methods of decontamination. Recent clinical studies have consistently shown that overdose patients treated with gastric lavage or syrup of ipecac do worse than those treated with charcoal [151,152,154]. Patients who receive lavage or ipecac in the emergency department stay there longer (prior to discharge or admission) and have a higher incidence of pulmonary aspiration (which sometimes necessitates admission of a patient who would otherwise be discharged). Hence, for most patients, activated charcoal alone is the preferred treatment [27,150–154,304–309]. The practice of routinely emptying the stomach via lavage or ipecac-induced emesis can no longer be considered a standard of care [179,304–316]. Gastric emptying procedures have no value as an aversive or punitive measure for reducing the likelihood of future overdoses in patients who have attempted suicide [317].

Gastric lavage and syrup of ipecac still have roles in the treatment of selected patients. They should be used when the ingested chemical is not well adsorbed by activated charcoal. Gastric lavage is also recommended for patients who are comatose or who are initially awake but deteriorate following a dose of charcoal. In the critically ill or comatose patient, a dose of charcoal can be given by an easily inserted nasogastric tube while diagnostic (e.g., ECG, laboratory, radiology) and supportive (e.g., airway, intravenous line, cardiac monitoring) measures are being accomplished and again following lavage. Syrup of ipecac, because of its widespread availability, continues to be useful for home management of asymptomatic patients (e.g., children) with accidental ingestions, reliable histories, and mild predicted toxicity.

Whole bowel irrigation should be considered in patients who have ingested chemicals that are slowly absorbed or not amenable to decontamination by other techniques. Endoscopy and surgery should be reserved for patients in whom alternative methods of treatment are unsuccessful or contraindicated.

ANTIDOTAL THERAPY. Antidotes are chemicals that directly or indirectly counteract the toxic effects of other chemicals. They can be classified as selective or nonselective. Selective antidotes act by competing with poisons for target sites or metabolic activation pathways, by neutralizing them as a result of antibody-antigen reactions or chemical binding (i.e., chelation), by promoting their metabolic detoxification, and by antagonizing their autonomic effects via activation or inhibition of opposing neuronal pathways. Nonselective antidotes act by correcting metabolic derangements or enhancing nonmetabolic elimination [13,14,318–321]. Only agents that act selectively are considered here. Nonselective antidotes are discussed in Provision of Supportive Care and Enhancement of Chemical Elimination.

Although antidotal therapies can reduce morbidity and mortality, few chemicals have antidotes (Table 128-6). In addition, most antidotes are potentially harmful, and reasonable diagnostic certainty and knowledge of the specific indications, contraindications, dosing, and potential complications are prerequisite to the safe and effective use of antidotal therapy. The reader is therefore referred to subsequent chapters and elsewhere [1,2,22,25,318–321] for the details of antidotal therapy for anticoagulants, arthropod and reptile envenomations, heavy metals, and the rat poison Vacor (PNU or N-3-pyridylmethyl-N'-p-nitrophenyl urea) [1,2,22,25,318–321].

ENHANCEMENT OF CHEMICAL ELIMINATION. The nonmetabolic elimination of most chemicals can be accelerated by therapeutic interventions such as diuresis, acidification or alkalization of the urine, GI dialysis (i.e., multiple-dose activated charcoal or WBI), and extracorporeal techniques. Enhanced elimination is also partly responsible for the therapeutic effect of some antidotes (e.g., chelating agents promote the urinary excretion of heavy metals and oxygen accelerates the dissociation of carbon monoxide from its binding sites and accelerates pulmonary elimination). Unfortunately, however, the pharmacokinetic and clinical efficacy of such interventions is often theoretical rather than proved. It is commonly accepted that a therapy must remove a significant fraction (i.e., ≥25%) of a chemical dose at a rate significantly greater (i.e., ≥25%) than that accomplished by intrinsic detoxification mechanisms to be considered effective from a pharmacokinetic standpoint. Clinical efficacy requires that an intervention shortens the duration of poisoning and improves patient outcome.

All enhanced elimination procedures are associated with complications, and some are expensive and require specialized equipment and technical expertise. Hence, reasonable or absolute (i.e., laboratory-confirmed) diagnostic certainty is generally a prerequisite to their use. The selection of which, if any, enhanced elimination procedure to use should be based on the actual or predicted severity of poisoning, its reversibility, the function of intrinsic detoxification mechanisms, the potential risks of the intervention, and its efficacy in removing the offending chemical. In general, invasive (i.e., extracorporeal) elimination procedures should be reserved for patients who would not otherwise have a favorable outcome. This category includes patients with severe poisoning who deteriorate or fail to improve despite aggressive supportive care, antidotal therapy, and noninvasive methods of chemical removal; patients with chemical levels, confirmed or reasonably certain exposure doses, or laboratory findings known to be associated with potentially irreversible, life-threatening, or prolonged toxicity (particularly when noninvasive measures are ineffective or less effective than invasive ones); patients who lack the capacity for intrinsic metabolic inactivation or excretion because of shock or liver or renal failure; and patients with underlying illnesses (e.g., severe cardiovascular or pulmonary disease) that adversely affect prognosis or are exacerbated by the effects of a chemical [322–325].

Diuresis and Manipulation of Urinary pH. Increasing the flow of urine enhances the excretion of chemicals by keeping the urine dilute and thus decreasing the passive distal tubular reabsorption of chemicals that have undergone glomerular filtration and proximal tubular secretion [323–328]. Increasing or decreasing the pH of urine (considered neutral at a pH of 6) can enhance the renal excretion of acidic or basic chemicals by the mechanism known as ion trapping [13,18,328]. Like all membranes, those of the nephron, particularly the distal tubule, are generally more permeable to nonionized and nonpolar molecules than to ionized and polar ones. After filtration and secretion, nonionized forms of weak acids or bases become ionized and hence trapped in an alkaline or acidic urine, respectively. Diuresis and manipulation of the urinary pH generally act synergistically [329]. The efficacy of these therapies in enhancing excretion of particular chemicals is reviewed in other chapters and elsewhere [2,3,25,323–328]. Only a brief summary is presented here.

Diuresis alone can enhance the renal excretion of alcohols, bromide, calcium, fluoride, lithium, meprobamate, potassium, and isoniazid. Except for calcium and potassium, however, the clinical benefits of such therapy remain to be proved.

Acidification of the urine (in conjunction with diuresis) can increase the renal elimination of amphetamines, chloroquine, cocaine, local anesthetics, phencyclidine, quinine, quinidine, strychnine, sympathomimetics, tocainide, and tricyclic antide-

Table 128-6. Chemicals and Toxic Syndromes with Specific Antidotes

Agent	Antidotes
Acetaminophen	N-acetylcysteine
Anticholinergic poisoning	Physostigmine
Anticoagulants	Phytonadione (vitamin K), protamine
Benzodiazepines	Flumazenil
Beta-adrenergic antagonists	Glucagon, calcium salts
Calcium channel blockers	Calcium salts, glucagon
Carbon monoxide	Oxygen, hyperbaric oxygen
Cholinergic syndrome	Atropine, pralidoxime
Cyanide	Nitrites, thiosulfate, hydroxycobalamine
Digoxin (digitalis)	Fab antibody fragments, magnesium
Dystonic reactions	Benztropine, diphenhydramine
Ethylene glycol	Ethanol, 4-methylpyrazole; pyridoxine, thiamine
Envenomations (arthropod, snake)	Antivenins
Fluoride	Calcium and magnesium salts
Heavy metals (arsenic, mercury, lead)	BAL (dimercaprol), dimercaptosuccinic acid (DMSA), D-penicillamine, calcium disodium EDTA
Hydrogen sulfide	Oxygen, nitrites
Iron	Deferoxamine
Isoniazid (hydrazines)	GABA agonists, pyridoxine
Methanol	Ethanol, 4-methylpyrazole; folate
Methemoglobinemia	Methylene blue
Opioids	Naloxone, nalmefene, naltrexone
Sympathomimetics	Adrenergic blockers
Vacor (PNU)	Nicotinamide (niacinamide)

pressants. However, the clinical efficacy of this intervention has not been documented and the risks of administering an acidifying agent such as ammonium chloride to patients who have or may develop rhabdomyolysis or acidosis (e.g., those with anoxia, shock, or seizures) include precipitation of myoglobinuric renal failure and exacerbation of cardiovascular, metabolic, and neurologic dysfunction. Hence, acid diuresis cannot be recommended for management of any poisoning.

Alkalinization of the urine (along with diuresis) can enhance the excretion of the chlorphenoxyacetic acid herbicide 2,4-D (and probably 2,4,5-T), chlorpropamide, diflunisal, fluoride, methotrexate, phenobarbital (and probably other long-acting barbiturates), sulfonamides, and salicylates. Only for phenobarbital and salicylate poisoning is its clinical efficacy accepted as proved.

The goal of diuresis is to achieve a urine flow of 3 to 8 ml/kg/hr and that of alkalinization is a urine pH of 7.5 or greater. The IV administration of 0.9% saline (sodium chloride) is the preferred method for inducing diuresis. An alkaline diuresis solution can be prepared by adding 1 to 3 ampules (44–132 mEq) of sodium bicarbonate to 1 liter of normal saline, half-normal saline, or D_5W such that the final solution is isotonic or slightly hypertonic. Fluids are administered roughly at the same rate as the desired urine output. Acetazolamide should not be used to produce an alkaline urine, since it may worsen toxicity by causing a concomitant systemic acidosis, resulting in an increase in the amount of un-ionized drug in the blood and enhanced tissue distribution [330]. It may also compete with acidic drugs for tubular secretion and thereby inhibit their elimination.

Acid-base, fluid, and electrolyte parameters as well as respiratory function and clinical response must be carefully monitored during therapy. All patients should have a Foley catheter in place. Fluid intake, urine output, and urine pH should be measured hourly. A loop diuretic (e.g., furosemide), osmotic diuretic (e.g., mannitol), or low-dose dopamine can be given if urine output fails to keep pace with fluid administration. For obvious reasons, diuresis is contraindicated in patients with congestive heart failure, renal failure, cerebral edema, pulmonary edema, or uncorrected electrolyte abnormalities.

Multiple-Dose Activated Charcoal. Activated charcoal administered intermittently and repetitively can enhance the elimination of previously absorbed chemicals by binding them within the GI tract as they are excreted in the bile, secreted by cells of the stomach or intestine, or passively diffuse back into the lumen (reverse absorption). The charcoal-chemical complex is then excreted with stool. Interruption of enterohepatic or enteroenteric recirculation appears to be the underlying mechanism of action for a minority of chemicals. In most cases, the surface of the entire gut acts as a dialysis membrane. Since activated charcoal keeps the concentration of free chemical in GI fluids near zero, chemicals merely diffuse from the blood perfusing the gut mucosa into the luminal fluids as a result of concentration gradients [69,305,306,331–335].

Multiple-dose activated charcoal (MDAC) is theoretically capable of enhancing the elimination of any chemical that can be absorbed by activated charcoal and can be absorbed from the GI tract. Its efficacy is likely to be greatest for chemicals with a high charcoal binding capacity and with physical and pharmacokinetic characteristics that make them amenable to removal by extracorporeal methods (see following section) [333]. It may be most effective for agents with a long intrinsic elimination half-life [336]. As with dialysis techniques, the ability of MDAC to enhance the elimination of a chemical is independent of the initial route of chemical absorption. It can enhance the elimination of chemicals administered IV [337–344] and intra-

peritoneally [345] as well as orally [85,86,87,93,107,111,112, 120,346–370].

From a pharmacokinetic standpoint, MDAC has been found to be effective in enhancing the elimination of most chemicals following their administration in both therapeutic doses and overdoses (Table 128-7). Since the gut has a relatively large surface area, the clearances achieved by MDAC therapy are comparable to those achieved by extracorporeal methods. Also, MDAC appears to enhance the elimination of organic solvents [371] and phencyclidine [372] and may be useful for removing agents with long elimination half-lives (e.g., amiodarone, isotretinoin, organochlorine pesticides, organic compounds containing heavy metals) [333]. It does not, however, significantly enhance the elimination of chlorpropamide, tobramycin, and possibly imipramine [104,373,374,375].

In contrast, the clinical efficacy of MDAC therapy in overdose patients remains open to debate [376]. Compared with historical controls (i.e., patients treated with GI decontamination and supportive measures), patients treated with MDAC clearly have shorter durations of toxicity. However, there are few prospective studies directly comparing patients treated with MDAC to those who are not, and MDAC is not without risk (see Activated Charcoal).

The efficacy of MDAC increases as the cumulative amount of charcoal administered increases, either by increasing the amount of charcoal given with each dose or increasing the frequency of dosing [377]. When the cumulative amount of charcoal remains constant, there is no difference in the efficacy of different dosing regimens (e.g., 25 gm in every 2 hours vs. 50 gm every 4 hours) [378]. Hence, the optimal amount of activated charcoal to administer should be as much as possible. From a practical standpoint, intrinsic bowel activity and the volume of charcoal that can be given are the limiting factors. In patients with normal bowel activity, doses of activated charcoal of 0.5 to 1 gm per kilogram every 4 hours are generally well tolerated. In those with decreased GI motility, smaller doses at more or less frequent intervals should be used. Alternatively, charcoal can be given by a slow continuous nasogastric infusion [379]. This method of administration may also be better for patients who cannot retain charcoal because of vomiting (e.g., those with theophylline poisoning). In the event of gastrostasis (i.e., the previous dose of charcoal is still present in the stomach when gastric aspiration is performed before administering the next dose), regurgitation, or abdominal distension, MDAC therapy should be discontinued. Although cathartics are often given along with charcoal, the use of multiple doses of magnesium salts should be avoided and the dose of cathartic must be carefully titrated to bowel activity to avoid

Table 128-7. Chemicals Whose Elimination Can Be Enhanced by Multiple-Dose Activated Charcoal Therapy

Amitriptyline	Nadolol
Carbamazepine	Nortriptyline
Chlordecone	Paroxetine
Cyclosporine	Phencyclidine
Dapsone	Phenobarbital
Diazepam	Phenylbutazone
Digitoxin	Phenytoin
Digoxin	Piroxicam
Dioxin (TCDD)	Propoxyphene
Disopyramide	Quinine
Doxepin	Salicylate
Glutethimide	Sotalol
Meprobamate	Theophylline
Methotrexate	Valproate

excessive diarrhea (see Cathartics). Complications of MDAC therapy are the same as for activated charcoal itself (see Activated Charcoal).

Extracorporeal Methods. Peritoneal dialysis, hemodialysis, hemoperfusion, hemofiltration, plasmapheresis, and exchange transfusion are theoretically capable of removing any chemical from the bloodstream [322,323,324,380–393]. Unfortunately, most chemicals undergo significant tissue distribution and only a fraction of the absorbed dose remains in the blood. Significant removal of chemical by these techniques is likely only if the volume of distribution is less than 1 liter per kilogram. In addition, with dialysis techniques, only chemicals that are small (i.e., molecular weight <500–1500 d), water-soluble, uncharged, and not highly bound to serum proteins readily diffuse across dialysis membranes. The ability of other extracorporeal methods to remove chemicals from the blood is less limited by chemical size, water solubility, or protein binding. The efficacy of these measures is also affected by blood flow, dialysate and membrane properties, and the type of hemoperfusion absorbent.

Clearance rates achieved by extracorporeal removal must be significantly greater than intrinsic total body clearance (i.e., the sum of metabolic, renal, and other routes of clearance) to be considered effective pharmacokinetically [394–397]. As with other treatments, the clinical efficacy of extracorporeal methods is based more on observation, experience, and retrospective comparisons than on controlled prospective studies. *Hemodialysis* is considered clinically as well as pharmacokinetically effective for enhancing elimination of barbiturates, bromide, chloral hydrate, ethanol, ethylene glycol, isopropyl alcohol, lithium, methanol, procainamide, theophylline, salicylate, and possibly heavy metals [27,322,323,324,388,394,395]. Except for bromide, heavy metals, lithium, and ethylene glycol, *hemoperfusion* is more effective in removing these chemicals than hemodialysis. However, since hemoperfusion is not as effective as hemodialysis in correcting acid-base and electrolyte abnormalities, hemodialysis remains the treatment of choice for patients with severe methanol and salicylate poisoning. *Hemoperfusion* is also considered effective in removing chloramphenicol, disopyramide, phenytoin, and lipophilic sedative-hypnotics such as ethchlorvynol, glutethimide, meprobamate, and methaqualone [323,324,388,396]. Hemoperfusion and hemodialysis in a tandem setup may be more effective than either technique alone [398]. Both techniques require central venous access and systemic anticoagulation. Hypotension, hypothermia, and bleeding are common complications. The usual complications of central venous cannulation may also be encountered. In addition, hemoperfusion frequently causes hemolysis, hypocalcemia, and thrombocytopenia. For chemicals that are removed by both techniques, the greater availability of and familiarity with hemodialysis may allow its more rapid initiation and outweigh the advantage of using hemoperfusion to achieve greater clearances.

Peritoneal dialysis is only 10 to 25 percent as effective as hemodialysis [323,324,380,381,389]. It may, however, be useful when hemodialysis and hemoperfusion are not available or technically difficult (e.g., in neonates) or when anticoagulation may be hazardous. Complications include infection, injury to intraabdominal organs, and hypothermia.

Exchange transfusion is a less effective alternative to hemodialysis and hemoperfusion [393]. It is also a useful treatment for hemolysis (e.g., arsine poisoning) and methemoglobinemia. Two blood-volume exchanges are usually performed using central or peripheral arteriovenous or venovenous access. Complications include transfusion reactions, hypothermia, and traumatic events related to blood vessel cannulation.

The roles of *hemofiltration* and *plasmapheresis* in the treatment of poisoning remain to be defined [389–392].

Extracorporeal techniques often remove chemicals from the blood faster than tissue redistribution can occur. A rebound increase in the blood concentration of a chemical and clinical relapse may occur following treatment. Patients and blood levels should therefore be closely monitored for several hours after the termination of extracorporeal therapies.

SAFE DISPOSITION. Most poisoned or potentially poisoned patients are initially evaluated and treated in the emergency department. As noted previously, the time between oral overdose and presentation to the hospital averages 1 to 3 hours. Patients who are admitted to the hospital spend an average of 2 to 4 hours in the emergency department [151,152,154,399], with length of stay in the emergency department tending to decrease with increasing severity of poisoning [399]. Those who are eventually discharged or referred for psychiatric evaluation spend roughly 6 to 8 hours in the emergency department [151,152,154]. It follows that many hours will have elapsed from the time of ingestion to the time of emergency department disposition in most patients. Even with exposures to toxic time bombs (see Prediction of Severity), this is usually more than sufficient time to observe directly or to evaluate and predict the ultimate severity of poisoning and the level of care needed [399,400].

Patients who have coma (grade 2 or greater), hypotension (systolic pressure 80 mm Hg), respiratory depression (PCO_2 > 45 mm Hg or intubated), seizures, or a nonsinus cardiac rhythm (including second- or third-degree atrioventricular block) in the emergency department will likely require further intensive care interventions and should be admitted to a full-service ICU [399,401]. The same can be said of patients with extremes of temperature, severe agitation, hallucinations, hypertension, or metabolic abnormalities and those who require antidotal or enhanced elimination therapy.

Patients who are less ill, stable, or even asymptomatic are frequently admitted to the ICU because of physician uncertainty, fear of late deterioration and potential litigation, and lack of acceptable alternatives (e.g., hospital policy that limits the time patients can spend in the emergency department, busy emergency department or no observation unit, appropriate level of nursing care unavailable outside the ICU). Such patients need close or continuous visual observation (e.g., one-to-one suicide precautions) and close or continuous monitoring of cardiac rhythm and vital signs to assure that they remain asymptomatic and recover without incident. Unless active interventions are likely to be necessary, admission to an intermediate care unit, telemetry unit, or emergency department observation unit is a more appropriate disposition for such patients, particularly when ICU beds are limited.

Patients with nontoxic exposures (Table 128-3) or mild clinical toxicity who become asymptomatic can often be discharged from the emergency department or referred for psychiatric evaluation. A 4- to 6-hour observation period and passage of a charcoal stool is generally sufficient to exclude the possibility of delayed toxicity.

PREVENTION OF RECURRENCE. The possibility of chemical reexposure and subsequent poisoning should always be assessed prior to discharge. If necessary, preventive measures should be addressed. As obvious as this is, physicians often forget to do this (especially in accidental and industrial poisonings) and subject themselves to potential litigation in the event of recurrence.

The environment of children should be "poison-proofed" [402]. Safety caps are helpful but are not always sufficient to prevent access. Alcoholic beverages, medications (including vitamins), nonedible plants, and automotive, cleaning, cosmetic, fuel, painting, pet care, and toiletry products should be stored out of reach or in cabinets with child-proof latches or locks. Family stress is a risk factor for accidental poisoning. Events such as a recent move, serious illness, pregnancy, parental anxiety, depression, separation, or unemployment may be responsible for lack of supervision of a child and should be investigated. Family counseling and social services should be offered if appropriate.

Suicidal patients require psychiatric assessment, disposition, and follow-up. If they are given prescriptions, the amount of drug should be limited to a 1- to 2-week supply and refills should be limited. Compliance with and response to therapy should be closely monitored. Substance abusers (recreational users as well as addicts) should be counseled regarding attendant medical risks and given the opportunity for rehabilitation through referral for behavior modification, supervised withdrawal, and abstinence or maintenance therapy.

Adults with accidental poisoning should be educated regarding the safe use of drugs and other chemicals. They should be advised to read labeling instructions carefully and to avoid future exposures. Assistance with the administration of medications may be required for visually impaired, elderly, retarded, or confused patients. Preventive education is a must for health care providers who have committed dosing errors or who are unaware of adverse drug interactions. When poisoning results from environmental or workplace exposure, the appropriate governmental agency (e.g., Environmental Protection Agency, Occupational Safety and Health Administration, National Institute of Occupational Safety and Health, or local, state, or federal health departments) should be notified. Unsafe working conditions should be brought to the attention of employers. Industrial hygiene and occupational health services should be offered if available. Finally, physicians have a duty to warn the general public (e.g., via press releases) of acute environmental hazards.

References

1. Veltri JC, McElwee NE, Schumacher MC: Interpretation and uses of data collected in poison control centres in the United States. *Med Toxicol* 2:389, 1987.
2. Goldfrank LR, Flomenbaum NE, Lewin NA, et al (eds): *Goldfrank's Toxicologic Emergencies*. 3rd ed. Norwalk, CT, Appleton-Century-Crofts, 1986.
3. Ellenhorn MJ, Bardeloux DG (eds): *Medical Toxicology: Diagnosis and Treatment of Human Poisoning*. New York, Elsevier, 1988.
4. Fazen LE, Lovejoy FF, Crone RK: Acute poisoning in a children's hospital: A 2-year experience. *Pediatrics* 77:144, 1986.
5. Soslow AR: Acute drug overdose: One hospital's experience. *Ann Emerg Med* 10:18, 1981.
6. Kozel NJ, Adams EH: Epidemiology of drug abuse: An overview. *Science* 234:970, 1986.
7. Woolf AD: The epidemiology of poisonings and drug abuse in adolescents and adults. *Clin Toxicol Rev* 10:1, 1988.
8. Woolf AD: Poisonings in the elderly. *Clin Toxicol Rev* 11:1, 1989.
9. Walton WW: An evaluation of the Poison Packaging Act. *Pediatrics* 69:363, 1982.
10. Litovitz TL, Clark LR, Soloway RA: 1993 Annual Report of the American Association of Poison Control Centers Toxic Exposure Surveillance System. *Am J Emerg Med* 12:546, 1994.
11. Chafee-Bahamon C: Epidemiology of serious poisonings. *Clin Toxicol Rev* 5:1, 1983.
12. Stern TA, Mulley AG, Thibault GE: Life-threatening drug overdose: Precipitants and prognosis. *JAMA* 251:1983, 1984.
13. Klassen CD, Amdur MO, Doull J (eds): *Casarett and Doull's Toxicology: The Basic Science of Poisons,* 3rd ed. New York, Macmillan, 1986.
14. Loomis TA: *Essentials of Toxicology*. 3rd ed. Philadelphia, Lea & Febiger, 1978.
15. Rosenberg J, Benowitz NL, Pond S: Pharmacokinetics of drug overdose. *Clin Pharmacokinet* 6:161, 1981.
16. Drew R: Applying pharmacokinetic principles to the management of drug poisoning. *Pediatr Ann* 16:913, 1987.
17. Albert A: *Selective Toxicity: The Physico-chemical Basis of Therapy*. 7th ed. New York, Chapman & Hall, 1985.
18. Gilman AG, Goodman LS, Rall TW, et al (eds): *Goodman and Gilman's The Pharmacological Basis of Therapeutics*. 7th ed. New York, Macmillan, 1985.
19. Levine RR: Factors affecting gastrointestinal absorptions of drugs. *Dig Dis* 15:171, 1970.
20. Nimmo WS: Drugs, diseases, and altered gastric emptying. *Clin Pharmacokinet* 1:189, 1976.
21. Baselt RC, Carvey RH: *Disposition of Toxic Drugs and Chemicals in Man*. 3rd ed. Chicago, Year Book, 1989.
22. Hayes WJ: *Pesticides Studied in Man*. Baltimore, Williams & Wilkins, 1982.
23. Clayton GD, Clayton FE (eds): *Patty's Industrial Hygiene and Toxicology*. 3rd ed. New York, Wiley, 1978.
24. Sullivan JB, Krieger GR: *Hazardous Materials Toxicology*. Baltimore, Williams & Wilkins, 1990.
25. Rumack BH (ed): *Poisindex Information System*. Denver, Micromedex, Updated quarterly.
26. Reynolds JEF (ed): *Martindale: The Extra Pharmacopoeia*. 29th ed. London, Pharmaceutical Press, 1989.
27. Goldberg MJ, Spector R, Park GD, et al: An approach to the management of the poisoning patients. *Arch Intern Med* 146:1381, 1986.
28. Spyker DA, Minocha A: Toxicodynamic approach to the management of the poisoned patient. *J Emerg Med* 6:117, 1988.
29. Kulig K: Initial management of ingestions of toxic substances. *N Engl J Med* 326:1677, 1992.
30. Hurst RE: Using federal standards to determine adequacy of consumer products precautionary labeling (abstract). *Vet Hum Toxicol* 28:471, 1986.
31. Alderman D, Burke M, Cohen B, et al: How adequate are warnings and first aid instructions on consumer product labels? An investigation. *Vet Hum Toxicol* 24:8, 1982.
32. Mrvos R, Dean BS, Krenzelok EP: An extensive review of commercial product labels: The good, bad, and ugly. *Vet Hum Toxicol* 28:67, 1986.
33. Dean BS, Krenzelok EP: Syrup of ipecac dosing: How much is a tablespoonful? *Vet Hum Toxicol* 28:155, 1986.
34. Watson WA, Bradford DC, Veltri JC: The volume of a swallow: Correlation of deglutition with patient and container parameters. *Am J Emerg Med* 3:278, 1983.
35. Saylor JH: Volume of a swallow: Role of orifice size and viscosity. *Vet Hum Toxicol* 29:79, 1987.
36. Merigian KS, Hedges JR, Roberts JR, et al: Use of an abbreviated mental status examination in the initial assessment of overdose patients. *Arch Emerg Med* 5:139, 1988.
37. Espelin DE, Done AK: Amphetamine poisoning: Effectiveness of chlorpromazine. *N Engl J Med* 278:1361, 1968.
38. Reed CE, Driggs MF, Foste CC: Acute barbiturate poisoning: A study of 300 cases based on a physiological system of classification of the severity of intoxication. *Ann Intern Med* 37:290, 1952.
39. Flanagan RJ, Heggett A, Saynor DA, et al: Value of toxicological investigation in the diagnosis of acute poisoning in children. *Lancet* 2:682, 1981.
40. Sullivan JB, Fisher JG: Proper use of the toxicology laboratory. *Emerg Med Rep* 5:125, 1984.
41. Hepler BR, Sutheimer CA, Sunshine I: Role of the toxicology laboratory in the treatment of acute poisoning. *Med Toxicol* 1:61, 1986.
42. Gaudreault P, Timberlake S: Toxic screens. I. *Clin Toxicol Rev* 12:1, 1989.
43. Gaudreault P, Timberlake S: Toxic screens. II. *Clin Toxicol Rev* 12:1, 1989.
44. Clemmesen C, Nilsson E: Therapeutic trends in the treatment of

barbiturate poisoning: The Scandinavian method. *Clin Pharmacol Ther* 2:220, 1961.

45. Aldrich T, Morrison J, Desario T: Aspiration after overdosage of sedative or hypnotic drugs. *South Med J* 73:456, 1980.

46. Shannon M, Lovejoy FH: Pulmonary consequences of severe tricyclic antidepressant poisoning. *Clin Toxicol* 25:443, 1987.

47. Roy TM, Ossorio MA, Dipolla LM, et al: Pulmonary complications after tricyclic antidepressant overdose. *Chest* 96:852, 1989.

48. Kulig K, Rumack BH, Rosen P: Gag reflex in assessing level of consciousness. *Lancet* 1:565, 1982.

49. McLeane DJ, Fisher M: Efficiency of high-volume, low-pressure cuffs in preventing aspiration. *Anaesth Intensive Care* 5:167, 1977.

50. Spray SB, Zuidema GD, Cameron JL: Aspiration pneumonia: Incidence of aspiration with endotracheal tubes. *Am J Surg* 131:701, 1976.

51. Torres A, Serva-Battles J, Ros E, et al: Pulmonary aspiration of gastric contents in patients receiving mechanical ventilation: The effect of body position. *Ann Intern Med* 116:540, 1992.

52. Mithoefer JC, Bossman OG, Thibeault DW, et al: The clinical estimation of alveolar ventilation. *Am Rev Respir Dis* 98:868, 1968.

53. Dobos JK, Phillips J, Covo GA: Acute barbiturate intoxication. *JAMA* 176:268, 1961.

54. Shubin H, Weil MH: The mechanism of shock following suicidal doses of barbiturates, narcotics, and tranquilizer drugs with observations on the effect of treatment. *Am J Med* 38:853, 1985.

55. Benowitz NL, Rosenberg J, Becker CE: Cardiopulmonary catastrophes in drug-overdosed patients. *Med Clin North Am* 63:267, 1979.

56. Blake KV, Massey KL, Hendeles L, et al: Relative efficacy of phenytoin and phenobarbital for the prevention of theophylline-induced seizures in mice. *Ann Emerg Med* 17:1024, 1988.

57. Snyder SH: Drug and neurotransmitter receptors: New perspectives with clinical reference. *JAMA* 261:3126, 1989.

58. McEvoy GK (ed): *American Hospital Formulary Service Drug Information.* Bethesda, MD, American Society of Hospital Pharmacists, 1989.

59. Klein DG, O'Malley P: Topical injury from chemical agents: Initial treatment. *Heart Lung* 16:49, 1987.

60. Rost KM, Jaeger RW, deCastro FJ: Eye contamination: A poison center protocol for management. *Clin Toxicol* 14:295, 1979.

61. Nelson JD, Kopietz LA: Chemical injuries to the eyes: Emergency, intermediate, and long-term care. *Postgrad Med* 81:62, 1987.

62. Herr RD, White GL, Bernhisel K, et al: Clinical comparison of ocular irrigation fluids following chemical injury. *Am J Emerg Med* 9:228, 1991.

63. Wester RC, Maibach HI: In vivo percutaneous absorption and decontamination of pesticides in humans. *J Toxicol Environ Health* 16:25, 1985.

64. Fredriksson T: Percutaneous absorption of parathion and paraoxon. IV. Decontamination of human skin from parathion. *Arch Environ Health* 3:67, 1961.

65. Walsh AC: Dog poisons man (letter). *JAMA* 249:253, 1983.

66. Cupit GC, Temple AR: Gastrointestinal decontamination in the management of the poisoned patient. *Emerg Med Clin North Am* 2:15, 1984.

67. Rodgers GC, Matyunas NJ: Gastrointestinal decontamination for acute poisoning. *Pediatr Clin North Am* 33:261, 1986.

68. Neuvonen PJ: Clinical pharmacokinetics of oral activated charcoal in acute intoxications. *Clin Pharmacokinet* 7:465, 1982.

69. Neuvonen PJ, Olkkala KT: Oral activated charcoal in the treatment of intoxications: Role of single and repeated doses. *Med Toxicol* 3:33, 1988.

70. Cooney DO: *Activated Charcoal in Medical Applications.* New York, Marcel Dekker, 1995.

71. Palatnick W, Tenenbein M: Activated charcoal in the treatment of drug overdose: An update. *Drug Saf* 7:3, 1992.

72. Tenenbein M: Whole bowel irrigation as a gastrointestinal decontamination procedure after acute poisoning. *Med Toxicol* 3:77, 1988.

73. Freedman GE, Pasternak S, Krenzelok EP: A clinical trial using syrup of ipecac and activated charcoal concurrently. *Am Emerg Med* 16:164, 1987.

74. Burton BT, Bayer MJ, Barron L, et al: Comparison of activated charcoal and gastric lavage in the prevention of aspirin absorption. *J Emerg Med* 1:411, 1984.

75. Decker WJ, Coombs HF, Corby DG: Absorption of drugs and poisons by activated charcoal. *Toxicol Appl Pharmacol* 13:454, 1968.

76. Mitchell RD, Walberg CB, Gupta RC: In vitro adsorption properties of activated charcoal with selected inorganic compounds (abstract). *Ann Emerg Med* 18:444, 1989.

77. Olkkola KT: Effect of charcoal-drug ratio on antidotal efficacy of oral activated charcoal in man. *Br J Clin Pharmacol* 19:767, 1985.

78. Olkkola KT: Factors affecting the antidotal efficacy of oral activated charcoal. Dissertation, Department of Clinical Pharmacology, University of Helsinki, 1985.

79. Chin L, Picchioni AL, Bourn WMN, et al: Optimal antidotal dose of activated charcoal. *Toxicol Appl Pharmacol* 26:103, 1973.

80. Neuvonen RJ, Olkkola KT: Effect of dose of charcoal on the absorption of disopyramide, indomethacin, and trimethoprim in man. *Eur J Clin Pharmacol* 26:761, 1984.

81. Neuvonen PJ, Kannisto H, Lankinen S: Capacity of two forms of activated charcoal to adsorb nefopam in vitro and to reduce its toxicity in vivo. *Clin Toxicol* 21:333, 1984.

82. Curd-Sneed CD, Bordelon JG, Parks KS, et al: Effects of activated charcoal and sorbitol on sodium pentobarbital absorption in the rat. *Clin Toxicol* 25:555, 1987.

83. Krenzelok EP, Heller MB: Effectiveness of commercially available aqueous activated charcoal products. *Ann Emerg Med* 16:1340, 1987.

84. Dillon EC, Wilton JH, Barlow JC, et al: Large surface area charcoal and the inhibition of aspirin absorption. *Ann Emerg Med* 18:547, 1989.

85. Crane P, Dowling S, Braithwaite RA: Effect of activated charcoal on absorption of nortriptyline. *Lancet* 2:1203, 1977.

86. Lin DT, Singh P, Nourtsis S, et al: Absorption inhibition and enhancement of elimination of sustained-release theophylline tablets by oral activated charcoal. *Ann Emerg Med* 15:1303, 1986.

87. Barone JA, Raia JJ, Huang YC: Evaluation of the effects of multiple dose charcoal on the absorption of orally administered salicylate in a simulated toxic ingestion model. *Ann Emerg Med* 17:34, 1987.

88. Levy G, Tsuchiya T: Effects of activated charcoal on aspirin absorption in man. *Clin Pharmacol Ther* 13:317, 1972.

89. Anderson HH: Medicinal charcoal in the treatment of poisoning: Treatment of experimentally poisoned pigs. *Ugeskr Laeg* 135:797, 1973.

90. Dordoni B, Willson RA, Thompson RPH, et al: Reduction of absorption of paracetamol by activated charcoal and cholestyramine: A possible therapeutic measure. *Br Med J* 3:86, 1973.

91. Dawling S, Crome P, Braithwaite R: Effect of delayed administration of activated charcoal on nortriptyline absorption. *Eur J Clin Pharmacol* 14:445, 1978.

92. Neuvonen PJ, Elfving SM, Elonen E: Reduction of absorption of digoxin, phenytoin, and aspirin by activated charcoal in man. *Eur J Clin Pharmacol* 13:213, 1978.

93. Neuvonen PJ, Elonen E: Effect of activated charcoal on absorption and elimination of phenobarbitone, carbamazepine, and phenylbutazone in man. *Eur J Clin Pharmacol* 17:51, 1980.

94. Neuvonen PJ, Vantiainen M, Tokola O: Comparison of activated charcoal and ipecac syrup in prevention of drug absorption. *Eur J Clin Pharmacol* 24:557, 1983.

95. Guay DRP, Meatherull RC, Macauley PA, et al: Activated charcoal adsorption of diphenhydramine. *Int J Clin Pharmacol Ther Toxicol* 22:395, 1984.

96. Olkkola KT, Neuvonen PJ: Do gastric contents modify antidotal efficacy of oral activated charcoal? *Br J Clin Pharmacol* 18:663, 1984.

97. Neuvonen PJ, Olkkola KT: Effect of purgatives on the antidotal efficacy of oral activated charcoal. *Hum Toxicol* 5:255, 1986.

98. Picchioni AL, Chin L, Verhulst HL, et al: Activated charcoal vs. "universal antidote" as an antidote for poisons. *Toxicol Appl Pharmacol* 8:447, 1966.

99. Phansalkar SV, Holt LE: Observations on the immediate treatment of poisoning. *J Pediatr* 72:683, 1968.

100. Chin L, Picchioni AL, Duplisse BR: Comparative antidotal effectiveness of activated charcoal, Arizona montmorillonite, and evaporated milk. *J Pharm Sci* 58:1353, 1969.

101. Tsuchiya T, Levy G: Drug adsorption efficacy of commercial activated charcoal tablets in vitro and in man. *J Pharm Sci* 61:624, 1972.
102. Hartel G, Manninen V, Reissell P: Treatment of digoxin intoxication. *Lancet* 2:258, 1973.
103. Boehm JJ, Brown TCK, Oppenheim RC: Reduction of pheniramine toxicity using activated charcoal. *Clin Toxicol* 12:523, 1978.
104. Neuvonen PJ, Karkkainen S: Effects of charcoal, sodium bicarbonate, and ammonium chloride on chlorpropamide kinetics. *Clin Pharmacol Ther* 33:386, 1983.
105. Neuvonen PJ, Kannisto H, Alanen T, et al: Effect of activated charcoal on the absorption of tolbutamide and valproate in man. *Eur J Clin Pharmacol* 24:243, 1983.
106. Galinsky RE, Levy G: Evaluation of activated charcoal-sodium sulfate combination for inhibition of acetaminophen absorption and repletion of inorganic sulfate. *Clin Toxicol* 22:21, 1984.
107. Karkkainen S, Neuvonen PJ: Effect of oral charcoal and urine pH on sotalol pharmacokinetics. *Int J Clin Pharmacol Ther Toxicol* 22:441, 1984.
108. Neuvonen PJ, Olkkola KT: Activated charcoal and syrup of ipecac in prevention of cimetidine and pindolol absorption in man after administration of metochlorpramide as an antiemetic agent. *Clin Toxicol* 22:103, 1984.
109. Neuvonen PJ, Olkkola KT, Alanen T: Effect of ethanol and pH on the adsorption of drugs to activated charcoal: Studies in vitro and in man. *Acta Pharmacol Toxicol* 54:1, 1984.
110. Olkkola KT, Neuvonen PJ: Effect of gastric pH on antidotal efficacy of activated charcoal in man. *Int J Clin Pharmacol Ther Toxicol* 22:565, 1984.
111. Karkkainen S, Neuvonen PJ: Effect of oral charcoal and urine pH on dextropropoxyphene pharmacokinetics. *Int J Clin Pharmacol Ther Toxicol* 23:219, 1985.
112. Karkkainen S, Neuvonen PJ: Pharmacokinetics of amitriptyline influenced by oral charcoal and urine pH. *Int J Clin Pharmacol Ther Toxicol* 24:326, 1986.
113. Neuvonen PJ, Kivisto K, Hirviselo EL: Effects of resins and activated charcoal on the adsorption of digoxin, carbamazepine, and furosemide. *Br J Clin Pharmacol* 25:229, 1988.
114. Eisen TF, Grbeich PA, Lacouture PG, et al: The adsorption of salicylates by a milk chocolate-charcoal mixture. *Ann Emerg Med* 20:143, 1991.
115. Decker WJ, Corby DG, Ibanez JD: Aspirin adsorption with activated charcoal. *Lancet* 1:754, 1968.
116. Decker WJ, Shpall RA, Corby DG, et al: Inhibition of aspirin absorption by activated charcoal and apomorphine. *Clin Pharmacol Ther* 10:710, 1969.
117. Fiser RH, Maetz VC, Treuting JJ, et al: Activated charcoal in barbiturate and glutethimide poisoning of the dog. *J Pediatr* 78:1045, 1971.
118. Alvan G: Effect of activated charcoal on plasma levels of nortriptyline after single doses in man. *Eur J Clin Pharmacol* 5:236, 1973.
119. Glab WN, Corby DG, Decker WJ, et al: Decreased absorption of propoxyphene by activated charcoal. *Clin Toxicol* 19:129, 1982.
120. Sheinin M, Virtanen R, Iisalo E: Effect of single and repeated doses of activated charcoal on the pharmacokinetics of digoxin. *Int J Clin Pharmacol Ther Toxicol* 23:38, 1985.
121. Rose SR, Gorman RL, Orderda GM, et al: Simulated acetaminophen overdose: Pharmacokinetics and effectiveness of activated charcoal. *Ann Emerg Med* 20:1064, 1991.
122. Curtis RA, Barone J, Giacona N: Efficacy of ipecac and activated charcoal/cathartic: Prevention of salicylate absorption in a simulated overdose. *Arch Intern Med* 144:48, 1984.
123. Tenenbein M, Cohen S, Sitar DS: Efficacy of ipecac-induced emesis, orogastric lavage, and activated charcoal for acute drug overdose. *Ann Emerg Med* 16:838, 1987.
124. Danel V, Henry JA, Glucksman E: Activated charcoal, emesis, and gastric lavage in aspirin overdose. *Br Med J* 296:1507, 1988.
125. McNamara RM, Aaron CK, Gemboys M, et al: Efficacy of charcoal cathartic versus ipecac in reducing serum acetaminophen in a simulated overdose. *Ann Emerg Med* 18:934, 1989.
126. Keller RE, Schwab RA, Krenzelok EP: Contribution of sorbitol combined with activated charcoal in prevention of salicylate absorption. *Ann Emerg Med* 19:654, 1990.
127. Lipscomb BJ, Widdop B: Studies with activated charcoal in the treatment of drug overdosage using the pig as an animal model. *Arch Toxicol* 34:37, 1975.
128. Arai K, Yamashita M, Sato S, et al: Utility of activated charcoal administered at 120 minutes after aspirin administration in man. *Jpn J Acute Med* 13:1001, 1989.
129. Kirschenbaum LA, Mathews SC, Sitar DS, et al: Whole-bowel irrigation versus activated charcoal in sorbitol for the ingestion of modified-release pharmaceuticals. *Clin Pharmacol Ther* 46:264, 1989.
130. Mayersohn M, Perrier D, Picchioni AL: Evaluation of charcoal mixture as an antidote for oral aspirin overdose. *Clin Toxicol* 11:561, 1977.
131. Esaom JM, Caraccio TR, Lovejoy FH: Evaluation of activated charcoal and magnesium citrate in the prevention of aspirin absorption in humans. *Clin Pharmacol* 1:154, 1982.
132. Sketris IS, Mowry J, Czajka PA, et al: Saline catharsis: Effect in aspirin bioavailability in combination with activated charcoal. *J Clin Pharm* 22:59, 1982.
133. Olkkola KT: Does ethanol modify antidotal efficacy of oral activated charcoal: Studies in vitro and in experimental animals, in Factors affecting the antidotal efficacy of oral activated charcoal in man. Dissertation, Department of Clinical Pharmacology, University of Helsinki, 1985.
134. Czajka PA, Konrad JD: Saline cathartics and the adsorptive capacity of activated charcoal for aspirin. *Ann Emerg Med* 15:548, 1986.
135. Wieland MJ, Ling LJ, Thompson JD: In vivo effects of excipient agents on the adsorptivity of activated charcoal (abstract). *Vet Hum Toxicol* 28:495, 1986.
136. Fillipone GA, Fish SS, Lacouture PG, et al: Reversible adsorption (desorption) of aspirin from activated charcoal. *Arch Intern Med* 147:1390, 1987.
137. Tsuchiya T, Levy G: Relationship between effect of activated charcoal on drug absorption in man and its drug adsorption characteristics in vitro. *J Pharm Sci* 61:586, 1972.
138. Lambert RJ, Kindler BL, Schaeffer DJ: The efficacy of superactivated charcoal in treating rats exposed to a lethal oral dose of potassium cyanide. *Ann Emerg Med* 17:595, 1988.
139. Anderson AH: Experimental studies on the pharmacology of activated charcoal. II. The effect of pH on the adsorption by charcoal from aqueous solutions. *Acta Pharmacol Toxicol* 3:199, 1947.
140. Smith RP, Gosselin RE, Henderson JA, et al: Comparison of the adsorptive properties of activated charcoal and Alaskan montmorillonite for some common poisons. *Toxicol Appl Pharmacol* 10:95, 1967.
141. Klein-Schwartz W, Oderda GM: Absorption of oral antidotes for acetaminophen poisoning (methionine and N-acetyl-cysteine) by activated charcoal. *Clin Toxicol* 18:283, 1981.
142. Rybolt TR, Burrell DE, Shults JM, et al: In vitro coadsorption of acetaminophen and N-acetyl-cysteine onto activated carbon powder. *J Pharm Sci* 75:904, 1986.
143. Hulten BA, Heath A, Mellstand T, et al: Does alcohol absorb to activated charcoal? *Hum Toxicol* 5:211, 1985.
144. Minocha A, Herold DA, Barth JT, et al: Activated charcoal in oral ethanol absorption: Lack of effect in humans. *Clin Toxicol* 24:225, 1986.
145. Katona BG, Siegel EG, Roberts JR, et al: The effect of "superactive" charcoal and magnesium citrate solution on blood ethanol concentrations and area under the curve in humans. *Clin Toxicol* 27:129, 1989.
146. North DS, Peterson RG, Krenzelok EP: Effect of activated charcoal administration on acetylcysteine serum levels in humans. *Am J Hosp Pharm* 38:1022, 1981.
147. Ekins BR, Ford DC, Thompson MB, et al: Effect of activated charcoal on N-acetyl-cysteine (NAC) absorption in normal subjects (abstract). *Vet Hum Toxicol* 26(suppl):45, 1984.
148. Renzi FP, Donovan JW, Martin TG, et al: Concomitant use of activated charcoal and N-acetyl-cysteine. *Ann Emerg Med* 14:568, 1985.
149. Krenzelok EP, Lush RM: Container residue after the administration of aqueous activated charcoal products. *Am J Emerg Med* 9:144, 1991.
150. Kulig K, Bar-Or D, Cantrill SV, et al: Management of acutely poisoned patients without gastric emptying. *Ann Emerg Med* 14:562, 1985.

151. Albertson TE, Derlet RW, Foulke GE, et al: Superiority of activated charcoal alone compared with ipecac and activated charcoal in the treatment of acute toxic ingestions. *Ann Emerg Med* 18:56, 1989.

152. Merigian KS, Woodard M, Hedges JR, et al: Prospective evaluation of gastric emptying in the self-poisoned patient. *Am J Emerg Med* 8:479, 1990.

153. Underhill TJ, Greene MK, Dove AR: A comparison of the efficacy of gastric lavage, ipecacuanha, and activated charcoal in the emergency management of paracetamol overdose. *Arch Emerg Med* 7:148, 1990.

154. Kornberg AE, Dolgin J: Pediatric ingestions: Charcoal alone versus ipecac and charcoal. *Ann Emerg Med* 20:648, 1991.

155. Minocha A, Herold DA, Bruns DE, et al: Effect of activated charcoal in 70% sorbitol in healthy individuals. *Clin Toxicol* 22:529, 1985.

156. Nau CA, Neal J, Stembridge V: A study of the physiological effects of carbon black. I. Ingestion. *Arch Ind Health* 17:21, 1957.

157. Yatzidis H: Activated charcoal rediscovered. *Br Med J* 7:51, 1972.

158. Nau CA, Neal J, Stembridge VA, et al: Physiological effects of carbon black. IV. Inhalation. *Arch Environ Health* 4:45, 1962.

159. Dockstader LL, Lawrence RA, Bresnick HL: Home administration of activated charcoal: Feasibility and acceptance (abstract). *Vet Hum Toxicol* 28:471, 1986.

160. Fish S, Munier-Sham J, Blansfield J: Activated charcoal/sorbitol preparations: Incidence of adverse effects (abstract). *Vet Hum Toxicol* 31:350, 1989.

161. Levy G: Charcoal for gastrointestinal clearance of drugs (letter). *N Engl J Med* 308:157, 1983.

162. Hoffman JR: Charcoal for gastrointestinal clearance of drugs (letter). *N Engl J Med* 308:157, 1983.

163. Watson WA, Cremer KF, Chapman JA: Gastrointestinal obstruction associated with multiple-dose activated charcoal. *J Emerg Med* 4:401, 1986.

164. Ray MJ, Padin R, Condie JD, et al: Charcoal bezoar: Small-bowel obstruction secondary to amitriptyline overdose therapy. *Dig Dis Sci* 33:106, 1988.

165. Olson KR, Pond SM, Verrier ED, et al: Intestinal infarction complicating phenobarbital overdose. *Arch Intern Med* 144:407, 1984.

166. Longdon P, Henderson A: Intestinal pseudo-obstruction following the use of enteral charcoal and sorbitol and mechanical ventilation with papaveretum sedation for theophylline poisoning. *Drug Saf* 7:74, 1992.

167. Pollack MM, Dunbar BS, Holbrook PR, et al: Aspiration of activated charcoal and gastric contents. *Ann Emerg Med* 10:528, 1981.

168. Menzies DG, Busuttil A, Prescott LF: Fatal pulmonary aspiration of oral activated charcoal. *Br Med J* 297:459, 1988.

169. Dunbar BS, Pollack MM, Shavari MB: Cardiorespiratory changes after charcoal aspiration (abstract). *Crit Care Med* 9:221, 1981.

170. Elliot CG, Colby TV, Kelly TM, et al: Charcoal lung: Bronchiolitis obliterans after aspiration of activated charcoal. *Chest* 96:672, 1989.

171. American Association of Poison Control Centers: Labeling of activated charcoal drug products. *Vet Hum Toxicol* 28:344, 1985.

172. Abdallah AH, Tye A: A comparison of the efficacy of emetic drugs and stomach lavage. *Am J Dis Child* 113:571, 1967.

173. Fane LR, Combs HF, Decker WJ: Physical parameters in gastric lavage. *Clin Toxicol* 4:389, 1971.

174. Auerbach PS, Osterloh J, Braun O, et al: Efficacy of gastric emptying: Gastric lavage versus emesis induced with ipecac. *Ann Emerg Med* 15:692, 1986.

175. Arnold FJ, Hodges JB, Barta PA, et al: Evaluation of the efficacy of lavage induced emesis in treatment of salicylate poisoning. *Pediatrics* 23:286, 1959.

176. Lanphear WF: Gastric lavage. *J Emerg Med* 4:43, 1986.

177. Burke M: Gastric lavage and emesis in the treatment of ingested poisons: A review and a clinical study of lavage in 10 adults. *Resuscitation* 1:91, 1972.

178. McDougel CB, Maclean MA: Modifications in the technique of gastric lavage. *Ann Emerg Med* 10:514, 1981.

179. Wheeler-Usher DH, Wanke LA, Bayer MJ: Gastric emptying: Risk versus benefit in the treatment of acute poisoning. *Med Toxicol* 1:142, 1986.

180. Vance MV, Selden BS, Clark RF: Optimal patient position for transport and initial management of toxic ingestions. *Ann Emerg Med* 21:243, 1992.

181. Watson WA, Leighton J, Guy J, et al: Recovery of cyclic antidepressants with gastric lavage. *J Emerg Med* 7:373, 1989.

182. Agocha A, Reyman L, Longmore W, et al: Can pills really fit through the lavage tubes? (abstract). *Vet Hum Toxicol* 28:494, 1986.

183. Agocha A, Wang R, Longmore W, et al: Drug disintegration time and its value in gastric lavage (abstract). *Vet Hum Toxicol* 28:493, 1986.

184. Rudolph JP: Automated gastric lavage and a comparison of 0.9% normal saline solution and tap water irrigant. *Ann Emerg Med* 14:1156, 1985.

185. Peterson CD: Electrolyte depletion following emergency stomach evacuation. *Am J Hosp Pharm* 36:1366, 1979.

186. Mathew H, Mackintosh TF, Tompsett SL, et al: Gastric aspiration and lavage in acute poisoning. *Br Med J* 1:1333, 1966.

187. Sharman JR, Cretney MJ, Scott RD, et al: Drug overdoses: Is one stomach washing enough? *N Z Med J* 81:195, 1975.

188. Thomas RT, Sterling ML, Salness K, et al: Absence of pulmonary aspiration in adults after gastric lavage without endotracheal intubation (abstract). *Vet Hum Toxicol* 23(suppl 1):57, 1981.

189. Pontoppidan H, Beecher HK: Progressive loss of protective reflexes in the airway with the advance of age. *JAMA* 174:2209, 1960.

190. Reid DHS: Treatment of the poisoned child. *Arch Dis Child* 45:428, 1970.

191. Tandberg D, Wood DA: Ipecac-induced emesis and gastric lavage are equally unpleasant. *Vet Hum Toxicol* 30:109, 1988.

192. Corby DG, Lisciandro RC, Lehman RH, et al: The efficacy of methods used to evacuate the stomach after acute ingestions. *Pediatrics* 40:871, 1967.

193. Tandberg D, Diven BG, McLeod JW: Ipecac-induced emesis versus gastric lavage: A controlled study in normal adults. *Am J Emerg Med* 4:205, 1986.

194. Boxer L, Anderson FP, Rowe DS: Comparison of ipecac-induced emesis with gastric lavage in the treatment of acute salicylate ingestion. *J Pediatr* 74:800, 1969.

195. Comstock EG, Faulkner TP, Boisaubin EV, et al: Studies on the efficacy of gastric lavage as practiced in a large metropolitan hospital. *Clin Toxicol* 18:581, 1981.

196. Pollack CV, Jordan RC, Carlton FB, et al: Gastric emptying in the acutely inebriated patient. *J Emerg Med* 10:1, 1992.

197. Saetta JP, Quinton DN: Residual gastric content after gastric lavage and ipecacuanha-induced emesis in self-poisoned patients: An endoscopic study. *J Roy Soc Med* 84:35, 1991.

198. Wright N: Common errors in the management of poisoning. *J R Coll Physicians Lond* 14:114, 1980.

199. Gough D, Rust D: Nasogastric intubation: Morbidity in an asymptomatic patient. *Am J Emerg Med* 4:511, 1986.

200. Coutselinis A, Plulos L, Boukis D, et al: A lethal complication of gastric lavage leading to malpractice suit: A case report. *Forensic Sci Int* 11:47, 1978.

201. Leclerc F, Martin V, Gandier B: Intoxication per l'eursecondaire au lavage d'estomac. *Nouv Press Med* 10:1149, 1981.

202. Scalzo AJ, Tominack RL, Thompson MW: Malposition of pediatric gastric lavage tubes demonstrated radiographically. *J Emerg Med* 10:581, 1992.

203. Calvanese JC: Midesophageal kinking and lodgement of a 34-F gastric lavage tube. *Ann Emerg Med* 14:1123, 1985.

204. Wald P, Stern J, Weiner B, et al: Esophageal tear following forceful removal of an impacted oral-gastric lavage tube. *Ann Emerg Med* 15:80, 1985.

205. Weiner BC: Management of oral-gastric lavage tube impaction of the esophagus. *Am J Gastroenterol* 81:1202, 1986.

206. Askenasi R, Abramowicz M, Jeanmart J, et al: Esophageal perforation: An unusual complication of gastric lavage. *Ann Emerg Med* 13:146, 1984.

207. Thompson AM, Robins JB, Prescott LF: Changes in cardiorespiratory function during gastric lavage for drug overdose. *Hum Toxicol* 6:215, 1987.

208. Justiniani FR, Hippalgoankar R, Martinez LO: Charcoal-containing empyema complicating treatment for overdose. *Chest* 87:404, 1985.

209. Chaudel S, Ducluzeau R, Pacheco Y, et al: Endoscopic gastric lesions after a gastric washing-out using the Faucher tube in intoxicated comatose patients (abstract). *Vet Hum Toxicol* 24:287, 1982.

210. Penner GE: Acid ingestion: Toxicology and treatment. *Ann Emerg Med* 9:374, 1984.
211. Friedman EM, Lovejoy FH: The emergency management of caustic ingestions. *Emerg Med Clin North Am* 2:77, 1984.
212. Howel JM: Alkaline ingestions. *Ann Emerg Med* 15:820, 1986.
213. Okada Y, Iway A, Kobayashi H: Gastric lavage solution for ingestion of corrosive agents. *Jpn J Acute Med* 11:75, 1987.
214. Seger DL: The hydrocarbon controversy. *Emerg Med Surv* 1:1, 1984.
215. Manno BR, Manno JE: Toxicology of ipecac: A review. *Clin Toxicol* 10:221, 1977.
216. King WD: Syrup of ipecac: A drug review. *Clin Toxicol* 17:353, 1980.
217. Stewart JJ: Effects of emetic and cathartic agents on the gastrointestinal tract and the treatment of toxic ingestion. *Clin Toxicol* 20:199, 1983.
218. Moran DM, Crouch DJ, Finkle BS: Absorption of ipecac alkaloids in emergency patients. *Ann Emerg Med* 13:1100, 1984.
219. Schofferman JA: A clinical comparison of syrup of ipecac and apomorphine use in adults. *JACEP* 5:22, 1976.
220. Gieseker DR, Troutman WG: Emergency induction of emesis using liquid detergent products: A report of 15 cases. *Clin Toxicol* 18:277, 1981.
221. Dabbous JA, Bergman AB, Robertson WD: The ineffectiveness of mechanically induced vomiting. *J Pediatr* 66:952, 1965.
222. American Association of Poison Control Centers: Labeling of ipecac syrup drug products. *Vet Hum Toxicol* 28:344, 1985.
223. Robertson WO: Syrup of ipecac: A slow or fast emetic? *Am J Dis Child* 103:136, 1962.
224. Thoman ME, Verhulst HL: Ipecac syrup in antiemetic ingestions. *JAMA* 196:147, 1966.
225. Manoquerra AS, Krenzelok EP: Rapid emesis from high-dose ipecac syrup in adults and children intoxicated with antiemetics and other drugs. *Am J Hosp Pharm* 35:1360, 1978.
226. Dean BS, Krenzelok EP: Syrup of ipecac: 15 ml versus 30 ml in pediatric poisonings. *Clin Toxicol* 23:165, 1985.
227. Bobbink S, Forrester H, Robertson WO: Syrup of ipecac induced emesis: Impact of fluids versus no fluids on time until emesis. *Vet Hum Toxicol* 28:580, 1986.
228. Grande GA, Ling LJ: The effect of fluid volume on syrup of ipecac emesis time. *Clin Toxicol* 25:473, 1987.
229. Grbcich PA, Lacouture PG, Lovejoy FH: Effects of fluid volume on ipecac-induced emesis. *J Pediatr* 110:970, 1987.
230. Uden DL, Davidson GJ, Kohen DP: The effect of carbonated beverages on ipecac-induced emesis. *Ann Emerg Med* 10:79, 1981.
231. Grbcich PA, Lacouture PG, Lewander WJ, et al: Effect of milk on ipecac-induced emesis. *J Pediatr* 110:973, 1987.
232. Spigiel RW, Abdouch I, Munn D: The effect of temperature on concurrently administered fluid on the onset of ipecac-induced emesis. *Clin Toxicol* 14:281, 1979.
233. Meester WD: Emesis and lavage. *Vet Hum Toxicol* 22:225, 1980.
234. Amitai Y, Mitchell AA, McGuigan MA, et al: Ipecac-induced emesis and reduction of plasma concentrations of drugs following accidental overdose in children. *Pediatrics* 80:364, 1987.
235. Vasquez TE, Evans DG, Ashburn WL: Efficacy of syrup of ipecac-induced emesis for emptying gastric contents. *Clin Nucl Med* 9:638, 1988.
236. Corby DG, Decker WJ, Moran MJ, et al: Clinical comparison of pharmacologic emetics in children. *Pediatrics* 42:361, 1968.
237. Tandberg D, Murphy LC: The knee-chest position does not improve the efficacy of ipecac-induced emesis. *Am J Emerg Med* 7:267, 1989.
238. Tandberg D, Liechty EJ, Fishbein D: Mallory-Weiss syndrome: An unusual complication of ipecac-induced emesis. *Ann Emerg Med* 10:521, 1981.
239. Knight KM, Doucet HJ: Gastric rupture and death caused by ipecac syrup. *South Med J* 80:786, 1987.
240. Robertson WO: Syrup of ipecac associated fatality: A case report. *Vet Hum Toxicol* 21:87, 1979.
241. Wolowodiuk OJ, McMicken DB, O'Brien P: Pneumomediastinum and retropneumoperitoneum: An unusual complication of syrup of ipecac-induced emesis. *Ann Emerg Med* 13:1148, 1984.
242. Klein-Schwartz W, Gorman RL, Oderda GM, et al: Ipecac use in the elderly: The unanswered question. *Ann Emerg Med* 13:1152, 1984.
243. Czajka PA, Russell SL: Nonemetic effects of ipecac syrup. *Pediatrics* 75:1101, 1985.
244. MacLeod J: Ipecac intoxication: Use of a cardiac pacemaker in management. *N Engl J Med* 268:146, 1963.
245. Adler AG, Walinsky P, Krall RA, et al: Death resulting from ipecac syrup poisoning. *JAMA* 243:1927, 1980.
246. Palmer EP, Guay AT: Reversible myopathy secondary to abuse of ipecac in patients with major eating disorders. *N Engl J Med* 313:1457, 1985.
247. Mateer JE, Farrell BJ, Chou SSM, et al: Reversible ipecac myopathy. *Arch Neurol* 42:188, 1985.
248. Pope HG, Hudson JI, Nixon RA, et al: The epidemiology of ipecac abuse. *N Engl J Med* 314:245, 1986.
249. Isner JM: Effects of ipecac on the heart. *N Engl J Med* 314:1253, 1986.
250. Rosenberg NL, Ringel SP: Myopathy from surreptitious ipecac ingestions. *West J Med* 145:386, 1986.
251. Schiff RJ, Wurzel CL, Brunson SC, et al: Death due to chronic syrup of ipecac abuse in a patient with bulimia. *Pediatrics* 78:412, 1986.
252. Berkner P, Kastner T, Skolnick L: Chronic ipecac poisoning in infancy: A case report. *Pediatrics* 82:384, 1988.
253. Sutphen JL, Saulsbury FF: Intentional ipecac poisoning: Munchausen syndrome by proxy. *Pediatrics* 82:453, 1986.
254. Day L, Kelly C, Reed G, et al: Fatal cardiomyopathy: Suspected child abuse by chronic ipecac administration. *Vet Hum Toxicol* 31:255, 1989.
255. Santangelo WC, Richey JE, Rivera L, et al: Surreptitious ipecac administration simulating intestinal pseudo-obstruction. *Ann Intern Med* 10:1031, 1989.
256. Beck DE, Harford FJ, DiPalma JA, et al: Bowel cleansing with polyethylene glycol electrolyte lavage solution. *South Med J* 78:1414, 1985.
257. Anonymous: Oral electrolyte solutions for colonic lavage before colonoscopy or barium enema. *Med Lett* 28:39, 1986.
258. Boba A: Management of drug overdose: Rapid whole gut evacuation. *IL Med J* 155:156, 1979.
259. Tennenbein M: Whole bowel irrigation for toxic ingestions. *Clin Toxicol* 23:177, 1985.
260. Tennenbein M: Whole bowel irrigation in iron poisoning. *J Pediatr* 111:142, 1987.
261. Rosenberg PJ, Livingstone DJ, McLellan BA: Effect of whole bowel irrigation on the antidotal efficacy of oral activated charcoal. *Ann Emerg Med* 17:681, 1988.
262. Tenenbein M, Cohen S, Sitar DS: Whole bowel irrigation as a decontamination procedure after acute drug overdose. *Arch Intern Med* 147:905, 1987.
263. Smith SW, Ling LJ, Halstenson CE: Whole-bowel irrigation as a treatment for acute lithium overdose. *Ann Emerg Med* 20:536, 1991.
264. Young TK, Lee SC, Tang CK: Diarrhea therapy of uremia. *Clin Nephrol* 11:86, 1979.
265. Porter RS, Baker EB: Drug clearance by diarrhea induction. *Am J Emerg Med* 3:182, 1985.
266. Brown CR, Becker CE, Osterlob JD, et al: Whole gut lavage in a simulated drug overdose (abstract). *Vet Hum Toxicol* 29:366, 1987.
267. Burkhart KK, Wuerz RC, Donovan JW: Whole bowel irrigation as an adjunctive treatment for sustained-released theophylline overdose. *Ann Emerg Med* 21:1316, 1992.
268. Palatnick W, Tenenbein M: Safety of treating poisoning patients with whole bowel irrigation. *Am J Emerg Med* 6:200, 1988.
269. Postuma R: Whole bowel irrigation in pediatric patients: A comparison of irrigating solutions. *J Pediatr Surg* 23:769, 1988.
270. Minocha A, Spyker DA: Acute overdose with sustained-release drug formulations: Perspectives in treatment. *Med Toxicol* 1:300, 1986.
271. Hoffman RS, Smilkstein MJ, Goldfrank LR: Whole bowel irrigation and the cocaine "body packer" (abstract). *Vet Hum Toxicol* 31:374, 1989.
272. Shah M, Nakanishi A: Polyethylene glycol-electrolyte solution for rectal sunflower seed bezoar. *Pediatr Emerg Care* 6:127, 1990.
273. Burkhart K, Kulig K, Rumack B: Whole bowel irrigation for zinc sulfate overdose. *Ann Emerg Med* 19:1167, 1990.

274. Roberge RJ, Martin TG: Whole bowel irrigation in an acute oral lead intoxication. *Ann J Emerg Med* 10:577, 1992.

275. Marsteller HJ, Gugler R: Endoscopic management of toxic masses in the stomach. *N Engl J Med* 296:1003, 1977.

276. Bartecchi CE: Removal of gastric drug masses. *N Engl J Med* 296:282, 1977.

277. Litovitz TL: Button battery ingestions. *JAMA* 249:2495, 1983.

278. Trent M, Kim U: Cocaine packet ingestion: Surgical or medical management. *Arch Surg* 122:1179, 1987.

279. Schwartz HS: Acute meprobamate poisoning with gastrotomy and removal of a drug-containing mass. *N Engl J Med* 295:1177, 1976.

280. Landsman J, Bricker J, Reid BS, et al: Emergency gastrostomy: Treatment of choice for iron bezoar. *J Pediatr Surg* 22:184, 1987.

281. Tenenbein M, Wiseman N, Yatscoff RW: Gastrotomy and whole bowel irrigation in iron poisoning. *Pediatr Emerg Care* 7:286, 1991.

282. Riegel JM, Becker CE: Use of cathartics in toxic ingestions. *Ann Emerg Med* 10:254, 1981.

283. Shannon M, Fish SS, Lovejoy FH: Cathartics and laxatives: Do they still have a place in management of the poisoned patient? *Med Toxicol* 1:247, 1986.

284. Tenenbein M: Cathartics for drug overdose. *Ann Emerg Med* 16:832, 1987.

285. Krenzelok EP, Keller R, Stewart RD: Gastrointestinal transit times of cathartics combined with charcoal. *Ann Emerg Med* 14:1152, 1985.

286. Minocha A, Wiley SH, Chabbra DQ, et al: Superior efficacy of sorbitol cathartics in poisoned patients (abstract). *Vet Hum Toxicol* 28:494, 1986.

287. Fish S, Munier-Sham J, Blansfield J: Activated charcoal/sorbitol preparations: Incidence of adverse effects (abstract). *Vet Hum Toxicol* 31:350, 1989.

288. Harchelroad F, Cottington E, Krenzelok EP: Gastrointestinal transit times of a charcoal-sorbitol slurry in overdose patients. *Clin Toxicol* 27:91, 1989.

289. Moses FF: Colonic perforation due to oral mannitol (letter). *JAMA* 260:640, 1988.

290. Morris ME, LeRoy S, Sutton SC: Absorption of magnesium from orally administered magnesium sulfate in man. *Clin Toxicol* 25:372, 1987.

291. Smilkstein MJ, Steedle D, Kulig KW, et al: Magnesium levels after magnesium-containing cathartics. *Clin Toxicol* 26:51, 1988.

292. Wiberg JJ, Turner GG, Nuttall FQ: Effect of phosphate or magnesium cathartics on serum calcium: Observations in normocalcemic patients. *Arch Intern Med* 138:1114, 1978.

293. Woodard JA, Shannon M, Lacouture PG, et al: Serum magnesium concentrations after repetitive magnesium cathartic administration. *Am J Emerg Med* 8:297, 1990.

294. Farley TA: Severe hypernatremic dehydration after use of an activated charcoal-sorbitol suspension. *J Pediatr* 109:719, 1986.

295. McCord MM, Okun AL: Toxicity of sorbitol-charcoal. *J Pediatr* 110:307, 1987.

296. Caldwell JW, Nova AJ, Dellaas DD: Hypernatremia associated with cathartics in overdose management. *West J Med* 147:593, 1987.

297. Brent J, Kulig K, Rumack BH: Iatrogenic death from sorbitol and magnesium sulfate during treatment for salicylism (abstract). *Vet Hum Toxicol* 31:334, 1989.

298. Sullivan JB, Krenzelok EP: Repetitive doses of the activated charcoal-sorbitol combination: A word of caution. *Am J Emerg Med* 6:201, 1988.

299. Jones J, Heiselman D, Dougherty J, et al: Cathartic-induced magnesium toxicity during overdose management. *Ann Emerg Med* 5:1214, 1986.

300. Gerard SK, Hernandez C, Khayem-Bashi H: Extreme hypermagnesemia caused by an overdose of magnesium-containing cathartics. *Ann Emerg Med* 17:778, 1988.

301. Garretts JC, Watson WA, Sweet DE: Magnesium toxicity secondary to catharsis during management of theophylline poisoning. *Am J Emerg Med* 7:34, 1989.

302. Gren J, Woolf A: Hypermagnesemia associated with catharsis in a salicylate-intoxicated patient with anorexia nervosa. *Ann Emerg Med* 18:200, 1989.

303. Dean BL, Peterson R, Garrettson LK, et al: American Association of Poison Control Centers' Policy Statement: Gastrointestinal dilution with water as a first aid procedure in poisoning. *Clin Toxicol* 19:531, 1982.

304. Spyker DA: Activated charcoal reborn: Progress in poison management. *Arch Intern Med* 145:43, 1985.

305. Park GD, Spector R, Goldberg MJ, et al: Expanded role of charcoal therapy in the poisoned and overdosed patient. *Arch Intern Med* 146:969, 1986.

306. Derlet RW, Albertson TE: Activated charcoal: Past, present, and future. *West J Med* 145:493, 1986.

307. Andelman RP: Changing priorities in GI decontamination in toxic ingestions. *Ann Emerg Med* 17:385, 1988.

308. Kulig KW: Gastric lavage in acute drug overdose. *JAMA* 262:1392, 1989.

309. Olson KR: Is gut emptying all washed up? *Am J Emerg Med* 8:560, 1990.

310. Rumack BH, Rosen P: Emesis: Safe and effective? *Ann Emerg Med* 10:551, 1981.

311. Decker WJ: Gastrointestinal decontamination. *Clin Toxicol* 20:III, 1983.

312. Proudfoot AT: Abandon gastric lavage in the accident and emergency department? *Arch Emerg Med* 2:65, 1984.

313. Tenenbein M: Inefficacy of gastric emptying procedures. *J Emerg Med* 3:133, 1985.

314. Rumack BH: Ipecac use in the home. *Pediatrics* 75:1148, 1985.

315. Vale JA, Meredith TJ, Proudfoot AT: Syrup of ipecac: Is it really useful? *Br Med J* 293:1321, 1986.

316. Flomenbaum NE, Hoffman R: GI evacuation: Is it still worthwhile? *Emerg Med* 22:80, 1989.

317. Kennedy P: Poisoning treatment centers. *Br Med J* 4:670, 1972.

318. Done AK: Clinical pharmacology of systemic antidotes. *Clin Pharmacol Ther* 2:750, 1961.

319. Linden CH: Antidotes in poisoning, in Callaham ML (ed): *Current Therapy in Emergency Medicine.* Philadelphia, BC Decker, 1990.

320. Goldfrank L, Cohen L, Flomenbaum N, et al: Newer antidotes and controversies in antidotal therapy, in Rund DA, Wolcott BW (eds): *Emergency Medicine Annual.* Vol 3. Norwalk, CT, Appleton-Century-Crofts, 1984, pp 223–266.

321. Litovitz TL: The anecdotal antidotes. *Emerg Med Clin North Am* 2:145, 1984.

322. Gelfand MC, Winchester JF: Hemoperfusion in drug overdose: A technique when conservative management is not sufficient. *Clin Toxicol* 17:583, 1980.

323. Pond SM: Diuresis, dialysis, and hemoperfusion: Indications and benefits. *Emerg Med Clin North Am* 2:29, 1984.

324. Peterson RG, Peterson LN: Cleansing the blood: Hemodialysis, peritoneal dialysis, exchange transfusion, charcoal hemoperfusion, forced diuresis. *Pediatr Clin North Am* 22:675, 1986.

325. Todd JW: Do measures to enhance drug removal save life? *Lancet* 1:331, 1984.

326. Barter DC: The pharmacological role of the kidney. *Drugs* 19:31, 1980.

327. Mudge GH, Silva P, Stibitz GR: Renal excretion by non-ionic diffusion. *Med Clin North Am* 59:681, 1975.

328. Garrettson LK, Geller RJ: Acid and alkaline diuresis: When are they of value in the treatment of poisoning? *Drug Saf* 5:220, 1990.

329. Morgan AG, Polak A: The excretion of salicylate in salicylate poisoning. *Clin Sci* 41:475, 1971.

330. Sweeney K, Chapron D, Brandt L, et al: Toxic interaction between acetazolamide and salicylate: Case reports and a pharmacokinetic explanation. *Clin Pharmacol Ther* 40:518, 1986.

331. Levy G: Gastrointestinal clearance of drugs with activated charcoal. *N Engl J Med* 307:676, 1982.

332. Mofenson HC, Caraccio TR, Greensher J, et al: Gastrointestinal dialysis with activated charcoal and cathartic in the treatment of adolescent intoxications. *Clin Pediatr* 24:678, 1985.

333. Pond SM: Role of repeated oral doses of activated charcoal in clinical toxicology. *Med Toxicol* 1:3, 1986.

334. Jones J, McMullen MJ, Dougherty J, et al: Repetitive doses of activated charcoal in the treatment of poisoning. *Am J Emerg Med* 5:205, 1987.

335. Anonymous: Repeated oral activated charcoal in acute poisoning (editorial). *Lancet* 1:1013, 1987.

336. Campbell JW, Chyka PA: Physiochemical characteristics of drugs

and response to repeat-dose activated charcoal. *Am J Emerg Med* 10:208, 1992.

337. Berg MJ, Berlinger WG, Goldberg MJ, et al: Acceleration of the body clearance of phenobarbital by oral activated charcoal. *N Engl J Med* 307:642, 1982.

338. Gadgil SD, Dainle SR, Advani SH, et al: Effect of activated charcoal on the pharmacokinetics of high-dose methotrexate. *Cancer Treat Rep* 66:1169, 1982.

339. Berlinger WG, Spector R, Goldberg MJ, et al: Enhancement of theophylline clearance by oral activated charcoal. *Clin Pharmacol Ther* 33:351, 1983.

340. Mahutte CK, True RJ, Michiels TN, et al: Increased serum theophylline clearance with orally administered activated charcoal. *Am Rev Respir Dis* 128:820, 1983.

341. Lalonde RL, Deshpande R, Hamilton PP, et al: Acceleration of digoxin clearance by activated charcoal. *Clin Pharmacol Ther* 37:367, 1985.

342. Wogan JM, Kulig K, Frommer DA: Multiple-dose activated charcoal in salicylate poisoning (abstract). *Ann Emerg Med* 15:651, 1986.

343. Mauro LS, Mauro VF, Brown DL, et al: Enhancement of phenytoin elimination by multiple-dose activated charcoal. *Ann Emerg Med* 16:1132, 1987.

344. Rowden AM, Spoor JE, Bertino JS: The effect of activated charcoal on phenytoin pharmacokinetics. *Ann Emerg Med* 19:1144, 1990.

345. Garaffini S: Hepatic toxicity with TCDD (abstract). National Academy of Sciences Workshop on Plans of Clinical and Epidemiological Follow-up After Areawide Chemical Contamination, Washington, DC, March 1980.

346. Schwartz CM, Sherman A: The treatment of tricyclic antidepressant overdose with repeated charcoal. *J Clin Psychopharmacol* 4:336, 1984.

347. Heath A, Van Loot G: Multiple dose oral activated charcoal therapy in carbamazepine overdose (abstract). XII International Congress of the European Association of Poison Control Centres, Brussels, August 1986.

348. Vale JA, Ruddock FS, Boldy DAR: Multiple doses of activated charcoal in the treatment of phenobarbitone and carbamazepine poisoning (abstract). XII International Congress of the European Association of Poison Control Centres, Brussels, August 1986.

349. Boldy DAR, Heath A, Ruddick S, et al: Activated charcoal for carbamazepine poisoning. *Lancet* 1:1027, 1987.

350. Wason S, Carolan P, Seigel R, et al: Carbamazepine toxicity: Pharmacokinetics with repetitive activated charcoal (abstract). *Vet Hum Toxicol* 31:333, 1989.

351. Guzelian PS: Therapeutic approaches for chlordecone poisoning in humans. *J Toxicol Environ Health* 8:757, 1981.

352. Honcharik N, Anthone S: Activated charcoal in acute cyclosporin poisoning. *Lancet* 2:1051, 1985.

353. Neuvonen PJ, Elonen E, Haapanen EJ: Acute dapsone intoxication: Clinical findings and effect of oral charcoal and hemodialysis on dapsone elimination. *Acta Med Scand* 214:215, 1983.

354. Treeger SM, Hang MT: Reduction of diazepam serum half life and reversal of coma by activated charcoal in a patient with severe liver disease. *Clin Toxicol* 24:329, 1986.

355. Pond S, Jacobs M, Marks J, et al: Treatment of digitoxin overdose with oral activated charcoal. *Lancet* 2:1177, 1981.

356. Lake KD, Brown DC, Peterson CD: Digoxin toxicity: Enhanced systemic elimination during oral activated charcoal therapy. *Pharmocotherapy* 4:161, 1984.

357. Boldy DAR, Smart V, Vale JA: Multiple doses of charcoal in digoxin poisoning. *Lancet* 2:1076, 1985.

358. Linden CH, Rumack BH: Enhanced elimination of meprobamate by multiple doses of activated charcoal (abstract). *Vet Hum Toxicol* 26(suppl 2):47, 1984.

359. Hassan E: Treatment of meprobamate overdose with repeated oral doses of activated charcoal. *Ann Emerg Med* 15:73, 1986.

360. DuSouich P, Caille G, LaRochelle P: Enhancement of nadolol elimination by activated charcoal and antibiotics. *Clin Pharmacol Ther* 33:585, 1983.

361. Goldberg MJ, Berlinger WG: Treatment of phenobarbital overdose with activated charcoal. *JAMA* 247:2400, 1982.

362. Linden CH, Lewis PK, Rumack BH: Phenobarbital overdosage:

363. Pond SM, Olson KR, Osterloh JD, et al: Randomized study of the treatment of phenobarbital overdose with repeated doses of activated charcoal. *JAMA* 251:3104, 1984.

364. Prescott LF, Boye GL, Simpson D: Rapid drug removal after overdosage by gastrointestinal dialysis with activated charcoal (abstract). III World Conference on Clinical Pharmacology and Therapeutics, Stockholm, July 1986.

365. Hillman RJ, Prescott LF: Treatment of salicylate poisoning with repeated oral charcoal. *Br Med J* 291:1472, 1985.

366. Kirshenbaum LA, Matthews SC, Sitar DS, et al: Does multiple-dose charcoal therapy enhance salicylate excretion? *Arch Intern Med* 150:1281, 1990.

367. Gal P, Miller A, McCue J: Oral activated charcoal to enhance theophylline elimination in an acute overdose. *JAMA* 251:3130, 1984.

368. True RJ, Berman JN, Mahutte CK: Treatment of theophylline toxicity with oral activated charcoal. *Crit Care Med* 12:113, 1984.

369. Ginoza GW, Strauss AA, Iskra MK, et al: Potential treatment of theophylline toxicity by high surface area activated charcoal. *J Pediatr* 111:140, 1987.

370. Shannon M, Amitai Y, Lovejoy FH: Multiple dose activated charcoal for theophylline poisoning in young infants. *Pediatrics* 80:368, 1987.

371. Laass W: Therapy of acute oral poisonings by organic solvents: Treatment by activated charcoal in combination with laxatives. *Arch Toxicol* 4(suppl):406, 1980.

372. Picchioni AL, Consroe PF: Activated charcoal: Aphencyclidine antidote, or hog in dogs. *N Engl J Med* 300:202, 1979.

373. Goldberg MJ, Park GD, Spector R, et al: Lack of effect of oral activated charcoal on imipramine clearance. *Clin Pharmacol* 38:350, 1985.

374. Watson WA, Jenkins TC, Velasquez N, et al: Repeated oral doses of activated charcoal and the clearance of tobramycin, a nonabsorbable drug. *Clin Toxicol* 25:171, 1987.

375. Roberts D, Honcharik N, Sitar DS, et al: Diltiazem overdose: Pharmacokinetics of diltiazem and its metabolites and effect of multiple dose charcoal therapy. *Clin Toxicol* 29:45, 1991.

376. Tenenbein M: Multiple doses of activated charcoal: Time for reappraisal? *Ann Emerg Med* 20:529, 1991.

377. Park GD, Radomski L, Goldberg MJ, et al: Effects of size and frequency of oral doses of charcoal on theophylline clearance. *Clin Pharmacol Ther* 34:663, 1983.

378. Ilkhanipourk K, Yealy DM, Krönzelok EP: The comparative efficacy of various multiple-dose activated charcoal regimens. *Am J Emerg Med* 10:298, 1992.

379. Ohning BL, Reed MD, Blumer JL: Continuous nasogastric administration of activated charcoal for the treatment of theophylline intoxication. *Pediatr Pharmacol* 5:241, 1986.

380. Golper TA: Drugs and peritoneal dialysis. *Dial Transplant* 8:41, 1979.

381. Exaire E, Trevino-Becerra A, Monteon F: An overview of treatment with peritoneal dialysis in drug poisoning. *Contrib Nephrol* 17:39, 1979.

382. Winchester JF, Gelfand MC, Knepschield JH, et al: Dialysis and hemoperfusion of poisons and drugs: Update. *Trans Am Soc Artif Intern Organs* 23:762, 1977.

383. Winchester JF, Gelfand MC, Tilstone WJ: Hemoperfusion in drug intoxication: Clinical and laboratory aspects. *Drug Metab Rev* 8:69, 1978.

384. Trafford A, Horn C, Sharpstone P, et al: Hemoperfusion in acute drug toxicity. *Clin Toxicol* 17:547, 1980.

385. Haapenen EJ: Hemoperfusion in acute intoxication: Clinical experience with 48 cases. *Acta Med Scand* 668(suppl):76, 1982.

386. Cohan SL, Winchester JF, Gelfand MC: Treatment of intoxication with charcoal hemoperfusion. *Drug Metab Res* 13:681, 1982.

387. Papadopoulou ZL, Novello AC: The use of hemoperfusion in children: Past, present, and future. *Pediatr Clin North Am* 29:1039, 1982.

388. Shannon M: Extracorporeal removal of toxins. *Clin Toxicol Rev* 12:1, 1990.

389. Shannon M: Extracorporeal drug removal. II. Other methods. *Clin Toxicol Rev* 12:1, 1990.

390. Golper TA, Bennet WM: Drug removal by continuous arteriovenous haemofiltration: A review of the evidence in poisoned patients. *Med Toxicol* 3:341, 1988.

391. Shumack KH, Rock GA: Therapeutic plasma exchange. *N Engl J Med* 310:762, 1984.

392. Jones JS, Dougherty J: Current status of plasmapheresis in toxicology. *Ann Emerg Med* 15:474, 1986.

393. Cropp GJA: Experience with a new isovolumetric exchange transfusion method. *J Pediatr* 71:332, 1967.

394. Watanabe AS: Pharmacokinetic aspects of the dialysis of drugs. *Drug Intell Clin Pharm* 2:407, 1977.

395. Takki S, Gambertoglio JC, Hondo DH, et al: Pharmacokinetic evaluation of hemodialysis in acute drug overdose. *J Pharmacokinet Biopharm* 6:427, 1978.

396. Pond S, Rosenberg J, Benowitz NL, et al: Pharmacokinetics of hemoperfusion for drug overdose. *Clin Pharmacokinet* 4:329, 1979.

397. Popovich RP, Moncrief JW: Kinetic modeling of peritoneal transport. *Contrib Nephrol* 17:59, 1979.

398. DeBroe ME, Verpooten GA, Christiaens MA, et al: Clinical experience with prolonged hemoperfusion-hemodialysis treatment of severe poisoning. *Artif Organs* 5:59, 1981.

399. Brett AS, Rothschild N, Gray R, et al: Predicting the clinical course of intentional drug overdose: Implications for use of the intensive care unit. *Arch Intern Med* 147:133, 1987.

400. Callahan M, Kassel D: Epidemiology of fatal tricyclic antidepressant ingestion: Implications for management. *Ann Emerg Med* 14:1, 1985.

401. Kulling P, Persson H: Role of the intensive care unit in the management of the poisoned patient. *Med Toxicol* 1:375, 1986.

402. Chafee-Bahamon C: Prevention of poisonings in young children. *Clin Toxicol Rev* 4:1, 1982.

129. Diagnosis and Differential Diagnosis of Poisoning

Christopher H. Linden

Introduction

The recognition of occult poisoning demands a constantly high index of suspicion. Although poisoning can cause a wide variety of nonspecific signs and symptoms, the diagnosis and etiology of poisoning can usually be established by the history, physical examination, routine and toxicologic laboratory evaluation, and the clinical course. Identification of the offending chemical or chemicals is necessary for prediction of potential toxicity and optimal patient management.

Recognition of Poisoning

Ideally, a diagnosis of poisoning requires analytic fulfillment of criteria similar to Koch's postulates for infectious disease: documentation of the presence of a chemical in or on the body in an amount known to cause the observed signs and symptoms within the reported time frame. In reality, the diagnosis is often made on the basis of a history of chemical exposure, a clinical course consistent with poisoning, and exclusion of other etiologies.

Making the diagnosis is relatively simple when a history of chemical exposure is available. Unfortunately, patients may be unaware of an exposure, unwilling to admit to one, or unable to give any history at all or they may give a history that is vague, confusing, or intentionally disguised. Victims of attempted murder, child or elder abuse, therapeutic misadventure, and chronic or insidious poisoning (e.g., that resulting from chemical exposure during hobby or vocational activities) may not relate an exposure to their present illness. Children, nonverbal patients, and those who are confused or comatose may not be capable of giving a history. Patients who have taken a chemical for the purpose of self-harm (e.g., suicide, Münchausen's syndrome), self-therapy (e.g., abortion, addiction, illness treatment with folk remedies or legitimate pharmaceuticals), or recreation may deny or disguise a history of exposure. Similarly, those who misuse chemicals at home may fear ridicule, and those who are exposed in the workplace may fear losing their jobs. In both instances, victims may be reluctant to admit to chemical exposure.

Circumstances that should arouse suspicion of occult poisoning include sudden or unexplained illness in a previously healthy individual (especially a young person); a history of psychiatric problems (particularly a past suicide attempt), alcoholism, or drug abuse; being a witness or victim of domestic violence (including isolation or neglect in the elderly); a recent change in health, economic status, or social relationships; and the onset of illness shortly after ingesting food, drink, or medication. Poisoning should always be considered in patients with metabolic abnormalities (especially acid-base disturbances), "gastroenteritis," or changes in behavior or mental status of unclear etiology. Leakage of illicit drug packets that have been ingested or concealed in body cavities should be suspected in patients with altered mental status or unusual behavior who have just arrived from abroad (especially Asia and South America) or who have recently been arrested or incarcerated for criminal activity [1,2,3]. Chemical use is also a risk factor for trauma and should be considered in patients with injuries that are unexplained or readily avoidable.

To avoid missing the diagnosis of poisoning, the physician must specifically inquire about chemical exposure. In suspicious but undocumented cases, the physician must assume the role of detective to elicit historical support for the diagnosis [4]. Paramedics, police, and family, friends, employer, pharmacist, or personal physician should be questioned regarding the circumstances and events surrounding the illness, particularly the availability of chemicals and the likelihood of exposure. A search of the patient's clothes or place of discovery may sometimes reveal a suicide note or containers of drugs or other chemicals. The garage, cellar, shed, refrigerator, and trash should be checked as well as more obvious locations, such as the bedside table and kitchen and bathroom cabinets. Any open or empty chemical containers should be brought to the hospital for inspection.

In the absence of a history of exposure, the characteristic clinical course of poisoning may also suggest the diagnosis. Characteristically, signs and symptoms develop within minutes to a hour of an acute exposure, progress to a maximum within several hours, and gradually resolve over a period of hours to a few days. In such situations, toxicology screening (see below) may allow for a positive diagnosis if signs and symptoms are consistent with the known toxicity of the chemical(s) detected and other etiologies have been excluded.

Identification of the Offending Chemical

HISTORY. As with the recognition of poisoning, the etiology of poisoning may or may not be disclosed by the history. Even when a history is available, its accuracy and reliability must be assessed. The identity of the chemical involved is incorrectly reported by up to 50 percent of patients with intentional ingestions [5,6]. The amount reportedly taken is also notoriously unreliable. Hence, in patients with intentional exposures, the history should always be approached with some degree of skepticism, and an attempt should be made to confirm it through a witness or investigation of the circumstances surrounding exposure, clinical findings, and toxicology screening. A particularly common and potentially fatal error is that resulting from patient confusion between acetaminophen and aspirin. Hence, the presence or absence of both drugs should always be confirmed by laboratory analysis when an overdose of either one is reported. Signs and symptoms must be consistent with the known toxicity of the chemical identified by the history and the laboratory to confirm the reported etiology of poisoning.

PILL, PRODUCT, PLANT, AND ANIMAL IDENTIFICATION. Drugs in pill form can often be identified by their imprint code and the alphabetical and numerical markings on tablets and capsules. In most states, imprinting of prescription drugs is required by law, and it is likely that imprinting of over-the-counter medications will be legislated in the near future. A listing of imprint codes with the corresponding trade name and ingredients of pills that they identify can be found in the Identidex portion of Poisindex [7]. Since Poisindex, a comprehensive compilation of chemical and product information (as well as management guidelines), is available at virtually all regional poison centers in the United States, the desired information can usually be obtained by a simple telephone call. Identidex also identifies street drugs by slang name. Poison centers can also provide this information and are usually knowledgeable in current or local street drug trends that may have not yet been reported in the literature. The pharmacy that dispensed a prescription drug may also be able to identify it by either prescription number or patient name and the date the prescription was filled. By law, the ingredients of currently marketed commercial products must be stated on their label. This information is not necessarily present on the label of many older products, however, and labels may be missing or unreadable. In such cases, the ingredients may be identified by consulting Poisindex or a regional poison center. Poisindex lists products by brand name

and provides detailed ingredient identities, amounts, and concentrations. Alternatively, if manufacturers or distributors and their location are known, these sources can be called to obtain information on drugs or products that they produce or distribute. This action may be particularly helpful if the product is an old formulation or a very recently reformulated or released one. Most large companies maintain 24-hour emergency telephone numbers for such purposes. Many companies also employ medical consultants who can provide management advice.

Drugs and chemical products manufactured or obtained in a foreign country may have a different generic or trade name than identical products available in the United States. Some foreign products are listed in Poisindex. Another useful reference is Martindale, the Extra Pharmacopeia [8], the European equivalent of the American Hospital Formulary Service Drug Information publication [9]. Drugs obtained in other parts of the world (e.g., Mexico, South America, Africa, India) can often be found in Martindale, since many of them are manufactured in Europe. This reference also can be a valuable source of information on drugs undergoing clinical trials in the United States, because it is common for them to have been previously studied or released for general use in Europe. Poison centers in other countries can also be called for information regarding products manufactured or obtained there; most have English-speaking staff or translators available.

Plants (including fungi or mushrooms), along with their active parts and chemical constituents, can be identified by their common and botanical names by consulting Poisindex. If the plant name is not known but a sample is available, a representative from a local nursery, horticultural or mycologic society, college or university botany department, or a botanical field guide may be of assistance in identifying it. Similarly, pet stores, zoos, veterinarians, amateur or academic entomologists, herpetologists, zoologists, or field guides can be helpful in identifying potentially venomous insects, reptiles, snakes, and other animals. Poison centers usually maintain lists of local experts who are willing to help with such identifications.

Direct identification of an available substance via chemical analysis (see Toxicology Screening) can also be attempted. This is particularly helpful in establishing the identity of street drugs. As previously noted, signs and symptoms must be consistent with the known toxicity of the identified agent to confirm the specific case.

CLINICAL MANIFESTATIONS. The etiology of poisoning can usually be narrowed to a few possibilities by the findings noted on physical examination and readily available ancillary tests [10–15]. The ECG, serum chemistries such as electrolytes, BUN, creatinine, glucose, and osmolality, and urinalysis can provide important diagnostic clues and are recommended in the routine evaluation of all patients with unknown or intentional overdoses, particularly those who are symptomatic.

Physical Examination. The mental status and vital signs provide the most useful information for identifying the cause of poisoning. Using these parameters, the first step is to characterize the physiologic state of the patient as excited (i.e., CNS excitation with increased blood pressure, pulse, respirations, and temperature), depressed (i.e., decreased level of consciousness and decreased vital signs), discordant (i.e., inconsistent, mixed or opposing CNS and vital sign abnormalities), or normal. The differential diagnosis can then be narrowed to the common or characteristic causes of these physiologic states. In this regard, it is helpful to consider the causes of each physiologic state first by the underlying cause or mechanism of action (i.e., sympathomimetic, cholinergic, metabolic acidosis) and then by chemical-specific etiology, as outlined in Table 129-1. Although plants and mushrooms are not listed, they are the source of most therapeutic agents and should also be included in every differential diagnosis.

The *excited state* is primarily caused by chemicals that act by directly or indirectly stimulating alpha- and beta-receptors of the sympathetic nervous system (sympathomimetics), those that block muscarinic receptors of the parasympathetic nervous system (anticholinergics), those that stimulate CNS receptors (hallucinogens), and those that cause CNS excitation when their use is abruptly terminated (withdrawal syndromes). The *depressed state* is primarily caused by chemicals that inhibit the sympathetic nervous system by their peripheral or central actions (sympatholytics), those that stimulate muscarinic receptors or parasympathetic ganglia directly or indirectly (cholinergics), those that stimulate opioid receptors (opioids), and those that directly or indirectly stimulate CNS inhibitory gamma-aminobutyric acid (GABA) receptors or depress neuronal membrane excitability in the CNS by other mechanisms (sedative-hypnotics). Chemicals that indirectly stimulate either division of the autonomic nervous system may promote the release of neurotransmitters, inhibit their degradation, or both. The *discordant state* is primarily due to chemicals that cause simple, cellular, or pulmonary irritation-induced asphyxia (asphyxiants), increased anion gap metabolic acidosis unrelated to hypoxia, shock, or seizures (low-lactate, increased anion gap metabolic acidosis), altered activity of excitable cell membranes (membrane active agents), and interference with the synthesis, metabolism or function of CNS dopamine, GABA, glycine, or serotonin neurotransmitters (CNS syndromes).

Sometimes agents listed under the excited or depressed categories (Table 129-1) may cause discordance among mental status and vital signs if they have activity that is selective for a receptor subtype, results in a compensatory or opposing autonomic response, or is dose-related. For example, hypotension may be accompanied by tachycardia if it is caused by an alpha-blocker, beta$_2$-agonist, or vasodilator. Conversely, hypertension may be accompanied by bradycardia if it is due to a selective alpha-adrenergic stimulant (e.g., phenylpropanolamine). Severe or high-grade stimulant or depressant poisoning can also cause discordant state (see Table 128-2). For example, prolonged seizures and extreme hyperthermia caused by sympathomimetics can eventuate in cardiovascular collapse as a consequence of anaerobic metabolism, acidosis, or depletion of neurotransmitters. Similarly, marked hypotension and hypoventilation caused by physiologic depressants can precipitate seizures and tachyarrhythmias as a result of ischemia, anoxia, and acidosis. In addition, the selective inhibition of cortical function by low doses of physiologic depressants can lead to paradoxical CNS excitation early in the course of poisoning by these agents. Finally, drugs that depress membrane excitability in therapeutic doses can destabilize membranes and induce arrhythmias or seizures at excessive doses. Although some discordance among the mental status and vital signs is present. In each of these instances, the correct physiologic state and underlying etiology can usually be identified by analyzing the clinical course and predominant manifestations.

A *normal physiologic state* may be due to presentation during the preclinical or absorptive phase of poisoning, the presence of a toxic time bomb (see Table 128-1), a nontoxic exposure (see Table 128-3), or psychopathology. The basic mechanisms are listed in Table 129-1. Psychogenic illness should be considered when symptoms are inconsistent with the reported exposure and cannot be substantiated by objective physical findings, laboratory abormalities, and toxicologic testing and other etiologies have been excluded [16].

For excited and depressed states, the mechanistic etiology can usually be identified by grading the severity of physiologic dysfunction (see Table 128-2) and by the nature of associated autonomic abnormalities. In the excited patient, marked vital sign abnormalities (e.g., severe hypertension with end-organ ischemia, tachyarrhythmias, marked hyperthermia, cardiovascular collapse) with relatively less pronounced mental status changes are almost always due to sympathomimetic poisoning. Conversely, marked mental status abnormalities with relatively minor increases in vital signs are characteristic of hallucinogen poisoning. Anticholinergic and withdrawal syndromes ususally cause moderate degrees of both vital sign and mental status excitation. Anticholinergic poisoning can be differentiated from sympathomimetic, hallucinogen, and withdrawal syndromes by the presence of dry, flushed, and hot skin, decreased or absent bowel sounds, and urinary retention; the other causes of excitation are usually accompanied by pallor, diaphoresis, and increased bowel or bladder activity . Similarly, in the depressed category, marked cardiovascular abnormalities with normal respirations and relatively clear sensorium suggest sympatholytic poisoning, whereas marked CNS and respiratory depression with minimal pulse and blood pressure abnormalities suggest opioid or sedative-hypnotic poisoning. Only after the development of deep coma with loss of most or all brainstem reflexes (e.g., corneals, calorics, doll's eyes, gag), deep tendon reflexes, and response to pain and with markedly decreased or absent respirations is significant cardiovascular depression seen with these latter agents. Cholinergic poisoning can cause all degrees of physiologic dysfunction but can usually be distinguished from other causes of physiologic depression by the presence of characteristic autonomic findings: *S*alivation, *L*acrimation, *U*rination, *D*efecation, *G*astrointestinal cramps, and *E*mesis (sludge syndrome). In addition, with cholinergic poisoning the skin is ususally pale and diaphoretic, whereas with other causes of physiologic depression it is generally warm and dry.

After assessing and categorizing the overall physiologic status and considering the underlying causes, the presence of specific signs and symptoms can sometimes help narrow the differential diagnosis further. Familiarity with the manifestations of commonly encountered poisons and toxic syndromes is essential. Extensive lists of the signs and symptoms of poisoning and their causes have been published elsewhere [7,10–15]. Manifestations of poisoning by specific chemicals not covered in subsequent chapters of this section can be found in a number of widely available toxicology references [7,12,13,17–23]. Only the most common and diagnostically useful findings are noted here. Because of limited specificity and sensitivity, the presence or absence of a particular sign or symptom cannot be used to confirm or exclude a given etiology with absolute certainty.

The *odor* of either the chemical or the patient's breath or vomitus may suggest the etiology of poisoning [24]. Unless the odor is recognized, however, it is of limited diagnostic value. Acetone, ammonia, arsenic (garlic), camphor, chloral hydrate, cyanide (bitter almond), ethanol, ethchlorvynol, hydrogen sulfide (rotten egg), isopropyl alcohol, marijuana, methyl salicylate (oil of wintergreen), naphthalene and paradichlorobenzene (mothballs), organophosphate insecticides (garlic), paraldehyde, petroleum distillates, phenol, phosphine (fishy), and thallium (garlic) are important poisons with characteristic odors.

Eye findings can sometimes help narrow the diagnostic possibilities. Although mydriasis can be caused by any agent or condition that results in physiologic excitation (Table 129-1), it is most pronounced in anticholinergic poisoning, where it is associated with minimal pupil response to light and accommodation. Similarly, although miosis is a nonspecific manifestation of physiologic depression, it is usually most pronounced

Table 129-1. Differential Diagnosis of Poisoning Based on Physiologic Abnormalities and Underlying Mechanistic and Specific Etiologies

Excited (CNS stimulation with increased vital signs)	Depressed (CNS depression with decreased vital signs)	Discordant (mixed CNS and vital sign abnormalities)	Normal

Sympathomimetics
  Amphetamines
  Bronchodilators (beta₂-agonists)
  Catecholamine analogs
  Cocaine
  Decongestants
  Ergot alkaloids
  Methylxanthines
  Monoamine oxidase inhibitors
  Thyroid hormones
	Sympatholytics
	  Alpha-adrenergic antagonists
	  Angiotensin converting enzyme inhibitors
	  Beta-adrenergic blockers
	  Calcium channel blockers
	  Clonidine/immiduzolin decongestants
	  Cyclic antidepressants (late, severe)
	  Digitalis
	  Neuroleptics
		Asphyxiants
		  Cytochrome oxidase inhibitors
		    Carbon monoxide
		    Cyanide
		    Hydrogen sulfide
		  Inert (simple) gases
		  Irritant gases, fumes, vapors
		
		  Methemoglobinemia
		  Oxidative phosphorylation inhibitors
		    Herbicides (nitrophenols)
			Agents with slow absorption[a]
			
			Agents with slow distribution[a]
			
			Agents that active metabolites[a]
			
			Agents that inhibit metabolism[a]
			
			Nontoxic exposure
			
			Psychogenic illness

Anticholinergics
  Antihistamines
  Atropine (belladonna alkaloids)
  Cyclic antidepressants (early, mild)
  Cyclobenzaprine
  Muscle relaxants
  Mydriatics (topical)
  Nonprescription sleep aids
  Parkinson's disease therapeutics
	Cholinergics
	  Carbamate insecticides
	  Myasthenia gravis therapeutics
	  Nicotine
	  Organophosphate insecticides
	
	  Physostigmine
	  Pilocarpine
	  Urecholine
		Low lactate increased anion gap metabolic acidosis
		  Alcoholic ketoacidosis
		  Ethylene glycol
		  Methanol (formaldehyde)
		  Paraldehyde
		  Phenformin (biguanide hypoglycemics)
		  Salicylate
		  Sulfur/sulfate
		  Toluene	

Hallucinogens
  LSD/tryptamine derivatives
  Marijuana
  Mescaline/amphetamine derivatives
  Psilocybin mushrooms
  Phencyclidine
	Opioids
	  Analgesics
	  Antidiarrheal drugs
	  Fentanyl and derivatives
	  Heroin
	  Opium
		Membrane active agents
		  Amantadine
		  Antiarrhythmics
		  Beta-blockers
		  Cyclic antidepressants (late, severe)
		  Fluoride
		  Heavy metals
		  Lithium
		  Local anesthetics
		  Meperidine/propoxyphene metabolites
		  Neuroleptics
		  Quinine (antimalarials)	

Withdrawal syndromes
  Beta-adrenergic blockers
  Clonidine
  Cyclic antidepressants
  Ethanol
  Sedative-hypnotics
	Sedative-hypnotics
	  Alcohols
	  Barbiturates
	  Benzodiazepines
	  Bromide
	  Ethchlorvynol
	  Gamma hydroxybutyrate
	  Glutethimide
	  Methyprylon
	  Muscle relaxants
		CNS syndromes
		  Disulfiram
		  Extrapyramidal (dystonic) reactions
		  Isoniazid (GABA lytic)
		  Neuroleptic malignant syndrome
		  Serotonin syndrome
		  Strychnine (glycinergic)
		  Volatile substances of abuse (hydrocarbons)	

[a] See Table 128-1
[b] See Table 128-3

in opioid poisoning. Notable miosis can, however, also be caused by cholinergic stimulants and sympatholytic agents with alpha-blocking effects (e.g., phenothiazines). Visual disturbances suggest anticholinergic, cholinergic, digitalis, hallucinogen, methanol, and quinine poisoning. Horizontal nystagmus and disconjugate gaze are nonspecific manifestations of sedative-hypnotic poisoning. However, vertical and rotary nystagmus are highly suggestive of phencyclidine intoxication. Although they can also be seen in patients with lithium and phenytoin poisoning, these etiologies should be readily distinguishable by assessing the physiologic state. Except for abnormalities due to topical chemical exposure, both eyes are equally affected. Although failure to respond to topical miotics has been said to be diagnostic of drug-induced pupillary dilatation, this has been shown to be true only for topical exposures [25]. Hence, unilateral findings should generally prompt evaluation for a structural lesion.

Dermatologic abnormalities may also be helpful in suggesting the etiology of poisoning. Flushed skin may be caused by anticholinergics, boric acid, a disulfiram-ethanol reaction, monosodium glutamate, niacin, scombroid (fish poisoning), and rapid infusion of vancomycin (red man's syndrome). Flushing should not be confused with the orange skin discoloration caused by rifampin. The skin is hot and dry in patients with anticholinergic poisoning but normal or moist in other conditions associated with flushing. Pallor and diaphoresis may be due to cholinergics, hallucinogens, hypoglycemics, sympathomimetics, and drug withdrawal (Table 129-1). As noted previously, manifestations of the sludge syndrome distinguish cholinergic poisoning from other etiologies. Cyanosis may be caused by cardiovascular depression, respiratory depression, methemoglobinemia, pneumonitis, or simple asphyxiants. When caused by methemoglobinemia, it may have a chocolate-brown or slate-gray hue and is unaffected by oxygen administration. Cyanosis should not be confused with the blue discoloration of the skin sometimes seen in patients taking amiodarone or that caused by topical exposure to blue dyes. The latter condition can be diagnosed by wiping the affected area with acetone or alcohol. Hair loss, mucosal pigmentation, and nail abnormalities are suggestive of heavy metal poisoning (e.g., arsenic, lead, mercury, thallium).

Finally, the presence of *neuromuscular abnormalities* may suggest certain etiologies. Seizures and tremors may occur in patients poisoned by agents that cause asphyxia, low lactate increased anion gap metabolic acidosis (see below), and cerebral hypoperfusion or hypoventilation (e.g., physiologic depressants) and by cholinergics, hypoglycemic agents, lithium, membrane-active agents, some narcotics (e.g., meperidine, propoxyphene), and most physiologic stimulants [24,25,26] (Table 129-1). Currently, the most common causes of seizures associated with poisoning and drug overdose are, in descending order, tricyclic antidepressants, cocaine and amphetamines, antihistamines, theophylline, and isoniazid [27–29]. Carbon monoxide, hypoglycemics, lithium, and theophylline can cause focal seizures [30–33]. However, since poisoning is usually associated with generalized neuromuscular dysfunction and since hypertensive and traumatic CNS hemorrhages are known complications of poisoning, the possibility of a structural lesion should generally be investigated if focal signs and symptoms are present.

Myoclonus suggests anticholinergic or sympathomimetic poisoning. Fasciculations are typical of cholinergic insecticide poisoning but can also be caused by sympathomimetics. Rigidity may be seen in patients with phencyclidine and sympathomimetic poisoning and those with CNS syndromes (Table 129-1). Dystonic posturing is most often caused by neuroleptics but is also a characteristic feature of strychnine poisoning.

Laboratory Findings. Acid-base, anion gap, serum osmolality, ketone, electrolyte, glucose, and organ function abnormalities identified by routine laboratory tests can be extremely helpful in the differential diagnosis of poisoning. As with clinical manifestations, the diagnostic sensitivity and specificity of a single laboratory abnormality are not sufficiently high for its presence or absence to confirm or exclude a specific etiology. Only those laboratory findings that are characteristic, common, or diagnostically important are discussed. Their use in the diagnosis of poisoning of unknown etiology is summarized in Figure 129-1.

An increased anion gap metabolic acidosis (AGMA) is particularly important because it may be due to advanced ethylene glycol, methanol, and salicylate poisoning. In this setting, prompt initiation of specific therapies is essential to prevent progressive, irreversible, or fatal poisoning [34–41]. The anion gap, calculated by subtracting the serum chloride and the serum bicarbonate concentrations from the serum sodium concentration, is normally 12 ± 4 mEq per liter. In ethylene glycol and methanol poisoning, AGMA is primarily due to the accumulation of their acid metabolites. In salicylate poisoning, it is caused by the accumulation of a variety of endogenous organic acids resulting from salicylate's interference with intermediary metabolism. Chemicals that cause hypoxemia, cellular asphyxia, seizures, shock, or extensive tissue necrosis can also cause an AGMA. In these instances, the accumulation of lactic acid generated by anaerobic metabolism is responsible for the AGMA.

Although the nature of the anion responsible for an AGMA is often suggested by associated clinical findings, measurement of the serum lactate level may sometimes be necessary. The lactate concentration is generally low (<5 mEq/L) or significantly less than the anion gap in ethylene glycol, methanol, and salicylate poisoning, whereas it is high (>5 mEq/L) or nearly equal to the anion gap in conditions associated with anaerobic metabolism. Ethanol can also disrupt intermediary metabolism in susceptible alcoholics and cause a low-lactate AGMA (i.e., alcoholic ketoacidosis [AKA]) [42]. Although rare, this metabolic picture can occur in poisoning by paraldehyde (presumably as a result of its metabolism to acetic acid [35]), formaldehyde (which is metabolized to formic acid [43]), toluene [44], elemental sulfur, and possibly sulfates [45,46]. An abnormally low anion gap may be seen in extreme hypercalcemia and hypermagnesemia and in severe bromide, iodine, lithium, and nitrate intoxication [35,36,40,41,47–51]. The low anion gap seen in halide and lithium intoxication results from spuriously elevated chloride levels, and that seen with nitrate poisoning is due to falsely elevated bicarbonate levels.

Measurement of the serum osmolality and serum ketones can be helpful in differentiating the toxic causes of a low lactate AGMA. An elevated serum osmolality or, more specifically, an increased osmolar gap may be seen early in the course of ethylene glycol and methanol but not salicylate poisoning when high serum levels of these alcohols are present [38]. In contrast, ketosis, as defined by a positive nitroprusside reaction, is relatively common in salicylate poisoning [52] but unusual in ethylene glycol and methanol poisoning. The serum osmolality is normally 290 ± 10 mOsm per kilogram of H_2O; the osmolar gap—the difference between the measured serum osmolality and the calculated serum osmolality—is normally less than 10. The simplest and most accurate way to calculate osmolality is to double the serum sodium concentration and add to this result the serum glucose and urea (BUN) concentrations [53]. This formula assumes that all concentrations are measured in millimoles per liter. If the glucose and BUN concentrations are measured in milligrams per deciliter, dividing them by 18 and 3, respectively, will give their approximate concentrations in millimoles.

An increased osmolar gap may also be caused by high levels

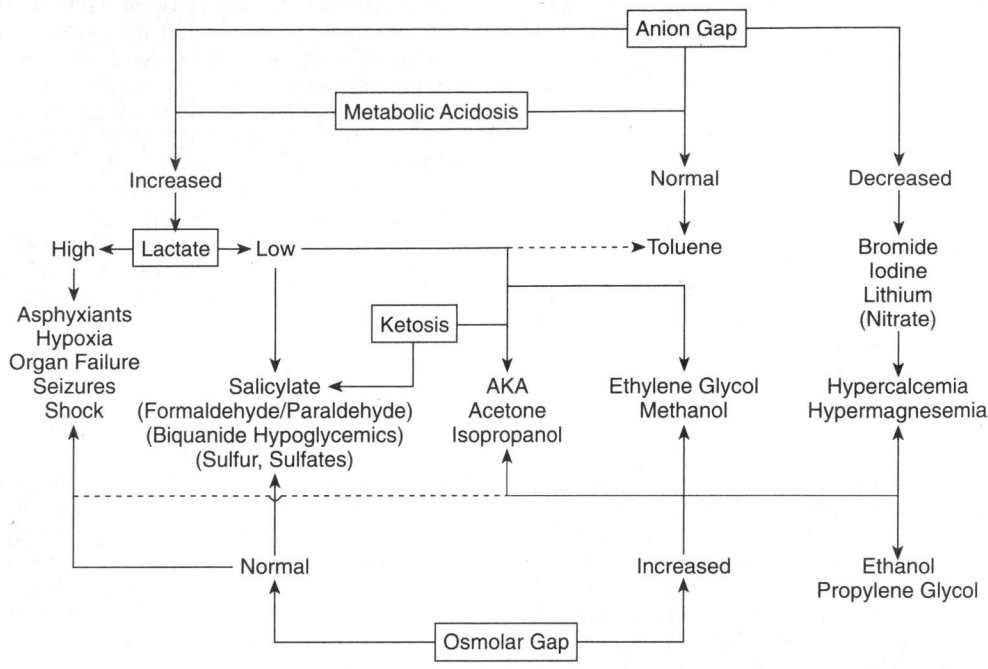

Fig. 129-1. Use of the anion gap, osmolar gap, and serum lactate and ketones in the diagnosis of poisoning.

of other low-molecular-weight solutes, such as acetone, ethanol, isopropyl alcohol, magnesium, mannitol, and propylene glycol [34,39,54–57]. The approximate concentration of these substances necessary to increase the serum osmolality by 1 mOsm per kilogram of H_2O, calculated on the basis of their molecular weights, is shown in Table 129-2. The serum osmolality must be measured by freezing point depression rather than the head space or vapor pressure method to detect the presence of volatile agents such as acetone and the alcohols. An increased osmolar gap has also been reported in patients with alcoholic ketoacidosis and lactic acidosis [58], and ketosis may also occur in AKA and in acetone and isopropyl alcohol poisoning [35].

The urinalysis, serum calcium concentration, and clinical manifestations can also be helpful in differentiating the toxic causes of a low lactate AGMA. Crystalluria, hypocalcemia, and

Table 129-2. Effects of Some Solutes on Serum Osmolality

Solute	Approximate concentration required to increase serum osmolality by 1 mOsm/kg
Alcohols, glycols, and ketones	
Acetone	5.8 mg/dl
Ethanol	4.6 mg/dl
Ethylene glycol	5.2 mg/dl
Isopropanol	6.0 mg/dl
Methanol	2.6 mg/dl
Propylene glycol	7.6 mg/dl
Electrolytes	
Calcium	4 mg/dl (1 mEq/L)
Magnesium	2.4 mg/dl (1 mEq/L)
Sugars	
Mannitol	18 mg/dl
Sorbitol	18 mg/dl

back pain or flank tenderness suggest ethylene glycol poisoning, visual symptoms implicate methanol, and tinnitus or impaired hearing point to salicylate poisoning [59,60]. As with other laboratory abnormalities, crystalluria and hypocalcemia are nonspecific. The former can also be seen in oxalate and primadone poisoning [61], and the latter may occur during fluoride intoxication [62].

Serum electrolyte and glucose abnormalities may sometimes provide clues regarding the etiology of poisoning [10–14]. Hypokalemia can be caused by barium, $beta_2$-adrenergic agonist, diuretic, methylxanthine, and toluene poisoning. Hyperkalemia is most often seen in patients with alpha-adrenergic agonist, beta-blocker, digitalis, and fluoride intoxication. Adrenergic influences on the movement of potassium across cell membranes are responsible for abnormalities caused by sympathomimetic and sympatholytic agents [63]. Hypoglycemia suggests poisoning by ethanol, beta-blockers, hypoglycemics, quinine, or salicylate, whereas hyperglycemia may be seen in patients with acetone, beta-agonist, calcium channel blocker, iron, and theophylline intoxication.

The most common chemical causes of acute liver dysfunction are acetaminophen, ethanol, halogenated hydrocarbons (e.g., carbon tetrachloride), heavy metals, and mushrooms (e.g., *Amanita phalloides* and related species) [64,65,66]. Acute renal toxicity is most often due to ethylene glycol, agents that cause hemolysis or rhabdomyolysis (see below), nonsteroidal antiinflammatory drugs, toluene, chemicals that cause acute liver dysfunction, and envenomations [67]. A spuriously elevated creatinine with a normal BUN can be seen in patients with severe isopropyl alcohol poisoning, since high serum levels of this alcohol interfere with colorimetric assays for creatinine [68]. Chemicals that cause acute hemolysis (in the absence of G-6-PD deficiency) include arsine gas, naphthalene, and agents that cause methemoglobinemia (see Chap. 129) [69]. Rhabdomyolysis can result from chronic toluene abuse, CNS syndromes (Table 129-1), or acute poisoning by any chemical that causes severe physiologic dysfunction (e.g., extreme agitation, deep or prolonged coma, hyperthermia, seizures) [70,71,72]. The most common offenders are amphetamines, cocaine, ethanol, heroin, and phencyclidine.

Electrocardiographic Findings. The electrocardiogram (ECG) may sometimes provide clues to the etiology of poisoning [14,15]. Sinus tachycardia and bradycardia are most often simply a reflection of generalized physiologic excitation or depression (Table 129-1). Ventricular tachyarrhythmias can be due to myocardial irritation (i.e., increased automaticity) or reentrant mechanisms (see Chap. 131). Myocardial irritants include sympathomimetics, digitalis, and "cardiac sensitizing" agents, such as chloral hydrate and aliphatic or halogenated hydrocarbons, which potentiate the activity of endogenous catecholamines [73,74]. Tachyarrhythmias caused by these agents occur in patients with otherwise normal QRS and Q–T intervals on the ECG. Reentrant arrhythmias are caused by agents that disturb cardiac membrane function (i.e., depolarization and repolarization) directly or indirectly (e.g., by inducing electrolyte abnormalities). Depolarization and repolarization abnormalities, reflected on the ECG by an increased QRS duration and prolonged Q–T interval, respectively, can occur in poisoning by amantadine, antiarrhythmics (primarily groups I and III), beta-blockers, fluoride, heavy metals (e.g., arsenic, thallium), magnesium, normeperidine (a metabolite of meperidine), organophosphate insecticides, potassium, psychotherapeutic agents (e.g., cyclic antidepressants, lithium, phenothiazines), and quinine and related antimalarials [14,75,76]. *Torsades de pointes* (polymorphous) ventricular tachycardia is strongly suggestive of poisoning by a chemical that prolongs the Q–T interval.

Atrioventricular conduction abnormalities (A–V block) and bradyarrhythmias can be caused by beta-blockers, calcium channel blockers, digitalis, membrane-active psychotherapeutic agents, organophosphate insecticides, and alpha-agonists such as phenylpropanolamine [14]. In the latter, they are a reflex (i.e., homeostatic) response to hypertension [77].

Radiologic Findings

Some chemicals can be visualized by radiography as radiopaque material within the GI tract. Hence, abdominal or kidney, ureter, and bladder (KUB) radiographs can occasionally be helpful in suggesting the identity of an unknown poison. Although a large variety of chemicals can be detected by radiography in vitro, relatively few are visible in vivo [14,78–82]. Agents most likely to be visible in actual patients can be remembered by the mnemonic CHIPES: *C*alcium salts (e.g., antacids) and *C*hlorinated *H*ydrocarbons (e.g., carbon tetrachloride, chloral hydrate); *H*eavy metals (e.g., arsenic, iron, lead, mercury, thallium); *I*odinated compounds (e.g., thyroid hormones); *P*acket of drugs, *P*lay-Doh, *P*otassium salts, and *P*sychotherapeutics (e.g., cyclic antidepressants, lithium, phenothiazines); *E*nteric-coated tablets; and *S*alicylates and *s*odium salts [13,59,83]. Ingested drug packets may appear as uniform, ovoid or round, marble-sized densities scattered along the GI tract [1,2]. Ingested hydrocarbons may sometimes appear as a gastric "double bubble" on abdominal films [84]. This finding represents the air-fluid and fluid-fluid interface lines created when less dense hydrocarbons layer on top of gastric fluids. As with other manifestations of poisoning, the sensitivity of plain films for detecting ingested chemicals is relatively low and a negative result does not rule out their presence.

Preliminary data suggest that abdominal ultrasound imaging may be helpful in the diagnosis and management of some cases of poisoning [85,86]. It may be able to detect pills, particularly enteric-coated and sustained-released formulations, in the GI tract and therefore be useful in confirming or refuting suspected ingestions when the history is unclear (e.g., children with possible exposures; adults with unexplained illness). Since the number of pills can also be determined, it may be useful in determining the need for and success of GI decontamination.

Abnormal findings on chest radiography can be caused by a wide variety of chemicals [10–14,87–92]. Diffuse or patchy infiltrates (i.e., pneumonitis or acute respiratory distress syndrome [ARDS]) can be seen in patients with acute poisoning caused by the inhalation of irritant gases (e.g., ammonia, chlorine, hydrogen sulfide, nitrogen oxides, phosgene, smoke, sulfur dioxide), fumes (e.g., beryllium, metal oxides, polymers), and vapors (e.g., acids, aldehydes, hydrocarbons, isocyanates, mercury). They can also be seen in patients who have ingested or injected cholinergic agents (e.g., carbamate and organophosphate insecticides), metabolic poisons (e.g., cyanide, carbon monoxide, heavy metals, hydrogen sulfide), paraquat, phencyclidine, salicylates, thiazide diuretics, and tocolytics, and in patients with envenomations. Aspiration pneumonitis is quite common and can occur in patients with coma or seizures of any etiology [93,94,95]. Acute respiratory distress syndrome can also develop in any patient with prolonged or pronounced anoxia, hyperthermia, or hypotension (e.g., those with severe narcotic, sedative-hypnotic, or sympathomimetic poisoning). Chronic chemical exposure can cause pulmonary fibrosis, granulomas, or pleural plaques [87,88] (see Chap. 71).

RESPONSE TO ANTIDOTES. The clinical response to antidotes can sometimes confirm or suggest the cause of poisoning. The prompt resolution of mental status changes and vital sign abnormalities following IV administration of dextrose, naloxone, and flumazenil is virtually diagnostic of hypoglycemia, opioid intoxication (see Chap. 151), and benzodiazepine poisoning (see Chap. 155), respectively. Similarly, the rapid reversal of dystonic posturing after IV administration of benztropine or diphenhydramine implicates a drug etiology (see Chap. 150). The reversal of both central and peripheral manifestations of anticholinergic poisoning (see Chap. 133) following an IV dose of physostigmine is diagnostic of this etiology of poisoning. However, physostigmine also has intrinsic nonspecific CNS stimulant effects and can cause arousal in patients with CNS depression of any etiology [96].

TOXICOLOGY SCREENING. Analysis of a sample of the chemical itself, urine, blood, gastric contents, or occasionally another body fluid can identify virtually any chemical. Urine is generally the best specimen to submit for analysis since large quantities can be obtained for chemical extraction procedures and many chemicals are normally concentrated in urine. Unfortunately, routinely available qualitative toxicology "screening tests" can detect only a small fraction of all chemicals (primarily drugs) and are not always reliable [97,98,99]. Although "drugs of abuse" immunoassay screens are inexpensive ($25 to $50) and results are available within minutes, they are only designed to detect five to ten agents. Comprehensive screens are expensive ($150 or more) and require 2 to 6 hours for completion (excluding transportation times). Finally, although the results may increase diagnostic certainty or specificity [100–104], toxicology screening is neither clinically useful (i.e., results rarely change disposition or treatment) nor cost-effective in overdose patients who are asymptomatic or who have signs and symptoms consistent with the reported history [105–111]. Noteworthy exceptions are acetaminophen and salicylate, poisons that are very common and often misidentified (for each other) by patients, require specific treatment, and can cause few or nonspecific early signs and symptoms. Hence, in many patients determination of quantitative acetaminophen and salicylate levels are the only screening tests required.

Toxicology screening is of greatest value in patients with severe or unexplained toxicity, such as coma, respiratory depression, seizures, cardiovascular instability, acid base abnormalities, multiple organ dysfunction, nonsinus cardiac rhythms, or cardiac conduction disturbances [108–111]. In these patients, a definitive diagnosis is essential for optimal management. Hence, patients who are sick enough to require admission to an intensive care unit should generally have comprehensive toxicology screening.

Knowledge of the methods used for chemical detection (e.g., colorimetric spot tests; thin layer paper or plate chromatography; gas or high-pressure liquid chromatography; absorbance, atomic absorption, flame ionization, or fluorimetric assays; enzyme-multiplied and radionuclide immunoassays; gas chromatography with mass spectrometry) is required for accurate interpretation of the results of screening tests [111–116]. A positive result on one assay should always be confirmed by repeat analysis using a different technique. The physician should speak directly with the laboratory technician to determine which chemicals can be detected by the screening methods used and the sensitivity and specificity of each assay [108,110,112,117]. In addition, directed analysis (e.g., coma, hallucinogen, or stimulant screen), with more rapidly available results, can be performed if the technician knows the patient's clinical status [117,118,119].

A negative result from a screen should never be used to exclude the diagnosis of poisoning when clinical findings suggest otherwise. It may simply mean a chemical is not detectable by the assay(s) used, its concentration is below the limit of detection of the assay(s), or its concentration is too low to be confirmed, and hence reported, as a positive result. It may also mean the time of sampling or the specimen submitted is inappropriate for chemical detection (e.g., the chemical may be undergoing absorption and not yet be present in urine or may already have been eliminated from the bloodstream). In such cases, repeating the screen on samples obtained at an earlier or later time may reveal the identity of the offending chemical. Again, only by direct communication will the physician and laboratory technician be able to take advantage of each other's knowledge and optimize the diagnostic utility of toxicology testing.

References

1. McCarron MM, Wood JD: The cocaine "body packer" syndrome: Diagnosis and treatment. *JAMA* 250:1417, 1983.
2. Carugna DS, Weinbach B, Goerg D, et al: Cocaine-packet ingestion: Diagnosis, management, and natural history. *Ann Intern Med* 10:73, 1984.
3. Roberts JR, Price D, Goldfrank L, et al: The bodystuffer syndrome: A clandestine form of drug overdose. *Am J Emerg Med* 4:24, 1986.
4. Fitzgerald FT, Tierney LM: The bedside Sherlock Holmes. *West J Med* 137:169, 1982.
5. Wright N: An assessment of the unreliability of the history given by self-poisoned patients. *Clin Toxicol* 16:381, 1980.
6. Soslow AR: Acute drug overdose: One hospital's experience. *Ann Emerg Med* 10:18, 1981.
7. Rumack BH (ed): *Poisindex Information System.* Denver, Micromedex, updated quarterly.
8. Reynolds JEF (ed): *Martindale: The Extra Pharmacopeia.* 29th ed. London, Pharmaceutical Press, 1989.
9. McEvoy GK (ed): *American Hospital Formulary Service Drug Information.* Bethesda, MD, American Society of Hospital Pharmacists, Inc., 1995.
10. Block JB: *The Signs and Symptoms of Chemical Exposure.* Springfield, IL, Charles C Thomas, 1980.
11. Done AK: The toxic emergency: Signs, symptoms, and sources. *Emerg Med* January 15, 42, 1982.
12. Arena JM, Drew RH: *Poisoning: Toxicology, Symptoms, Treatments.* 5th ed. Springfield, IL, Charles C Thomas, 1986.
13. Goldfrank LR, Flomenbaum NE, Lewin NA, et al (eds): *Goldfrank's Toxicologic Emergencies.* 4th ed. Norwalk, CT, Appleton-Century-Crofts, 1990.
14. Olson KR, Pentel PR, Kelley MT: Physical assessment and differential diagnosis of the poisoned patient. *Med Toxicol* 2:52, 1987.
15. Ashton CH, Teoh R, Davies DM: Drug-induced stupor: Some physical signs and their pharmacological basis. *Adverse Drug React Acute Poisoning Rev* 8:1, 1989.
16. Hutchesson EA, Volans GN: Unsubstantiated complaints of being poisoned: Psychopathology of patients referred to the national poisons unit. *Br J Psychiatry* 154:34, 1989.
17. Bryson PD: *Comprehensive Review in Toxicology.* 2nd ed. Rockville, MD, Aspen, 1989.
18. Haddad LM, Winchester JF: *Clinical Management of Poisoning and Drug Overdose.* 2nd ed. Philadelphia, WB Saunders, 1990.
19. Laupe KF, McCann MA (eds): *AMA Handbook of Poisonous and Injurious Plants.* Chicago, American Medical Association, 1985.
20. Rumack BH, Salzman E (eds): *Mushroom Poisoning: Diagnosis and Treatment.* West Palm Beach, CRC Press, 1978.
21. Hayes WJ, Laws ER (eds): *Handbook of Pesticide Toxicology.* San Diego, Academic, 1991.
22. Clayton GD, Clayton FE (eds): *Patty's Industrial Hygiene and Toxicology.* 3rd ed. New York, Wiley, 1978.
23. Sullivan JB, Kreiger GR: *Hazardous Materials Toxicology.* Baltimore, Williams & Wilkins, 1990.
24. Goldfrank LR, Weisman R, Flomenbaum N: Teaching the recognition of odors. *Ann Emerg Med* 11:684, 1982.
25. Thompson HS, Newsome DA, Lowenfeld IE: The fixed dilated pupil: Sudden iridoplegia or mydriatiatic drops? A simple diagnostic test. *Arch Ophthal* 86:21, 1971.
26. Woodbury DM: Convulsant drugs: Mechanisms of action. *Adv Neurol* 27:249, 1980.
27. Messing RO, Closson RG, Simon RP: Drug induced seizures: A 10 year experience. *Neurology* 34:1582, 1984.
28. Zaccara G, Muscas GC, Messori A: Clinical features, pathogenesis, and management of drug induced seizures. *Drug Saf* 5:109, 1990.
29. Olson KR, Kearney TE, Dyer JE, et al: Seizures associated with poisoning and drug overdose: Changing patterns of causes and poison center consultations. *Vet Hum Toxicol* 32: 361, 1990.
30. Durnin C: Carbon monoxide poisoning presenting with focal epileptiform seizures. *Lancet* 1:1319, 1987.
31. Andrade R, Matthew V, Morgenstern MJ, et al: Hypoglycemic hemiplegic syndrome. *Ann Emerg Med* 13:529, 1984.
32. Marshall SM, Kesson CM: Severe lithium poisoning. *Drug Intell Clin Pharm* 15:598, 1981.
33. Nakada T, Kwee IL, Lerner AM, et al: Theophylline induced seizures: Clinical and pathophysiologic aspects. *West J Med* 138:371, 1983.
34. Smithline N, Gardner KD: Gaps: Anionic and osmolal. *JAMA* 236:1594, 1976.
35. Emmett M, Narins RG: Clinical use of the anion gap. *Medicine* 56:38, 1977.
36. Oh MS, Carroll HJ: The anion gap. *N Engl J Med* 297:814, 1977.
37. Gabow PA, Kachny WD, Fennessey PV, et al: Diagnostic importance of an increased serum anion gap. *N Engl J Med* 303:854, 1980.
38. Jacobsen DJ, Bredesen JE, Eide I, et al: Anion and osmolal gaps in the diagnosis of methanol and ethylene glycol poisoning. *Acta Med Scand* 212:17, 1982.
39. Enger E: Acidosis, gaps, and poisoning. *Acta Med Scand* 212:1, 1982.
40. Oster JR, Perez GO, Materson BJ: Use of the anion gap in clinical medicine. *South Med J* 81:229, 1988.
41. Salem MM, Mujais SK: Gaps in the anion gap. *Arch Intern Med* 152:1625, 1992.
42. Levy LJ, Duga J, Girgis M, et al: Ketoacidosis associated with alcoholism in nondiabetic subjects. *Ann Intern Med* 78:213, 1973.
43. Eells JR, McMartin KI, Black K, et al: Formaldehyde poisoning: Rapid metabolism to formic acid. *JAMA* 246:1237, 1981.

44. Fischman CM, Oster JR: Toluene toxicity: A new cause of high anion gap metabolic acidosis. *JAMA* 241:1713, 1979.

45. Schwartz SM, Carroll HM, Schoschmidt LA: Sublimed (inorganic) sulfur ingestion: A cause of life-threatening metabolic high anion gap. *Arch Intern Med* 146:1437, 1986.

46. Newell GC: Self induced abortion and an elevated anion gap. *Hosp Pract* April 30, 1989, p 33.

47. Iberti TJ, Patterson BK, Fisher CJ: Prolonged bromide intoxication resulting from a gastric bezoar. *Arch Intern Med* 144:402, 1984.

48. Dyck KJ, Bear RA, Goldstein MB, et al: Iodine/iodide toxic reaction: Case report with emphasis on the nature of the metabolic acidosis. *Can Med Assoc J* 120:704, 1979.

49. Kelleher SP, Raciti A, Arbeit LA: Reduced or absent serum anion gap as a marker of severe lithium carbonate intoxication. *Arch Intern Med* 146:1839, 1986.

50. Senecal PE, Dyer JE, Osterloh JD: Nitrate as a cause of decreased anion gap. *Vet Hum Toxicol* 33:375, 1991.

51. Sporer KA, Mayer AP: Saltpeter ingestion. *Am J Emerg Med* 9:164, 1991.

52. Bartels PD, Lund-Jacobsen H: Blood lactate and ketone body concentrations in salicylate poisoning. *Hum Toxicol* 5:363, 1986.

53. Worthley LJG, Guerin M, Pain RW: For calculating osmolality, the simplest formula is the best. *Anaesth Intensive Care* 15:199, 1987.

54. Glasser L, Sternglanz PD, Combie J, et al: Serum osmolality and its application to drug overdose. *Am J Clin Pathol* 60:695, 1973.

55. Lund ME, Banner W, Finley PR, et al: Effect of alcohols and selected solvents on serum osmolality measurements. *Clin Toxicol* 20:115, 1983.

56. Gennari FJ: Serum osmolality: Uses and limitations. *N Engl J Med* 310:102, 1984.

57. Gerard SK, Hernandez C, Khayem-Bashi H: et al: Extreme hypermagnesemia caused by an overdose of magnesium-containing cathartics. *Ann Emerg Med* 17:728, 1988.

58. Schelling JR, Howard RL, Winter SD, et al: Increased osmolal gap in alcoholic ketoacidosis and lactic acidosis. *Ann Intern Med* 113:580, 1990.

59. Temple AR: Acute and chronic effects of aspirin toxicity and their treatment. *Arch Intern Med* 141:364, 1981.

60. Jacobsen D, McMartin KE: Methanol and ethylene glycol: Mechanism of toxicity, clinical course, diagnosis, and treatment. *Med Toxicol* 1:309, 1986.

61. Van Heijst ANP, deJong W, Seldenrijk R, et al: Coma and crystalluria: A massive primadone intoxication treated with hemoperfusion. *Clin Toxicol* 20:307, 1983.

62. Mayer TG, Gross PL: Fatal systemic fluorosis due to hydrofluoric acid burns. *Ann Emerg Med* 14:149, 1985.

63. Reid JL, Whyte KF, Struthers AD: Epinephrine-induced hypokalemia: The role of beta adrenoreceptors. *Am J Cardiol* 57:23F, 1986.

64. Dossing M, Andreason PB: Diagnosis of acute drug-induced liver injury: Usefulness of clinicopathological patterns and biochemical indices. *Med Toxicol* 1:77, 1986.

65. Kaplowitz N, Yee T, Simon FR, et al: Drug-induced hepatotoxicity. *Ann Intern Med* 104:826, 1986.

66. Lewis JH, Zimmerman HJ: Drug-induced liver disease. *Med Clin North Am* 73:775, 1989.

67. Abuelo JG: Renal failure caused by chemicals, foods, plants, animal venoms, and misuse of drugs: An overview. *Arch Intern Med* 150:505, 1990.

68. Hawley PC, Falke JM: "Pseudo" renal failure after isopropyl alcohol intoxication. *South Med J* 75:630, 1982.

69. Smith RP: Toxic responses of the blood, in Klaassen CD, Andur MO, Doull J (eds): *Casarett and Doull's Toxicology: The Basic Science of Poisons.* New York, Macmillan, 1986, pp 223–244.

70. Grossman RA, Hamilton RW, Morse BM, et al: Nontraumatic rhabdomyolysis and acute renal failure. *N Engl J Med* 291:807, 1974.

71. Gabow PA, Kaehny WD, Kelleher SP: The spectrum of rhabdomyolysis. *Medicine* 61:141, 1982.

72. Kunel RW, Wiggins WW: Toxic myopathies. *Neurol Clin* 6:593, 1988.

73. Bowyer K, Glasser SP: Chloral hydrate overdose and cardiac arrhythmias. *Chest* 77:232, 1980.

74. Boon NA: Solvent abuse and the heart. *Br Med J* 294:722, 1987.

75. Stratman HG, Kennedy HL: Torsade de pointes associated with drugs and toxins: Recognition and management. *Am Heart J* 113:1470, 1987.

76. Vukimir RB: Torsades de pointes: A review. *Am J Emerg Med* 9:250, 1991.

77. Pentel P: Toxicity of over-the-counter stimulants. *JAMA* 252:1898, 1984.

78. Handy CA: Radiopacity of oral nonliquid medications. *Radiology* 98:525, 1971.

79. Greensher J, Mofenson HC, Gavin WJ: The usefulness of abdominal x-rays in the diagnosis of poisoning. *Vet Hum Toxicol* 215:45, 1979.

80. Jaeger RW, Decastro FJ, Barry RC, et al: Radiopacity of drugs and plants in vivo: Limited usefulness. *Vet Hum Toxicol* 23:2, 1981.

81. O'Brien RP, McGedren PA, Helmeczi AW, et al: Detectability of drug tablets and capsules by plain radiography. *Am J Emerg Med* 4:302, 1986.

82. Savitt DL, Hawkins HH, Roberts JR: The radiopacity of ingested medications. *Ann Emerg Med* 16:331, 1987.

83. Wason S, Dalsey W, Billmire ME, et al: Radiological case of the month: Play-Doh in the gastrointestinal tract: Modify "CHIP" to "CHIPPED." *Am J Dis Child* 139:1149, 1985.

84. Daffner RH, Jimenez JP: The double gastric fluid level in kerosene poisoning. *Radiology* 106:383, 1973.

85. Anderson AC, Share JC, Woolf AD: The use of ultrasound in the diagnosis of toxic ingestions. *Vet Hum Toxicol* 32:355, 1990.

86. Amitai Y, Silver B, Leikin JG, et al: Detection of tablets in the gastrointestinal tract by ultrasound. *Am J Emerg Med* 10:18, 1992.

87. Rosenow EC: The spectrum of drug-induced pulmonary disease. *Ann Intern Med* 77:977, 1972.

88. Rigsby C, Swett HA, Sostman MD, et al: Roentgenographic features of drug-induced lung disease. *J Respir Dis* 4:60, 1983.

89. Cordasco EM, Stone FD: Pulmonary edema of environmental origin. *Chest* 64:182, 1973.

90. Shanies HM: Noncardiogenic pulmonary edema. *Med Clin North Am* 61:1319, 1977.

91. Coleman DL: Smoke inhalation. *West J Med* 135:300, 1981.

92. Reed CR, Glauser FL: Drug-induced noncardiogenic pulmonary edema. *Chest* 100:1120, 1991.

93. Huxley EJ, Viroshav J, Gray WR, et al: Pharyngeal aspiration in normal adults and patients with depressed consciousness. *Am J Med* 64:564, 1978.

94. Aldrich T, Marrison J, Desario T: Aspiration after overdosage of sedative or hypnotic drugs. *South Med J* 73:456, 1980.

95. Shannon M, Lovejoy FH: Pulmonary consequences of severe tricyclic antidepressant poisoning. *Clin Toxicol* 25:443, 1987.

96. Hershey LA: The use and abuse of physostigmine. *Drug Ther* 10:143, 1980.

97. Ingelfinger JA, Isakson G, Shine D, et al: Reliability of the toxic screen in drug overdose. *Clin Pharmacol Ther* 29:570, 1981.

98. Hansen HJ, Caudill SP, Boone J: Crisis in drug testing: Results of CDC blind study. *JAMA* 253:2382, 1985.

99. Davis KH, Hawks RL, Blanke RV: Assessment of laboratory quality in urine drug testing: A proficiency testing pilot study. *JAMA* 260:1749, 1988.

100. Horwitz JP, Hills HB, Andrzejewski D, et al: Adjunct hospital emergency toxicology service: A model for a metropolitan area. *JAMA* 235:1708, 1976.

101. Helliwell M, Harpel G, Sinclair E, et al: Value of emergency toxicology investigations in differential diagnosis of coma. *Br Med J* 2:819, 1979.

102. Bury RW, Mashford ML: Use of a drug-screening service in an inner-city teaching hospital. *Med J Aust* 1:132, 1981.

103. Flanagan RJ, Heggett A, Saynor DA, et al: Value of toxicological investigation in the diagnosis of acute poisoning in children. *Lancet* 2:682, 1981.

104. Taylor RL, Cohan SL, White JD: Comprehensive toxicology screening in the emergency department: An aid to clinical diagnosis. *Am J Emerg Med* 3:507, 1985.

105. Wiltbank TB, Sine HE, Brady BB, et al: Are emergency toxicology measurements really used? *Clin Chem* 20:116, 1974.

106. Qirbi AA, Poznanski WJ: Emergency toxicology in a general hospital. *Can Med Assoc J* 116:884, 1977.

107. Rygnestad T, Berg KJ: Evaluation of benefits of drug analysis in the routine clinical management of self poisoning. *Clin Toxicol* 22:51, 1984.

108. Kulig K: Utilization of emergency toxicology screens. *Am J Emerg Med* 3:574, 1985.
109. Kellermann AL, Fisher SD, LoGerfo JP, et al: Impact of drug screening in suspected overdose. *Ann Emerg Med* 16:1206, 1987.
110. Brett AS: Implication of discordance between clinical impression and toxicology analysis in drug overdose. *Arch Intern Med* 148:437, 1988.
111. Mahoney JD, Gross PL, Stern TA, et al: Quantitative serum toxic screening in the management of suspected drug overdose. *Am J Emerg Med* 8:16, 1990.
112. Sullivan JB, Fisher JG: Proper use of the toxicology laboratory. *Emerg Med Rep* 5:125, 1984.
113. AMA Council on Scientific Affairs: Scientific issues in drug testing. *JAMA* 257:3110, 1987.
114. Schwartz RH: Urine testing in the detection of drugs of abuse. *Arch Intern Med* 148:2407, 1988.
115. Gaudreault P, Timberlake S: Toxic screens. I. *Clin Toxicol Rev* 12:1, 1989.
116. Gaudreault P, Timberlake S: Toxic screens. II. *Clin Toxicol Rev* 12:1, 1989.
117. Hepler BR, Sutheimer CA, Sunshine I: Role of the toxicology laboratory in the treatment of acute poisoning. *Med Toxicol* 1:61, 1986.
118. Ashley DL, Needham U: Assessment of a scheme for prioritizing inorganic intoxicants by using signs-and-symptoms analysis. *Clin Toxicol* 24:375, 1986.
119. Nice A, Leikin JB, Maturen A: Toxidrome recognition to improve efficiency of emergency urine drug screens. *Ann Emerg Med* 17:676, 1988.

130. Acetaminophen Poisoning

Martin J. Smilkstein

Overview

PHARMACOLOGY. Acetaminophen (n-acetyl-para-aminophenol [APAP]) is an excellent antipyretic with significant analgesic action but almost no antiinflammatory effects. It belongs to the same drug family as phenacetin and acetanilid, the "coal tar" or aminobenzene analgesics [1,2]. Although APAP is the active metabolite of phenacetin, unlike phenacetin it rarely, if ever, causes nephrotoxicity and it does not cause methemoglobinemia and hemolytic anemia. Unlike aspirin, APAP has no "barrier-breaker" effect on the gastrointestinal tract, causes no platelet dysfunction, has a high therapeutic index, and has not been implicated as a factor in Reye's syndrome. As a result, APAP has gained wide acceptance as an alternative to aspirin when antiinflammatory action is not important, and its safety has led to markedly decreased aspirin use as well as the discontinuation of the use of phenacetin.

Acetaminophen is an active ingredient in several hundred products, including pure APAP formulations (e.g., Tylenol, Datril, Anacin 3, Panadol), combinations with opioid analgesics (e.g., Tylenol no. 3, Darvocet, Percocet), and numerous combination cough and cold preparations (e.g., Nyquil). It is also available in suppository form, but there is no commercial intravenous formulation.

Acetaminophen has a pK_a of 9.5 and is quickly and almost completely absorbed after ingestion of therapeutic doses (10–15 mg/kg every 4 hours), yielding peak plasma concentrations between 5 and 20 μg per ml within 30 to 120 minutes. Clinical effects are noted within 30 minutes. Liquid preparations are absorbed slightly faster than solid formulations. Rectal absorption is similar to that after oral ingestion. The volume of distribution of APAP is 0.9 to 1.0 liter per kilogram, and protein binding is negligible. Therapeutic plasma concentrations range from 10 to 20 μg per liter, and elimination after therapeutic dosing follows first-order kinetics, with an average half-life of 2 to 4 hours [1,3]. Elimination is slower in neonates and young infants [4], the elderly [2], and in patients with hepatic dysfunction [5]. Clinical effects persist for 3 to 4 hours after therapeutic doses.

TOXICOLOGY. The short- or long-term therapeutic use of APAP is rarely associated with adverse effects. Hypersensitivity reactions such as urticaria, fixed drug eruption, angioedema, laryngeal edema, and anaphylaxis are extremely rare [6]. Although high-dose APAP has been associated with chronic renal impairment [7], a cause-effect relationship is questionable. Idiosyncratic non-dose-related hepatotoxicity has been reported only twice [8,9].

Despite remarkable safety in appropriate doses, APAP can cause hepatic necrosis after overdosage. Fatal hepatotoxicity was first recognized in Europe in 1966 [10], and the first cases of toxicity in the United States were reported in 1975. Since that time, the incidence of APAP poisoning has increased dramatically in parallel with its increased availability and use: APAP is now the most common drug involved in exposures reported to U.S. poison control centers, accounting for more than 100,000 calls in 1991 [11]. The incidence of occult poisoning is unknown, but based on indirect information [12] some have estimated that 1 of every 500 overdose patients may have an unsuspected but potentially toxic APAP ingestion.

The metabolism of APAP explains its toxicity and the rationale for the current treatment of overdose (Fig. 130-1) [2]. After therapeutic doses, approximately 90 percent of APAP metabolism occurs by hepatic conjugation with sulfate or glucuronide to form inactive, nontoxic, renally eliminated metabolites. In adults, glucuronidation is the predominant route; in infants and young children, sulfation is the major pathway [3]. Less than 5 percent of APAP is eliminated unchanged in the urine.

The small remaining fraction (approximately 5%) undergoes oxidation by the P-450 mixed-function oxidase enzyme system to yield the highly reactive, potentially toxic, electrophilic intermediate n-acetyl-para-benzoquinoneimine (NAPQI) [13]. Under nonoverdose conditions, NAPQI is quickly detoxified by reduced glutathione (GSH) to form nontoxic cysteine and mercapturic acid conjugates that are excreted in the urine [14].

After overdose, the amount of drug metabolized by the P-450 route increases, both because of a greater total drug burden and because of saturation of alternative enzymatic pathways [15,16]. As a result, GSH utilization increases. If GSH regeneration is inadequate to meet demand it is significantly

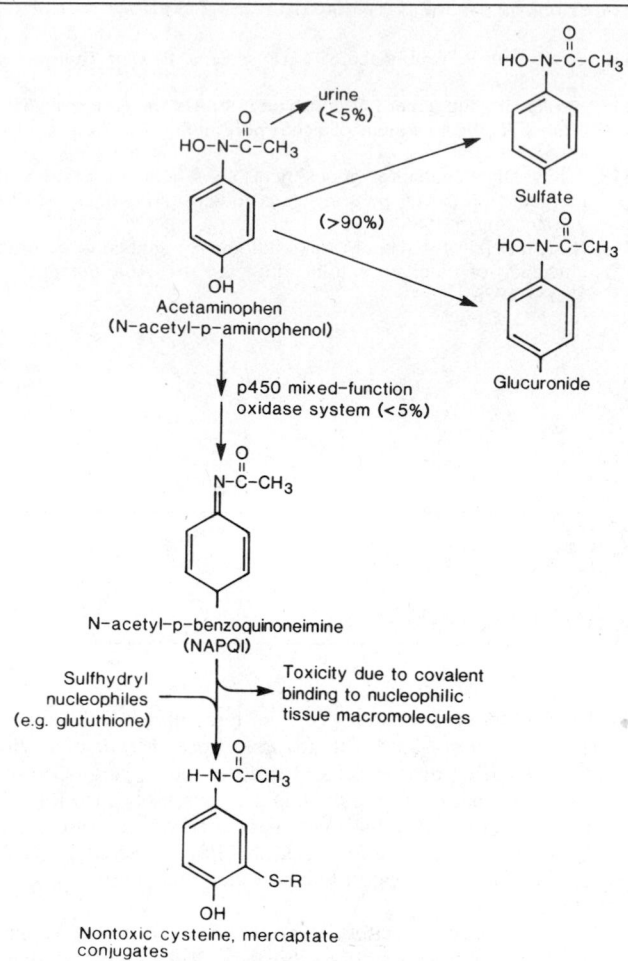

Fig. 130-1. Postulated metabolism of acetaminophen. Toxicity occurs when the supply of sulfhydryl nucleophiles (e.g., glutathione) is inadequate to prevent the persistence of n-acetyl-para-benzoquinoneimine (NAPQI) and subsequent binding to hepatocyte macromolecules.

depleted and NAPQI can then persist and react with hepatocyte macromolecules. In animal studies, hepatic injury occurs when GSH stores reach less than 30 percent of normal [14]. The destruction of hepatocytes by NAPQI is most pronounced in centrilobular areas of the liver. The degree of injury can range from asymptomatic elevations in aminotransferase levels to fulminant hepatic necrosis. Although far less common, the same process can occur in the kidney [17]. Very rarely, renal toxicity can occur in the absence of serious hepatotoxicity [18,19].

Pancreatitis, in some cases fulminant, can occur [20,21], and diffuse myocardial necrosis has been noted in fatal cases [22]. Very rarely, with massive ingestions, early coma and metabolic acidosis may be seen [23]. The mechanisms causing these atypical forms of toxicity are unknown, and it is unclear to what extent these effects are directly due to APAP.

The precise dosage required to produce toxicity is unknown and almost certainly varies to some degree with individual differences in P-450 activity, GSH stores, and capacity for GSH regeneration. Although retrospective data suggest that significant toxicity is likely only after acute overdoses of greater than 250 mg per kilogram [17], the possibility of toxicity at lower doses and skepticism regarding the accuracy of overdose his-

tories have led to acceptance of a more conservative definition of risk. Currently, single ingestions of greater than 7.5 gm in an adult or 140 to 150 mg per kilogram in children should be considered potentially toxic [2].

Toxicity has also been reported after repeated ingestions of therapeutic or slightly greater doses of APAP, especially in alcoholics [24,25], although the existence of "chronic" toxicity is still disputed. There is currently no valid estimation of the amount, frequency, or duration of the dosing that defines risk. It appears that after repeated doses, accumulation of APAP to concentrations associated with toxicity after acute overdose is not required and that sustained, moderate elevations are sufficient to cause GSH depletion and toxicity [26].

Toxicity occurs in several settings. Intentional acute overdose is the most common cause of toxicity and fatalities, but accidental therapeutic overdosing and the abuse of opioids with unintentional coingestion of APAP (e.g., with codeine, with propoxyphene) have also been reported. Therapeutic overdoses may result from dosing calculation errors, excessive self-treatment, the use of adult formulations or extra-strength formulations when lower-dosage formulations were intended, and errors involving substitution of higher-dose rectal suppositories for similar-appearing lower-dosage forms.

The importance of accurately diagnosing APAP toxicity soon after overdose extends beyond the high frequency with which it is encountered and its potential for causing morbidity and mortality. Acetaminophen is unique among common toxic exposures because effective treatment requires recognition of potential poisoning and initiation of therapy when no reliable clinical signs of overdose are present. Physicians must therefore consider occult APAP ingestion and liberally obtain APAP levels on all overdose patients to avoid missing the diagnosis.

Clinical Manifestations

Acetaminophen hepatotoxicity can be divided into four clinical stages based on the time interval following ingestion: stage I (0–24 hours), the latent period; stage II (24–48 hours), the onset of hepatotoxicity; stage III (72–96 hours), maximal hepatic injury; and stage IV (4 days to 2 weeks), recovery [2,17].

During stage I, patients may be completely asymptomatic but often experience nausea, vomiting, and malaise, which may be accompanied by pallor and mild diaphoresis. There is no known correlation between the presence or absence of early symptoms and the risk of hepatotoxicity. Although late in stage I very sensitive indicators of hepatic injury, such as gamma-glutamyltransferase (GGT) level, may be elevated, more widely used laboratory studies (e.g., asparate aminotransferase [AST], alanine aminotransferase [ALT], prothrombin time, bilirubin) are completely normal. Early coma and metabolic acidosis have been reported in patients with massive ingestions [23], but these findings are so atypical that other causes should be suspected. They should be attributed to APAP only if the APAP concentration is extremely high and other etiologies have been excluded.

Symptoms during stage II are typical of hepatitis and include right upper quadrant abdominal pain, nausea, fatigue, and malaise. Physical examination often reveals right upper quadrant tenderness and hepatomegaly. The first elevation of aminotransferase levels usually occurs between 24 and 36 hours after APAP ingestion, but in the most severe cases it can occur by 16 hours or earlier. Early in stage II, tests reflecting liver function, such as bilirubin and prothrombin time, are most often normal or only slightly elevated. Marked elevations of aminotransferase levels (>1000 IU/L) within 24 hours or bilirubin and prothrombin time within 36 hours should suggest that the time of ingestion was earlier than reported. Although unusual, in severe cases marked liver function abnormalities may be evident by 36 to 48 hours. Complications during stage II are directly related to the degree of liver injury and may include coagulopathy, encephalopathy, acidosis, and hypoglycemia. With few exceptions, life-threatening problems are not seen earlier than 48 hours, and death in this period is distinctly rare. Renal dysfunction, manifested by rising creatinine and an active urinary sediment, may become evident during this stage but usually lags somewhat behind the hepatic injury. The BUN may also be elevated, but it can be normal in the presence of hepatic failure and resultant decreased urea formation.

Biochemical evidence of liver injury becomes most pronounced during stage III. With successful treatment, however, peak aminotransferase levels may sometimes occur earlier (Fig. 130-2). The vast majority of patients, even those with markedly elevated aminotransferase levels, go on to recover fully. Most deaths occur 3 to 7 days after ingestion and result from intractable metabolic disturbances, secondary complications such as cerebral edema or dysrhythmias, or exsanguination due to coagulopathy. Oliguric or anuric renal failure may result from acute tubular necrosis and is sometimes accompanied by flank pain. Some degree of renal dysfunction occurs in approximately 25 percent of patients with significant hepatotoxicity [17]. Even when severe, renal failure is almost always reversible.

During stage IV, if sufficient hepatocytes remain viable and the patient survives, the liver regenerates. Recovery is often complete by day 5 or 6 in patients with minimal toxicity, but those with more serious poisoning may not be clinically normal for 2 weeks or more. It is interesting that even patients with severe toxicity who survive regain normal liver function. There are no known cases of chronic or persistent liver abnormalities from APAP poisoning. In those who ultimately die, a slow decline in aminotransferase levels without clinical improvement may be seen. Declining enzyme levels merely represent a "washout" of those released at the time of the initial insult, not a recovery of normal liver function. These patients can be identified by persistent or increasing marked elevations of bilirubin and prothrombin time. Although this pattern is occasionally seen in patients who recover, the vast majority of survivors do not have significant or persistent bilirubin or prothrombin time elevation after aminotransferase levels fall.

Because of variations in dosing patterns and patient characteristics, the time course of toxicity in patients with repeated ingestions is not well defined. With chronic toxicity, dose-response patterns differ from those of acute overdose but the clinical manifestations are the same.

Diagnostic Evaluation

The diagnostic evaluation can be divided into two separate phases: determination of the risk of potential toxicity and assessment of actual toxicity.

There are currently no available methods to assess GSH stores, P-450 activity, or NAPQI formation rapidly. Therefore, serum APAP concentration is used as an indirect predictor of toxicity. If the APAP concentration between 4 and 24 hours after ingestion falls on or above the acetaminophen treatment nomogram line (Fig. 130-3), the patient should be considered at risk for hepatotoxicity. When there is uncertainty about the exact time of ingestion, the worst-case scenario should be assumed. For example, if the ingestion was between 4 and 6 hours earlier, the 6-hour value on the nomogram should be used. If the APAP concentration is even slightly below the nomogram line, the antidote N-acetylcysteine (NAC) is not necessary. The original Matthew-Rumack nomogram line, which defined the risk of toxicity based on the natural course of untreated patients [27], was actually 25 percent higher than the line now used in the United States. Hence, the nomogram has

Fig. 130-3. Acetaminophen treatment nomogram. Patients with acetaminophen concentrations on or above the line require treatment with N-acetylcysteine. (Adapted from Rumack BH, Peterson RG, Koch GG, et al: Acetaminophen overdose: 662 cases with evaluation of oral acetylcysteine treatment. *Arch Intern Med* 141:380, 1981.)

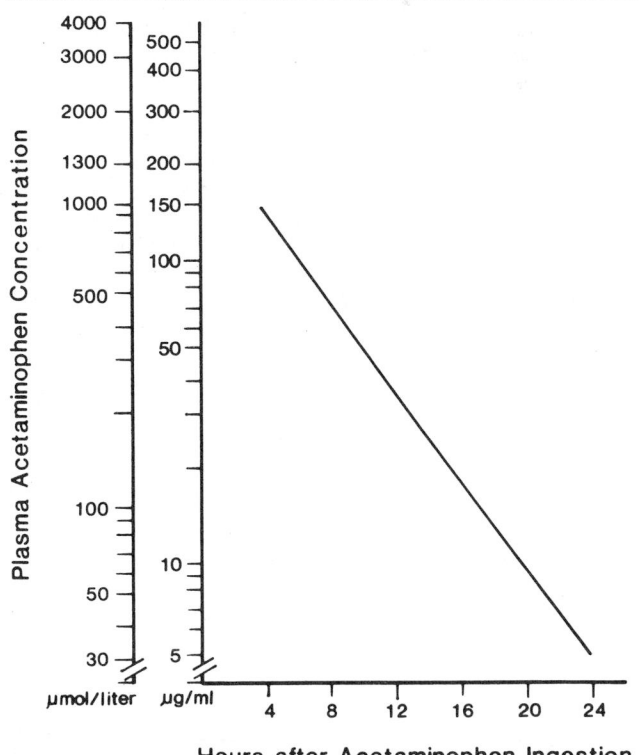

Fig. 130-2. Expected time course of aminotransferase elevation due to acetaminophen-induced hepatotoxicity. Solid line represents typical course, dashed line represents course of severe toxicity. (Adapted from Rumack BH, Peterson RG, Koch GG, et al: Acetaminophen overdose: 662 cases with evaluation of oral acetylcysteine treatment. *Arch Intern Med* 141:380, 1981.)

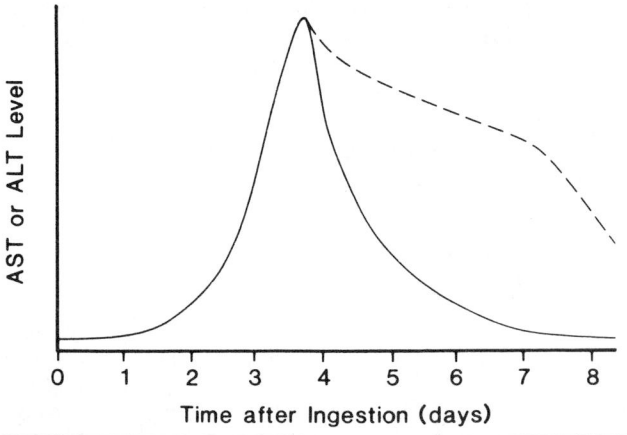

a 25 percent "safety margin" that allows one to be fairly rigid when using the nomogram to make treatment decisions.

A single APAP concentration within the time period specified by the nomogram is sufficient to plan appropriate therapy. With rare exceptions, there is no advantage of repeating APAP levels. While it is true that the elimination half-life of APAP is related to the likelihood of toxicity, half-lives should not be relied on in making therapeutic decisions. The observations that half-lives greater than 4 hours were associated with toxicity and that toxicity was negligible if APAP half-life was less than 4 hours [28] were based on multiple APAP determinations in untreated patients over a 36-hour period. Since treatment must be started as early as possible [29], and since treatment may alter APAP elimination [16], half-life determinations are not relevant to current standards of care. When the time of ingestion is unknown, treatment decisions should be based on a worst-case interpretation of the time of ingestion.

There are, however, two situations in which repeat measurements may be of value. The first is in the patient with a time of ingestion that is unknown but may have been within 4 hours. In this situation, an increasing APAP level indicates ongoing absorption from a recent ingestion. To detect a rising level and define the peak value, repeat determinations must be frequent (every 1–2 hours) until the level declines. This prevents underestimation of the peak value due to incomplete absorption at the time of the first level. It also may rule out toxicity by detecting a peak value less than 150 μg per milliliter. For practical purposes, if the second level is less than the first and the time of ingestion is completely unknown, it should be assumed that the first level was measured more than 4 hours since ingestion and the patient should be treated with NAC. Repeat APAP levels may also be of value in the patient with very high levels and slow elimination due to hepatotoxicity in whom it is possible that APAP may still be present at the completion of therapy. Antidotal treatment should not be discontinued while APAP is still present. Although this is rarely a consideration in patients who receive a 72-hour course of therapy, it may be a concern when using shorter courses.

In assessing the patient who is found to be at risk for toxicity and hence requires hospitalization and treatment, a complete blood count (CBC), electrolytes, BUN, creatinine, glucose, prothrombin time, aminotransferase levels, and bilirubin should be obtained at admission and repeated every 24 hours until resolution of toxicity is noted. If liver failure develops, laboratory values, particularly prothrombin time and glucose, must be obtained more frequently. Renal function, acid-base status, amylase, and electrocardiogram (ECG) may also need to be evaluated or repeated. Assessment of renal, pancreatic, and myocardial toxicity should follow the same guidelines as those for other etiologies.

Management

Treatment consists of three phases: gastrointestinal decontamination when appropriate antidotal treatment, and support of organ function. Unless clinically significant hepatic or renal failure develops, inpatient medical management consists only of antidote administration and monitoring of signs, symptoms, and laboratory parameters. Although this can be accomplished outside the ICU, patients often require monitoring or treatment for toxicity due to coingestions or constant observation because of suicide risk. As a result, most APAP overdose patients should initially be treated in the ICU. If significant hepatic failure ensues, ICU admission will be required for close monitoring and treatment of complications. Invasive monitoring is rarely required but may be useful if multisystem failure occurs.

GASTROINTESTINAL DECONTAMINATION. Gastrointestinal decontamination after APAP overdose has been controversial. In most cases, APAP is completely absorbed within 2 hours and the risk of gastric emptying after this time outweighs the potential benefit. Delayed absorption due to the coingestion of agents that slow GI motility has been suggested but not shown to be clinically significant. It is therefore advisable to consider gastric emptying after pure APAP overdose only within 2 hours of ingestion. Beyond 2 hours, gastric emptying decisions should be based on known or suspected coingestants. When gastric emptying is performed, gastric lavage is preferable to ipecac-induced emesis, because emesis may prevent or complicate subsequent antidotal therapy. The use of activated charcoal has generated tremendous debate. In vitro, activated charcoal clearly adsorbs NAC [30,31,32], thus causing concern that activated charcoal would decrease the bioavailability of NAC and diminish its efficacy. Although in vivo results have been somewhat conflicting, the coingestion of charcoal and NAC does decrease the total amount of NAC absorbed [33–36], but this decrease is unlikely to be clinically significant [33,34], particularly in view of the large NAC dose used in the United States. Therefore, it is recommended that activated charcoal be given if it is likely to be of benefit, regardless of the use of NAC. After pure APAP overdose, activated charcoal is likely to prevent APAP absorption only if it can be given within 4 hours of ingestion. After 4 hours, benefit is extremely unlikely, so there is no reason to complicate NAC therapy with the use of charcoal. Early administration of charcoal has no impact on NAC therapy because there is no need to start NAC until after evaluation of a 4-hour postingestion APAP concentration, as long as the result will be available within 8 hours of ingestion [29]. In patients with mixed or unknown overdoses, activated charcoal therapy should be used as appropriate for coingestants, regardless of the presence of APAP. When multiple doses of charcoal are used, the administration of NAC and charcoal should, if possible, be separated by 1 to 2 hours to minimize any potential interactions.

ANTIDOTAL TREATMENT. The observation that hepatotoxicity occurs only when GSH is depleted led to a search for agents that might increase available sulfhydryl groups either by increasing GSH or by providing alternative sulfhydryl sources. Exogenous GSH does not readily enter cells, so various precursors and substitutes, including cysteamine, methionine [37], and NAC [29,38], have been tried. Although all regimens are effective when started within 8 to 10 hours of ingestion, cysteamine was abandoned because of its toxicity and methionine has been replaced by NAC, which is more effective and probably carries less risk of worsening hepatic encephalopathy when liver failure is present.

There are several suggested mechanisms of action of NAC. In cells, NAC is converted to cysteine, a GSH precursor, and thus increases GSH stores [16,39,40]. Second, either NAC or cysteine can substitute directly for GSH because they have available sulfhydryl groups [41]. Third, NAC augments the sulfation of APAP to nontoxic metabolite by providing sulfur substrate [16,42]. Fourth, NAC may promote the back-conversion of NAPQI to its precursors [43], although this has not been demonstrated in humans. Finally, there is accumulating evidence that NAC may be beneficial even after liver injury has occurred, through mechanisms other than its effects on APAP metabolism [44,45,46]. Suggested mechanisms for these late effects of NAC include direct antioxidant action to modify postinflammatory radical-mediated destruction [47], restoration of enzyme function in injured tissue [48], and correction of microvascular function by restoring endothelial-derived relaxing factor [46]. It is likely that the relative importance of each of the above effects of NAC in any given patient varies with the severity of the overdose and the delay to NAC initiation. These variations may explain apparent differences in efficacy between different NAC protocols.

The only treatment regimen currently approved for use in the United States consists of a 72-hour course of oral NAC given as a 140 mg per kilogram loading dose, followed by 17 doses of 70 mg per kilogram every 4 hours beginning 4 hours after the loading dose, for a total NAC dose of 1330 mg per kilogram [49]. An experimental intravenous NAC protocol using the same loading dose but followed by only 12 maintenance doses over 48 hours, for a total NAC dose of 980 mg per kilogram, has been studied in the United States [50]. In Europe and Canada, standard treatment consists of a 20-hour course of IV NAC given as an initial bolus of 150 mg per kilogram, followed by continuous infusion of 50 mg per kilogram over the next 4 hours and 100 mg per kilogram over the remaining 16 hours, for a total NAC dose of 300 mg per kilogram [38].

For oral therapy NAC is usually supplied as a 20% solution (20 gm/100 ml), which should be diluted 3:1 to yield a 5% mixture with juice or a soft drink to increase its palatability and decrease GI side effects. Antiemetics (e.g., metoclopramide, 0.1–1 mg/kg IV, initial adult dose 10 mg; droperidol, 20–150 mcg/kg IV, initial adult dose 1.25 mg) 30 minutes prior to NAC dosing may be required to treat antecedent vomiting or vomiting due to NAC. Anecdotally, ondansetron (50–150 μg/kg IV, initial adult dose 4 mg) has shown promise when traditional antiemetics are ineffective. If antiemetics fail, NAC can be given by gastric or duodenal tube. Various other methods may prove helpful in decreasing emesis after dosing: chilling the solution with ice chips, using a straw and covering the container, diluting to a 10% solution, or administering the solution over 15 to 60 minutes instead of as a bolus. If vomiting occurs within 1 hour of any dose, that dose should be repeated.

In certain patients, intravenous NAC must be considered. In the United States, only a few centers have a supply of NAC approved for experimental IV use. The widely available oral preparation, which is not tested or guaranteed to be sterile or pyrogen-free, is not approved for IV administration. Nonetheless, it has been used in many instances to treat patients intravenously in unusual circumstances [51]. Despite apparent safety in these anecdotal reports, the use of an unapproved treatment should be restricted and considered only in certain settings. High-risk patients (by APAP concentration) with ongoing, refractory vomiting 12 to 16 hours after overdose warrant this consideration; it is probably also logical in patients with liver failure and perhaps in pregnant patients (see below). It is not justified within the first 8 hours or in patients whose APAP concentration is only slightly above the treatment nomogram line. Due to the complexity of this decision, consultation with a toxicologist or regional poison center is recommended before treating any patient intravenously with the formulation intended for oral use.

There are no well-documented serious side effects of oral NAC, although nausea and vomiting are extremely common [52]. Side effects from intravenous NAC are far less common but potentially more serious. There are several reports of serious or fatal anaphylactoid reactions (e.g., hypotension, bronchospasm, rash, death) to IV NAC during the 20-hour protocol, and minor dermatologic reactions are common [53–58]. It is important to recognize that adverse effects to IV NAC are not truly anaphylactic; they are dose- and concentration-dependent [57]. As a result, more dilute and slowly administered doses are far better tolerated [50]. Except for an anaphylactoid reaction in one patient after an NAC overdose, there have been no serious adverse reactions reported during the 48-hour IV protocol, but the incidence of transient skin rash is approximately 15 percent [50]. Skin reactions occurred during the loading dose and did not neccessitate discontinuing IV NAC. Experience with this protocol is limited; therefore the ultimate spectrum of side effects remains to be determined. It is also worth remembering that even though the protocol is safe, the consequences of dosing or administration errors by the IV route can be severe.

All three dosing protocols appear to be equivalent when NAC is started within 8 hours of ingestion. Efficacy decreases with longer delays in therapy, with apparent differences between the dosing regimens when NAC is started after 16 hours. With late treatment, 82 percent of high-risk patients treated with the 20-hour regimen developed aminotransferase values above 1000 IU per liter, an incidence not significantly different from the 89 percent incidence reported in untreated historical controls [38]. After treatment with 48 hours of IV NAC, only 58 percent of late-treated patients developed hepatotoxicity, a result that was significantly better than that with either the 20-hour course or no treatment [50]. After 72 hours of oral NAC, only 41 percent of late-treated patients developed hepatotoxicity [29], although this was not statistically different from the 48-hour protocol [50]. All of these studies included only patients receiving NAC within 24 hours of ingestion.

In the first controlled study of NAC started more than 24 hours after overdose, IV NAC started *after* onset of liver failure (median 53 hours after APAP) reduced cerebral edema, need for pressors, and mortality [45]. It is interesting that this study used the same NAC dosing that had earlier been found ineffective more than 15 hours after overdose [38], but instead of discontinuing NAC after 20 hours therapy was continued until either recovery or death.

The numerous actions of NAC may explain why various NAC protocols are equivalent when started early but not when started late. When started within 8 hours of overdose NAC probably exclusively affects APAP metabolism and glutathione turnover, and its role is preventative prior to glutathione depletion and NAPQI covalent binding. In this setting, NAC may be needed only until APAP metabolism is complete; thus shorter courses of NAC are effective. With further treatment delay, the role of NAC may increasingly be to ameliorate the effects of NAPQI covalent binding, and by 16 hours after ingestion this may be its sole action. This would explain why longer courses of NAC, continued during the period of maximal liver injury, appear to be superior. This theory has led to consideration of selective management, such as short-course NAC for those treated early who do not develop aminotransferase elevations by 36 hours and long-course NAC for any patient who develops liver injury. This approach deserves study; at present, however, only the 72-hour protocol is approved for use. Late NAC administration and other special considerations are discussed further below.

Cimetidine has been suggested as a possible antidote for APAP because of its inhibitory effect on P-450 activity [59]. Animal studies have shown efficacy of high-dose cimetidine given before or soon after APAP [60], but there is no evidence of efficacy in humans [61]. Even if the massive dose suggested by animal studies proved to be safe and effective in humans, its theoretical effect would require early administration, a setting in which NAC has already proven to be both safe and highly effective. In problematic cases, such as late presentation, there is no theoretical or experimental support for cimetidine use. In summary, while it is not contraindicated after APAP overdose, cimetidine has no proved role and should never be considered an alternative to NAC.

SUPPORTIVE CARE. The management of hepatic failure, renal failure, or other end-organ manifestations of APAP toxicity should be treated according to usual guidelines. In view of the increased availability and success of liver transplantation, the most severely ill patients deserve this consideration. Several successful transplants have been done following APAP overdose. The greatest challenge is early identification of patients destined for irreversible hepatic failure (see Prognosis and Outcome, below).

Special Considerations

ACUTE OVERDOSE IN ALCOHOLICS AND OTHER HIGH-RISK PATIENTS. Certain subgroups of patients appear to be at greater or lesser risk for APAP toxicity, but this fact is of more theoretical than practical value in the management of acute overdose. Higher risk is expected in patients with increased P-450 enzyme activity from chronic use of agents that induce this enzyme (e.g., ethanol, barbiturates, phenytoin, sedative-hypnotics, griseofulvin, haloperidol, tolbutamide) [62] or decreased GSH stores or low GSH turnover rates (e.g., malnourished patients or those with liver disease). Lower toxicity might be expected when P-450 activity is inhibited by chronic use of agents such as cimetidine or when a patient has coingested an agent that is metabolized via the P-450 system, thus competing with APAP and decreasing NAPQI formation [2].

Acute overdose studies in animals have demonstrated both increased toxicity after chronic ethanol use and decreased toxicity when ethanol and APAP were coingested [63]. The protective effect of ethanol coingestion appears to be due to competitive inhibition of NAPQI formation by P-450 ethanol metabolism [64,65], but debate continues as to whether chronic ethanol use worsens toxicity by P-450 induction [66] or by causing glutathione depletion [67].

Despite suggestions that some of these factors may be significant [68], these concepts have thus far proved too simplistic to be put to use. For example, a nutritionally deprived person might be expected to be at greater risk due to decreased GSH stores but at lesser risk because of lower P-450 activity. An alcoholic might have increased risk due to increased P-450 activity or glutathione depletion but may also be protected by acute coingestion of ethanol. Furthermore, the amount of chronic ethanol or drug use that is clinically significant is unknown and certain to be variable. Because of the interaction between these and many other variables, and because the treatment nomogram line is conservative, treatment decisions after acute overdose should be made in the same manner, regardless of the above factors. After repeated overdosing, these factors should be considered (see Chronic Overdose, below).

ACUTE OVERDOSE IN PEDIATRIC PATIENTS. Of 417 children with acute APAP overdose, 49 of whom had plasma APAP levels over the nomogram line, indicating potential toxicity, only 3 (6.1%) developed an AST or ALT greater than 1000 IU per liter [69]. This incidence is less than that reported in adults, leading to speculation that children are relatively protected from APAP toxicity.

Several pharmacokinetic differences between children and adults have been noted. The most consistent finding is that the ratio of APAP-sulfate to APAP-glucuronide is higher in children than in adults [3,4], but this difference in nontoxic routes of metabolism has not been shown to be associated with a decrease in production of NAPQI. Thus, increased sulfation has not been proved favorably to alter NAPQI formation. Decreased P-450 function, and thus decreased NAPQI formation, has also been postulated in children, but decreased P-450 activity is noted only in fetal and neonatal subjects [70]. The vast majority of APAP poisonings occur outside the newborn period, when P-450 activity may be even greater than in adults. Hence, this theory cannot explain a hepatoprotective effect in older children. If children are actually less susceptible to APAP toxicity, it may be because of an increased ability to regenerate glutathione [71], but this, too, is unproved.

Perhaps the most likely explanation is that pediatric overdoses are quantitatively less severe. In adults, particularly those treated late, the outcome is worse in patients with very high APAP levels [29]. Substantial toxicity has also developed in children with very high levels [72,73], but there are too few cases to allow for any conclusions. Until larger numbers of children with very high APAP levels are studied, patients of all ages with a significant overdose must still be considered at substantial risk and managed accordingly.

ACUTE OVERDOSE IN PREGNANCY. Although experience with overdose in pregnancy is limited [74], certain conclusions seem valid. First, there is clear evidence that APAP overdose can result in morbidity and mortality to both woman and fetus at all stages of pregnancy. Second, there currently is no evidence that NAC is harmful to either a pregnant woman or her fetus. Third, NAC is hepatoprotective to the woman. While it has been assumed that NAC is beneficial to the fetus this is not yet proved and has been questioned by one animal study [75]. Combining these observations, until further data are available, pregnant women should be treated according to standard guidelines regardless of gestational age of the fetus. The newborn infant who is born during a course of maternal NAC treatment should complete a course of NAC after delivery.

LATE TREATMENT. Treatment decisions in patients who present more than 24 hours after an overdose are problematic. Initial studies of the 20-hour IV NAC protocol suggested that NAC was of no value if started more than 12 to 15 hours after ingestion [38], and preliminary results of the 72-hour oral protocol indicated that treatment more than 16 hours after ingestion was ineffective [49]. As a result, studies of treatment initiated after 24 hours were not performed initially. Final analysis of patients treated with 72 hours of oral NAC has sparked new debate [29]. It revealed that patients first treated between 16 and 24 hours after overdose experienced less hepatotoxicity than untreated historical controls or historical controls treated late with a 20-hour course of IV NAC.

Subsequently, a series of studies has shown both theoretical [46,47,48,76] and clinical [44,45,46] benefit to late NAC administration. In the most remarkable of these, NAC started a median of 53 hours after ingestion and after evidence of severe liver injury reduced morbidity and mortality. While these studies have shown that late NAC can be beneficial, which cases warrant late treatment is not well defined. Until this is better defined, the following approach to the treatment of patients who present late is offered. If the APAP level is undetectable and aminotransferase levels are normal, NAC is not indicated, since the possibility of hepatotoxicity is extremely low. If hepatotoxicity is evident, NAC is indicated on the basis of studies showing benefit should severe toxicity develop. For patients who have detectable APAP levels and no hepatotoxicity, NAC therapy can be started and discontinued once the APAP concentration is negligible and 36 or more hours have elapsed without evidence of hepatotoxicity.

CHRONIC OVERDOSE. There are many reports of serious toxicity from chronic overdose in infants with acute, febrile illness [77–83]. Similarly, in alcoholics, chronic toxicity has been reported following doses only slightly higher than recommended and even with therapeutic doses [84]. There are no convincing reports of toxicity due to recommended doses in healthy individuals. Although the dosage required to produce toxicity is unknown and certainly variable, and some authors have questioned the validity of these reports [85,86], alcoholics do appear to be at greater risk for toxicity. In the absence of continued ethanol abuse, there is no evidence that therapeutic dosing carries an increased risk in patients with cirrhosis or other forms of chronic liver disease [87]. Based on current knowledge, there is no reason to avoid APAP in any of these groups, although patients must be clearly instructed to avoid repeated overdosing.

Patients with chronic overdose present the most difficult treatment decisions. In such cases, the nomogram has never been studied and has little or no validity. There are currently no reliable guidelines to assess risk. Evaluation of such patients should include a detailed history of the timing of doses, particularly the last dose, the amount ingested at each dose, possible increased risk factors (e.g., chronic alcoholism, use of other P-450 inducers), symptomatology, an APAP level at least 4 hours after the last dose, and aminotransferase levels. It is best then to consult with a toxicologist or regional poison center to determine the best course based on these data. One approach that deserves further study is to treat according to the guidelines discussed under Late Treatment (above). Using this approach, patients with elevated APAP levels and no hepatotoxicity are treated with NAC until their APAP level is negligible and it is clear that no hepatotoxicity has developed. Patients who develop hepatotoxicity should be given a full course of NAC.

Prognosis and Outcome

"Severe" hepatotoxicity after APAP overdose has traditionally been defined by an ALT or AST greater than 1000 IU per liter, although most patients with such elevations have no significant short- or long-term sequelae. Using this definition, the risk of hepatotoxicity can be estimated based on the initial APAP concentration. Without NAC therapy, hepatotoxicity develops in less than 8 percent of all overdose patients, in 60 percent of probable risk cases (APAP concentration above a nomogram line intersecting 200 μg/ml at 4 hours and 50 μg/ml at 12 hours), and in 89 percent of high-risk cases (APAP concentration above a nomogram line intersecting 300 μg/ml at 4 hours and 75 μg/ml at 12 hours) [17].

Far less toxicity occurs in patients treated with NAC, although outcome is dependent on both APAP concentration and the time NAC was started. Even in high-risk, late-treated cases, only 41 percent of patients treated with oral NAC for 72 hours developed toxicity. Most important is that regardless of APAP level, NAC is extremely effective when started within 8 hours [29]. Hepatotoxicity aoccurred in less than 5 percent of patients in this subset.

Death is unusual after APAP overdose. When patients at probable risk for hepatotoxicity are considered, the reported mortality rate in untreated cases varies from 5.3 percent [38] to 24 percent [88]. A mortality rate of 1.1 percent has been noted in similar patients treated with the 20-hour IV NAC protocol [46] and was found to be 0.68 percent in patients treated with the 72-hour oral NAC protocol [29]. In fact, even among high-risk cases first treated between 16 and 24 hours after overdose, the mortality rate was only 3.1 percent after oral NAC therapy [29].

It is not uncommon to see aminotransferase elevations greater than 10,000 IU per liter during stage III, with eventual complete recovery [2]. As a result, aminotransferase levels alone are inadequate to judge prognosis. Evidence of hepatic dysfunction, such as marked elevations in prothrombin time and bilirubin, or evidence of persistent hypoglycemia, lactic acidosis, or hepatic encephalopathy indicates true hepatic failure and a poor prognosis. Previous reports have suggested that a bilirubin greater than 4 mg per deciliter or a prothrombin time greater than twice control indicates a poor prognosis [89]. More recently, a pH less than 7.30, prothrombin time greater than 100 seconds, serum creatinine greater than 3.4 mg per deciliter, and grade III or higher encephalopathy have been used to define poor prognosis [90], as has the single criterion of an increasing prothrombin time on day 4 after overdose [91]. Unfortunately, these findings are evident late in the clinical course. In view of increased availability and success of liver transplantation, efforts have been made to establish early criteria that predict poor outcome, but these are not yet well established.

The presence or absence of aminotransferase elevation at the time of treatment initiation appears to be the most sensitive early prognostic indicator. To date, all reported patients who have died from APAP toxicity already had some degree of AST or ALT elevation at the time a 72-hour course of oral NAC was started [29]. Hence, all patients with liver enzyme values that are normal when oral NAC is started would be expected to survive.

References

1. Insel PA: Analgesic-antipyretics and anti-inflammatory agents: Drugs employed in the treatment of gout, in Gilman AG, Rall TW, Nies AS, et al (eds): *Goodman and Gilman's The Pharmacological Basis of Therapeutics,* 8th ed. New York, Permagon, 1990.
2. Linden CH, Rumack BH: Acetaminophen overdose. *Emerg Clin North Am* 2:103, 1984.
3. Miller RP, Roberts RJ, Fischer LJ: Acetaminophen elimination kinetics in neonates, children, and adults. *Clin Pharmacol Ther* 19:284, 1977.
4. Peterson RG, Rumack BH: Pharmacokinetics of acetaminophen in children. *Pediatrics* 62(suppl):877, 1978.
5. Andreasen PB, Hutters L: Paracetamol (acetaminophen) clearance in patients with cirrhosis of the liver. *Acta Med Scand* 624(suppl):99, 1979.
6. Stricker BH, Meyboom RH, Lindquist M: Acute hypersensitivity reactions to paracetamol. *Br Med J* 291:938, 1985.
7. Sandler DP, Smith JC, Weinberg CR, et al: Analgesic use and chronic renal disease. *N Engl J Med* 320:1238, 1989.
8. Johnson GK, Tolman KG: Chronic liver disease and acetaminophen. *Ann Intern Med* 87:302, 1977.
9. Bonkowsky HL, Mudge GH, McMurtry RJ: Chronic hepatic inflammation and fibrosis due to low doses of paracetamol. *Lancet* 1:1016, 1978.
10. Davidson DGD, Eastham WN: Acute liver necrosis following overdose of paracetamol. *Br Med J* 2:497, 1966.
11. Litovitz TL, Holm KC, Bariley KM, et al: 1991 annual report of the American Association of Poison Control Centers National Data Collection System. *Am J Emerg Med* 10:452, 1992.
12. Kulig KW, Bar-Or D, Cantrill SV, et al: Management of acutely

poisoned patients without gastric emptying. *Ann Emerg Med* 14:562, 1985.

13. Corcoran GB, Mitchell JR, Vaishnav YN, et al: Evidence that acetaminophen and N-hydroxyacetaminophen form a common arylating intermediate, N-acetyl-p-benzoquinoneimine. *Mol Pharmacol* 18:536, 1980.

14. Mitchell JR, Thorgeirsson SS, Potter WZ, et al: Acetaminophen-induced hepatic injury: Protective role of glutathione in man and rationale for therapy. *Clin Pharmacol Ther* 16:676, 1974.

15. Davis M, Simmons CJ, Harrison NG, et al: Paracetamol overdose in man: Relationship between pattern of urinary metabolites and severity of liver damage. *Q J Med* 45:181, 1976.

16. Slattery JT, Wilson JM, Kalhorn TF, et al: Dose-dependent pharmacokinetics of acetaminophen: Evidence of glutathione depletion in humans. *Clin Pharmacol Ther* 41:413, 1987.

17. Prescott LF: Paracetamol overdosage: Pharmacological considerations and clinical management. *Drugs* 25:290, 1983.

18. Gabriel R: Paracetamol-induced acute renal failure in the absence of fulminant liver damage. *Br Med J* 284:505, 1982.

19. Davenport A, Finn R: Paracetamol (acetaminophen) poisoning resulting in acute renal failure without hepatic coma. *Nephron* 50:55, 1988.

20. Coward RA: Paracetamol-induced acute pancreatitis. *Br Med J* 1:1086, 1977.

21. Gilmore IT, Touvras E: Paracetamol induced acute pancreatitis. *Br Med J* 2:753, 1977.

22. Sanerkin BH: Acute myocardial necrosis in paracetamol poisoning (letter). *Br Med J* 3:478, 1971.

23. Flanagan RJ, Mant TGK: Coma and metabolic acidosis early in severe acute paracetamol poisoning. *Hum Toxicol* 5:179, 1986.

24. Barker JD Jr, de Carle DJ, Anura S: Chronic excessive acetaminophen use and liver damage. *Ann Intern Med* 87:299, 1977.

25. Benson GD: Hepatotoxicity following the therapeutic use of antipyretic analgesics. *Am J Med* 75:85, 1983.

26. Smilkstein MJ, Hoffman RS, Foltin G, et al: Iatrogenic pediatric acetaminophen toxicity revisited (abstract). *Vet Hum Toxicol* 31:349, 1989.

27. Rumack BH, Matthew H: Acetaminophen poisoning and toxicity. *Pediatrics* 55:871, 1975.

28. Prescott LF, Roscoe P, Wright N, et al: Plasma paracetamol half-life and hepatic necrosis in patients with paracetamol overdosage. *Lancet* 1:519, 1971.

29. Smilkstein MJ, Knapp GL, Kulig KW, et al: Efficacy of oral N-acetylcysteine in the treatment of acetaminophen overdose: Analysis of the National Multicenter Study (1976–1985). *N Engl J Med* 319:1557, 1988.

30. Chinouth RW, Czajka PA, Peterson RG: N-acetylcysteine adsorption by activated charcoal. *Vet Hum Toxicol* 22:392, 1980.

31. Klein-Schwartz W, Oderda GM: Adsorption of oral antidotes for acetaminophen poisoning (methionine and N-acetylcysteine) by activated charcoal. *Clin Toxicol* 18:283, 1981.

32. Rybolt TR, Burrell DE, Shults JM, et al: In vitro coadsorption of acetaminophen and N-acetylcysteine onto activated carbon powder. *J Pharm Sci* 75:904, 1986.

33. North DS, Peterson RG, Krenzelok EP: Effect of activated charcoal administration on acetylcysteine serum levels in humans. *Am J Hosp Pharm* 38:1022, 1981.

34. Van de Graaf WB, Thompson WL, Sunshine I, et al: Adsorbent and cathartic inhibition of enteral drug absorption. *J Pharmacol Exp Ther* 221:656, 1982.

35. Renzi FP, Donovan JW, Martin TG, et al: Concomitant use of activated charcoal and N-acetylcysteine. *Ann Emerg Med* 14:568, 1985.

36. Ekins BR, Ford DC, Thompson MIB, et al: The effect of activated charcoal on N-acetylcysteine absorption in normal subjects. *Am J Emerg Med* 5:483, 1987.

37. Prescott LF, Sutherland GR, Park J, et al: Cysteamine, methionine, and penicillamine in the treatment of paracetamol poisoning. *Lancet* 2:109, 1976.

38. Prescott LF, Illingworth RN, Critchley JAJH, et al: Intravenous N-acetylcysteine: The treatment of choice for paracetamol poisoning. *Br Med J* 2:1097, 1979.

39. Miners JO, Drew R, Birkett DJ: Mechanism of action of paracetamol protective agents in vivo. *Biochem Pharmacol* 33:2995, 1984.

40. Corcoran GB, Todd EL, Racz WJ, et al: Effects of N-acetylcysteine on the disposition and metabolism of acetaminophen in mice. *J Pharmacol Exp Ther* 232:857, 1985.

41. Buckpitt AR, Rollins DE, Mitchell JR: Varying effects of sulfhydryl nucleophiles on acetaminophen oxidation and sulfhydryl adduct formation. *Biochem Pharmacol* 28:2941, 1979.

42. Lin JH, Levy G: Sulfate depletion after acetaminophen administration and replenishment by infusion of sodium sulfate or N-acetylcysteine in rats. *Biochem Pharmacol* 30:2723, 1981.

43. Lauterburg BH, Corcoran GB, Mitchell JR: Mechanism of action of N-acetylcysteine in the protection against the hepatotoxicity of acetaminophen in rats. *J Clin Invest* 71:980, 1983.

44. Harrison PM, Keays R, Bray GP, et al: Improved outcome in paracetamol-induced fulminant hepatic failure following late administration of acetylcysteine. *Lancet* 335:1572, 1990.

45. Keays R, Harrison PM, Wendon JA, et al: Intravenous acetylcysteine in paracetamol induced fulminant hepatic failure: A prospective controlled trial. *Br Med J* 303:1026, 1991.

46. Harrison PM, Wendon JA, Gimson AES, et al: Improvement by acetylcysteine of hemodynamics and oxygen transport in fulminant hepatic failure. *N Engl J Med* 324:1852, 1991.

47. Jaeschke H, Mitchell JR: Neutrophil accumulation exacerbates acetaminophen-induced liver injury (abstract). *FASEB J* 3:A920, 1989.

48. Bruno MK, Cohen SD, Khairallah EH: Antidotal effectiveness of N-acetylcysteine in reversing acetaminophen-induced hepatotoxicity: Enhancement of the proteolysis of arylated proteins. *Biochem Pharmacol* 37:4319, 1988.

49. Rumack BH, Peterson RC, Koch GC, et al: Acetaminophen overdose: 662 cases with evaluation of oral acetylcysteine treatment. *Arch Intern Med* 141:380, 1981.

50. Smilkstein MJ, Bronstein AC, Linden C, et al: Acetaminophen overdose: A 48-hour intravenous N-acetylcysteine protocol. *Ann Emerg Med* 20:1058, 1991.

51. Borys DJ, Jackson TW, Jacobs MR, et al: Intravenous N-acetylcysteine: Use of an unapproved drug product—A two year retrospective review. *Vet Hum Toxicol* 34:327, 1992.

52. Miller LF, Rumack BH: Clinical safety of high oral doses of acetylcysteine. *Semin Oncol* 10(suppl 1):76, 1983.

53. Walton NG, Mann TA, Shaw KM: Anaphylactoid reaction to N-acetylcysteine. *Lancet* 2:1298, 1979.

54. Vale JA, Wheeler DC: Anaphylactoid reactions to IV acetylcysteine. *Lancet* 2:988, 1982.

55. Mant TG, Tempowski JG, Volans GN, et al: Adverse reactions to acetylcysteine and effects of overdose. *Br Med J* 289:217, 1984.

56. Anonymous: Death after N-acetylcysteine. *Lancet* 1:1421, 1984.

57. Donovan JW, Javie D, Prescott LF, et al: Hypersensitivity reactions to N-acetylcysteine: A concentration-dependent phenomenon (abstract). Presented at the EAPCC Congress, Edinburgh, September 1988.

58. Dawson AH, Henry DA, McEwen J: Adverse reactions to N-acetylcysteine during treatment for paracetamol poisoning. *Med J Aust* 150:329, 1989.

59. Vendemiale G, Altomore E, Trizio T, et al: Effect of acute and chronic cimetidine administration on acetaminophen metabolism in humans. *Am J Gastroenterol* 82:1031, 1987.

60. Speeg KV Jr, Mitchell MC, Maldonado AL: Additive protection of cimetidine and N-acetylcysteine treatment against acetaminophen-induced hepatic necrosis in the rat. *J Pharmacol* 234:550, 1985.

61. Burkhart K, Janco N, Kulig KW, et al: Cimetidine as adjunctive treatment for acetaminophen overdose (abstract). *Vet Hum Toxicol* 31:337, 1989.

62. Coon MJ, Koop DR, Reeve LE, et al: Alcohol metabolism and toxicity: Role of cytochrome P-450. *Fundam Appl Toxicol* 4:134, 1984.

63. Tredger JM, Smith HM, Read RB, et al: Effects of ethanol ingestion on the metabolism of a hepatotoxic dose of paracetamol in mice. *Xenobiotica* 16:661, 1986.

64. Sato C, Lieber CS: Mechanism of the preventive effect of ethanol on acetaminophen-induced hepatotoxicity. *J Pharmacol Exp Ther* 218:811, 1981.

65. Thummel KE, Slattery JT, Nelson SD: Mechanism by which ethanol diminishes the hepatotoxicity of acetaminophen. *J Pharmacol Exp Ther* 245:129, 1988.

66. Dietz AJ Fr, Carlson JD, Khalil SKW, et al: Effects of alcoholism in acetaminophen pharmacokinetics in man. *J Clin Pharmacol* 24:205, 1984.

67. Lauterberg BH, Velez ME: Glutathione deficiency in alcoholics: Risk factor for paracetamol hepatotoxicity. *Gut* 29:1153, 1988.
68. Bray GP, Harrison PM, O'Grady JG, et al: Long-term anticonvulsant therapy worsens outcome in paracetamol-induced fulminant hepatic failure. *Hum Exp Toxicol* 11:265, 1992.
69. Rumack BH: Acetaminophen overdose in young children: Treatment and effects of alcohol and other additional ingestants in 417 cases. *Am J Dis Child* 138:428, 1984.
70. Roberts I, Robinson MJ, Mughal MZ, et al: Paracetamol metabolites in the neonate following maternal overdose. *Br J Clin Pharmacol* 18:201, 1984.
71. Lauterberg BH, Vaishnav Y, Stillwell WG, et al: The effects of age and glutathione depletion on hepatic glutathione turnover in vivo determined by acetaminophen probe analysis. *J Pharmacol Exp Ther* 213:54, 1980.
72. Arena JM, Rourk MH, Sibrack CD: Acetaminophen: Report of an unusual poisoning. *Pediatrics* 61:68, 1978.
73. Lieh-Lai MW, Sarnaik AP, Newton JF, et al: Metabolism and pharmacokinetics of acetaminophen in a severely poisoned young child. *J Pediatr* 105:125, 1984.
74. Riggs BS, Bronstein AC, Kulig KW, et al: Acute acetaminophen overdose during pregnancy. *Obstet Gynecol* 74:247, 1989.
75. Selden BS, Curry SC, Clark RF, et al: Transplacental transport of N-acetylcysteine in an ovine model. *Ann Emerg Med* 20:1069, 1991.
76. Devalia JL, Ogilvie RC, McLean AEM: Dissociation of cell death from covalent binding by flavones in a hepatocyte system. *Biochem Pharmacol* 31:3745, 1982.
77. Nogen AG, Bremner JE: Fatal acetaminophen overdosage in a child. *J Pediatr* 92:832, 1978.
78. Calvert LJ, Linder CW: Acetaminophen poisoning. *J Fam Pract* 7:953, 1978.
79. Weber JL, Cutz E: Liver failure in an infant. *Can Med Assoc J* 123:114, 1980.
80. Greene JW, Craft L, Ghishan F: Acetaminophen poisoning in infancy. *Am J Dis Child* 137:386, 1983.
81. Smith DW, Isakson G, Frankel LR, et al: Hepatic failure following ingestion of multiple doses of acetaminophen in a young child. *J Pediatr Gastroenterol Nutr* 5:822, 1986.
82. Blake KV, Bailey D, Zientek GM, et al: Death of a child associated with multiple overdoses of acetaminophen. *Clin Pharm* 7:391, 1988.
83. Henretig FM, Selbst SM, Forrest C, et al: Repeated acetaminophen overdosing: Causing hepatotoxicity in children. *Clin Pediatr* 28:525, 1989.
84. Seeff LB, Cuccherini BA, Zimmerman HG, et al: Acetaminophen hepatotoxicity in alcoholics: A therapeutic misadventure. *Ann Intern Med* 104:399, 1986.
85. Hall AH, Kulig KW, Rumack BH: Acetaminophen toxicity (letter). *JAMA* 256:1893, 1986.
86. Hall AH, Kulig KW, Rumack BH: Acetaminophen hepatotoxicity in alcoholics (letter). *Ann Intern Med* 105:624, 1986.
87. Benson GD: Acetaminophen in chronic liver disease. *Clin Pharmacol Ther* 33:95, 1983.
88. Hamlyn AN, Douglas AP, James O: The spectrum of paracetamol (acetaminophen) overdose: Clinical and epidemiological studies. *Postgrad Med J* 54:400, 1978.
89. Clark R, Thompson RPH, Borirakchanyavat V, et al: Hepatic damage and death from overdosage of paracetamol. *Lancet* 1:66, 1973.
90. O'Grady JG, Wendon J, Tan KC, et al: Liver transplantation after paracetamol overdose. *Br Med J* 303:221, 1991.
91. Harrison PM, O'Grady JG, Keays RT, et al: Serial prothrombin time as prognostic indicator in paracetamol induced fulminant hepatic failure. *Br Med J* 301:964, 1990.

131. Antiarrhythmic Poisoning

David N. Dunbar and Paul R. Pentel

Overview

Over the past 20 years, clinical and experimental electrophysiologic studies have increased our understanding of arrhythmia mechanisms and the effects of antiarrhythmic drugs. Despite these advances, adverse side effects from antiarrhythmic drugs are common; potentially lethal toxicity from proarrhythmic effects may occur in 5 to 15 percent of patients treated with these drugs [1]. Life-threatening toxicity associated with toxic drug concentrations may also result from accidental or suicidal overdose and from impaired drug elimination. The recognition, management, and prevention of antiarrhythmic drug toxicity requires an understanding of (1) arrhythmia mechanisms and their relationship to the underlying cardiac disease being treated (see Chap. 49); (2) the electrophysiologic effects of classes of antiarrhythmic drugs, since toxicity often presents as an exaggeration of these effects; (3) knowledge of specific drug pharmacokinetics with attention to drug interactions and disease states, which may affect antiarrhythmic drug metabolism and (4) principles of general supportive care and management of specific drug toxicity syndromes.

Actions of Antiarrhythmic Drugs

ELECTROPHYSIOLOGIC EFFECTS. Vaughan Williams proposed the most commonly used system for classifying antiarrhythmic drugs according to their electrophysiologic effects (see Chap. 207) [1,2]. The electrophysiologic effects of the class I drugs on conduction and repolarization are reflected in the changes of surface ECG intervals (Fig. 131-1). Class IA drugs moderately depress conduction, manifested by slight increases in the P–R and QRS intervals on the surface ECG. These drugs also prolong action potential duration, resulting in significant increases in the J–T interval. (The J point is the end of the QRS interval.) Class IB drugs have little effect on conduction or repolarization in normal cardiac tissues at normal rates. This is reflected in the lack of change in P–R, QRS, and J–T intervals with therapeutic levels. Class IB drugs act to depress conduction further in abnormal tissue. Class IC drugs markedly depress conduction, reflected by significant increases in the P–R and QRS intervals on the surface ECG. They have relatively little effect on repolarization, resulting in little change in the J–T interval. Antiarrhythmic drug toxicity may severely depress con-

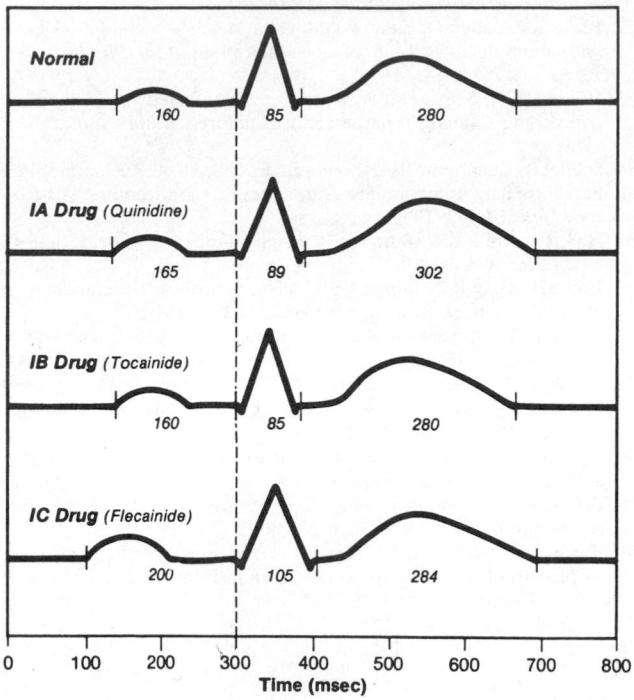

EFFECTS OF CLASS I ANTIARRHYTHMIC DRUGS ON SURFACE ECG INTERVALS
(Heart rate = 75)

Normal

IA Drug (Quinidine)

IB Drug (Tocainide)

IC Drug (Flecainide)

Fig. 131-1. Average P–R, QRS, and J–T intervals from normal patients and patients receiving quinidine, tocainide, and flecainide with intervals adjusted to reflect a heart rate of 75 beats per minute. Class IA drugs prolong only minimally. Class IB drugs do not prolong either the QRS or J–T intervals. Class IC drugs prolong the QRS complex substantially but have little effect on the J–T interval. (From Pentel PR, Dunbar DN: New cardiac antiarrhythmic agents, in Haddad LM, Winchester JF (eds): *Clinical Management of Poisoning and Drug Overdose.* 2nd ed. Philadelphia, WB Saunders, 1990, p 1382.)

duction, producing excessive QRS prolongation (≥50% widening of baseline values). Excessive J–T prolongation (Q–T interval >0.5 seconds) may be the first indication of an idiosyncratic response to class IA or IC drugs leading to *Torsades de pointes.*

MECHANISMS OF THERAPEUTIC AND PROARRHYTHMIA EFFECTS. Antiarrhythmic drugs may act to suppress or aggravate arrhythmias (proarrhythmia) through complex mechanisms that are difficult to define. Often, the tachyarrhythmia mechanism (e.g., automaticity or reentry) is uncertain. Even if the tachyarrhythmia mechanism is established, the potential electrophysiologic actions of drugs producing therapeutic or toxic effects are numerous and complex. For example, these drugs may have differing effects on automaticity, conduction, and refractoriness in normal and diseased myocardium even in the same patient. The electrophysiologic effects are further modified by factors such as heart rate, autonomic tone, electrolyte imbalances, and reversible ischemia. The margin of safety between the antiarrhythmic dose resulting in arrhythmia suppression and that resulting in toxicity is often quite narrow, producing toxicity when drug elimination is altered by hepatic or renal disease. Finally, the potential for proarrhythmia is profoundly influenced by the nature of the underlying heart dis-

ease. Nevertheless, therapeutic and toxic antiarrhythmic drug effects usually can be explained by the electrophysiologic effects of these drugs and underlying arrhythmia mechanisms.

Antiarrhythmic drugs may exert their therapeutic effects through the suppression of abnormal automaticity. They may decrease automaticity by decreasing the slope of phase 4 depolarization, causing the threshold potential to become more positive, or causing the resting membrane potential to become more negative (Fig. 131-2B, C, D) [3]. Thus, heart rate is slowed by increasing the time required for phase 4 depolarization to reach threshold. Antiarrhythmic drugs may also depress automaticity by prolonging action potential duration by slowing depolarization or repolarization [4]. The same drugs may produce proarrhythmic effects by excessive depression of sinus node automaticity, particularly in patients with underlying sinus node dysfunction or toxic drug levels. This may result in sinus bradycardia, sinus pauses, or asystole. Class IA and IC drugs depress automaticity relatively more than class IB drugs [4]. The direct depressant effects of quinidine and disopyramide on sinus node automaticity may be partially offset by their vagolytic effects.

Antiarrhythmic drugs may also induce inappropriate bradycardia by adversely altering conduction, especially in patients with underlying conduction system disease or toxic drug levels. Sinoatrial exit block and atrioventricular (A-V) block (usually infra-His) are more common with class IA or IC than with class IB drugs. Cardiac pacing may be adversely affected by loss of capture caused by significant increases in pacing threshold due to depressed membrane responsiveness and conduction [5]. Pacing problems are most common with massive antiarrhythmic drug overdose [6].

Antiarrhythmic drugs may suppress tachyarrhythmias that result from reentry by disturbing the critical relationship of unidirectional block, slow conduction, and refractoriness needed to sustain reentry. Class I drugs may further depress conduction to produce bidirectional block (Fig. 131-3B). Class IA and III drugs prolong action potential duration and refractoriness so that the reentry wavefront may be stopped by refractory tissue.

These same electrophysiologic properties can be proarrhythmic by creating new (or more stable) reentry circuits. Drugs may cause reentry by producing unidirectional block where only slow conduction was present before (Fig. 131-3C, D). Drugs may facilitate reentry by slowing conduction to allow more time for the pathway to recover in front of the advancing wavefront. Thus, the reentry wavefront does not encounter refractory tissue and the tachycardia is sustained. Drugs may convert nonsustained to sustained ventricular tachycardia in this manner [7]. This type of facilitation of reentry is likely responsible for the sustained and at times incessant ventricular tachycardia seen with class IC drugs, which markedly slow conduction but have little effect on refractory periods [8].

Incessant Ventricular Tachycardia. Incessant ventricular tachycardia is sustained ventricular tachycardia, which is difficult to terminate and frequently recurs after only several beats in sinus rhythm [9,10,11]. The rate is usually less than 150 beats per minute; QRS complexes are wide and at times sinusoidal. Incessant ventricular tachycardia may be polymorphic but is not associated with Q–T prolongation or pause-dependent initiation (as in *Torsades de pointes*) [9]. Incessant ventricular tachycardia is usually hemodynamically unstable and may be fatal [9]. It occurs most commonly in patients with a history of lethal ventricular arrhythmias and impaired left ventricular function treated with class IC antiarrhythmic drugs [9,10,12,13].

Torsades de Pointes. *Torsades de pointes* is a polymorphic ventricular tachycardia seen in the setting of Q–T prolongation

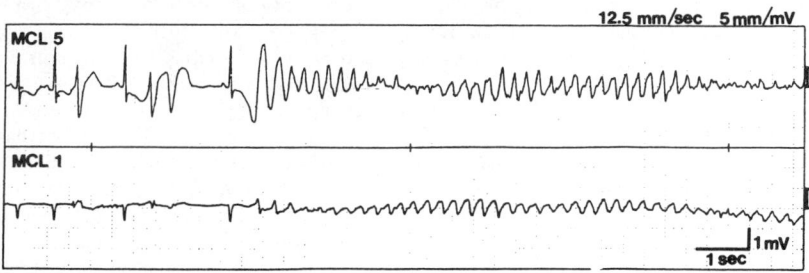

MCL 5

MCL 1

12.5 mm/sec   5 mm/mV

1 mV
1 sec

Fig. 131-2. Onset of *Torsades de pointes* in a 62-year-old woman with dilated cardiomyopathy and frequent ventricular premature beats 2 hours after receiving a single 325-mg dose of quinidine gluconate. Note the pause-dependent initiation after a ventricular couplet and the polymorphic QRS morphology, which appears to twist around the baseline.

[14–17]. With a rate of 150 to 300 beats per minute, this abnormality is characterized by QRS complexes of various amplitudes that appear to twist about the baseline, thus the descriptive name (Fig. 131-4) [15]. *Torsades de pointes* is most commonly associated with exposure to drugs, particularly class IA and class III antiarrhythmic drugs, that prolong repolarization [18]. It may also occur with noncardiac drugs, toxins, electrolyte disorders, and cardiac disorders [14,16,18]. Reports of *Torsades de pointes* with class IC drugs are rare. Although relatively few cases caused solely by amiodarone have been reported, one report described an incidence up to 4 percent [19]. The incidence of *Torsades de pointes* with sotalol is approximately 2 percent [20].

The incidence of *Torsades de pointes* with therapeutic doses of quinidine, procainamide, and disopyramide has been estimated to be less than 2 to 3 percent [21] and may vary with the severity of underlying heart disease. The incidence of quinidine-induced *Torsades de pointes* has ranged up to 8 percent in patients with atrial fibrillation and congestive heart failure, reflecting more severe underlying heart disease [20]. In contrast, no *Torsades de pointes* and a 0.9 percent incidence of excessive Q–T prolongation were reported in a population of 360 stable patients with benign or potentially lethal ventricular arrhythmias treated with quinidine [20]. Similar results are reported for sotalol [20]. *Torsades de pointes* occurs most often in patients with therapeutic or low, rather than toxic, plasma levels, sug-

gesting an idiosyncratic response for type I antiarrhythmic drugs [23,24,25]. In contrast, *Torsades de pointes* is a common manifestation with sotalol intoxication [26-29]. The influence of baseline Q–T interval on the incidence of *Torsades de pointes* is uncertain. One study reported that 14 of 32 patients who developed quinidine-induced *Torsades de pointes* had baseline Q–Tc prolongation greater than 0.45 seconds [23]. The magnitude of Q–T prolongation is highly variable in drug-induced *Torsades de pointes,* with approximately one-third of patients having Q–Tc intervals shorter than 0.48 seconds [14,25]. The minimal Q–T prolongation in these patients led one author to prefer the term *drug-induced polymorphic ventricular tachycardia* to *Torsades de pointes,* [25]. Hypokalemia, hypomagnesemia, and bradycardia may aggravate *Torsades de pointes* [23]. Approximately 50 percent of cases occur within the first 4

Fig. 131-4. A. Reentrant circuit with the antegrade impulse blocking in one pathway, conducting in the other pathway, and then propagating retrogradely through a segment with depressed conduction. The action potential is depicted as occurring in the depressed segment with slow phase 0 depolarization (V_{max}). B. An antiarrhythmic drug further depresses conduction so the segment is unexcitable, producing bidirectional block and terminating the arrhythmia. C. There is slight depression of conduction in a segment, but antegrade propagation persists. D. An antiarrhythmic drug has produced a proarrhythmic effect by further depressing conduction, producing unidirectional block and reentry. (From Rosen MR, Wit AL: Arrhythmogenic actions of antiarrhythmic drugs. *Am J Cardiol* 59:10E, 1987. With permission.)

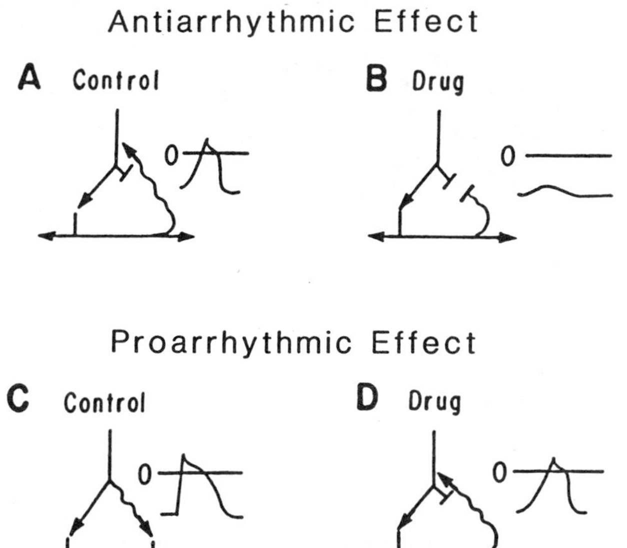

Fig. 131-3. Sinus node action potentials are depicted on this graph. A second action potential is produced when the gradual phase 4 depolarization reaches threshold potential (A). Sinus rate slows when the slope of phase 4 depolarization is decreased (B), when threshold potential is increased (C), or by a more negative resting membrane potential (D). (From Hoffman BF, Cranefield PF, Wallace AG: Physiological basis of cardiac arrhythmias: Part I. *Mod Concepts Cardiovasc Dis* 35:103, 1966. With permission.)

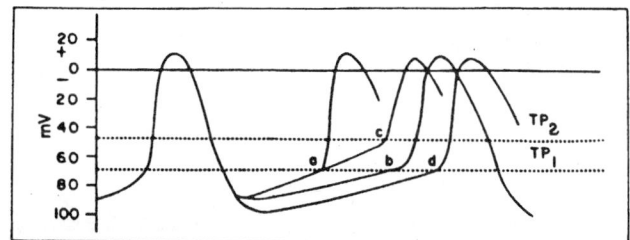

Antiarrhythmic Effect

A Control

B Drug

Proarrhythmic Effect

C Control

D Drug

days of treatment with antiarrhythmic drugs and another 30 percent within the first month of initiation of drug therapy [14,25].

PROARRHYTHMIA IDENTIFICATION AND RISK FACTORS. Distinguishing proarrhythmia effects from ineffective arrhythmia suppression by antiarrhythmic drugs can be difficult. Arrhythmia frequency can vary spontaneously or be affected by changes in underlying heart disease. A strong case for proarrhythmia can be made when new arrhythmias (e.g., sinus pauses or A–V block) develop soon after antiarrhythmic drug initiation or a dose increase. The diagnosis of proarrhythmia is more certain if this effect resolves with drug discontinuation or is reproduced with reexposure. New arrhythmias such as *Torsades de pointes* and incessant ventricular tachycardia are sufficiently characteristic to diagnose proarrhythmia. Proarrhythmia manifested only by increases in frequency of the underlying arrhythmia is more difficult to recognize. A 4-fold increase in ventricular premature beat (VPB) frequency and a 10-fold increase in repetitive form frequency were proposed as criteria for proarrhythmia, based on observations of spontaneous variability of ventricular arrhythmias using ambulatory monitoring [30]. Larger increases (up to ten-fold) have been proposed as criteria for proarrhythmia in patients with low VPB frequency because of greater spontaneous variability [31].

Although the overall incidence of proarrhythmia during drug treatment for ventricular arrhythmias is 5 to 15 percent, the incidence is modified by several factors [30,32]. Patients treated for lethal ventricular arrhythmias (history of sustained ventricular tachycardia or ventricular fibrillation) were 2.5 times more likely to develop proarrhythmia than patients treated for benign or potentially lethal arrhythmias (VPBs, nonsustained ventricular tachycardia) [32]. Increases in the incidence of serious proarrhythmia were reported with flecainide (6.6% vs. 0.4%) and encainide (8.5% vs. 4.2%) in patients with lethal versus nonlethal arrhythmias, respectively [12]. Patients treated with flecainide and encainide with structural heart disease had a twofold to threefold increased risk for proarrhythmia compared with those without structural heart disease [12]. Higher risks of proarrhythmia have been associated with more severe ventricular dysfunction [32]. Higher initial doses, more rapid escalation, and higher drug levels are associated with an increased risk of proarrhythmia in patients treated with flecainide and encainide [12]. Antiarrhythmic drug overdose can produce a similar spectrum of arrhythmias, including sinus node dysfunction, A-V block, and ventricular arrhythmias. Dose-related drug toxicity may be partially avoidable through close attention to pharmacokinetics, particularly in patients with hepatic or renal disease or congestive heart failure. Avoidance of dose escalation prior to steady state (4–5 elimination half-lives) and determination of plasma drug levels at steady state may help prevent dose-related toxicity.

General Management

TOXICITY DURING THERAPEUTIC DOSING. Non-life-threatening, dose-related side effects are common during antiarrhythmic drug treatment and can generally be managed by dose reduction or by switching to another drug if arrhythmia suppression is not achieved. Asymptomatic sinus bradycardia and Mobitz I A-V block can be observed under continuous rhythm monitoring with decreased dosing or discontinuation of the drug. Potential aggravating factors, such as myocardial is-

chemia or concurrent therapy with digoxin, calcium blockers, or beta-blockers, should be considered. Symptomatic bradycardia can be managed using intravenous atropine, isoproterenol, or an external cardiac pacemaker until temporary transvenous pacing can be performed.

Significant increases in ventricular ectopy or asymptomatic nonsustained ventricular tachycardia can be managed with drug discontinuation under continuous monitoring, again with attention to possible aggravating factors such as hypoxia, acidosis, myocardial ischemia, hypokalemia, and hypomagnesemia. Lidocaine can be used to suppress ventricular ectopy occurring during class IA, IC, and III antiarrhythmic drug therapy, because lidocaine shortens action potential duration and has little effect on conduction. Other class IA and IC drugs are generally contraindicated due to the potential for further arrhythmia aggravation. Direct current (DC) cardioversion may be needed for sustained ventricular tachycardia. Frequently recurring ventricular tachycardia may be converted by burst pacing through a temporary ventricular lead instead of repeated DC cardioversions. Pacing at rates of 90 to 110 beats per minute may be effective in suppressing recurrent ventricular tachycardia. Bretylium or beta-blockers may also be useful. Determination of plasma drug levels is also helpful. Subtherapeutic levels suggest that the arrhythmia may be caused by inadequate dosage or noncompliance. Therapeutic or high levels indicate the drug is ineffective or possibly proarrhythmic.

TOXICITY DUE TO ACUTE OVERDOSE. The signs, symptoms, and management of overdose toxicity are common to most antiarrhythmic drugs and are discussed together (Table 131-1). Unique aspects of antiarrhythmic drug toxicity and phar-

Table 131-1. Management of Life-Threatening Antiarrhythmic Drug Overdose

Supportive Care
  Gastric lavage/activated charcoal for acute oral ingestion
  Correct acidosis, hypoxia
  Diazepam for seizures

Enhancing drug elimination
  Hemoperfusion—disopyramide, NAPA (possible benefit—tocainide, procainamide)
  Hemodialysis—sotalol
  Urine acidification—flecainide, tocainide

Hypotension
  Fluid administration
  IM NaHCO$_3$ for class I drugs
  Inotropes, vasopressors
  Pulmonary artery catheter for monitoring
  Circulatory assist devices

Impaired conduction
  Temporary pacing
  IM NaHCO$_3$ for class I drugs
  Isoproterenol or epinephrine

Ventricular arrhythmias
  Torsade
    Temporary pacing
    MgSO$_4$
    Isoproterenol
  Monomorphic ventricular tachycardia
    Cardioversion if causing hypotension
    IM NaCHO$_3$ for class I drugs
    Lidocaine except for class IB drugs
    Overdrive pacing

NAPA = N-acetyl procainamide

macokinetics pertinent to each drug are discussed in later sections.

Supportive Care. Gastric lavage may be useful for patients who present within several hours of intentional drug overdose. Syrup of ipecac is contraindicated because coma and seizures can occur, and emesis could lead to aspiration. All overdose patients should receive oral activated charcoal, even if the ingestion was not recent, because the anticholinergic effects of some of these drugs may delay gastric emptying [26]. Patients with complications of therapeutic dosing may also benefit from oral activated charcoal to reduce absorption of a recently administered drug dose. Central nervous system (CNS) and respiratory depression are common with antiarrhythmic drug overdose and may be managed with endotracheal intubation and assisted ventilation. Seizures may result from class I (particularly IB) toxicity. No specific data regarding management are available. Diazepam is often used.

Hypotension. Hypotension may be caused by impaired cardiac contractility, vasodilation, or arrhythmia. Impaired contractility is most common with class IA or IC drugs but also may be seen with severe class IB drug toxicity. Quinidine has alpha-adrenergic antagonist properties that may produce vasodilation and hypotension. Intravenous procainamide can also produce significant hypotension, particularly during rapid infusions. Any antiarrhythmic drug may cause hemodynamically compromising bradycardia or tachycardia. Sotalol toxicity is also associated with hypotension due to adrenergic blockade.

Fluid administration is often effective for hypotension, particularly when vasodilation is present. Hypotension that does not respond readily to fluid administration is best treated by the use of a pulmonary arterial (Swan-Ganz) catheter. More fluid is indicated when hypotension is associated with low filling pressures. Hypotension associated with normal filling pressures and cardiac output but low systemic vascular resistance may be treated with pressors such as dopamine or norepinephrine. Cardiogenic shock is characterized by low cardiac output and elevated filling pressures. Inotropic agents, such as dopamine or dobutamine, can be used. Excessive doses of inotropic agents should be avoided because they may precipitate ventricular tachyarrhythmia. Early consideration should be given to circulatory assist devices for patients with cardiogenic shock. An intraatrial balloon pump has been used successfully to treat a patient with severe quinidine toxicity [27]. Cardiopulmonary bypass has been used to maintain circulation during massive lidocaine toxicity [28,29]. Extracorporeal circulatory assist devices that can be placed percutaneously are increasingly available for support during coronary angioplasty and could provide a quick and effective means of support during drug-induced cardiogenic shock. Assist devices may be more beneficial to these patients than to patients with cardiogenic shock due to primary myocardial disease, because of the reversibility of drug-induced cardiac dysfunction.

TOXICITY COMMON TO THERAPEUTIC DOSES AND OVERDOSES

Depression of Conduction and Automaticity: Role of Bicarbonate, Catecholamines, and Potassium. The depression of conduction and automaticity common to severe antiarrhythmic drug toxicity may be caused by a combination of direct electrophysiologic and secondary metabolic effects. Respiratory depression and shock may produce acidosis, hyperkalemia, and myocardial ischemia, which can further aggravate already depressed conduction. Cardiac manifestations include QRS prolongation, sinus node dysfunction, A-V block, ventric-

ular arrhythmias, and poor ventricular function. These derangements can culminate in intractable arrhythmias, cardiogenic shock, or death.

Observations that antiarrhythmic drug toxicity produced QRS widening similar to that observed with hyperkalemia led to the use of sodium lactate for quinidine and procainamide toxicity [33,34]. Although this rationale is now recognized to be incorrect, hypertonic (1 M) sodium lactate and sodium bicarbonate have been reported to decrease QRS prolongation with quinidine [33,34], procainamide [6,33], flecainide [35], and encainide [36] toxicity. The mechanism may be an increase in the pH and/or extracellular sodium concentration, leading to partial reversal of the sodium channel blockade [37,38]. Recent data suggest that extracellular sodium inhibits the binding of flecainide to myocardial sodium channels, a mechanism by which hypertonic sodium solutions may reduce the toxicity of class IA or IC drugs [39]. In vitro observations support additive roles of increasing sodium concentration and increasing pH in improving conduction [40]. In view of these experimental data as well as case reports of clinical improvement, sodium bicarbonate should be considered for class IA and IC toxicity. Repeat intravenous boluses of sodium bicarbonate can be given (50 mEq of 1 mEq/ml solution) to increase blood pH to 7.45 to 7.50.

Drug-induced depressant effects on automaticity and conduction may be partially reduced by catecholamines. Isoproterenol infusion has been shown to reverse depression of conduction and mortality in experimental quinidine overdose in animals and has been used in quinidine toxicity in humans [41,42]. Recently, epinephrine was shown to antagonize antiarrhythmic drug effects [43]. Thus, isoproterenol or epinephrine infusions may improve conduction in addition to their beneficial effects for bradyarrhythmia management.

Hyperkalemia can depress cardiac conduction. Potassium supplementation should probably not be given even with moderate hypokalemia in the presence of class I antiarrhythmic drug toxicity. Hypokalemia resulted in improved conduction in experimental quinidine toxicity in animals [44,45]. A case report described a patient with quinidine dialyzed with a 1.5 mEq potassium bath [39], resulting in substantial clinical improvement and QRS narrowing despite minimal reduction in quinidine levels. Clinical experience in using induced hypokalemia to treat antiarrhythmic drug toxicity, however, is quite limited, and this intervention is not recommended.

Incessant Ventricular Tachycardia. Management of incessant ventricular tachycardia typically consists of repeated cardioversions, cardiopulmonary resuscitation, pressor support, and mechanical ventilation [9,10,11,46–49]. Atrial and/or ventricular pacing is often attempted to suppress this rhythm disturbance. The goal of therapy is to support the patient by any means possible to allow time for elimination of the antiarrhythmic drug. Treatment with other class IA and IC antiarrhythmic drugs is generally not recommended, given the potential for further arrhythmia aggravation [9]. Intravenous lidocaine may be considered because it does not normally depress conduction, but it is often ineffective. Intravenous amiodarone suppressed incessant ventricular tachycardia induced by flecainide in one patient [50]. Improvement has been anecdotally described with sodium bicarbonate, which resulted in suppression of ventricular tachycardia and hemodynamic improvement [35,51,52].

Torsades de Pointes. Although *Torsades de pointes* commonly reverts to sinus rhythm spontaneously, it may degenerate into fatal ventricular fibrillation [53,54]. Direct current cardioversion is effective in terminating this arrhythmia, but it frequently recurs. Drug-induced *Torsades de pointes* is pause-dependent, characterized by long-short coupling intervals [24,53]. The typical sequence is a *long* compensatory pause following a ventricular premature beat, a supraventricular beat that usually has a more prolonged and bizarre Q–T interval, then a *short* cycle VPB initiating polymorphic ventricular tachycardia. The treatment of choice for pause-dependent *Torsades de pointes* is atrial or ventricular pacing at rates of more than 90 to 110 beats per minute, which is effective in more than 90 percent of patients [14,18,25]. In general, ventricular pacing is preferred over atrial pacing, due to a more stable lead position and to avoid pauses induced by nonconducted atrial premature beats or A-V block. Atrial pacing can be used in patients with decompensated congestive heart failure who may need A-V synchrony for hemodynamic reasons.

Isoproterenol infusion titrated to maintain heart rates greater than 90 beats per minute is the most effective pharmacologic therapy to suppress *Torsades de pointes*. It may suppress *Torsades* until a temporary pacemaker can be placed but has the disadvantage of increasing myocardial oxygen demand, which may pose a risk for patients with coronary artery disease. Atropine has been inconsistent in suppressing *Torsades de pointes*, mainly as a result of inconsistent increases in heart rate [14]. Magnesium sulfate administered as a 1- to 2-gm bolus in a 25% solution has suppressed drug-induced *Torsades de pointes* [17,55]. Lidocaine is the most frequently used antiarrhythmic drug for *Torsades de pointes* but also is inconsistently effective, with suppression in fewer than 50 percent of patients [14,18,25]. Similarly, bretylium is inconsistent or may actually increase frequency of *Torsades de pointes* [25]. Treatment with class IA antiarrhythmic drugs is contraindicated because further prolongation of repolarization and the Q–T interval may exacerbate *Torsades de pointes*. Attention should be given to correcting hypokalemia, but this alone is not often effective in suppressing *Torsades de pointes* [53].

Patients with *Torsades de pointes* should not receive other class IA agents and drugs known to prolong Q–T intervals, such as phenothiazines or tricyclic depressants, owing to a significant risk of recurrent *Torsades* [14,25]. Even if the *Torsades de pointes* (polymorphic ventricular tachycardia) is associated with minimal Q–T prolongation, other class IA antiarrhythmic drugs commonly produce ineffective suppression or arrhythmia aggravation [25,56]. Class IB antiarrhythmic drugs, which do not prolong repolarization, should be considered if antiarrhythmic therapy is required to suppress ventricular ectopy. The role of class IC drugs in this setting is poorly defined. Although amiodarone has been used successfully in patients with previous drug-mediated *Torsades de pointes* due to class IA agents [25,57], amiodarone-induced *Torsades* can occur [14]. Hemodialysis to enhance sotalol elimination has been described for sotalol-induced *Torsades de pointes* refractory to conventional management [29].

Enhancement of Drug Elimination. In general, maintenance of effective circulation to provide adequate hepatic and renal perfusion is the most effective way of eliminating antiarrhythmic drugs. Early improvement is probably due to drug distribution (to nontarget tissues) rather than drug elimination. Shock may markedly slow this drug distribution [58]. Attempts at accelerating drug removal should be considered when the usual routes of drug elimination are impaired by renal or hepatic disease or by circulatory collapse.

Because most antiarrhythmic drugs are weak bases, urine acidification can enhance drug excretion. However, this is generally not indicated. Administration of acid poses the risk of aggravating a systemic acidosis, depressing conduction, and worsening myoglobinuric renal failure in patients with rhabdomyolysis due to seizures. Moreover, for most drugs the magnitude of increased urinary excretion is small. Greatest benefit would be expected for flecainide (half-life 8 hours with acid urine and 33 hours with alkaline urine) and possibly tocainide [59].

Hemodialysis is of limited benefit for antiarrhythmic drug toxicity because drug clearance is limited by protein binding and high lipid solubility. Sotalol is an exception, in that hemodialysis shortens elimination half-life (from 33.9 hours to 5.8 hours in patients with renal insufficiency [60]) and has been used successfully to treat sotalol-induced *Torsades de pointes*. Hemoperfusion using charcoal resin with high absorptive capacity is generally superior. For hemoperfusion, the major limitation with regard to efficacy is the large volume of distribution of most antiarrhythmic drugs. Hemoperfusion is of greatest value for disopyramide [52] or N-acetyl procainamide (NAPA) [61] toxicity, but may be useful for other antiarrhythmic agents if other routes of elimination are impaired (see discussion of individual drugs).

Toxicity of Individual Agents

CLASS IA AGENTS. Quinidine, procainamide, and disopyramide are generally considered first-line agents for suppressing chronic ventricular ectopy, lethal ventricular arrhythmias, and primary atrial tachyarrhythmias. These drugs share characteristics of moderate sodium channel blockade, depression of conduction, and prolongation of repolarization.

Oral quinidine therapy is frequently limited by gastrointestinal (GI) side effects. Nausea, vomiting, and especially diarrhea occur in up to one-third of patients, even with therapeutic doses. Cinchonism with tinnitus, visual changes, and hearing loss is another potential dose-related side effect. Other adverse allergic or idiosyncratic reactions include fever, drug-induced hepatitis, thrombocytopenia, and anaphylaxis.

Therapeutic doses of oral quinidine have little adverse hemodynamic effect. Overdose and rapid IV administration may cause hypotension mediated by alpha-sympathetic blockade and/or depressed cardiac contractility. Quinidine can produce sinus node dysfunction and A-V block, but the direct depressant effects on sinus node automaticity and A-V nodal conduction are often offset by vagolytic effects. Vagolytic effects can cause ventricular rate acceleration owing to one-to-one A-V nodal conduction when atrial flutter is treated without concurrent medication such as digitalis to decrease A-V nodal conduction. Quinidine syncope is caused by *Torsades de pointes* [62], an idiosyncratic reaction occurring in 1 to 2 percent of patients treated with quinidine [21,23]. *Torsades de pointes* is commonly but not always associated with Q–T intervals longer than 0.5 seconds. QRS widening to greater than 25 percent of baseline is a sign of dose-related cardiotoxicity. Concerns over the safety of quinidine therapy for atrial fibrillation have arisen following the finding of excess mortality in patients treated with quinidine compared to placebo (2.9% vs. 0.8%) in a meta-analysis of randomized controlled trials [63].

Severe poisoning due to acute quinidine overdose is characterized by refractory hypotension, lethargy, seizures, and profound depression of cardiac contractility and conduction [11,39,64,65]. Hypotension may respond poorly even to high doses of norepinephrine, due to alpha blockade. In one case, an intra-aortic balloon pump was successful in providing circulatory support [11]. Repeated doses of oral activated charcoal (25–50 gm every 4 hours) may limit drug absorption after ingestion of slow-release formulations. Neither hemodialysis nor hemoperfusion is very effective for quinidine overdose, due to protein binding and the large volume of distribution [65,66].

Uncontrolled studies suggest that hypertonic sodium bicarbonate or lactate may be useful for quinidine cardiotoxicity; a trial of this therapy is warranted [33,34].

Procainamide. The usual oral dosage of procainamide is 2 to 6 gm per day, although higher doses have been used for recurrent ventricular tachycardia [69]. Gastrointestinal intolerance, with nausea, vomiting, bitter metallic taste, and especially anorexia, is usually the first sign of dose-related toxicity, appearing with procainamide levels of approximately 6 to 8 μg per milliliter. Weakness and general malaise are also common. Drug-induced leukopenia and agranulocytosis occur rarely. Drug-induced lupus erythematosus may occur in approximately 25 percent of patients with prolonged administration, particularly with high doses [67]. Symptoms include arthralgias, arthritis, pleuritis, pericarditis, fever, and rash [67,68]. Fluorescent antinuclear antibody studies (FANA) are abnormal in most patients with prolonged procainamide treatment and are not sufficient reason to discontinue therapy in the absence of symptoms.

Increasing toxicity is manifested by hypotension, QRS widening of more than 25 percent, conduction disturbances, and ventricular arrhythmias [6,63,69,70]. Renal insufficiency is the most common setting for chronic procainamide toxicity and is frequently caused by failure to adjust dosing or by dose increases before steady-state levels are achieved. Procainamide toxicity may also occur with development of prerenal azotemia induced by congestive heart failure or overdiuresis. Toxic NAPA levels (>25 μg/ml) may accumulate due to renal insufficiency, resulting in life-threatening *Torsades de pointes* [52,63].

Patients with signs of non-life-threatening procainamide toxicity and adequate renal function can be managed with supportive care, given the short elimination half-life of 3 hours. By analogy with quinidine toxicity, hypertonic sodium bicarbonate or lactate may be useful for procainamide toxicity [6,33]. This therapy would not be expected to benefit NAPA toxicity because NAPA is a class III drug. Hemodialysis or hemoperfusion is of little benefit in patients with normal renal function, due to rapid intrinsic cleaning. Hemoperfusion substantially increases NAPA (and to a lesser extent procainamide) clearance in patients with renal insufficiency and has been used for NAPA-induced *Torsades de pointes* [61,71].

Disopyramide. Signs of disopyramide toxicity commonly occur at levels of more than 7 μg per milliliter. Anticholinergic side effects are common, even within the therapeutic dosage range, consisting of dry mouth, blurry vision, urinary retention, constipation, and nausea [72]. Patients with glaucoma or benign prostatic hypertrophy are at particular risk for anticholinergic side effects. The signs of cardiotoxicity are similar to those of other class IA drugs (i.e., bradycardia, hypotension, conduction disturbances, QRS prolongation greater than 25 percent, and congestive heart failure). In contrast to other class IA agents, however, disopyramide has significantly more negative inotropic effect [73] and should not be used in patients with congestive heart failure or poor left ventricular function [74]. Cardiovascular collapse and death have been associated with disopyramide use in such patients, particularly when there is concomitant renal insufficiency [75].

Massive disopyramide overdose (ingestions of >2.5 gm) is characterized by early onset of cardiogenic shock accompanied by conduction disturbances [76]. Given the propensity for cardiogenic shock with disopyramide overdose, aggressive hemodynamic support with inotropes is indicated, along with early consideration of mechanical support, such as intraaortic balloon pump [77] or extracorporeal circulatory support. Because of its relatively small volume of distribution, disopyra-

mide clearance is substantially increased by hemoperfusion [52]. Hemodialysis is much less effective [26,78]. Adjunctive treatment with sodium bicarbonate may be considered (see Quinidine and Procainamide).

CLASS IB AGENTS. Lidocaine, the prototypic class IB antiarrhythmic drug, is a tertiary amine widely used as a local anesthetic. It is the drug of choice for the treatment of ventricular arrhythmias in the setting of acute myocardial infarction or ischemia. It has little efficacy for supraventricular arrhythmias. Tocainide and mexiletine are structural analogs of lidocaine used to suppress chronic ventricular ectopy. These drugs are commonly given in combination with class IA antiarrhythmic drugs to enhance arrhythmia suppression and to decrease the incidence of side effects [79,80]. The class IB drugs are weak sodium channel blockers with little effect on conduction in normal cells but greater effect on partially depolarized (e.g., ischemic) cells and little effect on repolarization.

Lidocaine. Most lidocaine toxicity is caused by errors in dosing and administration [81,82,83]. High peak concentrations from bolus (IV push) loading may cause transient adverse effects, usually neurologic symptoms. "Standard" loading doses of 150 to 200 mg or a maintenance dose of 3 mg per minute are inappropriate for small patients, particularly the elderly. Small stature has been identified as a risk factor for lidocaine toxicity, so maintenance doses based on weight were recommended (15–55 μg/kg/min) [83]. Toxicity may result from failure to adjust dosage when cardiac output (and therefore hepatic clearance) is decreased by congestive heart failure, shock, or advanced age or by the presence of cirrhosis [81,83]. Life-threatening overdose and death may result from massive overdoses with inadvertent injection of 20% lidocaine in prepackaged syringes intended for use in preparing maintenance infusions, rather than the 2% syringes meant for parenteral bolus injections [84,85]. Toxicity has also been described as a result of swallowing large amounts of viscous lidocaine used for topical oral anesthesia (especially in children receiving multiple doses) and as a result of large parenteral doses used for local, regional, or intravenous anesthesia [86].

Neurologic signs and symptoms usually precede cardiotoxicity, except in massive acute lidocaine overdose [87]. Symptoms may include light-headedness, visual disturbances, paresthesias, tinnitus, drowsiness, confusion, and psychosis. Neurologic signs may include muscle twitching, tremor, ataxia, dysarthria, and seizures. Massive overdose results in seizures, coma, respiratory arrest, and cardiovascular collapse. Nausea and vomiting also may occur with lidocaine therapy [82]. Adverse cardiac effects from lidocaine administration are unusual in the absence of severe underlying conduction system disease, acute myocardial ischemia, or massive overdose. Rare episodes of asystole have been reported after lidocaine administration during acute myocardial infarctions due to sinus node dysfunction [82,83] or suppression of junctional or idioventricular escape rhythms [88]. Patients with third-degree block should have a prophylactic pacemaker inserted prior to lidocaine administration. Acute lidocaine administration can result in complete A-V block in patients with very severe conduction system disease with a history of syncope (His-ventricular intervals generally >100 msec) [89,90]. However, lidocaine administration in asymptomatic patients with bundle branch block or intraventricular conduction disease carries a very low risk of induction of third-degree block [91]. Therapeutic doses of lidocaine have little negative inotropic effect and can be used with appropriately reduced doses in patients with congestive heart failure.

Patients with less non-life-threatening toxicity usually readily respond to reduction or discontinuation of the drug. Acute massive overdose can result in hypotension, third-degree A-V block, asystole, and coma, with death usually resulting from circulatory collapse [84,85,87]. Seizures can be managed using intravenous diazepam or phenytoin. Bradyarrhythmias may be temporized by isoproterenol infusion or external cardiac pacing until a temporary pacemaker is inserted. Hypotension and shock can be initially treated with fluid administration and pressors such as dopamine. Patients with massive lidocaine overdose causing circulatory collapse have survived through the use of extracorporeal circulatory assistance [28,29]. This technique supports the patient and maintains hepatic circulation to allow lidocaine elimination. Hemoperfusion is of little benefit, owing to lidocaine's high intrinsic hepatic clearance [92,93].

Tocainide. Adverse effects are common during tocainide therapy, with up to 50 percent of patients requiring dosage adjustments or discontinuation [94]. The most common side effects are nausea, vomiting, and anorexia and neurologic effects such as dizziness, paresthesias, tremor, ataxia, and confusion. Tremor may indicate that the maximal tolerable dose of tocainide is being approached. Rash early in the course of treatment has been noted in up to 8 percent of patients. Serious toxicity resulting from pulmonary fibrosis in up to 0.1 percent and agranulocytosis and leukopenia in 0.2 percent of patients has been reported [95]. Monitoring for clinical or laboratory signs of agranulocytosis has been recommended, particularly during the first 12 weeks of therapy with this drug. Tocainide has little hemodynamic effect in patients with acute myocardial infarction [96].

Case reports of a massive tocainide overdose are similar to those involving lidocaine, with loss of consciousness, seizures, third-degree block, asystole, and ventricular fibrillation [97,98,99]. Treatment considerations for tocainide overdose are similar to those with lidocaine. Although not reported, the use of repeated doses of oral activated charcoal might be useful due to tocainide's modest intrinsic clearance. Because 40 percent of tocainide elimination is renal, urine acidification might enhance tocainide elimination, but, again, data are lacking. Hemodialysis has been reported to shorten substantially tocainide's elimination half-life in patients with renal failure [99]. Hemodialysis or hemoperfusion may be useful in the management of acute toxicity even in patients without renal failure [100].

Mexiletine. The clinical use of mexiletine is limited mainly by the high incidence of GI and CNS side effects, which occur in approximately 30 percent of patients [101]. Anorexia, nausea, and epigastric discomfort are common and can be decreased somewhat by administering the drug with food. Dizziness, ataxia, and tremor are relatively common.

Mexiletine is generally well tolerated, with little effect on hemodynamics, even in patients with congestive heart failure [102]. It can depress sinus node function in patients with underlying sick sinus syndrome [103]. A fatal case of mexiletine overdose was described, with signs and symptoms similar to those of lidocaine overdose. After ingesting 4.4 gm of mexiletine, the patient developed convulsions, cyanosis, and severe bradycardia with third-degree A-V block progressing to asystole with no response to isoproterenol, epinephrine, or temporary pacing [104]. The plasma level was 34 μg per milliliter.

Management of mexiletine overdose is similar to that of lidocaine and tocainide overdose. Hemodialysis and hemoperfusion would not be expected to be helpful because of mexiletine's large volume of distribution.

CLASS IC AGENTS. Flecainide, encainide, and propafenone are recommended only for suppressing life-threatening ventricular arrhythmias. Flecainide and encainide were widely used to suppress ventricular ectopy until the Cardiac Arrhythmia Suppression Trial (CAST) study showed a significant increase in mortality and in life-threatening arrhythmic events in patients treated with these drugs after myocardial infarction compared with placebo [104]. Flecainide has been approved for the suppression of supraventricular arrhythmias refractory to other forms of medical management in patients without ischemic heart disease. The electrophysiologic effects of these drugs include potent slowing of atrial, A-V nodal, and ventricular conduction without significant effects on repolarization.

Flecainide. Central nervous system symptoms are common side effects, consisting of visual disturbances, dizziness, and ataxia. These symptoms usually respond to dosage reduction. Flecainide has moderate negative inotropic effects that may aggravate congestive heart failure in patients with significant left ventricular dysfunction [105]. Patients with left ventricular dysfunction are also at increased risk for proarrhythmia [12]. Flecainide is not recommended in patients with ischemic heart disease unless suppression of ventricular tachycardia has been demonstrated using electrophysiologic studies [104]. Flecainide can cause sinus node dysfunction or depressed A-V conduction, especially in patients with underlying conduction system disease [5]. Pacing thresholds can increase up to 200 percent during flecainide therapy [5]. Flecainide can aggravate ventricular arrhythmias, particularly in patients with a history of sustained ventricular tachycardia, poor ventricular function, or plasma levels greater than 1 μg per milliliter [10,13]. One review found no clear relationship between marked P–R or QRS prolongation with toxicity and recommended allowing asymptomatic patients to continue flecainide as long as the P–R interval remains less than 0.29 seconds and QRS duration less than 0.18 seconds [10]. Other authors have suggested that a 50 percent [51] or a 40 msec [106] increase in QRS duration indicates flecainide toxicity.

The management of incessant tachycardia is discussed above. In general, aggressive supportive care with mechanical ventilation, pressor support, cardiopulmonary resuscitation, and repeated cardioversions is often required. There have been reports of marked improvement with hypertonic (1 M) sodium bicarbonate or sodium lactate therapy [35,51] and a case report of suppression of incessant ventricular tachycardia with intravenous amiodarone [27]. Treatment with other antiarrhythmic agents is generally not recommended. Neither hemodialysis nor hemoperfusion provides much benefit, given the very large volume of distribution of this drug [51,107]. Urine acidification may be of modest benefit, particularly in patients with initially alkaline urine [59].

Encainide. Minor dose-related side effects are common, consisting of headache, dizziness, blurred vision, tremor, nausea, and confusion [108]. Encainide may have less negative inotropic effect than flecainide [109]. The most serious side effect associated with encainide is proarrhythmia, especially incessant ventricular tachycardia [9]. The risk of proarrhythmia increases with rapid dosage escalation and doses of more than 200 mg per day [12]. Marked QRS prolongation (i.e., >50 percent of baseline) may be associated with increased risk, but most patients with serious proarrhythmia have less pronounced QRS prolongation. Treatment of incessant ventricular tachycardia follows the principles outlined in the previous section. Hypertonic saline has been reported to terminate encainide-induced incessant ventricular tachycardia [52].

Acute encainide overdose may cause marked QRS prolongation, hypotension, bradycardia, seizures, and coma [36]. In general, the management of encainide toxicity is the same as that of flecainide toxicity, except that urinary acidification is of no value. No role for hemoperfusion has been established, although predictions of drug clearance are difficult because metabolite pharmacokinetics have not been fully described. Hypertonic sodium bicarbonate reduced QRS duration in one patient with acute encainide overdose [36].

Propafenone. Dose-related side effects include dizziness, taste disturbances, blurred vision, anorexia, nausea, and vomiting, which occur in up to 10 percent of patients. Neurologic side effects are more frequent when propafenone levels exceed 900 μg per milliliter and are therefore more common in slow metabolizers [110]. Propafenone can aggravate or produce congestive heart failure in patients with severe left ventricular dysfunction [111,112]. It can also produce sinus pauses and A-V block in patients with underlying conduction system disease [110,113]. As with other class IC drugs, incessant ventricular tachycardia or ventricular fibrillation can occur [48,112]. *Torsades de pointes* was described in one report [21]. Experience with acute propafenone overdose is limited. A 2-year-old child developed seizures, marked QRS prolongation, hypotension, bradycardia, and cardiac arrest. Resuscitation was successful with atropine, dopamine, and sodium bicarbonate [114]. The general approach outlined for flecainide is applicable to propafenone toxicity. Hemoperfusion was ineffective in one case of propafenone toxicity [114].

Moricizine. Neither efficacy nor toxicity has a consistent relationship to plasma concentration [115]. Moricizine is associated with GI or neurologic side effects in 15 to 25 percent of patients [116,117]. Dizziness, nausea, abdominal discomfort, and hypoesthesias are the most common side effects, with drug fever, thrombocytopenia, and elevated liver function tests infrequently reported [117]. Aggravation of congestive heart failure occurs infrequently and almost always in those patients with a preexisting history of it [118].

Moricizine has been reported to aggravate ventricular arrhythmias in 3 to 11 percent of patients [119,120]. In one review, 29 of 908 (3.2%) patients treated with moricizine had proarrhythmic effects [120]. Proarrhythmia was limited to patients with lethal or potentially lethal ventricular arrhythmias and occurred more frequently in patients with more structural heart disease. There was no relationship of dose to proarrhythmia. Proarrhythmia with moricizine is more common in patients with a history of congestive heart failure [121]. The Cardiac Arrhythmia Suppression Trial II, assessing the effect of ventricular premature beat suppression by moricizine on survival after myocardial infarction, was halted prematurely due to excess mortality with moricizine [122]. Seventeen of 665 patients treated with moricizine died or experienced cardiac arrest in the first 14-day treatment period, versus 3 of 60 patients in the placebo arm. There was no survival benefit with long-term ventricular ectopy suppression with moricizine in this study.

CLASS III AGENTS

Amiodarone. Pulmonary toxicity leading to pulmonary fibrosis is an important and potentially life-threatening side effect with long-term amiodarone therapy [123,124,125]. Approximately 5 to 15 percent of patients on long-term amiodarone therapy develop pulmonary toxicity, which is fatal in approximately 10 percent of these patients. Common presenting features are dyspnea, nonproductive cough, fever, and general malaise. A diffuse interstitial pattern on chest film is the most typical radiographic finding, which may be difficult to distinguish from congestive heart failure. A trial of diuresis or Swan-Ganz catheterization may be helpful in making a diagnosis. Symptoms usually resolve with withdrawal of amiodarone therapy. The role of corticosteroids in treatment is uncertain. Amiodarone pulmonary toxicity usually occurs with maintenance doses of 400 mg per day or greater [123,126].

Other noncardiac systemic side effects are common with chronic amiodarone treatment. Amiodarone interferes with T_4 to T_3 conversion, commonly causing significant elevations of T_4 and slight reductions in T_3 levels [115,127,128]. These patients are typically euthyroid with normal thyroid stimulating hormone (TSH) levels. The incidence of hypothyroidism is approximately 2 to 5 percent and hyperthyroidism approximately 2 percent. Amiodarone causes peripheral neuropathy in approximately 10 percent of patients and tremor and nervousness in up to 30 percent of patients [129,130]. Corneal microdeposits are present in almost all patients on long-term amiodarone therapy, but complaints of blurry vision and halos around objects are unusual. Dermatologic effects include increased photosensitivity and blue-gray skin discoloration with long-term amiodarone therapy. Gastrointestinal complaints are relatively common, and amiodarone-induced hepatitis can rarely occur [131].

Amiodarone generally does not produce congestive heart failure even in patients with poor ventricular function, because its vasodilator properties may offset negative inotropic effects [132,133]. Sinus bradycardia is common during amiodarone therapy, but symptomatic sinus pauses or sinus arrest occur in only 2 to 4 percent of patients. Atrioventricular block can also occur, particularly in patients with underlying conduction system disease. *Torsades de pointes* can occur, with an incidence up to 4 percent [19]. Exacerbation of monomorphic ventricular tachycardia is unusual.

A single case of amiodarone overdose has been reported [116]. Ingestion of 8 gm of amiodarone produced no clinical toxicity, and no specific therapy was required. A small decrease in heart rate and increase in Q-T interval was noted within hours of ingestion and persisted for 3 days. Experience in treating amiodarone-induced arrhythmias is limited. The usual measures used to control *Torsades de pointes* or monomorphic ventricular tachycardia should apply. Use of hemodialysis or hemoperfusion to enhance elimination with long-term amiodarone therapy is expected to be of no benefit, owing to the extensive volume of distribution. Hemoperfusion for acute amiodarone ingestion could possibly be of some benefit if initiated early, before extensive tissue distribution has taken place, but this has not been reported. Repeated doses of oral activated charcoal could potentially interrupt some enterohepatic recirculation, but this also has not been studied.

Sotalol. The incidence of side effects such as weakness, fatigue, depression, and lassitude is similar to the incidence with other beta-blockers [134]. Sotalol appears to be less likely to cause myocardial depression than other beta-blockers. The negative inotropic effects of beta blockade are partially offset by the positive inotropic effect of prolonging action potential duration, with greater calcium influx into the myocardial cells. Cardiac output is maintained with increased stroke volume due to increased preload and decreased afterload compensating for decreased heart rate [135]. Approximately 1 percent of patients discontinue sotalol due to exacerbation of congestive heart failure [135,136]. Proarrhythmic effects were reported in 4.3 percent of patients in a summary of controlled trials [136]. Symptomatic bradycardia led to discontinuation of sotalol therapy in

2.7 percent of patients. *Torsades de pointes* occurred in 1.9 percent of patients, generally within 1 week of initiation of therapy or a dose increase. *Torsades de pointes* was more common in patients with a history of ventricular tachyarrhythmias, and patients who developed *Torsades* had a longer baseline Q–T interval. In this series, DC cardioversion was required in six cases but there were no fatalities. Hypokalemia related to concomitant hydrochlorothiazide therapy was described in 12 of 13 patients with sotalol-induced *Torsades de pointes* [137].

Sotalol intoxication is characterized by bradycardia, hypotension, prolonged Q–T interval, and *Torsades de pointes* [26–29]. Hemodialysis was used to enhance sotalol elimination in one case refractory to conventional therapy [39]. A correlation between sotalol serum concentration and Q–T prolongation has been observed [138]. Supportive care with pressor or glucagon therapy as described for beta-blocker poisoning (Chap. 135) and measures described in this chapter for *Torsades de pointes* are indicated.

References

1. Vaughan Williams EM: Classification of antiarrhythmic drugs, in Sandoe E, Flendstod-Jensen E, Olesen K, (eds): *Cardiac Arrhythmias*. Sodertalje, Sweden, Ad Astra, 1970, p 449.
2. Harrison DC: Antiarrhythmic drug classification: New science and practical applications. *Am J Cardiol* 56:185, 1985.
3. Rosen MR, Danilo PD: Cellular electrophysiologic mechanisms of antiarrhythmic drug action, in Reiser HJ, Horowitz LN (eds): *Mechanisms and Treatment of Cardiac Arrhythmias: Relevance of Basic Studies to Clinical Management*. Baltimore-Munich, Urban & Schwarzenberg, 1985.
4. Campbell T: Differing electrophysiologic effects of class IA, IB, and IC antiarrhythmic drugs on guinea-pig sinoatrial node. *Br J Pharmacol* 91:395, 1987.
5. Hellestrand KJ, Nathan AW, Bexton RS, et al: Electrophysiologic effects of flecainide acetate on sinus node function, anomalous atrioventricular connections, and pacemaker thresholds. *Am J Cardiol* 53:30B, 1984.
6. Gay RJ, Brown DF: Pacemaker failure due to procainamide toxicity. *Am J Cardiol* 34:728, 1974.
7. Rinkenberger RL, Prystowsky EN, Jackman WM, et al: Drug conversion of nonsustained ventricular tachycardia to sustained ventricular tachycardia during serial electrophysiologic studies: Identification of drugs that exacerbate tachycardia and potential mechanisms. *Am Heart J* 103:177, 1982.
8. Levine JH, Morganroth J, Kadish AH: Mechanisms and risk factors for proarrhythmia with type IA compared with IC antiarrhythmic drug therapy. *Circulation* 80:1063, 1989.
9. Winkle RA, Mason JW, Griffin JC, et al: Malignant ventricular tachyarrhythmias associated with the use of encainide. *Am Heart J* 102:857, 1981.
10. Morganroth J, Horowitz LN: Flecainide: Its proarrhythmia effect and expected changes on the surface electrocardiogram. *Am J Cardiol* 53:89B, 1984.
11. Sellers TD, DiMarco JP: Sinusoidal ventricular tachycardia associated with flecainide acetate. *Chest* 85:647, 1984.
12. Morganroth J: Risk factors for the development of proarrhythmic events. *Am J Cardiol* 59:32E, 1987.
13. Morganroth J, Anderson J, Gentzkow G: Classification by type of ventricular arrhythmia predicts frequency of adverse cardiac events from flecainide. *J Am Coll Cardiol* 8:607, 1986.
14. Brachmann J, Scherlag BJ, Rosenshtraukh LV, et al: Bradycardia-dependent triggered activity: Relevance to drug-induced multiform ventricular tachycardia. *Circulation* 68:846, 1983.
15. Dessertenne F: La tachycardie ventriculaire à deux foyers opposés variables. *Arch Mal Coeur* 59:263, 1966.
16. Smith WM, Gallagher JJ: "Les Torsades de pointes": An unusual ventricular arrhythmia. *Ann Intern Med* 93:578, 1980.
17. Stern S, Keren A, Tzivoni D: Torsades de pointes: Definitions, causative factors, and therapy—Experience with sixteen patients. *Ann NY Acad Sci* 427:234, 1984.
18. Stratmann HG, Kennedy HL: Torsade de pointes associated with drugs and toxins: Recognition and management. *Am Heart J* 113:1470, 1987.
19. Jackman WM, Friday KJ, Anderson JL, et al: The long QT syndromes: A critical review, new clinical observations and a unifying hypothesis. *Prog Cardiovasc Dis* 31:115, 1988.
20. Soyka L, Wirtz C, Spangenberg R: Clinical safety profile of sotalol in patients with arrhythmia. *Am J Cardiol* 65:74A, 1990.
21. Hii J, Wyse G, Gillis A, et al: Propofenane-induced torsade de pointes: Cross-reactivity with quinidine. *PACE* 4:1568, 1991.
22. Zipes DP: Proarrhythmic effects of antiarrhythmic drugs. *Am J Cardiol* 59:26E, 1987.
23. Radford MD, Evans DW: Long-term results of DC reversion of atrial fibrillation. *Br Heart J* 30:91, 1968.
24. Morganroth J, Horowitz JN: Incidence of proarrhythmic effects from quinidine in the outpatient treatment of benign or potentially lethal ventricular arrhythmias. *Am J Cardiol* 56:585, 1985.
25. Roden D, Woosley R, Primm RK: Incidence and clinical features of the quinidine-associated long QT syndrome: Implications for patient care. *Am Heart J* 111:1088, 1986.
26. Neuvonen P, Elonen E, Tarssanen L: Sotalol intoxication, two patients with concentration-effect relationships. *Acta Pharmacol Toxicol* 45:52, 1979.
27. Neuvonen P, Elonen E, Vuorenzmau T, et al: Prolonged QT interval and severe tachyarrhythmias: Common features of sotalol intoxication. *Eur J Pharmacol* 20:85, 1981.
28. Kontopoulas A, Filindus A, Manaudis F, et al: Sotalol-induced torsade de pointes. *Postgrad Med J* 57:321, 1981.
29. Singh S, Lazin A, Cohen A, et al: Sotalol induced torsades de pointes successfully treated with hemodialysis after failure of conventional therapy. *Am Heart J* 121:601, 1991.
30. Velevit V, Podrid P, Lown B, et al: Aggravation and provocation of ventricular arrhythmias by antiarrhythmic drugs. *Circulation* 65:886, 1982.
31. Kay GN, Plumb VJ, Arciniegas JG, et al: Torsade de pointes: The long-short initiating sequence and other clinical features—Observations in 32 patients. *J Am Coll Cardiol* 2:806, 1983.
32. Nguyen PT, Scheinman MM, Seger J: Polymorphous ventricular tachycardia: Clinical characterization, therapy and the QT interval. *Circulation* 74:340, 1986.
33. Morganroth J, Michelson EL, Horowitz LN, et al: Limitations of routine long-term electrocardiographic monitoring to assess ventricular ectopic frequency. *Circulation* 58:408, 1978.
34. Podrid PJ, Lampert S, Graboys TB, et al: Aggravation of arrhythmia by antiarrhythmic drugs: Incidence and predictors. *Am J Cardiol* 59:38E, 1987.
35. Horn JR, Hughes ML: Disopyramide dialysability. *Lancet* 2:214, 1978.
36. Shub C, Gau GT, Sidell PM: The management of acute quinidine intoxication. *Chest* 73:173, 1978.
37. Freedman MD, Gal J, Freed CR: Extracorporeal pump assistance: Novel treatment for acute lidocaine poisoning. *Eur J Clin Pharmacol* 22:129, 1982.
38. Noble J, Kennedy DJ, Latimer RD, et al: Massive lignocaine overdose during cardiopulmonary bypass: Successful treatment with cardiac pacing. *Br J Anaesth* 56:1439, 1984.
39. Ranger S, Sheldon R, Fermini B, et al: Modulation of flecainide's cardiac sodium channel blocking actions by extracellular mechanisms for the action of sodium salts in flecainide cardiotoxicity. *J Pharmacol Exp Ther* 264:1160, 1993.
40. Wasserman F, Brodsky L, Dick MM, et al: Successful treatment of quinidine and procainamide intoxication: Report of three cases. *N Engl J Med* 259:797, 1958.
41. Bailey DJ Jr: Cardiotoxic effects of quinidine and their treatment: Review and case reports. *Arch Intern Med* 105:13, 1960.
42. Chouty F, Funck-Brentano C, Landau JM, et al: Efficacite de fortes doses de lactate molaire par voie veineuse lors des intoxications au flecainide. *Presse Med* 16:808, 1987.
43. Pentel PR, Goldsmith SR, Salerno DM, et al: Effect of hypertonic sodium bicarbonate on encainide overdose. *Am J Cardiol* 57:878, 1986.
44. Bellet S, Hamdan G, Somlyo A, et al: The reversal of cardiotoxic

effects of quinidine by molar sodium lactate: An experimental study. *Am J Med Sci* 237:165, 1959.

45. Keyler D, Pentel P: Hypertonic sodium bicarbonate partially reverses QRS prolongation due to flecainide in rats. *Life Sci* 45:1575, 1989.

46. Sasyniuk B, Jhamandas V: Mechanism of reversal of toxic effects of amitriptyline on cardiac Purkinje fibers by sodium bicarbonate. *J Pharmacol Exp Ther* 231:387, 1984.

47. Gottsegen G, Ostor E: Prevention of the cardiotoxic effect of quinidine by isoproterenol. *Am Heart J* 65:102, 1963.

48. Nickel SN, Thibaudeau Y: Quinidine intoxication treated by isoproterenol (Isuprel). *Can Med Assoc J* 85:81, 1961.

49. Caulkins H, Morady F: Reversal of antiarrhythmic drug effects by epinephrine. *Cardiovasc Rev Rep* 11:65, 1990.

50. Watanabe Y, Dreifus LS, Likoff W: Electrophysiologic antagonism and synergism of potassium and antiarrhythmic agents. *Am J Cardiol* 12:702, 1963.

51. Brandfonbrenor M, Kronholm J, Jones HR: The effect of serum potassium concentration on quinidine toxicity. *J Pharmacol Exp Ther* 154:250, 1966.

52. Gardner M, Brett-Smith H, Batsford W: Treatment of encainide proarrhythmia with hypertonic saline. *PACE* 13:1232, 1990.

53. Woie L, Oyri A: Quinidine intoxication treated with hemodialysis. *Acta Med Scand* 195:237, 1974.

54. Spirack C, Gottlieb S, Miura DS, et al: Flecainide toxicity. *Am J Cardiol* 53:329, 1984.

55. Nathan AW, Hellestrand KJ, Bexton RS, et al: The proarrhythmic effects of the new antiarrhythmic agent flecainide acetate. *Am Heart J* 107:222, 1984.

56. Nathan AW, Bexton RS, Hellestrand KJ, et al: Fatal ventricular tachycardia in association with propafenone: A new class IC antiarrhythmic agent. *Postgrad Med J* 60:155, 1984.

57. Buss J, Neuss H, Bidgin Y, et al: Malignant ventricular tachyarrhythmias in association with propafenone therapy. *Eur Heart J* 6:424, 1985.

58. Sagie A, Strasberg B, Kusniec J, et al: Rapid suppression of flecainide-induced incessant ventricular tachycardia with high dose intravenous amiodarone. *Chest* 93:879, 1988.

59. Winklemann BR, Leinberger H: Life-threatening flecainide toxicity. *Ann Intern Med* 106:807, 1987.

60. Blair A, Burgess E, Maxwell B, et al: Sotalol kinetics in renal insufficiency. *Clin Pharmacol Ther* 29:457, 1981.

61. Denes P, Gabster A, Huang SK: Clinical electrocardiographic and followup observations in patients having ventricular fibrillation during Holter monitoring: Role of quinidine therapy. *Am J Cardiol* 48:9, 1981.

62. Tzivoni D, Keren A, Cohen AM, et al: Magnesium therapy for torsades de pointes. *Am J Cardiol* 53:528, 1984.

63. Coplen S, Antman E, Berun J, et al: Efficacy and safety of quinidine therapy for maintenance of sinus rhythm after cardioversion: A meta-analysis of randomized control trials. *Circulation* 82:1106, 1990.

64. Minardo JD, Heger JJ, Miles WM, et al: Clinical characteristics of patients with ventricular fibrillation during antiarrhythmic drug therapy. *N Engl J Med* 319:257, 1982.

65. Mattioni TA, Zheutlin TA, Sarmiento JJ, et al: Amiodarone in patients with previous drug-mediated torsade de pointes. *Ann Intern Med* 111:574, 1989.

66. Chow MSS, Ronfeldt RA, Ruffet D, et al: Lidocaine pharmacokinetics during cardiac arrest and external cardiopulmonary resuscitation. *Am Heart J* 102:799, 1981.

67. Braden GL, Fitzgibbons JP, Germain MJ, et al: Hemoperfusion for treatment of N-acetylprocainamide intoxication. *Ann Intern Med* 105:64, 1986.

68. Swerdlow CD, Yu JO, Jacobson E, et al: Safety and efficacy of intravenous quinidine. *Am J Med* 75:36, 1983.

69. Selzer A, Wray HW: Quinidine syncope: Paroxysmal ventricular fibrillation occurring during treatment of chronic atrial arrhythmias. *Circulation* 30:17, 1964.

70. Finnegan TRL, Trounce JR: Depression of the heart by quinidine and its treatment. *Br Heart J* 16:341, 1954.

71. Reimold EW, Reynolds WJ, Fixler DE, et al: Use of hemodialysis in the treatment of quinidine poisoning. *Pediatrics* 52:95, 1973.

72. Haapanen EJ, Pellinen TJ: Hemoperfusion in quinidine intoxication. *Acta Med Scand* 210:515, 1981.

73. Drayer DE, Lewenthal DT, Woosley RL, et al: Accumulation of N-acetylprocainamide: An active metabolite of procainamide in patients with impaired renal function. *Clin Pharmacol Ther* 22:63, 1977.

74. Reidenberg MM, Drayer DE, Levy M, et al: Polymorphic acetylation of procainamide in man. *Clin Pharmacol Ther* 17:722, 1975.

75. Henningsen NC, Cederberg A, Hanson A, et al: Effect of long-term treatment with procainamide. *Acta Med Scand* 198:472, 1975.

76. Dubois EB: Procainamide induction of a systemic lupus erythematosus syndrome. *Medicine* 48:217, 1969.

77. Koch-Weser J, Klein SW: Procainamide dosage schedules, plasma concentrations and clinical effects. *JAMA* 215:1454, 1971.

78. Atkinson AJ Jr, Krumlovsky FA, Huang CM, et al: Hemodialysis for severe procainamide toxicity: Clinical and pharmacokinetic observations. *Clin Pharmacol Ther* 20:585, 1976.

79. Villalba-Pimental L, Epstein LM, Sellers EM, et al: Survival after massive procainamide ingestion. *Am J Cardiol* 32:727, 1973.

80. Raja R, Kramer M, Abvis R, et al: Resin hemoperfusion for severe N-acetylprocainamide toxicity in patients with renal failure. *Trans Am Soc Artif Intern Organs* 30:18, 1984.

81. Woosley R, Roden D: Pharmacologic causes of arrhythmogenic actions of antiarrhythmic drugs. *Am J Cardiol* 59:19, 1987.

82. Leach AJ, Brown JE, Armonstrong PW: Cardiac depression by intravenous disopyramide in patients with left ventricular dysfunction. *Am J Med* 68:839, 1980.

83. Podrid PJ, Shoeneberger A, Lown B: Congestive heart failure caused by oral disopyramide. *N Engl J Med* 302:614, 1980.

84. Desai JM, Scheinman MM, Hirschfeld D, et al: Cardiovascular collapse associated with disopyramide therapy. *Chest* 79:545, 1981.

85. Hayler AM, Hold DW, Volans GN: Fatal overdosage with disopyramide. *Lancet* 1:968, 1978.

86. Holt DW, Helliwell M, O'Keeffe B, et al: Successful management of serious disopyramide poisoning. *Postgrad Med J* 56:256, 1980.

87. Sevka MJ, Matthews SJ, Nightingale CH, et al: Disopyramide hemodialysis and kinetics in patients requiring long-term hemodialysis. *Clin Pharmacol Ther* 29:322, 1981.

88. Thomson AH, Kelman AW, de Vane PJ, et al: Changes in lignocaine disposition during long-term infusion in patients with acute ventricular arrhythmias. *Ther Drug Monit* 9:283, 1987.

89. Pfeifer HJ, Greenblatt DJ, Koch-Weser J: Clinical use and toxicity of intravenous lidocaine: A report from the Boston Collaborative Drug Surveillance Program. *Am Heart J* 92:168, 1976.

90. Rademaker AW, Kellen J, Tam YK, et al: Character of adverse effects of prophylactic lidocaine in the coronary care unit. *Clin Pharmacol Ther* 40:71, 1986.

91. Davison R, Parker M, Atkinson AJ: Excessive serum lidocaine levels during maintenance infusions: Mechanisms and prevention. *Am Heart J* 104:203, 1982.

92. Bryant CA, Hoffman JR, Nichtes LS: Pitfalls and perils of intravenous lidocaine. *West J Med* 139:528, 1983.

93. Burlington B, Freed C: Massive overdose and death from prophylactic lidocaine. *JAMA* 243:1036, 1980.

94. Hess GP, Walson PD: Seizures secondary to oral viscous lidocaine. *Ann Emerg Med* 17:725, 1988.

95. Denaro CP, Benowitz NL: Poisoning due to class IB antiarrhythmic drugs lignocaine, mexiletine and tocainide. *Med Toxicol Adverse Drug Exp* 4:416, 1989.

96. Cheng TO, Wadhwa K: Sinus standstill following intravenous lidocaine administration. *JAMA* 223:790, 1973.

97. Antonelli D, Bloch L: Standstill following lidocaine administration. *JAMA* 248:828, 1982.

98. Kuo C, Reddy P: Effect of lidocaine on escape rate in patients with complete atrioventricular block. *Am J Cardiol* 47:1315, 1981.

99. Lichstein E, Chadda K, Gupta P: Atrioventricular block with lidocaine therapy. *Am J Cardiol* 31:277, 1973.

100. Gupta P, Lichstein E, Chadde K: Lidocaine-induced heart block in patients with bundle branch block. *Am J Cardiol* 33:487, 1974.

101. Vaziri ND, Saiki JK, Hughes W: Clearance of lidocaine by hemodialysis. *South Med J* 72:1567, 1979.

102. Barber K, Chen SM, Ferguson R, et al: Lidocaine removal during resin hemoperfusion for phenobarbital intoxication. *Artif Organs* 8:229, 1984.

103. Roden DM, Woosley RL: Drug therapy: Tocainide. *N Engl J Med* 315:41, 1986.
104. Nyquist O, Forssell G, Nordlander R, et al: Hemodynamic and antiarrhythmic effects of tocainide in patients with acute myocardial infarction. *Am Heart J* 100:1000, 1980.
105. Shanks RG: Hemodynamic effects of mexiletine. *Am Heart J* 107:1065, 1984.
106. Roos JC, Paalman ACA, Dunning AJ: Electrophysiological effects of mexiletine in man. *Br Heart J* 38:1262, 1976.
107. Jequier P, Jones R, Mackintosh A: Fatal mexiletine overdose. *Lancet* 1:429, 1976.
108. Salerno DM, Granrud G, Sharkey P, et al: Pharmacodynamics and side effects of flecainide acetate. *Clin Pharmacol Ther* 40:101, 1986.
109. Braun J, Kollert JR, Gessler U, et al: Failure of haemoperfusion to reduce flecainide intoxication: A case study. *Med Toxicol* 2:463, 1987.
110. Woosley RL, Wood AJJ, Roden DM: Drug therapy: Encainide. *N Engl J Med* 318:1107, 1988.
111. Carey EL, Duff JH, Roden DM, et al: Encainide and its metabolites: Comparative effects in man on ventricular arrhythmia and cardiographic intervals. *J Clin Invest* 73:539, 1984.
112. Bergstrand RH, Wang T, Roden DM, et al: Encainide disposition in patients with renal failure. *Clin Pharmacol Ther* 40:64, 1986.
113. Wang T, Roden DM, Wolfenden HT, et al: Influence of genetic polymorphism on the metabolism and disposition of encainide in man. *J Pharmacol Exp Ther* 228:605, 1984.
114. Berchtold-Kanz E, Schwart G, Hust M, et al: Increased incidence of side effects after encainide: A newly developed antiarrhythmic drug. *Clin Cardiol* 7:493, 1984.
115. Bigger J: Cardiac electrophysiologic effects of moricizine hydrochloride. *Am J Cardiol* 65:15D, 1990.
116. Clyne C, Estes M, Wang P: Drug therapy: Moricizine. *N Eng J Med* 327:255, 1992.
117. Kennedy H: Noncardiac adverse effects and organ toxicity of moricizine during short- and long-term studies. *Am J Cardiol* 65:47D, 1990.
118. Pratt CM, Podrid P, Greatrix B, et al: Efficacy and safety of moricizine in patients with congestive heart failure: A summary of the experience in the United States. *Am Heart J* 119:1, 1990.
119. Wyndham C, Pratt C, Mann D, et al: Electrophysiology of ethmozine (moricizine HCl) for ventricular tachycardia. *Am J Cardiol* 60:67F, 1987.
120. Morganroth J, Pratt C: Prevalence and characteristics of proarrhythmia from moricizine (ethmozine). *Am J Cardiol* 63:172, 1989.
121. Podrid P, Bean S: Antiarrhythmic drug therapy for congestive heart failure with focus on moricizine. *Am J Cardiol* 65:56D, 1990.
122. The Cardiac Arrhythmia Suppression Trial II Investigators: Effect of the antiarrhythmic agent moricizine on survival after myocardial infarction. *N Engl J Med* 327:227, 1992.
123. Podrid PJ, Lown B: Propafenone: A new agent for ventricular arrhythmia. *J Am Coll Cardiol* 4:117, 1984.
124. Buss J, Neuss H, Bilgin Y, et al: Malignant ventricular tachyarrhythmias in association with propafenone treatment. *Eur Heart J* 6:424, 1985.
125. McHugh TP, Ferina DG: Propafenone ingestion. *Ann Emerg Med* 16:437, 1987.
126. Budde T, Beyer M, Breithardt G, et al: Therapy of severe propafenone poisoning: An attempt at elimination by hemoperfusion. *Zeitsch Kardiol* 75:764, 1986.
127. Dangman K, Hoffman B: Antiarrhythmic effects of ethmozin in cardiac Purkinje fibers: Suppression of automaticity and abolition of triggering. *J Pharmacol Exp Ther* 227:578, 1983.
128. Tsuji Y, Nishimura M, Osada M, et al: Membrane action of ethmozin on normoxic and hypoxic canine Purkinje fibers. *J Cardiovasc Pharmacol* 5:961, 1983.
129. Salerno DM, Ettinger A, Hodges M: The electrocardiographic effects of encainide, flecainide and moricizine in a subgroup of the cardiac antiarrhythmic suppression trial. *J Am Coll Cardiol* 17:56A, 1991.
130. Woosley R, Morganroth J, Forgoros R, et al: Pharmacokinetics of moricizine HCl. *Am J Cardiol* 60:35F, 1987.
131. Carnes C, Coyle J: Moricizine: A novel antiarrhythmic agent. *DICP Ann Pharmacother* 24:745, 1990.
132. Siddoway LA, Thompson KA, McAllister CB, et al: Polymorphism of propafenone metabolism and disposition in man: Clinical and pharmacokinetic consequences. *Circulation* 75:785, 1983.
133. Salerno D, Sharkey S, Granrud G, et al: Efficacy, safety, hemodynamic effects, and pharmacokinetics of high-dose moricizine during short- and long-term therapy. *Clin Pharmacol Ther* 42:201, 1987.
134. Singh B, Deedwania P, Nademanee K, et al: Sotalol: A review of its pharmacodynamic and pharmacokinetic properties and therapeutic use. *Drugs* 34:311, 1987.
135. Mahmarian J, Verani M, Pratt C: Hemodynamic effects of intravenous and oral sotalol. *Am J Cardiol* 65:28A, 1990.
136. Soyka L, Wirtz C, Spangenberg R: Clinical safety profile of sotalol in patients with arrhythmias. *Am J Cardiol* 65:74A, 1990.
137. McKibben J, Pocock W, Barlow J, et al: Sotalol, hypokalemia, syncope and Torsade de pointes. *Br Heart J* 51:57, 1984.
138. Neuvonen P, Elonen E, Tanskanen A, et al: Sotalol and prolonged QTC interval. *Lancet* 2:426, 1981.

132. Alcohols and Glycols

Marsha D. Ford

The consumption of alcohols, including those intended for human, industrial, or occupational use, poses a major health problem in the United States and other countries. According to 1992 American Association of Poison Control Centers data, ethanol ingestions were involved primarily or secondarily in 9.5 percent of 705 reported fatalities and methanol and ethylene glycol ingestions accounted for 2.8 percent of fatalities. Isopropanol ingestions were involved in three deaths [1]. Hospital discharge data indicate that ethanol use may be a factor in 10 to 50 percent of admissions [2] and 10 percent of annual fatalities, including death by accidents, fires, homicides, and suicides [3].

Acute Ethanol Intoxication

Ethanol in the form of beers, wines, and liquors is consumed socially by many people. Approximately one-third of the U.S. population can be categorized as moderate to heavy drinkers, consuming four or more drinks per week [4,5]. Of these, about 20 percent can be considered problem drinkers or alcoholics [4]. In 1984, an estimated 20 percent of U.S. hospital health care costs could be attributed to alcohol-related health care problems [6]. Besides the direct toxic effects of ethanol, alcohol contributes to increased health risks from trauma, criminal behavior, and suicides [4]. Ethanol is also a constituent of myriad colognes, perfumes, mouthwashes, aftershaves, and over-the-counter medicinals. Many of these products contain 50 to 99 percent ethanol and are sources for intoxication, especially for children [7].

Ethanol is an aliphatic alcohol, a slightly polar small molecule with a weak electric charge, miscible in both water and lipids [8]. It diffuses easily into all body tissues, assuming a distribution similar to that of body water. There is no consensus on its mechanism of action. Its properties may be due to alterations in intracellular calcium concentrations and calcium currents; to effects of the major metabolite, acetate, which secondarily increases CNS levels of adenosine (mimicking the effects of ethanol and sometimes increasing intracellular calcium); or to a potentiation of gamma-aminobutyric acid (GABA)-modulated chloride flux similar to that seen with benzodiazepines and barbiturates [9–12]. However, a specific ethanol receptor site has not been identified. Ethanol-induced changes in other neurotransmitters, electrolyte transport, and cerebral blood flow may also contribute to its effect [8].

Ethanol is readily absorbed from the gastrointestinal tract, with 80 percent of the absorption occurring in the small intestine. The type of beverage, concentration of ethanol, and presence of food can alter absorptive rates [4]. Peak ethanol levels typically occur 30 to 60 minutes after ingestion if the stomach is empty [7]. Compared to men, women have higher peak ethanol concentrations after a given dose, possibly due to diminished first-pass hepatic metabolism and reduced gastric mucosal alcohol dehydrogenase activity [13].

Metabolism occurs predominantly in the liver. Only 2 to 15 percent of unmetabolized ethanol is secreted via respiratory, renal, and perspiratory routes [4,14]. Three intrahepatic enzymatic systems degrade ethanol: alcohol dehydrogenase (ADH), the microsomal ethanol oxidizing system (MEOS), and catalase. Of these, ADH is the most important, normally being responsible for greater than 80 percent of ethanol metabolism at lower doses [15]. In the ADH metabolic pathway (Fig. 132-1), ethanol is oxidized to acetaldehyde and then to acetate in a process that reduces oxidized nicotinamide adenine dinucleotide (NAD^+) to NADH. The increased ratio of NADH to NAD^+ can inhibit NAD^+-dependent reactions, such as gluconeogenesis [8]. Acetate undergoes conversion to acetyl coenzyme A (CoA), which can then participate in the citric acid cycle, fatty acid synthesis, or ketone formation [14]. Genetic variations in alcohol dehydrogenase and aldehyde dehydrogenase may account for individual differences in ethanol metabolism [16]. Normally the MEOS and catalase systems play minor, less well-defined roles in ethanol metabolism [17,18,19]. Since the MEOS is inducible at higher ethanol levels or with chronic use, the MEOS plays a major role in ethanol metabolism [20] with chronic or heavy use. The chemical properties and kinetics of ethanol are summarized in Table 132-1.

Tolerance to ethanol's effects develops both acutely and after chronic consumption. With acute consumption, the physiologic effects at a given serum level of ethanol have been noted to be less when ethanol concentrations are declining rather than when levels are rising. Compared to inexperienced drinkers, chronic drinkers experience diminished effects to a given amount of ethanol [5]. Tolerance is accompanied by changes in cellular membranes [21].

CLINICAL PRESENTATION AND DIAGNOSTIC EVALUATION.

At high doses, ethanol functions as an anesthetic, causing CNS depression, autonomic dysfunction (e.g., hypotension,

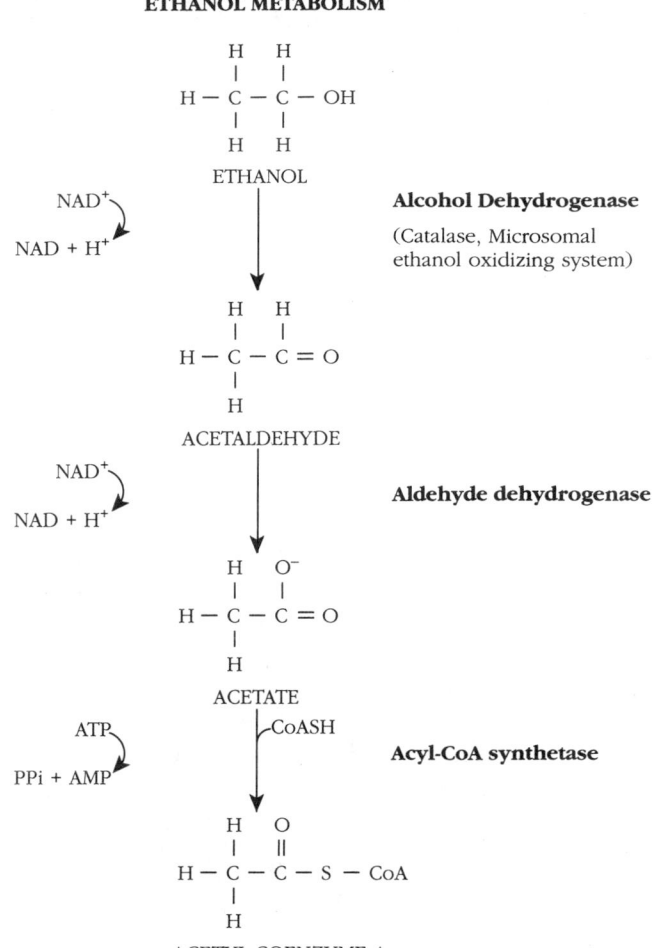

ETHANOL METABOLISM

Alcohol Dehydrogenase
(Catalase, Microsomal ethanol oxidizing system)

Aldehyde dehydrogenase

Acyl-CoA synthetase

Fig. 132-1. Ethanol metabolism.

hypothermia), coma, and death from respiratory depression and cardiovascular collapse. Ethanol levels at which this occurs vary among experienced and inexperienced drinkers but correlate roughly with the degrees of observed intoxication. For nontolerant individuals, initial symptoms of lethargy, ataxia, and muscular incoordination may be seen at serum levels of 150 mg per deciliter or greater, coma at approximately 250 mg per deciliter, and death with levels greater than 450 mg per deciliter [7,22]. Chronic drinkers can achieve higher levels before developing symptoms. Estimated LD_{50} doses are 5 to 8 gm per kilogram for adults and 3 gm per kilogram for children [7].

Patients may present with varying degrees of alteration of consciousness, including stupor and coma, usually with a strong odor of ethanol or its congeners on their breath. Little else about the physical assessment is specific for ethanol, and the physical examination should be directed toward evaluation of the airway and a search for complicating or contributing factors such as trauma, infection, and hemorrhage. Some of the differential diagnoses that must be considered are listed in Table 132-2.

Laboratory studies recommended in patients with moderate to severe poisoning include electrolytes, BUN, glucose, complete blood count, arterial blood gas, ethanol level, magnesium, calcium, phosphorus, liver function tests, prothrombin time, electrocardiogram, chest radiograph, and urinalysis. Further

Table 132-1. Comparative Data on the Toxic Alcohols and Glycols

Substance	Formula	Molecular weight	V_d L/kg	Elimination half-life	Boiling point °C	Odor	Onset to toxicity	Important metabolites
Ethanol	CH_3CH_2OH	46	0.6	Zero-order elimination, 15–30 mg/dl/hr	78.5	+	30–60 min	Acetaldehyde Acetic acid
Methanol	CH_3OH	32	0.7	Zero-order at 8.5 mg/dl/hr without ethanol. First-order at 46.5 hr with ethanol and 2.5 hr with hemodialysis	64.7	−	12–24 hr*	Formaldehyde Formic acid
Ethylene glycol	$\begin{array}{cc} CH_2\text{-}CH_2 \\ \mid \quad \mid \\ OH \ \ OH \end{array}$	62	0.7	2.5–4.5 hr without ethanol and with normal kidneys, 17 hr with ethanol, 2.5–3 hr with ethanol and hemodialysis, 11–14.75 hr with 4-MP	197.6	+	4–12 hr*	Glycolaldehyde Glyoxylic acid Glycolic acid Oxalic acid
Isopropanol	$\begin{array}{c} CH_3CHCH_3 \\ \mid \\ OH \end{array}$	60	0.6–0.7	2.5–3.5 hr	82.5	+ Fruity odor Secondary acetonemia	30–60 min	Acetone
Propylene glycol	$\begin{array}{c} CH_2CHCH_3 \\ \mid \\ OH \end{array}$	76	0.55	2–5 hr in adults, 19.3 hr in infants	188.2	?	Minutes with intravenous, ? with dermal	Pyruvate Lactate Acetate
Benzyl alcohol	CH_2OH	108	?	?	204.7	+	?	Benzoic acid Hippuric acid

* May be longer if ethanol coingested

Table 132-2. Differential Diagnoses for Acute Ethanol Intoxication

Metabolic
  Hypoglycemia
  Hyperglycemia
  Hyponatremia
  Hypothermia
  Hepatic encephalopathy
  Disulfiram reaction
  Hypercalcemia
  Hypoxia
Drug intoxication
  Phencyclidine
  Opioids
  Cyclic antidepressants
  Other alcohols (methanol, isopropanol, ethylene glycol)
  Other sedative-hypnotics (meprobamate, methaqualone, glutethimide, benzodiazepines, barbiturates, chloral hydrate, ethchlorvynol, methyprylon)
  Anticholinergics
  Carbon monoxide
Trauma
  Intracranial hemorrhage (subdural, epidural, intracerebral bleed)
Infectious
  CNS infections
  AIDS
  Sepsis
Neurologic
  Postictal
  Delirium tremens
  Wernicke's encephalopathy

Adapted from Adinoff B, Bone GHS, Linnoila M: Acute ethanol poisoning and the ethanol withdrawal syndrome. *Med Toxicol* 3:177, 1988. With permission

studies are dictated by the presence or absence of physical or laboratory abnormalities.

MANAGEMENT. In the presence of stupor or coma, the patient should be intubated, both to ensure a patent airway and to protect against pulmonary aspiration. Poor respiratory effort necessitates mechanical ventilatory support. Naloxone (2 mg) and thiamine hydrochloride (100 mg) should be given intravenously. Naloxone reverses opioids if they are present, while the thiamine many treat an underlying Wernicke's encephalopathy. If a bedside glucose test reveals hypoglycemia, intravenous dextrose (50 gm) should be administered.

A nasogastric tube may be placed to remove stomach contents in patients with large recent ingestions (<1–2 hours) and to evaluate for gastrointestinal bleeding. If coingestants are suspected, activated charcoal and a cathartic should be administered. Nutritional deficiencies should be corrected. Hypothermia, if present, is usually mild, unless environmental exposure has occurred. This can be managed with warm blankets. Although fructose has been used to increase ethanol elimination, possibly by enhancing hepatic blood flow and affecting a variety of metabolic reactions [23], it is not recommended because it can cause gastrointestinal irritation, hyperuricemia, and lactic acidosis [8].

Supportive care and monitoring should be continued until the patient is clinically stable and awake enough to protect the airway. Serum ethanol levels will decline by zero-order kinetics at approximately 15 to 30 mg per deciliter per hour [8]. If the level of consciousness does not correlate with the measured serum ethanol level or does not improve with diminishing levels, the physician should reconsider the differential diagnosis.

Alcoholic Ketoacidosis

Alcoholic ketoacidosis (AKA) develops as a result of hormonal, nutritional, metabolic, and intravascular volume changes caused by ethanol use (Fig. 132-2). Since ethanol retards ketogenesis, AKA usually occurs only when ethanol levels are low to absent [14]. The metabolism of ethanol produces acetate that is then converted to acetyl-CoA. Inadequate nutritional intake in alcoholics leads to depletion of glycogen stores and decreased intravascular volume secondary to vomiting. This in turn produces increased catecholamine levels that blunt insulin release [24]. These factors activate lipase, which converts triglycerides to free fatty acids (FFAs). The FFAs are transported to the liver, where they are either esterified to form triglycerides or oxidized. Glucagon-induced activation of the carnitine acyltransferase system produces long-chain fatty acids (LCFAs) capable of entering the mitochondria, where they are oxidized to acetyl-CoA [25], thus producing excess acetyl-CoA.

Acetyl-CoA is metabolized via three pathways: fatty acid synthesis, the citric acid cycle, or ketogenesis. The ketogenic pathway has the largest capacity for handling acetyl-CoA overload [25]. The liver, under constraint to metabolize ethanol in an energy-neutral fashion, can also metabolize a greater amount of ethanol per mole of adenosine triphosphate (ATP) produced via the ketogenic route [24]. Nutritional deficiencies do not favor the formation of triglycerides from acetyl-CoA, and the entrance of acetyl-CoA into the citric acid cycle may be retarded by both thiamine and magnesium depletion [14], thereby promoting the formation of ketone bodies. The resulting altered redox state favors an increased NADH-NAD$^+$ ratio, leading to preferential conversion of acetoacetate, a ketone body, to beta-hydroxybutyrate. This process leads to an acidosis.

Multiple other acid-base abnormalities may occur in alcoholic

Fig. 132-2. Mechanism of alcoholic ketoacidosis. (Adapted from Hoffman RS, Goldfrank LR: Ethanol-associated metabolic disorders. *Emerg Med Clin North Am* 7:943, 1989. With permission.)

MECHANISM OF ALCOHOLIC KETOACIDOSIS

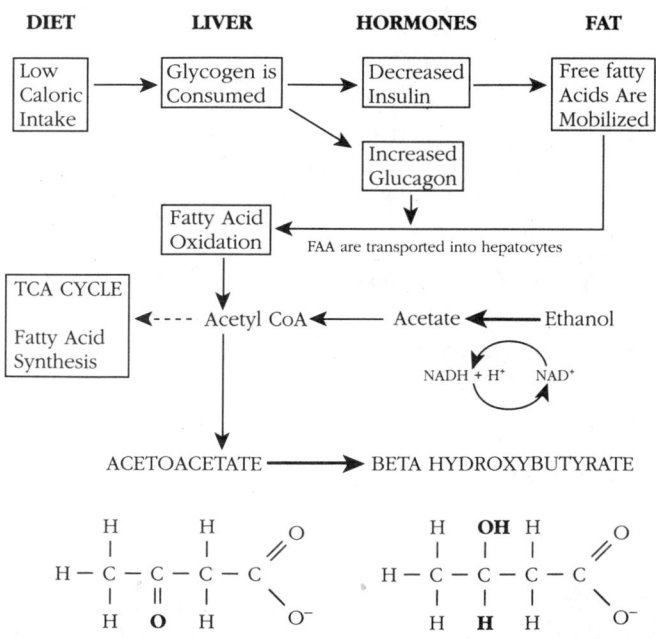

patients. Respiratory acidosis may be caused by either hypoglycemic or ethanol-induced respiratory depression [26]. Concomitant lactic acidosis can occur secondary to seizure activity, an increase in the NADH-NAD$^+$ ratio that favors the formation of lactate from pyruvate, an ethanol-induced decrease in the use of lactate to form glucose, thiamine deficiency that prevents the entry of pyruvate into the citric acid cycle, and decreased liver function with resultant depression of lactate metabolism [26]. Vomiting with extracellular volume contraction and hypokalemia may cause a metabolic alkalosis [24]. A mild acetic acidosis may be seen when acetate is incompletely oxidized by peripheral tissues [24]. Finally, an unexplained hyperchloremic metabolic acidosis has been observed in acutely intoxicated patients. [26].

CLINICAL PRESENTATION AND DIAGNOSTIC EVALUATION. Patients with alcoholic ketoacidosis usually present with a recent history of binge alcohol drinking and poor nutritional intake followed by vomiting. In the typical patient, the fruity odor of ketones may be present along with Kussmaul's breathing and signs of volume depletion, such as dry mucous membranes, tachycardia, orthostatic hypotension, and poor skin turgor [14,27]. Signs and symptoms of concomitant gastritis, pancreatitis, hepatitis, gastrointestinal hemorrhage, and vitamin and mineral deficiencies are commonly present.

Laboratory studies should include those listed for acute ethanol intoxication plus serum ketones, lactate, and osmolarity. Ethanol levels may be low to nondetectable, and hypoglycemia may be present [28]. Arterial blood gas and electrolyte measurements show an anion gap metabolic acidosis. A concomitant respiratory and/or metabolic alkalosis may be noted. For example, in 10 patients with 13 episodes of AKA, the mean anion gap was 34 ±3 mEq per liter, the mean serum pH was 7.29, and the average serum bicarbonate was 14 mEq per liter [24]. Serum ketones are present but at levels lower than expected, given the anion gap. This is due to the preferential formation of beta-hydroxybutyrate (rather than acetoacetate) caused by the increased NADH-NAD$^+$ ratio. The nitroprusside test is unable to detect beta-hydroxybutyrate because it lacks a ketone bond (C=O) [14]. Although patients may be potassium-depleted from vomiting, hypokalemia is uncommon, probably due to the extracellular shift of potassium associated with acidosis.

The differential diagnosis of an anion gap metabolic acidosis includes lactic acidosis, salicylate poisoning, uremia, diabetic ketoacidosis, and paraldehyde, iron, and toluene intoxication. Hypoxia and hypotension are the most common causes of lactic acidosis, but malignancies, leukemia, metformin therapy, and other toxins, such as cyanide and carbon monoxide, should also be considered [29]. Alcoholic ketoacidosis can usually be differentiated from diabetic ketoacidosis by the lack of significant hyperglycemia, a relatively mild acidosis, and rapid improvement with therapy.

MANAGEMENT. Supportive therapy is the same as that noted for acute intoxication. Intravenous volume repletion, glucose, and thiamine reverse the ketogenic process and are the mainstays of therapy. After an initial intravenous dextrose bolus of 50 gm, patients should receive a maintenance infusion of dextrose (5%) in normal saline [14]. Parenteral thiamine (100 mg) should be given to facilitate the entry of pyruvate into the citric acid cycle and to avoid precipitating Wernicke's encephalopathy [30]. Once normal renal function is ensured, potassium and magnesium replacement should begin. Due to increased glycolysis with carbohydrate refeeding, hypophosphatemia can develop. Levels should be monitored and potassium phosphate administered as necessary [28]. Hospitalization and refeeding of malnourished patients for days to weeks may be required to replete absent glycogen stores.

Ethanol-Related Hypoglycemia

Four types of hypoglycemia associated with or induced by ethanol have been delineated: (1) alcohol-induced fasting hypoglycemia, (2) reactive hypoglycemia of chronic alcoholism, (3) alcohol potentiation of drug- or exercise-induced hypoglycemia, and (4) alcohol-promoted reactive hypoglycemia [31]. Alcohol-induced fasting hypoglycemia is the best understood. Marginal nutritional status is the only requirement for its development, and it can occur in poorly nourished alcoholics as well as in young children, fasted normal subjects, patients on low-carbohydrate diets, and those with thyrotoxicosis and adrenocortical deficiency [28,31,32,33]. When these patients consume ethanol rather than food, their marginal glycogen stores are readily depleted by glycogenolysis. The body's next line of defense against hypoglycemia is gluconeogenesis. However, ethanol inhibits this reaction [32,33], probably by increasing the NADH-NAD$^+$ ratio that preferentially shunts pyruvate to lactate and thus blocks pyruvate from participating in gluconeogenesis or other reactions in which it is the key intermediate (Fig. 132-3) [14,34]. Ethanol may also directly block the first step in gluconeogenesis [35]. Contributory endocrinologic abnormalities may include impaired cortisol release and decreased growth hormone secretion due to hypothalamic-pituitary dysfunction [31,33,36]. Lactic acidosis may occur as a result of overproduction of lactate [32,33].

Fig. 132-3. Ethanol-induced hypoglycemia. (Adapted from Hoffman RS, Goldfrank LR: Ethanol-associated metabolic disorders. *Emerg Med Clin North Am* 7:943, 1989. With permission.)

The biochemical mechanisms underlying types 2 and 3 hypoglycemia are poorly understood [31,37]. Type 4 may be secondary to potentiation of insulin secretion by ethanol [31]. Liver disease is not necessary for the development of hypoglycemia [38].

CLINICAL PRESENTATION AND DIAGNOSTIC EVALUATION. Central nervous system depression ranging from confusion to coma and symptoms of increased sympathetic activity caused by catecholamine release, such as diaphoresis, anxiety, tremulousness, palpitations, and weakness, are the hallmarks of hypoglycemia. Hypothermia frequently occurs [31]. The CNS effects of hypoglycemia and ethanol intoxication can mimic one another, while hypoglycemia-induced adrenergic signs and symptoms can be mistaken for ethanol withdrawal. An inebriated individual left to sleep it off may slip imperceptibly into a hypoglycemic state without raising clinical suspicion [38]. The differential diagnoses are similar to those for acute ethanol intoxication (Table 132-2).

Laboratory evaluation is the same as that necessary to assess the patient with acute intoxication. If metabolic acidosis is present, the studies recommended for alcoholic ketoacidosis are also indicated. Glucose levels are usually less than 40 mg per deciliter, and low ethanol levels are frequently found [31]. Lactate levels may be elevated. In fasted males, ethanol infusion produced a rise in mean lactate from a steady-state level of 0.64 mM per liter to a mean peak level of 3.25 mM per liter [33].

Caution is advised when assessing glucose levels with rapid reagent strips. Levels may be affected by the age of the strips, by the accuracy of machines used to read them, and by visual overreading of borderline levels. The effect of varying ethanol levels on the accuracy of these strips has not been adequately studied [14]. Given the morbidity and mortality of severe hypoglycemia, the potential errors in strip interpretation, and the benign nature of intravenous glucose (except possibly in patients with cerebral anoxia), all patients should initially be treated with glucose, even if they have a normal or slightly elevated glucose by reagent strip [14].

ETHANOL-INDUCED HYPOGLYCEMIA

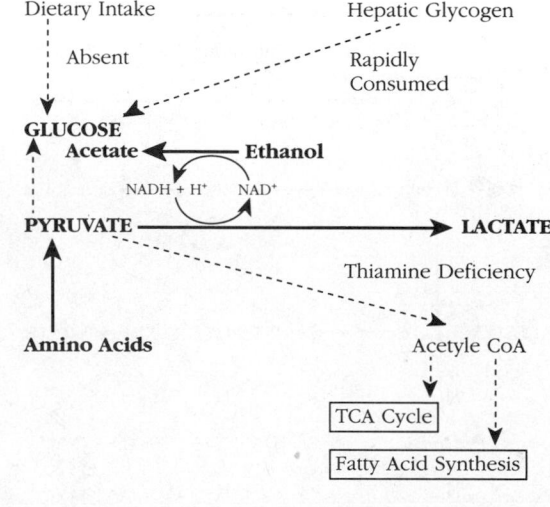

MANAGEMENT. Therapy for ethanol-induced hypoglycemia parallels that for acute ethanol intoxication. An intravenous bolus of 50 gm of dextrose (100 ml of $D_{50}W$, a 50% solution) should be followed by an infusion of 10% dextrose with frequent monitoring of glucose levels. In young children, 25% dextrose should be given in a bolus of 0.25 to 1.0 gm per kilogram, followed by a maintenance infusion of 4 to 6 mg per kilogram per minute [39]. Dextrose boluses should be repeated as necessary.

Most patients respond immediately to intravenous dextrose and return to normal levels of consciousness without major morbidity. Slow or partial response carries a worse prognosis. Posthypoglycemic encephalopathy and death have been reported [14,40].

Ethylene Glycol and Methanol

ETHYLENE GLYCOL. Found in many de-icers, antifreezes, detergents, polishes, cosmetics, paints, and lacquers, ethylene glycol (1,2-ethanediol) is a colorless, odorless, and slightly sweet liquid [41,42] that imparts a warm sensation to the tongue and esophagus when swallowed. Ingestions usually result from suicide attempts, intentional substitution of ethylene glycol for ethanol, or accidental exposure. The first reported deaths occurred in 1930 in two men who drank Prestone antifreeze, [43]. The many cases of renal failure and deaths that occurred during the Massengill Disaster of 1938 resulted from the use of a related glycol, diethylene glycol, as a vehicle for sulfanilamide [44]. By 1959, 40 to 60 deaths per year were ascribed to ethylene glycol [45]. In 1992, a total of 5225 glycol ingestions (e.g., ethylene glycol, propylene glycol, glycol ether) were reported, but only 7 resulted in death [1]. Improved therapy appears to be responsible for these better clinical outcomes.

Except for an ethanol-like intoxication, ethylene glycol causes little toxicity until it is metabolized in the liver to more harmful metabolites. During metabolism (Fig. 132-4), the parent compound undergoes oxidation by hepatic alcohol dehydrogenase to glycolaldehyde, which is rapidly transformed via aldehyde dehydrogenase to glycolic acid. Glycolic acid is converted to glyoxylic acid, whose most toxic metabolite is oxalic acid [42,46,47]. Glyoxylic acid is also metabolized via other pathways, some of which become therapeutically important when attempting to divert metabolism away from oxalic acid production. The two rate-limiting steps in metabolism are the conversion of ethylene glycol to glycolaldehyde and the conversion of glycolic acid to glyoxylic acid.

The anion gap metabolic acidosis seen in ethylene glycol poisoning derives predominantly from elevated glycolic acid levels [47–50]. While glyoxylate and glycolaldehyde are more toxic, glycolic acid is the only major intermediary that accumulates in significant concentrations [42,47,51]. Elevated glycolate levels are highly correlated to the anion gap, accounting for 96.1 percent of the increase [47]. Elevated lactic acid levels, ranging 1.4 to 7.1 mM per liter, may make small contributions to the acidosis [47,52,53,54]. The etiology of the increased lactate remains speculative [55]. Increased lactate levels have been documented in patients who were not hypoxic, hypotensive, or alcoholic [53,56]. The conversion of pyruvate to lactate may be promoted by the increased $NADH-NAD^+$ ratio produced by the metabolism of ethylene glycol [53,57]. Glyoxylate may uncouple mitochondrial respiration, but because of its short half-life and low concentrations it is an unlikely cause of increased lactate [42,47,49].

Pathologic effects are noted in the CNS, kidneys, lungs, heart,

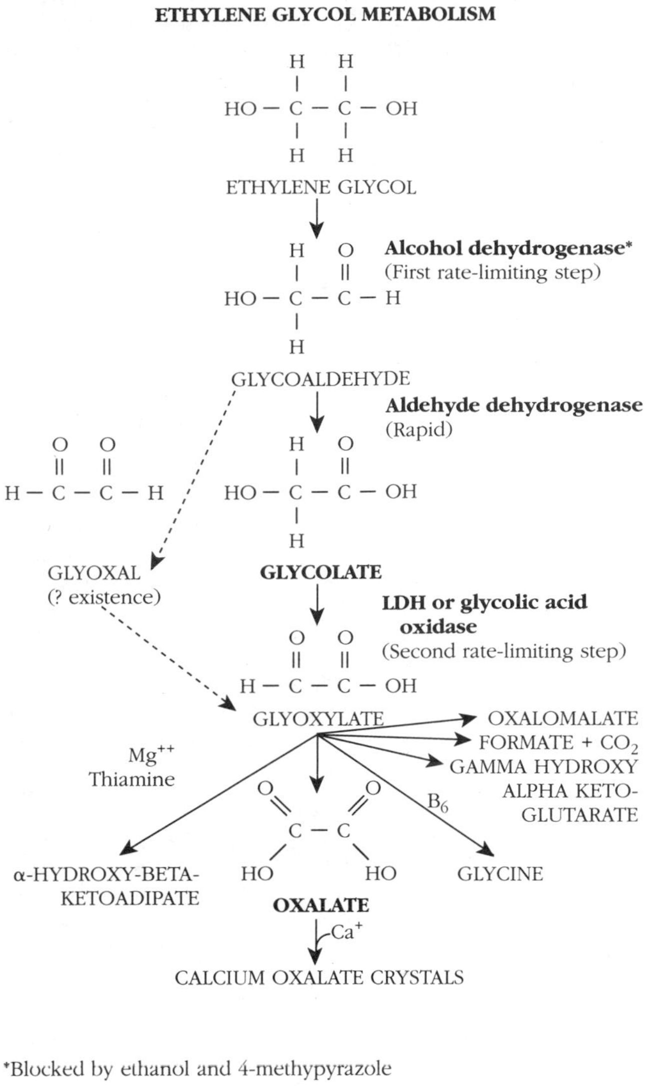

ETHYLENE GLYCOL METABOLISM

*Blocked by ethanol and 4-methypyrazole

Fig. 132-4. Ethylene glycol metabolism.

liver, muscles, and retina [51,58–61]. Renal findings include dilation of the proximal tubules with swelling and vacuolization of the epithelial cells, distal tubular dilation, intratubular deposition of calcium oxalate crystals, and interstitial edema. Pulmonary edema, interstitial pneumonitis, and hemorrhagic bronchopneumonia may occur. In some cases, interstitial myocarditis, skeletal muscle inflammation, and centrilobular hepatic fatty infiltration may occur. Central nervous system findings include cerebral edema, meningoencephalitis, and cerebellar changes, including focal loss of Purkinje's cells. An animal study demonstrated electrophysiologic and histologic changes in rabbit retinas associated with the depositon of calcium oxalate crystals [60].

Debate centers around whether these pathologic changes are attributable to the intracellular deposition of calcium oxalate crystals resulting from the complexation of calcium with oxalic acid, to direct cellular toxic effects of intermediary metabolites, or both. While renal tubular dilation is associated with tubular oxalosis, focal tubular epithelial necrosis can occur in the absence of crystalluria [51]. In rats, glycolaldehyde causes tubular epithelial cellular swelling, resulting in luminal obliteration while producing few crystals. Since maximal CNS depression coincides with peak aldehyde production, this metabolite may be primarily responsible for the CNS toxicity [62]. Deaths in rats correlate directly with the amount of urinary glycolate but are not related to the amounts of glycolaldehyde, glyoxylate, and oxalate produced. The role of each metabolite in the toxicopathologic process has not been clearly established.

Oral absorption of ethylene glycol occurs rapidly. Percutaneous absorption through intact skin is negligible, but ocular exposure can produce a chemical conjunctivitis and chemosis [58]. Due to a high boiling point (197.6°C), poisoning due to vapor inhalation does not occur. Distribution into total body water occurs rapidly. The apparent volume of distribution (V_d) of ethylene glycol ranges from 0.54 to 0.8 liter per kilogram, with 0.7 liter per kilogram commonly used for calculations [50,52,63]. The V_d glycolate is 0.55 liter per kilogram [47]. Serum protein binding does not occur. The elimination half-life of ethylene glycol in patients with normal renal function is 2.5 to 4.5 hours without ethanol therapy, 17 hours in patients treated with ethanol, and 2.5 to 3.0 hours during hemodialysis [41,42,63,64]. Renal failure can markedly prolong elimination [57,63]. During hemodialysis, the elimination half-life of glycolate has been reported as 2.4 hours [63].

The minimum lethal dose reported in humans is 1.6 gm per kilogram [46]. Hence, the estimated fatal dose in a 70-kg person is 112 ml of 100 percent (weight/volume) or 140 ml of 100% (volume/volume) ethylene glycol (Table 132-3). With intensive treatment, survival has been reported after a 700-ml ingestion (percent concentration unknown) [65].

METHANOL. Methanol is found in many cleaning materials, paints and varnishes, solvents, formaldehyde solutions, Sterno, antifreeze, duplicating fluid, and gasoline as a fuel extender [66,67,68]. A colorless liquid with a boiling point of 65°C, methanol has an odor distinct from that of ethanol [66,69]. Dietary sources and endogenous generation can produce methanol levels of approximately 1.5 mg per deciliter [66,70]. Poisonings occur as isolated events or in epidemics, usually as a result of substituting methanol for ethanol. In 1992, more than 2100 methanol ingestions were reported, with 11 deaths [1].

Like ethylene glycol, methanol must undergo metabolic transformation (Fig. 132-5) before toxicity occurs. Again, alco-

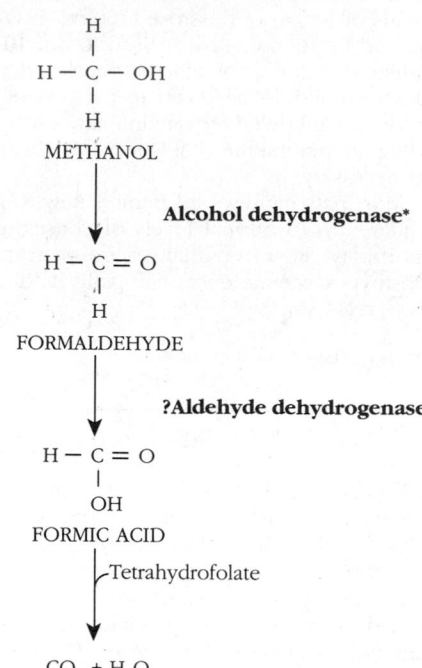

METHANOL METABOLISM

*Blocked by ethanol and 4-methypyrazole

Fig. 132-5. Methanol metabolism.

hol dehydrogenase, which catalyzes the formation of formaldehyde, is the rate-limiting enzyme. Formaldehyde is then converted to formic acid (formate). High levels of formic acid, an inhibitor of mitochondrial cytochrome oxidase, cause histotoxic hypoxia and are responsible for the characteristic metabolic acidosis and ocular toxicity seen with methanol poisoning [57,71,72]. Formaldehyde is also very toxic but has a very short elimination half-life and does not play a significant part in the toxicity of methanol.

Evidence for the role of formic acid in the acidosis comes from several studies. In methanol-intoxicated monkeys, blood concentrations of formate accounted for nearly all of the observed anion gap, with the other organic acids responsible for only a 2 to 3 percent decrease in the serum bicarbonate concentration [73]. In two human cases, an inverse correlation between serum formate and bicarbonate concentrations was noted [74]. Symptoms may also correspond better with formate than with methanol levels [75]. In 11 untreated patients with methanol poisoning, plasma formate concentrations correlated highly with the calculated anion gap, bicarbonate concentration, and negative base excess [76]. Lactic acidosis may be seen late in the course of methanol poisoning and may result from inhibition of the mitochondrial electron transport system [72,77] or from poor tissue perfusion [57]. Lactate levels of 11.5 and 23 mM per liter have been measured after an interval of 24 hours or more after ingestion [78,79].

Ocular toxicity results from the inhibition of cytochrome oxidase by formate in the optic nerve, leading to disruption of mitochondrial electron transport and decreased axoplasmic flow and electrical conduction [80,81]. Although this produces changes in the optic nerve head, direct retinal toxicity can also occur [82]. Primates infused with formate develop ocular toxicity, even when the acidosis is controlled with sodium bicar-

Table 132-3. Calculation of Ingested Alcohol Amounts

1. For alcohols whose weight by volume is known,
   Volume ingested (ml) × Weight by volume (gm/100 ml)
   = Amount ingested (gm)

Example: A patient gives a history of drinking 50 ml of a 60% (weight by volume) methanol windshield washing solution. How much methanol did he ingest?

Solution: 50 ml × 60 gm/100 ml = 30 gm

2. For alcohols whose volume by volume is known,
   A. Volume by volume × Specific gravity × 100
      = Weight by volume (gm/100 ml)
   B. Volume ingested (ml) × Weight by volume (gm/100 ml)
      = Amount ingested (gm)

Example: How many grams of ethylene glycol are contained in 50 ml of a de-icer that is 60% (volume by volume) ethylene glycol?

Solution: 0.60 vol/vol × 0.8 gm/ml × 100 = 48 gm/100 ml
          50 ml × 48 gm/ 100 ml = 24 gm

Specific gravity for ethanol, methanol and ethylene glycol is 0.8 grams/ml.

bonate [83]. Why the ocular nerve is particularly susceptible to the effects of formate remains unclear.

Methanol is absorbed orally, dermally, and through the respiratory tract [66,84,85]. The apparent volume of distribution of methanol is 0.7 liter per kilogram [86], while that of formate is 0.5 liter per kilogram [87]. Hepatic elimination predominates, with small amounts removed via the lungs and kidneys [66,71,88]. Methanol's metabolism is slower than that of ethylene glycol or ethanol [57,69,88], which may explain why toxicity develops more slowly with methanol. Elimination follows first-order kinetics at low doses and during hemodialysis, with reported elimination half-lives of 3 and 2.5 hours, respectively [89,90]. At higher doses, zero-order (Michaelis-Menten) kinetics prevail. In one untreated patient, methanol was eliminated at a rate of 8.5 mg/dl/hour [91]. The elimination half-life of formate in one untreated patient was 3.7 hours, compared with 1.1 hours in a patient who underwent hemodialysis [75].

Reported lethal doses vary considerably and are not well established. In the Atlanta epidemic, the minimal lethal dose was 15 ml of a 40 percent by weight methanol solution [69]. In an outbreak in Papua, New Guinea, one patient survived a 600-ml ingestion of pure methanol but had permanent sequelae, while another imbibed 500 ml without complications [92].

CLINICAL PRESENTATION

Ethylene Glycol. Symptoms of ethylene glycol poisoning usually occur 4 to 12 hours after ingestion (longer if ethanol was taken simultaneously). Patients may present alert, intoxicated with a mildly aromatic breath odor, or in a coma, depending on the time since ingestion and the amount of ethylene glycol and ethanol imbibed [42,47,52,57,58,93,94]. Vital signs can be normal or there may be mild elevations in blood pressure and temperature, varying degrees of tachycardia, and Kussmaul's respirations.

Three stages of ethylene glycol poisoning have been described [95]. During stage 1 (30 minutes to 12 hours after ingestion), CNS effects such as ethanol-like intoxication, stupor, coma, convulsions, nausea, and vomiting dominate the clinical picture. Stage 2 (12–24 hours after ingestion) is characterized by cardiovascular and pulmonary effects such as tachypnea, cyanosis, cardiogenic or noncardiogenic pulmonary edema, and death. During stage 3 (48–72 hours after ingestion), renal failure, manifested by flank pain and tenderness, proteinuria, anuria, and death from azotemia, is the major finding.

Seizures are usually generalized but do not occur in all cases. Jacksonian seizures have been reported, as have myoclonic jerks and tetanic contractions due to hypocalcemia [54,58,62]. Progressive CNS depression and prolonged seizures usually result from cerebral edema [57]. Transient nystagmus and bilateral sixth cranial nerve palsies were reported 24 hours after ingestion in a patient with cerebrospinal fluid (CSF) findings consistent with meningoencephalitis [62]. Autopsy studies have revealed both dilated and normal hearts in conjunction with pulmonary edema. Bronchopneumonia is a common complication [62]. A noncardiogenic etiology of pulmonary edema was recently documented by invasive monitoring [93]. Preterminal arrhythmias are rare. An idioventricular or junctional rhythm developed in a severely acidemic patient with normal serum potassium and calcium [54]. Acute renal failure occurs in nearly all untreated patients who manifest metabolic acidosis as a result of ingestion. Patients may also develop myositis with muscle tenderness and elevated creatine phosphokinase [42,57].

Methanol. Onset of toxicity usually occurs within 30 hours of ingestion [88]. In the Atlanta epidemic, involving 323 cases, a range of 40 minutes to 72 hours was reported [69]. Factors influencing time to symptoms include the amount ingested, concomitant ethanol intoxication, and the individual's folate status [66,86].

Neurologic, ophthalmologic, and gastrointestinal symptoms predominate [69,71,78,89,91,96–101]. Patients are frequently alert on admission and complain of headache and dizziness. Amnesia, restlessness, acute mania, lethargy, confusion, coma, and convulsions may be seen. Cases mimicking subarachnoid hemorrhage with severe headache, vomiting, hypertension, and bradycardia followed by loss of consciousness have been described [69].

Early on, many patients offer no visual complaints. Visual symptoms accompany the metabolic acidosis and are usually experienced acutely when the serum pH drops below 7.2, although patients presenting late may have a normal serum pH if the formic acid has been completely metabolized. Blurred vision, photophobia, scotomata, eye pain, partial or complete loss of vision, and visual hallucinations (e.g., bright lights, "skin over eyes," "snowstorm," dancing spots, flashes) have been reported.

Methanol can produce severe hemorrhagic gastritis and pancreatitis, causing upper abdominal pain, nausea, vomiting, and diarrhea. Liver function abnormalities have been documented in moderately to severely ill patients.

Back and flank pain as well as nuchal rigidity mimicking subarachnoid hemorrhage may occur. Dyspnea is an uncommon complaint.

Vital signs may reveal tachycardia and increased (e.g., Kussmaul's) respirations, but the blood pressure is usually maintained until death. Prior to the availability of current therapeutic modalities, patients died from sudden respiratory arrest [66,69]. The skin may be cool and diaphoretic, and rigidity of abdominal muscles without rebound tenderness has been seen [69].

The most notable physical findings are those discovered on ophthalmologic examination, but ocular abnormalities are not always present. Pupils may react sluggishly or be fixed and dilated [69,92]. Funduscopic examination may show hyperemia of the optic discs followed by retinal edema, which develops initially along the retinal vessels, then spreads to the central areas of the fundus. Retinal vessel engorgement accompanies the retinal edema [99]. Frank papilledema may occur [96]. Ophthalmologic findings do not correlate with visual complaints [69] but do parallel the severity of the toxicity.

DIAGNOSTIC EVALUATION. Poisoning by ethylene glycol and methanol should be suspected in all patients with a history of ingesting alcohol substitutes or who have an unexplained anion gap metabolic acidosis.

Ethylene Glycol. Baseline studies of arterial blood gases, CBC, electrocardiogram, serum electrolytes, glucose, BUN, creatinine, calcium, osmolarity, urinalysis, and ethanol, methanol, ethylene glycol, and isopropyl alcohol levels should be obtained. Early after ingestion, prior to significant metabolism of ethylene glycol, an osmol gap (Table 132-4) without a metabolic acidosis or an anion gap may be seen. As ethylene glycol is metabolized, the osmol gap, if present, decreases and an anion gap metabolic acidosis evolves. Patients who present late may have renal failure with normal osmol and anion gaps and no acidosis or measurable ethylene glycol levels.

Arterial pH measurements range from 6.72 to 7.37 [47,102]. One patient presented with a pH of 7.37 and a carbon dioxide tension (PCO_2) of 24 mm Hg but had an anion gap of 22 [102]. Ethylene glycol poisoning often results in higher anion gaps than other causes of this abnormality [53]. A gap of 58 mM per

Table 132-4. Osmol Gap

I. Determination of gap
  A. Measure serum osmolarity, sodium, glucose, BUN. Measure serum ethanol if applicable.
  B. Calculated osmolarity:

$$\frac{(1.86 \times Na^+) + \dfrac{Glucose}{18} + \dfrac{BUN}{2.8} + \dfrac{Ethanol}{4.6}}{0.93^*}$$

  B. Measured osmolarity − Calculated osmolality = Osmol gap
  C. See text for discussion of normal osmol gap

II. Causes of osmol gap [106,175]:
  A. Decreased serum water content (serum water coefficient range 0.90–0.93)
    Hyperlipidemia
    Hyperproteinemia
  B. Low-molecular-weight substances
    Mannitol
    Methanol
    Ethylene glycol
    Isopropanol
    Propylene glycol
    Other toxins with molecular weight <150
  C. Unknown substances accumulating in chronic renal failure; lactic acidosis and alcoholic ketoacidosis states
  D. Laboratory error

* Percentage of serum water

liter (58 mEq/L) has been reported [54]. The differential diagnosis of an increased anion gap metabolic acidosis is discussed in Chapter 129. In young children, child abuse and unrecognized disorders of amino acid and organic acid metabolism should be considered in the differential diagnosis [103,104]. Hyperkalemia may be seen in association with acidosis and with renal failure [42,58,62,93]. The creatinine and BUN are normal unless renal failure has supervened. Leukocytosis as high as 40,000 per cubic millimeter has been reported [105]. Calcium levels are usually normal initially but may drop significantly as tissue deposition of calcium oxalate occurs. The electrocardiogram may show ST–T wave and Q–Tc changes consistent with hypocalcemia and/or hyperkalemia.

Caution must be used when interpreting the osmol gap. Substances with low molecular weights and high serum concentrations are the primary contributors to serum osmolarity. The serum osmolarity can be measured by the freezing point depression or vapor pressure method. The former is preferred since most exogenous substances that cause significant osmol elevations are volatilized on heating and will not be measured by the vapor pressure method [106]. However, due to its high boiling point, ethylene glycol can produce an increased osmolarity using this technique [50].

Although an osmol gap is often cited as indirect evidence of the presence of an exogenous alcohol or glycol, other substances or conditions may be causative (Table 132-4). Conversely, failure to find an osmol gap may lead to the erroneous assumption that no exogenous substances are present. A small osmol gap may, however, represent a significant alcohol or glycol level.

One study found osmol gaps ranging from −9 to +5 mOsm per kilogram (mean − 0.89, S.D. ± 2.88) in normal patients and from −14 to +8 mOsm per kilogram (mean −0.86, S.D. ± 6.45) in overdose patients who had not taken ethanol, methanol, or isopropanol [107]. More recent studies have reported mean osmol gaps of −1.7 ± 1.7 mOsm per kilogram and −2 ± 6 mOsm per kilogram in groups of patients not known to have ingested or received osmotically active substances

[108,109]. An upper limit of 10 mOsm per kilogram was arbitrarily set for the normal osmol gap [110]. However, an osmol gap of 10 mOsm per kilogram in a patient whose baseline gap is 0 mOsm per kilogram could represent significant amounts of ethylene glycol (a serum level of 62 mg/dl) or methanol (a level of 32 mg/dL). One patient with an osmol gap of only 11 mOsm per kilogram had an ethylene glycol level of 38 mg per deciliter and subsequently developed renal failure [53], while another patient with an osmol gap of 7.2 mOsm per kilogram required hemodialysis for ethylene glycol toxicity [111]. As ethylene glycol and glycolaldehyde are metabolized, the osmol gap diminishes. Thus, an elevated osmol gap may be indirect evidence of the presence of an alcohol, but a normal gap does not rule it out [109,112].

Microscopic examination of the urine for crystals should be performed repetitively, since crystalluria may not be present initially [41,50]. Both calcium oxalate monohydrate and calcium oxalate dihydrate crystals can be seen (Fig. 132-6). Needle-shaped monohydrate crystals are the predominant form at all concentrations [113]. They may be confused with hippuric acid crystals [50,55]. The dihydrate crystals, morphologically resembling envelopes, tend to occur at higher concentrations and convert to the monohydrate form within 24 hours [113]. Other urinary findings can include low specific gravity, proteinuria, hematuria, and pyuria [62]. Some antifreeze manufacturers put fluorescein in their products to facilitate the detection of radiator leaks. Wood's lamp examination of the urine may demonstrate fluorescence and may provide indirect evidence of ethylene glycol ingestion.

Methanol. The baseline studies listed for ethylene glycol evaluation should be obtained. Methanol also causes an anion gap metabolic acidosis and may cause an osmolar gap [97], and the caveats noted under ethylene glycol apply equally to methanol. Elevated lactate levels, mild hypokalemia, and leukocytosis may occur. Amylase elevations and hypocalcemia can signify pancreatitis [91,92], although hyperamylasemia secondary to the salivary isoenzyme can occur. In one outbreak, 11 of 22 patients had amylase levels ranging from 400 to 1320 IU per liter [92].

A possible association between severity of methanol poisoning and changes in red blood cell (RBC) count indices has been reported [96]. Moderately to severely intoxicated patients had

Fig. 132-6. Morphology of calcium oxalate crystals.

CALCIUM OXALATE CRYSTALS

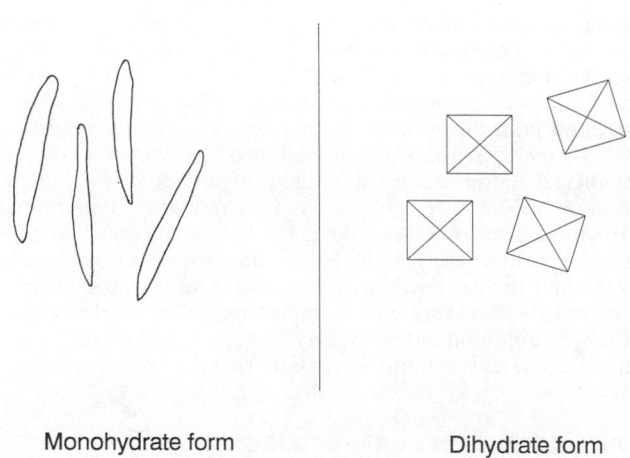

Monohydrate form   Dihydrate form

significantly elevated mean corpuscular volume (MCV) measurements (90–91 ± 1.5–1.9) compared to those with mild or no toxicity (82–83 ± 1.2–1.4). However, in vitro incubation of RBCs with methanol or formic acid did not alter the MCV, and underlying folate deficiency could not be invoked to explain this phenomenon.

MANAGEMENT. The treatment of patients with ethylene glycol and methanol poisoning is similar and includes supportive care, antidotal therapy, cofactor therapy, and measures to enhance elimination of the agent.

Supportive Care. Initial treatment includes airway management in the comatose patient, intravenous fluids, cardiac monitoring, and appropriate laboratory studies. All patients should have their gastric contents suctioned via a nasogastric or large-bore orogastric tube if coingested toxins are thought to be present, especially if they present within a few hours of ingestion. Although both substances normally have rapid GI absorption, the pharmacokinetics may be altered in overdose situations. In certain cases, delayed removal has been efficacious [69,114]. Oral activated charcoal is relatively ineffective but should be considered when coingestants are suspected.

Large doses of sodium bicarbonate may be required to control severe, life-threatening metabolic acidosis. Sodium bicarbonate is useful in ethylene glycol poisonings for two reasons. First, unlike the metabolites in lactic and ketoacidotic states, the metabolites of ethylene glycol cannot be transformed to regenerate bicarbonate [53] and the acidosis must be corrected by administration of exogenous alkali. Second, urinary alkalinization may slightly increase glycolic acid excretion through ion trapping, provided renal function remains normal [50]. However, hypocalcemia can occur as calcium complexes with oxalate and may be worsened by alkali administration. Calcium choloride should be administered intravenously to correct symptomatic hypocalcemia, but the indiscriminate use of calcium salts to correct a laboratory value should be avoided, since it may increase the precipitation of calcium oxalate crystals [57]. In methanol poisoning, increasing the serum pH may decrease the concentration of nonionized formic acid, thus diminishing formate access to the CNS and possibly ameliorating ocular toxicity [57]. The degree to which this happens is unclear. Given formate's pKa of 3.75, altering the serum pH from 7.0 to 7.4 would produce only a small increase in the nonionized form. Experiments in monkeys show that exposure to formate in the presence of a normal serum pH still results in ocular toxicity typical of methanol poisonings [83].

Seizures should initially be treated with standard anticonvulsants, such as diazepam and phenobarbital. Recurrent or persistent coma or seizures should prompt evaluation for underlying cerebral edema. Cerebral edema should be managed with hyperventilation, mannitol (provided renal function is intact), and possibly intracranial pressure monitoring. Cardiopulmonary complications may require pulmonary arterial pressure monitoring, inotropic agents, and vasopressors.

Antidotal Therapy. Ethanol is a preferential substrate for alcohol dehydrogenase [115], which competitively inhibits the initial step in the metabolism of these compounds to their initial metabolites and thus prevents formation of the more toxic compounds. Once alcohol dehydrogenase metabolism is blocked, methanol and ethylene glycol are eliminated slowly via pulmonary and renal excretion [66]. Ethanol has no effect on glycolate, oxalate, and formate metabolism, and preexisting metabolites produce end-organ damage and cause metabolic acidosis despite ethanol therapy.

Indications for ethanol therapy in cases of known or possible methanol or ethylene glycol intoxication include:

1. A history of ingestion when a serum level is not immediately available
2. A methanol or ethylene glycol level greater than 20 mg per deciliter, even if the patient is neither symptomatic nor acidotic
3. Unexplained metabolic acidosis with elevated anion and osmolar gaps and low lactate levels [66]
4. Unexplained coma with a high osmolar gap and low ethanol levels
5. Metabolic acidosis with elevated anion gap accompanied by visual signs and symptoms of urinary calcium oxalate crystals

Ethanol should be administered in doses sufficient to maintain serum ethanol concentrations between 100 and 150 mg per deciliter [75,89,116]. A loading dose is essential but should be adjusted if the patient has a known serum ethanol level (Table 132-5). Simultaneously, a constant ethanol infusion should be started. Maintenance dosages for ethanol range from 68 mg/kg/hr for nondrinkers to 200 mg/kg/hr for ethanol-tolerant individuals; hence, an initial infusion rate of 130 mg/kg/hr is recommended [116,117]. During hemodialysis, the maintenance infusion should be increased to 250 to 350 mg/kg/hr to compensate for the dialysis removal of ethanol [116]. Intravenous administration is preferable, using a dilute (5–10% ethanol) solution to minimize venous irritation [66]. If the intravenous form is unavailable, ethanol may be given orally, using a 20% to 30% concentration to decrease gastric irritation; however, vomiting and the presence of food may result in erratic absorption [117]. Serum ethanol levels should be monitored frequently to ensure adequate concentrations. The infusion should be continued until the ethylene glycol or methanol levels are undetectable. Since prolonged ethanol therapy can cause hypoglycemia, especially in children [14], glucose should be given and the ethanol and serum glucose levels checked frequently.

A more potent inhibitor of alcohol dehydrogenase, 4-methylpyrazole (4-MP), has been proposed as an alternative to ethanol therapy and all additional treatments [52,118,119]. Animal

---

Table 132-5. Ethanol Therapy for Ethylene Glycol and Methanol Poisoning

Loading dose of ethanol:
　0.8 g/kg (approximately 1 ml/kg) of 100% ethanol
　Oral or via nasogastric tube: use 20–30% concentration
　Intravenous: use 5–10% concentration

If ethanol is already present, the amount of ethanol required to achieve a serum ethanol level of 100 to 150 mg/dl may be calculated as follows:
　Amount ethanol (mg) = [Desired concentration (mg/dl) − Known concentration (mg/dl)] × Apparent volume of distribution of ethanol (0.6 L/kg) × Body weight (kg).

Maintenance doses of ethanol:
　Begin during administration of the loading dose. Give 130 mg/kg/hr of 100% ethanol (approximately 0.16 ml/kg/hr), orally or intravenously (as above). For a patient on hemodialysis, the maintenance dose should be higher—250–350 mg/kg/hr. Chronic alcoholics and patients given activated charcoal may also require higher doses. Due to potential hypoglycemia, glucose should be given along with ethanol and glucose levels must be frequently monitored.

Adapted from Goldfrank LR, Flomenbaum NE, Levin NA: *Goldfrank's Toxicologic Emergencies.* 3rd ed. Norwalk, CT, Appleton-Century-Crofts, 1986, p 464.

studies demonstrate blockade of ethylene glycol and methanol metabolism, and four human cases of ethylene glycol poisoning have been successfully treated with 4-MP [52,119,120,121]. 4-Methylpyrazole only diminishes catalase activity and may not block the MEOS enzymatic pathway [122]. These pathways, which may also play a role in metabolizing ethylene glycol and methanol, may remain active and possibly allow significant toxic metabolite production via these routes. However, current data do not support this concern [123,124]. The inhibitor 4-MP offers the advantages of oral administration, twice daily dosing, and no CNS depression. Unlike the more toxic pyrazole, which has been associated with weight loss, liver necrosis, and cytotoxicity in animals [121], the use of 4-MP has only been associated with a skin rash in one patient and possible eosinophilia and mild elevations in hepatic aspartate transaminase in two others [119]. There is no evidence that 4-MP induces ophthalmologic toxicity by interfering with retinol dehydrogenases involved in the visual rhodopsin cycle [125]. Further studies may establish 4-MP as preferential to ethanol for enzymatic blockade. Another inhibitor of ADH, 1,3-butylene glycol, proved superior to ethanol in a rodent study [126]. At this time both are investigational drugs.

Cofactor Therapy. Patients poisoned by ethylene glycol should receive pyridoxine (100 mg) and thiamine (100 mg) intravenously daily until ethylene glycol levels are unmeasurable and acidemia has cleared. Both vitamins are cofactors required to convert glyoxylic acid to nonoxalate compounds. Administering these cofactors may preferentially shunt metabolism away from the formation of oxalic acid [41,42,125], although this has not been documented in human poisonings.

Patients with methanol poisoning should be given intravenous folinic acid (leucovorin), 1 mg per kilogram (maximum dose 50 mg) every 4 hours for a total of six doses [57,75]. Folic acid, 1 mg per kilogram (maximum dose 50 mg) can be substituted if leucovorin is unavailable. Hepatic metabolism of formic acid occurs through a folate-dependent mechanism (Fig. 132-5), and exogenous folate may augment this metabolism. Although human data are not available, pretreatment of monkeys with either folate or 5-formyl tetrahydrofolic acid resulted in marked decreases in formate levels and degrees of metabolic acidosis following methanol administration [127]. In addition, 5-formyl tetrahydrofolic acid given after the onset of methanol poisoning diminished toxicity.

Enhanced Elimination. Hemodialysis effectively removes ethylene glycol, methanol, and their toxic metabolites and should be used along with ethanol therapy in nearly all cases of poisoning. Early hemodialysis can prevent the sequelae of these toxic substances, unless clinical manifestations are already consequential [101,113]. Addition of sodium bicarbonate to the dialysate can assist in control of the acidosis, and hemodialysis may assist in controlling volume status [65,128]. Ethanol dosing must be increased during hemodialysis to compensate for its removal, and serum ethanol levels should be frequently monitored to ensure that concentrations are sufficient to block alcohol dehydrogenase during this procedure.

Firm indications for hemodialysis have not been established. However, most authorities [57,66,71,116,129,130] recommend dialysis when one or more of the following conditions prevails:

1. A serum ethylene glycol or methanol level of 25 mg per deciliter or greater in an asymptomatic patient who is not acidotic
2. A history of ingesting at least 175 mg per kilogram of ethylene glycol or methanol when levels are not readily available
3. Ongoing metabolic acidosis (for both substances) or visual symptoms (in methanol exposures), regardless of the serum level
4. Unexplained metabolic acidosis with an anion gap and/or osmol gap when serum ethylene glycol or methanol levels are not readily obtainable

Ethylene glycol clearance rates of 156 and 210 ml per minute have been reported during hemodialysis, compared with a mean normal renal clearance of 27.5 ± 4.1 ml per minute and clearances of 1 to 4 ml per minute in patients with compromised renal function [64,131]. Glycolate is also readily removed by hemodialysis; its clearance has been measured at 105 ml per minute [47,53]. Hemodialysis elimination rates range from 142 to 286 ml per minute for methanol and 148 to 203 ml per minute for formate [71,87,91,96,117].

Hemodialysis should be continued until ethylene glycol or methanol levels are undetectable and acidemia has resolved or for a minimum of two 4-hour dialyses if levels are unknown [57]. Monitoring trends in the serum osmolar gap have been suggested [131], but the reliability of this method is unproved. Care must be taken to calculate the osmolar gap using simultaneously measured serum sodium, BUN, glucose, ethanol, and osmolarity, since dialysis alters the serum levels of all of these parameters. Rebounds in postdialysis methanol levels as high as 20 mg per deciliter have been documented [96]. In all cases, ethanol therapy should be continued until postdialysis ethylene glycol or methanol levels are found to be nondetectable.

Peritoneal dialysis is markedly inferior to hemodialysis [98]. Sorbent-based hemodialysis systems were inadvertently shown to be ineffective for methanol removal due to rapid saturation of the sorbent cartridge [132]. Charcoal cartridges also saturate within a few hours [65].

Patients with acute renal failure due to ethylene glycol poisoning may require hemodialysis for several months. Although permanent renal dysfunction has occurred in a few patients [62,114], recovery is usual [42,47,57]. Full neurologic recovery should be expected even after prolonged coma [62]. Several cases of transient cranial nerve palsies developing 6 to 14 days after ingestion have been reported [133,134].

Seizures, coma, and severe acidosis portend a poor prognosis in patients with methanol poisoning [97,98]. Cerebral edema is a common postmortem finding [130,135]. The development of dilated, unresponsive pupils carries a worse prognosis overall [99] and may result from optic nerve damage as well as cerebral edema. Other neurologic sequelae include a parkinsonianlike syndrome, spasticity, transient resting tremor, cognitive defects, and paraplegia. Computed tomography and autopsy studies document frontal lobe and basal ganglia hemorrhages and infarcts, especially in the putamen [135–141]. The etiology of these lesions remains uncertain, but they are likely due to the direct toxicity of methanol and/or its metabolites [139]. These abnormalities usually occur in severely acidemic patients with delayed presentation or diagnosis. Although it has been postulated that heparinization during hemodialysis predisposes the patient to hemorrhagic lesions [136], similar complications have occurred in nondialyzed patients [142].

Isopropyl Alcohol

Isopropyl alcohol (isopropanol) is a clear, colorless, volatile liquid with a disagreeable taste and characteristic odor [143,144]. It is available over the counter in 70% solutions of "rubbing alcohol," which may also contain ethanol as its chief constituent. Other sources include industrial or home cleaning products, antifreezes, skin lotions, and model cements [143]. Because of its ready availability at an inexpensive price, alcoholics often ingest isopropanol as an ethanol substitute. Cases of toxicity have been reported in small children who were sponge-bathed with the compound [145,146].

Isopropanol produces CNS depression, coma, and death from respiratory depression. In this respect it has twice the potency of ethanol [144,146,147,148], a phenomenon attributed to its higher molecular weight [143] and possibly the CNS depressant effects of its metabolite, acetone. Depending on individual tolerance, 150 to 240 ml of 100% isopropanol may be lethal. Serum levels of 150 mg per deciliter or greater may induce coma, and levels of 200 mg per deciliter or greater can be fatal, although lower concentrations may produce severe adverse effects [149].

Oral absorption occurs within 30 minutes but may be retarded in cases of overdose and in the presence of food. Cutaneous absorption has long been thought to be negligible, the toxicity from sponge bathing being attributed to vapor inhalation [143,144]. However, recent animal studies suggest significant dermal absorption [147]. Further research is needed to define whether dermal absorption is a possible route of toxicity in humans.

The apparent volume of distribution of isopropanol ranges from 0.6 to 0.7 liter per kilogram; maximal distribution usually occurs within 2 hours. Metabolism is hepatic, via an alcohol dehydrogenase, and produces acetone [143,148], but the specific mechanism has not been defined. Eighty percent of an absorbed dose is converted to acetone. Since isopropanol is a secondary (nonterminal) alcohol and the ketone moiety of acetone is located on the second carbon, further oxidation to an acid cannot occur (Fig. 132-7). Thus, metabolic acidosis is not a feature of isopropyl toxicity. Excretion of both acetone and unchanged isopropanol (20% of an absorbed dose) is predominantly renal, with some excretion by respiratory, gastric, and salivary routes [148]. Acetone can be detected in the urine 3 hours after ingestion [150]. Elimination half-lives measured in two ethanol-tolerant patients were 155 and 187 minutes [148]. Serum acetone levels frequently remain elevated after isopropyl levels are undetectable because it is eliminated slowly. The contribution of acetone to the prolonged duration of CNS depression remains speculative [143].

CLINICAL PRESENTATION AND DIAGNOSTIC EVALUATION. An "intoxicated" patient without acidemia yet with positive serum or urinary ketones and a fruity breath odor should

Fig. 132-7. Isopropyl alcohol metabolism.

ISOPROPYL ALCOHOL METABOLISM

ISOPROPANOL

? Alcohol dehydrogenase

ACETONE

raise suspicion of isopropanol intoxication. Symptoms usually begin within 30 minutes of ingestion and consist initially of mild intoxication with signs and symptoms of gastritis such as abdominal pain, nausea, vomiting, and possibly hematemesis [143]. Hemorrhagic tracheobronchitis may occur. As CNS depression progresses, patients become ataxic, dysarthric, confused, stuporous, and comatose. Pupils are typically miotic [143,145,151,152]. Hypotension may occur in severe intoxication [153].

Many patients who ingest isopropanol are alcoholics who have a multitude of diseases associated with ethanol abuse, including chronic liver disease, pancreatitis, traumatic injuries, and chronic obstructive pulmonary disease, which may complicate the clinical picture. Simultaneous exposure to isopropanol and carbon tetrachloride may potentiate the hepatic and renal toxicity of the latter [154].

Evaluation of patients with known or suspected isopropanol poisoning should include quantitative isopropanol and acetone serum levels as well as the baseline studies noted for acute ethanol intoxication. In patients who may also have ingested other toxic alcohols, serum osmolarity, ethanol, ethylene glycol, and methanol levels should also be obtained.

The differential diagnosis of isopropanol poisoning includes toxic and metabolic states in which ketonemia may develop, such as alcoholic, diabetic, and starvation ketoacidoses. Patients with these conditions have elevated levels of acetoacetate, beta-hydroxybutyrate, and acetone compared to the isolated acetonemia seen with isopropanol intoxication. Poisoning by salicylate, cyanide, and acetone itself, which is found in nail polish or super glue remover, should also be considered in the differential diagnosis of unexplained ketosis.

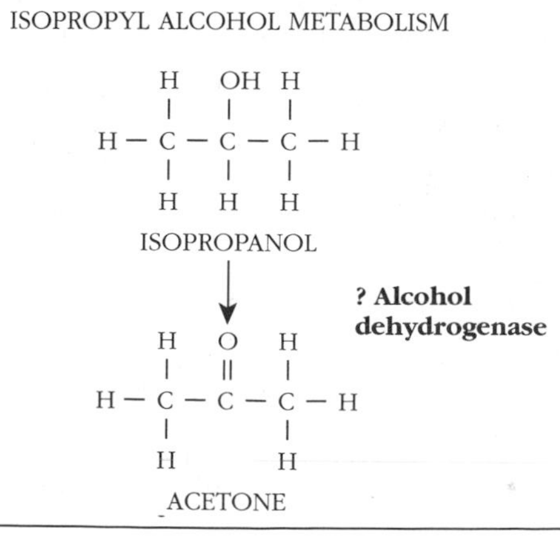

MANAGEMENT. Treatment is similar to that described for acute ethanol intoxication. Airway management and evaluation for hemorrhagic gastritis are particularly important. Delayed hypoglycemia may occur via the mechanism described for ethanol [143,145,149]. Hence, intravenous fluids should contain glucose and serum glucose levels should be periodically checked. Isopropanol and acetone are removed by hemodialysis [151,155]. No firm indications exist for using this therapy, although patients with cardiovascular instability may benefit [143].

Most patients, comatose or otherwise, recover with appropriate airway management and treatment of complicating factors. Pulmonary edema and hemorrhage are common findings on autopsy [149,153] and should be anticipated in severely ill patients. Central nervous system depression and volume depletion secondary to vomiting can cause hypotension, which is associated with an increased risk of mortality [143]. Because of the profound and prolonged cerebral depressive effects of isopropanol, comatose patients may develop compartment syndromes and rhabdomyolysis with myoglobinuria [153,156].

Propylene Glycol

Propylene glycol, or 1,2-propanediol ($HOCH_2CHOHCH_3$), is commonly used as a diluent for a number of pharmaceuticals, including intravenous formulations of chlordiazepoxide, diazepam, phenytoin, procainamide, nitroglycerin, and theophylline and topical silver sulfadiazine cream. Oral and dermal absorption are usually poor. However, toxic amounts may be absorbed through abraded or burned skin [157,158]. Fifty-five percent of a dose undergoes hepatic oxidation via alcohol dehydrogenase to pyruvate, lactate, and acetate; the remaining 45 percent is excreted unchanged in the urine [159].

Toxicity occurs in one of two ways. First, rapid intravenous infusion, as might occur during phenytoin loading, can cause prolonged P–R and QRS duration, idioventricular rhythms, and cardiorespiratory depression and arrest [160–163]. Infusion of smaller doses has also precipitated cardiac standstill [164]. Propylene glycol, rather than phenytoin (or other pharmaceuticals), is responsible for such toxicity [163]. Elderly patients, especially those with severe underlying cardiac disease, are at increased risk and should be infused with medications containing propylene glycol at rates slower than those usually recommended. Second, oral and dermal absorption through damaged skin has been associated with hyperosmolarity, hypoglycemia, lactic acidosis, seizures, and decreased consciousness level [157,165–168]. Propylene glycol can cause false positive readings for ethylene glycol when measured by the colorimetric method of Russell or gas chromatography using an OV-17 (gas chromotography) column. Use of an OV-1 column obviates this error [169].

Management consists of gastrointestinal decontamination with lavage and activated charcoal; if applicable, immediately stopping intravenous infusion or dermal application; and supportive therapy.

Benzyl Alcohol

A syndrome of gasping respirations, progressive metabolic acidosis, CNS depression, seizures, bradycardia, hypotension, and death has been described in neonates [170,171,172]. Many suffered intracranial hemorrhage prior to death. Large doses of benzyl alcohol (99–234 mg/kg/day) unwittingly administered in bacteriostatic solutions proved to be the toxicologic culprit. Benzyl alcohol is an aromatic alcohol. It undergoes hepatic oxidation to benzoic acid, which is then conjugated with glycine and excreted renally as hippuric acid [173]. Since newborns have limited hepatic metabolic capacity, they are unable to conjugate the large amounts of benzoic acid leading to benzyl alcohol and benzoic acid accumulation. This is presumed to be responsible for the observed toxicity [171,172]. To prevent further poisonings, the Food and Drug Administration, the Centers for Disease Control, and the American Academy of Pediatrics have recommended that benzyl alcohol be eliminated from flush solutions [174]. Management includes stopping the administration of solutions containing benzyl alcohol and supportive care.

References

1. Litovitz TL, Holm KC, Clancy C: 1992 Annual report of the American Association of Poison Control Centers Toxic Exposure Surveillance System. *Am J Emerg Med* 11:494, 1993.
2. Cyr MG, Wartman SA: The effectiveness of routine screening questions in the detection of alcoholism. *JAMA* 259:51, 1988.
3. West LJ, Maxwell DS, Noble EP, et al: Alcoholism. *Ann Intern Med* 100:405, 1984.
4. Eckardt MJ, Harford TC, Kaelber CT, et al: Health hazards associated with alcohol consumption. *JAMA* 246:648, 1981.
5. Tabakoff B, Cornell N, Hoffman PL: Alcohol tolerance. *Ann Emerg Med* 15:1055, 1986.
6. West LJ, Maxwell DS, Noble EP, et al: Alcoholism. *Ann Intern Med* 100:405, 1984.
7. Scherger DL, Wruk KM, Kulig KW, et al: Ethyl alcohol (ethanol)-containing cologne, perfume, and after-shave ingestions in children. *Am J Dis Child* 142:630, 1988.
8. Adinoff B, Bone GHA, Linnoila M: Acute ethanol poisoning and the ethanol withdrawal syndrome. *Med Toxicol* 3:172, 1988.
9. Carlen PL, Gurevich N, Durand D: Low dose ethanol augments calcium-mediated mechanisms measured intracellularly in hippocampal neurons. *Science* 215:306, 1982.
10. Carlen PL, Zhang L, Cullen N: Cellular electrophysiological actions of ethanol on mammalian neurons in brain slices. *Ann N Y Acad Sci* 265:17, 1991.
11. Nagy LE, Diamond I, Casso DJ, et al: Ethanol increases extracellular adenosine by inhibiting adenosine uptake via the nucleoside transporter. *J Biol Chem* 265:1946, 1990.
12. Wafford KA, Burnett DM, Dunwiddie TV, et al: Genetic differences in the ethanol sensitivity of $GABA_A$ receptors expressd in Xenopus oocytes. *Science* 249:291, 1990.
13. Frezza M, di Padova C, Pozzato G, et al: High blood alcohol levels in women: The role of decreased gastric alcohol dehydrogenase activity and first-pass metabolism. *N Engl J Med* 322:95, 1990.
14. Hoffman RS, Goldfrank LR: Ethanol-associated metabolic disorders. *Emerg Med Clin North Am* 7:943, 1989.
15. Geokas MC, Lieber CS, French S, et al: Ethanol, the liver, and the gastrointestinal tract. *Ann Intern Med* 95:198, 1981.
16. Li T-K, Bosron WF: Genetic variability of enzymes of alcohol metabolism in human beings. *Ann Emerg Med* 15:997, 1986.
17. Teschke R, Hasumura Y, Lieber CS: Hepatic microsomal alcohol-oxidizing system: Affinity for methanol, ethanol, propanol, and butanol. *J Biol Chem* 250:7397, 1975.
18. Lieber CS, DeCarli LM: The role of the hepatic microsomal ethanol oxidizing system (MEOS) for ethanol metabolism in vivo. *J Pharmacol Exp Ther* 181:279, 1972.
19. Oshino N, Jamieson D, Chance B: The properties of hydrogen peroxide production under hyperoxic and hypoxic conditions of perfused rat liver. *Biochem J* 146:53, 1975.
20. Lieber CS: Biochemical and molecular basis of alcohol-induced injury to liver and other tissues. *N Engl J Med* 319:1639, 1988.
21. Goldstein DB: Effect of alcohol on cellular membranes. *Ann Emerg Med* 15:1013, 1986.
22. Charness ME, Simon RP, Greenberg DA: Ethanol and the nervous system. *N Engl J Med* 321:442, 1989.
23. Brown SS, Forrest JAH: A controlled trial of fructose in the treatment of acute alcoholic intoxication. *Lancet* 2:898, 1972.
24. Halperin ML, Hammeke M, Josse RG, et al: Metabolic acidosis in the alcoholic: A pathophysiologic approach. *Metabolism* 32:308, 1983.
25. McGarry JD, Foster DW: Ketogenesis and its regulation. *Am J Med* 61:9, 1976.
26. Fulop M, Bock J, Ben-Ezra J, et al: Plasma lactate and 3-hydroxybutyrate levels in patients with acute ethanol intoxication. *Am J Med* 80:191, 1986.
27. Fulop M, Hoberman HD: Alcoholic ketosis. *Diabetes* 24:785, 1975.
28. Bluntzer ME, Blachley JD: Acid-base and electrolyte disturbances induced by alcohol. *J Crit Illness* 1:19, 1986.
29. Oliva PB: Lactic acidosis. *Am J Med* 48:209, 1970.
30. Watson AJS, Walker JF, Tomkin GH, et al: Acute Wernicke's encephalopathy precipitated by glucose loading. *Irish J Med Sci* 150:301, 1981.
31. Marks V: Alcohol and carbohydrate metabolism. *Clin Endocrinol Metab* 7:333, 1978.
32. Arky RA, Freinkel N: Alcohol hypoglycemia: Effects of ethanol on plasma. III. Glucose, ketones, and free fatty acids in "juvenile" diabetics: A model for "non-ketotic diabetic acidosis"? *Arch Intern Med* 114:501, 1964.
33. Wilson NM, Brown PM, Juul SM, et al: Glucose turnover and metabolic and hormonal changes in ethanol-induced hypoglycaemia. *Br Med J* 282:849, 1981.
34. Freinkel N, Cohen AK, Arky RA, et al: Alcohol hypoglycemia. II. A postulated mechanism of action based on experiments with rat liver slices. *J Clin Endocrinol* 25:76, 1965.
35. Ylikahri RH: Ethanol-induced hypoglycemia in thyroxine-treated rats. *Metabolism* 19:518, 1970.
36. Chalmers RJ, Bennie EH, Johnson RH, et al: The growth hormone response to insulin induced hypoglycaemia in alcoholics. *Psychiatr Med* 7:607, 1977.

37. Haight JSJ, Keating WR: Failure of thermoregulation in the cold during hypoglycaemia induced by exercise and alcohol. *J Physiol* 229:87, 1973.

38. Freinkel N, Singer DI, Arky RA, et al: Alcohol hypoglycemia. I. Carbohydrate metabolism of patients with clinical alcohol hypoglycemia and the experimental reproduction of the syndrome with pure ethanol. *J Clin Invest* 42:1112, 1963.

39. Hale DE, Lyen KR, Baker L: Endocrine emergencies, in Fleisher G, Ludwig S (eds): *Textbook of Pediatric Emergency Medicine.* 2nd ed. Baltimore, Williams & Wilkins, 1988, p 743.

40. Madison LL: Ethanol-induced hypoglycemia, in Levine R, Luft R (eds): *Advances in Metabolic Disorders.* vol 3. New York, Academic Press, 1968, p 95.

41. Haupt MC, Zull DN, Adams SL: Massive ethylene glycol poisoning without evidence of crystalluria: A case for early intervention. *J Emerg Med* 6:295, 1988.

42. Beasley VR, Buck WB: Acute ethylene glycol toxicosis: A review. *Vet Hum Toxicol* 22:255, 1980.

43. Anonymous: Possible death from drinking ethylene glycol ("Prestone"). *JAMA* 94:1940, 1930.

44. Geiling EMK, Cannon PR: Pathologic effects of elixir of sulfanilamide (diethylene glycol) poisoning. *JAMA* 111:919, 1938.

45. Haggerty RJ: Toxic hazards: Deaths from permanent antifreeze ingestion. *N Engl J Med* 261:1296, 1959.

46. Gessner PK, Parke DV, Williams RT: Studies in detoxication. *Biochem J* 79:482, 1961.

47. Jacobsen D, Steinar O, Ostborg J, et al: Glycolate causes the acidosis in ethylene glycol poisoning and is effectively removed by hemodialysis. *Acta Med Scand* 216:409, 1984.

48. Clay KL, Murphy RC: On the metabolic acidosis of ethylene glycol intoxication. *Toxicol Appl Pharmacol* 39:39, 1977.

49. Chou JY, Richardson KE: The effect of pyrazole on ethylene glycol toxicity and metabolism in the rat. *Toxicol Appl Pharmacol* 43:33, 1978.

50. Jacobsen D, Hewlett TR, Webb R, et al: Ethylene glycol intoxication: Evaluation of kinetics and crystalluria. *Am J Med* 84:145, 1988.

51. Bove KE: Ethylene glycol toxicity. *Am J Clin Pathol* 45:46, 1966.

52. Baud FJ, Galliot M, Astier A, et al: Treatment of ethylene glycol poisoning with intravenous 4-methylpyrazole. *N Engl J Med* 319:97, 1988.

53. Gabow PA, Clay K, Sullivan JB, et al: Organic acids in ethylene glycol intoxication. *Ann Intern Med* 105:16, 1986.

54. Scully RE, Galdabini JJ, McNeely BU: Case records of the Massachusetts General Hospital: Case 38-1979. *N Engl J Med* 301:650, 1979.

55. Jacobsen D: Organic acids in ethylene glycol intoxication (letter). *Ann Intern Med* 105:799, 1986.

56. Brown CG, Trumbull D, Klein-Schwartz W, et al: Ethylene glycol poisoning. *Ann Emerg Med* 12:501, 1983.

57. Jacobsen D, McMartin KE: Methanol and ethylene glycol poisonings: Mechanism of toxicity, clinical course, diagnosis and treatment. *Med Toxicol* 1:309, 1986.

58. Friedman EA, Greenberg JB, Merrill JP, et al: Consequences of ethylene glycol poisoning. *Am J Med* 32:891, 1962.

59. Pons CA, Custer RP: Acute ethylene glycol poisoning: A clinico-pathologic report of eighteen fatal cases. *Am J Med Sci* 211:544, 1946.

60. Rossa V, Weber U: Effect of ethylene glycol on rabbit retinas. *Ophthalmologica* 220:98, 1990.

61. Smith BJ, Anderson BG, Smith SA, et al: Early effects of ethylene glycol on the ultrastructure of the renal cortex in dogs. *Am J Vet Res* 51:89, 1990.

62. Parry MF, Wallach R: Ethylene glycol poisoning. *Am J Med* 57:143, 1974.

63. Jacobsen D, Hewlett TP, Webb R, et al: Ethylene glycol intoxication: Evaluation of kinetics and crystalluria. *Am J Med* 84:145, 1988.

64. Peterson CD, Collins AJ, Himes JM, et al: Ethylene glycol poisoning: Pharmacokinetics during therapy with ethanol and hemodialysis. *N Engl J Med* 304:21, 1981.

65. Linnanvuo-Laitinen M, Huttunen K: Ethylene glycol intoxication. *Clin Toxicol* 24:167, 1986.

66. Becker CE: Methanol poisoning. *J Emerg Med* 1:51, 1983.

67. Frederick LJ, Schulte PA, Apol A: Investigation and control of occupational hazards associated with the use of spirit duplicators. *Am Ind Hyg Assoc J* 45:51, 1984.

68. Wigg EE: Methanol as a gasoline extender: A critique. *Science* 186:785, 1974.

69. Bennett IL, Cary FH, Mitchell GL, et al: Acute methyl alcohol poisoning: A review based on experiences in an outbreak of 323 cases. *Medicine* 32:431, 1953.

70. Eriksen SP, Kulkarni AB: Methanol in normal human breath. *Science* 141:639, 1963.

71. Jacobsen D, Jansen H, Wilk-Larsen E, et al: Studies on methanol poisoning. *Acta Med Scand* 212:5, 1982.

72. Liesivuori J, Savolainen H: Methanol and formic acid toxicity: Biochemical mechanisms. *Pharmacol Toxicol* 69:157, 1991.

73. Clay KL, Murphy RC, Watkins WD: Experimental methanol toxicity in the primate: Analysis of metabolic acidosis. *Toxicol Appl Pharmacol* 34:49, 1975.

74. McMartin KE, Ambre JJ, Tephly TR: Methanol poisoning in human subjects: Role for formic acid accumulation in the metabolic acidosis. *Am J Med* 68:414, 1980.

75. Osterloh JD, Pond SM, Grady S, et al: Serum formate concentrations in methanol intoxication as a criterion for hemodialysis. *Ann Intern Med* 104:200, 1986.

76. Sejersted OM, Jacobsen D, Ovrebo S, et al: Formate concentrations in plasma from patients poisoned with methanol. *Acta Med Scand* 213:105, 1983.

77. Nicholls P: The effect of formate on cytochrome aa$_3$ and on electron transport in the intact respiratory chain. *Biochim Biophys Acta* 430:13, 1976.

78. Shahangian S, Ash KO: Formic and lactic acidosis in a fatal case of methanol intoxication. *Clin Chem* 32:395, 1986.

79. Smith SR, Smith SJM, Buckley BM: Combined formate and lactate acidosis in methanol poisoning (letter). *Lancet* 2:1295, 1981.

80. Martin-Amat G, Tephly TR, McMartin KE, et al: Methyl alcohol poisoning. II. Development of a model for ocular toxicity in methyl alcohol poisoning using the Rhesus monkey. *Arch Ophthalmol* 95:1847, 1977.

81. Hayreh MS, Hayreh SS, Baumbach GL, et al: Methyl alcohol poisoning: III. Ocular toxicity. *Arch Ophthalmol* 95:1851, 1977.

82. Eells JT: Methanol-induced visual toxicity in the rat. *J Pharmacol Exp Ther* 257:56, 1991.

83. Martin-Amat G, McMartin KE, Hayreh SS, et al: Methanol poisoning: Ocular toxicity produced by formate. *Toxicol Appl Pharmacol* 45:201, 1978.

84. Dutkiewicz B, Konczalik J, Karwacki W: Skin absorption and per os administration of methanol in men. *Int Arch Occup Environ Health* 47:81, 1980.

85. Kahn A, Blum D: Methyl alcohol poisoning in an 8-month-old boy: An unusual route of intoxication. *J Pediatr* 94:841, 1979.

86. Martensson E, Olofsson U, Heath A: Clinical and metabolic features of ethanol-methanol poisoning in chronic alcoholics. *Lancet* 1:327, 1988.

87. Jacobsen D, Ovrebo S, Sejersted OM: Toxicokinetics of formate during hemodialysis. *Acta Med Scand* 214:409, 1983.

88. Bartlett GR: Combustion of C$_{14}$ labeled methanol in intact rat and its isolated tissues. *Am J Physiol* 163:614, 1950.

89. McCoy HG, Cipolle RJ, Ehlers SM, et al: Severe methanol poisoning: Application of a pharmacokinetic model for ethanol therapy and hemodialysis. *Am J Med* 67:804, 1979.

90. Jones AW: Elimination half-life of methanol during hangover. *Pharmacol Toxicol* 60:217, 1987.

91. Jacobsen D, Webb R, Collins TD, et al: Methanol and formate kinetics in late diagnosed methanol intoxication. *Med Toxicol* 3:418, 1988.

92. Naraqi S, Dethlefs RF, Slobodniuk RA, et al: An outbreak of acute methyl alcohol intoxication. *Aust N Z J Med* 9:65, 1979.

93. Catchings TT, Beamer WC, Lundy L, et al: Adult respiratory distress syndrome secondary to ethylene glycol ingestion. *Ann Emerg Med* 14:594, 1985.

94. Jacobsen D, Ostby N, Bredesen E: Studies on ethylene glycol poisoning. *Acta Med Scand* 212:11, 1982.

95. Berman LB, Schreiner GE, Feys J: The nephrotoxic lesion of ethylene glycol. *Ann Intern Med* 46:611, 1957.

96. Swartz RD, Millman RP, Billi JE, et al: Epidemic methanol poison-

ing: Clinical and biochemical analysis of a recent episode. *Medicine* 60:373, 1981.

97. Jacobsen D, Bredesen JE, Eide I, et al: Anion and osmolal gaps in the diagnosis of methanol and ethylene glycol poisoning. *Acta Med Scand* 212:17, 1982.

98. Keyvan-Larijarni H, Tannenberg AM: Methanol intoxication: Comparison of peritoneal dialysis and hemodialysis treatment. *Arch Intern Med* 134:293, 1974.

99. Ingemansson S-O: Clinical observations on ten cases of methanol poisoning with particular reference to ocular manifestations. *Acta Ophthalmol* 62:15, 1984.

100. Dethlefs R, Naraqi S: Ocular manifestations and complications of acute methyl alcohol intoxication. *Med J Aust* 2:483, 1978.

101. Kane RL, Talbert W, Harlan J, et al: A methanol poisoning outbreak in Kentucky: A clinical epidemiologic study. *Arch Environ Health* 77:119, 1968.

102. Underwood F, Bennett WM: Ethylene glycol intoxication: Prevention of renal failure by aggressive management. *JAMA* 226:1453, 1973.

103. Woolf AD, Wynshaw-Boris A, Rinalso P, et al: Intentional infantile ethylene glycol poisoning presenting as an inherited metabolic disorder. *J Pediatr* 120:421, 1992.

104. Shoemaker JD, Lynch RE, Hoffman JW, et al: Misidentification of propionic acid as ethylene glycol in a patient with methylmalonic acidemia. *J Pediatr* 120:417, 1992.

105. Frommer JP, Ayus JC: Acute ethylene glycol intoxication. *Am J Nephrol* 2:1, 1982.

106. Walker JA, Schwartzbard A, Krauss EA, et al: The missing gap: A pitfall in the diagnosis of alcohol intoxication by osmometry. *Arch Intern Med* 146:1843, 1986.

107. Glasser L, Sternglanz PD, Combie J, et al: Serum osmolality and its applicability to drug overdose. *Am J Clin Pathol* 60:695, 1973.

108. Schelling JR, Howard RL, Winter SD, et al: Increased osmolal gap in alcoholic ketoacidosis and lactic acidosis. *Ann Intern Med* 113:580, 1990.

109. Hoffman RS, Smilkstein MJ, Howland MA, et al: Osmol gaps revisited: Normal values and limitations. *Clin Toxicol* 31:81, 1993.

110. Smithline N, Gardner KD: Gaps: Anionic and osmolal. *JAMA* 236:1594, 1976.

111. Steinhart B: Case report: Severe ethylene glycol intoxication with normal osmolal gap—"A chilling thought." *J Emerg Med* 8:583, 1990.

112. Lund ME, Banner W: Effect of alcohols and selected solvents on serum osmolality measurements. *J Toxicol Clin Toxicol* 20:115, 1983.

113. Burns JR, Finlayson B: Changes in calcium oxalate crystal morphology as a function of concentration. *Invest Urol* 18:174, 1980.

114. Stokes JB, Aueron F: Prevention of organ damage in massive ethylene glycol ingestion. *JAMA* 243:2065, 1980.

115. DaRoza R, Henning RJ, Sunshine I, et al: Acute ethylene glycol poisoning. *Crit Care Med* 12:1003, 1984.

116. Goldfrank LR, Flomenbaum NE, Lewin NA, et al: *Goldfrank's Toxicologic Emergencies*. 4th ed. Norwalk, CT, Appleton-Century-Crofts, 1990, pp 488–491.

117. Ekins BR, Rollins DE, Duffy DP, et al: Standardized treatment of severe methanol poisoning with ethanol and hemodialysis. *West J Med* 142:337, 1985.

118. Blomstrand R, Theorell H: Inhibitory effect on ethanol oxidation in man after administration of 4-methylpyrazole. *Life Sci* 9:631, 1970.

119. Baud FJ, Bismuth C, Garnier R, et al: 4-methylpyrazole may be an alternative to ethanol therapy for ethylene glycol intoxication in man. *Clin Toxicol* 24:463, 1986–1987.

120. Grauer GJ, Hull MA, Henre BA, et al: Comparison of the effects of ethanol and 4-methylpyrazole on the pharmocokinetics and toxicity of ethylene glycol in the dog. *Toxicol Lett* 35:307, 1987.

121. Blomstrand R, Ostling-Wintzell HA, et al: Pyrazoles as inhibitors of alcohol oxidation and as important tools in alcohol research: An approach to therapy against methanol poisoning. *Proc Natl Acad Sci USA* 76:4399, 1979.

122. Bradford BU, Seed CB, Handler JA, et al: Evidence that catalase is a major pathway of ethanol oxidation in vivo: Dose-response studies in deer mice using methanol as a selective substrate. *Arch Biochem Biophys* 303:172, 1993.

123. Makar AB, Mannering GJ: Role of the intracellular distribution of hepatic catalase in the perioxidative oxidation of methanol. *Mol Pharmacol* 4:484, 1968.

124. Blomstrand R, Ingemansson S-O: Studies on the effect of 4-methylpyrazole on methanol poisoning using the monkey as an animal model: With particular reference to the ocular toxicity. *Drug Alcohol Depend* 13:343, 1984.

125. Gibbs DA, Watts RWE: The action of pyridoxine in primary hyperoxaluria. *Clin Sci* 38:277, 1970.

126. Cox SK, Ferslew KE, Boelen LJ: The toxicokinetics of 1,3-butylene glycol versus ethanol in the treatment of ethylene glycol poisoning. *Vet Hum Toxicol* 34:36, 1992.

127. Noker PE, Eells JT, Tephly TR: Methanol toxicity: Treatment with folic acid and 5 formyl tetrahydrofolic acid. *Alcohol Clin Exp Res* 4:378, 1980.

128. Turk J, Morrell L, Alvioli LV: Ethylene glycol intoxication. *Arch Intern Med* 146:1601, 1986.

129. Ellenhorn MJ, Barceloux DG: *Medical Toxicology: Diagnosis and Treatment of Human Poisoning*. New York, Elsevier, 1988.

130. Cheng J-T, Beysolow TD, Kaul B, et al: Clearance of ethylene glycol by kidneys and hemodialysis. *Clin Toxicol* 25:95, 1987.

131. Gonda A, Gault H, Churchill D, et al: Hemodialysis for methanol intoxication. *Am J Med* 64:749, 1979.

132. Whalen JE, Richards CJ, Ambre J: Inadequate removal of methanol and formate using the sorbent based regeneration hemodialysis delivery system. *Clin Nephrol* 11:318, 1979.

133. Berger JR, Syyar DR: Neurological complications of ethylene glycol intoxication: Report of a case. *Arch Neurol* 38:724, 1981.

134. Factor SA, Lava NS: Ethylene glycol intoxication: A new stage in the clinical syndrome. *NY State J Med* 87:179, 1987.

135. McLean DR, Jacobs H, Mielke BW: Methanol poisoning: A clinical and pathological study. *Ann Neurol* 8:161, 1980.

136. Phang PT, Passerini L, Mielke B, et al: Brain hemorrhage associated with methanol poisoning. *Crit Care Med* 16:137, 1988.

137. Anderson TJ, Shuaib A, Becker WJ: Neurologic sequelae of methanol poisoning. *Can Med Assoc J* 136:1177, 1987.

138. Ley CO, Gali FG: Parkinsonian syndrome after methanol intoxication. *Eur Neurol* 22:405, 1983.

139. Guggenheim MA, Couch JR, Weinberg W: Motor dysfunction as a permanent complication of methanol ingestion. *Arch Neurol* 24:550, 1971.

140. Rosenberg NL: Methylmalonic acid, methanol, metabolic acidosis, and lesions of the basal ganglia (letter). *Ann Neurol* 22:96, 1987.

141. Aquilonius S-M, Askmark H, Enoksson P, et al: Computerised tomography in severe methanol intoxication. *Br Med J* 2:929, 1978.

142. Erlanson P, Fritz H, Hagstam K, et al: Severe methanol intoxication. *Acta Med Scand* 117:393, 1965.

143. LaCouture PG, Wason S, Abrams A, et al: Acute isopropyl alcohol intoxication: Diagnosis and management. *Am J Med* 75:680, 1983.

144. Grant DH: The pharmacology of isopropyl alcohol. *J Lab Clin Med* 8:382, 1923.

145. Lewin GA, Oppenheimer PR, Wingert WA: Coma from alcohol sponging. *JACEP* 6:165, 1977.

146. McFadden SW, Haddow JE: Coma produced by topical application of isopropanol. *Pediatrics* 43:622, 1969.

147. Martinez TT, Jaeger RW, deCastro FJ, et al: A comparison of the absorption and metabolism of isopropyl alcohol by oral, dermal and inhalation routes. *Vet Hum Toxicol* 28:233, 1986.

148. Daniel DR, McAnnalley BH, Garriott JC: Isopropyl alcohol metabolism after acute intoxication in humans. *J Anal Toxicol* 5:110, 1981.

149. Alexander CB, McBay AJ, Hudson RP: Isopropanol and isopropanol deaths: Ten years' experience. *J Forensic Sci* 27:541, 1982.

150. LaCouture PG, Heldreth DD, Shannon M, et al: The generation of acetonemia/acetonuria following ingestion of a subtoxic dose of isopropyl alcohol. *Am J Emerg Med* 7:38, 1989.

151. Rosansky SJ: Isopropyl alcohol poisoning treated with hemodialysis: Kinetics of isopropyl alcohol and acetone removal. *J Toxicol Clin Toxicol* 19:265, 1982.

152. Kelner M, Bailey DN: Isopropanol ingestion: Interpretation of blood concentrations and clinical findings. *J Toxicol Clin Toxicol* 20:497, 1983.

153. Adelson L: Fatal intoxication with isopropyl alcohol (rubbing alcohol). *Am J Clin Pathol* 38:144, 1962.

154. Folland DS, Schaffner W, Ginn HE, et al: Carbon tetrachloride toxicity potentiated by isopropyl alcohol. *JAMA* 236:1853, 1976.

155. Freireich AW, Cinque TJ, Xanthaky G, et al: Hemodialysis for isopropanol poisoning. *N Engl J Med* 277:699, 1967.

156. Juncos L, Taguchi JT: Isopropyl alcohol intoxication: Report of a case associated with myopathy, renal failure, and hemolytic anemia. *JAMA* 204:186, 1968.

157. Bekeris L, Baker C, Fenton J, et al: Propylene glycol as a cause of an elevated serum osmolality. *Am J Clin Pathol* 72:633, 1979.

158. Fligner CL, Jack R, Twiggs GA, et al: Hyperosmolality induced by propylene glycol: A complication of silver sulfadiazine therapy. *JAMA* 253:1606, 1985.

159. Ruddick JA: Toxicology, metabolism, and biochemistry of 1,2-propanediol. *Toxicol Appl Pharmacol* 21:102, 1972.

160. Unger AH, Sklaroff HJ: Fatalities following intravenous use of sodium diphenylhydantoin for cardiac arrhythmias. *JAMA* 200:335, 1967.

161. Zoneraich S, Zoneraich O, Siegal J: Sudden death following intravenous sodium diphenylhydantoin. *Am Heart J* 91:375, 1976.

162. Goldschlager AW, Karliner JS: Ventricular standstill after diphenylhydantoin for cardiac arrhythmias: Report of two cases. *JAMA* 200:335, 1967.

163. Louis S, Kutt H, McDowell F: The cardiocirculatory changes caused by intravenous Dilantin and its solvent. *Am Heart J* 74:523, 1967.

164. York RC, Coleridge ST: Cardiopulmonary arrest following intravenous phenytoin loading. *Am J Emerg Med* 6:255, 1988.

165. Arulanantham K, Genel M: Central nervous system toxicity associated with ingestion of propylene glycol. *J Pediatr* 93:515, 1978.

166. Cate JC, Hedrick R: Propylene glycol intoxication and lactic acidosis. *N Engl J Med* 303:1237, 1980.

167. Demey H, Daelemans R, DeBroe ME, et al: Propylene glycol intoxication due to intravenous nitroglycerin. *Lancet* 1:1360, 1984.

168. Martin G, Finberg L: Propylene glycol: A potentially toxic vehicle in liquid dosage. *J Pediatr* 77:877, 1970.

169. Robinson CA, Scott JW, Ketchum C: Propylene glycol interference with ethylene glycol procedures. *Clin Chem* 29:727, 1983.

170. Gershanik JJ, Boecler B, George W, et al: The gasping syndrome: Benzyl alcohol (BA) poisoning? *Clin Res* 29:895, 1981.

171. Gershanik J, Boecler B, Ensley H, et al: The gasping syndrome and benzyl alcohol poisoning. *N Engl J Med* 307:1384, 1982.

172. Brown WJ, Buist NRM, Gipson HTC, et al: Fatal benzyl alcohol poisoning in a neonatal intensive care unit. *Lancet* 1:1250, 1982.

173. Diack SL, Lewis HG: Studies in the synthesis of hippuric acid in the animal organism. VIII. A comparison of the rate of elimination of hippuric acid after the ingestion of sodium benzoate, benzyl alcohol, and benzyl esters of succinic acid. *J Biol Chem* 77:89, 1928.

174. Little GA, Harper RG, Levy LI, et al: Benzyl alcohol: Toxic agent in neonatal units. *Pediatrics* 72:356, 1983.

175. Gennari FJ: Serum osmolality: Uses and limitations. *N Engl J Med* 310:102, 1984.

133. Anticholinergic Poisoning

Robert P. Ferm

Introduction

Poisoning from anticholinergic agents is a relatively common toxicologic emergency that can be induced by a long list of compounds. Frequently the result is a relatively consistent and recognizable syndrome known as anticholinergic toxidrome. Although most cases are relatively benign, there is potential for serious and life-threatening manifestations that may require admission to an intensive care unit for appropriate monitoring and on-going therapy. As with any toxicologic emergency, supportive care is of paramount importance. In addition, for anticholinergic poisoning, an effective antidote, physostigmine, is usually readily available. However, controversy surrounds its appropriate use.

Epidemiology/Sources

In 1992 the American Association of Poison Control Centers Toxic Exposure Surveillance System (AAPCC TESS) reported 3729 exposures to pharmaceuticals classified as anticholinergic [1]. Based on the population base served by these poison control centers (PCCs) it can be estimated that the national incidence of potential anticholinergic poisoning was in excess of 4750 exposures. As not all cases of exposure or even significant poisoning are reported, the true incidence is undoubtedly substantially greater. The 1992 AAPCC data indicate that approxi-

mately 12 percent of reported cases had an outcome classified as moderate or greater in severity, including a case fatality rate of 1 per 1000 exposures. It is important to note that these figures include only pharmaceuticals classified by the AAPCC TESS as anticholinergics, and exclude many drugs that may have significant anticholinergic effects, including H_1-blockers (31,465 exposures with 15 deaths), anticholinergic antispasmodics (1,675 exposures, 2 deaths), cough and cold preparations (107,980 exposures, 15 deaths), and anticholinergic plant and mushroom exposures (949 and 25 exposures, respectively; no deaths).

This frequency of occurrence is not surprising, considering the wide distribution of compounds with anticholinergic activity. Agents with these effects are found in a large number of over-the-counter (OTC) and prescription medications as well as in a large number of plants. In some cases the anticholinergic effect is precisely the legitimate reason for using the drug (e.g., atropine to treat bradycardia, induce mydriasis, inhibit secretions). In other cases the anticholinergic action is an undesirable side effect (e.g., cyclic antidepressants, antihistamines). Some pharmaceuticals and plants are intentionally abused for the mind-altering consequence of excessive anticholinergic influence [2–5], most familiarly jimson weed tea. Table 133-1 provides a partial list of agents with anticholinergic effects. Anticholinergic poisoning has been attributed to exposures occurring by a number of different routes in addition to ingestion. Toxicity has been reported following inhalation of nebulized medication [6], inhalation of pyrolysis products [7,8], transdermal use [9,10], and ocular instillation [11,12].

Table 133-1. Agents That Cause Anticholinergic Syndrome*

Pharmaceuticals	Plants
Antihistamines (H₁-blockers)	Myristicaceae
Brompheniramine	*Myristica fragrans* (nutmeg)
Carbinoxamine	Solanaceae
Chlorpheniramine	*Atropa belladonna* (deadly
Clemastine	nightshade)
Cyclizine	*Brugmansia arborea* (angel's
Cyproheptadine	trumpet)
Dimenhydrinate	*Brugmansia suaveolens* (angel's
Diphenhydramine	trumpet)
Hydroxyzine	*Cestrum diurnum* (day-bloom-
Meclizine	ing jessamine)
Pyrilamine	*Cestrum nocturnum* (night-
Promethazine	blooming jessamine)
Tripelennamine	*Cestrum parqui* (willow-leaved
Antiparkinsonian drugs	jessamine)
Benztropine	*Datura metel* (downy thorn ap-
Biperiden	ple)
Ethopropazine	*Datura stramonium* (jimson
Procyclidine	weed)
Trihexyphenidyl	*Hyoscyamus niger* (black hen-
Antipsychotics	bane)
Acetophenazine	*Lycium halimifolium* (matrimony
Chlorpromazine	vine)
Chlorprothixene	*Physalis heterophylla* (ground
Fluphenazine	cherry)
Haloperidol	*Solanum carolinensis* (wild to-
Loxapine	mato)
Molindone	*Solanum dulcamara* (bitter-
Perphenazine	sweet)
Prochlorperazine	*Solanum nigrum* (black night-
Thiothixene	shade)
Thioridazine	*Solanum pseudocapsicum* (Jeru-
Trifluoperazine	salem cherry)
Antispasmodics	*Solanum tuberosum* (potato)
Anisotropine	Verbenaceae
Clidinium	*Lantana camara* (wild sage)
Dicyclomine	Mushrooms
Isometheptene	*Amanita muscaria* (fly agaric)
Methantheline	*Amanita pantheria* (panther
Propantheline	mushroom)
Stramonium	
Tridihexethyl	
Belladonna alkaloids and related	
synthetic congeners	
Atropine (racemic hyoscya-	
mine)	
Glycopyrrolate	
Hyoscine	
Ipatropium	
Methscopolamine	
Scopolamine	
Cyclic antidepressants	
Amitriptyline	
Amoxapine	
Desipramine	
Doxepin	
Imipramine	
Maprotiline	
Nortriptyline	
Protriptyline	
Trimipramine	
Zimelidine	
Muscle relaxants	
Cyclobenzaprine	
Orphenadrine	
Mydriatics	
Cyclopentolate	
Homatropine	
Tropicamide	

*Many of these agents have other significant toxic manifestations in addition to their anticholinergic effects.

Pharmacology

For a better understanding of the clinical presentation of poisoning by anticholinergic agents, it is useful to review relevant physiology and pharmacology. The anticholinergic compounds are by definition those agents that antagonize the effects of the endogenous neurotransmitter acetylcholine (ACh). Receptors for ACh are widely distributed in the body, including the central nervous system (CNS) and peripheral nervous system (PNS) (including sympathetic and parasympathetic ganglia, parasympathetic end terminals, and the motor end plate). Acetylcholine receptors are divided into two types—muscarinic and nicotinic—based on their ability to bind the naturally occurring alkaloids muscarine and nicotine. This division has a functional significance as well, best described in the PNS, where muscarinic receptors predominate in the parasympathetic end terminals while nicotinic receptors are associated with autonomic ganglia and the motor end plate. Additional subtypes of these receptors have been described, but their clinical significance has not yet been fully elucidated [13]. Although there may be some cross-over, especially at high doses or concentrations, most exogenous compounds have predominant effects on one of the two main types of ACh receptor.

Clinical Presentation/Diagnosis

Nicotinic agonists, such as the prototype drug nicotine, cause stimulation of the nicotinic receptors, leading to tachycardia, hypertension, muscle fasciculations and receptor fatigue, with consequent paralysis at high doses.

Nicotinic antagonists, such as the nondepolarizing muscle relaxants pancuronium and vecuronium, block the action of ACh at the motor end plate and produce paralysis of skeletal muscle. This chapter does not discuss nicotinic agonists/antagonists further but focuses on those drugs with predominant activity at the muscarinic receptors. Excessive stimulation of muscarinic receptors (e.g., in poisoning by cholinesterase inhibitors such as the organophosphate and carbamate insecticides) leads to the muscarinic cholinergic toxidrome recalled by the mnemonic *DUMB BELS*: *D*efecation, *U*rination, *M*iosis, *B*radycardia, *B*ronchorrhea, *E*mesis, *L*acrimation, and *S*alivation (see Chap. 137).

Blockade of ACh at muscarinic receptors may lead to the typical anticholinergic toxidrome. In a simplified version this has been described by the mnemonic:

> *Blind* as a bat
> *Hot* as Hades
> *Dry* as a bone
> *Red* as a beet
> *Mad* as a hatter

where reference is made to ciliary muscle paralysis, hyperthermia, anhydrosis, vasodilatation, and delirium. This toxidrome has been subdivided into those signs and symptoms due to quaternary amine (charged) anticholinergics (e.g., glycopyrrolate), which poorly penetrate the blood-brain barrier and give rise to the *peripheral anticholinergic syndrome,* versus those due to tertiary amine (uncharged) drugs (e.g., atropine), which more readily reach the CNS and result in the additional manifestations of the *central anticholinergic syndrome.* Table 133-2 provides a more complete listing of the symptoms attributable to peripheral and central antimuscarinic effects. The most commonly reported findings include sinus tachycardia, dry mucous membranes, mydriasis, urinary retention, and ileus. The most serious manifestations include agitated delirium, hyperthermia, seizures, and respiratory failure.

Table 133-2. Manifestations of the Anticholinergic Syndrome

Peripheral anticholinergic signs/symptoms
    Tachycardia
    Dry, flushed skin
    Dry mucous membranes
    Dilated pupils (variable)
    Hyperpyrexia
    Urinary retention
    Decreased bowel sounds
    Hypertension
    Hypotension (may be late finding)
Central anticholinergic signs/symptoms
    Confusion
    Disorientation
    Loss of short-term memory
    Ataxia
    Incoordination
    Psychomotor agitation
    Picking or grasping movements
    Extrapyramidal reactions
    Visual/auditory hallucinations
    Frank psychosis
    Coma
    Seizures
    Respiratory failure
    Cardiovascular collapse

Modified from Kirk M, Kulig K, Rumack BH: Anticholinergics, in Haddad LM, Winchester JF (eds): *Clinical Management of Poisoning and Drug Overdose.* 2nd ed. Philadelphia, WB Saunders, 1990, p 863. With permission.

The clinical presentation may be complicated by other pharmacologic actions of the ingested drug (e.g., type Ia antidysrhythmic, alpha-adrenergic blocking, and norepinephrine reuptake blocking effects of a cyclic antidepressant [CA]) or the actions of coingested compounds (e.g., salicylates, beta-adrenergic blockers, sympathomimetics). In the setting of CA (including cyclobenzaprine) overdose in particular, the anticholinergic effects (sinus tachycardia, hypertension) are the most commonly noted but of less clinical importance than the other pharmacologic actions (sodium channel blockade), necessitating a different therapeutic approach, such as sodium bicarbonate (see Chap. 140).

Evaluation and Treatment

Initial assessment and therapy must proceed rapidly and concurrently in the poisoned patient as in any critically ill patient. The first priority is evaluation and provision of support to the standard ABC's of airway, breathing, and circulation. In any potentially critically ill patient intravenous access should be obtained, supplemental oxygen provided, and cardiac monitoring initiated. Initial rapid assessment should include obtaining the six vital signs: temperature, heart rate, blood pressure, respiratory rate, pulse oximetry, and mental status. Any patient with alteration in mental status should also have rapid determination of the pulse oximetry or arterial blood gas status as indicated and rapid (bedside) determination of blood glucose concentration. If this is not immediately available, empiric treatment with $D_{50}W$ ($D_{25}W$ in infants) should be given. Accompanying glucose therapy with parenteral thiamine should be considered. In certain clinical settings, patients with altered mental status may receive naloxone (and possibly flumazenil). An electrocardiogram should be obtained on most patients with possible ingestion to evaluate for manifestations of potential cardiac toxins. A general toxicology screen is unlikely to be of

assistance, but a serum acetaminophen level should be considered. In certain settings quantitative levels of other drugs, such as salicylate, lithium, and theophylline, may prove helpful. In many cases, the toxicology screen is negative despite clear presence of an anticholinergic toxidrome [14]. Other potentially useful laboratory tests include serum electrolyte, renal function, and hemoglobin/hematocrit evaluation. Additional laboratory studies may be obtained as indicated but should not be ordered indiscriminately.

Gastrointestinal (GI) decontamination should be considered in all patients who present with anticholinergic poisoning following an ingestion. Due to delayed gastric emptying and impaired gut motility, this may prove beneficial even several hours after ingestion. Many toxicologists favor gastric lavage if gastric emptying is to be attempted; syrup of ipecac is rarely used in the hospital setting. Induction of emesis is specifically contraindicated in the patient with actual or potential obtundation, seizures, or other conditions leading to impairment of protective airway reflexes. Protection of the airway with a cuffed endotracheal tube may be necessary before orogastric lavage with a large-bore hose (e.g., 40 Fr. in an adult). A more complete discussion of the options for gastric emptying can be found in Chapter 128.

Activated charcoal (AC) is becoming the primary approach to GI decontamination in the hospital setting. In most cases of anticholinergic poisoning due to ingestion, even those presenting hours after ingestion, AC should be administered in the standard recommended dose of approximately 1 gm per kilogram of body weight (50–100 gm in the average adult). Multiple-dose AC may be considered, but repeated doses should not be given in the setting of ileus or obstruction due to the risk of impaction and/or aspiration. A cathartic should be given no more than once every 24 hours.

Patients displaying only minor signs (minor sinus tachycardia, dry mucous membranes) may be observed for 6 to 8 hours. If there is no progression of anticholinergic signs, the patient may be medically cleared for psychiatric evaluation or discharge, as appropriate. Patients with progression of signs and symptoms and those presenting with moderate or severe signs or symptoms (including delirium, hyperthermia, significant obtundation, convulsions, or hemodynamically unstable sinus tachycardia or other dysrhythmia), should have more aggressive treatment. Admission to an intensive care setting is appropriate.

Further interventions that may be indicated include placement of an indwelling catheter for bladder decompression, sedation with benzodiazepines (phenothiazines, butyrophenones, and other agents that have anticholinergic activity should be avoided), aggressive cooling measures (e.g., evaporative cooling with tepid sponging/fanning), anticonvulsant therapy with benzodiazepines and/or phenobarbital, and circulatory support with intravenous fluids and pressors.

Antidotal Therapy

Specific antidotal therapy with the acetylcholinesterase (AChE) inhibitor physostigmine may be indicated in limited circumstances. Physostigmine reversibly binds to AChE and prevents the action of this enzyme from degrading ACh, thereby allowing the neurotransmitter to persist and accumulate in more effective levels at its postsynaptic sites of action. Physostigmine, as opposed to similar drugs such as neostigmine and pyridostigmine, is a tertiary rather than a quaternary amine. This uncharged state allows more effective penetration across the blood-brain barrier, resulting in reversal of central as well as peripheral anticholinergic effects. When given in appropriate doses, physostigmine is clearly effective in reversing the effects of ACh blockade, including the CNS, cardiovascular, and GI effects.

Physostigmine, like any powerful drug, is not without risk. When administered in excessive amounts or to a patient not in an anticholinergic state, signs and symptoms of cholinergic excess may appear. These include potentially serious and life-threatening manifestations, such as bronchospasm, bronchorrhea, seizures, and asystole. Several case reports [15,16] and animal studies [17] describing adverse outcome with physostigmine have led to a reduction in its use. However, recently there has been interest in a more restrained role for physostigmine in specific clinical situations [18].

Specific indications for the use of physostigmine in anticholinergic toxicity include anticholinergic seizures, severe symptomatic hypertension with evidence of acute end organ injury, life-threatening arrhythmias with resultant cardiac ischemia or end organ hypoperfusion, and severe hallucinations or agitated delirium not responding to benzodiazepine sedation and requiring physical or excessive chemical restraint to protect the patient from self-harm or from harming others. Altered mental status or coma alone may be a relative indication.

Contraindications to the use of physostigmine [19] include asthma, gangrene, diabetes, cardiovascular disease, mechanical obstruction of the intestine or urogenital tract, any vagotonic state, or use of choline esters or depolarizing neuromuscular blocking agents (e.g., succinylcholine, decamethonium). Overly rapid administration of physostigmine has resulted in seizures and asystole.

Any patient receiving physostigmine must be on a cardiac monitor and under continuous careful observation. Recommendations for the safe use of physostigmine include dilution of the dose in 10 ml of D_5W or normal saline and slow intravenous infusion over 5 minutes or longer. The recommended dose for adults is a test dose of 0.5 mg followed by 1.5 mg infused over 5 minutes. If no reversal of anticholinergic effect has occurred after a 20-minute observation period and signs of cholinergic excess have not appeared, an additional 1 to 2 mg may be administered slowly. The recommended dose for a therapeutic trial in pediatric patients is 0.02 mg per kilogram up to 0.5 mg per minute administered by slow intravenous infusion. If toxic anticholinergic effects persist and there is no sign of cholinergic excess, the dosage may be repeated at 10- to 20-minute intervals until the therapeutic effect is achieved or a maximum dose of 2 mg is administered. The duration of action of physostigmine is 20 to 60 minutes, which is relatively short compared with many anticholinergic agents. If life-threatening anticholinergic signs or symptoms recur, additional doses of 1 to 4 mg (adult) or 0.02 mg per kilogram (pediatric) may be administered by slow intravenous infusion over 5 to 10 minutes. If physostigmine overdose occurs and the patient develops signs of cholinergic crisis, atropine can be used to reverse these signs. Atropine should be carefully titrated to effect; a dose of one-half the physostigmine dose has been recommended. As the duration of physostigmine's effect is so brief, atropine may not be needed unless major, life-threatening signs of cholinergic excess are present.

Summary

A wide variety of common prescription and over-the-counter medications as well as plants can cause anticholinergic poisoning. Most cases are mild and self-limited, requiring no specific therapy. The potential exists for severe life-threatening effects, and some patients need intensive care monitoring and administration of physostigmine as antidotal therapy.

References

1. Litovitz TL, Holm KC, Clancy C, et al: 1992 annual report of the American Association of Poison Control Centers Toxic Exposure Surveillance System. *Am J Emerg Med* 11:494, 1993.
2. Knable MB: Euphorigenic properties of anticholinergics (letter). *J Clin Psychiatry* 50:186, 1989.
3. Dilsaver SC: Antimuscarinic agents as substances of abuse. *J Clin Psychopharmacol* 8:14, 1988.
4. Chaconas NG: Jimson weed abuse. *Pharmacol Alert* 9:2, 1978.
5. Mikolich JR, Paulson GW, Cross CJ: Acute anticholinergic syndrome due to Jimson weed ingestion: Clinical and laboratory observation in six cases. *Ann Intern Med* 83:321, 1975.
6. Jannun DR, Mickel SF: Anisocoria and aerosolized anticholinergics. *Chest* 90:148, 1986.
7. Gowdy J: Stramonium intoxication: Review of symptomatology in 212 cases. *JAMA* 221:585, 1972.
8. Siegel RK: Herbal intoxication: Psychoactive effects from herbal cigarettes, tea, and capsules. *JAMA* 236:473, 1976.
9. Wilkinson JA: Side effects of transdermal scopolamine. *J Emerg Med* 5:389, 1987.
10. Ziskind AA: Transdermal scopolamine-induced psychosis. *Postgrad Med* 84:73, 1988.
11. Delberghe X, Zegers de Beyl D: Repeated delirium from homatropine eye-drops. *Clin Neurol Neurosurg* 89:53, 1987.
12. Reid D, Fulton JD: Tachycardia precipitated by topical homatropine (letter). *Br Med J* 299:795, 1989.
13. Gilman AG, Rall TW, Nies AS, Taylor P (eds): *Goodman and Gilman's The Pharmacological Basis of Therapeutics.* 8th ed. New York, Pergamon, 1990.
14. Goldfrank L, Flomenbaum N, Lewin N, et al: Anticholinergic poisoning. *J Toxicol Clin Toxicol* 19:17, 1982.
15. Walker WE, Levy RC, Hanenson IB: Physostigmine: Its use and abuse. *JACEP* 5:436, 1976.
16. Pentel P, Peterson CD: Asystole complicating physostigmine treatment of tricyclic antidepressant overdose. *Ann Emerg Med* 9:588, 1980.
17. Vance MA, Ross SM, Millington WR, Blumberg JB: Potentiation of tricyclic antidepressant toxicity by physostigmine in mice. *Clin Toxicol* 11:413, 1977.
18. Smilkstein MJ: Editorial. *J Emerg Med* 9:275, 1991.
19. Product information: Antilurium (physostigmine salicylate). *Physicians' Desk Reference.* 47th ed. Montvale, NJ, 1993.

134. Anticonvulsant Toxicity

Thomas E. Kearney and
Cynthia K. Aaron

Phenytoin

Phenytoin (diphenylhydantoin), introduced as an anticonvulsant in 1938, is the most commonly used antiseizure medication [1]. It is used in the treatment of generalized tonic-clonic, partial complex, and focal seizures [2] and in the treatment of trigeminal neuralgia. Although chemically related to the barbiturates, it is not a member of that class. Phenytoin has type IB antiarrhythmic properties and was the antiarrhythmic of choice for digitalis toxicity before the advent of digitalis Fab fragments [2] (see Chap. 141).

Phenytoin intoxications may occur accidentally, especially in children, or by deliberate overdose in older age groups [3–10]. Iatrogenic intoxications may occur with drug interactions, since the distribution, protein binding, and clearance of phenytoin are affected by other medications and disease states. Occasionally, toxicity may occur when the daily administered dose exceeds the patient's ability to metabolize and eliminate the drug [3,8,11]. Toxicity may result when switching dosage forms or between generic and proprietary forms of the drug because of different release and absorption characteristics. Finally, there are idiosyncratic and hypersensitivity reactions associated with therapeutic usage that are unrelated to dose; these are most commonly seen in patients with underlying neurologic disorders [12].

PHARMACOLOGY. Chemically, phenytoin is a weak acid, with a pKa of 8.5. It is soluble only in alkaline media, so the parenteral form must be prepared in a propylene glycol vehicle. This soluble form precipitates in an acidic medium but can be diluted into normal saline (pH 5.0) if administered immediately [3]. Phenytoin should not be administered as an intramuscular injection, because of the risk of musular necrosis, severe pain, and erratic absorption (see Chap. 213).

Since phenytoin is soluble in alkaline solutions, it is poorly absorbed in gastric acid [13]. Absorption occurs in the duodenum but depends on multiple factors, including dosage form, gastric emptying, and bowel motility. Peak levels are seen between 2.6 and 8.9 hours after oral dosing of an extended-release capsule. In overdosage, absorption may continue for up to 7 days, possibly due to decreased gastric motility and pharmacobezoar formation [4]. Phenytoin has a small volume of distribution (V_d 0.6 L/kg) and distributes preferentially into the brainstem and cerebellum [14]. It is highly protein-bound to albumin; decreased protein binding via receptor competition increases the free, pharmacologically active form of the drug. This increases free drug levels and the V_d. Since usually only total phenytoin levels are measured, toxicity from increased free phenytoin may occur at lower total phenytoin levels [11].

Hepatic metabolism occurs by enzymes that saturate at plasma levels of approximately 10 μg per milliliter [13]. Otherwise, metabolism follows first-order elimination kinetics, with an average half-life of 22 hours (range 7–55 hours). When plasma levels exceed 10 μg per milliliter, metabolism follows zero-order elimination kinetics, yielding a much longer half-life. The enzyme system may be induced or inhibited by other drugs, inherited genetic disturbances, or liver disease [15,16].

The anticonvulsant effects of phenytoin occur with plasma levels between 10 and 20 μg per milliliter. This can be achieved within 45 to 60 minutes by an intravenous loading dose of 15 to 20 mg per kilogram [3], by oral loading of 15 to 20 mg per kilogram over 24 hours, or by oral maintenance dosing over 5 to 7 days. The rate of intravenous administration should not exceed 50 mg per minute because of toxicity from propylene glycol [17]. Phenytoin has been successfully administered by the interosseus route in children with poor venous access. Maintenance dosing is usually 4 to 6 mg/kg/day in single or divided doses, although neonates may require higher doses (5–8 mg/kg/day) [18].

Single ingestions of more than 20 mg per kilogram have resulted in acute toxicity. Death from isolated phenytoin ingestions is unusual but has been reported in young children with ingestions of 100 to 220 mg per kilogram [7,19]. Survival has been reported with an ingestion of 249 mg per kilogram and a 70-hour level of 112 μg per milliliter in a child [9]. In adults, moderate CNS toxicity and recovery have occurred with ingestions of 12 to 25 gm and a maximum level of 96 μg per milliliter at 96 hours postingestion [20]. Death results from CNS depression with respiratory insufficiency and hypoxia-related complications.

CLINICAL PRESENTATION. Toxicity resulting from acute and chronic intoxication has a similar presentation. Initially, phenytoin affects the cerebellar and vestibular function. With increasing toxicity, cerebral function is affected. Between levels of 20 and 40 μg per milliliter, the patient is mildly intoxicated, with symptoms of dizziness, blurred vision, diplopia, and nausea. Signs include ataxia, tremor, lethargy, vomiting, slurred speech, normal to dilated pupils, and nystagmus in all directions [21]. The patient may be excited and agitated. As levels increase, the patient becomes confused, develops hallucinations, and may appear psychotic. Progressive CNS depression occurs and nystagmus may improve. Pupillary response then becomes sluggish and the deep tendon reflexes diminish [8]. Severe toxicity occurs with levels greater than 90 μg per milliliter and is associated with coma and respiratory depression [9]. Electroencephalograms (EEGs) performed during phenytoin intoxication document slowing of alpha wave activity. As toxicity increases, brainstem evoked potentials are suppressed and may be absent. In patients with underlying neurologic deficits, the presentation may be altered. "Paradoxical intoxication" has been reported in this population, with findings of dystonia, dyskinesia, choreoathetoid movements, decerebrate rigidity, and increased seizure activity [8,28]. Patients with baseline focal neurologic deficits may show contralateral abnormalities, including hemianopia, hemianesthesia, and hemiparesis. Patients recover completely if no anoxic or hypoxic complications develop during acute toxicity. However, there is a case report of cerebellar atrophy following acute intoxication with phenytoin that was not known to be attributed to hypoxia [23]. Recovery may take 1 week or longer, depending on the rate of drug elimination.

An adult on a chronic regimen of phenytoin developed a severe hypernatremic coma associated with high serum phenytoin levels. It was suspected that phenytoin inhibited ADH secretion [22]. In rare instances, chronic toxicity has resulted in encephalopathy and cerebellar degeneration [14]. Chronic use of phenytoin causes hyperglycemia, vitamin D deficiency and osteomalacia, folate depletion, and megaloblastic anemia. Peripheral neuropathy has occurred. Other side effects include altered collagen metabolism that causes hirsutism, gingival hyperplasia, keratoconus, and hypertrichosis [24,25].

Other non-dose-dependent phenytoin side effects include hypersensitivity reactions, such as fever, rash, eosinophilia, hepatitis, lymphadenopathy, myositis, a lupuslike syndrome, rhabdomyolysis, nephritis, vasculitis, and hemolytic anemia [12]. Phenytoin administration during pregnancy has resulted in fetal hydantoin syndrome [26].

Phenytoin-induced cardiac effects result predominately from propylene glycol toxicity during intravenous drug administration. If phenytoin is infused at a rate greater than 50 mg per minute, bradycardia, hypotension, ventricular fibrillation, conduction defects, congestive failure, respiratory arrest, and asystole may result. If the rate of infusion is slowed or temporarily halted, these effects usually resolve spontaneously but may persist for 1 to 2 hours [5,19]. Direct cardiac toxic effects from oral phenytoin toxicity are rare and occur in patients with underlying cardiac disorders.

ANCILLARY EVALUATION. Laboratory evaluation of the phenytoin-intoxicated patient should include a complete blood count (CBC), electrolytes, BUN, creatinine, glucose, serum protein, albumin, and liver function tests. Sequential serum phenytoin levels (free and total, if available) should be followed. Because of the long elimination half-life of phenytoin, levels will not fall rapidly and can be checked every 12 to 24 hours. A toxicology screen may be indicated, depending on the circumstances surrounding the intoxication; serum levels of other anticonvulsants should be ascertained if necessary. In all deliberate overdoses, an acetaminophen level should be obtained. An arterial blood gas will assist in evaluation of the patient's respiratory status. Chest radiography should be performed in patients at risk for aspiration, and a baseline electrocardiogram (ECG) should be obtained. If the etiology of an altered mental status is not clear, then computed tomography (CT) and lumbar puncture may be necessary.

DIFFERENTIAL DIAGNOSIS. The differential diagnosis of phenytoin intoxication is quite varied. Other drug intoxications with similar presentation include sedative-hypnotic agents, other anticonvulsants, phencyclidine (PCP), neuroleptic agents, and other CNS depressant drugs. Medical conditions such as sepsis, CNS infection, tumor, trauma, seizure disorders, extrapyramidal syndromes, and postictal states may mimic phenytoin intoxication. Diabetic ketoacidosis and hyperosmolar nonketotic coma may present with similar findings [12]. Nystagmus may be present with therapeutic phenytoin levels, PCP intoxication, and cerebellar abnormalities. Nystagmus is occasionally absent with toxicity.

MANAGEMENT. Patients presenting with phenytoin intoxication should have a rapid evaluation of respiratory status followed by intubation if hypoxia or risk of aspiration is present. As always on initial evaluation, the patient should have intravenous access established and be placed on a cardiac monitor. If the mental status is abnormal, then $D_{50}W$, thiamine, and naloxone should be administered, followed by the appropriate work-up. Patients who are hyperglycemic from phenytoin in-

toxication can be treated with discontinuation of the drug; insulin therapy is rarely required. Flumazenil, the benzodiazepine antagonist, should be avoided in patients with a preexisting seizure disorder. It has no apparent role in managing phenytoin intoxication even if benzodiazepines are part of the polypharmacy overdose. The use of flumazenil in this situation may increase the risk of status epilepticus.

Hypotension occurring during phenytoin infusion should be treated with discontinuation of the infusion and administration of crystalloids. If this is unsuccessful in increasing blood pressure, pressors may be necessary. Hypotension from phenytoin intoxication itself is rare and represents significant toxicity. Treatment is fluid administration and pressors as needed.

Cardiac arrhythmias are unusual during intoxication and occur in patients with underlying cardiac abnormalities. Treatment is supportive, with use of the appropriate antiarrhythmics when indicated. Type IB antiarrhythmic agents should be avoided [27].

Seizures should be treated with benzodiazepines and administration of a different anticonvulsant. Phenytoin should not be continued.

Since phenytoin has a long elimination half-life, measures to increase the rate of elimination should be considered. Gastrointestinal decontamination includes gastric lavage and oral activated charcoal administration. Phenytoin undergoes enterohepatic recirculation with active gut secretion; multiple-dose oral activated charcoal can increase the rate of elimination [28] (see Guidelines for Multiple-Dose Activated Charcoal Therapy for Anticonvulsant Poisoning, below). Large ingestions (> 0.1 gm/kg or 5–10 gm total phenytoin) may require extra doses of activated charcoal to maintain the desired charcoal to drug ratio of 10:1 (see Carbamazepine and Management). Because phenytoin has a high degree of protein binding and hepatic elimination, forced diuresis, hemodialysis, and hemoperfusion have not been shown to be useful [9,10]. It is anticipated that hemofiltration would not be useful for similar reasons. Hemoperfusion can increase clearance by a small amount, but the risk in this case outweighs the benefit [29].

DISPOSITION. Since the majority of patients with phenytoin poisoning do well with supportive therapy alone, determining the degree of toxicity is important. Patients presenting with phenytoin intoxication should have sequential levels checked in the emergency department. The interval between obtaining serum samples for determination of phenytoin levels should be based on several factors, including severity of intoxication, rate of rise of levels, and time since exposure. Intervals should be more frequent during the initial evaluation phase, while absorption is still occurring, than later during the postabsorptive rehabilitative phase. In the emergency department during the initial evaluation, it is justifiable to obtain sequential levels every 2 to 3 hours to aid in the disposition of the patient and to determine continued absorption. Intervals of 1 day or longer may be appropriate in stable patients whose levels have peaked or started to decline. After administration of activated charcoal, the patient should be evaluated for progression of toxicity. Patients who are not grossly ataxic, have no underlying cardiac arrhythmia, can feed themselves, and are not at risk of hurting themselves can be discharged, providing levels are not rising and a caretaker is available. Patients who do not meet these criteria should be admitted. Thus, patients with rising levels, suicidal patients, patients living alone, and those with severe toxicity require admission. Intoxicated patients on chronic therapy should also be evaluated for effects such as anemia, osteomalacia, and peripheral neuropathy. Patients with a seizure disorder should be placed on seizure precautions due to the possibility of paradoxical seizures during the acute intoxication phase or breakthrough seizures during the rehabilitative phase. Breakthrough seizures occur when phenytoin levels are allowed to drop into the subtherapeutic range. Serum levels of other concurrently administered anticonvulsants also decline when multiple-dose activated charcoal is administered, increasing the risk of breakthrough seizures. In general, an observation period is necessary to ensure establishment of a therapeutic anticonvulsant regimen and documentation of stable therapeutic serum levels even after passage of charcoal stools. Severely toxic patients, those with underlying cardiac or CNS disease, intubated patients, or patients with rapidly progressive signs of toxicity require intensive care monitoring. All other patients usually do not require cardiac monitoring but still should be carefully observed to prevent injury from falling and ataxic limb movements.

Valproic Acid

Valproic acid (VA) and its derivatives represent one of the newer anticonvulsants marketed in the United States since 1978. Consequently, the bulk of published clinical experience is from the 1980s. Structurally unique among the anticonvulsants, VA is a low-molecular-weight (144.21) branched-chain carboxylic acid with a pKa of 4.8. It is used as monotherapy for absence seizures and in conjunction with other anticonvulsants to manage several types of partial and generalized seizure disorders and as a secondary agent for refractory status epilepticus [30,31].

Valproic acid is marketed as a sodium salt in a 250-mg capsule (Depakene), in a syrup solution of 250 mg per 5 ml, and in a pro-drug form, divalproex sodium. The latter is a molecular complex that dissociates in the gastrointestinal tract into two molecules of VA. Divalproex sodium is available as enteric-coated tablets (Depakote), with VA equivalency doses of 125, 250, and 500 mg. There is no parenteral dosage form available [30,31]. Therapeutic dosing is initiated at 15 mg per kilogram daily, with increases of 5 to 10 mg/kg/day at weekly intervals until a therapeutic endpoint is achieved. The suggested maximum daily dosage is 60 mg per kilogram, but the average required daily dose for adults ranges from 1 to 1.6 gm per day in divided doses administered two to four times daily. Some patients require daily doses of up to 2.6 gm [30,31,32]. Patients achieve therapeutic serum levels of VA (50–100 µg/ml) with maintenance doses in the range of 1.2 to 1.5 gm per day [32]. Steady-state levels are usually achieved within 2 to 3 days after initiation of maintenance dosing.

Valproic acid is thought to mediate its anticonvulsant effect by increasing cerebral and cerebellar levels of the inhibitory neurotransmitter GABA [33,34,35]. It may increase GABA levels by blocking metabolism through inhibition of GABA transferase and succinic aldehyde dehydrogenase.

PHARMACOKINETICS. Valproic acid's pharmacokinetic profile is significantly altered in an overdose setting. Within its therapeutic serum level range of 50 to 100 µg per milliliter, it is 80 to 95 percent serum protein-bound [32,36,37]. The degree of protein binding decreases as VA levels exceed 90 µg per milliliter, due to saturation of protein binding sites [32,37]. The resultant increase in free VA levels allows more extensive distribution into target organ systems and better than predicted extracorporeal drug removal. This has been evidenced by a higher cerebrospinal fluid to serum level and hemodialysis ex-

traction ratios in the VA-poisoned patient [38,39]. Protein binding of VA may be decreased in uremia (as with phenytoin) or in the presence of other highly protein-bound agents, such as acetylsalicylic acid (ASA). These displace VA from its binding sites [40]. Whenever a higher free fraction of VA is present, the patient may manifest more pronounced clinical effects for a given serum level. Consequently, the small volume of distribution (0.13–0.22 L/kg) is confined to the extracellular space, and it increases as the serum protein binding of VA decreases [32,36].

Valproic acid is highly bioavailable, with the time to peak serum levels after ingestion dependent on the dosage form and VA species (e.g., salt, free-acid). In capsule form, VA itself achieves peak serum levels after 1 to 4 hours in therapeutic dosing, while peak serum levels may be delayed 4 to 5 hours after ingestion of the enteric-coated divalproex sodium tablets [36]. This may be explained by the enteric coating dissolution time and the sequential process of intestinal conversion of divalproex to the sodium salt. This is followed by the final conversion to the free-acid, the only form absorbed from the GI tract. There is no evidence suggesting formation of pharmacobezoars from large numbers of VA tablets.

Valproic acid is metabolized predominantly by the liver, with 1 to 4 percent excreted unchanged in the urine [32,36]. It undergoes omega and beta oxidation to several metabolities: hydroxyvalproate, 2-propylgluturate (2-PG), 2-propyl-pent-4-enoate (PP-4-E), 5-hydroxyvalproate (5-OH-VPA), and 4-hydroxyvalproate (4-OH-VPA). The metabolites undergo glucuronidation and biliary excretion, with a possible enterohepatic recirculation [38,41]. These metabolites have a significant impact on the evaluation and management of the overdose patient and have been implicated in the metabolic perturbations observed in overdose patients. The metabolites interfere with urine ketone determinations, may be the hepatotoxic mediators of VA, and are highly cross-reactive on Enzyme-Multiplied Immunoassay Technique (EMIT) assays for VA [38]. The extent of the contributory role of each of these in an overdose setting is not known. It has been suggested that certain metabolic pathways, such as omega oxidation, may saturate at high doses of VA, leading to a decrease in total body clearance [38]. At therapeutic levels, the elimination half-life for VA is in the range of 5 to 20 hours (average 10.6 hours), but in an overdose it may extend to 30 hours [30,36].

PHARMACODYNAMICS. Valproic acid can prevent pentylenetetrazol-induced seizures by increasing GABA levels [30,33,34]. The onset of therapeutic effect requires several days to a week, although VA may work rapidly with rectal administration during treatment of refractory status epilepticus. Valproic acid exhibits CNS depressant properties, resulting in a decreased level of consciousness. This may range from obtundation to deep coma, but it lacks the cerebellar-vestibular effects of the other anticonvulsants. Valproic acid disrupts amino acid and fatty acid metabolism [42,43]. This may result in encephalopathy associated with hyperammonemia at therapeutic levels of VA [44].

Serum VA levels may be inconsistent with clinical effect because of several variables. These include the chronicity of usage with different levels of tolerance, alterations in VA protein binding, the synergistic or additive influence of sedative-hypnotics, and the presence of other metabolic abnormalities. Mental status changes have been described in patients with levels of 113 to 120 µg per milliliter, while other patients have lacked any CNS symptomatology and require levels up to 150 µg per milliliter [45]. The widespread availability and use of the EMIT assay for VA also contributes to this variability, since the assay cross-reacts with metabolites in an overdose. There may be an overestimation of serum VA levels as high as 50 percent with the EMIT assay. This would not be seen with the more specific gas or liquid chromatography assays [38].

TOXICOLOGY. The adverse and toxic effects of VA are due to an interplay of multiple factors. These include CNS depressant activity leading to respiratory failure and pulmonary complications. It disrupts fatty acid and amino acid metabolism, which in turn may contribute indirectly to the CNS depressant effects acutely and to other target organ toxicity chronically. There may be a link between VA- and opiate-induced CNS toxicity because of their similar influence on the GABA-nergic systems [46,47]. Since VA and its metabolites are low-molecular-weight, branched-chain carboxylic acids, they may be used as substrates for several enzymatic processes. This leads to inhibition of critical biochemical pathways, such as the urea cycle, and subsequent fatalities in some sensitive patient populations. Death has occurred after therapeutic doses of VA in patients with a congenital deficiency of ornithine carbamoyltransferase [48]. In addition, a frequently fatal Reyes-like hepatitis has been observed in patients receiving therapeutic doses. Those at greatest risk appear to be very young patients (< 2 years of age), patients being treated with multiple anticonvulsants, and those with other long-term neurologic complications. The fatality rate is 1 of 500 in this patient population [49]. This hepatotoxic reaction occurs in chronic exposure and may be mediated by metabolites formed via the cytochrome P-450 pathway. These metabolites, in turn, depress fatty acid oxidation in the hepatocyte mitochondria [50]. This effect may parallel that seen after ingestion of ackee fruit containing hypoglycine, causing Jamaican vomiting sickness [50]. Valproic acid can produce a hyperammonemia and encephalopathy exclusive of the hepatotoxic reaction [44].

Valproate as the sodium salt provides a significant sodium load (13.8 mg sodium/100 mg VA) in overdose. Valproic acid and its metabolites are low-molecular-weight and osmotically active free-acid or anionic species. They may produce a slightly elevated osmolar gap and an elevated anion gap metabolic acidosis with a reduction in circulating endogenous cations, particularly calcium [38,42,51–54].

The morbidity and mortality from dose-related acute or acute superimposed on chronic VA poisoning appear to be related to hypoxic sequelae from respiratory failure, aspiration, or terminal cardiorespiratory arrest [38,51,52,53,55]. It has been speculated that VA has a direct irreversible neurotoxic effect. This has not been substantiated nor reproduced, and it is indistinguishable from hypoxic-related injury [53].

TOXICITY. The lowest reported acutely ingested fatal dose of VA is 15 gm (12 gm absorbed, or 750 mg/kg) in a 20-month-old child. Adults have survived ingestion of as much as 75 gm [42,51]. In a large series of VA poisonings, patients ingesting greater than 200 mg per kilogram were at high risk for significant CNS depression [56]. Patients dying from acute VA poisoning have had peak serum levels of VA ranging from 106 to 2728 μg per milliliter, while survival has been reported in a patient with a peak serum level of 2120 μg per milliliter [42,51,55]. In general, serum levels of 180 μg per milliliter or greater may be associated with coma and respiratory depression, whereas levels exceeding 1000 μg per milliliter are usually associated with serious CNS toxicity, including deep coma and apnea, and significant metabolic perturbations (acidosis, hypocalcemia) [42,51,55,57,58]. The duration of toxicity is dependent on the patient's body burden and peak serum level. Toxicity is influenced by methods to hasten VA elimination as well as the development of any secondary hypoxia-related complications. Based on normal population endogenous VA clearance, in a patient with a serum level greater than 1000 μg per milliliter it would take approximately 3 days for the serum level to drop within the therapeutic range. Most patients with serious acute VA poisoning manifest CNS toxicity for at least 24 hours, and this may extend to several days.

CLINICAL MANIFESTATIONS. The presentation of the VA-poisoned patient is similar in many respects to that of patients intoxicated with other anticonvulsants but is distinct in many other respects. The hallmarks of VA toxicity are global CNS-related depression in conjunction with unique metabolic changes. Non-dose-related toxicity (hepatic failure, pancreatitis, red cell aplasia, neutropenia, and alopecia) has not been reported in acute overdoses with high serum levels of VA. Pancreatitis is usually considered a non-dose-related effect but was observed in one case of severe VA intoxication (personal communication). Alopecia has been associated with both acute and chronic VA intoxication. In acute intoxications, vital signs may be abnormal, with hypotension, mild tachycardia, decreased respiratory rate, and elevated or depressed temperature. The mental status is altered, varying on a continuum from confusion and disorientation to obtundation and deep coma with respiratory failure. Patients with an underlying seizure disorder may have breakthrough seizures. Transient rises in serum transaminase levels have been observed without evidence of functional liver toxicity. Also reported are confusion, tremor, hallucinations, and hyperactivity. Another finding is miosis. Laboratory abnormalities observed in patients with high serum VA levels include an anion gap acidosis, hypocalcemia, hyperosmolality, and hypernatremia. Hyperammonemia associated with vomiting, lethargy, and encephalopathy may occur at therapeutic serum levels. Complications or delayed sequelae of severe intoxication include optic nerve atrophy, cerebral edema, acute respiratory distress syndrome (ARDS), and hemorrhagic pancreatitis. It has not been established whether these are direct VA effects or hypoxic-related sequelae, and they have been noted only in a few isolated case reports.

DIFFERENTIAL DIAGNOSIS. The differential diagnosis is broad and includes most CNS depressants. Valproic acid intoxication can be indistinguishable from opioid poisoning by signs and symptoms (coma, miosis, and respiratory depression), and VA-poisoned patients may occasionally respond to naloxone. Other causes of anion gap acidosis, especially ethylene glycol poisoning (anion gap, increased osmolar gap, and hypocalcemia), may present in a similar fashion but without nephrotoxicity. Since urine ketones are positive, aspirin toxicity, alcoholic ketoacidosis, and other causes of ketonuria are included in the differential diagnosis. Valproic acid should be included on the list of substances causing an increased anion gap metabolic acidosis (salicylate, methanol, uremia, diabetes, paraldehyde, phenformin, ibuprofen, iron, and isoniazid). It may also cause a false positive urine ketone determination, thereby misdirecting the clinician to causes of ketosis [42].

ANCILLARY EVALUATION. Laboratory evaluation of the VA-poisoned patient evolves around the quantitative VA serum level determinations and the patient's oxygenation status. Serial serum levels of VA are indicated, particularly after ingestion of the slowly dissolving enteric-coated dosage form, but it must be recognized that the EMIT assay may reflect a level 50 percent higher than actual. A serum panel should include electrolytes, BUN, creatinine, glucose, and calcium. Serum osmolality should be performed by freezing point depression. A quantitative arterial ammonia level may be useful. Potential alterations in VA protein binding caused by substances such as salicylate should always be considered and investigated. Liver function tests should be performed, and a coagulation profile assists in determining liver synthetic ability.

Arterial blood gas determinations are indicated to evaluate the progression of acidosis and hypoxemia from respiratory depression and ARDS. Although direct electrocardiographic changes are unusual, an ECG will help determine electrolyte abnormalities. A chest radiograph may be useful in the determination of ARDS. Since many of these patients have an underlying seizure disorder, comparison of their baseline EEG will be useful in evaluating seizure activity.

TREATMENT. As with any consequential ingestion, the patient requires immediate evaluation and airway management. Since VA is a respiratory depressant, early intubation and ventilation help prevent late hypoxic sequelae. Intravenous access and cardiographic monitoring should be established. Patients with an altered mental status should receive 25 to 50 gm of dextrose and 100 mg of thiamine intravenously.

Naloxone has been shown to increase the level of consciousness in selected patients with overdoses of VA [57,58]. In those case reports of VA poisoning in which there was a positive response to naloxone, the patients presented with profiles similar to that of opioid intoxication: miosis, coma, respiratory depression, and serum levels between 185 and 190 μg per milliliter. These patients were given 0.8 to 2.0 mg of naloxone intravenously. Patients with higher VA serum levels have not responded to larger doses of naloxone [55,59]. Naloxone has been shown experimentally to antagonize GABA, the inhibitory neurotransmitter increased by VA [46,47]. It is speculated that VA has an alternative mechanism of toxicity at higher serum levels; either the dose of naloxone necessary to influence GABA-nergic tone at high levels is much greater or those patients who responded may have had occult opiate intoxication. In all comatose patients with suspected VA poisoning, a trial of high-dose naloxone (up to 10 mg) is indicated, since the presentation of VA poisoning may mimic that of opioids. Flumazenil, the benzodiazepine antagonist, should be avoided in all patients with a preexisting seizure disorder. As with phenytoin, it has no apparent role in managing VA intoxication.

Patients with suspected VA ingestion should undergo a complete regimen of GI decontamination, even if several hours have elapsed since ingestion. Postmortem examination of a VA-poisoned decedent revealed several VA tablets in the stomach several hours after ingestion [60]. Gastric lavage and activated charcoal should be given (see Guidelines for Multiple-Dose Activated Charcoal Therapy, below). In the case of large ingestions (0.1 gm/kg or 5–10 gm total), additional doses of activated charcoal may be necessary to maintain the desired charcoal to drug ratio of 10:1 (see Carbamazepine Management).

After gut decontamination, additional methods to enhance elimination should be considered. In an overdose, the pharmacokinetic or toxicokinetic profile of VA changes, leading to a more favorable response to techniques that enhance elimination. This is attributed to an increase in the free serum circulating fraction (with a decrease in protein binding) and marked prolongation in elimination half-life. Theoretically, multiple-dose activated charcoal may enhance the clearance of VA by interrupting enterohepatic recirculation and gastrointestinal dialysis; however, to our knowledge, no data demonstrate the magnitude of its effect (see Multiple-Dose Activated Charcoal

Therapy). Severely poisoned patients may be treated with extracorporeal removal, such as hemodialysis or hemoperfusion. Valproic acid clearance in poisoned patients undergoing hemodialysis has been as high as 270 ml per minute, with a four to fivefold decrease in elimination half-life [39]. Hemodialysis has the added benefit of correction of metabolic disturbances secondary to VA and removal of its metabolites. In one such case report, in a patient with a level exceeding 2000 μg per milliliter, prompt institution of hemodialysis led to complete resolution of toxicity within 3 days, while a similar patient treated with supportive care only died [42,55]. The indications for hemodialysis are not clear, requiring a risk-benefit analysis on a case-by-case basis. In patients with levels exceeding 1000 μg per milliliter, extracorporeal drug removal should be seriously considered. In patients with levels exceeding 2000 μg per milliliter, it should certainly be considered a major form of treatment. Patients not responding to conventional therapy or who have severe metabolic abnormalities will benefit from hemodialysis. Prompt hemodialysis may greatly abbreviate a potentially prolonged comatose state and prevent any of the speculated direct neuropathic and metabolic disturbances that occur with very high body burdens of VA. Because of VA's extensive protein binding and predominate hepatic elimination, it is anticipated that forced diuresis, manipulation of urine pH, and hemofiltration would not be useful in the management of VA intoxication. Charcoal hemoperfusion used for VA intoxication has demonstrated clearance similar to that of hemodialysis [61, personal communication].

DISPOSITION. The disposition of the VA-poisoned patient is based on the severity of CNS toxicity, quantitative serum levels, evidence of hypoxic insult, and risk of secondary complications. The amount of VA ingested as determined by history may provide a rough estimate of the potential severity of the poisoning but should not solely dictate the final disposition. Ingestion of greater than 200 mg per kilogram of VA has the potential for significant CNS toxicity, but poor correlation exists between peak serum level and dose of VA ingested. In the reported case literature to date, all patients have manifested significant progressive toxicity within the first hour and did not demonstrate a cyclic vacillating pattern of symptoms. Patients with serum levels exceeding 150 μg per milliliter are at risk for CNS and respiratory depression and should be observed until levels return to the therapeutic range. Intoxicated patients with a seizure disorder should be placed on seizure precaution and observed until a stable anticonvulsant regimen can be established (see Phenytoin: Disposition). Patients with VA serum levels exceeding 1000 μg per milliliter are at high risk for serious prolonged toxicity and may require several days of intensive supportive care and extracorporeal treatment. The prognosis should be favorable if the patient has not suffered a hypoxic insult at some point during the clinical course.

Carbamazepine

Carbamazepine (CBZ), marketed as Tegretol, is an iminostilbene compound with a chemical structural backbone resembling that of the tricyclic antidepressants. It is stereochemically similar to phenytoin. It was first synthesized in the early 1950s and has long since been recognized as a well-tolerated and effective agent for the management of various types of seizure disorders, including generalized tonic-clonic, simple partial, and complex partial seizures. It is used for the treatment of trigeminal and glossopharyngeal neuralgias, tabetic pain, and affective disorders [62] (see Chap. 213).

PHARMACOKINETICS. The pharmacokinetics and toxicokinetics of CBZ are not well defined and are subject to significant inter- and intrapatient variability (see Chap. 213). Because of CBZ's physicochemical characteristics (un-ionized state and high lipophilicity), there is no parenteral dosage form, and the rate-limiting step for systemic absorption is tablet dissolution time [63]. Consequently, studies to determine bioavailability, volume of distribution, and clearance are extremely difficult to perform.

In overdose, systemic absorption of CBZ may be inconsistent over time. This leads to intermittent "surges" of drug released into the circulation and may cause unexpected clinical deterioration of patients. This may explain the "cyclic" coma associated with CBZ poisoning [64,65]. Patients have been reported to "relapse" into deep coma as late as 2 days after admission to the hospital; the relapse is coincident with a marked increase in plasma levels of CBZ, even after the patient has appeared to stabilize or improve clinically [64,66].

PHARMACOLOGY. Carbamazepine is approximately 80 percent protein-bound and may have twice the volume of distribution (V_d) of other anticonvulsants, such as phenytoin and phenobarbital. Carbamazepine's volume of distribution ranges from 1.4 to 3.0 liters per kilogram at toxic levels [67,68]. The difference in V_d is reflected in the peak and therapeutic range for CBZ being approximately half that of phenytoin or phenobarbital. Note that CBZ blood level prediction based on amount ingested and V_d may be unreliable; there is poor correlation between published accounts of amount ingested and peak blood levels.

Carbamazepine is predominantly metabolized in the liver, with 1 to 3 percent excreted unchanged in the urine. Endogenous clearance is reported as 0.6 to 1.3 ml/min/kg [62,67]. The variability in clearance may be attributed to alteration in the metabolic capabilities of hepatic enzymes, particularly the cytochrome P-450 system [62,69]. This system is subject to enhancement through autoinduction during chronic administration or, conversely, inhibition with concurrent administration of enzyme inhibitors such as erythromycin [70]. The elimination half-life of CBZ in naive users may exceed 24 hours, while in chronic users it may be less than 15 hours [62,63,67,71]. Half-life determinations of CBZ, especially in overdose, often are misleading due to erratic absorption and inability to determine the contribution of sustained absorption from the GI tract [71]. Most evidence suggests that CBZ undergoes first-order kinetics, although it is speculated that some of its metabolic pathways, such as epoxidation, may saturate at high levels [71].

Forty percent of CBZ is converted to the active metabolite CBZ-10,11-epoxide (CBZ-epoxide), further complicating the kinetic and toxicity profile of CBZ [62,65,66]. There is also an inactive metabolite formed. CBZ-epoxide has a shorter elimination half-life than CBZ (5–9.8 hours), and is, in turn, converted to the 10,11-dihydroxide [68,71]. CBZ-epoxide is much less protein-bound than the parent CBZ (50% vs. 80%) [71]. Steady-state serum levels of CBZ are achieved after 2 to 4 days of oral dosing. The therapeutic level is between 3 and 14 μg per milliliter. Within this range, side effects including nystagmus, ataxia, dizziness, and anorexia have been noted [67,72].

PHARMACODYNAMICS. Carbamazepine exerts its therapeutic effects in a manner parallel to that of phenytoin. Its side effect profile is similar to that of phenytoin. Carbamazepine is postulated to mediate its pharmacologic effects by several mechanisms, including reduction of neuronal ionic currents, alteration of neurotransmitter activity (norepinephrine, acetylcholine), enhancement of adenosine, stimulation of benzodiazepine receptors, and depression of evoked repetitive firings in neurons and the brainstem reticular formation [62]. Collectively, these account for the beneficial therapeutic effects of CBZ as an anticonvulsant, for specialized analgesic properties, and for management of affective disorders. Carbamazepine may be best described as a CNS depressant with anticholinergic activity and a proclivity for alteration of the cerebellar-vestibular brainstem function.

Carbamazepine has been incorrectly described as similar to tricyclic antidepressants (TCAs) in its toxicity profile [65,73, 74,75]. However, other than shared sedative and anticholinergic properties, there are significant differences between the two. These dissimilarities include CBZ's therapeutic index and inability to precipitate malignant cardiac arrhythmias and seizures in patients with a normal myocardium and without underlying neurologic deficits. The membrane-stabilizing properties and sequelae of the TCAs have not been reported for CBZ. However, in overdose with extremely high CBZ levels, arrhythmias have been reported.

TOXICOLOGY. Carbamazepine toxicity can be defined as either dose-dependent or non-dose-dependent. Non-dose-dependent toxicity includes idiosyncratic and immunologic-mediated reactions, which are responsible for the majority of CBZ-related fatalities [67,76,77] and are recognized in the course of chronic therapeutic dosing. Non-dose-dependent toxicity includes bone marrow suppression, hepatitis, tubulointerstitial renal disease, cardiomyopathy, hyponatremia, and exfoliative dermatitis [67,76,77,78]. Dose-related effects in sensitive populations include those with existing neurologic deficits and myocardial disease.

Dose-related toxicity has been reported in acute overdoses, with survival in adults after 80-gm ingestions. Death has been reported after ingestion of 60 gm acutely and after a 6-gm ingestion in a patient on chronic maintenance therapy [74, 79,80].

Life-threatening symptoms (respiratory depression) have been observed after acute ingestion of as little as 10 gm (50 tablets) in an adult [81]. In one child, a 148-mg per kilogram ingestion resulted in deep coma and seizures [68].

Significant neurologic toxicity and death have been described, with peak levels ranging from 20 to 65 μg per milliliter [64,66,68,72,74,75,80–89] At plasma levels in the range of 10 to 20 μg per milliliter, patients usually respond to verbal stimuli, unless other coexisting medical complications or additional sedative-hypnotic substances are present [72]. However, there is poor correlation between amount ingested and peak serum level. The reasons include acute or chronic ingestions, erratic CBZ absorption, the impact of GI decontamination procedures, the uncontrolled regimens used in determining serial blood levels, and differences in assay procedures.

Since levels and clinical outcome do not coincide, prognosis appears dependent on occurrence of respiratory depression and aspiration of gastric contents [65,66,72,74,75,80–84,87,88, 90]. All reported deaths occurred in patients with a history of seizure disorders. Surviving patients may have a protracted course (days to weeks) because of secondary complications arising from hypoxic-related sequelae from respiratory and CNS depression, prolonged GI absorption, and a prolonged elimination half-life. All of these variables may lead to an extremely deceptive course, with sudden deterioration occurring after admission [64,66].

The kinetics of CBZ toxicity are affected by the active metabolite, CBZ-epoxide, which may partially account for the lack of correlation between peak levels of the parent compound and the severity of symptoms. While the concentration of CBZ-epoxide is only 40 percent that of the parent compound, its concentration in the free unbound form may be equal to or greater than that of CBZ [91]. Carbamazepine-epoxide is less protein-bound and may be produced at higher rates in patients who have undergone autoinduction of the epoxidation process. It is probably a significant contributor to the toxicity observed during overdose, because CBZ and its epoxide have additive toxic effects [92,93]. The CBZ-epoxide has been shown to cross-react with the parent CBZ compound on EMIT assays. This does not occur with high-performance liquid chromatography (HPLC) [68].

Toxicity may occur by gradual accumulation of CBZ in patients receiving therapeutic dosing because of improper dosing protocols or as a result of a drug interaction with enzyme inhibitors such as erythromycin or verapamil [70]. Carbamazepine toxicity may result after accidental overdose in children, after deliberate overdose in patients with affective disorders, and by accidental misuse in patients with chronic pain syndromes [94,95].

CLINICAL MANIFESTATIONS AND DIAGNOSTIC EVALUATION.

Patients with acute and chronic exposures have similar findings, except for movement disorders in patients with preexisting neurologic deficits. Key findings suggestive of CBZ poisoning include the triad of coma, anticholinergic syndrome, and adventitious movements [75]. In patients without preexisting neurologic deficits, movement disorders have occurred but have been described as more choreoathetoid or ballismus in character [86].

Physical examination will reveal features consistent with sedative-hypnotic toxicity but with pronounced effects on the cerebellar-vestibular system, central and peripheral anticholinergic toxicity, and neuroleptic-type movement disorders. All other effects, including conduction defects, are not clearly reproducible and may be indirectly related to hypoxia or occur in specialized patient populations. Signs and symptoms include hypotension, hypothermia, respiratory depression, obtundation progressing to deep coma, diminished or exaggerated deep tendon reflexes, and dysarthria. Conversely, the patient may be agitated and restless, combative, or irritable, may experience hallucinations, or may have seizures. Signs consistent with cerebellar-vestibular dysfunction include nystagmus, ataxia, ophthalmoplegia, diplopia, absent doll's eyes, and absent caloric reflexes. Anticholinergic findings are hyperthermia, sinus tachycardia, hypertension, urinary retention, mydriasis, and ileus. Physical findings consistent with neurotransmitter imbalance include oculogyric crisis, dystonia, opisthotonus, choreoathetosis, and ballismus. Because CBZ has both prolonged absorption from the GI tract and a prolonged elimination half-life, the clinical course may be extremely protracted and deceptive, and sudden deterioration may occur days after admission [64,66].

Although seizures have been reported in CBZ overdose, their occurrence has never been fully elucidated. Many patients receiving CBZ have preexisting neurologic deficits; these patients may have threshold levels and a spectrum of neurologic effects that differ from those of a normal patient population. Anecdotal case reports suggest that seizures associated with high levels of CBZ occur predominantly in patients in this population. These seizures were self-limited or responded to intravenous diaze-

pam and phenytoin [68,82]. Other reports are unclear as to whether witnessed motor activity was a true seizure or if the seizure occurred primarily or was secondary to hypoxic insult [64,65,72,73,75,81,90]. Patients with neurologic deficits on chronic CBZ dosing may develop movement disorders with toxic CBZ levels. These movements range from initial intermittent dystonias and culminate in sustained opisthotonic posturing. All movement abnormalities resolved as blood levels declined [96].

A final adverse effect reported with CBZ toxicity relates to abnormal myocardial conduction. These conduction abnormalities include prolongation of the P–R, QRS, and Q–T intervals and complete heart block [65,81,87,89,97]. Patients with an underlying abnormal conduction system may be at particular risk for the development of complete heart block [98]. However, in the majority of published cases, no conduction defects were noted by ECG monitoring when CBZ levels were extremely high or peaking [73,74,75,86,88,90,92]. Either conduction disturbances occurred long after the patient suffered a significant hypoxic insult with a diminishing CBZ level or there was a borderline prolongation of the measured interval that did not progress to a malignant arrhythmia. None of the published cases of CBZ poisoning noted the need for antiarrhythmic therapy in their patients.

Evaluation of the patient with suspected CBZ poisoning should focus on identification of high risk for neurologic and cardiovascular toxicity as well as oxygenation status. Patients should be assessed for the presence of drug masses, or pharmacobezoars, in the GI tract. Procedures to evaluate these patients should be tailored to the individual case. Continuous ECG monitoring has been recommended for CBZ-poisoned patients [62,65,72,82]. Since significant cardiac arrhythmias may occur only in a special population, these patients should be identified as high risk and placed on routine ECG monitoring. Because pulmonary complications may be the best predictor of outcome, radiologic and arterial blood gas determinations should be made in obtunded patients and those with a history suggestive of aspiration risk or apneic episode, including postictal patients. Patients on chronic CBZ therapy may be at risk for non-dose-related CBZ toxicity and require a baseline CBC, serum electrolyte levels, and hepatic and renal function determinations. Patients with a preexisting seizure disorder presenting with adventitial movement activity or in a convulsive state may require a more specific and sensitive neurologic evaluation, including EEG monitoring. It may be useful to compare EEG findings with previous records and follow the EEG as the CBZ level declines or if other anticonvulsants are administered [85,99].

A crucial part of patient evaluation is determination of quantitative serum levels of CBZ and its active metabolite, CBZ-epoxide. Although the EMIT assay may be readily accessible, it has the disadvantage of cross-reactivity between the parent CBZ and CBZ-epoxide, resulting in a falsely elevated CBZ reading. However, the clinical consequence of this is debatable. The HPLC assay has the ability to resolve between the parent compound and metabolite. Using the ratio of CBZ concentration to CBZ-epoxide, an index can be generated that may reflect the rapidity of absorption of CBZ from the GI tract. A ratio greater than 2.5 is evidence of continuing absorption of drug from the GI tract. This should be monitored with serial levels. We suspect that in cases where patients appeared to relapse or deteriorate, this could be attributed to an abrupt increase in absorption occurring as late as 48 hours after the initial ingestion [64,66,74,82,89]. In cases where serial levels of the parent and metabolite were monitored, the ratio greatly increased just prior to and coincident with the clinical deterioration [64,66,89]. In patients at risk for delayed absorption of CBZ, attempts may be made to visualize masses of the drug in the GI tract by instilling a water-soluble contrast medium; CBZ itself is not radiopaque [80,100]. After GI decontamination, visualization is suggested for patients who have taken a large number of tablets or have clinical and laboratory evidence of continued absorption of CBZ from the GI tract.

The prognosis of CBZ-poisoned patients is complicated and must take into consideration the interplay of the potential sequelae of CNS and respiratory depression. Patients who have suffered a hypoxic insult, aspirated, had persistent or multiple seizures, been in a deep coma (serum levels >20 μg/ml), or harbored CBZ pharmacobezoars require several days to weeks of hospitalization. These are the patients at greatest risk for morbidity and mortality.

DIFFERENTIAL DIAGNOSIS. The differential diagnosis in CBZ intoxication is extensive because the clinical presentation mimics that of overdose of sedative-hypnotics, anticholinergic agents, and other anticonvulsants. In patients on CBZ for seizure control it may be difficult to distinguish between an exacerbation of their underlying disease state and CBZ toxicity. The definitive diagnosis of dose-dependent CBZ toxicity is made by quantitation and demonstration of high serum levels of CBZ and CBZ-epoxide. Random toxicology screening of blood or urine has rarely led to the diagnosis of CBZ toxicity; it is mainly a clinical diagnosis. In addition, there are no specific pharmacologic antagonists to aid in the diagnosis.

MANAGEMENT. The criteria for disposition and management of CBZ dose-related toxicity revolve around several factors, including the ability to predict and prevent GI absorption of ingested CBZ tablets, early airway protection, maintenance of oxygenation, and methods to shorten the duration of neurologic toxicity. These are the same principal concerns for sedative-hypnotic poisoning, but CBZ intoxication has the added problems of moderate anticholinergic potential and a physicochemical predilection for CBZ pharmacobezoar formation. Since CBZ displays erratic absorption, the decision should be in favor of admission and a prolonged observation period in an intensive care setting. This is especially true for any patient with a history suggestive of ingestion of a large number of tablets (acute ingestion of one or more times the maximal daily dosage) despite initial clinical presentation and CBZ serum level. If the exposure history, change in mental status, GI contrast studies, bowel motility, or serial serum levels suggest either remaining GI drug residue or on-going absorption after a 4- to 6-hour observation period, admission to an intensive care setting is recommended.

Patients at greatest risk for significant sequelae from CBZ poisoning and who require special consideration are those whose CBZ levels exceed 20 μg per milliliter, in whom levels are rapidly rising, are obtunded or comatose, have a potential risk for aspiration and/or respiratory failure, and exhibit persistent convulsive or involuntary movement activity. Adequate airway protection must be considered early, as poor outcomes with CBZ-poisoned patients are primarily attributable to pulmonary complications. The majority of patients at risk for significant sequelae require observation for a minimum 48 hours, which may be extended if there is a relapse or delayed absorption of ingested CBZ tablets.

Other supportive care therapies in CBZ poisoning include the use of additional anticonvulsant agents for patients with "paradoxical" seizures and crystalloid fluid challenges for hypotension. Pressor agents such as dopamine may be clinically indicated [64,74]. There is no specific recommended or proved antiarrhythmic regimen for CBZ toxicity, including systemic alkalinization unless the QRS is prolonged greater than 100 to 120 msec.

There is often evidence of continuing CBZ absorption several hours to days after ingestion, despite adequate GI decontamination with gastric lavage and instillation of activated charcoal and cathartic. A charcoal stool is not assurance of a CBZ-free GI tract. One-time routine activated charcoal doses (1 gm/kg) is not sufficient to bind all of the CBZ residues in the GI tract; a 10-fold or greater amount of activated charcoal is necessary to adsorb most compounds completely. The use of multiple-dose activated charcoal (MDAC) is necessary to "catch up" to unabsorbed gut CBZ and enhance elimination of systemically absorbed CBZ (see Guidelines for Multiple-Dose Activated Charcoal Therapy, below). However, although MDAC therapy for CBZ intoxication reduces serum levels, it has not been shown to improve patient outcome. The risk of this therapy should be weighed against the potential benefit and halted if any complications arise.

The risks of MDAC for CBZ intoxication include the potential for charcoal aspiration (necessitating airway protection) and bowel obstruction or impaction from the charcoal mass [88]. Obstruction may result from anticholinergic-induced decreased bowel motility progressing to ileus formation. In the presence of an adynamic ileus (not obstruction), a second cathartic dose or alternative cathartic should be considered. If this does not stimulate bowel activity or a charcoal stool within a short time period, MDAC is not advisable and the patient should be evaluated for bowel obstruction. Sorbitol should not be used in the presence of an ileus, since bowel flora ferments sorbitol, leading to gaseous distention. In the absence of a bowel obstruction and in patients with the potential for a CBZ concretion or pharmacobezoar, whole bowel irrigation (WBI) may be useful. This is accomplished with a polyethylene glycol electrolyte lavage solution (Golytely or Colyte) infused through a nasogastric tube at a rate of 2 liters per hour for adults and 0.5 to 1.0 liters per hour (25 ml/kg/hr) for children. Whole bowel irrigation has the theoretic risk of enhancing absorption by dissolving CBZ residues in the GI tract. There is no published experience with WBI in CBZ poisoning. One potential benefit of WBI is the ability to know when CBZ residues have been removed from the GI tract, which is indicated by a clear rectal effluent and follow-up contrast studies.

Antidotal Treatment. There is no proved pharmacologic antagonist for CBZ. However, there is one published case report of a CBZ-poisoned patient (serum level 27.8 μg/ml) who responded to a dose of the benzodiazepine antagonist flumazenil [85]. We believe flumazenil should be avoided in CBZ poisoning because it presents the risk of negating the anticonvulsant effect of benzodiazepines and may precipitate seizures in patients with seizure disorders. In a case report of CBZ poisoning in which the patient had repetitive episodes of dystonia, treatment with the anticholinesterase agent physostigmine was successful [73]. The same report suggests that since CBZ-induced dystonias are self-limiting the use of physostigmine may not be necessary [73]. Earlier cases showed no effect of physostigmine used as an analeptic agent [65,87]. Given the questionable efficacy and utility of physostigmine and its inherent eliptogenic risks in patients with seizure disorders, we do not recommend its use.

Enhanced Elimination. Attempts to hasten the elimination of systemically absorbed CBZ and shorten the duration of toxicity and sequelae from prolonged coma have led to the use of several techniques for hastening drug elimination. The indications for such procedures should be based on an evaluation of risk versus benefit. Patients with greatly elevated serum levels and concomitant deep comas should be considered candidates for enhanced elimination. Multiple-dose activated charcoal can prevent GI absorption of CBZ and approximately double total body CBZ clearance [101]. While MDAC is less invasive than extracorporeal methods of enhancing removal of CBZ, it does have the previously discussed side effects. One case series demonstrated that MDAC had no positive impact on the outcome of poisoning [102]. Furthermore, once CBZ levels decline into the therapeutic range, seizures have occurred in patients dependent on CBZ for seizure management [91]. Multiple-dose activated charcoal therapy must be used cautiously in this patient population and should be discontinued considerably earlier during the course of treatment.

The extensive protein binding of CBZ minimizes the effectiveness of peritoneal dialysis and hemodialysis. Hemoperfusion has been used in CBZ overdoses but enhances clearance only modestly, usually no more than the increase achieved by MDAC. In one case, it was equivalent to an increase in CBZ excretion of 200 mg per hour [74,83,84,87]. Hemoperfusion can be used to remove CBZ-epoxide but the literature is lacking on this. As most patients have favorable outcomes with good supportive care, the risk-benefit analysis usually does not favor hemoperfusion. Finally, because CBZ is a neutral compound and predominately metabolized, maneuvers to enhance elimination by forced diuresis and ion trapping with urine pH manipulation are not useful.

Newer Anticonvulsants

Several new anticonvulsants have recently been introduced in the United States. Felbamate (Felbatrol) has been approved for treatment of partial seizures in adults and seizures associated with Lennox-Gastaut syndrome in children [103]. Lamotrigine (Lamictal) is indicated for partial complex seizures [104]. Gabapentin (Neurontin) may be used in complex partial seizures and secondary generalized tonic-clonic seizures [104,105]. Other medications being studied include flunarizine, oxcarbazepine, remacemide, tiagabine, stiripentol, topiramate, and vigabatrin [105]. There are minimal data available on overdose of all of these; as they come into general use these data will become more available.

FELBAMATE. Felbamate is a phenyl dicarbamate with a structure similar to that of the sedative-hypnotic agent meprobamate. Its mechanism of action is not fully understood but it may have some indirect effect on the GABA_A receptor supramolecular complex [106,107]. It is believed to block repetitive neuronal firing and may affect the sodium channel on the neuronal membrane [103]. It is 90 percent absorbed orally, with peak effect at 1 to 3 hours after ingestion. The drug circulates as the free drug and is only 20 to 30 percent protein-bound. Absorption and elimination are linear and plateau at high levels. The drug undergoes partial hepatic metabolism with an inactive metabolite and renal excretion. Approximately 40 to 49 percent is excreted unmetabolized. The elimination half-life is 20 hours in both acute and chronic dosing. Felbamate does not induce its own metabolism [103,104,108].

Felbamate has significant drug interactions. It can both inhibit and induce the P-450 cytochrome system. This affects the metabolism of coadministered medications. Coadministration of felbamate and carbamazepine lead to a decrease in carbamazepine serum levels by approximately 30 percent but at the same time, by inhibition of epoxide hydrolase activity, increase the level of circulating carbamazepine-10,11 epoxide by 60 percent. Inhibition of epoxide hydrolase activity can lead to signs of CBZ toxicity with low to normal serum levels. The effect of felbamate on phenytoin and valproate is to increase serum levels of both agents. At the same time, the addition of CBZ to felbamate increases the clearance (decreases the level) of felbmate. The effect of valproate on felbamate metabolism is less clear, but valproate is thought to inhibit felbamate metabolism, leading to an increase in serum felbamate levels by 75 to 85 percent. Concomitant administration of felbamate, phenytoin, and CBZ increases the clearance of felbamate by approximately 36 percent. The net effect is the need to reduce the dose of phenytoin by 10 to 30 percent when adding felbmate and to increase the dose of felbamate in the presence of valproate. The effect of felbamate on metabolism takes roughly 2 to 3 weeks to clear after discontinuation of the drug [103,104,109].

Side effects of felbamate include headache, nausea, dyspepsia, vomiting, somnolence, anorexia, weight loss, and constipation or diarrhea. When felbamate is added to other anticonvulsants, there is an increase in ataxia and somnolence, which may be related to drug interaction. Rash, fever, agitation, and elevated hepatic transaminases have been reported, as have leukopenia, thrombocytopenia, agranulocytosis, and Stevens-Johnson syndrome. These last few effects have been reported only when felbamate is administered with other medications. The safety of felbamate use in pregnancy has not been established [103,104].

Since no overdose data are available, treatment of overdose should involve supportive care. Gut decontamination with activated charcoal would appear to be reasonable, although data on binding are lacking. Medications that alter protein binding (salicylates, coumarin) or affect the P-450 microsomal system (cimetidine, ciprofloxacin, erythromycin) should probably be avoided. There is no evidence that manipulation of the glomerular filtration rate or urinary pH affects felbamate clearance.

Unfortunately, in postmarketing surveillance, felbamate was associated with aplastic anemia and was withdrawn from general use. It is still available for limited use in patients whose seizures are unresponsive to other agents.

LAMOTRIGINE. Lamotrigine (LTG), or 3-5-diamino-6(2,3-dichlorophenyl)-1,2,4-triazine, is used to treat partial seizures. It was derived from medications that inhibit dihydrofolate reductase (e.g., phenytoin). The mechanism of action of LTG is believed to be similar to that of carbamazepine and phenytoin. It acts on the voltage-sensitive sodium channels and stabilizes neuronal membranes. Lamotrigine has no effect on the release of GABA, acetylcholine, norepinephrine, or dopamine. It may inhibit release of glutamate and aspartate evoked by sodium channel activation [104,106]. In oral dosing, LTG is rapidly and completely absorbed. Peak serum concentration is proportional to the oral dose at doses of 300 mg per day or less. Protein binding is approximately 55 percent and the volume of distribution ranges from 1.1 to 1.5 liters per kilogram. Lamotrigine is metabolized in the liver and excreted as the glucuronide metabolite. This is the rate-limiting step in metabolism [105]. Lamotrigine will not induce its own metabolism. The elimination half-life of the parent compound is 12 to 50 hours (mean 30 hours) [104].

Lamotrigine appears to be effective in treating refractory partial complex seizures. It also appears to have an effect in absence, atypical absence, and myoclonic seizures [104].

Side effects of LTG use include drowsiness, dizziness, headache, unsteady gait, tremor, and nausea. There have been no reported changes in cardiovascular, hematologic, and biochemical parameters [104].

Drug interactions are significant and are based on changes in metabolism. Both CBZ and phenytoin increase metabolism, leading to a shortened elimination half-life. Valproate inhibits LTG's metabolism, almost doubling LTG's half-life. Lamotrigine does not appear to have any effect on the metabolism of CBZ, valproate, phenytoin, primidone, and phenobarbital [104].

There are no overdose data available. In animals, LTG has a very high therapeutic index (effective dose $<<<$ toxic dose), which may carry over into humans. Since peak effect has a linear dependency on drug dose, oral activated charcoal may limit absorption of the drug. In the face of low protein binding, competition by other medications may not have much effect. Although at normal dosing there are no cardiovascular effects, LTG does affect voltage-dependent sodium channels. It remains to be seen whether high serum levels will cause aberrant cardiac conduction.

GABAPENTIN. Gabapentin (GBP) is an engineered molecule based on GABA and altered to increase membrane permeability and entrance through the blood-brain barrier. Essentially, GBP is GABA with a cyclohexane ring (1-[aminomethyl]-cyclohexane). It appears effective in treating complex partial seizures and secondary generalized tonic-clonic seizures. Its efficacy is said to be similar to that of CBZ and phenytoin, and it is synergistic with phenytoin, CBZ, valproate, and primidone in animal seizure models [104].

Gabapentin appears to bind to a specific site in the CNS but does not affect ligand binding to $GABA_A$, $GABA_B$, benzodiazepine, glutamate, glycine, and NMDA sites on the neuronal membrane. In the rat brain it increases GABA turnover. It does not appear to inhibit sustained repetitive firing of sodium-dependent action potentials [104,106].

Oral absorption of GBP depends on the active L-amino acid transport system. It is 60 percent bioavailable in oral dosing and is not protein-bound. The V_d is 1.0 liter per kilogram. There is a linear relationship of dose and time to peak serum effects with daily doses of 600 mg or less; at daily doses greater than 600 mg the kinetics are nonlinear. The serum peak concentration is achieved by 2 to 3 hours after ingestion, and the elimination half-life is 5 to 7 hours. In chronic dosing, the CSF concentration is approximately 7 to 35 percent of that in serum. There is no hepatic metabolism, and GBP is eliminated unchanged in the urine. Renal elimination and half-life are proportional to renal function. The elimination rate cannot be induced nor is the elimination half-life altered with repetitive dosing. Tolerance to drug effect has not been seen in chronic dosing [104,105].

There have been no reported drug interactions with CBZ, CBZ-epoxide, phenobarbital, phenytoin, and valproate [104].

Side effects include fatigue, nausea, somnolence, dizziness, slurred speech, and unsteady gait. At therapeutic dosing, there have been no reports of hematologic or biochemical abnormalities [104]. Animal carcinogenic data show an increase in pancreatic acinar cell tumors in male mice only, but a review by the National Institutes of Health concluded that this is not predictive of human carcinogenesis [104].

There are no overdose data. Supportive care appears to be the best form of treatment. There is no information on binding to activated charcoal, but it would seem reasonable to attempt to limit absorption by administering charcoal. Since GBP is a small molecule and relatively nonpolar, it may be amenable to hemodialysis, although the V_d of 1.0 liter per kilogram may make this difficult. There are no data on urinary manipulation.

FLUNARIZINE. Flunarizine is an extremely long-acting difluoro derivative of cinnarizine. Its efficacy is reported to be similar to that of phenytoin and CBZ. It has an oral bioavailability of approximately 86 percent, with tablets 10 percent less bioavailable than liquid and capsules. Peak serum levels occur within 2 to 4 hours. The V_d is 78 liters per kilogram and it is highly protein-bound. All of these factors contribute to its elimination half-life of 10 to 50 days. Steady-state serum levels are achieved by 8 weeks on oral dosing. It will induce its own hepatic metabolism. A very small amount is excreted in the urine. When flunarizine is added to CBZ and phenytoin, the serum level drops significantly [105].

OXCARBAZEPINE. Oxcarbazepine is the dihydro derivative of CBZ. It is almost 100 percent biotransformed during hepatic first-pass metabolism to 10,11-dihydro-10-hydroxycarbamazepine (MHD). It has the same anticonvulsant effect as CBZ. Both the parent and the metabolite are lipophilic and will pass into the CNS. Toxicity should be similar to that of CBZ [105].

REMACEMIDE. Remacemide is another engineered anticonvulsant designed to look and function like phenytoin. It has an active metabolite, which is the deglycine form. The half-life of the parent compound is 4 hours and of the metabolite is 15 hours. It has linear kinetics and undergoes hepatic induction. Toxicity data are lacking [105].

STIRIPENTOL. Stiripentol is a 3,4-methylenedioxyphenyl derivative that inhibits the P-450 microsomal system. It has dose-dependent nonlinear kinetics and undergoes accumulation kinetics. Its mean residence time in the serum is less than 30 minutes. It has a small bioavailability and crystallizes in the GI tract during oral dosing. It is extremely protein-bound, and less than 1 percent is free in the serum [105].

TIAGABINE. Tiagabine is derived from the GABA reuptake inhibitor nipecotic acid and a lipophic moiety designed to improve passage into the CNS. It is rapidly absorbed orally, with a peak level by 0.5 to 1 hour after ingestion. Kinetics are linear [105].

TOPIRAMATE. Topiramate is a sulphamate-substituted monosaccharide compound different from other anticonvulsants. It is being used for partial seizures. Oral absorption is rapid and increases in the presence of food. It is 70 to 97 percent eliminated unchanged in the urine. The elimination half-life is 19 to 23 hours, with a peak serum level at 1.8 to 4.3 hours. There have been no reported interactions with CBZ, phenytoin, and valproate [105].

VIGABATRIN. Vigabatrin is another engineered GABA-related anticonvulsant. Chemically, it is gamma-vinyl-GABA. It was designed to increase brain GABA concentration by inhibition of GABA transaminase. It is believed to decrease seizure activity by decreasing propagation of abnormal hypersynchronous discharges. Peak serum level occurs approximately 0.5 to 3 hours after ingestion and does not change with food intake. There is a large intrapatient variability in serum levels. The CSF level is approximately 0 to 15 percent of the serum level. There is no protein binding and no hepatic metabolism. It is eliminated unchanged in the urine [105].

Reported side effects include sedation, confusion, and ataxia [105]. There are no overdose data, and supportive therapy would be the most reasonable treatment.

Guidelines for Multiple-Dose Activated Charcoal Therapy for Anticonvulsant Poisoning

DOSAGE REGIMEN. An initial dose of 1 gm per kilogram activated charcoal is followed with 0.25 to 0.5 gm per kilogram every 2 hours, or 0.5 to 1.0 gm per kilogram every 4 hours administered either as a pulse dose or as a continuous infusion via nasogastric tube. Activated charcoal products *without* sorbitol should be used for multiple-dose therapy. Repeat doses of cathartics should be dictated by the frequency of charcoal stools and electrolyte and fluid balance. Cathartics should *not* be used with each dose of activated charcoal.

INDICATIONS. There is little controlled evidence that MDAC therapy shortens the duration of toxicity or improves outcome in patients with anticonvulsant poisoning. Not instituting MDAC therapy is an option even if a patient fulfills the criteria listed below, and MDAC may be halted if complications arise.

The indications for MDAC therapy are as follows.

1. Acute anticonvulsant ingestion history of greater than 0.1 gm per kilogram in which the routine initial dose of activated charcoal (1 gm/kg) would yield a charcoal to drug ratio less than 10:1
   AND/OR
2. Phenytoin
   a. Serum levels greater than 40 μg per milliliter* with moderate to severe neurologic toxicity
   b. Rising serum levels after emergency department gastric decontamination or other evidence of drug residues (pharmacobezoars) remaining in GI tract
3. Carbamazepine
   a. Serum levels greater than 20 μg per milliliter*
   b. Otherwise, same as 2b
4. Valproic acid
   a. Serum levels greater than 200 μg per milliliter*
   b. Otherwise, same as 2b

ENDPOINTS

1. Clinical—Amelioration of dose-related reversible neurologic symptoms that correspond to a decrease in serum levels; patients should be able to ambulate or sit up in bed, feed themselves, and carry out activities of daily living
2. Laboratory—Anticipate the rapidity of rate of decline of serum levels while patient is on MDAC therapy. As serum levels approach therapeutic range, MDAC therapy should be discontinued unless there is evidence of a pharmacobezoar in the GI tract. The effect of charcoal on clearance enhancement may persist for several hours. Clinical endpoint

---

* In the case of a polypharmacy ingestion containing an anticonvulsant or if the patient is a sensitive responder (e.g., novice user), then MDAC therapy at a lower serum level may be considered.)

---

achieved in the absence of pharmacobezoars should supersede a laboratory endpoint.
3. Other
   a. Patients should pass at least one charcoal stool prior to each repeat dose.
   b. Duration of MDAC therapy is usually 24 to 48 hours.

POTENTIAL COMPLICATIONS. The potential complications of MDAC therapy are the following.

Aspiration, empyema (need timely airway protection)
Bowel obstruction (Do not repeat dose of charcoal in patients who are not passing stools or who have an ileus.)
Hypermagnesemia with use of magnesium-containing cathartic, particularly in renal failure
Hypernatremic dehydration, particularly in young children or infants given potent cathartics such as sorbitol
"Breakthrough" seizures (Patients who require anticonvulsants therapeutically may seize if serum level drops or "overshoots" below the therapeutic range.)

RELATIVE CONTRAINDICATIONS. The relative contraindications to MDAC therapy are as follows.

Shock (loss of effectiveness of MDAC when there is decreased GI perfusion and loss of bowel motility)
Ileus, or diminished bowel activity or sounds (may attempt cathartic challenge)
GI tract dysfunction (includes hemorrhage, strictures, perforations, recent surgery, and esophageal varices)

References

1. Rall TW, Schleifer LS: Drugs effective in the therapy of the epilepsies, in Gilman AG, Goodman LS, Rall TW, et al (eds): *Goodman and Gilman's The Pharmacological Basis of Therapeutics*. 7th ed. New York, Macmillan, 1985, p 450.
2. Helfant RH, Seuffert GW, Patton RD: The clinical use of diphenylhydantoin (Dilantin) in the treatment and prevention of cardiac arrhythmias. *Am Heart J* 77:315, 1969.
3. Albertson TE, Fisher CJ, Shragg TA: Prolonged severe intoxication after ingestion of phenytoin and phenobarbital. *West J Med* 135:418, 1981.
4. Earnest MP, Marx JA, Drury LR: Complications of intravenous phenytoin for acute treatment of seizures: Recommendations for usage. *JAMA* 249:762, 1983.
5. Garrettson LK, Jsko WJ: Diphenylhydantoin elimination kinetics in overdosed children. *Clin Pharmacol Ther* 17:481, 1975.
6. Gill MA, Kern JW, Kaneko J, et al: Phenytoin overdose kinetics. *West J Med* 128:246, 1978.
7. Laubscher FA: Fatal diphenylhydantoin poisoning. *JAMA* 198:1120, 1966.
8. Patel H, Crichton JU: The neurologic hazards of diphenylhydantoin in childhood. *J Pediatr* 73:676, 1968.
9. Tenckhoff H, Sherrard DJ, Hickman O, et al: Acute diphenylhydantoin intoxication. *Am J Dis Child* 116:422, 1968.
10. Wilson JT, Huff JG, Kilroy AW: Prolonged toxicity following acute phenytoin overdose in a child. *J Pediatr* 95:135, 1979.
11. Reidenberg MM, Affrime M: Influence of disease on binding of drugs to plasma protein. *Ann NY Acad Sci* 226:115, 1973.
12. Powers NG, Carson SH: Idiosyncratic reactions to phenytoin. *Clin Pediatr* 26:120, 1987.
13. Woodbury DM, Swinyard EA: Diphenylhydantoin: Absorption, distribution, and excretion, in Woodbury DM, Penry JK, Schmidt RP, et al (eds): *Antiepileptic Drugs*. New York, Raven, 1972, p 113.

14. Kokenge R, Kutt H, McDowell FM: Neurological sequelae following Dilantin overdose in a patient and in experimental animals. *Neurology* 15:823, 1965.
15. Reynolds EH: Chronic antiepileptic toxicity: A review. *Epilepsia* 16:319, 1975.
16. Kutt H: Interactions of antiepileptic drugs. *Epilepsia* 16:393, 1975.
17. Louis S, Kutt H, McDowell F: The cardiocirculatory changes caused by intravenous Dilantin and its solvent. *Am Heart J* 74:523, 1967.
18. Borofsky LG, Louis B, Kutt H, et al: Diphenylhydantoin efficacy, toxicity, and dose-serum relationships in children. *J Pediatr* 81:995, 1972.
19. Petty CS, Muelling RJ, Sindell HW: Accidental poisoning with diphenylhydantoin (Dilantin). *J Forensic Sci* 2:279, 1957.
20. Blair AAD, Hallpike JF, Lascelles PT: Acute diphenylhydantoin and primidone poisoning treated by peritoneal dialysis. *J Neurol Neurosurg Psychiatry* 31:520, 1968.
21. Kutt H, Winters W, Kikenge R: Metabolism of diphenylhydantoin, blood levels, and toxicity. *Arch Neurol* 11:642, 1964.
22. Luschser TF, Siegenthaler-Zuber G, Kuhlmann U: Severe hypernatremic coma due to diphenylhydantoin intoxication. *Clin Nephr* 20:268, 1983.
23. Masur H, Elger CE, Ludolph AC, Galanski M: Cerebellar atrophy following acute intoxication with phenytoin. *Neurology* 39:432, 1989.
24. Wagner KJ, Zell M, Leiken JB: Metabolic effects of phenytoin toxicity. *Ann Emerg Med* 15:509, 1986.
25. Mauro LS, Mauro VF, Brown DL: Enhancement of phenytoin elimination by multiple-dose activated charcoal. *Am J Emerg Med* 16:1132, 1987.
26. Bodendorfer LG: Fetal effects of anticonvulsant drugs and seizures disorders. *Drug Intell Clin Pharm* 12:14, 1978.
27. Rizzon P, DiBiase M, Favales S, et al: Class 1B agents: Lidocaine, mexiletine, tocainide, phenytoin. *Eur Heart J* 8(suppl A):21-5, 1987.
28. Stillman N, Masden JC: Incidence of seizures with phenytoin toxicity. *Neurology* 35:1769, 1985.
29. Baechler RW, Work J, Smith W, et al: Charcoal hemoperfusion in the therapy of methsuximide and phenytoin overdose. *Arch Intern Med* 40:1466, 1980.
30. Pinder PM, Borgden RN, Speight TM: Sodium valproate: A review of its pharmacological properties and therapeutic efficacy in epilepsy. *Drugs* 13:81, 1977.
31. Covanis A, Gupton AK, Jeavons PM: Sodium valproate: Monotherapy and polytherapy. *Epilepsia* 23:693, 1982.
32. Chadwick DW: Concentration-effect relationships of valproic acid. *Clin Pharmacol* 10:155, 1985.
33. Faingold CL, Browning RA: Mechanism of anticonvulsant drug action. *Eur J Pediatr* 146:8, 1987.
34. Rimmer EM, Rickens A: An update on sodium valproate. *Pharmacology* 5:171, 1985.
35. Tamayo L, Contreras E: A dual action of valproic acid upon morphine analgesia and morphine withdrawal. *Pharmacology* 26:297, 1983.
36. Gugler R, von Unruh GE: Clinical pharmacokinetics of valproic acid. *Clin Pharmacol* 5:67, 1980.
37. Cramer JA, Mattson RH: Valproic acid: In vitro plasma protein binding and interaction with phenytoin. *Ther Drug Monit* 1:105, 1979.
38. Dupuis RE, Lichtman SN, Pollack GM: Acute valproic acid overdose, clinical course and pharmacokinetic disposition of valproic acid and metabolities. *Drug Saf* 5:65, 1990.
39. Brent J, Yanover M, Kulig K, et al: Valproic acid (VPA) poisoning treated by hemodialysis (abstract). AACT/AAPCC/ABMT/CAPCC Annual Scientific Meeting, Baltimore, 1988.
40. Goulden KJ, Dooley JM, Camfield PR, et al: Clinical valproate toxicity induced by acetylsalicylic acid. *Neurology* 37:1392, 1987.
41. Kingsley E, Tweedale R, Gray P: The role of toxic metabolites in the hepatotoxicity of valproic acid. *Gastroenterology* 79:511, 1980.
42. Mortensen PB, Hansen HE, Pederson B, et al: Acute valproate intoxication: Biochemical investigations and hemodialysis treatment. *Int J Clin Pharmacol Ther Toxicol* 21:64, 1983.
43. Mortensen PB: Inhibition of fatty acid oxidation by valproate. *Lancet* 1:856, 1980.
44. Coulter DL, Allen RJ: Hyperammonemia with valproic acid therapy. *J Pediatr* 99:317, 1981.
45. Chadwick DW, Cumming WJK, Livingstone I, et al: Acute intoxication with sodium valproate. *Ann Neurol* 6:552, 1979.
46. Hyden H, Capello A, Palu A: Naloxone reverses the inhibition by sodium valproate of GABA transport across the Deiters' neuronal plasma membrane. *Ann Neurol* 21:416, 1987.
47. Dingledine R, Iverson LL, Brecker E: Naloxone as a GABA antagonist. *Eur J Pharmacol* 47:19, 1978.
48. Kay JDS, Hilton-Jones D, Hyman N: Valproate toxicity and ornithine carbamoyltransferase deficiency. *Lancet* 2:1283, 1986.
49. Dreifuss FE, Santilli N, Langer DH, et al: Valproic acid hepatic fatalities. *Neurology* 37:379, 1987.
50. Gerbin N, Dickinson RG, Harland RC, et al: Reyes-like syndrome associated with valproic acid therapy. *J Pediatr* 95:142, 1979.
51. Schwabel R, Rambeck B, Jansson F: Fatal intoxication with sodium valproate. *Lancet* 1:221, 1984.
52. Janssen F, Rambeck B, Schnabel R: Acute valproate intoxication with fatal outcome in an infant. *Neuropediatrics* 15:235, 1985.
53. Bigler D: Neurological sequelae after intoxication with sodium valproate. *Acta Neurol Scand* 72:351, 1985.
54. Eeg-Olofsson O, Lindskog U: Acute intoxication with valproate. *Lancet* 2:1306, 1982.
55. Connacher AA, MacNab JP, Jung RT: Fatality due to massive overdose of sodium valproate. *Scot Med J* 32:85, 1987.
56. Garnier R, Boudignat O, Fournics PE: Valproate poisoning. *Lancet* 1:97, 1982.
57. Alberto G, Erickson T, Popiel R, et al: Central nervous system manifestations of valproic acid overdose responsive to naloxone. *Ann Emerg Med* 18:889, 1989.
58. Steinman GS, Woerpel RW, Sherwood ES: Treatment of accidental sodium valproate overdoses with an opiate antagonist. *Ann Neurol* 6:274, 1979.
59. Palatrick W, Honcharik N, Roberts D, et al: Coma, anion gap and metabolic derangements associated with massive valproic acid (abstract). AACT/AAPCC/ABMT/CAPCC Annual Scientific Meeting, Atlanta, October 1989.
60. Lokan RJ, Dinan AC: An apparent fatal valproic acid poisoning. *J Anal Toxicol* 12:35, 1988.
61. Van der Merwe AC, Albrecht CF, Brink MS, et al: Sodium valproate poisoning. *S Afr Med J* 67:735, 1985
62. Durelli L, Mussazza U, Cavallo R: Carbamazepine toxicity and poisoning: Incidence, clinical features, and management. *Med Toxicol Adv Drug Exp* 4:95, 1989.
63. Levy RH, Pitlick WH, Troupin AS, et al: Pharmacokinetics of carbamazepine in normal man. *Clin Pharmacol Ther* 17:657, 1975.
64. Sethna M, Solomon G, Cedarbaum J, et al: Successful treatment of massive carbamazepine overdose. *Epilepsia* 30:71, 1989.
65. Sullivan JB, Rumack BH, Peterson RG: Acute carbamazepine toxicity resulting from overdose. *Neurology* 31:621, 1981.
66. Dezeeuw RA, Westenberg HGM, Van der Kleijn E, et al: An unusual case of carbamazepine poisoning with a near-fatal relapse after two days. *Clin Toxicol* 14:263, 1979.
67. Rall TW, Schleifer LS: Drugs effective in the therapy of the epilepsies, in Gilman AG, Goodman LS, Rall TW, et al (eds): *Goodman and Gilman's The Pharmacological Basis of Therapeutics.* New York, Macmillan, 1985, p 457.
68. Deng J, Shipe JR, Rogol AD, et al: Carbamazepine toxicity: Comparison of measurement of drug levels by HPLC and EMIT and model of carbamazepine kinetics. *Clin Toxicol* 24:281, 1986.
69. Pynnonen S: Pharmacokinetics of carbamazepine in man: A review. *Ther Drug Monit* 1:409, 1979.
70. Goulden KJ, Camfield P, Dooley JM, et al: Severe carbamazepine intoxication after coadministration of erythromycin. *J Pediatr* 109:135, 1986.
71. Vree TB, Janssen TJ, Hekster YA, et al: Clinical pharmacokinetics of carbamazepine and its epoxy and hydroxymetabolites in humans after an overdose. *Ther Drug Monit* 8:297, 1986.
72. May DC: Acute carbamazepine intoxication: Clinical spectrum and management. *South Med J* 77:24, 1984.
73. O'Neal W, Whitten KM, Baumann RJ, et al: Lack of serious toxicity following carbamazepine overdosage. *Clin Pharm* 3:545, 1984.
74. Nilsson C, Sterner G, Idvall J: Charcoal hemoperfusion for treatment of serious carbamazepine poisoning. *Acta Med Scand* 216:137, 1984.
75. Fisher RS, Cysyk B: A fatal overdose of carbamazepine: Case report and review of literature. *Clin Toxicol* 26:447, 1988.

76. Hopen G, Nesthus I, Laerum OD: Fatal carbamazepine-associated hepatitis. *Acta Med Scand* 210:333, 1981.

77. Hart RG, Easton JD: Carbamazepine and hematological monitoring. *Ann Neurol* 11:309, 1982.

78. Ashton MG, Ball SG, Thomas TH: Water intoxication associated with carbamazepine treatment. *Br Med J* 1:113, 1977.

79. Noda S, Umezaki H: Carbamazepine-induced ophthalmoplegia. *Neurology* 32:1320, 1982.

80. Dennig DQ, Matheson L, Bryson SM, et al: Death due to carbamazepine self-poisoning: Remedies reviewed. *Hum Toxicol* 4:255, 1985.

81. Drenck NE, Risbo A: Carbamazepine poisoning: A surprisingly severe case. *Anaesth Intensive Care* 8:203, 1980.

82. Weaver DF, Camfield P, Fraser A: Massive carbamazepine overdose: Clinical and pharmacologic observations in five episodes. *Neurology* 38:755, 1988.

83. Leslie PJ, Heyworth R, Prescott LF: Cardiac complications of carbamazepine intoxication: Treatment by haemoperfusion. *Br Med J* 286:1018, 1983.

84. Chan K, Aguanno JJ, Jansen R, et al: Charcoal hemoperfusion for treatment of carbamazepine poisoning. *Clin Chem* 27:1300, 1981.

85. Zuber M, Elsasser S, Ritz R, et al: Flumazenil (Anexate) in severe intoxication with carbamazepine (Tegretol). *Eur Neurol* 28:161, 1988.

86. Lehrman SN, Bauman ML: Carbamazepine overdose. *Am J Dis Child* 135:768, 1981.

87. Gary NE, Byra WM, Eisinger RP: Carbamazepine poisoning: Treatment by hemoperfusion. *Nephron* 27:202, 1981.

88. Watson WA, Cremer KF, Chapman JA: Gastrointestinal obstruction associated with multiple-dose activated charcoal. *J Emerg Med* 4:401, 1986.

89. Rockoff S, Baselt RC: Severe carbamazepine poisoning. *Clin Toxicol* 18:935, 1981.

90. Kossoy AF, Weir MR: Therapeutic indications in carbamazepine overdose. *South Med J* 78:999, 1985.

91. Patsalos PN, Krishna S, Elyas AA, et al: Carbamazepine and carbamazepine-10, 11-epoxide pharmacokinetics in an overdose patient. *Hum Toxicol* 6:241, 1987.

92. Patsalos PN, Stephenson TJ, Krishna S, et al: Side effects induced by carbamazepine-10, 11-epoxide. *Lancet* 1:496, 1985.

93. Schoeman JF, Elyas AA, Brett EM, et al: Correlation between plasma carbamazepine-10, 11-epoxide concentration and drug side effects in children with epilepsy. *Dev Med Child Neurol* 26:756, 1984.

94. Mullally WJ: Carbamazepine-induced ophthalmoplegia. *Arch Neurol* 39:64, 1982.

95. Litovitz TL, Schmitz BF, Holm KC: 1988 Annual Report of the American Association of Poison Control Centers National Data Collection System. *Am J Emerg Med* 7:495, 1989.

96. Crosley CJ, Swender PT: Dystonia associated with carbamazepine administration: Experience in brain-damaged children. *Pediatrics* 63:612, 1979.

97. Beerman B, Edhag O, Vallen H: Advanced heart block aggravated by carbamazepine. *Br Heart J* 37:668, 1975.

98. Durelli L, Mutani R, Sechi GP: Cardiac side effects of phenytoin and carbamazepine: A dose related phenomenon? *Arch Neurol* 42:1067, 1985.

99. Hajnsek F, Sartorius N: A case of intoxication with Tegretol. *Epilepsia* 5:371, 1964.

100. Coutselinis A, Poulos L: An unusual case of carbamazepine poisoning with a near-fatal relapse after two days (letter). *Clin Toxicol* 16:385, 1980.

101. Neuvonen PJ, Elonen E: Effect of activated charcoal on absorption elimination of phenobarbitone, carbamazepine and phenylbutazone in man. *Eur J Clin Pharmacol* 17:51, 1983.

102. Wason S, Baker RC, Carolan P, et al: Carbamazepine overdose: The effects of multiple dose activated charcoal. *J Toxicol Clin Toxicol* 30:39, 1992.

103. Felbamate. *Med Lett* 35:107, 1993.

104. Ramsay RE: Advances in the pharmacotherapy of epilepsy. *Epilepsia* 34 (suppl 5):S9-16, 1993.

105. Biaker M: Comparative pharmacokinetics of the newer antiepileptic drugs. *Clin Pharmacokinet* 24:441, 1993.

106. MacDonald RL, Kelly KM: Antiepileptic drug mechanism of action. *Epilepsia* 34 (suppl 5):S1, 1993

107. White HS, Wolf HH, Swinyard EA, et al: A neuropharmacological evaluation of felbamate as a novel anticonvulsant. *Epilepsia* 33:564, 1992

108. Adusumalli VE, Gilchrist JR, Wichmann JK, et al: Pharmacokinetics of felbamate in pediatric and adult dogs. *Epilepsia* 33:955, 1992

109. Wagner ML, Remmel RP, Graves NM, Leppik IE: Effect of felbamate on carbamazepine and its major metabolites. *Clin Pharmacol Ther* 53:536, 1993

135. Beta-Blocker Poisoning

Laura Bilohrud and Kenneth W. Kulig

Introduction

HISTORY. Since 1958, when dichloroisoprenaline, the first beta-adrenergic blocker, was synthesized, more than a dozen beta-blockers have been introduced into the international pharmaceutical market [1]. Originally developed for the treatment of angina pectoris and dysrhythmias, beta-blockers are now used in a wide variety of disorders (Table 135-1). Intoxication may result from oral, parenteral, and even ophthalmic use [2,3,4]. Abrupt discontinuation of beta-blockers after long-term use may also have untoward effects [5,6,7].

PHARMACOLOGY. Beta-blockers act by competitively inhibiting the binding of epinephrine and norepinephrine to beta-adrenergic neuroreceptors in the heart (beta$_1$), blood vessels and bronchioles (beta$_2$), and other organs (Table 135-2). By reducing the activity of beta receptors, the production of cyclic AMP is decreased [7,8]. See Chapter 210 for a detailed discussion of therapeutic dosages in the United States.

Beta-blockers are usually rapidly absorbed after oral administration. Modified-release formulations, however, may be slowly absorbed, especially after overdose. The dose of beta-blocker required to produce a toxic effect is highly variable, depending on the sympathetic tone and metabolic capacity of the individual and the pharmacologic properties of the particular beta-blocker [9]. The first signs of toxicity can appear as early as 20 minutes after ingestion; peak effects typically occur 1 to 2 hours following an overdose [9]. This may occur later after overdose of sustained-release preparations. The duration of toxicity may be several days [7,9].

Table 135-1. Reported Indications for Beta-Adrenergic Receptor Blocking Drugs

Angina pectoris
Hypertension
Dysrhythmias
Reducing the risk of mortality and reinfarction in survivors of acute
    MI
Aortic dissection
Hyperacute phase of MI
Digitalis intoxication
Tetralogy of Fallot
Congestive cardiomyopathy
Mitral valve prolapse
Q–T interval prolongation
Neurocirculatory asthenia
Fetal tachycardia
Mitral stenosis
Glaucoma
Thyrotoxicosis
Migraine prophylaxis
Essential tremor
Portal hypertension and gastrointestinal bleeding
Anxiety and stage fright
Alcohol withdrawl
Hyperparathyroidism
Pheochromocytoma (used with alpha blockers)

MI = myocardial infarction.
Adapted from Frishman WH: Beta-adrenergic blockers. *Med Clin North Am* 72:37, 1988.

Table 135-2. Distribution and Function of Beta-Receptors

Receptor subtype	Location	Response to stimulation
Beta$_1$	Eye	Aqueous humor production
	Heart	Increased automaticity, conduction velocity, contractility and refractory period
	Kidney	Renin production
Beta$_2$	Blood vessels	Smooth muscle contraction
	Bronchioles	Smooth muscle contraction
	Fat	Lipolysis
	Liver	Gluconeogenesis, glycogenolysis
	Pancreas	Insulin release
	Skeletal muscle	Increased tone, potassium uptake
	Uterus	Smooth muscle relaxation

PHARMACOKINETICS. The pharmacokinetics of beta-blockers marketed in the United States are summarized in Chapter 210. Their half-lives vary widely, ranging from a few minutes to nearly a day. The half-life may be greatly prolonged in patients with depressed cardiac output as a result of decreased liver and kidney perfusion [9]. Intrinsic heart, kidney, and liver disease as well as the concomitant use of drugs with similar activity increases the risk of toxicity.

Beta-blockers vary greatly with respect to their lipid solubility, partial agonist activity (at beta$_1$ receptors), cardioselectivity (i.e., ability to block beta$_2$ as well as beta$_1$ receptors), and membrane-stabilizing or quinidinelike effects. Patients poisoned with beta-blockers possessing partial agonist activity can present with a normal heart rate or even tachycardia. Although cardioselectivity tends to be lost at high doses, the membrane-stabilizing effect, which appears to be of little significance at therapeutic doses, assumes an important role [7,9,10]. Membrane dysfunction may account for many of the central

nervous system (CNS) and myocardial depressant effects in patients poisoned by membrane-active drugs such as propranolol [7,10].

Clinical Toxicity

The major manifestations relate to the cardiovascular system and CNS. Respiratory, peripheral vascular, and metabolic (hypoglycemic and hyperkalemic) effects have been reported less frequently [9–12].

CARDIOVASCULAR EFFECTS. Disturbances of cardiac rhythm and cardiac conduction may occur. Most frequently, patients with severe poisoning present with hypotension and bradycardia [11]. However, tachycardia and hypertension have been reported with agents possessing intrinsic sympathomimetic activity, particularly pindolol [9,13,14]. Congestive heart failure and pulmonary edema have infrequently been reported and mainly occur in patients with underlying heart disease [15,16]. Electrocardiographic manifestations may include prolonged P–R interval, intraventricular conduction delay, progressive atrioventricular heart block, nonspecific S–T segment and T wave changes, early repolarization, and asystole [8, 10,17,18,19]. Sotalol poisoning may result in ventricular tachycardia (including *Torsades de pointes*), ventricular fibrillation, and multifocal ventricular extrasystoles [20,21,22]. These effects have been attributed to prolongation of the Q–T interval [20]. Labetalol, which also has mild alpha-receptor blocking properties, may cause profound hypotension, probably from decreased peripheral resistance [11].

CENTRAL NERVOUS SYSTEM EFFECTS. Depression in the level of consciousness, ranging from drowsiness to coma with seizures, is another common feature of beta-blocker poisoning [10]. Significant CNS depression has been reported in the absence of cardiovascular compromise [9] or hypoglycemia [11] and may be due to direct membrane effects [23]. However, cerebral hypoperfusion, hypoxia, and metabolic or respiratory acidosis frequently contribute to CNS toxiciy [10] Beta-blockers with high lipid solubility (propranolol, penbutolol, metoprolol) appear more likely to cause CNS effects than those with a low lipid solubility [23–26].

RESPIRATORY EFFECTS. Bronchospasm is a relatively rare consequence of beta-blocker poisoning and usually occurs more frequently in patients with preexisting reactive airway disease. In most instances, respiratory depression appears to be secondary to a CNS effect [11,27–32]. Cyanosis may be due to peripheral vascular as well as cardiopulmonary effects [10]. Peripheral cyanosis is believed to be due to blockade of beta$_2$ adrenoreceptor-mediated vasodilatation resulting in unopposed alpha vasoconstriction [10,11,33].

METABOLIC EFFECTS. Hypoglycemia is an infrequent complication of beta-blocker poisoning [8,16]. It appears to be more common in diabetics, children, and uremic patients [31] and is the consequence of blockade of the hyperglycemic effect of catecholamines. A blunted tachycardic response to hypoglycemia may be seen in patients poisoned by beta-blockers, although other symptoms of hypoglycemia appear unaffected [8].

OTHER EFFECTS. Oliguric renal failure has been reported as a complication of labetalol poisoning [34,35] Mesenteric ischemia and subsequent cardiovascular collapse has occurred following propranolol overdose [36].

WITHDRAWAL. Sudden discontinuation of long-term beta-blocker therapy may precipitate angina pectoris and myocardial infarction. This is the result of the so-called beta-blocker withdrawal phenomenon, explained by the theory that long-term beta-blocker therapy not only diminishes receptor occupancy by catecholamines but also increases the number of receptors sensitive to adrenergic stimulation. When beta-blockers are suddenly withdrawn, the increased pool of sensitive receptors responds more readily to the stimulation of circulating catecholamines [9].

Diagnostic Evaluation

HISTORY AND PHYSICAL EXAMINATION. The history should include the time, amount, and formulation of drug(s) ingested, the circumstances involved, time of onset and nature of any symptoms, and treatments rendered prior to arrival as well as underlying health problems. Beta-adrenergic blocker poisoning may be difficult to recognize, especially when multiple drugs have been ingested [9]. Beta-blocker poisoning should be suspected in a patient who suddenly develops hypotension or seizures or who has bradycardia resistant to the usual doses of chronotropic drugs [37]. Evaluation of patients with suspected beta-blocker poisoning should begin with a complete set of vital signs, continuous cardiac monitoring, and a 12-lead electrocardiogram (ECG). Physical examination should focus on the cardiovascular, pulmonary, and neurologic systems. Vital signs and physical examination should be repeated frequently.

ANCILLARY STUDIES. Serum drug levels may help confirm the diagnosis but are rarely available quickly enough to be clinically useful. In addition, differences in individual patient metabolism and sympathetic tone may make interpretation of blood levels difficult [9,12]. A serum specimen should be saved for later analysis in forensic cases such as nonaccidental poisoning in children or if the patient has committed a crime. Continuous cardiac rhythm monitoring, interpretation of 12-lead ECGs, and measurement of oxygen saturation should be routine. Laboratory evaluation of symptomatic patients should include complete blood count (CBC), electrolytes, blood urea nitrogen (BUN), creatinine, and glucose. Arterial blood gases and a chest film should also be assessed in patients with abnormal vital signs or altered level of consciousness.

DIFFERENTIAL DIAGNOSIS. Other causes of cardiovascular collapse to consider in the differential diagnosis of beta-blocker poisoning include anaphylactic, cardiogenic, hypovolemic, and septic shock. Poisoning by antiarrhythmic drugs, calcium channel blockers, cholinergic agents, clonidine, digitalis, narcotics, sedative-hypnotics, and tricyclic antidepressants may cause similar clinical toxicity.

Management

GENERAL. Treatment is primarily supportive and aimed at preventing or reducing drug absorption, enhancing elimination, and treating life-threatening CNS and cardiovascular abnormalities. An intravenous bolus of glucose (50 ml of $D_{50}W$ in adults; 4 ml/kg of $D_{25}W$ in children) as well as naloxone (2 mg) should be given to patients with altered mental status. Treatment of other consequences of beta-adrenergic blocker poisoning depends on the organ system involved and may include endotracheal intubation and mechanical ventilation for CNS or respiratory depression, anticonvulsants (e.g., diazepam, phenytoin, barbiturates) for seizures, and bronchodilators for wheezing. Peripheral and pulmonary artery pressure monitoring may be necessary in patients with hemodynamic instability.

GASTROINTESTINAL DECONTAMINATION. Activated charcoal and gastric lavage are the preferred methods for gastric decontamination [11,29,38,39]. Because seizures, obtundation, or hemodynamic compromise may occur suddenly after beta-blocker overdose, syrup of ipecac should not be given. Administration of atropine prior to lavage has been recommended to block increased vagal tone and potential cardiovasculant depressant effects [38]. Repeated doses of charcoal every 2 to 6 hours may enhance total body clearance and elimination of beta-blockers, especially those that are highly metabolized by the liver [34], in addition to preventing further drug absorption.

CARDIOVASCULAR SUPPORT. Of the number of agents used to treat hypotension and bradycardia, the one that seems most consistently effective in reversing these symptoms is glucagon [10,11,29,40–43]. Because glucagon has a half-life of only about 20 minutes, a continuous intravenous infusion of 1 to 5 mg per hour is recommended after an initial bolus of 3 to 10 mg for adults. In children, an initial intravenous dose of 0.05 mg per kilogram should be followed by a continuous infusion of 0.07 mg/kg/hr [9,11,12,40,44]. The dose should be tapered as the patient's clinical condition improves. The mechanism by which glucagon produces a positive inotropic and chronotropic effect on the heart is believed to be activation of the adenyl cyclase enzyme system independent of beta-receptors, thus augmenting contractility even in the presence of complete beta-adrenergic blockade [41]. It is recommended that glucagon be reconstituted in a solution of 5% dextrose in water or in preservative-free saline, rather than the diluent provided by the manufacturer, since the latter contains phenol, which may be toxic in large doses [40,45,46]. Non-phenol-containing high-dose glucagon preparations are now available [47].

Other agents used in the treatment of cardiovascular depression associated with beta-blocker overdose are atropine, isoproterenol, epinephrine, norepinephrine, dopamine, dobutamine, prenalterol [48], and calcium [49]. The simultaneous use of multiple agents may be effective when a single agent fails. Prenalterol, a beta1 agonist, is currently available only in Europe. Success in reversing bradycardia, hypotension, and heart block using these agents has been variable and inconsistent, frequently requiring very high doses to raise blood pressure and heart rate [9–12].

Transient blood pressure elevations caused by pindolol usually require no specific treatment. Short-acting agents such as nitroprusside should be used if marked blood pressure elevation occurs, especially if it is accompanied by organ ischemia. Ventricular dysrhythmias induced by sotalol have been treated with lidocaine, isoproterenol, magnesium, and cardioversion-defibrillation [12,20,50]. Electrical cardiac pacing may be needed if bradycardia, hypotension, and heart block fail to respond to pharmacologic therapy [9,10,11] or if ventricular tachydysrhythmias associated with a prolonged Q–T interval are difficult to control [20]. Intraaortic balloon pump counterpulsation [47] and extracorporeal circulation [51] have been successfully used for cardiovascular support.

HEMODIALYSIS/HEMOPERFUSION. Although the efficacy of hemodialysis in acute beta-blocker poisoning has not been studied in controlled clinical trials, it is theoretically useful in removing beta-blockers that are water-soluble and not significantly protein-bound. Hemodialysis appeared to be clinically useful in a single case of atenolol poisoning [52] and in a case of refractory *Torsades de pointes* due to sotalol [53]. Charcoal hemoperfusion has also been suggested as an adjunctive therapy in patients severely poisoned with beta-blockers, although experience is limited [54].

DISPOSITION. Patients with beta-blocker overdose who have abnormal vital signs, altered mental status, or dysrhythmias on presentation should be admitted to an intensive care unit. If vital signs can be supported, complete recovery can be expected within 24 to 48 hours. Patients with mild to absent toxicity who remain or become asymptomatic and have normal vital signs after 6 hours of observation in the emergency department can usually be referred for psychiatric evaluation (if the overdose was intentional) or discharged to the care of a reliable observer (if the overdose was accidental). Any symptoms should mandate longer observation or admission.

References

1. Powell CE, Slater IH: Blocking of inhibitory adrenergic receptors by a dichloro-analog of isoproterenol. *J Pharmacol Exp Ther* 122:480, 1958.
2. Fraunfelder FT: Ocular beta-blockers and systemic effects. *Arch Intern Med* 146:1073, 1986.
3. Nelson WL, Fraunfelder FT, Sills JM, et al: Adverse respiratory and cardiovascular events attributed to timolol ophthalmic solution. *Am J Ophthalmol* 102:606, 1986.
4. Hayes LP, Stewart CJ, Mohr J: Timolol side effects and inadvertent overdose. *J Am Geriatr Soc* 37:261, 1989
5. Miller RR, Olson HG, Amsterdam EA, et al: Propranolol withdrawal rebound phenomenon: Exacerbation of coronary events after abrupt cessation of anti-anginal therapy. *N Engl J Med* 293:416, 1975.
6. Prichard BNC, Walden RJ: The syndrome associated with the withdrawal of beta-blocking drugs. *Br J Clin Pharm* 13(suppl 2):3375, 1982.
7. Frishman WH: Beta-adrenergic blockers. *Med Clin North Am* 72:37, 1988.
8. Frishman WH: *Clinical Pharmacology of the Beta Adrenoceptor Blocking Drugs.* 2nd ed. Norwalk, CT, Appleton-Century-Crofts, 1984.
9. Frishman W, Jacob H, Eisenberg E, et al: Clinical pharmacology of the new beta-adrenergic blocking drugs. 8. Self-poisoning with beta-adrenoceptor blocking agents: Recognition and management. *Am Heart J* 98:798, 1979.
10. Critchley JA, Ungar A: The management of acute poisoning due to beta-adrenoceptor antagonists. *Med Tox Adverse Drug Exp* 4:32, 1989.
11. Weinstein RS: Recognition and management of poisoning with beta-adrenergic blocking agents. *Ann Emerg Med* 12:1123, 1984.
12. Prichard B, Battersby L, Cruickshank JM: Overdosage with beta-adrenergic blocking agents. *Adv Drug React Poison Rev* 3:91, 1984.

13. Thorpe P: Pindolol in hypertension. *Med J Aust* 58:1242, 1971
14. Offenstadt G, Hericord P, Amstutz P: Intoxication volontaire par le pindolol. *Nouv Presse Med* 5:1539, 1976.
15. Editorial: Self-poisoning with beta-blockers *Br Med J* 1:1010, 1978.
16. Favarel-Garrignes JC, Gbikpi-Benisson G, Poisot D, et al: Toxicite digue des beta-bloquants. *Bordeau Med* 11:2623, 1978.
17. Lagerfelt J, Matell G: Attempted suicide with 5.1 gm of propranolol. *Acta Med Scand* 199:517, 1976.
18. Khan A, Muscat Baron JM: Fatal oxprenolol poisoning. *Br Med J* 1:552, 1977.
19. Gwinup GR: Propranolol toxicity presenting with early repolarization, ST changes and peaked T waves on EKG. *Ann Emerg Med* 17:171, 1988.
20. Totterman KJ, Turto H, Pellinen T: Overdrive pacing as treatment of sotalol-induced ventricular tachyarrhythmias (torsade de pointes). *Acta Med Scand* 668(suppl):28, 1982.
21. Baliga BG: Beta-blocker poisoning: Prolongation of QT interval and inversion of T waves. *J Ind Med Assoc* 83:165, 1985.
22. Beattie JM: Sotalol-induced torsade. *Scot Med J* 29:240, 1984.
23. Turner P: Fatal oxprenolol poisoning. *Br Med J* 1:1084, 1977
24. Buiumsohn A, Eisenberg ES, Jacob H, et al: Seizures and intraventricular conduction defect in propranolol poisoning. *Ann Intern Med* 91:860, 1979.
25. Frishman W, Silverman R, Strom J, et al: Clinical pharmacology of the new beta-adrenergic drugs. 4. Adverse effect: Choosing a beta-adrenoceptor blocker. *Am Heart J* 98:256, 1979.
26. Frishman W: Clinical pharmacology of the new beta-adrenergic blocking drugs. 1. Pharmacodynamic and pharmacokinetic properties. *Am Heart J* 97:663, 1979.
27. Laake K, Kittang E, Refstadt S, et al: Convulsions and possible spasm of the lower oesophageal sphincter in a fatal case of propranolol intoxication. *Acta Med Scand* 210:137, 1981.
28. Mattingly PC: Oxprenolol overdose with survival. *Br Med J* 1:776, 1977.
29. Shore ET, Cepin D, Davidson MJ: Metoprolol overdose. *Ann Emerg Med* 10:524, 1981,
30. Wallin CJ, Hulting J: Massive metoprolol poisoning treated with prenalterol. *Acta Med Scand* 214:253, 1983.
31. Benowitz NL: Beta adrenoceptor blocker poisoning, in Haddad LM, Winchester JF (eds): *Clinical Management of Poisoning and Drug Overdose.* 2nd ed. Philadelphia, WB Saunders, 1990, p 1315.
32. Weinstein R, Cole S, Knaster H, et al: Beta-blocker overdose with propranolol and atenolol. *Ann Emerg Med* 14:161, 1985.
33. Lundvall J, Jahult J: Beta-adrenergic dilator component of the sympathetic vascular response in skeletal muscle. *Acta Physiol Scand* 96:180, 1976
34. Becker CE: Beta blocking agents, in Rumack BH (ed): *Poisindex.* Denver, Micromedex, 1990.
35. Korzets A, Danby P, Edmunds ME et al: Acute renal failure associated with a labetalol overdose. *Postgrad Med J* 66:66, 1990.
36. Pettei M, Levy J, Abramson S: Non occlusive mesenteric ischemia associated with propranolol overdose: Implications regarding splanchnic circulation. *J Pediatr Gastroenterol Nutr* 10:544, 1990.
37. Bekes C, Scott WE: Occult metoprolol overdose. *Crit Care Med* 13:871, 1985
38. Soni N, Baines D, Pearson IY: Cardiovascular collapse and propranolol overdose. *Med J Aust* 2:629, 1983.
39. Wilkinson J: Beta-blocker overdose. *Ann Emerg Med* 15:982,1986.
40. Illingworth RN: Glucagon for beta-blocker poisoning. *Practitioner* 223:863, 1979.
41. Kosinski EJ, Malindzak GS: Glucagon and isoproterenol in reversing propranolol toxicity. *Arch Intern Med* 132:840, 1973.
42. Parmley WW: The role of glucagon in cardiac therapy. *N Engl J Med* 285:801, 1971.
43. Robson RH: Glucagon for beta-blocker poisoning. *Lancet* 1:1357, 1980.
44. Agura ED, Wexler LF, Witzburg RA: Massive propranolol overdose: Successful treatment with high dose isoproterenol and glucagon. *Am J Med* 80:755, 1986.
45. Mofenson HC, Caraccio TR, Landano J: Glucagon for propranolol overdose (letter). *JAMA* 255:2025, 1986.
46. Cronk JD: Phenol with glucagon in cardiotherapy (letter). *N Engl J Med* 284:219, 1971.
47. Lane AS, Woodward AC, Goldman MR: Massive propranolol over-

dose poorly responsive to pharmacologic therapy: Use of the intraaortic-balloon pump. *Ann Intern Med* 16:1381, 1987.

48. Critchley J, Ungar A: The management of acute poisoning due to B adrenoceptor antagonists. *Med Toxicol* 4:32, 1989.

49. Brimacombe JR, Scully M, Swainston R: Propranolol overdose: A dramatic response to calcium chloride. *Med J Aust* 135:267, 1991.

50. Arstall M, Mii J, Lehman R, et al: Sotalol-induced *Torsades de pointes*: Management with magnesium infusion. *Postgrad Med J* 68:289, 1992.

51. Mcvey FK, Corke DF: Extracorporeal circulation in the management of massive propranolol overdose. *Anaesthesia* 46:744, 1991.

52. Saitz R, Williams B, Farber M: Atenolol-induced cardiovascular collapse treated with hemodialysis. *Crit Care Med* 19:116, 1991.

53. Singh S, Lazin A, Cohen A, et al: Sotalol-induced *Torsades de pointes* successfully treated with hemodialysis after failure of conventional therapy. *Am Heart J* 121:601, 1991.

54. Anthony T, Jastremski J, Elliott W, et al: Charcoal hemoperfusion for the treatment of a combined diltiazem and metoprolol overdose. *Ann Emerg Med* 15:1344, 1986.

136. Calcium Channel Blocker Poisoning

Christian Tomaszewski

Overview

Calcium channel blocker (CCB) poisoning can be life-threatening, and in certain susceptible individuals toxicity can occur with therapeutic doses [1–4]. In 1993, 6730 potentially toxic exposures involving CCBs were reported to the American Association of Poison Control Centers [5]. Of the 3802 cases evaluated at health care facilities, there were 182 cases of major poisoning and 35 deaths [5]. Diltiazem, nifedipine, and verapamil are among the top 20 drugs prescribed in the United States [6]. Opportunities for toxic exposures will increase with the introduction of new forms and indications for CCBs as well as aging of the U.S. population.

FORMULATIONS. The three most common CCBs, verapamil (Calan, Isoptin), diltiazem (Cardizem), and nifedipine (Procardia, Adalat), are used to treat a variety of conditions, including angina, hypertension, arrhythmias, congestive heart failure, Raynaud's syndrome, asthma, and migraine headaches [7]. All three agents have the ability to decrease coronary vascular resistance with an increase in coronary blood flow and decrease in myocardial oxygen demand [8]. Verapamil and diltiazem can also slow atrioventricular nodal conduction [9]. Although the dihydropyridines, of which nifedipine is the prototype, can inhibit calcium entry into vascular smooth muscle and myocardial tissue, they do not appear clinically to affect myocardial conduction and contractility at therapeutic doses.

A whole host of new CCBs was recently introduced, all of which are dihydropyridine derivatives. Most are approved for the treatment of angina and hypertension, and nimodipine is approved for cerebral vasospasm associated with subarachnoid hemorrhage. No overdose data are available for these agents, but the most common side effect is hypotension [10,11]. Unlike other dihydropyridines, isradipine can cause negative chronotropic effects because it has some selective inhibition of the sinoatrial node [12,13].

PHARMACOLOGY. The clinical effects of CCBs stem from their ability to prevent extracellular calcium from entering into cardiac and smooth muscle cells through calcium-specific membrane channels [14]. Calcium influx is necessary for the release of a larger intracellular pool of calcium, which combines with modulatory proteins interposed between actin and myosin [15]. The combination of calcium with the proteins allows the actin and myosin to interact and produce muscle contraction [16]. The end result is that CCBs decrease smooth muscle tone, with resulting systemic arteriolar and coronary artery vasodilation [8]. There also is a tendency for reduced myocardial contractility with these agents, compensated for by an increase in heart rate and decrease in afterload [17].

Calcium channels are also important in the pacemaker cells of the heart. In excitable tissues, depolarization is dependent on the rapid influx of sodium ions, followed by the slow influx of calcium ions. However, the sinoatrial and atrioventricular nodes are dependent on the latter, with the fast sodium channels inoperative at the lower resting membrane potentials of these cells [18]. Consequently, calcium channel blockade results in decreased impulse conduction at the sinoatrial and atrioventricular nodes [15,19,20].

Differences in structure influence the affinity of CCBs for calcium channels of various tissues and account for their diverse hemodynamic effects [21] (see Chap. 210). All of the CCBs have similar pharmacokinetic profiles (see Chap. 210). They are well absorbed from the small intestine, with an onset of action ranging from 15 to 30 minutes following ingestion [8,22]. Effects are noted within 5 minutes of "sublingual" nifedipine administration [8,22]. Verapamil is almost completely absorbed within 45 minutes of ingestion [23]. Sustained-release preparations are available of the original three CCBs (verapamil, diltiazem, and nifedipine) and some of the newer dihydropyridines.

The bioavailability of CCBs by the oral route is low because of extensive first-pass liver metabolism [24,25]. Verapamil is subjected to N-dealkylation in the liver to produce an active metabolite, norverapamil, having about 20 percent of the activity of the parent compound [26]. Diltiazem is deacetylated to deacetyldiltiazem, which is 50 to 75 percent less potent as a coronary vasodilator than the parent drug [27]. The principal metabolite of nifedipine, a methoxylcarbonylpyridine derivative, has minimal pharmacologic activity [28].

Clinical Manifestations

ACUTE TOXICITY. Cardiovascular toxicity is the primary effect of CCB poisoning. Hypotension, bradycardia, atrioventricular block, and asystole have all been reported following over-doses of verapamil [29–39] and diltiazem [30,34,40,41]. After overdose, verapamil, diltiazem, and nifedipine primarily cause hypotension. Of note, significant decreases in peripheral vascular resistance are not noted at doses of verapamil that cause hypotension [42]. It appears that the hypotension induced by verapamil and diltiazem stems from their negative inotropic effects [43]. In addition, diltiazem and to some extent verapamil interfere with reflexive tachycardia in response to hypotension [9]. Verapamil and diltiazem also decrease sinus node discharge and conduction through the atrioventricular node [44,45].

The primary symptom of nifedipine overdose is also hypotension [46]. However, canine studies demonstrate that nifedipine causes hypotension through direct peripheral vasodilation [14]. In contrast to diltiazem and verapamil, nifedipine overdoses are usually followed by tachycardia [46,47]. Cardiac conduction defects are seen less commonly with nifedipine toxicity than with toxicity from other CCBs [9,14,45,46]. However, several patients reported in the literature have developed bradycardia and atrioventricular block after isolated nifedipine overdose [46,48]. Animal studies show that high doses of nifedipine can cause conduction disturbances in addition to negative inotropic and chronotropic effects [49]. Overdoses of the other dihydropyridines have not yet been reported. Because of structural similarities, their toxicity is likely to be similar.

Other clinical effects of CCB overdose include confusion and lethargy, presumably secondary to hypotension [29,30,36,37,38]. Seizures have been described in children after verapamil overdose [29,50]. Nausea and vomiting are not uncommon [31,32]. Metabolic acidosis and hyperglycemia can occur but are usually self-limited [36,37,39,48]. One patient with hyperglycemia following diltiazem overdose required an intravenous insulin infusion [30]. Hyperglycemia is due to the inhibition of glucose-induced insulin release from pancreatic islet cells [51,52,53].

Patients without cardiac disease usually require supratherapeutic doses before manifesting toxicity. In a recent series, mean ingestions of the various CCBs in children that resulted in toxicity were as follows: verapamil 21 mg per kilogram, diltiazem 5.7 mg per kilogram, and nifedipine 8.0 mg per kilogram [46]. A 400-mg dose of verapamil was reported to cause hypotension, bradycardia, and seizures in an 11-month-old infant [50]. A 25-month-old boy died after ingesting 1.44 gm of a sustained-release verapamil preparation; his 24-hour verapamil blood level immediately prior to death was 3300 ng per milliliter [29].

In a recent series of 139 CCB overdoses, the smallest dose of CCB resulting in toxicity in adults was listed as verapamil 720 mg, diltiazem 420 mg, and nifedipine 50 mg [46]. Adults have survived ingestions of 3.2 and 16 gm of verapamil with peak measured verapamil levels of 4000 ng per milliliter and 1575 ng per milliliter, respectively, without permanent sequelae [54,55]. Ingestion of as little as 1.5 gm of diltiazem in a 74-year-old man resulted in asystole requiring cardiac pacing [30]. Two patients with nifedipine overdose of 300 and 900 mg recovered after treatment with intravenous saline, calcium, and pressors [47,48].

With routine preparations of these drugs, onset of toxicity is usually within 6 hours of ingestion [46]. Symptoms can be seen as early as 1 hour after verapamil overdose and may persist for 24 to 36 hours [31,34]. Duration of toxicity in most cases is less than 12 hours, with no reported case with toxicity beyond 48 hours [46]. With therapeutic doses of sustained-release verapamil, peak plasma level can be as late as 5 to 7 hours [56]. The onset of cardiovascular toxicity can be delayed 12 or more hours after overdose of sustained-release verapamil [46]. In overdose, symptoms can be both delayed in presentation and prolonged once they occur [57].

CHRONIC TOXICITY. Chronic toxicity with therapeutic use of CCBs is primarily seen in the elderly. This is partly due to underlying cardiac problems in this population. Therapeutic use of all of these drugs has resulted in hypotension [1]. In the case of diltiazem and verapamil, bradycardia and heart block requiring pacing have been reported [2,3,4]. Long-term use of CCBs can result in peripheral edema, especially with dihydropyridines [58].

Conditions that may exacerbate CCB toxicity include underlying liver disease and the concomitant use of other cardiac medications. Liver disease can reduce the elimination of verapamil [37,59]. Combined therapy with verapamil and beta-blockers has resulted in congestive heart failure, atrioventricular block, and even asystole [9,43,60,61]. Verapamil can also decrease the clearance of digoxin [62].

Diagnostic Evaluation

The initial work-up of a patient with CCB overdose should include a cardiac rhythm strip and 12-lead electrocardiogram. These are essential for documenting bradyarrhythmias and conduction defects and to serve as a baseline. A chest radiograph may be useful to rule out aspiration in the comatose patient or to check endotracheal tube placement. Pulmonary edema can occur with fluid resuscitation [48,63]. Laboratory evaluation should be dictated by severity of the clinical condition. Admitting blood work should include at least serum electrolytes and glucose. A serum calcium level may help guide subsequent therapy but is unaffected by CCBs. Seriously ill patients may also benefit from arterial blood gas, cell blood count, and renal and liver function tests. Serum levels of CCBs, although not routinely available, may be useful to confirm the overdose.

DIFFERENTIAL DIAGNOSIS. The differential diagnosis of a patient with hypotension, bradycardia, conduction delay, and altered mental status includes myocardial disease (i.e., infarction), cerebrovascular accident, anaphylaxis, hypovolemic shock, renal failure with hyperkalemia, and poisoning by other agents. Conduction block can be seen with acute digitalis intoxication; gastrointestinal distress is generally more severe, and hyperkalemia may be present [64]. Delayed cardiac conduction, hypotension, mental status changes, and vomiting can also be seen with beta-blocker overdose [65]. In contrast to the hyperglycemia noted with CCB poisoning, hypoglycemia may be associated with beta-blocker intoxication. Antiarrhythmics, clonidine, quinine, chloroquine, organophosphates, tricyclic antidepressants, narcotics, and sedative-hypnotics should also be considered in the differential diagnosis [66].

Management

GENERAL. Treatment of the patient with CCB poisoning should begin with routine airway management, establishment of an intravenous line of normal saline, and continuous cardiac monitoring. All patients should be observed for at least 6 hours; sustained-release preparations may require observation for 12 to 24 hours. Symptomatic hypotension should initially be treated with an intravenous fluid challenge of 0.5 to 1.0 liter (10 to 20 ml/kg in children) [67]. One canine study of verapamil poisoning found that rapid infusions of saline improved cardiac conduction and increased heart rate [68]. In cases where hypotension stems from bradycardia or atrioventricular blockade, atropine and electrical pacing can be attempted, though they are often ineffective [30,34,48,55,69]. Altered mental status should be treated presumptively with intravenous dextrose and naloxone.

Gastric decontamination should be accomplished using activated charcoal and lavage. The latter should be performed cautiously so as not to exacerbate bradycardia and heart block as a result of vagal effects. In the case of sustained-release preparations, multiple doses of charcoal or polyethylene glycol whole bowel irrigation may be useful [70]. Syrup of ipecac should be avoided because of the potential for decrease in mental status.

All symptomatic patients deserve frequent or continuous blood pressure monitoring. Central venous or pulmonary artery pressure evaluation may be necessary in patients with severe or persistent hypotension [38]. A central line also provides access for ventricular pacing, if needed [48]. All patients with hypotension, bradycardia, or atrioventricular block after CCB ingestion or overdose require admission to an intensive care setting.

CARDIOVASCULAR TOXICITY. The antidote of choice for CCB-induced hypotension is calcium [1,37,67,71,72]. Controlled human studies indicate that pretreatment with intravenous calcium can prevent the hypotension, but not the bradycardia, that occurs with intravenous verapamil therapy [73,74]. Multiple animal studies confirm calcium's ability to reverse the negative inotropic effects of CCB toxicity [42,68,75,76].

The effect of calcium salts on bradycardia and cardiac conduction is unclear. Animal studies have shown that calcium causes an increase in atrioventricular conduction after verapamil toxicity [68,77]. Improvement in heart rate after calcium infusions for CCB toxicity in humans has been reported [37,48,54,78]. Calcium in some instances has resulted in reversal of atrioventricular conduction disturbances [46,67].

The recommended dose of calcium chloride for the treatment of CCB toxicity in adults is 5 to 10 ml of a 10% solution and of calcium gluconate is 10 to 20 ml of a 10% solution [79,80,81]. The dose for children is 0.2 ml per kilogram of a 10% calcium chloride solution or 1 ml per kilogram of a 10% calcium gluconate solution [82]. Calcium chloride should be infused no faster than 1 to 2 ml/min with the patient monitored for cardiac dysrhythmias [80]. Rapid infusions of calcium have been reported to cause hypotension, bradycardia, arrhythmias, and cardiac arrest [83]. Following intravenous administration, it can take 0.5 to 2 hours for calcium serum levels to return to preinjection values [84]. A continuous calcium chloride infusion (1 ml/hr of 10% solution) was used with good response in a hypotensive nifedipine overdose patient [48]. Calcium chloride may be a better agent for CCB overdose than calcium gluconate, because the former provides three times as much calcium ion [84].

Hypotension often may not respond to calcium infusions [33,35,36,39,41,50,85]. If this occurs, pressors should be used in addition to intravenous fluids. One rat study suggested that sympathomimetic amines are superior to calcium at improving

pacemaker activity and cardiac conduction, as well as having inotropic action [75]. Both epinephrine and norepinephrine can indirectly increase the calcium available for cardiac and smooth muscle contraction [8]. In one patient, hypotension due to verapamil overdose was successfully treated with an epinephrine drip after calcium therapy corrected concomitant atrioventricular dissociation [35]. In an anesthetized dog model, epinephrine infusion improved survival and cardiac function after a lethal dose of intravenous verapamil [86].

Other catecholamines may be useful for treating CCB hypotension. Multiple case reports document the efficacy of dopamine for reversing hypotension due to CCB toxicity [36, 39,47,50]. In the canine model, sympathomimetic agents with beta-adrenergic activity (e.g., isoproterenol) were superior to atropine and sympathomimetic agents without beta activity (e.g., phenylephrine) in reversing myocardial depression from verapamil, partly through increasing heart rate [42]. Bradycardia and hypotension that failed to respond to calcium infusions have been successfully treated with isoproterenol [38,85]. Glucagon (3–5 mg IV) also has been shown to reverse myocardial depression and bradycardia in experimental verapamil toxicity [87,88,89]. Glucagon increases cyclic AMP concentrations through a receptor distinct from that of catecholamines [90]. Amrinone, another inotropic agent and potential treatment for CCB toxicity, is a phosphodiesterase inhibitor that increases intracellular cyclic AMP. Although only one case report attests to its usefulness [38], canine studies show its ability to improve cardiac dysfunction from verapamil toxicity [91,92].

NEW ANTIDOTES. There are several new experimental treatments for CCB toxicity. One promising drug is 4-aminopyridine (4-AP), a potassium channel blocker that indirectly increases calcium influx [93,94]. Studies of animals with verapamil toxicity show that 4-AP reverses bradycardia and negative inotropy [42] as well as increasing survival [95]. A patient who presented with hypotension, bradycardia, and third-degree block from chronic verapamil ingestion showed reversal of symptoms with two 10-mg infusions of 4-AP [78]. There is a whole class of calcium agonistic dihydropyridines that may be useful [96]. The prototype, Bay K 8644, was superior to 4-AP in reversing cardiac conduction problems and hypotension from verapamil intoxication in rabbits [97]. Finally, insulin treatment with a euglycemic clamp was found to provide protection from a lethal overdose of verapamil in a canine model [98]. As mentioned earlier, verapamil inhibits pancreatic secretion of insulin [51]. In addition, insulin may be necessary because of the heart's increased dependence on carbohydrates with verapamil toxicity [99].

OTHER MEASURES. Extracorporeal methods for drug elimination have been used with variable success for CCB overdoses. Charcoal hemoperfusion was claimed to be useful in a combined overdose of diltiazem and metoprolol, as it achieved diltiazem clearance rates averaging 67 ml per minute [100]. Hemodialysis used to treat a patient with a verapamil overdose was shown to have no impact on verapamil or norverapamil levels [78]. Because of their large volume of distribution and high protein binding, CCBs are not likely to be readily eliminated by extracorporeal procedures, and routine use of such therapy is not indicated. Intraaortic balloon pump or cardiac bypass pump support should be considered for refractory cases of CCB poisoning [101]. Most patients recover fully if vital signs can be supported until the drugs are eliminated.

References

1. Lipman J, Jardine I, Roos C: Intravenous calcium chloride as an antidote to verapamil-induced hypotension. *Intensive Care Med* 8:55, 1982.
2. McGraw BF, Wlaker SD, Hemberger JA, et al: Clinical experience with diltiazem in Japan. *Pharmacotherapy* 2:156, 1982.
3. Morris DL, Goldschlanger N: Calcium infusion for reversal of adverse effects of intravenous verapamil. *JAMA* 249:3212, 1983.
4. O'Mailia JJ, Sander GE, Giles TD: Nifedipine associated myocardial ischemia or infarction in the treatment of hypertensive urgencies. *Ann Intern Med* 107:185, 1987.
5. Litovitz TL, Clark LR, Soloway RA, et al: 1993 annual report of the American Association of Poison Control Centers Toxic Exposure Surveillance System. *Am J Emerg Med* 12:546, 1994.
6. Merz B: Pharmaceutical list tracks hit parade of prescriptions. *Am Med News* March 4: 4, 1991.
7. Weiner D: Calcium channel blockers. *Med Clin North Am* 72:83, 1988.
8. Conti CR, Pepine CJ, Feldman RL, et al: Calcium antagonists. *Cardiology* 72:297, 1985.
9. Mitchell LB, Schroeder JS, Mason JW: Comparative clinical electrophysiologic effects of diltiazem, verapamil, and nifedipine: A review. *Am J Cardiol* 49:629, 1982.
10. Scheidt S, LeWinter MM, Hermanovich J, et al: Nicardipine for stable angina pectoris. *Br J Clin Pharm* 20(suppl):178s, 1985.
11. Product information: Nimodipine. West Haven, CT, Miles. 1989.
12. Mauser M, Voelker W, Ickrath O, et al: Myocardial properties of the new dihydropyridine calcium antagonist isradipine compared to nifedipine with or without additional beta blockade in coronary artery disease. *Am J Cardiol* 63:40, 1989.
13. Van Den Berg EK, Dehmer GJ: Acute hemodynamic effects of intravenous isradipine. *Am J Cardiol* 61:1102, 1988.
14. Henry PD: Comparative pharmacology of calcium antagonists: Nifedipine, verapamil, and diltiazem. *Am J Cardiol* 46:1047, 1980.
15. Fleckenstein A: Specific pharmacology of calcium in myocardium, cardiac pacemakers, and vascular smooth muscle. *Annu Rev Pharmacol Toxicol* 17:149, 1977.
16. Winegrad S: Regulation of cardiac contractile proteins: Correlation between physiology and biochemistry. *Circ Res* 55:565, 1984.
17. Low RI, Takeda P, Mason DT, et al: The effects of calcium channel blocking agents on cardiovascular function. *Am J Cardiol* 49:547, 1982.
18. Schwartz DJ, Wasserstrom JA, Fozzard HA: Therapeutic uses of calcium-blocking agents: Verapamil, nifedipine, and diltiazem. *Compr Ther* 7:25, 1981.
19. Millard RW, Lathrop DA, Grupp G, et al: Differential cardiovascular effects of calcium channel blocking agents: Potential mechanisms. *Am J Cardiol* 49:499, 1982.
20. Das G: Fundamentals of calcium channel blockers. *Int J Clin Pharmacol Ther Toxicol* 26:575, 1988.
21. Snyder SH, Reynolds IJ: Caclium-antagonist drugs: Receptor interactions that clarify therapeutic effects. *N Engl J Med* 313:995, 1985.
22. McAllister RG: Clinical pharmacology of slow channel blocking agents. *Prog Cardiovasc Dis* 25:83, 1982.
23. Schomerus M, Spiegelhalder R, Stieren B, et al: Physiological disposition of verapamil in man. *Cardiovasc Res* 10:605, 1976.
24. Eichelbaum M, Dengler HJ, Somogyi A, et al: Superiority of stable isotope techniques in the assessment of the bioavailability of drugs undergoing extensive first pass elimination: Studies of the relative bioavailability of verapamil tablets. *Eur J Clin Pharmacol* 19:127, 1981.
25. Echizen H, Eichelbaum M: Clinical pharmacokinetics of verapamil, nifedipine and diltiazem. *Clin Pharmacokinet* 11:425, 1986.
26. Koike Y, Shimamura K, Shudo I, et al: Pharmacokinetics of verapamil in man. *Res Comm Chem Pathol Pharmacol* 24:37, 1979.
27. Morselli PL, Rovei V, Nitchand M, et al: Pharmacokinetics and metabolism of diltiazem in man, in Bing RJ (ed): *New Drug Therapy with Calcium Antagonist: Diltiazem Hakone Symposium 1978.* no. 487. Amsterdam, Excerpta Medica, 1978, p. 152.
28. Kroneberg G: Pharmacology of nifedipine, in Lochner W, Braasch W, Kroneberg G (eds): *Second International Adalat Symposium.* Berlin, Springer-Verlag, 1974, p 12.
29. Hendren WG, Schieber RS, Garrettson LK: Extracorporeal bypass for the treatment of verapamil poisoning. *Ann Emerg Med* 18:984, 1989.
30. Snover WS, Bocchino V: Massive diltiazem overdose. *Ann Emerg Med* 15:1221, 1986.
31. De Faire U, Lundman T: Attempted suicide with verapamil. *Eur J Cardiol* 6:195, 1977.
32. Candell J, Valle V, Soler M, et al: Acute intoxication with verapamil. *Chest* 75:200, 1979.
33. Da Silva OA, Ce Melo RA, Jorge Filho JPL: Verapamil acute self-poisoning. *Clin Toxicol* 14:361, 1979.
34. Immonen P, Linkola A, Waris E: Three cases of severe verapamil poisoning. *Int J Cardiol* 1:101, 1981.
35. Chimienti M, Previtali M, Medici A, et al: Acute verapamil poisoning: Successful treatment with epinephrine. *Clin Cardiol* 5:219, 1982.
36. Enyeart JJ, Price WA, Hoffman DA, et al: Profound hyperglycemia and metabolic acidosis after verapamil overdose. *J Am Coll Cardiol* 2:1228, 1983.
37. Zoghbi W, Schwartz JB: Verapamil overdose: Report of a case and review of the literature. *Cardiovasc Rev Rep* 5:356, 1984.
38. Goenen M, Col J, Compere A, et al: Treatment of severe verapamil poisoning with combined amrinone-isoproterenol therapy. *Am J Cardiol* 58:1142, 1986.
39. McMillan R: Management of acute severe verapamil intoxication. *J Emerg Med* 6:193, 1988.
40. Rey JL, Lecuyer D, Bernasconi P, et al: Intoxication volontaire par le diltiazem avec deficience sinusale et bloc auricoventriculaire. *Presse Med* 12:1873, 1983.
41. Jakubowski AT, Mizgala HF: Effect of diltiazem overdose. *Am J Cardiol* 60:932, 1987.
42. Gay RG, Alego S, Lee R, et al: Treatment of verapamil toxicity in intact dogs. *J Clin Invest* 77:1805, 1986.
43. Singh BN, Ellrodt G, Peter CT: Verapamil: A review of its pharmacological properties and therapeutic use. *Drugs* 15:169, 1978.
44. Antman EM, Stone PH, Muller JE, et al: Calcium channel blocking agents in the treatment of cardiovascular disorders. I. Basic and clinical electrophysiologic effects. *Ann Intern Med* 93:875, 1980.
45. Kawai C, Konishi T, Matsuyama E: Comparative effects of three calcium antagonists, diltiazem, verapamil and nifedipine, on the sinoatrial and atrioventricular nodes. *Circulation* 63:1035, 1981.
46. Ramoska EA, Spiller HA, Winter M, et al: A one-year evaluation of calcium channel blocker overdose: Toxicity and treatment. *Ann Emerg Med* 22:196, 1993.
47. Whitebloom D, Fitzharris J: Nifedipine overdose. *Clin Cardiol* 11:505, 1988.
48. Herrington DM, Insley BM, Weinmann GG: Nifedipine overdose. *Am J Med* 81:344, 1986.
49. Stone PH, Antman EM, Muller JE, et al: Calcium channel blocking agents in the treatment of cardiovascular disorders. II. Hemodynamic effects and clinical applications. *Ann Intern Med* 93:886, 1980.
50. Passal DB, Crespin FH: Verapamil poisoning in an infant. *Pediatrics* 73:543, 1984.
51. Devis G, Somers G, Ban Obberghen E, et al: Calcium antagonists and islet function. I. Inhibition of insulin release by verapamil. *Diabetes* 24:247, 1975.
52. DeMarinis L, Barbarino A: Calcium antagonists and hormone release. I. Effect of verapamil on insulin release in normal subjects and patients with islet-cell tumor. *Metabolism* 29:599, 1980.
53. Lewis JG: Adverse reactions to calcium antagonists. *Drugs* 25:196, 1983.
54. Perkins CM: Serious verapamil poisoning: Treatment with intravenous calcium gluconate. *Br Med J* 37:89, 1978.
55. Horowitz BZ, Rhee KJ: Massive verapamil ingestion: A report of two cases and a review of the literature. *Am J Emerg Med* 7:624, 1989.
56. Follath F, Ha HR, Schutz E, et al: Pharmacokinetics of conventional and slow-release verapamil. *Br J Clin Pharmacol* 21:149S, 1986.
57. Pearigan PD, Benowitz NL: Poisoning due to calcium antagonists: Experience with verapamil, diltiazem and nifedipine. *Drug Saf* 6:408, 1991.
58. Lynch P, Dargie H, Krikler S, et al: Objective assessment of antianginal treatment: A double-blind comparison of propranolol, nifedipine, and their combination. *Br Med J* 281:184, 1980.

59. Woodcock BG, Rietbrock I, Bohringer HF, et al: Verapamil disposition in liver disease and intensive care patients: Kinetics, clearance, and apparent blood flow relationships. *Clin Pharmacol Ther* 29:27, 1981.

60. Benaim ME: Asystole after verapamil. *Br Med J* 264:169, 1972.

61. Packer H, Meller J, Medina N, et al: Hemodynamic consequences of combined beta-adrenergic and slow calcium channel blockade in man. *Circulation* 65:660, 1982.

62. Klein HO, Lang R, Weiss E, et al: The influence of verapamil on serum digoxin concentration. *Circulation* 65:998, 1982.

63. Humbert VH, Munn NJ, Hawkins RF: Noncardiogenic pulmonary edema complication massive diltiazem overdose. *Chest* 99:258, 1991.

64. Bigger JT: Digitalis toxicity. *J Clin Pharmacol* 25:514, 1985.

65. Heath A: Beta-adrenoceptor blocker toxicity: Clinical features and therapy. *Am J Emerg Med* 2:518, 1984.

66. Rumack BH, Spoerke DG. POISONDEX® Information System. Denver, Micromedex, 1994.

67. Moroni F, Mannaioni PF: Calcium gluconate and hypertonic sodium chloride in a case of massive verapamil poisoning. *Clin Toxicol* 17:395, 1980.

68. Hariman RJ, Mangiardi LM, McAllister RG, et al: Reversal of the cardiovascular effects of verapamil by calcium and sodium: Differences between electrophysiologic and hemodynamic responses. *Circulation* 59:797, 1979.

69. Woodworth RS: Maximal contraction, "staircase" contraction, refractory period, and compensatory pause of the heart. *Am J Physiol* 8:213, 1902.

70. Buckley N, Dawson AH, Howarth D, et al: Slow-release verapamil poisoning: Use of polyethylene glycol whole-bowel lavage and high-dose calcium. *Med J Aust* 158:202, 1993.

71. Woie L, Storstein L: Successful treatment of suicidal verapamil poisoning with calcium gluconate. *Eur Heart J* 2:239, 1981.

72. Orr GM, Bodansky HJ, Dymond DS, et al: Fatal verapamil overdose. *Lancet* 1:1218, 1982.

73. Weiss AT, Lewis BS, Halon DA, et al: The use of calcium with verapamil in the management of supraventricular tachyarrhythmias. *Int J Cardiol* 6:193, 1988.

74. Haft JI, Habbab MA: Treatment of atrial arrhythmias: Effectiveness of verapamil when preceded by calcium infusion. *Arch Intern Med* 146:1085, 1986.

75. Strubelt O, Diederich K: Experimental investigations on the antidotal treatment of nifedipine overdosage. *Clin Toxicol* 24:135, 1986.

76. Zipes DP, Fischer JC: Effects of agents which inhibit the slow channel on sinus node automaticity and atrioventricular conduction in the dog. *Circ Res* 34:184, 1974.

77. Vick JA, Kandil A, Herman EH, et al: Reversal of propranolol and verapamil toxicity by calcium. *Vet Hum Toxicol* 25:8, 1983.

78. ter Wee PM, Kremer Hovinga TK, Uges DRA, et al: 4-aminopyridine and haemodialysis in the treatment of verapamil intoxication. *Hum Toxicol* 4:327, 1985.

79. AMA Department of Drugs: *AMA Drug Evaluations*. 5th ed. Chicago, American Medical Association, 1983.

80. Gilman AG, Goodman LS, Gilman A: *The Pharmacologic Basis of Therapeutics*. 6th ed. New York, Macmillan, 1983.

81. Hughes WS, Ruedy JR: Should calcium be used in cardiac arrest? *Am J Med* 81:285, 1986.

82. Benitz WE, Tatro DS: *The Pediatric Drug Handbook*. Chicago, Year Book, 1987.

83. Carlon GC, Howland WS, Goldner PL: Adverse effects of calcium administration. *Arch Surg* 113:882, 1978.

84. White RDD, Goldsmith RS, Rodrigues R: Plasma ionic calcium levels following injection of chloride, gluconate, and gluceptate salts of calcium. *J Thorac Cardiovasc Surg* 71:609, 1976.

85. Crump BJ, Holt DW, Vale JA: Lack of response to intravenous calcium in severe verapamil poisoning. *Lancet* 2:939, 1982.

86. Kline JA, Tomaszewski CA, Schroeder JD, et al: Insulin is a superior antidote for cardiovascular toxicity induced by verapamil in the anesthetized canine. *J Pharmacol Exp Therap* 267:744, 1993.

87. Jolly SR, Kipnis JN, Lucchesi BR: Cardiovascular depression by verapamil: Reversal by glucagon and interactions with propranolol. *Pharmacology* 35:249, 1987.

88. Zaloga GP, Malcolm D, Holladay J: Glucagon reverses the hypotension and bradycardia of verapamil overdose in rats. *Crit Care Med* 13:273, 1985.

89. Zaritsky AL, Horowitz M, Chernow B: Glucagon antagonism of calcium channel blocker induced myocardial dysfunction. *Crit Care Med* 16:246, 1988.

90. Murad F, Vaughan M: Effect of glucagon on rat heart adenyl cyclase. *Biochem Pharmacol* 18:1053, 1969.

91. Alousi AA, Canter JM, Fort DJ: The beneficial effect of amrinone on acute drug-induced heart failure in the anaesthetized dog. *Cardiovasc Res* 19:483, 1985.

92. Makela HMV, Kapur PA: Amrinone and verapamil-propranolol induced cardiac depression during isoflurane anesthesia in dogs. *Anesthesiology* 66:792, 1987.

93. Lundh H, Thesleff S: The mode of action of 4-aminopyridine and guanidine on transmitter release from motor nerve terminals. *Eur J Pharmacol* 42:411, 1977.

94. Yanagisawa T, Toira N: Positive inotropic effect of 4-aminopyridine on dog ventricular muscle. *Naunyn Schmiedebergs Arch Pharmacol* 307:207, 1979.

95. Agoston S, Maestrone E, van Hezik EJ, et al: Effective treatment of verapamil intoxication with 4-aminopyridine in the cat. *J Clin Invest* 73:1291, 1984.

96. Bechem M, Gross R, Hebisch S, et al: Ca-agonists: A new class of inotropic drugs. *Basic Res Cardiol* 84:105, 1989.

97. Korstanje C, Jonkman FA, Van Kemenade JE, et al: Bay k 8644, a calcium entry promoter, as an antidote in verapamil intoxication in rabbits. *Arch Int Pharmacodyn Ther* 287:109, 1987.

98. Reikeras O, Gunnes P, Sorlie D, et al: Haemodynamic effects of high doses of insulin during acute left ventricular failure in dogs. *Eur Heart J* 6:451, 1985.

99. Masters T, Duncan G: The effect of verapamil on myocardial metabolism. *J Molec Cell Cardiol* 15(suppl1):233, 1983.

100. Anthony T, Jastremski M, Elliot W: Charcoal hemoperfusion for the treatment of a combined diltiazem and metoprolol overdose. *Ann Emerg Med* 15:1344, 1986.

101. Martin TG, Menegazzi JJ, Perel HM, et al: Extraordinary medical therapy for severe verapamil overdose. *Ann Emerg Med* 21:627, 1992.

137. Cholinergic Agents

J. Edward Jackson and
Cynthia K. Aaron

Poisoning with cholinergic agents is common; approximately 20,000 organophosphate poisonings and 200 deaths are reported yearly in the United States [1,2]. Although several thousand organophosphates and carbamates have been synthesized, only about 50 compounds are used commercially in the United States. Their effectiveness as insecticides derives from their relative selectivity for insect cholinesterase and their rapid degradation in the environment or within the body [3]. This chapter focuses on management of poisoning by cholinesterase inhibitors, because these agents account for the vast majority of cholinergic poisonings.

Mechanism of Action

Most of the acute toxicity of cholinesterase inhibitors can be explained by inhibition of the enzyme acetylcholinesterase. Organophosphates cause irreversible inhibition of this enzyme by forming a covalent phosphate linkage with the serine residue of the active site. Carbamates (including physostigmine and neostigmine) and edrophonium (Tensilon) are reversible inhibitors of the enzyme, occupying, but not modifying, the catalytic region of acetylcholinesterase.

Inhibition of acetylcholinesterase allows the neurotransmitter acetylcholine to remain active in the synapse, resulting in sustained depolarization of the postsynaptic neuron. This effect occurs in the central nervous system (CNS) as well as at muscarinic sites in the peripheral nervous system, nicotinic sites in the sympathetic and parasympathetic ganglia, and nicotinic sites at the neuromuscular junction. Generally, effects at muscarinic sites are sustained, white nicotinic sites are stimulated and then depressed (hyperpolarization block).

An intermediate syndrome or type II toxicity has been described in a few patients (5–10%) beginning 24 to 96 hours after the initial serious cholinergic crisis. This intermediate syndrome is characterized by paralysis of proximal limb muscles, neck flexor, motor cranial nerves, and respiratory muscles, without prominent muscarinic findings [5,6]. This syndrome has been described exclusively in India and Sri Lanka and may represent a genetic pattern of either neurologic response or metabolism of certain organophosphates or an interaction of nutritional status with the toxin. This intermediate syndrome occurs with lipophilic, high-potency agents such as fenthion and may conceivably represent delayed elimination or redistribution of the organophosphate from tissue depots, although the relative paucity of muscarinic signs is difficult to explain [7]. Other authors suspect that the intermediate syndrome now represent partially treated organophosphate toxicity and need not be a new entry [8]. The intermediate syndrome appears to be reported predominately from countries with limited supplies of oximes. There are few cases of IMS reported from the Western countries, possibly related to early and aggressive use of oxime therapy. Since IMS is reported with fat-soluble organophosphorus agents, it is possible that symptoms result from prolonged absorption and redistribution of the agent with subsequent underdosing of the antidote [9,10,11].

In addition to these acute effects, some organophosphate compounds can cause a delayed neuropathy, which appears to be mediated by a specific esterase in peripheral neurons [8–15]. This specific esterase has been named "neurotoxic esterase." This peripheral neuropathy involves motor fibers almost exclusively, and pathology shows wallerian degeneration and secondary demyelination of long axons. There is one report of peripheral neuropathy following a severe carbamate poisoning, but sensory complaints were prominent, near complete recovery occurred, and other toxins were also ingested making inference about a causal relationship difficult [15]. In addition, carbamates are protective in animal models of organophosphate neuropathy [14].

Sources

Most anticholinesterase poisonings, especially agricultural exposures, involve insecticides, although significant numbers of pediatric and suicidal ingestions do occur. For example, in India organophosphates are the most common toxins involved in suicide attempts [6]. Cholinesterase inhibitors are found in flea collars, ant traps, flypapers, and spray cans and bottles as well as home and industrial insecticide concentrates. Many of these items are used or stored in places easily accessible to toddlers and small children. Almost all life-threatening intoxications are due to concentrated solutions that must be diluted before application.

Other potential settings for anticholinesterase insecticide poisoning include the home use of aerosol insecticides, indoor areas treated by professional exterminators, emergency workers exposed during fires and spills, outdoor workers exposed to pesticide drift, warehouse and transportation workers, and gardeners. In addition, there have been a number of outbreaks of food-borne anticholinesterase intoxication. These include "gingerjake" paralysis in the 1930s owing to contamination of moonshine whiskey with tri-o-cresyl phosphate (TOCP) leading to delayed neuropathy [3], and a large epidemic of mild to moderate symptoms related to use of a "systemic" carbamate, aldicarb, on watermelons [16,17].

A few reversible cholinesterase inhibitors, such as physostigmine, pyridostigmine, and neostigmine, are used clinically and may be iatrogenic toxins. Physostigmine and tetrahydroaminoacridine (THA) are being studied as treatments for Alzheimer's disease, and the future may see wider use of cholinergic agents in treating dementia, thus increasing the chances of accidental or intentional ingestions.

Routes of Exposure

The most common route of pesticide exposure is dermal. This accounts for the majority of occupational poisonings and a substantial number of accidental poisonings. There are cases of inadequately protected health care workers developing toxicity from transdermal absorption during decontamination and treatment of patients involved in pesticide spills of concentrated pesticides. Most suicide attempts and many pediatric poisonings are ingestions; attempted intravenous injection have been reported.

Pharmacodynamics

EFFECTS. The pharmacologic effects of anticholinesterase agents are quite predictable from their mechanism of action (Table 137-1). A number of mnemonics have been proposed to describe the signs of cholinergic excess, including DUMBELS (diarrhea, urination, miosis, bronchospasm, emesis, lacrimation, salivation) and SLUDGE (salivation, lacrimation, urination, defecation, emesis).

TIME COURSE. Symptoms usually begin minutes to hours after dermal, pulmonary, or oral exposure [3,4,18,19]. Onset, however, may be delayed with certain lipophilic compounds (e.g., fenthion, dichlofenthion, leptophos) when ingested or after prolonged dermal exposure, leading to accumulation of a toxic dose over time [20]. Some organophosphorus compounds require hepatic metabolism to increase their toxicity (parathion is metabolized to paraoxon). This may prolong onset of symptoms and duration of toxicity. In general, if symptoms begin more than 12 hours after exposure, it is unlikely that cholinesterase inhibitors are the cause.

Organophosphorus compounds (OPs). Because OPs are irreversible inhibitors of acetylcholinesterase, once symptoms develop they may persist for days to months, until adequate amounts of the enzyme regenerate. Generally, life-threatening symptoms abate within 1 to 3 days, although many cases requiring weeks of intensive care are reported.

The intermediate syndrome of proximal, bulbar, and respiratory weakness seen with some OPs begins 24 to 96 hours after poisoning and lasts 4 to 18 days [5,6].

Organophosphorus-ester-induced delayed neurotoxicity (OPIDN) is a separate entity caused by specific classes of OPs. It was first reported in the 1930s after an epidemic called "Jamaican ginger paralysis" or "ginger jake paralysis." The cause was found to be triorthocresyl phosphate (TOCP) [21]. There are several subsequent reports of large groups of people developing OPIDN from contaminated foodstuffs. Onset of symptoms from OPIDN is approximately 1 to 3 weeks after acute exposure, and symptoms may continue to worsen for several months. Neurologic symptoms have developed in people exposed chronically to low levels of fenthion or TOCP [3]. Patients initially report paresthesias that eventually progress to motor dysfunction [22,23]. Improvement is gradual over months to years, although most patients are left with residual weakness. In OPIDN, the membrane-bound esterase neurotoxic esterase (NTE) appears to be a marker for a delayed neuropathic effect. Certain organophosphorus esters, such as phosphates, phosphoraminates, and phosphonates, inhibit NTE and lead to axonal swelling. With time, this progresses to cell body death and axonal degeneration, or a "dying back" phenomenon [22–26]. The hen is used as the model for detecting OPIDN; there appears to be age and species specificity in determining toxicity [22]. Currently, development is proceeding on a human leukocyte and platelet assay for toxicity [22–28].

Carbamates. Because carbamates are reversible inhibitors of the cholinesterase enzyme, toxicity resolves more rapidly than with organophosphates. It is distinctly unusual for serious symptoms to persist beyond 12 to 24 hours. Continued symptoms raise the suspicion of continued absorption of the poison (inadequate decontamination).

DOSE RESPONSE. Anticholinesterase agents have a wide range of potencies and show a classic log-linear dose-response relationship in terms of pharmacologic and toxicologic effects. Lethal doses for adults range from a few milligrams for highly toxic agents, such as tetraethyl pyrophosphate (TEPP), phorate (Thimet), and ethylparathion, parathion, and thiophos (minimal lethal dose about 10 mg) to the 10- to 100-gm range for moderately toxic compounds, such as diazinon (Spectracide, minimal lethal dose about 25 gm) and malathion (minimal lethal dose about 50 gm) [29]. Some organophosphates require hepatic conversion of the parent compound to a more toxic intermediate (e.g., parathion to paraoxon), and this influences the stated toxicity of the compound.

Table 137-1. Pharmacologic Effects of Cholinesterase Inhibition Receptor Type

Location	Effects
Muscarinic (increased stimulation)	
Pupils	Miosis (constriction)
Ciliary body	Blurred vision
Exocrine glands	Increased secretions
Lacrimal	Tearing
Salivary	Salivation
Respiratory	Bronchorrhea, rhinorrhea
Heart	Bradycardia
Smooth muscle	Contraction
Bronchial	Bronchoconstriction
GI	Nausea, vomiting, abdominal cramps, diarrhea
Bladder	Incontinence, frequency
Sphincter of Oddi	Pancreatitis
CNS	Variable*
Nicotinic (stimulation then depression)	
Skeletal muscle	Weakness, cramps, fasciculation, paralysis
Sympathetic ganglia	Tachycardia, hypertension; then hypotension
CNS	Variable symptoms from anxiety and restlessness to confusion, obtundation, coma, and seizures*

* Relative contributions of nicotinic and muscarinic receptors to CNS effects unclear.
GI = gastrointestinal; CNS = central nervous system.

Toxicology

The toxicology of anticholinesterase agents is a direct extension of the pharmacology. Carbamates and other reversible cholinesterase inhibitors have onset of cholinergic symptoms within 2 hours and resolution in 12 to 24 hours. Organophosphates, being irreversible inhibitors of cholinesterase, cause symptoms of much longer duration. It is generally believed that inhibition of 50 to 60 percent of cholinesterase activity is required before acute symptoms appear [3,18,30,31]. One group suggested that moderate symptoms can occur with as little as 25 percent inhibition of cholinesterase in some individuals [32].

Organophosphates have two additional types of toxicity, for which the dose-response relationships are not clear:

1. Intermediate syndrome of proximal muscle, bulbar, and respiratory weakness without significant antimuscarinic signs, which occur 1 to 4 days after acute symptomatic poisonings (reported only with certain agents in India and Sri Lanka and not completely accepted as a distinct entity).
2. Peripheral neuropathy, which occurs 1 to 2 weeks after exposure to only certain agents, dependent on inhibition of "neurotoxic esterase."

Clinical Manifestations and Diagnosis

PRESENTATION OF ACUTE POISONING. Life-threatening cholinergic poisonings are not difficult to diagnose (Table 137-2). Not all of these symptoms need be present to lead to the diagnosis. Usually either a history of exposure or an odor of insecticide is present. Organophosphates are said by some to have a garlic odor, although often the hydrocarbon in which it is dissolved may be the predominant smell.

A definitive dignosis of anticholinesterase poisoning requires that four criteria be met:

1. Clinical picture of cholinergic symptoms
2. Onset within not more than 12 hours after exposure, with the exception of highly fat-soluble organophosphorus esters (fenthion, chlorfenthion)
3. Reduction of plasma and red blood cell cholinesterase to at least 50 percent below baseline values (Note that "normal range" is wide, so a postrecovery level may be needed to confirm the diagnosis.)
4. Reduced symptoms with atropine and relief of muscarinic symptoms by atropine

Many authors require, in addition, a definite history of exposure [30]. An increase in red blood cell cholinesterase following pralidoxime provides strong evidence of organophosphate exposure.

Table 137-2. Symptoms of Cholinergic Poisoning

Exposure only	Mild poisoning	Moderate poisoning	Severe poisoning
No symptoms	Can walk	Cannot walk	Unconscious
	Fatigue	Weakness	Unreactive pupils
	Headache	Difficulty	Fasciculations
	Dizzy	speaking	Flaccid paralysis
	Nausea	Fasciculations	Secretions
	Vomiting	Miosis	mouth/nose
	Numbness		Moist rales
	Sweating		Respiratory dis-
	Salivation		tress
	Chest tight-		Seizures
	ness		
	Abdominal		
	cramps		
	Diarrhea		
	ChE 20–	ChE 10–20%	ChE < 10% of
	50% of nl	of nl	nl

ChE = cholinesterase

Respiratory Symptoms. The immediate cause of death in cholinesterase inhibitor poisonings is respiratory failure due to muscle weakness. Such cases may present with noncardiogenic pulmonary edema, although the mechanism for this is less clear. The most probable hypothesis is capillary leak from a direct effect of augmented cholinergic input to the lungs, similar to that seen in neurogenic pulmonary edema. This is combined with exuberant mucus production, which, in the presence of markedly decreased respiratory muscle function, fills the pulmonary tree. Cholinergic input also directly causes spasm of the bronchial smooth muscle.

Already precarious respiratory status can be further compromised by aspiration of gastric contents following emesis. This can be compounded by hydrocarbon chemical pneumonitis if the insecticide was in a hydrocarbon solvent.

Neurologic Symptoms. After respiratory compromise, the most life-threatening consequences of anticholinesterase poisoning come from the neurologic effects. Seizures, coma, or delirium are the rule in serious cases, owing to direct effects of overwhelming cholinergic input in the midbrain and medulla. Cheynes-Stokes respiration and eventual depression of medullary respiratory and cardiovascular centers can occur. These striking CNS symptoms are more evident with organophosphates than with carbamates.

Dystonias and choreoathetoid movements have also been observed with anticholinesterase overdose (mechanism unclear) and seem to respond to atropine [33,34]. Less severe acute neurotoxicities include anxiety, agitation, emotional lability, headaches, insomnia, tremor, difficulty concentrating, slurred speech, ataxia, and hyperreflexia or hyporeflexia.

Fasciculations are the rule in severe cholinergic overdoses and may be an important point in the differential diagnosis.

In some cases, acute organophosphate poisoning may produce longer-lasting neuropsychiatric sequelae, although several studies in acute and chronic poisoning or exposure have not defined a consistent pattern of deficits. Generally, there is a tendency toward increased anxiety and emotional lability, possibly increased depression, and possibly subtle abstraction-problem solving difficulties [37]. These problems seem most severe following serious acute intoxications and generally resolve within 1 year [38].

As discussed previously, specific organophosphates (primarily the triaryl phosphates, including mipafox, trichlorphon, phytosol, tamaron, fenthion, and TOCP) can produce peripheral neuropathy. This is characterized clinically by paresthesias but more prominently by motor loss, with foot drop and the consequent high-stepping gait being common. This peripheral neuropathy becomes evident about 1 to 2 weeks after acute exposure.

Gastrointestinal Symptoms. Diarrhea and vomiting are seen almost universally with severe anticholinergic poisoning. Spasm of the sphincter of Oddi can lead to pancreatitis. This is diagnosed by elevated amylase, since such patients invariably have substantial abdominal pain from vigorous intestinal contraction, making differentiation of their abdominal pain difficult.

Cardiovascular Symptoms. Increased and unbalanced autonomic outflow (particularly vagal), augmented by increased nicotinic transmission at the cervical parasympathetic ganglia, probably is responsible for the arrhythmias seen in organophosphate and carbamate poisoning. These include both tachyarrhythmias and bradyarrhythmias and *Torsades de pointes* type ventricular tachycardia [35–38]. Almost all arrhythmias have been described.

Both hypotension and hypertension are seen, depending on

the balance between increased outflow from postganglionic sympathetic neurons (nicotinic stimulation) and depression of central vasomotor centers.

Increased Secretions. Increased secretions, tears, saliva, respiratory mucus, gastric acid, and sweat are all characteristic of anticholinesterase poisonings and are due to increased acetylcholine at the effector organs.

Metabolic Disturbances. Both hyperglycemia and hypoglycemia have been reported following anticholinesterase poisoning. Hyperglycemia is more common in several major series, occurring in the range of 1 to 10 percent [18,19,39]. Occasionally, this has led to misdiagnosis as diabetic hyperosmolar coma when an exposure history was not available [40].

PRESENTATION OF ORGANOPHOSPHORUS ESTER-INDUCED DELAYED NEUROTOXICITY.

Patients may present with OPIDN after exposure to aryl organophosphorus esters containing either a pentavalent phosphorus atom (type I, including derivatives of phosphoric acid, phosphonic, phosphoramidic acids, or phosphorofluoridates) or a trivalent phosphorus atom (type II or phosphorus acid derivatives) [23]. Patients initially recover from the acute OP toxicity but develop signs and symptoms of OPIDN 1 to 3 weeks after exposure. Symptoms develop slowly and can be divided into three phases: progressive, stationary, and improvement. During the progressive phase, patients develop a peripheral sensory neuropathy with complaints of burning, tightness, or pain in the legs and feet. This is followed by numbness and tingling. Following the sensory changes, motor weakness develops, with weakness and atropy of the peroneal muscles causing a foot drop. After approximately 1 week, the paresis may ascend symmetrically into the upper extremities. The sensory loss may occur in a stocking glove distribution and the patient loses proprioception. With time, there may be a positive Romberg and loss of lower extremity DTRs. Flaccid paralysis may occur in severe cases [23].

During the stationary phase, sensory complaints resolve within 2 to 9 weeks and motor findings cease to progress. This may occur over 3 to 12 months. Paresis may remain [23,27].

Once the patient enters the improvement phase (6–18 months after exposure), motor function begins to return in reverse order of loss. Motor function return may be partial or complete. During this phase, any central cord or brain lesions are unmasked and spasticity may develop. Permanent motor deficits may be left [23,27].

LABORATORY TESTS.

The primary diagnostic tests for evaluation of anticholinesterase poisoning are measurement of serum and red blood cell cholinesterase (RBC cholinesterase). The erythrocyte enzyme functions similarly to nervous tissue cholinesterase and is subject to fewer variations than the plasma cholinesterase (pseudocholinesterase). Red blood cell cholinesterase varies by about 10 percent on repeated testing in the same individual [41]. It regenerates at 0.5 to 1.0 percent per day based on production of new red cells. Thus, RBC cholinesterase may take several months to return to baseline following a severe poisoning with an irreversible inhibitor such as an organophosphate, although most cases are back within the normal range within 1 to 2 months.

Plasma cholinesterase (also called pseudocholinesterase, as it is nonspecific for acetylcholine) falls more rapidly and recovers more rapidly than the erythrocyte enzyme. It remains depressed typically for a maximum of 1 to 3 weeks [42]. Plasma

pseudocholinesterase is synthesized in the liver. Fluctuations in plasma cholinesterase have been reported with liver disease, chronic inflammation, malnutrition, pregnancy, and hypersensitivity reactions and with the use of morphine, codeine, and succinylcholine.

Only transient depressions of both RBC and plasma cholinesterase occur with carbamate poisoning, since these reversible inhibitors free the enzyme as they are metabolized.

In suspected cholinesterase inhibitor poisoning, plasma and RBC cholinesterase levels should be sent for laboratory determination initially and repeated if the clinical course is atypical. Blood for cholinesterase determination should be drawn into a serum separating tube (plasma pseudocholinesterase) or a heparinized tube (RBC cholinesterase). Samples that must be stored should be spun down and frozen. Blood drawn into fluoride tubes will show no activity, since fluoride inhibits cholinesterase activity. The assaying laboratory should be contacted to obtain specific drawing and storing instructions. Acute exposures are usually classified based on the degree of depression of RBC cholinesterase: mild (20–50% of baseline), moderate (10–20% of baseline), and severe (≤10% of baseline). Because the "normal range" for RBC cholinesterase is wide (substantial interindividual variation), an individual's baseline needs to be established if return to working with pesticides is a consideration. Workers should be removed from exposure until RBC cholinesterase is at least 75 percent of their baseline values [3,30].

p-Nitrophenol is a metabolite of several organophosphates that can be easily detected in the urine soon after poisoning. This can help verify exposure, although quantitation is not possible. Sophisticated gas chromatography-mass spectroscopy systems can quantify most organophosphate and carbamate insecticides in blood or serum, but the clinical usefulness of such assays is not apparent.

Other essential laboratory tests in serious poisonings include electrocardiogram, arterial blood gases, chest film, amylase, electrolytes, and glucose. Renal and liver function tests may be useful in following the patient's general recovery.

There are no laboratory tests per se for OPIDN. Electromyography and nerve conduction studies coupled with a history of organophosphorus ester exposure can help differentiate this disorder from other sensorimotor neuropathies. Work is continuing on a human leukocyte and platelet assay [23–27,42].

DIFFERENTIAL DIAGNOSIS.

Diagnosis of a serious cholinesterase-inhibitor poisoning is seldom difficult. Almost all patients show muscarinic symptoms (especially miosis, sweating, salivation, lacrimation, chest tightness, and abdominal symptoms), most show nicotinic symptoms (particularly fasciculations and weakness), and many show CNS symptoms (particularly difficulty walking or talking). Coma, rales, paralysis, and cardiovascular collapse in the presence of muscarinic findings and/or fasciculations should be considered anticholinesterase poisoning until proved otherwise. In serious cases, it is lethal to await laboratory confirmation of the poisoning. Cholinergic mushrooms and tetrodotoxin can produce pictures similar to that of cholinesterase-inhibitor poisonings, but there is almost always a distinctive history. The odor of the pesticide is often helpful. Difficulty arises when no history is apparent and the patient has a paucity of muscarinic signs with an altered mental status. Fasciculations should rapidly lead one to focus on cholinesterase inhibition.

CLINICAL COURSE.

Severe poisoning, with major respiratory, CNS, or cardiovascular compromise, is rapidly fatal if not treated aggressively. Asymptomatic exposures can be observed. Patients with mild and moderate poisonings should be hospitalized for careful observation, atropine treatment, and administration of pralidoxime if an organophosphate is known or suspected. Patients with mild to moderate poisonings almost always recover with proper treatment.

Once absorption of the poison has been stopped, clinical improvement should begin within several hours for carbamates and within days for organophosphates.

Management

INITIAL DISPOSITION. Careful history and detailed physical examination are key to staging the severity of an anticholinesterase poisoning. Patients with all but the mildest symptoms need to be admitted to an intensive care unit (ICU). In severe cases, intubation with ventilation is often required. Once a cholinesterase inhibitor intoxication is suspected, treatment with atropine should be instituted promptly, without waiting for cholinesterase results.

SUPPORTIVE CARE. The primary demands for supportive care relate to adequate ventilation, prevention of aspiration, and removal of respiratory secretions. This makes endotracheal intubation, suctioning, and ventilation necessary in most severe cases. Support of blood pressure, if needed (cautious use of direct-acting pressors such as norepinephrine), and control of seizures (atropine, followed by large doses of benzodiazepines or phenobarbital [loading 10–20 mg/kg] IV) are also important. Electrical pacing may rarely be needed to terminate ventricular arrhythmias, although sympathomimetics with beta-activity (e.g., norepinephrine, epinephrine, isoproterenol) substantially reduce the risk of *Torsades de pointes*.

Succinylcholine is metabolized by plasma pseudocholinesterase and has a long duration of action in the presence of cholinesterase inhibitors. It should not be used to aid intubation because prolonged (hours to days) paralysis may result [44,45]. Nondepolarizing neuromuscular blockers may have delayed onset and require larger doses for paralysis. The dose should be carefully titrated to effect.

DECONTAMINATION. Aggressive decontamination is critical in managing insecticide poisoning, since dermal exposure is common. All clothes should be removed and discarded, and skin should be washed thoroughly with soap. Leather items absorb the organophosphates and should be discarded. Tincture of green soap containing alcohol helps remove lipophilic compounds and is often recommended [37]. Use of a mildly alkaline soap or dilute hypochlorite solution (household bleach) inactivates the organophosphorus ester [46]. After the initial thorough cleansing, the entire area, including nails, intertriginous areas, and genitals, should be washed a second time.

For ingestions, gastric lavage and instillation of activated charcoal is indicated up to 6 hours after ingestion, and perhaps longer, to terminate absorption. Use of a cathartic is not necessary since many of these patients already have greatly decreased gastrointestinal transit time.

During the decontamination process, health care personnel should wear masks, aprons, and rubber gloves to avoid becoming poisoned themselves. For some very toxic organophos-

phates, absorption of even milligram quantities can produce severe poisoning.

ANTIDOTES
Atropine. Atropine is the mainstay of treatment for cholinergic poisonings. Adult doses should begin with 1 to 2 mg intravenously in mild to moderate cases and at least 2 to 5 mg in severe cases. Pediatric dosing starts at 0.02 to 0.05 mg per kilogram IV. Atropine should be continued every 10 to 30 minutes, until muscarinic signs (sweating, salivation, bronchorrhea) subside. Some authors suggest doubling the dose every 5 to 10 minutes until secretions cease. Tachycardia is not a contraindication to the use of atropine; it may reflect hypoxia or sympathetic stimulation. Pupils will dilate early and do not represent adequate atropinization.

A common pitfall is giving too little atropine during serious overdoses. Daily doses in the range of 100 mg are commonly required, with one patient requiring an average of nearly 1000 mg daily for several weeks [18,19,29,47,48]. Generally, more atropine is required during the first 24 hours, with doses decreasing dramatically if acetylcholinesterase can be reconstituted with pralidoxime. In all cases, careful titration of atropine to the individual patient is required, with frequent clinical re-evaluation. Atropine reverses *only* the muscarinic effects of these poisons and does not affect the nicotinic sites at skeletal muscle or the autonomic ganglia.

Pralidoxime. Pralidoxime (2-PAM, Protopam) specifically reactivates acetylcholinesterase by reversing phosphorylation of the active site on the enzyme. The details of this reaction are discussed by Taylor [4]. Pralidoxime acts synergistically with atropine. For moderate or severe organophosphate intoxications, including any case in which respiratory function is compromised or seizures or coma occur, pralidoxime is indicated. Other authors suggest the use of pralidoxime whenever atropine must be given. The rationale is that atropine competitively blocks the effects of acetylcholine on the postsynaptic muscarinic receptor but has no effect on regenerating the acetylcholinesterase. Pralidoxime regenerates the acetylcholinesterase. In mild cases, atropine may appear to treat the exposure completely because the effects of the small amount of inhibition are blocked long enough for endogenous metabolism, hydrolysis, and elimination to occur. While "aging" of the organophosphate-cholinesterase complex reduces the efficacy of pralidoxime after 24 to 48 hours, depending on the organophosphate involved, clinical benefit has been observed many days after exposure [50–55]. Delayed presentation of a symptomatic patient is *not* a contraindication to the use of pralidoxime. These patients may require continued dosing of pralidoxime, with reappearance of symptoms when the drug is withheld [50]. Pralidoxime is administered slowly intravenously, usually in an initial dose of 1 gm, in 150 ml of normal saline repeated in 30 minutes if no benefit or limited benefit is derived from the first dose. Too rapid injection may cause tachycardia, laryngeal spasm, muscle rigidity, and transient neuromuscular blockade. The initial dose is given over 5 to 30 minutes. Pralidoxime is metabolized by the liver, with renal excretion of active and inactive metabolites. There is the theoretical potential for accumulation and toxicity in the presence of renal failure. Nonetheless, pralidoxime is probably underused. Pediatric bolus dosing is 25 to 50 mg per kilogram IV. Some authors have recommended using a pralidoxime infusion (500 mg/hr of a 2.5% solution, adults, or 10–25 mg/kg/hr, pediatric). Alternatively, repeated boluses of 0.5 to 1 gm IV (25–50 mg/kg) can be administered every 6 to 8 hours if symptoms recur, based on the rationale that recurrence of symptoms implies repeat inhibition of the enzyme by organophosphates. This occurs possibly from tissue depots, hepatic activation of the organophosphate, or continued absorption. If large doses of pralidoxime are used, one should also consider cholinesterase inhibition by pralidoxime in the differential diagnosis of late recurrent symptoms. Although it does not enter the CNS well, a number of investigators have noted rapid improvement in coma or termination of seizures following pralidoxime administration [56].

Pralidoxime is relatively contraindicated in treatment of carbamate intoxication and may act as an additional competitive inhibitor. When faced with a serious anticholinesterase poisoning of unknown type, it is rational to use pralidoxime, since the adverse effect in a carbamate intoxication is small and the benefit in an organophosphate poisoning probably striking.

ENHANCED ELIMINATION. Although hemoperfusion can eliminate a number of anticholinesterase agents more rapidly than no treatment, the availability of specific antidotes for organophosphates and the relatively short course of carbamate intoxications make this issue moot.

PROGNOSIS AND SEQUELAE. As discussed previously, if a patient survives the first few hours, the prognosis is good, even in severe poisonings. Carbamates have a uniformly excellent prognosis because serious symptoms rapidly resolve as the reversible inhibitor is eliminated from the body. Organophosphates are more difficult because severe poisonings may require prolonged respiratory support, with its attendant complications. If pralidoxime is used early and aggressively with vigorous atropine, protection of the airway, and vigilant clinical monitoring, the outcome of patients who arrive in the emergency department alive should be good. The prognosis for OPIDN seen mainly with triaryl phosphates is not as promising, although most patients do improve substantially over the course of a year. Anoxic sequelae are the most troublesome, particularly those involving the CNS. These are not specific to cholinesterase inhibitors, but rather a consequence of respiratory arrest or prolonged hypoxia.

The future holds even more promising treatment options, with oximes more effective than pralidoxime [4] and "binary antidotes," which have antimuscarinic potency as well as protect the cholinesterase enzyme and interfere with the action of the neurotoxic esterase [49]. The ultimate solution, however, will come from the development of less toxic methods of pest control.

"NERVE AGENTS" USED IN WARFARE. During the Gulf War, there was concern about the potential use of "nerve agents" such as GA (Tabun), GB (Sarin), GD (Soman), GF, and VX. These chemicals are similar in structure and function to the organophosphorus insecticides but have a much greater potency. Since World War II, the only known use of "nerve agents" was in the Iran-Iraq War. There are, however, large stockpiles of these agents in the United States in the Commonwealth of Independent States, and possibly 21 other countries [57]. Middle Eastern countries such as Libya may have the potential to create them from insecticide precursors [46].

The nerve agents commonly exist as a liquid at room temperature but can be aerosolized by spraying or in an explosive blast from a shell. Although the G agents have relatively low vapor pressures, they are highly toxic, with as little as 1 mg being fatal. The G agents evaporate and will dissipate over several hours. VX is an oily liquid that persists in the environment for several weeks to months. It exerts its toxicity predominately through skin absorption [46,56,57].

Onset of symptoms from these agents is dependent on route of exposure and dose. In environmental conditions favoring aeorolization (hot, windy), onset is rapid after inhalation or skin contact [46]. Vapor rapidly afects the eyes, airways, and mucous membranes, leading to miosis, bronchospasm, bronchorrhea, dypsnea, and rhinorhea. If the vapor pressure is high, there will be loss of consciousness and seizures, paralysis, and respiratory arrest within seconds to minutes [58,59]. Absorption through the skin leads to a more delayed onset of signs and symptoms, with a latency lasting from 30 minutes to 18 hours [46,60]. If the "nerve agent" is ingested, onset may be within 30 minutes.

Initial treatment is the same as with organophosphorus ester pesticides, except the emphasis is on self-protection and decontamination. These agents penetrate most protective clothing, so a charcoal-impregnated sealed suit with a charcoal-sealed respirator are absolutely essential. The exposed person should be washed with an alkaline soap or 5% hypochlorite solution [60].

The remainder of treatment is supportive, with maintenance of an airway, breathing, and circulation. Antidote therapy should be started immediately. Oxime therapy with 2-PAM may be successful with Tabun and VX but may be ineffective with Soman and Sarin. Soman and Sarin cause the acetylcholinesterase-nerve agent complex to "age" almost immediately and be resistant to nucleophilic regeneration by pralidoxime [46,61,62]. In the event of an exposure, regardless of agent, atropine and pralidoxime should be immediately administered. Military personnel carry three 2-mg atropine self-injectors and three 600-mg pralidoxime self-injectors.

Since seizures are a significant risk after exposure to nerve agents, high-dose benzodiazepines should be administered at the first sign of CNS toxicity (diazepam in doses of 0.2–0.4 mg/kg). The most recent nonclassified studies suggest that there may be an additional action by organophosphorus esters on the N-methyl-D-receptor, affecting central GABA concentrations [46,61,63–67]. Use of oximes and benzodiazepines may be synergistic.

During the Gulf War, some high-risk military personnel were pretreated with carbamates to limit potential toxicity if exposed to the nerve agents. Organophosphorus esters cannot bind to acetylcholinesterase that is already bound to carbamates. Most carbamaylated acetylcholinesterase spontaneously hydrolyze back to functional acetylcholinesterase within a reasonable amount of time. Administration of pralidoxime will enhance the release of carbamates from acetylcholinesterase [46,61,63,68–73]. In addition, carbamates may possess direct nicotinic receptor ionic channel actions, contributing to their protective effect [68–71]. During the Gulf War, soldiers were pretreated with pyridostigmine effectively to bind approximately 30 percent of their cholinesterase; physostigmine was found to have too many side effects for use as a pretreatment.

Recent interest in the treatment of nerve agents has led to investigation into newer oxime agents with potential to protect again Soman and VX. The H-series oximes are superior in their ability to reactivate acetylcholine after Soman exposure; HI-6 is the most studied member of the group. HI-6 is effective against Soman exposure, probably is efficacious against the other three agents, and is relatively nontoxic [57,61,62,66,67,74–78]. HI-6 has both antimuscarinic and antinicotinic effects, but its effect is enhanced by atropine [79]. H-oximes, however, are relatively ineffective against seizures; a benzodiazepine must be administered with them [79].

Finally, new areas of development against "nerve gas" toxicity include injection of cholinesterase, a "scavenging vaccine," and neutralizing antibodies [63,79]. All of these areas deserve future attention.

References

1. Kahn E: Pesticide-related illnesses in California farm workers. *J Occup Med* 18:693, 1976.
2. Litovitz T, Veltri JD: 1984 annual report of the American Association of Poison Control Centers national data collection system. *Am J Emerg Med* 3:423, 1985.
3. Murphy SD: Toxic effects of pesticides, in Klassen CD, Amdur MO, Doull J (eds): *Casarett and Doull's Toxicology, The Basic Science of Poisons*. 3rd ed. New York, Macmillan, 1986, p 519.
4. Taylor P: Cholinergic agonists, anticholinesterase agents, in Goodman AG, Goodman LS, Gilman A, et al (eds): *The Pharmacological Basis of Therapeutics*. 7th ed. New York, Macmillan, 1985, p 110.
5. Senanayake N, Karalliedde L: Neurotoxic effects of organophosphorous insecticides: An intermediate syndrome. *N Engl J Med* 316:761, 1987.
6. Wadia RS, Chitra S, Amin RB: Electrophysiological studies in acute organophosphate poisoning. *J Neurol Neurosurg Psychiatr* 50:1442, 1987.
7. Mahieu P, Hassoun A, Van Binst R, et al: Severe and prolonged poisoning by fenthion: Significance of the determination of anticholinesterase capacity of plasma. *J Toxicol Clin Toxicol* 19:425, 1982.
8. Senanayake N, Johnson MK: Acute polyneuropathy after poisoning by a new organophosphate insecticide. *N Engl J Med* 306:155, 1982.
9. DeBleecker J, Van En Neucker K, Willems J: The intermediate syndrome in organophosphate poisoning: Presentation of a case and review of the literature. *Clin Toxicol* 30:321, 1992.
10. Haddad LM. Editorial comment: Organophosphate poisoning-Intermediate syndrome? *Clin Toxicol* 30:331, 1992.
11. De Bleecker J, Willems J, Van Den Neucker K, et al. Prolonged toxicity with intermediate syndrome after combined parathion and methyl parathion poisoning. *Clin Toxicol* 30:333, 1992.
12. Johnson MK: The target for initiation of delayed neurotoxicity by organophosphorus esters: Biochemical studies and toxicological applications. *Rev Biochem Toxicol* 4:141, 1982.
13. Dudek BR, Richardson RJ: Evidence for the existence of neurotoxic esterase in neural and lymphatic tissue of the adult hen. *Biochem Pharmacol* 31:1117, 1982.
14. Lotti M, Becker CE, Aminoff MJ: Organophosphate polyneuropathy: Pathogenesis and prevention. *Neurology* 34:658, 1984.
15. Dickoff DJ, Gerber O, Turovsky Z: Delayed neurotoxicity after ingestion of carbamate pesticide. *Neurology* 37:1229, 1987.
16. Green MA, Heumann MA, Wehr HM, et al: An outbreak of watermelon-borne pesticide toxicity. *Am J Public Health* 77:1431, 1987.
17. Centers for Disease Control: Aldicarb food poisoning from contaminated melons—California. *MMWR* 35:254, 1986.
18. Namba T, Nolte C, Jackrel J, et al: Poisoning due to organophosphate insecticides. *Am J Med* 50:495, 1970.
19. DuToit P, Muller F, Van Tonder W, et al: Experience with intensive care management of organophosphate insecticide poisoning. *S Afr Med J* 60:277, 1981.
20. Davies JE, Barquet A, Freed VH, et al: Human pesticide poisonings by a fat soluble organophosphate insecticide. *Arch Environ Health* 30:608, 1975.
21. Morgan JP: The Jamaica ginger paralysis. *JAMA* 248:1864, 1982.
22. Abou-Donia MB, Lapadula DM. Mechanisms of organophosphorus ester-induced neurotoxicity: Type I and Type II. *Ann Rev Pharmacol Toxicol* 30:405, 1990.
23. Baron RL (ed): Pesticide-Induced Delayed Neurotoxicity-Proceedings of a Conference. Co-sponsored by the Environmental Protection Agency and the National Institute for Environmental Health Sciences, February 19–20, 1976. EPA-600/1-76-025.
24. Johnson MK: The delayed neuropathy caused by some organophosphorus esters: Mechanisms and challenge. *CRC Crit Rev Toxicol* 3:289, 1975.
25. Stuart LD, Oehme FW: Organophosphorus delayed neurotoxicity:
A neuromyelopathy of animals and man. *Vet Hum Toxicol* 24:107, 1982.
26. Hierons R, Johnson MK: Clinical and toxicological investigation of a case of delayed neuropathy in man after acute poisoning by an organophosphorus pesticide. *Arch Toxicol* 40:279, 1978.
27. Nagymajtenyi L, Desi I, Lorencz R. Neurophysiological markers as early signs of organophosphate neurotoxicity. *Neurotoxicol Teratology* 10:429, 1988.
28. Metcalf RL, Swift TR, Sikes RK: Neurological findings among workers exposed to fenthion in a veterinary hospital: Georgia. *MMWR* 34:402, 1985.
29. Morgan DP: *Recognition and Management of Pesticide Poisonings*. 3rd ed. Washington, DC, US Environmental Protection Agency, 1982.
30. Ellenhorn MJ, Barceloux DG: *Medical Toxicology, Diagnosis and Treatment of Human Poisoning*. New York, Elsevier, 1988, p 167.
31. Summerford WT, Hayes WJ, Johnson JM, et al: Cholinesterase response and symptomatology from exposure to organic phosphorus insecticides. *Arch Ind Hyg Occup Med* 7:383, 1953.
32. Coye MJ, Barnett PG, Midling JE, et al: Clinical confirmation of organophosphate poisoning by serial cholinesterase analyses. *Arch Intern Med* 147:438, 1987.
33. Joubert J, Houbert PH, van der Spuy M, et al: Acute organophosphate poisoning presenting with choreo-athetosis. *Clin Toxicol* 22:187, 1984.
34. Moody SB, Terp DK: Dyntonic reaction possibly induced by cholinesterase inhibitor insecticides. *Drug Intell Clin Pharm* 22:311, 1988.
35. Wren C: Organophosphate poisoning and complete heart block. *J Roy Soc Med* 75:213, 1982.
36. Kiss Z, Fazekas T: Organophosphate and torsade de pointes ventricular tachycardia, letter. *J Roy Soc Med* 76:984, 1982.
37. Sharp DS, Eskenazi B, Harrison R, et al: Delayed health hazards of pesticide exposure. *Ann Rev Public Health* 7:441, 1986.
38. Gershon S, Shaw FH: Psychiatric sequelae of chronic exposure to organophosphate insecticides. *Lancet* 1:1371, 1961.
39. Hayes MM, van der Westhudize NG, Gelfand M: Organophosphate poisoning in Rhodesia: A study of clinical features and management of 105 cases. *S Afr Med J* 4:230, 1978.
40. Miller D, Fraser I, Kryger M: Hyperglycemia in anticholinesterase poisoning. *CMA J* 124:745, 1981.
41. Yeager J, McClean H, Hudes M, et al: Components of variability in blood cholinesterase assay results. *J Occup Med* 18:242, 1976.
42. Bertolazzi M, Caroldi S, Moretto A, Lotti M: Interaction of methamidophos with hen and human acetylcholinesterase and neuropathy target esterase. *Arch Toxicol* 65:580, 1991.
43. Midling JE, Barnett PG, Coye MJ, et al: Clinical management of field worker organophosphate poisoning. *West J Med* 142:514, 1985.
44. Selden BS, Burry SC: Prolonged succinylcholine-induced paralysis in organophosphate insecticide poisoning. *Ann Emerg Med* 16:215, 1987.
45. Manoguerra AS, Steiner RW: Prolonged neuromuscular blockade after administration of physostigmine and succinylcholine. *Clin Toxicol* 18:803, 1981.
46. Sidell FR, Borak J: Chemical warfare agents: II. Nerve agents. *Annals Emerg Med* 21:865, 1992.
47. Golsousidis H, Kokkas V: 19,590 mg of atropine during 24 days of treatment after a case of unusually severe parathion poisoning. *Hum Toxicol* 4:339, 1985.
48. LeBlanc FN, Benson BE, Gilg AD: A severe organophosphate poisoning requiring the use of an atropine drip. *Clin Toxicol* 24:69, 1986.
49. Leader H, Smejkal RM, Payne CS, et al: Binary antidotes for organophosphate poisoning: Aprophen analogues that are both antimuscarinics and carbamates. *J Med Chem* 32:1522, 1989.
50. Aaron CK, Smilkstein MJ: Organophosphate poisoning: Intermediate syndrome or inadequate therapy (abstract). *Vet Hum Toxicol* 30:370, 1988.
51. Amos WE Jr, Hall A: Malathion poisoning treated with protopam. *Ann Intern Med* 62:1013, 1965.
52. Borowitz SM: Prolonged organophosphate toxicity in a twenty-six-month-old child. *J Pediatr* 112:302, 1988.
53. Merrill DG, Mihm FG: Prolonged toxicity of organophosphate poisoning. *Crit Care Med* 10:550, 1982.

54. Namba T, Hiraki K: PAM (Pyridine-2-aldoxime methiodide) therapy for alkylphosphate poisoning. *JAMA* 166:1834, 1958.

55. Quinby GE: Further therapeutic experience with pralidoxime in organic phosphorus poisoning. *JAMA* 187:114, 1964.

56. Lotti M, Becker CE: Treatment of acute organophosphate poisoning: Evidence of direct effect on central nervous system by 2-PAM (pyridine-2-aldoxime methyl chloride). *J Toxicol Clin Toxicol* 19:121, 1982.

57. Gunderson CH, Lehmann CR, Sidell FR, Jabbari B. Nerve agents: A review. *Neurology* 42:946, 1992.

58. Comptom JAF. Military chemical and biological agents: Chemical and toxicologic properties. The Telford Press, Caldwell NJ, 1988.

59. Anzueto A, DeLemos A, Seidenfeld J, et al. Acute inhalational toxicity of soman and sarin in baboons. *Fundamental Appl Toxicol* 14:676, 1990.

60. Stewart CE, Sullivan Jr JB. Military munitions and antipersonnel agents. *In* Sullivan Jr JB, Krieger GR (eds): *Hazardous materials toxicology: Clinical Principles of Environmental Health.* Williams and Wilkins, Baltimore, 1992, pp 986–1014.

61. Dunn MA, Sidell F. Progress in medical defense against nerve agents. *JAMA* 262:649, 1989.

62. Lundy PM, Hansen AS, Hand BT, Boulet CA. Comparison of several oximes against poisoning by soman, tabun, and GF. *Toxicology* 72:99, 1992.

63. Rickett DJ, Glenn JF, Houston WE. Medical defense against nerve agents: New directions. *Military Medicine* 152:35, 1987.

64. McDonough JH, Jaax NK, Crowley RA, et al. Atropine and/or diazepam therapy protects against Soman-induced neural and cardiac pathology. *Fundamental and Appl Toxicol* 13:256, 1989.

65. McLeod CG. Pathology of nerve agents: Perspective on medical management. *Fundamental and Appl Toxicol* 5:S10, 1985.

66. Kusic R, Jovanovic S, Randjelovic S, et al. HI-6 in man: Efficacy of the oxime in poisoning by organophosphorus insecticides. *Human And Exptl Toxicol* 10:113, 1992.

67. Kusic R, Boskovic B, Vojvodic V, Jovanovic D. HI-6 in man: Blood levels, urinary excretion, and tolerance after intramuscular administration of the oxime to healthy volunteers. *Fundamental and Appl Toxicol* 5:S89, 1985.

68. Sidell FR, Groff WA. The reactivability of cholinesterase inhibited by VX and sarin in man. *Toxicol Appl Pharmacol* 27:241, 1974.

69. Albuquerque EX, Akaike A, Shaw K-P, et al. The interaction of acetylcholinesterase agents with the acetylcholine receptor-ionic channel complex. *Fundam Appli Toxicol* 4:S27, 1984.

70. Pascuzzo GJ, Akaike A, Maleque MA, et al. The nature of the interaction of pyridostigmine with the nicotinic acetylcholine receptor-ionic channel complex: I. Agonist, desensitizing, and binding properties. *Mol Pharmacol* 25:92, 1984.

71. Akaike A, Ikeda SR, Brookes N, et al. The nature of the interactions of pyridostigmine with the nicotinic acetylcholine receptor-ionic channel complex: II. Patch clamp studies. *Mol Pharmacol* 25:102, 1984.

72. Keeler JR, Hurst CG, Dunn MA. Pyridostigmine used as a nerve agent pretreatment under wartime conditions. *JAMA* 266:693, 1991.

73. Sharabi Y, Danon YL, Berkenstadt H, et al. Survey of symptoms following intake of pyridostigmine during the Persian Gulf War. *Israel J Med Sci* 27:656, 1991.

75. Shih T-M, Whalley C, Valdes J. A comparison of cholinergic effects of HI-6 and pralidoxime-2-chloride (2-PAM) in Soman poisoning. *Toxicol Lett* 55:131, 1991.

76. Weger N, Szinicz L. Therapeutic effects of the new oximes, benzctyzine, and atropine in Soman poisoning. Part I. Effects of various oximes in Soman, Sarin, and VX poisoning in dogs. *Fundam Appl Toxicol* 1:161,1981.

77. Wolfe AD, Rush RS, Doctor KP, et al. Acetylcholinesterase prophylaxis against organophosphate toxicity. *Fundam Appl Toxicol* 9:266, 1987.

78. DeJong LPA, Verhagen MAA, Langenberg JP, et al. The bispyridinium-dioxime HLo-7: A potent reactivator for acetylcholinesterase inhibited by the stereoisomers of Tabun and Soman. *Biochem Pharmacol* 38:633, 1989.

79. Rousseaux CG, Dua AK. Pharmacology of HI-6, and H-series oxime. *Can J Physiol Pharmacol* 67:1183, 1989.

80. Fischetti M. Gas vaccine. Bioengineered immunization could shield against nerve gas. *Scientific American* April 1991, 153.

138. Cocaine Poisoning

Francis Renzi

Cocaine is an alkaloid extracted from the leaves of the South American shrub *Erythroxylon coca*. Chemically, cocaine (benzoylmethylecgonine) is a tertiary amine ester of benzoic acid and ecgonine, an aminoalcohol base. The available forms and routes of administration of cocaine vary depending on the intent of use. Cocaine is used clinically by emergency physicians, otolaryngologists, and plastic surgeons as a topical anesthetic and vasoconstrictor (cocaine hydrochloride 4% and 10% solution and as TAC tetracaine-adrenaline-cocaine). The illicit forms of cocaine are produced as salts (cocaine hydrochloride, cocaine sulfate) or an alkaloid (freebase, crack).

Cocaine hydrochloride is readily absorbed from any mucosal surface (e.g., gut, vagina, urethra), although its most common route of administration is snorting (intranasal inhalation via a straw or coke spoon) [1]. Cocaine hydrochloride is water-soluble and can be administered by intravenous injection alone or in combination with other drugs such as heroin (a "speedball"). Cocaine sulfate ("pasta," "bazooka," "cocaine base") is a byproduct of coca leaf processing, is heat-stable, and can be smoked. This form of cocaine is popular in South America but

only sporadically used in the United States [2]. Alkalinization of cocaine hydrochloride can produce freebase or crack, depending on the method of extraction. These compounds are insoluble in water, are heat-stable, vaporize at temperatures greater than 200°F, and can be smoked [3].

Cocaine, like other amide local anesthetics, blocks initiation and conduction of nerve impulses by decreasing axonal membrane permeability to sodium ions [4]. Systemic effects result from cocaine's ability to promote the release of neurotransmitters such as dopamine, acetylcholine, and norepinephrine while blocking their reuptake in the central and sympathetic nervous systems [4,5,6].

Following absorption, cocaine is rapidly distributed in an apparent volume of 2 liters per kilogram [7]. Cocaine is rapidly metabolized by liver esterases and plasma cholinesterase (pseudocholinesterase) and by nonenzymatic hydrolysis [8,9] (Fig. 138-1). Only small amounts of cocaine (1–9%) are eliminated as unchanged drug in the urine [10].

The majority of the metabolites of cocaine are thought to be inactive, except for very small amounts (2.6–6.2%) of the active

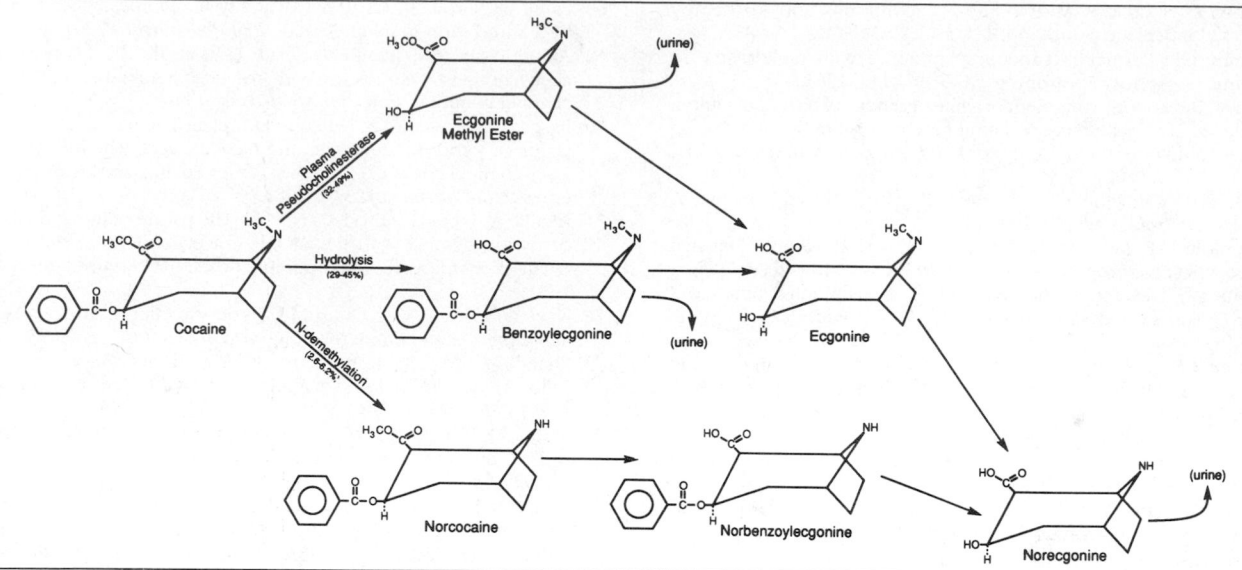

Fig. 138-1. Cocaine metabolism. (Courtesy of C.K. Aaron.)

metabolite, norcocaine. However, recurrent coronary vasoconstriction has been demonstrated to be temporally related in humans to increasing blood concentration of benzoylecgonine and ethyl methyl ecgonine [11,12]. The elimination half-life of cocaine is approximately 1 hour, whereas those of its metabolites range from 4 to 7 hours [13,14].

Alcohol is commonly used with cocaine to balance its central nervous system stimulatory effects. The concurrent use of alcohol and cocaine produces, by liver metabolism, cocaethylene, which also inhibits neurotransmitter uptake. The longer half-life of cocaethylene (2 hours) may help explain the delayed onset of cocaine-related complications such as myocardial infarction or stroke [15].

The onset and duration of effect varies with the dose, route of administration, rate of absorption, elimination, and individual's tolerance. After intravenous injection, a subjective euphoric response occurs in 3 to 5 minutes, with a cardiovascular response peaking in 8 to 12 minutes [16,17]. Both responses show parallel decreases, with a return to baseline in 30 to 40 minutes [16,17].

Following nasal insufflation (snorting), euphoric effects occur within 15 to 20 minutes after exposure, whereas maximal cardiovascular changes and peak plasma levels occur within 20 to 60 minutes [16,17]. Physiologic and subjective responses return to baseline within 60 to 90 minutes. Oral ingestion of cocaine produces peak plasma levels in 50 to 90 minutes and a subjective response after 45 to 90 minutes [16,17]. Subjective and cardiovascular responses from freebase smoking are similar to those from intravenous injection [16,17].

The recommended therapeutic dose of cocaine hydrochloride for local anesthesia should not exceed 1 mg per kilogram administered as a 4% solution [18,19]. Death has been reported with as little as 20 mg as an acute dose, whereas chronic abusers may tolerate up to 10 gm per day without toxic reactions [20,21]. Cocaine toxicity results from excessive adrenergic stimulation occurring both centrally (agitation, seizure) and peripherally (vasoconstriction). Primary sites of toxicity include the central nervous and cardiovascular systems [4,5,6,20]. Toxic reactions to the clinical use of cocaine can occur and may depend on individual tolerance to the drug or application of TAC (tetra-

caine, adrenaline, cocaine solution) to a mucosal surface [23,24]. The presence of adulterants, variation in cocaine content, and individual tolerance make prediction of a toxic reaction to illicit cocaine use difficult [25,26,27]. In the case of "body packers" (individuals who attempt to smuggle cocaine by ingesting wrapped packets of cocaine) and "body stuffers" (those who swallow or conceal loosely wrapped cocaine in body cavities when encountered by law enforcement agents), massive overdose may occur secondary to rupture or leakage of the packets [28,29,30]. Patients with pseudocholinesterase deficiency (genetic or acquired, as with opioid use or liver disease) may be at greater risk of toxicity from cocaine because of their reduced capacity for metabolism through the pseudocholinesterase pathway, although causality has yet to be determined [31]. Maternal cocaine use has been associated with abruptio placentae, spontaneous abortion, intrauterine growth retardation, preterm delivery, and fetal cerebrovascular injury [32]. Cocaine intoxication can occur in breast-fed infants of women who use this drug [33]. Although long-term outcomes are not yet known, infants exposed to cocaine exhibit impairment of orientation and motor behavior and an increased incidence of sudden infant death syndrome [34,35].

Clinical Manifestations and Diagnostic Evaluation

Important points to elicit in the history include route, amount, and time of cocaine use in relation to symptom onset. With mild cocaine intoxication, the patient may complain of headache, chest pain, nausea, or vomiting and demonstrate agitation and anxiousness. Vital signs may include normal or minimally increased pulse, blood pressure, temperature, and respiratory rate. Evidence of hyperreflexia, tremors, muscle twitching, diaphoresis, and mydriasis may be present.

Moderately intoxicated patients may complain of abdominal cramps, headache, chest pain, and formication (feeling of insects crawling on the skin). The patient may be anxious, agitated, and hyperactive and may be hallucinating. Vital sign abnormalities include tachycardia, hypertension, tachypnea, and hyperthermia. Patients may experience a brief generalized tonic-clonic seizure, usually within 2 hours of cocaine use but sometimes delayed up to 12 hours.

Severely intoxicated patients may present awake with an altered mental status, in status epilepticus, or comatose. Vital signs are abnormal, and the patient may be hypertensive or hypotensive, tachycardic or bradycardic, and demonstrate abnormal respirations, including Cheyne-Stokes respirations. Hyperthermia may result from hypothalamic stimulation, increased motor and metabolic activity, and peripheral vasoconstriction. The clinical picture may be clouded by the concomitant use of other drugs or by toxic reactions to common adulterants to cocaine (Table 138-1).

Toxicity has been demonstrated in all organ systems. Cerebrovascular toxicity includes cerebrovascular accidents, subarachnoid or intracerebral hemorrhage, and cerebral vasculitis [36,37]. Cardiovascular complications most frequently involve myocardial ischemia or infarct, aortic dissection, and ischemic bowel [38–44]. Cocaine-mediated hepatotoxicity may result from one of its metabolites, norcocaine nitroxide, which induces depletion of hepatic glutathione. In animals, N-acetylcysteine has offered protection against cocaine-induced hepatic damage [45]. Renal toxicity may be directly ischemic or related to vasculitis [39]. Skin and muscle necrosis has been reported; cocaine may have a direct muscular toxic effect [46]. Pulmonary infarcts may occur, as do bronchospasm, eosinophilia with granuloma formation, and noncardiogenic pulmonary edema [47,48]. Secondary complications may be specific to route of administration and include chronic rhinitis, epistaxis, septal perforation (intranasal use), pneumothorax, pneumomediastinum, pneumopericardium (inhalation) cellulitis, endocarditis, hepatitis, and acquired immunodeficiency syndrome (intravenous use) [49,50,51]. Manifestations of chronic cocaine abuse include anorexia, insomnia, impotence, paranoia, formication, depression, and psychosis.

Recent data suggest that cocaine-induced complications may occur temporally removed from actual cocaine use. Ambulatory electrocardiographic monitoring in cocaine-withdrawing patients revealed myocardial ischemia occurring up to 2 weeks after last cocaine use [52]. At least one case report documents cardiac ischemia with infarct 72 hours after cocaine use [53].

Patient Evaluation

Patients presenting with symptoms of cocaine toxicity should have a complete evaluation, with particular focus on the cardiac, pulmonary, and neurologic systems. Continuous electrocardiographic monitoring and frequent monitoring of vital signs, including core body temperature, are essential. Core temperature must be checked using a thermocouple, since standard thermometers may not read above 106°F. Patients may be hyperthermic even in the face of cool, clammy skin [54]. Evidence of the route of administration should be sought and remaining drug carefully removed to prevent further toxicity (e.g., powder in the nares).

Laboratory evaluation is not necessary when the history is clear and symptoms mild. However, when there is evidence of moderate to severe toxicity, routine laboratory evaluation should include a complete blood count, serum electrolytes, glucose, blood urea nitrogen, creatinine, arterial blood gas determination, urinalysis, and creatine phosphokinase. Expected laboratory abnormalities may include leukocytosis, hypokalemia, and hyperglycemia. Acidosis and an elevated creatine phosphokinase level suggest considerable toxicity. A qualitative toxicologic analysis of blood and urine for cocaine and metabolites may help confirm the diagnosis and identify other intoxicants. It must be remembered that serum cocaine determination is difficult, and a negative test does not rule out exposure. Cocaine metabolites remain detectable in the urine several days after exposure. An electrocardiogram (ECG) and chest radiograph should be obtained in patients with any cardiorespiratory sign or symptom. Serial cardiograms and cardiac enzyme determinations are necessary in patients with prolonged pressure or pain of suspected cardiac origin. Patients with a persistent or severe headache, abnormal neurologic examination, or prolonged seizures require computed tomography (CT) scan and lumbar puncture to rule out an intracranial lesion or infection. Hyperthermia must not be attributed solely to cocaine use, and occult infections should be excluded. Tea-colored urine should alert the physician to rhabdomyolysis, requiring close monitoring of renal function, since acute myoglobinuric renal failure may occur in up to one-third of these patients [55].

Prolonged toxicity (>4 hours) or progressive symptoms suggest continued drug absorption and require further investigation. Patients suspected of body packing or stuffing should be evaluated by cavity search and abdominal radiographs or contrast studies.

The differential diagnosis of acute cocaine intoxication includes poisonings with other sympathomimetics, methylxanthines, phencyclidine, hallucinogens, and anticholinergic agents. Medical conditions that may simulate cocaine use include thyrotoxicosis, malignant hypertension and hyperthermia, drug withdrawal, pheochromocytoma, hypoglycemia, and psychiatric illnesses such as mania or paranoid schizophrenia.

Table 138-1. Adulterants and Drugs Admixed with Street Cocaine

Local anesthetics—procaine, lidocaine, tetracaine, benzocaine
Stimulants—amphetamine, caffeine, methylphenidate, ergotamine, aminophylline, strychnine ("death hit")
Hallucinogens—LSD, hashish, marijuana, PCP
Opioids—codeine, heroin ("speedball")
Depressants—alcohol ("liquid lady"), methapyrilene
Inert substances—talc, flour, cornstarch, sugars (lactose, inositol, sucrose, maltose, mannitol)
Others—quinine, thiamine, tyramine, NaHCO, magnesium silicate, MgSO$_4$, salicylamide
Bacteria, fungi, and viruses may also contaminate the drug

From Goldfrank, L, Lewin N, Weisman RS: Cocaine. Reprinted with permission from *Hospital Physician*, May 1981.

Management

Management of cocaine-toxic patients consists predominantly of supportive care and symptomatic treatment of each complication. Airway, breathing, and circulation should be initially addressed. All patients should have continuous electrocardiographic monitoring and frequent vital sign checks, including core temperature. Patients with mild toxicity and a clear history can be managed with observation and reassurance. Laboratory evaluation is generally not necessary. Markedly agitated, anxious, or psychotic patients may be treated with a benzodiazepine, such as midazolam (2–10 mg IV), diazepam (2–10 mg IV), or lorazepam (2–4 mg IV). Tachycardia and mild hypertension in these patients are usually transient and resolve spontaneously. If treatment is necessary, benzodiazepine sedation may be sufficient to normalize vital signs. These patients usually become asymptomatic within several hours and may be discharged after 3 to 6 hours of observation.

Moderately or severely intoxicated patients require more aggressive therapy. In patients with an altered mental status, seizures, or coma, an adequate airway must be established. Supplemental oxygen, dextrose (25 gm IV), naloxone (2 mg IV), and thiamine (100 mg IV) should be administered. Hypertensive crisis or hemodynamically unstable tachycardia should be aggressively managed. These patients are often young and without the physiologic adaptations present in chronic hypertensives, which increases their risk for complications from elevated blood pressure. Systolic pressure greater than 140 mm Hg or diastolic pressure greater than 100 mm Hg should be cause for concern. Moderately hypertensive patients can be treated with benzodiazepine sedation or nifedipine. Severely symptomatic patients require titratable intravenous agents, such as phentolamine, nitroglycerin, and nitroprusside. The use of labetalol, esmolol, or other beta-blockers with these agents has been suggested, but recent animal and human data suggest that beta-blockers may worsen coronary artery vasoconstriction [56,57,58]. This study, however, did not evaluate beta-blockers combined with vasodilators. Hypotension is a premorbid event that requires active fluid resuscitation and, if necessary, vasopressor therapy. Since cocaine depletes neurotransmitters and prevents their reuptake, patients may be sensitive to small doses of vasopressors. A postsynaptic alpha agent, such as norepinephrine (Levophed), may be required. Inotropic agents such as dobutamine may be useful since hypotension can result from a direct depressant effect on the left ventricle independent of myocardial ischemia [59].

Isolated seizures may occur and require no treatment other than observation and neurologic evaluation. Status epilepticus must be treated aggressively with intravenous benzodiazepines, such as diazepam (0.1–0.3 mg/kg repeated as necessary). If seizures are refractory to high-dose benzodiazepines, consideration should be given to early paralysis while additional anticonvulsants such as short-acting barbiturates (amobarbital, thiopental, pentobarbital) are added to the therapy. Continued seizures and resulting hyperthermia and rhabdomyolysis are responsible for many of the complications resulting from cocaine intoxication [60,61,62]. A short-acting neuromuscular blocking agent, such as vecuronium (0.08–0.1 mg/kg) or pancuronium (0.06–0.1 mg/kg), can be given. Succinylcholine should be avoided because it may induce rhabdomyolysis with hyperkalemia, acidosis, and possibly pseudocholinesterase deficiency in chronic cocaine users [63]. Standard therapy with ice water sponging, fans, or ice water bath should be instituted for patients with hyperthermia. Cooling blankets alone are insufficient and should be used only with other modalities. Core temperatures as high as 114°F have been recorded [64]. Aggressive cooling should continue until the core temperature has decreased to 100 to 102°F. Early alkaline diuresis may help prevent renal failure in patients with rhabdomyolysis.

Chest pain related to cocaine use may be of cardiogenic origin regardless of the patient's age. The route of administration, coronary risk factors, angiographic absence of coronary artery disease, or an initial normal cardiogram do not identify those who will develop myocardial infarction after cocaine use. The onset of chest pain after cocaine use may be quite variable, occurring within 3 hours (range 1 minute to 4 days) in the majority of patients [65]. Since the etiology of cocaine-induced ischemic chest pain may be multifactorial (coronary artery spasm, direct myocardial toxicity, increased myocardial oxygen consumption, and nonatherosclerotic intimal proliferation), typical focal ischemic electrocardiographic changes may not be present. If the chest pain has features of myocardial ischemia,

it should be treated as such. Cocaine-related chest pain should be treated in the standard fashion (e.g., nitrates, opioids). Although coronary artery vasospasm, vasculitis, and platelet adhesiveness all may play a role in acute myocardial infarction following cocaine use, thrombolysis should be considered in all such patients. Beta-adrenergic blockade, on the other hand, may further decrease coronary artery diameter because of unopposed alpha-adrenergic blockade. Phentolamine, an alpha-adrenergic antagonist, has been used in humans to reverse cocaine-induced coronary artery vasoconstriction and appears to be effective in reducing myocardial oxygen demand and improving coronary blood flow [66,67]. Patients who have coronary artery disease and use alcohol and cocaine concurrently have 21.5 times the risk for sudden death of users of cocaine alone [15].

Ventricular dysrhythmias may be treated with lidocaine. Other antiarrhythmics, including bretylium, propranolol, and labetalol, may be used as alternatives, but consideration should be given to their risk-benefit ratio. Patients who present with ventricular tachycardia, fibrillation, or asystole should be treated using advanced cardiac life support recommendations.

Body packers or stuffers present a therapeutic challenge. Activated charcoal (1 gm/kg orally) should be given to all those who ingest cocaine. Emesis induced by syrup of ipecac should be avoided because of the possibility of bag rupture, seizures, and aspiration, although it has been done successfully within minutes after ingestion [68,69]. Asymptomatic patients who have ingested packets of cocaine may be treated with multiple-dose charcoal plus laxatives (sodium sulfate, magnesium sulfate, magnesium citrate, or sorbitol) or whole bowel lavage [69]. In vitro evidence implies a role for gastric alkalinization to increase the hydrolysis of cocaine liberated from packets [70]. Close observation with intravenous acccess and continuous electrocardiographic monitoring is necessary [29,30]. Endoscopic removal of intact packets must be performed with caution, since packet rupture can occur [71]. If signs or symptoms of cocaine toxicity are present or if intestinal obstruction occurs, immediate surgical intervention is indicated [72,73]. Enhanced elimination with acidification of the urine is impractical, because urinary excretion represents only a small fraction of the overall elimination and because of the short biologic half-life of cocaine [74]. Acidification may be dangerous since rhabdomyolysis is worsened in an acidic environment.

Death from cocaine intoxication usually occurs within minutes of exposure; the majority of patients who reach the hospital survive. Patients with mild cocaine intoxication who become asymptomatic after 3 to 6 hours of observation may be discharged. Those with moderate or severe toxicity or those who develop a secondary complication (e.g., myocardial infarction) require admission to an intensive care unit. All patients with prolonged toxicity or history of cocaine ingestion should be admitted and treated expectantly. Resolution of toxicity, passage of all packets, or radiographic evidence of a clear gastrointestinal tract all help determine when the patient can be safely discharged [30,75]. Drug abuse counseling and treatment should be offered to all patients.

References

1. Cregler LL, Mark H: Cardiovascular dangers of cocaine abuse. *Am J Cardiol* 57:1187, 1986.
2. Jeri FR, Sanchez C, Del Pozo T, et al: The syndrome of coca paste. *J Psychedelic Drugs* 132:225, 1975.

3. Loper KA: Clinical toxicology of cocaine. *Med Toxicol Adverse Drug Exp* 4:174, 1989.
4. Jaffe J: *The Pharmacologic Basis of Therapy.* 5th ed. New York, Macmillan, 1970.
5. Calligaro DO, Eldefrauir ME: Central and peripheral cocaine receptors. *J Pharmacol Exp Ther* 243:61, 1987.
6. Swanson KL, Albriquerque EX: Nicotinic acetylcholine receptor ion channel blockade by cocaine: The mechanism of synaptic action. *J Pharmacol Exp Ther* 243:1202, 1987.
7. Chow MJ, Ambre JJ, Ruo TL, et al: Kinetics of cocaine distribution, elimination and chronotropic effects. *Clin Pharmacol Ther* 38:318, 1985.
8. Misra AL, Nayak PK, Block R, et al: Estimation and deposition of [³H] benzoylecgonine and pharmacological activity of some metabolites. *J Pharm Pharmacol* 27:784, 1975.
9. Stewart DJ, Inaba T, Lucassen M, et al: Cocaine metabolism: Cocaine and norcocaine hydrolysis by liver and serum esterases. *Clin Pharmacol Ther* 25:464, 1979.
10. Fish F, Wilson W: Excretion of cocaine and its metabolites in man. *J Pharm Pharmacol* 21:135, 1969.
11. Inaba T, Stewart DJ, Kalow W: Metabolism of cocaine in man. *Clin Pharmacol Exp Ther* 23:547, 1978.
12. Brogan WC, Lange RA, Glamann, et al: Recurrent coronary vasoconstriction caused by intranasal cocaine: Possible role for metabolites. *Ann Intern Med* 116:556., 1992.
13. Wilkinson P, Wan Dyke C, Jatlow P, et al: Intranasal and oral cocaine kinetics. *Clin Pharmacol Ther* 27:386, 1980.
14. Chow MJ, Ambre JJ, Ruo TI et al: Kinetics of cocaine distribution, elimination and chronotropic effects. *Clin Pharmacol Ther* 38:318, 1985.
15. Randal T: Cocaine, alcohol mix in body to form even longer lasting, more lethal drug. *JAMA* 267:1043, 1992.
16. Javaid JL, Fischman MW, Schuster CR, et al: Cocaine plasma concentrations: Relation of physiological subjective effects in humans. *Science* 202:227, 1978.
17. Fischman MW, Schuster CR, Hatano Y: A comparison of the subjective and cardiovascular effects of cocaine and lidocaine in humans. *Pharmacol Biochem Behav* 18:123, 1983.
18. Adriani J, Campbell D: Fatalities following topical application of local anesthetics to mucous membranes. *JAMA* 162:1527, 1956.
19. Sawarese JJ, Covino BG: Basic and clinical pharmacology of local anesthetic drugs, in Ronald D. Miller (ed): *Anesthesia.* New York, Churchill Livingstone, 1986, pp 985–1014.
20. Adriani J, Filipenko J: Clinical effectiveness of drugs used for topical anesthesia. *JAMA* 188:711, 1964.
21. Price KR: Fatal cocaine poisoning. *J Forensic Sci Soc* 14:329, 1974.
22. Van Dyke C, Jaltlow P, Ungerer J, et al: Oral cocaine: Plasma concentrations and central effects. *Science* 200:211, 1978.
23. Doren S: Complications of TAC. *Ann Emerg Med* 12:333, 1982.
24. Dailey RH: Fatality secondary to misuse of TAC solution. *Ann Emerg Med* 17:159, 1988.
25. Goldfrank L, Lewin N, Weisman RS: Cocaine. *Hosp Physician* 26:26, 1981.
26. Siegel RK: Cocaine substitutes. *N Engl J Med* 302:817, 1980.
27. Insley BM, Grufferman S, Ayliffe E: Thallium poisoning in cocaine abusers. *Am J Emerg Med* 4:545, 1986.
28. Fishbain DA, Wetli CV: Cocaine intoxication delirium and death in a body packer. *Ann Emerg Med* 10:531, 1981.
29. Caruana DS, Weinbach B, Goerg D, Gardner LB: Cocaine packet ingestion. *Ann Intern Med* 100:73, 1984.
30. McCarron MM, Wood JD: The cocaine body packer syndrome. *JAMA* 250:1417, 1983.
31. Devenyi P: Cocaine complications and pseudocholinesterase. *Ann Intern Med* 110:167, 1989.
32. Chasnoff IJ, Burns WJ, Schnoll SH, et al: Cocaine use during pregnancy. *N Engl J Med* 313:666, 1985.
33. Chasnoff IJ, Lewis DE, Squires L: Cocaine intoxication in a breast-fed infant. *Pediatrics* 80:836, 1987.
34. Zuckerman B, Frank DA, Hingson R, et al: Effects of maternal marijuana and cocaine use on fetal growth. *N Engl J Med* 320:762, 1989.
35. Volpe JJ: Effect of cocaine use on the fetus. *N Engl J Med* 327:399, 1992.
36. Brust JCM, Richter RW: Stroke associated with cocaine abuse. *NY State Med* 77:1473, 1977.
37. Seaman ME: Acute cocaine abuse associated with cerebral infarction. *Ann Emerg Med* 19:34, 1990.
38. Barth CW, Bray M, Roberts WC: Rupture of the ascending aorta during cocaine intoxication. *Am J Cardiol* 57:496, 1986.
39. Sharff JA: Renal infarction associated with intravenous cocaine use. *Ann Emerg Med* 13:1145, 1984.
40. Texter EC Jr, Chou CC, Merill SL, et al: Direct effects of vasoactive agents on segmental resistance of the mesenteric and portal circulation: Studies with l-epinephrine, levarterenol, angiotensin, vasopressin, acetylcholine, methacholine, histamine, and serotonin. *J Lab Clin Med* 64:624, 1964.
41. Nalbandian H, Sheth N, Dietrich R, Georgiou J: Intestional ischemia caused by cocaine ingestion: Report of two cases. *Surgery* 97:374, 1985.
42. Cregler LL, Mark H: Relation of acute myocardial infarction to cocaine abuse. *Am J Cardiol* 56:794, 1985.
43. Cregler LL, Mark H: Medical complications of cocaine abuse. *N Engl J Med* 315:1438, 1986.
44. Isner JM, Estes M, Thompson PD, et al: Acute cardiac events temporally related to cocaine abuse. *N Engl J Med* 315:1438, 1986.
45. Suarez KA, Bhonsle P, Richardson DL: Protective effect of N-acetylcysteine pretreatment against cocaine induced hepatotoxicity and lipid peroxidation in the mouse. *Res Comm Substances Abuse* 7:7, 1986
46. Zamora-Quezada JL, Dinerman H, Stadecker MJ: Muscle and skin infarction after free-basing cocaine (crack). *Ann Intern Med* 108:564, 1988.
47. Kissner DG, Lawrence WD, Selis JE, Flint A: Crack lung-pulmonary disease caused by cocaine abuse. *Am Rev Respir Dis* 136:1250, 1987.
48. Cucco RA, Yoo OH, Cregler L, Chang JC: Nonfatal pulmonary edema after "freebase" cocaine smoking. *Am Rev Respir Dis* 136:179, 1987.
49. Vilensky W: Illicit and licit drugs causing perforation of the nasal septum. *J Forensic Sci* 27:958, 1982.
50. Aroesty DJ, Stanley RB, Crockett DM: Pneumomediastinum and cervical emphysema from the inhalation of "free based" cocaine: Report of three cases. *Otolaryngology* 94:372, 1986.
51. Adrouny A, Magnusson P: Pneumopericardium from cocaine inhalation. *N Engl J Med* 313:48, 1985.
52. Nademansee K, Gorelick DA, Josephson MA, et al: Myocardial ischemia during cocaine withdrawal. *Ann Intern Med* 111:876, 1989.
53. Aguila CD, Rosman H: Myocardial infarction during cocaine withdrawal. *Ann Intern Med* 112:712, 1990.
54. Loghmanee F, Tobak M: Fatal malignant hyperthermia associated with recreational cocaine and ethanol abuse. *Am J Forensic Med Pathol* 7:246, 1986.
55. Roth D, Alarcon FJ, Fernandez JA, et al: Acute rhabdomyolysis associated with cocaine intoxication. *N Engl J Med* 319:673, 1988.
56. Gay G, Loper K: The use of labetalol in the management of cocaine crisis. *Ann Emerg Med* 17:282, 1988.
57. Ramoska E, Sacchetti A: Propranolol induced hypertension in the treatment of cocaine intoxication. *Ann Emerg Med* 14:1112, 1985.
58. Lange RA, Cigarroa RG, Flores ED, et al: Potentiation of cocaine-induced coronary vasoconstriction by beta-adrenergic blockade. *Ann Intern Med* 112:897, 1990.
59. Fraker TD, Temesy-Armos PN, Brewster PS, Wilkerson RD: Mechanism of cocaine-induced myocardial depression in dogs. *Circulation* 81:1012, 1990.
60. Poque VA, Nurse HM: Cocaine associated acute myoglobinuric renal failure. *Am J Med* 86:183, 1989.
61. Roth DR, Alarcon FJ, Fernandez JA, et al: Acute rhabdomyolysis associated with cocaine intoxication. *N Engl J Med* 319:673, 1988.
62. Merrigian KS, Roberts JR: Cocaine intoxication: Hyperpyrexia, rhabdomyolysis, and acute renal failure. *Clin Toxicol* 25:135, 1987.
63. Hoffman RS, Henry GL, Weisman RS, et al: Association between plasma cholinesterase activity and cocaine toxicity (abstract). *Ann Emerg Med* 19:467, 1990.
64. Roberts JR, Quattrocchi E, Howland MA: Severe hyperthermia secondary to intravenous drug abuse. *Am J Emerg Med* 2:373, 1984.
65. Hollander JE, Hoffman RS: Cocaine induced myocardial infarction: An analysis and review of the literature. *J Emerg Med* 10:169, 1992.
66. Lange RA, Cigarroa RG, Yancy CW, et al: Cocaine-induced coronary-artery vasoconstriction. *N Engl J Med* 321:1557, 1989.

67. Hollander JE: Use of phentolamine for cocaine-induced myocardial ischemia. *N Engl J Med* 327:361, 1992.
68. Olson K, Benowitz NL, Pentel P, Gay G: Management of cocaine poisoning. *Ann Emerg Med* 12:655, 1983.
69. Hoffman RS, Chiang WK, Weisman RS, Goldfrank LR: Prospective evaluation of "crack-vial" ingestions. *Vet Hum Toxicol* 32:164, 1990.
70. Arks SE, VanderHoek TL, Hryhorczuk DO, et al: Cocaine liberation from body packets in an in vitro model. 21:1321, 1992.
71. Suarez CA, Arango A, Lester L: Cocaine-condom ingestion: Surgical treatment. *JAMA* 238:1391, 1977.
72. Nalbandian H, Sheth N, Dietrich R, et al: Intestinal ischemia caused by cocaine ingestion: report of two cases. *Surgery* 97:374, 1985.

73. Trent M, Kim U: Cocaine packet ingestion: Surgical or medical management. *Arch Surg* 122:1179, 1987.
74. Schwartz WK, Oderda GM: Management of cocaine intoxication. *Clin Toxicol Consult* 2:45, 1980.
75. Sinner WM: The gastrointestinal tract as a vehicle for drug smuggling. *Gastrointest Radiol* 6:319, 1981.
76. Woods JR, Plessinger MA, Clarke KE: Effect of cocaine on uterine blood flow and fetal oxygenation. *JAMA* 257:957, 1987.
77. Hoffman RS, Henry GL, Weisman RS, et al: Association between plasma cholinesterase activity and cocaine toxicity (abstract). *Ann Emerg Med* 19:467, 1990.

139. Corrosive Poisoning

Robert P. Dowsett and
Christopher H. Linden

Introduction

DEFINITIONS. Corrosives are compounds that cause tissue injury as a result of a chemical reaction. The term originally referred to acids that had the ability to corrode metals but is now used synonymously with *caustic,* originally applied only to a toxic base or alkali [1]. It also includes chemicals that react with cellular components by mechanisms other than acid-base reactions.

In solution, acids and bases react with water and donate or accept a proton to form their conjugate base or acid. In doing so, they alter the hydrogen ion concentration of the solution. The pH is defined as the negative logarithm of the H^+ ion concentration, expressed as moles per liter (M). Water, at 25°C, has a pH of 7 (signifying a hydrogen ion concentration of 10^{-7} M or 0.0001 mmol/L) and is considered "neutral." Acidic solutions, containing a higher concentration of free H^+ ions, have a pH less than 7. Conversely, basic solutions have a lower H^+ ion concentration and a pH greater than 7. Solutions with a pH of less than 2 or greater than 12 are considered strongly acidic or basic. The pH levels of some common solutions are listed in Table 139-1.

The relative strength of an acid or base can be defined by the ease with which it will donate or accept a proton and is measured by the dissociation constant (K) or its negative logarithm, the pK. The pK of an acid (pKa) is equal to the pH of a solution where half of the acid has lost a proton. For a strong acid, the pKa is low (<0). The pKb of an alkali is equal to the pOH of a solution where the base and conjugate are present in equal quantities. The strength of a base can also be expressed as the pKa of the conjugate, which is 14 minus the pKb. Strong alkalis are those with a high (>14) pKa (Table 139-2).

CHEMICAL REACTIONS. Although corrosives cause tissue injury primarily by reacting with organic molecules, disrupting cell membranes and function, they can also cause thermal burns if heat is generated when the chemical is neutralized or dissolved in an aqueous solution (e.g., in a body fluid). Reactions between strong acids and strong bases are usually highly exothermic. Adding a strong acid or base to water generates heat;

adding water to a strong acid or base may result in an explosively exothermic reaction. Metallic lithium, sodium, potassium, some aluminum and lithium salts, and titanium tetrachloride react violently when placed in water, producing large amounts of heat [2–5]. Chlorine reacts with water in an exothermic reaction to form hydrochloric (HCl) and hypochlorous (HClO) acids, elemental chlorine, and free oxygen radicals [6,7]. Similar reactions occur with bromine. Ammonia combines with water to form ammonium hydroxide in a reaction that liberates heat; the hydroxide formed is then responsible for corrosive effects [8]. Nitrogen dioxide reacts with water to release heat and produce nitric and nitrous acid.

The mixing of chemicals may result in reactions that liberate caustic gases. Mixing ammonia with hypochlorite (e.g., household bleach) generates chloramine gases (NH_2Cl and $NHCl_2$), which are highly irritating to mucosal epithelia [9–12]. Combin-

Table 139-1. Approximate pH of Some Common Solutions

Solution	pH
1.0 M HCl	0
Gastric juice	1.2–3.0
Battery acid (1% solution)	1.4
Domestic toilet cleaner (1%)	2.0
Citrus juices	1.8–4
Carbonated beverages	2.5–3.5
Wines	2.8–3.8
Black coffee	5.0
Saliva	6.4–6.9
Rainwater	6.5
Water (pure, at 25°C)	7.0
Bleach (1% solution)	9.5–10.2
Automatic dishwasher detergents	10.4–13
Laundry detergents	11.6–12.6
Domestic ammonium cleaners	11.9–12.4
Ammonia 10%	12.5
Drain cleaner	13.3–14
1 M NaOH	14
Saturated ammonia solution	15

Table 139-2. pKa of Corrosive Chemicals

Chemical	Formula	pKa
Acids		
Perchloric	$HClO_4$	−8
Hydrochloric	HCl	−3
Chromic	CrO_3	0.3
Bromic	$HBrO_3$	<1
Nitric	HNO_3	<1
Oxalic	$C_2H_2O_4$	1.5
Maleic	$C_4H_4O_4$	1.8
Sulfuric	H_2SO_4	1.9
Propiolic	C_3HO_2H	1.9
Phosphoric	$H_2P_2O_7$	2.1
Arsenic	H_3AsO_4	2.3
Malonic	$C_3H_4O_4$	2.8
Fumaric	$C_4H_4O_4$	3.0
Nitrous	HNO_2	3.3
Hydrofluoric	HF	3.4
Formic	CH_2O_2	3.8
Carbonic	H_2CO_3	3.8
Lactic	$C_3H_6O_3$	3.9
Acrylic	$C_2H_3CO_2H$	4.3
Methacrylic	$C_3H_5CO_2H$	4.7
Acetic	H_3C_2OOH	4.8
Isobutyric	$C_4H_8O_2$	4.8
Sulfurous	HSO_3	6.9
Hydrogen sulfide	H_2S	7.0
Ammonium ion	NH_4OH	9.3
Boric	H_3BO_3	9.2
Hydrogen peroxide	H_2O_2	11.6
Water	H_2O	15.8
Bases		
Calcium carbonate	$CaCO_3$	5.7
Hydrazine	N_2H_4	8
1,4-Butanediamine	$C_4H_{12}N_2$	9.2
Ammonia	NH_3	9.3
Ammonium hydroxide	NH_4	9.3
Ethanolamine	$NH_2C_2H_4OH$	9.5
Allylamine	C_3H_7N	9.7
Magnesium hydroxide	H_2MgO_2	10
Propylamine	C_3H_9H	10.6
Methylamine	CH_3NH_2	10.7
Ethylamine	$C_2H_5NH_2$	10.7
n-Butylamine	$C_4H_9HN_2$	10.7
Cyclohexylamine	$C_6H_{11}NH_2$	10.7
Zinc hydroxide	$Zn(OH)_2$	11
Calcium hydroxide	$Ca(OH)_2$	11.6
1,6-Hexanediamine	$NH_2C_6H_{12}NH_2$	11.8
Lithium hydroxide	$LiOH$	>14
Potassium hydroxide	KOH	>14
Sodium hydroxide	$NaOH$	>14
Calcium oxide	CaO	>14
Sodium carbonate	Na_2CO_3	>14
Potassium carbonate	K_2CO_3	>14
Sodium hypochlorite	$NaClO$	>14

ing bleach with acid (e.g., household toilet bowl and drain cleaners containing sulfuric acid or its sodium bisulfite salt) produces chlorine gas [13,14]. A number of metallic compounds react with acids, resulting in the liberation of potentially explosive hydrogen gas. Hydrogen sulfide and sulfur oxide gas result from the action of strong acids on sulfur-containing compounds such as orthopaedic plaster casting material [15]. Zinc hydroxide (present in soldering flux) is corrosive in an acidic environment [16].

EPIDEMIOLOGY. During 1992, more than 240,000 exposures to potentially corrosive chemicals were reported by poison cen-

ters in the United States; actual exposures are estimated to be several times greater [17,18]. Deaths due to ingestion of corrosive agents constituted 2.5 percent of all reported deaths due to poisoning [17]. Household cleaning products constitute the largest group of exposures, with bleaches and disinfectants most commonly identified. Ingestions by children younger than 6 years accounted for more than half of the reported cases. Only a few of these cases resulted in serious injury; there were no reported deaths and the incidence of significant injury was only one-fourth of that in adults, who, either by deliberate intent or because of concomitant intoxication, often ingest a larger amount of corrosive [19–24]. Deaths due to accidental ingestions of corrosives occurred exclusively in people older than 75 years and represented 22 percent of all deaths due to corrosive ingestion [17].

Before 1970, highly concentrated solutions of lye (sodium or potassium hydroxide) were available for domestic use and caused most of the serious injuries due to corrosive ingestions [25,26,27]. Although only moderately concentrated (<10%) liquid lye drain cleaners are currently available, they are still responsible for the largest number of severe gastrointestinal injuries [19,21,24,28–31]. Ingestion of acid toilet bowl cleaners now accounts for the same number of deaths as ingestion of alkaline drain cleaners [17]. Less commonly, severe alkali injuries may result from the ingestion of powdered automatic dishwasher detergents containing sodium carbonate [32]. Household ammonia, bleaches, and hydrogen peroxide solutions are generally much less potent than similar agents used in industry but can cause significant injury if ingested in large amounts. [19,31,33–37].

PATHOPHYSIOLOGY. Bases react with tissues to cause liquefaction necrosis, which results from the saponification of fats, dissolution of proteins, and emulsification of lipid membranes [38]. Cellular membranes are disrupted, resulting in cell death, tissue necrosis, and thrombosis of small vessels. The resultant tissue softening and sloughing (liquefaction) may allow the alkali to penetrate to deeper levels. Liquefaction necrosis is usually accompanied by heat production. Tissue injury progresses rapidly over the first few minutes but can continue for several hours [26,27,39,40]. Over the ensuing 4 days bacterial invasion and an inflammatory response can cause additional tissue injury. Granulation tissue then develops, but collagen deposition may not begin until the second week. The tensile strength of healing tissue is therefore lowest during the first 2 weeks following exposure. Epithelial repair may take weeks to months. Scar retraction begins in the third week and commonly continues for months as collagen is laid down and undergoes maturation. Scar retraction may result in stricture formation and shortening of the involved segment of the gastrointestinal tract.

Acid burns are characterized by coagulation necrosis. Protein is denatured and loses its water solubility, resulting in the formation of a firm coagulum or eschar. Characteristic findings are a white plaquelike appearance [27]. The resulting eschar may limit tissue penetration, but this does not appear to be a major variable in determining the extent of injury [8,27,31,41]. The release of thermal energy during this reaction is typically higher than for alkali reactions and the corrosive effects more prolonged [42,43]. The subsequent inflammatory response, tissue healing, and complications are similar to that seen with alkalis.

Hydrocarbons are solvents that may produce injury by dissolving lipids in cell membranes and coagulating cellular proteins. Significant damage usually occurs after prolonged contact [44,45,46]. Other chemicals cause tissue injury by reactions such as oxidation, reduction, denaturation, and alkylation.

DETERMINANTS OF SEVERITY. The severity of a chemical injury depends on the dose and formulation of the agent involved and the duration of contact [26,47]. Alkaline solutions with a pH greater than 12.5 are likely to cause mucosal ulceration, with deeper tissue necrosis resulting if the pH approaches 14 [40,48]. However, solutions with a pH less than 12.5 can cause significant injury, and solutions of different chemicals with the same pH can cause varying degrees of tissue damage [27,31,32,36,48,49]. Titratable alkaline or acidic reserve has been suggested as a better indicator of corrosive potency than pH [50]. Titratable reserve is expressed as the amount of hydrochloric acid or sodium hydroxide required to neutralize the pH of a basic or acidic solution. It depends on the valency and pK of the acid or base as well as the molar concentration and volume of the solution. Acids and bases are likely to produce tissue injury if they have a pKa less than 2 or greater than 12 [43,48]. While even small volumes of solutions with extremes of pH (<2 or >12) or containing a corrosive with extremes of pK should be considered highly corrosive, larger amounts of weaker acids and bases may also produce significant damage.

The physical state of a chemical also influences its toxicity. Corrosives that are gases or produce fumes at room temperature primarily affect the skin and mucous membranes of the eyes, airways, and lungs. Saturated acid solutions may liberate significant amounts of acid fumes, particularly if heated. Solid compounds may dissolve on contact with body fluids, producing highly concentrated solutions and causing severe but localized damage. Solutions with a high viscosity tend to cause deeper burns than those of lower viscosity, possibly by localizing the reaction in a manner similar to that for solids [48].

SYSTEMIC EFFECTS. Most systemic effects that occur following exposure to corrosives are secondary to local events such as tissue inflammation, acidosis, infection, and necrosis [51]. Massive fluid and electrolyte shifts can occur, resulting in hypovolemic shock, acidosis, and organ failure. Significant systemic absorption of corrosives is uncommon as the chemical is usually neutralized on contact with surface tissues. However, some chemicals (e.g., phenol, hydrazine, chromic acid) can be absorbed through intact skin or minor burns and cause systemic toxicity; a number of acids and a few bases can be absorbed and produce systemic effects following large ingestions or extensive dermal burns [16,44,49,52–63].

Clinical Toxicity

Corrosive injuries most commonly involve the epithelial surfaces of the skin, eyes, and gastrointestinal tract. The lungs may also be injured by the inhalation of gases or aspiration of ingested chemicals (see Chap. 71). Systemic effects may result from severe local tissue injury or systemic absorption of the corrosive.

EYE EXPOSURE. Chemical burns to the eye range from minor irritation to severe and permanent tissue damage [64,65]. Roper-Hall's classification of chemical injuries is generally recognized as having prognostic value (Table 139-3) [65]. Alkali injuries are said to be more severe than acid ones, but this has not been clearly established [66,67]. Eye pain and blepharospasm are a consistent feature of chemical burns. Decreased visual acuity may result from excessive tearing, corneal edema and ulceration, anterior chamber clouding, or lens opacities [68].

Table 139-3. Grading of Severity of Ocular Chemical Burns

Grade	Cornea	Limbal ischemia	Prognosis
I	Epithelial loss	None	Good
II	Stromal haze, iris details visible	< 1/3 of vessels affected	Good
III	Total epithelial loss, iris details obscured	1/3–1/2 of vessels affected	Doubtful, vision reduced
IV	Opaque, no view of iris or pupil	> 1/2 of vessels affected	Poor

Mild injuries are characterized by varying degrees of epithelial loss. Conjunctival hemorrhages and chemosis may be seen in all grades of injury. If the underlying stroma is exposed, the cornea will become opaque, obscuring details of the iris. In severe cases, the entire corneal epithelium is eroded and the pupil and iris are not visible. Severe burns can also result in increased intraocular pressure, blindness, and deformities and perforation of the globe [64,69]. The severity of a chemical burn can also be assessed by the degree of ischemia of conjunctival vessels at the limbus of the eye. If more than half of these vessels are thrombosed the prognosis is generally poor [65]. In such cases corneal scarring and opacification result in a severe loss of visual acuity [64]. Other chronic effects can include corneal denervation, replacement of ciliary body and iris tissue with granulation tissue, damage to tear-producing cells resulting in a dry eye, and lid eversion or inversion [69–72].

DERMAL EXPOSURE. Significant differences exist between thermal burns and those caused by corrosive chemicals. Although corrosives usually result in the immediate onset of pain, it may be delayed several hours [2,73–76]. Some agents, such as petroleum distillates, weak NaOH solutions, and cement typically do not produce burns unless allowed to remain in contact with the skin for prolonged periods (e.g., as a result of contamination of clothing or footwear). Although such exposures initially appear trivial, full-thickness skin burns can result [2,44,75,77,78]. High concentrations of acid or ammonia gases may also cause skin burns [79,80].

Most chemical burns involve less than 15 percent of the body surface [81,82]. Approximately half of all chemical burns seen at specialized centers are full-thickness burns, with a higher incidence of third-degree burns resulting from acids [81,82]. Assessing the depth of injury can be difficult. Chemical burns rarely blister and the affected skin is usually dark, insensate, and firmly attached, regardless of the burn depth [81]. Some specific color changes of the skin may be noted: green with hydrochloric acid, gray with sulfuric acid, and yellow with nitric acid [83]. With time the skin hardens and cracks, exposing the underlying dermis or subcutaneous tissue [81]. This may take up to 4 weeks. Healing generally takes longer than for thermal burns.

Some chemical warfare agents can cause severe dermal injury. Sulfur mustard, the most common antipersonnel agent used in military action, and Lewisite (chlorovinylarsine dichloride) are potent alkylating agents, resulting in severe vesication of the skin 4 to 12 hours after exposure. Phosgene oxide has a similar action but its effects are almost immediate. Respiratory burns are nearly always associated with sulfur mustard exposure [84,85]. When systemically absorbed, sulfur mustard acts as a cytotoxic on gastrointestinal mucosa and bone marrow [86]. White phosphorus is used in incendiary devices and in the manufacture of fertilizers and insecticides. It ignites spontaneously when exposed to air. Systemic absorption of white phosphorus results in hypocalcemia, hepatotoxicity, and renal failure [87]. Cardiac toxicity and sudden death may occur if more than 10 to 15 percent of the body surface is burned [88].

INGESTION. The ingestion of corrosives typically injures the oropharynx, esophagus, and stomach but may sometimes cause damage as distal as the proximal jejunum [30,41,89–93]. Areas most commonly affected are those at or immediately proximal to points of gastrointestinal tract narrowing: the cricopharyngeal area, diaphragmatic esophagus, and the antrum and pylorus of the stomach [19,83]. Multiple sites are affected in up to 80 percent of patients [90]. Esophageal lesions are seen predominantly in the lower half and gastric burns are usually most severe in the antrum [19,23,41,90,94,95,96]. In the presence of food, gastric injuries tend to be less severe and involve the lesser curve and pylorus [43]. In animal experiments, regurgitation occurs following gastric administration of strong corrosives, resulting in repeated reexposure of the esophagus and pharynx for several minutes [97]. In a clinical setting, vomiting is associated with a higher incidence of severe esophageal injuries [89]. Duodenal and more distal injuries are uncommon, even in the setting of severe gastric burns, probably due to pylorospasm [92].

Ingestion of an alkali is associated with a significantly higher incidence and severity of esophageal lesions than ingestion of an acid, which typically injuries the stomach [23,24,25,29,43,89]. There are, however, many exceptions to this generalization [19,21,23,41,89,92,98]. Experimentally, strong acids are at least as potent as strong alkali [27]. Alkaline agents have little taste, but acids are extremely bitter and more likely to be expelled if accidentally ingested [8]. The intentional (i.e., suicidal) ingestion of corrosives is significantly more likely to cause serious esophageal burns than is accidental ingestion [20,28].

Alkaline solids may adhere to mucosa of the oropharynx and cause oral pain that limits the quantity swallowed, thus sparing the esophagus [31,39,99]. If alkaline solids are swallowed, the stomach is uncommonly involved but severe upper esophageal burns are seen [39,100]. Shallow ulcers may result from ingestion of medications when tablets become lodged in the esophagus, usually at the level of the aortic arch or an enlarged left atrium [101,102,103]. In most cases, the injury is self-limiting and produces only transient retrosternal pain. However, hemorrhage and stricture formation may occur following esophageal impaction of potassium chloride, iron, quinidine, and antiinflammatory agents [96,103,104]. Ingestion of alkaline denture cleaning tablets and acidic Clinitest tablets is associated with a high incidence of esophageal perforation and stricture formation [24,29,94,105,106,107].

Common symptoms from corrosive ingestion are oropharyngeal pain, dysphagia, abdominal pain, vomiting, and drooling [28]. Less commonly, stridor, hoarseness, hematemesis, and melena are seen [28]. Patients who are asymptomatic on presentation are unlikely to have significant injuries, although this may be difficult to assess in children [28,29,30,32,89,108]. Vomiting, drooling, and stridor appear to be predictive of more severe injuries [28,29,31,89,108].

Mucosal burns are usually covered with a white to yellow membrane. Deeper burns are painful, appear gray or black, and bleed easily [39]. The absence of burns in the oropharynx does not exclude burns further along the gastrointestinal tract, nor is it predictive of less severe distal injuries [21,28,29,30,32,41,89,90,108,109]. Patients with laryngeal burns have a greater incidence and severity of esophageal lesions [89,110].

Massive hemorrhage, perforation, and fistula formation may occur in patients with full-thickness esophageal necrosis [90]. Signs of perforation and resultant mediastinitis include chest pain, respiratory distress, fever, subcutaneous emphysema of the chest or neck, pleural rub, and Hamman's sign. Chest radiograph findings include mediastinal widening, pleural effusion (usually left-sided), pneumomediastinum, and pneumothorax [111]. Peritonitis due to perforation of the abdominal esophagus, stomach, or small bowel may result in fever, abdominal tenderness, guarding and rebound, and ileus. Untreated, perforations may rapidly progress to septic shock, organ failure, and death. Some gastric perforations may become walled off by omentum to form an abscess around the liver or in the lesser sac. Rarely, perforation of the stomach may result from excessive CO_2 gas formation when ingested sodium bicarbonate reacts with stomach acid [112,113].

Extensions of severe gastric burns to the transverse colon, pancreas, spleen, small bowel, liver, and kidneys are occasionally seen [21,24,39,114]. Such injuries often produce massive fluid shifts manifest by abdominal distention and signs of hypovolemia. Perforation of the anterior esophageal wall may lead to formation of a tracheoesophageal fistula and extensive tracheobronchial necrosis [114–122]. This complication is usually fatal unless recognized early and surgically repaired. Tracheoesophageal aortic fistula, a rare and uniformly fatal complication, is suggested by hemoptysis and hematemesis in a patient with a tracheoesophageal fistula [117,118,122].

Burns to the larynx occur in up to 50 percent of patients and are the most common cause of respiratory distress [89,91,123,124]. Typically the epiglottis and aryepiglottic folds are edematous, ulcerated, or necrotic. The absence of respiratory symptoms on presentation does not exclude the presence of laryngeal burns that may eventually require intubation [89]. Respiratory distress may also be due to tracheitis and pneumonitis secondary to the aspiration of corrosives during their ingestion or emesis.

Esophageal strictures develop in up to 70 percent of acid and alkali ingestions that result in deep ulceration, whether discrete or circumferential, and most patients with areas of necrosis [21,90]. Strictures do not develop following superficial mucosal ulceration (i.e., those not penetrating through the muscularis mucosa layer) [24,41,92,110,125–128]. Strictures may become symptomatic as early as the end of the second week; half develop during initial hospitalization and 80 percent are evident within 2 months [31,91]. Those that develop early often rapidly progress to complete obstruction and require urgent intervention [31]. Gastric outlet strictures may also occur, but only 40 percent become symptomatic [21,23,41,90,91,129–132]. Strictures may also develop in the mouth and pharynx [133,134].

Esophageal pseudodiverticulum may occur in patients with esophageal stricture as early as 1 week following corrosive ingestions [135,136]. They appear to result from incomplete destruction of the esophageal wall and usually resolve with dilation of associated strictures [135]. Esophageal mucocele appears to be a similar phenomenon but is reported as a late complication in patients who have undergone total gastrectomy and colon interposition, occurring 1 to 5 years after surgery [137]. Surgical excision may be required if they enlarge and compress adjacent structures, such as the trachea. Esophageal carcinoma, usually squamous cell, is a well-documented complication of alkali, but not acid, burns [138,139]. It occurs most commonly at the level of the tracheal bifurcation and is estimated to be 1000 times more frequent in patients who have had corrosive injuries than in the general population [139]. Symptoms develop 22 to 81 years after the initial insult [138,139].

The prognosis for superficial esophageal burns is excellent, as they heal without complications [24,110,125–128]. All deaths occur in patients with extensive necrosis in the upper gastrointestinal tract [90]. Sepsis secondary to perforation is the most common cause of death; severe hemorrhage or aspiration may also contribute [5]. In one series, 5 of 20 patients who underwent total gastrectomy and terminal esophagostomy for repair of extensive necrosis or perforation ultimately died [95].

SYSTEMIC EFFECTS. Systemic toxicity has been reported following skin or gastrointestinal burns caused by acetic acid, arsenic and other heavy metals, cyanide, formic acid, fluoride, hydrazine, hydrochloric acid, nitrates, sulfuric acid, and phosphoric acid [16,44,49,52,54,55,56,58–62,140]. Severe acid burns may be accompanied by metabolic acidosis and hypotension; if uncorrected they may lead to myocardial ischemia, liver ischemia, and renal failure [54]. It is unclear whether metabolic acidosis is secondary to the absorption of an acid or results from extensive tissue necrosis. The anion gap is usually elevated, although a hyperchloremic acidosis may be seen in hydrochloric acid ingestion. Hyperphosphatemia and hypocalcemia have occurred with phosphoric acid ingestion [56]. Cardiovascular collapse is the most common cause of early death, following hydrochloric acid ingestion [54]. Other findings associated with severe acid injuries include hemolysis, hemoglobinuria, nephrotoxicity, and pulmonary edema [49,53,54,58,60,140].

Coma, bradycardia, hypotension, acidosis, pulmonary edema, liver dysfunction, and coagulopathy have been reported following ingestion and inhalation of ammonia [141, 142,143]. Following absorption ammonia is rapidly taken up by the liver, where it enters the urea cycle [79,80,141,144]. Systemic toxicity occurs when the rate of hepatic clearance is exceeded. Acute hemolysis, hyperkalemia, hypoxia, and cardiorespiratory arrest have occurred following the use of dialysis equipment and syringes sterilized with bleach [145,146]. Hydrazine can be absorbed through the skin, lungs, and gastrointestinal tract. Systemic toxicity is due to the inhibition of enzymes involved in intermediary metabolism and may be delayed up to 14 hours following initial exposure [147,148]. Hypotension, ataxia, coma, hypo- or hyperglycemia, hepatitis, renal tubular necrosis, hemolysis, and possibly methemoglobinemia may occur in severe cases of hydrazine poisoning [61,62,147,148].

Hydrocarbons, particularly toluene and xylene, can be absorbed through the skin on prolonged contact, but inhalation of vapors is usually the primary route of absorption [46]. Central nervous system depression is the main effect; pulmonary edema, cardiac arrhythmias, renal tubular acidosis, hypokalemia, and liver dysfunction may also be seen [46]. Systemic effects of phenol and related compounds may include hemolysis and renal failure [44,78,149]. Less commonly coma, convulsions, pulmonary edema, methemoglobinemia, and myocardial and respiratory depression are seen [44,149].

Evaluation

Decontamination and, if necessary, resuscitation should take priority over completing a detailed history and physical examination. Medical staff should wear protective clothing to avoid becoming secondary casualties. The duration of exposure, time of onset and nature of any symptoms, and details of prehospital decontamination treatments should be noted.

Identification of the compound(s) involved and any measures required for their safe handling can be established by a number of means: container labeling; Material Safety Data Sheets (MSDSs) and safety officers in cases of workplace exposure; Fire Department Hazardous Materials (Hazmat) Units; and regional poison information centers. Measuring the pH of any available chemical is always prudent.

If the exposure is the result of an industrial or transportation accident, the patient should be evaluated for traumatic injuries. Suicidal patients should be evaluated for other possible toxic exposures (e.g., ingestion of alcohol or medications). Pulmonary exposures should be evaluated as outlined in Chapter 71.

EYE EXPOSURE. The persistence of eye pain despite irrigation for at least 15 minutes indicates significant injury or incomplete decontamination. If pain is present, further irrigation takes priority over completing a detailed examination. Failure to irrigate the eye adequately or remove particles following chemical exposure is associated with chronic complications [71]. Up to one-third of patients with lime burns still have particles present in the eye on presentation [71]. Following treatment, assessment should include measurement of visual acuity and conjunctival pH and a slit lamp examination. Chemosis, conjunctival hemorrhages, corneal epithelial defects, stromal opacification, and loss of limbic vessels should be noted [64]. If injury to the anterior chamber is suspected, intraocular pressure should be measured.

DERMAL EXPOSURE. The assessment of any burn or area of discomfort is similar to that for thermal burns. Location, size, color, texture, and neurovascular status should be noted. If the affected area is greater than 15 percent of total body surface area or if systemic toxicity is possible, a complete physical examination with appropriate monitoring and laboratory testing should be performed.

INGESTION. The ability to swallow secretions and findings on examination of the oropharynx, neck, chest, and abdomen should be noted. Particular attention should be given to assessing the patency of the airway. Patients with signs and symptoms suggestive of esophageal or more distal injuries should have an ECG, arterial blood gas analysis, complete blood count, type and cross-match, coagulation profile, and biochemistry testing, including electrolytes, glucose, and liver and renal function. Radiologic studies should include a chest radiograph and an upright abdominal film to seek evidence of pneumonitis and free air. Upper gastrointestinal endoscopy should be performed in symptomatic patients. The absence of symptoms or signs does not preclude the presence of gastrointestinal burns in patients with accidental ingestions but, when present, are always of a minor nature, do not require treatment, and do not lead to complications [28,29,89,150]. However, endoscopy should be considered for patients who have intentionally ingested strong acids or bases, even if there are no symptoms or physical findings. The optimal timing of endoscopy appears to be 6 to 24 hours following exposure. Because injuries may progress over several hours, endoscopy performed earlier may not detect the full extent of injury and therefore may need to be repeated [16]. If performed later, the risk of perforation may be increased [90].

Contrast esophagography is less sensitive than endoscopy in visualizing mucosal lesions [22,133]. It has a role in the detection of perforation if this is suspected [31]. A water-soluble contrast agent should be used. Cine-esophagography can detect esophageal motility disorders, the pattern of which may predict the likelihood of stricture formation. Strictures can be expected to develop in all patients with an atonic dilated or atonic rigid esophagus and in some patients with abnormal uncoordinated contractions [151].

Due to concerns of producing a perforation, it has been suggested that endoscopy should not proceed beyond the first circumferential or full-thickness lesion [19,29,39,152]. However, iatrogenic perforation has been reported only with the use of rigid endoscopes, and not examining beyond the first significant lesion will result in failure to detect more distal lesions of the stomach or duodenum [23,127,153,154,155]. Careful use of a small-diameter (e.g., pediatric) flexible endoscope to assess the entire upper gastrointestinal tract is safe [83,90,123,156–159]. It is usually well tolerated, without the need for general anesthesia [19]. The endoscope should be advanced across the cricopharynx under direct vision to assess for the presence of laryngeal burns [90]. If laryngeal edema or ulceration is noted, the airway should be intubated before continuing with endoscopy. Examination should be done gently with minimal air insufflation, avoiding retroversion or retroflexion, and the procedure terminated if the endoscope cannot be easily passed through a narrowed area [90]. Attempts to dilate the esophagus on initial endoscopy carries a high risk of perforation and should be avoided [19,160]. Endoscopy should also be avoided during the subacute phase (5–15 days after ingestion), when the tensile strength of tissues is lowest [90].

A number of different systems for grading gastrointestinal burns have been proposed [19,24,41,90,161]. Some parallel grading systems used for thermal skin burns; others differentiate several levels of ulceration and necrosis (Table 139-4). The important findings are depth of ulceration and presence of necrosis. Injuries that consist of only mucosal inflammation or superficial ulceration, not penetrating through muscularis mucosa, are not at risk for stricture formation [64,90]. Deep ulceration, whether transmural or not, and discrete areas of necrosis can sometimes lead to stricture formation. Patients with full-thickness circumferential burns and extensive necrosis are at high risk for perforation and stricture formation.

SYSTEMIC TOXICITY. Evaluation of patients with symptoms and signs of systemic toxicity should include routine monitoring and ancillary testing. The extent and type of testing should be dictated by the nature and severity of clinical abnormalities, present or anticipated. Patients with significant exposure to some phenols (e.g., nitrophenol and pentachlorophenol) and to hydrazine should have methemoglobin level determination. Quantitative serum and urine heavy metal concentrations may be indicated.

Management

Advanced life support measures should be instituted as appropriate. Standard trauma and cardiac life support protocols should be followed. Decontamination is the next priority; procedures are specific to the route of exposure. Treatment of systemic poisoning is primarily supportive; in some cases antidotal therapy may also be necessary.

EYE EXPOSURE. Irrigation is the mainstay of first aid treatment and should be performed immediately. The procedure is described in Chapter 128. All cases where lesions are detected or eye symptoms persist after irrigation should be referred to an ophthalmologist. Management may consist of topical antibiotics, mydriatics, steroids, and eye patching. Hydrophilic contact lenses and drugs to lower intraocular pressure may also be used. The role of neutralization of chemical burns is currently under investigation. Ascorbic acid had been used to treat alkali burns, but its effectiveness has not been well studied and it cannot be recommended [64,162]. Most eye injuries can be managed on an outpatient basis.

DERMAL EXPOSURE. The initial treatment of known or suspected chemical burns is prompt and prolonged irrigation with copious amounts of water for at least 15 minutes for acid exposures and 30 minutes for alkaline exposures (see Chap. 179). Longer irrigation is recommended for alkalis, because they have detergent properties and require larger volumes of water to wash off the skin [75]. Failure to institute early first aid is associated with a greater incidence of full-thickness burns [3]. In experimental studies, tissue neutralization occurs in 10 minutes with acids and up to 1 hour with alkalis; therefore, even delayed irrigation may be beneficial [163]. Clothes act as a reservoir, and failure to remove them may result in full-thickness burns developing from even mildly corrosive chemicals [3,73,74,75]. Neutralization has been used, but data on the efficacy of such treatment are lacking and it cannot be recommended [164].

Water irrigation may sometimes be dangerous or ineffective. Since metallic lithium, sodium, potassium and cesium, titanium tetrachloride, and organic salts of lithium and aluminum react violently with water, burns caused by these agents should be inspected closely and any particles removed and placed in an anhydrous solution (oil) before the area is irrigated [3,4,165]. Alternatively, the area can be wiped with a dry cloth to remove particles and the skin then deluged with water to dissipate any heat [5]. Phenol is not water-soluble and dilution with water may aid its penetration into tissues, increasing systemic absorption [44,76]. Soaking the burn with isopropyl alcohol or polyethylene glycol in mineral oil is superior to rinsing with water to decrease the severity of experimental phenol burns [166]. This treatment does not necessarily decrease the systemic absorption of phenol [167]. In addition, application of isopropyl alcohol or polyethylene glycol to large burns may result in absorption of these agents [166]. Their use should therefore be followed by liberal washing with water. Ready-mixed concrete can be easily removed from skin by irrigating with 50 percent dextrose [168].

Application of a copper sulfate solution has been suggested to assist in identification and neutralization of white phosphorus particles on the skin, but systemic absorption of copper sulfate can result in massive hemolysis with acute renal failure and death [44,76,169,170,171]. The use of a Wood's lamp to detect embedded phosphorus particles, which fluoresce under ultra-

Table 139-4. Examples of Classifications for Grading Severity of Gastrointestinal Corrosive Injury

Grade I		Mucosal inflammation
Grade II	A	Hemorrhages, erosions and superficial ulceration
	B	Deep discrete or circumferential ulceration
Grade III	A	Small scattered areas of necrosis
	B	Extensive necrosis involving the whole esophagus
First degree:		Mucosal inflammation, edema or superficial sloughing
Second degree:		Damage extends to all layers of, but not through, the esophagus
Third degree:		Ulceration through to periesophageal tissues

violet light, is safer [44]. Such burns should be kept wet (e.g., with a saline-soaked gauze), as phosphorous will ignite in dry air.

As sulfur mustard is poorly water-soluble, a mild detergent should be used for its removal. Military decontamination kits contain chloramine wipes, which inactivate sulfur mustard [86]. British antilewisite, or Dimercaprol, is an effective chelator of lewisite and can be applied topically to the skin or eye [85].

Patients with second- or third-degree burns should be referred to a plastic or general surgeon for evaluation and treatment. Definitive management is the same as for thermal burns, although more aggressive use of early debridement and grafting is suggested [81]. Application of hydrocortisone cream is suggested to increase healing and reduce the complications of phenol burns, but it has not been studied in the treatment of other chemical burns [172].

INGESTION. Despite the rapidity of tissue injury, decontamination should be considered [26,27,47,173]. Rinsing with water or saline is recommended for oral exposures. Emesis is contraindicated, due to the risk of aspiration and its association with an increased severity of esophageal and laryngeal burns [89]. Dilution by drinking up to 250 ml (120 ml for a child) of water, milk, or a noncarbonated beverage is recommended for particulate ingestion, as the corrosive may adhere to the esophageal wall [174]. Although this procedure exposes the stomach to the corrosive agent, it will be diluted. The stomach, which has a thicker wall than the esophagus, may be less susceptible to full-thickness injury [31]. The role of dilution for liquid ingestion is less clear but it is usually recommended [174]. It may, however, promote emesis and reexpose the esophagus to corrosives, result in an exothermic reaction with some acids, and not be effective in limiting tissue damage unless undertaken within minutes of injury [26,27,39,43,175–178].

There is no consensus regarding the role of placing a nasogastric tube for gastric aspiration, dilution, or lavage [43, 152,179–183]. Esophageal perforation is a potential complication, but a review of more than 4200 reports of patients with corrosive ingestion revealed no perforations related to this procedure [83,152]. Placement of a gastric tube with fluoroscopic or endoscopic guidance has been suggested, but the blind, gentle introduction of a small-bore tube in a cooperative patient appears safe [19,31]. If inserted, the tube should be firmly taped in place to avoid motion. Gastric contents should be aspirated. Dilution or lavage with small aliquots (120–250 ml) of water can then be performed. There is insufficient evidence available to recommend neutralizing an ingested base with an acid solution, or vice versa [26,27,43,47,173,178]. Activated charcoal does not absorb significant amounts of inorganic acid and alkali, and because it interferes with endoscopic evaluation its administration is inadvisable [184]. It may, however, be indicated in patients who have ingested agents that have systemic effects. Patients should otherwise be given nothing by mouth until decisions regarding the need for endoscopy or other procedures are made.

The use of corticosteroids to reduce the incidence and severity of strictures is based on studies showing a decrease in collagen deposition and stricture formation in animals pretreated with steroids [38,40,160,185,186,187]. However, the applicability of this model to clinical circumstances is open to question. First-degree esophageal burns do not require the use of steroids, as strictures do not develop in this group [24,110,125–128]. The use of steroids in more severe burns is controversial. Most human studies have been retrospective and poorly controlled, with differing conclusions regarding the effect of steroids on stricture formation [20,110,125,127,128,

133,179,188–199]. Strictures that occur despite steroid therapy may be easier to dilate and have a lower requirement for surgery [197]. However, steroids may only delay the onset of stricture formation, which can occur within 2 to 3 weeks of ceasing therapy, even if given longer than 2 months [38,110]. Steroids may not influence the development of esophageal strictures following extensive deep ulceration or necrosis [125, 126,127,200]. In a meta-analysis of 10 retrospective and 3 prospective studies of 253 patients with second- or third-degree burns, a lower incidence of stricture formation was found in patients treated with steroids [57]. In contrast, a review of 14 studies and 2000 patients found no difference in the rate of stricture formation [200]. Controlled studies of steroid use in patients with second- or third-degree burns also came to differing conclusions [125,126]. A decrease in stricture formation was suggested in 9 adults treated with methylprednisolone but not in 25 children treated with prednisolone [125,126]. Both studies have been criticized for their methodology [201–204]. Although gastric ulcers are a side effect of steroid therapy, severe hemorrhage is uncommon and is associated with degree of injury rather than steroid use [20,125]. In a controlled prospective study steroid treatment had no effect on incidence of death, gastrointestinal hemorrhage, or esophageal perforation [126].

If steroids are administered, the recommended doses are 0.1 mg/kg/day of dexamethasone or 2 mg/kg/day of prednisolone or methylprednisolone for 3 weeks and then tapered [197,205,206]. To approximate experimental conditions showing a beneficial effect, the initial dose of steroids should be given on presentation. Active bleeding and perforation are contraindications to steroid use.

The rationale for routine antibiotic administration is based on their prophylactic use in patients receiving steroids and the high incidence of infection seen in animal studies [31,40,185]. Their use in a clinical setting has not been studied in a controlled manner, and opinions differ as to their value [39,133, 179,182,199]. Controlled animal experiments have shown a combination of steroids and antibiotic to give the best outcome [40,185]. Use of a broad-spectrum antibiotic, such as a first- or second-generation cephalosporin, should be considered, particularly if a patient is treated with steroids.

If initiated, the decision to continue or cease steroid and antibiotic therapy should be based on endoscopic findings. Patients with no visible injury or injuries limited to mucosal inflammation or small areas of superficial ulceration require supportive therapy only. Symptomatic relief can be provided with antacids, sucralfate, H2-blockers, or analgesics. As early endoscopy may not accurately grade mucosal burns, patients with persistent symptoms or inconclusive findings should be admitted for observation [25]. If symptoms persist, repeat endoscopy should be performed; otherwise patients may be discharged or referred for psychiatric care, providing they can tolerate fluids given orally. Patients should be able to swallow their own secretions before commencing oral fluids.

Patients with deep discrete ulceration, circumferential or extensive superficial ulceration, or small isolated areas of necrosis should remain in the hospital. All patients with these types of injuries are at risk of stricture formation and should be considered for steroids and prophylactic antibiotics. They should be given nothing by mouth and receive intravenous fluids. Symptomatic treatment should be provided, but no medications should be given orally. Patients with deep transmural ulceration or necrosis are at risk of perforation as well as stricture formation. The role of steroids in this group is less clear and possibly hazardous. Antibiotics should be given along with other supportive measures. Hyperalimentation, either parenteral or by jejunostomy feeding tube, should also be considered.

Surgical exploration is indicated if perforation or penetration is suspected clinically (e.g., by fever, progressive abdominal or chest pain, hypotension, or signs of peritonitis) or proved by endoscopic or radiographic findings [31]. Laparotomy and early excision have been suggested for patients with extensive full-thickness necrosis, but an advantage of this approach over more conservative treatment is not clear [23,156,207].

Placement of specialized nasogastric tubes, or stents, has lowered the rate of stricture formation in uncontrolled clinical trials and is superior to steroids in preventing strictures in animal experiments [16,24,208–212]. Oral sucralfate and H_2 blockers have no proved benefit in increasing tissue healing or reducing complications [213]. Lathyrogens, compounds such as beta-aminopropionitrile, D-penicillamine, and N-acetylcysteine, which interfere with the formation of covalent cross-links during collagen synthesis, have lessened the rate of stricture formation in animal experiments but have not been studied in humans [206,214–220].

Stricture formation is usually treated with bougienage beginning 3 to 4 weeks after ingestion. Surgical resection or colonic interposition may be required if attempts at dilation are unsuccessful. Early or prophylactic bougienage is of unclear benefit and has been associated with an increased risk of perforation [31].

SYSTEMIC TOXICITY. Supportive management is the mainstay of treatment for systemic toxicity. Heavy metal, cyanide, and hydrogen sulfide poisoning may require antidotal therapy (see Chaps. 145 and 157). Neurologic toxicity due to hydrazine may respond to intravenous pyridoxine, administered at an initial dose of 25 mg per kilogram repeated in several hours, if necessary [61,62] (see Chap. 146). Methemoglobinemia may require treatment with methylene blue (see Chap. 157). Hemodialysis may enhance the elimination of heavy metals and dichromate, particularly if renal failure develops [221].

References

1. Friedman EM: Caustic ingestions and foreign bodies in the aerodigestive tract of children. *Pediatr Clin North Am* 36:1403, 1989.
2. Siegers CP, Sullivan JB: Organometals and reactive metals, in Sullivan JB, Krieger GR (eds): *Hazardous Materials Toxicology: Clinical Principles of Enviromental Health*. Baltimore, Williams & Wilkins, 1992, pp 928–936.
3. Leonard LG, Scheulen JJ, Munster AM: Chemical burns: Effect of prompt first aid. *J Trauma* 22:420, 1982.
4. Herbert K, Lawrence JC: Chemical burns. *Burns* 15:381, 1989.
5. Chitkara DK, McNeela BJ: Titanium tetrachloride burns to the eye. *Br J Ophthalmol* 76:380, 1992.
6. Stair T: Chlorine, in Haddad LM, Winchester JF (eds): *Clinical Management of Poisoning and Drug Overdose*. 2nd ed. Philadelphia, WB Saunders, 1990, pp 1186–1220.
7. Wood BR, Colombo JL, Benson BE: Chlorine inhalation toxicity from vapours generated by swimming pool chlorinator tablets. *Pediatrics* 79:427, 1987.
8. Rothstein FC: Caustic injuries to the esophagus in children. *Pediatr Clin North Am* 33:665, 1986.
9. Reisz GR, Gammon RS: Toxic pneumonitis from mixing household cleaners. *Chest* 89:49, 1986.
10. Pinkus JL: Monochloramine hazard from a mixture of household cleaning solutions. *N Engl J Med* 272:1133, 1965.
11. Dooms-Gloossens A, Gevers D, Mertens A, et al: Allergic contact dermatitis due to chloramine. *Contact Dermatitis* 9:319, 1983.
12. Gapany-Gapanavicus M, Molho M, Tirosh ML: Chloramine induced pneumonitis from mixing household cleaning agents. *Br Med J* 285:1086, 1982.
13. Gapany-Gapanavicus M, Yellin A, Almog S, et al: Pneumomediastinum: A complication of chlorine exposure from mixing household cleaning agents. *JAMA* 248:349, 1982.
14. Philipp R, Shepherd C, Fawthrop F, et al: Domestic chlorine poisoning. *Lancet* 2:495, 1985.
15. Peters JW: Hydrogen sulfide poisoning in a hospital setting. *JAMA* 246:1588, 1981.
16. Wit J, Noack L, Gdanietz K, Vorpahl K: Experimental studies on caustic burns of the stomach by aggressive chemicals. *Prog Pediatr Surg* 25:68, 1990.
17. Litovitz TL, Holm KC, Clancy C, et al: 1992 annual report of the American Association of Poison Control Centers toxic exposure surveillance system. *Am J Emerg Med* 11:494, 1993.
18. Marchi AG, Messi G, Renier S: Epidemiology of children poisoning: Comparison between telephone inquiries and emergency room visits. *Vet Hum Toxicol* 34:402, 1992.
19. Sugawa C, Lucas CE: Caustic injury of the upper gastrointestinal tract in adults: A clinical and endoscopic study. *Surgery* 106:802, 1989.
20. Schild JA: Caustic ingestion in adult patients. *Laryngoscope* 95:1199, 1985.
21. Zargar SA, Kochhar R, Nagi B, et al: Ingestion of strong corrosive alkalis: Spectrum of injury to upper gastrointestinal tract and natural history. *Am J Gastroenterol* 87:337, 1992.
22. Mansson I: Diagnosis of acute corrosive lesions of the esophagus. *J Laryngol Otol* 92:499, 1978.
23. Marks IN, Bank S, Werbeloff L, et al: The natural history of corrosive gastritis: Report of five cases. *Am J Dig Dis* 8:509, 1963.
24. Estrera A, Taylor W, Mills LJ: Corrosive burns of the esophagus and stomach: A recommendation for an aggressive surgical approach. *Ann Thorac Surg* 41:276, 1986.
25. Allen RE, Thoshinsky MJ, Stallone RJ, et al: Corrosive injuries of the stomach. *Arch Surg* 100:409, 1970.
26. Leape LL, Ashcroft AW, Scarpelli DG, et al: Hazard to health: Liquid lye. *N Engl J Med* 284:578, 1971.
27. Ashcroft KW, Padula RT: The effect of dilute corrosives on the esophagus. *Pediatrics* 53:226, 1974.
28. Gorman RL, Khin-Maung-Gyi MT, Klein-Schwartz W, et al: Initial symptoms as predictors of esophageal injury in alkaline corrosive ingestions. *Am J Emerg Med* 10:189, 1992.
29. Crain EF, Gershel JC, Mezey AP: Caustic ingestions: Symptoms as predictors of esophageal injury. *Am J Dis Child* 138:863, 1984.
30. Previtera C, Giusti F, Guglielmi M: Predictive value of visible lesions (cheeks, lips, oropharynx) in suspected caustic ingestion: May endoscopy reasonably be omitted in completely negative pediatric patients? *Pediatr Emerg Care* 6:176, 1990.
31. Kikendall JW: Caustic ingestion injuries. *Gastroenterol Clin North Am* 20:847, 1991.
32. Kynaston JA, Patrick MK, Shepherd RW, et al: The hazards of automatic-dishwasher detergent. *Med J Aust* 151:5, 1989.
33. Klein J, Olsen KR, McKinney HE: Caustic injury from household ammonia. *Am J Emerg Med* 3:320, 1985.
34. Wason S, Stephan M, Breide C: Ingestion of aromatic ammonia "smelling salts" capsules (letter). *Am J Dis Child* 144:139, 1990.
35. Ernst RW, Leventhal M, Luna R, et al: Total esophagogastric replacement after ingestion of household ammonia. *N Engl J Med* 268:815, 1963.
36. Humberston CL, Dean BS, Krenzelok EP: Ingestion of 35% hydrogen peroxide. *J Toxicol Clin Toxicol* 28:95, 1990.
37. Lopez GP, Dean BS, Krenzelok EP: Oral exposure to ammonia inhalants: A report of 8 cases (abstract). *Vet Hum Toxicol* 30:350, 1988.
38. Johnson EE: A study of corrosive esophagitis. *Laryngoscope* 73:1651, 1963.
39. Kirsh MM, Ritter F: Caustic ingestion and subsequent damage to the oropharyngeal and digestive passages. *Ann Thorac Surg* 21:74, 1976.
40. Haller JR, Bachman K: The comparative effect of current therapy on caustic burns of the esophagus. *Pediatrics* 34:236, 1964.
41. Zargar SA, Kochhar R, Nagi B, et al: Ingestion of corrosive acids: Spectrum of injury to upper gastrointestinal tract and natural history. *Gastroenterology* 97:702, 1989.
42. Ritter FN, Newman MH, Newman DE: A clinical and experimental study of corrosive burns of the esophagus. *Ann Otol Rhinol Laryngol* 77:830, 1968.

43. Penner GE: Acid ingestion: toxicology and treatment. *Ann Emerg Med* 9:374, 1980.
44. Mozingo DW, Smith AA, McManus WF, et al: Chemical burns. *J Trauma* 28:642, 1988.
45. Papini RP: "Is all that's blistered burned?" A case of kerosene contact burns. *Burns* 17:415, 1991.
46. Matsumoto T, Koga M, Sata T, et al: The changes of gasoline compounds in blood in a case of gasoline intoxication. *J Toxicol Clin Toxicol* 30:653, 1992.
47. Fell SC, Denize A, Becker NH, et al: The effect of intraluminal splinting in the prevention of caustic stricture of the esophagus. *J Thorac Cardiovasc Surg* 52:675, 1966.
48. Vancura EM, Clinton JE, Ruiz E, et al: Toxicity of alkaline solutions. *Ann Emerg Med* 9:118, 1980.
49. Teixeira F, Morgan J, Kikeri D, et al: Hemolysis following 80% acetic acid ingestion. *Vet Hum Toxicol* 34:340, 1992
50. Hoffman RS, Howland MA, Kamerow HN, et al: Comparison of titratable acid/alkaline reserve and pH in potentially caustic household products. *J Toxicol Clin Toxicol* 27:241, 1989.
51. Okonek S, Bierbach H, Atzpodien W: Unexpected metabolic acidosis in severe lye poisoning. *Clin Toxicol* 18:225, 1981.
52. Linden CH, Berner JM, Kulig K, et al: Acid ingestion: toxicity following systemic absorption (abstract). *Vet Hum Toxicol* 25:282, 1983.
53. Husain MT, Hasanain J, Kumar P: Sulphuric acid burns: Report of a mass domestic accident. *Burns* 15:389, 1989.
54. Gosselin RE, Smith RP, Hodge HC (eds): *Clinical Toxicology of Commercial Products*. 5th ed. Baltimore, Williams & Wilkins, 1984.
55. Soni N, O'Rouke I, Pearson I: Ingestion of hydrochloric acid. *Med J Aust* 142:471, 1985.
56. Caraveti EM: Metabolic abnormalities associated with phosphoric acid ingestion. *Ann Emerg Med* 16:904, 1987.
57. Howell JM, Dalsey WC, Hartsell FW, et al: Steroids for the treatment of corrosive esophageal injury: A statistical analysis of past studies. *Am J Emerg Med* 10:421, 1992.
58. Greif F, Kaplan O: Acid ingestion: Another cause of disseminated intravascular coagulation. *Crit Care Med* 14:990. 1986.
59. Hazardous Substances Data Bank, National Library of Medicine, Bethesda.
60. Jefferys DB, Wiseman HM: Formic acid poisoning. *Postgrad Med* 56:761, 1980.
61. Keirklin JK, Watson M, Bondoc CC, et al: Treatment of hydrazine-induced coma with pyridoxine. *N Engl J Med* 249:938, 1976.
62. Harati Y, Naikan E: Hydrazine toxicity, pyridoxine therapy, and peripheral neuropathy. *Ann Intern Med* 104:727, 1986.
63. Terrill PJ, Gowar JP: Chromic acid burns: Beware, be aggressive, be watchful. *Br J Plast Surg* 43:699, 1990.
64. Beare JD: Eye injuries from assault with chemicals. *Br J Ophthalmol* 74:514, 1990.
65. Roper-Hall MJ: Thermal and chemical burns. *Trans Ophthalmol Soc UK* 85:631, 1965.
66. Shingleton BJ: Eye injuries. *N Engl J Med* 325:408, 1991.
67. Stern AL, Pamel GJ, Benedetto LG: Physical and chemical injuries of the eyes and eyelids. *Dermatol Clin* 10:785, 1992.
68. Smilkstein MJ: Ophthalmological principles, in Goldfrank LR, Fromenbaum NE, Lewin NA, et al (eds): *Goldfrank's Toxicologic Emergencies*. 4th ed. Norwalk, CT, Appleton and Lange, 1990, pp 219–225.
69. Highman VN: Early rise in intraocular pressure after ammonia burns. *Br Med J* 1:359, 1969.
70. Brent BD, Karcioglu ZA: Effect of topical corticosteroids on goblet-cell density in an alkali-burn model. *Ann Ophthalmol.* 23:221, 1991.
71. Rozenbaum D, Baruchin AM, Dafna Z: Chemical burns of the eye with special reference to alkali burns. *Burns* 17:136, 1991.
72. Lemp MA: Cornea and sclera. *Arch Ophthalmol* 92:158, 1974.
73. White A, Joseet M: Burns from iodine (letter). *Anaesthesia* 45:75, 1990.
74. Manoguerra AS: Full thickness skin burns secondary to an unusual exposure to diquat dibromide. *J Toxicol Clin Toxicol* 28:107, 1990.
75. Wilson GR, Davidson PM: Full thickness burns from ready-mixed cement. *Burns* 12:139, 1985.
76. Bentivegna PE, Deane LM: Chemical burns of the upper extremity. *Hand Clin* 6:253, 1990.
77. Lorette JL, Wilkinson JA: Alkaline chemical burn to the face requiring full-thickness skin grafting. *Ann Emerg Med* 17:739, 1988.
78. Schneider MS, Mani MM, Masters FW: Gasoline-induced contact burns. *J Burn Care Rehabil* 12:140, 1991.
79. National Institute for Occupational Safety and Health: *Occupational Exposure to Ammonia*. (criteria document for a recommended standard). DHEW 74-136. Washington, DC, Government Printing Office, 1974, pp 1–88.
80. International Programme on Chemical Safety: Ammonia, in *Enviromental Health Criteria*, 54. Geneva, World Health Organization, 1986, pp 1–210.
81. Sawhney CP, Kaushish R: Acid and alkali burns: Considerations in management. *Burns* 15:132, 1989.
82. Singer A, Sagi A, Ben Meir P, et al: Chemical burns: Our 10 year experience. *Burns* 18:250, 1992.
83. Linden CH: Inorganic acids and bases, in Sullivan JB, Krieger GR (eds): *Hazardous Materials Toxicology: Clinical Principles of Enviromental Health*. Baltimore, Williams & Wilkins, 1992, pp 762–774.
84. Newman-Taylor A, Morris AJ: Experience with mustard gas casualties (letter). *Lancet* 337:242, 1991.
85. Mellor S, Rice P, Cooper GJ: Vesicant burns. *Br J Plast Surg* 44:434, 1991.
86. Borak J, Sidell FR: Agents of chemical warfare: Sulfur mustard. *Ann Emerg Med* 21:303, 1992.
87. Ben-Hur N, Giladi A, Neuman Z, et al: Phosphorus burns: A pathophysiological study. *Br J Plast Surg* 22:238, 1972.
88. Bowen TE, Whelan TJ, Nelson TG: Sudden death after white phosphorus burns. *Ann Surg* 174:779, 1971.
89. Vergauwen P, Moulin D, Buts JP, et al: Caustic burns of the upper digestive and respiratory tracts. *Eur J Pediatr* 150:700, 1991.
90. Zargar SA, Kochhar R, Mehta S, et al: The role of fiberoptic endoscopy in the management of corrosive ingestion and modified endoscopic classification of burns. *Gastrointest Endosc* 37:165, 1991.
91. Sellars JA, Perry HD, McNamara TF, et al: Chemicals burns. *J Burn Care Rehabil* 7:404, 1986.
92. Dilawari JB, Singh S, Rao PN, et al: Corrosive acid ingestion in man: A clinical and endoscopic study. *Gut* 25:183, 1984.
93. Aitken RJ: The management of an ingested acid injury extending into the jejunum. *Burns* 12:132, 1985.
94. Warren JB, Griffen DJ, Olsen RC: Urine sugar tablet ingestion causing gastric and duodenal ulceration. *Arch Intern Med* 144:161, 1984.
95. Ribet ME: Esophagogastrectomy for acid injury (letter). *Ann Thorac Surg* 53:739, 1992.
96. Bott S, Prakash C, McCallum RW: Medication induced esophageal injury: Survey of the literature. *Am J Gastroenterol* 82:758, 1987.
97. Ritter FN, Gago O, Kirsh MM, et al: The rationale of emergency esophagogastrectomy in the treatment of liquid caustic burns of the esophagus and stomach. *Ann Otol Rhinol Laryngol* 80:513, 1971.
98. Lovejoy FH: Corrosive injury of the esophagus in children: Failure of corticosteroid treatment reemphasizes prevention (editorial). *N Engl J Med* 323:668, 1990.
99. Madarikan BA, Lari J: Ingestion of dishwasher detergent by children. *Br J Clin Pract* 44:35, 1990.
100. Einhorn A, Horton L, Altieri M, et al: Serious respiratory consequences of detergent ingestions in children. *Pediatrics* 84:472, 1989.
101. McCord GS, Clouse RE: Pill induced esophageal strictures: Clinical features and risk factors for development. *Am J Med* 88:512, 1990.
102. Perry PA, Dean BS, Krenzelok EP: Drug induced esophageal injury. *J Toxicol Clin Toxicol* 27:281, 1989.
103. Kikendall JW, Friedman AC, Oyewole MA: Pill-induced esophageal injury: Case reports and review of the medical literature. *Dig Dis Sci* 28:174, 1983.
104. Kikendall JW: Pill-induced esophageal injury. *Gastroenterol Clin North Am* 20:835, 1991.
105. Barclay GR, Finlayson ND: Severe esophageal injury caused by Steradent. *Postgrad Med J* 61:335, 1985.
106. Messersmith JK, Oglesby JE, Mahoney WD, et al: Gastric erosion from alkali ingestion. *Am J Surg* 119:740, 1970.

107. Lacouture PG, Gaudreault P, Lovejoy FH: Caustic burns by Clinitest tablets (abstract). *Vet Hum Toxicol* 25:282, 1983.

108. Gaudreault P, Parent M, Mcguigan MA, et al: Predictability of esophageal injury from symptoms and signs: A study of caustic ingestion in 378 children. *Pediatrics* 71:767, 1983.

109. Krenzelok EP, Clinton JE: Caustic esophageal and gastric erosion without evidence of oral burns following detergent ingestion. *J Am Coll Emerg Phys* 8:194, 1979.

110. Middlekamp JN, Ferguson TB, Roper CL, et al: The management and problems of caustic burns in children. *J Thorac Cardiovasc Surg* 57:341, 1969.

111. Leigh TF, Achord JL: Pharyngeal and esophageal perforations during instrumentation. *Am J Roentgenol Radiat Ther Nucl Med* 91:757, 1964.

112. Brismar B, Strandlberg A, Wiklund B: Stomach rupture following ingestion of sodium bicarbonate. *Acta Chir Scand* 530(suppl):97, 1986.

113. Mastrangelo MR, Moore EW: Spontaneous rupture of the stomach in a healthy adult man after sodium bicarbonate ingestion. *Ann Intern Med* 101:649, 1984.

114. Ray JR, Meyers W, Lawton BR: The natural history of liquid lye ingestion: Rationale for aggressive surgical approach. *Arch Surg* 109:436, 1974.

115. Sarfati E, Jacob L, Servant JM, et al: Tracheobronchial necrosis after caustic ingestion. *J Thorac Cardiovasc Surg* 103:412, 1992.

116. Rakic S, Gerzic Z: Esophagobronchial fistula associated with corrosive stricture of the esophagus. *Ann Thorac Surg* 53:142, 1992.

117. Singh AK, Kothawla LK, Karlson KE: Tracheoesophageal and aortoesophageal fistula complicating corrosive esophagitis. *Chest* 70:549, 1976.

118. McCabe RE, Scott JR, Knox G: Fistulization between the esophagus, aorta and trachea as a complication of acute corrosive esophagitis: Report of a case. *Am Surg* 35:450, 1969.

119. Burrington JD, Raffensperger JG: Surgical management of tracheoesophageal fistula complicating caustic ingestion. *Surgery* 84:329, 1978.

120. Shaw A, Garvey J, Miller B: Lye burn requiring total gastrectomy and colon substitution for esophagus and stomach in a two year old boy. *Surgery* 65:837, 1969.

121. Amoury RA, Harbovsky EE, Leonidis JC: Tracheoesophageal fistula after lye ingestion. *J Pediatr Surg* 10:273, 1975.

122. Rabinovitz M, Udekwu AO, Campbell WL, et al: Tracheoesophageal-aortic fistula complicating lye ingestion. *Am J Gastroenterol* 85:868, 1990.

123. Moulin D, Bertrand JM, Buts JP, et al: Upper airway lesions in children after accidental ingestion of caustic substances. *J Pediatr* 106:408, 1985.

124. Scott JC, Jones B, Eisele DW, et al: Caustic ingestion injuries of the upper aerodigestive tract. *Laryngoscope* 102:1, 1992.

125. Hawkins DB, Demeter MJ, Barness TE: Caustic ingestions: Controversies in management—A review of 214 cases. *Laryngoscope* 90:98, 1980.

126. Anderson KD, Rouse TM, Randolph JG: A controlled trial of corticosteroids in children with corrosive injury of the esophagus. *N Engl J Med* 323:637, 1990.

127. Webb WR, Koutras P, Eckker RR, et al: An evaluation of steroids and antibiotics in caustic burns of the esophagus. *Ann Thorac Surg* 9:95, 1970.

128. Cannon S, Chandler JR: Corrosive burns of the esophagus: Analysis of 100 patients. *Eye Ear Nose Throat Mon* 42:35, 1963.

129. Subbaro KS, Kakar AK, Chandrasekhar V, et al: Cicatrical gastric stenosis caused by corrosive ingestion. *Aust NZ J Surg* 58:143, 1988.

130. Broor SL, Kumar A, Chari ST, et al: Corrosive esophageal strictures following acid ingestion: Clinical profile and results of endoscopic dilatation. *J Gastroenterol Hepatol* 4:55, 1989.

131. Muhletaler CA, Gerlock AJ, de Soto L, et al: Acid corrosive esophagitis: Radiographic findings. *Am J Roentgenol* 134:1137, 1980.

132. Beg MH, Reyazuddin, Ansari MM: Corrosive pyloric obstruction without esophageal involvement in children: A report of two cases. *Ann Trop Pediatr* 10:223, 1990.

133. Borja AR, Ransdell HT, Thomas TV, et al: Lye injuries of the esophagus: Analysis of ninety cases of lye ingestion. *J Thorac Cardiovasc Surg* 57:533, 1969.

134. Rubin MM, Jui V, Cozzi GM: Treatment of caustic ingestion. *J Oral Maxillofac Surg* 47:286, 1989.

135. Kochhar R, Mehta SK, Nagi B, et al: Corrosive acid-induced esophageal intramural pseudodiverticulosis: A study of 14 patients. *J Clin Gastroenterol* 13:371, 1991.

136. Plavsic BM, Robinson AE: Intraluminal esophageal diverticulum caused by ingestion of acid. *Am J Roentgenol* 159:765, 1992.

137. Chambon JP, Robert Y, Remy J, et al: Esophageal mucocele complicating double exclusion of the esophagus after corrosive burns (French). *Ann Radiol* 33:270, 1990.

138. Appelqvist P, Salmo M: Lye corrosion carcinoma of the esophagus: A review of 63 cases. *Cancer* 45:2655, 1980.

139. Isolauri J, Markkula H: Lye ingestion and carcinoma of the esophagus. *Acta Chir Scand* 155:269, 1989.

140. Wang XW, Davies JWL, Sirvent RLZ, et al: Chromic acid burns and acute chromium poisonings. *Burns* 11:181, 1985.

141. Linden CH, Rumack BH, Galle SJ: Systemic toxicity following household ammonia ingestion (abstract). *Vet Hum Toxicol* 26(suppl 2):59, 1984.

142. Schmidt FC, Vallencourt DC: Changes in the blood following exposure to gaseous ammonia. *Science* 108:555, 1948.

143. Zitnik RS, Burchell HB, Shepherd JT: Hemodynamic effects of inhalation of ammonia in man. *Am J Cardiol* 24:187, 1969.

144. Eichler M: Psychological changes associated with induced hyperammonemia. *Science* 144:886, 1964.

145. Froner GA, Rutherford GW, Rokeach M: Injection of sodium hypochlorite by intravenous drug users (letter). *JAMA* 258:325, 1987.

146. Hoy RH: Accidental systemic exposure to sodium hypochlorite during hemodialysis. *Am J Hosp Pharm* 38:1512, 1981.

147. Comstock CC, Lawson LH, Green EA, et al: Inhalational toxicity of hydrazine vapour. *Arch Ind Hyg Occup Med* 10:476, 1954.

148. Reinhardt CF, Brittelli MR: Heterocyclic and miscellaneous nitrogen compounds, in Clayton GD, Clayton FE (eds): *Patty's Industrial Hygiene and Toxicology.* New York, Wiley, 1981, pp 2791–2800.

149. Lin CH, Yang JY: Chemical burn with cresol intoxication and multiple organ failure. *Burns* 18:162, 1992.

150. Muhlendahl KE, Oberdisse U, Krienke EG: Local injuries by accidental ingestions of corrosive substances by children. *Arch Toxicol* 39:299, 1978.

151. Kuhn JR, Tunell WP: Cine-esophagography in caustic burns of the esophagus. *Am J Surg* 146:804, 1983.

152. Graeber GM, Murray GF: Injuries of the esophagus. *Semin Thorac Cardiovasc Surg* 4:247, 1992.

153. Hollinger PH: Management of esophageal lesions caused by chemical burns. *Ann Otolaryngol Rhinol Laryngol* 77:819, 1968.

154. Thompson JN: Corrosive esophageal injuries. I. A study of nine cases of concurrent accidental caustic ingestion. *Laryngoscope* 97:1060, 1987.

155. Previtera C: Caustic ingestions (letter). *Pediatr Emerg Care* 7:126, 1991.

156. Chung RS, DenBestein L: Fibreoptic endoscopy in the treatment of corrosive injury of the stomach. *Arch Surg* 110:725, 1975.

157. Symbas PN, Vlasis SE, Hatcher CR: Esophagitis secondary to ingestion of caustic material. *Ann Thorac Surg* 36:73, 1983.

158. Sugawa C, Mullins RJ, Lucas CE, et al: The value of early endoscopy following caustic ingestion. *Surg Gynecol Obstet* 153:553, 1981.

159. Borjas JA, Quiros E: The value of emergency endoscopy in caustic esophagogastritis. *Am J Gastroenterol* 60:70, 1973.

160. Knox WG, Scott JR, Zintel HA, et al: Bouginage and steroids used singly or in combination in experimental corrosive esophagitis. *Ann Surg* 166:930, 1966.

161. DiConstanzo J, Noirelerc M, Jouglard J, et al: New therapeutic approach to corrosive burns of the upper gastrointestinal tract. *Gut* 21:370, 1980.

162. Haddox JL, Pfister RR, Yuille-Barr D: The efficacy of topical citrate after alkali injury is dependent on the period of time it is administered. *Invest Ophthalmol Vis Sci* 30:1062, 1989.

163. Gruber RP, Laub DR, Vistnes LM: The effect of hydrotherapy on the clinical course and pH of experimental cutaneous chemical burns. *Plast Reconstr Surg* 21:337, 1968.

164. Woodard D: Irrigation with acetic acid (letter). *Ann Emerg Med* 18:911, 1989.

165. Clare RA, Krenzelok: Chemical burns secondary to elemental metal exposure: Two case reports. *Am J Emerg Med* 6:355, 1988.

166. Hunter DM, Timerding BL, Leonard RB, et al: Effects of isopropyl alcohol, ethanol, and polyethylene glycol/industrial methylated spirits in the treatment of acute phenol burns. *Ann Emerg Med* 21:1303, 1992.

167. Pullin TG, Pinkerton NM, Johnston RV, et al: Decontamination of the skin of swine following phenol exposure: A comparison of the relative efficacy of water versus polyethylene glycol/industrial methylated spirits. *Toxicol Appl Pharmacol* 43:199, 1978.

168. Cuomo MD, Sobel RM: Concrete impaction of the external auditory canal. *Am J Emerg Med* 7:32, 1989.

169. Ben-Hur N, Giladi A, Applebaum J, et al: Phosphorus burns: The antidote—A new approach. *Br J Plast Surg* 22:245, 1972.

170. Goldman M, Karotkin RH: Acute potassium dichromate poisoning. *Am J Med Sci* 189:400, 1965.

171. Eldad A, Simon GA: The phosphorous burn: A preliminary comparative experimental study of various forms of treatment. *Burns* 17:198, 1991.

172. Altman MI, Suleskey C, Delisle R, et al: Silver sulfadiazine and hydrocortisone cream 1% in the management of phenol matricectomy. *J Am Podiatr Med Assoc* 80:545, 1990.

173. Krey H: On treatment of corrosive lesions of the esophagus: An experimental study. *Acta Otolaryngol* 102 (suppl):1, 1952.

174. Irritants/Caustics Specialty Board, in Rumack BH, Spoerke DG (eds): *POISINDEX Information System.* Denver, MICROMEDEX, 1988.

175. Homan CS, Maitra SR, Lane BP, et al: Effective treatment of acute alkaline injury of the esophagus with early saline dilution therapy. *Ann Emerg Med* 22:178, 1993.

176. Maull KI, Osmand AP, Maull CD: Liquid caustic ingestions: An in vitro study of the effects of buffer, neutralization, and dilution. *Ann Emerg Med* 14:1160, 1985.

177. Honcharuk L, Marcus S: Dilution in corrosive ingestions: Primum non nocere (abstract). *Vet Hum Toxicol* 31:338, 1989.

178. Rumack BH, Burrington JD: Caustic ingestions: A rational look at diluents. *Clin Toxicol* 11:27, 1977.

179. Bikhazi HB, Thompson ER, Shumrick DA: Caustic ingestion: Current status. *Arch Otolaryngol* 89:112, 1969.

180. Tucker JA, Yarington CT: The treatment of caustic ingestion. *Otolaryngol Clin North Am* 12:343, 1979.

181. Friedman EM, Lovejoy FH: The emergency management of caustic ingestions. *Emerg Med Clin North Am* 2:77, 1984.

182. Howell JM: Alkaline ingestions. *Ann Emerg Med* 15:820, 1986.

183. Wason S: Coping swiftly and effectively with caustic ingestion. *Emerg Med Rep* 10:25, 1989.

184. Decker WJ, Combs HF, Corby DG: Absorption of drugs and poisons by activated charcoal. *Toxicol Appl Pharmacol* 13:454, 1968.

185. Rosenberg N, Kunderman PJ, Vroman L, et al: Prevention of experimental lye strictures of the esophagus by cortisone, control of suppurative complications by penicillin. *Arch Surg* 63:147, 1951.

186. Weisskopf A: Effects of cortisone on experimental lye burn of the esophagus. *Ann Otol Rhinol Laryngol* 61:681, 1952.

187. McNeil RA, Wellborn RB: Prevention of corrosive stricture of the esophagus of the rat. *J Laryngol* 80:346, 1966.

188. Viscomi GJ, Beekhuis GJ, Whitten CF: An evaluation of early esophagoscopy and corticosteroid therapy in the management of corrosive injury of the esophagus. *J Pediatr* 59:356, 1961.

189. Cleveland WW, Thorton N, Chesney JG, et al: The effect of prednisolone in the prevention of esophageal stricture following the ingestion of lye. *South Med J* 51:861, 1958.

190. Feldman M, Iben AB, Hurley EJ: Corrosive injury to the oropharynx and esophagus: Eighty five consecutive cases. *Calif Med* 118:6, 1973.

191. Ferguson MK, Migliore M, Staszak VM, et al: Early evaluation and therapy for caustic esophageal injury. *Am J Surg* 157:116, 1989.

192. Middlekamp JN, Cone AJ, Ogura JH, et al: Endoscopic diagnosis and steroid and antibiotic therapy of acute lye burns of the esophagus. *Laryngoscope* 71:1354, 1961.

193. Cello JP, Fogel RP, Boland CR: Liquid caustic ingestion: Spectrum of injury. *Arch Intern Med* 140:501, 1980.

194. Ray ES, Morgan DL: Cortisone therapy of lye burns of the esophagus. *J Pediatr* 49:394, 1956.

195. Yarington CT, Bales GA, Frazer JP: A study of the management of caustic esophageal trauma. *Ann Otol* 72:1130, 1964.

196. Cardona JC, Daly JF: Current management of corrosive esophagitis: An evaluation of results in 239 cases. *Ann Otolaryngol* 80:521, 1971.

197. Haller JR, Andrews HG, White JJ, et al: Pathophysiology and management of acute corrosive burns of the esophagus: Results of treatment in 285 children. *J Pediatr Surg* 6:578, 1971.

198. Gundogdu HZ, Tanyel FC, Buyukpamukcu N, et al: Conservative treatment of caustic esophageal strictures in children. *J Pediatr Surg* 27:767, 1992.

199. Campbell GS, Burnett HF, Ransom JM, et al: Treatment of corrosive burns of the esophagus. *Arch Surg* 112:495, 1977.

200. Oakes DD, Sherck JP, Mark JB: Lye ingestion: Clinical patterns and therapeutic implications. *J Thorac Cardiovasc Surg* 83:194, 1982.

201. Hughes-Davies TH: Corticosteroids in children with corrosive injury of the esophagus (letter). *N Engl J Med* 324:418, 1991.

202. Anderson KD, Rouse TM, Randolph JG: Corticosteroids in children with corrosive injury of the esophagus (letter). *N Engl J Med* 324:419, 1991.

203. Wason S, Stephan M: Corticosteroids in children with corrosive injury of the esophagus (letter). *N Engl J Med* 324:418, 1991.

204. Temple RA: Corrosives-alkaline (management/treatment protocols), in Rumack BH, Spoerke DG (eds): *POISINDEX Information System.* Denver MICROMEDEX, Edition expires 2-28-94.

205. Marshall F: Caustic burns of the esophagus: Ten year results of aggressive care. *South Med J* 72:1236, 1979.

206. Saedi S, Nyhus LM, Gabrys BF, et al: Pharmacological prevention of esophageal stricture: An experimental study in the cat. *Am Surg* 39:465, 1973.

207. Meredith JW, Kon ND, Thomson JN: Management of injuries from liquid lye ingestion. *J Trauma* 28:1173, 1988.

208. Wijburg FA, Beukers MM, Heymans HS, et al: Nasogastric intubation as sole treatment of caustic esophageal lesions. *Ann Otol Rhinol Laryngol* 94:337, 1985.

209. Kirsh MM, Peterson A, Brown JW, et al: Treatment of caustic injuries of the esophagus: A ten year experience. *Ann Surg* 188:675, 1978.

210. Mills LJ, Estera AS, Platt MR: Avoidence of esophageal stricture following severe caustic burns by the use of an intraluminal stent. *Ann Thorac Surg* 28:60, 1979.

211. Reyes HM, Lin CY, Schlunk FF, et al: Experimental treatment of corrosive esophageal burns. *J Pediatr Surg* 9:317, 1974.

212. Wijburg FA, Heymans HSA, Urbanus NA: Caustic esophageal lesions in childhood: Prevention of stricture formation. *J Pediatr Surg* 24:171, 1989.

213. Reddy AN, Budrhaja M: Sucralfate therapy for lye-induced esophagitis. *Am J Gastroenterol* 85:868, 1990.

214. Cohen IK: Can collagen metabolism be controlled: Theoretical considerations. *J Trauma* 25:410, 1985.

215. Ehrenpreis ED, Leiken JB, Ehrenpreis S, et al: Use of sodium polyacrylate in rat gastrointestinal alkali burns. *Vet Hum Toxicol* 30:135, 1988.

216. Davis WM, Madden JW, Peacock EE: A new approach to the control of esophageal stenosis. *Ann Surg* 176:469, 1972.

217. Madden JW, Davis WM, Butler C, et al: Experimental esophageal lye burns: Correcting established strictures with beta-aminopropionitrile and bougienage. *Ann Surg* 179:277, 1973.

218. Barrow MV, Simpson CF: Caution against the use of iathyrogens. *Surgery* 71:309, 1972.

219. Kida K, Thurlbeck W: Lack of recovery of lung structure and function after the administraton of beta-amino-propionitrile in the postnatal period. *Am Rev Respir Dis* 122:465, 1980.

220. Liu AG, Richardson MA: Effects of N-acetylcysteine on experimentally induced esophageal injury. *Ann Otol Rhinol Laryngol* 94:477, 1985.

221. Kaufman DB, DiNicola W, McIntosh R: Acute potassium dichromate poisoning. *Am J Dis Child* 119:374, 1970.

140. Cyclic Antidepressant Poisoning

Cynthia K. Aaron

Cyclic antidepressants constitute a major component of reported drug overdoses requiring treatment in an intensive care setting [1]. These medications are freely available to patients who are at high risk for suicide or overdose. The consequences of overdose are severe and predominately affect the central nervous system (CNS) and cardiovascular system. Treatment of overdose is directed toward limiting drug absorption and managing complications of toxicity; there is no antidote for cyclic antidepressant toxicity.

History and Current Usage

Although iminodibenzyl was synthesized in the late nineteenth century, the pharmacology of iminodibenzyl derivatives was not detailed until the 1940s. These compounds were designed to have antihistaminic, sedative, analgesic, and antiparkinsonian properties. Imipramine, the first of the dibenzazepines, was synthesized as a phenothiazine derivative but was found to be ineffective as a neuroleptic agent. In the late 1950s, patients taking imipramine reported that the drug had mood elevating effects. Imipramine and later congeners have since been used in the treatment of endogenous depression. Other indications for cyclic antidepressants include therapy of enuresis in children (imipramine), treatment for migraine headaches (particularly the serotonergic active cyclic antidepressants), chronic pain control, and cocaine detoxification [2,3,4].

Available Forms

The classic cyclic antidepressants have a seven-membered central ring with a terminal nitrogen containing either three constituents (tertiary amines) or two constituents (secondary amines) [5]. Tertiary amines include amitriptyline, imipramine, doxepin, trimipramine, and chlorimipramine (clomipramine). Secondary amines include desipramine, protriptyline, and nortriptyline. Included with cyclic antidepressants are two dibenzoxazepine compounds that contain the central seven-membered ring with a heterocyclic constituent: loxapine and its demethylated metabolite amoxapine. Maprotiline, a dibenzobicyclooctadiene, is the only tetracyclic antidepressant available in the United States [6,7]. Mianserin, another tetracyclic antidepressant, is not available in the United States. Bicyclic compounds, such as viloxazine and zimeldine, are available only outside the United States. Trazodone and nefazadone are a triazolopyridine derivative structurally and pharmacologically different from the other cyclic antidepressants. Antidepressants recently released include bupropion, a unicyclic phenylaminoketone [8–16], and a large group of antidepressants called selective serotonergic reuptake inhibitors (SSRIs). Currently available SSRIs include fluoxetine, a straight chain phenylpropylamide; paroxetine, a phenylpiperidine derivative; sertraline, and venlafaxine. Other SSRIs under investigation include fluvoxamine, zimeldine, citalopram, tianeptine, and ritanserin [17–22]. Antidepressants not available in the United States because of side effects include mianserin (agranulocytosis), nomifensine

(hepatotoxicity and hemolytic anemia), lofepramine (hepatotoxicity and hyponatremia), and zimeldine (Guillain-Barré syndrome) [23–29]. All of the cyclic antidepressants are available for oral use. Imipramine and amitriptyline are available for intramuscular administration.

PHARMACOLOGY AND PHARMACOKINETICS

Classic Cyclic Antidepressants. The therapeutic effects of all of the cyclic antidepressants are relatively similar, but their pharmacology differs considerably. At therapeutic dosing, cyclic antidepressant effects depend on their relative affinity for different neurotransmitters. The cyclic antidepressants act as neurotransmitter postsynaptic receptor blockers for histamine, dopamine, acetylcholine, serotonin, and norepinephrine. They inhibit the reuptake of neurotransmitter biogenic amines and have quinidinelike membrane stabilizing effects (Tables 140-1 to 140-3) [2,5,6,7,17–29]. These agents may induce atrioventricular blocks [30–33] and have a direct negative cardiac inotropic effect, demonstrated by a decrease in the rate of change in left ventricular pressure and an increase in left ventricular end-diastolic pressure [21,34–38]. Central nervous system effects may be related to both neurotransmitter and direct membrane effects [37–41].

Table 140-1. Cyclic Antidepressant Effects on Neurotransmitters

Antidepressant	Effect
Receptor blockade	
Acetylcholine (antimuscarinic)	Sinus tachycardia, GI hypomotility, warm dry skin, urinary retention, mydriasis, lethargy, hallucinations, seizures, coma
Norepinephrine	Hypotension, reflex tachycardia, orthostasis, ?seizures
Histamine	"Antihistamine effects," sedation, hypotension
Serotonin	Hypotension, ejaculation disturbances
Dopamine	Endocrine disturbances (galactorrhea, impotence), dystonias
Biogenic amine reuptake blockade	
Dopamine	Hypotension, psychomotor retardation, antiparkinsonian effects
Norepinephrine	Transient hyperadrenergic state (tremor, tachycardia), adrenergic depletion (hypotension, antidepressant effects), ejaculation disturbances
Serotonin	Seizures, ejaculation disturbances, antidepressant effects

GI = gastrointestinal.
Data from references 2,5,7,17–29.

Table 140-2. Relative Potencies of Cyclic Antidepressants: Receptor Blockade

Compound	Anti-ACh	Anti-H$_1$	Alpha blockade	Anti-5-HT	Anti-DA
Tertiary amines					
Amitriptyline	+ + + +	+ + +	+ + + +	+ +	+
Imipramine	+ + +	+ +	+ +	+	+
Doxepin	+ + +	+ + + +	+ + + +	+ +	0
Secondary amines					
Nortriptyline	+ +	+ +	+ +	+	+
Protriptyline	+ + + +	+ +	+	+	±
Desipramine	+	+	+ +	0	0
Dibenzoxazepines					
Amoxapine	±	+ +	+ + +	0	+ +
Tetracyclics					
Maprotiline	±	+ + +	+ + +	+ +	+ +
Mianserin	0	+	+ +	+ +	+
Triazolopyridines					
Trazodone	0	+	+ + +	0	0
Bicyclics					
Viloxazine	+	+			
SSRIs					
Fluoxetine	±	±	±	+	0
Sertraline	0	0	0	0	0
Paroxetine	+ +		0	0	+
Others					
Bupropion	0	±	±		
Nomifensine	0	0	+	0	

ACh = acetylcholine (anticholinergic); H$_1$ = histamine$_1$ (antihistamine); 5-HT = serotonin (antiserotonergic); DA = dopaminergic (antidopaminergic).
Data from references 2,24,25,28,29,42,43,44,137.

Table 140-3. Relative Potencies of Cyclic Antidepressants: Biogenic Amine Pump Blockade

Substance	NE	5HT	DA	ACh
Tertiary amines				
Amitriptyline	+ +	+ + +	+	+ + +
Imipramine	+ +	+ + +	+	+ + +
Trimipramine	+	+	+	+ + + +
Doxepin	+ +	+ +	+	+ + +
Secondary amines				
Nortriptyline	+ + +	+ +	+ + +	+ + +
Desipramine	+ + + +	+ +	+	+ +
Clomipramine	+ +	+ + + +	+ + +	+ + +
Dibenzoxazepines				
Amoxapine	+ + +	+ +	+ + +	+ +
Tetracyclics				
Maprotiline	+ + +	+	+	±
Mianserin	+ +	+ + +	+	0
Triazolopyridines				
Trazodone	±	+ +	±	0
Bicyclics				
Viloxazine	+ +	0		0
SSRIs				
Fluoxetine	+	+ + +	+ + +	0
Sertraline	+	+ + + +	0	+
Paroxetine	0	+ + +	+	+
Others				
Bupropion	+	+	+ +	+
Nomifensine	+ + +	+ + +	+	

NE = norepinephrine; 5-HT = serotonin; DA = dopamine; NE selective = maprotiline, desipramine, protriptyline, doxepin, trimipramine, imipramine, amitriptyline; 5-HT selective = clomipramine, trazodone, fluoxetine, sertraline, paroxetine; DA selective = bupropion.
Data from references 24,25,26,28,42,43,44,137.

Selective Serotonergic Reuptake Inhibitors. Since the serotonergic system has gained prominence in the understanding of depression, agents are being developed that predominately affect serotonergic neurotransmission. Currently, there are at least nine identified 5-HT receptors. This class of antidepressants inhibits the reuptake of serotonin at the various receptor subtypes, whereas buspirone, a nonbenodiazepine sedative-hypnotic, is a 5-HT$_{1a}$ partial agonist [42]. 5-HT$_{1a}$ receptors are inhibitory on serotonin neuronal firing and have anxiolytic and antidepressant activity. Excessive stimulation can lead to hypotension. Antagonists at 5-HT$_{1c}$, such as ritanserin, may be anxiolytic. 5-HT$_{1d}$ receptor subtype stimulation leads to inhibition of neurotransmitter release. The agonist for the receptor is sumatriptan, an antimigraine medication. 5-HT$_2$ stimulation can cause vasoconstriction, and the antagonist ritanserin functions as an anxiolytic. 5-HT$_3$ antagonists have antiemetic and antipsychotic activity (ondansetron) [42–45]. Classic tricyclic antidepressants affect serotonin neurotransmission by enhancing the sensitivity of postsynaptic 5-HT$_{1a}$ postsynaptic receptors. The SSRIs alter the release of serotonin presynaptically, leading to an increase in the amount of serotonin available for neurotransmission without changing the sensitivity of the 5-HT$_{1a}$ postsynaptic receptors [44]. All tricyclic antidepressants increase the density of beta-adrenoreceptors. Some of the SSRIs, such as fluvoxamine, sertraline, and fluoxetine, function in a similar manner. Citalopram and paroxetine do not have this effect. In general, the SSRIs normalize the number and function of 5-HT$_{1a}$ and 5-HT$_2$ receptors [43,45].

Pharmacokinetics. Cyclic antidepressants are well absorbed orally in therapeutic dosing; peak serum levels occur 2 to 6 hours after ingestion [46]. In overdose, gastrointestinal (GI) absorption may be delayed secondary to the anticholinergic and antihistaminic properties of these drugs. Metabolism is predominately hepatic, with a small enterohepatic circulation [46–49]. Some cyclic antidepressants have active metabolites. The volume of distribution is large, with distribution occurring within the first several hours after ingestion [46,48,49]. Elimination half-life averages 8 to 30 hours but may be slightly prolonged in overdose [49,50,51]. Elimination is hepatic, with minimal renal involvement [50,52,53]. Cyclic antidepressants are extensively bound to serum proteins, particularly alpha$_1$ acid glycoprotein (AAG), and binding appears to be pH-dependent [54–57].

Toxicity

Toxicity from cyclic antidepressants results in abnormal mentation, seizures, hypotension, dysrhythmias, and conduction abnormalities [54–62]. Hyperthermia may occur as a result of increased muscle activity, seizures, and autonomic dysfunction [63]. These toxic effects are believed to have multiple causes, none of which have been fully elucidated.

Patients who ingest large amounts of cyclic antidepressants frequently present with hypotension. The etiology is unclear, but several mechanisms have been suggested, including direct negative inotropic effects [21,34,35,36] and dysrhythmias with subsequent decreases in filling time and cardiac output [63–66]. Receptor blockade produces vasodilation and autonomic dysfunction. In addition, blockade of the biogenic amine pump prevents adequate uptake and release of these neurotransmitters as active substances, thereby contributing to hypotension [18,25,28,31,58,59,64,64,67].

The CNS effects in cyclic antidepressant overdose can be quite profound. Although some of the newer cyclic antidepressants are less toxic in overdose, they can cause seizures and alteration in mental status [68,69,70]. The etiology of coma, seizures, and myoclonus is poorly understood; receptor blockade and direct membrane effects all may contribute to CNS derangements [2,3,5,6,29,40,41,68–77].

Dysrhythmias and conduction abnormalities often provide a clue to the recognition of cyclic antidepressant overdose. Action potential propagation, particularly in ventricular myocardial cells and the conduction system, is significantly affected by these drugs [78,79]. Cyclic antidepressants blunt phase 0 of the action potential depolarization by blocking the fast inward flux of sodium through the sodium channel [80]. This in turn slows the rate of rise of phase 0 ($\dot{V}_{max}$) and slows overall action potential depolarization. As ventricular conduction slows, the QRS complex widens [79–85]. This also contributes to unidirectional blocks and reentrant dysrhythmias [82,86]. Because inward sodium flux is coupled to the calcium excitation of myocardial cells, the myocardial cells are unable to contract fully and are less efficient [87]. A less toxic effect is seen on phase 4 of the action potential (spontaneous diastolic depolarization), leading to decreased automaticity [79,82,86,87,88]. Delayed repolarization occurs and may contribute to prolongation of the Q–T interval, with resultant *Torsades de pointes* [89–93]. Toxicity appears to be directly related to heart rate; in amitriptyline-poisoned dogs, increasing heart rate caused a decrease in $\dot{V}_{max}$ and widened the QRS complex [79–85, 94,95]. Interventions that slow the heart rate, such as beta-blockers, improved conduction but led to irreversible hypotension [82,85,92,95–97].

The decrease in $\dot{V}_{max}$ during phase 0 appears to be pH-sensitive [82,85,86,95]. Alkalinization with molar sodium lactate, sodium bicarbonate, or hyperventilation produces an increase in the rate of rise of the action potential ($\dot{V}_{max}$), narrows the QRS complex, decreases the incidence of ventricular tachycardia, and improves blood pressure [82,85,86,95–108]. Increasing the extracellular concentration of sodium in vitro has produced the same results. These studies also show that decreasing pH worsens conduction abnormalities, produces hypotension, and increases the incidence of dysrhythmias [82,85,86,95,96]. A combination of increased extracellular sodium and alkalosis (or hyperventilation plus sodium bicarbonate) in vitro has been shown to be equally and possibly more effective than either alone [82,95,96]. The use of lidocaine in animal studies decreased automaticity and ectopy and improved conduction. However, it did not have the same salutory effect on the blood pressure as alkalinization and may have worsened inotropy [95]. Finally, although binding of cyclic antidepressants to AAG is increased at an alkalotic pH, infusion of AAG in animals to increase serum protein binding has not been shown to be beneficial [54–57,109,110].

Presentation

The onset of symptoms from cyclic antidepressant overdose is rapid. Most patients who die from overdose do so before arriving at the hospital and after having ingested large (>1 gm) amounts of drug [59,77,110]. The majority of signs and symptoms usually occur within the first 6 hours after ingestion. Patients who survive the first 24 hours without hypoxic insult generally do well [110,111]. The progression of toxicity is rapid and unpredictable, with patients capable of deteriorating from an awake, alert state to seizures, hypotension, and dysrhythmias within 1 hour [59,77,110–121].

Vital signs on presentation may include tachycardia, although older patients taking beta-blockers or those with underlying conduction blocks may be bradycardic. Cyclic antidepressants without major anticholinergic effects, such as trazodone, may not cause significant tachycardia. Initial blood pressure may be mildly hypertensive but can rapidly change to normotensive or hypotensive values. The respiratory rate and body temperature may be elevated. If the patient develops marked myoclonus or seizures, severe hyperthermia may result [31,33,59,63,68, 77,110,111,112]. Cyclic antidepressants with prominent anticholinergic effects may cause mydriasis, urinary retention, ileus, and cutaneous vasodilation (Table 140-2). Absence of these signs does not eliminate cyclic antidepressant ingestion.

Progression of toxicity may be precipitous and lead to coma, hypotension, seizures, dysrhythmia, and finally death, although this is dependent on the ingested agent [59,82,111]. The newer agents (nefazadone, trazodone, the SSRIs, and bupropion) are unlikely to exhibit cardiovascular toxicity [59,68,69,70,113–121]. Maprotiline, amoxapine, and loxapine tend to cause CNS toxicity before cardiovascular toxicity [12,69,70,112,122–150]. Bupropion may cause seizures in therapeutic dosing [129–135]. It is unusual in all cases for patients to have hypotension and conduction disturbances without an altered mental status [49,58,59,77].

Cyclic antidepressant–induced seizures are generally single or brief flurries of motor activity. Status epilepticus, however, may occur without any prodrome. This is especially true with large ingestions or overdoses of amoxapine or loxapine. Status epilepticus can be very difficult to halt; if prolonged it will initiate an overall deterioration in the patient's condition [38,59,75,77].

Signs of cardiovascular toxicity may exist even with therapeutic dosing of classic cyclic antidepressants. A widened Q–Tc interval and mild sinus tachycardia may be observed on the electrocardiogram (ECG) in nonoverdose states [82,151]. Sinus tachycardia is usually the presenting dysrhythmia, whereas sinus tachycardia with aberrancy and ventricular tachycardia develops with increasing toxicity. As cardiovascular toxicity progresses, the axis shifts rightward. This is gradually followed by repolarization abnormalities, intraventricular conduction delays, ventricular dysrhythmia, high-grade atrioventricular blocks, profound bradycardias, and asystole [30,32,60,64,82,90,91,152–167]. Trazodone can cause marked prolongation of the Q–Tc interval and *Torsades de pointes* (polymorphous) ventricular tachycardia in the absence of other ECG abnormalities.

Attention has been placed on the early rightward axis changes that occur during therapy with these agents. The terminal 40 msec of the frontal plane QRS complex shifts to a rightward vector of 130 to 270 degrees. If computerized vector analysis is not available, a widened slurred S wave in leads I and aVL and an R wave in aVR represent this vector. Looking for these changes in overdosed or comatose patients may help in establishing a diagnosis. A small portion of the population normally has this unusual vector. Patients with extreme leftward axis deviation as a baseline may not show the rightward change with cyclic antidepressant toxicity [168,169]. The absence of this finding does not eliminate a classic cyclic antidepressant ingestion; finding it in conjunction with coma, seizures, arrhythmias, or hypotension is very suggestive of a cyclic antidepressant overdose [118,119].

The toxicity of SSRI agents is not fully understood. The majority of side effects from these agents involve the CNS or GI system. Reported effects include nausea, vomiting, diarrhea, lethargy and somnolence, tremor, headache, dizziness, and restlessness. Overdose data are limited; expected effects include seizures, coma, hypotension, movement disorders, myoclonus, muscle rigidity, and GI effects. These agents are ex-

pected to have minimal cardiac effects, although ritanserin may affect the Q–Tc. Animal experiments with paroxetine required much larger doses, compared to amitriptyline, to induce arrhythmias [11,16,42,43,44,123–150].

ADDITIONAL CONSIDERATIONS. Patients with cyclic antidepressant overdoses frequently develop secondary complications. These include noncardiogenic pulmonary edema, aspiration pneumonia, and rhabdomyolysis. Overdoses with agents that have prominent anticholinergic properties (e.g., amitriptyline) may cause urinary retention, ileus, and abdominal distention. Although rare, tardive dyskinesia, neuroleptic malignant syndrome, and the syndrome of inappropriate ADH secretion (SIADH) all have been reported in association with cyclic antidepressant overdose [31,35,57,58,63,170–178].

DRUG INTERACTIONS. In normal dosing, cyclic antidepressant agents and SSRIs may interact with other medications, increasing the effect of one or both agents. This effect may be magnified in the presence of an overdose. Drug interactions may alter metabolism, elimination, or the free fraction of the drug. Agents that stimulate the hepatic P-450 microsomal system (phenobarbital, carbamazepine, phenytoin, and rifampin) increase the clearance of cyclic antidepressants. Cigarette smoking may have the same effect. Cimetidine, as a competitor for the hepatic microsomal enzymes, leads to an increase in cyclic antidepressant levels. The coadministration of cyclic antidepressants and antipsychotic agents may lead to competitive inhibition of the metabolism of both drugs. Other medications that increase the steady-state levels of cyclic antidepressants include chloramphenicol and disulfiram, whereas erythromycin decreases the level. Finally, ethanol may decrease the metabolism of cyclic antidepressants, leading to markedly increased drug levels during acute ethanol intoxication [156].

Similar effects have been reported with paroxetine and the use of phenobarbital, cimetidine, and phenytoin. There is the potential for the potentiation of warfarin effect when administered in conjunction with paroxetine [44]. The interaction of fluoxetine and cyclic antidepressants causes an increase in serum levels of the cyclic antidepressant and can lead to cyclic antidepressant toxicity. Therapeutic administration of an SSRI and a cyclic antidepressant with strong serotonergic effects (e.g., clomipromine) may induce the serotonergic syndrome. Finally, the interaction of monoamine oxidase inhibitors and cyclic antidepressants may lead to significant and life-threatening toxicity, particularly with those antidepressants that have predominantly serotonergic effect (trazodone, clomipramine, and the SSRIs) [44,137,156,157].

Differential Diagnosis

Although many substances share some of the effects of cyclic antidepressants, duplicating the entire constellation of signs and symptoms is relatively unusual. Anticholinergic and antihistaminic medications produce some of the same peripheral findings, such as dilated pupils, GI hypomotility, confusion, and seizures. Phenothiazines share some of these physical signs and may increase the Q–Tc. Thioridazine and mesoridazine, two phenothiazines, prolong the QRS and Q–Tc. Other drugs that affect QRS width include type IA antiarrhythmics (quinidine, procainamide, disopyramide) and type IC antiarrhythmics (flecainide, encainide, and propofenone). Hyperkalemia and hypocalcemia widen the QRS complex, and patients with hypocalcemia develop muscle twitching and myoclonus. Beta-blockers, particularly propranolol, cause seizures and conduction abnormalities in overdose. Tramadol, a new opiate analgesic that also causes biogenic amine reuptake inhibition, may theoretically cause both opioid and cyclic antidepressant toxicity.

Ancillary Evaluation

Patients with suspected cyclic antidepressant overdose should have routine blood analyses. Although a complete blood count may not directly affect management, it may be useful in determining the differential diagnosis. Stress leukocytosis may occur with cyclic antidepressant overdoses, especially if seizures have occurred. Electrolyte, BUN, creatinine, and glucose levels should be determined, with special attention to the anion gap. Because rhabdomyolysis may occur, most frequently with seizures, creatinine kinase should be followed [63,174]. Frequent arterial blood gas evaluations are important in determining acid-base status and progression of noncardiogenic pulmonary edema. Urinalysis contributes to the diagnosis of rhabdomyolysis and possible myoglobinuric renal failure. Frequent ECGs are a necessity and should be done any time the patient has a change in status. A chest radiograph is useful for following the progression of noncardiogenic pulmonary edema and aspiration pneumonia. Although total tricyclic levels of more than 1000 ng per milliliter have been associated with significant toxicity [48,50,115–121,153,154,155], there is poor correlation between toxicity and serum level. Repeated levels during resolution of toxicity may be misleading; physical signs of toxicity abate prior to a significant drop in serum levels because of the prolonged elimination half-life and extensive protein binding [48]. A toxicology screen can be done at the discretion of the facility; an acetaminophen level and pregnancy test in a woman of childbearing age should always be checked.

Treatment

Patients who have ingested cyclic antidepressants require immediate evaluation and stabilization. Those who are awake and alert should receive an oral dose of activated charcoal. Patients who have ingested a classic cyclic antidepressant (amitriptyline, nortriptyline, imipramine, desipramine, clomipramine, doxepin, dothiepin, protriptyline, and maprotiline) may be safely observed in the emergency department if they are asymptomatic. An asymptomatic patient implies one with a normal ECG throughout the observation period, a mild sinus tachycardia that resolves within the first 1 to 2 hours, clear mental status, and a nontoxic acetaminophen level. This observation period is defined as a 6-hour interval during which the patient is on continuous ECG monitoring and has intravenous access in place [58,79,111,112,152–155,174–184]. In addition, these patients must have had adequate gastric decontamination and, preferably, have passed a charcoal stool. The patient should always be referred for psychiatric evaluation. Women of childbearing age should have a pregnancy test prior to discharge or transfer; pregnant women should be directed to prenatal counseling. There is no consensus on emergency department observation for patients with ingestions of bupropion, trazodone, and the

SSRIs (fluoxetine, paroxetine, sertraline) because of the paucity of overdose data for these medications [122–130,133,136,140, 146,147,148]. The author observes asymptomatic patients for 6 to 8 hours or until the ECG returns to normal or baseline. Any patient with signs or symptoms of toxicity is admitted to the ICU.

Symptomatic patients should have a rapid evaluation of their airway and, if obtunded or hypoventilating, be immediately intubated. Once an airway is established, the patient should be appropriately ventilated to prevent respiratory acidosis and subsequent deterioration of his or her condition.

Gastric decontamination is by gastric lavage only. Syrup of ipecac-induced emesis is contraindicated in cyclic antidepressant overdoses because of the rapid and unpredictable onset of coma, seizures, and dysrhythmias. Fifty to 100 gm of activated charcoal should be administered (1 gm/kg); use of a cathartic remains discretionary. If the patient has an altered mental status, a rapid bedside determination of serum glucose or administration of 25 to 50 gm of dextrose (0.5–1.0 gm/kg), 2 mg of naloxone, and 100 mg of thiamine should be given intravenously [44,48,49,52–55].

Because some cyclic antidepressants have a small enterohepatic circulation, an additional one to two doses of aqueous charcoal can be given every 4 hours until the patient awakens [48,52,55,185–188].This dose should not be administered in the presence of an ileus or gastric distension. Hemodialysis and hemoperfusion are not effective in reducing the toxic effects of these cyclic antidepressants [189–194].

Treatment is supportive. Single or brief flurries of seizures should be treated with adequate doses of a benzodiazepine [37,38,39,75,77,194]. Seizures are frequently isolated and the additional use of an anticonvulsant is not indicated in this situation. Status epilepticus, however, should be aggressively managed to prevent the development of acidosis, hyperthermia, and rhabdomyolysis [37,39]. Since cyclic cardiotoxicity worsens dramatically in the presence of an acidosis, prevention is paramount. Status epilepticus should be managed with large doses of benzodiazepines (e.g., 30–50 mg diazepam) [37,194]. Failing this, management becomes controversial. The author prefers to paralyze the patient with a nondepolarizing short-acting agent such as vecuronium, while simultaneously adding an anticonvulsant. The duration of action of vecuronium is approximately equal to the time it takes to load phenobarbital (15–20 mg/kg), thiopental (3–5 mg/kg), or phenytoin (18 mg/kg) intravenously. The transient chemical paralysis helps prevent development of hyperthermia, rhabdomyolysis, acidosis, and further deterioration. If available, continuous electroencephalographic monitoring should be used. If the patient continues to have seizure activity once the paralytic has worn off, an additional dose of vecuronium should be given and an alternative anticonvulsant or general anesthesia should be administered [37,49,59,194–201]. Once the patient fails the initial large benzodiazepine dose, the author prefers to go immediately to intravenous pentobarbital or thiopental (3–5 mg/kg). Alkalinization for abnormal cardiac conduction has no effect on halting seizure activity.

Hypotension frequently complicates cyclic antidepressant overdoses. It should be treated initially with fluid resuscitation. Because many patients have an acidosis or abnormal cardiac conduction in addition to hypotension, a bicarbonate solution can be used for both fluid resuscitation and serum alkalinization. A solution of 1000 ml of D_5W with 100 to 150 mEq of $NaHCO_3$ (roughly equivalent to 0.6% and 0.9% NaCl) is suggested. Twenty to 40 mEq of KCl should be added to the solution if renal function is adequate and serum potassium is not elevated. The rate of fluid administration should be adjusted to maintain a serum pH of 7.50 to 7.55 and prevent hypernatremia. In an adult, an initial rate of approximately 200 to 300 ml per hour (1.5–2 times maintenance fluids) is usually adequate. In the face of cardiotoxicity, invasive monitoring (arterial line, central venous pressure, or Swan-Ganz catheterization) may be necessary [59]. Pressor therapy with direct-acting sympathomimetics, such as norepinephrine (Levophed) or epinephrine, has been shown to be more effective than indirect-acting agents, such as dopamine [37,38,202–205]. If hypotension remains refractory, addition of an inotropic agent such as dobutamine may be required [31,67,202–206].

Abnormal conduction (QRS complex >100 msec in the limb leads) and ventricular dysrhythmias are treated with alkalinization. A combination of sodium bicarbonate infusion (previously described) and hyperventilation may be more useful than either alone, although hyperventilation is effective if the patient cannot tolerate a sodium load [81,82,85,95,96,98,99,103,104,105,202]. By combining the two modalities, the arterial CO_2 can be maintained at 24 to 26 mmHg, which prevents cerebral vasoconstriction, while serum sodium is kept within reasonable limits. Optimal arterial pH is between 7.45 and 7.55. Ventricular dysrhythmias not responsive to alkalinization may respond to lidocaine. Other than beta-adrenergic blockers, no antiarrhythmics have been studied, although phenytoin has been used anecdotally (see Controversies). In animal studies, propranolol was effective in improving conduction but led to intractable hypotension [81,85,92,95,96,97]. Other type IA and IC antiarrhythmics are contraindicated because they worsen cardiotoxicity. The use of bretylium in this situation has not yet been investigated. Magnesium is potentially useful, but was ineffective in the author's animal studies; data are not available to advocate its use. Overdrive pacing is a possibility but, again, well-controlled studies are lacking and it has been ineffective in the author's limited experience [87,89].

There is no specific therapy for overdose with SSRIs. Treatment is supportive. Early airway protection helps limit the secondary complications from aspiration. Seizure activity should be aggressively treated.

Disposition and Prognosis

Patients who survive the first 24 hours without any major complications (hypoxia, prolonged seizures, profound acidosis, and hyperthermia) generally do well. Most patients show some improvement within 24 hours. Once cardiac conduction improves (narrowing of QRS complex to 100 msec) alkalinization can be discontinued (usually within 12 hours) and the pH allowed to normalize. If the QRS complex again widens, alkalinization should be resumed and the weaning process repeated. Once the ECG has normalized without alkalinization, the patient should be monitored for an additional 12 to 24 hours in the ICU. The patient must be awake and alert and have passed a charcoal stool before transfer out of the unit. All overdose patients should be referred for psychiatric evaluation prior to discharge [31,77,108,110,111,113,114,116–119,121,152–155,158–169].

Controversies

PHENYTOIN. The use of phenytoin for cyclic antidepressant-induced abnormal cardiac condition and seizure control is controversial. Early studies advocating the use of phenytoin to improve cardiac conduction were empirically based on the prior use of phenytoin to improve conduction in digitalis toxicity. The studies utilizing phenytoin for cyclic antidepressants were poorly controlled and not reproducible [195,196,201,207–212]. Recent canine data suggest that phenytoin transiently facilitated conduction but then increased the incidence and duration of ventricular tachycardia and did not improve survival. The authors suggested that in their model the use of phenytoin was potentially detrimental [212]. The efficacy of phenytoin as an anticonvulsant for cyclic antidepressant-induced seizures is not clear. In some animal studies, phenytoin appeared to be beneficial, but in others, its efficacy has been questioned [99,197,199,204,212]. Anecdotally, phenytoin has been safely used for a number of years. In the author's experience and research, the negative inotropic effect outweighs any potential benefit.

PHYSOSTIGMINE. Physostigmine is a cholinesterase inhibitor that increases acetylcholine concentration at the postsynaptic receptor site. Physostigmine antagonizes only the anticholinergic-based sinus tachycardia and altered mental status [213–219]. Bradycardia and asystole have been reported with its use, and as a carbamate it may precipitate seizures [103,218,219]. Physostigmine is not advocated to treat cyclic antidepressant overdose [49,59,217].

PROPHYLACTIC ALKALINIZATION. Increasing the arterial pH improves abnormal cardiac conduction, but no studies have been done regarding prophylactic alkalinization prior to evidence of abnormal cardiac condition. The QRS width is used as a prognostic indicator, since an untreated narrow QRS complex can help determine the need for hospitalization. Once the pH has been altered, the QRS width is no longer a reliable predictor of cardiotoxicity. Alkalinization is not without risks, including hyperosmolality, cerebral vasoconstriction, and alterations in ionized calcium concentrations. There is no evidence to suggest that it affects seizure onset. There is no role for alkalinization without a prolonged QRS duration.

Future Developments

Two promising areas in the treatment of cyclic antidepressant overdose are being evaluated. In moribund patients in whom conventional therapy has failed, the use of mechanical circulatory support, such as intraaortic balloon pump assist or partial cardiac bypass, may be lifesaving. In this situation, the use of extracorporeal measures supports myocardial, hepatic, and cerebral perfusion while allowing the liver endogenously to detoxify the cyclic antidepressant [220,221,222].

The second area involves ongoing research in the use of immunotherapy for the treatment of this overdose. Fab fragments for cyclic antidepressants have been developed both as free fragments and bound to affinity columns for hemoperfusion [223,224]. The use of Fab fragments to treat desipramine toxicity in animal models has led to improvement in blood pressure and narrowing of the QRS complex. More recent data show that less than equimolar amounts of desipramine Fab fragments are required for this effect. Finally, the combination of hypertonic sodium bicarbonate and desipramine Fab fragments led to improved hemodynamic parameters compared with Fab fragments alone [225,226,227].

References

1. Litovitz TL, Smitz BF, Holm KC: 1988 Annual report of the American Association of Poison Control Centers National Data Collection System. *Am J Emerg Med* 7:495, 1989.

2. Richardson JW III, Richelson E: Antidepressants: A clinical update for medical practitioners. *Mayo Clin Proc* 59:330, 1984.

3. Kosten TR, Schumann B, Wright D, et al: A preliminary study of desipramine in the treatment of cocaine abuse in methadone maintenance patient. *J Clin Psychiatry* 48:442, 1987.

4. Fishman MW, Foltin RW: The effects of desipramine maintenance on cocaine self-administration in humans (abstract). *Psychopharmacol* 96:520, 1988.

5. Hollister LE: Tricyclic antidepressants (part I). *N Engl J Med* 299:1106, 1978.

6. Richelson E: Antimuscarinic and other receptor blocking properties of antidepressants. *Mayo Clin Proc* 58:40, 1983.

7. Richelson E: Tricyclic antidepressants and histamine H_1 receptors. *Mayo Clin Proc* 54:669, 1979.

8. Hollister LE: Current antidepressants. *Ann Rev Pharmacol Toxicol* 26:32, 1986.

9. Kulig K: Management of poisoning associated with "newer" antidepressant agents. *Ann Emerg Med* 15:1039, 1986.

10. Knudsen K, Heath A: Effects of self poisoning with maprotiline. *Br Med J* 288:601, 1984.

11. Hayes PE, Kristoff CA: Adverse reactions to five new antidepressants. *Clin Pharm* 5:471, 1986.

12. Cole J: Where are those new antidepressants we were promised? *Arch Gen Psychiatry* 45:193, 1988.

13. Stark P, Fuller RW, Wong DT: The pharmacologic profile of fluoxetine. *J Clin Psychiatry* 46:7, 1985.

14. Wernicke JF: The side effect profile and safety of fluoxetine. *J Clin Psychiatry* 46:59, 1985.

15. Bryant SG, Guernsey BG, Ingrim NB: Review of bupropion. *Clin Pharm* 2:525, 1983.

16. Settle EC: Bupropion: A novel antidepressant—Update 1989. *Int Drug Ther News* 24:29, 1989.

17. Hollister LE: Tricyclic antidepressants (part II). *N Engl J Med* 299:1168, 1978.

18. Collis MG, Shepherd JT: Antidepressant drug action and presynaptic alpha-receptors. *Mayo Clin Proc* 55:567, 1980.

19. Golden RN, Markey SP, Risby ED, et al: Antidepressants reduce whole-body norepinephrine turnover while enhancing 6-hydroxymelatonin output. *Arch Gen Psychiatry* 45:150, 1988.

20. Schwarz R, Esier M: Catecholamine levels in tricyclic antidepressant self-poisoning. *Aust NZ J Med* 4:479, 1974.

21. Follmer CH, Lum BKB: Protective action of diazepam and sympathomimetic amines against amitriptyline-induced toxicity. *J Pharmacol Exp Ther* 222:424, 1982.

22. Boakes AJ, Laurence DR, Teoh PC, et al: Interactions between sympathomimetic amines and antidepressant agents in man. *Br Med J* 1:311, 1973.

23. Wander TJ, Nelson A, Okazaki, Richelson E: Antagonism by antidepressants of serotonin S_1 and S_2 receptors of normal brain in vitro. *Eur J Pharmacol* 132:115, 1986.

24. Richelson E: The newer antidepressants: Structures, pharmacokinetics, pharmacodynamics, and proposed mechanisms of action. *Psychopharmacol Bull* 20:213, 1984.

25. Richelson E: Pharmacology of antidepressants. *Psychopathology* 20 (suppl 1):1, 1987.

26. Richelson E, Pfenning M: Blockade by antidepressants and related compounds of biogenic amine uptake into rat brain synaptosomes: Most antidepressants selectively block norepinephrine uptake. *Eur J Pharmacol* 104:277, 1984.

27. Snyder SH, Yamamura HI: Antidepressants and the muscarinic-acetylcholine receptor. *Arch Gen Psychiatry* 34:236, 1977.

28. Richelson E: Psychotropics and the elderly: Interactions to watch for. *Geriatrics* 39:30, 1984.

29. Richelson E, Nelson A: Antagonism by antidepressants of neurotransmitter receptors of normal human brain in vitro. *J Pharmacol Exp Ther* 230:94, 1984.

30. Freeman JW, Mundy GR, Beattie RR, Ryan C: Cardiac abnormalities in poisoning with tricyclic antidepressants. *Br Med J* 2:610, 1969.

31. Shannon M, Merola J, Lovejoy FH Jr: Hypotension in severe tricyclic antidepressant overdose. *Am J Emerg Med* 6:439, 1988.

32. Kantor SJ, Bigger JT, Glassman AH, et al: Imipramine-induced heart block: A longitudinal case study. *JAMA* 231:1364, 1975.

33. Jackson WK, Roose SP, Glassman AH: Cardiovascular toxicity of antidepressant medications. *Psychopathology* 20 (suppl 1):64, 1987.

34. Nicotra MB, Rivera M, Pool JL, Noall MW: Tricyclic antidepressant overdose: Clinical and pharmacologic observations. *Clin Toxicol* 18:599, 1981.

35. Jandhyala BS, Steenberg ML, Perel JM, et al: Effects of several tricyclic antidepressants on the hemodynamics and myocardial contractility of the anesthetized dogs. *Eur J Pharmacol* 42:403, 1977.

36. Rudorfer MV: Cardiovascular changes and plasma drug levels after amitriptyline overdose. *J Toxicol Clin Toxicol* 19:67, 1982.

37. Malatynska E, Knapp RJ, Ikeda M, Yamamura HI: Antidepressants and seizure-interactions at the GABA-receptor chloride ionophore complex. *Life Sci* 43:303, 1988.

38. Olson K, Benowitz N, Pentel P: Survey of causes and consequences of seizures during drug intoxication. *Vet Hum Toxicol* 24:23, 1982.

39. Roszkowski AP, Schuler ME, Schultz R: Augmentation of pentylenetetrazol induced seizures by tricyclic antidepressants. *Mater Med Pol* 2:141, 1976.

40. Freeman JM, Lietman PS: A basic approach to the understanding of seizures and the mechanism of action and metabolism of anticonvulsants. *Adv Pediatr* 20:291, 1973.

41. Weinberger J, Nicklas WJ, Berl S: Mechanism of action anticonvulsants. *Neurology* 26:162, 1976.

42. Rickels K, Schweizer E: Clinical overview of serotonin reuptake inhibitors. *J Clin Psychiatry* 51 (suppl B):9, 1992.

43. Leonard BE: Pharmacological differences of serotonin reuptake inhibitors and possible clinical relevance. *Drugs* 43 (suppl 2):3, 1992.

44. Dechant KL, Clissold SP: Paroxetine: A review of its pharmacodynamic properties and therapeutic potential in depressive illness. *Drugs* 41:225, 1991.

45. Dechant KL, Clissold SP: Sumatriptan: A review of its pharmacodynamic and pharmacokinetic properties and therapeutic efficacy in the acute treatment of migraine and cluster headache. *Drugs* 43:776, 1992.

46. Alexanderson B, Borga O, Alvan G: The availability of orally administered nortriptyline. *Eur J Clin Pharmacol* 5:181, 1973.

47. Bickel MH, Baggiolini M: Metabolism of imipramine and its metabolites by rat liver microsomes. *Biochem Pharmacol* 15:1155, 1966.

48. Gard H, Knapp D, Walle T, Gaffney T: Qualitative and quantitative studies on the disposition of amitriptyline and other tricyclic antidepressant drugs in man as it relates to the management of the overdosed patient. *Clin Toxicol* 6:571, 1973.

49. Pentel PR, Keyler DE, Haddad LM: Tricyclic, tetracyclic, and atypical antidepressants, in *Clinical Management of Poisoning and Drug Overdose*, 2nd ed. Philadelphia, WB Saunders, p 636.

50. Perry PJ, Pfohl BM, Holstad SG: The relationship between antidepressant plasma concentrations: A retrospective analysis of the literature using logistic regression analysis. *Med Toxicol* 13:381, 1987.

51. Gram LF, Bjerre M, Kragh-Sorenson P, et al: Imipramine metabolism in blood of patients during therapy and after overdose. *Clin Pharmacol Ther* 33:335, 1983.

52. Alvan G: Effect of activated charcoal on plasma levels of nortriptyline after single doses in man. *Eur J Clin Pharmacol* 5:236, 1973.

53. Crome P, Dawling S, Braithwaite RA, et al: Effect of activated charcoal on absorption of nortriptyline. *Lancet* 2:1203, 1977.

54. Freilich DI, Giardina E-GV: Imipramine binding to alpha-1-acid glycoprotein in normal subjects and cardiac patients. *Clin Pharmacol Ther* 35:670, 1984.

55. Javaid JI, Hendricks K, Davis JM: Alpha$_1$-acid glycoprotein involvement in high affinity binding of tricyclic antidepressants to human plasma. *Biochem Pharmacol* 32:1149, 1983.

56. Levitt MA, Sullivan JB, Owens SM, et al: Amitriptyline plasma protein binding: Effect of plasma pH and relevance to clinical overdose. *Am J Emerg Med* 4:121, 1986.

57. Seaberg DC, Weiss LD, Yealy DM, et al: Effects of alpha-1-acid glycoprotein on the cardiovascular toxicity of nortriptyline in a swine model. *Vet Hum Toxicol* 33:226, 1991.

58. Frommer DA, Kulig KW, Marx JA, Rumack B: Tricyclic antidepressant overdose: A review. *JAMA* 257:521, 1987.

59. Crome P: Poisoning due to tricyclic antidepressant overdosage: Clinical presentation and treatment. *Med Toxicol* 1:261, 1986.

60. Crome P, Newman B: Fatal tricyclic antidepressant poisoning. *J Roy Soc Med* 72:649, 1979.

61. Cassidy S, Henry J: Fatal toxicity of antidepressant drugs in overdose. *Br Med J* 295:1021, 1987.

62. Henry JA, Martin AJ: The risk-benefit assessment of antidepressant drugs. *Med Toxicol* 2:445, 1987.

63. Rosenberg J, Pentel P, Pond S, et al: Hyperthermia associated with drug intoxication. *Crit Care Med* 14:964, 1986.

64. Langou RA, VanDyke C, Tahan SR, Cohen LS: Cardiovascular manifestations of tricyclic antidepressant overdose. *Am Heart J* 100:458, 1980.

65. Janowsky D, Curtis G, Zisook S, et al: Trazodone-aggravated ventricular arrhythmias. *J Clin Psychopharmacol* 3:372, 1983.

66. Sigg EB, Osborne M, Korol B: Cardiovascular effects of imipramine. *J Pharmacol Exp Ther* 141:237, 1963.

67. Harvengt C, Desager JP, Vanderbist M, et al: Sympathetic nervous system response in acute cardiovascular toxicity induced by amitriptyline in conscious rabbits. *Toxicol Appl Pharmacol* 44:115, 1978.

68. Lesar T, Kingston R, Dahms R, Saxema K: Trazodone overdose. *Ann Emerg Med* 12:221, 1983.

69. Kulig K, Rumack BH, Sullivan JB Jr, et al: Amoxapine overdose: Coma and seizures without cardiotoxic effects. *JAMA* 248:1092, 1982.

70. Kulig K: Management of poisoning associated with "newer" antidepressant agents. *Ann Emerg Med* 15:1039, 1986.

71. Kuhn R: The discovery of modern antidepressants. *Psychiatr J Univ Ottawa* 14:249, 1989.

72. Baldessarini RJ: Drugs and the treatment of psychiatric disorders: Tricyclic antidepressants, in Goodman AG, Goodman LS, Rall TW, Murad F (eds): *Goodman and Gilman's The Pharmacological Basis of Therapeutics*, 7th ed. New York, Macmillan, 1985, p 413.

73. Dallos V, Heathfield K: Iatrogenic epilepsy due to antidepressant drugs. *Br Med J* 4:80, 1969.

74. Pincus JH, Grove I, Marino BB, Glaser GE: Studies on the mechanism of action of diphenylhydantoin. *Arch Neurol* 22:566, 1970.

75. Ellison DW, Pentel PR: Clinical features and consequences of seizures due to cyclic antidepressant overdose. *Am J Emerg Med* 7:5, 1989.

76. Trimble M, Anlezark G, Meldrum B: Seizure activity in photosensitive baboons following antidepressant drugs and the role of serotoninergic mechanism. *Psychopharmacology* 51:159, 1977.

77. Petti TA, Campbell M: Imipramine and seizures. *Am J Psychiatry* 132:538, 1975.

78. Pentel PR, Benowitz NL: Tricyclic antidepressant poisoning: Management of arrhythmias. *Med Toxicol* 1:101, 1986.

79. Connolly SJ, Mitchell LB, Swerdlow CD, et al: Clinical efficacy and electrophysiology of imipramine for ventricular tachycardia. *Am J Cardiol* 53:516, 1984.

80. Glassman AH: Cardiovascular effects of tricyclic antidepressants. *Ann Rev Med* 35:503, 1984.

81. Sasyniuk BI, Jhamandas V, Valois M: Experimental amitriptyline intoxication: Treatment of cardiac toxicity with sodium bicarbonate. *Ann Emerg Med* 15:1052, 1986.

82. Dumovic P, Burrows GD, Vohra J, et al: The effect of tricyclic antidepressants and the heart. *Arch Toxicol* 35:255, 1976.

83. Weld FM, Bigger JT Jr: Electrophysiological effects of imipramine on ovine cardiac Purkinje and ventricular muscle fibers. *Circ Res* 46:167, 1980.

84. Rawling DA, Fozzard HA: Effects of imipramine on cellular electrophysiological properties of cardiac Purkinje fibers. *J Pharmacol Exp Ther* 209:371, 1979.

85. Nattel S, Keable H, Sasyniuk BI: Experimental amitriptyline intoxication: Electrophysiologic manifestations and management. *J Cardiovasc Pharmacol* 6:83, 1984.

86. Pentel P, Benowitz N: Efficacy and mechanism of action of sodium bicarbonate in the treatment of desipramine toxicity in rats. *J Pharmacol Exp Ther* 230:12, 1984.

87. Tamargo J, Rodriguez S, Garcia de Jalon P: Electrophysiological effects of desipramine on guinea pig papillary muscles. *Eur J Pharmacol* 55:171, 1979.

88. Wit AL, Cranefield PF, Hoffman BF: Slow conduction and reentry in the ventricular conducting system. II. Single and sustained circus movement in networks of canine and bovine Purkinje fibers. *Circ Res* 30:11, 1972.

89. Davison ET: Amitriptyline-induced torsade de pointes. Successful therapy with atrial pacing. *J Electrocardiol* 18:299, 1985.

90. Hermann HC, Kaplan LM, Bierer BE: Q–T prolongation and torsades de pointes ventricular tachycardia produced by the tetracyclic antidepressant agent maprotiline. *Am J Cardiol* 51:904, 1983.

91. Krikler DM, Curry PVL: Torsade de pointes: An atypical ventricular tachycardia. *Br Heart J* 38:117, 1976.

92. Byrne JE, Gomoll AW: Differential effects of trazodone and imipramine on intracardiac conduction in the anesthetized dog. *Arch Int Pharmacodyn* 259:259, 1982.

93. Vlay SC, Friedling S: Trazodone exacerbation of VT. *Am Heart J* 106:604, 1983.

94. Nattel S: Frequency-dependent effects of amitriptyline on ventricular conduction and cardiac rhythm in dogs. *Circulation* 72:898, 1985.

95. Nattel S, Mittleman M: Treatment of ventricular tachyarrhythmias resulting from amitriptyline toxicity in dogs. *J Pharmacol Exp Ther* 231:430, 1984.

96. Sasyniuk BI, Jhamandas V: Mechanism of reversal of toxic effects of amitriptyline on cardiac Purkinje fibers by sodium bicarbonate. *J Pharmacol Exp Ther* 231:387, 1984.

97. Freeman JW, Loughhead MG: Beta blockade in the treatment of tricyclic antidepressant overdosage. *Med J Aust* 1:1233, 1973.

98. Hoffman JR, McElroy CR: Bicarbonate therapy for dysrhythmia and hypotension in tricyclic antidepressant overdose. *West J Med* 134:60, 1981.

99. Brown TCK: Sodium bicarbonate treatment for tricyclic antidepressant arrhythmias in children. *Med J Aust* 2:380, 1976.

100. Wasserman F, Brodsky L, Dick MM, et al: Successful treatment of quinidine and procaine amide intoxication: Report of three cases. *N Engl J Med* 259:797, 1958.

101. Bellet S, Hamden G, Somlyo A: Reversal of the cardiotoxic effects of quinidine by molar sodium lactate. *Clin Res* 6:226, 1958.

102. Bajaj AK, Woosley RL, Roden DM: Acute electrophysiologic effects of sodium administration in dogs treated with o-desmethylencainide. *Circulation* 80:994, 1989.

103. Kingston ME: Hyperventilation in tricyclic antidepressant poisoning. *Crit Care Med* 7:550, 1979.

104. Hedges JR, Baker PB, Tasset JJ, et al: Bicarbonate therapy for the cardiovascular toxicity of amitriptyline in an animal model. *J Emerg Med* 3:253, 1985.

105. Bessen HA, Niemann JT, Haskell RJ, Rothstein RJ: Effect of respiratory alkalosis in tricyclic antidepressant overdose. *West J Med* 139:373, 1983.

106. Bellet S, Hamdam G, Somlyo A, Lara R: The reversal of cardiotoxic effects of quinidine by molar sodium lactate: An experimental study. *Am J Med Sci* 237:165, 1959.

107. Bessen HA, Niemann JT: Improvement of cardiac conduction after hyperventilation in tricyclic antidepressant overdose. *Clin Toxicol* 23:537, 1986.

108. Tobis JM, Aronow WS: Cardiotoxicity of amitriptyline and doxepin. *Clin Pharmacol Ther* 29:359, 1981.

109. Pentel PR, Keyler DE: Effects of high dose alpha-1-acid glycoprotein on desipramine toxicity in rats. *J Pharmacol Exp Ther* 246:1061, 1988.

110. Goldberg RJ, Capone RJ, Hunt JD: Cardiac complications following tricyclic antidepressant overdose: Issues for monitoring policy. *JAMA* 254:1772, 1985.

111. Callaham M, Kassel D: Epidemiology of fatal tricyclic antidepressant ingestion: Implications for management. *Ann Emerg Med* 14:1, 1985.

112. Wedin GP, Oderda GM, Klein Schwartz W, Gorman RL: Relative toxicity of cyclic antidepressants. *Ann Emerg Med* 15:797, 1986.

113. Rasmussen J: Amitriptyline and imipramine poisoning (letter). *Lancet* 2:850, 1965.

114. Hayes PE, Kristoff CA: Adverse reactions to five new antidepressants. *Clin Pharm* 5:471, 1986.

115. Foulke GE, Albertson TE: QRS interval in tricyclic antidepressant

overdosage: Inaccuracy and a toxicity indicator in emergency settings. *Ann Emerg Med* 16:160, 1987.

116. Hulten B-A, Adams R, Askenasi R, et al: Predicting severity of tricyclic antidepressant overdosage. *Clin Toxicol* 30:161, 1987.

117. Hulten B-A, Heath A, Knudsen K, et al: Amitriptyline and amitriptyline metabolites in blood and cerebrospinal fluid following human overdose. *Clin Toxicol* 30:181, 1992.

118. Caravati EM, Bossart PJ: Demographic and electrocardiographic factors associated with severe tricyclic antidepressant toxicity. *Clin Toxicol* 29:31, 1991.

119. Groleau G, Jotte R, Barish R: The electrocardiographic manifestations of cyclic antidepressant therapy and overdose: A review. *J Emerg Med* 8:597, 1990.

120. Hulten B-A, Heath A, Knudsen K, et al: Severe amitriptyline overdosage: Relationship between toxicokinetics and toxicodynamics. *Clin Toxicol* 30:171, 1992.

121. Shannon MW: Duration of QRS disturbances after severe tricyclic antidepressant intoxication. *Clin Toxicol* 30:377, 1992.

122. Steinberg MI, Smallwood JK, Holland DR, et al: Hemodynamic and electrocardiographic effects of fluoxetine and its major metabolite, norfluoxetine, in anesthetized dogs. *Toxicol Appl Pharmacol* 82:70, 1986.

123. Fisch C: Effect of fluoxetine on the electrocardiogram. *J Clin Psychiatry* 46:42, 1985.

124. Benfield P, Heel RC, Lewis SP: Fluoxetine: A review of its pharmacokinetic properties, and therapeutic efficacy in depressive illness. *Drugs* 32:481, 1986.

125. Stark P, Fuller RW, Wong DT: The pharmacologic profile of fluoxetine. *J Clin Psychiatry* 46:7, 1985.

126. Lemberger L, Bergstrom RF, Wolen RL, et al: Fluoxetine: Clinical pharmacology and physiologic disposition. *J Clin Psychiatry* 46:14, 1985.

127. Wernicke JF: The side effect profile and safety of fluoxetine. *J Clin Psychiatry* 46:59, 1985.

128. Kim SW, Pentel PR: Flu-like symptoms associated with fluoxetine overdose: A case report. *Clin Toxicol* 27:389, 1989.

129. Bryant SG, Guernsey BG, Ingrim NB: Review of bupropion. *Clin Pharm* 2:525, 1983.

130. Van Wyck Fleet J, Manberg PJ, Miller LL, et al: Overview of clinically significant adverse reactions to bupropion. *J Clin Psychiatry* 44:191, 1983.

131. Settle EC: Bupropion: A novel antidepressant—Update 1989. *Int Drug Ther News* 24:29, 1989.

132. Sheehan DV, Welch JB, Fishman SM: A case of bupropion-induced seizure. *J Nerv Ment Dis* 174:496, 1986.

133. Davidson J: Seizures and bupropion: A review. *J Clin Psychiatry* 50:256, 1989.

134. Jefferson JW: Cardiovascular effects and toxicity of anxiolytics and antidepressants. *J Clin Psychiatry* 50:368, 1989.

135. Tucker WE: Preclinical toxicology of bupropion: An overview. *J Clin Psychiatry* 44:60, 1983.

136. Shopsin B: Second generation antidepressants. *J Clin Psychiatry* 41:45, 1980.

137. Cohen H, Hoffman RS, Howland MA: Cyclic antidepressant poisoning: A review and case report. *J Pharm Pract* 6:89, 1993.

138. Munger MA, Effron BA: Amoxapine cardiotoxicity. *Ann Emerg Med* 17:274, 1988.

139. Curtis RA, Giacona N, Burrows D, et al: Fatal maprotiline intoxication. *Drug Intell Clin Pharm* 18:716, 1984.

140. Knudsen K, Heath A: Effects of self poisoning with maprotiline. *Br Med J* 288:601, 1984.

141. Schatzberg AF, Dessain E, O'Neill P, et al: Recent studies on selective serotonergic antidepressants: Trazodone, fluoxetine, and fluvoxamine, *J Clin Psychopharmacol* 7:44S, 1987.

142. Mendels J: Clinical experience with serotonin reuptake inhibiting antidepressants. *J Clin Psychiatry* 48(suppl 3):26, 1987.

143. Burrows GD, McIntyre IM, Judd FK, Norman TR: Clinical effects of serotonin reuptake inhibitors in the treatment of depressive illness. *J Clin Psychiatry* 49(suppl 8):18, 1988.

144. Juvent M, Douchamps J, Delcourt E, et al: Lack of cardiovascular side effects of the new tricyclic antidepressant tianeptine: A double-blind, placebo-controlled study in young healthy volunteers. *Clin Neuropharmacol* 13:48, 1990.

145. Maguire KP, Norman TR, Burrows GD, Scoggins BA: A pharmacokinetic study of miaserin. *Eur J Clin Pharmacol* 21:17, 1982.

146. Burrows GD, Davies B, Hamer A, Vohra J: Effect of mianserin on cardiac conduction. *Med J Aust* 2:97, 1979.

147. Bateman DN, Chaplin S, Ferner RE: Safety of mianserin. *Lancet* Aug 13:401, 1988.

148. Lijeqvist J-A, Edvardsson N: Torsade de pointes, tachycardias induced by overdose of zimeldine. *J Cardiovasc Pharmacol* 14:666, 1989.

149. Nilsson BS: Adverse reactions in connection with zimeldine treatment: A review. *Acta Psychiatr Scand* 68 (suppl 308):115, 1983.

150. Burrows GD, Norman TR, Dennerstein L, Davies BM: Antidepressant therapy: Benefits and risks in perspective. *Acta Psychiatr Scand* 72 (suppl 320):43, 1985.

151. Borganelli M, Forman MB: Simulation of acute myocardial infarction by desipramine hydrochloride. *Am Heart J* 119:1413, 1990.

152. Pentel P: Incidence of late arrhythmias following tricyclic antidepressant overdose. *Clin Toxicol* 18:543, 1981.

153. Bramble MG, Lishman AH, Purdon J, et al: An analysis of plasma levels and 24-hour ECG recordings in tricyclic antidepressant poisoning: Implications for management. *Q J Med* 56:357, 1985.

154. Boehnert MT, Lovejoy FH: Value of the QRS duration versus the serum drug level in predicting seizures and ventricular arrhythmias after an acute overdose of tricyclic antidepressants. *N Engl J Med* 313:474, 1985.

155. Emerson TS: Inaccuracy of QRS interval as TCA toxicity indicator. *Ann Emerg Med* 16:1312, 1987.

156. Ereshefsky L, Tran-Johnson T, Davis CM, LeRoy A: Pharmacokinetic factors affecting antidepressant drug clearance and clinical effect: Evaluation of doxepine and imipramine—New data and review. *Clin Chem* 34:863, 1988.

157. Schmauss M, Kapfhammer P, Meyr P, Hoff P: Combined MAO-inhibitor and tri- (tetra) cyclic antidepressant treatment in therapy resistant depression. *Prog Neuropsychopharmacol Biol Psychiatry* 12:523, 1988.

158. Hedges JR, Otten EJ, Schroeder T, Tasset JJ: QRS duration in acute overdose of tricyclic antidepressants (letter). *N Engl J Med* 314:988, 1986.

159. Bishop MP, Briggs JH: QRS duration in acute overdose of tricyclic antidepressants (letter). *N Engl J Med* 314:989, 1986.

160. Nikolic G: QRS duration in acute overdose of tricyclic antidepressants (letter). *N Engl J Med* 314:989, 1986.

161. Cheng TS: QRS duration in acute overdose of tricyclic antidepressants (letter). *N Engl J Med* 314:989, 1986.

162. Schneider LS: QRS duration in acute overdose of tricyclic antidepressants (letter). *N Engl J Med* 314:989, 1986.

163. Giardina EGV: QRS duration in acute overdose of tricyclic antidepressants (letter). *N Engl J Med* 314:989, 1986.

164. Boehnert MT, Lovejoy FH: QRS duration in acute overdose of tricyclic antidepressants (letter). *N Engl J Med* 314:989,1986.

165. Salzman C: Clinical use of antidepressant blood levels and the electrocardiogram. *N Engl J Med* 313:512, 1985.

166. Thorstrand C: Clinical features in poisoning by tricyclic antidepressants with special reference to the ECG. *Acta Med Scand* 199:337, 1976.

167. Bengt-Ake H, Heath A: Clinical aspects of tricyclic antidepressant poisoning. *Acta Med Scand* 213:275, 1983.

168. Niemann JT, Bessen HA, Rothstein RJ, Laks MM: Electrocardiographic criteria for tricyclic antidepressant cardiotoxicity. *Am J Cardiol* 57:1154, 1986.

169. Wolfe TR, Caravati EM, Rollins DE: Terminal 40-ms frontal plane QRS axis as a marker for tricyclic antidepressant overdose. *Ann Emerg Med* 18:348, 1989.

170. Nosko MG, McLean DR, Chin W, Dat N: Loss of brainstem and pupillary reflexes in amoxapine overdose: A case report. *Clin Toxicol* 26:117, 1988.

171. Tao GK, Harada DT, Kootsikas ME, et al: Amoxapine-induced tardive dyskinesia. *Drug Intell Clin Pharm* 19:548, 1985.

172. Abbott R: Hyponatremia due to antidepressant medications. *Ann Emerg Med* 12:708, 1983.

173. Taylor NE, Schwartz HI: Neuroleptic malignant syndrome following amoxapine overdose. *J Nerv Ment Dis* 176:249, 1988.

174. Jennings AE, Levey AS, Harrington JT: Amoxapine-associated acute renal failure. *Arch Intern Med* 143:1525, 1983.

175. Roy TM, Ossorio MA, Cipolla LM, et al: Pulmonary complications after tricyclic antidepressant overdose. *Chest* 96:852, 1989.

176. Shannon M, Lovejoy FH: Pulmonary consequences of severe tricyclic antidepressant ingestion. *Clin Toxicol* 25:443, 1987.

177. Lydiard RB: Desipramine-associated SIADH in an elderly woman: Case report. *J Clin Psychiatry* 44:153, 1983.

178. Tasset JJ, Pesce AJ: Amoxapine in human overdose. *J Analyt Toxicol* 8:124, 1984.

179. Greenland P, Howe TA: Cardiac monitoring in tricyclic antidepressant overdose. *Heart Lung* 10:856, 1981.

180. Callaham M: Admission criteria for tricyclic antidepressant ingestion. *West J Med* 137:425, 1982.

181. McAlpine SB, Calabro JJ, Robinson MD, Burkle FM Jr: Late death in tricyclic antidepressant overdose revisited. *Ann Emerg Med* 15:1349, 1986.

182. Tokarski GF, Young MJ: Criteria for admitting patients with tricyclic antidepressant overdose. *J Emerg Med* 6:121, 1988.

183. Pentel P, Olson KR, Becker CE, Benowitz N: Late complications of tricyclic antidepressant overdose (letter). *West J Med* 138:423, 1983.

184. Pentel P, Olson KR, Becker CE, Benowitz N: Late complications of tricyclic antidepressant overdose (letter). *West J Med* 138:423, 1983.

185. Hulten B-A, Adams R, Askenasi R, et al: Activated charcoal in tricyclic antidepressant poisoning. *Hum Toxicol* 7:307, 1988.

186. Crome P, Adams R, Ali C, et al: Activated charcoal in tricyclic antidepressant poisoning: Pilot controlled clinical trial. *Hum Toxicol* 2:205, 1983.

187. Goldberg MJ, Park GD, Spector R, et al: Lack of effect of oral activated charcoal on imipramine clearance. *Clin Pharmacol Ther* 38:350, 1985.

188. Rinder HM, Murphy JW, Higgins GL: Impact of unusual gastrointestinal problems on the treatment of tricyclic antidepressant overdose. *Ann Emerg Med* 17:1079, 1988.

189. Diaz-Buxo JA, Farmer CD, Chandler JT: Hemoperfusion in the treatment of amitriptyline intoxication. *Trans Am Soc Artif Intern Organs* 24:699, 1978.

190. Comstock TJ, Watson WA, Jennison TA: Severe amitriptyline intoxication and the use of charcoal hemoperfusion. *Clin Pharm* 2:85, 1983.

191. Ryan R, Wians FH, Stigelman WH, et al: Imipramine poisoning in a child: Lack of efficacy of resin hemoperfusion. *Clin Pharm* 2:85, 1983.

192. Asbach HW, Holz F, Mohring K, Schuler HW: Lipid hemodialysis versus charcoal hemoperfusion in imipramine poisoning. *Clin Toxicol* 11:211, 1977.

193. Heath A, Wickstrom I, Martensson E, Ahlmen J: Treatment of antidepressant poisoning with resin hemoperfusion. *Hum Toxicol* 1:361, 1982.

194. Pentel PR, Bullock ML: Hemoperfusion for imipramine overdose, elimination of active metabolites. *J Toxicol Clin Toxicol* 19:239, 1982.

195. Beaubien AR, Carpenter DC, Mathieu LF, et al: Antagonism of imipramine poisoning by anticonvulsants in the rat. *Toxicol Appl Pharmacol* 38:1, 1976.

196. Blake KV, Massey KL, Hendeles L, et al: Relative efficacy of phenytoin and phenobarbital for the prevention of theophylline-induced seizures in mice. *Ann Emerg Med* 17:1024, 1988.

197. Young JA, Galloway WH: Treatment of severe imipramine poisoning. *Arch Dis Child* 46:353, 1971.

198. Bartholini G: GABA receptor agonists: Pharmacological spectrum and therapeutic actions. *Med Res Rev* 5:55, 1985.

199. Gerdes DA, Krenzelok EP: Seizure prophylaxis in amoxapine overdose. *Vet Hum Toxicol* 26:42, 1984.

200. Bender AS, Hertz L: Evidence for involvement of the astrocytic benzodiazepine receptor in the mechanism of action of convulsant and anticonvulsant drugs. *Life Sci* 43:477, 1988.

201. Hagerman GA, Hanashiro PK: Reversal of tricyclic-antidepressant-induced cardiac conduction abnormalities by phenytoin. *Ann Emerg Med* 10:82, 1981.

202. Hoffman JR, Votey SR, Bayer M, Silver L: Effect of hypertonic sodium bicarbonate in the treatment of moderate-to-severe cyclic antidepressant overdose. *Am J Emerg Med* 11:336, 1993.

203. Buchman AL, Dauer J, Geiderman G: The use of vasoactive agents in the treatment of refractory hypotension seen in tricyclic antidepressant overdose. *J Clin Psychopharmacol* 10:409, 1990.

204. Teba L, Schiebel F, Dedhia HV, Lazzell VA: Beneficial effect of norepinephrine in the treatment of circulatory shock caused by tricyclic antidepressant overdose. *Am J Emerg Med* 6:566, 1988.

205. Knudsen K, Abrahamsson J: Effects of epinephrine and norepinephrine on hemodynamic parameters and arrhythmias during a continuous infusion of amitriptyline in rats. *Clin Toxicol* 31:461, 1993.

206. Teba L, Schiebel F, Dedhia HV, Lazzel VA: Beneficial effect of norepinephrine in the treatment of circulatory shock caused by tricyclic antidepressant overdose. *J Emerg Med* 6:566, 1988.

207. Mayron R, Ruiz E: Phenytoin: Does it reverse tricyclic-antidepressant-induced cardiac conduction abnormalities? *Ann Emerg Med* 15:876, 1986.

208. Mayron R, Ruiz E: Tricyclic antidepressant overdose: Cardiac conduction abnormalities and the use of phenytoin for treatment. *EMS Stat MD*:341, 1986.

209. Boehnert M, Lovejoy FH Jr: The effect of phenytoin on cardiac conduction and ventricular arrhythmias in acute tricyclic antidepressant (TCA) overdose (abstract). *Vet Hum Toxicol* 28:297, 1985.

210. Uhl JA: Phenytoin: The drug of choice in tricyclic antidepressant overdose? *Ann Emerg Med* 10:270, 1981.

211. Kulig K, Bar-Or D, Wythe E, Rumack BH: Phenytoin as treatment for tricyclic antidepressant cardiotoxicity in a canine model. *Vet Hum Toxicol* 26:42, 1984.

212. Callaham M, Shumaker H, Pentel P: Phenytoin prophylaxis of cardiotoxicity in experimental amitriptyline poisoning. *J Pharmacol Exp Ther* 245:216, 1988.

213. Flect C, Braunlich H: Failure of physostigmine in intoxication with tricyclic antidepressants in rats. *Toxicology* 24:335, 1982.

214. Burks JS, Walker JE, Rumack BH, Ott JE: Tricyclic antidepressant poisoning: Reversal of coma, choreoathetosis, and myoclonus by physostigmine. *JAMA* 230:1405, 1974.

215. Lum BKB, Follmer CH, Lockwood RH, Thomas HM: Experimental studies on the effects of physostigmine and of isoproterenol on toxicity produced by tricyclic antidepressant agents. *J Toxicol Clin Toxicol* 19:51, 1982.

216. Slovis TL, Ott JE, Teitlebaum DT, Lipscomb W: Physostigmine therapy in acute tricyclic antidepressant poisoning. *Clin Toxicol* 4:451, 1971.

217. Pentel P, Peterson CD: Asystole complicating physostigmine treatment of tricyclic antidepressant overdose. *Ann Emerg Med* 9:588, 1980.

218. Goldberger AL, Curtis GP: Immediate effects of physostigmine on amitriptyline-induced QRS prolongation. *J Toxicol Clin Toxicol* 19:445, 1982.

219. Bigger JT Jr, Kantor SJ, Glassman AH, Perel JM: Is physostigmine effective for cardiac toxicity of tricyclic antidepressant drugs? (letter). *JAMA* 237:1311, 1977.

220. Martin TG, O'Connell JJ, Pentel PR, et al: Resuscitation from severe cyclic antidepressant toxicity using cardiopulmonary bypass (abstract). *Vet Hum Toxicol* 30:354, 1988.

221. Southall DP, Kilpatrick SM: Imipramine poisoning: Survival of a child after prolonged cardiac massage. *Br Med J* 4:508, 1974.

222. Freedberg RS, Friedman GR, Palu RN, Feit F: Antihistamine overdose: Reversal with intra-aortic balloon pump counterpulsation. *JAMA* 257:660, 1987.

223. Hursting MJ, Opheim KE, Raisys VA, et al: Tricyclic antidepressant-specific Fab fragments alter the distribution and elimination of desipramine in the rabbit: A model for overdose treatment. *Clin Toxicol* 27:53, 1989.

224. Liu D, Purssell R, Levy JG: Production and characterization of high affinity monoclonal antibodies to cyclic anti-depressant molecules. *Clin Toxicol* 25:527, 1987.

225. Brunn GJ, Keyler DE, Pond SM, Pentel PR: Reversal of desipramine toxicity in rats using drug-specific antibody Fab fragment: Effects on hypotension and interaction with sodium bicarbonate. *J Pharmacol Exp Ther* 260:1392, 1992.

226. Brunn GJ, Keyler DE, Ross CA, et al: Drug specific F(ab')2 fragment reduces desipramine cardiotoxicity in rats. *Int J Immunopharmacol* 13:841, 1991.

227. Bowles M, Johnson SC, Schoof DD, et al: Large scale production and purification of paraquat and desipramine monoclonal antibodies and their Fab fragments. *Int J Immunopharmacol* 10:537, 1988.

141. *Digitalis Poisoning*

Mark A. Kirk

Cardiac glycosides (CGs) are naturally occurring substances whose medicinal benefits have been recognized for more than 200 years [1]. Plants such as foxglove, lily of the valley, oleander, squill, and hellebore contain CGs. The major CG used for medicinal purposes today is digoxin, widely used in the treatment of congestive heart failure and supraventricular tachycardias [2]. Digoxin's ready availability in the home results in frequent accidental ingestions in children and intentional overdoses in suicidal adults. Those patients who benefit most from its therapeutic effects (i.e., patients with chronic illnesses and polypharmacy) have enhanced susceptibility to toxicity. In 1785, William Withering astutely recognized the toxic effects of CGs and vividly described them in his writings [1].

Identification of CG toxicity remains a challenge, because the clinical presentation is often subtle. A unique aspect of CG toxicity is the availability of a specific antidote that can reverse otherwise fatal toxicity. Hence, recognition of toxicity and early intervention can result in a favorable outcome in even the most critically ill patient.

EPIDEMIOLOGY. The incidence of digitalis toxicity with therapeutic doses has been reported to be as high as 23 percent in hospitalized patients [3]. Recent similar series have shown an incidence of less than 2 percent [4,5]. In 1991, 2309 acute CG exposures were reported by the American Association of Poison Control Centers. More than 250 (11%) were considered to have moderate to major effects, and 21 deaths (1%) were reported [6].

MECHANISM OF TOXICITY. Cardiac glycoside toxicity results from an exaggeration of its therapeutic action [7]. Cardiac glycosides bind to specific receptor sites, inactivating the sodium-potassium adenosine triphosphatase pump (Na^+/K^+ ATPase) on cardiac cell membranes [7,8]. This pump maintains the electrochemical membrane potential, vital to conduction tissues, by concentrating sodium extracellularly and potassium intracellularly. When the Na^+/K^+ ATPase is inhibited, the sodium-calcium exchanger removes accumulated intracellular sodium in exchange for calcium [7]. This exchange increases sarcoplasmic calcium and is the mechanism responsible for the positive inotropic effect of digitalis [7]. Increased vagal tone and direct atrioventricular (A-V) depression may produce conduction disturbances. The decreased refractory period of the myocardium increases automaticity [7,9,10]. Delayed afterdepolarization gives rise to triggered arrhythmias due to intracellular calcium overload [7].

PHARMACOLOGY. Cardiac glycosides are readily absorbed through the gastrointestinal tract: digoxin has up to 80 percent bioavailability and digitoxin has 100 percent bioavailability [7,11]. Digoxin is primarily eliminated by renal excretion and has a volume of distribution of 7 to 10 liters per kilogram. In contrast, digitoxin is eliminated through hepatic metabolism and has a volume of distribution of 0.54 liter per kilogram [2,11,12]. The half-lives of digoxin and digitoxin are 36 to 48 hours and 5 to 7 days, respectively [2,11]. Further details are provided in Chapter 207.

Clinical Presentation

Cardiac glycoside poisoning may result from acute or chronic overdosage. Chronic CG toxicity diagnosis may be difficult, because the presentation may mimic more common illnesses, such as influenza or gastroenteritis. Patients with chronic CG toxicity may present with gastrointestinal, psychiatric, or visual complaints that may not be recognized as signs of digitalis toxicity [12,13]. Symptoms most commonly reported include fatigue, weakness, nausea, anorexia, and dizziness [14,15,16]. Headache, weakness, vertigo, vomiting, syncope, and seizures have also been reported [14,17]. Psychiatric symptoms include memory loss, confusion, disorientation, delirium, depression, and hallucinations [18–22]. Cloudy, blurred vision or yellow-green halos are the most frequently reported visual disturbances [13,16,19].

CARDIAC TOXICITY. Cardiac manifestations of CG toxicity are common and frequently life-threatening. An extremely wide variety of arrhythmias have been reported [5,8,9,10,12,15,16,17,23–27]. Arrhythmias frequently associated with CG toxicity include ventricular premature beats, supraventricular tachycardia (e.g., paroxysmal atrial tachycardia or atrial fibrillation) with a conduction block, junctional tachycardia, sinus bradycardia, A-V nodal blocks, ventricular tachycardia, and ventricular fibrillation [8,9,10,12,15,16,17,23,24,27]. Atrial tachycardia (enhanced automaticity) with variable A-V block (impaired conduction), accelerated junctional rhythm (regularization of atrial fibrillation), and fascicular tachycardia are highly suggestive of CG toxicity [28,29]. Bidirectional ventricular tachycardia, a narrow-complex tachycardia with right bundle branch morphology, is specific for digitalis toxicity but extremely rare and hence not likely to be helpful diagnostically [10,30,31]. A helpful classification of digitalis-induced arrhythmias is shown in Table 141-1 [9].

FACTORS ENHANCING TOXICITY. A variety of factors increase susceptibility to CG toxicity. True end-organ sensitivity is seen with myocardial disease, myocardial ischemia, and metabolic or electrolyte disturbances [30,32]. Hypokalemia as well as hypomagnesemia and hypercalcemia predispose to increased toxicity [2,8,32–36]. The elderly are more susceptible to toxicity [1,3,13,32,37]. Alterations in renal function, hepatic disease, hypothyroidism, chronic obstructive pulmonary disease, and drug interactions alter sensitivity to CGs [1,8,30]. Drug interactions potentially resulting in CG toxicity include those with quinidine, calcium channel blockers, amiodarone, spironolactone, and indomethacin [7,8,38–41].

ACUTE VERSUS CHRONIC TOXICITY. Differences between the presentation of patients with poisoning due to single acute ingestion, both accidental and suicidal, and those with chronic toxicity resulting from excessive therapeutic doses are illustrated in Table 141-2.

Table 141-1. Digitalis-Induced Arrhythmias

1. Ectopic rhythms (reentry or enhanced automaticity or both)
    Atrial tachycardia with block
    Atrial fibrillation
    Atrial flutter
    Nonparoxysmal junctional tachycardia
    Ventricular premature complexes
    Ventricular tachycardia
    Ventricular flutter and fibrillation
    "Bidirectional" ventricular tachycardia
    Parasystolic ventricular tachycardia
2. Depression of pacemakers
    SA arrest
3. Depression of conduction
    SA block
    A-V block
    Exit block
4. Ectopic rhythms with depression of conduction
5. A-V dissociation (suppression of dominant pacemaker with escape pacemaker or inappropriate acceleration of lower pacemaker)
6. "Triggered" automaticity
    Accelerated junctional impulses after premature ectopic impulses
    Ventricular arrhythmias "triggered" by supraventricular arrhythmias
    Junctional tachycardia "triggered" by ventricular tachycardia

SA = sinoatrial; A-V = atrioventricular.

Table 141-2. Characteristics of Acute and Chronic Digitalis Toxicity

	Acute toxicity	Chronic toxicity
Gastrointestinal toxicity	Nausea, vomiting	Nausea, vomiting
CNS toxicity	Headache, weakness, dizziness, confusion, and coma	Confusion, coma
Cardiac toxicity	Bradyarrhythmias, supraventricular arrhythmias with A-V block	Virtually any arrhythmia (ventricular or supraventricular arrhythmias with or without A-V block)
	Ventricular arrhythmias are uncommon	Ventricular arrhythmias are common
Serum potassium	Elevated but may be normal (high levels correlated with toxicity)	Low or normal (hypokalemia secondary to concomitant diuretic use)
Serum digoxin level	Markedly elevated	May be within "therapeutic" range or minimally elevated

A-V = atrioventricular.
Adapted and combined from references 11,13,20,29,75.

Diagnostic Evaluation

Evaluation of patients with actual or potential CG poisoning should include a thorough history and focused physical examination. The intent of the overdose (suicidal or accidental), time of ingestion, and coingestants are important points. Physical examination should focus on accurate measurement of vital signs and evaluation of cardiac, gastrointestinal, and neurologic symptoms. Laboratory assessment should include serum calcium and magnesium levels, renal function tests, oxygen saturation or arterial blood gas analysis, a stat serum digoxin concentration and serial serum potassium levels. The patient should have continuous cardiac monitoring, a 12-lead electrocardiogram (ECG), and a chest radiograph.

SERUM DIGOXIN LEVELS. Measurement of serum digoxin and digitoxin concentrations by radioimmunoassay can assist in the diagnosis of CG toxicity [42]. The limitations of drug levels need to be thoroughly understood, because serum digoxin levels often do not serve as reliable indicators of toxicity [28]. Commonly accepted therapeutic levels of digoxin are 0.8 to 2.0 ng per milliliter [43]. A "therapeutic" level does not exclude toxicity, however, as predisposing factors can cause an individual to become poisoned despite a level within the therapeutic range. Conversely, levels above the upper limits of normal (>2 ng/ml) do not always cause toxicity [43].

Interpretation of the serum level must take into account the differences between acute and chronic poisoning. Although a review of 50 prospective and retrospective studies found that patients on chronic therapy who had clinical evidence of toxicity had two- to three-fold higher mean drug levels than those without toxicity, there was considerable overlap of drug levels between groups [1]. *Hence, levels should be interpreted in the overall clinical context and not relied on as the sole indicator of the presence or absence of chronic toxicity* [7,44]. A temporal correlation with clinical improvement and drug withdrawal or prompt termination of arrhythmias after Fab fragment administration confirms CG toxicity.

High digoxin levels following an acute ingestion are not always associated with clinical signs or symptoms of poisoning [37,45]. Digoxin follows a two-compartment model of distribution, with relatively rapid absorption into the plasma compartment and then slow redistribution into the tissue compartment [2,17,37,43]. Serum levels most reliably correlate with toxicity when obtained after distribution is complete, which occurs 6 hours or more after oral or intravenous administration of digoxin [2,43,46]. High serum levels may enhance renal clearance of digoxin and shorten its elimination half-life after an acute overdose [37].

Naturally occurring digitalis glycosides from plants and animals can also cross-react with the digoxin assay. The degree of cross-reactivity is unknown, and no correlation has been established between serum levels of these glycosides and toxicity [47,48,49]. A digoxinlike immunoreactive substance detected in neonates and patients with renal insufficiency, hepatic dysfunction, or third-trimester pregnancy may further limit the usefulness of serum digoxin measurements [50–55].

SERUM ELECTROLYTES. Laboratory parameters that may be abnormal in CG toxicity include serum potassium, magnesium, and calcium levels. Acute poisoning of the Na^+/K^+ ATPase pump may result in markedly elevated serum potassium levels [56]. A potassium level of 13 mEq per liter was reported in one acutely poisoned patient [56]. A 46 percent incidence of hyperkalemia has been noted in patients with severe acute poisoning [23]. In fact, serum potassium may be a better indicator of end-organ toxicity than the serum digoxin level in the acutely poisoned patient [37,57,58]. In contrast, hypokalemia and hypomagnesemia are commonly seen in the chronically intoxicated patient, presumably as a result of concomitant diuretic use.

Management

The management of CG poisoning includes supportive care, prevention of further drug absorption, enhanced drug elimination, antidotal therapy, and safe disposition. Meticulous attention to supportive care and a search for easily correctable conditions, such as hypoxia, hypoventilation, hypovolemia, hypoglycemia, and electrolyte disturbances, are top priorities. All patients should have an intravenous line established and continuous cardiac monitoring. Patients with clinical toxicity or elevated serum digoxin levels should be admitted to the intensive care unit (ICU).

GASTROINTESTINAL DECONTAMINATION. Prevention of further drug absorption should be addressed after life support measures have been initiated. Activated charcoal is the agent of choice [59]. It not only prevents absorption but also may enhance the elimination of digoxin and digitoxin by interrupting their enterohepatic and enteroenteric recirculation (i.e., "gastrointestinal dialysis") [60]. The half-life of digoxin is decreased from a mean time of 36 hours to 21.5 ± 6.5 hours when repeated doses of activated charcoal are given [61]. Elimination following both oral and intravenous digoxin administration is enhanced by administration of multiple doses of activated charcoal [61–65]. Digitoxin elimination is also increased by multiple-dose activated charcoal therapy [64,66].

The use of gastric lavage is controversial. Because activated charcoal is so effective, lavage has a limited role. In fact, asystole has occurred during this procedure in a digoxin-toxic patient [67]. Since vagal stimulation as a result of lavage was considered to be responsible, pretreatment with atropine prior to performing gastric lavage has been suggested [12,67]. Syrup of ipecac should be reserved for home treatment of children with minimal ingestions.

TREATMENT OF BRADYARRHYTHMIAS. Conventional treatment of bradyarrhythmias includes the use of atropine, isoproterenol, and cardiac pacing. Since CG-enhanced vagal activity is reversed by atropine sulfate, this agent has been used successfully in patients exhibiting A-V block [17,68,69]. Cardiac pacing has been advocated for bradyarrhythmias unresponsive to atropine [70,71]. However, with digitalis toxicity, cardiac tissue may be unresponsive to electrical pacing, the fibrillation threshold may be lowered, and the pacing wire may induce ventricular fibrillation [12,70,71].

TREATMENT OF VENTRICULAR ARRHYTHMIAS. The treatment of ventricular arrhythmias induced by CGs is different from treatment of those of other etiologies. The antiarrhythmic of choice is phenytoin; it increases the ventricular fibrillation threshold in the myocardium and enhances conduction through the A-V node [1,12,72]. Lidocaine has been advocated for treatment of ventricular arrhythmias due to digitalis toxicity, although it does not affect A-V nodal conduction [12,28]. Bretylium has been reported to be effective in suppressing arrhythmias in digitalis-toxic patients, but it has enhanced arrhythmias in digitalis-toxic animal models [73–76]. Amiodarone was reported to be effective in two cases refractory to other antiarrhythmics [40,77]. Quinidine and procainamide are contraindicated in digitalis toxicity because they depress A-V nodal conduction and may worsen cardiac toxicity [1,78]. Electrical cardioversion of the digitalis-toxic patient must be performed with extreme caution and considered only as a last resort. A low energy setting (e.g., 10–25 W-sec) should be used and preparations made to treat potential ventricular fibrillation [1,12,48,79].

TREATMENT OF METABOLIC ABNORMALITIES. Supplemental potassium may be beneficial in chronic digitalis toxicity when diuretic-induced hypokalemia is a factor. It should be given cautiously, as renal failure may be the cause of chronic digitalis toxicity. Potassium should not be routinely administered to the acutely poisoned patient, because hyperkalemia is common [37,80]. Patients with acute CG poisoning who exhibit hyperkalemia may be treated with glucose, insulin, and sodium bicarbonate, although these therapies may be ineffective [81]. The exchange resin, sodium polystyrene sulfonate, also should be considered. Hemodialysis may be of benefit in a CG-poisoned patient with uncontrolled hyperkalemia. Intravenous calcium to treat hyperkalemia is controversial in CG-poisoned patients, as hypercalcemia may enhance digitalis cardiac toxicity [15,82].

Hypomagnesemia has been reported in a significant number of patients with chronic CG toxicity [34,35,83]. Intravenous administration of magnesium has been shown to counteract ventricular irritability from digitalis toxicity [78,83–86]. The recommended dose of magnesium for malignant ventricular arrhythmias is 2 to 4 gm (10–20 ml of a 20% solution) given intravenously over 1 minute. It should be infused more slowly in patients with ectopy who are hemodynamically stable. Magnesium may also be helpful in treating hyperkalemia [87]. It should be used with extreme caution, if at all, in renal failure patients.

TREATMENT WITH DIGOXIN-SPECIFIC FAB FRAGMENTS. A milestone in the treatment of CG poisoning was the development of drug-specific antibodies. Digoxin-specific Fab (Digibind) is an antibody fragment produced by papain digestion of sheep immunoglobulin (IgG) antibodies to digoxin. Affinity chromatography is used to isolate these fragments further. Advantageous characteristics of Fab fragments over IgG itself include a larger volume of distribution with increased tissue penetration, decreased immunogenicity, and increased renal excretion [23,88,89,90].

Since the effect of digoxin on isolated human myocardium is reversed by Fab fragments, they appear to be capable of completely removing digoxin from binding sites [91]. Fab fragments can reverse digitalis-induced arrhythmias, conduction disturbances, myocardial depression, and hyperkalemia in severely poisoned patients [23,81,92–101]. In a multicenter study, 90 percent of 150 patients with digoxin or digitoxin toxicity had a complete or partial response to Fab fragment administration [81]. Most patients had an initial response to CG-toxic arrhythmias within 30 minutes of Fab administration [81]. Patients who responded had complete resolution by 4 hours [23,81,93]. Failure rates to administration of Fab fragments have ranged from 10 to 20 percent in clinical series [5,81,101]. These failures have been attributed to inadequate dosing, moribund clinical state prior to Fab fragment administration, and incorrect diagnosis of digitalis toxicity.

Toxicity has been reported from the ingestion of plants containing CG [48,49]. Animal studies and case reports have demonstrated the efficacy of Fab fragments to the CG contained in oleander [49,102]. Fab fragments have also been reported to be beneficial in digitoxin poisoning [23,81,96,103,104].

Adverse reactions to Fab administration have been few [5,81,99,101,105]. Hypersensitivity reactions have been a concern because Fab fragments are derived from sheep antibodies. Mild allergic reactions have been reported and include rash, flushing, and facial swelling. No cases of serum sickness or anaphylaxis have been reported [81,101]. Prior to Fab administration, an asthma and allergy history (especially allergic reactions to antibiotics) should be obtained; intradermal skin testing should be considered in high-risk patients [101]. Precipitous drop in serum potassium, development of cardiogenic shock in a patient dependent on digoxin for inotropic support, and recurrence of CG toxicity have also been reported [81,99,101,106]. Recurrent toxicity occurred in 3 percent of patients reported in a large observational surveillance study [101]. In most, it was attributed to inadequate Fab dosing. All patients who received a repeat dose of Fab had a partial response, with complete reversal of CG toxicity in most [101].

Fab fragment therapy is indicated for severely intoxicated patients who do not immediately respond to conventional therapies. Specifically, it should be given to patients with arrhythmias that threaten or result in hemodynamic compromise [29]. Patients with hyperkalemia following acute CG overdose should also be treated with Fab fragments [81,100]. Antibody therapy should be available at the bedside. Administer Fab when early signs of cardiac toxicity occur in patients presenting with acute massive CG ingestions or chronically poisoned patients with risk factors for severe toxicity, such as old age, preexisting cardiac disease, and renal impairment.

Although serum digoxin levels should not be the sole factor in determining the need to administer Fab [37,107], dosage calculations for Fab are based on the serum digoxin level or estimated body load of digoxin. It is assumed that equimolar doses of antibody fragments are required to achieve neutralization [23,93]. Forty milligrams of Fab (1 vial) will bind 0.6 mg of digoxin. The number of vials required can be calculated by dividing the total body burden by 0.6. The body burden can be estimated from the milligram amount of an acute ingestion or by multiplying the serum digoxin level (ng/ml) by 5.6 (0.56 for digitoxin) times the body weight (kg) and dividing by 1000. A median dose of 200 mg (5 vials, range 120–480 mg) was required to treat effectively 150 seriously digitalis-toxic patients with a mean serum digoxin level of 8.0 ng per milliliter [81]. A severely toxic patient in whom the quantity ingested acutely is unknown should be given 5 to 10 vials at a time and the clinical response observed. If cardiac arrest is imminent or has occurred, the dose can be given as a bolus. Otherwise, it should be infused over 30 minutes. In contrast, patients with chronic therapeutic overdose often have only mildly elevated digoxin levels and respond to one to two vials of antibody. The recommended dose for a given patient can be determined using the tables in the package insert or by contacting a regional poison center.

Free digoxin levels are decreased to zero within 1 minute of Fab fragment administration, but total serum digoxin levels are markedly increased (Fig. 141-1) [23,90,93,108,109]. Since the radioimmunoassay method measures both bound and free digoxin, very high digoxin levels are seen after Fab fragment therapy, but they have no correlation with toxicity [54,95]. Serum levels may be unreliable for several days after Fab treatment [108]. The digoxin-Fab complex is excreted in the urine and has a half-life of 16 to 20 hours [88,96,109]. In patients with renal failure, elimination of the digoxin-Fab complex is prolonged [110]. Dissociation or metabolism of this complex leads to free digoxin levels gradually increasing over hours (44–97 hours) after Fab administration [109–112]. Of 28 patients with renal impairment given Fab, only one has been reported to have recurrent CG toxicity, which occurred 10 days after Fab treatment and persisted for 10 days [110]. Hemodialysis does not enhance elimination of digoxin-Fab complex [109].

DISPOSITION. All patients who receive Fab fragments require continued monitoring in an ICU for at least 24 hours. All suspected suicidal patients should have a psychiatric evaluation prior to discharge. For the chronically poisoned elderly patient, modifying the outpatient treatment regimen by discontinuing the use of a CG or providing a more reliable method of drug

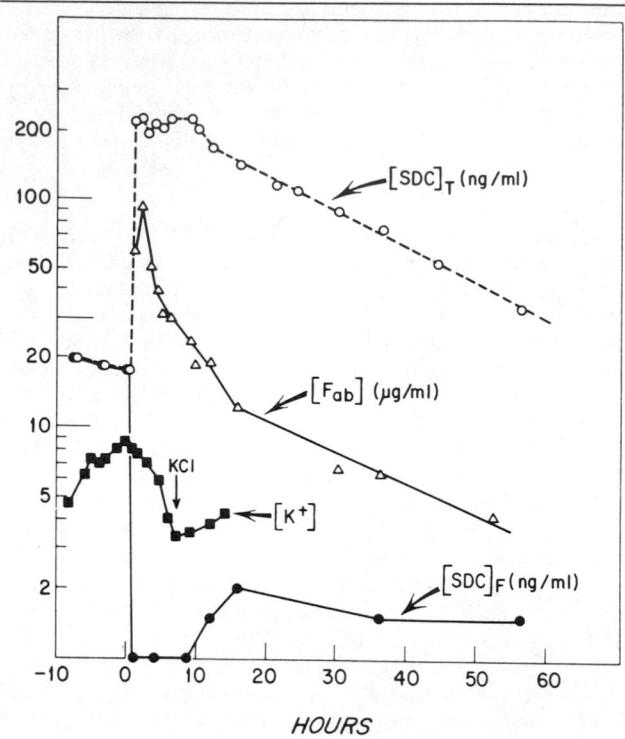

Fig. 141-1. Time course of serum potassium concentration in mEq per liter = [K⁻] (■—■); Total serum digoxin concentration = $[SDC]_T$ (O--O); free serum digoxin concentration = $[SDC]_F$ (●—●); and serum concentration of sheep digoxin-specific fab fragments = [Fab] (Δ–Δ). The scale on the vertical axis is logarithmic. On the horizontal axis, 0 denotes the time at which administration of digoxin-specific Fab fragments was started. (From Smith TW, Haber E, Yeatman L, et al: Reversal of advanced digoxin intoxication with Fab fragments of digoxin-specific antibodies. Reprinted by permission of the *New England Journal of Medicine* 294:797, 1976.)

administration with close clinical follow-up may avert further toxic episodes.

References

1. Smith TW, Antman EM, Friedman PL, et al: Digitalis glycosides: Mechanisms and manifestations. *Prog Cardiovasc Dis* 26:413, 1984.
2. Smith TW: Pharmacokinetics, bioavailability and serum levels of cardiac glycosides. *J Am Coll Cardiol* 5:43A, 1985.
3. Beller GA, Smith TW, Abelmann WH, et al: Digitalis intoxication: Prospective clinical study with serum level correlations. *N Engl J Med* 284:989, 1971.
4. Gheorghiade M, Roseman H, Mahdyoon H, et al: Incidence of digitalis intoxication. *Prim Cardiol* 1:5, 1988.
5. Mahdyoon H, Battilana G, Rosman H, et al: The evolving pattern of digoxin intoxication: Observations at a large urban hospital from 1980 to 1988. *Am Heart J* 120:1189, 1990.
6. Litovitz TT, Holm KC, Bailey KM, et al: 1991 annual report of the American Association of Poison Control Centers National Data Collection System. *Am J Emerg Med* 10:452, 1992.
7. Smith TW: Digitalis: Mechanisms of action and clinical use. *N Engl J Med* 318:358, 1988.
8. Bigger JT: Digitalis toxicity. *J Clin Pharmacol* 25:514, 1985.
9. Fisch C, Knoebel SB: Digitalis cardiotoxicity. *J Am Coll Cardiol* 5:91A, 1985.

10. Moorman JR, Pritchett EL: The arrhythmias of digitalis intoxication. *Arch Intern Med* 145:1289, 1985.
11. Doherty JE: Digitalis glycosides: Pharmacokinetics and their implications. *Ann Intern Med* 79:229, 1973.
12. Sharff JA, Bayer MJ: Acute and chronic digitalis toxicity: Presentation and treatment. *Ann Emerg Med* 11:327, 1982.
13. Wofford JL, Ettinger WH: Risk factors and manifestations of digoxin toxicity in the elderly. *Am J Emerg Med* 9:11, 1991.
14. Lely A, Van Enter C: Large scale digitoxin intoxication. *Br Med J* 3:737, 1970.
15. Elkins BR, Watanabe AS: Acute digoxin poisoning: Review of therapy. *Am J Hosp Pharm* 35:268, 1978.
16. Dubnow MH, Burchell HB: A comparison of digitalis intoxication in two separate periods. *Ann Intern Med* 62:956, 1965.
17. Smith TW, Willerson JT: Suicidal and accidental digoxin ingestion. *Circulation* 44:29, 1971.
18. Wambolt FS, Jefferson JW, Wambolt MZ: Digitalis intoxication misdiagnosed as depression by primary care physicians. *Am J Psychiatry* 143:219, 1986.
19. Closson RG: Visual hallucinations as the earliest symptom of digoxin intoxication. *Arch Neurol* 40:386, 1983.
20. Volpe BT, Soave R: Formed visual hallucinations as digitalis toxicity. *Ann Intern Med* 91:865, 1979.
21. Shear MK, Sacks MH: Digitalis delirium: Report of two cases. *Am J Psychiatry* 135:109, 1978.
22. Carney MWP, Rapp S, Pearace K: Digoxin toxicity presenting with psychosis in a patient with chronic phobic anxiety. *Clin Neuropharmacol* 8:193, 1985.
23. Wenger TL, Butler VP, Haber E, et al: Treatment of 63 severely digitalis-toxic patients with digoxin-specific antibody fragments. *J Am Coll Cardiol* 5:118A, 1985.
24. Rosen MR, Witt AL, Hoffman BF: Cardiac antiarrhythmic and toxic effects of digitalis. *Am Heart J* 89:391, 1975.
25. Smith TW, Haber E: Digitalis. *N Engl J Med* 289:945, 1973.
26. Gould L, Patel C, Betzu R, et al: Right bundle branch block: A rare manifestation of digitalis toxicity—case report. *Angiology* 37:543, 1986.
27. Dreifus LS, McNight EH, Katz M, et al: Digitalis intolerance. *Geriatrics* 18:494, 1963.
28. Kelly RA, Smith TW: Recognition and management of digitalis toxicity. *Am J Cardiol* 69:108G, 1992.
29. Marchlinski FE, Hook BG, Callans DJ: Which cardiac disturbances should be treated with digoxin immune Fab (ovine) antibody? *Am J Emerg Med* 9:24, 1991.
30. Friedman PL: Factors in individual sensitivity to cardiac glycosides and recognition of digitalis intoxication. *Prim Cardiol* 1:13, 1988.
31. Damato AN, Lau HS, Bobb GA: Digitalis induced bundle branch ventricular tachycardia studied by electrode catheter recordings of the specialized conducting tissues of the dog. *Circ Res* 28:16, 1971.
32. Akera T, Ng Y: Digitalis sensitivity of Na,K-ATPase, myocytes and the heart. *Life Sci* 48:97, 1991.
33. Mason DT, Zelis R, Lee G, et al: Current concepts and treatment of digitalis toxicity. *Am J Cardiol* 27:546, 1971.
34. Beller GA, Hood WB, Smith TW, et al: Prevalence of hypomagnesemia in a prospective clinical study of digitalis intoxication. *Am J Cardiol* 26:625, 1970.
35. Beller GA, Hood WB, Smith TW, et al: Correlation of serum magnesium levels and cardiac digitalis intoxication. *Am J Cardiol* 33:225, 1974.
36. Hall RJ, Gelbart A, Silverman M, et al: Studies on digitalis-induced arrhythmias in glucose- and insulin-induced hypokalemia. *J Pharmacol Exp Ther* 201:711, 1977.
37. Springer M, Olsen KR, Feaster W: Acute massive digoxin overdose: Survival without use of digitalis-specific antibodies. *Am J Emerg Med* 4:364, 1986.
38. Belz GG, Doering W, Munkes R, et al: Interaction between digoxin and calcium antagonist and antiarrhythmic drugs. *Clin Pharmacol Ther* 33:410, 1983.
39. Klein HO, Lang R, Segni ED, et al: Verapamil-digoxin interaction. *N Engl J Med* 303:160, 1980.
40. Maheswaran R, Bramble MG, Hardisty CA: Massive digoxin overdose: Successful treatment with intravenous amiodarone. *Br Med J* 287:392, 1986.
41. Bussey HI: The influence of quinidine and other agents on digitalis glycosides. *Am Heart J* 104:289, 1982.
42. Smith TW, Butler VA, Haber E: Determination of therapeutic and toxic digoxin concentrations by radioimmunoassay. *N Engl J Med* 281:1212, 1969.
43. Seltzer A: Role of serum digoxin assay in patient management. *J Am Coll Cardiol* 5:106A, 1985.
44. Ingelfinger JA, Goldman P: The serum digitalis concentration: Does it diagnose digitalis toxicity? *N Engl J Med* 294:867, 1976.
45. Lewander WJ, Gaudreault P, Einhorn A, et al: *Am J Dis Child* 140:770, 1986.
46. Walsh FM, Sode J: Significance of non-steady-state serum digoxin concentrations. *Am J Clin Pathol* 63:446, 1975.
47. Osterloh J: Cross-reactivity of oleander glycosides (letter). *J Anal Toxicol* 12:53, 1988.
48. Haynes BE, Bessen HA, Wightman WD: Oleander tea: Herbal draught of death. *Ann Emerg Med* 14:350, 1985.
49. Shumaik GM, Wu AW, Ping AC: Oleander poisoning: Treatment with digoxin-specific Fab antibody fragments. *Ann Emerg Med* 17:732, 1988.
50. Graves SW, Brown B, Valdes R: An endogenous digoxin-like substance in patients with renal impairment. *Ann Intern Med* 99:604, 1983.
51. Greenway OC, Nanji AA: Falsely increased results for digoxin in sera from patients with liver disease: Ten immunoassay kits compared (letter). *Clin Chem* 31:1078, 1985.
52. Shilo L, Shapito MS, Doley S, et al: Endogenous digoxin-like material in patients with liver disease (letter). *Ann Intern Med* 103:643, 1985.
53. Gervais A: Digoxin-like immunoreactive substance (DLIS) in liver disease: Comparison of clinical and laboratory parameters in patients with and without DLIS. *Drug Intell Clin Pharm* 21:540, 1987.
54. Stone JA, Soldin SJ: An update on digoxin. *Clin Chem* 35:1326, 1989.
55. Stone J, Bentur Y, Salstein E, et al: Effect of endogenous digoxin-like substances on the interpretation of high concentrations of digoxin in children. *J Pediatr* 117:321, 1990.
56. Reza MJ, Kovick RB, Shine KI, et al: Massive intravenous digoxin overdosage. *N Engl J Med* 291:777, 1974.
57. Bismuth C, Gaultier M, Conso F, et al: Hyperkalemia in acute digitalis poisoning: Prognostic significance and therapeutic implications. *Clin Toxicol* 6:153, 1973.
58. Citrin D, Stevenson IH, O'Malley K: Massive digoxin overdose: Observations on hyperkalemia and plasma digoxin levels. *Scott Med J* 17:275, 1972.
59. Neuvonen PJ, Elfving SM, Elonen E: Reduction of absorption of digoxin, phenytoin and aspirin by activated charcoal in man. *Eur J Clin Pharmacol* 13:213, 1978.
60. Levy G: Gastrointestinal clearance of drugs with activated charcoal. *N Engl J Med* 307:676, 1982.
61. Lalonde RL, Deshpande R, Hamilton PP, et al: Acceleration of digoxin clearance by activated charcoal. *Clin Pharmacol Ther* 37:367, 1985.
62. Boldy DA, Smart V, Vale JA: Multiple doses of charcoal in digoxin poisoning. *Lancet* 2:1076, 1985.
63. Lake KD, Brown DC, Peterson CD: Digoxin toxicity: Enhanced systemic elimination during oral activated charcoal therapy. *Pharmacotherapy* 4:161, 1984.
64. Park GD, Goldberg MJ, Spector R, et al: The effects of activated charcoal on digoxin and digitoxin clearance. *Drug Intell Clin Pharm* 19:937, 1985.
65. Caldwell JH, Cline CR: Biliary excretion of digoxin in man. *Clin Pharmacol Ther* 19:410, 1976.
66. Pond S, Jacobs M, Marks J, et al: Treatment of digitoxin overdose with oral activated charcoal. *Lancet* 2:1177, 1981.
67. Hobson JD, Zettner A: Digoxin serum half-life following suicidal digoxin poisoning. *JAMA* 223:147, 1973.
68. Duke M: Atrioventricular block due to accidental digoxin ingestion treated with atropine. *Am J Dis Child* 124:754, 1972.
69. Hansteen V, Jacobson D, Knudsen K, et al: Acute, massive poisoning with digitoxin: Report of seven cases and discussion of treatment. *Clin Toxicol* 18:679, 1981.
70. Bismuth C, Motte G, Conso F, et al: Acute digitoxin intoxication

treated by intracardiac pacemaker: Experience in sixty-eight patients. *Clin Toxicol* 10:443, 1977.

71. Citrin DL, O'Malley K, Hillis WS: Cardiac standstill due to digoxin poisoning successfully treated with atrial pacing. *Br Med J* 2:526, 1973.

72. Rumack BH, Wolfe RR, Gilfrich H: Diphenylhydantoin (phenytoin) treatment of massive digoxin overdose. *Br Heart J* 36:405, 1974.

73. Lipski JI, Donoso E, Friedberg CK: The effect of bretylium tosylate on the normal and digitalis-sensitized dog heart. *Am Heart J* 83:769, 1972.

74. Allen JD, Zaidi SA, Shanks RG, et al: The effects of bretylium on experimental cardiac dysrhythmias. *Am J Cardiol* 29:641, 1972.

75. Gillis RA, Clancy MM, Anderson RJ: Deleterious effects of bretylium in cats with digitalis-induced ventricular tachycardia. *Circulation* 47:974, 1973.

76. Vincent JL, Dufaye P, Berre J, et al: Bretylium in severe ventricular arrhythmias associated with digitalis intoxication. *Am J Emerg Med* 2:504, 1984.

77. Nicholls DP, Murtagh JG, Holt DW: Use of amiodarone and digoxin specific Fab antibodies in digoxin overdosage. *Br Med J* 53:462, 1985.

78. French JH, Thomas RG, Siskind AP, et al: Magnesium therapy in massive digoxin intoxication. *Ann Emerg Med* 13:562, 1984.

79. Hagemeijer F, Van Houwe E: Titrated energy cardioversion of patients on digitalis. *Br Heart J* 37:1303, 1975.

80. Warren SE, Fanestil DD: Digoxin overdose, limitations of hemoperfusion and hemodialysis. *JAMA* 242:2100, 1979.

81. Antman EM, Wenger TL, Butler VP, et al: Treatment of 150 cases of life-threatening digitalis intoxication with digoxin-specific Fab antibody fragments: Final report of a multicenter study. *Circulation* 81:1744, 1990.

82. Murphy DJ, Bremmer WF, Haber E, et al: Massive digoxin poisoning treated with Fab fragments of digoxin specific antibodies. *Pediatrics* 70:472, 1982.

83. Cohen L, Kitzes R: Magnesium sulfate and digitalis-toxic arrhythmias. *JAMA* 249:2808, 1983.

84. Neff MS, Mendelssohn S, Kim KE, et al: Magnesium sulfate in digitalis toxicity. *Am J Cardiol* 29:377, 1972.

85. Seller RH, Cangiano J, Kim K, et al: Digitalis toxicity and hypomagnesemia. *Am Heart J* 79:57, 1970.

86. Specter MJ, Schweizer E, Goldman RH: Studies on magnesium's mechanism of action in digitalis-induced arrhythmias. *Circulation* 52:1001, 1975.

87. Reisdorff EJ, Clark MR, Walters BL: Acute digitalis poisoning: The role of intravenous magnesium sulfate. *J Emerg Med* 4:463, 1986.

88. Smith TW, Lloyd BL, Spicer N, et al: Immunogenicity and kinetics of distribution and elimination of sheep digoxin-specific IgG and Fab fragments in the rabbit and baboon. *Clin Exp Immunol* 36:384, 1979.

89. Lloyd BL, Smith TW: Contrasting rates of reversal of digoxin toxicity by digoxin-specific IgG and Fab fragments. *Circulation* 58:280, 1978.

90. Shaumann W, Kaufman B, Neubert P, et al: Kinetics of the Fab fragments of digoxin antibodies and of bound digoxin in patients with severe digoxin intoxication. *Eur J Clin Pharmacol* 30:527, 1986.

91. Nabauer M, Erdmann E: Reversal of toxic and nontoxic effects of digoxin-specific Fab fragments in isolated human ventricular myocardium. *Klin Wochenschr* 65:558, 1987.

92. Clarke W, Ramoska EA: Acute digoxin overdose: Use of digoxin specific antibody fragments. *Am J Emerg Med* 6:465, 1988.

93. Smolarz A, Roesch E, Lenz E, et al: Digoxin specific antibody (Fab) fragments in 34 cases of severe digitalis intoxication. *Clin Toxicol* 23:327, 1985.

94. Leikin J, Vogel S, Graff J, et al: Use of Fab fragments of digoxin-specific antibodies in the therapy of massive digoxin poisoning. *Ann Emerg Med* 14:175, 1985.

95. Smith TW, Haber E, Yeatman L, et al: Reversal of advanced digoxin intoxication with Fab fragments of digoxin-specific antibodies. *N Engl J Med* 294:797, 1976.

96. Smith TW, Butler VP, Haber E, et al: Treatment of life-threatening digitalis intoxication with digoxin-specific Fab antibody fragments: Experience in 26 cases. *N Engl J Med* 307:1357, 1982.

97. Zucker AR, Lacina AJ, DasGupta DS: Fab fragments of digoxin-specific antibodies used to reverse ventricular fibrillation induced by digoxin ingestion in a child. *Pediatrics* 70:468, 1982.

98. Desantola JR, Marchlinski FE: Response of digoxin toxic atrial tachycardia to digoxin-specific Fab fragments. *Am J Cardiol* 58:1109, 1986.

99. Woolf AD, Wenger T, Smith TW, et al: The use of digoxin-specific Fab fragments for severe digitalis intoxication in children. *N Engl J Med* 326:1739, 1992.

100. Woolf AD, Wenger TL, Smith TW, et al: Results of multicenter studies of digoxin-specific antibody fragments in managing digitalis intoxication in the pediatric population. *Am J Emerg Med* 9:16, 1991.

101. Hickey AR, Wenger TL, Carpenter VP, et al: Digoxin immune Fab therapy in the management of digitalis intoxication: Safety and efficacy results of an observational surveillance study. *J Am Coll Cardiol* 17:590, 1991.

102. Clark RF, Selden BS, Curry SC: Digoxin-specific Fab fragments in the treatment of oleander toxicity in a canine model. *Ann Emerg Med* 20:1073, 1991.

103. Ochs HR, Smith TW: Reversal of advanced digitoxin toxicity and modification of pharmacokinetics by specific antibodies and Fab fragments. *J Clin Invest* 60:1303, 1977.

104. Hess T, Riesen W, Scholtysik G, et al: Digitoxin intoxication with severe thrombocytopenia: Reversal by digoxin-specific antibodies. *Eur J Clin Invest* 13:159, 1983.

105. Kirkpatrick CH: Allergic histories and reactions of patients treated with digoxin immune Fab (ovine) antibody. *Am J Emerg Med* 9:7, 1991.

106. Baud F, Bismuth CH, Pontal PG, et al: Time course of antidigitoxin Fab fragment and plasma digitoxin concentrations in an acute digitalis intoxication. *J Toxicol Clin Toxicol* 19:857, 1982.

107. Rollins DE, Brizgys M: Immunological approach to poisoning. *Ann Emerg Med* 15:1046, 1986.

108. Gibbs I, Adams PC, Parnham AJ, et al: Plasma digoxin: Assay anomalies in Fab-treated patients. *Br J Clin Pharmacol* 16:445, 1983.

109. Clinton GD, McIntyre WJ, Zannikos PN, et al: Free and total serum digoxin concentrations in a renal failure patient after treatment with digoxin immune Fab. *Clin Pharm* 8:441, 1989.

110. Wenger TL: Experience with digoxin immune Fab (ovine) in patients with renal impairment. *Am J Emerg Med* 9:21, 1991.

111. Ujhelyi MR, Colucci RD, Cummings DM, et al: Monitoring serum digoxin concentrations during digoxin immune Fab therapy. *Drug Intell Clin Pharm* 25:1047, 1991.

112. Allen NM, Dunham GD, Sailstad JM, et al: Clinical and pharmacokinetic profiles of digoxin immune Fab in four patients with renal impairment. *Drug Intell Clin Pharm* 25:1315, 1991.

142. Envenomations

Robert L. Norris, Jr.

Overview

"Their supreme arrogance, developed over millions of years as masters of their environment, commands respect out of all proportions to their size" [1].

While this statement was made in reference to snakes, it could easily be applied to any of the countless numbers of venomous creatures on the planet. In 1991, there were 72,331 calls to 73 poison control centers in the United States regarding animal bites or stings [2]. Few areas of medicine are immersed in such emotion and controversy as the management of envenomations. This chapter focuses on envenomations by snakes, spiders, and scorpions encountered in the United States and lends guidance to evaluation and treatment.

Snake Venom Poisoning

At least 120 species of snakes are native to the United States; 20 of these are venomous [3,4]. An estimated 8000 cases of venomous snakebite with 10 to 15 deaths occur each year [5,6,7].

All American venomous snakes belong to one of two families: Crotalidae (pit vipers) and Elapidae (coral snakes). There are three genera of pit vipers—*Crotalus* and *Sistrurus* (the rattlesnakes) and *Agkistrodon* (the copperheads and cottonmouth water moccasins)—and two genera of coral snakes—*Micrurus* (the Eastern and Texas coral snakes) and *Micruroides* (the Arizona coral snake). Venomous snakes are native to every state except Alaska, Hawaii, and Maine [6,8,9,10].

PIT VIPER VENOM POISONING. At least 99 percent of venomous snakebites in the United States are inflicted by pit vipers [6]. These snakes are characterized by an extremely sensitive, pitlike heat receptor located midway between and inferior to the nostril and eye. These receptors are important to the snake in aiming its strike and may play a role in determining the quantity of venom injected [5,8,11].

Pit viper venoms, containing as many as 15 enzymatic components and an undetermined number of nonenzymatic, low-molecular-weight polypeptides, are among the most complex venoms known [3,5,8,11–15]. Research is hampered by the fact that venom composition varies not only species to species, but also snake to snake within a species, and even in an individual snake depending on its age, size, and diet and the time of year [5,8,11,12,15].

The major enzymes in pit viper venoms include hyaluronidase (spreading factor), phospholipase A (responsible for cell membrane disruption), and various proteinases (which primarily cause local tissue destruction) [3,5,11,13,15,16]. Despite the impressive toxicity of such enzymes, the nonenzymatic, low-molecular-weight polypeptide fractions appear to be more lethal—up to 20 times more lethal, on a weight-for-weight basis, than crude venom [3,4,15,17]. The overall toxicity of pit viper venom is probably enhanced by the release of various auto-

pharmacologic compounds from damaged tissue (e.g., histamine, bradykinin, and serotonin) [3,4,5,13,15,16].

Clinical Manifestations. The envenomated patient typically experiences moderate to severe pain at the bite site within 5 to 10 minutes [3,4,5,8,18]. The pain is often described as burning and may radiate along the bitten extremity [8,18]. Swelling at the bite site soon follows and may progress along the entire extremity within hours [3,4,5,8,17]. There is often local ecchymosis due to disruption of blood vessels [3,4,5,8,18]. Since the venom is largely absorbed via the lymphatics, impressive lymphangitis may appear early [7].

Within the first 24 to 36 hours, hemorrhagic bullae or serous-filled vesicles may develop at the bite site and along the bitten extremity [3,4,5]. These are uncommon in bites treated early with adequate amounts of antivenin [3,4,5,17,19]. Petechiae or purpura may also be present, due to the anticoagulant effects of the venom [3,4,5].

Systemic manifestations of pit viper venom poisoning can involve virtually every organ system. Nausea and vomiting are common and when present early may indicate severe envenomation [3,4,18,20,21]. Also common are weakness, diaphoresis, fever and chills, dizziness, and syncope [3,4,5,8,17,20]. Some patients complain of a minty, rubbery, or metallic taste in their mouth and may also experience increased salivation [3,4,5]. Tingling or numbness in the scalp, face, or digits is an indication of a moderate to severe envenomation, as are fasciculations of the face, neck, back, or bitten extremity [3,5].

Systemic anticoagulation can lead to gingival bleeding, epistaxis, hemoptysis, hematuria, hematemesis, hematochezia, or melena [3,8,18,20]. Intraperitoneal, retroperitoneal, or intracranial hemorrhage may also occur [4,5,16]. Visual disturbances may result from retinal bleeding [20,22].

There may be an increase or decrease in heart rate, and blood pressure may be low [23]. Early shock is usually due to pooling of blood in the pulmonary and splanchnic vascular beds or in the bitten extremity [8,18,24]. Delayed shock is due to hypovolemia from bleeding or third spacing and hemolysis [5,8]. Pulmonary edema, common in severe envenomations, is due primarily to destruction of the intimal lining of pulmonary blood vessels and pooling of pulmonary blood [4,8,11,13]. Some venoms appear to contain a cardiodepressant factor that may contribute to pulmonary edema [11].

Renal failure is not uncommon. The major cause is hypotension, with hemoglobin, myoglobin, and fibrin deposition in renal tubules and direct venom effects contributing to nephrotoxicity [4,8,16].

Occasionally, paresis or even frank paralysis is seen, especially following envenomation by the Eastern diamondback (*Crotalus adamanteus*) or Mojave rattlesnake (*Crotalus scutulatus*) [3,5]. Neuromuscular respiratory failure is uncommon but can occur in severe poisoning by Mojave rattlesnakes [4,5,11]. The venom of this species is characteristically more neurotoxic than that of other North American pit vipers [3,8,11,17,22,25]. In contrast, however, there may be a paucity of local findings (e.g., swelling, ecchymosis, pain) after Mojave envenomations and a delay in onset of systemic symptoms [5,8,21,26].

Snake venoms do not appear to cross the blood-brain barrier to any significant extent. Seizures and coma are uncommon;

when they do occur they are likely secondary to hypotension or hypoxia [3,5].

Diagnostic Evaluation

HISTORY/PREHOSPITAL CARE. Initial evaluation involves obtaining a history of the circumstances surrounding the incident: Was the patient actually bitten by a snake? If so, was it venomous? Photographs of indigenous venomous snakes can help victims identify the offending serpent. The patient's symptoms and any first aid measures should be assessed.

In pit viper envenomations, the most commonly accepted first aid measure is application of a wide (> 1/2 inch) constricting band 2 to 4 inches above the bite site, only tight enough to occlude the superficial veins and lymphatics [8,11,27,28]. If applied within 30 minutes of the bite this may limit some central spread of venom [4,8,29]. An arterial tourniquet must be avoided. Any jewelry that could become a tourniquet as swelling progresses should be removed. If a patient arrives with a tourniquet in place, a constricting band should be placed more proximally and the tourniquet then released. There has been very little research evaluating the use of the compression/immobilization technique of limiting venom spread following pit viper bites (see Coral Snake Venom Poisoning) [30].

Incision and suction of the bite have been recommended as first aid measures [4,20,31–35] and may be beneficial when performed by a knowledgeable health care provider within a few minutes of the bite in a victim who is more than 30 to 60 minutes from the hospital [4,5,8,14,15,17,25,36,37]. The incisions should be parallel to the axis of the extremity and should be only approximately 6 mm long and 3 mm deep (intended to open the puncture wounds so that suction can be more effective [4,5,15,17,19,28]. Cross-cuts and multiple cuts should be avoided [11,27,36,38,39]. Mechanical suction (by a device similar to the "Extractor" found in the Sawyer First Aid Kit) is preferable to mouth suction, to avoid contamination of the wound with oral flora and prevent possible envenomation of the rescuer through breaks in the mucosa of the proximal gastrointestinal (GI) tract [8,36,40]. For maximal benefit suction should be maintained for approximately 30 to 60 minutes [4,5,17,19,20,28]. Incision and suction by uninformed rescuers can result in nerve, tendon, or major vessel lacerations.

Ice should be avoided [5,17,36,41]. The American Red Cross recommends that no cooling measures of any kind be used in venomous snakebite [42]. Cooling may actually drive some venom components deeper into the tissues [5]. Similarly, although high-voltage, low-amperage electrical shock has been used in managing snakebite victims in Ecuador [43], controlled animal studies have failed to demonstrate the efficacy of this technique [44–48]. Applying shock to snakebites using "stun guns," car batteries, or electric motors may have significant adverse effects and should not be performed [48,49,50]. First aid efforts are best directed at reassuring the victim, immobilizing and splinting the extremity at approximately heart level, and transporting the victim as quickly as possible to the hospital [5,27,41]. Victims should expend a minimum amount of energy getting to the hospital, to limit cardiac output and central spread of venom. Victims are rarely a great distance from medical care [5,51], but when they are, companions must weigh the risks and benefits of carrying the victim out, having the victim hike out, or going to bring back assistance.

Other important aspects of the history include the patient's past medical history, medications, allergies, and tetanus status. Any prior venomous snakebite, especially if antivenin therapy was used, should be noted. Patients who have received antivenin treatment previously may be at increased risk of an allergic reaction if antivenin is required again.

PHYSICAL EXAMINATION/SEVERITY ASSESSMENT. If a venomous snake is positively or presumptively identified, it must next be determined whether the bite resulted in envenomation: 20 to 30 percent of bites by U.S. pit vipers do not result in envenomation ("dry bites") [4,5,14,19,41,52]. If envenomation has occurred, its severity should be assessed. The grading scale in Table 142-1 summarizes the experience of a number of experts [3,5,14,16,17,20,40,52,53,54].

A dry bite may or may not have fang puncture marks, but there is no more pain than would be expected from simple puncture wounds. Swelling is absent. A mild or minimal envenomation yields moderate to severe pain and mild swelling. There are no systemic symptoms or signs and no laboratory abnormalities. Systemic manifestations and laboratory abnormalities begin to appear with moderate envenomations and become more pronounced with severe envenomations. The very severe category includes victims who have received deep intramuscular or intravascular envenomations or who have been bitten by exceptionally large snakes with tremendous venom deposition [20,55]. These patients may be in shock on

Table 142-1. Clinical Grading Scale and Recommended Dosage of Antivenin for Native U.S. Pit Viper Venom Poisoning[a]

	Nonenvenomation	Mild	Moderate	Severe	Very severe
Fang marks	±	+	+	+	+
Pain	None	Moderate	Severe	Severe	Very severe
Edema	None	Minimal (0–15 cm)[b]	Moderate (15–30 cm)[b]	Severe (>30 cm)[b]	Minimal or severe[c]
Erythema	None	+	+	+	+
Ecchymosis	None	±	+	+	+
Systemic signs and symptoms	None	None	Mild	Moderate to severe	Very severe
Laboratory values	NL	NL	Mildly abnormal	Very abnormal	Profoundly abnormal
Initial antivenin dose (number of vials)[d]	0	0 or 5	10	15	≥15

[a]Not applicable to coral snake or Mojave rattlesnake envenomations.
[b]Proximal spread of edema.
[c]Minimal swelling may occur with IM or IV envenomation [20].
[d]Larger doses may be required in some cases.
NL = normal

presentation [56]. It is important to keep in mind all aspects of the patient's condition (local findings, systemic complaints, laboratory abnormalities) when determining severity and to reassess these parameters continually. This system of grading does not apply to Mojave rattlesnake bites because of their different presentation and course [21,26].

Pit viper envenomation is a true emergency, with the potential for multisystem poisoning [4,41]. Good clinical judgment is more important than reliance on grading scales [4,5,56]. Consultation with an authority in the area of snake venom poisoning can be quite helpful. The University of Arizona Poison and Drug Information Center [telephone (520) 626-6016] maintains an around-the-clock consultant to advise physicians on the management of this problem. It also maintains a current index of locations of exotic snake antivenins and can assist physicians treating patients bitten by such snakes.

During the initial examination, several locations on the bitten extremity (at the bite site and at least two sites more proximal) should be marked and the circumferences measured. Measurements should be repeated every 15 minutes until swelling is no longer progressing and every 1 to 4 hours thereafter [3,4,5,28]. If swelling is progressive or systemic findings are present, the need for antivenin is likely [5,22]. If a pressure/immobilization device has been applied in the field so that the bite site is not visible for examination and the patient is not exhibiting systemic signs and symptoms, a constricting band should be applied more proximally, an intravenous line should be established, and the device should be slowly removed to allow assessment. If systemic manifestations appear, the device should be rapidly reapplied and antivenin therapy begun as outlined below. If systemic signs and symptoms are already present, the device should be left in place until antivenin therapy is started.

ANCILLARY STUDIES. Laboratory analysis should include a complete blood count with platelets; analysis of serum electrolytes, glucose, blood urea nitrogen, and creatinine; liver function studies; amylase; creatinine phosphokinase; prothrombin time (PT), partial thromboplastin time (PTT), fibrinogen and fibrin degradation products; arterial blood gases; and urinalysis and urine myoglobin. It is vital to obtain a sample for typing and cross-matching on the first blood drawn, as both direct venom effects and antivenin effects can interfere with later cross-matching [20]. An admission chest radiograph and electrocardiogram are indicated in moderate to severe cases and in patients older than 40 years [4,8,15]. It may also be useful to obtain soft tissue radiographs of the bite site to look for a retained fang. Laboratory evaluation should be repeated at frequent intervals during the acute phase to assess for progressive systemic toxicity.

DIFFERENTIAL DIAGNOSIS. The diagnosis of pit viper envenomation is usually clear-cut, given a history of a snakebite and the characteristic presentation. When patients present without having seen a snake and having no findings other than puncture wounds and mild pain, the differential diagnosis includes other animal or arthropod bites (e.g., nonvenomous snakes, centipedes, spiders), plant or thorn puncture wounds (e.g., cactus), and bacterial fasciitis or myonecrosis. A persistent bloody effluent from the wound suggests the presence of snake venom anticoagulants and should heighten concern regarding snake envenomation, as should the presence of pain out of proportion to the wound.

Management

INITIAL MEASURES. Initial management centers on assessing the airway, breathing, and circulatory status. Oxygen should be given to any envenomed patient and two large-bore intravenous lines of normal saline or Ringer's lactate established, preferably in a site other than the bitten extremity. Cardiac and pulse oximetry monitoring are also indicated.

ANTIVENIN THERAPY. The current standard of care for significant pit viper venom poisoning involves the judicious use of antivenin [3,4,9,25,57]. In the United States, the recommended product is an equine, polyvalent antiserum made by Wyeth labs (Antivenin [Crotalidae] Polyvalent). It is variably effective in reversing systemic effects of all North American pit viper venoms [25,53,58,59]. The venoms of four different pit vipers—the Eastern diamondback rattlesnake (*Crotalus adamanteus*), Western diamondback rattlesnake (*C. atrox*), fer-de-lance (*Bothrops atrox*), and South American rattlesnake (*C. durissus*)—are used to hyperimmunize horses in the preparation of this product. There is evidence that Wyeth antivenin is less protective in bites by some U.S. pit vipers, such as the prairie rattlesnake (*C. viridis*) [60,61], the Mojave rattlesnake [62], and probably the timber rattlesnake (*C. horridus horridus*). This is due to potent toxins in these snake venoms that are present in only low concentration in the venoms used for antivenin production [63]. For this reason, larger doses of antivenin may be required in treating bites by these species [59,62].

The efficacy of antivenin in limiting local wound necrosis is controversial, but it appears to be of benefit if given early [19,20,41,63–68]. Systemic abnormalities are most responsive to antivenin administered during the first 24 hours after envenomation [3,4,11,69]. After 24 hours it may be beneficial to patients with extremely severe systemic findings, especially coagulopathy [3,14,41,69]. Recommendations for initial dosages are outlined in Table 142-1.

The use of antivenin for mild envenomations is controversial. If used, at least five vials should be administered [5,19,25]. Children should receive at least the same dose as adults; due to the relatively greater venom load, they may occasionally require doses 50 percent larger than adults [8,20,25,36,53,70]. Bites to the head, neck, and digits also tend to require more antivenin [5,17,25,26,36,59].

While the antivenin package insert recommends a skin test to identify patients at risk for an allergic reaction, the test is neither sensitive nor specific. As many as 10 percent of patients with a negative skin test still have an immediate reaction to the antivenin infusion [71], and there are multiple reports of patients receiving antivenin after a positive skin test without developing a systemic reaction [71,72,73]. A positive skin test does not contraindicate the use of antivenin in a life-threatening envenomation [5,26,53]. Furthermore, it takes 15 to 30 minutes to apply and read the skin test, delaying antivenin treatment. The sooner adequate circulating levels of antivenin are achieved, the more protective it is. Once venom proteins bind to their target sites, the effects cannot be reversed [74]. In addition, it is possible for patients to develop an anaphylactic reaction to the skin test dose itself [75]. With all of these considerations in mind, it is wiser in circumstances where the need for antivenin is clear-cut to forego skin testing and proceed with intravenous administration, initially at a very slow rate, while observing closely for any signs of adverse reactions.

If a skin test is performed, epinephrine should be available for use in the event of a reaction. It is best to use 0.02 ml of a 1:10 dilution of reconstituted antivenin for the test dose, as opposed to the normal horse serum that comes in a separate vial with the antivenin. There is evidence that the constituent proteins in the antivenin differ from those in the normal horse serum, which may explain negative skin test results in some patients who subsequently have an antivenin reaction [76]. If there is a high likelihood of allergic reaction, a 1:100 dilution of antivenin can be used for the test [53,58].

Skin testing should never be performed unless the decision has already been made that the patient needs antivenin. This is due to a risk of anaphylaxis to the test dose and because the test may sensitize the patient to equine serums should such a product be necessary in the future.

Once the need for antivenin has been established, informed consent should be obtained from the patient, if possible. Each vial is diluted in 50 to 100 ml of normal saline, Ringer's lactate, or D_5W (this volume may be reduced in pediatric patients) [5,14,25,41,53]. Wyeth's antivenin comes in a lyophilized state and must be reconstituted before administration. This is best accomplished by releasing the vacuum in the vial with a sterile needle. Next, 10 ml of *warm* diluent is slowly injected into the vial and the mixture is gently agitated under warm water until the antivenin is in solution. This may take 15 minutes per vial, so reconstitution is begun as soon as the need for antivenin is recognized.

Antivenin is administered intravenously, preferably in an unbitten extremity [5,20,36]. There is no benefit in administering antivenin locally at the bite site, since the venom is rapidly bound to local tissue proteins [5,20,36]. A prophylactic dose of intravenous diphenhydramine (e.g., 50–100 mg over 5 minutes in an adult) may limit immediate reactions to the antivenin (see below) [26,41,53]. Adequate volume expansion prior to antivenin administration is important to limit early hypotensive responses [25]. Epinephrine should be immediately available and the physician must be at the bedside to observe for reactions. The antivenin infusion is started slowly (several drops per minute) and increased if there is no reaction, so that the total dose is administered within 2 to 4 hours [5, 25]. Antivenin administration should begin several minutes prior to removing constricting bands [15,36,41].

If an allergic reaction occurs during antivenin administration the infusion should be temporarily halted and diphenhydramine along with epinephrine and/or steroids administered as needed (see Chap. 83) [3,5,19,25]. Usually the infusion can then be restarted at a slower rate [3,5,19,25]. The antivenin can be further diluted if the patient can tolerate the volume load.

After the initial dose of antivenin is administered, the patient must be closely monitored for any progression of swelling, systemic symptoms, or abnormal laboratory values [25,41]. Should progression occur, further antivenin is given as needed (one to five vials every 30 minutes to 2 hours) [5,8,25]. With adequate antivenin administration, pain may be reduced, swelling should cease, systemic symptoms should improve, vital signs should normalize, and laboratory abnormalities should not worsen [5,36,40,41,77,78].

Management of envenomated patients with a history of horse serum allergy or a positive skin test can be difficult. If antivenin administration is deemed necessary in the face of a positive skin test or a reaction to the initial infusion, a prudent course would be to institute invasive hemodynamic monitoring (arterial line and pulmonary artery catheter) and administer large doses of intravenous antihistamines and steroids [25,79]. An intravenous epinephrine drip can be started in a different extremity (e.g., 1 mg epinephrine in 500 ml of diluent) and the dilute antivenin infusion started very slowly. If a reaction occurs, the antivenin should be temporarily halted, epinephrine infused until a sympathomimetic response is noted (increased heart rate), and then the antivenin restarted. By titrating the antivenin with the epinephrine, a sufficient amount of antivenin may be administered. Several authors have reported success using an alternating antivenin-epinephrine approach [8,71,79]. The antivenin package insert outlines a method of desensitizing patients [58], but this technique proves too slow to be clinically beneficial [8,11,17].

The adverse effects of antivenin can be divided into three major groups. The first reaction is an immediate, type I, IgE-mediated anaphylactic reaction that occurs in 3 to 25 percent of patients receiving antivenin (with approximately 50% of these being significant reactions) [71,80]. It is treated as outlined above. Although only a few deaths, possibly due to anaphylaxis, have been reported in almost 40 years of snake antivenin use in the United States, many more have occurred but gone unreported [9,40]. A second immediate reaction that can occur is a non-IgE-mediated, anaphylactoid response characterized by hypotension [25]. This occurs due to direct mast cell degranulation in response to rapid administration of foreign protein [25]. It can be limited by premedicating the patient with antihistamines, volume expansion, and administering the antivenin in a sufficiently dilute form or at a sufficiently slow rate [25]. The third and most common reaction is a delayed, type III, IgG- or IgM-mediated serum sickness response characterized by pruritus, fever, arthralgias, lymphadenopathy, and malaise, which occurs approximately 1 to 2 weeks after therapy [8,26,71]. Serum sickness is noted in approximately 30 to 75 percent of patients given antivenin (nearly 100% if they receive more than seven vials) [8,26,40,80]. Its occurrence is not predicted by skin test results [8,25,26,80]. This type of response is usually benign and easily treated with steroids, antihistamines, and nonsteroidal antiinflammatory drugs until symptoms resolve [17,26,53,80].

SUPPORTIVE MEASURES. Venom-induced hypotension should be treated by volume expansion. If it fails to respond promptly to crystalloid infusion (e.g. 1–2 liters in an adult or 20 ml/kg in a child), administration of albumin is advisable [5,11,24,41,81]. Pressors should be used only as a last resort [4,5,41,53]. Although envenomation can result in significant coagulopathies, the incidence of clinically significant bleeding is surprisingly low [16,25,57,81,82]. Management of coagulopathy in patients with evidence of clinically significant bleeding (other than hematuria or minor gingival bleeding) includes administration of appropriate blood products (packed red blood cells, platelets, fresh frozen plasma, cryoprecipitate) [4,5,25,83]. It is vital to begin antivenin administration prior to the infusion of such products to avoid adding fuel to a consumptive coagulopathy [84]. Therapy to prevent acute renal failure includes ensuring adequate hydration, closely monitoring urinary output, and possibly alkalinizing the urine in patients with rhabdomyolysis. If renal failure occurs, dialysis and electrolyte homeostasis maintenance may be required [4,5,22]. Dialysis does not, however, remove circulating venom components [5,19].

WOUND CARE. Wound care begins with cleansing the bite site with a suitable germicidal solution and covering it with a dry, sterile dressing. The extremity should be placed in a well-padded splint in a position of function with cotton between the digits and should be elevated after antivenin has been started or if antivenin is not required [4,5,8,11,28,41,85]. Routine use of antibiotic prophylaxis is controversial, but it is generally advisable for anything greater than a trivial envenomation [8,15,28]. A broad-spectrum antibiotic such as ampicillin, tetracycline, erythromycin, or a first-generation cephalosporin is sufficient [8,11,85,86]. Adequate tetanus prophylaxis is important [5].

The wound can be soaked several times each day in a 1:20 Burow's solution and bathed daily in a sterile whirlpool [4,5,8,11]. Necrotic areas are painted with triple dye solution (brilliant green 1:400, gentian violet 1:400, acriflavine 1:1000) several times each week [4,5,8]. Surgical debridement of the wound may also be required. Daily oxygen treatments to the bite site via oxygen tubing placed inside a vented plastic bag around the extremity have been recommended [4,5]. Hyperbaric oxygen may be beneficial in cases of severe necrosis [4,5]. Hemorrhagic blebs, vesicles, and superficial necrotic tissue should be debrided after 3 to 5 days [4,5,8,11,87]. Physical therapy, beginning after any required initial debridement, is vitally important to return the extremity to functional capacity [4,5,8,11].

SURGERY. The role of surgery in the management of pit viper envenomation remains controversial. The speed with which snake venom is absorbed makes routine excision of the bite site fruitless [16,88]. Routine exploration of the bite site does nothing to mitigate the systemic effects of the venom, may worsen the overall outcome by adding surgical trauma, and definitely prolongs hospitalization [5,16,41,81].

Some authors have recommended routine fasciotomy in pit viper envenomations [18,21,39,89]. The incidence of compartment syndrome following snake venom poisoning, however, appears to be quite low [5,57,90,91,92]. Muscle necrosis, when it occurs, is usually due to direct myonecrotic effects of venom, not vascular compromise from elevated intracompartmental pressures [5,64,90,91,93,94]. In combined series of nearly 2000 victims of pit viper envenomation, only 4 patients required fasciotomy (each of these patients received either inappropriate ice treatment or inadequate antivenin) [14,17,90,91]. Clinical findings in any envenomation can closely mimic those seen in a compartment syndrome—edema, tenderness, dusky coloration, dysesthesias, and pain on passive stretching of muscles [93]. If there is concern, intracompartmental pressures can be easily checked using readily available monitoring devices (e.g., Wick catheter). If the compartmental pressures exceed 30 to 40 mm Hg, fasciotomy is indicated in combination with appropriate antivenin administration [41,56,57,91].

OUTDATED INTERVENTIONS. Therapeutic modalities that have failed to prove clinically useful include cryotherapy, steroid therapy, heparin, and ethylenediaminetetraacetic acid (EDTA). Cryotherapy, popularized in the 1950s, consisted of packing the bitten extremity in ice water for 6 to 24 hours or longer [95,96,97]. This resulted in a large number of amputations and was subsequently abandoned [4,5,16,20,56]. While high-dose intravenous steroids have been used in the routine management of acute pit viper envenomations [18,39,56,89], this technique has never been proved to be efficacious [3,4,98,99] and there is concern that it might actually be harmful [5,11,19,41,53,56]. Heparin is not effective in reversing coagulopathy, despite the fact that this disorder bears resemblance to disseminated intravascular coagulopathy in some cases [3,5,14,41]. At one time EDTA was thought possibly to chelate proteases found in pit viper venoms [100,101]. However, no clinical studies have evaluated its effectiveness, and in animal studies it actually increased mortality when given intravenously [5].

DISPOSITION AND OUTCOME. Any patient with evidence of pit viper envenomation should be admitted to an intensive care unit (ICU) setting for at least 24 hours [15,17,25,36,53]. Proper disposition of the patient with an apparent dry bite is unclear. While some authors recommend observing these patients for 4 to 6 hours and then discharging them if no evidence of envenomation appears [3,9,15,41], a recent report of a few patients who had delayed findings of significant venom poisoning (including one death) is cause for concern [102]. It may be prudent to admit any patient bitten by a pit viper for 24 hours of observation, regardless of signs or symptoms. At the time of discharge, every patient should have appropriate follow-up arranged for continued wound care and physical therapy, and should be warned about the symptoms of serum sickness if antivenin was given [25,36]. If such symptoms occur, the patient should return promptly for appropriate therapy.

The incidence of functional disability following pit viper venom poisoning is unclear [16] but may be as high as 32 percent following upper extremity bites [56]. Death following pit viper venom poisoning is most likely to occur at 6 to 48

hours following envenomation (64% of deaths) [7,75]. Less than 17 percent of deaths occur within 6 hours and less than 4 percent within 1 hour [7,75]. There has been a significant reduction in mortality since the introduction of antivenin. Prior to the availability of antivenin, mortality rates ranged from 5 to 25 percent [5]. The mortality rate for patients treated with antivenin is approximately 0.28 percent, compared to 2.61 percent for patients who do not receive antivenin—a statistically significant difference [75]. The major reasons for poor outcome in pit viper venom poisoning are delayed presentation, inadequate fluid resuscitation, inappropriate use of vasopressors, and delayed administration or inadequate dosing of antivenin [3,28,41,80,103].

Pit viper envenomations will become less difficult when new techniques of antivenin production yield more potent agents with less risk of immunologic sequelae [104,105]. Clinical studies using such antivenins are in progress.

CORAL SNAKE VENOM POISONING. Coral snakes are reclusive animals that inflict only approximately 20 reported bites in the United States each year [2,106]. Native U.S. coral snakes can be identified by a characteristic red, yellow, and black banding pattern, with the red and yellow bands contiguous and the bands completely encircling the body ("red on yellow, kill a fellow; red on black, venom lack"). Coral snakes lack the heat receptor organs of pit vipers. Only approximately 40 percent of coral snake bites result in poisoning, due to their much less effective venom delivery mechanism [5,106].

Coral snake venoms are less complex than pit viper venoms [5]. They do not cause significant tissue necrosis but have major neurotoxic effects that appear to be due to low-molecular-weight polypeptides. Venom poisoning may result in a nondepolarizing, postsynaptic blockade similar to curare [8,107,108,109], but in contrast to curare the blockade seen with coral snake venom is quite prolonged [15,107]. It has been estimated that one large coral snake is capable of envenomating a human with four to five lethal doses of venom [110,111].

Clinical Manifestations. Difficulty in diagnosing envenomation following coral snake bites lies in the facts that there are few if any local findings at the bite site and the onset of systemic symptoms may be delayed for many hours [3,8,106,112]. The fang marks may be quite small and difficult to detect [3,5,112,113]. There is little or no pain or swelling at the site, and necrosis is notably absent [3,5,8,17,51,106,112]. The patient may complain of paresthesias at the site [5,8,17,19,112,113,114]. These may radiate proximally and may be associated with fasciculations [8,25,112]. The earliest findings may be drowsiness or euphoria [8,11,17,51]. Nausea and vomiting may be present, along with increased salivation [3,8,11,17,51,106,115]. Bulbar paralysis may occur as early as 90 minutes following the bite and can progress to peripheral paralysis [5,8,11,17, 51,106,114,115]. Findings may include extraocular muscle paresis, ptosis, pinpoint pupils, dysphagia, dysphonia, slurred speech, and laryngeal spasm [5,8,11,51,106,112,114,115]. Mild hypotension is not uncommon [5,8,11,25,106,115]. Death from coral snake envenomations is usually due to respiratory failure or cardiovascular collapse [4,7,8,75,106,107,112,116,117,118].

Diagnostic Evaluation

HISTORY/PREHOSPITAL CARE. The initial history obtained on patients reportedly bitten by coral snakes should be similar to that obtained in victims of pit viper poisoning. While there are no prehospital interventions of proved efficacy in coral snake bites [5,17], well-meaning rescuers may have attempted any number of first aid techniques. Most of the measures recommended for pit viper envenomation are of no benefit in coral snake venom poisoning, as coral snake venom is rapidly absorbed via the venous system [5]. Rapid transportation to a hospital is of utmost priority following coral snake bite [5].

In Australia, where all native venomous snakes are elapid relatives of the coral snake, a proved first aid technique is application of a compressive (elastic) bandage around the entire extremity combined with immobilization of the extremity [81,119,120]. This has been shown to decrease significantly the rate of absorption of elapid venoms [119,121–124]. While this has yet to be studied with coral snake venom, the technique is safe enough to be recommended in the initial management of coral snake bites and may well prove to be efficacious.

PHYSICAL EXAMINATION/ANCILLARY STUDIES. As with pit viper bites, attention is initially directed to the patient's airway, breathing, and circulatory status. Supplemental oxygen should be administered, cardiac and pulse oximetry monitoring should be established, and at least one intravenous line should be started. Impending respiratory failure is suggested by cyanosis, trismus, laryngeal or pharyngeal spasm, increased salivation, or any sign of bulbar paralysis [11,112]. If any of these findings are present, prophylactic intubation is indicated. Aspiration is common but can be prevented by intubating the patient prior to the onset of respiratory failure [112]. Once the airway and respiratory status appear stable, a more complete physical examination is performed. Swelling is infrequent, but if present it should be documented and observed for progression.

The clinical grading scale outlined for pit viper venom poisoning does not apply to coral snake bites due to the near total lack of local findings and the potential delay in onset of systemic symptoms [5,26]. There are no characteristic changes in routine laboratory tests in coral snake venom poisoning [5].

DIFFERENTIAL DIAGNOSIS. The differential diagnosis of coral snake venom poisoning is usually limited to bites by other brightly colored snakes, such as milk snakes and scarlet snakes. In these "coral snake mimics" the red and yellow bands are separated by black bands and the bands do not completely encircle the body. The remainder of the differential diagnosis is the same as for pit vipers.

Management

ANTIVENIN THERAPY. Definitive management of poisoning by the Eastern coral snake *(Micrurus fulvius fulvius)* and the Texas coral snake *(M. fulvius tenere)* centers around the use of another antivenin produced by Wyeth labs (Antivenin *[Micrurus fulvius]*) [5,8,36,53]. It is of no benefit in Arizona coral snake envenomations *(Micruroides euryxanthus),* but the venom of this snake is much less toxic and there have been no deaths reported after its bite [5,8,17,25,36,51,53,111].

Antivenin administration should be attempted in any patient who has clearly been bitten by a positively identified Eastern or Texas coral snake, even if no signs or symptoms are present [3,14,15,17,19,25,36,41,51,53,106,112]. Once signs and symptoms begin to appear, it may be difficult to reverse or halt their progression with antivenin [5,19,25,53,106,112].

Coral snake antivenin is administered following guidelines similar to those for pit viper antivenin: informed consent is obtained, a skin test may be performed, epinephrine is made available at the bedside, the patient is premedicated with antihistamines, and the infusion is begun slowly, and the rate gradually increased so that the total dose is given within 2 hours. The recommended starting dose is three to six vials, with each vial diluted in 50 to 100 ml of diluent [3,5,8,14,41,53,112]. If signs or symptoms subsequently appear or progress, three to five more vials should be given [3,14,41,53]. Rarely more than 10 vials is required [53]. As in pit viper envenomations, children often require larger doses of antivenin than adults [11,112]. The management of Arizona coral snake venom poisoning consists entirely of supportive care [125].

The complications of coral snake antivenin therapy are the same as those seen with pit viper antivenin. Proper management of an asymptomatic coral snake bite victim with a positive skin test or an immediate reaction to initial antivenin infusion is unclear. It may be prudent to withhold antivenin in this setting and rely on good supportive care [25,112]. If significant envenomation is suspected, the patient could be treated in a fashion similar to that outlined for pit viper envenomations, with alternating administration of antivenin and epinephrine by slow infusion. The risk of possible anaphylactic reaction must be weighed against the risks of respiratory failure with prolonged intubation and mechanical ventilation.

WOUND CARE. The wound from a coral snake bite should be washed with a germicidal solution and tetanus prophylaxis should be updated as necessary. Prophylactic antibiotics are unlikely to be beneficial, due to the superficial nature of the bite and the notable lack of tissue necrosis.

DISPOSITION AND OUTCOME. All patients with potential coral snake envenomation should be admitted to an ICU for close monitoring [53]. It has been estimated that prophylactic treatment of asymptomatic victims of coral snake bite results in approximately 25 percent receiving antivenin needlessly [112]. This is probably acceptable, considering that there have been no deaths in the United States since the antivenin became available [5,51] and that the projected case fatality rate in untreated cases is up to 10 percent [106,111]. Total resolution of all symptoms (e.g., weakness) may take several weeks [112,114].

Spider Venom Poisoning

At least 60 spider species have been implicated in bites to humans in the United States [126,127]. The two species of greatest medical importance are the widow spiders (*Latrodectus* sp.) and the brown spiders (*Loxosceles* sp.).

WIDOW SPIDER VENOM POISONING. Of five known species of widow spider in the United States [127], the black widows *(Latrodectus mactans, L. hesperus, L. variolus)* are the best known [128,129]. The female black widow is dark black and oval-shaped with a characteristic ventral red, orange, or yellow marking (typically hourglass-shaped) on the abdomen. The body is approximately 1.5 cm long, and the leg span up to 4 cm [129,130,131]. The other two species in the United States are the red-legged widow or red widow *(L. bishopi)* and the brown widow *(L. geometricus)* [127,128,129]. Widow spiders are found in all of the 48 contiguous states [127,130,132] and are responsible for the majority of spider-related deaths in the country [7]. Only the female is dangerous to humans; the male (a nondescript and much smaller brown spider) is incapable of delivering a bite through human skin [25,129,131,133].

The venoms of the various U.S. species of widow spiders appear to be very similar in composition and toxic effects [127,129,134]. On a volume-for-volume basis, they are more potent than pit viper venoms [131]. There appear to be at least six biologically active proteins in widow spider venom, with the most deleterious component being a potent neurotoxin that acts at nerve terminals, especially the neuromuscular junction [126,127,129,131,133,135]. It initially stimulates the release of neurotransmitters (acetylcholine and norepinephrine) and then blocks neurotransmission by depleting synaptic vesicles

[127,129,131,134,136–140]. Unlike pit viper venom and brown spider venom (see Brown Spider Venom Poisoning), the venom of the widow spider is incapable of producing dermonecrosis or hemolysis [135,141].

Clinical Manifestations. The widow spider bite often goes unnoticed by the patient; sometimes it is experienced as a pinprick sensation [127,129,131,133,134,142]. The bite site may be visible, with tiny fang marks approximately 1 mm apart, and the area may be slightly warm and blanched with a surrounding zone of erythematous induration [132,133,136,143,144]. Swelling is minimal [127,133].

Significant symptoms usually appear 10 minutes to 2 hours after envenomation [7,129,132,133]. The most prominent symptom is pain. It begins at the bite site as a dull ache or numbing sensation and spreads first to local muscle groups and then to larger regional muscle groups of the abdomen, back, chest, pelvis, and lower extremities [126,127,131,132,142,143,144]. The muscles go into spasm with resulting rigidity; a boardlike abdomen is common [127,130,132,136,142,144]. The severe, diffuse pain typically peaks after several hours [127,130–133,143]. Respirations may become labored, with significant tightness in chest muscles [126,131,132,133,142,144,145]. The respiratory rate may be increased and there may be associated tachycardia and hypertension (which can lead to cerebrovascular accidents, exacerbation of congestive heart failure, and myocardial ischemia) [131–134,142,144]. Cardiac dysrhythmias have been reported [132,135].

Associated signs and symptoms include fever, headache, diaphoresis, nausea and vomiting, restlessness and anxiety, periorbital edema, and skin rash [25,126,132,133,142,143]. Deep tendon reflexes may be increased [142,144]. Priapism has been reported [134,146].

Diagnostic Evaluation

HISTORY/PREHOSPITAL CARE. The history surrounding a widow spider bite may be confusing if a spider was not seen. A high index of suspicion must be maintained in patients presenting with compatible complaints. Prehospital interventions, such as analgesic use, should be noted. While there are no specific first aid measures effective in widow spider bites, temporary application of ice to the bite site may reduce pain [126,127,131]. Assessment of the victim's underlying medical conditions, such as hypertension and current pregnancy status, is vital. Allergies and tetanus immunization status must be documented.

PHYSICAL EXAMINATION/ANCILLARY STUDIES. The physical examination should consist of a good screening examination with particular attention to the vital signs, which should be checked at frequent intervals. Close examination for a bite site with a magnifying glass may be productive.

Routine admission laboratory values should be obtained. While there are no diagnostic changes, the white blood cell count and glucose are frequently elevated [25,129,133]. Serum creatinine phosphokinase values may be increased [129] and microscopic hematuria and proteinuria may be seen [133]. An admission electrocardiogram and chest radiograph should also be obtained.

DIFFERENTIAL DIAGNOSIS. The differential diagnosis includes envenomations by other arthropods, such as neurotoxic scorpions (see Scorpion Venom Poisoning), and systemic disorders, such as acute rhabdomyolysis, heat cramps, heat stroke, tetanus, and strychnine poisoning. Various etiologies for abdominal pain and rigidity should be considered, but peritonitis can usually be diagnosed by the presence of significant abdominal tenderness and rebound, which are notably absent in widow spider envenomations.

Management

INITIAL MEASURES. Hospital management of widow spider envenomation begins with ensuring an adequate airway, respirations, and circulatory status. After providing oxygen, initiating cardiac and pulse oximetry monitoring, and starting an intravenous line, attention can be directed to alleviating painful muscle spasms. The agent of choice for treating muscle spasms is unclear, but varying success has been obtained with the use of calcium gluconate, methocarbamol, diazepam, and narcotics [25,126,127,131,136,142,147]. Calcium gluconate (10% solution) can be given intravenously over 10 to 20 minutes and repeated every 3 to 4 hours as needed (adults 1.0 gm/dose; children 50 mg/kg/dose up to 250 mg/kg/day) [148]. If the first dose produces less than 1 hour of pain relief, repeat doses are unlikely to be beneficial [142]. Methocarbamol (10% solution) can be given intravenously over 5 to 10 minutes (adults 1.0 gm initially followed by 0.5–1.0 gm in 250–500 ml of D_5W over 3–4 hours; children 15 mg/kg every 6 hours) [148]. Diazepam and narcotics can be given in standard doses.

Hypertension usually responds to bed rest, muscle relaxants, analgesics, and sedation [131]. Specific antihypertensive agents can be used if necessary [131].

ANTIVENIN. Merck, Sharpe and Dohme manufactures a specific equine widow spider antivenin (Antivenin *Latrodectus mactans*) that is effective regardless of which *Latrodectus* species is involved [129,136,149]. It blocks the ability of the venom to bind to synaptic membranes [127,132,133]. The indications for use of this equine product are controversial. Its use is justifiable for significant envenomations in patients younger than 16 years or older than 60 years, pregnant patients, and those with a history of cardiovascular disease or other major medical problems [126,127,132,135,142,143,144]. Antivenin may be considered in the rare patient with signs of severe envenomation who is otherwise healthy [25,127,135,136]. Administration solely to reverse significant pain unrelieved by other measures is efficacious [25,150] but controversial, due to the risks of adverse drug reactions [132].

As with snake antivenin administration, informed consent should be obtained and epinephrine should be available at the bedside. A skin test is recommended by the manufacturer, but the drawbacks outlined for snake antivenin skin testing in cases of obviously severe envenomation apply. If the test is to be applied, 0.02 ml of a 1:10 dilution of normal horse serum is applied intradermally in the volar forearm [58]. A 0.02 ml normal saline control is applied simultaneously on the opposite side to aid in interpreting the test. If the skin test is negative or omitted, the patient is premedicated with an intravenous antihistamine and one vial of antivenin is administered in 50 to 100 ml of normal saline intravenously over 15 minutes [25,126] with the physician in immediate attendance to observe for any sign of reaction. Generally, one vial is adequate, but a second vial can be administered if necessary [25,126,127,136,142,143]. The dosage is the same for children [25,131,142]. The majority of symptoms usually resolve within a few hours of antivenin administration [127,142,143,145,151].

The adverse reactions to widow spider antivenin are essentially the same as for snake antivenins [25,132], but the risk of delayed serum sickness appears to be lower, due to the smaller total amount of foreign protein infused [127].

The clinical course of most patients with widow spider envenomation is benign [25,132], but significant pain and spasm can persist for 12 to 48 hours [127,130,131,150]. Most healthy adults can be treated with supportive measures alone [25,129,132].

DISPOSITION/OUTCOME. Patients who are symptomatic, particularly the very young, very old, and those with underlying medical problems, should generally be admitted for observation, even if antivenin is not used [126,131]. Adult patients in good health with normal vital signs and easily controlled symptoms can be discharged home with prescription for analgesics, muscle relaxants, and for bed rest with instructions to return if they get worse. The mortality rate from widow spider venom poisoning in the United States is less than 1 percent [132,134,152]. Recovery following widow spider envenomation may sometimes be slow, with weakness, fatigue, paresthesias, headache, and insomnia persisting for several months [129,131].

BROWN SPIDER VENOM POISONING. The brown spider (*Loxosceles* sp.) is also known as the fiddle-back or violin spider. Of the six species of brown spider found in the United States, the brown recluse (*L. reclusa*) is best known [153]. They are characterized by a violin-shaped marking on the dorsal aspect of the cephalothorax and three pairs of eyes (in contrast to the four pairs found in most spiders) [25,127, 130,143,154,155]. The adult body is 10 to 15 mm long and the leg span 2 to 3 cm [127,155]. Both the male and female spider are dangerous [155–158].

The brown recluse is found throughout the southern, south-central, and midwestern United States: other species are found in the western part of the country [25,127,128,129,133,140,154]. The fact that these spiders can be easily transported with household goods about the country, however, makes it possible for envenomations to occur in any state [130,140,143,159,160]. *Loxosceles reclusa* has gained a reputation for causing severe dermonecrosis (necrotic arachnidism), but all *Loxosceles* spiders as well as spiders of other genera indigenous to the United States can cause similar lesions [87,141,154]. The majority of brown spider bites actually result in insignificant lesions [136,161, 162,163].

The venoms of the different species of brown spider, though immunologically distinct, have similar toxic effects [127, 136,157,162]. They contain at least 10 different proteins, most of which demonstrate enzymatic activity [87,126,129, 154,160,164,165]. Brown spider venom is cytotoxic and hemolytic [155,166], but the precise component of *Loxosceles* venom responsible for these effects is unclear [126,129,140, 154,161,164,167,168]. There is evidence that sphingomyelinase D may be responsible [154,168,169,170]. It is also likely that venom activation of the complement cascade induces a series of autopharmacologic changes in the victim that amplify the degree of injury [127,128, 129,140,154,155,164,167].

The cutaneous changes seen following a brown spider bite are initiated by endothelial damage in small dermal vessels that become occluded with microthrombi, producing vascular stasis and infarction [25,87,129,140,154,156,160,165,171,172]. Polymorphonuclear leukocytes (PMNs) are attracted to the site via a chemotactic response and propagate the inflammatory necrotic reaction [25,87,127,129,140,154,156,165,171–174]. The accumulation of PMNs at the site appears to be a vital component of the dermonecrotic response and is probably related to complement activation [127,140,154,167,174].

Clinical Manifestations. The clinical manifestations of brown spider envenomation vary from mild, temporary irritation at the bite site to severe, potentially fatal systemic poisoning [140,153,160,161,165]. The bite is occasionally felt as a mild stinging sensation, though it may go completely unnoticed [126,133,160,175,176]. Over the next several hours there may be pruritus, tingling, mild swelling, and redness or blanching at the bite site [154,160,177]. Variable degrees of local pain and tenderness due to local vasospasm and ischemia occur with-

in 2 to 8 hours [141,154,165,175,176,177]. Within 12 to 18 hours, a small, central vesicle (clear or hemorrhagic) often develops at the site and is surrounded by an irregular zone of erythema or ecchymosis and edema [126,136,140, 154,160,165,175,176,177]. The bleb soon ruptures and the erythema gives way to violaceous discoloration [25,129,154,164]. In 5 to 7 days the bite site undergoes aseptic necrosis (dry, gangrenous slough), the center becomes depressed below the normal level of the skin, and a black eschar forms [87, 126,141,154,160]. The eschar later sloughs, leaving an open ulcer that heals over weeks to months [87,154,164]. Bites to fatty regions of the body, such as the buttocks, thighs, or abdomen, tend to be more severe, with undermining of of the skin and more extensive residual scarring [87, 127,154,160,161,176,178]. Rarely does necrosis involve deeper structures such as nerves, muscles, tendons, or ligaments [165,176,179]. Lesions destined to go on to develop significant necrosis usually demonstrate early evidence of local ischemia [140,141,177,180].

Systemic (viscerocutaneous) loxoscelism is rare but may be rapidly progressive and severe, particularly in children [127, 129,130,135,136,141,143,155,160,164,176]. Systemic symptoms generally start 24 to 72 hours after the bite and occasionally occur before cutaneous findings become impressive [133,143,153,154,160]. Symptoms are often flulike, with fever, chills, headache, malaise, weakness, nausea, vomiting, myalgias, and arthralgias [25,143,154,160,161,165,177]. Hemolytic anemia with hemoglobinemia, hemoglobinuria, jaundice, thrombocytopenia, disseminated intravascular coagulation, acute renal failure (secondary to hemoglobin deposition in renal tubules), shock, seizures, and coma has been reported [141,154,160,161,165,178,181,182,183]. The severity of systemic symptoms is directly related to the quantity of venom deposited but does not necessarily correlate with the severity of cutaneous changes [143,154,160,176]. In fact, it has been noted that the bite site is often more benign-appearing in cases of systemic loxoscelism [153].

Diagnostic Evaluation

HISTORY. It is extremely rare for a victim of a *Loxosceles* bite to see the offending spider, because the bite is relatively painless and a large percentage of bites occur while the victim is asleep [156,162,178]. Since the spider is rarely available for identification, determining the etiology of early lesions is often difficult [25,140,156,160,175]. The diagnosis of brown spider bite is presumptive in such cases, and care should be taken not to overdiagnose the lesion, especially in front of the patient [135,141,154,175]. The working diagnosis should be cutaneous necrosis if the cause is unknown and necrotic arachnidism if a biting spider was seen but not identified [154].

PHYSICAL EXAMINATION/ANCILLARY STUDIES. A good screening examination for any evidence of systemic loxoscelism should be performed. The severity of any lesion present should be assessed and any evidence of secondary infection noted.

Laboratory evaluation should include a complete blood count (including platelets) and urinalysis [154]. If there is any evidence of consumptive coagulopathy, hemolysis, or hemoglobinuria, further studies should include PT and PTT, electrolytes, blood urea nitrogen, creatine, blood sugar, liver function tests, serum haptoglobin, and type and cross-match [127, 129,135,141,154]. The white blood cell count may be as high as 20,000 to 30,000 per cubic millimeter and the hemoglobin may fall to as low as 4 gm per deciliter [127,141,154]. It is prudent to follow daily blood counts and urinalyses in patients with significant lesions, even if they are not admitted [154]. More frequent laboratory reevaluation is advised in patients with manifestations of systemic loxoscelism.

Attempts have been made to develop a technique to diagnose *Loxosceles* spider bites definitively [127,140,184]. While an in vitro lymphocyte transformation test can confirm such an envenomation approximately 6 weeks after the bite [162], there is no clinically available laboratory method of making the diagnosis early.

DIFFERENTIAL DIAGNOSIS. The differential diagnosis for *Loxosceles* envenomation includes bites or stings by other arthropods (e.g., spiders, ticks, scorpions, ants, fleas, kissing bugs, biting flies), superficial skin infections, diabetic ulcers, plant puncture wounds, sporotrichosis, toxic epidermal necrolysis, pyoderma gangrenosum, erythema nodosum, erythema chronicum migrans, herpes zoster, herpes simplex, erythema multiforme, purpura fulminans, and contact dermatitis [162,185,186].

Management

CUTANEOUS LESIONS. Proper management of the necrotic lesions seen with brown spider bites is highly controversial. The majority of cases require only local wound care, including cleansing of the bite site, application of a sterile dressing, immobilization with a well-padded splint, and tetanus prophylaxis as necessary [87,135,136,141,154]. Local application of ice or cold packs over the first few days to reduce sphingomyelinase activity may be beneficial [87,136,153,187]. If an ulcer develops, it should be cleaned several times each day with hydrogen peroxide or povidone-iodine solution [126,127,154], and frequent ice applications should continue until the wound heals [153]. Pruritus can be treated with diphenhydramine [140,143,154]. Antibiotics to prevent any secondary cellulitis may be beneficial, but this is controversial [87, 133,135,141,143,153,154,160].

It is important to understand and to caution patients that nothing has proved to decrease the extent of dermonecrosis after these bites and that the vast majority of lesions will heal quite satisfactorily with conservative management alone [25,141,154,180]. Controversial modalities for managing the wound include the use of steroids, dapsone, colchicine, and surgery. Steroids, either intralesional or systemic, are of no proved benefit to the cutaneous lesion [25,87,129,136,141,154,161,179,188]. Likewise, dapsone and colchicine are of uncertain efficacy [25,87,154,189]. The theory behind the use of these agents is that, as polymorphonuclear leukocyte inhibitors, they may limit the extent to which PMNs participate in the propagation of the local lesion. With dapsone, however, there are significant potential complications, including dose-dependent hemolytic anemia and methemoglobinemia [25,87,164]. Dapsone should be reserved for patients with severe gangrenous dermonecrotic lesions and should never be used in children [87,154]. The starting dosage should not exceed 50 to 100 mg per day (divided every 12 hours) orally, and it is advisable to test for glucose-6-phosphate dehydrogenase deficiency while beginning therapy [136,164]. The side effects of colchicine are less worrisome, but it has yet to be formally studied in brown spider bites. Hansen and Russell, using 1.2 mg initially followed by 0.6 mg every 2 hours for 2 days and 0.6 mg every 4 hours for 2 additional days, reported apparent efficacy with colchicine in a single case [189]. Routine use of these agents should be avoided until prospective, controlled studies prove that benefits outweigh risks. When such agents are started and are tolerated, it is important that therapy continues until the lesion heals or is grafted [153].

Early excision of the site is definitely not indicated, since it is impossible to predict the extent and severity of the lesion early [87,127,135,140,141,154,155,161]. Severe-appearing lesions commonly involute and regress spontaneously to minimal defects [25,161]. Any surgical procedure that might be required (e.g., skin grafting) should be postponed at least 6 to 8 weeks

to ensure that the necrotic process has been completed and to improve chances of healing [87,141,154,161]. Hyperbaric oxygen therapy may be useful in particularly severe wounds [87].

An experimental antivenin appears to decrease the extent of dermonecrosis following brown spider envenomations, but it is not commercially available [25,126,127,129,136,167,177]. Such an antivenin will be clinically useful only if an accurate laboratory test is developed to identify brown spider envenomations at the time of presentation [25].

SYSTEMIC POISONING. Initial management of systemic loxoscelism consists of ensuring adequate hydration, maintaining electrolyte balance, and administering antipyretics (avoid salicylates) and analgesics [141,154]. Though the use of systemic corticosteroids has yet to be studied in a controlled fashion, an early, short course of therapy may be beneficial in patients with hemolysis [25,135,141,143,145,154,161]. A reasonable regimen is 1 mg/kg/day of prednisone orally for 2 to 4 days [127,141,154]. Blood products are used as indicated to treat anemia or thrombocytopenia [127,141,154,160]. Heparin may be beneficial in treating disseminated intravascular coagulopathy [127,130,135,154,160,178,179]. If hemoglobinuria occurs, the urine should be alkalinized and adequate hydration becomes critically important [129,154]. If renal failure occurs, dialysis may be indicated [135,141,154,160,161]. Dialysis does not, however, remove venom or hemoglobin from the circulation [154,161].

DISPOSITION/OUTCOME. Admission is appropriate for patients with rapidly expanding lesions or evidence of systemic poisoning [140]. Patients who are not admitted should have daily wound checks and laboratory reevaluation for the first few days after envenomation. While there have been no reports of deaths in patients bitten by positively identified brown spiders in the United States [127,154], there is a significant risk of death from systemic loxoscelism, especially in children.

Scorpion Venom Poisoning

There are more than 1400 species of scorpions worldwide [190] but only one of major medical importance native to the United States—the bark scorpion (*Centruroides exilicauda*) [126,191,192]. This species is found throughout Arizona and immediately surrounding regions of neighboring states [126,133,191,193]. The bark scorpion is 13 to 75 mm long, usually yellow-brown and may have variable striping on the dorsum [191,193,194]. It is differentiated from other scorpions by a small tubercle at the base of the stinger [25,191,192,194]. Other scorpions of minimal medical significance can be found across the southern United States [190].

The venom of *C. exilicauda* is complex. It contains at least five distinct neurotoxins that cause a release of neurotransmitters from the autonomic nervous system and adrenal medulla and stimulate depolarization of neuromuscular junctions [25,140,195,196]. Its venom contains no major enzymatic components [197]. The venoms of the less toxic scorpions in the United States are poorly characterized.

Clinical Manifestations. Most *C. exilicauda* stings are minor, with the most serious envenomations usually occurring in children [25,133,136,140,194,195,197]. The sting is followed by intense pain at the site within several minutes [25,126,130, 136,191–195,197,198]. An interesting physical finding following envenomation is the presence of hyperesthesia, manifested by intense pain with mild palpation or tapping over the site (the "tap test") [140,192,193,194,197]. Pain or numbness may radiate up the extremity [25,192,193,194], but local pain may be absent in children younger than 10 years [193]. Soft tissue swelling and ecchymosis are notably absent in stings by this species, due to the lack of major venom enzymes [126,130,136,191,192,193,197].

Systemic symptoms, when they occur, reflect sympathetic, parasympathetic, and neuromuscular excitation [191,195]. Early on there may be restlessness or anxiety, followed by hypersalivation, a sensation of tongue thickening, dysphagia, difficulty focusing or temporary blindness, roving eye movements, tachypnea and respiratory distress, wheezing or stridor, involuntary voiding of stool or urine, muscle fasciculations and spasm, alternating opisthotonus and emprosthotonus, and paralysis [25,126,130,133,136,191–195,197,199]. Extreme neuromuscular hyperactivity may be mistaken for seizures [200]. Supraventricular tachycardia and hypertension have been reported [25,126,191,192,193,195], and the patient's temperature may reach 104° F [133,194]. The duration of symptoms appears to be inversely proportional to age and may persist for up to 30 hours [193].

Local consequences after envenomation by the nonneurotoxic scorpions in the United States consist of immediate, brief, intense burning or stinging, mild soft tissue swelling, and possibly mild ecchymosis [145]. Systemic manifestations are uncommon except in the rare instance when a victim is allergic to the venom [136].

Diagnostic Evaluation

HISTORY/PREHOSPITAL CARE. Patients stung by scorpions frequently see the offending organism. If the scorpion is brought in, it should be examined for the identifying tubercle at the base of the stinger.

A general medical history should be obtained, symptoms assessed, and prehospital treatments noted.

PHYSICAL EXAMINATION/ANCILLARY STUDIES. The victim's vital signs should be carefully noted and frequently monitored. The sting site should be examined and manifestations of sympathetic, parasympathetic, or neuromuscular excitation sought.

Routine admission laboratory evaluation should be obtained in significantly symptomatic patients suspected of *C. exilicauda* sting, but there are no tests of particular diagnostic benefit. The white blood cell count and serum glucose may be significantly elevated [195]. Increases in serum amylase, creatine phosphokinase, and renal function studies, mild abnormalities in coagulation parameters, and cerebral spinal fluid pleocytosis have been reported [199]. No laboratory tests are required in patients stung by other native U.S. scorpions.

DIFFERENTIAL DIAGNOSIS. The diagnosis is usually not difficult, as adults often relate the history of a scorpion sting, and in children the clinical picture following a *C. exilicauda* sting is rarely confused with other diagnoses [25,140,193]. The differential diagnosis includes central nervous system infection, widow spider envenomation, tetanus, dystonic drug reaction, intoxication (e.g., pesticides, anticholinergics, sympathomimetics, xanthines, propoxyphene, strychnine), drug withdrawal, anaphylaxis [200], and seizure disorder.

Management

SUPPORTIVE MEASURES. Patients stung by U.S. scorpions other than *C. exilicauda* can be treated with local cold therapy and mild analgesics. Tetanus status should be updated as necessary. The patient can be discharged if no signs of anaphylaxis are present.

The vast majority of *C. exilicauda* stings likewise can be treated with cold compresses and analgesics [25,191,193,195]. Patients with more severe envenomations should receive oxygen and have an intravenous line established and cardiac and pulse oximetry monitoring. The airway should be intubated if there are signs of respiratory failure or inability to handle secretions [199]. Anxiety, restlessness, muscular hyperactivity, and moderate hypertension can usually be treated with bed rest and sedation [25,130,135,136,140,191]. Modest doses of intravenous diazepam or phenobarbital can be used for sedation as long as respiratory status is closely monitored [25,126,130,136,193,195]. Beta-adrenergic blocking agents have been recommended for hemodynamically significant supraventricular tachycardia [25,195,196]. Antihypertensive agents can be used for severe blood pressure elevations [126]. A trial of calcium gluconate (10 ml of a 10% solution given slowly intravenously; 0.1 ml/kg in children) to treat severe muscle spasms can be attempted, though success with this approach is purely anecdotal [126,130,136,191]. Narcotics are avoided since they appear to have a synergistic neurotoxic effect [25,130,135,136,140,198].

ANTIVENIN. There is a goat-derived antivenin for *C. exilicauda* available in Arizona [196] but it is available for use only within that state and is not approved by the Food and Drug Administration (FDA) [25,195]. It appears anecdotally to be effective in severe envenomations in small children, but controlled clinical trials have not been performed [25,130,191,194,195,197,200]. It is a heterologous serum product, and is therefore associated with the same risks of anaphylaxis and delayed serum sickness as described for pit viper antivenin.

Adults stung by *C. exilicauda* should be observed for several hours; if significant toxicity appears they should be admitted to an ICU [193]. The vast majority of patients, however, can be safely treated at home [191,197]. It is extremely rare for envenomations in adults to be severe enough to require antivenin [191,200]. Symptomatic children should probably be admitted, and any child younger than 1 year or who has neurologic findings should be admitted to an ICU [140,193,195].

At one time, *C. exilicauda* caused more than twice as many deaths in Arizona as did all other venomous animals combined [192]. However, no deaths reported from this scorpion have been reported since 1968 [191,195], probably due to a combination of improved scorpion eradication techniques, public education, and advancements in supportive care [25,140,193]. The potential for a fatal outcome, however, should not be underestimated, especially in small children.

References

1. Mattison C: *Snakes of the World,* New York, Facts on File, 1986.
2. Litovitz TL, Holm KC, Bailey KM, et al: 1991 annual report of the American Association of Poison Control Centers National Data Collection System. *Am J Emerg Med* 10:452, 1992.
3. Russell FE, Picchioni AL: Snake Venom Poisoning. *Clin Toxicol Consul* 5:73, 1983.
4. Russell FE, Carlson RW, Wainschel J, et al: Snake venom poisoning in the United States: Experiences with 550 cases. *JAMA* 233:341, 1975.
5. Russell FE: *Snake Venom Poisoning.* 2nd ed. New York, Scholium, 1983.
6. Parrish HM: Incidence of treated snakebites in the United States. *Pub Health Rep* 81:269, 1966.
7. Parrish HM: Analysis of 460 fatalities from venomous animals in the United States. *Am J Med Sci* 245:129, 1963.
8. Wingert WA, Wainschel J: Diagnosis and management of envenomation by poisonous snakes. *South Med J* 68:1015, 1975.
9. Russell FE: AIDS, cancer, and snakebite: What do these three have in common? *West J Med* 148:84, 1988.
10. Parrish HM: Deaths from bites and stings of venomous animals and insects in the United States. *Arch Intern Med* 104:198, 1959.

11. Wingert WA: Poisoning by animal venoms. *Top Emerg Med* 2:89, 1980.
12. Jimenez-Porras JM: Biochemistry of snake venoms, in Minton SA (ed): *Snake Venoms and Envenomation.* New York, Marcel Dekker, 1971.
13. Russell FE, Puffer HW: Pharmacology of snake venoms, in Minton SA (ed): *Snake Venoms and Envenomation.* New York, Marcel Dekker, 1971.
14. Kunkel DB, Curry SC, et al: Reptile envenomations. *Clin Toxicol* 21:503, 1983-1984.
15. Van Mierop LHS: Poisonous snakebite: A review. 1. Snakes and their venom. *J Fla Med Assoc* 63:191, 1976.
16. Arnold RE: Controversies and hazards in the treatment of pit viper bites. *South Med J* 72:902, 1979.
17. Watt CH: Treatment of poisonous snakebite with emphasis on digit dermotomy. *South Med J* 78:694, 1985.
18. Glass TG: *Management of Poisonous Snakebite.* San Antonio, Thomas G. Glass, 1976.
19. Russell FE: Snake venom poisoning in the United States. *Ann Rev Med* 31:247, 1980.
20. McCollough NC, Gennaro JF: Evaluation of venomous snakebite in the Southern United States from parallel clinical and laboratory investigations: Development of treatment. *J Fla Med Assoc* 49:959, 1963.
21. Sprenger TR, Bailey WJ: Snakebite treatment in the United States. *Int J Dermatol* 25:479, 1986.
22. Arnold RE: Treatment of venomous snakebites in the Western hemisphere. *Mil Med* 149:361, 1984.
23. Glass TG: *First Aid for Snakebite.* San Antonio, Thomas G. Glass, 1981.
24. Schaeffer RC, Carlson RW, Puri VK, et al: The effects of colloidal and crystalloidal fluids on rattlesnake venom shock in the rat. *J Pharmacol Exp Ther* 206:687, 1978.
25. Banner W: Bites and stings in the pediatric patient. *Curr Probl Pediatr* 18:9, 1988.
26. Otten EJ, McKimm D: Venomous snakebite in a patient allergic to horse serum. *Ann Emerg Med* 12:624, 1983.
27. Stewart ME, Greenland S, Hoffman JR, et al: First-aid treatment of poisonous snakebite: Are currently recommended procedures justified? *Ann Emerg Med* 10:331, 1981.
28. Russell FE: Prevention and treatment of venomous animal injuries. *Experientia* 30:8, 1974.
29. Burgess JL, Dart RC, Egen NB, et al: Effects of constriction bands on rattlesnake venom absorption: A pharmacokinetic study. *Ann Emerg Med* 21:1086, 1992.
30. Sutherland SK, Coulter AR: Early management of bites by the Eastern diamondback rattlesnake *(Crotalus adamanteus):* Studies in monkeys *(Macaca fascicularis). Am J Trop Med Hyg* 30:497, 1981.
31. Jackson D: First aid treatment of snakebite. *Tex State J Med* 23:203, 1927.
32. Jackson D, Harrison WT: Mechanical treatment of experimental rattlesnake venom poisoning. *JAMA* 90:1928, 1928.
33. Jackson D: Treatment of snakebite. *South Med J* 22:605, 1929.
34. Jackson D, Githens TS: Treatment of *Crotalus atrox* venom poisoning in dogs. *Bull Antivenin Inst America* 5:1, 1931.
35. Minton SA: Snakebite: An unpredictable emergency. *J Trauma* 11:1053, 1971.
36. Watt CH: Poisonous snakebite treatment in the United States. *JAMA* 240:654, 1978.
37. Merriam TW, Leopold RS: Evaluation of incision and suction in venom removal. *Clin Res* 8:258, 1960.
38. Snyder CC, Pickins JE, Knowles RP, et al: A definitive study of snakebite. *J Fla Med Assoc* 55:330, 1968.
39. Glass TG: Early debridement in pit viper bites. *JAMA* 235:2513, 1976.
40. Sabback MS, Cunningham ER, Fitts CT: A study of the treatment of pit viper envenomization in 45 patients. *J Trauma* 17:569, 1977.
41. Russell FE, Banner W: Snake venom poisoning, in Rakel RE (ed): *Conn's Current Therapy.* Philadelphia, WB Saunders, 1988.
42. Watt CH: Treatment of poisonous snakebite with emphasis on digit dermotomy. *South Med J* 78:694, 1985.
43. Guderian RH, Mackenzie CD, Williams JF: High voltage shock treatment for snakebite. *Lancet* 2:229, 1986.
44. Howe NR, Meisenheimer JL: Electric shock does not save snakebitten rats. *Ann Emerg Med* 17:254, 1988.
45. Johnson EK, Kardong KV, Mackessy SP: Electric shocks are ineffective in treatment of lethal effects of rattlesnake envenomation in mice. *Toxicon* 25:1347, 1987.
46. Dart RC, Lindsey D, Schulman A: Snakebites and shocks. *Ann Emerg Med* 17:1262, 1988.
47. Stoud C, Amon H, Wagner T, et al: Effect of electric shock therapy on local tissue reaction to poisonous snake venom injection in rabbits. *Ann Emerg Med* 18:447, 1989.
48. Dart RC, Gustafson RA: Failure of electric shock treatment for rattlesnake envenomation. *Ann Emerg Med* 20:659, 1991.
49. Russell FE: Electroshock for snakebite (letter). *Vet Hum Toxicol* 29:320, 1987.
50. Bucknall NC: Electrical treatment of venomous bites and stings. *Toxicon* 29:397, 1991.
51. McCollough NC, Gennaro JF: Treatment of venomous snakebite in the United States. *Clin Toxicol* 3:483, 1970.
52. Parrish HM, Goldner JC, Silberg SL: Poisonous snakebites causing no venenation. *Postgrad Med* 39:265, 1966.
53. Otten EJ: Antivenin therapy in the emergency department. *Am J Emerg Med* 1:83, 1983.
54. Wood JT, Hoback WW, Green TW: Treatment of snake venom poisoning with ACTH and cortisone. *Va Med Mo* 82:130, 1955.
55. McCollough NC, Gennaro JF: Diagnosis, symptoms, treatment and sequelae of envenomation by *Crotalus adamanteus* and genus *Ancistrodon. J Fla Med Assoc* 55:327, 1968.
56. Grace TG, Omer GE: The management of upper extremity pit viper wounds. *Am J Hand Surg* 5:168, 1980.
57. Nelson BK: Snake envenomation: Incidence, clinical presentation and management. *Med Toxicol* 4:17, 1989.
58. *Physicians' Desk Reference.* 47th ed. Oradell, NJ, Medical Economics, 1993.
59. Russell FE, Lauritzen L: Antivenins. *Trans Roy Soc Trop Med Hyg* 60:797, 1966.
60. Ownby CL, Odell GV, Theakston RDG: Detection of antibodies to myotoxin a and prairie rattlesnake *(Crotalus viridis viridis)* venom in three antisera using enzyme-linked immunosorbent assay and immunodiffusion. *Toxicon* 21:849, 1983.
61. Ownby CL, Colberg TR, Odell GV: Ability of a mixture of antimyotoxin a serum and polyvalent (Crotalidae) antivenin to neutralize myonecrosis, hemorrhage and lethality induced by prairie rattlesnake *(Crotalus viridis viridis)* venom. *Toxicon* 23:317, 1985.
62. Ownby CL, Colberg TR, Claypool PL, Odell GV: *In vivo* test of the ability of antiserum to myotoxin a from prairie rattlesnake *(Crotalus viridis viridis)* venom to neutralize local myonecrosis induced by myotoxin a and homologous crude venom. *Toxicon* 22:99, 1984.
63. Ownby CL, Colberg TR: Ability of polyvalent (Crotalidae) antivenom to neutralize local myonecrosis induced by *Crotalus atrox* venom. *Toxicon* 24:201, 1986.
64. Garfin SR, Castilonia RR, Mubarak SJ, et al: The effect of antivenin on intramuscular pressure elevations induced by rattlesnake venom. *Toxicon* 23:677, 1985.
65. Russell FE, Ruzic N, Gonzalez H: Effectiveness of antivenin (Crotalidae) polyvalent following injection of *Crotalus* venom. *Toxicon* 11:461, 1973.
66. Ownby CL, Odell GV, Woods WM, et al: Ability of antiserum to myotoxin alpha from prairie rattlesnake *(Crotalus viridis viridis)* venom to neutralize local myotoxicity and lethal effects of myotoxin alpha and homologous crude venom. *Toxicon* 21:35, 1983.
67. Russell FE: Clinical aspects of snake venom poisoning in North America. *Toxicon* 7:33, 1969.
68. Lindsey D: Controversy in snakebite: Time for a controlled appraisal. *J Trauma* 25:462, 1985.
69. Parrish HM, Donnell HD: Bites by cottonmouths *(Ancistrodon piscivorus)* in the United States. *South Med J* 60:429, 1967.
70. Buntain WL: Successful venomous snakebite neutralization with massive antivenin infusion in a child. *J Trauma* 23:1012, 1983.
71. Jurkovich GJ, Luterman A, McCullar K, et al: Complications of Crotalidae antivenin therapy. *J Trauma* 28:1032, 1988.
72. Stueven H, Aprahamian C, Thompson B, et al: Cobra envenomation: An uncommon emergency. *Ann Emerg Med* 12:636, 1983.
73. Griffen D, Donovan JW: Significant envenomation from a preserved rattlesnake head (in a patient with a history of immediate hypersensitivity to antivenin). *Ann Emerg Med* 15:955, 1986.

74. Chippaux JP, Goyffon M: Principles and indications of antivenom serotherapy. *Toxicon* 30:498, 1992.

75. Parrish HM: *Poisonous Snakebites in the United States.* New York, Vantage, 1980.

76. Sullivan JB, Kulig K, Rumack BH, et al: Quantitative comparison of horse serum skin test, Wyeth Crotalidae Polyvalent Antivenin, and a purified affinity gel column antivenin. *Vet Hum Toxicol* 24(suppl):192, 1982.

77. Simon TL, Grace TG: Envenomation coagulopathy in wounds from pit vipers. *N Engl J Med* 305:443, 1981.

78. Riffler E, Curry SC, Gerkin R: Successful treatment with antivenin of marked thrombocytopenia without significant coagulopathy following rattlesnake bite. *Ann Emerg Med* 16:1297, 1987.

79. Loprinzi CL, Hennessee J, Tamsky L, et al: Snake antivenin administration in a patient allergic to horse serum. *South Med J* 76:501, 1983.

80. Corrigan P, Russell FE, Wainschel J: Clinical reactions to antivenin. *Toxicon* 16(suppl 1):457, 1978.

81. Hardy DL: *Snakebite Update: Crotalus Envenomation in Tucson, 1973-1980 and Comments on the New Australian Method of First Aid for Elapid Snakebites.* Presented to Annual Conference, American Association of Zoos, Parks and Aquariums, Scottsdale, Arizona, September 22, 1982.

82. Van Mierop LH, Kitchens CS: Defibrination syndrome following bites by the Eastern diamondback rattlesnake. *J Fla Med Assoc* 67:21, 1980.

83. Burgess JL, Dart RC: Snake venom coagulopathy: Use and abuse of blood products in the treatment of pit viper envenomation. *Ann Emerg Med* 20:795, 1991.

84. Sutherland SK: How good is the management of snakebite in Australia? *Aust Paediatr J* 14:237, 1978.

85. Wagner CW, Golladay ES: Crotalid envenomation in children: Selective conservative management. *J Pediatr Surg* 24:128, 1989.

86. Goldstein EJC, Citron DM, Gonzalez H, et al: Bacteriology of rattlesnake venom and implications for therapy. *J Infect Dis* 140:818, 1979.

87. Wasserman GS: Wound care of spider and snake envenomations. *Ann Emerg Med* 17:1331, 1988.

88. Allen FM: Observations of local measures in the treatment of snake bite. *Am J Trop Med* 19:393, 1939.

89. Glass TG: Early debridement in pit viper bite. *Surg Gynecol Obstet* 136:774, 1973.

90. Curry SC, Kraner JC, Kunkel DB, et al: Noninvasive vascular studies in management of rattlesnake envenomations to extremities. *Ann Emerg Med* 14:1081, 1985.

91. Garfin SR: Rattlesnake bites: Current hospital therapy. *West J Med* 137:411, 1982.

92. Hargens AR, Garfin SR, Mubarak SJ, et al: Edema associated with venomous snakebites. *Bibl Anat* 20:267, 1981.

93. Garfin SR, Castilonia RR, Mubarak SJ, et al: Role of surgical decompression in treatment of rattlesnake bites. *Surg Forum* 30:502, 1979.

94. Garfin SR, Castilonia RR, Mubarak SJ, et al: Rattlesnake bites and surgical decompression: Results using a laboratory model. *Toxicon* 22:177, 1984.

95. Stahnke HL: The L-C treatment of venomous bites or stings. *Am J Trop Med* 2:142, 1953.

96. Stahnke HL: *The Treatment of Venomous Bites and Stings.* Poisonous Animal Research Laboratory, Arizona State University, 1958.

97. Stahnke HL: *Sunday Edition of Arizona Days and Ways.* April 3, 1960.

98. Schottler WHA: Antihistamine, ACTH, cortisone, hydrocortisone and anesthetics in snake bite. *Am J Trop Med Hyg* 3:1083, 1954.

99. Russell FE, Emery JA: Effects of corticosteroids on the lethality of *Ancistrodon contortrix* venom. *Am J Med Sci* 241:507, 1961.

100. Deutsch HF, Diniz CR: Some proteolytic activities of snake venoms. *J Biol Chem* 216:17, 1955.

101. Philpot VB: Activation of venom proteases and reversal of chelating effects by sodium bicarbonate. *Proc Soc Exp Biol Med* 101:78, 1959.

102. Hurlbut KM, Dart RC, Spaite D, et al: Reliability of clinical presentation for predicting significant pit viper envenomation. *Ann Emerg Med* 17:438, 1988.

103. Hardy DL: Fatal rattlesnake envenomation in Arizona: 1969–1984. *Clin Toxicol* 24:1, 1986.

104. Russell FE, Sullivan JB, Egen NB, et al: Preparation of a new antivenin by affinity chromatography. *Am J Trop Med Hyg* 34:141, 1985.

105. Carroll SB, Thalley BS, Theakston RDG, et al: Comparison of the purity and efficacy of affinity purified avian antivenoms with commercial equine crotalid antivenoms. *Toxicon* 30:1017, 1992.

106. Parrish HM, Khan MS: Bites by coral snakes: Report of 11 representative cases. *Am J Med Sci* 253:561, 1967.

107. Lee CY: Elapid neurotoxins and their mode of action. *Clin Toxicol* 3:457, 1970.

108. Lee CY: Chemistry and pharmacology of polypeptide toxins in snake venoms. *Ann Rev Pharmacol* 12:265, 1972.

109. Chang CC: The action of snake venoms on nerve and muscle, in Lee CY (ed): *Snake Venoms.* New York, Springer-Verlag, 1979.

110. Fix JD: Venom yield of the North American coral snake and its clinical significance. *South Med J* 73:737, 1980.

111. Minton SA, Minton MR: *Venomous Reptiles.* New York, Scribner's, 1969.

112. Kitchens CS, Van Mierop LHS: Envenomation by the Eastern coral snake *(Micrurus fulvius fulvius):* A study of 39 victims. *JAMA* 258:1615, 1987.

113. Norris RL, Dart RC: Apparent coral snake envenomation in a patient without fang marks. *Am J Emerg Med* 7:402, 1989.

114. Pettigrew LC, Glass JP: Neurologic complications of a coral snake bite. *Neurology* 35:589, 1985.

115. Weis R, McIsaac RJ: Cardiovascular and muscular effects of venom from coral snake, *Micrurus fulvius. Toxicon* 9:219, 1971.

116. Neil WT: Some misconceptions regarding the eastern coral snake, *Micrurus fulvius. Herpetologica* 13:111, 1957.

117. Ramsey CF, Klickstein GD: Coral snake bite: Report of a case and suggested therapy. *JAMA* 182:949, 1962.

118. McCollough NC, Gennaro JF: Coral snake bites in the United States. *J Fla Med Assoc* 49:968, 1963.

119. Sutherland SK, Coulter AR, Harris RD: Rationalisation of first-aid measures for elapid snakebite. *Lancet* 1:183, 1979.

120. Edmondson KW: Treatment of snakebite. *Med J Aust* 2:257, 1979.

121. Murrell G: The effectiveness of the pressure/immobilization first aid technique in the case of a tiger snake bite. *Med J Aust* 2:295, 1981.

122. Pearn J, Morrison J, Charles N, et al: First-aid for snake-bite: Efficacy of a constrictive bandage with limb immobilization in the management of human envenomation. *Med J Aust* 2:293, 1981.

123. Balmain R, McClelland KL: Pantyhose compression bandage: First-aid measure for snakebite. *Med J Aust* 2:240, 1982.

124. Sutherland SK, Harris RD, Coulter AR, et al: First aid for cobra *(Naja naja)* bites. *Indian J Med Res* 73:266, 1981.

125. Russell FE: Bites by the Sonoran coral snake *Micruroides euryxanthus. Toxicon* 5:39, 1967.

126. Russell FE: *The Merck Manual of Diagnosis and Therapy.* 15th ed. Rahway, NJ, Merck Sharpe & Dohme, 1987.

127. Wong RC, Hughes SE, Voorhees JJ: Spider bites. *Arch Dermatol* 123:98, 1987.

128. Russell FE, Madon NB: New names for the brown recluse and the black widow. *Postgrad Med* 70:31, 1981.

129. Edlich RF, Rodeheaver GT, Feldman PS, et al: Management of venomous spider bites. *Curr Conc Trauma Care* Winter:17, 1985.

130. Biery TL, Moseley JC: Venomous arthropods in the United States: A review. *J Assoc Mil Dermatol* 2:8, 1976.

131. Kobernick M: Black widow spider bite. *Am Fam Physician* 29:241, 1984.

132. Moss HS, Binder LS: A retrospective review of black widow spider envenomation. *Ann Emerg Med* 16:188, 1987.

133. Hunt GR: Bites and stings of uncommon arthropods. 1. Spiders. *Postgrad Med* 70:91, 1981.

134. Maretic Z: Latrodectism: Variations in clinical manifestations provoked by *Latrodectus* species of spiders. *Toxicon* 21:457, 1983.

135. Anderson PC: Spider bites and scorpion stings, in Rakel RE (ed): *Conn's Current Therapy.* Philadelphia, WB Saunders, 1989.

136. King LE, Rees RS: Spider bites and scorpion stings, in Rakel RE (ed): *Conn's Current Therapy.* Philadelphia, WB Saunders, 1987.

137. Baba A, Cooper JR: The action of black widow spider venom on

cholinergic mechanisms in synaptosomes. *J Neurochem* 34:1369, 1980.

138. Smith JE, Clark AW, Kuster TA: Suppression by elevated calcium of black widow spider venom activity at frog neuromuscular junctions. *J Neurocytol* 6:519, 1977.

139. Gorio A, Mauro A: Reversibility and mode of action of black widow spider venom on the vertebrate neuromuscular junction. *J Gen Physiol* 73:245, 1979.

140. Harves AD, Millikan LE: Current concepts of therapy and pathophysiology in arthropod bites and stings. 1. Arthropods. *Int J Dermatol* 14:543, 1975.

141. Anderson PC: Necrotizing spider bites. *Am Fam Physician* 26:198, 1982.

142. Russell FE: Muscle relaxants in black widow spider *(Latrodectus mactans)* poisoning. *Am J Med Sci* 243:159, 1962.

143. Pascoe DJ: Bites and stings, in Pascoe DJ, Grossman M (eds): *Quick Reference to Pediatric Emergencies*. 2nd ed. Philadelphia, JB Lippincott, 1978.

144. Russell FE, Marcus P, Streng JA: Black widow spider envenomation during pregnancy: Report of a case. *Toxicon* 17:188, 1979.

145. Ellis MD: *Dangerous Plants, Snakes, Arthropods and Marine Life of Texas*. Galveston, Government Printing Office. 1975.

146. Stiles AD: Priapism following a black widow spider bite. *Clin Pediatr* 21:174, 1982.

147. Key GF: A comparison of calcium gluconate and methocarbamol (Robaxin) in the treatment of latrodectism (black widow spider envenomation). *Am J Trop Med Hyg* 30:273, 1981.

148. Bayer M, Kulig K: Black widow spider bite. *Emergindex System* 58:paragraph 6.1, 1988.

149. Harwood RF, James MT: *Entomology in Human and Animal Health*. 7th ed. New York, Macmillan, 1979.

150. Allen RC, Norris RL: Delayed use of antivenin in black widow spider *(Latrodectus mactans)* envenomation. *J Wild Med* 2:187, 1991.

151. Kunkel D: Editorial comment. *J Toxicol Clin Toxicol* 21:484, 1984.

152. Bogen E: Poisonous spider bites: Newer developments in our knowledge of arachnidism. *Ann Intern Med* 6:375, 1932.

153. Wilson DC, King LE: Spiders and spider bites. *Dermatol Clin* 8:277, 1990.

154. Wasserman GS, Anderson PC: Loxoscelism and necrotic arachnidism. *J Toxicol Clin Toxicol* 21:451, 1983–1984.

155. Jansen GT, Morgan PN, McQueen JN, et al: The brown recluse spider bite: Controlled evaluation of treatment using the white rabbit as a model. *South Med J* 64:1194, 1971.

156. Atkins JA, Wingo CW, Sodeman WA, et al: Necrotic arachnidism. *Am J Trop Med Hyg* 7:165, 1958.

157. Smith CW, Micks DW: A comparative study of the venom and other components of three species of *Loxosceles*. *Am J Trop Med Hyg* 17:651, 1968.

158. Morgan PN: Preliminary studies on venom from the brown recluse spider *Loxosceles reclusa*. *Toxicon* 6:161, 1969.

159. Schmaus LF: Case of arachnoidism (spider bite). *JAMA* 92:1265, 1929.

160. Arnold RE: Brown recluse spider bites: Five cases with a review of the literature. *JACEP* 5:262, 1976.

161. Anderson PC: What's new in loxoscelism—1978. *J Missouri State Med Assoc* 74:549, 1977.

162. Berger RS, Millikan LE, Conway F: An *in vitro* test for *Loxosceles reclusa* spider bites. *Toxicon* 11:465, 1973.

163. King LE, Rees RS: Dapsone treatment of a brown recluse bite. *JAMA* 250:648, 1983.

164. Iserson KV: Methemoglobinemia from dapsone therapy for a suspected brown recluse spider bite. *J Emerg Med* 3:285, 1985.

165. Auer AI, Hershey FB: Proceedings: Surgery for necrotic bites of the brown spider. *Arch Surg* 108:612, 1974.

166. Denny WF, Dillaha CJ, Morgan PN: Hemotoxic effects of *Loxosceles reclusus* venom: *In vivo* and *in vitro* studies. *J Lab Clin Med* 64:291, 1964.

167. Rees RS, O'Leary JP, King LE: The pathogenesis of systemic loxoscelism following brown recluse spider bites. *J Surg Res* 35:1, 1983.

168. Rees RS, Nanney LB, Yates RA, et al: Interaction of brown recluse spider venom on cell membranes: The inciting mechanism? *J Invest Dermatol* 83:270, 1984.

169. Forrester LJ, Barrett JT, Campbell BJ: Red blood cell lysis induced by the venom of the brown recluse spider: The role of sphingomyelinase D. *Arch Biochem Biophys* 187:355, 1978.

170. Kurpiewski G, Forrester LJ, Barrett JT, et al: Platelet aggregation and sphingomyelinase D activity of a purified toxin from the venom of *Loxosceles reclusa*. *Biochim Biophys Acta* 678:467, 1981.

171. Berger RS, Adelstein EH, Anderson PC: Intravascular coagulation: The cause of necrotic arachnidism. *J Invest Dermatol* 61:142, 1973.

172. Butz WC, Stacy LD, Heryford NN: Arachnidism in rabbits: Necrotic lesions due to the brown recluse spider. *Arch Pathol* 91:97, 1971.

173. Butz WC: Envenomation by the brown recluse spider (Aranae, Scytodidae) and related species: A public health problem in the United States. *Clin Toxicol* 4:515, 1971.

174. Smith CW, Micks DW: The role of plymorphonuclear leukocytes in the lesion caused by the venom of the brown spider, *Loxosceles reclusa*. *Lab Invest* 22:90, 1970.

175. Russell FE, Waldron WG, Madon MB: Bites by the brown spiders *Loxosceles unicolor* and *Loxosceles arizonica* in California and Arizona. *Toxicon* 7:109, 1969.

176. Hershey FB, Aulenbacher CE: Surgical treatment of brown spider bites. *Ann Surg* 170:300, 1969.

177. Rees R, Campbell D, Rieger E, et al: The diagnosis and treatment of brown recluse spider bites. *Ann Emerg Med* 16:945, 1987.

178. Anderson PC: Treatment of severe loxoscelism. *J Missouri State Med Assoc* 68:609, 1971.

179. Fardon DW, Wingo CW, Robinson DW, et al: The treatment of brown spider bite. *Plast Reconst Surg* 40:482, 1967.

180. Berger RS: Management of brown recluse spider bite. *JAMA* 251:889, 1984.

181. Nance WE: Hemolytic anemia of necrotic arachnidism. *Am J Med* 31:801, 1961.

182. James JA, Sellars WA, Austin OM, et al: Reactions following suspected spider bite. *Am J Dis Child* 102:395, 1961.

183. Vorse H, Seccareccio P, Woodruff K, et al: Disseminated intravascular coagulopathy following fatal brown spider bite (necrotic arachnidism). *J Pediatr* 80:1035, 1972.

184. Finke JH, Campbell BJ, Barrett JT: Serodiagnostic test for *Loxosceles reclusa* bites. *Clin Toxicol* 7:375, 1974.

185. Russell FE, Gertsch WJ: Letter to the editor. *Toxicon* 21:337, 1983.

186. Russell FE: A confusion of spiders. *Emerg Med* 18:8, 1986.

187. King LE: Brown recluse spider bites: Stay cool. *JAMA* 254:2895, 1985.

188. Berger RS: A critical look at therapy for the brown recluse spider bite. *Arch Dermatol* 107:298, 1973.

189. Hansen RC, Russell FE: Dapsone use for *Loxosceles* envenomation treatment. *Vet Hum Toxicol* 26:260, 1984.

190. Sissom WD: Systematics, biogeography, and paleontology, in Polis GA (ed): *The Biology of Scorpions*. Stanford, Stanford University Press, 1990.

191. Likes K, Banner W, Chavez M: *Centruroides exilicauda* envenomation in Arizona. *West J Med* 141:634, 1984.

192. Stahnke HL: *Scorpions* 2nd ed. Tempe, Poisonous Animals Research Laboratory, 1956.

193. Rimsza ME, Zimmerman DR, Bergeson PS: Scorpion envenomation. *Pediatrics* 66:298, 1980.

194. Stahnke HL: Arizona's lethal scorpion. *Ariz Med* 29:490, 1972.

195. Rachesky IJ, Banner W, Dansky J, et al: Treatments for *Centruroides exilicauda* envenomation. *Am J Dis Child* 138:1136, 1984.

196. Simard JM, Watt DD: Venoms and toxins, in Polis GA (ed): *The Biology of Scorpions*. Stanford, Stanford University Press, 1990.

197. Curry SC, Vance MV, Ryan PJ, et al: Envenomation by the scorpion *Centruroides sculpturatus*. *J Toxicol Clin Toxicol* 21:417, 1983-84.

198. Stahnke HL, Dengler AH: The effect of morphine and related substances on the toxicity of venoms: 1. *Centruroides sculpturatus* Ewing scorpion venom. *Am J Trop Med* 13:346, 1964.

199. Berg RA, Tarantino MD: Envenomation by the scorpion *Centruroides exilicauda (C. sculpturatus)*: Severe and unusual manifestations. *Pediatrics* 87:930, 1991.

200. Bond GR: Antivenin administration for *Centruroides* scorpion sting: Risks and benefits. *Ann Emerg Med* 21:788, 1992.

143. Hydrofluoric Acid Poisoning

Philip A. Edelman

Hydrofluoric acid (HF) is an inorganic acid produced when calcium fluoride (fluospar) reacts with sulfuric acid and heat. It is used in a large array of tasks, and new uses continue to be explored and implemented. Because of its ability to etch silicon dioxide (glass), it has been a mainstay in various industries, including the microelectronics industry, where it is used to etch computer chips (or wafers) and clean quartz furnace tubes. It is used in the oil refining industry as a catalyst to increase the octane rating of fuels and in the aerospace industry to mill titanium. In metallurgic applications it is used in the preparation of uranium compounds. It may be used in janitorial settings to clean porcelain, brick, and stone; in dental laboratories to clean and prepare porcelain prosthetic devices; in car detailing shops as a component of aluminum brighteners; and in laundries as a rust remover. Many electroplating shops use large vats and various concentrations of HF, depending on their plating technique. Hydrofluoric acid may be generated by pyrolysis or combustion of fluorinated compounds (Teflon, Freons). Carbonyl fluoride, the fluoride analog of phosgene, may be generated at that time.

Mechanism of Action

Although HF is an inorganic acid in the halogen series, its corrosivity is greater than expected from acidity alone. Hydrofluoric acid's dissociation constant (K_d) is about 1000 times less than that of hydrochloric acid, and although there is less hydrogen ion activity, the biologic activity of the fluoride ion is clearly far greater and more toxic than the other halides. Since it is less charged, HF is more capable of penetrating lipid barriers, including skin. Once absorbed into the tissue, the hydrogen fluoride equilibrates, freeing the fluoride ion. Since fluoride is the most electronegative element in the periodic chart, it attacks innumerable materials, including the proteins and lipids composing cell membranes; binds divalent cations, interrupting neural transport; blocks metal-containing enzymes; and inhibits glycolysis (enolase).

Routes of Exposure

The primary significant route of exposure is through skin contact. Pulmonary toxicity is minimal, unless HF is heated, aerosolized, in the gaseous or anhydrous state, or present in concentrations greater than 60 percent. However, fuming hydrofluoric acid (70%) or anhydrous material provides a serious route of exposure via inhalation and topical corrosion, leading to systemic toxicity. The vapor pressure of 70% solution at 26.7°C (80°F) is 150 mm Hg; at 20°C it is about 70 mm Hg [1].

Pharmacokinetics

The percent of absorption from dermal HF has not been adequately quantitated. Studies of dietary fluoride, however, have determined that approximately 50 percent of the ingested dose is excreted in the urine within 1 day [1]. Lesser portions are excreted in stool and sweat and a smaller percentage is incorporated into the bone and other body tissues. There is no metabolism of the fluoride ion. There is good concordance between airborne fluoride exposure and urinary concentrations [2]. In rats, limited data show good correlation between acute upper airway exposure and plasma ionic fluoride levels. Since fluoride is used as a dietary supplement, there is some background level in the population. It becomes obvious that there are levels of exposure below which there are no deleterious effects; in fact, these levels may be beneficial or therapeutic.

Presentation

Historically and pragmatically, HF exposures have been divided by concentration into three broad and overlapping categories [3]: dilute exposures (≤ 20%), moderate (20–40%), and concentrated solutions (40–70% and anhydrous hydrofluoric acid). These broad divisions have been recognized for several decades. Treatment and evaluation is generally based on the history of exposure in terms of duration of contact, latency to decontamination, effectiveness of decontamination, and concentration of the initial material. Whereas the effects of most chemical burns can be estimated within a few hours of presentation, this is not the case with HF because of its delayed toxicity, corrosivity, and subsequent delay in symptomatology. Its effects may not be immediately apparent due to lack of initial pain and warning properties associated with most other acids, especially when HF is in a nonconcentrated (< 40%) solution. Therefore, treatment is frequently effected on a basis of history rather than purely on clinical signs.

The most frequently involved area of the body burned by HF is the upper extremity, in particular the hands [4,5]. Most of these exposures occur due to failure to use protective equipment or protective clothing. Exposures to HF occur in all of the industries listed previously. Since dilute HF is commercially available as a rust remover, home exposures may also occur. Gloves should be worn during any contact with HF; however, small pinholes in the fingertips may allow leakage of HF into the glove. For workers using low-concentration HF, there may be no immediate warning symptoms, and the worker may have an exposure of several hours before he or she is aware of contact with HF.

DERMAL EXPOSURES. Patients may not present until 24 to 48 hours after contact with dilute HF. The skin may appear normal or mildly erythematous, although there may be pain out of proportion to the physical findings. Erythema, swelling, and rapid onset of disabling pain suggest exposure to higher concentrations or prolonged contact time with HF and signal the need for immediate treatment. Subjacent tissues may be affected by the penetration of HF, resulting in inflammation of the nerves, tendons, or related structures [6]. This may result in dysfunction due to pain syndromes or inflammatory reactions of the tendons or tendon sheaths. These changes occur even with minimal skin findings.

The longer the exposure to a dilute concentration of HF and the longer the latency between exposure and decontamination, the greater the penetration of HF and the greater the potential for injury. Exposures to moderate concentrations are more likely to lead to pain and other signs of burns in a shorter period. Clinical findings of a more significant burn include worsening erythema, transient blisters, or a white, waxy appearance. The white tissue generally has the appearance and feel of a tough, thickened callus. Sensation is frequently absent over the area. The patient complains of intense deep pain. Exposures to high concentrations or anhydrous HF lead to immediate pain and skin blanching. The deeper dermis may take on a blue-black appearance consistent with dermal hemorrhage. Skin that remains erythematous or develops superficial blisters usually recovers without grafting. Hemorrhagic or waxy-appearing skin is necrotic and may eventually slough. Deeper tissues, such as bone or muscle, may also necrose.

Significant dermal exposures can cause systemic effects. Tepperman [7] and Mayer and Gross [8] reported fatalities resulting from concentrated HF exposures to only 2.5 and 9 to 10 percent of the total body surface area (BSA). A patient with a skin burn of more than 1 percent of the BSA from a concentrated solution, especially when there has been a delay in decontamination, requires admission to an intensive care unit for close monitoring (hypocalcemia and arrhythmias) and treatment (principally calcium). All persons with extensive skin burns secondary to hydrogen fluoride gas, aerosol, or concentrated solutions should be evaluated for inhalation injury.

NONDERMAL EXPOSURES

Ocular. Ocular exposure may occur from contact with liquid, aerosol, or gaseous forms of HF and can lead to significant visual loss. The HF penetrates the cornea into the deeper structures of the eye. Patients may complain of pain, photophobia, tearing, blurred vision, or loss of vision in the affected eye. Clinically, the patient may have conjunctival or ciliary infection, tearing, and blepharospasm. The outer cornea may show blistering. With time, corneal opacification, with visual loss, perforation, scarring, and glaucoma, may occur [9,10,11]. However, brief exposures to lower concentrations may behave as a simple acid burn.

Pulmonary. Pulmonary edema and systemic toxicity may occur from inhalation of HF. Initially, the patient may complain of mild respiratory distress with pain, cough, hemoptysis, dyspnea, and bronchospasm. Airway edema, pulmonary hemorrhage, and pulmonary edema may rapidly occur [6,9,10].

Gastrointestinal. Ingestions of HF are extremely caustic and cause systemic illness. The patient may complain of burning, pain, and nausea. Clinically, the patient may vomit, develop hematemesis, and have diarrhea followed by severe systemic toxicity. Gastrointestinal caustic burns with later hemorrhage, necrosis, and perforation may occur [9,10].

SYSTEMIC TOXICITY. Systemic effects may occur following exposure to relatively small areas of the body to solutions of

HF greater than 20%. Burns from more dilute solutions that are not rapidly decontaminated and/or burns involving a large surface area may result in significant and potentially life-threatening fluoride absorption. Electrolyte imbalance and hypocalcemia can occur and may cause severe cardiac arrhythmia. Symptoms include anxiety, nausea, vomiting, and malaise. This is followed by a rapidly developing acidosis, hypocalcemia, hyperkalemia, coma, respiratory distress syndrome, ventricular arrhythmias, seizures, and death [9,10,12]. Since HF binds divalent cations, early signs of systemic hypocalcemia may be present. These include a widened Q–Tc, tetany, and Trousseau's and Chvostek's signs [12]. Hyperkalemia and hypocalcemia indicate severe biochemical toxicity and are usually premorbid findings.

Laboratory Studies

Blood and urine studies for fluoride are not clinically useful but can provide a good index of exposure. In serious exposures it is essential to monitor acid-base status, serum calcium (ionized and unionized), electrolytes, magnesium, BUN, creatinine, and liver functions [9,12,13]. Calcium and electrolytes, particularly potassium, should be performed serially every 2 to 6 hours for at least the first 24 hours in serious cases, although clinical signs of hypocalcemia precede laboratory abnormalities. Continuous electrocardiographic monitoring should be performed for suspected serious exposures to observe for increased Q–Tc intervals indicative of hypocalcemia. Chest radiograph and arterial blood gases are indicated for inhalation exposures or symptoms. Radiographs of osseous structures should be obtained as a baseline for possible lysis; seriously burned underlying tissue indicates serious injury.

Treatment

Immediate removal from exposure and decontamination are essential. Affected areas should be flooded with water for at least 15 minutes. In cases of serious exposure (≥5% BSA from dilute HF or >1% BSA from concentrated HF, inhalation, or gastrointestinal exposures), early parenteral calcium supplementation should be instituted [9,10]. Patients with renal or cardiac failure may need close observation to prevent hypercalcemia. Local treatments of exposed skin are aimed at decontamination and inactivation of the fluoride ion by complexing it with calcium, magnesium, or quaternary ammonium compounds. Severe cases may require aggressive support, including treatment of pulmonary edema (inhalation), arrhythmias and hypotension (all routes of exposure), and seizure control. In known or suspected ingestion, serious skin exposure, or inhalation, it is essential to treat the patient aggressively despite the initial benign appearance of the wound. The critical effects of hypocalcemia may be delayed for 2 to 24 hours.

DERMAL EXPOSURES. Dilute HF exposures that are immediately and thoroughly irrigated may require little or no therapy [14]. The presence of pain after thorough irrigation requires application of a calcium or magnesium salt. Prepared calcium gluconate gels, magnesium oxide pastes, and other preparations have been compared in various studies without convincing evidence of the superior nature of any agent [15].

Mild burns from exposure to dilute HF can be treated with calcium, magnesium, or quaternary ammonium salts (calcium chloride, calcium gluconate, magnesium sulfate, magnesium citrate, or Zephiran) applied as liquid, paste, or slurry. A 2.5% calcium gluconate gel is available and marketed in Europe and Canada as H-F Antidote Gel* but is not currently approved for use in the United States. Alternatively, a gel can be made by combining 3.5 gm calcium gluconate powder with 5 ounces of water-soluble lubricant. If powder is not available, ten 1-gm calcium gluconate tablets can be crushed into 20 ml of lubricant to make a 50% slurry [10]. Some authors have suggested using an occlusive dressing, such as a surgical glove [16], or combining the slurry with equal parts of dimethyl sulfoxide (DMSO) [17]. The use of DMSO is not recommended at this time. The use of calcium chloride in the gel is not recommended because of its irritative nature [10]. Henry and Hla [18] used regional intravenous administration of calcium gluconate to affected extremities using a method analogous to a Bier block. However, the results were not compelling. The authors have had good success with regional intravenous administration for nondigital hand and arm burns. We use a double tourniquet for the occlusion and dilute 1 gm calcium gluconate into 20 to 50 ml saline.

All bullae should be removed and the underlying tissues cleaned; calcium gluconate solution or gel should then be applied. Because the blister fluid is generally contaminated with HF, the blisters should not be left intact.

Skin burns may need local injection with 10% calcium gluconate solution if water decontamination and topical salts do not relieve the pain [4,5,6,14]. A 10% calcium gluconate solution is injected into the subcutaneous tissue using a 27- or 30-gauge needle. No more than 0.5 ml per square centimeter should be used [6,9]. Calcium chloride should *not* be used for local infiltration.

On injection, there is mild stinging with the infiltration for a few seconds; when this subsides the original pain from the HF is generally markedly diminished. Multiple small-volume injections into the subcutaneous tissues and deep dermis should be performed. A long spinal needle may be used for large surface area wounds. After placement under the wound, the needle is slowly withdrawn and the calcium gluconate injected continuously to infiltrate the entire tract. This is the definitive treatment. If the pain recurs after several hours, the injections should be repeated and extended over a greater area [14]. For large burn areas (>5–10%), the patient should be admitted, given intravenous calcium, and placed on continuous cardiac monitoring [19]. Large burn areas may be infiltrated with calcium gluconate, even in the absence of significant pain or redness, in an attempt to bind the available fluoride and decrease the likelihood and severity of hypocalcemia.

The fingers are the most frequently affected part of the body. Local infiltration should never exceed 0.5 ml of solution per phalanx, as pressure necrosis may occur. Injections of calcium gluconate solution into the skin and subcutaneous tissues of the fingers must not be circumferential and must be done only with careful judgment because of the possibility of the injection itself producing vascular impairment. The use of lidocaine in the calcium infusion is not recommended, as it may mask the resolution of pain occurring from complexation of fluoride with calcium. In the presence of periungual pain, redness, or subungual discoloration, the nail should be removed and the nail bed decontaminated and injected. The finger should be adequately anesthetized before fingernail removal.

---

* H-F Antidote Gel, Pharmascience, Montreal, Quebec, Canada, (514) 340-1114. H-F Antidote Gel, Moore & Company, Ltd., Rippleside Commercial Estate, Kenwick Road, Barking Essex 1G11 05D, England [10].

Alternatively, the patient should be referred for intraarterial calcium infusion [9,20,21,22]. Although more invasive, the results are clinically better, less painful, and less disfiguring, since the fingernails generally do not need to be removed [22]. The infusion, once started, is relatively painless and provides a higher concentration of calcium salts to all tissues, including bone. It does, however, require placement of an intraarterial catheter and has the risks of arterial line placement (arterial spasm and thrombosis); it should only be performed by someone experienced in placing intraarterial lines [9].

Intraarterial infusion requires placement of the catheter in the appropriate arterial supply, followed by a slow infusion of dilute calcium gluconate solution. It is not necessary to perform an arteriogram first [20,22]. Ten to 20 milliliters of 10% calcium gluconate are diluted into 50 to 100 ml of D_5W and infused over 4 hours. The infusion is repeated until pain relief is obtained, skin color is normalized, or a maximum of three infusions have been completed [9,10,20,21]. Local nerve blocks can be given, especially if necrosis has already occurred. Although poorly documented, this procedure has been used successfully in HF burns to the lower extremities. I do not use any regional anesthesia as I prefer to monitor the patient's discomfort to determine the effectiveness of treatment. Pain should be managed with parenteral narcotics, however, because the burns are exquisitely painful.

OCULAR EXPOSURES. The treatment of ocular exposures has been poorly studied. Immediate irrigation with isotonic sodium chloride or magnesium chloride remains the recommended therapy [10]. In McCully and co-workers' series, multiple irrigations increased the rate of corneal perforations [11]. Topical isotonic calcium chloride is not recommended because it is toxic to the eye [23]. Close follow-up with an ophthalmologist familiar with ocular caustic burns is recommended.

INHALATIONAL EXPOSURE. Pulmonary injury may be seen immediately after exposures to high concentrations or delayed if the exposure was more dilute. Acute upper airway embarrassment should be anticipated for 24 hours. Early laryngoscopy is recommended. Emergency tracheostomy or endotracheal intubation should be readily available and performed if there is any indication of airway edema.

Pulmonary edema may occur from inhalation; if by history this is a consideration, the patient should be monitored in a critical care setting for at least 24 hours. The onset of pulmonary edema may be delayed [9]. Pulmonary function testing, arterial blood gases, and diffusing capacity aid in determining the extent of airway trauma. Chest radiographs should be used as clinically indicated. Systemic toxicity should be anticipated.

Treatment is supportive and may require positive-pressure ventilation. The use of calcium gluconate by nebulization in a concentration of 2% to 3% has been suggested as therapy for inhalational exposure but it is of unproved efficacy [10].

GASTROINTESTINAL EXPOSURES. There are few data on decontamination of the gut. As HF is corrosive if ingested, it is best left in situ and complexed by the addition of calcium or magnesium salts (calcium gluconate, magnesium citrate or sulfate, calcium-containing antacids, or milk). Careful lavage after administration of oral calcium may be done, but this has not been studied. Limited experience has shown the devastating effects of HF on the untreated esophagus, which required colonic interposition in at least one patient. Early endoscopy after ingestion and gastroenterologic consultation are highly recommended. Systemic effects should be anticipated and treated expectantly. At least eight deaths have been reported from systemic toxicity resulting from HF ingestion. A unique case of an HF enema was recently reported with grossly necrotic bowel [24].

SYSTEMIC TOXICITY. Systemic effects may occur following exposure to relatively small areas of the body to solutions containing greater than 20% HF. Burns from more dilute solutions may result in significant and potentially life-threatening fluoride absorption if the area was not rapidly decontaminated or a large surface area is involved. Electrolyte imbalance and hypocalcemia can occur and cause severe cardiac arrhythmias. Hospitalization in a critical care setting is indicated for these patients. Calcium supplementation for hypocalcemia is essential [10,14]. Intravenous calcium chloride or calcium gluconate is advocated. Calcium chloride has a greater risk of local tissue injury in the event of extravasation but provides three times more calcium per weight than calcium gluconate.

Patients at high risk for systemic toxicity should have intravenous calcium started prophylactically prior to any evidence of hypocalcemia. Twenty milliliters of a 10% calcium salt solution should be added to the first liter of crystalloid [14]. Additional calcium should be given as clinically indicated. Once hypocalcemia is evident biochemically, the patient is usually in extremis and it may be difficult to provide sufficient calcium. Correction of acidosis and hyperkalemia may require large amounts of sodium bicarbonate or dialysis. Cardiovascular collapse is an ominous sign and should be treated supportively [9].

There is at least one case report of early excision of HF-burned tissue after onset of life-threatening systemic toxicity. The patient had burns on 5 percent of BSA from anhydrous HF and ventricular fibrillation; he survived after burn wound excision [25].

Controversies

Various agents and concentrations of agents have been used for topical application. There is no definitive treatise or study determining the best modality. However, calcium gluconate 2.5% gel, magnesium oxide paste, and magnesium sulfate solutions all have been standard treatment for many years. Some authors have insisted that iced water or alcohol is sufficient for burns, but most of these authors did not study a wide range of burns. It is generally accepted that local infiltration of the persistently painful burn wound is essential. Calcium gluconate is the standard modality. Other authors have suggested topical calcium carbonate [26] or the superiority of 5% calcium gluconate for injection [27]. However, the efficacy studies reviewed lack a validated model questioning their applicability. Some of the authors noted problems with variability in the burn at a given dose, necessitating the grouping of dosage subsets [27]. Our animal model research has found that skin preparation is critical (hair clippers, depilatory agents, skin cleaning, trauma, etc.) and the epidermal lipid layer is an important barrier to HF burns [28,29]. The breach of the lipid barrier due to a variety of factors results in serious dermal injury. As prior efficacy studies have not addressed the usual spectrum of HF exposure histories, and because their models have not been sufficiently validated, one is forced to conclude that these studies do not provide reliable information for establishing unequivocal treatment guidelines or recommendations.

Intraarterial perfusion of affected limbs has been successfully undertaken and may be a superior modality for the provision of calcium to the local tissues. One study evaluated DMSO as a topical carrier for calcium salts [17]. However, DMSO, even if effective for carrying calcium salts, would also carry other skin contaminants and affect the lipid barriers of the skin, potentially increasing HF penetration.

Calcium gluconate in a regional intravenous application (Bier block) has been tried, but a variety of problems with this technique remain, including the uncertain effect of prolonged circulatory stasis and diminished oxygen (with acidosis). Ultimately the calcium supply to the tissue is by diffusion rather than perfusion.

Calcium gluconate 1% as an eyewash is widely recommended for eye contamination, but thorough evaluations have not been published. The need to remove the fingernail when it is involved is unequivocal, unless intraarterial calcium is given. Early excision of burn wounds in patients with persistent, severe hypocalcemia has also been necessary [25]. The number of treatments, dose of calcium, and efficacy after a delay (> 12 hours) in treatment are untested parameters.

References

1. Sticht G: Fluorine, in Seilier HG, Sigel H (eds): *Toxicity of Inorganic Compounds.* New York, Marcel Dekker, 1988, p 283.
2. Dinman BD, Bovard WJ, Bonney TB, et al: Absorption and excretion of fluoride immediately after exposure. *J Occup Med* 18:7, 1976.
3. Division of Industrial Hygiene, National Institutes of Health: Hydrofluoric acid burns. *Ind Med* 12:634, 1943.
4. Blunt CP: Treatment of hydrofluoric acid skin burns by injection with calcium gluconate. *Ind Med* 33:869, 1964.
5. Iverson RE, Laub DR, Madison MS: Hydrofluoric acid burns. *Plast Reconstruct Surg* 48:107, 1971.
6. Edelman PA: Hydrofluoric acid burns. *State Art Rev Occup Med* 1:89, 1986.
7. Tepperman PB: Fatality due to acute systemic fluoride poisoning following a hydrofluoric acid skin burn. *J Occup Med* 22:691, 1980.
8. Mayer TG, Gross PL: Fatal systemic fluorosis due to hydrofluoric acid burns. *Ann Emerg Med* 14:149, 1985.
9. Caravati EM: Acute hydrofluoric acid exposure. *Am J Emerg Med* 6:143, 1988.
10. Hydrofluoric acid management, in *Poisindex.* 64th ed. Micromedex, May 1990.
11. McCully JP, Whiting DW, Petitt MG, et al: Hydrofluoric burns of the eye. *J Occup Med* 25:447, 1983.
12. McCulley JP: Ocular hydrofluoric acid burns: Animal model, mechanism of injury and therapy. *Trans Am Ophthalmol Soc* 88:649, 1990.
13. Grecco RJ, Hartford CE, Haith LR, et al: Hydrofluoric acid-induced hypocalcemia. *J Trauma* 28:1593, 1988.
14. Dibbell DG, Iverson RE, Jones W, et al: Hydrofluoric acid burns of the hand. *J Bone Joint Surg* 52A:931, 1970.
15. Bracken WM, Cuppage F, McLaury RL, et al: Comparative effectiveness of topical treatments for hydrofluoric acid burns. *J Occup Med* 27:733, 1985.
16. Bullock C: Hydrofluoric burns cooled with calcium carbonate slurry. *Emerg Med News* July 17-18, 1989.
17. Zachary LS, Reus W, Gottlieb J, et al: Treatment of experimental burns. *J Burn Care* 7:35, 1986.
18. Henry JA, Hla KK: Intravenous regional calcium gluconate perfusion for hydrofluoric acid burns. *J Toxicol Clin Toxicol* 30:203, 1992.
19. Trevino MA, Herrmann GH, Sprout WL: Treatment of severe hydrofluoric acid exposures. *J Occup Med* 25:861, 1983.
20. Velvart J: Arterial perfusion for hydrofluoric acid burns. *Hum Toxicol* 2:233, 1983.
21. Vance MV, Curry SC, Kunkel DB, et al: Digital hydrofluoric acid burns: Treatment with intraarterial calcium infusion. *Ann Emerg Med* 15:890, 1986.

22. Edelman PA: Intraarterial calcium gluconate for treatment of hydrofluoric acid burns of the extremities. Proceedings of the American Burn Association, Las Vegas, 1990.

23. Grant WM: *Toxicology of the Eye.* 3rd ed. Springfield, Ill, Charles C Thomas, 1986, p 490.

24. Cappell MS, Simon T: Fulminant acute colitis following a self-administered hydrofluoric acid enema. *Am J Gastroenterol* 88:122, 1993.

25. Buckingham FM: Surgery: A radical approach to severe hydrofluoric acid burns. *J Occup Med* 30:873, 1988.

26. Chick LR, Borah G: Calcium carbonate gel therapy for hydrofluoric acid burns of the hand. *Plast Reconstr Surg* 86:935, 1990.

27. Dunn BJ, MacKinnon MA, Knowlden NF, et al: Hydrofluoric acid dermal burns: An assessment of treatment efficacy using an experimental pig model—Survival following hydrofluoric acid ingestion. *J Occup Med* 21:1396, 1992.

28. Noonan T, Carter E, Kim J, et al: Epidermal lipids and the natural history of hydrofluoric acid (HF) injury. Proceedings of the American Burn Association, 1993.

29. Noonan T, Carter EJ, Edelman PA, Zawacki BE: Epidermal lipids and the natural history of hydrofluoric acid (HF) injury. *Burns* 20:202, 1994.

144. Hydrocarbons

William J. Lewander and
James G. Linakis

Hydrocarbons are a group of organic compounds composed entirely of hydrogen and carbon. Although often mixtures, hydrocarbons may be divided into three basic types: aliphatic (petroleum distillates), halogenated, and aromatic hydrocarbons.

Hydrocarbon exposures are frequent and account for an inordinate number of health care visits and hospital admissions. The American Association of Poison Control Centers reported 52,454 hydrocarbon exposures in 1988 [1]. Twenty-six percent of exposed individuals required treatment in a health care facility; and nearly 12 percent of these patients were considered to have suffered exposures of moderate or major severity. Over half of all exposures occur in children younger than 6 years of age, and the vast majority of all exposures are accidental. Nevertheless, intentional exposures are not uncommon and frequently have even greater potential for toxicity. Fortunately, only eight deaths were reported as a result of hydrocarbon exposure in 1988 [1].

This chapter addresses the toxicity, clinical manifestations, diagnostic evaluation, and management of aliphatic, halogenated, and aromatic hydrocarbons.

Petroleum Distillates

Petroleum distillates are produced from the fractional distillation of natural petroleum and contain varying amounts of aliphatic (straight chain) and aromatic (cyclic) hydrocarbons. Those classified predominantly as aliphatic hydrocarbons are discussed here. Common petroleum distillates include mineral spirits, naphtha, gasoline, kerosene, mineral seal oil, diesel oil, and fuel oil. Table 144-1 lists common petroleum distillates.

Petroleum distillates continue to be the most commonly reported hydrocarbon poisoning, accounting for more than 34,000 exposures in 1988, of which nearly one-third required treatment in a health care facility. Of these, approximately 8 percent resulted in moderate or major toxicity [1]. Unmarked, poorly stored containers or an attractive color or aroma are some of the factors that account for the high percentage of exposures in children younger than 6 years. In adults, poisoning generally occurs as a result of occupational exposure, intentional ingestion, or accidental aspiration during the siphoning of fuels. Ingestions in adults usually involve larger volumes, and there is a much greater likelihood of other coingested drugs or toxins. Although the most common route of exposure is by ingestion, inhalational, cutaneous, and even intravenous exposures have been described.

TOXICITY. The major toxicity of petroleum distillates is their potential to cause a fulminant and sometimes fatal chemical pneumonitis Central nervous system (CNS), gastrointestinal (GI), cardiovascular, hepatic, renal, hematologic, and cutaneous toxicity may also occur.

After oral ingestions, pulmonary toxicity occurs from aspiration rather than by hematogenous spread. Although vomiting often precedes and results in aspiration, lack of vomiting does not preclude the possibility that aspiration has occurred. The ratio of the oral LD_{50} of petroleum distillates when instilled intratracheally versus intragastrically is 1:140 in animals [2]. The aspiration of very small amounts may produce severe pulmonary toxicity; numerous studies have demonstrated that little or no systemic toxicity occurs even after large intragastric administration (12–18 ml/kg) in animals [3,4].

The potential for aspiration is determined by the physical properties of viscosity, surface tension, and volatility. The risk of aspiration increases with low viscosity, low surface tension, and high volatility. Viscosity, the tendency to resist flow, is the most important property determining aspiration potential [5]. Low viscosity permits deeper penetration into the distal airways. Viscosity is measured in Saybolt Seconds Universal (SSU). Substances with an SSU value less than 60 have a high aspiration potential (e.g., gasoline, mineral seal oil, kerosene), whereas those with an SSU value greater than 100 have a low potential for aspiration (e.g., mineral oil, fuel oil). Reduced surface tension may allow a substance to spread rapidly from the upper GI tract to the trachea, and high volatility (tendency of a liquid to become a gas) increases the likelihood of pulmonary absorption. When aspirated, petroleum distillates inhibit surfactant, resulting in alveolar collapse, ventilation/perfusion mismatch, and subsequent hypoxemia. In addition, bronchospasm and direct capillary damage lead to a chemical

Table 144-1. Common Petroleum Distillates

Product	Synonym	Main use
Gasoline	Petroleum spirits	Fuel
Petroleum naphtha fluid	Ligroin	Cigarette lighter
VM and P naphtha thinner	Varnish naphtha	Paint or varnish
Mineral spirits	Painter's naphtha	Dry cleaner
	Stoddard solvent	Solvent
	White spirits	Paint thinner
	Varsol	
	Mineral turpentine	
	Petroleum spirits	
Kerosene fluid	Coal oil	Charcoal lighter
		Solvent
		Fuel for stoves, lamps
Fuel oil	Home heating oil	Fuel
Diesel oil	Gas oil	Furniture polish

pneumonitis and hemorrhagic bronchitis/alveolitis [2,5,6,7]. In animals exposed to kerosene, Gross et al. demonstrated acute alveolitis, which peaked at 3 days and resolved by 10 days. Histologically, a chronic proliferative process occurred, peaking at 10 days and resolving over several weeks [8]. When highly viscous petroleum distillates are aspirated, a less inflammatory but more localized and indolent lipoid pneumonia may occur [9].

Systemic toxicity is limited by poor GI absorption. The CNS manifestations result principally from hypoxia and acidosis caused by pulmonary toxicity [7,10,11].

Although systemic toxicity is uncommon, it may be seen if the petroleum distillate is a vehicle for more toxic substances (e.g., heavy metal, pesticide), if it contains additives, or if a concomitant or massive ingestion has occurred [12]. Cardiovascular, hepatic, renal, and hematologic toxicity depend on the specific toxic substance involved.

Petroleum distillate inhalation abuse (e.g., gasoline sniffing) does not produce a chemical pneumonitis but instead leads to a complex toxicity caused by the combined effects of its many constituents (e.g., aromatic hydrocarbons, paraffins, naphthenes, and tetraethyl lead) [13,14].

CLINICAL MANIFESTATIONS AND DIAGNOSTIC EVALUATION. Presenting signs and symptoms following ingestion of petroleum distillates usually involve three main organ systems: pulmonary system, CNS, and GI system. Cardiovascular, renal, hematologic, and cutaneous toxicity have also been reported [15]. Although the majority of children who present to health care facilities after a petroleum distillate exposure remain asymptomatic, both adults and children who aspirate generally demonstrate symptoms within 30 minutes [16]. Initial coughing, gasping, and choking may progress during the first 24 hours to tachypnea with grunting respirations, nasal flaring, retractions, and cyanosis [12,16]. The odor of petroleum distillate may be apparent on the breath. Wheezing, rhonchi, and rales may be heard on auscultation. In severe cases, pulmonary edema and hemoptysis occur. Arterial blood gases may demonstrate hypoxemia from ventilation/perfusion mismatch and early hypocarbia, which progresses to hypercarbia and acidosis. Chest film abnormalities occur in up to 75 percent of hospitalized patients and appear within 2 hours in 88 percent of patients and by 12 hours in 98 percent [12,17,18]. Both radiographic abnormalities

and symptoms may be delayed several hours. Early radiographic abnormalities include unilateral but more commonly bilateral basilar infiltrates and fine punctate perihilar densities. Localized areas of atelectasis are often present, whereas pleural effusions, pneumatoceles, and pneumothoraces occur infrequently [17–20]. Pneumatoceles generally occur 3 to 15 days after ingestion and resolve over 15 days to 21 months [2,21]. Radiographic findings correlate poorly with clinical symptoms. Asymptomatic patients may have abnormal chest films, whereas symptomatic patients may have minimal or no radiographic abnormalities early in the course [12,22].

Within the first 24 to 48 hours, fever (38–39°C) and leukocytosis are common [16]. The persistence of fever beyond 48 hours suggests bacterial superinfection.

Central nervous system involvement occurs most commonly in the presence of aspiration-induced hypoxemia, toxic additives (e.g., aromatic hydrocarbons), and large intentional ingestions. Symptoms range from dizziness and lethargy (91%) to somnolence (5%) and rarely coma (3%) and convulsions (1%) [12,23]. Patients with moderate to severe respiratory involvement present with increasingly serious CNS manifestations.

Gastrointestinal symptoms, such as local irritation of the oropharynx (e.g., burning), nausea, vomiting, and abdominal pain, are commonly reported. Hematemesis and melena occur rarely [22]. Vomiting appears to increase the likelihood of aspiration [19,24].

Cardiovascular toxicity is uncommon, but dysrhythmias and sudden death after gasoline siphoning have been reported [25]. It is unclear whether hypoxia or gasoline absorption after aspiration may have sensitized the myocardium to endogenous catecholamines, resulting in fatal dysrhythmias [12,22].

Cases of acute renal tubular necrosis [26,27], hemoglobinuria secondary to intravascular hemolysis [28,29], severe burns following prolonged immersion in gasoline [30], and supraglottitis [31] have been reported.

Inhalation abuse of petroleum distillates (e.g., gasoline sniffing) has resulted in a range of acute CNS manifestations, including dizziness, incoordination, restlessness, excitement, confusion, and coma. There have been several reports of organo-lead poisoning [13,14,32,33]. Parenteral administration of petroleum distillates has caused local cellulitis, thrombophlebitis, and necrotizing myositis, with resultant compartment syndromes. Systemic effects include febrile reactions, hemorrhagic pneumonitis, pulmonary edema, seizures, and CNS depression [15,34,35].

Diagnostic evaluation includes a thorough history (e.g., identity, amount, and concentration of toxin, time of ingestion, and symptoms prior to presentation at health care facility) and a physical examination focusing on vital signs and the respiratory, central nervous, and GI systems. A chest film is indicated. In symptomatic patients or those who have ingested concomitant toxins or toxic additives, laboratory evaluation should include an arterial blood gas determination; complete blood count; electrolyte, BUN, creatinine, and glucose measurements; liver function tests; and urinalysis. Because the clinical course of most petroleum distillate exposures depends on the presence and quantity of toxin aspirated, patients who do not have symptoms of respiratory distress within 6 hours postexposure will remain asymptomatic [16].

If aspiration has occurred, respiratory symptoms should develop within 30 minutes to 6 hours and may progress and peak during a 24- to 48-hour period. In most cases symptoms resolve over the next 2 to 5 days with supportive care [16,19]. Most radiographic abnormalities progress and peak by 72 hours. The radiographic changes lag behind clinical improvement and may persist for several days to weeks after symptoms have resolved [17,19,21].

MANAGEMENT. Initial management of petroleum distillate exposure should focus on the clinical, radiographic, and laboratory assessment of respiratory distress. Patients who remain asymptomatic with a normal chest film (obtained 2 hours or more after exposure) may be discharged after 6 hours of observation. All symptomatic patients, those with abnormal chest films, and patients with suicidal intent should be hospitalized.

Gastric decontamination is not recommended in petroleum distillate ingestion because absorption and systemic toxicity are minimal, and spontaneous or induced vomiting increase the risk of aspiration and pneumonitis [23,37,38]. Gastric decontamination is recommended only if potentially toxic amounts of aromatic or halogenated hydrocarbons, pesticides, heavy metals, or other substances have been ingested. There is no uniform consensus on the management of these patients when they present awake and alert [18,23,39]. Two recent reviews recommended administration of ipecac syrup when GI decontamination is warranted in these patients [12,37], although the method of choice remains controversial. Patients who are unconscious, unable to protect the airway (e.g., poor or absent gag reflex), or deteriorating should be intubated with a cuffed endotracheal tube (in patients older than 6 years) and then lavaged. Administration of mineral or olive oil increases the risk of aspiration and is contraindicated [18]. Activated charcoal and cathartic are indicated only if a toxic additive is present or concomitant ingestion has occurred. If cutaneous exposure has occurred, contaminated clothing should be carefully removed and contaminated skin should be thoroughly washed with green soap and water [12].

All patients with respiratory symptoms should be given oxygen, placed on a cardiac monitor, and have intravenous access established. An arterial blood gas determination and chest film should be obtained. The need for intubation should be based on clinical assessment of respiratory distress and objective data from arterial blood gases or pulse oximetry. Although useful, chest films do not always correlate with clinical status and should not be used as the sole determinant for respiratory support. Continuous positive airway pressure may be necessary to maintain oxygenation, but the patient should be carefully monitored for the development of a pneumothorax. Bronchospasm should be treated with cardioselective bronchodilators because of potential myocardial sensitization to catecholamines [36].

Supportive care of serious petroleum distillate pneumonitis includes careful monitoring of acid-base, fluid, and electrolyte balance (e.g., cautious hydration to avoid pulmonary edema), serial arterial blood gases or pulse oximetry, and chest radiograph evaluation. Complete blood counts with differential, serial sputum, or tracheal aspirate Gram stains and cultures assist in determining whether bacterial superinfection has occurred. Baseline renal and liver function studies and a toxic screen should be obtained if toxic additives or concomitant ingestion is suspected. The regional poison center should be consulted.

Several animal and clinical investigations have failed to demonstrate any beneficial effect of steroid treatment [40,41,42]. Two animal studies indicate that they may be harmful [43,44,45]. In addition, prophylactic antibiotics have not been shown to be helpful [37,42,43]. Fever and leukocytosis secondary to chemical pneumonitis are commonly seen during the first 24 to 48 hours in the absence of superimposed bacterial pneumonia [12,18]. Antibiotics (e.g., penicillin or clindamycin) should be given only to patients with documented bacterial pneumonias (e.g., Gram stain or culture of sputum or tracheal aspirate) or worsening chest radiograph, chest pain, leukocytosis, and fever after the first 40 hours [12,22].

The vast majority of patients with petroleum distillate poisoning recover fully with supportive care. Despite the report of minor pulmonary function abnormalities in as many as 82 per-

cent of asymptomatic survivors of aspiration pneumonitis [46], most have no major sequelae. Long-term follow-up care with pulmonary function testing should be considered. When appropriate, the patient should receive psychiatric evaluation and poison prevention education prior to final disposition.

Halogenated Hydrocarbons

The halogenated hydrocarbons are a class of aliphatic and aromatic hydrocarbons containing one or more atoms of chlorine, bromine, fluorine, or iodine (Table 144-2). Although dozens of halogenated hydrocarbons are currently recognized, relatively few account for the majority of the toxicity caused by these compounds. Nevertheless, those that do cause significant toxicity represent an important source of morbidity and mortality. For example, in 1988, half of the hydrocarbon deaths reported to the American Association of Poison Control Centers National Data Collection System were due to halogenated hydrocarbons [1]. Although many of the halogenated hydrocarbons are an aspiration risk, similar to the aliphatic hydrocarbons, they represent a much greater risk of inducing systemic toxicity, most notably of the CNS, cardiovascular system, and hepatic and renal systems.

Halogenated hydrocarbons are used both in the household and in industry. They are frequently used as solvents, degreasers, dry cleaning agents, refrigerants, aerosol propellants, and fumigants. Toxic exposures occur most commonly through inhalation, and several halogenated hydrocarbons (e.g., trichloroethylene, methylene chloride, fluorocarbons) are intentionally inhaled for recreational purposes [47]. "Bagging" (spraying the solvent into a plastic bag and repeatedly inhaling the vapors) and "huffing" (spraying the solvent onto a cloth held to the mouth and nose) have been associated with a number of solvent abuse deaths.

Halogenated hydrocarbons are well absorbed from the GI tract and, occasionally, through the skin. Although specific values for volume of distribution are unavailable, animal studies indicate that most of these substances are concentrated in adipose tissue, liver, and kidney.

Metabolism and elimination of halogenated hydrocarbons vary according to the individual substance, with most undergoing at least some excretion through the lungs as unchanged parent compound and nearly all undergoing some degree of metabolism in the liver, with subsequent excretion of metabolites by the lungs and/or kidneys.

The large number of halogenated hydrocarbons precludes discussion of each individual substance. Certain solvents identified as prototypes for the clinical toxicology of this class of hydrocarbons are discussed in somewhat greater detail below.

CARBON TETRACHLORIDE. Previously used as a dry cleaning agent and antihelminthic, carbon tetrachloride (CCl_4) has

Table 144-2. Some Halogenated Hydrocarbons

Carbon tetrachloride	Ethylene dichloride
Chloroform	Halothane
Trichloroethylene (TCE)	Methyl chloride
1,1,1 Trichloroethane (TCA)	Prophylene dichloride
Methylene chloride	Tetrachloroethylene
Trichlorofluoromethane (Freon 11)	Trifluoromonobromomethane
Dichlorofluoromethane (Freon 12)	Trichlorotrifluoromethane
Methyl bromide	Methylene iodide
Ethylene dibromide	

been restricted by the Food and Drug Administration to those industrial products in which it is an intrinsic by-product. As a result, its use is now limited to industries manufacturing refrigerants, aerosol propellants, and solvents.

Carbon tetrachloride is well absorbed through the skin [48,49], lungs, and GI tract and concentrated in adipose tissue [50]. Approximately 50 percent of an absorbed dose is excreted unchanged by the lungs. The vast majority of the remainder is metabolized by the liver. It is thought that metabolism occurs primarily via microsomal cytochrome P-450 reductase and NADPH-dependent reductive pathways. Within these pathways, carbon tetrachloride is thought to be converted to reactive intermediates and/or free radicals, which covalently bind to proteins and induce lipid peroxidation, resulting in hepatocellular damage [51]. Ethanol, methanol, and isopropyl alcohol all increase carbon tetrachloride hepatotoxicity, presumably through enzyme induction [52].

Pathologically, at lower doses, fatty degeneration of the liver occurs; at higher concentrations, centrilobular necrosis results [53]. In addition to hepatic damage, carbon tetrachloride produces acute tubular necrosis of the kidney, affecting the proximal tubules and Henle's loop [54]. Although it has been assumed that this is the result of a direct nephrotoxic effect of carbon tetrachloride [55], there is evidence that in some patients, renal failure following carbon tetrachloride exposure is the result of volume contraction [56].

Clinically, inhalation exposure to carbon tetrachloride may produce mild CNS depression at concentrations of 150 to 300 ppm. Symptoms such as headache and drowsiness occur following exposure of 5 to 10 minutes to concentrations of 2000 ppm. Fatalities occur at concentrations of 20,000 ppm [50]. Although the estimated lethal dose of orally ingested carbon tetrachloride is 90 to 100 ml, deaths have occasionally been reported following much smaller doses.

Early signs and symptoms of carbon tetrachloride toxicity include nausea, vomiting, abdominal pain, diarrhea, drowsiness, and light-headedness, generally within a few hours of exposure, regardless of route of exposure. Although liver enzymes may start to rise on the first day after esposure, clinical evidence of hepatotoxicity generally occurs on days 2 to 4, with fever, elevated liver function tests, prolonged prothrombin time, liver tenderness and enlargement, and jaundice [57,58]. Gastrointestinal bleeding may occur secondary to a decrease in clotting factors.

Decline in renal function, as evidenced by azotemia, proteinuria, oliguria, and anuria, may occur concomitantly with hepatic dysfunction, although occasionally renal failure appears in the absence of hepatic failure [55,58]. The oliguric phase lasts, on average, 7 days (range 3–15 days), but with dialysis support recovery is generally complete [59]. Rarely, carbon tetrachloride toxicity is accompanied by coma, convulsions, or myocarditis.

Early fatalities are thought to be the result of respiratory depression or cardiac dysrhythmias caused by cardiac sensitization to circulating catecholamines. More commonly, death occurs as the result of hepatic or renal failure, generally within the first week. In nonfatal cases, liver function tests generally return to normal within 2 weeks; recovery is usually complete.

Diagnosis of carbon tetrachloride exposures is usually based on history, although abdominal radiographs may be helpful in confirming suspected ingestions, since carbon tetrachloride is radiopaque [60].

Treatment involves initial stabilization and monitoring for respiratory depression and cardiac dysrhythmias. Exposure should be interrupted by removing victims of inhalation from the exposure site; in dermal exposures, contaminated clothing should be removed and the skin washed thoroughly. Patients who ingest greater than 0.3 ml per kilogram should undergo gastric decontamination procedures within 3 to 4 hours of ingestion [61]. In patients with compromised upper airway protection, endotracheal intubation with a cuffed endotracheal tube is indicated prior to gastric lavage. There is no evidence regarding the utility of activated charcoal in adsorbing carbon tetrachloride. Although carbon tetrachloride appears not to be well removed by hemodialysis, dialysis may be required in cases of renal failure [59].

Animal studies suggest that hyperbaric oxygen may increase survival after intragastric administration of carbon tetrachloride [62], although few human data exist on this topic [63]. Additional experimental work is being conducted to examine the utility of N-acetyl-cysteine (NAC) in the reduction of carbon tetrachloride-induced hepatotoxicity. Because toxic intermediates of hepatic P-450 are throught to be responsible for carbon tetrachloride toxicity, it is thought that NAC may help prevent the development of liver failure [64]. Although human experience with this therapy is extremely limited in this setting and still considered experimental, a dosage schedule identical to that for acetaminophen is generally used.

Clinical outcome is usually determined in the first week after exposure. Patients should be followed carefully during this time for evidence of hepatic or renal failure. If no such evidence exists by 3 to 5 days after an acute exposure, the prognosis is excellent.

METHYLENE CHLORIDE. Methylene chloride is a colorless, volatile liquid commonly used as a solvent in aerosol products and as a degreaser and paint remover. It is well absorbed through the lungs and GI tract, but absorption through intact skin appears to be of a sufficiently low level as to avoid systemic toxicity [48]. The majority of an inhaled dose is metabolized by the liver to carbon dioxide (~65%) and carbon monoxide (~30%), with small amounts exhaled unchanged [65]. Methylene chloride is mildly hepatotoxic, but its main toxicity is to the CNS.

Concentrations of 1000 ppm of methylene chloride may produce mild light-headedness, whereas concentrations greater than 2000 ppm cause nausea and lethargy after 30 minutes [12]. An 8-hour exposure to 250 ppm of methylene chloride resulted in carboxyhemoglobin levels greater than 8 percent [66], and with large exposures carboxyhemoglobin levels up to 50 percent have been reported. Few cases of methylene chloride *ingestion* have been reported, although ingestion of 16 to 32 ounces of a methylene chloride-containing paint remover resulted in acidosis, coma, and intravascular hemolysis in an individual who ultimately survived [67].

Clinically, the toxicity caused by methylene chloride is the result of two factors: its direct effect on the CNS and the effects of elevated levels of carboxyhemoglobin. Central nervous system symptoms include light-headedness, headache, lethargy, syncope, irritability, gait disturbances, stupor, and coma. Seizures do not generally occur, but pulmonary edema has been reported. If high carboxyhemoglobin levels are present, signs and symptoms of carbon monoxide poisoning are also evident [68,69]. Cases of nephrotoxicity and hepatic toxicity have also been reported in association with methylene chloride exposure [70,71].

Treatment involves initial stabilization and monitoring for dysrhythmias. The patient should be removed from the source of inhalation exposure, and contaminated clothing should be removed. Exposed skin should be washed with soap and water. In cases of ingestion, gastric decontamination procedures should be carried out; in obtunded patients, however, endotracheal intubation should precede gastric lavage. The role of activated charcoal in methylene chloride ingestions is unclear

[72]. In all cases, carboxyhemoglobin levels should be determined and supplemental oxygen provided. Management is otherwise supportive. Because of the risk of hydrocarbon pneumonitis, patients should be observed for evidence of aspiration.

Although hyperbaric oxygen is commonly used in cases of severe carbon monoxide poisoning, its role in methylene chloride toxicity has not been delineated [69]. It would appear reasonable to institute hyperbaric therapy when elevated carboxyhemoglobin levels are documented.

TRICHLOROETHANE. 1,1,1 Trichloroethane (TCA) has been widely marketed as a safer alternative to carbon tetrachloride for use as a cleaning agent and degreaser. It is also used as a solvent in typewriter correction fluid and in some aerosol hairsprays, water repellants, and furniture polishes. In spite of its reputation for safety, there have been several TCA-related deaths in the past 25 years [73]. The great majority of these deaths resulted from inhalation exposures—either via occupational or household exposure or through intentional abuse of TCA-containing products [74,75].

Trichloroethane is rapidly absorbed through the lungs and GI tract. Under most circumstances cutaneous absorption appears unlikely to result in systemic toxicity [48]. Distribution is greatest to tissues with a high concentration of lipid, including the CNS. Most of an absorbed dose of TCA is excreted unchanged through the lungs, with smaller quantities metabolized in the liver and excreted by the kidneys [12].

The toxicity of TCA is predominantly on the CNS, with signs and symptoms ranging from dizziness, headache, fatigue, and ataxia with mild-moderate exposures to seizures, coma, apnea, and death at higher vapor concentrations. Coordination is affected after 15 minutes' exposure to 1000 ppm; anesthesia is obtained after 5 minutes' exposure to 10,000 to 26,000 ppm [12]. Ingestion of 600 mg per kilogram resulted in reversible CNS depression in one patient [76].

Trichloroethane has also been hypothesized to have direct effects on the cardiovascular system, which may be responsible for a number of the sudden deaths caused by the substance [77]. Premature ventricular contractions and S–T depression have been demonstrated in a number of individuals exposed to TCA [78]. Chronic cardiac toxicity has also been demonstrated after repeated inhalation abuse of TCA [79]; hepatic and renal toxicity rarely result from TCA exposures.

Treatment of intoxications resulting from TCA exposure is supportive. Patients with depressed respirations may require oxygen and ventilatory support. Hypotension should be corrected with fluid resuscitation. Cardiac monitoring is indicated in all but the most benign exposures, and adrenergic agonists should be used with extreme caution, since TCA may sensitize the myocardium to the actions of catecholamines. Decontamination measures should be undertaken as expeditiously as possible. In those patients in whom sudden death does not intervene, recovery is generally rapid and complete.

Aromatic Hydrocarbons

The aromatic hydrocarbons are a group of compounds containing one or more benzene rings. They include benzene, toluene, xylene, diphenyl, phenol, and styrene. Aromatic hydrocarbons are common constituents of glues, paints, paint removers, lacquers, degreasers, and adhesives. Although the aromatic hydrocarbons have aspiration risks similar to those of the other hydrocarbons, they also exhibit potentially severe systemic

toxicity. Exposure is primarily through inhalation and occurs in industry, the household, or via inhalant abuse. Benzene, toluene, xylene, and styrene are all liquids, and thus toxicity may result from ingestion. The toxicity of these compounds varies widely, both from substance to substance and from individual to individual. The toxicology of benzene, toluene, and xylene is best understood and most representative of the toxicity seen in this class of compounds.

BENZENE. Benzene is a colorless liquid used widely in the chemical industry and less commonly as a solvent. It is highly volatile and flammable and has a pleasant, aromatic odor. It is well absorbed through the lungs and GI tract, but absorption through the skin is limited [80]. Benzene is highly fat-soluble, and thus the highest postabsorption levels are found in lipid-containing tissues, including the bone marrow. The lungs excrete up to 50 percent of an absorbed dose of benzene unchanged, whereas most of the remaining amount (50–90%) is metabolized by the hepatic P-450 system to potentially cytotoxic metabolites. [50]. Most of an absorbed dose and its metabolites are eliminated within 48 hours of exposure.

Benzene has both acute and chronic toxicity. Central nervous system depression is the primary effect of acute exposures to high concentrations of the substance [12]. Initial euphoria is rapidly followed by nausea, dizziness, and headache; subsequent progression to ataxia, seizures, and coma may occur. In addition, patients may have persistent symptoms after recovery from the acute effects, including insomnia, anorexia, and headache.

Inhalation of high concentrations may lead to development of pulmonary edema; as with other solvents, cardiac dysrhythmias may develop, presumably as the result of myocardial sensitization to circulating catecholamines. Long-term exposure to benzene may result in a depression of bone marrow elements, which may progress to aplastic anemia [50,81]. Although symptoms generally occur during the height of exposure (usually after at least 3 months of exposure), occasionally they may not become evident for months to years. Epidemiologic studies also suggest an increased risk of acute myelocytic and monocytic leukemia in workers with prolonged exposure to benzene [82,83].

Initial management efforts after acute benzene exposure should focus on stabilizing the patient and monitoring for dysrhythmias. Patients should be removed from the exposure as rapidly as possible, and in cases of ingestion, gastric decontamination should be carried out up to 2 hours from the time of exposure. It is generally agreed that amounts in excess of 1 to 2 ml per kilogram should be removed from the GI tract, although some sources recommend GI decontamination of virtually any amount. Because of the potential for aspiration pneumonitis, the respiratory status requires careful attention, and airway protection with a cuffed endotracheal tube should be considered in any patient who is not totally alert. The role of activated charcoal in this setting is unproved [12,84]. Subsequent therapy is supportive.

TOLUENE. Toluene is a colorless, volatile, sweet-smelling liquid that is a common ingredient in paints, paint thinners, lacquers, and glues (e.g., "airplane glue"). Although toxicity may occur accidentally in industry or in the household, toluene is one of the most heavily abused solvents [85,86]. As with benzene, toluene is highly lipid-soluble, and on inhalation peak blood concentrations occur within 15 to 30 minutes [50]. While human data are lacking, animal studies suggest that *ingested* toluene is well absorbed from the GI tract, although peak blood concentrations occur somewhat later (1–2 hours after exposure) than with inhalation. Absorption through intact skin is slow.

Approximately 20 percent of an absorbed dose of toluene is exhaled unchanged. Most of the remainder is metabolized by the liver's cytochrome P-450 system. Elimination is biphasic, with an initial alpha phase having a half-life of 4 to 5 hours [85] and representing exhalation combined with distribution to fatty tissues. The beta phase has an apparent half-life of 15 to 20 hours and represents hepatic metabolism.

Toluene exerts its toxic effects on the CNS and peripheral nervous system as well as the kidney and heart. Electrolyte and metabolic disturbances may also result. Acute exposure to toluene has variable effects on the CNS, depending on the concentration and duration of exposure [86–90]. Initially toluene causes excitation, with euphoria and bizarre behavior. These effects may occur after inhalation of concentrations as low as 50 ppm. Subsequently, depression of the CNS ensues, with drowsiness, confusion, headache, and nausea occurring after exposure to 500 to 800 ppm. With continued exposure or exposure to higher concentrations (> 800 ppm), further depression may occur, resulting in increasing confusion, ataxia, and nystagmus, and in extreme cases, seizures and loss of consciousness. Peripheral neuropathy and skeletal muscle damage with rhabdomyolysis have been reported after chronic exposure [86].

Chronic toluene abuse is associated with a high incidence of renal dysfunction, including hematuria, proteinuria, and pyuria [91]. These abnormalities are the result of tubulointerstitial damage and are generally reversible on cessation of exposure. Metabolic acidosis and electrolyte disturbances have also been associated with toluene exposure [86,91,92]. The latter include hypokalemia, hypocalcemia, hypophosphatemia, and hyperchloremia and are thought to be the result of impaired renal function.

As with many other solvents, toluene inhalation has been associated with sudden cardiorespiratory arrest in a number of cases [93]. It has been speculated that the cardiac effects are secondary to myocardial sensitization to circulating catecholamines, although it has also been suggested that apnea due to marked CNS depression may be responsible [93].

The diagnosis of toluene poisoning is generally made on the basis of the history, with known exposure or solvent abuse the prominent features. Toluene toxicity should also be considered in any individual with altered mental status and metabolic acidosis of unclear etiology [94]. Laboratory studies should include electrolytes, BUN, creatinine, calcium, phosphate, CPK, arterial blood gases, and urinalysis. Serum toluene levels are not commonly available and are rarely helpful in patient management.

Treatment involves removal of the patient from the toluene exposure or gastric decontamination in cases of ingestion (with recognition of the aspiration risk). Cardiac monitoring is appropriate, and further care is primarily supportive, with special emphasis on correction of fluid and electrolyte imbalances. Serum calcium requires especially careful monitoring, and symptoms and hypocalcemia (e.g., tetany) should be treated with 10 to 20 ml of 10% calcium gluconate.

XYLENE. Xylene is a clear liquid that is widely used as a solvent in paints and lacquers, degreasers, adhesives, cleaning agents, and aviation fuel. It is rapidly absorbed by the pulmonary and GI systems, and to some extent through the skin, although the clinical significance of this route is unknown. It is distributed in highest concentrations to the adrenal gland, bone marrow, spleen, brain, and blood [50]. Small amounts of an absorbed dose of xylene are excreted unchanged through the lungs; most of the remainder is metabolized in the liver and metabolites excreted in the urine. Ethanol consumption delays the metabolic clearance of coingested xylene.

The primary clinical effects of xylene are on the CNS. As with other solvents, it has been speculated that xylene sensitizes the myocardium to circulating catecholamines, since its inhalation has been associated with sudden death, presumably secondary to cardiac dysrhythmias [95].

At low doses, xylene induces headache, nausea, light-headedness, and ataxia; at higher doses, confusion, coma, and respiratory depression may develop. Hepatic damage and Fanconi's syndrome have also been described in association with xylene exposure [95,96]. A young man who *ingested* a large quantity of xylene was found on postmortem examination to have pulmonary edema [97].

Treatment involves initial stabilization and supportive care. Because of the possibility of dysrhythmias, cardiac monitoring is recommended. Gastric decontamination is advisable in cases of xylene ingestion up to 2 hours after ingestion, although the risk of hydrocarbon aspiration pneumonitis should be recognized. Liver and renal function should be followed; care is otherwise supportive.

Terpenes

The aliphatic cyclic hydrocarbon group known as terpenes includes turpentine, pine oil, and camphor. Camphor is discussed elsewhere [12] and is outside of the scope of this chapter. Pine oil is, as its name suggests, the product of pine trees and is comprised primarily of terpene alcohols. It is a component of several household cleaners (e.g., Pine-Sol), normally in concentrations of 20 to 35 percent but occasionally in concentrations exceeding 60 percent. Turpentine is a pine tree distillate commonly used as a solvent for paint and varnish.

Because of their lower volatility, the aspiration risk for these compounds appears to be somewhat less than that of the more volatile hydrocarbons. Nevertheless, turpentine and pine oil carry the risk of aspiration and in addition produce more CNS and GI symptoms than the aliphatic hydrocarbons. Ingestions of more than 2 ml per kilogram of turpentine are considered potentially toxic [98] and 60 to 120 gm of pine oil is commonly cited as the lethal dose in adults; however, survival has been reported after ingestion of 400 to 500 gm [99]. The minimal lethal dose of pine oil reported in children is 14 gm [100].

Turpentine is well absorbed through the lungs and GI tract [98] and distributed throughout the body, with highest concentrations in the liver, spleen, brain, and kidney [101]. Although the specifics of its metabolism are unclear, turpentine or its metabolites are largely excreted through the kidney. Pine oil is also well absorbed from the GI tract and after absorption is metabolized by the epoxide pathway and excreted in the urine [100]. Although the volume of distribution is unknown, it is thought to be quite large, with high concentrations in the brain, kidney, and lung.

Both pine oil and turpentine produce GI irritation and CNS depression. Clinically, this may be manifest as nausea, vomiting, diarrhea, weakness, somnolence, or agitation. In severe cases, stupor or coma may result, although seizures appear to be uncommon [102]. Systemic toxicity, when it occurs, usually develops within 2 to 3 hours of exposure. In mild and moderate cases, GI and CNS symptoms generally resolve within 12 hours. Turpentine ingestion has been associated in a few cases with dysuria and hematuria occurring 12 hours to 3 days following exposure, thought to be secondary to hemorrhagic cystitis [103]. It is suggested that chemical pneumonitis may occur after pine oil *ingestion*, although this remains controversial.

Diagnosis of turpentine or pine oil exposures is generally made on the basis of history, although both substances have distinctive odors, which may provide an aid to diagnosis. Physical examination should concentrate on respiratory, GI, and central nervous systems. Although no specific laboratory tests assist in determination of the severity of exposure [98], arterial blood gases and a chest film should be obtained if aspiration is suspected.

Treatment of ingestion of terpenes depends on the amount of substance ingested, the time since ingestion, and the patient's level of consciousness at the time of treatment. When patients present within 2 hours of ingestion and are fully alert, quantities of turpentine greater than 2 ml per kilogram should be removed. Although the quantity of pine oil that should be lavaged is unclear, it is recommended that, in adults, amounts exceeding 5 ml of pure pine oil be removed [104]. Because of the risk of aspiration, airway protection should be considered in all but the most alert patients. Activated charcoal is probably not useful. Hemodialysis and hemoperfusion have not been extensively evaluated in this setting but appear to have little utility, presumably because of the large volume of distribution of terpenes.

Patients who remain asymptomatic for 6 hours and those with mild GI or CNS symptoms are unlikely to develop serious complications. Patients with pulmonary complications or severe CNS depression require ICU admission. Treatment is then primarily supportive.

References

1. Litovitz TL, Schmitz BF, Holm KC: 1988 annual reports of the American Association of Poison Control Centers National Data Collection System. *Am J Emerg Med* 5:495, 1988.
2. Gerarde HW: Toxicological studies in hydrocarbons vs kerosene. *Toxicol Appl Pharmacol* 1:462, 1959.
3. Wolfe B, Brodeur A, Shields J: The role of gastrointestinal absorption of kerosene in producing pneumonitis in dogs. *Pediatrics* 76:867, 1970.
4. Dice WH, Ward G, Kelley J, et al: Pulmonary toxicity following gastrointestinal ingestions of kerosene. *Ann Emerg Med* 11:138, 1982.
5. Gerarde HW: Toxicologic studies on hydrocarbons IX. The aspiration hazard and toxicity of hydrocarbons and hydrocarbon mixtures. *Arch Environ Health* 6:329, 1963.
6. Giammona ST: Effects of furniture polish on pulmonary surfactant. *Am J Dis Child* 13:658, 1967.
7. Truemper E, DeLaRocha SR, Atkinson SD: Clinical characteristics, pathophysiology, and management of hydrocarbon ingestion: Case report and review of the literature. *Pediatr Emerg Care* 3:187, 1987.
8. Gross P, McNerney JM, Babyale MA: Kerosene pneumonitis: An experimental study with small doses. *Am Rev Respir Dis* 88:656, 1963.
9. Beerman B, Christensson T, Moller P, et al: Lipoid pneumonia: An occupational hazard of fire-eaters. *Br J Med* 289:1728, 1984.
10. Mann MD, Pirie DJ, Wolfsdorf J: Kerosene absorption in primates. *J Pediatr* 91:495, 1977.
11. Wolfsdorf J: Kerosene intoxication: An experimental approach to the etiology of the CNS manifestations in primates. *J Pediatr* 88:1037, 1976.
12. Ellenhorn MJ, Barceloux DG: *Medical Toxicology; Diagnosis and Treatment of Human Poisoning.* New York, Elsevier, 1988, p. 940.
13. Fortenberry JD: Gasoline sniffing. *Am J Med* 79:740, 1985.
14. Edminster SC, Bayer MJ: Recreational gasoline sniffing: Acute gasoline intoxication and latent organolead poisoning. *J Emerg Med* 3:365, 1985.
15. Wason S, Greiner PT: Intravenous hydrocarbon abuse. *Am J Emerg Med* 4:543, 1986.
16. Anas N, Namasonthia V, Ginsburg CM: Criteria for hospitalizing children who have ingested products containing hydrocarbons. *JAMA* 246:840, 1981.
17. Eade NR, Taussig LM, Marks MI: Hydrocarbon pneumonitis. *Pediatrics* 54:351, 1974.
18. Beamon RF, Siegel CJ, Landers G, et al: Hydrocarbon ingestion in children: A six year retrospective study. *JACEP* 5:771, 1976.
19. Foley JC, Dreyer NB, Soule AB Jr, et al: Kerosene poisoning in young children. *Radiology* 62:817, 1954.
20. Ervin ME: Petroleum distillates and turpentine, in Haddad LM, Winchester JF (eds): *Clinical Management of Poisoning and Drug Overdose.* Philadelphia, WB Saunders, 1983, p. 771.
21. Bergeson PS, Hales SW, Lustgarten MD, et al: Pneumatoceles following hydrocarbon ingestion. *Am J Dis Child* 129:49, 1975.
22. Klein BL, Simon JE: Hydrocarbon Poisonings. *Pediatr Clin North Am* 33:411, 1986.
23. Press E, Adams WC, Chittenden RF, et al: Report of the subcommittee on accidental poisoning: Co-operative kerosene poisoning study. *Pediatrics* 29:648, 1962.
24. Bratton L, Haddow JE: Ingestion of charcoal lighter fluid. *J Pediatr* 87:633, 1974.
25. Bass M: Death from sniffing gasoline (letter). *N Engl J Med* 299:203, 1978.
26. Barrientos A, Ortuno MT, Morales JM, et al: Acute renal failure after use of diesel fuel as shampoo. *Arch Intern Med* 137:1217, 1977.
27. Crisp AJ, Bhalla AK, Hoffbrand BI: Acute tubular necrosis after exposure to diesel oil. *Br Med J* 2:177, 1979.
28. Adler R, Robinson RG, Binkin NJ: Intravascular hemolysis: An unusual complication of hydrocarbon ingestion. *J Pediatr* 89:679, 1976.
29. Stockman JA: More on hydrocarbon-induced hemolysis. *J Pediatr* 90:848, 1977.
30. Walsh WA, Scarpa FJ, Brown RS, et al: Gasoline immersion burn case report. *N Engl J Med* 291:830, 1974.
31. Grufferman S, Walker FW: Supraglottitis following gasoline ingestion. *Ann Emerg Med* 11:368, 1982.
32. Poklis A, Burkett CD: Gasoline sniffing: a review. *Clin Toxicol* 11:35, 1977.
33. Chessare JD, Wodarcyk K: Gasoline sniffing and lead poisoning in a child. *Am Fam Physician* 38:181, 1988.
34. Neeld EM, Limacher MC: Chemical pneumonitis after the intravenous injection of hydrocarbons. *Radiology* 129:36, 1978.
35. Tennenbein M: Hydrocarbon ingestion. *Curr Probl Pediatr* 16:221, 1986.
36. James FW, Kaplan S, Benzing G: Cardiac complications following hydrocarbon ingestion. *Am J Dis Child* 121:431, 1971.
37. Litovitz T, Green AE: Health implications of petroleum distillate ingestion. *Occup Med* 3:555, 1988.
38. Cachia EA, Fenech FF: Kerosene poisoning in children. *Arch Dis Child* 39:502, 1964.
39. Ng RC, Darwish H, Stewart DA: Emergency treatment of petroleum distillates and turpentine ingestion. *Can Med Assoc J* 111:537, 1974.
40. Hardman G, Tolson R, Baghdassarian O: Prednisone in the management of kerosene pneumonia. *Ind Pract* 13:615, 1960.
41. Schwartz SI, Breslau RC, Kutner F, et al: Effects of drugs and hyperbaric oxygen environment on experimental kerosene pneumonitis. *Dis Chest* 47:353, 1965.
42. Steele RW, Conklin RH, Mark HM: Corticosteroids and antibiotics for the treatment of fulminant hydrocarbon aspiration. *JAMA* 219:1424, 1972.
43. Brown J, Burke B, Dajani AS: Experimental kerosene pneumonia: Evaluation of some therapeutic regimens. *J Pediatr* 84:396, 1974.
44. Zieserl E: Hydrocarbon ingestion and poisoning. *Comp Ther* 5:35, 1979.
45. Marks MI, Chicoine L, Legere G, et al: Adrenocorticosteroid treatment of hydrocarbon pneumonia in children. A cooperative study. *J Pediatr* 81:366, 1972.
46. Gurwitz D, Kattan M, Levison H, et al: Pulmonary function abnormalities in asymptomatic children after hydrocarbon pneumonitis. *Pediatrics* 62:789, 1978.
47. Pointer J: Typewriter correction fluid inhalation: A new substance of abuse. *J Toxicol Clin Toxicol* 19:493, 1982.
48. Stewart RD, Dodd HC: Absorption of carbon tetrachloride, trichlo-

roethylene, tetrachloroethylene, methylene chloride and 1,1,1 trichloroethane through the human skin. *Am Ind Hyg Assoc J* 25:439, 1964.

49. Perez AJ, Courel M, Sobrado J, Gonzalez L: Acute renal failure after topical application of carbon tetrachloride. *Lancet* 1:515, 1987.

50. Bergman K: Whole body autoradiography and allied tracer techniques in distribution and elimination studies of some organic solvents. *Scand J Work Environ Health* 5(suppl 1):144, 1979.

51. Willis RJ: Possible role of endogenous toxigenic lipids in the carbon tetrachloride poisoned hepatocyte. *Fed Proc* 39:3134, 1980.

52. Cornish HH, Adofuin J: Potentiation of carbon tetrachloride toxicity by aliphatic alcohols. *Arch Environ Health* 14:447, 1967.

53. Moon HD: The pathology of fatal carbon tetrachloride poisoning with special reference to the histogenesis of the hepatic and renal lesions. *Am J Pathol* 26:1041, 1950.

54. Ehrenreich T: Renal disease from exposure to solvents. *Ann Clin Lab Sci* 7:6, 1977.

55. Schreiner GE, Maher JF: Toxic nephropathy. *Am J Med* 38:409, 1965.

56. Sinicrope RA, Gordon JA, Little JR, Schoolwerth AC: Carbon tetrachloride nephrotoxicity: A reassessment of pathophysiology based upon the urinary diagnostic indices. *Am J Kidney Dis* 3:362, 1984.

57. Alston WC: Hepatic and renal complications arising from accidental carbon tetrachloride poisoning in the human subject. *Clin Pathol* 23:249, 1970.

58. Stewart RD, Boettner EA, Southworth RR, et al: Acute carbon tetrachloride intoxication. *JAMA* 183:994, 1963.

59. Fogel RP, Davidman M, Poleski MH, Spanier AH: Carbon tetrachloride poisoning treated with hemodialysis and total parenteral nutrition. *Can Med Assoc J* 128:560, 1983.

60. Spiegel SM, Hyams BB: Radiographic demonstration of a toxic agent. *J Can Assoc Radiol* 34:204, 1984.

61. McGuigan MA: Carbon tetrachloride. *Clin Toxicol Rev* 9:1, 1987.

62. Burk RF, Reiter R, Lane JM: Hyperbaric oxygen protection against carbon tetrachloride hepatotoxicity in rats: Association with altered metabolism. *Gastroenterology* 90:812, 1986.

63. Truss CD, Killenberg PG: Treatment of carbon tetrachloride poisoning with hyperbaric oxygen. *Gastroenterology* 82:767, 1982.

64. Ruprah M, Mant TGK, Flanagan RJ: Acute carbon tetrachloride poisoning in 19 patients: Implications for diagnosis and treatment. *Lancet* 1:1027, 1985.

65. Rioux JP, Meyers RA: Methylene chloride: A paradigmatic review. *J Emerg Med* 6:227, 1988.

66. Lawwerys RR: *Industrial Chemical Exposure: Guidelines for Biological Monitoring.* Davis, CA, Biomedical Publications, 1983, p 83.

67. Roberts CJC, Marshall FPF: Recovery after "lethal" quantity of paint remover. *Br Med J* 1:20, 1976.

68. Fagin J, Bradley J, Williams D: Carbon monoxide poisoning secondary to inhaling methylene chloride. *Br Med J* 281:1461, 1980.

69. Horowitz BZ: Carboxyhemoglobin caused by inhalation of methylene chloride. *Am J Emerg Med* 4:48, 1986.

70. Miller L, Pateras V, Friederici H, Engel G: Acute tubular necrosis after inhalation exposure to methylene chloride. *Arch Intern Med* 145:145, 1985.

71. Cordes DH, Brown WD, Quinn KM: Chemically induced hepatitis after inhaling organic solvents. *West J Med* 148:458, 1988.

72. Soslow A: Methylene chloride. *Clin Toxicol Rev* 9:1, 1987.

73. King GS, Smialek JE, Troutman WG: Sudden death in adolescents resulting from the inhalation of typewriter correction fluid. *JAMA* 253:1604, 1985.

74. Jones RD, Winters DP: Two case reports of deaths on industrial premises attributed to 1,1,1-trichloroethane. *Arch Environ Health* 38:59, 1983.

75. Travers H: Death from 1,1,1-trichloroethane abuse: A case report. *Milit Med* 139:889, 1974.

76. Stewart RD, Andrews JT: Acute intoxication with methyl chloroform. *JAMA* 195:904, 1966.

77. Herd PA, Lipsky M, Martin HF: Cardiovascular effects of 1,1,1-trichloroethane. *Arch Environ Health* 28:277, 1974.

78. Dornette WHL, Jones JP: Clinical experiences with 1,1,1-trichloroethane: A preliminary report of 50 anesthetic administrations. *Anesth Analg* 39:249, 1960.

79. McLeod AA, Margot R, Monaghan MJ, et al: Chronic cardiac toxicity after inhalation of 1,1,1-trichloroethane. *Br Med J* 294:727, 1987.

80. Susten AS, Dames BL, Burg JR, et al: Percutaneous penetration of benzene in hairless mice: An estimate of dermal absorption during tire-building operations. *Am J Ind Med* 7:323, 1985.

81. Aksoy M, Dincol K, Akgun T, et al: Haematological effects of chronic benzene poisoning in 217 workers. *Br J Ind Med* 28:296, 1971.

82. Infante PF, Wagoner JK, Rinsky RA, et al: Leukemia in benzene workers. *Lancet* 2:76, 1977.

83. Yin S-N, Li G-L, Tain F-D, et al: Leukaemia in benzene workers: A retrospective cohort study. *Br J Ind Med* 44:124, 1987.

84. Laass W: Therapy of acute oral poisonings by organic solvents: Treatment by activated charcoal in combination with laxatives. *Arch Toxicol* 4(suppl):406, 1980.

85. Burgnone F, DeRosa E, Perbellini L, Bartolucci GB: Toluene concentrations in the blood and alveolar air of workers during the workshift and the morning after. *Br J Ind Med* 43:56, 1986.

86. Streicher HZ, Gabow PA, Moss AH, et al: Syndromes of toluene sniffing in adults. *Ann Intern Med* 94:758, 1981.

87. von Oettingen WF, Neal PA, Donahue DD: The toxicity and potential dangers of toluene: Preliminary report. *JAMA* 118:579, 1942.

88. Lazar RB, Ho SU, Melen O, Daghestani AN: Multifocal central nervous system damage caused by toluene abuse. *Neurology* 33:1337, 1983.

89. Boor JW, Hurtig HI: Persistent cerebellar ataxia after exposure to toluene. *Ann Neurol* 2:440, 1977.

90. Stollery BT, Flindt MLH: Memory sequelae of solvent intoxication. *Scand J Work Environ Health* 14:45, 1988.

91. Voigts A, Kaufman CE: Acidosis and other metabolic abnormalities associated with paint sniffing. *South Med J* 76:443, 1983.

92. Fischman CM, Oster Jr: Toxic effects of toluene. A new cause of high anion gap metabolic acidosis. *JAMA* 241:1713, 1979.

93. Bass M: Sudden sniffing death. *JAMA* 212:2075, 1970.

94. Shannon M: Toluene. *Clin Toxicol Rev* 9:1, 1987.

95. Morley R, Eccleston DW, Douglas CP, et al: Xylene poisoning: A report of one fatal case and two cases of recovery after prolonged unconsciousness. *Br Med J* 3:442, 1970.

96. Rastogi SP, Gold RM, Arruda JAL: Fanconi's syndrome associated with carburetor fluid intoxication. *Am J Clin Pathol* 82:124, 1984.

97. Abu Al Ragheb S, Salhab AS, Amr SS: Suicide by xylene ingestion: A case report and review of literature. *Am J Forensic Med Pathol* 7:327, 1986.

98. McGuigan MA: Turpentine. *Clin Toxicol Rev* 8:1, 1985.

99. Koppel C, Tenczer J, Tennesmann U, et al: Acute poisoning with pine oil: Metabolism of monoterpenes. *Arch Toxicol* 49:73, 1981.

100. Jill RM, Barer J, Leighton Hill L, et al: An investigation of recurrent pine oil poisoning in an infant by the use of gas chromatographic mass spectrometric methods. *J Pediatr* 87:115, 1975.

101. Sperling F: In vivo and in vitro toxicology of turpentines. *Clin Toxicol* 2:21, 1969.

102. Jacobziner H, Raybin HW: Turpentine poisoning. *Arch Pediatr* 78:357, 1961.

103. Klein FA, Hackler RH: Hemorrhagic cystitis associated with turpentine ingestion. *Urology* 16:187, 1980.

104. Brook MP, McCarron MM, Mueller JA: Pine oil cleaner ingestion. *Ann Emerg Med* 18:391, 1989.

145. Iron Poisoning

Milton Tenenbein

Iron poisoning is traditionally perceived as being limited to small children; indeed, it was recently identified as the most common cause of poisoning death in children younger than 6 years [1]. However, there appears to be an increasing number of severe purposeful iron ingestions in adolescents and adults, with resultant significant morbidity and mortality. National statistics reflect this observation (Table 145-1).

Iron poisoning is unique because, unlike most other toxicants, iron occurs naturally in the body. It is highly reactive and there are complex mechanisms for its absorption, transport, and storage. The capacity of these systems when presented with an acute overdose is unknown; it likely varies from individual to individual and with the state of iron stores. This contributes to the poor understanding of its toxicokinetics and to the many management controversies. Some of these controversies include the actual toxic dose, the best method of gastrointestinal decontamination, the effectiveness of various intragastric complexation therapies, and several issues regarding deferoxamine therapy (indications, dose, duration, and efficacy). This chapter reviews what is known of iron poisoning, elaborates on the above controversies, and recommends treatment guidelines.

Available Forms of Iron

Iron is prescribed for the treatment or prophylaxis of iron-deficiency anemia. It is routinely available as ferrous salts, either alone or in combination with other minerals and vitamins as a nutrition supplement. Its common salts are ferrous sulfate, fumarate, gluconate, and succinate, which are 20, 33, 12, and 35 percent elemental iron, respectively. These conversion factors are important because toxicity is based on the amount of elemental iron ingested. Thus, a 300-mg tablet of ferrous sulfate is equivalent to 60 mg of elemental iron. Iron is often marketed as a delayed-release pharmaceutical. There is no standard for dissolution time for delayed-release products, thus complicating the clinical course and management after toxic ingestion. In addition, product labeling is unclear as to whether the tablets are conventional or delayed-release.

Pharmacokinetics

Iron absorption, transport, and storage are well reviewed elsewhere [10–13]. Since there is no endogenous mechanism for iron excretion, iron stores are controlled by the absorptive process. Absorption occurs in the proximal small bowel, with approximately 10 percent of the ingested dose absorbed but with 10-fold variations, depending on iron stores and the amount ingested. The actual mechanism of iron absorption is not well understood but is believed to be an active process. Iron can also be passively absorbed once the active process saturates, such as occurs after massive overdose [14]. Even in such situations only a relatively small amount, approximately 15 percent, is actually absorbed [14].

Peak serum iron concentrations occur within 4 to 6 hours after an overdose of conventional tablets; however, the time to peak serum concentration is not known for delayed-release products. The half-life after therapeutic dosing is approximately 6 hours [11], with the rapid decline due to tissue distribution. In plasma, iron is bound to transferrin, a specific $beta_1$ globulin responsible for iron transport throughout the body. In iron overdose, transferrin binding capacity is exceeded, but free plasma iron does not truly exist. Iron complexes with other plasma proteins and organic ligands and is referred to as non-transferrin-bound plasma iron [15,16,17]. It is, however, only loosely bound and is quite available to produce structural damage and alteration of function within the body [15,16,17].

Toxicology

As in most poisonings, there are two typical overdose scenarios: accidental overdose by young children and purposeful overdose by adolescents and adults. Serious iron overdose in young children frequently involves the ingestion of a product intended for adults, typically a prenatal supplement that contains 60 mg of elemental iron per dosage form. Although ingestion of pediatric iron supplements such as multivitamin plus iron tablets is more common [18,19], these are unlikely to produce toxicity severe enough to warrant intensive care unit management, because of the low iron concentration per dosage form (as little as 4 mg). Liquid iron preparations, often found in homes with small infants and toddlers, rarely cause significant iron poisoning, because these children are too young to ingest these products independently and their older siblings do not find the liquid preparations attractive. Iron overdose is less common among teenagers and adults, but when it occurs it is typically more severe because of the larger amounts involved. Of particular note is the higher incidence of deliberate iron overdose during pregnancy [20], probably due to the greater likelihood of iron availability and increased life stressors associated with pregnancy.

Toxicity

Iron exerts both local and systemic toxicity. Locally, it irritates the gastrointestinal (GI) tract, resulting in nausea, vomiting, abdominal cramps, and diarrhea. These symptoms are produced by relatively small doses (20 mg/kg of elemental iron). The degree of systemic toxicity, however, is dose-related. Since most published data are anecdotal, specific values have not been established. In the pediatric literature, a dose greater than 60 mg per kilogram of body weight is quoted as necessary for the development of significant systemic toxicity [21,22], with a lethal dose being 200 to 250 mg per kilogram [22,23]. Both of these figures are likely overestimates, with a more realistic figure being 50 percent of these values. Toddlers have died after ingesting as little as 0.9 to 1.5 gm of elemental iron (75–125 mg/kg based on average weights) [24–27]. In adult patients there are insufficient data to establish the relative toxicity. My

Table 145-1. Iron Ingestions, 1984–1991: American Association of Poison Control Centers Data Base

Year	No. of iron ingestions	Iron ingestions/ total poisoning exposures (per 1000)	Iron ingestions by patients >6 yr (%)
1984	1738	2.4	20.4
1985	2013	2.2	23.7
1986	2574	2.3	24.4
1987	2910	2.5	24.9
1988	3699	2.7	27.4
1989	4279	2.7	28.8
1990	4448	2.6	29.5
1991	5144	2.8	29.7

Data are from references 2–9.

personal experience supports Olenmark and co-workers' opinion [27] that the published pediatric criteria underestimate the toxicity of iron in adults. Adults have died after ingestion of as little as 2.0 [28] and 5.0 gm [27] of elemental iron. In these case reports, the former patient had significant hepatic disease and the latter ingested 70 mg per kilogram, a value similar to the above revised pediatric figures. Any ingestion of 1.5 gm of elemental iron (twenty-five 300-mg ferrous sulfate tablets) by an adult should be cause for concern.

Contributing to this issue of the uncertainty of the toxic dose is that the amount of iron available to cause damage and destruction in the body after overdose is unknown because of iron's poor and unpredictable absorption and the unknown capacity for binding by as ferritin and hemosiderin. Although the size of this pool is unknown, it is likely very small, in the magnitude of milligrams even after gram quantities have been ingested. (Remember, the units of measurement of serum iron concentration are $\mu g/dl$.) This has implications for the dose and duration of deferoxamine therapy.

MECHANISM OF TOXICITY. Iron is a potent catalyzer of free radical formation, which results in highly reactive species that attack many cellular molecules [29]. Iron-generated free radical formation is thought to contribute to acute iron toxicity [23] and to be responsible for much of the damage and dysfunction of chronic iron overload [15,16,17]. Free radicals are highly reactive species that produce damage at their site of origin. Because of local detoxification pathways, a significant concentration of free radicals is required to cause damage. It then follows that those sites exposed to high iron concentrations will show greater local injury.

One such area is the GI tract. After ingestion, the gut lining is exposed to high iron concentrations. Local toxicity results, even though the ingested dose may be too low to produce systemic toxicity. Local damage includes GI mucosal necrosis and bleeding [30]. Iron itself is neither caustic nor corrosive; damage probably results from local free radical formation. Local toxicity can occur distally with proximal sparing [30] and may not occur even in the face of fatal systemic poisoning [14].

Systemic toxicity results when the absorbed iron is transported to target organs, such as the liver and heart. Non-transferrin-bound iron is rapidly cleared by the liver [31,32], putting this organ at risk for toxic damage [33,34,35].

Presentation of Acute Iron Poisoning

The amount and timing of the overdose and the type of the pharmaceutical preparation (conventional vs. delayed-release) are essential data for the estimation of degree and onset of toxicity. Traditionally, acute iron intoxication is divided into five clinical stages [21]: GI toxicity, relative stability, circulatory shock, hepatic necrosis, and GI scarring. Orderly progression through these stages is not necessary, and fatalities may occur without significant GI involvement [14]. Similarly, hepatotoxicity may not occur even in severe iron poisoning. Presenting signs and symptoms depend on the clinical stage.

The most common presentation is during stage I, when abdominal pain, vomiting, diarrhea, hematemesis, and hematochezia are seen. Gastrointestinal toxicity usually occurs within the first few hours of overdose. If enteric-coated tablets have been ingested, GI toxicity can be delayed as long as 12 hours. For such preparations, onset of GI toxicity is variable because of unpredictable gastric emptying and the lack of dissolution rate standards for these pharmaceuticals.

The severity of this stage is variable, and life-threatening hypovolemic shock may occur, especially if initial gut symptoms were mild or ignored. Occasionally, segmental intestinal infarction may occur, necessitating bowel resection [30]. It is unlikely that isolated hepatoxicity or GI obstruction would be the primary presentation of iron poisoning.

The second stage, a period of relative stability, follows significant GI symptoms and precedes the onset of circulatory shock and acidosis. Apparent improvement in the patient's clinical status should not lead to complacency. Patients are not completely asymptomatic: Careful assessment and repeated monitoring will document some degree of hypovolemia, circulatory shock, and acidosis.

Circulatory shock can occur within several hours of iron overdose or may be delayed as long as several days. Its pathogenesis is complex and poorly understood and is based on the results of limited experimental animal data [36–39]. Circulatory shock may be hypovolemic, distributive, or cardiogenic in nature or result from any combination of these elements. Shock occurring soon after the overdose would likely be hypovolemic and is chiefly due to fluid and blood loss from the GI tract. The early occurring hyperferremia-associated coagulopathy may aggravate this blood loss [40]. Distributive shock is dependent on iron absorption and usually occurs after hypovolemic shock, but they often overlap. It is speculated that distributive shock is due to decreased vascular tone or increased vascular permeability [38]. Suggested mechanisms include direct effects of iron or ferritin or an effect mediated by release of vasoactive substances. Cardiogenic shock usually occurs later, because its direct toxic effect is dependent on the presence of increased iron in myocardial cells. Anecdotal human examples [41] and strong experimental animal data [39] support its occurrence. Thus, the timing of the onset of shock can be somewhat helpful in elucidating its cause, but obviously there is considerable overlap of these three etiologies. Figure 145-1 depicts the multifactorial etiology of shock due to iron poisoning.

The acidosis of iron poisoning is usually discussed with circulatory shock but is only partially a consequence of hypoperfusion and usually precedes it. The acidosis can be quite profound, requiring large amounts of bicarbonate for treatment [39]. Acidosis is a direct toxic effect of iron poisoning that occurs after the plasma's capacity to bind the absorbed ferric ion has been exceeded. When this occurs, the ferric ion becomes hydrated and protons are released ($Fe^{3+} + 3H_2O \rightarrow FE(OH)_3 +$

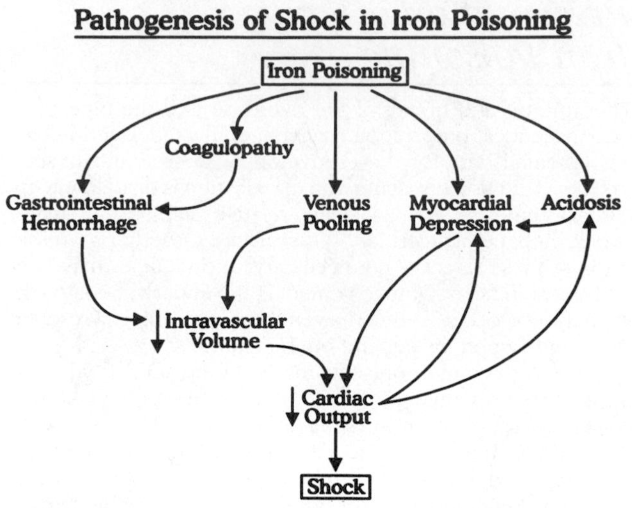

Pathogenesis of Shock in Iron Poisoning

Fig. 145-1. The multifactorial etiology of shock in iron poisoning.

$3H^+$). Thus each unbound iron ion generates three protons, accounting for the rather formidable acidosis. Another contributing factor is the interference with intracellular oxidative metabolism by iron, with subsequent generation of organic acids. Once shock occurs, hypoperfusion contributes to the acidosis.

Hepatotoxicity is a well-known consequence of iron poisoning [33,34,35] and is second only to shock as a cause of death. Its onset is unpredictable; it can occur any time during the first 72 hours after overdose. Its etiology is attributed to iron-catalyzed free radical production and subsequent lipid peroxidation of hepatic mitochondrial membranes [23].

Gastrointestinal scarring is the final consequence of iron's local action on the gut. Most cases involve the gastric outlet, but isolated strictures of distal intestine have been reported [30]. It occurs 2 to 4 weeks after overdose, but significant and protracted abdominal pain during the first few days is a prognosticator for its occurrence [30].

Iron Overdose During Pregnancy

Iron overdose during pregnancy deserves special mention because of its relatively high incidence [20]. The consequences for the woman are no different from those that occur in nonpregnant patients, but because transplacental iron passage is an energy-requiring saturable process, the fetus enjoys relative protection [42]. Treatment should be no different from that given a nonpregnant patient, since the woman's needs take precedence over those of the fetus. Deferoxamine should not be withheld, and its teratogenic risk is likely overstated [42].

Laboratory Evaluation

Key laboratory tests include abdominal radiographs, serum iron concentration studies, and blood gas determinations. An abdominal radiograph at presentation can be used to verify the iron overdose and to quantify the amount ingested [43,44,45]. However, it may not demonstrate the iron if enough time has passed for the tablets to have dissolved, if a liquid preparation has been ingested, or if there is a small amount of iron in each tablet, such as found in many pediatric iron-containing chewable multivitamins [46]. The abdominal radiograph may be used to judge the effectiveness of GI decontamination [47,48].

Serum iron concentration is the single most important test. It validates the ingestion, guides management, and provides prognostic information. Peak serum concentrations less than 500 μg per deciliter (90 μM/L) are usually associated with negligible to mild systemic toxicity; however, there may be significant GI symptoms. With peak concentrations of 500 to 1000 μg per deciliter (90–180 μM/L) moderate systemic toxicity is expected. A peak serum concentration greater than 1000 μg deciliter (180 μM/L) is regularly associated with severe toxicity consisting of profound acidosis, shock, hepatotoxicity, coma, and death. At serum concentrations greater than 10,000 μg per deciliter (1800 μM/L) almost 100 percent mortality is expected.

The timing of the serum iron concentration determination is very important. Peak concentration generally occurs 4 to 6 hours after an overdose of conventional tablets and several hours later for an overdose of the enteric-coated variety. Unfortunately, the type of preparation ingested is usually unknown at the time a patient seeks treatment and is surprisingly difficult to establish even after the fact [49]. Thus, serial serum iron concentration determinations are often needed during the early hours after overdose, especially if the last value is within the range of 300 to 500 μg per deciliter (55–90 μM/L). Levels should be obtained every 2 hours until a definite trend is established. Occasionally, concurrent abdominal radiographs are helpful. If many pills are seen on the radiograph, then the subsequent serum iron concentration will likely be greater. However, a negative radiographic study does not guarantee that the peak serum iron concentration has occurred. It is important to remember that treatment with deferoxamine can confound the laboratory determination of serum iron concentration [50,51] by producing falsely lower levels. Therefore, it is important to obtain specimens prior to initiation of chelation therapy. This problem should not delay treatment with deferoxamine, if indicated.

Blood gas determinations should be done early, because acidosis is the first objective indicator of significant iron toxicity. Frequency of repeat blood gas determinations is guided by previous values, the need for bicarbonate therapy, and clinical course. A pH less than 7.30 is indicative of significant toxicity, and these patients should be admitted to an intensive care unit.

Other important laboratory tests include assessments of blood coagulation and hepatic and renal function. A blood coagulation screen should be done early and repeated throughout the first few days following all significant iron poisonings, because of the potential for a biphasic coagulopathy [40]. Blood should be typed and cross-matched and kept available until after acute toxicity has subsided. Renal function should be monitored regularly, especially during deferoxamine therapy, because of the risk of acute renal failure [52]. Hepatic function should be monitored daily during the first 72 hours and longer if clinically indicated.

Notable because of its exclusion from this discussion is the recommendation for determination of the total iron binding capacity (TIBC). It is routinely recommended in the management of the iron overdose patient. Serum iron levels exceeding the TIBC have been used as an indication for initiation of deferoxamine therapy. This is based on the hypothesis that the iron overdose patient is at risk when the serum iron concentration exceeds the TIBC. The "free iron" would then be available to initiate tissue damage. However, this does not consider other protective factors, such as rapid hepatic uptake of iron with subsequent storage as ferritin. The occurrence of toxicity with minor excess of the TIBC has never been validated, and recent clinical data cast doubt on such a relationship [53]. Furthermore, routine methods for TIBC determination have been shown to be unreliable during hyperferremic states and are time-consuming [54]. Thus, the TIBC is not recommended in the management of iron overdose patients [53,54].

Another recommendation of questionable merit is the use of a battery of simple laboratory tests and symptoms as indicators of serum iron concentration greater than 300 μg per deciliter (55 μM/L). These include a white blood cell count greater than 15,000, a blood sugar level greater than 150 mg per deciliter (8.3 mM/L), and the presence of vomiting, diarrhea, and opacities on the abdominal radiograph. These were all found retrospectively to be associated with serum iron values greater than 300 μg per deciliter (55 μM/L) [55]. This association would be especially helpful when rapid serum iron concentrations are not available. However, subsequent studies were not supportive, [53,56,57], thus invalidating this approach [51].

Differential Diagnosis

Differential diagnosis becomes an issue only when the history of iron overdose is unknown. In such situations it can be quite problematic and is dependent on the chief clinical features at presentation (e.g., abdominal pain, GI hemorrhage, and shock).

Clinical Course

Because of the anecdotal nature of the published literature, it is difficult to predict outcomes accurately. Survival is expected with peak serum iron concentrations lower than 1000 μg per deciliter (180 μM/L) and appropriate supportive care. Chief causes of death are shock, followed by hepatic failure. Complications of iron poisoning include acute renal failure due to either shock or deferoxamine therapy without adequate volume replacement [52]. *Yersinia* septicemia, although rare, has been reported in patients treated with deferoxamine [58,59]. Late sequelae include GI obstruction, which presents 2 to 4 weeks after the overdose and is usually preceded by abdominal pain [30].

Management

The initial disposition of iron overdose patients presents a challenge for the physician because the patient often comes to the health care facility prior to the peaking of clinical toxicity. Many patients, especially young children, may be asymptomatic or only mildly ill. The challenge lies in identifying those who are at risk for significant toxicity in order to place them in an appropriate setting that can provide the anticipated level of care. The decision for the iron-overdosed, critically ill patient is straightforward. Table 145-2 provides guidelines for intensive care unit admission for those patients who are not critically ill.

GASTROINTESTINAL DECONTAMINATION. Over the past several years, the traditional methods of gastrointestinal decontamination, including ipecac-induced emesis and gastric lavage, have been questioned, and activated charcoal has be-

Table 145-2. Suggested Criteria for Admission of the Noncritically Ill Iron Overdose Patient to an Intensive Care Unit

	Admit to ICU	Strongly consider admission to ICU
Amount of elemental iron ingested		
Child (<6 yr)	>60 mg/kg	45–60 mg/kg
Adult (all others)	>3.0 gm	2.0–3.0 gm
Tablets seen in x-ray*		
Child (<6 yr)	1/kg	0.75–1/kg
Adult (all others)	>50	33–50
Peak serum iron concentrations	>1000 μg/dl	750–1000 μg/dl
	>180 μM/L	135–180 μM/L
Arterial pH	<7.30	7.30–7.35

* Assuming 60 mg elemental iron/tablet
Note: not all criteria need to be present.

come the primary recommended intervention [60–64]. Objective evidence supporting the ineffectiveness of ipecac-induced emesis and gastric lavage for iron overdose includes serial abdominal radiographs showing no change after gastric emptying [47,48]. In addition, activated charcoal does not adsorb iron [65], rendering it ineffective for this overdose.

Whole bowel irrigation (WBI) is recommended as the primary GI decontamination procedure for the iron overdose patient [48]. It is routinely done as preparation for colonoscopy and large bowel surgery and effectively irrigates the iron out of the GI tract. Large volumes of the specialized commercially available irrigating fluid, polyethylene glycol electrolyte lavage solution, are administered at a rapid rate through a small nasogastric tube. The rate for children 6 years of age or younger is 0.5 liter per hour and for teenagers and adults is 1.5 to 2.0 liters per hour. It should be initiated with history or radiologic documentation of elemental iron ingestions greater than 30 mg per kilogram of body weight and 1.0 gm in the above respective groups. Patients who have received prior treatment with syrup of ipecac will often not tolerate WBI; therefore its administration should be avoided. The endpoint is the passage of a clear rectal effluent. Contraindications are significant GI hemorrhage, bowel obstruction, perforation, or ileus. If emesis hampers effective WBI, intravenous metoclopramide is recommended because of its antiemetic and GI motility actions. Dosage of metoclopramide is 10 mg intravenously in adults and 0.1 mg per kilogram in children repeated every 6 hours as needed. Figure 145-2 provides an example of a patient with a potentially lethal iron overdose after the failure of both ipecac-induced emesis and gastric lavage but who was then successfully treated with WBI.

Iron can become adherent to the GI mucosa or may form tablet bezoars [66], the latter being primarily a problem with conventional iron tablets and not with the enteric-coated varieties. If either of these situations is documented to be present, WBI may not be effective but is not contraindicated. Gastrotomy for tablet removal has been reported [66–70] and should be considered in such situations. Initial radiographs in three planes (flat, upright, and decubitus) should identify whether either of these two situations is present. Gastroscopy may be considered if the above approach is inconclusive. Barium studies are unlikely to be helpful because of the anticipated lack of contrast between barium and iron. Surgical intervention must be done rapidly before the iron is absorbed, and the majority of the tablets must be in a localized area rather than scattered throughout the GI tract. A combined approach of gastrotomy

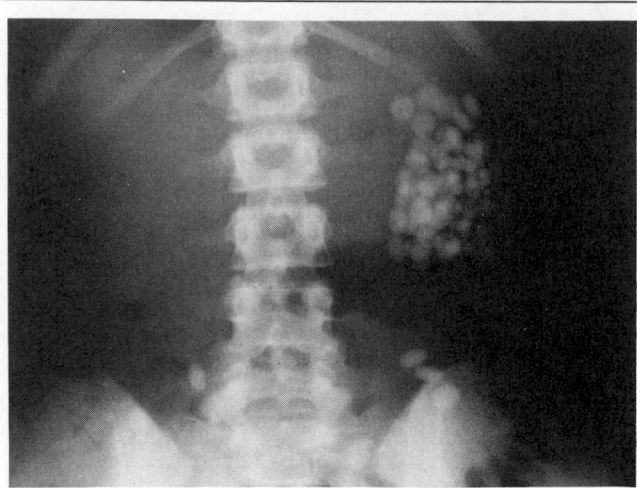

Fig. 145-2. Abdominal radiograph of a 16-year-old girl with a potentially lethal iron overdose, taken after syrup of ipecac-induced emesis and gastric lavage. Gastroscopy ruled out adherence of iron to stomach wall and medication concretion. She subsequently underwent whole bowel irrigation. Her peak serum iron concentration was 253 μg per deciliter (46 μM/L), and she was not treated with deferoxamine.

for tablet retrieval followed by WBI after surgery has been described [70]. The former removed the iron from the stomach and the latter removed it from the intestinal tract.

The oral administration of bicarbonate, phosphate, or deferoxamine has been advocated to decrease iron absorption by complexing it to these agents. In vitro [71] and rat in vivo [72] studies do not support either bicarbonate or phosphate administration, and the latter therapy has resulted in hypocalcemia and hypovolemia in iron overdose patients [73,74]. Neither is recommended.

Intragastric complexation with deferoxamine has provoked much discussion in the literature. Although there are proponents for its use [22,23], most authorites do not support this therapy. While deferoxamine is not appreciably absorbed from the GI tract, its chelant, ferrioxamine, is absorbed [21,37,75]. This compound is toxic and has been shown to be lethal in dogs [37] and mice [76]. Therefore, the enteral administration of deferoxamine is not recommended.

SUPPORTIVE CARE. Supportive care is provided concurrently with GI decontamination. Two intravenous lines are required, one for fluid resuscitation and bicarbonate administration and the other for deferoxamine therapy. Very large amounts of crystalloid and bicarbonate may be required [39], and occasionally colloid or blood may be necessary. Because of the complex nature of shock in iron poisoning, early placement of a Swan-Ganz catheter is needed both to help in diagnosis and to monitor the effectiveness of therapy. Early shock is usually hypovolemic, with or without a distributive component, and should respond to vigorous volume resuscitation; occasionally pressor therapy may be needed. Later shock is usually cardiogenic and requires inotropic support. Failure of inotropic support suggests the need for afterload reduction [41]; once a patient has reached this point, the prognosis is grave. An arterial catheter for blood gas determinations and a Foley catheter for monitoring urine output are necessary in all patients.

Parameters requiring serial monitoring include arterial blood gas measurements, hematocrit, serum electrolytes, renal and hepatic function, and blood coagulation factors. The frequency of these determinations is dependent on previous results, the patient's clinical condition, and specific intercurrent therapy.

Acute hepatic failure is managed by standard protocols. Acute renal failure may be a consequence of shock or deferoxamine therapy in a hypovolemic patient [52]. Hemodialysis may be required in such situations, especially if deferoxamine therapy is continued, since the chelate ferrioxamine is toxic and should be removed. Ferrioxamine is dialyzable. Coagulopathy may be biphasic [40]. The early stage occurs during the first few hours after overdose, depends on serum iron concentration, and is transient. Specific therapy is not recommended, and because deferoxamine lowers the serum iron concentration, initiation of deferoxamine therapy may hasten the resolution of this early coagulopathy [40]. The later presenting coagulation dysfunction occurs hours to a few days after overdose and is a manifestation of hepatic failure. Administration of fresh frozen plasma is recommended because vitamin K_1 is unlikely to be helpful.

ENHANCED ELIMINATION. Hemodialysis or hemoperfusion is not recommended specifically for iron removal because of the rapid intracellular distribution of the iron and its binding to plasma proteins as non-transferrin-bound iron [15,16,17]. However, if renal failure occurs during deferoxamine therapy, extracorporeal removal of ferrioxamine is recommended because of its toxicity.

CHELATION THERAPY. Deferoxamine, the specific treatment of choice for acute iron poisoning [21,22,23], is a naturally occurring siderophore isolated from *Streptomyces pilosus* and whose pharmacology was described in the early 1960s [77,78]. Its binding constant for ferric iron is 10^{31}, which compares to 10^{27} to 10^{29} for transferrin. It is capable of removing iron from ferritin and hemosiderin and to a very minor degree from transferrin, but not at all from hemoglobin or myoglobin.

Although deferoxamine is regarded as the treatment of choice, its effectiveness has been questioned [79]. Usual reasons cited are its limited chelation capacity and the small amount of iron recovered from the urine of deferoxamine-treated iron-poisoned patients [79]. The recommended daily deferoxamine dose of 6.0 gm is capable of chelating 510 mg of iron, or 8.5 ferrous sulfate tablets. This would seem to be of limited value for the patient who has ingested 50 tablets, but iron's poor absorption and the body's storage capabilities for this transition metal result in only a relatively small amount left to cause damage and destruction. Therefore, the chelation of small amounts of iron may be quite beneficial. Alternatively, 510 mg of iron is approximately 10 percent of the total amount of iron and approximately 35 percent of the non-heme iron in a 70-kg male [80]. Although only small amounts of iron have been found in the urine of deferoxamine-treated iron-poisoned patients, the assay's methodology was not stated and routine autoanalyzer methods would not detect this deferoxamine-bound iron [81]. Futhermore, this fails to account for the portion of ferrioxamine excreted into the gut [82–85].

Because placebo controlled trials are impossible, the efficacy of deferoxamine for acute iron poisoning will never be proved in humans, but animal data clearly support it as an effective agent [86,87]. In addition to chelating excess plasma iron, deferoxamine depletes the intracellular iron pool. This is well known in patients with chronic iron overload due to hypertransfusion, and ferrioxamine is found in the urine of iron-poisoned patients long after plasma iron concentrations have normalized.

Several practical but somewhat contentious issues remain with the use of this chelator. These include indications for its use and the dose, route of administration, and duration of therapy. Classic indications for the initiation of deferoxamine therapy include peak serum iron concentrations, a serum iron concentration greater than the TIBC, a positive chelation challenge test, and the patient's clinical condition. Recommendations based on peak serum iron concentration are empiric and range from 300 to 500 μg per deciliter (55–90 μM/L). Significant morbidity is unlikely with concentrations less than 500 μg per deciliter (90 μM/L) as long as this is the true peak serum iron concentration. Since one can never be certain of this, 400 μg per deciliter (75 μM/L) is a reasonable recommendation. Values at the lower end of the above range are based on the upper limit of normal for TIBC, which is not a valid indication. As discussed earlier, serum iron concentration greater than the TIBC, although theoretically attractive, is not recommended as an indication, because of the likelihood of laboratory error [54] and the lack of clinical correlation [53].

A positive chelation challenge test relies on visual detection of the rusty orange coloration of the urine caused by the presence of ferrioxamine after intramuscular administration of deferoxamine. The dose is empiric and not standardized, with 0.5 to 1.0 gm for young children and 1.0 to 2.0 gm for teenagers and adults being satisfactory. If the patient has been started on an intravenous infusion of deferoxamine without blood being drawn for a serum iron concentration, the iron to creatinine ratio can be used as an objective assessor of chelation challenge [81]. Clinical condition as an indication for initiation of deferoxamine therapy is useful only if the patient is iron-toxic at presentation. Certainly acidosis, shock, and coma are clear indicators. However, the goal is to identify patients prior to the development of clinical toxicity in order to initiate deferoxamine therapy with the hope of preventing or lessening the toxic effects of iron. Therefore, indications for initiation of deferoxamine therapy include a serum iron concentration greater than 400 μg per deciliter (75 μM/L), a positive chelation challenge test, or definite clinical evidence of iron toxicity.

Difficulties arise when choosing a route of administration of deferoxamine, because the manufacturer recommends intramuscular therapy unless the patient is in shock. Most likely, this indication is based on the concern for hypotension, which is associated with rapid intravenous administration. This complication is not seen with intravenous rates of 15 mg/kg/hr, and with modern infusion pumps the possibility of accidentally exceeding this rate is negligible. Furthermore, there is evidence in thalassemic patients that a continuous intravenous infusion is more effective. In these patients, a 750-mg intramuscular dose chelated 15 mg of iron, while a 750-mg infusion over 24 hours chelated 50 mg [88]. Therefore, the intramuscular route is not recommended. As discussed earlier, oral deferoxamine therapy for intragastric complexation is not recommended.

The dose of deferoxamine is also problematic. The manufacturer recommends a daily maximum total dosage of 6.0 gm given in divided doses. Robotham and Lietman [23] recommend a continuous infusion of 15 mg/kg/hr until 24 hours after the urine returns to its normal color. Neither recommendation is based on published data. The latter protocol exceeds the manufacturer's guidelines for any patient heavier than 17 kg but has been routinely used for more than 10 years; however, only 2 patients treated with 15 mg/kg/hr have been well described in the literature [89,90]. Recently, thalassemic patients with chronic iron overload developed pulmonary toxicity within 5 to 9 days after initiation of a similar dose of intravenous deferoxamine by continuous infusion [91]. Another recent report describes four patients with mild to moderate iron poisoning without evidence of shock, acidosis, or sepsis who received 15 mg/kg/hr of deferoxamine intravenously for 2 to 3 days and died of noncardiogenic pulmonary edema [92]. The pulmonary toxicity of prolonged deferoxamine therapy was recently confirmed in mice [76]. Hence, my preference is to infuse 15 mg/kg/hr until 6 gm has been administered and to repeat this dose daily if any of the above three indications for deferoxamine therapy remain present. In severe iron poisoning I give up to 12 gm per day, with careful monitoring of pulmonary status.

The usual recommendation for cessation of deferoxamine therapy is the return of urine color to normal. This is reasonable but creates problems for individuals with limited experience treating this poisoning. An objective criterion would be more desirable. Since the serum iron concentration can be inaccurate during deferoxamine therapy [50,51] and because it does not reflect the intracellular concentration, it is not recommended as a criterion for the cessation of deferoxamine therapy. A recent innovation, the urinary iron to creatinine ratio after pretreatment of the sample with a ferrioxamine cleaving agent, is a promising objective criterion, but more experience is required [81]. Until objective testing is available, a urine sample obtained prior to deferoxamine therapy should be saved. Later samples obtained during deferoxamine therapy can then be compared to the original sample. A positive urine, although classically defined as "vin-rose," is more of a rusty orange. However, urinary criteria are of no use if the patient is not producing urine. If the kidneys have failed, the plasma can be separated from a specimen of whole blood and examined for the rusty orange color of ferrioxamine.

Complications from short-term deferoxamine therapy are few but significant. Hypotension is associated with rapid administration and is prevented by adequate fluid resuscitation and by not exceeding an infusion rate of 15 mg/kg/hr. Acute renal failure can result if deferoxamine is administered to hypovolemic patients [52]. Therefore, expansion of the intravascular space is recommended prior to deferoxamine therapy. Pulmonary toxicity is associated with continuous intravenous therapy over several days [91,92]. Ocular toxicity has been reported with chronic use in thalassemia, and patients receiving deferoxamine may be at increased risk for *Yersinia* infections [58,59].

Potential Specific Future Therapies

Animal work with deferoxamine complexed to dextran and starch polymers is promising [93,94]. Its advantage lies in the ability to administer larger doses of deferoxamine safely and rapidly. The new iron chelator 1,2-dimethyl-3-hydroxypyrid-4-one shows promise for the treatment of chronic transfusional iron overload; its role in acute iron poisoning requires investigation [95]. The administration of free radical scavengers such as vitamin E to prevent tissue damage and dysfunction is theoretically attractive [96]. Another potential therapy is prostaglandin E_2, which in animals has been shown to confer a hepatocytic cytoprotective effect against both toxic [97] and infectious [98] insults. There is no published human experience with any of these three hypothetical therapies.

Final Disposition

Prior to discharge, a psychiatric assessment is indicated for all purposeful ingestions. The patient should be advised of the symptoms of bowel obstruction and to return immediately should they occur. A follow-up visit approximately 1 month later is recommended. At this time the patient's iron status and GI tract should be assessed. Chronic hepatic or cardiac sequelae do not seem to be complications of acute iron overdose.

References

1. Litovitz T, Manoguerra A: Comparison of pediatric poisoning hazards: An analysis of 38 million exposure incidents. *Pediatrics* 89:999, 1992.

2. Litovitz TL, Veltri JC: 1984 annual report of the American Association of Poison Control Centers National Data Collection System. *Am J Emerg Med* 3:423, 1984.

3. Litovitz TL, Normann SA, Veltri JC: 1985 annual report of the American Association of Poison Control Centers National Data Collection System. *Am J Emerg Med* 4:427, 1985.

4. Litovitz TL, Martin TG, Schmitz B: 1986 annual report of the American Association of Poison Control Centers National Data Collection System. *Am J Emerg Med* 5:405, 1986.

5. Litovitz TL, Schmitz BF, Matyunas N, Martin TG: 1987 annual report of the American Association of Poison Control Centers National Data Collection System. *Am J Emerg Med* 6:479, 1987.

6. Litovitz TL, Schmitz BF, Holm KC: 1988 annual report of the American Association of Poison Control Centers National Data Collection System. *Am J Emerg Med* 7:495, 1988.

7. Litovitz TL, Schmitz BF, Bailey KM: 1989 annual report of the American Association of Poison Control Centers National Data Collection System. *Am J Emerg Med* 8:394, 1990.

8. Litovitz TL, Bailey KM, Schmitz BF, et al: 1990 annual report of the American Association of Poison Control Centers National Data Collection System. *Am J Emerg Med* 9:461, 1991.

9. Litovitz TL, Holm KC, Bailey KM, Schmitz BF: 1991 annual report of the American Association of Poison Control Centers National Data Collection System. *Am J Emerg Med* 10:452, 1992.

10. Finch CA, Huebers HA: Iron metabolism. *Clin Physiol Biochem* 4:5, 1986.

11. Harju E: Clinical pharmacokinetics of iron preparations. *Clin Pharmacokinet* 17:69, 1989.

12. Bezkorovainy A: Biochemistry of nonheme iron in man. I. Iron proteins and cellular iron metabolism. *Clin Physiol Biochem* 7:1, 1989.

13. Bezkorovainy A: Biochemistry of nonheme iron in man. II. Absorption of iron. *Clin Physiol Biochem* 7:53, 1989.

14. Reissman KR, Coleman TJ, Budai BS, Moriarty LR: Acute intestinal iron intoxication. I. Iron absorption, serum iron and autopsy findings. *Blood* 10:35, 1955.

15. Hershko C, Peto TEA: Non-transferrin plasma iron. *Br J Haematol* 66:149, 1987.

16. Gutteridge JMC, Rowley DA, Griffiths E, Halliwell B: Low-molecular weight iron complexes and oxygen radical reactions in idiopathic haemochromatosis. *Clin Sci* 68:463, 1985.

17. Arouma OI, Bomford A, Polson RJ, Halliwell B: Nontransferrin-bound iron in plasma from hemochromatosis patients: Effect of phlebotomy therapy. *Blood* 72:1416, 1988.

18. Viets CA, Bilodeau N, Langstaff MJ: Children's chewable vitamins with iron: Their potential danger. *Can Fam Physician* 20:85, 1974.

19. Krenzelok EP, Hoff JV: Accidental childhood iron poisoning: A problem of marketing and labeling. *Pediatrics* 63:591, 1979.

20. Rayburn W, Aronow R, DeLancey B, Hogan MJ: Drug overdose during pregnancy: An overview from a metropolitan poison control center. *Obstet Gynecol* 64:611, 1984.

21. Banner W Jr, Tong TG: Iron poisoning. *Pediatr Clin North Am* 33:393, 1986.

22. Henretig FM, Temple AR: Acute iron poisoning in children. *Emerg Med Clin North Am* 2:121, 1984.

23. Robotham JL, Lietman PS: Acute iron poisoning. *Am J Dis Child* 134:875, 1980.

24. Spencer IOB: Ferrous sulphate poisoning in children. *Br Med J* 2:1112, 1951.

25. Thomson J: Two cases of ferrous sulphate poisoning. *Br Med J* 1:640, 1947.

26. Smith RP, Jones CW, Cochran EW: Ferrous sulfate toxicity. *N Engl J Med* 243:641, 1950.

27. Olenmark M, Biber B, Dottori O, Rybo G: Fatal iron intoxication in late pregnancy. *J Toxicol Clin Toxicol* 25:347, 1987.

28. Lavender S, Bell SA: Iron intoxication in an adult. *Br Med J* 2:406, 1970.

29. Halliwell B, Gutteridge JMC: Oxygen free radicals and iron in relation to biology and medicine: Some problems and concepts. *Arch Biochem Biophys* 246:501, 1986.

30. Tenenbein M, Littman C, Stimpson RE: Gastrointestinal pathology in adult iron overdose. *J Toxicol Clin Toxicol* 28:311, 1990.

31. Wright TL, Brissot P, Ma W, Weisiger RA: Characterization of non-transferrin-bound iron clearance by rat. *J Biol Chem* 261:10909, 1986.

32. Craven CM, Alexander J, Eldridge M, et al: Tissue distribution and clearance kinetics of non-transferrin-bound iron in the hypotransferrinemic mouse: A rodent model for hemochromatosis. *Proc Natl Acad Sci USA* 84:3457, 1987.

33. Luongo MA, Bjornson SS: The liver in ferrous sulfate poisoning. *N Engl J Med* 251:995, 1954.

34. deCastro FJ, Jaeger R, Gleason WA: Liver damage and hypoglycemia in acute iron poisoning. *Clin Toxicol* 10:287, 1977.

35. Gleason WA, deMello DE, deCastro FJ, Connors JJ: Acute hepatic failure in severe iron poisoning. *J Pediatr* 95:138, 1979.

36. Reissmann KR, Coleman TJ: Acute intestinal iron intoxication. II. Metabolic, respiratory and circulatory effects of absorbed iron salts. *Blood* 10:46, 1955.

37. Whitten CF, Chen Y, Gibson GW: Studies in acute iron poisoning: Further observations on desferrioxamine in the treatment of acute experimental iron poisoning. *Pediatrics* 38:102, 1966.

38. Whitten CF, Chen YC, Gibson GW: Studies in acute iron poisoning: The hemodynamic alterations in acute experimental iron poisoning. *Pediatr Res* 2:479, 1968.

39. Vernon DD, Banner W, Dean JM: Hemodynamic effects of experimental iron poisoning. *Ann Emerg Med* 18:863, 1989.

40. Tenenbein M, Israels SJ: Early coagulopathy in severe iron poisoning. *J Pediatr* 113:695, 1988.

41. Tenebein M, Kopelow ML, deSa DJ: Myocardial failure and shock in iron poisoning. *Hum Toxicol* 7:281, 1988.

42. Tenenbein M: Poisoning in pregnancy, in Koren G (ed): *Maternal-Fetal Toxicology: A Clinician's Guide.* New York, Marcel Dekker, 1990, p 89.

43. Staple TW, McAlister WH: Roentgenographic visualization of iron preparations in the gastrointestinal tract. *Radiology* 83:1051, 1964.

44. Hosking CS: Radiology in the management of acute iron poisoning. *Med J Aust* 1:576, 1969.

45. Ng RCW, Perry K, Martin DJ: Iron poisoning: Assessment of radiography in diagnosis and management. *Clin Pediatr* 18:614, 1979.

46. Everson GW, Oudjhane K, Young LW, Krenzelok EP: Effectiveness of abdominal radiographs in visualizing chewable iron supplements following overdose. *Am J Emerg Med* 7:459, 1989.

47. Tenenbein M: Inefficacy of gastric emptying procedures. *J Emerg Med* 3:133, 1985.

48. Tenenbein M: Whole bowel irrigation in iron poisoning. *J Pediatr* 111:142, 1987.

49. Boggs DR: Fate of a ferrous sulfate prescription. *Am J Med* 82:124, 1987.

50. Gevirtz NR, Wasserman LR: The measurement of iron and iron-binding capacity in plasma containing deferoxamine. *J Pediatr* 68:802, 1966.

51. Helfer RE, Rodgerson DO: The effect of deferoxamine on the determination of serum iron and iron-binding capacity. *J Pediatr* 68:804, 1966.

52. Koren G, Bentur Y, Strong D, et al: Acute changes in renal function associated with deferoxamine therapy. *Am J Dis Child* 143:1077, 1989.

53. Chyka PA, Brady AY: Assessment of acute iron poisoning by laboratory and clinical observations. *Am J Emerg Med* 11:99, 1993.

54. Tenenbein M, Yatscoff RW: The TIBC in iron poisoning: Is it useful? *Am J Dis Child* 145:437, 1990.

55. Lacouture PG, Wason S, Temple AR, et al: Emergency assessment

of severity of iron overdose by clinical and laboratory methods. *J Pediatr* 99:89, 1981.

56. Knansel AL, Collins-Barrow MD: Applicability of early indicators of iron toxicity. *J Natl Med Assoc* 78:1037, 1986.

57. Palatnick W, Tenenbein M: Leukocytosis, hyperglycemia, vomiting and positive x-rays are not markers for iron >300 ug/dl in adult iron overdose. *Vet Hum Toxicol* 34:330, 1992.

58. Melby K, Slordahl S, Gutteberg TJ, Nordbo SA: Septicemia due to *Yersinia enterocolitica* after oral overdoses of iron. *Br Med J* 285:467, 1982.

59. Mofenson HC, Caraccio TR, Sharieff N: Iron sepsis. *Yersinia enterocolitica* septicemia possibly caused by an overdose of iron. *N Engl J Med* 316:1092, 1987.

60. Kulig K, Bar-Or D, Cantrill SV, et al: Management of acutely poisoned patients without gastric emptying. *Ann Emerg Med* 14:562, 1985.

61. Tenenbein M, Cohen S, Sitar DS: Efficacy of ipecac-induced emesis, orogastric lavage, and activated charcoal for acute drug overdose. *Ann Emerg Med* 16:838, 1987.

62. Albertson TE, Derlet RW, Foulke GE, et al: Superiority of activated charcoal alone compared with ipecac and activated charcoal in the treatment of acute toxic ingestions. *Ann Emerg Med* 18:56, 1989.

63. Merigian KS, Woodard M, Hedges JR, et al: Prospective evaluation of gastric emptying in the self-poisoned patient. *Am J Emerg Med* 10:452, 1992.

64. Kulig K: Initial management of ingestions of toxic substances. *N Engl J Med* 326:1677, 1992.

65. Decker WJ, Combs HF, Corby DG: Adsorption of drugs and poisons by activated charcoal. *Toxicol Appl Pharmacol* 13:454, 1968.

66. Foxford R, Goldfrank L: Gastrotomy: A surgical approach to iron overdose. *Ann Emerg Med* 14:1223, 1985.

67. Peterson CD, Fifield GC: Emergency gastrotomy for acute iron poisoning. *Ann Emerg Med* 9:262, 1980.

68. Venturelli J, Kwee Y, Morris N, Cameron G: Gastrotomy in the management of acute iron poisoning. *J Pediatr* 100:768, 1982.

69. Landsman I, Bricker JT, Reid BS, Bloss RS: Emergency gastrotomy: Treatment of choice for iron bezoar. *J Pediatr Surg* 22:184, 1987.

70. Tenenbein M, Wiseman N, Yatscoff RW: Gastrotomy and whole bowel irrigation in iron poisoning. *Pediatr Emerg Care* 7:286, 1991.

71. Czajka PA, Konrad JD, Duffy JP: Iron poisoning: An in vitro comparison of bicarbonate and phosphate lavage solutions. *J Pediatr* 98:491, 1981.

72. Dean BS, Krenzelok EP: In vitro effectiveness of oral complexation agents in the management of iron poisoning. *Clin Toxicol* 25:221, 1987.

73. Bachrach L, Correa A, Levin R, Grossman M: Iron poisoning: Complications of hypertonic phosphate lavage therapy. *J Pediatr* 94:147, 1979.

74. Geffner M, Opas LM: Phosphate poisoning complicating treatment for iron ingestion. *Am J Dis Child* 134:509, 1980.

75. Whitten CF, Gibson GW, Good MH, et al: Studies in acute iron poisoning. I. Deferoxamine in the treatment of acute iron poisoning: Clinical observations, experimental studies and theoretical considerations. *Pediatrics* 36:322, 1965.

76. Adamson IYR, Sienko A, Tenenbein M: Pulmonary toxicity of deferoxamine in iron-poisoned mice. *Toxicol Appl Pharmacol* 120:13, 1993.

77. Moeschlin S, Schnider U: Treatment of primary and secondary hemochromatosis and acute iron poisoning with a new potent iron-eliminating agent (desferrioxamine B). *N Engl J Med* 269:57, 1963.

78. Keberle H: The biochemistry of desferrioxamine and its relation to iron metabolism. *Ann NY Acad Sci* 119:758, 1964.

79. Proudfoot AT, Simpson D, Dyson EH: Management of acute iron poisoning. *Med Toxicol* 1:83, 1986.

80. Worwood M: The clinical biochemistry of iron. *Semin Hematol* 14:3, 1977.

81. Yatscoff RW, Wayne EA, Tenenbein M: An objective criterion for the cessation of deferoxamine therapy in the acutely iron poisoned patient. *J Toxicol Clin Toxicol* 29:1, 1991.

82. Gevirtz NR, Tendler D, Lurinsky G, Wasserman LR: Clinical studies of storage iron with desferrioxamine. *N Engl J Med* 273:95, 1965.

83. Harker LA, Funk DD, Finch CA: Evaluation of storage iron by chelates. *Am J Med* 45:105, 1968.

84. Cumming RLC, Millar JA, Smith JA, Goldberg A: Clinical laboratory studies on the action of desferrioxamine. *Br J Haematol* 17:257, 1969.

85. Hershko C: Determinants of fecal and urinary iron excretion in desferrioxamine-treated rats. *Blood* 51:415, 1978.

86. Tripod J: A pharmacological comparison of the binding of iron and other metals, in Gross F (ed): *Iron metabolism: An International Symposium.* Berlin, Springer-Verlag, 1964, p 503.

87. Hosking CS: A pharmacological investigation of acute iron poisoning and its treatment. *Aust Paediatr J* 6:92, 1970.

88. Propper RD, Shurin SB, Nathan DG: Reassessment of the use of desferrioxamine B in iron overload. *N Engl J Med* 294:1421, 1976.

89. Peck MG, Rogers JF, Rivenbark JF: Use of high doses of deferoxamine (Desferal) in an adult patient with acute iron overdosage. *J Toxicol Clin Toxicol* 19:865, 1982.

90. Henretig FM, Karl SR, Weintraub WH: Severe iron poisoning treated with enteral and intravenous deferoxamine. *Ann Emerg Med* 12:306, 1983.

91. Freedman MH, Grisaru D, Olivieri N, et al: Pulmonary syndrome in patients with thalassemia major receiving intravenous deferoxamine infusions. *Am J Dis Child* 144:565, 1990.

92. Tenenbein M, Kowalski S, Sienko et al: Pulmonary toxic effects of continuous desferrioxamine administration in acute iron poisoning. *Lancet* 339:699, 1992.

93. Mahoney JR Jr, Hallaway PE, Hedlund BE, Eaton JW: Acute iron poisoning: Rescue with macromolecular chelators. *J Clin Invest* 84:1362, 1989.

94. Hallaway PE, Eaton JW, Panter SS, Hedlund BE: Modulation of deferoxamine toxicity and clearance by covalent attachment to biocompatible polymers. *Proc Natl Acad Sci USA* 86:10108, 1989.

95. Olivieri NF, Koren G, Hermann C, et al: Comparison of oral iron chelator L1 and desferrioxamine in iron-loaded patients. *Lancet* 336:1275, 1990.

96. Tollerz G, Lannek N: Protection against iron toxicity in vitamin E deficient piglets and mice by vitamin E and synthetic antioxidants. *Nature* 201:846, 1964.

97. Ruwart MJ, Rush BD, Friedle NM, et al: Protective effects of 16,16-dimethyl PGE_2 on the liver and kidney. *Prostaglandins* 21(suppl):97, 1981.

98. Abecasis M, Falk JA, Makowka L, et al: 16, 16 Dimethyl prostaglandin E_2 prevents the development of fulminant hepatitis and blocks the induction of monocyte/macrophage procoagulant activity after murine hepatitis virus strain 3 infection. *J Clin Invest* 80:881, 1987.

146. Isoniazid Poisoning

James B. Mowry and R. Brent Furbee

Overview

Since its introduction in 1952, isoniazid (isonicotinic acid hydrazide; INH) has become the cornerstone of treatment for patients with active tuberculosis and those whose purified protein derivative (PPD) skin tests become positive. As a bactericidal agent, INH interferes with lipid and nucleic acid biosynthesis in the growing *Mycobacterium* organism.

EPIDEMIOLOGY. A high incidence of INH overdose has been reported in the American Indian population in Alaska and in the Southwest, where tuberculosis is prevalent and suicide rates are high. In a 1975 study of an Apache Indian population of 55,000, there were 5553 suicide attempts using INH over a 30-month period. In this population, INH accounted for 7 percent of all suicide attempts; in the subpopulation of women between 15 and 29 years of age, 19 percent of suicide attempts involved INH [1]. In contrast, the incidence of INH overdose in the general population has been low compared to the more widely available drugs of misuse and abuse (e.g., opiates, sedative-hypnotics, CNS stimulants). However, the American Association of Poison Control Centers reported 2656 cases of INH intoxication in 1991, a 300 percent increase over 1990 [2]. The reason for this large increase is unknown but was seen primarily in accidental exposures and may be related to the recent increase in tuberculosis in the United States. Fifty-six percent of the cases involved adults, with 13 percent being intentional overdoses. Six deaths were reported in this series, and 5 percent of cases exhibited moderate to severe toxicity. In studies of American Indian populations, INH has produced significant morbidity, with a 20 to 30 percent incidence of neurologic sequelae among survivors of overdose [1].

AVAILABLE FORMS. Isoniazid is available under a variety of brand names in 50-, 100-, and 300-mg tablets, as an oral syrup (50 mg/5 ml), as an injectable solution (Nydrazid, 100 mg/ml), and in powder form. It is also available in combination with rifampin, pyridoxine, and other antitubercular drugs.

PHARMACOLOGY. Isoniazid is rapidly and nearly completely absorbed following oral administration, with peak plasma concentrations normally occurring within 1 to 2 hours [3]. The rate and extent of absorption are decreased by food. Isoniazid is widely distributed throughout the body, with a volume of distribution approximating that of total body water (0.67 ± 0.15 L/kg) [4]. Cerebrospinal fluid concentrations are generally 90 percent those of serum. Isoniazid also passes into breast milk and through the placental barrier. There is little protein binding.

Between 75 and 95 percent of a dose of INH is metabolized in 24 hours in the liver by acetylation to acetylisoniazid and by hydrolysis to isonicotinic acid and hydrazine [3]. Genetic variation in its metabolism significantly alters plasma concentration, elimination half-life, and toxicity. Rapid acetylators are most often found among Eskimos (95%) and American Indians, whereas the majority of black and white Americans are slow acetylators [5]. The elimination half-life is 0.5 to 1.5 hours in rapid acetylators and 2 to 4 hours in slow acetylators. The half-life can also be prolonged up to 6.7 hours with liver disease. Approximately 75 percent of an oral dose of 5 mg per kilogram of body weight is excreted in urine within 24 hours as metabolites and unchanged drug. Slow acetylators excrete approximately 10 percent of INH as unchanged drug, compared to approximately 2.5 percent in rapid acetylators [3]. In addition, slow acetylators may have a higher percentage of the dose metabolized to hydrazine, a potential hepatotoxin [6].

Range of Toxicity. The usual therapeutic dose of INH is 5 mg/kg/day for adults and 10 mg/kg/day in children up to a maximum of 300 mg per day. Acute ingestion of 1.5 to 3 gm in adults may be toxic, and 6 to 10 gm is uniformly associated with severe toxicity and significant mortality [7]. Adult ingestions of 35 to 45 mg per kilogram have been associated with seizures, although the range that produces severe toxicity is reported to be 50 to 180 mg per kilogram [7]. In patients with preexisting seizure disorders, convulsions have occurred with doses as low as 14 mg/kg/day; 19 mg/kg/day resulted in seizures in a 7-year-old child [7]. Limiting the daily dose of INH to 10 mg per kilogram and rifampin to 15 mg per kilogram may minimize hepatotoxicity in children [8].

Normal daily doses of INH (3–5 mg/kg/day) produce peak serum concentrations ranging from 1 to 7 μg per milliliter. Intermittent INH therapy (14 mg/kg biweekly) may produce concentrations in the range of 16 to 32 μg per milliliter. Retrospective analysis in acute intoxication shows that serum INH concentrations have ranged from 20 μg per milliliter to more than 710 μg per milliliter with no correlation to severity of intoxication [9–12].

TOXICOLOGY

Neurologic. The neurologic toxicity of INH involves gamma-aminobutyric acid (GABA), an inhibitory central nervous system (CNS) neurotransmitter whose receptor site is located in the neural cell walls in close association with picrotoxin-barbiturate and benzodiazepine receptors [13]. When GABA attaches to its receptor site, it activates a chloride influx, causing an increased negative charge within the cell. This negative charge prevents the action potential from reaching a sufficiently positive voltage to create a discharge. When the effect of GABA is blocked, neurons become more excitable and the seizure threshold is lowered. In animal models, seizure activity caused by INH poisoning is correlated with a decrease in synaptic GABA concentrations in the brain [13].

The enzyme L-glutamic acid decarboxylase (GAD) converts glutamic acid to GABA, with the active form of vitamin B_6, pyridoxal 5′ phosphate, as a coenzyme (Fig. 146-1). Isoniazid decreases GABA synthesis by at least three mechanisms: lowering pyridoxine concentrations in the body by forming isoniazid-pyridoxine hydrazones, which are rapidly excreted in the urine; competitively inhibiting the conversion of pyridoxine to pyridoxal 5′ phosphate; and inactivating pyridoxal phosphate-containing enzymes through the same hydrazone coupling mechanism [14].

Alcohol has been postulated to increase the metabolic deg-

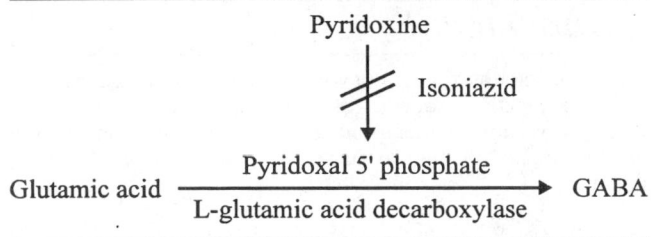

Fig. 146-1. Role of isoniazid (INH) in the reduction of gamma aminobutyric acid (GABA) synthesis. Pyridoxal 5′ phosphate acts as a coenzyme with L-glutamic acid decarboxylase to form GABA from glutamic acid. The INH blocks the conversion of pyridoxine to pyridoxal 5′ phosphate, resulting in decreased GABA formation and a decreased seizure threshold.

radation of pyridoxal 5′ phosphate and to potentiate the effects of INH. This has not been substantiated, since the presence of ethanol in experimental INH intoxication has been shown to have a mild anticonvulsant effect [15].

Metabolic. The severe metabolic acidosis seen in acute INH intoxication is primarily due to lactic acidosis resulting from seizure activity [16]. While INH may also interfere with nicotinamide-adenine dinucleotide (NAD)-mediated conversion of lactate to pyruvate, no acidosis was noted in animal experiments until seizures occurred, and correction of existing lactic acidosis occurred within 2 hours after seizures ceased [16]. Hyperglycemia may result from blockage of specific steps in the Krebs cycle that require NAD, as well as from stimulation of glucagon secretion [10].

Hepatic. The mechanism of action of INH-induced liver damage is not well defined. Hepatic damage may be due to hydrazine metabolites of INH covalently binding to liver macromolecules and producing necrosis [17]. Acetylhydrazine was first implicated as the causative agent for hepatic damage. Although rapid acetylators produce increased amounts of this metabolite, more rapid acetylation of acetylhydrazine to diacetylhydrazine results in lower concentrations of acetylhydrazine in this population (Fig. 146-2) [18,19]. Slow acetylators hydrolyze 3 percent of an isoniazid dose directly to isonicotinic acid and hydrazine, compared to only 0.3 percent in rapid acetylators [6]. Therefore, increased acetylhydrazine and/or hydrazine concentrations in slow acetylators may be responsible for the increased incidence of hepatotoxicity in these individuals [3,6].

Clinical Presentation

ACUTE TOXICITY. Symptoms appear within 30 minutes to 2 hours after acute INH ingestions. Nausea, vomiting, dizziness, slurred speech, blurring of vision, and visual hallucinations (bright colors, spots, strange designs) are among the first manifestations [7,9]. Stupor and coma can rapidly develop, followed by intractable tonic-clonic generalized or localized seizures, hyperreflexia or complete areflexia, and cyanosis [7,9]. In severe cases, cardiovascular and respiratory collapse can result in death. Oliguria progressing to anuria has been reported [7]. The metabolic alterations produced by INH intoxication are striking and include severe metabolic acidosis, hyperglycemia, glycosuria, ketonuria, and mild hyperkalemia [7,9,10]. The triad of metabolic acidosis refractory to sodium bicarbonate therapy,

seizures that are refractory to anticonvulsants, and coma suggests INH overdose.

CHRONIC TOXICITY. Hepatotoxicity due to toxic INH metabolites can present as clinical hepatitis or asymptomatic elevations in liver function tests [17]. From 15 to 20 percent of INH-treated patients may develop elevated serum aspartate amino transferase (AST) values within the first few months of therapy, although elevated AST concentrations can occur at any time. A 3.3 percent incidence of hepatotoxicity was reported in 430 children receiving INH and rifampin for tuberculosis [8]. Approximately 50 percent of reactions occurred during the first month of treatment; all reactions occurred during the first 10 weeks. Enzyme elevations usually return to normal with continued therapy, although some patients progress to hepatic necrosis.

Slow acetylator phenotype, increased age, alcohol consumption, and rifampin coadministration all increase the potential for liver damage. In one study, the incidence of INH-induced liver enzyme elevation in fast and slow acetylators was 3.7 percent and 13 percent in those younger than 35 years, and 13.2 percent and 37 percent in those older than 35 years [20]. It has been suggested that concomitant administration of rifampin and INH results in increased formation of hydrazine from

Fig. 146-2. Simplified metabolism of isoniazid and hepatotoxicity. A majority of isoniazid is acetylated to acetylisoniazid and then hydrolyzed to form acetylhydrazine. Rapid acetylators detoxify acetylhydrazine more rapidly to diacetylhydrazine, thereby avoiding accumulation of acetylhydrazine. In addition, slow acetylators hydrolyze 3% of an isoniazid dose to isonicotinic acid and hydrazine, compared to only 0.3% in rapid acetylators. Slow acetylators may accumulate hydrazine and/or acetylhydrazine, resulting in hepatotoxicity. (Modified from Sarma GR, Immanuel C, Kailasam S, et al: Rifampin-induced release of hydrazine from isoniazid. *Am Rev Respir Dis* 133:1072, 1986.)

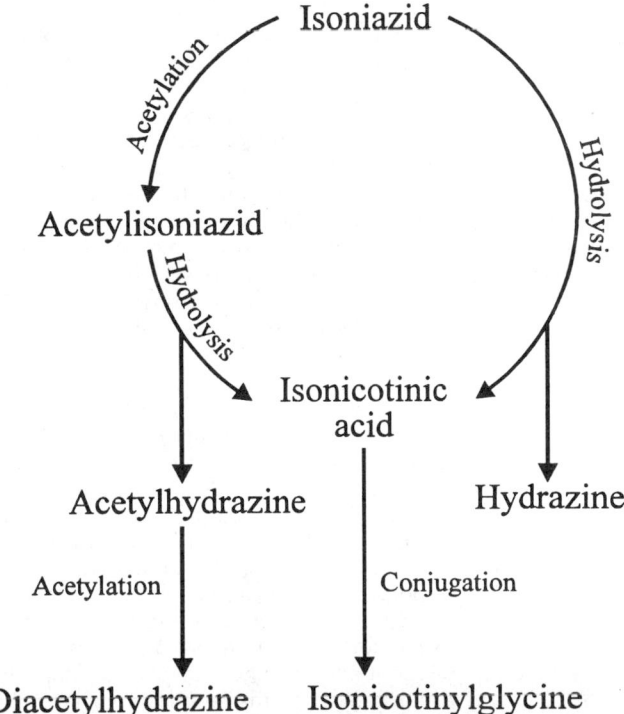

INH, especially in slow acetylators, resulting in increased toxicity [6,20]. Interestingly, a study of 3000 patients stratified as to acetylator phenotype failed to show any difference in incidence of hepatotoxicity between phenotypes [21].

Peripheral neuropathy, the most common toxic effect of chronic INH use, is related to pyridoxine deficiency. Other chronic effects include convulsions, encephalopathy, optic neuritis, optic atrophy, memory impairment, and psychosis [22]. Neural Wallerian degeneration of the myelin sheath and axon resulting in peripheral neuropathy occurs within 3 to 35 weeks after the start of therapy [23]. It is most often seen in slow acetylator phenotypes, uremia, malnourished patients, alcoholics, and diabetics and with INH doses greater than 6 mg/kg/day. Peripheral neuropathy rarely occurs in children, although 13 percent of children have pyridoxine deficiency while receiving INH, particularly those receiving doses greater than 10 mg/kg/day [24].

Diagnostic Evaluation

ANCILLARY TESTS. The initial laboratory evaluation of patients with acute INH intoxication should include blood for glucose, electrolytes, arterial blood gases with pH, and bicarbonate. Baseline electrocardiogram (ECG) and renal function tests (BUN, serum creatinine) are also recommended.

SERUM CONCENTRATIONS. The majority of laboratories capable of assaying INH quantitatively do so for research purposes. Qualitative analysis of urine or blood for the presence of INH may be helpful if there is question as to whether it has been ingested. Qualitative identification in the urine has been accomplished using reagent-impregnated paper strips sensitive to the metabolic products of INH [25].

DIFFERENTIAL DIAGNOSIS. Acute INH intoxication should be considered in the differential diagnosis of any patient presenting with unexplained neurologic symptoms, particularly intractable seizure activity [7,11]. Conditions that may resemble INH poisoning include trauma; tumors and infections of the CNS; electrolyte abnormalities; thyroid dysfunction; hypoglycemia; poisoning by CNS stimulants (anticholinergic, cholinergic, and adrenergic agents), sedative-hypnotics, meperidine (normeperidine), propoxyphene, carbon monoxide, or cyanide; and withdrawal syndromes. Because seizure activity alone can lead to acidosis, any agent that causes convulsions must be considered. The intractable nature of INH-induced seizures is relatively uncommon but may be shared by such agents as theophylline, amoxapine, maprotiline, cyanide, organophosphate insecticides, fluoride, and carbon monoxide, which often require treatment in addition to anticonvulsant therapy [26].

Other etiologies of an anion gap metabolic acidosis should also be considered. Diabetic ketoacidosis, ethylene glycol, methanol, and salicylates may present a similar clinical picture.

Ingestion of rifampin-INH combination products may produce, in addition to the symptoms of INH poisoning, a striking red-orange discoloration of the skin, urine, sclera, and mucous membranes; periorbital or facial edema; pruritus; and nausea, vomiting, or diffuse abdominal tenderness [27]. Transient elevations in total bilirubin and alkaline phosphatase indicating cholestasis may also be noted. Deaths from rifampin have been reported only in conjunction with other drugs [27].

Management

The management of a patient with acute INH overdose includes airway protection, support of respirations, treatment of seizures, correction of metabolic acidosis, minimization of drug absorption, and, in selected cases, enhancement of INH elimination.

DECONTAMINATION. Following stabilization, gastrointestinal decontamination using activated charcoal with or without gastric lavage should be performed. Because of the potential for rapid development of coma and seizures, syrup of ipecac is not recommended.

MONITORING. All patients treated with pyridoxine or who develop symptoms that do not resolve during 4 to 6 hours of observation should be admitted to an intensive care unit (ICU) for further management. Those who remain or become asymptomatic and who have not required interventions other than gastrointestinal decontamination may be discharged or referred for psychiatric evaluation.

NEUROLOGIC TOXICITY

Seizure Activity. Seizures are often refractory to most conventional anticonvulsants [15]. The anticonvulsant with the best activity, although still relatively ineffective, appears to be diazepam. Larger than usual doses are frequently required. Because some of INH's mechanisms of action involve pyridoxine and experimental work has demonstrated that supplemental pyridoxine lessens the effects of INH on GAD and GABA, this agent should be considered a specific antidote for neurologic toxicity.

It is recommended that pyridoxine (vitamin B_6) be administered in doses equal to the amount of INH ingested, to prevent or terminate seizure activity [7,9,28]. Five INH overdose patients treated with such doses of pyridoxine were compared with 41 historical controls; those treated with pyridoxine experienced no recurrent seizure activity (vs. 60% of controls), had a decreased duration of coma (7 hours vs. 24 hours), and had prompt resolution of their metabolic acidosis [11]. In a canine model, pyridoxine has a dose-related effectiveness against convulsions and prevents lethality at doses ranging from 75 to 300 mg per kilogram [29]. In another study, when the single-anticonvulsant regimens of pyridoxine, phenobarbital, pentobarbital, phenytoin, and diazepam were compared with the latter four anticonvulsants in combination with pyridoxine, pyridoxine was the only single agent that reduced the severity of convulsions and prevented death, although it did not completely block convulsions; the combination of other anticonvulsants with pyridoxine prevented both convulsions and lethality [15]. Hence, it is recommended that acute INH poisoning treatment include both pyridoxine and diazepam [29].

Asymptomatic patients who have ingested a potentially toxic dose of INH should be observed for at least 4 to 6 hours [7]. A dose of pyridoxine equal to the amount of INH ingested should be given at the first sign of neurologic toxicity. If the amount of INH is not reliably known, at least 5 gm of pyridoxine should be given [7,9]. In patients without seizures, the dose of pyridoxine should be administered intravenously over 30 to 60 minutes. In those with seizure activity, it may be given as a bolus over 3 to 5 minutes. Individual doses of pyridoxine may be repeated at 5- to 20-minute intervals until the INH dose is exceeded, seizures cease, or consciousness is regained [7]. Diazepam should also be administered, to potentiate the action of pyridoxine [7,15]. Seizures refractory to pyridoxine and diazepam have been successfully treated with thiopental-induced coma [30]. Brain damage should be suspected if coma persists more than 6 to 12 hours despite therapy, although complete reversal of coma after 36 and 42 hours has been temporally related to additional pyridoxine administration [31].

Peripheral Neuropathy. Prevention of peripheral neuropathy during chronic INH therapy can be accomplished by administration of pyridoxine, 15 to 50 mg per day, in high-risk patients [22]. Higher doses are unnecessary and may interfere with the antibacterial actions of INH. Doses of 500 to 2000 mg per day can result in peripheral and central sensory neuropathy characterized by numbness, burning, shooting or tingling pain, ataxia, muscle weakness, fasciculations, diminished reflexes, depression, headache, and irritability and are not recommended [32]. Pyridoxine prophylaxis in children is not usually necessary but should be considered in those who are debilitated or malnourished or who are taking larger than usual doses of isoniazid [22,24]. Peripheral neuropathy that develops during INH therapy is generally reversible on withdrawal of INH and treatment with high-dose pyridoxine (100–200 mg/day) [22]. The neuropathy may take months to a year or more to resolve and in some cases may be permanent.

METABOLIC ACIDOSIS. Treatment of metabolic acidosis should be guided by arterial blood gas and electrolyte measurements. In most cases, intravenous sodium bicarbonate will not correct acid-base abnormalities until seizure activity is terminated [11]. Bicarbonate should be given if the serum pH is lower than 7.2 or the acidosis does not rapidly resolve following seizure control.

HEPATIC TOXICITY. The management of INH-induced hepatotoxicity includes supportive care and cessation or reduction of INH administration. Patients should be instructed to report immediately any of the prodromal symptoms, such as fatigue, weakness, malaise, anorexia, nausea, or vomiting. If these symptoms appear or if signs suggestive of hepatic damage are detected, INH should be discontinued promptly. Even in asymptomatic patients, liver function tests should be routinely monitored. It is recommended that INH be discontinued in patients with transaminase concentrations three times the normal concentrations [20].

ENHANCED ELIMINATION. In the past, enhanced elimination procedures, along with megadoses of diazepam and sodium bicarbonate, were the mainstays of treatment for acute INH poisoning. The role of forced diuresis in the management of INH overdose is not clear. In a 20-gm ingestion, 11.52 gm of INH was recovered in 8 liters of urine over 4 hours [12]. In another case, 42.9 percent of a 2.3-gm absorbed dose was recovered in the urine over 72 hours. However, only small amounts of INH have been recovered in the urine of other patients: 144 mg in a 50-gm ingestion over 13 hours during hemodialysis and 6.2 mg in 9 liters over 24 hours during charcoal hemoperfusion [33,34].

Peritoneal dialysis removed 52.1 percent of a 2.3-gm absorbed dose over 72 hours, whereas exchange transfusion for an ingestion of 900 mg removed less than 4 percent of the dose [33,35]. Hemodialysis has decreased the elimination half-life from 2.3 to 1.1 hours and produced clearances of 76 ml per minute, but it resulted in removal of only 90.4 mg of INH in a person who reportedly ingested a 50-gm dose [34,36]. With charcoal hemoperfusion, an INH clearance of 140 ml per minute has been reported, with 360 mg eliminated in 4 hours and cerebrospinal fluid concentration decreases paralleling those in serum [34].

Considering the rapid elimination half-life of INH and the efficacy of current therapy using pyridoxine, measures to enhance the elimination of INH are no longer indicated in the routine management of INH intoxication. However, patients with intractable acid-base disturbances, persistent seizures, or liver or renal failure should still be considered candidates for hemodialysis or charcoal hemoperfusion. Unless the patient has suffered anoxia as a result of coma or seizures, complete recovery of neurologic function can be expected within 24 to 48 hours, despite severe poisoning.

References

1. Sievers ML, Cynamon MH, Bittker TE: Intentional isoniazid overdosage among Southwestern American Indians. *Am J Psychiatry* 132:662, 1975.
2. Litovitz TL, Holm KC, Bailey KM, et al: 1991 annual report of the American Association of Poison Control Centers National Data Collection System. *Am J Emerg Med* 10:452, 1992.
3. Ellard GA, Gammon PT: Pharmacokinetics of isoniazid metabolism in man. *J Pharmacokinet Biopharm* 4:83, 1976.
4. Benet LZ, Williams RL: Design and optimization of dosage regimens: Pharmacokinetic data, in Gilman AG, Rall TW, Nies AS, Taylor P (eds): *The Pharmacological Basis of Therapeutics*. 8th ed. New York, Pergamon, 1990, pp 1650–1735.
5. Jeans C, Schaefer O, Eidus L: Inactivation of isoniazid by Canadian Eskimos and Indians. *Can Med Assoc J* 106:331, 1972.
6. Sarma GR, Immanuel C, Kailasam S, et al: Rifampin-induced release of hydrazine from isoniazid: A possible cause of hepatitis during treatment of tuberculosis with regimens containing isoniazid and rifampin. *Am Rev Respir Dis* 133:1072, 1986.
7. Sievers ML, Herrier RN: Treatment of acute isoniazid toxicity. *Am J Hosp Pharm* 32:202, 1975.
8. O'Brien RJ, Long MW, Cross FS, et al: Hepatotoxicity from isoniazid and rifampin among children treated for tuberculosis. *Pediatrics* 72:491, 1983.
9. Brown CV: Acute isoniazid poisoning. *Am Rev Respir Dis* 105:206, 1972.
10. Terman DS, Teitelbaum DT: Isoniazid self-poisoning. *Neurology* 20:299, 1970.
11. Wason S, Lacouture PG, Lovejoy FH: Single high dose pyridoxine treatment for isoniazid overdose. *JAMA* 246:1102, 1981.
12. Sitprija V, Holmes JH: Isoniazid intoxication. *Am Rev Respir Dis* 90:248, 1964.
13. Wood JD, Peesker SJ: A correlation between changes in GABA metabolism and isonicotinic acid hydrazide induced seizures. *Brain Res* 45:489, 1972.
14. Miller J, Robinson A, Percy AK: Acute isoniazid poisoning in childhood. *Am J Dis Child* 134:290, 1980.
15. Chin L, Sievers ML, Herrier RN, et al: Potentiation of pyridoxine by depressants and anticonvulsants in the treatment of acute isoniazid intoxication in dogs. *Toxicol Appl Pharmacol* 58:504, 1981.
16. Chin L, Sievers ML, Herrier RN, et al: Convulsions as the etiology of lactic acidosis in acute isoniazid toxicity in dogs. *Toxicol Appl Pharmacol* 49:377, 1979.
17. Olin B: Isoniazid-induced hepatotoxicity (drug consult), in Gelman CR, Rumack BH (eds): *DRUGDEX Information System*. Denver, Micromedex (edition expires 8/31/95).
18. Mitchell JR, Thorgeirsson UP, Black M, et al: Increased incidence of isoniazid hepatitis in rapid acetylators: Possible relationship to hydrazine metabolites. *Clin Pharmacol Ther* 18:70, 1975.
19. Lauterburg BH, Smith CV, Todd EL, et al: Oxidation of hydrazine metabolites formed from isoniazid. *Clin Pharmacol Ther* 38:566, 1985.

20. Dickinson DS, Bailey WC, Hirschowitz BI, et al: Risk factors for isoniazid (INH)-induced liver dysfunction. *J Clin Gastroenterol* 3:271, 1981.
21. Gurumurthy P, Krishnamurthy MS, Nazareth O, et al: Lack of relationship between hepatic toxicity and acetylator phenotype in three thousand South Indian patients during treatment with isoniazid for tuberculosis. *Am Rev Respir Dis* 129:58, 1984.
22. Drug Information Analysis Service, University of California at San Francisco: Pyridoxine therapy of INH and hydralazine-induced peripheral neuropathy (drug consult), in Gelman CR, Rumack BH (eds): *DRUGDEX Information System.* Denver, Micromedex (edition expires 8/31/95).
23. Ochoa J: Isoniazid neuropathy in man: Quantitative electron microscope study. *Brain* 93:831, 1970.
24. Pellock JM, Howell J, Kendig EL, et al: Pyridoxine deficiency in children treated with isoniazid. *Chest* 87:658, 1985.
25. Kilburn JO, Beam RE, David HC, et al: Reagent-impregnated paper strip for detection of metabolic products of isoniazid in urine. *Am Rev Respir Dis* 106:923, 1972.
26. Olson K, Pentel P, Kelly M: Physical assessment and differential diagnosis of the poisoned patient. *Med Toxicol* 2:52, 1987.
27. Holdiness MR: A review of the redman syndrome and rifampin overdosage. *Med Toxicol Adverse Drug Exp* 4:444, 1989.
28. Wood JD, Peesker SJ: The effect on GABA metabolism in brain of isonicotinic acid hydrazide and pyridoxine as a function of time after administration. *J Neurochem* 19:1527, 1972.
29. Chin L, Sievers ML, Laird HE, et al: Evaluation of diazepam and pyridoxine as antidotes to isoniazid intoxication in rats and dogs. *Toxicol Appl Pharmacol* 45:712, 1978.
30. Bredemann JA, Krechel SW, Eggers GWN: Treatment of refractory seizures in massive isoniazid overdose. *Anesth Analg* 71:554, 1990.
31. Brent J, Vo N, Kulig K, et al: Reversal of prolonged isoniazid-induced coma by pyridoxine. *Arch Intern Med* 150:1751, 1990.
32. Dalton K, Dalton MJT: Characteristics of pyridoxine overdose neuropathy syndrome. *Acta Neurol Scand* 76:8, 1987.
33. Cocco AE, Pazourek LJ: Acute isoniazid intoxication: Management by peritoneal dialysis. *N Engl J Med* 269:852, 1963.
34. Konigshausen TH, Atrogge G, Hein D, et al: Hemodialysis and hemoperfusion in the treatment of most severe INH poisoning. *Vet Hum Toxicol* 21(suppl):12, 1979.
35. Katz BE, Carver MW: Acute poisoning with isoniazid treated by exchange transfusion. *Pediatrics* 18:72, 1956.
36. Jorgensen HE, Weith JO: Dialysable poisons: Hemodialysis in the treatment of acute poisoning. *Lancet* 1:81, 1963.

147. Lithium Poisoning

Kent R. Olson

Overview

Lithium was introduced in the nineteenth century for the treatment of gout, but toxicity was rarely encountered, apparently because of low recommended doses. In the 1940s, lithium chloride was briefly marketed as a salt substitute but was withdrawn after several cases of serious intoxication and death resulted from its use. In 1949, Cade reported its antimanic properties, and lithium has found increasingly wide psychiatric use since its approval by the Food and Drug Administration in 1970 [1,2].

THERAPEUTIC USE. In patients with mania, lithium reduces hyperactivity, irritability, pressured speech, assaultive behavior, and sleeplessness. These effects may require several days of therapy, during which time alternate medications are used. Lithium is very effective in reducing the recurrence of episodes of manic-depressive bipolar disorder and is used to treat some patients with unipolar depression and schizophrenia. Lithium induces neutrophilia (up to 1.5–2 times normal leukocyte counts), and is therefore often used to treat myelosuppressive-induced neutropenia [1,3].

Lithium is available in conventional tablets or capsules containing 300 mg (8.12 mEq) of lithium carbonate or sustained-release preparations containing 450 mg (12.18 mEq) of lithium carbonate. Liquid solutions of lithium citrate containing 8 mEq per 5 ml are also available [3].

PHARMACOLOGY. Lithium is the lightest alkali metal, occupying the same column in the periodic table as sodium and potassium, elements with which it shares some properties. However, it serves no known normal physiologic role. The exact mechanisms of lithium's therapeutic and toxic effects remain unknown. Lithium is known to affect ion transport and cell membrane potential by competing with sodium and potassium and possibly other cations. Unlike sodium and potassium, however, lithium cannot produce a large distribution gradient and therefore cannot maintain a significant membrane potential. Lithium may also enhance some effects of serotonin and acetylcholine. In addition, its inhibitory effects on second messengers, such as inositol phosphates, may reduce neuronal responsiveness to some neurotransmitters [1].

PHARMACOKINETICS. Lithium is readily absorbed from the gastrointestinal tract. The bioavailability of conventional tablets and capsules and the liquid solution is 95 to 100 percent; it is not affected by food. Normally, absorption is complete within 1 to 6 hours; peak levels are reached in 2 to 4 hours [1,3]. Sustained-release preparations (e.g., Lithobid) are less predictably (60–90%) absorbed, and peak levels may be delayed more than 4 to 12 hours [3]. Overdose has resulted in delayed peak levels or secondary peak levels as long as 148 hours after ingestion [4]. In one case, esophagoscopy at 84 hours revealed a 5- to 6-cm tablet and hair bezoar in the stomach [5].

Lithium initially occupies an apparent volume of distribution (V_d) of 0.3 to 0.4 liter per kilogram (extracellular water), but further distribution into various intracellular tissue compartments occurs over 6 to 10 hours and the final volume of distribution is approximately 0.7 to 1 liter per kilogram. This explains why initial serum lithium levels may be very high with few or no signs of toxicity. Following a single dose, the equilibrium serum lithium level can be expected to increase by 1.0 to 1.5 mEq per liter for each 1 mEq of lithium per kilogram of body weight. Steady-state tissue levels are achieved after about 3 to 4 days of therapy. Tissue distribution is uneven; whereas the cerebrospinal fluid (CSF) lithium concentration is only 40 to 60 percent that of plasma, the saliva concentration may be 2 to 3 times greater than that of plasma. Lithium is not bound to serum proteins and freely crosses the placenta [1,3].

Lithium is not metabolized. More than 95 percent of absorbed lithium is excreted by the kidney, with 4 to 5 percent eliminated in sweat and 1 percent in the feces. Lithium is also excreted in breast milk. Eighty percent of renally filtered lithium is reabsorbed in the proximal tubule, against a concentration gradient that does not distinguish lithium from sodium. Sodium depletion can result in as much as a 50 percent increase in lithium reabsorption. The usual renal clearance is approximately 15 to 30 ml per minute, but it may be 10 to 15 ml per minute or less in the elderly and in patients with reduced renal function [3]. The elimination half-life averages 20 to 24 hours; in patients with chronic intoxication, it may be as long as 47.6 hours [6]. The very slow terminal elimination phase may last up to 10 to 14 days, owing to gradual release from tissue storage sites such as bone and brain [1].

Therapeutic serum concentrations are usually considered to be 0.8 to 1.25 mEq per liter; prophylaxis against recurrent manic-depressive illness may be achieved with levels of 0.75 to 1 mEq per liter. Drug levels must be drawn at least 10 to 12 hours after the last dose to allow for complete tissue distribution. Onset of therapeutic effects usually requires 5 to 21 days after initiation of daily drug administration. Therapeutic levels are achieved by administration of 600 to 1200 mg of lithium carbonate (approximately 16–32 mEq of lithium) per day. Because of the low toxic-therapeutic ratio, careful monitoring of lithium levels is essential [3].

Toxicology

Lithium intoxication involves primarily the central nervous system and kidneys, although a variety of other organ systems are also affected (Table 147-1). Lithium intoxication may follow an

Table 147-1. Common Features of Lithium Intoxication

Features	Number	% of total
Confusion	19*	68
Agitation	17	61
Drowsiness	16*	57
Mutism	5	18
Coma (grades III–IV)	1	4
Convulsions	4	14
Hyperreflexia	22	79
Increased tone	16	57
Ankle clonus	4	14
Extensor plantar responses	3	11
Tremor	18	64
Ataxia	14	50
Dysarthria	10	36
Myoclonus	7	25
Vomiting	7	25
Diarrhea	4	14
Acute diabetes insipidus	3	11
Acute renal failure	2	7

* Excludes one patient who also took temazepam in overdose
From Dyson EH, Simpson D, Prescott LF, Proudfoot AT: Self-poisoning and therapeutic intoxication with lithium. *Hum Toxicol* 6:325, 1987. With permission.

acute overdose or may result from chronic accumulation, because of either an increase in dosage or a decrease in lithium elimination by the kidneys. Most serious toxicity occurs in patients with chronic intoxication.

Acute ingestion of at least 1 mEq per kilogram (approximately 40 mg/kg lithium carbonate) in a person not previously taking lithium would be required to produce a potentially toxic serum lithium level. The acutely toxic dose in a patient already taking lithium ("acute on chronic" overdose) depends on the prior lithium level. The dose required to produce chronic intoxication depends on the individual's rate of renal elimination of lithium.

CLINICAL MANIFESTATIONS OF POISONING. Signs and symptoms of mild poisoning include lethargy, fatigue, memory impairment, and fine tremor. Confusion, agitation, delirium, coarse tremor, hyperreflexia, hypertension, tachycardia, dysarthria, nystagmus, ataxia, muscle fasciculations, extrapyramidal syndromes, and choreoathetoid movements are manifestations of moderate intoxication. Bradycardia, coma, seizures, hyperthermia, and hypotension may be seen in severe poisoning. Permanent sequelae, including choreoathetosis, nystagmus, and ataxia, have been described [7].

Neurotoxic effects of lithium usually develop gradually and may become progressively severe over several days. Neurologic manifestations may worsen even as serum lithium levels are falling and may persist for days to weeks after cessation of therapy, in part due to slow movement of lithium into and out of intracellular brain sites.

Cardiovascular manifestations are nonspecific. The ECG changes are often similar to those occurring with hypokalemia and may result from displacement of intracellular potassium by lithium; U waves and flattened, biphasic, or inverted T waves can be seen with therapeutic doses as well as mild overdoses. Sinus and junctional bradycardia, sinoatrial and first-degree atrioventricular block, and QRS and Q–T interval prolongation may be seen with severe intoxication [8,9]. Life-threatening dysrhythmias are rare. Pulse and blood pressure abnormalities may be seen in moderate or severe poisoning but are usually not pronounced. Hypotension is more often due to dehydration, which can be a cause as well as a complication of lithium intoxication, than to direct cardiotoxicity [8,9].

Chronic lithium therapy has several important effects on renal function, including impaired urinary concentrating ability, nephrogenic diabetes insipidus, and even a sodium-losing nephritis [2]. These effects appear to be dose-related and usually correct within several weeks of discontinuing therapy [8]. Excessive water and sodium loss leads to increased proximal tubular reabsorption of lithium by transport mechanisms designed for sodium reabsorption. The accumulation of lithium may also be enhanced by illnesses that result in decreased glomerular filtration rate, such as fever with sweating, gastroenteritis, or heart failure, or by diuretic drugs that enhance distal tubular sodium and fluid loss. Rising lithium levels may further aggravate nephrotoxicity. A patient who has remained stable with a satisfactory lithium serum level at a constant daily dosage for years may suddenly develop life-threatening intoxication within days of entering such a vicious cycle [2].

Metabolic abnormalities reportedly associated with lithium use include hypercalcemia, hypermagnesemia, nonketotic hyperglycemia, transient diabetic ketoacidosis, and goiter. Frank hypothyroidism is rare [8].

Lithium is teratogenic in rats, mice, and rabbits, and human fetal malformations have been described, including cardiac defects such as Ebstein's anomaly [10].

DRUG INTERACTIONS. Several drugs may interact with lithium to alter its pharmacokinetics or directly to enhance its toxicity. Diuretics may promote fluid and sodium depletion, leading to enhanced tubular lithium reabsorption. This effect appears to be much less apparent with furosemide than with thiazide diuretics. Several agents (aminophylline, urea, bicarbonate, acetazolamide) may decrease serum lithium levels by increasing glomerular filtration rate. Nonsteroidal antiinflammatory agents may decrease glomerular filtration rate and lithium elimination. Antipsychotic medications may have additive central nervous system (CNS) depressant effects; in addition, lithium may enhance their dopamine-blocking effects and induce or aggravate rigidity and hyperthermia (possibly inducing neurologic malignant syndrome) [8].

Diagnostic Evaluation

The history should include the type of lithium preparation ingested, the amount(s) and time(s) of ingestion, and the nature of the symptoms. It is important to distinguish between chronic intoxication, acute overdose, and acute overdose in a patient using lithium chronically.

The physical examination should focus on the vital signs, neurologic function, and cardiovascular status. All patients should have an ECG and laboratory evaluation including serum electrolytes, glucose, blood urea nitrogen, creatinine, and serum lithium level. Lithium levels should be repeated at frequent (i.e., 2–4-hour) intervals following acute overdose until peak levels are observed. If the levels are elevated, they should be repeated until they fall below the toxic range and the patient becomes asymptomatic.

Patients with chronic intoxication are typically brought to medical attention by a family member or therapist because of neurologic symptoms. There is usually a recent history of excessive fluid loss caused by gastroenteritis, other flulike illness, or excessive urination. The severity of chronic intoxication generally correlates well with the serum lithium level [2,8]. In patients on chronic therapy, mild neurotoxic effects may occur even with levels less than 1.5 mEq per liter. Steady-state levels of 1.5 to 3.0 mEq per liter are associated with mild or moderate toxicity. With serum levels greater than 3 to 4 mEq per liter, severe poisoning and death may occur [2,6,8].

After acute overdose, the predominant initial symptoms are nausea and vomiting [2]. Because lithium is taken up slowly by the brain and other tissues, patients do not usually have significant neurologic manifestations despite high serum lithium levels during the first 12 hours or more after ingestion [6]. Levels as high as 9.8 mEq per liter without significant toxicity have been reported after acute overdose [11,12]. However, intoxication may develop over the subsequent 24 to 48 hours even as serum levels fall [13]. Levels drawn after acute or acute on chronic overdose cannot be used reliably to predict toxicity or to guide therapy (Fig. 147-1) [2,6]. Unfortunately, there does not appear to be any clinical variable that accurately predicts which patients will deteriorate. The use of CSF levels to estimate brain concentrations more closely has been advocated [14]. However, CSF concentrations do not reflect intracellular brain tissue levels or predict the level of coma (Fig. 147-2) [2,12,15].

Patients with acute on chronic overdose usually have a clinical course similar to those with acute ingestions. However, a smaller total dose may produce severe intoxication, depending on the preingestion therapeutic serum level.

Elevated BUN and creatinine reflect renal insufficiency and

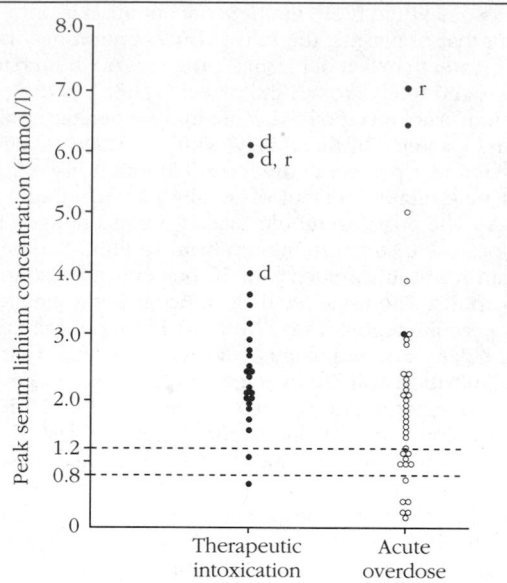

Fig. 147-1. Lack of correlation between serum levels and toxic manifestations in patients with acute intoxication. ● = features of toxicity present; ○ = no features of toxicity; d = diabetes insipidus; r = renal failure. (From Dyson EH, Simpson D, Prescott LF, Proudfoot AT: Self-poisoning and therapeutic intoxication with lithium. *Hum Toxicol* 6:325, 1987. With permission.)

suggest that intoxication results from gradual accumulation of lithium, rather than acute ingestion. Elevated creatinine may also be caused by cross-reactivity of the assay with creatine from muscle destruction and should prompt the measurement of serum creatine phosphokinase (CPK) and urinalysis for myoglobinuria.

Patients with lithium-induced nephrogenic diabetes insipidus usually have dilute urine with a low measured osmolality relative to serum. The diagnosis is confirmed by lack of response of the inappropriately dilute urine to administered vasopressin [8].

Leukocytosis may be seen in patients taking lithium. It is a nonspecific finding and does not reflect severity of intoxication. A reduced or absent anion gap may occur with severe lithium carbonate intoxication, probably because the carbonate anion (but not the lithium cation) is measured and used in calculating the anion gap.

Plain radiographs of the abdomen may or may not reveal radiopaque lithium tablets after acute ingestion. A negative radiograph should not be used to rule out acute ingestion [16].

DIFFERENTIAL DIAGNOSIS. Conditions such as hypoxia, hypoglycemia, temperature abnormalities (hypothermia, hyperthermia), electrolyte disturbances, CNS infection (meningitis, encephalitis), head trauma, and intracranial bleeding should be included in the differential diagnosis of any patient with altered mental status. In a patient with hyperthermia and rigidity who is also taking antipsychotic medications, neuroleptic malignant syndrome should be considered (see Chap. 73). Other drug intoxications should be considered (see Chap. 129), especially if CNS symptoms appear shortly after an acute overdose.

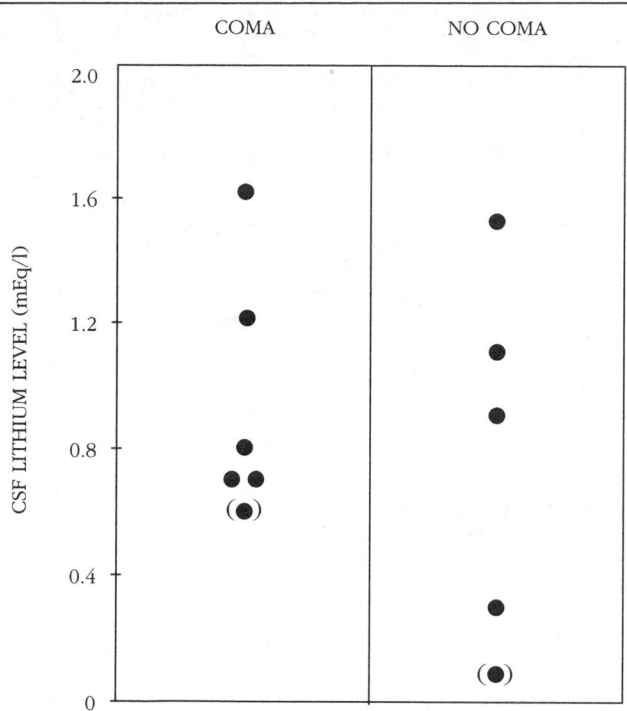

COMA   NO COMA

CSF LITHIUM LEVEL (mEq/l)

Fig. 147-2. Cerebrospinal fluid levels in patients with and without coma. (From Lee BL, Brown CR, Becker CE, et al: Lithium overdose: Factors that predict outcome in poisoned patients (abstract). *Vet Hum Toxicol* 28:505, 1986.)

Management

SUPPORTIVE CARE. In all patients with altered mental status, initial management should include assessment and stabilization of the airway, administration of oxygen, assisted ventilation if needed, insertion of an intravenous line, and administration of dextrose, naloxone, and thiamine. Diazepam, barbiturates, or phenytoin (see Chap. 186) should be administered to patients with seizures. If hyperthermia is present, immediate cooling measures should be instituted, including tepid sponging and fanning and neuromuscular paralysis if needed (see Chap. 73). Hypovolemia, if present, should be treated with IV crystalloids. Cardiac arrhythmias do not usually require treatment, but should respond to usual agents.

Asymptomatic patients with acute or acute on chronic overdose should be observed for a minimum of 6 hours after ingestion. Serial lithium levels must be obtained to confirm lack of significant absorption. Patients with mild overdoses can often be monitored and treated in the emergency department. Symptomatic patients, patients with a massive acute ingestion, and those whose levels continue to rise beyond 6 hours after ingestion should be admitted to an intensive care unit or similarly equipped observation area.

Lithium-induced nephrogenic diabetes insipidus does not respond to vasopressin but has been reported to improve with hydrochlorothiazide, amiloride, carbamazepine, and indomethacin [8].

GASTROINTESTINAL DECONTAMINATION. After acute ingestion, the gut should be decontaminated as soon as possible to prevent continued absorption of lithium. If the patient presents within 30 to 60 minutes following ingestion, emesis may be induced with syrup of ipecac. Alternately, and especially for patients who are obtunded, comatose, or convulsing, gastric lavage should be performed. Because activated charcoal does not effectively bind lithium, it should be given only if coingestion of another drug is suspected [17]. Whole bowel irrigation (see Chap. 110) may be useful for large ingestions, especially if they involve sustained-release tablets (e.g., Lithobid) [18]. If a tablet mass or concretion is suspected (e.g., because of sustained high levels after 2–3 days), radiographic contrast studies, ultrasound, or gastroduodenal endoscopy and endoscopic removal should be considered [5]. Preliminary evidence in animals and human volunteers suggests that sodium polystyrene sulfonate (Kayexalate) binds lithium and may enhance its elimination [19,20].

ENHANCEMENT OF LITHIUM ELIMINATION. In most patients with mild or moderate intoxication, intravenous fluid therapy is effective in restoring and maintaining renal elimination of lithium. A crystalloid solution (one-half normal or normal saline), 100 to 150 ml per hour, should be given after an initial bolus (10–20 ml/kg), depending on the degree of dehydration. Serum electrolytes should be followed closely, since hypernatremia may occur. To estimate the effectiveness of renal elimination, the lithium clearance can be estimated by obtaining simultaneous urine and serum lithium levels [21].

$$\text{Renal lithium clearance} = \frac{\text{Urine lithium}}{\text{Serum lithium}} \times \text{Urine flow rate (ml/min)}$$

If the clearance is below normal (15–30 ml/minute) in a patient without underlying cardiac or renal dysfunction, the rate of fluid administration should be increased, since this finding suggests low perfusion secondary to dehydration. The lithium clearance may be enhanced by administration of furosemide [7], although the effectiveness and safety of this treatment are unproved. There is no convincing evidence that excessive hydration (i.e., forced diuresis) increases lithium elimination.

Hemodialysis is the most efficient method for removing lithium; clearance rates of 100 to 150 ml per minute have been achieved [2,15,21]. Unfortunately, lithium is only slowly removed from intracellular tissue compartments, especially the brain, and rebound increases of serum lithium levels often occur within several hours following dialysis. Hemodialysis should be repeated frequently until the serum level drawn 6 to 8 hours after the last dialysis is 1 mEq per liter or less [2]. Despite repeated dialyses, however, patients with significant neurologic toxicity do not promptly improve, and recovery may take several days to weeks [2,14,15].

The indications for hemodialysis are not well established. It is generally agreed that patients with severe clinical toxicity and those with renal failure should undergo dialysis. Asymptomatic patients or those with mild to moderate intoxication who are otherwise healthy may be managed with intravenous fluids as long as they remain clinically stable or are improving and satisfactory lithium clearance (>15–20 ml/min) is achieved. Patients with chronic serum levels exceeding 3.5 to 4 mEq per liter and those with acute poisoning and peak levels exceeding 9 to 10 mEq/L (where significant toxicity is expected to occur with subsequent tissue distribution) should also be considered for hemodialysis.

Continuous arteriovenous hemodiafiltration (CAVH) has been reported to achieve a clearance of 20.5 ml/per minute. In one case, 14 hours of CAVH was estimated to achieve lithium elimination equivalent of 5.75 hours of hemodialysis [22]. This technique may be useful in cases where prolonged or repeated dialysis is required.

References

1. Baldessarini RJ: Drugs used in the treatment of psychiatric disorders, in Gilman AG, Goodman LS, Rall TW, et al (eds): *The Pharmacological Basis of Therapeutics*. 7th ed. New York, Macmillan, 1985, p 387.
2. Amdisen A: Clinical features and management of lithium poisoning. *Med Toxicol* 3:18, 1988.
3. McEvoy GK, McQuarrie GM (eds): *Drug Information 86*. Bethesda, MD, American Hospital Formulary Service, American Society of Hospital Pharmacists, 1986, p 1099.
4. Friedberg RC, Spyker DA, Herold DA: Massive overdoses with sustained-release lithium carbonate preparations: Pharmacokinetic model based on two case studies. *Clin Chem* 37:1205, 1991.
5. Thornley-Brown D, Galla JH, Williams PD, et al: Lithium toxicity associated with a trichobezoar. *Ann Intern Med* 116:739, 1992.
6. Dyson EH, Simpson D, Prescott LF, et al: Self-poisoning and therapeutic intoxication with lithium. *Hum Toxicol* 6:326, 1987.
7. Apte SN, Langston JW: Permanent neurological deficits due to lithium toxicity. *Ann Neurol* 13:453, 1983.
8. Simard M, Gumbiner B, Lee A, et al: Lithium carbonate intoxication: A case report and review of the literature. *Arch Intern Med* 149:36, 1989.
9. Mitchell JE, MacKenzie TB: Cardiac effects of lithium therapy in man: A review of the literature. *J Clin Psychiatry* 43:47, 1982.
10. Weinstein MR, Goldfield MD: Cardiovascular malformations with lithium use during pregnancy. *Am J Psychiatry* 132:529, 1975.
11. Lee BL, Brown CR, Becker CE, et al: Lithium overdose: Factors that predict outcome in poisoned patients. *Vet Hum Toxicol* 28:505, 1986.
12. Genser AS, Smith P, Honcharuk L, et al: Lithium overdose: When to dialyze? A report of 28 consecutive cases. *Vet Hum Toxicol* 30:355, 1988.
13. Rose SR, Klein-Schwartz W, Oderda GM, et al: Lithium intoxication with acute renal failure and death. *Drug Intell Clin Pharm* 22:691, 1988.
14. Clendenin NJ, Pond SM, Kaysen G, et al: Potential pitfalls in the evaluation of the usefulness of hemodialysis for the removal of lithium. *Clin Toxicol* 19:341, 1982.
15. Jaeger A, Sauder P, Kopferschmitt J, Jaegle ML: Toxicokinetics of lithium intoxication treated by hemodialysis. *Clin Toxicol* 23:501, 1985-1986.
16. Savitt DL, Hawkins HH, Roberts JR: The radiopacity of ingested medications. *Ann Emerg Med* 16:331, 1987.
17. Favin FD, Klein-Schwartz W, Oderda GM, Rose SR: In vitro study of lithium carbonate adsorption by activated charcoal. *J Toxicol Clin Toxicol* 26:443, 1988.
18. Smith SW, Ling LJ, Halstenson: Whole-bowel irrigation as a treatment for acute lithium overdose. *Ann Emerg Med* 20:536, 1991.
19. Tomaszewski C, Musso C, Pearson JR, Kulig K: Prevention of lithium absorption by sodium polystyrene sulfonate in volunteers (abstract). *Vet Hum Toxicol* 32:351, 1990.
20. Linakis JG, Eisenberg MS, Lacouture PG, et al: Multiple dose sodium polystyrene sulfonate in lithium intoxication: An animal model. *Pharmacol Toxicol* 70:38, 1992.
21. Jacobsen D, Aasen G, Frederichsen P, Eisenga B: Lithium intoxication: Pharmacokinetics during and after terminated hemodialysis in acute intoxications. *Clin Toxicol* 25:81, 1987.
22. Bellomo R, Kearly Y, Parkin G, et al: Treatment of life-threatening lithium toxicity with continuous arterio-venous hemodiafiltration. *Crit Care Med* 19:836, 1991.

148. Methylxanthines

Michael W. Shannon

Introduction

Theophylline (1,3-dimethylxanthine) is in wide therapeutic use as a bronchodilator for the management of reversible obstructive pulmonary diseases. It is also commonly used in the treatment of apnea of prematurity in neonates [1,2]. However, its potent pharmacologic actions, variable metabolic disposition in humans, and narrow therapeutic-toxic index combine to make theophylline a common cause of intoxication, especially in high-risk populations.

Three clinical circumstances account for most cases of theophylline poisoning: (1) unintentional ingestions by children, (2) suicide attempts by adolescents or adults, and (3) iatrogenic mismedication (miscalculation of dose, change in frequency of administration, lack of serum drug level monitoring, overdosing of a patient in whom chronic illness or an unrecognized drug-drug interaction leads to reduced clearance of theophylline) [3]. More than two-thirds of theophylline intoxications are unintentional [4].

Symptoms and signs of theophylline poisoning, referrable mainly to the gastric, cardiac, and neurologic systems, are frequently so severe as to require advanced medical management only available in the intensive care unit (ICU) setting.

Caffeine and theobromine are other naturally occurring methylxanthines in widespread use. As much as 180 mg of caffeine may be present in a single 5-ounce cup of coffee; soft drinks may contain 30 to 60 mg of caffeine per 12-ounce serving. Several over-the-counter diet aids or medications purporting to increase alertness may contain up to 200 mg of caffeine per tablet [5]. While severe toxicity from caffeine ingestion is rarely seen, case reports of serious poisoning in both children and adults are documented [6–11]. Clinical symptoms resemble those seen in theophylline intoxication, with cardiac, central nervous system (CNS), and gastrointestinal (GI) disturbances predominating. Because the profile of clinical toxicity resembles that of theophylline poisoning, the approach to management of caffeine intoxication is identical to that of theophylline.

Pentoxifylline is a methylxanthine vasodilator occasionally prescribed for intermittent claudication [12]. Epidemiologically, it is rarely involved in intoxications. As it is structurally similar to theophylline, the same manifestations of toxicity, including hypotension, cardiac disturbances, and metabolic derangements, appear after overdoses of pentoxifylline [13].

Pharmacokinetics

Theophylline, a bitter white powder, is available commercially in a variety of single and combination drug preparations (see Chap. 211). It is formulated as a liquid, in tablets, as sprinkles, in sustained-release preparations, in parenteral forms, and as suppositories. Significant variation in GI absorption has been documented [14,15]. However, oral preparations typically have greater than 95 percent bioavailability, with peak serum concentrations occurring in 1 to 2 hours (oral liquid), 2 to 4 hours (tablets), or 7 to 8 hours or longer (sustained-release). Stomach bezoars composed of slow-release theophylline capsules have been reported, associated with delays as long as 24 hours before absorption is complete [16]. Both antacids and food in the stomach are known to delay the absorption and metabolism of theophylline [17,18].

Theophylline has a volume of distribution (V_d) of 0.48 liter per kilogram and a pKa of 9.5 and is 58 to 70 percent bound to plasma proteins [19]. Its metabolism is exclusively hepatic, where it is oxidized or demethylated by multiple isoenzymes of the cytochrome P-450 system to form three inactive metabolites (1,3-dimethyluric acid, 1-methyluric acid, and 3-methylxanthine) [20]. Less than 15 percent of the drug is excreted unchanged in urine. At therapeutic doses, hepatic metabolism generally proceeds by first-order kinetics [21]. At therapeutic doses, the elimination half-life of theophylline varies widely with age: 30 hours in premature infants, 15 hours in newborns, 6 to 7 hours in infants 1 to 6 months old, 3.5 to 4 hours in children 6 months to 18 years old, and 4.5 to 5 hours in adults [22–26]. Corresponding clearance rates are also age-related, with rates of 0.3 ml/kg/min in premature neonates, 1 to 2 ml/kg/min in those 9 to 18 years old, and 0.7 ml/kg/min in adults [27]. The drug exhibits saturable kinetics, particularly in overdose, with the appearance of prolonged elimination half-lives, indicating Michaelis-Menten (saturable) kinetics.

Several mathematical models are used to predict steady-state serum theophylline concentrations [27,28]; however, because of wide individual variation, drug monitoring is necessary for all patients who receive theophylline chronically. The therapeutic serum concentration of theophylline is considered to be 10 to 20 μg per milliliter.

Although it was previously believed that the serum theophylline concentration could accurately predict symptoms of clinical toxicity, recent clinical research and experience largely discount this. Symptoms of severe intoxication may occur with steady-state levels of theophylline as low as 20 to 30 μg per milliliter (seizures have occurred in patients with levels as low as 17 μg/ml) [29,30]. Patients with chronic theophylline overmedication (particularly the elderly) are more likely to suffer severe toxicity at lower serum levels than patients with an acute single overdose [31]. Many drugs, chemicals, and medical conditions affect the steady-state serum concentration and elimination half-life of theophylline (Table 148-1) [32–45].

Pathophysiology

Theophylline intoxication is associated with a multitude of metabolic and clinical consequences. Although these complications have been well characterized clinically, their pathophysiology remains incompletely understood [46]. Three mechanisms of theophylline action, in both therapeutic and overdose contexts, have been theorized to produce toxic manifestations: disturbances in cyclic adenosine monophosphate (cyclic AMP) or cyclic guanosine monophosphate (cyclic GMP) activity, adenosine antagonism, and beta-adrenergic stimulation secondary to elevated levels of circulating plasma catecholamines [47,48].

Until recently all physiologic changes seen with therapeutic doses of theophylline (tachycardia, diuresis, bronchodilation, CNS stimulation) were thought to result from theophylline's inhibition of phosphodiesterase, the enzyme that breaks down

Table 148-1. Medical Conditions, Drugs, and Other Factors Affecting Serum Theophylline Concentrations

Action	Reference
Drugs lowering serum theophylline concentration	
Carbamazepine	31
Phenobarbital	32
Drugs raising serum theophylline concentration	
Norfloxacin	33
Oral contraceptives	34
Ciprofloxacin	35
Erythromycin	36
H_2-antagonists	37
Calcium channel blockers	38
Phenytoin	39
Propranolol	40
Conditions lowering serum theophylline concentration	
Cigarette smoking	41,42
Cystic fibrosis	43
Hyperthyroidism	43
Conditions raising serum theophylline concentration	
Hepatitis or cirrhosis	43
Congestive heart failure	43
Some viral infections	44

cyclic AMP to its inactive metabolite. This enzyme inhibition results in elevated intracellular cyclic AMP concentrations. As a "second messenger," cyclic AMP then effects many physiologic responses. The activity of a second intracellular nucleotide, cyclic GMP, is also increased by theophylline, although the physiologic consequence of this action has been less well characterized (Fig. 148-1) [49].

The role of cyclic AMP in the physiologic actions of theophylline has been questioned recently. In vitro data indicate that phosphodiesterase inhibition does not occur at therapeutic serum concentrations of theophylline, suggesting that increased cyclic AMP activity is not a major mechanism of its action. Whether the increased theophylline concentrations seen in the intoxicated patient are sufficient to inhibit phosphodiesterase activity has not been fully explored.

Investigation has also been directed at the role of adenosine receptor antagonism as a mechanism of theophylline action. Adenosine is a nucleoside that, among its actions, promotes smooth muscle constriction, slows cardiac conduction, and acts as an endogenous anticonvulsant [50]. Theophylline's structure is similar to that of adenine, and theophylline may compete with adenosine receptors at bronchial and vascular smooth muscle, cardiac, and CNS sites. However, adenosine antagonism alone does not provide a complete explanation for theophylline's pharmacologic effects [47,48].

Compelling data suggest that theophylline's action can be entirely accounted for by its stimulation of plasma catecholamines [51]. Recent data suggest that increased plasma catecholamine activity is universal after the administration of theophylline [52]. Circulating epinephrine, norepinephrine, and dopamine concentrations all rise after administration of theophylline. With therapeutic doses, plasma catecholamine activity typically increases four- to sixfold. After theophylline intoxication, plasma catecholamine activity may rise up to 30-fold [53,54]. Increased plasma catecholamines provide a ready explanation for many of theophylline's effects seen after therapeutic doses (increased pulse, widened pulse pressure, bronchodilation) and potentially mediate all the effects of theophylline intoxication.

Many metabolic derangements accompany theophylline in-

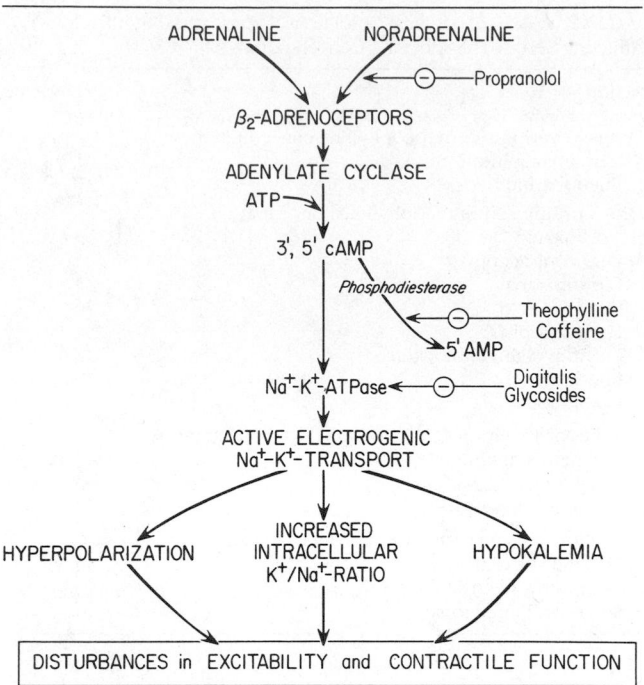

Fig. 148-1. Actions of theophylline and beta-adrenergic stimulation on cyclic AMP activity.

toxication including hyperglycemia, hypokalemia, hypercalcemia, hypophosphatemia, and metabolic acidosis [55]. Several of these metabolic consequences, particularly hypokalemia, hypercalcemia, and hypophosphatemia, have some correlation with increased cyclic AMP activity. In this regard, the hypokalemia of theophylline poisoning has been best studied.

Plasma catecholamines, particularly epinephrine, are capable of inducing hypokalemia, hyperglycemia, and metabolic acidosis. The latter results from increased oxygen consumption [53]. Epinephrine-induced hypokalemia appears to result from beta$_2$-adrenergic stimulation of Na$^+$/K$^+$ ATPase. Found in high concentrations in all excitable tissues including neurons, cardiac conduction tissue, and skeletal muscle, Na$^+$/K$^+$ ATPase leads to increased intracellular transport of potassium with preservation of total body potassium content (Fig. 148-1) [56,57,58]. Consistent with the theories of plasma catecholamine activity as the mediator of metabolic consequences is the observation that theophylline-induced hypokalemia can be inhibited by pretreatment with propranolol or reversed by propranolol once present [59,60,61].

The CNS effects of theophylline include respiratory stimulation, vomiting, and seizures. These may result from disturbances in CNS cyclic GMP activity, adenosine antagonism, or adrenergic neurotransmission. Changes in transmembrane potentials by any of these mechanisms would lower neuronal excitation thresholds. Theophylline administration has been associated with an abnormal electroencephalogram (EEG) pattern in 34 percent of children and 12 percent of adults [62,63].

Manifestations of Toxicity

Manifestations of theophylline intoxication are best placed into five categories: cardiac, CNS, GI, musculoskeletal, and metabolic. In severe cases, disturbances in all of these become clinically important and may be associated with life-threatening events [64,65].

The cardiovascular effects of theophylline intoxication consist of primary rhythm abnormalities as well as vascular disturbances. The hallmark of theophylline poisoning is tachycardia. Although theophylline-induced tachycardia usually has a sinus origin and is hemodynamically insignificant, supraventricular tachycardias often occur. Ventricular irritability may lead to the appearance of premature ventricular contractions, ventricular tachycardia, or ventricular fibrillation.

Blood pressure disturbances are also common. At lower ranges of intoxication, a mildly elevated blood pressure may be present, although severe hypertension is unusual in isolated theophylline poisoning. In severe cases, hypotension with a widened pulse pressure is seen in the face of an increased cardiac index [59,66,67]. Hypotension is associated with dramatic falls in systemic vascular resistance, typically without significant changes in central venous pressure or mean pulmonary artery wedge pressure [68]. Blood pressure depression is attributed to elevated plasma epinephrine concentrations.

The CNS effects of theophylline poisoning become prominent in severe overdose. Theophylline's stimulatory actions at the medullary respiratory center are responsible for the respiratory alkalosis that often accompanies intoxication. Patients commonly have extreme agitation and anxiety. Vomiting results, in part from stimulation of the vomiting center of the medullary chemoreceptor trigger zone.

The most severe CNS manifestation of theophylline intoxication is seizures. Theophylline-induced seizures are tonic-clonic in nature and may be focal; they may be single but are most commonly multiple and typically recalcitrant to conventional anticonvulsants. Seizures after theophylline intoxication are associated with a high frequency of adverse neurologic outcomes and a mortality that approaches 50 percent in elderly patients; they are a poor prognostic sign [62,69,70,71].

The GI effects of theophylline poisoning consist of vomiting, diarrhea, and hematemesis. Vomiting results not only from theophylline's stimulation of the CNS vomiting center but also from hypersecretion of gastric acid and the enzymes gastrin and pepsin [47]. These acids and digestive enzymes are mucosal irritants that can produce mucosal hemorrhage (occasionally manifested as hematemesis). Finally, theophylline is a potent relaxer of the lower esophageal sphincter; this action facilitates reflux of gastric contents.

Skeletal muscle tremor is a common feature of theophylline poisoning. These tremors are coarse and may include myoclonic jerks. Because they typically occur in association with hypokalemia, tremors are thought to result from disturbances in normal skeletal muscle depolarization secondary to increased intracellular concentrations of potassium (Fig. 148-1).

A number of metabolic disturbances accompany theophylline intoxication. These include metabolic acidosis, hypokalemia, hyperglycemia, hypophosphatemia, hypomagnesemia, and hypercalcemia [59,72–75]. Metabolic acidosis, which is predominantly a lactic acidosis, may appear late, but acidemia often does not occur because respiratory stimulation induces a respiratory alkalosis. Despite the normal pH, acidosis serves to exacerbate myocardial irritability. Hypokalemia and hyperglycemia correlate strongly with the degree of *acute* theophylline intoxication; their association has been used to predict serum theophylline concentration after theophylline poisoning [76]. The clinical consequences of hypokalemia are unclear. Although it has been speculated to increase the risk of cardiac disturbances, hypokalemia may be in some way protective, since patients with the greatest degree of hypokalemia have the highest serum theophylline concentration, often in the absence of severe toxic manifestations. Hypercalcemia and hypophosphatemia are common but not invariable disturbances. Their etiology is unclear, although theophylline (and epinephrine) have been shown to increase concentrations of parathyroid hormone and correction of theophylline-induced hypercalcemia has been reported after administration of propranolol [55].

Clinical manifestations of caffeine and pentoxifylline overdose are identical to those of theophylline, although both are associated with a significantly lower degree of toxicity than theophylline when taken in comparable doses. Toxic effects of caffeine have been correlated with doses of 80 to 100 mg per kilogram in children and 500 to 1000 mg in adults [6–11,77]; serum caffeine concentrations greater than 20 μg per milliliter are associated with irritability and tachycardia. Serum levels greater than 150 μg per milliliter may be fatal [16]. Caffeine intoxication has been associated with the development of rhabdomyolysis [77,78].

MODULATORS OF TOXIC MANIFESTATIONS

Method of Intoxication. Several recent studies have suggested that the metabolic and clinical consequences of theophylline intoxication vary depending on whether the poisoning occurs through a single ingestion (or single toxic intravenous dose), chronic overmedication (e.g., in the individual who is taking theophylline too frequently or has underlying abnormalities in theophylline clearance, such as hepatic disease), or acute on therapeutic ingestion (i.e., has maintained serum theophylline concentrations in the therapeutic range but then ingests a single toxic dose) [31]. The mechanism of these disparities may be related to increases in theophylline's volume of distribution after chronic intoxication such that the correlation between serum concentration and clinical effect becomes tenuous.

Acute Intoxication. The patient who ingests a single toxic dose of theophylline or who accidentally receives a toxic dose intravenously develops predictable clinical manifestations. With theophylline concentrations of 20 to 40 μg per milliliter, toxicity is generally confined to nausea, vomiting, and tachycardia. When theophylline concentrations approach 40 to 70 μg per milliliter, evidence of cardiac and neuromuscular irritability includes premature ventricular contractions, agitation, and tremor. At theophylline concentrations greater than 70 μg per milliliter, life-threatening events, including severe cardiac arrhythmias and intractable seizures, may appear [79,80].

Metabolic disturbances after acute theophylline intoxication also vary by method of intoxication. Hypokalemia can be profound after acute intoxication, with serum potassium concentrations falling to as low as 2.1 mEq per liter.

Chronic Intoxication. The features of chronic theophylline intoxication differ significantly from those of an acute overdose. Epidemiologically, victims of chronic theophylline intoxication are more likely to be elderly with underlying cardiac or hepatic disease. Such patients are also likely to be taking a number of different medications (which may, in fact, lead to theophylline toxicity, since several drugs inhibit theophylline clearance). These factors contribute to the greater morbidity and mortality observed after chronic theophylline intoxication [29,31].

The two most striking features of chronic theophylline intoxication are that: (1) there is *no correlation* between serum theophylline concentration and the appearance of life-threatening events after chronic theophylline intoxication; and (2) with chronic theophylline intoxication, seizures and arrhythmias may appear with serum theophylline concentrations in the therapeutic or mildly toxic range [81–84]. Therefore, serum theophylline concentration cannot be used to predict the appearance of these events, making decisions about the level of necessary intervention difficult.

Metabolic derangements are less striking after chronic theophylline intoxication. The incidence of both hypokalemia and hyperglycemia is low. Metabolic alkalosis is typically more common than metabolic acidosis after chronic theophylline poisoning.

Acute on Therapeutic Intoxication. In patients with acute on therapeutic theophylline intoxication, clinical and metabolic consequences are intermediate between those found with acute and chronic overdose. Clinical manifestations are somewhat predictable on the basis of peak serum theophylline concentration, with life-threatening events usually not appearing until serum theophylline concentrations exceed 60 μg per milliliter. Metabolic disturbances are not as severe as after acute theophylline intoxication and have little or no correlation with serum theophylline concentration.

Age. Patient age appears to be a significant risk factor in the development of life-threatening events after theophylline intoxication. The influence of age has been best characterized in patients with chronic theophylline poisoning, in which the extremes of age are more commonly associated with the development of seizures, severe cardiac arrhythmias, and death [69]. For example, after chronic overmedication patients older than 50 years have a greater than 10-fold risk of a life-threatening event than an adolescent with a comparable serum theophylline concentration [85]. Premature infants also may have a greater risk of severe toxicity [86,87]. Thus, in patients with chronic theophylline intoxication, age may be a better predictor of a life-threatening event than serum theophylline concentration.

Type of Theophylline Preparation. In patients with acute theophylline intoxication, toxic manifestations appear quickly after intravenous dosing errors. However, a delayed and unpredictable course is the rule after theophylline ingestion. This is the result of recent pharmaceutical changes that have made virtually all oral theophylline preparations sustained release in absorption. With ingestions of sustained-release preparations, serum theophylline concentrations may rise rapidly with the early onset of life-threatening events or may be delayed for 17 to 24 hours, resulting in severe toxic manifestations after an extended period of minor signs and symptoms.

Laboratory Assessment

In the emergency department or immediately on arrival in the ICU, the following laboratory assessment is necessary: serum theophylline concentration, serum electrolytes, arterial blood gas, anion gap, blood urea nitrogen, creatinine, calcium, magnesium, phosphorus, glucose, liver function panel, creatine phosphokinase (CPK), and complete blood count. Urine should be evaluated for the presence of myoglobin. An electrocardiogram (ECG) should be obtained on hospital arrival and the patient placed on continuous ECG monitoring.

Because ingestions of sustained-release preparations lead to delayed peaks in theophylline absorption, theophylline concentrations should be obtained every 1 to 2 hours until a plateau and subsequent decline have been documented. Serum electrolytes and creatine phosphokinase (CPK) should be monitored serially until all values have returned to normal. Urine should be evaluated frequently for evidence of myoglobinuria, particularly in patients who develop seizures.

Management

The management of theophylline intoxication involves four basic principles: gastric emptying, decreasing absorption, enhancing elimination, and supportive care (Table 148-2). With intoxications after acute ingestion, gastric emptying and decreasing absorption are the primary steps, followed by enhancement of elimination and supportive care. Treatment of chronic intoxication or intoxication after intravenous administration of theophylline bypasses intestinal decontamination and is aimed at the latter two stages of management.

GASTRIC EMPTYING. For acute or acute on therapeutic ingestions, the gastric contents should be evacuated. Ideally this is done on the patient's arrival in the emergency department. Should gastric evacuation be delayed or overlooked, it should be performed in the ICU. Gastric lavage with syrup of ipecac for gastric emptying remains controversial. For methylxanthine poisoning, lavage offers two advantages. First, because seizures may develop without warning, airway protection may be compromised by administration of an emetic whose time of onset may be delayed. Second, the vomiting induced by ipecac may last several hours, delaying successful administration of activated charcoal, the cornerstone in the treatment of theophylline intoxication [88]. Although the large size and nondissolvable matrix of sustained-release tablets may make lavage difficult, it remains the preferred method of gastric emptying.

What degree of delay makes gastric emptying nonproductive is not clear. Sustained-release tablets may coalesce, leading to prolonged and erratic absorption: peak serum theophylline concentrations are often not achieved for up to 17 hours after overdose. For this reason, gastric emptying should be undertaken as late as 8 to 10 hours following ingestion [89].

DECREASING ABSORPTION. Oral activated charcoal, with surface areas of up to 1500 m² per gram, is highly effective at decreasing absorption of theophylline [90,91]. The dose of activated charcoal is 50 to 60 gm in adults and 1 gm per kilogram in children. Ideally, based on in vitro data, a 10:1 ratio of charcoal to drug is preferred [92] but not always practical, because of patient weight, tolerance, or age or because of the amount of toxin ingested.

The concomitant use of a cathartic is recommended, though its efficacy at decreasing absorption or even enhancing elimination is controversial [93]. Magnesium citrate at a dose of 4 ml per kilogram in children (10–12 ounces in adults) or 70% sorbitol solution, 2 ml per kilogram in children and 75 to 150 ml in adults, is available. Whole bowel irrigation with polyethylene glycol electrolyte lavage (PEG-ELS, Golytely) may be effective at decreasing absorption by its efficient cleansing of entire bowel contents. Tenenbein [94] described the use of PEG-ELS in six children with iron intoxication and documented radiographic clearance of particulate from the stomach. The dose is 2 liters per hour by continuous nasogastric infusion (or 240 ml orally every 10 minutes) in adults and 0.5 liter per hour in children. Administration continues until the rectal effluent has the same appearance as the infusate.

ENHANCING ELIMINATION. Serial administration of activated charcoal is an important therapeutic measure for enhancing elimination of theophylline [66,95–98]. Both animal [95] and human studies [96,97] have demonstrated that repetitive doses of charcoal increase theophylline clearance more than twofold. Serial charcoal is as effective as hemodialysis, if not more so [97]. The mechanism of elimination enhancement by serial charcoal is referred to as GI dialysis. This principle is based on the apparent ability of the intestinal mucosa to act as a dialysis membrane when charcoal is in the gut lumen. Because of theophylline's low volume of distribution and relatively low protein binding, charcoal transit through the intestinal lumen appears to create a concentration gradient that favors theophylline diffusion out of the splanchnic circulation and into the lumen, where it is adsorbed to the activated charcoal and expelled in the feces.

Serial doses of oral activated charcoal are administered every 2 to 4 hours and continued until the theophylline level is less than 10 to 15 µg per milliliter. An alternative to boluses of charcoal is administration via continuous nasogastric infusion at a rate of 0.25 to 0.5 gm/kg/hour [99]. Another effective alternative is to give activated charcoal doses of 20 gm every 2 hours. Unfortunately, nausea with protracted emesis, present in up to 80 percent of patients with theophylline intoxication [64], may delay or preclude successful repetitive charcoal administration. Aggressive antiemetic therapy is therefore usually necessary and is directed at both the CNS and local origins of vomiting.

EXTRACORPOREAL DRUG REMOVAL. In severely intoxicated patients, rapid removal of theophylline is indicated. This is best accomplished by hemodialysis or hemoperfusion. When the need for extracorporeal drug removal is even entertained, a nephrologist should be involved early in the case. Because of the time and personnel required to initiate extracorporeal drug removal, early notification of personnel can expedite the process once the decision has been made. The decision to use extracorporeal drug removal should weigh the risks of hemoperfusion or hemodialysis against the significant morbidity and mortality associated with theophylline toxicity.

Charcoal Hemoperfusion. Charcoal hemoperfusion is the extracorporeal removal method of choice. It reduces the elimination half-life of theophylline to as low as 0.7 to 2.1 hours [100] and clearance is increased four- to sixfold [101]. Significant clinical improvement is typically observed after 4 hours of hemoperfusion [101]. Several cases have described serial charcoal administration or hemodialysis (to correct metabolic derangements) concurrent with hemoperfusion. An increase in plasma theophylline concentration may occur following termination of hemoperfusion, due to theophylline redistribution or continued absorption from slow-release products [100].

Hemoperfusion is invasive and has significant risks; medical centers with expertise in this process are few. The decision to institute hemoperfusion is therefore difficult, as it cannot always

Table 148-2. Principles of Theophylline Toxicity Management

1. Gastric emptying*
2. Decreasing absorption*
3. Enhancement of elimination
4. Supportive care

* Following acute ingestions.

be based on the serum theophylline concentration alone. Hemoperfusion is warranted for patients with protracted seizures or cardiovascular embarrassment unresponsive to medical therapy; however, outcome is consistently better in patients who undergo hemoperfusion before these life-threatening complications appear. Gaudreault and Guay [27] proposed several guidelines for charcoal hemoperfusion (Table 148-3): (1) persistently unstable hemodynamics or prolonged seizures (> 20 minutes[1] duration*) regardless of serum theophylline concentration; (2) in stable patients aged 6 months to 60 years, serum concentrations greater than 100 μg per milliliter following acute exposure; (3) serum theophylline concentrations greater than 60 μg per milliliter after chronic exposure. For patients younger than 6 months or older than 60 years and patients with a history of respiratory failure, congestive heart failure, or liver disease, hemoperfusion should be considered when theophylline concentration is greater than 40 μg per milliliter [30]. A low threshold for hemoperfusion is recommended for patients taking theophylline chronically, since serum concentrations in such a population are not predictive of onset or severity of symptoms and because these patients have the potential to develop life-threatening complications, often without warning, at low serum concentrations. Patients who have ingested a sustained-release product and have an early high level are at particular risk because of the kinetics of these preparations. Sudden and unpredictably large increases in levels are not unusual.

If hemoperfusion is performed, treatment should continue until serum concentrations are less than 15 μg per milliliter or clinical signs of theophylline intoxication have abated; serum concentrations should subsequently be monitored for at least 12 hours to allow for rebound from changes in theophylline redistribution [100].

Hemodialysis. When extracorporeal removal of theophylline is necessary and hemoperfusion is unavailable in the hospital or the patient's hemodynamic status precludes safe transport to a facility where hemoperfusion can be performed, hemodialysis is an effective therapy. Hemodialysis can double theophylline clearance, compared with endogenous clearance rates [87]. Hemodialysis, unlike hemoperfusion, also permits simultaneous correction of metabolic abnormalities.

There are several reports of combined modalities, such as hemodialysis and oral administration of activated charcoal or both hemoperfusion and hemodialysis, with evidence of increased clearance [102]. If the patient undergoes hemodialysis instead of hemoperfusion, continuing oral or nasogastric activated charcoal is indicated.

Other. Peritoneal dialysis is an ineffective mode of drug removal in theophylline intoxication and is not recommended. Exchange transfusion, formerly thought to have no role in theophylline poisoning, has been used successfully in neonates with severe intoxication. Other extracorporeal drug removal techniques, such as hemofiltration and plasmapheresis, have not been sufficiently evaluated to determine whether they have a potentially important role in the treatment of theophylline intoxication. Hemofiltration, because it is a slow, passive, cardiac output-dependent technique, is unlikely to effect the rapid removal of theophylline necessary in severe intoxications. Plasmapheresis would theoretically not be beneficial because theophylline has low protein-binding and might not be removed efficiently by a process that primarily removes plasma proteins

---

*The author recommends that prolonged seizures are defined as 10 minutes or greater.

Table 148-3. Suggested Indications for Hemoperfusion

1. Cardiovascular instability, despite medical therapy *or*
2. Prolonged seizures (10–20 min) *or*
3. Acute exposure
   a. >6 mo, <60 yr, plasma level >100 μg/ml
   b. <6 mo, >60 yr, plasma level >40 μg/ml
   or
4. Chronic exposure
   a. >6 mo, <60 yr, plasma level >60 μg/ml
   b. <6 mo, >60 yr, plasma level >40 μg/ml
   c. Patients with respiratory failure, congestive heart failure, or liver disease

and because plasmapheresis involves at least the same degree of technical difficulty and potential complications as hemodialysis, a clearly effective procedure. It therefore offers no advantages.

SUPPORTIVE CARE

Airway and Breathing. Airway protection is paramount, and the threshold for tracheal intubation in the patient with depressed mentation or an absent gag reflex should be low. Ventilation may be necessary if there is coingestion of a CNS depressant or if medications that depress respiratory drive, such as droperidol for vomiting or diazepam for seizures, are used in management.

Rhythm Disturbances. The most common arrhythmias are sinus tachycardia, supraventricular tachyarrhythmias, and ventricular irritability. The etiology of these rhythm abnormalities may be beta-adrenoceptor stimulation from catecholamine excess [11] in addition to the possible effect of theophylline on intracellular cyclic AMP in the cardiac tissue [54]. Though no controlled clinical studies are available, there has been much success in treating rhythm disturbances with beta-adrenergic antagonists, such as propranolol [30,59]. Propranolol counters tachycardia, restores coronary blood flow, and interrupts the reentry phenomena that often underlie theophylline-induced arrhythmias [54]. The dose of propranolol for adults is 1 to 3 mg given intravenously with repeated doses of 1 mg every 5 to 10 minutes until arrhythmias are corrected. In children the dose is 0.02 mg per kilogram with repeated doses as necessary every 5 to 10 minutes. The potential hazard in the use of propranolol is the risk of drug-induced bronchospasm; it therefore should be used cautiously, if at all, in patients receiving theophylline chronically for reversible airways disease. Esmolol, an ultra-short-acting beta$_1$ selective antagonist, has also been shown to alleviate theophylline-induced tachyarrhythmias [67]. A recent case report of caffeine intoxication describes successful control of multiple arrhythmias (and hypertension) using an esmolol infusion [103]. Esmolol's advantage lies in its ultrashort half-life (9 minutes), which allows titration of the dose to the desired effect, and cardioselectivity, which reduces the risk of bronchospasm. A disadvantage of esmolol is also found in its beta$_1$ selectivity: because hypotension and the metabolic derangements of theophylline overdose appear to be the result of beta$_2$ stimulation, they may not respond to beta$_1$ blockade by esmolol.

The recently approved antiarrhythmic agent adenosine has become the treatment of choice for supraventricular tachycardias and is an important therapeutic addition in the management of theophylline-induced tachyarrhythmias. Having a significant effect on atrioventricular node conduction, adenosine acts promptly in reversing supraventricular tachycardias. Moreover, because of the evidence that adenosine and theophylline compete for the same receptor, adenosine may be a specific "antidote" for theophylline-induced supraventricular tachycardia. In adults adenosine is administered as an initial 6-mg dose, followed by a 12-mg dose if the first infusion is ineffective. Children are given 50 to 100 μg per kilogram, increased as necessary by increments of 40 μg per kilogram. Because of adenosine's rapid elimination half-life (< 10 seconds), best effects occur when it is given by rapid intravenous infusion through the vein closest to the central circulation (e.g., antecubital). Adenosine has a wide margin of safety, with no absolute contraindications to its use.

Lidocaine is the recommended treatment of ventricular irritability associated with hemodynamic compromise. The dose in adults is 1.5 mg per kilogram given by slow intravenous push (rate ≤ 50 mg/min), followed by infusion of 2 to 4 mg per minute. In children, the dose is 1 mg per kilogram, followed by infusion of 10 to 20 μg/kg/min.

Hypotension. Hypotension with a wide pulse pressure is a characteristic feature of theophylline intoxication. If hypotension does not respond to an initial intravenous fluid bolus, propranolol may have a positive effect on blood pressure stabilization [30] and may be given in the doses stated previously. If a vasopressor is also required, an agent such as dopamine, which has some vasodilating properties at low doses, may be ineffective; alpha-adrenergic agents such as phenylephrine or norepinephrine may be more efficacious. Because these agents are removed during hemoperfusion and hemodialysis, increased infusion rates may be required during such procedures.

Seizures. Seizures are a grave sign and should be treated aggressively; however, they are frequently resistant to standard anticonvulsant therapy. Diazepam alone in the usual doses is rarely effective; doses up to 20 mg or larger may be necessary for seizure termination. Phenytoin was reported in several case reports to be ineffective [55,100,104] and in animal studies may have contributed to theophylline-induced seizures [105]. In animal studies phenobarbital is the most effective anticonvulsant [105]. Large doses may be required, since clearance of phenobarbital is increased with the use of activated charcoal, hemoperfusion, or hemodialysis. Should seizures become prolonged (>10 minutes), general anesthesia with a rapid-acting barbiturate, such as thiopental or pentobarbital, may be necessary. Neuromuscular blockade should be considered for seizures recalcitrant to the previously mentioned modalities, as significant morbidity may result from the rhabdomyolysis, hyperthermia, and acidosis seen with prolonged seizures. A short-acting agent, such as vecuronium, should be used to permit reassessment of the patient's status. There is some evidence that propranolol may help prevent or control theophylline-induced seizures [106].

Gastrointestinal Distress. As discussed previously, vomiting must be controlled in order to administer charcoal. Although no controlled clinical studies have investigated optimal antiemetic therapy, several investigators have reported success using droperidol for central emetic control [107] and the H₂-antagonist ranitidine for reduction of gastric hypersecretion [107,108]. Famotidine, a newer H₂-antagonist, does not appear to alter theophylline clearance [47] and should theoretically also be effective, although this agent has not been well studied in theophylline intoxication. Cimetidine is contraindicated in theophylline poisoning because it impairs endogenous theophylline clearance. The dose of droperidol is 2.5 to 10 mg given

intramuscularly or intravenously in adults and 0.088 to 0.165 mg per kilogram in children aged 2 to 12 years. This dose can be repeated every 30 minutes as needed. The dose of ranitidine is 50 to 100 mg given intravenously for adults and 0.1 to 0.8 mg per kilogram in children. Doses can be repeated every 6 to 8 hours. Metoclopramide also is an effective antiemetic that stimulates upper GI motility and increases lower esophageal tone without affecting theophylline clearance. The initial dose of metoclopramide is 10 mg given intravenously for adults or 0.1 mg per kilogram for children. This should be increased to a maximum of 1 mg per kilogram if necessary (although the risk of dystonia increases with increasing dose). Ondansetron, a newer antiemetic, offers the advantage of effective antiemesis with no alterations in mental status. Its use should be considered with severe vomiting, although its cost should limit liberal use. The phenothiazine antiemetics perchlorperazine and promethazine theoretically lower the seizure threshold and are not indicated.

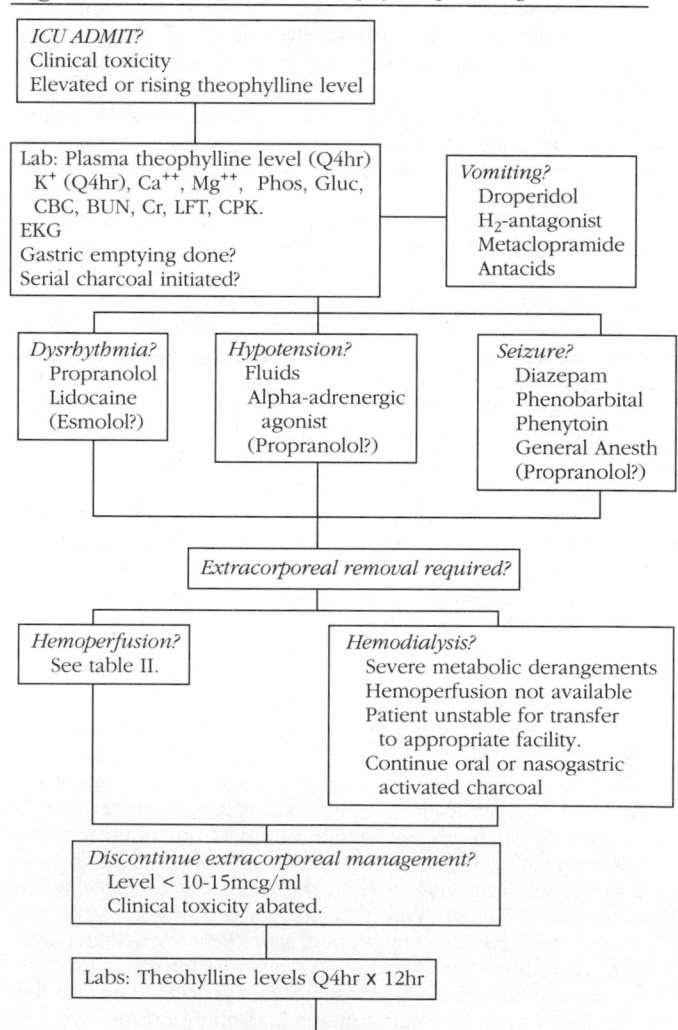

Fig. 148-2. Management of theophylline poisoning.

ICU ADMIT?
Clinical toxicity
Elevated or rising theophylline level

Lab: Plasma theophylline level (Q4hr)
K⁺ (Q4hr), Ca⁺⁺, Mg⁺⁺, Phos, Gluc,
CBC, BUN, Cr, LFT, CPK.
EKG
Gastric emptying done?
Serial charcoal initiated?

Vomiting?
Droperidol
H₂-antagonist
Metoclopramide
Antacids

Dysrhythmia?
Propranolol
Lidocaine
(Esmolol?)

Hypotension?
Fluids
Alpha-adrenergic
agonist
(Propranolol?)

Seizure?
Diazepam
Phenobarbital
Phenytoin
General Anesth
(Propranolol?)

Extracorporeal removal required?

Hemoperfusion?
See table II.

Hemodialysis?
Severe metabolic derangements
Hemoperfusion not available
Patient unstable for transfer
  to appropriate facility.
Continue oral or nasogastric
  activated charcoal

Discontinue extracorporeal management?
Level < 10-15mcg/ml
Clinical toxicity abated.

Labs: Theohylline levels Q4hr x 12hr

Transfer from ICU?
Level <10-15mcg/ml
Hemodynamically stable

Metabolic Derangements. Metabolic acidosis is most commonly seen in acute theophylline intoxication [73]. Treatment is conservative and is aimed at maintaining a normal serum pH.

Hypokalemia is also common in acute exposure. It is important to emphasize that because the hypokalemia represents predominantly cellular shifts of potassium and there are only minimal losses of total body potassium content through urine or vomitus, reversal of hypokalemia is best accomplished by lowering the theophylline concentration. Aggressive replacement of potassium may result in hyperkalemia [109]. Intravenous infusions of KCl or KPO$_4$ at 40 mEq per liter in a saline solution should be adequate; intravenous boluses are usually not indicated.

Hypophosphatemia, hypomagnesemia, hypercalcemia, and hyperglycemia rarely require correction.

Summary. Theophylline is a valuable compound with a variety of clinical applications at all ages; however, it has a narrow therapeutic index, and intoxication is commonly seen. The goal of successful management is enhanced elimination and supportive care (Fig. 148-2). The decision to use extracorporeal drug removal is difficult but should be influenced by the patient's history, age, theophylline level, and the type of preparation involved. Prolonged seizures or hemodynamic instability not responsive to medical therapy are indications for hemoperfusion regardless of history, age, or serum concentration. Morbidity and mortality are significantly lower if hemoperfusion is undertaken before the onset of life-threatening disturbances.

The patient may be transferred from the ICU once plasma levels are less than 20 μg per milliliter, provided all clinical signs of toxicity have abated and the patient has evidence of charcoal stools.

The natural history of theophylline intoxication is such that, provided seizures do not occur and management is aggressive, the patient should recover fully.

References

1. Aranda JV, Turmen T: Methylxanthines in apnea of prematurity. *Clin Perinatol* 6:87, 1979.
2. Avery ME: Respiratory failure, in Avery ME, First LR (eds): *Pediatric Medicine*. Baltimore, Williams & Wilkins, 1989, p 289.
3. Lam C, Ben-Zvi Z, Barnett S, et al: Pitfalls in the interpretation of serum theophylline levels. *Am J Dis Child* 136:345, 1982.
4. Litovitz T, Schmitz BF, Holm KC: 1988 annual report of the American Association of Poison Control Centers National Data Collection System. *Am J Emerg Med* 7:495, 1988.
5. Caffeine content evaluation, updated. *Drug Intell Clin Pharmacol* 18:94, 1985.
6. Zimmerman PM, Pulliam J, Schwengels J, et al: Caffeine intoxication: A near fatality. *Ann Emerg Med* 14:1227, 1985.
7. Garriott JC, Simmons IM, Piklis A, et al: Five cases of fatal overdose from caffeine-containing "look alike" drugs. *J Anal Toxicol* 9:141, 1985.
8. Jarboe CH, Hurst HE, Rodgers GC, et al: Toxicokinetics of caffeine elimination in an infant. *J Toxicol Clin Toxicol* 24:415, 1986.
9. Nagesh RV, Murphy KA: Caffeine poisoning treated by hemoperfusion. *Am J Kidney Dis* 12:316, 1988.
10. Dobmyer DJ, Stime RA, Leier CV, et al: The arrhythmogenic effects of caffeine in human beings. *N Engl J Med* 308:814, 1983.
11. Benowitz NL, Osterloh J, Goldschlager N, et al: Massive catecholamine release from caffeine poisoning. *JAMA* 248:1097, 1982.
12. Porter JM, Cutler BS, Lee BY, et al: Pentoxifylline efficacy in the treatment of intermittent claudication: Multicenter controlled double-blind trial with objective assessment of chronic occlusive arterial disease patients. *Am Heart J* 66:66, 1982.
13. Sznajder IJ, Bentur Y, Teitelman U: First and second-degree atrioventricular block in pentoxifylline overdose. *Br Med J* 288:26, 1984.
14. Rogers RJ, Kalisker A, Wiener MB, et al: Inconsistent absorption from a sustained-release theophylline preparation during continuous therapy in asthmatic children. *J Pediatr* 106:496, 1985.
15. Szefler SJ: Erratic absorption of theophylline from slow-release products in children. *J Allergy Clin Immunol* 78:710, 1986.
16. Cereda J, Scott J, Quigley EM: Endoscopic removal of pharmacobezoar of slow release theophylline. *Br Med J* 293:1143, 1986.
17. Myhre JF, Walstead RA: Influence of antacid on the absorption of two different sustained release formulations of theophylline. *Br J Clin Pharmacol* 15:683, 1983.
18. Pedersen S: Effects of food on the absorption of theophylline in children. *J Allergy Clin Immunol* 78:704, 1986.
19. Berdel D, Suverkrup R, Heimann G, et al: Total theophylline clearance in childhood: The influence of age-dependent changes in metabolism and elimination. *Eur J Pediatr* 146:41, 1987.
20. Van Dellen RG: Theophylline: Practical application of new knowledge. *Mayo Clin Proc* 54:733, 1979.
21. Lesko LJ: Dose-dependent elimination kinetics of theophylline. *Clin Pharmacokinet* 4:449, 1979.
22. Ishizaki T, Kubo M: Incidence of apparent Michaelis-Menten kinetic behavior of theophylline and its parameters (Vmax and Km) among asthmatic children and adults. *Ther Drug Monit* 9:11, 1987.
23. Aranda JV, Sitar DS, Parsons WD, et al: Pharmacokinetic aspects of theophylline in premature newborns. *N Engl J Med* 295:413, 1976.
24. Simons FER, Friesen FR, Simons KJ: Theophylline toxicity in term infants. *Am J Dis Child* 134:39, 1980.
25. Simons FER, Simons KJ: Pharmacokinetics of theophylline in infancy. *J Clin Pharmacol* 18:472, 1978.
26. Haley TJ: Metabolism and pharmacokinetics of theophylline in human neonates, children, and adults. *Drug Metab Rev* 14:295, 1983.
27. Gaudreault P, Guay J: Theophylline poisoning: Pharmacological considerations and clinical management. *Med Toxicol* 1:169, 1986.
28. Hoon TJ, Wood CA, Whidden MA, et al: The relative predictive performance of two theophylline pharmacokinetic dosing programs. *Pharmacotherapy* 8:82, 1988.
29. Bertino JS, Walker JW: Assessment of theophylline toxicity. *Arch Intern Med* 147:757, 1987.
30. Greenberg A, Piraino BH, Kroboth PD, et al: Severe theophylline toxicity. *Am J Med* 76:854, 1984.
31. Olson KR, Benowitz NL, Woo OF, et al: Theophylline overdose: Acute single ingestion versus chronic repeated overmedication. *Am J Emerg Med* 3:386, 1985.
32. Rosenberry KR, Defusco CJ, Mansmann HC, et al: Reduced theophylline half-life induced by carbamazepine therapy. *J Pediatr* 102:472, 1983.
33. Yazdani M, Kissling GE, Tran TH, et al: Phenobarbital increases the theophylline requirements of premature infants being treated for apnea. *Am J Dis Child* 141:97, 1987.
34. Ho G, Tierney MG, Dales RE: Evaluation of the effect of norfloxacin on the pharmacokinetics of theophylline. *Clin Pharmacol Ther* 44:35, 1988.
35. Roberts RK, Grice J, McGuffie C, et al: Oral contraceptive steroids impair the elimination of theophylline. *J Lab Clin Med* 101:821, 1983.
36. Rybak MJ, Bowles SK, Chandrasekar PH, et al: Increased theophylline concentrations secondary to ciprofloxacin. *Drug Intell Clin Pharmacol* 21:879, 1987.
37. Adebayo GI, Adewimi MO, Mabadeje AFB: Time-dependent inhibition of theophylline elimination by erythromycin stearate. *Biopharm Drug Dispos* 7:479, 1986.
38. Weinberger MM, Smith G, Milavetz G, et al: Decreased theophylline clearance due to cimetidine. *N Engl J Med* 304:672, 1981.
39. Sirmans SM, Peipers JA, Lalonde RL, et al: Effect of calcium channel blockers on theophylline disposition. *Clin Pharmacol Ther* 44:29, 1988.
40. Marquis J, Carruthers SG, Spence JD, et al: Phenytoin-theophylline interaction. *N Engl J Med* 307:1189, 1982.

41. Conrad KA, Nyman DW: Effects of metoprolol and propranolol on theophylline metabolism. *Clin Pharmacol Ther* 26:660, 1979.
42. Grygiel JJ, Birkett DJ: Cigarette smoking and theophylline clearance and metabolism. *Clin Pharmacol Ther* 30:491, 1981.
43. Hunt SN, Jusko WJ, Yurchak AM: Effect of smoking on theophylline disposition. *Clin Pharmacol Ther* 19:546, 1976.
44. Jenne JW: Effect of disease states on theophylline elimination. *J Allergy Clin Immunol* 78:727, 1986.
45. Chang KC, Lauer BA, Bell TD, et al: Altered theophylline pharmacokinetics during acute respiratory viral illness. *Lancet* 1:1132, 1978.
46. Bukowsky M, Nakatsu K, Munt PW: Theophylline reassessed. *Ann Intern Med* 101:63, 1984.
47. Fredholm BB: On the mechanism of action of theophylline and caffeine. *Acta Med Scand* 217:149, 1985.
48. Goodman, Gilman: Drugs used in the treatment of asthma, in Rall TW (ed): *The Pharmacological Basis of Therapeutics.* 8th ed. New York, Macmillan, 1990, pp 618–630.
49. Fenger M, Eriksen PB, Andersen O, et al: Plasma concentrations of the cyclic nucleotides, adenosine 3,5,-monophosphate and guanosine 3,5,-monophosphate, in healthy adults treated with theophylline. *Pharmacology* 24:215, 1982.
50. Blake KV, Massey KL, Hendeles L, et al: Relative efficacy of phenytoin and phenobarbital for the prevention of theophylline-induced seizures in mice. *Ann Emerg Med* 17:1024, 1988.
51. Higbee MD, Kumar M, Galant SP: Stimulation of endogenous catecholamine release by theophylline: A proposed additional mechanism of action for theophylline effects. *J Allergy Clin Immunol* 70:377, 1982.
52. Vestal RE, Eiriksson CE, Musser B, et al: Effect of intravenous aminophylline on plasma levels of catecholamines and related cardiovascular and metabolic responses in man. *Circulation* 67:162, 1983.
53. Shannon MW, Lovejoy FH Jr, Woolf A: Plasma catecholamines in acute vs. chronic theophylline intoxication. *Vet Hum Toxicol* 30:363, 1988.
54. Curry SC, Vance MV, Requa R, et al: The effects of toxic concentrations of theophylline on oxygen consumption, ventricular work, acid base balance, and plasma catecholamine levels in the dog. *Ann Emerg Med* 14:554, 1985.
55. McPherson ML, Prince SR, Atamer ER, et al: Theophylline-induced hypercalcemia. *Ann Intern Med* 105:52, 1986.
56. Clausen T, Flatman JA: Beta$_2$-adrenoceptors mediate the stimulating effect of adrenaline on active electrogenic Na-K-transport in rat soleus muscles. *Br J Pharmacol* 68:749, 1980.
57. DeFronzo RA, Bia M, Birkhead G: Epinephrine and potassium homeostasis. *Kidney Int* 20:83, 1981.
58. Clausen T: Adrenergic control of Na-K homeostasis. *Acta Med Scand* 672(suppl):111, 1983.
59. Biberstein MP, Ziegler MG, Ward DM: Use of β-blockade and hemoperfusion for acute theophylline poisoning. *West J Med* 141:485, 1984.
60. Brown MJ, Brown DC, Murphy MB: Hypokalemia from beta$_2$-receptor stimulation by circulating epinephrine. *N Engl J Med* 309:1414, 1983.
61. Amin DN, Henry JA: Propranolol administration in theophylline overdose. *Lancet* 2:520, 1985.
62. Richards W, Church JA, Brent DK: Theophylline-associated seizures in children. *Ann Allergy* 54:276, 1985.
63. Spector SL, Shucard DW: Central nervous system effects of anti-asthma medication: An EEG study. *Ann Allergy* 44:48, 1980.
64. Paloucek FP, Rodvoid KA: Evaluation of theophylline overdoses and toxicities. *Ann Emerg Med* 17:135, 1988.
65. Albert S: Aminophylline toxicity. *Pediatr Clin North Am* 34:61, 1987.
66. Greenberg A, Piraino BH, Kroboth PD, et al: Severe theophylline toxicity: Role of conservative measures, antiarrhythmic agents and charcoal hemoperfusion. *Am J Med* 76:854, 1984.
67. Gaar GG, Banner W, Laddu AR: The effects of esmolol on the hemodynamics of acute theophylline toxicity. *Ann Emerg Med* 16:1334, 1987.
68. Curry SC, Vance MV, Armstead R: Cardiovascular effects of toxic concentrations of theophylline in the dog. *Ann Emerg Med* 14:547, 1985.
69. Phung ND: Theophylline toxicity in ambulatory elderly patients. *Immunol Allergy Pract* 8:17, 1986.
70. Nakada T, Kwee IL, Lerner AM, et al: Theophylline-induced seizures: Clinical and pathophysiologic aspects. *West J Med* 183:371, 1983.
71. Zwillich CW, Sutton FD, Neff TA, et al: Theophylline-induced seizures in adults: Correlation with serum concentrations. *Ann Intern Med* 82:784, 1975.
72. Shannon MW, Lovejoy FH Jr: Hypokalemia after theophylline intoxication: The effects of acute versus chronic poisoning. *Arch Intern Med* 149:2725, 1989.
73. Sawyer WT, Caravati EM, Ellison MJ, et al: Hypokalemia, hyperglycemia and acidosis after intentional theophylline overdose. *Am J Emerg Med* 3:408, 1985.
74. Hall KW, Dobson KE, Dalton JG, et al: Metabolic abnormalities associated with intentional theophylline overdose. *Ann Intern Med* 101:457, 1984.
75. Amitai Y, Lovejoy FH Jr: Hypokalemia in acute theophylline poisoning. *Am J Emerg Med* 6:214, 1988.
76. Shannon MW, Lovejoy FH Jr: Prediction of serum theophylline concentration after acute theophylline intoxication. *Vet Hum Toxicol* 31:349, 1989.
77. Dalvi RR: Acute and chronic toxicity of caffeine: A review. *Vet Hum Toxicol* 28:144, 1986.
78. Wrenn KD, Oschner I: Rhabdomyolysis induced by a caffeine overdose. *Ann Emerg Med* 18:94, 1989.
79. Baker MD: Theophylline toxicity in children. *J Pediatr* 109:538, 1986.
80. Gaudreault P, Wason S, Lovejoy FH Jr: Acute pediatric theophylline overdose: A summary of 28 cases. *J Pediatr* 102:474, 1983.
81. Shannon M, Lovejoy FH Jr, Woolf A: Clinical and metabolic consequences of theophylline poisoning: The effects of acute vs. chronic intoxication. *Pediatr Emerg Care* 4:294, 1988.
82. Shannon M, Lovejoy FH Jr: Life-threatening events after theophylline intoxication: A prospective analysis of 144 cases. *Ann Emerg Med* 18:446, 1989.
83. Aitken ML, Martin TR: Life-threatening theophylline toxicity is not predictable by serum levels. *Chest* 91:10, 1987.
84. Covelli HD, Knodel AR, Heppner BT: Predisposing factors to apparent theophylline-induced seizures. *Ann Allergy* 54:411, 1985.
85. Shannon M, Lovejoy FH Jr: Risk analysis of age as a predictor of life-threatening events after chronic theophylline intoxication. *Vet Hum Toxicol* 31:331, 1989.
86. Woody RC, Laney M: A second case of infantile intracranial hemorrhage and severe neurological sequelae following theophylline overdose. *Dev Med Child Neurol* 28:120, 1986.
87. Walther FJ, Sims ME, Siassi B, et al: Cardiac output changes secondary to theophylline therapy in preterm infants. *J Pediatr* 109:874, 1986.
88. Tandberg D, Diven BG, McCleod JW: Ipecac-induced emesis vs. gastric lavage: A controlled study in normal adults. *Am J Emerg Med* 4:205, 1985.
89. Lim DT, Singh P, Nourtsis S, et al: Absorption inhibition and enhancement of elimination of sustained-release theophylline tablets by oral activated charcoal. *Ann Emerg Med* 15:1303, 1986.
90. Ginoza GW, Strauss AA, Iskra MK, et al: Potential treatment of theophylline toxicity by high surface area activated charcoal. *J Pediatr* 111:140, 1987.
91. Dillon EC, Wilton JH, Barlow JC, et al: Large surface area activated charcoal and the inhibition of aspirin absorption. *Ann Emerg Med* 18:547, 1989.
92. Neuvonen PF, Tokola O, Vartiamen M: Comparison of activated charcoal and ipecac syrup in prevention of drug absorption. *Clin Pharmacol Ther* 31:255, 1982.
93. Neuvonen PJ, Olkkola KT: Effect of purgatives of antidotal efficacy of oral activated charcoal. *Hum Toxicol* 5:255, 1986.
94. Tenenbein M: Whole bowel irrigation in iron poisoning. *J Pediatr* 111:142, 1987.
95. Kulig KW, Bar-Or D, Runack BH: Intravenous theophylline poisoning and multiple-dose charcoal in an animal model. *Ann Emerg Med* 16:842, 1987.
96. Shannon MW, Amitai YA, Lovejoy FH Jr: Use of multiple dose activated charcoal in very young infants with theophylline poisoning. *Pediatrics* 80:368, 1987.

97. Park GD, Radomski L, Goldberg MJ, et al: Effects of size and frequency of oral doses of charcoal on theophylline clearance. *Clin Pharmacol Ther* 34:663, 1983.

98. Goldberg MJ, Park GD, Berlinger WG: Treatment of theophylline intoxication. *J Allergy Clin Immunol* 78:811, 1986.

99. Ohning BL, Reed MD, Blumer JL: Continuous nasogastric administration of activated charcoal for the treatment of theophylline intoxication. *Pediatr Pharmacol* 5:241, 1986.

100. Heath A, Knudsen K: Role of extracorporeal drug removal in acute theophylline poisoning. *Med Toxicol* 2:294, 1987.

101. Park GD, Spector R, Roberts RJ, et al: Use of hemoperfusion for treatment of theophylline intoxication. *Am J Med* 74:961, 1983.

102. Russo ME: Management of theophylline intoxication with charcoal-column hemoperfusion. *N Engl J Med* 300:24, 1979.

103. Shannon M, Wernovsky G, Morris C. Exchange transfusion in the treatment of severe theophylline poisoning. *Pediatrics* 89:145, 1992.

104. Price KR, Fligner DJ: Treatment of caffeine toxicity with esmolol. *Ann Emerg Med* 19:44, 1990.

105. Sahney S, Abarzua J, Sessums L: Hemoperfusion in theophylline neurotoxicity. *Pediatrics* 71:615, 1983.

106. Stone WE, Javid MJ: Aminophylline and imidazone as convulsants. *Arch Int Pharmacodyn Ther* 345:120, 1980.

107. Schneider SM, Borok Z, Michelson EA: Beta-blockade for acute theophylline-induced seizures. *Vet Hum Toxicol* 29:451, 1987.

108. Amitai Y, Yeung AC, Moye J, et al: Repetitive oral activated charcoal and control of emesis in severe theophylline toxicity. *Ann Intern Med* 105:386, 1986.

109. Sessler CN: Poor tolerance of oral activated charcoal with theophylline overdose. *Am J Emerg Med* 5:492, 1987.

110. D'Angio R, Sabatelli F: Management considerations in treating metabolic abnormalities associated with theophylline overdose. *Arch Intern Med* 142:1837, 1987.

149. Monoamine Oxidase Inhibitor Toxicity

Diane Sauter

Overview

Monoamine oxidase inhibitors (MAOIs) have been in use since the 1950s. Initially marketed for the treatment of tuberculosis, then hypertension, they were noted to have mood-elevating properties and became widely used for treatment of endogenous depression [1]. Currently accepted indications for the use of these agents include neurotic illnesses with depressive features, treatment-resistant depression, atypical depression, eating disorders, anxiety, and phobias [2,3,4]. Three MAOIs are available for use in the management of psychiatric illness: phenelzine sulfate (Nardil), isocarboxazide (Marplan), and tranylcypromine sulfate (Parnate). In addition, the antitumor agent procarbazine (Matulane) has weak MAOI activity and is available for use in the treatment of Hodgkin's disease [1]. Selegilene (Deprenyl) is used to treat Parkinson's disease. Multiple other MAOIs (moclobemide, brofaromine, and tolaxotone) are currently undergoing investigation.

Monoamine oxidase (MAO) is a flavin-containing enzyme located in the mitochondrial membranes of almost all tissues [1]. Two distinct molecular types of MAO have been identified [5,6]: MAO-A and MAO-B. Human placenta contains exclusively MAO-A, whereas human platelets contain MAO-B. The brain and liver contain both forms [1]. Monoaminergic neurons contain predominantly MAO-A. Serotonergic neurons contain both [1]. Substrates metabolized by MAO-A include epinephrine (EPI), norepinephrine (NE), metanephrine, and 5-hydroxytryptophan (5-HT). Substrates metabolized exclusively by MAO-B include beta-phenylethylamine, phenylethanolamine, O-tyramine and benzylamine. Many substrates are metabolized by both MAO-A and MAO-B, including tyramine, octopamine and tryptamine [6].

Monoamine oxidase has two critical functions in the regulation of catecholamine metabolism. It mediates the oxidative deamination of the catecholamines EPI, NE, and dopamine (DA) and the indolealkylamine 5-HT intraneuronally [5,7]. Hepatic MAO functions along with catechol-O-methyl transferase (COMT) in the inactivation of circulating monoamines that are derived from the adrenal medulla or administered exogenously [8,9,10]. It also plays a critical role in the detoxification of ingested monoamines (tyramine, ethanolamine) that would otherwise be absorbed into the portal circulation [11,12].

The inhibition of MAO has diverse, poorly understood physiologic effects. It results in a decrease in the intraneuronal degradation of catecholamines and 5-HT within sympathetic nerve terminals [1,10]. This catecholamine storage pool becomes expanded and may be released following the administration of an indirectly acting sympathomimetic agent, such as dopamine [13,14]. The indirectly acting agents (Table 149-1) produce their pharmacologic effects by causing the release of stored catecholamines [1,4]. This is in contrast to the directly acting agents, such as NE (Levophed), which produce their effects by combining with postsynaptic receptors [15]. Tyramine, a naturally occurring, indirectly acting sympathomimetic agent found in many foods (Table 149-2), is normally inactivated by gut and liver MAO [11]. In MAO inhibition, dietary monoamines are readily absorbed into the portal circulation and cause release of the expanded pool of catecholamines. This results in a hypertensive crisis, the so-called "cheese reaction" [12,14]. In addition, once the normal metabolism of tyramine is chronically inhibited, tyramine metabolism is partially shunted into the production of the false neurotransmitter octopamine. Octopamine then replaces NE in the storage granules, and after the appropriate stimulus, is released instead of NE. Octopamine has no pressor effect. This may account for some of the hypotensive effects of the MAOIs [8].

In addition to its effect on MAO, the MAOIs have diverse physiologic effects unrelated to the inhibition of MAO. Multiple enzyme systems, including but not limited to decarboxylase, diamine oxidase, and pyridoxal phosphokinase, are inhibited by the MAOIs. The clinical implications of these effects are unknown [10].

The MAOIs currently available for use are nonselective, ir-

Table 149-1. Sympathomimetic Amines

Direct-acting
  Epinephrine
  Ethylnorepinephrine
  Isoetharine
  Isoproterenol
  Norepinephrine
  Phenylephrine
Indirect-acting
  Amphetamine*
  Benzphetamine
  Cocaine
  Fenfluramine
  Hydroxyamphetamine
  Methoxamine*
  Methylphenidate
  Phentermine
  Phenylpropanolamine*
  Propylhexadrine
  Ritodrine
  Tyramine*
Both direct and indirect effects
  Dopamine*
  Ephedrine*
  Mephentermine*
  Metaraminol*

* Hypertensive reactions have been reported with the use of MAOIs. Other indirect agents, or agents having both direct and indirect effects, are theoretically dangerous.

Table 149-2. Tyramine Content of Various Foods

High tyramine content—to be avoided
  Aged, mature cheeses
  Smoked or pickled, aged or putrefying meats, fish
  Yeast and meat extracts
  Red wines
  Italian broad beans
Moderate tyramine content—to be eaten in moderation
  Meat extracts
  Pasteurized light and pale beers
  Ripe avocados
Low tyramine content—permissible
  Distilled spirits
  Cottage, cream cheeses
  Chocolate and caffeine-containing beverages
  Fruits
  Soy sauce
  Yogurt, sour cream

reversible inhibitors of both MAO-A and MAO-B (phenelzine, isocarboxazide and tranylcypromine) and the MOA-B-selective inhibitor selegilene. The selective reversible inhibitor of MAO-A, moclobemide, is currently available for use in Europe but is under investigation in the United States [1].

The MAOIs are readily absorbed when given by mouth. No parenteral forms are available. Metabolism and inactivation occur through acetylation. Monoamine oxidase inhibitors are structurally related to amphetamine and have amphetaminelike activity unrelated to the inhibition of MAO [16,17,18]. Maximal MAO inhibition occurs within days, although antidepressant effects do not occur for 2 to 3 weeks [19]. Their biologic activity is prolonged due to the irreversible inactivation of MAO. Two weeks may be required for the normal activity of MAO to be restored following withdrawal of these agents. Mortality has been reported to occur with acute ingestion of as little as 170

to 650 mg of tranylcypromine, 375 to 1500 mg of phenelzine, and 5000 mg of nialamide [20].

Clinical Manifestations and Diagnostic Evaluation

The use of MAOIs may be associated with several adverse clinical effects, including acute toxicity, which occurs in patients taking overdoses of these agents, chronic toxicity, and multiple diverse drug and dietary interactions.

Understanding of the clinical presentation and natural history following an overdose of MAOIs is limited by the infrequency with which it has been reported [21–24]. The most recent report of the American Association of Poison Control Centers National Data Collection System [25] included four fatalities following the intentional ingestion of MAOIs. Two deaths followed ingestion of tranylcypromine sulfate alone. The other two fatalities resulted from ingestion of combined agents, including trifluperazine, thioridazine, tranylcypromine, phenelzine, lithium, and chlorpromazine. Acute overdose of MAOIs appears to be characterized by a delay in onset of clinical toxicity for as long as 24 hours following ingestion [22]. Mild toxicity is characterized by signs and symptoms of neuromuscular hyperactivity, such as hyperreflexia and myoclonus. Moderate toxicity is characterized by the same neuromuscular hyperactivity, altered mental status, and elevation of temperature, pulse, and blood pressure. Severe toxicity may result in seizures, central nervous system depression, respiratory depression, rigidity, hyperpyrexia, hypotension, cardiovascular collapse, and death. The duration of toxicity may be as long as 72 hours [22].

Patients with chronic toxicity may manifest tremors, insomnia, hyperhidrosis, agitation, hypomanic behavior, hallucinations, confusion, and seizures [1].

Avoidance of iatrogenic drug and dietary interactions is critical in the care of patients on MAOIs who are hospitalized as a result of other life-threatening processes. Information on the incidence of these interactions is unavailable.

The rational use of pressor agents in patients treated with MAOIs is well understood. In general, the indirectly acting sympathomimetic agents must be avoided, as hypertensive crisis is a well-known consequence. The agents specifically implicated in case reports or human studies include ephedrine [26,27], phenylephrine [26,28], dopamine [12], mephentermine [29], methylamphetamine [30], metaraminol [31], phenylpropanolamine [32,33], amphetamine [34], and tyramine. Animal studies confirm this drug interaction with MAOI and amphetamine [35], phenylethylamine, and tyramine [36]. This interaction does not occur with selegilene (when used in doses < 20 mg/day) [37] or moclobemide [38–55].

The clinical presentation of an adverse drug or tyramine reaction includes headache, hypertension, tachycardia (sometimes reflex bradycardia), diaphoresis, agitation, hypertonicity, hyperreflexia with myoclonus, rigidity, seizures, and coma. Intracranial hemorrhage and death may occur. The onset of toxicity is rapid (30–90 minutes) following ingestion or administration of sympathomimetic amines. The duration of effect is variable, but often resolves within a few hours.

Epinephrine, NE, and isoproterenol are pharmacologically active through a direct interaction with postsynaptic alpha- and beta-adrenergic receptors [15]. Theoretically, no potentiation of their effects should take place in the setting of MAO inhibition. In addition, these catecholamines are inactivated by COMT [9], an enzyme that is not affected by MAO inhibition. Lack of potentiation of the effects of EPI, NE, and isoproterenol has been reported in the setting of MAO inhibition [26,28,32,34,36].

A potentially fatal interaction between MAOIs and meperidine has been well described in case reports [56,57] and confirmed through animal studies [58–61]. A similar fatal reaction was described in a patient on an MAOI following the ingestion of a dextromethorphan-containing cold preparation [62]. The reaction is characterized by rapid onset of disorientation, muscular rigidity, severe hypertension or hypotension, coma, seizures, and death. While MAOIs are both competitive and noncompetitive inhibitors of meperidine-N-demethylation, this mechanism probably does not account for this drug interaction [58,63]. The effect is believed to result from a meperidine-induced exacerbation of MAOI-induced elevation in levels of central nervous system serotonin [64]. This well-described syndrome has been termed the serotonin syndrome [65,66,67]. Sinclair and Lo found that the ability of various agents to cause hyperthermia in rabbits pretreated with MAOIs was in direct proportion to each drug's ability to block the reuptake of serotonin [61]. These agents include fluoxetine (Prozac), meperidine, dextromethorphan, levorphanol (Levo Dromoran), and morphine. Relative potencies are as follows:

Fluoxetine > Meperidine = Dextromethorphan = Levorphanol > Morphine

In another animal model, morphine and pentazocine were found to lack potentiating effects [60]. Particular concern has been expressed concerning the combined use of the specific 5-HT receptor uptake inhibitor fluoxetine and the MAOIs. In clinical trials a very high incidence of adverse effects, including multiple deaths, has been reported [68,69]. Combined use of these agents is not recommended. In addition, a wash-out period of 5 weeks is recommended after stopping fluoxetine therapy and before initiating therapy with any of the MAOIs [68]. This effect is less pronounced and dose-dependent with moclobemide and the 5-HT reuptake inhibitors. However, this combination is not recommended [38].

Studies on the use of theophylline in MAO-inhibited animals have demonstrated significant toxic interactions [70,71]. Toxicity was found in rats pretreated with MAOIs and administered doses of theophylline and caffeine that were previously demonstrated to be safe. Another study demonstrated a significant reduction in the LD_{50} of both theophylline and caffeine following pretreatment with pargyline. The toxic reaction was characterized by marked hyperpyrexia, agitation, and tremors. The effects were blocked by inhibitors of serotonin synthesis [70,71]. Epinephrine, and the direct acting inhaled sympathomimetic agents should be safe in this setting.

Many reports exist of toxic reactions in patients treated with MAOIs who were given tryptophan for depression or levodopa for Parkinson's disease [7,16,72,73,74]. The reaction appears to be similar to the tyramine-MAOI interaction and includes hypertension, facial flushing, and a sensation of heat. This reaction has been attributed to the administration of precursor amino acids in the setting of decreased degradation. There are no reports of fatalities.

Potentiation of the hypoglycemic effects of insulin and sulfonylureas in the setting of MAO inhibition has been described in animal studies and human reports [75–79]. Tranylcypromine sulfate has been demonstrated to be a potent insulin secretagog. Doses of hypoglycemic agents should be adjusted or discontinued in this setting. The potentiation of the hypoglycemics has not been reported in patients treated in combination with moclobemide [38].

The MAOIs inhibit the mixed function oxidase enzyme systems involved in the metabolism and inactivation of codeine,

pentobarbitone, and hexobarbital [80,81]. Doses of these medications should be adjusted in patients on MAOIs. Phenylpropanolamine and dextromethorphan-containing over-the-counter cold preparations have a known toxicity in this setting and must be avoided.

Frequent reports of toxic or fatal interactions with the combination of MAOIs and imipramine [82–85] have appeared. The clinical picture includes restlessness, diaphoresis, excitability, opisthotonus, visual hallucinations, seizures, coma, and death. The etiology of this interaction is unclear. The combined use of lithium and MAOIs is reported by some to have greater therapeutic efficacy than the use of either agent alone. Lithium enhances serotonergic transmission at the presynaptic level [86]. Concerns of enhanced toxicity have been expressed [67] but rarely reported [25].

Doses of cocaine found to be nontoxic in an animal model resulted in severe toxicity when given to animals pretreated with MAOIs. These toxic signs included tremors, seizures, and death [87]. While cocaine is a known toxin, patients on MAOIs must be specifically warned about the life-threatening dangers associated with the use of this combination.

Differential Diagnosis

The differential diagnosis of the patient with an altered mental status and signs of sympathetic stimulation includes amphetamine and cocaine toxicity, over-the-counter sympathomimetics, such as appetite suppressants and decongestants, and withdrawal from sedative-hypnotics. Medical emergencies, such as hypoglycemia, hypoxemia, intracranial hemorrhage, meningitis, encephalitis, postictal states, and neuroleptic malignant syndrome, may have a similar clinical appearance.

Blood levels of MAOIs are generally unavailable and are not clinically useful. Abnormal laboratory findings are nonspecific but may include leukocytosis, hyperglycemia, elevated creatine phosphokinase, abnormal coagulation profile, and laboratory values reflective of renal impairment [22]. Toxicologic screening, when available, may be helpful. The MAOIs may not be identified on routine toxicologic screening.

Management

The management of any patient with an alteration of level or content of consciousness begins with stabilization of abnormal vital signs and empirical administration of oxygen, dextrose, and thiamine when indicated [88]. In some settings, the risks associated with syrup of ipecac or gastric lavage may be considered greater than the benefits [89]. The toxicity of MAOIs is great enough to warrant agressive gut decontamination with gastric lavage and administration of oral activated charcoal. Hyperpyrexia must be rapidly controlled. Reliance on antipyretic agents is inappropriate for patients who have pharmacologically induced temperature elevations. Patients with severe hyperpyrexia must be aggressively cooled with ice baths or wet sheets and fans. Iced gastric or urinary lavage may be performed but has minimal added effect. Hypothermia blankets are rarely adequate and should not be relied on to lower temperature rapidly.

Extreme agitation, neuromuscular hyperactivity, and seizures exacerbate hyperpyrexia and metabolic acidosis and may result in disseminated intravascular coagulation (DIC), rhabdomyolysis, and neurologic morbidity. Aggressive control with large doses of benzodiazepines, barbiturates, or a nondepolarizing paralyzing agent is appropriate. Phenothiazines and butyrophenones should be avoided in the treatment of agitation. Neuromuscular hyperactivity resulting in hyperpyrexia and rhabdomyolysis has been treated anecdotally with dantrolene and bromocriptine [90,91]. Bromocriptine should be avoided because of the potential for drug interactions [91,92]. Dantrolene is a muscle relaxant that functions peripherally by reducing calcium efflux into the sarcoplasm [92]. There are no controlled studies of the use of muscle relaxants in this setting. However, based on the mechanism of action of dantrolene, there appears to be no theoretical reason to anticipate a therapeutic effect with this mechanism of hyperpyrexia [93]; the author prefers the use of benzodiazepines.

Occasionally a question arises concerning the use of naloxone hydrochloride (Narcan), the specific opiate antagonist in patients who manifest serotonin syndrome following the combined use of an opiate and an MAOI. A single animal study demonstrated a significant exacerbation of temperature elevation in rats following the use of naloxone in an attempt to reverse serotonin syndrome. The same study found that the use of metoclopramide (Reglan) in these rats resulted in a significant attenuation of the temperature elevation following the onset of serotonin syndrome [94]. This single study suggests that naloxone may be contraindicated in this setting. In addition, there appears to be a role for the use of serotonin antagonists in serotonin syndrome management.

Seizures may require large doses of benzodiazepines. Phenobarbital (15–20 mg/kg) or phenytoin (18 mg/kg) can be used as anticonvulsants, although phenytoin may not be effective because of neurotransmitter excess. A nondepolarizing paralyzing agent, such as vecuronium or pancuronium, may be necessary if seizures persist.

Severe hypertension is most safely treated with a rapidly reversible antihypertensive agent, such as nitroprusside, nitroglycerin, or esmolol. The use of longer-acting agents (tolazoline, clonidine, phentolamine, and other beta-blockers) has been recommended [1,28]. These agents should be used with caution, as hypertension is often followed by severe hypotension. The continued activity of an antihypertensive agent that cannot be "turned off" may worsen the patient's condition.

Resuscitation of the hypotensive patient begins with volume replacement. A direct-acting pressor, such as NE, is preferred to agents such as DA. Indirect-acting agents such as DA require the release of intracellular amines and may lead to an exaggerated hypertensive response or hypotension.

Cardiac arrhythmias are generally a premorbid sign; when present, they should be treated with lidocaine, procainamide, or phenytoin. Bretylium causes release of stored catecholamines and should probably be avoided. Sinus tachycardia, in general, does not require treatment.

Diuresis, hemodialysis, and hemoperfusion are not effective in increasing clearance of the MAOIs. Hospitalized patients who have taken or are currently prescribed any of the irreversible nonselective MAOIs must have their diets carefully monitored. Specifically, foods high in tyramine content must be avoided (Table 149-2). In general, high-protein foods that are contaminated with decarboxylating bacteria or foods that are fermented should be avoided [95]. An excellent analysis of the tyramine content of several foods may be found in the review by DaPrada et al. [44].

Due to the potential for delayed toxicity, a reasonable suspicion of an MAOI overdose mandates extended observation in a monitored setting. Patients who develop clinical toxicity should be monitored until mental status and vital signs have returned to normal. This may require a prolonged period of intensive care management. Severely toxic patients frequently require intubation and mechanical ventilation. If intensive care monitoring is unavailable, arrangements for transfer to an institution with this capability should be made. Secondary sequelae from such an overdose may include DIC, acute respiratory distress syndrome, myoglobinuric renal failure, hepatic failure, and neurologic morbidity.

Patients with severe hypertension following drug or dietary interactions may be treated with a rapidly acting oral or parenteral agent, such as nifedipine, phentolamine, or tolazoline. These patients may not require hospital admission if the interaction has been mild and the resolution of symptoms complete. Patients with an altered mental status, seizures, or suspected intracranial hemorrhage must be aggressively managed and admitted to the hospital for further studies and/or observation.

Prior to discharge, patients require psychiatric evaluation if the problem is the result of an acute overdose. If a drug or dietary reaction is the cause, then careful education with regard to the food and pharmaceuticals to be avoided is required.

References

1. Baldessarini RJ: Drugs and the treatment of psychiatric disorder, in Goodman, Gilman A, Rall TW, Nies AS, Taylor P (eds): *Goodman and Gilman's The Pharmacological Basis of Therapeutics.* 8th ed. Elmsford, NY, Pergamon, 1990, pp 383–435.
2. Chaimowitz GA, Links PS, Padgett RW, et al: Treatment resistant depression: A survey of practice habits of Canadian psychiatrists. *Can J Psychiatry* 36:353, 1991.
3. Clary C, Mandos L, Schweizer E: Results of a brief survey on the prescribing practices for monoamine oxidase inhibitor antidepressants. *J Clin Psychiatry* 51:226, 1990.
4. Zisook S: A clinical overview of monoamine oxidase inhibitors. *Psychosomatics* 26:240, 1985.
5. Denny RM, Fritz RR, Patel NT, et al: Human liver MAO-A and MAO-B reported by immunoaffinity chromatography with MAO-B specific monoclonal antibody. *Science* 215:1400, 1982.
6. Wells DG, Bjorksten AR: Monoamine oxidase inhibitors revisited. *Can J Anaesth* 36:64, 1989.
7. Goldstein DS: Catecholamines in plasma cerebrospinal fluid: Sources and meaning, in Buckley JP, Ferrario CM (eds): *Brain Peptides and Catecholamines in Cardiovascular Regulation.* New York, Raven, 1987.
8. Axelrod J, Weinshilboum R: Catecholamines. *N Engl J Med* 287:237, 1972.
9. Axelrod J: O-Methylation of epinephrine and other catechols in vitro and in vivo. *Science* 126:400, 1957.
10. Sjoquist F: Psychotropic drugs. 2. Interaction between monoamine oxidase (MAO) inhibitors and other substances. *Proc Roy Soc Med* 58:967, 1975.
11. Blackwell B: Adverse effects of antidepressant drugs. I. Monoamine oxidase inhibitors and tricyclics. *Drugs* 21:201, 1981.
12. Horowitz D, Lovenberg W, Engleman K, et al: Monoamine oxidase inhibitors, tyramine, and cheese. *JAMA* 188:1108, 1964.
13. Norberg KA: Drug-induced changes in monoamine levels in the sympathetic adrenergic ganglion cells and terminals: A histochemical study. *Acta Physiol Scand* 65:221, 1965.
14. Smith CB: The role of monoamine oxidase in the intraneuronal metabolism of norepinephrine released by indirectly acting sympathomimetic amines or by adrenergic nerve stimulation. *J Pharmacol Exp Ther* 151:207, 1966.
15. Weiner N: Norepinephrine, epinephrine, and the sympathomimetic amines, in Gilman AG, Rall TW, Murad F (eds): *The Pharmacological Basis of Therapeutics.* 7th ed. New York, Macmillan, 1985, p 145.
16. Goldberg LI: Monoamine oxidase inhibitors: Adverse reactions and possible mechanisms. *JAMA* 190:132, 1964.
17. Keck PE Jr, Vuckovic A, Pope HG, et al: Acute cardiovascular response to monoamine oxidase inhibitors: A prospective assessment. *J Clin Psychopharmacol* 9:203, 1989.

18. Fallon B, Foote B, Walsh BT, et al: "Spontaneous" hypertensive episodes with monoamine oxidase inhibitors. *J Clin Psychiatry* 49:163, 1988.

19. Murphy DL, Sunderland T, Cohen RM: Monoamine oxidase-inhibiting antidepressants: A clinical update. *Psychiatr Clin North Am* 7:549, 1984.

20. Tolefson GD: Monoamine oxidase inhibitors: A review. *J Clin Psychiatry* 44:280, 1983.

21. Baldridge ET, Miller LV, Haverback BJ, et al: Amine metabolism after an overdose of a monoamine oxidase inhibitor. *N Engl J Med* 267:421, 1962.

22. Linden CH, Rumack BH, Strehilke C: Monoamine oxidase inhibitor overdose. *Am Emerg Med* 13:1137, 1984.

23. Midwinter RE: Accidental overdose of "Parstelin." *Br Med J* 2:1755, 1962.

24. Quill TE: Peaked T waves with tranylcypromine (Parnate) overdose. *J Psych Med* 11:155, 1981–1982.

25. Litovitz TL, Holm KC, Bailey KM, Schmitz BF: 1991 annual report of the American Association of Poison Control Centers National Data Collection System. *Am J Emerg Med* 10:452, 1992.

26. Elis J, Laurence DR, Mattie H, et al: Modification by monoamine oxidase inhibitors of the effect of some sympathomimetics on blood pressure. *Br Med J* 2:75, 1967.

27. Low Beer GA, Tidmarsh D: Collapse after "Parstelin." *Br Med J* 2:683, 1963.

28. Boakes AJ, Laurence DR, Teich PC, et al: Interactions between sympathomimetic amines and antidepressants on blood pressure. *Br Med J* 1:311, 1973.

29. Stark DCC: Effects of giving vasopressors to patients on MAO inhibitors. *Lancet* 2:1406, 1962.

30. Dally PJ: Fatal reaction with tranylcypromine and methylamphetamine. *Lancet* 1:1235, 1962.

31. Horler AR, Wynne NA: Hypertensive crisis due to pargyline and metaraminol. *Br Med J* 2:460, 1965.

32. Cuthbert MF, Vere DW: Potentiation of the cardiovascular effects of some catecholamines by a monoamine oxidase inhibitor. *Proc Br Pharm Soc* September 15–17, p 471, 1971.

33. Tonks CM, Lloyd AT: Hazards with monoamine oxidase inhibitors. *Br Med J* 1:589, 1965.

34. Trinker FR, Fearn HJ, McCulloch MW, et al: Experimental observations on the effects of adrenaline after treatment with antidepressant monoamine oxidase inhibitor (MAOI) drugs. *Aust Dent J* 12:297, 1967.

35. O'Dea K, Rand MJ: Interaction between amphetamine and monoamine oxidase inhibitors. *Eur J Pharmacol* 6:115, 1969.

36. Greisemer EC, Barsky J, Dragstedt CA, et al: Potentiating effects of iproniazid on the pharmacological action of sympathomimetic amines. *Proc Soc Exp Biol Med* 84:699, 1953.

37. Cedarbaum JM, Schleifer LS: Drugs for Parkinson's disease, spasticity and acute muscle spasms, in Goodman, Gilman A, Rall TW, Nies AS, Taylor P (eds): *Goodman and Gilman's The Pharamcological Basis of Therapeutics.* 8th ed. Elmsford, NY, Pergamon, 1990, pp 463–484.

38. Amrein R, Guntert J, Dingemanse T, et al: Interactions of moclobemide with concomitantly administered medication: Evidence from pharmacological and clinical studies. *Psychopharmacology* 106 (suppl):S24, 1992.

39. Berlin I, Zimmer R, Cournot A, et al: Determination and comparison of the pressor effect of tyramine during long-term moclobemide and tranylcypromine treatment in healthy volunteers. *Clin Pharmacol Ther* 46:344, 1989.

40. Bieck PR, Antonin KH: Oral tyramine pressor test and the safety of monoamine oxidase inhibitor drugs: Comparison of brofaromine and tranylcypromine in healthy subjects. *J Clin Psychopharmacol* 8:237, 1988.

41. Callingham BA, Ovens RS: Some in vitro effects of moclobemide and other MAO inhibitors on responses to sympathomimetic amines. *J Neural Transm* 26(suppl):17, 1988.

42. Chen DT: Safety of moclobemide in clinical use. *Clin Neuropharm* 15:428A, 1992.

43. Chouinard G, Saxena BM, Nair NPV, et al: Efficacy and safety of brofaromine in depression: A Canadian multicenter placebo controlled trial and a review of comparative controlled studies. *Clin Neuropharm* 15(suppl 1, pt A):426A, 1992.

44. Da Prada M, Zurchet G, Wuthrich I, et al: On tyramine, food, beverages and the reversible MAO inhibitor moclobemide. *J Neural Transm* 26(suppl):31, 1988.

45. Delker A, Gaertner HJ: Tolerability and antidepressive effect of brofaromine, a short-acting reversible MAO inhibitor: An open study. *Eur Neuropsychopharmacol* 1:177, 1991.

46. Gieschke R, Schmid-Burgk W, Amrein R: Interaction of moclobemide, a new reversible monoamine oxidase inhibitor with oral tyramine. *J Neural Transm* 26(suppl):97, 1988.

47. Korn A, Da Prada M, Raffesberg W, et al: Tyramine pressor effect in man: Studies with moclobemide, a novel, reversible monoamine oxidase inhibitor. *J Neural Transm* 26(suppl):57, 1988.

48. Laux G, Beckman H, Classen W, et al: Moclobemide and maprotiline in the treatment of inpatients with major depressive disorder. *J Neural Transm* 28(suppl):45, 1989.

49. Moll E, Hetzl W: Moclobemide (Ro 11-1163) safety in depressed patients. *Acta Psychiatr Scand Suppl* 360:69, 1990.

50. Muller T, Gieschke R, Ziegler WH: Blood pressure response to tyramine-enriched meal before and during MAO-inhibition in man: Influence of dosage regimen. *J Neural Transm* 26(suppl):105, 1988.

51. Provost JC, Funck-Bretano C, Rovei V, et al: Pharmacokinetic and pharmacodynamic interaction between toloxatone, a new reversible monoamine oxidase-A inhibitor, and oral tyramine in healthy subjects. *Clin Pharmacol Ther* 52:384, 1992.

52. Rafaelsen OJ: Cheese effects new reversible MAO A inhibitors: Summary. *J Neural Transm* 26(suppl):123, 1988.

53. Zimmer R, Fischback R, Breuel HP: Potentiation of the pressor effect of intravenously administered tyramine during moclobemide treatment. *Acta Psychiatr Scand Suppl* 360:76, 1990.

54. Zimmer R, Peuch AJ, Philipp F, Korn A: Interaction between orally administered tyramine and moclobemide. *Acta Psychiatr Scand Suppl* 360:78, 1990.

55. Zimmer R: Relationship between tyramine potentiation and monoamine oxidase (MAO) inhibition: Comparison between moclobemide and other MAO inhibitors. *Acta Psychiatr Scand Suppl* 360:81, 1990.

56. Cocks DP, Passmore-Rowe A: Dangers of monoamine oxidase inhibitors. *Br Med J* 2:1545, 1962.

57. Vigran IM: Dangerous potentiation of meperidine hydrochloride by pargyline hydrochloride. *JAMA* 187:953, 1964.

58. Eade NR, Renton KW: Effect of monoamine oxidase inhibitors on the N-dimethylation and hydrolysis of meperidine. *Bicochem Pharmacol* 19:2243, 1970.

59. Gong SNC, Rogers KJ: Role of brain monoamines in the fatal hyperthermia induced by pethidine or imipramine in rabbits pretreated with a monoamine oxidase inhibitor. *Br J Pharmacol* 48:12, 1973.

60. Penn RG, Rogers KJ: Comparison of the effects of morphine, pethidine and pentazocine in rabbits pretreated with a monoamine oxidase inhibitor. *Br J Pharmacol* 42:485, 1971.

61. Sinclair JG, Lo GF: The blockade of serotonin uptake and the meperidine monoamine oxidase inhibitor interaction. *Proc West Pharmacol Soc* 20:373, 1977.

62. Rivers N: Possible lethal reaction between nardil and dextromethorphan. *Can Med Assoc J* 103:85, 1970.

63. Clark B, Thompson JW: Analysis of the inhibition of pethidine N-demethylation by monoamine oxidase inhibitors and some other drugs with special reference to drug interactions in man. *Br J Pharmacol* 44:89, 1972.

64. Erspamer V: Recent research in the field of 5-hydroxytryptamine and related indolealkylamines. *Prog Drug Res* 3:307, 1961.

65. Nierenberg DW, Semprebon M: The central nervous system serotonin syndrome. *Clin Pharmacol Ther* 53:84, 1993.

66. Price WA, Zimmer B, Kucas P: Serotonin syndrome: A case report. *J Clin Pharmacol* 26:77, 1986.

67. Sternbach H: The serotonin syndrome. *Am J Psychiatry* 148:705, 1991.

68. Ciraulo DA, Shader RI: Fluoxetine drug-drug interactions. I. Antidepressants and antipsychotics. *J Clin Psychopharmacol* 10:48, 1990.

69. Feighner JP, Boyer WF, Tyler DL, et al: Adverse consequences of fluoxitine-MAOI combination therapy. *J Clin Psychiatry* 51:222, 1990.

70. Berkowitz BA, Tower JH, Spector S: Release of norepinephrine in

the central nervous system by theophylline and caffeine. *Eur J Pharmacol* 10:64, 1970.

71. Berkowitz BA, Spector S, Pool W: The interaction of caffeine, theophylline and theobromine with monoamine oxidase inhibitors. *Eur J Pharmacol* 16:315, 1971.

72. Friend DG, Bell WR, Kline NS: The action of L-dihydroxyphenylalanine in patients receiving nialamide. *Clin Pharmacol Ther* 6:362, 1965.

73. Pope HG, Jonas JM, Hudson JL, et al: Toxic reactions to the combination of monoamine oxidase inhibitors and tryptophan. *Am J Psychiatry* 142:491, 1985.

74. Teychene PF, Caine DB, Lewis PJ, et al: Interactions of levodopa with inhibitors of monoamine oxidase and L-aromatic acid decarboxylase. *Clin Pharmacol Ther* 18:273, 1975.

75. Adnitt PL: Hypoglycemic action of monoamine oxidase inhibitors (MAOIs). *Diabetes* 17:628, 1968.

76. Barrett AM: Modification of the hypoglycemic response to tolbutamide and insulin by mebanazine, an inhibitor of monoamine oxidase. *J Pharm Pharmacol* 17:19, 1965.

77. Bressler R, Vargas-Cordon M, Lebovitz HE: Tranylcypromine: A potent insulin secretagogue and hypoglycemic agent. *Diabetes* 17:617, 1968.

78. Cooper AJ, Ashcroft G: Potentiation of insulin hypoglycemia by monoamine oxidase in MAOI and antidepressant drugs. *Lancet* 1:407, 1966.

79. Wickstrom L, Pettersson K: Treatment of diabetes with monoamine oxidase inhibitors. *Lancet* 2:995, 1964.

80. Findlay JWA, Butz RF, Williams BB, et al: Effect of monoamine oxidase inhibitors on codeine disposition and pentobarbitone sleep-times in the rat. *J Pharm Pharmacol* 33:45, 1981.

81. LaRoche MJ, Brodie BB: Lack of relationship between monoamine oxidase and potentiation of hexabarbitol hypnosis. *J Pharmacol Exp Ther* 130:134, 1960.

82. Ayd FJ: Toxic somatic and psychopathologic reactions to antidepressant drugs. *J Neuropsy* 2:S119, 1961.

83. Brachfeld T, Wirtshaffer A, Wolfe S: Imipramine tranylcypromine incompatibility, near fatal toxic reaction. *JAMA* 183:1172, 1964.

84. Davies G: Side effects of phenelzine. *Br Med J* 2:1019, 1960.

85. Schopf J: Treatment of depressions resistant to tricyclic antidepressants, related drugs or MAO-inhibitors by lithium addition: Review of the literature. *Pharmacopsychiatry* 22:174, 1989.

86. Graham P, Potter JM, Paterson JW: Combination monoamine oxidase inhibitor/tricyclic antidepressant interaction. *Lancet* 2:440, 1982.

87. Christie J, Crow TJ: Behavior studies of the actions of cocaine, monoamine oxidase inhibitors and iminodibenzyl compounds on central dopamine neurones. *Br J Pharmacol* 47:39, 1973.

88. Flomenbaum NE, Goldfrank LR, Weisman RS, et al: General management of the poisoned or overdosed patient, in Goldfrank LR, Flomenbaum NE, Lewin NA, et al. (eds): *Goldfrank's Toxicologic Emergencies*. 4th ed. Norwalk CT, Appleton & Lange, 1990, pp 3–20.

89. Kulig K, Bar-Or D, Cantrill SV, et al: Management of acutely poisoned patients without gastric emptying. *Ann Emerg Med* 14:562, 1985.

90. Verrill MR, Salanga VD, Kozachuk WE, et al: Phenelzine toxicity responsive to dantrolene. *Neurology* 37:865, 1987.

91. Sheehan DV, Calycomb JB, Kouretas N: The monoamine oxidase inhibitors: Prescription and patient management. *Int J Psychiatry Med* 10:99, 1980–1981.

92. Guze BH, Baxter LR Jr: Neuroleptic malignant syndrome. *N Engl J Med* 313:163, 1985.

93. Vassallo SV, Delaney KA: Pharmacologic effects on thermoregulation: Mechanisms of drug-related heatstroke. *Clin Toxicol* 27:199, 1989.

94. Lakhanpal R, Azar A, Weinstein E, et al: Effects of naloxone and metoclopramide on the interaction of the monoamine oxidase inhibitor tranylcypromine with meperidine in an animal model (abstract). *Ann Emerg Med* 22:895, 1993.

95. Lippman SB, Nash K: Monoamine oxidase inhibitor update: Potential adverse food and drug interactions. *Drug Saf* 5:195, 1990.

150. Neuroleptic Agents

Ross S. Carol and
Christopher H. Linden

Overview

Neuroleptics, also known as antipsychotic agents and major tranquilizers, are primarily used in the therapy of schizophrenia, the manic phase of bipolar disorders, and agitated behavior. They are also used to treat nausea, vomiting, headaches, hiccoughs, and a variety of neurologic conditions (e.g., chorea, dystonias, hemiballismus, spasms, tics, torticollis). Neuroleptics are a structurally diverse group of compounds containing two, three, or four aliphatic, aromatic, or heterocyclic rings. They include butyrophenone, dibenzoxazepine, diphenylbutylpiperidine, dihydroindolone, phenothiazine, and thioxanthene derivatives (Table 150-1). Available formulations include tablet, capsule, liquid, and sustained-release oral preparations and suppository and injectable immediate-release and sustained-release (depot) solutions [1].

Poisoning may occur following ingestion of therapeutic doses or accidental or intentional overdosage. Poisoning in two infants resulted from treatment with topical promethazine cream [2]. Toxic effects include anticholinergic syndrome (see Chap. 133), extrapyramidal syndromes, neuroleptic malignant syndrome (see Chap. 73), and central nervous system (CNS) and cardiovascular depression [3,4]. Therapeutic use has been associated with fatal myocardial infarction, sleep apnea, sudden infant death syndrome, and sudden adult death [5,6,7]. Although abrupt cessation of neuroleptic therapy is generally without consequence, significant cachexia has been described [8,9]. Most deaths are the consequence of either suicidal overdose by psychotic or depressed adults or neuroleptic malignant syndrome.

Pharmacology

The mechanism of action of neuroleptic agents is complex and incompletely understood. Neuroleptic agents are known to block neuronal dopamine receptors (subtypes 1 and 2, which

Table 150-1. Neuroleptic and Related Agents

Structural class	Generic name	Trade name	Daily oral dose (adult, mg)
Butyrophenone	Droperidol	Inapsine	Parenteral only
	Haloperidol	Haldol	2–10
Dibenzoxazepine	Loxapine	Loxitane	20–200
Diphenylbutyl-piperidine	Pimozide	Orap	1–10
Indole	Molindone	Moban	15–335
Phenothiazine	Acetophenazine	Tindal	40–80
	Butaperazine	Repoise	30–50
	Carphenazine	Proketazine	25–400
	Chlorpromazine	Thorazine	100–1000
	Fluphenazine	Prolixin	0.5–20
	Mesoridazine	Serentil	50–400
	Perphenazine	Trilafon	8–64
	Piperacetazine	Quide	20–160
	Prochlorperazine	Compazine	10–100
	Promazine	Sparine	50–1000
	Promethazine[a]	Phenergan	50–150
	Triethylperazine[a]	Torecan	10–30
	Thiopropazate	Dartal	6–30
	Thioridazine	Mellaril	30–800
	Trifluoperazine	Stelazine	2–15
	Triflupromazine	Vesprin	Parenteral only
	Trimeprazine[b]	Temaril	2.5–10
Thioxanthene	Chlorprothixene	Taractan	50–600
	Thiothixene	Navane	20–30

[a] Antiemetic only
[b] Antipruritic only

respectively activate and inhibit adenylate cyclase when stimulated), histamine receptors (subtypes 1 and 2), alpha-adrenergic receptors (subtypes 1 and 2), muscarinic receptors, and serotonergic receptors [1,10]. Antipsychotic activity appears to be due to interference with cortical, limbic, and basal ganglia dopaminergic neurotransmission and has been correlated with affinity for dopamine-2 receptors [11]. Clozapine, however, may act primarily by blocking dopamine-1 receptors [12]. Antiemetic activity and the ability to increase prolactin secretion appear to result from a similar inhibition of dopaminergic receptors in the chemoreceptor trigger zone of the medulla and in the hypothalamus, respectively. Hypothalamic dysfunction may be responsible for disordered temperature regulation [1,13]. Anticholinergic effects (e.g., tachycardia, hypotension, ileus, mydriasis, urinary retention, dry mucous membranes) correlate directly with CNS depressant activity and inversely with the incidence of extrapyramidal reactions [3,13]. Chlorpromazine, chlorprothixene, and thioridazine have the greatest sedative activity, whereas fluphenazine, haloperidol, trifluoperazine, and triflupromazine are the agents most commonly associated with extrapyramidal toxicity. Agranulocytosis, cholestatic jaundice, photosensitivity reactions, and priapism are uncommon idiosyncratic reactions associated with phenothiazine therapy [3,10,13–17].

Hypotension miosis appears to be due to peripheral alpha$_1$-adrenergic blockade as well as to central effects [3,10]. Hypotension is primarily orthostatic and systolic in nature and tends to correlate in incidence and severity with sedative potency. Tachycardia usually occurs as a reflex response to hypotension. Concomitant therapy with a beta-adrenergic agonist (e.g., epinephrine) or antagonist (e.g., propranolol) can lead to severe hypotension [18,19]. Phenothiazines, particularly thioridazine and mesoridazine, also have local anesthetic, quinidinelike antiarrhythmic and myocardial depressant effects. Ventricular re-

polarization abnormalities, such as T wave changes, increased U wave amplitude, and prolongation of the Q–T interval, may be noted on the electrocardiogram (ECG) [20–24]. Conduction disturbances such as bundle branch, fascicular, intraventricular, and atrioventricular blocks and supraventricular and ventricular tachyarrthymias, including *Torsades de pointes* (polymorphic ventricular tachycardia), and ventricular fibrillation have also been reported [25,26,27]. Cardiac effects are dose-dependent but can occur with therapeutic as well as toxic doses. Ventricular tachyarrhythmias and asphyxia (due to seizures, aspiration, or respiratory depression) have been postulated as etiologies of sudden death in patients taking therapeutic doses of phenothiazines [28]. Many, but not all, antipsychotic agents have been found to lower the seizure threshold and can induce epileptiform discharge patterns on the electroencephalogram (EEG) [4].

Neuroleptic agents have a relatively flat dose-response curve [1]. Effective therapeutic doses vary over a wide range (Table 150-1). The optimal dose is determined by the clinical response, not by serum drug levels. Pharmacologic effects generally last 24 hours or more, allowing for once daily dosing.

The kinetics of neuroleptics are poorly understood [1]. Most agents have an unpredictable pattern of gastrointestinal absorption, with peak levels occurring 2 to 4 hours after ingestion. Their bioavailability following parenteral administration is 2 to 10 times greater than with oral dosing because of the lack of presystemic (gastrointestinal and hepatic) metabolism, which occurs only after ingestion. Hence, therapeutic intravenous or intramuscular doses are substantially less than oral ones. Following absorption, neuroleptic agents are highly bound to plasma proteins (90–99%). However, since they are also highly lipophilic, volumes of distribution are large (10–40 L/kg) and serum drug levels following therapeutic doses are quite low (one to several hundred nanograms per milliliter). Neuroleptics tend to accumulate in the brain and easily cross the placenta. Elimination occurs slowly by hepatic metabolism, with serum concentration half-lives averaging 20 to 40 hours. Small amounts (1–3%) are excreted unchanged by the kidney. As a rule, hepatic metabolism yields multiple metabolites, some of which are pharmacologically active (e.g., mesoridazine is an active metabolite of thioridazine) [29]. Metabolites are eliminated by urinary and, to some extent, biliary excretion and can be detected in the urine for several days following a single ingestion and for a month or more following cessation of chronic therapy [1]. Renal insufficiency may result in drug accumulation and toxicity [30].

Toxicology

OVERDOSAGE. The toxicity of neuroleptic drugs following overdosage results from exaggerated pharmacologic activity. Effects include CNS and consequent respiratory depression, cardiovascular depression, and, occasionally, delirium. Hypothermia may be due to peripheral vasodilatation as well as hypothalamic depression. Seizures are rare and occur mainly in patients with underlying epilepsy and those with loxapine overdoses [31]. Rhabdomyolysis may occur after prolonged convulsions. Cardiovascular effects include hypotension (initially with reflex tachycardia), cardiac conduction disturbances, tachyarrhythmias, bradyarrhythmias, and, rarely, pulmonary edema [32,33].

Of the thousands of neuroleptic overdoses reported each year, only 1 to 2 percent result in serious or fatal toxicity. Thioridazine, because of its greater cardiotoxicity, and mixed overdoses are responsible for the majority of fatal poisonings. Toxic doses are not well established. In general, acute ingestion of maximal therapeutic doses results in significant side effects and ingestions of greater than twice this amount are potentially serious. Death of an infant was reported following the ingestion of only 350 mg of chlorpromazine [3]. Adult fatalities have been reported following ingestions of 2 gm of chlorpromazine, 2.5 gm of loxapine and mesoridazine, and 1.5 gm of thioridazine [3]. Many patients, however, have survived much higher ingestions [3].

EXTRAPYRAMIDAL SYNDROMES. Extrapyramidal side effects of neuroleptics are movement disorders resulting from the interference with neurotransmitter (primarily dopamine-2 receptor blockade) function in the basal ganglia. They are more common in patients treated with high-potency agents and may occur early (i.e., within a few days to a few months) or late (i.e., after more than 3 months) in the course of therapy. Early pyramidal syndromes include acute dyskinesia (acute dystonic reactions), akathisia, and parkinsonism. Late disorders include tardive dyskinesia, tardive dystonia, and focal perioral tremor (Rabbit syndrome). Although extrapyramidal syndromes are relatively common in patients chronically treated with neuroleptics, they are distinctly unusual following acute overdose. Only the acute syndromes, those most likely to develop in the intensive care unit (ICU), are discussed.

Acute Dystonic Reactions. Acute dystonic reactions (ADRs) are reversible motor disturbances consisting of sustained, uncoordinated, and involuntary spasmodic movements of various muscle groups. Although ADRs most often occur following administration of therapeutic doses of neuroleptic drugs [34], they have also been described following administration of antihistamines (both H1 and H2 blockers) [35–40], anticholinergics (e.g., benztropine) [41], anticonvulsants (e.g., carbamazepine, phenytoin) [42,43], calcium channel blockers [44,45], metoclopramide [46,47,48] cyclic antidepressants [49,50,51], ketamine [52], and cholinergics (e.g., bethanechol, insecticides) [53,54] (Table 150-2). Acute dystonic reactions can also occur as a primary (non-drug-related) disorder [55].

The most accepted theory is that ADRs are caused by a disruption of activity in central cholinergic as well as dopaminergic neuronal pathways. In the CNS, acetylcholine is thought to be an excitatory neurotransmitter and dopamine is primarily an inhibitory one. Normal balance between these pathways is necessary for coordinated muscular activity. The blockage of dopaminergic receptors by various drugs and the resultant relative excess of cholinergic activity is postulated to be the underlying mechanism [55]. This theory best explains the observation that ADRs are most frequently associated with neuroleptics having high dopamine-2 and low muscaric receptor blocking activity [10]. Another theory proposes that drug-induced dopaminergic receptor blockade is directly responsible [56]. A third theory invokes both dopaminergic blockade and activation in the nigrostriatal dopamine system. After initial receptor blockade, increased dopamine synthesis and release and receptor "supersensitivity" may result in enhanced dopaminergic activity. This theory best explains the fact that ADRs usually do not occur until 12 to 24 hours after the first dose [57].

Although the absolute incidence of dystonic reactions is unknown, it is estimated to occur in 2 to 12 percent of all patients who take phenothiazines, 25 percent of patients treated with intramuscular depot preparations, and 16 percent of patients given haloperidol. Fifty percent of ADRs occur within 48 hours of initiating therapy and 85 percent within 4 days [58,59]. Phenothiazines that contain a piperazine side chain (i.e., prochlorperazine, trifluoperazine, perphenazine, fluphenazine, and ace-

Table 150-2. Additional Agents Associated with Acute Dystonic Reactions

Generic name	Common brand names	Classification
Amoxapine	Asendin	Antidepressant
Azatadine	Optimine	Antihistamine
Benztropine	Cogentin	Anticholinergic
Bethanechol	Urecholine	Cholinergic
Carbamazepine	Tegretol	Anticonvulsant
Chlorpheniramine	Chlor-Trimeton	Antihistamine
Cimetidine	Tagamet	Antihistamine
Diphenhydramine	Benadryl	Antihistamine
Ketamine	Ketalar	Anesthetic
Metoclopramide	Reglan	Antiemetic
Nifedipine	Procardia	Calcium channel blocker
Pheniramine	many	Antihistamine
Phenylephrine	NeoSynephrine	Decongestant
Phenylpropanolamine	many	Decongestant
Phenytoin	Dilantin	Antiepileptic
Trazodone	Desyrel	Antidepressant
Verapamil	Calan	Calcium channel blocker

tophenazine) are associated with a higher incidence of dystonic reactions than are other phenothiazines [58]. The likelihood of an ADR, however, is more dependent on individual susceptibility than on neuroleptic structure, potency, dose, and duration of therapy [59]. Acute dystonic reactions most commonly occur in men, patients 5 to 45 years of age (particularly those < 15 years), and those with a family history of dystonia or a personal history of drug or alcohol abuse [59,60,61].

Akathisia. Akathisia is a condition or subjective sensation of motor restlessness that occurs within hours to days after initiation of neuroleptic therapy or after an increase in drug dose [10]. About 20 percent of patients treated with neuroleptics develop this complication. It is most common with high-potency agents, such as fluphenazine, haloperidol, perphenazine, thiothixene, and trifluoperizine. In some patients, it occurs in association with severe parkinsonism [62]. Like ADRs, akathisia has been noted in patients treated with metoclopramide [46,47,48]. In contrast to ADRs, however, it occurs in patients of any age, and women are affected much more often than men [10].

Parkinsonism. Parkinsonism can occur early or late during the course of neuroleptic or metoclopramide therapy [10,46,47,48]. It occurs in about 13 percent of patients treated with neuroleptics and, like ADRs, is most common in those treated with agents having high dopamine-2 and low muscarinic receptor blocking activity. Like akathisia, it occurs in patients of all ages and affects women more often than men.

Clinical Presentation and Diagnostic Evaluation

OVERDOSAGE. Nausea and vomiting may develop soon after ingestion. However, CNS and cardiovascular effects usually dominate the clinical picture [2,3,4,25–28,63,64,65]. Findings in mild intoxication include ataxia, confusion, lethargy, slurred speech, tachycardia, and diastolic or orthostatic hypotension. Anticholinergic signs (e.g., dry skin and mucosa, decreased bowel sounds) and hyperreflexia may also be present. Electrocardiographic changes such as prolonged P–R and Q–T intervals, S–T segment depression, T wave abnormalities (biphasic, blunting, inversion, notching, widening), and increased U waves may be seen [20–26,66,67,68].

Signs and symptoms of moderate poisoning include low-grade coma (see Chap. 128), respiratory depression, and systolic hypotension. Miosis is common but mydriasis may also be seen. Internuclear ophthalmoplegia has been reported [69]. Paradoxic agitation, delirium, hallucinations, psychosis, and tachypnea may occur [70–73].

In severe cases, high-grade coma with loss of most or all reflexes, apnea, hypotension, and a variety of cardiac dysrhythmias may develop. Bradyarrhythmias include all degrees of atrioventricular (A-V) block, bundle branch block, nonspecific QRS widening, and asystole [21,25–28,74,75,76]. Tachyarrhythmias such as sinus tachycardia, supraventricular and ventricular premature beats, ventricular tachycardia and fibrillation, and *Torsades de pointes* may occur [21,77,78,79]. The latter arrhythmia typically occurs in the setting of Q–T interval prolongation. Occasionally, either hypothermia or hyperthermia may be seen [80]. Rare complications include pulmonary edema and seizures [32,33,70,71]. Although neuroleptic malignant syndrome is rare following acute overdose, hypertension, hyperthermia, and hypertonia have been described [80].

Loxapine poisoning results in an atypical clinical picture. Cardiovascular effects are mild or absent but convulsions are common and often lead to rhabdomyolysis and subsequent renal failure [31,81].

The maximal severity of poisoning is usually apparent within 2 to 6 hours of ingestion. The presentation is the same regardless of age and whether the overdose is acute or chronic. Children appear to be more sensitive than adults to the effects of neuroleptic agents [72]. Early deaths are due to dysrhythmias, shock, aspiration, and respiratory failure. Later complications include cerebral and pulmonary edema, disseminated intravascular coagulation, renal failure, and infection.

A complete history should be obtained from the patient as well as the person(s) who found or brought the patient (to corroborate the patient's history). As with all drug ingestions, the name, quantity, and time of ingestion of the drugs should be determined. In patients who become poisoned during chronic neuroleptic therapy, a recent medication or dose change or an illness may be responsible.

Physical examination should focus on the vital signs, respiratory function, and neurologic status. The patient should be examined for evidence of coexisting trauma. An initial rhythm strip and subsequent 12-lead ECG should be evaluated. Arterial blood gases and a chest radiograph should be ordered in patients with significant CNS depression. An abdominal radiograph showing radiopaque densities in the GI tract may suggest phenothiazine poisoning if the etiology of symptoms is unknown. The absence of this finding, however, does not rule out the possibility of phenothiazine poisoning. Routine laboratory evaluation should include a complete blood count (CBC), electrolytes, BUN, creatinine, and glucose. In patients with seizures, laboratory evaluation should include urinalysis (routine and for myoglobin), creatinine phosphokinase, calcium, magnesium, phosphate, and a coagulation profile.

Toxicologic analysis of the urine and serum by chromatography or immunoassay [82] should be obtained to confirm the identity of the offending agent and to rule out other ingestants. Quantitative drug levels are not helpful in predicting clinical toxicity or guiding treatment. Although neither sensitive nor specific nor readily available, the Forest, Mason, and Phenistix colorimetric tests are rapid urine screens that may be positive with phenothiazine ingestions [83]. These tests will not, however, detect nonphenothiazine neuroleptic agents.

EXTRAPYRAMIDAL SYNDROMES

Acute Dystonic Reactions. Dystonic reactions are characterized by abrupt onset, intermittent and repetitive nature, normal physical examination except for muscular findings, a history of recent drug use, and rapid response to anticholinergic drug therapy [60,63]. Muscle contractions may sometimes be sustained but usually last from seconds to minutes. They may be focal at the onset and then spread to contiguous muscles. Occasionally they are generalized [64]. Patients remain alert and oriented during these reactions.

Although dystonia may occur in any striated muscle, muscle groups in one of five areas are typically affected [60,63–67]. Acute dystonic reactions involving the muscles of the eye (oculogyric crisis) cause upward gazing, rotation of the eyes, and spasm of the lids. Those involving muscles of the tongue and jaw (buccolingual crisis) produce trismus, protrusion of the tongue, dysphagia, dysarthria, and facial grimacing. Contractions of muscles of the neck result in abnormal head positioning (torticollic reactions). Acute dystonic reactions involving the muscles of the back cause arching and twisting of the torso (opisthotonic posturing). When muscles of the abdominal wall are involved, patients present with abdominal wall pain and spasm, bizarre gait patterns, kyphosis, and lordosis (tortipelvic and gait crises). Buccolingual and torticollic ADRs are the most common [60].

Although ADRs are rarely life-threatening, those involving the tongue, jaw, neck, and chest can result in upper airway compromise and impaired respiratory mechanics [68,84]. Stridor can occur in those with buccolingual and torticollic reactions. Death from respiratory failure has been reported [68,85].

The patient should be questioned regarding current medications, previous ADRs, recreational drug use, and change in the dose of a neuroleptic or other medication associated with this syndrome. Dystonic reactions have occurred in drug abusers when Haldol has been confused with Valium, since both pills are similar in size, shape, and markings [61].

Akathisia. Patients with akathisia complain of feeling restless, jittery, and tense and that they cannot sit or stand still [10,62,86]. They are often unable to remain sitting and on standing may shift their weight from foot to foot as if walking in place. Examination may reveal semipurposeful or purposeless limb movements, especially of the legs and feet, frequent shifting of body position, and tremors of myoclonic jerking of the lower extremities. Vital signs are normal. The diagnosis is made on the basis of history of drug exposure and the physical examination.

Parkinsonism. Drug-induced parkinsonism is indistinguishable from other causes of this syndrome except by the history of drug exposure [46,47,48,86,87]. It is characterized by increased motor tone (rigidity), decreased motor activity (bradykinesia, masked facies), tremors (pill rolling) and postural instability [88]. Tremors typically occur in the forearm and hand, are present at rest, worsen with agitation or excitement, and disappear with sleep. Patients may complain of fatigue, stiffness, muscle aches, and incoordination or clumsiness. Examination may also reveal gait disturbances (e.g., shuffling with little or no arm swinging or retropulsion), cogwheel rigidity, limited upward gaze and convergence, positive glabellar, snout, and sucking reflexes. The diagnosis is based on the history and physical examination.

DIFFERENTIAL DIAGNOSIS. Poisoning by antiarrhythmic, anticholinergic, anticonvulsant, opioid, and sedative-hypnotic agents and the veterinary tranquilizer xylazine [89] may cause CNS and cardiovascular effects similar to those resulting from neuroleptic overdosage. It may be impossible to distinguish cyclic antidepressant poisoning from that due to thioridazine or mesoridazine without toxicologic analysis. Central nervous system infection and trauma should also be considered in the differential diagnosis.

The differential diagnosis of an acute dystonic reaction includes primary dystonias, seizures, cerebrovascular accident, encephalitis, tetanus, hypocalcemia, drug intoxication (especially strychnine and anticholinergic poisoning), hysterical conversion reactions, joint dislocations, meningitis, hypomagnesemia, and alkalosis [60,63].

Akasthisia may be misdiagnosed as anxiety or agitation related to an underlying psychiatric disorder.

Other etiologies of parkinsonism include encephalitis, carbon monoxide poisoning, CNS trauma and tumors, and possibly stroke (multiinfarct). Irreversible parkinsonism can occur in intravenous drug abusers exposed to an impurity (MPTP) in illicitly synthesized meperidine [90].

Management

OVERDOSAGE. The majority of patients with acute neuroleptic overdose remain asymptomatic or develop only mild poisoning and do not require hospitalization. All patients who are symptomatic should be observed until they are alert. Those with mild toxicity can often be managed in the emergency department or a similarly equipped observation unit. Those with hypotension, significant CNS depression, seizures, or arrhythmias should be admitted to an ICU. Patients with ECG abnormalities who are otherwise asymptomatic present a difficult disposition problem, since such findings, although they occur with therapeutic doses, have been implicated in sudden death. It seems safest to admit these patients for 24 hours of cardiac monitoring. Patients requiring transfer to a facility capable of providing intensive care should be accompanied by advanced life support personnel and have cardiac monitoring en route. Since treatment may require agents not included in standard advanced cardiac life support system protocols, it is advisable that a physician accompany the patient. Air and ground transportation are appropriate for this type of transfer.

Treatment is primarily supportive. The tempo and sequence of interventions depends on the clinical severity. Advanced life support measures should be instituted as necessary and underlying metabolic abnormalities corrected. All patients require cardiac and respiratory monitoring. Vital signs should be repeated frequently. Endotracheal intubation for airway protection or ventilatory support may be required. Patients with seizures or hyperthermia should have continuous (rectal or axillary probe) temperature monitoring. Those with altered mental status should receive supplemental oxygen and be given a diagnostic trial of naloxone (2 mg IV), dextrose (25 gm IV), and thiamine (100 mg IV). Although reversal of CNS depression following naloxone administration has been reported once [91], such a response is inconsistent with the pharmacology of neuroleptics and should not be expected.

Hypotension should be initially treated with several liters of intravenous normal saline. Norepinephrine and high-dose dopamine are the drugs of choice for refractory hypotension. Central venous, intraarterial, and pulmonary artery pressure monitoring may be necessary for optimal management of patients who are hemodynamically unstable.

Sinus and supraventricular tachycardias rarely require specific treatment. If they are associated with hypotension, correction of this abnormality is often all that is necessary. If these tachycardias are associated with other anticholinergic findings (see Chap. 133) and the QRS duration is normal, physostigmine (1–2 mg IV over 5 minutes) can be given. Ventricular tachyarrhythmias should be treated with lidocaine, phenytoin, and electrical cardioversion, depending on hemodynamic stability. Sodium bicarbonate (1 mEq/kg IV) may be tried if the QRS interval is prolonged. Type IA (i.e., disopyramide, quinidine, procainamide) and type II (i.e., beta-blockers) antiarrhythmic drugs should be avoided. *Torsades de pointes* ventricular tachycardia may respond to magnesium (50–100 mg/kg IV over 1 hour) or an increase in heart rate (overdrive pacing) using isoproterenol or electricity [27,78,92,93,94]. Increasing the heart rate may shorten a prolonged Q–T interval and thus facilitate conversion of this arrhythmia. The blood pressure should be carefully monitored during isoproterenol administration, as it may cause or worsen hypotension. Bradyarrhythmias associated with hemodynamic compromise should be treated with atropine or isoproterenol according to current advanced cardiac life support protocols. Complete heart block may require temporary cardiac pacing.

Seizures should be treated with incremental doses of diazepam or lorazepam (initial dose 0.05–0.1 mg/kg IV) followed by a loading dose of phenytoin (18 mg/kg IV at a maximal rate of 50 mg/min). A short-acting (e.g., amobarbital 10–15 mg/kg IV at a maximal rate of 100 mg/min) or long-acting barbiturate (e.g., phenobarbital, 20 mg/kg IV at a maximal rate of 30 mg/min) may sometimes be necessary. Refractory convulsions, as seen in loxapine poisoning [31,81], may require the use of a paralyzing agent to prevent complications such as hyperthermia and rhabdomyolysis. Since succinylcholine is potentially hazardous in patients with rhabdomyolysis and may itself cause malignant hyperthermia, a nondepolarizing neuromuscular blocker, such as pancuronium (0.06–0.1 mg/kg IV) or vecuronium (0.08–0.1 mg/kg IV), should be used. Continued treatment of seizures, as indicated by EEG monitoring, is necessary during therapeutic paralysis. Diuresis and alkalinization of urine may be useful in preventing myoglobinuric renal failure in patients with rhabdomyolysis (see Chap. 72).

After stabilization, GI decontamination should be performed in patients with acute ingestions. Activated charcoal and gastric lavage are the preferred methods. Because of the risk of aspiration in patients who may develop CNS depression, seizures, and acute dystonic reactions, syrup of ipecac should be reserved for asymptomatic patients who can be treated within 30 minutes of ingestion. Due to decreased GI motility resulting from poisoning, decontamination may be of benefit many hours after overdose. Although clinical improvement was reported during combined hemodialysis and charcoal hemiperfusion [95], the effect was transient and measures to enhance the elimination of neuroleptic agents, such as diuresis, dialysis, and hemoperfusion, have not been shown to be pharmacokinetically effective [95,96,97]. Repeated oral doses of activated charcoal are of potential, but unproved, benefit.

The vast majority of patients with neuroleptic poisoning recover completely within several hours to several days, depending on severity. Patients with intentional overdosage require psychiatric evaluation prior to discharge.

EXTRAPYRAMIDAL SYNDROMES

Acute Dystonic Reactions. Patients with respiratory distress should be given supplemental oxygen. Those with buccolingual and torticollic crises should be given nothing by mouth, since doing so could precipitate choking. In addition, since ADRs rarely result from an overdose, GI decontamination is usually not indicated and may, in fact, be hazardous because of the potential for airway complications.

Administration of an anticholinergic agent readily reverses ADRs, presumably by restoring the balance between cholinergic and dopaminergic pathways in the CNS [98]. Benztropine mesylate (Cogentin) 1 to 2 mg, or diphenhydramine (Benadryl) 50 to 100 mg, given intravenously over 1 to 2 minutes, can be used. Reversal of signs and symptoms usually occurs within a few minutes. In some cases, a second dose is needed for complete resolution. Benztropine appears to be more effective and is less likely to cause sedation and hypotension than diphenhydramine and is the preferred agent in adults [60,99]. Although it is contraindicated in children younger than 3 years of age because of its anticholinergic effects [100], this is precisely the desired effect, and its administration in small doses (e.g., 0.25–0.5 mg) is appropriate in this situation. Alternatively, diphenhydramine (1 mg/kg IV) can be used. Benztropine and diphenhydramine can also be given intramuscularly, but it may take 30 to 90 minutes for the ADR to resolve when this route is used. Acute dystonic reactions caused by metoclopramide can be relatively resistant to anticholinergic therapy. In such cases, administration of a muscle relaxant (e.g., an intravenous benzodiazepine) may be helpful.

Following intravenous therapy, an oral anticholinergic agent should be administered for 48 to 72 hours [98]. Without such therapy, the ADR may recur, since it may take several days to eliminate completely the agent that caused it and the duration of action of therapeutic drugs is much shorter. In addition to benztropine and diphenhydramine, biperiden (Akineton) and trihexyphenidyl (Artane) can be used for oral therapy. For reasons noted above, benztropine (1–2 mg twice per day) is the preferred agent for adults. Children younger than 3 years can be given diphenhydramine (1 mg/kg orally, three or four times per day). Although patients who have had an ADR are at increased risk for future ADRs, those requiring continued neuroleptic therapy can usually continue or resume taking the offending agent provided they are also maintained on anticholinergic therapy. Alternatively, they can be switched to a neuroleptic drug with less dopaminergic-blocking activity.

Akathisia. Patients who develop akathisia following a single therapeutic dose of neuroleptic or related agent should be reassured that the reaction will resolve within 24 hours. Specific therapy is usually not necessary. Akathisia in those who require continued neuroleptic therapy can be managed by reducing the dose of neuroleptic, switching to a lower potency agent (e.g., chlorpromazine, loxapine, thioridazine), or administering additional drug therapy [62,86,101]. If akathisia is accompanied by severe parkinsonism, an anticholinergic agent such as benztropine (see previous sections) may be effective [62]. Propranolol (10 mg orally three times per day) and clonidine (0.1 mg orally three times per day) have also been used successfully [88,102,103]. Propranolol, presumably because of its greater lipophilicity and greater CNS activity, is more effective than less lipophilic beta-blockers (e.g., atenolol, metoprolol, nadolol) [101]. Pindolol, a beta-blocker with intrinsic sympathomimetic activity, can be used in patients in whom propranolol could be hazardous (e.g., those with bradycardia, A-V block, or heart failure) [104]. Clonidine, because of its sedating and hypotensive side effects, is less well tolerated than propranolol [101].

Although benzodiazepines and short-acting barbiturates have also been used, they do not appear to be nearly as effective [62]. Since tolerance to akathisia may develop, drug therapy may be tapered once this side effect is controlled [86].

Parkinsonism. Neuroleptic-induced parkinsonism can be effectively treated by antimuscarinic agents such as benztropine, biperiden, diphenhydramine, and trihexyphenidyl [62,86]. Starting doses are the same as those listed for the treatment of acute dystonic reactions. Higher doses and chronic therapy may be necessary in patients who need continued neuroleptic treatment. Amantadine (Symmetrel), 100–400 mg/day orally, a dopaminergic agonist, is also effective and has fewer side effects [86]. However, its onset of action is slower and it may not be as effective as antimuscarinic agents in controlling rigidity [105].

References

1. Baldessarini RJ: Drugs and the treatment of psychiatric disorders, in Gilman AG, Rall TW, Nies AS, et al (eds): *Goodman and Gilman's The Pharmacological Basis of Therapeutics*. 8th ed. New York, Macmillan, 1990, p 83.
2. Shawn DH, McGuigan MA: Poisoning from dermal absorption of promethazine. *Can Med Assoc J* 130:1460, 1984.
3. McGuigan MA: Phenothiazines. *Clin Toxicol Rev* 3:4, 1981.
4. Zaratzian VL: Psychotropic drugs: Neurotoxicity. *Clin Toxicol* 17:231, 1980.
5. Laposata EA, Hale P, Poklis A: Evaluation of sudden death in psychiatric patients with special reference to phenothiazine therapy: Forensic pathology. *J Forensic Sci* 33:432, 1988.
6. Thorogood M, Cowen P, Mann J, et al: Fatal myocardial infarction and use of psychotropic drugs in young women. *Lancet* 340:1067, 1992.
7. Kahn A, Blum D: Phenothiazines and sudden infant death syndrome. *Pediatrics* 70:75, 1982.
8. Lacoursiere RB, Spohn HE, Thompson K: Medical aspects of abrupt neuroleptic withdrawal. *Compr Psychiatry* 17:285, 1976.
9. Mikkelsen EG, Albert LG, Updahaya A: Neuroleptic-withdrawal cachexia (letter). *N Engl J Med* 398:929, 1988.
10. Black JL, Richelson E: Antipsychotic drugs: Prediction of side effect profiles based on neuroreceptor data derived from human brain tissue. *Mayo Clin Proc* 62:369, 1987.
11. Richelson E: Neuroleptic affinities for human brain receptors and their use in predicting adverse effects. *J Clin Pyschiatry* 45:331, 1984.
12. Baldessarini RJ, Frankenburg FR: Clozapine: A novel antipsychotic agent. *N Engl J Med* 324:746, 1991.
13. Schwarcz G: A rational ordering of the actions of antipsychotic drugs. *J Family Pract* 14:263, 1982.
14. Trayle WH: Phenothiazine-induced agranulocytosis. *JAMA* 256:1957, 1986.
15. Herio T: Chlorpromazine photo-allergy: Co-existence of immediate and delayed type. *Arch Dermatol* 111:1469, 1975.
16. Fishbain DA: Priapism resulting from fluphenazine hydrochloride treatment reversed by diphenhydramine. *Ann Emerg Med* 14:600, 1985.
17. Gomez EA: Neuroleptic-induced priapism. *Texas Med* 81:47, 1985.
18. Gauttieri CT, Powell SF: Psychoactive drug interactions. *J Clin Psychiatry* 39:720, 1978.
19. Alexander HE, McCarty K, Giffen MB: Hypotension and cardiopulmonary arrest associated with concurrent haloperidol and propranolol therapy. *JAMA* 252:87, 1984.
20. Wendkos MH: The significance of electrocardiogenic changes produced by thioridazine. *J New Drugs* 4:322, 1964.
21. Fletcher GF, Kazamias TM, Wenger NK: Cardiotoxic effects of Mellaril: Conduction disturbances and supraventricular arrhythmias. *Am Heart J* 78:135, 1961.
22. Fowler ND, McCall D, Chou T, et al: Electrocardiographic changes

and cardiac arrhythmias in patients receiving psychotic drugs. *Am J Cardiol* 37:223, 1981.

23. Johnson RE, Ware JD, Moffit S, et al: Response to exercise in patients taking psychotropic drugs: Arrhythmias and the QT interval (QT wave peak). *Arch Intern Med* 142:755, 1982.

24. Flugelman MY, Tal A, Pollack S, et al: Psychotropic drugs and long QT syndromes: Case reports. *J Clin Psychiatry* 46:290, 1985.

25. Marris-Simon P, Zell-Kanter M, Kendzlerski D, et al: Cardiotoxic manifestations of mesoridazine overdose. *Ann Emerg Med* 17:1074, 1988.

26. Neimann JT, Stapczynski JS, Rothstein RJ, et al: Cardiac conduction and rhythm disturbances following suicidal ingestion of mesoridazine. *Ann Emerg Med* 10:585, 1981.

27. Trawn BL, Murphy ML: Case report: Successful treatment of ventricular tachycardia associated with thioridazine (Mellaril). *South Med J* 62:357, 1969.

28. Vertrees J, Siebel G: Rapid death resulting from mesoridazine overdose. *Vet Hum Toxicol* 29:65, 1987.

29. Heath A, Svensson C, Martensson E: Thioridazine toxicity: An experimental cardiovascular study of thioridazine and its major metabolites in overdose. *Vet Hum Toxicol* 27:100, 1985.

30. Dorson PG, Crisman ML: Chlorpromazine accumulation and sudden death in a patient with renal insufficiency. *Drug Intell Clin Pharm* 22:776, 1988.

31. Peterson C: Seizures induced by acute loxapine overdose. *Am J Psychiatry* 138:1089, 1981.

32. Mahutte CK, Nakassuto SK, Light RW: Haloperidol and sudden death due to pulmonary edema. *Arch Intern Med* 142:1951, 1982.

33. Li C, Gefter WB: Acute pulmonary edema induced by overdosage of phenothiazines. *Chest* 101:102,1992.

34. McGeer PL, Boulding JE, Gibson WC, et al: Drug-induced extrapyramidal reactions. *JAMA* 177:665, 1961.

35. Thach BT, Chase TN, Bosma JF: Oral facial dyskinesia associated with prolonged use of antihistaminic decongestants. *N Engl J Med* 293:486, 1975.

36. Romisher S, Felter R, Dougherty J: Tagamet-induced acute dystonia. *Ann Emerg Med* 16:1162, 1987.

37. Lavenstein BL, Cantor FK: Acute dystonia, an unusual reaction to diphenhydramine. *JAMA* 236:291, 1976.

38. Joske DJL: Dystonic reaction to azatidine. *Med J Aust* 141:449, 1984.

39. Powers JM: Decongestant-induced blepharospasm and orofacial dystonia. *JAMA* 247:3244, 1982.

40. Lewith GT, Davidson F: Dystonic reaction to Dimetapp elixir. *J Roy Coll Gen Pract* 31:241, 1981.

41. Howrie DL, Rowley AH, Krenzelok EP: Benztropine-induced acute dystonic reaction. *Ann Emerg Med* 15:594, 1986.

42. Choanard IA, Rosenbloom L: Focal dystonic reaction to phenytoin. *Dev Med Child Neurol* 26:677, 1984.

43. Arnstein E: Oculogyric crisis: A distinct toxic effect of carbamazepine. *J Child Neurol* 1:289, 1986.

44. Hicks CB, Abraham K: Verapamil and myocardial dystonia. *Ann Intern Med* 103:154, 1985.

45. DeMedina A, Biasini O, Rivera A, et al: Nifedipine and myoclonic dystonia. *Ann Intern Med* 104:125, 1986.

46. Bateman DN, Rawlins MD, Simpson JM: Extrapyramidal reactions with metoclopramide. *Br Med J* 291:930, 1985.

47. Miller LG, Jankovic J: Metoclopramide-induced movement disorders. *Arch Intern Med* 149:2486, 1989.

48. Gauzini L, Casey DE, Hoffman WF, et al: The prevalence of metoclopramide-induced tardive dyskinesia and acute extrapyramidal movement disorders. *Arch Intern Med* 153:1469, 1993.

49. Gardos G: Undiagnosed dystonic reaction secondary to amoxapine. *Psychosomatics* 25:66, 1984.

50. Kramer MS, Marcus DJ, DiFerdinado J, et al: Atypical acute dystonia associated with trazodone treatment. *J Clin Psychopharmacol* 6:117, 1986.

51. Finder E, Lin KM, Anath S: Dystonic reaction to amitriptyline. *Am J Psychiatry* 139:1220, 1982.

52. Felser JM, Orban DJ: Dystonic reaction after ketamine abuse. *Ann Emerg Med* 11:673, 1982.

53. Shafrir Y, Levy Y, Beharah A, et al: Acute dystonic reaction to bethanechol: A direct acetylcholine receptor agonist. *Dev Med Child Neurol* 28:646, 1986.

54. Moody SB, Terp DK: Dystonic reaction possibly induced by cho-

linesterase inhibitor insecticides. *Drug Intell Clin Pharm* 22:311, 1988.

55. Stahl SM, Berger PA: Bromocriptine, physostigmine, and neurotransmitter mechanisms in the dystonias. *Neurology* 32:889, 1982.

56. Baldessarini RJ, Tarsy D: Dopamine and the pathophysiology of dyskinesis induced by antipsychotic drugs. *Ann Rev Neurosci* 3:23, 1980.

57. Kolbe H, Clow A, Jenner P, et al: Neuroleptic-induced acute dystonic reactions may be due to enhanced dopamine release or to supersensitive postsynaptic receptors. *Neurology* 31:434, 1981.

58. Swett C: Drug-induced dystonia. *Am J Psychiatry* 132:532, 1982.

59. Ayd FJ: A survey of drug-induced extrapyramidal reactions. *JAMA* 175:1054, 1961.

60. Lee AS: Treatment of drug-induced dystonic reactions. *JACEP* 8:453, 1979.

61. Freed E: Alcohol-triggered neuroleptic-induced tremor, rigidity and dystonia. *Med J Aust* 2:44, 1981.

62. Brande WM, Barnes TRE, Gore SM: Clinical characteristics of akathisia: A systematic investigation of acute psychiatric inpatient admissions. *Br J Psychiatry* 143:139, 1983.

63. Feldman V: Serious reactions to phenothiamines. *J Pediatr* 89:163, 1976.

64. Hoffman AS, Schwartz HI, Novick RM: Catatonic reaction to accidental haloperidol overdose: An unrecognized drug abuse risk. *J Nerv Ment Dis* 174:428, 1986.

65. Fahn S: The varied clinical expressions of dystonia. *Neurol Clin* 2:541, 1984.

66. Jeste DV, Wisniewski AA, Wyatt RJ: Neuroleptic-associated tardive syndromes. *Psychiatr Clin North Am* 9:183, 1986.

67. Jankovic J: Drug-induced and other orofacial-cervical dyskinesias. *Ann Intern Med* 94:788, 1981.

68. Pollera CF, Cognetti F, Nardi M, et al: Sudden death after acute dystonic reactions to high-dose metoclopramide. *Lancet* 2:460, 1984.

69. Cook FE, Davis RG, Russo LS: Internuclear ophthalmoplegia caused by phenothiazine intoxication. *Arch Neurol* 38:465, 1981.

70. McKown CH, Verhulst HL, Crotty JJ: Overdose effects and danger from tranquilizing drugs. *JAMA* 185:425, 1963.

71. Barry D, Meyakens FL, Becker CE: Phenothiazine poisoning: a review of 48 cases. *Calif Med* 118:1, 1973.

72. Knight ME, Roberts RJ: Phenothiazine and butyrophenone intoxication in children. *Pediatr Clin North Am* 33:299, 1986.

73. McAllister CJ, Scowden EB, Stone WJ: Toxic psychosis induced by phenothiazine administration in patients with chronic renal failure. *Clin Nephrol* 10:191, 1978.

74. Axelsson R, Aspenstrom G: Electrocardiographic changes and serum concentrations in thioridazine-treated patients. *J Clin Psychiatry* 43:332, 1982

75. Thorton CC, Wendkos MH: EKG T-wave distortions among thioridazine-treated psychiatric inpatients. *Dis Nerv Syst* 32:320, 1971.

76. Elkayan U, Frishman W: Cardiovascular effects of phenothiazines. *Am Heart J* 100:397, 1980.

77. Tri TB, Combs DT: Phenothiazine induced ventricular tachycardia. *West J Med* 123:412, 1975.

78. Lumpkin J, Watanabe AS, Rumack BH, et al: Phenothiazine-induced ventricular tachycardia following acute overdose. *JACEP* 8:746, 1979.

79. Zee-cheng CS, Mueller CE, Seifert CF, et al: Haloperidol and torsades de pointes. *Ann Intern Med* 102:448, 1985.

80. Baker PB, Merigian KS, Roberts JR, et al: Hyperthermia, hypotension, hypertonia, and coma in a massive thioridazine overdose. *Am J Emerg Med* 6:346, 1988.

81. Tam CW, Olin BR, Ruiz AE: Loxapine-associated rhabdomyolysis and acute renal failure. *Arch Intern Med* 140:975, 1980.

82. Baselt RC, Carvey RH: *Disposition of Toxic Drugs and Chemicals in Man*. Chicago, Year Book, 1989.

83. Forrest FM, Forrest IS, Mason AS: Review of rapid urine tests for phenothiazine and related drugs. *Am J Psychiatry* 118:300, 1961.

84. Newton-John H: Acute upper airway obstruction due to supraglottic dystonia inducted by a neuroleptic. *Br Med J* 297:964, 1988.

85. Koek RJ, Edmond HP: Acute laryngeal dystonic reactions to neuroleptics. *Psychosomatics* 30:359, 1989.
86. Black JL, Richelson E, Richardson: Antipsychotic agents: A clinical update. *Mayo Clin Proc* 60:777, 1985.
87. Barbeau A: Parkinson's disease: Clinical features and etiopathology, in Vinton PJ, Bruyn GW, Klawans HL (eds): *Extrapyramidal Disorders: Handbook of Clinical Neurology*. vol. 49. Amsterdam, Elsevier, 1986, pp 87–152.
88. Lipinski JF, Zubenko GS, Barriera P, et al: Propranolol in the treatment of neuroleptic-induced akathisia (letter). *Lancet* 2:685, 1983.
89. Spoerke DG, Hall AH, Grimes MJ, et al: Human overdose with the veterinary tranquilizer xylazine. *Am J Emerg Med* 4:222, 1986.
90. Burns RS, LeWitt PA, Ebert MH, et al: The clinical syndrome of striatal dopamine deficiency: Parkinsonism induced by l-methyl-4-phenyl-1,2,3,6-tetrahydropyridine. *N Engl J Med* 312:1418, 1985.
91. Chandovasu O, Chatkupt S: Central nervous system depression from chlorpromazine poisoning: Successful treatment with naloxone. *J Pediatr* 106:515, 1985.
92. Pietri DA: Thioridazine-associated ventricular tachycardia and isoproterenol. *Ann Intern Med* 94:411, 1981.
93. Kemper A, Dunlop R, Pietro D: Thoridazine-induced torsades de pointes successful therapy with isoproterenol. *JAMA* 249:2931, 1983.
94. Tranum BL, Murphy ML: Successful treatment of ventricular tachycardia associated with thioridazine (Mellaril). *South Med J* 62:357, 1969.
95. Koppel C, Schirop T, Ibe K, et al: Hemoperfusion in chlorprothixene overdose. *Intensive Care Med* 13:358, 1987.
96. Donlon PT, Tupin JP: Successful suicides with thioridazine and mesoridazine. *Arch Gen Psychiatry* 34:955, 1977.
97. Hals PA, Jacobsen D: Resin hemoperfusion in levomepromazine poisoning: Evaluation of effect on plasma drug and metabolite levels. *Hum Toxicol* 3:497, 1984.
98. Corre K, Neimann J, Bessen H: Extended therapy for acute dystonic reactions. *Ann Emerg Med* 13:194, 1984.
99. Baillie GR, Nelson MV, Krenzelok EP, et al: Unusual treatment response of a severe dystonia to diphenhydramine. *Ann Emerg Med* 16:705, 1987.
100. Merck and Company: Cogentin, in *Physician Desk Reference*. Montvale, NJ, Medical Economics, 1993, p 1418.
101. Gelenberg AJ: Treating extrapyramidal reactions: Some current issues. *J Clin Psychiatry* 48 (suppl):24, 1987.
102. Adler L, Angrist B, Peselow E, et al: A controlled assessment of propranolol in the treatment of neuroleptic-induced akathisia. *Br J Psychiatry* 149:42, 1983.
103. Zubenko GS, Cohen BM, Lipinski JF, et al: Use of clonidine in treating neuroleptic-induced akathisia. *Psychiatry Res* 13:253, 1985.
104. Reiter S, Adler L, Erle S, et al: Neuroleptic-induced akathisia treated with pindolol (letter). *Am J Psychiatry* 144:383, 1987.
105. Dimascio A, Bernardo DL, Greenblatt DJ, et al: A controlled trial of amantadine in drug-induced extrapyramidal disorders. *Arch Gen Psychiatry* 33:599, 1976.
106. Kruesi M, Schaik JU: Illicit Haldol. *N Engl J Med* 305:769, 1981.

151. Opiate Overdose

Jay L. Schauben

Although the psychologic effects of opium may have been known as early as 4000 B.C., the first undisputed reference to the juice of the poppy plant appeared around the third century B.C. Opium, harvested from the unripened seed pods of *Papaver somniferum*, has been found to contain a myriad of alkaloidal substances. Of these, only morphine, codeine, and papaverine have proved medical utility. In time, we learned to manipulate the morphine and thebaine nucleus chemically to produce many other useful semisynthetic analgesic-anesthetic agents. Later, totally synthetic and structurally unrelated compounds were manufactured in the laboratory to imitate the pharmacologic properties of the traditional opium derivatives.

According to recent Drug Enforcement Administration (DEA) reports, the production of illegal street drugs by domestic clandestine laboratories is still on the rise. A 300 percent increase in the amount of dangerous drugs seized and a 60 percent increase in the number of street drug laboratories raided were reported between 1986 and 1988. In 1988, 810 clandestine laboratories operating in the United States were closed. Street chemists have produced exceedingly potent and toxic drugs as new manufacturing methods have been developed to circumvent the use of controlled or unavailable precursor compounds. Some of these drugs are field tested for the first time on the unsuspecting buyer. As government authorities place these products and their starting ingredients on the controlled substance list, new drugs and methods are "designed" to take their place [1].

We sometimes forget that street drug abuse does not always involve legitimately made and pharmaceutically pure compounds. In fact, a large share of today's street drugs are produced by these clandestine operations. We are not, therefore, dealing with the simple abuse of a specific substance, but rather with a wide variety of active ingredients, adulterants, and contaminants. The clinical syndromes seen in the abuser may be related either partly or wholly to these variables.

Pharmacology and Toxicology of Opiates

The opiate and opiatelike substances rely on their ability to interact with opiate receptors in the central nervous system (CNS) to produce their analgesic, euphoric, and sedative effects. On the basis of animal experiments, Martin et al. [2] proposed the existence of three opioid receptors in the CNS. Selective interaction with these receptors, designated mu, kappa, and sigma, produces variable degrees of pharmacologic effect (Table 151-1) [2–6]. Stimulation of the mu receptor results in miosis, analgesia, euphoria, and respiratory depression, whereas kappa receptor interaction results in analgesia and sedation. Dysphoria, delusions, and other psychogenic effects result from activation of the sigma receptor.

PHARMACOKINETICS AND PHARMACODYNAMICS. Most opioid analgesics are well absorbed from the gastrointes-

Table 151-1. Opiate Receptor System

	Mu	Kappa	Sigma

Agonists	Morphine
	Morphinelike
	  analgesics
		Pentazocine
		Nalorphine
		Cyclazocine
		Morphinelike
		  analgesics (?)
		Levallorphan (?)
			Pentazocine
			Cyclazocine
			Nalorphine
			Levallorphan (?)

Clinical effects	Analgesia Euphoria Respiratory depression Miosis	Analgesia Sedation Miosis	Dysphoria Delusions Hallucinations
Antagonists	Pentazocine Cyclazocine Nalorphine Naloxone Naltrexone Nalmefene	Naloxone Naltrexone Nalmefene	Naloxone Naltrexone Nalmefene

Adapted from Handel KA, Schauben JL, Salamone FR: Naloxone. *Ann Emerg Med* 12:438, 1983.

tinal (GI) tract as well as from various other sites of administration (e.g., musosal sites such as in the nose, pulmonary capillaries, intramuscular sites, and subcutaneous sites). Analgesia usually begins promptly following parenteral administration and within 15 to 30 minutes after oral dosing. Peak plasma levels are generally attained within 1 to 2 hours following therapeutic oral doses; however, acute toxic ingestions may produce pylorospasm and decreased peristalsis, resulting in prolonged absorption [3]. Therapeutic and toxic serum drug concentrations are not well established for the narcotic analgesics and thus play little more than a confirmatory role in management of opiate toxicity.

All of the opioids undergo hepatic biotransformation, including hydroxylation, demethylation, and glucuronide conjugation. Considerable first-pass metabolism accounts for the wide variations in oral bioavailability noted with compounds such as morphine and pentazocine. Only small fractions of free (parent) drug are excreted unchanged in the urine. Active metabolites contributing to the toxicologic profile of specific agents are discussed below. The major pharmacokinetic parameters for each compound are summarized in Chapter 215.

PHYSIOLOGIC AND PATHOPHYSIOLOGIC EFFECTS OF OPIATES.
In general, a drug classified as an opiate, or opioid-like, elicits the same overall physiologic effects as morphine, the prototype of this group. However, there are conspicuous differences noted among these agents.

Central Nervous System Effects. Administration of morphine in therapeutic amounts (5–10 mg) produces analgesia, usually without loss of consciousness, drowsiness, changes in mood, or mental clouding. Sometimes dysphoria rather than euphoria is manifest, resulting in mild anxiety or a fear reaction [3]. Nausea is frequently encountered, whereas vomiting is observed occasionally [3]. As one would expect, these effects become more pronounced as the dosage is increased (15–20 mg). Analgesia is stronger, lethargy and drowsiness progress to sleepiness, the euphoric and GI effects are accentuated, and the respiratory depressive effects are more pronounced. Slurred speech and significant motor incoordination are customarily absent [3].

Morphine and most of its congeners cause miosis in humans, the exact mechanism of which has not been clearly elucidated. Following overdose with the opioids, pupillary constriction is marked (predominantly a central effect) and is considered pathognomonic, with the exception of meperidine use and possibly with propoxyphene use, in the case of a mixed intoxication, or when metabolic or structural disorders are the result of respiratory depression-induced hypoxia [3].

Respiratory Effects. The most renowned side effect or toxic reaction from opiate administration is respiratory depression. Even in small doses, morphine depresses respiration by directly affecting the brainstem respiratory centers [3]. A decrease in both minute and alveolar ventilation occurs as a result of the depressant effects [7]. Arterial blood gas findings usually reflect hypoventilation: elevated partial pressure of carbon dioxide ($PaCO_2$), decreased arterial oxygen tension (PaO_2), and normal alveolar-arterial oxygen tension difference ($P(A-a)O_2$). The effect is dose-related, increasing progressively with escalation in dose. A reduction in responsiveness of the respiratory centers to an increase in carbon dioxide tension ($PaCO_2$) is the most generally accepted mechanism, although pontine and medullary effects are also postulated [3,7]. Respiratory rate and minute volume may be unreliable as indicators of the degree of respiratory depression in light of significantly altered CO_2 sensitivity of the respiratory center [3]. The peak respiratory depressant effect is usually noted within 7 minutes of intravenous morphine administration, but it may be delayed up to 30 minutes if the drug is administered intramuscularly [3]. Normal carbon dioxide sensitivity usually returns within 2 to 3 hours, while minute volume may remain considerably below normal for up to 4 to 5 hours following a therapeutic dose [3,8].

Cardiovascular Effects. Therapeutic doses of the opiates have little effect on heart rate, heart rhythm, or blood pressure [3]. Because the ability to accommodate to positional change is altered by peripheral vasodilatation, peripheral venous pooling, orthostatic hypotension, and fainting may occur in some patients [3,7]. Endogenous histamine release is the postulated cause of this peripheral vasodilatation. Even after a toxic dose, blood pressure is usually maintained if the patient remains supine. If the patient is allowed to hypoventilate, hypotension ensues, mainly as a result of hypoxia [3]. Cerebral circulation does not appear to be altered by the therapeutic administration of morphine, unless respiratory depression and carbon dioxide retention result in cerebral vasodilatation [7].

Gastrointestinal Effects. Morphine and related agents are known to cause a decrease in GI motility, delaying the passage of gastric contents through the duodenum up to 12 hours [3]. Propulsive contractions in the small and large intestines may also be markedly decreased. This may translate into a significantly prolonged absorption phase for an ingested overdose.

SEMISYNTHETIC AND SYNTHETIC OPIATES
Heroin. Produced from the diacetylation of morphine, heroin has two to five times the analgesic potency of morphine, with similar effects on the CNS [9]. Virtually all street heroin in the United States is produced in clandestine laboratories and therefore considered to be adulterated prior to use (Table 151-2). The purity of heroin on the street varies between 5 and 90 percent. Fatalities in the chronic user are very often due to the wide variation in potency [10]. Physiologically, the effects of

Table 151-2. Common Heroin Adulterants

Mannitol	Antipyrine
Dextrose	Boric acid
Lactose	Mercurous salts
Talc	Animal manure
Sodium bicarbonate	Cocaine
Quinine	Amphetamine
Strychnine	Methamphetamine
Caffeine	Barbiturates
Phenacetin	Flour
Procaine	Magnesium sulfate
Lidocaine	Antihistamines
Benzocaine	Phencyclidine
Tetracaine	

heroin administration are identical to those described for morphine. A 10-mg intravenous dose in a nonabusing adult produces miosis, drowsiness, respiratory depression, and small reductions in heart rate, blood pressure, and body temperature [11,12]. The drug can be administered intravenously or intranasally (snorted) and may be mixed with other drugs of abuse (e.g., amphetamine or cocaine for "speedballing"). Interindividual variation in sensitivity and tolerance makes correlation of serum levels with clinical symptoms difficult. Fatal overdoses with heroin have been reported with morphine serum levels as low as 0.1 and as high as 1.8 μg per milliliter [13].

The initial heroin "rush" is purportedly due to its high lipid solubility and rapid penetration of the blood-brain barrier [9]. The half-life of heroin in the plasma is only 5 to 15 minutes. The majority of its lasting effects are attributable to its metabolites 6-monoacetylmorphine (6-MAM) and morphine [14]. Initially deacetylated in the liver and plasma, it is renally excreted as a conjugate, with small amounts of morphine, diacetylmorphine, and 6-MAM also present [14].

The incidence of pulmonary edema among heroin overdose patients is reportedly 50 to 67 percent, resulting in death in 3 to 9 percent of these cases [15]. Interestingly, postmortem studies of patients who succumbed to heroin-induced pulmonary edema have revealed no gross cardiac pathologic findings [16]. The onset of the edema appears quite variable [17], and it is because of the possibilities of delayed onset and of recurrent respiratory depression that many clinicians recommend admission and/or observation for 24 hours or more. Smith et al. [18] have recently challenged these guidelines, advocating an observation period of 2 to 4 hours in pure intravenous heroin overdoses. In their series, hypoxic encephalopathy and pulmonary edema either were evident on admission or developed within 20 minutes of emergency department presentation. The mechanism for the increase in permeability of the alveolar capillary membranes remains controversial. Among the suggested hypotheses for the effect are profound hypoxemia secondary to heroin-induced hypoventilation and coma, hypersensitivity reactions, immune complex deposition in the alveolar capillary membrane, neurogenic manifestations, transient lymphatic pumping irregularities, and histamine-induced leakage [19–24].

Codeine. Codeine (methylmorphine), frequently prescribed for its potent analgesic and antitussive properties, is marketed as a sole ingredient and in combination with aspirin or acetaminophen. Fatal ingestions with codeine alone are rare, and it does not appear to be as commonly abused as some of the other opioid congeners. Nevertheless, illicit use and dependency has been described. Codeine's influence on the CNS is comparable, but less pronounced, than that of morphine. Codeine overdose manifests more CNS hyperirritability than does either morphine or heroin and may produce a mixture of stupor and delirium [3].

A dose of 120 mg of intramuscular codeine is equivalent in analgesic potency to 10 mg of morphine. It is rapidly and effectively absorbed by the oral route, producing a peak plasma level within 45 minutes to 1 hour of a therapeutic dose [25]. An estimated intravenous dose of 750 to 900 mg of codeine phosphate has been reported to produce symptoms similar to those seen with acute heroin overdose [26]. An approximate lethal dose in a nonabuser has been estimated to be 800 mg, with serum codeine levels ranging from 0.14 to 4.8 mg per 100 milliliters [27,28]. Although 15 mg per kilogram has been tolerated by children, 5 mg per kilogram may produce serious respiratory depression.

The major pathway of excretion involves metabolism and conjugation by the liver, with approximately 10 percent of the dose metabolized to morphine [29]. Both codeine and morphine may be detected in the urine within 24 to 72 hours after a codeine ingestion. Only morphine is found after approximately 96 hours [25]. A large number of deaths have been attributed to a street substitute for heroin that combined codeine and glutethimide [30].

Oxycodone. Oxycodone is a semisynthetic analog of codeine with considerably greater potency. It is available as a single entity or in combination with aspirin or acetaminophen. Ten to 15 mg of oxycodone has an analgesic potency comparable to that of 10 mg of morphine [3]. Oxycodone blood levels are barely detectable after a therapeutic dose, with the major metabolite noroxycodone found in the urine [31]. The abuse potential of oxycodone is thought to be significant, and clinical manifestations following significant acute ingestions parallel those outlined for codeine.

Hydromorphone. Administered parenterally or orally, hydromorphone elicits the same characteristic opioid syndrome in acute overdose as the other congeners in this group. It is reportedly associated with a significantly higher incidence of respiratory depression, hypotension, and coma when compared with morphine, codeine, or methadone, suggesting a greater toxic potential in comparison to other parenterally used narcotics [32].

Fentanyl. Fentanyl is a synthetic opioid of the phenylpiperidine class, with a potency approximately 200 times that of morphine [3]. Legitimate use is limited almost exclusively to anesthesia, and it is known to be commonly abused by hospital personnel. Large doses have produced muscular rigidity and seizures [33,34]. The recently marketed fentanyl transdermal delivery system presents an interesting facet to the management of toxic manifestations arising from the misuse or abuse of this product. The transdermal system establishes depot of drug in the upper skin layers, where it is then available for systemic absorption. On removal of the patch, and as with many of the transdermal delivery systems, drug absorption from the dermal reservoir continues. Consequently, the half-life of fentanyl following removal of the transdermal system is approximately 17 hours [35], versus 2 to 4 hours associated with the intravenous route. In these patients, the practitioner should expect a longer duration of pharmacologic or toxic effects and therefore rely on either repeated doses or continuous infusions of naloxone to maintain the desired degree of opiate antagonism.

Designer Fentanyl Derivatives. One of the more common groups of designer agents is related to the anesthetic-analgesic fentanyl. By manipulation of the chemical structure, alpha-methyl-fentanyl (China White), 3-methyl-fentanyl, and para-fluoro-fentanyl were produced and distributed on the street as heroin substitutes. These agents are 200 to 3000 times more potent than heroin [1]. More than 100 deaths from 3-methyl-fentanyl alone have been reported, primarily the result of minor errors in the measurement of dosage [36,37]. Government authorities found that alpha-methyl-acetyl-fentanyl, alpha-methyl-fentanyl acrylate, and benzyl fentanyl were synthesized with potencies up to 6000 times that of morphine. Since 1981 the DEA has identified at least nine fentanyl analogs.

Meperidine. Meperidine is a synthetic member of the phenylpiperidine class, chemically dissimilar to the traditional opiates. Although considered to possess strong analgesic properties when given by the parenteral route (80–100 mg equivalent to 10 mg of morphine), it is less than one-half as effective if given by the oral route [3,31,38]. It appears to be a common drug of abuse among medical personnel [39,40,41], yet there are few reports of meperidine poisoning or fatalities. Equianalgesic doses produce the same degree of sedation and euphoria as morphine, but meperidine has an increased propensity for dysphoric and hallucinogenic episodes as well as the ability to produce CNS excitation, tremors, muscle twitching, mydriasis and seizures with toxic doses [3,31,38,42,43,44]. A peak plasma level is reached approximately 1 minute following intravenous injection, 30 minutes after intramuscular administration, and approximately 1 to 2 hours following an oral dose [38]. The duration of action of meperidine is rather short (2–4 hours) in comparison to morphine [3,38].

Meperidine is metabolized primarily by N-demethylation to normeperidine, an active metabolite with approximately one-half the analgesic and euphoric potency of its parent but nearly twice the convulsant properties [3,45,46]. The seizures reported with meperidine overdose or abuse have been attributed to the accumulation of normeperidine, with a prolonged elimination half-life of 14 to 21 hours [3,38,42,45–49]. Repetitive meperidine abuse or acute ingestion of a large dose favors a high ratio of normeperidine to meperidine, producing a picture of mixed stupor and convulsions [3,42,44]. Meperidine and normeperidine may be detected in either urine or serum [50]. Excretion is primarily through the kidneys as conjugated metabolites [50].

Designer Meperidine Derivatives. Meperidine is the prototype for another series of potent street homologs. Methyl-phenyl-propionoxypiperidine (MPPP), a synthetic analog of meperidine, has been used as a heroin substitute. A new approach to its clandestine manufacture inadvertently produced MPPP contaminated with methyl-phenyl-tetrahydropyridine (MPTP). This contaminant led to an epidemic of parkinsonism among intravenous drug abusers within several days of repeated injections [51,52,53]. Hundreds of users are believed to have been exposed to MPTP and have various degrees of this irreversible drug-induced disease.

Diphenoxylate. Diphenoxylate is a meperidine congener with strong constipating effects. Its use, therefore, has been limited to the treatment of diarrhea. In therapeutic doses, the drug is devoid of morphinelike effects; higher doses (40–60 mg) invoke typical opioid activity [3]. This drug appears to be particularly toxic to children [54–59] with as little as 0.5 to 6 tablets causing serious toxicity [55,56]. Fatal ingestions have occurred with as little as 1.2 mg per kilogram in children [57]. Diphenoxylate (2.5 mg) is formulated with 0.025 mg of atropine sulfate (Lomotil),

which, following an overdose, often results in mild to moderate anticholinergic activity in addition to the opiate effects [3]. Symptoms arising from a toxic ingestion may be delayed up to 30 hours, owing to the anticholinergic-induced reduction in GI motility. For the same reason, symptoms may recur 24 to 36 hours after initial presentation.

Methadone. Methadone is a synthetic opioid with potent analgesic effects, used commonly for detoxification or maintenance of an opiate addict. It is frequently diverted from legal channels, accounting for the majority of acute opiate overdoses in certain areas of the United States [60,61]. Its analgesic, sedative, euphoric, and respiratory depressive effects are comparable to those seen with analogous doses of morphine [62,63]. As little as 40 to 50 mg may produce coma and respiratory depression in a nontolerant adult [64,65]. It is well absorbed orally, producing a peak plasma level within 2 to 4 hours of oral administration and a peak effect within 1 to 2 hours [66]. It differs from morphine in that it has an exceptionally prolonged duration of action [67]. The half-life averages 25 hours, with durations up to 52 hours reported during long-term maintenance therapy [68]. This translates into a serious and protracted course (24–48 hours) following an overdose [67]. Methadone and its inactive metabolite (an N-demethylated pyrolidine) may be detected in either urine or plasma [64].

Propoxyphene. Propoxyphene is structurally related to methadone. It was once the most commonly prescribed drug in the United States and is still widely used today for the treatment of mild to moderate pain [69]. It is available alone or in combination with aspirin or acetaminophen. Though once considered relatively harmless, propoxyphene has been involved in a large number of toxic ingestions that resulted in significant morbidity and mortality [70–74]. Oral administration is followed by rapid absorption, with peak levels achieved in the plasma in approximately 1 hour [75]. The clinical course following an overdose may be severe and rapidly progressive, with seizures and/or respiratory arrest developing within 15 to 45 minutes [76]. The plasma half-life of propoxyphene is approximately 6 to 12 hours. In contrast, the active metabolite norpropoxyphene exhibits a half-life of approximately 37 hours [77,78] and is the primary metabolic product excreted in the urine [79]. Norpropoxyphene's long duration of action is thought to play a role in the prolonged course seen after ingestion of toxic quantities [73].

The clinical picture following an acute large ingestion is similar to that seen with other opioid substances [76], with 180 mg causing the equivalent respiratory depression of 60 mg of codeine [80]. As little as 650 to 975 mg may be lethal in the untreated nontolerant adult, whereas chronic abusers may tolerate as much as 2600 mg per day [3,73]. Blood levels in fatal overdose have ranged from 0.1 to 2.5 mg per 100 milliliters [71]. In addition to opioid effects, propoxyphene intoxication has been associated with both focal and generalized seizures [3,76,81]. It also appears that norpropoxyphene and possibly propoxyphene may be directly cardiotoxic, producing nonspecific S–T and T wave abnormalities, widened QRS complexes with idioventricular rhythm, bigeminy, and bundle branch block [81–84].

Pentazocine. Pentazocine, a compound of the benzomorphan class, is a synthetic nonopiate analgesic developed as part of an effort to find an effective analgesic with little or no abuse potential [3,85]. Despite this original aspiration, pentazocine has been involved heavily in the drug abuse trade and is usually associated with significant toxicity [85]. In combination with the antihistamine tripelennamine (Pyribenzamine), forming a street product known as "T's and Blues," pentazocine was injected intravenously as a substitute for heroin [86]. Manifestations arising from acute overdosage of this combination have included the usual clinical syndrome of opiate intoxication as well as dyspnea, hyperirritability, mild to moderate hypertension, and seizures. It is believed that these effects may in fact be directly related to the dose of tripelennamine [86,87,88].

In an attempt to curtail its misuse further, Winthrop Laboratories reformulated their oral tablet (Talwin) in January 1983 to contain 0.5 mg of naloxone (Talwin-NX). The naloxone would presumably negate all opiatelike effects if the compound were used parenterally; in fact, it has resulted in the precipitation of a withdrawal reaction in opiate-addicted individuals [67]. It should be noted, however, that the duration of action of pentazocine exceeds that of the naloxone, and delayed respiratory depression may occur. If the tablet is ingested, the naloxone is rendered inactive.

Pentazocine has both agonist and weak antagonist activity at the opioid receptors, possessing about one-third the analgesic potency of morphine [3,85]. Orally administered, pentazocine achieves peak plasma levels within 1 hour [3,89] and is extensively metabolized in the liver [85,89], with the parent compound and metabolites detectable in either urine or plasma [85]. The physiologic effects associated with pentazocine administration are similar to those of morphine, with 30 to 50 mg of pentazocine equal in analgesic potency to 10 mg of morphine [3,85]. Anxiety, dysphoria, and hallucinations are reportedly more common with pentazocine than with any of the opiate derivatives [85].

Dextromethorphan. Dextromethorphan, an analog of codeine, is the principal component in a myriad of nonprescription cough and cold remedies. The predominant antitussive effect is generally attributed to the active metabolite dextrorphan, produced by first-pass hepatic metabolism [90]. Therapeutically, the duration of effect ranges from 3 to 6 hours, with a corresponding plasma half-life of 2 to 4 hours. Although rarely implicated in serious toxic human exposures, large ingestions may produce restlessness, hyperexcitability, mydriasis, and clonus, while extremely high doses result in the typical CNS and respiratory depression associated with opiate intoxication [91–96]. It has been suggested that ingestions of 10 mg per kilogram or more may produce prolonged CNS depression [94].

Within the therapeutic dosing range, dextromethorphan lacks analgesic, euphoriant, and physical dependence-producing properties [97]. Nevertheless, reports of dextromethorphan abuse have appeared sporadically over the past three decades, with references made to the appearance of psychologic rather than a physiologic dependence syndrome [97]. Abusers describe increased perceptual awareness, altered time perception, and visual hallucinations [98]. Easy over-the-counter access has been recounted as the primary reason for its popularity, although its abuse pattern seems to be self-limiting due to the development of undesirable effects, such as lethargy, somnambulism, and ataxia, after a few weeks of abuse [98].

Dextromethorphan is well absorbed from the GI tract, with peak plasma levels occurring 2.5 and 6 hours after ingestion of regular or sustained-release preparations, respectively. Any patient responding to naloxone administration should be observed for a minimum of 4 to 6 hours to determine whether further naloxone dosing is necessary. Since dextromethorphan is frequently found in combination with other active ingredients in cough and cold preparations, the contribution of these coingestants should be considered in assessing overdose or abuse

cases and in the degree of responsiveness to administration of naloxone.

Clinical Manifestations of Opiate Overdose

Coma, respiratory depression, miosis, and pulmonary edema are the hallmarks of opiate intoxication, with the magnitude of toxicity dependent on the dose and individual degree of tolerance. In general, the clinical effects encountered after an overdose with any one of the agents in this class are similar, although some very important differences between certain agents do exist. Large ingestions very often result in a prolonged clinical course, a result of the opiate-induced decrease in GI motility [67].

Miosis is considered a universal finding in opiate intoxication, unless severe acidemia, hypoxemia, or hypotension is present. If the offending agent is meperidine, diphenoxylate-atropine (Lomotil), or a mixed overdose with an anticholinergic or sympathomimetic drug, mydriasis may predominate [67]. Likewise, CNS depression is regarded as pathognomonic for opiate overdose, but codeine, meperidine, and dextromethorphan intoxications are noted for their ability to cause CNS hyperirritability, resulting in a mixed syndrome of stupor and delirium [3]. Meperidine may also manifest muscular twitching, spasticity, and tachypnea [3,32,38].

Pulmonary edema may complicate the clinical course of opiate overdose and is especially prevalent with heroin [99,100], codeine [27,28,101,102,103], methadone [104–107], and propoxyphene [82]. It may present within 2 hours of parenteral heroin use [108], up to 4 hours following intranasal heroin use [109], or up to 24 hours following significant oral methadone ingestion [110]. In most patients the lungs are initially clear to auscultation. Arterial blood gases usually reflect a moderate to severe hypoxemia and hypercapnia, with a mixed respiratory and metabolic acidosis [86,99]. Chest radiographs typically reveal bilateral fluffy alveolar infiltrates, occasionally unilateral in nature, and echo findings usually associated with pneumonia [100]. Normal capillary wedge pressures and slightly elevated pulmonary arterial pressures are seen with heroin-induced pulmonary edema [110]. In contrast, elevated systemic, pulmonary arterial, and pulmonary capillary wedge pressures as well as total peripheral resistance are seen with pentazocine intoxication [112,113]. This effect is believed to result from transient endogenous catecholamine release. Chest radiographs usually resolve within 24 to 48 hours in the recovering patient [67]. Significant pulmonary findings persisting beyond this time may indicate aspiration or bacterial pneumonitis, with atelectasis, fibrosis, bronchiectasis, granulomatous disease, or pneumomediastinum also possible [114]. It appears the injury is directed at the alveolar-capillary membrane, resulting in manifestations consistent with acute respiratory distress syndrome [102,115].

Common adulterants used in the manufacture of street opiates have long been recognized as potential pulmonary toxins. The injection of magnesium trisilicate (talc), a common additive, has produced granulomatosis in small pulmonary arteries [87,88,116,117,118], resulting in pulmonary hypertension and acute cor pulmonale [87,88,109]. Dyspnea, hypoxemia, and the presence of multiple reticulonodular infiltrates on chest film may in fact be directly caused by the presence of adulterants in the intravenous mixture used by chronic abusers [87,88,116–119]. A summary of the potential abuse-related pulmonary effects appears in Table 151-3.

Table 151-3. Common Pulmonary Problems Associated with Opiate Abuse

Pulmonary arteritis (cotton)
Pulmonary thrombosis (talc)
Pulmonary hypertension (talc)
Septic emboli
Lung abscess
Bacterial pneumonia
Aspiration pneumonitis
Pulmonary edema
Atelectasis
Respiratory arrest

Seizures and other focal neurologic signs are usually absent with opiate intoxication [120]. Convulsions could indicate the presence of a brain abscess [121] or subarachnoid hemorrhage [122], proconvulsive adulterants, or the chronic abuse-overdose of meperidine [3,45], propoxyphene [76,81], pentazocine (T's and Blues) [86], or fentanyl [34]. Meperidine-induced seizures are believed to be caused by the accumulation of the metabolite normeperidine and are often preceded by myoclonus, are of limited duration, respond to conventional therapy, and resolve on discontinuing meperidine abuse [42,47,48,49]. Propoxyphene-induced seizures have a similar presentation and may be related to norpropoxyphene accumulation. Both become more frequent in patients who chronically use meperidine or propoxyphene and have evidence of renal insufficiency. Propoxyphene seizures may respond to naloxone therapy.

Hypotension may be present in significant opiate overdose; pentazocine intoxication may manifest mild to moderate hypertension [86]. Acute changes in the electrocardiogram have been noted with heroin and propoxyphene. Nonspecific S–T segment and T wave changes [82], first-degree atrioventricular (A-V) block [116], atrial fibrillation [119], prolonged Q–T intervals, and ventricular dysrhythmias [81,83,84,123] have been reported. These cardiovascular findings may be the result of metabolic derangements associated with hypoxia [116], a direct effect of the abused agent, or possibly a reflection of the influence of common adulterants (e.g., quinine) found in street drugs [124].

The clinical course of an acute overdose may be complicated by rhabdomyolysis, severe hyperkalemia, myoglobinuria, and acute renal failure [125–128]. Three possible etiologies for this renal damage have been proposed: direct insult by the abused substance, adulterants found in the street drugs, and prolonged coma [125,126,127]. Acute tubular necrosis, a result of rhabdomyolysis and myoglobinuria, has been associated with impure heroin as well as prolonged seizure activity [129,130]. Rhabdomyolysis has occurred with intravenous, inhalational, and intranasal heroin abuse [131]. Glomerulonephritis and renal amyloidosis have occurred with parenteral opiate abuse and have been associated with concurrent bacterial infections [128,132].

Laboratory abnormalities, such as those described in the preceding discussion, reflect the primary and secondary toxic effects of opiate intoxication. The severity of these abnormalities correlates with variables such as dose, individual sensitivity, chronicity of exposure, prehospital course, and the specifics of therapeutic intervention. The chronic abuser may have elevations in creatine phosphokinase (CPK) (10,000–50,000 units/L), proteinuria, myoglobinuria, and urine sediment suggestive of acute renal tubular necrosis. Of interest, false-positive tests for syphilis have been reported with parenteral opioid abuse [67].

Although a discussion of the numerous infectious disorders common to the drug abuser (Table 151-4) is beyond the scope of this chapter, appropriate diagnostic studies and therapies geared to correct such problems are part of the total treatment plan.

Treatment

A diagnosis of opioid poisoning must be considered in all comatose patients, keeping in mind that the classic triad of opiate toxicity (coma, miosis, and respiratory depression) may be confounded by coingestion of other drugs. Resuscitation and stabilization of vital signs demand immediate attention. If protective airway reflexes are diminished or absent, tracheal intubation should accompany the routine administration of oxygen. Intravenous access should be established, and the patient should be placed on a cardiac monitor. Vital signs, including body temperature, need to be monitored frequently because rapid deterioration in clinical status may occur without warning. The empiric administration of a "coma cocktail" is the standard of care for patients presenting with coma of unknown etiology. Twenty-five to 50 gm of 50% dextrose is administered intravenously (if rapid bedside serum glucose evaluation is not available) along with 100 mg thiamine parenterally. Naloxone, the third component of the cocktail, can reverse the analgesia, respiratory depression, miosis, hyporeflexia, cardiovascular effects, and pulmonary edema associated with opiate toxicity [133]. It is also effective in terminating apomorphine-induced vomiting. Initially 2 to 4 mg is administered to adults (1–2 mg to children). Smaller doses can be used initially (0.1–0.5 mg) if the patient is known to be opiate-tolerant. Larger doses may precipitate withdrawal. If there is historical evidence of an opiate ingestion or parenteral exposure, a strong suspicion based on presenting symptoms, or a partial response to the initial naloxone dose, naloxone administration (IV bolus) is continued. Lack of response to approximately 10 mg is required to rule out the diagnosis of narcotic intoxication. Extremely high doses of naloxone are often required to antagonize methadone, pentazocine, propoxyphene, and diphenoxylate [134]. Administration of naloxone need not be delayed if intravenous access is not readily available. Intralingual, endotracheal, and perhaps intraosseous administration are acceptable alternatives [134,135,136]. Intramuscular and subcutaneous injections are less desirable in the emergent situation. Repeat bolus doses may be required every 20 to 60 minutes, due to the short half-life of naloxone (45–60 minutes) compared with that of most opiates. Flumazenil, a benzodiazepine antagonist, may be con-

Table 151-4. Common Infectious Problems in Intravenous Drug Abusers

Endocarditis	Aspergillosis
Bacterial meningitis	Cutaneous abscess
Mycotic aneurism	Cellulitis
Brain abscess	Lymphangitis
Subdural abscess	Lymphadenitis
Epidural abscess	Phlebitis
Viral hepatitis	Wound botulism
Tetanus	Osteomyelitis
AIDS	

AIDS = acquired immunodeficiency syndrome.

sidered in patients who fail to respond to the aforementioned agents after due consideration is given to the possibility of serious cyclic antidepressant poisoning or for chronic benzodiazepine use or abuse. Although physostigmine was once used for its "nonspecific arousal" effects in altered mental status patients, its use today is reserved for severe, life-threatening anticholinergic toxicity.

Hypotension not responsive to naloxone should be managed with Trendelenburg positioning, fluid administration, and vasopressors. Successive fluid boluses should be used with caution without adequate assessment of pulmonary capillary wedge pressure or central venous pressure, especially in light of the propensity for pulmonary edema in the overdosed patient.

Adult suicide attempts frequently involve multiple drugs. The clinician should persist in the identification of all possible coingestants. Prescription narcotics are often mixed with acetaminophen (Percocet, Tylox) or aspirin (Percodan). Alternative history sources, such as family or friends, should be employed to elicit as much history as possible concerning prior drug usage and current drug availability. The relative amounts of different opioids required to induce toxic effects vary due to differences in bioavailability, individual sensitivity, tolerance, and rates of metabolism. When there is doubt about the amount ingested, the worst-case scenario should always be assumed and management should be based on clinical findings rather than a possibly unreliable history.

Efforts to prevent further absorption of an orally administered drug are necessary once the vital signs have been stabilized. Gastric lavage (with protected airway) is the method of choice to empty the stomach. There is no role for ipecac-induced emesis in the hospitalized patient. Gastric emptying should be followed by administration of activated charcoal and cathartic. The benefits of multiple oral doses of activated charcoal are unproved in opiate poisoning, but charcoal is theoretically beneficial in light of the prolonged absorption phase usually encountered with opiate overdoses. Patients must be closely monitored for continued presence of bowel sounds and passing of charcoal-laden stool. Repeat charcoal doses should not be used in the absence of active bowel sounds or in the presence of an ileus. The use of a cathartic more than once or twice daily may do more harm than good.

A continuous infusion of naloxone should be considered in patients who (1) have a positive but inadequate response to the initial bolus dose, (2) require repeated bolus doses because of recurrent respiratory depression, or (3) are intoxicated with poorly antagonized (propoxyphene) or long-acting (methadone) drugs [138,139]. The current recommendation is to administer two-thirds of the initial reversal bolus dose hourly as an infusion. One-half of the initial reversal dose is repeated (IV bolus) 15 minutes after the infusion is started. For example, the IV bolus dose required to reverse opiate effects in a patient is determined to be 6 mg. An infusion consisting of 40 mg of naloxone in 1000 ml of 5% dextrose or normal saline is started at 100 ml per hour (4 mg/hr). Three mg of naloxone is administered IV push 15 minutes after the infusion is started. Hemodynamics should be closely monitored to avoid a net positive fluid balance. The naloxone infusion is titrated to the patient's clinical status, aiming for adequate reversal of hypoventilation. It is often desirable to maintain a mild degree of sedation to assist in the management of disruptive patients. Infusions can usually be tapered after several hours but may be needed for as long as 24 to 65 hours for long-acting drugs [140].

Naloxone has proved to be safe and effective, with minimal side effects. Up to 24 mg has been administered IV with no untoward effects [141]. Doses of 50 to 100 mg have been used in endorphin-mediated shock and spinal cord ischemia protocols. However, naloxone does not antagonize the convulsant effects of normeperidine, and addicted patients may be subject to the precipitation of narcotic withdrawal. Naloxone may antagonize norpropoxyphene-induced seizures [142]. A relative contraindication to the use of naloxone as part of the altered mental status protocol exists in the pregnant addict, in whom precipitation of the narcotic withdrawal state may induce premature labor or miscarriage. That does not preclude its use for severe respiratory depression or arrest in these patients. As a rule, addicts should receive 0.1- to 0.5-mg incremental doses of naloxone, with observation and titration for adequacy of respiratory effort. In the event of acute withdrawal, administration of additional opiates should be avoided. They invariably outlast the relatively short-acting antagonist, resulting in further CNS depression as the naloxone dose wears off in 20 to 45 minutes.

Naloxone-induced pulmonary edema has been receiving a moderate amount of attention in the recent literature [143–149]. The association of naloxone administration with the development of this adverse effect is somewhat controversial but appears to predominate in patients undergoing anesthesia with multiple agents and those with preexisting cardiac disease. Nevertheless, this reaction has also been described in healthy individuals. The consensus of opinion would seem to implicate a central release of endogenous catecholamines arising as a consequence of the rapid reversal of opioid analgesia, which in turn effects a sympathetic overdrive response [143,144,145,149]. A "neurogenic" form of pulmonary edema [145], a currently undescribed effect of naloxone on peripheral opiate receptors [149], and an unknown drug interaction [149] have also been suggested as possible causes. Of interest, naloxone administration does not appear to alter the vascular permeability of the lung directly [150]. Comparison of the incidence of pulmonary edema with the current rate of naloxone usage in altered mental status and overdose patients indicates that the safety profile of naloxone is still quite impressive.

The diagnostic interpretation of a positive response to naloxone in the comatose patient should be made with caution. Naloxone has been shown to reverse partially and inconsistently the CNS depression associated with exposure to ethanol, benzodiazepines, clonidine, and chlorpromazine [133,151,152,153]. Although a lack of response to an adequate naloxone trial should virtually rule out narcotic coma, a positive response may suggest several etiologies.

Other (partial) antagonists, such as nalorphine and levallorphan, are no longer recommended. Naltrexone is a potent, long-acting pure opiate antagonist that is effective orally. Its use is primarily limited to adjunctive therapy for the detoxification of an opiate addict trying to maintain an opiate-free state. It should not be used in the emergency department to reverse opioid effects in an addicted patient. Naltrexone can induce signs and symptoms of withdrawal lasting 72 hours.

Nalmefene, a currently investigational pure opiate antagonist, may also prove very useful for the reversal of opioid-induced CNS effects. Its half-life and dose-dependent duration of action are considerably longer than those of naloxone at 4 to 8 hours following IV administration [154,155]. Nalmefene, unlike naloxone, is also effective when administered orally. It has proved both safe and effective in its ability to reverse meperidine-induced sedation [156] and opiate overdose [157] in the emergency department. The principal advantage over naloxone is its considerably longer duration of antagonistic action, which translates into fewer complications arising from fluctuations in the level of consciousness, reduced incidence of resedation, better long-term control of longer-acting opiate ingestions, and fewer indications for naloxone infusions. Unfortunately, any withdrawal syndrome precipitated by the use of nalmefene would also be prolonged in nature. Nalmefene should not be used in addicted patients in the emergency department unless the patients will be observed for the duration of nalmefene's action. Discharged patients may attempt to override the opioid antagonism with larger and potentially longer acting opioids, resulting in respiratory depression after the nalmefene effect abates.

Pulmonary edema should be managed with oxygen, naloxone, and positive-pressure ventilation as needed. Inotropic agents and preload and afterload reducing agents appear to be of little value. Resolution in the recovering patient usually occurs within 2 to 4 days.

Seizures associated with propoxyphene toxicity should be treated with naloxone and standard anticonvulsant therapy. Normeperidine-induced seizure activity is usually short-lived, but repeated or prolonged seizures require short-term anticonvulsant therapy. Refractory seizures should suggest the possibility of multiple drug or toxin effects. For those agents with significant anticholinergic activity (e.g., Lomotil, antihistamine additives and substitutes), a trial of physostigmine may be indicated if seizures prove refractory to conventional therapy.

Observation and general supportive care are still the most important principles in the management of a drug overdose. Opiate serum levels are usually not warranted or helpful in the therapeutic plan. A general urine drug screen is usually not necessary in the naloxone-responsive patient with pure opiate intoxication. Forced diuresis, alteration of urine pH, and extracorporeal methods of drug removal are likewise not indicated.

Patients who require antagonist therapy for reversal of respiratory depression should be admitted to the hospital for a minimum of 24 hours. Those patients requiring naloxone infusions should be placed in a monitored setting and observed for at least 6 to 8 hours after the infusion is discontinued. Children who ingest any amount of diphenoxylate (Lomotil) need to be observed in an intensive care unit for at least 24 hours, regardless of symptoms [158].

References

1. Buchanan JF, Brown C: Designer drugs: A problem in clinical toxicology. *Med Toxicol* 3:1, 1988.
2. Martin WR, Eades CG, Thompson JA, et al: The effects of morphine and nalorphine-like drugs on the non-dependent and morphine-dependent chronic spinal dog. *J Pharmacol Exp Ther* 197:517, 1976.
3. Jaffe JH, Martin WR: Opioid analgesics and antagonists, in Gillman AG, Goodman LS, Rall TW (eds): *The Pharmacological Basis of Therapeutics,* 7th ed. New York, Macmillan, 1985, p 491.
4. Gilbert PE, Martin WR: The effects of morphine and nalorphine-like drugs in the non-dependent, morphine-dependent and cyclazocine-dependent chronic spinal dog. *J Pharmacol Exp Ther* 198:66, 1976.
5. Stoetling RK: Opiate receptors and endorphins: Their role in anesthesiology. *Anesth Analg (Cleve)* 59:874, 1980.
6. Snyder SH: The opiate receptor or morphine-like peptides in the brain. *Am J Psychiatry* 155:645, 1978.
7. Eckenhoff JE, Oech SR: The effects of narcotics and antagonists upon respiration and circulation in man. *Clin Pharmacol Ther* 1:483, 1960.
8. Eckenhoff JE, Helrich M, Hege M, et al: Respiratory hazards of opiates and other narcotic analgesics. *Surg Gynecol Obstet* 101:701, 1958.
9. Lasagna L: The clinical evaluation of morphine and its substitute as analgesic. *Pharmacol Rev* 16:47, 1964.
10. Louria DB, Hensle T, Rose J: The major medical complications of heroin addiction. *Ann Intern Med* 67:1, 1967.
11. Elliott HW, Parker KD, Wright JA, et al: Actions and metabolism of heroin administered by continuous intravenous infusion to man. *Clin Pharmacol Ther* 12:806, 1971.
12. Tress K, El-Sobsky A: Cardiovascular, respiratory and temperature responses to intravenous heroin (diamorphine) in dependent and nondependent humans. *Br J Clin Pharmacol* 10:477, 1980.
13. Nakamura GR: Toxicologic assessments in acute heroin fatalities. *Clin Toxicol* 13:75, 1978.
14. Boerner U, Abbott S, Roc RL: The metabolism of morphine and heroin in man. *Drug Metab Rev* 4:39, 1975.
15. Duberstein JL, Kaufman DM: A clinical study of an epidemic of heroin intoxication and heroin-induced pulmonary edema. *Am J Med* 51:704, 1971.
16. Lesry SB, Grimes ET: Pulmonary edema and heroin overdose in Vietnam. *Arch Pathol* 95:330, 1973.
17. Allen T: Narcotics, in Rosen P, Baker FJ, Barken RM, et al (eds): *Emergency Medicine.* St Louis, CV Mosby, 1988, pp 2125–2140.
18. Smith DA, Leake L, Loflin JR, et al: Is admission after intravenous heroin overdose necessary? *Ann Emerg Med* 21:1326, 1992.
19. Paranthaman SK, Khan F: Acute cardiomyopathy with recurrent pulmonary edema and hypotension following heroin overdosage. *Chest* 69:117, 1976.
20. Steinberg AD, Karliner JS: The clinical spectrum of heroin pulmonary edema. *Arch Intern Med* 122:122, 1968.
21. Duberstein JL, Kaufman KM: A clinical study of an epidemic of heroin intoxication and heroin induced pulmonary edema. *Am J Med* 31:704, 1971.
22. Halpern M, Rho YM: Deaths from narcotics in New York City. *NY State Med J* 66:2391, 1966.
23. Brecker WM: *Licit and Illicit Drugs.* Boston, Little, Brown, 1972, pp 101–114.
24. Smith WR, Glauser FL, Dearden LC, et al: Deposits of immunoglobulin and complement in the pulmonary tissue of patients with "heroin lung." *Chest* 73:471, 1978.
25. Soloman MD: A study of codeine metabolism. *Clin Toxicol* 7:255, 1974.
26. Huffman DH, Ferguson RL: Acute codeine overdose: Correspondence between clinical course and codeine metabolism. *Johns Hopkins Med J* 136:183, 1975.
27. Wright JA, Baselt R, Hine CH: Blood codeine concentrations in fatalities associated with codeine. *Clin Toxicol* 8:457, 1975.
28. Peat MA, Sengupta A: Toxicological investigations of cases of death involving codeine and dihydrocodeine. *Forensic Sci* 9:21, 1977.
29. Adler TK, Fukimotot JM, Way EL, et al: The metabolic fate of codeine in man. *J Pharmacol Exp Ther* 114:251, 1955.
30. Bailey DN, Shaw RF: Blood concentrations and clinical findings in nonfatal and fatal intoxications involving glutethimide and codeine. *Clin Toxicol* 23:557, 1985.
31. Weinstein SH, Gaylord JC: Determination of oxycodone in plasma and identification of a major metabolite. *J Pharm Sci* 68:827, 1978.
32. Miller RR, Jick HJ: Clinical effects of parenteral narcotics in hospitalized medical patients. *J Clin Pharmacol* 20:165, 1978.
33. Sokoll MD, Hoyt JL, Gergis SD: Studies in muscle rigidity, nitrous oxide, and narcotic analgesic agents. *Anesth Analg* 51:16, 1972.
34. Safwat AM, Daniel D: Grand mal seizure after fentanyl administration. *Anesthesiology* 59:78, 1983.
35. Product information: Duragesic, fentanyl. Piscataway, NJ, Janssen Pharmaceutica, 1991.
36. Ayers WA, Starsiak MJ, Sokolay P: The bogus drug: Three methyl and alpha methyl fentanyl sold as "china white." *J Psychedelic Drugs* 13:91, 1981.
37. Brittain JL: China white: The bogus drug. *J Toxicol Clin Toxicol* 19:1123, 1982.
38. Stambaugh JE, Wainer IW, Sanstead JK, et al: The clinical pharmacology of meperidine: Comparison of routes of administration. *J Clin Pharmacol* 16:245, 1976.
39. Putnam PL, Ellinwood EH: Narcotic addiction among physicians: A ten-year follow-up. *Am J Psychiatry* 122:745, 1966.
40. Ward CF, Ward GC, Saidman CJ: Drug abuse in anesthesia training programs: A survey, 1970–1980. *JAMA* 250:922, 1983.
41. Green RC, Carrol GJ, Buxton WD: Drug addiction among physicians: The Virginia experience. *JAMA* 235:1372, 1976.
42. Goetting MG: Neurotoxicity of meperidine. *Ann Emerg Med* 14:1007, 1985.

43. Morisy L, Platt D: Hazards of high dose meperidine. *JAMA* 255:467, 1986.

44. Kaiko R, Foley K, Heidrich G, et al: Normeperidine plasma levels and central nervous system irritability in cancer patients. *Fed Proc* 37:568, 1978.

45. Miller JW, Anderson HH: The effect of N-demethylation on certain pharmacologic actions of morphine, codeine, and meperidine in the mouse. *J Pharmacol Exp Ther* 112:191, 1954.

46. Hershley LA: Meperidine and central neurotoxicity. *Ann Intern Med* 98:548, 1983.

47. Mauro VF, Bonfiglio NF, Spunt AL: Meperidine-induced seizures in patients without renal dysfunction or sickle cell anemia. *Clin Pharm* 5:837, 1986.

48. Kaiko RF, Foley KM, Grabinski PY, et al: Central nervous system excitatory effects of meperidine in cancer patients. *Ann Neurol* 13:180, 1983.

49. Tang R, Shimomura SK, Rotblatt M: Meperidine-induced seizures in sickle cell patients. *Hosp Form* 15:764, 1980.

50. Mather LE, Tucker GT, Pglug AE, et al: Meperidine kinetics in man-intravenous injection in surgical patients and volunteers. *Clin Pharmacol Ther* 17:21, 1977.

51. Ballard PA, Tetrud JW, Lanston JW: Permanent human parkinsonism due to 1-methyl-4-phenyl-1,2,3,6-tetrahydropyridine (MPTP): Seven cases. *Neurology* 35:949, 1985.

52. Burns RS, LeWitt PA, Edbert MH, et al: The clinical syndrome of striatal dopamine deficiency: Parkinsonism induced by 1-methyl-4-phenyl-1,2,3,6-tetrahydropyridine (MPTP). *N Engl J Med* 312:1418, 1985.

53. Langston JW, Irwin I, Langston EB, et al: Chronic parkinsonism in humans due to a product of meperidine-analog synthesis. *Science* 219:979, 1983.

54. Rumack BH, Temple AP: Lomotil poisoning. *Pediatrics* 53:495, 1975.

55. Wasserman GS, Green VA, Wise GW: Lomotil ingestions in children. *Am Fam Physician* 11:93, 1975.

56. Henderson W, Psaila A: Lomotil poisoning. *Lancet* 1:306, 1969.

57. Ginsberg CM, Angle CR: Diphenoxylate-atropine (Lomotil) poisoning. *Cin Toxicol* 19:377, 1969.

58. Penfold P, Volans GN: Overdose from Lomotil. *Br Med J* 2:1401, 1977.

59. Curtis JA, Goel KM: Lomotil poisoning in children. *Arch Dis Child* 54:222, 1979.

60. Aronow R, Brenner SL, Wooley PV: An apparent epidemic: Methadone poisoning in children. *Clin Toxicol* 6:175, 1973.

61. Persky VW, Goldfrank LR: Methadone overdoses in a New York City hospital. *JACEP* 5:111, 1976.

62. Kreek MJ: Medical complications in methadone patients. *Ann NY Acad Sci* 311:110, 1978.

63. Norris JV, Don HF: Prolonged depression of respiratory rate following methadone analgesia. *Anesthesiology* 45:361, 1976.

64. Garriott JC, Sturner WQ, Mason MT: Toxicologic findings in six fatalities involving methadone. *Clin Toxicol* 6:163, 1973.

65. Gordon E: Treatment of methadone poisoning (letter). *JAMA* 220:728, 1972.

66. Berkowitz BA: The relationship of pharmacokinetics to pharmacological activity: Morphine, methadone and naloxone. *Clin Pharmacokinet* 1:219, 1976.

67. Goldfrank LR, Kulig K: Opioids/Opioid Antagonists (Management/treatment protocol), in Rumack BH (ed): *POISINDEX Information System.* Denver, Micromedex (edition expires 2/28/90).

68. Anggard E, Nilsson M, Holmstrand J, et al: Pharmacokinetics of methadone. *Eur J Clin Pharmacol* 16:53, 1979.

69. McBay AJ, Hudson P: Propoxyphene overdose deaths (letter). *JAMA* 233:1257, 1975.

70. Dougherty RJ: Propoxyphene overdose deaths (letter). *JAMA* 235:2716, 1976.

71. Sturner WQ, Garrioutt JC: Deaths involving propoxyphene: A study of 41 cases over a two-year period. *JAMA* 223:1125, 1973.

72. Hudson P, Barringer M, McBay AJ: Fatal poisoning with propoxyphene: Report from 100 consecutive cases. *South Med J* 70:938, 1977.

73. Baselt RC: *Disposition of Toxic Drugs and Chemicals in Man.* 2nd ed. Davis, CA, Biomedical Publications, 1982, p 670.

74. Carson DJL, Carson ED: Fatal dextropropoxyphene poisoning in Northern Ireland: Review of 30 cases. *Lancet* 1:894, 1977.

75. Wolen RL, Guber CM, Kiplinger GF, et al: Concentration of propoxyphene in human plasma following oral, intramuscular and intravenous infusion. *Toxicol Appl Pharmacol* 19:480, 1971.

76. Tennant FS: Complication of propoxyphene abuse. *Arch Intern Med* 132:191, 1973.

77. Gram LF, Schon J, May WL, et al: d-Propoxyphene kinetics after single oral and intravenous doses in man. *Clin Pharmacol Ther* 26:473, 1979.

78. Wolen RL, Zieye EA, Gurber CM: Determination of propoxyphene and norpropoxyphene by chemical ionization mass fragmentography. *Clin Pharmacol Ther* 17:15, 1975.

79. Verbely K, Inturrisi CE: Disposition of propoxyphene and norpropoxyphene in man after a single oral dose. *Clin Pharmacol Ther* 15:302, 1973.

80. Bellville JW, Seed JC: A comparison of the respiratory depressant effects of dextropropoxyphene and codeine in man. *Clin Pharmacol Ther* 9:428, 1968.

81. McCarthy WH, Keenan RL: Propoxyphene hydrochloride poisoning: A report of the first fatality. *JAMA* 187:460, 1964.

82. Bogartz LJ, Miller WC: Pulmonary edema associated with propoxyphene intoxication. *JAMA* 215:259, 1971.

83. Gary NE, Maher JF, DeMyttenaere MH, et al: Acute propoxyphene hydrochloride intoxication. *Arch Intern Med* 121:453, 1968.

84. Gustafson A, Gustafson B: Acute poisoning with dextropropoxyphene. *Acta Med Scand* 200:241, 1976.

85. Brogden RN, Speight TM, Avery GS: Pentazocine: A review of its pharmacological properties, therapeutic efficacy and dependence liability. *Drugs* 5:6, 1973.

86. Debard ML, Jagger JA: T's and B's: Midwestern heroin substitute. *Clin Toxicol* 18:1117, 1981.

87. Bhargavra HN: Mechanism of toxicity and rationale for use of the dependent subjects. *Clin Toxicol* 18:175, 1981.

88. Farber HW, Falls R, Glauser FL: Transient pulmonary hypertension from the intravenous injection of crushed, suspended pentazocine tablets. *Chest* 80:178, 1981.

89. Ehrnebo M, Boreus LO, Lonroth U: Bioavailability and first-pass metabolism of oral pentazocine in man. *Clin Pharmacol Ther* 22:888, 1977.

90. Silvasti M, Karttunen P, Tukiainen H, et al: Pharmacokinetics of dextromethorphan and dextrorphan: A single dose comparison of three preparations in human volunteers. *Int J Clin Pharmacol Ther Toxicol* 25:493, 1987.

91. Schneider SM, Michelson EA, Boucek CD, et al: Dextromethorphan poisoning reversed by naloxone. *Am J Emerg Med* 9:237, 1991.

92. Katona B, Watson S: Dextromethorphan danger (letter). *N Engl J Med* 314:993, 1986.

93. Shaul WL, Wandell M, Robertson WO: Dextromethorphan toxicity: Reversal by naloxone. *Pediatrics* 59:117, 1977.

94. Devlin KM, Hall AH, Smolinske SC, et al: Toxicity from long-acting dextromethorphan preparations (abstract). *Vet Hum Toxicol* 27:296, 1985.

95. Benson WM, Stefko PL, Randall LO: Comparative pharmacology of levorphan, racemorphan, and dextrorphan and related methyl ethers. *J Pharmacol Exp Ther* 109:189, 1953.

96. Pender ES, Parks BR: Toxicity with dextromethorphan-containing preparations: A literature review and report of two additional cases. *Pediatr Emerg Care* 7:163, 1991.

97. Bem JL, Peck R: Dextromethorphan: An overview of safety issues. *Drug Saf* 7:190, 1992.

98. McCarthy JP; Some less familiar drugs of abuse. *Med J Aust* 20:1078, 1971.

99. Dubenstein JL, Kaufman DM: A clinical study of an epidemic of heroin intoxication and heroin-induced pulmonary edema. *Am J Med* 51:704, 1971.

100. Jaffe RB, Koschmann EB: Intravenous drug abuse: Pulmonary, cardiac and vascular complications. *Am J Roentgenol* 109:107, 1970.

101. Pearson MA, Poklis A, Morrison RR: A fatality due to the ingestion of (methylmorphine) codeine. *Clin Toxicol* 15:267, 1979.

102. Sklar J, Timms RM: Codeine-induced pulmonary edema. *Chest* 72:230, 1977.

103. Winek CL, Collom WD, Wecht CH: Codeine fatality from cough syrup. *Clin Toxicol* 3:97, 1970.

104. Frand UI, Shim CS, Williams MH: Methadone-induced pulmonary edema. *Ann Intern Med* 76:975, 1972.

105. Schaaf JT, Spivack ML, Rath GS, et al: Pulmonary edema and adult respiratory distress syndrome following methadone abuse. *Am Rev Respir Dis* 107:1047, 1973.

106. Zyroff J, Slovis TL, Nagler J: Pulmonary edema induced by oral methadone. *Radiology* 112:567, 1974.

107. Presant S, Knight L, Klassen G: Methadone-induced pulmonary edema. *Can Med Assoc J* 113:966, 1975.

108. Duberstein JL, Kaufman DM: A clinical study of an epidemic of heroin intoxication and heroin-induced pulmonary edema. *Am J Med* 51:704, 1971.

109. Steinberg AD, Karlinger JS: The clinical spectrum of heroin pulmonary edema. *Arch Intern Med* 122:122, 1968.

110. Wilen SB, Ulreich S, Rabinowitz JG: Roentgenographic manifestations of methadone-induced pulmonary edema. *Radiology* 114:51, 1975.

111. Gopiathan K, Sajoja J, Speare R, et al: Hemodynamic studies in heroin induced acute pulmonary edema. *Circulation* 61(suppl III):44, 1970.

112. Lee G, DeMaria AN, Amsterdam EA, et al: Comparative effects of morphine, meperidine and pentazocine on cardiocirculatory dynamics in patients with acute myocardial infarction. *Am J Med* 60:949, 1976.

113. Tammisto T, Jaattela A, Nikki P, et al: Effect of pentazocine and pethidine on plasma catecholamine levels. *Ann Clin Res* 3:22, 1971.

114. Glassroth J, Adams GD, Schnoll S: The impact of substance abuse on the respiratory system. *Chest* 91:596, 1987.

115. Katz S, Aberman A, Frand UI, et al: Heroin pulmonary edema: Evidence for increased pulmonary capillary permeability. *Am Rev Respir Dis* 106:472, 1972.

116. Glauser FL, Downie RL, Smith WR: Electrocardiographic abnormalities in acute heroin overdosage. *Bull Narc* 29:85, 1977.

117. Pare JA, Fraser RG, Hogg JC, et al: Pulmonary mainline granulomatosis: Talcosis on intravenous methadone abuse. *Medicine* 58:229, 1979.

118. Sieniewicz, Nidecker AC: Conglomerate pulmonary disease: A form of talcosis in intravenous methadone abusers. *Am J Roentgenol* 135:697, 1980.

119. Labi M: Paroxysmal atrial fibrillation in heroin intoxication. *Ann Intern Med* 71:951, 1969.

120. Sternbach G, Moran J, Eliastam M: Heroin addiction: Acute presentation of medical complications. *Ann Emerg Med* 9:161, 1980.

121. Amine ARL: Neurosurgical complications of heroin addiction: Brain abscess and mycotic aneurysm. *Surg Neurol* 7:385, 1977.

122. Citron BP, Halpern M, Haverback BJ: Necrotizing angiitis associated with drug abuse: A new clinical entity. *Clin Res* 19:181, 1971.

123. Lipski J, Stimmel B, Donoso E: The effect of heroin and multiple drug abuse on the electrocardiogram. *Am Heart J* 86:663, 1973.

124. Perry DC: Heroin and cocaine adulteration. *Clin Toxicol* 8:239, 1975.

125. Pearce CJ, Cox JGC: Heroin and hyperkalemia. *Lancet* 2:923, 1980.

126. Richter RW, Challenor YN, Person J, et al: Acute myoglobinemia associated with heroin addiction. *JAMA* 216:1172, 1971.

127. Schwatzfarb D, Singh G, Marcus D: Heroin-associated rhabdomyolysis with cardiac involvement. *Arch Intern Med* 137:1255, 1977.

128. Cunningham EE, Zielenzny MA, Venuto RC: Heroin-associated nephropathy. *JAMA* 250:2935, 1983.

129. Nicholls K, Niall JF, Moran JE: Rhabdomyolysis and renal failure. *Med J Aust* 2:387, 1982.

130. Krige LP, Milne FJ, Margolius DA, et al: Rhabdomyolysis and renal failure: Unusual complications of drug abuse. *S Afr Med J* 64:253, 1983.

131. D'Agostino RS, Arnett EN: Acute myoglobinuria and heroin snorting. *JAMA* 241:277, 1979.

132. Dubrow A, Mittman N, Ghali V, et al: The changing spectrum of heroin-associated nephropathy. *Am J Kidney Dis* 5:36, 1985.

133. Handal KA, Schauben JL, Salamone FR: Naloxone. *Ann Emerg Med* 12:438, 1983.

134. Goldfrank LR: The several uses of naloxone. *Emerg Med* May 30:105, 1984.

135. Maio RF, Gaukel B, Freeman B: Intralingual naloxone injection for narcotic-induced respiratory depression. *Ann Emerg Med* 16:572, 1987.

136. Tandberg D, Abercrombie D: Treatment of heroin overdose with endotracheal naloxone. *Ann Emerg Med* 11:443, 1982.

137. O'Sullivan GF, Wade DN: Flumazenil in the management of acute drug overdosage with benzodiazepines and other agents. *Clin Pharmacol Ther* 42:254, 1987.

138. Goldfrank LR, Weisman RS, Errick JK, Lo MW: A dosing nomogram for continuous infusion intravenous naloxone. *Ann Emerg Med* 15:566, 1986.

139. Lewis JM, Klein-Schwartz W, Benson BE, et al: Continuous naloxone infusion in pediatric narcotic overdose. *Am J Dis Child* 138:944, 1984.

140. Romac DR: Safety of prolonged, high dose infusion of naloxone hydrochloride for severe methadone overdose. *Clin Pharm* 5:251, 1986.

141. Evans LE, Swainson CP, Roscoe P, et al: Treatment of drug overdosage with naloxone, a specific narcotic antagonist. *Lancet* 1:452, 1973.

142. Fiut RE, Picchioni AL, Chin L: Antagonism of convulsive and lethal effects induced by propoxyphene. *J Pharm Sci* 55:1085, 1966.

143. Flacke JW, Flacke WE, Williams GD: Acute pulmonary edema following naloxone reversal of high-dose morphine anesthesia. *Anesthesiology* 47:376, 1977.

144. Schwartz JA, Koenigsberg MD: Naloxone-induced pulmonary edema. *Ann Emerg Med* 16:1294, 1987.

145. Prough DS, Roy R, Bumgarner J: Acute pulmonary edema in healthy teenagers following conservative doses of intravenous naloxone. *Anesthesiology* 60:484, 1984.

146. Brimacombe J, Archdeacon J, Newell S, et al: Two cases on naloxone-induced pulmonary oedema: The possible use of phentolamine in management. *Anaesth Intensive Care* 19:578, 1991.

147. Olsen KS: Naloxone administration and laryngospasm followed by pulmonary edema. *Intensive Care Med* 16:340, 1990.

148. Taff RH: Pulmonary edema following naloxone administration in a patient without heart disease. *Anesthesiology* 59:576, 1983.

149. Pallasch TJ, Gill CJ: Naloxone-associated morbidity and mortality. *Oral Surg* 52:602, 1981.

150. Silverstein JH, Gintautas J, Tadoori P, et al: Effects of naloxone on pulmonary capillary permeability. *Prog Clin Biol Res* 328:389, 1990.

151. Jeffreys DB, Flanagan RJ, Volans GN: Reversal of ethanol-induced coma with naloxone. *Lancet* 1:308, 1980.

152. Kulig K, Duffy J, Rumack BH, et al: Naloxone for treatment of clonidine overdose. *JAMA* 247:1697, 1982.

153. Chandavasu O, Chatkupt S: Central nervous system depression from chlorpromazine poisoning: Successful treatment with naloxone. *J Pediatr* 106:515, 1985.

154. Dixon R, Howes J, Gentile J, et al: Nalmefene: Intravenous safety and kinetics of a new opioid antagonist. *Clin Pharmacol Ther* 39:49, 1986.

155. Gal TJ, Difazio CA: Prolonged antagonism of opioid action with intravenous nalmefene in man. *Anesthesiology* 64:175, 1986.

156. Barsan WG, Seger D, Danzl D, et al: Duration of antagonistic effects of nalmefene and naloxone in opiate-induced sedation for emergency department procedures. *Am J Emerg Med* 7:155, 1989.

157. Kaplan J, Marx J: Effectiveness and safety of intravenous nalmefene for emergency department patients with suspected narcotic overdose: A pilot study. *Ann Emerg Med* 22:187, 1993.

158. Rumack BH, Temple AR: Lomotil poisoning. *Pediatrics* 53:495, 1974.

152. Phencyclidine and Hallucinogens

Margaret M. McCarron

Overview

Phencyclidine (PCP) and psychedelic drugs such as lysergic acid diethylamine (LSD) are DEA Schedule 1 Controlled Substances often categorized as hallucinogens. Phencyclidine is best characterized, however, as a dissociative anesthetic. It produces a variety of alterations in consciousness and behavior, with hallucinations occurring in only about 10 percent of users [1]. In contrast, psychedelic agents intensify or distort sensory perception and commonly evoke hallucinations. Visual hallucinations caused by PCP are typically concrete and realistic (e.g., a blue fish), whereas those caused by psychedelic drugs are characteristically nebulous, rapidly changing, and unreal (e.g., streaks and blobs of color, kaleidoscopic multicolored shifting patterns). There are also significant differences between PCP and the psychedelic agents in the mechanism of toxicity, clinical effects, and treatment.

Phencyclidine

Phencyclidine is phenyl-cyclohexyl-piperidine, a synthetic compound chemically related to ketamine. It decreases pain perception and can produce anesthesia. It is a stimulant-type street drug used to obtain a "high." Phencyclidine may act on multiple chemical sites in the brain, and the resulting clinical effects are unpredictable. There are four major and five minor clinical patterns of PCP intoxication, and some patients may experience more than one pattern during an episode of intoxication. Treatment is aimed at counteracting cerebral stimulation and providing supportive care. Patients with major patterns of intoxication may have serious medical complications, including metabolic acidosis, seizures, rhabdomyolysis, and renal failure. Cardiac arrest may occur. Malignant hyperthermia with liver necrosis [2] and fatal hypertensive crisis [3] have been reported. Intracerebral hemorrhage may result from severe hypertension or concomitant head trauma. Death can occur from PCP toxicity or trauma sustained during intoxication.

AVAILABLE FORMS/USE. Phencyclidine has both an acid and an alkaloidal form. The acid form (PCP HCl) is a white crystalline substance sold as "angel dust" or incorporated into tablets. This form is usually taken orally or injected intravenously (IV); since it deteriorates when heated, PCP HCl is not suitable for smoking. Phencyclidine alkaloid is a grayish white amorphous powder, also called angel dust, which is smoked after incorporation into a marijuana or tobacco cigarette. More often, the alkaloid is dissolved in a liquid hydrocarbon and applied to the wrapper of a tobacco cigarette (e.g., More or Sherman brands). Many PCP-laced cigarettes contain only a few drops of PCP but some are saturated with it, making estimates of dosage impossible. Phencyclidine alkaloid is occasionally ingested or injected IV. In either form, PCP is odorless and nonvolatile. The ether-like odor surrounding some patients who have used PCP is the smell of the volatile hydrocarbon used to dissolve PCP alkaloid.

Several analogs of PCP are occasionally used as street drugs: PCE (cyclohexamine), PCPP (phenylcyclopentylpiperidine), PHP (phenylcyclohexylpyrrolidine), and TCP (thienylcyclohexylpiperidine). These analogs have pharmacologic actions so similar to those of PCP that they cannot be distinguished clinically. In addition, street PCP samples may be contaminated with 1-piperidinocyclohexane-carbonitrile (PCC), a toxic precursor of PCP that is more potent than PCP and capable of generating cyanide [4], although the clinical significance of this is unknown.

PHARMACOLOGY. The pharmacology of PCP has been extensively studied and many mechanisms of action have been identified. Phencyclidine acts by binding to various areas of the brain, with binding characteristics that differ from one area to another [5]. A principal action of PCP is antagonism at the dopamine type 2 receptor [6], thereby increasing the available dopamine in the brain by blocking the reuptake of dopamine and/or interfering with dopamine release by presynaptic dopaminergic neurons. Phencyclidine also releases catecholamines from brain neurons [7] and blocks sodium and potassium channels in brain cells [8]. There is evidence that PCP interferes with central serotonin activity [9]. It interacts with opioid receptors [10], especially the sigma subtype, but is not displaced from opioid receptors by naloxone [11]. In addition, PCP's structure allows binding at nicotinic [12] and muscarinic cholinergic receptors [13] in the brain and interaction with muscarinic receptors in cardiac cells [14]. Phencyclidine also has anticholinesterase activity.

Phencyclidine is well absorbed from the gastrointestinal (GI) tract and from the lungs. The drug has a large volume of distribution and concentrates in the brain, lungs, and liver; some PCP enters adipose tissues. The average serum half-life in controlled studies is about 17 hours [15]. The main route of PCP excretion is oxidative metabolism. At least two inactive metabolites (4-phenyl-4-piperidinocyclohexanol) and 1-1-phenylcyclohexyl-4-hydroxy-piperidine) are excreted in the urine as glucuronides [16]. Another metabolite (5-1-phenyl-cyclohexylamino valeric acid) has been found in the urine of asymptomatic users [17]. In one study, about 90 percent of PCP was metabolized and about 9 percent was excreted unchanged in the urine [15]. In another study, 30 to 50 percent of a labeled IV dose was eliminated in the urine after 72 hours, 4 to 19 percent of the dose as active drug and 25 to 30 percent as inactive metabolites [18]. Only 2 percent of PCP is excreted in the feces [18]. Small amounts of PCP are excreted in perspiration, saliva, and gastric juice.

CLINICAL MANIFESTATIONS

Acute Toxicity. The major manifestations of PCP toxicity are (1) alterations in sensorium (e.g., euphoria, lethargy, coma), cerebral excitement (e.g., nudism, pressured speech, severe agitation, violence), acute brain syndrome, toxic psychosis; (2) behavioral disturbances (e.g., bizarre or violent behavior, agitation, catatonia); (3) motor disturbances (e.g., seizures, generalized rigidity, localized dystonias, occasionally athetosis); (4) autonomic effects (e.g., hypersalivation, profuse diaphoresis, bronchorrhea, bronchospasm, urinary retention); and (5) alterations in vital signs (e.g., hypertension, tachypnea, tachycardia, hyperthermia) [19]. Findings may wax and wane. Hypertension and nystagmus are hallmarks of PCP intoxication, occurring in about 57 percent of cases [19]. Nystagmus may be horizontal, vertical, or even rotatory.

Chronic Toxicity. Chronic PCP intoxication has not been described, and there is no documentation of PCP flashbacks.

DIAGNOSTIC EVALUATION

History. The drug history should include the type of product, method of use, time of exposure, circumstances surrounding intoxication, and description of any effects witnessed by others or experienced by the patient. Particular attention should be paid to any abnormal behavior that might have resulted in nonapparent trauma (e.g., jumps or falls).

Drinking liquid PCP, injecting PCP intravenously, or swallowing the remnants of a PCP-soaked cigarette has resulted in severe intoxication within 1 hour.

Physical Examination. The physical examination should focus on the vital signs, sensorium, behavior, motor signs, and autonomic findings. The manifestations can be grouped into five minor and four major patterns of intoxication, based on the history and physical findings [1].

The minor patterns, which represent mild toxicity, are: (1) lethargy or stupor, (2) bizarre behavior, (3) violent behavior, (4) agitation, and (5) euphoria [1]. Except for lethargy or stupor, the minor patterns are characterized by a clear sensorium; patients are alert and oriented with no hallucinations or delusions. In patients with minor patterns of PCP toxicity, symptoms usually last less than 6 hours and medical complications are rare.

The major patterns represent moderate to severe toxicity and can include any combination of the symptoms and findings listed above. The major patterns are as follows [1].

1. Coma. Coma may occur suddenly and last for 2 hours to 3 weeks; the usual duration is 1 to 3 days. Disturbances in vital signs are common but variable. The patient is usually agitated but may be calm. Autonomic findings are usually prominent.
2. Organic Catatonic Syndrome. The criteria for diagnosing organic catatonic syndrome are (a) an episode of psychosocial withdrawal (most commonly the patient is immobile, mute, and staring but may be only oblivious to external stimuli), (b) at least one episode of agitation, (c) catalepsy (i.e., waxen flexibility of extremities), and (d) rigid muscles. The sensorium may be clear, obtunded, or confused; occasionally, the patient may exhibit hallucinations or delusions. Although the catatonic syndrome may last for several days, many patients recover in 6 to 8 hours.
3. Toxic Psychosis. This pattern consists primarily of psychiatric manifestations, such as hallucinations, delusions, or paranoid ideation, in patients who are not catatonic. The clinical presentation may be very similar to that seen in agitated schizophrenia. Violent, aggressive, and destructive behavior is common.
4. Acute Brain Syndrome. Acute organic brain syndrome is the most common manifestation of significant PCP intoxication. It is characterized by (a) disorientation or confusion, (b) lack of judgment, (c) loss of recent memory, and (d) inappropriate affect, without signs of toxic psychosis. The findings in this pattern often resemble those associated with delirium tremens.

Ancillary Tests. Routine laboratory tests and radiographs should be obtained as indicated. Severely ill patients should have arterial blood gases to rule out metabolic acidosis. A computed tomography (CT) head scan should be obtained if the patient is comatose or if head trauma or intracerebral bleeding is suspected. Patients with major patterns of intoxication require serum chemistries, including uric acid, creatinine, blood urea nitrogen, creatine phosphokinase (CK), and serum transaminases. Elevated uric acid and CK may be the first sign of rhabdomyolysis. The urine should be dip-tested; if the reaction is positive for blood, a microscopic urine examination should be done to determine whether red blood cells are present. The absence of red cells with a positive dip-test for blood suggests myoglobinuria secondary to rhabdomyolysis.

Complete toxicology screens, including urine assay for PCP, are recommended for all patients. Most urine assays for PCP cross-react with its metabolites and analogs and are not specific for unmetabolized PCP. Phencyclidine may be detected in the urine for 10 days following a single dose. The concentration of PCP in the blood does not correlate with the severity of intoxication [20].

Differential Diagnosis. The differential diagnosis of PCP intoxication includes cocaine, amphetamine, and tricyclic antidepressant poisoning; psychiatric illnesses; and sedative-hypnotic or alcohol withdrawal.

MANAGEMENT. The treatment of PCP intoxication depends on the severity of poisoning. Intramuscular haloperidol has been found to be effective in improving the overall toxic effects of PCP [21] and should be given promptly to all patients with signs and symptoms of central nervous system (CNS) excitation except seizures and for agitated or violent behavior. The blood pressure should be retaken 20 minutes after administration of haloperidol to detect potential hypotension resulting from administration of this drug. Some physicians prefer diazepam, because haloperidol is capable of producing malignant neuroleptic syndrome. Diazepam is the sedative of choice for stuporous or comatose patients with severe agitation, for seizures, and for patients with hyperthermia. The possibility of rhabdomyolysis should be considered in all cases. Treatment for severe intoxication consists of life support measures, symptomatic treatment, and monitoring for medical complications. Patients who have attempted suicide or have persistent signs of psychosis should have a psychiatric evaluation.

Decontamination. Most patients with minor patterns of PCP intoxication have smoked PCP, improve promptly after treatment for cerebral excitement, and are unlikely to benefit from GI decontamination. Gastric lavage and activated charcoal are indicated for comatose and catatonic patients and those who have PCP-induced life-threatening changes in vital signs or seizures or who are suspected of ingesting PCP or other drugs.

Routine Treatment and Monitoring. If it is impossible to examine the patient because he or she is violent, haloperidol (usual dose 5–10 mg IM) may be used for pharmacologic restraint; check for rigidity before administering haloperidol. Physical restraints with repositioning of the patient every 2 hours are recommended for 12 to 24 hours for violent patients. All patients with cerebral stimulation should be sedated with either haloperidol or diazepam (5–20 mg IV). Patients with altered mental status should receive an IV injection of 50% glucose. A trial of naloxone is recommended only if the patient has a respiratory rate of 10 breaths per minute or less, to avoid possible release of cerebral catecholamines by naloxone. Dystonic reactions may be treated with diphenhydramine (50 mg IV). The temperature should be taken as quickly as possible; plastic unbreakable thermometers and rectal measurement are preferred. Intravenous fluids should be administered to correct dehydration, electrolyte imbalances, or marked acidosis and to maintain brisk urine output.

Most patients with minor patterns of PCP intoxication may be sedated with haloperidol and observed in the emergency department. If a dipstick urinalysis result for myoglobin is negative, the patient may be discharged after symptoms clear. Patients with major patterns of intoxication usually require hospital admission, supportive care, and monitoring.

Cardiovascular. Moderate elevations in blood pressure often resolve without specific treatment or improve after administration of haloperidol. Intravenous labetalol is recommended for hypertensive urgencies and intravenous nitroprusside for hypertensive emergencies. Other beta-blockers and calcium channel blockers are not recommended for treatment of hypertension or arrhythmias.

Metabolic Abnormalities. For patients with temperatures of 102 to 104°F, cooling blankets, evaporative cooling measures, and rectal acetaminophen may be sufficient treatment. For patients with temperatures greater than 104°F, invasive cooling measures may be necessary (see Chap. 81).

Metabolic acidosis may be present early in the course of severe poisoning or with development of rhabdomyolysis or renal failure. For patients with suspected rhabdomyolysis who are not anuric or volume-depleted, a dose of furosemide (20–40 mg IV) followed by IV fluids (1–2 liters of normal saline at 200 ml/hr followed by 5% dextrose in water 150 ml/hr for 1 day) and oral fluids (if the patient is able to drink) are recommended. Intravenous fluids (2 liters of half normal saline in 5% dextrose and water and 1–2 liters of 5% dextrose in water per day) should be continued until the serum CK begins to drop. Fluid intake and output should be closely monitored. If the patient develops oliguric renal failure, fluids should be restricted and a nephrologist should be consulted regarding possible hemodialysis. Alkalinization of the urine is not recommended for the routine treatment of PCP rhabdomyolysis.

Antidotal Therapy. There is no antidote for PCP intoxication. Phencyclidine-specific Fab antibody fragments have been evaluated experimentally and significantly change the kinetics of PCP [22], but they are not commercially available or approved for clinical use. Intravenous administration of acidifying salts (i.e., ammonium chloride) is not recommended for ion trapping of PCP in the urine, as the primary route of PCP excretion is oxidative metabolism [15], and acidifying the urine is contraindicated if the patient has rhabdomyolysis. Charcoal hemoperfusion was found to be ineffective in altering the kinetics of PCP in dogs [23], since only a small amount of PCP is present in the blood.

Hallucinogens

The psychedelic hallucinogens are either synthetic indoleamines (derivatives of tryptamine), phenethylamines (derivatives of amphetamine), or plant products called organics. Many street preparations contain LSD or PCP in place of or in addition to the drug that was sold. Years ago, a few tablets were found to contain strychnine.

Hallucinogenic drugs cause two major groups of symptoms. The first is related to their mind-altering effects; the second results from physiologic disturbances. Homicide [24,25,26], self-destructive behavior [27], and accidental injuries may occur, and acute or chronic psychosis may be precipitated by the psychedelic experience. Physiologic effects vary from mild flushing to life-threatening alterations in vital signs, coma, seizures, and coagulopathies. Serious physiologic effects are rare and have been described only after large doses.

AVAILABLE FORMS/USE. Synthetic hallucinogens are sold as liquid, powder, tablets, capsules, microdots (dried drug residue) on printed paper, liquid-impregnated blotted paper, and as "window panes" (tiny translucent 3×3 mm gelatin squares).

The routes of administration are oral, intranasal, sublingual, conjunctival, smoking, or IV injection. Blotter paper is chewed and swallowed, whereas microdot paper is usually licked. Window panes are usually placed under the tongue or in the conjunctival sac but may also be swallowed.

PHARMACOLOGY. Psychedelic hallucinogens are capable of altering the normal function of serotonin, a central and peripheral neurotransmitter. In the brain, the actions of serotonin are complex and incompletely understood. The major central serotonin effect is inhibition of neurons that transmit sensory stimuli, thus providing a dampening effect on extraneous or irrelevant impulses and facilitating normal sensory perception. Serotonin also has a role in central regulation of body temperature [28].

The peripheral activity of serotonin is also complex. Its actions on nerves and smooth muscle are often opposite, resulting in stimulatory and inhibitory effects on the same organ. Vascular effects include both constriction and dilatation and can result in either hypertension or hypotension. The typical red "serotonin flush" is due to venous dilatation in the skin, particularly of the neck and face. This may be followed by venospasm, leading to engorgement of the tissues and a dusky appearance. Serotonin has both inotropic and chronotropic effects on the heart and, by an indirect action, can stimulate the vagus nerve. In the bowel, serotonin inhibits as well as stimulates contractions. Serotonin is manufactured by platelets and promotes platelet aggregation. In addition, high doses of serotonin cause secretion of catecholamines from the adrenal glands.

The tryptamine derivatives have been shown to act at presynaptic type 2 serotonin receptors (i.e., serotonin uptake sites) [29]. Some compounds appear to be partial agonists or agonist-antagonists at this receptor. Although derivatives of amphetamine are thought to have a different mechanism of action because of their amphetamine structure and monoamine oxidase-inhibiting properties, their main action is probably also on the serotonin system. Recent animal studies have shown that methylenedioxymethamphetamine (MDMA) produces a dose-related depletion of serotonin [30], and both methylenedioxyamphetamine (MDA) and MDMA selectively destroy serotonin uptake sites (i.e., serotonin type 2 receptors) in rodent and primate brains [31,32]. Although other factors may be involved, all of the actions of psychedelic drugs can be explained by direct or indirect stimulation or inhibition of serotonin receptors. Psychedelics do not cause physical dependence, but when used frequently they can produce tolerance and tachyphylaxis.

Hallucinogens are readily absorbed from the GI tract. Very little pharmacokinetic information is available in humans. Animal studies have shown that most psychedelics are rapidly and extensively metabolized to inactive products, and very little active drug is excreted in the urine. The clinical effects produced by different agents are very similar.

DERIVATIVES OF TRYPTAMINE.

Lysergic acid (LSD, or "acid"), a derivative of dimethyltryptamine, was originally synthesized from an alkaloid in ergot, the rye fungus. The usual street form is a 1-cm square piece of blotter paper (sometimes called "tabs"), with or without printed designs, containing approximately 20 to 80 μg of LSD. Occasionally, it is sold as design paper containing one or two microdots of LSD. It is also available as oral tablets and as window panes. The hallucinogenic dose is about 35 to 100 μg. Effects begin in about 30 minutes and usually last less than 12 hours. The plasma half-life is 3.0 to 4.0 hours [33]. Lysergic acid and its metabolites may be detected in the urine for 1 to 5 days after ingestion of a 300 μg oral dose [34]. Severe reactions to LSD have been reported in young children (i.e., panic associated with hyperactivity, tachycardia, and hyperventilation) [35,36]; in one case the reaction was described as "stark terror" [36]. Very high doses have been associated with severe autonomic disturbances in adults [37,38], although no deaths directly attributable to the toxic effects of LSD have been reported.

Dimethyltryptamine (DMT) occurs naturally in the body, in very small amounts, as a metabolite of serotonin; it is also found in some South American plants. Street DMT is a short-acting, rapidly metabolized hallucinogen available as liquid or yellow-tan powder that is sprinkled on tobacco, marijuana, or parsley and smoked. The usual dose is 50 to 150 μg. Effects are similar to those of LSD [39] but are milder, occur sooner, and last 30 minutes to 2 hours. Less than 1 percent of a dose is excreted unchanged in the urine over 24 hours [40].

Morning glory (*Ipomoea* and *Rivea* genus) seeds contain amides of lysergic acid [41] that are about one-tenth as potent as LSD. Popular varieties are Heavenly Blue, Pearly Gates, Flying Saucers, and Summer Skies. Toxic effects require chewing and ingesting about 200 to 300 seeds. Listlessness, apathy, and irritability appear about 30 to 90 minutes after ingestion, last several hours, and are usually followed by mild LSD-type effects, although severe psychedelic reactions have been reported [42,43,44]. In one case, a brown oily extract obtained by boiling the seeds was administered by IV injection, causing severe psychedelic effects [44].

Psilocybin and psilocin are substituted tryptamine derivatives found in *Psilocybe* and other hallucinogenic fungi (magic mushrooms). The dried mushroom may be sold whole or in small pieces, or as capsules or paper packets of brown powder. Pure psilocybin is also available in capsules of white powder. The toxic dose of psilocybin is 5 to 15 mg, equivalent to ingestion of one to five large mushrooms. Psilocybin effects are similar to those of LSD intoxication. Low doses produce psychedelic effects, GI symptoms, and myalgia. Prolonged psychedelic effects were reported after oral ingestion of about 200 mushrooms [45]. Systemic autonomic effects have occurred after IV injection of homemade extracts of *Psilocybe* mushrooms [46,47].

DERIVATIVES OF AMPHETAMINE.

Dimethoxymethylamphetamine (DOM or STP, for serenity, tranquility, and peace), although rarely used today, was believed during the 1960s to be a "mega-hallucinogen" with effects lasting as long as 3 days. It is about one-thirtieth as potent as LSD [48]. The drug is available in tablets containing 1 to 20 mg. In lower doses, DOM produces mild euphoria [48]. In doses greater than 3 mg, DOM effects are indistinguishable from those of LSD but last 5 to 8 hours [48]. About 20 percent of a 2- to 3-mg oral dose is excreted unchanged in the urine over 24 hours [48].

Dimethoxyamphetamine (DMA) is similar to DOM but less potent. It is available as powder in gelatin capsules. The hallucinogen dose is 20 to 50 mg.

Bromo-dimethoxyamphetamine, or dimethoxyamphetamine hydrobromide (DOB, "bromo STP," or "Blotter Blaze"), is also called "100×" because it is 100 times more potent than MDA. It is often sold as LSD. Like LSD, DOB is available as a dark spot on white blotter paper, on blotters with printed designs, or as capsules or tablets. The usual dose is 1 to 4 mg [49]. Onset of action occurs in about 1 hour; effects peak at 4 to 10 hours and last 12 to 36 hours [50]. Large doses of DOB may produce severe vascular spasm [49] and death [51].

Methylenedioxyamphetamine (MDA, "love drug") is usually sold as window panes but is available as liquid, tablets, or gelatin capsules containing about 100 to 150 mg. The hallucinogenic dose is 40 to 150 mg. It is also similar to LSD in its effects. Serious autonomic reactions have occurred with doses of about 500 mg [52]. Six nontraumatic deaths associated with MDA intoxication have been reported [53–58].

p-Methoxyamphetamine (PMA) is about three times more potent than MDA [59]. The psychedelic dose for an average adult is about 50 mg. It has been taken orally, sniffed, or injected. It is not as completely metabolized as other psychedelics: About 15 percent of a labeled dose was recovered as free drug in urine after 24 hours; 49 to 83 percent was recovered as free drug and metabolites [60]. At least nine deaths attributed to the action of PMA have been reported [61].

Methylenedioxymethamphetamine (MDMA, "ecstasy," "XTC," or "Adam"), an analog of MDA, was first synthesized in 1914 from oil of sassafras and oil of nutmeg for use as an appetite suppressant. The drug was never legally marketed. In the early 1980s, MDMA was used as an adjunct to psychotherapy. Its use then spread to the drug subculture. It is ingested as gelatin capsules or loose powder dissolved in fruit juice or followed by an orange juice chaser. The street dose is 100 to 200 mg. It is claimed that MDMA produces a mildly altered state of consciousness without hallucinations, dissolves psychologic and emotional barriers, and enhances communication. However, anecdotal reports of psychedelic reactions have appeared in the lay press [62], and four cases of severe toxicity have been documented [63,64]. Three patients developed confusional states, hyperpyrexia, and rhabdomyolysis after taking MDMA [64]. A patient with untreated Wolff-Parkinson-White syndrome died suddenly after taking MDMA [65]. One death probably due to MDMA and three deaths associated with MDMA use have been reported [66].

Methylenedioxyethamphetamine (MDEA, "Eve"), an analog of MDMA, is used as a substitute for MDMA. It is thought to have effects similar to those of MDMA but milder. It was found at autopsy in a 25-year-old patient who developed cardiac arrest after an auto accident; the role of MDEA in this death was not clear [66].

MESCALINE.

Mescaline is the psychedelic constituent of peyote (North American dumping cactus, *Lophophora williamsii*) and other cacti. Small segments of the crown of the cactus, known as "buttons" or "moons," may be swallowed whole or chopped into small pieces; the buttons have a bitter taste and are gritty. Ground peyote may be smoked. The hallucinogenic dose of mescaline is about 300 mg. The effects of mescaline do not differ significantly from those of LSD.

CLINICAL MANIFESTATIONS

Acute Toxicity. Psychedelic effects, known to users as a "trip" or "tripping," are characterized by changes in sensory perception. They include euphoria or dysphoria; increase in the intensity of sensory perception; distortions of time, place, and body image; visual hallucinations; synesthesias (i.e., "seeing sounds" and "hearing colors"); illusions; loss of spatial sense; and feelings of unreality. Visions and mystical experiences have been described [67]. The patient is usually awake and may appear hyperalert but is often uncommunicative and seems to be oblivious to surroundings or preoccupied with internal stimuli. For some patients, the psychedelic effects are frightening or terrifying, producing anxiety, extreme agitation, violence, or panic ("bad trip" or "bummer"). Other patients may be quiet, calm, and withdrawn and appear depressed.

Physiologic effects that commonly accompany psychedelic ones include facial flushing, mild tachycardia, mild to moderate hypertension, dilated pupils, nausea, vomiting, and diarrhea. Chills and myalgias may also occur [46].

Significant or life-threatening autonomic effects are rare and usually occur only after large overdoses. Manifestations include stupor or coma, bradycardia or tachycardia, shock or hypertension, malignant hyperthermia, seizures, muscle rigidity, coagulopathy, and dilated or constricted pupils. Mucous membranes may be dry. When pupils are dilated, mucous membranes are dry, the skin is flushed, and hypertension, tachycardia, and hyperthermia are present, the reaction can be mistaken for anticholinergic syndrome.

Hyperthermia was first reported following a large dose of LSD [37]. It has also been reported during intoxication with psilocybin [47], MDA [56], PMA [61], and MDMA [64]. Severe autonomic effects developed in eight people who had snorted pure LSD tartrate powder, thinking it was cocaine [38]. Findings included coma or toxic psychosis, hyperventilation, respiratory arrest, hypertension (up to 230/130 mm Hg), hyperthermia (up to 107.0°F), tachycardia (up to 200 beats per minute), athetosis, dystonic movements, and diarrhea. All eight had widely dilated and fixed pupils, emesis, flushing, sweating, and coagulopathy (inability to form firm clots and absence of clot retraction). There was evidence of bleeding in seven patients. All of the patients recovered after receiving supportive care only [38].

Flashbacks. After the drug effects have stopped, there may be recurrence of intrusive images (the flashback phenomenon). Flashbacks have been reported after intoxications with LSD [68], morning glory seeds [42,44], and psilocybin [45].

DIAGNOSTIC EVALUATION

History. A standard drug history should be obtained and should include a history of prior drug abuse and psychiatric illness. The patient may admit to using a particular product. Often, the name of the drug is not given but the route of intoxication and dosage form are described (e.g., "ate a paper," "chewed a button," "put acid in my eye"). Sometimes the only history is "on a trip."

Physical Examination. After obtaining the vital signs, the physical examination should focus on eliciting signs of altered sensory perception (e.g., synesthesias, illusions, hallucinations, delusions), abnormal behavior, and autonomic disturbances.

Ancillary Tests. Routine laboratory tests and radiographs should be obtained as indicated. Complete toxicology screens, including a urine assay for LSD [69], are recommended. Most laboratories use immunoassays screens or gas chromatography for the detection of other psychedelic substances.

MANAGEMENT. The standard recommendation of "talking down" patients with the psychedelic pattern of intoxication is often impractical and may be ineffective for severely disturbed or uncommunicative patients. Chlorpromazine (0.5–2 mg/kg IM) effectively ameliorates psychedelic symptoms [70]; the usual adult dose is 25 mg. Occasionally, repeat doses are needed at 4- to 6-hour intervals. Chlorpromazine was the most effective drug for sedation in a series of 60 hospital admissions for LSD intoxication [71].

Patients in a panic state need suicide precautions as well as sedation. Depressed and withdrawn patients are also unpredictable and should be kept under close observation in restraints. In both instances, the administration of chlorpromazine or diazepam may be of benefit.

Patients usually recover completely within 24 hours. If symptoms persist longer, it is likely that the psychedelic drug has precipitated a psychiatric condition that will require psychiatric therapy.

Decontamination. Gastric lavage or activated charcoal is indicated if the intoxicating substance is plant material, if multiple drug intoxication is suspected, or if the patient has significant autonomic manifestations. If lavage is performed, it should be followed by one dose of activated charcoal. Multiple doses of charcoal are not needed. The use of cathartics is not recommended because of the variable effects of psychedelic drugs on the GI tract.

Routine Treatment and Monitoring. As usual, IV dextrose (25–50 gm) should be given to patients with altered mental status or autonomic symptoms. Naloxone is not recommended unless the patient has respiratory depression, which is unlikely. Patients showing psychedelic symptoms may be treated with chlorpromazine (25–50 mg IM, repeated every 4–6 hours if needed) with monitoring of blood pressure for hypotension. Diazepam (5–10 mg IV) may be used instead of chlorpromazine.

Because of the complex pharmacology involved, the safest treatment of patients with significant physiologic abnormalities is intensive supportive care. Although the first reported cases of severe autonomic toxicity responded favorably to a dose of chlorpromazine (25 mg IM) [37], this agent is no longer recommended. If sedation is needed, diazepam is the agent of choice. Physostigmine should also be avoided, since there is no evidence that the autonomic effects are anticholinergic in etiology and some psychedelic products have anticholinesterase activity.

Cardiovascular. Nitroprusside may be needed to treat severe hypertension. Marked vagal effects, such as bradycardia with hypotension, may be treated with atropine and fluid administration.

Metabolic Effects. Hyperthermia requires prompt treatment (see Chap. 81). If a coagulopathy is present, a hematologist should be consulted. Rhabdomyolysis and renal failure should be managed as described in the PCP management section.

Antidotal Therapy. There are no antidotes for hallucinogenic intoxication.

References

1. McCarron MM, Schulze BW, Thompson GA, et al: Acute phencyclidine intoxication: Clinical patterns, complications, and treatment. *Ann Emerg Med* 10:290, 1981.
2. Armen R, Kanel G, Reynolds T: Phencyclidine-induced malignant

hyperthermia causing submassive liver necrosis. *Am J Med* 77:167, 1984.

3. Eastman JW, Cohen SN: Hypertensive crisis and death associated with phencyclidine poisoning. *JAMA* 231:1270, 1975.

4. Soine WH, Vincek WC: Phencyclidine contaminant generates cyanide. *N Engl J Med* 301:439, 1979.

5. Vincent JP, Vignon J, Kartalovski B, et al: Compared properties of central and peripheral binding sites for phencyclidine. *Eur J Pharmacol* 68:79, 1980.

6. Johnson SW, Haroldsen PE, Hoffer BJ, et al: Presynaptic dopaminergic activity of phencyclidine in rat caudate. *J Pharmacol Exp Ther* 229:322, 1984.

7. Boyorh MA, Zukowska-Grojec Z, Palkovits M, et al: Effect of phencyclidine (PCP) on blood pressure and catecholamine levels in discrete brain nuclei. *Brain Res* 321:315, 1984.

8. Tourneur Y, Romey G, Lazdunski M: Phencyclidine blockade of sodium and potassium channels in neuroblastoma cells. *Brain Res* 245:154, 1982.

9. Smith RC, Meltzer HY, Arora RC, et al: Effects of phencyclidine on catecholamines and serotonin uptake in synaptosomal preparations from rat brain. *Biochem Pharmacol* 26:1436, 1977.

10. Vincent JP, Cavey D, Kamenk JM, et al: Interaction of phencyclidines with the muscarinic and opiate receptors in the central nervous system. *Brain Res* 152:176, 1978.

11. Quirion R, Hammer RP, Herkenham M, et al: Phencyclidine (angel dust) sigma "opiate" receptor: Visualization by tritium-sensitive film. *Proc Natl Acad Sci USA* 78:5881, 1981.

12. Haring R, Kloog Y, Sokolovsky M: Localization of phencyclidine binding sites on alpha and beta subunits of the nicotinic acetylcholine receptor from *Torpedo ocellata* electric organ using azido phencyclidine. *J Neurosci* 4:627, 1984.

13. Paster Z, Maayani S, Weinstein H, et al: Cholinolytic action of phencyclidine derivatives. *Eur J Pharmacol* 25:270, 1974.

14. Fosset M, Renaud JF, Lenoie MC, et al: Interaction of molecules of phencyclidine series with cardiac cells: Association with the muscarinic receptor. *FEBS Lett* 103:133, 1979.

15. Cook CE, Brine DR, Jeffcoat AR, et al: Phencyclidine disposition after intravenous and oral doses. *Clin Pharmacol Ther* 31:625, 1982.

16. Wong LK, Beimann K: Metabolites of phencyclidine. *Clin Toxicol* 9:583, 1976.

17. Syracuse CD, Kuhnert BR, Golden NL, et al: Measurement of the amino acid metabolite of phencyclidine by selected ion monitoring. *Biomed Environ Mass Spectrom* 13:113, 1986.

18. Wall ME, Brine DR, Jeffcoat AR, et al: Phencyclidine metabolism and disposition in man following a 100 μg intravenous dose. *Res Commum Subst Abuse* 2:161, 1981.

19. McCarron MM, Schulze BW, Thompson GA, et al: Acute phencyclidine intoxication: Incidence of clinical findings in 1,000 cases. *Ann Emerg Med* 10:237, 1981.

20. Walberg CB, McCarron MM, Schulze BW: Quantitation of phencyclidine in serum by enzyme immunoassay: Results in 405 patients. *J Anal Toxicol* 7:106, 1983.

21. Giannini AJ, Eighan MS, Loiselle RH, et al: Comparison of haloperidol and chlorpromazine in the treatment of phencyclidine psychosis. *J Clin Pharmacol* 24:202, 1984.

22. Owens SM, Mayersohn M: *Modulation of Phencyclidine (PCP) Pharmacokinetics with PCP-Specific Fab Fragments.* National Institute of Drug Abuse Research Monograph 64, 1986, p 112.

23. Allen WR, O'Barr TP, Corby DG: Hemoperfusion of phencyclidine in the dog. *Int J Artif Organs* 8:101, 1985.

24. Knudsen K: Homicide after treatment with lysergic acid diethylamide. *Acta Psychiatr Scand* 180(suppl):389, 1965.

25. Klepfisz A, Racy J: Homicide and LSD. *JAMA* 223:429, 1973.

26. Reich P, Hepps R: Homicide during a psychosis induced by LSD. *JAMA* 219:869, 1972.

27. Thomas R, Fuller D: Self-inflicted ocular injury associated with drug use. *J SC Med Assoc* 68:202, 1972.

28. Feldberg W: The monoamines of the hypothalamus as mediators of temperature responses, in Robson JM, Stacey RS (eds): *Recent Advances in Pharmacology.* 4th ed. London, Churchill, 1968, pp 349–397.

29. Haigler HJ, Aghajanian GK: Lysergic acid diethylamide and serotonin: A comparison of effects on serotonergic neurons and neurons receiving a serotonergic input. *J Pharmacol Exp Ther* 188:688, 1974.

30. Ricaurte GA, Forno LS, Wilson MA, et al: 3,4-Methylenedioxymethamphetamine selectively damages central serotonergic neurons in nonhuman primates. *JAMA* 260:51, 1988.

31. Battaglia G, Yeh SY, O'Hearn E, et al: 3-4-Methylenedioxymethamphetamine and 3,4-methylenedioxyamphetamine destroy serotonin terminals in rat brain: Quantitation of neurodegeneration by measurement of (3H)paroxetine-labeled serotonin uptake sites. *J Pharmacol Exp Ther* 242:911, 1988.

32. Ricaurte GA, Bryan G, Strauss L, et al: Hallucinogenic amphetamine selectively destroys brain serotonin nerve terminals. *Science* 222:986, 1985.

33. Aghajanian GK, Bing OHL: Persistence of lysergic acid diethylamide in the plasma of human subjects. *Clin Pharmacol Ther* 5:611, 1964.

34. Peel HW, Boynton AL: Analysis of LSD in urine using radioimmunoassay: Excretion and storage effects. *Can Soc Forensic Sci J* 13:23, 1980.

35. Milman DH: An untoward reaction to accidental ingestion of LSD in a 5-year-old girl. *JAMA* 201:143, 1967.

36. Ianzito BM, Liskow B, Stewart MA: Reaction to LSD in a two-year-old child. *J Pediatr* 80:643, 1972.

37. Friedman SA, Hirsch SE: Extreme hyperthermia after LSD ingestion. *JAMA* 217:1549, 1971.

38. Klock JC, Boerner U, Becker CE: Coma, hyperthermia and bleeding associated with massive LSD overdose. *West J Med* 120:183, 1974.

39. Rosenberg DE, Isbell H, Miner EJ: Comparison of a placebo, N-dimethyltryptamine, and 6-hydroxy-N-dimethyltryptamine in man. *Psychopharmacologia* 4:39, 1963.

40. Kaplan J, Mandel LR, Stillman R, et al: Blood and urine levels of N,N-dimethyltryptamine following administration of psychoactive dosage in human subjects. *Psychopharmacology* 38:239, 1974.

41. Opp M: Beautiful but dangerous. *Med World News* 38, 1977.

42. Cohen S: Suicide after ingestion of morning glory seeds. *Am J Psychiatry* 120:1024, 1964.

43. Ingram AL: Morning glory seed reaction. *JAMA* 190:1133, 1964.

44. Fink PJ, Goldman MJ, Lyons I: Morning glory seed psychosis. *Arch Gen Psychiatry* 15:209, 1966.

45. Dewhurst K: Psilocybin intoxication. *Br J Psychiatry* 137:303, 1980.

46. Sivyer C, Dorrington L: Intravenous injection of mushrooms (letter). *Med J Aust* 140:182, 1984.

47. Curry SC, Rose MC: Intravenous mushroom poisoning. *Ann Emerg Med* 14:900, 1985.

48. Snyder SH, Faillace L, Hollister L: 2,5-dimethoxy-4-methyl-amphetamine (STP): A new hallucinogenic drug. *Science* 158:669, 1967.

49. Bowen JS, Davis GB, Kearney TE: Diffuse vascular spasm associated with 4-bromo-2,5-dimethoxyamphetamine ingestion. *JAMA* 249:1477, 1983.

50. Shulgin AT: Profiles of psychedelic drugs—DOB. *J Psychoactive Drugs* 13:99, 1981.

51. Winek CL, Collom WD, Bricker JD: A death due to 4-bromo-2,5-dimethoxyamphetamine. *Clin Toxicol* 18:267, 1981.

52. Richard KC, Borgstedt HH: Near fatal reaction to ingestion of the hallucinogenic drug MDA. *JAMA* 218:1826, 1971.

53. Finkle BS: MDA death. *Bull Int Assoc Forensic Toxicol* 6:4, 1969.

54. Cimbura G: 3,4-methylenedioxyamphetamine (MDA): Analytical and forensic aspects of fatal poisoning. *J Forensic Sci* 17:329, 1972.

55. Reed D, Cravey RH, Sedgwick PR: A fatal case involving methylenedioxyamphetamine. *Clin Toxicol* 5:3, 1972.

56. Lukaszewski T: 3,4-methylenedioxyamphetamine overdose. *Clin Toxicol* 15:405, 1979.

57. Poklis A, Mackell MA, Drake WK: Fatal intoxication from 3,4-methylenedioxyamphetamine. *J Forensic Sci* 24:70, 1979.

58. Simpson DL, Rumack BH: Methylenedioxyamphetamine: Clinical description of overdose, death, and review of pharmacology. *Arch Intern Med* 141:1507, 1981.

59. Shulgin AT, Sat T, Naranjo C: Structure-activity relationships of one-ring psychotomimetics. *Nature* 221:537, 1969.

60. Kitchen I, Tremblay J, Andre J, et al: Interindividual and interspecies variation in the metabolism of the hallucinogen 4-methoxyamphetamine. *Xenobiotica* 9:397, 1979.

61. Cimbura G: PMA deaths in Ontario. *Can Med Assoc J* 110:1263, 1974.

62. Corwin M: Psychiatrists defend new street drug for therapy. *Los Angeles Times,* May 27, 1985.

63. Brown C, Osterloh J: Multiple severe complications from recreational ingestion of MDMA ("ecstasy") (letter). *JAMA* 258:780, 1987.

64. Screaton GR, Cairns HJ, Sarner M, et al: Hyperpyrexia and rhabdomyolysis after MDMA ("ecstasy") abuse. *Lancet* 339:677, 1992.
65. Suarez RV, Riemersma R: "Ecstasy" and sudden cardiac death. *Am J Forensic Med Pathol* 9:339, 1988.
66. Dowling GP, McDonough ET III, Bost RO: "Eve" and "ecstasy": A report of five deaths associated with the use of MDEA and MDMA. *JAMA* 257:1615, 1987.
67. Pahnke WN, Jurland AA, Unger S, et al: The experimental use of psychedelic (LSD) psychotherapy. *JAMA* 212:1856, 1970.
68. Horowitz MJ: Flashbacks: Recurrent intrusive images after the use of LSD. *Am J Psychiatry* 126:565, 1969.
69. McCarron MM, Walberg CB, Baselt RC: Confirmation of LSD intoxication by analysis of serum and urine. *J Anal Toxicol* 14:165, 1990.
70. Schwarz BE, Bickford RB: Reversibility of induced psychosis with chlorpromazine. *Proc Staff Meetings Mayo Clin* 30:407, 1955.
71. Forest JAH, Tarala RA: 60 hospital admissions due to reactions to lysergide (LSD). *Lancet* 2:1310, 1973.

153. *Pesticide Poisoning*

William K. Chiang and Rick Y. Wang

Throughout history, humans have significantly altered the environment to suit their needs. Numerous pesticides have been formulated as one mechanism to help "control" the environment (Table 153-1), and pesticide usage has increased exponentially since the 1940s [1]. Some of the more notorious compounds include arsenicals, mercuric compounds, and dichlorodiphenyl trichloroethane (DDT). A pesticide is defined as an agent intended for killing, preventing, repelling, or mitigating any pest. *Pest* may be considered any "undesirable" animal, rodent, insect, plant, or fungus. Pesticides can be further classified by their intended targets or patterns of use, such as rodenticide, insecticide, herbicide, and fungicide. However, such classifications are not absolute, since many pesticides are used against more than one type of pest. There are more than 3,000 different formulations and 25,000 brand names of pesticides available in the United States [1]. An ideal pesticide would be an agent that is specific against only one species without causing any harm to humans or other living things. Unfortunately, such an agent does not exist: Most pesticides pose significant harm to other plant or animal species, including humans. With the increasing use of pesticides, environmental contamination and reports of epidemic poisonings are inevitable [1–6]. The consequences of long-term, low-level exposure—carcinogenesis [7,8,9], teratogenicity [10], fertility [11], and neurologic sequelae [12–14]—may be significant and immeasurable. In many countries where there are limited regulations on pesticide usage, pesticide ingestion is one of the leading forms of suicide and pesticides exposure is a major occupational risk [15,16,17]. Even in the United States, pesticides exposures remain a major public health problem [18,19,20]. The World Health Organization estimated that accidental pesticide poisonings worldwide account for 1.5 million cases and 28,000 deaths annually [21]. Suicide attempts from pesticide ingestions are responsible for 3 million hospitalizations and 220,000 deaths annually [15]. Because it is impossible to discuss every pesticide in this chapter, we review the most common and most clinically relevant pesticides. (Organophosphates are covered in Chapter 137.)

Organochlorines

Organochlorine compounds are commonly used as insecticides, soil fumigants, solvents, and herbicides. Human toxicity can result from acute exposure or chronic contact. Contamination typically occurs during production and application of the agents. Infants and toddlers are at risk for toxicity from bioaccumulation in foodstuffs, excretion in breast milk, and concentration in fetal tissues [22–26]. These toxins can cause a variety of systemic manifestations but are most notable for their central nervous system (CNS) effects. Organochlorides can be divided into four structural categories: DDT and related agents, the hexachlorocyclohexanes, the cyclodienes, and the toxaphenes [27]. Dichlorodiphenyl trichloroethane is one of the more well-known organochlorine compounds. It was a popular insecticide in the agricultural industry during the 1960s. The many environmental concerns related to the use of DDT, including carcinogenesis, bioaccumulation, and other health risks to humans and animals, led to banning of its use in the United States as of 1972, but it is still produced in the United States for exportation to other parts of the world [28]. Dicofol (a miticide) and methoxychlor are structurally related to DDT and have minimal toxicity. Human volunteers ingesting up to 2 mg/kg/day of methoxychlor for 8 weeks did not demonstrate any ill effects [27].

The cyclodienes include chlordane, heptachlor, endrin, aldrin, and dieldrin [27]. Chlordane is a common termiticide applied by soil injection. This form of application has resulted in home air and water contamination from soil runoff. Most deaths associated with chlordane have been from oral exposures in children [29–33]. Following these ingestions, there were prominent gastrointestinal (GI) and CNS symptoms. Autopsy demonstrated inflammation of the mucosa of the upper GI tract.

Aldrin is readily converted to dieldrin in the environment by epoxidation [34]. Dieldrin, however, is not easily biodegraded and persists in the environment. The use and manufacture of these two products has been banned since 1990. Inadvertent human exposures have been from pesticide spraying, which causes dermal and inhalational absorption [34].

Some of the other organochlorines that are structurally related to the cyclodienes include endosulfan, chlordecone, kelevan, and mirex [27]. Endosulfan is considered highly toxic and has been reported to cause pulmonary edema and death within 2 hours of ingestion [35,36]. Mirex was initially used against fire ants in the southern United States and is now used as a flame retardant [37]. Chlordecone (kepone) was introduced in 1965, but its production was quickly stopped because of resultant wide contamination of production workers and the surrounding environment [27,38]. Chlordecone is a recognized neurotoxin,

Table 153-1. Common Pesticides

Inorganic and organometal pesticides
Aluminum phosphide
Antimony potassium tartrate
Arsenical pesticides
Barium carbonate
Boric acid
Cadmium chloride
Copper sulfate
Elemental mercury
Elemental sulfur
Lead arsenate
Mercuric chloride
Methylmercury
Phophorus
Sodium chlorate
Sodium dichromate
Thallium sulfate
Zinc chloride
Zinc phosphide

Pyrethrins, pyrethroids, and plant-derived pesticides

Barthrin	Anabasine
Cyfluthrin	Nicotine
Cyfluthrinate	Sabadilla
Cyhalothrin	Cartap
Cypermethrin	Blasticidin-S
Decamethrin	Rotenone
Deltamethrin	Ricin
Phenothrin	Strychnine
Pyrethrins	Fluvalerate
Resmethrin	Fluvalinate
Tralocythrin	
Tralomethrin	

Fumigants and nematocides
Acryonitrile
Aluminum phosphide
Boron trifluoride
Carbon disulfide
Carbon tetrachloride
Chloropicrin
1,2-Dibromoethane
1,2-Dichloroethane
p-Dichlorobenzene
1,2-Dichloropropane
1,3-Dichloropropene
Epoxyethane
Hydrogen cyanide
Methylbromide
Naphthalene
1,1,1,-Trichloroethane
Trichloroethylene

Synthetic organic rodenticides
ANTU
Brodifacoum
Chloralose
Difenacoum
Diphacinone
Fluoroacetamide
Fluoroethanol
Norbormide
Pyriminil
Sodium fluoroacetate
Warfarin

Herbicides

Amitrole	Atrazine
Bromoxynil	Cycloate
Dicamba	Dichlobenil
Diuron	Diquat
Ioxynil	Mecoprop (MCPP)
MCPA	Molinate
Paraquat	Phenmedipham
Propanil	Propazine
Pyrazon	Silvex
Simazine	TCA

2,4-Dichlorophenoxyacetic acid (2,4-D)
2,3,5-Trichlorophenoxyacetic acid (2,3,5-T)

Fungicides and biocides

Benomyl	Captan
Captafol	1-Chlorodinitrobenzene
Dichloran	Diphenyl
Maneb	Organotins (tributyltin)
Quinotozene	Tetrachlorophthalide
Thiabendazole	Thiophante-methyl
Thiram	Ziram
Zineb	

Organochlorine pesticides

Aldrin	Chlordane
Chlordecone	Chlorobenzilate
Dicofol	Dieldrin
Endrin	Endosulfan
Ethylan	Heptachlor
Hexachlorobenzene	Isobenzan
Kelevan	Kelthane
Methoxychlor	Mirex
Toxaphene	TDE

DDT (Dichlorodiphenyl-trichloroethane)
Lindane (γ–Hexachlorocyclohexane)

Organophosphate Pesticides

Azinphos-methyl	Bromophos
Carbophenothion	Carejin
Chlorfenvinphos	Chlorphoxim
Chlorpyrifos	Demeton
Demeton-methyl	Dialifos
Diazinon	Dicapthon
Dichlofenthion	Dichlorvos
Dicrotophos	Dimefox
Dioxathion	Edifenphos
Endothion	Fenitrothion
Fensulfonthion	Fenthion
Fonofos	Formothion
Jodfenfos	Leptophos
Malathion	Merphos
Methidathion	Mevinphos
Mipafox	Monocrotophos
Naled	Oxydemeton-methyl
Parathion	Parathion-methyl
Phenthoate	Phorate
Phosalone	Phosphamidon
Phoxim	Pirimiphos-methyl
Schradan	Temephos
Thiometon	Trichlorfon

Carbamates

Aldocarb	Bendiocarb
Bufencarb	Carbaryl
Carbofuran	Dioxacarb
Isolan	Landrin
Methomyl	Mexacarbate
Oxamyl	Phencyclocarb
Promecarb	Propoxur

3-Isopropylphenyl-N-methylcarbamate
4-Benxiothielyn-N-methylcarbamate

Miscellaneous pesticides

Azoxybenzene	Busulfan
Chlorambucil	Chlordimeform
Chlorfenxon	5-Fluorouracil
Hexamethylmelamine	Metaldehyde
Methotrexate	Porfirmycin
Propargite	Thiotepa

N-N-Diethyl-m-toluamide (DEET)

Nitro compounds and related phenolic pesticides

Binapacryl	Dinocap
Dinoseb	2,4-Dinitrophenol
Pentachlorophenol	

TCDD (Tetrachlorodibenzo-dioxin)

ANTU = α-naphthylthiourea; MCPA = 4-chloro-2-methylphenoxyacetic acid; TCA = trichloroacetic acid; TDE = 1,1-dichloro-2,2-bis(4-chloro-phenyl) ethane.
Classifications adapted from Hayes WJ Jr, Laws ER (eds): *Handbook of Pesticide Toxicology.* San Diego, Academic, 1991.

causing peripheral neuropathies [39]. Other signs and symptoms of chlordecone toxicity include weight loss, opisthotonos, mental status changes, slurred speech, muscle tremors, weakness, arthralgias, and elevation of liver function tests [27,39].

PHARMACOKINETICS. The organochlorines are generally well absorbed from the GI tract [27]. This process is enhanced in the presence of a lipid-soluble medium. The serum half-lives of these chemicals are long, varying from days to months, because of their high lipid solubility. This allows these agents to be stored in fatty tissues with the resultant delay in total body clearance [27]. The distribution is greatest in the fatty tissues, followed, in decreasing order, by the brain, kidney, muscle, lungs, heart, spleen, liver, and blood [40,41]. The organochlorines are known to concentrate in breast milk and fetal tissue. At delivery, it has been shown that fetal blood and tissue had higher concentrations of lindane (Kwell) than maternal samples [22,23,24]. However, teratogenic effects have not been demonstrated in the limited number of animal studies performed [42,43].

Organochlorines are metabolized by the microsomal enzymes in the liver. Toxaphene, chlordane, DDT, and lindane (gamma-hexachlorocyclohexane) can induce microsomal enzyme activity and affect not only their own toxicity but also the effects of coadministered medications [27,44,45,46]. The toxicity of these agents can be diminished when microsomal enzyme induction leads to rapid metabolism to nontoxic metabolites; however, if these metabolites are active, then toxicity can be enhanced.

Chlordane has several metabolites, such as heptachlor, oxychlordane, and heptachlor epoxide [47]. Most of the available information on chlordane and metabolite tissue distribution is from case reports of accidental and suicidal exposures. Depending on the source, the elimination half-life of chlordane varies from 21 days to 88 days [48,49,50]. The majority of chlordane and metabolites are excreted by the biliary system [47]. Upon absorption into the body, aldrin is rapidly metabolized to the epoxide derivative, dieldrin [51]. Since very little of the aldrin remains, its toxicity is attributed to dieldrin. Dieldrin is stored in fatty tissues, and its elimination half-life in humans is approximately 266 days [34]. During physiologic stress (e.g., febrile reactions and weight loss), dieldrin can be mobilized from the fatty stores and into the plasma, resulting in clinical toxicity [34]. Endrin, an isomer of dieldrin, is rapidly metabolized in both humans and animals, with an elimination half-life of 2 to 6 days [27].

PATHOPHYSIOLOGY. There are several mechanisms of organochlorines toxicity. They can be considered axonal toxins that alter sodium and potassium channel movement across the membranes. In the instance of DDT, sodium ion transport is facilitated while potassium transport is inhibited. This results in the spontaneous firing and prolongation of action potentials and repetitive firing after a stimulus [52]. Dichlorodiphenyl trichloroethane also inhibits Na^+/K^+ ATPase and calmodulin activity, which reduces the rate of neuronal repolarization [52]. This may account for some of the neurologic manifestations, such as paresthesias, thought disturbances, myoclonus, and seizures. The cyclodienes, hexachlorocyclohexanes, and toxaphene manifest neurotoxicity by inhibiting gamma-aminobutyric acid receptor function in the CNS [53,54]. In the limbic system, lindane can directly excite neurons and result in agitation and seizures [53,55]. Abnormalities in respiratory rate patterns can result from direct medullary toxicity or pulmonary

Table 153-2. Organochlorines: Levels of Toxicity

High	Endrin, dieldrin, aldrin, endosulfan
Moderate	Chlordecone, heptachlor, chlordane, toxaphene, DDT, hexachlorobenzene
Low	Methoxychlor, perthane, kelthane, chlorobenzilate, mirex

DDT = dichlorodiphenyl trichloroethane.

aspiration. The level of toxicity of the various organochlorines can be categorized into high, moderate, and low (Table 153-2).

CLINICAL MANIFESTATIONS. Systemic toxicity can occur by ingestion, dermal absorption, or inhalation. The use of lindane in home vaporizers has resulted in significant inhalation toxicity [56]. Chemical absorption through the skin varies depending on the agent, amount applied, surface area involved, and skin integrity [57,58]. Generally, agents such as dieldrin, lindane, and kepone have good penetration [57]. Workers who directly handled lindane had health complaints of headaches, paresthesias, tremors, confusion, and memory impairment [59]. Seizures have also been reported in occupational surveys among sprayers and applicators of aldrin and dieldrin [34]. As little as two total body applications on two successive days of 1% lindane (Kwell), a common scabicide, resulted in seizures in an 18-month-old [60]. The peak concentration of lindane occurs 6 hours following dermal application [61]; thus delayed and prolonged manifestations of toxicity may occur from dermal absorption. Petroleum distillates are common additives in commercial preparations, and their odor can be noted on the patient's breath, vomitus, or skin after a significant exposure. Irritation of the nares, eyes, and mucous membranes of the oropharynx and esophagus may occur following contact [47]. Dermatitis has been reported with dicofol and methoxychlor [27]. Intradermal and subcutaneous injections of these agents can result in chemical dermatitis and sterile abscesses [62].

Seizures are the most prominent CNS effect of these agents. The seizures occur soon after exposure, may present without a prodrome, and can be quite protracted in frequency [27,63–66]. Late onset seizures may result from delayed gut or dermal absorption [27]. Acute exposures to DDT present initially with tremors, nausea, vomiting, muscle weakness, and confusion, which may progress to seizures [28]. However, seizures from cyclodiene toxicity can occur without any prodrome [67]. Among the organochlorines, both psychomotor agitation and CNS depression have been described. Chlordecone, mirex, endosulfan, and chlorbenzite are more likely to cause tremors and agitation than seizures [68]. Kelthane, perthane, methoxychlor, and lindane are more likely to cause CNS sedation than excitation [68]. Endrin is considered one of the most toxic of the chlordienes, with reports of hyperthermia and decerebrate posturing [27]. In 1984, an outbreak of endrin toxicity from contaminated foodstuffs occurred in Pakistan, where seizures resulted in a 10 percent mortality [69].

Neurologic symptoms resolve quickly due to rapid distribution of the organochlorines from blood to lipid stores. Since redistribution back into the blood pool can occur at a later time, continual observation of the patient for delayed toxicity may be warranted. Some of the long-term CNS effects (i.e., thought disturbances) following significant exposures may be due to direct chemical toxicity or anoxic encephalopathy from sustained seizures [36].

Nausea, vomiting, and diarrhea may occur following ingestions, especially if petroleum distillates are part of the preparation [65]. Pulmonary aspiration of these agents can cause tachypnea and significant respiratory distress, with resultant pulmonary edema [36,70]. When dicofol is heated or comes in contact with an acid, it decomposes to hydrogen chloride, which causes respiratory irritation [27]. Hypersensitivity pneumonitis may result from inhalational exposures when the organochlorine is mixed with pyrethrins [71].

Cardiac dysrhythmias, including ventricular fibrillation, have been reported from exposure to organochlorines [72]. Halogenated hydrocarbons sensitize the myocardium to catecholamines, which results in a variety of rhythm disturbances. Cardiotoxicity can be exacerbated by either stress-provoking events or the exogenous administration of catecholamines [73]. In severely ill patients, other etiologies of cardiac dysrhythmias, such as hypoxia and acidemia, should be considered.

Significant elevations in liver enzymes were reported in a group of 19 workers with a 10-year exposure to lindane [74]. Animal studies with acute oral exposures to lindane have resulted in fatty degeneration and necrosis of the liver [41]. From the few reports of human exposures to chlordane, there is little evidence of hepatotoxicity from this agent [33,75–78]. Microsomal enzyme induction has been demonstrated in animals that were orally administered chlordane [79]. Long-term exposure among 233 workers with aldrin, dieldrin, endrin, and kelodrin for 4 to 12 years failed to demonstrate any significant elevation of hepatic enzymes or hepatic enzyme induction [80].

Hematologic dyscrasias, including aplastic anemia, leukopenia, leukocytosis, granulocytopenia, granulocytosis, eosinophilia, thrombocytopenia, and pancytopenia, have been reported after repeated lindane exposures [41,56,81]. However, all of the involved preparations also contained benzene, which can account for such findings. Megaloblastic anemia and bone marrow depression have been associated with chlordane exposures [82,83].

There is no convincing evidence that the organochlorines are cancer-producing in humans. Workers exposed to DDT do not have a higher incidence of tumors than the general population [84]. Similarly, workers exposed to chlordane and heptachlor for 20 years or greater did not demonstrate an increase in mortality from cancer [85]. However, the lack of findings in these epidemiologic studies may be due to the limited ability of these investigations to detect small or delayed changes. It has been shown that tumors can be induced in mice by some of these agents [86,87]. Because animal data are convincing and human data are insufficient, agents such as DDT, aldrin, dieldrin, and toxaphene are classified by the Environmental Protection Agency as probable human carcinogens.

LABORATORY. Serum and urine levels of these organochlorines are provided by gas chromatography [88,89]. In obvious exposure, these levels are academic and would not alter clinical management. There are no correlations between concentrations in body tissues and specific health effects. If the diagnosis is in doubt, then these levels can at least confirm toxicity. The blood should be sampled if an acute exposure is in question, and fatty tissues and milk be evaluated if chronic exposure is of concern [90]. Alternatively, an acute exposure can be determined by a quantitative comparison of parent compound to metabolite. Because DDT and aldrin are rapidly metabolized on systemic absorption, their elevated presence in the blood would support recent exposure [91].

The organochlorines have no effect on either red blood cell or plasma cholinesterase.

Chlorinated hydrocarbons are radiopaque, and their radiopacity is directly related to the number of chlorine atoms per molecule [92]. Radiographs can assist in demonstrating aspiration pneumonia and gut burden.

MANAGEMENT. Initial management of organochlorine exposure involves limiting further chemical absorption by the patient and protection of rescue personnel. The patient should be removed from the scene, disrobed, and thoroughly and repeatedly washed with soap and water. Washing should include hair and fingernails. Rescue workers should be adequately gloved and gowned [58]. The patient's clothing and leather goods must be placed in a plastic bag and discarded because of the tenacious binding of these agents to leather. All wash water should be contained and discarded in a secure fashion.

The role of gastric decontamination depends on the clinical presentation. Immediately after an intentional ingestion and in asymptomatic patients without spontaneous emesis, gastric aspiration should be carefully performed with a small nasogastric tube. Emetics are contraindicated because the patient's mental status may rapidly deteriorate and pulmonary aspiration can occur. Activated charcoal should be administered as it can limit further gut absorption and enhance elimination by interrupting enterohepatic/enteroenteric circulation [27,93]. Cholestyramine may also interrupt enteric circulation and enhance elimination. Chlordecone and chlordane undergo enterohepatic circulation, and cholestyramine is indicated in symptomatic patients [46,94]. In a controlled trial, cholestyramine was administered as 16 gm per day to symptomatic factory workers exposed to chlordane. After 5 months, chlordane fecal elimination was shown to increase by 3.3 to 17.8 times, with neurologic symptoms improving as levels declined [94]. Milk and oil-based cathartics should be avoided, since their high lipid solubility can enhance gut absorption. Hemodialysis is not effective in enhancing elimination of these chemicals because of their high volume of distribution and protein binding [95]. Hemoperfusion is probably of no benefit [95].

Organochlorine-induced seizures should be managed with benzodiazepines and barbiturates. Phenytoin may be less effective as an anticonvulsant than barbiturates and may actually increase the incidence of these seizures [96,97]. For uncontrolled status epilepticus, muscle paralysis and general anesthesia may be necessary. Aggressive seizure control is warranted to limit further development of CNS damage, metabolic acidosis, hyperthermia, rhabdomyolysis, and myoglobinuric renal failure.

Respiratory distress due to bronchospasm is managed with humidified oxygen and nebulized bronchodilators. Parenteral administration of adrenergic amines is not recommended, since it may potentiate myocardial irritability [98]. Early administration of steroids and prophylactic use of antibiotics for pulmonary aspiration have not been demonstrated to improve patient outcome. The early use of antibiotics may predispose the selective growth of other bacterial organisms.

After appropriate decontamination, asymptomatic patients with oral exposure can be observed for 6 hours and then discharged if their clinical status remains unchanged. Patients presenting with cardiovascular, CNS, or persistent respiratory manifestations should be admitted for further therapy and observation.

Pyrethrins

Pyrethrum is a collection of naturally occurring insecticide esters from the chrysanthemum flower. The pyrethrin I ester has the greatest insecticidal activity and is subject to rapid environmental degradation. To enhance their effectiveness in commercial use, synthetic alternatives known as pyrethroids were developed that are more resistant to decay [99]. These compounds are present in more than 2000 consumer products, from flea and tick removers for pets to topical pediculicides [100]. The pyrethroids (including pyrethrins) delay closure of the sodium channel during the end of depolarization, with resultant insect paralysis [101]. Piperonyl butoxide is commonly added to commercial preparations to inhibit the insects' ability to metabolize the pyrethroid and prolong activity [102]. In mammals, these agents are relatively nontoxic because of the low concentration and mammalian metabolism [103]. However, people who are allergic to ragweed may develop hypersensitivity reactions to pyrethroids. The degree of this cross-sensitization has been reported to be as high as 46 percent [104]. Pyrethroids have no effects on cholinesterase activity and atropine and pralidoxime are not indicated in therapy.

The pyrethroids are readily absorbed from the GI tract. Dermal absorption varies depending on the type of agent and additive organic solvents. Systemic absorption is enhanced in the presence of petroleum distillates. These compounds are highly lipid-soluble and largely metabolized by the mixed-function oxidase enzymes in the liver [105,106]. Plasma pyrethroid levels are not useful.

CLINICAL MANIFESTATIONS. Neurologic manifestations and hypersensitivity reactions, including anaphylaxis, are the most common forms of systemic toxicity. Toxicity can occur from either inhalational, dermal, or oral exposures [107–111]. Neurologic findings are dependent on the type and concentration of the pyrethroid and may present as paresthesias, muscle fasciculations, coma, and seizures [108,111,112]. Nausea, vomiting, and diarrhea may occur after ingestion of pyrethroids [111].

MANAGEMENT. The management of pyrethroid exposures is very similar to that of the organochlorines (see Organochlorines). Gastrointestinal decontamination is as previously discussed. There is no role for repeat dose activated charcoal and cholestyramine therapy, since enterohepatic circulation has not been demonstrated for the pyrethroids. Hypersensitivity reactions, including anaphylaxis, should be managed with epinephrine, steroids, antihistamines, bronchodilators, and vasopressors, as indicated.

After appropriate decontamination, asymptomatic patients with oral exposures can be observed for 6 hours and medically cleared of toxicity if their clinical status remains unchanged. Patients presenting with cardiovascular, CNS, or persistent respiratory manifestations should be admitted for further therapy and observation.

Anticoagulants

Vitamin K antagonists were developed as a result of the serendipitous discovery of sweet clover disease in cattle, reported in 1924 [113]. Sweet clover disease is a bleeding disorder that resulted from the ingestion of spoiled clover silage [113]. Bishydroxycoumarin (dicumarol), the first anticoagulant, was isolated as the hemorrhagic agent in 1939 [114]. Numerous congeners, such as warfarin, have since been synthesized. Warfarin (3-alpha-acetonylbenzyl-4-hydroxycoumarin) has been used as

a rodenticide since 1948. Typically, for the bait to be effective, the rodent must consume it for 3 to 10 days; however, continuous feeding for 21 days may be necessary to achieve 100 percent mortality [115]. As rodents became increasingly resistant, different classes of warfarin derivatives were introduced and have supplanted warfarin [20,116–120]. These newer agents, "superwarfarins" or long-acting anticoagulants, include brodifacoum, difenacoum, and indanedione derivatives. The long-acting anticoagulants are approximately 100 times more potent than warfarin and have a much longer half-life [121,122]. A single consumption of a long-acting anticoagulant rodenticide is adequate to kill a mouse [121]. Most anticoagulant rodenticide is packaged with cereal or other food products as bait, with the amount of rodenticide in the product varying from 0.025 to 0.005 percent per weight [123]. Acute ingestions (accidental and suicidal) of warfarin-containing preparations are unlikely to cause significant toxicity in humans because of the limited dosage and potency. Accidental ingestion of a minimal amount of bait containing long-acting anticoagulants is not likely to cause toxicity [120,124]. However, a "mouthful" of a long-acting anticoagulant ingestion in an adult human has been reported to cause significant coagulopathy [125–131].

PHARMACOKINETICS. Warfarin and warfarin derivatives are oxidized by mixed-function oxidases into inactive metabolites in the liver [132]. The plasma half-life of warfarin is approximately 42 hours, with a duration of action of 2 to 5 days [132]. The long-acting anticoagulants are concentrated in the liver and have extremely long half-lives; brodifacoum has a half-life of 120 days in dogs, 61 hours in rabbits, and 156 hours in rats [133,134,135]. Because of significant interspecies variation, animal data cannot be extrapolated to humans. The half-life of long-acting anticoagulants may be affected by the dose. The exact half-life of long-acting anticoagulants in humans is unknown. Case reports in human exposures have reported a half-life of brodifacoum of 16 to 36 days and of chlorophacinone of 6 to 23 days [126,127]. However, the anticoagulant effects of these long-acting anticoagulants may persist even when they are no longer detectable in the blood. Clinical coagulopathy may persist as long as 42 to 300 days [125,129,131,136,137].

PATHOPHYSIOLOGY. Warfarin and warfarin derivatives inhibit vitamin K 2,3-epoxide reductase and, to a lesser extent, vitamin K reductase. These enzymes are responsible for the cyclic regeneration of vitamin K (Fig. 153-1) [138,139]. Vitamin K is the active coenzyme responsible for activation of clotting factors II, VII, IX, and X, as well as anticoagulant factors proteins C and protein S, by hepatic gamma carboxylation of glutamate residual on the N-terminal region of these proteins [138]. Once activated, vitamin K-dependent clotting factors can interact with calcium and phospholipids in the coagulation cascade [140]. Inhibition of vitamin K 2,3-epoxide reductase and vitamin K reductase results in the depletion of vitamin K and vitamin K-dependent clotting factors, resulting in coagulopathy and bleeding. The approximate half-lives of vitamin K-dependent clotting factors are: factor VII, 6 hours; factor IX, 24 hours; factor X, 36 hours; and factor II, 50 hours [113]. Because factor VII has the shortest half-life of the vitamin K-dependent clotting factors, increases in prothrombin time are not seen until a significant proportion of factor VII (approximately 50–70%) is cleared from the blood. In a normal individual, this change is not demonstrated until 24 to 48 hours after ingestion [124]. Clinical coagulopathy may not be evident until the other vitamin K-dependent factors are also depleted (several days) [141].

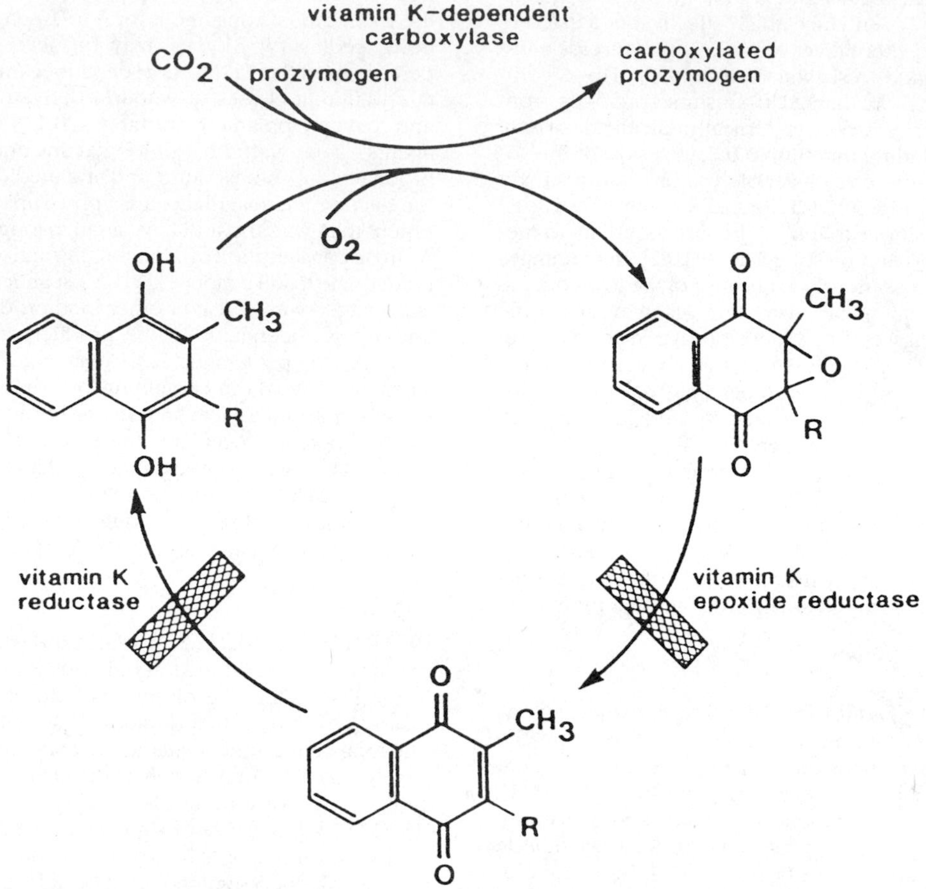

Fig. 153-1. Vitamin K cycle and its inhibition by warfarin and warfarin dervatives. Vitamin K, ingested as part of the normal diet, is converted to vitamin K hydroquinone by a vitamin K reductase. The reduced form of vitamin K, vitamin KH_2, is a substrate for the vitamin-dependent carboxylase/vitamin K epoxidase. With the carboxylation of glutamic acid residues on the protein substrate, vitamin K epoxide is formed. CO_2 and molecular oxygen are also requisite substrates. The vitamin K epoxide is recovered by a reaction catalyzed by the vitamin K epoxide reductase, and vitamin K is generated. The major site of warfarin and warfarin derivatives action (hatched) is the vitamin K epoxide reductase. Some vitamin K reductases are also inhibited. (From Furie B, Furie BC: Molecular basis of vitamin K-dependent gamma-carboxylation. *Blood* 75:1753, 1990. With permission.)

CLINICAL MANIFESTATIONS. The primary toxic manifestation of warfarin and warfarin derivatives is development of a coagulopathy. The most common symptoms are cutaneous bleeding, soft tissue ecchymosis, gingival bleeding, epistaxis, hematuria, and increased menstrual bleeding [128,142,143]. Gross hematuria, GI bleeding, hemoptysis, and diffuse alveolar bleeding may occur in patients with more significant symptoms [125,144–147]. Fatalities are uncommon and usually result from complications of cerebral hemorrhage [147,148].

MANAGEMENT. Gastric decontamination should be initiated for acute ingestions. Oral activated charcoal administration should be adequate for accidental ingestions. Gastric emptying with lavage or emesis should be considered for patients with intentional ingestion who present within 1 to 2 hours after ingestion. Clinical evaluations should be performed to assess other potential coingestions.

The most important laboratory analysis of anticoagulant ingestions is prothrombin time (PT). A baseline PT at presentation is expected to be normal; assays must be repeated at *48 hours* after exposure, since the onset of coagulopathy is delayed [124]. Any patient given empiric vitamin K supplementation may have an even further delay in PT abnormalities and may require longer coagulation profile monitoring. Clotting factor analysis, particularly for factor VII, may be a more sensitive and earlier indicator of coagulopathy [124]. However, factor analysis does not offer more useful information in most patients with minimal ingestions. Occasionally, serum analysis for warfarin and warfarin derivatives has demonstrated unsuspected exposures in coagulopathic patients of unknown etiology [127,128,149].

The primary treatment of anticoagulant toxicity is vitamin K replacement [150,151]. Warfarin and its congeners have much less effect on human than on rat vitamin K reductase, thus allowing vitamin K rescue therapy for anticoagulant toxicity in humans [151]. Since a single dose of vitamin K therapy cannot affect the prolonged toxicity of the long-acting anticoagulants, we do not recommend empiric vitamin K therapy unless the patient has a coagulopathy. Vitamin K is not immediately effective in reversing coagulopathy; fresh frozen plasma administration is the initial treatment of choice in patients with significant bleeding diathesis. Vitamin K is available in different forms, such as vitamins K_1, K_2, K_3, and K_4. Only vitamin K_1 (phytonadione) should be used; the other forms are ineffective in the treatment of anticoagulant toxicity [113,136,143,150]. Vitamin K_1 can be given orally, subcutaneously, intramuscularly, and intravenously. Intravenous administration has been associated with anaphylactoid reactions and may cause shock and fatality [152,153,154]. Furthermore, it offers no real advantage over other routes of administration. Intramuscular injection may cause hematoma formation in patients with coagulopathy. The authors believe subcutaneous administration of vitamin K_1 is the most advantageous route for initial therapy. Once the dose is adequately titrated, oral vitamin K_1 may be instituted. The amount required to reverse coagulopathy is variable, ranging from 100 to 200 mg per day [128,146]. The duration of vitamin K therapy and coagulopathy is also highly variable, from 40 to 300 days. Various methods have been proposed to decrease the duration of coagulopathy, including administration of hepatic enzyme inducers such as phenobarbital [133,134]. However, there is no concrete evidence to support any of these therapies.

Strychnine

Strychnine is an alkaloid primarily derived from *Strychnos nuxvomica*, a vine indigenous to India, Southern Asia, Australia, and Hawaii. The modern use of strychnine extract dates back to the sixteenth century, when the Phillipino St. Ignatius bean (*Strychnos ignatii*) was introduced as a rodenticide in Europe [155]. Strychnine was advocated as a tonic, cathartic, and aphrodisiac as late as 1970, and its use has resulted in numerous accidental deaths [156–159]. The only "legitimate" use of strychnine is as a pesticide for the control of mice, gophers, prairie dogs, squirrels, moles, porcupines, rabbits, birds, and predatory animals [160]. Because of its mechanism of action, strychnine is used in the study of neural transmission [161]. Strychnine is also found as an adulterant in various illicit drugs, such as cocaine and heroin.

PHARMACOKINETICS. Very limited data are available on strychnine metabolism in humans. It is rapidly absorbed through the nasal mucosa and orally in the small intestine [160]. The majority of strychnine (80–90%) undergoes hepatic oxidative transformation to unknown metabolites [162,163]. The remainder is excreted unchanged in the urine within 24 hours. The half-life of strychnine in humans is approximately 10 hours [164], and the volume of distribution is approximately 13 liters per kilogram [165].

PATHOPHYSIOLOGY. Strychnine antagonizes postsynaptic glycine inhibitory receptors at the spinal cord and, to a lesser degree, at the brainstem, cerebral cortex, and hippocampus [63,160,166,167,168]. Glycine receptors at the cerebral cortex and hippocampus are of a subtype insensitive to strychnine and are minimally affected [160]. The action of glycine is similar to that of gamma-aminobutyric acid (GABA), in that they enhance chloride ionic channel conduction, resulting in hyperpolarization of postsynaptic membrane and increased threshold for neurologic transmission [160,169]. The highest concentration of glycine receptors is found at the ventral horn motor neurons in the spinal cord [169]. Glycine antagonism reduces neuromuscular inhibition, including reciprocal inhibition between antagonistic muscles [63], resulting in contraction of both flexor and extensor muscle groups [170]. The pharmacologic effect of strychnine is quite similar to that of tetanus toxin, which inhibits the release of glycine at postsynaptic neurons in the spinal cord [171].

CLINICAL MANIFESTATIONS. The onset of strychnine toxicity is rapid, within 15 to 30 minutes after exposure. The lethal dose in adults is typically approximately 50 to 100 mg but it may be as little as 5 to 10 mg in children [123,172]. Diffuse muscle contractions and spasms are the primary manifestations of strychnine toxicity. Facial muscle spasms result in risus sardonicus (the sardonic smile) and trismus. Opisthotonos, abdominal muscle contractions, and tonic movements of the extremities may resemble convulsions [170,173]. Since glycine has limited effects in the higher CNS centers, seizures are unlikely and mental status is normally preserved until the patient is gravely ill and hypoxic [160,172]. The extensor muscles appear to be more affected than the flexor muscles, because they are the antigravity muscles and are generally stronger [160,170]. Of interest, in the sloth, where the antigravity muscles are the flexor muscles, strychnine toxicity causes more contractions of the flexor muscle groups [155]. Muscle contractions can be triggered or amplified by any stimulations, including auditory, tactile, and visual stimuli [63], and may lead to lactic acidosis, rhabdomyolysis, and hyperthermia [165,170,174,175,176]. Respiratory depression results from sustained chest and diaphragmatic muscle contractions and brainstem depression. Death is related to respiratory depression, anoxia, and complications from significant muscle contractions [165,172]. The clinical manifestations of strychnine toxicity are similar to those of tetanus infection, because both entities affect glycine transmission. However, the onset of symptoms in tetanus infection is more gradual and the duration of illness more prolonged [171].

MANAGEMENT. Securing the airway, assisting breathing, and maintaining the circulatory system are the immediate goals in symptomatic patients. Electrolytes, acid-base changes, oxygenation saturation, renal function, urine output, and temperature must be monitored carefully in any symptomatic patient. Gastrointestinal decontamination should be performed in any suspected strychnine ingestion. Because strychnine has a rapid onset of action, ipecac-induced emesis is contraindicated. Orogastric lavage followed by activated charcoal should be performed in all patients presenting within 1 to 2 hours after ingestion and all symptomatic patients. Activated charcoal should be administered after gastric decontamination. Asymptomatic patients presenting more than 2 hours after ingestion are unlikely to have significant toxicity from strychnine, and oral activated charcoal alone may suffice.

Enhanced elimination by urinary manipulation has no effect because of minimal renal elimination [162]. Extracorporeal removal (hemodialysis or charcoal hemoperfusion) is ineffective because of the large volume of distribution.

Termination of muscle contractions prevents or reverses lactic acidosis, rhabdomyolysis, hyperthermia, and respiratory depression. Benzodiazepines, because of their agonist GABA effects, are considered the agents of choice in terminating muscle contractions [176–181]. Barbiturates also are reported to be useful in treatment of strychnine toxicity. These agents, however, may not be completely effective in a massive strychnine exposure [182], and nondepolarizing muscle blockers may be required to terminate muscle contractions [170].

Strychnine toxicity usually resolves within 12 to 24 hours [162,170,178]. Supportive therapy should be continued until sufficient strychnine is eliminated by endogenous metabolism.

Sodium Monofluoroacetate (1080)

Sodium monofluoroacetate is a highly toxic pesticide developed during World War II. It is frequently referred as 1080, the number assigned to the compound during the initial investigation [183]. It is the primary toxic constituent in the South African Gifblaar (*Dichapetalum cymosum*) but is also present in other plants in South America and Australia [184,185]. Sodium monofluoroacetate is highly toxic to all mammals, and its use in the United States in limited to licensed exterminators. The congener sodium fluroacetamide (compound 1081), also used as a pesticide, has mechanisms and effects similar to those of fluoroacetate [186]. Sodium monofluoroacetate and fluoroacetamide are used in the extermination of rodents and larger mammals, such as coyotes, foxes, and feral pigs.

PHARMACOKINETICS. The pharmacokinetics of monofluoroacetate are extrapolated from animal models and clinical experience. It appears that monofluoroacetate is minimally absorbed cutaneously but rapidly absorbed from the GI tract [187]. Monofluoroacetate is metabolized to fluorocitrate in the tricarboxylic acid cycle (TCA). There are no other metabolites [188,189]. Approximately 12 percent of the ingested dose is excreted in the urine [189]. In animals with relative resistance to monofluoroacetate, a hepatic defluorination system cleaves the carbon-fluoride bond to detoxify the compound [190].

PATHOPHYSIOLOGY. Sodium monofluoroacetate is structurally similar to acetate and is incorporated into the tricarboxylic acid (TCA) cycle with the help of acetyl-CoA. Fluoroacetate combines with citrate to form fluorocitrate in the TCA cycle [188]. Fluorocitrate inhibits aconitase and succinate dehydrogenase and shuts down the TCA cycle (Fig. 153-2), halting cellular respiration and causing diffuse cellular death [185,187,188]. Organs with higher metabolic demands, such as the brain and heart, are affected immediately [191].

CLINICAL MANIFESTATIONS. Sodium monofluoroacetate exerts significantly different effects among different animal species [192]. Some animals (rabbits, goats, horse) manifest only cardiac arrhythmias or CNS toxicity (dogs), while others (monkeys, cats, pigs) manifest both CNS and cardiac toxicity [192]. The symptoms in humans are similar to those in primates, causing CNS and cardiac toxicity. Sodium monofluoroacetate is considered to be extremely toxic in humans, with the lethal dose estimated at 2 to 10 mg per kilogram [187,193]. The onset of toxicity is rapid, within 1 to 2 hours after exposure [194]. Initial symptoms are nausea and vomiting followed by cardiovascular and CNS toxicity [187,191,195,196]. Fatality is related to the CNS and cardiovascular toxicity [187,196]. The patient may present with agitation, lethargy, seizures, and coma [191,193,196,197]. Cardiovascular manifestations include tachycardia, premature ventricular contractions, S–T segment abnormalities, hypotension, ventricular tachycardia, and ventricular fibrillation [187]. Acute renal failure may be related to hypotension, rhabdomyolysis, and the direct toxic effects of monofluorophosphate on the kidney [191]. Laboratory abnormalities include significant metabolic acidosis and hypocalcemia from the fluoride ion.

MANAGEMENT. Gastric lavage should be performed in symptomatic patients and any patient with suspected exposure who presents within 2 hours after ingestion. Activated charcoal should be administered in all suspected ingestions.

General supportive measures are paramount and aimed at

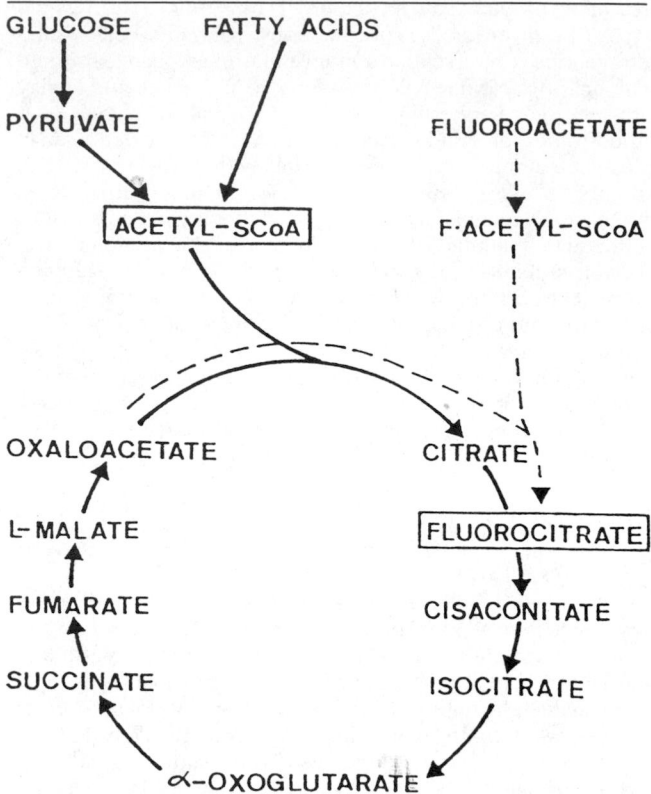

Fig. 153-2. Mechanism of action of fluoroacetate. Fluoroacetate is synthesized into fluorocitrate in the tricarboxylic acid cycle and will block the tricarboxylic acid cycle at the citrate stage. (From Egekeze JO, Oehme FW: Sodium monofluoroacetate: A literature review. *Vet Hum Toxicol* 21:413, 1979. With permission.)

maintaining the airway, breathing, and circulation. Seizures should be treated with benzodiazepines or barbiturates. Hypocalcemia and prolonged Q–Tc intervals may require calcium and magnesium supplementation. Various antidotes have been tested in animals [185,198,199,200]. The most useful agent appears to be glyceryl monoacetate, which provides excess acetate as a substrate for the TCA cycle [185,198]. However, the utility of glyceryl monoacetate in the management of monofluoroacetate toxicity in humans remains unproved.

N-3-Pyridylmethyl-N'-P-Nitrophenylurea

N-3-Pyridylmethyl-N'-p-nitrophenylurea (PNU; Vacor Rat-Killer) was marketed in 1975 as a safe, rapidly acting rodenticide [201,202]. As a rodenticide, PNU is effective with a single consumption and is effective against warfarin-resistant rats [201]. Soon after PNU was marketed, multiple human intoxications were reported [203–210], including death from ingestion of less than a single package (39 gm) [211]. Manufacture was voluntarily discontinued in 1979, without a public recall. Occasional poisonings were reported even after 1979 [209,212].

PHARMACOKINETICS. The pharmacokinetics of PNU in humans are unknown.

PATHOPHYSIOLOGY. N-3-Pyridylmethyl-N′-p-nitrophenyl-urea is structurally related to alloxan, streptozotocin, and pentamidine isethionate, all of which cause destruction of the pancreatic beta cells [213,214,215]. This leads to onset of acute and chronic symptoms of diabetes mellitus after significant exposure. The exact mechanism of action of PNU is still unknown, but it is probably related to the interference of nicotinamide adenine dinucleotide (NAD and NADH) synthesis [216]. Acute exposure to PNU may have diffuse adverse effects on the autonomic, peripheral, and central nervous systems [202, 203,204,207]. The mechanism through which PNU affects the nervous system is unclear. One postulated mechanism is destruction of the sympathetic nerve terminal, similar to the mechanism of 6-aminonicotinamide, a related compound, [207,217, 218]. The acute effects on the nervous system are too rapid to result from chemically induced diabetes.

CLINICAL MANIFESTATIONS. The onset of symptoms in PNU ingestion is within a few hours after ingestion. Significant nausea, vomiting, and abdominal pain are common because of direct corrosive GI effects of PNU [207]. Gastrointestinal perforations have been reported [215]. Derangement in glucose metabolism may occur within a few hours after ingestion. Hypoglycemia, occasionally seen in the initial presentation, may be related to insulin release from beta cell destruction [212]. The primary glucose derangement results from beta cell destruction and hypoinsulinemia; hyperglycemia and ketoacidosis can be clinically evident within hours [202,212]. Effects on the CNS are seen acutely and may became chronic. These effects include encephalopathy, orthostatic hypotension, and motor and sensory peripheral neuropathy [207,212]. Deaths from PNU exposure are related to ketoacidosis and GI perforation.

MANAGEMENT. Gastrointestinal decontamination should be performed in all suspected PNU exposures. Gastric lavage should be followed by activated charcoal administration. Serum glucose should be closely monitored; hypoglycemia in the initial phase of toxicity requires glucose supplementation. Subsequent hyperglycemia and ketoacidosis are managed much as in patients with diabetes mellitus and diabetic ketoacidosis. In animals niacinamide is an effective antidote; it prevents islet cell destruction when administered within 2 hours after toxic doses of PNU or streptozotocin [219–224]. Human data on the efficacy of niacinamide in antagonizing the toxic effect of PNU are limited. Niacinamide should not be confused with niacin and nicotinic acid, both of which are *not* effective antidotes [225]. Niacinamide has not been manufactured since PNU was withdrawn from the market [226], and very few medical facilities retain a supply. However, niacinamide remains the treatment of choice for PNU exposure and should be administered as soon as it is available [225]. The dose of niacinamide is 500 mg intravenously or intramuscularly initially, followed by 100 to 200 mg every 4 hours for up to 48 hours [225].

Aluminum and Zinc Phosphide

Aluminum and zinc phosphide (AlP, Zn_3P_2) are highly toxic insecticides and rodenticides commonly used as solid fumigants and grain preservatives. They are considered to be ideal pesticides for grain preservation because of the simplicity of application, low cost, and high efficacy without grain contamination [227]. These agents are widely available in many countries with minimal regulation; for example, aluminum phosphide is commonly used for home grain storage in Asia [228]. Aluminum phosphide has become the most common suicidal agent in India and other developing countries [229,230]. Phosphides are widely used in grain freighters and have emerged as the major maritime occupational health hazard [231]. Phosphine (hydrogen phosphide; PH_3) is used in the microchip industry as a doping agent and in the illicit manufacture of methamphetamine [232].

PHARMACOKINETICS. Phosphides react with water to form phosphine; the reaction may be accelerated in the acid environment of the stomach [232,229]. Phosphine is then readily absorbed in the stomach [232]. Phosphine itself can also be absorbed through the lungs. There is limited information on the pharmacokinetics and metabolism of phosphine, although it is known to be partly eliminated through the lungs [232].

PATHOPHYSIOLOGY. Phosphine is slowly liberated when phosphides react with moisture in an enclosed environment, as in grain freighters. The exact mechanisms of toxicity are not well elucidated; the most likely mechanism is related to inhibition of cytochrome oxidase [233]. As a cellular toxin, phosphine has deleterious effects on multiple organ systems, particularly organs with high metabolic demands.

CLINICAL MANIFESTATIONS. Inhalation of phosphine gas results in immediate eye and mucous membrane irritation and early onset of pulmonary symptoms [229,231]. Oral ingestion of phosphides causes profound GI symptoms, including nausea, vomiting, and abdominal pain [228,234,235,236]. Respiratory symptoms include cough, dyspnea, and chest tightness. Pulmonary edema and respiratory failure may be delayed for several hours after oral exposure to phosphides [229,236,237]. Fatalities are related to cardiovascular collapse from vasodilation and myocardial damage [235,236,238]. Histologic studies have demonstrated myocyte edema and focal myocardial necrosis [235]. Various electrocardiographic changes have been reported, including S–T segment elevation and depression, QRS prolongation, bundle branch blocks, atrioventricular nodal blockade, and supraventricular and ventricular tachycardia [238,239,240]. Central nervous system effects lead to headache, lethargy, and encephalopathy [235]. Other manifestations include severe metabolic acidosis, hepatitis, and renal failure [235]. Mortality varies from 37 to 100 percent in suicidal ingestions [234,235,236,238,241,242].

MANAGEMENT. The patient should be removed from the contaminated environment immediately after the rescuer is adequately protected. Airway, breathing, and circulatory support are important in the immediate management. Gastric lavage, while simultaneously protecting the staff from fume production, should be performed in any suicidal ingestion of phosphide because of the high morbidity and mortality. This should be followed by activated charcoal administration. Activated charcoal slurry should be mixed with sorbitol or magnesium citrate, rather than plain water, to reduce further liberation of phosphine in the GI tract [229]. Lavage with sodium bicarbonate (3–5% solution) or antacid has been advocated [229,243], but has not been studied in animal or human models.

Cardiac monitoring and electrocardiogram should be performed in suspected phosphine toxicity. Respiratory status should be monitored by continued clinical evaluation. Chest radiograph, pulse oximetry, and arterial blood gas should be obtained if clinically indicated. The diagnosis may be suggested from a decaying fish odor released by substituted phosphines and diphosphines [229]. Silver nitrate-impregnated paper blackens in the presence of phosphine in the gastric fluid [244].

There is no antidote for phosphine toxicity other than good supportive care. Hypomagnesemia has been reported with aluminum phosphide poisoning, and magnesium administration has been successful in abolishing various arrhythmias in some cases [239,245,246,247]. However, the prevalence of hypomagnesemia and the utility of magnesium therapy in phosphide poisoning remain unclear.

Methyl Bromide

Methyl bromide (CH_3Br) is a colorless halogenated hydrocarbon gas used primarily as a fumigant for the control of nematodes, insects, rodents, fungi, and weeds. Its use has became more prevalent since the abandonment of chlordane and acrylonitrile as fumigants [248]. Methyl bromide is one of the most widely used pesticides in California [249]. It is particularly popular in the food industry, since it is extremely effective, is able to diffuse into any empty spaces, and does not leave any residues after proper ventilation. Methyl bromide can be applied for space, soil, and structure fumigation. Space fumigation of fruits and tobacco can be performed in an airtight chamber (fumigation chamber). For soil fumigation, methyl bromide can be applied underground and sealed with an overlying tent or polyethylene cover. For structural fumigation, gas-proof tarpaulins are applied over the structure before the application of methyl bromide [250]. Methyl bromide was used in the past as a refrigerant and fire-extinguishing agent and is still used for the manufacture of chemicals such as aniline dyes. It has a musty chloroformlike odor at high concentrations, but is odorless at lower but still very toxic concentrations [251]. Since methyl bromide is heavier than air, it is particularly dangerous in an enclosed environment. Inadvertent exposures from accidents or inadequate ventilation have caused significant toxicities and fatalities [248,252–260].

PHARMACOKINETICS. Methyl bromide is primarily absorbed through the lungs. Cutaneous absorption is minimal. Methyl bromide easily penetrates and is retained in cloth, rubber, and leather [252,261]. It is eliminated unchanged in the lungs, but a small proportion is metabolized to 5-methylcysteine and inorganic bromide; these are excreted in the urine [262].

PATHOPHYSIOLOGY. The exact mechanism of toxicity is unclear. It is most likely related to the methylation of sulfhydryl groups in different intracellular enzymes, in a manner similar to heavy metal intoxications [263]. Low levels of bromide can be detected in the serum after significant exposure to methyl bromide, but they do not correlate well with toxicity [248,264]. The symptoms of methyl bromide toxicity are distinctly different from those of bromide toxicity [265,266].

CLINICAL MANIFESTATIONS. Acute toxicity is related to the central nervous and the pulmonary systems [248]. Most symptoms may be delayed for 1 to 6 hours or longer [250,259]. Exposures to concentrations of 2000 ppm or greater may produce immediate CNS depression and respiratory failure [250].

At 600 ppm at atmospheric pressure, fatality may occur with exposures over several hours. The current OSHA permissible exposure limit for methyl bromide is 5 ppm [267].

Mild toxicity may manifest as dizziness, headache, confusion, weakness, nausea, vomiting, and dyspnea [257]. Initial or mild symptoms are frequently dismissed as viral symptoms [258]. Skin irritation and burns commonly underlie clothes and rubber gloves where the methyl bromide gas is trapped [261,268]. After a significant exposure, the patient may present with tremor, myoclonus, and behavioral changes [252,254,268]. Severe toxicity may present with bronchitis, pulmonary edema, convulsions, and coma [252,259]. Fatality is related to pulmonary and CNS damage, although damage to different internal organs has been demonstrated [248,260,264]. Prolonged low-level methyl bromide exposure may cause subacute neurologic changes, including headaches, confusion, behavioral changes, visual disturbance, and motor and sensory deficits [253,256,264, 269]. Some residual neurologic deficits may remain after chronic exposure or significant acute exposure [260,264,270].

The only useful laboratory measurements in the management of methyl bromide intoxication are arterial blood gas or pulse oximetry monitoring. Chest radiography is useful in evaluating patients with pulmonary symptoms. Serum bromide analysis may confirm exposure but is not useful in determining the severity of exposure. Serum bromide levels varied from 4 to 65.6 mg per deciliter in methyl bromide fatalities [248,264,271]. When the serum bromide level is significantly elevated, an elevated chloride level may be observed due to cross-reactivity in the analysis [270].

MANAGEMENT. The management of methyl bromide toxicity consists of supportive therapy, particularly of the airway, breathing, and circulation. Since methyl bromide is a gas, GI decontamination is not relevant. Clothing should be removed and the skin washed with soap and water to eliminate potential methyl bromide residues. Various compounds with sulfhydryl groups, such as dimercaprol (BAL) and N-acetylcysteine, have been suggested as potential antidotes [252,270] but have not been demonstrated to be effective.

N,N-Diethyl-M-Toluamide

N,N-Diethyl-m-toluamide, (diethyltoluamide, or DEET) was initially synthesized in 1954 and marketed as an insect repellant in 1957 [272]. Currently, diethyltoluamide is the most effective and the most widely used insect repellant [273]. Use of diethyltoluamide will continue to increase with increasing public concern over Lyme disease transmission. Diethyltoluamide is effective against many types of insects, including mosquitoes, chiggers, ticks, fleas, gnats, and biting flies. Diethyltoluamide is the primary active ingredient in a number of commercial products, including Off, Deep Woods Off, Cutter Insect Repellant, Repel, Jungle Formula, and Muskol. The concentration of diethyltoluamide in the various products varies from 5 to 100 percent. Products with lower concentrations of diethyltoluamide (20–30%) are just as effective and safer than products containing 100 percent diethyltoluamide [273].

PHARMACOKINETICS. Diethyltoluamide is well absorbed through the skin, with approximately 48 percent of the applied dose absorbed within 6 hours [274]. The plasma concentration peaks 1 hour after dermal application [274]. Diethyltoluamide is primarily metabolized in the liver, and approximately 70 percent of the absorbed dose is excreted as metabolites within the first 24 hours [274]. Another 10 to 15 percent is excreted unchanged in the urine. Diethyltoluamide and its metabolites may accumulate in the fatty tissue, particularly after repeated applications [274].

PATHOPHYSIOLOGY. The mechanism of diethyltoluamide toxicity is unknown. Animal toxicity studies confirm typical CNS symptoms similar to those reported in humans [275]. Most human toxicities reported are in children [276], likely because children absorb a higher ratio of diethyltoluamide relative to their body weight. Initial reports of diethyltoluamide toxicity were almost exclusively in females. One case report was of a girl with ornithine-carbamoyl-transferase deficiency, an X-linked hereditary disease in ammonia transformation [277]. The initial theory suggested that patients with ornithine-carbamoyl-transferase deficiency may be particularly susceptible to diethyltoluamide toxicity. More recent reports have refuted this theory because a number of male patients have also developed diethyltoluamide toxicity [278,279].

CLINICAL MANIFESTATIONS. Diethyltoluamide may cause localized and systemic toxicity. Localized toxicity is primarily limited to skin irritation, contact dermatitis, skin necrosis, and urticaria [275,280,281]. Anaphylactic reactions have occasionally been reported with cutaneous application [281]. The systemic manifestations of diethyltoluamide vary from anxiety to behavioral changes, tremors, lethargy, ataxia, confusion, seizures, and coma [277,278,279,282–286]. Almost all of the case reports are related to application of concentrated diethyltoluamide preparations or repeated application of lower-concentration preparations [277,278,282,283].

MANAGEMENT. The management of diethyltoluamide toxicity is largely supportive. Patients with dermal exposure should have their skin washed with soap and water to prevent further systemic absorption. Seizures may be treated with benzodiazepines. Neurologic work-up may be required in many patients. The symptoms of diethyltoluamide toxicity should be distinguished from those of Reye's syndrome [277]. There is no antidote, and extracorporeal removal procedures are not helpful. Measures to prevent diethyltoluamide toxicity may be the most important treatment. These include avoidance of concentrated diethyltoluamide preparations. Products containing 20 to 30 percent diethyltoluamide are adequate and safer than those with higher concentrations. An additional agent, such as permethrin, can be applied to clothing and may decrease the need of diethyltoluamide [273]. The skin should be washed with soap when the insect repellant is no longer required, and the number of repeat applications should be limited.

Metaldehyde

Metaldehyde, a cyclic tetramer of acetaldehyde, is the primary active ingredient in slug and snail baits. In the United States the concentration of metaldehyde is limited to 4 percent by weight [287]. Other toxic ingredients, such as carbamates and organophosphates, are frequently found in some preparations. In Europe, the concentration of metaldehyde in molluscicides can be as high as 50 percent. Metaldehyde is also used as a portable solid fuel (Meta-fuel tablets) in Europe.

PHARMACOKINETICS. The pharmacokinetics of metaldehyde in humans are largely unknown; analytic assay has been reported in only one intoxicated patient [288]. It was once assumed that metaldehyde is rapidly hydrolyzed into acetaldehyde in the acidic environment in the stomach [287]. However, data from the single reported patient suggest that metaldehyde is absorbed and metabolized slowly in the body [288]. The plasma half-life of metaldehyde was reported to be approximately 27 hours [288]. Acetaldehyde metabolism in humans is extremely rapid unless acetaldehyde dehydrogenase is inhibited; therefore, minimal to no accumulation of acetaldehyde should be expected [289]. Animal studies and the human case report have not found significant acetaldehyde in the serum or urine [288,289].

PATHOPHYSIOLOGY. The mechanism of toxicity of metaldehyde is still unclear. It is postulated that the primary metabolite, acetaldehyde, is responsible by antagonizing the effect of GABA [291,292,293]. However, there is no evidence of any significant accumulation of acetaldehyde. In Antabuse (disulfiram) reactions, acetaldehyde is accumulated from acetaldehyde dehydrogenase inhibition [294]. Although some symptoms of the Antabuse reaction are similar to those of metaldehyde toxicity, seizures are extremely uncommon and prolonged coma has not been reported [295]. A more likely explanation is that metaldehyde itself causes direct CNS toxicity [290,296].

CLINICAL MANIFESTATIONS. Significant toxicity from metaldehyde exposure in the United States is uncommon because of the limited concentration. The clinical manifestations may be related to the amount of the exposure (Table 153-3) [292]. Patients with mild toxicity may present with salivation, facial flushing, nausea, vomiting, and abdominal pain. Central nervous system toxicity includes lethargy, coma, and convulsions [292,297]. Coma has been reported to last several days. Morbidity and mortality are related to prolonged and uncontrolled seizures [292,298]. Significant metabolic acidosis and hyperthermia are also reported with prolonged seizures [298,299].

MANAGEMENT. Patients with significant exposure (i.e., suicidal ingestion) should receive gastric lavage and activated charcoal. The most important management strategy is termi-

Table 153-3. Metaldehyde Poisoning: Relation Between Dose Ingested and Clinical Effects

Dose	Clinical effects
Traces (a few mg/kg)	Salivation, facial flushing, fever, abdominal cramps, nausea, vomiting
≤50 mg/kg	Drowsiness, tachycardia, spasms, irritability, salivation, abdominal cramps, facial flushing, nausea
50–100 mg/kg	Ataxia, increased muscle tone
100–150 mg/kg	Convulsions, tremor, hyperreflexia
150–200 mg/kg	Muscle twitching
Approximately 400 mg/kg	Coma, death

From Londstreth WT, Pierson DJ: Metaldehyde poisoning from slug bait ingestion. *West J Med* 137:135, 1982.

nation of seizure activity in symptomatic patients. Benzodiazepines are the agents of choice in terminating seizures [292]. There are no specific antidotes or specific therapy.

Pentachlorophenol

Pentachlorophenol was first synthesized in 1841 and was used as a pesticide in 1936 [300]. Although pentachlorophenol can be used as a insecticide, herbicide, fungicide, molluscicide, mildew retardant, and bactericide, it is primarily used as a wood preservative. Lumber treated with pentachlorophenol may be resistant to bacterial, fungal, and termite decay. Unlike creosote-treated lumber, pentachlorophenol does not alter the appearance, odor, and the ability to paint wood [301]. Unlike other types of pesticide toxicity in adults, poisonings from pentachlorophenol usually result from occupational exposures [302]. Occupational exposures to pentachlorophenol at wood-treating facilities frequently result from improper ventilation and inadequate engineering controls. Low-concentration, prolonged exposures to pentachlorophenol have been reported in log home residents from pentachlorophenol-treated wood [303]. Epidemics of infant poisoning have resulted from diapers improperly laundered with pentachlorophenol-containing antimicrobial soaps [304,305,306].

PHARMACOKINETICS. Pentachlorophenol can be absorbed via pulmonary, oral, and dermal routes, although pulmonary absorption is the most efficient route. The volume of distribution is approximately 0.35 liter per kilogram and the pKa is 5.0 [307]. Pentachlorophenol is primarily (74%) eliminated unchanged in the urine. A small proportion is oxidized to chlorohydroquinone, which is then eliminated in the urine. After a single oral exposure, the plasma half-life of pentachlorophenol is approximately 27 to 35 hours [307]. Because of the low pKa and significant renal elimination, pentachlorophenol elimination can be enhanced by alkalinization of the urine [308].

PATHOPHYSIOLOGY. The mechanism of toxicity of pentachlorophenol is similar to that of dinitrophenol: these agents uncouple oxidative phosphorylation by interfering with electron transport between flavoprotein and cytochrome P-450 [309,310]. Toxicity is mostly related to heat exhaustion and hyperthermia.

CLINICAL MANIFESTATIONS. Acute exposure to pentachlorophenol results in headache, diaphoresis, nausea, vomiting, weakness, abdominal pain, and fever [311]. With severe toxicity, significant hyperthermia (up to 108°F), coma, convulsions, cerebral edema, and cardiovascular collapse may occur [300,311,312,313]. Laboratory analysis may reveal a respiratory alkalosis and metabolic acidosis from significant exposures. Chronic exposures to pentachlorophenol have been reported to cause aplastic anemia, intravascular hemolysis, and pancreatitis [301,314,315,316]. Chloracne has also been reported because of dioxin contaminations [312].

MANAGEMENT. Gastric decontamination should be performed for oral exposure within several hours. Activated charcoal should also be administered. The skin should be decontaminated with soap and water. Initial management includes oxygen supplementation, airway support, fluid resuscitation, and cardiac monitoring. Core temperature should be frequently monitored, and external cooling should be initiated immediately for significant hyperthermia. Seizures should be treated immediately with benzodiazepines or barbiturates to prevent further temperature increase and rhabdomyolysis. Fluid administration should be adequate to maintain a urine output of 1 to 2 ml per minute. Alkalinization of the urine with sodium bicarbonate enhances elimination and should be performed in patients with significant toxicity [308,317]. However, the clinical efficacy of alkalinization has not been demonstrated.

Paraquat

Paraquat (1,1-dimethyl,4,4-bipyridyl dichloride) was developed in 1882 [318] and for many years was used as an oxidation-reduction indicator. An electron donation to the compound forms a blue free radical [319], hence paraquat was commonly called methyl viologen. The herbicidal properties of paraquat were discovered in 1955 and it was marketed as an herbicide in the 1962. Today, paraquat is most commonly used as a nonselective contact herbicide in many countries. Paraquat can be applied safely when used according to the manufacturer's guidelines [320]. Typically, it is available as a 10 to 30 percent concentrated solution for agricultural use. It is also available as a 5 percent powder for domestic use. Once diluted, paraquat has limited absorption through the skin [321] and by aerosolization into the respiratory system [322]. Paraquat is naturally inactivated in the soil and leaves little active residue in the environment. Despite its many desirable properties, however, the consequences of ingesting concentrated paraquat products are deadly. The LD$_{50}$ of paraquat is approximately 3 to 5 gm in adults [323]. As little as a mouthful (10–15 ml) of a 20 percent solution of paraquat is fatal. Paraquat ingestion is one of the leading methods of suicide in many countries, such as Taiwan, Japan, Malaysia, the West Indies, and Samoa. In Japan, 1200 to 1500 deaths per years from paraquat ingestions are reported [324].

PHARMACOKINETICS. Although oral exposure to paraquat is the most common route of toxicity, less than 5 percent of the ingested amount is actually absorbed [325]. Any recent food ingestion may decrease the amount of systemic absorption. The peak plasma level is reached within 1 to 2 hours after ingestion. Paraquat is almost completely eliminated unchanged via the renal system [325]. Plasma paraquat concentrations decline rapidly after peak absorption, due to tissue distribution. The terminal plasma half-life of paraquat is approximately 12 hours with normal renal function but may be as long as 120 hours as renal function deteriorates [326,327]. Limited data are available on the volume of distribution of paraquat, but the estimate from kinetic study in one patient is 2.75 liters per kilogram [328]. Paraquat is sequestered in different organ compartments, particularly the lungs and kidneys [325].

Dermal absorption of paraquat is minimal unless the exposure is prolonged with concentrated solutions [321]. Aerosolized paraquat particles have a diameter greater than 5 μm and do not reach the lower respiratory tree [322]. Concern about paraquat absorption from smoking marijuana is unfounded, since much of the paraquat is pyrolyzed during the smoking process [329]. Paraquat toxicity from marijuana smoking has not been reported.

PATHOPHYSIOLOGY. The primary organ of toxicity is the lungs, due to selective accumulation of paraquat. Paraquat is actively transported into type I and II alveolar cells through an existing transport system for different polyamines. Paraquat and polyamines share a common structural property: they have two positively charged quaternary nitrogen atoms separated by a distance of 6 to 7 nm (Fig. 153-3) [330]. Diquat, another related herbicide with different structural features, is not selectively taken up and does not cause pulmonary toxicity [330,331]. Inside the cells, paraquat undergoes a single electron reduction into paraquat free radical. This free radical reacts with oxygen to form superoxide free radicals (Fig. 153-4) [332], which then deplete NADPH, leading to lipid peroxidation and subsequent cellular destruction [332,333]. This mechanism of action is also responsible for the phytotoxic property of paraquat [334]. If the patient survives the initial insult, the acute alveolitis leads to pulmonary fibrosis and subsequent hypoxia [332,335]. The lungs accumulate paraquat, and, since they have a plentiful supply of oxygen and electrons for donation, are severely affected [323]. Paraquat is extremely corrosive to the GI tract. Other organs, such as the kidneys, heart, brain, and adrenal glands, are also affected [335,336,337].

CLINICAL MANIFESTATIONS. The symptoms and onset of symptoms of paraquat toxicity are largely determined by the amount of exposure. Patients who ingest greater than 40 mg per kilogram usually die within hours to a few days [336]. These patients develop multiple organ failure, including acute respiratory distress syndrome (ARDS), cerebral edema, myocardial necrosis, and hepatic and renal failure [335–340]. Death can be dramatic and may occur even before the development of significant chest radiograph abnormalities [336]. Patients who ingest 20 to 40 mg per kilogram of paraquat are most likely to die from pulmonary fibrosis, which progresses after a few days to a few weeks [341,342]. Ingestion of less than 20 mg per kilogram may lead to mild toxicity [336,341].

Paraquat is extremely corrosive to mucous membranes, and patients frequently complain of pain in the mouth, throat, esophagus, and abdomen [335,341]. The absence of significant ulcerations in the esophagus or stomach within the first 24 hours of exposure is a good prognostic indicator [335]. The development of renal failure is a poor prognostic indicator [326, 335,343]. This phenomenon cannot be fully explained by the decreased elimination of paraquat in the body, since the majority of the paraquat dose is eliminated within the first 24 hours, even in the setting of renal failure [326,327]. Conversely, renal failure may signify a large paraquat exposure. Almost all patients with renal failure from paraquat have significant pulmonary toxicity, but there are occasional reports of renal failure without significant pulmonary toxicity [338]. The prognosis for a patient with a paraquat ingestion can be determined by the measurement of plasma paraquat concentration and its relationship to time of ingestion. A nomogram initially was presented by Proudfoot et al. [344] and subsequently refined by Hart et al. (Fig. 153-4) [345]. While this nomogram has not been particularly helpful in managing paraquat toxicity, it may be a valuable tool in the study of different treatment modalities.

Fig. 153-3. Mechanism of toxicity of paraquat. 1 = structure of paraquat and putrescine, showing geometric standards of the distance between N atoms; 2 = putative accumulation receptor with a minimum separation of charge of approximately 0.5 nm (optimal distance unknown); 3 = redox cycling of paraquat utilizing NADPH; 4 = formation of OH· radical leading to lipid peroxidation; 5 = detoxification of H_2O_2 via glutathione reductase/peroxidase couple, utilizing NADPH. (From Smith LL: The toxicity of paraquat. *Hum Toxicol* 6:33, 1987. With permission.)

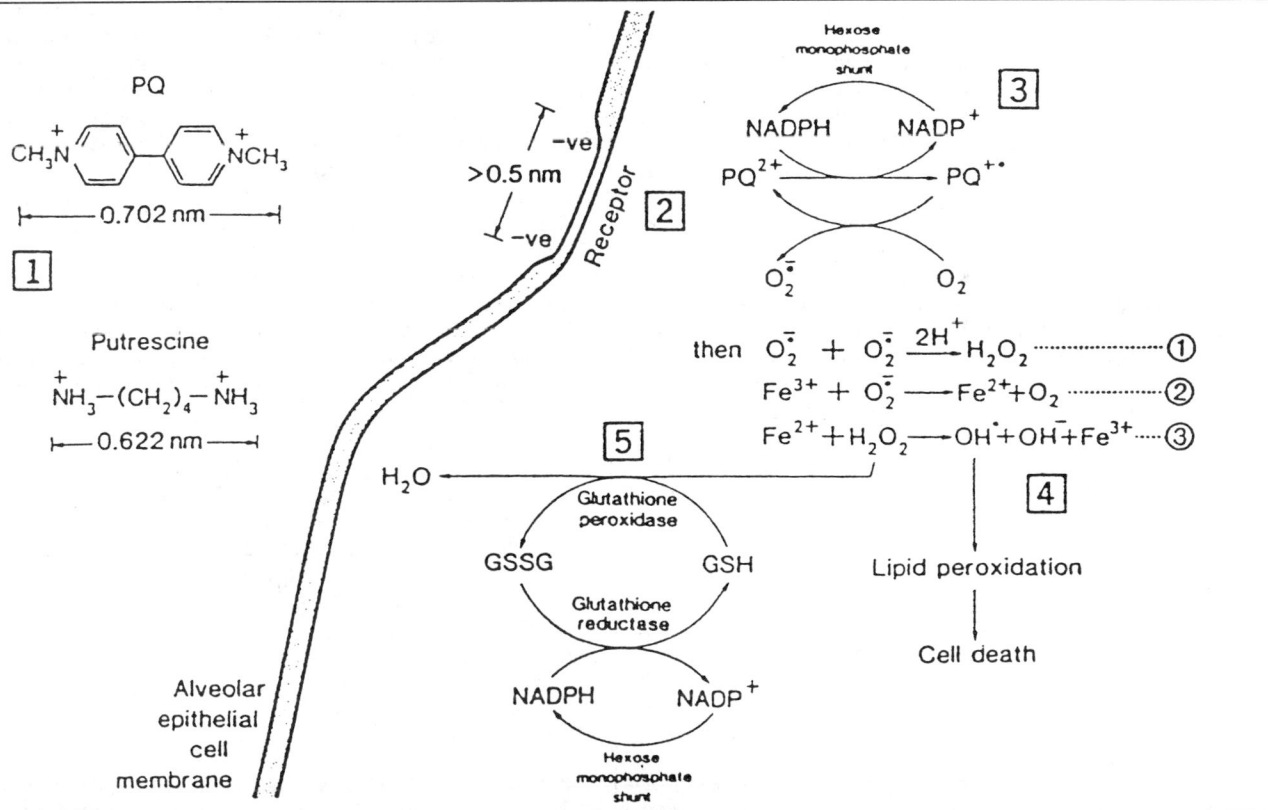

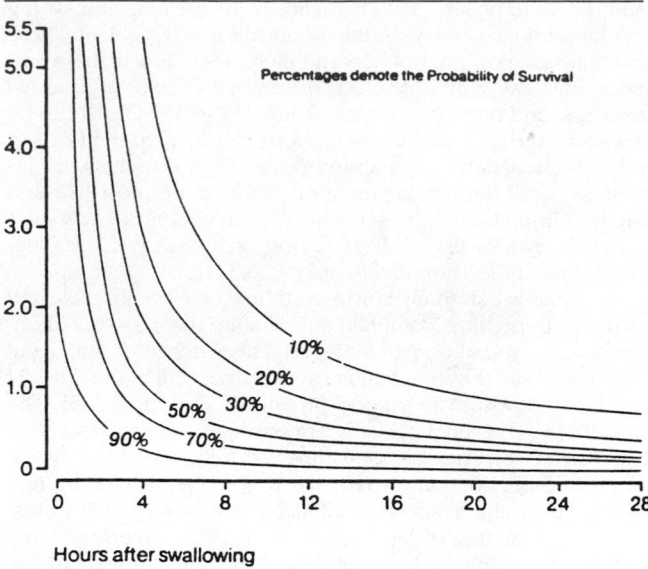

Fig. 153-4. Relation between plasma paraquat concentration (μg/ml), time of ingestion, and probability of survival. (From Hart TB, Nevitt A, Whitehead A: A new statistical approach to the prognostic significance of plasma paraquat concentrations. *Lancet* 1:1222, 1984. With permission.)

Although it is generally accepted that paraquat is not absorbed through the skin, it can be corrosive to the skin and nails [321,346,347]. Occasionally, dermal absorption and system toxicity may occur from prolonged exposure or exposure to concentrated products [346,348].

MANAGEMENT. The most important management strategy is to prevent systemic absorption of paraquat. Once ingested, it is rapidly absorbed and sequestered, frequently leading to death [336]. Gastrointestinal decontamination should be performed in any suspected paraquat ingestion. Orogastric lavage should be performed if the ingestion is within 1 to 2 hours. Fuller's earth (1–2 gm/kg) or activated charcoal should be administered with a cathartic agent as soon as possible to bind any residual paraquat in the GI tract [349,350,351]. Multiple doses of oral adsorbents should be continued until there is evidence of adsorbent in the stool. This is done to prevent desorption of the paraquat. Any dermal exposure should be thoroughly washed with soap. Plasma and urine assays for paraquat are useful to confirm the diagnosis and assess the prognosis; they are generally not useful in direct management of the patient. However, a rapid qualitative screen for paraquat exposure may be performed by the addition of sodium dithionite to urine under alkaline condition. A change in color to blue confirms paraquat absorption [352].

The treatment of paraquat toxicity consists of basic supportive therapy, particularly respiratory monitoring and support. Chest radiographs and oxygen monitoring of ARDS and impending respiratory failure are important in patients with significant exposure. Since the formation of paraquat free radicals requires oxygen, oxygen therapy should be administered only when it is necessary and should be maintained at the minimal required level [353].

Experimental therapies for paraquat toxicity have been formulated using various strategies. These include enhancement of paraquat elimination, neutralization of paraquat in the body, blockade of the cellular uptake of paraquat, prevention of free radical formation and lipid peroxidation, and prevention of pulmonary fibrosis [332,343]. Forced diuresis does not have significant effects on paraquat elimination. Hemodialysis and charcoal hemoperfusion can increase elimination. In an animal model, the institution of charcoal hemoperfusion within 2 hours after paraquat ingestion decreased the fatality rate [354]. Similarly, a follow-up animal study confirmed that delayed hemoperfusion (after 2 hours) did not alter the amount of paraquat in the central compartment [355,356]. Clinically, hemodialysis, charcoal hemoperfusion, and continuous arteriovenous hemofiltration have not altered mortality [357–380]. There are significant limitations in applying extracorporeal procedures. Because the volume of distribution of paraquat is relatively large and paraquat is sequestered into tissue compartments rapidly, extracorporeal removal must be performed during peak absorption (within 2 hours after ingestion) to alter the total body load of paraquat significantly. Since most patients present a number of hours after ingestion and the logistics of extracorporeal removal typically translate into an additional 1- to 2-hour delay, the amount of paraquat removed in most instances is insignificant.

Immunotherapy with monoclonal antibody fragments (Fab, Fv) against paraquat or against the active transport mechanism in the cells is intriguing [361,362] but will probably require that the therapy be administered before significant tissue redistribution. More research is required to assess the value of this therapy. Various agents, such as putrescine and spermidine (endogenous polyamines) [363,364], and beta-adrenergic receptor blockers [365], have been demonstrated to prevent active transport of paraquat into lung tissues but failed to provide any benefits in vivo.

Various antioxidants and free radical scavengers, such as vitamins C and E [333,343,366], deferoxamine [367], superoxide dismutase [368], clofibrate [343], selenium [369], glutathione peroxidase, and N-acetylcysteine [370,371], have been tested against paraquat toxicity. To date there has been no or insignificant improvement in animal models. One clinical study with significant design faults suggested that immunosuppressive agents, such as corticosteroids and cyclophosphamide, have some utility in altering the fatality of paraquat toxicity [372]. However, the results require further validation. Other agents that may alter pulmonary fibrosis, such as colchicine [373], nonsteroidal antiinflammatory agents, and collagen synthesis inhibitors [374], also require more study. Niacin, which increases NADPH synthesis, has some protective effects in rats, but it is unclear whether it is applicable to human toxicity [375]. Lastly, lung transplantation was unsuccessful in a number of patients. Because of the cellular accumulation of paraquat, any early lung transplantation results in fibrosis of the transplanted lungs [376,377,378].

Diquat

Diquat (1,1'-ethylene-2,2'-dipyridylium ion) is a contact herbicide with action and structure similar to that of paraquat. Both diquat and paraquat liberate hydrogen peroxide and oxygen free radical, resulting in toxicity to both plants and animals [379]. The use of diquat is more limited and hence results in fewer intoxications than paraquat.

PHARMACOKINETICS. The kinetics of diquat are unknown in humans. In animal models, less than 10 percent of the oral dose is absorbed. More than 90 percent of the absorbed dose is eliminated unchanged by the kidneys [380]. There are no known metabolites of diquat.

PATHOPHYSIOLOGY AND CLINICAL MANIFESTA-TIONS. In animal models, diquat is less toxic than paraquat [123]. However, human fatalities have been reported with approximately 20 to 50 ml of a 20 percent solution [381]. Similar to paraquat, diquat causes multiple organ damage. However, unlike paraquat, diquat normally spares the pulmonary system [381,382]. This is because diquat is not actively transported to and concentrated in the alveolar cells of the lungs [331]. The symptoms of diquat toxicity may be delayed several hours to 2 days [383]. Diquat toxicity may be characterized by toxicity to the GI tract, brain, and kidneys. Vomiting, abdominal pain, GI tract erosions, and paralytic ileus are common [381,384,385]. Acute renal failure may be related to hypovolemia and the direct toxic effects. The effects of diquat on the CNS may result in lethargy, seizures, and coma [381,384,386]. Brainstem infarctions may be specific to diquat toxicity. All patients who die have significant CNS manifestations before cardiovascular collapse [381,385].

MANAGEMENT. The management of diquat exposure is similar to that of paraquat. However, there are limited studies in the treatment of diquat toxicity compared to paraquat. Gastric lavage should be performed in any potential diquat ingestion within 2 hours. Fuller's earth or activated charcoal should be administered as soon as possible. The rest of the treatment is largely supportive. Hemodialysis or hemoperfusion has not been demonstrated to be effective for the treatment of diquat toxicity [381,385,387,388].

Chlorophenoxy Herbicides

Chlorophenoxy herbicides are used to control broad-leaf weeds and woody plants. At higher doses, they are used for total vegetation control. They exert their effects by mimicking the action of auxins (plant growth hormones) and cause overstimulation of plant growth [68]. Numerous derivatives are available for agricultural and domestic use [389]. The most commonly used agents include 2,4-dichlorophenoxyacetic acid (2,4-D), 2,4,5-trichlorophenoxyacetic acid (2,4,5-T), and 2-methyl-4-chlorophenoxypropionic acid (MCPP). Many preparations contain more than one chlorophenoxy herbicide or other types of herbicides. Despite extensive use of these agents, fatality and significant toxicity are limited. The chlorophenoxy herbicides are notorious due to the dioxin contamination of Agent Orange, a 1:1 mixture of 2,4-D and 2,4,5-T used extensively in the Vietnam War, so-named for the color of the drums used to store it. Agent Orange contained dioxin [2,3,7,9-tetrachlorodibenzo-dioxin (2,3,7,9-TCDD)], a contaminant in the synthesis of chlorophenoxy compounds and a potent teratogen in animals [9,68,390-394].

PHARMACOKINETICS. In general, chlorophenoxy herbicides are well absorbed orally. They have small volumes of distribution, large renal excretion, and a low pKa [389]

2,4-Dichlorophenoxyacetic Acid. 2,4-Dichlorophenoxyacetic acid [2,4-D) has a volume of distribution of 0.1 to 0.3 liter per kilogram and a pKa of 2.6 to 3.5 [395,396]. Oral doses of 5

mg per kilogram in human volunteers produce no ill effects. The peak serum concentration is achieved at approximately 4 to 12 hours [397]. Approximately 80 percent of the absorbed dose is eliminated unchanged in the urine, and 13 percent is eliminated as acid-labile conjugates. The plasma half-life is approximately 18 to 40 hours and varies with urine pH; it may range from 4 to 220 hours [385,397,398].

2,4,5-Trichlorophenoxyacetic Acid. 2,4,5-Trichlorophenoxyacetic acid (2,4,5-T) has a volume of distribution of 6.1 liters per kilogram. After oral administration of 5 mg per kilogram in volunteers, absorption of 2,4,5-T is nearly complete. 2,4,5-T is exclusively excreted unchanged in the urine, and the plasma half-life is approximately 11 to 23 hours [400].

PATHOPHYSIOLOGY. The mechanisms of toxicity in humans are uncertain. One potential mechanism may be related to uncoupling of oxidative phosphorylation (demonstrated in vitro and as mild heat exhaustion syndrome in case reports) [401,402,403]. There may be other direct toxic effects on the skeletal muscles and the peripheral nerves [404].

CLINICAL MANIFESTATIONS. Gastrointestinal symptoms are common with chlorophenoxy herbicide toxicity. Patients frequently develop nausea, vomiting, diarrhea, and abdominal pain [396,401]. Ulcerations may occur at the mouth and pharynx but are uncommon elsewhere in the GI tract [403]. A mild heat exhaustion syndrome consisting of fever, diaphoresis, and hyperventilation can be seen [396,401]. The CNS is particularly affected by the chlorophenoxy herbicides. The patient may present with confusion, lethargy, convulsions, and coma [396,405,406]. Prolonged coma (up to 4 days) has been reported with 2,4-D toxicity [407]. Myotonia, rhabdomyolysis, and chronic muscle weakness are also reported [408]. Renal complications result from rhabdomyolysis and myoglobinuria [408]. Hypocalcemia may occasionally be seen as a result of rhabdomyolysis and hyperphosphatemia [406,409]. Fatality is uncommon, and the etiology of death remains unclear [403,405,409–412].

The issue of carcinogenesis and chronic exposures to phenoxy herbicides remains controversial and conflicting. Several studies, though imperfect, suggested an increased risk for the development of soft tissue sarcoma, Hodgkin's disease, and non-Hodgkin's lymphoma with chronic phenoxy herbicide exposure [6,393,394,413,414].

MANAGEMENT. Gastric decontamination with lavage should be performed within a few hours of ingestion. Activated charcoal should be administered to all patients with acute oral exposure. Skin should be decontaminated with soap and water. Basic supportive therapies include the maintenance of good urine output with fluid resuscitation and external cooling for hyperthermia. Because of the low pKa and renal elimination of chlorophenoxy herbicides, renal elimination is related to the urine pH [389]. Alkalinization of the urine with sodium bicarbonate has been reported significantly to enhance renal excretion and decrease the plasma half-life of various chlorophenoxy herbicides [396]. Alkalinization of the urine may have potential benefits in preventing acute renal failure from myoglobinuria. However, both fluid and bicarbonate administration must be monitored closely, since renal dysfunction may develop from chlorophenoxy herbicide toxicity. The utility of extracorporeal removal procedures, such as hemodialysis and charcoal hemoperfusion, has not been studied. However, they may be useful for 2,4-D because of its small volume of distribution.

Chlorate Salts

Chlorate salts (sodium chlorate ($NaClO_3$), potassium chlorate ($KClO_3$)) are nonspecific herbicides. They are also used in the manufacture of explosives, dyestuffs, tanning agents, and matches. Toxic exposures are uncommon.

PATHOPHYSIOLOGY. Chlorates are strong oxidizing agents that result in hemolysis and methemoglobinemia. Chlorates have direct toxic effects on the kidneys and indirect nephrotoxicity from hemoglobinuria [123]. Since chlorates are primarily eliminated via the kidneys, nephrotoxicity further enhances their toxicity [415].

CLINICAL PRESENTATIONS. The acute lethal dose is approximately 25 to 35 gm [416]. Gastrointestinal symptoms are prominent within hours after an acute exposure and include nausea, vomiting, diarrhea, and abdominal pain [415,416,417]. Hemolytic anemia and methemoglobinemia result from the oxidizing effects. Both entities may result in a significantly decreased oxygen-carrying capacity and cellular hypoxia [415,418]. Cyanosis may be evident with significant methemoglobinemia. Acute renal failure typically develops within 48 hours after exposure [416,417,419,420]. Significant hyperkalemia from hemolysis is another potential fatal complication.

MANAGEMENT. Initial supportive therapies should be directed at the airway, breathing, and maintenance of circulation. Cardiac monitoring should be initiated. Hematocrit, serum electrolytes, methemoglobinemia, and renal function should be evaluated. Gastric decontamination should be performed within 2 hours after ingestion unless the patient already has significant vomiting. Activated charcoal should also be administered. Sodium thiosulfate (2–5 gm orally or intravenously) has been advocated to inactivate the chlorate ion but has not been proved clinically [421]. Methylene blue should be administered for methemoglobinemia but may not be effective in the setting of significant hemolysis, because intact intracellular enzymes are required for its activation [422]. Exchange transfusion may be required for refractory methemoglobinemia or when hemolysis is significant. Hemodialysis can remove chlorates and is recommended in patients with associated renal dysfunction [416,421].

References

1. Hayes WJ Jr: Introduction, in Hayes WJ Jr, Laws ER (eds): *Handbook of Pesticide Toxicology*. San Diego, Academic, 1991, pp 1–38.
2. Ferrer A, Cabral JPR: Epidemics due to pesticide contamination of food. *Food Addit Contam* 6(suppl):95, 1989.
3. Morgan JP: The Jamaica ginger paralysis. *JAMA* 248:1864, 1982.
4. Turnbull GJ: Pesticide residues in food: A toxicological view—Discussion paper. *J Roy Soc Med* 77:932, 1984.
5. Bakir F, Damiuji SF, Amin-Zaki, et al: Methylmercury poisoning in Iraq. *Science* 181:230, 1973.
6. Florentine MJ, Sanfilippo DJ: Elemental mercury poisoning. *Clin Pharm* 10:213, 1991.
7. Markovitz A, Crosby WH: Chemical carcinogenesis: A soil fumigant, 1,3-dichloropropene as possible cause of hematologic malignancies. *Arch Intern Med* 144:1409, 1984.
8. Pearce NE, Sheppard RA, Smith AH, et al: Non-Hodgkin's lymphoma and farming: An expanded case-control study. *Int J Cancer* 39:155, 1987.
9. Wiklund K, Dich J, Holm LE: Risk of malignant lymphoma in Swedish pesticide appliers. *Br J Cancer* 56:505, 1987.
10. Wilson JG: Environmental chemicals, in Wilson JG, Fraser FC (eds): *Handbook of Teratology. vol 1. General Principles and Etiology*. New York, Plenum, 1977, pp 357–385.
11. Donat H, Matthies J, Schwarz I: Fertility of workers exposed to herbicides and pesticides. *Andrologia* 22:401, 1990.
12. Rajput AH, Uitti RJ, Stern W, et al: Geography, drinking water chemistry, pesticides and herbicides and the etiology of Parkinson's disease. *Can J Neurol Sci* 14(suppl):414, 1987.
13. Semchuk KM, Love EJ, Lee RG: Parkinson's disease and exposure to agricultural work and pesticide chemicals. *Neurology* 42:1328, 1992.
14. Tanner CM, Langston JW: Do environmental toxins cause Parkinson's disease? A critical review. *Neurology* 40(suppl):17, 1990.
15. Jeyaratnam J: Acute pesticide poisoning: A major global health problem. *World Health Stat Q* 43:139, 1990.
16. Levine RS, Doull J: Global estimates of acute pesticide morbidity and mortality. *Rev Environ Contam Toxicol* 129:29, 1992.
17. Mehler LN, O'Malley MA, Krieger RI: Acute pesticide morbidity and mortality: California. *Rev Environ Contam Toxicol* 129:51, 1992.
18. Jackson RJ: Pesticides as a public health concern in California. *Prev Med Publ Health* 139:363, 1983.
19. Mahaney FX: Pesticide exposure in grain industry raises cancer rates. *J Natl Cancer Inst* 82:817, 1990.
20. Litovitz TL, Holm KC, Clancy C, et al: 1992 annual report of the American Association of Poison Control Centers Toxic Surveillance System. *Am J Emerg Med* 11:494, 1993.
21. Bodeker W: Suicidal pesticide poisoning. *World Health Forum* 12:208, 1991.
22. Saxena MC, Siddiqui MKJ, Bhargava AK, et al: Placental transfer of pesticides in humans. *Arch Toxicol* 48:127, 1981.
23. Saxena MC, Siddiqui MKJ: A comparison organochlorine insecticide contents in specimens of maternal blood, placenta, and umbilical cord blood from stillborn and live born cases. *J Toxicol Environ Health* 11:71, 1983.
24. Roncevic N, Pavkov S, Galetin-Smith R, et al: Serum concentrations of organochlorine compounds during pregnancy and the newborn. *Bull Environ Contam Toxicol* 38:117, 1987.
25. Takahasi W, Saidin D, Takei G, et al: Organochloride pesticide residues in human milk in Hawaii, 1979–1980. *Bull Environ Contam Toxicol* 27:506, 1981.
26. Stacey CI, Perriman WS, Whitney S: Organochlorine pesticide residue levels in human milk: Western Australia, 1979–1980. *Arch Environ Health* 40:102, 1985.
27. Hayes WJ: Chlorinated hydrocarbon insecticides, in Hayes WJ (ed): *Pesticides Studied in Man*. Baltimore, Williams & Wilkins, 1982, pp 172–283.
28. USPHS: *Toxicological Profile for p,p′-DDT, p,p′-DDE, p,p′-DDD*. Atlanta, Agency for Toxic Substances and Disease Registry, US Public Health Service. Government Printing Office, December 1989, p 75
29. Barnes R: Poisoning by the insecticide chlordane. *Med J Aust* 1:972, 1967.
30. Aldrich FD, Holmes JH: Acute chlordane intoxication in a child. *Arch Environ Health* 19:129, 1969.
31. Derbes VH, Dent JH, Forrest WW, et al: Fatal chlordane poisoning; Council on Pharmacy and Chemistry. *JAMA* 158:1367, 1955.
32. Dadey JL, Kammer AG: Chlordane intoxication. *JAMA* 153:723, 1953.
33. Kutz FW, Strassman SC, Sperling JF, et al: A fatal chlordane poisoning. *J Toxicol Clin Toxicol* 20:167, 1983.
34. USPHS: *Toxicological Profile for Aldrin/Dieldrin*. Atlanta, Agency for Toxic Substances and Disease Registry, US Public Health Service. Government Printing Office, 1989, p 71.

35. WHO: *Environmental Health Criteria 40: Endosulfan.* Geneva, World Health Organization, 1984.

36. Shemesh Y, Bourvine A, Gold D, et al: Survival after acute endosulfan intoxication. *J Toxicol Clin Toxicol* 26:265, 1988.

37. WHO: *Environmental Health Criteria 44: Mirex.* Geneva, World Health Organization, 1984.

38. Cannon SB, Veasey JM, Jackson RS, et al: Epidemic kepone poisoning in chemical workers. *Am J Epidemiol* 107:529, 1978.

39. Taylor J: Neurological manifestations in humans exposed to chlordecone: Follow up results. *Neurotoxicology* 6:231, 1985.

40. Ramachandran M, Banerjee M, Grover A, et al: DDT and HCH residues in the body fat and blood samples from some Delhi hospitals. *Ind J Med Res* 80:590, 1984.

41. USPHS: *Toxicological Profile for Hexachlorocyclohexane.* Atlanta, Agency for Toxic Substances and Disease Registry, US Public Health Service. Government Printing Office, December 1989, p 11.

42. Palmer AK, Cozens DD, Spicer EJF, et al: Effects of lindane upon reproduction function in a 3 generation study of rats. *Toxicology* 10:45, 1978.

43. Palmer AK, Bottomley AM, Worden AN, et al: Effect of lindane on pregnancy in the rabbit and rat. *Toxicology* 10:239, 1978.

44. Williams CH, Casterline JL: Effects on toxicity and on enzyme activity of the interactions between aldrin, chlordane, piperonyl butoxide and banol in rats. *Proc Soc Exp Biol Med* 135:46, 1970.

45. Conney AJ, Welch RM, Kuntzman R, et al: Effects of pesticides on drug and steroid metabolism. *Clin Pharmacol Ther* 8:1, 1966.

46. Garrettson LK, Guzelian PS, Blanke RV: Subacute chlordane poisoning. *Clin Toxicol* 22:565, 1984.

47. USPHS: *Toxicological Profile for Chlordane.* Atlanta, Agency for Toxic Substances and Disease Registry, US Public Health Service. Government Printing Office, December 1989, p 1.

48. Kutz FW, Strassman SC, Sperling JF, et al: A fatal chlordane poisoning. *J Toxicol Clin Toxicol* 20:167, 1983.

49. Curley A, Garrettson L: Acute chlordane poisoning, clinical and chemical studies. *Arch Environ Health* 18:211, 1969.

50. Olanoff L, Bristow W, Coloough J: Acute chlordane intoxication. *J Toxicol Clin Toxicol* 20:291, 1983.

51. Graham MJ, Williams FM, Rawlins MD: Metabolism of aldrin to dieldrin by rat skin following topical application. *Food Chem Toxicol* 29:701, 1991.

52. Narahashi T: Nerve membrane ionic channels as the target of insecticides, in Narahashi T (ed): *Neurotoxicology of Insecticides and Pheromones.* New York, Plenum, 1979, pp 211–243.

53. Shankland DL: Neurotoxic action of chlorinated hydrocarbon insecticides. *Neurobehav Toxicol Teratol* 4:805, 1982.

54. Matsumura F, Ghiasuddin SM: DDT sensitive Ca ATPase in the axonic membrane, in Narahashi T (ed): *Neurotoxicology of Insecticides and Pheromones.* New York, Plenum, 1979, pp 245–257.

55. Joy RM, Albertson TE: Lindane and limbic system excitability. *Neurol Toxicol* 2:193, 1985.

56. Morgan DP, Stockdale EM, Roberts RJ, et al: Anemia associated with exposure to lindane. *Arch Environ Health* 35:307, 1980.

57. Feldman RJ, Maibach HI: Percutaneous penetration of some pesticides and herbicides in man. *Toxicol Appl Pharmacol* 28:126, 1974.

58. Nitsche K, Lange M, Bauer E, et al: Quantitative distribution of locally applied lindane in human skin and subcutaneous fat in vitro: Dependence of penetration on the applied concentration, skin state, duration of action and nature and time of washing. *Derm Beruf Umwelt* 32:161, 1984.

59. Nigma SK, Karnik AB, Majumder SK, et al: Serum hexachlorocyclohexane residues in workers engaged at a HCH manufacturing plant. *Int Arch Occup Environ Health* 57:315, 1986.

60. Telch J, Jarvis DA: Acute intoxication with lindane. *Can Med Assoc J* 126:662, 1982.

61. Ginsburg CM, Lowry W, Reisch JS: Absorption of lindane in infants and children. *J Pediatr* 91:998, 1977.

62. Goldberg LH, Shupp D, Weitz HH, et al: Injection of household spray insecticide. *Ann Emerg Med* 11:626, 1982.

63. Klaassen CD: Nonmetallic environmental toxicants: Air pollutants, solvents and vapors, and pesticides. In Gilman AG, Rall TW, Nies AS, et al (eds): *Goodman and Gilman's The Pharmacocological Basis of Therapeutics.* 8th ed. New York, Pergamon, 1990, pp 1615-1639.

64. Acute convulsions with endrin poisoning. *MMWR* 33:687, 1986.

65. Wells WL, Milhorn HT: Suicide attempt by toxaphene ingestion: A case report. *J Miss State Med Assoc* 24:329, 1983.

66. Runhar EA, Sangster B, Greve PA, et al: A case of fatal endrin poisoning. *Hum Toxicol* 4:241, 1985.

67. Hayes WJ: *Clinical Handbook on Economic Poisons.* Public Health Service Publication no. 476. Washington, D.C., U.S. Government Printing Office, 1963.

68. Ecobichon DJ: Toxic effects of pesticides, in Amdur MP, Doull J, Klaassen CD (eds): *Casarett and Doull's Toxicology, The Basic Science of Poisons.* New York, Pergamon, 1991, p 575.

69. Rowley DL, Rab MA, Hardjotanojo W, et al: Convulsions caused by endrin poisoning in Pakistan. *Pediatrics* 79:928, 1987.

70. Jaeger V, Podczeck A, Haubenstock A, et al: Acute oral poisoning with lindane solvent mixtures. *Vet Hum Toxicol* 26:11, 1984.

71. Carlson JE, Villaveces JW: Hypersensitivity pneumonitis due to pyrethrum. *JAMA* 237:1718, 1977.

72. Kulig K, Rumack B: Hydrocarbon ingestion. *Curr Top Emerg Med* 3:1, 1981.

73. Bass M: Death from sniffing gasoline (letter). *N Engl J Med* 299:203, 1978.

74. Kashyap SK: Health surveillance and biological monitoring of pesticide formulations in India. *Toxicol Lett* 33:107, 1986.

75. Barnes R: Poisoning by the insecticide chlordane. *Med J Aust* 1:972, 1967.

76. Aldrich FD, Holmes JH: Acute chlordane intoxication in a child. *Arch Environ Health* 19:129, 1969.

77. Derbes VH, Dent JH, Forrest WW, et al: Fatal chlordane poisoning: Council on Pharmacy and Chemistry. *JAMA* 158:1367, 1955.

78. Dadey JL, Krammer AG: Chlordane intoxication. *JAMA* 153:723, 1953.

79. USPHS: *Toxicological Profile for Chlordane.* Atlanta, Agency for Toxic Substances and Disease Registry, US Public Health Service. Government Printing Office, December 1989, p 9.

80. Jager K: *Aldrin, Dieldrin, Endrin and Telodrin: An Epidemiological and Toxicological Study of Long Term Occupational Exposure.* New York, Elsevier, 1970, pp 121–131.

81. Berry DH, Brewster MA, Watson R, et al: Untoward effects associated with lindane abuse (letter). *Am J Dis Child* 14:125, 1981.

82. Furie B, Trubowitz S: Insecticides and blood dyscrasias: Chlordane exposure and self limited refractory megaloblastic anemia. *JAMA* 235:1720, 1976.

83. Mendeloff AI, Smith DE: Clinical pathologic conference: Exposure to insecticides, bone marrow failure, gastrointestinal bleeding, and uncontrollable infections. *Am J Med* 19:274, 1955.

84. Austin H, Keil JE, Cole P: A prospective follow up study of cancer mortality in relation to serum DDT. *Am J Public Health* 79:43, 1989.

85. Wang HH, McMahon B: Mortality of workers employed in the manufacture of chlordane and heptachlor. *J Occup Med* 21:745, 1979.

86. Sharp DS, Eskenazi B, Harrison R, et al: Delayed health hazards of pesticide exposure. *Ann Rev Public Health* 8:441, 1986.

87. Reuber MD: Carcinogenicity of heptachlor and heptachlor epoxide. *J Environ Pathol Toxicol Oncol* 7:85, 1987.

88. Saady JJ, Polkis A: Determination of chlorinated hydrocarbons pesticides by solid phase extraction and capillary GC with electron capture detection. *J Anal Toxicol* 14:301, 1990.

89. Salkinoja-Salonen MS, Jokela JK: Measurement of organic halogen compounds in urine as as indicator of exposure. *Scand J Work Environ Health* 17:75, 1991.

90. Frank R, Rasper J, Smout MS, et al: Organochlorine residues in adipose tissues, blood and milk from Ontario residents, 1976–1985. *Can J Public Health* 79:150, 1988.

91. USPHS: *Toxicological Profile for p,p'-DDT, p,p'-DDE, p,p'-DDD.* Atlanta, Agency for Toxic Substances and Disease Registry, US Public Health Service. Government Printing Office, December 1989, p 9.

92. Dally S, Garnier R, Bismuth C: Diagnosis of chlorinated hydrocarbon poisoning by x-ray examination. *Br J Ind Med* 44:424, 1987.

93. Morgan DP, Dotson TB, Lin LI: Effectiveness of activated charcoal, mineral oil, and castor oil in limiting gastrointestinal absorption of a chlorinated hydrocarbon pesticide. *Clin Toxicol* 11:61, 1977.

94. Cohn WJ, Boylan JJ, Blanke RV, et al: Treatment of chlordecone toxicity with cholestyramine. *N Engl J Med* 298:243, 1978.

95. Daerr W, Kaukel E, Schmoldt A: Hamoperfusion: Eine therapeutische alternative zue fruhbehandlung der akuten Lindan-intoxickation. *Dtsch Med Wochenschr* 110:1253, 1985.

96. Tilson HA, Hong JS, Mactutus CF: Effects of 5,5 diphenylhydantoin on neurobehavioral toxicity of organochlorine pesticides and permethrin. *J Pharmacol Exp Ther* 233:285, 1985.

97. Tilson MA, Shaw S, McLamb RL: The effects of lindane, DDT, and chlordecone on avoidance responding and seizure activity. *Toxicol Appl Pharmacol* 88:57, 1987.

98. Gleason MN, Gosselin RE, Hodge HC, et al: *Clinical Toxicology of Commercial Products.* 3rd ed. Baltimore, Williams & Wilkins, 1976.

99. Paton DL, Walker JS: Pyrethrin poisoning from commercial strength flea and tick spray. *Am J Emerg Med* 6:232, 1988.

100. Gleason MN, Gosselin RE, Hodge HC, et al: *Clinical Toxicology of Commercial Products.* 3rd ed. Baltimore, Williams & Wilkins, 1969, pp 196–197.

101. Dorman DC, Beasley VR: Neurotoxicology of pyrethrin and the pyretroid insecticides. *Vet Hum Toxicol* 33:238, 1991.

102. Casida JE, Gammon DW, Glockman AH, et al: Mechanism of selective action of pyrethroid insecticides. *Annu Rev Pharmacol Toxicol* 23:413, 1983.

103. Aldridge WN: Toxicology of pyrethroids, in Miyamoto J, Kearney PC (eds): *Pesticide Chemistry: Human Welfare and the Environment.* vol. 3. Oxford, Pergamon, 1983, pp 485–490.

104. Feinberg SM: Pyrethrum sensitization. *JAMA* 102:1557, 1934.

105. Shono T, Ohsawa K, Casida JE: Metabolism of trans and cis permethrin, trans and cis pypermethrin and decamethrin by microsomal enzymes. *J Agric Food Chem* 27:316, 1979.

106. Kulkarni AP, Hodgson E: The metabolism of insecticides: The role of monooxygenase enzymes. *Annu Rev Pharmacol Toxicol* 24:19, 1984.

107. He F, Sun J, Han K, et al: Effects of pyrethroid insecticides on subjects engaged in packaging pyrethroids. *Br J Ind Med* 45:548, 1988.

108. He F, Wang S, Liu L, et al: Clinical manifestations and diagnosis of acute pyrethroid poisoning. *Arch Toxicol* 63:54, 1989.

109. Wax PM, Hoffman RS, Goldfrank LR: Fatality associated with inhalation of a pyrethrin insecticide (abstract). *Vet Hum Toxicol* 33:363, 1991.

110. Newton JG, Breslin ABX: Asthmatic reactions to a commonly used aerosal insect killer. *Med J Aust* 1:378, 1983.

111. Poulos L, Athanaselis S, Courtselinis A: Acute intoxication with cypermethrin (letter). *J Toxicol Clin Toxicol* 19:519, 1982.

112. Tucker SB, Flanigan SA: Cutaneous effects from occupational exposure to fenvalerate. *Arch Toxicol* 54:195, 1983.

113. Majerus PW, Broze BJ, Miletich JP, et al: Anticoagulant, thrombolytic, and antiplatelet drugs, in Gilman AG, Rall TW, Nies AS, et al (eds): *Goodman and Gilman's The Pharmacocological Basis of Therapeutics.* 8th ed. New York, Pergamon, 1990, pp 1311–1331.

114. Link KP: The discovery of dicumarol and its sequels. *Circulation* 19:97, 1959.

115. O'Reilly RA, Aggeler PM: Determinants of the response to oral anticoagulant drugs in man. *Pharmacol Rev* 22:35, 1970.

116. Olson RE, Honser RM, Searcey MT, et al: Nature of vitamin K-dependent CO_2 fixation in microsomal membranes. *Fed Proc* 37:2610, 1978.

117. Bell RG: Metabolism of vitamin K and prothrombin synthesis: anticoagulants and the vitamin K-epoxide cycle. *FASEB J* 37:2599, 1978.

118. Hadler MR, Shadbolt RS: Novel 4-hydrocoumarin anticoagulants active against resistant rats. *Nature* 253:275, 1975.

119. O'Reilly RA, Pool JG, Aggeler PM: Hereditary resistance to coumadin anticoagulant drugs in man and rat. *Ann NY Acad Sci* 151:913, 1968.

120. Katona B, Wason S: Superwarfarin poisoning. *J Emerg Med* 7:627, 1989.

121. Lund M: Comparative effect of the three rodenticide warfarin, difenacoum, and brodifacoum on eight rodent species in short feeding periods. *J Hygiene* 87:101, 1981.

122. Leck JB, Park BK: A comparison study of the effect of warfarin and brodifacoum on the relationship between vitamin K_1 metab-

olism and clotting factor activity in warfarin-susceptible and warfarin-resistant rats. *Biochem Pharmacol* 30:123, 1981.

123. Ellenhorn MJ, Barceloux DG: Pesticides, in Ellenhorn MJ, Barceloux DG (eds): *Medical Toxicology: Diagnosis and Treatment of Human Poisoning.* New York, Elsevier, 1988, pp 1069–1108.

124. Smolinske SC, Scherger DL, Kearns PS, et al: Superwarfarin poisoning in children: A prospective study. *Pediatrics* 84:490, 1989.

125. Chen TW, Deng JF: A brodifacoum intoxication case of mouthful amount (abstract). *Vet Hum Toxicol* 28:488, 1986.

126. Burucoa C, Mura P, Robert R, et al: Chlorophacinone intoxication a biological and toxicological study. *Clin Toxicol* 27:79, 1989.

127. Weitzel JN, Sadowski JA, Furie BC, et al: Surreptitious ingestion of a long-acting vitamin K antagonist/rodenticide, brodifacoum: Clinical and metabolic studies of three cases. *Blood* 76:2555, 1990.

128. Chow EY, Haley LP, Vickars LM, et al: A case of bromaciolone (superwarfarin) ingestion. *Can Med Assoc J* 147:60, 1992.

129. Jones EC, Gershon GH, Sheldon NC: Prolonged anticoagulation in rat poisoning. *JAMA* 252:3005, 1984.

130. Barlow AM, Gay AL, Park BK: Difenacoum (Neosorexa) poisoning. *Br Med J* 285:541, 1982.

131. Watts RG, Castleberry RP, Sadowski JA: Accidental poisoning with a superwarfarin compound (brodifacoum) in a child. *Pediatrics* 86:883, 1990.

132. Baselt RC, Cravey RH: Warfarin, in *Disposition of Toxic Drugs and Chemical in Man.* 3rd ed. Chicago, Year Book, 1989, pp 851–854.

133. Bachmann KA, Sullivan TJ: Dispositional and pharmacodynamic characteristics of brodifacoum in warfarin-sensitive rats. *Pharmacology* 27:281, 1983.

134. Lipton RA, Klass EM: Human ingestion of a "superwarfarin" rodenticide resulting in a prolonged anticoagulant effect. *JAMA* 252:3004, 1984.

135. Breckenridge AM, Cholerton S, Hart JAD, et al: A study of the relationship between the pharmacokinetics and the pharmacodynamics of the 4-hydroxycoumarin anticoagulants warfarin, difenacoum, and brodifacoum in the rabbits. *Br J Pharmacol* 84:81, 1985.

136. Murdoch DA: Prolonged anticoagulation in chlorphacinone poisoning. *Lancet* 1:355, 1983.

137. Chong L, Chau W, Ho C: A case of "superwarfarin" rodenticide poisoning. *Scand J Hematol* 35:314, 1986.

138. Furie B, Furie BC: Molecular basis of vitamin-K-dependent gamma-carboxylation. *Blood* 75:1753, 1990.

139. Fasco MJ, Hildebrandt EF, Suttie JW: Evidence that warfarin anticoagulant action involves two distinct reductase activities. *J Biol Chem* 257:11210, 1982.

140. Wessler S, Gitel SN: Warfarin: From bedside to bench. *N Engl J Med* 311:645, 1984.

141. Hirsh J: Oral anticoagulant drugs. *N Engl J Med* 324:1865, 1991.

142. Greeff MC, Mashile O, MacDougall LG: "Superwarfarin" (bromodialone) poisoning two children resulting in prolonged anticoagulation. *Lancet* 2:1269, 1987.

143. O'Reilly RA, Aggeler PM: Covert anticoagulant ingestion: Study of 25 patients and review of world literature. *Medicine* 55:389, 1976.

144. Hoffman RS, Smilkstein MJ, Goldfrank LR: Evaluation of coagulation factor abnormalities in long-acting anticoagulant overdose. *Clin Toxicol* 26:233, 1988.

145. Ross GS, Zacharski LR, Robert D, et al: An acquired hemorrhagic disorder from long-acting rodenticide ingestion. *Arch Intern Med* 152:410, 1992.

146. Barnett VT, Bergmann F, Humphrey H, et al: Diffuse alveolar hemorrhage secondary to superwarfarin ingestion. *Chest* 102:1301, 1992.

147. Kruse JA, Carlson RW: Fatal rodenticide poisoning with brodifacoum. *Ann Emerg Med* 21:331, 1992.

148. Basehore LM, Mowry JM: Death following ingestion of superwarfarin rodenticide: A case report. *Vet Hum Toxicol* 29:459, 1987.

149. Wallace S, Worsnop C, Paull P, et al: Covert self poisoning with brodifacoum, a "superwarfarin." *Aust NZ J Med* 20:713, 1990.

150. Fitzgerald KT, Bronstein AC: Comparision of first and second generation anticoagulant rodenticide poisonings: Fourteen canine cases. *Vet Hum Toxicol* 29:476, 1987.

151. Wallin R, Martin LF: Vitamin K-dependent carboxylation and vitamin K-dependent carboxylation and vitamin K metabolism in the liver. *J Clin Invest* 76:1879, 1985.

152. Rich CE, Drage CN: Severe complications of intravenous phytadione therapy: Two cases with one fatality. *Postgrad Med* 72:303, 1982.

153. de la Rubia J, Grau E, Montserrat I, et al: Anaphylactic shock and vitamin K₁. *Ann Intern Med* 110:943, 1989.

154. Labatut A, Sorbette F, Virenque C: Shock states during injection of vitamin K₁. *Therapie* 45:58, 1988.

155. Kunkel DB: The toxic emergency: Strychnine is still with us. *Emerg Med* 17:81, 1985.

156. Stannard NW: Child death due to Easton's tablets. *Practitioner* 203:668, 1969.

157. Jackson G, Diggle G: Strychnine-containing tonics. *Br Med J* 2:176, 1973.

158. Campbell C: Dr. Mueller's strychnine cure of snakebite. *Med J Aust* 2:1, 1986.

159. Southby R: Fatal poisoning in children under five years of age: A survey in Victoria for the years 1955–1963. *Med J Aust* 1:533, 1965.

160. Hayes WJ Jr, Laws ER Jr: Botanical rodenticides, in Hayes WJ Jr, Laws ER Jr (eds): *Handbook of Pesticide Toxicology*. San Diego, Academic, 1991, pp 615–619.

161. Young AB, Zukin SR, Snyder SH: Interaction of benzodiazepines with central nervous glycine receptors: Possible mechanisms of action. *Proc Natl Acad Sci USA* 71:2246, 1974.

162. Baselt RC, Cravey RH: Strychnine, in *Disposition of Toxic Drugs and Chemical in Man*. 3rd ed. Chicago, Year Book, 1989, pp 760–762.

163. Adamson RH, Fouts JR: Enzymatic metabolism of strychnine. *Pharmacol Exp Ther* 127:87, 1959.

164. Edmunds M, Sheehan TMT, Van't Hoff W: Strychnine poisoning: Clinical and toxicological observations on a non-fatal case. *Clin Toxicol* 24:245, 1986.

165. Heiser JM, Daya MR, Magnussen AR, et al: Massive strychnine intoxication: Serial blood levels in a fatal case. *Clin Toxicol* 30:269, 1992.

166. Halsey MJ, Little HJ, Wardley-Smith B: Systemically administered glycine protects against strychnine convulsions, but not the behavioural effects of high pressure, in mice. *J Physiol* 408:431, 1989.

167. Ruiz-Gomez A, Morato E, et al: Localization of the strychnine binding site on the 48-kilodalton subunit of the glycine receptor. *Biochemistry* 29:7033, 1990.

168. Mackerer C: The binding of strychnine and strychnine analogs to synaptic membranes of rat brainstem and spinal cord. *J Pharmacol Exp Ther* 201:326, 1977.

169. Bloom FE: Drugs acting on the central nervous system, in Gilman AG, Rall TW, Nies AS, et al (eds): *Goodman and Gilman's The Pharmacological Basis of Therapeutics*. 8th ed. New York, Pergamon, 1990, pp 244–268.

170. Boyd RE, Brennan PT, Deng JF, et al: Strychnine poisoning: Recovery from profound lactic acidosis, hyperthermia, and rhabdomyolysis. *Am J Med* 74:507, 1983.

171. Bleck TP: Pharmacology of tetanus. *Clin Neuropharmacol* 9:103, 1986.

172. Perper JA: Fatal strychnine poisoning: A case report and review of the literature. *J Forensic Sci* 30:1248, 1985.

173. Smith BA: Strychnine poisoning. *J Emerg Med* 8:321, 1990.

174. Yamarick W, Walson P, DiTraglia J: Strychnine poisoning in an adolescent. *Clin Toxicol* 30:141, 1992.

175. Burn DJ, Tomson CRV: Strychnine poisoning as an unusual cause of convulsions. *Postgrad Med J* 65:563, 1989.

176. Jackson G, Ng SH, Diggle CE, et al: Strychnine poisoning successfully treated with diazepam. *Br Med J* 13:519, 1971.

177. O'Callaghan WG, Joyce N, Counihan HE, et al: Unusual strychnine poisoning and its treatment: Report of eight cases. *Br Med J* 285:478, 1982.

178. Maron BJ, Krupp JR, Tune B: Strychnine poisoning successfully treated with diazepam. *J Pediatr* 78:697, 1971.

179. Hardin JA, Griggs RC: Diazepam treatment in a case of strychnine poisoning. *Lancet* 2:372, 1971.

180. Lambert JR, Byrick RJ, Hammeke MD: Management of strychnine poisoning. *Can Med Assoc J* 124:1268, 1981.

181. Herishanu Y, Landau H: Diazepam in the treatment of strychnine poisoning. *Br J Anaesth* 44:747, 1972.

182. Gordon AM, Richards DW: Strychnine intoxication. *J Am Coll Emerg Physician* 8:520, 1979.

183. Kalmbach ER: "Ten-eighty": A war-produced rodenticide. *Science* 102:332, 1945.

184. Hall RJ: The distribution of organic fluoride in some tropical plants. *New Phytol* 71:855, 1972.

185. Chenoweth MB: Monofluoroacetatic acid and related compounds. *Pharmacol Rev* 1:383, 1949.

186. Allcroft R, Peters RA, Shorthourse M: Fluroacetamide poisoning. II. Toxicity in dairy cattle: A confirmation of diagnosis. *Vet Rec* 84:403, 1969.

187. Egekeze JO, Oehme FW: Sodium monofluoroacetate (SMFA, compound 1080): A literature review. *Vet Hum Toxicol* 21:411, 1979.

188. Peters R, Wakelin RW, Buffa P: Biochemistry of fluoroacetate poisoning: The isolation and properties of the flurotricarboxylic acid inhibitor of citrate metabolism. *Proc Roy Soc Lond* 140:497, 1953.

189. Baselt RC, Cravey RH: Fluroacetate, in *Disposition of Toxic Drugs and Chemical in Man*. 3rd ed. Chicago, Year Book, 1989, pp 358–360.

190. Kostyniak PJ, Defluorination: A possible mechanism of detoxification in rats exposed to fluoroacetate. *Toxicol Lett* 3:225, 1979.

191. Chung HM: Acute renal failure caused by acute monofluoroacetate poisoning. *Vet Hum Toxicol* 26:29, 1984.

192. Chenoweth MB, Gilman A: Studies on the pharmacology of fluroacetate. I. Species response to fluoroacetate. *J Pharmacol Exp Ther* 87:90, 1946.

193. Gajdusek DC, Luther G: Fluoroacetate poisoning: A review and report of a case. *Am J Dis Child* 79:310, 1950.

194. Reigart JR, Brueggeman JL, Keil JE: Sodium fluroacetate poisoning. *Am J Dis Child* 129:1224, 1975.

195. McTaggart DR: Poisoning due to sodium fluroacetate ("1080"). *Med J Aust* 2:641, 1970.

196. Brockmann JL, Mcdowell AV, Leeds WG: Fatal poisoning with sodium fluoroacetate: Report of a case. *JAMA* 159:1529, 1955.

197. Harrison JWE, Ambrus JL, Ambrus CM, et al: Acute poisoning with sodium fluoroacetate (compound 1080). *JAMA* 149:1520, 1952.

198. Chenoweth MB, Kandel A, Johnson LB, et al: Factors influencing fluroacetate poisoning: Practical treatment with glycerol monacetate. *J Pharmacol Exp Ther* 102:31, 1951.

199. Omara F, Sisodia CS: Evaluation of potential antidotes for sodium fluroacetate in mice. *Vet Hum Toxicol* 32:427, 1990.

200. Hutchens JO, Wagner H, Podolsky B, et al: The effect of ethanol and various metabolites on fluoroacetate poisoning. *J Pharmacol Exp Ther* 95:62, 1949.

201. Peardon DL: RH 787, A new selective rodenticide. *Pest Control* 42:14, 1974.

202. Miller LV, Stokes JD, Silipat C: Diabetes mellitus and autonomic dysfunction after Vacor ingestion. *Diabetes Care* 1:73, 1978.

203. Pont A, Rubino JM, Bishop D, et al: Diabetes mellitus and neuropathy following Vacor ingestion in man. *Arch Intern Med* 139:185, 1979.

204. Gallanosa AG, Spyker DA, Curnow RT: Diabetes mellitus associated with autonomic and peripheral neuropathy after vacor rodenticides: A review. *Clin Toxicol* 18:441, 1981.

205. Osterman J, Zmyslinski RW, Hopkins CB, et al: Full recovery from severe orthostatic hypotension after Vacor rodenticide ingestion. *Arch Intern Med* 141:1505, 1981.

206. Prosser PR, Karam JH: Diabetes mellitus following rodenticide ingestion in man. *JAMA* 239:1148, 1978.

207. LeWitt PA: The neurotoxicity of the rat poison Vacor: A clinical study of 12 cases. *N Engl J Med* 302:73, 1980.

208. Fretthold D, Sunshine I, Udinsky JR, et al: Postmortem findings for a Vacor poisoning case. *Clin Toxicol* 16:175, 1980.

209. Schum TR, Lachman BS: Effect of packaging and appearance on childhood poisoning: Vacor rat poison. *Clin Pediatr* 21:282, 1982.

210. Lee TH, Kang JC, Han MD, et al: A clinical analysis of rodenticide RH-787 intoxication in Korea. *Korean Diabetes J* 4:43, 1977.

211. Peoples SA, Maddy KT: Poisoning of man and animals due to ingestion of rodent poison, Vacor. *Vet Human Toxicol* 21:266, 1979.

212. Johnson D, Kubic P, Levitt C: Accidental ingestion of Vacor rodenticide: The symptoms and sequelae in a 25-month-old child. *Am J Dis Child* 134:161, 1980.

213. Rerup CC: Drugs producing diabetes through damage of insulin-secreting cells. *Pharmacol Rev* 22:485, 1970.

214. Shen M, Orwoll ES, Conte JE Jr: Pentamidine-induced pancreatic beta-cell dysfunction. *Am J Med* 86:726, 1989.
215. Kenney RM, Micheals IAL, Flomenbaum NE, et al: Poisoning with N-3-pyridylmethyl-N'-p-nitrophenyl urea (Vacor). *Arch Pathol Lab Med* 105:367, 1981.
216. Deckert FW, Moss JN, Sambuca AS, et al: Nutritional and drug interactions with Vacor rodenticide in rats. *Fed Proc* 36:990, 1977.
217. Sternberg SS, Philips FS: 6-Aminonicotinamide and acute degenerative changes in the central nervous system. *Science* 127:644, 1958.
218. Papasozomenos S: The rat poison Vacor. *N Engl J Med* 302:1146, 1980.
219. Ganda OP, Rossini AA, Like AA: Studies on streptozotocin. *Diabetes* 25:595, 1976.
220. Schein PS, Rakieten DA, Cooney RD, et al: Streptozotocin diabetes in monkeys and dogs, and its prevention by nicotinamide. *Proc Soc Exp Biol Med* 143:514, 1973.
221. Schein PS, Cooney DA, Vernon ML: The use of nicotinamide to modify the toxicity of streptozotocin diabetes without the loss of antitumor activity. *Cancer Res* 27:2324, 1967.
222. Stauffacher W, Burr I, Gulzeit D, et al: Streptozotocin diabetes: Time course of irreversible B-cell damage. *Proc Soc Exp Biol Med* 133:194, 1970.
223. Tjalve H, Wilander E: The uptake in the pancreatic islets of nicotinamide, nicotinic acid and tryptophan and their ability to prevent streptozotocin diabetes in mice. *Acta Endocrinol* 83:357, 1976.
224. Gunnarson R: Inhibition of insulin biosynthesis by alloxan, streptozotocin, and N-nitrosomethylurea. *Mol Pharmacol* 11:759, 1975.
225. Flomenbaum NE: Antidote in depth: Niacinamide for Vacor (PNU), alloxan, and streptozotocin poisoning, in Goldfrank LR, Flomenbaum NE, Lewin NA, et al (eds): *Goldfrank's Toxicologic Emergencies*. Norwalk, CT, Appleton Lange, 1990, pp 710–711.
226. Howland MA, Weisman R, Sauter D, et al: Nonavailability of poison antidotes. *N Engl J Med* 314:927, 1986.
227. Thomas PM: Aluminium phosphide: An ideal fumigant. *Pesticide* 12:15, 1973.
228. Sharma A, Gathwala G: Oral aluminium phosphide poisoning in Indian children. *J Trop Med Hyg* 95:221, 1992.
229. Chugh SN: Aluminium phosphide poisoning: Present status and management. *J Assoc Physicians India* 40:401, 1992.
230. Hedges C: Iran's old soldiers die, as suicides. *New York Times,* July 12, 1993.
231. Wilson R, Lovejoy FH, Jaeger RJ, et al: Acute phosphine poisoning aboard a grain freighter: Epidemiologic, clinical, and pathological findings. *JAMA* 244:148, 1980.
232. Baselt RC, Cravey RH: Phosphine, in *Disposition of Toxic Drugs and Chemical in Man*. 3rd ed. Chicago, Year Book, 1989, pp 693–694.
233. Chefurka W, Kashi KP, Bond EJ: The effect of phosphine on electron transport in mitochondria. *Pest Biochem Physiol* 6:65, 1976.
234. Singh S, Dilawari JB, Vashist R, et al: Aluminium phosphide ingestion. *Br Med J* 290:1110, 1985.
235. Chopra JS, Kalra OP, Malik VS, et al: Aluminium phosphide poisoning: A retrospective study of 16 cases in one year. *Postgrad Med J* 62:1113, 1986.
236. Chugh SN, Dushyand, Ram S, et al: Incidence and outcome of aluminium phosphide poisoning in a hospital study. *Indian J Med Res* 94:232, 1991.
237. Chugh SN, Ram S, Mehta LK, et al: Adult respiratory distress syndrome following aluminium phosphide ingestion: Report of 4 cases. *J Assoc Physicians India* 37:217, 1989.
238. Katira R, Eihence GP, Mehrotra ML, et al: A study of aluminium phosphide poisoning with special references to electrocardiographic changes. *J Assoc Physicians India* 38:471, 1990.
239. Chugh SN, Malhotra S, Malhotra KC: Successful reversion of supraventricular and ventricular tachycardia with magnesium sulphate in AIP poisoning. *J Assoc Physicians India* 39:642, 1991.
240. Raman R, Debery M: The electrocardiographic changes in Quickphos poisoning. *Indian Heart J* 37:193, 1985.
241. Jain SM, Baharani A, Sepaha GC, et al: Electrocardiographic changes in aluminium phosphide poisoning. *J Assoc Physicians India* 33:406, 1985.
242. Siwach SB, Yadar DR, Dalal S, et al: Acute aluminium phosphide poisoning: An epidemiological, clinical, and histopathological study. *J Assoc Physicians India* 36:594, 1988.
243. Rodenberg HD, Chang CC, Watson WA: Zinc phosphide ingestion: a case report and review. *Vet Hum Toxicol* 31:559, 1989.
244. Chugh SN, Ram S, Chugh K, et al: Spot diagnosis of aluminium phosphide ingestion: An application of a single test. *J Assoc Physicians India* 37:219, 1989.
245. Chugh SN, Juggal KL, Ram S, et al: Hypomagnesemic atrial fibrillation in a case of AIP poisoning. *J Assoc Physicians India* 37:548, 1989.
246. Ram A, Srivastava SSL, Ehlence GP, et al: A study of aluminium phosphide poisoning with special reference to therapeutic efficacy of magnesium sulphate. *J Assoc Physicians India* 36:23, 1988.
247. Suresh LV: Magnesium sulphate in aluminium phosphide poisoning. *J Assoc Physicians India* 37:482, 1989.
248. Marraccini JV, Thomas GE, Ongley JP, et al: Death and injury caused by methyl bromide: An insecticide fumigant. *J Forensic Sci* 28:601, 1983.
249. Kurtz PJ, Deskin R, Harrington RM: Pesticides, in Hayes AW (ed): *Principles and Methods of Toxicology*. 2nd ed. New York, Raven, 1989, pp 137–167.
250. Lowe J, Sullivan JB Jr: Fumigants, in Sullivan JB Jr, Krieger GR (eds): *Hazardous Materials Toxicology: Clinical Principles of Environmental Health*. Baltimore, Williams & Wilkins, 1992, pp 1053–1062.
251. Ruth J: Odor thresholds and irritant levels of several chemical substances: A review. *Am Ind Hyg Assoc J* 47:A142, 1986.
252. Rathus EM, Landy PJ: Methyl bromide poisoning. *Br J Ind Med* 18:53, 1961.
253. Collins RP: Methyl bromide poisoning: A bizarre neurologic disorder. *Calif Med* 103:112, 1965.
254. Shield LK, Coleman TL, Markesbery WR: Methyl bromide intoxication: Neurologic features, including simulation of Reye syndrome. *Neurology* 27:959, 1977.
255. Fuortes LJ: A case of fatal methyl bromide poisoning. *Vet Hum Toxicol* 34:240, 1992.
256. Drawneek W, O'Brien MJ, Goldsmith HJ, et al: Industrial methyl-bromide poisoning in fumigators. *Lancet* 2:855, 1964.
257. Unintentional methyl bromide gas release—Florida. *MMWR* 38:880, 1988.
258. Goldman LR, Mengle D, Epstein DM, et al: Acute symptoms in persons residing near a field treated with soil fumigant methyl bromide and chloropicrin. *West J Med* 147:95, 1987.
259. Bishop CM: A case of methyl bromide poisoning. *Occup Med* 42:107, 1992.
260. Viner N: Methyl bromide poisoning: A new industrial hazard. *Can Med Assoc J* 53:43, 1945.
261. Zwaverling JH, de Kort WLAM, Meulenbelt J, et al: Exposure of the skin to methyl bromide: A study of six cases occupationally exposed to high concentrations during fumigation. *Hum Toxicol* 6:491, 1987.
262. Baselt RC, Cravey RH: Methyl bromide, in *Disposition of Toxic Drugs and Chemical in Man*. 3rd ed. Chicago, Year Book, 1989, pp 542–544.
263. Lewis SE: Inhibition of SH enyzmes by methyl bromide. *Nature* 161:692, 1948.
264. Hines CH: Methyl bromide poisoning: A review of ten cases. *J Occup Med* 11:1, 1969.
265. Carney MWP: Five cases of bromism. *Lancet* 2:523, 1971.
266. Hanes F, Yates A: An analysis of four hundred instances of chronic bromide intoxication. *South Med J* 31:667, 1938.
267. NIOSH: *Pocket Guide to Chemical Hazards*. DHHS no. 90-117, Cincinnati, 1990, pp 146–147.
268. Wyers H: Methyl bromide intoxication. *Br J Ind Med* 2:24, 1945.
269. Chavez CT, Hepler RS, Straatsma BR: Methyl bromide optic atrophy. *Am J Ophthalmol* 99:715, 1985.
270. Zatuchni J, Hong K: Methyl bromide poisoning seen initially as psychosis. *Arch Neurol* 38:529, 1981.
271. Behrens RH, Dukes DCD: Fatal methyl bromide poisoning. *Br J Ind Med* 43:561, 1986.
272. Top rating for repellant. *Chemical Week* March 9, 1957, p 104.
273. Insect repellants. *Med Lett* 131:45, 1989.
274. Lurie AA, Gleiberman SE, Tsizin YS: Pharmacokinetics of insect repellent N, N-diethyltoluamide. *Med Parazitol* 47:72, 1979.
275. Ambrose AN: Pharmacologic and toxicologic studies on N,N-diethyltoluamide. *Toxicol Appl Pharmacol* 1:97, 1959.

276. Pronczuk de Garbino J, Laborde A: Toxicity of an insect repellent: N-N-diethyltoluamide. *Vet Hum Toxicol* 25:422, 1983.

277. Heick HMC, Shipman RT, Norman MG, et al: Reye-like syndrome associated with use of insect repellent in a presumed heterozygote for ornithine carbamoyl transferase deficiency. *J Pediatr* 97:471, 1980.

278. Seizures temporally assoicated with use of DEET insect repellent—New York and Connecticut. *MMWR* 38:678, 1989.

279. Lipscomb JW, Kramer JE, Leikin JB: Seizure following brief exposure to the insect repellent N,N-diethyl-m-toluamide. *Ann Emerg Med* 21:315, 1992.

280. Reuveni H, Yagupsky P: Dethyltoluamide-containing insect repellent: Adverse effects on worldwide use. *Arch Dermatol* 118:582, 1982.

281. Miller JD: Anaphylaxis associated with insect repellent. *N Engl J Med* 307:1341, 1982.

282. Gryboski J, Weinstein D, Ordway NK: Toxic encephalopathy apparently related to the use of an insect repellent. *N Engl J Med* 264:289, 1964.

283. Zadikoff CM: Toxic encephalopathy associated with use of insect repellant. *J Pediatr* 95:140, 1979.

284. Tenenbein M: Severe toxic reactions and death following the ingestion of diethyltoluamide containing insect repellant. *JAMA* 258:1509, 1987.

285. Roland EH, Jan JE, Rigg JM: Toxic encephalopathy in a child after brief exposure to insect repellents. *Can Med Assoc J* 132:155, 1985.

286. Edwards DL, Johnson CE: Insect-repellant-induced toxic encephalopathy in a child. *Clin Pharmacol* 6:496, 1987.

287. Baselt RC, Cravey RH: Metaldehyde, in *Disposition of Toxic Drugs and Chemical in Man*. 3rd ed. Chicago, Year Book, 1989, pp 509–510.

288. Moody JP, Inglis FG: Persistence of metaldehyde during acute molluscicide poisoning. *Hum Exp Toxicol* 11:361, 1992.

289. Brien JF, Loomis CW: Pharmacology of acetaldehyde. *Can J Physiol Pharmacol* 61:1, 1983.

290. Booze TF, Oehme FW: An investigation of metaldehyde and acetaldehyde toxicities in dogs. *Fundam Appl Toxicol* 6:440, 1986.

291. Dreisbach RH: *Handbook of Poisoning: Prevention, Diagnosis & Treatment*. 11th ed. Los Altos, CA, Lange, 1983, pp 202–205.

292. Longstreth WT Jr, Pierson DJ: Metaldehyde poisoning from slug bait ingestion. *West J Med* 137:134, 1982.

293. Homeida AM, Cooke RG: Anticonvulsant activity of diazepam and clonidine on metaldehyde-induced seizures in mice: Effects on brain gamma-aminobutyric acid concentrations and monoamine oxidase activity. *J Vet Pharmacol* 5:187, 1982.

294. Hald J, Jacobsen E: Formation of acetaldehyde in the organism after ingestion of Antabuse (tetraethylthiruramdisulphide) and alcohol. *Acta Pharmacol Toxicol* 4:305, 1948.

295. Kitson TM: The disulfiram-ethanol reaction. *J Stud Alcohol* 38:96, 1977.

296. Towne JC: Effect of ethanol and acetaldehyde on liver and brain monoamine oxidase. *Nature* 201:709, 1964.

297. Booze TF, Oehme FW: Metaldehyde toxicity: A review. *Vet Hum Toxicol* 27:11, 1985.

298. Lewis DR, Madel GA, Drury J: Fatal poisoning by "Meta Fuel" tablets. *Br Med J* 1:1283, 1939.

299. Spighel A, Ahoy-Spighel M: Metaldehyde poisoning. *Lancet* 2:1017, 1958.

300. Wood S, Rom WN, White GL, et al: Pentachlorophenol poisoning. *J Occup Med* 25:527, 1983.

301. Wood S: Pentachlorophenol, in Rom WN (ed): *Environmental and Occupational Medicine*. Boston, Little, Brown, 1983, pp 657–662.

302. Gasiewicz TA: Nitro compounds and related phenolic pesticides, in Hayes WJ Jr, Laws ER Jr (eds): *Handbook of Pesticide Toxicology*. San Diego, Academic, 1991, pp 1207–1216.

303. Pentachlorophenol in log homes—Kentucky. *MMWR* 29:431, 1980.

304. Brown BW: Fatal phenol poisoning from improperly laundered diapers. *Am J Public Health* 60:901, 1970.

305. Robson AM, Kissane JM, Elvick HN, et al: Pentachlorophenol poisoning in a nursery for newborn infants. I. Clinical features and treatment. *J Pediatr* 75:309, 1969.

306. Armstrong RW, Eichner ER, Klein DE, et al: Pentachlorophenol poisoning in a nursery for newborn infants. II. Epidemiologic and toxicologic studies. *J Pediatr* 75:317, 1969.

307. Baselt RC, Cravey RH: Pentachlorophenol, in *Disposition of Toxic Drugs and Chemical in Man*. 3rd ed. Chicago, Year Book, 1989, pp 646–649.

308. Uhl S, Schmid P, Schlatter C: Pharmacokinetics of pentachlorophenol in man. *Arch Toxicol* 58:182, 1986.

309. Parker UH: Effect of nitrophenols and halogenophenols on the enzymatic activity of rat-liver mitochondria. *Biochem J* 69:306, 1957.

310. Weinbach EC, Garbus J, Clagett EC: The interaction of uncoupling phenols with mitochondrial protein. *J Biol Chem* 240:1811, 1965.

311. Gordon D: How dangerous is pentachlorophenol. *Med J Aust* 2:485, 1956.

312. Exon JH: A review of chlorinated phenols. *Vet Hum Toxicol* 26:508, 1984.

313. Gray RE, Gilliland RD, Smith EE, et al: Pentachlorophenol intoxication: Report of a fatal case with comments on the clinical course and pathologic anatomy. *Arch Environ Health* 40:161, 1985.

314. Roberts HJ: Aplastic anemia due to pentachlorophenol. *N Engl J Med* 305:1650, 1981.

315. Cooper RG, Macaulay MB: Pentachlorophenol pancreatitis. *Lancet* 1:517, 1982.

316. Hassan NB, Seligmann H, Bassan HM: Intravascular haemolysis induced by pentachlorophenol. *Br Med J* 291:21, 1985.

317. Young JF, Haley TJ: A pharmacokinetic study of pentachlorophenol poisoning and the effect of forced diruresis. *Clin Toxicol* 12:41, 1978.

318. Weidel M, Rosso M: Studien uber das Pyridin. *Monatsschr Chem* 3:850, 1882.

319. Michaelis L, Hill ES: Potentiometric studies on semiquinones. *J Am Chem Soc* 55:1481, 1933.

320. Hart TB: Paraquat: A review of safety in agricultural and horticultural use. *Hum Toxicol* 6:13, 1987.

321. Smith JG: Paraquat poisoning by skin absorption: A review. *Hum Toxicol* 7:15, 1988.

322. Chester G, Ward RJ: Occupational exposure and drift hazard during aerial application of paraquat to cotton. *Arch Environ Contam Toxicol* 13:551, 1984.

323. Smith LL: The toxicity of paraquat. *Adv Drug React Acute Poison Rev* 1:1, 1988.

324. Onyon LJ, Volans GN: The epidemiology and prevention of paraquat poisoning. *Hum Toxicol* 6:19, 1987.

325. Baselt RC, Cravey RH: Paraquat, in *Disposition of Toxic Drugs and Chemical in Man*. 3rd ed. Chicago, Year Book, 1989, pp 637–639.

326. Bismuth C, Schermann JM, Garnier R, et al: Elimination of paraquat. *Hum Toxicol* 6:63, 1987.

327. Hawksworth GM, Bennett PN, Davies DS: Kinetics of paraquat elimination in the dog. *Toxicol Appl Pharmacol* 57:139, 1981.

328. Davies DS, Hawksworth GM, Bennett PN: Paraquat poisoning. *Proc Eur Soc Toxicol* 18:21, 1977.

329. Landrigan PJ, Powell KE, James LM, et al: Paraquat and marijuana: Epidemiologic risk assessment. *Am J Pubic Health* 73:784, 1983.

330. Gordonsmith RH, Brooke-Taylor S, Smith LL, et al: Structural requirements of compounds to inhibit pulmonary diamine accumulation. *Biochem Pharmacol* 32:3701, 1983.

331. Rose MS, Smith LL: Tissue uptake of paraquat and diquat. *Gen Pharmacol* 8:173, 1977.

332. Smith LL: Mechanism of paraquat toxicity in lung and its relevance to treatment. *Hum Toxicol* 6:31, 1987.

333. Yasaka T, Okudaira K, Fujito H, et al: Further studies of lipid peroxidation in human paraquat poisoning. *Arch Intern Med* 146:681, 1986.

334. Dodge AD: The mode of action of the bipyridilium herbicides, paraquat and diquat. *Endeavour* 30:130, 1971.

335. Bismuth C, Garnier R, Dally S, et al: Prognosis and treatment of paraquat poisoning: A review of 28 cases. *J Toxicol Clin Toxicol* 19:461, 1982.

336. Pond SM: Manifestations and management of paraquat poisoning. *Med J Aust* 152:256, 1990.

337. Russell LA, Stone BE, Rooney PA: Paraquat poisoning: Toxicologic and pathologic finding in three fatal cases. *Clin Toxicol* 18:915, 1981.

338. Florkowski CM, Bradberry SM, Ching GW, et al: Acute renal failure in a case of paraquat poisoning with relative absence of pulmonary toxicity. *Postgrad Med J* 68:660, 1992.

339. Dolan M, Danzl DF, Horowitz J, et al: Paraquat ingestion. *Ann Emerg Med* 12:612, 1984.

340. Oreopoulos DG, Soyannwo MAO, Sinniah R, et al: Acute renal failure in case of paraquat poisoning. *Br Med J* 1:749, 1968.

341. Vale JA, Meredith TJ, Buckley BM: Paraquat poisoning: Clinical features and immediate general management. *Hum Toxicol* 6:41, 1987.

342. Hudson M, Patel SB, Ewen, et al: Paraquat induced pulmonary fibrosis in three survivors. *Thorax* 46:201, 1991.

343. Bismuth C, Garnier R, Baud FJ, et al: Paraquat poisoning: An overview of the current status. *Drug Saf* 5:243, 1990.

344. Proudfoot AT, Stewart MS, Levitt T, et al: Paraquat poisoning: Significance of plasma paraquat concentrations. *Lancet* 2:330, 1979.

345. Hart TB, Nevitt A, Whitehead A: A new statistical approach to the prognostic significance of plasma paraquat concentration. *Lancet* 2:1222, 1984.

346. Tungsanga K, Israsema S, Chuslip S, et al: Paraquat poisoning: Evidence of systemic toxicity after dermal exposure. *Postgrad Med J* 59:338, 1983.

347. Samman PD, Johnston ENM: Nail damage associated with handling of paraquat and diquat. *Br Med J* 1:818, 1969.

348. Howard JK: Dermal exposure to paraquat. *Lancet* 1:1100, 1978.

349. Gaudreault P, Friedman PA, Lovejoy FH: Efficacy of activated charcoal and magnesium citrate in the treatment of oral paraquat intoxication. *Ann Emerg Med* 42:123, 1985.

350. Meredith TJ, Vale JA: Treatment of paraquat poisoning in man: Methods to prevent absorption. *Hum Toxicol* 6:49, 1987.

351. Nokata M, Tanaka T, Tsuchiya K, et al: Alleviation of paraquat toxicity by Kayexalate and Kalimate in rats. *Acta Pharmacol Toxicol* 55:158, 1984.

352. Braithwaiter RA: Emergency analysis of paraquat in biological fluids. *Hum Toxicol* 6:83, 1987.

353. Fisher HK, Humphries M, Bails R: Paraquat poisoning: Recovery from renal and pulmonary damage. *Ann Intern Med* 75:731, 1971.

354. Widdop BM, Medd RK, Braithwaite RA: Charcoal haemoperfusion in the treatment of paraquat poisoning. *Proc Eur Soc Toxicol* 18:156, 1976.

355. Hampson EC, Effeney DJ, Pond SM: Efficacy of single or repeated hemoperfusion in a canine model of paraquat poisoning. *J Pharmacol Exp Ther* 254:732, 1990.

356. Pond SM, Rivory LP, Hampson EC, et al: Kinetics of toxic doses of paraquat and the effects of hemoperfusion in the dog. *Clin Toxicol* 31:229, 1993.

357. Proudfoot AT, Prescott LF, Jarvie DR: Haemodialysis for paraquat poisoning. *Hum Toxicol* 6:69, 1987.

358. Hampson EC, Pond SM: Failure of haemoperfusion and haemodialysis to prevent death in paraquat poisoning: A retrospective review of 42 patients. *Med Toxicol* 3:64, 1988.

359. Pond SM, Johnston SC, Schoof DD, et al: Repeated hemoperfusion and continuous arteriovenous hemofiltration in a paraquat poisoned patient. *Clin Toxicol* 25:305, 1987.

360. Mascie-Taylor BH, Thompson J, Davidson AM: Haemoperfusion ineffective for paraquat removal in life-threatening poisoning. *Lancet* 2:1376, 1983.

361. Wright AF, Green TP, Robson RT, et al: Specific polyclonal and monoclonal antibody prevents paraquat accumulation into rat lung slices. *Biochem Pharmacol* 36:1325, 1987.

362. Pond SM, Chen N, Bowles MR: Prevention of paraquat toxicity in alveolar type II cells by paraquat-specific antibodies (abstract). *Vet Hum Toxicol* 35:332, 1993.

363. Dunbar AJ, Deluccia AJ, Acuff RV, et al: Prolonged intravenous paraquat infusion in rats. I. Failure of coinfused putrescine to attenuate pulmonary paraquat uptake, paraquat-induced biochemical changes, or lung injury. *Toxicol Appl Pharmacol* 2:207, 1988.

364. Smith LL: The identification of an accumulated system for diamines and polyamines into the lung and its relevance to paraquat toxicity. *Arch Toxicol* 5(suppl):1, 1982.

365. Fairshter RD, Rosen SM, Smith WR, et al: Paraquat poisoning: New aspects of therapy. *Q J Med* 180:551, 1976.

366. Redetzki M, Wood C, Grafton W: Vitamin E and paraquat poisoning. *Vet Hum Toxicol* 22:395, 1980.

367. Osherrof MR, Schaich KM, Drew RT, et al: Failure of desferoxamine to modify the toxicity of paraquat in rats. *J Free Radicals Biol Med* 1:71, 1985.

368. Frank L: Superoxide dismutase and lung toxicity. *Trends Pharmacol Sci* 14:124, 1983.

369. Glass M, Sutherland MW, Forman HJ, et al: Selenium deficiency potentiates lipid peroxidation in isolated perfused rat lung. *J Appl Physiol* 59:619, 1985.

370. Shum S, Hale TW, Habasang R: Reduction of paraquat toxicity by N-acetylcysteine. *Vet Hum Toxicol* 6:31, 1982.

371. Cramp TP: Failure of N-acetylcysteine to reduce renal damage due to paraquat in rats. *Hum Toxicol* 4:107, 1985.

372. Addo E, Poon-King DB: Leukocyte suppression in the treatment of 72 patients with paraquat poisoning. *Lancet* 1:1117, 1986.

373. Vincken W, Huyghen L, Schaedevyl W, et al: Paraquat poisoning and colchicine treatment. *Ann Intern Med* 95:391, 1981.

374. Akahori F, Oehme FW: Inhibition of collagen synthesis as a treatment of paraquat poisoning. *Vet Hum Toxicol* 25:321, 1983.

375. Brown OR, Heitkamp M, Song CS: Niacin reduces paraquat toxicity in rats. *Science* 212:1510, 1983.

376. Cooke NKJ, Flenley DC, Matthew H: Paraquat poisoning: Serial studies in lung function. *Q J Med* 42:683, 1973.

377. Kalmholz S, Veotj FJ, Mollenkopf F, et al: Single lung transplantation in paraquat intoxication. *NY State J Med* 84:81, 1984.

378. Toronto Lung Transplant Group: Sequential bilateral lung transplantation for paraquat poisoning: A case report. *J Thoracic Cardiovasc Surg* 89:734, 1985.

379. Stancliffe TC, Pirie A: Production of superoxide radicals in reactions of the herbicide diquat. *Fed Lett* 17:279, 1971.

380. Daniel JW, Gage JC: Absorption and excretion of diquat and paraquat in rats. *Br J Ind Med* 23:133, 1966.

381. Vanholder R, Colardyn F, DeReuck J, et al: Diquat intoxication: Report of two cases and review of the literature. *Am J Med* 70:1267, 1981.

382. Oreopoules DG, McEvoy J: Diquat poisoning. *Postgrad Med J* 45:635, 1969.

383. Baselt RC, Cravey RH: Diquat, in *Disposition of Toxic Drugs and Chemical in Man.* 3rd ed. Chicago, Year Book, 1989, pp 297–298.

384. Manoguerra AS: Full thickness skin burns secondary to an unusual exposure to diquat dibromide. *Clin Toxicol* 28:107, 1990.

385. McCarthy LG, Speth CP: Diquat intoxication. *Ann Emerg Med* 12:394, 1983.

386. Clark DG, Hurst EW: The toxicity of diquat. *Br J Ind Med* 27:51, 1970.

387. Okonek S, Hofmann A: On the question of extracoporeal hemodialysis in diquat intoxication. *Arch Toxicol* 33:251, 1975.

388. Powell D, Pond SM, Allen TB, et al: Hemoperfusion in a child who ingested diquat and died from pontine infarction and hemorrhage. *J Toxicol Clin Toxicol* 20:405, 1983.

389. Arnold EK, Beasley VR: The pharmacokinetics of chlorinated phenoxyacid herbicides: A literature review. *Vet Hum Toxicol* 31:121, 1989.

390. Suskind RR, Hertzberg VS: Human health effects of 2,4,5-T and its toxic contaminants. *JAMA* 251:2372, 1984.

391. The Center for Disease Control Veterans Health Studies: Serum 2,3,7,8-Tetrachlorodibenzo-p-dioxin levels in US army Vietnam-era veterans. *JAMA* 260:1249, 1988.

392. Hoffman RE, Stehr-Green PA, Webb KB, et al: Health effects of long-term exposure to 2,3,7,8-tetrachlorodibenzo-p-dioxin. *JAMA* 255:2031, 1986.

393. Hardell L, Sandstrom A: Case-controlled study: Soft tissue sarcomas and exposure to phenoxyacetic acid or chlorophenols. *Br J Cancer* 39:711, 1979.

394. Armstrong BK: Storm in a cup of 2,4,5-T. *Med J Aust* 144:284, 1986.

395. Baselt RC, Cravey RH: 2,4-Dichlorophenoxyacetic acid, in *Disposition of Toxic Drugs and Chemical in Man.* 3rd ed. Chicago, Year Book, 1989, pp 262–263.

396. Prescott LF, Park J, Darrien J: Treatment of severe 2,4-D and mecoprop intoxication with alkaline diuresis. *Br J Clin Pharmacol* 7:111, 1979.

397. Kohli JD, Khanna RN, Cupta BN, et al: Absorption and excretion of 2,4-dichlorophenoxyacetic acid in man. *Xenobiotica* 4:97, 1974.

398. Sauerhoff MW, Braun WH, Blau GE, et al: The fate of 2,4-dichlorophenoxyacetic acid (2,4-D) following oral administration to man. *Toxicology* 8:3, 1977.

399. Baselt RC, Cravey RH: 2,4,5-Trichlorophenoxyacetic acid, in *Disposition of Toxic Drugs and Chemical in Man*. 3rd ed. Chicago, Year Book, 1989, pp 831–832.

400. Gehring PJ, Kramer CG, Schweta BA, et al: The fate of 2,4,5-trichlorophenoxyacetic acid (2,4,5-T) following oral administration to man. *Toxicol Appl Pharmacol* 26:352, 1973.

401. Flanagan RJ, Meredith TJ, Ruprah M, et al: Alkaline diuresis for acute poisoning with chlorophenoxy herbicides and ioxynil. *Lancet* 335:454, 1990.

402. Brodie TM: Effect of certain plant growth substances on oxidative phosphorylation in rat liver mitochondria. *Proc Soc Exp Biol Med* 80:533, 1952.

403. Dickey W, McAleer JJA, Callender ME: Delayed sudden death after ingestion of MCPP and ioxynil: An unusual presentation of hormonal weedkiller intoxication. *Postgrad Med J* 64:681, 1988.

404. Friesen EG, Jones GR, Vaughan D: Clinical presentation and management of acute 2,4-D oral ingestion. *Drug Saf* 5:155, 1990.

405. Dudley Jr. AW, Thapar NT: Fatal human ingestion of 2,4-D, a common herbicide. *Arch Pathol* 94:270, 1972.

406. Meulenbelt J, Zwaveling JH, van Zoonen P, et al: Acute MCPP intoxication: Report of two cases. *Hum Toxicol* 7:289, 1988.

407. O'Reilly JF: Prolonged coma and delayed peripheral neuropathy after ingestion of phenoxyacetic acid weedkillers. *Postgrad Med J* 60:76, 1984.

408. Berwick P: 2,4-Dichlorophenoxyacetic acid poisoning in man: Some interesting clinical and laboratory findings. *JAMA* 214:1114, 1970.

409. Kancir CB, Andersen C, Olesen AS: Marked hypocalcemia in a fatal poisoning with chlorinated phenoxy acid derivatives. *Clin Toxicol* 26:257, 1988.

410. Neilsen K, Kaempe B, Jensen-Holm J: Fatal poisoning in man by 2,4-dichlorophenoxyacetic acid(2,4-D): Determination of agent in forensic science. *Acta Pharmacol Toxicol* 22:224, 1965.

411. Fraser AD, Isner AF, Perry RA: Toxicologic studies in fatal overdose of 2,4 D, mecoprop, and dicamba. *J Forensic Sci* 29:1237, 1984.

412. Osterloh J, Lotti M, Pond SM: Toxicologic studies in a fatal overdose of 2,4-D, MCPP and chlorpyrifos. *J Anal Toxicol* 7:125, 1983.

413. Hoar SK, Blair A, Holmes FF, et al: Agricultural herbicide use and risk of lymphoma and soft-tissue sarcoma. *JAMA* 256:1141, 1986.

414. Coggon D, Acheson ED: Do phenoxy herbicides cause cancer in man? *Lancet* 1:1057, 1982.

415. Jansen H, Zeldenrust J: Homicidal chronic sodium chlorate poisoning. *Forensic Sci* 1:103, 1972.

416. Jackson RC, Elder WJ, McDonnell H: Sodium-chlorate poisoning complicated by acute renal failure. *Lancet* 2:1381, 1961.

417. Stavrou R, Butcher R, Sakula A: Accidental self-poisoning by sodium chlorate weed killer. *Practitioner* 221:397, 1978.

418. Cunningham NE: Chlorate poisoning: Two cases diagnosed at autopsy. *Med Sci Law* 22:281, 1982.

419. Lee DBN, Brown DL, Baker LRI, et al: Haematological complications of chlorate poisoning. *Br Med J* 2:31, 1970.

420. Steffen C, Wetzel E: Pathologic aspects of chlorate poisoning. *Hum Toxicol* 4:541, 1985.

421. Helliwell M, Nunn J: Mortality in sodium chlorate poisoning. *Br Med J* 1:1119, 1979.

422. Curry S: Methemoglobinemia. *Ann Emerg Med* 11:214, 1987.

154. Salicylate and Other Nonsteroidal Antiinflammatory Drug Poisoning

Christopher H. Linden

Introduction

Nonsteroidal antiinflammatory drugs (NSAIDs) include aspirin, related salicylic acid derivatives (Table 154-1), and a variety of other aspirin-like drugs (see Chap. 215). All NSAIDs have analgesic and antipyretic as well as antiinflammatory activity. These effects are due to inhibition of the enzyme cyclo-oxygenase, resulting in decreased prostaglandin synthesis [1,2]. This mechanism of action is also responsible for the side effects of renal salt and water retention and gastric ulceration. Aspirin and, to a much lesser (i.e., clinically insignificant) extent, other salicylates and NSAIDs irreversibly inhibit platelet aggregation and prolong bleeding time. Platelet dysfunction may persist for as long as a week following exposure to aspirin. In high doses, salicylates can inhibit hepatic synthesis of clotting factor VII and, to some degree, factors IX and X and prolong the prothrombin time. This effect appears to be due to interference with the activity of vitamin K and can be reversed by administration of phytonadione (vitamin K_1).

PHARMACOKINETICS

Salicylates. Salicylates are available in oral, rectal, and topical formulations. Enteric-coated and sustained-release aspirin tablets are also marketed. Aspirin preparations frequently contain other drugs, such as anticholinergics, antihistamines, barbiturates, caffeine, decongestants, muscle relaxants, and opioids. The recommended pediatric dose of aspirin is 10 to 20 mg per kilogram of body weight every 6 hours, up to 60 mg/kg/day, and for adults is 1000 mg initially followed by 650 mg every 4 hours. Therapeutic doses of other salicylate salts are similar but depend on their salicylate content (Table 154-1) and formulation. Following a single oral dose of aspirin, therapeutic effects begin with 30 minutes, peak in 1 to 2 hours, and last about 4 hours [1,2].

Aspirin is a weak acid (pKa 3.5) that is predominantly nonionized, and therefore it is theoretically well absorbed in the stomach. However, gastric acidity slows the dissolution of tablets, and because of its larger surface area most absorption actually occurs in the small intestine [1]. Peak plasma or serum salicylate levels of 10 to 20 mg per deciliter occur 1 to 2 hours after ingestion of a single therapeutic dose. Levels up to 30 mg per deciliter can occur with chronic therapy and may be necessary for maximal antiinflammatory effects in some patients. Absorption is delayed or prolonged following ingestion of enteric-coated or sustained-release preparations and suppository use [3]. With overdosage, dissolution may be delayed, gastric drug concretions may form, pylorospasm may inhibit gastric emptying, and the absorption of aspirin may continue for 24 hours or longer following ingestion [4].

During absorption, aspirin is rapidly hydrolyzed by plasma esterases to its active metabolite, salicylic acid [1,4,5]. At physiologic pH, salicylic acid (pKa 3.0) is more than 99 percent

Table 154-1. Salicylate Preparations

Compound	Common/trade names	Percent salicylate
Acetylsalicylic acid	Aspirin	75
Bismuth subsalicylate	In Pepto-Bismol	37
Choline salicylate	Arthropan	56
Choline and magnesium salicylate	Trilisate	76
Difluorphenyl salicylic acid	Diflunisal	*
Homomenthyl salicylate	In sunscreens	51
Magnesium salicylate	Doan's Caplets, Magan	90
Methyl salicylate	Oil of wintergreen	89
Salicylic acid	In topical keratolytics	100
Salicylsalicylic acid	Salsalsate, Disalcid	96
Sodium salicylate	Pabalate	84
Trolamine salicylate	Aspercreme	48

* Not hydrolyzed to salicylic acid; may cause screening tests for salicylate to be falsely positive.

ionized to salicylate, which, in contrast to nonionized salicylic acid, diffuses poorly across cell membranes. The apparent volume of distribution of salicylate at pH 7.4 is only 0.15 liter per kilogram. Also responsible for the small apparent volume of distribution of salicylate is its extensive (90%) protein binding, primarily to serum albumin. Only free (i.e., unbound) salicylate is pharmacologically active.

Salicylate is unique in that its apparent volume of distribution does not remain constant. High drug levels (e.g., as a result of chronic therapeutic dosing or acute overdosage), low albumin levels, and the presence of other drugs that bind to albumin increase the amount and percentage of free salicylate and salicylic acid. When this occurs, the apparent volume of distribution may increase to 0.35 to 0.6 liter per kilogram. Acidemia, as a consequence of either concomitant illness or severe poisoning, may increase the fraction of nonionized, diffusible drug, promote its tissue penetration, and increase the apparent volume of distribution even more.

Following single therapeutic doses, salicylate is metabolized in the liver to the inactive metabolites salicyluric acid (75% of the dose), salicyl phenolic glucuronide (10%), salicylacyl glucuronide (5%), and gentisic acid (<1%). The remaining 10 percent of the dose is excreted unchanged in the urine. When serum concentrations exceed 20 mg per deciliter, the two main pathways of metabolism become saturated and elimination changes from first-order (i.e., proportional to the serum level) to zero-order (constant), as described by Michaelis-Menton kinetics. Hence, the half-life of salicylate is 2 to 3 hours after a single therapeutic dose, 6 to 12 hours with chronic therapeutic dosing (i.e., serum levels of 20–30 mg/dl), and 20 to 40 hours with overdosage (i.e., when levels exceed 30 mg/dl) [6]. Because of saturable metabolism, a small increase in the daily dose in patients chronically taking salicylates can lead to a large increase in serum drug levels, with the potential for unintentional poisoning [7].

Renal excretion of salicylate becomes the most important route of elimination when hepatic enzymes become saturated by overdosage [1]. Excretion is determined by the glomerular filtration of ionized salicylate and nonionized salicylic acid, active proximal tubular secretion of salicylate, and passive distal tubular reabsorption of salicylic acid. Alkalinization of the urine decreases the passive reabsorption of salicylic acid by converting it to ionized, nondiffusible salicylate and thereby increases drug excretion. Similarly, increasing the rate of urine flow (i.e., diuresis) increases the glomerular filtration of salicylic acid and

salicylate and decreases the distal tubular reabsorption of salicylic acid, leading to increased drug excretion. Combined alkalinization and diuresis can augment the renal elimination of salicylate by 20-fold or more [8]. Conversely, dehydration and aciduria (e.g., as a consequence of illnesses or febrile states and for which salicylates are often administered) decrease salicylate excretion and predispose the patient taking salicylates to intoxication. The dehydration and aciduria that result from salicylate poisoning itself also inhibit drug excretion and increase the duration of toxicity.

Salicylates readily cross the placenta and enter breast milk. Salicylate elimination in the fetus or infant may be prolonged because of immature metabolic pathways and renal function [9]. It may also be prolonged in patients with liver or renal disease.

Other NSAIDs. Despite their structural diversity, the pharmacokinetics of nonsalicylate NSAIDs are quite similar [10]. Like aspirin, they are weak acids, with pKa's ranging from 3.5 to 5.6 [11]. They are rapidly absorbed following ingestion, have small volumes of distribution (0.08–0.2 L/kg), and are 90 to 99 percent protein-bound [12]. Most nonsalicylate NSAID parent drugs are pharmacologically active and undergo hepatic metabolism to inactive metabolites that are then conjugated with glucuronic acid and excreted in the urine. Sulindac is an exception, in that its sulfide metabolite, rather than the parent drug, is the active form of the drug. Indomethacin, piroxicam, and sulindac undergo enterohepatic recirculation [10]. Small amounts of NSAIDs are excreted unchanged in the urine.

In contrast to salicylates, the metabolism of most nonsalicylate NSAIDs is not saturable and elimination follows first-order kinetics. An exception is phenylbutazone, whose elimination may follow Michaelis-Menton kinetics [10].

The pharmacokinetics of ibuprofen are representative. In adults, a 400-mg dose results in a mean peak plasma ibuprofen concentration of 29 μg per milliliter at 90 minutes [13]. The half-life of ibuprofen ranges from 0.86 to 3.06 hours and is not prolonged in overdose [14]. Therapeutic doses of other NSAIDs are shown in Chapter 215.

TOXICOLOGY

Salicylate. The pathophysiology of salicylate poisoning is multifactorial [5,15,16,17]. Early in the course of poisoning, direct stimulation of the respiratory center in the medulla by toxic salicylate concentrations results in a respiratory alkalosis. Increased carbon dioxide production may also be contributory. Alkalemia results in increased renal bicarbonate excretion (i.e., alkaluria). Respiratory stimulation can be blunted by concomitant ingestion of central nervous system (CNS) depressants [16]. Direct stimulation of the medullary chemoreceptor zone and irritant effects on the gastrointestinal tract are responsible for nausea and vomiting. Exaggerated antipyretic effects involving the hypothalamus may cause vasodilation and sweating [18]. Dehydration results from gastrointestinal, skin, and insensible fluid losses. The osmotic diuresis that occurs as bicarbonate is excreted also contributes to dehydration. Sodium and potassium depletion results from excretion of these electrolytes along with bicarbonate (in exchange for hydrogen ion reabsorption). A functional hypocalcemia (decreased ionized calcium) may accompany alkalemia and cause cardiac arrhythmias, tetany, and seizures.

The accumulation of salicylate in cells causes uncoupling of mitochondrial oxidative phosphorylation, inhibition of Krebs cycle enzymes, inhibition of amino acid metabolism, and stimulation of gluconeogenesis, glycolysis, and lipid metabolism during the intermediate stage of poisoning [19,20,21]. These derangements result in increased but ineffective metabolism, with increased glucose, lipid, and oxygen consumption and increased amino acid, carbon dioxide, glucose, ketoacid, lactic acid, and pyruvic acid production. It is the accumulation of organic acids, not the presence of large amounts of salicylate, that results in an increased anion gap metabolic acidosis. During this stage the renal excretion of organic acids may cause "paradoxical aciduria" (i.e., aciduria despite alkalemia, the latter due to persistent respiratory alkalosis). The accompanying osmotic diuresis may further accentuate fluid and electrolyte losses.

Late in the course of poisoning, if high salicylate levels are sustained, progressive dehydration and metabolic derangements and increasing levels of organic acids may result in acute renal failure (i.e., acute tubular necrosis) and increased capillary permeability [22], leading to pulmonary or cerebral edema. Hypoxia, CNS, respiratory, and cardiovascular depression and inability to excrete organic acids result in both metabolic and respiratory acidosis, with acidemia and aciduria. Capillary fragility and decreased platelet adhesiveness, thrombocytopenia, and liver dysfunction can result in bleeding problems, primarily in patients with chronic poisoning.

Other NSAIDs. Gastrointestinal irritation and renal dysfunction are probably due to the inhibition of prostaglandin synthesis. The acidosis that sometimes occurs with ibuprofen overdose appears to be due to high levels of the drug and its metabolites, rather than to interference with intrinsic metabolic pathways [23]. The mechanisms responsible for the CNS toxicity of nonsalicylate NSAIDs remain to be defined.

Clinical Manifestations and Diagnostic Evaluation

SALICYLATES. Salicylate poisoning may occur with acute as well as chronic overdose [1,15,16,17,24–34]. It almost always results from ingestion, but poisoning due to topical use has also been reported [35,36]. Infants may become poisoned by ingesting the breast milk of women chronically taking therapeutic doses of salicylate [37]. Neonatal poisoning resulting from the transplacental diffusion of maternal salicylate has also been described [38]. Whether poisoning is acute or chronic, it can be characterized as mild, moderate, or severe on the basis of signs, symptoms, and metabolic abnormalities (Table 154-2) [25]. Decisions regarding management should be based on direct assessment of severity, rather than serum salicylate level or the widely publicized Done nomogram. This nomogram, which attempted to correlate signs and symptoms with a timed salicylate level following acute ingestion [25], was never applicable to chronic poisoning and has been shown to have poor predictive value in acute poisoning [26].

Mild poisoning is defined by the presence of alkalemia (se-

Table 154-2. Severity of Salicylate Poisoning

Grade	Plasma pH	Urine pH	Underlying metabolic abnormality
Mild	>7.4	>6	Respiratory alkalosis
Moderate	≥7.4	<6	Combined respiratory alkalosis and metabolic acidosis
Severe	<7.4	<6	Metabolic acidosis with or without respiratory acidosis

rum pH >7.4) and alkaluria (urine pH >6). These findings typically develop 3 to 8 hours following an acute overdose of 150 to 300 mg of aspirin per kilogram, but can occur any time levels become toxic during chronic therapy. Signs and symptoms include nausea, vomiting, abdominal pain, headache, tinnitus, tachypnea (or subtle hyperpnea), ataxia, dizziness, agitation, and lethargy. Arterial blood gases show a pure respiratory alkalosis. The anion gap is normal until late in this stage, when compensatory renal bicarbonate excretion eventually lowers serum bicarbonate levels. Serum glucose, potassium, and sodium may be high, low, or normal. Despite total body fluid and electrolyte depletion and clinical dehydration, laboratory evidence of dehydration (e.g., hemoconcentration, increased serum blood urea nitrogen [BUN] and creatinine, increased urine specific gravity) may or may not be present.

Moderate poisoning is defined by the presence of a normal or alkaline serum pH and aciduria (urine pH <6). It typically occurs 12 to 24 hours after an acute overdose of 300 to 500 mg of aspirin per kilogram but may also occur in patients with chronic poisoning who delay seeking medical care for symptoms of mild poisoning and continue to take salicylate. Arterial blood gases reveal a combined respiratory alkalosis and metabolic acidosis, and electrolyte analysis demonstrates a low serum bicarbonate with an increased anion gap. Gastrointestinal and neurologic symptoms are more pronounced. There may be agitation, fever, asterixis, diaphoresis, deafness, pallor, confusion, slurred speech, disorientation, hallucinations, tachycardia, tachypnea, and orthostatic hypotension. Laboratory evaluation may show leukocytosis, thrombocytopenia, increased or decreased serum glucose and sodium, hypokalemia, and increased serum BUN, creatinine, and ketones.

Severe poisoning is defined by the presence of acidemia and aciduria. It occurs 24 hours or more after the acute ingestion of more than 500 mg of aspirin per kilogram. It may also be seen in progressive, unrecognized, or untreated chronic poisoning. Metabolic acidosis with inadequate respiratory compensation and a high anion gap is seen on arterial blood gas and electrolyte analysis. In cases with CNS and respiratory depression, shock, or noncardiogenic pulmonary edema (acute respiratory distress syndrome [ARDS]), there may be a concomitant respiratory acidosis. Dehydration may be severe. Other findings include coma, seizures, papilledema, hypotension, tachycardia, arrhythmias, congestive heart failure, oliguria, and hypothermia or hyperthermia. Rhabdomyolysis and multiple organ failure have also been noted [39,40]. Laboratory abnormalities are similar to those seen with moderate poisoning but are more pronounced. Hypoglycemia is relatively more common. The chest radiograph may show pulmonary edema with a normal-sized or enlarged heart [41,42,43]. Cerebral edema or hemorrhage may be seen on head computed tomography (CT). Electrocardiographic abnormalities other than sinus tachycardia reflect electrolyte abnormalities or the effects of coingested substances. Asystole frequently occurs as a terminal event [33,34,44].

Although an increased anion gap metabolic acidosis is often stated to be a hallmark of salicylate poisoning, the anion gap may be normal and acidosis may be absent in early or mild intoxication. The anion gap is rarely above 20 mEq per liter, even in patients with advanced poisoning [16]. Acid-base disturbances span a continuum from respiratory alkalosis to metabolic acidosis [16,32,33]. In adults, a combined respiratory alkalosis and metabolic acidosis is the most common finding (50–61%), followed by pure respiratory alkalosis (20–25%), pure metabolic acidosis (15–20%), and a combined respiratory and metabolic acidosis (5%) [16,34]. Children tend to progress more rapidly from mild to moderate to severe poisoning than adults [16,27,29,31], perhaps because of more rapid and extensive tissue distribution of drug [45]. Hence, metabolic acidosis is more common and respiratory alkalosis less common (and often absent) in children than in adults. Metabolic acidosis is also more common in patients with large acute ingestions, chronic intoxication, and delayed presentation or treatment [33].

Potential complications of both therapeutic and toxic doses of salicylate include gastrointestinal bleeding, increased prothrombin time, hepatic toxicity, pancreatitis, proteinuria, and abnormal urinary sediment [46–50]. Significant bleeding, gastrointestinal perforation, blindness, and inappropriate secretion of antidiuretic hormone are rare complications of acute poisoning. The overall mortality rate is less than 1 percent but with severe poisoning it may be as high as 15 percent [30,34].

In patients with acute overdose, the history should include time of ingestion, the specific product and amount ingested, and any concomitant ingestion or medication use. At least 25 percent of patients with chronic salicylism are initially undiagnosed [16,30,51]. These patients are typically elderly, have a variety of presenting complaints and underlying illnesses, and have been medicating themselves with aspirin. To avoid missing the diagnosis, all patients should be asked specifically about the use of nonprescription drugs.

The physical examination should focus on vital signs, neurologic and cardiopulmonary function, and assessment of the state of hydration. Vital signs should include an accurate (i.e., rectal) temperature and respiratory rate (i.e., counted for a full minute) and orthostatic measurements of pulse and blood pressure. The fundi should be examined for papilledema. Stool, urine, and vomitus should be tested for occult blood. Peritoneal signs should be sought on abdominal examination.

Initial laboratory evaluation should include arterial blood gases, electrolytes, glucose, BUN, creatinine, and urinalysis. In patients with moderate to severe poisoning, further evaluation should include determination of serum calcium, magnesium, and ketones; liver function tests; complete blood count; coagulation studies; and an ECG and chest radiograph. Since patients often confuse aspirin and acetaminophen, a toxicology testing should be performed to confirm the presence of salicylate and rule out the presence of acetaminophen (and possibly other agents). The presence of diflunisol may result in falsely elevated salicylate levels when measured by fluorescence polarization immunoassay or the Trinder colorimetric assay [52]. The ferric chloride spot test can be used to detect the presence of aspirin in the urine quickly. Several drops of 10% ferric chloride added to 1 ml of urine will turn purple if acetylsalicylic acid is present. False positive reactions may be caused by acetoacetic acid or phenylpyruvic acid.

Quantitative serum salicylate levels are useful for confirming the diagnosis of poisoning. As noted previously, however, severity and management should be assessed based on clinical and metabolic findings. Serum levels must be interpreted with respect to the duration (i.e., acute vs. chronic overdose) and time of ingestion. At similar salicylate levels, patients with chronic poisoning tend to be much sicker than those with acute poisoning [27,33,34]. Soon after an acute overdose, levels can be quite high (e.g., ≥60 mg/dl) in the absence of significant toxicity. Conversely, with chronic overdosage and late in the course of an acute overdose, moderate or severe toxicity may be present despite serum salicylate concentrations in the high therapeutic range. Finally, at similar salicylate levels, children, the elderly, and those with underlying disease tend to be sicker than otherwise healthy adults [27,31,45,53]. Poisoning in such patients, particularly if chronic, can occasionally be seen with therapeutic salicylate levels. Serial salicylate levels are useful for confirming the efficacy of gastrointestinal decontamination and enhanced elimination procedures but do not obviate the need for continued clinical and metabolic monitoring.

OTHER NSAIDs. Nonsalicylate NSAID poisoning usually results from acute overdose. However, renal toxicity can occur during chronic therapy, and some individuals cannot tolerate even single therapeutic doses because of gastrointestinal or CNS side effects. With the exception of the anthranilic acid and pyrazolone derivatives (see Chap. 215), acute overdose usually results in mild toxicity. Typical manifestations include nausea, vomiting, abdominal pain, headache, confusion, tinnitus, drowsiness, and hyperventilation [10,54,55]. Glycosuria, hematuria, and proteinuria are also common. These effects, and occasionally acute renal failure (acute tubular necrosis), can be caused by all nonsalicylate NSAIDs. Symptoms rarely last more than several hours, and acute renal toxicity is almost always reversible over a period of a few days to a few weeks.

A high incidence (30%) of muscle twitching and grand mal seizures has been reported in patients with mefenamic acid overdose [56]. Apnea, coma, and cardiac arrest can also occur [55]. Metabolic acidosis, coma, seizures, hepatic dysfunction, hypotension, and cardiovascular collapse are relatively common following large phenylbutazone overdoses [54,55,57,58,59]. With other nonsalicylate NSAIDs, severe poisoning is rare. Ibuprofen can cause coma, seizures, metabolic acidosis, and respiratory depression [13,14,23,60–63]; acute hepatic injury, thrombocytopenia, ARDS, and upper gastrointestinal bleeding of unclear etiology have also been reported [64]. Ketoprofen and naproxen poisoning can result in seizures [65,66]; metabolic acidosis has also been reported following naproxen overdose [66].

The spectrum of potential toxicity from NSAID overdose is the same in children and in adults [14,23,54,67]. Elderly patients are at increased risk of developing toxicity with both therapeutic doses and overdoses [71]. Even with severe poisoning, patients usually recover completely within 24 to 48 hours. Death has resulted from ibuprofen poisoning (alone or combined with other drugs) [13,68,69,70], but given the frequency of ibuprofen overdose, it is an extremely rare occurrence.

The minimum toxic and lethal doses for most nonsalicylate NSAIDs are not well defined. Little correlation was found between amount of ibuprofen reportedly ingested and symptoms in adults [14]. In the pediatric population, however, symptomatic patients had mean ingestions of 440 mg per kilogram, whereas asymptomatic ones had mean ingestions of 114 mg per kilogram [14]. For other nonsalicylate NSAIDs the ingestion of at least 5 adult doses in children and 10 therapeutic doses in adults is generally required to produce significant toxicity [54,55].

The diagnostic evaluation of patients with acute NSAID overdose is the same as for salicylates. Evaluation of acid-base, electrolyte, and renal parameters is particularly important. Additional ancillary testing is dictated by clinical severity. A toxicology screen may be useful for confirming the identity of the ingested agent and excluding other ingestions. Quantitative serum levels of nonsalicylate NSAIDs are neither routinely available nor necessary for treatment.

DIFFERENTIAL DIAGNOSIS. Occult salicylate poisoning should be considered in any patient with an unexplained acid-base disturbance, altered mental status, fever, dyspnea, vomiting, and pulmonary edema [16,51]. Other agents that cause an elevated anion gap acidosis include methanol, ethanol (alcoholic ketoacidosis), and ethylene glycol (see Chap. 132). Infection (particularly meningitis), CNS trauma and tumors, congestive heart failure, chronic obstructive pulmonary disease (COPD), carbon monoxide, isoniazid, lithium and valproate intoxication, and toxic gas inhalation should also be included in the differential diagnosis.

Salicylate poisoning in infants and children may be confused with inborn errors of metabolism. It may be particularly difficult to distinguish from Reye's syndrome, since they are not only similar in presentation but appear to be interrelated [72,73]. Fatty infiltration of the liver on pathologic examination of a biopsy specimen, low (i.e., subtherapeutic) cerebrospinal fluid (CSF) salicylate levels, and high alanine, glutamine, and lysine levels indicate Reye's syndrome rather than salicylate poisoning. Many medical conditions and other intoxications cause signs and symptoms similar to those seen in nonsalicylate NSAID poisoning. In the absence of a history of ingestion, the diagnosis is made by toxicology screening and exclusion of other etiologies. Radiopaque densities in the stomach on abdominal radiograph suggest the possibility of an enteric-coated or sustained-release formulation or a magnesium or bismuth salt of salicylate.

Management

SALICYLATES. Treatment should be tailored to the severity of poisoning. Advanced life support measures should be instituted as necessary. Since there is no antidote for salicylate poisoning, therapy is directed at limiting absorption, correcting dehydration and metabolic abnormalities, and enhancing elimination. Gastrointestinal decontamination should be performed in all patients with intentional overdoses and those with accidental ingestions of greater than 150 mg per kilogram. Decontamination may be effective for as long as 24 hours following overdose, even in patients with spontaneous vomiting, because of delayed absorption and concretion formation [4]. Gastric lavage, preceded and followed by a dose of activated charcoal, may be the most effective treatment for large overdoses [74]. Charcoal alone is preferable to ipecac for mild to moderate overdoses [75]. However, since charcoal binds neutral agents better than ionized ones, salicylate may be released from the charcoal, resulting in delayed absorption as the charcoal-drug complex moves from the acid milieu of the stomach to the alkaline environment of the small intestine, where salicylic acid becomes ionized [76]. This problem may be overcome by giving multiple oral doses of charcoal [77]. Whole bowel irrigation may be effective for decontamination of patients suspected of having concretions (e.g., with serum drug levels that continue to rise for more than 6 to 12 hours after overdose).

Therapy for dehydration should begin with 1 to 3 liters of intravenous D_5 1/2 NS or D_5 NS, with or without $NaHCO_3$ (1 amp/L) and potassium (10–20 mEq/L) over the first 1 to 2 hours. The degree of dehydration is often underestimated. The use of a dextrose-containing solution is important because CNS hypoglycemia may occur at normal serum glucose levels [78]. In patients with hypernatremia, a hypotonic solution should be used.

Electrolyte abnormalities should be corrected. In the presence of acidemia, the degree of hypokalemia is more severe than indicated by the serum level (by about 0.6 mEq/L for each 0.1 unit decrease in pH). Clinical tetany may require treatment with intravenous calcium chloride or calcium gluconate (10 ml of a 10% solution over 5–10 minutes) despite normal serum calcium levels if alkalemia is present, since this condition decreases the ionized (active) fraction of calcium. Coagulopathy should be treated with vitamin K. Fresh frozen plasma, red cell, and platelet transfusions may be required for patients with active bleeding or significant blood loss.

Central venous or pulmonary artery pressure monitoring may be necessary for optimal treatment of hypotension, especially if there is evidence of heart failure or pulmonary edema. Congestive heart failure can be treated by standard measures, but patients with noncardiac pulmonary edema should be treated with intubation and positive end-expiratory pressure (PEEP) rather than diuretics. Increased intracranial pressure due to cerebral edema may be reduced with head elevation, hyperventilation, and mannitol. Glucose as well as anticonvulsants (e.g., benzodiazepines, phenytoin, and barbiturates) should be given to patients with seizures. Hyperthermia should be treated with cooling blankets, ice packs, and evaporative methods (see Chap. 73).

Salicylate elimination can be enhanced by repeat oral doses of activated charcoal [77], urinary alkalinization and diuresis [1,14,27,79], and extracorporeal removal [80]. Recent evidence suggests that glycine administration enhances elimination of salicylate [31]. The clinical efficacy of multiple-dose charcoal therapy in overdose patients is unclear. In patients with acute overdose and salicylate levels less than 70 mg per deciliter, the mean salicylate half-life was reported to be 3.2 hours with multiple-dose charcoal [77]. However, these patients also received alkali therapy, since the brand of charcoal used (Medicoal) was an effervescent preparation containing bicarbonate. Since experimental studies have found therapy with multiple doses of noneffervescent charcoal to have little or no effect in simulated (i.e., <3 gm) overdoses in human volunteers [81,82,83], the oral administration of bicarbonate may have trapped salicylate in the gut or prevented its desorption from activated charcoal and accounted for the effectiveness of this treatment.

In a similar group of patients with acute poisoning and moderately elevated salicylate levels treated with alkaline diuresis, the mean salicylate half-life was 5.9 hours during the first 4 hours of therapy and 12.3 hours during the subsequent 12 hours [79]. This study also showed that urinary alkalinization alone was superior to diuresis alone and at least as effective as alkaline diuresis. However, patients in the alkalinization-only group actually received significant amounts (250 ml/hr vs. 500 ml/hr in the diuresis and alkaline diuresis groups, respectively) of intravenous and oral fluids. Although serum salicylate levels were similar, patients in the alkalinization-only group were treated much sooner after ingestion than those in the alkaline diuresis group, suggesting that the former group had lower peak drug levels. Since the treatment groups were not closely matched and the alkalinization-only group was, in fact, diuresed, the issue of whether alkalinization alone is as effective as alkaline diuresis remains to be resolved. Measures to enhance urinary salicylate excretion are likely to be less effective in patients with chronic salicylism or very high salicylate levels (i.e., >79 mg/dl) [84,85].

Indications for urinary alkalinization or alkaline diuresis include systemic symptoms, acid-base abnormalities, or salicylate levels greater than 30 mg per deciliter after an acute overdose. Patients with chronic overdoses may be symptomatic and require treatment despite "therapeutic" salicylate levels. The goal is to achieve a urine pH of 7.5 or greater. Although "forced" diuresis (e.g., 500 ml/hr in urine output in adults) has long been recommended [86], such therapy is potentially dangerous (see below) and of unproved benefit (see above). Hence, a moderate diuresis (2–3 ml/kg/hr) is recommended. All patients treated with alkaline diuresis need close monitoring in an intensive care unit or similar setting (e.g., emergency department observation unit). Bladder catheterization is essential because urine output and pH, as well as fluid intake, require frequent monitoring (every 1–2 hours). Furosemide can be given to enhance diuresis in adequately hydrated patients whose urine output falls below their fluid intake. Arterial blood gases and serum electrolytes, BUN, creatinine, and glucose should be rechecked at 2- to 6-hour intervals depending on previous findings and the response to therapy. Cardiac monitoring and frequent reevaluations of vital signs, mental status, and pulmonary function are also necessary during alkaline diuresis.

The aggressiveness of alkaline diuresis therapy should be based on the severity of poisoning (Table 154-3). Even in patients with mild poisoning who have alkalemia and alkaluria, bicarbonate and fluids should be given to replace ongoing renal losses. Alkalinization of the urine may be impossible to achieve in the presence of dehydration and hypokalemia, because hydrogen ions are excreted in exchange for reabsorbed sodium and potassium, respectively [87]. Therefore, correction of fluid and potassium deficits is critical. Carbonic anhydrase inhibitors (e.g., acetazolamide) should not be used to alkalinize the urine (especially without concomitant bicarbonate therapy) because they may cause a concomitant systemic acidosis, which may promote tissue distribution of salicylate and result in clinical deterioration [88]. In addition, the combined use of acetazolamide and salicylate may lead to acetazolamide poisoning [89].

Complications of alkaline diuresis include excessive alkalemia, hypokalemia, hypocalcemia, hypernatremia, and fluid overload with cerebral and pulmonary edema [31,85,86]. Young children, the elderly, and those with severe poisoning are most susceptible to such complications. Alkaline diuresis is contraindicated in patients with oliguric renal failure, congestive heart failure, and cerebral or pulmonary edema. Alkali therapy should be withheld if the serum pH is greater than 7.55.

Oral administration of glycine (28 gm dissolved in water initially, followed by 10 gm every 2 hours) or N-glycylglycine (8 gm dissolved in water, followed by 2 gm every 2 hours) has recently been used as an alternative to alkalinization [31,90]. Since the conjugation of salicylic acid with glycine to form salicyluric acid becomes saturated and glycine levels decrease in overdose patients, supplemental glycine can enhance the formation and excretion of this metabolite. To date, clinical experience with this therapy is limited, its comparative efficacy is unknown, and the side effects of nausea and vomiting have been problematic.

Hemodialysis is indicated in patients with severe poisoning and those with moderate poisoning who fail to respond to alkaline diuresis. It is essential for successful outcome in those with coma, seizures, cerebral or pulmonary edema, or renal failure [15]. High salicylate level (e.g., >80 mg/dl) is an indication for hemodialysis only if associated with severe or unresponsive clinical and laboratory toxicity. Conversely, patients with severe toxicity and lower salicylate levels should be treated with hemodialysis, particularly if they have significant underlying cardiorespiratory disease.

Drug extraction ratios during hemodialysis have been reported to be 0.2 to 0.7 [80]. Assuming a flow rate of 200 ml per minute, clearances of 40 to 140 ml per minute can be expected in adults. Clearance rates of 30 to 35 ml per minute have been reported in pediatric patients [90]. A high bicarbonate (e.g., 28–32 mEq/L) dialysate solution should be used. Potassium should also be added to the dialysate solution. Although hemoperfusion is also effective, hemodialysis has the advantage of being

able to correct fluid, electrolyte, and acid-base abnormalities and has fewer complications and is thus preferred [80,91]. A tandem setup, using hemoperfusion and hemodialysis in series (i.e., in the same circuit), has been suggested as optimal therapy but is impractical and, in most patients, unnecessary. If hemodialysis is unavailable or technically impossible, peritoneal dialysis (with 5% albumin added to bind salicylate) and exchange transfusion are less effective alternatives [92].

NONSALICYLATE NSAIDs. The treatment of nonsalicylate NSAID poisoning is supportive and symptomatic. Although most patients require only observation, advanced life support measures and invasive monitoring may be required in cases of severe poisoning. Interventions that may be necessary include airway protection, mechanical ventilation, fluid resuscitation, anticonvulsants for seizures, bicarbonate for acidosis, vitamin K or fresh frozen plasma for coagulopathy, antacids and H_2-receptor antagonists for gastritis, and blood products for gastrointestinal bleeding. Renal function should be monitored carefully in patients with abnormal urinalysis, underlying renal disease, or advanced age. Liver function tests should be followed in patients with severe phenylbutazone and piroxicam poisoning.

Gastrointestinal decontamination with gastric lavage and/or activated charcoal is recommended for patients who present within 4 hours of ingesting greater than 10 therapeutic doses in adults and more than 5 adult doses in children [54,55]. Because of the potential for CNS depression and seizures, especially in children and those with mefenamic acid or phenylbutazone poisoning, syrup of ipecac should be reserved for patients with mild to moderate overdoses who can be treated within 30 minutes of ingestion. Although charcoal hemoperfusion has been used to treat a patient with severe phenylbutazone poisoning who had impaired renal and hepatic function [57], extracorporeal elimination measures are unlikely to be effective for nonsalicylate NSAID poisoning because of the high protein binding and rapid intrinsic elimination of these agents. Similarly, although multiple-dose charcoal therapy was found to enhance the elimination of a therapeutic dose of phenylbutazone by 30% [93], kinetic data suggest that this therapy is unlikely to have significant clinical efficacy.

Table 154-3. Alkaline Diuresis Therapy of Salicylate Poisoning: Fluid and Electrolyte Therapy*

Grade	Intravenous solution	NaHCO₃ (amp/L)	Potassium (mEq/L)
Mild	D₅NS	1	20
Moderate	D₅½NS	2	40
Severe	D₅W	3	60–80

* Initial treatment should include hydration with 1 to 3 liters of a saline solution containing dextrose (see text).

References

1. Insel PA: Analgesic antipyretics and antiinflammatory agents: Drugs employed in the treatment of rheumatoid arthritis and gout, in Gilman AG, Rall TW, Niew AS, et al (eds): *Goodman and Gilman's The Pharmacological Basis of Therapeutics.* 8th ed. New York, Pergamon, 1990, pp 638–681.
2. McEvoy GK, Litvak K, Welsh OH, et al (eds): *American Hospital Formulary Service Drug Information.* Bethesda, American Society of Hospital Pharmacists, 1993.
3. Wortzman DJ, Grunfeld A: Delay absorption following enteric-coated aspirin overdose. *Ann Emerg Med* 16:434, 1987.
4. Matthew H, Mackintosh TF, Tompsett SL, Cameron JC: Gastric aspiration and lavage in acute poisoning. *Br Med J* 1:1333, 1966.
5. Levy G: Comparative pharmacokinetics of aspirin and acetaminophen. *Arch Intern Med* 141:279, 1981.
6. Snodgrass W, Rumack BH, Peterson RG, et al: Salicylate toxicity following therapeutic doses in young children. *Clin Toxicol* 18:247, 1981.
7. Levy G, Tsuchiya T: Salicylate accumulation kinetics in man. *N Engl J Med* 287:430, 1972.
8. Levy G: Pharmacokinetics of salicylate in man. *Drug Metab Rev* 9:3, 1979.
9. Garretson LK, Procknal JA, Levy G: Fetal acquisition and neonatal

elimination of a large amount of salicylate. *Clin Pharmacol Ther* 17:98, 1975.

10. Verbeeck RK, Blackburn JL, Loewen GR: Clinical pharmacokinetics of non-steroidal anti-inflammatory drugs. *Clin Pharmacokinet* 8:297, 1983.

11. Brown GR: Non-steroidal anti-inflammatory drugs. *Clin Toxicol Rev* 6:1, 1984.

12. Brater DL: Clinical pharmacology of NSAID. *J Clin Pharmacol* 28:518, 1988.

13. Adams SS, Bough RG, Cliffe EE, et al: Absorption, distribution and toxicity of ibuprofen. *Toxicol Appl Pharmacol* 15:310, 1969.

14. Hall AH, Smolinske SC, Conrad FL, et al: Ibuprofen overdose: 126 cases. *Ann Emerg Med* 15:1308, 1986.

15. Brenner BE, Simon RR: Management of salicylate intoxication. *Drugs* 24:335, 1987.

16. Gabow PA, Anderson RJ, Potts DE, et al: Acid base disturbances in the salicylate intoxicated adult. *Arch Intern Med* 138:1481, 1978.

17. Proudfoot AT: Toxicity of salicylates. *Am J Med* 75:99, 1983.

18. Lovejoy F: Aspirin and acetaminophen: A comparative view of their antipyretic and analgesic activity. *Pediatrics* 62(suppl):904, 1978.

19. Miyahara J, Karle R: Effect of salicylate on oxidative phosphorylation of mitochondrial fragments. *Biochem J* 97:194, 1965.

20. Smith M: The metabolic basis of the major symptoms in acute salicylate intoxication. *Clin Toxicol* 1:387, 1968.

21. Brody TM: Action of sodium salicylate and related compounds on tissue metabolism in vitro. *J Pharmacol Exp Ther* 117:39, 1956.

22. Hormaechea E, Carlson RW, Rogove H, et al: Hypovolemia, pulmonary edema, and protein changes in severe salicylate poisoning. *Am J Med* 66:1046, 1979.

23. Linden CH, Townsend PL: Metabolic acidosis after acute ibuprofen overdosage. *J Pediatr* 111:922, 1987.

24. Done AK: Aspirin overdosage: Incidence, diagnosis and management. *Pediatrics* 62(suppl):890, 1978.

25. Done AK: Salicylate intoxication: Significance of measurements of salicylates in blood in cases of acute ingestion. *Pediatrics* 26:800, 1960.

26. Dugandzic RM, Tierney ME, Dickinson GE, et al: Evaluation of the validitiy of the Done nomogram in the management of acute salicylate intoxication. *Ann Emerg Med* 18:1186, 1989.

27. Temple AR: Acute and chronic effects of aspirin toxicity and their treatment. *Arch Intern Med* 141:364, 1981.

28. Segar WE, Holliday MA: Physiologic abnormalities of salicylate intoxication. *N Engl J Med* 259:1191, 1958.

29. Goudrealt P, Temple AR, Lovejoy FH: The relative severity of acute versus chronic salicylate poisonings in children: A clinical comparison. *Pediatrics* 70:566, 1982.

30. McGuigan MA: A two-year review of salicylate deaths in Ontario. *Arch Intern Med* 147:510, 1987.

31. Notarianni L: A reassessment of the treatment of salicylate poisoning. *Drug Saf* 7:292, 1992.

32. Winters RW, White JS, Hughes MC, et al: Disturbances of acid base equilibrium in salicylate intoxication. *Pediatrics* 23:260, 1959.

33. Thisted B, Krantz T, Shrom J, et al: Acute salicylate poisoning in 177 consecutive patients treated in ICU. *Acta Anaesthesiol Scand* 31:312, 1987.

34. Chapman BJ, Proudfoot AT: Adult salicylate poisoning: Deaths and outcome in patients with high plasma salicylate concentrations. *Q J Med* 72:699, 1989.

35. Anderson JAR, Ead RD: Percutaneous salicylate poisoning. *Clin Exp Dermatol* 4:349, 1979.

36. Davies MG, Briffa DV, Graves MW: Systemic toxicity from topically applied salicylic acid. *Br Med J* 1:661, 1979.

37. Clark JH, Wilson WG: A 16 day old breast fed infant with metabolic acidosis caused by salicylate. *Clin Pediatr* 20:53, 1981.

38. Bond GR, Grebe TA, Arnold Capell PA: Transplacental salicylate poisoning masquerading as neonatal sepsis. *Vet Hum Toxicol* 31:364,1989.

39. Leventhal LJ, Kuritsky L, Ginsberg R, et al: Salicylate-induced rhabdomyolysis. *Am J Emerg Med* 7:409, 1989.

40. Leatherman JW, Schmitz PG: Fever, hyperdynamic shock, and multiple system organ failure. *Chest* 100:1391, 1991.

41. Heffner JE, Sahn SA: Salicylate-induced pulmonary edema. *JAMA* 95:405, 1981.

42. Walters JS, Woodring JH, Stelling CB, et al: Salicylate-induced pulmonary edema. *Radiology* 146:289, 1983.

43. Fisher CJ, Albertson TE, Foulke GE: Salicylate-induced pulmonary edema: Clinical characteristics in children. *Am J Emerg Med* 3:33, 1985.

44. Berk WA, Anderson JC: Salicylate-associated asystole: Report of two cases. *Am J Med* 86:505, 1989.

45. Nigogi SK, Rieders R: Salicylate poisoning: Differences in tissue levels and distribution between children and adults. *Eur J Toxicol* 2:234, 1969.

46. Miller MR: Suppression of urine in aspirin poisoning. *Lancet* 1:596, 1955.

47. Athreya BH, Gorske AL, Myers AR: Aspirin-induced abnormalities of liver function. *Am J Dis Child* 126:638, 1973.

48. Meyer OO, Howard B: Production of hypoprothrombinemia and hypocoagulability of the blood with salicylates. *Proc Soc Exp Biol Med* 53:243, 1943.

49. Rupp DJ, Seaton RD, Wiegmann TB: Acute polyuric renal failure after aspirin intoxication. *Arch Intern Med* 143:1237, 1983.

50. Kimberly RP, Plotz PH: Aspirin-induced depression of renal function. *N Engl J Med* 296:418, 1977.

51. Anderson RJ, Potts DE, Gabow PA: Unrecognized adult salicylate intoxication. *Ann Intern Med* 85:745, 1976.

52. Duffens KR, Smilkstein MJ, Bessen HA, et al: Falsely elevated salicylate levels due to diffusional overdose. *J Emerg Med* 5:499, 1987.

53. Bailey RB, Jones SR: Chronic salicylate intoxication: A common cause of morbidity in the elderly. *J Am Geriatr Soc* 37:556, 1989.

54. Vale JA, Meredith TS: Acute poisoning due to non-steroidal anti-inflammatory drugs: Clinical features and management. *Med Toxicol* 1:12, 1986.

55. Court H, Volans GN: Poisoning after overdose with nonsteroidal anti-inflammatory drugs. *Adverse Drug React Acute Poison Rev* 3:1, 1984.

56. Balali-Mood M, Proudfoot AT, Critchley JAJH, et al: Mefenamic acid overdose. *Lancet* 1:1354, 1981.

57. Berlinger WG, Spector R, Flanigan MJ: Hemoperfusion for phenylbutazone poisoning. *Ann Intern Med* 96:334, 1982.

58. Strong JE, Wilson J, Douglas JF, et al: Phenylbutazone self-poisoning treated by charcoal haemoperfusion. *Anaesthesia* 34:1038, 1979.

59. Okonek S, Reinecke H: Acute toxicity of pyrazolines. *Am J Med* 75(suppl A):94, 1983.

60. Hunt DP, Leigh RJ: Overdose with ibuprofen causing unconsciousness and hypotension. *Br Med J* 281:1458, 1980.

61. Chelluri L, Jastremski M: Coma caused by ibuprofen overdose. *Crit Care Med* 14:1078, 1986.

62. Menzies DG, Conn AG, Williamson FS, et al: Fulminant hyperkalemia and multiple complications following ibuprofen overdose. *Med Toxicol Adverse Drug Exp* 4:468, 1989.

63. Bennett RR, Dunleberg JC, Marks ES: Acute oliguric renal failure due to ibuprofen overdose. *South Med J* 78:490, 1985.

64. Lee CY, Finkler A: Acute intoxication due to ibuprofen overdose. *Pathol Lab Med* 110:747, 1986.

65. Bond GR, Curry SC, Arnold-Capell PA, et al: Generalized seizures and metabolic acidosis after ketoprofen overdose. *Vet Hum Toxicol* 31:369, 1989.

66. Martinez R, Smith DW, Frankel LR: Severe metabolic acidosis after acute naproxen sodium ingestion. *Ann Emerg Med* 18:1102, 1989.

67. Hall AH, Smolinske SC, Kulig KW, et al: Ibuprofen overdose: A prospective study. *West J Med* 148:653, 1988.

68. Barry WS, Meinzinger MM, Howse CR: Ibuprofen overdose and exposure in utero: Results from a postmarketing voluntary reporting system. *Am J Med* 77:35, 1984.

69. Court H, Streete P, Volans GN: Acute poisoning with ibuprofen. *Hum Toxicol* 2:381, 1983.

70. Litovitz TL, Schmitz BF, Holm KC: 1988 annual report of the American Association of Poison Control Centers National Data Collection System. *Am J Emerg Med* 7:495, 1989.

71. Woodhouse KW, Wynne H: The pharmacokinetics of non-steroidal anti-inflammatory drugs in the elderly. *Clin Pharmacokinet* 12:111, 1987.

72. Quint PA, Allman FD: Differentiation of chronic salicylism for Reye's syndrome. *Pediatrics* 74:1117, 1984.

73. Osterloh J, Cunningham W, Dixon A, et al: Biochemical relationships between Reye's and Reye's-like metabolic and toxicological syndromes. *Med Toxicol Adverse Drug Exp* 4:272, 1989.

74. Burton GT, Bayer MJ, Barron L, et al: Comparison of activated

charcoal and gastric lavage in the prevention of aspirin absorption. *J Emerg Med* 1:411, 1984.

75. Curtis RA, Barone J, Giacon N: Efficacy of ipecac and activated charcoal/cathartic: Prevention of salicylate absorption in a simulated overdose. *Arch Intern Med* 144:48, 1984.

76. Filippone G, Fish SS, Laconture PG, et al: Reversible adsorption (desorption) of aspirin from activated charcoal. *Arch Intern Med* 147:1390, 1987.

77. Hillman RJ, Prescott LF: Treatment of salicylate poisoning with repeated activated charcoal. *Br Med J* 291:1472, 1985.

78. Hobwach Thurston J, Pollock PG, et al: Reduced brain glucose with normal plasma glucose in salicylate poisoning. *J Clin Invest* 49:2130, 1970.

79. Prescott LF, Balali-Mood M, Critchley JAJH, et al: Diuresis or urinary alkalinization for salicylate poisoning? *Br Med J* 285:1383, 1982.

80. Winchester JF, Gelfand MC, Helliwell M, et al: Extracorporeal treatment of salicylate or acetaminopen poisoning: Is there a role? *Arch Intern Med* 141:370, 1981.

81. Ho JL, Tierney MG, Dickinson GE: An elevation of the effect of repeated doses of oral activated charcoal on salicylate elimination. *J Clin Pharmacol* 29:366, 1989.

82. Kirshenbaum LA, Matthew SC, Sitar DS, et al: Does multiple-dose charcoal therapy enhance salicylate excretion? *Arch Intern Med* 150:1281, 1990.

83. Mayer AL, Sitar DS, Tenenbein M: Multiple-dose charcoal and whole bowel irrigation do not increase clearance of absorbed salicylate. *Arch Intern Med* 152:393, 1992.

84. Coppack SW, Higgins CS: Algorithm for modified alkaline diuresis in salicylate poisoning. *Br Med J* 289:1452, 1984.

85. Elenbaas RM: Critical review of forced alkaline diuresis in acute salicylism. *Crit Care Q* 3:89, 1982.

86. Lawson AAH, Proudfoot AT, Brown SS, et al: Forced diuresis in the treatment of acute salicylate poisoning in adults. *Q J Med* 38:31, 1969.

87. Robin ED, Davis RP, Rees SB: Salicylate intoxication with special reference to the development of hypokalemia. *Am J Med* 26:869, 1959.

88. Hill JB: Experimental salicylate poisoning: Observations on the effects of altering blood pH on tissue and plasma salicylate concentrations. *Pediatrics* 47:658, 1971.

89. Sweeney K, Chapron D, Brandt L, et al: Toxic interaction between acetazolamide and salicylate: Case reports and a pharmacokinetic explanation. *Clin Pharmacol Ther* 40:518, 1986.

90. Spritz N, Fahey TJ, Thompson DD, et al: The use of extracorporeal hemodialysis in the treatment of salicylate intoxication in a 2-year-old child. *Pediatrics* 24:540, 1959.

91. Jacobsen O, Wiik-Larsen E, Bredesen JE: Haemodialysis or haemoperfusion in severe salicylate poisoning? *Hum Toxicol* 7:161, 1988.

92. Schlegel RJ, Altstatt LB, Canales L, et al: Peritoneal dialysis for severe salicylism: An evaluation of indications and results. *J Pediatr* 69:553, 1966.

93. Neuvonen PJ, Elonen E: Effect of activated charcoal on absorption and elimination of phenobarbitone, carbamazepine, and phenylbutazone in man. *Eur J Clin Pharmacol* 17:51, 1980.

155. Sedative-Hypnotic Poisoning

Cynthia K. Aaron, Mary C. Burke, Marc Restuccia, Constance Nichols, and Eric W. Schmidt

Sedative-hypnotic agents encompass a large number of medications, including benzodiazepines, barbiturates, nonbenzodiazepine nonbarbiturate sedative-hypnotics (NBNBs), and some muscle relaxants. The barbiturates (Veronal) and "bromides" were the first medications used as sedative-hypnotic agents. In the 1960s, the NBNBs, such as meprobamate (Miltown), were introduced and became popular. Once Roche introduced the benzodiazepines (diazepam and chlordiazepoxide), these medications and their congeners rapidly replaced NBNBs as the most commonly prescribed sedative-hypnotics (Table 155-1). This trend is now being reversed with the selective restrictions on benzodiazepine prescriptions in some states (e.g., New York).

Benzodiazepines

Benzodiazepines (BZDs) are one of the most widely prescribed classes of drugs. In the United States, multiple benzodiazepines and their derivatives are available to treat anxiety, depression, panic disorders, insomnia, musculoskeletal disorders, seizures, and alcohol withdrawal and as an adjunct for anesthesia [1,2].

PHARMACOLOGY. Benzodiazepines exert their therapeutic effect at specific benzodiazepine receptor sites in the central nervous system (CNS) [3] (see Chap. 209). The benzodiazepine receptor is located within the gamma-aminobutyric acid$_A$ (GABA$_A$) receptor supramolecular complex (GRSMC). Binding of GABA or GABA plus a BZD causes an allosteric change in the structure of the GRSMC. This activates the complex. Activation of the GRSMC leads to alteration in chloride channel permeability, with a subsequent increase in chloride flux and hyperpolarization. Gamma-aminobutyric acid is an inhibitory neurotransmitter and its receptors form an inhibitory bidirectional system with connections within many areas of the CNS. Once neurotransmission has been altered, there is a secondary effect on neurotransmitter release from the internuncial neurons. For the most part, activation of a GABA neuron leads to changes in dopamine release, although norepinephrine and acetylcholine may be involved. Serotonin effect is minimal except for neurons in the dorsal raphe [4]. Activation of GRSMC by a BZD potentiates synaptic GABA-mediated inhibition [5,6]. The GRSMCs are located throughout the brain and spinal cord area, with additional receptor complexes found on other organs including the adrenals, kidney, and pineal gland and on platelets [6,7,8]. The BZD receptors were initally described as central and peripheral, in an attempt to localize their function. These

Table 155-1. Sedative-Hypnotic Agents Available in the United States

Benzodiazepines	Barbiturates	Nonbenzodiazepine nonbarbiturates
Alprazolam	Amobarbital	Alpidem*
Bromazepam*	Aprobarbital	Buspirone
Brotizolam*	Butalbital	Chloral hydrate
Chlordiazepoxide	Mepthobarbital	Chlormethiazole*
Clobazam*	Pentobarbital	Ethinamate
Clorazepate	Phenobarbital	Ethchlorvynol
Diazepam	Secobarbital	Glutethimide
Estazolam	Thiopental	Methaqualone
Flunitrazepam		Methypylon
Flurazepam		Paraldehyde
Halazepam		Baclofen
Lorazepam		Meprobamate
Midazolam		Zolpidem
Nitrazepam		
Oxazepam		
Quazepam		
Triazolam		

* Investigational in the United States

receptors were recently redesignated as omega$_1$, omega$_2$, omega$_3$. Each of the omega subtypes tends to cluster in particular areas of the CNS, with a particular subtype being more common in some areas than others [4,7–14]. The omega subtypes are themselves heterogeneous, with six different subunit variants (alpha$_1$, alpha$_2$, alpha$_3$, alpha$_5$, beta$_2$, gamma$_2$). The particular combination of subunits determines which omega subtype is present [9,10]. The omega$_1$ subtype tends to predominate in the sensorimotor cortex and the omega$_2$ subtype seems to be increased in the limbic areas of the brain. Based on this localization, omega$_1$ subtype receptors may be predominately sedative-hypnotic and the omega$_2$ subtype receptors mostly anxiolytic and anticonvulsant. The function of the omega$_3$ sub-type is not understood. However, this crude delineation requires much more study before a distinction such as this can be made [4,6,8–13]. Some of the BZDs preferentially bind to different omega subtypes such as zolpidem and omega$_1$; alpidem prefers omega$_1$ and omega$_3$; flunitrazepam, flumazenil (BZD antagonist), diazepam, and other BZDs are mixed omega$_1$ and omega$_2$ [6–10].

Benzodiazepine absorption from the gastrointestinal tract is dependent on the intrinsic physiochemical properties and pharmaceutical formulation of each drug. Peak levels usually occur within 3 hours after ingestion; intramuscular absorption can be erratic and delayed. Duration of action is dependent on the lipophilicity of each compound: the more lipophilic, the shorter the duration of action. Lipophilic drugs tend to distribute into adipose tissue and rapidly partition between blood and brain. This decreases the effect on the CNS. Benzodiazepines are highly protein-bound (85–99%). The volume of distribution is dependent on the lipid solubility and can vary from chlordiazepoxide (V_d 0.26–0.58 L/kg) to diazepam (V_d 0.95–2 L/kg). Metabolism is hepatic and benzodiazepines are biotransformed via the microsomal oxidation system through N-dealkylation and glucuronification [15]. Benzodiazepines are classified on the basis of elimination half-life (Table 155-2) [16].

Benzodiazepines potentiate other CNS depressants and are themselves addititive to or synergistic with the effects of other sedative-hypnotics [17]. Since cimetidine inhibits hepatic drug microsomal activation, it reduces clearance of diazepam and prolongs diazepam drug effect. Oxazepam and lorazepam have different metabolic paths and should not be affected by cimetidine [17,18].

Lethal toxicity from pure benzodiazepine overdose has been reported infrequently. A retrospective review of 1239 overdose cases from a medical examiners' office revealed only two deaths solely related to diazepam overdose [19]. In chronic abusers, rapid clinical recovery after benzodiazepine overdose is believed to result from adaptation or tolerance to the depressant effects [20].

Table 155-2. Duration of Action and Elimination Half-Life of Benzodiazepines

Agent	Duration (hr)	Elimination t$^{1/2}$ (hr)	Peak effect (hr)	Active metabolites
Ultra short-acting	<10			
Midazolam (Versed)		2–5	0.3-0.8	−
Temazepam (Restoril)		10	2–3	−
Triazolam (Halcion)		1.7–3	0.5–1.5	+
Brotizolam		5	1	−
Short-acting	10–24			
Alprazolam (Xanax)		11–14	0.7–1.6	+
Lorazepam (Ativan)		10–20	2	−
Oxazepam (Serax)		3–21	1–2	−
Bromazepam		8–20	1–2	−
Flunitrazepam		20–30	2–8	+
Estazolam		10–24	1	−
Long-acting	>24	5–30	2–4	+
Chlordiazepoxide (Librium)		36–200	1–2.5	+
Clorazepate (Tranxene)		10–50	1–4	−
Clonazepam (Klonopin)		20–50	1–2	+
Diazepam (Valium)		50–100	3–6	+
Flurazepam (Dalmane)		26–200	6	+
Quazepam		11–77	1–3	+
Clobazam		14	1–3	+
Halazepam		Metabolites:50–100		+
Prazepam (Centrax)		25–41	6	+
		Metabolites:40–114		

CLINICAL PRESENTATION. Benzodiazepine overdose most commonly occurs as a part of polydrug overdoses. Benzodiazepines alone produce slurred speech, lethargy, ataxia, nystagmus, and coma. Loss of deep tendon reflexes and apnea are unusual in isolated benzodiazepine overdoses but may occur with massive overdose. Rare case reports have documented coma, cardiac arrest, acute respiratory distress syndrome (ARDS), and pulmonary edema [20–25]. Paradoxical reactions can occur and include tremulousness, apprehension, insomnia, suicidal ideation, severe anxiety, agitation, hallucinations, and manic responses [1].

Long-term and short-term use of benzodiazepines causes a clinically important withdrawal reaction. Symptoms include anxiety, tremor, headache, tension, diaphoresis, difficulty concentrating, insomnia, hallucinations, and fatigue [21,22]. The patient may appear to be hyperadrenergic, with tachycardia, tachypnea, hypertension, and hyperthermia. Benzodiazepine withdrawal may lead to seizures. Benzodiazepine withdrawal may occur after prolonged use of short-acting agents for sleep, especially in hospitalized patients. It should be considered in patients who complain of agitation, anxiety, or altered sleep patterns or who develop an altered mental status 2 to 5 days after cessation of drug or discharge from the hospital. Longer-acting agents, such as diazepam, when given at doses of 20 mg per day for more than 40 days, have led to tolerance and a subsequent withdrawal syndrome.

LABORATORY EVALUATION. The laboratory evaluation of benzodiazepine overdose should include metabolic, hematologic, urine, and arterial blood gas studies as clinically indicated. Since many benzodiazepines are involved in polydrug exposures, continuous ECG monitoring and a 12-lead ECG should be performed. Noninvasive end-capnography can help identify trends in respiratory insufficiency. Quantitative benzodiazepine levels are not useful in the clinical management of overdose cases [24,26].

TREATMENT. The most important aspect of benzodiazepine overdose management is supportive care. Airway management should precede all interventions, and intubation is indicated if the patient cannot adequately protect the airway. Intravenous access and administration of dextrose, thiamine, and naloxone are indicated if the mental status is abnormal. Gut decontamination with gastric lavage is suggested for overdoses presenting within 2 hours. Activated charcoal (1 gm/kg) with a cathartic should be administered [16]. If the patient remains symptomatic, then repeat-dose activated charcoal is given. Most patients do well solely with supportive care.

Treatment of benzodiazepine withdrawal is similar to that discussed for barbiturates and other nonbarbiturate sedative-hypnotics. Flumazenil (Mazicon; flumazepil or RO15-1788) is an imidazodiazepine that acts as a competitive inhibitor at the benzodiazepine receptor, reversing benzodiazepine sedative effect. It apparently binds to the GRSMC in the omega$_1$/omega$_2$ subtype binding areas [8,9]. Flumazenil has a half-life of 1 to 2 hours [27]. Flumazenil reverses the sedative and anxiolytic effect of benzodiazepines. In ongoing studies, flumazenil may reverse some of the findings associated with hepatic encephalopathy [28–31]. Its effects on respiratory rate are not clear; some researchers have found that flumazenil reverses benzodiazepine-induced respiratory depression, obviating the need for intubation, while others have not noted this effect [28–35]. Flumazenil has been described as having an inconsistent effect on reversing ethanol-induced sedation; consensus at this point is that it has minimal effect [28,32,35]. Of interest, flumazenil

does not appear to reverse fully the amnestic effects of benzodiazepines. Several authors have suggested that although the postoperative flumazenil-treated patient may appear awake and alert, subsequent recall of instructions is poor [29,33]. Side effects of flumazenil include anxiety, nausea, agitation, and crying. Use of flumazenil in benzodiazepine-tolerant patients causes an abrupt withdrawal syndrome with high potential for inducing seizures. Seizures that result from withdrawal may be treated with large doses of benzodiazepines (competitive antagonsim). Flumazenil should *not* be used in patients who are known to be benzodiazepine-tolerant or at risk for having developed tolerance [28,30,31,32,36]. Other patients at risk for seizures include those with polypharmacy overdoses in which reversal of benzodiazepine effect may unmask the elliptogenic effects of the other drugs. This includes but is not limited to cyclic antidepressants, isoniazid, and cocaine [30,31,32]. Patients with status epilepticus who have received a large dose of a benzodiazepine followed by flumazenil to reverse respiratory depression have had reoccurrance of seizures [31]. Finally, there is a suggestion that flumazenil will reverse the salutary effect of midazolam on reducing cerebral blood flow and should be used with caution in patients with head injury [30]. Suggested dosing of flumazenil is an initial dose of 0.2 to 0.5 mg intravenously followed by 0.1 to 0.2 mg every minute until the patient is awake or 1 to 2 mg has been administered. Failure to respond to 5 mg or greater suggests that benzodiazepines may not be the cause of coma [30].

Barbiturates

Barbiturates were the cornerstone of sedative-hypnotic therapy until the 1970s, when they were generally replaced by the less toxic benzodiazepines. Once common, barbiturate overdosage has declined in incidence with their diminishing use [37].

MECHANISM OF ACTION. Barbiturates and barbituric acid derivatives depress the activity of all excitable tissues. They enhance the GABA postexcitatory inhibition at the nerve terminal. They appear to have a binding site on the GRSMC, and their binding in conjunction with GABA leads to the same response of increased chloride flux. This seems to be the predominant mechanism of action, though a partial noradrenergic suppression has been postulated. The CNS is most sensitive, with skeletal and smooth muscle depression evident at higher doses.

Barbiturates are available in all forms, although most episodes of toxicity result from ingestion. Barbiturates have classically been divided into groups based on their duration of action. Ultra-short-acting barbiturates are highly lipid-soluble and rapidly partition into the CNS, with subsequent redistribution to all tissues. When administered parentally they have rapid onset with less than 1 hour duration; their predominant role is in induction of anesthesia.

Short- and intermediate-acting barbiturates are intermediate in lipid solubility and are used as anxiolytics and sedatives. Long-acting barbiturates have relatively low lipid solubility and are mainly used as anticonvulsants.

It is generally irrelevant which class is ingested, as the systemic toxicity is more a function of the drug's elimination half-life (Table 155-3).

Barbiturates are well absorbed from the gastrointestinal tract; levels and symptoms are detectable within 30 minutes and their peak effect is reached by 4 hours. The presence of food in the stomach slows the rate of absorption but does not decrease

Table 155-3. Duration of Action and Elimination Half-life of Barbiturates

	Duration (hr)	Elimination t½ (hr)
Ultra short-acting	<½	
Thiopental (Pentothal)		6–46
Thiamylal (Surital)		NA
Methohexital (Brevital)		1–2
Short-acting	3	
Hexobarbital (Sombulex)		3–7
Pentobarbital (Nembutal)		15–48
Secobarbital (Seconal)		19–34
Intermediate-acting	3–6	
Amobarbital (Amytal)		8–42
Aprobarbital (Alurate)		14–34
Butabarbital (Butisol)		34–42
Butalbital (Fiorinal, Esgic)		NA
Long-acting	6–12	
Barbital		48
Mephobarbital (Mebaral)		48–52
Phenobarbital (Luminal)		24–144
Primidone (Mysoline)		10–12

Source: Adapted from Ellenhorn MJ: Barbiturates, in Ellenhorn MJ, Barceloux DG (eds): *Medical Toxicology Diagnosis and Treatment of Human Poisoning.* New York, Elsevier, 1988, p 576, and Harves SC: Hypnotics and sedatives, in Goodman L, Gilman A (eds): *The Pharmacological Basis of Therapeutics,* ed 8, New York, Macmillan, 1990, p 357.

total absorption. Barbiturates are variably metabolized by the liver, with the majority of the highly lipid-soluble group excreted after glucuronidation. The longer-acting drugs are less metabolized by the liver and rely on urinary excretion for elimination (phenobarbital 25–33%, barbital 95%, primidone 15–42%, phenylthymolonamide [PEMA] 95%). Many metabolites are also active [38]. Overall barbiturate elimination follows a mixed-order kinetics: at low concentrations elimination follows first-order kinetics and at high concentrations zero-order kinetics predominate [39]. As tolerance develops, the half-life may decrease. Phenobarbital has a pKa of 7.2 and is predominately renally excreted. The combination of the pKa and metabolism means that its elimination can be enhanced by alkaline diuresis.

Barbiturates induce the P-450 system, which in turn induces their own metabolism and the metabolism other drugs. They may also increase the production of levulinic acid, precipitating acute porphyria in susceptible patients.

A dose-dependent sedation is produced by barbiturates (Table 155-4) [40]. Toxic dosages are in the range of 3 to 6 gm for the short-acting barbiturates and 6 to 10 gm for the long-acting ones. Most patients demonstrate some degree of sedation with levels of 8 μg per kilogram. Tolerance develops rapidly, and

Table 155-4. Sedative-Hypnotic Equivalents

Diazepam	5 mg	is equivalent to:	Oxazepam	30 mg
			Chlordiazepoxide	25 mg
			Flurazepam	15 mg
			Clorazepate	3.75 mg
			Lorazepam	1 mg
			Triazolam	0.5 mg
			Alprazolam	0.25 mg
Phenobarbital	30 mg	is equivalent to:	Pentobarbital	100 mg

Adapted from references 58–61

chronic users may require 5 to 10 times the normal dose for sedation. Other sedatives, especially ethanol, have an additive effect in lowering the toxic dose [41].

CLINICAL MANIFESTATIONS. The most common toxic scenario with barbiturates results from accidental or intentional oral ingestion by a seizure patient or a member of his or her family. Barbiturates may be involved in polypharmacy overdoses, particularly of butalbital, a component of several common headache medications. Substance abusers have been known to melt and inject barbiturates.

Most patients present with some degree of sedation evident within 30 minutes after ingestion. This may rapidly progress to coma, respiratory collapse, and hypotension. Peak effect usually occurs within 4 hours. The patient may be mildly hypothermic from loss of autonomic stability and decrease in overall muscle activity. The CNS depression is generalized, although there are many reports of focal findings [42,43,44]. Coma may be cyclic due to active metabolites [40].

Cardiovascular collapse with severe hypotension is thought to be secondary to direct myocardial suppression and vascular dilation. This is an indicator of a significant ingestion. Dysrhythmias are rare. The gut becomes atonic, producing delayed absorption or ileus, which may then progress to bowel necrosis. Approximately 6 percent of patients develop bullous skin lesions over pressure points within 24 hours of ingestion [45,46]. The lesions are tense clean bullae surrounded by erythema, and the bullae fluid has detectable amounts of barbiturate. The presence of bullae is not diagnostic, as other sedative-hypnotics, tricyclic antidepressants, methadone, and carbon monoxide may produce them. Crystalluria has been reported [47,48].

Withdrawal symptoms may occur after 1 to 2 months of chronic use. Symptoms usually present after 2 to 7 days of abstinence, depending on the drug, but usually after 4 to 5 elimination half-lives. Agitation, hyperreflexia, anxiety, and tremor are the most common symptoms, followed by confusion and hallucinations. In early withdrawal, up to 75 percent of patients experience seizures. Barbiturate withdrawal seizures are more severe than ethanol withdrawal seizures and may not respond to phenytoin. Effective treatment results from reinstitution of the particular barbiturate or equipotent doses of cross-tolerant medication, such as benzodiazepines (Table 155-4). Transplacental tolerance occurs, with neonatal irritability noted for months after birth [49,50].

Differential diagnosis includes all other sedative-hypnotics, phenothiazines, phencyclidine, antidepressants, narcotics, or carbon monoxide. Meningitis, head trauma, or CNS bleeds should be considered, especially with focal findings.

MANAGEMENT. The emergency management of barbiturate poisoning is supportive. Early airway management is imperative, as up to 40 percent of patients aspirate. All patients with an altered mental status should receive naloxone (2 mg), dextrose (25–50 gm), and thiamine (100 mg IV). Close monitoring of all vital signs, including rectal temperature, is indicated. A history of concurrent medical problems or coingestion should be sought. Since respiratory depression is common, an ABG or pulse oximetry with noninvasive end capnography should be obtained. Baseline electrolytes, arterial blood gas, barbiturate levels, ECG, salicylate and acetaminophen levels, and creatine kinase and liver function studies should be obtained. Foley catheterization with measurement of urine output should be used to guide fluid management. Gut decontamination is controversial, with the decision to do late lavage unresolved. Syrup of ipecac should never be used [51].

Multiple-dose charcoal dosage has been advocated in barbiturate overdose, starting with 1 gm per kilogram orally or via a nasogastric tube. This is followed by 25 to 50 gm every 4 to 6 hours for 3 to 4 days or until resolution of symptoms [52,53,54]. Assessment of the abdomen for decreased bowel sounds, a succession splash, or ileus is necessary before giving multiple doses of charcoal.

Hypotensive patients should receive a fluid challenge. Since hypotension is multifactorial, blood pressure unresponsive to 2 to 4 liters of fluids (20–30 ml/kg in children) should be followed by pressor therapy with dopamine or norepinephrine. Invasive monitoring of central venous pressure or pulmonary capillary wedge pressure may be necessary at this point to guide fluid therapy and maintenance of blood pressure of 90 mm Hg with an urine output of 100 to 200 ml per hour (1–2 ml/kg/hr).

Treatment of long-acting barbiturate ingestion (phenobarbital and barbituric acid) may be assisted by enhancing elimination. An alkaline diuresis may be achieved by the addition of 50 to 150 mEq (1–3 amp) of sodium bicarbonate to 1000 ml of D_5W infusing at 200 to 300 ml per hour after initial acid base abnormalities and hypotension have been corrected. The addition of 20 to 40 mEq of potassium chloride per liter of fluid is necessary to prevent bicarbonate ion retention. Inadequate potassium replacement is the primary reason for inability to maintain an alkaline urine. Some authors advocate a bolus of 1 to 2 mEq per kilogram of bicarbonate prior to instituting the infusion. The bicarbonate infusion must be accompanied by hourly urine pH monitoring. The urine pH should be maintained between 7.5 and 8.0.

Cardiovascular instability unresponsive to conservative measures is an indication for extracorporeal drug removal. Hemoperfusion (clearance 100–300 ml/min for phenobarbital) removes more drug than hemodialysis (clearance 60–75 ml/min), but hemodialysis is still effective, especially if combined with multiple-dose oral charcoal [55–58]. On completion of treatment, serum levels may rebound secondary to redistribution, and repeat hemodialysis/hemoperfusion may be necessary. Hypothermia requires rewarming. The patient should be monitored for development of aspiration pneumonia, ARDS, and electrolyte derangements.

A computed tomography (CT) scan and lumbar puncture should be considered if there are focal neurologic findings or an unclear history of ingestion. An isoelectric electroencephalogram (EEG) is not necessarily an indicator of poor outcome; barbiturates suppress brain electrical activity, and full recovery has been reported after an isoelectric tracing.

BARBITURATE WITHDRAWAL. Since almost all sedative-hypnotic agents are cross-tolerant, barbiturate withdrawal can be treated with reinstitution of either the same drug or another cross-tolerant sedative-hypnotic, such as benzodiazepines. The goal in therapy is to make the patient comfortable and suppress signs and symptoms of withdrawal. Ultimately, replacing the barbiturate with a long-acting substitute is indicated. Using an agent with a long duration of action maintains the serum concentration as close as possible to a steady state, limiting the side effects and cravings associated with falling levels. Barbiturate withdrawal should be attempted only in a controlled environment with adequate resuscitation equipment available, since withdrawal can precipitate seizures and subsequent cardiovascular collapse. In a sample withdrawal protocol, the patient is given sufficient amounts of the tolerant drug or phenobarbital equivalent to induce sedation, then the dose is decreased by 10 percent every 3 days. If the equivalent phenobarbital dose is not known, then 120 mg of phenobarbital can be administered every 1 to 2 hours until the appearance of drowsiness, nystagmus, ataxia, or resolution of withdrawal symptoms. This may be done orally or intravenously [59,60,61]. The long half-life of phenobarbital allows smooth withdrawal without additional medication [62].

Tolerance can be ascertained by the pentobarbital suppression test. The patient is given 200 mg of pentobarbital every 2 hours until sedation occurs. If after the initial 200 mg the patient is not sedated, then barbiturate tolerance is present. Patients who are tolerant to greater than 1200 mg will most likely experience withdrawal symptoms. Pentobarbital 100 mg is equivalent to 30 mg of phenobarbital (Table 155-4).

Nonbenzodiazepine, Nonbarbiturate Sedative-Hypnotics

This generally older class of medications has been mostly supplanted by the benzodiazepines, which have greater efficacy and a larger therapeutic ratio. These medications include glutethimide (Doriden), ethchlorvynol (Placidyl), meprobamate (Miltown), chloral hydrate (Noctec), methaqualone (Quaalude), methyprylon (Noludar), and the antispasmodic-muscle relaxants carisoprodol (Soma) and baclofen (Lioresal). In spite of their limited current clinical use, these medications remain a serious concern. Toxic effects and overdosages can be seen from both legitimate and illicit use. Newer agents have also been introduced, which vary in their toxicity in overdose. These include chlormethiazole derived from the thiazide moiety of thiamine, with sedative-hypnotic, anxiolytic, and anticonvulsant properties, which is used in Europe for ethanol withdrawal and eclampsia; buspirone, an azispirodecanedione that binds to 5-HT receptors; zopiclone, a cyclopyrrolone with sedative-hypnotic activity; zolpidem and alpidem, which are imidazopyridine sedative-hypnotic and anxiolytic agents, respectively; and ethinamate, a urethane-derived hypnotic agent used for insomnia [14,53–71]. Many of these medications have a high abuse potential secondary to their ability to induce tolerance and dependence. In addition, a large percentage of those who use and abuse these medications have a history of psychiatric disorders and concurrent ethanol use [53].

Most of these drugs induce sedation at low doses and induce general anesthesia at high doses [72]. Central nervous system depression is the hallmark of these drugs, with the exception of buspirone [54,55,56]. While low doses produce sedation, increasing doses lead to the slowing of mental functions, slurred speech, and ataxia. Higher doses lead to stupor, coma, respiratory depression, and death [73]. Tolerance does not develop to respiratory depression. This becomes a problem when dependent users increase their dosages, sometimes up to 10 to 20 times recommended [74].

All of these medications undergo hepatic metabolism through the microsomal enzyme system. They are capable of altering the biotransformation rate of themselves and other drugs cleared via the microsomal system.

CHLORAL HYDRATE. Chloral hydrate is one of the oldest known sedatives. It was first introduced in 1869 and is frequently utilized for sedation in pediatric patients [75].

Chloral hydrate is rapidly absorbed from the gastrointestinal tract, with onset of action occurring within 30 minutes [76]. The principal metabolite of chloral hydrate, trichloroethanol, is more active and has a longer half-life (4–12 hours) than the parent compound. The process of biotransformation occurs in the liver via the enzyme alcohol dehydrogenase and is accelerated by concomitant ethanol ingestion. Chloral hydrate is available as capsules in doses of 250 mg, 500 mg, and 1000 mg as well as an ethanol-containing elixir and suppositories.

The usual oral therapeutic dose is 500 mg to 1.0 gm. It has been used safely in pediatric and geriatric populations for sedation as well as in dentistry. Recent reports of significant toxicity in the pediatric population suggest that this drug is not quite so benign [77–82]. The manufacturer recommends doses less than 2.0 gm [82]. The lethal dose in adults is 5 to 10 gm, but as little as 1.25 gm has been fatal. Patients have survived doses as high as 36 gm [76].

Pharmacokinetics and Pharmacology. Chloral hydrate is hepatically reduced via alcohol dehydrogenase to trichloroethanol and either is oxidized again to trichloroacetic acid or undergoes glucuronidation. Both of these secondary metabolites are renally excreted. Chloral hydrate and its first metabolite, trichloroethanol, are lipid-soluble and have a high volume of distribution. The second metabolite of chloral hydrate metabolism is trichloroacetic acid [77]. The metabolism of chloral hydrate to trichloroethanol is age-related, with an increasing elimination half-life as the neonate ages to toddler [79]. In neonates, the glucuronidation pathway is still immature and chloral hydrate competes with bilirubin. In addition, renal clearance is limited due to immature kidney function. This can lead to direct hyperbilirubinemia in the neonate [79,80,81]. Finally, accumulation kinetics has been demonstrated in neonates and critically ill children [78,79]. All of these factors should be considered when chloral hydrate is administered to children. Saturation kinetics leading to prolonged elimination has been demonstrated in overdose [77].

Toxicity. Toxicity develops within 3 to 4 hours after ingestion. Clinically, this is manifested by significant gastrointestinal irritation, ranging from gastritis to hemorrhagic gastritis and perforation. Other findings include varying degrees of CNS depression, pinpoint pupils, hypothermia, hypotension, and respiratory depression. Paradoxical CNS excitation, particularly in children, has been reported coinciding with peak plasma levels (1–3 hours) [77,83]. Myocardial depression results from decreased myocardial contraction and decreased refractory period [77]. Cardiac arrhythmias have been reported and range from multifocal premature ventricular contractions (PVCs) to supraventricular arrhythmias and ventricular tachycardia [77,84]. Delayed manifestations of toxicity include dermal exfoliation, renal tubular necrosis, and hepatotoxicity [76].

In chronic abusers, tolerance and addiction can develop. The addicted patient may take very large doses of the drug and suffer a withdrawal syndrome similar to that from alcohol if it is suddenly discontinued [72]. Since this drug is hepatotoxic, the abuser may experience unexpected liver failure, leading to acute intoxication and death at doses that were previously tolerated.

Chloral hydrate interacts with multiple other medications. It displaces oral anticoagulants and furosemide from binding sites on albumin, enhancing hypoprothrombinemia and vasomotor instability [76,77]. It should not be used in patients with porphyria, since it affects porphyrin metabolism. Since chloral hydrate and ethanol compete for alcohol dehydrogenase, the addition of ethanol to chloral hydrate ("Mickey Finn") leads to enhanced sedative effects of both [77].

Laboratory Evaluation. The laboratory evaluation of the chloral hydrate-poisoned patient includes a complete blood count, liver function tests, BUN, creatinine, electrolytes, coagulation parameters, and arterial blood gases. Levels of trichloroethanol

may be of some value in determining the amount of chloral hydrate ingested [82].

Treatment. The cornerstone of treating the chloral hydrate-poisoned patient is supportive therapy. All patients with a suspected ingestion must have an intravenous line started, continuous electrocardiographic monitoring, and a secure airway. If the patency of the airway is questioned, the patient should be intubated with a cuffed endotracheal tube. This is followed by gut decontamination by gastric lavage with a large-bore orogastric hose. Induction of vomiting with ipecac is contraindicated because of the potential for a rapidly decreasing level of consciousness. Activated charcoal (1 gm/kg) can be instilled afterward. If the patient presents more than 2 to 3 hours after ingestion, activated charcoal can be administered via nasogastric tube.

Cardiac arrhythmias may not respond to standard antiarrhythmics, such as lidocaine; recent literature recommends the use of beta-blockers (propranolol 1.0 mg IV) [77,84]. Hypothermia can generally be treated with passive rewarming. Forced diuresis and urinary pH manipulation are of no value. Although some authors disagree [73], studies have shown increased drug clearance with hemoperfusion [85]. This should be considered in patients with prolonged coma, refractory arrhythmias, or hypotension. Trichloroethanol clearance by hemodialysis varies between 120 and 162 ml per minute. In one patient who ingested 38 gm, the half-life decreased from 35 to 6 hours after hemodialysis.

Admission criteria include the necessity for ventilatory or cardiovascular support, malignant cardiac arrhythmias, continued CNS depression, or ongoing suicide risk. No patient should be discharged with less than 4 to 6 hours of observation.

Because of the caustic nature of chloral hydrate, a small-bore nasogastric tube should be used when a liquid preparation has been ingested.

The outcome for chloral hydrate poisoning is excellent. Even those patients with the most severe manifestations of toxicity should recover with aggressive supportive therapy.

ETHCHLORVYNOL. Ethchlorvynol, first introduced in the late 1950s, is a hypnotic with muscle relaxant and anticonvulsant activities. Clinical effects are apparent within 15 to 30 minutes and peak levels are seen in 1 to 2 hours. This rapid onset of action results from rapid and complete absorption from the gastrointestinal tract. Ethchlorvynol is highly lipid-soluble and is stored in adipose tissue and the brain [86]. It has a unique half-life, being 10 to 25 hours in small or therapeutic ingestions but up to 100 hours in very large overdoses. Ninety percent of the drug is metabolized via the liver, with the remainder being excreted by the kidneys. Ethchlorvynol is available as 200-mg, 500-mg, and 750-mg capsules. The recommended dose of ethchlorvynol is 500 to 1000 mg at bedtime [87]. The lethal dose of the medication is quite variable. Fatalities have occurred after a 2.5-gm overdose, while those with ingestions as high as 50 gm have survived [76].

Clinically, the patient an ethchlorvynol overdose presents with an altered sensorium. This can range from dizziness to facial tingling, giddiness, excitement, dysarthria, ataxia, mydriasis, nystagmus, or areflexia with smaller doses. Patients ingesting larger doses may present with profound coma. Comatose patients may have a flat EEG with coma lasting greater than 200 hours [76]. Serum levels confirm but do not guide management. Seizures may occur following acute ethchlorvynol ingestion. Hypotension, bradycardia, and hypothermia have been reported. Pancytopenia, thrombocytopenia, and hemolysis are hematologic complications of ethchlorvynol use

[88]. Respiratory depression may be seen and is associated with increasing CNS depression. Noncardiogenic pulmonary edema has also been reported [89]. An interesting and sometimes clinically useful property of ethchlorvynol is its aromatic and quite pungent odor, described as similar to that of a new plastic shower curtain. It can be detected on the victim's breath and occasionally in the gastric aspirate.

As in other medications of this group, chronic abuse of ethchlorvynol results in tolerance and dependence. Abusers usually take large doses, up to 4.0 gm per day [72], and may appear to be intoxicated with alcohol. Sudden withdrawal can be confused with delirium tremens or an acute psychotic reaction.

There is no antidote to ethchlorvynol, and treatment is supportive. Establishment of an airway, respiratory support, and maintaining an adequate blood pressure are all necessary. Decontamination with repeated doses of charcoal is indicated secondary to the large volume of distribution. Hemoperfusion is extremely effective in clearing the drug [90]. Due to the drug's extensive lipid redistribution, however, repeated sessions of hemoperfusion may be necessary. Indications for hemoperfusion include acute ingestions of greater than 100 mg per kilogram, prolonged coma, and cardiovascular compromise refractory to conventional treatment [86].

The expected prognosis with ethchlorvynol poisoning is good, even in patients with the most severe symptoms. The mortality for patients with the most profound coma should be less than 5 percent with aggressive supportive therapy [91].

GLUTETHIMIDE. Glutethimide (Doriden, Dormtabs, Roletamide) is available as 0.25- and 0.5-gm tablets. The manufacturer's recommended dosage is 0.25 to 0.50 gm at bedtime. The toxic dose is greater than 3.0 gm, with a usual fatal dose being 10 to 20 gm [92]. It is very similar to the sedative-hypnotic methyprylon. Glutethimide is highly lipid-soluble and displays two-compartment kinetics with rapid intake in the brain followed by systemic distribution. It has a fairly rapid onset of action (20–30 minutes), but gastrointestinal absorption is erratic [93,94]. Peak effect is seen in 16 hours, and it has a long but variable duration of action. Glutethimide is metabolized in the liver to an active metabolite, 4-hydroxy-2-ethyl-2-phenylglutarimide [94], which has a longer duration of action and is more potent than the parent compound [95]. Glutethimide also stimulates the hepatic microsomal enzyme system and has considerable anticholinergic activity [72].

The most unique aspect of acute glutethimide intoxication is the fluctuating level of consciousness [86]. The reason for this is not well known, but theories include enterohepatic recirculation, prolonged absorption of the parent compound from an anticholinergic-induced paralytic ileus, or redistribution from adipose stores. The coma of glutethimide intoxication is very deep and quite prolonged [93]. Administration with alcohol has been shown to increase oral absorption of glutethimide [96,97].

Multiple authors note that the only predictable effect of this drug is its variability. Mildly toxic symptoms noted with therapeutic dosings include hangover, blurred vision, excitement, headache, gastric irritation, and occasional bone marrow suppression. As with the other sedative-hypnotics, acute intoxications lead to CNS and respiratory depression. In addition, increased intracranial pressure, seizures, areflexia, and muscular twitching may be seen. Cardiac arrest, shock, hypotension, hypothermia, and persistent acidosis have all been reported [86]. The anticholinergic actions of the drug cause xerostomia, paralytic ileus, atony of the urinary bladder, and mydriasis. Prolonged hyperthermia following a period of hypothermia has been documented [72,86].

The chronic use of glutethimide leads to tolerance and addiction, with a severe withdrawal syndrome. It is characterized by tremulousness, nausea, tachycardia, fever, and convulsions [72].

Glutethimide is frequently abused as a combination drug with codeine. Most preparations containing codeine also contain acetaminophen. This combination of glutethimide and Tylenol #3 or Tylenol #4 is called "loads" or "fours and doors." Suspicion of glutethimide usage should prompt a search for both codeine and acetaminophen abuse.

Treatment of the glutethimide-poisoned patient is similar to that for other medications in this group. Supportive measures aimed at maintaining an airway and blood pressure take precedence. Since there is an anticholinergic-induced delay in gastric emptying, late gut decontamination with gastric lavage may be effective. Treatment with multiple-dose activated charcoal is extremely efficacious because of glutethimide's extensive lipid distribution, delayed gastric emptying, and known enterohepatic circulation. Some authors have suggested an alkaline lavage solution to minimize absorption of this basic parent compound [96]. However, there is no literature to support this contention.

Hypotension should be treated with vasopressors, rather than large fluid volumes, since low blood pressure is most likely secondary to peripheral vasodilation. Aggressive fluid resuscitation may precipitate pulmonary edema [86].

Extracorporeal methods of removing glutethimide have not been shown to be effective in changing the course of intoxication. Glutethimide has a large V_d and high lipid solubility. This suggests that even with good clearance from the blood with hemoperfusion [97,98], large amounts of the drug cannot be adequately removed. Extracorporeal treatment is not recommended.

The prognosis in glutethimide poisoning is usually quite good. If there is no cardiopulmonary compromise, recovery occurs within 1 to 5 days [92]. Worsening prognosis is associated with pulmonary complications, increasing age, and increasing duration of coma.

METHYPRYLON. Methyprylon (Noludar) is another of the 1950s-era nonbarbiturate sedative-hypnotics that is no longer in widespread use. It is available as 200-mg and 300-mg tablets. The manufacturer's recommended dose is 200 to 400 mg, and it is not recommended for children younger than 12 years [87]. The lethal dose in humans is unknown, but deaths have been reported after ingestion of 6.0 gm. Patients have recovered after doses as high as 27 gm [72].

Almost all methyprylon is metabolized in the liver. The plasma half-life is 4 hours but can be prolonged in acute overdosages. The drug is highly protein-bound. Adverse effects from the drug are few but include nausea, vomiting, gastrointestinal irritation, headache, rash, diarrhea, esophagitis, neutropenia, and thrombocytopenia [72]. Depressed CNS and respiratory function, hyperactive reflexes, miotic pupils, nystagmus, and convulsions have been reported [99]. Hypotension, shock, and pulmonary edema can occur. The withdrawal syndrome may include insomnia, confusion, hallucinations, and seizures [72].

Treatment is supportive. Both hemodialysis and peritoneal dialysis are ineffective in removing significant amounts of the drug from the body.

MEPROBAMATE. Meprobamate (Equanil, Miltown, Bamate, Neuromate, and others) is an unusual member of this class of medications. It has sedative properties in addition to its antianxiety and muscle relaxant effects. Following its introduction in the 1950s, meprobamate enjoyed a period of considerable popularity. It has largely been supplanted by the benzodiazepines. Despite this, it is available through several companies in various formulations and strengths. It is available as 200-mg, 400-mg, and 600-mg tablets, as well as a 400-mg sustained-release capsule. The recommended dose is 1200 to 1600 mg per day in divided doses; dosages greater than 2400 mg are not recommended [87]. Toxicity can be seen in ingestions as small as 2.0 gm and fatalities with as little as 12 gm [99]. Survival has been documented with doses as high as 40 gm [99]. It is not a commonly abused street drug, but overdosages can be seen in elderly patients.

Meprobamate is rapidly and completely absorbed following an oral dose [72,100,101]. Peak effect is seen in 3 hours, with a half-life of 10 hours. The duration of action is dose-dependent. Most patients feel an effect for up to 36 hours [99]. The drug is largely metabolized in the liver, and its inactive metabolites are excreted in the urine. Very little of the drug is plasma protein-bound. The hepatic microsomal system is induced, leading to interactions with other medications.

Meprobamate increases the levels of delta aminolevulinic acid, a precursor of porphyrins. Its use in patients with porphyria is not recommended.

Clinical Manifestations. The clinical picture of meprobamate overdosage is similar to that of the other medications in this class. Central nervous system depression and impairment of respiratory system function dominate. This includes stupor, paresthesias, convulsions, and coma [86,87]. The cardiovascular effects of meprobamate include sudden hypotension, even after mild ingestion [102], arrhythmias, and palpitations [103]. Pulmonary edema occurs, especially following vigorous volume resuscitation. Extrapyramidal effects are possible, with nystagmus, tonic clonic reflexes, and ataxia [104].

Drug levels may be of some value in management of the meprobamate-poisoned patient. Since patients develop tolerance, the level may not reflect patient status. Levels greater than 20.5 to 22.5 mg per deciliter have been associated with CNS depression and coma [105,106].

A withdrawal-abstinence syndrome beginning 1 to 2 days after cessation can occur even after chronic daily ingestions of as little as 1.6 gm [46].

Treatment. Treating the meprobamate-poisoned person is identical to treatment for the other medications in this class. Airway management, support of blood pressure with early use of vasopressors, and avoidance of large volumes of infused fluids are indicated. Charcoal decontamination is efficacious. Meprobamate has a propensity for forming gastric concretions; repeated charcoal doses are probably of value [103]. Hemoperfusion has been shown to hasten drug clearance and should be used in all patients showing cardiovascular compromise and no sign of improvement despite aggressive supportive treatment.

The prognosis of patients with a meprobamate overdose is generally good with supportive treatment alone.

CARISOPRODOL AND BACLOFEN. Although not usually considered sedatives or hypnotics, the muscle relaxants carisoprodol and baclofen deserve mention. The presentation of these medications may mimic that of the sedative-hypnotic class and treatment is similar.

Baclofen (Lioresal) is a potent $GABA_B$ agonist. Its primary use is as an antispasmodic agent, decreasing flexor tone and spasm in certain neurologic diseases. Therapeutic doses of baclofen are 15 to 60 mg per day [104]. Baclofen is cleared by the kidney, with only a small portion hepatically transformed. Baclofen is well absorbed from the gastrointestinal tract. Elimination is via first-order elimination kinetics, with a half-life of 2 to 6 hours. Therapeutic levels are 0.08 to 0.1 mg per liter [105].

Both hypotension and hypertension have been reported with baclofen intoxications [106,107]. Psychosis, coma, seizures, apnea, and hypothermia can be seen [107]. Reported cardiac effects include conduction abnormalities, prolonged Q-T and P-R intervals, junctional escape beats, blocked premature atrial contractions, tachycardia, and bradycardia. Myoclonus and decreased deep tendon reflexes have occurred.

Treatment for a baclofen intoxication is supportive. As of 1986 all reported overdoses except one required mechanical ventilatory support [106]. The role of·charcoal is not clear. Baclofen in large overdose is more slowly absorbed from the gastrointestinal tract than with a single therapeutic dose, suggesting that charcoal is probably of value. Symptomatic bradycardia responds to atropine [108]. Intravenous fluids are adequate for hypotension; nitroprusside has been necessary for severe hypertension. The neurology literature suggests that physostigmine may be useful in intrathecal baclofen overdoses. Good controlled studies are lacking.

The outcome for baclofen-intoxicated patients is generally good. In a series from 1975 through 1986 only one reported death was attributable to baclofen overdose [109]. All remaining patients recovered full neurologic function. Ventilatory assistance was discontinued between 3 and 7 days after ingestion.

Carisoprodol (Soma, Rela) is a congener of meprobamate used as a muscle relaxant. Carisoprodol is metabolized in the liver and excreted in the urine, with an elimination half-life of 4 to 6 hours.

The predominant side effect of the drug is drowsiness. Rarely seen idiosyncratic reactions include asthenia, transient quadriplegia, dizziness, ataxia, diplopia, agitation, confusion, and disorientation [110]. Its toxicity and treatment are otherwise similar to those of meprobamate [102].

CHLORMETHIAZOLE. Chlormethiazole is a potent sedative-hypnotic, anxiolytic, and anticonvulsive agent that has weak action at the $GABA_A$ receptor. It potentiates GABA and glycine-mediated inhibition, probably via direct action at the chloride ionophore. It may have secondary effects on dopamine and serotonergic neurotransmission [14]. It is rapidly absorbed orally and has a short elimination half-life. It is the first-line drug for ethanol withdrawal in Europe. Overdose treatment is supportive. Since it does not bind to the $GABA_A$ receptor, it is unlikely to respond to flumazenil.

BUSPIRONE. Buspirone is an anxiolytic serotonergic and dopaminergic active drug with minimal sedative-hynotic effects during therapeutic dosing. It also has effects on acetylcholine and norepinephrine effects centrally. Its mechanism of action is not fully understood, but it appears to interact with exogenous and endogenous benzodiazepine, binding at the GRSMC. At low doses, it is predominately anxiolytic, although it may take several weeks to reach this effect. It does not have the immediate mood effects seen with benzodiazepines, so patients may feel that it is not working. At high doses, it can cause sedation similar to that seen with benzodiazepines (>20 mg/day), but the sedation is much less than that seen with an equivalent dose of the benzodiazepine. Buspirone has no anticonvulsant or muscle relaxant effect. It is well absorbed orally, and peak serum levels occur within 1 to 2 hours. It is hepatically metabolized, with an elimination half-life of 2 to 3 hours.

Side effects reported during therapeutic dosing include weakness, gastrointestinal distress, dysphoria, headache, and dizziness. Chronic dosing effects are not known, but in one study a single patient developed extrapyramidal effects. It may cause a withdrawal syndrome after prolonged use but does not cross-react with benzodiazepines in treating benzodiazepine withdrawal. Flumazenil will not reverse buspirone effect. Buspirone may have a limited additive effect with ethanol, but this is not clear.

There are no current overdose data for this drug. Based on its pharmacology, a reasonable observation period and supportive care may be adequate to treat overdose. There are minimal data on absorption of buspirone to charcoal; it seems reasonable to administer a 1 mg per kilogram dose of activated charcoal in the face of overdose [64,65,70].

ZOPICLONE. Zopiclone is a nonbenzodiazpine agent with sedative-hypnotic, anxiolytic, and muscle relaxant properties but is predominately marketed as a hypnotic agent. It appears to bind to the GRSMC, possibly with its own binding site. It has been found to displace diazepam and flunitrazepam from their benzodiazepine binding sites. It is well absorbed orally, with peak plasma concentration within 30 to 90 minutes. It undergoes first-order kinetics of distribution and is extensively metabolized. Elimination occurs via the kidneys and lungs. Absorption is significantly affected by gastric emptying. Side effects include a bitter taste in the mouth, and there is carryover sedation into the next day. There may be a morning-after amnesic effect. In chronic dosing, physical dependency and withdrawal have been reported. It may also have a potentiating sedative effect with ethanol.

Overdose data are minimal, but supportive care appears to be the mainstay of therapy. Since absorption is dependent on gastric emptying, oral activated charcoal may be useful in limiting absorption. In receptor binding studies, flumazenil displaces zopiclone. This suggests that flumazenil might reverse some of the effects of zopiclone sedation [66].

ZOLPIDEM AND ALPIDEM. Zolpidem and alpidem are imidazopyridime agents used as hypnotic and anxiolytic agents, respectively. Both bind to the GRSMC, zolpidem at the $omega_1$ and alpidem at the $omega_1/omega_3$ receptor binding sites. Neither agent has significant muscle relaxant effect at therapeutic dosing. Both agents are rapidly absorbed orally, highly protein-bound, and hepatically metabolized. Zolpidem has an elimination half-life of 2.5 to 5 hours and alpidem of 8 to 20 hours. Side effects of zolpidem include anxiety, dizziness, drowsiness, fatigue, headache, diplopia, diarrhea, and tremor. Side effects of alpidem are sedation, headache, dizziness, insomnia, nausea, and vomiting. Alpidem has been reported to increase serum transaminases. Zolpidem has been associated with a residual morning hangover and anterograde amnesia. Tolerance and dependency and subsequent withdrawal have been reported with zolpidem, although at high doses it causes signficant nausea and vomiting. Concomitant use of ethanol with zolpidem leads to a synergistic effect. Other drug interactions include increased sedation with the combination of zolpidem and imipramine or chlorpromazine.

Overdose data are limited for both agents. Death has been reported with the combination of overdose with zolpidem and other CNS depressants, although no deaths have yet been reported with zolpidem overdose alone. Treatment of overdose is predominately supportive. Activated charcoal has not yet been studied with these medications but may be useful in limiting absorption. Flumazenil reverses zolpidem effects. Flumazenil has reversed alpidem effects in receptor studies and may be useful in an alpidem overdose [65,66,71]

ETHAMINATE. Ethaminate (Valmid) is a rapid-acting hypnotic agent that is well absorbed orally. It has onset of action within 20 minutes of ingestion, with a duration of 3 to 5 hours. Elimination half-life is 2.5 hours. It is hepatically metabolized and renally eliminated. Its mechanism of action is unknown. Chronic use of ethaminate leads to rapid tolerance; sudden withdrawal after development of tolerance leads to a withdrawal syndrome. Reported side effects include drowsiness, gastrointestinal distress, skin rash, and excitation. Drug fever and thrombocytopenia purpura have been reported rarely with ethaminate. It has synergistic effects with other sedative-hypnotic agents. Treatment of overdose is supportive. Because of its rapid metabolism, activated charcoal is probably not indicated after an initial dose is given to limit absorption [69].

References

1. Abernathy DR, Laux G, Puryear DA: Benzodiazepines: Misuse, abuse, and dependency. *Am Fam Physician* 30:139, 1984.
2. Greenblat DJ, Shader RI, Abernathy DR, et al: Current status of benzodiazepines (second of two parts). *N Engl J Med* 309:410,1983.
3. Tallman JF, Paul PM, Skolnick P, et al: Receptors for the age of anxiety: Pharmacology of the benzodiazepines. *Science* 207:274, 1980.
4. Perrault G, Morel E, Sanger DJ, Zivkovic B: Differences in pharmacological profiles of a new generation of benzodiazepine hypnotics. *Eur J Pharmacol* 187:487, 1990.
5. Study RE, Barker JL: Cellular mechanisms of benzodiazepine action. *JAMA* 247:2147, 1982.
6. Dennis T, Dubois A, Benavides J, Scatton B: Distribution of central $omega_1$ (benzodiazepine$_1$) and $omega_2$ (benzodiazepine$_2$) receptor subtypes in the monkey and human brain: An autoradiographic study with [^{3}H] flunitriazepam and the $omega_1$ selective ligand [^{3}H] zolpidem. *J Pharmacol Exp Ther* 247:309, 1988.
7. Ruano D, Benavides J, Machado A, Vitorica J: Regional differences in the enhancement by GABA of [^{3}H] zolpidem binding to omega sites in rat membranes and sections. *Brain Res* 600:134, 1993.
8. Langer SZ, Arbilla S: Imidazopyridines as a tool for the characterization of benzodiazepine receptors: A proposal for a pharmacological classification of omega receptor subtypes. *Pharm Biochem Behav* 29:763, 1988.
9. Benavides J, Peny B, Durand A, et al: Comparative *in vivo* and *in vitro* ω(benzodiazepine) site ligands in inhibiting [^{3}H] flumazenil binding in the rat central nervous system. *J Pharmacol Exp Ther* 263:884, 1992.
10. Benavides J, Peny B, Ruano D, et al: Comparative autoradiographic distribution of central ω (benzodiazepine) modulatory site subtypes and high, intermediate, and low affinity for zolpidem and alpidem. *Brain Res* 604:240, 1993.
11. Goldberg ME, Salama AI, Patel JB: Malick JB: Novel non-benzodiazepine anxiolytics. *Neuropharmacology* 22:1499, 1983.
12. Sanger DJ, Zivkovic B: Differential development of tolerance to the depressant effects of benzodiazepine and non-benzodiazepine agons at the omega (BZ) modulatory sites of GABA$_A$ receptors. *Neuropharmacology* 31:693, 1992.
13. Lloyd KG, Danielou G, Thurcet F: Differentiation of activities within the GABA$_A$-chloride ionophore complex by means of ^{35}-S-TPS binding, in Biggio G, Costa E (eds): *Chloride Channels and Their Modulation by Neurotransmitters and Drugs.* NY, Raven, 1988, pp 199–207.
14. Ogren SO: Chlormethiazole-model of action. *Acta Psychiatr Scand* 2(suppl):13, 1986.
15. Greenblat DJ, Shader RI, Abernathy DR, et al: Current status of benzodiazepines (first of two parts). *N Engl J Med* 309:354, 1983.
16. Ellenhorn MJ, Baceloux DG: Benzodiazepines, in Ellenhorn MJ (ed): *Medical Toxicology: Diagnosis and Treatment of Human Poisoning.* New York, Elsevier, 1988, p 581.

17. Forrest AR, Marsh I, et al: Fatal temazepam overdoses. *Lancet* 2:226, 1986.

18. Greenblat DJ, Allen MD, Noel BJ, et al: Acute overdosage with benzodiazepine derivatives. *Clin Pharmacol Ther* 21:497,1977.

19. Finkle BS, McCloskey KL, Goodman LS, et al: Diazepam and drug associated deaths: A survey in the United States and Canada. *JAMA* 242:429, 1979.

20. Olson KR, Yin L, Osterloh J, et al: Coma caused by trivial triazolam overdose. *Am J Emerg Med* 3:210, 1985.

21. Sellers EM, Busto U, Sellers EM, et al: Withdrawal reaction after long-term therapeutic use of benzodiazepines. *N Engl J Med* 315:854, 1986.

22. Murphy SM: Withdrawal symptoms after six weeks' treatment with diazepam. *Lancet* 2:1389, 1984.

23. Berger R, Green G, Melnick A, et al: Cardiac arrest caused by oral diazepam intoxication. *Clin Pediatr* 14:842, 1975.

24. Stringer MD: Adult respiratory distress syndrome associated with fluorazepam overdose. *J Roy Soc Med* 78:74, 1985.

25. Richman S: Acute pulmonary edema associated with lubrium use. *Radiology* 103:57, 1979.

26. Jatlow P: Serum diazepam concentrations in overdose: Their significance. *Am J Clin Pathol* 72:571, 1979.

27. Lheureux P, Askenasi CU: Double-blind study of Anexate (flumazenil) in benzodiazepine intoxication. *Eur J Anesthesiol* (suppl 2):300, 1988.

28. Amrein R, Leishman B, Bentzinger C, Roncari G: Flumazenil in benzodiazepine antagonism: Actions and clinical use in intoxications and anaesthesiology. *Med Toxicol* 2:411, 1987.

29. Sanders LD, Piggott SE, Issac PA, et al: Reversal of benzodiazepine sedation with the antagonist flumazenil. *Br J Anaesth* 66:445, 1991.

30. Tefakis Karavokiros KA, Tsipis GB: Flumazenil: A benzodiazepine antagonist. *Ann Pharmacother* 24:976, 1990.

31. Spivey WH: Flumazenil and seizures: Analysis of 43 cases. *Clin Ther* 14:293, 1992.

32. Flumazenil in Benzodiazepine Intoxication Multicenter Study Group: Treatment of benzodiazepine overdose with flumazenil. *Clin Ther* 14:978, 1992.

33. Hommer D, Weingartner H, Breier A: Dissociation of benzodiazepine-induced amnesia from sedation by flumazenil pretreatment. *Psychopharmacology* 112:455, 1993.

34. Chern T-L, Hu S-C, Lee C-H, Deng J-F: Diagnostic and therapeutic utility of flumazenil in comatose patients with drug overdose. *Am J Emerg Med* 11:122, 1993.

35. Lheureux P, Fontaine J, Askenasi R: Effect of flumazenil in a model of acute alcohol intoxication in rats. *Hum Exp Toxicol* 12:177, 1993.

36. Ashton CH: Benzodiazepine overdose: Are specific agonists useful? *Br Med J* 290:805, 1985.

37. Litovitz TL, Normann SA, Veltri JC: 1985 annual report of the American Association of Poison Control Centers National Data Collection System. *Am J Emerg Med* 4:427, 1986.

38. Sumner DJ, Kalk J, Whiting B: Metabolism of barbiturate after overdosage. *Br Med J* 1:335, 1975.

39. Ellenhorn MJ: Barbiturates, in Ellenhorn MJ, Barceloux DG (eds): *Medical Toxicology: Diagnosis and Treatment of Human Poisoning.* New York, Elsevier, 1988, p 576.

40. McCarron MM, Schulze BW, Walberg CB, et al: Short acting barbiturate overdosage. *JAMA* 248:55, 1982.

41. Wilber GS, Coldwell BB, Trenholm HL: Toxicity of ethanol-barbiturate mixtures. *J Pharm Pharmacol* 21:232, 1969.

42. Yatzidis H: Bullous lesions in acute barbiturate poisonings. *JAMA* 27:211, 1971.

43. Winek CL, Collorn WD, Wecht CH, et al: Sustained release barbiturate risk. *Lancet* 2:155, 1967.

44. Carroll BJ: Barbiturate overdosage: Presentation with focal neurological signs. *Med J Aust* 1:1133, 1969.

45. Berveridge GW, Lawson AAH: Occurrence of bullous lesions in acute barbiturate poisoning. *Br Med J* 1:835, 1965.

46. Anonymous: Barbiturate coma and blisters. *Lancet* 1:733, 1972.

47. Van Heijst ANP, deJong W, Seldenrijk R, et al: Coma and crystalluria: A massive primidone intoxication treated with hemoperfusion. *J Toxicol Clin Toxicol* 20:307, 1983.

48. Cate JC, Tenser R: Acute primidone overdosage with massive crystalluria. *Clin Toxicol* 8:385, 1975.

49. Desmond MM, Schwanecte RP, Wilson GS, et al: Maternal barbiturate utilization and neonatal withdrawal symptomatology. *J Pediatr* 80:190, 1972.

50. Sullivan JY, Seller EM: Treating alcohol, barbiturate and benzodiazepine withdrawal. *Ration Drug Ther* 20:1, 1986.

51. Holzer P, Beubler B, Dirnhofer R: Barbiturate poisoning and gastrointestinal propulsion. *Arch Toxicol* 60:394, 1987.

52. Berg MJ, Berlinger WG, Goldber MJ, et al: Acceleration of the body clearance of phenobarbital by oral activated charcoal. *N Engl J Med* 307:642, 1982.

53. Goldberg MJ, Berlinger WG: Treatment of phenobarbital overdose with activated charcoal. *JAMA* 247:2400, 1982.

54. Boldy DAR, Vale JA, Prescott PI: Treatment of phenobarbitone poisoning with repeat oral administration of activated charcoal. *Q J Med* 235:997, 1986.

55. Jacobsen D, Wiik-Larsen E, Dahl T, et al: Pharmacokinetic evaluation of haemoperfusion in phenobarbital poisoning. *Eur J Clin Pharmacol* 26:109, 1984.

56. Zawada ET, Nappi J, Done G, et al: Advances in the hemodialysis management of phenobarbital overdose. *South Med J* 76:6, 1983.

57. DeBroc ME, Bismuth C, DeGroot G, et al: Haemoperfusion: A useful therapy for the severely poisoned patient? *Hum Toxicol* 5:11, 1986.

58. Pond SM: Renal principles, in Goldfrank LR, Flomenbaum NE, Lewin NA (eds): *Goldfrank's Toxicologic Emergencies.* 3rd ed. Norwalk, CT, Appleton-Century-Crofts, 1986, p 112.

59. Smith DE, Wesson DR: A new method for treatment of barbiturate dependence. *JAMA* 213:294, 1970.

60. Sellers EM: Alcohol, barbiturate and benzodiazepine withdrawal syndromes: Clinical management. *Can Med Assoc J* 139:113, 1988.

61. Harrison M, Busto U, Naranjo CA, et al: Diazepam tapering in detoxification for high-dose benzodiazepine abuse. *Clin Pharmacol Ther* 36:527, 1984.

62. Janecek E, Kapur B, Deveny P: Oral phenobarbital loading: A safe method of barbiturate and nonbarbiturate hypnosedative withdrawal. *Can Med Assoc J* 137:410, 1987.

63. Allgulander: History and current status of sedative-hypnotic drug use and abuse. *Acta Psychiatr Scand* 465, 1986.

64. Dommisse CS, DeVane CL Buspirone: A new type of anxiolytic. *Drug Intell Clin Pharm* 19:624, 1985.

65. Rickels K: Nonbenzodiazepine anxiolytics: Clinical usefulness. *J Clin Psychiatry* 44:38, 1983.

66. Goa KL, Heel RC: Zopiclone: A review of its pharmacodynamic and pharmacokinetic properties and therapeutic efficacy as a hypnotic. *Drugs* 32:48, 1986.

67. Zolpidem, in *Drugdex: Drug Evaluation Monographs.* Micromedex, vol. 77, 1993.

68. Alpidem, in *Drugdex: Drug Evaluation Monographs.* Micromedex, vol. 77, 1993.

69. Ethinamate, in *Drugdex: Drug Evaluation Monographs.* Micromedex, vol. 77, 1993.

70. Drugs for psychiatric disorders. *Med Lett Drugs Ther* 33:43, 1991.

71. Zolpidem for insomnia. *Med Lett Drugs Ther* 35:35, 1993.

72. Harvcy SC: Sedative hypnotics, in Goodman LS, Gilman AG (eds): *The Pharmacologic Basis of Therapy.* 7th ed. New York, Macmillan, 1985.

73. Bryson PD: Sedative-hypnotics, in *Comprehensive Review in Toxicology.* Rockville, MD, Aspen Publishers, 1989, p 345.

74. Mathew H: Barbiturates. *Clin Toxicol* 8:495, 1975.

75. Brow AM, Cade JF: Cardiac arrhythmias after chloral hydrate overdose. *Med J Aust* 1:28, 1980.

76. Ray VG: Chloral hydrate, in Noji EK, Kelen GO (ed): *Manual of Toxicologic Emergencies.* Chicago, Year Book, 1989, chap. 61.

77. Graham SR, Day RO, Lee R, Fulde GWO: Overdose with chloral hydrate: A pharmacological and therapeutic review. *Med J Aust* 149:686, 1988.

78. Anyebuno MA, Rosenfeld CR: Chloral hydrate toxicity in a term infant. *Dev Pharmacol Ther* 17:116, 1991.

79. Mayers DJ, Hindmarsh KW, Sankaran D, et al: Chloral hydrate disposition following single-dose administration to critically ill neonates and children. *Dev Pharmacol Ther* 16:71, 1991.

80. Lambert GH, Muraskas J, Anderson CL, Myers TF: Direct hyperbilirubinemia associated with chloral hydrate administration in the newborn. *Pediatrics* 86:277, 1990.

81. Reimche LD, Sankara K, Hindmarsh KW, et al: Chloral hydrate sedation in neonates and infants: Clinical and pharmacologic considerations. *Dev Pharmacol Ther* 12:57, 1989.
82. Jastak JT, Pallasch T: Death after chloral hydrate sedation: Report of a case. *J Am Dent Assoc* 116:345, 1988.
83. Millen RR, Greenblatt DJ: Clinical effects of chloral hydrate in hospitalized patients. *J Clin Pharmacol* 19:669, 1979.
84. Bowyer K, Gusser SP: Chloral hydrate overdose and cardiac arrhythmias. *Chest* 77:2, 1980.
85. Heath A, Delin K, Eden E, et al: Hemoperfusion with amberlite resin in the treatment of self poisoning. *Acta Med Scand* 207:455, 1980.
86. Bertino JS, Reed MD: Barbiturate and non-barbiturate sedative-hypnotic intoxication in children. *Pediatr Clin North Am* 3:703, 1986.
87. *Physicians Desk Reference*. 44th ed. Oradell, NJ, Medical Economics, 1990.
88. Teehan BP, Maher JF, Carey JT, et al: Acute ethchlorvynol intoxication. *Ann Intern Med* 72:875, 1970.
89. Glauser FL, Smith WR, Caldwell A: Ethchlorvynol induced pulmonary edema. *Ann Intern Med* 84:46, 1976.
90. Seyfart G: Ethchlorvynol, in Haddad LM, Winchester JF (eds): *Clinical Management of Poisoning and Drug Overdose*. Philadelphia, WB Saunders, 1983, p 516.
91. Ray VG: Ethchlorvynol, in Noji ER, Kelen GD (eds): *Manual of Toxicologic Emergencies*. Chicago, Year Book, 1989, chap. 58.
92. Ray VG: Glutethimide, in Nojii ER, Kelen GD (eds): *Manual of Toxicologic Emergencies*. Chicago, Year Book, 1989, chap. 59.
93. Banaclough BM: Are there safer hypnotics than barbiturates? *Lancet* 1:57, 1974.
94. Crow JW, Lain P, Bochner F, et al: Glutethimide and pharmacokinetics in man. *Clin Pharmacol Ther* 22:458, 1977.
95. Locket S: Glutethamide poisoning: A metabolite contributes to morbidity and mortality. *N Engl J Med* 292:250, 1975.
96. Curry SC, Hubbard JM, Gerkin R, et al: Lack of correlation between plasma 4-hydroxyglutethamide and severity of coma in acute glutethimide poisoning. *Med Toxicol* 2:309, 1987.
97. Locket S: Hemodialysis in the treatment of acute poisonings. *Proc Roy Soc Med* 63:427, 1970.
98. Seyfart G: Glutethimide, in Haddad LM, Winchester JF (eds): *Clinical Management of Poisoning and Drug Overdose*. Philadelphia, WB Saunders, 1983, p 531.
99. Baily DN, Jatlow PI: Methyprylon overdose. *Clin Toxicol* 6:563, 1973.
100. Ray VG: Meprobamate, in Noji ER, Kelen GD (eds): *Manual of Toxicologic Emergencies*. Chicago, Year Book, 1989.
101. Bailey DN: Meprobamate ingestion: A five year review of cases with serum concentrations and clinical findings. *Am J Clin Pathol* 75:102, 1981.
102. Greenblatt A: Meprobamate overdose: A continuing problem. *Clin Toxicol* 11:501, 1977.
103. Hassen E: Treatment of meprobamate overdose with repeated oral doses of activated charcoal. *Ann Emer Med* 15:73, 1986.
104. Bailey DN, Shaw RF: Interpretation of blood glutethimide, meprobamate and methylpyron concentrations in nonfatal and fatal intoxications involving a single drug. *J Clin Toxicol* 20:133, 1983.
105. Baselt RC: *Disposition of Toxic Drugs and Chemicals in Man*. Davis, CA, Biomed, 1982, p 350.
106. Nugent S, Katz MD, Little TE: Baclofen overdose with cardiac conduction abnormalities: Case report and review of the literature. *Clin Toxicol* 24:321, 1986.
107. Yassa RY, Iskandar HL: Baclofen induced psychosis: Two cases and a review. *J Clin Psych* 49:318, 1988.
108. Cohen MD, Gaily RA, McCoy GC: Atropine in the treatment of baclofen overdose. *Am J Emerg Med* 4:552, 1986.
109. Haubenstock A, Hruby K, Jage V, et al: Baclofen intoxication: Report of four cases and review of the literature. *J Toxicol Clin Toxicol* 229:59, 1983.
110. *AMA Drug Evaluations*. 4th ed. Chicago, American Medical Association, 1980, p 287.

156. Sympathomimetic Poisoning

Anthony S. Manoguerra

Overview

Sympathomimetic agents are structural analogs of catecholamines that have the ability to activate the sympathetic nervous system (Table 156-1). They also have potent central nervous system (CNS) effects that account for their high abuse potential. Amphetamines are DEA Class II or III "narcotics." They are rarely used in current medical practice but continue to be widely abused. Ephedrine, pseudoephedrine, and phenylpropanolamine are nonprescription drugs used primarily for ocular and nasal decongestion or as an adjunct in weight reduction programs. Tetrahydrozoline, naphazoline, oxymetazoline, and xylometazoline are topical agents available without prescription. They are found in vasoconstrictor eyedrops and nasal decongestant sprays and drops.

Amphetamines are now primarily obtained from illicit sources and are usually manufactured in clandestine, underground laboratories. This has not always been the case. In 1932, d,1-amphetamine inhalers were marketed as nasal decongestants [1]. Shortly thereafter, it was discovered that the potent CNS stimulant activity of this drug made it useful for the treatment of narcolepsy [2]. Over the next 30 years, amphetamines were used to treat a variety of unrelated disorders, particularly obesity and depression. Widespread abuse in the 1950s and 1960s led to legislation limiting the manufacture and distribution of amphetamines. The only current approved medical use for these drugs is the treatment of hyperkinetic behavior disorders in children and narcolepsy.

The most common amphetamines currently abused are racemic d,1-amphetamine, dextroamphetamine, and methamphetamine. Sporadically throughout the 1960s and 1970s, other amphetamine derivatives, such as 2,5-dimethoxy-4-methylamphetamine (STP or DOM) and 3-methoxy-4,5-methylenedeoxyamphetamine (MDA), were popular. At present, these drugs do not appear to be readily available.

Phenylpropanolamine is the most commonly abused over-the-counter sympathomimetic. During the late 1970s, two events resulted in an increase in phenylpropanolamine poisoning: the drug was approved for use as a nonprescription anorexiant, and mail order houses began selling large amounts of phenylpropanolamine-containing products as "body stimulants" or amphetamine look-alikes. In the past, anorexiant formulations also contained ephedrine and caffeine, but combination products were banned in 1984.

Propylhexedrine nasal decongestant inhalers were widely

Table 156-1. Commonly Available Sympathomimetic Agents

Generic name	Common trade name(s)	Therapeutic dose (mg)[a]
DEA schedule II or III agents		
Amphetamines		
Amphetamine	Benzedrine	5–10
Benzphetamine	Didrex	25–50
Dextroamphetamine	Dexadrine	5–15
Diethylpropion	Tenuate, Tepanil	25
Fenfluramine	Pondimin	20–40
Methamphetamine	Desoxyn	2.5–5
Methylphenidate	Ritalin	10–20
Phendimetrazine	Bontril, Phenazine	17.5–70
Phenmetrazine	Preludin	75[b]
Phentermine	Fastin, Ionamin, others	8–37.5
Nonprescription (OTC) agents		
Sympathomimetics		
Cinnamedrine	In Midol	5–15
Desoxyephedrine	Vicks Inhaler	Inhalation only
Ephedrine	Bronkaid, Primatene, others	25–50
Phenylpropanolamine	Allerest, Comtrex, Dexatrim, others	12.5–25
Propylhexedrine	Benzedrex Inhaler	Inhalation only
Pseudoephedrine	Novafed, Sudafed, others	30–60
Imidazolines		
Naphazoline	Clear Eyes, Naphcon, Privine, others	Topical only
Oxymetazoline	Afrin, Dristan, Nostrilla, others	Topical only
Tetrahydrozoline	Murine, Visine	Topical only
Zylometazoline	Neosynephrine II, Otrivin	Topical only

[a] Single oral adult dose
[b] Sustained-release formulation.

abused in the 1970s [3] and have sporadically resurfaced as drugs of abuse since then. The drug is found impregnated in a fibrous material in the inhaler. Abusers remove the material and ingest it or extract the propylhexedrine and inject it intravenously. Propylhexedrine produces effects and complications similar to those of other sympathomimetics.

Topical agents are not considered drugs of abuse. Poisoning primarily occurs when they are accidentally ingested by children.

During the Gulf War and the mid-1990s relief effort in Somalia, considerable interest was generated in the abuse of khat. This substance is the leaves of the *Catha edulis* and has been grown for centuries in East Africa and used throughout Africa and the Middle East for its stimulant effects. Acute and chronic use of khat produces sympathomimetic effects that closely resemble those seen with amphetamine. Three compounds have been isolated from the leaves: cathine, cathinone, and norephedrine. Cathinone has been shown closely to resemble amphetamine in its effects and is thought to be the primary ingredient responsible for the pharmacology of this plant [4,5].

Pharmacology

Amphetamines and sympathomimetics are phenylethylamine derivatives that appear to promote the release as well as block the reuptake of sympathetic neurotransmitters, primarily nor-

epinephrine and dopamine, in the sympathetic system and CNS [6,7,8]. However, their precise mechanisms of action remain unclear. Phenylpropanolamine is a relatively selective peripheral alpha-adrenergic receptor agonist. It can also cause the release of stored norepinephrine from presynaptic neurons. The net effect is typically pronounced alpha-adrenergic stimulation [6]. Tetrahydrozoline, naphazoline, oxymetazoline, and zylometazoline, like clonidine, are imidazoline derivatives that preferentially stimulate $alpha_2$-adrenergic receptors in the CNS, resulting in decreased sympathetic outflow. They are only partial $alpha_2$-agonists and can also stimulate peripheral alpha-receptors. Hence, clinical effects are variable and depend on the dose as well as the underlying level of sympathetic activity.

All of these agents are rapidly and completely absorbed from the gastrointestinal (GI) tract, with effects typically beginning in 30 minutes and peaking in 2 to 3 hours. Absorption is more rapid following nasal insufflation. A smokable form of methamphetamine known as "ice" has recently become popular. Smoking and intravenous (IV) injection provide almost instantaneous effects. The acute toxicity of these agents is due to exaggerated pharmacologic effects [1,9–14].

Following absorption, amphetamines and sympathomimetics undergo widespread distribution, with apparent volumes of distribution of 3 to 6 liters per kilogram of body weight. Amphetamines undergo extensive hepatic biotransformation with the production of active metabolites, some of which may play a role in the toxicity of these drugs [15]. For example, p-hydroxyamphetamine, a common active hepatic metabolite of amphetamine, is a potent hallucinogen and may be responsible for amphetamine-induced psychosis [16]. In contrast, ephedrine, pseudoephedrine, and phenylpropanolamine are resistant to degradation by peripheral and hepatic monoamine oxidase and are primarily eliminated by renal excretion. The kinetics of imidazoline derivatives are not well defined.

Since amphetamines and sympathomimetics are weak bases, their renal excretion is profoundly influenced by changes in urine pH [16,17,18]. Amphetamine has a pKa of 9.9, whereas that of other agents is between 8.8 and 10.4. In an acid urine (pH < 5), amphetamine exists almost totally in an ionized state, and drug that undergoes glomerular filtration cannot be reabsorbed in the distal renal tubules. Conversely, at a high urine pH, a significant fraction of drug is un-ionized and capable of being reabsorbed. Depending on urine flow rate and urine pH, the plasma half-life of amphetamine can vary between 7 and 34 hours. The renal disposition of other amphetamines is similarly variable. The half-lives of ephedrine, pseudoephedrine, and phenylpropanolamine, however, are significantly shorter, ranging from 2 to 4 hours. Hence, nonprescription agents are often marketed as sustained-release formulations.

Clinical Presentation

Poisoning results primarily in CNS and cardiovascular effects. Typical CNS manifestations include nausea, vomiting, headache, palpitations, anxiety, restlessness, nervousness, agitation, confusion, delirium, hyperactivity, muscle fasciculations and rigidity, hyperventilation, tremor, seizures, and coma. Severe hyperpyrexia is common in fatal poisonings [19,20]. In experimental animals, the pathologic and physiologic changes observed in fatal poisonings are similar to those seen in animals with experimentally induced hyperthermia [21].

Cardiovascular effects include systolic and diastolic hypertension and tachyarrhythmias. Hypertension may be more severe in the supine than the sitting or standing position [22]. In severe poisoning, cardiovascular collapse secondary to central vasomotor depression and catecholamine depletion may occur. Other effects include urinary retention, dilated but reactive pupils, and pale, dry skin.

The toxic dose of the amphetamines is not well defined. There is substantial variation between users as a result of tolerance. Extremely large doses may be used by chronic abusers before signs of toxicity become apparent [14]. In contrast, in nontolerant individuals, even "normal" or "therapeutic" doses may result in signs of toxicity [23].

The typical patient who has ingested a large amount of phenylpropanolamine is nervous, tremulous, and anxious. Seizures may occur abruptly [24]. Headache may or may not be present. Severe hypertension with a reflex bradycardia is common, although with ingestions of combination products or multiple drugs, tachycardia may be seen. Hypertensive crises with intracerebral hemorrhage or vasospasm and infarction have been reported [25,26,27]. Arrhythmias may include supraventricular tachycardia, premature ventricular contractions, and ventricular tachycardia. Acute renal failure secondary to rhabdomyolysis has been reported [28]. Poisoning has occurred following acute ingestions of 75 mg of nonsustained-release phenylpropanolamine in adults [28] and 8 to 10 mg per kilogram in children [29]. Severe (idiosyncratic) reactions to therapeutic doses have also been reported [25,26,30].

Pseudoephedrine has also been reported to produce severe hypertension [31] and intracranial hemorrhage in overdose [32]. Fenfluramine, a prescription anorexic agent, has produced agitation, seizures, coma, ventricular arrhythmias, and death [33]. Hypertension does not appear to be a predominant finding. Life-threatening effects may be evident 60 to 90 minutes following ingestion.

Imidazoline derivatives produce a unique syndrome of intoxication similar to that seen in clonidine poisoning. These substances produce paradoxical CNS depression, particularly in children, on ingestion of even small amounts [34,35,36]. Ingestion of as little as 2 to 5 ml of a 0.05% solution of tetrahydrozoline resulted in drowsiness, slowed respirations, and bradycardia in a 1-year-old child [37]. In other cases, periods of depression alternated with periods of agitation and hyperactivity. Effects on vital signs are variable. Hypertension with bradycardia appears to be the most common finding, but hypertension with tachycardia and hypotension with bradycardia have also been reported.

Death due to poisoning typically results from a cerebral vascular accident, cardiac event, or hyperthermia [38]. Hypertension and vasospasm may lead to ischemic damage of selected organs, whereas hyperthermia may result in generalized organ dysfunction. Cerebral vasospasm may lead to thrombotic events, whereas hypertension may result in intracerebral or subarachnoid hemorrhage [25,26,27,39,40,41]. Myocardial ischemia and infarction may occur [42,43,44]. Renal failure may result from renal ischemia or infarction or develop as a complication of rhabdomyolysis [45,46,47]. Hyperthermia may be due to a combination of hypothalamic dysfunction, metabolic or muscular hyperactivity, and seizures [10,21].

Chronic amphetamine abusers may develop a paranoid psychosis characterized by visual, tactile, and auditory hallucinations [48,49,50].

Diagnostic Evaluation

The evaluation of patients with potential poisoning should begin with a complete evaluation of vital signs and continuous cardiac monitoring. Often overlooked but very important is the accurate measurement of body temperature. A thorough history should be obtained to determine what substances are involved, by what route the patient was exposed, how much of the substance was involved, and when the exposure occurred. The physical examination should focus on neurologic and cardiovascular status. If the patient is symptomatic, a complete blood count, serum electrolytes, blood urea nitrogen, serum creatinine, blood glucose, urinalysis, and 12-lead electrocardiogram should be obtained. A urinalysis revealing hemoglobin in the absence of red blood cells suggests myoglobinuria. In patients with this finding, serum creatinine phosphokinase and liver function tests should be assessed. Patients with persistent coma, seizures, or focal neurologic findings should be evaluated for a structural lesion by a computed tomographic (CT) or magnetic resonance imaging (MRI) scan of the head. Other tests may be necessary to evaluate specific signs or symptoms (e.g., flank pain requires evaluation for possible renal infarction).

Quantitative blood levels of these agents are not clinically useful. A qualitative urine screen is sufficient to confirm exposure. Following methamphetamine exposures, urine samples may be positive for both methamphetamine and amphetamine, as the latter is formed by hepatic demethylation of the former.

Management

As with all drug overdoses, life support measures and stabilization of vital signs are of the utmost importance. Cardiac monitoring and an IV access line should be started on all patients. Activated charcoal should be given to patients with recent ingestions, particularly those involving sustained-release preparations of phenylpropanolamine. Charcoal has been shown to bind amphetamines avidly [51]. Syrup of ipecac-induced emesis should be avoided because of the risk of rapid onset of seizure activity with potential airway problems should vomiting occur.

All patients with major symptoms (hypertension, seizures, arrhythmias, hyperthermia, altered mental status, or hypotension) should be hospitalized in an ICU. Patients with mild tachycardia and general anxiety can be managed in the emergency department providing they were exposed to a short-acting agent only.

Seizures should initially be treated with IV diazepam. If seizures are refractory to diazepam, a short-acting barbiturate (e.g., amobarbital) may be tried. Although muscular activity may be controlled by paralyzing agents, paralysis alone is not adequate therapy, as occult seizure activity may continue and lead to CNS damage. Hence, electroencephalogram monitoring with continued treatment of seizures, using general anesthesia if necessary, is essential during paralysis.

Control of excessive muscular activity by sedation and paralysis is also extremely important if the patient is hyperthermic. Hyperthermia must also be treated vigorously with physical measures (see Chap. 73) [52]. The mechanism of hyperthermia due to sympathomimetic poisoning is different than that of anesthetic-induced malignant hyperthermia or neuroleptic malignant syndrome. There is no evidence that dantrolene or bromocriptine is effective in this setting.

Numerous agents have been advocated to control signs and symptoms of CNS excitation. Small, incremental doses of a benzodiazepine, such as diazepam or midazolam, are often effective and recommended as initial therapy [53]. For patients with extreme excitation and hallucinations that are unresponsive to benzodiazepines, haloperidol [54,55] or droperidol [56], which are adrenergic and dopaminergic receptor antagonists, may be used in conjunction with benzodiazepines [54,55,56].

Severe hypertension may require aggressive treatment. Traditionally, IV nitroprusside has been advocated. It is effective and easily titrated. Alpha-blockers, such as phentolamine and phenoxybenzamine, are also effective, but most clinicians have limited experience with their use. Chlorpromazine [11], diazoxide, and haloperidol [54,55] have been advocated, but these drugs are difficult to titrate and not recommended. The alpha- and beta-adrenergic receptor blocker labetalol has been used in patients who have both hypertension and tachycardia. Propranolol alone should be avoided: It slows the heart rate but also blocks vasodilatation and may result in unopposed alpha-mediated vasoconstriction with worsening hypertension. Urgent control of both heart rate and blood pressure can also be achieved with the combination of esmolol and sodium nitroprusside.

Ventricular arrhythmias should be treated with lidocaine or propranolol. A beta-blocker (with appropriate monitoring of blood pressure) or calcium channel blocker can be used for symptomatic supraventricular tachyarrhythmias. Myocardial infarction should be managed according to usual standards. Cardiovascular collapse is usually a preterminal event. Fluid resuscitation and vasopressors such as dopamine and norepinephrine should be administered, but therapy is unlikely to be successful.

The optimal treatment regimen for amphetamine and methamphetamine poisoning is not yet clear. Clinically, most patients do well with a combination of a benzodiazepine to control seizure activity and a short-acting beta-blocker and vasodilator to manage the cardiovascular toxicity. Animal research, however, has provided some interesting alternative results. In a study of d-amphetamine-poisoned rats [57], diazepam, haloperidol, yohimbine, and propranolol, when given alone, all failed to protect the rats from a lethal dose. The combination of diazepam and haloperidol was also ineffective. The combination of haloperidol and propranolol was most effective at preventing death in these animals. In another animal study [58], the same researchers found that diazepam protected animals against methamphetamine and d-amphetamine-induced seizures while propranolol reduced the incidence of methamphetamine-induced seizures only. Protection against amphetamine-induced death was afforded by haloperidol and propranolol in combination. None of the treatments was effective at decreasing death from methamphetamine. The applicability of these studies to humans remains to be determined. Of interest, the results reveal what may be significant differences in the mechanisms of toxicity between amphetamine and methamphetamine.

The use of acid diuresis to enhance the renal drug elimination has not been shown to alter the clinical course of poisoning; since it may produce adverse metabolic consequences (e.g., systemic acidemia), it is not recommended [16,18]. Acidification of the urine may precipitate renal failure in patients with myoglobinuria [59], a common complication of acute amphetamine poisoning [39,40].

Data concerning the use of extracorporeal elimination techniques are sparse. The amount of drug removed by these procedures compared to their total (metabolic and renal) clearance appears to be minimal [14] and does not appear to justify the routine use of such therapy. However, patients with severe poisoning who develop acute renal failure may theoretically benefit from these procedures.

The abrupt cessation of drug use in chronic amphetamine abusers is not life-threatening. Withdrawal effects include anxiety, abdominal pain and cramping, nausea, vomiting, diarrhea, sweating, and lethargy. Suicidal ideation and a marked increase in appetite are typical. Withdrawal effects peak 2 to 3 days after cessation of the drug. Subtle changes in rapid eye movement sleeping patterns have been shown to persist up to 8 weeks [60]. No specific medical management other than symptomatic care is needed for amphetamine withdrawal.

Psychiatric care and drug abuse treatment may be required for patients with intentional overdose, drug dependence, or withdrawal reactions.

References

1. Anderson RJ, Reed WG, Hillis JD, et al: History, epidemiology and medical complications of nasal inhaler abuse. *J Toxicol Clin Toxicol* 19:95, 1982.
2. Prinzmetal M, Bloomberger W: The use of benzedrine for the treatment of narcolepsy. *JAMA* 105:2051, 1935.
3. Garriott JC: Propylhexedrine: A new dangerous drug? *Clin Toxicol* 8:665, 1975.
4. *Khat Monograph: Lawrence Review of Natural Products.* St. Louis, Fact and Comparisons, 1993.
5. Drake PH: Khat chewing in the Near East. *Lancet* 1:532, 1988.
6. Gilman AG, Goodman LS, Rall TW, et al (eds): *The Pharmacological Basis of Therapeutics.* 7th ed. New York, Macmillan, 1985, p 146.
7. Baldessarini RJ: Pharmacology of the amphetamines. *Pediatrics* 49:694, 1972.
8. Caldwell J, Sever PS: The biochemical pharmacology of abused drugs. 1. Amphetamines, cocaines and LSD. *Clin Pharmacol Ther* 16:625, 1974.
9. Gunby P: Amphetamines may be banned for use in weight control. *JAMA* 242:1244, 1979.
10. Ginsberg MD, Hertzman M, Schmidt-Nowara WW: Amphetamine intoxication with coagulopathy, hyperthermia and reversible renal failure. *Ann Intern Med* 73:82, 1970.
11. Epselin DE, Done AK: Amphetamine poisoning: Effectiveness of chlorpromazine. *N Engl J Med* 278:1361, 1968.
12. Weiss SR, Raskind R, Morganstern NL, et al: Intracerebral and subarachnoid hemorrhage following use of methamphetamine. *Int Surg* 53:123, 1970.
13. Derlet RW, Rice P, Horowitz Z, et al: Amphetamine toxicity: Experience with 127 cases. *J Emerg Med* 7:157, 1989.
14. Zalis EG, Parmley LF: Fatal amphetamine poisoning. *Arch Intern Med* 112:60, 1963.
15. Baselt RC, Cravey RH: *Disposition of Toxic Drugs and Chemicals in Man.* 3rd ed. Chicago, Year Book, 1989, p 49.
16. Anggard E, Jonsson CE, Hogmark AL, et al: Amphetamine metabolism in amphetamine psychosis. *J Pharm Pharmacol* 17:628, 1965.
17. Beckett AH, Rowland M: Urinary excretion kinetics of amphetamine in man. *J Pharm Pharmacol* 17:628, 1965.
18. Davis TM, Kopin IJ, Lemberger L, et al: Effects of urinary pH on amphetamine metabolism. *Ann NY Acad Sci* 179:493, 1971.
19. Kojema T, Une I, Yashiki M, et al: A fatal methamphetamine poisoning associated with hyperpyrexia. *Forensic Sci Int* 24:87, 1984.
20. Jordan SC, Hampson F: Amphetamine poisoning associated with hyperpyrexia. *Br Med J* 2:844, 1960.
21. Zolis EG, Lundberg GD, Knutson RA: The pathophysiology of acute amphetamine poisoning with pathologic correlation. *J Pharmacol Exp Ther* 158:115, 1967.
22. Pentel P: Toxicity of over the counter stimulants. *JAMA* 252:1898, 1984.
23. Kramer JC, Fischman VS, Littlefield DC: Amphetamine abuse: Pattern and effects of high dose taken intravenously. *JAMA* 201:305, 1967.
24. Howrie DL, Wolfson JH: Phenylpropanolamine-induced hypertensive seizures. *J Pediatr* 102:143, 1983.
25. Kase CS, Foster TE, Rees JE, et al: Intracerebral hemorrhage and phenylpropanolamine use. *Neurology* 37:399, 1987.
26. Bernstein E, Diskant BM: Phenylpropanolamine: A potentially hazardous drug. *Ann Emerg Med* 11:311, 1982.
27. McDowell JR, LeBlanc HJ: Phenylpropanolamine-induced hypertensive seizures. *J Pediatr* 102:143, 1983.
28. Swenson RD, Golper TA, Bennett WM: Acute renal failure and rhabdomyolysis after ingestion of phenylpropanolamine-containing diet pills. *JAMA* 248:1216, 1982.

29. Ekins BR, Spoerke DG: An estimation of the toxicity of nonprescription diet aids from seventy exposure cases. *Vet Hum Toxicol* 25:81, 1983.

30. Edwards M, Russo L, Harwood-Nuss A: Cerebral infarction with a single dose of phenylpropanolamine. *Am J Emerg Med* 5:163, 1987.

31. Marianai PJ: Pseudoephedrine-induced hypertensive emergency: Treatment with labetalol. *Am J Emerg Med* 4:141, 1986.

32. Loizou LA, Hamilton JG, Tsementzis SA: Intracranial hemorrhage in association with pseudoephedrine overdose. *J Neurol Neurosurg Psychiatry* 45:471, 1982.

33. Veltri JC, Temple AR: Fenfluramine poisoning. *J Pediatr* 87:119, 1975.

34. Klein-Schwartz W, Gorman R, Oderda GM, et al: Central nervous system depression from ingestion of non-prescription eyedrops. *Am J Emerg Med* 2:217, 1984.

35. Hainsworth WC: Accidental poisoning with naphazoline hydrochloride. *Am J Dis Child* 75:76, 1948.

36. Waring JL, Charleston SC: Sedation as an unexpected systemic effect of Privine. *JAMA* 129:129, 1945.

37. Mindlin RL: Accidental poisoning from tetrahydrozoline eyedrops. *N Engl J Med* 275:112, 1966.

38. Kalant H, Kalant OJ: Death in amphetamine users: Causes and rates. *Can Med Assoc J* 112:299, 1975.

39. Chun KY: Acute subarachnoid hemorrhage. *JAMA* 233:55, 1975.

40. Conci F, D'Angelo V, Tampieri D, Vecchi G: Intracerebral hemorrhage and angiographic beading following amphetamine abuse. *Ital J Neurol Sci* 9:77, 1988.

41. Salanova V, Taubner R: Intracerebral hemorrhage and vasculitis secondary to amphetamine use. *Postgrad Med J* 60:429, 1984.

42. Lam D, Goldschlager N: Myocardial injury associated with poly substance abuse. *Am Heart J* 115:675, 1988.

43. Ozel JA: Acute myocardial infarction complicated by chronic amphetamine use. *Arch Intern Med* 142:644, 1982.

44. Rosenblum I, Wohl A, Stein A: Studies in cardiac necrosis. I Production of cardiac lesions with sympathomimetic amines. *Toxicol Appl Pharmacol* 7:1, 1965.

45. Scharff J: Renal infarction associated with intravenous cocaine use. *Ann Emerg Med* 13:1145, 1984.

46. Scandling J, Spital A: Amphetamine-associated myoglobinuric renal failure. *South Med J* 75:237, 1982.

47. Kendrick WC, Hull AR, Knochel JP: Rhabdomyolysis and shock after intravenous amphetamine administration. *Ann Intern Med* 86:381, 1977.

48. Alverno L, Larson C, Hieb E: Recognizing amphetamine psychosis. *Drug Ther* 4:92, 1975.

49. Hoffman BF: Diet pill psychosis: Followup after six years. *Can Med Assoc J* 129:1077, 1983.

50. Schaffer CB, Pauli MW: Psychotic reaction caused by proprietary oral diet pills. *Am J Psychiatry* 137:10, 1980.

51. Decker WJ, Combs HF, Corby DG: Adsorption of drugs and poisons by activated charcoal. *Toxicol Appl Pharmacol* 13:454, 1968.

52. Koppanyi T, Maling HM: Temperature-dependent toxicity of adrenergic agonists in mice as a basis for treating d-amphetamine poisoning. *Proc Soc Exp Biol Med* 144:575, 1973.

53. Linden CH, Kulig KW, Rumack BH: Amphetamines. *Top Emerg Med* 7:718, 1985.

54. Catravas JD, Waters IW, Davis WM, et al: Haloperidol for acute amphetamine poisoning: A study in dogs. *JAMA* 231:1340, 1975.

55. Davis WM, Logston DG, Hickenbottom JP: Antagonism of acute amphetamine intoxication by haloperidol and propranolol. *Toxicol Appl Pharmacol* 29:397, 1973.

56. Gary NE, Saidi P: Methamphetamine intoxication: A speedy new treatment. *Am J Med* 64:537, 1978.

57. Derlet RW, Albertson TE, Rice P: Protection against d-amphetamine toxicity. 8:105, 1990.

58. Derlet RW, Albertson TE, Rice P: Antagonism of cocaine, amphetamine and methamphetamine toxicity. *Pharmacol Biochem Behav* 36:745, 1990.

59. Eneas JF, Schonfield PY, Humphreys MH: The effect of infusion of mannitol-sodium bicarbonate on the clinical course of myoglobinuria. *Arch Intern Med* 139:801, 1979.

60. Oswald I, Thacore VR: Amphetamine and phenmetrazine addiction: Physiological abnormalities in the abstinence syndrome. *Br Med J* 2:427, 1963.

157. Systemic Asphyxiants

Alan H. Hall

Introduction and Definitions

Simple asphyxiants are gases or vapors that, in sufficiently high concentrations, displace oxygen from the breathing atmosphere, lowering the ambient FIO_2 by dilution and causing hypoxia. Simple asphyxiant effects occur primarily in enclosed spaces [11]. Air hunger, fatigue, decreased vision, mood disturbances, numbness of extremities, headache, confusion, decreased coordination and judgment, cyanosis, and coma may develop [1]. Signs of asphyxia are noted when atmospheric oxygen is displaced such that the oxygen concentration is 15 to 16 percent or less (normal atmospheric oxygen content 20.8 percent). Unconsciousness leading to death may be seen when the atmospheric oxygen concentration is decreased to 6 to 8 percent or less [1]. Examples of simple asphyxiants are flammable gases, such as ethane, ethylene, propylene, propane, hydrogen, butane, isobutane, liquified petroleum gas (LPG), and methane, and inert gases, such as helium, neon, and argon (see Chap. 58). Some of the acute effects of many chlorofluorocarbon compounds and other volatile hydrocarbons are also due to simple asphyxiation.

Systemic asphyxiants, in contrast, must be absorbed into the body to exert their effects. They act by preventing oxygen transport by hemoglobin or myoglobin, by inhibiting oxygen release from these proteins, or by blocking cellular utilization of oxygen. Although systemic asphyxiants in the gaseous or vapor state could also cause simple asphyxiation, these agents most often produce systemic toxicity at airborne concentrations insufficient to reduce the ambient FIO_2 to hypoxic levels. Systemic asphyxiants include carbon monoxide (see Chap. 58) as well as the agents discussed below.

Cyanide and Cyanogens

Cyanide is used in electroplating, jewelry cleaning, precious metal extraction, laboratory assays, and some photographic processes [2–6]. Imported cyanide-containing metal cleaning solutions have caused unintentional poisoning [7]. Hydrogen cyanide gas is used as a fumigant rodenticide [6,8]. Fatal cyanide poisonings have occurred from criminal tampering with over-the-counter capsules [3,9,10,11]. Chemists and laboratory workers may ingest cyanide compounds in suicide attempts [12,13].

Enclosed-space smoke inhalation victims may have cyanide poisoning as well as carbon monoxide toxicity, especially when plastic materials are pyrolized [14–18]. In aircraft accidents, inhalation of smoke and pyrolysis products including cyanide may rapidly incapacitate crew members and passengers, preventing their escape from the toxic cabin atmosphere [19].

Cyanide can be liberated from a number of compounds (e.g., cyanogen, cyanogen halides, calcium cyanide) by spontaneous or thermal decomposition or by chemical reaction with acids or acid fumes [2,3,6]. Cyanogen, cyanogen halides, and hydrogen cyanide gas have been considered for use as chemical warfare agents [20].

Certain cyanogenic compounds can release cyanide following hepatic metabolism (e.g., aliphatic nitriles, aliphatic thiocyanates) or chemical reaction and bacterial degradation in the gut following ingestion (e.g., Laetrile, amygdalin or other cyanogenic glycosides from plant sources) [3,21–32]. When bitter cassava (Manihot esculenta) or "gari" (a processed bitter cassava product) are improperly prepared and eaten, serious or even fatal acute poisoning may result from release of cyanide from the cyanogenic glycosides, linamarin and lotaustralin, found in this plant [33,34]. Symptom onset may be delayed for several hours after cassava is consumed [33,34].

Elevated whole blood cyanide levels have been documented in personnel performing autopsies on victims of suicidal cyanide ingestion [35]. The amount of cyanide remaining in the stomach may determine whether potentially toxic exposure may occur in this setting [36].

High-dose sodium nitroprusside therapy occasionally causes elevated blood cyanide levels, with or without clinical manifestations of cyanide poisoning [37–42]. There is little correlation between measured whole blood cyanide levels and the presence of cyanide poisoning symptoms during nitroprusside infusion [40,41]. Patients receiving high-dose nitroprusside therapy who suddenly develop otherwise unexplained central nervous system (CNS) dysfunction, elevated blood lactic acid levels, metabolic acidosis, or new-onset cardiovascular compromise may have nitroprusside-induced cyanide toxicity [41].

In most cases, only gastrointestinal distress follows ingestion of ferrocyanide or ferricyanide, as these compounds do not usually release significant amounts of cyanide [6]. Ingestion of potassium aurocyanide resulted in serious toxicity in one reported case, however [43]. Fatal poisonings have also occurred from inhaling fumes from silver cyanide sludge in an enclosed space [44] and from magnesium cyanide exposure [45].

PATHOPHYSIOLOGY. Cyanide binds to the ferric (Fe^{3+}) ion of mitochondrial cytochrome oxidase, inhibiting this enzyme, disrupting the electron transport chain, and decreasing or prohibiting oxidative phosphorylation [46]. This results in anaerobic metabolism, substantially decreased adenosine triphosphate (ATP) production, depletion of cellular energy stores, lactic acid generation, and an elevated anion gap metabolic acidosis [2].

Tissue hypoxia in cyanide poisoning has several etiologies. Until the stage of hypoventilation, the blood may be normally oxygenated, whereas the tissues are unable to extract and use this oxygen. Tissues with the highest oxygen utilization (myocardium and brain) are most severely and rapidly affected. Inhibition of the central respiratory centers then causes hypoventilation with decreased oxygen uptake. Stagnation hypoxia develops as myocardial depression results in decreased cardiac output.

Cyanide binding to cytochrome oxidase is reversible. The body's natural defense mechanism is the enzyme rhodanese, which catalyzes complexing of cyanide with sulfur, forming much less toxic thiocyanate ion (SCN^-). The body's sulfur pool is, however, quite limited, and the availability of sulfur thus constitutes the rate-limiting factor for endogenous cyanide detoxification. In the absence of exogenously supplied sulfur, rhodanese activity is too slow to prevent serious poisoning or death following significant cyanide exposure.

TOXICOKINETICS AND TOXICODYNAMICS. Toxicokinetic data are relatively sparse and are derived from animal experiments and human poisoning case reports. Cyanide is approximately 60 percent protein-bound in dog plasma [47]. Blood cyanide levels may be four or more times higher than serum levels, because cyanide is selectively concentrated in erythrocytes [48].

In dogs, cyanide has a volume of distribution (V_d) of 0.498 liter per kilogram [49]. In a single human potassium cyanide ingestion case, a similar V_d of 0.41 liter per kilogram was estimated following antidotal treatment [4]. In the same case, the initial elimination half-life was between 0.5 and 1 hour, while the terminal phase ($t_{1/2}$) was 19 hours [4]. A second patient who ingested potassium cyanide had a $t_{1/2}$ of 1 hour during the first 6 hours, followed by a $t_{1/2}$ of 6 hours thereafter [50]. In a case of suicidal acetonitrile ingestion, estimates of terminal half-lives were 32 hours for the parent compound and 15 hours for metabolically released cyanide [51]. Half-life values frequently quoted in the literature are 20 to 60 minutes [6,14]; in smoke inhalation cases, the $t_{1/2}$ was 1 hour [18]. The terminal elimination half-life may be shorter following inhalation than following ingestion. There may also be longer absorption and distribution phases following ingestion, compared to inhalation.

In dogs, there was only minimal urinary cyanide excretion in the first 3 hours after oral administration, despite about 95 percent absorption [47]. A single cyanide-poisoned patient not treated with specific antidotes had an average urinary cyanide excretion of only 0.64 mg per hour over nearly 40 hours [3]. The mean whole blood cyanide level 1 hour after ingestion in this case was 8.2 μg per milliliter, rising to a mean of 19.7 μg per milliliter at 3 hours and to 23.4 μg per milliliter at 9 hours after ingestion [3].

Without antidotal therapy, cyanide levels may continue to rise for hours after ingestion. When antidotes are administered, cyanide levels decrease more rapidly. In one patient who survived potassium cyanide ingestion following treatment with sodium nitrite/thiosulfate, the highest whole blood cyanide level was 15.68 μg per milliliter at 1.75 hours after ingestion, falling to 0.82 μg per milliliter by 5 hours [4]. A second patient who ingested potassium cyanide developed a whole blood cyanide level of 13 μg per milliliter over 1 hour; rapid clinical improvement followed administration of sodium nitrite/thiosulfate, and no blood cyanide was detectable 18 hours after ingestion [52]. A patient who survived cyanide poisoning (from propionitrile exposure) following treatment with hydroxocobalamin/sodium thiosulfate had a decrease in whole blood cyanide levels from 5.71 μg per milliliter 2 hours after exposure to 0.93 μg per milliliter 30 minutes later [28]. A child who ingested laetrile had a whole blood cyanide level of 16.3 μg per milliliter 6 hours after ingestion; following sodium nitrite/thiosulfate treatment, this blood level fell to 0.84 μg per milliliter at 15 hours [21]. An adult who injected potassium cyanide intravenously had a whole blood cyanide level of 4.4 μg per milliliter on admission; 12 hours after sodium nitrite/thiosulfate infusion, the level was 0.18 μg per milliliter [53]. In cases of acetonitrile exposure, however, "rebound" in whole blood cyanide levels may occur despite bolus doses of specific antidotes, due to continued metabolic cyanide release [27,52,54].

Without treatment, ingestion of 200 to 300 mg of sodium or potassium cyanide or 50 mg of hydrocyanic acid may be fatal in adults [55,56]. Serious acute poisoning has resulted from ingestion of 50 mg of potassium cyanide [57]. Inhalation of airborne cyanide concentrations of 200 to 300 mg per cubic meter (180–270 ppm) can rapidly be fatal [2]. In contrast, patients have survived inhalation exposure to 500 mg per cubic meter [58], ingestion of 1 gm or more of potassium cyanide [4,59], and total body immersion in cyanide salt solutions [60,61]. Significant poisoning symptoms may be seen when whole blood cyanide levels are 1.0 μg per milliliter or greater, and death may occur in untreated patients with whole blood cyanide levels of 3.0 μg per milliliter or higher [2]. Antidote-treated patients have survived with whole blood cyanide levels as high as 40 μg per milliliter [62].

CLINICAL MANIFESTATIONS AND DIAGNOSTIC EVALUATION.
Acute cyanide poisoning typically has a fairly rapid progression to coma, convulsions, shock, respiratory failure, and death [2,46]. Early findings include giddiness, headache, anxiety, tachycardia, hyperpnea, mild hypertension, and palpitations. Later findings in significant poisoning are nausea, vomiting, tachycardia or bradycardia, hypotension, generalized seizures, coma, apnea, dilated pupils (nonreactive or sluggishly reactive), and a variety of cardiac effects (e.g., supraventricular or ventricular tachyarrhythmias, atrioventricular blocks, ischemic ECG changes, and asystole) [2]. Noncardiogenic pulmonary edema has also been noted, even in cases of cyanide ingestion [63].

Retinal arteries and veins that appear nearly equally red have been described [64]. An odor of bitter almonds or a musty odor may be present on the breath or in the vomitus, but the ability to detect it is genetically determined and often lacking, making this an unreliable clinical sign [2]. Cyanosis usually develops only at the late stage of apnea and circulatory collapse. In spontaneously breathing or artificially ventilated patients with signs of severe hypoxia, the absence of cyanosis should suggest cyanide poisoning [2].

The onset of life-threatening symptoms may be delayed for 0.5 to 1 hour following cyanide salt ingestion [4]. A more delayed onset (1–5 hours) can follow laetrile or cyanogen ingestion [21,54]. Inhalation of high airborne cyanide concentrations may result in sudden loss of consciousness with only a few breaths [6,65]. Ingestion, inhalation, or dermal exposure to cyanogenic aliphatic nitrile compounds may not produce symptoms for up to 12 or more hours [26,27,51].

Ingestion of acetonitrile-based artificial glue-on nail remover has caused serious and prolonged cyanide poisoning, often with a delay of 12 hours or more in symptom onset [54,66–69]. The initial asymptomatic period after ingestion of such products by children, especially when confused with much less toxic acetone-based nail polish removers, has led to discharge before the onset of severe effects of cyanide poisoning. In all such cases, a period of several hours of close observation in a facility equipped to treat serious cyanide toxicity is warranted.

It has frequently been stated that systemic poisoning may occur following dermal exposure to cyanide compounds, but clinical cases—other than those from serious burns with molten cyanide salts [70] or hot solutions of hydrocyanic acid or potassium cyanide [71], complete immersion in vats of cyanide solutions (with potential ingestion and vapor inhalation) [60,61], or continued wearing of clothing soaked with concentrated

cyanide solutions in enclosed spaces [72]—are generally lacking. Significant absorption and systemic toxicity follow direct conjunctival instillation of cyanide salts in experimental animals [73]. No human cases of systemic poisoning from eye splashes have been reported.

Sequelae are rare in survivors of acute cyanide poisoning, but cases of delayed development of parkinsonianlike states or memory deficits and personality changes have been reported [74–81]. Lesions in the basal ganglia (bilaterally symmetric lesions in the putamen or globus pallidus) may be noted on computed tomography (CT), magnetic resonance imaging (MRI), or 6-fluoro-L-DOPA positron emission tomography (PET) scan [78,79,80].

The initial physical examination should focus on vital signs and respiratory, cardiovascular, and CNS function. Continuous lead II ECG and frequent vital signs monitoring are essential. While newer laboratory methods can provide rapid (30–45 minutes) measurement of blood cyanide levels [82], they are not generally available in the clinical setting. Whole blood cyanide levels determined by most methods available to clinicians take hours to obtain and thus cannot be used for acute diagnosis or to guide emergent therapy [2]. However, blood levels do confirm the diagnosis and document response to treatment. Lactic acid levels, serum electrolytes, and arterial blood gases should be monitored frequently to guide fluid, electrolyte, sodium bicarbonate, and respiratory therapy. A 12-lead ECG should be obtained initially and repeated if abnormal or if symptoms progress. A chest film should also be obtained on admission and repeated if evidence of pulmonary edema is present or develops later.

Nitrite antidotes have intrinsic toxicity and should not be used indiscriminately in cases in which the diagnosis is unclear. The presence of certain laboratory abnormalities may help increase diagnostic certainty such that it would be prudent to administer antidotes when cyanide poisoning is suspected but a definite history of exposure is not available [2,3]. Lactic acidosis, reflected in arterial blood gases as a decrease in pH not due to an elevated PCO_2 and in serum electrolytes as an elevated anion gap (anion gap = $Na - [Cl + CO_2]$; normal <12–16 mEq/L), is suggestive. A percent O_2 saturation gap (difference between measured and calculated arterial percent O_2 saturations) has been described [2,3]. However, it now appears that this "gap" may be due to the presence of methemoglobin from prior administration of amyl nitrite [52], and this finding cannot be reproduced in vitro [83]. Inhibition of oxygen extraction from the blood may be reflected as an increased (>40 mm Hg) peripheral venous PO_2 [21,68,69,84] or a narrowing of the difference between the measured arterial percent O_2 saturation and measured central venous or pulmonary artery percent O_2 saturation (a decrease in the arteriovenous percent O_2 saturation gap) [41,85]. Normal central venous percent O_2 saturation is about 70 percent.

Exactly how these parameters may be affected by supplemental oxygenation, if at all, is unclear. Hydrogen sulfide poisoning causes similar laboratory abnormalities, but since amyl and sodium nitrite are also used as hydrogen sulfide antidotes [86–90], this is not a serious drawback. In addition, although sodium thiosulfate has no efficacy in hydrogen sulfide poisoning [89], it is not harmful.

MANAGEMENT

Supportive Treatment. Antidotal therapy is not required for cyanide-exposed patients with only restlessness, anxiety, or hyperventilation [65,91]. Supplemental oxygen and careful monitoring until symptoms resolve are all that is necessary.

Rescuers must wear proper protective equipment and self-contained breathing apparatus when entering areas with high cyanide airborne concentrations, lest they become secondary victims. Mouth-to-mouth ventilation should be avoided whenever possible.

Amyl nitrite administered by inhalation (as a part of the Lilly Cyanide Antidote Kit) is the initial portion of specific antidotal therapy [2]. However, especially when combined with administration of supplemental oxygen, amyl nitrite inhalation may be properly considered as supportive therapy [21,92].

A satisfactory outcome in seriously poisoned patients may sometimes be seen with supportive measures alone [46,63,93–96]. However, administration of specific antidotes plus intensive supportive therapy have resulted in survival of patients with higher whole blood cyanide levels, more rapid resolution of coma and acidosis, and lesser requirements for sodium bicarbonate administration [3,4,21,23,52,62,97,98].

Supplemental oxygen should be administered to all patients with cyanide poisoning, because it has some antidotal activity of its own and is synergistic with available antidotes [99]. Endotracheal intubation and mechanical ventilation may be required when CNS or respiratory depression is present. Positive end-expiratory pressure (PEEP) may be needed if noncardiogenic pulmonary edema develops. Central venous or pulmonary artery pressure monitoring may be helpful in such cases. Standard antiarrhythmic and anticonvulsant drugs may be required; the medications commonly used for these indications are not contraindicated in cyanide poisoning. Atropine or vasopressors can be used to treat symptomatic bradycardia or hypotension. Metabolic acidosis can be corrected with sodium bicarbonate; serum sodium and osmolality should be monitored if large doses are needed.

Measures to decrease absorption may be useful but must not delay supportive or antidotal treatment. Exposed skin and eyes should be flushed copiously with water or normal saline. Contaminated clothing should be immediately removed and placed in an impervious container. Inducing emesis is *contraindicated*. Performing gastric lavage with a large-bore orogastric tube may be of benefit immediately after ingestion, but precautions must be taken to prevent pulmonary aspiration of gastric contents. Activated charcoal binds cyanide and decreases mortality in experimental animals [100,101]. Activated charcoal may be more effective if administered before as well as after gastric lavage and should be given as soon after ingestion as possible.

Antidotal Therapy. Specific antidotes currently available in the United States (e.g., amyl nitrite, sodium nitrite, sodium thiosulfate) are supplied in the Lilly Cyanide Antidote kit. Amyl nitrite pearls may be broken in gauze and held close to the nose and mouth of spontaneously breathing patients with significant symptoms or vital sign abnormalities. The pearls can also be placed into the lip of the face mask or inside the resuscitation bag when patients are apneic or hypoventilating [21,92]. Amyl nitrite should be inhaled for 30 seconds of each minute, with a fresh pearl used every 3 to 4 minutes.

When intravenous access has been established, amyl nitrite inhalation should be discontinued and sodium nitrite infused intravenously in an adult dose of 300 mg (one 10-ml ampule of 3% solution). The pediatric dose is 0.12 to 0.33 ml per kilogram. Children with anemia may require dosage adjustments, as described in the Lilly kit product information. Starting with lower doses is advised in children; further sodium nitrite should be titrated to the clinical response.

Sodium nitrite is a potent vasodilator; administering it too rapidly can result in significant hypotension [62,102,103]. Sodium nitrite should therefore be given either by slow intravenous push over no less than 5 minutes or by diluting the dose in 50 to 100 ml of normal saline or D_5W, starting with a slow infusion rate, and then increasing to the most rapid rate that does not produce or worsen hypotension. Blood pressure should be monitored frequently during sodium nitrite infusion.

A second potentially serious, although rare, side effect of sodium nitrite administration is induction of excessive methemoglobinemia. This complication is usually seen only with excessive doses, especially in children [24,62,91,103]. Methemoglobin levels should be monitored before and after sodium nitrite infusion, especially if multiple doses are required. Methemoglobin levels should always be kept less than 30 to 40 percent. Excessive methemoglobinemia may be treated with methylene or toluidine blue. Exchange transfusion and hyperbaric oxygen (HBO) therapy are alternatives in cases of life-threatening methemoglobinemia (see below).

Although administering enough sodium nitrite to produce a "therapeutic methemoglobin level" of 25 percent has sometimes been recommended [14,104], patients have fully recovered from severe acute cyanide poisoning following induction of no more than 2 to 9.2 percent measurable methemoglobinemia [4,52,53]. The clinical response is, therefore, the best determinant of adequate sodium nitrite dosing.

Sodium nitrite should be immediately followed with an intravenous bolus of sodium thiosulfate, given over several minutes in an adult dose of 12.5 gm (one 50-ml ampule of 25% solution). Children should be administered 1.65 ml per kilogram. No significant adverse effects from sodium thiosulfate administration as a cyanide antidote in humans have been reported in almost 60 years of clinical use [105]. However, in volunteer studies, sodium thiosulfate has caused nausea, vomiting, light-headedness, and localized discomfort at injection sites, especially with rapid intravenous infusion [106,107].

In some cyanide-poisoned patients, sodium thiosulfate combined with supplemental oxygen and intensive supportive measures may be sufficient therapy [13,105]. Repeat sodium nitrite and thiosulfate doses of one-half the initial amounts may be given 30 minutes after the first doses if the clinical response is inadequate.

In one severely poisoned patient, a continuous thiosulfate infusion at 1 gm per hour for 24 hours was associated with complete recovery [13]. With exposure to aliphatic nitrile compounds, continued metabolic release of cyanide may cause prolonged poisoning, requiring multiple doses of antidotes [27,54]. Sodium thiosulfate alone, either multiple bolus doses or as a continuous infusion, may be efficacious in such cases [51,54,69].

Low-dose hydroxocobalamin (1 mg/ml; total dose 100 mg) and sodium thiosulfate as a continuous intravenous infusion in a molar ratio of 1:5 (nitroprusside:thiosulfate; 2 ml of 0.15 gm/ml sodium thiosulfate added to nitroprusside solution and infused at 1 μg/kg/hr) have been used successfully to prevent sodium nitroprusside-induced cyanide poisoning [37,38,42]. When elevated blood cyanide levels are present in patients receiving high-dose sodium nitroprusside therapy but signs or symptoms of cyanide toxicity—particularly elevated lactic acid levels and metabolic acidosis—are absent, administration of specific cyanide antidotes is usually not necessary [40].

In smoke inhalation victims with combined carbon monoxide and cyanide poisoning, sodium thiosulfate and 100% supplemental oxygen should be administered first [102]. It is preferable to withhold sodium nitrite until the patient is being treated in an HBO chamber, at which time oxygen dissolved in plasma is adequate compensation for the loss of oxygen-transporting capacity caused by sodium nitrite-induced methemoglobinemia [15,102]. If HBO is not available, sodium nitrite may be administered, carefully observing the precautions described above [108].

Antidotes in clinical use in other countries—hydroxocobalamin, dicobalt-EDTA (Kelocyanor), and 4-dimethylaminophenol (4-DMAP)—are not available in the United States [2,33,44,46,81,107], although hydroxocobalamin as a 5% injectable solution (500 mg/ml) has previously undergone clinical trials [107]. As the hydroxocobalamin preparation generally available in the United States is quite dilute (1 mg/ml), the large volumes that would be required to treat cyanide poisoning prohibit its use.

Other Treatments. Oxygen at normobaric pressure is an efficacious therapy for cyanide poisoning [60]. In patients not responding to supportive and antidotal treatment, HBO may be considered, although there is limited and conflicting evidence for its efficacy in experimental animals and humans [97,99,109,110,111]. Smoke inhalation victims with significant carbon monoxide poisoning and possible cyanide toxicity should be treated with HBO when available [15,111].

Single cases of severe acute cyanide poisoning treated with hemodialysis or charcoal hemoperfusion, as well as supportive measures and specific antidotes, have been reported [7,112,113]. Although cyanide is theoretically dialyzable and might be removed by hemoperfusion [4,113], the clinical courses of these two reported patients were not different from those seen in other patients treated with only supportive measures and specific antidotes. It is therefore unlikely that either of these extracorporeal procedures contributed significantly to the favorable outcomes; thus they cannot be recommended as standard therapy.

DISPOSITION. Asymptomatic patients with minimal cyanide exposure should be observed in a controlled setting for at least 4 to 6 hours. The observation period should be at least 12 hours with exposure to acetonitrile or other aliphatic nitrile compounds. Patients with serious toxicity and those with lesser symptoms that persist more than 1 to 2 hours should be admitted to an intensive care unit (ICU) and carefully monitored for a minimum of 24 hours or until all signs and symptoms have fully resolved. To screen for potential CNS sequelae, periodic outpatient follow-up should be arranged for at least several weeks after significant cyanide or cyanogen exposure.

Hydrogen Sulfide

Hydrogen sulfide (H_2S) is a nonflammable, colorless, irritating gas with a strong odor of sulfur or rotten eggs that may be encountered in a wide variety of settings. The majority of exposures are due to its natural occurrence in petroleum, natural gas, volcanic gas, and some hot springs, as well as its frequent presence in sewer gas and swampy soils as a result of the decomposition of sulfur-containing organic materials [114–117]. In natural gas, hydrogen sulfide makes up from less than 1 to 90 percent of the sulfur-containing contaminants [118]. The largest reported series of cases involved mainly petrochemical workers [119].

Hydrogen sulfide is widely used as a reagent in analytical chemistry and is a by-product in a large number of industrial processes, including the manufacture of adhesives, barium salts, cellophane, depilatories, dyes and pigments, fertilizers, heavy water, lithophone, synthetic petroleum-based products, and viscose rayon [114,115,116]. It is also used or generated in some metallurgic processes, in making wood pulp and felt, as an agricultural disinfectant, in the purification of hydrochloric acid and phosphates, and in low-temperature coal carbonization [86,115]. Hydrogen sulfide may be generated in breweries, tanneries, and slaughterhouses and can be released during fat rendering or pelt processing, lithography, and photoengraving [115,120,121]. It is a source of elemental sulfur [114].

Poisonings have occurred from inhalation of fumes from cooling roofing asphalt [86] and in farm workers exposed to fumes from liquid manure [122,123,124]. Pouring hydrochloric acid into a rural well with a large amount of organic matter and a high iron content may generate hydrogen sulfide gas and cause poisoning, as may mixing alkaline and basic drain cleaners [125,126]. Breathing the fumes from sodium sulfite or an electrolytic bath containing sodium thiosulfate, sodium hypochlorite, and acetic acid has resulted in hydrogen sulfide intoxication [86,127]. Poisoning occurred in a worker attempting to clear a drain in a hospital cast room that contained calcium sulfite sludge from plaster of Paris [87].

Hydrogen sulfide is one of the major malodorous sulfur-containing air pollutants released from pulp and paper mills [128]. Residents in the vicinity of such mills have experienced an increased incidence of eye and mucous membrane irritation, mental symptoms (e.g., depression, anxiety), and headaches on days with high levels of hydrogen sulfide emissions [128].

PATHOPHYSIOLOGY. Hydrogen sulfide's major mechanism of toxicity is similar to that of cyanide: interaction with mitochondrial cytochrome oxidase and inhibition of the electron transport chain, resulting in cellular inability to use oxygen in aerobic metabolism [118,129,130,131]. Organs with a high oxygen demand (e.g., brain, myocardium) are most susceptible to hydrogen sulfide toxicity [118]. Hydrogen sulfide is well known for its rapid "knock-down" effects: unconsciousness may follow a single breath when the gas is present in sufficient concentration [116]. It is also a direct irritant of the eyes and mucous membranes of the respiratory tract [114,116,118, 121,132].

TOXICOKINETICS AND TOXICODYNAMICS. Coma and respiratory paralysis leading rapidly to death may occur with inhalation of 1000 ppm or more [116]. Unconsciousness, apnea, and death may occur less suddenly when concentrations of 500 to 1000 ppm are inhaled [114,118]. Concentrations of 50 to 500 ppm primarily cause respiratory tract irritation [114]. Prolonged exposure to concentrations greater than 250 ppm may result in pneumonitis or noncardiogenic pulmonary edema [114,116, 118]. Eye irritation has occurred at concentrations as low as 4 to 5 ppm in some cases [114], and more severe conjunctivitis or keratoconjunctivitis with corneal vesiculation may be noted at concentrations of 50 ppm or greater [116,118].

Although the threshold for perception of the odor of rotten eggs ranges from 0.003 to 0.02 ppm [118], olfactory fatigue occurs rapidly when airborne concentrations are 100 to 200 ppm or greater [116,118]. The loss of odor perception is often misinterpreted as meaning that the gas is no longer present, and workers may thus unintentionally remain in an area with dangerously high concentrations.

CLINICAL MANIFESTATIONS AND DIAGNOSTIC EVALUATION. With exposure to high airborne hydrogen sulfide concentrations, sudden onset of coma and respiratory depression leading rapidly to apnea and death are characteristic [86,119]. Neurologic effects, ranging from agitation to somnolence, may be noted [86,129]. Generalized seizures can also occur [119].

Noncardiogenic pulmonary edema is quite common in serious exposures, and metabolic acidosis may be present [86,119], although it is usually less severe than in cyanide poisoning. A variety of nonspecific effects, such as headache, nausea, vomiting, weakness, and fatigue, may be seen [86]. Irritant effects may be manifested as conjunctivitis, sore throat, dyspnea, cough, or hemoptysis [86,118,129].

In a series of 221 patients with occupational hydrogen sulfide poisoning, nearly 75 percent were rendered unconscious initially and 13 percent remained comatose at the time of emergency department presentation [119]. Noncardiogenic pulmonary edema was present in 20 percent of these workers. Overall, there was a 6 percent mortality in this group, with 5 percent of these patients pronounced dead on arrival at the emergency department [119].

Although many victims of acute hydrogen sulfide poisoning recover completely, chronic vegetative states and delayed onset of other neurologic sequelae (e.g., encephalopathies, motor dysfunction, disorders of hearing and vision, permanent retrograde amnesia) have been described following significant poisoning [86,88,118,125,133–136]. Neurologic sequelae have been reported in hydrogen sulfide-poisoned patients who did not lose consciousness [136]. One case of mild pulmonary fibrosis with dyspnea on exertion and mild decreases in lung volumes and carbon monoxide diffusing capacity developed 3 weeks following hydrogen sulfide poisoning with irritant effects but no loss of consciousness [137].

There are no specific laboratory assays available to diagnose hydrogen sulfide intoxication emergently, although blood sulfide levels may be measured to confirm the diagnosis, especially in fatal cases [118,138]. The laboratory abnormalities noted in cyanide poisoning may also be seen in hydrogen sulfide poisoning and should arouse suspicion for both diagnoses. An arterial percent O_2 saturation gap has been described in one hydrogen sulfide poisoning victim [86], although whether this was due to generation of sulfhemoglobin or some other abnormal hemoglobin in debatable [139].

A history of exposure to natural sources or industrial processes that use or generate hydrogen sulfide is the best clue to the diagnosis. An odor of rotten eggs or sulfur may be present on the breath, the patient's clothing, or a freshly drawn tube of blood.

MANAGEMENT

Supportive Treatment. Hydrogen sulfide poisoning victims should be rapidly removed from the toxic atmosphere to fresh air. Rescuers must wear a self-contained breathing apparatus when entering any area with possible high airborne hydrogen sulfide concentrations, to avoid becoming secondary victims [86,124,126]. Exposed eyes should be copiously flushed with tepid water or normal saline. An ophthalmologic examination should be done if significant conjunctival irritation or vesiculation is present.

Supplemental oxygen should be administered to all hydrogen sulfide-poisoned patients. Endotracheal intubation and assisted ventilation may be required. If noncardiogenic pulmonary edema develops, mechanical ventilation and PEEP may be necessary. Continuous ECG and frequent vital signs monitoring is essential. Seizures and pulse and blood pressure abnormalities should be treated with standard agents. Arterial blood gases and chest films should also be monitored. Sodium bicarbonate should be used to correct metabolic acidosis.

Antidotal Therapy. Amyl and sodium nitrite have been used as specific hydrogen sulfide antidotes [86], although this practice is somewhat controversial and some authors have stated that nitrites may be efficacious only if administered within a few minutes after hydrogen sulfide exposure [118]. Other authors have noted little benefit from nitrite administration in hydrogen sulfide-poisoned patients [119], and some have stated that supportive treatment and supplemental oxygen are sufficient [140]. The antidotal mechanism of action is presumably induction of methemoglobin, which has a greater affinity for hydrogen sulfide than cytochrome oxidase [131]. In in vitro studies, methemoglobin reversed cytochrome oxidase inhibition [131], although spontaneous dissociation of the methemoglobin-hydrogen sulfide complex occurs rapidly [141].

Mice and rats were protected against experimental sulfide poisoning by administration of sodium nitrite [89,90,142]. Hydrogen sulfide-poisoned patients have taken longer to regain consciousness when not administered nitrites, which suggests there is some efficacy of this treatment [86,87,88,140].

Amyl nitrite given by inhalation may be useful as a first aid measure. Sodium nitrite should be administered to hydrogen sulfide-poisoned patients who have not regained consciousness by the time of hospital arrival. The dosing regimens described above for cyanide poisoning should be used and the same precautions observed.

Other Treatments. Hyperbaric oxygen therapy has been suggested as a treatment for hydrogen sulfide poisoning. In experiments with rats, the best results were seen with a combination of sodium nitrite and HBO [142]. Four reported patients with hydrogen sulfide poisoning poorly responsive to other therapies were treated with HBO. Three of these victims were treated successfully, while the fourth had probably suffered brain death before arriving at the hospital [143–146]. Hyperbaric oxygen therapy should be reserved for patients not responding to supportive care and nitrite treatment.

Disposition. All patients rendered unconscious and those developing pneumonitis or pulmonary edema should be admitted to an ICU for monitoring and supportive treatment. Those with less severe toxicity should be observed in a controlled setting until all symptoms have resolved. Patients with severe poisoning, especially coma, should have periodic outpatient follow-up for several weeks to screen for possible neurologic or pulmonary sequelae. Neuropsychologic testing and measurement of the P-300 event-related potential latency may be helpful in evaluating patients with neurologic sequelae [134].

Methemoglobin Inducers

Methemoglobin is hemoglobin with the iron oxidized to the ferric (Fe^{3+}) state rather than in the normal, reduced ferrous (Fe^{2+}) state [47]. Methemoglobin is formed from deoxyhemoglobin and is incapable of binding and transporting oxygen [148]. Methemoglobinemia can be divided into three classes: physiologic, congenital, and acquired [149].

Physiologic methemoglobinemia is a normal condition, with approximately 1 percent of total hemoglobin in the oxidized or "met" state [150,151]. To maintain this normal 99:1 (hemoglobin:methemoglobin) ratio, two physiologic mechanisms operate. The first is reduction of oxidizing compounds by reactions with glutathione, sulfhydryl compounds, and ascorbic acid or by the enzymes glutathione reductase and catalase [152,153]. The second mechanism is the enzymatic reduction of methemoglobin back to normal hemoglobin, in which glutathione and ascorbic acid reactions play only a minor role [154,155].

The majority of methemoglobin reducing activity (67–95%)

normally resides in a nicotinamide adenine dinucleotide (NADH)-dependent methemoglobin reductase, with only about 5 percent or less of normal reducing capacity provided by a nicotinamide adenine dinucleotide phosphate (NADPH)-dependent methemoglobin reductase [154,156]. Methylene blue is a cofactor for the NADPH-dependent enzyme and can cause a marked increase in its normally insignificant activity [157,158]. The methemoglobin reductases may be either separate enzymes or two different active sites on the same molecule [159].

Congenital methemoglobinemias are rare, involving either an abnormal hemoglobin (hemoglobin M disease) or a deficiency of NADH-dependent methemoglobin reductase [157,160, 161,162]. Patients heterozygous for adult hemoglobin M disease maintain methemoglobin concentrations of 25 to 30 percent, and treatment with ascorbic acid or methylene blue is not effective [160,163]. Two rare cases of neonatal methemoglobinemia due to a mutant alpha-chain fetal hemoglobin M disease were reported; methemoglobinemia and cyanosis resolved at about 5 weeks of age in both patients, as alpha-chain synthesis was replaced by beta-chain synthesis [164]. Patients with NADH-dependent methemoglobin reductase deficiencies may have 10 to 50 percent methemoglobinemia and generally manifest no symptoms other than a cosmetically displeasing cyanosis, which responds to long-term ascorbic acid therapy [147,157].

Heterozygous forms of NADPH-dependent methemoglobin reductase deficiency exist but do not present with clinical cyanosis, because little of the normal physiologic methemoglobin reducing activity requires this enzyme [162]. Some treatment failures in acquired methemoglobinemia may be due to NADPH-dependent reductase deficiency, as methylene blue cannot function as a substitute cofactor when the enzyme itself is inactive [158–162].

PATHOPHYSIOLOGY. *Acquired methemoglobinemia* can be induced by a large number of drugs and chemicals in either therapeutic doses or overdose [147]. Some common methemoglobin-inducing compounds are listed in Table 157-1. These agents may be systemically absorbed following ingestion, inhalation, or dermal exposure [147,165–179]. Compounds that induce methemoglobin may be direct oxidants or may have oxidizing metabolites or intermediates. Concomitant alcohol consumption has been said to aggravate the development of occupational methemoglobinemia [166]. Small increases in the methemoglobin content of banked blood (mean 2.4%) have been noted over a 21-day period [80]. This might be of clinical significance in critically ill patients requiring massive blood transfusions [180], although no cases with such hematologic compromise have been reported.

Patients with the heterozygous form of NADH-dependent methemoglobin reductase deficiency may be predisposed to develop symptomatic methemoglobinemia following exposure to inducing agents [163,165,166,167,181]. Those with NADPH-dependent reductase deficiencies are not predisposed to develop symptomatic methemoglobinemia, because this enzyme normally accounts for only a minor portion of the normal physiologic reducing capacity [162].

Because methemoglobin cannot transport oxygen and causes a leftward shift of the oxyhemoglobin dissociation curve, methemoglobinemia can be considered a functional anemia. It causes decreased oxygen delivery and impairs oxygen unloading from normal oxyhemoglobin at the capillary level [149,182,183]. Clinically apparent cyanosis may be seen with only 1.5 gm of methemoglobin per deciliter of blood, representing about 10 to 20 percent of total hemoglobin in healthy patients [147,149]. In anemic patients, significant methemoglo-

Table 157-1. Some Reported Causes of Acquired Methemoglobinemia

Aniline and derivatives
Aminophenones
4-Aminopropiophenone
Antimalarials
   Chloroquine
   Primaquine
Cetrimide
Chlorates
Cocaine (adulterated with benzocaine)
Copper sulfate
Dapsone
4-Dimethylaminophenol
Exhaust fumes (truck)
Flutamide
Herbicides (some)
Hydroxylamine
Local/topical anesthetics
   Benzocaine
   Lidocaine
   Prilocaine
Metaclopramide
Methylene blue (clinically insignificant amounts)
Naphthalene
Nitrites/nitrates
   Amyl nitrite (inhalation, ingestion)
   Bismuth subnitrate
   Butyl nitrite (inhalation abuse)
   Isobutyl nitrite (inhalation abuse)
   Sodium nitrite
   Silver nitrate (burn therapy)
   Nitrite/nitrate meat preservatives
   Carrots/spinach (infants)
   Nitrate-contaminated well water (infants)
   Industrial nitrate salts
   Nitroglycerin
   Nitrite/nitrate medications
   Contaminated nitrous oxide
      anesthesia canisters
Nitrobenzene
Occupational exposure to:
   Aniline
   Chloroaniline
   Dichloroaniline
   Dinitrobenzene
   Nitroaniline
   Nitrobenzene
   4-Nitrobenzonitrile
   Nitrochlorobenzene
   Nitrotoluidine
   Orthotoluidine
   Paratoluidine
Para-aminosalicylic acid (PAS)
Phenacetin
Phenazopyridine
Resorcinol
Smoke inhalation (enclosed-space fires)
Sodium betanaphthol disulfonate (R salt)
Sulfonamides
Unknown (infants; rarely adults)

Data from references 147,165–179

binemia may occur without apparent cyanosis, and the condition may be more serious since there is a preexisting oxygen-transport deficiency. Metabolic acidosis and cardiac arrhythmias or ischemia may develop secondary to tissue hypoxia.

Most agents that induce methemoglobinemia can also cause hemolytic anemia. Oxidation of hemoglobin protein (*not* iron) causes its precipitation as Heinz bodies, leading to membrane fragility and hemolysis. "Bite cells" may be seen on the peripheral blood smear [184]. Patients with glucose-6-phosphate dehydrogenase (G-6-PD) deficiency do not respond to methylene blue therapy and may develop serious hemolysis if this drug is administered [158]. Some of the same agents that induce methemoglobin may also induce sulfhemoglobinemia [185,186]. Why some individuals develop methemoglobinemia and others develop sulfhemoglobinemia after exposure to the same agent is unknown.

Neonates younger than 4 months are more susceptible than adults to develop methemoglobinemia when exposed to oxidant stresses [187–191]. Fetal hemoglobin is more easily oxidized than adult hemoglobin [189]. The capacity of NADH-dependent methemoglobin reductase in neonates is only about 60 percent of that in adults, and the enzyme in the solubilized (and presumably more active) form is only present in the quantity of about 50 percent of that in normal adults [187]. Neonates may also have a different intestinal flora that more readily converts weak methemoglobin-inducing nitrates to more potent nitrites (the presumed cause of neonatal methemoglobinemia associated with the ingestion of nitrate-contaminated well water) [187,190,192]. In infants, diarrhea increases the rate of nitrite production from nitrate, as well as increasing systemic nitrite absorption, and can contribute to the development of methemoglobinemia [191].

While methemoglobin levels in neonates born to women who have had prilocaine pudendal anesthesia are usually not clinically significant [193,194], one case of neonatal methemoglobinemia was attributed to a maternal pudendal bock [95]. In another report development of neonatal methemoglobinemia was attributed to a combination of maternal lidocaine and prilocaine epidural infusion and use of prilocaine as a local anesthetic for repair of a facial laceration suffered during delivery by cesarean section in the infant [170].

An unexplained syndrome of methemoglobinemia, metabolic acidosis, leukocytosis, vomiting, and diarrhea has been described in 2- to 4-week-old infants [88]. No abnormal hemoglobins, methemoglobin reductase deficiencies, or known exposure to methemoglobin-inducing agents were found in these neonates [188].

TOXICOKINETICS AND TOXICODYNAMICS. Knowledge of the half-life and dose of the methemoglobin-inducing agent may be useful to predict the potential duration of methemoglobinemia, as well as to estimate whether prolonged hospital observation and repeated administration of methylene blue may be required. Doses of agents that may induce methemoglobinemia, however, are generally quite low (e.g., very small amounts of chemical agents; therapeutic or slightly greater amounts of pharmaceuticals).

CLINICAL MANIFESTATIONS AND DIAGNOSTIC EVALUATION. At methemoglobin concentrations of 10 to 15 percent, the only findings may be a dark or chocolate brown appearance of the blood and central cyanosis involving the proximal limbs and trunk [86]. This cyanosis is not associated with evidence of cardiac or respiratory compromise and does not respond to administration of 100% oxygen [149]. Patients usually appear much less ill than would be expected with a similar degree of cyanosis due to cardiac or respiratory compromise.

In healthy workers, methemoglobin levels as high as 50 to 65 percent have been associated with only headache and dizziness [147,166]. More commonly, dyspnea, fatigue, lethargy, dizziness, headache, and syncopal episodes are seen with levels between 20 and 45 percent, and increasing impairment of the sensorium may occur at 45 to 55 percent [147,149]. Conversely, one patient with severe cardiopulmonary disease and anemia secondary to AIDS developed cyanosis and marked respiratory distress with a methemoglobin level of only 8.2 percent while being treated with dapsone; substantial improvement followed treatment with methylene blue [196]. Patients with anemia or cardiopulmonary compromise may be more severely affected than individuals with normal cardiopulmonary status or normal hemoglobin concentrations [149,196].

Patients with methemoglobin concentrations ranging from 55 to 70 percent can develop coma, generalized seizures, hemodynamic instability, and cardiac arrhythmias [147,149]. A high incidence of fatality is seen in patients, especially children, with levels in excess of 70 percent [147,149,168,197]. Hemolytic anemia may occur concomitantly or be delayed in onset for 2 to 3 days; hemolysis can produce jaundice or renal failure.

Sulfhemoglobinemia is most often a benign condition in persons with hemoglobin A but could cause sickling in those with hemoglobin S [198]. Clinical cyanosis may be seen in patients with a sulfhemoglobin concentration of 5 percent or greater [199].

A presumptive diagnosis of methemoglobinemia can be made by examining a freshly drawn tube of blood for a dark or chocolate brown color or by placing a drop of the patient's blood alongside a normal control on filter paper; when greater than 15 percent methemoglobin is present, the patient's sample will dry to a deep brown compared with normal blood. It may, however, be difficult to appreciate such subtle color differences, which could lead to delayed diagnosis [200]. Another bedside test involves bubbling oxygen through a blood sample; those containing deoxyhemoglobin rapidly turn bright red, while samples with methemoglobin will not. Alternatively, a venous blood sample may be diluted by 1:100 with de-ionized water and a crystal of potassium cyanide added; in the presence of methemoglobin, the cyanide reacts, producing bright pink cyanmethemoglobin [197].

When clinical suspicion of methemoglobinemia exists, methemoglobin levels should be measured with a co-oximeter. Sulfhemoglobin is usually falsely reported as methemoglobin by this instrument [199,201,202]. A false positive methemoglobinemia may be found if normal blood specimens are heated, as this can produce a measurable increase in methemoglobin levels, followed by a slow decline [203]. Samples should be analyzed as soon as possible, because methemoglobin is rapidly reduced by erythrocyte methemoglobin reductase unless samples are stored frozen [204]. However, when samples are stored at $-30°C$ without a cryoprotectant, autoxidation and generation of low levels of methemoglobin may occur; storage at $-30°C$ with a cryoprotectant or at $-80°C$ or $-196°C$ without a cryoprotectant prevents artefactual methemoglobin formation [204].

An arterial percent O_2 saturation gap (a difference between calculated percent O_2 saturation and co-oximeter-measured percent O_2 saturation) is a clue to the presence of some non-oxygen-transporting hemoglobin derivatives, such as carboxyhemoglobin, methemoglobin, or sulfhemoglobin [79]. Arterial percent O_2 saturations measured by pulse oximeters or blood gas instruments other than co-oximeters may be unreliable, especially following administration of methylene blue [177,201, 205–210].

Arterial blood gases should be followed closely in all patients with suspected methemoglobinemia. Because of the possible development of hemolytic anemia, hemoglobin and hematocrit, urinalysis, renal function tests, and plasma free hemoglobin levels should be monitored in patients with clinically significant methemoglobin levels or serious illness.

Measuring blood levels of methemoglobin-inducing agents is usually of no value in guiding therapy. However, identification of the offending substance should be attempted so the patient can be warned to avoid future contact. Blood nitrate levels are usually elevated in children with infantile methemoglobinemia, although the relationship between nitrate and methemoglobin levels is not linear at lower nitrate concentrations [191].

MANAGEMENT

Supportive Treatment. Supplemental oxygen should be administered to all patients with methemoglobinemia to maximize tissue oxygen delivery by remaining functional hemoglobin. Restricted activity is advisable, as exertion can exacerbate symptoms. Asymptomatic or only mildly symptomatic patients with methemoglobin levels of 30 percent or less may not require further interventions, as methemoglobin will be reduced back to normal hemoglobin over approximately 24 to 72 hours. In mild cases secondary to therapeutic drug administration, simply discontinuing the offending medication may be adequate treatment [184].

Gastrointestinal decontamination procedures might help prevent further absorption of ingested methemoglobin-inducing agents. Multiple-dose activated charcoal may increase the elimination rate of dapsone. Patients exposed by inhalation should be moved from the toxic atmosphere as rapidly as possible and administered supplemental oxygen with assisted ventilation, if required. Exposed skin should be thoroughly decontaminated with repeated soap and water washes.

Serial methemoglobin levels should be monitored. For accurate results, they must be assayed as soon as blood is obtained, because methemoglobin will be reduced back to normal hemoglobin over a few hours by erythrocyte methemoglobin reductase [204]. Continuous ECG and frequent vital signs monitoring is necessary in patients with moderate to severe symptoms. Pulse oximetry is unreliable for monitoring oxygenation in this situation [201,205–210]. A brisk urine output should be maintained and the patient observed for possible jaundice or renal injury if hemolysis develops.

Standard anticonvulsant or antiarrhythmic therapy may be needed in severe poisonings. If exposure to a local anesthetic has caused methemoglobinemia, it is advisable to choose an antiarrhythmic agent other than lidocaine. Airway support and mechanical ventilation may be necessary if coma or circulatory collalpse develops. Metabolic acidosis should be corrected with sodium bicarbonate.

Antidotal Therapy. Specific therapy for methemoglobinemia is administration of intravenous methylene blue (tetramethylthionine chloride), in a dose of 0.1 to 0.2 ml per kilogram of a 1% solution (1–2 mg/kg) over 5 minutes [147,151,201]. The similarity of the numerical values of these different units makes 10-fold dosing errors possible; calculations should be carefully checked before the drug is administered. The average adult requires one to two 100-mg ampules of methylene blue. In refractory cases or when methemoglobinemia recurs, additional doses may be administered as needed. The total dose of methylene blue usually should not exceed 7 mg per kilogram [211].

A continuous methylene blue infusion at a rate of 1 mg/kg/hr was used in one case of dapsone-induced methemoglobinemia [212]. Continuous infusions are not routinely recommended. Methylene blue may itself induce clinically insignificant levels of methemoglobin (up to 7%) [213,214], but this is not a reason to withhold indicated therapy. Toluidine blue is an alternate antidote used in some European countries.

Methylene blue is not effective in individuals with G-6-PD or NADPH-dependent methemoglobin reductase deficiency [158]. It may provoke serious hemolytic anemia if given to patients with G-6-PD deficiency and is contraindicated in such patients [158]. Other side effects include blue or green urine discoloration, dysuria, anxiety, and substernal chest discomfort [213]. Patients with sulfhemoglobinemia also do not respond to methylene blue administration [185,186,198,199]. Only the normal processes of red cell destruction and replacement will resolve sulfhemoglobinemia [215].

Long-term oral therapy with ascorbic acid is useful for treating cosmetically displeasing cyanosis in patients with NADH-dependent methemoglobin reductase deficiency. Ascorbic acid alone is not useful for the acute treatment of acquired methemoglobinemia because its action is too slow [191]. It has been used in conjunction with methylene blue in some cases, although with questionable efficacy [216].

Other Treatments. Transfusion or exchange transfusion may be necessary if massive hemolysis occurs. In severe methemoglobinemia, exchange transfusion can be lifesaving, especially in children with methemoglobin levels in excess of 70 percent and in chlorate poisoning, which may be poorly responsive to methylene blue therapy. Hyperbaric oxygen therapy also can be used in severe cases, because sufficient oxygen can be dissolved directly in the plasma to support life [15].

DISPOSITION. Patients with methemoglobinemia should be observed in a controlled setting until all signs and symptoms have fully resolved and methemoglobin levels are decreasing without specific therapy. All patients should be rechecked 3 to 5 days following the initial insult for the presence of hemolysis. If CNS or respiratory depression, circulatory instability, or cardiac arrhythmias are present, the patient should be admitted to an ICU. Those with suicidal intent require close observation and psychiatric evaluation. Patients must be cautioned to avoid further contact with the offending agent. Infants developing methemoglobinemia from nitrate-contaminated wells must have an alternate source of drinking water [187,190,191]. Patients with confirmed methemoglobinemia who do not respond to methylene blue therapy should be evaluated for the presence of hemoglobin M disease, methemoglobin reductase deficiency, or G-6-PD deficiency [149].

References

1. Kizer KW: Toxic inhalations. *Emerg Med Clin North Am* 2:649, 1984.
2. Hall AH, Rumack BH: Clinical toxicology of cyanide. *Ann Emerg Med* 15:1067, 1986.
3. Hall AH, Rumack BH, Schaffer MI, Linden CH: Clinical toxicology of cyanide: North American clinical experiences, in Ballantine B, Marrs TC (eds): *Clinical and Experimental Toxicology of Cyanides.* Bristol, Weight, 1987, p 312.
4. Hall AH, Doutre WH, Ludden T, et al: Nitrite/thiosulfate treated acute cyanide poisoning: Estimated kinetics after antidote. *Clin Toxicol* 25:121, 1987.

5. Blanc P, Hogan M, Mallin K, et al: Cyanide intoxication among silver-reclaiming workers. *JAMA* 253:367, 1985.
6. Hartung R: Cyanides and nitriles, in Clayton GD, Clayton FE (eds): *Patty's Industrial Hygiene and Toxicology.* vol. 2. 3rd ed. New York, Wiley, 1982, p 4845.
7. Krieg A, Saxena K: Cyanide poisoning from metal cleaning solutions. *Ann Emerg Med* 16:582, 1987.
8. Haasnoot K, van Vught AJ, Meulenbelt J, et al: Acute cyanide poisoning in an infant. *Ned Tijdschr Geneeskd* 133:1753, 1989.
9. Wolnik KA, Fricke FL, Bonnin E, et al: The Tylenol tampering incident: Tracing the source. *Anal Chem* 56:466, 1984.
10. Murphy DH: Cyanide-tainted Tylenol: What pharmacists can learn. *Am Pharm* ES26:19, 1986.
11. Cyanide poisonings associated with over-the-counter medication—Washington State, 1991. *MMWR* 40:161, 1991.
12. Binder L, Fredrickson L: Poisonings in laboratory personnel and health care professionals. *Am J Emerg Med* 9:11, 1991.
13. Heintz B, Bock TA, Kierdorf H, et al: Cyanid-intoxikation: Behandlung mit hiperoxigenation und natriumthiosulfat. *Dtsch Med Wochenschr* 115:1100, 1990.
14. Jones J, McMullen MJ, Dougherty J: Toxic smoke inhalation: Cyanide poisoning in fire victims. *Am J Emerg Med* 5:317, 1987.
15. Hart GB, Strauss MB, Lennon PA, Whitcraft DD: Treatment of smoke inhalation by hyperbaric oxygen. *J Emerg Med* 3:211, 1985.
16. Clark CJ, Campbell D, Reid WH: Blood carboxyhaemoglobin and cyanide levels in fire survivors. *Lancet* 1:1332, 1981.
17. Symington IS, Anderson RA, Thomson I, et al: Cyanide exposure in fires. *Lancet* 2:91, 1978.
18. Baud FJ, Barriot P, Toffis V, et al: Elevated blood cyanide concentrations in victims of smoke inhalation. *N Engl J Med* 325:1761, 1991.
19. Mayes RW: The toxicological examination of the victims of the British Air Tours Boeing 737 accident at Manchester in 1985. *J Forensic Sci* 36:179, 1991.
20. Barr SJ: Chemical warfare agents. *Top Emerg Med* 7:62, 1985.
21. Hall AH, Linden CH, Kulig KW, Rumack BH: Cyanide poisoning from laetrile: Role of nitrite therapy. *Pediatrics* 78:269, 1988.
22. Sayre JW, Kaymakcalan S: Cyanide poisoning from apricot seeds among children in central Turkey. *N Engl J Med* 270:1113, 1964.
23. Rubino MJ: Cyanide toxicity: Report of a case. *Poison Info Bull* 3:1, 1978.
24. Lasch EE, El Shawa R: Multiple cases of cyanide poisoning by apricot kernals in children from Gaza. *Pediatrics* 68:5, 1981.
25. Shragg TA, Albertson TE, Fisher CJ: Cyanide poisoning after bitter almond ingestion. *West J Med* 136:65, 1983.
26. Amdur ML: Accidental group exposure to acetonitrile: A clinical study. *J Occup Med* 1:627, 1959.
27. Dequidt J, Furon D, Wattel F, et al: Les intoxications par l'acetonitrile: A propos d'un cas mortel. *J Eur Toxicol* 7:91, 1974.
28. Bismuth C, Baud FJ, Djeghout H, et al: Cyanide poisoning from propionitrile exposure. *J Emerg Med* 5:191, 1987.
29. Cameron GR, Doniger CR, Hughes AWM: The toxicity of lauryl thiocyanate and n-butyl-carbitol-thiocyanate (Lethane 384). *J Pathol Bacteriol* 49:363, 1939.
30. Coulter E, Creery RDG: "Lethane" poisoning: Report of a fatal case. *Br Med J* 1:379, 1953.
31. Guy AG: Aspiration pneumonia due to "Lethane" hair oils. *Br Med J* 2:94, 1951.
32. von Oettingen WF, Heuper WC, Deichmann-Gruebler W: The pharmacological action and pathological effects of alkyl rhodanates in relation to their chemical constitution and physical-chemical properties. *J Ind Hygiene* 18:310, 1936.
33. Espinoza OB, Perez M, Ramirez MS: Bitter cassava poisoning in eight children: A case report. *Vet Hum Toxicol* 34:65, 1992.
34. Akintonwa A, Tunwashe OL: Fatal cyanide poisoning from cassava-based meal. *Hum Exp Toxicol* 11:47, 1992.
35. Andrews JM, Sweeney ES, Grey TC, et al: The biohazard potential of cyanide poisoning during postmortem examination. *J Forensic Sci* 34:1280, 1989.
36. Forrest ARW, Galloway JH, Slater DN: The cyanide poisoning necropsy: An appraisal of risk factors. *J Clin Pathol* 45:544, 1992.
37. Cottrell JE, Casthely P, Brodie JD, et al: Prevention of nitroprusside-induced cyanide toxicity with hydroxocobalamin. *N Engl J Med* 298:809, 1978.
38. Schulz V, Gross R, Pasch T, et al: Cyanide toxicity of sodium nitroprusside in therapeutic use with and without sodium thiosulfate. *Klin Wochenschr* 60:1393, 1982.
39. Vessey CJ, Cole PV, Linnell JC, Wilson J: Some metabolic effects of sodium nitroprusside in man. *Br Med J* 2:140, 1974.
40. Linakis JG, Lacouture PG, Woolf A: Monitoring cyanide and thiocyanate concentrations during infusion of sodium nitroprusside in children. *Pediatr Cardiol* 12:214, 1991.
41. Curry SC, Arnold-Capell P: Nitroprusside, nitroglycerin, and angiotensin-converting enzyme inhibitors. *Crit Care Clin* 7:555, 1991.
42. Lundquist P, Rosling H, Tyden H: Cyanide release from sodium nitroprusside during coronary bypass in hypothermia. *Acta Anaesthesiol Scand* 33:686, 1989.
43. Wright IH, Vesey CJ: Acute poisoning with gold cyanide. *Anesthesia* 41:936, 1986.
44. Singh BM, Coles N, Lewis P, et al: The metabolic effects of fatal cyanide poisoning. *Postgrad Med* 65:923, 1989.
45. Fernando GC, Busuttil A: Cyanide ingestion: Case studies of four suicides. *Am J Forensic Med Pathol* 12:241, 1991.
46. Vogel SN, Sultan TR, Ten Eyck RP: Cyanide poisoning. *Clin Toxicol* 18:367, 1982.
47. Christel D, Eyer P, Hegemann M, et al: Pharmacokinetics of cyanide poisoning in dogs, and the effects of 4-dimethylaminophenol or thiosulfate. *Arch Toxicol* 38:177, 1977.
48. Ballantyne B: Artifacts in the definition of toxicity by cyanide and cyanogens. *Fundam Appl Toxicol* 3:400, 1983.
49. Sylvester DM, Hayton WL, Morgan RL, Way JL: Effects of thiosulfate on cyanide pharmacokinetics in dogs. *Toxicol Appl Pharmacol* 69:265, 1983.
50. Selden BS, Clark RF, Curry SC: Elimination kinetics of cyanide after acute KCN ingestion (abstract). *Vet Hum Toxicol* 32:361, 1990.
51. Michaelis HC, Clemens C, Kijewski H, et al: Acetonitrile serum concentrations and cyanide blood levels in a case of suicidal oral acetonitrile ingestion. *J Toxicol Clin Toxicol* 29:447, 1991.
52. Johnson WS, Hall AH, Rumack BH: Cyanide poisoning successfully treated without "therapeutic methemoglobin levels." *Am J Emerg Med* 7:437, 1989.
53. DiNapoli J, Hall AH, Drake R, Rumack BH: Cyanide and arsenic poisoning by intravenous injection. *Ann Emerg Med* 18:308, 1989.
54. Turchen SG, Manoguerra AS, Whitney C: Severe cyanide poisoning from the ingestion of acetonitrile-containing cosmetic. *Am J Emerg Med* 9:264, 1991.
55. Bonnichsen R, Maely AC: Poisoning by volatile compounds. *J Forensic Sci* 11:516, 1966.
56. Baselt RC, Cravey RH: *Disposition of Toxic Drugs and Chemicals in Man.* 3rd ed. Chicago, Year Book, 1989.
57. Racle JP, Chausset R, Dissait F, Fontanella JM: L'intoxication cyanhydrique aigue: Aspects toxicologiques, cliniques et therapeutiques. (Rapport d'une observation traitée avec succès par hydroxocobalamine). *Rev Med Clermont-Ferrand* 5:371, 1976.
58. Bonsall JL: Survival without sequelae following exposure to 500 mg/m^3 of hydrogen cyanide. *Hum Toxicol* 5:57, 1984.
59. Yacoub M, Faure J, Morena H, et al: L'intoxication cyanhydrique aigue: Données actuelles sur le metabolisme du cyanure et le traitement par hydroxocobalamine. *J Eur Toxicol* 7:22, 1974.
60. Bismuth C, Cantineau J-P, Pontal P, et al: Priorité de l'oxygenation dans l'intoxication cyanhydrique: A propos de 25 cas. *J Toxicol Med* 4:107, 1984.
61. Dodds C, McKnight C: Cyanide toxicity after immersion and the hazards of dicobalt edetate. *Br Med J* 291:785, 1985.
62. Feihl F, Domenighetti G, Perret C: Intoxication massive au cyanure avec evolution favorable. *Schweiz Med Wochenschr* 112:1280, 1982.
63. Graham DL, Laman D, Theodore J, Robin ED: Acute cyanide poisoning complicated by lactic acidosis and pulmonary edema. *Arch Intern Med* 137:1051, 1977.
64. Buchanan IS, Dhamee MS, Griffiths FED, Yeoman MB: Abnormal fundus appearance in a case of poisoning by a cyanide capsule. *Med Sci Law* 16:29, 1976.
65. Peden NR, Taha A, McSorley PD, et al: Industrial exposure to hydrogen cyanide: Implications for treatment. *Br Med J* 293:538, 1986.
66. Carvati EM, Litovitz TL: Pediatric cyanide intoxication and death from an acetonitrile-containing cosmetic. *JAMA* 260:3470, 1988.

67. Kurt TL, Day LC, Reed WS, Gandy W: Cyanide poisoning from glue-on nail remover. *Am J Emerg Med* 9:271, 1991.

68. Losek JD, Rock AL, Boldt RR: Cyanide poisoning from a cosmetic nail remover. *Pediatrics* 88:337, 1991.

69. Geller RJ, Ekins BR, Iknoian RC: Cyanide toxicity from acetonitrile-containing false nail remover. *Am J Emerg Med* 9:268, 1991.

70. Bourrelier J, Paulet G: Intoxication cyanhydrique consecutive à des brulures graves par cyanure de sodium fondu: Sur trois cas traites par EDTA cobaltique. *Presse Med* 22:1013, 1971.

71. Murray VSG, Volans GN, Gillis C: Cyanide poisoning: The United Kingdom National Poisons Unit experience, 1963–1984, in Ballantyne B, Marrs TC (eds): *Clinical and Experimental Toxicology of Cyanides.* Bristol, Wright, 1987, pp 334–347.

72. Bryson DD: Acute industrial cyanide intoxication and its treatment, in Ballantyne B, Marrs TC (eds): *Clinical and Experimental Toxicology of Cyanides.* Bristol, Wright, 1987, pp 348–358.

73. Ballantyne B: Acute systemic toxicity of cyanide by topical application to the eye. *J Toxicol Cutan Ocular Toxicol* 2:119, 1983.

74. Jouglard J, Nava G, Botta A, et al: A propos d'une intoxication aigue par le cyanure traite par l'hydroxocobalamine. *Marseille Med* 12:617, 1974.

75. Jouglard J, Fagot G, Dequigne B, Arlaud J-A: L'intoxication cyanhydrique aigue et son traitement d'urgence. *Marseille Med* 9:571, 1971.

76. Uitti RJ, Rajput AH, Ashenhurst EM, Rozdilsky B: Cyanide-induced parkinsonism: A clinicopathologic report. *Neurology* 35:921, 1985.

77. Carella F, Grassi MP, Savoiardo M, et al: Dystonic-Parkinsonian syndrome after cyanide poisoning: Clinical and MRI findings. *J Neurol Neurosurg Psychiatry* 51:1345, 1988.

78. Rosenberg NL, Myers JA, Martin WRW: Cyanide-induced parkinsonism: Clinical, MRI, and 6-fluorodopa PET studies. *Neurology* 39:142, 1989.

79. Grandas F, Artieda J, Obeso JA: Clinical and CT scan findings in a case of cyanide intoxication. *Mov Disord* 4:188, 1989.

80. Feldman JM, Feldman MD: Sequelae of attempted suicide by cyanide ingestion: A case report. *Int J Psychiatry Med* 20:173, 1990.

81. Tassan H, Joyon D, Richard T, et al: Potassium cyanide poisoning treated with hydroxocobalamin. *Ann Fr Anesth Reanim* 9:383, 1990.

82. Lundquist P, Sorbo B: Rapid determination of toxic cyanide concentrations in blood. *Clin Chem* 35:617, 1989.

83. Curry SC, Patrick HC: Lack of evidence for a percent saturation gap in cyanide poisoning. *Ann Emerg Med* 20:523, 1991.

84. Johnson RP, Mellors JW: Arteriolization of venous blood gases: A clue to the diagnosis of cyanide poisoning. *J Emerg Med* 6:401, 1988.

85. Paulet G: Valeur et mechanisme d'action de l'oxygenotherapie dans le traitement de l'intoxication cyanhydrique. *Arch Int Physiol Biochem* 63:340, 1955.

86. Hoidal CR, Hall AH, Robinson MD, et al: Hydrogen sulfide poisoning from toxic inhalations of roofing asphalt fumes. *Ann Emerg Med* 15:826, 1986.

87. Peters JW: Hydrogen sulfide poisoning in a hospital setting. *JAMA* 246:1588, 1981.

88. Stine RJ, Slosberg B, Beachman BE: Hydrogen sulfide intoxication: A case report and discussion of treatment. *Arch Intern Med* 85:756, 1976.

89. Smith RP, Kruszyna R, Kruszyna H: Management of acute sulfide poisoning: Effects of oxygen, thiosulfate, and nitrite. *Arch Environ Health* 166:166, 1976.

90. Scheler W, Kabisch R: Uber die Antagonistiche Beeinflussung der Akutan H$_2$S Vergiftung bei der Mass Durch Methamoglobinbildner. *Acta Biol Med Ger* 11:194, 1963.

91. Berlin CM: Treatment of cyanide poisoning in children. *Pediatrics* 46:793, 1970.

92. Wurzburg H: Treatment of cyanide poisoning in an industrial setting (abstract). *Vet Hum Toxicol* 33:373, 1991.

93. Brivet F, Delfraissy JF, Duche M, et al: Acute cyanide poisoning: Recovery with non-specific supportive therapy. *Intensive Care Med* 9:33, 1983.

94. Ortega JA, Creek JE: Acute cyanide poisoning following administration of laetrile enemas. *J Pediatr* 93:1059, 1978.

95. Moertel CG, Ames MM, Kovack JS, et al: A pharmacological and toxicological study of amygdalin. *JAMA* 245:591, 1981.

96. Morse LD, Boros L, Findley PA: More on cyanide poisoning from laetrile. *N Engl J Med* 301:892, 1979.

97. Litovitz TL, Larkin RF, Myers RAM: Cyanide poisoning treated with hyperbaric oxygen. *Am J Emerg Med* 1:94, 1983.

98. Moss M, Khalil N, Gray J: Deliberate self-poisoning with laetrile. *Can Med Assoc J* 124:1126, 1981.

99. Way JL, End E, Sheehy MH, et al: Effects of oxygen on cyanide intoxication. IV. Hyperbaric oxygen. *Toxicol Appl Pharmacol* 22:415, 1972.

100. Anderson AH: Experimental studies on the pharmacology of activated charcoal. *Acta Pharmacol* 2:69, 1946.

101. Lambert RJ, Kindler BL, Schaeffer DJ: The efficacy of superactivated charcoal in treating rats exposed to a lethal oral dose of potassium cyanide. *Ann Emerg Med* 17:595, 1988.

102. Hall AH, Kulig KW, Rumack BH: Suspected cyanide poisoning in smoke inhalation: Complications of sodium nitrite therapy. *J Toxicol Clin Exp* 9:3, 1989.

103. Viana C, Cagnoli H, Cedan J: L'action du nitrite de sodium dans l'intoxication par les cyanures. *Compt Rend Soc Biol* 115:1649, 1934.

104. Birse GS: Cyanide poisoning. *J Am Osteopath Assoc* 83:811, 1984.

105. Perrson H, Meredith TJ, Jacobsen D et al (eds): *Antidotes for Poisoning by Cyanide.* Cambridge, Cambridge University Press, 1993.

106. Ikankovich AD, Braverman B, Stephens TS, et al: Sodium thiosulfate disposition in humans: Relation to sodium nitroprusside toxicity. *Anesthesiology* 58:11, 1983.

107. Forsyth JC, Mueller PD, Becker CE, et al: Hydroxocobalamin as a cyanide antidote: Safety, efficacy, and pharmacokinetics in heavily smoking normal volunteers. *Clin Toxicol* 31:277, 1993.

108. Kirk M, Kulig K, Rumack BH: Methemoglobin and cyanide kinetics in smoke inhalation (abstract). *Vet Hum Toxicol* 31:353, 1989.

109. Trapp W: Massive cyanide poisoning with recovery: A Boxing Day story. *Can Med Assoc J* 102:517, 1970.

110. Takano T, Miyazaki Y, Nashimoto I, Kobayashi K: Effect of hyperbaric oxygen on cyanide intoxication: In situ changes in intracellular oxidation reduction. *Undersea Biomed Res* 7:191, 1980.

111. Meyer GW, Hart GB, Strauss MB: Hyperbaric oxygen therapy for acute smoke inhalation injuries. *Postgrad Med* 89:221, 1991.

112. Wesson DE, Foley R, Sabatini S, et al: Treatment of acute cyanide intoxication with hemodialysis. *Am J Nephrol* 5:121, 1985.

113. Gonzales J, Sabatini S: Cyanide poisoning: Pathophysiology and current approaches to therapy. *Int J Artif Organs* 12:347, 1989.

114. ACGIH: *Documentation of the Threshold Limit Values and Biological Exposure Indices.* 5th ed. Cincinnati, American Conference of Governmental Industrial Hygienists, 1986, p. 318.

115. Sitting M: *Handbook of Toxic and Hazardous Chemicals and Carcinogens.* 2nd ed. Park Ridge, NJ, Noyes, 1985, p 512.

116. Hathaway GJ, Proctor NH, Hughes JP, et al: *Chemical Hazards of the Workplace.* 3rd ed. New York, Van Nostrand Reinhold, 1991, pp 339–340.

117. Deng J-F, Chang S-C: Hydrogen sulfide poisonings in hot-spring reservoir cleaning: Two case reports. *Am J Ind Med* 11:447, 1987.

118. Reiffenstein RJ, Hulbert WC, Roth SH: Toxicology of hydrogen sulfide. *Ann Rev Pharmacol Toxicol* 32:109, 1992.

119. Burnett WW, King EG, Grace M, Hall WF: Hydrogen sulfide poisoning: Review of 5 years' experience. *Can Med Assoc J* 117:1277, 1977.

120. Audeau FM, Gnanaharan C, Davey K: Hydrogen sulphide poisoning associated with pelt processing. *NZ Med J* 98:145, 1985.

121. Luck J, Kaye SB: An unrecognized form of hydrogen sulphide keratoconjunctivitis. *Br J Ind Med* 46:748, 1989.

122. Donham KJ, Knapp LW, Monson R, Gustafson K: Acute toxic exposure to gases from liquid manure. *J Occup Med* 24:142, 1982.

123. Morse DL, Woodbury MA, Rentmeester K, Farmer D: Death caused by fermenting manure. *JAMA* 245:63, 1981.

124. Osbern LN, Cralpo RO: Dung lung: A report of toxic exposure to liquid manure. *Ann Intern Med* 95:312, 1981.

125. Thomas M: Sewer gas: Hydrogen sulfide intoxication. *Clin Toxicol* 2:383, 1969.

126. Oderda GM: Fatality produced by accidental inhalation of drain cleaner fumes. *Clin Toxicol* 8:547, 1975.

127. Gann P, Roseman J: Hazards of metal processing (letter). *JAMA* 248:1580, 1982.

128. Haahtela T, Marttila O, Vilkka V, et al: The South Karelia air pol-

lution study: Acute health effects of malodorous sulfur air pollutants released by a pulp mill. *Am J Public Health* 82:603, 1992.

129. Smith RP, Gosselin RE: Hydrogen sulfide poisoning. *J Occup Med* 21:93, 1979.

130. Nicholls P, Kim J-K: Sulphide as an inhibitor and electron donor for the cytochrome C oxidase system. *Can J Biochem* 60:613, 1982.

131. Smith L, Kruszyna H, Smith RP: The effect of methemoglobin on the inhibition of cytochrome C oxidase by cyanide, sulfide or azide. *Biochem Pharmacol* 26:2247, 1977.

132. Tavris DR, Field L, Brumback CL: Outbreak of illness due to volatilized asphalt coming from a malfunctioning fluorescent lighting fixture. *Am J Public Health* 74:614, 1984.

133. Matsuo F, Cummins JW, Anderson RE: Neurological sequelae of massive hydrogen sulfide inhalation (letter). *Arch Neurol* 36:451, 1979.

134. Wasch HH, Estrin WJ, Yip P, et al: Prolongation of the P-300 latency associated with hydrogen sulfide exposure. *Arch Neurol* 46:902, 1989.

135. Tvedt B, Edland A, Skyberg K, et al: Delayed neuropsychiatric sequelae after acute hydrogen sulfide poisoning: Affection of motor function, memory, vision and hearing. *Acta Neurol Scand* 84:348, 1991.

136. Tvedt B, Skyberg K, Aaserud O, et al: Brain damage caused by hydrogen sulfide: A follow-up study of six patients. *Am J Ind Med* 20:91, 1991.

137. Parra O, Monso E, Gallego M, et al: Inhalation of hydrogen sulphide: A case of subacute manifestations and long term sequelae. *Br J Ind Med* 48:286, 1991.

138. Jappinen P, Tenhunen R: Hydrogen sulphide poisoning: Blood sulphide concentration and changes in haem metabolism. *Br J Ind Med* 47:283, 1990.

139. Curry SC, Gerkin RD: A patient with sulfhemoglobin? (letter). *Ann Emerg Med* 16:828, 1987.

140. Ravizza AG, Carugo D, Cierchiari EL, et al: The treatment of hydrogen sulfide intoxication: Oxygen versus nitrites. *Vet Hum Toxicol* 24:241, 1982.

141. Beck JF, Bradbury CM, Connors AJ, Donini JC: Nitrite as an antidote for acute hydrogen sulfide intoxication? *Am Ind Hyg Assoc J* 42:805, 1981.

142. Bitterman N, Talmi Y, Lerman A, et al: The effect of hyperbaric oxygen on acute experimental sulfide poisoning in the rat. *Toxicol Appl Pharmacol* 84:325, 1986.

143. Whitcraft DD, Bailey TD, Hart GB: Hydrogen sulfide poisoning treated with hyperbaric oxygen. *J Emerg Med* 3:23, 1985.

144. Smilkstein MJ, Bronstein AC, Pickett IIM, Rumack BH: Hyperbaric oxygen therapy for severe hydrogen sulfide poisoning. *J Emerg Med* 3:27, 1985.

145. Vicas I, Fortin S, Uptigrove OJ, et al: Hydrogen sulfide exposure treated with hyperbaric oxygen (HBO) (abstract). *Vet Hum Toxicol* 31:353, 1989.

146. Al-Mahasneh QM, Cohle SD, Haas E: Lack of response to hyperbaric oxygen in a fatal case of hydrogen sulfide poisoning: A case report (abstract). *Vet Hum Toxicol* 31:353, 1989.

147. Hall AH, Kulig KW, Rumack BH: Drug- and chemical-induced methaemoglobinaemia: Clinical features and management. *Med Toxicol* 1:253, 1986.

148. Strauch B, Buch W, Grey W, Laub D: Successful treatment of methemoglobinemia secondary to silver nitrate therapy. *N Engl J Med* 281:257, 1969.

149. Curry S: Methemoglobinemia. *Ann Emerg Med* 11:214, 1982.

150. Shapiro BA, Cane RD, Harrison RA, et al: Methemoglobin levels in the patient population of an acute general hospital. *Intensive Care Med* 8:295, 1982.

151. Smith RP, Olson MV: Drug-induced methemoglobinemia. *Semin Hematol* 10:253, 1973.

152. Bodansky O: Methemoglobinemia and methemoglobin producing compounds. *Pharmacol Rev* 3:144, 1951.

153. Rossi-Fanelli A, Antonini E, Mondovi B: Ferrihemoglobin reduction in normal and methemoglobinemic subjects. *Clin Chim Acta* 2:476, 1954.

154. Scott EM: Congenital methemoglobinemia due to DPNH-diaphorase, in Buetler E (ed): *Hereditary Disorders of Erythrocyte Metabolism.* New York, Grune & Stratton, 1968, p 102.

155. Mills GC: Hemoglobin catabolism II. The protection of hemoglobin from oxidative breakdown. *J Biol Chem* 229:189, 1957.

156. Scott EM, Duncan IW, Ekstrand V: Reduction of methemoglobin. *Fed Proc* 22:467, 1963.

157. Jaffe E: Hereditary methemoglobinemia associated with abnormalities in the metabolism of erythrocytes. *Am J Med* 41:786, 1966.

158. Rosen PJ, Johnson C, McGehee WG, Beutler E: Failure of methylene blue treatment in toxic methemoglobinemia: Association with glucose-6-phosphate dehydrogenase deficiency. *Ann Intern Med* 75:83, 1971.

159. Miale JB: *Laboratory Medicine Hematology.* St. Louis, CV Mosby, 1977, p 528.

160. Easley JL, Condon BF: Phenacetin-induced methemoglobinemia and renal failure. *Anesthesiology* 41:99, 1974.

161. Jaffe E, Hsieh H-S: DPNH-methemoglobin reductase deficiency and hereditary methemoglobinemia. *Semin Hematol* 8:417, 1971.

162. Sass MD, Caruso CJ, Farhangi M: TPNH-methemoglobin reductase deficiency: A new red-cell enzyme defect. *J Lab Clin Med* 70:760, 1967.

163. O'Donohue WJ, Moss LM, Angelillo VA: Acute methemoglobinemia induced by topical benzocaine and lidocaine. *Arch Intern Med* 140:1508, 1980.

164. Priest JR, Watterson J, Jones RT, et al: Mutant fetal hemoglobin causing cyanosis in a newborn. *Pediatrics* 83:734, 1989.

165. Rumack BH, Spoerke DG: Methemoglobinemia inducers, in *POISINDEX Information System.* (CD-ROM Version). Denver, Micromedex, 1993.

166. Sekimpi DK, Jones RD: Notifications of industrial chemical cyanosis poisoning in the United Kingdom 1961–1980. *Br J Ind Med* 43:272, 1986.

167. Wilson CM, Bird SG, Bocash W, et al: Methemoglobinemia following metaclopramide therapy in an infant. *J Pediatr Gastroenterol Nutr* 6:640, 1987.

168. Ellis M, Hiss Y, Shenkman L: Fatal methemoglobinemia caused by inadvertent contamination of a laxative solution with sodium nitrite. *Isr J Med Sci* 28:289, 1992.

169. Hoffman RS, Sauter D: Methemoglobinemia resulting from smoke inhalation. *Vet Hum Toxicol* 31:168, 1989.

170. Lloyd CJ: Chemically induced methaemoglobinaemia in a neonate. *Br J Oral Maxillofac Surg* 30:63, 1992.

171. Laney RF, Hoffman RS: Methemoglobinemia secondary to automobile exhaust fumes. *Am J Emerg Med* 10:426, 1992.

172. Schott AM, Vial T, Gozzo I, et al: Flutamide-induced methemoglobinemia. *DICP* 25:600, 1991.

173. Monechi G, Fabrizi de Biani G, Colasanti L: A case of methemoglobinemia due to 4-nitrobenzonitrile exposure. *Med Lav* 82:137, 1991.

174. McKinney CD, Postiglione KF, Herold DA: Benzocaine-adulterated street cocaine in association with methemoglobinemia. *Clin Chem* 38:596, 1992.

175. Muchmore EA, Dahl BJ: One blue man with mucositis. *N Engl J Med* 327:133, 1992.

176. Severinghaus JW, Fa-Di X, Spellman MJ: Benzocaine and methemoglobin: Recommended actions (letter). *Anesthesiology* 74:385, 1991.

177. White CD, Weiss LD: Varying presentations of methemoglobinemia: Two cases. *J Emerg Med* 9:45, 1991.

178. Nigam A, Ruddy J, Robin PE: BIPP induced methaemoglobinaemia. *J Laryngol Otol* 105:74, 1991.

179. Forsyth RJ, Moulden A: Methaemoglobinaemia after ingestion of amyl nitrite. *Arch Dis Child* 66:152, 1991.

180. Uchida I, Tashiro C, Koo YH, et al: Carboxyhemoglobin and methemoglobin levels in banked blood. *J Clin Anesth* 2:86, 1990.

181. Cohen RJ, Sachs JR, Wicker DJ, Conrad ME: Methemoglobinemia provoked by malarial chemoprophylaxis in Vietnam. *N Engl J Med* 279:1127, 1968.

182. Wintrobe M (ed): *Clinical Hematology.* 5th ed. Philadelphia, Lea & Febiger, 1981, p 97.

183. Lukens JN: The legacy of well-water methemoglobinemia. *JAMA* 257:2793, 1987.

184. Yoo D, Lessin LS: Drug-associated "bite cell" hemolytic anemia. *Am J Med* 92:243, 1992.

185. Kneezel LD, Kitchens CS: Phenacetin-induced sulfhemoglobine-

mia: Report of a case and review of the literature. *Johns Hopkins Med J* 139:175, 1976.

186. Tursz TH, Bernard JF, Verdier F, Boivin P: Sulfhemoglobine et deficit en glutathione peroxydase. *Nouv Presse Med* 3:1487, 1974.

187. Johnson CJ, Bonrud PA, Dosch TL, et al: Fatal outcome of methemoglobinemia in an infant. *JAMA* 257:2796, 1987.

188. Yano SS, Danish EH, Hsia YE: Transient methemoglobinemia with acidosis in infants. *J Pediatr* 100:415, 1982.

189. Committee on Nutrition: Infant methemoglobinemia: The role of dietary nitrate. *Pediatrics* 46:475, 1970.

190. Comly HH: Cyanosis in infants caused by nitrates in well water. *JAMA* 129:112, 1945.

191. Kross BC, Ayebo AD, Fuortes LJ: Methemoglobinemia: Nitrate toxicity in rural America. *Am Fam Physician* 46:183, 1992.

192. Terblance APS: Health hazards of nitrate in drinking water. *Water SA* 17:77, 1991.

193. Kirschbaum M, Biscoping J, Bachmann B, et al: Fetal methemoglobinemia caused by prilocaine: Is use of prilocaine for pudendal block still justified? *Geburtshilfe Frauenheilkd* 51:228, 1991.

194. Biscoping J, Bachmann B, Kirschbaum M, et al: Does the development of methemoglobin in the newborn infant affect the suitability of prilocaine for pudendal anesthesia? A clinical study in the peripartum phase. *Reg Anaesth* 12:50, 1989.

195. Hrgovic Z: Methemoglobinemia in a newborn infant following pudendal anesthesia with prilocaine: A case report. *Anaesthesiol Intensivther Notfallmed* 25:172, 1990.

196. Gallant GE, Hoehn-Saric E, Smith MD: Respiratory insufficiency from dapsone-induced methemoglobinemia. *AIDS* 5:1392, 1991.

197. Done AK: The toxic emergency. *Emerg Med* 18:283, 1976.

198. Park CM, Nagel RL: Sulfhemoglobinemia: Clinical and molecular aspects. *N Engl J Med* 310:1579, 1984.

199. Lambert M, Sonnet J, Mahieu P, Hassoun A: Delayed sulfhemoglobinemia after acute dapsone intoxication. *J Toxicol Clin Toxicol* 19:45, 1982.

200. Henretig FM, Gribetz B, Kearney T, et al: Interpretation of color change in blood with varying degree of methemoglobinemia. *Clin Toxicol* 26:293, 1988.

201. Seger DL: Methemoglobin forming chemicals, in Sullivan JB, Krieger GR (eds): *Hazardous Materials Toxicology: Clinical Principles of Environmental Health.* Baltimore, Williams & Wilkins, 1992, pp 800–806.

202. Zwart A, Buursma A, Oeseburg B, Zijlstra WG: Determination of hemoglobin derivatives with the IL 282 co-oximeter as compared with a manual spectrophotometric five-wavelength method. *Clin Chem* 27:1903, 1981.

203. Fechner GGP, Gee DJ: Study on the effects of heat on blood and on the post-mortem estimation of carboxyhaemoglobin and methaemoglobin. *Forensic Sci Int* 40:63, 1989.

204. Sato K, Tamaki K, Tsutsumi H, et al: Storage of blood for methemoglobin determination: Comparison of storage with a cryoprotectant at −30°C and without any additions at −80°C or −196°C. *Forensic Sci Int* 45:129, 1990.

205. Barker SJ, Tremper KK, Hyatt J, Zaccari J: Effects of methemoglobinemia on pulse oximetry and mixed venous oximetry. *Anesthesiology* 67:A171, 1987.

206. Rieder HU, Frei FJ, Zbinden AM, Thomson DA: Pulse oximetry in methaemoglobinaemia: Failure to detect low oxygen saturation. *Anaesthesia* 44:326, 1989.

207. Kulick RM: Pulse oximetry. *Pediatr Emerg Care* 3:127, 1987.

208. Marks LF, Desgrand D: Prilocaine associated methemoglobinemia and the pulse oximeter. *Anaesthesia* 46:703, 1991.

209. Schweitzer SA: Spurious pulse oximeter desaturation due to methaemoglobinaemia. *Anesth Intensive Care* 19:269, 1991.

210. Delwood L, O'Flaherty D, Prejean EJ, et al: Methemoglobinemia and its effect on pulse oximetry. *Crit Care Med* 19:988, 1991.

211. Harvey JW, Keitt AS: Studies of the efficacy and potential hazards of methylene blue therapy in aniline-induced methemoglobinemia. *Br J Haematol* 54:29, 1983.

212. Berlin G, Brodin B, Hilden J-O: Acute dapsone intoxication: A case treated with continuous infusion of methylene blue, forced diuresis, and plasma exchange. *J Toxicol Clin Toxicol* 22:537, 1985.

213. Nadler JE, Green H, Rosenbaum A: Intravenous injection of methylene blue in man with reference to its toxic symptoms and effect on the electrocardiogram. *Am J Med Sci* 188:15, 1934.

214. Whitwam JG, Taylor AR, White JM: Potential hazard of methylene blue. *Anaesthesia* 34:181, 1979.

215. Schmitter CR: Sulfhemoglobinemia and methemoglobinemia: Uncommon causes of cyanosis. *Anesthesiology* 43:586, 1975.

216. Bolyai JZ, Smith RP, Gray GT: Ascorbic acid and chemically induced methemoglobinemias. *Toxicol Appl Pharmacol* 21:176, 1972.

158. Withdrawal Syndromes

Paul M. Wax

Physicians who care for critically ill patients need to be familiar with the various manifestations and treatment of drug withdrawal, particularly that associated with chronic sedative-hypnotic (including ethanol) and opioid use. Anticipation and recognition of early signs of sedative-hypnotic withdrawal in the suspected or unsuspected sedative-hypnotic abuser allows timely treatment and prevents development of serious withdrawal manifestations, such as seizures, hyperthermia, and delirium. Recognition and treatment of the less life-threatening signs and symptoms of opioid withdrawal avoids unnecessary investigation of the frequently severe gastrointestinal (GI) symptoms and makes the patient more comfortable and able to cooperate. Since ethanol and other sedative-hypnotic withdrawal may have life-threatening manifestations, patients with signs of significant sedative-hypnotic withdrawal are placed in the intensive care unit (ICU) for stabilization and monitoring. In addition, drug-dependent patients admitted to the ICU for

management of other serious medical or surgical problems may subsequently enter withdrawal in this substance-free environment [1]. Managing a significant withdrawal syndrome superimposed on a serious underlying illness will challenge the most seasoned intensivist.

Clinical withdrawal implies the presence of physical tolerance and dependency. Factors contributing to the development of dependency include dose of the drug, duration of effect, frequency of administration, and duration of abuse. Shorter-acting drugs require more frequent administration to produce dependency and are associated with more acute and severe withdrawal symptoms than longer-acting drugs. Tolerance is defined as a decreased physiologic response elicited by a given dose of the drug. Clinical examples of tolerance are familiar. A patient who chronically ingests large amounts of alcohol may not be sedated by a dose that would render a nondrinker comatose. A heroin abuser who has been drug-free during a year's imprisonment may suffer fatal respiratory depression from a dose of heroin that would previously have provided only mild sedation. This physiologic tolerance to drug effect that occurs with chronic use may arise from changes in drug metabolism, such as increased activity of hepatic microsomal enzyme systems and changes in drug effect at the cellular level [2]. Cross-tolerance occurs when the chronic ingestion of one substance decreases the response to a second substance. Cross-dependency allows one drug to be substituted for another to prevent withdrawal symptoms. Ethanol, the barbiturates, and nonbarbiturate sedative-hypnotic agents are cross-tolerant and cross-dependent with one another, but not with other sedating drugs, such as opiates, neuroleptics, or antihistamines. These factors have important therapeutic implications.

Alcohol Withdrawal

PHARMACOLOGY AND PATHOPHYSIOLOGY. The clinical neurologic effects of ethanol—relaxation, euphoria, disinhibition, slurred speech, ataxia, sedation, stupor, coma, and respiratory depression—are familiar to most observers (see Chap. 132). The biochemical events that promote these effects at a cellular level contribute to understanding of what happens to the nervous system when ethanol is suddenly withdrawn. Whereas the opiates bind to a specific high-affinity receptor, a specific ethanol receptor has yet to be identified. It has been suggested that ethanol acts, in part, by altering the lipid matrix of cell membranes [3]. Others have postulated that ethanol may interact with the inhibitory neurotransmitter gamma-aminobutyric acid (GABA) receptor complex, affecting ion fluxes through chloride channels [4]. Although it was not recognized until the 1950s that delirium was a manifestation of ethanol withdrawal, rather than toxicity, it is now clear that the hallmarks of ethanol and other sedative-hypnotic intoxication are distinctly different from the manifestations of withdrawal from these agents [5,6].

Ethanol withdrawal produces a hyperadrenergic state characterized by intense autonomic stimulation. This may be due in part to compensatory central nervous system (CNS) mechanisms that counteract the depressant effects of ethanol intoxication. During withdrawal these compensatory mechanisms are unopposed, resulting in increased neural stimulation [7]. In support of this theory, elevated levels of plasma and urinary catecholamines have been demonstrated in withdrawing patients [8]. A decrease in the inhibitory activity of presynaptic alpha$_2$-receptors has been demonstrated in withdrawing patients and may explain, in part, the increase in norepinephrine levels [9]. In addition, an increase in beta-adrenergic receptors during withdrawal has been exhibited [10]. A recent study demonstrated an increase in plasma levels of the dopamine metabolite homovanillic acid in patients presenting with delirium tremens [11]. While the authors suggest that elevated levels of this metabolite may be a possible predicator of severe ethanol withdrawal, the utility of this finding awaits further study.

Another theory of the pathogenesis of ethanol withdrawal suggests that the abrupt withdrawal of the GABA potentiating effects of ethanol leads to a "disinhibition" of neural pathways in the CNS [12]. Hypomagnesemia and respiratory alkalosis, both of which are associated with central and peripheral hyperirritability, have also been proposed as possible explanations for withdrawal [13,14]. Whether they really play any consequential role in the pathogenesis of the withdrawal state remains to be clarified.

Ethanol withdrawal occurs when a dependent patient suddenly stops drinking or drinks at a slower rate than he or she has been accustomed to. In either case, a significant drop in the serum ethanol level occurs. In the chronic alcoholic, signs of withdrawal are commonly present even when ethanol levels are 100 mg per deciliter (mg/100 ml) or greater [15]. Patients admitted to the ICU with ethanol withdrawal often have significant underlying disease that has led to an inability to obtain or maintain an ethanol intake adequate to prevent withdrawal. Alcoholic gastritis, hepatitis, pancreatitis, and pneumonia commonly precipitate decreased ethanol use and withdrawal. These patients typically present to the hospital after 24 to 48 hours of abdominal pain or fever and may be tremulous or have had a withdrawal seizure. Another type of ICU patient prone to withdrawal is one who continued to imbibe ethanol nearly to the moment of arrival at the hospital. Intoxicated patients are prone to suffer traumatic events and arrive in the operating room, recovery room, or ICU still intoxicated. A history of ethanol abuse or previous withdrawal may not be available in the postoperative or intubated patient when initial signs of withdrawal occur. Failure to recognize ethanol withdrawal in the seriously ill or injured patient may lead to prolonged complications [7].

CLINICAL MANIFESTATIONS

Presentation. Clinical manifestations of ethanol withdrawal encompass a variety of presentations that vary in severity and duration. In their landmark paper, Victor and Adams described withdrawal as a "tremulous-hallucinating-epileptic-delirious" state [6]. While this description is often used to divide ethanol withdrawal syndrome into four stages, it is important to remember that the various manifestations of ethanol withdrawal form a progressive continuum of severity. A patient in ethanol withdrawal may exhibit one or more of these manifestations. The sequence of clinical events may be inconsistent. The severity of the withdrawal is often dose-dependent, with more severe reactions associated with heavier and longer periods of drinking [15]. It has been suggested that repeated withdrawal episodes produce a kindling effect, such that each subsequent withdrawal elicits increasingly more severe reactions [9,15,16].

Tremulousness and seizures are the most common clinical manifestations of ethanol withdrawal. They tend to occur early and are generally considered mild to moderate ethanol withdrawal symptoms. Alternatively, delirium tremens is a late manifestation of ethanol withdrawal and constitutes the most serious clinical presentation. While dramatic and life-threatening, delirium tremens is but one aspect of ethanol withdrawal and affects 1 in 20 withdrawal patients [17].

Acute Alcoholic Tremulousness. Mild ethanol withdrawal is usually characterized by a period of acute tremulousness (the "shakes"). It begins 6 to 8 hours after a reduction in ethanol intake [15,18]. Patients usually complain of tremulousness, nausea, vomiting, anorexia, anxiety, and insomnia. Physical examination reveals evidence of mild CNS and autonomic hyperactivity, including tachycardia, mild hypertension, hyperreflexia, irritability, and a resting tremor. Occasionally significant tremor may not be appreciated despite the patient's complaint of feeling "shaky inside." While patients in delirium tremens have evidence of significant disorientation, this milder form of withdrawal is characterized by a clear sensorium, although the patient may have a minor disorientation to time. Symptoms of mild ethanol withdrawal usually peak between 24 and 36 hours, and 75 to 80 percent of these patients recover uneventfully in a few days. Twenty to 25 percent of patients presenting with symptoms of mild ethanol withdrawal progress to more serious manifestations, including seizures, hallucinations, and/or delirium tremens. Unfortunately, it is impossible to predict reliably which patients will progress [15].

Alcoholic Related Seizures. Seizures that occur in alcoholics may or may not be due to ethanol withdrawal. While ethanol withdrawal accounts for many of these seizures, other common causes include preexisting idiopathic epilepsy and posttraumatic epilepsy [5,6]. Other complications of ethanol abuse not necessarily associated with withdrawal, such as hypoglycemia, hypomagnesemia, and hyponatremia, may also precipitate seizure activity [19]. Ethanol intoxication itself is not thought to be proconvulsant [20]. Alcoholic patients with a prior history of epilepsy appear to have a greater incidence of seizures than those without a preexisting seizure disorder. Failure to comply with anticonvulsant regimens may, in part, account for this. Brief abstinence (even overnight) may also lower the seizure threshold sufficiently to provoke seizures in susceptible patients. Since management strategies differ depending on whether there is a history of previous seizure disorder unrelated to ethanol withdrawal, differentiating between them becomes quite important [21].

Early studies showed that approximately one-quarter to one-third of patients in ethanol withdrawal demonstrate seizure activity [5,6]. Most alcohol withdrawal seizures ("rum fits") occur between 7 and 48 hours after cessation or relative abstinence from drinking [22]. Mild to moderate signs of withdrawal may precede the seizures or the seizure may herald the onset of ethanol withdrawal. They are short generalized tonic-clonic seizures, 40 percent of which are limited to a single isolated event. Often a short burst of two to six seizures with normal sensorium between seizures occurs over a few hours. Patients with withdrawal seizures usually have normal baseline electroencephalograms, in contrast to those with underlying seizure disorders. Status epilepticus or recurrent seizure activity lasting longer than 6 hours is distinctly uncommon in ethanol withdrawal and suggests another diagnosis [23].

Alcohol withdrawal seizures may foreshadow the development of delirium tremens. In Victor and Brausch's series of patients with ethanol withdrawal seizures, one-third developed delirium tremens [22]. In some patients, postictal confusion blended imperceptibly into delirium tremens. Approximately 40 percent of patients who subsequently developed delirium tremens exhibited an initial clearing followed by the onset of delirium tremens 12 hours to 5 days later.

Alcoholic Hallucinations. Victor and Adams noted that approximately one of four tremulous patients in early withdrawal also exhibited some disordered perception characterized by hallucinations and nightmares. The hallucinations were predominantly visual in nature, auditory only in 20 percent of cases, and rarely tactile or olfactory [6]. Commonly described visual phenomena in this setting may include the graphic depiction of bugs crawling on the walls or bed [24].

A subset of hallucinating patients does not demonstrate tremulousness or other signs of sympathetic hyperactivity. This less common clinical presentation, known as acute alcoholic hallucinosis, is a distinct manifestation of ethanol withdrawal that usually begins within 8 to 48 hours of cessation of drinking. It is characterized by disabling auditory hallucinations, often of a persecutory nature. These patients display no evidence of formal thought disorder, have no personal or family history of schizophrenia, and are usually oriented to person and place. In most cases symptoms last 1 to 6 days, although they may persist for months and come to resemble chronic paranoid schizophrenia. These symptoms usually respond to therapy with cross-tolerant agents such as benzodiazepines [6,25].

Delirium Tremens. The hallmark of delirium tremens is a significant alteration of sensorium associated with dramatic autonomic and CNS hyperactivity. Only 5 percent of patients who exhibit any of the previously discussed manifestations of ethanol withdrawal progress to delirium tremens. Delirium tremens appears to be more common in patients with a prior history of significant withdrawal and a long history of ethanol use. Patients who develop delirium tremens may not have demonstrated earlier signs of withdrawal. Other patients who had had withdrawal seizures or hallucinations may deceptively improve prior to the onset of delirium tremens. The onset of delirium tremens is rarely seen before 48 to 72 hours after cessation or reduction in drinking, and may be delayed as long as 5 to 14 days [6,18]. These patients are truly delirious, exhibiting disorientation, global confusion, hallucinations, and delusions. Speech is unintelligible. Psychomotor disturbances, such as picking at bedclothes, significant restlessness, and agitation, are common and often require the use of physical restraints. Autonomic disturbances, such as tachycardia, hypertension, tachypnea, hyperpyrexia, diaphoresis, and mydriasis, are present. Cardiac arrhythmias may also occur [26]. Seizures rarely occur during delirium tremens [18]. Concomitant illness, trauma, seizures, or therapeutic drugs may mask or modify the typical presentation.

Reported mortality rates for delirium tremens vary with the presence of significant underlying disease. Higher mortality rates are associated with superimposed pneumonia, meningitis, pancreatitis, GI bleeding, and major trauma. In the untreated patient without serious coexisting medical disease, mortality usually is a consequence of severe dehydration and/or hyperthermia precipitating cardiovascular collapse [27]. Before adequate therapeutic agents were available, a 24 to 35 percent mortality rate was cited in the literature [28]. This had decreased to 5 to 10 percent with the use of barbiturates and paraldehyde [29]. With the availability of benzodiazepines and aggressive ICU monitoring and earlier recognition of this problem, mortality should now be much lower in the absence of significant underlying disease [12].

DIFFERENTIAL DIAGNOSIS. The differential diagnosis of ethanol withdrawal includes other causes of a hyperadrenergic state. Most importantly, ethanol-related hypoglycemia needs to be differentiated from withdrawal. Clinically, these two conditions may appear remarkably similar, although only hypoglycemia improves rapidly following the empirical intravenous administration of 50 gm of glucose [30].

Intoxication with sympathomimetic agents such as cocaine or amphetamine shares many features with ethanol withdrawal, including signs and symptoms of adrenergic excess. Monoamine oxidase inhibitors, phencyclidine, anticholinergic, and lithium overdose, as well as neuroleptic malignant syndrome, may all demonstrate marked agitation and confusion [31]. In the elderly patient, almost any therapeutic drug may be associated with delirium [32]. Withdrawal from other sedative-hypnotics, such as benzodiazepines, barbiturates, ethchlorvynol, glutethimide, and meprobamate, may precipitate a delirium tremens-like state (see following).

Significant underlying metabolic, traumatic, and infectious disorders should be excluded in the patient with altered mental status associated with ethanol withdrawal. Differentiation may require lumbar puncture, laboratory tests, and computed tomography (CT) scan. These include CNS emergencies, such as subdural and epidural hematoma, subarachnoid hemorrhage, meningitis and encephalitis; metabolic causes, including hypoxia, hypercarbia, sepsis, thiamine deficiency, sodium and calcium abnormalities; and endocrine disturbances, such as thyroid storm and pheochromocytoma. Distinguishing between delirium tremens and hepatic encephalopathy may be particularly difficult, especially since these conditions often coexist [33].

MANAGEMENT. A successful strategy in treating ethanol withdrawal must address several key goals: alleviation of symptoms, prevention of progression of withdrawal to a more serious stage, avoidance of complications, treatment of coexisting medical problems, and planning for long-term rehabilitation and drug independence [18]. Initial treatment involves securing the ABCs. Patients with an altered level of consciousness require oxygen and IV administration of 100 mg of thiamine and 50 gm of glucose. The latter two substrates are particularly important, as Wernicke's encephalopathy and hypoglycemia may be confused or coexist with ethanol withdrawal. Severely agitated patients may initially require physical restraints to prevent injury and facilitate sedation. Prolonged use of physical restraints without adequate sedation, however, may be detrimental, since agitated patients quite often continue to struggle against their restraints. Such activity perpetuates the risk for hyperthermia, muscle destruction, and resultant myoglobinuric renal failure. Volume resuscitation, correction of electrolyte abnormalities, and vigilance in the diagnosis and treatment of coexisting medical and surgical disorders are vital in reducing morbidity and mortality in the patient with delirium tremens [29,34].

Achievement of adequate sedation is the cornerstone of successful treatment of ethanol withdrawal. Sedation alleviates the excitatory manifestations of withdrawal and prevents progression to delirium tremens. Sedation prevents common complications of agitation, including trauma, rhabdomyolysis, and hyperthermia. While many agents have been used over the years, benzodiazepines have proved the most effective [35,36,37]. Benzodiazepines, unlike the neuroleptics, are cross-tolerant with ethanol and thereby function as a replacement drug for the short-acting ethanol. Benzodiazepines appear to produce less drowsiness and respiratory depression than other sedative-hypnotic agents. Dosages are easier to titrate, and the effects are more predictable. Diazepam (Valium), chlordiazepoxide (Librium), and lorazepam (Ativan) are the most commonly used parenteral agents. All three agents can easily be given IV to facilitate rapid sedation and titration of effect. Of these agents, only lorazepam can be given intramuscularly. Diazepam and chlordiazepoxide are poorly absorbed after intramuscular administration [15,38]. These benzodiazepines also have an intermediate to long half-life, avoiding the need for frequent dosing associated with shorter-acting agents. Diazepam and chlordiazepoxide have active metabolites that prolong their therapeutic effect. Lorazepam has no active metabolites and is better tolerated in the elderly and patients with hepatic dysfunction. In some patients lorazepam may be the preferred agent [7,29,39].

The dose of benzodiazepines needed to achieve adequate sedation varies considerably depending on the patient's tolerance. While oral therapy may be appropriate in patients with very mild withdrawal, patients with significant signs of withdrawal require IV treatment. Therapy with an IV benzodiazepine is titrated to the patient's needs by the use of frequent boluses. This method helps avoid undertreatment or excessive sedation. For example, 5 to 20 mg of diazepam can be administered to the patient every 5 minutes until the patient is quietly sleeping but easily awakened. Initial safe titration of benzodiazepines requires continual reevaluation by an observer at the bedside. Failure to obtain adequate sedation with standard doses of the chosen agent should not prompt a switch to a second drug. Some patients require very high doses to achieve

sedation; cases of patients receiving greater than 1000 mg of diazepam over 24 hours have been reported [40]. The use of a continuous intravenous infusion of midazolam, a short-acting benzodiazepine, has also been recommended in the treatment of delirium tremens [41]. The approach, however, requires more vigilant monitoring, especially in the nonintubated patient, and does not provide the advantages of a long-acting benzodiazepine that is gradually eliminated over several days.

Adequate early treatment suppresses significant manifestations of withdrawal and prevents progression to delirium tremens. If delirium tremens is already manifest, sedation with a benzodiazepine does not completely reverse mental status abnormalities. This may be a consequence of benzodiazepine's incomplete cross-tolerance with ethanol or perhaps of the lack of immediate reversibility of some of the CNS effects of withdrawal [42].

Barbiturates, particularly intermediate and long-acting agents such as pentobarbital and phenobarbital, are an alternative class of cross-tolerant sedative-hypnotic agents that may be used in the treatment of ethanol withdrawal [43]. While excess sedation and a greater tendency to produce respiratory depression may be more of a concern with barbiturates as compared with benzodiazepines, the drugs are still titrated until the patient is quietly asleep but easily awakened [44]. Dosages of phenobarbital up to 20 mg per kilogram or greater may be required. Withdrawal patients with idiopathic or posttraumatic epilepsy who require maintenance anticonvulsant levels may particularly benefit from this alternative strategy.

Two other sedative-hypnotics of historical interest in the treatment of ethanol withdrawal are paraldehyde and ethanol itself. Prior to the development of the safer benzodiazepines, paraldehyde was widely used. It is considerably more toxic than benzodiazepines and is very difficult to titrate due to variable rates of absorption. Overdosage and underdosage are equally likely. Other disadvantages include hepatotoxicity, gastritis when given orally, sterile abscesses when given intramuscularly, and proctitis following rectal administration. Intravenous administration requires glass syringes and metal needles, since paraldehyde may dissolve plastic tubing. It also has a notoriously unpleasant odor [44].

Ethanol administered intravenously or orally has also been used to suppress withdrawal [45]. Recent advocacy for prophylactic use of ethanol in hospitalized patients can be found in the surgical literature [46,47,48]. However, there are several problems with the use of ethanol in the treatment of ethanol withdrawal. It has a very short duration of action and is difficult to titrate [44], and its CNS and hepatotoxicity are well known [12,34]. Continued IV use of ethanol intensifies the biochemical abnormalities associated with ethanol metabolism, shifting energy production toward lactate and ketogenesis [49]. Finally, extravasation of ethanol may cause local tissue necrosis, which in a recent report required excision and grafting [48]. There is no indication to use either paraldehyde or ethanol in the treatment of ethanol withdrawal.

The use of phenothiazines and butyrophenones to treat ethanol withdrawal has been associated with excessive fatalities [34,49,50]. Despite their potent sedative effects, these neuroleptic drugs are not cross-tolerant with ethanol and do not prevent or suppress ethanol withdrawal [44,51,52]. In addition, both phenothiazines and butyrophenones have been shown to lower the seizure threshold, induce hypotension, impair thermoregulation, and precipitate dystonic reactions [53,54,55]. These drugs have no role in the management of sedative-hypnotic withdrawal and should not be used in agitated patients unless the presentation is clearly from a primarily psychiatric etiology [56].

Recently, beta-blockers and central adrenergic agonists have been promoted as both primary agents and adjuncts to sedative-hypnotics in the treatment of ethanol withdrawal [57]. These agents, while not cross-tolerant with ethanol, appear to ameliorate the catecholamine excess characteristic of withdrawal. Rapid normalization of vital signs and reduction in tremor have been demonstrated in patients with mild withdrawal [58,59,60]. These agents do not prevent agitation, hallucinations, confusion, and seizures [37,43]. Side effects from propranolol, such as hallucinations and delirium, may be potentiated by alcohol withdrawal [61]. Since tachycardia, hypertension, and tremor are useful clinical indicators to gauge the adequacy of sedation in the withdrawing patient, suppression of these signs with sympatholytic agents in the patient with serious withdrawal may mask a deteriorating clinical situation due to inadequate dosing of a benzodiazepine [62]. Use of sympatholytic agents should be limited to outpatient therapy of mild withdrawal. A role for sympatholytic agents in management of the seriously ill patients has not been demonstrated.

In cases of mild withdrawal, beta-blockers used in conjunction with benzodiazepines have been shown to decrease total sedative requirements [59]. A daily oral dose of 50 to 100 mg of atenolol per day has been recommended. Controlling elevations in blood pressure and pulse rate with the addition of a beta-blocker may be of particular help in managing ethanol withdrawal patients with primary hypertension or coronary artery disease [44]. Beta-blockers should be used very cautiously in patients with congestive heart failure, asthma, or diabetes mellitus.

Alpha$_2$-receptor agonists such as clonidine and lofoxedine have also been used in the treatment of ethanol withdrawal [63]. They act centrally to attenuate sympathetic outflow from the locus ceruleus [9,15]. Reduction in plasma catecholamine levels in patients treated with these agents has been demonstrated [64]. Problems with orthostatic hypotension have been reported [65], and questions regarding clonidine exacerbation of withdrawal seizures remain unanswered [66]. While alpha$_2$-agonists may help relieve mild symptoms of withdrawal, such as tremor, diaphoresis, and tachycardia [67,68], there is no evidence that they actually prevent delirium tremens [69]. Failure to recognize the onset of delirium tremens in a patient with mixed opiate and sedative-hypnotic dependency was reported in a patient treated with clonidine for opiate withdrawal [70].

There continues to be much controversy and confusion regarding the use of anticonvulsants (primarily phenytoin) in the management of ethanol withdrawal seizures [7]. Patients who have had an ethanol withdrawal seizure are at risk of progression to delirium tremens and should be sedated with benzodiazepines or barbiturates, as discussed previously. Adequate sedation of the patient with early signs of withdrawal prevents the development of withdrawal seizures and progression to delirium tremens. There is no evidence that phenytoin has any therapeutic efficacy in the treatment or prevention of seizures secondary to ethanol withdrawal [18,71]. Two recent studies failed to show any significant benefit of IV phenytoin when compared with placebo in the prevention of subsequent withdrawal seizures [72,73].

The use of anticonvulsants to prevent or treat seizures in ethanol withdrawal should be limited to patients with an underlying chronic seizure disorder who require maintenance anticonvulsant therapy [21]. These patients often seize at the onset of mild withdrawal secondary to poor compliance with their anticonvulsant regimen and require restoration of adequate serum levels with an anticonvulsant such as phenytoin. Patients who present with an apparent ethanol withdrawal seizure but do not have a history of either chronic seizure disorder or previous ethanol withdrawal seizures require a full seizure work-up. For those rare patients in ethanol withdrawal who

develop status epilepticus, aggressive anticonvulsant treatment is indicated, and phenytoin and/or phenobarbital may be used in addition to the benzodiazepines. Since status epilepticus and seizures during delirium tremens are very rare sequelae of ethanol withdrawal, their occurrence requires a search for underlying traumatic injuries and infection, regardless of any previous history of ethanol withdrawal seizures.

Benzodiazepines

Since their introduction in the early 1960s, benzodiazepines have replaced the barbiturates as the most widely prescribed sedative-hypnotic agents. Initially these newer agents were not thought to have the same serious withdrawal problems associated with the barbiturates [74]. Subsequent experience has shown that withdrawal from benzodiazepines may be as severe as withdrawal from barbiturates or ethanol. It is estimated that 10 to 20 percent of adults in the United States use benzodiazepines on a regular basis [75]. The early signs of withdrawal from benzodiazepines are the same as those of ethanol withdrawal. Differences include delayed time of onset, depending on the duration of action of the agent involved, and the presence or absence of active metabolites. When a hospitalized patient develops delayed tachycardia, hypertension, and irritability, prior benzodiazepine abuse should be suspected.

PATHOPHYSIOLOGY. Signs and symptoms of benzodiazepine withdrawal occur when tolerant patients experience a decline in brain benzodiazepine levels. Individuals who have not developed tolerance will not experience symptoms of withdrawal. Patients who have taken therapeutic amounts of these drugs over an extended period may experience withdrawal (therapeutic dose withdrawal) [76,77], although more commonly it occurs in patients who have been regularly taking higher than recommended antianxiety doses. A high daily dose and long duration of benzodiazepine use correlate with a greater risk of developing a moderate to severe withdrawal syndrome [75,78]. While withdrawal usually occurs following abrupt discontinuation of these medications, it may occur to a lesser extent during drug tapering [74].

Although the exact mechanism responsible for benzodiazepine tolerance is unknown, several theories have been postulated. The most commonly accepted theory suggests that increases in the number or sensitivity of benzodiazepine receptors in the brain occur during chronic exposure, and this may be associated with the development of tolerance. Withdrawal symptoms occur when a decrease in the availability of exogenous benzodiazepine leaves an abundance of unoccupied receptor sites, causing unopposed nervous system stimulation and an increase in agitation and anxiety [79].

Variability in the time course and severity of withdrawal among the various benzodiazepines can be explained by their differing pharmacokinetic properties [80]. Drug half-life and the presence of active metabolites correlate with the onset, frequency, and severity of withdrawal symptoms. The onset of withdrawal from shorter-acting agents without active metabolites, such as lorazepam or alprazolam, may be precipitous, with marked symptoms as early as 24 hours following cessation of the drug [81]. Signs of withdrawal from longer-acting agents, such as diazepam, which has an extended elimination half-life for the parent compound in addition to active metabolites, may be delayed up to 8 days or longer. Withdrawal symptoms from long-acting benzodiazepines may persist for months [82,83].

Concurrent use of other cross-tolerant sedative-hypnotic substances, such as ethanol, barbiturates, chloral hydrate, glutethimide, ethchlorvynol, or meprobamate, along with benzodiazepines increases the probability of developing withdrawal on abrupt discontinuation of these substances.

The recent introduction of the benzodiazepine competitive antagonist flumazenil raises the spectrum of flumazenil-induced iatrogenic benzodiazepine withdrawal. Flumazenil was recommended for its ability to reverse sedation in the settings of benzodiazepine overdose, intravenous conscious sedation, and general anesthesia [84] and was suggested as an adjunct in the weaning of patients from mechanical ventilation [85]. Unfortunately, benzodiazepine-dependent patients are at risk of developing withdrawal manifestations on administration of flumazenil. A history of benzodiazepine use and dependence may not be available when unconscious patients are admitted to the ICU. Benzodiazepine withdrawal syndromes, seizures, and death have been reported after the use of flumazenil [86,87,88]. Furthermore, flumazenil has not been proved effective in the treatment of benzodiazepine-induced respiratory depression [84]. Flumazenil, if it is to be used at all in the ICU, should probably be used only in selected cases of oversedation from benzodiazepine conscious sedation. Patients with a history of benzodiazepine dependence or risk factors for seizures, such as the use of potentially proconvulsant medications (tricyclic antidepressants, neuroleptics, isoniazid), head trauma, or previous seizure history, should not be given flumazenil.

PRESENTATION. Benzodiazepine withdrawal is characterized by CNS excitation and autonomic hyperactivity. Mild early manifestations of withdrawal include psychologic symptoms such as anxiety, apprehension, irritability, mood swing, dysphoria, and insomnia. Somatic complaints commonly include nausea, palpitations, tremor, diaphoresis, and muscle twitching.

Benzodiazepine withdrawal may be difficult to diagnose, since the underlying anxiety symptomatology may be indistinguishable from that of withdrawal itself [89]. The time course of the symptoms helps distinguish these two diagnoses. Withdrawal symptoms often worsen rapidly in the early period, followed by gradual improvement and resolution. Unmasked anxiety disorders tend not to deteriorate significantly and persist with time. Perceptual disturbances, not generally associated with underlying anxiety disorders, are commonly found during early withdrawal and may also help distinguish withdrawal from the return of anxiety [82]. These disturbances include paresthesia, tinnitus, visual abnormalities, vertigo, metallic taste, depersonalization, and derealization [77].

More severe signs of withdrawal include vomiting, cramps, tachycardia, postural hypotension, and hyperthermia. Significant neuromuscular hyperactivity manifested as fasciculations, myoclonic jerks, and seizures also occurs [90]. Agitated delirium accompanied by hallucinations and paranoid delusions has been described [89].

Patients taking clonazepam, a benzodiazepine used chiefly as an anticonvulsant, may develop withdrawal symptoms 3 to 4 days after cessation of therapy. Clonazepam withdrawal may be provoked and/or accentuated by concomitant neuroleptic therapy [91]. Seizures, agitation, and paranoid psychosis have been described as manifestations of clonazepam withdrawal [91,92].

TREATMENT. Treatment strategies for benzodiazepine withdrawal are similar to those used for ethanol withdrawal. Reinstitution of the drug at a dose that relieves withdrawal symptoms followed by slow withdrawal over a period of 2 to 4 weeks minimizes symptoms and effects the desired decrease in CNS tolerance. Alternatively, a similar cross-tolerant agent may be used. A long-acting benzodiazepine with active metabolites, such as diazepam or chlordiazepoxide, is preferred. Shorter-acting agents are disadvantageous because serum drug levels are maintained for a much shorter time, necessitating more frequent drug administration to prevent recurrent withdrawal. In patients with moderate to severe symptoms (e.g., seizures, delirium), small intravenous boluses, such as 5 mg of diazepam, should be given until adequate sedation is obtained. Patients experiencing more mild symptomatology may be treated by the oral route. Barbiturates such as pentobarbital and phenobarbital may also be used in the treatment of benzodiazepine withdrawal [93,94].

Alternatively, beta-blockers and clonidine have been effectively employed in the treatment of benzodiazepine withdrawal [95]. Propranolol (10–40 mg every 6 hours) may help ameliorate tremor, muscle twitching, tachycardia, and hypertension. It has little effect on subjective signs of anxiety, agitation, and dysphoria [75]. Clonidine use has also been advocated, although its efficacy in modulating the intensity, severity, and duration of withdrawal was recently questioned [96]. As with ethanol withdrawal, it is important to realize that blocking peripheral manifestations of withdrawal may obscure early warnings of impending delirium and cloud the assessment of adequacy of sedation achieved with concurrent cross-tolerant medications. Phenothiazines and butyrophenones exhibit no cross-tolerance to the benzodiazepines and do not have a role in the treatment of benzodiazepine withdrawal, for the same reasons seen in ethanol withdrawal [97].

Few data are available on the treatment of flumazenil-induced benzodiazepine withdrawal. Since flumazenil has a relatively short half-life (about 1 hour) supportive care should be sufficient in the treatment of mild withdrawal symptoms. The precipitation of seizure activity may require additional dosing with a benzodiazepine or barbiturate. Due to receptor blockade from flumazenil, a higher dose of one of these GABAnergic agonists may be required.

Opiates

Opiate withdrawal is commonly encountered in the ICU. Unlike withdrawal from sedative-hypnotic agents [98], the manifestations of opiate withdrawal are not usually life-threatening. Recognition of the problem facilitates optimum management of the critically ill patient.

PATHOPHYSIOLOGY. Opiate withdrawal occurs when a tolerant individual experiences a decline in CNS levels of a chronically used opioid. Opiate receptors in the locus ceruleus bind exogenous opiates, such as heroin, methadone, or codeine, as well as endogenous opiatelike substances known as endorphins and enkephalins. Stimulation of opiate receptors reduces the firing rate of locus ceruleus noradrenergic neurons, resulting in the inhibition of catecholamine release [99,100]. The stimulation of inhibitory adrenergic receptors, also found in the locus ceruleus, causes a similar reduction in sympathetic outflow. Chronic opiate use may produce an increase or upregulation of these adrenergic receptors. Subsequent withdrawal of opiates results in increased sympathetic discharge and noradrenergic hyperactivity.

The time course of the withdrawal syndrome depends on pharmacokinetic parameters of the individual opiates [99].

Withdrawal symptoms usually appear about the time of the expected next dose [101]. Withdrawal from heroin, which has a short half-life, begins 4 to 8 hours after the last dose, while withdrawal from methadone, with a long half-life, is delayed until 36 to 72 hours after the last dose. Withdrawal symptoms are more intense if the opiate has a shorter half-life, while symptoms are less dramatic but often more prolonged if the abused opiate has a long half-life. Typically heroin withdrawal will peak at 36 to 72 hours, with symptoms subsiding by 7 to 10 days. Methadone withdrawal may not peak until the sixth day of abstinence and may persist for weeks.

PRESENTATION. Early signs of opiate withdrawal include mydriasis, lacrimation, rhinorrhea, diaphoresis, yawning, piloerection, anxiety, and restlessness [102]. With time these symptoms may worsen and be accompanied by mild elevation in pulse, blood pressure, and respiratory rate. Fever cannot be attributed to withdrawal from opiates. Myalgias, vomiting, diarrhea, anorexia, abdominal pain, and dehydration accompany more severe withdrawal. While these patients may become extremely restless, central agitation, such as seizures (except in cases of neonatal withdrawal) and mental status alteration, are not seen. An intense craving for the drug accompanies withdrawal. This may result in clinically puzzling pain syndromes in an attempt to obtain relief. Recognition of these signs and symptoms in the ICU patient will obviate the need for extensive evaluation of the GI symptoms and put clinically puzzling pain complaints in perspective. Appropriate therapy alleviates the patient's discomfort and facilitates management of more pressing ICU problems. Following the resolution of most of the objective signs of withdrawal, subjective symptoms, especially dysphoria, may persist for weeks [100].

The sudden onset of opiate withdrawal may occur in the opiate-dependent patient after receiving naloxone [103]. This iatrogenic withdrawal often occurs after naloxone is given to the unsuspected dependent patient who is lethargic or comatose. Naloxone-induced withdrawal may also occur in dependent patients after use of naloxone to reverse the effects of an opiate employed during conscious sedation. Vomiting and subsequent aspiration in the unconscious patient are the major complications arising from this problem. This abstinence syndrome is of brief duration due to the short half-life of naloxone, lasting 20 to 60 minutes, and treatment with additional opiate to reverse the unwarranted effects of naloxone is not indicated. Naloxone, if required, should not be withheld in the dependent patient. A small starting dose of 0.04 to 0.1 mg should be used, titrated until the desired effect is achieved or mild signs of withdrawal occur. Coma or hypoventilation that persists following the onset of withdrawal signs is not reversed by administration of additional naloxone. Naltrexone, an orally activating opiate antagonist, however, will induce withdrawal symptoms for up to 48 hours. A less commonly recognized cause of opiate withdrawal is the use of agonist-antagonist in the opiate-dependent person. Drugs with agonist-antagonist activity include pentazocine (Talwin), nalbuphine (Nubaine), and butorphanol (Stadol).

TREATMENT. Treatment of opiate withdrawal is a two-tier approach, using both cross-tolerant opiate replacement and/or sympatholytic therapy (e.g., clonidine). The benzodiazepines are not cross-tolerant with opioids. Their role is limited to the management of significant anxiety associated with opiate withdrawal.

The substitution of long-acting methadone for heroin has played a prominent role in the management of opiate addiction

[98]. It is useful in treating the uncomfortable symptoms in patients who are dependent on any opiate. The dose should be judiciously titrated to relieve symptoms but avoid oversedation. A safe initial dose is 20 mg orally or 10 mg intramuscularly (IM). The IM route guarantees absorption in the vomiting patient [102]. Relief of symptoms usually occurs within 30 to 60 minutes when given parenterally and longer when given orally. A second 10 mg IM dose may be given if significant relief is not obtained 1 hour following the first IM dose. Ten to 20 mg IM will block most manifestations of physiologic withdrawal, although some patients may require dosages of 20 to 40 mg daily or divided twice per day to avoid psychologic withdrawal. In general, dosing for withdrawal requires considerably less drug than dosing for methadone maintenance. Opioid withdrawal in patients who have used large doses of methadone for the treatment of chronic pain, a practice often seen among cancer patients, may require additional methadone to keep the patient comfortable and suppress withdrawal symptomatology. Heroin-dependent patients may be tapered with methadone over 1 week. Methadone-dependent patients require 4 weeks or more of gradually decreasing dosages.

Every attempt should be made to minimize significant withdrawal manifestations in the opiate-dependent pregnant patient. Withdrawal in these patients may adversely affect the developing fetus, causing fetal distress and even intrauterine death [104]. Oral methadone maintenance is more compatible with maternal and fetal well-being than continued heroin abuse [105,106], and would likely also decrease the risk of intrauterine acquisition of acquired immunodeficiency syndrome (AIDS). Cautious treatment of these patients with sufficient methadone to avoid withdrawal may avert these additional complications. Following delivery, the neonate must be hospitalized and withdrawn from the drug.

The use of clonidine, a central alpha$_2$-agonist, to treat opiate withdrawal has received much attention [107,108]. Clonidine binds to the adrenergic alpha$_2$-receptors in the locus ceruleus. This results in feedback inhibition of the norepinephrine activity, decreasing the firing rate of the noradrenergic neurons. These noradrenergic neurons also possess opiate receptors whose stimulation produces a similar reduction in sympathetic activity through the same intracellular messenger system [101]. Replacing the withdrawn opiate with clonidine may then prevent the development of symptoms of opiate withdrawal. Clonidine (0.1–0.2 mg every 4–6 hours) used without the addition of a replacement opiate has successfully treated opiate withdrawal. Treatment should continue for 5 to 10 days and then be slowly tapered by 0.2 mg per day. Tachyphylaxis to the antiwithdrawal effects of clonidine develops by 10 to 14 days [99]. The most concerning side effect of clonidine is hypotension, especially with the first dose. This requires close monitoring.

Concomitant disease stemming from complications of opiate abuse should not be overlooked when treating the withdrawing patient. Complications of bacterial endocarditis and thrombophlebitis, and AIDS, often prove much more debilitating than the withdrawal itself.

References

1. Fruensgaard K: Withdrawal psychosis: A study of 30 consecutive cases. *Acta Psychiatr Scand* 53:105, 1976.
2. Tabakoff B, Cornell N, Hoffman PL: Alcohol tolerance. *Ann Emerg Med* 15:1005, 1986.
3. Goldstein DB: Effect of alcohol on cellular membranes. *Ann Emerg Med* 15:1013, 1986.

4. Charness ME, Simon RP, Greenberg DA: Ethanol and the nervous system. *N Engl J Med* 321:442, 1989.
5. Isbell H, Fraser HF, Wikler A, et al: An experimental study of the etiology of "rum fits" and delirium tremens. *Q J Stud Alcohol* 16:1, 1955.
6. Victor M, Adams RD: The effects of alcohol on the nervous system. *Proc Assoc Res Nerv Ment Dis* 32:526, 1953.
7. Sellers EM, Kalant H: Alcohol intoxication and withdrawal. *N Engl J Med* 294:757, 1976.
8. Castaneda R, Cushman P: Alcohol withdrawal: A review of clinical management. *J Clin Psychiatry* 50:278, 1989.
9. Linnoila M: Alcohol withdrawal and noradrenergic function. *Ann Intern Med* 107:875, 1987.
10. Hawley RJ, Major LF, Schulman EWA, Lake CR: CSF levels of norepinephrine during alcohol withdrawal. *Arch Neurol* 38:289, 1981.
11. Sano H, Suzuki Y, Ohara K, et al: Circadian variation in plasma homovanillic acid level during and after alcohol withdrawal in alcoholic patients. *Alcohol Clin Exp Res* 16:1047, 1992.
12. Adinoff B, Bone GH, Linnoila M: Acute ethanol poisoning and the ethanol withdrawal syndrome. *Med Toxicol Adverse Drug Exp* 3:172, 1988.
13. Victor M: The role of hypomagnesemia and respiratory alkalosis in the genesis of alcohol-withdrawal symptoms. *Ann NY Acad Sci* 215:235, 1973.
14. Wolfe SM, Victor M: The relationship of hypomagnesemia and alkalosis to alcohol withdrawal symptoms. *Ann NY Acad Sci* 162:973, 1969.
15. Mendelson JH, Mello NK: Biological concomitants of alcoholism. *N Engl J Med* 301:912, 1979.
16. Rosenbloom AJ: Optimizing drug treatment of alcohol withdrawal. *Am J Med* 81:901, 1986.
17. Lerner WD, Fallon HJ: The alcohol withdrawal syndrome. *N Engl J Med* 313:951, 1985.
18. Brown CG: The alcohol withdrawal syndrome. *Ann Emerg Med* 11:276, 1982.
19. Johnson R. Alcohol and fits. *Br J Addict* 80:227, 1985.
20. Simon RP: Alcohol and seizures. *N Engl J Med* 319:715, 1988.
21. Morris JC, Victor M: Alcohol withdrawal seizures. *Emerg Med Clin North Am* 5:827, 1987.
22. Victor M, Brausch C: The role of abstinence in the genesis of alcoholic epilepsy. *Epilepsia* 8:1, 1967.
23. Thompson WL: Management of alcohol withdrawal syndromes. *Arch Intern Med* 138:278, 1978
24. Turner R, Lichstein PR, Peden JG, et al: Alcohol withdrawal syndromes: A review of pathophysiology, clinical presentation, and treatment. *J General Med* 4:432, 1989.
25. Surawicz FG: Alcoholic hallucinosis: A missed diagnosis. *Can J Psychiatry* 25:57, 1980.
26. Fisher J, Abrams J: Life-threatening ventricular tachyarrhythmias in delirium tremens. *Arch Intern Med* 137:1238, 1977.
27. Tavel ME, Davidson W, Batterton TD: A critical analysis of mortality associated with delirium tremens. *Am J Med Sci* 242:18, 1961.
28. Moore M, Gray MG: Delirium tremens: A study of cases at the Boston City Hospital 1915–1936. *N Engl J Med* 220:953, 1939.
29. Rosenbloom A: Emerging treatment options in the alcohol withdrawal syndrome. *J Clin Psychiatry* 49(suppl 12):28, 1988.
30. Victor M, Adams RD, Collins GH: *The Wernicke-Korsakoff Syndrome.* Philadelphia, FA Davis, 1971, p 66.
31. Goldfrank LR, Flomenbaum NE, Lewin NA, et al: Substance withdrawal, in Goldfrank LR, Flomenbaum NE, Lewin NA, et al (eds): *Goldfrank's Toxicologic Emergencies,* 4th ed. Norwalk, CT, Appleton & Lange, 1990, pp 535–545.
32. Drugs that cause psychiatric symptoms. *Med Lett Drugs Ther* 31:113, 1989.
33. Lichtigfeld FJ: Hepatic encephalopathy and delirium tremens: Double jeopardy. *South Afr Med J* 67:880, 1985.
34. Delaney KA, Goldfrank K: Delirium assessment and management in the critical care environment. *Probl Crit Care* 1:78, 1987.
35. Moscowitz G, Chalmers TC, Sacks HS, et al: Deficiencies of clinical trials of alcohol withdrawal. *Alcoholism* 7:42, 1983.
36. Thompson WL, Johnson AD, Maddrey WL, et al: Diazepam and paraldehyde for treatment of delirium tremens. *Ann Intern Med* 82:175, 1975.
37. Liskow BI, Goodwin DW: Pharmacologic treatment of alcohol intoxication, withdrawal and dependence: A critical review. *J Stud Alcohol* 48:356, 1987.
38. Wartenberg AA: Treatment of alcohol withdrawal syndrome. *JAMA* 250:1271, 1983.
39. Miller WC, McCurdy L: A double-blind comparison of the efficacy and safety of lorazepam and diazepam in the treatment of acute alcohol withdrawal syndrome. *Clin Ther* 6:364, 1984.
40. Nolop KB, Natow A: Unprecedented sedative requirements during delirium tremens. *Crit Care Med* 13:246, 1985.
41. Lineaweaver WC, Anderson K, Hing DN: Massive doses of midazolam infusion for delirium tremens without respiratory depression. *Crit Care Med* 16:294, 1988.
42. Aaronson LA, Hinman DJ, Okamoto M: Effects of diazepam on ethanol withdrawal. *J Pharmacol Exp Ther* 221:319, 1982.
43. Young GP, Rores C, Murphy C, et al: Intravenous phenobarbital for alcohol withdrawal and convulsions. *Ann Emerg Med* 16:847, 1987.
44. Holloway HC, Hales RE, Watanabe HK: Recognition and treatment of acute alcohol withdrawal syndromes. *Psychiatr Clin North Am* 7:729, 1984.
45. Faillace LA, Flamer RN, Imber SD, Ward RF: Giving alcohol to alcoholics. *Q J Stud Alcohol* 33:85, 1972.
46. Gower WE, Kersten H: Prevention of alcohol withdrawal symptoms in surgical patients. *Surg Gynecol Obstet* 151:382, 1980.
47. Hansbrough JF, Zapata-Sirvent RL, Carroll WJ, et al: Administration of intravenous alcohol for prevention of withdrawal in alcoholic burn patients. *Am J Surg* 148:266, 1984.
48. Hansbrough JF: Massive doses of midazolam infusion for delirium tremens. *Crit Care Med* 17:597, 1989.
49. Golbert TM, Sanz CJ, Rose HD, et al: Comparative evaluation of treatments of alcohol withdrawal syndromes. *JAMA* 201:99, 1967.
50. Thomas DW, Freedman DX: Treatment of the alcohol withdrawal syndrome: Comparison of promazine and paraldehyde. *JAMA* 188:316, 1964.
51. Schwarz L, Schmidt H, Stern J: A double blind trial of the efficacy of promazine in the treatment of alcohol withdrawal syndrome. *Dis Nerv Syst* 27:173, 1968.
52. Kaim S, Klett C, Rothfeld B: Treatment of the acute alcohol withdrawal state: A comparison of four drugs. *Am J Psychiatry* 125:54, 1969.
53. Blum K, Eubanks JD, Wallace JE, et al: Enhancement of alcohol withdrawal convulsions in mice by haloperidol. *Clin Toxicol* 9:427, 1976.
54. Greenblatt DJ, Gross PL, Harris J, et al: Fatal hyperthermia following haloperidol therapy of sedative-hypnotic withdrawal. *J Clin Psychiatry* 39:673, 1978.
55. Sereny G, Kalant H: Comparative clinical evaluation of chlordiazepoxide and promazine in treatment of alcohol-withdrawal syndrome. *Br Med J* 1:92, 1965.
56. Gilman MA, Lichtigfeld FJ: The drug management of severe alcohol withdrawal syndrome. *Postgrad Med J* 66:1005, 1990.
57. Horwitz RI, Gottlieb LD, Kraus ML: The efficacy of atenolol in the outpatient management of the alcohol withdrawal syndrome. *Arch Intern Med* 149:1089, 1989.
58. Baumgartner GR, Rowen RC: Clonidine vs chlordiazepoxide in the management of acute alcohol withdrawal syndrome. *Arch Intern Med* 147:1223, 1987.
59. Kraus ML, Gottlieb LD, Horwitz RI, et al: Randomized clinical trial of atenolol in patients with alcohol withdrawal. *N Engl J Med* 313:905, 1985.
60. Zilm DH, Sellers EM, MacLeod SM, et al: Propranolol effect on tremor in alcoholic withdrawal. *Ann Intern Med* 83:234, 1975.
61. Jacob MS, Zilm DH, MacLeod SM, et al: Propranolol-associated confused states during alcohol withdrawal. *J Clin Psychopharmacol* 3:185, 1983.
62. Liskow B, Reed J: Atenolol for alcohol withdrawal. *N Engl J Med* 314:783, 1986.
63. Cushman P, Sowers JR: Alcohol withdrawal syndrome: Clinical and hormonal responses to alpha-2-adrenergic agonist treatment. *Alcoholism* 13:361, 1989.
64. Cushman P, Forbes R, Lerner W, et al: Alcohol withdrawal syndromes: Clinical management with lofexidine. *Alcoholism* 9:1103, 1985.

65. Robinson BJ, Robinson GM, Maling TJ, et al: Is clonidine useful in the treatment of alcohol withdrawal? *Alcoholism* 13:95, 1989.
66. Blum K, Briggs AH, DeLallo L: Clonidine enhancement of alcohol withdrawal in mice. *Subst Alcohol Actions Misuse* 4:59, 1983.
67. Wilkins AJ, Jenkins WJ, Steiner JA: Efficacy of clonidine in treatment of alcohol withdrawal state. *Psychopharmacology* 81:78, 1983.
68. Bjorkqvist SE: Clonidine in alcohol withdrawal. *Acta Psychiatr Scand* 52:256, 1975.
69. Treatment of alcohol withdrawal. *Med Lett Drugs Ther* 28:75, 1986.
70. Hughes PL, Morse R: Use of clonidine in a mixed-drug detoxification regimen: Possibility of masking of clinical signs of sedative withdrawal. *Mayo Clin Proc* 60:47, 1985.
71. Gessner PK: Is diphenylhydantoin effective in treatment of alcohol withdrawal? *JAMA* 219:1072, 1972.
72. Alldredge BK, Lowenstein DH, Simon RP: Placebo-controlled trial of intravenous diphenylhydantoin for short-term treatment of alcohol withdrawal seizures. *Am J Med* 87:645, 1989.
73. Chance JF: Emergency department treatment of alcohol withdrawal seizures with phenytoin. *Ann Emerg Med* 20:520, 1991.
74. Tyrer P, Owen R, Dawling S: Gradual withdrawal of diazepam after long-term therapy. *Lancet* 1:1402, 1983.
75. Mackinnon GL, Parker WA: Benzodiazepine withdrawal syndrome: A literature review and evaluation. *Am J Drug Alcohol Abuse* 9:19, 1982.
76. Winokur A, Rickels K, Greenblatt DJ, et al: Withdrawal reaction from long-term low-dosage administration of diazepam. *Arch Gen Psychiatry* 37:101, 1980.
77. Petursson H, Lader MH: Withdrawal from long-term benzodiazepine treatment. *Br Med J* 283:643, 1981.
78. Lukas SE, Griffiths RR: Precipitated diazepam withdrawal in baboons: Effects of dose and duration of diazepam exposure. *Eur J Pharmacol* 100:163, 1984.
79. Scharf MB, Feil P: Acute effects of drug administration and withdrawal on the benzodiazepine receptor. *Life Sci* 32:1771, 1983.
80. Benzer D, Cushman P: Alcohol and benzodiazepines: Withdrawal syndromes. *Alcoholism* 4:243, 1980.
81. Noyes R, Clancy J, Coryell WH, et al: A withdrawal syndrome after abrupt discontinuation of alprazolam. *Am J Psychiatry* 142:114, 1985.
82. Busto U, Sellers EM, Naranjo CA, et al: Withdrawal reaction after long-term therapeutic use of benzodiazepines. *N Engl J Med* 315:854, 1986.
83. Ashton H: Benzodiazepine withdrawal: An unfinished study. *Br Med J* 288:1135, 1984.
84. *Mazicon Product Monograph*. Nutley, NJ, Hoffmann-La Roche, 1992.
85. Kleinberger G, Grimm G, Laggner A, et al: Weaning patients from mechanical ventilation by benzodiazepine antagonist Ro 15-1788. *Lancet* 2:268, 1985.
86. Lopez A, Rebello J: Benzodiazepine withdrawal syndrome after a benzodiazepine antagonist. *Crit Care Med* 18:1480, 1990.
87. Burr W, Sandham P: Death after flumazenil. *Br Med J* 293:1712, 1989.
88. Lheureux P, Vrankx M, Askenasi R: Administration of flumazenil. *Ann Emerg Med* 20:592, 1991.
89. Owen RT, Tyrer P: Benzodiazepine dependence: A review of the evidence. *Drugs* 25:385, 1983.
90. De Bard ML: Diazepam withdrawal syndrome: A case with psychosis, seizure and coma. *Am J Psychiatry* 136:104, 1979.
91. Gharirian AM, Gauthier S, Wong T: Convulsions in patients abruptly withdrawn from clonazepam while receiving neuroleptic medication. *Am J Psychiatry* 144:686, 1987.
92. Jaffe R, Gibson E: Clonazepam withdrawal psychosis. *J Clin Psychopharmacol* 6:193, 1986.
93. Preskorn SH, Denner LJ: Benzodiazepines and withdrawal psychosis. *JAMA* 237:36, 1977.
94. Wikler A: Diagnosis and treatment of drug dependence of the barbiturate type. *Am J Psychiatry* 125:758, 1968.
95. Abernethy DR, Greenblatt DJ, Shader RI: Treatment of diazepam withdrawal syndrome with propranolol. *Ann Intern Med* 94:354, 1981.
96. Goodman WK, Charney DS, Price LH, et al: Ineffectiveness of clonidine in the treatment of benzodiazepine withdrawal syndrome: Report of three cases. *Am J Psychiatry* 143:900, 1986.
97. Dysken MW, Chan CH: Diazepam withdrawal psychosis: A case report. *Am J Psychiatry* 134:573, 1977.
98. Khantzian EJ, McKenna GJ: Acute toxic withdrawal reactions associated with drug use and abuse. *Ann Intern Med* 90:361, 1979.
99. Freitas PM: Narcotic withdrawal in the emergency department. *Am J Emerg Med* 3:456, 1985.
100. George CF, Robertson D: Clinical consequences of abrupt drug withdrawal. *Med Toxicol Adv Drug Exp* 2:367, 1987.
101. Flemenbaum A, Boza R, Slater VL, et al: Clonidine opiate withdrawal. *Res Staff Physician* 35:111, 1989.
102. Fultz JM, Senay EC: Guidelines for the management of hospitalized narcotic addicts. *Ann Intern Med* 82:815, 1975.
103. Goldfrank LR: The several uses of naloxone. *Emerg Med* 16:105, 1984.
104. Zuspan FP, Gumpel JA, Mejia-Zelaya A, et al: Fetal stress from methadone withdrawal. *Am J Obstet Gynecol* 122:43, 1975.
105. Fraser AC: Drug addiction in pregnancy. *Lancet* 2:896, 1976.
106. Kandall SR: Managing neonatal withdrawal. *Drug Ther* 6:47, 1976.
107. Gold MS, Redmond DE, Kleber HD: Clonidine blocks acute opiate withdrawal symptoms. *Lancet* 2:599, 1978.
108. Gold MS, Pottash AC, Sweeney DR, et al: Opiate withdrawal treatment using clonidine. *JAMA* 243:343, 1980.

XI. Surgical Problems in the Intensive Care Unit

Section Editor
Mitchell P. Fink

159. Diagnosis and Management of Intraabdominal Sepsis

Joseph S. Solomkin
and Jonathan S. Moulton

Intraabdominal infections are commonly encountered in general medical/surgical intensive care units. Perhaps the largest group consists of patients identified as having intraabdominal infection who have recently undergone or will shortly undergo some form of an interventional procedure. The primary set of problems surrounding their care concerns the extent of preoperative diagnostic and resuscitative efforts and the timing of intervention. A second group consists of patients resident in intensive care units for whom intraabdominal infection may represent a source of occult sepsis. There are significant numbers of patients with clinical findings suggestive of infection, often with unexplained ileus, in whom no source of nosocomial infection can be identified by routine investigations. In patients who have recently undergone elective or emergent abdominal operation, concern for the appearance of abscesses is often sufficient to lead to empiric treatment for this working diagnosis. Such an approach can result in overlooking other, less common causes of infection. A more sinister group of patients is made up of those ultimately found to have bowel ischemia, pseudomembranous colitis, or pancreatitis.

Pathophysiology of the Local and Systemic Response to Intraabdominal Infections

Patients with intraabdominal infections may be viewed as a unique subset of sepsis syndrome patients. In an era in which laboratory advances suggest the possibility of pharmacologic intervention beyond antibiotics, this material is of interest in suggesting points for disease-specific intervention. The defense mechanisms of the peritoneal cavity help explain the specific pattern of response seen. There are well-defined systems for rapid mechanical clearance of forign particulates and solutes from the intraperitoneal space. Diaphragmatic lymphatic channels provide a means for the entry of peritoneal fluid (and any bacteria and proinflammatory mediators) through the thoracic duct into the venous circulation (Fig. 159-1). Lymphatic capillaries are distributed in the subperitoneal connective tissue of the diaphragm. Mesothelial cells are organized into two discrete populations: cuboidal cells and flattened cells. Gaps (stomata) between neighboring cells of the peritoneal mesothelium are abundant in the peritoneal mesothelium [1]. The stomata are found only among cuboidal cells [2]. The average area of a stoma is about 10^2 μm. Peritonitis increases the width of these stomata [3]. Inspiration decreases intrathoracic pressure relative to intraabdominal pressure, creating a pressure gradient favoring fluid movement out of the abdomen. Entry of proinflammatory substances into the vascular space would be expected to produce many of the hemodynamic and respiratory findings of severe sepsis. Positive-pressure ventilation likely attenuates this process but has not been well studied as a therapeutic maneuver [4].

Other peritoneal defense mechanisms include resident peritoneal macrophages and large recruitable pools of circulating neutrophils and monocytes. These cell types participate in abscess formation. Ingestion of microorganisms by these cells may result in secretion of a variety of proinflammatory molecules, including cytokines, lipid derivatives, oxidants, and lysosomal enzymes. Manipulation of the number and function of these resident and recruited cells is now possible through the use of colony-stimulating factors but has not been examined in clinical trials.

The contribution of proinflammatory products released into mesenteric, lymphatic, and vascular channels to the systemic septic response has not been fully addressed. Liver dysfunction is common during the course of intraabdominal infection and occasionally progresses to fatal hepatic failure [5,6]. There is considerable evidence that various macrophage products, including IL-1, IL-6, and TNF-α, substantially alter hepatocyte function [7]. Aside from conversion of hepatic synthetic function to acute phase reactants, serum chemistries reveal evidence of ductal epithelial cytotoxicity, including elevated alkaline phosphatase levels and elevated bilirubin levels. The large number of fixed tissue phagocytes (Kuppfer cells) in the liver capable of responding to endotoxin absorbed from systemic or mesenteric blood vessels represents a potentially important source of cytokines and other hepatocyte regulatory substances, although portal endotoxemia has not been detected in humans [8,9].

The bacteriology of mixed flora infections, encompassing aerobic, anaerobic, and facultative gram-negative organisms, explains at least part of the local histopathology of intraabdominal infection. Facultative and aerobic gram-negative organisms express and release endotoxin and endotoxin-associated proteins spontaneously, and such shedding is likely intensified by administration of antibiotics [10]. Aside from the potential for inducing the release of cytokines and other inflammatory mediators, these substances induce local thrombosis through a variety of endothelial and macrophage-mediated processes. Synergistic interactions between certain anaerobes, most notably *Bacteroides fragilis,* and endotoxin-bearing gram-negative organisms suppress local host defense mechanisms and facilitate the establishment of infection [11–14]. *Bacteroides fragilis* produces a capsular polysaccharide that interferes with complement activation and inhibits leukocyte function [15]. These phenomena are thought to restrict the delivery of phagocytes to the site of infection, permitting a more rapid rate of bacterial growth than would otherwise be seen.

Clinical Aspects of Care for Patients with Intraabdominal Infections

INITIAL THERAPEUTIC GOALS. Acute perforations of the gastrointestinal tract with peritonitis commonly present with

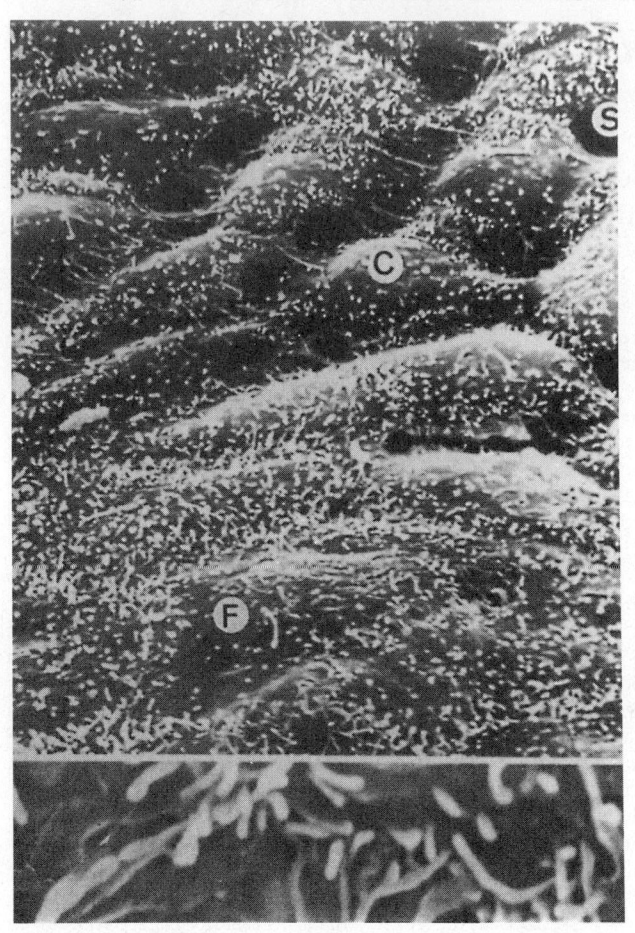

A

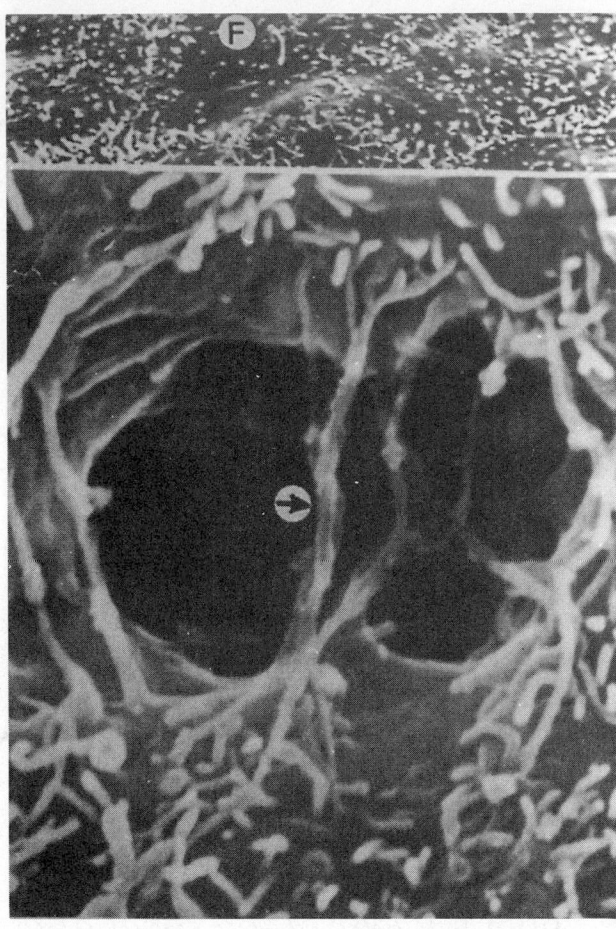

B

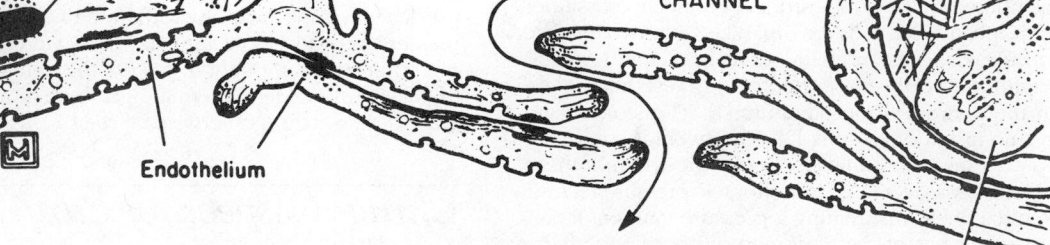

PERITONEAL CAVITY

Basement Membrane

Tight Junction

Mesothelium

Nucleus

Gap Junction

Collagen

STOMA

Microfibrils

Elastic Fibers

CHANNEL

Endothelium

LUMEN OF THE LACUNA

Fibroblast

C

Fig. 159-1. A. There are two kinds of cells, cuboidal cells (C) and flattened cells (F), on the peritoneum of the muscular portion of the diaphragm. Stomata (S) are detected among cuboidal cells. ×1,650. (Source: *Acta Anatomica,* J.J.-Chang, 141:26–30, 1991, with permission.) B. There are some of the filamentous projections (↑) across the stoma, which is quite a deep pore on the tendinous portion of the diaphragmatic peritoneum, ×8,300. (Source: *Acta Anatomica,* J.J. Chang, 141:26–30, 1991, with permission.) C. Diagram of a typical stoma and underlying channel linking the peritoneal cavity with the lumen of a lymphatic lacuna. Lacunar mesothelial cells forming the stoma and flaplike endothelial processes that bridge the channel contain actin filaments. Where lacunar mesothelial cells and lacunar endothelial cells meet, their apposed plasma membrane lack junctional specializations. Both types of cells lack a basement membrane. The connective tissue adjacent to the channel contains abundant microfibrils. A pseudopod of a fibroblast contacts an endothelial cells. (Source: *The American Journal of Anatomy* 180:195, 1987, with permission.)

clinical evidence of infection severe enough to mandate initial treatment in an intensive care environment. Physical findings and the patient's history routinely provide sufficient diagnostic weight to obviate further diagnostic testing. Plain radiographs of the abdomen may reveal free air, a uniform indicator of visceral perforation in the absence of prior intervention. Other findings from plain radiographs that support the diagnosis of intraabdominal infection include pneumatosis intestinalis, bowel obstruction, and a mass effect. There are rare benign causes of pneumatosis [16]. More dramatic but less common findings are air in the portal vein or extraluminal gas collections indicative of an abscess; these radiographic signs are sufficiently specific to justify immediate intervention. Patients with serious intraabdominal infections have the same general problems as patients with other forms of sepsis but, in addition, require some form of physical intervention to control infection.

Perforations of the upper gastrointestinal tract cause impressive physical findings of peritonitis but rarely manifest evidence of septic shock. Conversely, perforations of the colon result in such substantial bacterial contamination as to be routinely accompanied by a hypotensive reaction. In either setting, progressive clinical deterioration cannot be controlled until continued soiling of the peritoneal cavity is terminated. This issue puts important limits on the extent to which resuscitation should be pursued prior to operative intervention. Patients with acute perforations of the gastrointestinal tract should be sufficiently resuscitated to be able to undergo induction of anesthesia, but resuscitation should continue during operation. The primary point is rapid volume loading to counter the vasodilatory effects of anesthetics. More refined parameters of completed resuscitation, such as maximization of cardiac output or oxygen delivery, should not be employed until patients have undergone intervention. Many units have developed protocols for the transport of critically ill patients to radiology suites. These include descriptions of accompanying personnel and support equipment. Resuscitation should continue as radiologic diagnostic and therapeutic efforts are undertaken.

In addition to intravascular volume loading, certain other maneuvers are of value in protecting patients from intraoperative hypotension. Infusing low doses of dopamine is thought to improve renal blood flow and reduce the incidence of acute renal failure, although hard data supporting this conclusion are lacking. In general, positive end-expiratory pressure (PEEP) should be used sparingly, since this maneuver decreases venous return and can compromise cardiac output. High inspired oxygen concentrations should be used as needed to maintain adequate arterial oxygen saturation until intravascular volume has been satisfactorily restored.

SURGICAL MANAGEMENT OF DIFFUSE PERITONITIS.

Operative management of peritonitis involves immediate evacuation of all purulent collections, with particular attention to subphrenic, subhepatic, interloop, and pelvic collections. It is well established that the perforated bowel should be resected. This notion has evolved from studies over several decades of mortality rates following surgical treatment of perforated diverticulitis [17,18]. Resection with end colostomy was shown to significantly decrease acute mortality as compared to transverse loop colostomy and drainage. The complication rates from primary anastomosis are staggering. In one study, mortality from primary anastomosis was 23 percent, with most of this mortality attributed to anastomotic leakage [19].

Controversies in the operative management of peritonitis primarily surround wound closure techniques and scheduled relaparotomies. Patients with diffuse peritonitis secondary to colonic perforation or anastomotic dehiscence typically develop abdominal wall edema as part of a generalized syndrome of increased capillary permeability. This syndrome is exacerbated by the accepted need to provide aggressive restoration of intravascular volume. Primary closure of the abdominal incision in such patients may be difficult or even unwise. Increased intraabdominal pressure can result in compression of mesenteric and renal veins, leading in some instances to acute renal failure or bowel necrosis. This situation can be handled by insertion of a fascial prosthesis. A variety of materials have been employed, including Marlex, Silastic, and polytetrafluoroethylene (PTFE) [20,21]. Each material has its own virtues and problems. Impermeable materials can exacerbate peritonitis and should be used only if planned relaparotomies are to be undertaken.

It is important to recognize the high mortality rates and the high recurrence rate both of abscesses and, less commonly, persisting peritonitis in patients with diffuse peritonitis. These patients usually manifest a continued septic picture with varying degrees of renal and hepatic dysfunction, and there is little satisfaction with current approaches for operative management. This has led surgeons to try various mechanical approaches to reduce mortality. These generally have been premised on the notion that failure of host defense mechanisms of the peritoneal cavity may lead to persisting infection, often with fungal and gram-positive organisms [22,23]. Of these newer approaches, perhaps the most attractive is planned relaparotomy. Patients treated with this method undergo standard operative management of their infection, but the fascia is not closed. A prosthetic material is sewn to the fascia as a temporary closure, and at intervals of 24 to 48 hours the mesh is opened and the peritoneal cavity debrided and irrigated. Early reports were quite positive, but used historical controls [24,25]. Unfortunately, more recent reports have not found that survival is substantially improved or that the incidence of late abscess formation is reduced. Occasional fistulas have occurred.

We have used planned relaparotomy in conjunction with prosthetic fascial closure for a small number of patients with septic shock and colon-derived peritonitis. The obvious benefits relate to absence of wound tension and the ability to obtain sequential microbiologic data to guide antimicrobial therapy. Once the prosthetic mesh is in place, the surgical team can decide to perform relaparotomy on a scheduled basis, or as dictated by the patient's clinical course and the results of adjunctive tests, particularly computed tomography. The latter, more conservative approach seems worthwhile for patients who recover from their initial episode of shock and who do not manifest progressive organ failure. In such patients, abdominal wall and visceral edema typically resolves over the first week, at which time definitive closure of the abdomen can be performed.

INDICATIONS FOR DIAGNOSTIC IMAGING FOR SUSPECTED INTRAABDOMINAL INFECTIONS: PERCUTANEOUS ABSCESS DRAINAGE.

In the absence of physical findings of diffuse peritonitis, diagnostic imaging with either computed tomography (CT) or ultrasound should be routinely performed in seriously ill patients with intraabdominal infection. The urgency of investigation is dictated by the degree of hemodynamic instability present. Most patients should be evaluated within hours of clinical diagnosis. Interventional radiology has replaced operative treatment for many localized processes, including diverticular abscesses.

CT is the single best modality for fully evaluating the extent of disease in most situations. Ultrasound is also quite versatile and has the added advantage of being portable, allowing certain procedures to be performed in the ICU [26,27]. Ultrasonography is limited by bowel gas, body habitus, and lower sensitivity for retroperitoneal processes and parenchymal infection. Usually the choice of modality is based on the experience and preference of the interventional radiologist.

When feasible, nonoperative (i.e., percutaneous) drainage of pus is preferable to open surgical intervention. This is because of the initial deterioration that almost always occurs following operative manipulation of intraabdominal infection. The exact basis for this is unclear, but a substantial proportion of patients undergoing emergency operation for intraabdominal infection suffer acute hemodynamic compromise in the early postoperative period. When used for appropriate indications, percutaneous abscess drainage (PAD) is at least as effective as operation and is associated with less morbidity [28,29].

PERCUTANEOUS DRAINAGE PROCEDURES FOR INTRAABDOMINAL ABSCESSES.

PAD and operative intervention are best viewed as complementary rather than competitive techniques. There are many situations for which PAD is the definitive procedure of choice, others for which surgery alone is indicated, and some for which both techniques are applicable, alone or in conjunction. Inflammation may manifest as a phlegmon (viable inflamed tissue), a liquefied abscess, infected necrotic (nonviable) tissue, or a combination. Liquefied abscesses are drainable, whereas phlegmonous and necrotic tissue is not. Decisions regarding which modality to employ are largely based on CT findings and require experience, clinical judgment, and careful consideration of underlying and coexistent disease processes. Close cooperation between the surgeon, interventional radiologist, and other physicians involved in the patient's care is mandatory. Specific indications for PAD have expanded significantly over the past decade and now include many conditions previously thought undrainable, such as multiple and/or multiloculated abscesses, abscesses with enteric communication, and infected hematomas [30].

It is important to define the goals of the procedure in evaluating indications and success. Potential outcomes include cure, temporization, palliation, and failure [31,32,33]. A *cure* is achieved when the abscess is resolved by the drainage procedure. *Temporization* refers to resolution of an abscess and clinical improvement, with operative intervention needed to treat the underlying cause. *Palliation* refers to improvement in the patient's condition due to abscess drainage, despite the presence of a rapidly fatal underlying condition. We consider temporizing and palliative results to represent success.

The basic requirements for PAD include a safe route of percutaneous access and the presence of a fluid collection of drainable consistency. Bleeding dyscrasias are a relative contraindication, as is the case for any interventional procedure. Safe percutaneous access is attainable in most cases. It is generally possible to distinguish drainable fluid from phlegmonous or necrotic tissue using a combination of imaging and fine-needle aspiration. Not all fluid collections require drainage, although it is generally required for those that are infected and for sterile collections that cause symptoms based on their mass effect. This determination must be made on an individual basis.

It is important to consider the possibility of underlying neoplastic disease in the setting of enteric perforation, especially in elderly patients. Significant soft tissue thickening of the bowel wall, especially if localized and noncircumferential, should raise the possibility of underlying tumor, as should the demonstration of potential metastatic disease such as adenopathy or liver lesions. A "target" appearance, with circumferential low-attenuation submucosal thickening sandwiched between the enhancing mucosa and submucosa, is felt to be specific for inflammatory disease. To fully exclude the possibility of neoplasia, follow-up imaging is needed to document resolution, or confirmatory tests such as barium studies or endoscopy may be performed.

Technical Aspects. Excellent imaging is a key element for successful PAD. Imaging permits precise localization and characterization of disease, appropriate access route planning, and immediate assessment of technical success. Imaging also is needed for adequate follow-up to identify problems and gauge outcome. It is important that the drainage route not cross a sterile fluid collection or other infected space due to the risk of cross-contamination. Crossing the pleural space for thoracic and upper abdominal drainage carries the risk of empyema formation. Thus, collections in the upper abdomen often require an angled subcostal or low intercostal approach [34]. It is acceptable to cross the peritoneal space in order to drain an extraperitoneal abscess. Placement of a catheter through the small bowel or colon should always be avoided. Transgastric drainage of lesser sac pseudocysts has been advocated by some authors and appears to be safe, although this approach remains controversial [30]. Lesser sac collections also can be approached transhepatically through the left lobe of the liver [35], although traversing solid organs should be avoided whenever possible. Obviously, it is important to be aware of, and avoid, major vascular structures.

In most cases drainage is performed following fine-needle (18–22 gauge) aspiration, with the aspirate being used to document infection and gauge the viscosity of the fluid. Immediate gram stain of the fluid is useful to determine the need for drainage. In some situations, single-step aspiration of the fluid may suffice, without the need for tube placement. Examples include clearly aseptic collections, small abscesses (2–3 cm) into which tube placement would be difficult, and relatively nonviscous collections that can be completely evacuated. However, for most collections, a drain should be placed to ensure complete evacuation and minimize the chance of recurrence. The aspiration needle can be used for placement of a guidewire or as a guide for tandem insertion of the drain. If the patient is not already on antimicrobial therapy, this should be instituted prior to the drainage procedure to minimize the infectious complications of contaminating sterile tissue.

A wide variety of techniques and equipment are available for catheter placement, the majority falling into one of two categories. The trocar technique involves the one-step insertion of a catheter that is loaded coaxially onto a stiffening cannula and needle. This is the technically simpler approach and is applicable to most superficial and large collections. The Seldinger technique is preferable for deep abscesses with difficult access, for drainages whose access route crosses exceptionally firm tissue, and for placement of catheters larger than 14 Fr. A needle is first inserted into the collection. A guidewire is then passed through the needle and the needle is withdrawn. The tract is sequentially dilated over the guidewire until it is possible to insert the catheter.

There are a multitude of catheters available for percutaneous insertion. The choice of catheter size is determined primarily by the viscosity of the fluid to be drained. In the majority of cases, 8 to 12 Fr. drains are sufficient [36,37]. Larger drains may be needed for collections containing debris or more viscous fluid. Drains of larger caliber can be placed, if needed, by exchange over a guidewire. There is no absolute limit on the number of drains that can be placed. While most abscesses can be drained with a single catheter, there should be no hesitation in placing as many drains as are needed to effectively evacuate the abscess(es).

Following catheter placement, the cavity should be evacuated as completely as possible and irrigated with saline until the fluid is clear. Initial manipulation of the catheter(s) and irrigation should be done as gently as possible to minimize the induction of bacteremia. Immediate imaging determines the need for repositioning of the catheter, placing a large-bore catheter, or for placing additional drains. For cavities that are completely evacuated at the initial drainage and for which there are no abnormal communications to viscera, simple gravity drainage generally suffices. For larger or more viscous collections and those with ongoing output due to fistulous connections, suction drainage with sump catheters is more effective [35,36,38]. Thoracic drains always should be placed to water-seal suction.

Proper catheter management following the initial placement is a critical determinant of success and requires the interventional radiologist to become an active member of the management team [39]. Drains should be checked regularly (at least daily) to monitor the volume and nature of the output, ensure adequate function and clinical response, and quickly recognize and correct any catheter-related problems. Most authorities recommend periodic irrigation of the drains, once or several times per day, with sterile saline [40]. This may be performed by either physicians or trained nurses. In general, irrigation with proteolytic agents (e.g., acetylcysteine) or antibiotics is of no value, although fibrinolytic agents may be useful for evacuation of fibrinous or hemorrhagic collections. There is no standard protocol for follow-up imaging. Repeat imaging studies and catheter injections are frequently used to document progress and identify problems. Occasionally, it may be necessary to replace or reposition tubes or add additional catheters. The need for follow-up imaging studies should be determined on a case-by-case basis by monitoring clinical progress and drainage output.

Catheters should be removed when criteria for abscess resolution are met. Clinical criteria of success include resolution of symptoms and indicators of infection (fever, leukocytosis). Catheter-related criteria include a decrease in daily drainage to less than 10 ml and a change in the character of the drainage from purulent to serous. Radiographic criteria include documentation of abscess resolution and closure of any fistulous communications. If catheters are maintained until these criteria are satisfied, the likelihood of recurrence of the abscess will be minimized. Although some authorities recommend gradual catheter removal over several days [40], we usually remove the drain in one step and have had no significant problem with recurrence. For sterile fluid collections, the drain should be removed as soon as possible, generally within 24 to 48 hours, to minimize the risk of superinfection [40].

Causes of Failure. In evaluating the causes of PAD failure, a number of factors are consistently identified. Among these are fluid that is too viscous for drainage or the presence of phlegmonous or necrotic debris. Technical modifications such as increasing the drain size and irrigation can salvage some of these procedures. Recognition of phlegmonous or necrotic tissue on follow-up imaging studies may lead to cessation of attempts at PAD or a modification of the expected goal. Multiloculated collections and multiple abscesses are another cause of failure that can be minimized by using an adequate number of catheters along with mechanical disruption of adhesions with a guidewire. Fistulous communications, either unrecognized or persistent, are yet another potential cause of failure, as is drainage of a necrotic tumor mistaken by imaging to represent an abscess. Recognition of a significant soft-tissue component, maintenance of a high index of suspicion, and the use of percutaneous biopsies can minimize the risk of failing to appreciate the presence of tumor. Suspicious fluid also may be sent for cytology. The success rate for PAD tends to be lower in immunocompromised patients. Lambiase et al. found a cure rate of 53 percent in immunocompromised patients (including those with alcoholism, AIDS, diabetes, renal failure, or steroid use) as compared to 73 percent in immunocompetent patients [31].

Management of Specific Intraabdominal Infections

MANAGEMENT OF ABSCESSES. In cases with abscesses complicating diverticulitis, PAD usually permits stabilization and allows time to optimally prepare the patient for operative therapy [41,42]. Subsequent operation is required in most, but not all, patients and is generally simplified to a one-step procedure (Fig. 159-2). In some patients who remain asymptomatic following drainage, such as those with other ultimately fatal diseases, subsequent colectomy may be avoided. It is important to perform follow-up radiographic studies to exclude the possibility of a perforated neoplasm. Initial concerns regarding persistent fecal fistulas have not been borne out by clinical experience.

The results of PAD for abscesses complicating Crohn's disease are less positive. Patients without fistulous communications to the bowel are usually cured by PAD, whereas those with fistulas generally required bowel resection [43–46]. Among patients requiring operation, initial PAD usually leads to significant clinical improvement and permits performance of a one-stage operation. There are no reports of iatrogenic enterocutaneous fistulas.

Low pelvic abscesses in contact with the rectum or vagina may be treated surgically by incision and drainage through these organs. The same approach can be taken using sonographic guidance, and recent advances in endoluminal ultrasound techniques have facilitated such procedures [47,48]. Experience with ultrasound-guided transrectal and transvaginal drainage is growing, and these procedures appear to be effective and well-tolerated. Good success also has been achieved in the management of tuboovarian abscesses complicating pelvic inflammatory disease that are refractory to medical management. In many such cases, the need for hysterectomy and oophorectomy has been obviated [49].

INFECTIONS COMPLICATING ACUTE PANCREATITIS. Infections superimposed on acute pancreatitis are among the most difficult intraabdominal infections to manage (see Chap.

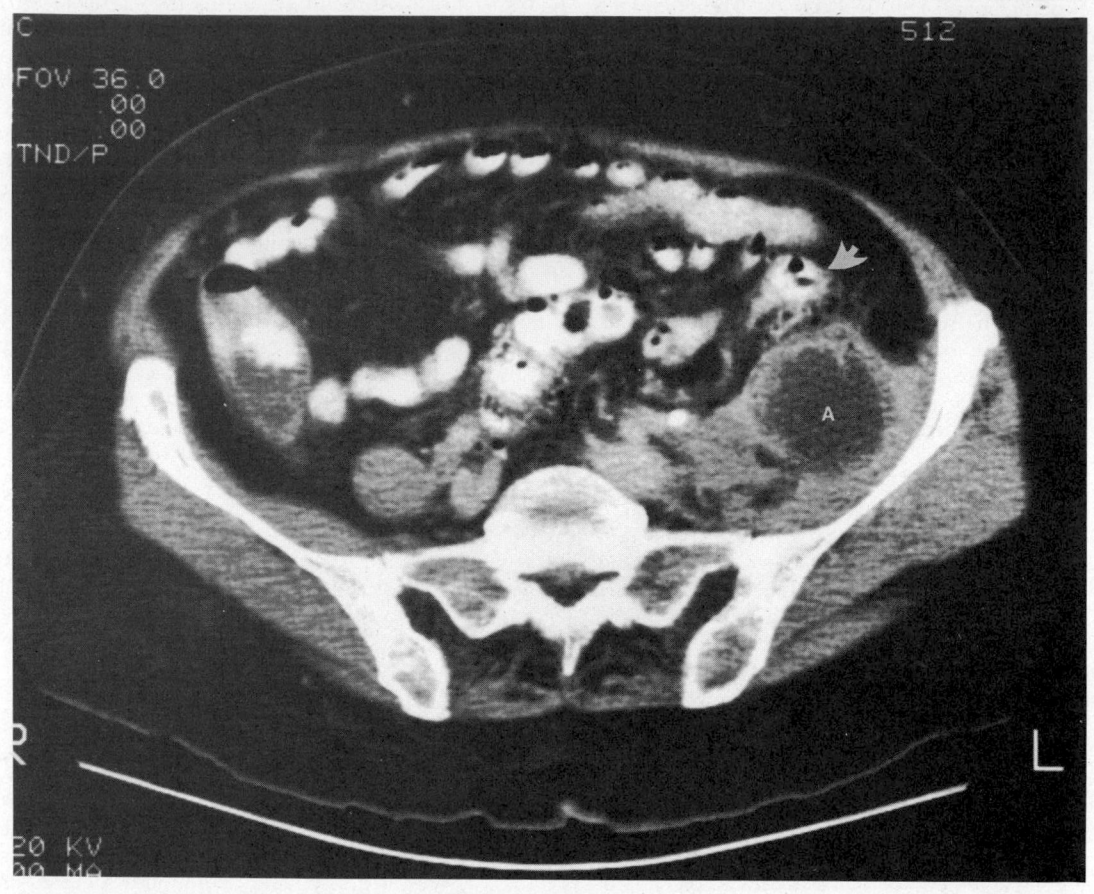

A

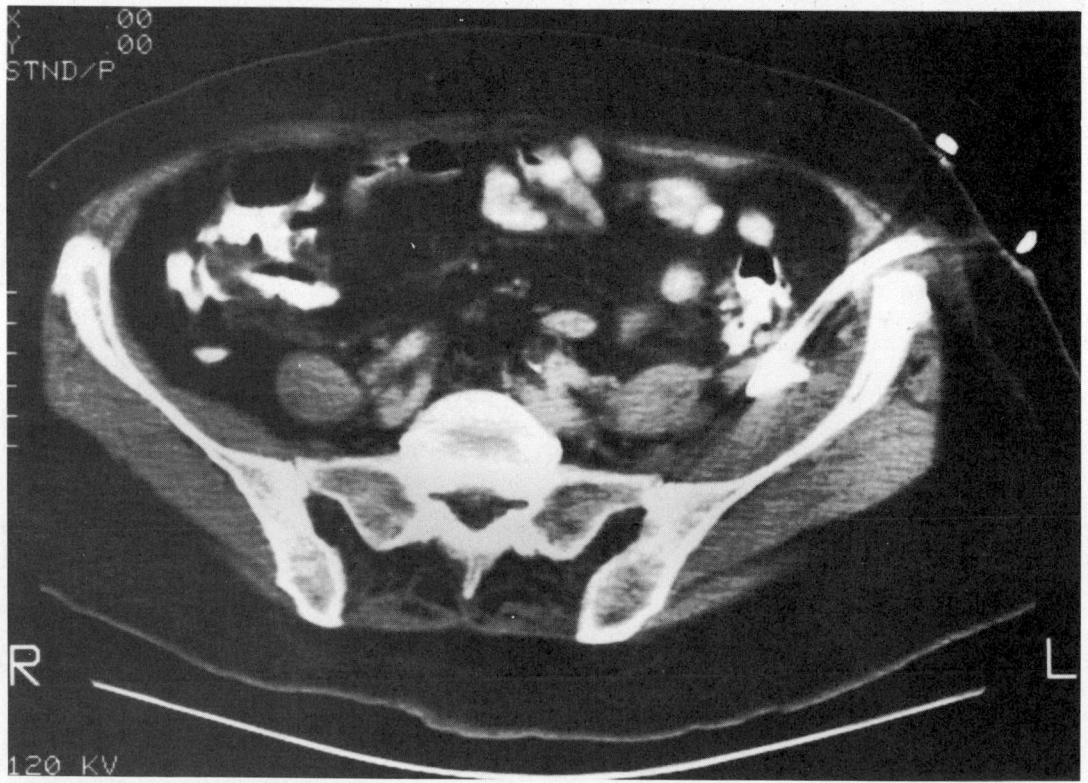

B

Fig. 159-2. An 85-year-old female with diverticulitis and persistent fever after 1 week of antibiotic therapy. A. Computed tomography (CT) scan shows an abscess (A) in the left psoas muscle, adjacent to an inflamed sigmoid colon with diverticula (white arrow). B. CT scan after 1 month of percutaneous drainage shows resolution of the abscess and associated inflammation. A low-volume colonic fistula remained open and the patient underwent an uneventful single-stage left hemicolectomy. Source: *New Horizons,* J. S. Moulton, Vol. 1, pps 231–245, May 1993, with permission.

160). Discrete abscesses or infected pseudocysts are not particularly complicated problems, but no satisfactory approach exists to lesser sac collections with pancreatic necrosis [50,51]. Current surgical therapy consists of repetitive scheduled debridement at 48-hour intervals [52,53,54]. This approach has improved outcome but results in prolonged stays in the ICU.

For pancreatic debridement, we use a bilateral subcostal (chevron) incision to avoid exposure of the small bowel. The lesser sac is entered and the stomach and colon retracted cephalad and caudad, respectively. Blunt dissection is used to remove necrotic pancreas and open loculated abscesses. The pancreatic bed is often packed with gauze. The value of using packing material has not been established by clinical studies and probably has little physiologic merit. Foreign material incites an inflammatory response and prolongs the time needed to clear the infection. Failure to remove packing within 48 hours results in recurrent fever and other findings of infection. The use of topical antibiotic solutions is not recommended since parenteral antibiotics penetrate sites of inflammation well and topical solutions may produce unwanted adverse systemic effects.

As a general guide, three or four reexplorations suffice to remove necrotic tissue and produce a granulating wound. At this time, prosthetic material used to facilitate abdominal reentry should be removed and the fascia closed. Patients should be monitored closely for evidence of recurrent infection and undergo computed tomographic scanning if infection is suspected.

For localized (acute or chronic) fluid collections, percutaneous drainage is successful in 78 to 91 percent of cases [55,56]. Fistulous communications to the pancreatic duct are commonly present but may be difficult to document radiographically. To minimize the risk of recurrence with pancreatic fluid collections, it is especially important to document complete cessation of drainage (<5 ml/day) prior to removing drains. Endoscopic retrograde cholangiopancreatography (ERCP) is valuable to document patency of the pancreatic duct, since fistulas associated with downstream obstruction are unlikely to heal and generally require operation [57].

Computed tomography is the procedure of choice for localizing and characterizing complications of acute pancreatitis, and fine-needle aspiration is invaluable in documenting infection [58–62]. Percutaneous drainage is a therapeutic option for evacuation of infected fluid but is not capable of removing infected necrotic tissue [63,64,65]. Percutaneous drainage can be used to temporize and allow for a delayed definitive necrosectomy (Fig. 159-3). Factors that would mitigate against this approach include the presence of multiple small lesser sac abscesses or concern about erosion of the inflammatory mass into the colon or major blood vessels. Two recent series detailing the use of PAD for severe complicated pancreatitis reported success rates of only 37 percent and 47 percent [66,67]. Although the fluid collections associated with pancreatitis can usually be drained percutaneously, operation is required for debridement of infected necrotic tissue. Drainage of central (pancreatic bed and lesser sac) collections is less often successful than is drainage

of peripheral collections, due to the frequent presence of phlegmon and necrosis in the central regions [67].

There is no general consensus regarding the optimal means of managing patients with infections complicating acute pancreatitis; management must be individualized. Most authorities recommend some combination of percutaneous drainage and surgical debridment [30,55,57,66,67]. One possible approach is to perform PAD initially, followed by operation for necrosectomy. This carries the risk of unduly delaying definitive surgical therapy in critically ill patients, if temporization is not achieved. An alternative approach is to perform early surgical debridement of the central necrotic tissues and to utilize PAD, if needed, for peripheral or residual fluid collections.

Antimicrobial chemotherapy for patients with infections complicating pancreatitis should be guided by cultures of the pancreatic bed. Often patients are sequentially infected with gram-negative enteric flora, then gram-positive, methicillin-resistant organisms, and finally *Candida* species.

BILIARY INFECTIONS, INCLUDING ACALCULOUS CHOLECYSTITIS. Ascending cholangitis, which results from biliary obstruction and secondary bacterial infection, typically presents with the clinical triad of fever, chills, and jaundice. Relief of obstruction should be performed on an emergency basis. Imaging is performed to document biliary obstruction and identify the cause. The diagnosis of biliary obstruction is based on demonstration of abnormal dilatation of the common bile duct and/or its tributaries. Ultrasound is the best modality for demonstrating biliary dilatation. Ultrasound also may demonstrate ancillary findings such as ductal wall thickening or intraluminal gas or pericholecystic fluid collections [68,69]. Intravenous contrast administration is needed to document biliary dilatation with computed tomography.

Common causes of biliary obstruction include ductal calculi, benign strictures, adenopathy, and neoplastic diseases (pancreatic carcinoma, cholangiocarcinoma). Ultrasound is extremely sensitive in detecting stones in the gallbladder, but is less sensitive (55%) in detecting common duct calculi [70]. Computed tomography is less sensitive than ultrasound in identifying stones, as stones often have the same radiographic density as the surrounding bile [71]. Computed tomography is superior to ultrasound for demonstrating underlying pancreatic diseases, whether inflammatory or neoplastic. There are several pitfalls in the diagnostic imaging of cholangitis. Early obstruction may present without demonstrable biliary dilatation. Conversely, a dilated bile duct may not be functionally obstructed, but rather the dilatation may be due to prior biliary obstruction with resultant ectasia. Clinical and laboratory signs of biliary obstruction (i.e., jaundice, hyperbilirubinemia, elevated serum alkaline phosphatase activity) are generally adequate to distinguish between obstructive and nonobstructive biliary dilatation. Patients who have undergone prior biliary bypass or sphincterotomy may have gas in the biliary tree without infection.

Direct visualization of the biliary tree, via percutaneous transhepatic cholangiography (PTC) or ERCP, is often utilized for both diagnostic and therapeutic purposes. A thorough discussion of the relative merits of these two techniques is beyond the scope of this chapter. In most cases, cross-sectional imaging is sufficient for diagnostic purposes, and intervention is utilized for therapy. If biliary obstruction is strongly suspected on clinical grounds and imaging does not demonstrate dilatation, direct visualization of the duct may be warranted to identify early nondilated obstruction. Both studies (ERCP and PTC) require transportation of the patient to a fluoroscopy suite. ERCP is less invasive and generally is the initial procedure of choice for distal obstruction, whereas PTC may be more useful for proxi-

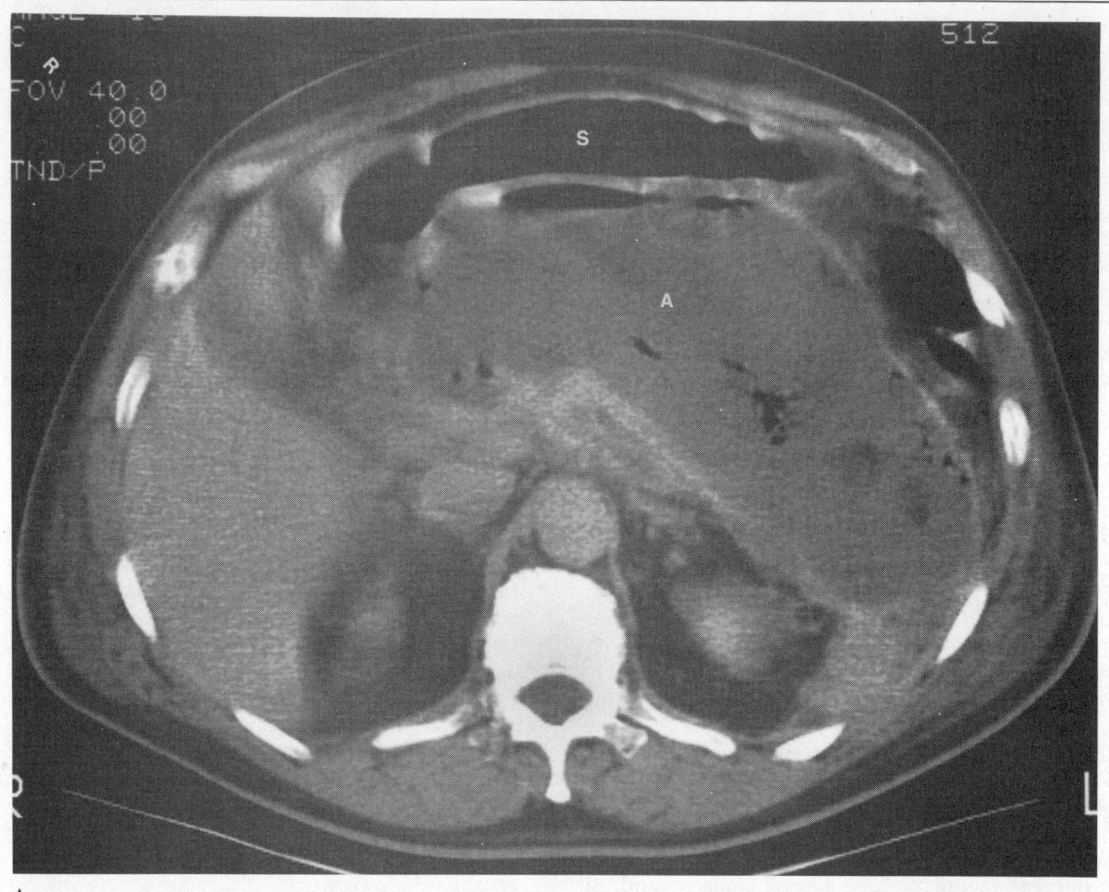

A

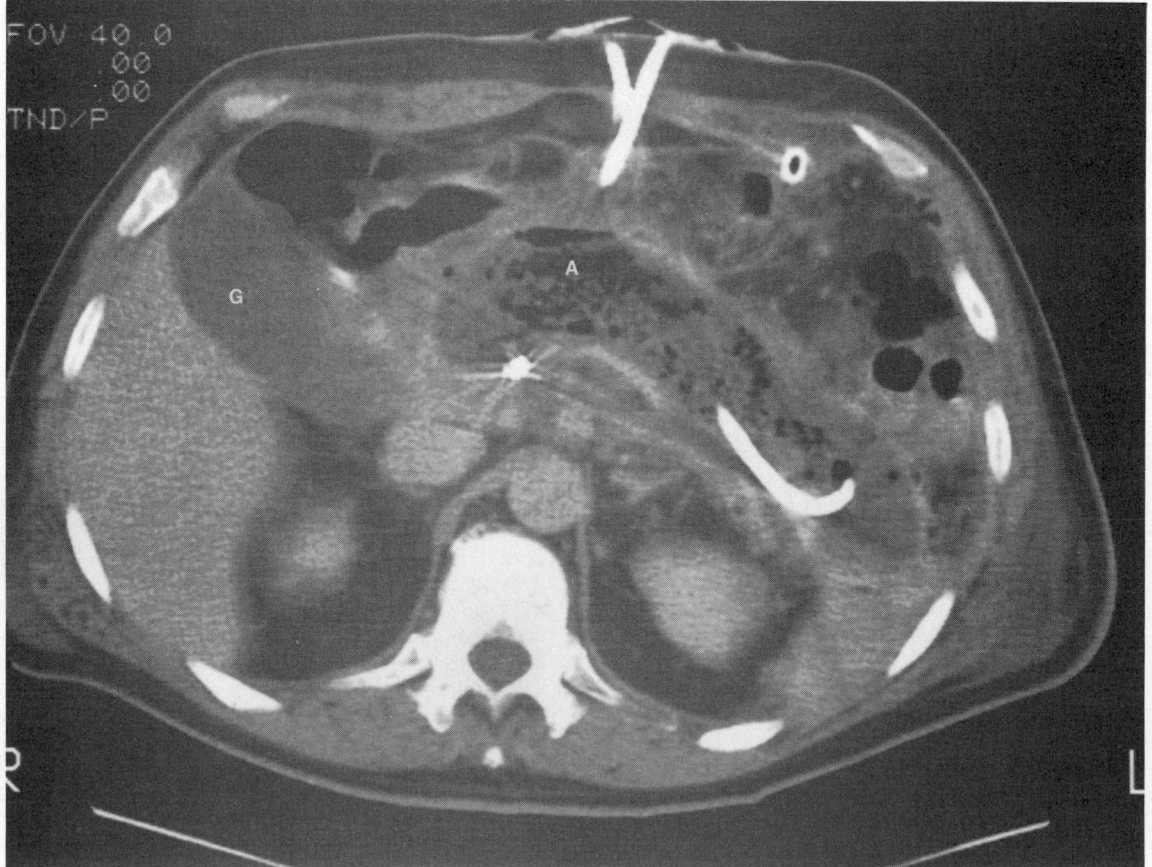

B

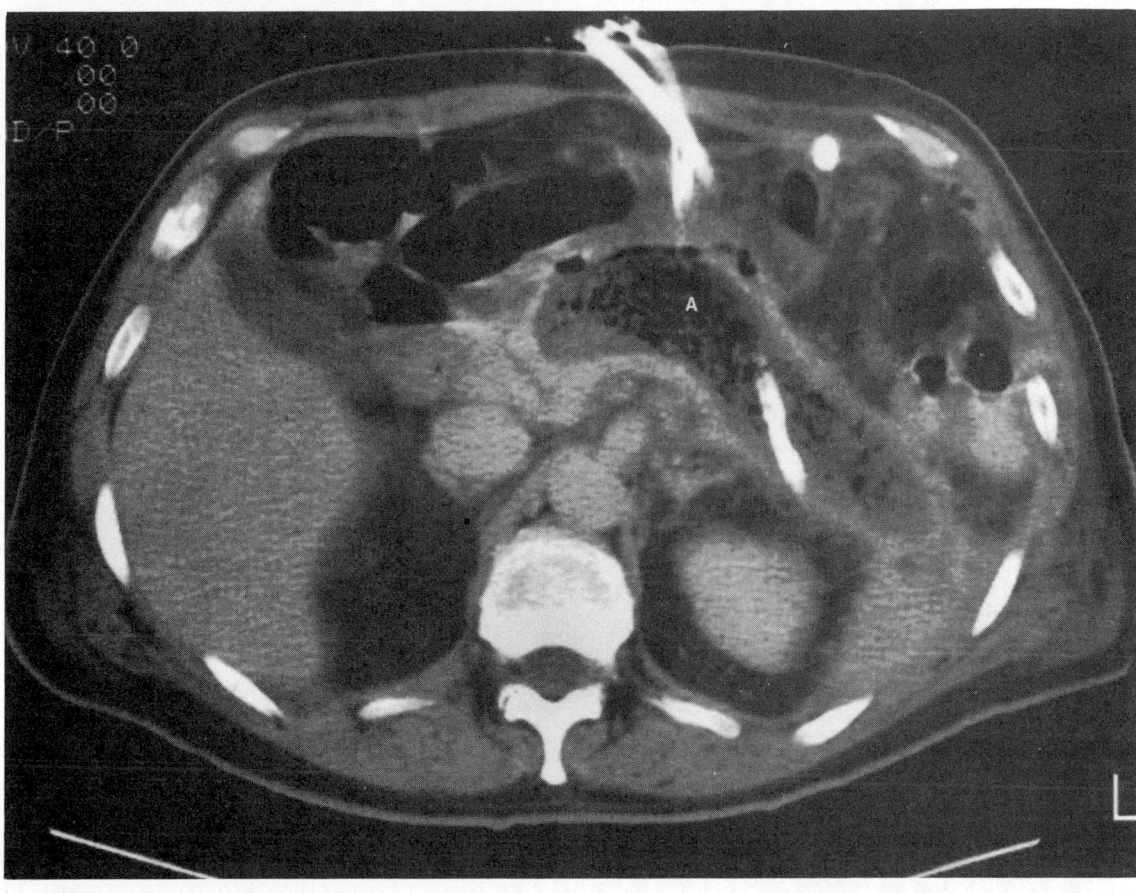

C

Fig. 159-3. A 66-year-old male transferred from an outside institution after 2 months of hospitalization for severe pancreatitis. A. Contrast-enhanced computed tomography (CT) scan at the time of transfer shows infected pancreatic necrosis with a water-density mass (A) containing gas bubbles, completely replacing the normal pancreas (S, stomach; L, liver). B. CT scan 10 days after placement of two 16 Fr Sump drains in the pancreatic bed shows significant reduction in the amount of fluid but persistence of a pancreatiform mass (A) of infected necrotic tissue (G, gallbladder). C. CT scan after an additional 3 weeks of drainage shows no further resolution of the infected necrotic mass. The patient had significantly improved clinically and underwent subsequent operative necrosectomy. Source: *New Horizons,* J. S. Moulton, Vol. 1, pps 231–245, May 1993, with permission.

mal obstructions. To a large extent, the choice of modalities rests with the expertise of available personnel.

Acute Cholecystitis as a Complication of Intensive Care.

Acute cholecystitis in the ICU is a different disease than that seen in ambulatory populations. Most cases are acalculous and likely represent complications of microvascular and mucosal dysfunction [14,15]. This condition often presents as occult sepsis, with or without physical findings of right upper quadrant tenderness [15,20,22,23,72]. Liver chemistries are abnormal in about half of the patients and therefore are not reliable as screening tests.

Ultrasound is used most commonly to identify this condition. Sonographic findings include diffuse or focal increases in wall thickness, striated intramural gallbladder lucencies, pericholecystic fluid, and/or sonolucency. Increased gallbladder wall thickness beyond 3 mm can be due to a variety of benign conditions, including hypoalbuminemia and right heart failure. Wall thickness alone is a poor indicator of acute cholecystitis [24]. Intramural lucencies reflect subserosal inflammation and are therefore believed to be relatively specific for acute cholecystitis [14,24,25,73]. Similarly, pericholecystic fluid is specific but uncommon.

Computed tomography, often used as an early diagnostic test for patients with unidentified postoperative sepsis, is both sensitive and specific for acute cholecystitis [74]. As with ultrasound, increased gallbladder wall thickness, intramural low-attenuation areas, and pericholecystic fluid collections in the absence of ascites are important findings [75,76].

There has been great interest in percutaneous cholecystostomy for patients suspected of having this condition. The current debate centers on the utility of this procedure when other sources of sepsis have been excluded [12,21]. We reserve cholecystostomy for patients with some evidence of biliary disease.

INTESTINAL ISCHEMIA. Ischemic disease of the bowel may result from arterial or venous occlusion or from a nonocclusive low-flow state in the mesenteric vessels [77]. Enteric ischemia is a frequent diagnostic consideration in the acutely ill septic patient. Plain radiography always should be performed first to seek evidence of advanced ischemia such as pneumatosis or portal vein gas. When enteric ischemia is strongly suspected, angiography is the procedure of choice for confirmation and

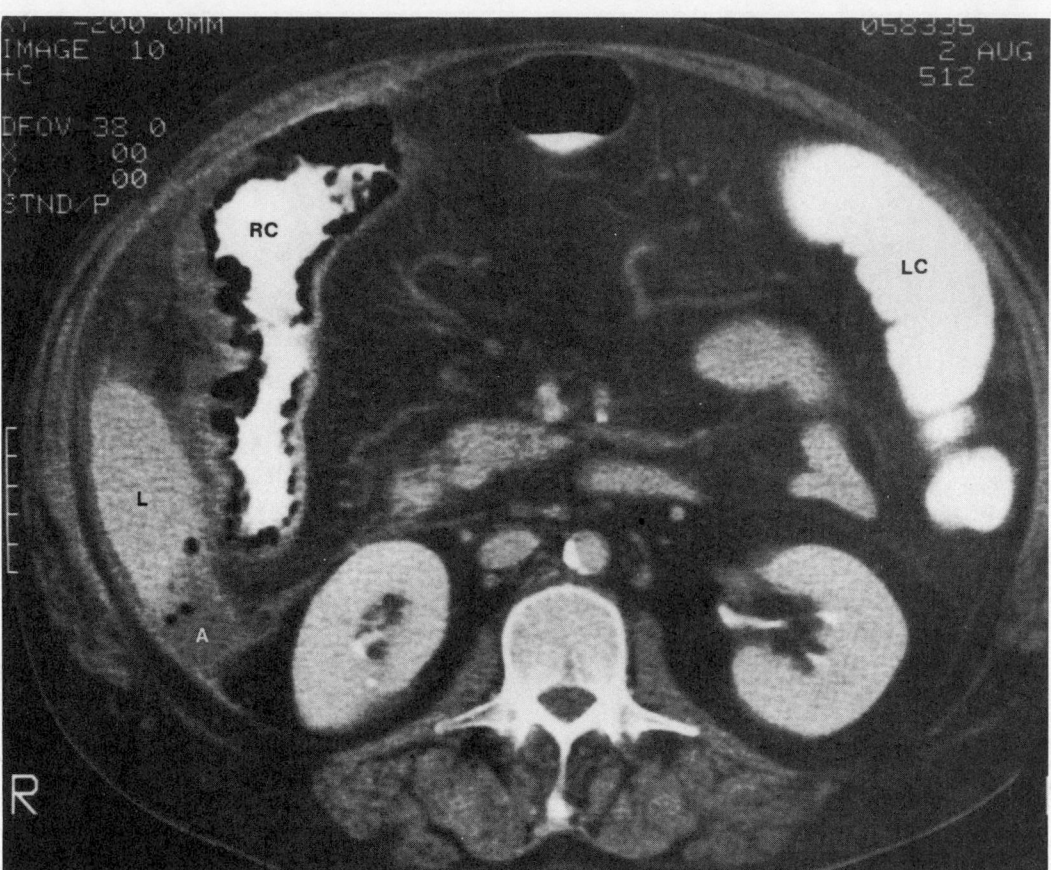

Fig. 159-4. Ischemic colitis. A 56-year-old male with severe ischemic cardiac disease who presented with acute abdominal pain, fever, and leukocytosis. Abdominal CT demonstrates mural thickening and extensive pneumatosis of the right colon (RC) that is most consistent with ischemic colitis. A localized abscess (A) is present in the paracolic gutter, indicating perforation. The patient initially responded to antibiotic therapy and percutaneous drainage of the abscess. Recurrence of symptoms led to a right hemicolectomy, which confirmed the diagnosis of ischemic colitis. LC, normal left colon; L, liver. Source: *New Horizons,* S. E. Braley, Vol. 1, pps 214–230, May 1993, with permission.

identification of the site and cause of ischemia. In patients whose symptomatology is less specific, computed tomography is a very useful modality for evaluating suspected enteric ischemia [16], as well as for identifying strangulation complicating closed-loop intestinal obstruction [78]. The earliest changes of ischemia are nonspecific and include bowel dilatation and mural thickening. With transmural ischemia, inflammatory changes are seen in the perienteric fat. Unfortunately, these findings are nonspecific, and computed tomography has limited sensitivity for detecting early and potentially reversible cases of mesenteric ischemia. The imaging findings are more specific when transmural necrosis has developed and include air within the bowel wall and portal venous system (Fig. 159-4). Computed tomography can also identify perforation with abscess formation or free peritonitis or demonstrate clot within a mesenteric vessel. If ischemic disease is suspected on the basis of the clinical evaluation or imaging studies, but the findings remain nonspecific, angiography should be performed [79,80]. The oral and intravenous contrast used for computed tomography may compromise the subsequent performance of angiography. However, computed tomography can detect other forms of pathology in the abdomen and is less invasive. Accordingly, the choice between computed tomography and angiography depends on the degree of clinical suspicion of ischemia.

INTRAABDOMINAL INFECTIONS IN POSTOPERATIVE PATIENTS. Postoperative peritonitis generally is a consequence of anastomotic dehiscence. This is a highly lethal condition, in part because it often is diagnosed late because of reluctance to entertain the possibility of a suture-line leak. This diagnosis should be considered in any patient with signs of sepsis who has undergone a gastrointestinal anastomosis. Typical findings of diffuse abdominal tenderness may be masked by incisional pain. Because laparotomy itself introduces free air into the abdominal cavity, pneumoperitoneum is a nonspecific finding in patients during the first few days after celiotomy. The most common error is to ascribe clinical deterioration to pulmonary processes that often are a consequence of peritonitis.

Ultrasound or computed tomography will reveal peritoneal fluid, which, if present, should lead to ultrasound-guided aspiration for diagnostic purposes. A Gram stain that reveals white cells or bacteria is an indication for immediate laparotomy. Surgical treatment should include either reanastomosis (small bowel) or end colostomy (colon). Postoperative abscesses are managed as detailed above.

MANAGEMENT OF ENTERIC FISTULAS. Intestinal fistulas present some of the more difficult diagnostic and therapeutic problems following intraabdominal operation. The most common source is the small intestine, followed by colon, stomach, duodenum, biliary tract, and pancreas. The initial finding in most patients is that of occult sepsis, and the systemic response is due to the inflammation surrounding the nascent fistula. Commonly, radiographic evaluation suggests an abscess.

Abscesses with fistulous communication to the alimentary canal, biliary tree, or pancreatic duct represent a special problem for percutaneous drainage. Fistulas are loosely characterized as high (>100 ml/day) or low (<100 ml/day) output. Low-output fistulas can be managed easily with PAD in most cases, and most high-output fistulas can be quickly converted to low-output ones [81].

Recognizing the presence of a fistula is the first important step in management. In several series only 26 percent of fistulas were identified (range 17–40%) at the time of initial drainage [81–84]. Presumably, the abnormal communication is initially occluded with debris, or adequate maneuvers to demonstrate the leak are not performed in order to minimize tissue manipulation. A sudden change in the character of drainage or persistent output greater than 50ml per day should alert the clinician to the presence of a fistula. Injection of contrast into the drainage catheter or other contrast studies (upper gastrointestinal contrast study, barium enema, ERCP, or radionuclide biliary scan) are useful for demonstrating a fistula, assessing the adequacy of catheter placement, and later documenting closure of the fistula.

It is important to place a catheter as close as possible to the site of leakage, using additional catheters as needed for abscess drainage. In general, suction drainage should be used to gain control of the leak. Later, after the abscesses have resolved and the tract has matured, drainage can be changed to a gravity system. At that time, slowly withdrawing the drain may promote tract closure, although the catheter should not be removed until drainage stops. Some authors recommend a trial of capping the drain prior to removal, followed by imaging, to exclude fluid reaccumulation.

In five reported series, the success rate of PAD with fistulas range from 67 to 85 percent [31,81–84]. A significant number of patients not cured were temporized by the procedure, simplifying subsequent surgery to cure the underlying disease. When the involved bowel (or duct) is otherwise normal, as commonly occurs with postoperative fistulas, the vast majority of drainages are successful. The presence of active underlying inflammatory disease (e.g., Crohn's disease, diverticulitis), ischemia, or neoplasia is associated with a higher rate of failure, and temporization in these cases is often a more reasonable goal. It is important to exclude downstream obstruction, as this invariably prevents closure of the fistula. Proximal diversion of bowel contents to diminish flow (by means of gastric or intestinal tube suction) and maintenance of nutrition (intestinal tube feeding distal to fistula or parenteral nutrition) are critical determinants of success. Proximal diversion is recommended for all gastroduodenal and small bowel fistulas and for all high-volume leaks. Some low-volume distal colonic fistulas can be managed by simply eliminating oral intake.

The importance of aggressive nutritional support cannot be overemphasized. If possible, enteric nutrition should be provided through catheters placed distal to the fistula. For high-output fistulas, parenteral nutrition is often required. Somatostatin appears useful in the management of patients with fistulas. In one randomized study, patients treated with total parenteral nutrition plus somatostatin had the fistulas close within a significantly shorter period of time. Moreover, this treatment was associated with a significantly lower morbidity [85,86].

Antimicrobial Therapy for Intraabdominal Infections

The goals of antibiotic therapy for intraabdominal infections that will be treated by either percutaneous or operative intervention are to hasten the elimination of infecting microorganisms and thereby minimize the risk of recurrent intraabdominal infection and (perhaps) shorten the clinical manifestations of infection. Since the surgical wound is heavily contaminated by the infecting microorganisms, it is important that effective antimicrobial therapy be begun prior to operation. Necrotizing fasciitis and other forms of extension of infection to the surgical wound represent catastrophic failures of antimicrobial treatment.

In patients with localized abscesses, antibiotics reduce fever and other manifestations of systemic response, but only over a 24- to 36-hour interval. Antibiotics should be administered *after* fluid resuscitation has been initiated to restore adequate visceral perfusion and provide better drug distribution. Particularly in the case of aminoglycosides, nephrotoxicity is exacerbated by impaired renal perfusion.

In practice, antimicrobial agents are often begun when the diagnosis of intraabdominal infection is suspected. This is often prior to the establishment of an exact diagnosis and before results of appropriate cultures are available. Accordingly, the clinician must anticipate the pathogens most likely to be encountered at the site of infection. Antibiotics used for intraabdominal infections should be active against enteric gram-negative facultative and obligate anaerobic bacilli (Table 159-1). The microbiology of intraabdominal infection has been well defined [87]. The identity and density of microorganisms depend on the site of the gastrointestinal tract perforation. In general, gastric, duodenal, and proximal jejunal perforations release small numbers of gram-positive aerobic and gram-negative anaerobic organisms into the peritoneal cavity. These organisms are generally susceptible to beta-lactam antibiotics and are rapidly eradicated by defense mechanisms in intact hosts. *Candida albicans* or other fungi are cultured from about 20 percent of patients with acute perforations of the gastrointestinal tract [88]. Even when fungi are recovered, antifungal agents are unnecessary unless the patient has recently received immunosuppressive therapy for neoplasm, transplantation, or inflammatory disease, or has recurrent intraabdominal infection.

Cultures from patients with distal small bowel perforations grow gram-negative facultative organisms with variable density. Perforations of the distal small bowel often evolve to localized abscess formation and present with peritonitis only after rupture of the abscess. Colonic anaerobes such as *Bacteroides fragilis* are variably present. Patients with colon-derived intraabdominal infections contaminate the peritoneal cavity with large numbers of facultative and obligate anaerobic gram-negative organisms.

Subsequent decisions regarding antimicrobial therapy should be guided by the results of intraoperative cultures. Fluid collections, particularly if purulent, should be sampled for Gram stain smears and culture. Specimens of infected intraabdominal fluid should either be sent to the laboratory in a capped airless syringe with no needle or collected in appropriate (separate) aerobic and anaerobic transport media. If the gram-stained smear reveals a predominance of gram-positive cocci, which may indicate that enterococci or other fecal streptococci are significant copathogens at the site of infection, the clinician should consider alterations in the antibiotic regimen to include agents specifically active against enterococci [89].

Although the appropriate role of anti-enterococcal therapy is controversial, most authorities believe that specific anti-enter-

Table 159-1. Bacteria Commonly Encountered in Intraabdominal Infections

Facultative Gram-Negative Bacilli	Obligate Anaerobes	Facultative Gram-Positive Cocci
Escherichia coli	*Bacteroides fragilis*	Enterococci
Klebsiella species	*Bacteroides* species	*Staphylococcus* species
Proteus species	*Fusobacterium* species	*Streptococcus* species
Enterobacter species	*Clostridium* species	
Morganella morganii	*Peptococcus* species	
Other enteric gram-negative bacilli	*Peptostreptococcus* species	
	Lactobacillus species	
Aerobic gram-negative bacilli		
Pseudomonas aeruginosa		

ococcal therapy should be given only when enterococci are the only organisms isolated or are isolated from blood. Isolation of enterococci as part of a mixed gram-positive and gram-negative flora should not prompt addition of ampicillin or vancomycin to the antibiotic regimen. The incidence of treatment failure for patients harboring enterococci and not treated for it is the same as for patients treated with imipenem or other agents effective against enterococci. Enterococci are very low-level pathogens, meaning that they incite little host response and do not cause invasive infection in intact hosts. However, patients who have had one major episode of sepsis are sufficiently immunosuppressed so that isolation of enterococci from a second infectious site (including recurrent infection within the abdomen) should mandate specific anti-enterococcal therapy. If the smear reveals gram-negative bacilli, failure to isolate either facultative or obligate anaerobes on culture does not obviate the need to continue providing antimicrobial agents against both. Antimicrobial susceptibility patterns within each hospital should be heeded in selecting initial empiric therapy [90,91].

RATIONALE FOR SELECTION OF ANTIBACTERIAL AGENTS. In vitro data, especially antimicrobial susceptibility tests, are predictive of the in vivo response of infecting bacteria to particular antibacterial agents. While a variety of susceptibility testing techniques are available, disk or automated testing is appropriate for bacteria isolated from intraabdominal infections except in extraordinary circumstances. Table 159-2 summarizes the in vitro susceptibilities of important pathogens to antiinfective agents commonly used for treating intraabdominal infections.

Evidence from in vitro data, animal studies, and clinical trials has led to widespread acceptance of the need to provide empiric antimicrobial therapy directed against *Escherichia coli* and other common members of the family Enterobacteriaceae and *B. fragilis* [92,93]. *B. fragilis* and *E. coli* are the most common isolates from intraabdominal infections and are the organisms most likely to cause bacteremia in abdominal sepsis, further attesting to their pathogenicity.

The evidence in support of broadening therapy to cover organisms other than common facultative and obligate anaerobes such as *E. coli* and *B. fragilis* is more controversial. In a study by Yellin et al., initial empiric coverage of *Pseudomonas aeruginosa* was associated with a decreased likelihood of persistent or recurrent abdominal infection when these organisms were isolated from the site of infection [94]. Other clinical trials, however, using antiinfectives not effective against *P. aeruginosa* have not found a high incidence of treatment failure when this organism was isolated [95].

A large number of agents are broadly active against the bacteria found in intraabdominal infection. These are best discussed as classes of drugs and include aminoglycosides, car-

bapenems, cephalosporins, penicillins plus beta-lactamase inhibitors, and quinolones. Aztreonam can be considered as a cephalosporin-class agent.

Aminoglycosides have been the mainstay of therapy for serious gram-negative infections for the past 30 years. Due to their potential for nephrotoxicity and ototoxicity, there has been considerable movement away from aminoglycosides as first-choice agents for community-acquired intraabdominal infections. The use of beta-lactam antibiotics with clindamycin or metronidazole, beta-lactams combined with beta-lactamase inhibitors, or single-agent imipenem/cilastatin in mixed flora infections has given clinical results equivalent to or better than those seen with aminoiglycoside-based combinations [96]. Aminoglycosides no longer represent the "gold standard" for therapy of intraabdominal infections and need not be used for community-acquired intraabdominal infections. Some data, however, suggest that hypotensive patients with gram-negative bacteremias have higher survival rates if treated at least initially with aminoglycoside-based combination therapy [13]. Approximately one third of patients with nonappendiceal intraabdominal infection are bacteremic. Although gram-negative organisms are not as likely as *Staphylococcus aureus* to cause endocarditis on normal valves or metastatic abscess formation, aminoglycoside-containing regimens may result in more rapid clearance of organisms and abbreviate host deterioration. We believe that aminoglycosides should be used in combination with an appropriate beta-lactam agent for the initial treatment of patients with major intraabdominal infection and hypotension.

There has been considerable movement toward high-dose intermittent therapy with aminoglycosides. Patients with major infections have expanded volumes of distribution for aminoglycosides and commonly require 2.5 mg per kilogram of gentamicin or tobramycin to achieve therapeutic levels [97]. Recently, we and others have evaluated regimens involving high doses (10 mg/kg) of gentamicin or tobramycin given once every 24 hours. The rationale for this form of treatment is based on two key antimicrobial properties of aminoglycosides: dose-dependent killing and a post-antibiotic effect [98,99]. If cultures reveal organisms sensitive to a nonaminoglycoside use, single-agent anti–gram-negative therapy may be continued after 48 hours.

"First-generation" cephalosporins, including cefazolin, cephapirin and cephalothin, have excellent gram-positive activity, moderate gram-negative activity, and no anaerobic activity. Cefonocid, cefamandole, and cefuroxime may be grouped with these agents because none have anaerobic activity. The "second-generation" agents, including cefoxitin, cefotetan, and cefmetazole, all have some anaerobic activity, improved facultative gram-negative activity, and less gram-positive coverage. The anaerobic activity of these agents against *B. fragilis* is unimpressive; in general surveys, about a third to a half of tested

Table 159-2. Antimicrobial Sensitivities of Commonly Encountered Pathogens to Parenteral Antibiotics Used in Abdominal Infection[a]

	Gram-Negative Bacilli	Gram-Positive Cocci		Gram-Negative Bacilli	Gram-Positive Bacilli	Gram-Positive Cocci
		Enterococci	Other *Streptococcus* species			
Penicillin	0	+ +	+ + +	+	+ + +	+ + +
Ampicillin	+	+ + +	+ + +	+	+ + +	+ + +
Piperacillin	+ + +	+ + +	+ + +	+ +	+ + +	+ + +
Ticarcillin[b]	+ +	+ +	+ + +	+ +	+ +	+ +
Cefazolin[c]	+ +	0	+ + +	+	+ + +	+ + +
Cefamandole[d]	+ +	0	+ + +	+	+ +	+ + +
Cefoxitin[e]	+ +	0	+ +	+ +	+ + +	+ + +
Cefotaxime[f]	+ + +	0	+ +	+	+ +	+ + +
Imipenem	+ + +	+ +	+ + +	+ + +	+ + +	+ + +
Aztreonam	+ + +	0	0	0	0	0
Aminoglycosides[g]	+ + +	0	0	0	0	0
Clindamycin	0	0	+ +	+ + +	+ + +	+ + +
Metronidazole	0	0	0	+ + +	+ + +	+ + +
Beta-lactamase inhibitor– Beta-lactam combinations						
Ampicillin/Sulbactam	+ +	+ + +	+ + +	+ + +	+ + +	+ + +
Ticarcillin/Clavulanic acid	+ +	+ +	+ + +	+ + +	+ + +	+ + +
Piperacillin/Tazobactam	+ + +	+ + +	+ + +	+ + +	+ + +	

[a] 0 = little or no activity; + = some activity, + + = moderate to good activity; + + + = excellent activity.
[b] Azlocillin, mezlocillin, and carbenicillin have similar spectra.
[c] Includes cephalothin, cephapirin, and cephradine.
[d] Includes cefuroxime, cefonicid, cefotiam, and ceforanide.
[e] Includes cefotetan and cefmetazole.
[f] Includes ceftriaxone, ceftazidime, cefoperazone, and ceftizoxime.
[g] Includes gentamicin, tobramycin, netilmicin, and amikacin.

isolates are resistant [100,101]. Because of the high incidence of *B. fragilis* and relatively large inoculum loads encountered in colon-derived infections, these agents are best used for prophylaxis and for treatment of low-inoculum infections such as appendicitis.

The "third-generation" agents, cefotaxime, ceftizoxime, cefoperazone, ceftriaxone, and ceftazidime, have considerable facultative gram-negative activity but no anaerobic and limited gram-positive coverage. Aztreonam, termed a monobactam, has activity against facultative gram-negative organisms equivalent to third-generation cephalosporins. It has no gram-positive or anaerobic activity. Metronidazole has remained highly effective against *Bacteroides* species, in contradistinction to clindamycin, and is now the preferred agent for combination therapy.

The specific choice of one third-generation cephalosporin or aztreonam over another is not a major issue. As clinical experience with these agents has widened, it has become apparent that the differences between agents do not affect outcome. Many hospitals have therefore taken the position that cephalosporins can be grouped into classes and that within each class the agents are therapeutically interchangeable. Commonly, acquisition costs now determine which cephalosporin is used within each class. Ceftazidime is not recommended for general empiric therapy because broad usage of this agent is associated with decreasing susceptibility of *P. aeruginosa,* and this agent is the only cephalosporin reliably effective against this pathogen. Additionally, ceftazidime therapy is associated with an increased incidence of enterococcal superinfections.

An alternative strategy to the use of beta-lactamase–resistant cephalosporins is to utilize currently available beta-lactams in combination with beta-lactamase inhibitors, such as sulbactam, clavulanic acid, and tazobactam. These agents are potent inhibitors of beta-lactamases from gram-positive and anaerobic organisms. They have less activity against the chromosomal beta-lactamases seen in many strains of Enterobacteriaceae and do not completely compensate for the marginal gram-negative activity of the penicillin derivative. The primary concern has to do with organisms that constitutively express beta-lactamases [102]. Organisms that typically do this include *Enterobacter* species, *P. aeruginosa, Citrobacter, Serratia* and *Acinetobacter* species. These particular organisms are most commonly encountered in nosocomial infections but are also present in about 15 percent of community-acquired infections. Clinical trials with these agents for intraabdominal infections have been generally confined to patients with acutely perforated gastroduodenal ulcers and acute appendicitis. These inhibitors add considerable anti-staphylococcal and anti-*Bacteroides* activity to the base antibiotic.

Imipenem, a carbapenem derivative, has broad activity against facultative and obligate gram-negative anaerobes and excellent gram-positive activity (excepting methicillin-resistant staphylococci). This agent is formulated with cilastatin, a renal dehydropeptidase inhibitor that prevents renal tubal epithelial metabolism of the drug. In situations where plasma accumulation of the drug occurs (high dose levels or renal failure), the drug can cause seizures. With lower dose levels (500 mg every 6 hours) and appropriate adjustments for renal failure, seizures have not been a problem. Other carbapenems without equivalent neurotoxicity are undergoing clinical testing. These agents, meropenem and biapenem, have antibacterial activity similar to that of imipenem and somewhat decreased neurotoxicity.

As clinical experience has accumulated, quinolone antibiotics appear to be potentially useful for intraabdominal infections. These agents act by inhibiting DNA replication and have shown similar activity to imipenem in clinical trials for pneumonia and intraabdominal infection. Available quinolones have little anti–*B. fragilis* activity and should be combined with metronidazole. Quinolones are attractive because serum levels following oral absorption parallel those seen with intravenous infusion. In patients with anatomically extensive infections, such as diffuse peritonitis, prolonged therapy with oral quinolones may be an attractive strategy.

Dosing of cephalosporin, penicillin, carbapenem, and quinolone antibiotics should be optimized based on the known pharmacodynamics of these agents. Cell-wall–active agents are effective at the minimum inhibitory concentration (MIC) of the drug for the organisms being treated [103,104]. Increasing the drug concentration substantially above about two to four times the MIC does not increase the rate of killing. Once the drug level falls below the MIC, the organisms begin regrowth immediately. Dosage regimens for cell-wall–active agents in critically ill patients should involve dosing intervals sufficiently short to maintain serum levels above the MIC. Therefore, the general rule with these agents should be to give relatively small doses frequently to maintain the trough levels above the MIC and avoid the costs and toxicities seen with high doses. This is best accomplished by administering these drugs every four half-lives, with adjustments as needed for renal compromise. There has been interest in infrequent drug dosing with beta-lactams. This is likely to succeed primarily in mild to moderate infections in otherwise intact hosts.

References

1. Oya M, Shimada T, Nakamura M, Uchida Y: Functional morphology of the lymphatic system in the monkey diaphragm. *Arch Histol Cytol* 56:37, 1993.
2. Li JC, Yu SM: Study on the ultrastructure of the peritoneal stomata in humans. *Acta Anat* 141:26, 1991.
3. Levine S, Saltzman A: Postinflammatory increase of lymphatic absorption from the peritoneal cavity: Role of diaphragmatic stomata. *Microcirc Endothelium Lymphatics* 4:399, 1988.
4. Elk JR, Adair T, Drake RE, Gabel JC: The effect of anesthesia and surgery on diaphragmatic lymph vessel flow after endotoxin in sheep. *Lymphology* 23:145, 1990.
5. Banks J, Foulis A: Liver function in septic shock. *J Clin Pathol* 35:1249, 1982.
6. Gimson AE: Hepatic dysfunction during bacterial sepsis. *Intensive Care Med* 13:162, 1987.
7. Cerra FB: Multiple organ failure syndrome. *Dis Mon* 26:816, 1992.
8. van Deventer SJ, Knepper A, Landsman J, et al: Endotoxins in portal blood. *Hepatogastroenterology* 35:223, 1988.
9. Moore FA, Moore EE, Poggetti R: Gut bacterial translocation via the portal vein: A clinical perspective with major torso trauma. *J Trauma* 31:629, 1991.
10. Shenep JL, Flynn PM, Barrett FF, et al: Serial quantitation of endotoxemia and bacteremia during therapy for Gram-negative bacterial sepsis. *J Infect Dis* 157(3):565, 1988.
11. Onderdonk AB, Bartlett JG, Louie T, et al: Microbial synergy in experimental intra-abdominal abscess. *Infect Immun* 13:22, 1976.
12. Lindemann SR, Tung G, Silverman SG, et al: Percutaneous cholecystostomy. *Semin Interventional Radiology* 5:179, 1988.
13. Salacata A, Chow JW: Cephalosporin therapeutics for intensive care infection, in Solomkin JS (ed): *New Horizons*. Baltimore, Williams & Wilkins, 1993, pp 181–186.
14. Boland G, Lee MJ, Mueller PR: Acute cholecystitis in the intensive care unit, in Solomkin JS (ed): *New Horizons*. Baltimore, Williams & Wilkins, 1993, pp 246–260.
15. Frazee RC, Nagorney DM, Mucha P: Acute acalculous cholecystitis. *Mayo Clin Proc* 64:163, 1989.
16. Alpern MB, Glazer GM, Francis IR: Ischemic or infarcted bowel: CT findings. *Radiology* 166:149, 1988.
17. Wachs ME, Wolfgang HS: Primary intestinal anastomosis is unsafe in the presence of generalized peritonitis, in Simmons RL, Udekwu AO (eds): *Debates in Clinical Surgery*. St. Louis, Mosby-Year Book, 1991, pp 228–239.
18. Liebert C, Deweese BM: Primary resection without anastomosis for perforation of acute diverticulitis. *Surg Gynecol Obstet* 152:30, 1981.
19. Debas H, Thomson FB: A critical review of colectomy with anastomosis. *Surg Gynecol Obstet* 135:747, 1972.
20. DuPriest RW, Khaneja SC, Cowley RA: Acute cholecystitis complicating trauma. *Ann Surg* 189:84, 1979.
21. Lee ML, Saini S, Brink JA: Treatment of critically ill patients with sepsis of unknown cause: Value of percutaneous cholecystostomy. *Am J Surg* 156:1163, 1991.
22. Devine RM, Farnett MB, Mucha P: Acute cholecystitis as a complication in surgical patients. *Arch Surg* 119:1389, 1984.
23. Flancbaum L, Majerus TC, Cox EF: Acute posttraumatic acalculous cholecystitis. *AJR* 150:252, 1985.
24. Cohan RH, Mahoney BS, Bowie JD, et al: Striated intramural gallbladder lucencies on US studies: Predictors of acute cholecystitis. *Radiology* 164:31, 1987.
25. Marchal GT, Casaer M, Baert AL, et al: Gallbladder wall sonolucency in acute cholecystitis. *Radiology* 133:429, 1979.
26. Jeffrey RB Jr, Wing VC, Laing FC: Real-time sonographic monitoring of percutaneous abscess drainage. *AJR* 144:469, 1985.
27. McGahan JP: Aspiration and drainage procedures in the intensive care unit: Percutaneous sonographic guidance. *Radiology* 154:531, 1985.
28. Pruett TL, Simmons RL: Status of percutaneous catheter drainage of abscesses. *Surg Clin North Am* 68:89, 1988.
29. Johnson WC, Gerzof SG, Robbins AH, et al: Treatment of abdominal abscesses: Comparative evaluation of operative drainage versus percutaneous catheter drainage guided by computed tomography or ultrasound. *Ann Surg* 194:510, 1981.
30. vanSonnenberg E, D'Agostino HB, Casola G, et al: Percutaneous abscess drainage: Current concepts. *Radiology* 181:617, 1991.
31. Lambiase RE, Deyoe L, Cronan JJ, et al: Percutaneous drainage of 335 consecutive abscesses: Results of primary drainage with 1-year follow-up. *Radiology* 184:167, 1992.
32. vanSonnenberg E, D'Agostino HB, Sanchez RB, et al: Percutaneous abscess drainage: Editorial comments. *Radiology* 184:27, 1992.
33. vanSonnenberg E, Wing VW, Casola G, et al: Temporizing effect of percutaneous drainage of complicated abscesses in critically ill patients. *AJR* 142:821, 1984.
34. Neff CC, Mueller PR, Ferrucci JT Jr, et al: Serious complications following transgression of the pleural space in drainage procedures. *Radiology* 152:335, 1984.
35. Mueller PR, Ferrucci JR Jr, Simeone JF, et al: Lesser sac abscesses and fluid collections: Drainage by transhepatic approach. *Radiology* 155:615, 1985.
36. vanSonnenberg E, Mueller PR, Ferrucci JR et al: Sump catheter for percutaneous abscess and fluid drainage by trocar or Seldinger technique. *AJR* 139:613, 1982.
37. Gobien RP, Stanley JH, Schabel SI, et al: The effect of drainage tube size on adequacy of percutaneous abscess drainage. *Cardiovasc Intervent Radiol* 8:100, 1985.
38. Golden GT, Roberts TL, Rodeheaver G, et al: A new filtered Sump tube for wound drainage. *Am J Surg* 129:716, 1975.
39. Goldberg MA, Mueller PR, Saini S, et al: Importance of daily rounds by the radiologist after interventional procedures in the abdomen and chest. *Radiology* 180:767, 1991.
40. vanSonnenberg E, Ferrucci JR Jr, Mueller PR, et al: Percutaneous drainage of abscesses and fluid collections: Technique, results, and applications. *Radiology* 142:1, 1982.
41. Neff CC, vanSonnenberg E, Casola G, et al: Diverticular abscesses: Percutaneous drainage. *Radiology* 163:15, 1987.
42. Mueller PR, Saini S, Wittenburg J, et al: Sigmoid diverticular abscesses: Percutaneous drainage as an adjunct to surgical resection in 24 cases. *Radiology* 164:321, 1987.
43. Casola G, vanSonnenberg E, Neff CC, et al: Abscesses in Crohn disease: Percutaneous drainage. *Radiology* 163:19, 1987.
44. Safrit HD, Mauro MA, Jaques PF: Percutaneous abscess drainage in Crohn disease. *AJR* 148:859, 1987.
45. Doemeny JM, Burke DR, Meranze SG: Percutaneous drainage of abscesses in patients with Crohn's disease. *Gastrointest Radiol* 13:237, 1988.
46. Lambiase RE, Cronan JJ, Dorfman GS, et al: Percutaneous drainage of abscesses in patients with Crohn disease. *AJR* 150:1043, 1988.
47. Nosher JL, Needell GS, Amorosa JK, et al: Transrectal pelvic abscess drainage with sonographic guidance. *AJR* 146:1047, 1986.

48. vanSonnenberg E, D'Agostino HB, Casola G, et al: US-guided transvaginal drainage of pelvic abscesses and fluid collections. *Radiology* 181:53, 1991.

49. Casola G, vanSonnenberg E, D'Agostino HB, et al: Percutaneous drainage of tubo-ovarian abscesses. *Radiology* 182:399, 1992.

50. Bassi C, Vesentini S, Nifosi F, et al: Pancreatic abscess and other pus-harboring collections related to pancreatitis: A review of 108 cases. *World J Surg* 14:505, 1990 (Discussion).

51. Bittner R, Block S, Buchler M, Beger HG: Pancreatic abscess and infected pancreatic necrosis. Different local septic complications in acute pancreatitis. *Dig Dis Sci* 32:1082, 1987.

52. Hughes CJ, Ramsey-Stewart G, Storey DW: Sequential laparotomy and zipper closure in the management of gross peripancreatic sepsis. *Aust NZ J Surg* 60:467, 1990.

53. Lumsden A, Bradley E III: Secondary pancreatic infections. *Surg Gynecol Obstet* 170:459, 1990.

54. Bradley E III, Olson RA: Current management of pancreatic abscess. *Adv Surg* 24:361, 1991.

55. vanSonnenberg E, Wittich GR, Casola G, et al: Complicated pancreatic inflammatory disease: Diagnostic and therapeutic role of interventional radiology. *Radiology* 155:335, 1985.

56. vanSonnenberg E, Wittich G, Casola G, et al: Percutaneous drainage of infected and noninfected pancreatic pseudocysts: Experience in 101 cases. *Radiology* 170:757, 1989.

57. Freeny PC, Lewis GP, Traverso LW, et al: Infected pancreatic fluid collections: Percutaneous catheter drainage. *Radiology* 167:435, 1988.

58. Beger HG, Maier W, Block S, Buchler M: How do imaging methods influence the surgical strategy in acute pancreatitis? in Malfertheiner P, Ditschuneit H (eds): *Diagnostic Procedures in Pancreatic Disease.* Berlin, Springer-Verlag, 1986, pp 54–60.

59. Balthazar EJ: CT diagnosis and staging of acute pancreatitis. *Radiol Clin North Am* 27:19, 1989.

60. vanSonnenberg E, Casola G, Varney RR, Wittich GR: Imaging and interventional radiology for pancreatitis and its complications. *Radiol Clin North Am* 27:65, 1989.

61. Bradley E III, Murphy F, Ferguson C: Prediction of pancreatic necrosis by dynamic pancreatography. *Ann Surg* 210:495, 1989.

62. Balthazer EJ, Robinson DL, Megibow AJ, Ranson JH: Acute pancreatitis: Value of CT in establishing prognosis. *Radiology* 174:331, 1990.

63. Adams DB, Harvey TS, Anderson MC: Percutaneous catheter drainage of infected pancreatic and peripancreatic fluid collections. *Arch Surg* 125:1554, 1990.

64. Stanten R, Frey CF: Comprehensive management of acute necrotizing pancreatitis and pancreatic abscess. *Arch Surg* 125:1269, 1990 (Discussion).

65. Rotman N, Mathieu D, Anglade MC, Fagniez PL: Failure of percutaneous drainage of pancreatic abscesses complicating severe acute pancreatitis. *Surg Gynecol Obstet* 174:141, 1992.

66. Steiner E, Mueller PR, Hahn PF, et al: Complicated pancreatic abscesses: Problems in interventional management. *Radiology* 167:443, 1988.

67. Lee MJ, Rattner DW, Legemate DA, et al: Acute complicated pancreatitis: Redefining the role of interventional radiology. *Radiology* 183:171, 1992.

68. Doust BD, Quiroz F, Stewart JM: Ultrasonic distinction of abscesses from other intra-abdominal fluid collections. *Radiology* 125:213, 1977.

69. Doust BD, Thompson R: Ultrasonography of abdominal fluid collections. *Gastrointest Radiol* 3:273, 1978.

70. Korobkin M, Callen PW, Filly RA, et al: Comparison of computed tomography, ultrasonography, and Ga-67 scanning in the evaluation of suspected abdominal abscesses. *Radiology* 129:59, 1978.

71. Barakos JA, Ralls PW, Lapin SA, et al: Cholelithiasis: Evaluation with CT. *Radiology* 162:415, 1987.

72. Johnson LB: The importance of early diagnosis of acute acalculus cholecystitis. *Surg Gynecol Obstet* 164:197, 1987.

73. Ekberg O, Weiber S: The clinical importance of a thick-walled, tender gallbladder without stones on ultrasonography. *Clin Radiol* 44:38, 1991.

74. Mirvis SE, Vainright JR, Nelson AW, et al: The diagnosis of acute acalculous cholecystitis: A comparison of sonography, scintigraphy, and CT. *AJR* 147:1171, 1986.

75. Kane RA, Costello P, Duszlak E: Computed tomography in acute cholecystitis: New observations. *AJR* 141:697, 1983.

76. Terrier F, Becker CD, Stoller C, et al: Computed tomography in complicated cholecystitis. *J Comput Assist Tomogr* 8:58, 1984.

77. Clark RA, Gallant TE: Acute mesenteric ischemia: Angiographic spectrum. *AJR* 142:555, 1984.

78. Balthazar EJ, Birnbaum BA, Megibow AJ, et al: Closed-loop and strangulating intestinal obstruction: CT signs. *Radiology* 185:769, 1992.

79. Clark RA: Computed tomography of bowel infarction. *J Comput Assist Tomogr* 11:757, 1987.

80. Boley SJ, Brandt LT, Veith FJ: Ischemic disorders of the intestines. *Curr Probl Surg* 15:1, 1978.

81. Lambiase RE, Cronan JJ, Dorfman GS, et al: Postoperative abscesses with enteric communication: Percutaneous treatment. *Radiology* 171:497, 1989.

82. Kerlan RK, Jeffrey RB Jr, Pogany AC, et al: Abdominal abscess with low-output fistula: Successful percutaneous drainage. *Radiology* 155:73, 1985.

83. Papanicolaou N, Mueller PR, Ferrucci JT Jr, et al: Abscess-fistula association: Radiologic recognition and percutaneous management. *AJR* 143:811, 1984.

84. Ercoli FR, Milgram LM, Nosher JL, et al: Percutaneous catheter drainage of abscesses associated with enteric fistulae. *Am Surg* 54:45, 1988.

85. Prickett D, Montgomery R, Cheadle WG: External fistulas arising from the digestive tract. *South Med J* 84:736, 1991.

86. Torres AJ, Landa JI, Moreno Azcoita M, et al: Somatostatin in the management of gastrointestinal fistulas. A multicenter trial. *Arch Surg* 127:97, 1992.

87. Lorber B. Swenson RM: The bacteriology of intra-abdominal infections. *Surg Clin North Am* 55:1349, 1975.

88. Solomkin JS: Pathogenesis and management of *Candida* infection syndromes in non-neutropenic patients, in Solomkin JS (ed): *New Horizons.* Baltimore, Williams & Wilkins, 1993, pp 202–213.

89. Barie PS, Christou NV, Dellinger EP, et al: Pathogenicity of the enterococcus in surgical infections. *Ann Surg* 212:155, 1990.

90. Thornsberry C: Review of in vitro activity of third-generation cephalosporins and other newer beta-lactam antibiotics against clinically important bacteria. *Am J Med* 79(2A):14, 1985.

91. Cornick NA, Cuchural GJJ, Snydman DR, et al: The antimicrobial susceptibility patterns of the *Bacteroides fragilis* group in the United States, 1987. *J Antimicrob Chemother* 25:1011, 1990.

92. Berne TV, Yellin AE, Appleman MD, et al: Surgically treated gangrenous or perforated appendicitis. A comparison of aztreonam and clindamycin versus gentamicin and clindamycin. *Ann Surg* 205:133, 1987.

93. Lau WY, Fan ST, Yiu TF, et al: Prophylaxis of postappendecectomy sepsis by metronidazole and cefotaxime; A randomized, prospective and double blind trial. *Br J Surg* 70:670, 1983.

94. Yellin AE, Heseltine PN, Berne TV, et al: The role of *Pseudomonas* species in patients treated with ampicillin and Sulbactam for gangrenous and perforated appendicitis. *Surg Gynecol Obstet* 161:303, 1985.

95. Malangoni MA, Condon RE, Spiegel CA: Treatment of intra-abdominal infections is appropriate with single-agent or combination antibiotic therapy. *Surgery* 98:648, 1985.

96. Solomkin JS, Dellinger EP, Christou NV, Busuttil RW: Results of a multicenter trial comparing imipenem/cilastatin to tobramycin/clindamycin for intra-abdominal infections. *Ann Surg* 212:581, 1990.

97. Beckhouse MJ, Whyte IM, Blyth PL, et al: Altered aminoglycoside pharmacokinetics in the critically ill. *Anaesth Intensive Care* 16:418, 1988.

98. Kapusnik JE, Hackbarth CJ, Chambers HF, et al: Single, large, daily dosing versus intermittent dosing of tobramycin for treating experimental pseudomonas pneumonia. *J Infect Dis* 158:7, 1988.

99. Gilbert DN: Once-daily aminoglycoside therapy. *Antimicrob Agents Chemother* 35:399, 1991.

100. Bieluch VM, Cuchural GJ, Snydman DR, et al: Clinical importance of cefoxitin-resistant *Bacteroides fragilis* isolates. *Diagn Microbiol Infect Dis* 7:119, 1987.

101. Jacobus NV, Cuchural GJ Jr, Tally FP: In-vitro susceptibility of the *Bacteroides fragilis* group and the inoculum effect of newer beta-

lactam antibiotics on this group of organisms. *J Antimicrob Chemother* 24:675, 1989.

102. Sanders WEJ, Sanders CC: Inducible beta-lactamases: Clinical and epidemiologic implications for use of newer cephalosporins. *Rev Infect Dis* 10:830, 1988.

103. Leggett JE, Fantin B, Ebert S, et al: Comparative antibiotic dose-effect relations at several dosing intervals in murine pneumonitis and thigh-infection models. *J Infect Dis* 159:281, 1989.

104. Vogelman B, Gudmundsson S, Leggett J, et al: Correlation of antimicrobial pharmacokinetic parameters with therapeutic efficacy in an animal model. *J Infect Dis* 158:831, 1988.

160. Acute Pancreatitis

Michael L. Steer

Definition, Classification, and Pathology

Pancreatitis, an inflammatory disease of the pancreas, can be classified as *acute* or *chronic* on the basis of either clinical or morphologic/functional criteria. The classification of any particular patient's disease may depend on the criteria being used. Clinically, acute pancreatitis is defined as a process that is of rapid onset and usually associated with pain and alterations in exocrine function. With successful treatment, complete resolution can be expected. Chronic pancreatitis, on the other hand, is usually associated with repeated episodes of pain and/or diminished exocrine function that recur even after successful treatment of an attack. The morphologic/functional classification of pancreatitis, which has been the subject of several international symposia [1,2,3], also distinguishes between an acute and a chronic form of the disease, but that distinction is based on the reversibility of morphologic and/or functional changes in the pancreas. According to this scheme, acute pancreatitis is defined as an inflammatory process that occurs in a gland that was both morphologically and functionally normal prior to the attack and that can return to that state after resolution of the attack. In contrast, chronic pancreatitis is defined as an inflammatory disease involving a pancreas that was morphologically and/or functionally abnormal prior to the onset of symptoms or that will remain abnormal even after the attack has resolved. For the most part, the term *acute pancreatitis* will be used in this chapter in its clinical rather than its morphologic/functional context. For reasons of completeness, however, the pathologic, etiologic, and therapeutic issues that are of particular relevance to morphologically and/or functionally defined chronic pancreatitis also will be discussed.

The pathologic changes associated with acute pancreatitis vary, to a great extent, with the severity of an attack. Mild acute pancreatitis is associated with interstitial edema, a mild infiltration of inflammatory cells, and evidence of intrapancreatic and/or peripancreatic fat necrosis. In contrast, severe attacks of acute pancreatitis are usually associated with acinar cell necrosis, which may be either focal or diffusely distributed throughout the gland. In addition, thrombosis of intrapancreatic vessels, vascular disruption with intraparenchymal hemorrhage, and abscess formation may be noted. Since chronic pancreatitis involves inflammation in a previously diseased gland, areas of scarring with fibrosis, along with atrophy of acinar tissue, can be seen even in tissue taken during the early stages of an attack. Varying degrees of acute inflammation are usually observed to be superimposed on these more chronic changes.

Etiology

Pancreatitis is associated with a number of other disease states or conditions that are, collectively, referred to as the "etiologies" of pancreatitis [4]. In developed countries, 70 to 80 percent of patients with pancreatitis have that disease in association with either ethanol abuse or biliary tract stone disease. Another 10 to 20 percent of patients have no identifiable cause of pancreatitis and are considered to have idiopathic pancreatitis. The remaining 5 to 10 percent of patients develop pancreatitis in association with one of the various etiologies listed in Table 160-1. In the less well developed countries, particularly those in Africa and Asia, a significant fraction of the patients with acute pancreatitis develop that disease as a result of malnutrition and/or ingestion of potentially toxic agents (e.g., cassava root) [5,6,7]. Their pancreatitis has been termed "nutritional" pancreatitis.

BILIARY TRACT STONE DISEASE. Biliary tract stones are the most frequent cause of morphologic and functionally defined acute pancreatitis and, along with ethanol abuse, account for 60 to 80 percent of patients with clinically acute pancreatitis. The frequency of either biliary tract stones or ethanol abuse among any group of patients being evaluated with acute pancreatitis depends on the socioeconomic composition of that group, i.e., in affluent suburban groups, biliary tract stones account for more attacks, whereas ethanol abuse is more commonly found to be associated with pancreatitis when inner-city and poorer patients are studied [4]. Biliary tract stone disease is a frequent cause of acute pancreatitis among Native Americans, who are prone to develop stones, and among many Asian groups, who have a high incidence of stone formation as a consequence of chronic bactobilia.

Reports by Acousta and Ledesma [8,9] as well as others have indicated that the onset of pancreatitis that is associated with biliary tract stones is related to the passage of those stones through the terminal biliopancreatic duct and into the duodenum. The mechanism by which stone passage triggers this so-called gallstone pancreatitis has been the subject of considerable speculation and experimental investigation. Three theories have been proposed. The first was the "common channel" theory proposed by Opie in 1901 after he noted gallstones impacted in the ampulla of Vater when patients who had died of gallstone pancreatitis underwent autopsy examination. He suggested that such stones might create a common biliopancreatic channel proximal to the stone-induced obstruction and that, as

Table 160-1. Miscellaneous Etiologies of Acute Pancreatitis

Trauma
Postoperative
    Common duct exploration
    Sphincteroplasty
    Distal gastrectomy
    Cardiopulmonary bypass
    Cardiac or renal transplantation
ERCP
Translumbar aortography
Metabolic
    Hyperparathyroidism
    Hyperlipoproteinemias Types I, IV, V
Penetrating ulcer
Connective tissue disorders
Scorpion bite
Renal failure
Hereditary

a consequence, bile could reflux into the pancreatic ductal system [10]. He reasoned that bile reflux would be injurious to the pancreas and trigger pancreatitis. Subsequent investigations by many groups, however, have cast considerable doubt on the validity of this theory since (1) pancreatic duct pressure normally exceeds biliary duct pressure and, therefore, pancreatic juice reflux into the biliary tract rather than bile reflux into the pancreas would be expected if an obstruction were to create a common channel [11]; (2) many patients develop pancreatitis but lack a common channel that could permit reflux [12]; and (3) bile perfused into the pancreatic duct at normal pressure does not induce pancreatitis [13]. The second theory proposed to explain gallstone-induced pancreatitis suggested that the stone passing through the sphincter of Oddi could render that sphincter incompetent and, as a result, permit reflux of duodenal juice containing activated digestive enzymes into the pancreas [14]. This "duodenal reflux" would seem an unlikely explanation for the development of pancreatitis since it is now clear that neither endoscopic nor surgical procedures that make the sphincter of Oddi incompetent lead to subsequent attacks of acute pancreatitis. The third theory suggests that either the stone or edema and inflammation resulting from stone passage cause pancreatic duct obstruction and that pancreatic duct obstruction is the event that triggers acute pancreatitis. Recently completed studies using a model of acute necrotizing biliary pancreatitis induced in opossums would support this theory [15] and, with exclusion of the other two hypotheses for reasons listed above, it would seem most likely that pancreatic duct obstruction is, indeed, the event that triggers pancreatitis.

The pancreas synthesizes and secretes a large array of potentially harmful digestive enzymes, and the pathologic appearance of the pancreas during acute pancreatitis suggests that an autodigestive injury has occurred. Most of the digestive enzymes that are secreted by the pancreas are not activated until they reach the duodenum, where the brush border enzyme enterokinase activates trypsinogen and trypsin activates the remaining zymogens. Pancreatic duct obstruction cannot, by itself, be sufficient to explain the mechanism for gallstone pancreatitis since, for the most part, the enzymes present in the ductal space would be expected to be inactive zymogens. Recent studies using a number of dissimilar models of experimental pancreatitis have indicated that, during the early stages of each of these models, digestive enzyme zymogens become colocalized with lysosomal hydrolases within intracellular organelles. Since the lysosomal hydrolase cathepsin B can activate trypsinogen, these studies may have provided the needed explanation for the mechanism by which pancreatic duct obstruction triggers pancreatitis. They suggest that, after duct obstruction, lysosomal hydrolases activate digestive enzymes within acinar cells of the pancreas, and this leads to cell injury [16,17,18].

ETHANOL ABUSE. The majority of patients with ethanol-associated pancreatitis develop their first clinical attack of pancreatitis after many years of ethanol abuse. The incidence of pancreatitis is related to the logarithm of alcohol consumption, but there is no threshold below which alcohol ingestion is not associated with an increased incidence of pancreatitis. The mean consumption of ethanol among patients with ethanol-associated pancreatitis is 150 to 175 gm per day. The mean duration of consumption prior to the first attack is 18 ± 11 years for men and 11 ± 8 years for women [19]. Ethanol-associated pancreatitis, like ethanol abuse itself, is more common among men than among women. Epidemiologic studies have suggested that ethanol-associated pancreatitis is most common among those ingesting a high-protein diet with either high or low fat content [19]. The mechanism by which chronic ethanol abuse leads to chronic pancreatic injury is not clear, although some studies have suggested that injury may result from secretion of a juice that is high in proteolytic enzyme content and low in proteolytic enzyme inhibitors and that contains lysosomal hydrolases capable of activating trypsin either within acinar cells or in the pancreatic ductal space [20,21,22]. Some patients with ethanol-induced pancreatitis develop disease after only one or several exposures to ethanol. This observation, along with the finding that a substantial number of patients dying of ethanol-associated disease do not have pancreatic fibrosis at autopsy [23], has suggested that ethanol might be a cause of morphologic/functional as well as clinical acute pancreatitis. The mechanism by which ethanol might cause acute injury to the pancreas is not clear. Some suggested possibilities include a direct toxic, drug-like effect on acinar cells or, alternatively, induction of ductal hypertension as a result of stimulating both exocrine secretion and sphincteric contraction.

DRUGS. Exposure to certain drugs represents perhaps the third most common cause of acute pancreatitis (see Table 160-2) [24,25,26]. The relationship between drug exposure and the development of pancreatitis can be categorized as definite, probable, or equivocal on the strength of the data that indicate that that specific drug actually causes pancreatitis. The former

Table 160-2. Drugs Associated with Acute Pancreatitis

Definite	
Thiazide diuretics	Valproic acid
Ethacrynic acid	Estrogens
Furosemide	Tetracycline
Azathioprine	Sulfonamides
Dideoxyinosine	Pentamidine
Probable	
Methyl dopa	Iatrogenic hypercalcemia
L-Asparaginase	Procainamide
Chlorthalidone	Phenphormin
Equivocal	
Isoniazid	Rifampin
Acetaminophen	Steroids
H-2 blockers	Propoxyphene

category includes those drugs whose use is associated with an increased incidence of pancreatitis and that, on specific re-challenge, have been found to induce the disease. On the other hand, drugs in the equivocal category include those anecdotally associated with the disease but never demonstrated, in prospective studies, to be capable of inducing pancreatitis. Historically, diuretic agents such as the thiazides, ethycrynic acid, and furosemide were considered the most likely drugs to cause pancreatitis. More recently, however, drug-related pancreatitis has been reported to be most common among individuals with AIDS or AIDS-related complex receiving dideoxyinosine [27], pentamidine, or related compounds and among transplant patients receiving immunosuppressant agents such as azothio-prine. Although previously considered to cause pancreatitis, H-2 blockers and steroids are not currently believed to be capable of causing acute pancreatitis.

PANCREATIC DUCT OBSTRUCTION. Obstruction of the pancreatic duct is considered by most investigators to be the mechanism by which biliary tract stones trigger acute pancreatitis. Other events or processes that cause pancreatic duct obstruction also can cause pancreatitis. Thus, pancreatitis may be caused by duodenal, ampullary, biliary duct, or pancreatic tumors that obstruct the duct or by inflammatory lesions (e.g., peptic ulcer, duodenal Crohn's disease, periampullary diverticulitis) that interfere with pancreatic duct drainage [4]. Pancreatic cysts and pseudocysts as well as periampullary diverticula filled with food and debris can interfere with duct drainage and, as a consequence, precipitate pancreatitis. Ductal strictures, frequently the result of traumatic duct injury or previous pancreatitis, can be a cause of obstructive pancreatitis. Finally, certain parasites such as *Ascaris* and *Clonorchis* can trigger pancreatitis by physically obstructing the pancreatic duct [4,28].

MISCELLANEOUS CAUSES OF ACUTE PANCREATITIS. The remaining "miscellaneous" causes of pancreatitis are listed in Table 160-1. Traumatic pancreatitis usually follows blunt abdominal trauma during which the body of the pancreas is compressed against the vertebral column. As a result, the gland is "cracked" and the duct either partially or completely transected [29]. Lesser degrees of blunt trauma may be associated with pancreatic contusion, whereas penetrating injury can affect any portion of the pancreas. Traumatic injury to the pancreas also can be associated with surgical procedures performed on or near the pancreas [30,31,32]. Postoperative pancreatitis is also frequently associated with procedures performed on or near the sphincter of Oddi (duct exploration, sphincteroplasty, distal gastrectomy), procedures associated with hypoperfusion or atheroembolism of the pancreatic circulation (cardiopulmonary bypass, cardiac transplantation, renal transplantation, translumbar aortography) [33,34], or procedures involving pancreatic duct injection (ERCP) [35].

IDIOPATHIC PANCREATITIS. Approximately 5 to 10 percent of patients with acute pancreatitis have that disease in the absence of biliary tract stones, ethanol abuse, or any other identifiable etiology. Recent reports suggest that many of these patients have biliary sludge, that their attacks can be prevented by cholecystectomy, and that they actually have biliary rather than idiopathic pancreatitis [36]. Approximately 40 percent of individuals with chronic pancreatitis neither abuse ethanol nor have malnutrition. As a result, they are considered to have idiopathic chronic pancreatitis [37]. Recent studies in Europe and the United States have suggested that those individuals can

be divided into a juvenile group with an onset of disease at a median age of 18 and a senile group whose disease begins at a mean age of 60. Disease in the former group is characterized by pain, whereas that in the senile group is most often painless and associated with calcifications and/or diabetes mellitus [38].

Clinical Presentation (Table 160-3)

SYMPTOMS. The symptoms of acute pancreatitis include abdominal pain, nausea, and vomiting [4,28,39,40,41]. The pain is typically localized to the epigastrium but frequently involves one or both upper quadrants. On occasion, it may be felt in the lower abdomen, one or both shoulders, or in the lower chest. The pain is usually described as being of rapid onset, slowly increasing to a maximal severity, and then remaining constant. It usually lacks the waxing and waning character of intestinal or ureteral colic, but it may be diminished by assuming an upright position, leaning forward, or lying on the side with the knees drawn upward. The pain may have a pleuritic component and be associated with rapid but shallow respirations. Frequently, the pain is described as being a boring or knife-like sensation that passes straight through to the mid-central back from the epigastrium.

Nausea and vomiting are commonly noted in patients with acute pancreatitis. The vomiting typically persists even after the stomach has been emptied and may result in gastroesophageal tears with bleeding (i.e., Mallory-Weiss syndrome). The vomiting and retching may be relieved by passage of a nasogastric tube, but neither the vomiting nor gastric decompression results in reduction of the abdominal pain.

PHYSICAL EXAMINATION. Patients with acute pancreatitis typically appear anxious and ill. They may be diaphoretic and hyperthermic. Tachycardia, tachypnea, and hypotension are common. Patients often roll or move around in search of a more comfortable position. In this respect, they are quite unlike those with peritonitis caused by a perforated viscus who remain motionless because movement exacerbates their pain. Most patients with acute pancreatitis have a clear sensorium, but some may have mild or even severe alterations in their mental status as a result of drug or ethanol exposure, hypoxemia, hypotension, or release of circulating toxic agents from the inflamed pancreas. Jaundice is common, even in patients with nonbiliary pancreatitis among whom the hyperbilirubinemia may reflect nonobstructive cholestasis. The abdominal examination of patients with acute pancreatitis usually reveals abdominal tender-

Table 160-3. Signs and Symptoms of Acute Pancreatitis

Observation	Incidence (%)
Pain	95
Guarding	50
Nausea/vomiting	80
Pain radiating to back	50
Distention	75
Abdominal mass	15
Jaundice	20
Hematemesis	3
Melena	4

ness and both voluntary and involuntary guarding. These findings may be limited to the epigastrium or diffusely present throughout the abdomen. A mass may be felt in the epigastrium and/or left upper quadrant of the abdomen. Direct, percussion, and rebound tenderness usually can be elicited. Abdominal distention also can be seen. Hypovolemia and dehydration are commonly present and can be detected by the presence of hypotension, tachycardia, collapsed neck veins, dry skin, dry mucous membranes, and decreased subcutaneous elasticity. Bowel sounds are often diminished or absent. Flank ecchymoses (Grey-Turner's sign) or other evidence of retroperitoneal bleeding (Cullen's sign) may be noted. Examination of the chest may reveal evidence of pleural effusion that may be on either or both sides but is most commonly present on the left. Because of pleuritic pain as well as abdominal pain, deep breathing is difficult, and atelectasis, particularly at the bases, is common. Examination of the skin may reveal areas of tender subcutaneous induration and erythema, which resembles erythema nodosum. These lesions are believed to result from fat digestion by circulating pancreatic lipases.

Laboratory Tests and Radiologic Examinations

ROUTINE BLOOD TESTS. Acute pancreatitis is associated with significant losses of intravascular fluid. A substantial amount of fluid is lost as a result of the anorexia, nausea, and vomiting that accompany the disease. In addition to these fluid losses, large volumes of fluid can be sequestered in the retroperitoneum as a result of the pancreatic inflammatory process. In addition, a systemic "capillary leak" process may result in additional fluid sequestration. Taken together, these losses of fluid from the intravascular compartment can cause the hematocrit, hemoglobin, blood urea nitrogen, and serum creatinine to rise. Hypoalbuminemia is common but the serum electrolytes may remain normal unless vomiting has been significant. Because of the pancreatic inflammatory process, the white blood cell count is usually elevated and the differential may show a shift to the left. Hyperglycemia, which is commonly noted, may result from the combined effects of elevated circulating catecholamines, decreased insulin release, and hyperglucagonemia [42,43]. A mild rise in serum bilirubin, which is the result of nonobstructive cholestasis, is frequently seen even in nonbiliary acute pancreatitis. When the disease is induced by the passage of gallstones, the hyperbilirubinemia is even more marked, and superimposed cholangitis with bacteremia and positive blood cultures can occur [44]. Markedly elevated circulating triglyceride levels always are seen in individuals whose pancreatitis is caused by hyperlipoproteinemia [45], but hypertriglyceridemia with lactescent serum also can be seen in alcohol-induced acute pancreatitis [46]. Hypocalcemia is relatively common among individuals with acute pancreatitis [47]. For the most part, the hypocalcemia is caused by hypoalbuminemia and, as a result, the ionized calcium level is actually normal. Some patients, however, can develop hypocalcemia that is out of proportion to the degree of hypoalbuminemia and that reflects a true decrease in circulating ionized calcium levels. Some of these patients may develop tetany and carpopedal spasm as well as other complications of their hypocalcemia. Marked hypocalcemia has been considered a sign of a poor prognosis. Patients with severe pancreatitis may develop disseminated intravascular coagulation [48], and, as a result, they may have thrombocytopenia, elevated levels of fibrin degradation prod-

ucts, decreased fibrinogen levels, and prolongations of both the partial thromboplastin and prothrombin times.

AMYLASE. The serum amylase concentration is usually, but not always, elevated during an attack of pancreatitis. The magnitude of that rise is not dependent on the severity of pancreatitis, and some reports have indicated that as many as 10 percent of patients with normal or near-normal serum amylase levels may have lethal pancreatitis [49]. To a great extent, this may reflect the fact that amylase elevations during pancreatitis are typically transient, with an increase 2 to 12 hours after the onset of an attack and a decline in serum amylase values to near-normal levels 3 to 6 days after the attack has begun. Thus, patients presenting long after the onset of an attack may have normal or only slightly increased serum amylase levels. Serum amylase activity also may be increased in a number of diseases other than pancreatitis [40,50] (Table 160-4). Amylase may be synthesized at extrapancreatic sites (e.g., salivary glands, fallopian tube, lung) or produced by nonpancreatic tumors (e.g., lung, prostate, ovary), and release of the nonpancreatic amylase into the circulation may result in hyperamylasemia. Patients with these nonpancreatic causes for hyperamylasemia are rarely confused with those having pancreatitis because the clinical features of pancreatitis are usually absent in the former group. On the other hand, some patients with disorders that might be clinically confused with acute pancreatitis also may have hyperamylasemia. This is particularly true for patients with acute cholecystitis, perforated gastric or duodenal ulcers, small bowel obstruction, intestinal ischemia, and intestinal infarction. It may also be true for some patients passing common bile duct stones into the duodenum who do not have pancreatitis. The overall sensitivity and specificity of amylase determination in the diagnosis of pancreatitis depend on the value chosen as the cut-off level [51] and the presence or absence of clinical features of pancreatitis. Patients with hyperamylasemia but not pancreatitis usually have mild elevations of the circulating amylase level (approximately 200 IU/L) and/or lack clinical features of pancreatitis, whereas those with pancreatitis usually manifest profound hyperamylasemia (greater than 1000 IU/L) in association with clinical features of the disease.

Approximately 0.5 percent of individuals have a condition referred to as macroamylasemia in which amylase is bound to an abnormal circulating protein and, as a result, is not cleared

Table 160-4. Causes of Hyperamylasemia

Pancreatic
    Pancreatitis, pseudocyst, ascites
    Pancreatic cancer
    Pancreatic duct obstruction
    Pancreatic trauma
    ERCP
Non-pancreatic Intraabdominal
    Perforated hollow viscus
    Bowel obstruction
    Cholangitis, cholecystitis
    Mesenteric infarction
    Ovarian cyst
    Renal failure
    Ruptured ectopic pregnancy
Extraabdominal
    Salivary gland tumors, trauma, infection, obstruction
    Lung tumors
    Burns
    Diabetic acidosis
    Pneumonia

by the kidney [40,52,53]. Some of these individuals may develop abdominal pain and be incorrectly suspected of having pancreatitis. In this setting, measurement of urinary amylase activity may be particularly helpful since, in macroamylasemia, urinary amylase levels are usually very low. Renal clearance of amylase also may be reduced as a result of renal failure, and this reduced clearance can lead to mild hyperamylasemia. On the other hand, enhanced renal clearance of amylase can occur in pancreatitis, and this phenomenon can result in an increase in the clearance ratio for amylase compared with creatinine [53,54]. Unfortunately, measurement of the so-called amylase-to-creatinine clearance ratio has not been helpful in the diagnosis of pancreatitis. Alterations of this ratio appear to represent a nonspecific response to an acute illness. Thus, the clearance ratio may be elevated in many patients who do not have pancreatitis but may be normal in many who have pancreatitis [55–58].

OTHER ENZYME ASSAYS AND BLOOD TESTS. The urine amylase level may remain elevated long after serum amylase levels have returned to normal. As a result, measurement of urinary amylase activity may be particularly helpful in patients who are first seen several days after an attack of pancreatitis and who are found to have normal or near-normal serum amylase activity [40]. Hyperlipasemia also may persist after serum amylase levels have returned to normal, and, in such patients, measurement of serum lipase activity may be useful [40,49]. Circulating levels of other pancreatic enzymes (trypsinogen, chymotrypsinogen, phospholipase, elastase) also can be measured, but there is little or no evidence to suggest that these determinations will be more helpful in the diagnosis of pancreatitis than the simpler measurement of serum amylase activity [41,49]. Acute pancreatitis also can be associated with methemalbuminemia [59] as well as with increased circulating levels of several lymphokines and acute phase reactants (e.g., c-reactive protein) [60,61]. The magnitude and duration of these changes may have some prognostic value in pancreatitis, but these changes are not specific to pancreatitis and are therefore of little diagnostic value.

ROUTINE RADIOGRAPHY. Routine chest radiographs may reveal basal atelectasis as a result of splinted respiration and/or elevated diaphragms. A pleural effusion, more common on the left than on the right, also can be seen. Abdominal films may reveal pancreatic calcifications in patients with chronic pancreatitis. These calcifications result from calcium precipitation in the proteinaceous intraductal stones that may develop in chronic pancreatitis. In general, plain abdominal films reveal evidence of a paralytic ileus, whereas contrast gastrointestinal studies may reveal displacement of peripancreatic organs by pancreatic masses. Retroperitoneal air may be seen when pancreatic abscess is caused by a gas-forming organism. In general, however, the value of routine radiographs when pancreatitis is suspected lies in the failure of those films to reveal evidence of nonpancreatic diseases that might mimic acute pancreatitis (e.g., pneumonia, perforated hollow viscus, and mechanical bowel obstruction).

ULTRASONOGRAPHY. The ultrasound examination of patients with acute pancreatitis is usually limited by the presence of intestinal gas in the upper abdomen during the early stages of the disease. Even in this setting, ultrasound may be helpful in detecting gallbladder stones and/or bile duct dilatation. Later during the course of pancreatitis, ultrasound examination may be very useful in detecting and monitoring pancreatic inflammatory masses and pseudocysts [62].

COMPUTED TOMOGRAPHY. In acute pancreatitis, particularly during the early stages of the disease, CT is the most useful imaging modality because it can actually define the gross features of the pancreas and peripancreatic organs without being limited by the presence of distended gas-filled loops of bowel in the upper abdomen [63]. The pancreas may be normal or slightly swollen in appearance on CT in mild cases of pancreatitis. Evidence of peripancreatic inflammation, including streaking in the retroperitoneal and transverse mesocolic fat, also may be seen. With more severe attacks, peripancreatic and intrapancreatic fluid collections can be detected. Dynamic CT, performed by rapidly imaging the pancreas during bolus injection of contrast material, can define areas of pancreatic necrosis since those areas will not enhance as a result of contrast administration [64,65]. Detection of some of these changes may be of prognostic value in acute pancreatitis (see following), but their major value in the early stages of the disease lies in the fact that their presence confirms the diagnosis of acute pancreatitis. Conversely, the finding of a normal pancreas without signs of peripancreatic inflammation on the CT scan of a patient suspected of having severe pancreatitis, particularly if that patient's condition is deteriorating, should suggest that the patient does not, in fact, have pancreatitis.

DIFFERENTIAL DIAGNOSIS. The differential diagnosis of acute pancreatitis includes other processes that may cause upper abdominal pain, nausea, vomiting, and abdominal tenderness. The serum amylase and/or lipase is usually elevated in acute pancreatitis and normal or near normal in many other processes that may cause similar symptoms. On the other hand, serum levels of pancreatic enzymes may be elevated in some states that can mimic acute pancreatitis (Table 160-5). For the most part, those states are associated with only one- to twofold elevations in circulating enzyme levels and with a normal appearance of the pancreas and peripancreatic tissues on CT examination. On occasion, however, the diagnosis may be uncertain and operative intervention may be indicated to establish the diagnosis, particularly in patients whose condition is deteriorating despite aggressive nonoperative therapy.

Prognosis

Most patients with acute pancreatitis have a relatively mild self-limited attack that will resolve with only supportive treatment. On the other hand, roughly 5 to 10 percent of patients in most series have a severe attack that is associated with considerable morbidity and a mortality rate that can approach 40 percent. Certain clinical features have been identified that are associated with a poor prognosis. These include age over 60, a "first at-

Table 160-5. Differential Diagnosis of Acute Pancreatitis

Perforated hollow viscus
Cholecystitis/cholangitis
Bowel obstruction
Mesenteric ischemia/infarction

tack" of pancreatitis, postoperative pancreatitis, hypocalcemia, methemalbuminemia, and the presence of either Grey Turner's or Cullen's sign [66]. Investigators in New York and in Glasgow have evaluated large groups of patients with pancreatitis and identified clinical and laboratory features available during the initial 48 hours of diagnosis that can be used to define the prognosis of an attack. These criteria, frequently referred to as the Ranson [67] and Imrie [68] criteria, are listed in Tables 160-6 and 160-7, respectively. The presence of fewer than three of the Ranson criteria is associated with mild pancreatitis, little morbidity, and a mortality rate of less than 1 percent. In contrast, many patients with three or more of these prognostic signs have severe pancreatitis, with a 34 percent incidence of septic complications and a mortality rate that, with 7 to 8 prognostic signs, may reach 90 percent. Using the Imrie criteria, severe pancreatitis has been found when three or more of the criteria are present, whereas mild pancreatitis is associated with fewer of the prognostic signs. While the criteria developed by the New York and Glasgow groups have proved of considerable value in allowing for prospective trials in the evaluation of new therapies and interventions for acute pancreatitis, these prognostic criteria are not particularly helpful in the management of an individual patient and should never be used as criteria for the diagnosis of pancreatitis. Recently, it has been suggested that the APACHE-2 system [69] might be a useful method for evaluating the severity of an attack, predicting its risk of morbidity as well as mortality, and comparing groups of patients with acute pancreatitis. It is likely that reports using this system will appear in the future and that the APACHE-2 system will replace the Ranson and the Imrie systems for evaluating the prognosis of acute pancreatitis because it allows for ongoing modifications in the grading of severity as the disease progresses.

The morbidity of an individual attack of pancreatitis is closely related to the presence of peripancreatic fluid collections demonstrable by CT. Ranson and coworkers [70], in a prospective

study involving 83 patients with acute pancreatitis, noted that those with two or more peripancreatic fluid collections seen on CT had a 61 percent incidence of late pancreatic abscess, those with only one fluid collection and/or inflammation confined to the pancreas and peripancreatic fat had a 12 to 17 percent incidence of pancreatic abscess, and those either with no CT changes of pancreatitis or with only pancreatic enlargement on CT had a zero incidence of pancreatic abscess. The morbidity, incidence of abscess formation, and mortality rate of an attack of pancreatitis also have been shown to be related to the amount of pancreatic tissue that is not enhanced on CT after bolus administration of contrast material during dynamic CT. Beger and associates [65] have suggested that patients might benefit from surgical intervention and necrosectomy of the pancreas when dynamic CT indicates that considerable portions of the pancreas are poorly perfused or nonperfused (i.e., necrotic).

Treatment of Acute Pancreatitis

INITIAL MANAGEMENT. During the early stages of an acute attack of pancreatitis, efforts should be made to confirm the diagnosis, control pain, and support fluid as well as electrolyte needs. Establishing the diagnosis of acute pancreatitis may be difficult and, at times, impossible without exploratory laparotomy. Usually the clinical picture combined with hyperamylasemia, a convincing CT scan, and favorable response to aggressive nonoperative therapy is sufficient but, when doubt persists, exploration may be warranted if the dire consequences of an overlooked bowel perforation, infarction, or obstruction are to be avoided. On the other hand, there have been reports suggesting that laparotomy may increase the incidence of septic complications in pancreatitis [71] and, therefore, exploration should be avoided if possible.

TREATMENT OF PAIN. The pain of pancreatitis is often severe and difficult to control. Most patients require narcotic medications. Demerol rather than morphine would appear to be the narcotic drug of choice for gallstone pancreatitis since it relaxes the sphincter of Oddi whereas morphine causes sphincteric contraction [72].

FLUID AND ELECTROLYTE REPLACEMENT. The early stage of severe acute pancreatitis is characterized by major fluid and electrolyte losses. External losses, caused by repeated episodes of vomiting and exacerbated by nausea and diminished fluid intake, can lead to hypochloremic alkalosis. Internal losses caused by leakage of intravascular fluid into the inflamed retroperitoneum, pulmonary parenchyma, and soft tissues elsewhere in the body contribute to hypovolemia. The most sensitive indicator of the magnitude of fluid loss during this stage of pancreatitis is the hematocrit, since serum electrolytes may remain normal because the electrolyte composition of the lost fluid is similar to that in plasma. On the other hand, the blood pH may fall as hypovolemia and poor tissue perfusion lead to metabolic acidosis. Hypoalbuminemia and hypomagnesemia, caused by preexisting malnutrition in chronic alcoholics and/or losses during the early stages of pancreatitis, may warrant replacement therapy. Tetany, carpopedal spasm, or other manifestations of hypocalcemia are rare but, when they occur, should prompt aggressive calcium replacement.

Table 160-6. Ranson's Prognostic Signs

On admission
  Age over 55 years
  White blood cell count over 16,000/mm³
  Blood glucose over 200 mg/dL
  Lactate dehydrogenase over 350 IU/L
  Glutamic oxaloacetic transaminase above 250 SFU/dL
During initial 48 hours
  Hematocrit decrease over 10%
  Blood urea nitrogen rise greater than 5 mg/dL
  Serum Ca^{2+} below 8 mg/dL
  PaO_2 below 60 mm Hg
  Base deficit over 4 mEq/L
  Fluid sequestration over 6 L

Table 160-7. Imrie's Prognostic Signs

Age over 55 years
White blood cell count over 15,000/mm³
Blood glucose over 10 mmol/L
Serum urea over 16 mmol/L
PaO_2 below 60 mm Hg
Serum Ca^{2+} below 2.0 mmol/L
Lactic dehydrogenase over 600 µg/L
Asparate aminotransferase/alanine aminotransferase over 100 µg/L
Serum albumin below 32 gm/L

The hemodynamic parameters during severe pancreatitis may resemble those during septic shock [73]. Thus, heart rate, cardiac output, and cardiac index rise and total peripheral resistance falls. The arterial–venous oxygen difference and intrapulmonary shunt rise, and marked hypoxemia may result. The basis for these changes is, most likely, multifactorial and includes hypovolemia, atelectasis, and the release of vasoactive agents and cytokines.

Treatment requires meticulous management of fluid and electrolyte needs. A fluid balance flow sheet may prove extremely useful in this regard. Endotracheal intubation and mechanical ventilatory support may be needed. For the most part, patients with severe pancreatitis should be in an intensive care unit where facilities for close monitoring are available. Volume status can best be followed using a Swan-Ganz catheter to track filling pressures and an indwelling urethral catheter to monitor urine output. Arterial oxygenation can be followed using an indwelling arterial catheter and frequent blood gas determinations.

OTHER TREATMENTS. The role of prophylactic antibiotics in the management of acute pancreatitis is not clear. Early randomized studies, performed primarily in patients with mild alcohol-induced pancreatitis, suggested that prophylatic antibiotics did not alter the incidence of septic complications or the mortality resulting from pancreatitis [74,75]. More recent studies, focusing on patients with severe gallstone-induced pancreatitis, have indicated that prophylactic treatment with broad-spectrum agents, such as imipenem, may be of benefit to these patients [76].

The peritoneal exudate that develops during acute pancreatitis contains a number of potentially harmful vasoactive agents and enzymes. It is believed that these substances are absorbed from the peritoneal cavity into the circulation and contribute to the morbidity of pancreatitis by causing complications such as vasomotor collapse, myocardial depression, adult respiratory distress syndrome (ARDS), and renal failure [77–80]. Peritoneal lavage has been used in an attempt to remove these substances, and early anecdotal reports suggested that peritoneal lavage was beneficial [71,81–84]. Recently, however, a large multi-institutional prospectively randomized and controlled trial in the United Kingdom indicated that short-term peritoneal lavage did not alter the morbidity or mortality of pancreatitis [85]. On the other hand, Ranson and co-workers recently reported the results of a study in which peritoneal lavage was performed for a prolonged period in a small group of severely ill patients with pancreatitis. They concluded that prolonged peritoneal lavage might, indeed, be of value in the management of such patients [86]. Thus, at present, the actual value as well as the ideal method of performing peritoneal lavage in this setting remain unclear.

Many other methods of treating pancreatitis have been examined, but, to date, no controlled trials have been reported that demonstrate a beneficial effect of these forms of therapy in pancreatitis (Table 160-8). Nasogastric suction has not been shown to alter the morbidity or mortality of pancreatitis, yet many clinicians, including this author, believe that it improves patient comfort. H-2 blockers and/or antacids may diminish the risk of stress ulcers, but these drugs do not alter the severity or course of pancreatitis. Agents that reduce pancreatic function (atropine, glucagon, calcitonin, somatostatin), inhibit inflammation or cytotoxic response (indomethacin, steroids, prostaglandins), inhibit digestive enzymes (procainamide, gabexate, aprotinin), or improve flow in the pancreatic microcirculation (isoproterenol, heparin, dextrans) have not been found to alter

Table 160-8. Treatments of Limited or Unproven Value

Nasogastric suction	Prostaglandins
H₂ blockers	Procainamide
Antacids	Gabexate mesilate
Atropine	Aprotinin
Glucagon	Isoproterenol
Calcitonin	Heparin
Somatostatin	Dextran
Indomethacin	Vasopressin
Steroids	Propylthiouracil
Hypothermia	Epsilon amino caproic acid
Thoracic duct drainage	Peritoneal lavage
Plasmapheresis	

the course of pancreatitis in humans, although many of these approaches have been found to be of benefit if begun early in the course of experimental pancreatitis in laboratory animals [87,88].

THE ROLE OF SURGERY AND ENDOSCOPY IN GALLSTONE PANCREATITIS. Most patients with biliary tract stone–induced pancreatitis recover quickly and uneventfully as the offending stone either is passed into the duodenum or disimpacts itself from the ampulla of Vater by moving proximally in the duct. The role of early interventions designed to remove obstructing stones in this disease has been extremely controversial. Acosta et al. [89] and Stone et al. [90] concluded that early surgical intervention could reduce the severity of pancreatitis and shorten hospitalization times. In contrast, Kelly and Wagner [91] found that early surgical intervention was associated with greater morbidity and mortality than was delayed surgery. Recently, two prospectively randomized controlled trials have evaluated the benefit of early endoscopic sphincterotomy and stone extraction in the management of patients with gallstone pancreatitis [44,92]. Both studies concluded that early intervention did not alter the course of mild pancreatitis but that the morbidity of severe pancreatitis was reduced by early stone removal. It would appear that early stone removal by endoscopic sphincterotomy benefits these patients by reducing the incidence of associated cholangitis. Based on currently available data, it would seem most appropriate that patients with mild pancreatitis not undergo either early surgical or endoscopic intervention. On the other hand, early intervention would seem warranted for patients with severe gallstone pancreatitis, and that intervention could be either surgical or endoscopic, depending on the local availability of expertise in these areas. It is possible that the benefit of early surgical or endoscopic intervention could also be achieved by the use of prophylactic antibiotics designed to prevent cholangitis, but a trial evaluating this approach has not been reported.

Recurrent attacks of gallstone pancreatitis may develop if stones either in the gallbladder or biliary ducts remain after resolution of the index attack. For that reason, most clinicians recommend that some form of treatment designed to prevent recurrent attacks be administered before discharge of the patient from hospital. This might be accomplished by laparoscopic or open cholecystectomy combined with surgical or endoscopic duct clearance. Alternatively, in patients whose only symptoms are those of duct disease and who lack symptoms of cholecystolithiasis, endoscopic sphincterotomy and duct clearance may be sufficient, particularly if the patients are poor surgical risks.

Treatment of Systemic Complications

Systemic complications of acute pancreatitis include cardiovascular collapse, respiratory failure, renal failure, metabolic encephalopathy, disseminated intravascular coagulation, and gastrointestinal bleeding (Table 160-9). For the most part, the pathogenesis and management of these manifestations of acute pancreatitis are identical to those involved when these processes are superimposed on other diseases that result in severe peritonitis and hypovolemic shock. In other words, there may be nothing specific about these systemic complications of pancreatitis although these complications may be made worse by circulating vasoactive agents, activated digestive enzymes, and protein breakdown fragments absorbed from the inflamed pancreas.

Treatment of the cardiovascular collapse of acute pancreatitis requires aggressive and meticulous fluid and electrolyte administration. Measurement of venous filling pressures, hematocrit, cardiac output, and urinary output may be extremely helpful in gauging fluid needs. There is a growing consensus that aggressive fluid and electrolyte therapy actually may be the most effective method of preventing the appearance of pulmonary and renal failure in these patients. Theoretically, peritoneal dialysis, by removing the yet unabsorbed but potentially harmful agents released by the inflamed pancreas, and plasmaphoresis, which could permit removal of circulating harmful agents, may also prevent or reduce the severity of these systemic complications of pancreatitis, but the value of these modalities has not been shown by good prospective randomized studies.

Treatment of the atelectasis and ARDS associated with acute pancreatitis is similar to the treatment of these problems when they are associated with other causes of peritonitis. Thus, good pulmonary toilet and close monitoring of pulmonary function by measurement of mechanics and blood gases are indicated. With deterioration in function, intubation and respiratory support may be needed. Similarly, the management of the renal failure of pancreatitis is not different from that of acute renal failure caused by other diseases. The renal failure of pancreatitis is prerenal and, when it occurs, is associated with a poor prognosis. Dialysis, usually in the form of hemodialysis, may be needed in the most severely affected.

Disseminated intravascular coagulation, manifested by decreased platelet counts and fibrinogen levels, prolonged pro-

Table 160-9. Complications of Acute Pancreatitis

Systemic
  Cardiovascular collapse
  Respiratory failure
  Renal failure
  Metabolic encephalopathy
  Disseminated intravascular coagulation
  Gastrointestinal bleeding
Local
  Acute fluid collection
  Pancreatic necrosis ± infection
  Pancreatic pseudocyst
  Pancreatic abscess
  Pancreatic ascites
  Pancreatic-pleural fistula
  Duodenal obstruction
  Bile duct obstruction
  Splenic vein thrombosis
  Pseudoaneurysm + hemorrhage

thrombin and partial thromboplastin times, and increased circulating levels of fibrin split products, occurs in some patients with severe acute pancreatitis. Bleeding caused by disseminated intravascular coagulation, however, is rare. Thus, prophylactic anticoagulation with heparin in patients with biochemical evidence of disseminated intravascular coagulation is not indicated and may, in fact, be associated with significant problems, including retroperitoneal hemorrhage.

The gastrointestinal bleeding sometimes seen in patients with pancreatitis usually results from stress-induced gastroduodenal lesions. Thus, prophylaxis with either antacids or H-2 blockers may be useful in preventing this problem. Rarely, massive bleeding may result from injury to gastrointestinal structures by the inflammatory process in the peripancreatic retroperitoneum. Thus, thrombosis of gastrointestinal vessels may lead to ischemic injury and bleeding from the stomach, intestine, or colon. In extreme cases, infarction and perforation of the viscus may occur. The inflammatory process may lead to erosion into retroperitoneal vessels near the pancreas. Treatment, in these situations, is dictated by the lesions present but usually involves resection of nonviable tissues.

Local Complications of Pancreatitis (Table 160-9)

Definitions. Considerable confusion has surrounded the terminology used to describe the local complications of an acute attack of pancreatitis. At a recent symposium in Atlanta [93], an international group of clinicians and scientists attempted to resolve this confusion by proposing use of the following definitions.

1. *Acute pancreatic and peripancreatic fluid collections:* Fluid collections in or near the pancreas that occur early in the course of acute pancreatitis and that lack a wall of granulation or fibrous tissue.
2. *Pancreatic necrosis:* An area of nonviable pancreatic tissue that may be diffuse or focal and that is typically associated with peripancreatic fat necrosis. Pancreatic necrosis may be either *sterile* or *infected.*
3. *Pancreatic pseudocyst:* A collection of pancreatic juice that is usually rich in digestive enzymes and that is enclosed by a nonepithelialized wall of fibrous or granulation tissue (Figs. 160-1 and 160-2). It is usually round or ovoid in shape and is not present before 4 to 6 weeks have elapsed since the onset of acute pancreatitis. Prior to this time, the fluid collection usually lacks a defined wall and may be either an "acute fluid collection" or a localized area of "pancreatic necrosis." Bacteria may be present in a pseudocyst as a result of contamination, but, in this setting, clinical infection is usually absent. When pus is present, however, the lesion should be referred to as a *pancreatic abscess.* Leakage of pseudocysts into the peritoneal cavity or chest leads to the development of *pancreatic ascites* or *pancreatic-pleural fistula,* respectively.
4. *Pancreatic abscess:* A circumscribed intraabdominal collection of pus, usually in proximity to the pancreas, that contains little or no necrotic pancreatic tissue but that arises as a consequence of either acute pancreatitis or pancreatic trauma (Fig. 160-3) (see Chap. 159). The relative absence of necrosis distinguishes *pancreatic abscess* from *infected pancreatic necrosis.*

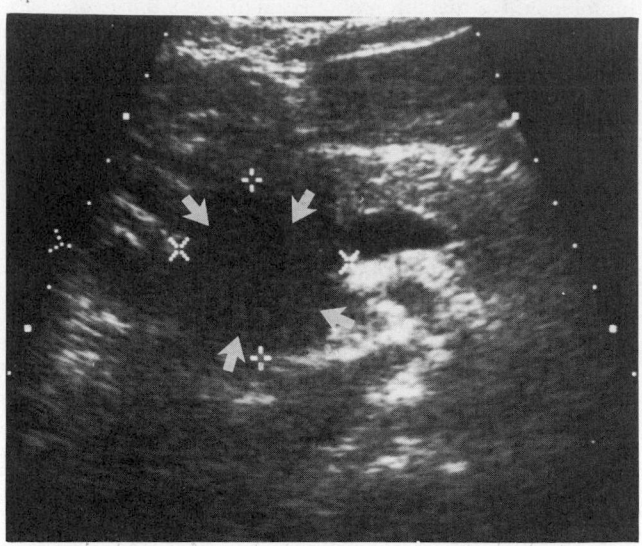

Fig. 160-1. Ultrasound showing pancreatic pseudocyst. The area of the pseudocyst is indicated by the white arrows.

DIAGNOSIS. Patients with uncomplicated pancreatitis usually are judged by the various prognostication schemes to have mild pancreatitis at the time of diagnosis and they usually recover uneventfully within the subsequent 1 to 2 weeks. In contrast, patients with severe pancreatitis, who remain ill for longer periods, frequently have one or more of the local complications of pancreatitis. In the past, these lesions were identified on the basis of physical examination, contrast radiography, and blood chemistry studies. For the most part, these relatively crude and inaccurate methods have been replaced by the techniques of ultrasound and computed tomography. Both ultrasound and CT can be used to accurately diagnose and define the extent of

Fig. 160-2. CT scan showing pancreatic pseudocyst. The area of the pseudocyst in the pancreatic head is indicted by the white arrows.

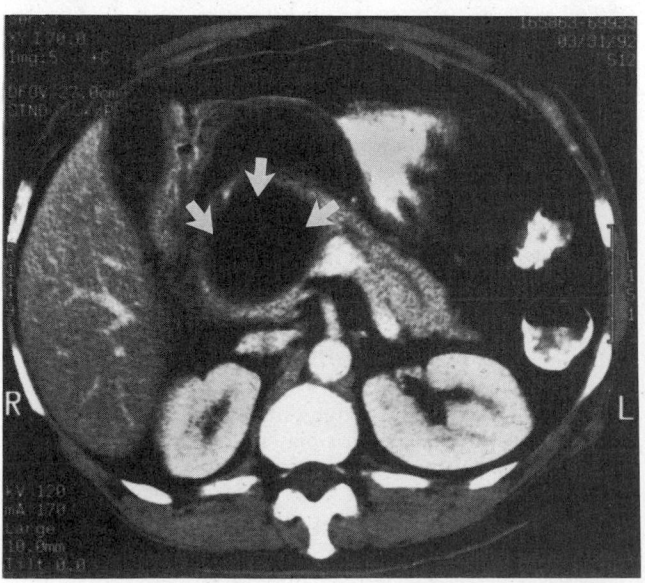

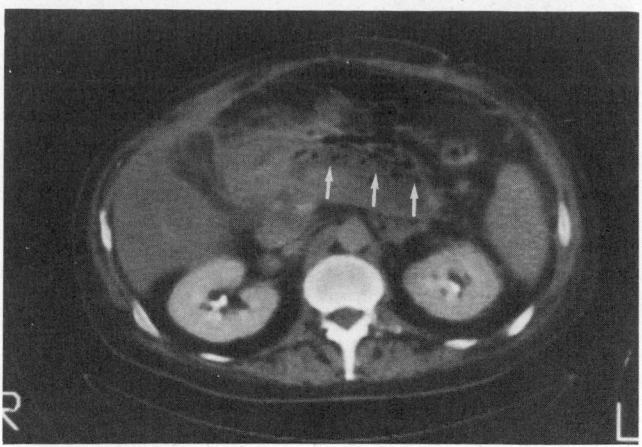

Fig. 160-3. CT scan showing area of infected pancreatic necrosis. Air in the peripancreatic area is indicated by the white arrows.

acute fluid collections and pseudocysts. Both techniques can be used to follow the progression of these lesions and determine whether or not a wall, which distinguishes a pseudocyst from an acute fluid collection, is present. Dynamic contrast-enhanced CT is the most accurate means of identifying and quantitating areas of pancreatic necrosis, whereas ERCP may be useful in determining whether fluid collections communicate with the main pancreatic duct. In addition, ERCP can be used to localize the point of duct rupture in patients with either pancreatic ascites or pancreatic-pleural fistulas. The presence of extraintestinal gas on either ultrasound or CT is diagnostic of either infected necrosis or abscess, but this finding is only occasionally noted. More often, patients with either infected necrosis or abscess are found to have poorly enhanced areas on dynamic CT and/or fluid collections on ultrasound in a clinical setting of suspected sepsis. When doubt about the presence or absence of infection persists, fine needle aspiration of these areas, under either ultrasound or CT guidance, may yield material that, on Gram stain, reveals the presence of bacteria [94,95].

MANAGEMENT

1. *Acute fluid collections* generally require no specific treatment. They usually resolve spontaneously within several weeks of an attack. Attempts to drain these collections either by percutaneously placed catheters or early surgical intervention should be discouraged.

2. *Sterile necrosis,* particularly when it involves large portions of the pancreas, has been treated by surgical necrosectomy combined with postoperative lavage of the peripancreatic area [96]. However, there is considerable controversy surrounding the question of whether surgical intervention is needed in patients with sterile necrosis even if large areas of necrosis are present [97]. It has been the author's practice to intervene only when the status of a patient was observed to be deteriorating in spite of aggressive nonoperative treatment but to manage most patients with sterile pancreatic necrosis nonoperatively. Surgical intervention in such patients may be associated with considerable morbidity. It may even result in secondary infection of the inflamed but previously sterile pancreas. On the other hand, the absence of infection does not guarantee that recovery is possible without debridement. Thus, when forced

by a deteriorating clinical course, surgical intervention should include aggressive debridement of necrotic tissue. Repeated reexploration and debridement may be needed. For this purpose, some have advocated either leaving the abdomen open between explorations [98] or using a "zipper" closure [99] to permit reexploration and packing in the intensive care unit rather than in the operating room. The author has preferred, in this setting, to close the abdomen and, if necessary, reexplore the patient in the operating room where facilities for exposure, suctioning, and debridement are better. Continuous lavage rather than reexploration and debridement may be a reasonable alternative to this approach.

3. *Infected necrosis* is always an indication for surgical intervention whether it is detected by the presence or extra-intestinal gas on CT examination or by fine needle aspiration of an area of pancreatic necrosis (see Chap. 159). Organisms recovered in areas of infected pancreatic necrosis are usually those present in the gastrointestinal tract (*Klebsiella* sp., *Pseudomonas* sp., *Escherichia coli, Enterococcus, Proteus* sp.) [100]. In addition, yeast such as *Candida albicans* may be encountered. It is believed that most of these organisms reach the inflamed pancreas via transmigration from adjacent segments of the intestine. Antibiotic therapy, while indicated, by itself represents an inadequate approach to the management of infected pancreatic necrosis. Similarly, because of the presence of large amounts of necrotic putty-like material, percutaneous drainage of these areas using indwelling catheters is almost always unsuccessful. For the most part, patients with infected necrosis require aggressive and repeated surgical debridement and drainage. The mortality rate for untreated or inadequately treated infected pancreatic necrosis may approach 100 percent.

Pseudocysts may cause symptoms either because they are themselves tender or because they cause obstruction of adjacent organs such as the stomach, duodenum, and bile duct. On occasion, pancreatic pseudocysts contribute to the progression of pancreatitis by causing pancreatic duct obstruction. On the other hand, many pseudocysts do not cause symptoms. Until relatively recently, the general consensus of opinion was that pseudocysts should be treated regardless of their size or whether they caused symptoms [101]. Several recent reports, however, have indicated that chronic pseudocysts, even those greater than 6 cm in diameter, can be safely observed and that treatment is needed only for those that become symptomatic [102,103]. Several methods of treating pseudocysts have been proposed, including internal surgical drainage (cystogastrostomy, cystoduodenostomy, Roux-y-cystojejunostomy), endoscopic drainage (cystogastrostomy, cystoduodenostomy), and percutaneous drainage (aspiration, aspiration followed by administration of somatostatin, and catheter drainage, with or without administration of somatostatin) [104]. The author's experience with percutaneous drainage has, to a great extent, been disappointing because of a considerable incidence of either recurrence after aspiration or infection after catheter drainage. In fit surgical candidates, internal surgical drainage would seem an appropriate first choice for the treatment of symptomatic pseudocysts, whereas an attempt at endoscopic drainage would seem appropriate for poor surgical risk patients.

Patients with *pancreatic ascites* or *pancreatic-pleural fistulas* may respond to nonoperative therapy with bowel rest, parenteral nutrition, and administration of somatostatin or other agents designed to inhibit pancreatic secretion [105–112]. Most, however, fail this method of treatment and some form of intervention is needed. An ERCP should be performed to identify the site of duct disruption [113,114,115], which, if in the pancreatic tail, can be treated easily by distal pancreatectomy. Alternatively, anastomosis of a Roux-en-Y loop of jejunum to the

site of rupture, particularly if it is in the head or neck of the gland, may be preferable. A recent report suggested that endoscopically placed stents may be used to prevent leakage of juice from the duct and that this nonoperative approach might be useful in the management of these complications [116].

Pancreatic abscess, like infected pancreatic necrosis, always requires some form of intervention, but since pancreatic abscesses contain liquid pus rather than the paste-like material in pancreatic necrosis, percutaneous drainage of pancreatic abscesses might be considered (see Chap. 159). Alternatively, surgical intervention and placement of drainage catheters in the abscess may also be appropriate. The author has, for the most part, treated such patients with surgical drainage, but recent advances in the field of invasive radiology may permit successful nonoperative management of such patients in the future.

References

1. Sarles H: Introduction and proposal adopted unanimously by the participants of the symposium, in Sarles H (ed): *Pancreatitis—Symposium, Marseilles, 1963.* Basel, Verlag S. Karger, 1965, pp VI–VIII.
2. Sarner M, Cotton PB: Classification of pancreatitis. *Gut* 25:756, 1984.
3. Singer MV, Gyr K: Revised classification of pancreatitis—Marseilles 1984. *Gastroenterology* 89:683, 1985.
4. Steer ML: Etiology and pathophysiology of acute pancreatitis, in Go VLW, Gardner JD, Brooks EP, et al (eds): *The Exocrine Pancreas: Biology, Pathobiology, and Diseases.* New York, Raven Press 1986, pp 465–474.
5. Pitchumoni CS: Special problems of tropical pancreatitis. *Clin Gastroenterol* 13:541, 1984.
6. Narendranathan M: Chronic calcific pancreatitis of the tropics. *Trop Gastroenterol* 2:40, 1981.
7. Pitchumoni CS, Jain NK, Lowenfels AF, et al: Chronic cyanide poisoning. Unifying concept for alcoholic and tropical pancreatitis. *Pancreas* 3:220, 1988.
8. Acosta JL, Ledesma CL: Gallstone migration as a cause for acute pancreatitis. *N Engl J Med* 290:484, 1974.
9. Acosta JL, Ross R, Ledesma CL: The usefulness of stool screening for diagnosing cholelithiasis in acute pancreatitis: A description of the technique. *Am J Dig Dis* 22:168, 1977.
10. Opie EL: The etiology of acute hemorrhagic pancreatitis. *Bull Johns Hopkins Hosp* 12:182, 1901.
11. Menguy RB, Hallenbeck GA, Bollman JL, et al: Intraductal pressures and sphincteric resistance in canine pancreatic and biliary ducts after various stimuli. *Surg Gynecol Obstet* 106:306, 1958.
12. Mann FC, Giordano AS: The bile factor in pancreatitis. *Arch Surg* 6:1, 1923.
13. Robinson TM, Dunphy JE: Continuous perfusion of bile protease activators through the pancreas. *JAMA* 183:530, 1963.
14. McCutheon AD: Reflux of duodenal contents in the pathogenesis of pancreatitis. *Gut* 5:260, 1964.
15. Larch MM, Saluja AK, Runzi M, et al: Pancreatic duct obstruction triggers acute necrotizing pancreatitis in the opossum. *Gastroenterology* 104:853, 1993.
16. Steer ML, Meldolesi J, Figarella C: Pancreatitis: The role of lysosomes. *Dig Dis Sci* 29:934, 1984.
17. Steer ML: How and where does acute pancreatitis begin? *Arch Surg* 127:1350, 1992.
18. Steer ML, Meldolesi J: The cell biology of experimental pancreatitis. *N Engl J Med* 316:144, 1987.
19. Sarles H: Chronic pancreatitis: Etiology and pathophysiology, in Go VLW, Gardner JD, Brooks EP, et al (eds): *The Exocrine Pancreas: Biology, Pathobiology, and Diseases.* New York, Raven Press, 1986, p 37.
20. Steer ML, Glazer G, Manabe T: Direct effects of ethanol on exocrine secretion from the in-vitro rabbit pancreas. *Dig Dis Sci* 24:769, 1979.

21. Rinderknecht H, Renner IG, Koyama HH: Lysosomal enzymes in pure pancreatic juice from normal healthy volunteers and chronic alcoholics. *Dig Dis Sci* 24:180, 1979.

22. Figarella C, Amouric M, Guy-Crotte O: Role of lysosomes in pancreatic disease. *Int J Pancreatol* 3:S9, 1988.

23. Renner IG, Savage WT 3rd, Pantoja JL, et al: Death due to acute pancreatitis, a retrospective analysis of 405 autopsy cases. *Dig Dis Sci* 30:1005, 1985.

24. Thomas FB: Drug-induced pancreatitis: Facts vs fiction. *Drug Ther Hosp* 7:60, 1982.

25. Greenberger NJ, Toskes P, Isselbacher KJ: Diseases of the pancreas, in Braunwald E, et al (eds): *Harrison's Principles of Internal Medicine.* New York, McGraw-Hill, 1988, p 1372.

26. Mallory A, Kern F: Drug-induced pancreatitis: A critical review. *Gastroenterology* 78:813, 1980.

27. Lambert JS, Seidlin M, Reichman RC, et al: 2', 3'-Dideoxyinosine (ddI) in patients with the acquired immunodeficiency syndrome of AIDS-related complex. A Phase I trial. *N Engl J Med* 322:1333, 1990.

28. Durr GH: Acute pancreatitis, in Howatt HT, Sarles H (eds): *The Exocrine Pancreas.* London, WB Saunders, 1979, p 292.

29. Wilson RH, Moorehead RJ: Current management of trauma to the pancreas. *Br J Surg* 78:1196, 1991.

30. Bardenheier JA, Kaminski DL, William VL: Pancreatitis after biliary tract surgery. *Am J Surg* 16:773, 1968.

31. Peterson LM, Collins JJ, Wilson RE: Acute pancreatitis occurring after operation. *Surg Gynecol Obstet* 127:23, 1968.

32. White TT, Morgan A, Hopton D: Postoperative pancreatitis: A study of seventy cases. *Am J Surg* 120:132, 1970.

33. Adiseshia M: Acute pancreatitis after cardiac transplantation. *World J Surg* 7:519, 1983.

34. Feiner H: Pancreatitis after cardiac surgery. *Am J Surg* 131:684, 1976.

35. Cotton PB: Progress report. ERCP. *Gut* 18:316, 1977.

36. Lee SP, Nicholls JF, Park HZ: Biliary sludge as a cause of acute pancreatitis. *N Engl J Med* 326:589, 1992.

37. Owyang C, Levitt M: Chronic pancreatitis, in Yamada T, et al (eds): *Textbook of Gastroenterology.* Philadelphia, JB Lippincott, 1991, pp 1874–1893.

38. Layer P, Kalthoff L, Clain JE, et al: Nonalcoholic chronic pancreatitis—two diseases? *Dig Dis Sci* 30:980, 1985.

39. Silen W: *Cope's Early Diagnosis of the Acute Abdomen.* 15th ed. New York, Oxford University Press, 1979.

40. Leavitt MD, Edkfeldt JH: Diagnosis of acute pancreatitis, in Go VLW, Gardner JD, Brooks EP, et al (eds): *The Exocrine Pancreas: Biology, Pathobiology, and Diseases.* New York, Raven Press, 1986, p 481.

41. Banks PA: Acute pancreatitis: Clinical presentation, in Go VLW, Gardner J, Brooks EP, et al (eds): *The Exocrine Pancreas: Biology, Pathobiology, and Diseases.* New York, Raven Press, 1986, p 475.

42. Solomon SS, Duckworth WC, Jallepalli P, et al: The glucose intolerance of acute pancreatitis. *Diabetes* 29:22, 1980.

43. Drew SI, Joffe B, Vinik A, et al: The first 24 hours of acute pancreatitis. *Am J Med* 64:795, 1978.

44. Fan ST, Lai ECS, Mok FPT, et al: Early treatment of acute biliary pancreatitis by endoscopic papillotomy. *N Engl J Med* 328:228, 1993.

45. Frederickson DS, Lees RS: Familial hyperlipoproteinemia, in Stanbury JB, Wyngaarden JB, Fredrickson DS (eds): *The Metabolic Basis of Inherited Disease.* New York, McGraw-Hill, 1966, pp 429–485.

46. Cameron JL, Crisler C, Margolis S, et al: Acute pancreatitis with hyperlipemia. *Surgery* 70:53, 1971.

47. Imrie CW, Beastall GH, Allam BF, et al: Parathyroid hormone and calcium homeostasis in acute pancreatitis. *Br J Surg* 65:717, 1978.

48. Ranson JHC, Lackner H: Coagulopathies, in Bradley EL (ed): *Complications of Pancreatitis.* Philadelphia, WB Saunders, 1982, pp 154–175.

49. Steer ML: Actue pancreatitis, in Yamada, T, et al (eds): *Textbook of Gastroenterology.* Philadelphia, JB Lippincott, 1991, pp 1859–1874.

50. Salt WB, Schenker S: Amylase—its clinical significance: A review of the literature. *Medicine* (Baltimore) 55:269, 1976.

51. Steinberg WM, Goldstein SS, Davis ND, et al: Diagnostic assays in acute pancreatitis. A study of sensitivity and specificity. *Ann Intern Med* 102:576, 1985.

52. Berk JE, Kizu H, Wilding P: A newly recognized cause for elevated serum amylase activity. *N Engl J Med* 277:941, 1967.

53. Levitt MD, Rapoport M, Cooperband SR: The renal clearance of amylase in renal insufficiency, acute pancreatitis, and macroamylasemia. *Ann Intern Med* 71:919, 1969.

54. Warshaw AL, Fuller AF: Specificity of increased renal clearance of amylase in diagnosis of acute pancreatitis. *N Engl J Med* 292:325, 1975.

55. McMahon MJ, Playforth MJ, Rashid SA, et al: The amylase-to-creatinine clearance—a nonspecific response to acute illness? *Br J Surg* 69:29, 1982.

56. Levitt MD, Gross JB Jr: Postoperative elevation of amylase/creatinine clearance ratio in patients without pancreatitis. *Gastroenterology* 77:497, 1979.

57. Levin RJ, Galuser FL, Berk JE: Enhancement of the amylase-creatinine clearance ratio in disorders other than acute pancreatitis. *N Engl J Med* 292:329, 1975.

58. Morton WJ, Tedesco FJ, Harter HR, et al: Serum amylase determinations and amylase to creatinine clearance ratios in patients with chronic renal insufficiency. *Gastroenterology* 71:594, 1976.

59. Bank S, Barbezat GO, Marks IN, et al: Methemalbuminaemia in acute abdominal emergencies. *Br Med J* 2:86, 1968.

60. Buchler M, Malfertheiner P, Beger HG: Correlation of imaging procedures, biochemical parameters and clinical stage in acute pancreatitis, in Malfertheiner P, Ditschuneit H (eds): *Diagnostic Procedures in Pancreatic Disease.* Berlin, Springer-Verlag, 1986, pp 123–129.

61. Mayer AD, McMahon MJ, Bowen M, et al: C-reactive protein; an aid to assessment and monitoring of acute pancreatitis. *J Clin Pathol* 37:207, 1984.

62. Lees WR: Pancreatic ultrasonography. *Clin Gastroenterol* 13:763, 1984.

63. Freeny PC: Radiology of acute pancreatitis: Diagnosis, detection of complications, and interventional therapy, in Glazer G, Ranson JHC (eds): *Acute Pancreatitis.* London, Bailliere Tindall, 1988, pp 275–302.

64. Kivisarri L, Somer K, Standertskjold-Nordenstam C-G, et al: A new method for the diagnosis of acute hemorrhagic-necrotizing pancreatitis using contrast-enhanced CT. *Gastrointest Radiol* 9:27, 1984.

65. Beger HG, Krautzberger W, Bittner R, et al: Results of surgical treatment of necrotizing pancreatitis. *World J Surg* 9:972, 1985.

66. Ranson JHC: Prognostication in acute pancreatitis, in Glazer G, Ranson JHC (eds): *Acute Pancreatitis.* London, Bailliere Tindall, 1988, pp 303–330.

67. Ranson JHC, Rifkind KM, Roses DF, et al: Prognostic signs and the role of operative management in acute pancreatitis. *Surg Gynecol Obstet* 139:69, 1974.

68. Imrie CW, Benjamin IS, Ferguson JC, et al: A single-centre double-blind trial of Trasylol therapy in primary acute pancreatitis. *Br J Surg* 65:337, 1978.

69. Larvin M, McMahon MJ: Apache-2 score for assessment and monitoring of acute pancreatitis. *Lancet* 2:201, 1989.

70. Ranson JHC, Balthazar E, Caccavale R, et al: Computed tomography and the prediction of pancreatic abscess in acute pancreatitis. *Ann Surg* 201:656, 1985.

71. Ranson JHC, Spencer FC: The role of peritoneal lavage in severe acute pancreatitis. *Ann Surg* 187:565, 1978.

72. Thune A, Baker RA, Saccone GT, et al: Differing effects of pethidine and morphine on human sphincter of Oddi motility. *Br J Surg* 77:992, 1990.

73. Beger HG, Bittner R, Buchler M, et al: Hemodynamic data pattern in patients with acute pancreatitis. *Gastroenterology* 90:70, 1986.

74. Finch WT, Sawyers JL, Schenker S: A prospective study to determine the efficacy of antibiotics in acute pancreatitis. *Ann Surg* 183:667, 1976.

75. Howes R, Zuidema GD, Cameron J: Evaluation of prophylactic antibiotics in acute pancreatitis. *J Surg Res* 18:197, 1975.

76. Bassi C, Vesentini S, Abbas H, et al: Result of the Italian Multicenter Trial with Imipenum (I) in necrotizing pancreatitis (NP). *Pancreas* 7:732, 1992.

77. McMahon MJ, Lankisch PG: Peritoneal lavage and dialysis for the

treatment of acute pancreatitis, in Beger HG, Buchler M (eds): *Acute Pancreatitis.* Berlin, Springer-Verlag, 1987, pp 278-284.

78. Frey CF, Wong HN, Hickman D, et al: Toxicity of hemorrhagic ascitic fluid associated with hemorrhagic pancreatitis. *Arch Surg* 117:401, 1982.
79. Traverso LW, Pullos TG, Frey CF: Haemodynamic characterisation of porcine hemorrhagic pancreatitis ascites fluid. *J Surg Res* 34:254, 1983.
80. Ellison EC, Pappas TN, Johnson JA, et al: Demonstration and characterisation of the hemoconcentrating effect of ascitic fluid that accumulates during haemorrhagic pancreatitis. *J Surg Res* 30:241, 1981.
81. Geokas MC, Olsen H, Barbour B, et al: Peritoneal lavage in the treatment of acute hemorrhagic pancreatitis. *Gastroenterology* 58:950, 1970.
82. Wall AJ: Peritoneal dialysis in the treatment of severe acute pancreatitis. *Med J Aust* 2:281, 1965.
83. Bolooki H, Gliedman ML: Peritoneal dialysis in the treatment of acute pancreatitis. *Surgery* 64:466, 1978.
84. Lasson A, Balldin G, Genell S, et al: Peritoneal lavage in severe acute pancreatitis. *Acta Chir Scand* 150:479, 1984.
85. Mayer AD, McMahon MJ, Corfield AP, et al: Controlled clinical trial of peritoneal lavage for the treatment of severe acute pancreatitis. *N Engl J Med* 312:339, 1985.
86. Ranson JH, Berman RS: Long peritoneal lavage decreases pancreatic sepsis in acute pancreatitis. *Ann Surg* 211:708, 1990.
87. Goebell H, Singer MV: Acute pancreatitis: Standards of conservative treatment, in Beger HG, Buchler M (eds): *Acute Pancreatitis.* Berlin, Springer-Verlag, 1987, pp 259–265.
88. Steinberg WM, Schlesselman SN: Treatment of pancreatitis. Comparison of animal and human studies. *Gastroenterology* 93:1420, 1987.
89. Acosta JM, Rossi R, Galli OMR, et al: Early surgery for acute gallstone pancreatitis: Evaluation of a systemic approach. *Surgery* 83:367, 1978.
90. Stone HH, Fabian TC, Dunlop WE: Gallstone pancreatitis. Biliary tract pathology in relation to time of operation. *Ann Surg* 194:305, 1981.
91. Kelly TR, Wagner DS: Gallstone pancreatitis: A prospective randomized trail of the timing of surgery. *Surgery* 104:600, 1988.
92. Neoptolemos JP, Carr-Locke DL, London NJ, et al: Controlled trial of urgent endoscopic retrograde cholangiopancreatography and endoscopic sphincterotomy versus conservative treatment for acute pancreatitis due to gallstones. *Lancet* 2:979, 1988.
93. Bradley EL: A clinically based classification system for acute pancreatitis. Summary of the International Symposium on Acute Pancreatitis, Atlanta, GA, Sept. 11–13, 1992. *Arch Surg* 128:586, 1993.
94. Gerzoff SG, Banks PA, Robbins AH, et al: Early diagnosis of pancreatic infection by computed tomography-guided aspiration. *Gastroenterology* 93:1315, 1987.
95. Banks PA, Gerzoff SG: Indications and results of fine needle aspiration of pancreatic exudate, in Beger HG, Buchler M (Eds): *Acute Pancreatitis.* Berlin, Springer-Verlag, 1987, p 171.
96. Beger HG, Buchler M, Bittner R, et al: Necrosectomy and postoperative local lavage in necrotizing pancreatitis. *Br J Surg* 75:207, 1988.

97. Bradley EL, Allen K: A prospective longitudinal study of observation versus surgical intervention in the management of necrotizing pancreatitis. *Am J Surg* 161:19, 1991.
98. Bradley EL, Fulenwider JT: Open treatment of pancreatic abscess. *Surg Gynecol Obstet* 159:509, 1984.
99. Garcia-Sabrido JL, Tallado JM, Chistou NV, et al: Treatment of severe intraabdominal sepsis and/or necrotic foci by an "open-abdomen" approach. Zipper and Zipper-mesh techniques. *Arch Surg* 123:152, 1988.
100. Pemberton JH, Nagorney DM, Dozois RR: Pancreatic abscess, in Go VLW, Garden JD, Brooks EP, et al (eds): *The Exocrine Pancreas: Biology, Pathobiology, and Diseases.* New York, Raven Press, 1986, pp 513–525.
101. Bradley EL, Clements JL, Gonzales AC: The natural history of pancreatic pseudocysts: A unified concept of management. *Am J Surg* 137:135, 1979.
102. Yeo CJ, Bastidas JA, Lynch-Nyhan A, et al: The natural history of pancreatic pseudocysts documented by computed tomography. *Surg Gynecol Obstet* 170:411, 1990.
103. Vitas GJ, Sarr MG: Selected management of pancreatic pseudocysts: Operative versus expectant management. *Surgery* 111:123, 1992.
104. Morali GA, Braverman DZ, Shemesh D, et al: Successful treatment of pancreatic pseudocysts with a somatostatin analogue and catheter drainage. *Am J Gastroenterol* 86:515, 1991.
105. Sankaran S, Walt AJ: Pancreatic ascites: Recognition and management. *Arch Surg* 111:430, 1976.
106. Cameron JL, Kieffer RS, Anderson WJ, et al: Internal pancreatic fistulas: Pancreatic ascites and pleural effusions. *Ann Surg* 184:587, 1976.
107. Kavin H, Sobel JD, Dembo AJ: Pancreatic ascites treated by irradiation of pancreas. *Br Med J* 2:503, 1971.
108. DeWale B, Van der Spek P, Devis G: Peritoneovenous shunt for pancreatic ascites. *Dig Dis Sci* 32:550, 1987.
109. Variyam EP: Central vein hyperalimentation in pancreatic ascites. *Am J Gastroenterol* 78:178, 1983.
110. Ward PA, Raju S, Suzuki H: Preoperative demonstration of pancreatic fistula by endoscopic pancreatography in a patient with pancreatic ascites. *Ann Surg* 185:232, 1977.
111. Cameron JL, Brawley RK, Bender HW, et al: The treatment of pancreatic ascites. *Ann Surg* 170:668, 1969.
112. Gislason H, Growbech JE, Soreide O: Pancreatic ascites: Treatment by continuous somatostatin infusion. *Am J Gastroenterol* 86:519, 1991.
113. Sankaran S, Sugawa C, Walt AJ: Value of endoscopic retrograde pancreatography in pancreatic ascites. *Surg Gynecol Obstet* 148:185, 1979.
114. Rawlings W, Bynum TE, Pasternak G: Pancreatic ascites: Diagnosis of leakage site by endoscopic pancreatography. *Surgery* 81:363, 1977.
115. Levine JB, Warshaw AL, Falchuk KR, et al: The value of endoscopic retrograde pancreatography in the management of pancreatic ascites. *Surgery* 81:360, 1977.
116. Kozarek RA, Ball TJ, Paterson DJ, et al: Endoscopic transpapillary therapy for disrupted pancreatic duct and peripancreatic fluid collections. *Gastroenterology* 100:1362, 1991.

161. Necrotizing Fasciitis and Other Soft Tissue Infections

David H. Ahrenholz

The skin is the largest organ of the human body, and one of its primary functions is to provide a barrier to infection. After birth, the skin is colonized by a variety of mostly nonpathogenic bacteria, unless the infant remains hospitalized [1,2]. Normal adult bacterial flora include *Staphylococcus epidermidis* and various *Corynebacterium, Propionibacterium, Lactobacillus,* and *Micrococcus* species. These number about 10^3 per cm^2, rising to 10^6 per cm^2 in the axilla and groin [1].

Any minor break in the skin allows bacteria to reach underlying soft tissue. These contaminating bacteria multiply and colonize the wound within a few hours, but an infection occurs only when bacteria invade surrounding viable tissue. Bacteria that have this capability are functionally defined as pathogens [3]. But even minimally virulent bacteria can establish an infection if the local or systemic defenses of the host are impaired. Local trauma, with tissue edema, hematoma, ischemic tissue, or a foreign body, increases the risk of infection [4]. Systemic conditions associated with more virulent disease include diabetes mellitus, cirrhosis, collagen vascular disease, malignancies, malnutrition, major trauma, advanced age, atherosclerosis, neutropenia, and use of steroids or other antiinflammatory agents [3–6].

Terminology for Soft Tissue Infections

Soft tissue infections include a spectrum of diseases ranging from folliculitis to life-threatening clostridial myonecrosis. Most physicians are confounded by the multiplicity and inconsistency of terms applied to serious infections. A practical classification system defines infections by the deepest level of tissue penetration [4,7,8]. A few specific terms can then be used to describe the most common soft tissue infections (Table 161-1).

Cutaneous cellulitis is a nonpyogenic infection limited to the skin and superficial subcutaneous tissue (level 1) and characterized by spreading erythema and edema. This superficial infection is adequately treated with antibiotics combined with local heat and elevation to resolve the edema [9]. Surgical intervention is not indicated. Deep necrotizing infections can have an external appearance identical to that of typical cellulitis, but the outcome is frequently fatal if surgical treatment is delayed.

The most common soft tissue infection is a subcutaneous abscess (level 2), which resolves rapidly with simple incision and drainage [10]. Adjunctive antibiotics are indicated only if the patient has some underlying chronic disease state or evidence of poorly localized infection [11].

Necrotizing fasciitis is the generic term used to describe an infection that spreads along the fascia (level 3) [12]. It may begin around a deep abscess, chronic ulcer, puncture wound, or surgical incision. At the fascial plane there is little resistance to the lateral spread of bacteria, so extensive areas become rapidly involved with minimal cutaneous signs. Aggressive surgical debridement is required to control the infection.

Muscular infections (level 4) can be life-threatening, especially when caused by bacteria such as *Clostridium perfringens,* which produce potent exotoxins [13]. Necrotizing muscular infections mandate surgical exploration, radical debridement, and, in the most severe cases, amputation. Hyperbaric oxygen is helpful as well [14].

These four terms comprise a surprisingly useful vocabulary to describe common soft tissue infections. More significantly, they emphasize a consistent treatment plan, based on the anatomic planes affected (see Table 161-1).

Other terms have been a source of confusion for clinicians. "Gas gangrene" is a popular term for clostridial myonecrosis, but the presence of gas is neither mandatory nor diagnostic in this condition. Other infections of the soft tissue associated with gas production include "clostridial abscess" and many cases of nonclostridial myonecrosis [15,16]. Gas also occurs in tissue after surgical manipulation, irrigation with pressure devices or hydrogen peroxide, disruption of the esophagus or trachea, and factitious injection of air [4,15,16].

Nor is dermal necrosis (gangrene) pathognomonic of an infection (Table 161-2). Dermal infarction is found in such diverse disease states as ischemic dermal necrosis (dry gangrene), synergistic ulcerating skin lesions (Meleney cutaneous gangrene), streptococcal necrotizing fasciitis (streptococcal gangrene), and life-threatening clostridial myonecrosis ("gas gangrene") [4]. Dermal necrosis is an adequate description of this cutaneous finding, regardless of the underlying cause.

Table 161-1. Common Soft Tissue Infections and Their Treatment

Tissue Level	Term	Common Pathogen	Treatment
Epidermis/dermis	Cellulitis	*S. pyogenes*	Antibiotics, heat, elevation
Subcutaneous tissue	Abscess	*S. aureus*	Above plus incision and drainage*
Fascia	Necrotizing fasciitis	Mixed flora	Above plus debridement of necrotic tissue
Muscle	Myonecrosis	*C. perfringens*	Above plus radical debridement or amputation; hyperbaric oxygen for anaerobic infections

* Antibiotics for poorly localized infections only.

Table 161-2. Causes of Dermal Necrosis

Anoxia
   Thrombosis
   Embolism
   Vasculitis
   Atherosclerosis
Toxins
   Envenomation
   Bacterial toxins
   Extravasation
      Hypertonic solutions
      Cytotoxic agents
      Vasoconstrictors
Trauma
   Heat or cold injury
   Mechanical injury

Pathogens Associated with Skin Infections

The majority of serious soft tissue infections are caused by six groups of bacteria, some of which produce a variety of soft tissue infections, determined by the tissue level affected (Table 161-3) [4,8]. Surprisingly, for a given level of tissue invasion, the clinical picture is often the same regardless of the organisms involved [4,17,18].

Group B beta-hemolytic *Streptococcus pyogenes* is a highly-virulent pathogen in soft tissue, usually producing a marked cellulitis (erysipelas) and sparing underlying soft tissue. The intense red color and sharply demarcated borders are hallmarks of this disease [19]. However, *S. pyogenes* also produces ecthyma contagiosum, a superficial infection characterized by superficial dermal ulcerations similar to impetigo [8]. Streptococcal lymphangitis, in which bacteria spread along dermal lymphatics as a visible red line, can lead to streptococcal septicemia. In the preantibiotic era this "blood poisoning" had a very high mortality rate, and immediate amputation was considered life-saving.

Streptococcal infections at the fascial level can spread widely beneath normal-appearing skin as streptococcal necrotizing fasciitis [20,21]. Ultimately cutaneous erythema and edema and patchy dermal necrosis appear (streptococcal gangrene) [21,22]. Muscular infection (streptococcal myositis) is uncommon, typically caused by anaerobic streptococci after major trauma [22].

Staphylococcus aureus, the most common cause of skin infections, is a much less invasive organism [10]. It can produce cellulitis but usually elicits an intense inflammatory exudate of phagocytic cells, called pus [23]. Common terms for staphylococcal pyogenic infections include *folliculitis* for pustules of the dermis, *superficial abscess* for pus limited to superficial soft tissue, and *carbuncle* for more widespread burrowing infection (see Table 161-3). Staphylococcal muscular infection (pyomyositis) usually occurs from hematogenous spread of bacteria to an intramuscular hematoma after trauma [24].

The most serious muscular infections are caused by a few clostridial species, including *Clostridium perfringens, C. novi,* and *C. septicum,* which are gram-positive, spore-forming, obligate anaerobes not typically found on the skin [18]. Within ischemic muscle, the bacteria multiply and release potent exotoxins, which intensify local tissue necrosis and cause the severe systemic intoxication associated with clostridial myonecrosis [25].

Not all clostridial infections occur in muscle. In traumatized or ischemic subcutaneous tissue, these bacteria produce a spreading subcutaneous and fascial level infection (clostridial necrotizing fasciitis), characterized by a musky odor; watery, brownish drainage; abundant gas production; and minimal systemic toxicity [18]. Morbidity and mortality are uncommon.

Three combinations of bacteria are also commonly isolated from soft tissue infections (see Table 161-3). The clinical presentation in these mixed infections is largely determined by the depth of bacterial invasion [17,18]. For example, streptococci and staphylococci cause a necrotizing fasciitis that is clinically identical to that produced by oral or enteric bacteria [26].

Recent work by Scal and Kingston [27] has defined the synergistic effects of staphylococcal alpha-lysin and *Streptococcus pyogenes* in an animal model of necrotizing fasciitis, confirming the pioneering studies of Meleney in 1932 [28]. Other experimental animal work has clearly demonstrated synergistic effects among the aerobic and anaerobic enteric flora [29] and to a lesser degree between the various oral pathogens [30]. The mechanisms of bacterial synergism are reviewed elsewhere [31].

The enteric bacteria of the lower gastrointestinal (GI) tract that produce synergistic infections include the facultative gram-negative bacteria of the group *Enterobacteriaceae* (*Escherichia coli, Klebsiella, Enterobacter, Proteus*), group D streptococci (enterococci), and anaerobes such as *Clostridium* and *Bacteroides* species [31]. These bacteria readily induce a perineal abscess after a break in the rectal mucosa, or an infection that spreads along fascial planes as necrotizing fasciitis.

Table 161-3. Infection Syndromes Defined by Organism and Tissue Level

	Level of Infection			
Pathogens	Skin	Subdermis	Fascia	Muscle
Streptococcus pyogenes	Ecthyma contagiosum, erysipelas, cellulitis	Lymphagitis	Streptococcal necrotizing fasciitis	Streptococcal myositis
Staphylococcus aureus	Folliculitis, cellulitis (rare)	Abscess	Carbuncle	Pyomyositis
Clostridium perfringens		Clostridial abscess		Clostridial myonecrosis
Combinations				
Staphylococci and Streptococci	?Impetigo	Meleney's ulcer	Necrotizing fasciitis	Nonclostridial myonecrosis
Oral flora	Human bite cellulitis	Head and neck abscesses, noma	Necrotizing fasciitis	Nonclostridial myonecrosis
Enteric flora	Neutropenic perineal cellulitis	Perineal abscess, tropical ulcer	Necrotizing fasciitis	Nonclostridial myonecrosis

The human mouth contains a number of virulent bacterial species as well. The bacterial counts of saliva are quite low, and the majority of pathogenic organisms reside in the gingival cleft, including *Prevotella* (*melaninogenica*), *Fusobacterium* species, spirochetes, and oral streptococci [32]. Human bites inoculate these bacteria into soft tissue, where they cause an intense cellulitis [33]. Neglected wounds may produce tendon sheath abscesses, requiring surgical debridement [34]. Occasionally only *Eikenella corrodens* is isolated from such infections [35].

Breaks in the oral mucosa can produce deep head and neck abscesses, requiring surgical drainage [7,36]. Necrotizing fasciitis is rare because of the excellent blood supply of the head and neck [5]. However, in tropical countries where hygiene and nutrition are poor, the oral bacteria produce a chronic ulcerating, burrowing facial lesion called *noma,* a disease almost unknown in the United States [37]. Meleney described similar burrowing, ulcerating lesions of the extremities caused by a mixture of streptococci and staphylococci [38], but enteric or soil bacteria are also implicated, especially in patients with diabetes [8]. There is a zone of intense erythema and a central area of leathery eschar. Wide surgical excision combined with antibiotics is curative. This disease is typically limited to immunologically impaired persons.

Thus, Table 161-3 lists a spectrum of soft tissue infections caused by a limited number of bacteria or bacterial combinations. In many cases neglect or misdiagnosis will allow progression of localized disease to a deeper level of infection. Aggressive early treatment is required to reduce the risk of this complication.

Infections Responding to Antibiotics

Most superficial infections are so common and respond so readily to conventional treatment that little is written about their management. Cellulitis caused by *Streptococcus pyogenes* occurs commonly after an insect bite, blister, or other minor break in the skin. Oral penicillin or a cephalosporin quickly resolves these infections [39].

Cellulitis caused by mixed oral flora results from human bite wounds, but *Eikenella corrodens* is sometimes the only pathogen isolated [33]. It is sensitive to cephalosporins and penicillin but resistant to dicloxacillin [35]. Similarly, cellulitis after animal bites or scratches is usually caused by *Pasteurella multocida* [40]. This organism is susceptible to penicillin, cephalosporins, and tetracycline. In both cases early treatment with splinting, elevation, and parenteral antibiotics may obviate the need for surgical debridement [34].

Many textbooks have advocated aggressive needle aspiration and culture to identify the causative organisms of cellulitis, but several recent studies report a recovery rate of less than 30 percent [9,41–44]. Other authors have performed cultures of skin biopsies, with similar poor yields [39,45]. Neither procedure is probably justified in healthy adults, in whom the usual pathogens are streptococci or staphylococci [39]. Aggressive cultures are justified in children, who have an increased risk of *Haemophilus influenzae* cellulitis [46]. Similarly, cultures of open wounds have a somewhat higher recovery rate and are probably warranted in specific patients [41].

Most subcutaneous abscesses caused by *Staphylococcus aureus* resolve rapidly after drainage, even without antibiotics [10,11,47]. The typical presentation is of a fluctuant area of redness, which yields purulent material on aspiration or incision. Antibiotics are given only if the host has poor defenses or if there is evidence of spreading infection [11].

Both human and animal bite wounds occasionally produce subcutaneous abscesses, which require surgical drainage, especially if a tendon sheath is involved. Tendon sheath abscess is suspected when there is severe pain on motion of the affected digit [34,48]. After debridement, prolonged treatment with cephalosporin antibiotics and intensive physical therapy are necessary to regain full hand function [34].

Abscesses in the perineal area are typically caused by mixed enteric organisms. Infections usually arise in an infected Bartholin's or pilonidal cyst or from a break in the rectal mucosa, causing a perirectal abscess. Cultures yield mixed aerobic and anaerobic organisms. Antibiotics are indicated if the patient has surrounding inflammation or poor host defenses (diabetes, obesity, advanced age, malnutrition, or malignancy). Neglected abscesses are a common cause of perineal necrotizing fasciitis (see later section) [49,50].

Infections Requiring Surgical Debridement

SUPERFICIAL INFECTIONS. Although bite infections involving joints or tendon sheaths require surgical debridement, most other superficial infections resolve with appropriate parenteral antibiotics and rigorous measures to reduce edema. However, some chronic pyogenic infections also require surgical debridement. A carbuncle is a widespread staphylococcal infection with multiple draining sinuses, sometimes invading to the fascial level [4]. Once rather common, this infection is now rare, usually the result of an inadequately treated primary infection in a person with diabetes. The infection resolves after wide surgical debridement to remove all necrotic subcutaneous tissue, combined with parenteral antistaphylococcal antibiotics. Skin flaps can sometimes be salvaged, but delayed skin grafting is typically required [51].

Similarly, hidradenitis suppurativa is a chronic burrowing infection of the axilla or groin found usually in diabetics or the massively obese. Cultures grow mixed aerobic and anaerobic flora [51]. The tissue is excised after instituting broad-spectrum antibiotics. Local flaps or skin grafts can be used to close the defects [52], but a cosmetically acceptable scar results from healing by secondary intention [53].

An additional form of ulcerating lesion deserves discussion. The synergistic bacterial ulcer described by Meleney is a chronic burrowing ulcer with necrotic leathery skin edges but little spread along fascial planes [38]. Causative organisms of these phadenie ulcers include oral flora (noma) [37], enteric flora (tropical ulcer) [8], and staphylococci and streptococci (Meleney ulcer) [38]. All three forms are exceedingly rare in developed countries but sporadically complicate surgical wound infections or diabetic foot ulcers [22]. The ulcers look indolent but rarely heal if limited debridement is attempted. Extensive tissue loss occurs in chronic cases with secondary infection of bones or joints. Complete surgical excision of the affected area combined with antibiotics effective against the organisms involved is curative [22,54].

Clinicians associate clostridia with deep muscular infections, but inappropriate closure of contaminated skin wounds can produce an infection described variously as "clostridial cellulitis" or "clostridial abscess." Intravenous drug abusers are also at risk [25]. The opened wound reveals a musky odor; watery, brownish discharge; and profuse soft tissue gas [55]. Wound pain is variable [18,55]. Gram stain demonstrates large numbers of gram-positive rods and few phagocytic cells. The process is localized to subcutaneous tissue and fascia, and there are few systemic symptoms, since the bacteria produce exotoxins only in anaerobic conditions. The infection resolves with debridement of the affected tissue and parenteral penicillin [22]. Hyperbaric oxygen and amputation are not indicated in treatment of this disease.

NECROTIZING FASCIITIS. Necrotizing fasciitis describes any necrotizing soft-tissue infection spreading at the level of the fascia, with or without overlying erythema and edema. It was first described as hospital gangrene in 1871 [56]. Meleney [20] described the clinical syndrome caused by *Streptococcus pyogenes,* but McCafferty [57] and associates identified spread at the fascial level as the hallmark of this infection. Wilson [12] was the first to use necrotizing fasciitis generically for fascial level infections. It is a syndrome recognized with increasing frequency, and over 650 cases have been reported in the last 25 years [4,58,95].

Etiology. Necrotizing fasciitis may begin at the site of a minor wound or chronic ulcer. The causative organism may be *Streptococcus pyogenes* alone or a combination of bacteria [58]. Intravenous drug abusers also develop infections caused by gram-positive organisms because the injected agents are so frequently contaminated by saliva [59,60]. Infections caused by enteric organisms begin in perineal sites or after inappropriate primary wound closure of contaminated abdominal operations [49,50,61,62]. However, necrotizing fasciitis can complicate any surgical procedure, including laparoscopy [63], endoscopic gastrostomy [64], tube thoracostomy [65], thoracotomy [66], and suction lipectomy [67]. Spontaneous infections may herald perforated diverticulitis [68] or may occur via hematogenous seeding of ecchymoses after blunt trauma [69]. Reports in children are very rare, but infants can develop infections of the umbilicus or scalp [70,71,72]. There are case reports of factitious infections in malingerers or the emotionally disturbed [73].

Pathogenesis. Bacteria proliferating at the fascial level encounter few barriers to lateral spread. Initially the overlying skin appears little affected except for the scrotum, which readily develops dermal necrosis (Fournier syndrome) [74]. This is commonly the first sign of perineal necrotizing fasciitis from urologic or colorectal sites of infection [75]. Most cases of perineal necrotizing fasciitis result from neglected or inadequately treated perineal abscesses [49,50]. Oncologists have also reported an increased risk of perineal sepsis in patients with granulocytopenia from chemotherapy treatment for malignancy [76,77].

Necrotizing fasciitis also arises from a break in the skin or at the site of a chronic ulcer. Chronic wound colonization by pathogenic bacteria may precede tissue invasion [78]. These are frequently less acute infections, usually involving the extremity and demonstrating a serous discharge but little systemic toxicity.

Intravenous drug abusers may have a surprisingly benign presentation [79]. Perhaps they delay treatment because the narcotics mask the initial wound pain. The importance of human immunodeficiency virus (HIV) infection in the clinical course of these infections is unknown [59].

Alcoholics are susceptible to severe necrotizing fasciitis caused by virulent marine vibrios, especially *Vibrio vulnificus,* probably because of an immunologic defect. Septicemia and death are common [80,81].

Diagnosis. The early diagnosis of deep surgical soft tissue infections remains a challenge. Pain, edema, fever, and leuko-

cytosis are the typical presenting findings in most large series [58,82–95]. Table 161-4 lists some of the features that increase the risk of a hidden septic process.

Some patients have a subacute form of infection and attenuated symptoms. Initially there is a thin, reddish drainage from an undermined wound edge. A spreading area of cutaneous anesthesia develops after initial wound tenderness, although peripheral neuropathy may mask these symptoms in diabetics [78]. The patient is not toxic, and the surrounding skin has slowly developing edema. Erythema and dermal necrosis rarely appear. Gram-stained smears reveal neutrophils and mixed bacterial species. The diagnosis is made by slipping an instrument without resistance along the fascial plane [22].

Streptococcal necrotizing fasciitis follows a more fulminant course [20,21,96]. Initially there is localized wound redness and edema with a watery drainage. The patient has pain, fever, tachycardia, and leukocytosis. As the inflammation spreads, there is blistering of the skin, which turns dusky. Dermal infarction is secondary to cutaneous vascular thrombosis. Blood cultures may be positive for streptococcal organisms [57].

Necrotizing fasciitis occurring in a neglected perineal abscess or complicating a surgical wound infection presents with local pain over a period of days, followed by the rapid onset of systemic symptoms, including fever, chills, leukocytosis, and even hypotension [49,58]. The overlying skin is tender and slightly reddened, and edema may extend widely over the perineum, buttocks, or trunk. Scrotal skin infarction (Fournier syndrome) is pathognomonic of perineal necrotizing fasciitis [74,75].

The diagnosis of necrotizing fasciitis is easy in the presence of scrotal necrosis. More commonly, the infection must be differentiated from a severe cellulitis, which the clinician believes will resolve rapidly with antibiotics. Delay in aggressive surgical therapy may have a fatal outcome. Such infection is associated with diabetes, severe malnutrition, steroid use, or malignancy [4]. Patients with uncomplicated cellulitis rarely have high fever, tachycardia, or hyperglycemia [97]. Similarly, intense pain or paresthesias of the skin, dusky mottling, and a watery or malodorous drainage from an open wound are alarming signs [4].

Plain radiographs occasionally demonstrate soft tissue gas in necrotizing fasciitis, even in the absence of clostridia [15,16,98]. Wound sonography or computed tomography may demonstrate soft tissue fluid or gas, prompting surgical exploration and debridement [99,100]. The high-resolution images possible with magnetic resonance imaging may further facilitate early diagnosis [101,102].

Needle aspiration of the inflamed area may recover infected fluid, but negative aspiration is insufficient to exclude deep necrotizing infection [93]. The gold standard is surgical explo-

Table 161-4. Indications for Surgical Exploration

Systemic
  Confusion/obtundation
  Tachycardia/tachypnea
  Hyperglycemia/keroacidosis
  Hypovolemic shock
  Thrombocytopenia
Local
  Cyanosis, bronzing, blistering or necrosis of skin
  Severe pain or spreading areas of anesthesia
  Cellulitis
    Spreading despite antibiotics
    In any surgical wound or hematoma
  Abscess with multiple tracts
  Thin, reddish drainage from wound with undermined edges
  Crepitus (or radiographic gas)

ration of the wound. Melluzzo et al. [103] perform bedside biopsy under local anesthesia and repeat it if the diagnosis is inconclusive. Similarly, Stamenkovic and Lew [93] reduced the mean time to diagnosis from 6 days to 21 hours after bedside biopsy with frozen section examination of the tissue. Rimailho et al. [6] reported catastrophic clinical courses in five patients with misdiagnosed necrotizing fasciitis whose initial pain symptoms were treated with nonsteroidal antiinflammatory agents. Any delay in diagnosis of these severe infections increases the risk of morbidity and mortality [104].

Treatment. Early surgical debridement is critical to control these infections [17,18,104]. Adequate fluid resuscitation is required in dehydrated patients, and extensive preoperative radiographic studies are contraindicated in the face of spreading infection. Preoperative antibiotics are based on the Gram stain results of the wound drainage. Intraoperative aerobic and anaerobic cultures of tissue and fluid are used to determine subsequent antibiotic therapy.

If Gram stain and cultures of the wound indicate only *Streptococcus pyogenes* or *Clostridia,* high-dose penicillin G is the agent of choice [51]. Otherwise the initial antibiotics should be effective against the facultative and anaerobic enteric organisms [31]. Single agents include cefoxitin, defotetan, and the semisynthetic penicillins, which are most useful in stable patients. The role of new combination agents such as ampicillin/sulbactam, ticarcillin/clavulanate, or imipenem/cilastatin is unknown, but preliminary reports indicate a high success rate [105,106]. In toxic or unstable patients, many clinicians choose a combination of antibiotics, such as an aminoglycoside, combined with clindamycin, metronidazole, or a semisynthetic penicillin [51,105]. Large doses may be required to achieve therapeutic, but not toxic, levels [107].

At operation the skin is edematous and drains copious fluid. The appearance of the fascia is highly variable. In early or subacute cases, the skin flaps separate easily by blunt dissection from the fascia, which appears intact. Incisions are extended to the limits of the edematous skin. Debridement is minimal, and the wound is packed open with antiseptic- or antibiotic-soaked gauze [4]. The edema and erythema resolve completely within 24 to 48 hours with appropriate antibiotics. The skin flaps heal by secondary intention. This pattern is most common with localized infections of the extremity.

When treatment is delayed in streptococcal necrotizing fasciitis, the skin blisters and appears dusky [104]. At operation there is extensive liquefaction necrosis of the subcutaneous tissue. The fascia has a stringy, grayish appearance, but the muscle is unaffected. Wound fluid shows gram-positive cocci in chains. The soft tissue is meticulously debrided to viable margins at the time of primary exploration. The thin skin flaps rarely survive, and soft tissue defects require delayed skin grafting. Amputation is occasionally necessary to control spreading infection [21].

Infections of the perineum caused by mixed aerobic and anaerobic organisms often show extensive subcutaneous spread. Incisions reveal foul-smelling, cloudy pus and grayish necrotic fascia. The skin and soft tissue are edematous but appear free of necrosis. All tissue planes are opened primarily and any necrotic tissue excised. Diverting colostomy reduces subsequent perineal soiling but may not be necessary in all cases [77,90,108].

A subset of these patients has bacterial invasion of the subcutaneous fat, presenting as marbled areas of greenish-black necrosis [4]. The areas affected may be massive, including the genitalia, buttocks, and trunk. All areas of soft tissue containing necrotic tissue must be completely excised at the primary operation. Failure to remove completely the necrotic tissue results in persistent sepsis and a rapidly fatal course [95].

Patients with postoperative necrotizing fasciitis have a high incidence of intraabdominal sepsis as well [61]. After radical debridement of necrotic fascia, abdominal wall defects are initially covered with Marlex mesh [94]. Mesh removal before definitive wound coverage reduces chronic sinus tract formation [61].

Aggressive enteral or parenteral nutritional support is always required [94]. The patient should undergo daily operative debridement until no additional necrotic areas are encountered. As the patient stabilizes, whirlpool treatments facilitate daily dressing changes. Eventually remaining skin flaps adhere to the granulating wound bed, and skin grafts are used to close residual tissue defects.

In patients with exposed tendons, bone, or neurovascular structures, early soft tissue coverage helps to preserve function and prevent osteomyelitis. Debridement of the necrotic scrotal skin in Fournier syndrome exposes the testicles, which can be later placed in thigh pockets or covered with local rotation flaps [75,108,109].

Prognosis. A collective review [4] of 15 papers published between 1980 and 1986 records a mortality of 38 percent for necrotizing fasciitis, unchanged since a similar review of cases from the previous decade [58], but recent reports indicate a decreasing mortality rate (Table 161-5). Males presenting with scrotal necrosis from a perineal infection (Fournier syndrome) also have a better prognosis, probably because the diagnosis is made earlier [110]. Stephens et al. [111] in 1993 tabulated a mortality for males of 19 percent (55/320). Females in the same review article presenting with skin necrosis had a 59 percent mortality (20/41), with obstetric infections causing the excess deaths.

Adjunctive hyperbaric oxygen also has beneficial effects in mixed infections containing anaerobes, noted clinically by Grainger, who treated Meleny ulcers [112]. The mechanisms are reviewed elsewhere [111]. Gozal et al. [81] found just 2 of 16 patients died who were treated with hyperbaric oxygen after surgical debridement of necrotizing fasciitis. Only a few more recent clinical series have been reported [83,89,91], but the data are encouraging (see Table 161-4). Randomized, stratified clinical trials have not been performed.

Francis et al. [91] have identified a number of risk factors for mortality in fascial level infections, including age greater than

Table 161-5. Mortality of Necrotizing Fasciitis

Study	Deaths	Patients
Casali et al [61]	4	12
Kaiser and Cerra [17]	8	20
Freeman et al [81]	4	14
Oh et al [82]	10	28
Rouse et al [83]	20	27
Majeski and Alexander [84]	10	30
Miller [86]	4	15
Walker and Hall [87]	3	8
Adinolfi et al [49]	3	11
Lamb and Juler [75]	4	12
Spirnak et al [74]	9	20
Stamenkovic and Lew [88]	8	19
Freischlag et al [89]	5	9
Pessa and Howard [90]	11	33
Barzlai et al [91]	4	11
Gozal et al [92]	2	16
Sudarsky et al [93]	2	33
Mortality	111	318
	35%	

50 years and presence of diabetes mellitus, malnutrition, hypertension, or drug abuse. Presence of three or more risk factors increased the mortality from 17 percent to 79 percent compared to those with two or fewer risk factors. Delay in diagnosis also markedly reduces survival [89,93,94].

Pessa and Howard [95] recorded the acute physiology and chronic health evaluation (APACHE) scores prospectively in 33 patients treated aggressively for necrotizing fasciitis. The mean admission score was higher for nonsurvivors than for survivors, but the individual score increased by day 3 in each nonsurvivor and decreased by day 3 for each survivor. Although Francis et al. [91] were not able to confirm these findings using APACHE II scores, every effort must be made to control sepsis immediately in these very ill patients.

NONCLOSTRIDIAL MYONECROSIS. Stone and Martin [113] in 1972 first described a series of patients with infections extending into muscle as "synergistic necrotizing cellulitis." There are no unique signs or symptoms; the clinical syndrome is indistinguishable from necrotizing fasciitis, but at operation skeletal muscle is blackened and nonviable. Control of the infection is difficult, and the mortality is high.

Etiology. The invading organisms are mixed enteric bacteria like those recovered from the wounds of patients with necrotizing fasciitis. Rarely infection with *Aeromonas hydrophila* in diabetics causes a fulminant nonclostridial myonecrosis [114]. *Bacillus cereus* has also been implicated [115].

Pathogenesis. This disease represents the end stage of necrotizing fasciitis, usually in patients with impaired host defenses due to advanced age, diabetes, renal failure, obesity, or atherosclerosis [113]. One series describes the typical patient as an obese diabetic treated for a perineal abscess with oral antibiotics for several days [116]. Less commonly the infection occurs in extremity ulcers, surgical wounds, or after deep penetrating trauma.

Once the bacteria breach the fascia, they spread longitudinally along muscle bundles. Muscular edema and, in many cases, profuse gas production increase muscle compartment pressure and local ischemia, fostering further anaerobic growth [16].

Diagnosis. Preoperatively this disease presents as necrotizing fasciitis, but the patients are usually older and have more concurrent diseases. Radiographs may demonstrate gas outlining muscle bundles [98]. At operation the fascia is necrotic, with irregular areas of blackened muscle extending longitudinally within a fascial sheath. The disease is differentiated from clostridial myonecrosis by the finding of mixed organisms on Gram stain as well as the usually lesser degree of systemic toxicity.

Treatment. All areas of infected and necrotic tissue are excised at the primary operation, and skin flaps are rarely spared. In the most severe cases, extremity amputation or disarticulation is required. Inadequate primary excision is followed by clinical deterioration and death.

Prognosis. Stone and Martin [113] reported a mortality rate of 76 percent; almost all survivors had extremity infections. Young age and absence of diabetes or obesity are also associated with a higher survival rate. In the series of Skiles et al. [116], 11 of 17 patients with nonclostridial myonecrosis died, compared with 5 of 15 with clostridial myonecrosis. Diabetes did not increase mortality, but none of the nonclostridial infections were debrided before transfer to their referral center; all six

patients with clostridal infections who were debrided before transfer survived. Other series of "nonclostridial gas gangrene" describe chiefly gas-producing infections in diabetic foot ulcers, which have a very low mortality [78,117].

CLOSTRIDIAL MYONECROSIS. Perhaps the most feared of all soft tissue infections, clostridial myonecrosis has a fulminant clinical course and high mortality if treatment is delayed. With aggressive treatment, the survival rate exceeds 75 percent in collected series [14,118].

Etiology. Wartime injuries, farm machinery accidents, and motor vehicle accidents produce deep tissue wounds contaminated by soil organisms including clostridia. But these deep muscular infections typically occur only when wounds are inadequately debrided or inappropriately closed. The bacteria also may be inoculated into surgical wounds after operations on the GI or biliary tract [119]. In the past, clostridial infections complicated up to 1 percent of all criminal abortions [14].

Not all species of clostridia cause myonecrosis. *Clostridium perfringens* is the most frequent pathogen and can produce the greatest variety of toxins, but *C. novi* and *C. septicum* are also virulent organisms [18]. *C. septicum* often occurs as a spontaneous muscular infection in patients with occult malignancy [120,121]. Other clostridial species rarely produce myonecrosis except in mixed infections [14,25].

Pathogenesis. The fascia is an excellent barrier to bacterial invasion, but if trauma introduces clostridial spores into ischemic tissue, they germinate and release a variety of lethal exotoxins. Rarely spores may lie inactive for long periods in healthy tissue, and clostridial infections have occurred in acutely contused wounds, years after presumed primary spore inoculation [122].

In an anaerobic environment, the growing bacteria may produce a dozen discrete toxins, including the lethal alpha toxin, which causes hemolysis and muscle necrosis and has direct depressant effects on cardiac muscle [14]. Local gas production increases muscle ischemia and spreads the infection with startling rapidity.

Diagnosis. The infection usually presents with severe wound pain, accompanied by tachycardia and apathy or mental confusion [55]. Woody skin edema is evident, followed by darkening of the wound edges and formation of hemorrhagic bullae. The patient may exhibit sudden cardiovascular collapse and death, mediated primarily by the circulating exotoxins, rather than the toxic effects of muscle necrosis. Opened wounds produce a brownish discharge containing gram-positive rods and few phagocytic cells, and soft tissue gas is present in perhaps 40 percent of cases [22]. Hemolysis with anemia and hematuria implies a grave prognosis [13]. Furste et al. [123] recommend serum creatine kinase determinations as an indicator of severe myonecrosis. Clostridial myonecrosis is differentiated from other wound infections by the presence of severe systemic toxicity, marked local pain, woody skin edema, and gram-positive rods in the wound fluid.

Treatment. Clostridial myonecrosis is a surgical emergency. Surgical exploration is undertaken after fluid resuscitation with the aid of Swan-Ganz and arterial monitoring catheters. Parenteral penicillin G in large doses, commonly 12 to 20 million units per day, is started immediately, although experimental work indicates other agents such as clindamycin may be even more effective [124,125]. Polyvalent clostridial antitoxin was of questionable efficacy and is no longer available in the United States.

At operation incisions are extended to include wide fasciotomies, and all pale, noncontracting muscle is aggressively debrided. The wounds are packed open and redebrided daily until infection is controlled. Rising creatine kinase levels suggest uncontrolled muscular sepsis [123]. Intensive supportive measures are required, including blood transfusions to replace major operative losses or occasional toxin-induced hemolysis [16,119]. Hyperbaric oxygen, when available, suppresses toxin formation but does not inactivate circulating toxins [14,18]. Emergency limb amputation may be life-saving, especially in the debilitated or elderly.

Prognosis. The overall mortality for collected series from institutions with hyperbaric oxygen facilities is 22 to 25 percent [14,118]. This may represent a selected patient population that survives long enough to permit transfer to a referral center. The overall incidence of this disease, even in war wounds, is declining with the widespread use of prophylactic antibiotics and the emphasis on aggressive debridement [55,126]. Open treatment of contaminated wounds further reduces the risk of clostridial infection.

Summary

A variety of soft tissue infections are encountered in clinical practice. The terminology used to describe them has been confusing and even contradictory, but a few generic terms can be used to describe most infections and even suggest their clinical management.

Deep soft tissue sepsis may have a benign presentation, but any delay in diagnosis increases morbidity and mortality. Only a high index of suspicion and early surgical exploration, combined with aggressive nutritional and hemodynamic support, will reduce the morbidity and mortality of these difficult infections.

References

1. Mackowaik PA: The normal human microflora. *N Engl J Med* 307:83, 1982.
2. Goldman DA, Leclair J, Macone A: Bacterial colonization of neonates admitted to an intensive care environment. *J Pediatr* 93:288, 1978.
3. Howard RJ: Microbes and their pathogenicity, in Howard RJ, Simmons RL (eds): *Surgical Infectious Diseases*. 2nd ed. Norwalk, CT, Appleton & Lange, 1988, p 1.
4. Ahrenholz DH: Necrotizing soft tissue infections. *Surg Clin North Am* 68(1):199, 1988.
5. Balcerak RJ, Sisto JM, Bosak RC: Cervicofacial necrotizing fasciitis: Report of three cases and literature review. *J Oral Maxillofac Surg* 46:450, 1988.
6. Rimailho A, Riou B, Richard C, et al: Fulminant necrotizing fasciitis and nonsteroidal anti-inflammatory drugs. *J Infect Dis* 155:143, 1987.
7. Klabacha ME, Stankiewicz JA, Clift SE: Severe soft tissue infection of the face and neck: A classification. *Laryngoscope* 92:1135, 1983.
8. Seal DV, Leppard B: Necrotizing fasciitis—a disease of temperate and warm climates. *Trans R Soc Trop Med Hyg* 76:392,1982.
9. Lutomski DM, Trott AT, Runyon JM, et al: Microbiology of cellulitis. *J Fam Pract* 26:45, 1988.
10. Macfie J, Harvey J: The treatment of acute superficial abscesses: A prospective clinical trial. *Br J Surg* 64:264, 1977.
11. Llera JL, Levy RC: Treatment of cutaneous abscess: A double-blind clinical study. *Ann Emerg Med* 14:15, 1985.
12. Wilson B: Necrotizing fasciitis. *Am Surg* 18:416, 1952.
13. MacLennan JD: The histotoxic clostridial infections of man. *Bacteriol Rev* 26:177, 1962.
14. Hart GB, Lamb RC, Strauss MB: Gas gangrene: I. A collective review. *J Trauma* 23:991, 1983.
15. Nichols RL, Smith JW: Gas in the wound: What does it mean? *Surg Clin North Am* 55:1289, 1975.
16. Van Beek A, Zook E, Yaw P, et al: Nonclostridial gas-forming infections. *Arch Surg* 108:552, 1974.
17. Kaiser RE, Cerra FB: Progressive necrotizing surgical infections—a unified approach. *J Trauma* 21:349, 1981.
18. Dellinger EP: Severe necrotizing soft-tissue infections: Multiple disease entities requiring a common approach. *JAMA* 246:1717, 1981.
19. Sverdrup B, Blomback M, Borlgund E, et al: Blood coagulation and fibrinolytic systems in patients with erysipelas and necrotizing fasciitis. *Scand J Infect Dis* 13:29, 1981.
20. Meleney FL: Hemolytic streptococcus gangrene. *Arch Surg* 9:317, 1924.
21. Aitken DR, Mackett MCT, Smith LL: The changing pattern of hemolytic streptococcal gangrene. *Arch Surg* 117:561, 1982.
22. Baxter CR: Surgical management of soft tissue infections. *Surg Clin North Am* 52:1483, 1972.
23. Sheagren JN: Treatment of skin and skin structure infections in the patient at risk. *Am J Med* 76(Suppl 5A):180, 1984.
24. Levin M, Gardner P, Waldvogel FA: "Tropical pyomyositis": An unusual infection due to *Staphylococcus aureus*. *N Engl J Med* 284:196, 1971.
25. Gorbach G, Thadepalli H: Isolation of clostridium in human infections: Evolution in 114 cases. *J Infect Dis* 131:5, 1975.
26. Giuliano A, Lewis F Jr, Hadley K, et al: Bacteriology of necrotizing fasciitis. *Am J Surg* 134:52, 1977.
27. Seal DV, Kingston D: Streptococcal necrotizing fasciitis: Development of an animal model to study its pathogenesis. *Br J Exp Pathol* 69:813, 1988.
28. Meleney FL: A differential diagnosis between certain types of infectious gangrene—with particular reference to haemolytic streptococcus gangrene and bacterial synergism. *Surg Gynecol Obstet* 56:847, 1933.
29. Onderdonk AB, Bartlett JG, Louie T, et al: Microbial synergy in experimental intra-abdominal abscess. *Infect Immun* 13:22, 1976.
30. Socransky SS, Gibbons RL: Required role of *Bacteroides melaninogenicus* in mixed anaerobic infection. *J Infect Dis* 115:247, 1965.
31. Ahrenholz DH, Simmons RL: Mixed and synergistic infections, in Howard RJ, Simmons RL (eds): *Surgical Infectious Diseases*. 3rd ed. Norwalk, CT, Appleton & Lange, 1994.
32. Liljemark WF, Bloomquist CG: Normal microbial flora of the human body, in Newman MG, Nisengard R (eds): *Oral Microbiology and Immunology*. Philadelphia, WB Saunders, 1988, p 135.
33. Goldstein EJC, Citron DM, Wiels B, et al: Bacteriology of human and animal bite wounds. *J Clin Microbiol* 8:667, 1978.
34. Basadre JO, Parry SW: Indications for surgical debridement in 125 human bites to the hand. *Arch Surg* 126:65, 1991.
35. Schmidt DR, Heckman JD: *Eikenella corrodens* in human bite infections of the hand. *J Trauma* 23:478, 1983.
36. Linder HH: The anatomy of the fasciae of the face and neck with particular reference to the spread and treatment of intraoral infections (Ludwig's) that have progressed into adjacent fascial spaces. *Ann Surg* 204:705, 1988.
37. Ghosal SP, Sen Gupta PC, Mukherjee, et al: *Noma neonatorum*: Its aetiopathogenesis. *Lancet* 2:289, 1978.
38. Meleney FL: Bacterial synergism in disease processes with confirmation of synergistic bacterial etiology of certain types of progressive gangrene of the abdominal wall. *Ann Surg* 94:961,1931.
39. Bernard P, Bedane C, Mounier M, et al: Streptococcal cause of erysipelas and cellulitis in adults. *Arch Dermatol* 125:779, 1989.
40. Arons MS, Fernando L, Polayes IM: *Pasturella multocida*—the major cause of hand infections following domestic animal bites. *J Hand Surg* 7:47, 1982.
41. Newell PM, Norden CW: Value of needle aspiration in bacteriologic diagnosis of cellulitis in adults. *J Clin Microbiol* 26:401, 1988.
42. Sigurdsson AF, Gudmundsson S: The etiology of bacterial cellulitis

as determined by fine-needle aspiration. *Scand J Infect Dis* 21:537, 1989.

43. Kielnhofner MA, Brown B, Dall L: Influence of underlying disease process on the utility of cellulitis needle aspirates. *Arch Intern Med* 148:2451, 1988.

44. Hook EW, Hooton MT, Horton CA, et al: Microbiologic evaluation of cutaneous cellulitis in adults. *Arch Intern Med* 146:195, 1986.

45. Duvanel T, Auckenthaler R, Rohner P, et al: Qualitative cultures of biopsy specimens from cutaneous cellulitis. *Arch Intern Med* 149:293, 1989.

46. Goetz JP, Tafari N, Boxerbaum B: Needle aspiration in *Haemophilus influenzae* type B cellulitis. *Pediatrics* 54:504,1974.

47. Meislin HW: Pathogen identification of abscesses and cellulitis. *Ann Emerg Med* 15:329, 1986.

48. Goldstein EJC: Infections following human bites. *Infection Surg* 4:849, 1985.

49. Adinolfi MF, Voros DC, Moustoukas NM, et al: Severe systemic sepsis resulting from neglected perineal infections. *South Med J* 76:746, 1983.

50. Frolich EP, Schein M: Necrotizing fasciitis arising from Bartholin's abscess. Case report and review of the literature. *Isr J Med Sci* 25:644, 1989.

51. Simmons RL, Ahrenholz DH: Infections of skin and soft tissue, in Howard RJ, Simmons RL (eds): *Surgical Infectious Diseases*. 3rd ed. Norwalk, CT, Appleton & Lange, 1994.

52. Watson JD: Hidradenitis suppurativa—a clinical review. *Br J Plast Surg* 38:567, 1985.

53. Silverburg B, Smoot CE, Landa SJF, et al: Hidradenitis suppurativa: Patient satisfaction with wound healing by secondary intention. *Plast Reconstr Surg* 79:555, 1987.

54. Mbonu O, Nwako FA: Synergistic bacterial gangrene and allied lesions: A unified etiological theory. *Int Surg* 68:323, 1983.

55. Weinstein L, Barza MA: Gas gangrene. *N Engl J Med* 289:1129, 1973.

56. Jones J: Investigation upon the nature, cause, and treatment of hospital gangrene as it prevailed in confederate armies, 1861–1865. New York, US Sanitary Commission Surgical Memoirs of the War of the Rebellion, 1871.

57. McCafferty EL, Lyons C: Suppurative fasciitis as the essential feature of hemolytic streptococcal gangrene. *Surgery* 24:438, 1948.

58. Janevicius RV, Hann SE, Batt MD: Necrotizing fasciitis. *Surg Gynecol Obstet* 154:97, 1982.

59. Orangio GR, Pitlick SD, Della Latta P, et al: Soft tissue infections in parenteral drug abusers. *Ann Surg* 199:97, 1984.

60. Biderman P, Hiatt JR: Management of soft-tissue infections of the upper extremity in parenteral drug abusers. *Am J Surg* 154:526, 1987.

61. Casali RE, Tucker WE, Petrino RA, et al: Postoperative necrotizing fasciitis of the abdominal wall. *Am J Surg* 140:787,1980.

62. Farrell LD, Karl SR, Davis PK, et al: Postoperative necrotizing fasciitis in children. *Pediatrics* 82:874, 1988.

63. Sotrel G, Hirsch E, Edelin KC: Necrotizing fasciitis following diagnostic laparoscopy. *Obstet Gynecol* 62(Suppl):67s,1983.

64. Cave DR, Robinson WR, Brotschi EA: Necrotizing fasciitis following percutaneous endoscopic gastrostomy. *Gastrointest Endosc* 32:294, 1986.

65. Pingleton SK, Jeter J: Necrotizing fasciitis as a complication of tube thoracostomy. *Chest* 83:925, 1983.

66. Van de Sadt J, Rocmans P, Thys JP: Synergistic necrotizing cellulitis after pneumonectomy. *Intensive Care Med* 11:158, 1985.

67. Alexander J, Takeda D, Sanders G, et al: Fatal necrotizing fasciitis following suction-assisted lipectomy. *Ann Plast Surg* 20:562, 1988.

68. Galbut DL, Gerber DL, Belgraier AH: Spontaneous necrotizing fasciitis. Occurrence secondary to occult diverticulitis. *JAMA* 238:2302, 1977.

69. Svensson LG, Brookstone AJ, Wellsted M: Necrotizing fasciitis in contused areas. *J Trauma* 25:260, 1985.

70. Goldberg GN, Hansen RC, Lynch PJ: Necrotizing fasciitis in infancy: Report of three cases and review of the literature. *Pediatr Dermatol* 2:55, 1984.

71. Lally KP, Atkinson JB, Woolley MM, et al: Necrotizing fasciitis. A serious sequela of omphalitis in the newborn. *Ann Surg* 199:101, 1984.

72. Gibboney W, Lemons JA: Necrotizing fasciitis of the scalp in neonates. *Am J Perinatol* 3:58, 1986.

73. Aduan RP, Fauci AS, Dale DC, et al: Facticious fever and self-induced infection: A report of 32 cases and a review of the literature. *Ann Intern Med* 90:230, 1979.

74. Spirnak JP, Resnick MI, Hampel N, Persky L: Fournier's gangrene: Report of 20 patients. *J Urol* 131:289, 1984.

75. Lamb RC, Juler GL: Fournier's gangrene of the scrotum. A poorly defined syndrome or misnomer? *Arch Surg* 118:38, 1983.

76. Berg A, Armitage JO, Burns CP: Fournier's gangrene complicating aggressive therapy for hematologic malignancy. *Cancer* 57:2291, 1986.

77. Hiatt JR, Kuchenbecker SL, Winston DJ: Perineal gangrene in the patient with granulocytopenia: The importance of early diverting colostomy. *Surgery* 100:912, 1986.

78. Sapico FL, Witte JL, Canawati HN, et al: The infected foot of the diabetic patient: Quantitative microbiology and analysis of clinical features. *Rev Infect Dis* 6(Suppl 1):S171, 1984.

79. Schecter W, Meyer A, Schecter G, et al: Necrotizing fasciitis of the upper extremity. *J Hand Surg* 7:15, 1982.

80. Howard RJ, Bennet NT: Infections caused by halophilic marine *Vibrio* bacteria. *Ann Surg* 217:525, 1993.

81. Gozal D, Ziser A, Shupak A, et al: Necrotizing fasciitis. *Arch Surg* 121:233, 1986.

82. Sudarsky LA, Laschinger JC, Coppa GF, et al: Improved results from a standardized approach in treating patients with necrotizing fasciitis. *Ann Surg* 206:661, 1987.

83. Umbert IJ, Winkelman RK, Oliver GF, Peters MS: Necrotizing fasciitis: A clinical, microbiologic, and histopathologic study of 14 patients. *J Am Acad Dermatol* 20:774, 1989.

84. Kent RB, Richards JJ: Fournier's perineal gangrene. *Surg Rounds* p.33, May, 1989.

85. Riseman JA, Zamboni WA, Curtis A, et al: Hyperbaric oxygen therapy for necrotizing fasciitis reduces mortality and the need for debridements. *Surgery* 108:847, 1990.

86. Patino JF, Castro D, Valencia A, et al: Necrotizing soft tissue lesions after a volcanic cataclysm. *World J Surg* 15:240,1991.

87. Ward RG, Walsh MS: Necrotizing fasciitis: 10 years' experience in a district general hospital. *Br J Surg* 78:488,1991.

88. Asfar SK, Baraka A, Juma T, et al: Necrotizing fasciitis. *Br J Surg* 78:838, 1991.

89. Wang KC, Shih CH: Necrotizing fasciitis of the extremities. *J Trauma* 32:179, 1992.

90. Iorianni P, Oliver GC: Synergistic soft tissue infections of the perineum. *Dis Colon Rectum* 35:640, 1992.

91. Francis KR, Lamaute HR, Davis JM, Pizzi WF: Implications of risk factors in necrotizing fasciitis. *Am Surgeon* 59:304, 1993.

92. Maisel RH, Karlen R: Cervical necrotizing fasciitis. *Laryngoscope* (in press).

93. Stamenkovic I, Lew PD: Early recognition of potentially fatal necrotizing fasciitis. The use of frozen-section biopsy. *N Engl J Med* 310:1689, 1984.

94. Majeski JA, Alexander JW: Early diagnosis, nutritional support, and immediate extensive debridement improve survival in necrotizing fasciitis. *Am J Surg* 145:784, 1983.

95. Pessa ME, Howard RJ: Necrotizing fasciitis. *Surg Gynecol Obstet* 161:357, 1985.

96. Riefler J, Molavi A, Schwartz D, et al: Necrotizing fasciitis in adults due to Group B streptococcus. Report of a case and review of the literature. *Arch Intern Med* 148:727, 1988.

97. Hautekeete ML, Nagler JM, Mertens AH, et al: Necrotizing fasciitis precipitating diabetic ketoacidotic coma. *Intensive Care Med* 12:383, 1986.

98. Fisher JR, Conway MJ, Takeshita RT, et al: Necrotizing fasciitis. Importance of roentgenographic studies for soft-tissue gas. *JAMA* 241:803, 1979.

99. Begley MG, Shawker TH, Robertson CN, et al: Fournier gangrene: Diagnosis with scrotal ultrasound. *Radiology* 169:387,1988.

100. Rogers JM, Gibson JV, Farrar WE, et al: Usefulness of computerized tomography in evaluating necrotizing fasciitis. *South Med J* 77:782, 1984.

101. Beltran J, Noto AM, McGhee RB, et al: Infection of the musculoskeletal system: High-field-strength MR imaging. *Radiology* 164:449, 1987.

102. Durham JR, Lukens ML, Campanini DS, et al: Impact of magnetic resonance imaging on the management of diabetic foot infections. *Am J Surg* 162:150, 1991.
103. Melluzzo PJ, Willscher M, Mason W, et al: Necrotizing fasciitis in narcotic addicts. *Am Surg* 42:251, 1976.
104. Meleney FL: Hemolytic streptococcus gangrene. Importance of early diagnosis and early operation. *JAMA* 92:2009, 1929.
105. Sanders CV, Aldridge KE: Current antimicrobial therapy of anaerobic infections. *Eur J Clin Microbial Infect Dis* 11:999, 1992.
106. Karam GH, Sanders CV, Aldridge KE: Role of newer antimicrobial agents in treatment of mixed aerobic and anaerobic infection. *Surg Gynecol Obstet* 172 (Suppl):17, 1991.
107. Bakker-Woudenber IA, Roosendaal R: Impact of dosage schedule of antibiotics on the treatment of serious infections. *Intensive Care Med* 16:S229, 1990.
108. Clayton MD, Fowler JE, Sharifi R, et al: Causes, presentation and survival of fifty-seven patients with necrotizing fasciitis of the male genitalia. *Surg Gynecol Obstet* 170:49, 1990.
109. Banks DW, O'Brien DP, Amerson JR, et al: Gracilis musculocutaneous flap scrotal reconstruction after Fournier gangrene. *Urology* 28:275, 1986.
110. Paty R, Smith AD: Gangrene and Fournier's gangrene. *Urol Clin North Am* 19(1):149, 1992.
111. Stephens BJ, Lathrop JC, Rice WT, Gruenberg JC: Fournier's gangrene: Historic (1764–1978) versus contemporary (1979–1988) differences in etiology and clinical importance. *Am Surg* 59:149, 1993.
112. Grainger RW, MacKenzie DA, McLachlin AD: Progressive bacterial synergistic gangrene: Chronic undermining ulcer of Meleney. *Can J Surg* 10:439, 1967.
113. Stone HH, Martin JD: Synergistic necrotizing cellulitis. *Ann Surg* 175:702, 1972.
114. Hennessy MJ, Ballon-Landa GR, Jones JW, et al: *Aeromonas hydrophila* gas gangrene: A case report of management with surgery and hyperbaric oxygen. *Orthopedics* 11:289, 1988.
115. Johnson DA, Aulicino PL, Newby JG: *Bacillus cereus*-induced myonecrosis. *J Trauma* 24:267, 1984.
116. Skiles MS, Covert GK, Fletcher HS: Gas-producing clostridial and non-clostridial infections. *Surg Gynecol Obstet* 147:65, 1978.
117. Bessman AN, Wagner W: Nonclostridial gas gangrene. *JAMA* 233:958, 1975.
118. Roding B, Groeneveld PH, Boerima I: Ten years of experience in the treatment of gas gangrene with hyperbaric oxygen. *Surg Gynecol Obstet* 134:579, 1972.
119. McSwain B, Sawyers JL, Lawler MR Jr: Clostridial infections of the abdominal wall. *Ann Surg* 163:859, 1966.
120. Kolbeinsson ME, Holder WD, Aziz S: Recognition, management, and prevention of *Clostridium septicum* abscess in immunosuppressed patients. *Arch Surg* 126:642, 1991.
121. Kudsk KA: Occult gastrointestinal malignancies producing metastatic *Clostridium septicum* infections in diabetic patients. *Surgery* 112:765, 1992.
122. Stevens DL, Laposky LL, McDonald P, et al: Spontaneous gas gangrene at a site of remote injury—localization due to circulating antitoxin. *West J Med* 148:204, 1988.
123. Furste W, Lobe TE, Botros NN: Gangrenous soft tissue infections. *Infect Surg* 4:837, 1985.
124. Stevens DL, Maier KA, Laine BM, et al: Comparison of clindamycin, rifampin, tetracycline, metronidazole and penicillin for efficacy in prevention of experimental gas gangrene due to *Clostridium perfringens. J Infect Dis* 155:220, 1987.
125. Stevens DL, Bryant AE, Adams K, et al: Evaluation of therapy with hyperbaric oxygen in clostridial myonecrosis. *Clin Infect Dis* 17:231, 1993.
126. Altemeier W, Fullen W: Prevention and treatment of gas gangrene. *JAMA* 217:806, 1971.

162. Management of the Postoperative Cardiac Surgical Patient

Alan Lisbon, Thomas J. Vander Salm, and Marc S. Visner

The management of the postoperative cardiac surgical patient has had a great impact on the way modern intensive care unit (ICU) technology and care have evolved. Cardiac surgical patients are heavily monitored and dependent on mechanical ventilation, often require cardiovascular support, and have a propensity for rapid physiologic changes. The care of the postoperative adult cardiac surgical patient is best handled using a system-oriented approach [1].

Cardiac Subsystem

MONITORING AND INITIAL ASSESSMENT. The restoration and maintenance of normal physiologic homeostasis without injuring the heart is the most important goal in the care of the postoperative cardiac surgical patient and requires proper patient monitoring. An arterial cannula, usually in the radial artery, permits easy access to blood for various laboratory tests (see Chap. 3) and provides the ability to continuously measure systemic blood pressure. At least one lead of the surface electrocardiogram (ECG) also should be displayed, with several leads being monitored for ST segment changes. The waveforms representing pulmonary artery pressure, central venous pressure, and, in those cases where indicated, left atrial pressure also should be displayed. A triple-lumen pulmonary artery catheter inserted via an internal jugular vein permits measurement of the right atrial, pulmonary artery, and pulmonary capillary wedge (PCW) pressures and the determination of cardiac output by thermodilution.

Pulse oximetry allows assessment of O_2 saturation and reduces the need for arterial blood gases. The end-tidal CO_2 monitor may provide useful physiologic information about the adequacy of ventilation and pulmonary blood flow and also provides an additional alarm to signal ventilator malfunction or disconnection. Special pulmonary artery catheters with an oximeter probe at the distal end allow continuous monitoring and tracking of mixed venous O_2 saturation.

Cardiac output is usually normalized to cardiac index by dividing it by the patient's body surface area. Systemic vascular resistance (SVR) and pulmonary vascular resistance (PVR) can be calculated from the cardiac output and the pressure gradients across the appropriate vascular beds.

$$SVR \ (dyne\text{-}sec/cm^5) = [map^* - CVP^\dagger]/CO \times 80$$

$$PVR \ (dyne\text{-}sec/cm^5) = [MPAP\ddagger - MLAP^\S]/CO \times 80$$

In unstable patients and in patients in whom complex hemodynamic interventions (valve replacement procedures and some reoperations) are needed, a left atrial catheter is often used for measuring cardiac filling pressures rather then relying on the PCW pressure to assess left ventricular preload. Left atrial and PCW pressures often do not correlate during the first 12 hours postoperatively, particularly in the presence of left ventricular failure. The PCW pressure usually exceeds the left atrial pressure, probably due in part to an elevation of the former by the increased interstitial pulmonary water [2]. Body temperatures should be recorded frequently during the early postoperative period when the patient is hypothermic and is rewarming. Fluid balance monitoring requires hourly measurements of urine output and chest tube drainage; nasogastric tube drainage also should be measured.

A brief but systematic physical examination of the patient is mandatory on arrival in the ICU. Inspection of the skin and extremities may reveal intraoperative injuries, infiltration or disconnection of intravenous infusions, absence of pulses, signs of drug or transfusion reactions, or evidence of hypoperfusion. Auscultation of the chest may reveal unilateral absence of breath sounds due to malposition of the endotracheal tube or pneumothorax. Auscultation of the heart should document normal heart sounds, normal prosthetic valve sounds, and the absence of regurgitant murmurs. The abdomen should be inspected to ensure that there is no abdominal distention. Mediastinal and chest tubes should be examined for drainage.

Initial laboratory studies should include both arterial oxygen tension (PaO_2) and carbon dioxide tension ($PaCO_2$), as well as pH, hematocrit, sodium, potassium, glucose, calcium, magnesium, prothrombin time (PT), partial thromboplastin time (PTT), and platelet count. A portable chest roentgenogram and a 12-lead ECG with atrial electrograms should be obtained immediately on admission to the ICU. The postoperative chest roentgenogram should be inspected with specific attention to the following:

1. Pneumothorax and mediastinal shift
2. Position of the endotracheal tube, nasogastric tube, and intravascular catheters
3. Size and contour of the mediastinal silhouette
4. Pleural and extrapleural fluid collections

PHYSIOLOGIC PRINCIPLES OF CARDIAC FUNCTION.
Cardiac function (the ability of the heart to fill with blood during diastole without generating excessive pulmonary venous pressure and the ability to eject a stroke volume during systole sufficient to supply adequate oxygen to the tissues) is determined by intrinsic myocardial properties as well as by ambient loading conditions (see also Chap. 171). The passive viscoelastic properties of the myocardium are important determinants of the diastolic compliance of the two ventricles. The inotropic

state (contractility) of the myocardium during systole is a determinant of systolic stroke volume. Systolic function also is determined by ambient hemodynamic conditions (heart rate, preload, and afterload). The conceptual framework that provides maximal information about intrinsic myocardial properties, as well as the inter-relationships among systolic contractility, preload, and afterload, is represented in cartesian coordinates by the ventricular pressure-volume relationship (Fig. 162-1). There are four phases of the cardiac cycle:

1. Passive ventricular filling during diastole (which in Fig. 162-1 has been extended as a curvilinear line to describe the distensibility of the ventricle beyond the range of the illustrated cardiac cycle)
2. Isovolumic systole (before aortic valve opening)
3. Systolic ejection
4. Isovolumic relaxation

The stroke volume for an individual cardiac cycle can be obtained by subtracting end-systolic ventricular volume from the volume at end-diastole. The systolic ejection fraction can be determined from the fractional relationship between stroke volume and end-diastolic volume. The external stroke work done by the ventricle during each cardiac cycle is equal to the integrated area inscribed within the pressure-volume loop.

This framework aids in conceptualizing and predicting the effects of changes in loading conditions and contractility on measurable hemodynamic parameters. Clinically, ventricular volume and intracavitary pressure are rarely measured, although the latter can be assessed indirectly from measurements of pulmonary artery, aortic, and central venous pressures.

Peak ejection phase pressure in the pulmonary artery is assumed to be equal to the peak systolic pressure in the right ventricle, and peak ejection phase systemic arterial pressure is assumed to be equal to left ventricular peak systolic pressure (in the absence of significant valvular or subvalvular obstruction). Central venous pressure closely reflects right ventricular diastolic pressure; left atrial pressure reflects left ventricular diastolic pressure. Left atrial pressure can be measured, or its mean can be estimated by the measurement of pulmonary capillary wedge pressure or pulmonary diastolic pressure. These three pressures are equal only under ideal circumstances. Generally, pulmonary diastolic pressure exceeds pulmonary artery wedge pressure, which exceeds mean left atrial pressure. These differences are determined by gravitational effects related to

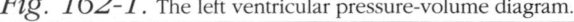

Fig. 162-1. The left ventricular pressure-volume diagram.

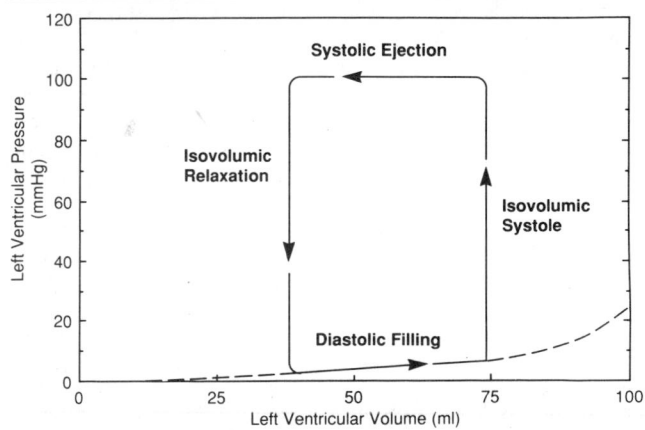

---

pulmonary artery catheter position and by diastolic pressure gradients in the pulmonary vasculature.

Although the systolic stroke volume (SV) of the left ventricle is not measured directly, it can be determined from measurements of cardiac output and heart rate. If left ventricular systolic ejection fraction (EF) is determined (using radionuclide imaging or transesophageal echocardiography), then the end-diastolic volume (EDV) and end-systolic volume (ESV) of the left ventricle can be determined:

EDV = SV/EF, and ESV = EDV − SV

Preload is an estimation of average end-diastolic myocardial fiber length and correlates best with ventricular EDV. As the left ventricle distends, EDV, rather than end-diastolic pressure, is a highly predictive determinant of systolic function. The relationship between diastolic ventricular pressure and diastolic ventricular volume is exponential in form, differs from one patient to another, and may vary from one time to another in any given patient. The position and configuration of this relationship (representing ventricular diastolic compliance) is determined primarily by the intrinsic viscoelastic properties of the myocardium.

Mechanical interaction between the two ventricles and between each ventricle and the surrounding mediastinal and thoracic structures also can influence ventricular distensibility. For example, acute distention of the right ventricle by pressure overload may cause a leftward shift of the interventricular septum and a decrease in the diastolic chamber compliance of the left ventricle. Left ventricular end-diastolic pressure (rather than EDV) can be used to monitor preload only when those factors that alter ventricular distensibility are constant. When ventricular distensibility is changing (due, for example, to the loss of myocardial compliance that occurs with transient ischemia), the measurements or estimates of ventricular diastolic pressure will not accurately represent preload. Under conditions in which ventricular compliance is known to be reduced, higher than usual filling pressures need to be maintained in order to achieve optimal preload.

The term *afterload* usually is used to describe the hydraulic energetics at the ventricular outlet. Afterload describes forces that retard the ventricular ejection of blood. The afterload of the right ventricle and that of the left ventricle are determined primarily by the resistive and capacitive characteristics of the pulmonary and systemic circulations. As blood is ejected from the ventricle, the actual afterload forces that oppose the shortening of myocardial fibers are distributed as stresses throughout the ventricular walls. Therefore, factors that either increase the hydraulic impedance opposing the ejection of blood (e.g., increased vascular input impedance) or increase systolic wall stress (ventricular dilatation) increase the afterload facing myocardial contraction.

A theoretical index of intrinsic myocardial contractility that is independent of preload, afterload, and heart rate has been sought for many years. Two conceptualizations have emerged that presently have limited clinical usefulness but are important investigative tools. An understanding of these principles is useful in predicting the hemodynamic outcome of therapeutic interventions. The Frank-Starling principle is usually illustrated by the curvilinear relationship between ventricular stroke work (y-axis) and ventricular end-diastolic pressure (x-axis). When preload is represented by end-diastolic volume, rather than by end-diastolic pressure, this relationship becomes linear and is minimally affected by afterload and heart rate [3]. The slope of this relationship is a sensitive indicator of intrinsic myocardial performance and responds appropriately to inotropic interven-

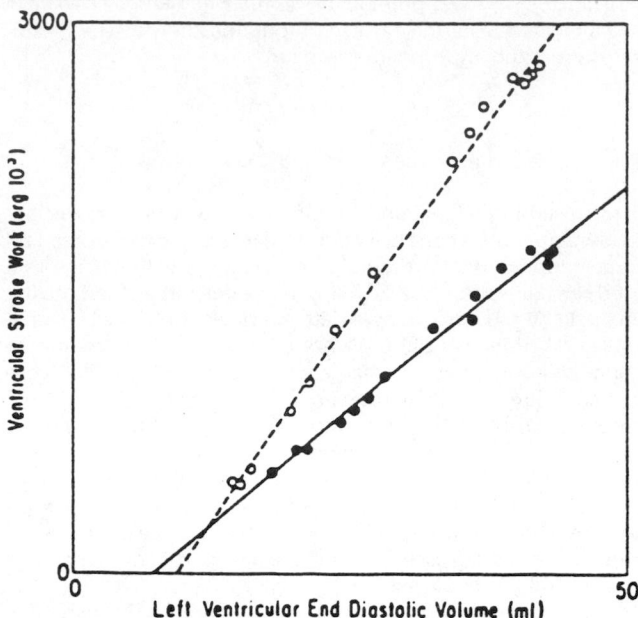

Fig. 162-2. The preload recruitable stroke work relationship for the left ventricle. The slope of this relationship (the increase in stroke work per unit increase in end-diastolic volume) is sensitive to inotropic interventions and is increased by the infusion of calcium. Glower DD, Spratt JA, Snow ND, et al. (From *Circulation* 71:1003, 1985 by permission of the American Heart Association, Inc.)

tions. The augmentation of stroke work by increases in preload is referred to as *preload recruitable stroke work* (Fig. 162-2).

Left ventricular systolic performance also can be assessed by generating the relationship between end-systolic ventricular pressure and end-systolic ventricular volume over a range of loading conditions. If the ratio of ventricular pressure to volume is viewed as the time-varying elastance of the ventricle, elastance is maximal (E_{max}) at end-systole (Fig. 162-3) [4]. For cardiac cycles executed under different loading conditions but at an equal inotropic state, the end-systolic points lie on a line. The slope of this line is the end-systolic elastance (E_{es}) of the ventricle and characterizes the intrinsic contractility of the myocardium. This parameter can be determined by defining the linear relationship between end-systolic pressure (P_{es}) and volume (V_{es}): $E_{es} = P_{es}/(V_{es} - V_o)$, where V_o is the x-intercept and has no clearly defined physical equivalent. This framework of analysis clearly demonstrates the inverse relationship between afterload (a determinant of P_{es}) and stroke volume (see Fig. 162-3). For any given end-diastolic volume of the left ventricle, an increase in P_{es} causes a proportional increase in end-systolic volume and a decrease in stroke volume.

Increases in cardiac output, afterload, preload, inotropic state, and heart rate are all achieved at the expense of increased myocardial oxygen demand. Several models have been used to describe the balance between myocardial oxygen demand and myocardial oxygen supply. Suga has extended the analysis of time-varying systolic elastance to predict myocardial oxygen requirements based on mechanical energy expenditure [5]. In this conceptualization, potential (or internal) energy remains in the ventricular myocardium at end-systole and is expended as heat during the cardiac cycle. This potential energy, when added to the external work performed during each cardiac cycle (the integrated area of the pressure-volume loop), has

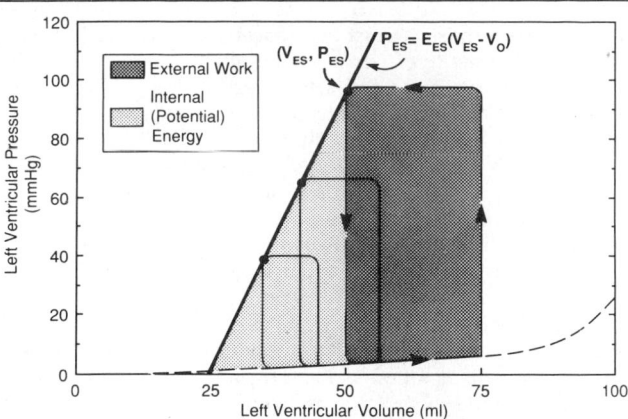

Fig. 162-3. The left ventricular end-systolic pressure-volume relationship. End-systole is defined as that moment when the slope of this relationship is maximal. This slope (Emax) is determined by identifying end-systole for cardiac cycles at variable loading. Emax is an index of the inotropic state of the left ventricle. The area lying to the left of the pressure-volume loop that is bounded above by the end-systolic pressure-volume relationship and below by the diastolic pressure-volume relationship is equal to the potential energy lost as heat during each cardiac cycle.

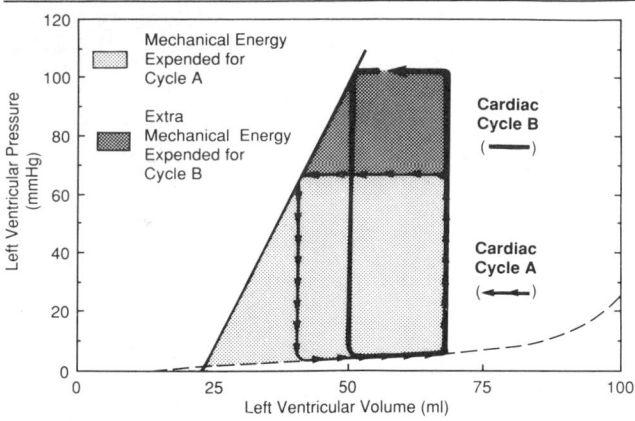

Fig. 162-4. When afterload is increased (resulting in an increase in end-systolic pressure), there is an increase in total energy expenditure for each cardiac cycle. This is represented by the sum of external work plus potential energy. This increase in total energy occurs despite the fact that the ventricle may perform little or no external work at the higher afterload.

been correlated with myocardial oxygen consumption. Suga and his colleagues have proposed that the area lying to the left of the external work loop (beneath the end-systolic pressure-volume relationship and above the diastolic pressure-volume relationship) is equal to the potential energy lost as heat during each cardiac cycle (see Fig. 162-3). Their experiments in supported blood-perfused heart preparations have demonstrated a high correlation between total mechanical energy calculated in this fashion and myocardial oxygen consumption.

By conceptualizing the mechanical energy requirements of the ventricle in this way, one can predict the energy cost of manipulating the preload, afterload, and inotropic state. This model clearly predicts the large energy cost of increasing afterload (Fig. 162-4). At any given level of contractility (defined by a single end-systolic pressure-volume relationship), an increase in afterload (at a fixed preload) results in a taller and narrower (smaller stroke volume) loop. However, the total energy expenditure for this contraction (external work plus potential energy) is considerably greater than for a contraction with a smaller afterload and greater stroke volume.

The clinical goal of greatest importance in caring for cardiac surgical patients immediately postoperatively is to ensure that blood pressure and cardiac output are adequate to perfuse all organs (particularly the heart) without causing undue myocardial energy expenditure. This is not always a simple matter, since the heart is the only organ that must feed itself and, therefore, depends on its own work for its blood supply. If that work is too great or the blood supply too small, myocardial ischemia, failure, and infarction result. The driving force for myocardial blood flow is the aortic pressure minus the intramyocardial pressure. During systole, the left ventricular endocardium—the portion of the myocardium most vulnerable to ischemia—has an intramyocardial pressure nearly equal to aortic pressure and hence receives little, if any, blood flow. During diastole, myocardial blood flow depends on the gradient between aortic pressure and intramyocardial pressure. Myocardial oxygen consumption (MVO₂) is determined by myocardial blood flow (MBF) and myocardial oxygen extraction:

$MVO_2 = MBF (aO_2 - vO_2)$, where aO_2 and vO_2 are the coronary arterial and venous oxygen contents, respectively. An important feature of myocardial oxygen consumption is that oxygen extraction is nearly maximal at rest, so that increases in myocardial oxygen consumption can be achieved only by increases in coronary blood flow. Increased afterload is, to a degree, self-compensatory in that increased diastolic coronary perfusion pressure tends to increase coronary blood flow. Increases in inotropic state also may be associated with increases in myocardial blood flow as a result of increases in diastolic aortic pressure. However, inotropic stimulation usually also depends on coronary vasodilation to meet the increased metabolic demands.

One model for conceptualizing how hemodynamic changes can affect the balance between myocardial oxygen demand and myocardial oxygen supply is the endocardial viability ratio (EVR) [6]. This conceptual framework requires the determination of the diastolic pressure-time index and the systolic pressure-time index by integration over time of the area between the aortic pressure tracing and the left ventricular pressure tracing during diastole (DPTI) and the area beneath the left ventricular pressure tracing during systole (SPTI) (Fig. 162-5). The DPTI tends to reflect the supply of oxygen to the myocardium, since the integrated pressure difference between aortic diastolic pressure and left ventricular diastolic pressure approximates the time-averaged driving force for blood flow to the myocardium. Decreases in the DPTI due to reductions in aortic pressure or abbreviated diastolic duration must be balanced by coronary vasodilation to maintain myocardial blood flow. The time-integral of SPTI is an estimate of the myocardial requirements for oxygen based on the pressure component of work performed during the cardiac cycle. The ratio of DPTI-SPTI is the EVR, and for a healthy heart this is 0.8 to 1.2. When the EVR decreases to values less than 0.8, endocardial ischemia results.

Many of the manipulations used to increase cardiac output or blood pressure decrease the EVR. Increases in heart rate and left ventricular end-diastolic pressure both decrease DPTI. With coronary artery disease, DPTI overestimates coronary blood flow and O₂ supply, and with aortic stenosis, SPTI underesti-

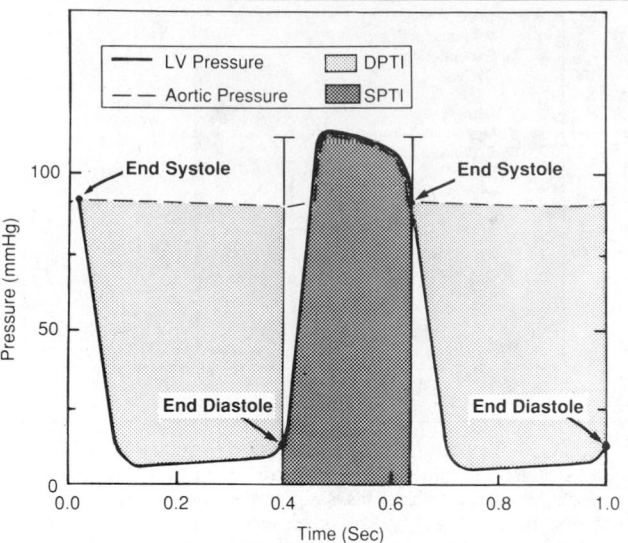

Fig. 162-5. The diastolic and systolic pressure-time indices for the left ventricle. Integration over time is a means of time averaging the pressure gradient driving myocardial blood flow during diastole (DPTI) and the systolic ventricular pressure that is a determinant of myocardial oxygen demand during systole (SPTI).

mates myocardial O_2 requirements. If, in raising blood pressure or cardiac output, EVR falls much below 0.8, the resultant myocardial ischemia leads to increasing left ventricular diastolic pressure, myocardial failure, and further decreases in DPTI and EVR. If this cycle is uninterrupted, the imbalance between myocardial oxygen demand and myocardial oxygen supply leads to hypotension, decreased perfusion, acidosis, and ultimately, cardiac death.

INITIAL STATUS. On arrival in the ICU, most patients are hypothermic. Peripheral vasoconstriction commonly occurs as a result of deliberate systemic cooling during cardiopulmonary bypass. During rewarming, the periphery often lags behind, and while the core temperature may be 37 to 38°C at the completion of cardiopulmonary bypass, the still cold extremities leach out heat from the core as they rewarm. Thus, core temperatures in the 34 to 36°C range are commonly seen in the ICU. Peripheral vasoconstriction persists as a result of the cold limbs and as a result of elevated angiotensin levels in the immediate postoperative period [7]. Shivering during rewarming increases metabolic and circulatory demands, increases CO_2 production, and complicates ventilator management. Shivering can be eliminated with paralyzing agents and sedation [8]. These maneuvers reduce the need for inotropic support [9]. The patient is generally maximally warm by 6 to 8 hours postoperatively.

The cardiac index is often low as a result of several factors. Intraoperative ischemia and myocardial edema both cause myocardial depression. The blood pressure is an insensitive indicator of cardiac function. Peripheral vasoconstriction increases resistance and further reduces cardiac index or raises blood pressure, or both. Intravascular hypovolemia often exists at this stage, further reducing cardiac output. The cold patient has a lowered metabolic rate and decreased demand for blood flow [10]. Nevertheless, an initial cardiac index of 1.5 liters per square meter per minute or less, and a cardiac index 12 hours later of 2 liters per square meter per minute or less portend an increased

risk of death [11,12]. When the cardiac index is below these limits, efforts to raise it must be vigorous.

No single measure of perfusion is sufficient in assessing the adequacy of tissue perfusion. Each must be viewed in the context of the whole patient. Mixed venous oxygen saturation (SvO_2) gives a numerical indication of tissue oxygenation adequacy but only of perfused tissue. For a normal recovery, SvO_2 should be 60 percent or greater. If SvO_2 is less than 50 percent, a high likelihood of death exists [10,13]. The SvO_2 should be interpreted in light of the cardiac index and hemoglobin. In the worst situation, and the one often leading to death, the SvO_2 may be adequate only because so much of the peripheral tissues are unperfused [10]. In this case, however, the cardiac index also will be reduced. The monitoring of SvO_2 does not describe the balance of oxygen supply and demand in vascular beds, in which O_2 extraction is fixed. The kidney, skin, and resting muscle can maintain viability during reduced blood flow by augmenting oxygen extraction. The heart and brain, on the other hand, extract oxygen nearly maximally at rest, and their vulnerability to ischemia is not reflected by widened O_2 extraction.

The clinical correlates of reduced cardiac index are pale and cool skin, cyanotic mottling of the skin (occurring first over the knees), decreased urine output, and deterioration of mental status or slowness in awakening from anesthesia. A low cardiac output and decreased peripheral perfusion also cause a metabolic acidosis (from lactic acid accumulation in poorly perfused tissues) (see Chap. 80), which, to a mild degree, occurs even after routine operations.

Postoperative hypertension is common, particularly after routine operations that are not associated with significant injury to the myocardium. Hypertension may be a consequence of several factors, such as inadequate sedation, hypoxemia, hypercarbia, activation of cardiogenic reflexes, vasoactive drug administration, and withdrawal of beta-blocking agents, but intense vasoconstriction accounts for most of the hypertension. Regardless of the cause, hypertension must be aggressively controlled in patients who have suture lines in the ascending aorta (which includes nearly every patient having a cardiac operation). Failure to control the blood pressure increases the risk of aortic tear or rupture. Aortic wall tension is proportional to the product of radius and pressure. Since increasing pressure increases radius, wall tension increases geometrically as blood pressure increases. Also, increased pressure elevates myocardial oxygen demand, leading to the possibility of decreased subendocardial perfusion and ischemia.

A clinically obvious "postpump syndrome" occurs in a few patients. In its most severe form, these patients have a coagulopathy, pulmonary dysfunction with hypoxia, renal and cerebral insufficiency, and a diffuse inflammatory response that is characterized by increased capillary permeability and leakage of fluid into the interstitial space with diffuse edema, fever, and leukocytosis. The cause of these derangements may be activation of complement during cardiopulmonary bypass [14,15]. Both C3 and C5 are activated during cardiopulmonary bypass [14].

As a consequence of fluid administration, the patient seen in the ICU just after a cardiopulmonary bypass operation usually weighs 2 to 5 kg more than he or she did preoperatively. Urine output is typically high in patients with good left ventricular function. If urine output is low, intravascular volume or cardiac output may be low. Inappropriate antidiuretic hormone (ADH) excretion commonly exists as a consequence of operative trauma. The patient is frequently treated with intravenous nitroglycerin and other afterload-reducing and venodilating agents, which shift blood volume to the periphery and consequently decrease preload. These factors tend to reduce urine output.

The postcardiac patient almost routinely has a widened alveolar-arterial oxygen tension gradient. This pulmonary shunting is accompanied by decreased functional residual capacity and microatelectasis.

TREATMENT OF LOW CARDIAC OUTPUT. Low cardiac output in the postoperative period is associated with a higher incidence of respiratory, renal, hepatic, and neurologic failure. Treatment of low cardiac output first requires an analysis of possible causes (Table 162-1) [10]. Operative maloccurrences, such as coronary graft closure, inadequate revascularization, poor myocardial protection, valve malfunction, or paravalvular leak, can cause pump dysfunction. Graft closure or acute coronary occlusion can have immediate hemodynamic effects (a fall in cardiac output and a rise in left-sided filling pressures). Early graft failures are usually the result of technical factors, but perioperative myocardial infarction due to coronary spasm also can occur and may lead to sudden, unexpected ventricular fibrillation. Spasm can occur in operated or in nonoperated vessels [16]. The closure of a graft or graft spasm should be suspected when hemodynamic deterioration occurs early and suddenly and is associated with dramatic changes in the ST segments on the ECG. When the diagnosis of spasm is entertained, aggressive management with nitroglycerin and sublingual nifedipine should be instituted [17]. If these drugs are unsuccessful in reversing the hemodynamic deterioration, cardiac catheterization and/or reexploration with inspection of the grafts should be considered [18]. Functional myocardial depression (lasting about 12–24 hours) occurs as a result of the operation in most patients, including those who ultimately will have a normal recovery. Common causes of perioperative pump dysfunction include arrhythmias, tamponade, hypovolemia, myocardial infarction, systemic acidosis, electrolyte imbalance, and hypoxia.

Early graft patency is an important determinant of postoperative ventricular function and performance on stress tests. On the other hand, the occurrence of perioperative myocardial infarction without hemodynamic compromise has not been shown to be significantly related to graft patency, late survival, or cardiac performance status [19]. The significance of perioperative myocardial infarction probably depends ultimately on its effect on postoperative ventricular function. The treatment of perioperative infarction consists of therapy to maintain cardiac output. Supportive therapy should include afterload reduction, especially with nitroglycerin and beta blockade if tolerated.

If an easily correctable or mechanical cause of low cardiac output is not identified, an orderly systematic approach toward optimizing pump function should be undertaken (Table 162-2). An easy way to organize this approach is by examining rate, rhythm, preload, afterload, and contractility. Since cardiac output is the product of stroke volume and heart rate (CO = SV × HR), either can be increased.

Initially, the clinician should next optimize cardiac rate and rhythm. Every effort should be made to maintain sinus rhythm. A properly timed atrial contraction may improve cardiac output by as much as 25 percent. Following cardiac surgery, sinus bradycardia and first-degree, second-degree, or third-degree heart block can occur. These arrhythmias are usually transient

Table 162-1. Causes of Low Cardiac Output

A. Inadequate preload
  1. Volume deficit
  2. Excessive positive end-expiratory pressure
B. Increased afterload
  1. Vasoconstriction from endogenous catecholamines (sympathetic stimulation)
    a. Painful stimuli
    b. Nonpulsatile flow during cardiopulmonary bypass
    c. Hypothermia
    d. Preexisting hypertension
  2. Vasoconstriction from exogenous catecholamines
  3. Aortic stenosis
  4. Idiopathic hypertrophic subaortic stenosis
C. Myocardial depression
  1. Uncorrected mechanical lesions
    a. Incomplete coronary revascularization
    b. Valvular stenosis or insufficiency
    c. Mechanical valve malfunction
  2. Functional depression (lasts about 24 hr)
  3. Coronary spasm
  4. Inadequate myocardial protection intraoperatively
    a. Myocardial edema
    b. Myocardial ischemia
    c. Myocardial necrosis-infarct
D. Metabolic derangement
  1. Hypocalcemia
  2. Hypomagnesemia
  3. Hypoxia
  4. Acidosis
E. Arrhythmias
F. Conduction defects
G. Tamponade
H. Pharmacologic depression
  1. Anesthetic agents
  2. Quinidine
  3. Procainamide
  4. Lidocaine
  5. Beta-blockers
  6. Calcium channel blockers

Table 162-2. Treatment of Low Cardiac Output

A. Treat or exclude complications
  1. Valve malfunction (reoperate)
  2. Coronary graft occlusion (reoperate)
  3. Tamponade (reoperate)
  4. Bleeding (reoperate)
  5. Coronary spasm (nifedipine 10 mg sublingually)
B. Treat arrhythmias by optimizing heart rate
  1. Increase rate to 90–100
  2. Atrial pacing if no heart block
  3. A-V pacing if heart block
C. BP (systolic) ≥100, or BP (MAP) ≥85
  1. Low LAP (<15 mm Hg)
    a. Give volume (packed cells) if Hct <25%
    b. Give Ringer's lactate or hetastarch if Hct ≥25%
    c. Continue step-wise treatment with volume and dilators until CI adequate (≥2.5): do not allow LAP to remain >15 mm Hg or BP to remain <100
  2. High LAP (≥15 mm Hg): begin nitroprusside* or nitroglycerin 0.2–0.6 μg/kg/min and increase until desired effect obtained
D. BP (systolic) <100 or BP (MAP) <85
  1. Low LAP (<15 mm Hg)
    a. Give volume (packed cells) if Hct <25%
    b. Give Ringer's lactate or hetastarch if Hct ≥25%
  2. High LAP (≥15 mm Hg): if BP still low.
    a. Give dopamine* 3–5 μg/kg/min; increase gradually with 15 μg/kg/min maximum; dobutamine
    b. When BP ≥100, begin nitroprusside* 0.2–0.6 μg/kg/min; increase until desired effect obtained.
E. If BP and CO still low, insert IABP

*See text for alternative drugs.
A-V = atrioventricular; BP = blood pressure; LAP = left atrial pressure; Hct = hematocrit; CI = cardiac index; CO = cardiac output; IABP = intraaortic balloon pump; MAP = mean arterial pressure.

and may be related to perioperative beta blockade, hyperkalemic damage during the administration of cardioplegia, or unprotected ischemia of the conduction system [20,21]. Permanent injury to the conduction system is usually the result of surgically induced trauma during intracardiac procedures.

Optimal pacing, using temporary atrial and ventricular wires inserted at the time of surgery, must be individualized. Simple atrial pacing (at a rate of 80 to 100) for the treatment of sinus bradycardia may effectively augment cardiac output. However, underlying first degree heart block is often aggravated by atrial pacing. Therefore, the advantage of an increase in heart rate may be mitigated by the introduction of atrioventricular dyssynchrony. In this situation, atrioventricular sequential pacing should be attempted. The optimal atrioventricular interval is usually in the range of 100 to 175 msec, depending on the heart rate. The advantage of atrial pacing over atrioventricular sequential pacing is the maintenance of the normal anatomic pattern of ventricular activation. Loss of the normal sequence of activation depresses ventricular function by approximately 10 to 15 percent. When temporary pacing is not possible, bradyarrhythmias can be treated with atropine and isoproterenol, by introducing a transvenous pacing wire, or, as a last resort, by using a transthoracic stimulator.

Next, hypovolemia should be corrected. Volume replacement can be provided easily using continuous autotransfusion; the infusion of other products may be required as well. Normal saline and lactated Ringer's solution are commonly used. Serum albumin (25% solution) can be infused but must recruit extravascular fluid to result in effective volume replacement. Hydroxyethyl starch (Hetastarch) generally provides plasma volume expansion for more than 24 hours. Urticarial and anaphylactoid reactions as well as pancreatitis can occur with the use of this product [22]. Coagulation abnormalities associated with each of these agents are usually related to hemodilution rather than to specific anticoagulant effects.

Stroke volume may be augmented by increasing contractility or reducing systemic vascular resistance (SVR). Vasodilator therapy is usually warranted because most patients are cold and vasoconstricted (Table 162-3). Decreasing SVR decreases the heart's oxygen demand, but if aortic diastolic pressure drops too much, the decrease in DPTI may be proportionally greater than the decrease in SPTI. In patients with relatively normal left ventricular function, nitroprusside reliably decreases SVR and

increases cardiac output, whereas nitroglycerin may lower cardiac output, perhaps as a result of too great a decrease in cardiac preload (left atrial pressure). In the presence of left ventricular failure, however, both of these agents effectively increase cardiac output and decrease left ventricular pressures.

Theoretically, the pressure-volume relationship of the left ventricle can be used to predict improvements in stroke volume secondary to reductions in afterload. The therapeutic results depend on the inotropic state of the ventricle (as characterized by the end-systolic pressure-volume relationship). Ventricles with the poorest contractility benefit the most from afterload reduction. If the ventricle is operating on an end-systolic pressure-volume relationship with a shallow slope (depressed contractility), reducing afterload (and end-systolic pressure) will result in a relatively large increase in stroke-volume (Fig. 162-6). Afterload reduction is also beneficial when residual mitral regurgitation and aortic insufficiency are present.

An excellent strategy in the postoperative patient with a low cardiac output is to give increasing doses of nitroprusside, taking care to ensure that blood pressure remains adequate. Cardiac index and stroke volume rise as filling pressures and blood pressure fall. Eventually, decreasing preload causes cardiac index to fall. At this point, cardiac output will increase substantially if volume is infused to bring the left atrial pressure back to the pretreatment level. When high-dose nitroprusside therapy is needed, but cannot be tolerated, alternative parenteral agents can be considered. Sublingual nifedipine also may be used and has the least depressive effect on myocardial performance of the calcium channel blockers [23].

Intravenous nitroglycerin and nitroprusside have similar effects, but nitroglycerin, being a more potent venous dilator, decreases ventricular preload to a greater extent. However, in the presence of ischemia or an acute myocardial infarction, nitroglycerin increases regional myocardial flow and decreases ischemic ST segments toward normal, whereas nitroprusside may have an opposite and deleterious effect [24,25]. Nitroprusside also must be used with caution because of its potential for causing cyanide and/or thiocyanate poisoning. Its breakdown product, cyanide, complexes with, and inactivates, cytochrome oxidase interfering with oxidative phosphorylation. This acute toxicity results in metabolic acidosis. Cyanide is inactivated by reacting with thiosulfate to yield thiocyanate. Accumulation of this by-product results in chronic toxicity manifested by fatigue,

Table 162-3. Vasodilators Used in Postoperative Cardiac Surgery Patients

Drug	Dosage Range*	Activity Arterial	Activity Venous	Onset	Duration	Mechanism	Comments	Toxicity
Nitroprusside (Nipride)	0.2–5 μg/kg/ min	+3	+2	Immediate	Immediate	Direct vasodilator	May increase myocardial ischemia	Cyanide and thiocyanate
Nitroglycerin	0.3–5 μg/kg/ min	+1	+4	Immediate	30 min	Direct vasodilator	Improves myocardial ischemia	—
Trimethaphan (Arfonad)	3–90 μg/kg/min	+3	+2	Immediate	10–30 min	Ganglionic blockade	Sympathetic and parasympathetic blockade: tachycardia common, tachyphylaxis	Histamine release may exacerbate allergies
Prostaglandin E₁	0.03–1 μg/kg/ min	Pulmonary arterial dilator		Immediate	Immediate	Direct vasodilator	May require norepinephrine via left arterial line	Inhibits platelet aggregation
Hydralazine	5–10 mg IV 10–20 mg IM	+4	0	15–30 min 20–80 min	2–6 hr	Direct vasodilator	Reflex increases CO and HR; may cause angina in ischemic heart	None short-term

*Initiate treatment at low end of dosage range.

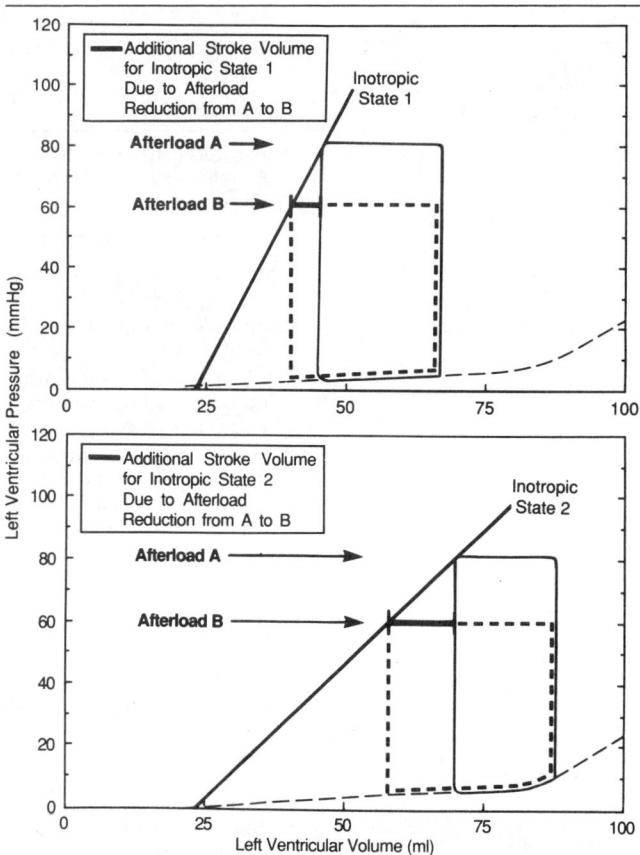

Fig. 162-6. The improvement in stroke-volume that can be achieved with a reduction in afterload (and consequently, a reduction in end-systolic pressure) depends on the inotropic state of the myocardium. There is more to be gained by afterload reduction in a ventricle with depressed inotropic state (a smaller slope of the end-systolic pressure-volume relationship).

nausea, psychosis, and even convulsions. Nitroprusside infusions generally should not exceed 8 μg/kg/min (see Table 162-3).

Left ventricular depression commonly occurs after the operation. If it is sufficiently severe, treatment with vasodilators alone may be unsuccessful because of the induced hypotension. Ventricular contractility must be augmented. Preload must be optimized first. If too high, it reduces myocardial blood flow, which is determined by the difference between the aortic diastolic and left ventricular diastolic pressures. High biventricular filling pressures also compromise pulmonary, renal, hepatic, and cerebral function and result in hypoxia, azotemia, jaundice, and obtundation. Nitroglycerin reduces left ventricular and right ventricular filling pressures quickly and effectively.

Improvement in cardiac function with inotropic agents is generally at the expense of increased myocardial oxygen demand. Inotropic agents, therefore, should be used only when manipulations of heart rate, rhythm, preload, and afterload are ineffective. When left ventricular depression and low output persist, inotropic therapy must be used. A number of drugs and drug regimens can be used including dopamine, dobutamine, epinephrine, isoproterenol, norepinephrine, and amrinone (Table 162-4). Dopamine, a norepinephrine precursor, usually causes a small increase in heart rate, although in some patients heart rate increases markedly and deleteriously. Dopamine increases cardiac index by stimulating beta-adrenergic receptors.

At doses less than 3 μg/kg/min, dopamine causes renal, splanchnic, coronary, and cerebral arterial vasodilatation via the activation of dopaminergic receptors. When dopamine is infused at a rate below 7.5 μg/kg/min, it causes little change in systemic vascular resistance; above this rate, systemic vasoconstriction, due to stimulation of alpha-adrenergic receptors, increases. The usual dose range for dopamine is 1 to 10 μg/kg/min.

Dobutamine, a synthetic congener of isoproterenol, has minimal alpha-adrenergic activity but pronounced beta$_1$- and beta$_2$-adrenergic activity. It increases cardiac output by increasing ventricular contractility and rate as well as causing peripheral vascular dilatation. For patients with a low cardiac output and marked peripheral vasoconstriction, dobutamine is preferable to dopamine, when the latter is used alone. Nevertheless, because dobutamine is a vasodilator, use of this drug in the presence of hypotension may lead to cardiovascular collapse. The usual doses for dobutamine are 5 to 20 μg/kg/min.

Epinephrine is an alpha- and beta-receptor agonist. It increases myocardial contractility and rate. It also increases ventricular irritability. Peripherally, its beta-mediated effects (vasodilation) predominate at low doses, whereas alpha-mediated effects (vasoconstriction) predominate at high doses. Although epinephrine has been supplanted to some extent by dopamine because of the lesser risk of myocardial ischemia with the newer drug, it still remains an excellent agent, especially when dopamine produces severe tachycardia. The usual epinephrine dose is 1 to 10 μg per minute (0.015–0.15 μg/kg/min).

Isoproterenol is not commonly used. It is a pure beta-adrenergic agonist; it increases heart rate and contractility and produces peripheral vasodilatation. Blood pressure changes depend on the balance between increased cardiac output and decreased systemic vascular resistance. A marked increase in myocardial oxygen demand limits its usefulness in patients with coronary disease. However, it is useful postoperatively in patients with pure mitral valvular disease. Because it causes pulmonary vasodilatation, isoproterenol is also useful in patients with pulmonary hypertension. It may also be useful in lowering pacing thresholds. The usual dose is 1 to 4 μg per minute (0.015–0.06 μg/kg/min).

Norepinephrine has both alpha- and beta-adrenergic activity; the former effect predominates, causing peripheral vasoconstriction, especially at higher doses. However, at doses of less than about 2 μg per minute, cardiac beta-effects usually increase cardiac output with little change in systemic vascular resistance. Internal mammary grafts remain innervated and are responsive to vasoactive drugs. Saphenous vein grafts are not. Norepinephrine has been shown to decrease flow in internal mammary grafts less than phenylephrine in the early postoperative period and is our drug of choice when a vasoconstrictor is needed [26]. The usual dose is 4 to 10 μg per minute (0.06–0.150 μg/kg/min).

Amrinone is an agent that reportedly increases myocardial contractility, produces peripheral vasodilatation, and may produce coronary vasodilatation. The inotropic activity of this agent is the subject of some controversy [27,28]. Amrinone is a member of a class of noncatecholamine inotropic agents that act by inhibiting an intracellular phosphodiesterase and thereby increasing intracellular concentrations of cyclic adenosine monophosphate (cAMP). Although the pharmacologic effects of amrinone are similar to those of dobutamine, tachyphylaxis is occasionally a problem with the latter agent, but not with the former one [29]. Therapy with amrinone is initiated with a bolus dose (0.75 mg/kg) that can be repeated every 5 minutes for three doses. A constant infusion (5–20 μg/kg/min) is then titrated to obtain the required response. Amrinone does not generally induce tachycardia, but it does increase cardiac output

Table 162-4. Inotropic Agents Used in Postoperative Cardiac Surgery Patients

Drug	Dose range	Activity Alpha	Beta	Onset	Offset (min)	Heart rate[a]	Comments
Dopamine	1–3 μg/kg/min	Plus renal and mesenteric vasodilatation, dopaminergic	Same as alpha	Immediate	Few	Increase of 20–30% non–dose related (rate: idiopathic increase to 50–70%)	Minimal PVR at dose <10 μg/kg/min; renal blood flow at low dose[b]
	1–10 μg/kg/min		+2				
	>10 μg/kg/min	+2	+2				
Dobutamine	1–10 μg/kg/min	0	+4	Immediate	2–3	25–30%	Very similar to isoproterenol; tachyphylaxis[b]
Epinephrine	1–2 μg/min	0	+2	Immediate	2–3	+1	Predominant effect varies with dose, marked vasoconstriction at high doses
	2–10 μg/min	+2	+2				
	>10 μg/min	+2	0				
Norepinephrine	2–16 μg/min	+4	+2	Immediate	2–3	0	Pronounced vasoconstriction increases myocardial work; valuable in vasodilated patient or in use with vasodilator; may reduce renal perfusion, especially at higher doses[b]
Isoproterenol	1–4 μg/min	0	+4	Immediate	2–3	+2	Excellent pulmonary vasodilator, most useful in RV failure; dangerous in ischemia because of tachycardia; ventricular dysrhythmia possible[b]
Amrinone	10–30 μg/kg/min[c]			2–10 min	60–90	0	Increases output and decreases SVR; no tachyphylaxis; may cause thrombocytopenia
Calcium chloride (CaCl₂)	100–200 mg	Restores ionized Ca^{2+} and acts synergistically with inotropic catecholamines	Same as alpha	Immediate	15	0	

[a]Depends on balance of direct cardiac effect vs. reflex effects.
[b]May all decrease EVR (DPTI/SPTI)
[c]Initiate amrinone with 0.75 mg/kg bolus over 5 min; repeat up to 2 times if necessary. Next, titrate infusion to increase cardiac index 25–40%.
PVR = pulmonary vascular resistance, RV = right ventricular; SVR = systemic vascular resistance, EVR = endocardial ratio; DPTI = diastolic pressure time index; SPTI = systolic pressure time index.

while decreasing systemic resistance. Thrombocytopenia has been reported with its use. Amrinone has also been reported to markedly increase intrapulmonary shunting [30]. Hence, the improvement in cardiac output induced by this agent may not lead to a corresponding decrease in the arteriovenous oxygen content difference.

For patients who have just received blood products, excess citrate can chelate ionic calcium, and this phenomenon may contribute to myocardial depression. Administration of calcium chloride (100–200 mg IV) can augment contractility. Care must be taken that the patient is neither hypokalemic nor digitalis-toxic before calcium is administered. Calcium infusions can cause major disturbances in cardiac rhythm, including sinus arrhythmias, bradycardia, and atrioventricular dissociation.

Epinephrine and norepinephrine are partially metabolized and bound in the lung. Administration of these drugs through a left atrial catheter therefore allows a smaller dose to create the same cardiac and peripheral effect that a larger dose would when given intravenously [31,32]. An advantage of this approach is that pulmonary vasoconstriction is lessened.

All the agents that increase myocardial contractility can decrease EVR by increasing SPTI, decreasing DPTI, or both. Thus, all these agents can further injure an already damaged left ventricle. In some cases, cardiac output remains inadequate even after optimizing preload, afterload, and contractility. In these instances, energy must be added to the system from without. The most common method to achieve this is the insertion of an intraaortic balloon pump (IABP), percutaneously via a femoral artery (see Chap. 9) . By raising aortic diastolic pressure, the IABP increases DPTI. Because the IABP decreases afterload, it allows better ventricular emptying, which decreases left ventricular diastolic pressure, thus further increasing DPTI. Furthermore, because of the systolic unloading, SPTI falls. Coronary flow and cardiac output increase. Proper balloon pump function requires synchronization with the cardiac cycle using the ECG or intraarterial pressure tracing. Supraventricular and ventricular arrhythmias can interfere with synchronization. Weaning is usually accomplished by gradually reducing the proportion of augmented beats from 1:1 to 1:3 or by reducing balloon volume.

Most patients undergo insertion of the IABP either preoperatively, typically for unstable angina or left ventricular failure, or intraoperatively for inability to wean from bypass. Rarely, patients who have been successfully weaned from cardiopulmonary bypass require the intraaortic balloon postoperatively. In these patients, the clinician should suspect a mechanical cause of left ventricular failure, such as coronary graft closure, valve malfunction, paravalvular leak, or new myocardial infarction. The IABP has a high complication rate. Complications include aortic dissection, arterial perforation, femoral artery occlusion or thrombosis with leg ischemia, arterial emboli, and wound infection [33]. Although extremely rare, spinal cord ischemia resulting in paraplegia has been reported [34]. Blood seen in the lumen of the IABP signals rupture of the balloon. In this situation, the balloon should be turned off and removed immediately. Percutaneous introduction of the intraaortic balloon is technically easier than exposing the femoral artery, but the incidence of vascular complications with this method may be higher than with direct surgical insertion [35].

Rarely, patients may require even more mechanical assistance than can be provided with the IABP. In these cases, an option is the use of a left ventricular assist device (LVAD) [36,37]. The LVAD actually pumps blood around the injured left ventricle, something the IABP cannot do. While its experimental use is restricted to a few investigating centers, it may be a device that will find wider use in the future. The Hemopump, a catheter-mounted hydraulic pump that drives blood from the left ventricle into the aorta, is capable of supporting nearly the entire output of the left ventricle (4 L/min). This device can be introduced surgically through a femoral artery or the aorta. The initial experience with this device has been quite favorable [38].

HYPOTENSION. Treatment decisions for hypotension often parallel those for a low cardiac output (see Chap. 171), but the two processes may occur independently. Causes for hypotension (MAP < 70) include those for low cardiac output (see Table 162-1), but "decreased afterload" should be substituted for "increased afterload." Other possible causes of decreased afterload include pharmacologic vasodilatation or sepsis. In most cases, treatment of hypotension follows diagnosis (Table 162-5). For catastrophic hypotension, treatment must be instituted immediately because marked coronary hypoperfusion can lead to arrhythmias, ventricular malfunction, and death. Immediate treatment consists of norepinephrine (about 4–10 μg/min) and volume repletion.

In evaluating hypotension, one should measure cardiac index, heart rate, and right and left atrial filling pressures. Bradycardia, especially in the presence of a poorly compliant postoperative ventricle, causes hypotension because the ventricle is unable to compensate by augmenting stroke volume. Hypovolemia presents with low filling pressures and low cardiac output. Left ventricular depression presents with high left atrial and, sometimes, right atrial pressures and a very low cardiac output.

Tamponade. Cardiac tamponade is the result of fluid or clotted blood occupying space within the mediastinum and restricting diastolic filling of both ventricles. The findings associated with tamponade in the immediate postoperative period include:

1. Elevation and equalization of the central venous pressure, pulmonary diastolic pressure, left atrial pressure (pulmonary artery capillary wedge pressure), and right ventricular diastolic pressure (central venous pressure)
2. Low urine output
3. Excessive chest tube drainage (or a sudden decrease in chest tube drainage)
4. Mediastinal widening on chest x-ray
5. Low cardiac output and hypotension

The treatment for cardiac tamponade is early reoperation. The patient may temporarily respond to some simple supportive measures such as reducing airway pressure (using smaller tidal volumes and eliminating positive end-expiratory pressure), infusing intravascular volume expanders, and providing inotropic support. Myocardial dysfunction and myocardial edema reduce the amount of space occupied by fluid and clot required to cause tamponade physiology [39]. In cases of severe myocardial edema and dysfunction, the patient may not even tolerate approximation of the sternum·at the conclusion of the initial operative procedure.

Although cardiac tamponade usually presents within the first 24 hours postoperatively, it can present as a subacute syndrome as late as several weeks following surgery. The symptoms are often nonspecific and reflect the ongoing inflammatory process by which retained fluid and clot are reabsorbed and digested in the mediastinum. Symptoms can include malaise, low-grade fever, diaphoresis, dyspnea, chest pain, and anorexia. Transesophageal or transthoracic echocardiography may demonstrate retained clot and blood or wall motion abnormalities characteristic of tamponade (diastolic collapse of the right atrium and right ventricle). On occasion, right-sided heart catheterization may be necessary to establish the diagnosis (equalization and elevation of filling pressures). Treatment of tamponade consists of reopening the sternotomy, evacuating the clot, and controlling any bleeding site.

Arrhythmias, as a cause of hypotension, are usually obvious from the electrocardiographic monitor. Technical problems with prosthetic valves may be seen with transesophageal echocardiography. Sepsis often presents as hypovolemia and fever. Vasodilating drugs are commonly used in the cardiac surgical ICU, and an inadvertently large dose can cause hypotension and should be considered as a possible etiology.

Treatment of hypotension begins with optimization of rate (Table 162-6). If the rate is too slow, atrial (or, in the presence of complete heart block, atrioventricular) pacing should be used to bring the rate up to 90 to 100, depending on the response. Arrhythmias should be treated promptly (see Arrhythmias, following, and Chap. 49). Intravascular volume should be

Table 162-5. Diagnosis of Hypotension

Cause	CVP	LAP or PCW	CI
Hypovolemia			
Vasodilatation			
Myocardial failure			
Tamponade			

CVP = central venous pressure; LAP = left atrial pressure; PCW = pulmonary capillary wedge; CI = cardiac index; = low; = variable (equilibration); = high.

Table 162-6. Management of Bradycardia

Diagnosis	Treatment
Sinus or nodal	Atrial pacing at 80–100
A-V block	A-V sequential pacing at 80–100 (? digoxin toxic)
Atrial fibrillation	Ventricular pacing (? digoxin excess)

A-V = atrioventricular.

optimized. Ventricular filling pressures in the early postoperative patient routinely need to be higher than normal in order to maximize stroke volume, because the ventricle is stiff and dysfunctional following cardiopulmonary bypass.

If tamponade is absent, and intravascular volume and heart rate are optimized, then continued hypotension mandates treatment with vasoactive drugs.

In some patients with severe left ventricular failure vasodilators alone may increase blood pressure paradoxically if the improvements in left ventricular function and cardiac index more than offset the decrease in peripheral resistance. If none of these modalities proves successful, and if no correctable mechanical cause can be found, insertion of an IABP may be necessary (see Chap. 9).

HYPERTENSION. Hypertension frequently occurs in the postoperative period after coronary artery bypass grafting (CABG) in patients with good left ventricular function. Postoperative hypertension is also common after corrective surgery for aortic stenosis or idiopathic hypertrophic subaortic stenosis (IHSS). Postoperative hypertension is a common problem in patients with a history of hypertension. Hypertension may also be caused by hypoxemia, hypercarbia, shivering, or anxiety. Hypertension is potentially deleterious because it increases myocardial work and increases wall tension, which may result in rupture of aortic suture lines. The treatment of choice for systolic blood pressures over 150 mm Hg is nitroprusside at an initial dose of 0.2 to 0.6 μg/kg/min. The infusion rate should be increased as necessary to achieve the desired effect, setting an upper limit of 8 μg/kg/min. Beta-blockers may be added for additional blood pressure reduction.

In some patients with a hyperdynamic left ventricle (normal stroke volume and increased peripheral resistance), however, sodium nitroprusside treatment may be ineffective. In this group, nitroprusside reduces peripheral resistance, which causes reflex sympathetic stimulation. This unmasks the underlying hyperdynamic heart, and stroke volume, pulse pressure, and heart rate increase [40]. In these patients, nitroprusside decreases EVR, since DPTI falls (due to reduced diastolic pressure and increased heart rate) while SPTI rises (due to increased systolic pressure and increased heart rate). In these instances, nitroprusside must be discontinued.

Beta-blockers are also effective in controlling hypertension in the cardiac surgical patient; esmolol may be given as a 500 μg per kilogram loading dose and an infusion of 50 to 300 μg/kg/min [41]. Sublingual nifedipine, 10 to 20 mg, also may be useful. Diuretics are valuable for managing patients with difficult-to-control hypertension. If the hypertension existed preoperatively, long-term antihypertensive agents should be restarted (see Chaps. 52 and 210).

ARRHYTHMIAS. Arrhythmias cause trouble primarily by reducing cardiac output and blood pressure. At Beth Israel Hospital in Boston, all cardiac surgical patients undergo placement of temporary epicardial pacing wires—two ventricular and two atrial electrodes. The wires are used diagnostically or therapeutically in about 80 percent of patients. Atrial wires facilitate the diagnosis of supraventricular tachycardia when the underlying atrial rhythm is obscure. The previously hidden atrial rhythm becomes obvious when amplified P waves are recorded directly from the atrial wires. The atrial electrical activity can be recorded on a unipolar precordial (V) lead while standard limb leads are in place; the atrial wires can be attached to the right and left arm leads (with standard leg leads in place) and the electrical signals recorded on a bipolar (I) lead or unipolar (II or III) lead.

The atrial wires also can be used for overdrive pacing to convert supraventricular tachycardias, especially atrial flutter. By pacing at a rate faster than the intrinsic atrial rate, the atrium becomes entrained. The critical entrainment rate is evidenced by lead II P waves changing from negative to positive. When the critical entrainment rate has been reached for the critical duration (usually 10–20 sec), the atrial pacer may be slowed and then stopped; atrial rhythm follows the slowing and then converts to sinus mechanism [42]. Alternatively, the pacer may be turned off abruptly. Atrial flutter with an atrial rate of 240 to 340 breaks more easily than a more rapid atrial flutter [42].

The primary use of the pacing wires postoperatively is to increase a slow heart rate (see Table 162-6). For sinus bradycardia, atrial pacing should be used. For a junctional slow rhythm, atrial pacing should be tried, but if any atrioventricular block exists, sequential atrial and ventricular pacing will be necessary. For complete heart block, sequential atrial and ventricular pacing should be used. Postoperatively, cardiac output is 30 percent higher with atrial than with ventricular pacing. In patients with left ventricular hypertrophy, the difference is 40 percent [43], since these patients have a greater need for atrial systole to fill the poorly compliant, hypertrophied ventricle.

TREATMENT OF SPECIFIC ARRHYTHMIAS. Ventricular extrasystoles may be caused by myocardial ischemia, hypokalemia, hypomagnesemia, hypoxia, acidosis, sympathetic stimulation, or irritation related to malpositioned intracardiac catheters. Initial treatment should be directed at eliminating any of the above exacerbating causes. Atrial pacing at a more rapid rate may exceed the rate of firing of an ectopic ventricular focus and then suppress its emergence. In the early postoperative period, ventricular ectopy often occurs when the serum potassium concentration is in the low normal range. Keeping the potassium concentration between 4.5 and 5 mEq per liter and the magnesium greater than 2 mEq per liter tends to suppress ectopic beats [44]. Prophylaxis with lidocaine against ventricular ectopy is not generally necessary [45]. It is not necessary to treat isolated premature ventricular contractions (PVCs). However, if PVCs are causing hemodynamic compromise, lidocaine (50–100 mg bolus intravenously, followed by an intravenous infusion of 2–3 mg/min) usually suppresses them. Since the hepatic metabolism of lidocaine is reduced in the presence of congestive heart failure, the dose should be adjusted downward as the degree of failure increases (Table 162-7) (see Chap. 207). It never has been shown convincingly that nonsustained asymptomatic ventricular extrasystoles justify chronic pharmacologic therapy. Among the risks of treatment are the proarrhythmic effects of most available agents [46].

Ventricular tachycardia (VT) can occur at a relatively slow

Table 162-7. Lidocaine Dosage in Congestive Heart Failure (CHF)*

	Infusion rate (maximal–minimal)	
Class CHF	μg/kg/min	70-kg man (mg/min)
I	88–35	6.2–2.5
II	35–12	2.5–0.8
III + IV	12–5	0.8–0.3

*To achieve therapeutic serum levels at 2.4–6 μg/ml.

rate and depress blood pressure minimally, or it can occur at a rapid rate, leading to severe left ventricular depression. In either case, VT can degenerate into ventricular fibrillation. When VT markedly depresses blood pressure, DC cardioversion should be performed immediately. Cardioversion should be performed using a synchronized (with the QRS) mode with 200 joules, escalating if necessary to 400 joules. In hemodynamically stable patients, lidocaine sometimes terminates VT and obviates the need for cardioversion (see Chap. 207).

Ventricular fibrillation is fatal if not treated immediately. This arrhythmia mandates immediate electrical defibrillation (asynchronous mode) using the same energy levels mentioned above (see Chap. 6). An overall approach to ventricular arrhythmias in the postoperative cardiac surgery patient is found in Table 162-8.

Supraventricular tachycardias occur commonly during the first few postoperative days. Premature atrial contractions often progress to either atrial flutter or atrial fibrillation. These arrhythmias occur in 25 to 33 percent of postoperative cardiac surgical patients and may be due to unprotected atrial ischemia, atrial stretch, administration of hyperkalemic cardioplegic solutions, or pericarditis secondary to surgery [47]. Prophylactic treatment of all postoperative heart surgery patients with propranolol reduces the incidence of atrial fibrillation [48,49]. Patients who were taking beta-blocking agents preoperatively benefit more from propranolol prophylaxis than do patients who were not taking beta-blockers before operation. Procainamide (Procan SR 750 mg orally every 6 hours) can be useful, especially if atrial fibrillation has already occurred. Patients with preoperative atrial fibrillation, especially in the presence of mitral valvular disease, often revert to atrial fibrillation within 2 to 4 days postoperatively whether or not prophylactic drugs are administered.

Atrial fibrillation is usually obvious from the standard ECG. Other supraventricular tachycardias may be more difficult to diagnose, and the diagnosis is sometimes facilitated by examining an atrial wire ECG. When junctional tachycardia occurs, the rapid rate causes inadequate ventricular diastolic filling. In addition, the lack of a normal atrioventricular delay causes mitral and tricuspid regurgitation, because the ventricles contract before the mitral and tricuspid valves have closed. Treatment is directed at slowing atrioventricular conduction by administering digoxin or verapamil (2.5–5 mg IV bolus) followed by atrioventricular sequential pacing.

Atrial flutter often can be treated effectively with atrial overdrive pacing (either by entrainment or by nonspecific rapid stimulation). Atrial fibrillation ordinarily cannot be treated using overdrive pacing. Indeed, atrial fibrillation can be induced when these techniques fail to convert atrial flutter to sinus rhythm. The ventricular response to atrial fibrillation, however, is sometimes slower and better tolerated than that of the ventricular response to atrial flutter. Pharmacologic therapy for atrial flutter has two goals: (1) blockade of the atrioventricular node to decrease ventricular response and (2) conversion to sinus rhythm. Intravenous digoxin (1 mg loading dose), intravenous verapamil (2.5–5 mg) [50], or esmolol (500 μg/kg loading dose and an infusion of 50–300 μg/kg/min) slows the rate by increasing the degree of atrioventricular block. Esmolol may be more effective in restoring sinus rhythm [51]. Beta-blockers and calcium channel blockers should not be used concomitantly. With the atrioventricular node blocked to reduce ventricular rate, quinidine sulfate or procainamide (see Chap. 207) may convert the rhythm to sinus mechanism. Electrical cardioversion may be used if pharmacologic therapy fails to convert atrial flutter.

Atrial fibrillation is treated in the same way as atrial flutter except that overdrive pacing is ineffective. Should ventricular rate be very rapid with adverse hemodynamic effects, immediate electrical cardioversion is necessary. Drug treatment should be initiated concomitantly [52].

An overall approach to supraventricular arrhythmias in the postoperative cardiac surgery patient is found in Table 162-9.

Respiratory Subsystem

Cardiac operations reduce functional residual capacity (FRC), cause alveolar and small airway closure and microatelectasis [53], increase shunting, and decrease arterial oxygenation. The alveolar-arterial oxygen tension gradient typically widens on both the day of and the day after surgery, but then the gradient usually narrows. Positive end-expiratory pressure (PEEP) of 5 cm H_2O helps to restore FRC toward normal [54].

Almost all patients arrive in the cardiac surgical ICU on a ventilator (see Chap. 66). The initial ventilator settings are typically as follows: tidal volume 10 to 15 ml per kilogram; rate 8 to 10 breaths per minute; fractional inspired oxygen concentration (FIO_2) is set at 1.0. After the first set of arterial blood gas measurements returns, the FIO_2 is decreased to maintain the

Table 162-8. Management of Ventricular Arrhythmias

Diagnosis	Treatment
Premature ventricular contractions	Atrial pacing to suppress automatic focus; lidocaine bolus 50–100 mg + lidocaine drip; keep K^+ 4.5–5; eliminate acidosis; $Mg^{2+} > 2$
Ventricular tachycardia	If BP adequate: lidocaine bolus 50–100 mg + lidocaine drip; keep K^+ 4.5–5; eliminate acidosis ischemia; if tachycardia persists, electrical cardioversion $Mg^{2+} > 2$ If BP low; immediate electrical cardioversion, followed by lidocaine, maintain K^+ 4.5–5
Ventricular fibrillation	Immediate defibrillation

BP = blood pressure.

Table 162-9. Management of Supraventricular Arrhythmias

Diagnosis	Treatment
Premature atrial contractions	Atrial pacing at faster rate; digoxin and propranolol ± quinidine
Atrial flutter	If markedly ↓ BP or ischemia: DC cardioversion, followed by digoxin + procainamide If BP adequate and no ischemia: Digoxin + procainamide; overdrive pacing; if heart rate >120 beats/min, verapamil or esmolol to slow
Atrial fibrillation	If markedly ↓ BP or ischemia: DC cardioversion, followed by digoxin + quinidine If BP adequate and no ischemia: Digoxin, followed by procainamide; if heart rate >120 beats/min, verapamil or esmolol

↓ = low; BP = blood pressure; DC = direct current.

PO_2 at 70 to 100 mm Hg; minute volume is regulated to keep PCO_2 at about 40 mm Hg. Oxygen consumption and CO_2 will increase as the patient warms. PEEP is added to keep FIO_2 below 0.5. High levels of PEEP may be necessary when there is a large intrapulmonary shunt.

Controversy exists over the optimal duration of mechanical ventilation. Extubation in the first few hours postoperatively simplifies respiratory management and, in most patients, works satisfactorily; however, at the Beth Israel Hospital, we generally continue mechanical ventilation until the morning after operation. This approach has many advantages. If narcotics were the main anesthetic agent, as is usually the case, duration of anesthesia is not easily predictable and may be many hours. Premature extubation can lead to inadequate ventilation and respiratory collapse. The use of opioid antagonists to reverse the effects of narcotics should be avoided. Narcotic antagonists can cause marked agitation and dangerous hypertension. If there is hemodynamic instability, controlled ventilation allows better control of arterial pH and PCO_2 as well as more vigorous fluid administration without as much worry about adverse pulmonary effects. In the presence of excessive mediastinal bleeding, continued mechanical ventilation permits a smoother return to the operating room if reexploration is necessary. (see Bleeding, following.)

Weaning and extubation are performed in accordance with standard criteria (Table 162-10) (see Chap. 67). Weaning is easiest using intermittent mandatory ventilation (IMV) mode, reducing the rate gradually until the patient is breathing spontaneously. During weaning, arterial blood gases should be measured periodically. Minimal criteria for extubation include a PaO_2 greater than 80 mm Hg with an FIO_2 less than or equal to 0.5, a pH greater than or equal to 7.35, a vital capacity greater than or equal to 15 ml per kilogram, and a maximal inspiratory force greater than or equal to 35 cm H_2O. Additionally, the patient should be alert and awake. The best predictor of success in weaning from mechanical ventilation has been shown to be the ratio of respiratory rate to spontaneous tidal volume. A ratio of less than 100 has been shown to be an accurate predictor of success [55]. Contraindications to weaning from mechanical ventilation include unstable hemodynamics, excessive bleeding, severe acid-base abnormalities, unstable arrhythmias, and patients who are still warming. In patients who are doing well from both cardiac and respiratory standpoints, the presence of an IABP is not a contraindication to weaning and extubation. A complete discussion of the management of mechanical ventilation is found in Chapters 66 and 67.

Rarely, the postoperative course is complicated by fulminant, noncardiogenic pulmonary edema. Left atrial pressures are low, and the protein content of the edema fluid is high—70 to 96 percent that of plasma [56]. The etiology of this phenomenon

appears to be allergic or may be due to white blood cell aggregation and complement activation. Various drugs have been implicated, including protamine and plasma protein fractions [57].

In addition to the pulmonary edema, severe bronchospasm may occur. Generalized edema occurs, with a vivid *peau d'orange* being the cutaneous response. Myocardial edema leads to left ventricular depression and decreased ventricular compliance. The lungs become so stiff and often so overdistended that inadequate space exists in the chest for both heart and lungs; accordingly, attempted sternal closure can cause cardiac tamponade. Reinstitution of cardiopulmonary bypass may be necessary [58]. If this syndrome begins in the ICU, it can be fatal. Treatment is supportive and empirical, consisting of PEEP, diuretics, steroids, antihistamines, and pulmonary vasodilators. If the PEEP interferes excessively with cardiac function, insertion of an IABP may help improve cardiac output.

After extubation, cardiac surgical patients are usually mildly hypoxic on room air. Oxygen therapy is usually required for several days because of increased lung water and the development of atelectasis, pleural effusions, and other pulmonary complications. Pulse oximetry is useful for determining whether supplemental oxygen therapy can be safely discontinued.

Pneumonia is generally not seen in this group of patients until 48 to 72 hours postoperatively. Other causes of hypoxemia include aspiration and atelectasis. Pulmonary embolus is unusual in the early postoperative period.

The phrenic nerve may be injured at the time of surgery both by surgical manipulation and by cooling [59]. In a patient with good pulmonary function preoperatively, the postoperative course will not be affected. However, in the patient with marginal reserves, prolonged ventilatory support may be necessary. Poor diaphragmatic function must be suspected if there is paradoxical breathing when weaning, elevated diaphragm on x-ray, or decreased vital capacity. The diagnosis can usually be made with fluoroscopy.

Renal Subsystem

Renal function reflects cardiac function. With adequate cardiac output, most postcardiac surgical patients have a high urine output, usually greater than 50 ml per hour. When urine output is lower, the clinician should suspect poor renal function caused by low cardiac output, low blood pressure, or locally obstructed renal arteries.

Many patients exhibit a marked diuresis in the immediate postoperative period, with urine outputs of 200 to 500 ml per hour. The cause of this diuresis is multifactorial. Hypothermia diminishes flow to the outer renal cortex, decreases the free water clearance, and increases the filtration fraction [60]. Atrial distention may promote the release of atrial natriuretic factor and inhibit the release of vasopressin. Hypothermia may cause redistribution of blood volume more centrally. A marked diuresis is generally not seen in those patients who have acute reductions in chronically elevated left atrial pressures [61].

Salt and water, accumulated during the intraoperative and early postoperative periods, are excreted over the first several days postoperatively. In patients who are healthy, the diuresis usually begins on the second postoperative day.

Renal failure following heart surgery occurs infrequently, but it carries a high mortality rate (27–47%) [62,63]. Postoperative renal failure is associated with preoperative renal insufficiency, advanced age, prolonged operation, prolonged cardiopulmonary bypass, and perioperative left ventricular dysfunction. Fac-

---

Table 162-10. Criteria for Extubation

1. PaO_2 > 80 mm Hg with FIO_2 ≤ 0.5
2. pH ≥ 7.35 (no respiratory acidosis)
3. VC ≥ 15 cc/kg
4. MIF ≥ 35 cm H_2O
5. Demonstrated satisfactory ventilation on CPAP/T-piece
6. Alert, awake, able to protect airway
7. No excessive bleeding, hemodynamic instability, unstable arrhythmias
8. Normothermic

PaO_2 = arterial oxygen tension; FIO_2 = fraction of oxygen in inspired air; CPAP = continuous positive airway pressure; VC = vital capacity; MIF = maximal inspiratory force.

tors that increase the risk of perioperative renal failure include exposure to contrast media, perioperative use of aminoglycosides, nonsteroidal antiinflammatory agents, or angiotensin-converting enzyme inhibitors. At present, there is little evidence that low doses of dopamine prevent or modify established renal failure. Lasix and dopamine may, however, make management easier by allowing removal of fluid and electrolytes.

Fluid Administration

Despite an increase in total body water many postoperative patients also are intravascularly volume depleted during the first few hours in the ICU. The rewarming that occurs over the early postoperative hours causes progressive peripheral vasodilatation and relative hypovolemia. Rapid volume repletion is often required. The best fluid to use for resuscitation remains controversial. Deficiencies in red cell mass call for administration of packed red blood cells. If hematocrit is adequate (23–27%), then one can infuse any of several acellular volume expanders, including balanced salt solutions, albumin, or hydroxyethyl starch.

Bleeding

The most common and potentially the most serious immediate postoperative problem is excessive bleeding. Control of excessive bleeding begins in the preoperative period when potential causes are sought. A careful history provides the best clue to intrinsic bleeding problems. Patients taking aspirin or antiinflammatory drugs usually have some degree of platelet dysfunction. Screening tests include PT, PTT, platelet count, and bleeding time. Specific abnormalities require further evaluation and correction before performing elective heart surgery (see Chap. 118). Preoperative use of antiplatelet agents, thrombolytic agents, and heparin increases the incidence of preoperative coagulation defects and the probability of excessive postoperative bleeding.

Intraoperative factors can predispose to bleeding. Inadequate heparin administration results in excessive consumption of clotting factors. Inadequate neutralization of heparin with protamine leaves residual heparin activity. Improved titration of heparin and protamine can be achieved by assaying heparin activity either indirectly with an activated clotting time (ACT) or directly with a heparin analyzer [64–68]. Prolonged cardiopulmonary bypass causes platelet dysfunction and depletion and dilution of clotting factors. The resultant increase in bleeding causes further loss of clotting factors, and thus a vicious cycle may ensue where bleeding causes further bleeding.

When evaluating excessive postoperative bleeding, the possibility of surgical bleeding always must be considered. Abnormalities of systemic clotting include residual heparin activity, excessive fibrinolysis, excessive clotting factor consumption, and thrombocytopenia. These abnormalities must be corrected rapidly to reduce bleeding and to allow determination of the need to reoperate on patients for surgical bleeding. Nevertheless, disseminated intravascular coagulation (DIC) occurs rarely, while a substantial body of evidence suggests that some primary fibrinolysis occurs routinely during cardiopulmonary bypass (see Chap. 118).

A standard battery of screening tests enables an assessment of postoperative clotting mechanisms. We routinely obtain a PT, PTT, and platelet count in the postoperative period. If residual heparin effect is suspected, a thrombin time (TT) and reptilase time are obtained. A systematic analysis of clotting disorders may be based on Table 162-11. Platelets may be deficient in function as well as in number; cardiopulmonary bypass causes both defects [65].

Treatment is based on the diagnosis, although the diagnosis may not be straightforward because the pathogenesis of abnormal clotting may be mixed. Residual heparin effect is a common problem. Even though heparin was fully reversed after the operation, heparin rebound can occur as heparin that was stored in body fat elutes into the blood. Heparin rebound is the most common cause for prolonged PTT and TT [66]. A normal reptilase time establishes this diagnosis, and additional protamine treats it.

Table 162-11. Excessive Bleeding from Clotting Abnormalities in the Postoperative Cardiac Surgery Patient

	Tests							
Cause	PT	PTT	TT	Platelet count	RT	FIB	FSP	Treatment
Heparin excess	N–			N	N	N	N	Protamine sulfate titrated with ACT or heparin assay
Excessive primary fibrinolysis		N–Sl		N		N–		EACA 4–8 gm IV over 10 min followed by 1 gm/hr infusion for 5–8 hr (until clotting factors N); FFP to regulate clotting factors
Compensated[a]	N							
Uncompensated[a]				N				
Excessive consumption[b]								Treat cause: FFP, cryoprecipitate, platelets
Thrombocytopenia or platelet dysfunction[c]	N	N	N		N	N	N	Platelets
"Undefined"[d]	Sl		Sl	N	N	N	N	FFP, cryoprecipitate, ? EACA

[a] *Compensated* refers to a minor fibrinolysis under which the body can keep up with the deficiencies; *uncompensated* refers to a rapid process under which the body cannot keep up with the fibrinolysis.
[b] Rare excessive consumption (also known as *diffuse intravascular coagulation* [DIC]) always has associated secondary fibrinolysis.
[c] Platelets may be reduced in function as well as number.
[d] This group, probably of mixed etiology, occurs frequently.
PT = prothrombin time; PTT = partial thromboplastin time; TT = thrombin time; RT = reptilase time; FIB = fibrinogen; FSP = fibrin-split products; ACT = activated clotting time; EACA = epsilon-aminocaproic acid; FFP = fresh-frozen plasma; N = normal; Sl = slightly; = elevated; = very elevated; = low; = very low.

Excessive primary fibrinolysis and excessive consumption may be indistinguishable by the tests listed, although the latter condition is usually characterized by a lower platelet count. Treatment of DIC should be aimed at its cause. Treatment of primary fibrinolysis consists of repleting clotting factors and infusing an antifibrinolytic agent, epsilon-aminocaproic acid (EACA). Cryoprecipitate is the cold-insoluble protein fraction of plasma and is rich in factor V, factor VIII, von Willebrand factor, and fibrinogen. It is more concentrated than fresh-frozen plasma, but, because it is a pooled product, it carries a higher risk of transfusion-related infection. Fresh-frozen plasma contains all of the clotting factors, as well as anti-erythrocyte antibodies. It is given as a type-specific product, and is available only after a thawing period of 45 minutes.

When platelet dysfunction is suspected, either on the basis of preoperative aspirin intake or prolonged cardiopulmonary bypass, platelets should be transfused. Although there has been some enthusiasm in recent years for administering desmopressin acetate (DDAVP) to either all cardiac surgical patients or to those with excessive bleeding after heparin reversal, the majority of controlled trials have not supported routine use of this drug [69]. We use DDAVP in those patients undergoing complex cardiac operations [70].

In some centers, PEEP is used to help control bleeding after cardiac surgery. Some studies have shown a marked diminution of bleeding with levels of PEEP from 10 to 20 cm H_2O [71,72], whereas others have not [73].

Bleeding in most patients is successfully controlled by these measures. In those who continue to bleed excessively, a surgically correctable cause must be sought and repaired. The definition of *excessive bleeding* varies with each patient. As a general guideline, however, bleeding is excessive when drainage from chest tubes is greater than 400 ml per hour for the first hour, 300 ml per hour for the first 2 hours, 200 ml per hour for the first 3 consecutive hours, or 100 ml per hour over the first 6 hours. A sudden increase in bleeding suggests an arterial source and mandates reexploration. Bleeding that will flow uphill in the mediastinal tubes indicates that the patient should be reexplored. Bleeding sufficient to cause marked hypotension or tamponade also requires reexploration. Massive bleeding necessitates emergency reexploration, regardless of any clotting abnormalities.

When bleeding is so rapid that cardiac arrest occurs or is imminent, the patient should *not* be brought back to the operating room to control bleeding. Instead, the sternotomy should be reopened immediately in the ICU, where finger pressure on the obvious site of bleeding almost always controls it. Transfusions are administered to increase blood volume and blood pressure. With the bleeding temporarily controlled, the patient and the operation are transferred to the operating room for definitive control. Patients with emergency exploration for bleeding in the ICU have a survival of 60 percent and a wound infection rate of 5 percent [74].

The increasing use of autotransfusion over the past 15 years has reduced requirements for transfusing homologous blood. Two methods of autotransfusion are widely available. In the first, a closed system is created in which shed blood is collected in a reservoir. An outlet port of the reservoir is connected to the patient's intravenous access, and a peristaltic pump is used to infuse the blood. The pump is adjusted each hour to return the previous hour's losses. With the second method, blood for autotransfusion is collected in a removable chamber that is part of the standard chest drainage system. If and when autotransfusion is required, this chamber is removed from the system, and the contents are reinfused by gravity drainage, much like a homologous transfusion. With either method, 20 μM filtering is required. It has been demonstrated that autotransfused blood is extensively defibrinated [75]. While the plasma component of the transfusate is very deficient in clotting factors (platelets, factor VII, fibrinogen), there is no evidence to suggest that autotransfusion compromises the function of circulating clotting factors or is a cause of fibrinolysis.

Fever and Antibiotics

Systemic warming before the termination of cardiopulmonary bypass brings the core temperature to 37°C, but cooling subsequently occurs as heat transfers to the cool extremities. Patients routinely have temperatures in the 34 to 36°C range when they arrive in the ICU. Warming, shivering, and vasodilatation occur during the first several hours, and a temperature overshoot commonly occurs after 6 to 12 hours. Temperatures in the 38 to 39°C range at this time should be expected and require no further evaluation. However, fever during subsequent days is abnormal and requires the usual investigation (see Chap. 84).

Prophylactic antibiotic usage is widely recommended because of the extraordinary seriousness of infections of mediastinum, sternum, cardiac suture lines, and prosthetic valves. Although staphylococcal infections are the greatest concern, antibiotics with broad-spectrum coverage are generally used in preference to specific antistaphylococcal antibiotics [76]. Antibiotics should be stopped within 2 days; administration for a longer period offers no advantage and may result in more serious infections [77]. Low serum antibiotic levels at the end of surgery correlate with an increased incidence of infection [77].

One-third of all hospital-acquired bacteremias and most candidemias are associated with vascular catheters [78]. One and one-half percent of vascular catheters yield positive cultures, and pulmonary artery catheters have the highest rate of colonization (2.1%) [79]. Catheter-related sepsis is most commonly due to coagulase-negative staphylococci and cannot be treated successfully with antibiotics unless the catheter is removed. A 7- to 10-day course of systemic antibiotics is then usually sufficient, although 4 to 6 weeks is necessary for cases of septic venous thrombosis. Infection from invasive lines is best prevented by removing invasive lines as soon as they are no longer needed.

Mediastinal infections are seen in about 1 percent of postoperative cardiac surgical patients. Risk factors include long operation, re-operation, low cardiac output, and prolonged mechanical ventilation [80]. Mental status changes, fever, rising white blood cell count, drainage from chest wounds, sternal click, or new pneumonia, all may signal development of such an infection. These patients should be returned to the operating room for debridement and irrigation with dilute povidone-iodine solution.

Psychological and Neurologic Dysfunction

Both central and peripheral nervous system dysfunction occur postoperatively. The former can be far more serious and range from minor transient ischemic episodes to frank strokes. These events may be caused by emboli of air, clot, or other particulate matter (e.g., calcified pieces of debrided valve) and are associated with prior carotid bruits [81]. Diffuse metabolic encephalopathy also occurs in very sick patients and improves as overall condition improves.

Peripheral neuropathies occur in the legs from bleeding in the groin leading to femoral nerve compression and from pressure on the peroneal nerve, usually in patients operated on in a frog-legged position to facilitate removal of the saphenous vein. Both neuropathies are preventable. Dysfunction in the distribution of C_8-T_1 occurs from lower cord brachial plexus injury during the operation [82,83]. Sternal retraction can force the first rib into the brachial plexus [83] or break the rib, with resultant penetration of the plexus by a sharp fragment [82]. These neuropathies improve with time.

Postoperative psychological dysfunction occurs in 40 to 60 percent of patients [84,85]. Three types have been described: (1) an organic syndrome, which corresponds to the central metabolic neurologic dysfunction described above; (2) a postcardiotomy delirium, occurring after a lucid interval; and (3) a postcardiotomy depressive syndrome [86]. Multiple risk factors for the latter two syndromes have been identified, including increased use of anticholinergic drugs [86], elevated preoperative blood urea nitrogen or decreased body weight [85], decreased body temperature while on cardiopulmonary bypass [84], and increased magnitude of overall preoperative sickness [84]. Patients undergoing valve operations are affected more commonly than are patients undergoing coronary revascularization. The incidence seems to be higher in the elderly. Postulated pathogenic mechanisms include cerebral microemboli, cerebral red cell sludging, and sensory deprivation [84].

Treatment of the depressed patient begins with frequent reassurance. Antidepressant drugs may be useful in severe cases. In patients with postcardiotomy delirium, helpful measures include frequent contact with relatives, general reassurance, and provision of adequate sleep. Removing the patient from the ICU is desirable. The most effective short-term management is the administration of small doses of intravenous haloperidol (1–2 mg or more).

Gastrointestinal Complications

A nasogastric tube is placed in the operating room and used routinely to prevent postoperative gastric distention. It is placed to suction, but it is clamped for 1 1/2 hours after administering medications through the tube. In most cases the tube can be removed on the first postoperative day after endotracheal extubation. If gastric distention develops, the nasogastric tube should be replaced promptly.

Approximately half of the patients with gastrointestinal complications following cardiac surgery have a history of previous gastrointestinal disease. Depressed gastrointestinal motility is often related to low cardiac output and the resultant redistribution of blood flow away from the splanchnic bed (see Chaps. 163 and 171). Diminished peristalsis can lead to potentially fatal complications. Cecal distention can lead to cecal necrosis. Aggressive management is indicated when cecal diameter exceeds 12 cm. Colonoscopic decompression is usually successful, although operative diversion or resection is sometimes necessary. Bowel ischemia and bowel infarction can be caused by embolism or low mesenteric flow. Emboli can originate from the heart, from an atherosclerotic aorta, or from suture lines communicating with the systemic circulation. Atrial fibrillation predisposes to the formation of atrial thrombi and embolization. Low cardiac output, alpha-adrenergic pressors, and digoxin all increase the risk of low mesenteric flow (see Chap. 163). When bowel ischemia or infarction is suspected, laparotomy should be performed urgently.

Postoperative cholecystitis and cholangitis are difficult to diagnose because upper abdominal pain and tenderness are commonly related to the surgical incision and mediastinal tubes. Mild hyperbilirubinemia is also common in the postoperative period. An enlarged acalculous gallbladder may be the only finding on ultrasonography. Nuclear scans (HIDA) must be interpreted cautiously in patients with no oral intake.

To prevent upper gastrointestinal ulceration and bleeding, the gastric pH should be maintained above 4.0. Both H-2 blockers and antacids may be required. Sucralfate is also an effective prophylactic agent and, because it does not reduce acidity, may decrease colonization of the upper gastrointestinal tract with gram-negative organisms [87]. The early institution of enteral feedings may also reduce the incidence of gastrointestinal bleeding [88].

Pancreatitis is a potentially lethal complication of cardiac surgery. Its occurrence is probably related to reduced splanchnic blood flow, and therefore it tends to occur in patients with associated cardiac complications. In approximately one-third of cardiac surgical patients, there is a significant rise in the level of serum amylase (>300 IU/L) by the second postoperative day [89]. However, clinically overt pancreatitis occurs in only approximately 2 percent of patients. Nonpancreatitic hyperamylasemia is associated with increased mortality. The cause is unknown [90].

Mesenteric ischemia secondary to embolism or poor perfusion must be suspected in the cardiac surgical patient with a metabolic acidosis, low SVR, and increased white blood cell count in the postoperative period.

Endocrine Complications

The most common endocrine abnormality requiring postoperative management is diabetes mellitus. In known diabetics, insulin requirements increase during the postoperative period due to increases in the serum levels of counter-regulatory hormones [91]. Patients are most easily managed with a continuous insulin infusion. During cardiac operations, insulin requirements under hypothermia are low but increase dramatically during rewarming. Insulin requirements usually decrease by the third postoperative day as the stress of surgery diminishes. However, intensive management of diabetes may be necessary when the patient resumes an oral diet. It is not uncommon for non–insulin-dependent diabetics to require insulin at the time of discharge.

Thyroid dysfunction can occur in seriously ill patients who were euthyroid preoperatively. The perioperative determination of thyroid function is difficult because of abnormalities in T_4 binding and the fact that thyroid-stimulating hormone responds sluggishly to decreased T_3 and T_4 levels in critically ill patients. The possibility of hypothyroidism should be entertained in any postoperative patient who has unexplained hemodynamic dysfunction and is experiencing a prolonged and complicated postoperative course.

Miscellaneous Therapeutic Measures

The incidence of coronary graft occlusion over the first year postoperatively can be reduced by perioperative treatment and then chronic treatment with aspirin and dipyridamole [92]. This regimen does not cause increased bleeding, but these drugs should not be given to patients with peptic ulcer disease.

References

1. Kirklin JW: *Systems Analysis in Surgical Patients (The Macewen Memorial Lectures, 15)*. Glasgow, University of Glasgow, 1970.
2. Mammana RB, Hiro S, Levitsky S, et al: Inaccuracy of pulmonary capillary wedge pressure when compared to left atrial pressure in the early postsurgical period. *J Thorac Cardiovasc Surg* 84:420, 1982.
3. Glower DD, Spratt JA, Snow ND, et al: Linearity of the Frank-Starling relationship in the intact heart: The concept of preload recruitable stroke work. *Circulation* 71:994, 1985.
4. Suga H, Sagawa K: Instantaneous pressure-volume relationships and their ratio in the excised, supported canine left ventricle. *Circ Res* 35:117, 1974.
5. Suga H: Total mechanical energy of a ventricle model and cardiac oxygen consumption. *Am J Physiol* 236:H, 1979.
6. Hoffman JIE, Buckberg GD: The myocardial supply:demand ratio—A critical review. *Am J Cardiol* 41:327, 1978.
7. Taylor KM, Morton JJ, Brown JJ, et al: Hypertension and the renin-angiotensin system following open-heart surgery. *J Thorac Cardiovasc Surg* 74:840, 1977.
8. Rodriguez JL, Weissman C, Damask MC, et al: Physiologic requirements during rewarming: Suppression of the shivering response. *Crit Care Med* 11:490, 1983.
9. Zwischenberger JB, Kirsh MM, Dechert RE, et al: Suppression of shivering decreases oxygen consumption and improves hemodynamic stability during postoperative rewarming. *Ann Thorac Surg* 43:428, 1987.
10. Kirklin JK, Kirklin JW: Management of the cardiovascular subsystem after cardiac surgery. *Ann Thorac Surg* 32:311, 1981.
11. Applebaum A, et al: Early risks of open heart surgery for mitral valve disease. *Am J Cardiol* 37:201, 1976.
12. Dietzman RH, Ersek RA, Lillehei CW, et al: Low output syndrome. Recognition and treatment. *J Thorac Cardiovasc Surg* 57:138, 1969.
13. Parr GVS, Blackstone EH, Kirklin JW: Cardiac performance and mortality early after intracardiac surgery in infants and young children. *Circulation* 51:867, 1975.
14. Chenoweth DE, Cooper SW, Hugli TE, et al: Complement activation during cardiopulmonary bypass. Evidence for generation of C3a and C5a anaphylatoxins. *N Engl J Med* 304:497, 1981.
15. Moore FD Jr, Warner KG, Assousa S, et al: The effects of complement activation during cardiopulmonary bypass. *Ann Surg* 208:95, 1988.
16. Zeff RH, Iannone LA, Kongtahworn C, et al: Coronary artery spasm following coronary artery revascularization. *Ann Thorac Surg* 34:196, 1982.
17. Kopf GS, Riba A, Zito R: Intraoperative use of nifedipine for hemodynamic collapse due to coronary artery spasm following myocardial revascularization. *Ann Thorac Surg* 34:457, 1982.
18. Lemmer JH Jr, Kirsch MM: Coronary artery spasm following coronary artery surgery. *Ann Thorac Surg* 46:108, 1988.
19. Codd JE, Wiens RD, Kaiser GC, et al: Late sequelae of perioperative myocardial infarction. *Ann Thorac Surg* 26:208, 1978.
20. Smith PK, Buhrman WC, Ferguson TB Jr, et al: Conduction block following cardioplegic arrest: Prevention by augmented atrial hypothermia. *Circulation* (Suppl) 68:II-1, 1983.
21. Smith PK, Buhrman WC, Ferguson TB Jr, et al: Relationship of atrial hypothermia and cardioplegic solution potassium concentration to postoperative conduction defects. *Surg Forum* 34:304, 1983.
22. Simpson MB Jr: Adverse reactions to transfusion therapy: Clinical and laboratory aspects, in Koepke JA (ed): *Laboratory Hematology*. New York, Churchill Livingstone, 1984, Vol 2, Chap 44.
23. Mullen JC, Miller DR, Weisel RD, et al: Postoperative hypertension: A comparison of diltiazem, nifedipine, and nitroprusside. *J Thorac Cardiovasc Surg* 96:122, 1988.
24. Chiariello M, Gold HK, Leinbach RC, et al: Comparison between the effects of nitroprusside and nitroglycerin on ischemic injury during acute myocardial infarction. *Circulation* 54:766, 1976.
25. Kaplan JA, Finlayson DC, Woodward S: Vasodilator therapy after cardiac surgery: A review of the efficacy and toxicity of nitroglycerin and nitroprusside. *Can Anaesth Soc J* 27:254, 1980.
26. Dinardo JA, Bert A, Schwartz MJ, et al: Effects of vasoactive drugs on flows through internal mammary artery and saphenous vein grafts in man. *J Thorac Cardiovasc Surg* 102:730, 1991.
27. Ko W, Zelano JA, Fahey AL, et al: The effects of amrinone versus dobutamine on myocardial mechanics and energetics after hypothermic global ischemia. *J Thorac Cardiovasc Surg* 105:1015, 1993.
28. Goto Y, Slinker BK, LeWinter MM: Effects of amrinone and isoproterenol on mechanoenergetics of blood-perfused rabbit heart. *Am J Physiol* 262:H719,1992.
29. Klein NA, Siskind SJ, Frishman WH, et al: Hemodynamic comparison of intravenous amrinone and dobutamine in patients with chronic congestive heart failure. *Am J Cardiol* 48:170, 1981.
30. Prielipp RC, Butterworth JF, Zaloga GP, et al: Effects of amrinone on cardiac index, mixed venous oxygen saturation and venous admixture in patients recovering from cardiac surgery. *Chest* 99:820, 1991.
31. McEnany MT, Morgan RJ, Mundth ED, et al: Circumvention of detrimental pulmonary vasoactivity of exogenous catecholamines in cardiac resuscitation. *Surg Forum* 26:98, 1975.
32. D'Ambra MN, La Raia PJ, Philbin DM, et al: Prostaglandin E1—A new therapy for refractory right heart failure and pulmonary hypertension after mitral valve replacement. *J Thorac Cardiovasc Surg* 89:567, 1985.
33. Isner JM, Cohen RS, Virmani R, et al: Complications of the intraaortic balloon counterpulsation device: Clinical and morphologic observations in 45 necropsy patients. *Am J Cardiol* 46:260, 1980.
34. Harris RE, Reimer KA, Crain BJ, et al: Spinal cord infarction following intra-aortic balloon support. *Ann Thorac Surg* 42:206, 1986.
35. Goldberg MJ, Rubenfire M, Kantrowitz A, et al: Intra-aortic balloon pump insertion: A randomized study comparing percutaneous and surgical techniques. *J Am Coll Cardiol* 9:515, 1987.
36. Bernhard WF, Berger RL, Stetz JP, et al: Temporary left ventricular bypass: Factors affecting patient survival. *Circulation* 60(2 Pt 2):131, 1979.
37. Norman JC, Igo SR: Mechanical circulatory assistance: Established (IABP) and evolving (LVAD). A narrative summary. *Thorac Cardiovasc Surg* 33:133, 1985.
38. Frazier OH, Wampler RK, Davian SM, et al: First human use of the Hemopump, a catheter-mounted ventricular assist device. *Ann Thorac Surg* 49:299, 1990.
39. Shabetai R: Changing concepts of cardiac tamponade. *J Am Coll Cardiol* 12:194, 1988.
40. Sladen RN: Management of the adult cardiac patient in the intensive care unit, in Ream AK, Fogdall RP (eds): *Acute Cardiovascular Management Anesthesia and Intensive Care*. Philadelphia, JB Lippincott, 1982.
41. Gray RJ, Bateman TM, Czer LSC, et al: Comparison of esmolol and nitroprusside for acute post-surgical hypertension. *Am J Cardiol* 59:887, 1987.
42. Waldo AL, Wells JL Jr, Plumb VJ, et al: Studies of atrial flutter following open heart surgery. *Annu Rev Med* 30:259, 1979.
43. Friesen WG, Woodson RD, Ames AW, et al: A hemodynamic comparison of atrial and ventricular pacing in postoperative cardiac surgical patients. *J Thorac Cardiovasc Surg* 55:271, 1968.
44. England MR, Gordon G, Salem M, et al: Magnesium administration and dysrhythmias after cardiac surgery: A prospective controlled, double blind, randomized trial. *JAMA* 68:2395, 1992.
45. Johnson RG, Goldberger AL, Thurer RL, et al: Lidocaine prophylaxis in coronary revascularization patients: A randomised, prospective trial. *Ann Thorac Surg* 55:1180, 1993.
46. Zipes DP: Proarrhythmic events. *Am J Cardiol* 61:70A, 1988.
47. Smith PK, Buhrman WC, Levett JM, et al: Supraventricular conduction abnormalities following cardiac operations: A complication of inadequate atrial preservation. *J Thorac Cardiovasc Surg* 85:105, 1983.
48. Stephenson LW, MacVaugh H 3rd, Tomasello DN, et al: Propranolol for prevention of postoperative cardiac arrhythmias: A randomized study. *Ann Thorac Surg* 29:113, 1980.
49. Mohr R, Smolinsky A, Goor DA: Prevention of supraventricular

tachyarrhythmia with low-dose propranolol after coronary bypass. *J Thorac Cardiovasc Surg* 81:840, 1981.

50. Plumb VJ, Karp RB, Kouchoukos NT, et al: Verapamil therapy of atrial fibrillation and atrial flutter following cardiac operation. *J Thorac Cardiovasc Surg* 83:590, 1982.

51. Platia EV, Michelson EL, Porterfield JK, et al: Esmolol versus verapamil in the acute treatment of atrial fibrillation or atrial flutter. *Am J Cardiol* 63:925, 1989.

52. Lauer MS, Eagle KA: Atrial fibrillation following cardiac surgery, in Falk RH, Podrid PJ (eds): *Atrial Fibrillation: Mechanisms and Management*. New York, Raven Press, 1992.

53. Matthay M, Wiener-Kronish JP: Respiratory management after cardiac surgery. *Chest* 95:424, 1989.

54. Downs JB, Mitchell LA: Pulmonary effects of ventilatory pattern following cardiopulmonary bypass. *Crit Care Med* 4:295, 1976.

55. Tobin MJ, Yang KL: A prospective study of indexes predicting the outcome of trials of weaning from mechanical ventilation. *N Engl J Med* 324:1445, 1991.

56. Culliford AT, Thomas S, Spencer FC: Fulminating noncardiogenic pulmonary edema: A newly recognized hazard during cardiac operations. *J Thorac Cardiovasc Surg* 80:868, 1980.

57. Olinger GN, Becker RM, Bonchek LI: Noncardiogenic pulmonary edema and peripheral vascular collapse following cardiopulmonary bypass: Rare protamine reaction? *Ann Thorac Surg* 29:20 1980.

58. Maggart M, Stewart S: The mechanisms and management of noncardiogenic pulmonary edema following cardiopulmonary bypass. *Ann Thorac Surg* 43:231, 1987.

59. Espositio RA, Spencer FC: The effect of pericardial insulation on hypothermic phrenic nerve injury during open-heart surgery. *Ann Thorac Surg* 43:303, 1987.

60. Utley JR, Wachtel C, Cain RB, et al: Effects of hypothermic, hemodilution, and pump oxygenation on organ water content, blood flow and oxygen delivery, and renal function. *Ann Thorac Surg* 31:121, 1981.

61. Shannon RP, Libby E, Elahi D, et al: Impact of acute reduction in chronically elevated left atrial pressure on sodium and water excretion. *Ann Thorac Surg* 46:430, 1988.

62. Gailiunas P Jr, Chawla R, Lazarus JM, et al: Acute renal failure following cardiac operations. *J Thorac Cardiovasc Surg* 79:241, 1980.

63. Holper K, Struck E, Sebening F: The diagnosis of acute renal failure (ARF) following cardiac surgery with cardio-pulmonary bypass. *Thorac Cardiovasc Surg* 27:231, 1979.

64. Kaul TK, Crow MJ, Rajah SM, et al: Heparin administration during extracorporeal circulation. Heparin rebound and postoperative bleeding. *J Thorac Cardiovasc Surg* 78:95, 1979.

65. Van Oeveren W, Kazatchkine MD, Descamps-Latsha B, et al: Deleterious effects of cardiopulmonary bypass. A prospective study of bubble versus membrane oxygenation. *J Thorac Cardiovasc Surg* 89:888, 1985.

66. Pifarre R, Babka R, Sullivan HJ, et al: Management of postoperative heparin rebound following cardiopulmonary bypass. *J Thorac Cardiovasc Surg* 81:378, 1981.

67. Bull BS, et al: Heparin therapy during extracorporeal circulation: I. Problems inherent in existing protocols. *J Thorac Cardiovasc Surg* 69:674, 1975.

68. Bull BS, Huse WM, Brauer FS, et al: Heparin therapy during extracorporeal circulation: II. The use of a dose-response curve to individualize heparin and protamine dosage. *J Thorac Cardiovasc Surg* 69:685, 1975.

69. Rocha E, Llorens R, Paramo JA, et al: Does desmopressin acetate reduce blood loss after surgery in patients on cardiopulmonary bypass? *Circulation* 77:1319, 1988.

70. Salzman EW, Weinstein MJ, Weintraub RM, et al: Treatment with desmopressin acetate to reduce blood loss after cardiac surgery. *N Engl J Med* 314:1402, 1986.

71. Ilabaca PA, Ochsner JL, Mills NL: Positive end-expiratory pressure in the management of the patient with a postoperative bleeding heart. *Ann Thorac Surg* 30:281, 1980.

72. Hoffman WS, Tomasello DN, MacVaugh H: Control of post-cardiotomy bleeding with PEEP. *Ann Thorac Surg* 34:71, 1982.

73. Zurick AM, Ursua J, Ghattas M, et al: Failure of positive end-expiratory pressure to decrease postoperative bleeding after cardiac surgery. *Ann Thorac Surg* 34:608, 1982.

74. Fairman RM, Edmunds LH Jr: Emergency thoracotomy in the surgical intensive care unit after open cardiac operation. *Ann Thorac Surg* 32:386, 1981.

75. Hartz RS, Smith JA, Green D: Autotransfusion after cardiac operation. *J Thorac Cardiovasc Surg* 96:178, 1988.

76. Kreter B, Woods M: Antibiotic prophylaxis for cardiothoracic operations: Meta-analysis of thirty years of clinical trials. *J Thorac Cardiovasc Surg* 104:590, 1992.

77. Goldmann DA, Hopkins CC, Karchmer AW, et al: Cephalothin prophylaxis in cardiac valve surgery: A prospective, double-blind comparison of two-day and six-day regimens. *J Thorac Cardiovasc Surg* 73:470, 1977.

78. Maki DG: Infections associated with intravascular lines, in Remington JS, Swartz MN (eds): *Current Clinical Topics in Infectious Diseases*. New York, McGraw-Hill, 1982.

79. Damen J, Verhoef J, Bolton DT, et al: Microbiologic risk of invasive hemodynamic monitoring in patients undergoing open-heart operations. *Crit Care Med* 13:548, 1985.

80. Grossi EA, Culliford AT, Krieger KH, et al: A survey of 77 major infectious complications of median sternotomy: A review of 7,949 consecutive operative procedures. *Ann Thorac Surg* 40:214, 1985.

81. Reed GL 3rd, Singer DE, Picard EH, et al: Stroke following coronary bypass surgery: A case control estimate of the risk from carotid bruits. *N Engl J Med* 319:1246, 1988.

82. Vander Salm TJ, Cereda JM, Cutler BS. Brachial plexus injury following median sternotomy. *J Thorac Cardiovasc Surg* 80:447, 1980.

83. Kirsh MM, Magee KR, Gago O, et al: Brachial plexus injury following median sternotomy incision. *Ann Thorac Surg* 11:315, 1971.

84. Dubin WR, Field HL, Gastfriend DR: Postcardiotomy delirium: A critical review. *J Thorac Cardiovasc Surg* 77:586, 1979.

85. Huse-Kleinstoll G, Dahme B, Flemming B, et al: Open-heart surgery: Somatic predictors of post-operative psychopathology. *Thorac Cardiovasc Surg* 27:271, 1979.

86. Summers WK: Psychiatric sequelae to cardiotomy. *J Cardiovasc Surg* 20:471, 1979.

87. duMoulin GC, Paterson DG, Hedley-Whyte J, et al: Aspiration of bacteria in antacid treated patient: A frequent cause of post-operative colonization of the airway. *Lancet* 1:242, 1982.

88. Pingleton SK, Hadzima SK: Enteral alimentation and gastrointestinal bleeding in mechanically ventilated patients. *Crit Care Med* 11:13, 1983.

89. Svenson LG, Decker G, Kinsley RB: A prospective study of hyperamylasemia and pancreatitis after cardiopulmonary bypass. *Ann Thorac Surg* 39:409, 1985.

90. Rattner DW, Guz Y, Vlahakes GJ: Hyperamylasemia after cardiac surgery. Incidence, significance, and management. *Ann Surg* 209:279, 1989.

91. Crock PA, Ley CJ, Martin IK, et al: Hormonal and metabolic changes during hypothermic coronary artery bypass surgery in diabetic and nondiabetic subjects. *Diabetic Med* 5:47, 1988.

92. Chesebro JH, Clements IP, Fuster V, et al: A platelet-inhibitor-drug trial in coronary artery bypass operations. Benefit of perioperative dipyridamole and aspirin therapy on early postoperative vein graft patency. *N Engl J Med* 307:73, 1982.

163. Mesenteric Ischemia

Anne C. Mosenthal and Peter E. Rice

In the past, the term *mesenteric ischemia* has been used to describe the clinical entity of infarcted intestine, first described by Virchow in 1840 [1]. It is now known that mesenteric ischemia encompasses a spectrum of pathophysiologic changes that result when oxygen delivery to the gut is inadequate to meet metabolic demands. These changes range from subtle and reversible mucosal injury to frank transmural infarction of the intestine. While mesenteric venous or arterial thrombosis can lead to mesenteric ischemia, most cases are caused by embolism or nonocclusive hypoperfusion [2]. The clinical presentation varies from no apparent signs or symptoms to the classic picture of severe abdominal pain that is out of proportion to physical findings. Critically ill patients, particularly those suffering from burns, sepsis, shock, or cardiac disease, are likely to have a net decrease in oxygen delivery to the gut, putting them at risk for mesenteric ischemia. Transient mucosal ischemia in this setting may promote the systemic absorption of enteric flora or trigger the release of gut-derived mediators. This may elicit a systemic inflammatory response, which ultimately causes multiple organ failure and nosocomial infection, two leading causes of mortality in the intensive care unit [3,4,5].

Etiology

NONOCCLUSIVE ISCHEMIA. In critically ill patients, mesenteric ischemia is most commonly due to a functional derangement in the regulation of arteriolar tone in the mesenteric bed rather than mechanical occlusion of the superior mesenteric artery or its primary branches. The presence of cardiac disease, in particular congestive heart failure, pericardial tamponade, or cardiogenic shock, leads to release of vasoconstrictive mediators, which shunt blood flow away from the mesenteric circulation [6,7]. Nonpulsatile cardiopulmonary bypass perfusion predisposes to intestinal ischemia by a similar mechanism [8,9]. Pharmacologic agents such as digitalis, propranolol, alpha-adrenergic agonists, or arginine vasopressin, which are often prescribed in the critical care setting, also can lead to mesenteric hypoperfusion [10–13]. Shock due to sepsis, burns, or trauma may be associated with the release of inflammatory mediators that cause mesenteric hypoperfusion. Nonocclusive mesenteric ischemia probably is often clinically inapparent, being manifest only by a systemic inflammatory response. Some cases, however, go on to demonstrate clinically evident ischemia and even infarction, requiring surgical intervention [14].

OCCLUSIVE ISCHEMIA. Occlusive mesenteric ischemia is a result of acute embolism or thrombosis of the superior mesenteric artery or thrombosis of the mesenteric veins. In the majority of cases embolization is secondary to atrial fibrillation, valvular disease, myocardial infarction, or cardiomyopathy [15,16]. A large embolus may lodge in the proximal superior mesenteric artery, or multiple small emboli may travel more distally to the middle colic and intestinal branches.

Thrombotic arterial occlusion is an acute event superimposed on chronic atherosclerotic occlusive disease of the celiac, superior mesenteric, and inferior mesenteric arteries. Thrombosis of one or more of these vessels may be precipitated by vasoconstriction or hypercoagulable states due to shock, surgery, sepsis, or cancer. Small vessel thrombosis may occur secondary to collagen vascular disease, hematologic disorders, or diabetes mellitus [17–20].

Mesenteric venous occlusion is a rare entity. Hypercoagulable states, chronic renal failure, cancer, and myeloproliferative disorders may all predispose patients to this potentially catastrophic illness [21,22].

Pathophysiology

Blood is supplied to the small and large intestine by the superior and inferior mesenteric arteries. The superior mesenteric artery supplies the midgut, from the proximal jejunum to the splenic flexure of the colon. The inferior mesenteric artery supplies the hindgut, including the descending colon, sigmoid colon, and upper one-third of the rectum. The superior and inferior mesenteric arteries anastomose via the marginal artery of Drummond and the arc of Riolan. In patients with extensive arteriosclerotic disease, the inferior mesenteric artery may be occluded, the left colon being supplied entirely by the superior mesenteric artery via the marginal artery of Drummond. Embolic occlusion of the superior mesenteric artery in these cases may cause left colonic as well as small bowel ischemia.

Approximately 25 percent of the cardiac output goes to the splanchnic circulatory bed. The major mesenteric arteries branch to form segmental arteries that in turn divide to form the vasa recta. The vasa recta penetrate the bowel wall and form two networks, the submucosal plexus and the serosal plexus. While the muscularis propria is supplied by both these plexi [23], the mucosa is supplied only by arterioles of the submucosal plexus. This may account for the relative resistance to ischemia of the muscularis as compared to the mucosa. A single arteriole penetrates each villus and courses its length. It then anastomoses with a network of surface vessels, as well as a central vein [24–28]. It is theorized by some that this system allows for a diffusional counter-current exchange of oxygen and other solutes [29,30]. Small changes in perfusion may therefore render the villus hypoxic.

The precapillary arterioles are the resistance vessels that control local blood flow. Postcapillary venules and veins are capacitance vessels; during hypovolemia or shock they can autotransfuse blood from the splanchnic bed to the systemic circulation. The control of splanchnic vascular resistance is by the arterioles. A reduction in perfusion pressure will, during normal autoregulation, lead to compensatory dilation of the resistance arterioles, thereby preserving local blood flow to the intestine. Blood flow during physiologic changes in perfusion is also controlled by local metabolites produced by focally ischemic intestine. Adenosine, carbon dioxide, and hydrogen ion are vasodilators that contribute to autoregulatory control of splanchnic blood flow [31,32,33].

During pathologic conditions, such as cardiogenic or hemorrhagic shock, nonocclusive ischemia results because extrinsic systemic mediators released in response to shock override autoregulation. Angiotensin II and, to a lesser degree, vasopressin are the most important mediators of splanchnic vasoconstriction during cardiogenic shock or low-flow states [9,34,35,36]. Angiotensin II has a direct vasoconstrictive effect on the mesenteric resistance arterioles; angiotensin receptors are present in mesenteric arteries [37,38]. Blockade of the renin-angiotensin axis in animal models of shock ameliorates splanchnic ischemia [35]. Nonpulsatile cardiopulmonary bypass also is associated with activation of the renin-angiotensin system, which probably accounts for nonocclusive mesenteric ischemia under these conditions [39]. Alpha-adrenergic stimulation during shock has an important vasoconstrictive effect on the postcapillary resistance vessels, serving to shunt blood to the central circulation. Adrenergic mechanisms, however, are not an important factor leading to nonocclusive mesenteric ischemia.

Mesenteric ischemia during sepsis is not completely understood. It is likely mediated in a different manner. In some models of septic shock, hypoperfusion is responsible, at least in part, for mucosal injury [40,41]. This, in turn, is mediated by thromboxane A_2 and the leukotrienes [42,43,44]. Prostaglandins F_2 and D_2 and leukotrienes C_4 and D_4 are known to cause mesenteric vasoconstriction [45].

How mesenteric ischemia leads to injury is incompletely understood. Hypoxia can cause both depletion and net hydrolysis of ATP, resulting in intracellular acidosis [46,47]. It is not the hypoxia itself, but rather the reperfusion of ischemic tissue, that may be the more important cause of injury. Reperfusion after only 2 hours of ischemia leads via the xanthine oxidase pathway to formation of toxic oxygen metabolites, such as hydroxyl, hydrogen peroxide, and superoxide [48]. Infiltration and adherence of neutrophils to damaged gut tissue further injure cells by release of proteases and more toxic oxygen metabolites [49,50]. Administration of xanthine oxidase inhibitors or free radical scavengers ameliorates gut injury in animal models of ischemia/reperfusion [51].

Regardless of the mechanism, intestinal ischemia and mucosal injury increase the permeability of the intestine to various substances. Multiple mediators are released from the gut, which in turn lead to the systemic sequelae of this illness. Histamine, prostaglandins, bradykinin, myocardial depressant factor(s), and possibly cytokines contribute to the deleterious systemic response seen in clinical intestinal ischemia [52,53]. The cardiovascular system is further activated by prostaglandin-mediated stimulation of visceral afferent nerves [54,55].

Pathology

The pathologic changes of intestinal ischemia have been well documented. Following superior mesenteric arterial occlusion, gross arterial pulsations are absent and the bowel is spastic and aperistaltic. Necrosis begins in the mucosa and extends to all layers after several hours of complete ischemia. Full-thickness infarction occurs after 8 to 10 hours of severe ischemia [56]. Perforation may be a late finding. Incomplete ischemia may result in late stricture formation if muscular damage has occurred.

Histologically, mucosal injury is visible after only 10 minutes of ischemia; the epithelium is separated from the basement membrane and glandular cells [57,58]. The villi are exquisitely susceptible to ischemic injury, possibly due to the countercurrent architecture of the villous microvasculature. With increasing periods of ischemia, evidence of injury (necrosis, invasion of inflammatory cells, and fibrin deposition) extends from the villi through all layers of the intestine, producing submucosal edema and hemorrhage. Hypoperfusion of the intestine without complete arterial occlusion reproduces these same histologic changes but over a longer time course [59]. Mucosal injury without epithelial crypt or full-thickness damage may be reversible on reperfusion [60,61]. Reperfusion itself has been shown to increase mucosal injury following ischemia. It leads to marked inflammatory infiltration, edema, and sequestration of fluid in the intestinal lumen. Ischemia reperfusion produces more extensive necrosis of villi and crypts than does ischemia alone [62].

Diagnosis

CLINICAL PRESENTATION. The presentation of mesenteric ischemia may range from subtle signs and symptoms to severe abdominal pain and gastrointestinal bleeding. The physician must have a high index of suspicion to make the diagnosis, particularly in critically ill patients in whom symptoms may be masked. While the history is rarely pathognomonic, clinical circumstances may suggest the diagnosis. Those at high risk tend to be elderly or have cardiac disease, arrhythmias, or hypotension secondary to sepsis, hemorrhage, or pancreatitis. New onset of abdominal pain in these patients should suggest the possibility of mesenteric ischemia.

Severe abdominal pain is the most common presenting symptom. In cases of arterial embolization, abdominal pain typically is acute in onset. In cases of nonocclusive or thrombotic ischemia, abdominal pain may develop more slowly. Classically, pain is very severe but objective physical findings such as abdominal tenderness, rebound tenderness, or guarding are minimal or absent. If pain is absent, as it may be in 25 percent of cases, symptoms such as bloody diarrhea or abdominal distention or nonspecific signs such as mental status changes, tachycardia, or fever may be the only clues to the diagnosis. The development of peritonitis and acidemia usually implies transmural infarction; absence of these signs, however, does not exclude this possibility. The severity of signs and symptoms in mesenteric ischemia often does not correlate with the extent of intestinal injury.

LABORATORY TESTS. Considerable effort has been directed at the identification of markers that would permit the early diagnosis of mesenteric ischemia. Peripheral blood leukocyte counts [63,64,65], amylase concentration [15], alkaline phosphatase concentration [66], lactate dehydrogenase concentration [67], aspartate transferase concentration [67], and creatine kinase concentration [68] all may be elevated in mesenteric ischemia. These tests, however, are neither sensitive nor specific. Measurements of more unusual serum enzymes, including hexosaminidase [69], porcine ileal peptide [70], and diamine oxidase [71], have not been shown to be diagnostic for mesenteric ischemia any earlier than traditional laboratory tests. Metabolic acidosis and hemoconcentration are both late findings, reflecting infarcted intestine.

RADIOLOGIC TESTS. Standard radiologic tests also have proved to be of little predictive value in the early diagnosis of mesenteric ischemia. The radiographic finding of "thumbprinting" caused by submucosal bowel edema is considered the hallmark of bowel ischemia [72], but invariably indicates advanced disease [73]. Standard abdominal films may be helpful, however, in ruling out other disease, such as a perforated viscus. Computed tomography may demonstrate more specific findings of mesenteric ischemia, such as venous gas and occluded arterial vessels, but absence of these findings does not exclude the diagnosis [74]. In cases of mesenteric venous thrombosis, computed tomography with intravenous contrast may demonstrate clot within the vessel [75]. As with plain films, computed tomography has its greatest use in excluding other etiologies of abdominal pain.

VASCULAR IMAGING. Arteriography is considered by many to be the single best test for the diagnosis of mesenteric ischemia, as well as being a useful therapeutic adjunct. Arteriography is useful for differentiating between occlusive and nonocclusive types of mesenteric ischemia [76,77] or distinguishing between embolization and thrombosis of the superior mesenteric artery. However, the presence of atherosclerotic disease of the superior mesenteric and/or celiac arteries does not necessarily correlate with acute ischemia unless an embolus can be demonstrated. Nonocclusive ischemia is suggested by the presence of vasoconstriction or "pruning" of smaller mesenteric vessels, but these findings do not reveal any information about the extent of intestinal injury. If nonocclusive ischemia is diagnosed, then infusion of papaverine directly into the superior mesenteric artery may have some therapeutic benefit [78]. Arteriography has no role in the evaluation of patients who already demonstrate obvious signs of peritonitis and intestinal infarction, since exploratory surgery is already mandated.

Noninvasive vascular imaging with Doppler and color-flow duplex ultrasonography of the superior mesenteric artery is a diagnostic tool that holds promise for the evaluation of suspected mesenteric ischemia. It has been shown to be accurate in the diagnosis of hemodynamically significant superior mesenteric or celiac arterial stenosis in patients with chronic mesenteric ischemia [79]. Currently, the clinical usefulness of this modality is confined to screening symptomatic patients for chronic mesenteric arterial occlusive disease. It does not provide information regarding blood flow to the intestine via collaterals, nor does it predict the level of ischemia or injury present in the tissue [80,81].

ENDOSCOPY AND LAPAROSCOPY. Endoscopic evaluation of the colon has been used extensively to diagnose ischemic colitis. This is the diagnostic method of choice in patients in whom colonic rather than small bowel ischemia is suspected, such as those with predominantly left-sided abdominal pain and bloody diarrhea or those who have recently undergone abdominal aortic surgery.

Colonoscopy can reveal a spectrum of mucosal changes. Acute injury is manifested by hyperemic mucosa alternating with pale areas and areas with petechial hemorrhage. Subacute injury appears as ulcerations with submucosal hemorrhage. More severe injury appears as pseudomembranes with exudates [82]. Frank intestinal gangrene appears black or green through the endoscope. Only those patients with grossly necrotic mucosa are at significant risk for perforation and, accordingly, are the only patients who require surgical exploration [83]. Patients with lesser degrees of injury at the time of the initial colonoscopy should be followed with repeat endoscopic examinations, because injury may progress over time. It should be emphasized that the degree of histologic mucosal injury often does not correlate with the endoscopic appearance of the mucosa. Furthermore, abnormal endoscopic findings cannot always predict transmural viability since only the mucosa can be evaluated.

In most instances, mesenteric ischemia occurs in the part of the gastrointestinal tract supplied by the superior mesenteric artery (i.e., the small intestine and right colon). Unfortunately,

the small intestine is beyond the reach of the conventional endoscope. It is possible, however, to evaluate the right colon, which also is supplied by the superior mesenteric artery, by colonoscopy. Future development of newer techniques of enteroscopy may permit evaluation of the small bowel as well.

The recent enthusiasm for laparoscopic surgery has produced several reports of the use of this new methodology to diagnose mesenteric ischemia [84,85]. Unfortunately, a negative laparoscopic examination may not exclude the diagnosis, since transmural infarction is a late finding and the mucosa is not visible by laparoscopy [86]. The judicious use of laparoscopy and endoscopy together may improve the diagnostic accuracy in cases of mesenteric ischemia.

TONOMETRY. In the research laboratory, tonometric estimation of mucosal CO_2 tension has proved to be a valid method for measuring intramucosal pH [87]. Mucosal acidosis is a reliable indicator of tissue ischemia. Tonometry permits diagnosis of ischemia before other evidence of disease is apparent in patients. For example, it has been shown that ischemic colitis following aortic aneurysm resection can be predicted days before clinical signs appear by the tonometric detection of mucosal acidosis on the day of surgery [88]. Gastric tonometry has been used following cardiac surgery to detect changes in splanchnic perfusion and predict complications [89]. However, the usefulness of tonometry in the diagnosis of clinically significant mesenteric ischemia of the small bowel has not been proven at this time. Placement of a tonometer into the small bowel is difficult. Although an endoscopic method has been used in experimental animals [90], this approach has not been validated in the clinical setting.

DIFFERENTIAL DIAGNOSIS. The diagnosis of mesenteric ischemia can be difficult. Certainly, the sudden onset of severe abdominal pain in the presence of minimal physical findings in a patient with arrhythmias should prompt the clinician to strongly suspect embolization of the superior mesenteric artery. The majority of cases of mesenteric ischemia, however, are more insidious, particularly in patients who already are critically ill. Perforated viscus, pancreatitis, peptic ulcer disease, bowel obstruction, and acute biliary disease all may present with similar findings. Routine laboratory studies and plain abdominal roentgenograms should be helpful in excluding the majority of these other diagnoses. Occasionally, acute myocardial infarction, aortic dissection, or aneurysm rupture may present with abdominal pain and acidosis, thereby suggesting the diagnosis of mesenteric ischemia. The electrocardiogram, careful physical examination, and computed tomography should reveal these entities, and computed tomography may be helpful in differentiating these diagnoses.

Ischemic colitis usually presents with left-sided abdominal pain and bloody diarrhea. The differential diagnosis includes inflammatory bowel disease with or without toxic megacolon, *Clostridium difficile* colitis or other infectious colitides, and, rarely, diverticulitis. Abdominal roentenograms, stool cultures, and barium enema may aid in differentiating these entities. Endoscopy is useful, but the mucosal appearance of several of these problems may mimic ischemic colitis. Mucosal biopsies may be helpful.

Management

The hardest part of the management of patients with suspected mesenteric ischemia is establishing the diagnosis before irre

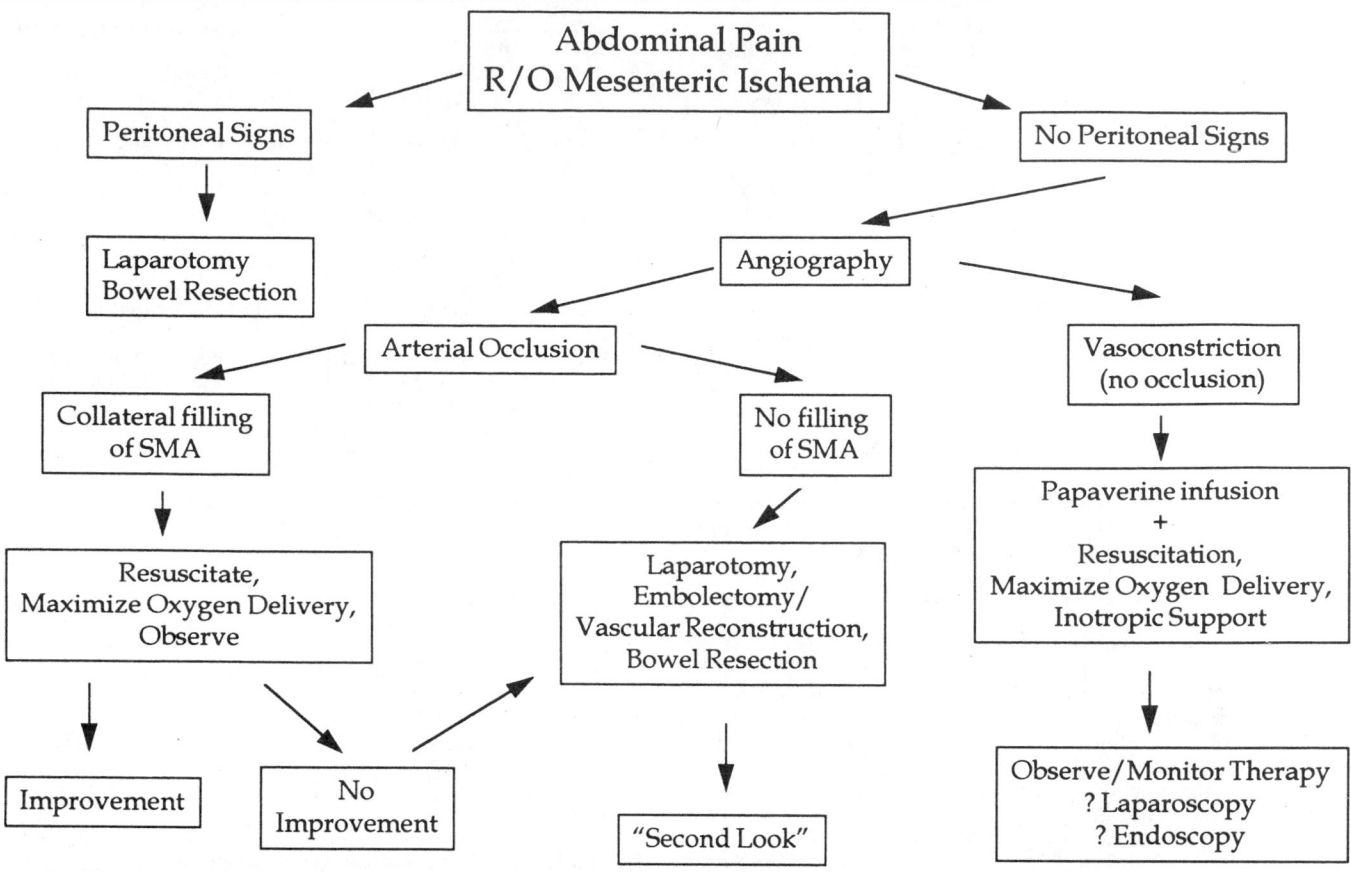

Fig. 163-1. Management of suspected mesenteric ischemia.

versible infarction occurs. The early use of visceral angiography in all high-risk patients in whom the diagnosis is entertained has been advocated by Boley and others [78,91,93]. The early use of mesenteric arteriography seems especially prudent when the clinical presentation makes the diagnosis of superior mesenteric artery embolization likely [78,92,93]. However, if there is evidence of frank peritonitis, transmural infarction probably already is present and delaying definitive surgery to perform an angiogram is unwise (see Fig. 163-1). If angiography reveals occlusion of the superior mesenteric artery without collateral circulation, a finding suggestive of an acute event (rather than chronic occlusion), urgent surgery for vascular reconstruction and possible bowel resection is mandated. If the arteriogram reveals nonocclusive ischemia, intraarterial papaverine can be infused to reverse vasoconstriction [78]. In cases of nonocclusive ischemia, the most important aspect of management is aggressive medical therapy directed at maximizing perfusion and oxygen delivery to the mesenteric circulation. Measures to improve mesenteric perfusion may include intravascular volume loading (guided, if necessary, by invasive hemodynamic monitoring), infusion of inotropic agents, treatment with angiotensin-converting enzyme inhibitors (to block mesenteric vasospasm induced by angiotensin II), and discontinuing digoxin (since this drug has been implicated as a mesenteric vasoconstrictor). Invasive hemodynamic monitoring in the intensive care unit is recommended to evaluate the effectiveness of ongoing therapy as is frequent measurement of blood lactate levels and arterial pH. Gastric tonometry may play a role in monitoring the adequacy of splanchnic oxygen delivery, as it appears to be a more sensitive means for detecting tissue ischemia than are other tests. All medications that cause mesenteric vasoconstriction, such as digitalis or vasopressin, should be discontinued. Prevention of reperfusion injury also may be important. The use of free radical scavengers and xanthine oxidase inhibitors, although theoretically beneficial, has not been shown to improve outcome in the clinical setting. Frequent reexamination of the abdomen as well repeat angiography should be done. If abdominal findings progress despite maximal medical therapy, exploratory laparotomy is indicated to resect infarcted bowel.

Patients who present with left-sided abdominal pain and bloody diarrhea can be managed differently, since ischemic colitis is the most likely diagnosis. A history of recent aortic surgery should prompt immediate evaluation for colonic ischemia in this setting. Endoscopy, rather than angiography, is the diagnostic method of choice; repeat endoscopic examinations may be necessary to monitor ongoing or progressive ischemia to determine if and when surgery is required. Only gross mucosal necrosis puts the patient at risk and mandates surgery [83]. Nevertheless the endoscopic findings should be interpreted in the clinical context; the presence of acidosis, leukocytosis, and/or peritoneal signs should prompt exploration regardless of the appearance of the mucosa.

References

1. Virchow RLK: Über die akute Entzundung der Arterien. *Virchows Arch Pathol Anat* 1:272, 1847.

2. Kaleya RN, Sammartano RJ, Boley SJ: Aggressive approach to intestinal ischemia. *Surg Clin North Am* 157, 1992.

3. Shires GT, Dineen P: Sepsis following burns, trauma and intra-abdominal infection. *Arch Intern Med* 142:2012, 1982.

4. Border JR, Hassett J, LaDuca J, et al: The gut origin septic states in blunt multiple trauma (ISS-40) in the ICU. *Ann Surg* 206:42, 1987.

5. Deitch EA, Bridges RM: Effect of stress and trauma on bacterial translocation from the gut. *J Surg Res* 42:563, 1987.

6. Porter JM, Sussman MS, Bulkley GB: Splanchnic vasospasm in circulatory shock, in Marston A, Bulkley GB, Fiddian-Green RG, Haglund UH (eds): *Splanchnic Ischemia and Multiple Organ Failure.* London, Edward Arnold 73, 1989.

7. Reilly PM, Bulkley GB: Vasoactive mediators and splanchnic perfusion. *Crit Care Med* 21:S55, 1993.

8. Krasna MJ, Flancbaum L, Trooskin SZ, et al: Gastrointestinal complications after cardiac surgery. *Surgery* 104:773, 1988.

9. Leitman IM, Paull DE, Barie PS, et al: Intra-abdominal complication of cardiopulmonary bypass operations. *Surg Gynecol Obstet* 165:251, 1987.

10. Bynum TE, Hanley HG: Effects of digitalis on estimated splanchnic blood flow. *J Lab Clin Med* 99:84, 1982.

11. Pettei MJ, Levy J, Abramson S: Nonocclusive mesenteric ischemia associated with propranolol overdose: Implications regarding splanchnic circulation. *Ped Gastroenterol Nutr* 10:544, 1990.

12. Banks RO, Callavan RH, Zinner MJ, et al: Vasoactive agents in control of mesenteric circulation. *Fed Proc* 44:2743, 1985.

13. McNeill JR, Wilcox WC, Pang CCY: Vasopressin and angiotensin: Reciprocal mechanism controlling mesenteric conductance. *Am J Physiol* 232:H260, 1977.

14. Desai MH, Herndon DN, Rutan RL, et al: Ischemic intestinal complications in patients with burns. *Surg Gynecol Obstet* 172:257, 1991.

15. Wilson C, Gupta R, Gilmour DG, et al: Acute superior mesenteric ischemia. *Br J Surg* 74:279, 1987.

16. Pierce GE, Brockenbrough EG: The spectrum of mesenteric infarction. *Am J Surg* 119:233, 1970.

17. Jordan PH, Boulafendis D, Guinn GA: Factors other than major vascular occlusion that contribute to intestinal infarction. *Ann Surg* 171:189, 1970.

18. Fauci AS, Haynes BF, Katz P: The spectrum of vasculitis. Clinical, pathological, immunologic and therapeutic consideration. *Ann Intern Med* 89:660, 1978.

19. Ferrari BT, Ray JE, Robertson HD, et al: Colonic manifestation of collagen vascular disease. *Dis Colon Rectum* 23:473, 1980.

20. Whelan MA, Karm P: Mesenteric complication in a patient with polycythemia vera. *Am J Gastroenterol* 77:526, 1982.

21. Pokorney BH, Eyster ME, Jeffries GH: Antithrombin III deficiency appearing as mesenteric vein thrombosis. *Am J Gastroenterol* 76:534, 1981.

22. Balz J, Minton JP: Mesenteric thrombosis following splenectomy. *Ann Surg* 181:126, 1976.

23. Brockus JG, Moffat DB: The intrinsic blood vessels of the pelvic colon. *J Anat* 92:52, 1958.

24. Jacobson LF, Noer RF: The vascular pattern of the intestinal villi in various laboratory animals and man. *Anat Rec* 114:85, 1952.

25. Marston A: Basic structure and function of the intestinal circulation. *Clin Gastroenterol* 1:429, 1972.

26. Griffiths JD: Extramural and intramural blood supply of the colon. *BMJ* 1:323, 1961.

27. Baulter PS, Parks AG: Submucosal vascular patterns of the alimentary tract and their significance. *Br J Surg* 47:546, 1959.

28. Parks DA, Jacobsen ED: Physiology of the splanchnic circulation. *Arch Intern Med* 145:1278, 1985.

29. Lundgren O: Studies on blood distribution and countercurrent exchange in the small intestine. *Acta Physiol Scand* (Suppl) 303:1, 1967.

30. Hallback DA, Hulten L, Jodal M, et al: Evidence for the existence of a countercurrent exchanger in the small intestine in man. *Gastroenterology* 74:683, 1978.

31. Haglund U: The small intestine in hypotension and hemorrhage. *Acta Physiol Scand* 387(Suppl):1, 1973.

32. Granger DN, Valleau JP, Parker RD: Effects of adenosine on intestinal hemodynamics, oxygen delivery and capillary fluid exchange. *Am J Physiol* 4:H707, 1978.

33. Martillaro NA, Mustafa SJ: Possible role for adenosine in intestinal reactive hyperemia. *Abst Fed Proc* 37:874, 1978.

34. McNeil JR, Wilcox, Pang CCY: Intestinal vasoconstriction after hemorrhage. The roles of vasopressin and angiotensin. *Am J Physiol* 219:I342, 1970.

35. Bailey RW, Bulkley GB, Hamilton SR, et al: Protection of the small intestine from nonocclusive mesenteric ischemia injury due to cardiogenic shock. *Am J Surg* 153:108, 1987.

36. Bailey RW, Bulkley GB, Hamilton SR, et al: Pathogenesis of nonocclusive ischemic colitis. *Am Surg* 203:509, 1986.

37. Gunther S, Gimbrone MA, Alexandrew RW: Identification and characterization of the high affinity vascular angiotensin II receptor in rat mesenteric artery. *Circ Res* 47:278, 1980.

38. Tuerker RK, Ercan ZS: High degree of conversion of angiotensin I to angiotensin II in the mesenteric circulation of the isolated perfused terminal ileum of the cat. *Arch Int Physiol Biochim* 83:845, 1970.

39. Watkins L, Lucas SK, Gardner TJ, et al: Angiotensin II levels during cardiopulmonary bypass: A comparison of pulsatile and non-pulsatile flow. *Surg Forum* 30:229, 1979.

40. Fink MP, Kaups KL, Wang H, et al: Maintenance of superior mesenteric arterial perfusion prevents increased intestinal mucosal permeability in endotoxic pigs. *Surgery* 110:154, 1991.

41. Navaratnam NRL, Morris SE, Traber DL, et al: Endotoxin (LPS) increases mesenteric vascular resistance (MVR) and bacterial translocation (BT). *J Trauma* 30:1104, 1990.

42. Temple GE, Cook JA, Wise WC, et al: Improvement in organ blood flow by inhibition of thromboxane synthetase during experimental endotoxic shock in the rat. *J Cardiovasc Pharmacol* 8:514, 1986.

43. Fink MP, Rothschild HR, Deniz YF, et al: Systemic and mesenteric O_2 metabolism in endotoxic pigs, effect of ibuprofen and meclofenamate. *J Appl Physiol* 67:1950, 1989.

44. Cohn SM, Fink MP, Lee PC, et al: LY171883 preserves mesenteric perfusion in porcine endotoxic shock. *J Surg Res* 49:37, 1990.

45. Chapnick BM, Feigen LP, Hyman AL: Differential effects of prostaglandins in mesenteric vascular bed. *Am J Physiol* 235:H326, 1978.

46. Mosenthal AC, Wang H, BelleIsle JM, et al: Mesenteric hypoperfusion and decreased mucosal ATP in porcine endotoxicosis. *Surg Forum* 42:39, 1991.

47. Hochachka PW, Mommsen TP: Protons and anaerobiosis. *Science* 219:1391, 1983.

48. Granger DN, Rutile G, McCord JM: Superoxide radicals in feline intestinal ischemia. *Gastroenterology* 81:22, 1981.

49. Parks DA, Bulkley GB, Granger DN, et al: Ischemic injury in the cat small intestine. Role of superoxide radicals. *Gastroenterology* 82:9, 1982.

50. Grisham MB, Hernandez LA, Granger DN: Adenosine inhibits ischemia reperfusion induced leukocyte adherence and extravasation. *Am J Physiol* 257:H1334, 1989.

51. Granger DN, McCord JM, Parks DA, et al: Xanthine oxidase inhibitors attenuate ischemia induced vascular permeability changes in the cat intestine. *Gastroenterology* 90:80, 1986.

52. Haglund U: Systemic mediators released from the gut in critical illness. *Crit Care Med* 21:S15, 1993.

53. Deitch EA: Cytokines yes, cytokines no, cytokines maybe? *Crit Care Med* 21:817, 1993.

54. Stahl GL, Halliwell B, Longhhurst JC: Hydrogen peroxide-induced cardiovascular reflexes, role of hydroxyl radicals. *Circ Res* 71:295, 1992.

55. Longhurst JC, Toto DM, Kaufman MP, et al: Chemically sensitive abdominal visceral afferents: Response to cyclo-oxygenase blockade. *Am J Physiol* 261:H2075, 1991.

56. Marston A: Causes of death in mesenteric arterial occlusion. *Ann Surg* 58:952, 1963.

57. Ahren C, Haglund UH: Mucosal lesions in the small intestine of the cat during low flow. *Acta Physiol Scand* 88:1, 1973.

58. Chiu CJ, McCardle C: Intestinal mucosal lesions in low-flow states. *Arch Surg* 101:489, 1970.

59. Haglund U, Hulten L, Ahren C, et al: Mucosal lesions in the human small intestine in shock. *Gut* 16:979, 1975.

60. Gorey TF: The recovery of intestine after ischemic injury. *Br J Surg* 67:699, 1980.

61. Glotzer DJ, Villegase EH, Anekayema S, et al: Healing of the intestine in experimental bowel infarction. *Ann Surg* 155:183, 1962.

62. Parks DA, Granger DN: Contribution of ischemia and reperfusion to mucosal lesion formation. *Am J Physiol* 250:G749, 1986.

63. Jenson C, Smith G: A clinical study of 51 cases of mesenteric infarction. *Surgery* 40:930, 1956.
64. Ottinger L, Austen G: A study of 136 patients with mesenteric infarction. *Surg Gynecol Obstet* 124:251, 1967.
65. Ghanem M, Goodale RL, Spanos P, et al: Value of leukocyte counts in the recognition of mesenteric infarction and strangulation of shorter intestinal lengths. An experimental study. *Surgery* 68:635, 1970.
66. Williams R, Wilson S: Correlation of alkaline phosphatase with submucosal blood flow and morbid histology of the ischemic colon. *Surg Gynecol Obstet* 151:412, 1980.
67. DeToma G, Marayaro D, Salvatore P, et al: Enzymatic and metabolic changes in the peripheral serum after superior mesenteric artery ligation in dogs. *J Surg Sci* 13:269, 1983.
68. Graeber G, Cafferty P, Reardon M, et al: Elevations of serum creatinine phosphokinase in experimental mesenteric infarction. *Surg Forum* 31:148, 1980.
69. Cobe T, Schwartz M, Richardson J et al: Hexosaminidase: A marker for intestinal gangrene in necrotizing enterocolitis. *J Pediatr Surg* 18:449, 1983.
70. Marks W, Salvino C, Newell K, et al: Circulating concentrations of porcine ileal peptide but not hexosaminidase are elevated following one hour of mesenteric ischemia. *J Surg Res* 45:134, 1988.
71. Bounous G, Echave V, Vobecky S, et al: Acute necrosis of the intestinal mucosa with high serum levels of diamine oxidase. *Dig Dis Sci* 29:872, 1984.
72. Schwartz S, Boley SJ, Robinson K, et al: Roentgenologic features of vascular disorders of the intestines. *Radiol Clin North Am* 2:71, 1964.
73. Tomchik FS, Wittenberg J, Ottinger LW: The roentgenographic spectrum of bowel infarction. *Ann Surg* 96:249, 1970.
74. Smerud MJ, Johnson CD, Stephens DH: Diagnosis of bowel infarction: A comparison of plain films and CT scans in 23 cases. *AJR* 154:99, 1990.
75. Franquet T, Bescos JM, Reparaz B: Noninvasive methods in the diagnosis of isolated superior mesenteric vein thrombosis: Ultrasound and CT scan. *Gastrointest Radiol* 14:321, 1989.
76. Clark RH, Gallant TE: Acute mesenteric ischemia angiographic spectum. *AJR* 142:555, 1984.
77. Siegelman SS, Sprayregen S, Boley SJ: Angiographic diagnosis of mesenteric arterial vasoconstriction. *Radiology* 122:533, 1974.
78. Boley SJ, Sprayregen S, Siegelman SS, et al: Initial results from an aggressive roentgenological and surgical approach to acute mesenteric ischemia. *Surgery* 82:848, 1977.
79. Harward TRS, Smith S, Seeger JM: Detection of celiac axis and superior mesenteric artery occlusive disease with use of abdominal duplex scanning. *J Vasc Surg* 17:738, 1993.
80. Moneta GL, Yeager RA, Dalman R, et al: Duplex ultrasound criteria for diagnosis of splanchnic artery stenosis or occlusion. *J Vasc Surg* 14:511, 1993.
81. Bowersox JC, Zwolak RM, Walsh DB, et al: Duplex ultrasonography in the diagnosis of celiac and mesenteric artery occlusive disease. *J Vasc Surg* 14:780, 1991.
82. Scowcroft CW, Sanowski RA, Kozarek RA: Colonoscopy in ischemic colitis. *Gastrointest Endosc* 27:156, 1981.
83. Scherpenisse J, van Hess P: The endoscopic spectrum of colonic mucosal injury following aortic aneurysm resection. *Endoscopy* 21:174, 1986.
84. Iberti J, Salky B, Omefrey D: Use of bedside laparoscopy to identify intestinal ischemia in post-operative cases of aortic reconstruction. *Surgery* 105:686, 1989.
85. Jabbari M, Cherry R, Goresky C: The endoscopic diagnosis of mesenteric venous thrombosis. *Gastrointest Endosc* 31:405, 1985.
86. Serreyn RF, Schoofs PR, Barterns PR, et al: Laparoscopic diagnosis of mesenteric venous thrombosis. *Endoscopy* 18:249, 1986.
87. Antonsson JB, Boyle CC, Kruithoff KL, et al: Validation of tonometric measurement of gut intramucosal pH during endotoxemia and mesenteric occlusion in pigs. *Am J Physiol* 259:G519, 1990.
88. Fiddian-Green RG, Amelin F, Hermann JB, et al: Prediction of the development of sigmoid ischemia on the day of operation. Indirect measurement of intramural pH in the colon. *Arch Surg* 121:654, 1986.
89. Fiddian-Green RG, Baker S: Predictive value of the stomach wall pH for complication after cardiac operation. Comparison with other monitoring. *Crit Care Med* 15:153, 1987.
90. Schonholtz S, Pleatman M, Kasserman D, et al: Endoscopic tonometric assessment of intestinal perfusion in a canine model. *Gastrointest Endosc* 135:425, 1989.
91. Batellier J, Kieny R: Superior mesenteric artery embolism: Eighty-two cases. *Ann Vasc Surg* 2:112, 1990.
92. Levy PJ, Krausz MM, Manny J: Acute mesenteric ischemia: Improved results—a retrospective analysis of ninety-two patients. *Surgery* 107:372, 1990.
93. Sachs SM, Morton JH, Schwartz SI: Acute mesenteric ischemia. *Surgery* 92:646, 1982.

164. *Noncardiac Surgery in the Cardiac Patient*

Ira S. Ockene and Thomas A. Holly

In the United States, cardiovascular diseases account for approximately half of all deaths. Three-quarters of these cardiovascular deaths are related to ischemic heart disease [1]. In the Framingham study, the chance of developing cardiovascular disease by age 65 was 37 percent for men and 18 percent for women [2]. After age 65 these percentages increase sharply. It is therefore common for the physician to have to deal with the problem of noncardiac surgery in a cardiac patient. This may be a patient with overt heart disease, an asymptomatic patient who has a history of a cardiac event in the past, or an individual who is felt to be at high risk for cardiac disease. These patients present a problem to the primary physician or consultant who

must make a decision about the risk–benefit ratio and timing of elective (or semielective) operations, the surgeon who must evaluate the patient and perform the operation, and the anesthesiologist whose responsibility it is to have the patient in the best possible physiologic state before, during, and after surgery.

It is useful to begin by considering the stresses that surgery imposes on the cardiovascular system and how these may precipitate overt manifestations of cardiovascular disease. When considering how any given factor affects the heart, it is helpful to consider it with reference to the determinants of myocardial oxygen consumption, as the work of the heart is closely related to this parameter. This approach is appropriate because it is most commonly ischemic heart disease with which we are concerned, and because it is myocardial oxygen delivery that is limited in this disorder.

Myocardial oxygen consumption is essentially determined by four factors: (1) preload, (2) afterload, (3) myocardial contractility, and (4) heart rate. *Preload* is that load, or stretch on a muscle fiber, that exists before contraction begins. In the human this translates to end-diastolic volume, and in the clinical setting the parameter that most closely relates to preload is left ventricular filling pressure, most commonly measured via the pulmonary capillary wedge pressure obtained through a pulmonary artery balloon flotation catheter. Increasing preload increases myocardial oxygen demand. *Afterload* is the resistance against which the left ventricle must contract once the aortic valve is open. Clinically, this translates into the peripheral vascular resistance. Increasing afterload also increases myocardial oxygen consumption. *Myocardial contractility* is the innate contractile state of the myocardium. Increases in contractility are associated with increases in myocardial oxygen consumption. Many drugs affect myocardial contractility, either increasing or decreasing it. Elevated catecholamine levels also increase myocardial contractility. Finally, increases in *heart rate* are correlated with increases in myocardial oxygen demand.

The stresses of surgery may be divided into three categories: preoperative, intraoperative, and postoperative, as shown in Table 164-1. The metabolic changes associated with surgery significantly stress the cardiovascular system. Some of the physiologic alterations induced by surgery may affect both the supply and demand sides of the myocardial oxygen supply equation. For example, hypotension tends to reduce myocardial oxygen demand, but it also can be associated with reduced

myocardial oxygen delivery. The net effect may be difficult to predict. Hypotension during surgery is often associated with ischemia, yet controlled hypotension, induced with agents such as morphine, is beneficial during certain types of surgery. Hypothermia reduces systemic and myocardial oxygen demands during surgery, but an intraoperative temperature drop of 0.3 to 1.2°C was found to be associated with a doubling of postoperative oxygen consumption [3]. Shivering during rewarming may cause a tripling or quadrupling of postoperative cardiac output [4].

Anesthetic agents frequently have important myocardial depressant and arrhythmogenic effects. Manipulations such as intubation or intraabdominal traction can cause a parasympathetic discharge that leads to bradycardia and hypotension. On the other hand, hypoxia and hypercapnia can stimulate the release of catecholamines, resulting in arrhythmias and hypertension.

Coronary Artery Disease and Noncardiac Surgery

A number of studies have examined the relationship between coronary artery disease, especially antecedent myocardial infarction, and the risk of surgery. In 1962, Knapp et al. reported their experience with noncardiac surgery in 8964 men over 50 years of age, of whom 427 (4.8%) had had a prior myocardial infarction (MI) [5]. Of the 8557 men who had no history of MI, only 59 (0.7%) suffered a postoperative MI, with a mortality rate of 19 percent. On the other hand, among the 427 patients with a history of MI, the perioperative infarction rate was 6.1 percent and the mortality among these patients was a striking 58 percent. The highest reinfarction rate occurred among those men who had had a recent infarction.

In 1964, the Cornell group reported an extension of their data [6], examining 12,712 male surgical patients over the age of 50, selected from a total 5-year (1959–1963) surgical population of 35,937 persons. Their findings are summarized in Tables 164-2 and 164-3. In this study, anesthetic agent, type of surgery, or duration of surgery appeared to play no significant role in determining the risk of postoperative MI. The risk was greatest for those with the shortest interval between the prior infarction and subsequent surgery (see Table 164-3). Most of the excess risk was seen in those with less than a 2-year period between infarction and surgery.

These studies reported data collected in the late 1950s and early 1960s. Since that time, surgical and anesthetic techniques have improved; techniques of intensive care, such as the use of pulmonary artery pressure monitoring, have been devel-

Table 164-1. Surgical Stresses

1. Preoperative
   a. Anxiety—increases BP, heart rate, catecholamine levels
   b. Sedation—may impair ventilation
2. Intraoperative
   a. Anesthesia—can cause myocardial depression
   b. Impaired ventilation—decreases oxygenation and causes acid-base disturbances
   c. Blood pressure fluctuations—may cause myocardial ischemia due to decreased coronary blood flow (hypotension) or increased myocardial oxygen demand (hypertension)
   d. Blood loss—decreases myocardial oxygen delivery
   e. Compromised function of vital organs, especially secondary to hypotension
   f. Acid-base disturbances
   g. Reactions to drugs, blood products
   h. Volume overload—increases preload; decreases oxygenation secondary to pulmonary congestion
   i. Hypovolemia—decreases cardiac output; decreases flow to myocardium and other vital organs
   j. Hyper- or hypothermia, shivering—increases myocardial oxygen demand
3. Postoperative
   a. Hypovolemia related to blood loss, vomiting, diaphoresis, poor intake, excessive diuresis
   b. Anemia secondary to blood loss—decreases myocardial oxygen delivery
   c. Volume overload from excessive transfusion, fluid infusions
   d. Sepsis—markedly increases myocardial oxygen demands
   e. Venous or arterial thrombosis related to postoperative clotting factor changes and immobility
   f. Endocarditis—can directly affect cardiac valvular function, as well as increasing metabolic demands
   g. Reactions to drugs, blood products
   h. Anxiety

Table 164-2. Incidence and Mortality of Postoperative Myocardial Infarction

Class	Total no. patients	No. (%) of patients with postop MI	No. (%) mortality
No previous history of MI	12,054	79(0.66)	21(26.5)
Previous history of MI	658	43(6.5)	31(70.0)
Total	12,712	122(0.95)	52(42.0)

Source: From Topkins MJ, Artusio JF Jr: Myocardial infarction and surgery: A five year study. *Anesth Analg* 43:716, 1964, with permission.

Table 164-3. Relationship of Incidence of Postoperative Myocardial Infarction to Time Between Antecedent Myocardial Infarction and Surgery

Time between MI and surgery	No. of patients with preop MI	No. (%) of patients with postop MI
<6 mo	22	12(54.5)
6–12 mo	36	9(25.0)
1–2 yr	49	11(22.4)
2–3 yr	51	3 (5.9)
>3 yr	493	5 (1.0)
Age unclear; MI at autopsy	7	3(43.0)
Total	658	43(6.5)

Source: From Topkins MJ, Artusio JF Jr: Myocardial infarction and surgery. A five year study. *Anesth Analg* 43:716, 1964, with permission.

Table 164-4. Myocardial Reinfarction and Mortality

Time between prior MI and surgery (mo)	No. patients	No. (%) postop reinfarctions	No. (%) deaths
0–3	15	4(27)	4(100)
4–6	18	2(11)	1(50)
7–12	31	2(6)	2(100)
13–18	30	1(3)	0(0)
19–24	17	1(6)	1(100)
>25	383	15(4)	8(53)
Unknown	93	11(12)	9(82)
Total	587	36(6.1)	25(69)

Source: From Steen PA, Tinker JH, Tarhan S: Myocardial reinfarction after anesthesia and surgery. *JAMA* 239:2566, June 1978. By permission of Mayo Foundation.

oped; and potent new drugs, such as the loop diuretics and the newer intravenous inotropic agents, have become available. Older studies, therefore, may give an unnecessarily pessimistic view of the risks of surgery in the post-MI patient. There is little evidence, however, that improved techniques have brought about a concomitant reduction in the risk of surgery in patients with a history of MI. Two studies from the Mayo Clinic specifically addressed this issue. In the first, Tarhan et al. reported on a total of 32,877 patients who underwent general anesthesia during the years 1967 and 1968 [7]. Of these, 422 had a history of a previous myocardial infarction. Twenty-eight patients (6.6%) experienced another infarction within the first postoperative week, with a mortality rate of 54 percent. This contrasts with a 0.13 percent postoperative infarction rate among those patients without a prior history of MI and is very similar to the earlier statistics reported by the Cornell group [5,6].

The second study from the Mayo Clinic was an extension of their earlier paper. In this paper Steen et al. reviewed the records of 73,321 patients who underwent anesthesia and noncardiac surgery at the Mayo Clinic during the years 1974 and 1975; 587 of these patients had suffered *previous* MIs [8]. Thirty-six (6.1%) had a reinfarction, and 25 of the 36 (69%) died. This paper, published 16 years after the paper of Knapp et al., reported the same perioperative infarction rate for patients with a history of prior infarction as was seen in the earlier study (6.1% in both). Mortality rates for those with infarctions were similar (69% in the newer study, 58% in the study of Knapp et al.). Thus, despite the introduction of newer anesthetic agents and techniques, major changes in medical management, and sophisticated postoperative monitoring, the risk of general anesthesia and surgery continues to be increased in patients with a history of MI.

The relationship of morbidity and mortality to the length of time between infarction and surgery in the study of Steen et al. is shown in Table 164-4 [8]. This study also addressed a number of other factors of interest. *Sex* and *age* were not found to be significant factors. The incidence of reinfarction among the 121 women (6.6%) was not significantly different from that seen in the 466 men (6.0%). The difference in reinfarction rate between patients older or younger than 60 years of age also failed to reach statistical significance (p<0.1). The presence of *diabetes* did not alter the risk of postoperative infarction, nor did the presence of preoperative *angina. Hypertension,* on the other hand, was a definite risk factor for recurrent infarction. Patients with preoperative hypertension requiring medical treatment had a significantly greater reinfarction rate than normotensive patients (9.4% vs. 4.7%; p<0.05). Site of previous infarction did

not correlate with reinfarction rate or mortality, nor did the type of general anesthetic used.

Blood pressure changes during surgery were important. Sixty-five patients had a 30 percent or greater rise in systolic pressure for 10 minutes or more at least once during anesthesia. In these patients, the reinfarction rate was higher than among patients who did not have such a hypertensive episode (9.2% vs. 4.4%), but the difference did not achieve statistical significance (p<0.15). Among 145 patients who experienced a decrease in systolic pressure of at least 30 percent for 10 minutes or more at least once during anesthesia, the reinfarction rate was significantly higher (15.2% vs. 3.2%; p<0.001) than it was for patients who did not have such episodes. Of course, these data only establish an association; they do not allow us to know if the hypotensive episode caused the infarction or rather was a consequence of an infarction already occurring.

The subgroups of patients undergoing surgery on the great vessels, having noncardiac thoracic surgery, or undergoing upper abdominal surgery had significantly greater reinfarction rates (16%, 13%, and 8%, respectively).

The reinfarction rate for the entire group increased significantly with increasing duration of *anesthesia,* from 1.9 percent for procedures lasting less than 1 hour to 16.7 percent for procedures lasting more than 6 hours (p<0.001) (Fig. 164-1).

Fig. 164-1. Relationship of myocardial infarction to duration of anesthesia. (From Steen PA, Tinker JH, Tarhan S: Myocardial reinfarction after anesthesia and surgery. *JAMA* 239:2566, 1978, with permission.)

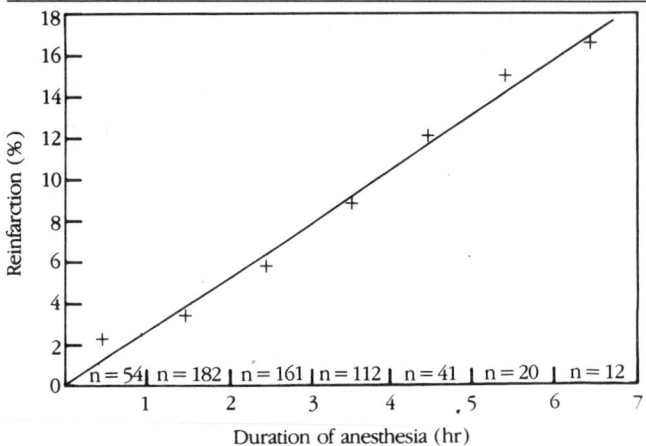

Patients cared for in an intensive care unit (ICU) postoperatively suffered an excess incidence of reinfarction, but when appropriate corrections were made for the different types of patients selected for postoperative ICU care (patients with great-vessel operations comprised 39% of the ICU admissions, and patients who had other intrathoracic surgery made up an additional 15%), the incidence of reinfarction in patients admitted to an ICU was no different from that in the overall group. These relationships are summarized in Table 164-5.

The authors of this study cautioned that they did not separate stable from unstable angina, nor mild from severe diabetes, noting that patients with more severe disease may not have been sent for elective or semi-elective surgery. They also did not evaluate the impact of congestive heart failure on postoperative MI. The authors concluded that elective surgery should not be done within 6 months of an MI.

Although patients with recent MI are at high risk, patients with other manifestations of heart disease also present a problem. In 1970, Mauney et al. reported on 365 selected patients who underwent noncardiac surgery at the Duke University Medical Center [9]. In this prospective study, patients over the age of 50 who were undergoing major surgery were selected on the basis of abnormal ECGs showing one or more of the following: (1) previous MI; (2) bundle branch block, left ventricular strain, or hypertrophy; or (3) S–T segment evidence of subendocardial injury. Patients with evidence of prior MI were entered into the study only if there was no clinical evidence of infarction within the preceding 24 months. Most of the procedures were over 2 hours in length, and 90 percent were done under general anesthesia.

Sixty-four (18%) patients had ECG changes of new or additional ischemia. Thirty-four of these 64 had S–T changes without clinical evidence of myocardial injury. Two of these 34 died and were found to have new MIs at autopsy. Thirty of the 365 (8%) suffered postoperative MIs; 16 of the 30 (53%) died. Fifteen percent of patients in this select population who sustained an intraoperative fall in systolic blood pressure of 30 percent for at least 10 minutes developed postoperative infarction. There was no relationship between postoperative MI and the presence of diabetes or old (>2 yr) infarction. There was, however, a direct correlation between the incidence of postoperative MI and the length of the operative procedure.

Perhaps the most comprehensive study of cardiac risk for patients undergoing noncardiac surgical procedures was reported by Goldman et al. in 1977 [10]. In this prospective study from the Massachusetts General Hospital, 1001 patients over 40 years of age who underwent surgery in 1975 and 1976 were included. Excluded were minor operations under local anesthesia, uncomplicated endoscopies, and transurethral resec-

tions of the prostate. Members of the study team saw each patient, usually before surgery, and took a history of cardiac risk factors and examined the patient. An anesthesiologist also assigned each patient a Dripps-American Society of Anesthesiologists classification, a widely used method for preoperatively assessing surgical risk [11].

Postoperative pulmonary edema, MI, and ventricular tachycardia were defined as life threatening, and each was associated with a 25 percent or greater incidence of cardiac death. Other cardiac complications were associated with a substantially lower chance of cardiac death and were defined as minor. A multivariate discriminant analysis was used to evaluate the relative importance of the various risk factors for cardiac complications.

Of the 1001 operations, 804 were elective and 197 were emergent. Fifty-seven percent of the patients were men. Dyspnea was present in 224 and was thought to be cardiac in origin in 103. Classic angina was present in 69, atypical angina in another 69, and hypertension in 280. Nineteen patients suffered postoperative cardiac deaths. Thirty-nine other patients suffered one or more life-threatening cardiac complications but did not die of cardiac causes. The discriminant analysis identified 9 factors that had statistically independent correlations with cardiac outcome; these are listed in Table 164-6.

The discriminant analysis was used to develop a point system that could be used to predict risk. These point values are shown in Table 164-6. Based on point totals, patients were separated into four risk categories (Table 164-7). Progression from class I to class IV was associated with incremental increase in the percentage of patients suffering cardiac complications or cardiac death. Those patients in the highest risk category had an extraordinarily high risk of these complications.

The Dripps-American Society of Anesthesiologists class had a strong univariate correlation with cardiac outcome but did not add a statistically significant increment in classification power to the 9-factor index according to the discriminant analysis.

The authors concluded that only lifesaving procedures should be performed on class IV (score ≥26) patients and that patients with preoperative scores of 13 to 25 (class III) should be considered to have sufficient risk to warrant preoperative medical consultation. If at all possible, surgery should be postponed until 6 months after an MI, but even within this time

Table 164-5. Postoperative Reinfarction Related and Nonrelated Factors

1. Related factors
   a. Interval from previous infarction to surgery
   b. Hypertension on medical therapy
   c. Hypotension during surgery
   d. Surgical site (great-vessel, intrathoracic, or upper abdominal)
   e. Duration of anesthesia
2. Nonrelated factors
   a. Age
   b. Sex
   c. Diabetes
   d. Prior presence of angina
   e. Anesthetic technique
   f. Site of previous infarction
   g. Postoperative ICU admission

Table 164-6. Preoperative Factors Related to Postoperative Cardiac Outcome (in order of decreasing significance)

Factors	No. points
1. S_2 gallop or jugular venous distention	11
2. Myocardial infarction in the preceding 6 mo	10
3. Rhythm other than sinus, or premature atrial contraction on the preoperative electrocardiogram	7
4. >5/min premature ventricular contractions at any time before surgery	7
5. Intraperitoneal, intrathoracic, or aortic operation	3
6. Age >70 yr	5
7. Significant valvular aortic stenosis	3
8. Emergency surgery	4
9. Poor general medical condition (PO_2 <60 mm Hg, PCO_2 >50 mm Hg, K <3.0 or HCO_2 <20 mEq/L, BUN >50 or creatinine >3.0 mg/dl, elevated SGOT, signs of chronic liver disease, or patient bedridden from noncardiac causes)	3

Source: From Goldman L, Caldera DL, Nussbaum SR, et al: Multifactorial index of cardiac risk in noncardiac surgical procedures. *N Engl J Med* 297:845, 1977. By permission of the New England Journal of Medicine.

Table 164-7. Cardiac Risk Index

Class	Point total	No. (%) of only minor complication	No. (%) life-threatening complication	Cardiac death
I (N = 537)	0–5	532(99)	4(0.7)	1(0.2)
II (N = 316)	6–12	295(93)	16(5)	5(2)
III (N = 130)	13–25	112(86)	15(11)	3(2)
IV (N = 18)	>26	4(22)	4(22)	10(56)

N = number of patients studied.
Source: From Goldman L, Caldera DL, Nussbaum SR, et al: Multifactorial index of cardiac risk in noncardiac surgical procedures. *N Engl J Med* 27:845, 1977. By permission of the New England Journal of Medicine.

period, use of the index permits separation of patients into high- and low-risk categories.

Variables that were not found to be significant in their analysis included hyperlipidemia, smoking, diabetes, hypertension, peripheral vascular disease, stable angina, old MI by history or ECG, S–T segment or T-wave changes, cardiomegaly, mitral valve disease, bundle branch blocks, and congestive heart failure (CHF) in the absence of an S_3 or jugular venous distention. The number of patients, however, in some of these categories was small.

Subsequently, Detsky et al. [12] carried out a validation study using Goldman's index and found that modifying it by adding categories for angina and for past history of pulmonary edema improved its predictive power. Their study also differed in that it applied the score obtained on the multifactorial index (patient characteristics) to the pre-test probability of a cardiac complication to give a final, post-test probability. The pre-test probability is based on the average risk of a cardiac complication and is dependent on the procedure, the institution, and referral bias, among other factors.

PATIENTS WITH CORONARY RISK FACTORS BUT WITHOUT CLINICAL HEART DISEASE. In addition to the millions of patients with clinical evidence of heart disease, there are large numbers of surgical patients who have subclinical heart disease, i.e., coronary artery disease that has not yet caused symptoms. It has been suggested [13] that it may be useful to identify these patients by the use of a cardiovascular risk profile such as that developed by the Framingham study [14]. In a follow-up to their original paper, however, Goldman et al. emphasized the lack of a relationship between the general cardiovascular risk factors, such as cigarette smoking and hyperlipidemia, and the risk of noncardiac surgery, despite the importance of these factors in the general prediction of coronary artery disease [15].

SPECIAL TYPES OF SURGERY. Certain types of surgery are known to be associated with a low risk of cardiac complications, even in patients with preexistent heart disease. Operations done under local anesthesia and uncomplicated endoscopies fall into this category. An operation of special interest is transurethral prostatic resection. This operation is performed on elderly men, frequently with coexistent cardiac disease. The operation has nonetheless been shown to be relatively safe even in this high-risk group [16]. Furthermore, Thompson et al. showed that in a group of 192 men who underwent transurethral prostatic resection and who had a history of MI, the mortality was no greater in patients operated on within 6 months of infarction than it was for the group as a whole [17]. Low spinal anesthesia was employed in 171 of these patients, with intra-

venous thiopental (sometimes in combination with halothane by inhalation) used in the remainder. In the group as a whole, however, 11 of 192 (5.7%) patients suffered perioperative MIs, with a 63 percent mortality rate (7 of 11 cases).

Specific Cardiovascular Problems

ANESTHESIA. Anesthetic agents have two major harmful effects on the heart: myocardial depression and promotion of dysrhythmias. All anesthetic agents are myocardial depressants [13]. Of the inhaled agents, halothane is the most and nitrous oxide the least depressant. These agents also are peripheral vasodilators and can cause blood pressure to fall. Ketamine and cyclopropane stimulate adrenergic activity, which tends to counteract their direct negative inotropic and vasodilator qualities. In contrast, halothane decreases autonomic activity in addition to its direct effects on the heart and circulation. Narcotics have a variable effect. Morphine and fentanyl are minimally depressant, whereas meperidine is a potent cardiac depressant. Morphine, in particular, has been extensively used in cardiac surgery and has been found by Lowenstein et al. to increase cardiac and stroke index and to decrease systemic vascular resistance [18]. The authors point out that these findings are in agreement with the results of animal experiments, which have shown that morphine is a potent peripheral vascular dilator with only minimal direct cardiac effects. They suggest that morphine should be considered as the agent of choice in patients with poor circulatory reserve who require major surgery that is likely to require postoperative ventilatory support.

Barbiturates are primarily venodilators, with little activity as myocardial depressants except in large doses. Diazepam, very frequently used for preoperative sedation, is usually free of major circulatory effects unless given by rapid IV injection [19]. Lorazepam has few cardiovascular effects [20], and midazolam has been shown to be safe in patients with coronary artery disease [21].

The other major complication of anesthesia is the induction of arrhythmias. Intubation, induction, and extubation are often associated with significant autonomic nervous system effects, blood pressure changes, ischemia, and arrhythmias [22,23]. In one study, 5013 patients were monitored during operations under halothane anesthesia [24]. Operative arrhythmias were found to be more often associated with the presence of known heart disease than with the presence of preoperative arrhythmias. Patients on digitalis were more likely to have intraoperative arrhythmias, but it is possible that the taking of this drug is a marker for the presence of underlying heart disease rather than a cause of the arrhythmias. Arrhythmias may be of almost any type. Serious ventricular arrhythmias may be induced by autonomic imbalance, especially excess catecholamine release. Hypoxia and hypercapnia also may induce arrhythmias. Intraoperative ventricular arrhythmias often respond to lightening the anesthesia, improving ventilation, or controlling factors causing ischemia (blood loss, hyper- or hypotension). Ventricular arrhythmias sometimes require specific therapy. In this setting, lidocaine, an agent with only minimal negative inotropic activity, is the preferred antiarrhythmic drug. Mechanical stimulation by tracheal intubation, intraabdominal traction, or ocular manipulation can cause excessive parasympathetic activity that can lead to bradycardia and hypotension, requiring atropine for control. Atropine itself, however, may induce an excessive tachycardia that can lead to myocardial ischemia in patients with coronary artery disease.

There is little evidence that spinal or epidural anesthetic techniques are safer for the cardiac patient [5,7,8,10,15]. Both spinal and epidural anesthesia can cause hypotension secondary to sympathetic blockade; furthermore, these techniques are not as easily reversible as is general anesthesia. Recently, it has been suggested that continuous spinal anesthesia may be a safer technique for patients with underlying cardiovascular disease [25]. Sutter et al. compared the use of continuous spinal anesthesia with continuous epidural anesthesia in 731 patients undergoing surgery. Although the patients undergoing continuous spinal anesthesia were at higher anesthetic risk, significantly fewer had a decrease in mean arterial pressure of greater than 30 percent (44% versus 65%; p<0.0001) or needed vasopressor support (65% versus 77%; p<0.01). The authors concluded that the use of continuous spinal anesthesia results in greater cardiovascular stability. Regional anesthesia is usually quite safe, but local anesthetics are absorbed systemically and can cause myocardial toxicity when used in excessive amounts [26].

In patients with known depressed myocardial function, it is preferable to use agents with minimal negative inotropic activity, such as intravenous morphine and nitrous oxide by inhalation, or agents with adrenergic activity, such as ketamine. The combination of morphine and nitrous oxide is frequently used in cardiac surgery and can be utilized with equal effectiveness and safety in patients with heart disease undergoing noncardiac surgery.

CONDUCTION DEFECTS. Patients with complete heart block should have pacemakers placed prior to surgery. It is also generally agreed that patients with advanced second-degree atrioventricular (A-V) block (Mobitz type II) and a wide QRS pattern should have temporary pacing. Patients with first-degree A-V block, second-degree A-V block with Wenckebach pauses, and right or left bundle branch block do not require prophylactic pacemakers [27].

The management of patients with bifascicular block is more controversial. Here too, however, the weight of evidence is on the side of conservatism. A study of 98 patients with bifascicular block who underwent measurement of H-V intervals prior to surgery revealed no evidence of intraoperative or postoperative complete heart block, although the P-R interval was prolonged in 25 [28]. In another study, 44 patients with right bundle branch block and left axis deviation were studied prospectively as they underwent a total of 52 operations [29]. All patients were monitored continuously during induction of anesthesia, operation, and recovery. Only one episode of transient complete heart block occurred, and that was by a type I mechanism during intubation (i.e., P-R prolongation occurred before a higher-degree block developed). Significant pacer-related ventricular irritability developed in two of the six patients in whom temporary pacemakers had been placed. The authors concluded that prophylactic pacing is rarely indicated in patients with bifascicular block.

In patients with permanent pacemakers, the type of pacemaker and its response to rapid electrical stimulation (such as can occur during the use of electric cautery) should be known prior to surgery. Most new pacemakers are well shielded and convert to fixed-rate mode when subjected to excess stimuli. Some older pacemakers, however, are suppressed by the external stimulation of electrocautery. Many of these can be converted to fixed-rate mode by the use of a magnet.

HYPERTENSION. Patients with hypertension present special problems when undergoing surgery [30]. A study of the risk of surgery in the hypertensive patient was done by Goldman and Caldera [31]. They prospectively analyzed 676 consecutive operations in a series of patients over 40 years of age and found

that neither the preoperative in-hospital systolic or diastolic pressure correlated with perioperative blood pressure lability or the development of arrhythmias, ischemia, heart failure, or postoperative renal failure. Goldman and Caldera concluded that effective intraoperative management may be more important than the degree of preoperative control of hypertension in terms of decreasing clinically significant blood pressure lability and cardiovascular complications in patients with mild to moderate hypertension.

VALVULAR HEART DISEASE. Patients who are significantly symptomatic from valvular heart disease are likely to require corrective valve surgery prior to other forms of elective surgery. Patients with mitral stenosis who have exertional dyspnea or who have had paroxysmal nocturnal dyspnea or orthopnea can be assumed to have a severely stenotic valve. Further evaluation would include chest roentgenograms and echocardiography. These patients are at increased risk for perioperative pulmonary edema, as well as supraventricular arrhythmias, especially atrial fibrillation. They tolerate tachycardia poorly because of their need for adequate diastolic filling time and are sensitive to relatively small fluid shifts in either direction.

Chronic mitral insufficiency is generally well tolerated and adds little to risk in an asymptomatic patient; however, preoperative assessment should include careful evaluation of the ECG, chest roentgenogram, and echocardiogram. Evidence of atrial fibrillation, cardiomegaly, increased left atrial size, pulmonary congestion, or impaired ventricular function (on the echocardiogram) suggest the presence of hemodynamically significant mitral insufficiency that would increase surgical risk. Doppler echocardiography provides a qualitative measure of the degree of insufficiency. If doubt still remains, a gated radioventriculogram (RVG) permits assessment of ventricular dimensions and ejection fraction. A low ejection fraction (<30%) is associated with a marked increase in surgical risk.

Mitral valve prolapse is very common but is only rarely a cause of significant heart disease [32]. As with other forms of mitral regurgitation, the chest roentgenogram and the echocardiogram are the best noninvasive tools for assessing the hemodynamic significance of mitral valve dysfunction.

Aortic ejection murmurs are very common in the elderly. Most, however, are not caused by significant aortic stenosis, but rather are associated with hemodynamically insignificant irregularities of the aortic valve and root. The most helpful finding on physical examination for detecting hemodynamically significant aortic stenosis is slowing of the carotid upstroke. Echocardiography is most useful if a normal aortic valve is seen, in which case significant aortic stenosis is essentially ruled out; however, two-dimensional echocardiographic evidence of an abnormal aortic valve with a diminished opening and increased echodensity may or may not be associated with significant aortic stenosis. Continuous wave and pulsed Doppler echocardiography have been used to measure the aortic valve area noninvasively, and results are well correlated with data obtained by cardiac catheterization [33,34]. If syncope, heart failure, or angina is related to aortic stenosis, the risk of surgery is significantly increased, and one should consider valve replacement or dilatation by valvuloplasty before elective or semielective surgery is carried out.

Aortic insufficiency can be difficult to evaluate. More than any other valvular lesion, it can cause insidious deterioration of cardiac function without producing symptoms [35]. If cardiomegaly is found on the chest roentgenogram, echocardiography and, if needed, RVG should be obtained to evaluate cardiac function.

Acute regurgitation of either the mitral or aortic valves,

whether caused by trauma, infection, aotic dissection, or idiopathic rupture of mitral chordae, is a generally catastrophic occurrence with the abrupt onset of left ventricular failure and pulmonary congestion. When there is an associated need for noncardiac surgery, the valve must be replaced first or, if time does not permit, concomitantly.

Prophylactic antibiotics for the prevention of bacterial endocarditis need to be given to patients with valvular heart disease when such patients undergo surgery involving unsterile areas of the body. A suggested program of prophylactic antibiotics is given in Table 164-8 [36].

PERIPHERAL VASCULAR DISEASE. Patients with peripheral vascular disease (PVD) present a particularly interesting problem. These patients have a high incidence of associated coronary artery disease (CAD), but because the ability to exercise is limited by claudication, they may have little or no angina. Routine coronary arteriography in patients with PVD has shown that the incidence of significant (but often asymptomatic) CAD may be over 30 percent [37,38]. In a study of 1000 cases from the Cleveland Clinic, Hertzer et al. [38] found that 34 percent of patients undergoing peripheral vascular surgery and clinically suspected of having CAD as well as 14 percent of those without clinical evidence for CAD had "severe, correctable" CAD documented by catheterization.

In 1981, Cutler et al. [39] showed that ECG stress testing was especially valuable in the preoperative assessment of patients with PVD. Either treadmill or arm ergometry testing was used. In the lowest risk group (35 of 130 patients, who achieved >75% of maximum predicted heart rate and had no ischemic ECG changes), there were no postoperative cardiac complications. In contrast, in the highest risk group (26 patients with an ischemic ECG response at <75% of maximum predicted heart rate), there were 10 postoperative cardiac complications (38%), including 7 MIs (27%), 5 of which were fatal. Based on these results, the authors suggested that aortoiliac disease patients falling into the highest risk group should more often be given extraanatomic grafts (axillofemoral or femorofemoral). The authors also suggested that patients with strongly positive exercise tests should have preoperative coronary arteriography and some may require coronary artery bypass surgery prior to their indicated vascular procedure, if they have operable severe CAD.

Dipyridamole-thallium testing has become an established noninvasive alternative to conventional stress testing for patients at high risk for CAD who cannot exercise because of PVD or orthopedic problems [40–46]. Boucher et al. [41] were the first group to report on the utility of dipyridamole-thallium imaging in the preoperative assessment of cardiac risk. Forty-eight patients with suspected CAD were evaluated before they underwent vascular surgery. Sixteen of these patients had thallium redistribution. All 8 perioperative cardiac events occurred in patients who had preoperative thallium redistribution. The 32 patients with normal scans or only persistent thallium defects had no cardiac complications.

Leppo et al. [42] followed this with a study in which dipyridamole-thallium imaging was performed on 100 consecutive patients admitted for elective peripheral vascular surgery. Eleven patients were referred for cardiac angiography based on the results of noninvasive testing. Of the remaining 89 patients, postoperative MI occurred in 15, 14 of whom had thallium redistribution. Among the many variables examined, the presence of thallium redistribution was the most significant predictor of serious cardiac events.

Although its sensitivity for detecting patients at increased risk is excellent, one of the criticisms of using dipyridamole-thallium imaging for preoperative screening is that its specificity is low. In order to improve the specificity and positive predictive value, some investigators have tried combining clinical markers with noninvasive testing while others have demonstrated that quantifying the amount of myocardium at risk can better define the patients at risk for perioperative cardiac events.

Eagle et al. [43] performed preoperative dipyridamole-thallium testing and clinical evaluation in 254 patients prior to major vascular procedures. Surgery was subsequently performed in 200. Of these 200 patients, 30 (15%) had early postoperative ischemic events; there were 6 deaths (3%) and 9 nonfatal MIs (4.5%). Thallium *redistribution* was highly predictive of subsequent events, as were five clinical variables (Q waves on ECG, history of ventricular ectopic activity, diabetes, age >70 years, angina). Use of both the clinical and thallium data yielded significantly higher specificity with no loss of sensitivity. The authors noted that for nearly half of the patients, very low or very high operative risk could be predicted on the basis of clinical variables alone, making dipyridamole-thallium imaging unnecessary (Fig. 164-2).

In a group of patients undergoing major general and vascular surgery, Lette et al. [44] showed that there was a strong correlation between the extent and severity of reversible thallium defects and the risk of cardiac death or MI. Levinson et al. [45] examined the impact of dividing the thallium images into 15 myocardial segments. Patients with redistribution in four or more segments, two of three views, and two of three coronary territories had the greatest perioperative risk. Of note is that there were no cardiac events in patients with redistribution seen in only one view. More recently, Brown and Rowen [46] developed a method to stratify perioperative risk based on the number of segments (out of a total of 9; see Fig. 164-3) with transient thallium defects and a history of diabetes mellitus (see

Table 164-8. Regimens for Genitourinary/Gastrointestinal Procedures

Drug	Dosage regimen*
Standard Regimen	
Ampicillin, gentamicin, and amoxicillin	Intravenous or intramuscular administration of ampicillin, 2.0 gm, plus gentamicin, 1.5 mg/kg (not to exceed 80 mg), 30 min before procedure; followed by amoxicillin, 1.5 gm, orally 6 h after initial dose; alternatively, the parenteral regimen may be repeated once 8 hr after initial dose
Ampicillin/Amoxicillin/Penicillin—Allergic Patient Regimen	
Vancomycin and gentamicin	Intravenous administration of vancomycin, 1.0 gm, over 1 hr plus intravenous or intramuscular administration of gentamicin, 1.5 mg/kg (not to exceed 80 mg), 1 hr before procedure; may be repeated once 8 hr after initial dose
Alternate Low-Risk Patient Regimen	
Amoxicillin	3.0 gm orally 1 hr before procedure; then 1.5 gm 6 hr after initial dose

* Initial pediatric doses are as follows: ampicillin, 50 mg/kg; amoxicillin, 50 mg/kg; gentamicin, 2.0 mg/kg; and vancomycin, 20 mg/kg. Follow-up doses should be half the initial dose. **Total pediatric dose should not exceed total adult dose.**
From: Dajani AS, Bisno AL, Chung KJ, et al: Prevention of bacterial endocarditis. Recommendations of the American Heart Association. *JAMA,* 264:2919, 1990.

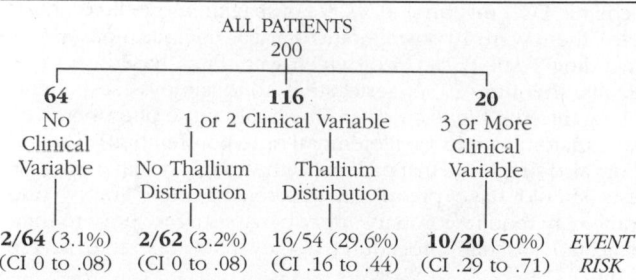

Fig. 164-2. Algorithm for using clinical variables and results of dipyridamole-thallium imaging to stratify cardiac risk as applied to this group of 200 patients. Event refers to postoperative cardiac ischemic events, including unstable angina, ischemic pulmonary edema, myocardial infarction, and cardiac death. Clinical variables are Q wave on ECG, age > 70 years, history of angina, history of ventricular ectopic activity requiring treatment, and diabetes mellitus requiring treatment. (From Eagle KA, et al: *Ann Intern Med* 110:859, 1989, used with permission.)

Table 164-9. Perioperative Risk Subgroups Based on the Number of Segments with Transient Thallium-201 Defects and a History of Diabetes Mellitus

	History of diabetes mellitus		No history of diabetes mellitus	
Risk	No. of segments with TD	Perioperative risk of CD/ NFMI	No. of segments with TD	Perioperative risk of CD/ NFMI
Low	0	<5%	0–2	≤5%
Medium	1–2	10%–20%	3–4	10%–20%
High	≥3	>25%	≥5	>25%

CD = cardiac death; NFMI = nonfatal myocardial infarction; TD = transient thallium-201 defects. From Brown KA, Rowen M: Extent of jeopardized viable myocardium determined by myocardial perfusion predicts perioperative cardiac events in patients undergoing noncardiac surgery. *J Am Coll Cardiol* 21:325, 1993.

Table 164-9). The impact of combining these methods with clinical indices such as those described by Eagle et al. has not been tested.

Ambulatory ECG monitoring also has been shown to identify ischemia in symptomatic patients with normal 12-lead ECGs and negative exercise tolerance tests [47] and in patients with silent ischemia [48]. It is less expensive and more widely available than dipyridamole-thallium imaging [40]. Raby et al. [49] prospectively studied 176 patients undergoing elective vascular surgery. Thirty-two patients had S–T segment depression on preoperative ambulatory ECG monitoring. Of these, 12 patients had postoperative ischemic events (MI, unstable angina, or ischemic pulmonary edema) as compared with only one of 144 patients who did not have preoperative ischemia on ambulatory monitoring. The sensitivity of S–T depression on ambulatory monitoring was 92 percent, specificity was 88 percent, positive predictive value was 38 percent, and negative predictive value was 99 percent.

Dobutamine stress echocardiography (DSE) has been used recently to identify patients at risk for cardiac complications of surgery. Several papers [50,51] have described this modality's usefulness in diagnosing CAD. A recent study by Poldermans et al. [52] demonstrated the ability of DSE to identify patients at high and low risk for surgery. DSE was used to screen 136 consecutive patients admitted for elective vascular surgery. Adequate, complete studies were obtained in 131 (96%). All 15 patients with perioperative cardiac events had positive tests (new or worsened wall motion abnormality), and no one with a negative DSE (96 patients) had an event. This gives a positive predictive value of 42 percent and a negative predictive value of 100 percent. These results are similar to data presented by Lalka et al. with a smaller group of patients undergoing aortic surgery (PPV* = 29%, NPV* = 95%) [53]. DSE would seem to be a promising new tool that deserves further investigation with more widespread use.

Treatment

PREOPERATIVE ASSESSMENT. Based on the foregoing, preoperative assessment of the patient is generally easily carried out, with history, physical examination, ECG, and chest roentgenogram being all that are necessary in the large majority of patients. Using some form of risk assessment criteria such as those described by Goldman, Detsky, and Eagle may be helpful and may select out patients in whom further functional or anatomic information may be needed. Exercise testing (ECG monitored or thallium), dipyridamole-thallium imaging, echocardiography, dobutamine stress echocardiography, ambulatory ECG monitoring, radioventriculography, and cardiac catheterization provide additional information in those situations where

* PPV = positive predictive value;
NPV = negative predictive value.

Fig. 164-3. Schematic representation of how anterior, left anterior oblique, and left lateral images were divided into three segments per view for a total of nine myocardial segments. AI = apical inferior; AL = anterolateral; ANT = anterior; AP = apical; INF = inferior; LAO = left anterior oblique; P = posterior; S = septal. (From Brown KA, Rowen M: *J Am Coll Cardiol* 21:325, 1993.)

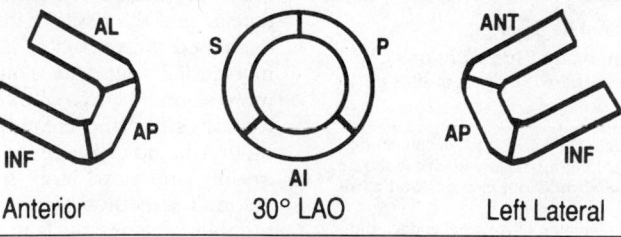

the expense and risk (in the case of catheterization) can be justified.

The place of coronary artery bypass surgery (CABG) and percutaneous transluminal coronary angioplasty (PTCA) in the preoperative management of the patient with coronary artery disease undergoing noncoronary surgery is unsettled, although there are many who feel that under appropriate circumstances, CABG or PTCA prevents ischemic morbidity and mortality during subsequent noncardiac surgery. Four studies that have addressed the issue of CABG are worth noting. McCollum et al. reported on 60 patients (average age 60.4 years) who underwent CABG prior to a major noncardiac procedure. Twenty-three of the 60 underwent both procedures during the same admission (average interval between operations, 17 days) [54]. There were no deaths or MIs associated with the noncardiac procedures. Although this was not a controlled study, the authors suggested that myocardial revascularization should be performed prior to major noncardiac surgery in CAD patients with documented ischemia.

The second study, by Mahar et al., examined the incidence of postoperative MIs in 148 patients with known CAD who underwent 226 noncardiac surgical procedures [55]. In 99 patients who underwent coronary artery bypass grafting prior to their noncardiac procedure(s), there were no perioperative MIs, whereas in 49 patients who did not undergo prior myocardial revascularization, there were 3 MIs (p<0.02), all of which occurred in individuals with three-vessel CAD. This study, although also not controlled, again suggests a possible role for myocardial revascularization in the management of these patients.

In the third study, Arous et al. [56] reviewed the records of 135 patients who had an ischemic response on exercise testing done before peripheral vascular surgery. The patients were divided into four groups.

Group I (n = 56): peripheral vascular surgery despite positive stress test
Group II (n = 23): alternate surgery chosen
Group III (n = 10): coronary artery bypass grafting done in addition to peripheral vascular surgery
Group IV (n = 46): surgery cancelled

Within 5 years of follow-up, 32% of group I (18/56), 17% of group II (4/23), 22% in group IV (10/46), but none in group III developed MIs.

The fourth study was an analysis of data from the coronary artery surgery study (CASS) [57]. A total of 1600 patients underwent major noncardiac procedures during the course of the study. They were divided into three groups.

Group I (n = 399): Patients without significant CAD. The operative mortality was 0.5% (2/399).
Group II (n = 743): Patients with significant CAD who had CABG performed prior to noncardiac surgery. The subsequent operative mortality was 0.9 percent (7/743) (group I versus group II; p = 0.42).
Group III (n = 458): Patients with significant CAD undergoing noncardiac surgery without a prior CABG procedure. The operative mortality was 2.4 percent (11/458) (p = 0.009, Group III versus Groups I and II).

The incidence of perioperative MI and arrhythmia was similar in the three groups.

Two recent studies have examined the use of PTCA before noncardiac surgery. Huber et al. [58] looked at the incidence of perioperative MI and death in a group of 50 high-risk patients undergoing 54 operations a median of 9 days after angioplasty. The overall frequency of perioperative MI was 5.6 percent, and the mortality was 1.9 percent. Although there was no control group, they concluded that patients who have had successful PTCA for severe coronary artery disease have a low risk of major cardiac complications associated with noncardiac surgery.

Another study from the Mayo Clinic compared the cardiac morbidity, mortality, and survival of patients who underwent PTCA (n = 14) or CABG (n = 86) prior to abdominal aortic aneurysm repair [59]. The rate of perioperative MI was 0 for the PTCA group and 5.8 percent for the CABG group, and no hospital deaths occurred in either group. Of note, the 3-year survival was not statistically different between groups.

In summary, although none of these studies were randomized prospective trials, the weight of evidence strongly suggests that antecedent mechanical intervention is indicated in selected, high-risk patients who are scheduled to undergo a major noncardiac operation, bearing in mind the morbidity and mortality of the myocardial revascularization procedure itself.

DRUG THERAPY. The management of drug therapy deserves special comment. Many surgical patients are taking antihypertensives, beta-blocking agents for ischemia, or digitalis. Antihypertensive therapy is a relatively straightforward issue. Antihypertensives should be continued up to the time of surgery, and perioperative hypertension should be controlled by judiciously using diuretics and potent intravenous agents, such as nitroprusside [30]. As soon as possible, the patient's normal oral medications should be resumed.

The prophylactic use of digitalis in patients with heart disease undergoing surgery is controversial. Some data suggest that digitalis controls the ventricular response rate in patients who develop postoperative supraventricular tachycardias [60]; however, the general consensus is that routine prophylactic use of this agent is not indicated [61]. On the other hand, preoperative administration of digitalis is clearly indicated in patients with congestive heart failure or a definite propensity toward supraventricular arrhythmias [62].

Perhaps the most controversial class of drugs in patients with cardiac disease undergoing noncardiac surgery is the beta-adrenergic blockers, typified by propranolol. It was feared that continuation of propranolol therapy would blunt the necessary metabolic and hemodynamic responses to the stress of surgery [63]. Subsequent work, however, has shown that hemodynamic responses usually remain appropriate despite continued therapy with propranolol [64]. Thus, heart rate and arterial blood pressure increase appropriately in response to such stresses as endotracheal intubation. Indeed, it is now clear that it is dangerous to withdraw beta-blocker therapy from patients who may then become ischemic [65,66]. It is generally agreed that propranolol (or a similar agent) should be continued to the morning of surgery in those patients who were receiving it to treat angina or hypertension.

The prophylactic use of beta-blockers may actually decrease the occurrence of perioperative ischemia. Only a few studies have been published, but some have indicated a decrease in intraoperative ischemic episodes [67,68,69], and one demonstrated a decrease in perioperative MI [69]. There are even fewer data regarding the use of other antianginals during surgery, and no clear consensus has been reached about the use of these agents.

PERIOPERATIVE MANAGEMENT. The skill of the anesthesiologist is critical to the management of these patients. Anesthesiologists who are familiar with the care of patients undergoing cardiac surgery will bring those same skills to the care of the cardiac patient undergoing noncardiac surgery [27]. Certain patients with a history of CHF or significant angina should have arterial as well as pulmonary artery pressure monitoring lines placed at the time of surgery. By monitoring filling pressures, systemic arterial pressure, and cardiac output, impending fluid overload, hypotension, or cardiac decompensation can be quickly detected and treated in the operating room or ICU.

Postoperative arrhythmias are common and should not be overtreated. Ventricular premature beats (VPBs) often are a sign of hypoxia or electrolyte disturbance, especially potassium depletion, and these abnormalities should be sought and aggressively treated. Pain also should be well controlled, as the hemodynamic response to pain (tachycardia and hypertension) may precipitate or exacerbate ischemia, leading to arrhythmias. When specific therapy of VPBs is indicated, a limited course of intravenous lidocaine usually suffices. Supraventricular arrhythmias are often indicative of pulmonary or infectious complications, and correction of the underlying abnormality often corrects the arrhythmia. Even when the supraventricular arrhythmia is of direct cardiac origin, it is often a marker of increasing congestive failure, and treatment directed at improving cardiac hemodynamics is of greater value than is antiarrhythmic therapy.

The physician must remain vigilant during the first week after surgery. Mobilization, decreasing sedation, increasing anemia because of inadequate replacement of blood loss, and infection can all place additional stresses on the cardiovascular system, resulting in postoperative infarction. A level of anemia that would be entirely acceptable in the noncardiac patient may lead to ischemia in the patient with a limited ability to augment myocardial oxygen delivery, and in these patients the hematocrit should not be allowed to fall much below 30 percent. Minidose heparin (5000 units subcutaneously 2 hr prior to surgery and q8–12h for 4 or 5 days postoperatively) is recommended to prevent deep venous thrombosis and pulmonary embolism in most cases [70]. In those patients at greater risk (orthopedic surgery), higher, adjusted doses of heparin or perioperative warfarin therapy is appropriate [71].

Cardiac patients undergoing noncardiac surgery present a challenge to the health care team. With modern tools, however, the cardiac patient should be able to undergo noncardiac surgery with only a small increase in risk beyond that of the patient without heart disease.

References

1. Arteriosclerosis 1981: Report of the Working Group on Arteriosclerosis of the National Heart, Lung and Blood Institute. Washington, DC, National Institutes of Health, NIH publication 81:2034, 1981.
2. Kannel WB, McGee D, Gordon T: A general cardiovascular risk profile: The Framingham study. Am J Cardiol 38:46, 1976.
3. Roe CF, Goldberg MJ, Blair CS, et al: The influence of body temperature on early postoperative oxygen consumption. Surgery 60:85, 1966.
4. Bay J, Nunn JF, Prys-Roberts C: Factors influencing arterial pO$_2$ during recovery from anesthesia. Br J Anaesth 40:398, 1966.
5. Knapp RB, Topkins MJ, Artusio JF Jr: The cerebrovascular accident and coronary occlusion in anesthesia. JAMA 182:106, 1962.
6. Topkins MJ, Artusio JF Jr: Myocardial infarction and surgery: A five year study. Anesth Analg 43:716, 1964.
7. Tarhan S, Moffit EA, Taylor WF, et al: Myocardial infarction after general anesthesia. JAMA 220:1451, 1972.
8. Steen PA, Tinker JH, Tarhan S: Myocardial reinfarction after anesthesia and surgery. JAMA 239:2566, 1978.
9. Mauney FM Jr, Ebert PA, Sabiston DA Jr: Postoperative myocardial infarction: A study of predisposing factors, diagnosis and mortality in a high risk group of surgical patients. Ann Surg 172:497, 1970.
10. Goldman L, Caldera DL, Nussbaum SR, et al: Multifactorial index of cardiac risk in noncardiac surgical procedures. N Engl J Med 297:845, 1977.
11. Dripps RD, Lamont A, Eckenhoff JE: The role of anesthesia in surgical mortality. JAMA 178:261, 1961.
12. Detsky AS, Abrams HB, McLaughlin JR, et al: Predicting cardiac complications in patients undergoing non-cardiac surgery. J Gen Intern Med 1:211, 1986.
13. Rose SD, Corman LC, Mason DT: Cardiac risk factors in patients undergoing noncardiac surgery. Med Clin North Am 63:1271, 1979.
14. Kannel WB, McGee D, Gordon T: A general cardiovascular risk profile: The Framingham study. Am J Cardiol 38:46, 1976.
15. Goldman L, Caldera DL, Southwick FS, et al: Cardiac risk factors and complications in non-cardiac surgery. Medicine 57:357, 1978.
16. Erlik D, Valero A, Birkhan J, et al: Prostatic surgery and the cardiovascular patient. Br J Urol 40:53, 1968.
17. Thompson GJ, Kelalis PP, Connolly DC: Transurethral prostatic resection after myocardial infarction. JAMA 182:908, 1962.
18. Lowenstein E, Hallowell P, Levine FH, et al: Cardiovascular response to large doses of intravenous morphine in man. N Engl J Med 281:1389, 1969.
19. Stanley TH, Bennett GM, Lorser EA, et al: Cardiovascular Anesth 44:255, 1976.
20. Ameer B, Greenblatt DJ: Lorazepam: A review of its clinical pharmacologic properties and therapeutic uses. Drugs 21:161, 1981.
21. Marty J, Nitenberg A, Blanchet F, et al: Effects of midazolam on the coronary circulation in patients with coronary artery disease. Anesthesiology 64:206, 1986.
22. Katz RL, Bigger JT Jr: Cardiac arrhythmias during anesthesia and operation. Anesthesiology 33:193, 1970.
23. Rosen M, Mushin WW, Kilpatrick GS, et al: Study of myocardial ischemia in surgical patients. BMJ 2:1415, 1966.
24. Massumi RA, Mason DT, Amsterdam EA, et al: Ventricular fibrillation and tachycardia after intravenous atropine for treatment of bradycardias. N Engl J Med 287:336, 1972.
25. Sutter PA, Gamulin Z, Forster A, et al: Comparison of continuous spinal and continuous epidural anaesthesia for lower limb surgery in elderly patients—a retrospective study. Anaesthesia 44:47, 1989.
26. McCaughey W: Adverse effects of local anesthetics. Drug Safety 7:178, 1992.
27. Logue B, Kaplan JA: The cardiac patient and noncardiac surgery. Curr Probl Cardiol 7:1, 1982.
28. Belloci F, Santarelli P, DiGennaro M, et al: The risk of cardiac complications in surgical patients with bifascicular block: A clinical and electrophysiologic study of 98 patients. Chest 77:3, 1980.
29. Pastore JO, Yurchak PM, Janis KM, et al: The risk of advanced heart block in surgical patients with right bundle branch block and left axis deviation. Circulation 57:677, 1978.
30. Foex P, Prys-Roberts C: Anaesthesia and the hypertensive patient. Br J Anaesth 46:575, 1974.
31. Goldman L, Caldera DL: Risks of general anesthesia and elective operation in the hypertensive patient. Anesthesiology 50:285, 1979.
32. Procacci PM, Savran SV, Schrieter SL, et al: Prevalance of clinical mitral valve prolapse in 1169 young women. N Engl J Med 294:1086, 1976.
33. Skjaerpe T, Hegrenaes L, Hatle L: Noninvasive estimation of valve area in patients with aortic stenosis by Doppler ultrasound and two-dimensional echocardiography. Circulation 72:810, 1985.
34. Agatston AS: Doppler diagnosis of valvular aortic stenosis. Echocardiography 3:3, 1986.
35. O'Rourke RA, Crawford MH: Timing of aortic valve replacement in patients with chronic aortic regurgitation: Editorial. Circulation 61:493, 1980.
36. Dajani AS, Bisno AL, Chung KJ, et al: Prevention of bacterial endocarditis: Recommendations by the American Heart Association. JAMA 264:2919, 1990.
37. Tomatis LA, Fierens EE, Verbrugge GP: Evaluation of surgical risk in peripheral vascular disease by coronary arteriography. Series of 100 cases. Surgery 71:429, 1972.
38. Hertzer NR, Beven EG, Young JR, et al: Coronary artery disease in peripheral vascular patients. Ann Surg 199:223, 1984.

39. Cutler BS, Wheeler HB, Paraskos JA, et al: Applicability and interpretation of electrocardiographic stress testing in patients with peripheral vascular disease. *Am J Surg* 141:501, 1981.

40. Eagle KA, Boucher CA: Cardiac risk of noncardiac surgery. *N Engl J Med* 321:1330, 1989.

41. Boucher CA, Brewster DC, Darling RC, et al: Determination of cardiac risk by dipyridamole-thallium imaging before peripheral vascular surgery. *N Engl J Med* 312:389, 1985.

42. Leppo J, Plaja J, Gionet M, et al: Noninvasive evaluation of cardiac risk before elective vascular surgery. *J Am Coll Cardiol* 9:269, 1987.

43. Eagle KA, Coley CM, Newell JB: Combining clinical and thallium data optimizes preoperative assessment of cardiac risk before major vascular surgery. *Ann Intern Med* 110:859, 1989.

44. Lette J, Waters D, Lapointe J, et al: Usefulness of the severity and extent of reversible perfusion defects during thallium-dipyridamole imaging for cardiac risk assessment before noncardiac surgery. *Am J Cardiol* 64:276, 1989.

45. Levison JR, Boucher CA, Coley CM, et al: Usefulness of semiquantitative analysis of dipyridamole-thallium-201 redistribution for improving risk stratification before vascular surgery. *Am J Cardiol* 66:406, 1990.

46. Brown KA, Rowen M: Extent of jeopardized viable myocardium determined by myocardial perfusion imaging predicts perioperative cardiac events in patients undergoing noncardiac surgery. *J Am Coll Cardiol* 21:325, 1993.

47. Stern S, Tzivoni D: Early detection of silent ischemic heart disease by 24-hour electrocardiographic monitoring of active subjects. *Br Heart J* 36:481, 1974.

48. Cohn PF: Silent myocardial ischemia: Classification, prevalence, and prognosis. *Am J Med* 79(Suppl 3A)2, 1985.

49. Raby KE, Goldman L, Creager MA, et al: Correlation between preoperative ischemia and major cardiac events after peripheral vascular surgery. *N Engl J Med* 321:1296, 1989.

50. Sawada SG, Segar DS, Ryan T, et al: Echocardiographic detection of coronary artery disease during dobutamine infusion. *Circulation* 83:1605, 1991.

51. Marcovitz PA, Armstrong WF: Accuracy of dobutamine stress echocardiography in detecting coronary artery disease. *Am J Cardiol* 69:1269, 1992.

52. Poldermans D, Fioretti PM, Forster T, et al: Dobutamine stress echocardiography for assessment of perioperative cardiac risk in patients undergoing major vascular surgery. *Circulation* 87:1506, 1993.

53. Lalka SG, Sawada SG, Dalsing MC, et al: Dobutamine stress echocardiography as a predictor of cardiac events associated with aortic surgery. *J Vasc Surg* 15:831, 1992.

54. McCollum CH, Garcia-Rinaldi R, Graham JM, et al: Myocardial revascularization prior to subsequent major surgery in patients with coronary artery disease. *Surgery* 81:302, 1977.

55. Mahar LJ, Steen PA, Tinker JH, et al: Perioperative myocardial infarction in patients with coronary artery disease with and without aortocoronary bypass grafts. *J Thorac Cardiovasc Surg* 76:533, 1978.

56. Arous EJ, Baum PL, Cutler BS: The ischemic exercise test in patients with peripheral vascular disease. *Arch Surg* 119:780, 1984.

57. Foster ED, Davis KB, Carpenter JA, et al: Risk of noncardiac operation in patients with defined coronary disease: The coronary artery surgery study (CASS) registry experience. *Ann Thorac Surg* 41:42, 1986.

58. Huber KC, Evans MA, Bresnahan JF, et al: Outcome of noncardiac operations in patients with severe coronary artery disease successfully treated preoperatively with coronary angioplasty. *Mayo Clin Proc* 67:15, 1992.

59. Elmore JR, Hallett JW, Gibbons RJ, et al: Myocardial revascularization before abdominal aortic aneurysmorrhaphy: Effect of coronary angioplasty. *Mayo Clin Proc* 68:637, 1993.

60. Goldman L: Supraventricular tachyarrhythmias in hospitalized adults after surgery: Clinical correlates in patients over 40 years of age after major noncardiac surgery. *Chest* 73:450, 1978.

61. Selzer A, Kelly JJ, Gerbode F, et al: Case against routine use of digitalis in patients undergoing cardiac surgery. *JAMA* 195:549, 1966.

62. Goldman L: Cardiac risks and complications of noncardiac surgery. *Ann Intern Med* 98:504, 1983.

63. Viljoen JF, Estafanous FG, Kellner GA: Propranolol and cardiac surgery. *J Thorac Cardiovasc Surg* 64:826, 1972.

64. Kopriva CJ, Brown ACD, Pappas G: Hemodynamics during general anesthesia in patients receiving propranolol. *Anesthesiology* 48:28, 1978.

65. Miller RR, Olson HG, Amsterdam E, et al: Propranolol withdrawal rebound phenomenon: Exacerbation of coronary events after abrupt cessation of antianginal therapy. *N Engl J Med* 293:416, 1975.

66. Slogoff S, Keats AS, Ott E: Preoperative propranolol therapy and aortocoronary bypass operation. *JAMA* 240:1487, 1978.

67. Stone JG, Foex P, Sear JW, et al: Myocardial ischemia in untreated hypertensive patients: Effect of a single small oral dose of a beta-adrenergic blocking agent. *Anesthesiology* 68:495, 1988.

68. Pasternack PF, Grossi EA, Baumann FG, et al: Beta blockade to decrease silent myocardial ischemia during peripheral vascular surgery. *Am J Surg* 158:113, 1989.

69. Pasternack PF, Imparato AM, Baumann FG, et al: The hemodynamics of β-blockade in patients undergoing abdominal aortic aneurysm repair. *Circulation* 76(Suppl 3):III-1, 1987.

70. Kakkar VV, Corrigan TP, Fossard DP: Prevention of fatal postoperative pulmonary embolism by low doses of heparin: An international multicentre trial. *Lancet* 2:45, 1975.

71. Clagett GP, Anderson FA, Levine MN, et al: Prevention of venous thromboembolism. *Chest* 102(4 Suppl):391S, 1992.

165. Arterial Diseases of the Extremities

Michael J. Rohrer and
David F. Giansiracusa

A variety of pathophysiologic processes can impair arterial perfusion of the extremities. The key factors determining the clinical presentation and outcome are the size of the affected artery, the rapidity of arterial occlusion, the degree of the underlying vascular disease, and the extent of collateral circulation. Acute arterial embolization and thrombosis, chronic arterial occlusive disease, atheroembolization, and iatrogenic vascular complications are discussed in this chapter. Conditions causing primarily digital symptoms such as systemic vasculitis and Raynaud's phenomenon are discussed in Chapter 220.

Acute Limb Ischemia

ETIOLOGY

Arterial Emboli. Acute arterial insufficiency of the lower extremities is a common clinical problem. From 50 to 75 percent of cases of acute lower extremity ischemia are due to embolic arterial occlusion [1–4]. In the upper extremities, embolic arterial occlusion accounts for an even greater majority of cases of acute arterial insufficiency, since symptomatic acute thrombotic occlusive disease is very uncommon in this anatomic location [5].

Approximately 80 percent of arterial emboli have a cardiac source [6]. This percentage has decreased over the years as the prevalence of rheumatic valvular heart disease has diminished. The greatest single risk factor for the development of arterial emboli is atrial fibrillation, since thrombus forms in the relative static pool of blood in the fibrillating atrium. Atrial fibrillation is associated with two-thirds to three-fourths of cases of peripheral thromboembolism [1,2,3]. Although embolization can occur spontaneously, conversion to sinus rhythm markedly increases the risk of embolization [7].

The second most frequent condition predisposing to peripheral embolization is myocardial infarction in which an akinetic and acutely infarcted myocardial wall can serve as a nidus for thrombus formation. Thromboembolism occurs in up to 5 percent of acute anterior wall infarcts [8,9,10]. Peripheral embolization can be the initial manifestation of "silent" myocardial infarction; thus, evidence of myocardial infarction must be sought in patients with acute limb ischemia, especially those without atrial fibrillation [8].

Peripheral thromboemboli can originate from thrombus formed in a ventricular aneurysm [11]. Other less common cardiac sources of emboli include thrombi on prosthetic heart valves [8,12] and fragments of intracardiac tumors, particularly left atrial myxomata [13,14].

Noncardiac sources of emboli account for approximately 10 percent of cases of embolization [15]. Most originate from mural thrombi within a proximal arterial aneurysm (Fig. 165-1) [16]. Other arterial sources of emboli include ulcerated atherosclerotic plaques (see later). Thromboemboli originating in the venous system can flow through a patent atrial septal defect into the left side of the heart and be ejected into the arterial circulation. This phenomenon, called "paradoxical embolization," is possible when right atrial pressures exceed left atrial pressures

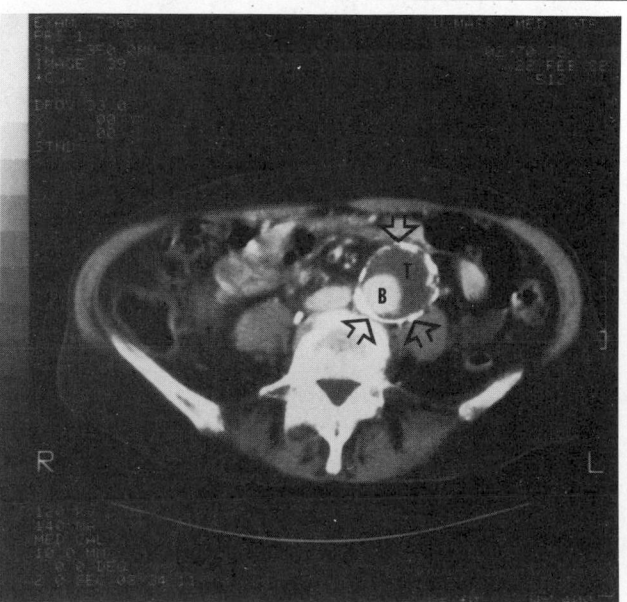

Fig. 165-1. The calcified outer wall of a 4-cm abdominal aortic aneurysm is outlined by three open arrows on this CT scan image. The contrast-enhanced column of flowing blood (*B*) is surrounded by the commonly seen laminated thrombus (*T*), which may be a source of embolic material.

and is most common in patients with pulmonary hypertension secondary to previous pulmonary emboli [17,18].

In 5 to 10 percent of patients with acute peripheral arterial emboli, no source can be identified [1,2,6,19–22]. Some of these emboli undoubtedly arise from an undiagnosed cardiac source. Echocardiography can fail to recognize intracardiac thrombi, especially within the atrial appendage [23]. Some cases of "thromboembolism" are probably due to in situ arterial thrombosis.

Acute Arterial Thrombosis. Acute arterial thrombosis in the lower extremity almost always occurs at the site of a preexisting stenosis and may account for up to 50 percent of episodes of acute lower limb ischemia [24]. Symptomatic acute thrombosis of the upper extremity arteries is rare since atherosclerotic occlusive disease is relatively infrequent in these vessels and, when occlusive disease is present, collateral circulation is typically extensive [5].

Atherosclerosis is the most common predisposing factor for in situ arterial thrombosis of the large arteries of the extremities [25]. Acute thrombosis usually occurs in those arterial segments that are frequently affected with atherosclerotic lesions, primarily the iliac arteries and the superficial femoral arteries at the level of the adductor hiatus (Fig. 165-2) [8].

Acute thrombosis of a previously stenotic arterial segment is often precipitated by a low cardiac output state, such as congestive heart failure, shock, or dehydration [6,26]. Another condition that predisposes to acute arterial thrombosis is the presence of an arterial aneurysm. In contrast to abdominal aortic aneurysms, peripheral aneurysms rarely rupture but often present with acute thrombosis, resulting in severe leg ischemia [27].

Clinical suspicion for traumatic arterial occlusion in an extremity is usually raised by the clinical history and the presence of associated bone fractures or penetrating injuries [28]. Injury to the popliteal artery, however, can occur in association with dislocation of the knee [29], and, unless the knee is specifically examined for stability, the diagnosis of popliteal artery injury can be overlooked. Arterial injuries occur in nearly half of cases of knee dislocation [29]; therefore, arteriography is always indicated (Fig. 165-3).

Inherited or acquired hypercoagulable states are unusual, but antithrombin III deficiency, protein C deficiency, protein S deficiency, and homocysteinuria can result in acute arterial ischemia secondary to thrombosis [30]. Polycythemia, thrombocytosis, and cryoglobulinemia also predispose patients to acute arterial thrombosis [31,32]. Arterial thrombosis associated with the antiphospholipid antibody syndrome is discussed in Chapter 220.

Vasospasm. Vasospastic disorders can result in acute limb ischemia in the absence of arterial thrombosis. Vasospasm induced by ergot alkaloids can cause actue limb ischemia and even limb loss (Fig. 165-4) [33–36]. Intense vasoconstriction leading to tissue necrosis (usually involving the digits) is a recognized complication of therapy with high doses of alpha-adrenergic vasopressor.

Aortic Dissection. Aortic dissection can present with acute upper or lower extremity ischemia. Occlusion of the branches of the aorta occurs most commonly by extrinsic compression of the true lumen by the false lumen (Fig. 165-5) [37]. Although chest and back pain is usually present [38–41], dissection can occur in the absence of complaints other than those associated with acute limb ischemia [37].

CLINICAL PRESENTATION AND DIAGNOSIS. The clinical manifestations of acute arterial occlusion depend on the loca-

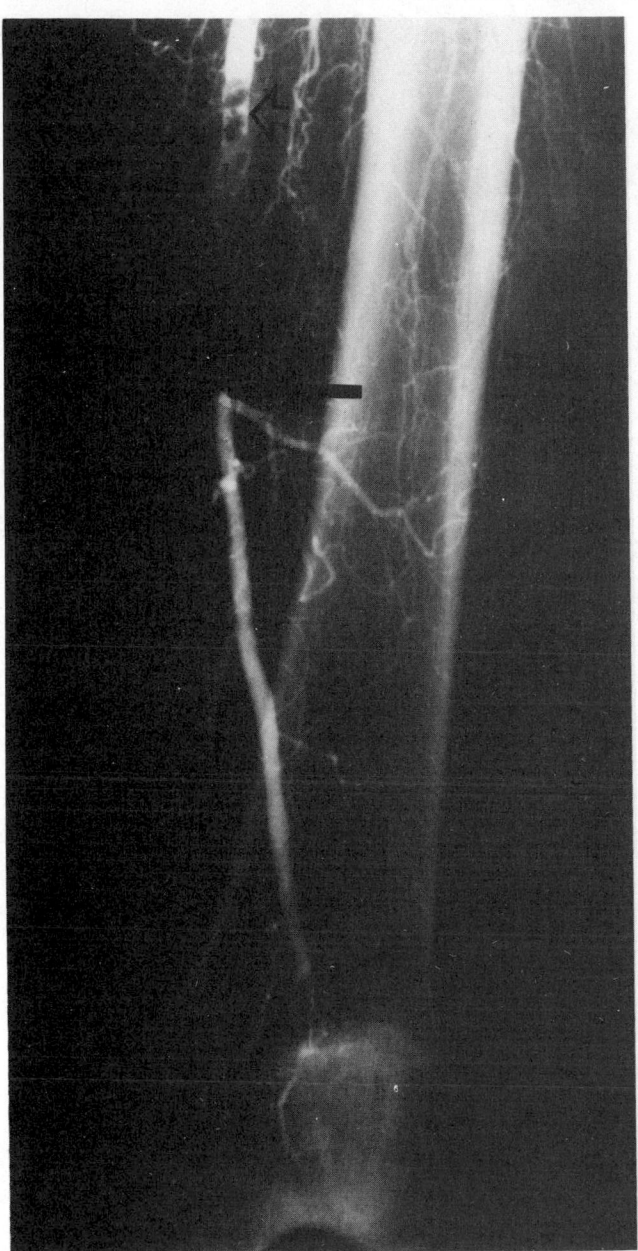

Fig. 165-2. Angiogram of a patient with an acutely ischemic left leg showing acute occlusion of the superficial femoral artery near the adductor hiatus (*solid arrow*) with proximal and distal acute arterial thrombosis (*open arrows*).

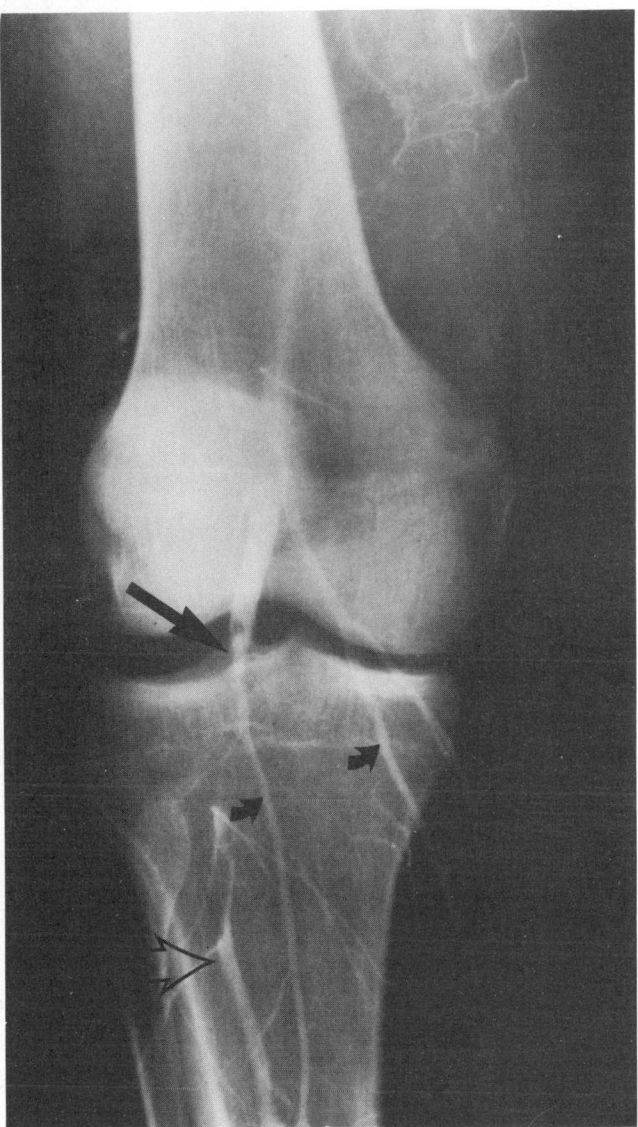

Fig. 165-3. Angiogram of a patient with a right knee dislocation and absent distal pulses with an acutely ischemic leg. The popliteal artery is thrombosed at the level of the knee joint (*large solid arrow*). The tibioperoneal trunk is seen to reconstitute distally (*open arrow*) because of flow of contrast through geniculate collateral vessels (*small curved arrows*).

tion and extent of the occlusion, the size of the artery occluded, the adequacy of collateral circulation, the extent of distal clot propagation, and arterial spasm [42,43]. Patients with abrupt embolic arterial obstruction as well as approximately 50 percent of individuals with acute arterial thrombosis present with abrupt onset of extremity coldness, pain, paresthesias, pallor, paralysis, and absence of palpable peripheral pulses [44]. These are findings indicative of a nonviable extremity. The remaining patients with acute arterial thrombosis present with claudication that progressively worsens over several hours [45].

In more than 50 percent of cases of acute arterial occlusion, the initial symptom is pain, which can range in intensity from dull and aching to excruciating. In other cases, coolness, numbness, loss of strength, and dysesthesias occur before pain is experienced [44]. As the thrombus extends over the course of several hours, pain may develop or intensify [45]. The severity of pallor, the extent of sensory and motor dysfunction, and the magnitude of muscle tenderness and rigidity depend on the degree of ischemia. Mottling, cyanosis, and pallor may not be apparent until the leg is elevated to 45 degrees for 1 to 2 minutes [45].

Specific clinical syndromes are suggested by the patient's clinical presentation. For example, acute thrombotic or embolic occlusion of the terminal aorta generally causes the sudden onset of severe bilateral leg pain and paresis. In this syndrome, pulses below the umbilicus are absent, and the skin of the lower

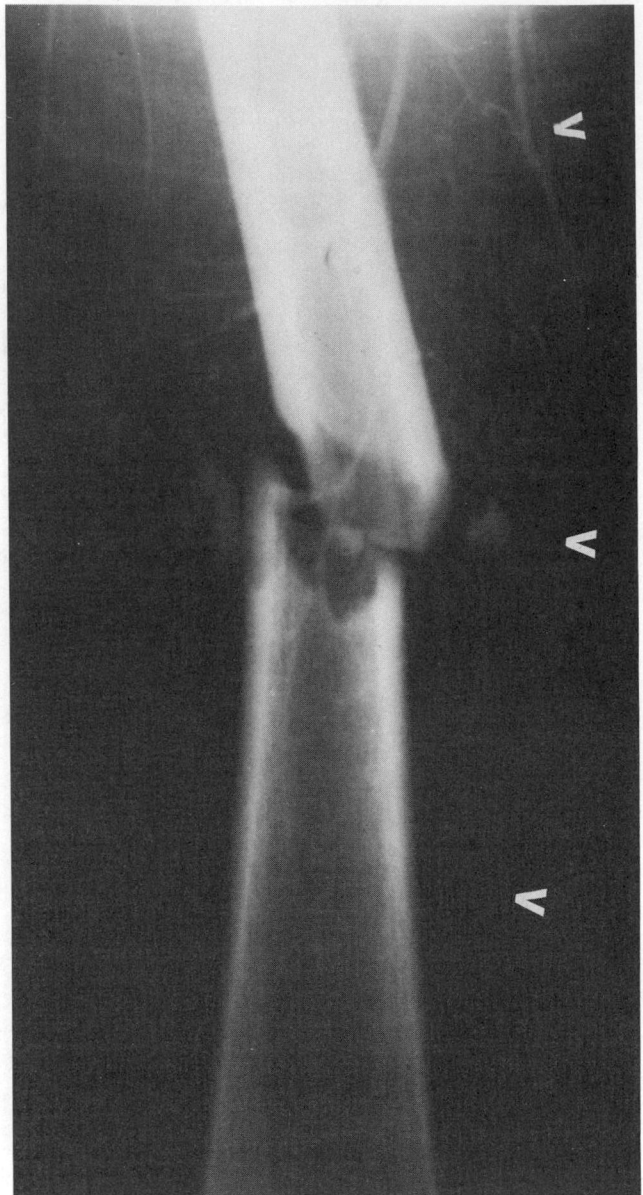

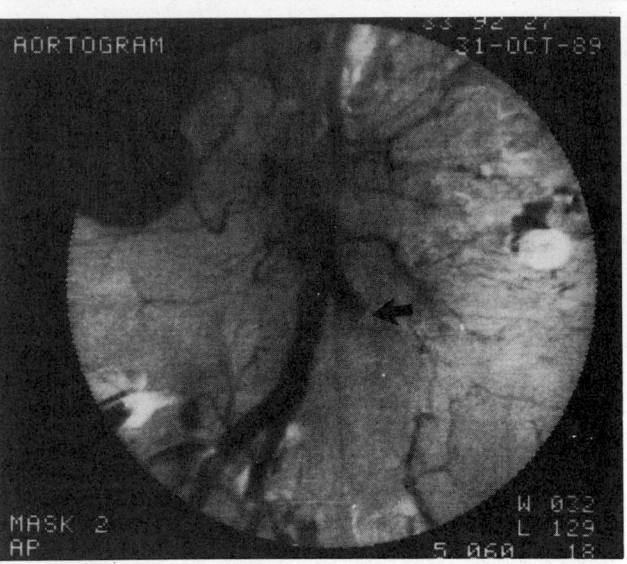

Fig. 165-5. A 55-year-old hypertensive man presented with symptoms of an acutely ischemic left leg and severe back pain. This digital subtraction angiogram shows absent perfusion of the left kidney and occlusion of the left iliac artery (*arrow*).

Fig. 165-4. Angiogram of a young patient with a right femur fracture who developed acutely ischemic and nonviable lower extremities 4 days after his injury. He had recently received a deep venous thrombosis prophylaxis regimen containing ergotamine. Severe spasm of the superficial femoral artery is seen (*white arrows*).

abdomen and buttocks is mottled and cyanotic. In most cases of acute aortic thrombosis, there is a history of arterial insufficiency in the lower extremities [46].

Arterial embolization and acute arterial thrombosis may be difficult to differentiate [45,47]. Because the management of arterial thrombosis (i.e., arteriography and reconstructive surgery under general anesthesia) differs from the management of acute arterial embolism (i.e., embolectomy under local anesthesia without prior arteriography), it is important to make the distinction [48]. There is a readily identifiable source (e.g., the fibrillating atrium) in most cases of arterial embolization. Patients with acute arterial thrombosis typically have a clear his-

tory of atherosclerotic peripheral occlusive disease and/or bruits and diminished arterial pulses in multiple locations. Aortic dissection should be considered in the differential diagnosis of acute arterial occlusion, especially when there is evidence for a generalized process involving multiple, seemingly unrelated organ systems [37]. Thus, the simultaneous presence of chest pain (in the absence of myocardial infarction) and a cold pulseless leg strongly suggests aortic dissection. In this case, management should focus on the acute life-threatening aortic dissection rather than considering only local treatment of the ischemic leg [37].

Diagnosis of acute thrombosis of a popliteal aneurysm can be a difficult to make preoperatively because the characteristic wide pulse of the aneurysm can be absent as a result of the thrombosis. This diagnosis is suggested, however, by palpation of the popliteal fossa of the opposite leg, since popliteal aneurysms are bilateral in more than 50 percent of patients [49,50].

A history of recent trauma may be relevant, even in the absence of bony fractures. Ligamentous injury resulting in knee dislocation may result in a stretch injury to the popliteal artery, leading to intimal disruption and immediate or delayed popliteal artery thrombosis (see Fig. 165-3) [29].

Arteriography helps to differentiate arterial thrombosis from embolic occlusion. In situ arterial thrombosis most commonly occurs in atherosclerotic vessels, and, therefore, arteriographic findings indicative of atherosclerosis suggest thrombotic occlusion. Embolism is suggested when the arteriogram shows a generally patent artery with smooth walls and an abrupt cutoff at the site of the occlusion (Fig. 165-6) [51].

TREATMENT. Management of acute thrombotic arterial occlusion includes assessment of the severity of the ischemia and treatment of the systemic and local factors. The initial symptoms of acute arterial occlusion, including pain, paresthesias, and paralysis, are secondary to neuronal ischemia [52] and are completely reversible if treated promptly. Unless acute aortic dissection is a very strong diagnostic possibility, intravenous hep-

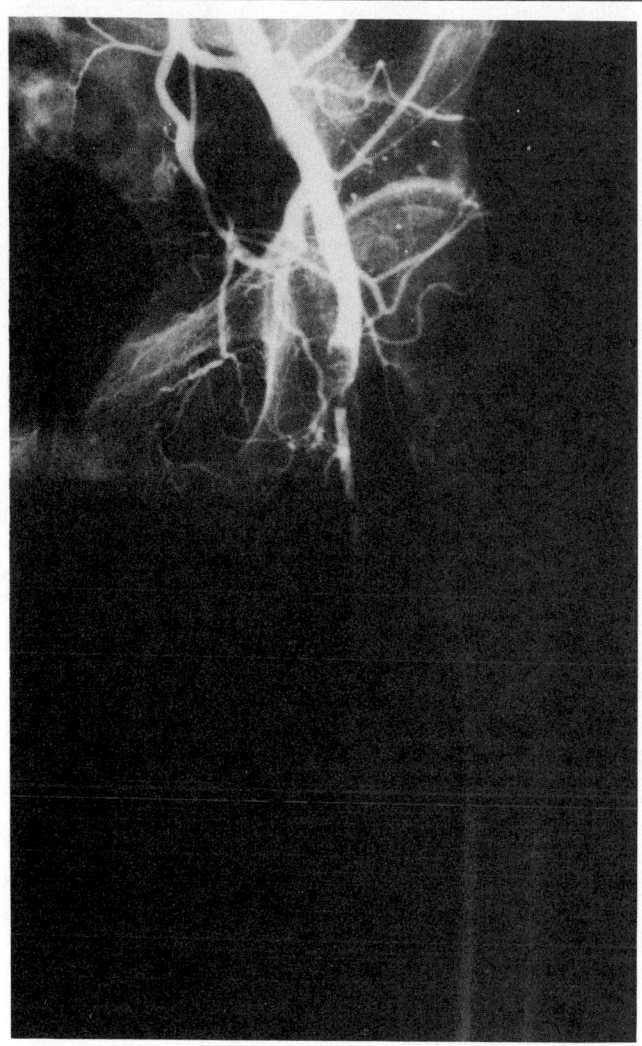

Fig. 165-6. The left leg arteriogram demonstrates the abrupt left common femoral artery occlusion at the level of the femoral bifurcation characteristic of an embolus. There is some contrast seen beyond the embolus in the superficial femoral artery.

arin (100 units/kg) should be administered immediately to prevent propagation of thrombus proximal and distal to the site of occlusion [6]. A constant heparin infusion (15–20 units/kg/hr) should be started to maintain the partial thromboplastin time (PTT) at least twice the control value.

Other medical measures are of relatively little importance in managing acute limb ischemia. The extremity should be protected from extremes of temperature and from physical trauma by bulky loose dressings [53]. Prompt evaluation and treatment of metabolic, cardiovascular, and pulmonary disorders should be carried out to prepare the patient for an operation.

Arteriography is indicated when acute thrombosis is suspected, when the etiology of the limb ischemia is in doubt, or when thrombolytic therapy with urokinase or streptokinase is being considered. An aortogram performed to make the diagnosis of an aortic dissection should include the entire aortic arch and abdominal aorta to define the initial area of the intimal tear and associated arch and visceral and lower extremity arterial involvement.

When a clinical diagnosis of an extremity embolus has been made, delay for preoperative arteriography is unnecessary, and

the patient should be taken directly to the operating room. An embolectomy can almost always be accomplished using local anesthesia for a femoral or brachial artery exploration. A balloon-tipped Fogarty catheter is passed proximally and distally to remove both embolic and thrombotic material and, thereby, restore perfusion to the extremity. Occasionally, when distal pulses are not palpable following embolectomy, intraoperative arteriography is indicated. If residual thrombus is present, the therapeutic options include repeat passage of the embolectomy catheter, local arterial exploration, and intraoperative thrombolytic therapy [54].

Emboli retrieved at the time of operation should be submitted for pathologic examination. Rarely, an embolus will consist of a fragment of a cardiac tumor, which otherwise might remain undiagnosed.

Anticoagulation should be continued postoperatively using heparin and warfarin. Life-long anticoagulation with warfarin is indicated, unless the risk factors for embolus formation can be eliminated [6,8].

When the lower extremity is ischemic secondary to an acute thrombotic occlusion of a previously stenotic artery, a balloon catheter thrombectomy may initially restore limited patency, but reocclusion of the stenotic artery is a certainty. Therefore, some form of arterial reconstruction is warranted. When limb viability is acutely threatened, bypass grafting may be required because it is the most expeditious means to restore lower extremity perfusion. When immediate revascularization is not mandatory for limb salvage, thrombolytic therapy using urokinase or streptokinase may be used to recanalize the recently thrombosed arterial lumen [55]. Operative intervention may be further avoided by the use of percutaneous balloon angioplasty [55]. Although arterial patency with this approach is not as durable as with surgical reconstruction [56,57], it may be in the patient's best interest to avoid an emergency operation. Complications of thrombolytic therapy are common [55], however, and the contraindications to this modality of treatment must be considered (Table 165-1).

Limb ischemia in the setting of an acute aortic dissection is an indication for surgical repair of the dissection [11]. Surgical management of acute aortic dissection not only directly ad-

Table 165-1. Contraindications to Thrombolytic Therapy

Absolute Contraindications
  Active internal bleeding
  Recent (within 2 months) cerebrovascular accident or other active
    intracranial process
Relative Major Contraindications
  Recent (<10 days) major surgery, obstetrical delivery, organ bi-
    opsy, previous puncture of noncompressible vessels
  Recent serious gastrointestinal bleeding
  Recent serious trauma
  Severe arterial hypertension (≥ 200 mm Hg systolic or ≥ 110 mm
    Hg diastolic)
Relative Minor Contraindications
  Recent minor trauma, including cardiopulmonary resuscitation
  High likelihood of a left heart thrombus, e.g., mitral disease with
    atrial fibrillation
  Bacterial endocarditis
  Hemostatic defects including those associated with severe hepatic
    or renal disease
  Pregnancy
  Age over 75 years
  Diabetic hemorrhagic retinopathy

Source: *Data from* NIH consensus development conference on thrombolytic therapy in thrombosis: A National Institutes of Health consensus development conference. *Ann Intern Med* 93:141, 1980.

dresses the life-threatening process, but may also restore perfusion to the limb and obviate the need for peripheral vascular reconstruction [11].

Many of the systemic and metabolic features of acute arterial occlusion affecting the extremities are the sequelae of muscle ischemia and rhabdomyolysis [44–47,58,59]. The viability of muscle cells is compromised by prolonged periods of ischemia. Further damage occurs during reperfusion owing to the generation of toxic reactive oxygen species [60–63]. The combined effects of ischemia and reperfusion injury lead to edema formation, which can cause a compartment syndrome, myonecrosis, and rhabdomyolysis (see Chaps. 180 and 161) [64]. Fasciotomy and debridement of necrotic muscle may be necessary to salvage the extremity.

Chronic Arterial Occlusive Disease

ETIOLOGY. Chronic occlusive disease of the lower extremities is extremely common and in North America is almost always due to atherosclerosis. Although arterial occlusive disease of the upper extremities is much less common, atherosclerotic disease is still the most common cause of chronic arterial insufficiency in the upper extremities [65]. Other causes of chronic occlusive disease involving large and medium arteries include Takayasu's arteritis and thromboangiitis obliterans. Small-vessel occlusive disease is often due to vasculitis (see Chap. 220).

Atherosclerosis is pathologically characterized by thickening of the intima, focal accumulation of lipid and fibrous tissue within the intima, deposition of calcium in the intima, loss of arterial elasticity, and reduction of vessel caliber [66]. The earliest microscopic lesion is proliferation of intimal smooth muscle cells, particularly at arterial branch points [67]. Hemodynamic or mechanical stress may lead to endothelial cell injury, resulting in platelet aggregation. The interaction of platelets with the arterial wall causes the platelets to release a substance that stimulates smooth muscle cell proliferation in the intima [68–71] and may contribute to atherogenesis.

Progression of the atherosclerotic process is characterized by the appearance of lipid, first in intimal cells and later in extracellular spaces. Grossly, this is evidenced by the presence of fatty streaks in the well of the vessel. Studies using a hypercholesterolemic rat model of atherosclerosis suggest that fatty streaks originate from mononuclear cells. In this rat model, mononuclear cells (approximately 90% monocytes and 10% lymphocytes) adhere to the aortic intima, migrate into the subendothelial spaces, and transform into foam cells associated with fatty streaks [72].

Cholesterol deposition is accelerated by lipoprotein receptors on fibroblasts and smooth muscle cells [73]. Cholesterol is esterified by an enzyme, microsomal cholesterol ester synthetase [74]. Decreased activity of cholesterol ester hydrolase, a lysosomal enzyme in the vessel wall, allows cholesterol esters to accumulate in the atheromatous lesions [75]. Later, fibrous tissue and calcium appear in the lesions and are associated with thrombus formation. Fragmentation of the elastic elements in the wall of the vessel leads to the formation of ulcerated lesions and atheromata and the development of aneurysms. Further narrowing of the lumen can result from hemorrhage into the vessel wall, enlargement of atheromata, and/or formation of mural thrombus [76].

CLINICAL PRESENTATION AND DIAGNOSIS

Atherosclerosis Obliterans. An early and characteristic symptom of chronic arterial occlusive disease is intermittent claudication, characterized by exercise-induced aching, cramping, numbness, and fatigue in the extremity. Claudication results when blood flow is inadequate to meet the metabolic demand of the muscle, which is increased during exercise. The symptoms characteristically resolve after several minutes of rest.

The clinical feature of more severe chronic arterial obstruction is ischemic rest pain. Dull and aching in character, rest pain is generally most intense at night when cardiac output falls. Ischemic neuropathy is manifested by steady or paroxysmal shocklike pain, burning paresthesias, and numbness [77]. Signs of chronic limb-threatening lower extremity ischemia include dependent rubor, thinning and dryness of skin, loss of leg hair, muscle atrophy, loss of subcutaneous fat, decreased skin temperature, and dry gangrene [26]. Dry gangrene usually begins in the most distal portion of the toes and results from thrombosis of small nutrient arteries. Tissue necrosis can be precipitated by factors that increase the oxygen requirements of the tissue such as trauma or infection.

The gradual progression of atherosclerotic occlusive disease is accompanied by the development of collateral circulation; therefore, complete occlusion of the native vessel is usually a clinically silent event. Angiograms of atherosclerotic vessels typically demonstrate varying degrees of arterial involvement and intermittent areas of vascular occlusion. More distal vessels can be imaged because contrast fills them via collateral routes (Fig. 165-7).

Takayasu's Arteritis. Takayasu's arteritis can involve any segments of the aorta as well as its major branches and can lead to cerebrovascular and visceral ischemia as well as obliteration of the palpable pulses in the extremities [78,79]. Pathologically, transmural arterial inflammation and luminal compromise are observed.

Thromboangiitis Obliterans. Thromboangiitis obliterans, also known as Buerger's disease, is an inflammatory disorder of peripheral arteries and veins. It generally affects men younger than 50 years of age; most patients are 20 to 35 years old [80]. Smoking plays a definite role in the initiation and progression of the disease [81].

The most common presenting symptoms are claudication and foot pain. Other manifestations include cutaneous ulcers and distal gangrene. Ischemic sequelae also can involve the upper extremities, primarily the hands and fingers, and include Raynaud's phenomenon, digital ulcers, and hyperhidrosis [82,83,84]. Unlike atherosclerosis obliterans, thromboangiitis obliterans is associated with venous thrombophlebitis in 50 to 60 percent of individuals [84].

Pathologic specimens of acute lesions of thromboangiitis obliterans demonstrate intimal proliferation, giant intimal cells, infiltration of the vessel wall with histiocytes and polymorphonuclear leukocytes, and the presence of organized clot within the lumen of affected arteries and veins. Sterile microabscesses within luminal thrombi are a specific pathologic feature of the disease [85]. The arterial lesions are segmental and are separated by normal regions. With time, all layers of the vessel wall become involved. The arteries and veins become thickened and bound together, and the thrombi recanalize [86].

Angiography can provide useful diagnostic information. The earliest changes of thromboangiitis obliterans occur in the arteries of the feet. Thromboangiitis obliterans affects intermediate-sized and small peripheral arteries, most commonly the popliteal posterior tibial, anterior tibial, and peroneal arteries of the lower extremities and the ulnar, radial, and digital arteries in the upper extremities [87,88]. In contrast to atherosclerosis obliterans, thromboangiitis obliterans rarely affects the femoral or aortoiliac arteries [84,86]. Angiographic features include seg-

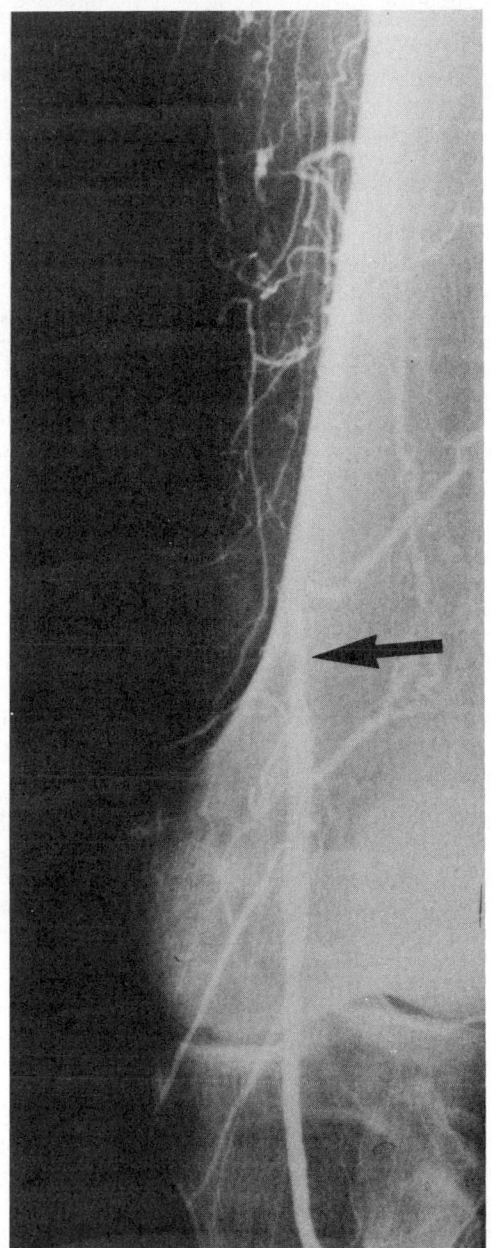

Fig. 165-7. The superficial femoral artery is occluded with reconstitution of the popliteal artery (*arrow*). The well-developed proximal collateral vessels are typical in the setting of a chronic occlusive process.

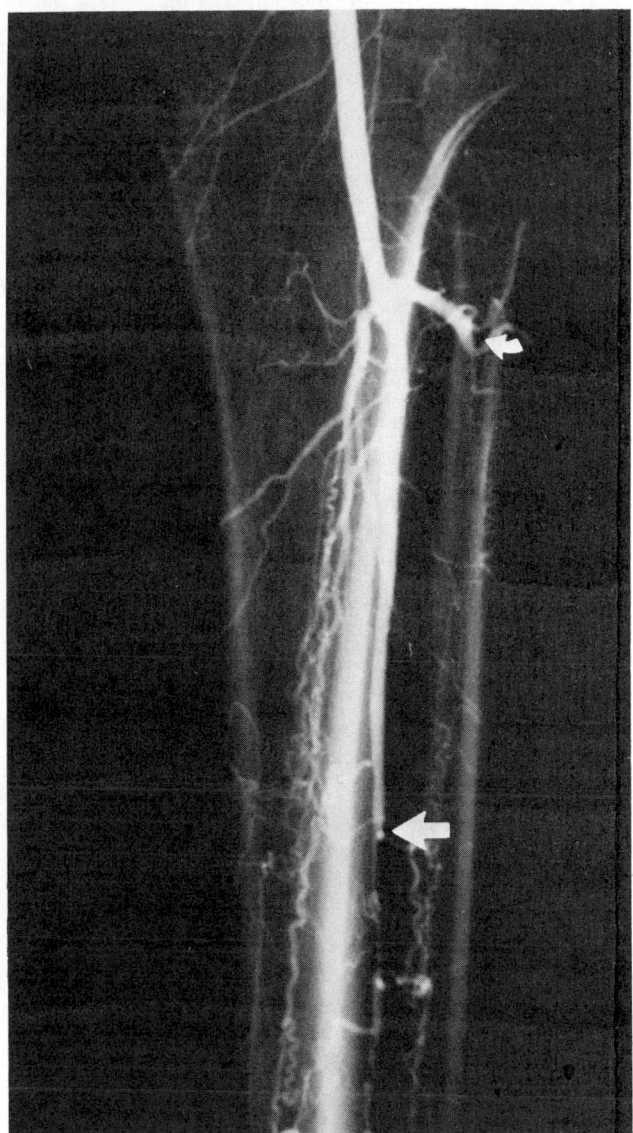

Fig. 165-8. Arteriogram of the left leg of a patient with pathologically proved thromboangiitis obliterans. The arteriogram demonstrates a normal popliteal artery with smooth arterial walls, an abrupt occlusion of the anterior tibial artery (*curved arrow*), a total occlusion of the peroneal artery (*straight arrow*), and an extensive network of collateral arteries.

mental symmetrical narrowing of affected arteries and progressive, abrupt tapering and complete obstruction without signs of plaques in arterial walls. These findings contrast with the diffuse pattern of eccentric filling defects seen on arteriograms of atherosclerotic vessels (Fig. 165-8) [87,88]. Although clinical features help to distinguish thromboangiitis obliterans from antherosclerosis, the diagnosis is established by histologic examination of biopsy specimens of the artery or by the characteristic angiographic findings [84,88].

TREATMENT. Interventions to prevent progression of atherosclerosis include treatment of hypercholesterolemia and hy-

pertriglyceridemia, control of diabetes mellitus and polycythemia, and avoidance of tobacco. Measures to optimize collateral blood flow include avoidance of smoking and vasoconstricting drugs (including beta-adrenergic blockers), maintenance of a warm environment, sleeping with the head of the bed elevated on 12- to 16-inch blocks (reverse Trendelenburg position), and exercise [89]. Sympathetic denervation, performed either surgically or by percutaneous injection of absolute ethanol or phenol, may alleviate rest pain and aid in healing of ulcers [89]. Little evidence is available to support the use of a vasodilator for chronic atherosclerosis [90].

Meticulous local care is an important aspect of the management of chronic limb ischemia. The affected limb should be washed daily with lukewarm water and a nonalkaline, non-medicated soap, followed by thorough drying and application of lanolin to prevent skin fissures. Concentrated heat and strong antiseptics should be avoided. If skin breakdown occurs, the area should be gently cleansed and covered with sterile dressings. Adhesive tape should not be applied to the skin. Pressure points should be protected with soft padding. Corns or calluses should not be trimmed. Fungal and bacterial infections should be promptly treated with appropriate antibiotics, and purulent or necrotic material should be debrided [91,92].

Arteriography for evaluation of chronic lower extremity ischemia is indicated when surgical intervention is being considered to improve circulation. The presence of ischemic rest pain or tissue necrosis is an indication for revascularization. Claudication does not necessarily reflect limb-threatening ischemia, but if it impairs the patient's life-style significantly and the patient is a reasonable operative risk, claudication may be an indication for surgical treatment, especially in the case of aortoiliac occlusive disease.

In general, proximal atherosclerotic occlusive disease should be treated before more distal disease. Bypass of aortoiliac occlusive disease restores normal perfusion to the femoral level and frequently provides symptomatic relief, even in the presence of superficial femoral artery occlusion. Although surgical revascularization is sometimes accomplished by endarterectomy, bypass of the occluded arterial segment, using either a prosthetic graft or autogenous saphenous vein, is more common. Other modalities include balloon angioplasty of stenotic segments, catheter atherectomy, and laser arterial recanalization.

Medical management of Takayasu's arteritis involves control of the inflammatory process with corticosteroids. Once the inflammatory component of the disease is quiescent, symptomatic arterial insufficiency can be surgically corrected [78].

Treatment of thromboangiitis obliterans consists of cessation of smoking and local care of the ischemic lesions [86]. Surgical reconstruction is of limited benefit [93].

Complications of Intraarterial Procedures

Intraarterial procedures are commonly performed in the critical care setting for monitoring purposes as well as for access to the arterial circulation for diagnostic and therapeutic peripheral arterial and cardiac procedures. These arterial interventions are frequently of great value to the patient and in some cases help to avoid a surgical procedure, such as in the case of angiographic embolization of bleeding sites or percutaneous transluminal angioplasty of the coronary or peripheral arteries. These interventions, however, are associated with a real risk of serious morbidity.

ATHEROEMBOLIZATION. Although atheroembolization can occur spontaneously, it is frequently iatrogenic, occurring as a result of surgical manipulation of an atheromatous aorta or intraarterial catheterization [94–97]. Atheroemboli may also occur after warfarin anticoagulation [98] and after thrombolytic therapy [99]. Atheroemboli are typically small enough to flow out to the terminal arterioles of the fingers and toes and cause digital ischemia. Atheromatous material can also embolize to organs throughout the body. Because the most common sources of atheroemboli are atherosclerotic lesions in the aorta and the iliac sand femoral arteries, the sites most frequently affected are the abdominal viscera, kidneys, and lower extremities [100,101].

Microemboli consisting of cholesterol crystals and other atherosclerotic debris from atheromatous plaques occlude arterioles with diameters of 50 to 900 µ, often in more than one organ [102]. The clinical presentation of atheromatous microemboli is fairly consistent [103–108]. Patients often have cyanotic, severely painful toes, often with bluish patches and hemorrhagic areas resulting from occlusion of digital arterioles; this is the so-called blue-toe syndrome [109]. Livedo reticularis (i.e., cutaneous mottling with a blotchy, netlike [reticular] reddish blue appearance) appears most commonly on the lower extremities and occasionally on the trunk and is due to occlusion of arterioles of the skin [110–113]. Microemboli can also shower the kidneys, the most frequently affected visceral organs [103,104,114]. Evidence of renal involvement is manifested by impairment of renal function [104,105,106,115–119], hypertension [106,110,117,120,121], microscopic hematuria, leukocyturia, and proteinuria without red cell casts [106].

The chronology of impaired renal function after angiography can help distinguish contrast-induced renal failure from renal failure due to atheromatous microemboli. Renal failure caused by contrast agents typically appears soon after the study and reaches maximal severity within 7 to 10 days. Renal function then improves, returning to baseline over the next several weeks. Renal failure due to atheromatous microemboli generally develops over 1 to 4 weeks following the angiographic procedure [122]. In the case of severe renal impairment secondary to atheroemboli, dialysis may allow time for renal function to improve [106].

Showers of microemboli can cause ischemic tissue injury presenting as ulceration and gangrene, most commonly of the toes [100,123], but infarction of tissue may not occur if adequate collateral circulation is present. Pedal pulses may be normal even in the presence of severe toe ischemia, a sign that helps to distinguish atheroemboli from other forms of vascular obstruction [100].

Laboratory features of atheromatous embolization are nonspecific but often include elevated erythrocyte sedimentation rates and transient eosinophilia [103,114,117,118,124] as well as microhematuria, leukocyturia, and proteinuria, without red cell casts [100,105,114–117,123].

The pathologic features of atheromatous embolization to small arteries and arterioles include endothelial and fibroblastic proliferation, foreign body giant cell response to the cholesterol crystals, and lymphocytic perivascular infiltration [125]. Atheromatous emboli have been documented in interlobar, arcuate, and intralobular renal arteries [94], as well as in larger [103] and smaller vessels [116]. Occasionally, necrotizing angiitis of small arteries occurs, being characterized by polymorphonuclear leukocytic infiltration and fibrinoid necrosis of the walls of the involved vessels [110,126].

The differential diagnosis of the "blue toe syndrome" and of other clinical features of atheromatous embolization includes cardiac embolism (infective endocarditis, nonbacterial thrombotic endocarditis, cardiac myxoma), hyperviscosity syndromes (cryoglobulinemia, cryofibrinogenemia, cold agglutinins, polycythemia vera, leukemias, macroglobulinemia), hypercoagulable states (malignancy, antiphospholipid antibody syndrome, diabetes mellitus, essential thrombocythemia, disseminated intravascular coagulation, erythromelalgia), and vasculitis (polyarteritis and other forms of necrotizing arteritis) [97].

The diagnosis of atheromatous embolization is suggested by the clinical features cited earlier and the presence of a proximal aortic aneurysm or an ulcerated arterial plaque [127,128]. The diagnosis of atheromatous embolization, however, is established by the demonstration, in biopsy or postmortem specimens, of characteristic biconvex needle-shaped clefts that remain in vessels after dissolution of cholesterol crystals during routine histologic preparation of the affected tissue, be it kidney [104,129], skin [130,131], muscle [112,132,133,134], or other tissue [103,106,107,108,135–138]. If special techniques are used to preserve the cholesterol crystals during histologic preparation of tissue specimens, the crystals can be identified under polarized microscopy by their double refractile nature [139].

Treatment of the atheromatous embolization syndrome consists of controlling pain and blood pressure and instituting measures to increase local blood flow with topical glyceryl trinitrate (2% Nitrol) ointment and sympathetic blockade [140,141]. Definitive treatment involves identification and surgical resection of the arterial source of atheromatous emboli. Endarterectomy may be adequate for relatively localized atheromatous intimal lesions. Excision and grafting are generally necessary when there is extensive atheromatous involvement of the aorta or arterial aneurysmal disease [142,143,144].

An important aspect of treatment of atheromatous embolism is prevention. The incidence or severity of atheromatous embolization may be decreased by one or more of the following: (1) increasing the awareness of clinicians of the risks of atheromatous embolization associated with surgical manipulation and angiographic studies of atheromatous vessels, (2) minimizing intraarterial procedures in atherosclerotic aortas and femoral arteries, (3) using the brachial rather than the femoral artery approach for cardiac catheterization in patients with atherosclerotic disease of the aorta and iliac arteries, (4) minimizing catheter manipulation during angiographic procedures, and (5) using softer, more flexible catheters [122].

The use of heparin to treat atheroembolization is controversial. In spite of the presence of ischemic tissue, some argue that the drug is contraindicated because it may prevent the formation of an organized thrombus over ulcerated plaques and, therefore, allow continued embolization of atheromatous material [145,146,147]. A case of anticoagulation-induced multisystem disease due to well-documented atheroemboli has been reported. In this case, the patient clearly improved when anticoagulation was discontinued [146]. Anticoagulation also can increase hemorrhage into tissues infarcted by atheromatous emboli [148].

RADIAL ARTERY THROMBOSIS. Factors that contribute to symptomatic thrombosis of the radial artery secondary to intraarterial procedures include (1) prolonged duration of cannulation, (2) repeated arterial punctures, (3) low systemic perfusion pressure, (4) use of a more thrombogenic material (polyethylene) instead of less thrombogenic material (Teflon) for the cannula [149], and (5) the absence of a complete palmar arch, which occurs in approximately 1.6 percent of the population [150]. The Allen test should be used to evaluate flow in the palmar arch prior to radial artery cannulation.

Following removal of the radial artery catheter, hand ischemia may improve with heparin therapy and/or cervicodorsal sympathetic block. Critical ischemia may be treated by thrombectomy [151].

BRACHIAL ARTERY THROMBOSIS. Thrombosis, bleeding, false aneurysm formation, and arterial perforation are potential complications of brachial artery catheterization [152]. The overall incidence of brachial artery thrombosis as a result of catheterization is approximately 16 percent (range of 4–28%) [153,154,155]. Factors that contribute to thrombosis are (1) mul-

tiple arterial punctures, (2) elevation of an intimal flap, (3) use of an excessively large catheter, and (4) multiple catheter changes. A study of brachial artery thrombosis in 20 patients identified prolonged catheterization time, delay in diagnosis of brachial artery thrombosis, and failure to use systemic heparinization at the time of diagnosis as factors that contributed to the morbidity of brachial artery catheterization [156]. Evaluation of postcatheterization brachial artery thrombosis includes examination of arterial integrity and clinical assessment of the degree of hand ischemia by examination of the distal ulnar and radial pulses, evaluation of skin temperature, and performance of Doppler studies.

Patients with postcatheterization brachial artery thrombosis who are treated conservatively may present later with chronic disability due to intermittent exercise-induced pain of the arm or hand or even limb-threatening ischemia. Therefore, arterial patency should be restored surgically. The proper procedure depends on the findings at the time of operation. If the vessel is relatively normal and surgery is performed within 12 to 48 hours, simple thrombectomy under local anesthesia without preoperative arteriography is usually sufficient [157]. If significant atherosclerotic disease is present in the brachial artery, resection of the thrombosed portion and end-to-end anastomosis or graft interposition may be necessary [157].

THROMBOTIC COMPLICATIONS OF PERCUTANEOUS FEMORAL ANGIOGRAPHY. Complications of femoral angiography that may result in arterial occlusion are (1) thrombosis at the site of femoral arterial puncture; (2) thrombosis along the catheter, with embolization of thrombus; and (3) embolization of material from the atheromatous plaques within the femoral, iliac, and aortic walls (see previous section). Factors that predispose patients to femoral artery thrombosis include (1) intimal disruption and laceration, (2) preexistent arterial disease, and (3) severe arterial spasm, which is more common in women and children than in men [158].

Clinical features of femoral artery thrombosis are the onset of severe and constant pain within hours of the procedure, coolness of the affected leg, paresthesias, and numbness. Femoral and more distal pulses are absent. In the case of embolization to the popliteal artery, this artery may be palpable, but the pedal pulses may be absent [155].

Treatment of femoral artery thrombosis consists of anticoagulation to prevent propagation of clot, followed by urgent thrombectomy. Because the majority of thrombi develop at the site of arterial puncture, preoperative arteriography is usually not necessary, and thrombectomy can be performed using local anesthesia [159]. If severe atherosclerotic disease is found during femoral artery exploration, thromboendarterectomy or bypass with an interposition graft may be necessary. Arterial blood flow is almost always restored, particularly if femoral artery thrombosis is recognized and surgically removed within 24 hours of onset [160].

ISCHEMIC COMPLICATIONS OF INTRAAORTIC BALLOON PUMPING. Since its introduction in 1968, the intraaortic balloon pump (IABP) has been used extensively as a cardiac assist device for cardiogenic shock and unstable angina (see Chap. 9). Unfortunately, many patients requiring support with the IABP have atherosclerotic peripheral vascular disease. Vascular complications have been reported to occur in up to 36 percent of cases [161] and include thrombotic episodes, retrograde aortic dissection, retroperitoneal aortoiliac perforation with hemorrhage, and arterial embolism [161,162]. One study reported vascular complications in 11 of 23 (47%) individuals with preexisting peripheral atherosclerosis obliterans who were treated with IABP [162]. Thrombus often develops around the shaft of the catheter in the iliac artery and to a lesser extent around the balloon, despite therapy with dextran or heparin [163].

The status of peripheral pulses in the lower extremities should be documented before insertion of the IABP. While the IABP is in place, lower extremity blood flow should be monitored frequently by examination of distal pulses and Doppler studies.

Management of thrombotic and embolic complications of the IABP includes intravenous heparin therapy beginning when the balloon is inserted. Arterial thrombosis with limb ischemia requires removal of the balloon and thrombectomy or creation of a femorofemoral crossover graft.

References

1. Abbott WM, Maloney RD, McCabe CC, et al: Arterial embolism: A 44 year perspective. *Am J Surg* 143:460, 1982.
2. Darling RC, Austen WG, Linton RR: Arterial embolism. *Surg Gynecol Obstet* 124:106, 1967.
3. Fogarty TJ, Daily PO, Shumway NE, et al: Experience with balloon catheter technic for arterial embolectomy. *Am J Surg* 122:231, 1971.
4. Dale WA: Differential management of acute peripheral arterial ischemia. *J Vasc Surg* 1:269, 1984.
5. Haimovici H: Cardiogenic embolism of the upper extremity. *J Cardiovasc Surg* 23:214, 1982.
6. Smith GJ, Holcroft JW, Blaisdell FW: Acute arterial insufficiency, in Wilson SE, Veith FJ, Hobson RW, Williams RA (eds): *Vascular Surgery: Principles and Practice.* New York, McGraw-Hill, 1987, p 325.
7. Josephson ME, Buxton AE, Marchlinski FE: The tachyarrhythmias, in Braunwald E, Isselbacher KJ, Petersdorf RG, et al (eds): *Harrison's Principles of Internal Medicine.* 11th ed. New York, McGraw-Hill, 1987, p 923.
8. Brewster DC, Chin AK, Fogarty TJ: Arterial thromboembolism, in Rutherford RB (ed), *Vascular Surgery.* 3rd ed. Philadelphia, WB Saunders, 1989, p 548.
9. Asinger RW, Mikell FL, Elsperger J, et al: Incidence of left ventricular thrombus after acute transmural myocardial infarction: Serial evaluation by two-dimensional echocardiography. *N Engl J Med* 305:297, 1981.
10. Keating EC, Gross SA, Schlamowitz RA: Mural thrombi in myocardial infarction. *Am J Med* 74:989, 1983.
11. Loop FD, Effler DB, Navia JA, et al: Aneurysm of the left ventricle: Survival and results of a ten-year surgical experience. *Ann Surg* 177:767, 1973.
12. Perier P, Bessau JP, Swanson JS, et al: Comparative evaluation of aortic valve replacement with Starr, Bjork, and porcine valve prostheses. *Circulation* 72(Suppl II):140, 1985.
13. Brewster DC: How can you best identify and treat arterial embolism? *J Cardiovasc Med* 7:354, 1982.
14. Bulkely BH, Hutchins GM: Atrial myxomas: A fifty year review. *Am Heart J* 97:639, 1979.
15. Abbott WM, Maloney RD, McCabe CC, et al: Arterial embolism: A 44 year perspective. *Am J Surg* 143:460, 1982.
16. Lord JW Jr, Rossi G, Daliana M, et al: Unsuspected abdominal aortic aneurysm as the cause of peripheral arterial occlusive disease. *Ann Surg* 177:767, 1973.
17. Gazzaniga AB, Dalen JE: Paradoxical embolism: Its pathophysiology and clinical recognition. *Ann Surg* 171:137, 1970.
18. Laughlin RA, Mandel SR: Paradoxical embolization: Case report and review of the literature. *Arch Surg* 112:648, 1977.
19. Elliott JP Jr, Hageman JH, Szilagyi DE, et al: Arterial embolization: Problem of source, multiplicity, recurrence and delayed treatment. *Surgery* 88:833, 1980.
20. Hight DW, Tilney NL, Couch NP: Changing clinical trends in patients with peripheral arterial emboli. *Surgery* 79:172, 1976.
21. Sheiner NM, Zelter J, MacIntosh E: Arterial embolectomy in the modern era. *Can J Surg* 25:373, 1982.
22. Thompson JE, Sigler L, Raut RS, et al: Arterial embolectomy: A 20 year experience. *Surgery* 67:212, 1970.
23. Shrestha NK, Moreno FL, Narcisco FV, et al: Two dimensional echocardiographic diagnosis of left atrial thrombus in rheumatic heart disease: A clinicopathologic study. *Circulation* 67:341, 1983.
24. Dale WA: Differential management of acute peripheral arterial ischemia. *J Vasc Surg* 1:269, 1984.
25. Humphries AW, Young JR Jr: The severely ischemic leg. *Curr Probl Surg* Jun:4, 1970.
26. Fairbairn JF II, Joyce JW, Pairolero PC: Acute arterial occlusion of the extremities, in Juergens JL, Spittell JA Jr, Fairbairn JF II (eds): *Peripheral Vascular Diseases.* Philadelphia, WB Saunders, 1980, p 385.
27. Vermilion BD, Kimmins SA, Pale WG, et al: A review of 147 popliteal aneurysms with long-term follow-up. *Surgery* 90:1009, 1981.
28. Snyder WH III, Thal ER, Perry MO: Vascular injuries of the extremities, in Rutherford RB (ed): *Vascular Surgery.* 3rd ed. Philadelphia, WB Saunders, 1989, p 613.
29. Green NE, Allen BL: Vascular injuries associated with dislocation of the knee. *J Bone Joint Surg* 59[A]:236, 1977.
30. Horker LA, Stichter SJ, Scott CR, et al: Hemocytopenia: Vascular injury and arterial thrombosis. *N Engl J Med* 291:537, 1974.
31. Smith SB, Sikin C: Hypofibrinogenemia: Incidence, clinical correlations, and review of the literature. *Am J Clin Pathol* 58:524, 1972.
32. Edwards EA, Cooley MH: Peripheral vascular symptoms as the initial manifestations of polycythemia vera. *JAMA* 214:1463, 1970.
33. Andersen PK, Christensen KN, Hole P, et al: Sodium nitroprusside and epidural blockade in treatment of ergotism. *N Engl J Med* 296:1271, 1977.
34. Maples M, Mulherin JL, Harris J, et al: Arterial complications of ergotism. *Am J Surg* 47:224, 1981.
35. Kempczinski RF, Buckley CJ, Darling RC: Vascular insufficiency secondary to ergotism. *Surgery* 79:597, 1976.
36. Merhoff GC, Porter JM: Ergot intoxication: Historical review and description of unusual clinical manifestations. *Ann Surg* 180:773, 1974.
37. Sarris GE, Miller DC: Peripheral vascular manifestations of acute aortic dissection, in Rutherford RB (ed): *Vascular Surgery.* 3rd ed. Philadelphia, WB Saunders, 1939, p 942.
38. Miller DC: Surgical management of aortic dissections: Indications, perioperative management and long-term results, in Doroghazi RM, Slater EE (eds): *Aortic Dissection.* New York, McGraw-Hill, 1983, p 193.
39. Bickershoff LK, Pairolero PC, Hollier LH, et al: Thoracic aortic aneurysms: A population based study. *Surgery* 92:1103, 1982.
40. Slater EE, DeSanctis RW: The clinical recognition of dissecting aortic aneurysm, *Am J Med* 60:625, 1976.
41. Slater EE: Aortic dissection: Presentation and diagnosis, in Doroghazi RM, Slater EE (eds): *Aortic Dissection.* New York, McGraw-Hill, 1983, p 61.
42. Haimovici H: Acute atherosclerotic thrombosis, in Haimovici H (ed): *Vascular Emergencies.* New York, Appleton-Century-Crofts, 1982, p 316.
43. Fairbairn JF II, Joyce JW, Pairolero PC: Acute arterial occlusion of the extremities, in Juergens JL, Spittell JA Jr, Fairbairn JF II (eds): *Peripheral Vascular Diseases.* Philadelphia, WB Saunders, 1980, p 386.
44. Fairbairn JF II, Joyce JW, Pairolero PC: Acute arterial occlusion of the extremities, in Juergens JL, Spittell JA Jr, Fairbairn JF II (eds): *Peripheral Vascular Diseases.* Philadelphia, WB Saunders, 1980, p 388.
45. Haimovici H: Acute atherosclerotic thrombosis, in Haimovici H (ed): *Vascular Emergencies.* New York, Appleton-Century-Crofts, 1982, p 216.
46. Danto LA, Fry WJ, Kraft RI: Acute aortic thrombosis. *Arch Surg* 106:66, 1971.
47. Abramson DI: *Circulatory Diseases of the Limbs: A Primer.* New York, Grune & Stratton, 1978, p 145.
48. Fairbairn JF II, Joyce JW, Pairolero PC: Acute arterial occlusion of the extremities, in Juergens JC, Spittell JA Jr, Fairbairn JF II (eds): *Peripheral Vascular Diseases.* Philadelphia, WB Saunders, 1980, p 385.
49. Evans WE, Hayes JP: Atherosclerotic popliteal aneurysms, in Ernst

CB, Stanley JC (eds): *Current Therapy in Vascular Surgery.* Toronto, BC Decker, 1987, p 151.

50. Wychulis AP: Popliteal aneurysms. *Surgery* 68:942, 1970.
51. Abramson DI: *Circulatory Diseases of the Limbs: A Primer.* New York, Grune & Stratton, 1978, p 77.
52. Khalil IM: Bilateral compartment syndrome after prolonged surgery in the lithotomy position. *J Vasc Surg* 5:879, 1987.
53. Falk K, Rayyes AN, David DS, et al: Myoglobinuria with reversible acute renal failure. *Ny State J Med* 73:537, 1973.
54. Parent FN III, Bernhard VM, Pabst TS III, et al: Fibrinolytic treatment of residual thrombus after catheter embolectomy for severe lower limb ischemia. *J Vasc Surg* 9:153, 1989.
55. Berkowitz HD, Hargrove WE III, Roberts B: Thrombolysins in vascular disease, in Wilson SE, Veith FJ, Hobson RW, Williams RA (eds): *Vascular Surgery: Principles and Practice.* New York, McGraw-Hill, 1987, p 251.
56. Borozan PC, Schuler JJ, Spigus DG, Flanigan DP: Long-term hemodynamic evaluation of lower extremity percutaneous translumenal angioplasty. *J Vasc Surg* 2:785, 1985.
57. Blair JM, Gewertz BC, Moosa H, et al: Percutaneous translumenal angioplasty versus surgery for limb-threatening ischemia. *J Vasc Surg* 9:698, 1989.
58. Bywater EGL, Stead JK: Thrombosis of femoral artery with myohemoglobinuria and low serum potassium concentration. *Clin Sci* 5:19, 1945.
59. Haimovici H: Arterial embolism myoglobinuria and renal tubular necrosis. *Arch Surg* 100:639, 1970.
60. Rutherford RB: Nutrient bed projection during lower extremity arterial reconstruction. *J Vasc Surg* 5:529, 1987.
61. Perry MO, Shires GT III, Albert SA: Cellular changes with graded limb ischemia in reperfusion. *J Vasc Surg* 1:536, 1984.
62. Presta M, Ragnotti G: Quantification of damage to striated muscle after normothermic or hypothermic ischemia. *Clin Chem* 27:297, 1981.
63. McCord JM: Oxygen derived free radical in post-ischemic tissue injury. *N Engl J Med* 313:154, 1985.
64. Perry MO: Compartmental syndrome and reperfusion injury. *Surg Clin North Am* 68:853, 1988.
65. Sumner DS: Evaluation of acute and chronic ischemia of the upper extremity, in Rutherford RB (ed): *Vascular Surgery.* 3rd ed. Philadelphia, WB Saunders, 1989, p 815.
66. Fuster V, Kottke BA, Juergens JL: Atherosclerosis, in Juergens JL, Spittell JA Jr, Fairbairn JF II (eds): *Peripheral Vascular Diseases.* Philadelphia, WB Saunders, 1980, p 219.
67. National Heart and Lung Institute Task Force on Arteriosclerosis: *Arteriosclerosis.* Publication No (NIH) 72-219, Vol 2. Washington DC, US Department of Health, Education and Welfare, Public Health Service, 1971.
68. Ross R, Glomset J, Kariya B, et al: A platelet-dependent serum factor that stimulates the proliferation of arterial smooth muscle cells in vitro. *Proc Natl Acad Sci USA* 71:1207, 1974.
69. Goldsmith HL: Blood flow and thrombosis. *Thromb Diath Haemorrh* 32:35, 1974.
70. Rutherford RB, Ross R: Platelet factors stimulate fibroblasts and smooth muscle cells quiescent in plasma serum to proliferate. *J Cell Biol* 69:196, 1976.
71. Fuster V, Lewis JC, Kottke BA, et al: Platelet factor 4-like activity in the initial stages of atherosclerosis in pigeons. *Thromb Res* 10:169, 1977.
72. Joris I, Zand T, Nunnari JT, et al: Studies on the pathogenesis of atherosclerosis. I: Adhesion and emigration of mononuclear cells in the aorta of hypercholesterolemic rats. *Am J Pathol* 113:341, 1983.
73. Bierman EL, Albers JJ: Lipoprotein uptake by cultured human arterial smooth muscle cells. *Biochim Biophys Acta* 388:198, 1975.
74. Fuster V, Kottke BA, Juergens JL: Atherosclerosis, in Juergens JL, Spittell JA Jr, Fairbairn JF II (eds): *Peripheral Vascular Diseases.* Philadelphia, WB Saunders, 1980, p 226.
75. Sloan HR, Frederickson DS: Enzyme deficiency in cholesterol ester storage disease. *J Clin Invest* 51:1923, 1972.
76. Haimovici H: Atherogenesis: Recent biological concepts and clinical implications. *Am J Surg* 134:174, 1977.
77. Abramson DI: *Circulatory Diseases of the Limbs: A Primer.* New York, Grune & Stratton, 1978, p 77.
78. Gewertz BL: Arteritis and dysplastic arterial lesions, in Wilson SE,

Veith FJ, Hobson EW, Williams RA (eds): *Vascular Surgery: Principles and Practice.* New York, McGraw-Hill, 1987, p 42.
79. Bloss RS, Duncan JM, Cooley DA, et al: Takayasu's arteritis: Surgical considerations. *Ann Thorac Surg* 27:579, 1978.
80. Jurgens JL: Thromboangiitis obliterans, in Rutherford RB (ed): *Vascular Surgery.* Philadelphia, WB Saunders, 1980, p 469.
81. McPherson JR, Juergens SL, Gifford RW Jr: Thromboangiitis obliterans and arteriosclerosis obliterans: Clinical and prognostic differences. *Ann Intern Med* 59:228, 1963.
82. Shionoya S, Ban I, Nakata Y, et al: Diagnosis, pathology, and treatment of Buerger's disease. *Surgery* 75:695, 1974.
83. Brown H, Sellwood RA, Harrison CV, et al: Thromboangiitis obliterans. *Br J Surg* 56:59, 1969.
84. Goodman RM, Elion B, Moyes M, et al: Buerger's disease in Israel. *Am J Med* 39:601, 1965.
85. Williams G: Recent views on Buerger's disease: A distinct clinical and pathologic entity. *JAMA* 181:5, 1962.
86. Shinoya S, Ban I, Nakata Y, et al: Diagnosis, pathology and treatment of Buerger's disease. *Surgery* 75:695, 1974.
87. Hirai M, Shinoya S: Arterial obstruction of the upper limb in Buerger's disease: Its incidence and primary lesion. *Br J Surg* 66:124, 1979.
88. McKusick VA, Haris WS, Ottesen OE, et al: Buerger's disease: A distinct clinical and pathologic entity. *JAMA* 181:5, 1962.
89. Fairbairn JF II, Joyce JW, Pairolero PC: Acute arterial occlusion of the extremities, in Juergens JL, Spittell JA Jr, Fairbairn JF II (eds): *Peripheral Vascular Diseases.* Philadelphia, WB Saunders, 1980, p 275.
90. Coffman JD: Vasodilator drugs in peripheral vascular disease. *N Engl J Med* 300:713, 1974.
91. Abramson DI: *Circulatory Diseases of the Limbs: A Primer.* New York, Grune & Stratton, 1978, p 97.
92. Fairbairn JF II, Joyce JW, Pairolero PC: Acute arterial occlusion of the extremities, in Juergens JL, Spittell JA Jr, Fairbairn JF II (eds): *Peripheral Vascular Diseases.* Philadelphia, WB Saunders, 1980, p 277.
93. Shinoya S, Ban I, Nakata Y, et al: Vascular reconstruction in Buerger's disease. *Br J Surg* 63:841, 1976.
94. Thrulbeck WM, Castleman B: Atheromatous emboli to the kidneys after aortic surgery. *N Engl J Med* 257:442, 1957.
95. Roscher AA, Endlich HL: Atheroembolization, a complication of vascular surgery and/or diagnostic angiography. *Int Surg* 56:82, 1971.
96. Stout C, Hartsuck JM, Howe J, et al: Atheromatous embolization after aortofemoral bypass and aortic ligation. *Arch Pathol Lab Med* 93:271, 1972.
97. O'Keefe ST, Woods B O'B, Breslin DJ, Tsapatsaris NP: Blue toe syndrome: Causes and management. *Arch Intern Med* 152:2197, 1992.
98. Feder W, Auerbach R: "Purple toes": An uncommon sequela of oral coumadin drug therapy. *Ann Intern Med* 55:911, 1961.
99. Ridker PM, Michel T: Streptokinase therapy and cholesterol embolization. *Am J Med* 87:357, 1989.
100. Carvajal JA, Anderson WR, Weiss L, et al: Atheroembolism: An etiologic factor in renal insufficiency, gastrointestinal hemorrhages, and peripheral vascular diseases. *Arch Intern Med* 119:593, 1967.
101. Tunick PA, Culliford AT, Lamparello PJ, Kronzen I: Atheromatosis of the aortic arch as an occult source of multiple systemic emboli. *Ann Intern Med* 114:391, 1991.
102. Haimovici H: Atheroembolism, in Haimovici H (ed): *Vascular Emergencies.* New York, Appleton-Century-Crofts, 1982, p 203.
103. Gore I, Collins DP: Spontaneous atheromatous embolization. *Am J Clin Pathol* 33:416, 1960.
104. Retan JW, Miller RE: Microembolic complications of atherosclerosis. *Arch Intern Med* 118:534, 1966.
105. Case 50-1977, Case records of the Massachusetts General Hospital: Weekly clinicopathological exercises. *N Engl J Med* 297:1337, 1977.
106. Smith MC, Ghose MK, Henry AR: The clinical spectrum of renal cholesterol embolization. *Am J Med* 71:174, 1981.
107. Darsee JR: Cholesterol embolism: The great masquerader. *South Med J* 72:174, 1979.
108. Case 33-1974, Case records of the Massachusetts General Hospital: Weekly clinicopathological exercises. *N Engl J Med* 291:406, 1974.

109. Karmody AM, Powers SR, Monaco VJ, et al: "Blue-toe" syndrome: An indication for limb salvage surgery. *Arch Surg* 3:1263, 1976.

110. Fisher ER, Hellstrom HR, Myers JD: Disseminated atheromatous emboli. *Am J Med* 29:176, 1960.

111. Kazmier FJ, Sheps SG, Bernatz PE, et al: Livedo reticularis and digital infarcts: A syndrome due to cholesterol emboli arising from atheromatous abdominal aneurysms. *Vasc Dis* 3:12, 1966.

112. Haygood TA, Fessel J, Strange DA. Atheromatous microembolism stimulating polymyositis. *JAMA* 203:423, 1968.

113. Hoye SJ, Teitelbaum S, Gore I, et al: Atheromatous embolization: A factor in peripheral gangrene. *N Engl J Med* 261:128, 1959.

114. Bloom MG, Winthrop LH, Sarosi GA: Spontaneous cholesterol embolic renal failure. *Minn Med* 55:1099, 1972.

115. Case 25-1967, Case records of the Massachusetts General Hospital: Weekly clinicopathological exercises. *N Engl J Med* 276:1268, 1967.

116. Greendyke RM, Akamatus Y: Atheromatous embolism as a cause of renal failure. *J Urol* 83:231, 1960.

117. Kassirer JP: Atheroembolic renal disease, in Strauss HB, Welt LB (eds): *Disease of the Kidney*. 2nd ed. Boston, Little, Brown & Co, 1971, p 1031.

118. Schipper H, Hordon H, Berris B: Atheromatous embolic disease. *Can Med Assoc J* 113:640, 1975.

119. Ford RG, Siekert RG: Central nervous system manifestations of periarteritis nodosa. *Neurology* 15:114, 1965.

120. Handler FP: Clinical and pathologic significance of atheromatous embolization with emphasis on etiology of renal hypertension. *Am J Med* 20:366, 1956.

121. Palakos TG, Streeter DPH, Jones D, et al: "Malignant" hypertension resulting from atheromatous embolization predominantly of one kidney. *Am J Med* 57:135, 1974.

122. Harrington JT, Summers SC, Kassirer JP: Atheromatous emboli with progressive renal failure. Renal angiogram as the probable inciting factor. *Ann Intern Med* 68:152, 1968.

123. Kempczinski R: Lower extremity arterial emboli from ulcerated atherosclerotic plaques. *JAMA* 241:807, 1979.

124. Richards AM, Eliot RS, Kanjuh VI, et al: Cholesterol embolism: A multiple system disease masquerading as polyarteritis nodosa. *Am J Cardiol* 15:696, 1972.

125. Snyder HE, Shapiro JI: A correlative study of atheromatous embolism in human beings and experimental animals. *Surgery* 49:195, 1961.

126. Taylor NS, Gueft B, Lebowich RJ: Atheromatous embolization: A cause of gastric ulcers and small bowel necrosis. *Gastroenterology* 47:97, 1964.

127. Maurizi CP, Barker AE, Trueheart RE: Atheromatous emboli: A postmortem study with special reference to lower extremities. *Arch Pathol* 86:528, 1968.

128. Anderson NR, Richards AM: Evaluation of lower extremity muscle biopsies in the diagnosis of atheroembolism. *Arch Pathol* 86:535, 1968.

129. Jones DB, Iannaccone PM: Atheromatous emboli in renal biopsies. *Am J Pathol* 78:261, 1975.

130. Maurizi CP, Barker AE, Trueheart RE: Atheromatous embolism: A post-mortem study with special reference to lower extremities. *Arch Pathol* 86:528, 1968.

131. Calhoun P: Cholesterol emboli causing gangrene of extremities. *Arch Dermatol* 111:1373, 1975.

132. Carvajal JA, Anderson WR, Weiss L, et al: Atheroembolism: An etiologic factor in renal insufficiency, gastrointestinal hemorrhages, and peripheral vascular diseases. *Arch Intern Med* 119:593, 1967.

133. Anderson RW: Necrotizing angiitis associated with embolization of cholesterol. *Am J Clin Pathol* 43:65, 1965.

134. Perdue GD, Smith RB: Atheromatous microemboli. *Ann Surg* 169:954, 1969.

135. Eliot RS, Kanjuh VI, Edwards JE: Atheromatous embolism. *Circulation* 30:611, 1964.

136. Werger NK, Bauer S: Coronary embolism, a review of the literature and presentation of 15 cases. *Am J Med* 25:549, 1958.

137. Probstein JG, Joshi RA, Blumenthal HT: Atheromatous embolization: Etiology of acute pancreatitis. *Arch Surg* 75:566, 1957.

138. Flory CM: Arterial occlusions produced by emboli from eroded aortic atheromatous plaques. *Am J Pathol* 21:549, 1945.

139. Mehigan JT, Stone FJ: Lower extremity atheromatous embolization. *Am J Surg* 132:163, 1976.

140. Shannon FL, Rutherford RB: Lumbar sympathectomy: Indications and technique, in Rutherford RB (ed): *Vascular Surgery*. 3rd ed. Philadelphia, WB Saunders, 1989, pp 764–773.

141. Lee BY, Brancato RF, Thoden WR, Madden JL: Blue digit syndrome: Urgent indication for digit salvage. *Am J Surg* 147:418, 1984.

142. Brenowitz JB, Edwards WS: The management of atheromatous emboli in the lower extremities. *Surg Gynecol Obstet* 143:941, 1976.

143. Kwaan JMM, Connolly JE: Peripheral atheroembolism. *Arch Surg* 112:987, 1977.

144. Kempczinski RF: Lower extremity arterial emboli from ulcerating atherosclerotic plaques. *JAMA* 241:807, 1979.

145. Moldveen-Geroniums M, Merriam JC Jr: Cholesterol embolization from pathological curiosity to clinical entity. *Circulation* 35:946, 1967.

146. Bruns FJ, Segel DP, Adler S: Control of cholesterol embolization by discontinuation of anticoagulant therapy. *Am J Med Sci* 275:105, 1978.

147. Wagner RB: Peripheral atheroembolism: Confirmation of a clinical concept with a case report and review of the literature. *Surgery* 73:353, 1973.

148. Walter JR, Ryan RW: Atheromatous embolism of the central retinal artery. *Arch Ophthalmol* 87:301, 1972.

149. Downs JB, Chapman RL, Hawkins IF: Prolonged radial artery catheterization. *Arch Surg* 108:671, 1974.

150. Little JM, Zylstra PL, West J, et al: Circulation in the normal hand. *Br J Surg* 60:562, 1973.

151. Haimovici H: Iatrogenic acute arterial thrombosis, in Haimovici H (ed): *Vascular Emergencies*. New York, Appleton-Century-Crofts, 1982, p 228.

152. Haimovici H: Iatrogenic acute arterial thrombosis, in Haimovici H (ed): *Vascular Emergencies*. New York, Appleton-Century-Crofts, 1982, p 229.

153. Armstrong PW, Parker JO: The complications of brachial arteriotomy. *J Thorac Cardiovasc Surg* 61:24, 1971.

154. Page CP, Hapgood CO, Kemmerer WT: Management of postcatheterization brachial artery thrombosis. *Surgery* 72:619, 1972.

155. Brener BJ, Couch NP: Peripheral arterial complication of left heart catheterization and their management. *Am J Surg* 125:521, 1973.

156. Nicholas GG, DeMuth WE: Long-term results of brachial thrombectomy following cardiac catheterization. *Ann Surg* 183:436, 1976.

157. Haimovici H: Iatrogenic acute arterial thrombosis, in Haimovici H (ed): *Vascular Emergencies*. New York, Appleton-Century-Crofts, 1982, p 226.

158. Haimovici H: Iatrogenic acute arterial thrombosis, in Haimovici H (ed): *Vascular Emergencies*. New York, Appleton-Century-Crofts, 1982, p. 228.

159. Haimovici H: Iatrogenic acute arterial thrombosis, in Haimovici H (ed): *Vascular Emergencies*. New York, Appleton-Century-Crofts, 1982, p. 229.

160. Yellin AE, Shore EM: Surgical management of arterial occlusion following percutaneous femoral angiogram. *Surgery* 73:772, 1973.

161. Alpert J, Braktan EK, Gielchinsky I, et al: Vascular complications of intra-aortic balloon pumping. *Arch Surg* 111:1190, 1976.

162. Pace PD, Tilney NL, Lesch M, et al.: Peripheral arterial complications of intra-aortic balloon counterpulsation. *Surgery* 82:685, 1977.

163. Haimovici H: Iatrogenic acute arterial thrombosis, in Haimovici H (ed): *Vascular Emergencies*. New York, Appleton-Century-Crofts, 1982, p 230.

166. Pressure Sores

Gary M. Fudem and
Robert L. Walton, Jr.

Pressure sores are the result of unrelieved pressure over bony prominences that causes tissue injury, resulting in inflammation, necrosis, ulceration, and fibrosis. These wounds occur most commonly in patients suffering from neurologic impairment and in the elderly. Over half of all pressure sores are hospital-acquired and occur within the first two weeks of hospitalization. The incidence of pressure sores is 3 percent in acute-care facilities and a staggering 45 percent in long-term care facilities [1]. It is unfortunate that the treatment of pressure sores is given so little attention despite the adverse effects these injuries have on the overall well-being and clinical recovery of patients. Although most pressure sores are perceived as nuisances that parasitically coexist with certain disease states, they frequently dominate the aftermath of therapeutics, giving rise to prolongation of hospitalization and increased morbidity. The costs of treating pressure sores soberly reflect their economic impact on today's health care system; it is estimated that the cost of each pressure sore admission averages approximately $78,000—a figure that is nearly seven times that observed a decade ago [2]. National estimates show 1.7 million patients annually develop pressure ulcers, with associated health care costs of $8.5 billion [3]. The incidence of pressure sores will probably continue to increase, largely owing to the increased survival and mobility of spinal cord injury patients and the progressive increase in the number of elderly persons in our society. For these reasons, it is important that all practitioners be aware of this ubiquitous problem and some important aspects of its prevention and treatment.

Etiology and Pathophysiology

Although the development of pressure sores is multifactorial, the single major cause is pressure. Pressure on tissue produces ischemia, and this can lead to tissue necrosis. Theoretically, the minimal pressure necessary to impede blood flow is the end venule pressure, which is only 11 mm Hg. In time, obstructed capillary outflow and the resultant edema cause functional occlusion of the end capillaries (mean pressure = 20 mm Hg), then the beginning capillaries (mean pressure = 40 mm Hg), and finally the arterial system (mean pressure = 100 mm Hg). In this scenario, time and pressure are the key determinants for producing pressure injury. The critical pathophysiologic process leading to tissue necrosis is ischemia-induced endothelial cell separation. Platelet thrombi fill the cellular gaps and serve as a nidus for total vascular occlusion due to thrombosis [4].

In addition to the localized ischemia produced by lack of blood flow, increased capillary pressure results in capillary leakage, edema, and eventually autolysis [5]. Compression of local lymphatics leads to accumulation of toxic metabolic waste products, further propagating the insult to the surrounding tissues [6]. Experimentally, edema and reactive hyperemia occur after several minutes of pressure injury. Moderate pressure (100 mm Hg for 2 hours) causes patchy congestion of skin vessels, subcutaneous edema, and a moderate inflammatory infiltrate. Sustained pressure (100 mm Hg for 6 hours) causes an intense inflammatory infiltrate and degeneration of muscle fibers characterized by the loss of cross-striations and swelling of the myofibrils [7].

Approximately 87 percent of pressure sores occur on the lower body, with 67 percent involving the hip–buttock area and 29 percent the lower limbs [8]. Pressure measurements taken in the supine position show 40 to 60 mm Hg at the occiput, spine, sacrum, and heels. Pressure measurements in the prone position show 50 mm Hg at the knees and costal margins. Femoral trochanteric readings are 70 to 95 mm Hg when subjects lie on their side. Measurements sitting on a padded chair average 75 mm Hg on the ischii (60 mm Hg if the feet are hanging free and 100 mm Hg if the feet are supported). A harder surface affords a smaller area of weight distribution, thus increasing the effective pressure in an unpadded wooden chair to 300 mm Hg [9,10,11].

In the clinical setting, intermittent pressure is tolerated much better than sustained pressure. Pressure-relief intervals as short as 5 minutes every 2 hours in the recumbent patient and 10 seconds every 10 minutes in the seated patient significantly decrease tissue ischemia and subsequent injury [12]. The inability to perceive pressure and/or to shift the body mechanically off pressure points seriously predisposes to pressure injury. For this reason, Vilain referred to the bed as the most dangerous splint ever devised [1].

Fat and resting muscle resist pressure injury less well than does the skin [13]. Teleologically, this may account for the observation that no muscles traverse major bony pressure points either in the sitting or in the recumbent position.

Other forces predisposing to ulcer formation are shear and friction forces. Shear forces are directed tangentially across bony prominences, causing stretching and torsion of the soft tissues. This effect is most pronounced at the juncture of the subcutaneous and deep fascial planes, and it results in thrombosis of the important blood vessels that traverse these planes to supply the skin, thereby accentuating the ischemic effect of the pressure injury. Elevation of the head of a supine patient more than 30 degrees predisposes to shearing in the sacral and coccygeal areas. The addition of a shear factor decreases the perpendicular pressure needed to produce ulceration by 83 percent [14]. Friction forces also occur tangentially to the underlying bony prominence. Their effects, however, are more superficial than those observed for shear forces and are characterized primarily by the formation of skin abrasions. These superficial abrasions are commonly caused by dragging an unsupported patient across a sheet. Abrasions cause disruption of the keratin layer of the epidermis and predispose the underlying soft tissues to bacterial invasion.

Other Predisposing Factors

Predisposing factors for pressure injury include mental or physical debilitation, malnutrition, age, and any disease state that alters the body's ability to respond to injury. Diabetes and collagen vascular diseases negatively influence immune responses and wound healing. Major trauma and burns are associated with immune dysfunction and protein wasting. Furthermore, these patients are often immobilized, predisposing them to pressure injury. Depression decreases immune competence [15].

Poorly perfused tissues are vulnerable to pressure injury. Mechanical impedance to blood flow, as in patients with cardiovascular disease or localized vascular injury, increases the risk for pressure injury. Stress alone can predispose to pressure sore formation by increasing catecholamine release and peripheral vasoconstriction.

Other than pressure, the most consistent, potentially preventable factor predisposing to pressure ulcers is malnutrition. Holmes [16] studied 36 hospitalized patients considered at risk for pressure injury and found that 75 percent of the patients with a serum albumin level below 3.5 gm per deciliter developed pressure sores. Of those with a serum albumin level greater than 3.5, only 16.6 percent developed pressure sores [16]. Takeda et al. experimentally studied pressure sores in food-deprived rabbits. The healing process was strongly suppressed with reduction in fibroblast proliferation, capillary formation, macrophage infiltration, and epidermal cell proliferation [17]. Admittedly, there may have been other variables making poorly nourished patients more vulnerable to ulceration; however, negative nitrogen balance clearly impairs immune responsiveness and decreases the rate of wound healing. Subcutaneous tissue loss also effectively exaggerates bony prominences.

With increased age, the skin thins and becomes much less elastic. Peripheral perfusion is often decreased in older patients, making their tissues more fragile and less resistant to friction, shear, and direct pressure insults. In the extreme case, an aged patient suffering mental and physical debilitation and incontinence has a fivefold increased risk for the development of pressure sores [18]. Maceration and skin breakdown were shown to be highly correlated in a biomechanical study, indicating that overhydration and inadequate aeration increase the level of friction against the skin while simultaneously reducing the mechanical protective properties of the stratum corneum [19].

Denervated tissue is no more vulnerable to pressure injury than is sensate tissue. Similarly, denervation alone does not alter the cellular or vascular inflammatory response to ischemia [12]. It has been demonstrated, however, that collagenase levels in uninjured denervated tissues are elevated [20]. The clinical significance of this finding is unknown, but it suggests that scar maturation and collagen turnover resulting from the reparative processes in denervated tissues might be altered.

Clinical Grading of Pressure Sores

Shea [21] suggested a clinical grading system for pressure sores. Grade I pressure sores are characterized by involvement of the epidermis only. These present as erythema, blistering, or superficial epidermal ulceration over a point of pressure injury. Grade II pressure sores involve the full thickness of the skin, including the dermis. Grade III sores involve the skin and subcutaneous tissues. These frequently present as ulcerations but also may present as adherent patches of tenacious eschar directly overlying the site of pressure injury. Grade IV pressure sores extend to and involve the underlying bone (Fig. 166-1). Aside from direct clinical observation of bone involvement, grade IV pressure sores frequently reveal radiographic signs of osteitis or osteomyelitis.

Although convenient, the above grading system may be somewhat inaccurate in terms of the categorization of pressure sores from a pathophysiologic perspective. A study using monolithic silicon pressure sensors by Le et al. [22] demonstrated

that tissue pressure increases with proximity to bony prominences. This suggests that pressure sores develop from within and progress outward and helps to explain the common clinical finding of a small skin ulcer overlying a much larger area of soft tissue destruction.

Differential Diagnosis

Not all ulcers are caused by pressure, and therefore not all ulcers will respond to relief of pressure. Other etiologies for ulceration include arterial insufficiency, hypertensive ischemia, pyoderma gangrenosum, venous stasis, vasculitis, infection, and self-inflicted wounds/infections [23]. Arterial insufficiency, although a common denominator to the end stage of many vascular lesions, rarely results in an ulcer de nova. Early in their course, hypertensive ischemic ulcers have a central necrotic area surrounded by satellite infarcts. Livedo reticularis can be associated with cutaneous infarcts usually on the toes secondary to cholesterol embolization. Pyoderma gangrenosum appears as multiple purplish ulcers often associated with ulcerative colitis or Cushing's syndrome. Venous stasis ulcers usually result from venous hypertension. Classic venous stasis changes include edema, hyperpigmentation, and loss of hair. Vasculitic ulcers may start as purpura and are often associated with polyarteritis nodosa or systemic lupus erythematosus. Infectious ulcers appear in the distribution of the lymphatic chain. They often are caused by fungal infections such as sporotrichosis or blastomycosis. Factitious ulcers have an unlikely history and often very irregular borders with sharp edges. Most organic ulcers have rounded smooth edges secondary to thrombosis of involved vessels supplying a discrete skin area. Marjolin's ulcers or carcinomas arising in pressure sores are notable for their short latency period, fulminant clinical course, and high rate of metastases [24].

The location of an ulcer also may aid in diagnosis. Pressure ulcers usually occur over known pressure points, e.g., sacrum, ischii, occiput, heels. Upper extremity ulcers are almost never caused by venous disease, excluding arteriovenous malformations or major venous occlusion. Hypertensive ulcers usually occur proximal to the ankles, whereas arterial insufficiency ulcers are often distal. Diabetic ulcers are usually beneath weight-bearing areas (e.g., metatarsal heads); both pressure and abnormal healing capacity are factors predisposing to their development.

Prevention

The appearance of a pressure sore in a hospitalized patient often raises questions about the quality of nursing care, yet pressure sores sometimes develop even with the best of care. In the intensive care unit, where most attention is directed to life support, it is difficult, if not impossible, to avoid exceeding capillary perfusion pressures on dependent surfaces. Immobility, combined with low perfusion states and/or peripheral vasoconstriction, sets the stage for the development of tissue necrosis and ulcer formation. In these situations, extraordinary measures are required to avoid the development of pressure injury. Aside from standard therapeutic adjuncts, such as optimizing nutrition and body hygiene, new measures recently have been introduced to help disperse the pressure of recumbency.

If the weight of a 68-kg man could be evenly distributed, the

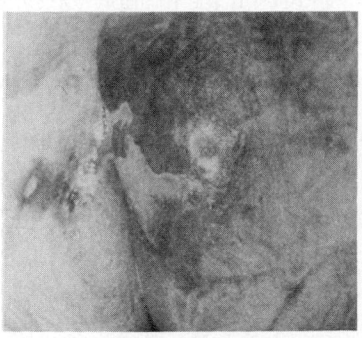 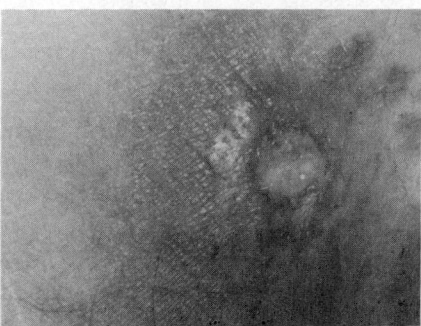 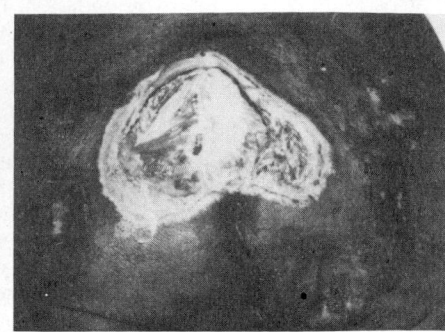

Fig. 166-1. Pressure injury manifests on a spectrum between cutaneous erythema and bony erosion, as seen from these sacral wounds.

skin pressure would be less than 18 mm Hg [25]. Special beds have been designed for pressure dispersion. The common types available are air-fluidized beds (air is pumped through a bed of fine silicone beads), mud beds (a viscous fluid medium imparts greater stability than air or water beds), and low-air-loss beds (columns of regulated air support the patient). Each type of bed has its advantages and disadvantages, but most can maintain skin pressures below 30 mm Hg when properly used [26,27]. Air-fluidized beds tend to cause dehydration and wound desiccation because of convective currents that increase insensible fluid losses. Therefore, these beds may be undesirable in elderly patients or those with large open wounds. In addition, we have observed devitalization and resultant deepening of skin graft donor sites when exposed to the desiccating effects of air-fluidized beds. Interposition between the patient and the bed sheet of an air-impervious barrier such as a disposable bed pad inhibits the evaporative and concomitant heat loss side effects of convection-type beds. Care must be taken to change these frequently to avoid maceration. Most bed companies supply partially impervious bed pads that may suit the situation best if there is an exudative wound that would benefit from some drying effect. The standard air mattress is relatively inefficient in the dispersion of pressure. When compared with air-fluidized beds in the management of established pressure sores, air mattresses are less effective for promoting wound healing. Current beds are very expensive and cumbersome and some are quite noisy. Despite their shortcomings, specialized beds in the context of good nursing care are of value in the prophylactic management of high-risk patients.

When pressure-dispersion beds are unavailable or economically unfeasible, strict attention must be paid to changing patient position at least every 2 hours. Horseshoe-shaped padding of a vulnerable pressure point is sometimes of use in preventing pressure injury. This technique involves placing padding in the configuration of a horseshoe around a bony prominence, with the open end of the horseshoe providing an avenue for lymphatic egress. This method should not be confused with padding directly beneath the bony prominence because the latter tends to increase pressure and focus it at the weight-bearing site. Similarly, constructing a doughnut-shaped padding to surround a bony prominence decreases pressure but impedes lymphatic drainage.

Viscoelastic gel pads are quite effective in dispersing pressure over bony prominences. When used as seat cushions, they reduce pressure by as much as 75 mm Hg over the ischii [28]. Although effective in reducing pressure, these pads do not diminish it below capillary perfusion pressure. Thus, even with these adjuncts, it is still necessary to relieve the pressure for at least 10 seconds every 10 minutes to avoid pressure injury.

Treatment

Given our current understanding of the pathophysiology of pressure-induced injury, it is interesting that the treatment of pressure sores varies so greatly from institution to institution and from specialty to specialty. The constant barrage of so-called cures for pressure sores that find their way into our therapeutic armamentarium is astounding. Currently available topical ointments, salves, creams, and dressings promise as much as those available only 10 years ago; the main difference is that they are nearly 10 times more expensive. Vilain accurately observed that anything can be put on a pressure ulcer except the patient [29].

Optimal treatment of the pressure sore requires that three primary therapeutic criteria be satisfied. These are relief of pressure, debridement of necrotic tissue, and control of infection. The elimination of necrotic debris in the wound should be performed surgically, unless only a superficial dry eschar exists, which may serve as a biologic dressing beneath which epithelial cells can migrate. Leaving a necrotic eschar over the wound allows the risk of infection and causes the inability to evaluate accurately the condition of the wound. Enzymatic debridement can be employed as an excellent, atraumatic technique for removing superficial devitalized tissue [30]. Care must be exercised, however, when using enzymatic agents because they may expose the wound to bacterial invasion and thus promote infection. Sutilains ointment (proteolytic enzymes derived from *Bacillus subtilis*) can be used effectively in conjunction with topical antimicrobials such as silver sulfadiazine to diminish the likelihood of infectious complications.

There is no sound rationale for the use of the common "wet-to-dry" dressing. A wet gauze, when applied to an open wound and allowed to dry, adheres to dead tissue and facilitates its removal when the gauze is pulled away. This rather crude method is effective in debriding the wound. Unfortunately, these dressings also can do a lot of harm to the wound. If one allows the gauze to dry, the underlying wound surface also dries and the tissue desiccates and dies. Each dressing change, in effect, reinjures the wound. This prolongs healing and is obviously undesirable. Remnants of the gauze material remain attached to the wound surface after the dressing is removed and incite further inflammation and increase the fibroblastic response in the wound. Wet-to-dry dressing changes also cause pain, stress, and occasional bleeding. For all these reasons, wet-to-dry dressing changes have no role in the biologic management of pressure sore wounds. Reports that these dressings reduce bacterial counts in wounds must be tempered with the realization that almost any therapy applied to the wound, including simple daily irrigations, will also diminish bacterial counts.

Pressure causes a full-thickness injury. The concept that pressure sores develop from within, directly adjacent to bony prominences, and progress outward has significant therapeutic implications [7]. Pathogenic bacteria localize at sites of pressure injury and tissue necrosis [13]. Infection results from a combination of factors; bacterial contamination from surface and systemic sources and impaired host resistance are the most important. There is a high degree of cross-contamination between infected pressure sores and the urinary and respiratory tracts [31]. The most common organisms encountered are *Staphylococcus aureus* and gram-negative bacilli [1], especially *Bacteroides fragilis* [32]. Simple treatment of surface wounds without consideration for the insult inflicted on deeper tissues can result in the failure to identify a deeper infection. This is not a trivial point; systemic sepsis, if caused by pressure ulcers, carries a 50 percent mortality rate despite debridement and administration of intravenous antibiotics [33,34].

Diagnosis of infection in pressure sores sometimes cannot be based on direct clinical observation. A high level of clinical suspicion must be exercised. In neurologically disabled or elderly patients, there is often a scarcity of symptoms, and the usual signs of fever and leukocytosis may be absent. Radionuclide scanning is of little value in these patients. Standard radiographs, contrast-enhanced sinograms, and computed tomography are perhaps the most helpful adjuncts for making the diagnosis. The only definitive approach to diagnosis is direct biopsy of soft tissue and bone for quantitative bacterial analysis [35].

In acute situations such as septicemia or cellulitis, systemic antimicrobial therapy constitutes the first line of therapy. If it is at all possible, the infecting organism should be identified prior to instituting systemic antimicrobial therapy. Qualitative and quantitative wound cultures, Gram stains of wound drainage specimens, and cross-checks of urine, sputum, and stool cultures are employed to obtain the necessary information on potentially infecting pathogens. Quantitative cultures are obtained by excising approximately 1 gm of tissue after cleansing the wound of surface contamination [36,37]. These give the most accurate information to guide antibiotic therapy, since surface swab cultures correlate poorly with tissue cultures [38]. Wound infection is present if there are greater than 10^5 colony-forming units of a single organism per gram of tissue. Beta-hemolytic streptococcus requires only 10^2 organisms per gram of tissue to represent a virulent wound infection. In some cases, the offending organism cannot be determined, and empirical treatment, with antimicrobials having broad-spectrum coverage for gram-positive and gram-negative organisms, is warranted.

Topical antibiotics should be employed on all pressure ulcers until the necrotic tissue has been removed. Silver sulfadiazine and mafenide acetate are two commonly used, broad-spectrum topical creams with mild penetrating ability. Topical metronidazole has been advocated to effectively control the odor from anaerobic colonization of pressure sores [39,40].

The theory that a pressure ulcer is different from other wounds because it is missing something such as a trophic factor has never been proved. Systemic deficiencies interfering with wound repair are almost always related to malnutrition [41]. Positive nitrogen balance must be attained, preferably via the enteral route. Topical therapies aimed at correcting deficiencies in wound repair or nutrition have included antibiotics, elements and simple compounds, hormones, foam sponges, plasma, ultrasound and electricity, brine, enzymes, sugar, tannic acid, and

many more. Attempts have been made to apply topical nutrients with poultices of carrots, turnips, and honey. Moist exudative wounds have been treated with bread, dextran polymers, and hair dryers. Gelfoam has been placed in wounds as a matrix for cell migration. Hyperbaric oxygen and topical insulin have been used to augment local anabolism [42]. The future may reveal more sophisticated biochemical manipulation of the wound milieu, as a study by Robson suggests that topically applied recombinant growth factors improved the healing of chronic pressure sores [43,44].

What should be placed in the open pressure sore once adequate debridement of infected and necrotic tissue has been accomplished? An old adage suggests that one should not place into the wound anything that cannot be placed safely into the conjunctival sac of the eye. From a biologic perspective, this makes good sense. Wounds heal at a maximal rate only if allowed to do so. Ideally, the wound should be kept moist, and there should exist some method for removing exudate from the wound. Few substances are available that fit these criteria. Although infrequently employed, dextran polymers are excellent adjuncts in the temporary management of open pressure sores. These agents effectively absorb toxic exudates without leaving a foreign body residue and do not adversely affect the wound healing process [45,46]. Relatively new calcium alginate dressings exchange calcium ions on their fibers for sodium ions in wound fluid, causing the fibers to swell as they absorb wound exudate. Until it becomes saturated, this dressing forms a hydrogel that keeps wounds moist without macerating surrounding healthy skin. As a semiocclusive dressing it decreases pain and is changed every 2 to 3 days when it becomes saturated. Its use cannot be recommended on infected or highly contaminated wounds that require close monitoring and strong topical antimicrobial therapy.

Occlusive dressings are desirable in the management of pressure sores because they promote wound healing [47], require little attention beyond their initial application, significantly decrease pain, and can be left in place for days. Examples include adhesive hydrocolloid occlusive dressings (Duoderm), polyurethane film dressings (Op-Site), cadaver allografts, and xenografts. The major drawback to these adjuncts, however, is that they interfere with the detection of necrotic debris in the wound. The result is predictable: a wound infection. Necrotic tissue, hermetically sealed by occlusive dressings in a warm, humid environment, is the perfect substrate for bacterial proliferation and infection. To be effective, therefore, occlusive dressings should be used only on wounds that have been thoroughly debrided of all nonviable elements.

Surgical management of pressure ulcers begins with removal of necrotic tissue. If there is only a small amount of superficial necrotic debris, this may be done in the office or at the bedside. Enzymatic agents also may be used in conjunction with a topical antimicrobial, as discussed earlier. More often, the surface ulcer is only the tip of the iceberg (Fig. 166-2). Beneath the surface lies a widely undermined area of necrotic tissue, possibly infected bursae, and sinus tracts leading to infected joints and osteomyelitis in 25 to 50 percent of infected pressure sores [48]. These types of wounds should be debrided and drained in the operating room. Bursae that are normally found over bony prominences suffer ischemic and infectious insults like any other soft tissue and respond with either intense inflammation or necrosis. Damaged bursae often become thick-walled and calcific, thus increasing the effective projection of bony prominences. These infected, calcified bursae must be excised to allow coaptation of the tissue planes and primary healing. In some cases sinograms are helpful in demonstrating a tract between the ulcer and an infected joint, the urethra, or intestines.

Infected and necrotic bone should be thoroughly debrided

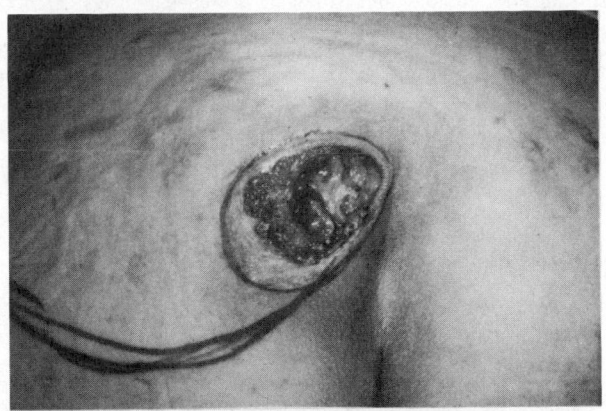

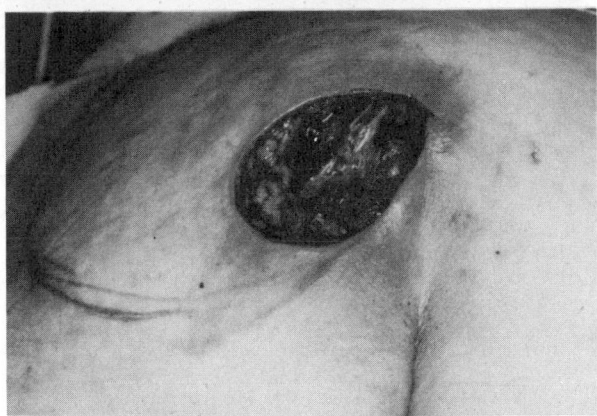

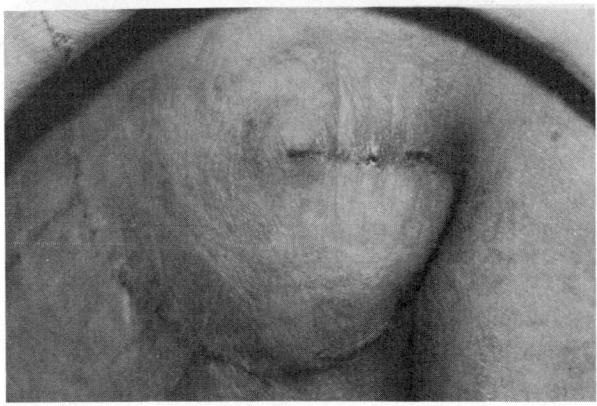

Fig. 166-2. Wide debridement of all necrotic tissue and granulation tissue containing bacteria was necessary before rotation flap closure of this sacral ulcer.

based on clinical assessment of its viability. With adequate debridement, it is usually not necessary to systemically treat bone infections longer than the standard therapeutic period of 5 to 7 days [35]. Unusual configurations of heterotopic bone and accentuated bony prominences are excised with care, making efforts to analyze whether forces are truly being dispersed or merely shifted to another focal point where pressure ulceration will soon occur [49]. Closure of large pressure sores is ideally performed at the time of surgical debridement with a well-vascularized flap or directly by primary closure, provided that the suture line does not lie in the line of weight-bearing [50,51].

Early closure of the wound obliterates dead space, improves blood supply (and delivery of systemic antibiotics), and pro-

motes healing of the wound. In cases of pressure sore infection characterized by cellulitis or septicemia, wound closure should be delayed until the infection has been resolved. Interim treatment of the delayed wound should consist of combined systemic and topical antimicrobial therapy. Concurrent with debridement and cleansing of the infected pressure ulcer, optimization of patient nutrition and other physiologic and immune functions should be emphasized.

In choosing a method of wound closure, one should seek simple methods first followed by more sophisticated methods as the wound conditions dictate. The first option on this *reconstructive ladder* is nonsurgical therapy. Conservative management is successful in achieving eventual wound closure, provided that three important criteria are met: total relief of pressure, positive nutritional balance, and modification of patient behavior such that recurrence is prevented. Conway and Griffith [51] reviewed the nonsurgical treatment of pressure sores and found that although an average of 55 percent healed in 3 to 6 months, over 50 percent recurred.

Because recurrence is the rule rather than the exception, surgical management must emphasize behavior modification both preoperatively and postoperatively. If the patient is psychologically motivated and physically able to prevent a recurrence, surgery can effect a cure. The health care team must educate and evaluate each individual patient. Disa et al. reviewed 40 patients with 68 pressure sores operated on between 1981 and 1989. Only 80 percent were healed at the time of discharge. Moreover, 61 percent of the sores and 69 percent of the patients had recurrent ulceration, within a mean of 9.3 months. Recurrence was most common in young posttraumatic paraplegics and cerebrally compromised elderly patients [52]. The goals of surgical therapy are to reduce protein losses from a large exudative wound, prevent progressive osteomyelitis and sepsis, reduce hospital and patient costs, and improve the quality of life. If these indications are not present, for example in the case of a small pressure sore in an institutionalized, organically demented patient, conservative therapy with daily dressing changes may be indicated. Frantz retrospectively reviewed the nonsurgical treatment costs of 240 pressure sores in an 830-bed long-term care facility over a 5-year period. The mean treatment cost was $5.35/pressure ulcer/day [53].

Primary closure of pressure sores is quite effective if the cause of ulceration is due to an acutely debilitated state that no longer presents as a danger for recurrence and if significant dead space and tissue tension do not prohibit this choice. Skin grafting rarely meets the requirements of long-term durability or ability to contour to irregularly shaped, undermined wounds. Fasciocutaneous flaps and musculocutaneous flaps fill large irregular defects, bring in new blood supply, and provide padding (Figs. 166-3 and 166-4). These flaps have revolutionized our ability to treat large and/or multiple pressure sores. Flaps should be of sufficient size to be readvanced in case of recurrence and should not violate adjacent flap territories. Multiple ulcers may require multiple flaps. Often flap donor sites must be skin grafted. Tissue expansion has been proposed as a means of delivering sensate coverage [54]. Other neurosensory flaps may help prevent recurrence [55,56,57].

Postsurgical management requires suction drains to improve tissue apposition and flap adherence and for aspirating serosanguineous collections, constipation for 5 days when treating perianal wounds, and systemic antibiotics for 3 to 5 days. Occasionally, fecal and urinary diversion may be indicated to allow healing of pressure sores and provide a simpler method of personal hygiene [58]. Postoperative complications include hematoma, infection, and partial or total flap loss.

While young, active paraplegics must take responsibility for the prevention of pressure sores, chronically debilitated nursing

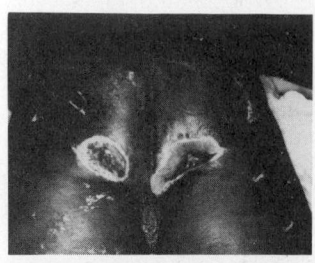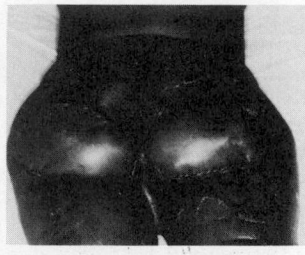

Fig. 166-3. Posterior thigh skin, fat, and fascia are transposed to close bilateral ischial pressure sores. Tissue laxity in this area allows primary closure of the donor sites.

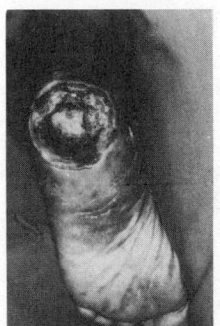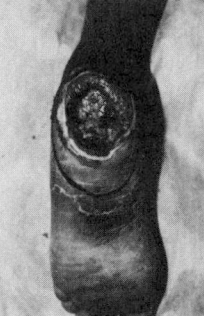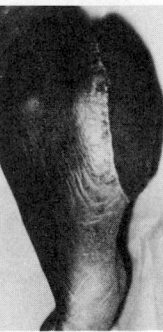

Fig. 166-4. After soft tissue and bony debridement of this heel wound, a posterior calf fasciocutaneous free flap was used to repair the defect.

home patients or acutely debilitated intensive care patients must rely on the knowledge and attentiveness of physicians and nurses to avoid this oftentimes preventable problem.

References

1. Kenedi RM, Cowden JM, Scales JT (eds): *Bedsore Biomechanics.* Baltimore, University Park Press, 1976.
2. Manley MT: Incidence, contributory factors and costs of pressure sores. *S Afr Med J* 53:147, 1978.
3. Kuhn BA, Coulter SJ: Balancing the pressure ulcer cost and quality equation. *Nursing Economics* 10:353, 1992.
4. Barton A: Pressure sores viewed by electron microscope and thermographically. *Geriatrics* 28:143, 1973.
5. Guyton AC, Granger HJ, Taylor AE: Interstitial fluid pressure. *Physiol Rev* 51:527, 1971.
6. Krouskop TA, Reddy NP, Spencer WA, Sacor JW: Mechanisms of decubitus ulcer formation—an hypothesis. *Med Hypotheses* 4:37, 1978.
7. Husain T: An experimental study of some pressure effects on tissues, with reference to the bedsore problem. *J Pathol* 66:347, 1953.
8. Dansereau JG, Conway H: Closure of decubiti in paraplegics. *Plast Reconstr Surg* 33:474, 1964.
9. Bush CA: Study of pressure over skin under the ischial tuberosities and thighs during sitting. *Arch Phys Med Rehabil* 50:207, 1959.
10. Kosiak M, Kubicek WG, Olson M, et al: Evaluation of pressure as a factor in the production of ischial ulcers. *Arch Phys Med Rehabil* 39:623, 1958.
11. Lindan O: Etiology of decubitus ulcers: An experimental study. *Arch Phys Med Rehabil* 42:774, 1961.
12. Kosiak M: Etiology and pathology of ischemic ulcers. *Arch Phys Med Rehabil* 40:62, 1959.
13. Groth KE: Klinische Beobachtungen und experimentelle Studien über die Entstehung des Dekubitus. *Acta Chir Scand* 87(Suppl 76):1, 1942.
14. Dinsdale SM: Decubitus ulcers: Role of pressure and friction in causation. *Arch Phys Med Rehabil* 55:147, 1974.
15. Carstensen LL, Neale JM (eds): *Mechanisms of Psychological Influence on Physical Health: With Special Attention to the Elderly.* New York, Plenum Press, 1989.
16. Holmes R: Nutrition know-how: Combating pressure sores nutritionally. *Am J Nurs* 87:1301, 1987.
17. Takeda T, Koyama T, Izawa Y, et al: Effects of malnutrition on development of experimental pressure sores. *J Dermatol* 19:602, 1992.
18. Reuter JB, Cooney TG: The pressure sore: Pathophysiology and principles of management. *Ann Intern Med* 94:661, 1981.
19. Flam E: Skin maintenance in the bed-ridden patient: Implications for plastic surgery. University of Medicine and Denistry of New Jersey, Robert Wood Johnson Medical School, 1989.
20. Peacock EE: Repair of skin wounds, in Peacock E, Van Winkle W: *Wound Repair.* Philadelphia, WB Saunders, 1976, pp 204–270.
21. Shea JD: Pressure sores: Classification and management. *Clin Orthop* 112:89, 1975.
22. Le KM, Madsen BL, Barth PW, et al: An in-depth look at pressure sores using monolithic silicon sensors. *Plast Reconstr Surg* 74:745, 1984.
23. Constantian MB: *Pressure Ulcers, Principles and Techniques of Management.* Boston, Little, Brown & Co, 1980, p 25.
24. Mustoe T, Upton J, Marcellino V, et al: Carcinoma in chronic pressure sores: A fulminant disease process. *Plast Reconstr Surg* 77:116, 1986.
25. Trumble HC: Skin tolerance for pressure and pressure sores. *Med J Aust* 2:724, 1930.
26. Redfern SJ, Jeneil PA, Gillingham ME, Lunn HF: Local pressures with ten types of patient-support systems. *Lancet* 1:277, 1973.
27. Allman RM, Walker JM, Hart MK, et al: Air-fluidized beds or conventional therapy for pressure sores. *Ann Intern Med* 107:641, 1987.
28. Houle RJ: Evaluation of seat devices designed to prevent ischemic ulcers in paraplegic patients. *Arch Phys Med Rehabil* 50:587, 1969.
29. Ursu G: Bedsores treated with negative air-ions. *Paraplegia* 8:182, 1970.
30. Lee LK, Ambrus JL: Collagenase therapy for decubitus ulcers. *Geriatrics* 30:91, 1975.
31. Sugarman B, Brown D, Musher D: Fever and infection in spinal cord injury patients. *JAMA* 248:66, 1982.
32. Rissing JP, Crowder JG, Dunfee T, et al: Bacteroides bacteremia from decubitus ulcers. *South Med J* 67:1179, 1974.
33. Galpin JE, et al: Sepsis associated with decubitus ulcers. *Am J Med* 61:346, 1976.
34. Bryan CS, Dew CE, Reynolds KL: Bacteremia associated with decubitus ulcers. *Arch Intern Med* 143:2093, 1983.
35. Lewis VL Jr, Bailey HM, Pulawski G, et al: The diagnosis of osteomyelitis in patients with pressure sores. *Plast Reconstr Surg* 81:229, 1988.
36. Robson MC, Lea CE, Dalton JB, et al: Quantitative bacteriology and delayed wound closure. *Surg Forum* 19:501, 1968.
37. Heggars JP, Robson MC, Doran ET: Qualitative assessment of bacterial contamination of open wounds by a slide technique. *Mil Med* 134:666, 1969.
38. Robson MC: George H. Monks Memorial Lecture. Boston, September, 1989.
39. Rice TT: Metronidazole use in malodorous skin lesions. *Rehabilitation Nursing* 17(5):244, 255, 1992.
40. Witkowski JA, Parish LC: Topical metronidazole gel. The bacteriology of decubitus ulcers. *Int J Dermatol* 30(9):660, 1991.
41. Hunt TK: Nutritional requirements of repair, in Ballinger WF (ed): *Manual of Surgical Nutrition.* Philadelphia, WB Saunders, 1975.
42. Morgan EJ: Topical therapy of pressure ulcers. *Surg Gynecol Obstet* 141:945, 1975.
43. Robson MC, Phillips LG, Lawrence WT, et al: The safety and effect of topically applied recombinant basic fibroblast growth factor on the healing of chronic pressure sores. *Ann Surg* 216(4):401, 1992.
44. Robson MC, Phillips LG, Thomason A, et al: Platelet-derived growth

factor BB for the treatment of chronic pressure ulcers. *Lancet* 339:23, 1992.
45. Pace WE: Beads of a dextran polymer for the local treatment of cutaneous ulcers. *J Dermatol Surg Oncol* 4(9):678, 1978.
46. Sawyer PN, Dowbak, Sophie Z, et al: A preliminary report of the efficacy of Debrisan (dextranomer) in the debridement of cutaneous ulcers. *Surgery* 85:201, 1979.
47. Zitelli J: Wound healing for the clinician. *Adv Dermat* 2:243, 1987.
48. Blocksma R, Kostrubala JG, Greeley PW: The surgical repair of decubitus ulcers in paraplegics: Further observations. *Plast Reconstr Surg* 4:123, 1949.
49. Karaca AR, Binns JH, Blumenthal FS: Complications of total ischiectomy for the treatment of ischial pressure sores. *Plast Reconstr Surg* 62:96, 1978.
50. Kostrubala JG, Greeley PW: The problem of decubitus ulcers in paraplegics. *Plast Reconstr Surg* 2:403, 1947.
51. Conway H, Griffith BH: Plastic surgery for closure of decubitus ulcers in patients with paraplegia: Based on experience with 1000 cases. *Am J Surg* 91:946, 1956.

52. Disa JJ, Carlton JM, Goldberg NH: Efficacy of operative cure in pressure sore patients. *Plast Reconstr Surg* 89(2):272, 1992.
53. Frantz RA, Gardner S, Harvey P, Specht J: The cost of treating pressure ulcers in a long-term care facility. *Decubitus* 4(3):37, 1991.
54. Neves RI, Kahler SH, Banducci DR, Manders EK: Tissue expansion of sensate skin for pressure sores. *Ann Plast Surg* 29(5):433, 1992.
55. Kuhn W, Luscher NJ, de Roche R, et al: The neurosensory musculocutaneous tensor fasciae latae flaps: Long term results. *Paraplegia* 30(6):396, 1992.
56. Hauge EN: The anatomical basis of a new method for re-innervation of the gluteal region in paraplegics. *Acta Physiol Scand* 603(Suppl):19, 1991.
57. Lesavoy MA, Dubrow TJ, Korn HN, et al: "Sensible" flap coverage of pressure sores in patients with meningomyelocele. *Plast Reconstr Surg* 85(3):390, 1990.
58. Bejany DE, Chao R, Perito PE, Politano VA: Continent urinary diversion and diverting colostomy in the therapy of non-healing pressure sores in paraplegic patients. *Paraplegia* 31(4):242, 1993.

167. *Management of Pain in the Critically Ill*

Donald S. Stevens and
W. Thomas Edwards

Many patients with a critical illness are in pain. Although there are only a few studies that scientifically document this problem, the facts are clear that pain is a major problem for patients hospitalized in intensive care units [1,2,3].

When traditional (pro re nata [PRN]) analgesia is prescribed, a complicated and time-consuming ritual ensues. The nurse must be located, the narcotic keys obtained, the medication drawn up and charted, the patient drug administration records double-checked, and, finally, the medication administered. This procedure can result in a patient remaining in pain up to 80 minutes out of every 4-hour cycle of drug dosing [4].

Physicians may think that today we do a much better job of providing analgesia than was done 25 or 30 years ago, but as can be seen in Table 167-1, this is not the case. In the 1950s, 33 percent of patients had insufficient analgesia after surgery [5,6,7]. Multiple reports from the 1970s and 1980s show the same complaint from 31 to 41 percent of patients [8–15]. Even more striking are recent data indicating that 58 percent of medical-surgical patients experience "excruciating pain" during their hospitalization [14]. Ineffectiveness of opioid analgesia in intensive care settings is probably more related to the manner in which the drugs are used than to the properties of the analgesics themselves.

There are many reasons for the undertreatment of pain in the hospital setting. Traditionally, the treatment of pain has depended on the judgment of the nurse caring for the patient. Pain is frequently undertreated because of fears of depressing spontaneous ventilation, inducing opioid dependence, or precipitating cardiovascular instability. Unfortunately, little attention has been paid to developing appropriate skills for evaluating and treating pain during the basic clinical education of physicians and nurses [16]. As a result, the methods for assessing pain, the tactics for aggressively treating pain, and the results of effective pain management are poorly understood by most clinicians [17–26]. Correct treatment begins with a proper understanding of the source of the patient's complaint. A rational plan is then developed, which culminates in satisfactory treatment of the problem. Ultimately, this leads to resolution of the patient's pain, which in turn facilitates recovery. It is important to remember that pain is a totally subjective phenomenon. When the patient says "I hurt" it is true, regardless of whether the observer feels that the amount of pain reported is appropriate.

A Conceptual Framework for the Management of Pain

The terms listed here will be used in the following discussion of the management of pain:

1. *Pain:* an unpleasant sensory and emotional experience associated with actual or potential tissue damage, or described in terms of such damage [27].
2. *Suffering:* the reaction of an organism to the experience of pain [28].
3. *Pain-Related Behavior:* behavior that leads an observer to conclude that pain and suffering are being experienced [29].
4. *Acute Pain:* pain that has an identifiable temporal and causal relationship to the occurrence of an injury. This is in distinction to *chronic pain,* which persists beyond the time of

Table 167-1. Incidence of Therapeutic Failures when Conventional Intramuscular Injections of Opiates Are Given for Postoperative Pain Relief

Reference	Number of patients	Insufficient analgesia, moderate or severe pain (%)
Papper et al. (1952)	286	33
Lasagna & Beecher (1954)	122	33
Keats (1965)	?	26–53
Keeri-Szanto & Heaman (1972)	106	20
Cronin et al. (1973)	100	42
Banister (1974)	437	12–26
Tammisto (1978)	100	24
Cohen (1980)	109	75
Tamsen et al. (1982)	56	38
Donovan (1983)	200	31
Sriwatanakul et al. (1983)	81	41

Reprinted by permission: Harmer M, Rosen M, Vickers MD: *Patient Controlled Analgesia.* Cambridge, Blackwell Scientific, 1985.

healing of an injury and for which there may not be any clearly identifiable cause [29].

5. *Noxious Stimulus:* a stimulus that is inimical or potentially inimical to the integrity of tissue [28].
6. *Nociception:* the process of detecting and signaling the presence of a noxious stimulus [28].

The representation that best characterizes the relationship among the components of acute pain is shown in Figure 167-1. The observer cannot tell the relative sizes of the circles because all that can be observed is the "pain-related behavior." Certainly, a more extensive surgical dissection or trauma resulting in greater tissue damage is likely to cause the release of

Fig. 167-1. The multifaceted model of Acute Pain derived from the Multifaceted Model of Pain originally presented by J. Loeser [362]. (From Loeser JD: Concepts of pain, in Stanton-Hicks M, Boas R (eds): *Chronic Low Back Pain.* New York, Raven Press, 1982, p 146.)

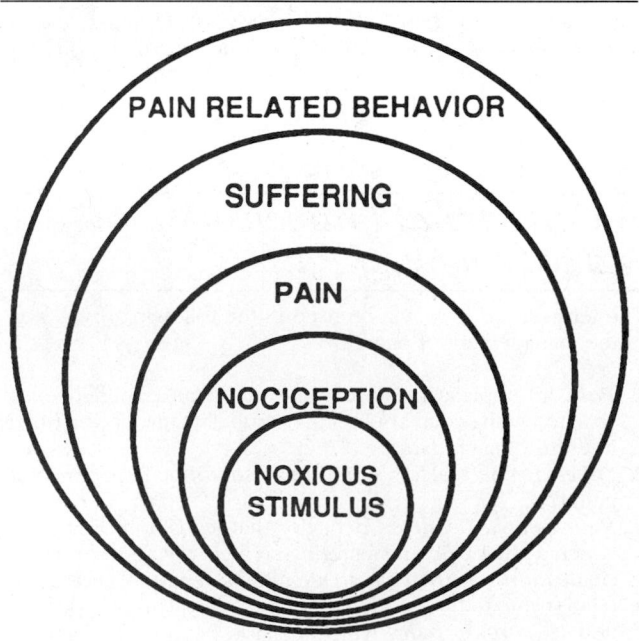

greater quantities of the various components of the inflammatory response and other pain-causing substances (algogens). It is common, however, for two patients who have undergone similar operations with similar anesthetics to experience markedly different degrees of pain. The difference in pain often results in pejorative terms being applied to the patient who seems to have greater pain.

Nociception, however, is modulated by many things, including ethnocultural background, learned behaviors, and the meaning of the particular experience for the individual [22,23]. In general, the most successful approach for treating pain takes into consideration both pharmacologic and nonpharmacologic factors.

The successful management of acute pain is based on four principles [28]:

1. The clinician must establish the correct *diagnosis* of the source and magnitude of nociception.
2. The clinician must *understand* the relationship of ongoing nociception with the other components of pain (including anxiety, ethnocultural factors, situational meaning, prior experience, etc.).
3. *Treatment* should be based on establishing and maintaining drug levels at active sites to achieve and maintain appropriate levels of analgesia and anxiolysis.
4. The clinician should continually *reevaluate* therapy for its effectiveness and modify the approach as needed.

Acute Pain Pathways

The anatomy of the pain pathway is presented in schematic form in Figure 167-2. Acute pain begins with damage to the skin or deeper structures. Algogens (including small peptides, prostaglandins, and other compounds), which are produced or released locally, sensitize or stimulate peripheral nociceptors. These are "pain-specific," small, thinly myelinated or unmyelinated fibers. The signal is propagated along the nociceptor fibers into the dorsal horn of the spinal cord (or, in the case of cranial nerves, into the sensory nuclei). Modulation (either amplification or attenuation) of the signal can take place before the signal is transmitted into pain-specific areas of the deep brain structures and cerebral cortex.

Reflexes are generated all along the pain pathway, resulting in responses that can be beneficial (e.g., withdrawal from the noxious stimulus) or deleterious (e.g., sympathetic discharge causing neuroendocrine changes characteristic of the stress response) to the injured organism [30]. One of the reflex responses associated with trauma or surgery is increased skeletal muscle tone and localized spasm, which increases oxygen consumption and lactic acid production. Increased sympathetic outflow causes tachycardia and increased stroke volume, cardiac work, and myocardial oxygen consumption. Supraspinal reflex responses to pain result in hypothalamic stimulation, increased sympathetic tone, increased release of catecholamines and other "stress" hormones (cortisol, adrenocorticotropic hormone [ACTH], arginine vasopressin, growth hormone, glucagon, aldosterone, renin, angiotensin II), and decreased secretion of anabolic hormones (insulin, testosterone). The postsurgical catabolic state can be worsened if the process continues.

Each separate part of the pain pathway can be influenced so that the nociceptive signal is diminished or eliminated. Appropriate tailoring of the analgesic technique to meet the needs of the individual patient is both desirable and possible.

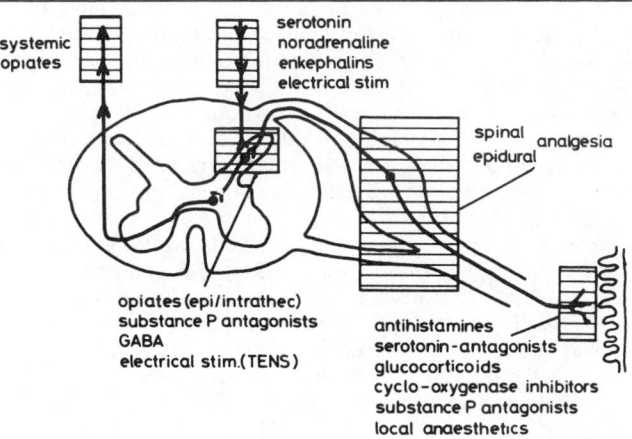

Fig. 167-2. A "map" of the path of nociceptive information from the periphery to the central nervous system. Modification of that information can be effected at any point of information transfer. (From Cousins MJ, Phillips GD: *Acute Pain Management.* New York, Churchill-Livingstone, 1986, p 52, with permission.)

Formulating a Treatment Plan: Questions That Need to be Asked

Acute pain usually remits spontaneously. The intensity of pain is greatest at the onset, immediately after injury. As healing and stabilization of the injured part occur, the intrinsic-pain modulation system continues to be active, and there is a reduction in the amount of algogens released. This gradually reduces the amount of pain. This is true of most types of "simple" acute pain, such as postoperative, trauma, or burn pain. During different stages of the recovery process, the character of the pain often changes from sharp or cutting to deep and aching. There also may be a concomitant change from well-localized myotomal or dermatomal pain to poorly localized pain. It is therefore important to ask several questions about the pain when one is designing a treatment plan.

WHERE DOES IT HURT? Is the location of the pain appropriate for the injury sustained or for the surgery performed, or is it in another location entirely? If nociception is not accounted for by the injury, surgical procedure, or deep visceral process, then a secondary source must be investigated. The pain may result from intraoperative malpositioning and be myofascial in origin. Neuropathic pain can arise from the interruption of peripheral nerve fibers (deafferentation pain) subsequent to nerve injury. Pain may have nothing to do with the current acute problem in patients with underlying problems with chronic pain. There may be another (unrecognized) source of acute pain, such as another injury in victims of multiple trauma.

HOW MUCH PAIN? Each patient should be asked to try to quantify his or her pain level. If possible, in the case of postoperative pain, this should be done by using a system that was taught before surgery. Visual or verbal analog scales are useful for this purpose (Fig. 167-3) [31]. With these measurements, each patient serves as his or her own control, and the response to treatment is best measured as a change from the baseline value. A numerical scale without the visual analog also can be used effectively by asking the patient to assign a number to the

TECHNIQUES FOR GRADING PAIN BEFORE AND AFTER TREATMENT

Five Point Global Scale	NONE=0 A LITTLE=1 SOME=2 A LOT=3 THE WORST=4
Verbal Quantitative	0 . . . . 5 . . . . 10 none worst imaginable
Visual Pain Analog Scale (VPAS)	no worst ――――――――――――― pain pain

Place a mark on the line
to show where your pain is now.

Fig. 167-3. Several scales that can be useful for the evaluation of patient "self reports" of pain before and after treatment.

pain from 0 to 10, where 0 is no pain at all and 10 is the worst pain you could possibly imagine. Although this type of scale may not be as accurate as a visual scale, it has the advantage of being simple and can even be taught while putting in a patient's intravenous line preoperatively.

During the patient's hospital course, other scales can be added. Sensory and affective components of pain can be assessed using the short form of the McGill Pain Questionnaire [32,33]. Pain in intubated patients can be assessed even if they are unable to communicate. Various markers of sympathetic activity, such as restlessness, sweating, tachycardia, lacrimation, pupillary dilatation, and hypertension, can be graded as signs of pain intensity, although any one of these is not an adequate measure of pain intensity by itself [34]. It is crucial that measurements be made and recorded in the chart both before and after treatment. This permits an accurate assessment of changes in pain level with therapy [20].

WHAT DOES IT FEEL LIKE? The quality of the sensation is important. If the pain is sharp, it is probably due to direct nociception (e.g., incisional pain). Dull aching sensations that respond well to opioids are typical of pain arising from deeper structures. Pulling or tugging sensations can be caused by the sutures in the wound or visceral stimulation.

Buzzing, stinging, "pins and needles" sensations, or a sensation of electricity indicate abnormal neural function. These sensations are minimal and short-lived following regional anesthesia. When they occur in the postoperative or trauma setting, they are indicative of neural compression and reestablishment of neural function. Painful dysesthesias can occur as part of a preexisting medical condition, as is seen in patients with peripheral neuropathies.

Formulating a Treatment Plan: Approaches to Therapy

Figure 167-2 shows the different levels of the pain pathway. It also lists some of the different techniques that can be used at each different level to eliminate or lessen the nociceptive signal. The choice of therapeutic approach is made based on the type and location of the patient's pain.

1. Techniques can be used that interfere with nociception in the *periphery*. These include the use of nonsteroidal antiinflammatory drugs, infiltration with local anesthetics, and peripheral nerve blockade.
2. Techniques can be used that interfere with the first integration of the nociceptive information at the *spinal cord level*. These include epidural and intrathecal infusions of local anesthetics, opioids, or a combination thereof, as well as transcutaneous electrical nerve stimulation.
3. Techniques can be used that modify higher orders of integration of the nociceptive information throughout the nervous system. This *systemic approach* includes the use of systemic opioids administered by depot injection (intramuscularly or subcutaneously), transdermal delivery system, bolus or continuous IV infusion, or patient-controlled analgesia (PCA).

When one is choosing a therapeutic modality, consideration should be given to the availability of knowledge, skills, equipment, personnel, and medications, as well as the expected advantages to the patient and the anticipated risks of the modality selected [29].

Specific Analgesic Techniques: The Periphery

NONSTEROIDAL ANTIINFLAMMATORY DRUGS. Nonsteroidal antiinflammatory drugs (NSAIDs) interfere with the production of prostaglandins, which are algogens that can produce hyperalgesia [35]. NSAIDs may diminish the inflammatory response to trauma or surgery and thereby diminish nociceptive input. One of their most common uses is to augment analgesia from opioids. Some of these compounds, including acetylsalicylate [36], diclofenac [37], dipyrone [38], indoprofen [39], and ketorolac [40], are available in parenteral formulations in Europe. None except ketorolac tromethamine (Toradol, Syntex Laboratories, Palo Alto, CA) are currently available in the United States in parenteral form.

Ketorolac has been shown to be effective in reducing opioid requirement after major surgery [41]. It also can be administered intravenously [42,43]. One great advantage of parenteral ketorolac is that it does not depress the respiratory drive, as do the opioids [44]. The addition of ketorolac to an opioid regimen can provide analgesia while maintaining respiration. This is useful for the patient whose pain is not relieved by opioids before respiratory depression occurs. Another use for ketorolac is in patients after thoracic surgery. Even with dense epidural blockade, chest and shoulder pain may not be relieved after lung resection. Ketorolac has been shown to be effective in controlling this type of pain [45]. When prescribing ketorolac, the physician must remember that it also has the same side effects of other NSAIDs, including nausea, peptic ulceration, and inhibition of platelet function [46]. Severe bronchospasm may also occur in patients with asthma, nasal polyposis, and allergy to aspirin or other NSAIDs [46,47]. Appropriate caution should be observed when prescribing ketorolac in the unconscious patient. Ketorolac is contraindicated in the presence of acute or chronic renal failure and in the presence of hypovolemia. Ketorolac should not be given for more than five days.

LOCAL ANESTHETIC TECHNIQUES

Local Infiltration. The action of local anesthetics sometimes persists far beyond the expected length of time. In a recent study of the severity of postoperative pain after elective herniorrhaphy, patients received general anesthesia, general anesthesia plus local anesthetic infiltration of the incision, or spinal anesthesia [48]. The severity of pain during rest, during movement, or with pressure on the wound was evaluated for each group. There was a significant decrease in the severity of each type of pain when local anesthetic was used. Local infiltration (with general anesthesia) was better than spinal anesthesia, which was better than general anesthesia alone. The effect of the local anesthetic appeared to last at least 48 hours postoperatively. The prolonged analgesic effect may occur because blockage of nociceptive afferent impulses prevents an increase in the excitability of the neurons of the intraspinal pain pathway [49]. This effect is termed "preemptive analgesia" [50]. Local anesthetics also inhibit leukocyte migration, which may result in fewer leukocytes in the surgical site and smaller amounts of algogens being released [51]. This would result in less inflammatory response and less incisional pain.

Intercostal Blocks. Repeated intermittent intercostal nerve blocks have been used for many years to provide analgesia for thoracic injuries such as fractured ribs, as well as for treating postoperative pain. This technique provides analgesia without widespread sympathetic blockade or weakness of major muscle groups, disadvantages that are seen with epidural local anesthetics. Nerve blocks provide analgesia without sedation or respiratory depression, in contrast to analgesia obtained with opioids administered either epidurally or parenterally [52,53]. Disadvantages of the intercostal block technique include the need for repeated injections [54], the risk of pneumothorax (0.073–19%) [55], and the possibility of systemic toxic reactions to the local anesthetic if excessive amounts are used. This technique may not be appropriate in anticoagulated patients because of the risk of bleeding and hematoma formation subsequent to laceration of an intercostal vessel [56].

Intercostal nerve blocks can be performed under direct vision during thoracotomy [57,58]. The intercostal nerve sheaths at the level of the incision and one or two ribs above and below this level are injected with 4 to 5 ml of a long-acting local anesthetic. This is usually performed close to the vertebra, where the nerves first appear visible through the parietal pleura. Additionally, one or two levels may be blocked at the site of the thoracostomy tube.

Opinions are divided regarding this method of treatment. Some authors feel that intraoperative intercostal blocks help patients during the postoperative period by relieving pain and improving pulmonary function [58]. Other authors disagree [57]. The transient nature of the relief provided by a single injection is the main point of controversy. However, as previously discussed, perhaps even a single injection can "preempt" spinal cord level integration of the nociceptive impulses and therefore relieve pain longer than would be expected on the basis of the pharmacology of the local anesthetic.

The main problem with the use of single intercostal blocks is that they need to be repeated to provide long-lasting analgesia. To avoid this drawback, a continuous technique for intercostal nerve block has been developed [59,60,61]. A plastic catheter is inserted into a single intercostal space through a Tuohy needle. A bolus of 5 to 10 ml of local anesthetic can then be injected through the catheter to provide analgesia to several intercostal segments. Potential problems with this technique include difficulty with catheter placement [62] and chest wall hematoma formation [63,64]. Some attempts at continuous intercostal catheter placement have resulted in an interpleural catheter placement [65] (see the following section on interpleural analgesia).

Studies have been performed to determine where local anesthetics work to cause intercostal blockade. The distribution of intercostal injectate has been assessed using various markers, including India ink [66,67,68], iodinated contrast agents [69,70,71], liquid latex [69], and radioactive tracers [72]. Data from these studies suggest that injection into an intercostal space causes spread both peripherally and centrally along the same intercostal space. Spreading into the paravertebral space can be demonstrated if enough volume is injected. Alternatively, as illustrated in Figure 167-4, spreading also can occur between the parietal pleura and the internal aspect of the ribs. Spread of the injected material into the epidural space [72] as well as to the contralateral paravertebral space [62] has been demonstrated, explaining the appearance of bilateral blocks [72]. Horner's syndrome can occur following intercostal blockade at the level of the ninth rib, presumably due to rostral spread of the local anesthetic in the paravertebral space to the level of the cervicothoracic sympathetic ganglion [73].

The analgesia produced through intercostal blockade, whether by multiple injections or through a continuous catheter, is excellent in comparison to the analgesia achieved with traditional methods of parenteral opioid administration [74,75]. Some data suggest that continuous intercostal blockade improves pulmonary function relative to treatment with systemic opioids in postthoracotomy patients [61,75,76,77]. The intercostal block technique is most appropriate for treating unilateral thoracic or upper abdominal pain.

Paravertebral Block. Analgesia for pain in the thorax or abdomen can be provided by paravertebral nerve blockade. This can be performed with either a single injection of local anes-

thetic or a continuous catheter technique [78]. To perform the block, the patient is placed in the lateral position, with the side to be blocked uppermost. If possible, the block should be performed at the level of the pain. The point of injection is located 3 cm lateral to the top edge of the posterior spinous process of the appropriate vertebra. A 3½-inch, 22-gauge spinal needle is used. An appropriately sized Tuohy needle can be used, if a catheter is to be placed. The needle is introduced perpendicular to the skin in all planes and is advanced until bone is contacted, usually at a depth of 1 to 1½ inches (Fig. 167-5). A syringe filled with air is attached. The needle is redirected cephalad to pass above the bone (rib or transverse process). A loss of resistance to the injection of air is felt as the needle passes through the superior costotransverse ligament into the paravertebral space. Care must be taken not to direct the needle medially, because the epidural space can be entered. Aspiration should also be done to make sure that the needle has not entered pleura, lung, blood vessel, or a dural cuff [78].

If this block is performed as a single injection, the recommended dose of local anesthetic is 15 ml of 0.375% bupivacaine [78]. For the continuous catheter technique, a Tuohy needle is used, and a catheter is advanced through the needle 1 to 3 cm into the paravertebral space. Rotation of the needle may be necessary to allow passage of the catheter. Initial doses of local anesthetic ranging from 25 to 30 ml of 0.25% bupivacaine with epinephrine 1:200,000 have been used effectively through a paravertebral catheter [78].

Injection into a paravertebral catheter causes flow laterally into an intercostal space as well as up and down the ipsilateral paravertebral space [79]. Several intercostal nerves are thus bathed with anesthetic, providing analgesia over several dermatomal levels.

The advantages of paravertebral block are similar to those of the intercostal technique. Analgesia can be obtained without widespread cardiovascular effects, because only unilateral sympathetic blockade is produced. Analgesia is produced over several dermatomes with only one injection. Because the site of injection is medial to the scapula, this block is easier to perform at high thoracic levels than are intercostal blocks. Finally, in contrast to routine intercostal blocks, the posterior primary ramus of the intercostal nerve is covered by this block, providing

Fig. 167-4. Lateral radiograph of contrast injected through an intercostal catheter. Note the distention of the extrapleural space with spread over multiple intercostal spaces (arrows). (From Hord AH, Wang JM, Pai UT, Raj PP: Anatomic spread of India ink in the human intercostal space with radiographic correlation. *Reg Anesth* 16:13, 1991, with permission.)

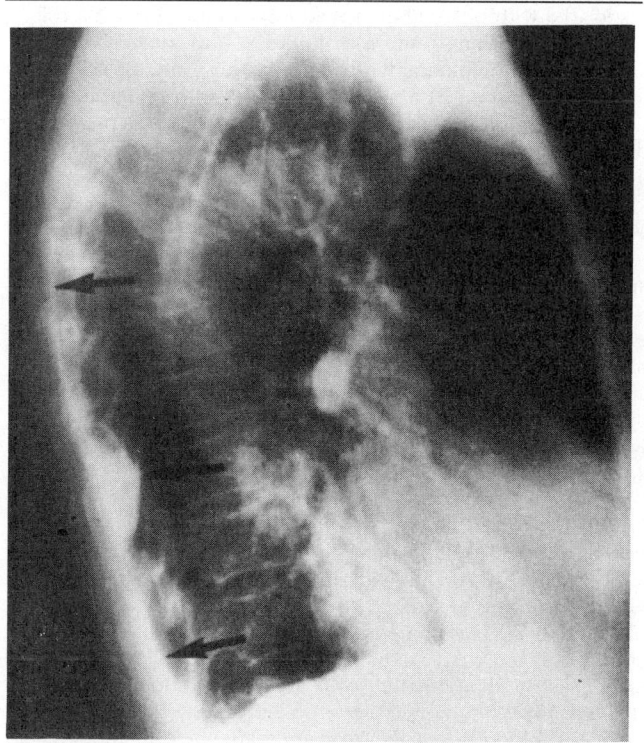

Fig. 167-5. Direction of needle: (1) initial to strike transverse process or rib; (2) angled to pass through superior costotransverse ligament. (From Eason MJ, Wyatt RL: Paravertebral thoracic block—A reappraisal. *Anaesthesia* 34:638, 1979, with permission).

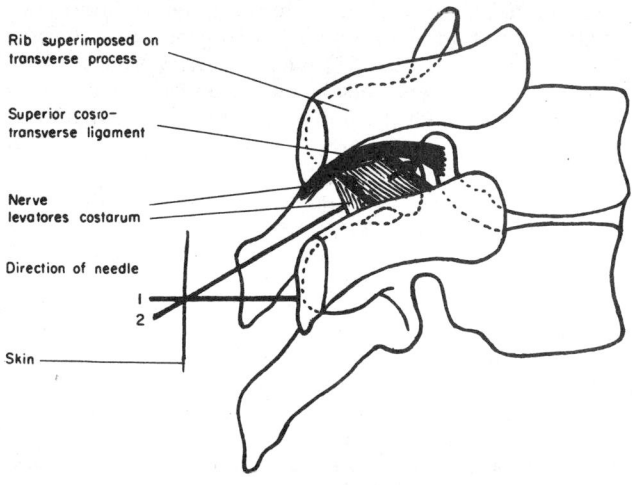

analgesia to the posterior spinal muscles and the costovertebral ligaments.

Risks of this technique include pneumothorax, epidural blockade, and inaccurate catheter placement [80]. Use of a loss of resistance technique minimizes the chance of pneumothorax. Gradual injection of the local anesthetic allows early detection of an epidural blockade. A test dose of the anesthetic should be administered to detect intravascular catheter placement, although intravascular placement is nearly impossible with the technique described.

Paravertebral catheters can be placed during thoracotomy, just prior to closing the incision [81]. Normal saline is used for the loss of resistance test. The surgeon should be able to see a bubble of saline outside the parietal pleura after the loss of resistance has been obtained. Ten milliliters of saline should then be injected to allow easier threading of the catheter.

Interpleural Analgesia. Interpleural analgesia has been used to manage various types of pain in the thorax and upper abdomen. Interpleural block has been used after renal surgery [82], unilateral mammary surgery [82,83,84], cholecystectomy [82,83], thoracotomy [85], and esophagectomy (performed through a thoracoabdominal incision) [86]. It also has been used to provide analgesia for patients with multiple rib fractures [87]. Pain from pancreatitis [88,89] and from pancreatic cancer [89] has been treated using this technique, as has pain from hepatic metastases [90].

In this technique, a conventional epidural catheter is placed into the interpleural space (between the parietal and visceral pleurae) using a Tuohy needle [82,83]. The usual point of injection is at the angle of the rib, approximately 8 to 10 cm lateral to the posterior midline. The technique is similar to that used for thoracentesis (i.e., the needle is "walked off" the superior border of the rib). The bevel of the needle is directed cephalad. Entry into the interpleural space is detected by a "hanging drop" technique, in which the "negative pressure" upon entry into the interpleural space is recognized when a drop of saline placed on the hub of the needle is sucked inward [91]. An epidural catheter is then advanced 5 to 10 cm into the interpleural space. Once the catheter is in place, either intermittent injections or a continuous infusion of local anesthetic may be used. Care must be exercised with the use of a continuous infusion to avoid accumulating a toxic dose of local anesthetic.

If a posterior approach is not possible, an anterior approach may also be used. The catheter also may be positioned in the interpleural space under direct vision during thoracotomy [92].

It is uncertain how interpleural analgesia works. Possibilities include diffusion of local anesthetic through the parietal pleura either superficially to block the intercostal nerves or posteromedially to reach the paravertebral area to block nerve roots and sympathetic ganglia [92,93]. Intercostal nerves are anesthetized [94], but to a lesser extent than with standard percutaneous intercostal techniques [93]. Sympathetic blockade also has been reported, which may account for the relief of visceral pain seen with this technique [88,95–99]. The block tends to be denser in dependent areas, which may require patients to be in the lateral position when each top-up dose is given [83,94,95].

Bupivacaine is the local anesthetic most commonly used to provide interpleural analgesia. However, the preferred dose and method of administration (bolus vs. continuous infusion) have not been determined. Bupivacaine is absorbed very rapidly from the interpleural space [82,85]. It is unclear if epinephrine slows this absorption [85,92,100]. The use of doses of 20 ml of 0.25% or 0.5% bupivacaine with or without epinephrine repeated every 6 hours appears to be safe. One report examined continuous interpleural infusion of 0.25% or 0.5% bupivacaine at 5 ml per hour [101]. A plateau in serum bupivacaine

was not reached during the 24 hours of the study, indicating that toxic serum levels might eventually be reached. Systemic toxicity has been reported with a continuous interpleural infusion of 2% lidocaine with epinephrine 1:200,000 at 15 to 20 ml per hour [102].

A case of bupivacaine toxicity was reported following a single interpleural injection of 30 ml of 0.5% bupivacaine with 1:200,000 epinephrine [103] in a patient with a pleural effusion and a recent history of pneumonia. Thus, a recent thoracic infection with concomitant pleuritis should be considered a relative contraindication to the use of interpleural analgesia.

Inaccurate catheter placement has been a major problem with interpleural analgesia. Use of a loss of resistance to injection technique for detection of entry into the interpleural space was used initially but resulted in a high incidence of incorrect catheter placement, including placement into lung tissue [100]. The "hanging-drop" technique may be the most accurate method [91]. Although pneumothorax can occur, interpleural air is easily evacuated through the catheter [104].

Inadequate analgesia may occur with interpleural blockade in the presence of a thoracostomy tube, because drainage may remove a large amount of the anesthetic agent from the interpleural space [105]. A thoracostomy tube should clamped for 20 minutes after injection of interpleural local anesthetic, to keep the medication in the interpleural space. If a patient cannot tolerate having a thoracostomy tube clamped, another method of analgesia should be chosen.

Analgesia may be inadequate if this technique is applied to patients with bilateral pain. It is probably best used only if one side of the thorax or upper abdomen is involved [106]. To circumvent this problem, *bilateral* interpleural catheters can be placed, using reduced doses of bupivacaine (10–20 ml of 0.25%–0.375% on each side) [107,108]. Because of concerns about local anesthetic toxicity and bilateral thoracic sympathetic blockade, other methods of analgesia are preferable in patients with bilateral pain, and bilateral interpleural catheters are *not* recommended. The possibility of ipsilateral phrenic nerve blockade with interpleural blockade contributes to the hazards associated with bilateral interpleural blockade [108,109,110].

Contraindications to the use of interpleural analgesia include (1) fibrosis of the pleura, which may make it difficult to identify the pleural space; (2) blood or fluid within the pleural space, which may be indicative of pleural inflammation (as previously discussed) or may dilute the local anesthetic; and (3) recent thoracic infection, which may cause rapid absorption of the local anesthetic, leading to toxicity (as previously discussed). The usual contraindications to regional anesthesia (patient refusal, anticoagulation, localized infection at the site of injection) are applicable to this technique.

Interpleural analgesia is a relatively simple technique. Unfortunately, it does not give a dense enough sensory block to allow many patients to improve pulmonary function. If there is a contraindication to placement of a thoracic epidural catheter, then this technique should be considered, but many patients will still require additional analgesia beyond interpleural blockade.

Other Regional Blocks. Brachial plexus anesthesia has long been a part of the anesthesiologist's armamentarium. "Single shot" brachial plexus blocks can provide hours of analgesia for vigorous turning in bed, chest physiotherapy, and other activities that would be limited by upper extremity pain. Use of a continuous brachial plexus technique can provide prolonged analgesia or sympathetic blockade for an upper extremity [111,112,113]. Sympathectomy may be of benefit by providing increased blood flow to an extremity after reimplantation surgery and also may prevent the development of a sympathetically maintained pain syndrome in a traumatized extremity. Blockade of both the nociceptive afferents and the sympathetic efferents may prevent the development of phantom pain in a limb following amputation.

Placement of a brachial plexus catheter in the axillary sheath can be verified radiographically [114] or clinically by obtaining the expected response to a local anesthetic injection. Bupivacaine is the most commonly used local anesthetic. After blockade is established with a bolus of local anesthetic (with appropriate monitoring and precautions), a continuous infusion of 0.125% bupivacaine is started at 7 to 10 ml per hour. The rate of infusion or the concentration of bupivacaine may need to be increased if tachyphylaxis develops. Catheters can be kept from being dislodged by carefully suturing them in place, and they can function for 4 to 7 days. Analgesia can be maintained with extremely low doses of bupivacaine with this technique.

Continuous femoral nerve block has been reported, using a catheter placed in the femoral nerve sheath and an infusion of 0.125% bupivacaine at 6 to 10 ml per hour [115,116]. This procedure may be of benefit for patients who have localized knee or thigh pain, especially those who cannot tolerate systemic opioids. It may facilitate nursing care of patients with femur fractures. It has the added advantage of producing very limited sympathectomy and cannot mask the occurrence of compartment syndrome in the lower leg in patients with multiple lower extremity injuries.

Specific Analgesic Techniques: Spinal Cord Level

TRANSCUTANEOUS ELECTRICAL NERVE STIMULATION. Although the mechanism whereby transcutaneous electrical nerve stimulation (TENS) produces analgesia is incompletely understood, it is probable that this technique works by down-modulating the afferent nociceptive signal at the spinal cord or brainstem level [117,118,119]. When TENS is used alone, adequate analgesia may not be produced; nevertheless, multiple studies have clearly documented a benefit when TENS is combined with other methods of analgesia for the treatment of acute pain problems.

Various types of waveforms are available, but regardless of the configuration of the waveform, it is important that current be delivered equally in both phases of the wave to prevent electrolysis in the skin [117]. It appears that high-frequency (80–100 Hz), low-intensity stimulation is the best type for postoperative pain [117].

TENS units are relatively easy to use. Patients are taught how to set the amplitude of the signal so that the current is just high enough to cause a tingling or buzzing sensation. After surgery, sterile electrodes are applied to the skin on either side of the incision approximately 1 cm from the suture line. Sterile dressings are placed over the pads, and the signal amplitude is set to the level determined preoperatively [117].

The effect of TENS has been evaluated after a variety of procedures, including knee surgery [118,119], appendectomy [120], cholecystectomy [121], lumbar laminectomy [122,123,124], thoracotomy [125,126], and cardiac surgery [127]. Some studies were unable to demonstrate analgesic efficacy [120,121,123,124,126], whereas others showed a decrease in opioid requirements and a decrease in postoperative pain [118,119,122,125,127]. Most of the studies yielding negative results did not use patient satisfaction or patient evaluation of pain (such as by use of a visual analog scale) as part of their evaluation.

There is a trend toward reduced frequency of postoperative nausea and vomiting with TENS [126]. The incidence of atelectasis and postoperative ileus may be decreased as well [128,129]. TENS may be beneficial in other acute pain states, including rib fractures [130], burns [131], and chronic stable severe angina pectoris [132,133].

CENTRAL CONDUCTION BLOCK—EPIDURAL OR SUBARACHNOID

General Considerations. The transmission of afferent nociceptive information also can be altered at a central level by more invasive techniques. Afferent conduction can be blocked at the nerve root or spinal cord level with local anesthetics. Nociceptive signals can be down-modulated centrally by intraspinal opioids acting on specific opiate receptors in the dorsal horn of the spinal cord. Regional analgesia techniques used for central conduction blockade include epidural or subarachnoid administration of local anesthetics, opiates, or mixtures of local anesthetics and opiates. These techniques can be used with intermittent dosing or with continuous infusion of the analgesic agent.

Subarachnoid Techniques: Local Anesthetics. Although subarachnoid (spinal) anesthesia is commonly used for many surgical procedures, analgesia from a single injection of local anesthetics does not last long enough to be useful for postoperative pain relief. Continuous spinal anesthesia is a useful technique for surgical procedures [134]. The use of continuous intrathecal (spinal) local anesthetics for postoperative analgesia has been reported [135,136]. Continuous monitoring at the bedside by an anesthetist may be necessary because of the potential for profound sympathectomy and hemodynamic instability [137]. The potential for central nervous system infection through prolonged use of an intrathecal catheter has been raised, but modern techniques appear to be safe for at least 48 hours [138,139].

Subarachnoid Techniques: Opioids. Some studies suggest that intrathecal opioid analgesia is a useful technique [140,141], but the duration of analgesia is always less than 24 hours. Patients receiving 10 µg per kilogram of intrathecal morphine after transsternal thymectomy have been reported to have improved pulmonary function for the first 24 hours postoperatively [142], but this dose can be associated with side effects [143,144]. The relative merit of a single injection of intrathecal morphine for the intensive care unit patient is therefore open to question [145,146].

Continuous intrathecal infusions of opioids (with or without local anesthetics) have been used to treat pain from cancer, without neurologic side effects [147,148]. Recent reports describe a similar technique for the management of postoperative pain. Continuous intrathecal catheters have been used to administer intermittent doses of morphine [149,150], or continuous infusions of morphine [151], fentanyl [151], diamorphine [152], morphine with lidocaine [153], or fentanyl with lidocaine [154]. Patient-controlled analgesia (discussed later in this chapter) has also been reported for administration of intrathecal fentanyl [155], and intrathecal bupivacaine with or without sufentanil [156]. A continuous intrathecal technique can provide excellent analgesia, but side effects and technical problems may make it impractical [157]. A combined spinal-epidural technique has been reported, which may offer the advantages of both techniques [158,159,160].

Epidural Techniques: Catheter Placement. Continuous epidural analgesia is an effective method for providing pain relief.

Epidural catheters can be placed either preoperatively before or after induction of general anesthesia or postoperatively prior to emergence from general anesthesia or in the intensive care unit. It is preferable to place the catheter while the patient is responsive. Paresthesias and the early symptoms of intravascular injection are difficult or impossible to detect in unresponsive patients. Moreover, sympathectomy-induced hypotension is the only way to detect correct positioning of the catheter in an unresponsive patient.

The loss of resistance technique is commonly used for locating the epidural space. Air and saline have both been used to detect the loss of resistance to injection, but we recommend the use of saline. Several potential problems may arise if air is injected epidurally. During general anesthesia, nitrous oxide will diffuse into an epidural air bubble, which may cause mechanical compression of intraspinal structures. Pneumoencephalos and neurologic symptoms have been reported after inadvertent intrathecal introduction of air during "loss of resistance" testing, followed by general anesthesia that included nitrous oxide [161]. Lumbar root compression and paraplegia have been reported with the injection of large volumes of air epidurally [162,163]. Use of air for loss of resistance has been implicated as the cause for spotty epidural blockade [164,165]. Air is not sterile and, therefore, should *not* be used in immunocompromised patients.

Careful consideration should be given to the level at which the catheter is placed. If a local anesthetic is used, either alone or in a mixture with an opioid, the epidural catheter should be placed at an interspace close to the center of the dermatomal segments needing analgesia. If opioids alone are used, a more caudad approach may be adequate, particularly if morphine is the opioid chosen. Rostral spread of morphine in the cerebrospinal fluid covers a more cephalad dermatomal site. Lumbar epidural [166] and even caudal epidural [167] morphine has been shown to provide adequate analgesia after thoracotomy, provided that the doses of morphine are adequate. More lipid-soluble opioids (e.g., fentanyl or sufentanil) should be given through a catheter placed as for segmental anesthesia. Thoracic analgesia may not be reliable if any opioid other than morphine is used via a lumbar epidural catheter.

Continuous lumbar epidural catheters are placed routinely by anesthetists, and this technique is relatively easy to master. However, placement of thoracic epidural catheters should be done only by an anesthetist already well experienced in epidural techniques [168]. The epidural space between T_3 and T_1 is more difficult to find than the epidural space in the lumbar region because of the extreme angulation of the long posterior spinous processes at these levels. A paramedian approach to the epidural space may be easier than a midline approach between T_3 and L_1, but this technique should be mastered in the lumbar interspaces first. A paramedian approach may allow for easier threading of the epidural catheter once the epidural space has been located. Above L_2 the epidural space gradually becomes smaller because of the size of the spinal cord, so greater care must be taken at more cephalad levels [169].

Epidural catheters must be properly tested for correct placement, even if postoperative pain relief is the sole indication [170]. When testing a catheter with local anesthetic, one must be prepared to treat sympathetic blockade and hypotension. Significant segmental blockade and sympathectomy can result from the usual test dose of 4 or 5 ml of 1.5% lidocaine with epinephrine 1:200,000, especially if the epidural catheter has been placed at a thoracic level.

Epidural Techniques: Local Anesthetic Infusion. Once a catheter has been placed into the epidural space and is functioning appropriately, adequate postoperative analgesia can be provided by the continuous infusion of local anesthetics. Rapid onset of analgesia can be obtained by using 1% lidocaine, or longer-lasting analgesia can be obtained with 0.25% bupivacaine. An initial dose of 3 ml of either medication is recommended if the catheter is located at or above the T_{10} level, and 5 ml is recommended if the catheter is located at or below T_{11}. If adequate analgesia is not obtained, the dose can be repeated after waiting at least 15 minutes. If analgesia is still not obtained, correct catheter placement should be verified by checking for a definite decrease to pinprick or cold sensation. If the catheter is not functioning correctly, it should be replaced.

Once adequate analgesia is obtained, a continuous infusion of local anesthetic can be administered for prolonged analgesia. The use of a low concentration of bupivacaine is preferable, because motor function tends to be spared with this agent. A routine starting dose is 6 to 8 ml per hour of 0.125% bupivacaine (without epinephrine) administered with an infusion pump.

Tachyphylaxis to bupivacaine occurs commonly and may occur as early as 24 hours after initiation of the block. This can be handled by increasing the volume infused each hour or by increasing the concentration of the bupivacaine infused while keeping the volume the same. Our usual protocol is to increase the volume in 2 ml per hour steps to a maximum of 14 to 16 ml per hour. At the maximum volume, if there is inadequate analgesia, the concentration of bupivacaine is increased to 0.25%, and the infusion rate is slowed to 8 ml per hour. Further escalation in bupivacaine dosage again can be achieved by increasing the rate of infusion. The next increase in bupivacaine concentration should be to 0.375%. Each increase in infusion rate should be preceded by reinforcement of the block, as at the outset, so that adequate analgesia is obtained. Although firm pharmacokinetic data do not exist, clinical experience indicates that a maximum infusion rate of 0.5 to 1 mg/kg/hour appears to be safe for up to 48 hours. Patients should be examined routinely for symptoms of local anesthetic toxicity when these maximum rates are used.

Continuous epidural infusion of local anesthetics allows prolonged analgesia [171,172], but hypotension, presumably due to sympathetic blockade, is a frequent problem [173,174]. Upper thoracic epidural blockade decreases cardiac output, primarily by decreasing heart rate but also by decreasing contractility [175]. Hypotension usually can be managed by expanding intravascular volume [171]. In cases where fluid overload may be a problem, sympathetic tone can be maintained by infusing a small dose of an alpha-adrenergic agent (e.g., phenylephrine at 10–20 μg/min).

Use of a continuous epidural infusion of local anesthetics for anesthesia and for postoperative analgesia has been associated with a reduction in postoperative complications in high-risk patients [176]. Other studies using thoracic epidural analgesia in patients with unstable angina pectoris [177] or acute myocardial infarction [178] indicate that hypotension occurs in almost every case, but myocardial perfusion is not adversely affected. Therefore, in the routine postoperative patient, hypotension is not a cause for alarm, provided that vital signs are monitored carefully and measures to restore blood pressure are instituted and treated promptly. With sympathetic blockade, orthostatic hypotension can be precipitated by changes in the patient's position. This may limit the mobility of the patient and may restrict the use of this technique to nonambulatory patients.

Epidural Techniques: Opioids. Epidural opioids are extremely effective when they are used properly to produce postoperative analgesia. A number of factors determine the amount of opioid required to produce adequate analgesia. These include the spinal level of administration, the location of the pain, the age of the patient, and the lipid solubility of the opioid involved [179,180].

The opioid most commonly used is morphine. Because of its low lipid solubility, morphine tends to stay dissolved in the cerebrospinal fluid (CSF) instead of being absorbed by the spinal cord structures or taken up into the circulation. There is much more rostral migration with morphine than with more lipid-soluble opioids such as fentanyl, which tend to be absorbed into lipid-containing structures close to the site of injection. Thus, morphine can be administered at lumbar levels for thoracic analgesia [166,181,182], but the more lipid-soluble agents need to be given closer to the involved segments.

Rostral spread may be responsible for the side effects peculiar to epidural opioids, including nausea, pruritus, urinary retention, and so-called late respiratory depression. When the catheters are placed in the thoracic region, lower doses are recommended to limit rostral spread of the analgesic and, therefore, side effects.

Relatively fast onset of analgesia is achieved when lipid-soluble opioids such as fentanyl are used. A simultaneous dose of epidural morphine can be given, allowing for the slower onset of analgesia with morphine. Alternatively, a subsequent dose of epidural morphine can be given after the effect of the fentanyl has been determined. Analgesia is then maintained with bolus doses of morphine only.

Dosing schedules should be adjusted according to the patient's response to the medication. The need for a second dose of epidural morphine about 6 hours after surgery is common. Dosing every 8 hours may be needed for the first 1 to 2 postoperative days. Most patients require dosing every 12 hours, but occasional patients, particularly elderly ones, need only one dose per day to achieve good analgesia. Timed (rather than PRN) reinjection is preferable, and the optimal dosing interval can usually be determined within the first 24 hours. Tables 167-2 and 167-3 provide guidelines for dosing with the most commonly used intraspinal opioids and suggestions for modifying dosing to account for age and catheter position. It is important to remember that both the duration of analgesia and the incidence of all complications rise as the dose of opioid is increased.

In most patients, epidural catheters remain in place about 2 to 3 days. Beyond this time, patients usually have less pain and are taking fluids orally; thus, their analgesic needs can be met adequately with oral medications. Epidural catheters can be left in place indefinitely, however, if there are no signs of inflammation and there is a need for continued aggressive analgesia.

Table 167-2. Intraspinal Opioids for Postthoracotomy Pain

Drug	Single dose[a]	Infusion[b]	Onset (min)	Duration (hr)[c]
Epidural				
Morphine	1–6 mg	0.1–1.0 mg/hr	30	6–24
Meperidine	20–150 mg	2–20 mg/hr	5	6–8
Fentanyl	25–150 μg	25–100 μg/hr	5	3–6
Sufentanil	10–60 μg	10–50 μg/hr	5	2–4
Subarachnoid				
Morphine	0.1–0.3 mg		15	8–24
Fentanyl	5–25 μg		5	3–6

[a] Doses must be carefully adjusted for patient age and catheter position. (See Table 167-3 for suggested epidural morphine doses.)
[b] When using epidural infusion, adjust concentration to allow infused volume to be approximately 10 ml/hr for accuracy and convenience of administration. For infusion with bupivacaine, use 0.0625% bupivacaine solution.
[c] Duration of analgesia is variable. It tends to increase with dose and patient age.

Table 167-3. Starting Doses of Epidural Morphine for Thoracic Analgesia*

Patient Age (yr)	Dosage with Catheter Tip at T4–T11 Level (mg)	Dosage with Catheter Tip at T12–L4 Level (mg)
15–44	4	6
45–65	3	5
66–75	2	4
76 and older	1	2

* Careful consideration must be given to the presence of other concurrent disease and to the response seen with these suggested initial doses.

Studies have compared the analgesic effectiveness of intravenous or intramuscular opioids, intercostal blocks, epidural morphine, and epidural local anesthetics [183,184,185]. Patients were the most alert and mobile with segmental epidural blocks with local anesthetics, but the potential for hypotension required close monitoring, and, occasionally, vasopressors were required to restore blood pressure [183]. Epidural opioids allowed easier ambulation and did not impair bowel or bladder function. Even a single dose of epidural morphine provided more prolonged analgesia than a single intercostal block [184]. Compared to parenteral morphine, epidural morphine may provide not only better analgesia but also better preservation of pulmonary function in postthoracotomy patients [185].

The common side effects of epidural opioids (nausea, pruritus, urinary retention) are rarely life-threatening. These side effects can be treated with medications that are specific for the symptom (e.g., metoclopramide or prochlorperazine for nausea, diphenhydramine for pruritus) or with parenteral opioid antagonists such as naloxone [186]. Systemic administration of a mixed opioid agonist-antagonist (e.g., nalbuphine, butorphanol) may be effective in reversing side effects without reversing analgesia [187,188]. Intraspinal administration of butorphanol also has been reported to decrease the occurrence of pruritus and nausea without affecting analgesia, respiratory function, or alertness [189].

Depression of sensorium and concomitant respiratory depression is the most serious potential side effect of epidural opioids, but this complication can occur with parenteral (IV or IM) opioids as well. One study examined the frequency and severity of oxyhemoglobin desaturation in 49 patients after cesarean section, who were treated with IM meperidine, epidural morphine, or meperidine by patient-controlled analgesia (PCA) [190]. Sixty-three percent of the patients receiving IM meperidine had episodes of desaturation to less than 85 percent. In the epidural group, 71 percent of patients had similar episodes of desaturation to less than 85 percent. Both of these groups had "more frequent episodes of severe desaturation" compared with the PCA group, which had "prolonged periods of mild desaturation." The authors of this study concluded that "caesarian section patients receiving opioids by *any* of the methods studied may be at risk for respiratory depression." We agree with this statement and feel certain that the true incidence of respiratory depression with IM opioids is *much* higher than is commonly assumed. Assessing the patient's condition frequently remains the most important way to avert potential problems, regardless of the method used to administer analgesics.

The incidence of clinically significant respiratory depression with epidural morphine is low—0.9 percent in one review [186] and 0.6 percent in another [177]. There are two peaks of respiratory depression, one within 1 to 2 hours of epidural morphine administration and another about 6 to 12 hours later. The early peak appears to correspond with systemic absorption of the opioid from the epidural space. The later peak appears to correspond to rostral spread of the opioid. Most reports describe the gradual onset of respiratory depression, corresponding to rostral migration. Most patients become sedated prior to developing respiratory insufficiency. Thus, patients should be observed for sedation, rather than for decreased respiratory rate, as the earliest sign of impending respiratory depression [179].

Some institutions have established guidelines for instituting respiratory monitoring (Table 167-4) [179]. Because of concerns about respiratory depression, some institutions do not allow the use of intraspinal opioids anywhere except in an intensive care unit. However, intraspinal opioids can be safely used in ward settings if appropriate guidelines for selection of patients, dosing, and monitoring are followed [191,192].

It is better to prevent complications than to treat them [193,194]. The use of a planned dosage scale based on catheter location, surgical site, and the age of the patient may prevent respiratory depression. It is especially important to ensure that additional systemic opioids are not given unless there has been discussion with a pain management specialist familiar with the use of epidural opioids. Summation of the gradually increasing central effect of the epidural opioid with the systemic effect of additional opioids can cause severe respiratory depression. Other medications such as sedatives and tranquilizers (e.g., benzodiazepines) also can interact with epidural opioids in this fashion.

Clinically significant respiratory depression should be treated with incremental doses of an opioid antagonist (e.g., divided doses of naloxone 0.1–0.2 mg IV or 0.4–0.8 mg IM). An ampule of naloxone should be kept at the patient's bedside at all times. To prevent respiratory depression, some authors recommend continuous intravenous infusion of naloxone or nalbuphine [195,196,197].

Epidural Techniques: Continuous Opioid Infusions. In an effort to provide smoother analgesia, continuous techniques using various opioids have been described. Morphine was the first opioid so used. One study of epidural analgesia techniques compared bolus dosing with 0.5% bupivacaine, bolus dosing with morphine, and continuous infusion of morphine at 0.1 mg per hour in postthoracotomy patients [198]. Bupivacaine was associated with severe hypotension in 23 percent of patients.

Table 167-4. Criteria for Determining When to Use a Respiratory Monitor*

Respiratory monitor is not required when all the following criteria are met:
   Age < 50
   ASA physical status is determined to be level I or II
   All surgical sites except thorax or upper abdomen
   Duration of surgery < 4 hr
   Anesthetic—little or no narcotics or other long-acting central nervous system depressants used before or during surgery
   Epidural morphine dose is 6 mg or less; subarachnoid morphine dose is 0.5 mg or less

OR

Postoperative care location provides continuous nursing surveillance

* These are only guidelines. A respiratory monitor may be ordered for any patient at the discretion of the operating room anesthesiologist, the Acute Pain Service, or the Unit Charge Nurse.
Reprinted by permission from Ready LB, Oden R, Chadwick HS, et al: Development of an anesthesiology-based postoperative pain management service. *Anesthesiology* 68:102, 1988.

Bolus dosing with morphine resulted in urinary retention in 100 percent, pruritus in 40 percent, and depressed consciousness in 27 percent of patients. Administering morphine by continuous infusion resulted in good analgesia and a low incidence of side effects (depressed level of consciousness, 0%; urinary retention, 7%; pruritus, 3%). Although this study is open to criticism on several points, it nevertheless supports the notion that continuous epidural infusion of morphine is a useful technique. Continuous epidural infusion of morphine (0.1 mg/hour) was recently shown to improve pain relief and decrease the length of intensive care unit stay in patients with blunt chest trauma [199].

Continuous epidural infusion of fentanyl has been used to treat postoperative pain. Because of its greater lipid solubility, fentanyl should cause fewer side effects than morphine (see the preceding section on Epidural Techniques: Opioids) [200]. One series compared a continuous epidural infusion of fentanyl with IM papaveretum in patients after abdominal surgery [201]. An epidural catheter was placed at the seventh thoracic interspace, and an infusion at 6 ml per hour of a 10 µg per milliliter fentanyl solution was used. Patients receiving epidural fentanyl had better analgesia and were more alert than patients receiving the IM opioid. Respiratory function was significantly better in the epidural group. There were more complaints of nausea in the epidural group, but urinary retention was not observed. Twenty percent of the patients in the epidural group developed pruritus. In another study a continuous epidural infusion of fentanyl was more effective than cryoanalgesia for postthoracotomy pain [202].

Although one might predict that highly lipid-soluble opioids would cause less respiratory depression than morphine, epidural fentanyl, whether given by bolus dose or continuous infusion, is capable of causing respiratory depression [203,204]. One study examined the effect of continuous epidural fentanyl on minute ventilation, respiratory rate, tidal volume, arterial carbon dioxide tension, and the ventilatory response to a carbon dioxide challenge [205]. Except for the ventilatory response to carbon dioxide (which decreased), none of the measured parameters changed from control measurements. Nevertheless, the tests used may not have been sensitive enough to show subclinical effects of the opioid on central respiratory drive.

The main site of action of epidural fentanyl given by infusion may not be intraspinal. Several studies have shown that identical doses of fentanyl given either by intravenous or by epidural infusion result in similar fentanyl serum levels and similar pain scores [206–210]. A slow continuous epidural infusion may be just another form of parenteral injection. Absorption of opioids can occur from many locations, including the interpleural space [211]. However, other studies indicate that an intraspinal effect is important for at least part of the analgesic action of epidural fentanyl, especially when a bolus of fentanyl is given [212,213,214]. Therefore, with continuous epidural fentanyl infusion, both intraspinal receptors close to the site of injection and other central opioid receptors may be involved in the production of analgesia. With other agents that are less lipid-soluble (e.g., morphine) less systemic absorption may take place, making the intraspinal action more important.

Epidural Techniques: Combined Local Anesthetic-Opioid Infusions. Combining a local anesthetic with an opioid can give the benefits of each medication, without the severity of side effects observed when either class of drug is used alone. One approach is to use bolus doses of epidural morphine for analgesia, adding intermittent bolus doses of bupivacaine to allow greater movement [215]. In one series of 50 patients with chest trauma, excellent analgesia was obtained in 96 percent using this technique.

Continuous infusions of a local anesthetic mixed with an opioid have also been used. The initial studies were performed with morphine and bupivacaine. One study evaluated this technique in patients after major abdominal surgery [216]. With a continuous epidural infusion of 0.5% bupivacaine, sensory analgesia gradually regressed with time and, after 16 hours, analgesia was inadequate in 90 percent of patients. The addition of epidural morphine (0.5 mg/hour) to the same infusion gave excellent analgesia in 100 percent of the patients at 16 hours after surgery. Another study compared continuous epidural infusions of bupivacaine, morphine, or a mixture of bupivacaine and morphine for analgesia in postthoracotomy patients [217]. This study found no difference in the analgesia obtained with morphine compared with that obtained with morphine plus bupivacaine, but found both the morphine and the morphine/ bupivacaine groups to have better analgesia than the group that received only bupivacaine.

The combination of a local anesthetic and an opioid for epidural infusion may be synergistic. One study in mice examined the antinociceptive effects of local anesthetics, opioids, and combinations of the two types of medications and documented potentiation of the effects of opioids by local anesthetics and vice versa [218]. Intensity, but not duration, of analgesia was increased. Extremely low doses of a local anesthetic and an opioid in combination produced analgesia, suggesting that synergistic action may allow doses of drugs to be used that are low enough to avoid major side effects.

Fentanyl also has been used in combination with bupivacaine for epidural infusion. Studies have indicated the effectiveness of thoracic epidural infusion of 0.2% bupivacaine with 0.001% (10 μg/ml) fentanyl in providing analgesia after thoracotomy or abdominal aortic surgery [219,220]. In both studies, the group given a bupivacaine/fentanyl mixture had better analgesia than groups given just fentanyl or just bupivacaine by infusion. Epidural infusion of 0.25% bupivacaine with 0.00125% (12.5 μg/ ml) fentanyl has been used to control leg pain for several weeks in a patient with Guillain-Barré syndrome [221]. However, the use of lumbar epidural infusion of 0.1% bupivacaine with 0.001% (10 μg/ml) fentanyl was not effective for analgesia after total knee joint replacement [222]. The dose of bupivacaine in this study may have been too low to block the somatic pain experienced after a peripheral orthopedic procedure. Visceral pain may be blocked by lower concentrations of local anesthetics, allowing more dilute bupivacaine to be effective for pain relief after intraabdominal procedures.

Other opioids have been used in combination with bupivacaine for continuous epidural infusion. A comparison of the infusion of bupivacaine, sufentanil, and bupivacaine with sufentanil was reported in postthoracotomy patients [223]. The best analgesia, especially with exercise, was reported in the group that received both bupivacaine and sufentanil. Another study reported excellent analgesia in patients after thoracotomy, when sufentanil was given either epidurally or intravenously to supplement an epidural bupivacaine infusion [224]. Serum sufentanil levels during the first 24 hours of this study were significantly less with epidural administration than with intravenous administration, indicating a spinal action. Epidural diamorphine infusion also has been reported to supplement epidural bupivacaine for analgesia after major gynecologic surgery [225,226].

Overall, the use of combinations of local anesthetics with opioids for continuous epidural infusion appears to be an effective technique for postoperative analgesia. There seem to be fewer side effects with this technique than with the use of either local anesthetics or opioids alone.

Subarachnoid and Epidural Techniques: Other Agents. The selective modulation of nociceptive signals at the spinal cord level is thought to be the method of action of intraspinal opioids. However, a variety of spinal cord receptors produce analgesia by modifying the response to noxious stimuli [227,228.229]. Much recent research has been directed toward finding substances that are analgesic when administered intraspinally. The hope is to be able to use small doses of medications that exert additive or synergistic analgesic effects when combined with opioids, but that do not have clinically significant side effects at the doses used [230].

Clonidine is the medication that has received the most study [231,232]. It is an alpha$_2$-adrenergic agonist that has been used for treatment of hypertension for over 20 years. Recently, it has been found to have both sedative and analgesic effects. Only the specific effects related to analgesia are considered here. Clonidine, when administered intrathecally with a local anesthetic, prolongs the duration of sensory and motor block with hyperbaric tetracaine [233] and isobaric bupivacaine [234]. The use of 150 μg of clonidine in this fashion does not have major hemodynamic effects [233,234]. Epidural clonidine potentiates the duration of 2% lidocaine or 0.25% bupivacaine given for epidural anesthesia [235,236]. This may be due to an epinephrine-like action that slows lidocaine absorption from the epidural space [237]. When given with epidural morphine, clonidine potentiates the intensity but not the duration of analgesia [238,239]. Unfortunately, the intensity of respiratory depression due to epidural morphine is also increased [238]. Clonidine has intrinsic analgesic activity when given epidurally [240]. This effect is dose-dependent; higher doses (700–900 μg) give longer-lasting analgesia than lower doses (100–300 μg) [241]. Its physicochemical characteristics suggest that the clinical behavior of clonidine should be similar to that of fentanyl in onset and duration [241]. Almost all patients have hemodynamic changes when clonidine is administered. Mild bradycardia and hypotension are common [241]. In the periphery, clonidine increases blood pressure via alpha$_2$-receptor–mediated vasoconstriction [242]. Thus, clonidine-induced hemodynamic changes paradoxically are often greater with lower doses of intraspinal (subarachnoid or epidural) clonidine because less systemic absorption occurs.

Oral clonidine does not increase the duration of subarachnoid bupivacaine anesthesia [243] but does increase the duration of action of subarachnoid tetracaine [244]. Achieving sustained clonidine levels with an oral loading dose followed by a transdermal patch has only a short postoperative effect on epidural morphine analgesia [245], but it may have a more long-term effect on IV morphine administered with a patient-controlled analgesia device [246]. A continuous infusion of IV clonidine after a bolus loading dose also appears to decrease postoperative parenteral morphine requirements [247]. One concern is that clonidine is apparently a respiratory depressant [248,249]. Sedation occurs at the same time as respiratory depression.

Another agent that modulates impulses at the spinal cord level is ketamine, but this drug has been ineffective in relieving postoperative pain in a number of studies, when doses were low enough to avoid systemic effects [250–253]. Ketamine is currently the only clinically available N-methyl D-aspartate (NMDA) receptor antagonist and therefore may be of benefit for preemptive analgesia by blocking the production of central hyperexcitability after peripheral injury [254,255]. Somatostatin exerts analgesic effects only when toxic neurologic changes are seen [256,257]. Other agents such as dexmedetomidine [258], serotonin [259], midazolam [260,261] and baclofen [262] are undergoing investigation.

Specific Analgesic Techniques: Systemic Approach

NONOPIOID SYSTEMIC ANALGESICS. Because of the potential complications of high doses of opioids, adjuvant therapy with systemic agents that are not opioids is an attractive therapeutic alternative.

Nonsteroidal Antiinflammatory Agents. Although these medications are given systemically, they act in the periphery. Their use has therefore been discussed under that earlier heading.

Inhaled Anesthetic Agents. Subanesthetic doses of inhaled anesthetics have been used in various clinical situations to provide analgesia. Examples include the use of nitrous oxide for patients with tetanus [263] and methoxyflurane for patients in labor [264]. However, prolonged exposure to low levels of volatile anesthetics can cause complications, including bone marrow suppression (nitrous oxide) [263], teratogenesis (nitrous oxide) [265], and fluoride toxicity from anesthetic metabolism [266]. Thus, the role of these agents in managing critically ill patients is limited. Occasional use during short painful procedures might be of benefit. An example is the use of nitrous oxide during dressing changes in burn patients [267].

Medications Used for Sedation. Benzodiazepines, barbiturates, phenothiazines, and butyrophenones have been given in conjunction with opioids [268]. These drugs should be used for anxiolysis, sedation, and production of amnesia, but not for analgesia, because they have no analgesic properties. When used for anxiolysis, they can depress consciousness and ventilation and sometimes necessitate endotracheal intubation and mechanical ventilation. These drugs are useful for patients who will need prolonged ventilatory assistance and in those in whom sedation will be helpful during the first 24 to 48 hours postoperatively. They also can be used for anxiolysis during painful bedside procedures (see Chap. 28 on Anesthesia for Bedside Procedures).

Systemic Opioid Analgesia. The traditional approach to opioid administration is intramuscular or subcutaneous injection. The medication is then absorbed and redistributed according to many variables, including blood flow to the tissue in which the depot is placed and the intrinsic chemistry of the drug itself. If intramuscular or subcutaneous depot administration is used, it should be done on a basis that is consistent with the uptake, redistribution, and elimination kinetics of the medication chosen. This type of administration is not recommended in the intensive care unit, however, because of the extreme delay in attaining therapeutic drug levels and, therefore, pain relief. In addition, perfusion of muscle and subcutaneous tissue can be quite variable in critically ill patients, so absorption can be erratic or delayed. Use of small intravenous doses of opioids is preferable.

A relatively new approach to opioid delivery is transdermal fentanyl (TTS-fentanyl, ALZA Corp., Palo Alto, CA). In this approach, a patch containing a store of fentanyl is worn on the skin and functions as a depot from which the drug is metered to and absorbed through the skin. Various rates of delivery can be chosen by selecting different patches. Because the drug is slowly deposited into the skin, from which absorption takes place, the fentanyl is functionally in an intradermal depot. A delay of approximately 12 to 16 hours occurs after patch placement before effective analgesic fentanyl concentrations are achieved in plasma [269–272]. The final plateau in serum fentanyl concentration may not be reached for 36 to 48 hours [270]. One recent study examined the use of this system after upper abdominal surgery [273]. The transdermal fentanyl patch decreased demand for additional opioid, which was provided by a patient-controlled analgesia (PCA) device. Peak expiratory flow rates were improved when compared with controls, who used only the PCA device. Other studies also have found a decreased demand for supplemental opioids when a transdermal fentanyl system was used [274,275,276].

The rationale for use of a transdermal delivery system is to produce relatively constant serum fentanyl levels that exceed the minimum effective analgesic concentration (MEAC) and therefore achieve relatively constant pain relief. The potential danger with this technique is choosing the wrong dose and giving the patient too much medication. Because there is a fairly large store of drug in the skin, fentanyl is absorbed into the circulation for an extended period after the patch is removed [277]. Therefore, the usual side effects of opioid excess can gradually worsen and persist longer than expected. Respiratory depression may gradually develop [278]. Perhaps because of altered pharmacokinetics, cancer patients using transdermal fentanyl became severely obtunded when they developed other unrelated medical complications [279]. Prolonged sedation of intubated intensive care unit patients has been provided using this technique instead of continuous IV fentanyl [280].

Continuous intravenous infusion of opioids is a relatively simple technique, but it is often overlooked or used incorrectly. Opioids used systemically must be front-loaded in order to achieve a MEAC in a reasonable length of time. If opioids are administered without front-loading, MEAC will not be achieved for at least three elimination half-lives [281], during which time patients experience unrelieved pain. Table 167-5 provides some simple guidelines for front-loading the opioid drugs commonly used in postoperative pain management [17].

Therapeutic blood opioid levels can be maintained by continuous infusion. The rate of infusion can be determined using a fairly simple calculation: (1) most conventionally used opioid drugs have an elimination half-life of about 3 hours; (2) the dose required during each half-life to maintain the level of analgesia achieved during front-loading will be one-half the dose required to produce analgesia during front-loading; (3) therefore the hourly requirement can be calculated and infused continuously to maintain a therapeutic level.

Example: A patient requires 7.5 mg of IV morphine sulfate to obtain analgesia following a hysterectomy. A continuous infusion is to be used. In one elimination half-life, 7.5 mg/2 = 3.75 mg will be eliminated. Therefore, every 3 hours, 3.75 mg is eliminated, or 3.75 mg per 3 hours (1.25 mg/hr) is required.

This approximation tends to underestimate the hourly requirements because the elimination half-life is actually less than 3 hours. As a first approximation, however, it usually yields fairly good results and makes the calculation of continuous infusion rates more than just a guess.

Increasing the infusion rate in a patient who has experienced breakthrough pain leaves the patient with nontherapeutic levels for at least three drug half-lives. Breakthrough pain therefore must be dealt with as new-onset pain, and the opioid *must* be titrated to effect before the new infusion rate is established.

Patient-Controlled Analgesia. PCA is a technique for the administration of small doses of opioid intravenously on a demand basis. This is truly the ideal melding of the continuous IV infusion principle with "need-driven" administration. There are two major differences between conventional PRN regimens and PCA [17]:

Table 167-5. Guidelines for Front-loading Intravenous Analgesics

Drug	Total front-load dose (mg/kg)	Increments	Cautions
Morphine	0.08–0.12	0.03 mg/kg every 10 minutes	Histamine effects; nausea; biliary colic; reduce dose for elderly
Meperidine	1.0–1.5	0.30 mg/kg every 10 minutes	Reduce dose or change drug for impaired renal function
Codeine	0.5–1.0	One-third of total every 15 minutes	Nausea
Methadone	0.08–0.12	0.03 mg/kg every 15 minutes	Do not administer maintenance dose after analgesia achieved; accumulation; sedation
Levorphanol	0.02	50–75 μg/kg every 15 minutes	Similar to methadone
Hydromorphone	0.02	25–50 μg/kg every 10 minutes	Similar to morphine
Pentazocine	0.5–1.0	One-half of total every 15 minutes	Psychomimetic effects; may cause withdrawal in narcotic-dependent patients
Nalbuphine	0.08–0.15	0.03 mg/kg every 10 minutes	Less psychomimetic effect than pentazocine; sedation
Butorphanol	0.02–0.04	0.01 mg/kg every 10 minutes	Sedation; psychomimetic effects like nalbuphine
Buprenorphine	up to 0.2	One-quarter of total every 10 minutes	Long-acting like methadone and levorphanol; may precipitate withdrawal in narotic-dependent patients; safe to give subcutaneous maintenance after analgesia—different from methadone.

1. The route of administration is IV. This obviates the lag induced in the feedback loop by uptake and redistribution from a subcutaneous or intramuscular depot.
2. The patient's request for medication is almost immediately answered. The time-consuming ritual described earlier that must be followed by a medication nurse is therefore avoided.

Removing these two delays by using a fixed prescription of opioid delivered by a microprocessor-controlled pump makes a rapid return to MEAC possible. When the circulating opioid level becomes subtherapeutic, analgesia can be reestablished within seconds rather than within minutes (which seems like hours to a patient in pain).

Since PCA is basically a modified IV infusion technique, many of the same principles are used as in the calculation of infusion rates. The problem with both PCA and continuous infusions is that requirements for the opioid are highest at the beginning of therapy. Even front-loading does not cover all eventualities in this regard because of factors such as the diminishing effects of general anesthetic agents in the early postoperative period and the redistribution of analgesic drugs, which takes place most dramatically during the first 24 hours of therapy. When establishing the upper limit for PCA (i.e., the 1-hr or 4-hr dosage limit required by the instrument as an alarm condition), it is best to take into account as much as a fivefold increase in need during the early postoperative period [282,283]. Therefore, if one predicts that 1.5 mg per hour should be infused to maintain MEAC for morphine in a particular patient, the 1-hour limit should be set at 7.5 mg per hour. This allows the patient to titrate his or her own increased requirement during the early phase. Maintenance (demand) doses should generally not exceed 0.02 mg of morphine (or its equivalent) per kilogram of body weight, or 1.5 mg of morphine per dose in most adult patients. The usual lockout interval (5–10 min) accounts for the time required for an adequate concentration of the opioid to be established at the active site before another dose is given. Breakthrough pain necessitates another loading dose before a new prescription is started. PCA is useful for maintaining established analgesia but not for establishing it in the first place.

Overdose with PCA is rare because patients tend to titrate themselves into the therapeutic range and keep themselves out of the toxic range. Most patients choose not to eliminate pain entirely, but instead maintain a satisfactory level of analgesia, which is individually determined [284–287]. If the maintenance (demand) dose is overestimated, patients become sleepy with each dose and do not request additional medication.

Overdose is a more significant risk if a continuous background (basal) infusion is added to PCA. Some machines do not allow background infusion, but if one is used in an effort to provide longer pain-free periods, *no more than one-half of the predicted hourly requirement (PHR) should be supplied in this way.* THIS IS NOT THE 1-HOUR OR 4-HOUR LIMIT! Recall that alarm limits are deliberately set high. Because patients do not control the background infusion, accumulation is possible if the continuous background infusion is set too high. Therefore, if the PHR determined by calculation is 2 mg per hour, no more than 1 mg per hour should be given by background infusion.

There are problems with PCA, as with any therapeutic technique. Lack of adequate analgesia results from inadequate dosing. This can occur because the patient fails to understand the technique, the equipment malfunctions, or there are programming errors. Overdosing can be caused by equipment malfunctions or programming errors [282]. An unusual problem is the administration of the drug by someone other than the patient. This occurs most often in pediatric patients for whom patient-controlled analgesia becomes parent-controlled, but it has also been reported once in an adult as a result of spouse-controlled analgesia [288]. One recent report examined parent-assisted PCA, in which the doses for children 5 to 10 years of age were intentionally (for study purposes) administered by a parent [289]. Most patients apparently achieved good analgesia, with minimal sedation. The danger inherent in this type of maneuver is that the parent might administer too much medication to the patient, since the built-in safety feature of not dosing when the patient is sedated is removed. This practice (i.e., allowing someone other than the patient to control dosing) is *not* recommended under most circumstances. Other studies have shown that pediatric patients 5 years of age and older can understand and use the PCA technique themselves with good success [290,291]. However, most centers restrict PCA to patients older than 10 years of age.

The very nature of PCA requires that patients be awake and cooperative. This technique is not suitable for unconscious, drowsy, or uncooperative patients who cannot reliably activate the demand switch. Recently, however, some centers have begun using a novel variation of PCA in some critically ill ventilated patients. A PCA pump is programmed in a manner similar to that for patient use, but the control of the demand switch is given to the critical care nurse who activates the pump for analgesic administration. This may be done on patient request, arbitrarily or prophylactically before nursing procedures, or at times when a nurse might ordinarily utilize a routine "PRN morphine" order such as is commonly written in intensive care units. The use of a PCA pump to carry out these tasks reduces the time and effort the nurse must expend to administer an analgesic (and thus increases the likelihood of its occurring) and automatically provides an accurate record of opioid dose and time of administration.

There is still no scientific evidence regarding whether patients with a history of drug abuse can use PCA effectively, and there is considerable controversy surrounding this issue. If PCA is considered for use in patients with a history of drug-seeking behavior, it must be done with extremely careful monitoring of total opioid consumption and the use of low 1-hour or 4-hour limits. Objective signs of opioid effect (slowing of respiratory rate, pupillary constriction) may be useful for monitoring serum opioid concentrations in these patients [292,293,294]. At the present time, PCA is not routinely recommended for patients with a history of drug-seeking behavior. It is important that societal judgments not be brought to bear on critically ill patients, however. In the presence of critical illness or injury, patients with known opioid dependence must have their opioid needs replaced to avoid the occurrence of acute abstinence syndromes. This includes patients with iatrogenic opioid dependence as well as those who present with true addiction. The sympathetic hyperactivity resulting from abstinence syndrome can be misinterpreted easily as new medical or surgical pathology leading to inappropriate therapy. The setting of acute illness or injury is an inappropriate time to consider detoxification from opiate dependence.

Recently, PCA has been used to give epidural medications (so-called patient controlled epidural analgesia, or PCEA) [295]. In an initial study, postoperative patients obtained excellent analgesia from continuous epidural morphine plus additional small bolus doses of the drug given on demand by the anesthesiology staff [296]. Subsequent studies used PCA devices for the administration of demand doses with the lockout intervals set between 15 and 30 minutes [297,298]. These studies found PCEA to be effective, requiring less opioid than when continuous epidural opioid infusion was performed alone [298]. Therefore, use of this technique may avoid side effects seen with larger doses of epidural opioids.

PCEA has been used to deliver local anesthetics, alone or in combination with opioids [299,300,301]. This technique has been found to work well for patients in labor [299,300]. Another study of postsurgical and trauma patients (age 6–18 years) showed that PCEA, using a dilute solution of morphine with or without bupivacaine, provides excellent analgesia without complications or side effects other than those expected with epidural morphine [301].

PCA also has been used to administer intrathecal medications through a continuous intrathecal catheter. Reports have been made of the effective use of fentanyl [154] or isobaric bupivacaine with or without sufentanil [155] for postoperative analgesia.

Influence of Pain Control on Complications, Outcome, and Length of Stay

PULMONARY FUNCTION AND PULMONARY COMPLICATIONS. The prevention of postoperative pulmonary complications is one of the major goals of providing adequate postoperative analgesia. The major pulmonary complications generally considered include atelectasis, lung infections, and arterial hypoxemia [302]. These complications have been re-lated to decreases in vital capacity and to a reduced ability to cough and to clear secretions [193]. The magnitude of postoperative decreases in forced vital capacity (FVC) and forced expiratory volume at 1 second (FEV_1) depends on the site of the surgical incision [303]. Postthoracotomy patients treated with traditional analgesic techniques typically experience a decrease in both FVC and FEV_1 to 25 percent of preoperative values on the first postoperative day.

A reduction in functional residual capacity (FRC) is the most important mechanical abnormality linked to pulmonary complications [304]. Atelectasis occurs when the FRC falls below closing volume (the lung volume at which small airway closure occurs). Stasis of secretions also occurs, which increases the risk of pulmonary infection [305].

A simple maneuver that improves FRC is changing the position of the patient, since FRC is higher in the sitting position than in the supine position, and changing to the sitting position can raise FRC above closing volume [306]. One of the advantages of the analgesic techniques described here is that they can provide enough pain relief to allow patients to assume the sitting position earlier, reducing the likelihood of pulmonary complications due to airway closure and atelectasis [307].

Splinting due to incisional pain decreases FRC. Intercostal nerve blocks limit the decrease in FVC and FEV_1 seen after thoracotomy [308]. This effect lasts for the entire first week after thoracotomy [309]. The use of interpleural bupivacaine limits the decrease in FVC and FEV_1 after cholecystectomy [310]. The use of epidural local anesthetics improves FVC relative to control patients after upper abdominal surgery [311,312]. Some data suggest that the incidence of atelectasis in patients using epidural local anesthetics is lower in comparison to the incidence in patients receiving traditional IM or IV opioid analgesia [185,313,314]. In contrast to these data, some studies failed to find evidence for a statistically significant decrease in complications after surgery when aggressive analgesia was provided [315–318].

In patients with multiple rib fractures, epidural morphine analgesia clearly lessens the incidence of tracheostomy and shortens the duration of mechanical ventilation and intensive care unit stay [199]. Comparisons have been made between central regional analgesic techniques and the use of morphine by parenteral injection, continuous IV infusion, or PCA [319,320]. If used aggressively, the other analgesic techniques described in this chapter appear to provide the same beneficial pulmonary effects as does epidural opioid administration. This may explain the lack of a decrease in complications seen in some studies comparing various analgesic techniques [317,318].

ENDOCRINE AND METABOLIC STRESS RESPONSE. Surgical trauma is a form of injury, and both local and systemic responses to the injury are seen [321]. There is a local inflammatory reaction, which is considered beneficial for healing and for defense against infection. A systemic hypermetabolic state follows the surgical insult characterized by increases in both substrate mobilization and the rate of most biochemical reactions [321]. This is referred to as the stress response.

The stress response may be beneficial. However, if prolonged, the stress response may have adverse nutritional consequences. The reader is referred to recent reviews for an in-depth analysis of the individual hormonal responses involved [321,322,323].

Only major regional anesthesia is beneficial in preventing or diminishing the stress response to a surgical procedure [320]. Very deep levels of general anesthesia do not have much effect on the stress response to surgery [321]. Even high-dose opioid techniques have only a mild effect of short duration.

The beneficial effect of regional anesthesia on the stress response can continue into the postoperative period if a regional technique with local anesthetic is used to provide postoperative analgesia. This has been shown for lower abdominal procedures and procedures on the lower extremities [321]. Two recent studies indicated that there was a definite nitrogen-sparing effect when epidural analgesia was used during and after lower abdominal surgery [324,325]. Regional techniques are less successful in blocking the endocrine and metabolic stress responses to surgery when the procedure is performed either on the upper abdomen or thorax. Nevertheless, some evidence suggests that epidural bupivacaine blocks the stress response during the first day after upper abdominal surgery [326]. Intercostal blocks can block the rise in glucose seen after thoracotomy [327]. Continuous spinal anesthesia with bupivacaine infusion continued postoperatively also has been reported to be effective in diminishing the metabolic stress response after colonic surgery [328].

The relative ineffectiveness of regional analgesia-anesthesia in blocking the stress response to procedures cephalad to the lower abdomen may be because there is limited blockade of fast-conducting afferent nerve fibers with thoracic epidural analgesia, even with the use of 0.5% bupivacaine [329]. Incomplete blockade of somatic sensory fibers may allow the stress response to occur. Because it is easier to achieve a more complete somatic sensory block in a more caudad location, more complete interruption of the sensory afferent triggers of the stress response is possible with regional anesthesia for lower abdominal surgery than for thoracic surgery. Incomplete blockade of either the sympathetic or parasympathetic efferents also may allow the stress response to proceed [321].

The use of parenteral opioid analgesics in the postoperative period does not reduce the stress response [321]. However, one study documented decreased energy expenditure in critically ill, mechanically ventilated patients treated with IV morphine [330]. This may represent a reduction in the hypermetabolic state associated with the stress response. When continuous epidural bupivacaine with or without sufentanil was compared with IV morphine, analgesia was better in the epidural infusion group but there was no difference among groups in the stress response to surgery [331,332].

Other medications have the potential to reduce the stress response. A preliminary study indicates that epidural clonidine may block the cortisol response to abdominal surgery [333].

GASTROINTESTINAL FUNCTION. Postoperative ileus, the slowing of gastrointestinal function after surgery, is a routine postoperative finding. Opioids inhibit gastrointestinal motility. This phenomenon occurs with parenteral opioids [334,335] but can also be seen with epidural opioids [335,336].

Studies have examined the effect of postoperative epidural analgesia with bupivacaine on postoperative paralytic ileus. In healthy volunteers, thoracic epidural morphine (4 mg) delayed gastric emptying, but thoracic epidural bupivacaine (0.5%, enough to block T_6-T_{10}) did not [336]. In patients after cholecystectomy, thoracic epidural morphine (4 mg) similarly delayed gastric emptying, but thoracic epidural bupivacaine 0.25% infused at 6 to 8 ml per hour did not [337]. In patients after hysterectomy, a significantly shorter duration of ileus was seen in patients who received epidural bupivacaine as compared with patients treated with an IM opioid (ketobemidone) [338].

One study compared patients 1 day after cholecystectomy treated with intrathecal morphine (0.8 mg) or IM papaveretum [339] and found that gastric emptying was significantly greater in the intrathecal morphine group.

Analgesia with epidural local anesthetics may produce the least amount of gastrointestinal slowing. Intrathecal opioids may have as good an effect, but their use is limited to the first 12 to 24 hours postoperatively. Longer duration of ileus is seen with epidural opioids than with epidural local anesthetics, but this is still better than the duration seen with parenteral opioid analgesic therapy [336]. PCA would be expected to produce the same amount of gastrointestinal slowing as an equivalent dose administered parenterally via conventional means.

HEMODYNAMIC STABILITY. Painful stimuli evoke a generalized sympathetic response [340]. With sympathetic stimulation, the major determinants of myocardial oxygen consumption (heart rate, contractility, wall stress) are all increased. This can set the stage for myocardial ischemia, especially in patients with marginal coronary perfusion. Treatment of the underlying pain is necessary to reverse this situation.

Although analgesic techniques other than major regional anesthesia do not prevent the endocrine and metabolic stress response to surgery, intraoperative administration of epidural opioids can blunt the sympathetic response following major surgery. One recent study examined the effect of epidural morphine on plasma catecholamine levels and the incidence of postoperative hypertension in patients undergoing operations on the abdominal aorta [341]. Control patients received epidural saline, whereas study patients received one dose of epidural morphine intraoperatively. All patients were given IV morphine for analgesia in the postoperative period. Patients who received epidural morphine received 50 percent less parenteral morphine in the first 24 hours following surgery and had lower pain scores. Plasma epinephrine levels were not different in the two groups, but plasma norepinephrine levels were lower in the epidural morphine group. Most importantly, once the patients regained normothermia, there was a lower incidence of hypertension requiring treatment in the epidural morphine group (33%) than in the control group (75%). It appears that even though the stress response to surgery may not be eliminated by epidural opioids, there is enough of a reduction in sympathetic nervous system activation to make this analgesic technique worthwhile for improving hemodynamic stability, especially for the first few hours after surgery. Our clinical experience suggests that intraoperative administration of epidural opioids also makes the intraoperative course smoother.

LENGTH OF HOSPITAL STAY. Postcholecystectomy patients who received intercostal blocks for analgesia were found to ambulate more quickly and go home sooner than control patients treated with IM meperidine for analgesia [342]. The use of PCA in postthoracotomy patients shortens length of hospitalization by 22 percent as compared with controls treated with conventionally administered parenteral analgesics [343,344]. A study in patients after cesarean section indicated that patients receiving intrathecal morphine for analgesia were discharged from the hospital significantly earlier than patients who received epidural morphine [345]. Of note is that the epidural morphine group was not discharged earlier than the control group, whose members received systemic opioids for analgesia. Possible explanations for this may be that earlier ambulation occurred with intrathecal morphine or that there were fewer problems with postoperative ileus in this group.

A number of studies also have reported decreased length of hospitalization with use of epidural analgesia postoperatively, with the use of either epidural opioids or local anesthetic infusions. Patients receiving epidural analgesia were discharged sooner than controls receiving IM or IV opioids, after anterior cruciate ligament repair [346], radical retropubic prostatectomy with pelvic lymphadenectomy [347], major vascular surgery [348], major cancer surgery [349], or total knee replacement [350]. Patient controlled epidural analgesia with opioids has also been reported to decrease hospital stay after nephrectomy [351] or cesarean section [352].

In summary, there definitely appears to be a positive effect on the length of hospital stay if more advanced analgesic techniques are used. For the patient in the intensive care unit, the avoidance of pulmonary, cardiovascular, or gastrointestinal complications is most important, so that the length of intensive care unit stay can be kept to a minimum.

Conclusion

The overall goals of postoperative pain management must always be:

1. To provide maximum patient comfort consistent with well-being
2. To hasten recovery by reducing rates of complication
3. To do 1 and 2 above in the most efficient, cost-effective way possible

It is clear that advanced techniques for analgesia can make a significant difference in overall patient outcome. Totally apart from the issue of providing better patient comfort, these techniques appear to be able to shorten the length of recovery time. Due to their knowledge of pharmacokinetics, their experience with the clinical pharmacology of analgesics, and their experience with block procedures, anesthesiologists who are specially trained in advanced pain management are in a unique position to influence the clinical course of critically ill patients. At our institutions and in several others that employ the acute pain service concept [179], it is almost routine for patients who have undergone major chest surgery or have experienced major trauma to receive a consultation from and intervention by the acute pain management service at the request of the responsible surgeon.

References

1. Hewitt PB: Subjective follow-up of patients from a surgical intensive therapy ward. *Br Med J [Clin Res]* 4:669, 1970.
2. Marks RM, Sachar EJ: Undertreatment of medical inpatients with narcotic analgesics. *Ann Intern Med* 78:173, 1973.
3. Jones J, Hoggart B, Withey J, et al: What the patients say: A study of reactions to an intensive care unit. *Intensive Care Med* 5:89, 1979.
4. Ferrante FM, Orav EJ, Rocco AG, et al: A statistical model for pain in patient-controlled analgesia and conventional intramuscular opioid regimens. *Anesth Analg* 67:457, 1988.
5. Papper EM, Brodie BB, Rovenstine EA: Postoperative pain: Its use in the comparative evaluation of analgesics. *Surgery* 32:107, 1952.
6. Lasagna L, Beecher H: The optimal dose of morphine. *JAMA* 156:230, 1954.
7. Keats AS: Postoperative pain: Research and treatment. *J Chronic Dis* 4:72, 1956.
8. Keeri-Szanto M, Heaman S: Postoperative demand analgesia. *Surg Gynecol Obstet* 134:647, 1972.
9. Cronin M, Redfern PA, Utting JE: Psychometry and postoperative complaints in surgical patients. *Br J Anaesth* 45:879, 1973.
10. Banister EHD: Six potent analgesic drugs. A double-blind study in postoperative pain. *Anaesthesia* 29:158, 1974.
11. Tammisto T: Analgesics in postoperative pain relief. *Acta Anaesthesiol Scand (Suppl)* 70:47, 1978.
12. Cohen FL: Postsurgical pain relief: Patients' status and nurses' medication choices. *Pain* 9:265, 1980.
13. Tamsen A, Hartvig P, Fagerlund C, et al: Patient-controlled analgesic therapy: Clinical experience. *Acta Anaesthesiol Scand (Suppl)* 74:157, 1982.
14. Donovan M, Dillon P, McGuire L: Incidence and characteristics of pain in a sample of medical-surgical inpatients. *Pain* 30:69, 1987.
15. Sriwatanakul K, Weis OF, Alloza JL, et al: Analysis of narcotic usage in the treatment of postoperative pain. *JAMA* 250:926, 1983.
16. Pilowsky I: An outline curriculum on pain for medical schools. *Pain* 33:1, 1988.
17. Edwards WT: Optimizing opioid treatment of postoperative pain. *Journal of Pain and Symptom Management* 5:S24, 1990.
18. Oden RV: Acute postoperative pain: Incidence, severity, and etiology of inadequate treatment. *Anesthesiol Clin North Am* 7:1, 1989.
19. Fields HC: Sources of variability in the sensation of pain. *Pain* 33:195, 1988.
20. Egan K: Psychological issues in postoperative pain. *Anesthesiol Clin North Am* 7:183, 1989.
21. Austin KL, Stapleton JV, Mather LE: Multiple intramuscular injections: A major source of variability in analgesic response to meperidine. *Pain* 8:47, 1980.
22. Bates MS: Ethnicity and pain, a biocultural model. *Soc Sci Med* 24:47, 1987.
23. Bates MS, Edwards WT, Anderson KO: Ethnocultural influences on variation in chronic pain perceptions. *Pain* 52:101, 1993.
24. Wallace LM: Preoperative state of anxiety as a mediator of psychological adjustment to and recovery from surgery. *Br J Med Psychol* 59:253, 1986.
25. Parkhouse J, Lambrechts W, Simpson BRJ: The incidence of postoperative pain. *Br J Anaesth* 33:345, 1961.
26. Benedetti UC, Bonica J, Bellucci G: Pathophysiology and therapy of postoperative pain; a review. *Advances in Pain Research and Therapeutics* 7:373, 1984.
27. Merskey H, Albe-Fessard DG, Bonica JJ, et al: Pain terms: A list with definition and notes on usage. *Pain* 7:249, 1979.
28. Edwards WT, Breed RJ: The treatment of acute postoperative pain in the post-anesthesia care unit. *Anesthesiol Clin North Am* 8:235, 1990.
29. Ready LB, Edwards WT: IASP Task Force on Acute Pain. The management of acute pain, a practical manual. Seattle, IASP Publications, 1992.
30. Kehlet H: The stress response to anaesthesia and surgery: Release mechanism and modifying factors. *Clin Anaesth* 2:215, 1984.
31. Huskisson EC: Visual analog scales, in Melzack R (ed): *Pain Measurement and Assessment*. New York, Raven Press, 1983, p 33.
32. Melzack R: The short form McGill Pain Questionnaire. *Pain* 30:191, 1987.
33. Puntillo KA, Wilkie DJ: Assessment of pain in the critically ill, in Puntillo KA (ed): *Pain in the Critically Ill*. Gaithersburg, Maryland Aspen Publishers, Inc., 1991, Chapter 4.
34. Rawal N, Tandon B: Epidural and intrathecal morphine in intensive care units. *Intensive Care Med* 11:129, 1985.
35. Ferreira SH: Prostaglandin hyperalgesia and the control of inflammatory pain, in Bonta IL, Bray MA, Parham MJ (eds): *Handbook of Inflammation: The Pharmacology of Inflammation*, vol 5. New York, Elsevier, 1985, p 107.
36. Tammisto T, Tigerstedt I, Korttila K: Comparison of lysine acetylsalicylate and oxycodone in postoperative pain following upper abdominal surgery. *Ann Chir Gynaecol* 69:287, 1980.
37. Tigerstedt I, Janhunen L, Tammisto T: Efficacy of diclofenac in a single prophylactic dose in postoperative pain. *Ann Clin Res* 19:18, 1987.
38. Lal A, Pandey K, Chandra P: Dipyrone for treatment of post-operative pain. *Anaesthesia* 28:43, 1973.
39. Rigamonti G, Zanella E, Lampugani R: Dose-response with indoprofen as an analgesia in postoperative pain. *Br J Anaesth* 55:513, 1983.
40. Gillies GW, Kenny GN, Bullingham BE: The morphine-sparing effect of ketorolac tromethamine. *Anaesthesia* 42:727, 1987.
41. O'Hara DA, Fragen RJ, Kinzer M, et al: Ketorolac tromethamine as compared with morphine sulfate for treatment of postoperative pain. *Clin Pharmacol Ther* 41:556, 1987.

42. Oberlander T, Berde C: Ketorolac: Raising the roof on ceiling effects for NSAIDs. *IASP Newsletter* Sept/Oct: 2, 1991.

43. Vega H, McGory R, Schwenzer KJ: Is intravenous ketorolac safe in critically ill patients? *Anesth Analg* 74:S333, 1992.

44. Bravo LJCB, Mattie H, Spierdik J, et al: The effects on ventilation of ketorolac in comparison with morphine. *Eur J Clin Pharmacol* 35:491, 1988.

45. Burgess FW, Anderson DM, Colonna D, et al: Ipsilateral shoulder pain following thoracic surgery. *Anesthesiology* 78:365, 1993.

46. Zikowski D, Hord AH, Haddox D, et al: Ketorolac-induced bronchospasm. *Anesth Analg* 76:417, 1993.

47. Haddow GR, Riley E, Isaacs R, et al: Ketorolac, nasal polyposis, and bronchial asthma: A cause for concern. *Anesth Analg* 76:420, 1993.

48. Tverskoy M, Cozacov C, Ayache M, et al: Postoperative pain after inguinal herniorrhaphy with different types of anesthesia. *Anesth Analg* 70:29, 1990.

49. Woolf CJ: Recent advances in the pathophysiology of acute pain. *Br J Anaesth* 63:139, 1989.

50. Yaksh TL, Abram SE: Preemptive analgesia—a popular misnomer, but a clinically relevant truth? *APS Journal* 2:116, 1993.

51. Eriksson AS, Sinclair R, Cassuto J, et al: Influence of lidocaine on leukocyte function in the surgical wound. *Anesthesiology* 77:74, 1992.

52. Rawal N, Sjostrand U, Christofferson E, et al: Comparison of intramuscular and epidural morphine for postoperative analgesia in the grossly obese: Influence on postoperative ambulation and pulmonary function. *Anesth Analg* 63:583, 1984.

53. Faust RG, Nauss LA: Post-thoracotomy intercostal block: Comparison of its effects on pulmonary function with those with intramuscular meperidine. *Anesth Analg* 55:542, 1976.

54. Gibbons J, James O, Quail A: Relief of pain in chest injury. *Br J Anaesth* 45:1136, 1973.

55. Moore DC: Intercostal nerve block for postoperative somatic pain following surgery of thorax and upper abdomen. *Br J Anaesth* 47:284, 1975.

56. Nielsen CH: Bleeding after intercostal nerve block in a patient anticoagulated with heparin. *Anesthesiology* 71:162, 1989.

57. Galway JE, Caves PK, Dundee JW: Effect of intercostal nerve blockage during operation on lung function and the relief of pain following thoracotomy. *Br J Anaesth* 47:730, 1975.

58. Delilkan AE, Lee CK, Yong NK, et al: Post-operative local analgesia for thoractomy with direct bupivacaine intercostal blocks. *Anaesthesia* 28:560, 1973.

59. O'Kelly E, Garry B: Continuous pain relief for multiple fractured ribs. *Br J Anaesth* 53:989, 1981.

60. Murphy DF: Intercostal nerve blockade for fractured ribs and postoperative analgesia, description of a new technique. *Reg Anesth* 8:151, 1983.

61. Murphy DF: Continuous intercostal nerve blockade for pain relief following cholecystectomy. *Br J Anaesth* 55:521, 1983.

62. Mowbray A, Wong KKS, Murray JM: Intercostal catheterization. *Anaesthesia* 42:958, 1987.

63. Baxter AD, Flynn JF, Jennings FO: Continuous intercostal nerve blockade. *Br J Anaesth* 56:665, 1984.

64. Moore DC: Intercostal blockade. *Br J Anaesth* 57:543, 1985.

65. Graziotti PJ, Smith GB: Multiple rib fractures and head injury—an indication for intercostal catheterization and infusion of local anaesthetics. *Anaesthesia* 43:964, 1988.

66. Nunn JF, Slavin G: Posterior intercostal nerve block for pain relief after cholecystectomy, anatomical basis and efficacy. *Br J Anaesth* 52:253, 1980.

67. Moore DC: Intercostal nerve block: Spread of India ink injected to the rib's costal groove. *Br J Anaesth* 53:325, 1981.

68. Murphy DF: Continuous intercostal nerve blockade: An anatomical study to elucidate its mode of action. *Br J Anaesth* 56:627, 1984.

69. Moore DC, Bush WH, Scurlock JE: Intercostal nerve block: A roentgenographic anatomic study of technique and absorption in humans. *Anesth Analg* 59:815, 1980.

70. Hosie HE, Crossley AWA: A radiographic study of intercostal nerve blockade in healthy volunteers. *Br J Anaesth* 58:129P, 1986.

71. Hord AH, Wang JM, Pai UT, et al: Anatomic spread of india ink in the human intertcostal space with radiographic correlation. *Reg Anesth* 16:13, 1991.

72. Middaugh RE, Menk EJ, Reynolds WJ, et al: Epidural block using large volumes of local anesthetic solution for intercostal nerve block. *Anesthesiology* 63:214, 1985.

73. Brown RH, Tewes PA: Cervical sympathetic blockade after thoracic intercostal injection of local anesthetic. *Anesthesiology* 70:1011, 1989.

74. Rawal N, Sjostrand UH, Dahlstrom B, et al: Epidural morphine for postoperative pain relief: A comparative study with intramuscular narcotic and intercostal nerve block. *Anesth Analg* 61:93, 1982.

75. Baxter AD, Jennings FO, Harris RS, et al: Continuous intercostal blockade after cardiac surgery. *Br J Anaesth* 59:162, 1987.

76. Murphy DF: Postoperative intercostal block. *Br J Anaesth* 61:370, 1988.

77. Lyles R, Skurdal D, Stene J, et al: Continuous intercostal catheter techniques for treatment of post-traumatic thoracic pain. *Anesthesiology* 65:A205, 1986.

78. Eason NJ, Wyatt R: Paravertebral thoracic block—a reappraisal. *Anaesthesia* 34:638, 1979.

79. Conacher ID, Kokri M: Postoperative paravertebral blocks for thoracic surgery. *Br J Anaesth* 59:155, 1987.

80. Purcell-Jones G, Pither CE, Justins DM: Paravertebral somatic nerve block: A clinical, radiographic, and computed tomographic study in chronic pain patients. *Anesth Analg* 68:32, 1989.

81. Govenden V, Mattews P: Percutaneous placement of paravertebral catheters during thoracotomy. *Anaesthesia* 43:246, 1988.

82. Kvalheim L, Reiestad F: Interpleural catheter in the management of postoperative pain. *Anesthesiology* 61:A231, 1984.

83. Reiestad F, Stromskag KE: Interpleural catheter in the management of postoperative pain, a preliminary report. *Reg Anesth* 11:89, 1986.

84. Schlesinger TM, Laurito CE, Bauman VL, et al: Interpleural bupivacaine for mammography during needle localization and breast biopsy. *Anesth Analg* 68:394, 1988.

85. Kambam JR, Handte RE, Flanagan J, et al: Intrapleural anesthesia for post thoracotomy pain relief. *Anesth Analg* 66:S90, 1987.

86. Tartiere J, Delassus P, Sillard B, et al: Intrapleural bupivacaine analgesia, after thoracoabdominal incision for esophagectomy. *Anesthesiology* 71:A664, 1989.

87. Rocco A, Reiestad F, Gudman J, et al: Intrapleural administration of local anesthetics for pain relief in patients with multiple rib fractures, preliminary report. *Reg Anesth* 12:10, 1987.

88. Sihota MK, Ikuta PT, Holmblad BR, et al: Successful pain management of chronic pancreatitis and post herpetic neuralgia with intrapleural technique. *Reg Anesth* 13(Suppl 2):40, 1988.

89. Ahlburg P. Noreng M, Mølgaard J et al: Treatment of pancreatic pain with interplenral bupivacine: An open trial. *Acta Anaesth Scand* 34:156, 1990.

90. Waldman SD, Allen ML, Cronen MC: Subcutaneous tunneled intrapleural catheters in the long-term relief of right upper quadrant pain of malignant origin. *Journal of Pain and Symptom Management* 4:86, 1989.

91. Squier RC, Morrow JS, Roman R: Hanging-drop for intrapleural analgesia. *Anesthesiology* 70:2, 1989.

92. Kambam JR, Hammond J, Parris WCV, et al: Intrapleural analgesia for postthoracotomy pain and blood levels following bupivacaine intrapleural injection. *Can J Anaesth* 36:106, 1989.

93. Covino BG: Interpleural regional analgesia. *Anesth Analg* 67:427, 1988.

94. Riegler FX, Pelligrino DA, VadeBoncoeur TR: An animal model of intrapleural analgesia. *Anesthesiology* 69:A365, 1988.

95. Sihota MK, Holmblad BR: Horner's syndrome after intrapleural anesthesia with bupivacaine for post-herpetic neuralgia. *Acta Anaesthesiol Scand* 32:593, 1988.

96. Parkinson SK, Mueller JB, Rich TJ, et al: Unilateral Horner's syndrome associated with interpleural catheter injection of local anesthetic. *Anesth Analg* 68:61, 1989.

97. Reiestad F, McIlvaine WB, Kvalheim L, et al: Interpleural analgesia in treatment of upper extremity reflex sympathetic dystrophy. *Anesth Analg* 69:671, 1989.

98. Morrow JS, Squier RC: Sympathetic blockade with interpleural analgesia. *Anesthesiology* 71:A662, 1989.

99. Durrani Z, Winnie AP, Ikuta P: Interpleural catheter analgesia for pancreatic pain. *Anesth Analg* 67:479, 1988.

100. Denson D, Sehlhorst CS, Schultz REG, et al: Pharmacokinetics of Intrapleural bupivacaine: Effects of epinephrine. *Reg Anesth* 13(Suppl 1):47, 1988.

101. van Kleef JW, Logeman EA, Burm AGL, et al: Continuous interpleural infusion of bupivacaine for postoperative analgesia after surgery with flank incisions: A double-blind comparison of 0.25% and 0.5% solutions. *Anesth Analg* 75:268, 1992.

102. El-Baz N, Faber LP, Ivankovich AD: Intrapleural infusion of local anesthetic: A word of caution. *Anesthesiology* 68:809, 1988.

103. Seltzer JL, Larijani GE, Goldberg ME, et al: Intrapleural bupivacaine—a kinetic and dynamic evaluation. *Anesthesiology* 67:798, 1987.

104. Brismar B, Pettersson N, Tokics L, et al: Postoperative analgesia with intrapleural administration of bupivacaine-adrenaline. *Acta Anaesthesiol Scand* 31:515, 1987.

105. Chan VWS, Arthur GR, Ferrante FM: Intrapleural bupivacaine administration for pain relief following thoracotomy. *Reg Anesth* 13(Suppl 2):70, 1988.

106. Raj P: Intrapleural anesthesia—applications and contraindications. *Anesthesiol Alert* 1:1, 1988.

107. Aguilar JL, Montero A, Vidal LF, et al: Bilateral interpleural injection of local anesthetics. *Reg Anesth* 14:93, 1989.

108. Aguilar JL, Montero A, Vidal LF, et al: Intrapleural analgesia and phrenic nerve palsy. *Reg Anesth* 15:45, 1990.

109. Kowalski SE, Bradley BD, Greengrass RA, et al: Effects of interpleural bupivacaine (0.5%) on canine diaphragmatic function. *Anesth Analg* 75:400, 1992.

110. Lauder GR: Interpleural analgesia and phrenic nerve paralysis. *Anaesthesia* 48:315, 1993.

111. Selander D: Catheter technique in axillary plexus block. *Acta Anaesth Scand* 21:324, 1977.

112. Sada T, Kobayashi T, Murakami S: Continuous axillary brachial plexus block. *Can Anaesth Soc J* 30:201, 1983.

113. Haynsworth RF, Heavner JE, Racz GB: Continuous brachial plexus blockade using an axillary catheter for treatment of accidental intra-arterial injections. *Reg Anesth* 10:187, 1985.

114. Gaumann DM, Lennon RL, Wedel DJ: Continuous axillary block for postoperative pain management. *Reg Anesth* 13:77, 1988.

115. Hord AH, Roberson JR, Thompson WF, et al: Evaluation of continuous femoral nerve analgesia after primary total knee arthroplasty. *Anesth Analg* 70:S164, 1990.

116. Edwards ND, Wright EM: Continuous low-dose 3-in-1 nerve blockade for postoperative pain relief after total knee replacement. *Anesth Analg* 75:265, 1992.

117. Tyler E, Caldwell C, Ghia JN: Transcutaneous electrical nerve stimulation: An alternative approach to the management of postoperative pain. *Anesth Analg* 61:449, 1982.

118. Wolf SL: Neurophysiologic mechanisms in pain modulation: Relevance to T.E.N.S., in Mannheimer JS, Lampe JN (eds): *Clinical Transcutaneous Nerve Stimulation*. Philadelphia, FA Davis, 1984, p 41.

119. Ottoson D, Lundeberg T: *Pain Treatment by Transcutaneous Electrical Nerve Stimulation (TENS), A Practical Manual*. New York, Springer-Verlag, 1988.

120. Conn IG, Marshall AH, Yadav S, et al: Transcutaneous electrical nerve stimulation following appendectomy: The placebo effect. *Ann R Coll Surg Engl* 68:191, 1986.

121. Reus R, Cronen P, Abplanalp L: Transcutaneous electrical nerve stimulation for pain control after cholecystectomy: Lack of expected benefits. *South Med J* 81:1361, 1988.

122. Schuster GD, Infante MC: Pain relief after low back surgery: The efficacy of transcutaneous electrical nerve stimulation. *Pain* 8:299, 1980.

123. Zahl K, Bray C, Taylor L, et al: Does transcutaneous electrical nerve stimulation provide pain relief after lumbar laminectomy? *Anesth Analg* 67:S264, 1988.

124. McCallum MID, Glynn CJ, Moore RA, et al: Transcutaneous electrical nerve stimulation in the management of acute postoperative pain. *Br J Anaesth* 61:308, 1988.

125. Rooney SM, Jain S, Goldiner PL: Effect of transcutaneous nerve stimulation on postoperative pain after thoracotomy. *Anesth Analg* 62:1010, 1983.

126. Stubbing JF, Jellicoe JA: Transcutaneous electrical nerve stimulation after thoracotomy. *Anaesthesia* 43:296, 1988.

127. Navarathnam RG, Wang IYS, Thomas D, et al: Evaluation of the transcutaneous electrical nerve stimulator for postoperative analgesia following cardiac surgery. *Anaesth Intensive Care* 12:345, 1984.

128. Hymes AC, Yonehiro EG, Raab DE, et al: Electrical surface stimulation for treatment and prevention of ileus and atelectasis. *Surg Forum* 25:222, 1974.

129. Hymes A: The therapeutic value of postoperative T.E.N.S. (case study), in Mannheimer JS, Lampe JN (eds): *Clinical Transcutaneous Nerve Stimulation*. Philadelphia, FA Davis, 1984, p 497.

130. Sloan JP, Muwanga CL, Waters EA, et al: Multiple rib fractures: Transcutaneous nerve stimulation versus conventional analgesia. *J Trauma* 26:1120, 1986.

131. Kimball KL, Drews JE, Walker S, et al: Use of TENS for pain reduction in burn patients receiving Travase. *J Burn Care Rehabil* 8:28, 1987.

132. Mannheimer C, Carlsson CA, Vedin A, et al: Transcutaneous electrical nerve stimulation (TENS) in angina pectoris. *Pain* 26:291, 1986.

133. Mannheimer C, Emanuelsson H, Waagstein F: The effect of transcutaneous electrical nerve stimulation (TENS) on catecholamine metabolism during pacing-induced angina pectoris and the influence of naloxone. *Pain* 41:27, 1990.

134. Hurley RJ: Continuous spinal anesthesia. *Int Anesthesiol Clin* 27:46, 1989.

135. Ansbro FP, Latteri FS, Blundell AE, et al: Prolonged spinal anesthesia (seven, eleven and fourteen days). *Anesthesiology* 15:569, 1954.

136. Bevacqua BK, Slucky AV, Adusumilli SB: Post operative analgesia with continuous intrathecal lidocaine infusion. *Reg Anesth* 16(1S):44, 1991.

137. Peterson DO, Borup JL, Chestnut JS: Continuous spinal anesthesia. *Reg Anesth* 8:109, 1983.

138. Kamsler PM: Study of changes in spinal fluid cell count during spinal anesthesia. *Anesth Analg (Curr Res)* 30:103, 1951.

139. Bevacqua BK, Slucky AV: Is post operative intra-thecal catheter use associated with CNS infections? *Reg Anesth* 16(1S):12, 1991.

140. Kennedy BM: Intrathecal morphine and fractured ribs. *Br J Anaesth* 57:1266, 1985.

141. Stoelting RK: Intrathecal morphine—an underused combination for postoperative pain management. *Anesth Analg* 68:707, 1989.

142. Nilsson E, Perttunyn K: Intrathecal morphine for poststernotomy pain in patients with myasthenia gravis. *Anesthesiology* 77:A857, 1992.

143. Jacobson L, Chabal C, Brody MC, et al: Intrathecal methadone and morphine for postoperative analgesia: A comparison of the efficacy, duration and side effects. *Anesthesiology* 70:742, 1989.

144. Dickson GR, Sutcliffe AJ: Intrathecal morphine and multiple fractured ribs. *Br J Anaesth* 58:1342, 1986.

145. Fromme GA, Gray JR: A comparison of intrathecal and epidural morphine for treatment of post-thoracotomy pain. *Anesth Analg* 64:214, 1985.

146. Gray JR, Fromme GA, Nauss LA, et al: Intrathecal morphine for post-thoracotomy pain. *Anesth Analg* 65:873, 1988.

147. Follett KA, Hitchon PW, Piper J, et al: Response of intractable pain to continuous intrathecal morphine: A retrospective study. *Pain* 49:21, 1992.

148. Sjöberg M, Karlsson PA, Nordborg C, et al: Neuropathologic findings after long-term intrathecal infusion of morphine and bupivacaine for pain treatment in cancer patients. *Anesthesiology* 76:173, 1992.

149. Sethna NF, Berde CB: Continuous subarachnoid analgesia in two adolescents with severe scoliosis and impaired pulmonary function. *Reg Anesth* 16:333, 1991.

150. Stasic A, Davis R, Chapple I, et al: Opioid administration via intrathecal catheter for children undergoing spinal fusion. *Anesth Analg* 74:S306, 1992.

151. Niemi L, Pitkänen MT, Tuominen MK, et al: Comparison of intrathecal fentanyl infusion with intrathecal morphine infusion or bolus for postoperative pain relief after hip arthroplasty. *Anesth Analg* 77:126, 1993.

152. Burchett KR, Denny NM: Initial experience of continuous subarachnoid diamorphine infusion for postoperative pain relief. *Reg Anesth* 16:253, 1991.

153. Bevacqua BK, Slucky AV, Nemec D: Intrathecal lidocaine/morphine infusion for postoperative pain ablation. *Anesth Analg* 74:S25, 1992.

154. Bevacqua BK, Slucky AV: Intrathecal lidocaine/fentanyl infusion for post-operative analgesia. *Anesth Analg* 72:S20, 1991.

155. Domsky M, Tarantino D: Patient-controlled spinal analgesia for postoperative pain control. *Anesth Analg* 75:453, 1992.
156. Geernaert K, Vandeput D, Vercauteren M, et al: Spinal PCA using isobaric bupivacaine with or without sufentanil: preliminary results. *Reg Anesth* 18(2S):20, 1993.
157. Crul BJP, Delhaas EM: Technical complications during long-term subarachnoid or epidural administration of morphine in terminally ill cancer patients. *Reg Anesth* 16:209, 1991.
158. Campbell C: Epidural opioids—the preferred route of administration. *Anesth Analg* 68:710, 1989.
159. Eldor J, Gozal Y, Guedj P, et al: Combined spinal-epidural anesthesia with a specialized needle. *Reg Anesth* 16:348, 1991.
160. Eldor J, Guedj P, Gozal Y: Combined spinal-epidural anesthesia using the CSEN. *Anesth Analg* 74:169, 1992.
161. Katz Y, Markovits R, Rosenberg B: Pneumoencephalos after inadvertent intrathecal air injection during epidural block. *Anesthesiology* 73:1277, 1990.
162. Kennedy TM, Ullman DA, Harte FA, et al: Lumbar root compression secondary to epidural air. *Anesth Analg* 67:1184, 1988.
163. Nay PG, Milaszkiewicz R, Jothilingam S: Extradural air as a cause of paraplegia following lumbar analgesia. *Anaesthesia* 48:402, 1993.
164. Dalens B, Bazin J, Haberer J: Epidural bubbles as a course of incomplete analgesia during epidural anesthesia. *Anesth Analg* 66:679, 1987.
165. Valentine SJ, Jarvis AP, Shutt LE: Comparative study of the effects of air or saline to identify the extradural space. *Br J Anaesth* 66:224, 1991.
166. Fromme GA, Steidl LJ, Danielson DR: Comparison of lumbar and thoracic epidural morphine for relief of post-thoracotomy pain. *Anesth Analg* 68:710, 1985.
167. Brodsky JB, Kretzschmar KM, Mark JBD: Caudal epidural morphine for post-thoracotomy pain. *Anesth Analg* 67:409, 1988.
168. Cousins MJ, Bromage PR: Epidural neural blockade, in Cousins MJ, Bridenbaugh PO (eds): *Neural Blockade in Clinical Anesthesia and Management of Pain.* 2nd ed. Philadelphia, JB Lippincott, 1988, p 253.
169. Blomberg RG, Jaanivald A, Walther S: Advantages of the paramedian approach for lumbar epidural analgesia with catheter technique. *Anaesthesia* 44:742, 1989.
170. Moore DC, Batra MS: The components of an effective test dose prior to epidural block. *Anesthesiology* 55:693, 1981.
171. Griffiths DPG, Diamond AW, Cameron JD: Postoperative extradural analgesia following thoracic surgery: A feasibility study. *Br J Anaesth* 47:48, 1975.
172. Shuman RL, Peters RM: Epidural anesthesia following thoracotomy in patients with chronic obstructive airway disease. *J Thorac Cardiovasc Surg* 71:82, 1976.
173. Conacher ID, Paes ML, Jacobson L, et al: Epidural analgesia following thoracic surgery. *Anaesthesia* 78:546, 1983.
174. James EC, Kolberg HL, Iwen GW, et al: Epidural analgesia for postthoracotomy patients. *J Thorac Cardiovasc Surg* 82:898, 1981.
175. Otton PE, Wilson EJ: The cardiopulmonary effects of upper thoracic epidural analgesia. *Can Anaesth Soc J* 13:541, 1966.
176. Yeager MP, Glass DD, Neff RK, et al: Epidural anesthesia and analgesia in high risk surgical patients. *Anesthesiology* 66:729, 1987.
177. Blomberg S, Emanuelsson H, Ricksten SE: Thoracic epidural anesthesia and central hemodynamics in patients with unstable angina pectoris. *Anesth Analg* 69:558, 1989.
178. Toft P, Jorgensen A: Continuous thoracic epidural analgesia for the control of pain in myocardial infarction. *Intensive Care Med* 13:388, 1987.
179. Ready LB, Oden R, Chadwick HS, et al: Development of an anesthesiology-based postoperative pain management service. *Anesthesiology* 68:100, 1988.
180. Klinck JR, Lindop MJ: Epidural morphine in the elderly. *Anaesthesia* 37:907, 1982.
181. Larsen VH, Iversen AD, Christenson P, et al: Postoperative pain treatment after upper abdominal surgery with epidural morphine at thoracic or lumbar level. *Acta Anaesthesiol Scand* 29:566, 1985.
182. Hakanson E, Bengtsson M, Rutberg H, Ulrick AM: Epidural morphine by the thoracic or lumbar routes in cholecystektomy. Effect on postoperative pain and respiratory variables. *Anaesth Intensive Care* 17:166, 1989.
183. Bromage PR, Camporesi E, Chestnut D: Epidural narcotics for postoperative analgesia. *Anesth Analg* 59:473, 1980.
184. Rawal R, Sjostrand UH, Dahlstrom B, et al: Epidural morphine for postoperative pain relief: A comparative study with intramuscular narcotic and intercostal nerve block. *Anesth Analg* 61:93, 1982.
185. Shulman M, Sandler AN, Bradley JW, et al: Postthoracotomy pain and pulmonary function following epidural and systemic morphine. *Anesthesiology* 61:569, 1984.
186. Stenseth R, Sellevold O, Breivil H: Epidural morphine for postoperative pain: Experience with 1085 patients. *Acta Anaesthesiol Scand* 29:148, 1985.
187. Henderson SK, Cohen C: Nalbuphine augmentation of analgesia and reversal of side effects following epidural hydromorphone. *Anesthesiology* 65:216, 1986.
188. Miguel R, McNelis M: Intravenous butorphanol decreases the incidence of epidural morphine induced pruritus in cancer patients. *Anesth Analg* 70:S267, 1990.
189. Lawhorn CD, McNitt JD, Fibuch EE, et al: Epidural morphine with butorphanol for postoperative analgesia after cesarean delivery. *Anesth Analg* 72:53, 1991.
190. Brose WG, Cohen SE: Oxyhemoglobin saturation following caesarian section in patients receiving epidural morphine, PCA, or IM meperidine analgesia. *Anesthesiology* 70:948, 1989.
191. Ready LB, Edwards WT: Postoperative care following intrathecal or epidural opioids II. *Anesthesiology* 72:213, 1990.
192. Mott JM, Eisele JH: A survey of monitoring practices following spinal opiate administration. *Anesth Analg* 65:S105, 1986.
193. Egbert LD, Laver MB, Bendixen HH: The effect of site of operation and type of anesthesia upon the ability to cough in the postoperative period. *Surg Gynecol Obstet* 44:161, 1964.
194. Etches RC, Sandler AN, Daley MD: Respiratory depression and spinal opioids. *Can J Anaesth* 36:165, 1989.
195. Rawal N, Wattwil M: Respiratory depression after epidural morphine—an experimental and clinical study. *Anesth Analg* 63:8, 1984.
196. Rawal N, Schott U, Dahlstrom B, et al: Influence of naloxone infusion on analgesia and respiratory depression following epidural morphine. *Anesthesiology* 64:194, 1986.
197. Baxter AD, Samson B, Penning J, et al: Prevention of epidural morphine induced respiratory depression with intravenous nalbuphine infusion in post-thoracotomy patients. *Can J Anaesth* 36:503, 1989.
198. El-Baz NM, Faber LP, Jensik RJ: Continuous epidural infusion of morphine for treatment of pain after thoracic surgery: A new technique. *Anesth Analg* 63:757, 1984.
199. Ullman D, Fortune SB, Greenhouse BB, et al: The treatment of patients with multiple rib fractures using continuous thoracic epidural narcotic infusion. *Reg Anesth* 14:43, 1989.
200. Cousins MJ, Mather LE: Intrathecal and epidural administration of opioid. *Anesthesiology* 61:276, 1984.
201. Welchew EA, Thornton JA: Continuous thoracic epidural fentanyl. *Anaesthesia* 37:309, 1982.
202. Gough JD, Williams AB, Vaughan RS, et al: The control of postthoracotomy pain. A comparative evaluation of thoracic epidural fentanyl infusions and cryo analgesia. *Anaesthesia* 43:780, 1988.
203. Renaud B, Brichant JF, Clergue F, et al: Continuous epidural fentanyl: Ventilatory effects and plasma kinetics. *Anesthesiology* 63:A234, 1985.
204. Ahuja BR, Strunin L: Respiratory effects of epidural fentanyl. *Anaesthesia* 40:949, 1985.
205. Renaud B, Brichant JF, Clergue F, et al: Ventilatory effects of continuous epidural infusion of fentanyl. *Anesth Analg* 67:971, 1988.
206. Loper KA, Ready LB, Downey M, et al: Epidural and intravenous fentanyl infusions are clinically equivalent after knee surgery. *Anesth Analg* 70:72, 1990.
207. Ellis DJ, Millar WL, Reisner LS: A randomized double-blind comparison of epidural versus intravenous fentanyl infusion for analgesia after cesarean section. *Anesthesiology* 72:981, 1990.
208. Glass PSA, Estok P, Ginsburg B, et al: Use of patient-controlled analgesia to compare the efficacy of epidural to intravenous fentanyl administration. *Anesth Analg* 74:345, 1992.
209. Sandler AN, Stringer D, Panos L, et al: A randomized, double-blind comparison of lumbar epidural and intravenous fentanyl infusions for postthoracotomy pain relief. *Anesthesiology* 77:626, 1992.
210. Guinard JP, Mavrocordatos P, Chiolero R, et al: A randomized

comparison of intravenous versus lumbar and thoracic epidural fentanyl for analgesia after thoracotomy. *Anesthesiology* 77:1108, 1992.

211. Fineman SP: Long-term post-thoracotomy cancer pain management with interpleural bupivacaine. *Anesth Analg* 68:694, 1989.
212. Lomessy A, Magnin C, Viale JP, et al: Clinical advantages of fentanyl given epidurally for postoperative analgesia. *Anesthesiology* 61:466, 1984.
213. Grant GJ, Ho I, Winter E, et al: Epidural versus intravenous fentanyl during cesarean section. *Anesth Analg* 72:S92, 1991.
214. Salomäki TE, Laitinen JO, Nuutinen LS: A randomized double-blind comparison of epidural versus intravenous fentanyl infusion for analgesia after thoracotomy. *Anesthesiology* 75:790, 1991.
215. Rankin APN, Comber REH: Management of five cases of chest injury with a regimen of epidural bupivacaine and morphine. *Anaesth Intensive Care* 12:311, 1984.
216. Hjortso NC, Lund C, Mogensen T, et al: Epidural morphine improves pain relief and maintains sensory analgesia during continuous epidural bupivacaine after abdominal surgery. *Anesth Analg* 65:1033, 1986.
217. Logas WG, El-Baz N, El-Ganzouri A, et al: Continuous thoracic epidural analgesia for postoperative pain relief following thoracotomy: A randomized prospective study. *Anesthesiology* 67:787, 1987.
218. Akerman B, Arwestrom E, Post C: Local anesthetics potentiate spinal morphine antinociception. *Anesth Analg* 67:943, 1988.
219. George KA, Wright PMC, Chisakuta A: Continuous thoracic epidural fentanyl for post-thoracotomy pain relief: With or without fentanyl? *Anaesthesia* 46:732, 1991.
220. George KA, Chisakuta AM, Gamble JAS, et al: Thoracic epidural infusion for postoperative pain relief following abdominal aortic surgery: Bupivacaine, fentanyl or a mixture of both? *Anaesthesia* 47:388, 1992.
221. Ali MJ, Hutfluss R: Epidural fentanyl-bupivacaine infusion for management of pain in the Guillain-Barré syndrome. *Reg Anesth* 17:171, 1992.
222. Badner NH, Reimer EJ, Komar W, et al: Low-dose bupivacaine does not improve postoperative fentanyl analgesia in orthopedic patients. *Anesth Analg* 72:337, 1991.
223. Mourisse J, Hasenbos WM, Gielen MJM, et al: Epidural bupivacaine, sufentanil or the combination for post-thoracotomy pain. *Acta Anaesthesiol Scand* 36:70, 1992.
224. Harbers JBM, Hasenbos MAWM, Gort C, et al: Ventilatory function and continuous high thoracic epidural administration of bupivacaine with sufentanil intravenously or epidurally: A double-blind comparison. *Reg Anesth* 16:65, 1991.
225. Lee A, Simpson D, Whitfield A, et al: Postoperative analgesia by continuous extradural infusion of bupivacaine and diamorphine. *Br J Anaesth* 60:845, 1988.
226. Lee A, McKeown D, Brockway M, et al: Comparison of extradural and intravenous diamorphine as a supplement to extradural bupivacaine. *Anaesthesia* 46:447, 1991.
227. Yaksh TL, Aimone L: The central pharmacology of pain transmission, in Wall PD, Melzack R (eds): *Textbook of Pain*. Edinburgh, Churchill-Livingstone, 1989, p 181.
228. Maze M, Tranquilli W: Alpha-2 adrenoceptor agonists: defining the role in clinical anesthesia. *Anesthesiology* 74:581, 1991.
229. Sosnowski M, Yaksh TL: Role of spinal adenosine receptors in modulating the hyperesthesia produced by spinal glycine receptor antagonism. *Anesth Analg* 69:587, 1989.
230. Kitahata LM: spinal analgesia with morphine and clonidine. *Anesth Analg* 68:191, 1989.
231. Bloor BC: Clonidine and other alpha-2 adrenergic agonists: An important new drug class for the perioperative period. *Sem Anesth* 3:170, 1988.
232. Franz DN, Wong KC: The potential use of clonidine in anesthesia. *Literature Scan: Anesthesiology* 3:2, Dec 1989.
233. Bonnet F, Brun-Buisson V, Saada M, et al: Dose-related prolongation of hyperbaric tetracaine spinal anesthesia by clonidine in humans. *Anesth Analg* 68:619, 1989.
234. Bonnet F, Diallo A, Saada M, et al: Prevention of tourniquet pain by spinal isobaric bupivacaine with clonidine. *Br J Anaesth* 63:93, 1989.
235. Tzeng JI, Wang JJ, Mok MS, et al: Clonidine potentiates lidocaine-induced epidural anesthesia. *Anesth Analg* 68:S298, 1989.

236. Carabine UA, Milligan KR, Moore J: Extradural clonidine and bupivacaine for postoperative analgesia. *Br J Anaesth* 68:132, 1992.
237. Veillette Y, Orhant E, Benhamou D, et al: Addition of clonidine decreases lidocaine absorption after epidural injection. *Anesthesiology* 71:A267, 1989.
238. Petit J, Oskenheindler G, Colas G, et al: Comparison of the effects of morphine, clonidine and a combination of morphine and clonidine administered epidurally for postoperative analgesia. *Anesthesiology* 71:A647, 1989.
239. Motsch J, Gräber E, Ludwig K: Addition of clonidine enhances postoperative analgesia from epidural morphine: a double-blind study. *Anesthesiology* 73:1067, 1990.
240. Carabine UA, Milligan KR, Mulholland D, et al: Extradural clonidine infusions for analgesia after total hip replacement. *Br J Anaesth* 68:338, 1992.
241. Eisenach JC, Lysak SZ, Viscomi CM: Epidural clonidine analgesia following surgery: Phase I. *Anesthesiology* 71:640, 1989.
242. Langer SZ, Duval N, Massingham R: Pharmacologic and therapeutic significance of alpha-adrenoceptor subtypes. *J Cardiovasc Pharmacol* 7(Suppl 8):1, 1985.
243. Bonnet F, Brun-Buisson V, Francois Y, et al: Effects of oral and subarachnoid clonidine on spinal anesthesia with bupivacaine. *Reg Anesth* 15:211, 1990.
244. Ota K, Namiki A, Ujike Y, et al: Prolongation of tetracaine spinal anesthesia by oral clonidine. *Anesth Analg* 75:262, 1992.
245. Curletta JD, Coyle RJ, Ghignone M: Systemically administered clonidine enhances postoperative epidural opiate analgesia. *Anesth Analg* 68:S66, 1989.
246. Segal IS, Jarvis DA, Duncan SR, et al: Perioperative use of transdermal clonidine as an adjunctive agent. *Anesth Analg* 68:S250, 1989.
247. Bernard JM, Hommeril JL, Passuti N, et al: Postoperative analgesia by IV clonidine. *Anesthesiology* 75:577, 1991.
248. Rouge P, Dureuil B, Loiseau A, et al: Effects of clonidine on the ventilatory response to CO_2. *Anesthesiology* 71:A1090, 1989.
249. Penon C, Ecoffey C, Cohen SE: Ventilatory effects of epidural clonidine. *Anesthesiology* 71:A649, 1989.
250. Ravat F, Dorne R, Baechle JP, et al: Epidural ketamine or morphine for postoperative analgesia. *Anesthesiology* 66:819, 1987.
251. Kawana Y, Sato H, Shimada H, et al: Epidural ketamine for postoperative pain relief after gynecologic operations. *Anesth Analg* 66:735, 1987.
252. Mori K, Shingu K: Epidural ketamine does not produce analgesia. *Anesthesiology* 68:296, 1988.
253. Peat SJ, Bras P, Hamma MH: A double-blind comparison of epidural ketamine and diamorphine for postoperative analgesia. *Anaesthesia* 44:555, 1989.
254. Dubner R: Pain and hyperalgesia following tissue injury: new mechanisms and new treatments. *Pain* 44:213, 1991.
255. Nagasaka H, Nagasaka I, Sato I, et al: The effects of ketamine on the excitation and inhibition of dorsal horn WDR neuronal activity induced by bradykinin injection into the femoral artery in cats after spinal cord transection. *Anesthesiology* 78:722, 1993.
256. Gaumann DM, Yaksh TL: Intrathecal somatostatin in rats: Antinociception only in the presence of toxic effects. *Anesthesiology* 68:733, 1988.
257. Gaumann DM, Yaksh TL, Post C, et al: Itrathecal somatostatin in cat and mouse studies on pain, motor behavior, and histopathology. *Anesth Analg* 68:623, 1989.
258. Aho M, Lehtinen AM, Erkola O, et al: The effect of intravenously administered dexmedetomidine on perioperative hemodynamics and isoflurane requirements in patients undergoing abdominal hysterectomy. *Anesthesiology* 74:997, 1991.
259. Nakagawa I, Murata K, Omote K, et al: Serotonergic mediation of spinal analgesia and its interaction with noradrenergic systems. *Anesthesiology* 69:A644, 1988.
260. Rattan AK, Gudehithlu KP, McDonald JS, et al: Differential effect of intrathecal midazolam on morphine analgesia. *Anesthesiology* 69:A681, 1988.
261. Edwards M, Serrao JM, Gent JP, et al: On the mechanism by which midazolam causes spinally mediated analgesia. *Anesthesiology* 73:273, 1990.
262. Loubser P, Donovan W, Narayan RK: Control of spasticity and pain with intrathecal baclofen—a GABA analog. *Anesthesiology* 71:A111, 1989.

263. Lassen HC, Henriksen E, Neukirch F: Treatment of tetanus: Severe bone marrow depression after prolonged nitrous oxide anaesthesia. *Lancet* 1:527, 1956.

264. Marx GF, Chen LK, Tabora JA: Experience with a disposable inhaler for methoxyflurane analgesia during labor: Clinical biochemical results. *Can Anaesth Soc J* 16:66, 1969.

265. Corbett TH, Cornell RG, Endres JL, et al: Birth defects among children of nurse anesthetists. *Anesthesiology* 41:341, 1974.

266. Truog RD, Rice SA: Inorganic fluoride and prolonged isoflurane anesthesia in the intensive care unit. *Anesth Analg* 69:843, 1989.

267. Wilson GR, Tomlinson P: Pain relief in burns—how we do it. *Burns* 14:331, 1988.

268. Mather LE, Phillips GD: Opioids and adjuvants: Principles of use, in Cousins MJ, Phillips GD (eds): *Acute Pain Management.* New York, Churchill-Livingstone, 1986, p 77.

269. Varvel JR, Shafer SL, Hwang SS, et al: Absorption characteristics of transdermally administered fentanyl. *Anesthesiology* 70:928, 1989.

270. Gourlay GK, Kowalski SR, Plummer JL, et al: The transdermal administration of fentanyl in the treatment of postoperative pain: Pharmacokinetics and pharmacodynamic effects. *Pain* 37:193, 1989.

271. Gourlay GK, Kowalski SR, Plummer JL, et al: The efficacy of transdermal fentanyl in the treatment of postoperative pain: A double-blind comparison of fentanyl and placebo systems. *Pain* 40:21, 1990.

272. Lehmann KA, Zech D: Transdermal fentanyl: Clinical pharmacology. *J Pain Symptom Management* 7:S8-S16, 1992.

273. Rowbotham DJ, Wyld R, Peacock JE, et al: Transdermal fentanyl for the relief of pain after upper abdominal surgery. *Br J Anaesth* 63:56, 1989.

274. Holley FO, Van Stennis C: Postoperative analgesia with fentanyl: Pharmacokinetics and pharmacodynamics of constant-rate IV and transdermal delivery. *Br J Anaesth* 60:608, 1988.

275. Caplan RA, Ready LB, Oden RV, et al: Transdermal fentanyl for postoperative pain management. *JAMA* 261:1036, 1989.

276. Sevarino FB, Naulty JS, Sinatra R, et al: Transdermal fentanyl for postoperative pain management in patients recovering from abdominal gynecologic surgery. *Anesthesiology* 77:463, 1992.

277. Bell SD, Goldberg ME, Lerigani GE, et al: Evaluation of transdermal fentanyl for multi-day analgesia in postoperative patients. *Anesth Analg* 68:S22, 1989.

278. Torjman M, Bartkowski RR, Marr A, et al: Respiratory effects of a fentanyl transdermal delivery system compared to fixed interval IM morphine following spinal surgery. *Anesthesiology* 75:A1101, 1991.

279. Miser AW, Narang PK, Dothage JA, et al: Transdermal fentanyl for pain control in patients with cancer. *Pain* 37:15, 1989.

280. Chauvin M, Strumza P, Levron JC, et al: Plasma fentanyl concentrations during transdermal delivery. *Anesthesiology* 71:A717, 1989.

281. Stanski DR, Watkins DW: *Drug Disposition in Anesthesia.* Orlando, Fla., Grune and Stratton, 1982.

282. Mather LE, Owen H: The pharmacology of patient-administered opioids, in Ferrante FM, Ostheimer GW, Covino BG (eds): *Patient-Controlled Analgesia.* Cambridge, England, Blackwell Scientific, 1990, p 27.

283. White PF: Patient-controlled analgesia: A new approach to management of postoperative pain. *Sem Anesth* 4:255, 1985.

284. Thompson CC, Bailey MK, Conroy JM, et al: Patient-controlled analgesia—advances in the last five years. *Anesthesiol Rev* 3:14, 1989.

285. Tamsen A: Patient characteristics influencing pain relief, in Harmer M, Rosen M, Papper EM (eds): *Patient-Controlled Analgesia.* Oxford, England, Blackwell Scientific, 1985, p. 30

286. Johnson LR, Magnani B, Chan V, et al: Modifiers of patient-controlled analgesia efficacy, 1. Locus of control. *Pain* 39:17, 1989.

287. Bennett RL, Batenhorst RL, Graves DA: Morphine titration in postoperative laparotomy patients using patient-controlled analgesia. *Curr Ther Res* 32:45, 1982.

288. Wakerlin G, Larson CP Jr: Spouse-controlled analgesia. *Anesth Analg* 70:119, 1990.

289. Broadman LM, Rice LJ, Vaughan M, et al: Parent-assisted "PCA" for postoperative pain control in young children. *Anesth Analg* 70:S34, 1990.

290. Dodd E, Wang J: Patient controlled analgesia for post-surgical pediatric patients ages 6-16 years. *Reg Anesth* 13(Suppl 2):41, 1988.

291. Broadman LM, Brown RE, Rice LJ, et al: Patient controlled analgesia in children and adolescents: A report of postoperative pain management in 150 patients. *Anesthesiology* 71:A1171, 1989.

292. Fedder IL, Vlasses PH, Mojaverian P, et al: Relationship of morphine-induced miosis to plasma concentration in normal subjects. *J Pharmaceutical Sciences* 73:1496, 1984.

293. Tress KH, El-Soky AA: Pupil responses to intravenous heroin (diamorphine) in dependent and non-dependent humans. *Br J Clin Pharm* 7:213, 1979.

294. Peacock JE, Henderson PD, Nimmo WS: Changes in pupil diameter after oral administration of codeine. *Br J Anaesth* 61:598, 1988.

295. Sinatra R: Patient-controlled epidural analgesia. *ASRA News* October 1992, pp. 2–3.

296. Chrubasik J, Wiemers K: Continuous-plus-on-demand epidural infusion of morphine for postoperative pain relief by means of a small, externally worn infusion device. *Anesthesiology* 62:263, 1985.

297. Sjöstrom S, Hartvig D, Tamsen A: Patient-controlled analgesia with extradural morphine or pethidine. *Br J Anaesth* 60:358, 1988.

298. Marlowe S, Engstrom R, White PF: Epidural patient-controlled analgesia (PCA): An alternative to continuous epidural infusions. *Pain* 37:97, 1989.

299. Gambling DR, Yu P, Cole C, et al: A comparative study of patient controlled epidural analgesia (PÇEA) and continuous infusion epidural analgesia (CIEA) during labour. *Can J Anaesth* 35:249, 1988.

300. Lysak S, Eisenach JC, Dobson CE: Patient-controlled epidural analgesia during labor: A comparison of three solutions with a continuous infusion control. *Anesthesiology* 72:44, 1990.

301. Bellamy CD, McDonnell FJ, Colclough GW, et al: Epidural infusion/PCA for pain control in pediatric patients. *Anesth Analg* 70:S19, 1990.

302. Ali J, Weisel RD, Layug AB, et al: Consequences of postoperative alterations in respiratory mechanics. *Am J Surg* 128:376, 1974.

303. Johnson WC: Postoperative ventilatory performance: Dependence upon surgical incision. *Am Surg* 41:615, 1975.

304. Craig DB: Postoperative recovery of pulmonary function. *Anesth Analg* 60:46, 1981.

305. Bishop MJ, Cheney FW: Respiratory complications of anesthesia and surgery. *Sem Anesth* 2:91, 1983.

306. Craig DB, Wahba WM, Don HF, et al: "Closing volume" and its relationship to gas exchange in seated and supine position. *J Appl Physiol* 31:717, 1971.

307. Rawal N, Sjostrand U, Christoffersson E, et al: Comparison of intramuscular and epidural morphine for postoperative analgesia in the grossly obese: Influence on postoperative ambulation and pulmonary function. *Anesth Analg* 63:583, 1984.

308. Kaplan JA, Miller ED, Gallagher EG: Postoperative analgesia for thoracotomy patients. *Anesth Analg* 54:773, 1975.

309. Toledo-Pereyra LH, DeMeester TR: Prospective randomized evaluation of intrathoracic intercostal nerve block with bupivacaine on postoperative ventilatory function. *Ann Thorac Surg* 27:203, 1979.

310. VadeBoncouer TR, Riegler FX, Gautt RS, et al: A randomized, double blind comparison of the effects of intrapleural bupivacaine and saline on morphine requirements and pulmonary function after cholecystectomy. *Anesthesiology* 71:339, 1989.

311. Simpson BR, Parkhouse J, Marshall R, et al: Extradural analgesia and the prevention of postoperative respiratory complications. *Br J Anaesth* 33:628, 1961.

312. Wahba WM, Craig DB, Don HF: Postoperative epidural analgesia: Effect on lung volumes. *Can Anaesth Soc J* 22:519, 1975.

313. Hasenbos M, van Egmond J, Gielen M, et al: Postoperative analgesia by high thoracic epidural versus intramuscular nicomorphine after thoracotomy, Part III. The effect of pre and post operative analgesia on morbidity. *Acta Anaesthesiol Scand* 31:608, 1987.

314. Bennett R, Batenhorst RL, Foster TS, et al: Postoperative pulmonary function with patient-controlled analgesia. *Anesth Analg* 61:171, 1982.

315. Pflug AE, Murphy TM, Butler SH, et al: The effects of postoperative peridural analgesia on pulmonary therapy and pulmonary complications. *Anesthesiology* 41:8, 1974.

316. Hjortso NC, Neumann P, Frosig F, et al: A controlled study on the effect of epidural analgesia with local anesthetics and morphine on morbidity after abdominal surgery. *Acta Anaesthesiol Scand* 29:790, 1985.

317. Jayr C, Thomas H, Rey A, et al: Postoperative pulmonary complications, epidural analgesia using bupivacaine and opioids versus parenteral opioids. *Anesthesiology* 78:666, 1993.

318. Cohen SE, Subak LL, Brose WG, et al: Analgesia after cesarean delivery: patient evaluations and costs of five opioid techniques. *Reg Anesth* 16:141, 1991.

319. Cheng EY, Wang-Cheng RW: Postoperative analgesia and respiratory function. *Anesthesiology* 71:A663, 1989.

320. Cuschieri RJ, Morran CG, Howie JC, et al: Postoperative pain and pulmonary complications: Comparison of three analgesic regimens. *Br J Surg* 72:495, 1985.

321. Kehlet H: Modification of responses to surgery by neural blockade: Clinical implications, in Cousins MJ, Bridenbaugh PO (eds): *Neural Blockade in Clinical Anesthesia and Pain Management,* ed 2. Philadelphia, Lippincott, 1988, p 145.

322. Kehlet H: Pain relief and modification of the stress response, in Cousins MJ, Phillips GD (eds): *Acute Pain Management.* New York, Churchill-Livingstone, 1986, p 49.

323. Weissman C: The metabolic response to stress: an overview and update. *Anesthesiology* 73:308, 1990.

324. Vedrinne C, Vedrinne JM, Guiraud M, et al: Nitrogen sparing effect of epidural administration of local anesthetics in colon surgery. *Anesth Analg* 69:354, 1989.

325. Carli F, Webster J, Pearson M, et al: Protein metabolism after abdominal surgery: effect of 24-h extradural block with local anesthetics. *Br J Anaesth* 67:729, 1991.

326. Rutberg H, Hakanson E, Andenberg B, et al: Effects of the extradural administration of morphine, or bupivacaine, on the endocrine response to upper abdominal surgery. *Br J Anaesth* 56:233, 1984.

327. Pother CE, Bridenbaugh LK, Reynolds F: Preoperative intercostal nerve block: Effect on the endocrine metabolic response to surgery. *Br J Anaesth* 60:730, 1988.

328. Webster J, Barnard M, Carli F: Metabolic response to colonic surgery: extradural vs continuous spinal. *Br J Anaesth* 67:467, 1991.

329. Lund JC, Hansen OB, Mogensen T, et al: Effect of thoracic epidural bupivacaine on somatosensory evoked potentials after dermatomal stimulation. *Anesth Analg* 66:731, 1987.

330. Swinamer DL, Phang PT, Jones RL, et al: Effect of routine administration of analgesia on energy expenditure in critically ill patients. *Chest* 92:4, 1988.

331. Scott NB, Mogensen T, Bigler D, et al: Continuous thoracic extradural 0.5% bupivacaine with or without morphine: Effect on quality of blockade, lung function and the surgical stress response. *Br J Anaesth* 62:253, 1989.

332. Zwarts SJ, Hasenbos MAMW, Gielen MJM, et al: The effect of continuous epidural analgesia with sufentanil and bupivacaine during and after thoracic surgery on the plasma cortisol concentration and pain relief. *Reg Anesth* 14:183, 1989.

333. Arnold DE, Coombs DW, Yeager MP, et al: Single blend comparison of epidural clonidine epidural morphine and parenteral narcotic analgesia upon postabdominal surgery neuroendocrine stress response (cortisol). *Anesth Analg* 68:S11, 1989.

334. Scheinin B, Asantila R, Orko R: The effect of bupivacaine and morphine on pain and bowel function after colonic surgery. *Acta Anaesthesiol Scand* 31:161, 1987.

335. Konturek SJ: Opiates and the gastrointestinal tract. *Am J Gastroenterol* 74:285, 1980.

336. Thorén T, Wattwil M: Effects on gastric emptying of thoracic epidural analgesia with morphine or bupivacaine. *Anesth Analg* 67:687, 1988.

337. Thören SE, Wattwil M, Näslund I: Postoperative epidural morphine, but not epidural bupivacaine, delays gastric emptying on the first day after cholecystectomy. *Reg Anesth* 17:91, 1992.

338. Wattwil M, Thorén T, Hennerdal S, et al: Epidural analgesia with bupivacaine reduces postoperative paralytic ileus after hysterectomy. *Anesth Analg* 68:353, 1989.

339. England DW, Davis JJ, Timmins AE, et al: Gastric emptying: A study to compare the effects of intrathecal morphine and IM papaveretum analgesia. *Br J Anaesth* 59:1403, 1987.

340. O'Gara PT: The hemodynamic consequences of pain and its management. *J Intensive Care Med* 3:3, 1988.

341. Breslow MJ, Jordan DA, Christopherson R, et al: Epidural morphine decreases postoperative hypertension by attenuating sympathetic nervous system hyperactivity. *JAMA* 261:3577, 1989.

342. Bridenbaugh PO: Anesthesia and influence on hospitalization time. *Reg Anesth* 7:S151, 1982.

343. Finley RJ, Kerri-Szanto M, Boyd D: New analgesic agents and techniques shorten postoperative hospital stay. *Pain* 2(Suppl): S397, 1984.

344. Ross EL, Perumbetti P: PCA: Is it cost effective when used for postoperative pain management? *Anesthesiology* 69:A710, 1988.

345. Stenkamp SJ, Easterling TR, Chadwick HS: Effect of epidural and intrathecal morphine on the length of hospital stay after caesarean section. *Anesth Analg* 68:66, 1989.

346. Bellamy CD, McDonnell FJ, Colclough GW: Postoperative epidural pain management results in shorter hospital stay than IV PCA morphine: A comparison in anterior cruciate ligament repair. *Anesthesiology* 71:A685, 1989.

347. Lamer TJ: Postoperative pain management with epidural narcotics results in shorter hospital stay than IV or IM narcotics. *Reg Anesth* 15(1S):83, 1990.

348. Tuman KJ, McCarthy RJ, March R, et al: Epidural anesthesia/analgesia improves outcome after major vascular surgery: A hypothesis revisited. *Anesth Analg* 72:S302, 1991.

349. de Leon-Casasola OA, Parker B, Schwartz C, et al: Postoperative epidural analgesia decreases length of hospitalization and ICU stays in high risk surgical patients. *Anesthesiology* 77:A899, 1992.

350. Ganz SD, Williams-Russo P, Heim LH, et al: Does epidural anesthesia enhance the rate of rehabilitation following total knee arthroplasty? *Reg Anesth* 18(2S):5, 1993.

351. Walmsley PNH, Colclough GW, Mazloomdoost M, et al: Epidural PCA/infusion for postnephrectomy pain: Shorter hospitalization. *Anesthesiology* 71:A683, 1989.

352. Grass JA, Zuckerman RL, Tsao H, et al: Patient-controlled epidural analgesia results in shorter hospital stay after cesarean section. *Reg Anesth* 15(1s):26, 1990.

168. Epistaxis

Daniel Y. Kim

General Considerations

Although frequently minor and self-limiting, epistaxis can at times be profuse and life-threatening. The vast majority of nosebleeds stop spontaneously and are never seen by a physician. Depending on the site of bleeding, epistaxis can be broadly classified as anterior or posterior. The majority of nosebleeds are anterior and involve the anterior portions of the nasal septum, or turbinates. These bleeds are usually relatively minor and can be easily controlled by applying pressure for several minutes. Some require cauterization or simple anterior packing. Posterior nosebleeds are more difficult to control and, in almost all cases, require posterior packing. Nosebleeds are always a frightening experience for the patient. In some severe cases of epistaxis, a large amount of blood can be lost in a short period of time, and the bleeding can have grave consequences. In general, younger patients are more likely to have an anterior bleeding point. Venous epistaxis is characterized by constant bleeding, ranging from mild oozing to moderately heavy bleeding. With arterial bleeding, there is usually a history of episodic bleeding, with each episode being quite profuse.

Because of the superficial location of the blood vessels in the nasal mucosa, minimal trauma can initiate epistaxis. Dryness, irritation, digital manipulation, bleeding tendencies, hypertension, and nasal or facial trauma are other common factors associated with epistaxis. Whatever the etiology, a vessel ruptures and bleeds. In patients with no obvious nasal trauma, the possibility of coagulopathy should be excluded by obtaining a careful personal and family history, including history of aspirin or anticoagulant use. Hematologic neoplasms, which decrease platelet counts and/or clotting factors, can lead to susceptibility for epistaxis. Chronic liver dysfunction can have a similar effect. Other less common causes include tumors within the nasal cavity, the paranasal sinuses, or the nasopharynx. In a young male teenager with a history of recurrent massive epistaxis without an obvious cause, the possibility of juvenile nasopharyngeal angiofibroma should be considered in the differential diagnosis. In such a case, the evaluation should include nasopharyngoscopy and radiologic studies.

Blood tests should include a complete blood count, prothrombin time, partial thromboplastin time, platelet count, and serum electrolyte panel. If there is a history of extensive blood loss, or if the hematocrit is depressed below 30, the patient should be typed and cross-matched and transfused as the situation warrants. An electrocardiogram should be obtained. Vital signs should be monitored to identify hypertension or hypovolemic hypotension. All underlying medical conditions should be treated aggressively [1].

Blood Supply

Five arteries supply the internal nose on either side of the body. The anterior ethmoidal artery and posterior ethmoidal artery are branches of the ophthalmic artery. The sphenopalatine artery and the greater palatine artery are branches of the internal maxillary artery. The septal branch of the superior labial artery is a branch of the facial artery (Fig. 168-1B). Thus, the nose is

supplied by branches of both the internal and external carotid arteries. However, it is the external carotid artery system that plays a dominant role in epistaxis [2].

Three of the five arteries divide into lateral and medial, or septal, branches: the anterior ethmoidal artery, the posterior ethmoidal artery, and the important sphenopalatine artery (Fig. 168-1). The sphenopalatine artery enters the nose from the pterygopalatine fossa by way of the sphenopalatine foramen and divides into lateral and septal branches. The lateral branch supplies all of the lateral wall of the nose, including the turbinates and the meati of the sinuses. The septal branch crosses the anterior wall of the sphenoid sinus and supplies most of the middle and posterior portions of the septum, and contributes to Kisselbach's plexus on the anterior and inferior portion of the nasal septum [3] (Fig. 168-1B). Most posterior nosebleeds are due to rupture of this artery.

Of the ethmoidal arteries, the anterior ethmoidal artery is the larger and contributes more significantly to both the septum and the lateral wall of the nose (Fig. 168-1). The greater palatine artery travels from the pterygopalatine fossa through the greater palatine canal to emerge from the greater palatine foramen on its way to the palate. It then travels anteriorly where its terminal branch travels through the incisive canal into Kisselbach's area to supply the septum. The septal branch of the superior labial artery supplies the medial wall of the vestibule of the nose and contributes to Kisselbach's area.

Causes of Epistaxis

Direct trauma to the nose either by digital manipulation or external force is a common cause of epistaxis. Drying of the nasal mucosa caused by dry air due to central heating, wood-burning stove, or fireplace is a frequent cause of nosebleeds in the winter. Septal deformity with alteration of normal airflow patterns within the nasal cavity can cause excessive drying of the nasal mucosa, leading to epistaxis. Benign and malignant tumors of the nose, sinuses, or nasopharynx, as well as granulomatous diseases such as Wegener's granulomatosis, tuberculosis, and sarcoidosis, can lead to bleeding.

Systemic causes of epistaxis include use of aspirin and anticoagulants, thrombocytopenia of any cause, and hereditary diseases such as hemophilia and Osler-Weber-Rendu disease. In such patients, the underlying coagulopathy must be corrected before reasonable control of bleeding can be expected. As long as the basic pathophysiology is active, the bleeding will continue unabated. Infusion of vitamin K, platelets, fresh-frozen plasma, or clotting factors should be instituted when indicated. In some cases, no obvious cause can be found [4].

Instruments and Materials

Effective control of epistaxis requires the availability and use of a variety of instruments and materials such as suction, bayonet forceps, headlight, topical cocaine solution or a mixture of phenylephrine and tetracaine hydrochloride, cotton balls, cottonoid

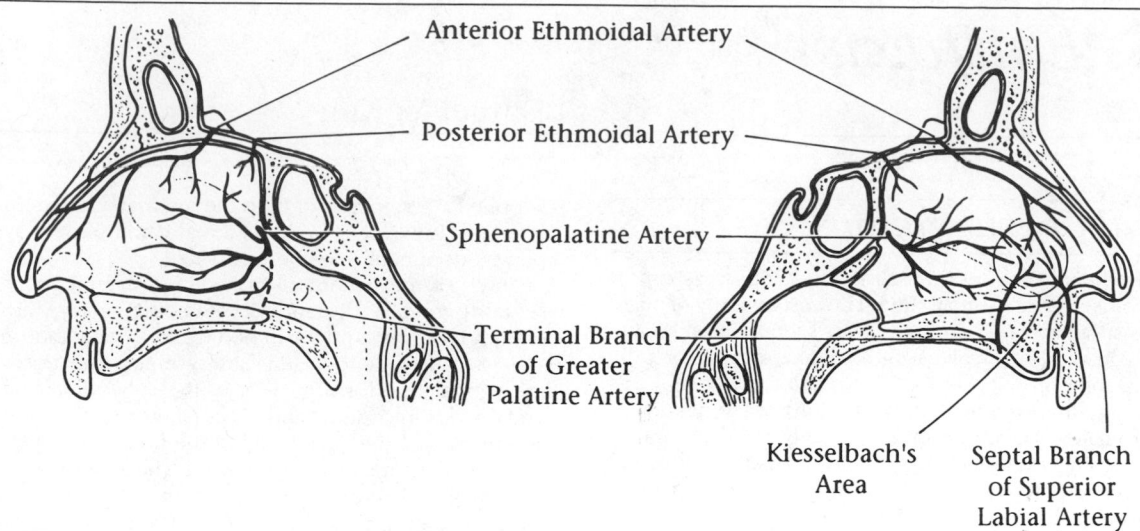

Fig. 168-1. *A*, Blood supply to the lateral wall of nose. *B*, Blood supply to the nasal septum.

pledgets, a variety of nasal packing materials such as petrolatum gauze strips, preformed nasal tampons, and nasal balloons (Fig. 168-2), as well as Gelfoam, Surgicel, Oxycel, and thrombin. The key to successful management of most nosebleeds lies in identification and visualization of the bleeding point.

Anterior Epistaxis

The most common site of anterior epistaxis is Kisselbach's plexus (Little's area), located on the anterior-inferior portion of the nasal septum. Ninety percent of all nosebleeds occur in this

Fig. 168-2. *A*, Petrolatum gauze packing. *B*, Merocel nasal tampon. *C*, Epistat nasal balloon.

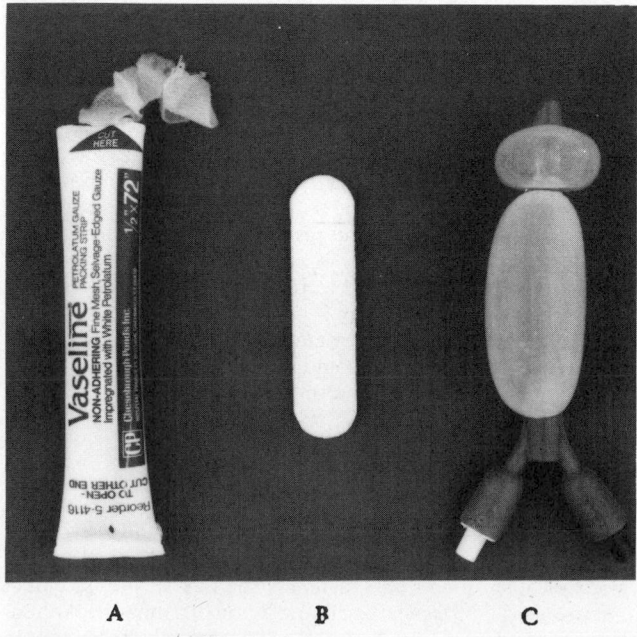

area, which contains a plexus of vessels representing the end branches of vessels supplying the septum (i.e., the sphenopalatine, anterior ethmoidal, greater palatine, and superior labial arteries). The posterior ethmoidal artery supplies a small portion of the posterior-superior nasal septum and does not contribute to any significant degree to the plexus. Other sites of anterior nosebleeds are the anterior portion of the inferior turbinate, the inferior meatus, and the superior portion of the septum.

Anterior bleeds are usually mild and self-limiting and can be easily controlled by applying digital pressure over the mobile lower half of the nose by the thumb and the index finger. When there is active bleeding, a concerted effort should be made to locate and visualize the bleeding point. The patient should be placed in a sitting or a semierect position, and the patient's head should be tilted slightly forward to minimize bleeding into the nasopharynx and oropharynx. All clots should be carefully suctioned out of the nostrils while minimizing trauma from instrumentation. The source of bleeding may be visible after this simple maneuver. If there is significant oozing or bleeding, cotton strips or cottonoids saturated with either 4% cocaine or a 50/50 mixture of 2% tetracaine hydrochloride and 0.25% phenylephrine should be placed gently in the nostrils for approximately 10 minutes. Two or three strips are usually required to cover the anterior, posterior, and superior portions of the septum and lateral wall. This procedure can be repeated several times as needed. This maneuver provides both nasal mucosal anesthesia and vasoconstriction of nasal vessels, which slows down the bleeding. This allows easy visualization of the exact bleeding site so that cauterization with silver nitrate sticks or electrocautery can be accomplished.

If the vessels continue to ooze after this maneuver or appear to be unstable, anterior packing may be necessary. Either half-inch petrolatum gauze (Fig. 168-2*A*) or a preformed packing such as Merocel surgical sponge (Fig. 168-2*B*) can be used. The preformed sponges can be trimmed to size prior to insertion. The packing must be placed firmly enough to tamponade the bleeding points. If gauze strips are used, the first strip should be placed along the floor of the nose and advanced posteriorly as far as it will go into the choana. Subsequent strips should be laid over the preceding strip in an anterior to posterior direction and packed down firmly until the entire nasal cavity is packed from the floor to the roof (Fig. 168-3). The end of the gauze strip should be brought out anteriorly and placed in an easily accessible portion of the nose for subsequent removal of the

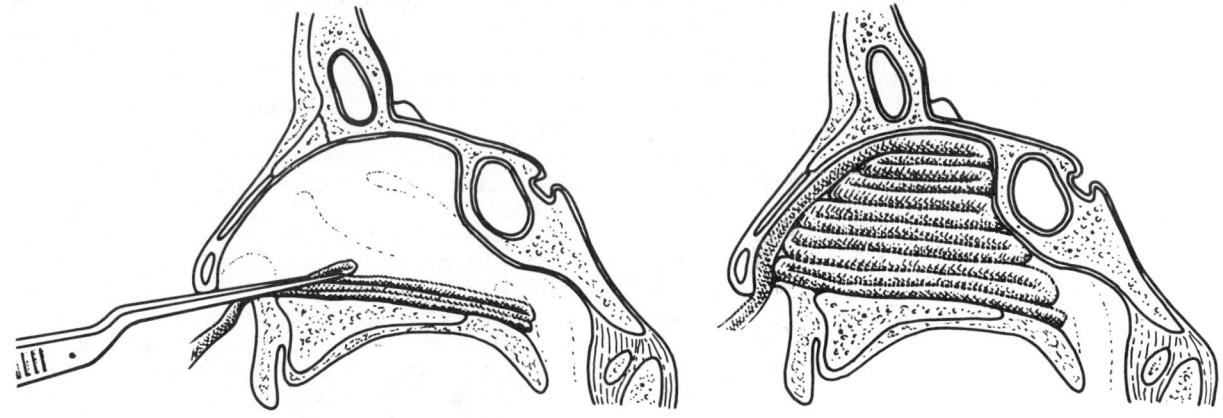

A. Start packing along the floor of the nose

B. Fully packed nose

Fig. 168-3. A, Start packing along the floor of the nose. *B,* Fully packed nose.

packing in an orderly fashion. The strips should be left in place for 24 to 48 hours, and the patient should be placed on oral broad-spectrum antibiotics until the packing is removed. The blood in the packing material makes an excellent culture medium for bacteria.

If the bleeding appears to be from the superior portion of the nose, it is likely due to ethmoidal arteries. In such cases, the bleeding point will be difficult to visualize. These bleeds are best treated with nasal packing as described above. The superior-most portions of the nose are better packed with gauze strips than with the preformed variety of packs. Surgicel, Oxycel, Gelfoam, and Avitene can aid in control of bleeding when placed directly on the bleeding areas and should be used accordingly.

Unless there is a medical contraindication, patients can be sent home and asked to return in a day or two for removal of packing. They should be instructed to keep the head elevated 30 to 45 degrees while sleeping, to avoid bending over or lifting heavy objects, to avoid any strenuous activity, and to use humidification. Blowing of the nose and digital manipulation should be strictly avoided.

Posterior Epistaxis

Difficult nosebleeds generally involve posterior portions of the nose and are usually due to bleeding from the sphenopalatine artery and its branches. Patients with posterior epistaxis are usually older, may be hypertensive or debilitated, or have systemic problems. Bleeding is usually very brisk and can be intermittent. The bleeding point is usually not visualized, and active bleeding can be seen going down the back of the nose into the pharynx.

The initial treatment should be the same as for anterior epistaxis. The patient should be placed in an erect position with the head tilted slightly forward, and all clots should be suctioned out of the nostrils and pharynx. Good vasoconstriction and topical anesthesia should be obtained by careful and exact placement of cotton strips soaked in cocaine or tetracaine hydrochloride/phenylephrine solution, as outlined earlier for an-

terior epistaxis. It is important to place these strips as far posteriorly as possible. However, most posterior bleeds will not be effectively controlled by this method and will require posterior packing.

For all practical purposes, the traditional posterior gauze packing has been replaced by balloon catheters. Surgical sponges with posterior portions designed to flare out into the nasopharynx are also commercially available. Although Foley catheters were used for posterior packing in the past, these too have been replaced by commercial epistaxis balloons designed specifically for this purpose. The Epistat nasal balloon (Fig. 168-2C) has both anterior and posterior chambers, which can be inflated independently with either air or water. These devices are easy to insert and allow quick control of brisk posterior and/or anterior bleeding. Before insertion, the balloons should be tested to ensure that they are working properly and to obtain an estimate of how much air or water is required to inflate them to desired size. One should keep in mind that air can leak out of the balloons after a time. In addition, the weight of the water in the balloons can pull the balloon away from the site of bleeding.

The technique for inserting these devices is the same as for inserting a nasogastric tube. The device should be coated with lubricant and inserted gently along the floor of the nose into the nasopharynx. This can sometimes be difficult in a patient with severe septal deviation but can be managed in most instances. The posterior balloon should then be inflated with 10 to 15 ml of air or water. When the balloon is inflated, all patients will feel extreme discomfort—and sometimes pain—within the nasopharynx, and the actual extent of inflation should be titrated to the tolerance of the patient. The soft palate can bulge slightly, but the balloon should not be inflated to the extent that it can be seen bulging into the oropharynx. Next, with gentle anterior traction placed on the device, the anterior balloon should be inflated. This usually requires 15 to 30 ml of air or water. Again, the extent of inflation should be titrated to the tolerance of the patient. The balloon should be large enough to cause tamponade and to prevent posterior displacement, but not so large as to cause unbearable pain. Individual differences in the size of the nasal cavity, as well as any septal deviation, should be taken into account. It is also well to remember that the anterior nasal septum is cartilaginous and quite flexible, which will tend to make it bulge into the opposite nasal cavity. As such, the opposite nasal cavity may need to be packed with petrolatum gauze to maintain some counterpressure and support. In some severe cases, a second device may need to be inserted on the opposite side in order to control the posterior epistaxis. Care should be taken to ensure that the stem of the device does not rest on the nasal ala, which can cause pressure necrosis. This can be accomplished by wrapping a soft material such as Xeroform or gauze around the stem. In the rare instance that bleeding is not controlled by this method, the classic posterior pack made of a gauze sponge should be placed transorally into the nasopharynx and secured anteriorly over a gauze stent with a silk suture or umbilical tape.

All patients with posterior epistaxis should be admitted to the hospital and placed on bed rest in a semi-Fowler's position. The packings should remain in place for about 3 days, during which time the patients should be maintained on broad-spectrum antibiotics to prevent sinusitis. Patients with posterior packs will experience some degree of alteration in respiratory physiology. Typically, they will experience a lowering of PO_2 with or without a rise in PCO_2 [5]. These changes are postulated to be due to a "nasopulmonary reflex" resulting in a decrease in pulmonary compliance [6,7,8]. Furthermore, with their nostrils obstructed with packing and clots, they become obligate mouth breathers, which will dry out the oropharyngeal and hypopharyngeal mucosa, resulting in irritation and sore throat. Therefore, humidified oxygen via an open face mask should be provided. Some of the preformed sponges and balloons have built-in nasal airways, but it is still a good idea to provide humidification and oxygen. Analgesia and sedation can decrease the discomfort associated with a posterior pack and should be used as needed. The patient should be observed for signs of hypoxemia, hypoperfusion, and nitrogen retention. After about 3 days, the packings are removed and the patient is observed for 24 hours before discharge.

Persistent or Recurrent Bleeding

Despite good packing and appropriate medical care, some patients will have persistent or recurrent bleeding. Surgery in the form of arterial ligation may be indicated in some of these patients. Surgical intervention should be considered earlier in elderly patients in poor health and in patients with poor cardiopulmonary reserve. As a rule, debilitated patients tolerate nasal packing less well and are more prone to complications, not only from the bleeding but also from the packing. There is a higher morbidity associated with posterior packing than with surgical interruption of the blood supply [9].

Surgery involves ligation of the internal maxillary artery and its branches through the transmaxillary approach. This will effectively stop the bleeding in most patients by interrupting the blood supply of sphenopalatine and greater palatine arteries [10,11,12]. The external carotid artery can be ligated in certain selected cases. In rare cases, especially when bleeding is from the superior nasal cavity, the ethmoidal arteries may need to be ligated selectively or in addition to the internal maxillary artery. These are supplied by the ophthalmic artery, which is a branch of the internal carotid system [13].

The surgical approach for internal maxillary artery ligation is through an incision in the upper gingivolabial sulcus, as in the Caldwell-Luc procedure. The anterior wall of the maxillary sinus is exposed by reflecting the overlying cheek soft tissues superiorly. The sinus is entered with a chisel, and the opening is enlarged with rongeurs. The posterior wall of the sinus is then exposed and the bony wall is removed widely to expose the contents of the pterygomaxillary fossa. The internal maxillary artery and its branches are dissected and ligated with vascular clips. The morbidity from this procedure is surprisingly low. These patients do extremely well and are able to go home within a day or two of the operation.

An alternative approach for exposure of the internal maxillary artery is via the intraoral route. This method provides surgical access to the first and second portions of the artery as it travels behind the ramus of the mandible [14]. The technique does not require a Caldwell-Luc operation and can be used in patients with maxillary fractures or malignancies within the maxillary sinus or in the soft tissues of the cheek. The incision is made at the gingivobuccal sulcus at the level of the third molar and extended inferiorly along the ramus of the mandible. After removing or retracting buccal fat, the maxillary artery is identified in the space created between the mandibular ramus and temporalis muscle, and medium size vascular clips are applied.

A surgical alternative to internal maxillary artery ligation is mobilization and lateral displacement of the nasal septum from the maxillary crest. This maneuver permits excellent visualization of the lateral nasal wall and posterior nasal cavity, which allows electrocoagulation of bleeding sites [15].

Surgical control of ethmoidal arteries is approached through a Lynch incision midway between the medial canthus of the eye and the bridge of the nose. The periosteum of the medial orbital wall is incised and reflected posteriorly. With the orbit retracted medially, the anterior and posterior ethmoidal arteries are identified in a strict anatomical dissection, and they are either ligated with vascular clips or cauterized [16].

An alternative to surgery is embolization of the internal maxillary artery and its branches in certain selected cases [17,18]. However, these embolized vessels tend to recanalize with time and may require either reembolization or surgical ligation. Nevertheless, this can be a viable alternative in a patient who is not a good surgical candidate.

References

1. Chapnik JS, Noyek AM: Medical therapy in rhinology. *Otolaryngol Clin North Am* 17:662, 1984.
2. Shaheen OH: Epistaxis, in Scott-Brown's Otol, vol 4, 5th ed. Boston, Butterworths, 1987, Chapter 16, pp 272–282.
3. Paff GH: *Anatomy of the Head and Neck.* Philadelphia, WB Saunders, 1973.
4. Ballenger JJ: Epistaxis, rhinophyma, nasal septal perforation, and choanal atresia, in Ballenger JJ (ed): *Diseases of the Nose, Throat, Ear, Head, and Neck.* 14th ed. Philadelphia, Lea & Febiger, 1991, Chapter 8, pp 150–157.
5. Ogura JH, Unno T, Nelson JR: Baseline values in pulmonary mechanics for physiologic surgery of the nose: Preliminary report. *Ann Otol* 78:369, 1968.
6. Cassisi NJ, Biller HF, Ogura JH: Changes in arterial oxygen tension and pulmonary mechanics with the use of posterior nasal packing. *Laryngoscope* 81:1261, 1971.
7. Ogura J, Harvey J: Nasopulmonary mechanics: Experimental evidence of the influence of the upper airway upon the lower. *Acta Otolaryngol* 71:123, 1971.
8. Ogura J: Physiologic relationship of the upper and lower airways. *Ann Otolaryngol* 79:495, 1970.
9. Schaitkin B, Strauss M, Houch Jr: Epistaxis: Medical versus surgical therapy: A comparison of efficacy, complications and economic considerations. *Laryngoscope* 97:1392, 1987.
10. Pearson BW, MacKenzie RG, Goodman WS: The anatomical basis of transantral ligation of the maxillary artery in severe epistaxis. *Laryngoscope* 79:969, 1969.
11. Simpson PJ, Janfaza P, Becker JD: Transantral sphenopalatine artery ligation. *Laryngoscope* 92:1001, 1982.
12. Gergely Z: Transmaxillary ligature of the arteria maxillaris interna (Seiffert's method). *Acta Otolaryngol* 22:142, 1935.
13. Kirchner JA, Yanagisawa E, Crelin FS Jr: Surgical anatomy of the ethmoidal arteries: A laboratory study of 150 orbits. *Arch Otolaryngol* 74:382, 1961.
14. Maceri DR, Makielski KH: Intraoral ligation of the maxillary artery for posterior epistaxis. *Laryngoscope* 94:737, 1984.

15. Anderson RG, Shannon DN, Schaefer SD, Raney LA: A surgical alternative to internal maxillary artery ligation for posterior epistaxis. *Otolaryngol Head Neck Surg* 92:427, 1984.
16. Weddell G, MacBeth RG, Sharp HS, Calver CA: The surgical treatment of severe epistaxis in relation to the ethmoidal arteries. *Br J Surg* 33:387, 1946.
17. Robertson GH, Reardon EJ: Angiography and embolization of the internal maxillary artery for posterior epistaxis. *Arch Otolaryngol* 105:333, 1979.
18. Vanwyck LG, Vinuela F, Heeneman H: Therapeutic embolization for severe epistaxis. *J Otolaryngol* 11:271, 1982.

169. Esophageal Perforation and Mediastinitis

Frank W. Sellke

Overview

Although the management of many illnesses has been improved and defined over the past decades, the treatment of esophageal perforation and acute mediastinitis continues to be controversial and a challenge to physicians and surgeons. A documented case of esophageal perforation was first described in 1724 by Boerhaave [1]. In an extensive and complete description of clinical and pathologic findings, Boerhaave described the distal esophageal perforation in Admiral Baron de Wessenaer after a long night of overindulgence of food and alcohol, culminating in repeated forceful retching. Although the Baron's clinical course resulted in his death, the past several decades have seen significantly more favorable, yet far less than perfect, rates of survival after perforation.

With the rapid development and expansion of cardiac surgery over the past 50 years, the occurrence of postoperative wound infection and mediastinitis, unfortunately, has become a common complication associated with prolonged length of hospital stay, great expense, and significant mortality. Descending pharyngeal infection, which was formerly the most common cause of mediastinitis, still presents on occasion even in the present era of potent systemic antibiotics.

This chapter describes the presenting signs and diagnostic modalities involved in the management of perforation of the esophagus and acute mediastinal infection and presents the various methods of management of these serious and challenging clinical problems.

Esophageal Perforation

ETIOLOGY. Esophageal perforation is a potentially life-threatening condition that requires rapid diagnosis and immediate treatment in order to prevent catastrophic consequences. While spontaneous rupture of a normal esophagus may occur during retching or other conditions associated with increased intraesophageal pressure [1], the more common scenario is related to instrumentation with or without associated esophageal pathology.

Perforation of the cervical esophagus may occur in patients with bony spurs of the cervical vertebrae that perforate the posterior aspect of the esophageal wall at the time of rigid esophagoscopy due to a crush-type injury [2,3]. In addition, perforation may occur as a result of a direct "spearing" of the organ with a rigid or flexible esophagoscope during an examination. While rigid esophagoscopy in the past was a frequent cause of esophageal perforation, flexible endoscopy today is more frequently utilized and probably results in a lower relative incidence of perforation. This type of perforation generally occurs at the level of the cricopharyngeal muscle [3,4]. The other leading cause of iatrogenic esophageal perforation is dilation of a stricture with either pneumatic or conventional dilators. Perforations secondary to dilation generally occur in the mid to distal portion of the esophagus, since it is in this region that diseases such as achalasia and esophageal reflux cause strictures. Perforation following esophagoscopy, dilatation, or other instrumentation of the mid or distal esophagus usually occurs in association with a stricture, obstructing malignancy, or foreign body. The absence of a serosal layer in the esophageal wall renders this tubular structure more prone to rupture at lower pressures than the remainder of the alimentary tract. Perforations of the lower esophagus frequently occur into the left thoracic cavity and manifest with a left pleural effusion. Perforations of the mid esophagus tend to cause right pleural effusions. These paths are followed since only small amounts of mediastinal tissue surround the organ in these respective regions to support and buttress the esophagus [5]. Rare causes of esophageal perforation include blunt [6] or penetrating trauma, foreign bodies [7], and chronic pressure with erosion due to an inflated endotracheal tube cuff or other instrument [8–11]. Finally, inadvertent esophageal perforation may occur during thyroidectomy [12], proximal gastric vagotomy [13,14], or other procedures in the neck or mediastinum [5] (Table 169-1).

CLINICAL MANIFESTATIONS AND DIAGNOSIS. Except under conditions in which the patient is heavily sedated or under general anesthesia, the manifestations of acute esophageal perforation are usually apparent immediately and are frequently catastrophic. Nevertheless, esophageal perforation may be confused with other disorders, such as perforated peptic ulcer, pancreatitis, myocardial infarction, or aortic dissection [5,15]. Since esophageal perforation in the cervical region most frequently occurs during or following instrumentation, any abnormal sensation following the procedure should alert the clinician to the possibility of an esophageal injury. Early signs include neck pain or stiffness, difficulty swallowing, cough, or the presence of cervical emphysema [15,16]. Because of the relative spatial discontinuity of the cervical esophagus with the

Table 169-1. Causes of Esophageal Perforation

I. Spontaneous
   A. During increased intraesophageal pressure
   B. Esophageal carcinoma
   C. Peptic ulceration
II. Traumatic
   A. Gunshot wound
   B. Laceration due to knife injury
   C. Blunt trauma
   D. Foreign body
   E. Swallowed caustic agents
III. Instrumentation
   A. Dilation
   B. Esophagoscopy
     1. Rigid
     2. Flexible
   C. Intubation
IV. Postsurgical
   A. Anastomotic leak
   B. Inadvertent injury during operation
     1. Vagotomy
     2. Thyroidectomy
     3. Esophageal myotomy
     4. Aortic surgery

mediastinum, the patient with perforation may not develop signs of serious illness for several hours after the procedure.

In contrast to cervical esophageal perforation, perforation of the intrathoracic esophagus generally results in a more rapid progression to acute illness due to the quick spread of infection, the rapid development of mediastinal inflammation and fluid sequestration [15,16], and the mechanisms of injury. Contamination of the pleural space occurs early, resulting in pleural effusion. Gastric, duodenal, and esophageal secretions may accumulate within the mediastinum, causing further inflammation, fluid sequestration, and signs of systemic illness. Chest pain occurs immediately or within minutes, and dyspnea is frequently a prominent feature. Intraabdominal esophageal perforations result in signs of peritonitis and epigastric pain. Systemic signs of peritonitis and sepsis generally occur within several minutes or hours of perforation.

A delay in the diagnosis of esophageal perforation following instrumentation is unfortunately frequent. This may occur due to confusion with other illnesses or a denial of this possible complication following instrumentation. Plain roentgenograms may show the presence of cervical, mediastinal, intrapleural, or intraabdominal free air. In addition, increased soft tissue densities may be seen within the mediastinum or within the cervical tissue planes [17]. Fluid obtained by thoracentesis that shows the presence of food particles and an elevated amylase level, or a pH less than 6, is highly suggestive if not pathognomonic of esophageal perforation [18]. In the event of a suspected perforation, esophageal contrast studies should be performed promptly. A water-soluble contrast medium should be used initially to prevent contamination of the mediastinum, pleural cavity, or peritoneal cavity with barium [19]. If these studies fail to show an injury, the examination may be repeated with a barium-containing contrast medium if the diagnosis is still in doubt and a small perforation is suspected [4,20]. Laboratory findings frequently include an elevation of the white blood count and hematocrit, the latter reflecting fluid sequestration. However, these laboratory findings are nonspecific. Esophageal endoscopy is rarely needed to confirm the diagnosis [16] and may lead to an enlargement of the perforation. However, some feel that this is an underutilized modality in the evaluation of esophageal perforation. [21,22]. Computed tomography may be useful if the diagnosis remains in doubt [18,22], especially if

there is a delay in the diagnosis of the suspected perforation. Findings suggestive of perforation or associated mediastinitis include soft tissue emphysema in the mediastinum surrounding the esophagus or cervical region, air–fluid levels and abscess cavities adjacent to the esophagus, or the actual demonstration of a perforation [18,22]. In addition, computed tomography may be used to direct catheter drainage following surgical intervention and to assess the progression of infection or inflammation following surgical treatment [23,24].

MANAGEMENT. Once the diagnosis of acute esophageal perforation is confirmed, the initiation of broad-spectrum intravenous antibiotics, which cover the multitude of both aerobic and anaerobic bacterial species in the oral cavity and the esophagus, should be immediate. In addition, hydration and other resuscitative measures should be instituted without delay. Definitive treatment options for esophageal perforation traditionally have been surgical, although nonoperative management may be utilized in selected cases if the perforation is small, extra-esophageal contamination is limited [25–29], and a surgeon trained in the management of esophageal disease is involved in the decision-making.

Surgical treatment of perforation of the cervical esophagus is approached through an incision anterior to the left sternomastoid muscle and anterior to the carotid sheath [30]. Perforations of the upper thoracic esophagus can be approached through a right posterolateral thoracotomy in the fourth or fifth interspace. Perforations of the distal intrathoracic esophagus are best approached through a thoracotomy in the left sixth or seventh interspace [15,16]. Abdominal esophageal perforations may be approached either through a low left thoracotomy or a laparotomy. If the perforation is recent and associated with little destruction of esophageal tissue and minimal surrounding inflammation is present, primary closure should be attempted. If possible, the mucosal and muscular layers should be closed separately and the closure reinforced with surrounding tissue such as pleura [31,32]. If the diagnosis has been delayed, if the perforation has resulted in substantial esophageal tissue destruction, or if gross inflammation has developed, wide external drainage may be required with or without an attempt at primary closure. Large drainage tubes should be placed in proximity to the esophageal perforation but away from large vascular structures to avoid the possibility of vascular erosion and exsanguinating hemorrhage. In the case of cervical perforation, a soft Penrose drain or flat, closed drain should be placed in the area of the repair. In the case of perforations associated with malignant obstruction, massive esophageal necrosis, or lye ingestion, esophageal resection may be necessary. In the latter case, resection may be performed either through a thoracotomy or via a transhiatal non-thoracotomy approach. If the stomach is available for use in reconstruction, primary reconstruction should be attempted if the patient is not so unstable that a large and possibly prolonged operation is contraindicated. Otherwise, a delayed reconstruction using either the stomach or colon may be performed after initial control of the fistula and infection. Perforations associated with functional obstruction such as with achalasia are best repaired by primary closure and the performance of a myotomy opposite the perforation. An anti-reflux procedure is generally not required [5]; however, a Belsey-type operation may offer the advantage of reinforcing the closure, especially if the perforation occurs distally [33]. In the event of massive tissue destruction in a gravely ill patient who would not likely survive a primary reconstruction, thoracotomy and drainage with irrigation may be indicated. A T-tube may be placed through the perforation to create a controlled esophagocutaneous fistula [34]. Alternatively, the area of the perforation may be excluded and a proximal diverting loop and cervical esophagostomy may be created [35,36]. To prevent gastroesophageal reflux, ligation of the distal gastroesophageal junction with an absorbable suture may be warranted [35]. A gastrostomy or feeding jejunostomy tube should be placed to provide access for enteral nutrition.

When esophageal perforation is due to instrumentation and results in limited contamination and minimal systemic signs, nonoperative management may be instituted. The justification for this approach is that (1) perforations are now usually due to instrumentation and are generally more limited and associated with less tissue inflammation and contamination; (2) antibiotics have been found to be effective in controlling infection; (3) diagnostic modalities such as computed tomography provide the ability to closely monitor the degree of inflammation and tissue destruction and provide a method to drain the thoracic cavity through percutaneous methods; and (4) methods of enteral and parenteral nutrition may be utilized to maintain nutritional status during recovery [15,24,25,26,37,38].

Nonoperative therapy is best used when esophageal perforation is due to instrumental manipulation and the perforation is small and pleural contamination is limited [25–29]. When perforation occurs during dilation for peptic stricture or other conditions associated with periesophageal sclerosis and fibrosis, contamination tends to be more limited than when perforation occurs in a nondiseased organ. In addition, patients with esophageal perforation diagnosed several days after injury and with minimal symptoms may be treated nonoperatively. When distal esophageal obstruction is present, nonoperative management is unlikely to succeed. According to Cameron et al. [26], the criteria for attempting nonoperative management of esophageal perforations include the following:

1. The perforation should be diagnosed quickly, or if the presentation is late, there should be evidence that the infection is walled off.
2. The infected cavity should be well drained, with minimal intrathoracic soilage.
3. There should be no intake of food between the time of injury and the time of diagnosis.
4. No distal obstruction by tumor or stricture should be present.
5. The patient should not have clinical manifestations of acute illness such as fever or severe pain.
6. Signs of sepsis or other significant physiologic derangements should be absent.

Nonoperative management generally includes nasogastric drainage and chest tube drainage of the pleural space on the side of the perforation, in addition to broad-spectrum antibiotics. Patients should be given parenteral nutrition for at least 10 days while they are given nothing by mouth. If the patient's condition fails to improve or deteriorates within 24 hours of initiation of nonoperative treatment, strong consideration should be given to operative management.

CLINICAL OUTCOME. The factors predicting a poor clinical result following treatment of esophageal perforation have been identified in several published series [39–42]. The most consistent factors predicting a poor prognosis are (1) poor general medical condition, most notably the presence of esophageal cancer; (2) spontaneous perforation (as compared to instrumental or traumatic esophageal perforation); (3) intrathoracic or intraabdominal perforation (as compared to cervical perforation); and (4) greater than 24-hour delay prior to diagnosis and initiation of treatment. Recently Jones and Ginsberg [15] reviewed and summarized 13 series of patients [42–53] treated

for esophageal perforation. The mortality rates in the series ranged from 0 to 54 percent, and averaged 15 percent. A more favorable outcome was associated with reinforced, primary repair compared with an unreinforced primary closure. A relatively poor outcome was predicted by treatment with exclusion and diversion, drainage only, or esophageal resection. However, these higher rates of mortality are likely related, in large part, to the inclusion of more complicated and advanced cases. Interestingly, nonoperative treatment was associated with a 22 percent mortality rate in these series, whereas previous reports on the results of operatively treated cases have shown a mortality between 12 and 38 percent [15,45,52,53]. Again, these comparisons are difficult since most reported series of nonoperatively treated patients are small, include a disproportionate number of pediatric and instrumental perforations, and have a high success rate.

Acute Mediastinitis

ETIOLOGY. Acute mediastinitis is a serious condition most frequently related to the perforation of a thoracic viscus, a descending cervical infection, or following median sternotomy and cardiac surgery. Prior to the development of widespread cardiac surgery, the most common causes of acute mediastinitis were esophageal perforation secondary to instrumentation and descending infections from peritonsillar abscesses, dental infections, or Ludwig's angina [30].

Occurring along with the rapid expansion of cardiac surgery through a median sternotomy incision, sternal wound infection with associated mediastinitis is all too common and occurs after 0.16 to 8.4 percent of all cardiac operations [54,55]. Although the organisms responsible for the infection are varied, *Staphylococcus* species and other gram-positive organisms are the most frequent isolates [56]. Perioperative risk factors for postcardiotomy sternal infection include poor tissue handling [54,57], obesity [58,59], low cardiac output syndrome and excessive bleeding after surgery [56,60], prolonged ventilator support [59,61], and poor nutritional status [62]. Suspected but controversial factors predisposing to postoperative mediastinitis include the use of one or two internal mammary artery grafts [56,58,59,61], diabetes [58,59,61,63], and the duration of the operation [60,64]. Patient mortality associated with postcardiotomy mediastinitis approaches 20 percent or greater, largely due to concomitant medical problems. Loop et al. [58] reported that the cost of caring for a cardiac surgery patient who develops mediastinitis is 2.8 times that of patients with an uncomplicated postoperative course and noted a mean hospitalization of 6 weeks.

Mediastinitis due to noninstrumental esophageal perforation is usually due to spontaneous perforation (Boerhaave's syndrome) or leakage from an esophageal suture line. Rarely, acute mediastinitis may be caused by perforation of the esophagus by a foreign body [16].

CLINICAL MANIFESTATIONS AND DIAGNOSIS. Acute mediastinitis following esophageal perforation may present with pain without other clinical manifestations, as described above. However, over the ensuing hours, increasing chest pain, dysphasia, diaphoresis, and systemic manifestations of sepsis should prompt immediate suspicion and evaluation for a perforation. Intrathoracic perforations present with a rapidly progressive course [16]. On occasion, mediastinitis occurs following a dental infection or as the result of postanginal sepsis [30]. A history of head and neck infection, neck swelling, or a recent dental or pharyngeal infection is important. Mediastinitis following cardiac surgery may present in an indolent fashion. The presence of an unstable sternum with wound drainage, either serous or purulent, should immediately alert the clinician to the possibility of acute mediastinal infection. Plain x-ray films may show the presence of mediastinal or pleural air or intrapleural effusion. X-ray films of the neck may show loss of normal cervical spine contour as well as the presence of increased soft tissue density and air within the fascial spaces. Mediastinal anatomy is disrupted and plain x-ray films may be nondiagnostic following cardiac operation. Computed tomography recently has been advocated for use in the acute diagnosis of mediastinitis following cardiac surgery and to evaluate the presence of sternal osteomyelitis [65]. However, mediastinal air is not an unusual finding soon after cardiac operations. Thus, although computed tomography may aid in the diagnostic evaluation, it should not be relied on to provide definitive confirmation or exclusion.

MANAGEMENT. Treatment of acute mediastinitis nearly always involves surgical intervention. In the case of esophageal perforation, treatment should be directed toward repairing the perforation and providing adequate drainage, with or without a proximal diversion or exclusion procedure. In the case of a descending pharyngeal infection causing acute mediastinitis, adequate cervical and retrovisceral mediastinal drainage should be performed along with pleural drainage on the side of the pleura effusion [2]. Immediate transthoracic mediastinal exploration may not be necessary, although in the author's experience, delayed intervention for residual abscesses or for the control of sepsis is often required.

Following cardiac surgery, a strong suspicion for mediastinal infection necessitates reopening the sternotomy incision and performing debridement of necrotic and devascularized tissue [66]. While the primary placement of muscular [67–70], myocutaneous [71], or omental [72–75] flaps has been advocated by some, we have found it unnecessary as an initial step unless a sternectomy is required due to extensive sternal osteomyelitis, a large residual dead space is present following debridement, or if the infection is of long duration. Placement of irrigation catheters and drains has been advocated in the treatment of mediastinitis following cardiac operation. An antibiotic solution is instilled for several days to a week following exploration [66]. Although controversial because of wound healing considerations, a dilute iodine solution also may be used [76]. The fascia and skin usually can be safely closed. In most cases of postcardiotomy mediastinitis, initial primary muscle flap closure or the instillation of antibiotic solution and catheter drainage are equally effective techniques [77].

In addition to local debridement and wound care, all patients with poststernotomy mediastinitis should receive systemic antibiotics. The type of antibiotics should be chosen according to initial Gram staining and later altered according to the results of culture and sensitivity testing. The duration of the systemic antibiotic treatment has been controversial and should be individualized in each case, but generally ranges from 2 to 6 weeks.

The use of prophylactic antibiotics during cardiac surgery has become an accepted medical practice. The choice of drug and the length of therapy have also been topics of debate. However, a cephalosporin active against *Staphylococcus* species has been advocated in the absence of a penicillin allergy [78,79,80]. In the presence of a penicillin allergy, vancomycin is an appropriate alternative [79,80].

As with most operative complications, post-cardiac surgery mediastinitis is best treated with preventive measures. However, despite aseptic technique, careful tissue handling, the use of prophylactic perioperative antibiotics, and an expedient operation, mediastinal infection remains a complication resulting in great expense and inconvenience, if not a catastrophic outcome for the patient and the physician as well.

References

1. Boerhaave H: *Atrocis, nec descripti prius, morbi historia secundem artis leges conscripta, lugduni batavorum, bontes teniana.* Medici, 1724, pp 1-60, Leiden, Boutesteniana.
2. Seybold WD, Johnson MA, Learly WV: Perforation of the esophagus. *Surg Clin North Am* 30:1155, 1950.
3. Kirby TJ, Ginsberg RJ: Complications of endoscopy: Bronchoscopy, esophagoscopy, and mediastinoscopy, in Waldhausen JA, Orringer MB (eds): *Complications in Cardiothoracic Surgery.* St. Louis, Mosby–Year Book, 1991.
4. Orringer MB: Complications of esophageal surgery and trauma, in Greenfield LJ (ed): *Complications in Surgery and Trauma.* Philadelphia, JB Lippincott, 1984.
5. Ellis FH Jr: Disorders of the esophagus in the adult, in Sabiston DC Jr, Spencer FC (eds): *Surgery of the Chest.* Philadelphia, WB Saunders, 1990.
6. Vauthey JN, Lerut J, Laube M, et al: Blunt oesophageal perforation: Treatment with surgical exclusion and percutaneous drainage under computed tomographic guidance. *Eur J Surg* 158(9):509, 1992.
7. Nashef SA, Klein C, Martigne C, et al: Foreign body perforation of the normal oesophagus. *Eur J Cardiothorac Surg* 6(10):565, 1992.
8. Johnson KG, Hood DD: Esophageal perforation associated with endotracheal intubation. *Anesthesiology* 64:281, 1986.
9. Blair GK, Filler RM, Theodorescu D: Neonatal pharyngoesophageal perforation mimicking esophageal atresia: Clues to diagnosis. *J Pediatr Surg* 22:770, 1987.
10. Dubost C, Kaswin D, Durante A, et al: Esophageal perforation during attempted endotracheal intubation. *J Thorac Cardiovasc Surg* 78:44, 1979.
11. Jackson RH, Payne K, Bacon BR: Esophageal perforation due to nasogastric intubation. *Am J Gastroenterol* 85:439, 1990.
12. Witte J, Pratschke E: Esophageal perforations, in Baue AE, Geha AS, Hammond GL, et al (eds): *Glenn's Thoracic and Cardiovascular Surgery.* 5th ed. Norwalk, CT, Appleton & Lange, 1991.
13. McBurney RP: Perforation of the esophagus: A complication of vagotomy or hiatal hernia repair. *Ann Surg* 169:851, 1969.
14. Postlethwait RW, Kim SK, Dillon ML: Esophageal complications of vagotomy. *Surg Gynecol Obstet* 128:481, 1969.
15. Jones WG II, Ginsberg RJ: Esophageal perforation: A continuing challenge. *Ann Thorac Surg* 53:534, 1992.
16. Shields TW, Vanecko RM: Trauma to the esophagus, in Shields TW (ed): *General Thoracic Surgery.* 3rd ed. Philadelphia, Lea & Febiger, 1989.
17. Han SY, McElvein RB, Aldrete JS, et al: Perforation of the esophagus: Correlation of site and cause with plain film findings. *AJR* 145:537, 1985.
18. Backer CL, LoCicero J III, Hartz RS, et al: Computed tomography in patients with esophageal perforation. *Chest* 98:1078, 1990.
19. Foley MJ, Ghahremani GG, Rogers LF: Reappraisal of contrast media used to detect upper gastrointestinal perforations: Comparison of ionic water soluble media with barium sulfate. *Radiology* 144:231, 1982.
20. Phillips LG, Cuningham J: Esophageal perforation. *Radiol Clin North Am* 22:1607, 1984.
21. Moghissi K, Pender D: Instrumental perforations of the oesophagus and their management. *Thorax* 43:642, 1988.
22. White CS, Templeton PA, Attar S: Esophageal perforation: CT findings. *AJR* 160(4):767, 1993.
23. Endicott JN, Molony TB, Campbell G, et al: Esophageal perforations: The role of computerized tomography in diagnosis and management decisions. *Laryngoscope* 96:751, 1986.
24. Maroney TP, Ruiz EJ, Gordon RL, et al: Role of interventional radiology in the management of esophageal leaks. *Radiology* 170:1055, 1989.

25. Shaffer HA Jr, Valenzuela G, Mittal RK: Esophageal perforation. A reassessment of the criteria for choosing medical or surgical therapy. *Arch Intern Med* 152(4):757, 1992.
26. Cameron JL, Kieffer RF, Hendrix TR, et al: Selective non-operative management of contained intrathoracic esophageal disruptions. *Ann Thorac Surg* 27:404, 1979.
27. Mollitt DL, Schulinger JN, Santulli TV: Selective management of iatrogenic esophageal perforation in the newborn. *J Pediatr Surg* 16:989, 1981.
28. Mengold LR, Klassen KP: Conservation management of esophageal perforation. *Arch Surg* 91:232, 1965.
29. Vantrappen G, Hellemans J: Treatment of achalasia and related motor disorders. *Gastroenterology* 79:144, 1980.
30. Jamplis RW, McFadden PM: Infections of the mediastinum and the superior vena caval syndrome, in Shields TW (ed): *General Thoracic Surgery*. 3rd ed. Philadelphia, Lea & Febiger, 1989.
31. Skinner DB: Perforation of the esophagus: Spontaneous (Boerhaave's syndrome), traumatic, and following esophagoscopy, in Sabiston DC (ed): *Textbook of Surgery*. 13th ed. Philadelphia, WB Saunders, 1986.
32. Grillo HC, Wilkins EW Jr: Esophageal repair following late diagnosis of intrathoracic perforation. *Ann Thorac Surg* 20:387, 1975.
33. Miller RE, Tiszenkel HL: Esophageal perforation due to pneumatic dilation for achalasia. *Surg Gynecol Obstet* 166:458, 1988.
34. Abbott OA, Mansour KA, Logan WD Jr, et al: Atraumatic so-called "spontaneous" rupture of the esophagus. A review of 47 personal cases with comments on a new method of surgical therapy. *J Thorac Cardiovasc Surg* 59:67, 1970.
35. Urschel HC, Razzuk MA, Wood RE, et al: Improved management of esophageal perforation: Exclusion and diversion in continuity. *Ann Surg* 179:587, 1974.
36. Johnson J, Schwegman CW, Kirby CK: Esophageal exclusion for persistent fistula following spontaneous rupture of the esophagus. *J Thorac Surg* 32:827, 1956.
37. Swedlund A, Traube M, Siskind BN, et al: Non-surgical management of esophageal perforation from pneumatic dilatation in achalasia. *Dig Dis Sci* 34:379, 1989.
38. Trastek VF: Esophageal perforation: A reassessment of the criteria for choosing medical or surgical therapy (letter). *Arch Intern Med* 152:693, 1992.
39. Bladergroen MR, Lowe JE, Postlethwait RW: Diagnosis and recommended management of esophageal perforation and rupture. *Ann Thorac Surg* 42:235, 1986.
40. Attar S, Hankins JR, Suter CM, et al: Esophageal perforation: A therapeutic challenge. *Ann Thorac Surg* 50:45, 1990.
41. Richardson JD, Martin LF, Borzotta AP, et al: Unifying concepts in the treatment of esophageal leaks. *Am J Surg* 149:157, 1985.
42. Flynn AE, Verrier ED, Way LW, et al: Esophageal perforation. *Arch Surg* 124:1211, 1989.
43. Goldstein LA, Thompson WR: Esophageal perforations: A 15-year experience. *Am J Surg* 143:495, 1982.
44. Sarr HG, Pemberton JH, Payne WS: Management of instrumental perforations of the esophagus. *J Thorac Cardiovasc Surg* 84:211, 1982.
45. Larsen K, Skov Jensen B, Axelsen F: Perforation and rupture of the esophagus. *Scand J Thorac Cardiovasc Surg* 17:311, 1983.
46. Ajalat GM, Mulder DG: Esophageal perforations, the need for an individualized approach. *Arch Surg* 119:1318, 1984.
47. Borgeskov S, Brynitz S, Siemenssen O: Perforation of the esophagus. Experience from a department of thoracic surgery. *Scand J Thorac Cardiovasc Surg* 18:93, 1984.
48. Radmark T, Sandberg N, Pettersson G: Instrumental perforation of the oesophagus. A ten year study from two ENT clinics. *J Laryngol Otol* 100:461, 1986.
49. Brewer LA, Carter R, Mulder GA, et al: Options in the management of perforations of the esophagus. *Am J Surg* 152:62, 1986.
50. Nesbitt JC, Sawyers JL: Surgical management of esophageal perforation. *Am Surg* 53:183, 1987.
51. Gouge TH, Depan HJ, Spencer FC: Experience with the Grillo pleural wrap procedure in 18 patients with perforation of the thoracic esophagus. *Ann Surg* 209:612, 1989.
52. Erwall C, Ejerblad S, Lindholm CE, et al: Perforation of the oesophagus. A comparison between surgical and conservative treatment. *Acta Otolaryngol* (Stockh) 97:1850, 1984.
53. Skinner DB, Little AG, DeMeester TR: Management of esophageal perforation. *Am J Surg* 139:760, 1980.
54. Nishida H, Grooters RK, Soltanzadeh H, et al: Discriminate use of electrocautery on the median sternotomy incision. *J Thorac Cardiovasc Surg* 101:488, 1991.
55. Fairchild PG, Gantz NN: Mediastinal and sternal infections, in Vander Salm TJ (ed): *Cardiac Surgery: State of the Art Reviews*. Philadelphia, Hanley & Belfus, 1988.
56. Ulicny KS Jr, Hiratzka LF: The risk factors of median sternotomy infection: A current review. *J Card Surg* 6(2):338, 1991.
57. Baffes TG, Blazek WV, Fridman JL: Postoperative infections in 1,136 consecutive cardiac operations. *Surgery* 68:791, 1970.
58. Loop FD, Lytle BW, Cosgrove DM, et al: Sternal wound complications after isolated coronary artery bypass grafting: Early and late mortality, morbidity, and cost of care. *Ann Thorac Surg* 49:179, 1990.
59. Kouchoukos NT, Wareing TH, Murphy SF, et al: Risks of bilateral internal mammary artery bypass grafting. *Ann Thorac Surg* 49:210, 1990.
60. Culliford AT, Cunningham JN, Zeff RH, et al: Sternal and costochondral infections following open-heart surgery. A review of 2,594 cases. *J Thorac Cardiovasc Surg* 72:714, 1976.
61. Demmy TL, Park SB, Liebler GA, et al: Recent experience with major sternal wound complications. *Ann Thorac Surg* 49:458, 1990.
62. Rich MW, Keller AJ, Schechtman KB, et al: Increased complications and prolonged hospital stay in elderly cardiac surgery patients with low serum albumin. *Am J Cardiol* 63:714, 1989.
63. Rutledge R, Applebaum RE, Kim BJ: Mediastinal infection after open heart surgery. *Surgery* 97:88, 1985.
64. Macmanus Q, Okies JE: Mediastinal wound infection and aortocoronary graft patency. *Am J Surg* 132:558, 1976.
65. Goodman LR, Haasler GB: Mediastinal and sternal infection: Imaging strategies, in Vander Salm TJ (ed): *Mediastinal and Sternal Infections. Cardiac Surgery: State of the Art Reviews*. Philadelphia, Hanley & Belfus, 1988.
66. Culliford AT, Rosenfeld K: Role of antibiotic lavage and radical debridement in the treatment of acute mediastinal wound infections following sternotomy, in Vander Salm TJ (ed): *Mediastinal and Sternal Infections, Cardiac Surgery: State of the Art Reviews*. Philadelphia, Hanley & Belfus, 1988.
67. Voegele LD, Metcalf MM, Prioleau WH Jr, et al: Median sternotomy infection. Management and reconstruction. *Am Surg* 51:645, 1985.
68. Jurkiewicz MJ, Bostwick JB III, Hester TR, et al: Infected median sternotomy wound: Successful treatment of muscle flaps. *Ann Surg* 191:738, 1980.
69. Walton RL, Gonzalez F, Chick LR: The rectus abdominis flap in reconstruction of sternal wounds, in Vander Salm TS (ed): *Mediastinal and Sternal Infections. Cardiac Surgery: State of the Art Reviews*. Philadelphia, Hanley & Belfus, 1988.
70. Kohman LJ, Auchincloss JH, Gilbert R, et al: Functional results of muscle flap closure for sternal infection. *Ann Thorac Surg* 52:102, 1992.
71. Herrera RA, Ginsberg ME: The pectoralis major myocutaneous flap and omental transposition for closure of infected median sternotomy wounds. *J Plast Reconstr Surg* 70:465, 1982.
72. Belcher P, McLean N, Breach N, et al: Omental transfer in acute and chronic sternotomy wound breakdown. *Thorac Cardiovasc Surg* 38:186, 1990.
73. Lovich SF, Iverson LI, Young JN, et al: Omental pedicle grafting in the treatment of postcardiotomy sternotomy infection. *Arch Surg* 124:1192, 1989.
74. Kutsal A, Ibrisim E, Catav Z, et al: Mediastinitis after open heart surgery. Analysis of risk factors and management. *J Cardiovasc Surg* (Torino) 32(1):38, 1991.
75. Mainwaring RD, Lamberti JJ, Kirkpatrick SE: Omental transfer for the treatment of mediastinitis in an infant. *J Card Surg* 7(3):269, 1992.
76. Thurer RJ, Bognolo D, Vargas A, et al: The management of mediastinal infection following cardiac surgery: An experience utilizing continuous irrigation with povidone-iodine. *J Thorac Cardiovasc Surg* 68:962, 1974.
77. Scully HE, Leclerc T, Martin RD, et al: Comparison between antibiotic irrigation and mobilization of pectoral muscle flaps in treat-

ment of deep sternal infections. *J Thorac Cardiovasc Surg* 90:523, 1984.

78. Kreter B, Woods M: Antibiotic prophylaxis for cardiothoracic operations. Meta-analysis of thirty years of clinical trials. *J Thorac Cardiovasc Surg* 104(3):590, 1992.

79. Woods M, Tillman D: Antibiotic prophylaxis in cardiothoracic surgery. 1990: Results of a third survey. *Hosp Pharm* 27:404, 1992.

80. Maki DG, Bohn MJ, Stolz SM, et al: Comparative study of cefazolin, cefamandole, and vancomycin for surgical prophylaxis in cardiac and vascular operations. A double-blind randomized trial. *J Thorac Cardiovasc Surg* 104:1423, 1992.

170. Obstetric Problems in the Intensive Care Unit

Jonathan F. Critchlow

Despite its everyday occurrence, pregnancy involves significant risk to the mother even in developed countries. Pregnancy-associated mortality rates have declined from 50 per 100,000 live births to less than 10 per 100,000 live births over the past 35 years in the United States owing to the declining deaths from direct obstetric causes—eclampsia, hemorrhage, infection, and cardiac disease [1,2]. Deaths due to trauma, pulmonary embolism, and poor antenatal care have now become most prevalent (Table 170-1) [3]. Improvements in obstetric, anesthetic, and intensive care are probably partially responsible for the general decline of mortality and the shift in responsible causes. The patient population seen in the intensive care unit setting has also changed; today, there are fewer septic obstetric patients and more patients with hypertension and concurrent medical illnesses.

The management of the acutely ill pregnant patient presents challenges to the intensive care unit team due to disease states unique to pregnancy, concurrent anatomic changes in the mother, and the altered cardiopulmonary physiology of mother and fetus. Obstetric critical care is the support of *two* patients (i.e., the mother and the fetus) with differing physiologic profiles. The basic changes in maternal and fetal physiology during pregnancy are reviewed in this chapter. General considerations with respect to diagnosis and treatment of mother and fetus are discussed. Disease states specific to pregnancy—bleeding, eclampsia and preeclampsia, trauma, and infection—are covered. Specifics related to the diagnosis and treatment of respiratory failure in pregnancy (pneumonia, amniotic fluid embolus, pulmonary embolus, etc.) are thoroughly addressed in Chapter 59.

Maternal/Fetal Physiology

A number of hemodynamic changes occur during pregnancy to increase oxygen delivery to the placenta during gestation and delivery (Table 170-2). Cardiac output increases during the first trimester and peaks in the second trimester to almost 50 percent above normal. This is accomplished by an increase in heart rate and stroke volume and accompanied by a decrease in systemic vascular resistance (SVR) [4,5]. The decrease in SVR may be secondary to elevated prostacyclin levels. During later pregnancy, assuming the supine position causes caval compression by the gravid uterus, which may markedly decrease

venous return, leading to a marked decrease in cardiac output [6]. During labor, uterine contraction increases venous return but also markedly increases afterload; the latter effect can be detrimental to patients with underlying cardiac disease.

Blood volume increases in the first trimester and peaks at 140 percent of the nonpregnant state by the third trimester. Both red cell mass and total blood volume increase, but because red cell mass does not increase at the same rate as plasma volume, a modest dilutional anemia is present due to excess extracellular water [7]. Hematocrits of 30 to 35 percent and serum albumin concentrations of 3.0 to 3.5 are considered normal in pregnancy.

Marked changes in the lung, ventilatory control, and respiratory mechanics also occur [8,9]. Chronic compensated hyperventilation with a resultant PCO_2 of 30 to 35 mm Hg results

Table 170-1. Cause-Specific Maternal Mortality Rates in Massachusetts, 1954 through 1957, 1966 through 1969, and 1982 through 1985.

Cause of death	Period 1954–57	1966–69	1982–85
	Deaths/100,000 Live Births		
All causes	50	29	10
Trauma	0.5	1.6	1.9
Pulmonary embolus	3.4	1.9	1.2
Pregnancy-induced hypertension	5.0	1.1	0.9
Intracranial hemorrhage	2.9	3.4	0.9
Infection	8.8	4.5	0.6
Amniotic-fluid embolus	0.7	1.1	0.6
Ectopic pregnancy	1.4	0.8	0.6
Hemorrhage	3.8	1.1	0.3
Cardiac disease	5.6	2.4	0.3
Anesthetic accident	2.3	1.9	0.3
Abortion	1.4	0.3	0.3
Central nervous system disorder (excluding hemorrhage)	0.7	0	0.3
Cancer	3.2	2.1	0
Ruptured uterus	1.6	1.3	0
Other and unspecified	1.6	0.8	0.9

Source: From Sachs B, Brown D, Driscoll DJ, et al: Maternal Mortality in Massachusetts. *N Engl J Med* 316:669, 1987. Reprinted by permission of *The New England Journal of Medicine*.

Table 170-2. Changes in the Cardiopulmonary System During Normal Pregnancy

Hemodynamics	I	II	III
Heart rate	⟷	↑ by 5–10%	↑ by 15–20%
Blood pressure	⟷	↓ Systolic	⟷ (except preeclampsia)
		↓ Diastolic	
Cardiac output	↑ by 20%	↑ by 40%	↑ by 30% (position may ↓ by 40–50%)
Blood Volumes			
Plasma volume	↑	↑	↑ by 50%
HCT	⟷	↓	↓ to 30–35%
Respiratory Function			
Respiratory rate	⟷	↑ by 10%	↑ by 15%
Tidal volume	↑ by 10%	↑ by 20%	↑ by 40%
PCO_2	↓ (mild)	↓	↓ to 30 mm Hg

from increases in respiratory rate and tidal volume. These ventilatory changes precede the increases in oxygen requirements from the placenta and fetus and may be a response to elevated progesterone levels [10]. Pregnancy is associated with small decreases in total lung volume and functional residual capacity. In early pregnancy, tidal volume increases by 30 percent but later may decrease as the diaphragm rises due to an upward shift of intraabdominal contents.

Fetal oxygen delivery is a function of arterial oxygen content, the flow of blood through the uterine arteries, placental transfer, and the special attributes of fetal hemoglobin. Uterine blood vessels are normally maximally dilated. Thus, uterine blood flow is not self-regulating and flow is directly related to maternal blood pressure [11]. Blood flow to the placenta may be adversely affected by alkalosis, diminished maternal cardiac output or blood pressure, uterine contractions, or increased sympathetic tone. Despite the relative inefficiency of placental oxygen transfer, the greater oxygen affinity of fetal hemoglobin affords the fetus a blood oxygen content very close to that of maternal blood, even though the PO_2 is substantially lower.

General Considerations in Diagnosis and Therapy

MONITORING. Although pregnant patients are usually young, healthy women with normal cardiac function, invasive monitoring with central venous pressure lines or Swan-Ganz catheters can, on occasion, be helpful in management [12,13]. Despite the normally elevated cardiac output during pregnancy, filling pressures are usually in the range seen in the nonpregnant state, and left ventricular function is well preserved in most obstetric patients, even those with significant preeclampsia. In patients with preeclampsia, or in cases of simple blood loss, a central venous pressure line may provide adequate monitoring of intravascular volume. However, in patients with cardiac failure, refractory pulmonary edema, severe underlying cardiac or pulmonary disease, nonhemorrhagic shock, or acute respiratory distress syndrome (ARDS), pulmonary artery catheterization may be quite beneficial. Insertion techniques, risks, and complications are similar to those encountered in the non-pregnant population [14].

Continuous fetal monitoring is useful in situations where de-

cisions will be based on the results. This most often occurs in later pregnancy (over 28 weeks) when early delivery may be expected to yield a potentially viable fetus. Fetal monitoring also may be valuable in the assessment of resuscitative efforts, especially after trauma, where reaching normal hemodynamic endpoints in the mother may not be adequate to ensure fetal survival [15]. Tocographic monitoring is most helpful after trauma or surgery to demonstrate premature contractions, which may warn of premature labor or placental abruption.

RADIATION EXPOSURE. Radiography is often essential in the diagnosis and management of the critically ill patient, but in pregnant women one must be concerned about radiation exposure to the fetus. The risks to the fetus of death, malformation, or later childhood cancers depend on gestational age at the time of exposure and the amount of radiation delivered. In the first weeks of pregnancy, radiation doses of 10 cGy may cause fetal death. During the first 12 weeks of gestation, the period of fetal organ development, the fetus is more vulnerable to developmental abnormalities. Exposures of several cGy appear to be safe. The clinician should be concerned about exposures of 5 to 10 cGy; the risk of malformations is much increased at doses above 15 cGy [16]. For gestations beyond 15 weeks, the "acceptable" level of radiation exposure is probably much higher. A chest roentgenogram exposes the maternal lungs to approximately 0.5 cGy and the shielded fetus to much less ionizing radiation. A single film of the pelvis yields less than 1 cGy to the fetus. Abdominopelvic computed tomography (CT) scans deliver a larger radiation dose, between 5 and 10 cGy, to the fetus [17]. Therefore, plain films necessary for diagnosis and safe care of the pregnant patient should be obtained without undue concern over fetal exposure. Although CT scans have been performed in pregnant patients without obvious sequelae [18], the role of CT scanning, especially in early pregnancy, remains controversial.

CARDIOPULMONARY RESUSCITATION. In the event of cardiopulmonary arrest, closed chest resuscitation should begin immediately. The uterus should be shifted off of the inferior vena cava by tilting the abdomen or with manual pressure [19]. The Trendelenburg position is of little benefit to patients with advanced pregnancy. If there is no response to standard measures, cesarean section should be performed within minutes [20]. Emptying the uterus relieves vena caval compression and may aid in resuscitation. This is most effective for mother and fetus if done within 5 minutes of arrest and should be undertaken only in later pregnancy, when the potential benefits of relieving uterine compression and the chances for fetal viability are greatest.

INTUBATION AND MECHANICAL VENTILATION. The indications for intubation and mechanical ventilation are identical to those used in nonpregnant adults—airway protection, pulmonary toilet, treatment of severe hypoxia, and management of ventilatory failure manifested by significant noncompensated respiratory acidosis (see Chaps. 1 and 66). Due to pregnancy-related increases in blood flow and congestion of mucous membranes, a smaller endotracheal tube may be required and nasotracheal intubation should either be avoided or done with great care. The increased oxygen consumption seen in pregnancy, coupled with a decreased functional residual capacity, predisposes pregnant women to rapid arterial desaturation during periods of apnea. The ventilator should be set with tidal volumes of 10 to 15 ml per kg of body weight and rates of 10 to 18, with an aim of mimicking the mild compensated respiratory alkalosis of pregnancy (i.e., PCO_2 = 30–35 mm Hg). Greater degrees of hyperventilation should be avoided, as marked hypocarbia may decrease uterine blood flow. Fractional inspired oxygen concentration should be adjusted up to 50 percent to keep arterial PO_2 greater than 90 mm Hg. Some patients will require positive end-expiratory pressure (PEEP) to ensure an adequate arterial PO_2.

DRUGS

Analgesics and Anxiolytics. Morphine and related opiates have not been associated with fetal malformations [21]. Transfer across the placenta is rapid, and prolonged use may lead to fetal withdrawal, which is usually seen only in addicted mothers. Large doses of morphine or other opiates given near delivery may cause fetal respiratory depression. Diazepam, though once thought to be associated with cleft lip, seems to be free of teratogenic effects [22]. However, neonatal depression at delivery may be seen if large doses are given. (See Chaps. 209 and 215.)

Antibiotics. The penicillins and cephalosporins have been used frequently during pregnancy and have established safety records. The aminoglycosides have been implicated in cases of ototoxicity to the fetus, but this effect has been demonstrated only with streptomycin and kanamycin and has not been reported with gentamicin [23]. Nonetheless, because of concern about ototoxicity and because aminoglycosides have been reported to potentiate $MgSO_4$-induced neuromuscular weakness in neonates [24], use of these agents is generally restricted to severe infections. Sulfonamides are contraindicated near term, because these drugs affect bilirubin metabolism in neonates and can increase the risk of neonatal kernicterus. Chloramphenicol, when given in large doses near delivery, has been implicated in cases of the "gray syndrome" (neonatal cardiovascular collapse) [23]. Tetracycline is contraindicated due to teratogenic effects (especially to bone and teeth) [25]. Clindamycin and vancomycin appear to be safe, although some concerns have been raised regarding possible toxicity to the fetal kidney and eighth nerve from vancomycin [23,25]. (See Chap. 85.)

Anticoagulants. Heparin does not cross the placenta and has not been shown to be teratogenic. Although it has been thought that long-term use may be associated with an increased rate of stillbirth, more recent studies suggest that heparin therapy has no significant effect on fetal outcome [26]. Warfarin is associated with a distinct syndrome of developmental defects and should be avoided especially in early pregnancy [21,27]. (See Chap. 121.)

Antihypertensives. Hydralazine and alphamethyldopa are the most commonly used agents for treating hypertension associated with pregnancy [28]. Nitroglycerin (NTG) has been used as well, and this drug may increase uterine blood flow [29]. However, decreased preload may lower maternal cardiac output, and the antihypertensive effect of NTG may be minimal in severely preeclamptic patients receiving intravenous fluids [30]. Sodium nitroprusside crosses the placenta and may lead to elevated fetal cyanide levels [31], and, therefore, this drug should either be avoided or used only for very short periods close to delivery. (See Chap. 210.)

Vasoconstrictor and Inotropic Agents. Hypotension refractory to fluids and postural changes may require vasoconstrictor and inotropic therapy, which should be guided by invasive monitoring techniques. Of the agents with alpha activity, ephedrine seems to best preserve uterine blood flow [32]. Use of phenylephrine in treating hypotension due to spinal or epidural anesthesia for *elective* cesarean section [33] seems safe, but its excessive alpha activity makes it less attractive in the critically ill patient. Beta-agonists such as isoproterenol or dopamine may diminish uterine blood flow if maternal hypotension ensues.

Nutrition

Just as good nutrition is emphasized during normal pregnancy, nutritional support also is important in the stressed critically ill patient. Maternal malnutrition may contribute to intrauterine growth retardation. Experiments in rats with low body energy stores have shown that nutrients are preferentially channeled to the mother rather than to the fetus during periods of starvation or semistarvation [34]. This observation is supported by outcomes of pregnancy in humans during periods of food shortage and famine where infants of lower birth weight have been documented [35].

Nutritional support should commence early. The enteral route is preferable. Aspiration of nasogastric feedings is of great concern, however, due to the anatomic and physiologic effects of pregnancy—progesterone decreases lower esophageal sphincter pressure and delays gastric emptying; the gravid uterus displaces the stomach upward, increasing abdominal pressure; and low gastric pH is seen in pregnancy due to the effects of placental gastrin [36]. Total parenteral nutrition (TPN) has been successfully utilized in pregnancy complicated by malnutrition and inability to eat and has been shown to enable normal fetal development [37,38]. Due to concerns over macrosomia and other adverse effects of hyperglycemia, glucose levels should be maintained at less than 120 mg per deciliter. Large quantities of intravenous lipid (greater than 40% of calories) should be avoided because of experimental evidence showing fatty infiltration of the placenta in animals given 50 percent of calories intravenously as fat [39]. (See Chap. 200.)

Hypertensive Disorders of Pregnancy

Hypertension during pregnancy may be due to chronic hypertension, preeclampsia/eclampsia, chronic hypertension complicated by preeclampsia, or transient hypertension. Chronic essential hypertension does not seem to affect pregnancy adversely unless it is severe. Transient hypertension, which occurs very late in pregnancy, is also most often benign. Preeclampsia and eclampsia, however, may have profound effects on mother and fetus. These syndromes are complex multisystem disorders involving the maternal vasculature and are commonly characterized by hypertension.

Preeclampsia is defined as hypertension occurring after the twentieth week of pregnancy with proteinuria (greater than 2 gm/day) and peripheral edema. Preeclampsia is most often seen in nulliparous women. It occurs in 10 percent of all pregnancies and may be associated with varying end-organ manifestations, such as acute renal failure, cardiac or pulmonary failure, disseminated intravascular coagulation (DIC), hemolysis, elevated liver enzymes, and thrombocytopenia [28,40,41]. Occasionally other end organ manifestations of preeclampsia may be present without hypertension [41,42]. Eclampsia is defined as the onset of seizures unrelated to a known seizure disorder or anatomic focus.

Arteriolar vasospasm seems to be the underlying pathologic lesion of preeclampsia. Arteriolar constriction leads to a generalized increase in peripheral vascular resistance, which, in turn, causes hypertension, diminished circulating blood volume and flow to essential organs, and microangiopathy. Although total body water is increased secondary to salt and water retention, the actual circulating blood volume is significantly lower in preeclamptic patients than it is in patients with uncomplicated pregnancy [43,44]. Circulating albumin concentrations and plasma oncotic pressures are also lower in preeclampsia than during normal pregnancy [45]. Renal function is impaired by decreased renal blood flow, endothelial cell swelling, and fibrin deposition in glomeruli [41]. Proteinuria is seen, and there is plugging of the renal tubules by proteinaceous casts. The central nervous system (CNS) in preeclampsia is irritable; hyperreflexia is common. In true eclampsia, grand mal seizures occur. Although the mechanisms responsible for CNS dysfunction in eclampsia have not been clearly elucidated, it seems probable that systemic hypertension exceeds the protective capacity of the cerebral autoregulation system and causes hypertensive encephalopathy, cerebral vasospasm, and cerebral edema [46,47]. Although full-blown DIC is rare in preeclampsia, a hypercoagulable state does commonly exist, and more subtle signs of intravascular coagulation are often seen in the kidney, lungs, liver, and placenta.

A particular combination of end-organ abnormalities affecting preeclamptic mothers, consisting of hemolysis, elevated liver function tests, and thrombocytopenia, has been described. Termed the HELLP syndrome (H—hemolysis, EL—elevated liver enzymes, LP—low platelets) by Weinstein [48], this entity affects 2 to 12 percent of severely preeclamptic patients. Typical early manifestations include nonspecific malaise, weight gain, and right upper quadrant discomfort. Hypertension may be absent in as many as 50 percent of patients in the early stages of the syndrome. Although not totally proven, the pathogenesis of this syndrome involves vasospasm, which triggers endothelial cell damage and microangiopathic hemolysis. Platelet consumption and fibrin deposition occur. The liver is primarily involved, with fibrin deposits leading to areas of necrosis and occasional subcapsular hematoma formation. Although criteria may vary, the diagnosis is made by documentation of hemolysis on the peripheral smear and elevated circulating lactate dehydrogenase levels (greater than 600 U/L), elevated liver function tests (alanine aminotransferase greater than 70 IU/L), and a platelet count less than 100,000 [42,49]. A decrease in fibrinogen levels and elevation of fibrin degradation products, prothrombin time, and partial thromboplastin time may occur, but these are usually very late findings. These coagulation abnormalities *follow* the anemia and thrombocytopenia in HELLP as opposed to being an early prominent feature of the DIC that often results from other complications of pregnancy (placental abruption, acute fatty liver of pregnancy, thrombotic thrombocytopenic purpura, or hemolytic uremic syndrome) with which this syndrome may be confused [42] (Table 170-3).

Management

Since the definitive treatment of preeclampsia is delivery, the majority of patients must be stabilized and then delivered shortly thereafter. If the fetus is very immature, stabilization and observation, if possible, are the best route [50]. After admission, a full physical examination, including neurologic and pelvic examinations, should be performed. The patient should be

Table 170-3. MHA and Thrombocytopenia: Predominant Clinical features

Clinical feature	HELLP	TTP	HUS
Anemia	Yes	Yes	Yes
Thrombocytopenia	Yes	Yes	Yes
Increased LDH	Yes	Yes	Yes
Increased IND BIL	Yes	Yes	Yes
Red cell fragments	Yes	Yes	Yes
Decreased haptoglobin	Yes	Yes	Yes
Kidney: prime target	No	No	Yes
Liver: prime target	Yes	No	No
Hypertension	Yes	Not usually	Yes
Neurologic symptoms	Sometimes	Yes	Rarely
Hyaline thrombi	No	Yes	Yes
BUN	Mild increase	Mild increase	Marked increase

Source: From Martin JM, Steadman CM: Imitators of pre-eclampsia and HELLP syndrome. *Obstet Gynecol Clin North Am* 18(2):187, 199.

placed on bed rest and given vigorous intravenous fluid therapy. Standard blood tests should be performed, paying special attention to results of urinalysis for protein, blood smear for hemolysis, platelet count, coagulation profile, and tests of renal and hepatic function. As volume depletion is the rule in pregnancy-induced hypertension, patients not exhibiting pulmonary edema should be volume loaded. The use of invasive monitoring should be dictated by the severity of symptoms and associated health problems [28,51]. Blood pressure should be controlled with vasodilators—hydralazine and/or alphamethyldopa are most often used [52]. Sodium nitroprusside is used only in severe cases for short time periods due to concerns over fetal cyanide toxicity [31]. In the absence of pulmonary edema, diuretics should be avoided as they may further decrease circulating blood volume and blood flow to the uterus. Although somewhat controversial, $MgSO_4$ remains the most commonly used prophylactic anticonvulsant in the United States [28,46,47,53]. A loading dose of 2 to 4 gm is given, followed by a maintenance infusion of 1 to 2 gm per hour, aiming for serum levels of 4 to 6 mEq per liter. Although relatively safe, an overdose of $MgSO_4$ may lead to hypoventilation and respiratory or cardiac arrest. Because magnesium is primarily cleared by renal excretion, adequate urine output must be maintained. Though it is a mild vasodilator, vasodilation does not seem to be its major mode of action. Magnesium decreases uterine tone, which may be beneficial in cases of premature labor but may be detrimental around the time of delivery. The efficacy of $MgSO_4$ as a prophylactic or therapeutic agent has been questioned [46,47].

Treatment of eclamptic seizures is best accomplished with intravenous diazepam (5–10 mg) [46,47]. Vigorous antihypertensive therapy should continue, and treatment to prevent further seizures should be instituted. Intravenous $MgSO_4$ is used by some [52,54], although others would immediately begin therapy with phenytoin (10 mg/kg IV over 20 minutes) [46,47,55]. Despite being potentially teratogenic in early pregnancy, phenytoin seems to have little effect on the developed fetus.

Treatment of the HELLP syndrome is similar to that given for severe preeclampsia [42]. Patients should be stabilized, coagulation profiles checked and corrected, and the fetus evaluated for well-being and maturity. Patients with fetuses dated at greater than 35 weeks or with mature lungs should be prepared for delivery, which can be accomplished vaginally in most cases. If necessary, steroids may be given to accelerate lung maturity. If the fetus is immature, expectant management may be attempted although there is some risk for placental abruption, DIC, acute renal failure, or rupture of a subcapsular liver hematoma. Bed rest, intravenous fluids (with or without albumin), and antihypertensives are key. There are anecdotal reports of improvement or reversal of HELLP with aspirin, dipyridamole, or dazoxiben (a thromboxane synthetase inhibitor). [49]. However, the true utility of these drugs remains unclear. The possible benefits of greater fetal maturity must be weighed against the real risk to the mother and fetus of the complications of a worsening syndrome. Patients presenting with severe abdominal pain in the right upper quadrant, shoulder pain, or shock may have the rare complication of rupture of a subcapsular hepatic hematoma. Immediate operation is required for patients in shock. Evaluation by ultrasound or CT may be beneficial in the diagnosis and management of more stable patients.

Hemorrhage

Despite a significant decline in mortality due to hemorrhage over the past three decades, bleeding is still a significant cause of maternal morbidity and mortality and of fetal wastage. Although improvements in obstetric, anesthetic, and critical care have brought about these gratifying changes in mortality, hemorrhage remains a common occurrence, placing both mother and unborn child in jeopardy.

As outlined previously, natural physiologic changes occur during pregnancy, which increase circulating blood volume, decrease hematocrit, and increase cardiac output. Near term, cardiac output may significantly decline with postural changes. Coagulation is generally accelerated in pregnancy. Circulating levels of most coagulation factors increase; fibrinogen levels are 50 to 80 percent above the prepregnancy state [56]. The platelet count may be constant or slightly decreased. The teleologically beneficial response of accelerated coagulation may be markedly altered by DIC or DIC-like states brought about by preeclampsia, HELLP syndrome, thrombotic thrombocytopenic purpura (TTP), amniotic fluid embolus, uteroplacental trauma, or placental abruption.

Blood loss at the time of delivery is a normal phenomenon. A normal vaginal delivery can be expected to be accompanied by a 500-ml blood loss, which may increase to 1 liter during a routine cesarean section [57]. This degree of blood loss is usually offset by the preexistent increase in blood volume; therefore, the overall effect of delivery or cesarean section on the mother's circulatory status is most often minimal. However, pregnancy-related bleeding disorders—abruptio placentae, placenta previa, and postpartum bleeding—may occur, leading to massive bleeding.

Antepartum Hemorrhage

Most significant antepartum bleeding (other than ectopic pregnancy or abortion) occurs in later pregnancy and is due to placenta previa or abruptio placentae. In placenta previa, areas of the placenta overlie the cervical os and may bleed through the cervix. In abruption, a normally located placenta separates from the uterine wall, causing either intrauterine and/or external bleeding.

Placenta Previa

Placenta previa is relatively common, occurring at a rate of 1 in 200 pregnancies [58]. The severity of the condition may be graded by ultrasound according to the amount of placental tissue that impinges on or covers the cervical os. Bleeding is usually painless and usually occurs as multiple sporadic bleeds from the lower uterine segment through the os. Diagnosis is most readily made by history, ultrasound examination, and then digital examination, which, if done, should be performed with great care in the operating room because it may initiate severe bleeding.

As with most disorders of pregnancy, the key factors in therapeutic decision-making and management are the establishment of an accurate diagnosis, determination of the stage of gestation of the fetus, and assessment of the severity of symptoms of the mother. Severe hemorrhage is fortunately relatively rare. In these cases, immediate cesarean section is indicated. If the fetus has matured beyond 35 weeks and bleeding continues in the relatively stable patient, delivery should be accomplished without delay. Controversy exists over whether women with mild bleeding and small amounts of placenta abutting the os (low-lying placenta or marginal placenta previa) should be induced and allowed to deliver vaginally or whether cesarean section should be undertaken in all symptomatic patients with ultrasonically confirmed placenta previa.

Patients carrying less developed fetuses present thornier judgment issues. Attempts should be made to expectantly manage these patients to allow for further fetal maturation [59]. Patients should be placed on bed rest, with both mother and fetus monitored, and supported with fluid and blood therapy as needed. Delivery should be accomplished at a time when fetal maturity is judged by ultrasound and lecithin/sphingomyelin ratios to be sufficient for independent survival.

Abruptio Placentae

Placental abruption is the premature separation of the placenta from the uterus. The anatomic location and severity of abruption may lead to hemorrhage, which can either be contained or visible through the os. Abruption may occur in up to 1 in 100 pregnancies, with a maternal mortality of several percent. As many as 25 to 40 percent of infants may die as a consequence of this problem. Most patients present with pain, which increases with contractions. External bleeding may be present or absent. Because the majority of blood loss may be intrauterine, the degree of maternal volume depletion may not correlate with observed blood loss even in patients who present with vaginal bleeding. A history of antecedent trauma is relatively rare but may be present. Hypertension during pregnancy is relatively common. A predelivery diagnosis of abruption is most often made on clinical grounds and by excluding placenta previa. Ultrasound can easily identify placenta previa but may not accurately diagnose an abruption. Postpartum, diagnosis may be made by observing areas of clot on the placenta.

Treatment of placental abruption includes resuscitation and stabilization with intravenous fluids and blood as necessary. Invasive monitoring with central venous catheterization or Swan-Ganz monitoring may be helpful to assess the degree of blood loss. Fetal monitoring is essential, because there is a high incidence of fetal distress. Because of the possibility of fetal abruption-induced DIC, coagulation studies should be done and coagulation factors repleted as required.

Since the only therapy for this problem is delivery and removal of the placenta, the issues of maternal and fetal stability and fetal maturity arise [60]. A mother with mild blood loss carrying a term fetus without distress may be induced for vaginal delivery. Emergent cesarean section is indicated for maternal or fetal distress. If the fetus is immature, supportive measures should be continued unless maternal or fetal health is in danger.

Following delivery or cesarean section, bleeding usually ceases. However, some patients may exhibit continuing bleeding from various, and often multiple, causes. Some form of DIC occurs in 15 to 30 percent of cases [61]. Although DIC is probably overdiagnosed it is common in placental abruption and may be related to a number of causes [62]. Release of tissue thromboplastin during abruption causes activation of the extrinsic clotting cascade and also probably increases the rate of fibrinolysis. There also may be increased consumption of clotting factors from a large intrauterine clot. The diagnosis of DIC is supported by documentation of decreased levels of clotting factors, platelets, and fibrinogen and increased levels of fibrin degradation products. In practice, it is often quite difficult to differentiate DIC from (the more common) simple dilutional coagulopathy, as similar coagulation profiles may be seen after severe hemorrhage with both conditions. Uterine atony may also contribute to continued bleeding.

The treatment of patients with refractory bleeding involves vigorous repletion of clotting factors, especially platelets, and removal of all placental fragments. Heparin therapy is not useful and may be harmful. On occasion hysterectomy or even hypogastric artery ligation or embolization may be necessary to control severe bleeding.

Postpartum Hemorrhage

Given the tremendous vascularity of the uterus and the degree of trauma encountered even in uncomplicated delivery, it is a wonder that significant hemorrhage occurs in only 2 to 5 percent of pregnancies. Conditions that prohibit adequate contraction of the uterus are the most common causes of postpartum hemorrhage. These conditions include fragments or clot, overdistention of the uterus, lacerations, idiopathic uterine atony, and use of certain drugs, such as terbutaline or $MgSO_4$ [63]. Disorders of coagulation such as DIC or dilutional coagulopathy from antepartum hemorrhage also may be contributory.

Medical treatment is based on maneuvers to improve uterine contraction and correct coagulopathy. The treatment of DIC and dilutional coagulopathy has been discussed. Compression or massage of the uterus may be all that is necessary to stimulate adequate contraction and decrease hemorrhage. If this is not effective, oxytocin may be administered as a continuous infusion to increase contractions. Intramuscular injections of ergonovine are also effective in inducing contraction of the uterus and decreasing hemorrhage. However, the use of this agent is limited in patients with pregnancy-induced hypertension due to the potent vasoconstrictive properties of ergonovine and the observation that this agent has been implicated in cases of intracerebral hemorrhage [64]. Prostaglandin F_2 alpha also may be used for its oxytocic properties. It is often given as an intrauterine injection via either the transabdominal or cervical route. A 15 methyl $PGF_{2\alpha}$ analog has been administered intramuscularly with good success [65]. Maternal hypertension is less commonly seen with prostaglandins than with ergonovine, but has been reported.

Postpartum bleeding that continues after oxytocic therapy must be treated surgically. If the uterus contracts and bleeding persists, a search must be made for other causes of bleeding, such as lacerations, retained placental fragments, and coagulopathy. Repair of lacerations and evacuation of placental fragments are accomplished surgically. Curettage is necessary for the adequate removal of retained placenta. Refractory bleeding may require hysterectomy and/or hypogastric artery ligation [66]. We have found that a number of patients admitted follow-

ing surgery for postpartum hemorrhage have required another procedure. Angiographic transcatheter embolization therapy either prior to or following surgical therapy occasionally may be of benefit [67].

Trauma

Trauma in pregnancy is common and complicates 6 to 7 percent of pregnancies, although well less than 1 percent of pregnant women require hospitalization [68]. Trauma has been identified as the most common nonobstetric cause of maternal death in several studies. It was the most common cause of maternal mortality in Massachusetts, where the incidence has actually increased over 30 years, whereas maternal death rates secondary to all other causes have declined [3] (see Table 170-1). Maternal injury has been associated with an increased incidence of premature labor, spontaneous abortion, abruptio placentae, fetomaternal hemorrhage, and intrauterine fetal demise. The incidence of fetal death exceeds that of maternal death by three- to ninefold [69].

The physiologic and anatomic changes that occur during pregnancy alter both the types of injuries seen and the maternal response to accompanying blood loss. The previously mentioned increase in blood volume that accompanies gestation may improve tolerance for hemorrhage but may significantly delay the appearance of signs until severe shock is manifested. As fetal well-being depends on uterine blood flow, which is not self-regulating, moderate decreases in maternal cardiac output and blood pressure, which are insufficient to cause maternal shock, still may be detrimental to the fetus. As the uterus grows and becomes an abdominal organ, it becomes more vulnerable to direct trauma. Upward displacement of the bladder also makes this organ more prone to injury. The shift of other abdominal organs also may affect pertinent physical findings.

Most maternal injuries during pregnancy are due to blunt trauma, with automobile accidents being most common [70]. Serious injuries do not seem to carry a higher mortality in pregnant women than in young women who are not pregnant. Head injury and hemorrhagic shock account for the majority of maternal deaths. Significant abdominal injury, especially in late pregnancy, may cause uterine rupture, but this is fortunately quite rare, with an incidence of less than 1 percent of all cases of maternal trauma. Maternal death rates approach 10 percent with this entity, usually secondary to coexistent injuries, whereas fetal loss is almost universal. Placental abruption is relatively rare after minor trauma, but rates rise dramatically after more severe injuries. Abruption carries a much graver prognosis to the fetus than to the mother. Because the fetus is well protected in the pelvis and cushioned by amniotic fluid, direct fetal injuries due to blunt trauma are rare.

Fetomaternal hemorrhage may occur after trauma from transplacental transfer of fetal blood into the maternal circulation. This occurs much more commonly in injured than in noninjured mothers, but it does not seem to correlate with the severity of injury or the length of gestation. Its complications include Rh sensitization of the mother, neonatal anemia, and fetal death. Therefore, assessment of fetomaternal hemorrhage by the Kleinhaur-Betke assay should be considered in all pregnancies complicated by trauma [71].

Resuscitation and Assessment

The initial resuscitation and primary survey of the injured pregnant woman should follow guidelines outlined by the American

College of Surgeons Committee on Trauma Advanced Trauma Life Support Program [72]. Concerns over a competent airway, functional breathing, and adequate circulation are of first priority. Because of the increased vascularity of the nasal passages in pregnancy, nasotracheal intubation should be done with great care. Standard fluid and blood resuscitation should be used to restore circulating blood volume, keeping in mind the requirement for an increased blood volume in pregnancy and ensuring that the fetal circulation is also well supported. If possible, the pregnant woman should be transported and cared for lying on the left side to improve venous return to the heart. The pneumatic antishock garment (PASG) may have deleterious effects on blood volume by compressing the uterus against the inferior vena cava, especially late in pregnancy.

The secondary survey should then ensue. If felt to be necessary, peritoneal lavage (DPL) may be performed, if the incision is made well above the fundus and an open technique is used. DPL may be preferable to CT for assessing intraabdominal bleeding because there is no radiation exposure with the former technique [72]. The surgeon should perform a formal examination of the uterus and vagina, looking for signs of trauma, bleeding, or ruptured membranes. Fetal assessment should include evaluation of fetal movement, auscultation of fetal heart tones by Doppler, and tocographic monitoring. Although fetal radiation exposure should be minimized, essential radiographs must be obtained, with appropriate shielding if possible. Significant effects on the fetus should be rare with exposures of 1 to 2 cGy, especially if the fetus is over 12 weeks gestation [16]. CT delivers 5 to 10 cGy [17], raising more concern with respect to fetal radiation exposure. However, scans occasionally have been used in pregnancy without reported ill effects [18]. Blood should be drawn and sent for standard tests as well as for blood typing, Rh screening, and the Kleihaur-Betke test. Rh immunization should be given within 72 hours to Rh-negative mothers sustaining more than the most trivial of trauma. During the first trimester, 50 μg of Rh immune globulin should be administered. The dose should be increased to 300 μg in more advanced pregnancy. Additional doses of immune globulin may be necessary in cases where large volumes of fetomaternal hemorrhage or continued fetal blood are seen in serial Kleihaur-Betke assays [15].

Ultrasound may be helpful in the assessment of gestational size, the determination of fetal movement and cardiac activity in cases of uncertain Doppler monitoring results, the quantification of amniotic fluid in cases of suspected ruptured membranes, and the final confirmation of suspected fetal demise.

Both mother and fetus should have continuous monitoring. It is important that the fetus have cardiotocographic monitoring because fetal demise is much more common than maternal death. Increasing risk of fetal death is associated with high maternal injury severity scores, severe head injury, maternal acidosis, shock, and hypoxia [73]. Unfortunately the most commonly followed standard maternal clinical parameters, such as blood pressure, heart rate, hematocrit, and arterial PCO_2, are not predictive of fetal survival [15]. Although fetal heart rate on admission may not be predictive of fetal outcome, cardiotocographic monitoring may allow for earlier detection of fetal distress. Increased uterine contractual activity (greater than 8 contractions per hour) is often seen as an early warning of impending placental abruption. As abruption most often occurs soon after injury, a 4- to 24-hour period of continuous monitoring should be predictive with respect to posttraumatic abruption [74,75].

The definitive therapy rendered the pregnant trauma victim should mirror that given those who are not pregnant (see Chap. 174). Because of the increased vascularity around the uterus, pelvic fractures should be aggressively stabilized. Special consideration should be given to cesarean section in situations of fetal distress and in states of refractory maternal shock [19,20,76]. Removal of the fetus may be lifesaving to the child and to the mother, and the increase in venous return following delivery may improve resuscitative efforts.

References

1. Kaunitz AM, Hughes JM, Grimes D, et al: Causes of maternal mortality in the United States. *Obstet Gynecol* 65:605, 1985.
2. Varner MW: Maternal mortality in Iowa from 1952 to 1986. *Surg Gynecol Obstet* 168:555, 1989.
3. Sachs B, Brown D, Driscoll DJ, et al: Maternal mortality in Massachusetts. *N Engl J Med* 316:667, 1987.
4. Veland K, Novy MJ, Peterson EN, et al: Maternal cardiovascular dynamics. IV. The influence of gestational age on the maternal cardiovascular response. *Am J Obstet Gynecol* 104:856, 1969.
5. Mashin IS, Albazzaz SJ, Feidel, ME: Serial non-invasive evaluation of cardiovascular hemodynamics during pregnancy. *Am J Obstet Gynecol* 156:1208, 1987.
6. Veland K, Hansen JM: Maternal cardiovascular dynamics. II. Posture and uterine contractions. *Am J Obstet Gynecol* 103:1, 1969.
7. Pritchard JA: Changes in the blood volume during pregnancy and delivery. *Anesthesiology* 26:393, 1965.
8. Weinberger SE, Weiss ST, Cotton WR, et al: Pregnancy and lung. *Am Rev Respir Dis* 121:559, 1980.
9. Novy MJ, Edwards MJ: Respiratory problems in pregnancy. *Am J Obstet Gynecol* 99:1024, 1967.
10. Machida H: Influence of progesterone on arterial blood and CSF acid-base balance in women. *J Appl Physiol* 51:1433, 1981.
11. Wilkening RB, Meschia G: Fetal oxygen uptake, oxygenation and acid-base balance as a function of uterine blood flow. *Am J Physiol* 244:H749, 1983.
12. Berkowitz RL, Rafferty TD: Invasive hemodynamic monitoring in critically ill patients: Role of Swan-Ganz catheterization. *Am J Obstet Gynecol* 137:127, 1980.
13. Helmkamp BF, Civetta JM, Girtanner R, et al: The Swan-Ganz catheter and its application in the gynecologic patient. *Am J Obstet Gynecol* 139:628, 1981.
14. Berkowitz RL: The Swan-Ganz catheter and colloid osmotic pressure determinations, in Berkowitz RL (ed): *Critical Care of the Obstetric Patient*. New York, Churchill Livingstone, 1983, pp 1–20.
15. Kissinger DP, Rozycki GS, Morris JA, et al: Trauma in pregnancy. Predicting pregnancy outcome. *Arch Surg* 126:1079, 1991.
16. Brent RL: The effects of embryonic and fetal exposure to x-ray, microwaves and ultrasound. Counseling the pregnant and nonpregnant patient. *Semin Oncol* 16:347, 1989.
17. Wagner LK, Archer BR, Zeck OT: Conceptus dose from two state-of-the-art CT scanners. *Radiology* 159:787, 1986.
18. Esposito RJ, Gans DR, Gerber-Smith L, et al: Evaluation of blunt abdominal trauma occurring during pregnancy. *J Trauma* 29:1628, 1989.
19. Lee RV, Rodgers BD, White CM, et al: Cardiopulmonary resuscitation of pregnant woman. *Am J Med* 81:311, 1986.
20. Katz VL, Dotters DJ, Droegnueller W: Postmortem caesarean delivery. *Obstet Gynecol* 68:571, 1986.
21. Kalter H, Warkany J: Congenital malformations. *N Engl J Med* 308:491, 1983.
22. Rosenberg L, Mitchell AA, Persells JL, et al: Lack of relation of oral clefts to diazepam use during pregnancy. *N Engl J Med* 309:1282, 1983.
23. Briggs CG, Freeman RK, Yaffee SJ: *Drugs in Pregnancy and Lactation*. Baltimore, Williams & Wilkins, 1986.
24. L'Hommideau CS, Nicholas D, Armas DA, et al: Potentiation of $MgSO_4$ induced neuromuscular weakness by gentamicin, tobramycin, and amikacin. *J Pediatr* 102:629, 1983.
25. Chow AW, Jewesson RJ: Pharmacokinetics and safety of antimicrobial agents in pregnancy. *Rev Infect Dis* 7:278, 1985.
26. Ginsberg B, Hirsch J, Turner C, et al: Risks to the fetus of anticoagulant therapy during pregnancy. *Thromb Haemost* 61:197, 1989.

27. Hall JG, Paul RM, Wilson KM: Maternal and fetal sequelae of anticoagulants during pregnancy. *Am J Med* 68:122, 1978.
28. Berkowitz RL: The management of hypertensive crisis during pregnancy, in Berkowitz RL (ed): *Critical Care of the Obstetric Patient*. New York, Churchill Livingstone, 1983, pp 299–334.
29. Wheeler AJ, James FM III, Meis PJ, et al: Effect of nitroglycerin and nitroprusside in the uterine vasculature of gravid ewes. *Anesthesiology* 52:390, 1980.
30. Cotton DB, Longmire S, Jones MM, et al: Cardiovascular alterations in severe pregnancy-induced hypertension: Effects of intravenous nitroglycerin coupled with blood expansion. *Am J Obstet Gynecol* 154:1053, 1986.
31. Naulty J, Cefalo RC, Lewis PE: Fetal toxicity of nitroprusside in the pregnant ewe. *Am J Obstet Gynecol* 139:708, 1981.
32. Ralston DH, Shnider SM, deLorimer AA: Effect of equipotent ephedrine, metaraminol, mephentermine and methoxamine on uterine blood flow in the pregnant ewe. *Anesthesiology* 40:354, 1974.
33. Moran DH, Perillo M, LaPorta RF, et al: Phenylephrine in prevention of hypotension following spinal anesthesia for cesarean delivery. *J Clinic Anesth* 3:301, 1991.
34. Berg BN: Dietary restriction and reproduction in the rat. *J Nutr* 87:344, 1965.
35. Rosso P: Nutrition and maternal-fetal exchange. *Am J Clin Nutr* 34:744, 1981.
36. James CF, Gibbs CP, Banner T: Postpartum perioperative risk of aspiration pneumonia. *Anesthesiology* 61:756, 1984.
37. Martin R, Blackburn G: Hyperalimentation during pregnancy, in Berkowitz RL (ed): *Critical Care of the Obstetric Patient*. New York, Churchill Livingstone, 1983, pp 133–163.
38. Lee RV, Rodgers BD, Young C, et al: Total parenteral nutrition during pregnancy. *Obstet Gynecol* 68(4):563, 1968.
39. Heller L: Clinical and experimental studies in complete parenteral nutrition. *Scand J Gastroenterol* 4(Suppl 4):7, 1968.
40. Sibai BM: Pitfalls in diagnosis and management of pre-eclampsia. *Am J Obstet Gynecol* 159:1, 1988.
41. Maikranz P, Katz A: Acute renal failure in pregnancy. *Obstet Gynecol Clin North Am* 18(2):333, 1991.
42. Martz JN, Stedman CM: Imitators of pre-eclampsia and HELLP syndrome. *Obstet Gynecol Clin North Am* 18(2):181, 1991.
43. Pritchard JA, Baldwin RM, Dickey JC: Blood volume changes in pregnancy and puerperium. *Am J Obstet Gynecol* 84:1271, 1962.
44. Sattronor EC, Kartmann BM, Connaufrton JF: Intravascular volume determinations and fetal outcome in hypertensive diseases of pregnancy. *Am J Obstet Gynecol* 127:4, 1977.
45. Benedotti TJ, Carlson RW: Studies of colloid oncotic pressure in pregnancy-involved hypertension. *Am J Obstet Gynecol* 135:308, 1979.
46. Donaldson JO: Eclamptic hypertensive encephalopathy. *J Neurol* 8:230, 1988.
47. Donaldson JO: Neurologic emergencies in pregnancy. *Obstet Gynecol Clin North Am* 18(2):199, 1991.
48. Weinstein L: Syndrome of hemolysis, elevated liver enzymes and low platelet count. A severe consequence of hypertension in pregnancy. *Am J Obstet Gynecol* 142:159, 1982.
49. Barton JR, Sibai BM: Care of the pregnancy complicating HELLP syndrome. *Obstet Gynecol Clin North Am* 18(2):165, 1991.
50. Goldenberg RL, Nelson KG, David RO, et al: Delay in delivery: Influence of gestational age and the duration of delay on perinatal outcome. *Obstet Gynecol* 64:480, 1984.
51. Sullivan JM, Ramanathan A: Management of medical problems in pregnancy—severe cardiac disease. *N Engl J Med* 66:491, 1984.
52. Cunningham FG, Pritchard JA: How should hypertension during pregnancy be managed? *Med Clin North Am* 68:505, 1984.
53. Pritchard JA, Cunningham FG, Pritchard SA: The Parkland Memorial Hospital protocol for treatment of eclampsia: Evaluation of 245 cases. *Am J Obstet Gynecol* 148:951, 1984.
54. Sibai BM: Magnesium sulfate is the ideal anticonvulsant in pre-eclampsia/eclampsia. *Am J Obstet Gynecol* 162:1141, 1990.
55. Kaplan PW, Lesser RP, Fisher RS, et al: A continuing controversy: Magnesium sulfate in the treatment of eclamptic seizures. *Arch Neurol* 47:1031, 1990.
56. Stirling Y, Woolf L, North WRS, et al: Haemostasis in normal pregnancy. *Thromb Haemost* 52:176, 1984.
57. Pritchard JA, Baldwin RM, Dickey JC: Blood volume changes in pregnancy and puerperium. *Am J Obstet Gynecol* 84:1271, 1962.
58. Clark S: Placenta previa accreta and prior cesarean section. *Obstet Gynecol* 66:89, 1985.
59. Brenner WE, Edelmar DA, Hendricks CA: Characteristics of patients with placenta previa and results of expectant management. *Am J Obstet Gynecol* 132:180, 1978.
60. Hurd WW, Miodovnik M, Hertzberg V, et al: Selective management of abruptio placentae: A prospective study. *Obstet Gynecol* 61:467, 1983.
61. Pritchard JA, Brekken AL: Clinical and laboratory studies on severe abruptio placentae. *Am J Obstet Gynecol* 97:681, 1967.
62. Romero R: The management of acquired hemostatic failure during pregnancy, in Berkowitz RL (ed): *Critical Care of the Obstetric Patient*. New York, Churchill Livingstone, 1983, pp 219–284.
63. Luca WE: Postpartum hemorrhage. *Clin Obstet Gynecol* 23:637, 1980.
64. Casady GN, Moore DL, Bridenbaugh D: Postpartum hypertension after use of vasoconstrictor and oxytocic drugs: Etiology, incidences, complications and treatment. *JAMA* 172:101, 1960.
65. Hayashi RH, Castillo MS, Noah ML: Management of severe postpartum hemorrhage due to uterine atony using an analogue of prostaglandin F₂. *Obstet Gynecol* 58:426, 1981.
66. Schwartz PE: The surgical approach to severe postpartum hemorrhage, in Berkowitz RL (ed): *Critical Care of the Obstetric Patient*. New York, Churchill Livingstone, 1983, pp 285–297.
67. Pais SO, Glickman M, Schwartz P, et al: Embolization of pelvic arteries for control of postpartum hemorrhage. *Obstet Gynecol* 55:754, 1980.
68. Peckham AF, King RA: A study of intercurrent conditions observed during pregnancy. *Am J Obstet Gynecol* 87:609, 1963.
69. Drost RF, Rosemary AS, Sherman HF, et al: Major trauma in pregnant women: Maternal/fetal outcome. *J Trauma* 30:576, 1990.
70. Lavin JP Jr, Polsy SS: Abdominal trauma during pregnancy. *Clin Perinatol* 10:424, 1983.
71. Pearlman MD, Tintinalli JE, Lorenz RP: Blunt trauma during pregnancy. *N Engl J Med* 323(23):1609, 1990.
72. Committee on Trauma, American College of Surgeons: *Advanced Trauma Life Support Program for Physicians*. Chicago, American College of Surgeons, 1993.
73. Hoff WS, D'Ameko LF, Tinkoff GH: Maternal predictors of fetal demise in trauma during pregnancy. *Surg Gynecol Obstet* 172(3):175, 1991.
74. Pearlman MD, Tinitalli JE, Lorenz RP: A prospective controlled study of trauma during pregnancy. *Am J Obstet Gynecol* 162:1502, 1990.
75. Higgins SD, Gantz D: Late abruptio placenta in trauma patients: Implications for monitoring. *Obstet Gynecol* 63:105, 1984.
76. Buschbaum HJ, Crukshank DP: Postmortem cesarean section, in Buschbaum HJ (ed): *Trauma in Pregnancy*. Philadelphia, WB Saunders, 1979.

XII. Shock and Trauma

Section Editor
Mitchell P. Fink

171. Shock: An Overview

Mitchell P. Fink

Definition

HISTORICAL PERSPECTIVE. *Shock* as an English language medical term was apparently first used in 1743 in a translation by Sparrow of Henri Francois Le Dran's second French edition of "A Treatise of Reflections Drawn from Experience with Gunshot Wounds" [1]. Beginning with this work and continuing until the end of the 19th century, shock was defined purely on the basis of clinical description. For example, in 1895, John Collins Warren considered shock to be a "momentary pause in the act of death" characterized by "cold, clammy sweat" and a "weak, thread-like" radial pulse [2]. During the early part of the current century, when blood pressure measurement was introduced into routine clinical practice, the term *shock* was generally used as a synonym for systemic arterial hypotension caused by trauma or hemorrhage. However, as early as 1899, Crile emphasized the role of inadequate venous return in the pathophysiology of shock and documented the beneficial effect of treating shock by infusing saline [3]. The notion that shock is a manifestation of hypoperfusion rather than simply arterial hypotension was subsequently further delineated in the writings of clinicians and scientists, such as Cannon [4], Keith [5], Blalock [6], and Cournand et al. [7].

MODERN DEFINITIONS. Currently, shock is usually defined as a syndrome (i.e., a complex of symptoms, signs, and laboratory abnormalities) precipitated by a systemic derangement in perfusion leading to widespread cellular hypoxia and vital organ dysfunction. Global perfusion, however, is often normal or even supranormal in patients with shock attributable to sepsis [8,9,10]. Nevertheless, patients with septic shock typically manifest many of the metabolic and clinical features (e.g., hyperlactatemia, oliguria, confusion) associated with other forms of shock. The basis for "shock" in sepsis despite normal or high cardiac output is discussed in greater detail below and in Chapters 173 and 199.

SUPPLY-DEPENDENT OXYGEN UPTAKE. Except for oxymyoglobin found in muscle cells, oxygen is not stored by tissues. Therefore, oxidative metabolism depends on the constant delivery of oxygen by the bloodstream. In most tissues, oxygen uptake (VO_2) is determined by metabolic demand and is not regulated or determined by its availability; this is Pfluger's law [11,12,13]. If oxygen delivery (DO_2) decreases in the setting of constant metabolic demand, extraction of oxygen increases and VO_2 remains constant until extraction is maximized. If DO_2 decreases to less than this critical level (called DO_{2crit}), then VO_2 decreases as well; i.e., VO_2 is rendered supply dependent. This relationship between DO_2 and VO_2 has been termed "O_2 regulation" [13a]. In anesthetized humans undergoing cardiac surgery, systemic DO_{2crit} is approximately 300 to 330 ml/min/ M^2 [15,16]. When DO_2 is less than DO_{2crit}, oxygen consumption is regulated by availability and not metabolic demand and, thus, an oxygen deficit exists. When VO_2 is supply dependent, anaerobic metabolism and lactate production increase and metabolic acidosis ensues. If the oxygen deficit is sufficiently large or prolonged, then intracellular stores of high-energy phosphates (adenosine triphosphate [ATP] and phosphocreatine)

decrease enough to result in derangements in key biochemical processes, such as the functioning of membrane ion pumps. These biochemical events lead to membrane depolarization, intracellular edema, impaired regulation of intracellular calcium ion concentration, loss of membrane integrity, and ultimately cell death [17].

In many forms of shock, the precipitating event (e.g., massive hemorrhage or rupture of the mitral valve apparatus) clearly leads to a low cardiac output state and, on that basis, supply dependency of systemic VO_2. In patients with septic shock, however, systemic DO_2 and VO_2 are often both supranormal. Nevertheless, there is evidence that an oxygen deficit is present in many septic patients despite "adequate" systemic DO_2 [18–21]. It has been hypothesized that peripheral oxygen extraction is deranged in septic shock and that VO_2 in this syndrome is pathologically supply dependent [22,23]. The mechanisms underlying the apparent pathologic supply dependency of VO_2 in septic shock are poorly understood, although it has been hypothesized that abnormalities at the microvascular level lead to maldistribution of perfusion, such that regions of hyperfusion and hypoperfusion coexist.

Making matters more complicated are clinical data, which call into question the notion of pathologic supply dependency of VO_2 in septic shock [24–27]. Furthermore, recent experimental data suggest that tissue oxygenation in sepsis is not impaired [28]. Accordingly, other mechanisms have been suggested to account for metabolic acidosis, hyperlactatemia, and organ system failure in septic shock, because these findings are indicative of energy starvation at the cellular level. Some data suggest that organ system dysfunction in septic shock is not a consequence of cellular hypoxia per se, but is caused by an uncoupling of mitochondrial oxidative phosphorylation so that intracellular energy stores decline despite normal or supranormal VO_2 [29,30]. Other recent studies suggest that mediators released in sepsis (cytokines, lipopolysaccharide, and nitric oxide) can impair the activity of key mitochondrial enzymes [31,32]. Alternatively, intracellular high-energy phosphate stores may be adequate in septic shock, but other derangements in regulation of the intracellular milieu may be responsible for key clinical features of the syndrome. For example, data suggest that sepsis leads to hyperlactatemia by altering the activity of an enzyme complex, pyruvate dehydrogenase, that is an important regulatory point in intermediary metabolism (see Chap. 156) [33,34]. Recent studies suggest that organ dysfunction caused by sepsis may be caused, at least in part, by dysregulation of the release of calcium ions from intracellular stores [35].

Pathophysiology

During the early stages of shock, it is usually possible to identify a single primary cause of the circulatory disturbance. Because avoiding the adverse sequelae of shock depends on the prompt recognition and reversal of the primary problem, shock syndromes traditionally have been classified on the basis of the initiating pathophysiologic derangement (*vide infra*). Although this approach is both clinically useful and mechanistically valid, it is important to emphasize that there is a great deal of overlap among the various shock syndromes. This is particularly true when the initiating problem goes uncorrected and the shock syndrome is permitted to evolve. Major subcellular events (particularly membrane depolarization and ion pump dysfunction) are very similar in all forms of shock [17]. Furthermore, fundamentally different shock syndromes overlap considerably even at the organ system level. For example, impaired myocardial performance, the initiating event in primary cardiogenic shock, is clearly present in septic shock and is probably also a factor in several other kinds of shock; inadequate preload caused by hypovolemia is the precipitating event in hemorrhagic shock, but absolute or relative hypovolemia is also often a factor contributing to the circulatory derangements observed in septic shock; bloodstream invasion by microbes or microbial products is the usual precipitating event in septic shock, but recent data suggest that blood cultures are also often positive for enteric organisms in cases of hemorrhagic shock.

DETERMINANTS OF CARDIAC OUTPUT.

In most forms of shock, the fundamental problem is that systemic DO_2 is inadequate to meet metabolic demand. Systemic DO_2 is determined by four factors: hemoglobin concentration, arterial oxygen saturation, arterial PO_2, and cardiac output. Most often, inadequate DO_2 in shock occurs because cardiac output precipitously or progressively declines. Low (or relatively low) cardiac output may be an important problem even in septic shock.

In the absence of regurgitant flow, cardiac output is equal to left ventricular stroke volume (LVSV) times heart rate. LVSV, in turn, is a function of three variables: preload, afterload, and contractility.

Preload. In many shock states, the primary problem is low cardiac output attributable to inadequate preload. The term *preload* derives from in vitro experiments using mammalian myocardial tissue (papillary muscle, trabeculae carneae, or atrial myocardium) (Fig. 171-1). One end of the muscle is mounted to a force transducer and the other to a lever arm. The other end of the lever arm is attached to a pan. Small weights (preload) are added to the pan to stretch the muscle before triggering contraction with an electrical stimulus. Although preload is typically measured in units of force (i.e., the force generated when gravity acts on the mass in the pan), it is the initial muscle *length* that is the major determinant of the force generated when the muscle contracts. Similarly, in the intact ventricle, force of contraction is determined by end-diastolic *volume* (EDV) and not end-diastolic pressure (EDP), although the latter is often used as a proxy for the former in clinical practice. The relationship between EDV (dependent variable) and EDP (independent variable) depends on the diastolic compliance (distensibility) of the ventricle. Diastolic compliance is decreased by myocardial ischemia [36] and hypertrophy [37]. Thus, in some pathophysiologic conditions

Fig. 171-1. Schematic representation of in vitro apparatus for studying the effects of preload and afterload on myocardial performance.

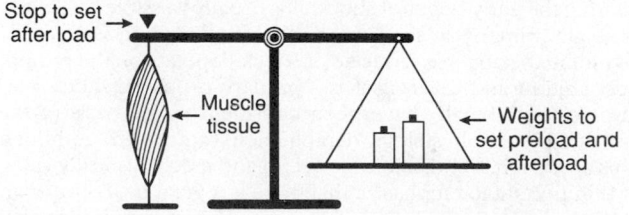

(e.g., coronary artery occlusive disease), measuring a "normal" central venous pressure (CVP) or pulmonary capillary wedge pressure (PCWP) may not rule out inadequate preload as a cause of shock.

INTRAVASCULAR VOLUME. Most frequently shock secondary to inadequate preload is a consequence of decreased venous return caused by loss of intravascular volume (i.e., "hypovolemia"). Hypovolemia can be caused by external or internal losses of whole blood (i.e., hemorrhagic shock); contraction of the (cell-free) intravascular space caused by external fluid losses (e.g., diarrhea or inappropriate polyuria); contraction of the intravascular fluid compartment caused by internal (so-called third-space) sequestration; or some combination of the above (as in "traumatic shock").

SYSTEMIC VASCULAR RESISTANCE. Several factors other than total intravascular volume also affect venous return. Of these, systemic vascular resistance (SVR) is the most important, venous return and SVR being inversely related. Thus, for example, exercise and anemia decrease SVR and increase venous return (and, hence, cardiac output) [38]. In septic shock, SVR is typically markedly diminished [8]. Because myocardial systolic performance is clearly impaired in septic shock [39], low SVR is presumably the major factor permitting the maintenance or even elevation of cardiac output in this setting.

VENOUS VASOMOTOR TONE. Venous return, and hence preload, also depend on vasomotor tone in venous capacitance vessels. Venodilation, by lowering effective intravascular volume, decreases venous return and cardiac output [40]. This mechanism is of pathophysiologic importance in neurogenic and anaphylactic shock and may also play a role in some cases of septic shock [41].

INTRATHORACIC PRESSURE. Venous return is adversely affected by increasing intrathoracic pressure. This is the primary mechanism leading to shock and hypotension in patients with tension pneumothorax. Intrathoracic pressure is also increased to a variable extent by intermittent positive pressure ventilation (IPPV) and the application of positive end-expiratory pressure (PEEP). Because IPPV tends to *diminish* afterload (*vide infra*), the effect of IPPV on cardiac output in any particular patient is difficult to predict a priori and depends on several factors, particularly intravascular volume status and pulmonary compliance.

When intravascular volume is low (as in hypovolemic shock), the adverse effect of positive pressure ventilation on preload predominates and cardiac output diminishes. Clinicians must be cognizant of this phenomenon when converting a marginally compensated but hypovolemic patient from spontaneous to positive pressure ventilation. When intravascular volume is normal or high (as in some cases of cardiogenic shock), the beneficial effect of positive intrathoracic pressure on afterload may predominate and cardiac output may improve. This is particularly true when intrinsic myocardial contractility is impaired. Oftentimes, the beneficial effect of positive pressure ventilation on cardiac output goes unrecognized until it is withdrawn. Thus, intubated and mechanically ventilated patients with poor intrinsic cardiac performance may remain adequately compensated until ventilatory support is withdrawn, but then suddenly (and unexpectedly) "crash" shortly after extubation, manifesting signs and symptoms of low output and pulmonary edema. Increased intrathoracic pressure synchronized to the cardiac cycle is undergoing investigation as a way to use mechanical ventilation to reduce afterload and augment cardiac output without paying a penalty in terms of preload [42,43].

Pulmonary compliance determines the effect of PEEP on intrathoracic pressure. When compliance is low (i.e., the lungs are "stiff"), as in severe acute respiratory distress syndrome (ARDS), a given level of PEEP results in less expansion of the lungs and a smaller increase in intrathoracic pressure than occurs when compliance is normal.

INTRAPERICARDIAL PRESSURE. Markedly elevated intrapericardial pressure (i.e., pericardial tamponade) impedes venous return by decreasing the apparent diastolic compliance of the ventricles.

VENTRICULAR INTERACTION. Venous return to the left ventricle also can be adversely affected by changes in ventricular geometry induced by shifts in the intraventricular septum. Volume or pressure overload of the right ventricle can lead to encroachment of the septum on the left ventricular cavity. This leads to a shift of the left ventricular pressure-volume relationship (i.e., decreased left ventricular compliance). The effect of ventricular interaction on left ventricular filling is particularly prominent when the pericardium is intact [44]. Septal shift may be a factor contributing to diminished cardiac output in acute pulmonary hypertension caused, for example, by pulmonary embolism, sepsis, or ARDS.

LOSS OF ATRIAL "KICK." Atrial contraction, if coordinated and properly timed, augments ventricular diastolic filling [45]. In some supraventricular dysrhythmias, the effectiveness of atrial augmentation is lost. If myocardial performance is already impaired, for example, because of inadequate circulating volume, impaired contractility, or increased diastolic stiffness, then loss of atrial augmentation can precipitate low-output shock.

TACHYARRHYTHMIA. As noted already, heart rate is a determinant of cardiac output. Ordinarily, increasing heart rate increases output by simply increasing the number of ejections per unit time. In addition, increasing heart rate typically also increases contractility [46,47]. When heart rate is very high, however, the diastolic interval is short enough to interfere with ventricular filling, and hence, cardiac output is compromised. In the clinical setting, rapid ventricular rates often occur in patients with preexisting ischemic heart disease, and in this situation, tachyarrhythmias can also adversely affect cardiac output by upsetting the balance between myocardial DO_2 and VO_2, leading to impaired contractility on the basis of ischemia.

Afterload. Excessive ventricular afterload is occasionally the primary problem leading to shock. More often, therapeutic measures directed at decreasing afterload are essential to the optimal management of shock, even when "excessive" afterload is not the primary initiating derangement. Like preload, the term *afterload* derives from studies of myocardial function performed in vitro (see Fig. 171-1). After resting length is adjusted by adding weights to the pan, a stop is positioned against the lever so that adding additional weight to the pan will not further stretch the muscle. More weight is then added. The force generated by gravity acting on the total mass in the pan (i.e.,

the afterload) is the load that the muscle must move to perform external work. Studies performed in vitro indicate that increasing afterload decreases the velocity and extent of contraction [48,49].

Considerable controversy exists regarding the correct in vivo correlate of afterload. According to some authorities, ventricular afterload is best expressed in terms of intracavitary pressure [50]. Because intracavitary (or aortic root) pressure depends in a major way on ventricular contraction, this definition implies that the ventricle, to a large extent, creates its own afterload. Thus, other authorities regard "vascular input impedance" as the appropriate in vivo measure of ventricular afterload [51,52].

Although clinicians frequently equate SVR and vascular input impedance, this is an oversimplification. SVR represents the impediment to flow in the vascular circuit under conditions of nonpulsatile flow. In contrast, vascular input impedance is a complex term that is determined by several factors, including frequency (i.e., heart rate and higher-order harmonics of heart rate), arterial compliance, pulse wave reflection, blood inertia, *and* SVR [50]. When frequency is zero (i.e., flow is nonpulsatile), impedance equals SVR. However, frequency is never zero in living subjects, and thus input impedance is inevitably multifactorial.

Decreased compliance of the aorta, caused for example by aging or atherosclerosis, increases input impedance and hence afterload. Pulse wave reflection, a phenomenon that can magnify aortic root and intracavitary pressures during ejection, is a complex phenomenon that is, in part, a function of SVR; maneuvers that decrease SVR also tend to decrease the magnitude of pulse wave reflection [53,54]. Thus, lowering SVR by infusing an arteriolar vasodilator lowers input impedance (and afterload) in two ways: by lowering SVR and by decreasing the magnitude of pulse wave reflection.

In the systemic circulation, vascular resistance is determined primarily by the degree of vasomotor tone in the precapillary arteriolar smooth muscle sphincters. Other factors, however, also effect SVR, including hematocrit and plasma fibrinogen concentration (anemia and hyperfibrinogenemia both decrease SVR).

In the pulmonary circulation, intravascular pressures are low, and the vessels are thin-walled and surrounded by the thoracic cavity or alveolar airspaces. Thus, elements in the pulmonary circulation have the characteristics of a Starling resistor, which is a collapsible tube surrounded by a pressurized compartment (Fig. 171-2). In a system with a Starling resistor, changes in driving pressure have a minimal effect on flow, and changes in flow have a minimal effect on pressure. To conceptualize this, it is helpful to consider the mechanical model of a Starling resistor shown in Figure 147-2 [54]. If inflow increases, then the size of the orifice increases without any substantial elevation in upstream pressure. Conversely, if downstream pressure decreases while inflow from the faucet remains constant, then the

Fig. 171-2. A Starling resistor (A) and a mechanical analog (B). The great veins in the chest and the pulmonary vasculature manifest the hemodynamic characteristics of a Starling resistor (see text).

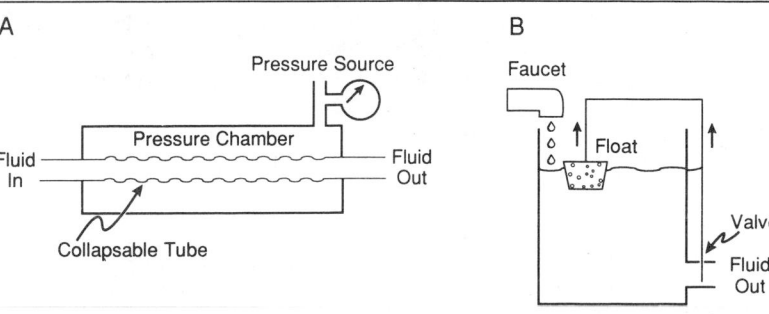

level in the reservoir will decrease slightly and the area of the orifice will decrease, causing flow to remain constant despite the larger upstream-to-downstream pressure gradient. In the pulmonary circulation, the consequence of this phenomenon is that vascular resistance tends to be inversely related to cardiac output and pulmonary artery pressure.

AORTIC STENOSIS. Tight aortic stenosis leading to shock is a particularly difficult problem. In this disease, left ventricular wall tension is high, and this increases myocardial oxygen demand. Cardiac output is compromised by excessive impedance to ejection, but attempts to decrease afterload using agents like sodium nitroprusside can dangerously lower diastolic blood pressure and compromise coronary perfusion without greatly affecting left ventricular wall tension or oxygen demand. Thus, pharmacotherapy with afterload-reducing agents can precipitate myocardial ischemia, arrhythmias, and cardiac arrest. Inotropic agents can increase wall tension and myocardial oxygen demand, and in aortic stenosis caused by asymmetric septal hypertrophy (see Chap. 33), actually exacerbate the obstruction to ventricular ejection. Thus, correction or amelioration of the mechanical problem in the operating room or cardiac catheterization laboratory is often the only satisfactory approach for treating shock caused by critical aortic stenosis.

PULMONARY EMBOLISM. Massive pulmonary thromboembolism is a rare but important cause of shock (see Chap. 60). Obstruction of the pulmonary artery by blood clot can be a direct mechanical impediment to right ventricular ejection. In addition, in cases of diffuse embolization of smaller thrombi, mediators (e.g., thromboxane A_2 and serotonin) are released that cause marked pulmonary vasoconstriction and on that basis excessively afterload the right ventricle [55,56,57]. As noted already, pressure overload of the right ventricle can increase left ventricular diastolic elastance (stiffness) and compromise preload in the systemic ventricle.

Contractility.

Shock is frequently caused by deterioration in the intrinsic performance of the heart irrespective of loading conditions. This can be attributable to outright loss of contractile tissue (i.e., myocardial infarction), diminished contractility of viable myocardial tissue, regurgitant flow, or some combination of the above. Most often, acute deterioration of myocardial performance is a complication of acute myocardial infarction. Another fairly common cause is "myocardial stunning" after an episode of transient myocardial ischemia followed by reperfusion (such as occurs during and after cardiopulmonary bypass) [58,59,60]. Other causes, however (e.g., viral myocarditis), are occasionally encountered.

Assessing myocardial contractility in vitro is straightforward because it is possible to ensure that loading conditions (i.e., preload and afterload) remain constant. If loading is constant, changes in myocardial work are attributable to changes in contractility. However, in vivo, it is generally impossible to fix preload and afterload. Indeed, in the clinical setting, it is cumbersome to reliably measure preload (end-diastolic volume), and afterload is usually estimated by calculating systemic or pulmonary vascular resistance, which, as already suggested, overly simplifies a complex parameter.

Currently, clinicians typically use myocardial performance (Frank-Starling) curves or ejection phase parameters to estimate contractility. For example, in discussing a patient in cardiogenic shock with high PCWP, clinicians sometimes refer to the patient's "flat" Starling curve, indicating by this terminology that augmenting PCWP (a proxy for preload) leads to little improvement in stroke work or stroke volume (measures of pump performance). Alternatively, in this clinical scenario, reference might be made to the patient's low left ventricular ejection fraction, implying that this is evidence of poor myocardial contractility.

Although their clinical utility is not disputed, it is still essential to recognize that estimates of contractility using ventricular performance curves or ejection fraction are influenced by loading conditions. It is noteworthy, therefore, that load-independent estimators of contractility have been described that use the end-systolic pressure-dimension relationship [61]. According to this theoretic model, the ventricle can be viewed as a distensible chamber. The elastance (i.e., the reciprocal of the compliance) of this chamber varies over time during each cardiac cycle. Ventricular elastance is maximal at the end of systole. It has been shown that end-systolic elastance (E_{es}) is a load-independent measure of ventricular contractility [61]. Moreover, both theoretical studies [62], studies in animals [63], and studies in patients [64] have shown that ventricular efficiency (i.e., the ratio of stroke work to myocardial oxygen consumption) and maximal left ventricular output depend on the ratio of E_{es} to "effective arterial elastance," a term that is related to vascular input impedance (*vide supra*). In other words, myocardial performance depends on the proper coupling between the viscoelastic properties of the ventricle and the arterial tree. Although not currently used to monitor ventricular performance in the critically ill, E_{es} can be measured in patients [65,66] and can provide useful insights into pathophysiology.

OTHER CAUSES OF LOW CARDIAC OUTPUT LEADING TO SHOCK. Occasionally, bradyarrhythmias diminish cardiac output sufficiently to cause shock. Although cardiac arrest caused by ventricular fibrillation, asystole, or electrical-mechanical dissociation is the ultimate low-output state, this problem is usually not discussed in the context of shock but is considered as a separate topic (see Chap. 32). Regurgitant flow attributable to acute ventricular septal perforation, papillary muscle dysfunction or rupture, or aortic valvular insufficiency can precipitate shock. When shock is caused by regurgitant flow, the problem is lack of forward cardiac output caused by the presence of a low-impedance shunt diverting flow away from the systemic circulation. Although repair of the mechanical problem is usually required, patients in shock from regurgitant flow can sometimes be stabilized medically by using inotropic agents to increase contractility and arteriolar vasodilators to decrease systemic vascular input impedance.

COMPENSATORY RESPONSES TO SHOCK. The progression of shock is classically divided into two or three stages. From a clinical standpoint, a three-stage classification scheme is probably most useful. The first stage is variously called *early, reversible,* or *compensated* shock and is characterized by normally functioning compensatory mechanisms and the absence of damage to vital tissues. If the primary problem is successfully corrected during this stage, full recovery with minimal morbidity is the expected outcome. During the second stage of shock, microvascular and cellular derangements become manifest. Although patients often survive if shock is successfully treated during this stage, recovery is usually protracted and complicated by failure of one or more organ systems. The third stage is called *late, irreversible,* or *decompensated* shock. By the time shock has progressed to this stage, there has been irrevocable damage to vital tissues, and even instituting vigorous therapy cannot prevent the inevitable progression to death.

With the notable exception of septic shock and a few other rare shock syndromes, the compensatory responses to shock are sufficiently similar to warrant presenting a general summary.

In most shock states, compensatory mechanisms (1) act to preserve coronary and cerebral perfusion at the expense of perfusion to skin, skeletal muscle, kidneys, and splanchnic viscera; (2) attempt to defend cardiac output by increasing heart rate and myocardial contractility; (3) act to partially restore effective intravascular volume by venoconstriction and transcapillary refill [67].

Autonomic Nervous System. In most conditions leading to shock, the initial circulatory perturbation that induces compensatory autonomic responses is decreased arterial pressure caused by a decrement in cardiac output [68]. Decreased arterial pressure initiates the baroreceptor reflex through high-pressure stretch receptors located in the carotid sinus, aortic arch, and splanchnic vasculature [67,69]. If hypovolemia is present, reflex pathways are also triggered by low-pressure (volume) receptors in the right atrium [67]. These baroreceptor reflexes are rapidly responsive to even small changes in pressure. They function under both physiologic conditions (e.g., changes in posture) and pathophysiologic circumstances (e.g., hemorrhage). The baroreflexes are mediated primarily by activation of the sympathetic nervous system, although decreased parasympathetic traffic also plays a role. Activation of the sympathetic nervous system leads to numerous actions, including (1) arteriolar constriction in several vascular beds, resulting in increased vascular inflow impedance and redistribution of blood flow away from skeletal muscle and splanchnic viscera [67,70]; (2) augmentation of heart rate and myocardial contractility [67]; (3) constriction of venous capacitance vessels, particularly in the splanchnic bed, augmenting venous return [67,71]; (4) release of adrenomedullary hormones, including epinephrine and [met]enkephalin [72,73]; (5) activation of the renin-angiotensin axis [74].

Renin-Angiotensin System and Arginine Vasopressin. In addition to the sympathoadrenal axis, two other neurohumoral mechanisms aid in defending blood pressure in shock. These are the renin-angiotensin system and the release of arginine-vasopressin (AVP) by the posterior pituitary. In shock, secretion of renin by renal juxtaglomerular cells is triggered by increased adrenergic traffic in the renal nerves [75] and the local renal barostat mechanism [74]. Renin enzymatically acts on renin substrate, generating a decapeptide called angiotensin (A)I, which is subsequently converted to AII by angiotensin-converting enzyme [76]. Although the renin-angiotensin axis is usually thought of as a humoral system, data indicate that AII also can be generated locally at its site of action and thus functions as a paracrine mediator [77,78].

AII acts to restore or defend arterial blood pressure by increasing arteriolar vasomotor tone, primarily in the mesenteric bed [79,80]. In addition, AII has other less important actions, including increasing sympathetic outflow and AVP release from the central nervous system [81], stimulating the release of catecholamines by the adrenal medulla [76], and increasing myocardial contractility [76]. AII also increases release of aldosterone by the adrenal cortex, promoting the conservation of salt and water. Whereas this last action of AII is of utmost importance in the long-term regulation of blood pressure, it is largely irrelevant in the acute response to shock.

AVP is another peptide hormone that is important in the acute response to volume-depleted states, such as hemorrhage and dehydration. By binding to so-called V_1 receptors, AVP increases vascular resistance in the splanchnic and other vascular beds [82]. Whereas arterial baroreceptors are the major drive for autonomic regulation of blood pressure during hemorrhage, signals from cardiac stretch receptors provide the major afferent

stimulus for the release of AVP [83]. Because there are three major pressor systems (autonomic, renin-angiotensin, and AVP), there is considerable redundancy in the compensatory response to shock. Despite this redundancy, all three mechanisms appear to be important, at least under certain circumstances [84].

Transcapillary Refill. Several parameters affect the movement of fluid from the intravascular compartment to the interstitial compartment (or vice versa). These parameters are related by the equation initially described by Starling and subsequently modified by others [85]:

$$\dot{Q} = Kf[(Pmv - Pt) - \sigma(\pi mv - \pi t)] \qquad \text{Equation 1}$$

where $\dot{Q}$ = flow (volume/unit time) across the capillary wall
Kf = filtration coefficient
Pmv = microvascular (i.e., capillary hydrostatic) pressure
Pt = tissue interstitial fluid hydrostatic pressure
σ = osmotic reflection coefficient
πmv = capillary colloid osmotic pressure
πt = tissue interstitial fluid colloid osmotic pressure

The osmotic reflection coefficient (σ) is an expression of the permeability of the capillary wall to solutes. It ordinarily ranges from 0 for very small molecules to almost 1 for large proteins, although under pathologic conditions that are characterized by microvascular "leakiness," σ approaches zero for all proteins.

From the above equation, it is clear that the rate and *direction* of net fluid movement across the capillary is heavily influenced by the hydrostatic pressure gradient between the microvascular and the interstitial spaces. In the compensatory response to shock, precapillary vasoconstriction decreases Pmv, promoting the net movement of fluid from the interstitial compartment into the vascular compartment [86]. In addition, early metabolic changes release glucose and other glycolytic products into the interstitial compartment, favoring the expansion of interstitial volume and pressure at the expense of intracellular dehydration [86]. Increased interstitial hydrostatic pressure then further promotes the restitution of intravascular volume. This expansion of intravascular volume by hydrostatic and osmotic forces is a process termed transcapillary refill and represents an important compensatory mechanism in many shock states.

DECOMPENSATORY MECHANISMS IN SHOCK. If shock is allowed to persist sufficiently long, the syndrome becomes refractory to efforts designed to correct the hemodynamic derangements; this is the irreversible or decompensated phase of shock. Numerous mechanisms apparently contribute to the development of irreversibility.

Peripheral Vasomotor Decompensation. In animal models of hemorrhagic shock, the onset of irreversibility is signaled by vasodilation of precapillary sphincters [87]. The loss of compensatory vasoconstriction exacerbates hypotension, worsens myocardial and central nervous system ischemia, and promotes transudation of fluid from the vascular into the interstitial space. Several mechanisms seem to be responsible for peripheral vascular decompensation, including (1) release of counterregulatory (i.e., vasodilating) prostaglandins [88]; (2) derangements in the recycling and uptake of catecholamines leading to catecholamine depletion [89,90]; (3) decreased sympathetic outflow as a result of central nervous system ischemia [91]; and induction of the production of the potent endogenous vasodilator, nitric oxide [92]. The local accumulation of vasodilatory metabolic end products (e.g., adenosine) does not appear to be important [87].

Another mechanism contributing to cardiovascular decompensation in shock is the release of endogenous opioid peptides. This mechanism was first brought to light by studies in rats showing that naloxone, an opioid peptide antagonist, improves arterial blood pressure in hemorrhagic [93] and endotoxic [94] shock. Subsequent studies demonstrated that naloxone therapy improves survival in certain models of experimental shock from hemorrhage or endotoxin [95,96]. In addition, data are available indicating that circulating levels of opioid peptides (beta endorphin and met-enkephalin) are elevated in shock states [97–100]. Questions remain regarding the role played by endogenous opioid peptides in the decompensatory response to shock. Nevertheless, the weight of evidence suggests that their primary action is to decrease sympathetic outflow from the central nervous system [101,102]. The pressor response to naloxone seems to be attributable to increased vascular input impedance rather than to improved myocardial performance [103].

Neutrophil-Endothelial Cell Interactions. In addition to the development of unfavorable precapillary-to-postcapillary resistance ratios, microcirculatory failure in shock occurs as a result of other important phenomena, including increased capillary permability; microvascular plugging by platelet and leukocyte aggregates; decreased deformability of erythrocytes; and endothelial cell swelling.

A large body of data suggest that late shock is accompanied by increased microvascular permeability; i.e., σ in Equation 1 approaches 0. Two main mechanisms probably play major roles in the development of increased microvascular permeability in late shock. First is the release of various vasoactive and permeability-enhancing mediators, including histamine [104,105], bradykinin [106], platelet-activating factor [107], the sulfidopeptide leukotrienes [107], and cytokines [108–112]. Second is endothelial injury mediated by oxygen-derived free radicals generated by activated polymorphonuclear leukocytes or the xanthine oxidase system [113].

Another factor contributing to microvascular failure in late shock may be the plugging of capillary networks by aggregates of activated leukocytes and platelets. Disseminated intravascular coagulation and leukostasis in shock are triggered by complex mechanisms, including the activation of the complement cascade by traumatized or ischemic tissue or lipopolysaccharide, the activation of the intrinsic coagulation cascade, and the release of cytokines and thromboxane A_2.

The attachment of neutrophils to the microvasculature in shock is mediated by various adhesion molecules found on leukocytes and endothelial cells. These adhesion molecules can be grouped into three main families: the *selectins,* members of the *immunoglobulin superfamily,* and the *integrins* [114].

Three selectins, namely E-selectin (also called ELAM-1), P-selectin (also called GMP-140, PADGEM, or CD62), and L-selectin (also called LECAM-1), are thought to play a role in endothelial-neutrophil interactions. The natural ligands for these selectins are carbohydrates, namely, the Lewis x and sialylated Lewis x antigens. E-selectin is found on endothelial cells, which have been stimulated by exposure to cytokines or endotoxin. P-selectin is present on platelets, and endothelial cells stimulated by thrombin or histamine. L-selectin is found on leukocytes. Both P- and L-selectin apparently are important in causing neutrophils to begin rolling along the endothelial surface of capillaries, which is the first step in the process leading to microvascular sequestration of neutrophils.

The intercellular adhesion molecules (ICAM-1 and ICAM-2) are proteins belonging to the immunoglobulin superfamily. ICAM-1 (also called CD54) is a natural ligand for the integrins, LFA-1 and Mac-1 (see below). Although expressed constitutively on endothelium, ICAM-1 expression can be upregulated by exposure to certain cytokines.

The integrins [115] are a family of cell-surface glycoproteins that consist of two subunits (α and β). The integrin, Mac-1 (also called CD11b/CD18 and CR3), is present mainly on neutrophils and monocytes and appears to play a critical role in the firm attachment of neutrophils to the endothelial surface of capillaries. Besides being the receptor for ICAM-1, Mac-1 is also the natural binding site on leukocytes for one of the products of complement activation (C3bi), which is important in the opsonization of particulate antigens.

The importance of the sequestration of activated neutrophils in the microvasculature in the pathogenesis of irreversibility or organ failure in shock is evidenced by data from several recent studies. For example, granulocytopenia has been shown to dramatically improve survival in a rat model of hemorrhagic shock [116], and the extent of neutrophil activation (assessed using the nitro blue tetrazolium test) has been shown to correlate with survival in this model [117]. Delayed organ system dysfunction is ameliorated in baboons when a monoclonal antibody against the CD18 component of Mac-1 is administered just before resuscitation after 90 minutes of hemorrhagic shock [118]. Presumably, leukosequestration adversely affects microvascular flow by increasing the input impedance of capillaries [119]. Furthermore, activated neutrophils generate a variety of toxic and destructive substances, including oxidants and granular enzymes, that are capable of injuring capillary endothelium.

Altered Red Cell Deformability. There is increasing interest in the role of altered erythrocyte deformability as a factor contributing to microcirculatory failure in shock states, particularly those caused by sepsis [120]. The normal diameter of human erythrocytes is 7 μ, and the mean diameter of capillaries is 4.5 μ. It is apparent, therefore, that normal microcirculatory function depends on the capability of red blood cells to alter their shape and squeeze through capillary networks. Convincing data suggest that erythrocyte deformability decreases in hemorrhagic, septic, and endotoxic shock [120,121,222]. Although the mechanisms responsible are not well defined, it seems probable that peroxidation of lipids in the red cell membrane by oxygen free radicals plays a role in this phenomenon.

Cellular Depolarization. Since the seminal work by Shires and colleagues [125], it has been known for many years that shock states are associated with a lessening of the normal transmembrane electrochemical potential gradient in myocytes and other cell types. Cellular depolarization is associated with disturbances in the regulation of intracellular concentrations of key ions, including sodium, chloride, and potassium [124,125]. Although cellular depolarization has been attributed solely to decreased intracellular concentrations of ATP [126], some data have suggested that a circulating factor might also play a role in the pathogenesis of this phenomenon [127]. Recently, Gann and colleagues [128,129] have identified a factor in the plasma of hemorrhaged rats and dogs that induces depolarization of a variety of cell types. This protein appears to have a molecular weight of 78 kD and does not appear to be tumor necrosis factor [128,129].

Myocardial Failure. There is increasing evidence that derangements in cardiac performance contribute to irreversibility in most shock states, even those not initially caused by impaired myocardial contractility. Animal or clinical studies have provided evidence of depressed myocardial contractile function in shock caused by hemorrhage [130,131], anaphylaxis [132], thermal injury [133,134], intestinal ischemia [135], and sepsis [136].

Despite intense investigation, the mechanisms underlying the cardiac derangements in shock remain incompletely understood. In some shock states, data suggest that coronary perfusion is inadequate to meet the metabolic demands of the myocardium [137,138]. Coronary perfusion is jeopardized in shock by lowered diastolic blood pressure, particularly when there are atherosclerotic occlusive lesions in the coronary circulation. It is partly for this reason that the risk of mortality attributable to shock is higher for elderly patients and patients with atherosclerotic vascular disease. Myocardial perfusion in shock is further compromised by the release of various lipid mediators that are coronary vasoconstrictors, most notably the peptidoleukotrienes [139] and platelet-activating factor [139]. Recent studies also suggest that intrinsic regulation of coronary vasomotor tone is impaired by hemorrhagic shock [140].

Myocardial ischemia, however, is not the only mechanism contributing to cardiac dysfunction in shock; indeed, in septic shock, the best available data suggest that coronary perfusion is generally adequate to meet the metabolic demands of the heart. Accumulating data strongly support the notion that myocardial performance in shock states is impaired by circulating depressant substances [139,141,142,143]. Experiments performed in animals have implicated ischemic intestine [142,143] and pancreas [144] as the source of these substances. Other data suggest that certain monokines known to be released in shock, particularly tumor necrosis factor, are myocardial depressants [105,105a,105b]. Recent data suggest that cytokine-induced myocardial depression is mediated via the local generation of nitric oxide (or a closely related species) [148, 149,150].

Bradycardia. In some cases, severe hemorrhage leads to paradoxical bradycardia. This phenomenon has been observed in both experimental animals [151,152] and patients [153] with hypotension due to hemorrhage. Some data suggest that paradoxical bradycardia in hemorrhagic shock is caused by the activation of inhibitory cardiac vagal afferents, perhaps due to the vigorous contraction of the heart around nearly empty chambers [152]. Recent data suggest that central serotonergic inhibitory pathways are critically important in this phenomenon [152].

EFFECT OF SHOCK ON ORGAN SYSTEMS

Lungs. Early shock is characterized by tachypnea, increased minute ventilation, and hypocapnia. This response is probably mediated by pulmonary J-receptors responding to vasoactive agents [154]. As shock evolves, tachypnea and hypocapnia persist as a compensatory response to metabolic acidosis. In severe and prolonged shock, ventilatory failure occurs, primarily as a result of respiratory muscle fatigue due to ischemia [155]. A common complication of septic shock is the acute respiratory distress syndrome (ARDS), which is discussed in detail in Chapter 55.

Heart. The effect of shock on coronary perfusion and the elaboration of myocardial depressant substances have been discussed above. Myocardial dysfunction in sepsis is discussed in greater detail in Chapter 173. The effect of ischemia on myocardial performance is discussed in Chapter 42.

Kidneys. Because of the renin-angiotensin system, the kidneys play a vital role in the compensatory response to shock. The kidneys are also frequently damaged in shock states; indeed, the most common cause of acute renal failure is renal hypo-

perfusion caused by hemorrhage, dehydration, or trauma [156,157]. Acute renal failure is discussed in greater detail in Chapter 81.

Moderate increments in arterial perfusion pressure have only a minimal effect on renal blood flow; this phenomenon is called *autoregulation* [158]. In severe shock, however, total renal blood flow decreases dramatically. This effect is mediated by both sympathetic traffic in the renal nerves and humoral mediators (AII and vasopressin) [159–162]. Resistance increases in both afferent (preglomerular) and efferent (postglomerular) arterioles. Glomerular filtration rate (GFR) decreases, but to a lesser extent than renal plasma flow; i.e., filtration fraction increases [161,162,163]. Through several humoral, neural, and biophysical mechanisms, there is increased reabsorption of tubular fluid along several segments of the nephron [158]. Thus, oliguria, which is a characteristic clinical feature of most shock syndromes, is attributable to two factors: decreased GFR and increased tubular reabsorption of salt and water.

Numerous studies using experimental animals have documented that hemorrhagic hypotension prompts a redistribution of renal blood flow from outer cortical to medullary nephrons [164,165]. It has been speculated that this corticomedullary redistribution of perfusion may be an adaptive response designed to defend the delivery of oxygen to the medullary interstitium, because tissue oxygen tension in the medulla is very low even under normal conditions, and the medullary part of the thick ascending limb of Henle seems to be at particular risk for ischemic injury [166].

Splanchnic Organs. Splanchnic vasoconstriction plays a major role in the defense of blood pressure in low-flow states (*vide supra*). Nevertheless, the resulting splanchnic ischemia is probably a factor leading to a variety of visceral complications of shock, including erosive gastritis, pancreatitis, acalculous cholecystitis, and derangements in the barrier function of the gastrointestinal tract (see Chapter 199) [79].

Ischemia-induced alterations in the integrity of the gastrointestinal tract may be instrumental in permitting the systemic absorption of gut-derived microbes and microbial products (notably lipopolysaccharide). Although most of the data regarding the adverse effects of gut ischemia on mucosal permeability have been obtained using animal models [167,168], investigators in one study found that a large percentage of patients with hemorrhagic shock have positive blood cultures for enteric bacteria [169]. These data suggest that the movement of bacteria from the lumen of the gut into the systemic circulation (a process called *translocation*) occurs in shock in humans as well as animals. Other data, however, have called into question the idea that trauma and shock are associated with increases in translocation in humans [170,171]. In some instances, absorption of lipopolysaccharide or bacteria from the gut may play a role in the development of irreversibility in shock. More often, derangements in the barrier function of the gut may be instrumental in the pathophysiology of the slowly progressive failure of multiple organ systems often observed after "successful" resuscitation from shock (see Chap. 199) [172]. As already noted, the venous effluent from ischemic intestine and pancreas has been implicated as containing substances capable of depressing myocardial contractility.

Liver. In low-flow states, such as that induced by pericardial tamponade, both hepatic portal and hepatic arterial blood flow decrease out of proportion to the decrease in cardiac output [173]. The liver, therefore, is a potential target of ischemic injury in shock syndromes. Indeed, massive centrilobular hepatic necrosis (also called ischemic hepatitis or shock liver) is occasionally seen after an episode of major hemorrhage or cardiogenic shock [174–177]. Clinically, shock liver is characterized by slight elevations in serum bilirubin and alkaline phosphatase and marked by transient elevations of serum transaminase values. Although transaminase levels typically increase by 8- to 10-fold, the values return to normal within 3 to 12 days. The clinical course is quite variable, depending in part on the history of the patient. The histopathologic lesion is massive loss of centrilobular hepatocytes with sparing of cells in the portal regions.

Although dramatic, massive centrilobular hepatic necrosis is rare in current clinical practice. More commonly, deranged hepatic function after shock is characterized by hyperbilirubinemia with no or only mild changes in serum transaminase levels. The histopathology of this lesion is unimpressive, showing primarily evidence of intrahepatic cholestasis. This form of postshock liver dysfunction is a common component of the multiple organ failure syndrome (MOFS) and is discussed in greater detail in Chapter 199.

Central Nervous System. Clinically, central nervous system manifestations are common in shock, ranging from restlessness and agitation to stupor and coma. In compensated shock, however, perfusion of the central nervous system is well preserved. Thus, alterations in mental status in early shock are probably caused by poorly defined factors other than ischemia. With profound shock, blood flow to the brain decreases markedly [70,178], and, as already mentioned, ischemic injury to the central nervous system apparently contributes to the development of irreversibility.

Clotting, Reticuloendothelial, and Immune Systems. As alluded to previously, pathologic intravascular thrombosis is a characteristic feature of some shock syndromes. In endotoxic and septic shock, one of the mechanisms favoring intravascular coagulation may be the consumption of two key natural circulating anticoagulants (protein C and antithrombin III) [179,180,181]. Another mechanism may be lipopolysaccharide-induced enhancement of tissue factor expression on endothelial cells coupled with diminished expression of thrombomodulin activity [182].

In contrast to endotoxic or septic shock, pure hemorrhagic shock (in the absence of tissue trauma) does not lead to disseminated intravascular coagulation [183]. Some experimental studies indicate that hemorrhagic shock leads to significant changes in circulating activities of coagulation proteins [184,185]. Dilution may play a role in this phenomenon. From a clinical standpoint, diffuse clotting dysfunction in massively transfused patients is usually caused by a deficiency of platelets (i.e., dilutional thrombocytopenia) [186] or hypothermia [187]. Because patients in shock requiring multiple transfusions are often hypothermic, it is noteworthy that recent data suggest that another factor contributing to diffuse bleeding in multiply transfused patients may be a reversible form of platelet dysfunction induced by subnormal body temperature [188].

The central role in shock of the *reticuloendothelial system* (RES) has long been recognized [189]. The RES, consisting of sessile macrophages in the liver, spleen, lungs, peritoneum, and bone marrow, functions to remove bacteria, tumor cells, senescent blood cells, denatured proteins, fibrin thrombi, and other particulates from the vascular compartment. Shock leads to transient functional derangements in the ability of this network of phagocytic cells to clear bloodborne particulate material [190,191]. In time, after successful resuscitation, RES function is restored and actually manifests hyperactivity. In contrast, in irreversible shock, RES function remains depressed until death. The importance of RES function in the response to shock has been emphasized by studies showing that prior impairment of

phagocytic function decreases survival in animal models of shock [192].

Convincing evidence has been presented to support the idea that RES failure in shock is caused by depletion of plasma fibronectin [189]. Fibronectin is a complex glycoprotein that is found in soluble form in plasma and lymph and in insoluble form in the extracellular tissue matrix. Fibronectin has binding sites for collagen, fibrin, actin, C1q (a complement fragment), heparin, DNA, and other molecules. Soluble fibronectin functions as a circulating "nonspecific" opsonin to permit the clearance by phagocytic cells of circulating particulates. In shock, depletion of fibronectin is presumably caused by consumption in excess of synthetic capacity.

Shock and trauma lead to marked derangements in multiple facets of immune function. Whereas shock-induced immunosuppression probably has little effect on the acute response to shock, there can be little doubt that depressed host resistance to infection after successful resuscitation is a major cause of delayed morbidity and mortality [193]. Shock-induced immunosuppression is a complex topic, and it is difficult to sort out which effects are attributable to shock per se and which effects are caused by tissue injury. Nevertheless, experimental data suggest that hemorrhagic shock, even in the absence of tissue trauma, leads to numerous abnormalities in immune function, including: (1) generation of functionally active suppressor cells [194]; (2) derangements in lymphokine and cytokine production (upregulation in some instances, downregulation in others) [195,196]; (3) impaired ability to mount an inflammatory response [197]; (4) decreased responsiveness to mitogens [198]; (5) diminished neutrophil chemotaxis [199]; and (6) increased susceptibility to sepsis [200,201]. Clinical data also support the notion that shock impairs immunocompetence [202]. Recent data suggest that hemorrhage-induced derangements in immunocompetence are caused, at least in part, by ATP depletion in macrophages or other immunocytes [203].

Diagnosis and Differential Diagnosis

GENERAL CONSIDERATIONS. Five major issues assume importance in the management of shock: (1) prompt recognition of shock, optimally while the syndrome is still in the compensatory phase; (2) early institution of general supportive measures, often before the precise etiologic diagnosis is established with certainty; (3) determination of the underlying primary problem leading to shock; (4) early correction (if possible) of the primary underlying cause; and (5) management of the complications of shock (e.g., acute renal failure).

DIAGNOSIS. Making the diagnosis of shock frequently requires nothing more than measuring low arterial blood pressure or feeling a thready, rapid pulse. Often the underlying problem is instantly apparent (e.g., massive surgical bleeding in the operating room or massive upper gastrointestinal hemorrhage). However, as noted previously, shock and systemic arterial hypotension are not synonymous terms; the former can be present in the absence of the latter. Optimally, shock should be recognized and treated during the compensatory phase, before systemic arterial hypotension becomes manifest. Thus, more subtle symptoms and signs of altered perfusion must be recognized and evaluated. These clinical findings include oliguria, altered mental status, peripheral cyanosis or pallor, and cool skin temperature. Associated clinical findings that sometimes support the diagnosis of shock include tachycardia, tachypnea, and hyperthermia or hypothermia.

The most important laboratory findings suggestive of shock are metabolic acidosis and elevated blood lactate concentration [204,205,206]. Because alveolar hyperventilation is a frequent finding in early shock, arterial blood gases are often indicative of a mixed acid-base disturbance (i.e., primary metabolic acidosis plus primary respiratory alkalosis). Arterial hypoxemia from ARDS occurs commonly in septic shock. Because transcapillary refill requires time, measuring a normal hematocrit or blood hemoglobin concentration does not rule out the possibility of hemorrhagic shock; conversely, an acute decrease in hematocrit is diagnostic of hemorrhage or hemolysis. Leukocytosis is a nonspecific finding indicative of infection, and in conjunction with other clinical parameters can suggest the presence of septic shock; leukopenia is occasionally observed in patients with septic shock. Thrombocytopenia frequently occurs in septic shock, even in the absence of frank disseminated intravascular coagulation [207]. A 12-lead electrocardiogram may support the diagnosis of cardiogenic shock by showing evidence of cardiac ischemia, infarction, or dysrhythmia. The chest roentgenogram may provide important information, being diagnostic for tension pneumothorax and providing supportive data in cases of septic shock (e.g., infiltrates indicative of pneumonia or ARDS) or cardiogenic shock (e.g., cardiomegaly, pulmonary edema, or pleural effusions). Cultures and Gram-stained smears of purulent secretions and body fluids may support the diagnosis of septic shock. In many cases, a single clinical observation or laboratory value in isolation is not very helpful, whereas serial changes over several hours are often of paramount importance in establishing the diagnosis and cause of shock. "Prophylactic" use of pulmonary artery catheterization *may* be of value in certain high-risk patients because routine clinical parameters may not be sufficiently sensitive to detect early (i.e., normotensive) shock states.

CLASSIFICATION OF SHOCK. The classical classification system for shock proposed by Hinshaw and Cox uses four categories: (1) hypovolemic (i.e., shock attributable to inadequate circulating volume, as after hemorrhage); (2) cardiogenic (i.e., shock caused by pump failure, as with decreased myocardial contractility); (3) distributive (i.e., shock from "maldistribution" of blood volume and flow, as in sepsis); and (4) obstructive (i.e., shock attributable to extracardiac obstruction to blood flow, as in tamponade) [208]. Although this classification scheme has merit, it tends to oversimplify the issues; e.g., the pathophysiology of septic shock is far more complex than simply a maldistribution of blood volume and flow. The classification system adopted here divides shock into three main categories: "hypovolemic," "cardiogenic," and "other."

Hypovolemic Shock. In hypovolemic shock syndromes, the primary initial derangement is a loss of circulating volume. This category is further subdivided into hemorrhagic hypovolemic shock and nonhemorrhagic hypovolemic shock.

HEMORRHAGIC SHOCK. Hemorrhagic shock is discussed in greater detail in Chapter 172. The diagnosis of shock from hemorrhage is usually straightforward, being based on obvious external blood loss. External hemorrhage can be manifested in many ways, including bleeding from the skin and soft tissue lacerations; surgical bleeding during operations; blood loss through pleural or mediastinal tubes after trauma or thoracic surgery; blood loss through abdominal, pelvic, or soft tissue

drains after various surgical procedures; upper or lower gastrointestinal bleeding; or vaginal bleeding after pelvic surgery or complicating pregnancy.

In some instances, bleeding is occult (i.e., internal) but nonetheless sufficiently massive to cause shock. Occult bleeding is a frequent cause of shock in trauma patients. Internal hemorrhage occasionally leads to shock in the early postoperative period. These topics are discussed in greater detail below. In the absence of trauma or recent surgery, occult bleeding can be caused by a variety of problems that are usually intraabdominal, including ruptured aortic or visceral artery aneurysm and ruptured hepatic adenoma. In these cases, the initial history is often helpful; e.g., abdominal and low back pain caused by contained rupture of an abdominal aortic aneurysm. Physical examination may demonstrate absent bowel sounds, abdominal tenderness, abdominal distension, or an expansile, pulsatile abdominal mass. An electrocardiogram and chest roentgenogram are helpful in ruling out a primary cardiac problem or occult intrathoracic bleeding. CVP is typically low (<5 mm Hg). Occasionally, special studies (e.g., computed tomography [CT] scan) are helpful in these cases; usually, however, these patients are sufficiently unstable that immediate exploration is warranted based on the history, physical examination, and laboratory findings indicative of an intraabdominal catastrophe.

NONHEMORRHAGIC HYPOVOLEMIC SHOCK. Inadequate circulating volume can result from the loss of cell-free fluid from the intravascular compartment. Commonly this is caused by global dehydration secondary to excessive (or inadequately replaced) gastrointestinal or urinary losses, or excessive evaporative losses through perspiration. In addition, contraction of intravascular volume can occur as a result of transudation of asanguinous fluid into the extravascular extracellular compartment. Massive sequestration of so-called third-space fluid occurs commonly in a variety of conditions, including burns, extensive soft tissue injuries, bowel obstruction, and acute pancreatitis. Excessive capillary permeability leading to hypovolemia is pathophysiologically important in septic and anaphylactic shock, although these syndromes are considered separately because other mechanisms are important as well. Findings supporting the diagnosis of nonhemorrhagic hypovolemic shock include one or more of the following: poor skin turgor; dry mucous membranes; marked hyperthermia; elevated hematocrit; low (<5 mm Hg) CVP or PCWP; marked hyperglycemia; hypernatremia; glucosuria; and inappropriately dilute urine.

Cardiogenic Shock. In cardiogenic shock syndromes, the primary problem is pump failure. Causes of cardiogenic shock include loss of contractile tissue (i.e., infarction), diminished myocardial contractility, dysrhythmias, ventricular septal perforation, valvular heart disease, tamponade, tension pneumothorax, and excessive right ventricular afterload (caused by pulmonary embolism or pulmonary hypertension).

Most often, cardiogenic shock is a complication of acute myocardial infarction (MI) or surgery requiring cardiopulmonary bypass; these topics are discussed later in this chapter and also in Chapter 42. Tamponade is most commonly a complication of trauma, cardiac surgery, or MI; it is discussed under those headings below and in Chapter 24. Ventricular septal perforation and acute mitral regurgitation are complications of MI and are discussed under that heading below. Some other causes of cardiogenic shock are discussed here.

ACUTE AORTIC REGURGITATION. Acute aortic regurgitation is most commonly caused by infective endocarditis; other causes include aortic dissection and trauma. In contrast to chronic aortic valvular insufficiency, there is insufficient time to permit compensatory dilation of the left ventricular cavity [209,210]. As a result, forward stroke volume is markedly diminished and left ventricular end-diastolic pressure is markedly elevated. The diagnosis of acute aortic regurgitation is suggested by auscultatory findings (early diastolic murmur) and is confirmed by echocardiography [211], Doppler echocardiography [212], and cardiac contrast angiography (see also Chap. 37).

PULMONARY EMBOLISM. Occasionally, massive pulmonary thromboembolism can present as cardiogenic shock. Cardiac output decreases because of excessive afterloading of the right ventricle caused by mechanical obstruction of the pulmonary arterial tree or the release of secondary mediators that promote pulmonary hypertension (vide supra). Findings that support the diagnosis of shock caused by massive pulmonary embolism include low cardiac output, pulmonary hypertension, and high CVP with normal PCWP. Arterial hypoxemia is a nonspecific finding that supports the diagnosis of pulmonary embolism; only 5 percent of patients with angiographically documented pulmonary embolism have a PO_2 of more than 80 mm Hg [213], and the degree of hypoxemia correlates with size of the embolism [214]. Because MI (particularly involving the right ventricle) and tamponade are in the differential diagnosis, suspicion of pulmonary embolism should be heightened in the absence of electrocardiographic, echocardiographic, or serum enzyme changes that suggest the former problems. The diagnosis is confirmed by pulmonary arteriography (see also Chap. 60.)

TENSION PNEUMOTHORAX. In tension pneumothorax, the great veins in the chest are collapsed by high intrapleural pressure leading to inadequate venous return and shock. Although occurring occasionally as an isolated spontaneous problem, tension pneumothorax occurs most commonly in the setting of trauma (vide infra).

Other Causes of Shock

ANAPHYLACTIC SHOCK. Severe anaphylactic reactions are often a complication of diagnostic studies or drug therapy in the hospital, although insect stings are another common cause [215,216]. Severe anaphylactic reactions leading to shock typically occur shortly after exposure to the offending agent and are characterized by one or more of the following features: sensation of being unable to breathe, generalized dermatologic abnormalities (erythema, urticaria, angioedema, etc.), bronchospasm, laryngeal or pharyngeal edema, and wheezing. Rarely, shock can occur without any of the above findings. Inadequate preload is a major factor leading to shock in anaphylaxis [217]. In rare cases where the diagnosis is in question, findings suggestive of anaphylaxis include elevated hematocrit, low CVP, low PCWP, and low cardiac output (see Chap. 217).

SEPTIC SHOCK. Septic shock is discussed in detail in Chapter 173. In most instances, the diagnosis of septic shock is straightforward. Frequently, signs of shock (e.g., hypotension, altered mental status, oliguria) in patients with infections are attributable to the superimposed effects of sepsis per se and hypovolemia. Often, the hypovolemic component is assessed and treated simultaneously by administering an intravascular volume challenge. The main considerations in the differential diagnosis of septic shock are occult hemorrhage, other causes of hypovolemia, massive pulmonary embolism, and myocardial infarction. In difficult cases, data obtained by Swan-Ganz catheterization are helpful in establishing the diagnosis of septic shock. In contrast to most other forms of shock, SVR is almost always low in sepsis [8].

The toxic shock syndrome (Chap. 91) is a specific syndrome closely associated with infections by several strains of toxin-producing Staphylococcus aureus. Most patients are menstruating women. The diagnosis is suggested by history (use of tampons; recent infection with S. aureus), high fever, rash (usually red and macular), and desquamation (particularly on the palms and soles).

DIFFERENTIAL DIAGNOSIS OF SHOCK IN COMMON CLINICAL SETTINGS

Shock in the Setting of Acute Traumatic or Thermal Injury.
The differential diagnosis of shock in the setting of acute trauma or burn injury includes (1) external or occult hemorrhage; (2) hypovolemia caused by massive transudation of cell-free fluid from the intravascular compartment to the extravascular extracellular compartment (i.e., traumatic or burn shock); (3) tension pneumothorax; (4) tamponade; (5) cardiogenic shock caused by myocardial contusion or infarction; or (6) spinal shock.

External hemorrhage is almost always obvious. Findings indicative of occult hemorrhage include expanding abdominal girth; abdominal pain and tenderness; low CVP or PCWP (<5 mm Hg); acutely low or falling hematocrit; paracentesis yielding gross blood; peritoneal lavage fluid containing greater than 100,000 erythrocytes μl [218]; CT scan showing major intraabdominal or retroperitoneal hemorrhage; presence of femur or major pelvic fractures; or pleural fluid on chest roentgenogram.

Hypovolemia without hemorrhage is the usual problem in burn patients; the diagnosis of this problem is supported by a normal or elevated hematocrit and low (<5 mm Hg) CVP. The resuscitation of burn patients is discussed in greater detail in Chapter 155. Shock in patients with major soft tissue or crush injuries is inevitably multifactorial, being caused at least in part by the combined effects of hemorrhage and third-space sequestration of cell-free fluid.

Both tension pneumothorax and pericardial tamponade are suggested by the presence of shock despite high (>15 mm Hg) CVP. In both conditions, neck veins are prominent. Plethora of the upper chest and face suggests pericardial tamponade. Tracheal deviation suggests tension pneumothorax. Diminished breath sounds and hyperresonance to chest percussion are indicative of tension pneumothorax; however, these auscultatory findings are unreliable in the usual noisy emergency room or ICU environment. Muffled heart sounds suggest pericardial tamponade. The diagnosis of tension pneumothorax can be confirmed by chest roentgenogram. However, when tension pneumothorax is strongly suspected, valuable time should not be wasted waiting for radiographs to be obtained and developed. Rather, a large-bore needle or chest tube should be inserted into the pleural space, the diagnosis of tension pneumothorax being confirmed when the procedure is rewarded by a gush of air and a favorable clinical response. The diagnosis of pericardial tamponade is strongly supported by echocardiographic evidence of pericardial fluid; however, clinical circumstances rarely permit the luxury of obtaining this study. Rather, pericardial tamponade is typically confirmed by pericardiocentesis yielding blood and a favorable clinical response. Some authorities advocate performing a diagnostic subxyphoid pericardial window rather than pericardiocentesis [219].

Shock caused by myocardial contusion or infarction should be suspected when the mechanism of injury is appropriate (i.e., there is evidence of direct blunt trauma to the chest) or the medical history is indicative of ischemic heart disease. Electrocardiographic changes consistent with injury, ischemia, or infarction and echocardiographic evidence of wall motion abnormalities support these diagnoses.

Spinal shock is rare. In the setting of trauma, all other causes of shock must be excluded before attributing shock to spinal cord injury. In the presence of cord trauma above T5, findings that support the diagnosis of spinal shock include bradycardia and low SVR [220,221].

Shock Complicating Acute Myocardial Infarction. Shock occurs in approximately 15 percent of patients hospitalized with acute MI [222]. Possible mechanisms include (1) rupture of the ventricular free wall; (2) acute development of a mechanical defect leading to regurgitant flow; (3) rhythm disturbances; or (4) severe left, right, or biventricular dysfunction.

Rupture of the ventricular free wall usually involves the left ventricle and typically occurs 3 to 6 days after the infarct. Survival depends on immediate recognition and surgical repair [223–226]. Acute rupture of the ventricular free wall presents as tamponade with shock (often leading rapidly to electrical-mechanical dissociation) and elevated CVP and PCWP. The diagnosis is confirmed by pericardiocentesis [227] or, rarely, echocardiography.

Rupture of the intraventricular septum occurs with greater frequency after anterior as compared with inferior infarcts [228]. The onset of shock is often preceded by the development of a new, harsh holosystolic murmur. The diagnosis is confirmed by placing a Swan-Ganz catheter and documenting arterialization of right ventricular blood (i.e., left-to-right shunt). The diagnosis also can be confirmed echocardiographically.

Rupture of a left ventricular papillary muscle results in acute mitral regurgitation. Total rupture of a left ventricular papillary muscle is invariably fatal [229]. As in patients with acute ventricular septal perforation, the onset of shock in patients with acute partial papillary muscle rupture is usually preceded by the development of a new holosystolic murmur. The diagnosis of papillary muscle rupture is made echocardiographically [230]. The presence of large V waves in the PCWP tracing supports the diagnosis of mitral regurgitation, although large V waves are seen in other conditions as well.

Rhythm disturbances leading to decreased cardiac output and cardiogenic shock are diagnosed by 12-lead electrocardiography.

Isolated right ventricular dysfunction is suggested when CVP is elevated out of proportion to the increase in PCWP [231] in the setting of electrocardiographic changes indicative of right ventricular involvement in patients with an inferior or inferior-posterior wall infarction [232,233]. The diagnosis of right-sided dysfunction is supported by echocardiographic evidence of abnormal right ventricular wall motion or dilatation [234].

Left ventricular dysfunction is suggested by the presence of signs and symptoms of pulmonary edema, elevated PCWP, roentgenographic evidence of left ventricular failure, and echocardiographic data showing poor left ventricular contractility. Shock caused by left ventricular dysfunction implies destruction of more than 40 percent of the myocardium.

Biventricular decompensation is suggested by a combination of the findings typical of isolated right- and left-sided dysfunction. The hemodynamic profile of profound acute biventricular decompensation is very similar to that observed with acute tamponade (i.e., low cardiac output, high CVP, high PCWP). Echocardiographic data excluding the presence of pericardial fluid are sometimes essential to make the differential diagnosis.

Shock After Cardiopulmonary Bypass. The adequacy of cardiac output in the early postoperative period after cardiopulmonary bypass is a major determinant of outcome. If cardiac index is persistently less than 1.2 l/min/m², mortality exceeds 90 percent [235]. Shock after cardiopulmonary bypass is often multifactorial, having both cardiogenic and hypovolemic components.

Hypovolemia can be caused by inadequate replacement of third-space losses, hemorrhage, or both. Ongoing hemorrhage is usually obvious, being recognized as excessive bleeding from pleural or mediastinal tubes. Occasionally, major postoperative bleeding into the pleural space can be occult, requiring chest radiography and thoracentesis for diagnosis. The role of preload is usually assessed by performing a therapeutic trial, cardiac output being determined before and after an intravenous volume challenge. Even when PCWP is normal or elevated, derangements in diastolic compliance may necessitate infusion of additional volume to ensure adequate preload.

Cardiogenic shock after cardiopulmonary bypass can be due to dysrhythmias, pericardial tamponade, myocardial "stunning," or myocardial infarction. Rhythm disturbances are easily diagnosed electrocardiographically. Tamponade should be suspected when the development of shock is temporally associated with an acute decrement in the volume of mediastinal tube drainage. The diagnosis of tamponade is supported by observing high (and nearly equal) right- *and* left-sided filling pressures, although this characteristic hemodynamic profile also can be observed with acute biventricular failure. If time permits, the diagnosis of tamponade is confirmed echocardiographically. Frequently, however, the diagnosis of tamponade is confirmed by reopening the chest, either in the intensive care unit or, preferably, in the operating room.

Myocardial stunning is a term used to denote reversible depression of contractility after a period of ischemia and reperfusion [58,59]. In the absence of tamponade or dysrhythmia, generally it should be assumed that some element of contractile dysfunction contributes to low cardiac output after cardiopulmonary bypass. Thus, management consists of optimizing preload and afterload and infusing inotropic drugs. From a practical management standpoint, it generally matters little whether diminished contractility is caused by stunning or frank infarction, because therapy is the same.

Rarely, right ventricular dysfunction secondary to acute pulmonary hypertension complicates the postoperative course after cardiopulmonary bypass. Patients undergoing mitral valve replacement seem to be at particular risk for this problem [236]. Acute pulmonary hypertension resulting in right heart failure is also occasionally caused by apparent allergic reactions to the protamine used to reverse anticoagulation after cardiopulmonary bypass [237,238]. Excessive right ventricular afterload is diagnosed by measuring very high pulmonary artery and central venous pressures despite low or normal left atrial or pulmonary capillary wedge pressures.

Shock in the Early Perioperative Period. Shock during operations and in the early postoperative period is almost always attributable to hypovolemia secondary to hemorrhage, third-space losses, or both. Occasionally, when the operation is performed as part of the treatment for an infection (e.g., empyema or peritonitis), shock in the perioperative period is caused by sepsis; even then, however, a component of hypovolemia is almost always present. Rarely, shock in the early perioperative period is caused by myocardial infarction or massive pulmonary embolism.

Management

MONITORING. Numerous studies support the notion that the magnitude of oxygen deficit is a key predictor determining outcome in patients with shock [239]. The goal of effective therapy, therefore, must be to optimize tissue oxygenation. In general, careful physiologic monitoring is necessary to achieve this objective.

Blood Lactate Levels. When oxygen delivery is inadequate to support mitochondrial oxidative phosphorylation, anaerobic glycolysis is used to generate ATP. Lactate is an end product of anaerobic metabolism of glucose, and, in low-flow shock states, blood lactate concentrations increase in proportion to the systemic oxygen deficit [240]. Blood lactate levels are also often elevated in hyperdynamic sepsis, perhaps because of alterations in the activity of pyruvate dehydrogenase, an enzyme complex that plays a key role in the regulation of intermediary metabolism [33].

Several studies have shown that high blood lactate levels prognosticate mortality in patients with shock [205,206]. In one recent study of trauma patients, blood lactate levels, which remained elevated after 12 hours of resuscitative efforts, were highly correlated with the subsequent development of MOFS [190a]. Moreover, elevated blood lactate levels seem to correlate with other data indicative of supply dependency of systemic VO_2 [21,242,243]. Thus, serial measurements of blood lactate concentration can provide useful information about the adequacy of resuscitation in patients with shock [244,245,246], although in patients with shock caused by sepsis, changes in lactate levels do not necessarily correlate with changes in systemic DO_2 [245].

Indices of Oxygen Transport. The most direct way to assess the progress of resuscitation in shock is to measure indices of systemic oxygen transport. As noted previously, cardiac output is a major determinant of survival after cardiopulmonary bypass; in one large series, mortality was less than 2 percent when cardiac index was maintained in excess of 2.1 liters per minute per square meter [235]. In an extensive series of studies in high-risk *surgical* patients, Shoemaker and colleagues have provided data suggesting that the median values of three key indices of oxygen transport are higher in survivors as compared with non-survivors [247,248,249]. The indices are CI, DO_2, and VO_2, and the median values for surviving patients are 4.5 l/min/m², 600 ml/min/m², and 170 ml/min/m², respectively. In a randomized, prospective trial, Shoemaker et al. reported significantly improved survival in high-risk surgical patients who were resuscitated using these "supranormal" values of oxygen transport as therapeutic goals in an algorithm-driven resuscitation protocol [250]. In another randomized prospective trial, Shoemaker and colleagues showed that titration to "supranormal" values of CI, DO_2, and VO_2 improves survival and shortens the duration of ICU stay in trauma patients [251]. Other recent studies, however, have failed to document significantly improved outcome when critically ill patients have been titrated to "supranormal" indices of oxygen transport [252,253].

Although accumulating data support the notion of using supranormal indices of oxygen transport as therapeutic goals in disease states characterized by hypermetabolism (notably trauma and sepsis), there is no evidence that this approach is either helpful or safe in other shock states, particularly those associated with acute MI.

Central Venous Pressure. CVP measurements often provide useful diagnostic information in the early evaluation of shock, permitting, for example, the rapid differentiation in blunt trauma of tamponade or tension pneumothorax, characterized by high CVP, from hypovolemia, characterized by low CVP. However, because CVP is affected by many variables (including intravascular volume, venous vasomotor tone, intrathoracic pressure, and right ventricular diastolic compliance), the diagnostic value of CVP is limited; CVP readings between 5 and 15 mm Hg are not helpful in distinguishing shock caused primarily by hypovolemia from shock attributable to other causes.

Swan-Ganz Catheterization. Although the value of bedside pulmonary artery catheterization has been questioned [254], the thermistor-tipped Swan-Ganz catheter remains the "gold-standard" device for measuring cardiac output in the clinical setting. Other, less invasive methods of measuring cardiac output have been evaluated [255–258]; but, at present, none enjoy widespread acceptance. Furthermore, in addition to permitting reliable measurements of cardiac output, the Swan-Ganz catheter allows measurements of CVP, pulmonary artery pressures, mixed venous oxygen saturation (and content), and PCWP (see also Chap. 4).

In most patients with shock, cardiac output and systemic DO_2 should be optimized by intravascular volume loading until PCWP approaches 18 to 20 mm Hg. Even higher left-sided filling pressures are occasionally required in patients with poor left ventricular diastolic compliance, such as patients with aortic stenosis or some patients after cardiopulmonary bypass. Although additional cardiac output often can be recruited by further increasing preload, very high PCWPs can promote the formation of pulmonary edema, impairing oxygenation and overall oxygen transport. Thus, when PCWP approaches 18 to 20 mm Hg, the potential beneficial effects of further augmentation of preload must be titrated against the potentially adverse effects of this maneuver on pulmonary function.

Arterial Pressure. The prime variable in the management of shock is perfusion, not blood pressure. Nevertheless, cardiac output and blood pressure often correlate in shock patients, and, given current technology, continuous monitoring of blood pressure is more practical than is continuous monitoring of cardiac output. Blood pressure should be monitored in shock using an indwelling arterial catheter because sphygmomanometric measurements are frequently inaccurate in patients with markedly increased arteriolar vasomotor tone [259]. In addition, when caring for patients in shock, it is usually necessary to obtain multiple blood samples to measure arterial blood gases, lactate levels, hemoglobin concentrations, and numerous other laboratory parameters. Frequent blood sampling, particularly of arterial blood, is greatly facilitated by placing an intraarterial catheter.

Urine Output. Placing an indwelling urinary (Foley) catheter is essential for managing patients in shock. Whereas normal urine flow rates (i.e., >0.5 ml/kg/hr) do not insure that renal perfusion is optimal, oliguria in patients with previously normal renal function is an important warning that perfusion to the kidneys is inadequate.

Pulse Oximetry. The adequacy of oxygen transport depends not only on perfusion, but also on arterial hemoglobin content and saturation. The latter variable can be assessed continuously using pulse oximetry [260]. This noninvasive technology is in widespread use in clinical medicine, being a standard component of intraoperative monitoring. Because derangements in pulmonary function commonly occur in shock states, continuous monitoring of arterial saturation using pulse oximetry should be used routinely in the management of these patients. Occasionally, when pulse pressure is very low in patients with profound shock, this methodology fails to provide satisfactory data (see also Chap. 19).

Other Measures of Tissue Perfusion. Regional derangements in blood flow are probably pathophysiologically important in many shock states. Hence, measuring cardiac output may provide an incomplete assessment of the adequacy of perfusion at the organ or tissue level. For this reason, there is a great deal of interest in the clinical use of methods that permit assessing perfusion or oxygenation at the tissue level. Methods under investigation include transcutaneous PO_2 measurement

[261,262], tonometric measurement of subcutaneous PO_2 [263], polarographic measurement of skeletal muscle PO_2 [264], measurement of conjunctival PO_2 [265], and, especially, tonometric measurement of gastric intramural pH [266,267,268].

THERAPY

Asanguinous Intravenous Fluids. Unless it is certain that (absolute or relative) hypovolemia is not a contributing factor, all patients in shock should be treated initially with an intravenous asanguinous fluid challenge. The amount of fluid necessary is unpredictable, and fluid administration should be guided by monitoring arterial blood pressure, cardiac output, cardiac filling pressures, indices of oxygen transport, and urine output.

The optimal asanguinous fluid to administer remains the subject of much controversy. The osmotic reflection coefficient in Equation 1 is 0 for ions (e.g., Na^+ and Cl^-) and small molecules (e.g., lactic acid) in crystalloid solutions. Therefore, crystalloid solutions (e.g., normal saline, Ringer's lactate) rapidly diffuse from the intravascular into the interstitial compartment. The osmotic reflection coefficient for large molecules (e.g., albumin, hydroxyethyl starch, dextran) in colloid solutions approximates 1.0 under normal conditions, although in some shock states associated with increased microvascular permeability, the value of σ may be considerably less than unity. In general, it is possible to expand the intravascular compartment by infusing either colloid or crystalloid solutions; when resuscitation is titrated to a defined hemodynamic end point, the volume of crystalloid infused is typically twofold to fourfold higher than the volume of colloid required to achieve the same end point [69]. Infusing crystalloid results in greater tissue (including lung) edema, but, in general, data showing that this is deleterious are lacking [85].

Some data in the literature support the use of colloid solutions; other results strongly favor the use of crystalloid solutions. In a recent review of the crystalloid versus colloid controversy, Haupt concluded that "both fluid types appear to be safe" [85]. Haupt further stated that "in the severely hypovolemic patient with signs of circulatory shock and anaerobic metabolism, the ability of colloids to cause a rapid and sustained expansion of intravascular volume may be advantageous." We agree with this view, although a meta-analysis of data from many clinical trials concluded that trauma patients should be resuscitated with crystalloids [269].

There is a great deal of interest in the use of hypertonic crystalloid solutions for the resuscitation of shock caused by hemorrhage or burns. A variety of beneficial effects have been attributed to the use of hypertonic solutions, including decreased tissue edema [270,271,272], lower incidence or shorter duration of ileus [271,272], prevention of intracranial hypertension [273–276], enhanced myocardial performance [270, 271,277], and blunted "stress" hormonal response to injury [278]. Results from several recent clinical trials suggest that resuscitation with a 7.5% (weight/volume) solution of sodium chloride (with or without added dextran 70) is safe and may improve survival in trauma patients, particularly those requiring emergency operations or with head trauma [279–282].

Blood. Hemoglobin is essential for optimal oxygen transport. The effects of hemodilution on oxygen transport and use have been extensively studied. Although several reports suggest that tissue oxygenation is not impaired by moderate normovolemic hemodilution [283,284,285], other studies suggest that oxygen uptake by certain tissues, notably the stomach and intestine, is impaired under these circumstances [286]. Thus, it is impossible to provide rigid guidelines for red blood cell transfusion. In general, young, well-resuscitated, hemodynamically stable patients tolerate hematocrits as low as 20 to 25 percent. Older patients with atherosclerotic occlusive disease and patients in profound shock require higher hematocrits to prevent or limit ischemic injury to the heart and other organs; in these high-risk patients, we generally attempt to maintain the hematocrit at about 30 percent (see also Chap. 172).

Oxygen and Mechanical Ventilation. Virtually all patients in shock should receive supplemental oxygen. Although not always necessary, most patients in shock require endotracheal intubation and mechanical ventilation. Data from studies using animal models suggest that controlled mechanical ventilation plus neuromuscular paralysis improves visceral perfusion by shunting blood flow away from the diaphragm [287].

In addition, there are convincing data indicating that, under certain conditions, IPPV can improve cardiac output by decreasing left ventricular afterload [42,43]. The effects of IPPV are complicated, however, and, particularly in hypovolemic shock, IPPV can adversely affect preload, and hence, cardiac output and systemic DO_2. Thus, careful monitoring is necessary when mechanical ventilation (and PEEP) are used in patients in shock (see Chap. 66).

Inotropes and Vasopressors. Inotropic agents are of paramount importance in the management of cardiogenic shock. It is increasingly apparent that these drugs also can be of considerable value in septic shock. Most inotropic agents also have peripheral vascular effects; some are vasodilators, others are vasoconstrictors, and some (e.g., dopamine) are both, depending on the dose of the drug infused. Inotropic agents fall into three broad categories: cardiac glycosides, sympathomimetic amines, and other newer drugs.

CARDIAC GLYCOSIDES (DIGITALIS, DIGOXIN, AND OTHERS). Digoxin, the most widely used compound in this class, is also discussed in Chapter 207. Digoxin is a positive inotrope in both normal and failing heart muscle [288]. Digoxin is not commonly used in cardiogenic shock because of its complicated pharmacokinetics and narrow therapeutic margin. In addition, digoxin may worsen splanchnic ischemia in low-flow states [289,290]. In septic shock, however, digoxin may be more effective than dobutamine in improving cardiac output and systemic DO_2 [291].

SYMPATHOMIMETIC AMINES. Catecholamines and related drugs are widely used in the treatment of shock. Dopamine and dobutamine are the most commonly employed agents, although epinephrine and norepinephrine are employed occasionally.

Dopamine. Dopamine is an endogenous catecholamine that is capable of stimulating cardiac beta$_1$ receptors, peripheral alpha receptors, and dopaminergic receptors in the splanchnic, renal, and other vascular beds [292,293]. The effects of dopamine are dose dependent [292]. At low doses (2–3 μg/kg/min), dopamine increases renal blood flow and glomerular filtration rate (GFR) in normal human volunteers [294]. Recent studies, however, suggest that "low-dose" dopamine may not increase GFR in patients [295]. Moreover, in a recent randomized, double-blind, prospective trial, "low-dose" dopamine failed to affect urine output or GFR in patients undergoing coronary artery bypass surgery [296]. Interestingly, in another clinical study, prophylactic therapy with "low-dose" dopamine prevented the development of renal dysfuncton in cancer patients treated with a toxic cytokine (recombinant human interleukin-2) [297]. Thus, the clinical role for "low-dose" dopamine as a means for preserving renal function remains controversial.

At higher doses (~5 μg/kg/min), dopamine increases contractility and cardiac output through the activation of cardiac beta$_1$ receptors. At high doses (>10 μg/kg/min), peripheral alpha-adrenergic and cardiac beta-adrenergic effects become more prominent and heart rate and blood pressure increase substantially. At very high doses, peripheral alpha-adrenergic effects predominate. Dose-response curves for dopamine (and other sympathomimetic amines) may be shifted to the right in septic shock [298].

Dopamine has several undesirable attributes. Dopamine can increase PCWP [299,300,301], although this effect is not always observed [302]. Dopamine has been reported to induce angina and coronary vasospasm, particularly when administered at higher dosages [303]. Even in the absence of coronary vasoconstriction, dopamine-induced tachycardia may be undesirable because of the adverse effect of increased heart rate on myocardial oxygen demand. Dopamine increases intrapulmonary shunt, although this effect is observed with other inotropes as well [299,304]. Finally, dopamine can inhibit the release of prolactin, a phenomenon that may have adverse effects on immune responsiveness in critically ill patients [305].

Despite these undesirable attributes, dopamine remains a valuable part of the clinical armamentarium, primarily because of its ability to augment visceral (i.e., renal and splanchnic) perfusion. The strategy of combining dopamine with other agents for the treatment of shock is reasonable and finds support in the literature [299,306,307]. Data from animal studies suggest that renal vasodilation induced by "low-dose" dopamine is evident even when pressor doses of norepinephrine are infused simultaneously [308].

Dobutamine. Dobutamine is a synthetic catecholamine that binds to alpha$_1$, beta$_1$, and beta$_2$ adrenergic receptors. Dobutamine is structurally related to isoproterenol, and in studies using in vitro myocardial preparations, dobutamine and isoproterenol have similar chronotropic and inotropic actions [309,310]. In vivo, however, dobutamine exerts powerful inotropic effects, but, unlike isoproterenol, is only a weak chronotrope [311]. Because increasing heart rate increases myocardial oxygen demand, marked tachycardia is usually undesirable in the management of shock, particularly in patients with coronary occlusive disease. The mechanisms responsible for dobutamine's favorable inotropic/chronotropic ratio are incompletely understood; available data, however, suggest that the inotropic effects of dobutamine are mediated by activation of both cardiac beta$_1$- and alpha$_1$-adrenergic receptors [312,313]. Although the predominant cardiac adrenoreceptor is of the beta$_1$ subtype [314], cardiac alpha$_1$ receptors also exist [315], and stimulation of these latter receptors increases contractility without increasing heart rate [314,315]. Compared with most other sympathomimetic amines in clinical use, dobutamine has relatively minimal effects on peripheral vasomotor tone, perhaps because of off-setting alpha$_1$ (vasoconstricting) and beta$_2$ (vasodilating) effects. Nevertheless, the increase in cardiac output induced by dobutamine clearly is partly caused by decreased vascular input impedance (i.e., afterload reduction caused by peripheral vasodilation) leading to improved ventricular-vascular coupling [316,317].

Dobutamine has been widely used for treating cardiogenic shock complicating myocardial infarction or cardiopulmonary bypass [299,318,319,320]. Studies comparing dopamine and dobutamine in these settings favor the latter agent, indicating that cardiac filling pressures are lower with dobutamine [319,320]. Accumulating data suggest that dobutamine can improve systemic oxygen transport in some cases of septic shock, and thus, this agent may be beneficial in this setting as well [321,322].

Epinephrine. Epinephrine is an endogenous catecholamine with both alpha- and beta-adrenergic activity. Epinephrine is the drug of choice for the treatment of anaphylactic shock, primarily because of the extensive experience with this agent for this indication. Epinephrine is occasionally used to treat low-output states after cardiopulmonary bypass, but its superiority over other agents for this indication is not well documented.

Norepinephrine. Norepinephrine is another endogenous catecholamine with alpha- and beta-adrenergic activity. Because it is a potent vasoconstrictor, clinicians have been reluctant to use norepinephrine for the treatment of shock, being concerned about adverse effects on visceral, particularly renal, blood flow. Nevertheless, there is increasing evidence that judicious use of norepinephrine may be valuable in certain shock states, especially those characterized by hypotension and right ventricular pressure overload [323]. In the setting of right ventricular failure, norepinephrine, carefully titrated, may improve right ventricular perfusion and function without adversely affecting peripheral perfusion [324]. Results from several studies show that use of norepinephrine can improve urine output in septic, oliguric patients [306,325–328]. In septic shock characterized by marked hypotension and relatively normal cardiac output, results from one study suggest that norepinephrine may be preferable to dopamine for providing cardiovascular support [329], whereas results from another study suggest that norepinephrine and dopamine are similarly effective [330]. According to one study of septic shock, norepinephrine was deleterious in a subgroup of patients with elevated blood lactate levels [327].

Dopexamine. Dopexamine is a synthetic catecholamine that stimulates D$_1$ and D$_2$ dopaminergic and β_2 adrenergic receptors, but is devoid of α or β_1 adrenergic effects [331]. In patients with left ventricular failure, dopexamine has been shown to decrease systemic vascular resistance and increase cardiac output, stroke volume, and heart rate [332,333]. Dopexamine also has been shown to increase cardiac output in animals and patients with septic shock or endotoxicosis [334,335,336].

NONCATECHOLAMINE INOTROPES. In the United States, amrinone is the only currently available nondigitalis noncatecholamine intravenous inotropic agent. Amrinone is a synthetic bipyridine with inotropic and vasodilator effects [337]. Its physiologic actions mimic those obtained by simultaneous infusion of dobutamine (inotrope) and sodium nitroprusside (vasodilator). Amrinone is an inhibitor of phosphodiesterase III and it apparently acts by raising the intracellular concentration of cyclic adenosine monophosphate (cyclic AMP) [338,339]. Although some studies have provided clear evidence that amrinone is a positive inotrope [340], other data suggest that the beneficial effects of this drug on cardiac output are due primarily to afterload reduction [341]. Amrinone appears to be useful in cardiogenic shock complicating myocardial infarction [342] and cardiopulmonary bypass [343]. Other phosphodiesterase III inhibitors have been used investigationally to treat cardiogenic [344,345] and septic shock [346]. Studies using animal models further support the notion that this new (phosphodiesterase inhibitor) class of inotrope/vasodilator drugs may be beneficial in septic shock [347,348].

Vasodilators. Afterload reduction is widely used in the management of cardiogenic shock, particularly when the primary problem is acute aortic or mitral regurgitation or ventricular septal defect (see Chaps. 37 and 38). Obviously, vasodilator therapy must be used with careful monitoring and extreme care in patients who are already hypotensive. Sodium nitroprusside is the most widely employed vasodilator. It has a rapid onset of action and is short acting; therefore, it is relatively easy to titrate. Sodium nitroprusside is a so-called balanced vasodilator, affecting arteriolar resistance and venous capacitance vessels more or less equally. It is often used in combination with an inotropic agent (e.g., dopamine or dobutamine). Nitroglycerin affects primarily capacitance vessels, although this agent also decreases arteriolar resistance and is capable of improving cardiac output [349]. Angiotensin-converting enzyme (ACE) inhibitors prevent the formation of AII, and thus are potent afterload-reducing agents. In view of the data implicating AII as the key mediator of excessive splanchnic vasoconstriction in low-output states, ACE inhibitors would seem to be ideal agents for reducing afterload and improving visceral perfusion. Unfortunately, these drugs tend to be long acting and hence difficult to titrate in patients with an unstable or rapidly changing hemodynamic status.

Mechanical Devices. The use of mechanical devices to augment cardiac output is discussed in Chapters 9 and 10. Mechanical devices include the intraaortic balloon pump (IABP), right and left ventricular assist devices (LVAD and RVAD, respectively), and mechanical hearts, used as a temporary bridge pending cardiac transplantation.

The use of the IABP to treat low-output states after cardiopulmonary bypass is well established. Conversely, there is some controversy regarding the use of the IABP in cardiogenic shock complicating acute MI unless there is a clear-cut surgically correctable problem (e.g., mitral regurgitation). Although improvements of 15 to 20 percent in cardiac output can be achieved with insertion of the IABP in patients with MI and no surgically treatable problem, weaning from the device is invariably difficult or impossible, and survival is not affected [350,351].

References

1. Hardaway RM, Adams WH: Shock. *Problems in Critical Care* 3:1, 1989.
2. Warren JC: *Surgical Pathology and Therapeutics*. Philadelphia, WB Saunders, 1895.
3. Crile GW: *An Experimental Research into Surgical Shock*. Philadelphia, JB Lippincott, 1899.
4. Cannon WB: *Traumatic Shock*. New York, Appleton, 1923.
5. Keith NM: *Blood Volume Changes in Wound Shock and Primary Hemorrhage*. Special report series No. 27. London, Great Britain Medical Research Council, 1919.
6. Blalock A: Experimental shock, the cause of the low blood pressure produced by muscle injury. *Arch Surg* 20:959, 1930.
7. Cournand A, Riley RL, Bradley SE, et al: Studies of the circulation in clinical shock. *Surgery* 13:964, 1943.
8. Abraham E, Bland RD, Cobo JC, et al: Sequential cardiorespiratory patterns associated with outcome in septic shock. *Chest* 85:75, 1984.
9. Gunnar RM, Loeb RS, Winslow EJ, et al: Hemodynamic measurements in bacteremia in septic shock in man. *J Infect Dis* 128:S295, 1973.
10. Siegal JH, Greenspan M, Del Guercio LRM: Abnormal vascular tone, defective oxygen transport in myocardial failure in human septic shock. *Ann Surg* 65:504, 1967.
11. Pfluger E: Uber die diffusion des sauerstoffs, den ort und die gesetze des oxydationsprozesses des tierischen organismus. *Arch Ges Physiol* 6:43, 1872.
12. Warburg O, Kubowitz F: Atmung bein sehr kleinen sauerstoff drucken. *Biochem Zeit* 214:5, 1929.
13. Kleiber M: Respiratory exchange and metabolic rate, in Fenn WO, Rahn H (eds): *Handbook of Physiology*, section 3: *Respiration*. Washington, DC, American Physiological Society, 1965, vol 2, p 927.
14. Hochachka PW: Metabolic suppression and oxygen availability. *Can Z Zool* 66:152, 1987.
15. Komatsu T, Shibutani K, Okamoto K, et al: Critical level of oxygen delivery after cardiopulmonary bypass. *Crit Care Med* 15:194, 1987.
16. Shibutani K, Komatsu T, Kubal K, et al: Critical level of oxygen delivery in anesthetized man. *Crit Care Med* 11:640, 1983.
17. Sayeed MM: Ion transport in circulatory and/or septic shock. *Am J Physiol* 252:R809, 1987.
18. Bihari D, Smithies M, Gimson A, et al: The effect of vasodilation with prostacyclin on oxygen delivery and uptake in critically ill patients. *N Engl J Med* 317:397, 1987.
19. Wolf YG, Cotev S, Perel A, et al: Dependence of oxygen consumption on cardiac output in sepsis. *Crit Care Med* 15:198, 1987.
20. Astiz ME, Rackow EC, Falk JL, et al: Oxygen delivery and consumption in patients with hyperdynamic septic shock. *Crit Care Med* 15:26, 1987.
21. Haupt MC, Gilbert EM, Carlson RW: Fluid loading increases oxygen consumption in septic patients with lactic acidosis. *Am Rev Respir Dis* 131:912, 1985.
22. Cain SM: Peripheral oxygen uptake and delivery in health and disease. *Clin Chest Med* 4:139, 1983.
23. Nelson DP, Bayer C, Samsel RW, et al: Pathological supply dependence of O_2 uptake during bacteremia in dogs. *J Appl Physiol* 63:1487, 1987.
24. Carlile PV, Gray BA: Effect of opposite changes in cardiac output and arterial pO_2 on the relationship between mixed venous pO_2 and oxygen transport. *Am Rev Respir Dis* 140:891, 1989.
25. Vermeij CG, Feenstra BWA, Adrichem WJ, et al: Independent oxygen uptake and oxygen delivery in septic and postoperative patients. *Chest* 99:1438, 1991.
26. Ronco JJ, Fenwick JC, Wiggs BR, et al: Oxygen consumption is independent of increases in oxygen delivery by dobutamine in septic patients who have normal or increased plasma lactate. *Am Rev Respir Dis* 147:25, 1993.
27. Ronco JJ, Phang PT, Walley KR, et al: Oxygen consumption is independent of changes in oxygen delivery in severe adult respiratory distress syndrome. *Am Rev Respir Dis* 143:1267, 1991.
28. Hotchkiss RS, Karl IE: Reevaluation of the role of cellular hypoxia and bioenergetic failure in sepsis. *JAMA* 267:1503, 1992.
29. Mela L, Bacalzo LV, Miller LD: Defective oxidative metabolism of rat liver mitochondria in hemorrhagic and endotoxin shock. *Am J Physiol* 220:571, 1971.
30. Greer GG, Milazzo FH: *Pseudomonas aeruginosa* lipopolysaccharide: An uncoupler of mitochondrial oxidative phosphorylation. *Can J Microbiol* 21:877, 1975.
31. Stadler J, Bentz BG, Harbrecht BG, et al: Tumor necrosis factor alpha inhibits mitochondrial respiration. *Ann Surg* 216:539, 1992.
32. Stadler J, Billiar TR, Curran RD, et al: Effect of exogenous and endogenous nitric oxide on mitochondrial respiration of rat hepatocytes. *Am J Physiol* 260:C910, 1991.
33. Vary TC, Siegel JH, Nakatani T, et al: Effect of sepsis on activity of pyruvate dehydrogenase complex in skeletal muscle and liver. *Am J Physiol* 250:E634, 1986.
34. Vary TC, Martin LF: Potentiation of decreased pyruvate dehydrogenase activity by inflammatory stimuli in sepsis. *Circ Shock* 30:299, 1993.
35. Song S-K, Karl IE, Ackerman JJH, et al: Increased transcellular Ca^{2+}: A critical link in the pathophysiology of sepsis? *Proc Natl Acad Sci USA* 90:3933, 1993.
36. Mann T, Goldberg S, Mudge GH, et al: Factors contributing to altered left ventricular diastolic properties during angina pectoris. *Circulation* 59:14, 1979.
37. Lorell BH, Wexler LF, Momomura SI, et al: The influence of pressure overload left ventricular hypertrophy on diastolic properties during hypoxia in isovolumically contracting rat hearts. *Circ Res* 58:653, 1986.
38. Braunwald E, Sonnenblick EH, Ross J, Jr: Mechanisms of cardiac contraction and relaxation, in Braunwald E: *Heart Disease: A Textbook of Cardiovascular Medicine*. Philadelphia, WB Saunders, 1988, p 408.
39. Parrillo JE: The cardiovascular pathophysiology of sepsis. *Annu Rev Med* 40:469, 1989.
40. Pouleur H, Covell JW, Ross J Jr: Effects of nitroprusside on venous return and central blood volume in the absence and presence of acute heart failure. *Circulation* 61:328, 1980.

41. Bressack MA, Morton NS, Hortop J: Group B streptococcal sepsis in the piglet: Effects of fluid therapy on venous return, organ edema, and organ blood flow. *Circ Res* 61:659, 1987.

42. Beyar R, Halperin HR, Tsitlik JE, et al: Circulatory assistance by intrathoracic pressure variations: Optimization and mechanisms studied by a mathematical model in relation to experimental data. *Circ Res* 64:703, 1989.

43. Pinsky MR, Matuschak GM, Bernardi L, et al: Hemodynamic effects of cardiac cycle specific increases in intrathoracic pressure. *J Appl Physiol* 60:604, 1986.

44. Glantz SA, Misbach GA, Moores WY, et al: The pericardium substantially affects the left ventricular diastolic pressure volume relationship in the dog. *Circ Res* 42:433, 1978.

45. Braunwald E, Frahm CJ: Studies on Starling's law of the heart. IV. Observations on hemodynamic functions of left atrium in man. *Circulation* 24:633, 1961.

46. Koch-Weser J, Blinks JR: The influence of the interval between beats on myocardial contractility. *Pharmacol Rev* 15:601, 1963.

47. Mitchell JH, Wallace AG, Skinner NS Jr: Intrinsic effects of heart rate on left ventricular performance. *Am J Physiol* 205:41, 1963.

48. Sonnenblick EH: Force-velocity relations in mammalian heart muscle. *Am J Physiol* 202:931, 1962.

49. Strobeck JE, Kruger JW, Sonnenblick EH: Load and time considerations in the force-length relation of cardiac muscle. *Fed Proc* 39:175, 1980.

50. O'Rourke MF: Vascular impedance in studies of arterial and cardiac function. *Physiol Rev* 62:570, 1982.

51. Milnor WR: Arterial impedance as ventricular afterload. *Circ Res* 36:565, 1975.

52. Hausknecht MJ, Brin KP, Weisfeldt ML, et al: Effects of left ventricular loading by negative intrathoracic pressure in dogs. *Circ Res* 62:620, 1988.

53. Laskey WK, Kussmaul WD: Arterial wave reflection in heart failure. *Circulation* 75:711, 1987.

54. Permutt S, Riley RL: Hemodynamics of collapsible vessels with tone: The vascular waterfall. *J Appl Physiol* 18:924, 1963.

55. Thompson JA, Millen JE, Glauser FL, et al: Role of 5-HT$_2$ receptor inhibition in pulmonary embolization. *Circ Shock* 20:299, 1986.

56. Utsonomiya T, Krausz MM, Levine L, et al: Thromboxane mediation of cardiopulmonary effects of embolism. *J Clin Invest* 70:361, 1982.

57. Horgan MJ, Fenton JW, Malik AB: α-thrombin-induced pulmonary vasoconstriction. *J Appl Physiol* 63:1993, 1987.

58. Braunwald E, Kloner RA: The stunned myocardium: The long, postischemic ventricular dysfunction. *Circulation* 66:1146, 1982.

59. Opie LH: Reperfusion injury and its pharmacologic modification. *Circulation* 80:1049, 1989.

60. Heyndrickx GR, Wijns W, Vogelaers D, et al: Recovery of regional contractile function and oxidative metabolism in stunned myocardium induced by 1-hour circumflex coronary artery stenosis in chronically instrumented dogs. *Circ Res* 72:901, 1993.

61. Suga H, Sugawa K: Instantaneous pressure-volume relationship and their ratio in the excised, supported canine left ventricle. *Circ Res* 35:117, 1974.

62. Burkhoff D, Sagawa K: Ventricular efficiency predicted by an analytical model. *Am J Physiol* 250:R1021, 1986.

63. Little WC, Cheng C: Left ventricular-arterial coupling in conscious dogs. *Am J Physiol* 261:H70, 1991.

64. Starling MR: Left ventricular-arterial coupling relations in the normal human heart. *Am Heart J* 125:1659, 1993.

65. Fifer MA, Braunwald E: End-systolic pressure-volume and stress-length relations in the assessment of ventricular function in man. *Adv Cardiol* 32:36, 1985.

66. Mehmel HC, Stockins B, Ruffman K, et al: The linearity of the end-systolic pressure-volume relationship in man and its sensitivity for the assessment of the left ventricular function. *Circulation* 63:1216, 1981.

67. Chien S: Role of the sympathetic nervous system in hemorrhage. *Physiol Rev* 47:214, 1967.

68. Green HD: Circulatory systems: Physical principals, in Glasser O (ed): *Medical Physics*. Chicago, Yearbook Publishers, 1950, vol 2, p 228.

69. Bond RF, Green HD: Cardiac output redistribution during bilateral common carotid occlusion. *Am J Physiol* 216:393, 1969.

70. Forsyth RP, Hoffbrand BI, Melmon KL: Redistribution of cardiac output during hemorrhage in the unanesthetized monkey. *Circ Res* 27:311, 1970.

71. Rothe BF: Reflex controls of veins and vascular capacitance. *Physiol Rev* 63:1281, 1983.

72. Hanbauer I, Giovoni S, Majane EA, et al: In vivo regulation of the release of met-enkephalin-line peptides from dog adrenal medulla. *Adv Biochem Psychopharmacol* 33:209, 1982.

73. Bereiter DA, Zaid AM, Gann DS: Effect of rate of hemorrhage on sympathoadrenal catecholamine release in cats. *Am J Physiol* 250:E69, 1986.

74. Davis JO, Freeman RH: Mechanisms regulating renin release. *Physiol Rev* 56:1, 1976.

75. Abboud FM, Thames MD: Interaction of cardiovascular reflexes in circulatory control, in *Handbook of Physiology. The Cardiovascular System. Peripheral Circulation and Organ Blood Flow*. Bethesda, MD, American Physiological Society, 1984, section 2, vol III, part 2, chap 19, p 675.

76. Peach MJ: Renin-angiotensin system: Biochemistry and mechanisms of action. *Physiol Rev* 57:313, 1977.

77. Desjardins-Giasson S, Gutkowska J, Garcia R, et al: Renin substrate in rat mesenteric artery. *Can J Physiol Pharmacol* 59:528, 1981.

78. Malik MU, Nasjletti A: Facilitation of adrenergic transmission by locally generated angiotensin II in rat mesenteric arteries. *Circ Res* 38:26, 1976.

79. Porter JM, Sussman MS, Bulkley GB: Splanchnic vasospasm in circulatory shock, in Marston A, Bulkley GB, Fiddian-Green RG, et al (eds): *Splanchnic Ischemia and Multiple Organ Failure*. London, Edward Arnold, 1989, p 73.

80. Reilly PM, MacGowan S, Miyachi M, et al: Mesenteric vasoconstriction in cardiogenic shock in pigs. *Gastroenterol* 102:1968, 1992.

81. Klingbeil CK, Keil LC, Chang D, et al: Role of vasopressin in stimulation of ACTH secretion by angiotensin II in conscious dogs. *Am J Physiol* 251:E52, 1986.

82. Liard JF: Vasopressin in cardiovascular control: Role of circulating vasopressin. *Clin Sci* 67:473, 1984.

83. Quail AW, Woods RL, Korner PI: Cardiac and arterial baroreceptor influences in release of vasopressin and renin during hemorrhage. *Am J Physiol* 252:H1120, 1987.

84. Brand PH, Metting PJ, Britton SL: Support of arterial blood pressure by major pressor systems in conscious dogs. *Am J Physiol* 255:H483, 1988.

85. Haupt MT: The use of crystalloidal and colloidal solutions for volume replacement in hypovolemic shock. *Crit Rev Clin Lab Sci* 27:1, 1989.

86. Gann DS, Carlson DE, Byrnes GJ, et al: Role of solute in the early restitution of blood volume after hemorrhage. *Surgery* 94:439, 1983.

87. Bond RF, Johnson G III: Vascular adrenergic interactions during hemorrhagic shock. *Fed Proc* 44:281, 1985.

88. Bond RF, Bond CH, Peissner LC, et al: Prostaglandin modulation of adrenergic vascular control during hemorrhagic shock. *Am J Physiol* 241:H85, 1981.

89. Hift H, Campos HA: Changes in the subcellular distribution of cardiac catecholamines in dogs dying in irreversible hemorrhagic shock. *Nature* 196:678, 1962.

90. Coleman B, Glaviano VV: Tissue levels of norepinephrine in hemorrhagic shock. *Science* 139:54, 1962.

91. Koyama S, Aibiki M, Kanai K, et al: Role of central nervous system in renal nerve activity during prolonged hemorrhagic shock in dogs. *Am J Physiol* 254:R761, 1988.

92. Thiemermann C, Szabo C, Mitchell JA, et al: Vascular hyporeactivity to vasoconstrictor agents and hemodynamic decompensation in hemorrhagic shock is mediated by nitric oxide. *Proc Natl Acad Sci USA* 90:267, 1993.

93. Faden AI, Holaday JW: Opiate antagonists: A role in the treatment of hypervolemic shock. *Science* 205:317, 1979.

94. Holaday JW, Faden AI: Naloxone reversal of endotoxin hypotension suggests role of endorphins in shock. *Nature* 275:450, 1978.

95. Vargish T, Reynolds DG, Gurll NJ, et al: Naloxone reversal of hypovolemic shock in dogs. *Circ Shock* 7:31, 1980.

96. Reynolds DG, Gurll NJ, Vargish T, et al: Blockade of opiate receptors with naloxone improves survival and cardiac performance in canine endotoxic shock. *Circ Shock* 7:39, 1980.

97. Vargish T, Beamer K: Hemodynamic effects of naloxone in early canine hypovolemic shock. *Circ Shock* 17:45, 1985.

98. Evans SF, Medbak S, Hines CJ, et al: Plasma levels in biochemical characterizations of circulatory met-enkephalin in canine endotoxin shock. *Life Sci* 34:1481, 1984.

99. Shatney EH, Cohen RM, Cohen MR, et al: Endogenous opioid activity in clinical hemorrhagic shock. *Surg Gynecol Obstet* 160:547, 1985.

100. Pasi A, Moccetti T, Legler M, et al: Elevation of blood levels of beta-endorphin-like immunoreactivity in patients with shock. *Res Commun Chem Pathol Pharmacol* 42:509, 1983.

101. Schadt JC, Gaddis RR: Endogenous opiate peptides may limit norepinephrine release during hemorrhage. *J Pharmacol Exp Ther* 232:656, 1985.

102. Schadt JC, York DH: Involvement of both adrenergic and cholinergic receptors and the cardiovascular effects of naloxone during hemorrhagic hypotension in the conscious rabbit. *J Auton Nerv Syst* 6:237, 1982.

103. Schadt JC, McKown MD, McKown DP, et al: Hemodynamic effects of hemorrhage and subsequent naloxone treatment in conscious rabbits. *Am J Physiol* 247:R497, 1984.

104. Hinshaw LB, Jordan MM, Vick JA: Histamine release and endotoxin shock in the primate. *J Clin Invest* 40:1631, 1961.

105. Nagy S, Nagy A, Adamicza A, et al: Histamine level changes in the plasma and tissues in hemorrhagic shock. *Circ Shock* 18:227, 1986.

106. O'Donnel TF, Clowes GHA, Talamo RC, et al: Kinin activation in the blood of patients with sepsis. *Surg Gynecol Obstet* 143:539, 1976.

107. Lefer AM: Significance of lipid mediators in shock states. *Circ Shock* 27:3, 1989.

108. Ayala A, Wang P, Ba ZF, et al: Differential alterations in plasma IL-6 and TNF levels after trauma and hemorrhage. *Am J Physiol* 260:R167, 1991.

109. Abraham E, Richmond NJ, Chang YH: Effects of hemorrhage on interleukin-1 production. *Circ Shock* 25:33, 1988.

110. Pelicane JV, DeMaria EJ, Abd-Elfattah A, et al: Interleukin-1 receptor antagonist improves survival and preserves organ adenosine-5'-triphosphate after hemorrhagic shock. *Surgery* 114:278, 1993.

111. Hoch RC, Rodriguez R, Manning T, et al: Effects of accidental trauma on cytokine and endotoxin production. *Crit Care Med* 21:839, 1993.

112. Tan LR, Waxman K, Scannell G, et al: Trauma causes early release of soluble receptors for tumor necrosis factor. *J Trauma* 34:634, 1993.

113. Carden DL, Smith JK, Zimmerman BJ, et al: Reperfusion injury following circulatory collapse: The role of reactive oxygen metabolites. *J Crit Care* 4:294, 1989.

114. Williams TJ, Hellewell: Endothelial cell biology: Adhesion molecules involved in the microvascular inflammatory response. *Am Rev Respir Dis* 146:S45, 1992.

115. Ruoslahti E: Integrins. *J Clin Invest* 87:1, 1991.

116. Barroso-Aranda J, Schmid-Schonbein GW, Zweifach BW, et al: Granulocytes and no-reflow phenomenon in irreversible hemorrhagic shock. *Circ Res* 63:437, 1988.

117. Barroso-Aranda J, Schmid-Schonbein GW: Transformation of neutrophils as indicator of irreversibility in hemorrhagic shock. *Am J Physiol* 257:H846, 1989.

118. Mileski WJ, Winn RK, Vedder NB, et al: Inhibition of CD18-dependent neutrophil adherence reduces organ injury after hemorrhagic shock in primates. *Surgery* 108:206, 1990.

119. Sutton DW, Schmid-Schonbein GW: Elevation of organ resistance due to leukocyte perfusion. *Am J Physiol* 262:H1646, 1992.

120. Hurd TC, Dasmahapatra KS, Rush BF Jr, et al: Red blood cell deformability in human and experimental sepsis. *Arch Surg* 123:217, 1988.

121. Powell RJ, Machiedo GW, Rush BF Jr: Decreased red blood cell deformability and impaired oxygen utilization during human sepsis. *Am Surg* 59:65, 1993.

122. Chien S, Usami J, Dellenback J, et al: Blood rheology after hemorrhage and endotoxin. *Adv Surg* 8:75, 1984.

123. Campion DS, Lynch LJ, Rector FC, Jr, et al: Effect of hemorrhagic shock on transmembrane potential. *Surgery* 66:1051, 1969.

124. Cunningham JN Jr, Shires GT, Wagner Y: Cellular transport defects in hemorrhagic shock. *Surgery* 70:215, 1971.

125. Shires GT, Cunningham JN, Baker CRF, et al: Alterations in cellular membrane function during hemorrhagic shock in primates. *Ann Surg* 176:288, 1972.

126. Chaudry IH, Clemens MG, Baue AE: Alterations in cell function with ischemia and shock. *Arch Surg* 116:1309, 1981.

127. Trunkey DD, Illner H, Arango A, et al: Changes in cell membrane function following shock and cross perfusion. *Surg Forum* 25:1, 1974.

128. Evans JA, Darlington DN, Gann DS: A circulating factor(s) mediates cell depolarization in hemorrhagic shock. *Ann Surg* 213:549, 1991.

129. Boulanger BR, Evans JA, Lilly MP, et al: A circulating protein that depolarizes cells increases after hemorrhage in dogs. *J Trauma* 34:591, 1993.

130. Horton JW: Hemorrhagic shock depresses myocardial contractile function in the guinea pig. *Circ Shock* 28:23, 1989.

131. Horton JW, Mitchell JH: Left ventricular dimensions during hemorrhagic shock measured by biplane cinefluorography. *Am J Physiol* 263:H1559, 1992.

132. Correa E, Mink S, Unruh H, et al: Left ventricular contractility is depressed in IgE-mediated anaphylactic shock in dogs. *Am J Physiol* 260:H744, 1991.

133. Kaufman TM, Horton JW: Burn-induced alterations in cardiac β-adrenergic receptors. *Am J Physiol* 262:H1585, 1992.

134. Horton JW, White DJ: U-74,500A inhibition of burn-induced cardiac dysfunction. *J Surg Res* 52:251, 1992.

135. Nightingale LM, Tambolini WP, Kish P, et al: Depression of left ventricular performance during canine splanchnic artery occlusion shock. *Circ Shock* 14:93, 1984.

136. Cunnion RE, Parrillo JE: Myocardial dysfunction in sepsis. *Crit Care Clin* 5:99, 1989.

137. Sarnoff SJ, Case RB, Waitag PE, et al: Insufficient coronary flow and myocardial failure as a complicating factor in late hemorrhagic shock. *Am J Physiol* 176:439, 1954.

138. Horton J, Landreneau R, Tuggle D: Cardiac response to fluid resuscitation from hemorrhagic shock. *Surg Gynecol Obstet* 160:444, 1985.

139. Lefer AM: Interaction between myocardial depressant factor and vasoactive mediators with ischemia and shock. *Am J Physiol* 252:R193, 1987.

140. Dignan RJ, Wechsler AS, DeMaria EJ: Coronary vasomotor dysfunction following hemorrhagic shock. *J Surg Res* 52:382, 1992.

141. Parrillo JE, Burch C, Shelhamer JH, et al: A circulating myocardial depressant substance in humans with septic shock: Septic shock patients with a reduced ejection fraction have a circulating factor that depresses in vitro myocardial cell performance. *J Clin Invest* 76:1539, 1985.

142. Lundgren O, Haglund U, Isaksson, et al: Effects on myocardial contractility of blood-borne material released from the feline small intestine in simulated shock. *Circ Res* 38:307, 1976.

143. Horton JW, White JD: Lipid peroxidation contributes to cardiac deficits after ischemia and reperfusion of the small bowel. *Am J Physiol* 264:H1686, 1993.

144. Lefer AM: Properties of cardioinhibitory factors produced in shock. *Fed Proc* 37:2734, 1978.

145. Natanson C, Eichenholz PW, Danner RL, et al: Endotoxin and tumor necrosis factor challenges in dogs simulates the cardiovascular profile of human septic shock. *J Exp Med* 169:823, 1989.

146. Pagani FD, Baker LS, Hsi C, et al: Left ventricular systolic and diastolic dysfunction after infusion of tumor necrosis factor-α in conscious dogs. *J Clin Invest* 90:389, 1992.

147. Heard SO, Perkins MW, Fink MP: Tumor necrosis factor-α causes myocardial depression in guinea pigs. *Crit Care Med* 20:523, 1992.

148. Finkel MS, Oddis CV, Jacob TD, et al: Negative inotropic effects of cytokines on the heart mediated by nitric oxide. *Science* 257:387, 1992.

149. Brady AJB, Poole-Wilson PA, Harding SA, et al: Nitric oxide production within cardiac myocytes reduces their contractility in endotoxemia. *Am J Physiol* 263:H1963, 1992.

150. Balligand J-L, Ungureanu D, Kelly RA, et al: Abnormal contractile function due to induction of nitric oxide synthesis in rat cardiac myocytes follows exposure to activated macrophage-conditioned medium. *J Clin Invest* 91:2314, 1993.

151. Skoog P, Mansson J, Thoren P: Changes in sympathetic outflow

during hypotensive haemorrhage in rats. *Acta Physiol Scand* 125:655, 1985.

152. Morgan DA, Thoren P, Wilczynski EA, et al: Serotonergic mechanisms mediate renal sympathoinhibition during severe hemorrhage in rats. *Am J Physiol* 255:H496, 1988.

153. Sander-Jensen R, Secher NH, Bie P, et al: Vagal slowing of the heart during hemorrhage: Observations from twenty consecutive hypotensive patients. *Br Med J* 295:365, 1986.

154. Douglas ME, Downs JB, Dannemiller FJ, et al: Acute respiratory failure and intravascular coagulation. *Surg Gynecol Obstet* 143:555, 1976.

155. Roussos C, Macklem PT: The respiratory muscles. *N Engl J Med* 307:786, 1982.

156. Rasmussen HH, Ibels LS: Acute renal failure: Multivariate analysis of causes and risk factors. *Am J Med* 73:211, 1982.

157. Menashe PI, Ross SA, Gottlieb JE: Acquired renal insufficiency in critically ill patients. *Crit Care Med* 16:1106, 1988.

158. Badr KF, Ichikawa I: Prerenal failure: A deleterious shift from renal compensation to decompensation. *N Engl J Med* 319:623, 1988.

159. Henrich WL, Berl T, McDonald KM, et al: Angiotensin II, renal nerves, and prostaglandins in renal hemodynamics during hemorrhage. *Am J Physiol* 235:F46, 1978.

160. Oliver JA, Sciacca RR, Pinto J, et al: Participation of the prostaglandins in the control of renal blood flow during acute reduction of cardiac output in the dog. *J Clin Invest* 67:229, 1981.

161. Yared A, Kon V, Ichikawa I: Mechanism of preservation of glomerular perfusion and filtration during acute extracellular fluid volume depletion: Importance of intrarenal vasopressin-prostaglandin interaction for protecting kidneys from constrictor action of vasopressin. *J Clin Invest* 75:1477, 1985.

162. Kon V, Yared A, Ichikawa I: Role of renal sympathetic nerves in mediating hypoperfusion of renal cortical microcirculation in experimental congestive heart failure and acute extracellular fluid volume depletion. *J Clin Invest* 76:1913, 1985.

163. Heller BI, Jacobson WE: Renal hemodynamics in heart disease. *Am Heart J* 39:188, 1950.

164. Carriere S, Thurnburn GD, O'Morcho CC, et al: Intrarenal distribution of blood flow in dogs during hemorrhagic hypotension. *Circ Res* 19:167, 1966.

165. Grandchamp A, Ayer G, Truniger B: Pathogenesis of redistribution of intrarenal blood flow in hemorrhagic hypotension. *Eur J Clin Invest* 1:271, 1971.

166. Brezis M, Rosen S, Silva P, et al: Renal ischemia: A new perspective. *Kidney Int* 26:375, 1984.

167. Rush BF Jr, Redan JA, Flanagan JJ Jr, et al: Does the bacteremia observed in hemorrhagic shock have clinical significance? A study in germ-free animals. *Ann Surg* 210:342, 1989.

168. Deitch EA, Bridges W, Baker J, et al: Hemorrhagic shock-induced bacterial translocation is reduced by xanthine oxidase inhibition or inactivation. *Surgery* 104:191, 1988.

169. Rush BF Jr, Sori AJ, Murphy EF, et al: Endotoxemia and bacteremia during hemorrhagic shock. *Ann Surg* 207:549, 1988.

170. Moore FA, Moore EE, Poggetti R, et al: Gut bacterial translocation via the portal vein: A clinical perspective with major torso trauma. *J Trauma* 31:629, 1991.

171. Peitzman AB, Udekwu AO, Ochoa J, et al: Bacterial translocation in trauma patients. *J Trauma* 31:1083, 1991.

172. Meakins JL, Marshal JC: The gut as the motor of multiple system organ failure, in Marston A, Bulkley GB, Fiddian-Green RG, et al (eds): *Splanchnic Ischemia and Multiple Organ Failure*. London, Edward Arnold, 1989, p 339.

173. Bulkley GB, Oshima A, Bailey RW: Pathophysiology of hepatic ischemia in cardiogenic shock. *Am J Surg* 151:87, 1986.

174. Nunes G, Blaisdel FW, Margaretten W: Mechanism of hepatic dysfunction following shock and trauma. *Arch Surg* 100:546, 1970.

175. Champion HR, Jones RT, Trump BF, et al: A clinicopathologic study of hepatic dysfunction following shock. *Surg Gynecol Obstet* 142:657, 1976.

176. Birgens HS, Henriksen J, Matzen P, et al: The shock liver. *Acta Med Scand* 204:417, 1978.

177. Gibson PR, Dudley FJ: Ischemic hepatitis: clinical features, diagnosis and prognosis. *Aust N Z J Med* 14:822, 1984.

178. Kaihara S, Rutherford RB, Schwentker EP, et al: Distribution of

179. Taylor FB Jr, Chang A, Esmon CT, et al: Protein C prevents the coagulopathic and lethal effects of *Escherichia coli* infusion in the baboon. *J Clin Invest* 79:918, 1987.

180. Hauptman JG, Hassouna HI, Bell TG, et al: Efficacy of antithrombin III in endotoxin-induced disseminated intravascular coagulation. *Circ Shock* 25:111, 1988.

181. Taylor FB Jr, Emerson TE Jr, Jordan R, et al: Antithrombin-III prevents the lethal effect of *Escherichia coli* infusion in baboons. *Circ Shock* 26:227, 1988.

182. Moore KL, Andreoli SP, Esmon NL, et al: Endotoxin enhances tissue factor and suppresses thrombomodulin expression of human vascular endothelium in vitro. *J Clin Invest* 79:124, 1987.

183. Garcia-Barreno P, Balibrea JL, Aparicio P: Blood coagulation changes in shock. *Surg Gynecol Obstet* 147:6, 1978.

184. Martin DJ, Lucas CE, Ledgerwood AM, et al: Fresh frozen plasma supplement to massive red blood cell transfusion. *Ann Surg* 202:505, 1985.

185. Lucas CE, Ledgerwood AM: Clinical significance of altered coagulation tests after massive transfusion for trauma. *Am Surg* 47:125, 1981.

186. Counts RB, Haisch C, Simon TL, et al: Hemostasis in massively transfused trauma patients. *Ann Surg* 190:91, 1979.

187. Rohrer MJ, Natale AM: Effect of hypothermia on the coagulation cascade. *Crit Care Med* 20:1402, 1992.

188. Valeri CR, Cassidy K, Khuri S, et al: Hypothermia-induced reversible platelet dysfunction. *Ann Surg* 205:175, 1977.

189. Saba TM: Fibronectin: Relevance to phagocytic post-response to injury. *Circ Shock* 29:257, 1989.

190. Altura BM, Hershey SG: Reticuloendothelial function in experimental injury and tolerance to shock. *Adv Exp Med Biol* 33:545, 1973.

191. Kaplan JE, Saba TM: Humoral deficiency and reticuloendothelial depression after traumatic shock. *Am J Physiol* 230:7, 1976.

192. Zweifach BW, Benacerraf B, Thomas L: Relationship between the vascular manifestation of shock produced by endotoxin, trauma, and hemorrhage. II. The possible role of the RES in resistance to each type of shock. *J Exp Med* 106:403, 1957.

193. Abraham E: Host defense abnormalities after hemorrhage, trauma, and burns. *Crit Care Med* 17:934, 1989.

194. Abraham E, Chang Y-H: Generation of functionally active suppressor cells by haemorrhage and haemorrhagic serum. *Clin Exp Immunol* 72:238, 1988.

195. Abraham E, Freitas AA: Hemorrhage produces abnormalities in lymphocyte function and lymphokine generation. *J Immunol* 142:899, 1989.

196. Zapata-Sirvent RL, Hansbrough JF, Cox MC, et al: Immunologic alterations in a murine model of hemorrhagic shock. *Crit Care Med* 20:508, 1992.

197. Abraham E, Chang Y-H: Effects of hemorrhage on inflammatory response. *Arch Surg* 119:1154, 1984.

198. Abraham E, Chang Y-H: Cellular and humoral bases of hemorrhage-induced depression of lymphocyte function. *Crit Care Med* 14:81, 1986.

199. Davis JM, Stevens JM, Peitzman A, et al: Neutrophil laboratory activity in severe hemorrhagic shock. *Circ Shock* 10:199, 1983.

200. Stephan RN, Kupper TS, Geha AS, et al: Hemorrhage without tissue trauma produces immunosuppression and enhances susceptibility to sepsis. *Arch Surg* 122:62, 1987.

201. Fink MP, Gardiner WM, MacVittie TJ: Sublethal hemorrhage impairs the acute peritoneal inflammatory response in the rat. *J Trauma* 25:234, 1985.

202. Baker CC, Miller CL, Trunkey DD: Correlation of traumatic shock with immunocompetence and sepsis. *Surg Forum* 30:20, 1979.

203. Mechanism of increased susceptibility to infection following hemorrhage. *Am J Surg* 165:59S, 1993.

204. Weil MW, Afifi AA: Experimental and clinical studies on lactate and pyruvate as indicators of acute circulatory failure. *Circulation* 16:989, 1970.

205. Tuchschmidt J, Fried J, Swinney R, et al: Early hemodynamic correlates of survival in patients with septic shock. *Crit Care Med* 17:719, 1989.

cardiac output in experimental hemorrhagic shock in dogs. *J Appl Physiol* 27:218, 1969.

206. Henning RJ, Weil MH, Weiner F: Blood lactate as a prognostic indicator of survival in patients with acute myocardial infarction. *Circ Shock* 9:307, 1982.

207. Wilson JJ, Neame PB, Kelton JG: Infection-induced thrombocytopenia. *Semin Thromb Hemost* 8:217, 1982.

208. Hinshaw LB, Cox BG: *The Fundamental Mechanisms of Shock.* New York, Plenum Press, 1972, p 13.

209. Benotti JR: Acute aortic insufficiency, in Dalen JE, Alpert JS (eds): *Valvular Heart Disease.* 2nd ed. Boston, Little, Brown and Company, 1987, p 319.

210. Dervan J, Goldberg S: Acute aortic regurgitation: pathophysiology and management, in Frankl WS, Breast AN (eds): *Cardiovascular Clinics. Valvular Heart Disease: Comprehensive Evaluation and Management.* Philadelphia, FA Davis, 1986, p 281.

211. Meyer T, Sareli P, Pocock WA, et al: Echocardiographic and hemodynamic correlates of diastolic closure of mitral valve and diastolic opening of aortic valve in severe aortic regurgitation. *Am J Cardiol* 59:1144, 1987.

212. Grayburn PA, Smith MD, Handshoe R, et al: Detection of aortic insufficiency by standard echocardiography, pulsed Doppler echocardiography and auscultation. *Ann Intern Med* 104:599, 1986.

213. Urokinase-pulmonary embolism trial: A national cooperative study. *Circulation* 47(suppl 2):2, 1973.

214. McIntyre KM, Sasahara AA: The hemodynamic response to pulmonary embolism in patients without prior cardiopulmonary disease. *Am J Cardiol* 28:288, 1971.

215. Steel K, Gertman PM, Crescenzi C, et al: Iatrogenic illness on a general medical service at a university hospital. *N Engl J Med* 304:638, 1981.

216. Bernard JH: Studies of 400 hymenoptera sting deaths in the United States. *J Allergy Clin Immunol* 52:259, 1973.

217. Carlson RW, Schaeffer BC, Puri VK, et al: Hypovolemia in permeability pulmonary edema associated with anaphylaxis. *Crit Care Med* 9:883, 1981.

218. Sherman JC, Delaurier GA, Hawkins ML, et al: Percutaneous peritoneal lavage in blunt trauma patients: A safe and accurate diagnostic method. *J Trauma* 29:801, 1989.

219. Brewster SA, Thirlby RC, Snyder WH: Subxiphoid pericardial window and penetrating cardiac trauma. *Arch Surg* 123:937, 1988.

220. Troll GF, Dohrmann GJ: Anesthesia of the spinal cord-injured patient: Cardiovascular problems and their management. *Paraplegia* 13:162, 1975.

221. Mackenzie CF, Shin B, Krishnaprasad D, et al: Assessment of cardiac and respiratory function during surgery on patients with acute quadriplegia. *J Neurosurg* 62:843, 1985.

222. Wackers FJ, Lie KI, Becker AE: Coronary artery disease in patients dying from cardiogenic shock or congestive heart failure in the setting of acute myocardial infarction. *Br Heart J* 38:906, 1976.

223. London RE, London SB: Rupture of the heart: A critical analysis of 47 consecutive autopsy cases. *Circulation* 31:202, 1965.

224. Bjorck G, Mogensen L, Nyquist O, et al: Studies of myocardial rupture with cardiac tamponade in acute myocardial infarction. *Chest* 61:4, 1972.

225. Balakumaran K, Verbaan CJ, Essed CE, et al: Ventricular free wall rupture: Sudden, subacute, slow, sealed and stabilized varieties. *Eur Heart J* 5:282, 1984.

226. McMullan MH, Kilgore TL, Dear HD, et al: Sudden blowout rupture of the myocardium after infarction: Urgent management. *J Thorac Cardiovasc Surg* 89:259, 1985.

227. Cohn LH: Surgical management of acute and chronic cardiac mechanical complications due to myocardial infarction. *Am Heart J* 102:1049, 1981.

228. Radford MJ, Johnson RA, Dagget WM, et al: Ventricular septal rupture: A review of clinical and physiologic features and an analysis of survival. *Circulation* 64:545, 1981.

229. Wei JY, Hutchins GM, Bulkley BH: Papillary muscle rupture in fatal acute myocardial infarction. *Ann Intern Med* 90:149, 1979.

230. Come PC, Riley MF, Weintraub R, et al: Echocardiographic detection of complete and partial papillary muscle rupture during acute myocardial infarction. *Am J Cardiol* 56:787, 1985.

231. Coma-Canella I, Lopez-Sendon J, Gamallo C: Low output syndrome in right ventricular infarction. *Am Heart J* 98:613, 1978.

232. Chou T, Van Der Bel-Chan J, Allen J, et al: Electrocardiographic diagnosis of right ventricular function. *Am J Med* 70:1175, 1981.

233. Croft CH, Nicod P, Corbett JR, et al: Detection of acute right ventricular infarction by right precordial electrocardiography. *Am J Cardiol* 50:421, 1982.

234. Jugdutt BI, Sussez BA, Sivaram CA, et al: Right ventricular infarction: Two-dimensional echocardiographic evaluation. *Am Heart J* 107:505, 1984.

235. Sturm JT, McGee MG, Fuhrman TM, et al: Treatment of postoperative low output syndrome with intraaortic balloon pumping: Experience with 419 patients. *Am J Cardiol* 41:1033, 1980.

236. D'Ambra MN, LaRaia PJ, Philbin DM, et al: Prostaglandin E_1: A new therapy for refractory right heart failure and pulmonary hypertension after mitral valve replacement. *J Thorac Cardiovasc Surg* 89:567, 1985.

237. Morel DR, Lowenstein E, Nguyeneuy T, et al: Acute pulmonary vasoconstriction and thromboxane release during protamine reversal of heparin anticoagulation in awake sheep: Evidence for the role of reactive oxygen metabolites following nonimmunological complement activation. *Circ Res* 62:905, 1988.

238. Lowenstein E, Johnston WE, Lappas DG, et al: Catastrophic pulmonary vasoconstriction associated with protamine reversal of heparin. *Anesthesiology* 59:470, 1983.

239. Vincent J-L, de Backer D: Initial management of circulatory shock as prevention of MSOF. *Crit Care Clin* 5:369, 1989.

240. Cain SM: Appearance of excess lactate in anesthetized dogs during anemic and hypoxic hypoxia. *Am J Physiol* 209:604, 1965.

241. Moore FA, Haenel JB, Moore EE, et al: Incommensurate oxygen consumption in response to maximal oxygen availability predicts postinjury multiple organ failure. *J Trauma* 33:58, 1992.

242. Annat G, Viale JP, Percival C, et al: Oxygen delivery and uptake in the adult respiratory distress syndrome: Lack of relationship when measured independently in patients with normal blood lactate concentrations. *Am Rev Respir Dis* 133:999, 1986.

243. Gilbert EM, Haupt MT, Mandanas RY, et al: The effect of fluid loading, blood transfusion, and catecholamine infusion on oxygen delivery and consumption in patients with sepsis. *Am Rev Respir Dis* 134:873, 1986.

244. Vincent J-L, Dufaye P, Berre' J, et al: Serial lactate determinations during circulatory shock. *Crit Care Med* 11:449, 1983.

245. Groeneveld ABJ, Kester ADM, Nauta JJP, et al: Relation of arterial blood lactate to oxygen delivery and hemodynamic variables in human shock states. *Circ Shock* 22:35, 1987.

246. Mizock BA, Falk JL: Lactic acidosis in critical illness. *Crit Care Med* 20:80, 1992.

247. Shoemaker WC, Montgomery ES, Kaplan E, et al: Physiologic patterns in surviving and nonsurviving shock patients. *Arch Surg* 106:630, 1973.

248. Shoemaker WC, Czer LSC: Evaluation of the biologic importance of various hemodynamic and oxygen transport variables. *Crit Care Med* 7:424, 1979.

249. Shoemaker WC, Appel P, Bland R: Use of physiologic monitoring to predict outcome and to assist in clinical decisions in critically ill postoperative patients. *Am J Surg* 146:43, 1983.

250. Shoemaker WC, Appel PL, Kram HB: Prospective trial of supranormal values of survivors as therapeutic goals in high risk surgical patients. *Chest* 94:1176, 1988.

251. Fleming A, Bishop N, Shoemaker W, et al: Prospective trial of supranormal values as goals of resuscitation in severe trauma. *Arch Surg* 127:1175, 1992.

252. Yu M, Levy MM, Smith P, et al: Effect of maximizing oxygen delivery on morbidity and mortality rates in critically ill patients: A prospective, randomized, controlled study. *Crit Care Med* 21:830, 1993.

253. Tuchschmidt J, Fried J, Astiz M, et al: Elevation of cardiac output and oxygen delivery improves outcome in septic shock. *Chest* 102:216, 1992.

254. Robin ED: The cult of the Swan-Ganz catheter: Overuse and abuse of pulmonary flow catheters. *Ann Intern Med* 103:445, 1985.

255. Preiser JC, Daper A, Parquier J-N, et al: Transthoracic electrical bioimpedance versus thermodilution technique for cardiac output measurement during mechanical ventilation. *Intensive Care Med* 15:221, 1989.

256. Gotshall RW, Wood VC, Miles DS: Comparison of two impedance cardiographic techniques for measuring cardiac output in critically ill patients. *Crit Care Med* 17:806, 1989.

257. Singer M, Clarke J, Bennett ED: Continuous hemodynamic monitoring by esophageal Doppler. *Crit Care Med* 17:447, 1989.

258. Bernstein DP: Noninvasive cardiac output, Doppler flowmetry, and gold-plated assumptions. *Crit Care Med* 15:886, 1987.

259. Cohn J: Blood pressure measurement in shock: Mechanism of inaccuracy in auscultatory and palpatory methods. *JAMA* 199:972, 1967.

260. Tremper KK: Pulse oximetry. *Chest* 94:713, 1989.

261. Tremper KK, Barker SJ, Hufstedler SM, et al: Transcutaneous and liver surface P_{O_2} during hemorrhagic hypotension and treatment with phenylephrine. *Crit Care Med* 17:537, 1989.

262. Tremper KK, Waxman K, Shoemaker WC: Effects of hypoxia and shock on transcutaneous P_{O_2} values in dogs. *Crit Care Med* 7:526, 1979.

263. Chang N, Goodson WH, Gottrup F, et al: Direct measurement of wound and tissue oxygen tension in postoperative patients. *Ann Surg* 197:470, 1983.

264. Beerthuizen GIJM, Goris RJA, Bredee JJ, et al: Muscle oxygen tension-hemodynamics and oxygen transport after extracorporeal circulation. *Crit Care Med* 16:748, 1988.

265. Abraham E, Oye RK, Smith M: Detection of blood volume deficits through conjunctival oxygen tension monitoring. *Crit Care Med* 12:931, 1984.

266. Fiddian-Green RG, Baker S: The predictive value of measurements of pH in the wall of the stomach for complications after cardiac surgery: A comparison with other forms of monitoring. *Crit Care Med* 15:153, 1987.

267. Guitierrez G, Palizas F, Doglio G, et al: Gastric intramucosal pH as a therapeutic index of tissue oxygenation in critically ill patients. *Lancet* 339:195, 1992.

268. Maynard N, Bihari D, Beale R, et al: Assessment of splanchnic oxygenation by gastric tonometry in patients with acute circulatory failure. *JAMA* 270:1203, 1993.

269. Velanovich V: Crystalloid versus colloid fluid resuscitation: A meta-analysis of mortality. *Surgery* 105:65, 1989.

270. Bowser-Wallace BH, Caldwell FT: A prospective analysis of hypertonic lactated saline vs. Ringer's lactate-colloid for the resuscitation of severely burned children. *Burns* 12:402, 1986.

271. Caldwell FT, Casali RE, Flanigan WA, et al: What constitutes the proper solution for resuscitation of the severely burned patient? *Am J Surg* 122:655, 1971.

272. Shackford SR, Fortlage DA, Peters RM, et al: Serum osmolar and electrolyte changes associated with large infusions of hypertonic sodium lactate for intravascular volume expansion of patients undergoing aortic reconstruction. *Surg Gynecol Obstet* 164:127, 1987.

273. Prough DS, Johnson JC, Poole GV, et al: Effects of intracranial saline versus lactated Ringer's solution. *Crit Care Med* 13:407, 1985.

274. Prough DS, Johnson JC, Stullken EH, et al: Effects on cerebral hemodynamics of resuscitation from endotoxic shock with hypertonic saline versus lactated Ringer's solution. *Crit Care Med* 13:1040, 1985.

275. Gunnar WP, Merlotti GJ, Jonasson O, et al: Resuscitation from hemorrhagic shock: Alterations in the intracranial pressure after normal saline, 3% saline and dextran-40. *Ann Surg* 204:686, 1986.

276. Ducey JP, Mozingo DW, Lamiell JM, et al: A comparison of the cerebral and cardiovascular effects of complete resuscitation with isotonic and hypertonic saline, hetastarch, and whole blood following hemorrhage. *J Trauma* 29:1510, 1989.

277. Peters RM, Shackford SR, Hogan JS, et al: Comparison of isotonic and hypertonic fluids in resuscitation from hypovolemic shock. *Surg Gynecol Obstet* 163:219, 1986.

278. Cross JS, Gruber DP, Gann DS, et al: Hypertonic saline attenuates the hormonal response to injury. *Ann Surg* 209:684, 1989.

279. Vassar MJ, Perry CA, Gannaway WL, et al: 7.5% sodium chloride/dextran for resuscitation of trauma patients undergoing helicopter transport. *Arch Surg* 126:1065, 1991.

280. Vassar MJ, Holcroft JW: Use of hypertonic-hyperoncotic fluids for resuscitation of trauma victims. *J Intensive Care Med* 7:189, 1992.

281. Younes RN, Aun F, Accioly CQ, et al: Hypertonic solutions in the treatment of hypovolemic shock: A prospective, randomized study

in patients admitted to the emergency room. *Surgery* 111:380, 1992.

282. Vassar MJ, Perry CA, Holcroft JW: Prehospital resuscitation of hypotensive trauma patients with 7.5% NaCl versus 7.5% NaCl with added dextran: A controlled trial. *J Trauma* 34:622, 1993.

283. Biro GP, Beresford-Kroeger D: Myocardial blood flow and O_2-supply following dextran-hemodilution and methaemoglobin anemia in the dog. *Cardiovasc Res* 13:459, 1979.

284. Messmer KL, Sunder-Plassmann L, Jesch F, et al: Oxygen supply to the tissues during limited normovolemic hemodilution. *Res Exp Med* 159:152, 1973.

285. Baer RW, Vlahakes GJ, Uhlig PN, et al: Maximal myocardial oxygen transport during anemia and polycythemia in dogs. *Am J Physiol* 252:H1086, 1987.

286. Kiel JW, Riedel GL, Shepherd AP: Effects of hemodilution on gastric and intestinal oxygenation. *Am J Physiol* 256:H171, 1989.

287. Hussain SNA, Roussos C: Distribution of respiratory and organ blood flow during endotoxic shock in dogs. *J Appl Physiol* 59:1802, 1985.

288. Lewis RP: Digitalis: A drug that refuses to die. *Crit Care Med* 18:S5, 1990.

289. Bynum TE, Hanley HG: Effect of digitalis on estimated splanchnic blood flow. *J Lab Clin Med* 99:84, 1982.

290. Ferrer MI, Bradley SE, Sheeler HO: The effect of digoxin in the splanchnic circulation in ventricular failure. *Circ Res* 32:524, 1965.

291. Nasraway SA, Rackow EC, Astiz ME, et al: Inotropic response to digoxin and dopamine in patients with severe sepsis, cardiac failure, and systemic hypoperfusion. *Chest* 95:612, 1989.

292. Goldberg LI: Dopamine: Clinical uses of an endogenous catecholamine. *N Engl J Med* 291:707, 1974.

293. Goldberg LI, Rajfer SI: Dopamine receptors: Applications in clinical cardiology. *Circulation* 72:245, 1985.

294. Olsen NV, Hansen JM, Kanstrup IL, et al: Renal hemodynamics, tubular function, and response to low-dose dopamine during acute hypoxia in humans. *J Appl Physiol* 74:2166, 1993.

295. Gravees TA, Cioffi WG, Vaughan GM, et al: The renal effects of low-dose dopamine in thermally injured patients. *J Trauma* 35:97, 1993.

296. Myles PS, Buckland MR, Schenk NJ, et al: Effect of "renal-dose" dopamine on renal function following cardiac surgery. *Anaesth Intensive Care* 21:56, 1993.

297. Palmieri G, Morabito A, Lauria R, et al: Low-dose dopamine induces early recovery of recombinant interleukin-2-impaired renal function. *Eur J Cancer* 29A:1119, 1993.

298. Breslow MJ, Miller CF, Parker SD, et al: Effect of vasopressors on organ blood flow during endotoxin shock in pigs. *Am J Physiol* 252:H291, 1987.

299. Richard C, Richome JL, Rimailho A, et al: Combined hemodynamic effects of dopamine and dobutamine in cardiogenic shock. *Circulation* 67:620, 1983.

300. Francis GS, Sharma B, Hodges M: Comparative hemodynamic effects of dopamine and dobutamine in patients with acute cardiogenic circulatory collapse. *Am Heart J* 103:995, 1982.

301. Leier CV, Heban PT, Huss P, et al: Comparative systemic and regional hemodynamic effects of dopamine and dobutamine in patients with cardiomyopathic heart failure. *Circulation* 58:466, 1978.

302. Mueller HS, Evans D, Ayres SM: Effect of dopamine on hemodynamics and myocardial metabolism in shock following acute myocardial infarction in man. *Circulation* 57:361, 1978.

303. Crea F, Chierchia S, Kaski JC, et al: Provocation of coronary spasm by dopamine in patients with active variant angina pectoris. *Circulation* 74:262, 1986.

304. Regnier B, Kapin M, Gory G, et al: Hemodynamic effects of dopamine in septic shock. *Intensive Care Med* 3:47, 1977.

305. Devins SS, Miller A, Herndon BL, et al: Effects of dopamine on T-lymphocyte proliferative responses and serum prolactin concentrations in critically ill patients. *Crit Care Med* 20:1644, 1992.

306. Desjars P, Pinaud M, Bugnon D, et al: Norepinephrine therapy has no deleterious renal effects in human septic shock. *Crit Care Med* 17:426, 1989.

307. Uretsky BF, Hua J: Combined intravenous pharmacotherapy in the treatment of patients with decompensated congestive heart failure. *Am Heart J* 121:1879, 1991.

308. Schaer GL, Fink MP, Parrillo JE: Norepinephrine alone versus norepinephrine plus low-dose dopamine: Enhanced renal blood flow with combination pressor therapy. *Crit Care Med* 13:492, 1985.

309. Bodem R, Skelton CL, Sonnenblick EH: Inotropic and chronotropic effects of dobutamine on isolated cardiac muscle. *Eur J Cardiol* 2:181, 1974.

310. Lumley P, Broadley KJ, Levy GP: Analysis of the inotropic: Chronotropic selectivity of dobutamine and dopamine in anesthetized dogs and guinea pig isolated atria. *Cardiovasc Res* 11:17, 1977.

311. Tuttle RR, Mills J: Dobutamine: Development of a new catecholamine to selectively increase cardiac contractility. *Circ Res* 36:185, 1975.

312. Kenakin TP: An in vitro quantitative analysis of the α-adrenoreceptor partial agonist activity of dobutamine and its relevance to inotropic selectivity. *J Pharmacol Exp Ther* 216:210, 1981.

313. Ruffolo RR Jr, Spradlin TA, Pollock GD, et al: Alpha and beta adrenergic effects of the stereoisomers of dobutamine. *J Pharmacol Exp Ther* 219:447, 1981.

314. Broadley KJ: Cardiac adrenoreceptors. *J Auton Pharmacol* 2:119, 1982.

315. Schumann HJ, Wagner J, Knorr A, et al: Demonstration in human atrial preparations of α-adrenoreceptors mediating positive inotropic effects. *Naunyn Schmiedebergs Arch Pharmacol* 302:333, 1978.

316. Binkley PF, VanFossen DB, Nunziata E, et al: Influence of positive inotropic therapy on pulsatile hydraulic load and ventricular-vascular coupling in congestive heart failure. *J Am Coll Cardiol* 15:1127, 1990.

317. Binkley PF, Murray KD, Watson KM, et al: Dobutamine increases cardiac output of the total artificial heart: Implications for the vascular contribution of inotropic agents to augmented ventricular function. *Circulation* 84:1210, 1991.

318. Fowler MB, Timmis AD, Crick JP, et al: Comparison of haemodynamic responses to dobutamine and salbutamol in cardiogenic shock after acute myocardial infarction. *Br Med J Clin Res* 284:73, 1982.

319. DiSesa VJ, Gold JP, Shemin RJ, et al: Comparison of dopamine and dobutamine in patients requiring postoperative circulatory support. *Clin Cardiol* 9:253, 1986.

320. Tyden H, Nystrom SO: Dopamine versus dobutamine after open heart surgery. *Acta Anaesthesiol Scand* 27:193, 1983.

321. Vincent J-L, Van der Linden P, Domb M, et al: Dopamine compared with dobutamine in experimental septic shock: Relevance to fluid administration. *Anesth Analg* 66:565, 1987.

322. Tell B, Majerus TC, Flancbaum L: Dobutamine in elderly septic shock patients with refractory to dopamine. *Intensive Care Med* 13:14, 1987.

323. Mathru M, Dries DJ: Is levorphed lethal? *Chest* 95:1177, 1989.

324. Angle MR, Molloy DW, Penner B, et al: The cardiopulmonary and renal hemodynamic effects of norepinephrine in canine pulmonary embolism. *Chest* 95:1333, 1989.

325. Desjars P, Pinaud M, Potel G, et al: A reappraisal of norepinephrine therapy in human septic shock. *Crit Care Med* 15:134, 1987.

326. Hesselvik JF, Brodin B: Low dose norepinephrine in patients with septic shock and oliguria: Effects on afterload, urine flow, and oxygen transport. *Crit Care Med* 17:179, 1989.

327. Fukuoka T, Nishimura M, Imanaka H, et al: Effects of norepinephrine on renal function in septic patients with normal and elevated serum lactate levels. *Crit Care Med* 17:1104, 1989.

328. Cesare JF, Ligas JR, Hirvela ER: Enhancement of urine output and glomerular filtration in acutely oliguric patients using low-dose norepinephrine. *Circ Shock* 39:207, 1993.

329. Martin C, Papazian L, Perrin G, et al: Norepinephrine or dopamine for the treatment of hyperdynamic septic shock? *Chest* 103:1826, 1993.

330. Schreuder WO, Schneider AJ, Groeneveld ABJ, et al: Effect of dopamine vs. norepinephrine on hemodynamics in septic shock. Emphasis on right ventricular performance. *Chest* 95:1282, 1989.

331. Smith GW, O'Connor SE: An introduction to the pharmacologic properties of Dopacard (dopexamine hydrochloride). *Am J Cardiol* 62:406, 1988.

332. Colardyn FA, Vandenbogaerde JF: Use of dopexamine hydrochloride in intensive care patients with low-output left ventricular heart failure. *Am J Cardiol* 62:68C, 1988.

333. Gollub SB, Elkayam U, Young JB, et al: Efficacy and safety of a short-term (6-h) intravenous infusion of dopexamine in patients with severe congestive heart failure: A randomized, double-blind, parallel, placebo-controlled multicenter study. *J Am Coll Cardiol* 18:383, 1991.

334. Tighe D, Moss R, Haywood G, et al: Dopexamine hydrochloride maintains portal blood flow and attenuates hepatic ultrastructural changes in a porcine peritonitis model of multiple system organ failure. *Circ Shock* 39:199, 1993.

335. van Lambalgen AA, van Kraats AA, Mulder MF, et al: Organ blood flow and distribution of cardiac output in dopexamine- or dobutamine-treated endotoxemic rats. *J Crit Care* 8:117, 1993.

336. Colardyn FA, Vandenbogaerde JF, Vogelaers DP, et al: Use of dopexamine hydrochloride in patients with septic shock. *Crit Care Med* 17:999, 1989.

337. Braunwald E: Introduction—A symposium on amrinone. *Am J Cardiol* 56(3):1B, 1985.

338. Chatterjee K: Newer oral inotropic agents: Phosphodiesterase inhibitors. *Crit Care Med* 18:S34, 1990.

339. Colucci WS, Wright RF, Braunwald E: New positive inotropic agents in the treatment of congestive heart failure. Mechanisms of action and recent clinical developments. *N Engl J Med* 314:349, 1986.

340. Ko W, Zelano JA, Fahey AL, et al: The effects of amrinone versus dobutamine on myocardial mechanics and energetics after hypothermic global ischemia. *J Thorac Cardiovasc Surg* 105:1015, 1993.

341. Goto Y, Slinker BK, LeWinter MM: Effects of amrinone and isoproterenol on mechanoenergetics of blood-perfused rabbit heart. *Am J Physiol* 262:H719, 1992.

342. Taylor SH, Verma SP, Hussain M, et al: Intravenous amrinone in left ventricular failure complicated by acute myocardial infarction. *Am J Cardiol* 56:29B, 1985.

343. Goenen M, Pedemonte O, Baele P, et al: Amrinone in the management of low cardiac output after open heart surgery. *Am J Cardiol* 56:33B, 1985.

344. Vincent J-L, Carlier E, Berre J, et al: Administration of enoximone in cardiogenic shock. *Am J Cardiol* 62:419, 1988.

345. Thuillez C, Richard C, Teboul JL, et al: Arterial hemodynamics and cardiac effects of enoximone, dobutamine, and their combination in severe heart failure. *Am Heart J* 125:799, 1993.

346. Vincent J-L, Van Reeth O, Van Borgaert E, et al: Use of the new inotropic agent ARL-115 BS to treat severe myocardial depression in septic shock. *Crit Care Med* 14:661, 1986.

347. Vincent J-L, Domb M, Van der Linden P, et al: Amrinone administration in endotoxic shock. *Circ Shock* 25:75, 1988.

348. de Boelpaepe C, Vincent J-L, Contempre B, et al: Combination of norepinephrine and amrinone in the treatment of endotoxin shock. *J Crit Care* 4:202, 1989.

349. Ribner HS, Breshnan D, Hsieh A, et al: Acute hemodynamic responses to vasodilator therapy in congestive heart failure. *Prog Cardiovasc Dis* 25:1, 1982.

350. Miller MG, Weintraub RM, Hedley-Whyte J, et al: Surgery for cardiogenic shock. *Lancet* 2:1342, 1974.

351. Mundth ED, Buckley MJ, Daggett WM, et al: Intra-aortic balloon pump assistance and early surgery in cardiogenic shock. *Adv Cardiol* 15:159, 1975.

172. Hemorrhage and Resuscitation

Steven A. Gould, Barry Rosen,
Arthur L. Rosen, Hansa L. Sehgal,
Lakshman R. Sehgal, and
Gerald S. Moss

Shock is defined by the inability of the circulation to provide adequate oxygen substrate for the metabolic requirements of the tissues (see Chap. 170). Successful treatment of hemorrhagic shock depends on increasing oxygen delivery to the tissues via intravascular volume repletion, augmentation of the oxygen-carrying capacity of the circulation, and prevention of further blood loss. Accordingly, resuscitation from hemorrhagic shock can be divided into three phases: volume expansion, red blood cell (RBC) replacement, and correction of clotting deficiencies.

Phase 1: Intravascular Volume Expansion

The infusion of fluid is the fundamental treatment of acute hypovolemia. All commercially available intravenous (IV) fluids (human bovine, recombinant, and transgenic) share the ability to replenish the circulation once appropriate IV access is established. The challenge inherent with the use of these solutions is to promote the prompt and adequate restoration of cardiac filling pressures to optimum values without compromising ventilation secondary to fluid overload. Regardless of the fluid used for resuscitation, it is therefore imperative to use physiologic endpoints to gauge the initial response to treatment and to adjust the therapy to meet the individual needs of the patient.

Controversy surrounding the appropriate IV solution to use in the management of hemorrhagic shock centers on their ultimate distribution after IV administration, which, in turn, is dependent on their composition. To understand their fate, it is necessary to review the physiology of normal fluid exchange.

NORMAL FLUID DYNAMICS. On examination of the fluid distribution in adults, approximately two-thirds of the total body water is intracellular; the remaining one-third present in the extracellular compartment is distributed between the interstitial and intravascular spaces at a ratio of 3:1. The movement of fluids between the major compartments of the body is governed by the number of particles, or osmoles, in solution. Under steady-state conditions, the osmolality of the intracellular and extracellular compartments is maintained between 280 to 300 mOsm by the Na-K ATPase pump. In contrast, the distribution of fluid between the intravascular and extravascular spaces, as defined by the Starling equation, is dependent on the transcapillary hydrostatic and oncotic pressures, and the relative permeability of the capillary membranes that separate these spaces. Although controversy exists regarding the absolute values of these forces, the net effect is a small efflux of fluid into the interstitium, which is returned to the circulation by the lymphatics.

CRYSTALLOID SOLUTIONS. The osmolality of a solution is dependent on the number of particles in solution. The functional osmolality, or tonicity, of a solution is defined by the ability of the particles in solution to permeate cell membranes. Accordingly, isotonic solutions such as 0.9% sodium chloride and Ringer's lactate freely equilibrate between the intravascular and interstitial spaces but do not promote intracellular fluid shifts. In contrast, the osmotic pressure exerted at the cell membrane by the infusion of hypertonic saline solutions leads to the redistribution of intracellular fluid into the extracellular compartment.

Isotonic crystalloid solutions are universally recognized as the primary fluid for acute intravascular volume expansion. When care is taken to titrate total infusion volume to physiologic endpoints, resuscitation is usually successful without the development of pulmonary edema. A concern with isotonic fluids is the large volume often required for resuscitation. This usually results in peripheral edema, which clears within several days. The large volume requirements may also represent a logistical problem in some settings. For these reasons, hypertonic saline solutions have been studied.

The theoretic advantage of hypertonic saline solution relates to the total infusion volume required for adequate resuscitation. The greater the sodium concentration, the less total volume is necessary for satisfactory resuscitation when compared with isotonic saline solution. In addition to the osmotic effects, hypertonic solutions are believed to exert a positive inotropic effect on the myocardium and a direct effect on the peripheral vasculature leading to vasodilation [1,2,3]. The principal disadvantage of hypertonic saline is the danger of hypernatremia. Serum sodium levels above 170 mEq per liter produce extreme brain dehydration and can be fatal [4].

The primary mechanism for the maintenance of relatively constant serum sodium levels in the face of hypertonic infusions involves the movement of intracellular water into the extracellular compartment. Thus, the infusion of exogenous hypertonic saline solution is always accompanied by an endogenous infusion of free water into the extracellular space. A simple method of calculating the expected endogenous infusion is to examine the ratio of the infused fluid to the normal serum sodium concentration. For example, a solution containing 300 mEq per liter of sodium would produce a 2:1 endogenous infusion, whereas a solution containing 1200 mEq per liter of sodium would produce a 7:1 infusion volume. The safety of hypertonic solutions depends on how much of the intracellular volume can be safely transferred to the extracellular compartments without injuring cell function or leading to hypernatremia in a given clinical situation.

COLLOID SOLUTIONS. IV colloidal solutions share the presence of large molecules that are relatively impermeable to the capillary membranes. These oncotically active particles produce an effective volume expansion with little loss into the interstitial space, as occurs with the simple salt solutions. In addition, the intravascular persistence of these molecules increases their duration of action. The net effect of colloid administration is a marked reduction in the volume of infusate necessary to expand the intravascular space, as compared with isotonic saline solutions.

One of the most commonly used colloid preparations is 5% albumin. It is prepared from normal donor plasma that is heat treated to eliminate the potential for disease transmission. Once administered, it leads to an effective intravascular volume expansion of approximately one-half of the volume infused, with a duration of action of 24 hours. Side effects include the rare occurrence of anaphylactic reactions (0.5%) and inhibition of hemostasis [5].

The high cost and limited availability of albumin solutions led to the development of synthetic colloid preparations such as 6% hetastarch and 6% dextran solutions. Hetastarch is an amylopectin-derived polymer with an average molecular weight of 450,000 daltons. Dextran 70 is a polysaccharide formed by bacterial growth and digestion in sucrose media. Administration of these solutions leads to a plasma volume expansion and duration of action approximately 50 percent greater than 5% albumin. Side effects of these solutions are similar to albumin, with the exception of the documented inhibition of platelet aggregation and interference with red blood cell cross-matching with dextran 70. In addition, concern has been raised over the long-term effects that these synthetic macromolecules might have on immune function secondary to their incomplete elimination by the reticuloendothelial system.

Theoretically, fresh frozen plasma also can be used as a volume expander. It is similar to 5% albumin in electrolyte concentration and oncotic pressure. In addition, it contains all the naturally occurring immunoglobulins and all the clotting factors except platelets. At first glance, it appears to be an ideal volume expander. Unfortunately, as is the case with all currently used blood components, the risk of hepatitis and acquired immunodeficiency syndrome (AIDS) is real, and neither risk can be totally eliminated by current screening techniques. Accordingly, its use after acute blood loss should be limited to the treatment of clinically significant coagulopathies after large volume resuscitation, as discussed later in this chapter.

EXPERIMENTAL COMPARISONS OF INTRAVENOUS SOLUTIONS

Laboratory Studies. There has been considerable controversy over the role of resuscitation with crystalloid or colloid solutions in the subsequent development of deranged pulmonary function after major nonthoracic trauma. Proponents of colloid therapy cite the following points derived from laboratory studies:

1. Resuscitation with colloid leads to a more rapid and effective correction of the intravascular volume deficits that follow acute hemorrhage [6].
2. Colloid resuscitation prevents pulmonary edema formation through maintenance of the intravascular colloid osmotic pressure [7].
3. Crystalloid resuscitation dilutes the plasma protein pool, thereby reducing plasma oncotic pressure and setting the stage for the development of pulmonary edema [8,9].
4. The peripheral edema that follows large volume crystalloid infusions may impair wound healing and nutrient transport [10].

Crystalloid proponents cite the following:

1. Crystalloid administration most effectively replaces the interstitial fluid deficits that follow hemorrhagic shock [11].
2. The rapid intravascular-extravascular fluid equilibrium that follows crystalloid resuscitation may reduce the incidence of pulmonary edema by promoting a less rapid rise in the pulmonary artery occlusion pressure [12].
3. Albumin normally enters the pulmonary interstitium rela-

tively freely and is returned to the circulation via the lymphatic system. The exogenous administration of colloid solutions increases the albumin pool in the pulmonary interstitium, promoting the accumulation of interstitial fluid [13,14].

It is evident from this discussion that the arguments supporting either treatment regimen are in direct conflict with respect to the physiologic changes that are believed to follow resuscitation with either crystalloid or colloid solutions. Much of this conflict stems from the divergent study conditions employed to answer these questions in the laboratory setting. Nevertheless, numerous clinical studies designed to compare the efficacy and safety of these resuscitation regimens after acute blood loss have failed to demonstrate a clear advantage of colloid administration to justify its cost. The following section reviews these clinical trials, with particular emphasis on the resuscitation from hemorrhagic shock.

Randomized Trials in Human Subjects

CRYSTALLOID VERSUS COLLOID. One of the first trials comparing crystalloid and colloid resuscitation was reported by Skillman et al. [7], in which 16 patients undergoing elective abdominal aortic operations received either colloid or crystalloid in the perioperative period. They noted a significant difference during the immediate postoperative period in plasma colloid oncotic pressure between the Ringer's lactate–treated group and the colloid-treated group (22 and 27 mm Hg, respectively) but no alveolar-arterial oxygen tension difference. They also reported a significant correlation between the amount of infused sodium and the alveolar-arterial oxygen difference in the Ringer's lactate–treated group but not in the albumin-treated group. It was concluded that albumin-rich fluid was perferable because it reduced the amount of sodium-containing fluid required for adequate resuscitation. This study does not represent a strong argument for albumin-rich fluids, because both groups received albumin in the form of whole blood administered intraoperatively. Furthermore, the test fluid was given by formula rather than by titration to physiologic endpoints. The positive correlation between infused sodium and pulmonary function was not confirmed in several subsequent studies by other investigators.

Another study involving patients undergoing elective vascular operations was published in 1979 by Virgilio et al. [12]. During the operation, patients received either Ringer's lactate (14 patients) or 5% albumin in Ringer's lactate (15 patients) to maintain preoperative filling pressures, cardiac output, and urine output. Blood loss was replaced by packed cells. Patients assigned to the Ringer's lactate–treated group received approximately 11 liters of test fluid on the day of operation, whereas those in the albumin-treated group received 6 liters. Both groups required approximately 6.5 units of packed RBCs. Patients receiving Ringer's lactate gained 10 percent of their original body weight and had a 40 percent reduction in plasma colloid oncotic pressure.

During the study, no deaths occurred in either group. No difference was noted between groups in regard to the intrapulmonary shunt on any day of the study. Furthermore, no correlation was found between the intrapulmonary shunt and the plasma colloid oncotic pressure-hydrostatic pressure gradient. Mean postoperative ventilator time was 23 hours in both groups. Pulmonary edema developed in two patients receiving albumin. No patients treated with Ringer's lactate manifested evidence of pulmonary edema despite reduced colloid oncotic pressures. It was concluded that safe resuscitation without albumin could be achieved in patients undergoing elective vascular operations.

Numerous clinical trials have compared the effects of crystalloid or colloid administration in the resuscitation of trauma patients. In 1977, Lowe et al. [15] reported a clinical trial in 141 trauma victims from Cook County Hospital in Chicago. Thirty-six of these patients were in shock on admission. Patients received, in random sequence, either Ringer's lactate (84 patients) or 4% albumin solution (55 patients) in volumes sufficient to restore normal vital signs and urine output. This was the first report in the literature of a group of human subjects resuscitated without any albumin. RBC losses were replaced with washed RBCs. These patients received an average of 5.5 liters of test fluid and 2 units of RBCs before operation.

Three deaths occurred in each group. Eight patients (14%) in the albumin-treated group required ventilatory support after operation, whereas three (3.6%) assigned to the Ringer's lactate–treated group required ventilatory support. There were no changes in the results of a battery of pulmonary function tests, including intrapulmonary shunt fraction and alveolar-arterial oxygen tension difference. In addition, no correlation was found between the amount of sodium infused and any pulmonary function test result in either group. Lowe et al. [15] concluded that the addition of albumin in Ringer's lactate was unnecessary to achieve successful resuscitation in this group of patients. A criticism of this study was that too few patients were in shock on admission, so the failure to find differences in mortality or pulmonary function with either test fluid was not surprising [16].

In 1981, further findings in the 36 patients at Cook County Hospital who were in shock on admission were published by Moss et al. [17]. Twenty patients were assigned to the Ringer's lactate–treated group and 16 received albumin. These patients received an average of 8 units of packed RBCs and 9 liters of test fluid, indicating severe injury and blood loss. Only one death occurred. Two patients in each group required ventilatory support, and no differences were noted in the pulmonary function test results. Once again, no evidence could be found that albumin added to Ringer's lactate was necessary to prevent acute respiratory distress syndrome.

In an effort to determine the relative mortality after resuscitation with either crystalloid or colloid solutions, Velanovich [18] pooled the results of these and other clinical trials and compared the mortality rates by meta-analysis. On examination of results from clinical trials derived from trauma patients, the mortality rate was 12 percent lower for those that received crystalloid. In contrast, the relative difference in mortality from studies performed on nontrauma patients was 8 percent in favor of colloid treatment. Based on these results it was concluded that crystalloid administration may be more efficacious than colloids in the trauma setting.

HYPERTONIC SALINE SOLUTIONS. Hypertonic saline solution is an attractive fluid in the treatment of burn resuscitation because peripheral edema is frequently seen after conventional resuscitation and may complicate local burn tissue management. If resuscitation with hypertonic saline solution resulted in a smaller infusion volume and less peripheral edema, then this would constitute an argument in favor of its use in burns. The effect of varying the concentration of sodium in resuscitative fluids for burn victims has been reported [19]. Three groups of patients were studied. One group was given saline solution with sodium concentrations of 116 to 149 mEq per liter, the second group was given saline solutions with sodium concentrations between 150 and 199 mEq per liter, and the third group was given saline solutions with sodium concentrations of 200 to 250 mEq per liter. The total volume infused decreased as the sodium concentration in the infusate increased. No increase was seen in sodium loading. However, in two instances, the serum sodium concentration increased to greater than 170 mEq

per liter. Similar results with hypertonic saline solution have been reported in young and aged burn victims [20,21]. Weight gain was noted to be minimal in children treated with hypertonic saline solution, and the problem of hypernatremia was avoided by serial monitoring of serum sodium levels. Hypertonic saline solution has become an acceptable form of therapy in burn resuscitation.

Clinical studies of hypertonic saline solutions for resuscitation of hemorrhage have been reported. In a study of 58 patients undergoing vascular operations, Shackford et al. [22] showed that the hypertonic saline solution group required less fluid during operation than did the isotonic saline solution group (4.5 and 9.5 liters, respectively) and gained less weight. They concluded that the use of hypertonic saline solution during operation resulted in a reduction in infusion volume but demanded careful monitoring of serum osmolarity to avoid hypernatremia. In a clinical study in trauma victims, 1 group of 10 patients received 3 percent saline solution at a volume of 4 ml per kilogram for no more than 3 hours, whereas the control group received isotonic saline solution [23]. The hypertonic saline solution group required less fluid and produced more urine than the isotonic saline solution group.

Phase II: Restoration of the Oxygen-Carrying Capacity

The traditional approach to transfusion of the critically ill patient is to maintain the hemoglobin concentration above 10 gm per deciliter by transfusion of homologous blood. This dogma has rarely been questioned in the past because a patient is unlikely to die of anemia at this level. However, the recent concern over the safety of all blood components as related to disease transmission, blood compatibility, and immunogenicity has led to a reassessment of traditional transfusion practices.

It is clear that after acute massive blood loss red cell transfusions are indicated for the restoration of the blood's oxygen-carrying capacity. Nevertheless, the use of the hemoglobin concentration as the sole indicator of the need for RBC replacement, the so-called transfusion trigger [24], may lead to the unnecessary administration of homologous blood products. Indeed, clinical and laboratory studies have clearly demonstrated that hemoglobin concentrations far below 10 gm per deciliter may be well tolerated after acute normovolemic anemia [25,26,27]. Accordingly, transfusion therapy should be instituted based on the patient's physiologic needs, as determined by their oxygen demand, rather than by an arbitrary hemoglobin value. To understand the appropriate indications for a blood transfusion, the basic principles of oxygen transport should be briefly reviewed.

NORMAL OXYGEN TRANSPORT. Oxygen delivery is defined as the product of blood flow (cardiac output; CO) and arterial oxygen content ($[O_2]_a$):

$$O_2 \text{ delivery} = CO \times [O_2]_a$$

Although the $[O_2]_a$ depends on several variables, hemoglobin is the principal determinant. A fall in hemoglobin, and therefore $[O_2]_a$, leads to one of two outcomes: a fall in oxygen delivery if CO does not change, or an increase in CO to maintain oxygen delivery. For anemic patients with good cardiac function, this increased CO does occur, and it is the justification used by advocates of purposeful hemodilution. This response has been observed during normovolemic hemodilution in baboons [28]. Other authors also have documented this ability of the cardiovascular system to compensate for significant reductions in hemoglobin [29,30,31]. Tissue oxygenation is well maintained by hematocrits as low as 20 to 25 percent as long as the blood volume remains normal [25]. These observations are further evidence that hemoglobin alone is not an adequate parameter for determining whether a red cell transfusion is required.

The important issue then becomes the adequacy of oxygen supply at any given hemoglobin. The actual utilization of oxygen by the tissues is the oxygen consumption, which can be calculated as the product of CO and the difference in oxygen content between the arterial and venous blood:

$$O_2 \text{ consumption} = CO \times ([O_2]_a - [O_2]_v)$$

Tissue oxygen tension is the appropriate monitor of oxygen supply [32]. The mixed venous PO_2 (PVO_2) is the oxygen tension of the venous blood when oxygen unloading has been completed and is the best indication of mean tissue oxygen tension. PVO_2 thus becomes a key measurement for assessing the adequacy of oxygen transport, and whether an anemic patient requires red cells. The normal value for PVO_2 is 40 mm Hg.

The authors have evaluated the oxygen extraction ratio (ER) as another physiologic indication of transfusion need. The oxygen ER is the ratio of oxygen consumption to oxygen delivery:

$$ER = \frac{O_2 \text{ consumption}}{O_2 \text{ delivery}}$$
$$= \frac{CO \times ([O_2]_a - [O_2]_V)}{CO \times [O_2]_a}$$
$$= \frac{[O_2]_a - [O_2]_V}{[O_2]_a}$$

Because the normal $[O_2]_a = 20$ vol percent, and the normal arteriovenous oxygen content difference = 5 vol percent, the normal ER = 25 percent. In other words, the available oxygen is four times the oxygen normally consumed, leaving a large oxygen reserve.

The authors have performed an analysis of changes in PVO_2 and ER in extreme normovolemic anemia [33]. Animals survive normovolemic exchange transfusion to hematocrits of 5 percent. PVO_2 falls and ER increases as soon as the hematocrit begins to fall, but no hemodynamic instability is evident until the hematocrit is below 10 percent or the hemoglobin is 3.5 gm per deciliter. At this point the PVO_2 is less than 25 mm Hg, and the ER is greater than 50 percent. The PVO_2 and ER may thus represent indicators of the compensation for any level of hemoglobin.

CLINICAL IMPLICATIONS. Patients with a low PVO_2 can be categorized as being in a stable or an unstable condition based on the adequacy of their hemodynamics, ventilation, urine output, and acid-base status. If a patient's condition is stable with a low PVO_2, no therapy is indicated unless a true critical value is reached (≤ 25 mm Hg). If a patient is unstable with a low PVO_2, therapeutic intervention is indicated.

In practical terms, we consider a patient with a changing PVO_2 value to be undergoing significant alterations of the oxygen transport system, which may be explained by many different conditions, only a few of which may actually be manipulated. A patient with normal lungs will have a normal saturation, and a patient with significant pulmonary disease

may be quite refractory to attempts to improve his or her hypoxia. Likewise, a healthy person can easily compensate for a fall in hemoglobin by an increase in CO. The cardiac patient with a CO that cannot be augmented might benefit from a blood transfusion when PVO_2 is reduced or ER is increased, despite an "acceptable" hemoglobin concentration. In effect, a life-threatening anemia might exist despite only a modest reduction in hemoglobin mass.

In sum, we believe the hemodynamic stability of the patient, the PVO_2, and the ER might be more appropriate indicators of the need for RBC transfusion than hemoglobin concentration alone. Conversely, use of this analysis may lead to a reduction in the transfusion trigger, thus contributing to a reduction in exposure to homologous blood [34].

The current recommendations set forth by the National Institutes of Health Consensus Conference on Perioperative Red Cell Transfusions [35] reflect these changing attitudes toward red cell need, as follows.

1. If hemoglobin is greater than 10 gm per deciliter, transfusion is rarely indicated.
2. If the hemoglobin is less than 7 gm per deciliter, transfusion is usually indicated.
3. If the hemoglobin is greater than 7 but less than 10 gm per deciliter, the clinical status, PVO_2, and ER will be helpful in assessing transfusion need.

TRANSFUSION. Once a need for restoration of the oxygen-carrying capacity of the blood has been established, a number of alternative interventions exist. The most common method employed to increase RBC mass is through the administration of homologous blood (see Chap. 124). Autologous blood represents a viable alternative to homologous transfusions, when applicable. A third alternative currently undergoing laboratory and clinical evaluation is the use of RBC substitutes.

Homologous Blood. The identification of the major isoagglutinins of human blood by Landsteiner made safe transfusions possible by the development of principles of blood grouping and compatibility. With the evaluation of blood component therapy, there has been a steady decline in the number of transfusions given in the form of whole blood. Whereas as much as 30 percent of homologous blood administered in the United States a decade ago was in the form of whole blood [36], the theoretical and practical advantages of component therapy have made whole blood's use and availability limited at the present time.

Component therapy consists of fractionation of whole blood at the time of collection into RBCs, platelets, and plasma. The use of packed cells rather than whole blood to restore oxygen-carrying capacity is specific treatment, allows more efficient use of the other limited commodities (platelets and plasma), and avoids the undesirable effects often seen after the administration of platelet and white blood cell (WBC) debris [37]. The argument that a patient bleeding whole blood must undergo blood replacement with whole blood is no longer acceptable.

After separating the RBCs from the other blood components, they may be stored and used in three separate ways:

PACKED RED BLOOD CELLS. A concentrated suspension of RBCs is obtained by removing the supernatant plasma from the whole blood after settling or centrifugation. The RBC mass is the same as in 1 unit of whole blood. The plasma citrate level and volume of plasma are substantially reduced.

WASHED RED BLOOD CELLS. After the RBCs have been obtained by settling or centrifugation, they are washed with sterile isotonic saline solution. This process results in a still lower plasma citrate level than is present in a unit of nonwashed cells. The only disadvantage is the additional preparation time required and the possibility of bacterial contamination.

FROZEN RED BLOOD CELLS. The use of frozen RBCs has been an important addition to blood component therapy. A major concern with the use of the liquid preserved blood has been the outdating of blood because of the limited shelf life (21–28 days). Despite progress in the development of better preservatives, 28 days is still a relatively brief period. Frozen RBCs can be stored indefinitely, with no apparent loss of safety or efficacy after thawing and administration. In addition to providing an indefinite shelf life, frozen blood facilitates the application of autologous blood usage, permits stockpiling of all blood groups, particularly those that are difficult to obtain, maintains normal levels of 2,3-diphosphoglycerate (2,3-DPG) and P50, and may be associated with a lower risk of hepatitis transmission [38], although the latter issue remains unsettled.

Autologous Blood. The risks inherent with the use of homologous blood products have led to the evaluation of numerous strategies designed to limit exposure to homologous blood. The reinfusion of the patient's own blood, autologous blood transfusion, clearly represents the safest form of transfusion therapy. Three established methods are available for the use of autologous blood: preoperative autologous blood donation (ABD) programs; immediate preoperative collection and hemodilution; and intraoperative autotransfusion. A fourth method that is currently under laboratory and clinical investigation is the pharmacologic acceleration of endogenous erythropoiesis with hematopoietic growth factors.

PREOPERATIVE AUTOLOGOUS BLOOD DONATION PROGRAMS. This technique was developed in the 1960s as a means of obtaining blood for patients with rare antibodies that were difficult to cross-match. The real and perceived risks of blood-borne infection transmission from homologous transfusions have led to an exponential rise in the use of ABD programs before elective operations. In a recent national survey of transfusion practices in the United States during the 1980s, ABDs increased from 30,000 units in 1982 to 397,000 in 1987 [39]. Nevertheless, the application of this procedure to the treatment of hemorrhagic shock is limited to those situations where acute blood loss is anticipated.

The criteria used for donor acceptability for ABD programs are variable from institution to institution. The American Association of Blood Banks recommends a minimum hematocrit value of 34 percent and a hemoglobin of 11 gm per deciliter for autologous donation [40]. Donations are most commonly scheduled 7 days apart [41]. A recent review has shown that after the above criteria 96 percent of patients could donate at least three units of blood before operative intervention [42]. The most common reasons cited for the limitation of this procedure in the elective surgical setting are physician underutilization, insufficient time intervals for collection before surgery, and the limited erythropoietic reserve of patients subjected to repeated phlebotomy [43].

IMMEDIATE PREOPERATIVE COLLECTION AND HEMODILUTION. This technique is based on the cardiovascular changes that occur during the induction of normovolemic anemia. Blood is withdrawn to acutely reduce the hematocrit to 30 percent, and blood volume is maintained with Ringer's lactate, dextran, or other volume expanders. A healthy individual maintains oxygen delivery during this period of normovolemic anemia by increasing CO. Messmer et al. [25] showed that tissue oxygenation remains normal, and advocates of purposeful hemodilution actually believe that a hematocrit of 30 percent is optimal.

This method can provide approximately 3 units of whole blood for intraoperative use. Although the technique has been used widely in Europe, in the United States it has been primarily limited to patients undergoing open heart operations. Because open heart operations are responsible for a large proportion of our homologous blood demand [44], wide use of this method could have a substantial influence on the availability of blood.

INTRAOPERATIVE AUTOTRANSFUSION. Autotransfusion represents an efficient means of reducing homologous blood requirements through the recycling of red cells lost during intraoperative hemorrhage. Although the potential of autotransfusion is appealing, there are certain practical limitations to its use. The theoretical problem of bacterial contamination limits its use in a variety of settings in which it might be most helpful, such as major trauma. A second concern is the required logistic support necessary to implement this expensive technique on a 24-hour basis. Lastly, air embolism during reinfusion is a rare but troublesome complication.

ACCELERATION OF ERYTHROPOIESIS. Approximately two-thirds of all red cell transfusions are administered in the perioperative period [35]. Loss of blood is the most common cause of anemia in the surgical patient and occurs in one of two settings: elective surgery (planned blood loss) or emergency surgery (unplanned blood loss). Effective preoperative autologous donation and rapid postoperative recovery both depend on brisk erythropoietic responses. The pharmacologic stimulation of erythropoiesis thus represents an attractive means of increasing red cell recovery after acute blood loss.

The advent of recombinant DNA technology has led to the isolation and cloning of numerous hematopoietic growth factors that promote bone marrow cellular proliferation. Erythropoietin, a glycoprotein normally released by the kidney in response to tissue hypoxia, is known to be the primary regulator of bone marrow red cell proliferation. Preclinical [45,46] and clinical [47] studies with exogenously administered recombinant-human erythropoietin (rHuEPO) have demonstrated its efficacy in increasing the number of autologous units collected before elective operations and enhancing erythropoietic recovery when given before acute blood loss. However, when rHuEPO is administered after acute blood loss, clinically significant effects are not evident until 1 week after therapy is initiated [48]. Accordingly, in the setting of nonanticipated blood loss, rHuEPO's therapeutic potential is limited. Nevertheless, laboratory studies are underway investigating the application of other erythropoietic growth factors that may further accelerate the endogenous response after acute blood loss.

Red Blood Cell Substitutes. Efforts to develop a safe and effective red cell substitute have continued for many decades. The goal has been to obtain a product that would transport oxygen and carbon dioxide adequately enough to replace the primary function of the red cell in the setting of temporary unavailability of blood. The recent focus on the risks associated with homologous transfusion has stepped up efforts to develop a sterile red cell substitute as an alternative to homologous blood. Perfluorochemical emulsions and hemoglobin solutions are the two potential products that have been most extensively evaluated.

PERFLUOROCHEMICAL EMULSIONS. Considerable progress has been made in research with perfluorochemicals since they were first described by Clark and Gollan in 1966 [49]. Perfluorochemicals are organic liquids that have the unique property of carrying large amounts of oxygen in physically dissolved form. The solubility of oxygen in the pure perfluorochemicals is actually 10- to 20-fold greater than in water. It was Clark and Gollan's liquid breathing experiment with mice that so vividly demonstrated this remarkable property and led to the potential application of perfluorochemicals as clinically useful oxygen carriers. The next important event was the report by Geyer [50], who demonstrated that rats could survive a total exchange transfusion with perfluorochemicals to a zero hematocrit. The important stipulation, however, was that the rats breathe supplemental oxygen, because the perfluorocarbons required a high partial pressure of oxygen to carry adequate amounts of oxygen. This requirement continues to be a limiting factor with all perfluorochemicals.

Considerable efforts were then devoted to developing a product that would be suitable for clinical testing. The commercially prepared product, Fluosol-DA, 20 percent (Green Cross Corporation, Japan) was the first product to be introduced into clinical testing. Several brief studies eventually led to clinical studies with Fluosol in the United States, including the trial at Michael Reese Hospital and Medical Center in Chicago [26].

In the trial, the safety and efficacy of Fluosol-DA as a red cell substitute in acute anemia were assessed. Twenty-three surgical patients with blood loss and religious objections to receiving blood transfusions were evaluated. Fifteen moderately anemic patients with a mean hemoglobin level ($\pm$ SE) of 7.2 ± 0.5 gm per deciliter had no evidence of a physiologic need for increased arterial oxygen content and did not receive Fluosol-DA. Eight severely anemic patients with a mean hemoglobin level of 3.0 ± 0.4 gm per deciliter met our criteria of need and received the drug until the physiologic need disappeared or a maximal dose of 40 ml per kilogram of body weight was reached. All patients breathed supplemental oxygen. No adverse reactions to Fluosol-DA were observed. The average peak increment in arterial oxygen content with the drug was only 0.7 ± 0.1 ml per deciliter. This is equivalent to an increase in hemoglobin concentration of only 0.5 gm per deciliter. There were no appreciable beneficial effects of Fluosol-DA, perhaps because of the small increase in arterial oxygen content, the brief half-life of the drug (24.3 ± 4.3 hours) and the limited total dose. Six of the eight patients receiving Fluosol-Da died. One of the survivors received red cell transfusions against his wishes, under a court order, after his total Fluosol-DA dose. Fourteen of the 15 moderately anemic patients lived.

These data suggest that after blood loss, Fluosol-DA is unnecessary in moderate anemia and ineffective in severe anemia. Efforts are continuing to develop other modifications that would have higher concentrations of perfluorochemicals and a longer intravascular biologic half-life. In the near future, however, there does not appear to be any perfluorochemical that will likely be an effective red cell substitute.

HEMOGLOBIN SOLUTIONS. There is considerable interest in the development of a hemoglobin-based oxygen carrier that would be a clinically useful red cell substitute. It has long been recognized that free hemoglobin is able to load and unload oxygen in a manner similar to hemoglobin contained within the red cell. The potential benefits of such a hemoglobin solution include universal compatibility and immediate availability, convenient and prolonged storage capability, and freedom from infectious disease transmission.

There are several properties that must be considered when describing the nature of a hemoglobin solution. The first is the source of the hemoglobin starting material (Table 172-1). Human blood is the best known source, based on its long and well-described clinical experience. Although some consider a bovine source to be of benefit when trying to obtain larger volumes of starting material, there is little experience to support this approach. Recombinant and transgenic sources are intriguing because of their use of genetic engineering technology. However, there is no evidence to suggest any physiologic or functional benefit. In fact, the choice of source has not been a crucial issue in the development of a red cell substitute.

The limiting factor in this field has been the safety of the hemoglobin solution. It is now evident that unmodified tetrameric hemoglobin is unsafe because of the associated toxicities of renal dysfunction and vasoconstriction. Therefore, the most important property of a hemoglobin solution is the nature of the hemoglobin preparation itself. Unmodified tetramer dissociates into dimers and monomers when removed from the red cell. The renal dysfunction is thought to be due to filtration of dimers and monomers through the kidney. Vasoconstriction is thought to reflect extravasation of the tetramer beyond the endothelial cell barrier to the vascular muscle layer, where it is bound by endothelial-derived relaxing factor, or nitric oxide. The end result is the observed vasoconstriction.

The efforts to eliminate these toxicities have consisted of attempts to stabilize the simple unmodified tetramer. Table 172-2 shows the various approaches. It is now accepted that an unmodified tetrameric solution will not be acceptable in the clinical setting. Each attempt uses a different approach, and only human testing will eventually resolve the issue of safety. The issue of source material is less important than the actual hemoglobin preparation.

The third characteristic of any hemoglobin solution is the intended clinical use (Table 172-2). Although there are numerous potential applications for a safe and effective acellular oxygen carrier, it is likely that the major role will be as red cell substitute for use in acute blood loss.

There are numerous clinical trials underway in both volunteers and patients using human polymerized hemoglobin, human cross-linked tetramer, bovine polymer, and recombinant cross-linked tetramer. The trials are at an early stage, but the next several years should provide important information regarding the potential role of these oxygen carriers in transfusion therapy.

The remainder of this section deals with the authors' attempts to develop a hemoglobin solution. The starting material is outdated human blood.

Various techniques have been used to separate the hemoglobin from the red cell membrane to prepare this stroma-free hemoglobin (SFH) solution. The first generation of this unmodified tetrameric form or "stripped" hemoglobin solution had a hemoglobin concentration of only 7 gm per deciliter, and a P50 of 12 to 14 mm Hg (normal 26 mm Hg). Although SFH can be prepared with a hemoglobin level of 14 gm per deciliter, the solution has a colloid osmotic pressure (COP) of greater than 60 mm Hg. This hyperoncotic solution would not be acceptable for clinical use. The hemoglobin of 7 gm deciliter is therefore required to maintain an iso-oncotic product. The low P50 is

Table 172-1. Hemoglobin Preparation

- Unmodified tetramer
- Conjugated tetramer
- Cross-linked tetramer
- Polymer
- Encapsulation

Table 172-2. Hemoglobin Clinical Use

- Acute blood loss
- Hemodilution
- Ischemia
- Cardioplegia
- Organ preservation

caused by the loss of 2,3-DPG from the solution. Despite these limitations, SFH supports life in primates at a zero hematocrit reading, documenting effective oxygen transport in the absence of red cells [28]. Subsequent efforts have attempted to develop a product with a normal oxygen-carrying capacity [51]. The P50 issue was the first problem to be corrected. Pyridoxal phosphate is an alternative organic phosphate ligand that can be permanently bound to the hemoglobin molecule. The resulting pyridoxylated hemoglobin or SFH-P has a P50 of 20 to 22 mm Hg. Although this was an improvement compared with the stripped hemoglobin, the product still has a low hemoglobin concentration.

The authors' approach to the problem of the hemoglobin concentration was to use a polymerized product that would permit a normal hemoglobin concentration and a normal COP. SFH-P is initially prepared with a hemoglobin of 14 gm per deciliter. Polymerization of this hyperoncotic product reduces the total number of molecules while increasing the average molecular size. However, no hemoglobin mass is lost. The COP is lowered to an iso-oncotic range (20 mm Hg), because the COP is proportional only to the actual number of particles (molecules). Polymerized pyridoxylated hemoglobin solution, or Poly SFH-P, therefore achieves the goal of both a normal hemoglobin concentration of 15 gm per deciliter and a normal COP of 20 mm Hg. The P50 is 28 to 30 mm Hg. Thus we have a product that has virtually the same properties as a bag of red cells. In addition to these physiologic improvements, the product has a half-life of 24 to 48 hours [52] in animal studies.

The authors have evaluated the efficacy of Poly SFH-P. The results document that Poly SFH-P supports life in a primate at a zero hematocrit reading [53,54]. Furthermore, the observations indicate that this product is more effective in maintaining hemodynamic and oxygen transport values than were any of our earlier hemoglobin modifications [55]. We believe that Poly SFH-P is indeed an effective oxygen carrier, and are therefore enthusiastic about its potential clinical applications.

The limiting factor before clinical testing is concern about the safety of Poly SFH-P. The main uncertainty is the effect of this product on renal function. The key observation was a 1978 study by Savitsky et al. [56], in which tetrameric hemoglobin solution was given to human volunteers. The study showed that small infusions of hemoglobin solution produced transient, but significant, changes in renal function, and vasoconstriction. The authors have developed a sensitive and reproducible animal model that virtually duplicates these findings [57]. Infusion of tetrameric hemoglobin solution into unanesthetized primates produces the same changes in hemodynamics and renal function that were observed in humans. It is our hypothesis that because the polymerized hemoglobin molecule does not traverse the renal tubules, it may not produce these same effects.

We have recently completed the first clinical evaluation of Poly SFH-P in acutely bleeding patients. In this study no significant differences between preinfusion and postinfusion measures of renal function and no evidence of vasoconstriction occurred. There were no clinically significant abnormalities in routine chemical and hematologic variables throughout a 6-week follow-up. Although these results are encouraging, the efficacy of this therapy is dependent on further studies in anemic patients after acute blood loss.

SUMMARY OF PHASE II. In conclusion, the restoration of the oxygen-carrying capacity of the circulation is a fundamental adjunct to volume expansion in the treatment of hemorrhagic shock. The risks associated with homologous transfusion necessitate the adoption of a multitiered approach to red cell replacement, encompassing both the reduction in the transfu-

sion trigger and the increased use of the various autologous techniques, so as to reduce homologous blood exposure. Finally, further developments with red cell substitutes hold promise that exposure to homologous transfusions may be avoided altogether.

Phase Three: Component Therapy of Hemostatic Defects

The components most frequently used are platelets and fresh frozen plasma (FFP). This section reviews the indications for the use of these two components in massive transfusion.

In most patients with acute reduction in circulating volume, treatment with crystalloid solutions followed by RBC transfusions, when indicated, will achieve successful resuscitation. In the case of massive transfusion, defined as blood volume replacement greater than $1\frac{1}{2}$ times the recipient volume, abnormal bleeding may occur. This hemostatic defect is characterized by oozing from the operative wound, mucous membranes, and IV puncture sites. The probability of developing a hemostatic defect is roughly related to the volume of infused blood and fluids.

Investigations of massively transfused patients with a hemostatic defect usually demonstrate the following changes in the coagulation profile: (1) reduced platelet count, (2) increased bleeding time, (3) increased prothrombin time (PT), (4) increased activated partial prothrombin time (PTT), and (5) decreased fibrinogen levels. In addition, studies of the coagulation profile after a 3-liter plasma exchange in normal apheresis donors demonstrated similar changes.

For these reasons, the traditional explanation for the hemostatic defect after massive transfusion has been dilution of the various clotting elements. Recommendations for coagulopathy prophylaxis include administration of platelet concentrations and FFP during resuscitation and before the onset of oozing. An established coagulopathy is treated with either platelet concentrates or FFP, or both, depending on the coagulation profile. This approach is logical but should be reexamined for several reasons.

First, both platelets and FFP may transmit non-A, non-B hepatitis. Exposure to more than 2 units carries an estimated 10 percent risk of hepatitis [58]. It is important to emphasize that this often takes the form of chronic liver inflammation. The risk is likely to be the same as for whole blood. These components should therefore be used with the same precautions used for any other blood components.

Second, in the case of FFP, the observation that PT and activated PTT is abnormal in the presence of a coagulopathy is not, in itself, evidence that administration of FFP will correct the hemostatic defect. It is well known that normal clotting can still occur when the various clotting protein concentrations are substantially reduced. Furthermore, the infusion of FFP in patients who are oozing after massive transfusion and who have abnormal PT and PTT frequently fails to stop the bleeding despite normalization of PT and PTT [59]. Also, prophylactic use of FFP (and platelets) has failed to reduce the incidence of coagulopathy after massive transfusion [60].

Third, regarding platelets, there is no doubt that after the loss of more than 1 blood volume, platelet counts of 100,000 or less may be seen. In addition, the bleeding time will be abnormal in almost all massively transfused patients. However, the bleeding time and platelet count in such patients without coagulopathy may also be abnormal and not different from those in patients who bleed. This is particularly evident in patients with hypothermia, a known cause of elevated bleeding times. Furthermore, spontaneous bleeding from thrombocytopenia rarely occurs when the platelet count is greater than 20,000, a level infrequently seen in massive transfusion.

On the basis of these observations, we recommend the following approach to component use in the third phase of resuscitation:

1. Platelet count, PT, and PTT should be measured frequently during massive resuscitation.
2. Bleeding times may not be useful, particularly in the hypothermic patient.
3. Administration of components prophylactically during resuscitation is not helpful and exposes the patient unnecessarily to the risk of hepatitis.
4. If a coagulopathy develops during massive resuscitation, platelet infusions will be helpful if the platelet count is less than 100,000.
5. FFP will not be helpful in most cases of a coagulopathy. If the PT and PTT are substantially prolonged (greater than $1\frac{1}{2}$ times control), FFP infusion may be helpful.

The clinical value of FFP has been summarized in a National Institutes of Health consensus statement as follows [61]:

1. Approximately 90 percent of current FFP use is inappropriate.
2. The risk of hepatitis with FFP is similar to that associated with any other blood component.
3. The use of FFP has risen tenfold during the last decade for no apparent reason.
4. Unacceptable indications for FFP use include the following:
   a. Volume expander
   b. Source of immunoglobin except in rare instances
   c. Source of nutrition
   d. Source of fibronectin.
5. Acceptable indications include the following:
   a. Treatment of postresuscitation clotting defect when a major decrease in clotting problems can be demonstrated
   b. Treatment of life-threatening coumadin intoxication.

References

1. Templeton GH, Mitchell JH, Wildenthal K: Influence of hyperosmolarity on left ventricular stiffness. *Am J Physiol* 222:1406, 1972.
2. Wildenthal KD, Mierzwiak DS, Mitchell JH: Acute effects of increased serum osmolality on left ventricular performance. *Am J Physiol* 216:898, 1969.
3. Marshall RJ, Shepherd JT: Effect of injections of hypertonic solutions on blood flow through the femoral artery of the dog. *Am J Physiol* 97:951, 1959.
4. Kleeman CR: CNS manifestations of disordered salt and water balance. *Hosp Pract* 14:59, 1979.
5. Lucas CE, Ledgerwood AM, Mammen EF: Altered coagulation protein content after albumin resuscitation. *Ann Surg* 196, 1982.
6. Shoemaker MC, Schluchter M, Hopkins JA, et al: Fluid therapy in emergency resuscitation; Clinical evaluation of colloid and crystalloid regimens. *Crit Care Med* 9:367, 1981.
7. Skillman JJ, Restall DS, Salzman EW: Randomized trial of albumin vs. electrolyte solutions during abdominal aortic operations. *Surgery* 78:291, 1975.
8. Moore FD, Lyons JH, Pierce EC: *Posttraumatic Pulmonary Insufficiency*. Philadelphia, WB Saunders, 1969.
9. Rackow EC, Falk JL, Fein IA, et al: Fluid resuscitation in circulatory shock: A comparison of the cardiorespiratory effects of albumin, hetastarch, and saline solutions in patients with hypovolemic and septic shock. *Crit Care Med* 11:839, 1983.
10. Hauser CJ, Shoemaker WC, Turpin 1, et al: Oxygen transport re-

sponses to colloids and crystalloids in critically ill surgical patients. *Surg Gynecol Obstet* 150:811, 1980.
11. Shires GT, Braun FT, Canizaro PC, et al: Distributional changes in extracellular fluid during acute hemorrhagic shock. *Surg Forum* 11:115, 1960.
12. Virgilio RW, Rice CL, Smith DE, et al: Crystalloid vs. colloid resuscitation: Is one better? *Surgery* 85:129, 1979.
13. Siegal DC, Moss GS, Cochin A: Pulmonary changes following treatment for hemorrhagic shock: Saline versus colloid infusion. *Surg Forum* 21:17, 1970.
14. Lucas CE, Denis R, Ledgerwood AM, et al: The effect of hespan on serum and lymphatic albumin, globulin and coagulant protein. *Ann Surg* 207:416, 1988.
15. Lowe RJ, Moss GS, Jilek J, et al: Crystalloid vs. colloid in the etiology of pulmonary failure after trauma: A randomized trial in man. *Surgery* 81:676, 1977.
16. Shoemaker WC, Hauser CJ: Critique of crystalloid vs. colloid therapy in shock and shock lung. *Crit Care Med* 7:117, 1979.
17. Moss GS, Lowe RJ, Jilek J, et al: Colloid or crystalloid in the resuscitation of hemorrhagic shock: A controlled clinical trial. *Surgery* 89:434, 1981.
18. Velanovich V: Crystalloid versus colloid fluid resuscitation: A meta-analysis of mortality. *Surgery* 105:65, 1989.
19. Monafo WW, Halverson JD, Schechtman K: The role of concentrated sodium solutions in the resuscitation of patients with severe burns. *Surgery* 95:129, 1984.
20. Bowser-Wallace B, Caldwell FT Jr: A prospective analysis of hypertonic lactated saline vs. Ringer's lactate-colloid for the resuscitation of severely burned children. *Burns* 12:402, 1986.
21. Bowser-Wallace B, Cone JB, Caldwell FT Jr: Hypertonic lactated saline resuscitation of severely burned patients over 60 years of age. *J Trauma* 25:22, 1985.
22. Shackford SR, Sise MJ, Fridlund PH, et al: Hypertonic sodium lactate versus lactated Ringer's solution for intravenous fluid therapy in operations on the abdominal aorta. *Surgery* 94:41, 1983.
23. Holcroft JW, Vassar MJ, Blaisdell FW: Resuscitation of severely injured patients with a 3 percent NaCl solution. *Ann Surg* 206:279, 1987.
24. Friedman BA, Burns TL, Schork MA: An analysis of blood transfusion of surgical patients by sex: A quest for the transfusion trigger. *Transfusion* 20:179, 1980.
25. Messmer K, Sunder-Plassman L, Jesch F, et al: Oxygen supply to the tissues during limited normovolemic hemodilution. *Res Exp Med* 159:152, 1973.
26. Gould SA, Rosen AL, Sehgal LR, et al: Fluosol-DA as a red cell substitute in acute anemia. *N Engl J Med* 314:1653, 1986.
27. Carson JL, Spence RK, Poses RM, et al: Severity of anemia and operative mortality and morbidity. *Lancet* 1:727, 1988.
28. Moss GS, DeWoskin R, Rosen AL, et al: Transport of oxygen and carbon dioxide by hemoglobin-saline solution in the red cell-free primate. *Surg Gynecol Obstet* 142:357, 1976.
29. Carey JS: Determinants of cardiac output during experimental therapeutic hemodilution. *Ann Surg* 181:196, 1975.
30. Geha AS: Coronary and cardiovascular dynamics and oxygen availability during acute normovolemic anemia. *Surgery* 80:47, 1976.
31. Gump TE: Anemia in surgical patients, in Collins JA, Lundsgaard Hansen P (eds): *Surgical Hemotherapy*. Basel, S. Karger, 1980, p 105.
32. Finch CA, Lenfant C: Oxygen transport in man. *N Engl J Med* 286:407, 1972.
33. Wilkerson DK, Rosen AL, Gould SA, et al: Oxygen extraction ratio: A valid indicator of myocardial metabolism in anemia. *J Surg Res* 42:629, 1987.
34. Levine EA, Rosen AL, Sehgal LR, et al: Physiologic effects of acute anemia: Implications for a reduced transfusion trigger. *Transfusion* 30:11, 1990.
35. Consensus Conference: Perioperative red blood cell transfusion. *JAMA* 260:2700, 1988.
36. Kahn RA, Staggs SD, Miller WV, et al: Use of plasma products with whole blood and packed RBC's. *JAMA* 242:2087, 1979.
37. Chaplin H: Current concepts: Packed red blood cells. *N Engl J Med* 281:364, 1969.
38. Valeri CR: Viability and function of preserved red cells. *N Engl J Med* 284:81, 1971.

39. Surgenor DN, Wallace EL, Hao SHS, et al: Collection and transfusion of blood in the United States, 1982-88. *N Engl J Med* 322:646, 1990.

40. Holland PV, Schmidt PJ: *Standards for Blood Banks and Transfusion Services,* ed 12. Arlington, VA, American Association of Blood Banks, 1987, p 38.

41. Council on Scientific Affairs: Autologous blood transfusions. *JAMA* 256:2378, 1986.

42. Goodnough LT: Autologous blood donation. *JAMA* 259:2405, 1988.

43. Goodnough LT, Wasman J, Corlucci K, et al: Limitations to donating adequate autologous blood prior to elective orthopedic surgery. *Arch Surg* 124:494, 1989.

44. Roche JK, Stengle JM: Open-heart surgery and the demand for blood. *JAMA* 225:1516, 1973.

45. Levine EA, Rosen AL, Gould SA, et al: Recombinant human erythropoietin and autologous blood donation. *Surgery* 104:365, 1988.

46. Levine EA, Gould SA, Rosen AL, et al: Perioperative recombinant human erythropoietin. *Surgery* 106:432, 1989.

47. Goodnough LT, Rudnick S, Price TH, et al: Increased perioperative collection of autologous blood with recombinant human erythropoietin therapy. *N Engl J Med* 321:1163, 1989.

48. Levine EA, Rosen AL, Sehgal LR, et al: Treatment of acute postoperative anemia with recombinant human erythropoietin. *J Trauma* 19:1134, 1989.

49. Clark LC, Gollan F: Survival of mammals breathing organic liquids equilibrated with oxygen at atmospheric pressure. *Science* 152:1755, 1966.

50. Geyer RP: Whole animal perfusion with fluorocarbon dispersions. *Fed Proc* 29:1758, 1970.

51. Moss GS, Gould SA, Sehgal LR, et al: Hemoglobin solution: From tetramer to polymer. *Surgery* 95:249, 1984.

52. Sehgal LR, Gould SA, Rosen AL, et al: Polymerized pyridoxylated hemoglobin: A red cell substitute with normal O_2 capacity. *Surgery* 95:433, 1984.

53. Gould SA, Sehgal LR, Rosen AL, et al: Polyhemoglobin: An improved red cell substitute. *Surg Form* 36:30, 1985.

54. Gould SA, Rosen AL, Sehgal LR, et al: Is polyhemoglobin an effective O_2 carrier? *J Trauma* 26:903, 1986.

55. Gould SA, Sehgal LR, Rosen AL, et al: The efficacy of polymerized pyridoxylated hemoglobin solution as an O_2 carrier. *Ann Surg* 211:394, 1990.

56. Savitsky JP, Doczij J, Black J, et al: A clinical safety trial of stroma-free hemoglobin. *J Clin Pharmacol Ther* 23:73, 1978.

57. Rosen AL, Sehgal LR, Gould SA, et al: Renal response to hemoglobin solutions (abstract). *Physiologist* 29:161, 1986.

58. Alter HJ: The dominant role of non-A, non-B in the pathogenesis of post-transfusion hepatitis: A clinical assessment. *Clin Gastroenterol* 9:155, 1980.

59. Miller RD, Robbins TO, Tong MJ, et al: Coagulation defects associated with massive blood transfusions. *Ann Surg* 174:794, 1971.

60. Counts RB, Haisch C, Simon TL, et al: Hemostasis in massively transfused patients. *Ann Surg* 190:91, 1979.

61. National Institutes of Health, Consensus Conference: Fresh-frozen plasma: Indications and risks. *JAMA* 253:551, 1985.

173. Septic Shock

Margaret M. Parker and Mitchell P. Fink

Definitions

The literature dealing with the systemic consequences of severe infection is complicated by the imprecise use of myriad, partially overlapping, terms such as sepsis, septicemia, and endotoxic shock. To a certain extent, the lack of precision in the use of these terms has hampered the progress of clinical investigation into the pathophysiology of septic shock and related problems.

For the purposes of the current discussion, *bacteremia, fungemia,* and *viremia* denote the presence of positive blood cultures for bacteria, yeast, and viruses, respectively. *Sepsis* refers to a constellation of symptoms, signs, and abnormal laboratory values associated with serious infections. To emphasize that sepsis is a constellation of findings rather than a specific disease, the term *sepsis syndrome* has been employed [1,2]. There has not been unanimous agreement on the definitions of sepsis, and particularly septic shock, and other terms and definitions have been proposed [3,4,5]. Representatives of the American College of Chest Physicians and the Society of Critical Care Medicine held a consensus conference and proposed that the following terms be adopted [4]:

1. The Systemic Inflammatory Response Syndrome (SIRS) is defined by the presence of two or more of the following findings: (a) fever or hypothermia, (b) tachycardia, (c) tachypnea, (d) alteration of white blood cell count. SIRS can be triggered by both infectious and noninfectious processes. Examples of the latter include severe trauma and necrotizing pancreatitis.

2. Sepsis is the systemic inflammatory response (i.e., SIRS) caused by infection.

3. Severe sepsis is sepsis associated with organ dysfunction.

4. Septic shock is severe sepsis with hypotension (defined as a systolic blood pressure <90 mm Hg) persisting despite adequate fluid resuscitation.

5. Septicemia is an imprecise term that is not recommended for current usage.

In addition to the terms defined above, two other terms are commonly used. *Endotoxic shock* is a syndrome induced in laboratory animals by infusing large doses of lipopolysaccharide (LPS, endotoxin), a component of the cell wall of gram-negative bacteria. *Endotoxemia* is defined by the presence of circulating endotoxin and has been documented in many patients with sepsis and septic shock (see the section on mediators).

Epidemiology

Septic shock is currently one of the most common causes of mortality in intensive care units. Data from the Centers for Disease Control (CDC) indicate that sepsis is the 13th leading cause of death in the United States and accounts for 5 to 10 billion dollars of health care costs annually [6]. According to the CDC, the mortality rate for "septicemia" was 25.3 percent in 1987 [6]. From 1979 through 1987, the sepsis rate in the United States increased 139 percent from 73.6 cases per 100,000 persons to 175.9 cases per 100,000 persons. Although the rate of sepsis increased among all age groups, the increase was largest among the group aged 65 or older.

Numerous factors probably have contributed to the increasing incidence of septic shock [7]. Immunosuppressive therapy for malignancies, organ transplants, or inflammatory diseases places patients at increased risk for infectious complications. Patients predisposed to infection because of other diseases (such as diabetes mellitus, renal failure, and cancer) are living longer because of improvements in therapy. Invasive medical devices (such as intravascular catheters, prosthetic heart valves, vascular grafts, and respiratory equipment) are being used with increasing frequency. The clustering of critically ill patients in special care units, although beneficial in many ways, undoubtedly fosters the development of nosocomial infections.

Microbiology

Septic shock can be caused by infections attributable to a variety of different organisms. Gram-negative bacilli are most commonly implicated, but serious infections from gram-positive bacteria, fungi, viruses, and even protozoa can be associated with hypotension and signs of visceral hypoperfusion [8–12]. Although some data suggest that the hemodynamic response is different for gram-negative as compared with gram-positive bacteremia [13], most data suggest that the cardiovascular manifestations of serious infections are independent of the type of infecting organism [8–12,14,15].

Clinical Manifestations of Septic Shock

DERANGED TEMPERATURE REGULATION. Temperature instability is a cardinal feature of sepsis [1]. Most septic patients are febrile, although hypothermia is occasionally observed, particularly in very old or very young patients. Fever is probably mediated by the release of interleukin-1 (IL-1), tumor necrosis factor alpha (TNFα), or other cytokines with activity as "endogenous pyrogens" [16]. Hypothermia has been associated with a worse prognosis [17,18].

CARDIAC MANIFESTATIONS. Tachycardia is virtually always present in septic patients, unless they are receiving beta-blocker therapy. Tachycardia (defined as a heart rate greater than 90 beats per minute) has been used as an entry criterion for clinical trials of adjuvant therapy for sepsis [1]. In one series, only 9 of 48 patients with septic shock had an initial heart rate less than 106 beats per minute [14]. Fungal sepsis has been associated with bradycardia and a serum factor, which is a negative chronotrope in some patients [19].

Cardiac output is typically normal or elevated in adequately resuscitated patients with septic shock [7,9,14,20–27]. Cardiac output is similarly well maintained in a variety of animal models of septic [28–31] and endotoxic [32,33,34] shock. Despite these findings, it is now clearly established that myocardial performance is profoundly depressed in patients with septic shock

[23,35–40]. Biventricular depression of the ejection fraction (EF) associated with ventricular dilatation occurs during the first few days after sepsis-induced hypotension and resolves over 10 to 14 days as the patient recovers (Fig. 173-1) [23,24,37]. As noted in Chapter 171, EF is not an unambiguous index of the inotropic state of the heart, because it is affected by factors other than contractility, especially vascular input impedance. In septic shock, however, systemic vascular resistance index (SVRI), a proxy for vascular input impedance, is almost always abnormally low (see the section on Peripheral Vascular Manifestations that follows) and, hence, depressed left ventricular (LV) EF in this setting provides strong evidence of diminished myocardial contractility.

In addition to depressed EF, patients with septic shock manifest other findings indicative of deranged cardiac function. For example, in one study that examined the effect of a volume challenge in patients with and without sepsis, the observed increases in LV end-diastolic volume index and LV stroke work index were smaller in the septic group, although the augmen-

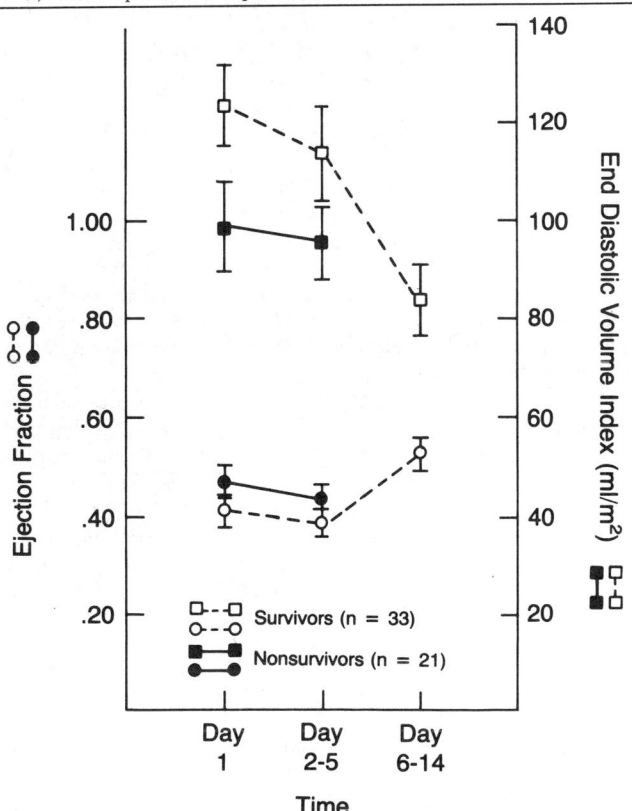

Fig. 173-1. Serial mean ejection fraction (circles) and serial mean end-diastolic volume index (squares) in 33 survivors (open symbols) and 21 nonsurvivors (closed symbols) of septic shock. The survivors have an initial mean ejection fraction that is significantly lower than that of critically ill, nonseptic control patients and an initial mean end-diastolic volume index that is significantly greater than that of control patients. The nonsurvivors have initial mean ejection fraction and end-diastolic volume index values that do not differ significantly from those of control patients. In the survivors, the mean ejection fraction and end-diastolic volume index values returned to normal 6 to 14 days after the onset of septic shock. (Source: Parker MM, Suffredini AF, Natanson C, et al: Responses of left ventricular function in survivors and nonsurvivors of septic shock. *J Crit Care* 4:19, 1989. Reprinted with permission.)

tation of pulmonary artery wedge pressure due to the fluid load was similar in both groups [41]. In another study of the effect of fluid loading in patients with septic shock, increases in LV stroke work index were smaller in nonsurvivors than in survivors [21].

The mechanism(s) responsible for myocardial depression in septic shock are not completely understood. Some investigators have proposed that myocardial function is impaired on the basis of decreased coronary perfusion leading to myocardial ischemia [42–45]. Two studies, however, have documented that coronary blood flow and myocardial oxygen consumption are not decreased in patients with septic shock [46,47]. Moreover, in patients with septic shock, the heart is a lactate consumer rather than a lactate producer [47]. These observations are inconsistent with the hypothesis that impaired myocardial performance in sepsis is on the basis of ischemia.

Currently, the best available data suggest that depression of cardiac function in septic shock is caused by the presence of circulating substances that decrease myocardial contractility [48–56]. Studies employing videomicroscopy to assess the performance of spontaneously beating rat myocardial cells have shown that a myocardial depressant substance is present in serum from septic patients (but not appropriate controls) and that the extent of myocardial depression observed in vitro correlates with the degree of depression of EF (as assessed by radionuclide ventriculography) observed in vivo [55]. Although the identity of the myocardial depressant substance remains elusive, accumulating data suggest that it is a cytokine, such as TNFα [57–61]. Recent data suggest that the negative inotropic effects of LPS or cytokines, like TNFα, are mediated via the induction of nitric oxide formation [61,62,63]. Additional mechanisms, which may be partly responsible for myocardial depression in sepsis, include beta-adrenergic receptor dysfunction [64,65] and shortening of the duration of the action potential [66].

PERIPHERAL VASCULAR MANIFESTATIONS. Regulation of peripheral vasomotor tone is markedly deranged in septic shock. In contrast to most other shock states (see Chap. 171), systemic vascular resistance is abnormally low in most cases of septic shock [7,9,14,26,27]. Indeed, low SVRI is usually the major factor responsible for hypotension in patients with overwhelming infections. In one study of human septic shock, peripheral vasomotor "failure" was shown to be a major determinant of mortality, because SVRI was persistently lower in nonsurvivors as compared with survivors, whereas cardiac output was similar in both groups [27]. Other studies have confirmed the notion that very low SVRI contributes to mortality in patients with sepsis [67].

Several mechanisms seem to be responsible for vasodilation in sepsis. Some data suggest that low SVRI in sepsis and septic shock is caused by the release of vasodilating mediators, particularly prostacyclin (PGI$_2$) [68–71] and bradykinin [72,73]. However, other data do not support this idea [74–77].

It seems likely that excessive release of nitric oxide is a major cause of vasodilation in sepsis. Nitric oxide, which is a highly reactive free-radical gas, causes vasodilation by activating a soluble guanylate cyclase in vascular smooth muscle cells [78,79]. Nitric oxide is derived from the amino acid, arginine, via the action of a class of enzymes called nitric oxide synthases [78,79]. Both constitutive and inducible forms of nitric oxide synthase have been described [78,79].

Several lines of evidence support the notion that nitric oxide is a key mediator of sepsis-induced vasodilation. First, elevated levels of nitrite and nitrate, end-products of nitric oxide metab-

olism, have been detected in patients with sepsis [80,81]. Second, in experimental animal models of sepsis, arterial hypotension and low SVRI can be reversed by the administration of various competitive inhibitors of nitric oxide synthesis [82–85]. Third, inhibitors of nitric oxide synthesis have been shown to ameliorate endotoxin- or cytokine-induced derangements in vascular smooth muscle contractility assessed in vitro [86,87].

Vascular endothelium is capable of synthesizing and releasing nitric oxide; indeed, nitric oxide, or some closely related compound, has been identified as the endothelial-derived relaxing factor (EDRF) [78,79]. Initially, it was thought that endothelial-derived nitric oxide was responsible for the loss of vascular reactivity to endogenous and exogenous vasopressors in sepsis [88]. More recent data, however, suggest that exposure to LPS actually decreases nitric oxide release by vascular endothelium [89,90]. Thus, the endothelium probably is not a major source of excessive nitric oxide release in sepsis or endotoxicosis; rather, based on recently reported findings, it seems likely that the vascular smooth muscle itself releases excess quantities of nitric oxide during sepsis [91].

TNFα and IL-1, cytokines suspected of being pathophysiologically important in sepsis, cause vasodilation in vivo [92,93] and diminish vascular smooth muscle contractility in vitro [94–97]. These phenomenona appear to be mediated, at least in part, by the induction nitric oxide synthase, particularly in vascular smooth muscle [91].

As noted above, administration of nitric oxide synthase or guanylate cyclase inhibitors can reverse hypotension in experimental models of sepsis. Indeed, anecdotal reports suggest that the same effects can be observed in humans with septic shock [98,99]. However, based on results obtained in studies using animals [100–103], pharmacologic inhibition of nitric oxide synthesis in sepsis actually may be deleterious, possibly as a result of excessive vasoconstriction leading to visceral ischemia or other effects (e.g., increased microvascular thrombosis).

In addition to nitric oxide, other factors that may contribute to vasodilation in sepsis include: opening of ATP-sensitive K$^+$ channels in vascular smooth muscle cells [104]; release of calcitonin gene-related peptide, a potent vasodilator [105]; and alterations in adrenergic signal transduction by vascular smooth muscle cells [105].

RENAL MANIFESTATIONS. Kidney function is frequently deranged in septic shock; oliguria and azotemia are common clinical findings [22,106,107,108]. Inappropriate polyuria also has been reported in patients with sepsis [109]. As many as 50 percent of cases of acute renal failure are attributable to septic shock [110]. Although high fractional excretion of filtered sodium (FE$_{Na}$) is frequently used to help differentiate acute (intrinsic) renal failure from "prerenal azotemia" [111], FE$_{Na}$ is often low (<1%) in patients with acute renal failure caused by sepsis [112] as well as other conditions; thus, the value of the FE$_{Na}$ test has been questioned [113].

Relatively little is known regarding the mechanisms responsible for sepsis-induced acute renal failure. In compensated (nonhypotensive) sepsis, renal blood flow is typically elevated [109]. Administration of "pyrogens" to human volunteers also increases renal blood flow [114]. The effect of decompensated sepsis (i.e., septic shock) on renal perfusion in humans is not known, although data from recent studies using clinically relevant animal models of septic shock suggest that renal perfusion is markedly diminished [31,33]. Data from one study indicate that renal dysfunction in sepsis is due to excessive activation of the sympathetic nervous system leading to renal vasoconstriction [115].

GASTROINTESTINAL MANIFESTATIONS. In the classic canine model of endotoxic shock, bloody diarrhea is a prominent feature of the syndrome. In humans, however, this finding is distinctly unusual, although ileus is common, and nausea and vomiting sometimes occur [106,108]. Alterations in the barrier function of the gastrointestinal tract have been implicated as playing a central role in the pathophysiology of the multiple organ failure syndrome (MOFS) (see Chap. 199).

In patients with *compensated* sepsis, total hepatosplanchnic perfusion (i.e., hepatic vein blood flow) increases substantially [116,117]. Nevertheless, hepatosplanchnic oxygen extraction also increases, so that total oxygen uptake across this visceral bed is markedly elevated [116]. There are no data regarding the effects on splanchnic perfusion of septic shock in humans. However, in a normodynamic porcine model of septic shock, mesenteric blood flow decreases almost 50 percent (Fig. 173-2) [75,118]. This phenomenon seems to be mediated, at least in part, by the release of sulfidopeptide leukotrienes, lipid mediators known to possess potent mesenteric vasoconstrictor activity [119,120].

Gastrointestinal mucosal acidosis has been documented in both clinical [121] and experimental [75,118,119,120] studies of septic shock. In septic patients, development of gastric mucosal acidosis correlates with early death [121] and the development of the multiple organ dysfunction syndrome (MODS) [122]. Thus, monitoring mucosal pH may be of value in the care of patients with septic shock. This topic is discussed in greater detail in Chapters 171, 181, and 199.

HEPATIC MANIFESTATIONS. Jaundice is a frequent occurrence in severe sepsis [106,123,124,125]. Rarely, patients with septic shock subsequently develop massive centrilobular hepatic necrosis, evidenced by marked elevations in circulating transaminases. Most often, however, sepsis-induced hepatocellular dysfunction is manifested as cholestatic jaundice, without evidence of extrahepatic biliary obstruction. It is becoming increasingly apparent that sepsis-induced derangements in hepatocyte function are mediated, at least in part, by the release of nitric oxide from LPS-stimulated Kupffer's cells [83,126–131]. Nevertheless, inhibition of nitric oxide synthesis in experimental endotoxicosis exacerbates hepatic dysfunction [102,103]; thus, nitric oxide seems to have both deleterious and beneficial effects on hepatocyte function in sepsis.

HEMATOLOGIC MANIFESTATIONS. Abnormalities of the clotting system, ranging from mild prolongation of the prothrombin time (PT) and partial thromboplastin time (PTT), to profound thrombocytopenia or frank disseminated intravascular coagulation (DIC), are common in patients with septic shock [17,132,133]. In one study, the mean PTs in nonbacteremic and bacteremic septic patients were 22 and 17 seconds, respectively [1]. In this study, the mean platelet counts in these two groups were significantly lower in bacteremic as compared with nonbacteremic patients (195,910 and 233,850 cell/μl, respectively). In another study of 48 septic adults, activation of the coagulation system was observed in all patients, as was inhibition of the fibrinolytic system [134]. Compared with survivors, nonsurviving patients showed evidence of greater activation of coagulation and more intense inhibition of fibrinolysis [134]. DIC, discussed in greater detail in Chapter 118, results in fibrin deposition and microthrombi in many organs, phenomena that may contribute to the development of MOFS [135,136].

The triggers that lead to activation of the coagulation system in septic shock remain incompletely understood [137]. Nevertheless, the results of recent studies of acute endotoxemia and cytokinemia in human volunteers suggest that initial activation of the coagulation cascade in sepsis depends, for the most part, on initiation of the extrinsic (tissue-factor) pathway [137]. In vitro, TNFα induces the expression of tissue factor on mononuclear cells [138]. Tissue factor, in turn, activates factor VII to form factor VIIa. A complex of VIIa and tissue factor can activate factor X to factor Xa and thereby initiate the conversion of prothrombin to thrombin. The importance of tissue factor upregulation (and the DIC that results from it) in the pathogenesis of sepsis is illustrated by the demonstration that treatment with a monoclonal antibody to tissue factor prevents death in baboons infused with a lethal dose of gram-negative bacteria [139]. Another factor that contributes to intravascular thrombosis in sepsis is downregulation of a key normal system for inhibiting coagulation, i.e., the protein C/protein S/thrombomodulin system [137]. The fibrinolytic system also seems to play a role in the pathogenesis of sepsis. It has been shown that injecting normal volunteers with LPS results in the release of tissue plasminogen activator, followed by the release of plasminogen-activator inhibitor [140]. Thus, it is possible that early activation of the fibrinolytic system may act to prevent intravascular fibrin deposition; subsequent release of plasminogen-activator inhibitor may serve to control fibrinolytic activity.

CENTRAL NERVOUS SYSTEM MANIFESTATIONS. The CNS is commonly affected in septic shock. Altered mental status, ranging from mild confusion and lethargy to stupor and even coma, is a frequent finding [1,141]. In one study, 126 (70%) of 179 patients with the sepsis syndrome had evidence of altered mentation [1]. In another study, 307 (23%) of 1333 patients with positive blood cultures had acute encephalopathy diagnosed [142]. The presence and degree of encephalopathy have been shown to correlate with mortality in patients with sepsis [142,143]. It has been suggested that alterations in cerebral blood flow may contribute to abnormalities in cerebral function

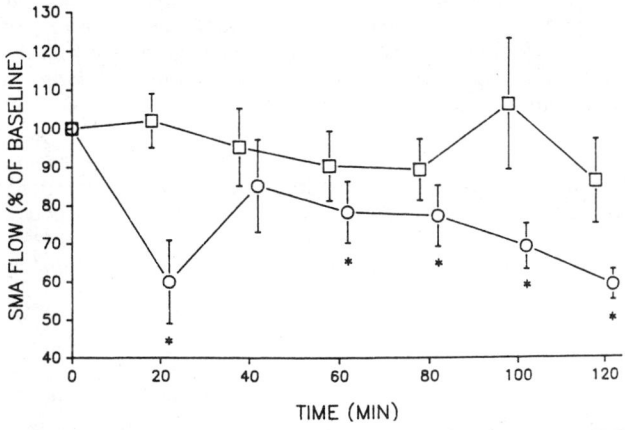

Fig. 173-2. Effect of lipopolysaccharides on superior mesenteric arterial (SMA) blood flow in resuscitated endotoxic pigs (circles) compared with saline-treated controls (squares). Symbols are means +/− standard error. Asterisks represent points that are significantly different from baseline (p < 0.05). (Source: Fink MP, Cohn SM, Lee PC, et al: Effect of lipopolysaccharide on intestinal intramucosal hydrogen ion concentration in pigs: Evidence of gut ischemia in a normodynamic model of septic shock. *Crit Care Med* 17:641, 1989. Reprinted with permission.)

in sepsis [141–146]. Although data from animal models regarding this issue are conflicting [29,147], recent data obtained in humans with septic shock support this theory [141]. Other mechanisms that have been implicated as producing encephalopathy in septic patients include abnormalities in the blood-brain barrier and changes in the concentrations of circulating amino acids [148,149,150].

PULMONARY MANIFESTATIONS. Tachypnea is another common feature in sepsis or septic shock, and this finding is typically associated with respiratory alkalosis [1,151]. In one study of patients with the sepsis syndrome, the average respiratory rate was approximately 30 breaths per minute; the average carbon dioxide tension (PCO_2) was 35 mm Hg in the nonbacteremic subgroup and 33 mm Hg in the bacteremic subgroup [1]. The mechanism(s) responsible for respiratory alkalosis are poorly understood. The acute respiratory distress syndrome (ARDS) is one of the major complications of septic shock. ARDS is discussed in great detail in Chapter 55.

Mediators

LIPOPOLYSACCHARIDE. Gram-negative bacteria contain within their cell walls a macromolecular glycolipid, LPS, that is composed of two components: the O-specific chain and the core [152]. The terms endotoxin and LPS are not strictly synonymous; LPS refers to the purified glycolipid, whereas bacterial endotoxins contain small amounts of cell wall proteins, lipids, lipoproteins, and polysaccharides in additon to LPS. The O-specific chain is a polymer of oligosaccharide units and accounts for the antigenic diversity among species and strains of gram-negative bacteria. The core is composed of an oligosaccharide bound to a glycolipid called lipid A. The core region is subdivided into an "outer" region (adjacent to the O-specific chain) and an "inner" region (adjacent to lipid A). The inner core region contains a unique 8-carbon sugar, 2-keto-3-deoxyoctonate (KDO). The lipid chains in the lipid A moiety are bound to a disaccharide backbone consisting of two N-acetyl glucosamine residues. The toxicity of LPS resides in the lipid A moiety.

In contrast to the O-specific chain, the structure of the core region of LPS is relatively constant across species and strains of bacteria. Certain strains of bacteria (e.g., the J5 mutant of *Escherichia coli*) lack key enzymes, and hence are unable to add sugar residues to the core region. The availability of these mutant strains and the constancy of the core region across genera have prompted the development of (polyclonal and monoclonal) antibodies that recognize shared core epitopes and thus may be useful for adoptive immunotherapy against a wide range of gram-negative endotoxins. This topic is discussed further below and in Chapter 199.

Recent studies have provided new insights into the mechanisms whereby LPS initiates the inflammatory responses characteristic of sepsis. LPS binds to a circulating protein, called lipopolysaccharide-binding protein (LBP). Synthesized by hepatocytes, LBP is released into the circulation as a 60-kD glycoprotein [153,154]. Complexes of LPS and LBP bind to a cell-surface receptor on macrophages called CD14, and this interaction stimulates the production of cytokines such as TNFα [155].

The precise role of LPS in the pathogenesis of human sepsis and septic shock remains incompletely defined. The classic model of canine endotoxic shock (induced by infusing a large bolus dose of LPS) is characterized by low cardiac output, elevated SVRI, and bloody diarrhea [156,157]. Bolus injections of LPS lead to a low-output vasoconstricted state in other species as well [158,159]. Because these findings are markedly different from those observed in most cases of human septic shock, concerns were raised about the clinical relevance of experimental "endotoxic shock," and the importance of LPS in the pathophysiology of the human syndrome was called into question [160].

Other findings also call into question the role of LPS in human septic shock: (1) gluconeogenesis is suppressed and hypoglycemia occurs in acute experimental endotoxicosis [161,162], whereas the opposite occurs in human sepsis [163]; (2) in some studies, measurements of circulating endotoxin correlated poorly with clinical findings, microbiologic status, or outcome [164,165]; (3) human volunteers rendered tolerant to LPS by repeated injections still manifest fever and other signs of acute toxicity when infected with viable gram-negative bacteria [166]; (4) an inbred strain of mice (C3H/HeJ) that are genetically very hyporesponsive to LPS manifest increased (not decreased) susceptibility to the lethal effects of infections caused by certain gram-negative bacteria [167]; (5) in a clinically relevant animal model of septic shock, the cardiovascular perturbations are similar for infections caused by *Escherichia coli* (associated with detectable levels of endotoxin in blood) and *Staphylococcus aureus* (not associated wtih measurable endotoxemia) [168]; and (6) (as mentioned earlier) the hemodynamic and metabolic manifestations of septic shock are independent of the infecting organism.

Despite these observations, accumulating data support the notion that LPS is pathophysiologically important in at least some cases of human septic shock. In one study, circulating LPS was detectable in 43 of 100 patients with proven or suspected sepsis, but detectable endotoxin was present in plasma in only 1 of 10 patients with shock from other causes such as hemorrhage or adrenal insufficiency [169]. In another study of 473 febrile patients, 15 of 19 who subsequently met rigid criteria for sepsis had detectable levels of LPS in their blood, whereas only 16 of 454 who failed to meet criteria for sepsis had detectable levels of endotoxemia [170]. In patients with fulminant meningococcal sepsis, circulating LPS levels are significantly associated with both mortality and the development of organ system failure [171].

Additional support for the idea that endotoxin is pathophysiologically important in human sepsis and septic shock derives from studies using normal volunteers injected with very small doses of LPS. In normal subjects, low doses of LPS elicit hemodynamic, metabolic, and hematologic effects that are qualitatively similar to those observed in septic shock, including fever, tachycardia, elevated cardiac output, hypotension, decreased SVRI, leukocytosis, lymphopenia, elevated levels of "stress" hormones (corticotropin, cortisol, growth hormone, catecholamines), elevated oxygen consumption, and widened alveolar-arterial oxygen tension gradient [172,173,174].

INFLAMMATORY MEDIATORS. In many ways, septic shock represents the normal inflammatory response to an infection run amok. It seems probable that LPS is only one of several possible initiators of the inflammatory cascade that is ultimately responsible for the clinical manifestations of sepsis and septic shock. The inflammatory mediators implicated in the pathogenesis of septic shock include cytokines, particularly TNFα, interleukin-1 (IL-1), interleukin-6 (IL-6), interleukin-8 (IL-8); eicosanoids, including thromboxane A_2, prostacyclin, leukotriene B_4 (a potent chemoattractant and activator of neutrophils), and the sulfidopeptide leukotrienes C_4, D_4, and E_4 (the slow-reacting substance(s) of anaphylaxis); platelet-activating factor; brady-kinin; complement and complement-derived peptides, especially C5a; polymorphonuclear leukocytes (PMNL) and products derived from these cells (e.g., elastase); reactive oxygen metabolites such as hydrogen peroxide and hydroxyl radical; and nitric oxide. The role of these various inflammatory mediators in sepsis and the multiple organ failure syndrome is discussed at length in Chapter 199.

Management

DIAGNOSIS. The diagnosis and differential diagnosis of shock are discussed in Chapter 171. As emphasized in that chapter, it is important to establish the diagnosis of shock promptly so as to initiate appropriate therapy without delay. Accumulating data suggest that the risk of MODS is determined (at least in part) by the duration of shock [175]. The classic early findings in septic shock include fever, tachycardia, systemic arterial hypotension, tachypnea, warm skin, altered sensorium, leukocytosis, respiratory alkalosis, and hyperlactic acidemia. The diagnosis is supported by the presence of thrombocytopenia or evidence of DIC. Septic shock always should be considered when signs of hypoperfusion (with or without frank hypotension) are present in patients with risk factors for overwhelming infection. These risk factors include profound neutropenia; immunosuppression induced by drugs or other causes; the presence of a known or suspected focus of infection; the presence of prosthetic intravascular devices; and the necessity for intubation and mechanical ventilation for other reasons.

Patients with septic shock do not always present with classic findings. The placement of a pulmonary arterial (Swan-Ganz) catheter provides valuable diagnostic and monitoring information in many cases of shock (see Chap. 4). The diagnosis of septic shock is supported by observing a hyperdynamic hemodynamic profile. If the calculated SVRI is low, the diagnosis of other forms of shock should be questioned. Alternatively, if the calculated SVRI is high, the diagnosis of septic shock should be considered less likely (although not excluded entirely).

Blood cultures should be obtained routinely in cases of suspected or proved septic shock. In untreated patients with subsequently documented bacteremia, the cumulative rate of positive blood cultures is nearly 100 percent when only three sets of blood cultures are drawn [176]. Because low-level bacteremia is common, it is important that at least 10 ml (and, preferably, 20–30 ml) of blood be obtained for each culture [176,177]. Although it has been recommended that blood cultures never be obtained with intravascular catheters, recently published data suggest that such cultures are very reliable (96% sensitivity and 98% specificity), provided that the following steps are followed: (1) the infusion fluid is temporarily discontinued; (2) the stopcock or sampling port is disinfected with povidone-iodine followed by 70% isopropyl alcohol; and (3) the first 3-ml blood sample is discarded [178]. Because patients are often already receiving antibiotics when bacteremia is suspected, efforts have been made to develop methods to inhibit the effects of antibiotics in blood samples for culture [177]. In general, the use of antibiotic-adsorbent resins has not been very beneficial [177] and we do not routinely use these devices in our institutions.

Urine cultures also should be performed routinely. Cultures of other fluids (e.g., sputum and cerebral spinal fluid) should be performed if clinically indicated. Other obviously or potentially infected sites or fluids (e.g., bile in cases of infective cholangitis) should be cultured if feasible.

ANTIBIOTICS. Rapid institution of empiric antibiotic therapy is an essential early step in the management of patients with septic shock. Withholding treatment until culture results are available is rarely, if ever, the appropriate course of action in patients with shock known or presumed to be caused by sepsis. Sometimes patients develop septic shock while they are already receiving antimicrobial chemotherapy. In this situation, the clinician usually must assume that the infecting organism is resistant to the current antibiotic regimen and make appropriate adjustments in therapy. Patients who do not receive appropriate antibiotics (i.e., agents that are active against the implicated organism(s)) have a significantly worse prognosis than patients who are treated appropriately [179]. Thus, it is important to institute therapy with drugs with excellent activity against all likely pathogens.

The precise choice of agents is dictated by numerous factors, including (1) the presumed focus of infection; (2) the patterns of antimicrobial resistance in the particular hospital; (3) recent hospital epidemiologic data regarding the likelihood of nosocomial infection with certain pathogens, such as *Pseudomonas aeruginosa,* multiply resistant *Enterobacter* species, or methicillin-resistant *Staphylococcus aureus.* Empiric antifungal therapy should be strongly considered in patients who develop septic shock while already receiving broad-spectrum antibacterial coverage, particularly if evidence of colonization with *Candida* species is already evident from preexisting recent sputum, catheter-tip, or urine cultures.

Multiple drug antibacterial therapy is usually employed for the early empiric management of septic shock, the regimen being simplified or modified later when definitive culture and sensitivity data are available from the clinical microbiology laboratory [180]. The decision to use a multiple-drug regimen is typically based on several considerations: (1) combination chemotherapy using appropriate agents ensures excellent coverage against a broad spectrum of potential pathogens; (2) multidrug regimens may delay or prevent the emergence of resistant strains by preventing the proliferation of small subpopulations that are resistant to one but not both antibiotics in the combination [181]; (3) some drugs manifest synergistic antibacterial activity when administered in combination, and this phenomenon may be an important factor in determining outcome, particularly in neutropenic patients with bacteremia [182,183].

Most multidrug regimens for sepsis or septic shock in medical patients combine an aminoglycoside with an antipseudomonal beta-lactam [183,187]. The standard empiric regimens for overwhelming surgical infections (e.g., intraabdominal sepsis and necrotizing fasciitis) consist of an aminoglyoside and an agent with excellent activity against obligate anaerobes (e.g., metronidazole or clindamycin) plus, in some instances, ampicillin to provide coverage against enterococcal species [188,189,190]. Some empiric multidrug regimens add vancomycin for grampositive coverage [191]; others substitute a second beta-lactam antibiotic for the aminoglycoside component present in most two- or three-drug combinations [183,184].

The question of whether combination antibiotic therapy is truly necessary has been addressed in several recent randomized, prospective clinical trials. In one study comparing single-agent therapy (with ceftazidime) with combination therapy (with cephalothin plus carbenicillin plus gentamicin) for fever in neutropenic patients, the incidence of fatal gram-positive superinfections was increased for the group of patients treated with the one-drug regimen [192]. In another study of neutropenic cancer patients with documented gram-negative bacteremia, treatment with ceftazidime plus a long (9-day) course of amikacin was more successful than was treatment with either ceftazidime plus a short (3-day) course of amikacin or azlocillin plus a long course of amikacin [187]. Thus, the results from these two studies suggest that combination regimens are superior to monotherapy. In contrast, data from another study of febrile neutropenic patients suggest that single-agent therapy with ceftazidime is as effective as a multidrug regimen consisting of carbenicillin plus cephalothin plus gentamicin [193]. In this latter study, however, relatively few patients had documented bacteremia.

Although aminoglycosides are useful against a wide range of gram-negative bacilli [194], shock is a recognized risk factor for aminoglycoside-induced nephrotoxicity [195,196]. Thus, consideration should be given to using regimens that avoid these agents, particularly when other risk factors for aminoglycoside-induced nephrotoxicity such as preexisting renal or hepatic insufficiency and old age [195,196] are known to be present. The recent introduction of new classes of antibiotics, particularly the thienamycins and the fluoroquinolones, may decrease the need for aminoglycosides in these high-risk patients. Some data suggest that beta-lactam–based regimens are as effective as aminoglycoside-based regimens for patients with intraabdominal sepsis, even when significant risk factors for an adverse outcome are present [188].

OTHER ANTIINFECTIVE MEASURES. In addition to antibiotic therapy, other steps to eradicate sources of infection should be pursued aggressively. Collections of pus such as abscesses or empyemas must be identified and drained. Any indwelling device that is a potential source of infection such as an intravascular catheter or transvenous pacemaker should be removed. If prosthetic graft sepsis is suspected, surgical removal of the foreign material must be strongly considered. Above all, the patient must be carefully examined for any clues as to the source of the infection. Commonly overlooked sources include perirectal abscesses and sinus infections.

FLUID RESUSCITATION. Fluid resuscitation is the first step in the management of hypotension caused by septic shock. Patients with sepsis often require enormous volumes of intravenous fluids to maintain adequate levels of preload. Data have been presented supporting the idea that a pulmonary artery wedge pressure (PAWP) of approximately 12 mm Hg produces the maximum response in cardiac function in patients with septic shock [197,198,199]. It is not possible, however, to provide a target value for PAWP that will apply to all patients in septic shock, because the relationship between LV end-diastolic volume (the true measure of preload) and PAWP can be distorted by changes in LV compliance and, particularly, the effects of high levels of positive end-expiratory pressure (PEEP).

The choice of fluids to be used for resuscitation remains the subject of considerable controversy. In patients with anemia (hematocrit <30%), packed red blood cells are an optimal component of fluid therapy. The relative merits of various asanguinous fluids are discussed in greater detail in Chapter 171, but, in brief, no study of septic shock has demonstrated a difference in outcome based on whether colloid or crystalloid fluids are used for resuscitation.

VASOPRESSORS, VASODILATORS, AND INOTROPES. When fluid resuscitation alone fails to reverse hypotension or restore adequate urine flow, it is usually necessary to administer drugs with vasopressor or inotropic activity. Inotropic therapy may be warranted even in the absence of hypotension or oliguria, if there are findings indicative of relative hypoperfusion,

such as low systemic oxygen uptake and hyperlactacidemia (see Chaps. 171, 181, and 199).

The clinical pharmacology of the various vasopressors, vasodilators, and inotropic agents commonly used in the treatment of shock states is discussed at length in Chapter 171. Brief mention is made here of several agents widely used in the management of septic shock.

Dopamine is the initial vasopressor recommended by many clinicians for the management of septic shock that is refractory to intravascular volume loading [9,200,201]. Low doses of dopamine (1–5 μg/kg/min) have inotropic and renal vasodilating effects that may be beneficial in improving cardiac performance and renal blood flow. Higher doses of dopamine exert alpha-adrenergic effects that tend to increase blood pressure, an important goal in patients with profound hypotension.

Norepinephrine (levarterenol) is a potent alpha-adrenergic agonist. It is usually effective in raising blood pressure in patients with septic shock who have not responded to fluids and dopamine [200,202]. Several recent reports suggest that norepinephrine can be used without adversely affecting peripheral (and particularly renal) perfusion in patients with septic shock [202–210]. Indeed, in some hypotensive and oliguric septic patients, norepinephrine seems to improve renal function and urine flow [202–208]; however, one report cautioned that norepinephrine can adversely affect kidney function in patients with septic shock and elevated blood lactate levels [205]. In a recent, randomized, double-blind, prospective clinical trial, norepinephrine was shown to be more effective and reliable than dopamine in reversing the hemodynamic abnormalities (including oliguria) characteristic of septic shock [204]. Concurrent administration of low-dose dopamine may help preserve renal perfusion during the administration of norepinephrine [211], although this notion has never been validated in the clinical setting. In the surgical intensive care unit at Beth Israel Hospital in Boston, norepinephrine is the vasoactive agent most commonly used for managing patients with septic shock.

As noted above, myocardial performance is clearly impaired in septic shock. Therefore, a reasonable case can be made for using an inotropic agent like dobutamine to improve cardiac output and oxygen delivery [212–215]. However, dobutamine is capable of causing beta-adrenergically mediated vasodilation and this may be undesirable in septic patients with profound hypotension. Dopexamine [216], an experimental dopaminergic and beta-adrenergic agonist, and digoxin [217], a well-studied noncatecholamine inotropic agent, are two other drugs that may be of value in selected cases of septic shock. Epinephrine, a potent alpha- and beta-adrenergic agonist, may produce an increase in blood pressure, even in patients who are refractory to norepinephrine [218]. Like dopamine, it often produces tachycardia and may provoke tachyarrhythmias. Phenylephrine is an alpha-adrenergic agonist that may be helpful in maintaining perfusion without increasing heart rate in some patients with septic shock [219].

Drugs with predominant activity as vasodilators may be of value in selected cases of septic shock characterized by low cardiac output and high SVRI (i.e., a hemodynamic profile similar to that observed in cardiogenic shock) [220]. Therapy with vasodilators also may improve oxygen delivery and uptake in compensated normotensive sepsis, even when cardiac output is well preserved [221]. This approach, however, remains investigational and cannot be advocated at present. Certainly, vasodilators should not be used in the management of profoundly hypotensive septic patients with low SVRI.

STEROIDS. The use of corticosteroids in the treatment of septic shock was controversial for many years. Support for the idea derived, in part, from studies showing that the administration of very large doses of methylprednisolone markedly improves survival in several animal models of endotoxic and septic shock [222–226]. Although many of these experiments used a pretreatment design, other studies documented that survival is improved even when methylprednisolone is administered after the initiation of the septic challenge, which is a more clinically realistic scenario [223,224]. Other data suggested that the beneficial pharmacologic effects of corticosteroids in experimental septic shock are attributable to their ability to inhibit the activation of the complement cascade [227,231]. Finally, in 1976, Shumer reported that high-dose steroid therapy significantly improves survival in human septic shock [232]; this study, however, was open to criticism on several counts [233].

Recently, several large, well-controlled, randomized, prospective trials have convincingly demonstrated that large doses of corticosteroids are not beneficial, even when used early in septic shock [234–238]. Furthermore, there is evidence that in certain subsets of patients—i.e., patients with diminished renal function [235] or ARDS [238]—steroids significantly worsen outcome. High-dose steroids may also worsen hepatic or renal function in patients with septic shock [239]. Thus, the routine use of corticosteroids in the treatment of septic shock is not recommended. Obviously, if adrenal insufficiency is proved or suspected, then physiologic (not pharmacologic) doses of cortisol, or another glucocorticoid, should be administered.

NALOXONE. In 1978, the opioid antagonist, naloxone, was shown to reverse hypotension in a rat model of endotoxic shock [240]. This observation was subsequently confirmed and extended in an extensive series of experiments using laboratory models of endotoxic and septic shock. In some animal studies, naloxone was shown to improve survival [241]. Based on these promising results, there was considerable enthusiasm regarding the use of naloxone as an adjunctive measure in the management of septic shock in humans. This enthusiasm was fostered by early anecdotal data suggesting that large doses of naloxone (0.4–1.2 mg) are beneficial in hypotensive, septic patients [242]. Later reports, however, failed to support the idea that naloxone is of value in the management of human septic shock [243,244,245]. Indeed, major adverse reactions (hypotension, seizures, pulmonary edema) have been observed in septic patients treated with naloxone [244]. Therefore, adjuvant therapy with naloxone in human septic shock cannot be advocated, although further studies may better delineate the circumstances in which this agent is likely to be of benefit [246].

CYCLOOXYGENASE AND THROMBOXANE SYNTHASE INHIBITORS. As noted above, cyclooxygenase-derived metabolites of arachidonic acid (e.g., thromboxane A_2 and prostacyclin) have been implicated as important mediators of some of the pathophysiologic events occurring in septic shock. The data supporting this view are summarized in Chapter 199; it is sufficient to say here that drugs that inhibit cyclooxygenase (i.e., nonsteroidal antiinflammatory agents, such as ibuprofen) have been shown to improve survival in experimental endotoxic and septic shock. One recent, randomized, double-blind, multicenter trial of ibuprofen demonstrated good antipyretic effects with no significant toxicity [247]. In this study, there were no differences between the ibuprofen- and the placebo-treated groups with respect to hemodynamic or respiratory parameters or survival. In another, small-scale, randomized, double-blind, placebo-controlled trial of ibuprofen, patients in the ibuprofen (but not the control) group experienced significant declines in peak airway pressure, heart rate, and temperature [248]. Prompted

by these encouraging results, a large-scale, multicenter trial of ibuprofen in sepsis has been organized. At the time of this writing, this study has enrolled more than half of the targeted number of patients. As yet, however, no results have been reported.

Although thromboxane A_2 has been implicated as being an important mediator in the pathogenesis of sepsis and sepsis-induced ARDS (see Chap. 56), two early studies of dazoxiben, a thromboxane synthase inhibitor, in established ARDS yielded negative results [249,250]. Nevertheless, another drug with activity as a thromboxane synthase inhibitor, ketoconazole, may be able to decrease the incidence of ARDS in patients with sepsis when it is administered in a prophylactic fashion. Ketoconazole is an imidazole derivative, which is available for enteral administration as an antifungal agent. In 1986, Slotman et al. reported that enteral administration of ketoconazole (200 mg daily) significantly decreased the incidence of ARDS in high-risk patients [251]. Recently, Yu et al. conducted a prospective, randomized, placebo-controlled, double-blind trial of ketoconazole (400 mg daily) in 54 patients with sepsis [252]. Treatment with ketoconazole decreased the incidence of ARDS from 64 percent in the placebo group to 15 percent in the treated group (p = 0.002). Mortality was 39 percent in the placebo group versus 15 percent in the treated group. These data suggest that this relatively inexpensive and relatively nontoxic agent warrants more extensive evaluation as an adjuvant for the treatment of patients with sepsis.

MONOCLONAL ANTIBODIES, RECOMBINANT INTERLEUKIN-1 RECEPTOR ANTAGONIST, RECOMBINANT SOLUBLE TNFα RECEPTOR FUSION PROTEINS. Passive immunization using monoclonal antibodies has been investigated as a therapeutic adjunct in the management of septic shock [253]. Several avenues of immunotherapy using monoclonal antibodies are undergoing active investigation, including (1) decreasing PMNL-mediated organ damage by limiting the attachment of these cells to the endothelium by administering antibodies against a functional epitope on the PMNL membrane glycoprotein complex (CD11/CD18) that permits these cells to adhere to each other and to endothelial cells [254]; (2) neutralizing TNFα by administering antibodies to this monokine [255]; (3) blocking the effects of the complement fragment C5a by infusing antibodies to this mediator [256]; (4) neutralizing the effects of LPS by using antibodies directed against epitopes in the core region of the molecule that are shared among many genera of gram-negative bacteria (see the preceding section on Mediators).

The widest clinical experience is with the last approach listed. In animals, antisera raised against the J5 mutant of *E. coli* enhance survival when shock is induced by bacteria of several strains [257,258]. In a 1982 report describing the results of a randomized, prospective trial, Ziegler and colleagues showed that passive immunization with a human polyclonal anti-J5 antiserum significantly improved survival in cases of human gram-negative bacteremia and shock [259]. Another clinical study of passive immunization with polyclonal anti-J5 antibodies was unable to document improved outcome [260]. A prophylactic trial of anti-J5 antiserum in high-risk surgical patients documented a lower incidence of shock and mortality in the treated group [261]. Results have been reported from two separate multicenter, randomized, prospective trials of monoclonal anti-J5 antibodies for gram-negative sepsis. One study examined HA-1A, and one examined E5. Both studies reported a beneficial effect in some subgroups with gram-negative infections, but no benefit in overall survival [262,263]. Although each of these agents has been evaluated in a second randomized multicenter trial, results from these later trials have not been published as yet. Neither drug has been approved by the FDA. A polyclonal immunoglobulin preparation also has been reported to improve survival in patients with early septic shock [264]. Confirmatory trials must be done before these agents are put into general use.

Several monoclonal anti-TNFα antibodies have been evaluated in clinical trials. Results from one early-phase trial have been published [265]. In this early phase study, which evaluated several different dosing regimens for the anti-TNFα antibody, no survival benefit was apparent when all patients were analyzed.

Other anti-cytokine strategies also have been evaluated in clinical trials. Interleukin-1 receptor antagonist (IL-1ra) is a naturally occurring polypeptide that binds to the IL-1 receptor but is devoid of agonist activity. In animal models of sepsis, treatment with IL-1ra has been shown to be protective [266]. Two clinical trials of recombinant human IL-1ra have been completed, but the results of these trials have not yet been reported in the peer-reviewed literature.

There are two distinct receptors for TNFα, which are referred to as p60 and p80. The extracellular ligand-binding domains of these TNFα receptors are shed into the circulation during a variety of inflammatory illnesses. The p80 soluble TNFα receptor (sTNFR) has been fashioned into a divalent construct by fusing the receptor with the Fc region of human IgG1. This divalent construct (sTNFR:Fc) has been shown to bind TNFα in vitro and in vivo and to provide protection against LPS-induced mortality in mice [267]. This recombinant protein has been evaluated in an early phase clinical trial in humans, but the results of this study have yet to be published.

Prognostication

A variety of systems for assessing severity of illness in critically ill patients have been described [268,269]. This topic is discussed at length in Chapter 231. Several scoring systems have been developed that are intended to be used specifically in patients with sepsis [270–275]. Several standard scoring systems have been found to be useful in patients with septic shock as well, including the Multiorgan Failure Scoring System, APACHE II, and the Acute Organ Failure Scoring System [276]. Many studies have examined hemodynamic parameters in an attempt to identify those that are prognostic indicators in patients with septic shock. Most studies suggest that on initial presentation, the hemodynamic profile does not distinguish between patients who will survive and those who will not [9,14,27]. The trend in hemodynamics over the first day after the onset of septic shock, however, seems to provide valuable prognostic information. Normalization of key hemodynamic parameters (i.e., decrease in heart rate and cardiac output, increase in SVRI) tends to portend a favorable outcome [14]. Extremely high cardiac output has been reported to be associated with a poor prognosis [26], as has persistently low SVRI [27].

References

1. Bone RC, Fisher CJ, Clemmer TP, et al: Sepsis syndrome: A valid clinical entity. *Crit Care Med* 17:389, 1989.
2. Pepe PE, Potkin RT, Reus DH, et al: Clinical predictors of the adult respiratory distress syndrome. *Am J Surg* 144:124, 1982.
3. Benjamin E, Liebowitz AB, Oropello J, et al: Systemic hypoxic and inflammatory syndrome: An alternative designation for "sepsis syndrome." *Crit Care Med* 20:680, 1992.
4. American College of Chest Physicians/Society of Critical Care Medicine Consensus Conference: Definitions for sepsis and organ failure and guidelines for the use of innovative therapies in sepsis. *Crit Care Med* 20:864, 1992.
5. Sibbald WJ, Marshall J, Christou N, et al: "Sepsis": Clarity of existing terminology . . . or more confusion? *Crit Care Med* 19:996, 1991.
6. *MMWR* 39:31, 1990.
7. Parker MM, Parrillo JE: Septic shock: Hemodynamics and pathogenesis. *J Am Med Assoc* 250:2324, 1983.
8. Wiles JB, Cerra FB, Siegel JH, et al: The systemic septic response: Does the organism matter? *Crit Care Med* 8:55, 1980.
9. Winslow EJ, Loeb HS, Rahimtoola SH, et al: Hemodynamic studies and results of therapy in 50 patients with bacteremic shock. *Am J Med* 54:421, 1973.
10. Parker MM, Shelhamer JH, Ognibene FP, et al: Severe *Pneumocystis carinii* pneumonia produces a hyperdynamic profile similar to bacterial pneumonia with sepsis. *Crit Care Med* 22:50, 1994.
11. Deutschman CS, Konstantinides FN, Tsai M, et al: Physiology and metabolism in isolated viral septicemia: Further evidence of an organism-independent host-dependent response. *Arch Surg* 122:21, 1987.
12. Okrent DG, Abraham E, Winston D: Cardiorespiratory patterns in viral septicemia. *Am J Med* 83:681, 1987.
13. Gunnar RM, Loeb HS, Winslow EJ, et al: Hemodynamic measurements in bacteremic and septic shock in man. *J Infect Dis* 128:287, 1973.
14. Parker MM, Shelhamer JH, Natanson C, et al: Serial cardiovascular variables in survivors and nonsurvivors of human septic shock: Heart rate as an early predictor of prognosis. *Crit Care Med* 15:923, 1987.
15. Ahmed AJ, Kruse JA, Haupt MT, et al: Hemodynamic responses to gram-positive versus gram-negative sepsis in critically ill patients with and without circulatory shock. *Crit Care Med* 19:1520, 1991.
16. Dinarello CA, Cannon JG, Wolff SM: New concepts on the pathogenesis of fever. *Rev Infect Dis* 10:168, 1988.
17. Harris RL, Musher DM, Bloom K, et al: Manifestations of sepsis. *Arch Intern Med* 147:1895, 1987.
18. Clemmer TP, Fisher CJ, Bone RS, et al: Hypothermia in the sepsis syndrome and clinical outcome. *Crit Care Med* 20:1395, 1992.
19. Rosenfeld BA, Bosnjak ZK, Shapiro RM, et al: Negative chronotropic factor in patients with fungemia. *Crit Care Med* 20:327, 1992.
20. Wilson RF, Thal AP, Kindling PH, et al: Hemodynamic measurements in septic shock. *Arch Surg* 91:121, 1965.
21. Weisel RD, Vito L, Dennis RC, et al: Myocardial depression during sepsis. *Am J Surg* 133:512, 1977.
22. MacLean LD, Mulligan WG, McLean APH, et al: Patterns of septic shock in man: A detailed study of 56 patients. *Ann Surg* 166:543, 1967.
23. Parker MM, Shelhamer, JH, Bacharach SL, et al: Profound but reversible myocardial depression in patients with septic shock. *Ann Intern Med* 100:483, 1984.
24. Parker MM, Suffredini AF, Natanson C, et al: Responses of left ventricular function in survivors and nonsurvivors of septic shock. *J Crit Care* 4:19, 1989.
25. Abraham E, Shoemaker WC, Bland RD, et al: Sequential cardiorespiratory patterns in septic shock. *Crit Care Med* 11:799, 1983.
26. Baumgartner JD, Vaney C, Perret C: An extreme form of the hyperdynamic syndrome in septic shock. *Intensive Care Med* 10:245, 1984.
27. Groeneveld ABJ, Bronsveld W, Thijs LG: Hemodynamic determinations of mortality in human septic shock. *Surgery* 99:140, 1986.
28. Natanson C, Fink MP, Ballantyne HK, et al: Gram-negative bacteremia produces both severe systolic and diastolic cardiac dysfunction in a canine model that simulates human septic shock. *J Clin Invest* 78:259, 1986.
29. Lang CH, Bagvy GJ, Ferguson JL, et al: Cardiac output and redistribution of organ blood flow in hypermetabolic sepsis. *Am J Physiol* 246:R331, 1984.
30. Carroll GC, Snyder JV: Hyperdynamic severe intravascular sepsis depends on fluid administration in cynomolgus monkeys. *Am J Physiol* 243:R131, 1982.
31. Schaer GL, Fink MP, Chernow B, et al: Renal hemodynamics and

prostaglandin E_2 excretion in a nonhuman primate model of septic shock. *Crit Care Med* 18:52, 1990.

32. Fink MP, Fiallo V, Stein KL, et al: Systemic and regional hemodynamic changes after intraperitoneal endotoxin in rabbits: Development of a new model of the clinical syndrome of hyperdynamic sepsis. *Circ Shock* 22:73, 1987.

33. Breslow MJ, Miller CF, Parker SD, et al: Effect of vasopressors on organ blood flow during endotoxin shock in pigs. *Am J Physiol* 252:H291, 1987.

34. Fink MP, Rothschild HR, Deniz YF, et al: Complement depletion with *Naje haje* cobra venom factor limits prostaglandin release and improves visceral perfusion in porcine endotoxin shock. *J Trauma* 29:1076, 1989.

35. Ellrodt AG, Riedinger MS, Kimchi A, et al: Left ventricular performance in septic shock: Reversible segmental and global abnormalities. *Am Heart J* 110:402, 1985.

36. Kimchi A, Ellrodt GA, Berman DS, et al: Right ventricular performance in septic shock: A combined radionuclide and hemodynamic study. *J Am Coll Cardiol* 4:945, 1984.

37. Parker MM, McCarthy KE, Ognibene FP, et al: Right ventricular dysfunction and dilatation, similar to left ventricular changes, characterize the cardiac depression of septic shock in humans. *Chest* 97:126, 1990.

38. Raper R, Sibbald WJ, Driedger AA, et al: Relative myocardial depression in normotensive sepsis. *J Crit Care* 4:9, 1989.

39. Mitsuo T, Shimazaki S, Matsuda H. Right ventricular dysfunction in septic patients. *Crit Care Med* 20:630, 1992.

40. Vincent J-L, Gris P, Coffernils M, et al: Myocardial depression characterizes the fatal course of septic shock. *Surgery* 111:660, 1992.

41. Ognibene FP, Parker MM, Natanson C, et al: Depressed left ventricular performance response to volume infusion in patients with sepsis and septic shock. *Chest* 93:903, 1988.

42. Adiseshiah M, Baird RJ: Correlation of the changes in diastolic myocardial tissue pressure and regional coronary blood flow in hemorrhage and endotoxin shock. *J Surg Res* 24:20, 1978.

43. Postel J, Schloerb PR: Cardiac depression in bacteremia. *Ann Surg* 186:74, 1977.

44. Elkins RC, McCurdy JR, Brown PP, et al: Effects of coronary perfusion pressure on myocardial performance during endotoxin shock. *Surg Gynecol Obstet* 137:991, 1973.

45. Peyton MD, Hinshaw LB, Greenfield LJ, et al: The effects of coronary vasodilatation on cardiac performance during endotoxin shock. *Surg Gynecol Obstet* 143:533, 1976.

46. Cunnion RE, Schaer GL, Parker MM, et al: The coronary circulation in human septic shock. *Circulation* 73:637, 1986.

47. Dhainaut JF, Huyghebaert MF, Monsallier JF, et al: Coronary hemodynamics and myocardial metabolism of lactate, free fatty acids, glucose, and ketones in patients with septic shock. *Circulation* 75:533, 1987.

48. Lefer AM, Martin J: Origin of myocardial depressant factor in shock. *Am J Physiol* 218:1423, 1970.

49. Lovett WL, Wangensteen SL, Glenn TM, et al: Presence of a myocardial depressant factor in patients in circulatory shock. *Surgery* 70:223, 1971.

50. McConn R, Greineder JK, Wasserman F, et al: Is there a humoral factor that depresses ventricular function in sepsis? *Circ Shock* (Suppl)1:9, 1979.

51. Maksad KA, Cha JC, Stuart CR, et al: Myocardial depression in septic shock: Physiologic and metabolic effects of a plasma factor on an isolated heart. *Circ Shock* (Suppl)1:35, 1979.

52. Santis DD, Phillips P, Spath MA, et al: Delayed appearance of a circulating myocardial depressant factor in burn patients. *Ann Emerg Med* 10:22, 1981.

53. Okada K, Kosugi I, Tanokura Y, et al: MDF: Its participation in the pathophysiology of shock, in Lefer AM, Schumer W (eds): *Molecular and Cellular Aspects of Shock and Trauma.* New York, AR Liss, 1983, p 125.

54. Lefer AM: Mechanisms of cardiodepression in endotoxin shock. *Circ Shock* (Suppl)1:1, 1979.

55. Parrillo JE, Burch C, Shelhamer JH, et al: A circulating myocardial depressant substance in humans with septic shock. *J Clin Invest* 76:1539, 1985.

56. Reilly JM, Cunnion RE, Burch-Whitman C, et al: A circulating myocardial depressant substance is associated with cardiac dys-

57. function and peripheral hypoperfusion (lactic acidemia) in patients with septic shock. *Chest* 95:1072, 1989.

57. Natanson C, Eichenholz PW, Danner RL, et al: Endotoxin and tumor necrosis factor challenges in dogs simulate the cardiovascular profile of human septic shock. *J Exp Med* 169:823, 1989.

58. Heard SO, Perkins MW, Fink MP: Tumor necrosis factor-α causes myocardial depression in guinea pigs. *Crit Care Med* 20:523, 1992.

59. Pagani FD, Baker LS, Hsi C, et al: Left ventricular systolic and diastolic dysfunction after infusion of tumor necrosis factor-α in conscious dogs. *J Clin Invest* 90:389, 1992.

60. Eichenholz PW, Eichacker PQ, Hoffman WD, et al: Tumor necrosis factor challenges in canines: patterns of cardiovascular dysfunction. *Am J Physiol* 263:H668, 1992.

61. Finkel MS, Oddis CV, Jacob TD, et al: Negative inotropic effect of cytokines on the heart mediated by nitric oxide. *Science* 257:387, 1992.

62. Balligand J-L, Ungureanu D, Kelly RA, et al: Abnormal contractile function due to induction of nitric oxide synthesis in rat cardiac myocytes follows exposure to activated macrophage-conditioned medium. *J Clin Invest* 91:2314, 1993.

63. Brady AJB, Poole-Wilson PA, Harding SE, et al: Nitric oxide production with cardiac myocytes reduces their contractility in endotoxemia. *Am J Physiol* 263:H1963, 1992.

64. Campbell KL, Forse RA: Endotoxin-exposed atria exhibit G protein-based deficits in inotropic regulation. *Surgery* 114:471, 1993.

65. Silverman HJ, Penaranda R, Orens JB, et al: Impaired-adrenergic receptor stimulation of cyclic adenosine monophosphate in human septic shock: Association with myocardial hypo-responsiveness to catecholamines. *Crit Care Med* 21:31, 1993.

66. Hung J, Lew WYW: Cellular mechanisms of endotoxin-induced myocardial depression in rabbits. *Circulation Res* 73:125, 1993.

67. Baumgartner J-D, Bula C, Vaney C, et al: A novel score for predicting the mortality of septic shock patients. *Crit Care Med* 20:953, 1992.

68. Morel DR, Huttemeier PC, Skoskiewicz MJ, et al: Dose-dependent effects of a pyridaquinazoline thromboxane synthetase inhibitor on arachidonic acid metabolites and hemodynamics during *E. coli* endotoxemia in anesthetized sheep. *Prostaglandins* 33:879, 1987.

69. Nishijima MK, Breslow MJ, Miller CF, et al: Effect of naloxone and ibuprofen on organ blood flow during endotoxic shock in pigs. *Am J Physiol* 255:H177, 1988.

70. Hanly PJ, Sianko A, Light RB: Role of prostacyclin and thromboxane in the circulatory changes of acute bacteremic *Pseudomonas* pneumonia in dogs. *Am Rev Respir Dis* 137:700, 1988.

71. Slotman GJ, Burchard KW, Williams JJ, et al: Interaction of prostaglandins, activated complement, and granulocytes in clinical sepsis and hypotension. *Surgery* 99:744, 1986.

72. O'Donnell TF, Clowes JHA, Talamo RC, et al: Kinin activation in the blood of patients with sepsis. *Surg Gynecol Obstet* 143:539, 1976.

73. Mason JW, Kleeberg U, Dolan P, et al: Plasma kallikrein and Hageman factor in gram-negative bacteremia. *Ann Intern Med* 73:545, 1970.

74. Fink MP, Morrissey PE, Stein KL, et al: Systemic and regional hemodynamic effects of cyclooxygenase and thromboxane synthetase inhibition in normal and hyperdynamic endotoxemic rabbits. *Circ Shock* 26:41, 1988.

75. Fink MP, Rothschild HR, Deniz YF, et al: Systemic and mesenteric O_2 metabolism in endotoxic pigs: Effect of ibuprofen and meclofenamate. *J Appl Physiol* 67:1950, 1989.

76. Janssen HF, Pugh JL, Lange DL: Bradykinin does not contribute to hypotension in early canine endotoxemia. *Circ Shock* 23:197, 1987.

77. Mann R, Woodson LC, Traber LD, et al: The role of bradykinin in ovine endotoxemia. *Circ Shock* 34:224, 1991.

78. Nathan C: Nitric oxide as a secretory product of mammalian cells. *FASEB J* 6:3051, 1992.

79. Palmer RMJ: The discovery of nitric oxide in the vessel wall: a unifying concept in the pathogenesis of sepsis. *Arch Surg* 128:396, 1993.

80. Ochoa JB, Udekwu AO, Billiar TR, et al: Nitrogen oxide levels in patients after trauma and during sepsis. *Ann Surg* 214:621, 1991.

81. Evans T, Carpenter A, Kinderman H, et al: Evidence of increased

nitric oxide production in patients with the sepsis syndrome. *Circ Shock* 41:77, 1993.

82. Lorrente JA, Landin L, Renes E, et al: Role of nitric oxide in the hemodynamic changes of sepsis. *Crit Care Med* 21:759, 1993.

83. Meyer J, Traber LD, Nelson S, et al: Reversal of hyperdynamic response to continuous endotoxin administration by inhibition of NO synthesis. *J Appl Physiol* 73:324, 1992.

84. Thiemermann C, Vane J: Inhibition of nitric oxide synthesis reduces the hypotension induced by bacterial lipopolysaccharide in the rat in vivo. *Eur J Pharmacol* 182:591, 1990.

85. Kilbourn RG, Jubran GA, Gross SS, et al: Reversal of endotoxin-mediated shock by NG-methyl-L-arginine, an inhibitor of nitric oxide synthesis. *Biochem Biophys Res Commun* 172:1132, 1990.

86. Vallance P, Palmer RMJ, Moncada S: The role of induction of nitric oxide synthesis in the altered responses of jugular veins from endotoxaemic rabbits. *Br J Pharmacol* 106:459, 1992.

87. Julou-Schaeffer G, Gray GA, Fleming I, et al: Loss of vascular responsiveness induced by endotoxin involves L-arginine pathway. *Am J Physiol* 259:H1038, 1990.

88. Salvemini D, Korbut R, Anggard E, et al: Lipopolysaccharide increases release of a nitric oxide-like factor from endothelial cells. *Eur J Pharmacol* 171:135, 1989.

89. Aoki N, Siegfried M, Lefer A: Anti-EDRF effect of tumor necrosis factor in isolated, perfused cat carotid arteries. *Am J Physiol* 256:H1509, 1989.

90. Myers PR, Wright TF, Tanner MA, et al: EDRF and nitric oxide production in cultured endothelial cells: Direct inhibition by *E. coli* endotoxin. *Am J Physiol* 262:H710, 1992.

91. Beasley D, Schwartz JH, Brenner BM: Interleukin 1 induces prolonged L-arginine-dependent cyclic guanosine monophosphate and nitrite production in rat vascular smooth muscle cell. *J Clin Invest* 87:602, 1991.

92. Vicaut E, Hou X, Payen D, et al: Acute effects of tumor necrosis factor on the microcirculation in rat cremaster muscle. *J Clin Invest* 87:1537, 1991.

93. Pagani FD, Baker LS, Knox MA, et al: Load-insensitive assessment of myocardial performance after tumor necrosis factor-α in dogs. *Surgery* 111:683, 1992.

94. McKenna TM: Enhanced vascular effects of cyclic GMP in septic rat aorta. *Am J Physiol* 254:R436, 1988.

95. McKenna TM, Lueders JE, Titius WAW: Monocyte-derived interleukin 1: Effects on norepinephrine-stimulated aortic contraction and phosphoinositide turnover. *Circ Shock* 28:131, 1989.

96. Beasley D, Cohen RA, Levinsky NG: Interleukin-1 inhibits contraction of vascular smooth muscle. *J Clin Invest* 83:331, 1989.

97. Hollenberg SM, Cunnion RE, Parrillo JE: The effect of tumor necrosis factor on vascular smooth muscle: *in vitro* studies using rat aortic rings. *Chest* 100:1133, 1991.

98. Petros A, Bennett D, Vallance P: Effect of nitric oxide synthase inhibitors on hypotension in patients with septic shock. *Lancet* 338:1557, 1991.

99. Schneider F, Lutun Ph, Hasselmann M, et al: Methylene blue increases systemic vascular resistance in human septic shock: Preliminary observations. *Intensive Care Med* 18:309, 1992.

100. Cobb JP, Natanson C, Hoffman WD, et al: N^w-amino-L-arginine, an inhibitor of nitric oxide synthase, raises vascular resistance but increases mortality rates in awake canines challenged with endotoxin. *J Exp Med* 176:1175, 1992.

101. Schultz PJ, Raij L: Endogenously synthesized nitric oxide prevents endotoxin-induced glomerular thrombosis. *J Clin Invest* 90:1718, 1992.

102. Harbrecht BG, Billiar TR, Stadler J, et al: Nitric oxide synthesis serves to reduce hepatic damage during acute murine endotoxemia. *Crit Care Med* 20:1568, 1992.

103. Frederick JA, Hasselgren PO, Davis S, et al: Nitric oxide may upregulate in vivo hepatic protein synthesis during endotoxemia. *Arch Surg* 128:152, 1993.

104. Landry DW, Oliver JA: The ATP-sensitive K$^+$ mediates hypotension in endotoxemia and hypoxic lactic acidosis in dog. *J Clin Invest* 89:2071, 1992.

105. Joyce CD, Fiscus RR, Dries DJ, et al: Calcitonin gene-related peptide levels are elevated in patients with sepsis. *Surgery* 108:1097, 1990.

105a. Carcillo JA, Litten RZ, Suba EA, et al: Alterations in rat aortic alpha$_1$-adrenoreceptors and alpha$_1$-adrenergic stimulated phosphoinositide hydrolysis in intraperitoneal sepsis. *Circ Shock* 26:331, 1988.

106. Udhoji VN, Weil MH: Hemodynamic and metabolic studies on shock associated with bacteremia. *Ann Intern Med* 62:966, 1965.

107. Kreger BE, Craven DE, McCabe WR: Gram-negative bacteremia. *Am J Med* 68:344, 1980.

108. Weil MH, Shubin H, Biddle M: Shock caused by gram-negative microorganisms. *Ann Intern Med* 60:384, 1964.

109. Lucas CE, Rector FE, Werner M, et al: Altered renal homeostasis with acute sepsis: Clinical significance. *Arch Surg* 106:444, 1973.

110. Beaman M, Turney JH, Rodger RSC, et al: Changing patterns of acute renal failure. *Q J Med* 237:15, 1987.

111. Espinel CH: The FE$_{Na}$ test. *JAMA* 236:2096, 1976.

112. Vaz AJ: Low fractional excretion of urine sodium in acute renal failure due to sepsis. *Arch Intern Med* 143:738, 1983.

113. Pru C, Kjellsternd CM: The FE$_{Na}$ test is of no prognostic value in acute renal failure. *Nephron* 36:20, 1984.

114. Gombos EA, Lee TH, Solinas J, et al: Renal response to pyrogen in normotensive and hypertensive man. *Circulation* 36:555, 1967.

115. Cumming AD, Kline R, Linton AL: Association between renal and sympathetic responses to nonhypotensive systemic sepsis. *Crit Care Med* 16:1132, 1988.

116. Dahn MS, Lange P, Lobdell K, et al: Splanchnic and total body oxygen consumption differences in septic and injured patients. *Surgery* 101:69, 1987.

117. Dahn MS, Lange P, Wilson RF, et al: Hepatic blood flow and splanchnic oxygen consumption measurements in clinical sepsis. *Surgery* 107:295, 1990.

118. Fink MP, Cohn SM, Lee PC, et al: Effect of lipopolysaccharide on intestinal intramucosal hydrogen ion concentration in pigs: Evidence of gut ischemia in a normodynamic model of septic shock. *Crit Care Med* 17:641, 1989.

119. Cohn SM, Kruithoff KL, Rothschild HR, et al: LY203647, a selective leukotriene (LT) D$_4$/E$_4$ antagonist, improves pulmonary function and mesenteric perfusion in a porcine model of septic shock and ARDS. *Surg Forum* 40:105, 1989.

120. Cohn SM, Fink MP, Lee PC, et al: LY171883, a leukotriene D$_4$/E$_4$ receptor antagonist, preserves mesenteric perfusion and ameliorates intestinal intramucosal acidosis in porcine endotoxic shock. *J Surg Res* 49:37, 1990.

121. Gys T, Hubbens A, Neels H: The prognostic value of gastric intramural pH in surgical intensive care patients. *Crit Care Med* 16:1222, 1988.

122. Marik PE: Gastric intramucosal pH: a better predictor of multiorgan dysfunction syndrome and death than oxygen-derived variables in patients with sepsis. *Chest* 104:225, 1993.

123. Franson TR, Hierholzer WJ Jr, LaBrecque DR: Frequency and characteristics of hyperbilirubinemia associated with bacteremia. *Rev Infect Dis* 7:1, 1985.

124. Banks JG, Foulis AK, Ledingham I McA, et al: Liver function in septic shock. *J Clin Pathol* 35:1249, 1982.

125. Nolan JP: Endotoxin, reticuloendothelial function, and liver injury. *Hepatology* 5:458, 1981.

125a. West MA, Keller GA, Cerra FE, et al: Killed *Escherichia coli* stimulates macrophage-mediated alterations in hepatocellular function during *in vitro* co-culture: A mechanism of altered liver function in sepsis. *Infect Immun* 49:563, 1985.

126. Billiar TR, Curran RD, Stuehr DJ, et al: Evidence that the activation of Kupffer cells results in the production of L-arginine metabolites that release cell-associated iron and inhibit hepatocyte protein synthesis. *Surgery* 106:364, 1989.

127. Billiar TR, Curran RD, Stuehr DJ, et al: An L-arginine dependent mechanism mediates Kupffer cell inhibition of hepatocyte protein synthesis in vitro. *J Exp Med* 169:1467, 1989.

128. Billiar TR, Curran RD, West MA, et al: Kupffer cell cytotoxicity to hepatocytes in coculture requires L-arginine. *Arch Surg* 124:1416, 1989.

129. Stadler J, Bentz BG, Harbrecht BG, et al: Tumor necrosis factor alpha inhibits hepatocyte mitochondrial respiration. *Ann Surg* 216:539, 1992.

130. Stadler J, Billiar TR, Curran RD, et al: Effect of exogenous and endogenous nitric oxide on mitochondrial respiration of rat hepatocytes. *Am J Physiol* 260:C910, 1991.

131. Harbecht BG, Billiar TR, Stadler J, et al: Nitric oxide synthesis

serves to reduce hepatic damage during acute murine endotoxemia. *Crit Care Med* 20:1568, 1992.

132. Corrigan JJ Jr: Vitamin K-dependent coagulation factors in gram-negative septicemia. *Am J Dis Child* 138:240, 1984.

133. Wilson JJ, Neame PB, Kelton JG: Infection-induced thrombocytopenia. *Semin Thrombosis Hemostasis* 8:217, 1982.

134. Lorente JA, Garcia-Frade LJ, Landin L, et al: Time course of hemostatic abnormalities in sepsis and its relation to outcome. *Chest* 103:1536, 1993.

135. Coalson JJ: Pathology of sepsis, septic shock, and multiple organ failure, in Sibbald WJ, Sprung CL (eds): *Perspectives on Sepsis and Septic Shock*. Fullerton, Calif., Society of Critical Care Medicine, 1986, p 27.

136. McGovern VJ: Shock revisited. *Pathol Ann* 19:15, 1984.

137. Levi M, ten Cate H, van der Poll T, et al: Pathogenesis of disseminated intravascular coagulation in sepsis. *JAMA* 270:975, 1993.

138. Conkling PR, Greenberg CS, Weinberg JB: Tumor necrosis factor induces tissue factor-like activity in human leukemia cell line U937 and peripheral blood monocytes. *Blood* 72:128, 1988.

139. Taylor FB Jr, Chang A, Ruf W, et al: Lethal *E. coli* septic shock is prevented by blocking tissue factor with monoclonal antibody. *Circ Shock* 33:127, 1991.

140. Suffredini AF, Harpel PC, Parrillo JE: Promotion and subsequent inhibition of plasminogen activation after administration of intravenous endotoxin to normal subjects. *N Engl J Med* 320:1165, 1989.

141. Bowton DL, Bertels NH, Prough DS, et al: Cerebral blood flow is reduced in patients with sepsis syndrome. *Crit Care Med* 17:399, 1989.

142. Sprung CL, Peduzzi PN, Shatney CH, et al: Impact of encephalopathy on mortality in the sepsis syndrome. The Veterans Administration Systemic Sepsis Cooperative Study Group. *Crit Care Med* 18:801, 1990.

143. Young GB, Bolton CF, Austin TW, et al: The encephalopathy associated with septic illness. *Clin Invest Med* 13:297, 1990.

144. Parker JL, Emerson TE: Cerebral hemodynamics, vascular reactivity, and metabolism during canine endotoxic shock. *Circ Shock* 4:41, 1977.

145. Ekstrom-Jodal B, Haggendal E, Larsson LE: Cerebral blood flow and oxygen uptake in endotoxic shock. An experimental study in dogs. *Acta Anaesthesiol Scand* 26:163, 1982.

146. Miller CF, Breslow MJ, Shapiro RM, et al: Role of hypotension in decreasing cerebral blood flow in porcine endotoxemia. *Am J Physiol* 253:H956, 1987.

147. Fish RE, Lang CH, Spitzer JA: Regional blood flow during continuous low-dose endotoxin infusion. *Circ Shock* 18:267, 1986.

148. Jeppson B, Freund HR, Gimmon Z, et al: Blood-brain barrier derangement in sepsis: Cause of septic encephalopathy? *Am J Surg* 141:136, 1981.

149. Freund HR, Ryan JA, Fischer JE: Amino acid derangements in patients with sepsis. *Ann Surg* 188:423, 1978.

150. Sprung CL, Cerra FB, Freund HR, et al: Amino acid alterations and encephalopathy in the sepsis syndrome. *Crit Care Med* 19:753, 1991.

151. Clowes GHA Jr: Pulmonary abnormalities in sepsis. *Surg Clin North Am* 54:993, 1974.

152. Rietschel ETH, Schade U, Jensen M, et al: Bacterial endotoxin: Chemical structure, biological activity and role in septicemia. *Scand J Infect Dis* 31(Suppl):821, 1982.

153. Ramadori G, Meyer zum Buschenfelde KH, Tobias PS, et al: Biosynthesis of lipopolysaccharide-binding protein in rabbit hepatocytes. *Pathobiology* 58:89, 1990.

154. Schumann RR, Leong SR, Flaggs GW, et al: Structure and function of lipopolysaccharide binding protein. *Science* 249:1429, 1990.

155. Wright SD, Ramos RA, Tobias PS, et al: CD14, a receptor for complexes of lipopolysaccharide (LPS) and LPS binding protein. *Science* 249:1431, 1990.

156. Hinshaw LV, Solomon LA, Holmes DD: Comparison of canine responses to *Escherichia coli* organisms and endotoxin. *Surg Gynecol Obstet* 127:981, 1968.

157. D'Orio V, Wahlen C, Rodriguez L-M, et al: A comparison of *Escherichia coli* endotoxin single bolus injection with low-dose endotoxin infusion on pulmonary and systemic vascular changes. *Circ Shock* 21:207, 1987.

158. Wyler F, Neutze JM, Rudolph AM: The effects of endotoxin on distribution of cardiac output in unanesthetized rabbits. *Am J Physiol* 219:246, 1970.

159. Law WR, Ferguson JL: Naloxone alters organ perfusion during endotoxin shock in conscious rats. *Am J Physiol* 255:H1106, 1988.

160. Wichterman KA, Baue AE, Chaudry IH: Sepsis and septic shock: A review of laboratory models and a proposal. *J Surg Res* 29:189, 1980.

161. Buchanan BJ, Filkins JP: Hypoglycemic depression of RES function. *Am J Physiol* 231:265, 1976.

162. Filkins JP, Cornell RP: Depression of hepatic gluconeogenesis and the hypoglycemia of endotoxin shock. *Am J Physiol* 227:778, 1974.

163. Wilmore DW, Goodwin CW, Aulick LM, et al: Effect of injury and infection on visceral metabolism and circulation. *Ann Surg* 192:491, 1980.

164. Elin RJ, Robinson RA, Levine AS, et al: Lack of clinical usefulness of the limulus test and the diagnosis of endotoxemia. *N Engl J Med* 292:521, 1975.

165. Stumacher RJ, Kovnat MJ, McCabe WR: Limitations of the usefulness of the limulus assay for endotoxin. *N Engl J Med* 288:1261, 1973.

166. Greisman SE, Hornick RB, Wagner HN Jr, et al: The role of endotoxin during typhoid fever and tularemia in man. IV. The integrity of the endotoxin tolerance mechanism during infection. *J Clin Invest* 48:613, 1969.

167. Hagberg L, Hull R, Hull S, et al: Difference in susceptibility to gram-negative urinary tract infection between C3H/HeJ C3H/HeN mice. *Infect Immun* 46:839, 1984.

168. Natanson C, Danner RL, Elin RJ, et al: Role of endotoxemia in cardiovascular dysfunction and mortality: *Escherichia coli* and *Staphylococcus aureus* challenges in a canine model of human septic shock. *J Clin Invest* 83:243, 1989.

169. Danner RL, Elin RJ, Hosseini JM, et al: Endotoxemia in human septic shock. *Chest* 99:169, 1991.

170. Van Deventer SJH, Buller HR, ten Cate JW, et al: Endotoxaemia: An early predictor of septicaemia in febrile patients. *Lancet* 1:605, 1988.

171. Brandtzaeg P, Kieruff P, Gaustad P, et al: Plasma endotoxin as a predictor of multiple organ failure and death in systemic meningococcal disease. *J Inf Dis* 159:195, 1989.

172. Revhaug A, Michie HR, Manson J McK, et al: Inhibition of cyclooxygenase attenuates the metabolic response to endotoxin in humans. *Arch Surg* 123:162, 1988.

173. Suffredini AF, Fromm RE, Parker MM, et al: The cardiovascular response of normal humans to the administration of endotoxin. *N Engl J Med* 321:280, 1989.

174. Suffredini AF, Shelhamer JH, Newmann RD, et al: Pulmonary oxygen transport effects of intravenously administered endotoxin in normal humans. *Am Rev Respir Dis* 145:1398, 1992.

175. Vincent J-L, de Backer D: Initial management of circulatory shock as prevention of MSOF. *Crit Care Clin* 5:369, 1989.

176. Aronson MD, Bor DH: Blood cultures. *Ann Intern Med* 106:246, 1987.

177. Washington JA II, Ilsturp DM: Blood cultures: Issues and controversies. *Rev Infect Dis* 8:792, 1986.

178. Wormser GP, Onorato IM, Preminger TJ, et al: Sensitivity and specificity of blood cultures obtained through intravascular catheters. *Crit Care Med* 18:152, 1990.

179. Bryant RE, Hood AF, Hood CE, et al: Factors affecting mortality of gram-negative rod bacteremia. *Arch Intern Med* 127:120, 1971.

180. Gribble MJ, Chow AW, Naiman SC, et al: Prospective randomized trial of piperacillin monotherapy versus carboxypenicillin-aminoglycoside combination regimens in the empirical treatment of serious bacterial infections. *Antimicrob Agents Chemother* 24:388, 1983.

181. Klatersky J, Cappel R, Daneau D: Clinical significance of in vitro synergism between antibiotics in gram-negative infections. *Antimicrob Agents Chemother* 2:470, 1972.

182. Klatersky J, Meunier-Carpentier F, Prevost J-M: Significance of antimicrobial synergism for the outcome of gram negative sepsis. *Am J Med Sci* 273:157, 1977.

183. Winston DJ, Barnes RC, Ho WG, et al: Moxalactam plus piperacillin versus moxalactam plus amikacin in febrile granulocytopenic patients. *Am J Med* 77:442, 1984.

184. Feld R, Louie TJ, Mandell L, et al: A multicenter comparative trial of tobramycin and ticarcillin vs moxalactam and ticarcillin in febrile neutropenic patients. *Arch Intern Med* 145:1083, 1985.

185. De Jongh CA, Wade JC, Schimpff SC, et al: Empiric antibiotic therapy for suspected infection in granulocytopenic cancer patients: A comparison between the combination of moxalactam plus amikacin and ticarcillin plus amikacin. *Am J Med* 73:89, 1982.

186. Wade JC, Schimpff SC, Newman KA, et al: Piperacillin or ticarcillin plus amikacin: A double-blind prospective comparison of empiric antibiotic therapy for febrile granulocytopenic cancer patients. *Am J Med* 71:983, 1981.

187. The EORTC International Antimicrobial Therapy Cooperative Group. Ceftazidime combined with a short or long course of amikacin for empirical therapy of gram-negative bacteremia in cancer patients with granulocytopenia. *N Engl J Med* 317:1692, 1987.

188. Hackford AW, Talley FP, Reinhold RB, et al: Prospective study comparing imipenem-cilastatin with clindamycin and gentamicin for the treatment of serious surgical infections. *Arch Surg* 123:322, 1988.

189. Stellato TA, Danziger LH, Hau T, et al: Moxalactam vs tobramycin-clindamycin: A randomized trial in secondary peritonitis. *Arch Surg* 123:714, 1988.

190. Canadian Metronidazole-Clindamycin Study Group: Prospective, randomized comparison of metronidazole and clindamycin, each with gentamicin for the treatment of serious intra-abdominal infection. *Surgery* 93:221, 1983.

191. Schenep JL, Hughes WT, Roberson PK, et al: Vancomycin, ticarcillin, and amikacin compared with ticarcillin-clavulanate and amikacin in the empirical treatment of febrile, neutropenic children with cancer. *N Engl J Med* 319:1053, 1988.

192. Kramer BS, Ramphal R, Rand KH: Randomized comparison between two ceftazidime-containing regimens and cephalothin-gentamicin-carbenicillin in febrile granulocytopenic cancer patients. *Antimicrob Agents Chemother* 30:64, 1986.

193. Pizzo PA, Hathorne JW, Hiemenz J, et al: A randomized trial comparing ceftazidime alone with combination antibiotic therapy in cancer patients with fever and neutropenia. *N Engl J Med* 315:552, 1986.

194. Pancoast SJ: Aminoglycoside antibiotics in clinical use. *Med Clin North Am* 72:581, 1988.

195. John JF Jr: What price success? The continuing saga of the toxic: Therapeutic ratio in the use of aminoglycoside antibiotics. *J Infect Dis* 158:1, 1988.

196. Moore RD, Smith CR, Lipsky JJ, et al: Risk factors for nephrotoxicity in patients treated with aminoglycosides. *Ann Intern Med* 100:352, 1984.

197. Rackow EC, Kaufman BS, Falk JL, et al: Hemodynamic response to fluid repletion in patients with septic shock: Evidence for early depression of cardiac performance. *Circ Shock* 22:11, 1987.

198. Packman MI, Rackow EC: Optimum left heart filling pressure during fluid resuscitation of patients with hypovolemic and septic shock. *Crit Care Med* 11:165, 1983.

199. Kaufman BS, Rackow EC, Falk JL: The relationship between oxygen delivery and consumption during fluid resuscitation of hypovolemic and septic shock. *Chest* 85:336, 1984.

200. Parker MM, Parrillo JE: Septic shock and other forms of distributive shock, in Parrillo JE (ed): *Current Therapy in Critical Care Medicine.* Philadelphia, BC Decker, 1987, p 44.

201. Wilson RF, Sibbald WJ, Jaanimagi JL: Hemodynamic effects of dopamine in critically ill septic patients. *J Surg Res* 20:163, 1976.

202. Desjars P, Pinaud M, Burnon D, et al: Norepinephrine therapy has no deleterious renal effects in human septic shock. *Crit Care Med* 17:426, 1989.

203. Cesare JF, Ligas JR, Hirvela ER: Enhancement of urine output and glomerular filtration in acutely oliguric patients using low-dose norepinephrine. *Circ Shock* 39:207, 1993.

204. Martin C, Papazian L, Perrin G, et al: Norepinephrine or dopamine for the treatment of hyperdynamic septic shock? *Chest* 103:1826, 1993.

205. Fukuoka T, Nishimura M, Imanaka H, et al: Effects of norepinephrine on renal function in septic patients with normal and elevated serum lactate levels. *Crit Care Med* 17:1104, 1989.

206. Martin C, Eon B, Saux P: Renal effects of norepinephrine used to treat septic shock patients. *Crit Care Med* 18:282, 1990.

207. Hesselvik JF, Brodin B: Low dose norepinephrine in patients with septic shock and oliguria: Effects on afterload, urine flow, and oxygen transport. *Crit Care Med* 17:179, 1989.

208. Desjars P, Pinaud M, Potel G, et al: A reappraisal of norepinephrine therapy in human septic shock. *Crit Care Med* 15:134, 1987.

209. Meadows D, Edwards JD, Wilkins RG, et al: Reversal of intractable septic shock with norepinephrine therapy. *Crit Care Med* 16:663, 1988.

210. Schreuder WO, Schneider AJ, Groeneveld ABJ, et al: Effect of dopamine vs norepinephrine on hemodynamics in septic shock. *Chest* 95:1282, 1989.

211. Schaer GL, Fink MP, Parrillo JE: Norepinephrine alone versus norepinephrine plus low-dose dopamine: Enhanced renal blood flow with combination pressor therapy. *Crit Care Med* 13:492, 1985.

212. Jardin F, Sportiche M, Bazin M, et al: Dobutamine: A hemodynamic evaluation in human septic shock. *Crit Care Med* 9:329, 1981.

213. Vincent J-L, Van der Linden P, Domb M, et al: Dopamine compared with dobutamine in experimental septic shock: Relevance to fluid administration. *Anesth Analg* 66:565, 1987.

214. Tell BE, Majerus TC, Flancbaum L: Dobutamine in elderly septic shock patients refractory to dopamine. *Intensive Care Med* 13:14, 1987.

215. Bakker J, Vincent JL: Effects of norepinephrine and dobutamine on oxygen transport and consumption in a dog model of endotoxic shock. *Crit Care Med* 21:425, 1993.

216. Colardyn FC, Vandenbogaerde JF, Vogelares DP, et al: Use of dopexamine hydrochloride in patients with septic shock. *Crit Care Med* 17:999, 1989.

217. Nasraway SA, Rackow EC, Astiz ME, et al: Inotropic response to digoxin and dopamine in patients with severe sepsis, cardiac failure, and systemic hypoperfusion. *Chest* 95:612, 1989.

218. Moran JL, O'Fathartaigh MS, Peisach AR, et al: Epinephrine as an inotropic agent in septic shock: A dose profile analysis. *Crit Care Med* 21:70, 1993.

219. Gregory JS, Bonfiglio MF, Dasta JF, et al: Experience with phenylephrine as a component of the pharmacologic support of septic shock. *Crit Care Med* 19:1395, 1991.

220. Cerra FB, Hassett J, Siegel JH: Vasodilator therapy in clinical sepsis with low output syndrome. *J Surg Res* 25:180, 1978.

221. Bihari D, Smithies M, Gimson A, et al: The effect of vasodilation with prostacyclin on oxygen delivery and uptake in critically ill patients. *N Engl J Med* 317:397, 1987.

222. Hinshaw LB, Archer LT, Beller-Todd BK, et al: Survival of primates in LD_{100} septic shock following steroid/antibiotic therapy. *J Surg Res* 28:151, 1980.

223. Hinshaw LB, Archer LT, Beller-Todd BK, et al: Survival of primates in lethal septic shock following delayed treatment with steroid. *Circ Shock* 8:291, 1981.

224. Beller BK, Archer LT, Passey RB, et al: Effectiveness of modified steroid-antibiotic therapies for lethal sepsis in the dog. *Arch Surg* 118:1293, 1983.

225. Hollenbach SJ, DeGuzman LR, Bellamy RF: Early administration of methylprednisolone promotes survival in rats with intra-abdominal sepsis. *Circ Shock* 20:161, 1986.

226. White GL, Archer LT, Beller BK, et al: Increased survival with methylprednisolone treatment in canine endotoxin shock. *J Surg Res* 25:357, 1978.

227. O'Flaherty JT, Craddock PR, Jacob HS: Mechanism of anti-complementary activity of corticosteroids in vivo: Possible relevance in endotoxin shock. *Proc Soc Exp Bio Med* 154:206, 1977.

228. Heideman M, Kaijser B, Gelin LE: Complement activation early in endotoxin shock. *J Surg Res* 26:74, 1979.

229. Leon C, Rodrigo MJ, Tomasa A, et al: Complement activation in septic shock due to gram-negative and gram-positive bacteria. *Crit Care Med* 10:308, 1982.

230. Hammerschmidt DE, White JG, Craddock PR, et al: Corticosteroids inhibit complement-induced granulocyte aggregation: A possible mechanism for their efficacy in shock states. *J Clin Invest* 63:798, 1979.

231. Skubitz KM, Craddock PR, Hammerschmidt DE: Corticosteroids block binding of chemotactic peptide to its receptor on granulocytes and cause disaggregation of granulocyte aggregates in vitro. *J Clin Invest* 68:13, 1981.

232. Shumer W: Steroids in the treatment of clinical septic shock. *Ann Surg* 184:333, 1976.
233. Shine KI, Kuhn M, Young LS, et al: Aspects of the management of shock. *Ann Intern Med* 93:723, 1980.
234. Sprung CL, Caralis PV, Marcial EH, et al: The effects of high-dose corticosteroids in patients with septic shock: A prospective, controlled study. *N Engl J Med* 311:1137, 1984.
235. Bone RC, Fisher CJ, Clemmer TP, et al: A controlled clinical trial of high-dose methylprednisolone in the treatment of severe sepsis and septic shock. *N Engl J Med* 317:653, 1987.
236. The Veterans Administration Systemic Sepsis Cooperative Study Group: Effect of high-dose glucocorticoid therapy on mortality in patients with clinical signs of systemic sepsis. *N Engl J Med* 317:659, 1987.
237. Bernard GR, Luce JM, Sprung CL, et al: High-dose corticosteroids in patients with adult respiratory distress syndrome. *N Engl J Med* 317:1565, 1987.
238. Bone RC, Fisher CJ, Clemmer TP, et al: Early methylprednisolone treatment for septic syndrome and the adult respiratory distress syndrome. *Chest* 92:1021, 1987.
239. Slotman GJ, Fisher CJ, Bone RC, et al: Detrimental effects of high-dose methylprednisolone sodium succinate on serum concentrations of hepatic and renal function indicators in severe septic shock. *Crit Care Med* 21:191, 1993.
240. Holiday JW, Faden AI: Naloxone reversal of endotoxin hypotension suggests role of endorphins in shock. *Nature* 275:450, 1978.
241. Reynolds DG, Gurll NJ, Vargish T, et al: Blockade of opiate receptors with naloxone improved survival and cardiac performance in canine endotoxic shock. *Circ Shock* 7:39, 1980.
242. Peters WP, Johnson MW, Friedman PA, et al: Pressor effect of naloxone in septic shock. *Lancet* 1:529, 1981.
243. Bonnet F, Lhoste BF, Mankikian LH, et al: Naloxone therapy of human septic shock. *Crit Care Med* 13:972, 1985.
244. Rock P, Silverman H, Plump D, et al: Efficacy and safety of naloxone in septic shock. *Crit Care Med* 13:28, 1985.
245. DeMaria A, Heffernan JJ, Gridlinger GA, et al: Naloxone versus placebo in treatment of septic shock. *Lancet* 1:1363, 1985.
246. Napolitano L, Chernow B: Endorphins in circulatory shock. *Crit Care Med* 16:566, 1988.
247. Haupt MT, Jastremski MS, Clemmer TP, et al: Effects of ibuprofen in patients with severe sepsis: A randomized double-blind, multicenter study. *Crit Care Med* 1339, 1991.
248. Bernard GR, Reines HD, Halushka PV, et al: Prostacyclin and thromboxane A₂ formation is increased in human sepsis syndrome: effects of cyclooxygenase inhibition. *Am Rev Respir Dis* 144:1095, 1991.
249. Leeman M, Boeynaems J, Degaute J, et al: Administration of dazoxiben, a selective thromboxane synthetase inhibitor, in the adult respiratory distress syndrome. *Chest* 87:726, 1986.
250. Reines HD, Halushka PV, Olanoff LS, et al: Dazoxiben in human sepsis and adult respiratory distress syndrome. *Clin Pharmacol Ther* 37:391, 1985.
251. Slotman GJ, Burchard KW, D'Arezzo A, et al: Ketoconazole prevents acute respiratory failure in critically ill surgical patients. *J Trauma* 28:648, 1988.
252. Yu M, Tomasa G: A double-blind, prospective, randomized trial of ketoconazole, a thromboxane synthetase inhibitor, in the prophylaxis of adult respiratory distress syndrome. *Crit Care Med* 21:1635, 1993.
253. Larrick JW: Antibody inhibition of the immunoinflammatory cascade. *J Crit Care* 4:211, 1989.
254. Vedder NB, Winn RK, Rice CL, et al: A monoclonal antibody to the adherence promoting leukocyte glycoprotein CD18 reduces organ injury and improves survival from hemorrhagic shock and resuscitation in rabbits. *J Clin Invest* 81:939, 1988.
255. Tracey KJ, Fong Y, Hesse DG, et al: Anti-cachectin/TNF monoclonal antibodies prevent septic shock during lethal bacteremia. *Nature* 330:662, 1987.
256. Stevens JH, O'Hanley P, Shapiro JM, et al: Effects of anti-C5a antibodies on the adult respiratory distress syndrome in septic primates. *J Clin Invest* 77:1812, 1986.
257. Ziegler EJ, Douglas H, Sherman JE, et al: Treatment of *E. coli* and *Klebsiella* bacteremia in agranulocytic animals with antiserum to a UDP-Gal epimerase-deficient mutant. *J Immunol* 111:433, 1973.
258. Ziegler EJ, McCutchan JA, Douglas H, et al: Prevention of lethal *Pseudomonas* bacteremia with epimerase-deficient *E. coli* antiserum. *Trans Assoc Am Phys* 88:101, 1975.
259. Ziegler EJ, McCutchan JA, Fierer J, et al: Treatment of gram-negative bacteremia and shock with human antiserum to a mutant *Escherichia coli*. *N Engl J Med* 307:1225, 1982.
260. McCutchan JA, Wolf JL, Ziegler EJ, et al: Ineffectiveness of single-dose human antiserum to core glycolipid (*E. coli* J5) for prophylaxis of bacteremic, gram-negative infections in patients with prolonged neutropenia. *Schweiz Med Wochenschr* 113(Suppl 14):40, 1987.
261. Baumgartner JD, Glauser MP, McCutchan JA, et al: Prevention of gram-negative shock and death in surgical patients by antibody to endotoxin for glycolipid. *Lancet* 2:59, 1985.
262. Ziegler EJ, Fisher CJ Jr, Sprung CL, et al: Treatment of gram-negative bacteremia and septic shock with HA-1A human monoclonal antibody against endotoxin: A randomized, double-blind, placebo-controlled trial. *N Engl J Med* 324:429, 1991.
263. Greenman RL, Schein RMH, Martin MA: A controlled clinical trial of E5 murine monoclonal IgM antibody to endotoxin in the treatment of gram-negative sepsis. *JAMA* 266:1097, 1991.
264. Schedel I, Dreikhausen U, Nentwig B, et al: Treatment of gram-negative septic shock with an immunoglobulin preparation: A prospective, randomized clinical trial. *Crit Care Med* 19:1104, 1991.
265. Fisher CJ Jr, Opal SM, Dhainaut J-F, et al: Influence of an anti-tumor necrosis factor monoclonal antibody on cytokine levels in patients with sepsis. *Crit Care Med* 21:318, 1993.
266. Alexander HR, Doherty GM, Venzon DJ, et al: Recombinant interleukin-1 receptor antagonist (IL-1ra): Effective therapy against gram-negative sepsis in rats. *Surgery* 112:188, 1992.
267. Mohler KM, Torrance DS, Smith CA, et al: Soluble tumor necrosis factor (TNF) receptors are effective therapeutic agents in lethal endotoxemia and function simultaneously as both TNF carriers and TNF antagonists. *J Immunol* 151:1548, 1993.
268. Knaus WA, Draper EA, Wagner DP, et al: APACHE II-a severity of disease classification system. *Crit Care Med* 13:818, 1985.
269. Lemeshow S, Teres D, Pastides H, et al: A method for predicting survival and mortality of ICU patients using objectively derived weights. *Crit Care Med* 13:519, 1985.
270. Jordan DA, Miller CF, Kubos KL, et al: Evaluation of sepsis in a critically ill surgical population. *Crit Care Med* 15:897, 1987.
271. Elebute EA, Stoner HB: The grading of sepsis. *Br J Surg* 70:29, 1983.
272. Knaus WA, Sun X, Nystrom P-O, et al: Evaluation of definitions for sepsis. *Chest* 101:1656, 1992.
273. D'Orio V, Mendes P, Saad G, et al: Accuracy in early prediction of prognosis of patients with septic shock by analysis of simple indices: Prospective study. *Crit Care Med* 18:1339, 1990.
274. Hebert PC, Drummond AJ, Singer J, et al: A simple multiple system organ failure scoring system predicts mortality of patients who have sepsis syndrome. *Chest* 104:230, 1993.
275. Baumgartner J-D, Bula C, Vaney C, et al: A novel score for predicting the mortality of septic shock patients. *Crit Care Med* 20:953, 1992.
276. Arregui LM, Moyes DG, Lipman J, et al. Comparison of disease severity scoring systems in septic shock. *Crit Care Med* 19:1165, 1991.

174. Trauma: An Overview

Jean-Denis Yelle and Arthur L. Trask

Traumatic injury has reached epidemic proportions in North America. Trauma is the leading cause of death for those younger than 45 years of age and is the third leading cause of death for all ages, exceeded only by cardiovascular diseases and cancer [1]. In 1989, the total cost of accidents was estimated to be in excess of $148.5 billion, including $23.7 billion in medical expenses, $28.4 billion in insurance, $37.7 billion in lost wages, $38.2 billion in vehicle and fire loss, and $22.4 billion in indirect work loss. Most of these injuries were a result of falls (12 million) and motor vehicle collisions (MVC) (5.3 million). Most of the traumatic deaths (155,665) were secondary to MVC, with 1,173,000 total person-years of life lost, exceeding cardiovascular diseases and cancer combined [2].

Prevention of traumatic injury is the only adequate solution. A good prevention program should include two components: First, educational activities that focus on high-risk behaviors, such as drinking while driving and not using seat belts and other protective equipment, are required to control the frequency of trauma. Second, research should become a priority in trauma care. Systematic collection and analysis of trauma data should be linked directly to the design of prevention programs and to the manufacture of protective equipment.

Experience has shown that traumatic deaths follow a trimodal distribution [3]. When mortality is plotted as a function of time after injury, three peaks can be identified that correspond to immediate death, early death, and late death. Immediate deaths occur at the scene and represent almost one-half of all trauma related deaths. Major vascular injury, brain injury, and cardiac injury are the usual causes, and these deaths will only decrease with effective prevention programs. Early deaths occur within a few hours after injury. Hemorrhage and airway or respiratory problems are usually the cause. Shackford et al. [4] have shown a decrease in mortality for this second peak when a trauma system is in place and a short transport time is possible. The optimal transport time is often referred to as "the golden hour" because as many as 20% of patients who had previously been classified as dead on arrival can be resuscitated in the emergency room and eventually leave the hospital without permanent neurologic sequelae [5]. Late deaths occur between 3 and 4 days (e.g., severe head injury complicated by uncontrolled increased intracranial pressure) and 3 and 4 weeks (e.g., multiple organ dysfunction) postinjury. Baker et al. [5] have shown that late deaths accounted for 25 percent of all trauma deaths before the institution of trauma systems. The institution of trauma care systems has reduced this rate to 10 percent.

Etiology

Exposure to risk is directly related to frequency of injury. Traumatic injury results from the application of mechanical energy, electricity, heat, cold, chemicals, or radiation to the human body. Typically, injuries are characterized as penetrating or blunt. A penetrating injury involves application of a force focused over a small area of the body. Common penetrating injuries are stab wounds and gunshot wounds. Less common penetrating injuries result from the fragmentation of agents such as metal, glass, or wood.

The damage caused by a penetrating injury is directly related to the kinetic energy carried by the projectile at impact. Velocity of the projectile is the major determinant of the amount of tissue destruction. Another important factor is the elasticity of the injured tissues (more damage is caused in bone or muscle than lung or skin). The absorption of kinetic energy initiates a sequence of traumatic events, beginning with a crush injury in the primary cavity and followed by a stretching of the tissues causing a secondary temporary cavity commonly called the "blast effect." Every penetrating injury has the potential of sending secondary projectiles, such as fragments of a missile or of bone, to surrounding tissues, spreading the damage.

Blunt trauma distributes energy over a larger surface area than a penetrating injury and is associated with rapid acceleration (e.g., a pedestrian struck by a car) or rapid deceleration (e.g., collisions and falls). Because of rapid acceleration, tissues fixed at different points are stretched. The rate of tissue stretching is the major determinant of tissue damage (e.g., aortic arch disruption distal to the left subclavian artery where it is attached to the ligamentum arteriosum). In addition to the tissue deformation and compression that occurs at the point of impact, more tissue damage can occur along the axis to which the forces are applied. Injuries from blunt traumatic impact are generally more difficult to diagnose and more complex to manage than penetrating injuries. Falls from height account for 50 percent and motor vehicle collisions for another 25 percent of all blunt traumatic injuries [2].

Trauma Care Systems

DEFINITION. A trauma care system is a comprehensive, organized approach to managing the injured patient. The system is composed of internal and external elements (Fig. 174-1). Optimal trauma care includes unencumbered access to prehospital care, hospital care, family support, and extensive rehabilitation care. Continuous quality improvement (CQI) activities provide the essential feedback for educational, research, and preventive strategies of trauma management. To optimize trauma care, the planners of the local trauma system must consider the external factors in *each* community. These factors include the public's awareness and demands, the local economy and geography, the volume and types of injuries, and the demographic patterns of the community. Ultimately, the goals of the trauma care system are to assure access to comprehensive trauma care for all victims, to decrease death and disability, and to contain cost of trauma care through efficiency and greater economies of scale. A comprehensive and regional trauma care system can significantly reduce death and disability [6,7].

Trauma Care System Components

PREHOSPITAL. Prehospital care in North America exists along a continuum. In rural areas, there may be long delays in re-

TRAUMA SYSTEMS

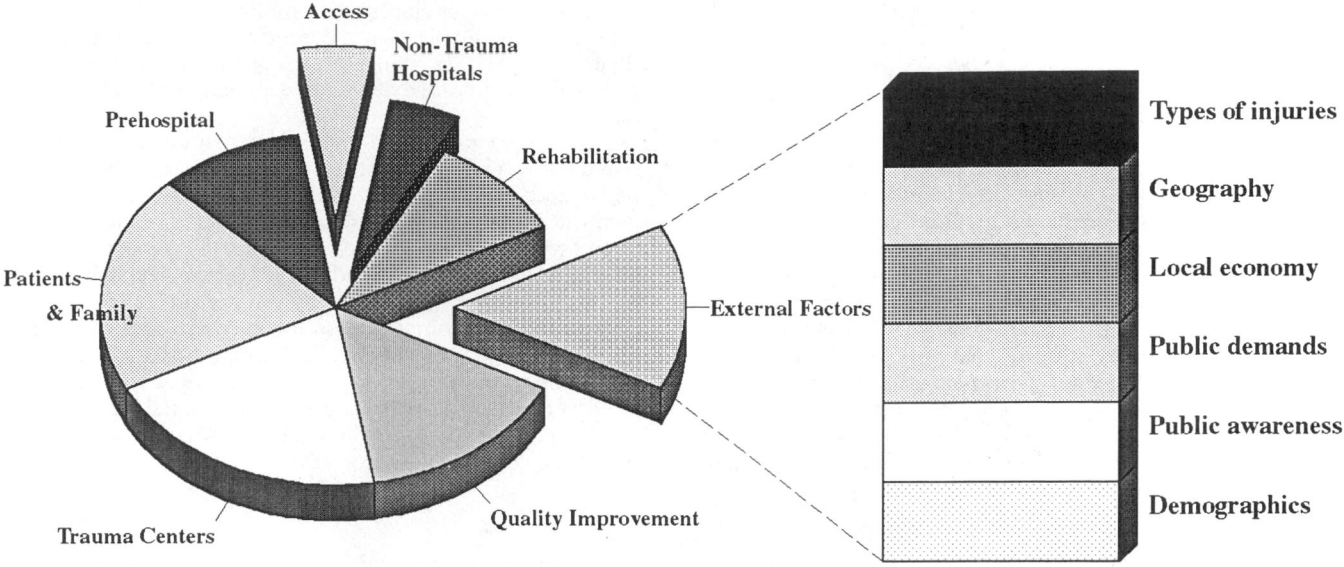

COMPONENTS

Fig. 174-1. Components of trauma system.

sponse because of geography, lack of health care providers, lack of equipment, or weather conditions. In large urban areas, prehospital care is totally integrated into the system, and advanced life support personnel (paramedics) can respond in less than 5 minutes, regardless of the weather or the time of day. Transport may be by ground transportation, by air transportation, or even by boat. Air transport should be activated when ground transport time is greater than 30 minutes or when the casualties exceed the capability of the ground transport system.

A communication network is a basic requirement of prehospital care. Prompt entry into the trauma care system is directly related to this network. A state-wide 911 dialing system allows reporting of an accident to the Emergency Operating Center (EOC). The communication system keeps the prehospital provider in contact with a medical expert. This is a multidirectional transmission of information between the different components of the trauma system. The goal of prehospital care is to bring the patient to the *appropriate* medical facility quickly and safely. The receiving facility should be alerted to the severity of the injury and be prepared to deal with all aspects of the situation.

TRAUMA CENTERS AND NONTRAUMA HOSPITALS. There is no need for 85 to 90 percent of injured patients to receive specialized trauma care. For the remaining 10 to 15 percent of patients, specialized trauma care is desirable. Trauma centers should be certified by the state Emergency Medical System (EMS) agencies or by the Committee on Trauma of the American College of Surgeons (ACS). Three levels of trauma

hospitals now exist [8]. A fourth level for specialized rural settings soon may be added.

A Level I trauma center is a regional resource. It can provide 24-hour, immediately available care by an in-hospital trauma team. Such centers have teaching and research responsibilities and serve as a leader for prevention programs in the communities they serve. These centers are qualified to care for the most severely injured patients.

A Level II trauma center provides a level of patient care similar to a Level I center, but with less commitment to research and education. There also may be gaps in coverage for special injuries, such as burns and reimplantation. A Level II center ideally has prearranged transfer agreements to a regional center for these special needs.

A Level III center is a smaller community hospital that provides assessment and stabilization followed by local surgical treatment or transport to a higher-level center. As in Level II centers, prearranged patient transfer agreements should be negotiated for the definitive care of burns, multiple systems injuries, traumatic brain injuries, spinal cord injuries, organ reimplantation or even pediatric trauma.

The nontrauma community hospitals receive the bulk of injured patients and must be integrated into the system. They must *recognize* the potential for serious injury in any patient brought to them and expeditiously arrange for transfer to an appropriate trauma center when indicated.

REHABILITATION. A trauma center should have access to state-of-the-art rehabilitation programs. Unfortunately, rehabilitative services are often lacking. Recent advances in vocational rehabilitation programs and technology have substantially reduced residual disability and have shortened the time to independent living for a select group of injured patients. Rehabilitation personnel consulting in the ICU can increase these beneficial effects. Rehabilitation should start early after admission to the hospital and should be continued with a personalized plan through discharge. Further, outcome studies examining the cost-to-benefit ratio for these services are urgently needed.

A specialized social work staff is needed to introduce the concept of injury to the family and to prepare them for accepting the medical prognosis when it is presented to them by the trauma team leader. They also will identify the appropriate community services available and will be involved in the patient's disposition early in the patient's treatment.

Finally, every trauma center should have an organ procurement program to facilitate organ donation. For example, if a patient with a low Glasgow Coma Score (GCS) has potentially irreversible brain injury, the trauma team physicians in the trauma ICU should be alert to the possibility of organ donation. When brain death has been determined and the tasks of the attending physician have been completed, the organ procurement team should then introduce organ donation to the family to maximize the chances for consent for organ retrieval [9].

Scoring Techniques

The idea of scoring systems for trauma patients was introduced early in the 1970s. A scoring system is important to (1) attain the appropriate level of care for the injured patient; (2) quantify expected outcomes; (3) assess results of trauma care; (4) compare large groups of patients; (5) guide CQI activities; and, more recently, (6) facilitate reimbursement of care.

Scoring systems for trauma are useful tools for the analysis and evaluation of patient cohorts. However, one should remember their limitations when applied to individual patients. Although scoring systems can derive a probability of survival for an individual patient, clinical science should not be replaced by blind submission to numerical algorithms. A list of currently used scoring techniques includes the Glasgow Coma Score [10], the Trauma Score [11], the Revised Trauma Score [11], the Crams Score [12], the Injury Severity Score [13], Triss [14], and Ascot [11]).

Trauma Center Response

The quality of a trauma center's response to traumatic injury is essential for patient outcome. The major quality components are the organization of the trauma service, the nature of the trauma team response, and the management of the trauma care.

TRAUMA SERVICES ORGANIZATION. The most comprehensive trauma services are offered by a Level I trauma center. The director of a Level I trauma center should be a general surgeon with a special expertise in trauma care developed either through experience or through a trauma fellowship. The director must be able to coordinate the needs of the trauma team and consultants with administration and other members of the hospital staff.

Trauma surgeons must be board certified and have adequate training in both trauma and critical care. All trauma surgeons should have satisfactorily completed an Advanced Trauma Life Support (ATLS) Provider Course, and most should be ATLS instructors. Surgeons should participate in continuing medical education programs emphasizing trauma and critical care. They also should be involved in the education and training of residents and medical students. An interest in research and publication also is indicative of a strong commitment to trauma care [8].

Ideally, the trauma service should be composed of a trauma coordinator, a researcher, a data entry specialist, and administrative and secretarial support. The trauma coordinator, usually a critical care or emergency department nurse, coordinates activities with the trauma director and is involved with prehospital care, CQI activities [15], and outcome management for the trauma program. The researcher's main goal is to implement a comprehensive program of protocol design and evaluation, standard data collection techniques, and database maintenance. This information supports CQI efforts. Finally, a trauma service needs a dedicated administrative and secretarial staff to assure smooth and efficient functioning on a daily basis. Level II or III trauma centers have less extensive staff.

TRAUMA TEAM RESPONSE. When a trauma code is received from the prehospital provider to the hospital, a trauma response is initiated at all levels of the trauma center. The most common type of response is to have a preselected team of persons to respond to the code. In most centers, this team includes a trauma surgeon, surgical house staff if a training program is a part of the center, an emergency department physician, an anesthesiologist or respiratory care technician, an x-ray technician, trauma nurses, an emergency department technician, a laboratory technician, a social worker, and other specially trained persons, depending on the type of injury or special needs of the patient. In many centers, the trauma team includes 15 or more responders.

Fifty percent of patients do not require all members of this team [8,16], and so a second option is to base the immediate hospital response on the communicated field assessment. A detailed examination of the local trauma experience may distinguish traumatic injuries that require a full team response from those that do not. If the primary assessment suggests that a patient's status has changed, the trauma code can be upgraded or downgraded as required. Dekeyser et al. [17] have shown that this two-tier system reduces the cost per patient by approximately $1000 without reducing quality of care.

Trauma centers should have an operating room available 24 hours a day. In Level I centers, this room should be capable of accommodating more than one surgical team at a time. All persons involved in patient care should have proper attire for protection from blood-borne diseases and tuberculosis.

The ICU is essential for trauma care. The care of the seriously injured patient is different from that of other critically ill patients because the trauma patient typically does not have a premorbid condition. Common problems encountered in the ICU care of trauma patients include central nervous system injury, coagulopathy and hypothermia, pulmonary or cardiac injuries, and other potentially life-threatening injuries. To ensure continuity of care, an ICU nurse should be present in the trauma bay with the most seriously injured patients. The nurse then can become a resource person for the patient and be involved in the subsequent decision-making process in the ICU. If multiple disciplines are involved with patient care, weekly multidisciplinary rounds are recommended to ensure a coordinated approach among all specialties.

Trauma Management

The Committee on Trauma of the ACS has standardized the early care of the trauma patient through the implementation of Advanced Trauma Life Support (ATLS) [18]. Early management involves four phases: primary survey, resuscitation, secondary survey, and definitive management. This protocol is now used throughout the world.

In a well-run trauma system, the prehospital personnel perform a primary survey at the site of the incident. Hypoxia is the primary reason for early death or subsequent central nervous system dysfunction in trauma patients. Airway management is essential at the scene because death occurs long before a patient can be transported to the appropriate facility if the airway is not controlled. Most advanced life support personnel and some basic life support personnel are trained in advanced airway management, including nasotracheal and oral tracheal intubation. Some may be trained to perform rapid-sequence intubation, transtracheal jet insufflation, or cricothyrotomy. For trauma patients, protection of the cervical spine while the airway is being controlled is imperative.

Once the airway is controlled, either in the field or in the emergency department, further assessment of breathing is done. Rapid, labored breathing, abdominal respiratory movements, or cyanosis suggest the presence of potentially life-threatening chest trauma. Tension pneumothorax rarely occurs in the field unless there is positive pressure ventilation, but simple pneumothorax and flail chest are frequently identified. The rapid insertion of bilateral closed thoracostomy tubes is indicated if a tension pneumothorax is suspected on clinical grounds alone, even in the absence of radiographic confirmation. These tubes may aid diagnosis in addition to providing therapy for major breathing problems. If a large gush (1000–1500 ml) of blood is obtained, immediate transport to the operating room is indicated.

Once airway and breathing problems have been diagnosed and treated, efforts to assess and control cardiovascular performance assume paramount importance. In the past, placement of large bore intravenous lines (16 gauge or larger) was performed by cutdown, but today most busy trauma centers use the "Seldinger technique" to place even larger (8–10 French) central catheters. Rapid infusion devices are now available that simultaneously warm and deliver fluid at up to 1700 ml/per minute. Clinical evaluation of blood loss is taught as part of the ATLS course and will guide the caregiver on the timing of blood replacement.

Blood replacement continues to be essential for management of major trauma patients. Until a suitable asanguinous oxygen transporter is developed, the appropriate use of blood and blood products is key to resuscitation when blood loss is the source of cardiovascular instability. Many trauma surgeons believe that an adequate blood pressure, pulse, and urine output are not suitable measures of cellular resuscitation. Measuring oxygen delivery (DO_2) and increasing DO_2 to greater than normal levels is advocated by some clinicians [19].

Once the primary survey and resuscitation have been completed, a more comprehensive secondary survey should be obtained, which should include a systematic evaluation of the head, neck, thorax, abdomen, pelvis, back, all extremities (including circulatory status), and a more complete neurologic examination. Usually during the primary survey, a very quick assessment of mental status and motor activity is done, particularly if it is necessary to paralyze and intubate the patient for airway and breathing purposes.

Information derived from the primary and secondary surveys influences the definitive care strategy of the trauma surgeon and the prioritization of further diagnostic or surgical efforts. An incorrect plan can result in an unfavorable outcome. Because experience and knowledge are critical to the process, the most senior physician is commonly in charge.

The definitive management process is illustrated by the following example. A patient arrives in the trauma bay as a result of a high-speed motor vehicle collision. The patient, who was not belted and was thrown from the vehicle after impact, is hemodynamically unstable with the following obvious injuries:

Open unstable pelvic fracture with blood and stool issuing from the perineum
Contusion of chest and left upper quadrant of the abdomen
Open fracture of left arm
Glasgow Coma Score of 9

Initial chest radiograph shows a widened mediastinum, fracture of the first rib on left, and an indistinct left cardiac border.

What should be done first? After assuring that the patient had a clear airway and was breathing satisfactorily, placement of a 40 French chest tube on the left will establish whether the patient is bleeding into his thorax. If a massive amount of blood (i.e., 1500 ml) is obtained, the patient must go to the operating room immediately for a left thoracotomy. If the patient has a lesser degree of bleeding from the left chest, the next most likely cause for the hypotension must be hemorrhage associated with pelvic fractures.

Should an angiogram of the pelvic vessels be performed before doing a head CT or a thoracic aortogram? Massive bleeding associated with pelvic fractures may take priority and require embolization to control. Conversely, if the patient stabilizes rapidly with a minimal amount of blood and fluid, perhaps a limited head CT should be done before the thoracic aortogram. There are traumatologists who advocate emergency department placement of external fixators for this type of pelvic fracture, whereas others believe MAST trousers are appropriate to temporarily control hemorrhage. This patient requires operative treatment of the pelvic fracture and the open upper extremity fracture after the diagnosis and treatment of blood loss and after the possibility of a central nervous system mass lesion has been ruled out.

The use of algorithms for management is becoming more prominent in today's literature. Penetrating injuries, typically less challenging to prioritize, most frequently need operative intervention. Nonetheless, the presence of multiple missile injuries requires clinical judgment to determine which injury should be dealt with first. For example, if a patient presents with an abdominal wound and with a wound to the lower extremity with absent distal pulses, what should be done first? The life-threatening injuries are most likely to be found in the abdomen, but delay in revascularization of a lower extremity may present significant chances for subsequent disability or limb loss. When in the sequence of evaluation should an angiogram be performed to determine the extent of the injury? Some experts suggest doing a limited arteriogram in the trauma bay, which may provide necessary information rapidly. In some centers, two teams may be used to deal simultaneously with the abdominal and extremity injuries. This strategy makes sense if the operating room is large enough and adequate resources are available.

Future Problems

Three major problems confront trauma care systems. The first problem is economic. Major inner-city trauma centers treat and provide care to a large population of indigent and uninsured patients. The high costs of trauma care and relatively poor reimbursement have decreased the commitment and allocation of resources for trauma. The experiences in Miami, Chicago, and Los Angeles, where many trauma centers have closed, illustrate this problem.

The second problem reflects the population density in rural communities. The identification and timely transport of injured patients to the appropriate trauma facilities is difficult in rural communities. The low population density typically translates into relatively low revenues from taxation and hence insufficient resources to maintain a costly trauma system.

The third problem is the difficulty in recruiting dedicated and qualified physicians to provide trauma care. Because of its impact on lifestyle and reimbursement, physicians today have indicated that they may not be willing to continue providing trauma care. Furthermore, a majority of new physicians completing surgical training also have stated that trauma care is not in their professional plans for the future [19,20].

Summary

To optimize management of the trauma patient, a complete and well-run system is necessary. Excluding one component or not giving sufficient attention to all aspects results in patients dying unnecessarily or sustaining long-term or permanent disability. We continue to improve as more research and CQI data are fed back into the system. There will not be improvement in early trauma deaths until effective prevention programs are implemented and tested. Those who manage trauma patients in the ICU must have an understanding of all aspects of the trauma care systems to facilitate optimal critical care.

References

1. Cales RH, Heilig RW: *Trauma Care Systems*, Rockville, MD, Aspen Publishers, 1986.

2. U.S. Bureau of the Census: *Statistical Abstract of the United States: 1991*. 112th ed. Washington, DC, 1992.
3. Trunkey DD, Blaisdell FW: American College of Surgeons, Care of the surgical patient. *Sci Am* 1:1, 1993.
4. Shackford SR, Hollingsworth-Fridlund P, Cooper GF, et al: The effect of regionalization upon the quality of trauma care as assessed by concurrent audit before and after institution of trauma system. *J Trauma* 16:812, 1986.
5. Baker CC, Oppenheimer L, Stephens B, et al: Epidemiology of trauma deaths. *Am J Surg* 140:144, 1980.
6. Cales RH, Trunkey DD: Preventable trauma deaths, a review of trauma care systems development. *JAMA* 254:1059, 1985.
7. West JG, Cales RH, Gazzaniga: Impact of regionalization: The Orange County Experience. *Arch Surg* 118:740, 1983.
8. Committee on Trauma, American College of Surgeons: *Resources for Optimal Care of the Injured Patient*. Chicago, American College of Surgeons, 1990.
9. Garrison RN, Bentley RF, Raque GH, et al.: There is an answer to the shortage of organ donors. SG&O 173:391, 1991.
10. Teasdale G, Jennell B: Assessment of coma and impaired consciousness: A practical scale. *Lancet* 2:81, 1974.
11. Wisner DH: History and current status of trauma scoring systems. *Arch Surg* 127:111, 1992.
12. Gormican SP: CRAMS Scale: Field triage of trauma victims. *Ann Emerg Med* 11:132, 1992.
13. Baker SP, O'Neill B, Haddon W, et al: The Injury Severity Score. *J Trauma* 14:187, 1974.
14. Champion HR, Sacco WJ, Hunt TK: Trauma severity scoring to predict mortality. *World J Surg* 7:4, 1983.
15. American College of Emergency Physicians: Trauma care systems quality improvement guidelines. *Ann Emerg Med* 21:736, 1992.
16. O'Rourke B, Bade RH, Drezner T: Trauma triage: A nine-year experience. *Ann Emerg Med* 21:686, 1992.
17. Dekeyser FG, Paratore A, Seneca RP, Trask A: Decreasing cost of trauma care: A system of secondary, in-hospital triage. *Ann Emerg Med* (Accepted for publication).
18. American College of Surgeons Committee on Trauma: *Advanced Life Support Course Student Manual*. Chicago, American College of Surgeons, 1989.
19. Fleming A, et al: Prospective trial of supranormal values as goals of resuscitation in severe trauma. *Arch Surg* 127:1175, 1992.
20. Richardson JR, Miller F: Will future surgeons be interested in trauma care? Results of a resident survey. *J Trauma* 32:229, 1992.

175. Head Trauma

Shailendra Joshi, Faustino Guinto, and Donald S. Prough

Trauma causes more deaths in persons aged 1 to 44 years than all other diseases combined [1]. Head injury is present in 60 percent of fatalities secondary to motor vehicle accidents and causes or contributes to nearly nine-tenths of fatal outcomes [2]. Of the 410,000 severe head injuries (an intermediate estimate) that occur in the United States per year, 300,000 result in hospitalizations, 18,000 produce moderate to severe disabilities, and 2000 result in persistent vegetative states [3]. Despite the mortality and morbidity associated with head injury, definitive treatment of trauma victims is hindered in many localities by inadequate transport systems and by delayed transfer to trauma centers.

Brain trauma is produced by closed or penetrating head injuries. Head trauma is further subdivided into *severe* (from which patients are rendered comatose, i.e., unable to obey simple verbal commands), *moderate* (after which patients either require cranial surgery or are rendered comatose, if only briefly), and *minor* (after which patients neither require surgery nor lose consciousness). Although primary brain injury may not be remediable, preventable secondary insults such as hypotension, hypercarbia, hypoxemia, or intracranial hypertension may worsen injury [4,5]. Intensive care of head trauma victims is aimed toward prevention of these secondary insults. This chapter reviews the current treatment of head injury and describes therapies actively under investigation.

Epidemiology

Head injury, which occurs in the United States every 7 seconds and produces a fatality every 5 minutes [6], is the leading cause of death in persons younger than 24 years of age, with the peak incidence occurring in males 15 to 24 years old [7]. The most common circumstances leading to severe head injury in adults are traffic accidents, assaults, and falls [8], often associated with alcohol or drug abuse. Although the overall incidence of head injury–associated death is nearly identical for blacks and whites, blacks outnumber whites among the estimated 16,500 annual civilian deaths from cerebral gunshot wounds [8]. From an epidemiological standpoint, the most effective way of controlling the cost of head injury is by prevention. Proposed measures include redesigned roads and vehicles, stricter control of alcohol, reduced speed limits, higher licensure age, and stricter gun control. Full front-seat air bags would reduce the incidence and severity of brain injuries by 25 percent [9].

Clinical Profile of Head Trauma

Head injuries commonly are complicated by intoxication and by associated injuries. Intoxication may compromise initial neurologic assessment. In adults, unlike children, shock rarely accompanies isolated closed head injuries. Many patients (35–40%) with severe head injuries resulting in coma have associated facial, thoracic, abdominal, or extremity injuries [10]. The mortality rate of comatose patients is 48 percent if associated with one extracerebral injury and 78 percent with four associated injuries; the incidence of shock in these two groups is 44 percent and 100 percent, respectively [10]. Cervical spine injuries must be diagnostically excluded in any moderate or severe head injury. An estimated 20 percent to 25 percent of comatose, head-injured patients also have thoracic injuries. Overall, 42 percent of patients having head injury with unconsciousness, flail chest, and pulmonary contusion fail to survive [10]. Other associated thoracic injuries include myocardial contusion, thoracic aortic disruption, and thoracic spine injury. Abdominal injuries associated with head trauma usually present initially as hypovolemic shock. Associated orthopedic trauma can worsen outcome by causing hemorrhagic shock, by predisposing to complications such as infection, thromboembolism, and fat embolism, and by restricting chest physiotherapy and physical therapy.

Pathology

BIOMECHANICS OF HEAD TRAUMA. Head injuries are described as direct or indirect. Direct injuries, which occur when the head strikes or is struck by another object, disseminate force throughout the cranial vault, resulting in skull fractures, contusions, and intraaxial and extraaxial hematomas. Indirect injuries occur when cranial motion is abruptly arrested. The intracranial contents undergo rapid acceleration and deceleration, creating differential movement and compression of the intracranial contents relative to the skull. The inertial forces also stretch tissues and shear surface vessels. Indirect trauma results in concussions, subdural hematomas, *contra coup* injuries, and diffuse axonal injuries.

Pathologists categorize fatal traumatic brain injuries [11] as either *diffuse*, which include diffuse axonal injury, hypoxic brain damage, diffuse brain swelling, and diffuse punctate brain hemorrhages, or *focal*, including contusions, avulsions, hematomas, hemorrhages, infarctions, and infections. During initial clinical assessment, comatose trauma patients are also classified as having diffuse or focal injury. Those who demonstrate no signs of an intracranial hematoma by computed tomography (CT) or magnetic resonance imaging (MRI) have diffuse brain injury [12].

Focal and diffuse injuries produce unconsciousness by different mechanisms: focal injuries by brain compression, brain shift, or herniation and diffuse injuries through damage to multiple sites in the brainstem or cerebral cortex. Patients with diffuse brain injury are much less likely than those with focal injuries to have sustained a skull fracture or cerebral contusion, to develop signs of sustained intracranial hypertension, or to demonstrate a "lucid" interval after injury before becoming comatose [5,11,13].

Diffuse Brain Injury. The pathogenesis of diffuse axonal injury, defined as widespread damage to the axons in the cerebral hemispheres, corpus callosum, brainstem, or cerebellum [14], is believed to be stretching and shearing of axons as a result of elastic deformation of the brain. Diffuse axonal injury is assigned three pathologic grades: Grade I, without focal lesions; grade II, focal lesions in the corpus callosum; grade III, focal lesions in the corpus callosum and dorsolateral quadrant of the rostral brainstem [14].

Histologically, diffuse axonal injury is characterized by axonal ballooning, microglial stars, long-tract degeneration, or diffuse gliosis [14]. Axonal ballooning is typically seen between 12 and 24 hours. Microglial stars, small clusters of hypertrophied microglia, are usually seen within 24 to 48 hours. Long-tract degeneration, which occurs weeks to months after injury, affects both the ascending and the descending tracts, particularly the corticospinal tracts, the medial lemnisci, the superior cerebellar peduncles, and the pyramidal tracts in the spinal cord. Diffuse gliosis of the white matter, particularly in the brainstem, is a late finding. Focal lesions that accompany diffuse injury are hemorrhagic in the acute phase, later to become cystic and discolored with hemosiderin.

Other forms of diffuse brain injury include hypoxic damage, diffuse swelling, cerebral edema, and intraparenchymal hemorrhage. Hypoxic cerebral damage, a common postmortem finding after blunt head trauma [15,16], is associated with arterial hypoxemia or cerebral hypoperfusion occurring as a consequence of shock, sustained intracranial hypertension, or cerebral arterial spasm. Cerebral arterial spasm often predicts vegetative survival after severe head injury [17]. Bilateral, diffuse cerebral swelling, which represents vascular congestion rather than cerebral edema, typically occurs after head trauma in young children [18]. The cardinal diagnostic feature on CT scan is symmetric compression of the lateral ventricles and cisterns, and normal or increased white matter density. Vasogenic cerebral edema occurs when damage to the blood-brain barrier results in increased interstitial water accumulation. Cerebral edema may surround intracerebral hematomas or may develop after evacuation of an ipsilateral intracranial hematoma. Patients with diffuse injury who die within a few days after trauma usually demonstrate multiple intraparenchymal brain hemorrhages [11], probably occurring adjacent to small vessels damaged by abrupt acceleration or deceleration. In the few patients who survive this type of injury, the multiple petechial hemorrhages are gradually reabsorbed and replaced by cystic scars.

Focal Lesions. Focal brain injury may be isolated or may accompany diffuse injury. The most common focal injuries are intraaxial (within the substance of the neuraxis) hematomas, extraaxial hematomas, and cerebral contusions. Often associated with skull fractures [19], extraaxial hematomas include subdural and epidural hematomas. Ten percent of patients with a Glasgow Coma Scale (GCS) score of 13 require surgery for intracranial lesions [20]. Extraaxial hematomas rarely are detected in patients who have a GCS of 15 and no focal neurologic deficits [21]. Because skull fracture increases the risk of intracranial hematoma, patients who have a skull fracture and score <15 on the GCS should have a CT scan within 24 hours of injury [22].

Contusions usually result from contact between the brain surface and bony intracranial prominences. Immediately after contusion, disruption of the blood-brain barrier leads to sequestration of blood cells and serum proteins [23]. Edema, evident within minutes and fully manifested by 24 hours after injury, is both vasogenic and cytotoxic. Edema may lead to failure of the microcirculation in neighboring regions. Microscopic hemorrhages, which occur almost immediately in the perivascular areas, attain maximal size in 24 hours. Neutrophilic infiltration, evident within 48 hours, may last for a month. Axonal ballooning may be seen in the first 1 to 2 days. Neuronal death appears to occur in two waves: severely damaged neurons are lost within 24 to 48 hours; those less severely injured are lost around day 7. Myelin degeneration may begin within hours but continue for months. As macrophages clear dead and dying cells, repair begins. Synaptic regeneration is evident by the fourth or fifth posttraumatic day. New capillaries are seen by the end of the first week and are maximal by the third week. Astrocytic reaction is seen by the 10th day, with subsequent glial scar formation.

Pathophysiology

PATHOPHYSIOLOGY OF CLOSED TRAUMATIC BRAIN INJURY. To characterize the pathophysiology of head injury, three approaches are used to separate graded and reproducible subcomponents. The first approach replicates the mechanical forces using synthetic subcomponents with physical properties similar to those of the intracranial contents. The second approach uses cell cultures to provide insight into the cellular response to mechanical injury and enables manipulation of the cellular environment and avoids the confounding effects of anesthetic drugs [24]. In the third approach, production of head injuries in intact animals, confounding variables include species variations, anesthetic agents, muscle relaxants, interlaboratory reproducibility, and the requirement for postinjury intensive care.

Gennarelli and Thibault [25] have categorized current models of injury in intact animals into four groups: (1) free head-impact acceleration (which produces skull fractures and contusions); (2) angular acceleration without impact (the "Penn model"), which produces graded, diffuse injury; (3) fluid-percussion injury, which produces primarily diffuse injuries; and (4) penetrating injury. Fluid-percussion injury produces a graded and reproducible injury that has been adapted for cats [26] and rats [27]. Recent studies of fluid-percussion injury have clarified metabolic responses [28], pathologic changes, such as regional edema [29], loss and recovery of blood-brain barrier function [30], changes in regional cerebral blood flow [31,32], dysfunction of the brainstem [26] and the hippocampus [33], functional recovery of axons [34], impaired recovery from shock [35], and the effects of aging on injury [36]. Immediate physiologic responses to injury include apnea, the duration of which varies directly with the severity of the injury, hypertension, bradycardia, and transient intracranial hypertension. Such models have also been used for evaluation of drugs [37], and treatments such as fetal cell transplantation [38].

The clinical spectrum of anatomic findings in minor, moderate, and severe diffuse brain injuries is best reproduced by either the Penn model or by fluid-percussion injury. Outcome from experimental head trauma correlates with the degree of injury to brain parenchyma, especially the extent of primary axonal injury [25,39]. Axoplasmic transport is impaired even in the absence of axonal "shearing" injuries. Using these animal data, and the clinical pathologic findings of Pilz [40], Povlishock et al. have theorized that traumatic brain injury can be graded histologically in terms of a predictable range of axonal injury patterns [39].

Traumatic brain injury is also associated with gross and microscopic changes in the brain vasculature. Even minor head injury typically disrupts the blood-brain barrier [41]. Blood-brain barrier disruption may represent the most fundamental response of the brain vasculature to injury. Indeed, Povlishock et al. have hypothesized that loss of blood-brain barrier integrity may represent the morphologic substrate for concussion [42].

PATHOPHYSIOLOGY OF PENETRATING BRAIN INJURY. The pathophysiology of penetrating brain injury is best described in reference to specific injury models. In missile-injured cats [43], the duration of injury-induced apnea increased in proportion to the muzzle energy of the projectile. Cats that had suffered penetrating brain injury exhibited transient bradycardia; declining arterial pH and PaO_2; and increased $PaCO_2$, blood glucose, and hematocrit. In missile-wounded monkeys [44], intracranial pressure (ICP) increased immediately to 40 to 60 mm Hg and remained at that level for at least 10 minutes. Blood pressure increased immediately after injury, then quickly declined to hypotensive levels. As cerebral perfusion pressure (CPP) fell, cerebral blood flow (CBF) declined to approximately 60 percent of baseline. In a feline model of fronto-occipital wounding, missile injury led to transient bradypnea, hypertension, and bradycardia in four surviving animals; apnea caused or contributed to death in 10 of the 11 nonsurvivors [45]. Cardiac output and CBF decreased precipitously; ICP abruptly increased sufficiently to produce negative CPP.

Physiologic Responses to Clinical Brain Injury

EXTRACEREBRAL RESPONSES

Systemic Circulatory Responses. Clinical head injury is associated with hypertension, tachycardia, and increased cardiac output. Elevated plasma norepinephrine levels and tachycardia inversely correlate with the initial GCS in patients suffering isolated head injury [46]. Spontaneous extensor (decerebrate) posturing is associated with prominent increases in arterial epinephrine concentrations and cardiac index [47]. Woolf et al. [48] suggested that increased circulating levels of norepinephrine and epinephrine identify patients with low GCS scores who are unlikely to improve rapidly. Beta-adrenergic blockade reduces heart rate and cardiac index and also reduces circulating catecholamines in head-injured patients [49].

In addition to the characteristic hyperdynamic response associated with head injury, hypertension also accompanies severe increases in ICP, a phenomenon first described by Cushing [50]. If permitted to progress, increasing ICP results in medullary failure and hypotension. Management of the Cushing response consists of therapy to reduce ICP, thereby interrupting the reflex response. If systemic hypertension is secondary to the Cushing response, attempts to control blood pressure using vasodilators may both reduce mean arterial pressure and increase ICP, thereby further compromising CPP.

General Metabolic Response to Head Injury.

Head-injured patients typically have stress-induced hyperglycemia and undergo accelerated protein wasting, potentiated by exogenous corticosteroids [51]. Young et al. [52] have described an acute-phase response consisting of leukocytosis, increased hepatic synthesis of acute-phase proteins, and changes in serum levels of zinc, iron, and copper. The frequent occurrence of fever and hypoalbuminemia has been attributed to endothelial cell injury [53].

Pulmonary Effects of Head Injury.

Acute head injury is associated with a variety of respiratory problems [54–58], some of which are potentially fatal. Head injury sufficiently severe to produce coma precipitates apnea in experimental animals and humans [54]. Coma is associated with mechanical upper airway obstruction. Impaired airway reflexes may predispose patients to aspiration of vomitus. Decreased central respiratory responses to hypoxia and hypercarbia may contribute to raised ICP. Patients with multiple injuries may develop impaired gas exchange as a consequence of fat embolism, pulmonary contusion, or hemopneumothorax. Despite absent auscultatory or radiographic evidence of pulmonary compromise, head-injured patients may be hypoxemic, apparently because of failure of mechanisms that regulate ventilation-perfusion matching [57]. Hypoxemia correlates with the location and magnitude of head injury, is associated with increased morbidity and mortality [56], and can potentially magnify head injury [56]. One life-threatening complication of head injury, central neurogenic pulmonary edema, is characterized by the sudden onset of profuse, protein-rich edema [55,58]. Proposed mechanisms include hydrostatic pulmonary edema, secondary to sympathetically mediated systemic and pulmonary hypertension, and changes in capillary permeability [58]. The treatment strategy for neurogenic pulmonary edema requires immediate reduction of ICP (if possible), accompanied by respiratory support, judicious fluid therapy, and blood pressure reduction with agents that do not increase ICP.

Coagulopathy.

Coagulopathy commonly complicates experimental and clinical brain injury [59,60], presumably because thromboplastins, plentiful in brain tissue, are released into the systemic circulation [61]. Laboratory evidence of disseminated intravascular coagulation is reported in nearly one quarter of head-injured patients [62]. Elevated levels of fibrin degradation products correlate with the extent of brain tissue damage and may detect tissue damage that is below the limits of sensitivity of CT scans [63]. Patients with higher concentrations of fibrin degradation products have poorer functional outcomes and are more likely to develop the acute respiratory distress syndrome

[64]. Abnormal hemostasis, particularly prolongation of the activated partial thromboplastin time, correlates with unfavorable outcome and death [65]. Abnormal prothrombin times, partial thromboplastin times, or platelet counts are seen in 55 percent of patients who develop delayed intracranial hematomas [66]. Therefore, Stein et al. recommended early CT follow-up of patients with coagulation abnormalities [66].

CEREBRAL CIRCULATORY RESPONSES TO ACUTE HEAD INJURY.

Pathologic examination of humans dying after head injury discloses evidence of ischemic damage in nearly 90 percent of cases [67]. Many severely head-injured patients have subnormal CBF within the first 8 hours of injury, as determined by measurements using xenon 133 (^{133}Xe) clearance [68]. Cerebral ischemia seems to be an acute cerebrovascular response that tends to resolve within 24 hours [68]. However, many older patients, especially those with diffuse brain injury, demonstrate persistently subnormal CBF of 15 to 20 ml/100 gm/min [69]. The cause of cerebral ischemia remains speculative; however, an 18 to 39 percent incidence of cerebral vasospasm has been documented by angiography [70,71]. One potential implication of this observation is that aggressive treatment of systemic hypertension in the first day after trauma may critically impair pressure-dependent cerebral perfusion. In some head-injured patients, despite apparently adequate CBF, cerebral lactate production is increased; these patients may subsequently progress to cerebral infarction as determined by CT [72]. After traumatic brain injury, the brain becomes even more dependent than is the case normally on aerobic and anaerobic metabolism of glucose [73]; head-injured patients appear to use other cerebral metabolic substrates such as acetoacetate and beta-hydroxybutyrate poorly. Through metabolic autoregulation, pressure autoregulation, CO_2 response, and viscosity autoregulation, the human brain has considerable ability to ensure adequate substrate availability; that ability appears to be compromised by acute trauma.

The uninjured cerebral circulation is responsive to changes in metabolic demand, cerebral perfusion pressure, $PaCO_2$, and PaO_2. Human acute head injury sufficiently severe to produce coma is associated with markedly depressed cerebral metabolic oxygen consumption ($CMRO_2$), moderately decreased CBF, and highly variable autoregulation and reactivity to $PaCO_2$ and PaO_2. Metabolic demand varies directly with body temperature and with the level of brain activation, as evidenced by increases in $CMRO_2$ produced by fever, seizures, or pain. Approximately 50 percent of cerebral energy consumption is required to maintain structural integrity; thus, a $CMRO_2$ of less than 1.6 ml/100 gm/min under normothermic conditions represents a potential threshold for ischemic damage.

Some patients with head injury demonstrate depressed levels of both $CMRO_2$ and CBF, whereas others demonstrate uncoupling, with CBF substantially in excess of $CMRO_2$ [74]. In the majority of comatose, closed-head trauma patients, CBF was less than the normal value of 50 ml/100 gm/min and $CMRO_2$ was well below the normal value of 3.5 ml/100 gm/min [75]. Hyperemia, i.e., CBF exceeding metabolic demand or even exceeding normal values, is common in younger head-injured patients. Nearly 90 percent of patients younger than 18 years of age demonstrate cerebral hyperemia at some point during intensive monitoring [76]. Hyperemia increases cerebral blood volume and decreases intracranial compliance [68].

Those patients in whom reduced CBF appears to represent the expected coupling between low $CMRO_2$ and low CBF may be vulnerable to excessive vasoconstriction during acute hyperventilation. Nearly 20 percent of patients develop a wide cerebral A-VDO_2 during hyperventilation, suggesting that hyperventilation therapy should be accompanied by an estimate of the adequacy of cerebral perfusion [74]. In some patients with severely reduced $CMRO_2$, acute hyperventilation actually increases $CMRO_2$ [77]. Occasionally, hyperventilation may result in local, paradoxic increases in CBF, or a so-called inverse steal [78]. If increased ICP develops in patients with a wide cerebral A-VDO$_2$, mannitol may be more appropriate than further hyperventilation [79]. If CBF measurements are unavailable, calculation of cerebral oxygen extraction or lactate extraction may provide clinically useful information regarding the adequacy of cerebral perfusion [80].

Pressure autoregulation maintains nearly constant CBF over a range of CPP from approximately 50 to approximately 130 mm Hg and helps to preserve CBF despite decreasing CPP. Trauma tends to disrupt pressure autoregulation [68]. DeWitt et al. have demonstrated impaired regional and global autoregulation after experimental fluid-percussion injury [81]. In head-injured patients, CBF may not increase to normal levels even if CPP is high [82]. The integrity of autoregulation cannot be predicted based on ICP, neurologic status, or baseline CBF [75], although intracranial mass lesions are associated with defective autoregulation [75], as are abnormally high or abnormally low CBF in children [83]. In patients with diffuse cortical injuries, CBF is directly proportional to CPP and inversely proportional to ICP [84]. In head-injured patients in whom autoregulation is intact, mannitol reduces ICP and does not change CBF; if autoregulation is defective, ICP changes little and CBF increases [82]. This observation has resulted in speculation regarding whether the normal cerebral circulation also autoregulates in response to changing blood viscosity [82].

In healthy individuals, $PaCO_2$ and PaO_2 exert powerful control over cerebrovascular resistance. Over the range of $PaCO_2$ from 20 to 80 mm Hg, CBF will be acutely halved if $PaCO_2$ is halved and will double if CBF doubles. That relationship, intact in most head-injured patients, necessitates careful monitoring and control of $PaCO_2$. Hyperventilation has been used after head injury to decrease CBF and therefore to decrease cerebral blood volume and ICP. However, the effects of hyperventilation are transient. Moreover, hyperventilation also could reduce CBF below levels necessary to meet metabolic demand or could redistribute CBF away from brain regions that are poorly perfused. PaO_2 exerts little effect on CBF until PaO_2 declines below 60 mm Hg (hemoglobin saturation <90%). Below that level, CBF increases abruptly.

The regional distribution of CBF is more variable in head-injured patients than in healthy individuals [85]. Patients who will die of their injuries or survive in a persistent vegetative state frequently demonstrate regional CBF values less than 20 ml/100 gm/min, especially in the frontal and parietal lobes [85]. Low flow in arterial boundary regions in the frontoparietal cortex, often secondary in high ICP, contributes to poor neurologic outcome [86]. Even in patients who ultimately progress to good recovery, however, CBF may be less than 20 ml/100 gm/min in some brain regions.

Initial Care of the Head Trauma Patient

STABILIZATION. Rapid interventions are critical to the outcome of patients with acute head injury to prevent secondary brain damage. Secondary insults such as anemia, hypotension, hypoxemia, and hypercarbia, alone or in combination, occur in 48 percent of comatose, head-injured patients (Table 175-1) [5]. Respiratory depression and the risk of hypoxemia immedi-

Table 175-1. Influence of Remediable Causes of Secondary Injury on Outcome After Head Injury

Secondary insult	Definition	Poor outcome (%)*
Hypoxemia	PaO$_2$<60 mm Hg	59
Hypotension	SBP<90 mm Hg	65
Anemia	Hct<30%	62
Hypercarbia	PaCO$_2$>45 mm Hg	78
Intracranial	ICP>20, reducible	45
hypertension	ICP>20, not reducible	95

* Poor outcome = severe disability, persistent vegetative state, or death.
Source: Modified from Miller JD, Butterworth JF, Gudeman SK, et al: Further experience in the management of severe head injury. *J Neurosurg* 54:289, 1981, with permission.

ately follow both clinical and experimental severe head injury. Because of impaired cerebral autoregulation after trauma, hypovolemic hypotension that would not otherwise reduce CBF may lead to brain ischemia [87]. Thus, prompt application of basic life support, i.e., tracheal intubation, positive-pressure ventilation with oxygen, and intravenous fluid resuscitation, may limit secondary hypoxic brain damage [54].

Intubation may be difficult because of distortion of normal anatomic landmarks or trismus. Facial fractures constitute a relative contraindication to nasotracheal intubation. Fiberoptic intubation, cricothyroidotomy, transcricothyroid oxygen insufflation, or formal tracheostomy may be required. The laryngeal mask airway, though no protection against aspiration of vomitus, merits evaluation as a tool in emergency airway management of head-injured patients. Whether prehospital emergency personnel should attempt to facilitate endotracheal intubation through the use of relaxants and sedatives, which could further impair ventilation and confound subsequent neurologic evaluation, is controversial.

There is legitimate concern that the depolarizing muscle relaxant succinylcholine may aggravate intracranial hypertension [88,89]. However, clinicians caring for acutely injured patients should not lose sight of the overall goal of preventing secondary hypoxic brain damage. If the more rapid onset of succinylcholine, compared with nondepolarizing muscle relaxants, appears necessary for immediate intubation of an unstable patient, it should be used. After intubation, the patient should be ventilated with an oxygen-enriched gas mixture. Minute ventilation should be adjusted to maintain $PaCO_2$ at 40 mm Hg or less (see the following section). Although routine hyperventilation has been advocated, current data suggest that this practice may be deleterious [90].

In patients with multiple trauma and head injury, no resuscitation fluid has proved ideal. Animal studies have demonstrated lower ICP or higher CBF when hypertonic saline solutions are substituted for isotonic fluids (Fig. 175-1) [91–95]. Clearly, hypotonic solutions, which increase brain tissue volume, should be avoided. In this regard, lactated Ringer's solution is slightly hypotonic relative to plasma, whereas 0.9% saline is slightly hypertonic. The role of colloid-containing solutions is also controversial. Administration of dextran-40 for resuscitation of animals with intracranial mass lesions and hemorrhagic shock increases ICP to the same extent as saline solutions, although the increase occurs later with dextran-40 [93].

Whether hypotension in the setting of severe traumatic brain injury should be treated temporarily using pneumatic antishock trousers remains unclear. Studies indicate that inflation of antishock trousers modestly increases ICP in head trauma patients in whom ICP is less than 20 mm Hg [96]. In *conscious* trauma

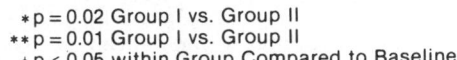

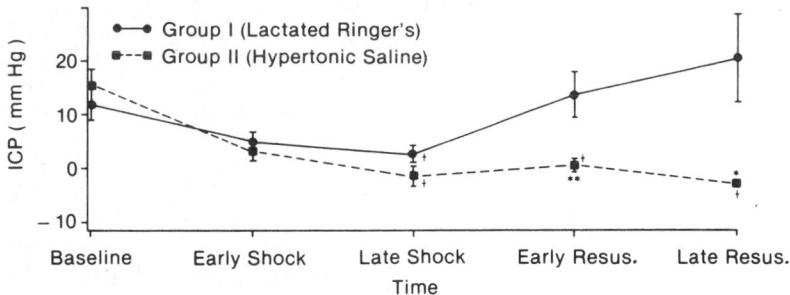

Fig. 175-1. Response of ICP to resuscitation from shock with lactated Ringer's solution or 7.5% hypertonic saline. After a 30-minute interval of hemorrhagic shock at a mean arterial pressure of 50 mm Hg, extending from early shock to late shock, rapid resuscitation with 6.0 ml per kilogram of 7.5% saline maintained ICP at the levels present during shock. In contrast, resuscitation with 60 ml per kilogram of lactated Ringer's solution increased ICP to a level in excess of baseline. (From Prough DS, Johnson JC, Stump DA, et al: Effects of hypertonic saline versus lactated Ringer's solution on cerebral oxygen transport during resuscitation from hemorrhagic shock. *J Neurosurg* 64:627, 1986, with permission.)

victims (who rarely demonstrate intracranial hypertension), the device seems suitable for short-term support of blood pressure. In contrast, ICP may exceed 20 mm Hg in 60 percent of *comatose* patients [5]. However, the acutely injured brain is extremely vulnerable to inadequate perfusion, whether from intracranial hypertension (which is not detected readily in the field) or arterial hypotension (which is easily diagnosed). Therefore, antishock trousers may be justified while the hypotensive head trauma victim is transported to a trauma center for definitive evaluation and treatment.

DIAGNOSTIC ASSESSMENT. Initial neurologic assessment provides information about the site and location of injury, the need for urgent therapeutic intervention, and prognosis. Skull fractures indicate considerable impact, provide an important marker of the site of injury, and increase the possibility of an intracranial hematoma. Skull fractures also may serve as the site of CSF leaks and bacterial contamination, may produce cranial nerve palsies, and may become the site of brain tissue herniation. Basilar skull fractures produce a variety of clinical signs: hemotympanum (blood behind the tympanic membrane), Battle's sign (ecchymosis over the mastoid), or the raccoon sign (periorbital ecchymosis). Basilar skull fractures can damage cranial nerves, transect the hypothalamic hypophyseal axis, and cause CSF rhinorrhea, CSF otorrhea, or meningitis. Compound skull fractures predispose to meningitis and thus require prompt surgical debridement.

The neurologic examination, preferably conducted before induction of neuromuscular paralysis, should include the GCS, a reliable index of overall brain function and level of consciousness with minimal interobserver variability (Table 175-2) [97]. Response to pain is essential in assessing patients who make no verbal responses. Because consciousness waxes and wanes, the painful stimuli must be severe enough to elicit a response. Motor responses are lost in the following sequence: obeying commands, localization of pain, withdrawal to pain, flexion to pain, and extension to pain. The likelihood of severe morbidity

and mortality increases substantially in patients who have abnormal posturing. Neurologic outcome may be better in children than in adults who have abnormal posturing, although this assertion has been challenged [98].

Because the GCS does not provide information regarding brainstem functions, pupillary responses, corneal reflexes, ocular muscle function, and respiratory function also should be assessed. Pupillary light responses in comatose patients assist in establishing prognosis [97,99,100]. In paralyzed, intubated patients, the pupillary reaction provides the only clinical means for neurologic assessment. Transtentorial herniation compresses the superficial parasympathetic fibers of the third nerve, resulting in ipsilateral pupillary dilation. Bilateral dilated pupils constitute a grave prognostic sign. Pupillary examination may be difficult in the presence of an associated orbital hematoma or erroneous with direct ocular or optic trauma. Corneal reflexes, important for protection of the eyes, are lost early after traumatic brain injury and have little prognostic significance.

Both the oculovestibular and the oculocephalic reflexes require the integrity of the third, fourth, and sixth cranial nerves, the medial longitudinal fasciculus, the eighth nerve afferents, and an intact brainstem. The oculocephalic reflex requires movement of the neck and is hence inappropriate in the pres-

Table 175-2. Glasgow Coma Scale

Component	Response	Score
Eye opening	Spontaneously	4
	To verbal command	3
	To pain	2
	None	1
		Subtotal: 1–4
Motor response (best extremity)	Obeys verbal command	6
	Localizes pain	5
	Flexion-withdrawal	4
	Flexor (decorticate posturing)	3
	Extensor (decerebrate posturing)	2
	No response (flaccid)	1
		Subtotal: 1–6
Best verbal response	Oriented and converses	5
	Disoriented and converses	4
	Inappropriate words	3
	Incomprehensible sounds	2
	No verbal response	1
		Subtotal: 1–5
		Total: 3–15

ence of a cervical spine injury. The normal oculocephalic response, tested by abruptly rocking the head from right to left, is maintenance of the direction of gaze despite a shift in head position. If a normal oculocephalic ("doll's eyes") response cannot or should not be elicited, the normal vestibuloocular (ice-water caloric) response of a comatose patient to irrigation of the external ear canal with 10 to 20 ml of ice-cold water should be tonic gaze deviation of both eyes to the ipsilateral side [101]. The oculovestibular response requires a patent external auditory canal. Initial syringing with measured cold saline should be performed with the head in a neutral position if cervical spine injury is a consideration; however, neck flexion of 30 degrees may be required if the reflex is impaired. Impaired oculocephalic and oculovestibular reflexes are grave prognostic signs.

Diagnostic priorities for patients who obey commands after head injury should proceed as indicated by the description of the traumatic event and by the general physical examination. In all comatose, head-injured patients, unless they are known to have suffered *only* an isolated head injury, diagnostic peritoneal lavage [102] or abdominal CT scan should be performed to detect occult intraabdominal injury. Likewise, a radiologic survey is helpful to exclude unsuspected skeletal injury [103]. Because 7 percent of patients with severe head injury have a coincident cervical spine injury [104], patients should be considered to have cervical spine fractures until this possibility has been excluded by a cross-table lateral neck radiograph (or a cervical CT scan) that adequately shows all cervical vertebrae. Clearly, the highest priority for comatose, head-injured patients is to determine the need for craniotomy. Patients who require evacuation of subdural hematomas but in whom craniotomy is delayed have a far worse outcome than those patients in whom hematomas are promptly evacuated [105].

Shock accompanying head trauma is a diagnostic challenge (see Chap. 171). Although shock sometimes occurs in association with an isolated head injury, other causes of hypotension must be excluded [102]. These include intraabdominal hemorrhage (evaluated by CT scan or diagnostic peritoneal lavage), intrathoracic hemorrhage (evaluated by chest radiography, CT scan, or aortography), long-bone fractures (assessed using the skeletal survey), myocardial ischemia or cardiac decompensation (evaluated using electrocardiography or pulmonary arterial catheterization), pericardial tamponade (suggested by a paradoxical pulse, central venous or pulmonary artery pressure monitoring, chest radiography, echocardiography, or pericardiocentesis), and, particularly in children, intracranial or scalp hemorrhage (evident from CT scan or inspection).

Occasionally during initial diagnostic evaluation, neurologic function may abruptly deteriorate. If the diagnosis of epidural hematoma is highly likely (e.g., a temporal bone fracture with a dilated ipsilateral pupil and contralateral hemiparesis), it may be appropriate to place a burr hole empirically while still in the emergency department. More often, preferable management consists of an emergent "single cut" CT scan to visualize the lateral ventricles and any brain shift (and, perhaps, the clot producing the brain shift), followed by immediate transport to the operating room for a craniotomy under controlled circumstances. If the diagnosis is correct, empirical drainage of an epidural hematoma may be lifesaving. If incorrect, burr hole placement may delay definitive diagnostic studies and treatment of other lesions (e.g., bilateral intracranial hematomas), thereby endangering the patient.

CLINICAL ESTIMATION OF INTRACRANIAL PRESSURE. The symptoms and signs of raised ICP are not uniformly reliable. A patient able to follow simple commands, even if stupor-

ous or lethargic, rarely has a raised ICP, but 40 to 50 percent of head-injured patients with altered consciousness have intracranial hypertension. In unconscious patients, the probability of increased ICP is lower if the patient withdraws to painful stimuli, moans, or grimaces. A frankly raised ICP is likely to be encountered with a GCS score of 4 to 6. Severe increases in ICP may present as Cushing's triad of hypertension, bradycardia, and respiratory irregularity. Pupillary dilatation may herald transentorial herniation, but is a late manifestation of central herniation [101].

Transport of Head-Injured Patients

Trauma patients require transport from accident scenes to hospitals and often require transfer from one institution to another or from one department to another (i.e., from the Emergency Department to Radiology). During transport, problems such as hypoxemia or hypotension can produce secondary brain injury, influence the choice of diagnostic procedures, or alter therapeutic interventions. It is reasonable to assume that any patient reaching the hospital with a GCS score ≤ 8 has a severe, bilateral, cortical injury or an intracranial mass lesion and is at risk for intracranial hypertension. Therefore, the goal during transport of head-injured patients is to prevent further deterioration from preventable secondary insults. Activities during transport are directed at stabilization of vital signs, close observation of neurologic status, and preservation of adequate CPP and pulmonary gas exchange. The logistics of transport should minimize transportation time from the scene to the hospital, between hospitals, or within hospitals.

INTERINSTITUTIONAL TRANSPORT. Gentleman and Jennett audited interinstitutional transfers and concluded that the major cause of avoidable deaths occurred within the hospital system itself and not during prehospital care [106]. They found a 15 percent incidence of hypoxia, a 7 percent incidence of hypotension, and a failure to diagnose extracranial injuries. Forty-two percent of comatose patients did not have an endotracheal tube when transferred to a referral head injury center. These authors advocated a checklist for interinstitutional transfers (Table 175-3).

INTRAHOSPITAL TRANSPORT. For neurosurgical patients who require transport from an intensive care unit to another location in the hospital, high-quality intensive care must be maintained throughout transport. Adequate ventilation and oxygenation must be assured, often with the use of a portable ventilator. Invasive vascular and ICP monitoring must be continued; transducers must be "zeroed" and calibrated in positions appropriate for transport.

Radiology of Head Trauma

Head-injured patients must undergo prompt assessment of the nature and extent of injury so that appropriate treatment can be instituted. The choice among radiologic studies depends on the clinical presentation. Skull radiographs have a very limited

Table 175-3. Checklist Before Transfer of Severely Head-Injured Patients

System	Checklist
Respiration	Airway adequately protected? $PaO_2 \geq 100$ mm Hg? $PaCO_2 \leq 40$ mm Hg? Airway clear?
Circulation	Systolic BP ≥ 120 mm Hg? Peripheral perfusion adequate? Reliable venous access?
Head injury	Glasgow Coma Scale score? Trend of GCS score? Focal neurologic signs?
Other injuries	Cervical spine injury, chest injury, pneumothorax, broken ribs? Suspected intrathoracic or intraabdominal bleed? Pelvic or long-bone fractures? Have extracranial injuries been splinted? (e.g. cervical collar, limb splints)
Escort	Escorting personnel experienced? Escorting personnel familiar with the patient? Appropriate drugs and equipment? Records available?

Modified from Gentleman D, Jennett B: Audit of transfer of unconscious head-injured patients to a neurosurgical unit. *Lancet* 335:330, 1990, with permission.

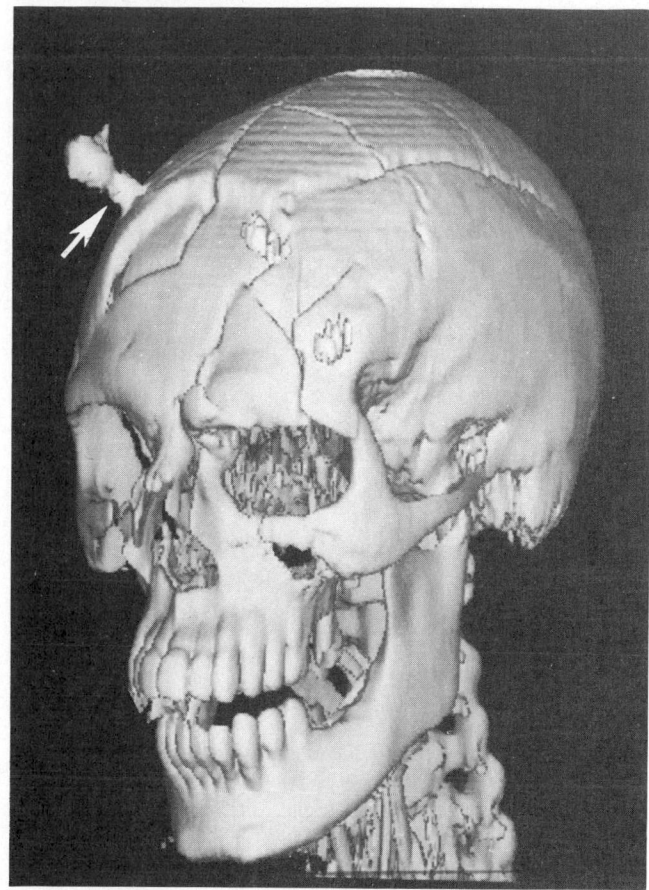

Fig. 175-2. Three-dimensional reconstructions of computed tomographic skull images can clearly illustrate skull fractures. The arrow indicates the location of an intracranial pressure monitor. Just inferior to the monitor is a large depressed skull fracture.

role in evaluating skull fractures [107,108]; they have now been supplanted by CT. With improvement in software technology, reformatted and three-dimensional images of the skull can be obtained if necessary (Fig. 175-2). Patients who have lost consciousness, but subsequently have a completely normal neurologic examination, do not need a CT scan in the absence of other clinical indications (e.g., clinical evidence of skull fracture). All patients who do not obey simple commands (in the absence of drug or alcohol intoxication) are severely injured and require prompt CT scanning to exclude intracranial hematoma. The management of patients who fall between these two conditions is problematic [109]. In North America, most such patients receive a CT scan [20,21].

For high-risk patients, emergency CT examination and neurosurgical consultation are indicated [110]. CT remains the undisputed initial step in determining whether surgical evacuation of a hematoma is indicated [111–114]. However, CT cannot resolve nonhemorrhagic sequelae of trauma such as shearing injuries of the white matter, small infarcts of the hypothalamus and brainstem, and small superficial cortical contusions; MRI has proven superior to CT in demonstrating these abnormalities [115–118]. The limitations of MRI are related to availability, longer scanning time, difficulty in monitoring critically ill patients who are on life-support devices, and inability to reliably demonstrate acute subarachnoid hemorrhage with conventional pulsing techniques [119,120].

SKULL FRACTURES. Skull fractures do not imply brain injury, although depressed skull fractures are notorious for causing cortical contusions and lacerations. Skull fractures that are significant because of their nature and location include fractures through the frontal sinus and cribriform plate, which serve as a pathway for infection, and basal skull fractures, which may cause cranial nerve impingement resulting in nerve palsies [121] or may cause damage to the entering vertebral or carotid arteries [122].

SUBDURAL HEMATOMA. Subdural hematoma results from rupture of veins that bridge the subdural space between the cortex and dural sinus. The lack of firm adherence of the arachnoid membrane to dura allows the hematoma to spread and assume a crescentic shape (Fig. 175-3). The CT appearance of a subdural hematoma is hyperdense during the acute phase (1–3 days), becomes isodense during the subacute stage (3–14 days), and then becomes lucent in the chronic phase (≥ 2 weeks). Subdural hematomas develop most frequently over the frontoparietal convexity and less commonly over the subtemporal, peritentorial interhemispheric, and vertex areas. On MRI scans, subdural hematomas are best demonstrated during the subacute and chronic stages, when the hematoma appears bright on the T1-weighted image [123] (Fig. 175-4).

EPIDURAL HEMATOMA. A fracture that tears a meningeal artery results in hemorrhage between the inner table of the skull and dura, producing an epidural hematoma. Rarely, epidural hematoma is the result of a venous bleed [124]. The close adherence of the dura to the inner table of the skull resists peripheral enlargement, thereby imparting the characteristic lenticular configuration [125], bulging inward toward the brain (Fig. 175-5).

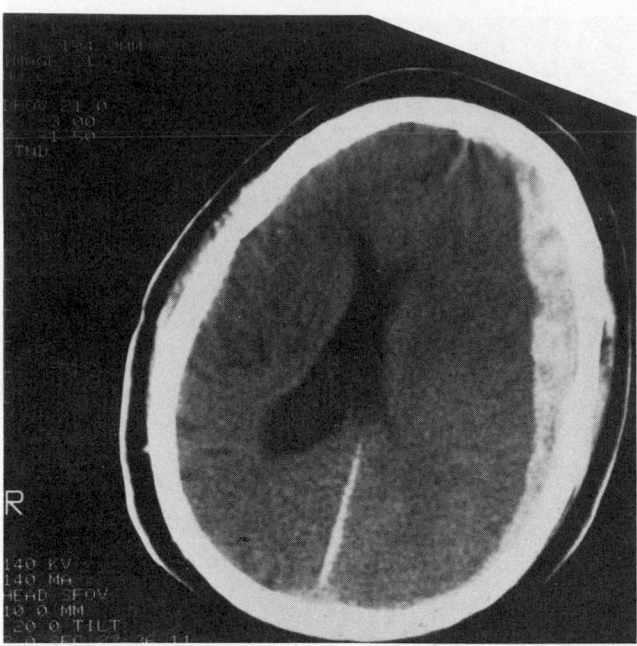

Fig. 175-3. On a computed tomographic scan, a large, posttraumatic subdural hematoma adjacent to the left cerebral hemisphere illustrates the typical crescentic shape. Note the compression of the left lateral ventricle and the shift of the midline structures toward the right side. (Courtesy of Dr. John Howard, Department of Radiology, Bowman Gray School of Medicine.)

CONTUSION. Contusions are superficial cortical bruises characterized by petechial hemorrhages and torn capillaries, along with evidence of mechanical damage to adjacent neurons [121,126]. Commonly found adjacent to roughened edges of the inner table of the skull, contusions appear on CT scans as multiple punctate blood-density lesions with prominent zones of surrounding edema (Fig. 175-6). MRI detects 98 percent of brain contusions compared with only 56 percent by CT [127].

INTRACEREBRAL HEMATOMA. Hematoma formation deep in the parenchyma may be an extension of a contusion or may arise from rupture of corticomedullary vessels [128]. Intracerebral hematomas are easily demonstrated with either CT or MRI.

SUBARACHNOID HEMORRHAGE. As a consequence of contusional injury, veins and arteries on the pia and arachnoid membrane may rupture and bleed into the subarachnoid space. This type of hemorrhage is best demonstrated with CT.

DELAYED INTRACRANIAL HEMATOMA. Lipper et al. [129] reported an incidence of 8.4 percent and a death rate of 50 percent in patients who develop delayed intracranial hematomas, as compared with an overall 30 percent mortality in a series of head-injured patients. The mechanism suggested for development of delayed hematoma is a local failure, owing to contusion, of the mechanisms that regulate CBF [130]. Figure 175-7 illustrates a hematoma recognized 1 week after head injury.

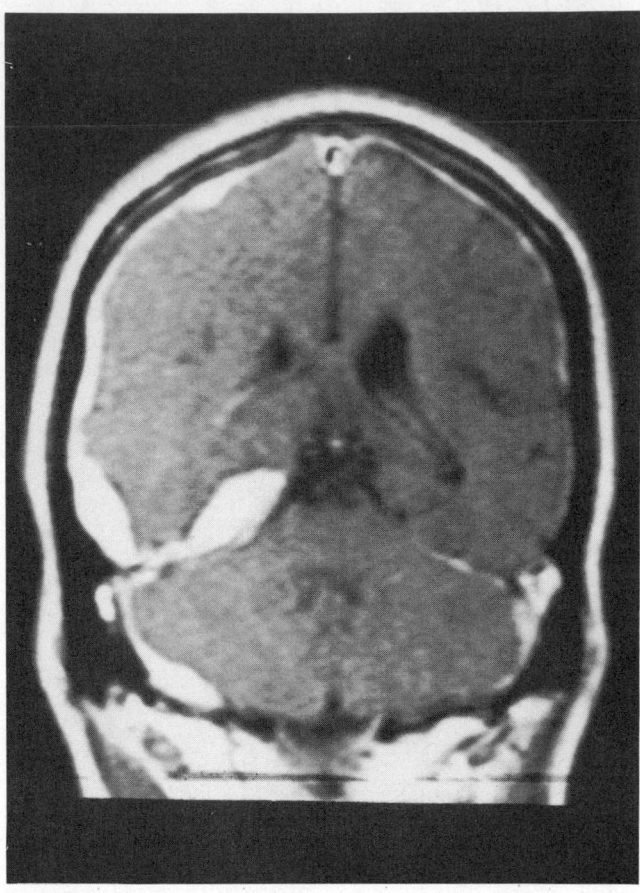

Fig. 175-4. On a T1-weighted magnetic resonance image, a subacute subdural hematoma appears brightly silhouetted adjacent to the right cerebral hemisphere.

BRAIN EDEMA. After mechanical trauma to the brain, there is often loss of vascular integrity with extravasation of plasma proteins and fluid into the extracellular space [131]. Brain edema becomes manifest on CT as early as 3 to 5 hours after insult but appears most intense in 12 to 24 hours [132]. The most reliable sign of brain edema is obliteration of the mesencephalic cistern [133].

DESCENDING TRANSTENTORIAL HERNIATION. Uncal herniation can directly compress the brainstem, causing hemorrhage, and may compress the posterior cerebral artery as it crosses the free margin of the tentorium, leading to occipital lobe infarction [134,135]. Hematomas within or adjacent to the temporal lobe are more likely to cause transtentorial herniation than those located in a more remote site. The CT manifestations of uncal herniation include dislocation of the brainstem and its accompanying blood vessels along with distortion of the adjacent cisterns. An indirect but reliable sign of herniation is dilatation of the contralateral temporal horn [136].

POSTERIOR FOSSA TRAUMA. Although traumatic hematomas of the posterior fossa are relatively rare (3.3% incidence) [137], even small acute mass lesions can severely compromise

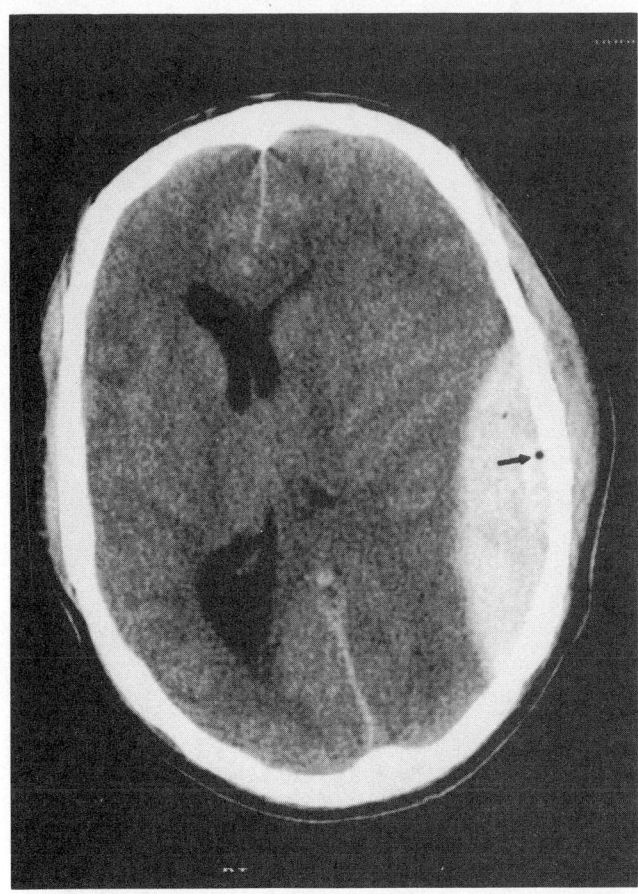

Fig. 175-5. On a computed tomographic scan, a left epidural hematoma assumes the classic biconvex lenticular shape adjacent to the left hemisphere. The arrow shows the approximate location of the middle meningeal artery.

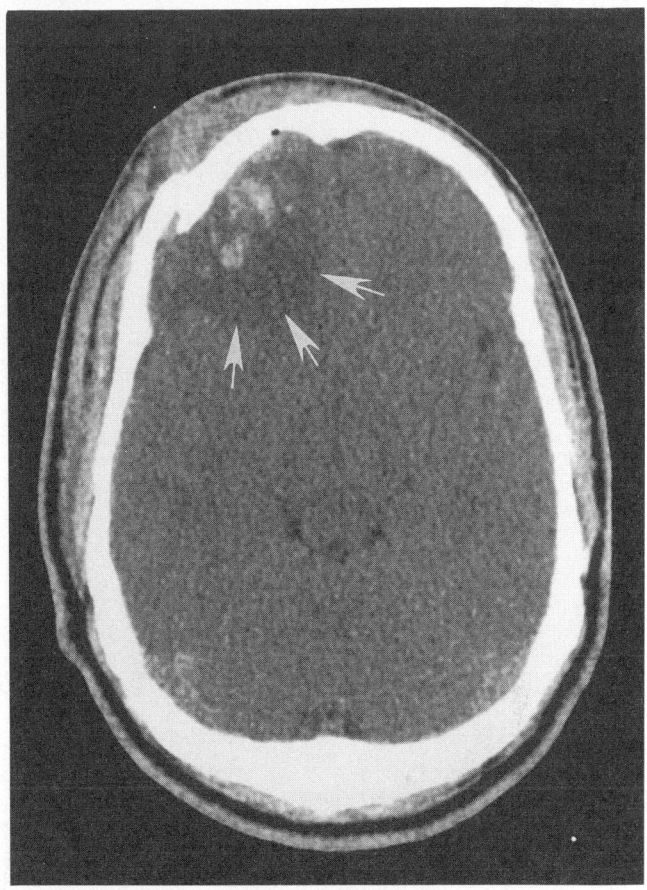

Fig. 175-6. On a computed tomographic scan, a right cortical contusion includes both punctate blood-density lesions and surrounding edema (arrows).

brainstem functions, resulting in rapid neurologic deterioration. Therefore, hematomas in this location represent neurosurgical emergencies [138–142]. Parenchymal and extraaxial hematomas of the posterior fossa are easily recognized on CT.

RADIOLOGY OF PEDIATRIC HEAD TRAUMA. The pattern of brain injury in younger children differs from that occurring in older persons because of differences in mechanisms, injury thresholds, and the frequency of child abuse [143]. The child's skull is malleable and the brain is more deformable, allowing for greater distortion to occur between the cranium and the cerebral hemispheres [121]. This mechanism may explain the greater frequency of hematoma formation in the posterior fossa and peritentorial areas among these children [144].

The so-called whiplash type of injury often associated with child abuse is a major cause of brain damage in children younger than 2 years of age [145]. Subdural hematoma in the interhemispheric fissure (Fig. 175-8), bilateral or multiple skull fractures, and fractures that cross the sutures are characteristic radiologic features of this syndrome [146–149]. CT remains the primary screening method to demonstrate lesions amenable to surgery.

PROGNOSTIC VALUE OF RADIOGRAPHIC PROCEDURES. Eighty percent of patients who have a normal CT scan on admission have good outcomes; 67 percent of patients who have both intraparenchymal and extraparenchymal lesions on CT have poor outcomes; and 75 percent of patients with bilateral hemorrhagic lesions progress to a persistent vegetative state or death [150]. Other ominous CT or MRI findings are large hematomas [151], acute brain edema in children [133], and shearing injuries of the corpus callosum and brainstem [152].

Management in the ICU

The survival of patients with severe closed head injury, with or without injuries to other organ systems, depends on prolonged, high-quality intensive care. The primary goals of management in the ICU are to prevent secondary neurologic injury and limit complications that develop in other organ systems. By preventing secondary brain damage, the percentage of "good recoveries" in patients with GCS scores ≥4 can be increased from 15 percent to 52 percent [153].

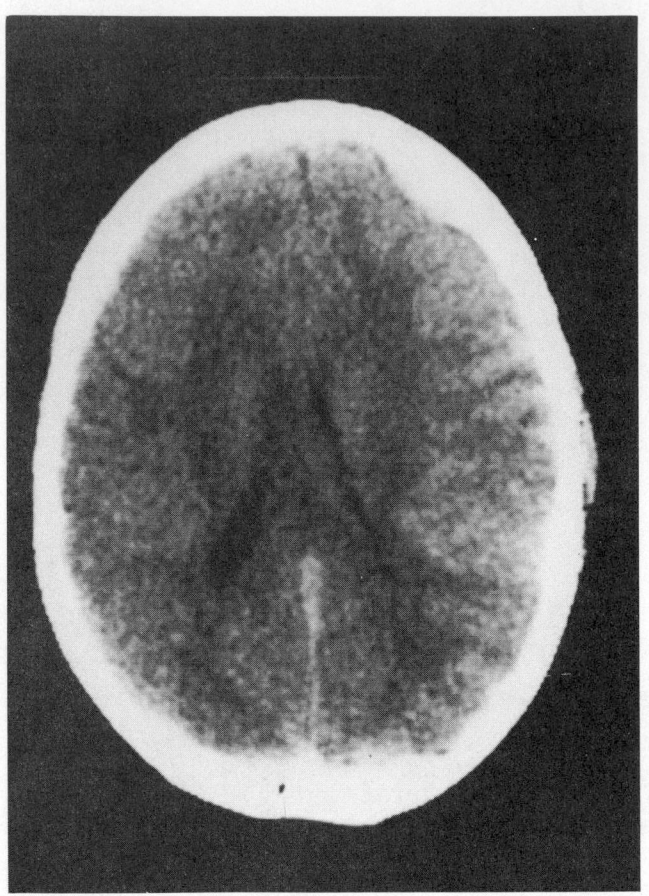

A

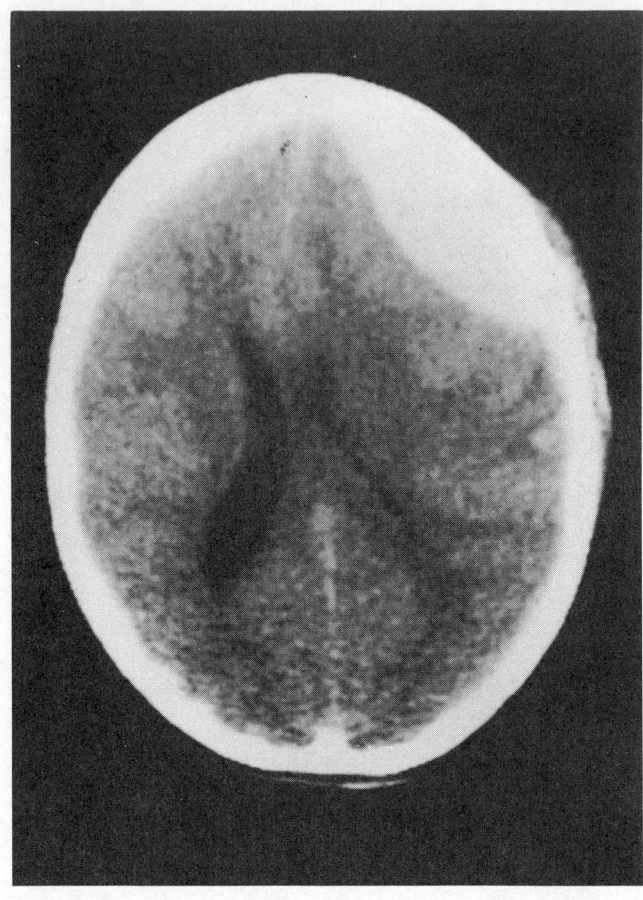

B

Fig. 175-7. On an immediate postadmission computed tomographic scan, no hematoma is evident (A); on a scan 1 week later, a delayed hematoma is evident (B).

GENERAL SUPPORTIVE CARE. The essential elements of general supportive care include airway support, administration of fluids, provision of sedation and analgesia, careful head positioning, and frequent turning. If airway reflexes are impaired by brainstem injury or coma, intubation may prevent aspiration and reduce the likelihood of hypoxemia or hypocapnia, both potentially deleterious to the injured brain. Pulse oximetry and capnography facilitate prompt detection of hypoxemia or hypercarbia. Most clinicians restrict fluids to 50 to 75 percent of calculated maintenance, despite the lack of evidence that the rate of administration of maintenance fluids exerts clinically important effects on ICP. Because agitation or pain increases $CMRO_2$ and CBF and can precipitate intracranial hypertension, adequate analgesia is particularly important in head-injured patients with other painful injuries, such as surgical wounds or fractured long bones or ribs. Neuromuscular blockade necessitates generous, empirical administration of sedatives and analgesics.

The head should not be rotated excessively. Although compression of the jugular venous system by head rotation produces no change in ICP in normal individuals, it may impede cerebral venous drainage and increase ICP in those with reduced intracranial compliance. Despite the possibility that head elevation will reduce CPP [154], most clinicians maintain patients with acute head injury in a 15 to 30 degrees head-up position.

An essential aspect of the nursing care of head-injured patients is frequent, systematic turning from the right lateral decubitus position to the supine to the left lateral decubitus position. This reduces decubitus ulceration and pulmonary retention of secretions. If increases in ICP, induced by turning, prevent adequate positioning, the use of a laterally rotating kinetic bed may both facilitate pulmonary toilet and limit the incidence of decubitus ulcers. Continuous rotation therapy does not result in deleterious increases in ICP in brain-injured patients [155]. In patients who do not require the kinetic bed, appropriate skin care includes the use of a low-pressure mattress pad.

CEREBRAL CIRCULATORY CONSIDERATIONS. As noted previously, the traumatized brain is uniquely vulnerable to hypoxemia and hypotension and may have markedly disturbed, regionally variable responses to changes in blood pressure. Although much of the management of acute head injury patients is intended to maintain appropriate levels of CBF, neither CBF nor any other cerebral circulatory variable, such as jugular venous bulb PaO_2 or hemoglobin saturation, is routinely measured. Most cerebral circulatory information is inferred from mean arterial pressure (MAP), $PaCO_2$, and ICP. Measurement

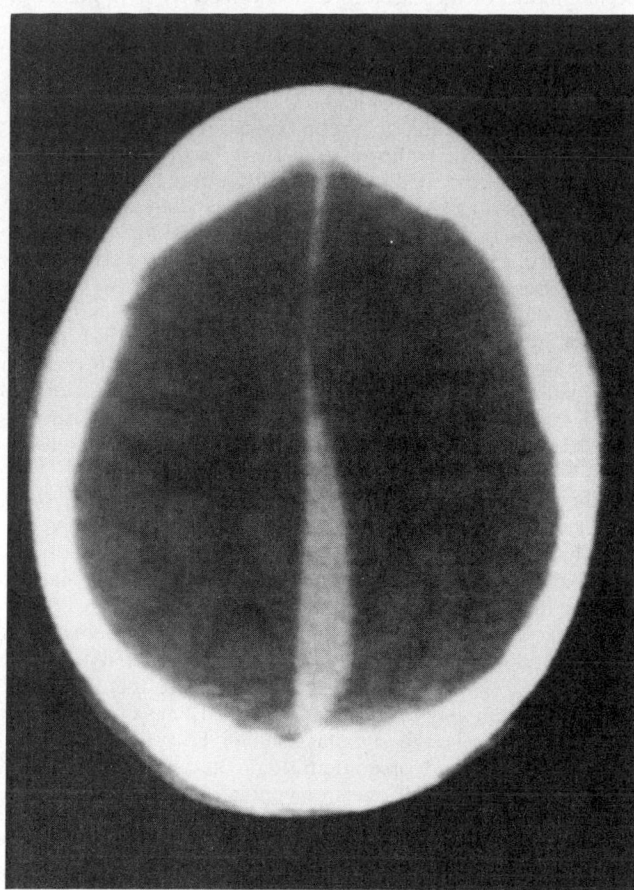

Fig. 175-8. On a computed tomographic scan, an interhemispheric hematoma is evident in a child who was a victim of suspected child abuse.

of ICP, combined with measurement of MAP, permits calculation of CPP according to the equation:

$$CPP = MAP - ICP$$

Rosner and Daughton [156] have suggested that therapy of head-injured patients should be directed toward maintaining CPP, with proportionately less attention directed at reducing ICP.

MANAGEMENT OF INTRACRANIAL HYPERTENSION. Because the skull is rigid, and brain, cerebrospinal fluid, and blood are incompressible, addition of sufficient volume to the intracranial compartment ultimately exceeds the limited compensatory capacity of the cranial vault and increases ICP. Langfitt et al. [157] originally described the brain elastance curve produced by gradually adding volume to the intracranial space. Lundberg et al. [158] popularized the concept that ICP monitoring could be used to facilitate management of patients at risk for intracranial hypertension. Through extensive monitoring of ventricular fluid pressure in patients who had chronic intracranial mass lesions, they demonstrated that ICP is subject to periodic wave phenomena. The most dangerous, plateau waves, which often precipitate acute neurologic deterioration, appear

to result from cerebral vasodilation (Fig. 175-9) [159] and increased cerebral hemispheric blood volume, resulting subsequently in a decline in CBF [160]. In more than one third of patients, ICP with severe brain trauma exceeds 20 mm Hg during monitoring and is an important correlate of increased morbidity and death [161]. Consequently, 20 mm Hg is commonly employed as a threshold for intervention. ICP monitoring has been associated by some investigators with more favorable outcome in patients with severe head injury [5,13,161,162,163]. Others are more skeptical about the value of ICP monitoring in improving outcome after acute head trauma in many types of patients [164,165]. No definitive randomized trial has compared outcome with and without ICP monitoring.

The perceived risk of ventricular cannulation inhibited widespread application of ICP monitoring until the development of the subarachnoid bolt [166]. Although the subarachnoid bolt occasionally generates erroneous information [167,168], measurement of ICP is usually considered to be a fundamental part of the care of patients with severe closed head injury (GCS ≤8) [169]. Measurement at any supratentorial site appears to provide equivalent information [170]. A practical, reliable fiberoptic ICP monitor has been developed (Camino Laboratories, San Diego, CA). This transducer-tipped monitor works well as an intraventricular, subdural, or brain tissue monitor [171] and demonstrates relatively little drift of calibration over periods of 5 days or less [172].

Numerous authors have investigated ways in which the clinical value of ICP monitoring could be enhanced. The pressure volume index (PVI) can be calculated by removing or adding volume to CSF through a ventricular cannula according to the equation:

$$PVI = \frac{V}{\log P_0/P_{m \text{ or } p}}$$

Fig. 175-9. Plateau wave during intracranial pressure recording. Shortly after receiving Pavulon (pancuronium) 0.4 mg IV, systemic arterial pressure declined slightly. Almost immediately, intracranial pressure increased dramatically, causing a marked decline in cerebral perfusion pressure. (From Rosner MJ, Becker DP: Origin and evolution of plateau waves: Experimental observations and a theoretical model. *J Neurosurg* 60:312, 1984, with permission.)

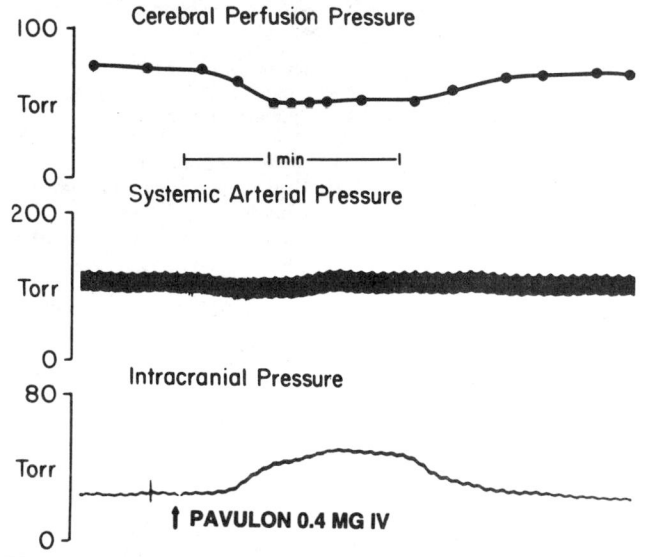

where V = the volume withdrawn or injected; P_0 = the pressure before withdrawing or injecting fluid; P_m = the minimum pressure after fluid withdrawal, and P_p = the peak pressure after volume addition. A lower PVI, implying reduced brain compliance, is associated with the subsequent development of intracranial hypertension and with poorer neurologic outcome [173]. The critical value for PVI appears to be approximately 13 ml, below which level treatment is likely to be necessary either to reduce ventricular fluid pressure or to improve compliance [174]. If the PVI is less than 10 ml, reduction of ICP is nearly always required. Robertson et al. [175] correlated the PVI with a computerized frequency analysis of the ICP waveform in 55 severely head-injured patients and determined that this continuous technique provided information that correlated very highly with the PVI, provided earlier evidence of changes in intracranial compliance than ICP alone, and did not require manipulation of intracranial fluid volume.

Intracranial hypertension or reduced intracranial compliance can be managed using a variety of strategies, all of which are based on the central concept that reduction of ICP or improvement of intracranial compliance can be accomplished by reducing one of the three intracranial constituents: blood volume, tissue volume, or cerebrospinal fluid volume (Table 175-4).

Increased intracranial blood volume can increase ICP primarily and also may increase the "tightness" of brain tissue (decrease brain elastance). Cerebral blood volume can be reduced using several techniques. Endotracheal intubation limits

Table 175-4. Strategies for Controlling ICP

Strategy	Mechanism
Reduction of cerebral blood volume	
Endotracheal intubation*	Prevent hypoxemia or hypercarbia
Passive hyperventilation*	Reduce CBF
Neuromuscular blockade*	Prevent increased cerebral venous volume secondary to coughing or straining
Head elevation*	Facilitate cerebral venous drainage
Sedation/analgesia*	Reduce increased CMRO$_2$ and CBF secondary to noxious stimuli
Fever control	Avoid CMRO$_2$ and CBF increases
Barbiturates*	Reduce CMRO$_2$, CBF, and ICP
Reduction of brain tissue volume	
Osmotic diuresis	Reduce brain water in normal bain
Fluid restriction†	Limit accumulation of brain water
Temporal lobectomy	Removed contused brain tissue
Hypertonic saline*	Reduced brain water in normal brain
Glucocorticoids†	Decrease brain edema (ineffective)
Reduction of CSF volume	
Ventricular cannulation*	Remove CSF
Acetazolamide†	Limit CSF production
Increase cranial compliance	
Subtemporal decompression*	Reduce brain volume and provide alternate route for herniation of edematous brain

* Controversial.
† Little or no demonstrable benefit.
ICP = intracranial pressure; CBF = cerebral blood flow; CMRO$_2$ = cerebral metabolic rate for oxygen; CSF = cerebrospinal fluid.

the likelihood of increases in CBF induced by hypoxemia or hypercarbia. Neuromuscular blockade prevents increases in cerebral venous volume as a consequence of coughing, straining, or actively exhaling. Head elevation facilitates cerebral venous drainage and, in volume-replete patients, does not adversely affect CPP, CBF, or cerebral metabolic parameters [176]. However, in hypovolemic patients, by reducing venous return, cardiac output, and MAP, head elevation may actually reduce CPP [154]. Adequate sedation and analgesia attenuate increases in CMRO$_2$ and CBF produced by painful or noxious stimulation.

Control of fever limits increases in CMRO$_2$ and the accompanying increases in CBF. The CMRO$_2$ may increase dramatically in decerebrate patients during fever [177]. Stress responses, infections, pontine injuries, or autonomic dysfunction accompanying bilateral frontal damage may cause fever, but other causes must be considered. Recently, as a result of experimental evidence that hypothermia reduces neurologic injury, therapeutic interest in cerebral hypothermia is increasing [178,179].

Although hypocarbia acutely reduces CBF, cerebral blood volume, and ICP, the therapeutic value of routine hyperventilation has been debated. The popularity of hyperventilation has been based on the circular assumption that hyperventilation, by reducing CBF, will reduce ICP, thereby preserving CPP and CBF. Although there is little question that severe increases in ICP may reduce CPP sufficiently to produce regional or global cerebral hypoperfusion, there is also evidence that excessive hyperventilation may lead to inadequate CBF, as evidenced by excessive cerebral oxygen extraction [74]. Empirical hyperventilation may actually worsen neurologic outcome and mortality compared with normal levels of ventilation [90]. Because the loss of CSF bicarbonate that occurs over 8 to 24 hours of hyperventilation limits the duration of ICP reduction, the buffer tromethamine (THAM) has been added to hyperventilation in a controlled, randomized, clinical trial comparing normal ventilation (PaCO$_2$ 35 ± 2 mm Hg) with hyperventilation (PaCO$_2$ 25 ± 2 mm Hg), with or without THAM [90]. THAM prevented the hyperventilation-associated deterioration in the Glasgow Outcome Score at 3, 6, and 12 months after injury [90], but did not improve outcome in patients who were managed at a PCO$_2$ of 33 ± 2 mm Hg [181].

Barbiturate therapy is an intuitively logical means of reducing CBV in patients who fail to respond adequately to other means of controlling ICP. Barbiturates in sufficient doses suppress both CMRO$_2$ and CBF in conjunction with profound electrophysiologic suppression [182]. The reduction in CBF does not occur in all patients; those who have poor CO$_2$ reactivity respond minimally to barbiturates [183], as do those with low baseline levels of CMRO$_2$.

Because experimental data and the results of anecdotal reports were encouraging, barbiturates have been used to control ICP in head-injured patients. In 25 patients with refractory intracranial hypertension, barbiturate therapy controlled ICP in 19, and was associated with return to productive life in 10 of the 19 [184]. In a subsequent, well-designed, randomized clinical trial, however, Ward et al. [185] used prophylactic barbiturates in 53 severely head-injured patients who were predicted to be at higher risk of intracranial hypertension. Barbiturates did not reduce the incidence of intracranial hypertension or improve outcome; in fact, the occurrence of barbiturate-induced hypotension prompted the authors to suggest caution. Pentobarbital, the most commonly used barbiturate for reduction of ICP in head-injured patients, is a potent myocardial depressant and vasodilator that substantially reduces stroke volume index and mean arterial pressure [186]. Barbiturates also have been associated with pulmonary, renal, and hepatic complications and perhaps with an increased incidence of opportunistic infections [187]. Of 38 patients who received thiopental for 1 to 15 days to control ICP, hypotension developed in 58 percent, hypokalemia in 82 percent, respiratory complications in 76 percent, hepatic dysfunction in 87 percent, renal dysfunction in 47 percent, and infections in 55 percent. Twenty patients died with intractably increased ICP [188]; one fatality was attributed to barbiturate therapy.

Barbiturates still may have a role in selected patients. Of 925 head-injured patients, 80 patients who had refractory intracranial hypertension were randomized to receive high-dose pentobarbital in addition to conventional therapy or to receive conventional therapy alone [189]. Those in whom pentobarbital controlled ICP had a lower mortality than those in whom barbiturates did not control ICP. The large number of patients who crossed over from conventional therapy to barbiturate therapy precluded a definitive analysis of the efficacy of barbiturates. If pentobarbital is used to control ICP, the dose should be adjusted using electroencephalographic burst suppression rather than serum concentrations, because of the poor correlation between CSF and serum levels of pentobarbital [190].

Increased brain tissue volume may be caused by disruption of the blood-brain barrier (vasogenic edema), cellular swelling owing to ischemia (cytotoxic edema), or cellular changes after excitotoxic injury, recently termed neurotoxic edema. Reduction of brain tissue volume is conventionally achieved by diuresis. Osmotic diuresis, usually accomplished using mannitol, reduces brain water primarily in normal brain. A continuous intravenous infusion of mannitol significantly increases regional CBF without increasing blood pressure or reducing ICP [191]. The effect of mannitol on CBF depends on the integrity of autoregulation [82]. If autoregulation is intact, mannitol does not increase CBF; if autoregulation is defective, mannitol increases CBF but does not influence cerebral blood volume. Although most clinicians use mannitol to treat acute increases in ICP, empirical treatment with mannitol in a dose of 0.25 gm/ kg every 2 hours does not change morbidity and mortality compared with patients in whom mannitol is infused only in response to increased ICP [192]. Maximal reduction of ICP appears to be achieved by larger doses of mannitol administered rapidly, particularly if followed by furosemide [193]. Cruz et al., using fiberoptic jugular venous oximetry, have demonstrated the benefit of mannitol therapy when ICP treatment with hyperventilation resulted in oligemic cerebral hypoxia [79].

Fluid restriction, a conventional part of therapy, does not reduce brain tissue volume or ICP in experimental animals. Because the blood-brain barrier is poorly permeable to sodium, hypertonic saline reduces brain water and ICP. Experimental resuscitation after TBI using 7.5 percent hypertonic saline in 6 percent Dextran-70 lowered ICP and improved CBF. The response could be sustained for 6 hours with repeated injections [194]. In an anecdotal clinical report, small volumes of a solution (approximating 30% NaCl in water) produced prolonged reductions in ICP and improved prerenal azotemia in two patients [195].

Temporal lobectomy has been employed to debulk the brain, particularly if the temporal tip is severely contused. If intracranial hypertension is refractory to pharmacologic therapy, subtemporal decompression may reduce mortality [196].

From a pharmacologic standpoint, the most disappointing agents for reduction of cerebral edema and ICP have been the glucocorticoids. In 20 consecutive patients with severe head injury, methylprednisolone, 40 mg every 6 hours, failed to reduce ICP or improve intracranial compliance [197]. Cooper et al. [198], in a randomized, prospective, double-blind study, failed to show any benefit of either low-dose (16 mg/day) or

high-dose dexamethasone (96 mg/day) [198]. Saul et al. [199] demonstrated that methylprednisolone in a dose of 5 mg/kg/ day produced no difference in outcome compared with conventional therapy. In experimental animals, the neuroprotective effect of methylprednisolone in brain injuries depended on a narrow therapeutic range, equivalent to a synaptosomal concentration of 100 μM; higher or lower concentrations were less effective [200]. Investigational compounds, the 21-aminosteroids [200,201], may exert therapeutic effects without the undesirable side effects of glucocorticoids.

SYSTEMIC CIRCULATORY MANAGEMENT. Management of hypertension and tachycardia frequently represents a challenge because of high circulating levels of catecholamines. Treatment of hypertension requires careful distinction of the occasional Cushing response from hypertension associated with the typical hyperdynamic response to head injury. If systemic hypertension is not secondary to intracranial hypertension, reduction of MAP may reduce CBF in brain that does not autoregulate normally and thereby reduce cerebral blood volume and ICP. Moreover, many commonly used antihypertensive agents, including sodium nitroprusside, nitroglycerin, and hydralazine, may increase ICP. Although those drugs may be acceptable in patients if ICP is monitored carefully, alternative agents, such as propranolol or labetalol, a long-acting alpha-adrenergic and beta-adrenergic antagonist, may be preferable. Labetalol reduces blood pressure without increasing ICP. For acute, short-term control of MAP, esmolol may provide rapidly reversible control of blood pressure and heart rate. Adequate sedation and analgesia may also reduce the hyperdynamic circulatory response to head injury.

PULMONARY AND VENTILATORY MANAGEMENT. Two-fifths of severely head-injured patients develop pulmonary complications, with the peak incidence occurring 2 to 4 days after injury [202]. Hypoxemia may aggravate acute head injury and may interfere with appropriate compensation for the additional systemic oxygen demand associated with posttraumatic hypermetabolism [56]. Patients with severe head injury are also at risk for aspiration pneumonitis, noncardiac pulmonary edema, pulmonary embolism, and mechanical complications of ventilatory support such as pneumothorax. Prevention of aspiration after admission to the ICU requires gastric decompression and the use of an appropriately inflated, cuffed endotracheal tube. Overgrowth of pathogenic bacteria in the stomach may play a role in the genesis of pneumonia secondary to aspirated oropharyngeal material [203,204]. Pneumonia may develop as a consequence of secretion retention, atelectasis, and secondary infection. As noted above, compulsive turning is essential if the incidence of this complication is to be minimized. Early internal fixation of skeletal trauma has been recommended to permit turning and reduce the risk of the fat embolism syndrome [205].

The ventilatory management of patients with severe head trauma necessitates decisions regarding the type of ventilatory support to be provided, the desired level of $PaCO_2$, and the use of neuromuscular blockers. Many patients with severe head injury ventilate and oxygenate normally if they are provided with a secure airway. In fact, many spontaneously hyperventilate.

Regardless of whether head-injured patients are ventilated to a normal or reduced level of $PaCO_2$, many North American clinicians routinely paralyze patients for at least the first several days of intensive care. The alleged advantages of neuromuscular blockade include prevention of posturing and active expiration, which are associated with increases in MAP, central venous pressure, and ICP. The primary disadvantage of neuromuscular blockade is that it interferes with clinical neurologic examination and thereby necessitates the use of other more invasive indicators, such as ICP monitoring, and more frequent transportation for CT scanning.

An occasional patient with severe head injury develops the acute respiratory distress syndrome, secondary either to infection or severe intracranial injury, in which case the syndrome is often called central neurogenic pulmonary edema. The management of hypoxemia in the acute respiratory distress syndrome consists of ventilatory support with positive end-expiratory pressure (PEEP) and relief of intracranial hypertension, if present. Increases in intrathoracic pressure secondary to PEEP may increase cerebral venous pressure and ICP. Although ICP increases in some patients after the application of PEEP [206,207], increases in ICP are avoided both clinically and experimentally by head elevation [208,209]. If PEEP reduces cardiac output, subsequent volume expansion may increase ICP [210].

Because virtually all patients with severe head injury require an artificial airway, clinicians should anticipate the need for weaning from mechanical ventilatory support and artificial airway support. For patients who remain comatose or in whom airway reflexes remain inadequate to maintain airway patency or prevent aspiration, a decision must be made regarding continuation of endotracheal intubation versus tracheostomy. If airway support appears likely to be prolonged, early tracheostomy has been advised, because the duration of intubation correlates strongly with the development of complications [211].

Severe head injury predisposes patients to deep venous thrombosis, with or without pulmonary embolism, for several reasons, including immobility, lower limb trauma, protracted vascular infusions, and surgery. The recognition of deep venous thrombosis in neurosurgical patients depends on the diagnostic criteria, such as whether the diagnosis was based on clinical findings (10%), symptoms (17%), or the use of radiolabeled fibrinogen (29–41%) [212,213,214]. Bedside diagnostic tests include impedance plethysmography and venous Doppler ultrasonography. Definitive diagnosis of pulmonary embolism requires ventilation/perfusion scanning, which is often nondiagnostic in critically ill patients, or pulmonary angiography. The diagnosis of deep venous thrombosis or pulmonary embolism poses a therapeutic dilemma because full anticoagulation is relatively contraindicated in patients after acute trauma, recent surgery, or in those likely to need surgical intervention in the near future, although some clinicians suggest that anticoagulation may be undertaken 5 days after uncomplicated craniotomy [215]. An alternative in patients at high risk for bleeding is interruption of the inferior vena cava. Methods of prevention of deep venous thrombosis include the use of intermittent pneumatic compression stockings, which do not influence ICP or CPP in brain-injured patients [216], and antithrombotic doses of heparin.

GASTROINTESTINAL COMPLICATIONS. Acute head injury predisposes patients to stress-induced gastrointestinal bleeding, the incidence of which is directly proportional to the severity of injury [217,218]. Because stress ulceration and erosive gastritis are associated with high gastric acidity [219], treatment with antacids or H_2 blockers has been used to minimize the incidence of these complications. Aggressive antacid therapy or frequent administration of H_2 blockers may be necessary to control gastric pH; however, recent data demonstrate that gas-

tric bacterial overgrowth is common if gastric pH is increased in an effort to prevent stress gastritis [203,204]. Because of the increased risk of passive regurgitation of gastric contents with subsequent aspiration and infection, sucralfate may be preferable for ulcer prophylaxis [220].

NUTRITION. Patients with acute head injury have substantially increased metabolic needs. Patients with a GCS score of 4 to 5 require nearly 70 percent more nutritional support than predicted resting metabolic requirements [221]. Heart rate, temperature, and the days elapsed after head injury also correlate significantly with measured energy expenditure [222]. Hypermetabolism and the effects of fever on metabolism are most marked in patients who exhibit abnormal posturing. Because of intense catabolism after head injury and inadequate caloric intake, protein-calorie malnutrition can develop within a few days, potentially leading to immunocompromise and infection, hypoalbuminemia, poor wound healing, and skin breakdown [223]. Loss of amino acids from skeletal muscle produces muscle wasting and weight loss [224]. The medical management of head-injured patients may also affect nutritional requirements. Glucocorticoids increase nitrogen wasting in head-injured patients without increasing metabolic rate [225]. Because of the extraordinary requirements for both calories and nitrogen, positive nitrogen balance may be difficult to achieve [226,227]. Aggressive enteral nutrition containing 22 percent protein may be sufficient in some patients to promote nitrogen equilibrium, however [228] (see Chap. 201).

High circulating levels of catabolic hormones initiate increased gluconeogenesis and reduce glucose tolerance [229]. Hyperglycemia may occur despite increased insulin levels. Therefore, when feeding head-injured patients, the possibility of hyperglycemia should be anticipated, and glucose should be controlled. Although only descriptive data implicate hyperglycemia as a cause of worse neurologic outcome after head trauma [230,231], considerable experimental and clinical data suggest that hyperglycemia worsens injury in some, but not all, models of focal and global neurologic ischemia and in patients with cardiac arrest or stroke [232–236].

Although patients with severe head injury remain hypermetabolic for prolonged intervals, the appropriate level of nutritional support has yet to be defined [237]. Undernutrition of head-injured patients may be unrecognized [223]. Although recent reports suggest caution [237], some investigators report improved mortality in patients who receive early parenteral nutrition, as opposed to early enteral nutrition, after head trauma [238,239]. Some patients with acute head injury tolerate enteral feeding poorly, with the greatest difficulty encountered in those patients with more severe injury and intracranial hypertension [240]. The intolerance for enteral feeding may be related to delayed gastric emptying, reduced intestinal motility, or increased susceptibility to diarrhea [240]. Nevertheless, many centers prefer enteral feeding, which does not require central venous catheterization and may benefit gut integrity and immune competence. Hyperglycemia is less frequent; the incidence of regurgitation and aspiration can be reduced by head elevation and by insuring that feeding tubes are placed within the duodenum. Early enteral nutrition may also improve function of the immune system [239].

In 1984, Gadisseux et al. [241] lamented the lack of guidelines for nutrition in head trauma patients and the absence of definitive answers to many questions regarding nutritional support. Many questions remain unanswered. Most clinicians tend to initiate either enteral or parenteral nutrition as soon as possible after acute head injury, generally preferring enteral nutrition if tolerated. An appropriate strategy is to provide sufficient calories and nitrogen to prevent catabolism without causing hyperglycemia. To avoid hyperglycemia, nonglucose calorie sources, including short-chain fatty acids, merit evaluation. Neurologic recovery from head injury may occur with prompt, aggressive nutritional support [239].

FLUID AND ELECTROLYTE IMBALANCE. Electrolyte abnormalities occurred at least once in 59 percent of 734 patients enrolled in the Trauma Coma Data Bank, although such disorders infrequently altered outcome [202]. Abnormalities of sodium and potassium are most common. Head-injured patients frequently develop hyponatremia, occasionally as the result of the syndrome of inappropriate antidiuretic hormone secretion (SIADH) [242] or more commonly as a consequence of sodium losses from the gastrointestinal tract complicated by administration of free water. The treatment of hyponatremia depends on its cause (see Chap. 79). Hyponatremia may be associated with a contracted, normal, or expanded intravascular volume. An occasional patient develops hypovolemic hyponatremia after head trauma from excessive urinary sodium excretion as a consequence of circulating natriuretic factors [243]. Hyponatremia associated with hypovolemia should be managed with intravenous (isotonic or mildly hypertonic) fluid administration. In the normovolemic hyponatremia of SIADH, the diagnosis is confirmed by demonstrating high urinary sodium concentration despite hypoosmolality. Differentiation of SIADH from cerebral salt wasting is necessary because fluid restriction, usually adequate therapy for SIADH, may exacerbate hypovolemia in cerebral salt wasting. Occasionally, demeclocycline may be necessary to correct SIADH [244]. Rapid correction of hyponatremia is unnecessary and dangerous, especially if hyponatremia is chronic, because of the risk of central pontine myelinosis. Hypervolemic hyponatremia, usually seen in edematous states, usually reflects intercurrent diagnoses such as congestive heart failure or cirrhosis.

Diabetes insipidus may result from trauma or transection of the pituitary stalk [245,246]. Typically, traumatic diabetes insipidus follows a three-phase course, with polyuria occurring initially, followed by reduced urinary output as stored antidiuretic hormone is released from the damaged pituitary, followed finally by prolonged diabetes insipidus [245]. Partial deficits of antidiuretic hormone also occur. The diagnosis of diabetes insipidus necessitates the demonstration that polyuria is unphysiologic, which is usually confirmed by the development of hypovolemia or hypernatremia. When diabetes insipidus develops, the free-water deficit should be corrected slowly. Antidiuretic hormone replacement can be provided in the form of either aqueous vasopressin (5–10 units every 6–8 hours IM), lysine vasopressin, or desmopressin (DDAVP) 0.1 ml every 12 to 24 hours administered intranasally. Occasionally, a continuous infusion of synthetic arginine vasopressin, 1 to 2 units per hour, permits better control of diuresis.

INFECTIOUS COMPLICATIONS. Patients with severe head injury are at risk for nonpulmonary as well as pulmonary infections because defense barriers must be violated in the course of care. Cell-mediated immunity is impaired in some children (and presumably in some adults) after severe head injury; testing of immune status has been recommended to identify those in whom immune compromise increases the risk of infection [247]. Urinary tract infection may result from prolonged bladder catheterization. Maxillary sinusitis is surprisingly common among nasotracheally intubated, head trauma patients [248],

although the incidence may be no greater than in orally intubated patients. Otitis media occurs in one-sixth of intubated, head-injured patients [249]. Ventriculitis and meningitis complicate penetrating trauma, surgical procedures that violate the dura, and indwelling intraventricular monitoring devices. Most clinicians believe that ventricular cannulae are acceptable in patients with head trauma for limited periods, provided that strict asepsis is maintained [250]. The risk of intracranial infection appears to be less with subarachnoid bolts than with ventriculostomies.

SEIZURE PROPHYLAXIS. The majority of patients with severe closed head injury are at risk for posttraumatic seizures. Although the overall incidence is low, most clinicians provide seizure prophylaxis in the acute interval after head injury, particularly for those patients with skull fractures or intracranial hematomas [251]. In adults, the prophylactic seizure medication most commonly employed is phenytoin, in a dose of 100 mg three times daily. This is usually sufficient to produce a therapeutic serum concentration of 10 to 20 mg/per milliliter. Phenobarbital is commonly added. For the management of acute seizures, diazepam, lorazepam, or phenytoin is usually chosen [252].

Evolving Therapies

BIOCHEMICAL ALTERATIONS ASSOCIATED WITH BRAIN INJURY. Secondary brain injury strongly influences outcome after brain trauma. Evidence of cerebral tissue hypoxia is present in 90 percent of fatal head injuries [67]. Four mechanisms, contusion, hematoma, diffuse axon injury, and hypoxia, appear to contribute to progressive neural damage. Because of the hope that identification of biochemical factors potentiating brain injury could lead to specific medical therapy, studies of the biochemical consequences of experimental brain injury have been extensive [253–284].

EXPERIMENTAL BIOCHEMICAL INTERVENTIONS. Promising interventions, most of which have not been tested in humans or have only been tested in preliminary clinical trials, are based on those mediators that appear to be important in the progression of damage after brain trauma. These include THAM [285], free radical scavengers, [286,287], excitotoxin antagonists [253,263,279,280] calcium entry blockers [265,288,289], magnesium [267], cholinergic blockers [273,290], prostaglandin inhibitors [291], opioid antagonists [284,290,292,293] and antagonists of polyamines [275].

Pediatric Brain Injury

An estimated 100,000 to 250,000 children with acute head injuries, most suffered in motor vehicle accidents, are admitted annually to U.S. hospitals [294]. Pediatric head injury differs from adult injury because of incomplete skull and brain development in children. Among other differences, the brain increases from 25 to 70 percent of adult weight in the first 4 years of life; the glial cell population increases in the first 3 years; myelinization, most rapid in the first year, is not complete until the second decade; dendritic arborization and synaptic connections develop primarily in the first and the second postnatal years; and the skull remains thin and pliable with unfused sutures [294]. It is commonly believed that the immature brain, in contrast to the adult, responds differently to injury and tends to have a better outcome.

Primary head injuries involve the scalp, the skull, and the brain. Scalp lacerations may require no surgical intervention, but scalp contusions always require close inspection to rule out an underlying fracture. Most skull fractures in children are linear. Potentially serious linear fractures include those that cross the middle meningeal artery or the dural sinuses, or those involving the occipital bone, the base of the skull, or the lambdoid suture. Fractures peculiar to the pediatric age-group include ping-pong fractures and growing skull fractures. A growing skull fracture is an enlarging bone associated with a palpable, soft, pulsating mass, neurologic deficts, and seizures. The cause is thought to be the incarceration of arachnoid membrane subsequently associated with an enlarging leptomeningeal cyst, causing a bony defect. In infants, concussive injuries may manifest as benign posttraumatic seizures, vomiting, diaphoresis, pallor, and lethargy. Concussion in a young child may present only as a history of transient loss of consciousness; an older child may present with complaints of headache, dizziness, fatigue, or behavioral changes.

Subdural hematomas, more frequent than epidural hematomas in children [293], commonly result from tears in bridging cortical veins. Symptoms include drowsiness, lethargy, irritability, and seizures. Bleeding can be severe enough to cause anemia and shock. On examination, a tense, bulging, nonpulsatile fontanelle, sutural separation, and retinal hemorrhage may be evident.

Posttraumatic epidural hematomas are relatively rare in children, probably because the close apposition of the dura to the periosteum restricts dissection of blood [294]. Moreover, because the middle meningeal artery does not imbed in the skull until about 2 years of age, it may escape laceration if the temporal bone fractures. Clinically, a lucid interval may not be seen in children who suffer epidural hematomas. A lucid interval followed by decompensation is more likely in children to result from generalized cerebral swelling, or cerebral hyperemia, rather than from an increasing intracranial mass [294].

Rapid evaluation of head-injured children follows the same priorities as in adults, which include cardiorespiratory evaluation and support, and evaluating the possibility of other injuries and causes of coma. In preverbal children, a modified Glasgow Coma Scale (Table 175-5) is useful.

Recovery from Traumatic Brain Injury

Recovery proceeds differently after minor than after severe head trauma, reflecting differences in pathophysiology. In addition, early recovery after traumatic injury probably results from different mechanisms (e.g., recovery of function in injured, but structurally intact brain cells) whereas late recovery may represent development of new neuronal connections and pathways [295,296].

Severely injured patients first evidence recovery from coma by spontaneous eye opening [109]. Subsequently they may begin to obey commands and speak. Later agitation may necessitate sedation or restraint, which may in turn further exacerbate agitation. Gradually patients become less noisy, less excitable, and more cooperative, but may remain disoriented. Amnesia

Table 175-5. Children's Coma Scale (CCS) Modified from Glasgow Coma Scale (GCS)

Eye opening
  4 Spontaneous
  3 Reaction to speech
  2 Reaction to pain
  1 No response

Best motor response
  6 Spontaneous (obeys verbal command)
  5 Localizes pain
  4 Withdraws in response to pain
  3 Abnormal flexion in response to pain (decorticate posture)
  2 Abnormal extension in response to pain (decerebrate posture)
  1 No response

Best of verbal response

(GCS subscore)		(CCS subscore)	
Oriented	5	Smiles, oriented to sound, follows objects, interacts	
Confused/disordered	4	*Crying*	*Interacts*
		Consolable	Inappropriate
Inappropriate words	3	Inconsistently consolable	Moaning
Incomprehensible sounds	2	Inconsolable	Irritable, restless
No response	1	No response	No response

Reproduced from Hahn YS, Chyung C, Barthel MJ, et al: Head injuries in children under 36 months age. *Child Nerv Syst* 4:34, 1988, with permission.

often persists until higher mental functions, e.g., judgment and reasoning, begin to return. The duration of posttraumatic amnesia often has been used as an indication of the severity of brain injury [109].

Even after minor head injury, many patients complain of headache, fatigue, dizziness, and inability to concentrate, which collectively have been termed the postconcussion syndrome. Although in some cases these symptoms may be prompted by secondary gain (e.g., workers' compensation or pending litigation), these symptoms occur so ubiquitously that they should be considered part of the usual recovery process [297]. There often appears to be an inverse relationship between the severity of headache and the severity of the precipitating head injury [298].

MENTAL SEQUELAE. Brain function often improves most dramatically within the first week after acute head injury. Subsequent recovery is usually more gradual. Unfortunately, patients who regain good neurologic function often demonstrate persistent cognitive or emotional deficits or personality changes [299], particularly if posttraumatic coma results from diffuse brain injury rather than discrete focal lesions. Changes in personality, distressingly common after severe head injury [299,300,301], are exceedingly difficult to quantify. Brooks et al. [302,303] have performed serial intelligence tests on a large population of head trauma survivors, confirming different patterns of recovery between verbal and performance intelligence quotient (IQ). Recovery from verbal impairment usually begins within a few months and reaches a steady-state level more rapidly than performance IQ, which may continue to improve for a year or more [302,303,304]. In some patients, organic motor dysfunction, e.g., decreased speed of finger tapping, may be associated with behavioral alterations.

One common pattern of brain injury includes orbitofrontal,

anterior and inferior temporal contusions, and diffuse axonal injury, which also involves the corpus callosum, superior cerebellar peduncles, basal ganglia, and the periventricular white matter. Cognitive impairment is diffuse and higher functions, including memory, rate of information processing, problem solving, attentiveness, and cognitive flexibility, are most frequently affected [305]. Intellect, language, and perceptual skills are relatively preserved [305]. The involvement of frontal, temporal and limbic areas results in prominent impulsivity, affective instability, disinhibition, and problems with impulse control. These result in the "personality change" of traumatic brain injury, with problems arising from substance abuse, sexual expression, and aggression [305]. Neuropsychiatric problems are often associated with even minor or mild head injuries; the underlying mechanisms may be linked to alterations in structural, functional, or chemical alterations in the neurons. Psychotic and depressive disorders are common sequelae of head injury but the incidence of manic disorder has not been established [305]. The role of head trauma in Alzheimer's disease and Parkinson's disease has been debated [306]. However, dystonic movements [307], tremors [308], and ataxia [309] may occur.

Some focal lesions may lead to specific deficits. For example, left hemispheric lesions often are associated with dysphasia, learning difficulties, and cognitive deficits [109,297], whereas right hemispheric lesions of apparently equal severity may produce less obvious perceptual deficits or emotional effects. Frontal lobe lesions may lead to antisocial behaviors, such as aggression or inappropriate sexual drive; conversely, frontal lobe injury may result in loss of initiative and lassitude [300,301]. Memory deficits, which may lead to severe social stress and unemployability, commonly occur after all degrees of head injury. Usually memory deficits persist only briefly after minor injuries. In contrast, patients with severe injuries, particularly those involving both temporal lobes, may have persisting, profound difficulty with both long-term and short-term memory [302]. Neuropsychiatric syndromes that follow traumatic brain injury may be difficult to classify in conventional diagnostic terms [305].

PHYSICAL SEQUELAE. The most common major neurologic findings in patients who survive head injury are a consequence of unilateral cerebral hemispheric dysfunction and cranial nerve palsies [109]. Some survivors demonstrate hemiparesis or dysphasia. Roughly one in five develop epilepsy [310]. Cranial nerve involvement may be isolated or multiple [311]. Among cranial nerve deficits, damage to the optic nerve is most common, followed by the auditory, oculomotor, trochlear, and olfactory nerves. Posttraumatic hydrocephalus, either "normal pressure" or obstructive (communicating), is common after severe injury. The diagnosis is established by CT scanning followed by cisternography, to distinguish hydrocephalus from cerebral atrophy and ventricular enlargement, also common findings after head trauma.

Late traumatic epilepsy, i.e., that developing weeks after injury, is relatively common after missile injuries to the brain but uncommon after closed head injuries [312]. Factors associated with an increased risk of epilepsy after closed head injury include intracranial hematomas and depressed skull fractures. Jennett [310] has shown that of those patients who develop seizures within 5 years of injury, nearly 75 percent will have their first seizure during the first year after injury. Thus, prophylactic antiepileptic drugs (usually phenobarbital and phenytoin) should be discontinued after 12 months if the electroencephalogram is satisfactory and no seizures have occurred [310].

Outcome of Traumatic Brain Injury

Over the past two decades, opinion has shifted from a fatalistic view of cranial trauma to one in which intensive management is the standard of care. Without question, the efficacy of many individual components of intensive care regimens remain unproven. Perhaps intensive management may alter the outcome of only a subset of all severely injured patients. Nevertheless, most clinicians now favor a program consisting of early diagnosis and evacuation of hematomas, controlled ventilation, ICP monitoring, and aggressive supportive care to prevent medical complications. By following such a program, good to moderate recovery can be anticipated for approximately 50 percent of adult patients [5,162,163]. Much better results can be anticipated for children [5,313].

To standardize terminology, many clinicians describe neurologic outcome in terms of the Glasgow Outcome Scale (GOS) (Table 175-6) [314]. The GOS has been updated [315] by subdividing the best three categories into graded levels. Other scales [316] have been proposed, but the GOS remains the most widely used. In individual patients, the neurologic examination can help predict outcome, particularly in those who have no mass lesions on admission [99,100]. Overall, the level of consciousness (as assessed by the GCS) and brainstem reflexes (pupillary light responses and vestibuloocular or oculocephalic reflexes) are well correlated with patient outcome [5,99,100]. Studies consistently demonstrate increasing mortality with declining GCS scores [5,99,100,317]. However, in children, in the absence of hypoxic and ischemic injuries, GCS scores of 3 to 5 are compatible with recovery of function [318]. Bilaterally impaired pupillary light responses or impaired eye movements are associated with a mortality rate exceeding 75 percent [5,99,100]. The initial neurologic examination is of less prognostic value for patients with intracranial hematomas because signs of brainstem failure (which would ordinarily predict a dismal outcome) may reverse rapidly after evacuation of a hematoma [5,99,100,319]. A more flexible approach in evaluating outcome uses a prediction tree [320]. Using 23 prognostic factors, patients are ranked into eight groups, giving an overall predictive accuracy of 77.7 percent with accurate predictions in 89 and 90.1 percent, respectively, of patients in groups 1 and 8 [320].

Factors unrelated to the neurologic examination that adversely influence outcome include increasing age (which also correlates with an increasing risk of medical complications);

Table 175-6. Glasgow Outcome Scale

Grade 1	Good recovery. Those normal or minimally impaired patients who have returned to school, university, former occupation, or are capable of managing their households.
Grade 2	Moderately disabled. Patients who can perform the tasks of daily living, but are no longer able to work or attend school.
Grade 3	Severely disabled. Patients who require assistance to perform the tasks of daily living but do not require institutional care.
Grade 4	Vegetative.
Grade 5	Dead.

Source: From Jennett B, Bond M: Assessment of outcome after severe brain damage. *Lancet* 1:480, 1975, with permission.

hypoxemia, hypocarbia, hypotension, or anemia on admission to the hospital; and the presence of an intracranial mass lesion on CT scan [5,99,100]. Measurements of "multimodality" evoked potentials (visual, auditory, and somatosensory) may provide some limited assistance in establishing prognosis [76,100,321]. Unfortunately these techniques may not be readily accessible to most critically ill patients. In comatose patients, the presence of fever, diffuse sweating, disturbances of adrenocorticotropic hormone release, abnormal motor reactivity, respiratory disturbances, non-neurologic injuries, late-onset epilepsy, and communicating hydrocephalus also correlate with poor recovery from coma [322]. Non-neurologic diagnostic tests also correlate with outcome. Poor outcome is associated with high circulating levels of the BB isotype of creatine kinase (CK) [323], a blood sugar exceeding 250 mg/dl [231,324], an abnormal clotting profile, and thrombocytopenia. Endocrine changes associated with adverse prognosis after head injury include depressed and unchanged insulin levels, high fasting and fluctuating serum glocose levels, and high circulating cortisol and decreased epinephrine levels.

Patients who sustain focal lesions more frequently require surgical evacuation and tend to have a worse outcome than those presenting with diffuse injury and a similar level of consciousness (Table 175-7) [13,19]. Subdural hematoma results in death in nearly three quarters of patients who present with an initial GCS score of 3 to 5, whereas diffuse brain injury with a similar GCS score is associated with only 30 percent mortality [325]. Prompt surgical evacuation of extraaxial hematomas exerts a powerful effect on outcome. Patients whose subdural hematomas are evacuated within four hours have a 30 percent mortality rate; those operated on later have a 90 percent mortality rate [105].

Epidural hematoma is associated with a more favorable outcome than subdural hematoma, because there is usually less underlying brain injury. More timely diagnosis using CT appears to have reduced the mortality associated with epidural hematoma [326]. Those patients requiring surgery within 12 hours of injury do less well than those who require surgery 12 to 48 hours after injury, presumably because larger, more rapidly developing hematomas produce more severe brain compression before evacuation [327]. Intracranial hypertension after hematoma evacuation worsens outcome.

The severity and duration of intracranial hypertension, reflecting the severity of brain injury, also strongly influence patient outcome. For example, patients in whom ICP consistently exceeds 20 mm Hg have a mortality rate exceeding 50 percent, whereas patients in whom ICP remains continuously less than 20 mm Hg have a mortality rate of only 16 percent [5,162,163]. Mortality approaches 100 percent if intracranial hypertension cannot be controlled medically.

The relationship between posttraumatic CBF and neurologic outcome has been extensively investigated. The normal distribution of regional CBF, in which front flow exceeds posterior flow, is frequently reversed in head-injured patients, but this pattern, which often normalizes as consciousness is regained, may be a consequence rather than a cause of reduced mental activity [328]. Patients who have been hyperemic while in coma show greater chronic impairment of intellectual and memory function than patients in whom CBF has been lower than normal [329]. Posttraumatic $CMRO_2$ tends to be higher in patients who subsequently have better outcomes [330].

Regardless of the quality of intensive care and the extent of physiologic monitoring, it is clear that intensive management cannot improve outcome from some severe lesions. Likewise, intensive management cannot influence most benign injuries. Colohan et al. [164] have recently compared head injury mortality rates in Charlottesville, Virginia (where controlled ventilation and ICP monitoring are employed), and New Delhi, India (where neither controlled ventilation nor ICP monitoring is employed). Mortality rates in the two cities were remarkably similar except among comatose patients who demonstrated a purposeful response to a painful stimulus (GCS motor score = 5). Thus, only patients with coma, but without an abnormal motor response, appeared to have a more favorable outcome if provided intensive therapy. Jennett et al. [331] reported a similar lack of influence of steroids, intubation, and ICP monitoring on mortality of patients with a GCS score of 8 or less [331]. Among survivors, use of these techniques was associated with greater disability.

To increase cost effectiveness, future research should identify those patients who are so severely impaired that intensive therapy offers no benefit. Toward that end, Butterworth et al. [317] have shown that the few survivors among patients who were admitted with GCS score of 3 had no mass lesions on admission CT scans, whereas those with mass lesions consistently had an unfavorable outcome. Likewise, Gibson and Stephenson [332] have tested a prognostic scale that successfully predicted a fatal outcome (without a single falsely pessimistic prediction) in 23 of 52 severely head-injured patients. If confirmed in larger studies, such data would permit physicians to make informed, ethical decisions to withhold therapy from certain well-defined categories of patients, thereby more effectively allocating decreasing resources.

Acute brain trauma is an unfortunately common cause of death and disabilty. With early diagnosis, rapid evacuation of hematomas (if present), control of intracranial hypertension, and aggressive treatment and prevention of medical complications, more than half of brain-injured patients make a moderate to good recovery.

Table 175-7. Comparative Outcome After Brain Injury*

Lesion	Outcome at 3 months or more (% of patients)				
	Good recovery	Moderate disability	Severe disability	Vegetative	Dead
ALL HEAD INJURIES	36	24	8	2	30
Diffuse brain injury	40	26	7	3	23
All intracranial mass lesions	29	21	8	2	40
Acute epidural hematoma	75	17	0	0	8
Acute subdural hematoma	23	27	4	4	42
Acute intracerebral mass lesion	12	17	17	0	54

* Based on 160 patients who received intensive therapy.
Source: From Becker DP, Miller JD, Ward JD, et al: The outcome from severe head injury with early diagnosis and intensive management. *J Neurosurg* 47:491, 1977, with permission.

References

1. Harrison CL, Dijkers M: Traumatic brain injury registries in the United States: An overview. *Brain Inj* 6:203, 1992.
2. Gennarelli TA, Champion HR, Sacco WJ, et al: Mortality of patients with head injury and extracranial injury treated in trauma centers. *J Trauma* 29:1193, 1989.
3. Lacqua MJ, Sahdev P: Effective management of penetrating head injury. *Hosp Pract* 27:30, 1992.
4. Miller JD, Sweet RC, Narayan R, et al: Early insults to the injured brain. *JAMA* 240:439, 1978.
5. Miller JD, Butterworth JF, Gudeman SK, et al: Further experience in the management of severe head injury. *J Neurosurg* 54:289, 1981.
6. White RJ, Likavec MJ: The diagnosis and initial management of head injury. *N Engl J Med* 327:1507, 1992.
7. Kalsbeek WD, McLaurin RL, Harris BSH III, et al: The national head and spinal cord injury survey: Major findings. *J Neurosurg* 53:S19, 1980.
8. Sosin DM, Sacks JJ, Smith SM: Head injury-associated deaths in the United States from 1979 to 1986. *JAMA* 262:2251, 1989.
9. Jagger J: Prevention of brain trauma by legislation, regulation, and improved technology: A focus on motor vehicles. *J Neurotrauma* 9:S313, 1992.
10. Pitts LH, Trunkey DD: The multiple trauma patient in the NICU, in Wirth FP, Ratcheson RA (eds): *Neurosurgical Critical Care.* Baltimore, Williams & Wilkins, 1987, pp 215-230.
11. Adams JH, Graham DI, Gennarelli TA: Contemporary neuropathological considerations regarding brain damage in head injury, in Becker DP, Povlishock JT (eds): *Central Nervous System Trauma Status Report.* Bethesda, MD, National Institutes of Health, 1985, pp 65-77.
12. Bruce DA, Schut L, Bruno LA, et al: Outcome following severe head injuries in children. *J Neurosurg* 48:679, 1978.
13. Becker DP, Miller JD, Ward JD, et al: The outcome from severe head injury with early diagnosis and intensive management. *J Neurosurg* 47:491, 1977.
14. Crooks DA: The pathological concept of diffuse axonal injury: Its pathogenesis and the assessment of severity. *J Pathol* 165:5, 1991.
15. Graham DI, Adams JH: Ischaemic brain damage in fatal head injuries. *Lancet* 1:265, 1971.
16. Adams JH, Graham DI, Scott G, et al: Brain damage in fatal nonmissile head injury. *J Clin Pathol* 33:1132, 1980.
17. Graham DI, McLellan D, Adams JH, et al: The neuropathology of the vegetative state and severe disability after non-missile head injury. *Acta Neurochir Suppl* 32:65, 1983.
18. Bruce DA, Alavi A, Bilaniuk L, et al: Diffuse cerebral swelling following head injuries in children: The syndrome of "malignant brain edema." *J Neurosurg* 54:170, 1981.
19. Chan K-H, Mann KS, Yue CP, et al: The significance of skull fracture in acute traumatic intracranial hematomas in adolescents: A prospective study. *J Neurosurg* 72:189, 1990.
20. Stein SC, Ross SE: The value of computed tomographic scans in patients with low-risk head injuries. *Neurosurgery* 26:638, 1990.
21. Feuerman T, Wackym PA, Gade GF, et al: Value of skull radiography, head computed tomographic scanning, and admission for observation in cases of minor head injury. *Neurosurgery* 22:449, 1988.
22. Miller JD: Assessing patients with head injury. *Br J Surg* 77:241, 1990.
23. Cervós-Navarro J, Lafuente JV: Traumatic brain injuries: Structural changes. *J Neurol Sci* 103:S3, 1991.
24. Lucas JH: In vitro models of mechanical injury. *J Neurotrauma* 9:117, 1992.
25. Gennarelli TA, Thibault LE: Biological models of head injury, in Becker DP, Povlishock JT (eds): *Central Nervous System Trauma Status Report.* Bethesda, National Institutes of Health, 1985, pp 391-404.
26. Shima K, Marmarou A: Evaluation of brain-stem dysfunction following severe fluid-percussion head injury to the cat. *J Neurosurg* 74:270, 1991.
27. Dixon CE, Lyeth BG, Povlishock JT, et al: A fluid percussion model of experimental brain injury in the rat. *J Neurosurg* 67:110, 1987.
28. Andersen BJ, Marmarou A: Post-traumatic selective stimulation of glycolysis. *Brain Res* 585:184, 1992.
29. Soares HD, Thomas M, Cloherty K, et al: Development of prolonged focal cerebral edema and regional cation changes following experimental brain injury in the rat. *J Neurochem* 58:1845, 1992.
30. Tanno H, Nockels RP, Pitts LH, et al: Breakdown of the blood-brain barrier after fluid percussive brain injury in the rat. Part 1: Distribution and time course of protein extravasation. *J Neurotrauma* 9:21, 1992.
31. DeWitt DS, Prough DS, Taylor CL, et al: Reduced cerebral blood flow, oxygen delivery, and electroencephalographic activity after traumatic brain injury and mild hemorrhage in cats. *J Neurosurg* 76:812, 1992.
32. Yamakami I, McIntosh TK: Alterations in regional cerebral blood flow following brain injury in the rat. *J Cereb Blood Flow Metab* 11:655, 1991.
33. Taft WC, Yang K, Dixon CE, et al: Hypothermia attenuates the loss of hippocampal microtubule-associated protein 2 (MAP2) following traumatic brain injury. *J Cereb Blood Flow Metab* 13:796, 1993.
34. Erb DE, Povlishock JT: Neuroplasticity following traumatic brain injury: A study of GABAergic terminal loss and recovery in the cat dorsal lateral vestibular nucleus. *Exp Brain Res* 83:253, 1991.
35. Yuan X-Q, Wade CE, Clifford CB: Suppression by traumatic brain injury of spontaneous hemodynamic recovery from hemorrhagic shock in rats. *J Neurosurg* 75:408, 1991.
36. Hamm RJ, Jenkins LW, Lyeth BG, et al: The effect of age on outcome following traumatic brain injury in rats. *J Neurosurg* 75:916, 1991.
37. McIntosh TK: Pharmacologic strategies in the treatment of experimental brain injury. *J Neurotrauma* 9:S201, 1992.
38. Soares H, McIntosh TK: Fetal cortical transplants in adult rats subjected to experimental brain injury. *J Neural Transplant Plast* 2:207, 1991.
39. Povlishock JT, Becker DP, Cheng CL, et al: Axonal change in minor head injury. *J Neuropathol Exp Neurol* 42:225, 1983.
40. Pilz P: Axonal injury in head injury. *Acta Neurochir Suppl* 32:119, 1983.
41. Povlishock JT, Kontos HA: Continuing axonal and vascular change following experimental brain trauma. *Cent Nerv Syst Trauma* 2:285, 1985.
42. Povlishock JT, Becker DP, Miller JD, et al: The morphopathologic substrates of concussion. *Acta Neuropathol* 47:1, 1979.
43. Carey ME, Sarna GS, Farrell JB, et al: Experimental missile wound to the brain. *J Neurosurg* 71:754, 1989.
44. Crockard A, Johns L, Levett J, et al: "Brainstem" effects of experimental cerebral missile injury, in Popp AJ, Bourke RS, Nelson LR, Kimelberg KH (eds): *Neural Trauma.* New York, Raven Press, 1979, pp 19-25.
45. Torbati D, Jacks AF, Carey ME, et al: Cerebral cardiovascular and respiratory variables after an experimental brain missile wound. *J Neurotrauma* 9:S143, 1992.
46. Clifton GL, Ziegler MG, Grossman RG: Circulating catecholamines and sympathetic activity after head injury. *Neurosurgery* 8:10, 1981.
47. Clifton GL, Robertson CS, Kyper K, et al: Cardiovascular response to severe head injury. *J Neurosurg* 59:447, 1983.
48. Woolf PD, Hamill RW, Lee LA, et al: The predictive value of catecholamines in assessing outcome in traumatic brain injury. *J Neurosurg* 66:875, 1987.
49. Robertson CS, Clifton GL, Taylor AA, et al: Treatment of hypertension associated with head injury. *J Neurosurg* 59:455, 1983.
50. Cushing H: The blood-pressure reaction of acute cerebral compression, illustrated by cases of intracranial hemorrhage. *Am J Med Sci* 125:1017, 1903.
51. Deutschman CS, Konstantinides FN, Raup S, et al: Physiological and metabolic response to isolated closed-head injury: Part 2: Effects of steroids on metabolism. Potentiation of protein wasting and abnormalities of substrate utilization. *J Neurosurg* 66:388, 1987.
52. Young AB, Ott LG, Beard D, et al: The acute-phase response of the brain-injured patient. *J Neurosurg* 69:375, 1988.
53. McClain CJ, Hennig B, Ott LG, et al: Mechanisms and implications

of hypoalbuminemia in head-injured patients. *J Neurosurg* 69:386, 1988.

54. Levine JE, Becker D, Chun T: Reversal of incipient brain death from head-injury apnea at the scene of accidents. *N Engl J Med* 301:109, 1979.

55. Baigelman W, O'Brien JC: Pulmonary effects of head trauma. *Neurosurgery* 9:729, 1981.

56. Demling R, Riessen R: Pulmonary dysfunction after cerebral injury. *Crit Care Med* 18:768, 1990.

57. Schumacker PT, Rhodes GR, Newell JC, et al: Ventilation-perfusion imbalance after head trauma. *Am Rev Respir Dis* 119:33, 1979.

58. Malik AB: Mechanisms of neurogenic pulmonary edema. *Circ Res* 57:1, 1985.

59. van der Sande JJ, Emeis JJ, Lindeman J: Intravascular coagulation: A common phenomenon in minor experimental head injury. *J Neurosurg* 54:21, 1981.

60. Goodnight SH, Kenoyer G, Rapaport SI, et al: Defibrination after brain-tissue destruction: A serious complication of head injury. *N Engl J Med* 290:1043, 1974.

61. Kaufman HH, Moake JL, Olson JD, et al: Delayed and recurrent intracranial hematomas related to disseminated intravascular clotting and fibrinolysis in head injury. *Neurosurgery* 7:445, 1980.

62. Kumura E, Sato M, Fukuda A, et al: Coagulation disorders following acute head injury. *Acta Neurochir* 85:23, 1987.

63. van der Sande JJ, Veltkamp JJ, Boekhout-Mussert RJ, et al: Hemostasis and computerized tomography in head injury: Their relationship to clinical features. *J Neurosurg* 55:718, 1981.

64. Crone KR, Lee KS, Kelly DL Jr: Correlation of admission fibrin degradation products with outcome and respiratory failure in patients with severe head injury. *Neurosurgery* 21:532, 1987.

65. Olson JD, Kaufman HH, Moake J, et al: The incidence and significance of hemostatic abnormalities in patients with head injuries. *Neurosurgery* 24:825, 1989.

66. Stein SC, Young GS, Talucci RC, Greenbaum BH, et al: Delayed brain injury after head trauma: Significance of coagulopathy. *Neurosurgery* 30:160, 1992.

67. Graham DI, Ford I, Adams JH, et al: Ischaemic brain damage is still common in fatal non-missile head injury. *J Neurol Neurosurg Psychiatry* 52:346, 1989.

68. Bouma GJ, Muizelaar JP. Cerebral blood flow, cerebral blood volume, and cerebrovascular reactivity after severe head injury. *J Neurotrauma* 9:S333, 1992.

69. Cold GE, Jensen FT: Cerebral blood flow in the acute phase after head injury. Part 1: Correlation to age of the patients, clinical outcome and localisation of the injured region. *Acta Anaesthesiol Scand* 24:245, 1980.

70. Suwanwela C, Suwanwela N: Intracranial arterial narrowing and spasm in acute head injury. *J Neurosurg* 36:314, 1972.

71. Macpherson P, Graham DI: Correlation between angiographic findings and the ischaemia of head injury. *J Neurol Neurosurg Psychiatry* 41:122, 1978.

72. Robertson CS, Grossman RG, Goodman JC, et al: The predictive value of cerebral anaerobic metabolism with cerebral infarction after head injury. *J Neurosurg* 67:361, 1987.

73. Robertson CS, Clifton GL, Grossman RG, et al: Alterations in cerebral availability of metabolic substrates after severe head injury. *J Trauma* 28:1523, 1988.

74. Obrist WD, Langfitt TW, Jaggi JL, et al: Cerebral blood flow and metabolism in comatose patients with acute head injury. *J Neurosurg* 61:241, 1984.

75. Bruce DA, Langfitt TW, Miller JD, et al: Regional cerebral blood flow, intracranial pressure, and brain metabolism in comatose patients. *J Neurosurg* 38:131, 1973.

76. Muizelaar JP, Marmarou A, DeSalles AF, et al: Cerebral blood flow and metabolism in severely head-injured children: Part 1: Relationship with GCS score, outcome, ICP, and PVI. *J Neurosurg* 71:63, 1989.

77. Obrist WD, Clifton GL, Robertson CS, et al: Cerebral metabolic changes induced by hyperventilation in acute head injury, in Meyer JS (ed): *Cerebral Vascular Disease*. New York, Elsevier Science Publishers, 1987, pp 251-255.

78. Darby JM, Yonas H, Marion DW, et al: Local "inverse steal" induced by hyperventilation in head injury. *Neurosurgery* 23:84, 1988.

79. Cruz J, Miner ME, Allen SJ, et al: Continuous monitoring of cerebral oxygenation in acute brain injury: Injection of mannitol during hyperventilation. *J Neurosurg* 73:725, 1990.

80. Robertson CS, Narayan RK, Gokaslan ZL, et al: Cerebral arteriovenous oxygen difference as an estimate of cerebral blood flow in comatose patients. *J Neurosurg* 70:222, 1989.

81. DeWitt DS, Prough DS, Taylor CL, et al: Regional cerebrovascular responses to progressive hypotension after traumatic brain injury in cats. *Am J Physiol* 32:H1276, 1992.

82. Muizelaar JP, Lutz HA III, Becker DP: Effect of mannitol on ICP and CBF and correlation with pressure autoregulation in severely head-injured patients. *J Neurosurg* 61:700, 1984.

83. Muizelaar JP, Ward JD, Marmarou A, et al: Cerebral blood flow and metabolism in severely head-injured children. Part 2: autoregulation. *J Neurosurg* 71:72, 1989.

84. Cold GE: Cerebral blood flow in the acute phase after head injury. Part 2: Correlation to intraventricular pressure (IVP), cerebral perfusion pressure (CPP), PaCO$_2$, ventricular fluid lactate, lactate/pyruvate ratio and pH. *Acta Anaesthesiol Scand* 25:332, 1981.

85. Overgaard J, Mosdal C, Tweed WA: Cerebral circulation after head injury. Part 3: Does reduced regional cerebral blood flow determine recovery of brain function after blunt head injury? *J Neurosurg* 55:63, 1981.

86. Overgaard J, Tweed WA: Cerebral circulation after head injury. Part 4: Functional anatomy and boundary-zone flow deprivation in the first week of traumatic coma. *J Neurosurg* 59:439, 1983.

87. DeWitt DS, Prough DS, Whitley JM, et al: Cerebral hypoperfusion after fluid resuscitation from hemorrhage in head injured cats (abstract). *Crit Care Med* 17:S148, 1989.

88. Lanier WL, Iaizzo PA, Milde JH: Cerebral function and muscle afferent activity following intravenous succinylcholine in dogs anesthetized with halothane: The effects of pretreatment with a defasciculating dose of pancuronium. *Anesthesiology* 71:87, 1989.

89. Lanier WL, Milde JH, Michenfelder JD: Cerebral stimulation following succinylcholine in dogs. *Anesthesiology* 64:551, 1986.

90. Muizelaar JP, Marmarou A, Ward JD, et al: Adverse effects of prolonged hyperventilation in patients with severe head injury: A randomized clinical trial. *J Neurosurg* 75:731, 1991.

91. Prough DS, Johnson JC, Stump DA, et al: Effects of hypertonic saline versus lactated Ringer's solution on cerebral oxygen transport during resuscitation from hemorrhagic shock. *J Neurosurg* 64:627, 1986.

92. Prough DS, Whitley JM, Taylor CL, et al: Regional cerebral blood flow following resuscitation from hemorrhagic shock with hypertonic saline. *Anesthesiology* 75:319, 1991.

93. Gunnar W, Jonasson O, Merlotti G, et al: Head injury and hemorrhagic shock: Studies of the blood brain barrier and intracranial pressure after resuscitation with normal saline solution, 3% saline solution, and dextran-40. *Surgery* 103:398, 1988.

94. Whitley JM, Prough DS, Brockschmidt JK, et al: Cerebral hemodynamic effects of fluid resuscitation in the presence of an experimental intracranial mass. *Surgery* 110:514, 1991.

95. Gunnar W, Kane J, Barrett J: Cerebral blood flow following hypertonic saline resuscitation in an experimental model of hemorrhagic shock and head injury. *Brazilian J Med Biol Res* 22:287, 1989.

96. Gardner SR, Maull KI, Swensson EE, et al: The effects of the pneumatic antishock garment on intracranial pressure in man: A prospective study of 12 patients with severe head injury. *J Trauma* 24:896, 1984.

97. Teasdale G, Jennett B: Assessment of coma and impaired consciousness. *Lancet* 2:81, 1974.

98. Bricolo A, Turazzi S, Alexandre A, et al: Decerebrate rigidity in acute head injury. *J Neurosurg* 47:680, 1977.

99. Braakman R: Injuries of the brain and skull: Part 1, in Vinken PJ, Bruyn GW (eds): *The Handbook of Clinical Neurology*. New York, American Elsevier, 1975.

100. Narayan RK, Greenberg RP, Miller JD, et al: Improved confidence of outcome prediction in severe head injury: A comparative analysis of the clinical examination, multimodality evoked potentials, CT scanning, and intracranial pressure. *J Neurosurg* 54:751, 1981.

101. Plum F, Posner JB: The diagnosis of stupor and coma, in Plum F, McDowell FH (eds): *Contemporary Neurology Series* 2nd ed. Philadelphia, F.A. Davis, 1972, pp 39-52.

102. Butterworth JF IV, Maull KI, Miller JD, et al: Detection of occult abdominal trauma in patients with severe head injuries. *Lancet* 2:759, 1980.
103. Mackersie RC, Shackford SR, Garfin SR, et al: Major skeletal injuries in the obtunded blunt trauma patient: A case of routine radiologic survey. *J Trauma* 28:1450, 1988.
104. Michael DB, Guyot DR, Darmody WR: Coincidence of head and cervical spine injury. *Neurotrauma* 6:177, 1989.
105. Seelig JM, Becker DP, Miller JD, et al: Traumatic acute subdural hematoma: Major mortality reduction in comatose patients treated within four hours. *N Engl J Med* 304:1511, 1981.
106. Gentleman D, Jennett B: Audit of transfer of unconscious head-injured patients to a neurosurgical unit. *Lancet* 335:330, 1990.
107. Masters SJ: Evaluation of head trauma: Efficacy of skull films. *AJNR* 1:329, 1980.
108. Thornbury JR, Campbell JA, Masters SJ, et al: Skull fracture and the low risk of intracranial sequelae in minor head trauma. *AJR* 143:661, 1984.
109. Jennett B, Teasdale G: Management of head injuries, in Plum F, McDowell FH, Barringer JR (eds): *Contemporary Neurology Series #20.* Philadelphia, F.A. Davis, 1981.
110. Masters SJ, McClean PM, Arcarese JS, et al: Skull x-ray examinations after head trauma: Recommendations by a multidisciplinary panel and validation study. *N Engl J Med* 316:84, 1987.
111. Ambrose J: Computerized transverse axial scanning (tomography): Part 2: Clinical application. *Br J Radiol* 46:1023, 1973.
112. Housefield GN: Computerized transverse axial scanning (tomography). Part 1: Description of system. *Br J Radiol* 46:1016, 1973.
113. Dublin AB, French BN, Rennick JM: Computed tomography in head trauma. *Radiology* 122:365, 1977.
114. Zimmerman RA, Bilaniuk LT, Gennarelli T, et al: Cranial computed tomography in diagnosis and management of acute head trauma. *Am J Roentgenol* 131:27, 1978.
115. Zimmerman RA, Bilaniuk LT, Hackney DB, et al: Head injury: Early results of comparing CT and high-field MR. *AJNR* 7:757, 1986.
116. Sato Y, Yuj WTC, Smith WL, et al: Head injury in child abuse: Evaluation with MR imaging. *Radiology* 173:653, 1989.
117. Kelly AB, Zimmerman RD, Snow RB, et al: Head trauma: Comparison of MR and CT—Experience in 100 patients. *AJNR* 9:699, 1988.
118. Gentry LR, Godersky JC, Thompson BH: Traumatic brain stem injury: MR imaging. *Radiology* 171:177, 1989.
119. Shellock FG, Crues JV: Safety considerations of magnetic resonance imaging. *MRI Decisions* 2:25, 1988.
120. Crow W: Aspects of neuroradiology of head injury. *Neurosurg Clin North Am* 2:321, 1991.
121. Zimmerman RA: Craniocerebral trauma, in Lee SH, Rao KCVG, Zimmerman RA (eds): *Cranial MRI and CT.* 3rd ed. New York, McGraw-Hill, 1992, pp 509-538.
122. Rumbaugh CL, Bergeron RT, Kurze T: Intracranial vascular damage associated with skull fractures: Radiographic aspects. *Radiology* 104:81, 1972.
123. Bradley WG, Jr: MRI of hemorrhage and iron in the brain, in Stark DD, Bradley WG, Jr. (eds): *Magnetic Resonance Imaging.* St. Louis, The C.V. Mosby Company, 1988, pp 359-374.
124. Munro D, Maltby GL: Extradural hemorrhage: A study of forty-four cases. *Ann Surg* 113:192, 1941.
125. Radcliffe WB, Guinto FC, Jr., Scatliff JH: Cerebral and extracerebral hematomas. *Semin Roentgenol* 6:103, 1971.
126. Lindenberg R: Pathology of craniocerebral injuries, in Newton TH, Potts DG (eds): *Radiology of the Skull and Brain. Anatomy and Pathology.* St. Louis, The C.V. Mosby Company, 1977, pp 3049-3087.
127. Hesselink JR, Dowd CF, Healy ME, et al: MR imaging of brain contusions: A comparative study with CT. *AJR* 150:1133, 1988.
128. Scatliff JH, Williams AL, Krigman MR, et al: CT recognition of subcortical hematomas. *AJNR* 2:49, 1981.
129. Lipper MH, Rad FF, Kishore PRS, et al: Delayed intracranial hematoma in patients with severe head injury. *Radiology* 133:645, 1979.
130. Baratham G, Dennyson WG: Delayed traumatic intracerebral haemorrhage. *J Neurol Neurosurg Psychiatry* 35:698, 1972.
131. Klatzo I: Neuropathological aspects of brain edema. *J Neuropathol Exp Neurol* 26:1, 1967.
132. Koo AH, LaRoque RL: Evaluation of head trauma by computed tomography. *Radiology* 123:345, 1977.
133. Aldrich EF, Eisenberg HM, Saydjari C, et al: Diffuse brain swelling in severely head-injured children: A report from the NIH traumatic coma data bank. *J Neurosurg* 76:450, 1992.
134. Osborn AG: Diagnosis of descending transtentorial herniation by cranial computed tomography. *Radiology* 123:93, 1977.
135. Sunderland S: The tentorial notch and complications produced by herniations of the brain through that aperture. *Br J Surg* 45:422, 1958.
136. Stovring J: Contralateral temporal horn widening in unilateral supratentorial mass lesions: A diagnostic sign indicating tentorial herniation. *J Comput Assist Tomogr* 1:319, 1977.
137. Tsai FY, Teal JS, Itabashi HH, et al: Computed tomography of posterior fossa trauma. *J Comput Assist Tomogr* 4:291, 1980.
138. Shalen PR, Handel SF: Diagnostic challenges in closed head trauma. *Radiol Clin North Am* 19:53, 1981.
139. Little JR, Tubman DE, Ethier R: Cerebellar hemorrhage in adults: Diagnosis by computerized tomography. *J Neurosurg* 48:575, 1978.
140. Garza-Mercado R: Extradural hematoma of the posterior cranial fossa. *J Neurosurg* 59:664, 1983.
141. Fisher RG, Kim JK, Sachs E, Jr.: Complications in posterior fossa due to occipital trauma—Their operability. *JAMA* 167:176, 1958.
142. Andrews BT, Chiles BW III, Olsen WL, et al: The effect of intracerebral hematoma location on the risk of brain-stem compression and on clinical outcome. *J Neurosurg* 69:518, 1988.
143. Duhaime A-C, Gennarelli TA, Thibault LE, et al: The shaken baby syndrome: A clinical, pathological, and biomechanical study. *J Neurosurg* 66:409, 1987.
144. Lau LSW, Pike JW: The computed tomographic findings of peritentorial subdural hemorrhage. *Radiology* 146:699, 1983.
145. Duhaime AC, Alario AJ, Lewander WJ, et al: Head injury in very young children: Mechanisms, injury types, and ophthalmologic findings in 100 hospitalized patients younger than 2 years of age. *Pediatrics* 90:179, 1992.
146. Meservy CJ, Towbin R, McLaurin RL, et al: Radiographic characteristics of skull fractures resulting from child abuse. *AJNR* 8:455, 1987.
147. Caffey J: The whiplash shaken infant syndrome: Manual shaking by the extremities with whiplash-induced intracranial and intraocular bleedings, linked with residual permanent brain damage and mental retardation. *Pediatrics* 54:396, 1974.
148. Zimmerman RA, Bilaniuk LT: L'examen scanographique en traumatologie cranio-céphalique pédiatrique. *J Neuroradiol* 8:257, 1981.
149. Zimmerman RA, Bilaniuk LT, Bruce D, et al: Computed tomography of craniocerebral injury in the abused child. *Radiology* 130:687, 1979.
150. Lipper MH, Kishore PRS, Enas GG, et al: Computer tomography in the prediction of outcome in head injury. *AJNR* 6:7, 1985.
151. Kido DK, Cox C, Hamill RW, et al: Traumatic brain injuries: Predictive usefulness of CT. *Radiology* 182:777, 1992.
152. Zimmerman RA, Bilaniuk LT, Gennarelli T: Computed tomography of shearing injuries of the cerebral white matter. *Radiology* 127:393, 1978.
153. Wärme P-E, Bergström R, Persson L: Neurosurgical intensive care improves outcome after severe head injury. *Acta Neurochir* 110:57, 1991.
154. Rosner MJ, Coley IB: Cerebral perfusion pressure, intracranial pressure, and head elevation. *J Neurosurg* 65:636, 1986.
155. Tillett JM, Marmarou A, Agnew JP, et al: Effect of continuous rotational therapy on intracranial pressure in the severely brain-injured patient. *Crit Care Med* 21:1005, 1993.
156. Rosner MJ, Daughton S: Cerebral perfusion pressure management in head injury. *J Trauma* 30:933, 1990.
157. Langfitt TW, Weinstein JD, Kassell NF, et al: Transmission of increased intracranial pressure. I. Within the craniospinal axis. *J Neurosurg* 21:989, 1964.
158. Lundberg N, Troupp H, Lorin H: Continuous recording of the ventricular fluid pressure in patients with severe acute traumatic brain injury. *J Neurosurg* 22:581, 1965.
159. Rosner MJ, Becker DP: Origin and evolution of plateau waves: Experimental observations and a theoretical model. *J Neurosurg* 60:312, 1984.

160. Hayashi M, Kobayashi H, Handa Y, et al: Brain blood volume and blood flow in patients with plateau waves. *J Neurosurg* 63:556, 1985.

161. Miller JD, Becker DP, Ward JD, et al: Significance of intracranial hypertension in severe head injury. *J Neurosurg* 47:503, 1977.

162. Marshall LF, Smith RW, Shapiro HM: The outcome with aggressive treatment in severe head injuries. *J Neurosurg* 50:20, 1979.

163. Saul TG, Ducker TB: Effect of intracranial pressure monitoring and aggressive treatment on mortality in severe head injury. *J Neurosurg* 56:498, 1982.

164. Colohan AR, Alves WM, Gross CR, et al: Head injury mortality in two centers with different emergency medical services and intensive care. *J Neurosurg* 71:202, 1989.

165. Stuart GG, Merry GS, Smith JA, et al: Severe head injury managed without intracranial pressure monitoring. *J Neurosurg* 59:601, 1983.

166. Vries JK, Becker DP, Young HF: A subarachnoid screw for monitoring intracranial pressure. *J Neurosurg* 39:416, 1973.

167. Miller JD, Bobo H, Kapp JP: Inaccurate pressure readings for subarachnoid bolts. *Neurosurgery* 19:253, 1986.

168. Allen R: Intracranial pressure: A review of clinical problems, measurement techniques and monitoring methods. *J Med Eng Tech* 10:299, 1986.

169. Ward JD: Intracranial pressure monitoring, in Fuhrman BP, Shoemaker WC (eds): *Critical Care. State of the Art.* Fullerton, CA, The Society of Critical Care Medicine, 1989, pp 173–185.

170. Yano M, Ikeda Y, Kobayashi S, et al: Intracranial pressure in head-injured patients with various intracranial lesions is identical throughout the supratentorial intracranial compartment. *Neurosurgery* 21:688, 1987.

171. Ostrup R, Luerssen TG, Marshall LF, et al: Continuous monitoring of intracranial pressure with a miniaturized fiberoptic device. *J Neurosurg* 67:206, 1987.

172. Crutchfield JS, Narayan RK, Robertson CS, et al: Evaluation of a fiberoptic intracranial pressure monitor. *J Neurosurg* 72:482, 1990.

173. Maset AL, Marmarou A, Ward JD, et al: Pressure-volume index in head injury. *J Neurosurg* 67:832, 1987.

174. Tans JTJ, Poortvliet DCJ: Intracranial volume-pressure relationship in man. Part 2: Clinical significance of the pressure-volume index. *J Neurosurg* 59:810, 1983.

175. Robertson CS, Narayan RK, Contant CF, et al: Clinical experience with a continuous monitor of intracranial compliance. *J Neurosurg* 71:673, 1989.

176. Feldman Z, Kanter MJ, Robertson CS, et al: Effect of head elevation on intracranial pressure, cerebral perfusion pressure, and cerebral blood flow in head-injured patients. *J Neurosurg* 76:207, 1992.

177. van Hilten JJ, Roos RAC: Posttraumatic hyperthermia: A possible result of frontodiencephalic dysfunction. *Clin Neurol Neurosurg* 93-3:223, 1991.

178. Dietrich WD: The importance of brain temperature in cerebral injury. *J Neurotrauma* 9:S475, 1992.

179. Clifton GL, Jiang JY, Lyeth BG, et al: Marked protection by moderate hypothermia experimental traumatic brain injury. *J Cereb Blood Flow Metab* 11:114, 1991.

180. Jiang JY, Lyeth BG, Kapasi MZ, et al: Moderate hypothermia reduces blood-brain barrier disruption following traumatic brain injury in the rat. *Acta Neuropathol* 84:495, 1992.

181. Wolf AL, Levi L, Marmarou A, et al: Effect of THAM upon outcome in severe head injury: A randomized prospective clinical trial. *J Neurosurg* 78:54, 1993.

182. Michenfelder JD: The interdependency of cerebral functional and metabolic effects following massive doses of thiopental in the dog. *Anesthesiology* 41:231, 1974.

183. Cold GE: Measurements of CO_2 reactivity and barbiturate reactivity in patients with severe head injury. *Acta Neurochir* 98:153, 1989.

184. Marshall LF, Smith RW, Shapiro HM: The outcome with aggressive treatment in severe head injuries. Part II: Acute and chronic barbiturate administration in the management of head injury. *J Neurosurg* 50:26, 1979.

185. Ward JD, Becker DP, Miller D, et al: Failure of prophylactic barbiturate coma in the treatment of severe head injury. *J Neurosurg* 62:383, 1985.

186. Todd MM, Drummond JC, U HS: Hemodynamic effects of high dose pentobarbital: Studies in elective neurosurgical patients. *Neurosurgery* 20:559, 1987.

187. Sato M, Tanaka S, Suzuki K, et al: Complications associated with barbiturate therapy. *Resuscitation* 17:233, 1989.

188. Schalén W, Messeter K, Nordström C-H: Complications and side effects during thiopentone therapy in patients with severe head injuries. *Acta Anaesthesiol Scand* 36:369, 1992.

189. Eisenberg HM, Frankowski RF, Contant CF, et al: High-dose barbiturate control of elevated intracranial pressure in patients with severe head injury. *J Neurosurg* 69:15, 1988.

190. Winer JW, Rosenwasser RH, Jimenez F: Electroencephalographic activity and serum and cerebrospinal fluid pentobarbital levels in determining the therapeutic end point during barbiturate coma. *Neurosurgery* 29:739, 1991.

191. Jafar JJ, Johns LM, Mullan SF: The effect of mannitol on cerebral blood flow. *J Neurosurg* 64:754, 1986.

192. Smith HP, Kelly DL, Jr., McWhorter JM, et al: Comparison of mannitol regimens in patients with severe head injury undergoing intracranial monitoring. *J Neurosurg* 65:820, 1986.

193. Roberts PA, Pollay M, Engles C, et al: Effect on intracranial pressure of furosemide combined with varying doses and administration rates of mannitol. *J Neurosurg* 66:440, 1987.

194. Walsh JC, Zhuang J, Shackford SR: A comparison of hypertonic to isotonic fluid in the resuscitation of brain injury and hemorrhagic shock. *J Surg Res* 50:284, 1991.

195. Worthley LI, Cooper DJ, Jones N: Treatment of resistant intracranial hypertension with hypertonic saline: Report of two cases. *J Neurosurg* 68:478, 1988.

196. Gower DJ, Lee KS, McWhorter JM: Role of subtemporal decompression in severe closed head injury. *Neurosurgery* 23:417, 1988.

197. Gudeman SK, Miller JD, Becker DP: Failure of high-dose steroid therapy to influence intracranial pressure in patients with severe head injury. *J Neurosurg* 51:301, 1979.

198. Cooper PR, Moody S, Clark WK, et al: Dexamethasone and severe head injury: A prospective double-blind study. *J Neurosurg* 51:307, 1979.

199. Saul TG, Ducker TB, Saloman M, et al: Steroids in severe head injury: A prospective randomized clinical trial. *J Neurosurg* 54:596, 1981.

200. Braughler JM, Hall ED: Current application of "high-dose" steroid therapy for CNS injury. *J Neurosurg* 62:806, 1985.

201. McIntosh TK, Thomas M, Smith D, et al: The novel 21-aminosteroid U74006F attenuates cerebral edema and improves survival after brain injury in the rat. *J Neurotrauma* 9:33, 1992.

202. Piek J, Chesnut RM, Marshall LF, et al: Extracranial complications of severe head injury. *J Neurosurg* 77:901, 1992.

203. Craven DE, Kunches LM, Kilinsky V, et al: Risk factors for pneumonia and fatality in patients receiving continuous mechanical ventilation. *Am Rev Respir Dis* 133:792, 1986.

204. Driks MR, Craven DE, Celli BR, et al: Nosocomial pneumonia in intubated patients given sucralfate as compared with antacids of histamine type 2 blockers: The role of gastric colonization. *N Engl J Med* 317:1376, 1987.

205. Poole GV, Miller JC, Agnew SG, et al: Lower extremity fracture fixation in head-injured patients. *J Trauma* 32:654, 1992.

206. Shapiro HM, Marshall LF: Intracranial pressure responses to PEEP in head-injured patients. *J Trauma* 18:254, 1978.

207. Burchiel KJ, Steege TD, Wyler AR: Intracranial pressure changes in brain-injured patients requiring positive end-expiratory pressure ventilation. *Neurosurgery* 8:443, 1981.

208. Frost EAM: Effects of positive end-expiratory pressure on intracranial pressure and compliance in brain-injured patients. *J Neurosurg* 47:195, 1977.

209. Toung TJ, Miyabe M, McShane AJ, et al: Effect of PEEP and jugular venous compression on canine cerebral blood flow and oxygen consumption in the head elevated position. *Anesthesiology* 68:53, 1988.

210. Doblar DD, Santiago TV, Kahn AU, et al: The effect of positive end-expiratory pressure ventilation (PEEP) on cerebral blood flow and cerebrospinal fluid pressure in goats. *Anesthesiology* 55:244, 1981.

211. Lanza DC, Parnes SM, Koltai PJ, et al: Early complications of airway management in head-injured patients. *Laryngoscope* 100:958, 1990.

212. Valladares JB, Hankinson J: Incidence of lower extremity deep vein thrombosis in neurosurgical patients. *Neurosurgery* 6:138, 1980.

213. Joffe SN: Incidence of postoperative deep vein thrombosis in neurosurgical patients. *J Neurosurg* 42:201, 1975.

214. Cerrato D, Ariano C, Fiacchjno F: Deep vein thrombosis and low-dose heparin prophylaxis in neurosurgical patients. *J Neurosurg* 49:378, 1978.

215. Stern WE: Preoperative evaluation: Complications, their prevention, and treatment, in Youmans JR, (ed): *Neurological Surgery*. Philadelphia, PA, W.B. Saunders, 1982, pp 65 75.

216. Davidson JE, Willms DC, Hoffman MS: Effect of intermittent pneumatic leg compression on intracranial pressure in brain-injured patients. *Crit Care Med* 21:224, 1993.

217. Kamada T, Fusamoto H, Kawano S, et al: Gastrointestinal bleeding following head injury: A clinical study of 433 cases. *J Trauma* 17:44, 1977.

218. Kamada T, Fusamoto H, Kawano S, et al: Acute gastroduodenal lesions in head injury: An endoscopic study. *Am J Gastroenterol* 68:249, 1977.

219. Fitts CT, Cathcart RS III, Artz CP, et al: Acute gastrointestinal tract ulceration: Cushing's ulcer, steroid ulcer, Curling's ulcer and stress ulcer. *Am Surg* 37:218, 1971.

220. Tryba M: Risk of acute stress bleeding and nosocomial pneumonia in ventilated intensive care unit patients: Sucralfate versus antacids. *Am J Med* 83:117, 1987.

221. Robertson CS, Clifton GL, Grossman RG: Oxygen utilization and cardiovascular function in head-injured patients. *Neurosurgery* 15:307, 1984.

222. Sunderland PM, Heilbrun MP: Estimating energy expenditure in traumatic brain injury: Comparison of indirect calorimetry with predictive formulas. *Neurosurgery* 31:246, 1992.

223. Godbole KB, Berbiglia VA, Goddard L: A head-injured patient: Caloric needs, clinical progress and nursing care priorities. *J Neurosci Nurs* 23:290, 1991.

224. Young B, Ott L, Phillips R, et al: Metabolic management of the patient with head injury. *Neurosurg Clin North Am* 2:301, 1991.

225. Robertson CS, Clifton GL, Goodman JC: Steroid administration and nitrogen excretion in the head-injured patient. *J Neurosurg* 63:714, 1985.

226. Clifton GL, Robertson CS, Grossman RG, et al: The metabolic response to severe head injury. *J Neurosurg* 60:687, 1984.

227. Clifton GL, Robertson CS, Choi SC: Assessment of nutritional requirements of head-injured patients. *J Neurosurg* 64:895, 1986.

228. Clifton GL, Robertson CS, Contant CF: Enteral hyperalimentation in head injury. *J Neurosurg* 62:186, 1985.

229. Hadfield JM, Little RA, Jones RAC: Measured energy expenditure and plasma substrate and hormonal changes after severe head injury. *Injury* 23:177, 1992.

230. Prough DS, Coker LH, Lee S, et al: Hyperglycemia and neurologic outcome in patients with closed head injury (abstr). *Anesthesiology* 69(suppl 3a):A584, 1988.

231. Lam AM, Winn HR, Cullen BF, et al: Hyperglycemia and neurological outcome in patients with head injury. *J Neurosurg* 75:545, 1991.

232. Lanier WL, Stangland KJ, Scheithauer BW, et al: The effects of dextrose infusion and head position on neurologic outcome after complete cerebral ischemia in primates: Examination of a model. *Anesthesiology* 66:39, 1987.

233. Longstreth WT, Jr., Diehr P, Inui TS: Prediction of awakening after out-of-hospital cardiac arrest. *N Engl J Med* 308:1378, 1983.

234. Longstreth WT, Inui TS: High blood glucose level on hospital adminisson and poor neurological recovery after cardiac arrest. *Ann Neurol* 15:59, 1984.

235. Longstreth WT, Jr., Diehr P, Cobb LA, et al: Neurologic outcome and blood glucose levels during out-of-hospital cardiopulmonary resuscitation. *Neurology* 36:1186, 1986.

236. Pulsinelli WA, Levy DE, Sigsbee B, et al: Increased damage after ischemic stroke in patients with hyperglycemia with or without established diabetes mellitus. *Am J Med* 74:540, 1983.

237. Kaufman HH, Bretudiere J-P, Rowlands BJ, et al: General metabolism in head injury. *Neurosurgery* 20:254, 1987.

238. Rapp RP, Young B, Twyman D, et al: The favorable effect of early parenteral feeding on survival in head-injured patients. *J Neurosurg* 58:906, 1983.

239. Young B, Ott L, Twyman D, et al: The effect of nutritional support on outcome from severe head injury. *J Neurosurg* 67:668, 1987.

240. Norton JA, Ott LG, McClain C, et al: Intolerance to enteral feeding in the brain-injured patient. *J Neurosurg* 68:62, 1988.

241. Gadisseux P, Ward JD, Young HF, et al: Nutrition and the neurosurgical patient. *J Neurosurg* 60:219, 1984.

242. Doczi T, Tarjanyi J, Huszka E, et al: Syndrome of inappropriate secretion of antidiuretic hormone (SIADH) after head injury. *Neurosurgery* 10:685, 1982.

243. Kiwit JC, Schroders C, Wambach G: Plasma ANP levels and its relation to electrolyte and water regulation in neurosurgical intensive care patients. *Z-Kardiol* 77:119, 1988.

244. Singer I, Rotenberg D: Demeclocycline induced nephrogenic diabetes insipidus: In-vivo and in-vitro studies. *Ann Intern Med* 79:679, 1973.

245. Geheb MA: Clinical approach to the hyperosmolar patient. *Crit Care Clin* 2:797, 1987.

246. Moses AM, Blumenthal SA, Streeten DHP: Acid-base and electrolyte disorders associated with endocrine disease: Pituitary and thyroid, in Arieff AI, DeFronzo RA (eds): *Fluid, Electrolyte and Acid-Base Disorders*. New York, Churchill Livingstone, 1985, pp 851-892.

247. Wilson NW, Gooding A, Peterson B, et al: Anergy in pediatric head trauma patients. *Am J Dis Child* 145:326, 1991.

248. Humphrey MA, Simpson GT, Grindlinger GA: Clinical characteristics of nosocomial sinusitis. *Ann Otol Rhinol Laryngol* 96:687, 1987.

249. Christensen L, Schaffer S, Ross SE: Otitis media in adult trauma patients: Incidence and clinical significance. *J Trauma* 31:1543, 1991.

250. Mayhall CB, Archer NH, Lamb VA, et al: Ventriculostomy-related infections: A prospective epidemiologic study. *N Engl J Med* 310:553, 1984.

251. Jennett B, Miller JD, Braakman R: Epilepsy after nonmissile depressed skull fracture. *J Neurosurg* 41:208, 1974.

252. Riela AR: Management of seizures. *Crit Care Clin* 5:863, 1989.

253. Yoshino A, Hovda DA, Kawamata T, et al: Dynamic changes in local cerebral glucose utilization following cerebral concussion in rats: Evidence of a hyper- and subsequent hypometabolic state. *Brain Res* 561:106, 1991.

254. Wagner KR, Tornheim PA, Eichhold MK: Acute changes in regional cerebral metabolite values following experimental blunt head trauma. *J Neurosurg* 63:88, 1985.

255. Unterberg AW, Anderson BJ, Clarke GD, et al: Cerebral energy metabolism following fluid-percussion brain injury in cats. *J Neurosurg* 68:594, 1988.

256. Yang MS, DeWitt DS, Becker DP, et al: Regional brain metabolite levels following mild experimental head injury in the cat. *J Neurosurg* 63:617, 1985.

257. Inao S, Marmarou A, Clarke GD, et al: Production and clearance of lactate from brain tissue, cerebrospinal fluid, and serum following experimental brain injury. *J Neurosurg* 69:736, 1988.

258. Ishige N, Pitts LH, Hashimoto T, et al: Effect of hypoxia on traumatic brain injury in rats: Part 1. Changes in neurological function, electroencephalograms, and histopathology. *Neurosurgery* 20:848, 1987.

259. Ishige N, Pitts LH, Pogliani L, et al: Effect of hypoxia on traumatic brain injury in rats: Part 2: Changes in high energy phosphate metabolism. *Neurosurgery* 20:854, 1987.

260. Ishige N, Pitts LH, Berry I, et al: The effects of hypovolemic hypotension on high-energy phosphate metabolism of traumatized brain in rats. *J Neurosurg* 68:129, 1988.

261. Anderson BJ, Unterberg AW, Clarke GD, et al: Effect of posttraumatic hypoventilation on cerebral energy metabolism. *J Neurosurg* 68:601, 1988.

262. Brown SA, Hall ED: Role of oxygen-derived free radicals in the pathogenesis of shock and trauma, with focus on central nervous system injuries. *J Am Vet Med Assoc* 200:1849, 1992.

263. Faden AI, Demediuk P, Panter SS, et al: The role of excitatory amino acids and NMDA receptors in traumatic brain injury. *Science* 244:798, 1989.

264. McBurney RN, Daly D, Fischer JB, et al: New CNS-specific calcium antagonists. *J Neurotrauma* 9:S531, 1992.

265. Okiyama K, Smith DH, Thomas MJ, et al: Evaluation of a novel calcium channel blocker, (S)-emopamil, on regional cerebral edema and neurobehavioral function after experimental brain injury. *J Neurosurg* 77:607, 1992.

266. Arrigoni E, Cohadon F: Calcium-activated neutral protease activities in brain trauma. *Neurochem Res* 16:483, 1991.

267. Vink R. Magnesium and brain trauma. *Magnes Trace Elem* 10:1, 1991.

268. Pappius HM: Brain injury: New insights into neurotransmitter and receptor mechanisms. *Neurochem Res* 16:941, 1991.

269. Shohami E, Nates JL, Glantz L, et al: Changes in brain polyamine levels following head injury. *Exp Neurol* 117:189, 1992.

270. Hayes RL, Pechura CM, Katayama Y, et al: Activation of pontine cholinergic sites implicated in unconsciousness following cerebral concussion in the cat. *Science* 223: 301, 1984.

271. Lyeth BG, Dixon CE, Hamm RJ, et al: Effects of anticholinergic treatment on transient behavioral suppression and physiological responses following concussive brain injury to the rat. *Brain Res* 448:88, 1988.

272. Hayes RL, Stonnington HH, Lyeth BG, et al: Metabolic and neurophysiologic sequelae of brain injury: A cholinergic hypothesis. *Cent Nerv Syst Trauma* 3:163, 1986.

273. Jenkins LW, Lyeth BG, Lewelt W, et al: Combined pretrauma scopolamine and phencyclidine attenuate posttraumatic increased sensitivity to delayed secondary ischemia. *J Neurotrauma* 5:275, 1988.

274. Lindsberg PJ, Hallenbeck JM, Feuerstein G: Platelet-activating factor in stroke and brain injury. *Ann Neurol* 30:117, 1991.

275. Gilad GM, Gilad VH: Polyamines in neurotrauma: Ubiquitous molecules in search of a function. *Biochem Pharmacol* 44:401, 1992.

276. Wei EP, Christman CW, Kontos HA, et al: Effects of oxygen radicals on cerebral arterioles. *Am J Physiol* 248:H157, 1985.

277. Wei EP, Kontos HA, Christman CW, et al: Superoxide generation and reversal of acetylcholine-induced cerebral arteriolar dilation after acute hypertension. *Circ Res* 57:781, 1985.

278. Lewelt W, Jenkins LW, Miller JD: Autoregulation of cerebral blood flow after experimental fluid percussion injury of the brain. *J Neurosurg* 53:500, 1980.

279. McIntosh TK, Vink R, Soares H, et al: Possible role of excitatory amino acid neurotransmitters in pathophysiology of experimental brain injury (abstract). *J Cereb Blood Flow Metab* 9:S77, 1989.

280. Katayama Y, Becker DP, Tamura T, et al: Massive increases in extracellular potassium and the indiscriminate release of glutamate following concussive brain injury. *J Neurosurg* 73:889, 1990.

281. Nilsson P, Hillered L, Pontén U, et al: Changes in cortical extracellular levels of energy-related metabolites and amino acids following concussive brain injury in rats. *J Cereb Blood Flow Metab* 10:631, 1990.

282. DeWitt DS, Kong DL, Lyeth BG, et al: Experimental traumatic brain injury elevates brain prostaglandin E_2 and thromboxane B_2 levels in rats. *J Neurotrauma* 5:303, 1988.

283. McIntosh TK, Head VA, Faden AI: Alterations in regional concentrations of endogenous opioids following traumatic brain injury in the cat. *Brain Res* 425:225, 1987.

284. McIntosh TK, Hayes RL, DeWitt DS, et al: Endogenous opioids may mediate secondary damage after experimental brain injury. *Am J Physiol* 253:E565, 1987.

285. Rosner MJ, Becker DP: Experimental brain injury: Successful therapy with the weak base, tromethamine. With an overview of CNS acidosis. *J Neurosurg* 60:961, 1984.

286. Hall ED, Yonkers PA, McCall JM, et al: Effects of the 21-aminosteroid U74006F on experimental head injury in mice. *J Neurosurg* 68:456, 1988.

287. Levasseur JE, Patterson JL, Ghatak NR, et al: Combined effect of respirator-induced ventilation and superoxide dismutase in experimental brain injury. *J Neurosurg* 71:573, 1989.

288. Bailey I, Bell A, Gray J, et al: A trial of the effect of nimodipine on outcome after head injury. *Acta Neurochir* 110:97, 1991.

289. Teasdale G, Bailey I, Bell A, et al: The effect of nimodipine on outcome after head injury: A prospective randomised control trial. *Acta Neurochir Suppl* 51:315, 1990.

290. Lyeth BG, Hayes RL: Cholinergic and opioid mediation of traumatic brain injury. *J Neurotrauma* 9:S463, 1992.

291. Kim HJ, Levasseur JE, Patterson JL, Jr., Jackson GF, et al: Effect of indomethacin pretreatment on acute mortality in experimental brain injury. *J Neurosurg* 71:565, 1989.

292. Hayes RL, Lyeth BG, Jenkins LW, et al: Possible protective effect of endogenous opioids in traumatic brain injury. *J Neurosurg* 72:252, 1990.

293. Bruce DA, Gennarelli TA, Langfitt TW: Resuscitation from coma due to head injury. *Crit Care Med* 6:254, 1978.

294. Vernon-Levett P. Head injuries in children. *Crit Care Nurs Clin North Am* 3:411, 1991.

295. Grady MS, Jane JA, Steward O: Synaptic reorganization within the human central nervous system following injury. *J Neurosurg* 71:534, 1989.

296. Steward O: Reorganization of neuronal connections following CNS trauma: Principles and experimental paradigms. *J Neurotrauma* 6:99, 1989.

297. Brooks N: Cognitive deficits after head injury, in Brooks N (ed): *Closed Head Injury: Psychological, Social, and Family Consequences.* Oxford, Oxford University Press, 1984, pp 44-73.

298. Yamaguchi M: Incidence of headache and severity of head injury. *Headache* 32:427, 1992.

299. Brooks N: Head injury and the family, in Brooks N (ed): *Closed Head Injury: Psychological, Social, and Family Consequences.* Oxford, Oxford University Press, 1984, pp 123-147.

300. Oddy M: Head injury and social adjustment, in Brooks N (ed): *Closed Head Injury: Psychological, Social, and Family Consequences.* Oxford, Oxford University Press, 1984, pp 108-122.

301. Bond M: The psychiatry of closed head injury, in Brooks N (ed): *Closed Head Injury: Psychological, Social, and Family Consequences.* Oxford, Oxford University Press, 1984, pp 148-178.

302. Brooks DN: Disorders of memory, in Rosenthal M (ed): *Rehabilitation of the Head Injured Adult.* Philadelphia, F.A. Davis, 1983, p 185.

303. Brooks DN, Aughton ME, Bond MR, et al. Cognitive sequelae in relationship to early indices of severity of brain damage after severe blunt head injury. *J Neurol Neurosurg Psychiatry* 43:529, 1980.

304. Capruso DX, Levin HS: Cognitive impairment following closed head injury. *Neurol Clin* 10:879, 1992.

305. McAllister TW: Neuropsychiatric sequelae of head injuries. *Psychiatry Clin North Am* 15:395, 1992.

306. Goetz CG, Pappert EJ: Trauma and movement disorders. *Neurol Clin* 10:907, 1992.

307. Krauss JK, Mohadjer M, Braus DF, et al: Dystonia following head trauma: A report of nine patients and review of the literature. *Mov Disord* 7:263, 1992.

308. Johnson SL, Hall DM: Post-traumatic tremor in head injured children. *Arch Dis Child* 67:227, 1992.

309. Goetz CG, Stebbins GT: Effects of head trauma from motor vehicle accidents on Parkinson's disease. *Ann Neurol* 29:191, 1991.

310. Jennet B: *Epilepsy After Non-Missile Head Injuries.* 2nd ed. London: Heinemann, 1975.

311. Yadav YR, Khosla VK: Isolated 5th to 10th cranial nerve palsy in closed head trauma. *Clin Neurol Neurosurg* 93-1:61, 1991.

312. Caveness WF, Walker AE, Ascroft PB: Incidence of posttraumatic epilepsy in Korean veterans as compared with those from World War I and World War II. *J Neurosurg* 19:122, 1962.

313. Pascucci RC: Head trauma in the child. *Intensive Care Med* 14:185, 1988.

314. Jennett B, Bond M: Assessment of outcome after severe brain damage. *Lancet* 1:480, 1975.

315. Jennett B, Snoek J, Bond MR, et al: Disability after severe head injury: Observations on the use of the Glasgow Outcome Scale. *J Neurol Neurosurg Psychiatry* 44:285, 1981.

316. Giacino JT, Kezmarsky MA, DeLuca J, Cicerone KD: Monitoring rate of recovery to predict outcome in minimally responsive patients. *Arch Phys Med Rehabil* 72:897, 1991.

317. Butterworth JF IV, Selhorst JB, Greenberg RP, et al: Flaccidity after head injury: diagnosis, management, and outcome. *Neurosurgery* 9:242, 1981.

318. Lieh-Lai MW, Theodorou AA, Sarnaik AP, et al: Limitations of the Glasgow Coma Scale in predicting outcome in children with traumatic brain injury. *J Pediatr* 120:195, 1992.

319. Seelig JM, Greenberg RP, Becker DP, et al: Reversible brain-stem dysfunction following acute traumatic subdural hematoma: A clinical and electrophysiological study. *J Neurosurg* 55:516, 1981.

320. Choi SC, Narayan RK, Anderson RL, et al: Enhanced specificity of prognosis in severe head injury. *J Neurosurg* 69:381, 1988.

321. Obrist WD, Gennarelli TA, Segawa H, et al: Relation of cerebral blood flow to neurological status and outcome in head-injured patients. *J Neurosurg* 51:292, 1979.

322. Sazbon L, Groswasser Z: Outcome in 134 patients with prolonged posttraumatic unawareness. Part 1: Parameters determining late recovery of consciousness. *J Neurosurg* 72:75, 1990.
323. Hans P, Albert A, Franssen C, et al: Improved outcome prediction based on CSF extrapolated creatine kinase BB isoenzyme activity and other risk factors in severe head injury. *J Neurosurg* 71:54, 1989.
324. Michaud LJ, Rivara FP, Longstreth WT, Jr., Grady MS: Elevated initial blood glucose levels and poor outcome following severe brain injuries in children. *J Trauma* 31:1356, 1991.
325. Gennarelli TA, Spielman GM, Langfitt TW, et al: Influence of the type of intracranial lesion on outcome from severe head injury. *J Neurosurg* 56:26, 1982.
326. Rivas JJ, Lobato RD, Sarabia R, et al: Extradural hematoma: Analysis of factors influencing the courses of 161 patients. *Neurosurgery* 23:44, 1988.
327. Lobato RD, Rivas JJ, Cordobes G, et al: Acute epidural hematoma: an analysis of factors influencing the outcome of patients undergoing surgery in coma. *J Neurosurg* 68:48, 1988.
328. Deutsch G, Eisenberg HM: Frontal blood flow changes in recovery from coma. *J Cereb Blood Flow Metab* 7:29, 1987.
329. Uzzell BP, Obrist WD, Dolinskas CA, et al: Relationship of acute CBF and ICP findings to neuropsychological outcome in severe head injury. *J Neurosurg* 65:630, 1986.
330. Jaggi JL, Obrist WD, Gennarelli TA, et al: Relationship of early cerebral blood flow and metabolism to outcome in acute head injury. *J Neurosurg* 72:176, 1990.
331. Jennett B, Teasdale G, Galbraith S, et al: Severe head injuries in three countries. *J Neurol Neurosurg Psychiatry* 40:291, 1977.
332. Gibson RM, Stephenson GC: Aggressive management of severe closed head trauma: Time for reappraisal. *Lancet* 2:369, 1989.

176. Spinal Cord Trauma

Brian J. Kelly and John M. Luce

Spinal cord injury remains a devastating disorder in the United States. Annually, approximately 10,000 Americans are rendered paraplegic or quadriplegic by spinal cord injury [1]. Additionally, it is estimated that there are approximately 177,000 people in the United States, alive, with sequelae from spinal cord injury [2]. The most common causes of spinal cord injury in the United States are motor vehicle accidents (40%), falls (20%), and gunshot wounds (13.6%). In a recent study of major trauma in the United States, approximately 2.6% of trauma victims had acute spinal cord injuries [3]. Although the prognosis for spinal cord injury patients has improved in recent years, the mortality from spinal cord injury remains high [3]. For patients with isolated spinal cord injury, the present mortality rate is 6.9 percent [3]. However, almost 80 percent of patients with traumatic spinal cord injury have multiple injuries; for these patients the hospital mortality rate is 19.8 percent [3].

The keys to improving the outcome of spinal cord injuries are twofold. Most importantly, educational programs targeted to reduce the number of head and spinal cord injuries by proper use of seat belts and safe driving habits are paramount. Preliminary data from the National Head and Spinal Cord Injuries Prevention Program of the American Association of Neurologic Surgeons and the Congress of Neurologic Surgeons have suggested that a national education program does have a favorable impact on the incidence of spinal cord injury [4]. Secondly, appropriate early management of spinal cord injuries with attention toward preventing respiratory and medical complications can positively affect patient outcome. Furthermore, there is now excellent evidence that the early use of high-dose methylprednisone improves neurologic recovery after spinal cord injury [5].

This chapter has been prepared to help critical care physicians understand the pathophysiology and mechanisms in spinal cord injuries and to deal with the medical complications of this disorder. Additionally, the current recommended therapies, as well as future experimental therapies for the management of spinal cord injuries, are discussed.

Anatomy of the Vertebral Column and Spinal Cord

The spinal anatomy can be best understood by dividing it into three categories: the bony vertebral column, the spinal cord itself, and the blood vessels of the spinal cord (the spinal vascular unit). Although traumatic injuries to the spinal cord often affect several of these units in an interrelated manner, it is useful to consider each unit separately.

VERTEBRAL UNIT. The vertebral unit consists of the vertebral body, its posterior elements, and its attendant ligaments and muscles. The vertebral column consists of 7 cervical, 12 thoracic, 5 lumbar, 5 fused sacral, and the coccygeal vertebral bodies. The mobility of the human body is made possible because of the ability of the adjacent vertebral bodies to articulate by virtue of the intravertebral discs and by the posterolateral apophyseal (facet) joints. Although movement at each joint is limited, the human body's wide range of movement occurs because of the additive effect of movement at subsequent vertebral levels.

Figures 176-1 and 176-2 demonstrate the anatomy of the vertebral unit. Stability is achieved by the vertebral bodies, the intravertebral discs, the posterior elements, and the various ligaments that connect these structures. Of these ligaments, the posterior longitudinal ligament and the flaval ligament (or ligamentum flavum) are particularly important. Additional support is provided by the anterior longitudinal ligament, the intraspinous ligament, and the nuchal ligament or supraspinal ligaments.

An important concept in injuries to the vertebral bony unit is that of clinical stability. Clinical stability is defined as "the ability of the spine under physiologic loads to prevent initial or additional neurologic damage, severe, intractable pain or gross de-

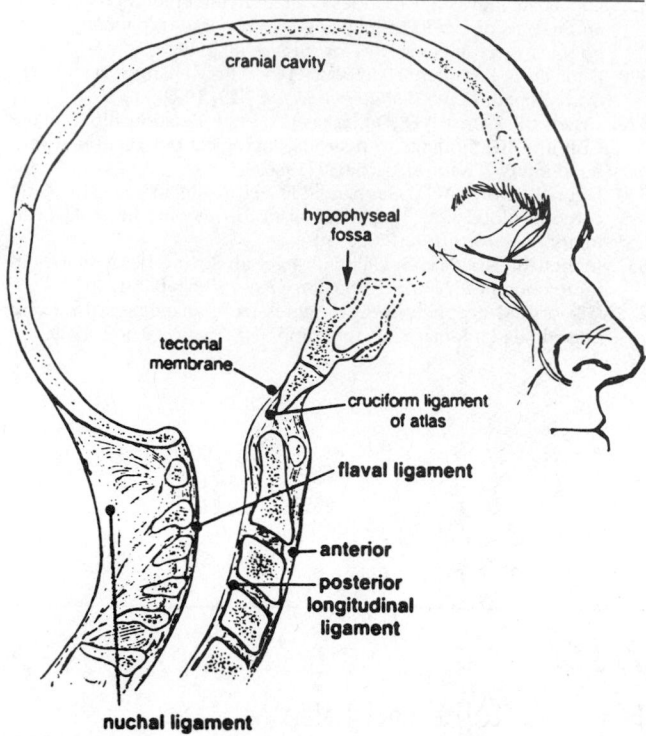

Fig. 176-1. A sagittal view of the cervical vertebrae and ligaments. (Reproduced with permission, from *Melloni's Illustrated Medical Dictionary*. Baltimore, Williams & Wilkins)

formity" [7]. Because of the potential for further neurologic injury to the spinal cord, identifying patients with unstable spinal injuries is crucial. To aid in the identification of unstable spine injuries, Denis developed his three column theory of spinal stability [8]. In this theory, the vertebral units are divided up into three theoretical columns. The anterior column is formed by the anterior longitudinal ligament, the anterior annulus fibrosus, and the anterior part of the vertebral body. The middle column is formed by the posterior longitudinal ligament, the posterior annulus fibrosis, and the posterior wall of the vertebral column. The posterior column is formed by the posterior bony complex (posterior arch) and the posterior ligamentous complex formed by the supraspinous and intraspinous ligaments, the apophyseal joints' capsules, and the ligamentum flavum. According to Denis, if two of these three columns are disrupted, instability is present [8]. Additionally, isolated damage to the middle column, although clinically rare, does have the potential for being unstable because of herniation of disc or bony material into the spinal canal.

SPINAL CORD UNIT. The spinal cord is a cylindrical extension of the brain that stretches from the foramen magnum to its termination in the filum terminale at approximately the L1–L2 bony vertebral level (Fig. 176-3). The spinal cord is anchored in place by the nerve roots that exit at each vertebral level and by the suspensory ligaments of the spinal cord, the dentate ligaments.

The spinal cord is covered by three membranes that are collectively known as the spinal meninges. The thickest of these, the spinal dura, is a continuous extension of the cranial dura and extends from the foramen magnum to the filum ter-

minale. The space between the spinal dura and the bony vertebral column is a true space called the epidural space. The epidural space contains fat, ligaments, and numerous venous plexus, as well as the spinal nerve roots and vascular structures supplying the spinal cord. In addition to the dura, the spinal cord is covered by a closely adherent layer called the pia mater and a loosely arranged thin membrane called the arachnoid.

Similar to other structures in the central nervous system, the spinal cord is somatotopically organized. Figures 176-4 and 176-5 illustrate the anatomy and blood supply of the cervical spinal cord. As is evident from Figure 176-4, the spinal cord can be divided into a central rim of gray matter with surrounding white matter tracts that are composed of ascending and descending axons.

SPINAL VASCULAR UNIT. The spinal cord receives its blood supply from multiple radicular arteries that form the anterior spinal and two posterior spinal arteries. As illustrated in Figure 176-5, the anterior spinal artery provides the major blood supply to the spinal cord, supplying the anterior commissure, the adjacent white matter of the ventral columns, the anterior horns, the base of the posterior horns, Clark's columns, the corticospinal and spinothalamic tracts, and the ventral parts of the posterior columns. The posterior spinal arteries each distribute blood to the posterior third of the spinal cord on their respective sides.

It is important to realize that the radicular arteries supplying the anterior and posterior spinal arteries vary greatly in size. Only approximately eight of these radicular arteries are of a significant enough caliber to provide meaningful perfusion to the spinal cord. As a result, areas of the spinal cord are a great distance from the radicular arteries and therefore are susceptible to ischemia. These areas can be considered watershed areas, and studies have demonstrated that these are most likely to occur in the lower cervical region [9,10].

Recent work has also demonstrated that, similar to the brain, the spinal cord autoregulates blood flow over a wide range of blood pressure. Between mean arterial blood pressures (MAP) of 60 and 120 mm Hg, spinal cord blood flow is maintained at a constant level. However, when the MAP is less than 60 mm Hg, spinal cord blood flow falls directly with MAP and spinal cord ischemia results [11].

Pathophysiology of Spinal Cord Injury

Spinal cord injury results when the muscles, ligaments, and bony structures surrounding the spinal cord fail to dissipate the energy generated by flexion, extension, vertical compression, or rotation [12,13]. The spinal cord can be injured directly in trauma from any of these force vectors, as well as by shearing [14]. Vertical compression classically produces burst fractures and ligamentous ruptures. Severe flexion injuries cause characteristic anterior subluxation or dislocations to the vertebral bodies with disruption of the posterior longitudinal ligaments and herniation of the intravertebral discs. Extreme hyperextension is associated with transverse fractures of the vertebra, disruption of the anterior longitudinal ligaments, and posterior dislocations [1]. Although these patterns are those classically described, most spinal cord injuries result from a combination of different vector forces. Additionally, because the alignment of the facet joints is very different between the cervical spine and the lumbar spine, the resulting injury from a similarly ap-

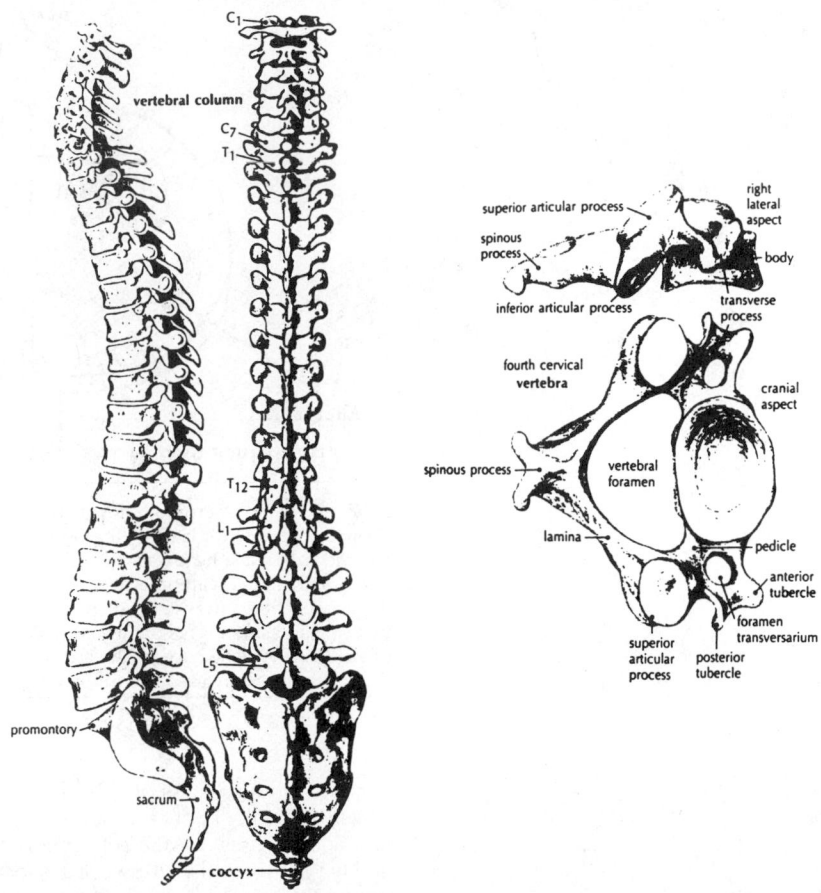

Fig. 176-2. (Left) Lateral and posterior views of the bony vertebral column. *(Right)* A lateral and superior view of the fourth cervical
vertebra. (Reproduced with permission, from *Melloni's Illustrated Review of Human Anatomy.* Philadelphia, J.B. Lippincott Co.)

plied force to these areas can vary greatly [15]. Therefore, it is
extremely difficult to classify fracture patterns seen radiographically by mechanism [15]. The spinal cord can also be injured
without evidence of injury to the vertebral column [14]. Ligaments can rupture without bony structures failing. These injuries are most common in elderly patients with cervical spon-
dylosis [16].

The actual initial cause of traumatic damage to the spinal
cord is controversial [17,18]. One theory, the neuronal theory,
states that the direct trauma to the neuronal membranes leads
to a cascade of biochemical events that cause the initial injury
[17]. The other leading theory, the vascular theory, states that it
is the initial vascular insult to the spinal cord's blood supply
that is the primary cause of neuronal damage [18].

Histologically, soon after injury, the small intramedullary vessels within the central gray matter of the cord are damaged and
hyperemia and hemorrhage occur in this area [1]. This hemorrhage often progresses to central hemorrhagic necrosis. Later,
small hemorrhages are seen in the corticospinal tracts, and the
white matter tracts become edematous [19]. Numerous studies
have also demonstrated that there is an initial acute decrease
in the blood flow to the central gray matter [20,23]. Blood flow,
however, to the white matter is variable and an increase in flow
is sometimes found [23,24]. This increased blood flow may be
related to transient hypertension seen immediately after injury

and may increase hemorrhage and edema formation. As time
progresses, the central gray matter is invaded with polymorphonuclear leukocytes, which produce cavitation, and glial
cells proliferate in the white matter tracts, forming glial scars
[25].

Although the initial damage to the spinal cord may not be
amenable to therapy, much research over the past decade has
demonstrated that secondary injuries caused by a cascade of
biochemical and rheologic events may occur and be more treatable. Because complete transection of the spinal cord is rare,
therapy now is targeted at preventing this secondary cascade
to save any viable neurons and axons. Even small amounts of
preservation of white matter tracts are important because viability of as little as 10 percent of these tracts can be associated
with significant recovery [14].

The cascade of secondary events leading to neuronal death
is similar to that described for other areas of the central nervous
system [26]. After injury, there is a decrease in tissue PO_2 and
cellular adenosine triphosphate (ATP) stores. This leads to a
depolarization of the cells with the subsequent block of nerve
impulses. Excitotoxins such as glutamate are released and result
in the influx of large amounts of sodium, calcium, and water
into the neurons [26]. This influx of calcium activates phospho-
lipases, which further degrade neuronal and cell membranes
[27]. As these membranes are broken down, polyunsaturated
fatty acids are liberated in high concentrations and serve as
precursors for various leukotrienes. Several of these leukotrienes (thromboxane A_2 and leukotrienes C4 and D4) are potent
vasoconstrictors and promote platelet aggregation and poly-

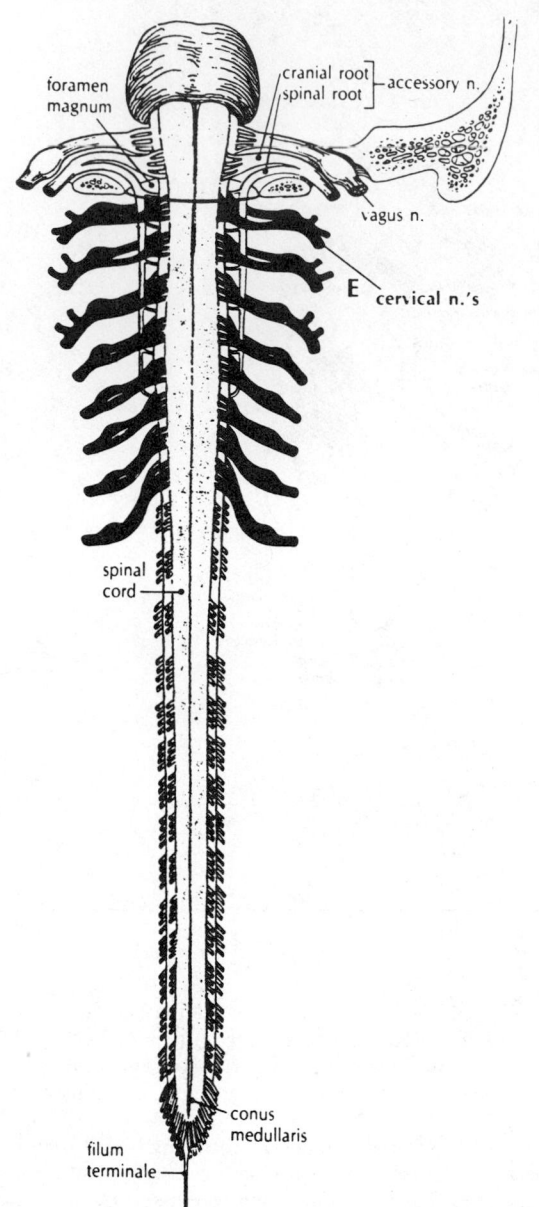

Fig. 176-3. The anatomy of the spinal cord. (Reproduced with permission, from *Melloni's Illustrated Review of Human Anatomy.* Philadelphia, J.B. Lippincott Co.)

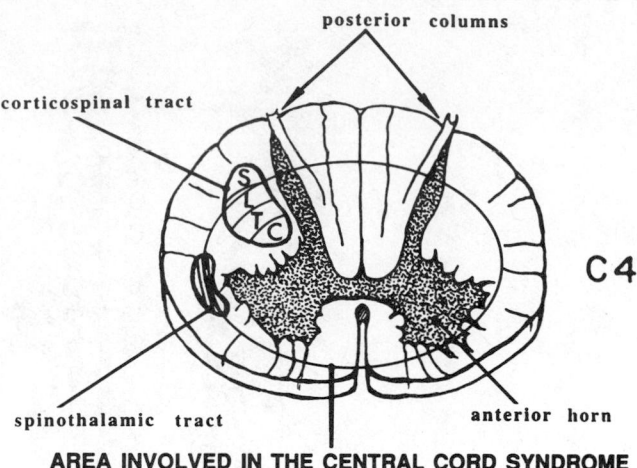

AREA INVOLVED IN THE CENTRAL CORD SYNDROME

Fig. 176-4. A cross-sectional view of the cervical spinal cord showing the anterior horns, the posterior columns, and the corticospinal and spinothalamic tracts. Note the somatotopic organization of the corticospinal tract with the fibers from the sacrum most lateral and the cervical fibers most medial. The spinothalamic tract is organized in a similar fashion. This organization accounts for the phenomenon of *sacral sparing* (see text). The area enclosed in the solid circle is the region clinically involved in the *central cord syndrome* (see text).

decrease perfusion. As previously described, spinal cord blood flow is normally kept constant through autoregulation at mean arterial pressures (MAPs) between 60 and 120 mm Hg [11]. This ability to autoregulate, however, is lost in traumatic spinal cord injury. The onset of spinal shock with its resulting hypotension can further decrease spinal cord perfusion and worsen ischemia. Therefore, it is essential to maintain adequate perfusion to the spinal cord in the early initial hours after injury.

Patterns of Spinal Cord Injury

Complete spinal cord lesions block all neuronal transmission across the injured cord segments. Clinically, the patient has no sensation or voluntary motor function below the level of cord injury. However, spinal cord reflexes such as deep tendon reflexes and single reflex arcs such as the bulbocavernous reflex are present. Incomplete spinal cord injuries spare some of the motor or sensory pathways across the injured segment with partial loss of sensation or motor function. The most common of these patterns in the cervical spinal cord is the central cord syndrome. This syndrome is due to bleeding and edema within the central gray matter of the cord. The areas involved are illustrated in Figure 176-4. The clinical syndrome that results is characterized by lower motor neuron dysfunction in the upper extremities caused by the involvement of the cervical anterior horn cells, variable degrees of upper motor neuron signs in the lower extremities caused by involvement of the corticospinal tracts, bilateral loss of pain and temperature caused by the involvement of the spinothalamic tracts, and a variable degree of dorsal column dysfunction.

Another classically described syndrome is that of the anterior spinal artery. This syndrome often is not attributable to traumatic compression, but rather to ischemic infarction or embolization of the anterior spinal artery. It usually occurs around

morphonuclear leukocyte infiltration [28,29]. The infiltration of leukocytes and the presence of calcium in the mitochondria also cause the generation of free radicals. These free radicals are highly unstable compounds that can cause more lipid membrane degradation and further neuronal damage [30].

A variety of other mediators have been implicated in spinal cord injury. Catecholamines may cause vasoconstriction and worsen ischemia [31]. Faden and colleagues have shown that certain opioid receptors (probably the kappa subtype) may also be important mediators in spinal cord injury [32,33,34].

Ischemia in the hours after spinal cord injury may be the most important mechanism underlying the secondary injury phenomenon [35]. Hemorrhage into the gray matter and vasogenic edema increase tissue pressure within the spinal cord and

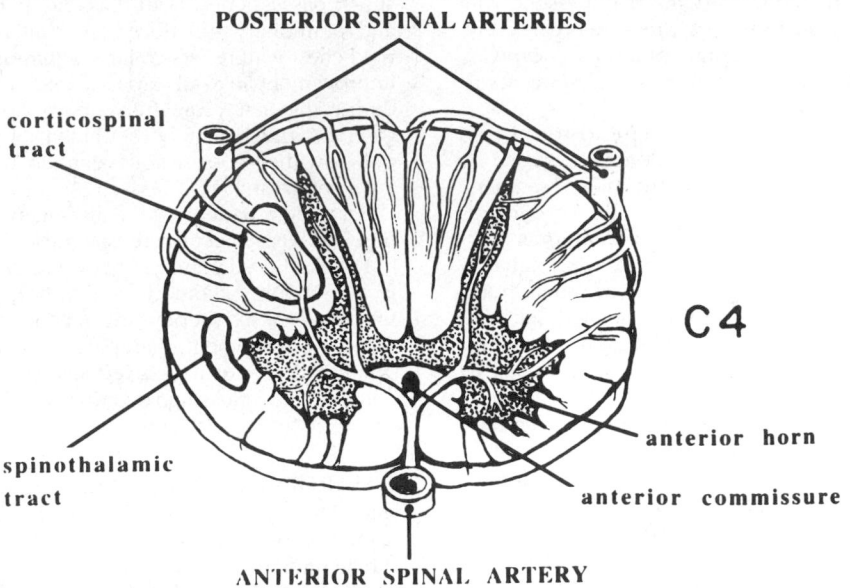

POSTERIOR SPINAL ARTERIES

corticospinal tract

C4

spinothalamic tract

anterior horn

anterior commissure

ANTERIOR SPINAL ARTERY

Fig. 176-5. A cross-sectional view of the cervical spinal cord demonstrating its arterial blood supply. The anterior spinal artery provides the major blood supply to the cord, supplying the anterior commissure, the adjacent white matter of the ventral columns, the anterior horns, the base of the posterior horns, Clark's columns, the corticospinal and spinothalamic tracts, and the ventral parts of the posterior columns. The posterior spinal arteries each distribute blood to the posterior third of the spinal cord on their respective sides.

spinal level C5–C6 and is characterized by the loss of pain, temperature, and lower motor neuron function in the arms, upper motor neuron weakness below the level of the lesion, and total sparing of dorsal column function. Although other spinal cord syndromes such as the Brown-Sequard syndrome are well described, these are unusual after spinal cord trauma.

Prognostically, there are major differences between complete and incomplete spinal cord injuries. With the exception of those with anterior spinal artery syndromes, patients with incomplete spinal cord syndromes often regain significant amounts of neurologic function [36]. Unfortunately, most patients with complete spinal cord injury do not recover significant neurologic function. Therefore, the initial clinical assessment is extremely important. If the patient has any voluntary motor function or sensation below the level of the lesion, this is important to note. Sensation should be tested around the perineum because the phenomenon of "sacral sparing" implies an incomplete lesion. Sacral sparing refers to preserved sensation in the perineum after spinal cord injury. It is caused by the normal anatomic distribution of sensory fibers in the ascending spinothalmic tracts. The fibers from the perineum and lower extremities are located in the lateral aspects of the spinal cord. Therefore, central cord lesions affect these fibers last, and these fibers are often spared in incomplete lesions.

An important entity to keep in mind in performing this initial assessment, however, is that of spinal shock. After spinal cord trauma, there is an absence of sensorimotor function and the presence of flaccidity below the injured segment. Spinal cord reflexes such as the deep tendon reflexes, bulbocavernous reflex, and the anal wink are absent. Spinal cord shock can last from minutes to days, and its exact cause is unknown. Some physicians hypothesize that it is related to an increase in extracellular potassium at the level of injury that results in an axonal

conduction block [37]. Others maintain that it is caused by a disruption of the balance of spinal cord inhibitory and facilatory pathways [38]. Clinically, a spinal cord injury cannot be diagnosed as complete in the presence of spinal shock. One must therefore wait until spinal reflexes such as the deep tendon reflexes, the bulbocavernous reflex, and the anal wink have returned to document a lesion as complete.

Clinical Manifestations of Spinal Cord Injury

CARDIOVASCULAR EFFECTS. Cardiovascular complications of spinal cord trauma are characterized by autonomic hyperactivity and hyporeactivity [1]. Studies indicate that the immediate response to spinal cord trauma is a period of hypertension usually accompanied by bradycardia [39,40,41]. This period is usually accompanied by electrocardiographic evidence of left ventricular strain and ventricular ectopy and is presumably mediated by the sympathetic nervous system, because it can be blocked by alpha-adrenergic blockers such as phentolamine and phenoxybenzamine [39,40,41].

Pulmonary edema is a well-recognized complication of spinal cord injury [42,43]. The cause of this pulmonary edema is complex. In some patients, it is clearly caused by fluid overload during volume resuscitation [42]. However, it can occur in the absence of volume overload [43]. The occurrence of pulmonary edema after spinal cord trauma probably is attributable in large part to an acute massive sympathetic discharge at the time of injury. Albin has described increases in pulmonary capillary wedge pressure and mean arterial blood pressure after spinal cord transection [39]. Additionally, various electrocardiographic changes, dysrhythmias, and blood pressure changes have been described after central nervous system injury [44,45,46]. These changes can cause left ventricular failure and disrupt pulmonary capillary endothelium, setting the stage for the development of cardiac and noncardiac pulmonary edema [12]. Other factors released during spinal cord injury may also affect left ventricular function [47]. Therefore, pulmonary edema may be seen with an elevated pulmonary capillary wedge pressures (caused by left ventricular failure) or with normal pulmonary capillary wedge pressures (caused by increased pulmonary microvascular leak) [12].

Although hypertension is the initial response to spinal cord trauma, most patients rapidly develop hypotension causd by loss of sympathetic tone below the level of the injured segment. If the injured spinal segment is above level T1, bradycardia progressing to complete heart block and poikilothermia sufficient to reduce the core body temperature to approximately 34°C may occur, and are collectively referred to as spinal shock. Systemic vascular resistance is low during spinal shock with cardiac output either normal or increased [42]. These patients may manifest significant orthostatic hypotension and must be moved carefully.

Although most quadriplegic patients continue to manifest low or normal blood pressure and pulse for weeks to months after their injuries, more than 50 percent of patients with lesions above level T7 exhibit periodic episodes of autonomic dysreflexia. These episodes consist of severe hypertension, bradycardia, headache, sweating, and flushing or pallor associated with vasodilatation triggered most frequently by distension of visceral organs, especially the urinary bladder and bowels [47,48]. In such patients, noxious stimuli below the level of the neurologic lesion can cause the massive activation of the sympathetic nervous system with the release of high levels of norepinephrine into the bloodstream [47,48,49]. This release occurs because of dysfunctional supraspinal regulatory control of the autonomic nervous system [47].

RESPIRATORY EFFECTS. Spinal cord injury is often associated with profound respiratory compromise. Injuries at or above the cord segments C3–C5 result in partial or complete bilateral hemidiaphragmatic paralysis. In addition, intercostal muscle paralysis below the lesion limits the normal outward expansion of the middle and upper rib cage, further compromising inspiration. Active expiration is also greatly reduced because of paralysis of abdominal and other expiratory muscles. Although sternocleidomastoid, scalene, and trapezoid muscle activities persist in high cord injuries, their efficiency is greatly reduced.

Because of their extensive respiratory muscle dysfunction, high cervical quadriplegics are unable to generate an adequate vital capacity because of reduced inspiratory and expiratory function [50]. Hypoxemia is common and results from both hypoventilation and microatelectasis [51].

Quadriplegic patients with lesions in the lower cervical spinal cord below level C3–C5, which spare the phrenic nerve nuclei, can contract the diaphragm to a variable extent. However, they lack the intercostal muscle activity necessary to stabilize the rib cage so the diaphragm can function properly; as a result their inspiratory function is mildly compromised. Like high-level quadriplegics, these patients have also lost the use of their abdominal and other expiratory muscles. This combination of respiratory and inspiratory weakness prevents them from coughing and clearing secretions, placing them at high risk for respiratory tract infection.

A large percentage of patients with acute cervical spinal cord injury require ventilatory support [50]. The vital capacity is reduced and is commonly between 1.2 and 1.5 liters after these injuries and is accompanied by reductions in the maximal inspiratory pressure and, to a greater extent, the maximal expiratory pressure [52]. The higher the spinal cord lesion, the more profound the respiratory failure. Fortunately, the need for ventilatory support is often temporary. As the initial phase of spinal shock passes, chest wall flaccidity is replaced with spasticity, and pulmonary function significantly improves as the more rigid chest wall resists collapse. Pulmonary function tests show improvement in vital capacity and resting breathing patterns during the first year after cervical spinal cord injury [53,54]. Overall, approximately 80 percent of patients with injuries at or below the C4 level can eventually be weaned from mechanical ventilation [54].

Paraplegic patients generally maintain diaphragmatic function and have intact intercostal muscles at or above the level of their spinal cord injury. However, they may manifest the same lack of abdominal muscle activity as quadriplegics, if they have thoracic lesions. Depending on the extent of the abdominal muscle involvement, paraplegics may exhibit impaired diaphragmatic performance, reduced vital capacity, and problems coughing and clearing secretions [1,55].

GASTROINTESTINAL EFFECTS. Ileus and gastric atony frequently accompany spinal cord injury and may lead to gastric aspiration or compromised ventilation by pushing upwards on the hemidiaphragms. The use of steroids, decreased gastric emptying, and unopposed parasympathetic innervation all predispose spinal cord injury patients to a variety of gastrointestinal complications [56]. Furthermore, symptoms and signs of intraabdominal pathology may be masked in these patients. Recently, there has been a significant decrease in the incidence of gastrointestinal bleeding after spinal cord injury, probably because of better stress ulcer prophylaxis [56]. Esophageal perforation has also been associated with cervical spinal cord injuries [57]. Clinical manifestations of this injury may be subtle and include fever of unknown origin, leukocytosis, and unexplained persistent tachycardia.

Finally, the exaggerated catabolic state and immobilization of spinal cord injury patients may cause severe hypoalbuminemia, hypocalcemia, and other deficiencies unless adequate nutrition is provided.

GENITOURINARY EFFECTS. Genitourinary function is often severely affected in spinal cord injury. During spinal shock, the bladder becomes flaccid but does not empty. This can result in overdistension and autonomic dysreflexia. Quadriplegic patients do not sense bladder distension and cannot effectively exert abdominal pressure on their bladder to void. This may result in urinary stasis and urinary tract infections. These may lead to pyelonephritis and acute or chronic renal failure.

Initial Management of Spinal Cord Injury

The management of the patient with spinal cord injury begins at the scene where the injury occurred [14]. Symptoms such as weakness, paralysis, sensory disturbances, laceration or abrasions on the head or neck, or spinal tenderness suggest the presence of spinal cord injury. Most patients with cord lesions do not lose consciousness and can testify to numbness or paralysis. Unconscious patients should be considered to have a spinal cord injury until proven otherwise.

Proper early care of the spinal cord injury patient is critical to minimize the chance of an incomplete lesion progressing to a complete one. The airway should be assessed and if not patent, an oral airway or esophageal obturator should be inserted. Supplemental oxygen should be administered. If ventilation is inadequate, the patient should be intubated immediately. This can be performed by the blind nasotracheal method or by direct laryngoscopy, without unduly extending the neck. In the field, this is usually performed by immobilizing the spine with manual in-line traction. Several recent reviews of oral tracheal intubation in patients with spinal cord injury have documented that if performed properly, the risk of exacerbating spinal cord injury during oral intubation with in-line traction is small [58,59].

The blood pressure should be assessed as soon as possible. If hypotension is present, neurogenic spinal shock must be differentiated from hemorrhagic shock [14]. Because up to 80 percent of patients with spinal cord injury have other associated injuries, a quick survey for sites of obvious hemorrhage is indicated [3]. Actively bleeding sites should be treated with compression and appropriate amounts of intravenous fluids. If the spinal cord level of injury is above T6, and the patient is hypotensive and bradycardic, the presence of spinal shock should be considered. Because overly aggressive hydration of these patients can result in pulmonary edema, initial volume resuscitation should be limited. These patients should be treated by mild elevation of the legs to decrease venous pooling, careful volume expansion, and if necessary, the administration of vasopressors (see below).

The spine should be immobilized as completely as possible. This is best accomplished with a full-length spine board with the head taped in the midline position and sand bags placed on each side of the neck. If the patient's head is initially flexed, gentle in-line traction should be applied, and the neck should be aligned with the rest of the body. The patient should be logrolled gently onto a long spine board. It is important to immobilize the entire vertebral column because there is approximately a 5 to 15 percent incidence of noncontiguous fractures of the spinal column [60].

The patient should be transferred to the nearest facility qualified to manage spinal cord injuries. Because aspiration and shock are the most common causes of death associated with spinal cord injuries, the patient should be transported in the Trendelenburg position at a 20° to 30° tilt [14].

Emergency Room Management of Spinal Cord Injury

On initial presentation to the emergency room, the airway and breathing should be reassessed, and intubation should be performed if necessary. Pressures should be normalized with the judicious administration of fluid and vasopressors, if necessary (see below). Consultation with a general or trauma surgeon is essential to exclude other injuries and causes of hypotension. A Foley catheter should be inserted to monitor urine outflow and prevent overdistension of the bladder and autonomic dysreflexia. A nasogastric tube should be inserted to minimize the risk of aspiration and respiratory compromise from an ileus. If open wounds are present, tetanus prophylaxis and broad-spectrum antibiotics should be administered [14].

Once the patient is stabilized, a thorough neurologic examination should be performed. Mental status and cranial nerve examination should be completed. Abnormal results suggest intracranial pathology. The presence of a Horner's syndrome or unilateral neck or facial pain may indicate a carotid dissection, whereas symptoms or signs of brainstem ischemia may suggest damage to the vertebral arteries. In these cases, angiography or magnetic resonance angiography should be performed. The spine should be palpated for malalignment of the spinous processes or a boggy gap of the supraspinous ligaments suggesting disruption of the posterior column [15]. A detailed motor and sensory examination should be performed to document the level of spinal cord injury. Any voluntary motor function or sensation below the level of the lesion implies that the lesion is incomplete and is of important prognostic significance. The ability to voluntarily contract the anal sphincter or the presence of intact sensation in the perineum implies sacral sparing, and also implies an incomplete lesion. Deep tendon reflexes and cremasteric and abdominal reflexes should be tested. Their absence, like that of the bulbocavernous reflex, implies the presence of spinal shock [61].

The initial radiographic films that should be performed for a trauma victim include an anteroposterior (AP) view of the chest and pelvis and a lateral cervical spine film. It is mandatory that all cervical vertebrae including the top of the first thoracic vertebra be visualized by either pulling the arms down or using a swimmer's view. In addition to the lateral cervical spine film, an anterior view and open-mouth view of the cervical spine are recommended. Other additional radiograph are based on clinical findings. The radiograph should be examined closely for the configuration and alignment of the vertebral bodies, the alignment of the facets and posterior vertebral bodies, and the interspinous distances [15]. Complete radiographic survey of the spinal column is necessary to rule out the presence of noncontiguous fractures, which are known to occur in 5 to 15 percent of patients [62].

If a fracture or dislocation is present and bone impinges into the spinal canal, the normal anatomic alignment must be aggressively restored [14]. Neurosurgical consultation in these patients is mandatory. Generally, closed reduction is attempted through traction with Gardner-Wells tongs or a halo ring. Many patients' fractures can be reduced with closed reduction; however, if reduction cannot be obtained, the patient should be studied with computed tomography (CT) myelography [14]. Computed tomography can also be used to study the head, chest, abdomen, and pelvis; these studies should be coordinated to minimize patient transfers. Recently, magnetic resonance imaging has been used to study acute spinal cord injured patients safely [63,64]. Magnetic resonance imaging offers rapid visualization of the extent and degree of spinal cord deformity and associated bony injuries and may help determine the need for acute surgical intervention in specific cases of spinal cord injury [63]. Unfortunately, the maintenance of proper spine stabilization requires the use of nonferromagnetic skull traction devices, and hemodynamic monitoring is difficult in the multiple-injured trauma patient undergoing this procedure.

The final therapy that should be initiated in the emergency room is the administration of high-dose methylprednisolone. Although early studies failed to show a beneficial effect from its administration [65,66,67], the second national acute spinal cord injury study (NASCIS-2) showed that high-dose methylprednisolone administered within 8 hours of the injury resulted in significant improvement in motor function and sensory function compared with placebo [6]. If the treatment was initiated more than 8 hours from the time of injury, however, neurologic outcome was similar to placebo. Additionally, mortality and major morbidities did not differ with the administration of methylprednisolone [6].

A bolus of 30 mg/kg of body weight of methylprednisolone followed by an infusion at 5.4 mg/kg/hr for 23 hours should be given as soon as possible [6]. Stress ulcer prophylaxis should be concurrently administered in these patients. Although the mechanisms of action of methylprednisolone may be multiple, the primary mechanism is probably through a reduction of injury-induced, free radical-catalyzed lipid peroxidation [68].

Intensive Care Unit Management of Spinal Cord Injury

CARDIOVASCULAR MANAGEMENT. When persistent hypotension is associated with clinical signs of organ hypoperfusion or an ascending temperature gradient in the lower extremities, therapeutic intervention is necessary [12]. Because spinal cord–injured patients are systemically vasodilated, their effective intravascular volume is low. Therefore, initial careful volume resuscitation is indicated. Studies of acutely quadriplegic patients have demonstrated that a pulmonary capillary wedge pressure of 18 torr produces optimal left ventricular function [69]. Because these patients are subject to pulmonary edema, the use of a pulmonary artery catheter in the hypotensive spinal cord–injured patient facilitates management, although it is not obligatory. Albin advocates repeated administration of fluid challenges until evidence of hypoperfusion reverses or until the pulmonary artery capillary wedge pressure exceeds 18 mm Hg and does not fall to lower levels within 5 minutes of completion of the fluid challenge [12]. If fluid therapy fails because of increasing lung water, or if the arterial blood pressure remains low despite a high pulmonary capillary wedge pressure, vasopressors such as dopamine, dobutamine, or phenylephrine are then added. This approach minimizes the risk of pulmonary edema and maintains arterial blood pressure and therefore minimizes the chance of secondary spinal cord hypoperfusion during the critical early period after spinal cord injury.

RESPIRATORY MANAGEMENT. Intubated patients should receive supplemental oxygen and be placed on mechanical ventilation. For those patients not initially intubated, continuous careful assessment of ventilatory status is essential. Many patients develop respiratory failure gradually over the initial days of hospitalization. Serial measurements of vital capacity (VC) and maximum inspiratory and expiratory pressures (P_{IMAX}, P_{EMAX}) should be monitored closely. Hypercapnia occurs at VC < 10 cc per kilogram of body weight and at a P_{IMAX} < 20 cm H_2O [52]. A P_{EMAX} < 40 cm H_2O preludes effective coughing.

Quadriplegic and high paraplegic patients lose their ability to cough and clear secretions and are prone to progressive atelectasis. Quad coughing, in which the therapist pushes forcefully on the abdomen, is useful to generate the positive airway pressure necessary to expel mucus. Suctioning with a nasal trumpet also may facilitate secretion removal in these patients. Nevertheless, many of these patients require intubation and the temporary use of mechanical ventilation. As previously mentioned, most spinal cord–injured patients with lesions below the C4 level can be weaned from ventilation eventually.

Prophylactic antibiotics should be avoided, because they may contribute to the emergence of resistant organisms. However, antibiotics should be promptly administered if the patient develops fever, leukocytosis, an infiltrate on chest radiograph, and purulent sputum.

Thromboembolic disease is a major cause of morbidity and mortality in patients with spinal cord injury; approximately 16.3 percent of such patients suffer clinically apparent thromboembolic disease [70,71]. However, when they are prospectively studied using objective tests such as fibrinogen uptake, impedance plethysmography, and venography, 79 percent of patients with spinal cord injury have evidence of thromboembolic disease [70]. Patients with complete paralysis are at particularly high risk for deep venous thrombosis, and elderly patients are more prone to pulmonary emboli [71] (see Chap. 60).

Recently, a consensus conference on deep venous thrombosis and spinal cord injury recommended that all patients with spinal cord injury and motor paralysis receive prophylaxis for thromboembolic disease by means of compression devices, anticoagulant drugs, or vena caval filters [70–77]. Compression devices are safe, but there is still a significant risk of thromboembolic disease despite their use. The early use of compression devices plus low-dose heparin therapy with prolongation of the prothrombin time to 1.3 to 1.5 times the control value beginning at 72 hours seems to be effective. However, once the compression devices are removed, then the dose of heparin needs to be increased. Vena cava filters should be inserted only in patients who cannot be fitted with compression devices or are not candidates for anticoagulation [72]. Anticoagulant prophylaxis should be discontinued in patients who have return of motor function and are able to ambulate. In those with persistent paralysis, 3 months of therapy is the usual duration of therapy.

GASTROINTESTINAL MANAGEMENT. Spinal cord–injured patients should be maintained on nasogastric suction to prevent abdominal distension and ileus. Tube feedings should begin only when gastric and intestinal activity has been restored. Metoclopramide may improve gastrointestinal motility in some patients, but most require the return of autonomic function [1]. Hyperalimentation may be indicated if atony is prolonged. Stool softeners should be considered to avoid constipation and autonomic dysreflexia.

GENITOURINARY MANAGEMENT. A Foley catheter should be maintained during the initial ICU period to facilitate fluid management and avoid overdistension of the bladder. Colonization of the bladder may occur and does not require medical treatment. However, a urinary tract infection should be treated with antibiotics in the face of gross pyuria, fever, and other symptoms [1].

OTHER MANAGEMENT ISSUES. Meticulous nursing care with attention to avoiding pressure sores and hypothermia is essential. The use of a Rotorest bed for the multiple-injured patient greatly facilitates nursing management. Most centers are not routinely using the Stryker frame because of its potential to exacerbate respiratory fatigue and cause cardiac complications and the risk of hyperextension to the cervical spine with turning [78]. If long-term mechanical ventilation is likely, early tracheostomy should be considered to facilitate communication. Finally, these patients require immense emotional support during their acute injury [79].

Experimental and Future Therapies for Spinal Cord Injury

A host of various compounds and therapies have been studied over the past decade in spinal cord injury. Many of these have shown improvement in neurologic outcome or spinal cord blood flow in experimental models [80–88]. Most of these therapies target one or more of the biochemical steps that lead to permanent neuronal injury or facilitate spinal cord blood flow. These therapies include various leukotrienes and prostaglandin inhibitors, N-methyl-D-aspartate receptor inhibitors, various opioid antagonists, thyrotropin-releasing hormone, and inhibitors of lipid peroxidation [80–87].

Recently, a small study of GM-1 ganglioside in human acute spinal cord injury was completed and showed that GM-1 ganglioside enhanced neurologic recovery after 1 year [89]. Although the mechanism of action of GM-1 ganglioside is unknown, it probably acts by enhancing neuronal survival in white matter tracts. Presently, human studies are in progress looking at tirilazad, a 21-aminosteroid inhibitor of lipid peroxidation, in spinal cord injury.

References

1. Luce JM: Medical management of spinal cord injury. *Crit Care Med* 13:126, 1985.
2. Harvey C, Rothschild BB, Asmann AJ, et al: New estimates of traumatic SCI prevalence: A survey-based approach. *Paraplegia* 28(9):537, 1990.
3. Burney RE, Maio RF, Maynard F, et al: Incidence, characteristics, and outcome of spinal cord injury at trauma centers in North America. *Arch Surg* 128(5):596, 1993.
4. Stover SL, Fine PR: *Spinal Cord Injury: The Facts and Figures.* Birmingham, AL, University of Alabama, 1986.
5. National Head and Spinal Cord Injury Prevention Program of the American Association of Neurological Surgeons and the Congress of Neurological Surgeons. *J Neurotrauma* 9(Suppl 1):S307, 1992.
6. Bracken MB, Shepard MJ, Collins WF, et al: A randomized, controlled trial of methylprednisolone or naloxone in the treatment of acute spinal cord injury. *N Engl J Med* 322(20):1407, 1990.
7. White AA, Panjabi MM: The role of stabilization in the treatment of cervical spine injuries. *Spine* 9:512, 1984.
8. Denis F: The three column spine and its significance in the classification of acute thoracolumbar spinal injuries. *Spine* 8(8):817, 1983.
9. Manners T: Vascular lesion in the spinal cord in the aged. *Geriatrics* 21:151, 1966.
10. Jellinger K: Spinal cord arteriosclerosis and progressive vascular myelopathy. *J Neurol Neurosurg Psychiatry* 30:195, 1967.
11. Hickey R, Albin M, Bunegin L, et al: Autoregulation of spinal cord and cerebral blood flow: Is the spinal cord a microcosm of the brain? *Stroke* 17:1183, 1987.
12. Albin MS: Acute spinal cord trauma, in Shoemaker WC, Ayres S, Grenvik A, et al. (eds): *Textbook of Critical Care. 2nd ed.* Philadelphia, WB Saunders Co, 1989, pp 1277–1285.
13. Bunegin L, Hung TK, Chang GL: Biomechanics of spinal cord injury. *Crit Care Clin* 3:453, 1987.
14. Sonntag VKH, Douglas RA: Management of cervical spinal cord trauma. *J Neurotrauma* 9(Suppl 1):S385, 1992.
15. Johnson GE: Spine injuries, in Hall JB, Schmidt GA, Wood LD (eds): *Principles of Critical Care.* New York, McGraw-Hill, 1987, pp 715–724.
16. Tator CH: Spine-spinal cord relationships in spinal cord trauma. *Clin Neurosurg* 30:479, 1983.
17. Kobrine AI: The neuronal theory of experimental traumatic spinal cord injury. *Surg Neurol* 3:261, 1975.
18. Nelson E, Gertz SD, Rennels ML, et al: Spinal cord injury: The role of vascular damage in the pathogenesis of central hemorrhagic necrosis. *Arch Neurol* 34:332, 1977.
19. White RJ: Pathology of spinal cord injury in experimental lessons. *Clin Orthop* 112:16, 1975.
20. Griffiths IR: Spinal cord blood flow after acute experimental cord injury in dogs. *J Neurol Sci* 27:247, 1976.
21. Rivlin AS, Tator CH: Regional spinal cord blood flow in rats after severe cord trauma. *J Neurosurg* 40:52, 1974.
22. Senter HJ, Venes JL: Altered blood flow and secondary injury in experimental spinal cord trauma. *J Neurosurg* 49:844, 1978.
23. Eidelberg E: The pathophysiology of spinal cord injury. *Radiol Clin North Am* 15:241, 1977.
24. Kobrine AI, Doyle TF, Martins AM: Local spinal cord blood flow in experimental traumatic myelopathy. *J Neurosurg* 42:144, 1975.
25. Yashon D: Pathogenesis of spinal cord injury. *Orthop Clin North Am* 9:247, 1978.
26. Kelly BJ, Luce JM: Current concepts in cerebral protection. *Chest* 103:1246, 1993.
27. Siesjo BK, Bengtsson F: Calcium fluxes, calcium antagonists, and calcium related pathology in brain ischemia, hypoglycemia, and spreading depression: A unifying hypothesis. *J Cereb Blood Flow Metab* 9:127, 1989.
28. Wolfe LS: Eicosanoids, prostaglandins, thromboxanes, leukotrienes, and other derivatives of carbon-20 unsaturated fatty acids. *J Neurochem* 38:1, 1982.
29. Rosemblum WI: Constricting effects of leukotrienes on cerebral arterioles of mice. *Stroke* 16:262, 1985.
30. Hallenbeck JM, Dutka AJ: Background review and current concepts of reperfusion injury. *Arch Neurol* 47:1245, 1990.
31. Simon RP, Swan JH, Griffiths T, et al: Blockade of N-methyl-D-aspartate receptors may protect against ischemic damage in brain. *Science* 226:850, 1984.
32. Faden AI, Jacobs TP, Holaday JW: Opiate antagonist improves neurologic recovery after spinal injury. *Science* 211:493, 1981.
33. Faden AI, Molineaux CJ, Rosenberger JG, et al: Endogenous opioid immunoreactivity in rat spinal cord following traumatic injury. *Ann Neurol* 17:386, 1985.
34. Faden AI, Jacobs TP, Mougey E, et al: Endorphins in experimental spinal injury: Therapeutic effect of naloxone. *Ann Neurol* 10:326, 1981.
35. Weeks EJ, Fiandaca MS: Spinal cord injury, in Rippe JM, Irwin RS, Alpert JS, et al. (eds): *Intensive Care Medicine.* Boston, Little, Brown and Co, 1991, pp 1478–1489.
36. Chehrazi B, Wagner FC, Collins WF, et al: A scale for the evaluation of spinal cord injury. *J Neurosurg* 54:310, 1981.
37. Eidelberg E, Sullivan J, Brigham A: Immediate consequences of spinal cord injury: Possible role of potassium in axonal conduction block. *Surg Neurol* 3:317, 1975.
38. Bach-Y-Rita P, Illis LS: Spinal shock: Possible role of receptor plasticity and nonsynaptic transmission. *Paraplegia* 31(2):82, 1993.
39. Albin MS, Bunegin L, Wolf S: Brain and lungs at risk after cervical spinal cord transection: Intracranial pressure, brain water, blood-brain barrier permeability, cerebral blood flow, and extravascular lung water changes. *Surg Neurol* 24:191, 1985.
40. Alexander S, Kerr FWL: Blood pressure responses in acute compression of the spinal cord. *J Neurosurg* 21:485, 1964.
41. Eidelberg EE: Cardiovascular responses to experimental spinal cord compression. *J Neurosurg* 38:326, 1973.
42. Meyer GA, Berman IR, Doty DB, et al: Hemodynamic responses to acute quadriplegia with or without chest trauma. *J Neurosurg* 34:168, 1971.
43. Poe RH, Reisman JL, Rodenhouse TG: Pulmonary edema in cervical spinal cord injury. *J Trauma* 18(1):71, 1978.
44. Evans DE, Kobrine AI, Rizzoli HV: Cardiac arrhythmias accompanying acute compression of the spinal cord. *J Neurosurg* 52:52, 1980.
45. Natelson BH: Neurocardiology: An interdisciplinary area for the 80s. *Arch Neurol* 42:178, 1985.
46. Talman WT: Cardiovascular regulation and lesions of the central nervous system. *Ann Neurol* 18:1, 1985.
47. Colachis SC: Autonomic hyperreflexia with spinal cord injury. *J Am Paraplegia Soc* 15(3):171, 1992.
48. Trop CS, Bennett CJ: The evaluation of autonomic dysreflexia. *Semin Urol* 10:95, 1992.
49. Sell GH, Naftchi NE, Lowman EW, et al: Autonomic hyperreflexia and catecholamine metabolites in spinal cord injury. *Arch Physiol Med* 53:415, 1972.
50. Kelly BJ, Luce JM: The diagnosis and management of neuromuscular diseases causing respiratory failure. *Chest* 99:1485, 1991.
51. Schmidt-Nowara WW, Altman AR: Atelectasis and neuromuscular respiratory failure. *Chest* 85:792, 1984.
52. Mansel JK, Norman JR: Respiratory complications and management of spinal cord injuries. *Chest* 97:1446, 1990.
53. Ledsome JR, Sharp JM: Pulmonary function in acute cervical cord injury. *Am Rev Respir Dis* 124:41, 1985.
54. Wicks AB, Menter RR: Long-term outlook in quadriplegic patients with initial ventilator dependency. *Chest* 90(3):406, 1986.
55. Loveridge B, Sanii R, Dubo HI: Breathing pattern adjustments during the first year following cervical spinal cord injury. *Paraplegia* 30:479, 1992.
56. Albert TJ, Levine MJ, Balderston RA, et al: Gastrointestinal complications in spinal cord injury. *Spine* 16:S522, 1991.

57. English GM, Hsu SF, Edgar, et al: Esophageal trauma in patients with spinal cord injury. *Paraplegia* 30:903, 1992.

58. Rhee KJ, Green W, Holcroft JW, et al: Oral intubation in the multiply injured patient: The risk of exacerbating spinal cord damage. *Ann Emerg Med* 19(5):511, 1990.

59. Suderman VS, Crosby ET, Lui A: Elective oral tracheal intubation in cervical spine-injured adults. *Can J Anaesth* 38(6):785, 1991.

60. Reiss SJ, Raque GH, Shields GB, et al: Cervical spine fractures with major associated trauma. *Neurosurgery* 18:327, 1986.

61. Rengachary SS: Examination of the motor and sensory systems and reflexes, in Wilkins RH, Rengachary SS (eds.): *Neurosurgery (Volume I)*. New York, McGraw-Hill, 1985, pp 122–147.

62. Brant-Zawadski M, Miller EM, Federle C: CT in the evaluation of spine trauma. *AJR* 136:369, 1981.

63. Kalfas I, Wilberger J, Goldberg A, et al: Magnetic resonance imaging in acute spinal cord trauma. *Neurosurgery* 23(3):295, 1988.

64. Chakeres DW, Flickinger F, Bresnahan JC, et al: MR imaging of acute spinal cord trauma. *AJNR* 8:5, 1987.

65. Kuchner EF, Hansebout RR: Combined steroid and hypothermia treatment of experimental spinal cord injury. *Surg Neurol* 6:371, 1976.

66. Green BA, Kahn T, Klose KJ: A comparative study of steroid therapy in acute experimental spinal cord injury. *Surg Neurol* 13:91, 1980.

67. Bracken MB, Collins WF, Freeman DF, et al: Efficacy of methylprednisolone in acute spinal cord injury. *JAMA* 251(1):45, 1984.

68. Hall ED, Braughler JM: Glucocorticoid mechanisms in acute spinal cord injury: A review and therapeutic rationale. *Surg Neurol* 18(5):320, 1982.

69. Mackenzie CF, Shin B, Krisnaprasad D, et al: Assessment of cardiac and respiratory function during surgery on patients with acute quadraplegia. *J Neurosurg* 62:843, 1985.

70. Weingarden SI: Deep venous thrombosis in spinal cord injury: Overview of the problem. *Chest* 102(6):636S, 1992.

71. Waring WP, Karunas RS: Acute spinal cord injuries and the incidence of clinically occurring thromboembolic disease. *Paraplegia* 29:8, 1991.

72. Green D, Hull RD, Mammen EF, et al: Deep vein thrombosis in spinal cord injury: Summary and recommendations. *Chest* 102(6):633S, 1992.

73. Mammen EF: Pathogenesis of venous thrombosis. *Chest* 102(6):640S, 1992.

74. Yao JS: Deep vein thrombosis in spinal cord-injured patients. Evaluation and assessment. *Chest* 102(6):645S, 1992.

75. Green D: Prophylaxis of thromboembolism in spinal cord-injured patients. *Chest* 102(6):649S, 1992.

76. Merli GJ: Management of deep vein thrombosis in spinal cord injury. *Chest* 102(6):652S, 1992.

77. Hull RD: Venous thromboembolism in spinal cord injury patients. *Chest* 102(6):658S, 1992.

78. Schnieber ME: Cardiac complications of the Stryker frame. *Crit Care Nurse* 10:73, 1990.

79. Brackett TO, Condon N, Kindelan KM, et al: The emotional care of a person with a spinal cord injury. *JAMA* 252(6):793, 1984.

80. Hallenback JM, Jacobs TP, Faden AT: Combined PGI$_2$, indomethacin, and heparin improves neurological recovery after spinal trauma in cats. *J Neurosurg* 58:749,1983.

81. Lux WE, Feurstein G, Faden AI: Alteration of leukotriene D$_4$ hypotension by thyrotropin releasing hormone. *Nature* 302:822, 1983.

82. Bakshi R, Faden AI: Competitive and non-competitive NMDA antagonists limit dynorphin A-induced rat hindlimb paralysis. *Brain Res* 507:1, 1990.

83. Faden AI, Jacobs TP, Smith MT: Thyrotropin-releasing hormone in experimental spinal injury: Dose response and late treatment. *Neurology* 34:1280, 1984.

84. Faden AI, Jacobs TP, Holaday JW: Thyrotropin-releasing hormone improves neurologic recovery after spinal trauma in cats. *N Engl J Med* 305(18):1063, 1981.

85. Faden AI, Jacobs TP: Opiate antagonist WIN 44,441-3 stereospecifically improves neurologic recovery after ischemic spinal injury. *Neurology* 35:1311, 1985.

86. Hall ED: Effects of the 21-aminosteroid U74006F on posttraumatic spinal cord ischemia in cats. *J Neurosurg* 68:462, 1988.

87. Anderson DK, Braughler JM, Hall ED, et al: Effects of treatment with U-74006F on neurological outcome following experimental spinal cord injury. *J Neurosurg* 69:562, 1988.

88. Albin MS, White RJ, Acost-Rua G, et al: Study of functional recovery produced by delayed localized cooling after spinal cord injury in primates. *J Neurosurg* 29:113, 1968.

89. Geisler FH, Dorsey FC, Coleman WP: Recovery of motor function after spinal cord injury: A randomized, placebo controlled trial with GM-1 ganglioside. *N Engl J Med* 324(26):1829, 1991.

177. Thoracic Trauma

A. Thomas Pezzella and
Thomas J. Vander Salm

Epidemiology

It is estimated that over 250,000 individuals per year in the United States require hospital admission for chest-related injuries [1]. Twenty-five percent of trauma-related deaths are associated with injuries to the thorax [2]. The in-hospital mortality for isolated chest trauma is 4 to 8 percent; mortality increases to 10 to 15 percent when one other organ system is involved; and mortality is 35 percent when multiple systems are involved [3]. Penetrating injuries constitute approximately 30 percent of thoracic trauma cases; the remainder are attributable to blunt mechanisms of injury [4]. In a recent review from the Maryland Institute of Emergency Medical Services (MIEMS), 71 percent of 515 blunt chest injuries occurred as a result of motor vehicle accidents [5]. Overall mortality in this study was 15.5 percent.

Of interest is the increase in minor chest wall injuries in seatbelt wearers [6]. Penetrating chest trauma is seen in both civilian and military practice. In the civilian setting, stab wounds account for 60 to 70 percent of penetrating thoracic injuries. These injuries carry a low mortality (2–3%). In contrast, thoracic gunshot wounds are associated with a 14 to 20 percent mortality rate [7].

Pathophysiology

In blunt trauma, thoracic injuries occur as a result of several mechanisms [8]. Deformation of the chest wall can cause sternal or rib fractures, as well as compression of internal structures.

Organs can be damaged by forces causing anterior or posterior deceleraton, torsion, or shearing. Shearing occurs when there are differences in the degree of fixation or mobility of adjacent tissues and, hence, differing rates of deceleration. Compression or decompression injuries to the lung and airways can occur if the chest is deformed when the glottis is closed. Blast injuries occur from explosions that transmit energy in the form of a shock wave. The primary blast causes disruption of tissue when the pressure wave passes through a transition zone between a dense medium (e.g., liquid) and a less dense medium (e.g., air). Such a transition zone exists in the alveoli. Injury patterns in penetrating trauma are difficult to predict, as missiles can deflect off bony surfaces. Factors affecting the degree of tissue injury in penetrating trauma are discussed in Chapter 170.

Diagnosis

HISTORY AND PHYSICAL EXAMINATION. The initial history and physical examination are often abbreviated because the focus during the primary survey and resuscitation phases is the identification and correction of immediately life-threatening problems. During the secondary survey, however, a complete history should be obtained and a thorough physical examination performed. Details regarding the mechanism of injury and medical history should be obtained, using sources other than the patient if necessary. Key details regarding the injury may include the height of the fall, the speed of the automobile(s), the extent of damage to the vehicles(s), the time required for extrication, the number of fatalities, the presence or absence of damage to the steering wheel, and whether the victim was thrown from the vehicle. The time that the injury occurred and the time the patient arrived at the trauma center should be documented in the record. Photos taken at the scene can be of help. Knowledge of the weapons in penetrating trauma is extremely valuable. Important findings on physical examination include air hunger or use of accessory muscles of ventilation (evidence of airway obstruction or pneumothorax); tracheal deviation (evidence of tension pneumothorax); cyanosis or dilated neck veins (evidence of tension pneumothorax or pericardial tamponade); major defects in the chest wall ("sucking chest wounds"); unilaterally diminished breath sounds or hyperresonance to percussion (evidence of closed pneumothorax or tension pneumothorax); diminished heart sounds (evidence of pericardial tamponade); location of foreign bodies; and location of entry and exit wounds.

CHEST ROENTGENOGRAM. The chest roentgenogram remains the single most valuable diagnostic study for the recognition and continuing assessment of chest trauma. Interpretation of the chest roentgenogram is discussed in greater detail in Chapter 70. The anteroposterior (AP) supine chest roentgenogram is commonly performed first. However, pneumothoraces are sometimes missed on the supine AP film and mediastinal widening can be artifactual.

Chest radiographs should be inspected for subcutaneous air, foreign bodies, bony fractures, widening or shift of the mediastinum, pneumothorax, pneumomediastinum, pleural fluid, abnormalities in the cardiac silhouette, and pulmonary parenchymal abnormalities (infiltrates, atelectasis, collapse, abscesses, cysts). Radiopaque skin markers are useful for identifying entry and exit wounds. The plain chest radiograph is invaluable for assessing the position of endotracheal tubes, nasogastric or orogastric tubes, central venous pressure (CVP) lines, Swan-Ganz catheters, and chest tubes. Serial chest roentgenograms permit recognition of delayed pneumothoraces, missed rib and vertebral fractures, progressive widening of the mediastinum, increasing size of pleural collections, and progressive pulmonary parenchymal abnormalities. On upright films, pleural air is best seen superiorly and laterally outlining the thin visceral pleural margin. On supine films, pleural air tends to be seen medially, laterally, in the minor fissure, and caudal to the bases.

Fluoroscopy is occasionally useful for documenting movement of foreign bodies or impaired diaphragmatic function. Inspiration-expiration films can help demonstrate small pneumothoraces as well as air trapping on expiration because of airway occlusion by aspirated foreign bodies.

COMPUTED TOMOGRAPHY. CT is a valuable diagnostic study in chest trauma. It can unmask subtle or unsuspected injuries, and when used in a serial fashion, can aid in monitoring various pathologic processes (Fig. 177-1). Thoracic injuries are frequently noted on an abdominal CT scan [9]. Chest CT aids in the diagnosis and precise localization of numerous lesions, including rib and sternal fractures, sternoclavicular dislocations, foreign bodies, retrosternal hematomas, vertebral injuries, anteromedial and subpulmonic pneumothoraces, posterior fluid or blood collections, and pulmonary contusions. The location of chest tubes in relation to undrained pleural collections is better appreciated by CT than with plain chest films. Intraparenchymal placement of chest tubes, often missed on plain films, is obvious by chest CT. Collections of blood or fluid in the pericardium can be appreciated on CT, even in the absence of widening of the cardiac silhouette on plain films. When intravenous contrast is used, CT is helpful for evaluating intrathoracic vascular structures and, particularly, for detecting mediastinal hemorrhage and periaortic hematomas, findings suggestive of aortic rupture (Fig. 177-2) [10]. CT is also valuable for evaluating infectious complications such as empyema, lung abscess, and infected pulmonary pseudocyst [11,12]. In some instances, needle or catheter drainage of infected collections can be performed under CT guidance [13]. An exciting area is CT scanning in the evaluation and classification of pulmonary contusion [14]. A classification of pulmonary laceration (I–IV) and quantification of air space consolidation yield a predicted need for mechanical ventilation and more invasive procedures.

Fig. 177-1. Chest computed tomography scan with atelectasis of the right lung and multiloculated pleural collections.

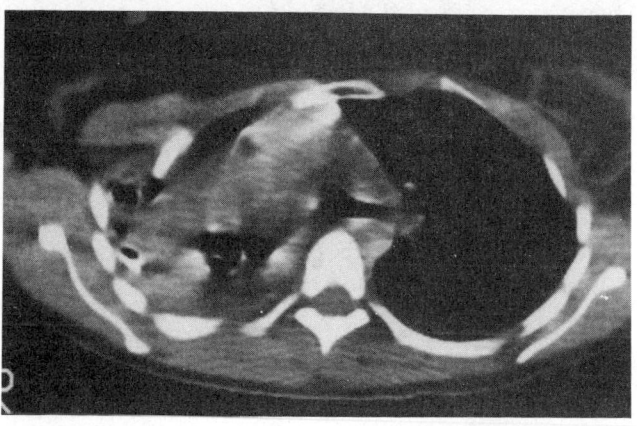

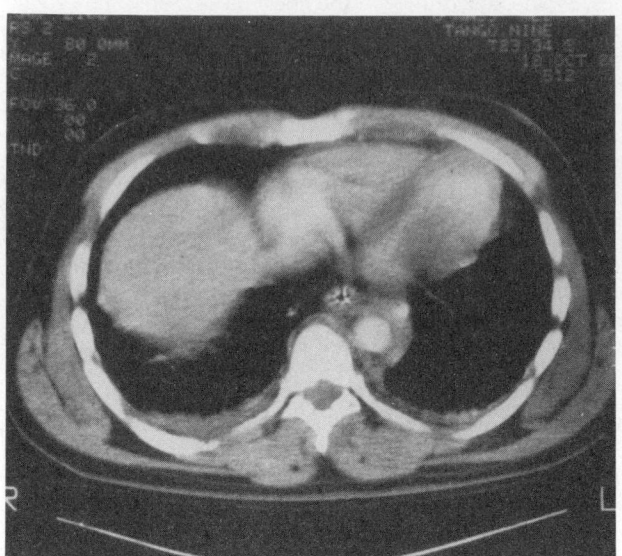

Fig. 177-2. Periaortic hematoma of descending aorta on abdominal computed tomography scan above the diaphragm.

ECHOCARDIOGRAPHY. Portable transthoracic echocardiography is frequently invaluable for evaluating cardiac wall motion and valve function and diagnosing the presence of foreign bodies and pericardial fluid or blood. Transesophageal echocardiography adds a new and exciting dimension both for blunt cardiac injuries and acute aortic transection [15,16] (see Chap. 7).

ELECTROCARDIOGRAPHY. Abnormal electrocardiographic (ECG) findings, particularly in older patients, may suggest the presence of preexisting cardiac disease. Indeed, myocardial infarction is occasionally the antecedent cause of a motor vehicle accident. In one study, ECG abnormalities were present in 63 percent of 240 patients with blunt trauma. The most common ECG abnormalities in thoracic trauma are S-T and T wave changes and findings indicative of bundle branch block [17].

ANGIOGRAPHY. Angiography remains the "gold standard" for diagnosing and defining major thoracic vascular injuries [18]. Angiography is indicated whenever vascular injury (e.g., torn thoracic aorta) is suspected, but may need to be postponed when clinical circumstances place higher priority on another study (e.g., head CT) or procedure (e.g., celiotomy). Cardiac catheterization is required in rare instances to evaluate subtle or delayed complications of cardiac trauma.

BRONCHOSCOPY. Bronchoscopy (also discussed in Chap. 12) plays a major role in the management of chest trauma. Indications for bronchoscopy include evaluation of airway injury, evaluation of hemoptysis, evaluation and treatment of segmental or lobar collapse, and removal of aspirated foreign bodies. Fiberoptic bronchoscopy is adequate in most cases; however, foreign bodies are generally removed more readily and safely using a rigid bronchoscope. Massive hemoptysis may preclude the use of a flexible bronchoscope and necessitate

rigid bronchoscopy and the use of a Fogarty occluding catheter [19]. In a recent review of 50 blunt chest trauma cases, bronchoscopy was thought to be valuable in 28 patients [20]. In this study, bronchoscopy was particularly useful for identifying tracheal or bronchial injuries.

SUBXYPHOID WINDOW. Creation of a subxyphoid pericardial window has been advocated as a means for diagnosing and (temporarily) treating pericardial tamponade [21,22,23]. In a recent review of 108 patients with penetrating chest wounds who underwent creation of a pericardial window, pericardial blood was present in approximately 10 percent of asymptomatic patients [23]. The management of pericardial tamponade is discussed in greater detail below.

General Supportive Measures

RESUSCITATION. The choice of asanguinous fluid for resuscitation of hypovolemic patients is discussed elsewhere (Chaps. 171 and 172). Although some authors have suggested that crystalloid resuscitation worsens respiratory function in pulmonary contusion [24,25], recent data do not support this view [26].

ANTIBIOTICS. There is a bias toward the value of "prophylactic" antibiotics in chest trauma requiring tube thoracostomy [27]. In a randomized, prospective, double-blind trial, clindamycin (300 mg q6h for approximately 5 days) reduced the incidence of septic complications (pneumonia, empyema, fever, positive blood cultures) in victims of penetrating chest trauma [28]. In another study, the incidence of infectious complications after tube thoracostomy was decreased by the administration of cefoxitin (1 gm q6h) started before chest tube placement and continued until 12 hours after chest tube removal [29].

Perioperative antibiotics also are indicated when thoracotomy is required for esophageal injury, bronchial injury, or control of cardiac bleeding. Clindamycin (300 mg IV q6h) for 5 days or until the chest tubes are removed is recommended [30].

PAIN CONTROL. Thoracic injuries, particularly rib fractures, are very painful. Splinting, due to pain, decreases vital capacity and functional residual capacity and promotes the development of atelectasis. Thus, **pain** control is of paramount importance in the management of thoracic trauma. This topic is discussed in detail in Chapter 167.

Specific Injuries

CHEST WALL PROBLEMS. Significant chest wall injuries occur in more than one-third of patients with blunt multiple trauma [10]. Chest wall contusions are common.

Rib Fractures. Rib fractures are the most common blunt thoracic injury [31]. The extent of intrathoracic trauma and mortality correlates directly with the number of rib fractures [10]. Rib fractures, though less common in children than adults because of the more compliant thoracic cage, are being seen with increased frequency [32].

Because the shoulder girdle tends to protect the first three ribs from injury, fractures of the first, second, or third ribs are evidence that a large amount of energy was transferred to the chest at the time of the injury. The clinician should suspect the presence of serious internal thoracic injuries [33,34,35]. This concept, however, was recently challenged on the basis of data collected in a review of 1393 blunt trauma patients with first or second rib fractures [36]. In this study, the incidence of injuries to the thoracic aorta was 6.2 percent, and the incidence of injuries to the great vessels was 4.5 percent. These incidence rates are similar to those previously reported for victims with severe blunt chest trauma, irrespective of the presence of upper rib fractures [37].

Fractures of the 10th, 11th, or 12th ribs are often associated with blunt injuries involving the spleen, liver, kidneys, and diaphragm [36]. Fractures involving three or more ribs are commonly associated with pulmonary contusion (see below) and typically necessitate hospitalization.

Sternal Fractures. Sternal fractures are being seen more commonly [38]. The presence of a sternal fracture should increase suspicion of visceral injury, especially myocardial contusion or rupture of the great vessels [39,40]. Undisplaced and partially displaced transverse fractures with paradoxical motion warrant early operative repair [41]. After 2 weeks, scarring and fixation may make operative repair more difficult [41].

Clavicular Fractures and Dislocations. In some cases, the fractured ends of the clavicle cause injury to the subclavian vessels or brachial plexus. Callus formation at the site of the fracture can compress the subclavian artery. Anterior dislocation can occur at the sternoclavicular joint. The rarer posterior displacement of the medial clavicle can cause serious injury to the trachea or innominate vessels [30].

Scapular Fractures. Isolated scapular fractures are rare. More than 50 percent of scapular fractures are associated with rib fractures and pulmonary contusion; 10 to 20 percent are associated with pneumothorax; and more than 10 percent are associated with brachial plexus or major arterial injuries [42]. Thus, the presence of a scapular fracture should prompt a search for other major ipsilateral thoracic injuries.

Flail Chest. Flail chest denotes the paradoxical movement of a portion of the chest wall with inspiration and expiration. A flail segment can result from multiple rib fractures, costochondral separation, sternal fracture, or a combination of these injuries. The major physiologic insult in flail chest is contusion of the underlying lung and decreased vital capacity [43,44]. The pendelluft phenomenon (i.e., useless to-and-fro movement of air from one lung to the other) is no longer considered to be an important pathophysiologic mechanism [45].

With appropriate analgesia and physiotherapy, approximately 50 percent of the cases of flail chest can be managed without mechanical ventilation [46]. The remainder require intubation and mechanical ventilation, typically for about 1 to 3 weeks [47,48]. The chest wall usually stabilizes within 1 to 2 weeks. Operative internal fixation has been advocated by some authors [49,50,51]. We use this approach at our institution infrequently.

Subcutaneous Emphysema. Subcutaneous emphysema occurs when air is forced into the subcutaneous tissue. The source of air is usually a pneumothorax associated with rib fractures or flail chest, although air can also dissect from the mediastinum secondary to injuries involving the larynx, tracheobronchial tree, or esophagus. Hence, subcutaneous emphysema should prompt the clinician to suspect the presence of one of these serious injuries. Another common source of subcutaneous emphysema is a malpositioned chest tube that permits air to leak out of a side hole improperly placed in the chest wall instead of the pleural space.

Subcutaneous emphysema presents as crepitus on palpation of the skin of the thorax or neck. Subcutaneous air on chest roentgenogram confirms the diagnosis. The treatment of subcutaneous emphysema is correction of the underlying problem(s); venting with skin incisions, needle aspiration, or cervical mediastinotomy are rarely indicated. If the source of air is a poorly positioned chest tube, applying an airtight occlusive dressing usually corrects the problem. In any event, the original chest tube should not be advanced further in to the chest, because of the unacceptable risk of pleural contamination. If an occlusive dressing fails to solve the problem, a new chest tube (in a new site) should be inserted. Subcutaneous emphysema in the absence of pneumothorax is not an indication for placing a chest tube, unless positive pressure ventilation will be necessary for some other reason (e.g., generally anesthesia or acute respiratory failure).

Traumatic Asphyxia. Traumatic asphyxia occurs as a result of sustained blunt anteroposterior chest wall compression [52,53,54]. Prolonged compression of the thorax results in increased superior vena caval pressure and obstruction of flow through the valveless veins of the innominate and jugular system. The clinical findings are craniocervical cyanosis and edema, subconjunctival hemorrhage or petechia, and distension of the cervical neck veins. Commonly associated injuries include pulmonary contusion and hemothorax. Treatment is directed at the associated injuries.

PLEURAL SPACE PROBLEMS

Closed Pneumothorax. Air in the pleural space (pneumothorax) results in partial or total collapse of the ipsilateral lung. Closed pneumothorax can occur as a result of either penetrating or nonpenetrating chest trauma. Pneumothorax caused by penetrating trauma or rib fractures is usually associated with blood in the pleural space (hemothorax). In the absence of tension pneumothorax (see below), partial or even total collapse of one lung is usually well tolerated, because pulmonary blood flow is preferentially directed to well-aerated segments by virtue of hypoxic pulmonary vasoconstriction. The diagnosis of closed pneumothorax is suggested by decreased breath sounds, hyperresonance to percussion, and diminished chest wall motion. The diagnosis of closed pneumothorax (without tension) is confirmed by chest roentgenogram. The diagnosis may be missed on a supine anterior-posterior (AP) film; an expiratory upright chest roentgenogram may be necessary to establish the diagnosis. Tube thoracostomy is the treatment of choice, although small, isolated, uncomplicated pneumothoraces can sometimes be managed with needle aspiration or percutaneous catheter drainage [55].

Chest tubes are sometimes warranted even in the absence of radiographic confirmation of pneumothorax. This is particularly true in patients with subcutaneous emphysema requiring emergency surgery under general anesthesia with positive pressure ventilation. In this situation, the risks associated with tube thoracostomy are small compared with the potentially devastating consequences of tension pneumothorax developing under general anesthesia. Asymptomatic pneumothorax seen on CT scan alone has been treated with observation alone [56].

If the lung expands incompletely after placing a chest tube, several possible problems should be considered: (1) the chest tube may be improperly positioned (e.g., the lung may be trapped and the pneumothorax loculated away from the site of the chest tube), (2) suction may be inadequate, (3) the tube may be occluded by clot or exudate, and (4) the airways may be occluded by blood or secretions. Operative removal of the pleural clot, aggressive pulmonary physiotherapy or therapeutic bronchoscopy, or insertion of another chest tube may be required to obtain full expansion of the lung.

In general, chest tubes placed for traumatic pneumothoraces (especially penetrating trauma) should be kept in place for a minimum of 3 to 5 days and not removed until full lung expansion and absence of air leak occurs.

Tension Pneumothorax. Tension pneumothrax is an immediately life-threatening problem. Although typically present at the time of the primary survey, tension pneumothorax also can present as a delayed problem in patients receiving positive pressure ventilation. Tension pneumothorax results when a flap valve effect allows air to enter the pleural space but prevents its escape. Shock results because increased intrapleural pressure collapses the great veins, decreasing cardiac return, and hence, decreasing preload (see Chap. 170). Mediastinal shift (away from the involved hemithorax) can further diminish venous return. Increased intrapleural pressure also interferes with ventilation of the contralateral lung.

Findings indicative of tension pneumothorax include hypotension, distended neck veins, elevated central venous pressure (CVP), tracheal deviation (away from the involved side), hyperresonance to percussion (on the involved side), and diminished breath sounds (on the involved side). Unexplained sudden deterioration of ventilation (e.g., high peak airway pressures and diminished arterial oxygen tension [PO_2]), systemic arterial hypotension, or low cardiac output during general anesthesia or positive pressure ventilation should raise the suspicion of tension pneumothorax. Radiographic findings include collapse of the ipsilateral lung, mediastinal shift, and widening of the intercostal spaces on the involved side. *Tension pneumothorax, however, is a clinical diagnosis, not a radiographic one; it is a true surgical emergency.* If the diagnosis is suspected, a needle should be rapidly inserted in the ipsilateral second intercostal space in the midclavicular line. A gush of air from the needle (or easy aspiration of air from the needle) confirms the diagnosis and is followed by tube thoracostomy. If the patient's condition does not improve after thoracostomy, then the diagnosis of pericardial tamponade (*vide infra*) should be considered. Note that if a tension pneumothorax is not present, needle thoracostomy can injure the lung and create a pneumothorax.

Open Pneumothorax. This is an infrequent problem [57]. Although a true emergency, the diagnosis is usually obvious. Audible air rushes in and out through a gaping hole in the chest wall, producing a sucking sound. Because of the open communication between the ipsilateral pleural space and the atmosphere, the lung on the involved side is totally collapsed. Moreover, much of the expansion of the chest on the contralateral side serves only to ventilate the open pleural space; hence alveolar air exchange is markedly embarrassed. Treatment consists of immediate application of an occlusive dressing on the wound. Leaving one side of the dressing untaped provides a flap valve effect, allowing air to escape from but not to leak back into the pleural space [58]. After application of the occlusive dressing, tube thoracostomy should be performed through a separate site and suction applied to allow reexpansion of the lung on the involved side. Definitive treatment consists of operative debridement and closure of the defect plus pleural drainage.

Hemothorax. The incidence of hemothorax and hemopneumothorax is 60 to 70 percent in blunt chest trauma [5,7] and 50 to 60 percent in penetrating chest trauma [59,60]. Sources of blood include lacerated vessels in the chest wall (including intercostal arteries), lacerations of the lung, and injuries to the heart or great vessels. Massive hemothorax, defined as greater than 1500 ml of blood in the pleural space [58], compromises perfusion on the basis of both hypovolemia and compression of the great veins. Massive hemothorax also embarrasses ipsilateral pulmonary function by limiting alveolar expansion and gas exchange.

Although diminished breath sounds and dullness to percussion are usually evident in patients with hemothorax, the diagnosis usually is made by chest roentgenogram. In massive hemothorax, the neck veins can be flat or distended.

The treatment of massive hemothorax is chest tube drainage and intravascular volume resuscitation. Thoracotomy is indicated for the 10 to 15 percent of cases of hemothorax that drain in excess of 1500 mL of blood initially or manifest ongoing blood loss through the chest tube(s) in excess of 200 mL per hour for 3 to 4 hours.

Posttraumatic Empyema. The risk of empyema after trauma is increased by failure to achieve complete expansion of the lung and adequate drainage of the pleural space [61]. The risk is further enhanced by the presence of persistent air leak from the lung or bronchi. Posttraumatic empyema is often diagnosed by CT and CT-guided needle aspiration of suspicious collections. Treatment options include placement of multiple chest tubes, CT- or ultrasound-guided catheter placement, and thoracotomy with drainage and decortication [62,63]. Early decortication (i.e., within 3 weeks of the time of injury) should be considered under the following circumstances: (1) evidence of retained or clotted hemothorax; (2) pleural air-fluid levels in the presence of sepsis; (3) persistently collapsed lung despite aggressive pulmonary toilet and adequate chest tube placement and suction; (4) residual loculated pleural collections, especially if known or likely to be infected [63].

Posttraumatic Chylothorax. Chylothorax is a rare complication of chest trauma, usually occurring as a result of hyperextension of the spine or surgical procedures performed in the vicinity of the thoracic duct [64]. Normally, 2 to 4 liters of lymph flows through the thoracic duct and drains into the venous system [65]. If the thoracic duct is injured, lymph leaks into the pleural space. Chylothorax, therefore, presents as a pleural effusion. Aspiration of milky pleural fluid should cause the clinician to suspect the diagnosis. The diagnosis is confirmed if the fluid contains numerous lymphocytes and is sterile, alkaline, high in triglycerides, and positive for fat by Sudan stain [65]. Repeated needle-catheter thoracentesis may be therapeutic, but tube thoracostomy is preferred. Most chylous leaks stop spontaneously, if lymph flow is decreased by instituting total parenteral nutrition and discontinuing enteral feeding. If the drainage is persistent but less than 0.25 ml per kilogram per hour, then chest tube drainage should not be abandoned for at least 3 to 4 weeks [65]. However, if chylous drainage persists for longer than a month or if the volume exceeds 0.25 ml/kg/hr, then thoracotomy and ligation of the thoracic duct should be undertaken [65].

PULMONARY PARENCHYMAL INJURIES. Lung injury in trauma occurs in several ways: the lung can be directly injured as a result of contusion, laceration, or aspiration; the lung can be injured as a result of secondary infection of normal or already damaged pulmonary parenchyma; and the lung can be injured indirectly as a result of fat embolism, thromboembolism, or the acute respiratory distress syndrome (ARDS). In trauma patients, these several causes can occur singly or in combination, leading to acute respiratory failure and the necessity for mechanical ventilation and prolonged care in an ICU.

Pulmonary Contusion. Pulmonary contusion occurs in 30 to 40 percent of patients sustaining blunt chest trauma [46]. The contused lung is hemorrhagic, edematous, and consolidated. Hypoxemia is usually present within 24 to 36 hours after the injury. Plain films of the chest show localized, peripheral, homogenous infiltrates within 4 to 24 hours. They can be focal or diffuse [66]. Pulmonary contusions can be evident on chest CT before they are demonstrable on conventional roentgenograms [13]. The treatment of pulmonary contusion is supportive and depends on the degree of pulmonary dysfunction. Many cases are adequately managed with supplemental oxygen without intubation or mechanical ventilation. Care should be taken to avoid unnecessarily overhydrating patients with pulmonary contusions, although fear of pulmonary edema should not lead to the inadequate resuscitation of hypovolemic trauma victims. Although corticosteroids have been advocated in the past [67], their use in pulmonary contusion has never been shown to improve outcome in a well-designed clinical trial and cannot be advocated. Prophylactic positive end-expiratory pressure (PEEP) is similarly of no value [68]. Most uncomplicated contusions resolve in 10 to 14 days with complete resolution on chest roentgenogram.

Pulmonary Laceration. Pulmonary lacerations are commonly associated with hemopneumothorax and hemoptysis and are most often adequately managed with simple tube thoracostomy. Occasionally, pneumothorax can be delayed, resulting from central necrosis of lung parenchyma and subsequent leakage of air into the pleural space. Other complications include the formation of intraparenchymal hematomas or cystic cavities. Lacerations are sometimes diagnosed during a thoracotomy that was performed for other reasons. At operation, most lacerations are managed with simple control of bleeding, suturing or stapling of air leaks, and pleural drainage. Occasionally, extensive parenchymal tears with involvement of the hilum necessitate extensive repair, resection, or even pneumonectomy [69,70].

Pulmonary Hematoma. Uncomplicated hematomas usually resolve in 3 to 4 weeks. Large hematomas resulting from high-velocity missile wounds may require thoracotomy and local resection [71].

Posttraumatic Pulmonary Cavitary Lesions. Posttraumatic cysts, pseudocysts, or pneumatoceles are cavitary lesions within the lung parenchyma filled with fluid, blood, or air [11,72,73,74]. Although cavities are sometimes evident on early plain films of the chest, these lesions usually appear later after reabsorption of blood and tissue debris. CT is very useful for identifying and localizing posttraumatic cavitary lesions [11]. Although most resolve spontaneously, some posttraumatic cavities become secondarily infected, necessitating aggressive management with antibiotics, CT-guided aspiration, and, in some instances, thoracotomy and pulmonary resection [11].

Miscellaneous Parenchymal Injuries. Traumatic pulmonary arteriovenous fistulae have been described [75]. Diagnosis of this problem is by pulmonary angiography. Torsion of the lung is a rare complication of trauma [76]. It is evidenced on chest film by opacification of the affected hemithorax, mediastinal shift toward the contralateral side, and reversal of the bronchoalveolar markings of the affected side with the major pulmonary vessels coursing cephalad instead of caudad. Treatment is urgent thoracotomy.

Acute Respiratory Distress Syndrome. This is discussed at length in Chapter 55.

AIRWAY PROBLEMS

Hemoptysis. Fortunately, posttraumatic massive hemoptysis (>600 ml/24 hr) is very rare [77]. In the severely traumatized patient, hemoptysis can be aggravated by factors that affect coagulation (particularly, hypothermia and thrombocytopenia) (see Chap. 172). Bronchoscopy can aid in identifying the source of the bleeding. Double-lumen endotracheal tubes, bronchial blockers, and selective bronchial artery embolization are modalities to better define and treat the severely hemoptysising patient.

Air Embolism. Air embolism occurs during mechanical ventilation when pressurized air from disrupted bronchi leaks into torn, low-pressure pulmonary veins. The air bubbles flow into the left ventricle and are ejected into the systemic circulation. The magnitude of the problem is determined by several factors, including airway pressures, degree of bronchial disruption, and proximity between the torn airway and the torn pulmonary vein. Clinically, air embolization typically presents as stroke or cardiac failure caused by dissemination of bubbles into the cerebral and coronary circulations. If the diagnosis is made, treatment consists of discontinuing positive pressure ventilation (if possible) and immediate thoracotomy to control the bronchopulmonary venous fistula [78]. Established cerebral air emboli patients have responded to hyperbaric oxygen therapy [79] (see Chap. 68).

Laryngeal Trauma. Laryngeal trauma usually occurs as a result of blunt trauma to the anterior neck in motor vehicle accidents, although other mechanisms of injury, including penetrating trauma, are sometimes seen [80]. The clinical features of laryngeal trauma include local tenderness, ecchymoses and swelling, subcutaneous emphysema, and hoarseness. Laryngeal trauma is a cause of acute airway obstruction and is one of the surgical emergencies that must be recognized during the primary survey. Findings indicative of airway obstruction caused by laryngeal injury include inspiratory stridor, air hunger, and use of the accessory muscles of ventilation. Urgent endotracheal intubation (under direct vision) or cricothyroidotomy may be necessary to establish or maintain a patent airway. With complete separation of the larynx or the trachea, it is necessary to perform a cervical exploration and intubate the distal tracheal segment.

Tracheal and Bronchial Injuries. The distal trachea and bronchi are well protected within the bony thorax, but the proximal trachea is vulnerable to injury in the neck [80,81]. Nevertheless, tracheal injuries are uncommon, and most are attributable to penetrating trauma [81]. Cough, dyspnea, hemoptysis, subcutaneous emphysema, and pneumomediastinum on chest roentgenogram should suggest the possibility of tracheal injury. In blunt trauma, the posterior membranous portion of the trachea is usually involved, whereas in penetrating trauma, injuries can occur anywhere, depending on the course of the missile or penetrating object [80]. In penetrating trauma deep to the platysma, cervical exploration is warranted in most instances because of possible carotid injury or asphyxia secondary to aspirated blood [81].

Most injuries to the distal trachea and mainstem bronchi are caused by blunt trauma. Ruptures or tears are usually transverse, involving part or all of the circumference between cartilaginous rings and resulting in varying degrees of separation [8]. Commonly associated clinical findings include rib fractures, subcutaneous emphysema, pneumomediastinum, and pneumothorax. A persistent air leak after tube thoracostomy for pneumothorax suggests the possibility of a tracheobronchial injury. The diagnosis is made by early bronchoscopy; immediate operative repair should be undertaken once the diagnosis is established. Complex injuries may even require cardiopulmonary bypass for complete and safe repair [82].

Posttraumatic Tracheoesophageal Fistula. Acquired cervical posttraumatic tracheoesophageal fistula (TEF) is usually a complication of prolonged endotracheal, tracheal, nasogastric, or orogastric intubation. Blunt trauma can cause formation of a midesophageal fistula into the membranous trachea at the level of the carina.

Findings that suggest the presence of TEF include subcutaneous emphysema, suctioning of tube feedings from the endotracheal or tracheostomy tube, gastric distention with positive pressure ventilation despite gastric suction, and an inability to obtain an adequate seal around the cuff on the endotracheal or tracheostomy tube. In most instances, the diagnosis is made by fiberoptic bronchoscopy and esophagoscopy. Some authorities favor early repair [83], whereas others prefer to wait until the patient has been weaned from mechanical ventilatory support [84]. Esophageal diversion with the creation of a reverse gastric tube may be indicated for complicated, large, or distal fistulas [85].

Posttraumatic Tracheoinnominate Fistula. This devastating problem is a rare complication of prolonged tracheostomy or tracheal reconstruction [86]. Posttraumatic tracheoinnominate fistula (TIF) carries an overally mortality of 75 to 80 percent [86]. Massive hemorrhage from the tracheostomy ultimately occurs but is often heralded by lesser bleeding. All patients with a long-standing tracheostomy should be suspect for TIF when sudden bleeding occurs. Investigation of the stoma site and distal flexible bronchoscopy through the tracheostomy can rule out local or distant bleeding sources. For massive bleeding, control should be obtained by passing a cuffed endotracheal tube beyond the site of bleeding, using the cuff of the tube to tamponade the bleeding and control the distal airway and thus prevent the patient from drowning in blood. Patients then should be transferred immediately to the operating room. Blunt dissection of the tissue deep to the suprasternal notch and anterior to the trachea permits occlusion of the innominate artery by digital pressure against the sternum, a potentially life-saving maneuver [87]. Definitive repair requires median sternotomy and ligation and division of the innominate artery [81]. Of 22 collected patients with innominate interruption, only one neurologic deficit was noted [88].

Diaphragmatic Injuries. Blunt disruption of the diaphragm occurs when abruptly increased intraabdominal pressure tears this muscular organ. The left hemidiaphragm is ruptured more commonly than is the right, presumably because the liver buttresses and protects the diaphragm on the right side [89]. The most common pattern is a radial tear along the posterolateral aspect of the left side of the diaphragm, but avulsion from the anterior chest wall also occurs [89]. Symptoms vary from none to severe respiratory compromise caused by the displacement of abdominal viscera into the chest. The diagnosis is most often made when the chest roentgenogram (with a nasogastric or orogastric tube in place) shows the stomach in the left hemithorax. However, herniation sometimes is delayed or consists of displacement of the liver in the right hemithorax; in these cases, the diagnosis is typically made at the time of laparotomy (for other indications), or is established by abdominal CT or a chest roentgenogram performed after the initial study. Acute ruptures are repaired through the abdomen; late repairs (i.e., beyond several weeks) are performed either through the abdomen or chest [89]. A transthoracic approach allows easier release of visceral adhesions from thoracic structures.

Penetrating diaphragmatic wounds are more common than blunt ones [90]. Initial herniation of abdominal viscera is unusual, but associated intraabdominal injuries are common. The initial finding is usually hemoperitoneum. The early experience with thoracoscopy offers a promising diagnostic modality when conventional efforts fail to yield a diagnosis [91].

Posttraumatic paresis or paralysis of the diaphragm occurs as a result of injury to the phrenic nerve in the neck or chest. Phrenic nerve damage can be attributable to neck trauma, penetrating thoracic trauma, or stretch injury to the nerve in blunt trauma [92,93]. Bilateral involvement (as in cervical cord injuries) can lead to severe embarrassment of ventilatory function and even ventilator dependence.

Esophageal Trauma. Because of its protected posterior location, trauma to the esophagus is relatively rare [94]. Iatrogenic trauma is most common [95]. Ingestion of lye, particularly the liquid solutions, causes extensive damage to the pharynx, hypopharynx, esophagus, and even stomach (see Chap. 139). Perforation of the esophagus leads to contamination and eventually infection, which is initially confined to the mediastinum but eventually extends into the pleural space [96]. Cervical perforations are less often fatal than are thoracic perforations [95].

Esophageal perforation is suggested by pain, subcutaneous emphysema, pneumomediastinum and pleural effusion on chest roentgenogram, and signs of sepsis (i.e., fever, leukocytosis, tachycardia). The diagnosis is confirmed by contrast study, thoracic CT using oral contrast, or fiberoptic esophagoscopy. Treatment consists of resuscitation, broad-spectrum antibotics, and, in most instances, operative intervention. Most cervical and virtually all intrathoracic esophageal perforations require surgical exploration, operative debridement, repair, and drainage [88]. When surgical repair is not feasible, temporary diversion with cervical esophageal and gastric drainage is recommended [97]. Mortality is about 10 to 25 percent for injuries treated within 24 hours, but increases to 25 to 60 percent if therapy is delayed longer than that [98].

CARDIAC TRAUMA

Cardiac Tamponade. Cardiac tamponade caused by trauma virtually always results from bleeding from the heart, although delayed posttraumatic tamponade from pericardial effusion has been reported [99]. Tamponade results when elevated intrapericardial pressure decreases the transmural (distending) pressure on the cardiac chambers, thus effectively decreasing end-diastolic volume (e.g., preload) (see Chaps. 24 and 147). Diminished preload leads to low cardiac output, shock, and ultimately death. *Cardiac tamponade is a true surgical emergency; it must be recognized and treated during the primary survey.* Cardiac tamponade is suggested by these findings: systemic arterial hypotension, muffled heart sounds, cyanosis of the upper thorax and face, paradoxical pulse, distended neck veins, and elevated CVP. Although a dilated cardiac silhouette is sometimes present on the chest roentgenogram, absence of this finding should not diminish suspicion that tamponade is occurring if other findings suggestive of the diagnosis are present. Echocardiography can confirm the presence of pericardial fluid noninvasively, but the exigencies of the clinical situation rarely afford the luxury of obtaining such confirmation. Therefore, the diagnosis is usually established by pericardiocentesis, a procedure that is both diagnostic and therapeutic. Once the presence of tamponade is established, the patient should be transferred immediately to the operating room. General anesthesia should not be induced until the patient is prepared and draped and ready for subxiphoid window or median sternotomy.

CARDIAC PERFORATION. Most often, cardiac perforation results from penetrating thoracic trauma [100,101], although cases of atrial or ventricular perforation or rupture attributable to blunt mechanisms are recorded [102]. In order of decreasing frequency, the areas injured are the right ventricle, left ventricle, right atrium, left atrium, and great vessels [100]. Approximately 25 to 50 percent of victims of penetrating cardiac trauma die early because of tamponade or hemorrhage or both. An aggressive approach to penetrating cardiac trauma, including emergency thoracotomy, is advocated [103].

Myocardial Contusion. The true incidence of myocardial contusion is unknown, because no gold standard method currently exists for establishing this diagnosis. Cardiac contusion most often involves the anteriorly situated right ventricle. Most cases have associated thoracic injuries [104]. The diagnosis of cardiac contusion is suggested by clinical suspicion, serial ECGs, cardiac enzymes, two-dimensional (2D) echocardiogram, and nuclear scanning techniques [105]. Currently, the best evidence of myocardial contusion is 2D echocardiographic documentation of abnormal wall motion and pericardial effusion [106]. Coronary angiography is potentially indicated if coronary laceration is suspected, although we have never had occasion to use this invasive study for this indication.

In the absence of frank cardiac decompensation due to massive damage to the myocardium, the diagnosis of myocardial contusion rarely affects outcome or management in trauma patients. The necessity for prolonged ECG monitoring to detect arrhythmias has been questioned [107]. If myocardial contusion has been well documented and operative therapy under general anesthesia is necessary for another problem, then consideration should be given to perioperative invasive hemodynamic monitoring, as would be appropriate after recent myocardial infarction. Rare delayed sequelae of myocardial contusion include ventricular aneurysm, ventricular septal perforation, pericardial effusion, constrictive pericarditis, and coronary artery fistula [43,99,108]. Posttraumatic pericarditis warrants treatment with nonsteroidal antiinflammatory agents and, if there is associated tamponade, catheterization or open drainage of the pericardium. Massive myocardial contusion leading to cardiogenic shock occurs rarely and should be managed by optimizing preload, inotropic agents, and perhaps providing temporary support with an intraaortic balloon pump [109].

INJURIES INVOLVING THE THORACIC AORTA AND GREAT VESSELS

Penetrating Injuries. Most intrathoracic major vascular injuries result from gunshot or stab wounds [110]. Subsequent uncontrolled hemorrhage into the mediastinum or pleural space is usually fatal. Aortic lacerations usually present with massive bleeding into the left pleural cavity, requiring immediate thoracotomy [111]. These patients are rarely stable enough to undergo angiography. Penetrating injuries to the arch vessels can present with bleeding from the skin wound, hemothorax, widening of the mediastinum or apical infiltrate on chest roentgenogram, thoracic murmur or bruit, or an expanding neck mass. Intact distal pulses in the upper extremities do not rule out major arterial injury within the thorax, because bleeding may be temporarily controlled and flow maintained by the formation of a pseudoaneurysm consisting of intact adventitial tissue and mediastinal pleura. New central nervous system deficits suggest the presence of innominate or carotid arterial injury. If the patient is hemodynamically stable, angiography is helpful to confirm the diagnosis and aid in planning of the operative approach.

Blunt Injuries. Most patients with traumatic tears of the thoracic aorta caused by blunt trauma die of exsanguination at the scene of the accident. Approximately 15 percent survive long enough to reach the hospital alive, the tear being contained by the adventitial wall of the aorta [2]. The tear is at the aortic isthmus in over 80 percent of initial survivors [112]. Findings indicative of mediastinal hemorrhage on the plain film of the chest include mediastinal widening greater than 8 cm, a ratio of mediastinal width to chest width greater than 0.25, abnormality of aotic contour, opacification of the aortopulmonary window, depression of the left main stem bronchus, deviation of the trachea to the right, deviation of the nasogastric tube to the right, presence of an apical cap, widening of the right paratracheal stripe, and left hemothorax [113]. These findings are sensitive, but specificity is poor. If the mechanism of injury is appropriate and the plain film of the chest has findings that increase suspicion for traumatic aortic rupture, then urgent angiography is indicated. This practice necessarily results in the performance of numerous negative arteriograms [37], but is necessary to avoid missing potentially correctable lesions. Some studies have advocated chest CT in the evaluation of thoracic aortic injury [114], but this approach is not widely practiced and our view is that CT is not sufficiently reliable to rule out the diagnosis of aortic disruption.

In general, once the diagnosis is established, urgent operative repair is indicated. Occasionally patients will have other associated problems, particularly massive pulmonary contusion and acute respiratory distress syndrome, severe burns, extensive head injury, that render general anesthesia, thoracotomy, and collapse of a lung excessively risky. In this situation, we and others have delayed operative repair until the physiologic status of the patient improves, using antihypertensive agents to maintain arterial blood pressure in the low normal range [115].

Operative mortality approaches 15% [116]. Major postoperative complications include hypertension and paraplegia. The incidence of paraplegia ranges to as high as 24% [117]. Paraplegia results from anterior spinal cord ischemia during cross-clamping of the aorta. Sodium nitroprusside should be avoided during aortic repair, because use of this agent may decrease spinal cord perfusion [118].

References

1. Ross SE, Cernaianu: Epidemiology of thoracic injuries: Mechanisms of injury and pathophysiology. *Topics Emerg Med* 12:1, 1990.
2. Matox KL: Thoracic great vessel injury. *Surg Clin North Am* 68:693, 1988.
3. Shires GT: *Principles of Trauma Care.* New York, McGraw-Hill, 1985.

4. LoCicero J, Mattox KL: Epidemiology of chest trauma. *Surg Clin North Am* 69:15, 1989.

5. Shorr RM, Crittenden M, Indeck M, et al: Blunt thoracic trauma. *Ann Surg* Aug:200, 1987.

6. Newman RJ, Jones IS: A prospective study of 413 consecutive car occupants with chest injuries. *J Tauma* 24:129, 1984.

7. Zuidema GD, Rutherford RB, Ballinger WF II: *The Management of Trauma.* Philadelphia, WB Saunders, 1985.

8. Magnusson AR, Schriver JA: Mechanisms of injury: Pathophysiology of blunt, blast, and penetrating injury of the chest. *Topics Emerg Med* 10(2):1, 1988.

9. Rhea JT, Novelline RA, Lawrason J, et al: The frequency and significance of thoracic injuries detected on abdominal CT scans of multiple trauma patients. *J Trauma* 29(4):502, 1989.

10. Pate JW: Chest wall injuries. *Surg Clin North Am* 69:59, 1989.

11. Willeford ME, Godwin JD: Computed tomography of lung abscess and empyema. *Radiol Clin North Am* 21:575, 1983.

12. Carroll K, Cheeseman SH, Fink MP, et al: Secondary infection of post-traumatic pulmonary cavitary lesions in adolescents and young adults: Role of computer tomography and operative debridement and drainage. *J Trauma* 29(1):109, 1989.

13. Van Sonnenberg E, Nakamoto SK, Mueller PR, et al: CT and ultrasound-guided catheter drainage of empyemas after chest-tube failure. *Radiology* 151:349, 1984.

14. Wagner RB, Jamieson PM: Pulmonary contusion: Evaluation and classification by computed tomography. *Surg Clin North Am* 69:31, 1989.

15. Brooks SW, Young JC, Cmolik B: The use of transesophageal echocardiography in the evaluation of chest trauma. *J Trauma* 32:761, 1992.

16. Plotnick GD, Hamilton S, Lee YC: The cardiologist and the trauma patient: Noninvasive testing. *Semin Thorac Cardiovasc Surg* 4:168, 1992.

17. Berk WA: ECG findings in nonpenetrating chest trauma: A review. *J Emerg Med* 5:209, 1987.

18. Thomas AN, Goodman PC, Roon AJ: Role of angiography in cervicothoracic trauma. *J Thorac Cardiovasc Surg* 76(5):663, 1987.

19. Hurst JM, Davis K, Branson RD: Early care of the injured patient, in Moore EE (ed): *The Thorax.* Philadelphia, Decker, 1990, pp 155-156.

20. Hara KS, Prakash UBS: Fiberoptic bronchoscopy in the evaluation of acute chest and upper airway trauma. *Chest* 96(3):627, 1989.

21. Trinkle JK, Marcos J, Grover FL, et al: Management of the wounded heart. *Ann Thorac Surg* 17:230, 1974.

22. Arom KV, Richardson JD, Webb G, et al: Subxiphoid pericardial window in patient with suspected traumatic pericardial tamponade. *Ann Thorac Surg* 23:545, 1977.

23. Brewster SA, Thirlby RC, Snyder WH: Subxiphoid pericardial window and penetrating cardiac trauma. *Arch Surg* 123:937, 1988.

24. Trinkle JK, Furman RW, Hishaw MA, et al: Pulmonary contusion. *Ann Thorac Surg* 16:568, 1973.

25. Fulton RL, Peter ET: Physiologic effects of fluid therapy after pulmonary contusion. *Am J Surg* 126:773, 1973.

26. Bongard FS, Lewis FR: Crystalloid resuscitation of patients with pulmonary contusion. *Am J Surg* 148:145, 1984.

27. Fallon WF, Wears RL: Prophylactic antibiotics for the prevention of infectious complications including emphysema following tube thoracostomy for trauma: Results of meta analysis. *J Trauma* 33:110, 1992.

28. Grover FL, Richardson JD, Fewel JG, et al: Prophylactic antibiotics in the treatment of penetrating chest wounds. *J Thorac Cardiovascular Surg* 74(4):528, 1977.

29. Locurto JJ, Tischler CD, Swan KG, et al: Tube thoracostomy and trauma—Antibiotics or not? *J Trauma* 26(2):1067, 1986.

30. Kaiser AB: Use of antibiotics in cardiac and thoracic surgery, in Sabiston DC, Spencer FC, (eds): *Surgery of the Chest.* 5th ed. Philadelphia, WB Saunders, 1990.

31. Carrero R, Wayne M: Chest trauma emergency. *Med Clin North Am* 7:389, 1989.

32. Meller JL, Little AG, Shermeta DW: Thoracic trauma in children. *Pediatrics* 74(5):813, 1984.

33. Richardson JD, McElvern RB, Trinkle JK: First rib fracture: A hallmark of severe trauma. *Ann Surg* 181:251, 1975.

34. Wilson JM, Thomas AN, Goodman PC, et al: Severe chest trauma. *Arch Surg* 113:846, 1978.

35. Albers JE, Rath RK, Glaser RS, et al: Severity of intrathoracic injuries associated with first rib fractures. *Ann Thorac Surg* 33:614, 1982.

36. Poole GV: Fracture of the upper ribs and injury to the great vessels. *Surg Gynecol Obstet* 169:275, 1989.

37. Gundry SR, Williams S, Burney RE, et al: Indications for aortograph, radiography after blunt chest trauma: A reassessment of the radiographic findings associated with traumatic rupture of the aorta. *Invest Radiol* 18:230, 1983.

38. Sturm JT, Luxenberg MG, Moudry BM, et al: Does sternal fracture increase the risk for aortic rupture? *Ann Thorac Surg* 48:697, 1989.

39. Harley DP, Mena I: Cardiac and vascular sequelae of sternal fractures. *J Trauma* 26(6):553, 1986.

40. Buckman R, Trooskin SZ, Flanchbaum L, et al: The significance of stable patients with sternal fractures. *Surg Gynecol Obstet* 164:261, 1987.

41. Carey S, Pezzella AT, Gilliam H: Traumatic sternal fractures: Current concepts in diagnosis and management. *Military Med* 153(9):451, 1988.

42. Fischer RP, Flynn TC, Miller PW, et al: Scapular fractures and associated major ipsilateral upper-torso injuries. *Current Concepts in Trauma Care* Fall:14, 1985.

43. Maylan JA: *Trauma Surgery.* Philadelphia, JB Lippincott, 1988.

44. Trinkle JK, Richardson JD, Franz JL, et al: Management of flail chest without mechanical ventilation. *Ann Thorac Surg* 19(4):355, 1975.

45. Maloney JV, Schmutzer KJ, Raschke E: Paradoxical respiration and "pendelluft." *J Thorac Cardiovasc Surg* 41:291, 1961.

46. Richardson JD, Adams L, Flint LM: Selective management of flail chest and pulmonary contusion. *Ann Surg* 196(4):481, 1982.

47. Lewis F, Thomas AN, Scholobohm RM: Control of therapy in flail chest. *Ann Thorac Surg* 20:170, 1975.

48. Hankins JR, Shin B, McAslan TC, et al: Management of flail chest: An analysis of 99 cases. *Am Surg* 43:176, 1979.

49. Champion HR, Robbs JV, Trunkey DD: *Rob & Smith's Operative Surgery, Trauma Surgery Part I.* 4th ed. London, England, Butterworths, 1989.

50. Thomas AN, Blaisdell W, Lewis FR Jr, et al: Operative stabilization for flail chest after blunt trauma. *J Thorac Cardiovasc Surg* 75(6):793, 1978.

51. Menard A, Testart J, Philippe JM, et al: Treatment of flail chest with Judet's struts. *J Thorac Cardiovasc Surg* 86:300, 1983.

52. Shewmake KB, Wagner CW, Golladay ES: Traumatic asphyxia. *Contemp Surg* 35:13, 1989.

53. Lee MC, Wong SS, Chu JJ: Traumatic asphyxia. *Ann Thorac Surg* 51:86, 1991.

54. Jongewaard WR, Cogbill TH, Landercasper J: Neurologic consequences of traumatic asphyxia. *J Trauma* 32:28, 1992.

55. Obeid FN, Shapiro MJ, Richardson HH, et al: Catheter aspiration for simple pneumothorax (CASP) in the outpatient management of simple traumatic pneumothorax, *J Trauma* 25:882, 1985.

56. Collins JC, Levin G, Waxman K: Occult traumatic pneumothorax: Immediate tube thoracostomy versus expectant management. *Am Surg* 58:743, 1992.

57. Trunkey DD: Torsion trauma. *Curr Probl Surg* 24:209, 1987.

58. *Advanced Trauma Life Support Instructor Manual.* American College of Surgeons, 1989.

59. Gerami S, Cousar JE, Davis JM, et al: The management of gunshot wounds of the chest. *Ann Thorac Surg* 5:189, 1968.

60. Hirschberg A, Thomson SR, Bade PG, et al: Pitfalls in the management of penetrating chest trauma. *Am J Surg* 157:372, 1989.

61. Wilson JM, Thomas AN, Goodman PC, et al: Severe chest trauma. *Arch Surg* 113:846, 1978.

62. Villalba M, Lucas CE, Ledgerwood AM, et al: The etiology of post-traumatic empyema and the role of decortication. *J Trauma* 19(6):414, 1979.

63. Coselli JS, Mattox KL, Beall AC Jr: Reevaluation of early evaluation of clotted hemothorax. *Am J Surg* 148:786, 1984.

64. Keen G: *Chest Injuries.* Bristol, England, Wright, 1984.

65. Hix WR, Aron BL: *Residua of Thoracic Trauma.* Mount Kisco, NY, Futura Publishing, 1987.

66. Mirvis SE, Templeton PA: Imaging of thoracic trauma. *Semin Thorac Cardiovasc Surg* 4:177, 1992.

67. Franz JL, Richardson JD, Grover FL, et al: Effect of methylprednisolone sodium succinate on experimental pulmonary contusion. *J Thorac Cardiovasc Surg* 68:842, 1975.

68. Pepe PE, Hudson LD, Carrico CJ: Early application of positive end-expiratory pressure in patients at risk for the adult respiratory distress syndrome. *N Engl J Med* 311:281, 1984.

69. Trunkey DD, Lewis BC: *Current Therapy of Trauma, 1984-1985.* Philadelphia, Decker, 1984.

70. Hankins JR, McAslan TC, Shin B, et al: Extensive pulmonary laceration caused by blunt trauma. *J Thorac Cardiovasc Surg* 74(4):519, 1977.

71. Fischer RP, Geiger JP, Guernsey JM: Pulmonary resections for severe pulmonary contusions secondary to high-velocity missile wounds. *J Trauma* 14:293, 1974.

72. Ganske JG, Dennis DL, Venderveer JB Jr: Traumatic lung cyst: Case report and literature review. *J Trauma* 21(6):493, 1981.

73. Kato R, Horinouchi H, Maenaka Y: Traumatic pulmonary pseudocyst. *J Thorac Cardiovasc Surg* 97:309, 1989.

74. Moore FA, Moore EE, Haenel JB, et al: Post-traumatic pulmonary pseudocyst in the adult: Pathophysiology, recognition, and selective management. *J Trauma* 29(10):1380, 1989.

75. Arom KV, Lyons GW: Traumatic pulmonary arteriovenous fistula. *J Thorac Cardiovasc Surg* 70(5):918, 1975.

76. Moser ES Jr, Proto AV: Lung torsion: Case report and literature review. *Radiology* 162(3):639, 1987.

77. Garzon AA, Cerruti MM, Golding ME: Exsanguinating hemoptysis. *J Thorac Cardiovasc Surg* 84:829, 1982.

78. Yee ES, Verrier ED, Thomas AN: Management of air embolism in blunt and penetrating thoracic trauma. *J Thorac Cardiovasc Surg* 85:661, 1983.

79. Orebaugh SL: Venous air embolism: Clinical and experimental considerations. *Crit Care Med* 20:1169, 1992.

80. Mathisen DJ, Grillo H: Laryngotracheal trauma. *Ann Thorac Surg* 43:254, 1987.

81. Pate JW: Tracheobronchial and esophageal injuries. *Surg Clin North Am* 69(1):111, 1989.

82. Symbas PN, Justicz AG, Ricketts RR: Rupture of the airways from blunt trauma: treatment of complex injuries. *Ann Thorac Surg* 54:177, 1992.

83. Bartlett RH: A procedure for management of acquired tracheoesophageal fistula in ventilator patients. *J Thorac Cardiovasc Surg* 71(1):89, 1976.

84. Hildenberg AD, Grillo HC: Acquired nonmalignant tracheoesophageal fistula. *J Thorac Cardiovasc Surg* 85:492, 1983.

85. Utley JR, Dillon ML, Todd EP: Giant tracheoesophageal fistula. *J Thorac Cardiovasc Surg* 75(3):373, 1978.

86. Courcy PA, Rodriquez A, Garrett HE: Operative technique for repair of tracheoinnominate artery fistula. *J Vasc Surg* 2(2):332, 1988.

87. Utley JR, Singer MM, Roe BB, et al: Definitive management of innominate artery hemorrhage complicating tracheostomy. *JAMA* 220(4):577, 1972.

88. Jones JW, Reynolds M, Hewitt RL, et al: Tracheoinnominate artery erosion: Successful surgical management of a devastating complication. *Ann Surg* 184(2):194, 1976.

89. Sharma OP: Traumatic diaphragmatic rupture: Not an uncommon entity—Personal experience with collective review of the 1980's. *J Trauma* 29(5):678, 1989.

90. Symbas PN, Vlasis S, Hatcher C Jr: Blunt and penetrating diaphragmatic injuries with or without herniation of organs into the chest. *Ann Thorac Surg* 42:158, 1986.

91. Ochsner MG, Rozycki GS, Lucente F, et al: Prospective evaluation of thoracoscopy for diagnosing diaphragmatic injury in thoracoabdominal trauma: A preliminary report. *J Trauma* 34:704, 1993.

92. Iverson LI, Mittal A, Dugan DJ, et al: Injuries to the phrenic nerve resulting in diaphragmatic paralysis with special reference to stretch trauma. *Am J Surg* 132:263, 1976.

93. Gastinne H, Venot J, Dupuy JP, et al: Unilateral diaphragmatic dysfunction in blunt chest trauma. *Chest* 93(3):518, 1988.

94. Glatterer MS Jr, Toon RS, Ellestad C, et al: Management of blunt and penetrating external esophageal trauma. *J Trauma* 25(8):784, 1985.

95. Cohn HE, Hubbard A, Patton G: Management of esophageal injuries. *Ann Thorac Surg* 48:309, 1989.

96. Pate JW: Esophageal injuries. *Surg Clin North Am* 69:118, 1989.

97. Graeber GM, Murray GF: Injuries of the esophagus. *Semin Thorac Cardiovasc Surg* 4:247, 1992.

98. Wilson RF, Steiger Z: *Esophageal injuries.* Rob & Smith, 1989.

99. Gabram SG, Devavanney J, Jones D, et al: Delayed hemorrhagic pericardial effusion: case reports of a complication from severe blunt chest trauma. *J Trauma* 32:794, 1992.

100. Evans J, Gray LA Jr, Rayner A, et al: Principles for the management of penetrating cardiac wounds. *Ann Surg* 189(6):777, 1979.

101. Jebara VA, Saade B: Penetrating wounds to the heart: A wartime experience. *Ann Thorac Surg* 47:250, 1989.

102. Baillot R, Dontigny L, Verdant A, et al: Intrapericardial trauma: Surgical experience. *J Trauma* 29:736, 1989.

103. Attar S, Suter CM, Hankins JR, et al: Penetrating cardiac injuries. *Ann Thorac Surg* 51:711, 1991.

104. Kudsk KA, Voeller GR, Mangiante EC, et al: Myocardial contusion: Diagnosis and management. *Contemp Surg* 35:11, 1989.

105. Soutter DI, Rodriquez A: Cardiac contusion: Diagnosis and management. *TQ* 4(2):16, 1988.

106. Reid CL, Kawanishi DT, Rahimtoola SH, et al: Chest trauma: Evaluation by two-dimensional echocardiography. *Am Heart J* 113:971, 1987.

107. Holness R, Waxman K: Diagnosis of traumatic cardiac contusion utilizing single photon-emission computed tomography. *Crit Care Med* 18:1, 1990.

108. Goldstein S, Yu PN: Constrictive pericarditis after blunt chest trauma. *Am Heart J* 69(4):544, 1965.

109. Orlando R III, Drezner AD: Intra-aortic balloon counterpulsation in blunt cardiac injury. *J Trauma* 23(5):424, 1983.

110. Mavroudis C, Roon AJ, Baker CC, et al: Management of acute cervicothoracic vascular injuries. *J Thorac Cardiovasc Surg* 80:342, 1980.

111. Richardson JD, Polk HC Jr, Flint LM: *Trauma, Clinical Care & Pathophysiology.* Chicago, Year Book Medical Publishing, 1987.

112. Parmley LF, Mattingly TW, Manion WC, et al: Nonpenetrating traumatic injury of the aorta. *Circulation* 17:1086, 1958.

113. Woodring JH, Dillon ML: Radiographic manifestations of mediastinal hemorrhage from blunt chest trauma. *Ann Thorac Surg* 37:171, 1984.

114. Heibert E, Wolverson MK, Sundaram M, et al: CT in aortic trauma. *Am J Roentgenol* 140:1119, 1983.

115. Akins GW, Mortimer JB, Dagget W, et al: Acute traumatic disruption of the thoracic aortic: A ten-year experience. *Ann Thorac Surg* 31(4):305, 1981.

116. Mattox KL: Approaches to trauma involving the major vessels of the thorax. *Surg Clin North Am* 69(1):77, 1989.

117. Laschinger JC: Spinal cord injury following surgical correction of acute aortic disruption. *Semin Thorac Cardiovasc Surg* 4:217, 1992.

118. Marini CP, Grubbs PE, Toporoff B, et al: Effect of sodium nitroprusside on spinal cord perfusion and paraplegia during aorta cross-clamping. *Ann Thorac Surg* 47:379, 1989.

178. Abdominal Trauma

Stephen M. Cohn and Gerard A. Burns

Abdominal trauma occurs in about 20 percent of civilian injuries requiring operation [1]. It is estimated that one-half of all preventable trauma deaths are related to inappropriate management of abdominal trauma [2].

Abdominal injuries should be suspected in all patients sustaining major trauma. Patients with nonpenetrating trauma caused by vehicular crashes or falls are at particular risk. Extraabdominal injuries are often clues to the presence of injuries within the abdomen. For example, almost 50 percent of patients with gunshot wounds to the chest have abdominal injuries [1].

Diagnostic Methods

Findings indicative of abdominal trauma include bruises or abrasions over the abdomen (e.g., markings caused by seat belts or tires), abdominal pain or tenderness, guarding, absent bowel sounds, or unexplained hypotension. Physical examination findings, however, are often equivocal or misleading. Peritoneal signs are absent in 40 percent of patients with significant intraabdominal injuries; conversely, 20 percent of patients with positive physical findings have no injuries detected at laparotomy [1]. The absence of physical findings is a particularly unreliable observation in patients with an abnormal sensorium secondary to head trauma, spinal cord injury, or intoxication. The unreliability of physical examination as a means for identifying intraabdominal injury has prompted the development of a variety of supplementary diagnostic methods, including diagnostic peritoneal lavage (DPL); local exploration of penetrating wounds; abdominal computed tomography (CT) scanning; bedside abdominal ultrasonography; laparoscopy; and serial observation.

MANDATORY EXPLORATION. Abdominal exploration is mandatory in patients with abdominal gunshot wounds, because visceral injury is present in more than 90 percent of cases [3], and other modes of evaluation are unreliable in this setting [4]. In patients with stab wounds, exploration is mandated by the presence of peritoneal signs, hemodynamic instability, overt signs of visceral injury, or evisceration of abdominal contents. Mandatory abdominal exploration of trauma patients may be appropriate at institutions that rarely evaluate abdominal trauma but leads to an increase in morbidity associated with the nontherapeutic operations [5].

LOCAL EXPLORATION. Local exploration of stab wounds effectively identifies cases in which the wound does not penetrate the peritoneum; these patients can be expeditiously discharged from busy emergency departments [6,7]. If local exploration shows that the peritoneal cavity has been violated, then DPL should be performed (*vide infra*).

DIAGNOSTIC PERITONEAL LAVAGE AND ABDOMINAL COMPUTED TOMOGRAPHY. DPL is useful for evaluating patients with abdominal stab wounds [8] or suspected blunt abdominal trauma [9]. DPL is not indicated in abdominal gunshot wounds, because 25 percent of patients have a falsely negative study [4]. The test is considered positive when the lavage fluid contains greater than or equal to 100,000 red blood cells (RBC) per cubic millimeter, bilirubin or amylase in concentrations higher than plasma, bacteria, or food particles. Elevation in white blood cell count greater than 500 per cubic millimeter is no longer considered an absolute indication for laparotomy [10,11,12]. DPL successfully identifies most injuries after stab wounds [13], although hollow viscus injuries, retroperitoneal (e.g., duodenal or pancreatic) injuries, and diaphragmatic injuries are sometimes missed [14,15]. The threshold for mandatory laparotomy in stab wounds to the subcostal area (intrathoracic abdomen) has been lowered to 5000 RBC per cubic millimeter, in an effort to identify diaphragmatic lacerations [15].

DPL is more reliable than abdominal CT for identifying the presence of intraabdominal injuries after blunt trauma, the accuracy of the two modalities being greater than 90 percent and about 75 percent, respectively [16,17,18]. The two methods are considered complementary. CT may be particularly helpful in patients with pelvic fractures, whereas DPL has a high (29%) false-positive rate [19]. CT is also useful for identifying retroperitoneal injuries [20,21] and selecting certain patients with splenic or hepatic trauma for nonoperative management (*vide infra*). Abdominal CT scanning has little role in the evaluation of penetrating abdominal trauma, except in patients with flank or back wounds [22,23]. Both DPL and abdominal CT scans evaluate the abdomen at a single point in time; therefore, follow-up DPL [24] or CT scans may be helpful in revealing evolving or overlooked lesions.

SERIAL OBSERVATION. Serial observation can be used as a primary diagnostic modality in selected patients with abdominal stab wounds [25,26,27]. This approach is quite accurate, but applicable only in patients with normal mentation and requires experienced personnel to perform the examinations.

ULTRASONOGRAPHY AND LAPAROSCOPY. The bedside abdominal ultrasound can detect blood within the peritoneal cavity with substantial accuracy (94–96%) [28,29]. This technique has the advantages of being noninvasive, portable, rapid, and inexpensive, but accuracy is dependent on the skill of the operator. The utility of laparoscopy in the setting of abdominal trauma is still under investigation. Initial reports suggest this modality is of particular benefit in identifying the entrance into the peritoneal cavity of tangential gunshot wounds or flank stab wounds [30]. In addition, laparoscopy may be helpful in excluding diaphragmatic lacerations in stab wounds of the intrathoracic abdomen [31].

Specific Injuries

SPLEEN

Diagnosis. The spleen is commonly injured in both blunt and penetrating trauma. Manifestations of splenic injury include hemodynamic instability caused by hemorrhage, left upper quadrant abdominal pain and tenderness, and left shoulder pain caused by diaphragmatic irritation by blood. Pain and tenderness may be absent, particularly in patients with altered mentation from head injuries or intoxication. DPL followed by laparotomy remains the "gold standard" for diagnosing splenic injury, but abdominal CT scanning is clearly useful for both identifying damage to the spleen and predicting the likelihood of splenic salvage [32,33,34].

Splenic Preservation. It is increasingly apparent that the spleen plays an important role in the host's defenses against infection [35]. Asplenic individuals appear to be at increased risk for developing sudden and often lethal bacterial infections [36]. This syndrome, termed overwhelming postsplenectomy infection (OPSI), is usually caused by encapsulated organisms, particularly *Streptococcus pneumoniae, Haemophilus influenzae, or Neisseria meningitidis* [37]. OPSI is characterized by a fulminant course, with death frequently occurring less than 24 hours after the onset of the syndrome. The true incidence of OPSI is unknown, but it appears to be less than 1 percent overall [38,39]. The risk of OPSI appears to be much greater in the pediatric age-group [40,41]. The increased susceptibility to infection noted in adults after splenectomy is much less than that seen in children [42,43] (see Chap. 91).

Concerns about OPSI have led to an increased emphasis on preserving splenic tissue after traumatic injury whenever possible. Grading systems have been devised to provide a framework for intraoperative decision making, leading to salvage of the spleen in more than 50 percent of cases of splenic trauma [33,44,45]. Established methods of surgical repair of the injured spleen (splenorrhaphy) [46] in addition to a myriad of advanced techniques such as argon beam coagulation [47,48], fibrin glue [49,50], and absorbable mesh wrap [51,52], may further improve the rate of splenic preservation. Complications of splenorrhaphy, such as intraabdominal abscess or rebleeding, are infrequent [45]. One group had a 12 percent postsplenorrhaphy complication rate and stressed that the risk of this procedure may have been underestimated in earlier reports [53]. The benefit of splenic autotransplantation, in preventing OPSI after total splenectomy, has not been demonstrated in clinical trials [54,55].

Another approach for preserving splenic tissue is nonoperative management of the injured spleen. Nonoperative therapy has been successfully used in children [56,57] and carefully selected adults [33] with splenic trauma. Nonoperative therapy is more often successful in pediatric patients as compared with adults, possibly because the chest wall is more elastic and the splenic capsule is relatively thicker in children. The role of nonoperative therapy of splenic trauma is now well established in selected cases, but is applicable to only about 15 percent of patients [33]. In adults, nonoperative management should be used only if the following criteria are satisfied: CT evidence of minimal splenic trauma [32,33,34]; no evidence of other intraabdominal injuries requiring operative correction or evaluation; absolute hemodynamic stability; minimal or absent peritoneal findings; and a maximal transfusion requirement (to maintain a hematocrit in excess of 30%) of less than or equal to 2 units of blood [34]. Age older than 54 years recently has been proposed as an additional independent predictor of failure of nonoperative management [58]. The risks of transfusion-related hepatitis [38] and missed intraabdominal injury [59] appear to be less significant than previously postulated in patients with minimal splenic injury [60]. If nonoperative management is selected, then patients should be observed carefully in a monitored setting for 48 to 72 hours. During this period, blood pressure should be monitored continuously, hematocrit measured every

6 hours, and abdominal examination repeated serially. Recently, the use of transcatheter arterial embolization of the splenic artery in stable patients with angiographic evidence of bleeding has been proposed as a method of avoiding laparotomy and improving splenic salvage [61]. We routinely perform a follow-up abdominal CT scan before hospital discharge on all patients managed nonoperatively. Progressive healing of the spleen occurs over a 6-week period [62], but CT may identify patients who develop occult enlarging subcapsular hematomas [63].

Postoperative Considerations. For patients undergoing splenectomy or splenorrhaphy, the serum amylase concentration should be determined daily for several days in an effort to detect unrecognized pancreatic injury or posttraumatic pancreatitis (Table 178-1). Because drainage of the splenic bed does not increase the risk of postoperative infection when drains are left in place less than 48 hours [64], drains should be removed in the early postoperative period (unless there is a very large volume of drainage or the amylase concentration of the drainage is elevated). We routinely administer perioperative antibiotics (e.g., cefotetan). Persistent leukocytosis, fever, or prolonged ileus should suggest the possibility of intraperitoneal sepsis, particularly left subphrenic abscess. Abdominal CT scanning is often useful for diagnosing splenic fossa collections. Left pleural effusions occur commonly (88%) after mesh splenorrhaphy [51] and are generally self-limited.

Long-term prophylactic antibiotics and antipneumococcal vaccination may be effective in preventing OPSI [65], but the efficacy of these approaches has not been substantiated by controlled clinical trials. We routinely administer Pneumovax to patients who have undergone traumatic splenectomy, usually waiting until just before discharge from the hospital. Thrombocytosis occurs routinely after splenectomy, and, occasionally, platelet counts in excess of 1,000,000 per cubic millimeter are recorded. In general, postsplenectomy thrombocytosis is not associated with increased risk of thrombotic complications [66] and does not warrant therapy.

LIVER AND PORTA HEPATIS

Epidemiology and Diagnosis. Liver injuries occur in 15 to 20 percent of blunt and about 40 percent of penetrating trauma victims. The liver is the second most commonly injured organ in abdominal trauma (after the spleen in blunt trauma and after the small intestine in penetrating trauma). Mortality is about 11 percent after hepatic injury and results from exsanguinating hemorrhage in 80 percent of cases [67]. The presence of hepatic injury is established by DPL followed by laparotomy or, in selected instances, by abdominal CT scanning.

Table 178-1. Complications of Splenic Injury

Nonoperative management
  Missed concurrent intraabdominal injury
  Persistent hemorrhage
  Delayed splenic rupture
After splenectomy or splenorrhaphy
  Overwhelming postsplenectomy sepsis
  Pancreatitis
  Intraabdominal abscess
  Rebleeding
  Thrombocytosis
  Necrosis of gastric wall

Classification. A six-level scheme for hepatic trauma has been proposed [68]: classes I to III include minor capsular tears or small nonruptured intraparenchymal hematomas that generally require minimal suturing or hemostatic agents; classes IV to VI are severe injuries such as ruptured intraparenchymal hematomas, major (>25%) lobar destruction, hepatic venous injuries, and hepatic avulsion that often require extensive efforts at repair or debridement and may necessitate vascular isolation, major resection, or packing. Most deaths attributable to hepatic trauma occur in patients with severe injuries, and it is typically these patients who develop major problems, including hypothermia, coagulopathy, intraabdominal abscesses, biliary leakage, and late hemorrhage [67,69].

Management. Nonoperative management of liver trauma in hemodynamically stable adults is usually indicated, if abdominal CT findings indicate nonbleeding hepatic injuries and the absence of other significant intraabdominal injuries [70,71,72]. Observation is undertaken with extreme caution as the abdominal CT scan significantly underestimates the degree of liver injury in almost one-third of cases [73]. Patients undergoing nonoperative management should be observed in a monitored setting for at least 72 hours. Expectant management should be abandoned if the patient requires multiple transfusions for ongoing hepatic hemorrhage; the patient becomes hemodynamically unstable; abdominal CT indicates expansion of hematomas; a bile leak is identified; or there is suspicion of a septic focus within the liver [70,71,72].

Complications. The most common complications occurring in survivors of liver injury are bleeding, bile leakage, and abdominal infection (Table 178-2) [67,69]. Manifestations of bleeding include sanguinous drainage from drains or the incision; falling hematocrit; expanding abdominal girth; or hemodynamic instability. Utilization of heat exchangers for blood rewarming and intraoperative autotransfusion can help minimize the hypothermia, acidosis, and coagulation defects seen in patients with severe hepatic trauma [69]. In cases of continued bleeding, efforts should be made to rewarm the patient and correct metabolic abnormalities before reoperation is performed to place (or replace) packs and ligate or coagulate active bleeding sites. Fluids and blood products should be warmed and heating blankets applied. Platelet transfusions and fresh frozen plasma should be administered, as indicated by appropriate laboratory studies. Selective hepatic artery embolization may be a useful adjunct in hemodynamically stable patients with continued bleeding [74].

Table 178-2. Complications of Hepatic Injury

Nonoperative management
  Missed concurrent intraabdominal injury
  Persistent hemorrhage
  Expansion of hematoma
  Hepatic abscess
  Hepatic rupture
  Hemobilia
  Biliary leakage
After hepatorrhaphy or hepatic resection and packing
  Hypothermia
  Coagulopathy
  Hypoglycemia
  Rebleeding
  Intraabdominal sepsis
  Biliary leakage
  Hemobilia

Intraabdominal sepsis is the leading cause of delayed mortality after traumatic liver injury, accounting for 10 to 20 percent of all deaths caused by hepatic trauma. Abscesses occur in approximately 10 percent of patients with liver injuries [75]. A number of factors increase the likelihood of abdominal infections: (1) The severity of liver injury is clearly a major factor, with perihepatic abscesses complicating the course of about 10 percent of serious injuries, twice the rate seen with minor (Grade I and II) lesions; (2) Concomitant hollow viscus injuries also result in peritoneal soilage and increase the risk of sepsis after liver trauma; (3) Drainage of the peritoneal cavity after injury to the liver increases the likelihood of infection, if sump suction drainage systems are employed; (4) Blood transfusion volume appears to correlate well with the development of septic complications; and (5) use of perihepatic packing markedly increases infectious morbidity [75]. Thus, it is apparent that victims of major hepatic trauma require intensive surveillance for the development of intraabdominal infections. It is imperative to rapidly recognize and aggressively drain infected perihepatic collections. Percutaneous CT-guided drainage is useful in selected patients, but many cases are better handled by reoperation.

Biliary leakage occurs in approximately 25 percent of patients with major hepatic trauma but is self-limited in 80 percent of cases [75]. Biliary leakage is caused by bile duct disruption and should be suspected when bilious fluid exits drains or there is an unexplained infection associated with direct hyperbilirubinemia. Abdominal CT can be useful for identifying perihepatic biliary collections and, in many instances, percutaneous techniques can implement placement of drains. Posttraumatic hepatic biliary fistulae usually close spontaneously in 2 to 3 weeks if adequate drainage is provided.

Hemobilia (i.e., bleeding into the biliary tract) is a rare but serious complication of hepatic trauma. The triad of right upper quadrant abdominal pain, jaundice, and GI hemorrhage are present in only one-third of patients with hemobilia. Other findings include right upper quadrant abdominal mass and abnormal liver function tests. Arteriography is the diagnostic procedure of choice, and angiographic embolization of the involved artery is the preferred treatment, carrying a lower mortality than hepatic resection [76,77].

Porta Hepatis Structures. Traumatic injuries to structures in the porta hepatis (gallbladder, extrahepatic bile ducts, hepatic artery, and portal vein) are uncommon. Injuries to these structures are usually recognized intraoperatively because the vast majority (90%) of these patients present with hemorrhagic shock [78]. Mortality in these patients is high (25–50%) and is often attributable to uncontrolled bleeding from the portal venous system [78,79]. The portal vein should be repaired when possible, but ligation is compatible with survival and rarely results in long-term problems with portal hypertension [78]. Partial lacerations of extrahepatic bile ducts should be repaired. Complete lacerations, however, are best managed by biliary-enteric bypass and stenting [78]. Injuries to the gallbladder occur rarely in blunt trauma and are accompanied by injuries to the liver in 80 percent of cases [80]. Cholecystectomy is the treatment of choice for traumatic injuries to the gallbladder. Hepatic artery lacerations can be managed by repair or ligation. The latter approach rarely, if ever, results in hepatic necrosis.

SMALL INTESTINE

Epidemiology, Diagnosis, and Intraoperative Management. Small bowel disruption occurs in about 15 percent of patients requiring celiotomy for blunt trauma. The small intestine is the most commonly injured organ in penetrating abdominal trauma. Mechanisms leading to intestinal rupture after blunt trauma include crushing of the gut between the abdominal wall and vertebral column; sudden increase in intraluminal pressure; shearing forces; and devascularization by injury to the mesenteric circulation. In gunshot wounds to the abdomen, laparotomy is mandatory, and therefore the diagnosis of small bowel injury is made in the operating room. In blunt trauma and stab wounds to the abdomen, however, identification of intestinal disruption may be difficult. The contents of the small intestine have a neutral pH and contain relatively few bacteria. Thus, spillage of small bowel contents may not elicit abdominal findings for many hours after the injury. Therefore, it is of paramount importance to maintain a high index of suspicion for small bowel injury.

Serial physical examinations [25] and DPL [81,82] continue to play an important role in the identification of intestinal disruption. DPL is diagnostic in about 95 percent of patients with intestinal injury [81,82]. Identification of isolated hollow viscus injury by DPL has been enhanced by the addition of enzyme determinations (amylase and alkaline phosphatase) [83]. Abdominal CT scanning [16,18,84] and laparoscopy [31] are unreliable methods of delineating small bowel injury. Early recognition of small bowel disruption is essential as delay contributes to septic morbidity and mortality [85,86,87]. Intraoperative management usually consists of primary repair, but more extensive small bowel injuries may require segmental resection with primary anastomosis. Rarely, in the face of massive contamination or hemodynamic instability, creation of an enterostomy is warranted.

Postoperative Considerations. Patients sustaining isolated small intestinal injuries do not routinely warrant critical care management unless there are severe associated injuries. Major postoperative concerns include prolonged ileus, bowel obstruction, suture line breakdown, fistula formation, abscess formation, delayed hemorrhage, and missed injury. Septic complications, fortunately, are rare after isolated small intestinal trauma.

DUODENUM

Epidemiology. Duodenal injuries occur infrequently but carry a substantial (18%) mortality [88,89]. Early deaths are invariably attributable to hemorrhage resulting from injuries to nearby vital structures such as the liver and major vessels [89]. Mortality in patients surviving the initial 24 hours is usually caused by generalized infection [89]. Early recognition is imperative because mortality increases fourfold when operations are delayed for more than 24 hours [90]. The mortality rate for gunshot wounds (31%) is substantially higher than for blunt trauma (10%) or stab wounds (6%) [89]. Complex duodenal injuries (i.e., those associated with concomitant pancreatic trauma) are particularly serious, carrying a mortality ten times higher than simpler injuries [91].

Diagnosis and Management. Expeditious identification of duodenal injury is key in determining outcome, but accurate diagnosis is often difficult. The duodenum is frequently injured in its retroperitoneal portion, and, thus, leakage of intraluminal contents may not cause peritoneal irritation until late. In fact more than one-third of duodenal injuries go undetected for more than 24 hours [90]. Hyperamylasemia is an inconsistent finding, occurring in 50 percent of blunt duodenal injuries and only 25 percent of duodenal injuries attributable to gunshot wounds [87]. Because duodenal injuries are frequently retroperitoneal, DPL is often unreliable. Findings on abdominal CT

(retroperitoneal air or extravasation of contrast) are often subtle and easily missed by inexperienced observers.

Duodenal injuries are commonly classified as follows: type I, seromuscular tear, intramural hematoma, or contusion; type II, full-thickness laceration; type III, duodenal injury with any pancreatic injury; and type IV, combined severe pancreaticoduodenal injury [90]. Although simple closure is adequate for relatively minor duodenal injuries [87], failure to divert gastric contents in type III and IV injuries is associated with high mortality [88,92]. A popular method of diversion is the pyloric exclusion procedure, in which the pylorus is oversewn and gastrojejunostomy performed [88]. For about 3 weeks the gastric contents are excluded from bathing the injured duodenum, thereby decreasing the release of pancreatic and biliary secretions during the healing process. The use of decompressive tube duodenostomy to minimize the risk of uncontrolled fistula formation remains controversial [89,93,94]. Most patients require prolonged nasogastric decompression and total parenteral or enteral (feeding jejunostomy) nutrition.

Duodenal intramural hematoma formation, invariably the result of blunt abdominal trauma, is rare in all age-groups but occurs more commonly in children. The lesion is manifested by partial or complete duodenal obstruction secondary to the submucosal mass caused by the hematoma. Common findings include nausea, bilious vomiting, abdominal pain, and epigastric tenderness. The diagnosis is supported by elevated serum amylase concentrations in about one-third of patients [95], and confirmed by upper GI contrast radiography. Although the classic roentgenographic finding is the "stacked coin sign," dilation of the duodenum proximal to an obstruction is more commonly observed [96]. Abdominal CT should be performed to exclude concomitant pancreatic injury, found in 21 percent of cases [97]. Nonoperative management, consisting of nasogastric suction and total parenteral nutrition, is almost always successful. Operation should be reserved for cases that show no resolution of obstruction after 2 weeks or have evidence of perforation. Operative treatment of duodenal intramural hematoma (without perforation) consists of simple evacuation of the clot [97].

Complications. Abdominal infection is the leading cause of postoperative mortality after duodenal injury, accounting for 43 percent of deaths in one series (Table 178-3) [88]. Gastric, duodenal, or pancreatic fistulae, which occur in about 6 percent of cases [88], must be controlled by adequate external drainage to prevent the development of sepsis. It is crucial that all drains and tubes be meticulously maintained, because their accidental dislodgement can lead to major morbidity. Elevated serum amylase concentrations, leukocytosis, fever, or abdominal tenderness may be indicative of pancreatitis, suture line dehiscence, fistula formation, or the development of intraabdominal abscesses. Abdominal CT (with intraluminal contrast) or conventional upper GI contrast radiography may be helpful in delineating leaks or fluid collections. Drainage can be obtained either percutaneously under CT (or ultrasound) guidance or by reoperation, the choice depending on the number, size, and character of the collections.

PANCREAS

Epidemiology. Injuries to the pancreas occur in only 1 to 2 percent of patients sustaining abdominal trauma and are caused by penetrating wounds in about two-thirds of cases [98]. Although relatively rare, pancreatic injuries are associated with a high mortality and morbidity [98]. Three main factors affect outcome in patients with pancreatic wounds: (1) the magnitude of associated injuries; (2) the presence or absence of major ductal injury; (3) and the presence or absence of combined

Table 178-3. Complications of Duodenal and Pancreatic Injury

Intraabdominal abscess
Duodenal and pancreatic fistulae
Pancreatitis
Pancreatic pseudocyst and abscess
Duodenal suture-line dehiscence

pancreatic and duodenal injury. Associated abdominal injuries are common in pancreatic trauma; 42 percent of patients have major vascular injuries; 50 percent have accompanying liver injury; and 21 percent have accompanying duodenal injury [98].

Diagnosis. The diagnosis of injury to the pancreas is generally established at the time of abdominal exploration for penetrating injury. In the setting of blunt abdominal trauma, however, diagnosis can be difficult. Because the pancreas is retroperitoneal, peritoneal irritation may be absent and DPL results are frequently falsely negative. Amylase determinations are not helpful in predicting the presence of pancreatic injury for a number of reasons: hyperamylasemia is absent in 75 percent of penetrating pancreatic wounds and 30 percent of blunt pancreatic wounds [98]; amylase isoenzyme studies are misleading [99]; serial amylase determinations lead to a critical delay in operative intervention [100]; and amylase values are often elevated because of acute alcohol intoxication, a common clinical finding in trauma victims [101]. Endoscopic retrograde cholangiopancreatography (ERCP) has been abandoned as a diagnostic adjunct in most centers [98]. The most valuable study in blunt trauma for establishing the diagnosis of pancreatic injury is abdominal CT scanning, which may identify peripancreatic fluid or pancreatic transection [102]. Early diagnosis is imperative, because untreated pancreatic wounds often lead to pseudocyst and fistula formation, and failure to provide adequate debridement and drainage fosters the development of intraabdominal sepsis.

Classification and Management. Pancreatic injuries are classified as follows: type I, contusion, hematoma, or peripheral laceration with an intact duct; type II, distal transection or distal injury with duct disruption; type III, proximal transection or injury with probable duct disruption; type IV, combined severe pancreaticoduodenal injury. The essential principles of operative management in pancreatic injury are control of hemorrhage, excision of necrotic tissue, control of exocrine secretions, and preservation of endocrine function. Fortunately, only 21 percent of patients with pancreatic wounds require resection or special procedures. Most injuries are operatively treated using simple repair and drainage [98]. Type III and IV injuries represent a major operative challenge and may require resection or diversion of gastric contents and extensive drainage [103]. Rarely is a pancreaticoduodenectomy (Whipple procedure) needed [104]. Closed suction drains are used after pancreatic trauma in an effort to control secretions and minimize the risk of intraabdominal abscess formation [105]. These drains should be left in place at least 10 days and removed only if output is minimal (i.e., <50 ml/day) and low in amylase content. Persistently high amylase concentrations in drainage fluid suggest pancreatic ductal disruption (or duodenal suture line dehiscence). Maintaining adequate drainage is critical in determining outcome under these circumstances.

Patients with pancreatic injuries typically have a long and complicated postoperative course (see Table 178-3). As with duodenal injury, nasogastric suction is routinely required for extended periods, and all drains must be meticulously secured and maintained. Nutritional support, either parenteral or enteral (via jejunostomy tube), must be initiated early. A 24-hour (perioperative) course of antibiotics is warranted, but extended administration of antibiotics is indicated only for the treatment of defined infections [106]. Frequent determinations of amylase concentration in serum and drainage fluids aid in the early diagnosis of pancreatitis and fistula formation.

Complications. Death occurs in 19 percent of patients sustaining pancreatic injury and is most frequently caused by hemorrhage (55%) and sepsis (11%) [98]. Complications such as fistula, abscess, pancreatitis, and pseudocyst are common after pancreatic trauma, occurring in more than one-third of patients [98]. Fistulae, although the most common complication (20%), rarely lead to death and generally close spontaneously with nonoperative treatment [98]. The administration of somatostatin analogue may hasten the closure of pancreatic fistulae [107]. In patients with established peripancreatic infections, CT-guided percutaneous techniques may be an adjunct to operative management in selected cases [108]. Postoperative pancreatic insufficiency is rare unless more than 80 percent of the pancreas is resected.

COLON AND RECTUM

Epidemiology and Diagnosis. Colonic injury, common in penetrating trauma (15–39% of cases) [109], is relatively rare in blunt trauma (<1% of cases) [110]. Penetrating colonic injuries are usually diagnosed at laparotomy. DPL misses 30 percent of penetrating wounds of the large intestine [111] and is unreliable in this setting. Abdominal CT with intraluminal contrast may be of value in stab wounds of the flank and back, but colonic injuries are sometimes missed with this study as well [23].

Blunt colonic injuries result from shearing forces, devascularization, increased intraluminal pressure in temporarily "closed" loops, and direct contusion. These wounds are usually secondary to direct impact or compression by seat belts or steering wheels and are frequently accompanied by injuries to other intraabdominal organs [110]. A high index of suspicion for this lesion is necessary after major blunt abdominal trauma to avoid delay in diagnosis and subsequent severe abdominal infections.

Rectal injuries are usually caused by pelvic fractures, abdominal gunshot wounds, or perineal avulsion injuries. In patients with these injuries, proctosigmoidoscopy must be performed to exclude rectal laceration because gross rectal blood or occult blood in the stool may be absent [112]. Failure to make an early diagnosis of rectal trauma almost invariably leads to pelvic infection.

Classification and Management. Penetrating colonic injuries are classified by the severity of tissue destruction and the degree of peritoneal soilage [113]. In a prospective trial, Stone and Fabian demonstrated that selected civilian penetrating colon wounds can be safely closed at the initial operation without creation of a colostomy [114]. Subsequent studies have demonstrated that primary closure of colonic injuries does not increase the risk of postoperative infectious complications, even in unselected patients (including those with hemorrhagic shock, contamination, associated abdominal injuries, and delayed operation) [115,116]. In patients with colonic injuries attributable to blunt or penetrating trauma, diversion of the fecal stream is indicated only in the setting of tenuous physiologic status, gross fecal contamination, or technical difficulties [110,115].

In World War I, rectal wounds were lethal in 45 percent of cases, whereas during the Vietnam conflict, mortality was reduced to 14 percent. The improved survival has been attributed to the use of antibiotics, pelvic drainage, routine diversion of the fecal stream, and washout of the distal (rectal) segment [117]. Civilian wounds of the rectum may be managed with fecal diversion without rectal washout [118,119], but a subset of patients with complicated blunt pelvic-perineal trauma or high-velocity missile injuries should be managed as in wartime [120]. Distal washout may decrease the likelihood of pelvic sepsis by reducing translocation (i.e., transmural migration) of intraluminal bacteria [121].

Complications. Infection is the most important complication of colonic or rectal trauma. Most studies indicate that rates of infection (25–33%) and death (4%) are not dependent on the anatomic site of colonic injury [122,123]. Numerous authors have related the incidence of infection to the presence or absence of associated injuries, transfusion requirement, and patient age [123,124]. In wounds of the colon, a 12-hour [125] or 24-hour [106] course of perioperative antibiotics is as effective as a 5-day regimen in lowering the incidence of infectious complications. Single-agent therapy with cefoxitin or cefotetan appears to be effective in providing adequate perioperative gram-negative aerobic and anaerobic coverage [106]. The use of intraperitoneal drains in these contaminated procedures should be avoided [114], although pelvic drainage should be provided in rectal injuries. Retained missiles that have passed through the colon may increase the likelihood of major septic complications and should be removed whenever possible [126].

Genitourinary Trauma

KIDNEY

Epidemiology and Diagnosis. Urinary and genital injuries occur in 10 to 15 percent of patients with abdominal trauma [1]. Blunt trauma accounts for about 80 percent of all cases of renal trauma [1]. The diagnosis of renal injury is usually suggested by gross hematuria and is confirmed by intravenous pyelography (IVP) or contrast-enhanced abdominal CT in more than 90 percent of cases [114,115]. Radiography should be utilized, in the setting of blunt trauma, for patients with gross hematuria or marked microscopic hematuria (> 30 red blood cells per high power field) [127]. Kidney trauma requiring operative intervention is unlikely in hemodynamically stable patients in the absence of gross hematuria, flank hematoma, or penetrating wounds that could reasonably injure the genitourinary tract [128]. Renal pedicle and collecting system injuries are occasionally present in the absence of hematuria [129,130,131], and these lesions should be suspected in patients absorbing particularly large amounts of kinetic energy, such as victims of falls or pedestrians hit by rapidly moving vehicles.

Management. Renal contusion is by far the most common type of renal injury. Most renal injuries, therefore, are managed nonoperatively with bed rest and liberal fluid administration to promote a brisk diuresis. Operative management is reserved for penetrating injuries, after blunt trauma in hemodynamically unstable patients, and in those individuals with major renal lacerations, shattered or devitalized kidneys, or pedicle injuries [132,133,134]. Associated injuries are common in patients with blunt renal trauma, particularly in those requiring operative intervention [135,136]. The diagnosis of renovascular injury should be aggressively pursued, because preservation of renal function is apparently sometimes possible even when therapy is substantially delayed (more than 12 hours) [137].

Complications. Although major complications after surgery for renal injury occur in one-third of patients [138], azotemia and renal failure are unusual (11% of cases) and appear to be related to the extent of renal injury and the type of repair performed [138]. Most patients who subsequently develop renal insufficiency present in shock and have multiple associated injuries. Other major complications directly related to renal surgery include delayed bleeding, abscess formation, urinoma, necessity for prolonged urinary drainage, and arteriovenous fistula formation [138]. Urinary leaks (with reabsorption of urea) lead to azotemia despite a normal glomerular filtration rate. Urinary fistulae are detected by measuring higher concentrations of creatinine in drainage fluids than plasma. When adequately drained, urinary leaks are generally self-limited. If urinary leakage persists longer than 5 to 7 days despite adequate drainage, an IVP should be obtained to rule out distal ureteral obstruction by blood clot or stent [1].

Bladder. The bladder is the most frequently injured organ in patients with pelvic fractures. Conversely, more than three-fourths of patients with bladder injuries have associated pelvic fractures [139,140]. The death rate with bladder rupture is high (12–22%), reflecting the severity of associated injuries [139,140,141]. Essentially all patients with bladder injuries have gross hematuria or physical evidence of pelvic fractures [141]. The diagnosis of bladder rupture is confirmed by cystography. This study is extremely accurate, but many (13%) require a postdrainage film to identify bladder ruptures [142]. Pelvic CT is inaccurate in the diagnosis of bladder trauma and is not recommended [143,144].

The bladder injury is repaired in conjunction with suprapubic cystostomy. Urinary drainage should be provided until a repeat cystogram performed at 7 to 10 days documents complete healing. Selected patients with extraperitoneal bladder rupture and sterile urine can be managed nonoperatively with urinary drainage alone, although complications (e.g., infection of pelvic hematomas and development of persistent urinary extravasation requiring operative closure) have been reported in up to 20 percent of cases managed in this manner [139,140].

Urethra. Urethral injury is found in about 5 percent of patients with pelvic fractures [145,146]. A high index of suspicion is required, because more than 50 percent of patients with urethral injury have no physical signs (blood at the urethral meatus, perineal hematoma, or high-riding prostate). A retrograde urethrogram confirms the diagnosis of urethral tear. These injuries generally are managed initially with suprapubic cystostomy, definitive reconstruction being performed at a later date [147,148,149].

Reproductive Tract. Uterine injuries are uncommon and typically involve the gravid organ, because enlargement renders the uterus more vulnerable to trauma [150].

Vaginal injuries are rare (<4% of pelvic fractures) but are not trivial problems, because delayed diagnosis can lead to catastrophic complications, including pelvic infection. Penetration by bony fragments, tearing caused by lateral forces on the perineum in straddle injuries, and trauma caused by foreign bodies are proposed mechanisms of vaginal laceration [151]. Major perineal-pelvic lacerations should be managed conservatively with serial dressing changes under anesthesia. Creation of a diverting colostomy is frequently warranted to prevent fecal soilage.

Trauma to male genitalia is unusual and is generally managed by early conservative debridement and dressing changes with delayed definitive repair [152].

PELVIC FRACTURES

Epidemiology and Diagnosis. Pelvic fracture is the third most common injury in motor vehicle crash fatalities [153]. Mortality is increased in patients with initial hemodynamic instability [153]. Open pelvic fractures or severe crushing injuries have been reported to carry a mortality of almost 50 percent [154]. Hemorrhage is the leading cause of death in these patients, and an adoption of an early aggressive multidisciplinary approach to arrest pelvic bleeding has lowered overall mortality to under 10 percent [155,156]. Delayed septic complications remain the second most important cause of death [157].

Pelvic fractures are identified by evidence of pelvic instability or peripelvic ecchymosis on physical examination. Diagnosis is confirmed radiographically. Digital rectal examination to exclude rectal injury (bloody stool or bony spicules) and urethral injury (high-riding prostate) is mandatory. Proctosigmoidoscopy and contrast urethrogram and cystogram are essential in identifying associated injuries.

Classification and Management. There are numerous classification schemes for pelvic fractures. The Kane modification of the Key-Conwell system is as follows: type I, fractures of individual bones not involving the pelvic ring; type II, a single break of the pelvic ring through both ipsilateral rami or other ring fractures not involving displacement of the fracture segment; type III, double breaks in the pelvic ring; type IV, acetabular fractures [158]. Patients with hemodynamically unstable pelvic fractures, defined as injuries requiring transfusion of more than 6 units of blood in 24 hours, typically require management in an ICU environment. More than 60 percent of hemodynamically unstable patients with pelvic fractures can be managed successfully using conventional resuscitative measures, including Swan-Ganz catheter monitoring [153]. Twenty percent of patients with pelvic fractures require transfusion of 10 or more units of blood. The average transfusion requirement for surviving, but initially hemodynamically unstable, patients is 18.4 units [157,158].

Exclusion of life-threatening intraabdominal hemorrhage in these patients is imperative, and DPL is the diagnostic study of choice. DPL has a high false-positive rate (29%), but a low false-negative rate [19]. If DPL is grossly positive, then urgent laparotomy is performed [157]. If DPL is negative and initial efforts to achieve hemodynamic instability are unsuccessful, then the patient should be placed in a pneumatic antishock garment (PASG) and transferred to the operating room for external skeletal fixation [155,159]. The PASG helps to tamponade bleeding from torn pelvic veins, and assists in control of hemorrhage in two-thirds of patients [160,161]. Angiography with selective embolization is reserved for the few patients with ongoing bleeding after bony alignment is obtained, and is successful in controlling hemorrhage if a specific bleeding site is identified [162].

Complications. The acute respiratory distress syndrome occurs in about 15 percent of patients with complex pelvic fractures; this is possibly related to the frequent occurrence of associated thoracic injuries, multiple blood transfusion, shock, and fat embolization [153]. Late complications are primarily related to infection.

Patients with pelvic fractures are at greatly increased risk for the development of deep venous thrombosis (DVT) because of stasis resulting from prolonged bed rest and venous endothelial damage from frequently associated lower-extremity injuries. Conventional prophylaxis against DVT is often contraindicated or impossible in patients with pelvic fractures and concurrent injuries. Thus, subcutaneous heparin is relatively contraindicated in the presence of a pelvic hematoma and is absolutely contraindicated when intracranial or spinal injuries are present.

Pneumatic compression boots cannot be applied if lower-extremity fractures are stabilized with casts or external fixators. Simple surveillance measures are probably inadequate in trauma patients confined to bed rest because DVT occurs so commonly, being detected in one study in 67 percent of patients not receiving prophylaxis [163]. Therefore, we routinely place inferior vena caval filters in patients with major pelvic fractures who cannot wear bilateral pneumatic compression boots.

References

1. Moore EE, Mattox KL, Feliciano DV: *Trauma.* Norwalk, CT, Appleton & Lange, 1991.
2. Kreis DJ Jr, Plasencia G, Augenstein D, et al: Preventable trauma deaths: Dade County, Florida. *J Trauma* 26:649, 1986.
3. Moore EE, Moore JB, Van Duzer-Moore S, et al: Mandatory laparotomy for gunshot wounds penetrating the abdomen. *Am J Surg* 140:847, 1980.
4. Thal ER, May RA, Beesinger D: Peritoneal lavage. *Arch Surg* 115:430, 1980.
5. Weigelt JA, Kingman RG: Complications of negative laparotomy for trauma. *Am J Surg* 156:544, 1988.
6. Thompson JS, Moore EE, Van Duzer-Moore S, et al: The evolution of abdominal stab wound management. *J Trauma* 20:478, 1980.
7. Oreskovich MR, Carrico CJ: Stab wounds of the anterior abdomen. *Ann Surg* 198:411, 1983.
8. Nance FC, Wennar MH, Johnson LW, et al: Surgical judgment in the management of penetrating wounds of the abdomen. *Ann Surg* 179(5):639, 1974.
9. Fischer RP, Bevelin BC, Engrav LH, et al: Diagnostic peritoneal lavage. *Am J Surg* 136:701, 1978.
10. Jacobs DG, Angus L, Rodriguez A, et al: Peritoneal lavage white count: A reassessment. *J Trauma* 30(5):607, 1990.
11. D'Amelio LF, Rhodes M: A reassessment of the peritoneal lavage leukocyte count in blunt abdominal trauma. *J Trauma* 30(10):1291, 1990.
12. Soyka JM, Martin M, Sloan EP, et al: Diagnostic peritoneal lavage: Is an isolated WBC count ≥ 500/mm³ predictive of intra-abdominal injury requiring celiotomy in blunt trauma patients? *J Trauma* 30(7):874, 1990.
13. Feliciano DV, Bitondo CG, Steed G, et al: Five hundred open taps or lavages in patients with abdominal stab wounds. *Am J Surg* 148:772, 1984.
14. Jackson GL, Thal ER: Management of stab wounds of the back and flank. *J Trauma* 19:660, 1979.
15. Henneman PL, Marx JA, Moore EE, et al: Diagnostic peritoneal lavage: Accuracy in predicting necessary laparotomy following blunt and penetrating trauma. *J Trauma* 30(11):1345, 1990.
16. Marx JA, Moore EE, Jorden RC, et al: Limitations of computed tomography in the evaluation of acute abdominal trauma: A prospective comparison with diagnostic peritoneal lavage. *J Trauma* 25:933, 1985.
17. Fabian TC, Mangiante EC, White TJ, et al: A prospective study of 91 patients undergoing both computed tomography and peritoneal lavage following blunt abdominal trauma. *J Trauma* 26:602, 1986.
18. Meyer DM, Thal ER, Weigelt JA, et al: Evaluation of computed tomography and diagnostic peritoneal lavage in blunt abdominal trauma. *J Trauma* 29:1168, 1989.
19. Hubbard SG, Bivins BA, Sachatello CR, et al: Diagnostic errors with peritoneal lavage in patients with pelvic fractures. *Arch Surg* 114:844, 1979.
20. Sorkey AJ, Farnell MB, Williams HJ, et al: The complementary roles of diagnostic peritoneal lavage and computed tomography in the evaluation of blunt abdominal trauma. *Surgery* 106:794, 1989.
21. Kearney PA, Vahey T, Burney RE, et al: Computed tomography and diagnostic peritoneal lavage in blunt abdominal trauma. *Arch Surg* 124:344, 1989.
22. Meyer DM, Thal ER, Weigelt JA, et al: The role of abdominal CT

in the evaluation of stab wounds to the back. *J Trauma* 29:1226, 1989.

23. Phillips T, Sclafani JA, Goldstein A, et al: Use of the contrast-enhanced CT enema in the management of penetrating trauma to the flank and back. *J Trauma* 26:593, 1986.
24. Alyono D, Perry JF: Significance of repeating diagnostic peritoneal lavage. *Surgery* 91:656, 1982.
25. Zubowski R, Nallathambi M, Ivatury R, et al: Selective conservatism in abdominal stab wounds: The efficacy of serial physical examination. *J Trauma* 28:1665, 1988.
26. Robin AP, Andrews JR, Lange DA, et al: Selective management of anterior abdominal stab wounds. *J Trauma* 29(12):1684, 1989.
27. Shorr RM, Gottlieb MM, Webb K, et al: Selective management of abdominal stab wounds. *Arch Surg* 123:1141, 1988.
28. Tso P, Rodriguez A, Cooper C, et al: Sonography in blunt abdominal trauma: A preliminary progress report. *J Trauma* 33(1):39, 1992.
29. Hoffmann R, Nerlich M, Nuggia-Sullam M, et al: Blunt abdominal trauma in cases of multiple trauma evaluated by ultrasonography: A prospective analysis of 291 patients. *J Trauma* 32(4):452, 1992.
30. Ivatury RR, Simon RJ, Weksler B, et al: Laparoscopy in the evaluation of the intrathoracic abdomen after penetrating injury. *J Trauma* 33(1):101, 1992.
31. Livingston, DH, Tortella BJ, Blackwood J, et al: The role of laparoscopy in abdominal trauma. *J Trauma* 33(3):471, 1992.
32. Resciniti A, Fink MP, Raptopoulos V, et al: Nonoperative treatment of adult splenic trauma: Development of a computed tomographic scoring system that detects appropriate candidates for expectant management. *J Trauma* 128:828, 1988.
33. Cogbill TH, Moore EE, Jurkovich GJ, et al: Nonoperative management of blunt splenic trauma: A multicenter experience. *J Trauma* 29(10):1312, 1989.
34. Buntain WL, Gould HR, Maull KI: Predictability of splenic salvage by computed tomography. *J Trauma* 28:24, 1988.
35. Llende M, Santiago-Delpin EA, Lavergne J: Immunological consequences of splenectomy: A review. *J Surg Res* 40:85, 1986.
36. King H, Schumacker HB: Splenic studies. *Ann Surg* 136:239, 1952.
37. Diamond LK: Splenectomy in childhood and the hazard of overwhelming infection. *Pediatrics* 43:886, 1969.
38. Luna GK, Dellinger EP: Nonoperative observation therapy for splenic injuries: A safe therapeutic option? *Am J Surg* 153:462, 1987.
39. Lucas CE: Splenic trauma: Choice of management. *Ann Surg* 213(2):98, 1991.
40. Eraklis AJ, Filler RM: Splenectomy in childhood: A review of 1413 cases. *J Pediatr Surg* 7:382, 1972.
41. Holdsworth RJ, Irving AD, Cuschieri A: Postsplenectomy sepsis and its mortality rate: Actual versus perceived risks. *Br J Surg* 78(9):1031, 1991.
42. Green JB, Shackford SR, Sise MJ, et al: Late septic complications in adults following splenectomy for trauma: A prospective analysis in 144 patients. *J Trauma* 26:999, 1986.
43. Cullingford GL, Watkins DN, Watts ADJ, et al: Severe late postsplenectomy infection. *Br J Surg* 78:716, 1991.
44. Shackford SR, Sise MJ, Virgilio RW, et al: Evaluation of splenorrhaphy: A grading system for splenic trauma. *J Trauma* 21:538, 1981.
45. Feliciano DV, Spjut-Patrinely V, Burch JM: Splenorrhaphy - The alternative. *Ann Surg* 211(5):569, 1990.
46. Buntain WL, Lynn HB: Splenorrhaphy: Changing concepts for the traumatized spleen. *Surgery* 86:748, 1979.
47. Dowling RD, Ochoa J, Yousem A, et al: Argon beam coagulation is superior to conventional techniques in repair of experimental splenic injury. *J Trauma* 31(5):717, 1991.
48. Dunham CM, Cornwell III EE, Militello P: The role of the argon beam coagulator in splenic salvage. *SGO* 173:179, 1991.
49. Kram HB, del Junco T, Clark SR: Techniques of splenic preservation using fibrin glue. *J Trauma* 30(1):97, 1990.
50. Ochsner MG, Maniscalco-Theberge ME, Champion HR: Fibrin glue as a hemostatic agent in hepatic and splenic trauma. *J Trauma* 30(1):884, 1990.
51. Lange DA, Zaret P, Merlotti GJ, et al: The use of absorbable mesh in splenic trauma. *J Trauma* 28(3):269, 1988.
52. Rogers FB, Baumgartner NE, Robin AP, et al: Absorbable mesh splenorrhaphy for severe splenic injuries: Functional studies in an animal model and an additional patient series. *J Trauma* 31(2):200, 1991.
53. Beal SL, Spisso JM: The risk of splenorrhaphy. *Arch Surg* 123:1158, 1988.
54. Holdsworth RJ: Regeneration of the spleen and splenic autotransplantation. *Br J Surg* 78:270, 1991.
55. Traub A, Giebink GS, Smith C: Splenic reticuloendothelial function after splenectomy, spleen repair, and spleen autotransplantation. *N Eng J Med* 317(25):1559, 1987.
56. Lally KP, Rosario V, Mahour GH, et al: Evolution in the management of splenic injury in children. *Surg Gynecol Obstet* 170:245, 1990.
57. King DR, Lobe TE, Haase GM, et al: Selective management of injured spleen. *Surgery* 90:677, 1981.
58. Smith JS, Wengrovitz MA, DeLong BS: Prospective validation of criteria, including age, for safe, nonsurgical management of the ruptured spleen. *J Trauma* 33(3):363, 1991.
59. Traub AC, Perry JF: Injuries associated with splenic trauma. *J Trauma* 21:840, 1981.
60. Flaherty L, Jurkovich J: Minor splenic injuries: Associated injuries and transfusion requirements. *J Trauma* 31(12):1618, 1991.
61. Scalfani SJ, Weisberg A, Scalea TM, et al: Blunt splenic injuries: Nonsurgical treatment with CT, arteriography, and transcatheter arterial embolization of the splenic artery. *Radiology* 181(1):189, 1991.
62. Dulchavsky SA, Lucas CE, Ledgerwood AM, et al: Wound healing of the injured spleen with and without splenorrhaphy. *J Trauma* 27(10):1155, 1987.
63. Do HM, Cronan JJ: CT appearance of splenic injuries managed nonoperatively. *AJR* 157:757, 1991.
64. Pachter HL, Hofstetter SR, Spencer FC: Evolving concepts in splenic surgery: Splenorrhaphy versus splenectomy and post-splenectomy drainage: Experience in 105 patients. *Ann Surg* 194:262, 1981.
65. Powell RW, Blaylock WE, Hoff CJ, et al: The efficacy of postsplenectomy sepsis prophylactic measures: The role of penicillin. *J Trauma* 28:1285, 1988.
66. Boxer MA, Braun J, Ellman L: Thromboembolic risk of postsplenectomy thrombosis. *Arch Surg* 113:808, 1978.
67. Feliciano DV, Jordan GL, Bitondo CG, et al: Management of 1000 consecutive cases of hepatic trauma (1979-1984). *Ann Surg* 204:438, 1986.
68. Moore EE, Shackford SR, Pachter HL, et al: Organ injury scaling: Spleen, liver and kidney. *J Trauma* 24:1664, 1989.
69. Cogbill TH, Moore EE, Jurkovich GJ, et al: Severe hepatic trauma: A multicenter experience with 1,335 liver injuries. *J Trauma* 28:1433, 1988.
70. Knudson MM, Lim RC, Oakes DD, et al: Nonoperative management of blunt liver injuries in adults: The need for continued surveillance. *J Trauma* 30(12):1494, 1990.
71. Hollander MJ, Little JM: Nonoperative management of blunt liver injuries. *Br J Surg* 78(8):968, 1991.
72. Bynoe RP, Bell RM, Miles WS, et al: Complications of nonoperative management of blunt hepatic injuries. *J Trauma* 32(3):308, 1992.
73. Croce MA, Fabian TC, Kudsk KA, et al: AAST organ injury scale: Correlation of CT-graded liver injuries and operative findings. *J Trauma* 31(6):806, 1991.
74. Fandrich BL, Gnanadev DA, Jaecks R, et al: Selective hepatic artery embolization as an adjunct to liver packing in severe hepatic trauma: Case Report. *J Trauma* 29:1716, 1989.
75. Fabian TC, Croce MA, Stanford GG, et al: Factors affecting morbidity following hepatic trauma. *Ann Surg* 213(6):540, 1991.
76. Heimbach DM, Ferguson GS, Harley JD: Treatment of traumatic hemobilia with angiographic embolization. *J Trauma* 18:221, 1978.
77. Clouse ME: Hepatic artery embolization for bleeding and tumors. *Surg Clin North Am* 69(2):419, 1989.
78. Sheldon GF, Lim RC, Yee ES, et al: Management of injuries to the porta hepatis. *Ann Surg* 202:539, 1985.
79. Busuttil RW, Kitahama A, Cerise E, et al: Management of blunt and penetrating injuries to the porta hepatis. *Ann Surg* 191:641, 1980.
80. Soderstrom CA, Maekawa K, DuPriest RW, et al: Gallbladder injuries resulting from blunt abdominal trauma. *Ann Surg* 193:60, 1981.
81. Dauterive AH, Flancbaum LL: Blunt intestinal trauma. *Ann Surg* 201:198, 1985.

82. Wisner DH, Chun Y, Blaisdell FW: Blunt intestinal injury. *Arch Surg* 125:1319, 1990.

83. McAnena OJ, Marx JA, Moore EE: Peritoneal lavage enzyme determinators following blunt and penetrating abdominal trauma. *J Trauma* 31:1161, 1991.

84. Sherck JP, Oakes DD: Intestinal injuries missed by computed tomography. *J Trauma* 30(1):1, 1990.

85. Robbs JV, Moore SW, Pillay SP: Blunt abdominal trauma with jejunal injury: A review. *J Trauma* 20:308, 1980.

86. Schenk WG, Lonchyna V, Moylan J: Perforation of the jejunum from blunt abdominal trauma. *J Trauma* 23:54, 1983.

87. Donahue JH, Crass RA, Trunkey DD: The management of duodenal and other small intestinal trauma. *World J Surg* 9:904, 1985.

88. Martin TD, Feliciano DV, Mattox KL, et al: Severe duodenal injuries. *Arch Surg* 118:631, 1983.

89. Cogbill TM, Moore EE, Feliciano DV et al: Conservative management of duodenal trauma: A multicenter perspective. *J Trauma* 30:1469, 1990.

90. Lucas CE, Ledgerwood AM: Factors influencing outcome after blunt duodenal injury. *J Trauma* 15:839, 1975.

91. Levison MA, Petersen SR, Sheldon GF, et al: Duodenal trauma: Experience of a trauma center. *J Trauma* 24:475, 1984.

92. Berne CJ, Donovan AJ, White EJ, et al: Duodenal "diverticulization" for duodenal and pancreatic injury. *Am J Surg* 127:503, 1974.

93. Snyder WH, Weigelt JA, Watkins WL, et al: The surgical management of duodenal trauma. *Arch Surg* 115:422, 1980.

94. Stone HH, Fabian TC: Management of duodenal wounds. *J Trauma* 19:334, 1979.

95. Woolley MM, Mahour GH, Sloan T: Duodenal hematoma in infancy and childhood. *Am J Surg* 136:8, 1978.

96. Fullen WD, Selle JG, Whitely DH, et al: Intramural duodenal hematoma. *Ann Surg* 179:549, 1974.

97. Jewett TC, Caldarola V, Karp MP, et al: Intramural hematoma of the duodenum. *Arch Surg* 123:54, 1988.

98. Howard JM, Jordan GL, Reber HA: *Surgical Diseases of the Pancreas*. Philadelphia, Lea & Febiger, 1987.

99. Bouwman DL, Weaver DW, Walt AJ: Serum amylase and its isozymes: A clarification of their implications in trauma. *J Trauma* 24(7):573, 1984.

100. Wisner DM, Wold RC, Frey CF: Diagnosis and treatment of pancreatic injuries. *Arch Surg* 1250:1109, 1990.

101. Bloch RS, Weaver DW, Bouwman DL: Acute alcohol intoxication: Significance of the amylase level. *Ann Emerg Med* 12(5):294, 1983.

102. Cogbill TM, Moore EE, Morris JA, et al: Distal pancreatectomy for trauma: A multicenter experience. *J Trauma* 31:1600, 1991.

103. Feliciano DV, Martin TD, Cruse PA, et al: Management of combined pancreatoduodenal injuries. *Ann Surg* 205:673, 1987.

104. Eastlick L, Fogler RJ, Shaftan GW. Pancreaticoduodenectomy for trauma: Delayed reconstruction: A case report. *J Trauma* 30:503, 1990.

105. Fabian TC, Kudsk KA, Croce MA, et al: Superiority of closed suction drainage for pancreatic trauma. *Ann Surg* 211:724, 1990.

106. Fabian TC, Croce MA, Payne LW, et al: Duration of antibiotic therapy for penetrating abdominal trauma: A prospective trial. *Surgery* 112(4): 788, 1992.

107. Prinz RA, Pickleman J, Hoffman JP: Treatment of pancreatic cutaneous fistulas with a somatostatin analog. *Am J Surg* 155:36, 1988.

108. Adams DB, Harvey B, Anderson MC. Percutaneous catheter drainage of infected pancreatic and peripancreatic fluid collectors. *Arch Surg* 125:1554, 1990.

109. Corman ML: *Colon and Rectal Surgery*. Philadelphia, J.B. Lippincott, 1989.

110. Ross SE, Cobean RA, Hoyt DB, et al: Blunt colonic injury: A multicenter review. *J Trauma* 33(3):379, 1992.

111. Obeid FN, Sorensen V, Vincent G, et al: Inaccuracy of diagnostic peritoneal lavage in penetrating colonic trauma. *Arch Surg* 119:906, 1984.

112. Levine H, Simon RJ, Smith TR, et al: Guaiac testing in the diagnosis of rectal trauma: What is its value? *J Trauma* 32(2):210, 1992.

113. Flint LM, Vitale GC, Richardson JD, et al: The injured colon: Relationships of management to complications. *Ann Surg* 193:619, 1981.

114. Stone HH, Fabian TC: Management of perforating colon trauma. *Ann Surg* 190:430, 1979.

115. Chappuis CW, Frey DJ, Dietzen CD, et al: Management of penetrating colon injuries: A prospective randomized trial. *Ann Surg* 213(5):492, 1991.

116. Burch JM, Martin R, Richardson RJ, et al: Evolution of the treatment of the injured colon in the 1980s. *Arch Surg* 126:97, 1991.

117. Lavenson GS, Cohen A: Management of rectal injuries. *Am J Surg* 122:226, 1971.

118. Robertson HD, Ray JE, Ferrari BT, et al: Management of rectal trauma. *Surg Gynecol Obstet* 154:161, 1982.

119. Burch JM, Feliciano DV, Mattox KL: Colostomy and drainage for civilian rectal injuries: Is that all? *Ann Surg* 209:600, 1989.

120. Kusminsky RE, Shbeeb I, Makos G, et al: Blunt pelviperineal injuries. *Dis Colon Rectum* 25:787, 1982.

121. Shannon FL, Moore EE, Moore FA, et al: Value of distal colon washout in civilian rectal trauma: Reducing gut bacterial translocation. *J Trauma* 28:989, 1988.

122. Thompson JS, Moore EE, Moore JB: Comparison of penetrating injuries of the right and left colon. *Ann Surg* 193:414, 1981.

123. Dawes LG, Aprahamian C, Condon RE, et al: The risk of infection after colon injury. *Surgery* 100:796, 1986.

124. Nichols RL, Smith JW, Klein DB, et al: Risk of infection after penetrating abdominal trauma. *N Engl J Med* 311:1065, 1984.

125. Dellinger EP, Wertz MJ, Lennard ES, et al: Efficacy of short-course antibiotic prophylaxis after penetrating intestinal injury. *Arch Surg* 121:23, 1986.

126. Porte HA III, Fabian TC, Croce MA, et al: Analysis of septic morbidity following gunshot wounds to the colon: The missile is an adjuvant for abscess. *J Trauma* 31(8):1088, 1991.

127. Klein S, Johs S, Fujitani R, et al: Hematuria following blunt abdominal trauma. *Arch Surg* 123:1173, 1988.

128. Guice K, Oldham K, Eide B, et al: Hematuria after blunt trauma: When is pyelography useful? *J Trauma* 23:305, 1983.

129. Presti JC, Carroll PR, McAninch JW: Ureteral and renal pelvic injuries from external trauma: Diagnosis and management. *J Trauma* 29:370, 1989.

130. Stables DP, Fouche RF, DeVilliers VanNiekerk JP, et al: Traumatic renal artery occlusion: 21 cases. *J Urology* 115:229, 1976.

131. Cass AS, Bubrick M, Luxenberg M, et al: Renal pedicle injury in patients with multiple injuries. *J Trauma* 25:892, 1985.

132. Corriere JN Jr, McAndrew JD, Benson GS: Intraoperative decision-making in renal trauma surgery. *J Trauma* 31(10):1390, 1991.

133. Atala A, Miller FB, Richardson JD, et al: Preliminary vascular control for renal trauma. *SGO* 172:386, 1991.

134. Husmann, DA, Morris JS: Attempted nonoperative management of blunt renal lacerations extending through the corticomedullary junction: The short-term and long-term sequelae. *J Urol* 143:682, 1990.

135. Sagalowsky AI, McConnell JD, Peters PC: Renal trauma requiring surgery: An analysis of 185 cases. *J Trauma* 23:128, 1983.

136. Knudson MA, McAninch JW, Gomez R: Hematuria as a predictor of abdominal injury after blunt trauma. *Am J Surg* 164:482, 1992.

137. Ivatury RR, Zubowski R, Stahl WM: Penetrating renovascular trauma. *J Trauma* 29:1620, 1989.

138. Carroll PR, Klosterman PW, McAninch JW: Surgical management of renal trauma: Analysis of risk factors, technique, and outcome. *J Trauma* 28:1071, 1988.

139. Cass AS: The multiple injured patient with bladder trauma. *J Trauma* 24:731, 1984.

140. Corriere JN, Sandler CM: Management of the ruptured bladder: Seven years of experience with ill cases. *J Trauma* 26:830, 1986.

141. Carroll PR, McAninch JW: Major bladder trauma: Mechanisms of injury and a unified method of diagnosis and repair. *J Urol* 132:254, 1984.

142. Carroll PR, McAninch JW: Major bladder trauma: The accuracy of cystography. *J Urol* 130:887, 1983.

143. Mee SL, McAninch JW, Federle MP: Computerized tomography in bladder rupture: Diagnostic limitations. *J Trauma* 137:207, 1987.

144. Rehm CG, Mure AJ, O'Malley KF, et al: Blunt traumatic bladder rupture: The role of retrograde cystogram. *Ann Emerg Med* 20(8):845, 1991.

145. Weems WL: Management of genitourinary injuries in patients with pelvic fractures. *Ann Surg* 189:717, 1979.

146. Lowe MA, Mason JT, Luna GK, et al: Risk factors for urethral injuries in men with traumatic pelvic fractures. *J Urol* 140:506, 1988.

147. Cass AS: Urethral injury in the multiple-injured patient. *J Trauma* 24:901, 1984.
148. Turner-Warwick R, Oxon DM: Prevention of complications resulting from pelvic fracture urethral injuries—and from their surgical management. *Urol Clin North Am* 16(2):335, 1989.
149. Jenkins BJ, Badenoch DF, Fowler CG, et al: Long-term results of treatment of urethral injuries in males caused by external trauma. *Br J Urol* 70:73, 1992.
150. Quast DC, Jordan GL: Traumatic wounds of the female reproductive organs. *J Trauma* 4:389, 1964.
151. Niemi TA, Norton LW: Vaginal injuries in patients with pelvic fractures. *J Trauma* 25:547, 1985.
152. Bertini JE, Corriere JN: The etiology and management of genital injuries. *J Trauma* 28:1278, 1988.
153. Mucha P, Farnell MB: Analysis of pelvic fracture management. *J Trauma* 24:379, 1984.
154. Sinnott R, Rhodes M, Brader A: Open pelvic fracture: An injury for trauma centers. *Am J Surg* 163:283, 1992.
155. Flint LM, Babikian G, Anders M, et al: Definitive control of mortality from severe pelvic fracture. *Ann Surg* 211(6):703, 1979.
156. Burgess AR, Eastridge BJ, Young JWR, et al: Pelvic ring disruptions: Effective classification system and treatment protocols. *J Trauma* 30(7):848, 1990.
157. Evers BM, Cryer HM, Miller FB: Pelvic fracture hemorrhage. *Arch Surg* 124:423, 1989.
158. Cryer HM, MIller FB, Evers BM, et al: Pelvic fracture classification: Correlation with hemorrhage. *J Trauma* 28:973, 1988.
159. Moreno C, Moore EE, Rosenberger A, et al: Hemorrhage associated with major pelvic fracture: A multispecialty challenge. *J Trauma* 26:987, 1986.
160. Flint LM, Brown A, Richardson JD, et al: Definitive control of bleeding from severe pelvic fractures. *Ann Surg* 189:709, 1979.
161. Panetta T, Sclafani SJA, Goldstein AS, et al: Percutaneous transcatheter embolization for massive bleeding from pelvic fractures. *J Trauma* 25:1021, 1985.
162. Mucha P Jr, Welch TJ: Hemorrhage in major pelvic fractures. *Surg Clin North Am* 68(4):757, 1989.
163. Kudsk KA, Fabian TC, Baum S, et al: Silent deep vein thrombosis in immobilized multiple trauma patients. *Am J Surg* 158:515, 1989.

179. Burn Management

Edwin A. Deitch

In the United States, it is conservatively estimated that each year 2.5 million people seek medical care for thermal injuries. More than 100,000 thermally injured patients are hospitalized each year, and 12,000 burn victims die of their injuries [1]. The care of the burn victim has progressed rapidly over the last 50 years. Before World War II, the average burn size associated with a 50 percent mortality rate in healthy young adults was less than 30 percent of the total body surface area (TBSA). Today the mean burn size associated with a 50 percent mortality rate ranges from 65 to 75 percent TBSA [2,3]. This major advance in burn survival is attributable to multiple factors, including: (1) a better understanding of the pathophysiology of the burn injury, leading to improvements in all aspects of critical care; (2) improved methods of volume resuscitation to prevent the development of burn shock and acute renal failure; (3) the development of topical antimicrobial agents, such as silver sulfadiazine and mafenide acetate, to reduce the incidence of burn wound infections; (4) the development and implementation of improved methods of nutritional support to optimize burn wound healing and increase resistance to infection; and (5) the understanding that early surgical removal of the burn wound with immediate skin grafting shortens the period of physiologic stress.

Nonetheless, burn injuries still remain a common cause of death. Only motor vehicle accidents cause more accidental deaths than do burns [4]. The three major causes of death in burn victims are cardiopulmonary failure, uncontrolled infection, and the development of the multiple organ failure syndrome. Only by understanding the deleterious effects of thermal injury on normal host defenses and homeostatic systems will it be possible to develop and use effective therapeutic regimens to improve survival. Therefore, the major goal of this chapter is to integrate basic physiologic concepts with clinical practice to aid in the diagnosis and treatment of the burn victim.

Classification of Thermal Injury

The three most important prognostic variables used in predicting survival after thermal injury are the patient's age, the size and depth of the burn injury, and whether an inhalation injury has occurred [2,5]. Burns generally are classified as first-, second- or third-degree. First-degree burns involve only the epidermis. The skin is red and painful, but blisters are not present. These burns heal in less than 1 week and rarely result in permanent scars. Second-degree burns can be superficial or deep. In superficial second-degree burns, damage is limited to the epidermis and the uppermost portion of the dermis. These burns are painful and characterized by the formation of blisters. Underneath the blisters, the skin is moist, pink, and tender. These burns generally heal spontaneously over a 2-week period. In contrast, deep second-degree burns spare only the deepest portion of the dermis. These burns are less painful, because the cutaneous nerves have been destroyed along with the dermis and epidermis. Deep second-degree burns may take over 3 weeks to heal or may require skin grafts for wound closure. Third-degree burns are full-thickness injuries. The entire dermis and epidermis is destroyed. They are nonpainful, dry, and have a milky white or tanned leather appearance. Third-degree burns do not heal spontaneously, and skin grafting is required in most cases.

Many charts and nomograms are available to assist in determining the extent of the body surface area that has been burned. One of the easiest to remember and thus most commonly used systems of estimating the burn size in adults is the Rule of Nines. In this system, each portion of the body is divided into a multiple of nine. For example, each upper extremity is 9 percent of the body surface area, and each lower extremity is 18 percent. Although determination of burn size using the Rule

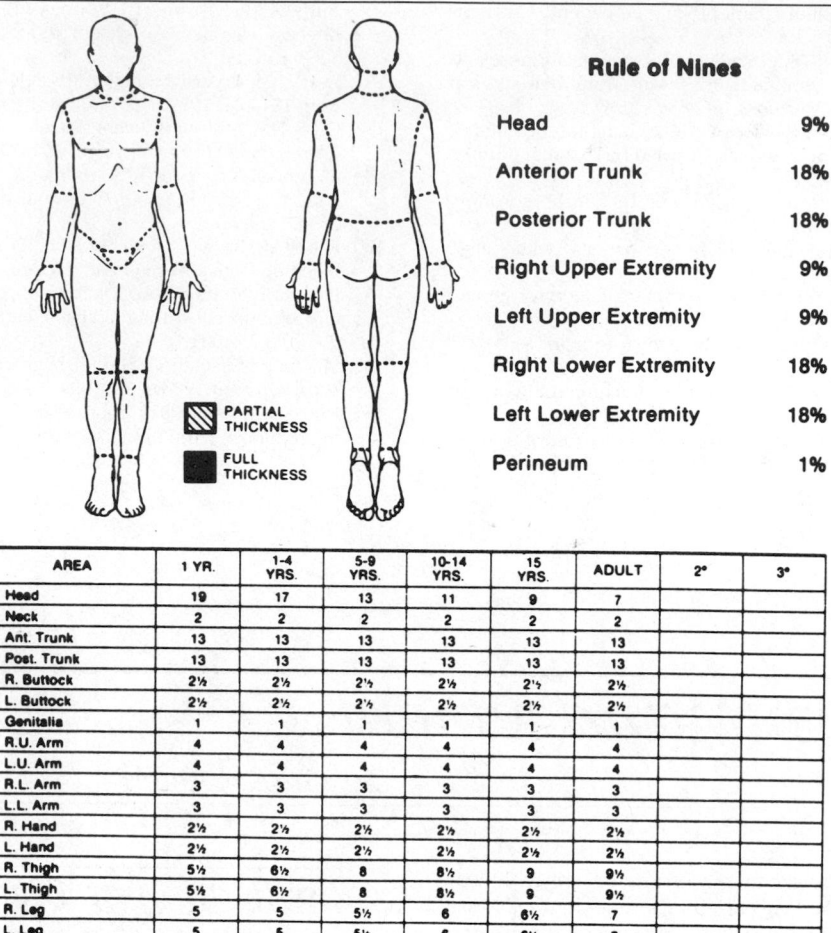

Rule of Nines

Head	9%
Anterior Trunk	18%
Posterior Trunk	18%
Right Upper Extremity	9%
Left Upper Extremity	9%
Right Lower Extremity	18%
Left Lower Extremity	18%
Perineum	1%

PARTIAL THICKNESS

FULL THICKNESS

AREA	1 YR.	1-4 YRS.	5-9 YRS.	10-14 YRS.	15 YRS.	ADULT	2°	3°
Head	19	17	13	11	9	7		
Neck	2	2	2	2	2	2		
Ant. Trunk	13	13	13	13	13	13		
Post. Trunk	13	13	13	13	13	13		
R. Buttock	2½	2½	2½	2½	2½	2½		
L. Buttock	2½	2½	2½	2½	2½	2½		
Genitalia	1	1	1	1	1	1		
R.U. Arm	4	4	4	4	4	4		
L.U. Arm	4	4	4	4	4	4		
R.L. Arm	3	3	3	3	3	3		
L.L. Arm	3	3	3	3	3	3		
R. Hand	2½	2½	2½	2½	2½	2½		
L. Hand	2½	2½	2½	2½	2½	2½		
R. Thigh	5½	6½	8	8½	9	9½		
L. Thigh	5½	6½	8	8½	9	9½		
R. Leg	5	5	5½	6	6½	7		
L. Leg	5	5	5½	6	6½	7		
R. Foot	3½	3½	3½	3½	3½	3½		
L. Foot	3½	3½	3½	3½	3½	3½		
TOTAL								

Fig. 179-1. The Rule of Nines and the Lund and Browder methods for calculating the extent of burn injury in adults and in children.

of Nines is relatively accurate in adults, it is not accurate in children, because the body proportions of children change as they grow. For this reason, most burn centers use the Lund-Browder chart to determine burn percentage in children as well as in adults (Fig. 179-1). By knowing the percentage of the body that has been burned, the depth of the burns, and the patient's age, it is possible to estimate the predicted mortality of the injury [2,5]. Additionally, by knowing the percentage of the body that has been burned and the patient's approximate weight, it is possible to estimate the volume of fluid required to resuscitate the patient.

Volume Resuscitation: Pathophysiology and Management

FIRST 24 HOURS. A thermal injury alters normal homeostasis in many ways. It induces a metabolic stress response, causes major fluid shifts, and places increased demands on the cardiac, pulmonary, and renal systems. After a thermal injury, multiple vasoactive mediators are released that alter the permeability of

the vascular endothelium, resulting in the leakage of intravascular fluid into the interstitial space. These vasoactive mediators include kinins, serotonin, histamine, prostaglandins, and oxygen radicals and their lipid peroxidation products [6,7,8]. The accumulation of fluid in the interstitial space results in the rapid formation of edema within the area of the burn wound [9]. However, after a major thermal injury, edema can also form in nonburned tissues. In contrast to the burned tissue, edema formation in nonburned tissue is not primarily caused by altered capillary permeability, but instead is related to the severe hypoproteinemic state of the patient [10]. Because the cells at the site of the thermal injury are injured, they swell, and more fluid leaves the intravascular space to enter these injured, swollen cells. What this means physiologically is that the edema and cell swelling that occur after a thermal injury result in the depletion of the fluid normally contained within the intravascular space [9]. The body's initial response to a decrease in intravascular volume is vasoconstriction. By constricting the blood vessels, the injured patient is initially able to maintain a normal blood pressure. However, as more fluid is lost from the intravascular space, the body's ability to maintain a normal blood pressure by vasoconstriction ultimately fails. The patient becomes hypotensive and develops burn shock. Unless these fluid losses are corrected, the uncompensated loss of fluid from the intravascular space results in systemic hypotension, organ hypoperfusion, and ultimately death. Thus, the ultimate goal of the resuscitation of a burn victim is to prevent hypotension and organ hypoperfusion by restoring the intravascular volume to a normal level.

Several factors must be considered in calculating the composition and volume of the fluid that needs to be administered to restore the intravascular volume. These factors include the extent of the burn, the age and weight of the patient, and the patient's physiologic status, including the effects of other injuries [11,12]. These calculations must be accurate to provide enough fluids to prevent intravascular volume depletion without causing overhydration and the subsequent development of pulmonary edema or excessive peripheral edema. By maintaining homeostasis in all of the body's fluid compartments, cardiac, renal, and pulmonary functions are optimized. Furthermore, by ensuring adequate cardiopulmonary function and limiting unnecessary edema, oxygenation of the injured tissue is maintained and wound healing fostered.

Although many fluid resuscitation regimens have been proposed to volume-resuscitate the burn victim, the most commonly used fluid regimen, and the one used by the author, is the Parkland formula [1]. The Parkland formula calls for the patient to receive 4 ml per kilogram of Ringer's lactate per percent of burn during the first 24-hour postburn period. One half of the fluid regimen must be given within the first 8 hours *after* the burn, and the remaining one half is infused at a constant rate over the next 16 hours. The following example illustrates the use of the Parkland formula to compute estimated fluid needs.

A 70-kg man sustaining a 50 percent body surface area burn will require 14,000 ml of Ringer's lactate (70 kg × 50% × 4 ml = 14,000). However, it is important to keep in mind that these calculated fluid needs are only estimates. Some patients require more fluid than calculated, and others can be adequately resuscitated with less than the calculated volume [11]. It is necessary to monitor the patient closely to prevent overhydration or underhydration. Thus, during resuscitation, the patient's pulse, urine output, blood pressure, and sensorium must be monitored to assess the patient's response to fluid therapy (Table 179-1). Because excessive edema within the burn wound may limit oxygen diffusion to injured cells and thereby promote further cell death [13,14], attempts to prevent overresuscitation are warranted. In about 20 percent of our patients, the volume of fluid initially administered (based on the Parkland formula) overestimates the patient's actual needs. A high urine output (greater than 2 ml/kg/hr) in a hemodynamically stable patient is frequently the first clinical indication that the volume of fluid administered exceeds the patient's actual fluid requirements. In this situation, the hourly rate of fluid administration is reduced by 25 percent, and the patient's urine output and hemodynamic status are followed over the next 2 to 4 hours. If the patient remains hemodynamically stable and the urine output remains above 0.5 ml/kg/hr, this new fluid infusion rate is maintained. If the urine output remains high, the infusion rate is decreased in further increments of 25 percent. However, before decreasing the infusion rate, it is necessary to ensure that the increased urine output is not attributable to a glucose-mediated osmotic diuresis. Occasionally in the nondiabetic, and more commonly in the diabetic patient, increased urine output is attributable to a stress-induced hyperglycemic state and not to the excess administration of fluids.

Although most patients can be adequately resuscitated using the Parkland formula, about 10 percent of the patients are refractory to standard measures to restore intravascular volume. This group of patients includes elderly patients with limited cardiovascular reserve as well as patients with preexisting cardiac disease [15]. Because of the presence of limited cardiac reserve or cardiac disease, these patients may not be able to increase their cardiac output sufficiently to meet the increased metabolic demands of a burn injury [16]. When this occurs, cardiotonic drugs, such as dopamine or dobutamine, should be instituted prophylactically to augment cardiac output and prevent cardiac failure [17]. If empiric use of these cardiotonic drugs in combination with full-volume resuscitation fails, a Swan-Ganz catheter should be placed to measure the patient's pulmonary wedge pressure, cardiac output, and peripheral vascular resistance. Subsequent fluid and drug therapy are based on these measurements. Although some investigators suggest inserting Swan-Ganz catheters prophylactically [17,18], we do not routinely place them in these patients because the risk of infection and other complications is increased in burn patients [19]. Instead, these monitoring catheters are placed only in patients who do not respond to volume resuscitation in combination with cardiotonic drugs. Although there is evidence that early colloid administration improves the patient's hemodynamic response [20], the use of colloid immediately postburn remains controversial, because it has not been documented to improve survival [21]. Even when all of these modalities are used, these are some patients who do not have adequate cardiac function to survive their injury. The urine output of these patients is never satisfactory, and they ultimately develop and die with a refractory metabolic acidosis.

Because of the increasing evidence that oxidants may play a role in both the early and later phases of tissue injury and organ failure after major traumatic or inflammatory insults, the use of resuscitative regimens containing anti-oxidants is an area of intense study [22]. Based on the results of these and future studies, it is likely that future resuscitative regimens will focus on techniques aimed at decreasing oxidant-mediated injury as well as volume resuscitation.

FLUID THERAPY BEYOND 24 HOURS POSTBURN. By 24 hours postburn, the increased vascular permeability to protein (but not to sodium) has largely returned to normal [9,11,16]. Because the effective intravascular volume can be better maintained with colloid (albumin or plasma) than crystalloid, and microvascular permeability protein is relatively normal, the intravenous fluids are changed from Ringer's lactate to 5% dextrose (D_5W) plus colloid. Although the exact hourly infusion rate of D_5W and the amount of colloid required to maintain hemodynamic stability may vary, the following formula is a good starting point:

D_5W at 2ml/kg/%burn + plasma (or plasma equivalent) at 0.3 to 0.5 ml/kg/%burn

In patients with burns of less than 20 percent TBSA, including children and infants, it is frequently possible to switch the patient partially or totally from intravenous fluids to oral fluid resuscitation during the second postburn day.

Table 179-1. Clinical Response to Resuscitation

	Acceptable	Unacceptable
Sensorium	Alert	Altered
Blood pressure	Systolic > 100	Systolic < 100
Pulse	<120	>120
Respiratory rate	<24	>24
Urine output	0.5–1 cc/kg/hr	<0.5 cc/kg/hr or >2 cc/kg/hr

By the third postburn day, vascular permeability generally has continued to return toward normal, and the previously administered water and sodium are beginning to enter the intravascular space from the interstitial and intracellular spaces. These physiologic responses are mirrored clinically by decreased edema and increased urine output. This period of increased mobilization of sequestered extravascular fluid and increased urine output is known as the diuretic phase of resuscitation. Intravenous fluids should now be adjusted to maintain a stable urine output. During this phase, large amounts of potassium must be administered intravenously to maintain normal serum potassium levels. Supplemental potassium is required, not only because potassium has been lost in the urine, but also because potassium will move from the intravascular to the intracellular space as the injured cells recover. Thus, potassium is infused parenterally at a constant rate to avoid hypokalemia, cardiac arrhythmias, and decreased intestinal motility. It is not uncommon for patients who have sustained large burn injuries (50% TBSA or greater) to require 10 mEq of potassium per hour to maintain a normal serum potassium level during this third 24-hour period.

During the remainder of the patient's hospitalization, attention must be directed toward maintaining a normal circulating volume and electrolyte balance; additionally, the patient's serum albumin level and red cell mass must be monitored. A common potential fluid and electrolyte problem that must be guarded against until the patient's burns have healed is the development of hypernatremia. Hypernatremia frequently occurs if these patients do not receive adequate amounts of salt-free fluids (free water), because insensible evaporative water loss is much greater across the burn wound than through intact skin. In fact, patients with large burns may lose up to 5 liters of water per day from their burn wounds (1 ml/kg/%burn). Therefore, D_5W should be administered in sufficient quantity to maintain the serum sodium level within a normal range.

Although capillary leakage has now largely ceased and protein is no longer lost from the intravascular space, the liver does not synthesize enough albumin to maintain a normal oncotic pressure [23]. Therefore, in patients with burns larger than 20 percent, albumin or plasma must be periodically administered in sufficient quantities to maintain a serum albumin of at least 2 to 2.5 gm per deciliter to prevent intestinal and peripheral edema.

The patient's hemoglobin levels should be monitored at least biweekly, because after a major thermal injury red cell survival is decreased and anemia is common [24]. Because of the increased rate of red blood cell destruction, it is not uncommon for patients with major burn injuries to become severely anemic. However, because of the risks of transfusions, a selective transfusion policy, in which burn patients are not routinely transfused prophylactically to maintain an arbitrary hemoglobin concentration (i.e., 10 gm/dl), appears beneficial. Using this approach, patients are transfused only when their hemoglobin levels fall below 6.0 to 6.5 gm per deciliter or they manifest signs of anemia-related hemodynamic instability or inadequate oxygen delivery [25]. This policy is based on the recognition of the risks of transfusions and physiologic information indicating that anemia in the absence of signs or symptoms of cardiopulmonary distress or evidence of inadequate oxygen delivery does not mandate prophylactic blood transfusions [25].

Smoke Inhalation Injury

Burn victims who sustain inhalation injuries represent a group of patients with special problems. The presence of an inhalation injury superimposed on a cutaneous burn significantly increases the mortality rate of these patients, regardless of the size of the burn [26,27]. Moreover, the physiologic effects of an inhalation injury are not limited to the lungs. Patients with inhalation injuries frequently require up to 50 percent more fluid to be resuscitated adequately during the first 24-hour postburn period [28,29]. Thus, it may be necessary to administer fluids at rates up to 6 ml per kilogram per percent burn. Although it is tempting to try to resuscitate these patients with less than their calculated fluid needs to minimize the amount of fluid sequestered in the injured lungs, this is the wrong approach. Recent studies suggest that the amount of lung water is higher in underresuscitated patients than in fully resuscitated patients [29].

Any patient burned in a closed space where smoke can accumulate should be treated as having a smoke-inhalation injury, and supplemental oxygen should be administered. Most patients who have sustained a severe inhalation injury are hoarse and may have difficulty ventilating. The presence of a facial burn, singed nasal hairs, or soot in the airways are signs of a potential inhalation injury. Because the incidence of smoke-inhalation injury is several times higher than previously thought, routine fiberoptic bronchoscopy or xenon ventilation-perfusion scanning should be performed in patients believed to have an inhalation injury [30]. Because there are no ways of accurately predicting the magnitude of the pulmonary injury, early endotracheal intubation and mechanical ventilation with positive end-expiratory pressure should be considered at the first sign of respiratory distress [31].

The presence of an endotracheal tube stents the partially patient airway and prevents the development of complete airway occlusion as progressive edema of the hypopharynx develops. These patients should be intubated with the largest endotracheal tube possible to allow optimal pulmonary toilet and diagnostic and therapeutic bronchoscopy. In the absence of bronchoscopically verified lower airway injury, most patients can be safely extubated 3 or 4 days postburn when the upper airway edema has resolved. In contrast, patients with smoke inhalation injuries of their lower airways frequently require prolonged periods of intubation. Patients with lower airway injuries should routinely receive humidified air to prevent drying of secretions as well as frequent pulmonary toilet to prevent atelectasis and the subsequent development of pneumonia. Positive end-expiratory pressure (PEEP) is also a critical part of the respiratory regimen, because in the absence of adequate levels of PEEP, alveolar collapse will almost certainly occur [31]. A minority of patients require systemic bronchodilator therapy because of smoke-induced irritation of the airways causing bronchospasm. In the past, some clinicians have recommended the prophylactic use of steroids to prevent pulmonary damage in patients with documented lower airway smoke inhalation injuries. However, it is now clear that steroid therapy is not beneficial in these patients. In fact, in a randomized study on the use of steroid therapy in burned children with inhalation injury, the mortality rate of children receiving steroids was more than four times higher (56%) than that of children not receiving steroids (13%) [32]. Because the incidence of systemic infections in the steroid-treated patients was three times higher than the non-steroid–treated group, the increased mortality rate associated with the use of steroids appears to be attributable to its immunosuppressive effects. Similar deleterious effects of steroids on survival have been documented in adults [33].

Recently, because it has become increasingly recognized that high levels of peak inspiratory pressure (PIP) as well as as high levels of PEEP may result in significant barotrauma, new ventilatory strategies have been employed to keep PIP levels less than 40 cm H_2O in patients with thermal injuries [34]. These options include variations of jet ventilation and most recently pressure-controlled inverse ratio ventilation.

Metabolic and Nutritional Considerations

The hypermetabolic response that occurs after a thermal injury is greater than that observed after any other form of trauma or during severe sepsis [35]. The magnitude and duration of the hypermetabolic response parallels the severity of the burn injury and reaches a maximum when the burn size reaches 60 percent TBSA [35]. This hypermetabolic state is associated with increased heat production and a 2° to 3°F increase in core temperature attributable to a resetting of the hypothalmic temperature set point. Several factors have been implicated in the cause of the increased metabolic response after thermal injury. These factors include (1) wound-generated mediators, such as interleukin-1, tumor necrosis factor, prostanoids, and oxygen-free radicals and their products [36]; (2) hormonal mediators, especially the counter-regulatory hormones, catecholamines, cortisol, and glucagon [37,38]; (3) evaporative water loss from the burn wound [39]; and (4) the escape of bacteria or their products (endotoxin) from the burn wound [40] or intestine [41,42]. The recently emerging concept that endotoxemia is the trigger for the hypermetabolic response is attractive, because endotoxin induces fever by the same hypothalmic mechanisms as a thermal injury. In addition, the hormonal and cytokine changes observed during endotoxemia are very similar to those observed after thermal injury. Regardless of the cause, it has been documented that total energy expenditure can be reduced by maintaining the patient in a more thermoneutral environment (ambient temperature 30°C or higher) [43]. Thus, patients should be treated in a warm environment (30°C).

Metabolically, a major thermal injury is characterized by increased skeletal muscle proteolysis, lipolysis, and gluconeogenesis [33]. The amino acids released from the skeletal muscle are shunted to the liver, where they are used in gluconeogenesis and the synthesis of acute phase reactants. The newly synthesized glucose is shunted to the burn wound, where it is anaerobically metabolized to lactate. The wound-generated lactate is then shunted back to the liver, where it is converted back to glucose (Cori cycle) [44]. The energy for these metabolic processes is derived largely from fat oxidation.

Because the burn patient is hypermetabolic and severely catabolic, massive weight and nitrogen losses occur unless adequate exogenous calories and protein are administered. Failure to meet the metabolic needs of the burn patient results in muscle wasting, decreased immunologic reserve, and impaired wound healing. Monitoring of the nutritional status of the burn victim is difficult, because traditional serum (i.e., albumin or transferrin) and immunologic (i.e., skin test reactivity or total lymphocyte count) markers of nutritional status are all directly altered by the burn injury and thus are not accurate predictors of the patient's nutritional status. Similarly, daily weights and nitrogen balance studies are fraught with error in these patients. Daily weights are frequently inaccurate because of the presence of dressings and the occurrence of fluid shifts, whereas nitrogen balance studies are confounded by the fact that large amounts of protein are lost through the burn wound. Thus, the best method of monitoring the nutritional status of the burn victim is by monitoring the daily administration of calories and protein.

Although there is some controversy over the optimal nutritional regimen for the burn victim, many points are clear. First, these patients require both increased amounts of calories and protein, and because the burn wound is an obligate glucose consumer, at least 50 to 60 percent of the calories administered must be carbohydrate calories. The increased requirements for glucose is reflected in the finding that blood flow to the burn wound is tenfold higher than that to an equivalent area of uninjured skin [45]. Secondly, it is clear that patients administered a high-protein diet (calorie-to-nitrogen ratio of 100:1) have an improved survival over patients receiving a more standard diet (protein-to-calorie ratio 150:1), especially when at least some of the nutrient mix is administered enterally [46]. Our approach to the nutritional support of the adult burn patient is outlined in Table 179-2. Essentially, we compute the patient's basal energy needs with the Harris-Benedict equation [47] and use a combination of enteral and parenteral nutrition to meet these nutritional needs. As GI function returns, we increase the amount of nutritional support administered through the gut. Although glucose is the major energetic substrate administered, it is important not to exceed the patient's ability to metabolize the administered glucose. Studies by Burke

Table 179-2. Nutritional Requirements in Adult Burn Patients

Basal energy expenditure (BEE)			
Male: BEE = 66 (13.7 × Wt) + (5 × Ht) − (6.8 × A) Wt = Weight (kg)			
Ht = Height (cm)			
Female: BEE = 655 + (9.6 × Wt) + (1.9 × Ht) − (4.7 × A) A = Age (yr)			

Postburn alterations			
Burn category	BEE	Protein (gm/kg)	Carbohydrate
Moderate burn (15–30% TBSA)	1.5 × Normal	1.5	1.5–2 × Normal
Major burn (31–45% TBSA)	1.5–1.8 × Normal	1.5–2.0	2–2.5 × Normal
Massive burn (> 46% TBSA)	1.8–2.2 × Normal	2.0–2.3	3 × Normal

Massive burn

Example 70-kg man = 1750 cal × 2 BEE = 3500 cal
Protein: 140–210 gm protein = 560 − 840 cal
Carbohydrate: 500 gm glucose = 2000 cal
Fat: Remainder as enteral feeding
(Never exceed 20–25% of total calories with fat)

et al. [48] clearly indicate that the maximal amount of glucose that can be metabolized is 5 to 7 mg/kg/min (this represents 1800–2200 cal/day). If the amount of glucose administered exceeds this level, several problems generally occur. These problems include glucose intolerance, increased carbon dioxide production, increased fat synthesis, and the development of a fatty liver. Because fat synthesis is an energy-requiring process, overfeeding glucose is energetically inefficient. Because early wound closure does not immediately reverse the increased metabolic rate to normal, as was once hoped [49], nutritional support must continue throughout the patient's hospital course (see Chaps. 200–202).

Infection and Immunity, Including Burn Wound Sepsis

Once the patient has been successfully resuscitated, the major threat to survival is infection, and sepsis remains the major cause of death in patients with adequate physiologic reserve to survive the acute resuscitative phase of burn injury [50]. Most bacterial infections are caused by organisms that are already colonizing the patient, some of which are hospital acquired. These infections tend to originate at sites of mucosal damage, ciliary dysfunction, or integumentary damage. Because the local mechanical defenses of the skin and the respiratory tract are most frequently injured in the burn victim, it is not surprising that the lungs and the burn wound are the most frequent foci of fatal infection. However, many therapeutic maneuvers, such as the use of intravenous catheters, Swan-Ganz catheters, Foley catheters, or endotracheal tubes, facilitate bacterial penetration across mechanical barriers and thus potentially predispose the burn victim to an increased risk of infection. Even though urinary tract and intravenous line infections are relatively common in these patients, they are rarely fatal if diagnosed early. Burn wound sepsis and pneumonia are the most frequent causes of lethal infections in the burn victim [51,52] and therefore are discussed individually.

Although the originating site or focus of infection can be identified in most patients, in an increasing number of patients with bacteremia a source of infection is never identified [51,52]. On the basis of experimental studies, it appears that the intestine may serve as a primary reservoir for life-threatening infections after thermal injury [53,54]. The process by which bacteria escape from the GI tract to infect systemic organs and tissues has been termed "bacterial translocation" [42,53]. We have documented that bacterial translocation can be induced in one of three general ways: (1) by disrupting the ecology of the normal GI microflora, resulting in overgrowth with certain gram-negative, enteric bacilli, (2) by impairing host immune defenses, or (3) by physically disrupting the gut mucosal barrier [42]. It is hoped that, as more attention is directed toward preserving intestinal barrier function, the risk of gut-derived septic states will be reduced.

Multiple organ system failure is being recognized as a leading cause of death in these patients. Although infection is the primary initiator of the hyperdynamic state and subsequent multiple organ failure, it now appears that devitalized tissues (uncontrolled inflammatory response) can also initiate and perpetuate a mediator-induced response that may lead to organ failure in the absence of bacteremia or the presence of an identifiable focus of infection [55]. Burn-induced failure of intestinal mucosal barrier function leading to systemic endotoxemia [56] or the postburn liberation of cytokines or other immunoinflammatory mediators may help explain why circulating bacteria cannot be detected in a large number of burned patients who die of what appears to be sepsis [42,57].

BURN WOUND SEPSIS. Burn victims develop multiple defects in their immune system that predispose them to an increased risk of infection [50,58]. These include alterations in immunoglobulin levels, changes in the concentrations and activities of components of both the classical and alternate complement pathways, reduced circulating plasma fibronectin levels, depressed serum opsonic activity, and impairment of lymphocyte, neutrophil, and reticuloendothelial system activity [50]. These acquired defects in systemic antibacterial host defenses plus local failure of the immune system at the burn wound [59] result in the burn victim becoming profoundly immunocompromised. This immunocompromised state in combination with loss of the normal barrier function of the skin results in the burn patient being uniquely susceptible to infections originating from bacteria colonizing the burn wound. Thus, much attention has focused on the use of topical antimicrobial agents, such as silver sulfadiazine or Sulfamylon, local wound care, and strict infection control practices to reduce the incidence of burn wound sepsis by preventing or limiting the extent of colonization of the burn wound by potential pathogens [60,61].

Although excellent wound care reduces the incidence of burn wound sepsis, it does not totally eliminate them. Because the local signs of burn wound infection may be subtle, these early signs are frequently not appreciated until the patient has developed obvious signs of systemic sepsis. Therefore, the development of any of the local wound signs listed in Table 179-3 should alert one to the possibility that the burn wound has become infected. At the first indication of burn wound infection, biopsies should be done of the suspicious areas for histologic and bacteriologic analysis to confirm or refute the diagnosis of burn wound infection and to identify the infecting microorganism [62]. One common mistake that must be avoided is the unnecessary use of systemic antibiotics in patients who are not infected, because the systemic administration of broad-spectrum antibiotics can result in the emergence of antibiotic-resistant bacteria. Yet, because of the potentially lethal nature of burn wound sepsis, it is not always appropriate to wait for bacteriologic confirmation of infection before the administration of antibiotics. This dilemma is compounded by the fact

Table 179-3. Burn Wound Sepsis: Signs and Diagnosis

Signs of burn wound sepsis
Focal or diffuse areas of discoloration (black, brown, or violet)
Presence of purulent fluid draining from the eschar
Signs of cellulitis (edema and erythema) at unburned margins of the burn wound
Too rapid eschar separation

Diagnosis of burn wound sepsis
Clinical criteria
Change in sensorium
Development of ileus
Change in appearance of burn wounds
Laboratory criteria
Development of glucose intolerance
Burn wound biopsy evidence of infection
Positive blood cultures
Fever and leukocytosis are not reliable indicators of infection

that, because a burn injury is associated with extensive tissue injury, fever and leukocytosis are present in most patients even in the absence of infection. For these reasons, clinical judgment plays a major role in the treatment of these patients. Table 179-3 lists the most reliable clinical and laboratory indicators of burn wound sepsis [50,60,61]. Patients clinically thought to be infected are treated with a short course of antibiotics while awaiting the results of bacteriologic tests. The choice of which antibiotics to use initially is primarily based on the results of surveillance cultures of the burn wounds or knowledge of the microbial flora of the unit. However, antibiotic choice must be modified to fit the individual patient.

Although antibiotics may be effective in the eradication of infections originating in partial thickness burns, in most cases of burn wound sepsis, antibiotics play only a supportive role. To control the infection, the infected tissue must be surgically excised. Details of the various surgical procedures used to excise and graft the burn wound are beyond the scope of this chapter [63,64]. However, it is important to realize that these operations are hemodynamically stressful and are associated with major blood loss (up to 100 ml of blood per percent body excised and grafted). Therefore, before undertaking a major excision, it is critical to verify that the patient is in the best hemodynamic status possible. In the septic burn patient requiring emergency surgery, the frequent presence of peripheral edema and sinus tachycardia makes an accurate assessment of volume status by physical diagnosis difficult. Because peripheral vasodilatation manifested as low systemic vascular resistance is common, fluids may be required even in the grossly edematious patient. Once the patient has been hemodynamically stabilized, total surgical excision of the infected burn wound is performed when the infected area is less than 15 to 20 percent of the total body surface. However, if larger areas are involved, then staged operative procedures are performed separated by a period of 1 to 3 days. Because it is clearly better to prevent burn wound sepsis than to treat it, many burn centers have adopted a policy of early burn wound excision and grafting beginning within a few days of admission [15,65]. The goal of early burn wound excision and grafting is to remove the burn wound before the occurrence of infection as well as to shorten the hospital course.

PNEUMONIA. Pneumonia is emerging as a more frequent cause of infectious death in burn victims as the incidence of burn wound sepsis decreases [26,27,51,52]. There are many reasons why the burn victim, even in the absence of an inhalation injury, is predisposed to the development of pneumonia. These include the fact that burn victims are profoundly immunosuppressed, have a poor cough because of skeketal muscle wasting, and require frequent operations under general anesthesia. The presence of an inhalation injury further increases the risk of pneumonia by directly damaging the lung parenchyma and impairing the normal ciliary action of the tracheobronchial mucosa. Pneumonias also can be hematogenous and secondary to contaminated IV lines or the burn wound. There also appears to be a relationship between the incidence of hematogenous pneumonias and the magnitude of the cutaneous burn. This association was verified in a recent study by Shirani et al. [26] documenting that the incidence of pneumonia increased with increasing burn size.

The prophylactic use of antibiotics to prevent pneumonia in high-risk burn victims has not been effective and may be dangerous because of the emergence of antibiotic-resistant bacteria [66]. Pneumonias occurring within the first 3 days postburn are generally caused by penicillin-resistant *Staphylococcus*, whereas those occurring later are most commonly attributable to gram-negative, enteric bacilli or *Pseudomonas*. Knowledge of the most likely causative organism is critical in choosing the appropriate empiric antimicrobial regimen while awaiting culture results. The best way to prevent pneumonias is through the combination of good aseptic technique and maneuvers to minimize bacterial contamination of the lower airways. This is especially true during the operative and postoperative periods when the patient is intubated and his or her mechanical defenses are compromised. Other therapies directed toward the prevention of pneumonia include ambulation and physical therapy to prevent atelectasis, respiratory therapy and bronchodilators to improve pulmonary toilet and help in the clearance of secretions, and aggressive nutritional therapy to supply adequate protein and energy to help the patient maintain a good cough. In the intubated patient, there is evidence that the risk of developing pneumonia can be reduced by using sucralfate rather than antacids or H_2 blockers, such as cimetidine, for stress ulcer prophylaxis [42,67].

Once pneumonia has developed, therapeutic options are limited. Treatment includes respiratory support, including mechanical ventilation when necessary, pulmonary toilet, bronchodilators in patients with chronic lung disease, nutritional support, and antibiotics. To limit the emergence of antibiotic-resistant strains of bacteria, we treat our patients with as short a course of antibiotics as possible. Antibiotics can be discontinued after 5 to 7 days in most patients who respond to treatment. A more difficult question is what to do in patients who are not responding to maximal medical therapy. If pulmonary toilet is not adequate, then endotracheal intubation and mechanical ventilation are mandatory. In patients who are already intubated, tracheostomy may be required. In some patients, it is not clear whether the primary infection has originated in the lungs or in the burn wound. In this situation, surgical excision of the burn wound may be necessary, even though the risk of surgery and anesthesia are increased. There are no easy answers to this clinical problem.

Future Directions and Summary

Improvement in the care of the burn victim must await further advances in several fields, including a better understanding of wound healing, host immune defenses, the stress response, cardiovascular physiology, and metabolism. For example, further study of host immune defenses is required because, in spite of the development of successive generations of more powerful antibiotics, sepsis remains a common cause of death in the burn patient. This is not surprising, because it is of little importance which organism is causing the infection if the patient's intrinsic antibacterial defenses cannot respond. Only by paying attention to both the host and the pathogen will we be able to reduce the risk of infection. Thus, our therapeutic maneuvers must be directed not only toward eradication of the invading bacteria, but also at strategies to increase the host's resistance to infection. For example, by debriding necrotic tissue (policy of early burn wound excision) and controlling bacterial contamination (aseptic technique and topical antimicrobial agents), it is possible not only to remove the milieu in which bacteria multiply, but also to improve the delivery of host resistance factors to the burn wound [50]. Another area of importance is the judicious use of oral and systemic antibiotics to reduce the incidence of antibiotic-resistant bacterial and fungal overgrowth in the GI tract and other areas.

Because most of the abnormalities of host defenses documented in the burn victim can be caused by protein-calorie malnutrition, aggressive nutritional support, especially by the enteral route, is mandatory. In fact, recognition that an exaggerated cytokine-mediated inflammatory response not only may lead to organ injury but may mediate (potentiate) the hypermetabolic response has resulted in clinical studies investigating the cytokine response to burn injury. Although to some extent the results of these studies are confusing and in some cases contradictory, as a whole they do indicate that certain cytokine patterns are of prognostic importance. For example, persistent elevations in IL-6 levels were associated with increased mortality in one study [68], whereas the inability to maintain elevated IL-1β levels was a poor prognostic sign in a second study [69]. Interestingly, the administration of physiologic amounts of cytokines, such as interleukin-1, interleukin-2, tumor necrosis factor, and the family of colony stimulating factors as immunoadjuvants to bolster host defenses has improved survival in burned or shocked rodents subjected to an infectious challenge [70,71,72].

Work continues on techniques to aid in closure of the burn wound, because by closing the burn wound, evaporative water and heat loss through the burn wound are reduced, the hypermetabolic response begins to return to normal, and resistance to burn wound infection is increased. Therefore, much effort has been directed toward the development of temporary or permanent skin substitutes [73]. Some of the most promising approaches that have been tested clinically are the use of cultured cadaver skin allografts [74], cultured epithelial autografts [75], artificial dermis [76], or a composite graft composed of cultured autologous keratinocytes and fibroblasts attached to a collagen-glycosaminoglycan substrate [77] to achieve wound closure.

References

1. *Reports on the Epidemiology and Surveillance of Injuries.* U.S. Dept. of Health, Education, and Welfare publication No. (HSM) 73-10001, Atlanta, Centers for Disease Control, 1982.
2. Feller I, Tholen D, Cornell RG: Improvement in burn care, 1965 to 1979. *JAMA* 244:2074, 1980.
3. Herndon DN, Curreri PW, Abston S, et al: Treatment of burns. *Curr Probl Surg* 24:341, 1987.
4. *Accident facts.* Chicago, National Safety Council, 1983.
5. Zawacki BE, Azen SP, Impus SH, et al: Multifactorial probit analysis of mortality in burned patients. *Ann Surg* 189:1, 1979.
6. Harms BA, Bodai BI, Smith M, et al: Prostaglandin release and altered microvascular integrity after burn injury. *J Surg Res* 31:274, 1981.
7. Carvajal HF, Brouhard BH, Linares HA: Effect of antihistamine-antiserotonin and ganglionic blocking agents upon increased capillary permeability following burn trauma. *J Trauma* 15:969, 1975.
8. Saez JC, Ward PH, Gunther B, et al: Superoxide radical involvement in the pathogenesis of burn shock. *Circ Shock* 12:229, 1984.
9. Baxter CR: Fluid volume and electrolyte changes in the early postburn period. *Clin Plast Surg* 1:693, 1974.
10. Demling RH, Kramer G, Harms B: Role of thermal injury-induced hypoproteinemia on fluid flux and protein permeability in burned and non-burned tissue. *Surgery* 95:136, 1984.
11. Baxter CR, Shires GT: Physiological response to crystalloid resuscitation of severe burns. *Ann NY Acad Sci* 150:874, 1968.
12. Mason AD Jr: The mathematics of resuscitation: 1980 presidential address, American Burn Association. *J Trauma* 20:1015, 1980.
13. Mangalore P, Hunt TK: Effect of varying oxygen tension on healing of open wounds. *Surg Gynecol Obstet* 135:756, 1972.
14. Remensnyder TP: Topography of tissue oxygen tension changes in acute burn edema. *Arch Surg* 105:477, 1972.
15. Deitch EA. A policy of early excision and grafting in elderly burn patients shortens the hospital stay and improves survival. *Burns* 12:109, 1985.

16. Pruitt BA Jr: Advances in fluid theory and the early care of the burn patient. *World J Surg* 2:139, 1978.
17. Aikawa N, Ishikari K, Naito C, et al: Individualized fluid resuscitation based on hemodynamic monitoring in the management of extensive burns. *Burns* 8:249, 1982.
18. Agarwal N, Petro J, Salisbury RE: Physiologic profile monitoring in burned patients. *J Trauma* 23:577, 1983.
19. Ehrie M, Morgan A, Moore FD, et al: Endocarditis with the indwelling balloon tipped pulmonary artery catheter in burn patients. *J Trauma* 18:664, 1978.
20. Burke JF: Fluid therapy to reduce morbidity. *J Trauma* 19:865, 1979.
21. Goodwin CW, Dorethy J, Lam V, Pruitt BA Jr: Randomized trial of efficacy of crystalloid and colloid resuscitation on hemodynamic response and lung water following thermal injury. *Ann Surg* 197:520, 1983.
22. Youn YK, LaLonde C, Demling R: Use of antioxidant therapy in shock and trauma. *Circ Shock* 35:245, 1991.
23. Dickson PW, Bannister D, Schreiber G: Minor burns lead to major changes in synthesis rates of plasma proteins in the liver. *J Trauma* 27:283, 1987.
24. Loebl EC, Marvin JA, Curreri W, et al: Erythrocyte survival following thermal injury. *J Surg Res* 16:96, 1974.
25. Deitch EA, Sittig KM: A serial study of the erythropoietic response to thermal injury. *Ann Surg* 217:293, 1993.
26. Shirani KZ, Pruitt BA, Mason AD: The influence of inhalation injury and pneumonia on burn mortality. *Ann Surg* 205:92, 1987.
27. Thompson PB, Herndon DN, Traber DL, et al: Effect on mortality of inhalation injury. *J Trauma* 26:163, 1986.
28. Navar PD, Saffle JR, Warden GD: Effect of inhalation injury on fluid resuscitation requirements after thermal injury. *Am J Surg* 150:716, 1985.
29. Herndon DN, Traber DL, Traber LD: The effect of resuscitation on inhalation injury. *Surgery* 100:248, 1986.
30. Moylan JA: Smoke inhalation: Diagnostic techniques and steroids. *J Trauma* 19:917, 1979.
31. Venus B, Matsuda T, Copiozo JB, et al: Prophylactic intubation and continuous positive airway pressure in the management of inhalation injury in burn victims. *Crit Care Med* 9:519, 1981.
32. Moylan JA, Alexander LC Jr: Diagnosis and treatment of inhalation injury. *World J Surg* 2:185, 1978.
33. Levine BA, Petroff PA, Slade LC, et al: Prospective trials of dexamethasone and aerosolized gentamycin in the treatment of inhalation injury in the burned patient. *J Trauma* 18:188, 1978.
34. Rodelberg DA, Maschinot NE, Housinger TA, et al: Decreased pulmonary barotrauma with the use of volumetric diffusive respiration in pediatric patients with burns. *J Burn Care Rehabil* 13:506, 1992.
35. Wilmore DW, Aulick LH: Metabolic changes in burned patients. *Surg Clin North Am* 58:1173, 1978.
36. Herndon D: Mediators of metabolism. *J Trauma* 21:701, 1981.
37. Wilmore DW, Long JM, Mason AD Jr, et al: Catecholamines: Mediator of the hypermetabolic response to thermal injury. *Ann Surg* 180:653, 1974.
38. Bessey PQ, Watters JM, Aoke TT, et al: Combined hormonal infusion simulates the metabolic response to injury. *Ann Surg* 200:264, 1984.
39. Caldwell FT Jr, Bowser BH, Crabtree JH: The effect of occlusive dressings on the energy metabolism of severely burned children. *Ann Surg* 193:579, 1981.
40. Aulick LH, Wroczyski FA, Coil JA, et al: Metabolic and thermoregulatory responses to burn wound colonization. *J Trauma* 29:478, 1989.
41. Mochizuki H, Trocki O, Dominioni L, et al: Mechanism of prevention of postburn hypermetabolism and catabolism by early enteral feeding. *Ann Surg* 200:297, 1984.
42. Deitch EA: Does the gut protect us or injure us when ill in the ICU, in Cerra F (ed): *Perspectives in Critical Care.* St. Louis, Quality Medical Publishers, 1988.
43. Wilmore DW, Mason AD Jr, Johnson DW, et al: Effect of ambient temperture on heat production and heat loss in burn patients. *J Appl Physiol* 38:593, 1975.
44. Wolfe RR, Durkot MJ, Allsop JR, et al: Glucose metabolism in severely burned patients. *Metabolism* 28:1031, 1979.
45. Wilmore DW, Aulick LH, Mason AD Jr, et al: Influence of the burn wound on local and systemic responses to injury. *Ann Surg* 186:444, 1977.

46. Alexander JW, MacMillan BG, Stinnett JD, et al: Beneficial effects of aggressive protein feeding in severely burned children. *Ann Surg* 192:505, 1980.

47. Harris J, Benedict F: *A Biometric Study of Basal Metabolism in Man.* Washington, DC, Carnegie Institute, 1919.

48. Burke JF, Wolfe RR, Mullany CS, et al: Glucose requirements following burn injury. *Ann Surg* 190:274, 1979.

49. Rutan TC, Herndon DN, van Osten T, et al: Metabolic rate alterations in early excision and grafting versus conservative treatment. *J Trauma* 26:140, 1986.

50. Deitch EA: Infection in the compromised host. *Surg Clin North Am* 68:181, 1988.

51. Sittig K, Deitch EA: Effects of bacteremia on mortality after thermal injury. *Arch Surg* 123:1367, 1988.

52. Mason AD Jr, McManus AT, Pruitt BA Jr: Association of burn mortality and bacteremia. *Arch Surg* 121:1027, 1986.

53. Deitch EA, Maejima K, Berg RD: Effect of oral antibiotics and bacterial overgrowth on the translocation of the GI-Tract microflora in burned rats. *J Trauma* 25:385, 1985.

54. Deitch EA, Berg R: Endotoxin but not malnutrition promotes bacterial translocation from the gut in burned mice. *J Trauma* 27:161, 1987.

55. Deitch EA: Multiple organ failure: Pathophysiology and potential future therapy. *Ann Surg* 216:117, 1992.

56. Deitch EA, Ma L, Ma JW, et al: Inhibition of endotoxin-induced bacterial translocation in mice. *J Clin Invest* 84:36, 1989.

57. Aikawa N, Shinozawa Y, Ishibiki K, et al: Clinical analysis of multiple organ failure in burned patients. *Burns* 13:103, 1987.

58. Deitch EA, Gelder F, McDonald JC: Sequential prospective analysis of the nonspecific host defense system after thermal injury. *Arch Surg* 119:83, 1984.

59. Deitch EA, Bridges RM, McDonald JC, Dobke M: Burn wound sepsis may be promoted by a failure of local immunity. *Ann Surg* 206:340, 1987.

60. Harnar TJ, Canizaro PC: Controlling infection in major burns. *Infections in Surgery* 14:31, 1984.

61. Hansbrough JF: Burn wound sepsis. *J Intensive Care Med* 2:313, 1987.

62. Pruitt BA Jr, Foley FD: The use of biopsies in burn patient care. *Surgery* 73:887, 1973.

63. Janzekovic Z: A new concept in the early excision and immediate grafting of burns. *J Trauma* 10:1103, 1970.

64. Deitch EA: Prospective study of the effect of the recipient bed on skin graft survival after thermal injury. *J Trauma* 25:118, 1985.

65. Gray DT, Pine PW, Harnar JT, et al: Early surgical excision vs. conventional therapy in patients with 20 to 40 per cent burns: A comparative study. *Am J Surg* 144:76, 1982.

66. Herndon DN, Thompson PB, Traber DL: Pulmonary injury in burned patients. *Crit Care Clin* 1:79, 1985.

67. Craven DE, Kunches LM, Kilinsky V, et al: Risk factors for pneumonia and fatality in patients receiving continuous mechanical ventilation. *Am Rev Respir Dis* 133:792, 1986.

68. Schluter B, Konig B, Bergmann U, et al: Interleukin 6—A potential mediator of lethal sepsis after major thermal trauma: evidence for increased IL-6 production by peripheral blood mononuclear cells. *J Trauma* 31:1663, 1991.

69. Cannon JG, Friedberg JS, Gelfand JA et al: Circulating interleukin-1β and tumor necrosis factor-α concentrations after burn injury in humans. *Crit Care Med* 20:1414, 1992.

70. Livingston DH, Malangoni MA, Sonnenfeld G: Immune enhancement by tumor necrosis factor-alpha improves antibiotic efficacy after hemorrhagic shock. *J Trauma* 29:967, 1989.

71. Silver GM, Gamelli RL, O'Reilly M: The beneficial effect of granulocyte colony-stimulating factor (G-CSF) in combination with gentamicin on survival after Pseudomonas burn wound infection. *Surgery* 106:452, 1989.

72. O'Riordain MG, Collins KH, Pilz M, et al: Modulation of macrophage hyperactivity improves survival in a burn-sepsis model. *Arch Surg* 127:152, 1992.

73. Pruitt BA Jr, Levine NS: Characteristics and uses of biologic dressings and skin substitutes. *Arch Surg* 119:312, 1984.

74. Madden MR, Finkelstein JL, Staiano-Coico L, et al: Grafting of cultured allogeneic epidermis on second- and third-degree burn wounds on 26 patients. *J Trauma* 26:955, 1986.

75. Odessey R: Multicenter experience with cultured epidermal autograft for treatment of burns. *J Burn Care Rehabil* 13:174, 1992.

76. Heimbach D, Luterman A, Burke J, et al: Artificial dermis for major burns: A multi-center randomized clinical trial. *Ann Surg* 208:313, 1988.

77. Hansbrough JF, Boyce ST, Cooper ML, et al: Burn wound closure with cultured autologous keratinocytes and fibroblasts attached to a collagen-glycosaminoglycan substrate. *JAMA* 262:2125, 1989.

180. Compartment Syndromes

Michael J. Rohrer

Elevated compartment pressure involving an extremity is rarely an immediate threat to survival. Nevertheless, this problem must be recognized promptly and treated properly to maximize the likelihood of salvaging a useful, sensate limb. When neglected, untreated compartment syndrome can rapidly lead to life-threatening complications secondary to the systemic effects of extensive muscle necrosis.

Definition

The muscles of the extremities are divided into distinct groups or "compartments," each having its own nerve and blood supply. These muscular compartments are delineated by a tough layer of noncompliant fascia. A "compartment syndrome" oc-

curs when increased interstitial pressure within a myofascial compartment compromises capillary perfusion and hence neuromuscular function [1–5]. In theory, elevated compartmental pressure can result from a reduction in the size of the compartment, such as after repair of a fascial hernia [1]. In practice, however, compartment syndromes are almost always caused by an increase in the volume of the tissue in the compartment as a result of edema caused by mechanical or ischemic injury. The fascial covering of the compartment is usually the limiting factor preventing the edematous tissues from swelling, although in some instances the skin or externally applied bandages or casts are the constricting layer [6].

Compartment syndromes can present as both acute and chronic conditions. Chronic compartment syndromes are not limb threatening and are most commonly seen secondary to muscle hypertrophy in highly conditioned athletes who present with exercise-induced extremity pain that is relieved by rest

[6,7,8]. Acute compartment syndromes are limb- and life-threatening conditions that are common in the critical care setting and are the focus of this discussion.

Pathophysiology

The clinical events that may precipitate an acute compartment syndrome are numerous, but the common mechanism in each case involves an elevation of the pressure within the extremity muscular compartments leading to impaired perfusion of the tissues within that compartment. The resulting neuronal and muscular ischemia is responsible for the symptoms of pain and weakness that are the hallmarks of the early symptom complex [9]. Usually swelling within a compartment is caused by interstitial edema fluid, although compartmental hypertension also can be caused by bleeding and hematoma formation [10,11].

Normal precapillary and postcapillary microvascular blood pressures are approximately 25 and 16 mm Hg, respectively [12]. The resulting 9 mm Hg pressure gradient across the capillary bed is the driving force responsible for maintaining perfusion. Despite being flaccid conduits, the postcapillary venules and veins ordinarily remain patent because normal compartmental (interstitial) pressures are close to zero [13], and hence, intraluminal venous hydrostatic pressure exceeds interstitial hydrostatic pressure [14,15,16]. However, as interstitial hydrostatic pressure increases, transmural distending pressure decreases and ultimately leads to partial or complete microvascular venous obstruction. Continued arterial inflow with impaired venous outflow changes the Starling forces (see Chap. 170) within the capillary, favoring the transudation of fluid and the further elevation of compartmental pressure. Thus, a vicious cycle is created that progressively compromises microvascular perfusion. Complete cessation of tissue perfusion in the extremities has been documented to occur when compartmental pressure exceeds 64 mm Hg in the forearm and is as low as 35 mm Hg in the calf [17], well below the average diastolic blood pressure. Therefore, compartmental ischemia and cell death can occur even if distal pulses remain palpable [18,19].

Recent studies using magnetic resonance spectroscopy have improved our understanding of the relationship between compartment pressure and oxidative metabolism within muscles [20]. Data from these studies suggest that the threshold for the onset of anaerobic metabolism is defined not by the absolute value of the tissue pressure within the compartment but by the gradient between mean arterial pressure and compartmental pressure. Anaerobic metabolism ensues when this gradient is less than 30 mm Hg in normal muscle or less than 40 mm Hg in traumatized muscle.

In experimental models, ischemic neuronal dysfunction is evident after as little as 15 minutes of limb compression [21]. If recognized and treated early, the ischemic changes are entirely reversible. Prolonged compartmental hypertension, however, inevitably leads to cell death. Intracellular ions and proteins, such as potassium and myoglobin, are released after as few as 4 hours of ischemia [22]. Irreversible damage to nerves and muscles generally occurs after 12 hours of inadequate perfusion [11].

Ischemia-induced cellular injury occurs during periods of both hypoperfusion and reperfusion. Indeed, several studies suggest that reperfusion-mediated events are the major component contributing to muscular injury [23,24]. Injury during the reperfusion phase is mediated by reactive oxygen species [25] (see Chap. 156). Adenosine triphosphate (ATP) is normally metabolized to adenosine diphosphate (ADP) and adenosine monophosphate (AMP). During periods of ischemia, insuffi-

cient oxygen is available to regenerate ATP through oxidative phosphorylation, and intracellular AMP concentrations increase. AMP is then further degraded to adenosine, inosine, and hypoxanthine. In addition to promoting the degradation of nucleotides, ischemia also leads to conversion of the enzyme purine dehydrogenase to another enzyme, xanthine oxidase, that catalyzes the metabolism of hypoxanthine to xanthine, and xanthine to uric acid. The two reactions catalyzed by xanthine oxidase result in the production of reactive oxygen species ("free radicals") that are capable of damaging cell membranes and intracellular constituents such a proteins and nucleic acids [26]. Reperfusion-mediated cellular injury can lead to further edema and compartmental hypertension.

Compartment syndromes occur most commonly in the leg and are rare in the thigh, buttock, arm, or forearm [27]. There are several reasons for this. First, acute vascular insufficiency is relatively common in the arteries supplying the compartments of the leg. Second, compartmental hypertension is common after tibial fractures and crush injuries to the leg. Third, the fascial compartments of the leg are small and noncompliant, and the muscle bulk of the leg is relatively large [27]. The compartments of the thigh are larger and more compliant; therefore, swelling can occur to a greater extent in the thigh before interstitial pressures exceed the critical level that compromises tissue perfusion [10,27].

Clinical Presentation

Numerous clinical events can precipitate an acute compartment syndrome (Table 180-1). Most compartment syndromes occur in the leg as a result of tibial fractures or muscle contusion [29] or the reestablishment of perfusion after acute lower-extremity arterial occlusion [30]. Other, less common compartment syndromes occur in certain characteristic circumstances. For example, patients obtunded by drug or alcohol intoxication can present with gluteal or thigh compartment syndromes secondary to prolonged muscle compression while unconscious in the sitting position. Crush injuries are common in disasters associated with mass casualties such as earthquakes and explosions in which extremities are injured by heavy debris, and extrication is often prolonged [31]. One should also consider gluteal or thigh compartment syndrome in the differential diagnosis of acute sciatic nerve palsy [32]. Compartment syndromes involving the foot are very unusual but can occur after a crush or ischemic injury. Pedal compartment syndromes present with paresthesias and dysfunction of the intrinsic muscles of the foot manifested by inability to spread the toes [33,34,35].

Compartment syndromes are sometimes iatrogenic. One common precipitating event is the application of circumferential dressings or casts that are too tight [6,35]. Anticoagulation

Table 180-1. Etiologies of Compartment Syndromes

Ischemia
Tibial fractures
Crush injuries
Muscle overuse, forced march [2,27]
Hemorrhage within extremity
Snake bite [2]
MAST trouser application
Dysfunction of automated blood pressure cuff
Dysfunction of intermittent compression boot
Compression dressing, cast
After lithotomy position
After tetany [28]

is commonly implicated as an iatrogenic contributing factor in compartment syndromes caused by bleeding after muscular injuries [11] or blood drawing [6,36,37]. Iatrogenic cases of compartment syndrome have been caused by dysfunction of intermittent compression boots [38] and automated sphygmomanometers [39]. Lower-extremity compartment syndromes have also been caused by the application of pneumatic antishock garments for as short as 140 minutes [12,13,40–43]. Compartment syndromes have also occurred in the calves after prolonged operations in the lithotomy position [9,44] and in the thighs after operations performed on a fracture table [45]. These iatrogenically induced compartment syndromes are often diagnosed late because, in the absence of an obvious traumatic or ischemic event, the index of suspicion for the diagnosis is typically low.

Diagnosis

In the alert patient the diagnosis of compartment syndrome can be made on clinical grounds alone [6,46]. The key findings are pain, tenderness, hypoesthesia, weakness, and tenseness of the affected compartment. The pain is severe, tends to increase over time, and is out of proportion to what would be expected from the clinical situation in the absence of a compartment syndrome. Pain is induced or exacerbated by passive stretch of the muscles within the involved compartment; thus, for example, in a patient with an anterior compartment syndrome in the leg, pain is elicited or increased by passive plantar flexion of the foot. Hypoesthesia is noted in the distribution of the sensory nerves compressed in the involved compartment. In the leg, hypoesthesia in the interdigital cleft between the first and second metatarsals is an early finding that reflects dysfunction of the deep peroneal nerve that traverses the anterior compartment [2,47]. In one study, the earliest sensory abnormality in patients with compartment syndromes was a decreased ability to detect vibratory stimulation at 256 Hz [48]. The muscles in the involved compartment are weak. Finally, the compartment is tense and tender on palpation.

Making the diagnosis of compartment syndrome is much more difficult in the sedated, obtunded, or unconscious patient. Although the examiner can still palpate a tense muscular compartment, key subjective findings, such as pain and hypoesthesia, are absent. Although the assessment of peripheral pulses and capillary refill is an important part of the physical examination, the findings of palpable pulses and good capillary refill do not rule out the possibility of compartment syndrome [1,3]. Pulselessness and pallor are very late findings in compartment syndrome and are indicative of extensive neuromuscular damage [21]. For the same reason, arteriography is not a useful test to establish the diagnosis of compartment syndrome [10].

Thus, an objective, reliable test for confirming the diagnosis of compartment syndrome is needed, particularly when the patient is unable to provide essential subjective data. The two best objective tests are measurement of nerve conduction velocity and measurement of compartmental pressure [1]. The measurement of nerve conduction velocity has the advantage of being a functional test, reflecting the adequacy of compartmental perfusion and neuromuscular function [21]. This test can even document viability of muscle by demonstrating muscular contraction [10]. However, measurement of nerve conduction velocity is performed only by specially trained individuals and requires expert interpretation. Furthermore, it is rarely available on an emergency basis. Finally, a false-positive examination can result from the presence of a nerve injury attributable to causes other than a compartment syndrome [21].

Direct measurement of compartmental pressures is the most practical and widely used objective diagnostic test to document the presence of a compartment syndrome. Several different techniques for measuring compartmental pressure are available, including the slit catheter technique described by Whitesides et al. [19] and various approaches using a central venous pressure manometer. It is faster, more convenient, and more reproducible, however, to measure compartment pressure electronically using a strain-gauge transducer-amplifier analogous to those routinely employed in the intensive care unit to monitor intraarterial pressure [49,50]. The pressure transducer and noncompliant tubing assembly can be attached to a 20-gauge needle, taking care to flush air from the system. The skin is sterilely prepared over the relevant compartment, and local anesthesia can be obtained by injecting lidocaine intradermally and subcutaneously at the proposed needle insertion site. Once the needle has been inserted into the compartment, numerical pressure readings are obtained from the digital monitor. If an oscilloscope display is available, it is possible to assess the effect of passive leg movement and manual compression on compartmental pressure. Using this technique, it is a simple matter to document the compartment pressures in all four compartments of the leg in a matter of minutes. Moreover, the process can be repeated as frequently as is clinically indicated.

Although the measurement of compartment pressures is straightforward, interpretation of the values derived is more controversial. All authorities agree that patients with compartment pressures below 30 mm Hg are unlikely to sustain any pressure-related neuromuscular injury [6,18,51,52]. Mubarak et al. [47] recommend that fasciotomy be performed when compartment pressures exceed 30 to 35 mm Hg in a normally perfused patient, whereas Patman and others recommend fasciotomy when compartment pressures exceed 40 mm Hg [18,51,52]. Matsen et al. [18] noted that patients with compartment pressures that remain below 50 mm Hg usually sustain no neuromuscular deficit, but those with interstitial pressures greater than 60 mm Hg consistently develop evidence of neuromuscular dysfunction.

As previously noted, it may be more appropriate to base clinical decisions on the magnitude of the gradient between diastolic arterial and compartmental pressure, although this approach is somewhat more complex than simply interpreting the absolute value of the interstitial pressure. Whitesides et al. [19] consistently noted neuromuscular dysfunction when the diastolic arterial to compartment pressure gradient was less than 10 to 30 mm Hg. Others have noted the development of compartment syndromes at lower absolute compartment pressures when patients are hypotensive or in shock [1,6].

In a given situation, the physician must make a decision based on the clinical information available. Judgment must be based, in part, on knowledge regarding the natural history of the disease process and the clinical course of the patient. For example, the clinician can expect to observe further elevations in compartment pressure over the next several hours if compartment pressure is already 35 mm Hg only 1 hour after delayed arterial embolectomy. In this case, urgent fasciotomy is a rational decision despite the "equivocal" pressure reading of 35 mm Hg. Conversely, if the same compartment pressure was noted 48 hours after a tibial fracture, the appropriate decision might be to observe the patient and repeat the pressure measurements in several hours. In this case, it is reasonable to expect that compartment pressures will fall, and the morbidity of fasciotomy avoided.

Other ancillary tests, particularly serum creatine kinase (CK) levels and urine myoglobin assays, may help make the diagnosis of compartment syndrome. In the presence of dead skeletal muscle, CK levels are typically dramatically elevated up to levels in the tens of thousands IU per liter (normal <125 IU/L). Because both elevated CK levels and myoglobinuria are a reflection of myonecrosis, these are very late findings and should not be relied on to make the clinical diagnosis of a compartment syndrome.

Revascularization of an acutely ischemic limb is a well-recognized cause for the development of compartment syndrome; however, compartment syndromes after lower-extremity bypass surgery for chronic limb-threatening ischemia are very unusual, even though significant swelling of the extremities is a common finding [53,54]. On average, compartment pressures increase to only about 10 mm Hg in these patients, usually peaking on the second postoperative day [55]. Clinically, these patients rarely manifest signs or symptoms suggestive of compartment syndrome. The swelling of extremities after revascularization for chronic ischemia is probably caused by impaired lymphatic drainage and increased capillary filtration. It occurs primarily in the subcutaneous tissue superficial to the deep fascia, not in the myofascial compartments [54].

Management

It is critical that the developing compartment syndrome be recognized early, because the neuromuscular dysfunction of a compartment syndrome is fully reversible when promptly treated. Once the diagnosis of a compartment syndrome has been made, fasciotomy should be performed promptly, because the duration of compartment syndrome before surgical decompression is the major factor influencing the functional outcome [30]. Generally, permanent damage to nerves and muscles occurs in 6 to 12 hours [21,26,56–59]. Only 31 percent of patients who undergo fasciotomy within 12 hours of the onset of a compartment syndrome have a residual neuromuscular deficit. Conversely, 91 percent of patients with compartment syndromes for greater than 12 hours have residual deficits, and 20 percent require amputation [1]. In a review of 125 fasciotomies performed for trauma, 75 percent of the cases that came to amputation experienced a delay in performing the fasciotomy or an incomplete or inadequate fascial decompression [60].

Preoperative management of the patient with a compartment syndrome includes such general measures as removing casts and circumferential dressings to release externally applied pressure. Although intuitively one might imagine that the leg should be elevated to improve venous drainage and lessen edema, elevation has been shown to impair arterial perfusion [1,61], and therefore, the extremity should be maintained in a level position.

It may be possible to pharmacologically limit reperfusion injury in compartment syndromes. The data supporting the feasibility of this approach derive from experiments using animal models of muscle ischemia. Thus, postischemic damage to muscle in dogs has been ameliorated by administering allopurinol (an inhibitor of xanthine oxidase) or agents that scavenge free radicals (e.g., dimethyl sulfoxide and superoxide dismutase) [62]. Mannitol, usually thought of as an osmotic diuretic, also has activity as a free radical scavenger, and in experimental animals, infusing this compound decreases vascular resistance and improves oxygen uptake by muscle during reperfusion [63,64]. These results suggest that pharmacotherapy to prevent reperfusion injury may have an important role in the clinical management of compartment syndromes. Unfortunately, not all studies have yielded data as encouraging as those just cited. Although free radical scavengers do limit damage to muscle

during reperfusion, their use has not resulted in an improvement in postischemic neuromuscular function or overall clinical outcome [65,66]. Thus, free radical scavengers or xanthine oxidase inhibitors remain experimental forms of therapy, and these agents cannot be recommended for routine clinical use.

The surgical fasciotomy should (1) remove all of the potentially constricting layers of soft tissue around the swollen muscle groups to relieve compartmental hypertension; (2) assure that arterial perfusion is adequate; and (3) debride all obviously necrotic muscle. The fascia in each compartment is the least compliant and most constricting layer, and incision of the fascia is the most important step leading to relief of compartmental hypertension. A complete epidermotomy, however, is also an important part of the procedure. In most compartment syndromes the muscular swelling is so extensive that, if left undivided, skin overlying the incised fascia would limit muscular expansion and cause continued pressure elevation within the compartment [1,6]. Thorough skin and fascial incisions also permit complete inspection and debridement of the muscle tissue.

Several surgical techniques have been described for fasciotomy of the leg [6,67,68]. Each involves dividing the fascial constraints to achieve decompression of all four compartments. Fibulectomy accomplishes this goal through a single lateral incision and is associated with no long-term orthopedic morbidity (Fig. 180-1) [16,67,68]. Fibulectomy, however, requires an extensive dissection that may lead to hemorrhage, especially from the adjacent peroneal artery and veins. Decompression through a single lateral incision also limits the ability to inspect and debride the muscles of the posterior compartments.

A second technique of fasciotomy uses a medial calf incision to decompress the superficial and deep posterior compartments, and a lateral incision to decompress the anterior and lateral compartments (Fig. 180-2). Although this technique requires two skin incisions, it permits the surgeon to thoroughly inspect and debride all of the muscles in the leg. This technique also makes it relatively easy to inspect each of the three tibial

Fig. 180-1. Fibulectomy can be performed through a single lateral calf incision to accomplish decompression of all four calf compartments. A = anterior compartment; L = lateral compartment; DP = deep posterior compartment; SP = superficial posterior compartment.

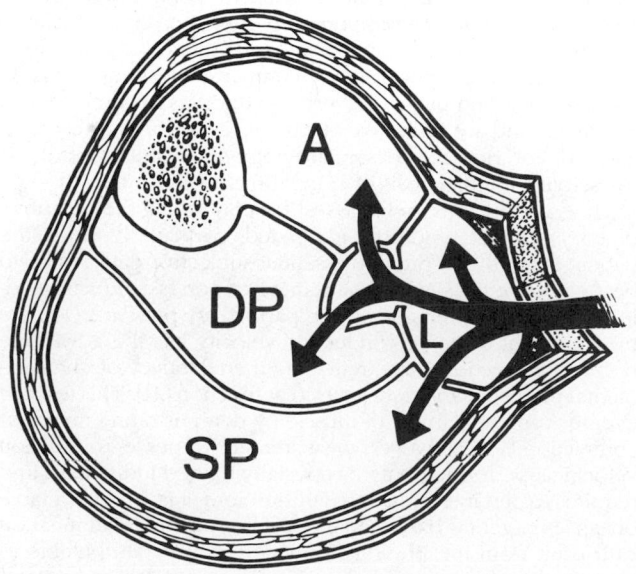

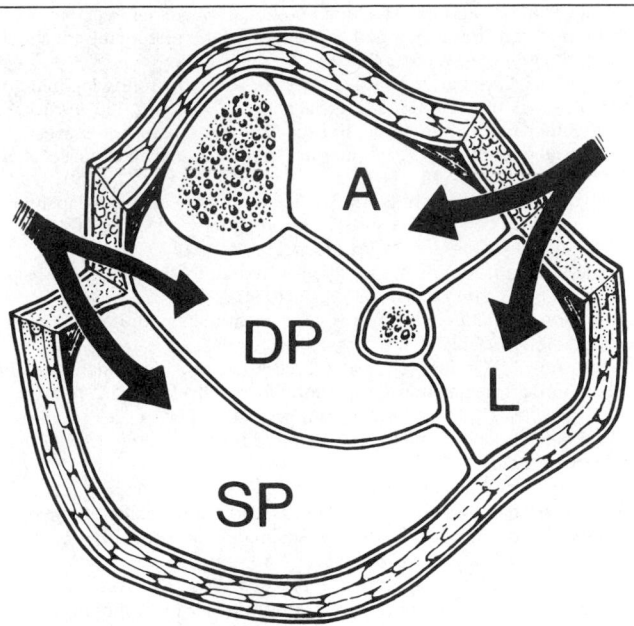

Fig. 180-2. A medial incision can be used to decompress the two posterior compartments, and anterior and lateral compartments can be released from a lateral incision. A = anterior compartment; L = lateral compartment; DP = deep posterior compartment; SP = superficial posterior compartment.

arteries. This procedure can be performed expeditiously and with minimal hemorrhage.

Techniques of fasciotomy for relief of local compartment syndromes have also been described for the buttocks [31,69], the three compartments of the thigh [41,42,45,70,71], the ankle and foot [33,34,35], and the arm and forearm [46].

When acute arterial insufficiency and a compartment syndrome coexist, it is generally better to perform the fasciotomy before the revascularization procedure. The fasciotomy is a brief procedure, whereas revascularization is typically a long one. Promptly decompressing a compartment syndrome is more desirable than permitting compartmental hypertension to persist during a prolonged arterial reconstruction. A preliminary fasciotomy may also prevent misinterpretation of operative arteriograms, improve arterial outflow, and help preserve patency of bypass grafts.

Once all of the involved fascial compartments are decompressed, the muscles should be thoroughly examined for evidence of viability. At the time of the initial procedure, only obviously necrotic muscle should be debrided, because decompressing the compartment and restoring perfusion may allow compromised but viable muscle to recover [30,72,73]. Muscle that is gray, fails to contract when stimulated with electrocautery, and does not bleed when incised is nonviable [3,31] and should be debrided because of the very high risk of infection in necrotic muscle [10]. Furthermore, dead muscle releases intracellular potassium and myoglobin, and failure to obtain adequate debridement may lead to life-threatening complications. In general, skin is highly resistant to ischemic damage. Only very rarely does cutaneous necrosis necessitate debridement of skin in a limb that is otherwise salvageable [31].

Reexamination of the muscle in the involved compartments should be performed 12 to 24 hours after the initial fasciotomy. When any doubt exists regarding the viability of remaining muscle, the muscle should be reexamined in the operating room and necrotic tissue debrided. If, after fasciotomy, the patient develops the metabolic sequelae of massive myonecrosis (metabolic acidosis, hyperkalemia, and myoglobinuria), immediate radical debridement or amputation of the extremity should be considered [74].

There are reports of using contrast-enhanced computed tomography (CT) scans to identify the presence of nonviable muscle groups [75]. Direct inspection of the muscle, however, has been a satisfactory technique and does not involve administration of nephrotoxic intravenous contrast agents to patients already at risk for renal failure attributable to myoglobinuria. The continued presence of nonviable muscle within the extremity is suggested by persistently elevated serum CK levels.

The wounds after fasciotomy should be left open and covered with sterile dressings moistened with isotonic saline. Once perfusion has been restored, the leg should be elevated to help lessen edema. Physical therapy with passive range of motion exercises is important to maintain joint mobility. Wounds usually can be closed within a week of fasciotomy either by secondary skin reapproximation or by split-thickness skin grafting [1].

Complications

Inevitable complications of a neglected compartment syndrome include ischemic neuropathy, myonecrosis, and fibrosis resulting in the characteristic appearance seen in Volkman's ischemic contracture [2]. Even if nerve regrowth occurs [76,77], muscular fibrosis and contraction cause permanent loss of function in the limb [72]. Persistent pain, weakness, and paresthesia occasionally necessitate late amputation [78]. Some patients are afflicted with incapacitating postischemic causalgia [26].

The recommendation for the liberal use of fasciotomy is predicated, of course, on the assumption that the potential complications of the procedure (e.g., infection, paresthesias, and edema) are not long-term disabling problems. In one study, 85 patients who underwent 39 upper-extremity fasciotomies and 57 lower-extremity fasciotomies were examined 5 to 11 years after their procedures. Only 11 extremities required amputation, and in no case was the fasciotomy causally related to limb loss [78]. The major postfasciotomy complications, infection and myoglobinuria, can be prevented or limited in most cases by thoroughly debriding necrotic tissue and obtaining early wound closure.

Reperfusion of ischemic or necrotic muscle after fasciotomy may lead to the release of intracellular constituents resulting in systemic metabolic consequences such as myoglobinemia, myoglobinuria, hyperphosphatemia, metabolic acidosis, coagulation defects, and ultimately shock [3,4,79,80,81]. Leakage of fluid into the interstitium of muscular compartments decreases circulating volume, ultimately resulting in decreased tissue perfusion, prerenal azotemia, and hypotension [4]. Myoglobinemia, which peaks approximately 3 hours after circulation is restored [82,83], is a primary cause of acute renal failure, although the mechanisms underlying myoglobin-induced renal failure are incompletely understood [84]. The release of large quantities of intracellular potassium into the systemic circulation can lead to arrhythmias and cardiac arrest [58,85,86]. Diminished renal function caused by hypovolemia or myoglobinuria can impair the patient's ability to clear the large potassium load.

Often the earliest diagnostic clue suggesting the presence of rhabdomyolysis is the appearance of dark "tea" or "cola" colored urine. The urine characteristically tests positively for blood on the "dipstick" urinalysis, but microscopic examination shows no red blood cells [3]. Physical examination shows the swollen and tense muscle groups responsible for the rhabdomyolysis.

Laboratory findings consistent with the diagnosis of rhabdomyolysis include hyperkalemia, hyperphosphatemia, and metabolic acidosis. The hematocrit may be elevated secondary to the loss of (cell-free) intravascular volume, but the possibility of hemorrhage associated with the predisposing trauma makes this a variable finding. The confirmatory laboratory tests for myoglobinemia or myoglobinuria are rarely available soon enough to be useful for clinical decision making. Serum CK levels, however, are often promptly available and are characteristically markedly elevated.

Intravascular volume should be rapidly restored and metabolic acidosis corrected with sodium bicarbonate. Hyperkalemia can be managed temporarily by administering glucose and insulin; cation exchange resins and even dialysis are sometimes necessary when the case is complicated by oliguria or anuria.

Based on data obtained in uncontrolled studies, it seems probable that the risk of myoglobin-induced acute renal failure is reduced by establishing a brisk diuresis using an osmotic diuretic such as mannitol, and alkalinizing the urine to a pH greater than 6.5 by administering intravenous sodium bicarbonate [4,31,87]. These measures help to prevent the precipitation of myoglobin, which tends to occur in a concentrated acidic urine [87].

The role of fasciotomy in preventing or lessening the systemic effects of rhabdomyolysis is not well delineated. Fasciotomy, however, clearly provides the opportunity to halt ongoing muscle necrosis and debride nonviable muscle tissue [3]. Amputation of the extremity or radical muscle debridement has been advocated if severe myoglobinuria persists for more than 6 hours [88].

Even with aggressive and appropriate management, myoglobin-induced acute renal failure secondary to rhabdomyolysis is a common occurrence [81,89,90]. Renal function apparently recovers in most patients if supportive measures, including dialysis, are provided during the acute phase of the syndrome [91,92].

References

1. Matsen FA III, Krugmire RB: Compartmental syndromes. *Surg Gynecol Obstet* 147:943, 1978.
2. Hyde GL, Peck D, Powell DC: Compartment syndromes: Early diagnosis and a bedside operation. *Am Surg* 49:563, 1983.
3. Mubarak S, Owen CA: Compartmental syndrome and its relation to the crush syndrome: A spectrum of disease. *Clin Orthop* 113:81, 1975.
4. Kikta MJ, Meyer JP, Bishara RA, et al: Crush syndrome due to limb compression. *Arch Surg* 122:1078, 1987.
5. Mubarak SJ, Hargens AR, Owen CA, et al: The wick catheter technique for measurement of intramuscular pressure: A new research and clinical tool. *J Bone Joint Surg [Am]* 58A:1016, 1976.
6. Bourne RB, Rorabeck CH: Compartment syndromes of the lower leg. *Clin Orthop* 240:97, 1989.
7. Awbrey BJ, Sienkiewicz PS, Mankin HJ: Chronic exercise-induced compartment pressure elevation measured with a miniaturized fluid pressure monitor: A laboratory and clinical study. *Am J Sports Med* 16:610, 1988.
8. Kutz JE, Singer R, Lindsay M: Chronic exertional compartment syndrome of the forearm: A case report. *J Hand Surg* 10A:302, 1987.
9. Khalil IM: Bilateral compartmental syndrome after prolonged surgery in the lithotomy position. *J Vasc Surg* 5:879, 1987.
10. Perry MO: Compartmental syndromes and reperfusion injury. *Surg Clin North Am* 68:853, 1988.
11. Annouchi YS, Parker RD, Seitz WH: Posterior compartment syndrome of the calf resulting from misdiagnosis of a rupture of the medial head of the gastrocnemius. *J Trauma* 27:678, 1987.
12. McLellan BA, Phillips JH, Hunter GA, et al: Bilateral lower extremity amputation after prolonged application of the pneumatic antishock garment: A case report. *Can J Surg* 30:55, 1987.
13. Maull KI, Capehart JE, Cardea JA, et al: Limb loss following military anti-shock trousers (MAST) application. *J Trauma* 21:60, 1981.
14. Kjellmer I: An indirect method for estimating tissue pressure with special reference to tissue pressure in muscle during exercise. *Acta Physiol Scand* 62:30, 1964.
15. Ryder HW, Molle WE, Ferris EB: The influence of the collapsibility of veins on venous pressure, including a new procedure for measuring tissue pressure. *J Clin Invest* 23:333, 1944.
16. Duomarco J, Rimini R: Energy and hydraulic gradients along systemic veins. *Am J Physiol* 178:215, 1954.
17. Ashton H: Critical closing pressure in human peripheral vascular beds. *Clin Sci* 22:79, 1961.
18. Matsen FA, Winquist RA, Krugmire RB: Diagnosis and management of compartment syndromes. *J Bone Joint Surg [Am]* 62:286, 1980.
19. Whitesides TE, Haney TC, Morimotok, et al: Tissue pressure measurements as a determinant of the need for fasciotomy. *Clin Orthop* 113:43, 1975.
20. Heppenstall RB, Sapega AA, Scott R, et al: The compartment syndrome: An experimental and clinical study of muscular energy metabolism using phosphorus nuclear magnetic resonance spectroscopy. *Clin Orthop* 226:138, 1988.
21. Matsen FA, Mayo KA, Krugmire RB, et al: A model compartmental syndrome in man with particular reference to the quantification of nerve function. *J Bone Joint Surg [Am]* 59:648, 1977.
22. Matsen FA III: Compartmental syndrome: A unified concept. *Clin Orthop* 113:8, 1975.
23. Perry MO, Shires GT III, Albert SA: Cellular changes with graded limb ischemia in reperfusion. *J Vasc Surg* 1:536, 1984.
24. Presta M, Ragnotti G: Quantification of damage to striated muscle after normothermic or hypothermic ischemia. *Clin Chem* 27:297, 1981.
25. Bulkley GB: Pathophysiology of free radical mediated reperfusion injury. *J Vasc Surg* 5:512, 1987.
26. Rutherford RB: Nutrient bed protection during lower extremity arterial reconstruction. *J Vasc Surg* 5:529, 1987.
27. Viegas SF, Rimoldi R, Scarborough M, et al: Acute compartment syndrome in the thigh: A case report and review of the literature. *Clin Orthop* 234:232, 1988.
28. Lees AJ: Anterior tibial compartment syndrome following prolonged tetany. *J Neurol Neurosurg Psychiatry* 39:406, 1976.
29. Gershuni DH, Mubarak SJ, Yaru NC: Fracture of the tibia complicated by acute compartment syndrome. *Clin Orthop* 217:221, 1987.
30. Matsen FA III, Veith RG: Compartmental syndromes in children. *J Pediatr Orthop* 1:33, 1981.
31. Reis ND, Michaelson M: Crush injury to the lower limbs: Treatment of the local injury. *J Bone Joint Surg [Am]* 68:414, 1986.
32. Petrik ME, Stambough JL, Rothman RH: Posttraumatic gluteal compartment syndrome: A case report. *Clin Orthop* 231:127, 1988.
33. Ascer E, Strauch B, Calligro KD, et al: Ankle and foot fasciotomy: An adjunctive technique to optimize limb salvage after revascularization for acute ischemia. *J Vasc Surg* 9:594, 1989.
34. Ziv I, Mosheiff R, Zeligowski A, et al: Crush injury of the foot with compartment syndrome: Immediate one-stage management. *Foot Ankle* 9:185, 1989.
35. Meyerson MS: Experimental decompression of the fascial compartments of the foot: The basis for fasciotomy in acute compartment syndromes. *Foot Ankle* 8:308, 1988.
36. Nixon RG, Brinkley GW: Hemophilia presenting as compartment syndrome in the arm following venipuncture: A case report and review of the literature. *Clin Orthop* 244:176, 1989.
37. Halpein AA, Mochizuki R, Long CE III: Compartment syndrome of the forearm following radial artery puncture in a patient treated with anticoagulants. *J Bone Joint Surg [Am]* 60:1136, 1978.
38. Werbel GB, Shybut GT: Acute compartment syndrome caused by a malfunctioning pneumatic compression boot. *J Bone Joint Surg [Am]* 68:1445, 1986.
39. Celoria G, Dawson JA, Teres D: Compartment syndrome in a patient monitored with an automated blood pressure cuff. *J Clin Monit* 3:139, 1987.
40. Templeman D, Lange R, Harms B: Lower extremity compartment syndrome associated with use of pneumatic antishock garments. *J Trauma* 27:79, 1987.

41. Bass RR, Alison EJ Jr, Reines HD, et al: Thigh compartment syndrome without lower extremity trauma following application of pneumatic antishock trousers. *Ann Emerg Med* 12:382, 1983.
42. Kunkel JM: Thigh and leg compartment syndrome in the absence of lower extremity trauma following MAST application. *Am J Emerg Med* 5:118, 1987.
43. Williams TM, Knopp R, Ellyson JH: Compartment syndrome after anti-shock trouser use without lower extremity trauma. 22:595, 1982.
44. Leff RG, Shapiro SR: Lower extremity complications of the lithotomy position: Prevention and management. *J Urol* 122:138, 1979.
45. McLaren AC, Ferguson JH, Minaci A: Crush syndrome associated with use of the fracture-table: A case report. *J Bone Joint Surg [Am]* 69:1447, 1987.
46. Carter PR: Crush injury of the upper limb: Early and late management. *Orthop Clin North Am* 14:719, 1984.
47. Mubarak SJ, Owen CA, Hargens AR, et al: Acute compartment syndromes: Diagnosis and treatment with the aid of a wick catheter. *J Bone Joint Surg [Am]* 60:1091, 1978.
48. Phillips JH, MacKinnon SE, Beatty SE, et al: Vibratory sensory testing in acute compartment syndromes: A clinical and experimental study. *Plast Reconstr Surg* 79:796, 1987.
49. Russell WL, Apyan PM, Burns P: Electronic technique for compartment pressure measurement using the wick catheter. *Surg Gynecol Obstet* 161:173, 1985.
50. Mubarak SJ, Hargens AR: Acute compartment syndrome. *Surg Clin North Am* 63:539, 1983.
51. Patman RD: Fasciotomy: Indications and technique, in Rutherford RB (ed): *Vascular Surgery*. Philadelphia, WB Saunders, 1984, p 513.
52. Russell WL, Burns RP: Acute upper and lower extremity compartment syndromes, in Bergan JJ, Yao JST (eds): *Vascular Surgical Emergencies*. Orlando, Grune & Stratton, 1987, p 203.
53. Skillman JJ, Dohlman LE, Gerhart TN, et al: Compartmental pressure monitoring after arterial reconstruction lacks clinical relevance. *J Vasc Surg* 3:871, 1986.
54. Scott DJA, Allen MJ, Bell PRF, et al: Does oedema following lower limb revascularization cause compartment syndromes? *Ann R Coll Surg Engl* 70:372, 1988.
55. Melberg PE, Styf J, Biber B, et al: Muscular compartment pressure following reconstructive arterial surgery of the lower limbs. *Acta Chir Scand* 150:129, 1984.
56. Matsen FA, Clawson DK: The deep posterior compartment syndrome of the leg. *J Bone Joint Surg [Am]* 57:34, 1975.
57. Sheridan GW, Matsen FA: An animal model of the compartmental syndrome. *Clin Orthop* 113:36, 1975.
58. Sheridan GW, Matsen FA: Fasciotomy in the treatment of the acute compartment syndrome. *J Bone Joint Surg [Am]* 58:112, 1976.
59. Sheridan GW, Matsen FA, Krugmire RB: Further investigations on the pathophysiology of the compartmental syndrome. *Clin Orthop* 123:226, 1977.
60. Feliciano DV, Crus PA, Spjut-Patrinely V: Fasciotomy after trauma to the extremities. *Am J Surg* 156:533, 1988.
61. Ashton H: The effect of increased tissue pressure on blood flow. *Clin Orthop* 113:15, 1975.
62. Korthuis RJ, Granger DN, Townsley MI, et al: The role of oxygen-derived free radicals in ischemia-induced increases in canine skeletal muscle vascular permeability. *Circ Res* 57:599, 1985.
63. Buchbinder D, Karmody N, Leather R, et al: Hypertonic mannitol: Its use in the prevention of revascularization syndrome after acute arterial ischemia. *Arch Surg* 116:414, 1981.
64. Perry MO, Fantini G: Ischemia: Profile of an enemy. *J Vasc Surg* 6:231, 1987.
65. Ricci MA, Graham AM, Corbisiero R, et al: Are free radical scavengers beneficial in the treatment of compartment syndrome after acute arterial ischemia? *J Vasc Surg* 9:244, 1989.
66. Hutton M, Rhodes RS, Chapman G: The lowering of post-ischemic compartment pressures with mannitol. *J Surg Res* 32:239, 1982.
67. Ernst CB, Kaufer H: Fibulectomy-fasciotomy: An important adjunct in the management of lower extremity arterial trauma. *Trauma* 11:365, 1971.
68. Furman RW, Hyde GL, Playforth RH, et al: Fibulectomy: A radical decompression of the post-ischemic leg. *Am Surg* 37:750, 1971.
69. Owen CA, Woody PR, Mubarak SJ, et al: Gluteal compartment syndromes: A report of three cases and management utilizing the wick catheter. *Clin Orthop* 132:57, 1978.
70. Clancey GJ: Acute posterior compartment syndrome in the thigh: A case report. *J Bone Joint Surg [Am]* 12:1278, 1985.
71. Tarlow SD, Achterman CA, Hayhurst J, et al: Acute compartment syndrome in the thigh complicating fracture of the femur: A report of three cases. *J Bone Joint Surg [Am]* 68:1439, 1986.
72. Sanderson RA, Foley RK, McIvor GWD, et al: Histological response of skeletal muscle to ischemia. *Clin Orthop* 113:27, 1975.
73. Vracko R, Benditt EP: Basal lamina, the scaffold for orderly cell replacement: Observation on regeneration of injured skeletal muscle fibers and capillaries. *J Cell Biol* 55:406, 1972.
74. Matsen FA: *Compartmental Syndromes*. New York, Grune & Stratton, 1980, p 122.
75. Vukanovic S, Hauser H, Wettstein P: CT localization of myonecrosis for surgical decompression. *AJR* 135:1298, 1980.
76. Lundborg G: Limb ischemia and nerve injury. *Arch Surg* 104:631, 1972.
77. Miller HH, Welch CS: Quantitative studies on the time factor in arterial injuries. *Ann Surg* 130:428, 1949.
78. Vitale GC, Richardson JD, George SM Jr, et al: Fasciotomy for severe blunt and penetrating trauma of the extremity. *Surg Gynecol Obstet* 166:397, 1988.
79. Bywaters EGL: Ischemic muscle necrosis. *JAMA* 24:1103, 1944.
80. Knochel JP: Rhabdomyolysis and myoglobinuria, in Suki WN, Eknoyan G (eds): *The Kidney in Systemic Diseases*. 2nd ed. New York, John Wiley and Sons, 1981, pp 263–284.
81. Gabow PA, Kaehny WD, Kelleker SP: The spectrum of rhabdomyolysis. *Medicine* 61:141, 1982.
82. Montagnani CA, Simeone FA: Observations on the liberation and elimination of myoglobin and of hemoglobin after release of muscle ischemia. *Surgery* 34:169, 1953.
83. Schreiber SN, Liebowitz MR, Bernstein LH: Limb compression and renal impairment (crush syndrome) following narcotic and sedative overdose. *J Bone Joint Surg [Am]* 54:1683, 1972.
84. Weeks SR: The crush syndrome. *Surg Gynecol Obstet* 127:369, 1968.
85. Coupland GAE: Anterior tibial syndrome following restoration of arterial flow. *Aust N Z J Surg* 41:338, 1972.
86. Allister C: Cardiac arrest after crush injury. *Br Med J* 287:531, 1983.
87. Ron D, Taitelman V, Michaelson M, et al: Prevention of acute renal failure in traumatic rhabdomyolysis. *Arch Intern Med* 144:277, 1984.
88. Baxter CR: Present concepts in the management of major electrical injury. *Surg Clin North Am* 50:1401, 1970.
89. Santangelo ML, Usberti M, DiSalvo E, et al: A study of the pathology of the crush syndrome. *Surg Gynecol Obstet* 154:372, 1982.
90. Eneas JF, Schonfeld PY, Humphreys MH: The effect of infusion of mannitol-sodium bicarbonate on the clinical course of myoglobinuria. *Arch Intern Med* 139:801, 1979.
91. Grossman RA, Hamilton RW, Morse BM, et al: Nontraumatic rhabdomyolysis and acute renal failure. *N Engl J Med* 291:807, 1974.
92. Koffler A, Friedler RM, Massry SG: Acute renal failure due to nontraumatic rhabdomyolysis. *Ann Intern Med* 85:23, 1976.

181. Derangements of Oxygen Transport in Shock States and Sepsis

Guillermo Gutierrez

The process of oxygen transport from the atmosphere to the mitochondria is the most basic and important of all body functions. Without oxygen the cells die because they cannot generate sufficient energy to maintain an adequate transmembrane gradient for calcium and other anions. Paradoxically, oxygen is poisonous to the cells through the formation of O_2 radical species, and it has taken millions of years of evolution to tame the great potential energy derived from this molecule. Moreover, as organisms progressed from unicellular to multicellular entities, simple gas diffusion alone was not sufficient to assure the required flow of O_2 from the surrounding environment into each cell's mitochondria. Different species developed mass transport processes to carry O_2 from the periphery to the interior of the organism. For example, some insects have small tubes that carry air deep inside their bodies. Vertebrates have a complex O_2 delivery system composed of a gas exchange organ, a blood-borne oxygen carrier, a pump to impel blood, and an intricate network of blood vessels to bring hemoglobin in proximity to the cells from where O_2 diffuses into the cells and CO_2 moves in the opposite way.

Present knowledge of the normal functioning of this transport system is, at best, rudimentary. This knowledge is mostly related to mechanisms of blood pressure and flow control by α and β adrenergic and dopaminergic receptors. Precious little is known of the microcirculation, where the bulk of flow control occurs. This region is characterized by local regulation of blood flow resulting in the phasic opening and closing of terminal arterioles, the phenomenon of vasomotion [1]. It is this local regulation of blood flow that perhaps is most affected by sepsis and other conditions affecting the critically ill patient.

Basic Principles of Oxygen Transport

DEFINITIONS. Before we discuss the possible derangements in O_2 transport in shock states and sepsis, it may be useful to review some of the basic principles governing the transport of O_2 to the tissues and its relationship to O_2 consumption. O_2 transport to an organ is defined as

$$TO_2 = \text{Blood flow} \times \text{arterial blood } O_2 \text{ concentration}$$

where the blood O_2 concentration (C_aO_2) is a function of the total hemoglobin concentration, its fractional saturation with O_2, and the PO_2,

$$C_aO_2 = 1.34 \times \text{Hemoglobin concentration} \times O_2 \text{ saturation} + 0.003 \times PO_2$$

Under steady-state conditions, oxygen consumption for an organ can be calculated using Fick's equation:

$$VO_2 = \text{Blood flow} \times (C_aO_2 - C_vO_2)$$

where C_vO_2 is the venous blood O_2 concentration. For the body as a whole, cardiac output should be substituted for blood flow and mixed venous O_2 concentration for C_vO_2.

Ordinarily, oxygen consumption by an organ, or by the body as a whole, is proportional to its level of energy expenditure. Most of this O_2 consumption is used in the aerobic production of energy in the form of adenosine triphosphate (ATP). A small portion is used in the formation of O_2 free radical species, such as superoxide, hydrogen peroxide, and hydroxyl radicals. The fraction of TO_2 used in this manner is difficult to quantitate and ordinarily ranges [2] from 2% to 5%, but it may be higher in some organs, such as the lung, during inflammatory states.

Energy requirements at rest remain relatively constant, regardless of the supply of O_2 reaching the tissues. To maintain O_2 utilization constant when faced with reductions in TO_2, the tissues extract a greater fraction of O_2 from capillary blood. This is expressed as the O_2 extraction ratio, or ERO_2. Calculation of the ERO_2 does not require knowledge of blood flow, because

$$ERO_2 = (C_aO_2)/(C_aO_2 - C_vO_2)$$

Increases in ERO_2 occur as formerly closed capillaries are recruited, decreasing the diffusion distance from the red blood cell to the mitochondria [3,4]. Organs with the greatest capacity for capillary recruitment, such as skeletal muscle, have the capacity to extract more O_2. Control of the microvasculature occurs primarily through the action of potent vasoactive substances released by endothelial cells in response to local changes in cellular metabolism. Among these are potent vasodilators nitric oxide and adenosine.

THE RELATIONSHIP OF O_2 CONSUMPTION TO O_2 TRANSPORT. The relationship of O_2 transport to O_2 consumption in an organ such as skeletal muscle is nonlinear [3]. This is schematically illustrated in Figure 181-1, where VO_2 is shown as a function of TO_2. This figure shows a biphasic function composed of an O_2 supply-independent region and an O_2 supply-dependent region. Changes in TO_2 in the O_2 supply-independent region do not produce changes in VO_2. The constancy of VO_2 is the result of microvascular adaptations that increase ERO_2 as formerly closed capillaries are recruited, decreasing the diffusion distance from the red blood cell to the mitochondria [4,5]. Control of capillary recruitment occurs primarily through the action of potent vasoactive substances released by endothelial cells in response to local changes in cellular metabolism. Among these are the vasodilators nitric oxide and adenosine. The ability of the tissues to cope with decreases in TO_2 by increasing ERO_2 varies among different organs. Organs with the greatest capacity to recruit capillaries, such as skeletal muscle, also have the greatest capacity to extract capillary O_2. Other organs, such as the gut, have a limited capacity to recruit capillaries and are more dependent on increases in blood flow when exposed to decreases in TO_2.

With progressive decreases in TO_2, a point is reached where the tissues cannot increase ERO_2 further and VO_2 begins to fall

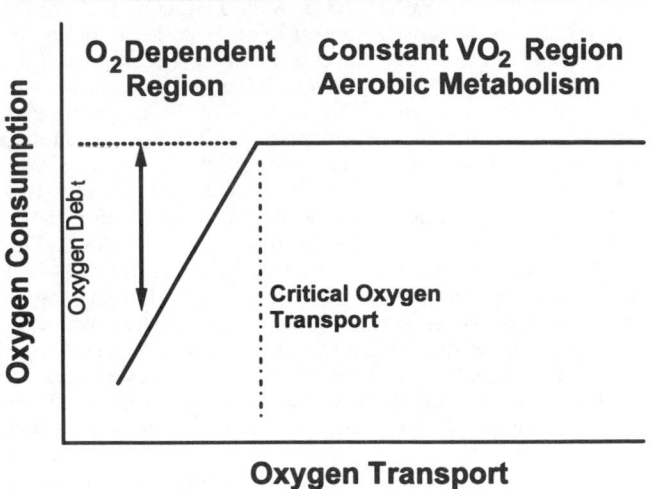

Fig. 181-1. The relationship of O_2 transport (TO_2) to O_2 consumption (VO_2) as observed in experimental animal studies. VO_2 remains constant until a critical level of TO_2 is reached. VO_2 becomes dependent on decreases in TO_2 below TO_{2crit}.

below the "plateau" value. This level of TO_2, also called the "critical" TO_2 (TO_{2crit}), demarcates the transition from full aerobic metabolism, to a region in which anaerobic sources of energy are requried to supplement aerobic ATP production.

The nonlinear or biphasic TO_2-VO_2 function, where VO_2 remains constant in spite of decreases in TO_2, has been defined as oxygen regulation [6]. This type behavior is characteristic of most mannalian species, including humans. In contrast, the situation in which linear decreases in VO_2 occur in response to decreases in TO_2 is defined as oxygen conformity. It occurs in certain species such as the goldfish and the freshwater turtle [7]. Except for diving mammals, who employ the diving reflex to apportion O_2 storages to vital organs, mammals lack mechanisms to decrease energy requirements during hypoxia.

PATHOLOGIC O_2 SUPPLY DEPENDENCY. Numerous experimental studies have shown that the TO_{2crit} is a variable parameter. The value of TO_{2crit} for a given experimental condition depends on factors governing tissue O_2 diffusion and metabolic rate. Hypothermia, with its lower metabolic rates, results in significantly lower levels of TO_{2crit} [8]. Increases in hemoglobin O_2 affinity impair the release of O_2 by hemoglobin in the tissue capillaries, resulting in greater TO_{2crit} [9]. Sepsis also increases the TO_{2crit}, perhaps by interference with microvascular control mechanisms [10].

The results of studies performed in critically ill patients differ from those obtained in laboratory animals. The basic difference is that critically ill patients behave as conformers [11], with a linear TO_2-VO_2 relationship, rather than exhibiting the familiar biphasic TO_2-VO_2 curve. With the exception of the work of Shibutani et al. [12], who found a biphasic TO_2-VO_2 relationship in 58 patients undergoing cardiac surgery, all published clinical studies show a straight-line relationship between TO_2 and VO_2. In a now classic study, Danek et al [13] measured TO_2, VO_2, and mixed venous PO_2 in 20 patients with acute respiratory distress syndrome (ARDS) and 12 others with various diseases. In all but one of the patients, the TO_2-VO_2 relationship was linear and had a positive slope even when TO_2 was as high as 50 ml/min/kg, three times that of normal subjects at rest.

The proportional relationship between TO_2 and VO_2 in patients with sepsis and ARDS has been confirmed by others [13,14]. Dorinsky et al. [15] noted that this behavior also extends to patients with congestive heart failure and chronic obstructive pulmonary disease, although the dependency phenomenon appears to be stronger in patients with ARDS than in those with pulmonary failure from other causes [16]. In a prospective study on a heterogeneous patient population, Gutierrez and Pohil [17] fitted six different mathematical functions to each patient's TO_2-VO_2 data using regression analysis and concluded that a linear function was an accurate representation of the TO_2-VO_2 relationship in acutely ill patients, regardless of their diagnosis. Perhaps even more interesting to the clinician, the patients were divided into two groups according to the slope of their TO_2-VO_2 relationship (Fig. 181-2). In one group (group A), changes

Fig. 181-2. The relationship of O_2 consumption to O_2 transport and O_2 extraction ratio measured in two groups of critically ill patients. Group A exhibited O_2 supply dependency and had a mortality of 70 percent. Group B maintained constant O_2 consumption by increases in O_2 extraction ratio. This group had a mortality of only 30 percent. From: Gutierrez G, Pohil R: Oxygen consumption is linearly related to O_2 supply in critically ill patients. *J Crit Care* 1:45, 1986. Reproduced by permission.

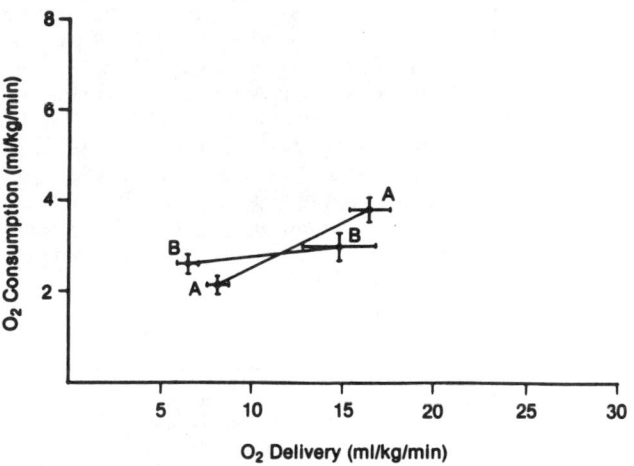

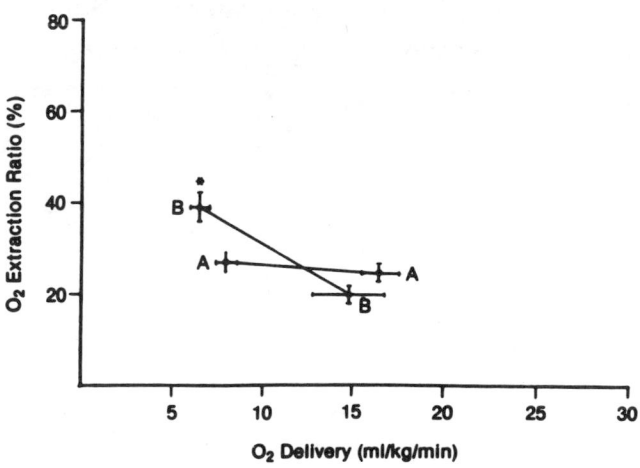

in VO_2 were dependent on changes in TO_2, whereas in the other (group B) VO_2 varied little with alterations in TO_2. As one would expect, the correlation between TO_2 and VO_2 was dependent on the ability of the tissue to extract oxygen from blood. Patients in group A had a 70 percent mortality rate. They suffered from disorders associated with alterations in microvascular control, such as ARDS, sepsis, and acute bleeding. Group B had a mortality rate of only 30 percent, and mostly consisted of patients with heart failure. These data suggest that patients who retain the ability to control tissue perfusion and increase ERO_2 when faced with decreased TO_2 have a better prognosis.

Among the many hypothesis that may explain the lack of a biphasic TO_2-VO_2 relationship in clinical studies, the one with the widest acceptance is the one offered by Kreuzer and Cain [18]. They proposed that the biphasic curve is the true physiologic behavior of the O_2 transport system in humans. The linear dependency of VO_2 on TO_2 was explained on the basis of an increased basal VO_2 in patients with ARDS, combined with a decreased ability to extract O_2 from blood. This results in a pathologic TO_2-VO_2 function that has a higher plateau and is shifted to the right of the physiologic condition (Fig. 181-3). This condition is defined as pathologic supply dependency.

The notion that septic patients may have "pathologic supply dependency" is supported by animal experiments showing that infusion of *Escherichia coli* bacteria or endotoxin to anesthetized dogs impairs their ability to extract O_2 from blood [10,18]. The clinical basis for the concept of "pathologic supply dependency" hypothesis can be found in the work of Gutierrez and Pohil [17] and in the study by Bihari et al [19]. The latter noted increases in VO_2 in a group of critically ill patients after the infusion of prostacyclin, a potent vasodilator. This was taken as evidence of a covert tissue hypoxia that ultimately proved fatal for these patients. Bihari and colleagues [19] proposed the use of an "oxygen flux" test, in which increases in VO_2 in response to rapid increases in TO_2 is proof that a "supply-dependent" state exists and that the patient may benefit from a sustained increase in TO_2.

Fig. 181-3. Comparison of the physiologic behavior of the TO_2-VO_2 relationship found in experimental animals (solid line) to the O_2 supply dependency hypothesis of Kreuzer and Cain [18] for patients with sepsis and the acute respiratory distress syndrome. The pathologic curve is characterized by a flatter O_2 extraction slope and a higher VO_2 plateau.

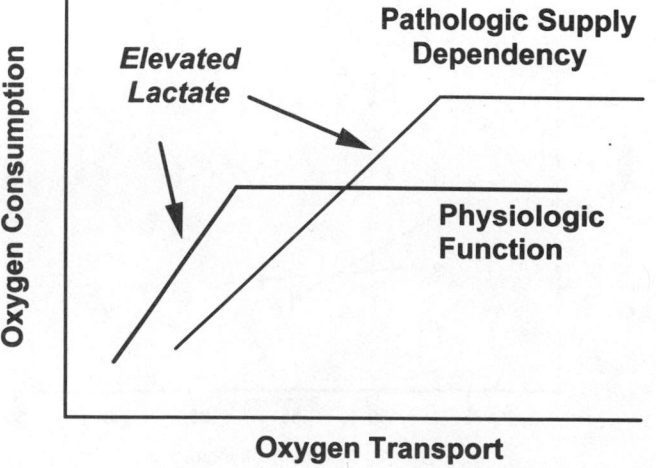

IS O_2 SUPPLY DEPENDENCY A PATHOLOGIC CONDITION? Studies dispute the existence of "pathologic supply dependency." These studies have as a common denominator the measurement of VO_2 independently from cardiac output, that is, where VO_2 is measured by analysis of the expired gases. The idea is to eliminate the possibility of mathematical coupling of data as the cause of O_2 supply dependency. Because both TO_2 and VO_2 are calculated variables that include the measurement of cardiac output by thermodilution, random errors in this measurement could result in spurious linear functions. This problem was mathematically analyzed by Moreno et al [20], who concluded that mathematical coupling, although present, probably plays a minor role in the genesis of the linear TO_2-VO_2 function, as long as changes in TO_2 are sufficiently large. This may not be the case when data for a given patient are analyzed, and several studies now show that "supply dependency" disappears once independent measurements of TO_2 and VO_2 are used.

Annat et al [21] measured VO_2 in eight mechanically ventilated patients with ARDS using the expired gas method. They decreased TO_2 by applying positive end-expiratory pressure and found no change in VO_2 or increases in blood lactate. They concluded that these patients were capable of increasing O_2 extraction to meet cellular O_2 requirements. Furthermore, they also found that the basal VO_2 of these patients was similar to that of other mechanically ventilated patients. Ronco et al [22] also measured VO_2 by the expired gases method in patients with ARDS and increased TO_2 by blood transfusion. Although there were significant increases in TO_2, there were no changes in baseline VO_2, even in patients with initial elevations in plasma lactate. Conversely, when VO_2 was calculated using Fick's equation, they found that increases in TO_2 for the same data set were accompanied by increases in VO_2. They concluded that the finding of O_2 supply dependency may be the result of methodologic error when the calculation of TO_2 and VO_2 involves shared variables.

Another possibility is that the TO_2-VO_2 relationship in patients may represent the normal physiologic response of the system, instead of an abnormal manifestation of impaired oxygen extraction [23]. During an experiment, a healthy animal preparation is exposed for a relatively short time to reductions in TO_2 produced by one of three methods: decreases in O_2 saturation, cardiac output, or hemoglobin concentration. Under these conditions, VO_2 is clearly the dependent variable, while TO_2 is the manipulated variable. This is not the case in the clinical setting, where TO_2 is not a manipulated variable; instead, changes in TO_2 occur spontaneously in response to changes in the patient's metabolic rate. Therefore, it is possible that sometimes TO_2 may lie below the critical point, and VO_2 may be dependent on TO_2, whereas at other times, TO_2 is dependent on VO_2. That is, increases in VO_2 in response to agitation, fever, increased work of breathing, etc., result in an appropriate increase in TO_2. This physiologic response of TO_2 to increases in VO_2 is akin to that which normally occurs during exercise. A consensus is emerging among investigators, that "pathologic O_2 supply dependency" cannot be taken as evidence of covert tissue hypoxia, and that regional monitoring of oxygenation and metabolic parameters is needed to ascertain the adequacy of tissue oxygenation.

INCREASES IN O_2 TRANSPORT AS THERAPY FOR O_2 SUPPLY DEPENDENCY. The condition defined as O_2 supply dependency has been interpreted as evidence that O_2 transport in most critically ill patients is below the critical point, and therefore inadequate to meet tissue O_2 demands. Therapy based on this hypothesis calls for potent cardiac stimulating drugs to augment cardiac output and blood transfusions, with the ultimate aim of increasing O_2 transport to supernormal levels. The effect of such therapy on patient outcome is unknown.

Shoemaker et al [24] found better postoperative survival rates in nonseptic patients in whom pulmonary artery catheters (PA) were used to help maximize cardiac output, VO_2, and TO_2. This was a prospective, randomized study comparing three groups: a group treated according to the information derived from central venous lines (CVP-control), a group using PA catheters to achieve normal values of oxygenation parameters as therapeutic goals (PA-control), and a protocol group, where patients with PA catheters were treated with fluids and catecholamines (mainly dobutamine) in efforts to reach supernormal levels of VO_2 and TO_2 as therapeutic end points (PA-protocol). Hospital mortality rates were 38 percent, 23 percent, and 4 percent for the CVP-control, PA-control, and PA-protocol groups, respectively, suggesting that prevention of an oxygen debt improved mortality in this group of patients.

Application of this concept to critically ill patients has met with variable success. Russell et al. [25] studied 29 patients with ARDS and found that survivors (n = 13) had greater levels of TO_2 and VO_2 within the first 24 hours of onset of ARDS. No effort was made in this study to increase TO_2 to supernormal levels. Conversely, Gutierrez et al. [26] found lower TO_2 and VO_2 in survivors in a heterogeneous group of critically ill patients. There are few studies in which a consistent effort has been applied to maintain greater than normal values of TO_2 in critically ill patients. In the prostaglandin E_1 trial for treatment of ARDs [27], the study group had significantly greater TO_2 than control, but survival was similar. Tuchschmidt et al [28] prospectively studied a group of patients with septic shock (n = 26) in whom cardiac index was increased to 6.0 L/min/m² for 72 hours using dobutamine. This group was compared with a normal treatment control with cardiac indices averaging 3.6 L/min/m². They found no difference in mortality between the groups (p < 0.14), although their sample may not have had sufficient power to detect a significant difference. Other investigators have found increases in VO_2 in response to catecholamines and fluid loading in septic patients [29–33], but the effect of increasing VO_2 on mortality could not be assessed from these studies.

Microvascular Disturbances in Sepsis

There is overwhelming evidence that blood flow is redistributed among the different organs in sepsis, not always to the ultimate benefit of the organism as a whole. After the injection of endotoxin in rabbits, there are decreases in flow to the kidney and hepatic artery [34], whereas in pigs [35] and monkeys [36] endotoxin reduces blood flow to the cerebrum, kidney, spleen, and skeletal muscle. Endotoxin exerts a profound effect on the rat diaphragmatic microvasculature, manifested by constriction of arterioles and impaired capillary perfusion [37]. In a rat Langendorff preparation exposed to endotoxin, Rumsey et al. [38] found diminished capacity of the heart's vasculature to adjust blood flow to energy needs. They also noted a *hyperdynamic, hypermetabolic* state characterized by increases in myocardial O_2 consumption.

Several experimental studies have singled out the intestines as a target organ of sepsis. It appears that the ability of the gut to extract O_2 is impaired in sepsis. Drazenovic et al [39] infused

E. coli endotoxin to an exteriorized segment of dog small intestine labeled with colloidal carbon and found decreased perfused capillary density in the mucosal villi and crypts of the septic gut segments. There may be a differential microvascular response to sepsis among tissues, with skeletal muscle being more resilient than the gut. Gutierrez et al. [40] examined the effect of *E. coli* endotoxin administration on rabbit hindlimb skeletal muscle oxygenation measured with surface PO_2 microelectrodes. They noted decreased O_2 transport with endotoxin and the development of tissue hypoxia, but the distribution of the tissue PO_2 histograms remained constant for 2 hours after the infusion of endotoxin, implying that increases in skeletal muscle microcirculatory heterogeneity do not increase in early sepsis. These findings agree with those of Kopp et al [41], who measured muscle PO_2 in pigs and concluded that microcirculatory changes do not take place in skeletal muscle during the first 2 hours of septic shock.

It is not clear how endotoxin or other septic mediators alter the microvascular response to sepsis. The role played by endothelial-derived vascular mediators has received considerable attention recently. Beasley et al [42] measured smooth muscle contractility in intact and endothelial-denuded thoracic aortic rings from rats. They found an endothelium-dependent inhibition to contraction after a 1-hour exposure to endotoxin. In contrast, after a 3-hour exposure to endotoxin, aortic ring contraction was inhibited to a similar degree in rings with or without endothelium.

It appears that endothelium-derived nitric oxide may play an important role in vascular reactivity during sepsis, perhaps by the activation of soluble guanylate cyclase into guanosine $3',5'$-cyclic monophosphate [43,44], a potent intracellular mediator of vasodilation [45]. Evidence is accumulating pointing toward NO-induced guanylate cyclase activation as the mediator of the vascular manifestations of sepsis. Should this prove to be the case, substances that inhibit endothelial NO synthesis may prove to be the "magic bullets" in the treatment of sepsis. On the basis of this hypothesis, that is, that vascular changes in sepsis are related to the overproduction of NO, Kilbourn et al [46,47] infused N^G-methyl-L-arginine, an inhibitor of NO synthesis, in dogs after the administration of either *E. coli* endotoxin or tumor necrosis factor-α (TNFα). In both cases they noted the reversal of the hypotensive response to these agents. Meyer et al [48] found that the intravenous administration of N^ω-nitro-L-arginine methyl ester to septic ewes increased mean arterial pressure and decreased the pulmonary shunt fraction. It appears that NO also may exert a direct effect on myocardial contractility in sepsis [49]. Isolated guinea pig cardiac ventricular myocytes from endotoxin treated animals show decreased contractility. This effect of endotoxin is reversed by N^G-methyl-L-arginine.

Although preliminary data are promising, there are no studies demonstrating improved animal mortality, or a reduction in organ system failure, resulting from the administration of inhibitors of NO synthesis during sepsis. Moreover, inhibitors of NO synthesis produce decreases in cardiac output [50], perhaps by an acute increase in afterload. This implies that the restoration of blood pressure by inhibitors of NO synthesis during sepsis may be the result of nonselective systemic vasoconstriction, perhaps to the detriment of nutritive flow to individual tissues. NO probably plays a very important role in mediating the systemic vasodilation of sepsis; however, these vascular abnormalities may be the manifestation, not the cause, of cellular metabolic damage set in motion by sepsis related cytokines. In other words, the initial insult is directed to the tissue cells, which in turn signal the endothelium to produce NO and perhaps other vasodilator substances.

Therapeutic Principles in the Treatment of Sepsis and Other Shock States

THE "FLIGHT OR FIGHT" REACTION HYPOTHESIS. Sepsis results in a fairly predictable pattern of hemodynamic and metabolic alterations. These changes occur under conditions of O_2 transport and tissue oxygenation that ordinarily are adequate for most organs. Perhaps the cytokines associated with endotoxemia, TNFα, Il-1, etc., set in motion a series of intracellular events leading to a generalized "flight or fight" cellular reaction to stress. This reaction is manifested primarily by a hyperdynamic condition with redistribution of the cardiac output to organs involved in locomotion, skeletal muscle, the heart, the adrenal glands, and the brain, to the detriment of "less vital" organs such as the gut and kidneys. Therefore, it is possible that the systemic manifestations of sepsis represent a maldirected effort of the organism to flee from danger. This concept may be useful in our efforts to treat patients with sepsis.

THERAPEUTIC GOALS IN THE TREATMENT OF SEPSIS.

The main therapeutic goal in the treatment of sepsis should be the maintenance of adequate levels of cellular oxygenation in all organs. With the loss of microvascular control during sepsis, capillary beds open, and peripheral vascular resistance decreases. As a consequence, control of cardiac output distribution is lost, resulting in overperfusion of some organs while others receive less than their share of blood flow. Increasing systemic TO_2, primarily by increasing cardiac output, is the mainstay of septic shock therapy. The therapeutic goal is to achieve a level of systemic TO_2 capable of satisfying the O_2 requirements of all organs. Obviously, this is a grossly inefficient way to accomplish this goal, but there are no selective vasoactive agents to redirect cardiac output, although animal experiments suggest that dopexamine hydrochloride, a potent β_2 adrenergic and dopaminergic agonist, may be useful in this respect [51]. Cain and Curtis [52] treated a group of dogs with a combination of dextran and dopexamine after the infusion of *E. coli* endotoxin and found greater gut VO_2 and less gut lactate efflux in that group when compared with a control group treated with dextran only.

MONITORING TISSUE HYPOXIA.

The question remains, how best to monitor the adequacy of tissue oxygenation in sepsis? To answer this question we must have the means to determine the adequacy of tissue oxygenation in those organs most vulnerable to hypoxia, the gastrointestinal tract and the kidney [53]. In the case of the gut, this question has an even greater import. Gut mucosal ischemia may result in the loss of the mucosal barrier, which in turn may promote the translocation of cytokines from the gut lumen into the bloodstream, perpetuating the septic state and leading to the syndrome of multiple systems organ failure [54]. The mucosa is vulnerable to decreases in perfusion or hypoxia because of the close proximity of the arteriole to the venule in the intestinal villus. This creates a countercurrent shunt of O_2 from arteriole to venule resulting in a decreasing PO_2 gradient from base to tip [55].

Among the methods clinically available to gauge the state of aerobic metabolism in a septic patient are the arterial lactate concentration and tonometrically measured gastric mucosal pH.

Arterial Lactate. Arterial lactate has been proposed as a marker of inadequate TO_2 in critically ill patients [56]. Rashkin

et al. [57] used blood lactate as an indicator of hypoxia in patients with ARDS and found that levels of TO_2 below 8 ml/kg/min resulted in decreased survival (14%) and elevated lactate levels. Although an elevated blood lactate usually signifies generalized tissue hypoxia, a normal value is not prima facie evidence of adequate oxygenation in all organs. Arterial or mixed venous lactate concentrations reflect the pooling of blood from several tissue beds, and elevations in venous lactate derived from underperfused organs may be lost in the normality of blood from overperfused tissues. Therefore, it is not surprising that a clear relationship between lactate levels and the energy status of the patient may be difficult to establish, except in obvious cases of systemic hypoperfusion [58].

Lactate production for individual organs is by far a more reliable index of anaerobic metabolism. It can be calculated from measurements of the organ blood flow and the arteriovenous lactate difference. However, the measurement of whole-body lactate production may misrepresent the true state of anoxic tissues because this parameter is influenced by changes in tissue lactate accumulation and washout [59]. Moreover, the kinetics of lactate accumulation in blood are difficult to predict, because lactate is released by the liver in response to circulating catecholamines while simultaneously being metabolized by various organs. Furthermore, the results from recent experimental studies suggest that the relationship between tissue lactate release and regional tissue hypoxia in sepsis may be more complicated than was previously appreciated [60,61,62].

Various investigators have attempted to combine information derived from the TO_2-VO_2 relationship and elevations in blood lactate to test for the existence of covert tissue hypoxia in critically ill patients. Haupt et al [63] noted that VO_2 could be increased in septic patients who also had lactic acidosis by the infusion of colloidal fluids. In a subsequent study [64], these investigators found that the infusion of fluids or blood increased VO_2 in patients with sepsis who also had blood lactate > 2.2 mM. In contrast, dobutamine raised VO_2 in septic patients with or without lactic acidosis. They concluded that fluid or blood infusion could be used to predict the presence of anaerobic metabolism in sepsis, whereas dobutamine was not as useful, because this catecholamine appeared to exert a direct positive effect on metabolic rate. Conversely, Vincent et al [65] noted increases in VO_2 in response to an infusion of 5 μg/kg/min only in a septic group with lactic acidosis. They concluded that, at the dose used, dobutamine does not increase VO_2 in critically ill patients, unless there is coexisting tissue hypoxia evidenced by lactic acidosis. They proposed a short-term trial of dobutamine to disclose an oxygen uptake/supply dependency condition in sepsis. More recently, Ronco et al [66] measured VO_2 by the expired gases method and found no changes in VO_2 in response to increase in TO_2 produced by dobutamine, regardless of the level of lactic acidosis. They concluded that the plasma concentration of lactate does not predict O_2 supply dependency.

Measurements of arterial lactate concentration continue to be useful to the clinician, because a high lactate concentration is compatible with severe global hypoperfusion. However, a normal lactate cannot be taken as evidence of adequate tissue oxygenation.

Gastric Tonometry. The tonometric measurement of intestinal or gastric mucosal pH (pH_i) provides noninvasive metabolic information from an organ exquisitely sensitive to hypoxia. A tonometer consists of a Silastic balloon filled with saline inserted in the gastric or intestinal lumen [67]. After sufficient time is allowed for equilibration between the PCO_2 in the balloon and that of the mucosal layer, the tonometered saline is removed and PCO_2 measured with a standard blood gas analyzer. An approximation to the mucosal pH can be obtained by applying the Henderson-Hasselbalch equation to the tonometrically measured PCO_2 and a simultaneous measurement of arterial HCO_3. Gastric mucosa pH_i is not related to luminal pH, and it is normally greater than 7.30.

Gastric tonometry appears to be an excellent prognostic indicator of survival in critically ill patients. Measurements of gastric pH_i are highly predictive of morbidity [68,69] and of mortality [70,71,72,73]. Patients admitted to an ICU with a low gastric mucosal pH (<7.32), who maintain a low pH_i during the first 12 to 24 hours after admission have a significantly, and substantially, greater risk of death than those who maintained normal pH_i during that time [70,73].

The efficacy of pH_i as a guide to therapy directed toward increases in TO_2 was tested in a multicenter, prospective, randomized study [74] in which gastric pH_i was measured at 6-hour intervals in 260 patients admitted to the ICU with APACHE II scores between 15 and 25. Decreases in pH_i below 7.35 were treated with therapy aimed at increasing TO_2, including fluids, blood transfusions, and the infusion of dobutamine. Patients admitted with pH_i < 7.35 did not benefit from this resuscitation protocol. Conversely, patients admitted with pH_i ≥ 7.35, in whom pH_i-guided resuscitation was actively pursued whenever pH_i decreased below 7.35, had a 58 percent survival rate, compared with 42 percent for the control group (Fig. 181-4).

Gastric tonometry is a new monitoring modality that appears to yield reliable and important information regarding the oxygenation state of an "early warning" organ, the gastric mucosa. Although intense research on tonometry is still under way in defining the utility of this device, the accumulated data provide a compelling case for its routine use in the ICU to monitor tissue oxygenation in patients with sepsis.

GUIDELINES FOR TREATMENT. The successful treatment of septic shock is a formidable task. Given the multiplicity of initiating conditions, as well as the heterogeneity of the patient population, it is impossible to devise a detailed therapeutic algorithm for this condition. Therefore, treatment should be guided by broad guidelines revolving around the principle of adequate tissue oxygenation [75,76,77].

In addition to the use of antibiotics and the removal of an infecting source of cytokines, it is important to assure the ventilation of the lungs by establishing a patent airway. Given the hemodynamic instability of these patients, as well as the frequency with which ARDS is associated with the septic state, most septic patients require mechanical ventilation. The smooth coupling between the patient's respiratory efforts and ventilator-driven breaths, to minimize the work of breathing, cannot be overemphasized.

Hemodynamic and oxygenation parameters must be monitored on a regular basis. The use of pulmonary catheters, pulse oximetry, and gastric tonometry is strongly encouraged. If the patient has relatively normal lungs, the measurement of end-expired PCO_2 may be useful to monitor changes in ventilation. The placement of an arterial line will allow continuous monitoring of the systemic blood pressure and also will serve to sample arterial blood for blood gases. Measurements of TO_2, VO_2, ERO_2, and pH_i every 4 to 6 hours should provide sufficient information on the oxygenation-metabolic state of the patient. Unlike changes in blood pressure and temperature, which can occur abruptly, alterations in tissue oxygenation and metabolism may not be manifested by changes in hemodynamic profile or in end organ function for several hours. This provides the clinician with an early warning period that should be used judiciously if organ failure is to be avoided. Important questions

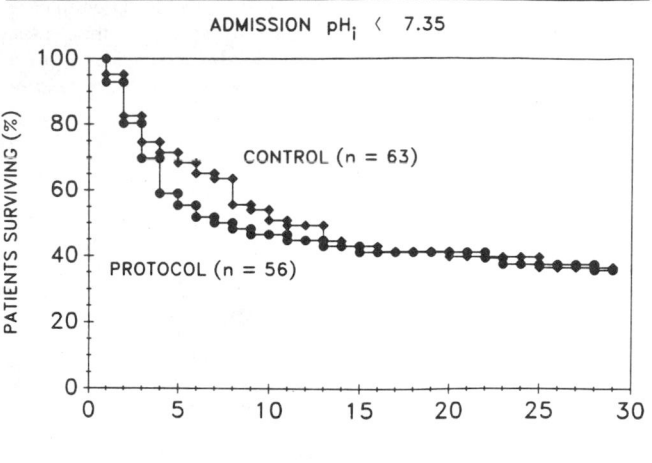

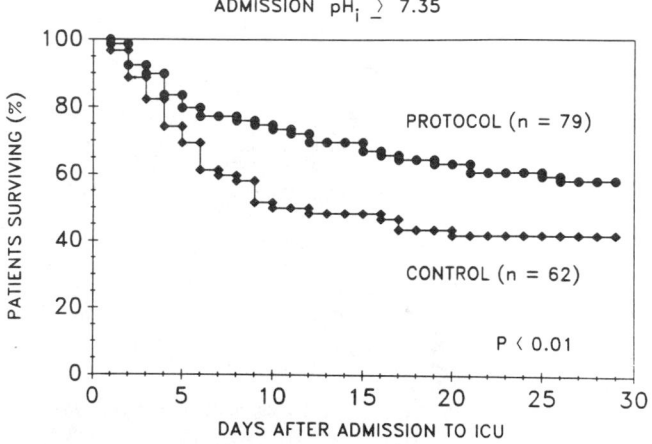

Fig. 181-4. Kaplan-Meier curves showing hospital survival rates for the control and pH_i-guided protocol for patients with initial pH_i < 7.35 (no effect on survival) and those with initial pH_i ≥ 7.35 (16% greater survival in the protocol-treated group). From: Gutierrez G, Palizas F, Doglio G, et al: Gastric intramucosal pH as a therapeutic index of tissue oxygenation in critically ill patients. *Lancet* 339:195, 1992. Reproduced by permission.

that must be answered during that time are: what are the causes of inadequate oxygenation? Are the data correct? Is it a local or a global phenomenon? Is the cardiac output adequate? Is the patient bleeding and hemoglobin falling? Is there a continuing source of cytokine release, such as an abscess, still present?

Until more data become available, pharmacologic increases in TO_2 to supernormal levels should not be attempted in every patient. Many patients will have perfectly adequate perfusion at relatively low levels of TO_2, provided that control of the microvasculature is not impaired. Only in response to increases in arterial lactate concentration, a fall in pH_i, or changes in organ function, such as with deteriorating renal function, should increases in TO_2 be attempted. This can be accomplished by infusing fluids or blood products, or by increasing concentrations of dobutamine. Usually 5 to 10 μg/kg/min is sufficient to reverse a low pH_i [78,79], although greater concentrations may be required in individual cases.

Finally, close attention to the patient's nutritional requirements, frequent changes of intravenous and intraarterial lines, and a high level of nursing care are paramount to improving the patient's chances of survival. These are complex clinical cases and only by the coordinated action of the ICU health care team, composed of physicians, nurses, respiratory therapists, dietitians, etc., can we improve the odds of survival from a syndrome that has become a major cause of death in our intensive care units.

References

1. Messmer K: Blood rheology factors and capillary blood flow, in Gutierrez G, Vincent JL (eds): *Tissue Oxygen Utilization.* Berlin, Springer-Verlag, 1991.
2. Grisham MB, McCord JM: Chemistry and cytotoxicity of reactive oxygen metabolites, in Taylor AE, Matalon S, Ward P (eds): *Physiology of Oxygen Radicals.* Bethesda, American Physiological Society, 1986.
3. Stainsby WN, Otis AB: Blood flow, oxygen tension, oxygen uptake, and oxygen transport in skeletal muscle. *Am J Physiol* 206:858, 1964.
4. Lindbom L, Tuma RF, Arfors KE: Influence of oxygen on perfused capillary density and capillary red cell velocity in rabbit skeletal muscle. *Microvasc Res* 19:197, 1980.
5. Morff RJ: Contribution of capillary recruitment to regulation of tissue oxygenation in rat cremaster muscle. *Microvas Res* 36:150, 1988.
6. Hochachka PW, Guppy M: *Metabolic Arrest and the Control of Biological Time.* Cambridge, Harvard, 1987, pp 10–35.
7. Hochachka PW: Defense strategies against hypoxia and hypothermia. *Science* 231:234, 1986.
8. Gutierrez G, Warley A, Dantzker D: Oxygen delivery and utilization in hypothermic dogs. *J Appl Physiol* 60:751, 1986.
9. Warley A, Gutierrez G: Chronic administration of sodium cyanate decreases O_2 extraction ratio in dogs. *J Appl Physiol* 64:1584, 1988.
10. Nelson DP, Samsel RW, Wood L, et al: Pathological supply dependence of systemic and intestinal O_2 uptake during endotoxemia. *J Appl Physiol* 64:2410, 1988.
11. Nishimura N: Oxygen conformers in critically ill patients. *Resuscitation* 12:53, 1984.
12. Shibutani K, Komatsu T, Kubal K, et al: Critical level of oxygen delivery in anesthetized man. *Crit Care Med* 11:640, 1983.
13. Danek SJ, Lynch JP, Weg JG, et al: The dependence of oxygen uptake on oxygen delivery in the adult respiratory distress syndrome. *Am Rev Respir Dis* 122:387, 1980.
14. Mohsenifar A, Goldbach P, Tashkin DP, et al: Relationship between O_2 delivery and O_2 consumption in the adult respiratory distress syndrome. *Chest* 84:267, 1983.
15. Dorinsky PM, Costello JL, Gadek JE: Relationship of oxygen uptake and oxygen delivery in respiratory failure not due to the adult respiratory distress syndrome. *Chest* 93:1013, 1988.
16. Lorente JA, Renes E, Gomez-Aguinaga MA, et al: Oxygen delivery-dependent oxygen consumption in acute respiratory failure. *Crit Care Med* 19:770, 1991.
17. Gutierrez G, Pohil R: Oxygen consumption is linearly related to O_2 supply in critically ill patients. *J Crit Care* 1:45, 1986.
18. Kreuzer F, Cain S: Regulation of peripheral vasculature and tissue oxygenation in health and disease. *Crit Care Clin* 1:453, 1985.
19. Bihari D, Smithies M, Gimson A, Tinker J: The effects of vasodilation with prostacyclin on oxygen delivery and uptake in critically ill patients. *New Engl J Med* 317:397, 1987.
20. Moreno LF, Stratton HH, Newell JC, et al: Mathematical coupling of data: Correction of a common error for linear calculations. *J Appl Physiol* 60:335, 1986.
21. Annat G, Viale J, Pereival C, et al: Oxygen delivery and uptake in the adult respiratory distress syndrome. *Am Rev Respir Dis* 133:999, 1986.
22. Ronco JJ, Phang PT, Walley JR: Oxygen consumption is independent of changes in oxygen delivery in severe adult respiratory distress syndrome. *Am Rev Respir Dis* 143:1267, 1991.
23. Dantzker DR, Foresman B, Gutierrez G: Oxygen supply and utilization relationships: A reevaluation. *Am Rev Respir Dis* 143:675, 1991.
24. Shoemaker W, Appel P, Kram H, et al: Prospective trial of supranormal values of survivors as therapeutic goals in high risk surgical patients. *Chest* 94:1176, 1988.
25. Russell JA, Ronco JJ, Lockhat D, et al: Oxygen delivery and consumption and ventricular preload are greater in survivors than in nonsurvivors of the adult respiratory distress syndrome. *Am Rev Respir Dis* 141:659, 1990.
26. Gutierrez G, Bismar H, Dantzker D, et al: Comparison of gastric intramucosal pH with measures of oxygen transport and consumption in critically ill patients. *Crit Care Med* 20:451, 1992.
27. Bone RC, Slotman G, Maunder RJ, et al: Randomized double-blind, multicenter study of prostaglandin E_1 in patients with the adult respiratory distress syndrome. *Chest* 96:114, 1989.
28. Tuchschmidt J, Fried J, Swinnery R, et al: Early hemodynamic correlates of survival in patients with septic shock. *Crit Care Med* 17:719, 1989.
29. Kaufman BS, Rackow EC, Falk JL: The relationship between oxygen delivery and consumption during fluid resuscitation of hypovolemic and septic shock. *Chest* 85:336, 1984.
30. Wolf YG, Cotev S, Perel A, et al: Dependence of oxygen consumption on cardiac output in sepsis. *Crit Care Med* 15:198, 1987.
31. Edwards JD, Brown GC, Brown S, et al: Use of survivors' cardiorespiratory values as therapeutic goals in septic shock. *Crit Care Med* 17:1098, 1989.
32. Haupt M, Gilbert E, Carlson R: Fluid loading increases oxygen consumption in septic patients with lactic acidosis. *Am Rev Respir Dis* 131:912, 1985.
33. Gilbert E, Haupt M, Mandanas R, et al: The effect of fluid loading, blood transfusion, and catecholamine infusion on oxygen delivery and consumption in patients with sepsis. *Am Rev Respir Dis* 134:873, 1986.
34. Fink MP, Fiallo V, Stein KL, et al: Systemic and regional hemodynamic changes after intraperitoneal endotoxin in rabbits. *Circ Shock* 22:73, 1987.
35. Nishijima MK, Breslow MJ, Miller CF, et al: Effect of naloxone and ibuprofen on organ blood flow during endotoxin shock in pig. *Am J Physiol* 255:H177, 1988.
36. Weiner DE: Effects of endotoxin on cerebral blood flow in the monkey. *Am J Physiol* 218:160, 1970.
37. Boczkowski J, Vicaut E, Aubier M: In vivo effects of *Escherichia coli* endotoxemia on diaphragmatic microcirculation in rats. *J Appl Physiol* 72:2219, 1992.
38. Rumsey WL, Kilpatrick L, Wilson DF, et al: Myocardial metabolism and coronary flow: effects of endotoxemia. *Am J Physiol* 255:H1295, 1988.
39. Drazenovic R, Samsel RW, Wylam ME, et al: Regulation of perfused capillary density in canine intestinal mucosa during endotoxemia. *J Appl Physiol* 72:259, 1992.
40. Gutierrez G, Lund N, Palizas F: Rabbit skeletal muscle PO_2 during hypodynamic sepsis. *Chest* 99:244, 1991.
41. Kopp KH, Sinagowitz E, Muller H: Oxygen supply of skeletal muscle in experimental septic shock, in Lubbers DW, Acker H, Leniger-Follert E, Goldstick TK (Eds): *Oxygen Transport to Tissue,* Vol V. New York, Plenum, 1984, pp 467–476.
42. Beasley D, Cohen R, Levinsky N: Endotoxin inhibits contraction of vascular smooth muscle in vitro. *Am J Physiol* 258:H1187, 1990.
43. Beasley D: Interleukin 1 and endotoxin activate soluble guanylate cyclase in vascular smooth muscle. *Am J Physiol* 259:R38, 1990.
44. Lamas S, Michel T, Brenner BM, et al: Nitric oxide synthesis in endothelial cells: Evidence for a pathway inducible by TNF-α. *Am J Physiol* 261:C634, 1991.
45. Murad F: Cyclic guanosine monophosphate as a mediator of vasodilation. *J Clin Invest* 78:1, 1986.
46. Kilbourn RG, Jubran A, Gross SS, et al: Reversal of endotoxin-mediated shock by N^G-Methyl-L-arginine, an inhibitor of nitric oxide synthesis. *Biochem Biophys Res Commun* 172:1132, 1990.
47. Kilbourn RG, Gross SS, Jubran A, et al: N^G-Methyl-L-arginine inhibits tumor necrosis factor-induced hypotension: Implications for the involvement of nitric oxide. *Proc Natl Acad Sci USA* 87:3629, 1990.
48. Meyer J, Traber LD, Nelson S, et al: Reversal of hyperdynamic response to continuous endotoxin administration by inhibition of NO synthesis. *J Appl Physiol* 73:324, 1992.
49. Brady AJB, Poole-Wilson PA, Harding SE, et al: Nitric oxide production within cardiac myocytes reduces their contractility in endotoxemia. *Am J Physiol* 263:H1963, 1992.
50. Meyer J, Traber LD, Nelson S, et al: Reversal of hyperdynamic response to continuous endotoxin administration by inhibition of NO synthesis. *J Appl Physiol* 73:324, 1992.

51. Bredle DL, Cain SM: Systemic and muscle oxygen uptake/delivery after dopexamine infusion in endotoxic dogs. *Crit Care Med* 19:198, 1991.

52. Cain SM, Curtis SE: Systemic and regional oxygen uptake and lactate flux in endotoxic dogs resuscitated with dextran and dopexamine or dextran alone. *Circ Shock* 38:173, 1992.

53. Dantzker DR: The gastrointestinal tract. The canary of the body? *JAMA* 270:1247, 1993.

54. Deitch EA, Morrison J, Berg R, et al: Effect of hemorrhagic shock on bacterial translocation, intestinal morphology, and intestinal permeability in conventional and antibiotic-decontaminated rats. *Crit Care Med* 18:529, 1990.

55. Shepherd AP, Kiel JW: A model of countercurrent shunting of oxygen in the intestinal villus. *Am J Physiol* 262:H1136, 1992.

56. Kruse J, Haupt M, Puri V, et al: Lactate levels as predicators of the relationship between oxygen delivery and consumption in ARDS. *Chest* 98:959, 1990.

57. Rashkin MC, Bosken C, Baughman RP: Oxygen delivery in critically ill patients: Relationship to blood lactate and survival. *Chest* 87:580, 1985.

58. Weil MH, Afifi AA: Experimental and clinical studies on lactate and pyruvate as indicators of the severity of acute circulatory failure (shock). *Circulation* 41:989, 1970.

59. Connett RJ, Gayeski TE, Honig CR: Lactate accumulation in fully aerobic working dog gracilis muscle. *Am J Physiol* 246:H120, 1984.

60. Hurtado FJ, Gutierrez AM, Silva N, et al: Role of tissue hypoxia as the mechanism of lactic acidosis during *E. coli* endotoxemia. *J Appl Physiol* 72:1895, 1992.

61. Curtis SE, Cain SM: Regional and systemic oxygen delivery/uptake relations and lactate flux in hyperdynamic, endotoxin-treated dogs. *Am Rev Respir Dis* 145:348, 1992.

62. Hotchkiss RS, Karl IE: Reevaluation of the role of cellular hypoxia and bioenergetic failure in sepsis. *JAMA* 267:1503, 1992.

63. Haupt M, Gilbert E, Carlson R: Fluid loading increases oxygen consumption in septic patients with lactic acidosis. *Am Rev Respir Dis* 131:912, 1985.

64. Gilbert E, Haupt M, Mandanas R, et al: The effect of fluid loading, blood transfusion, and catecholamine infusion on oxygen delivery and consumption in patients with sepsis. *Am Rev Respir Dis* 134:873, 1986.

65. Vincent JL, Roman A, De Backer D, et al: Oxygen uptake/supply dependency. Effect of short-term dobutamine infusion. *Am Rev Respir Dis* 142:2, 1990.

66. Ronco JJ, Fenwick JC, Wiggs BR, et al. Oxygen consumption is independent of increases in oxygen delivery by dubutamine in septic patients who have normal or increased plasma lactate. *Am Rev Respir Dis* 147:25, 1993.

67. Fiddian-Green RG, Gantz NM: Transient episodes of sigmoid ischemia and their relation to infection from intestinal organisms after abdominal aortic operations. *Crit Care Med* 15:835, 1987.

68. Fiddian-Green RG, McGough E, Pittenger G, et al: Predictive value of intramural pH and other risk factors for massive bleeding from stress ulceration. *Gastroenterology* 85:613, 1983.

69. Fiddian-Green RG, Baker S: The predictive value of measurements of pH in the wall of the stomach for complications after cardiac surgery: a comparison with other forms of monitoring. *Crit Care Med* 15:153, 1987.

70. Doglio G, Pusajo J, Egurrola M, et al: Gastric mucosa pH as a prognostic index of mortality in critically ill patients. *Crit Care Med* 19:1037, 1991.

71. Gutierrez G, Bismar H, Dantzker DR, et al: Comparison of gastric intramucosal pH with measures of oxygen transport and consumption in critically ill patients. *Crit Care Med* 20:451, 1992.

72. Marik PE: Gastric intramucosal pH: A better predictor of multiorgan dysfunction syndrome and death than oxygen-derived variables in patients with sepsis. *Chest* 104:225, 1993.

73. Maynard N, Bihari D, Beale R, et al: Assessment of splanchnic oxygenation by gastric tonometry in patients with acute circulatory failure. *JAMA* 270:1203, 1993.

74. Gutierrez G, Palizas F, Doglio G, et al: Gastric intramucosal pH as a therapeutic index of tissue oxygenation in critically ill patients. *Lancet* 339:195, 1992.

75. American College of Chest Physicians/Society of Critical Care Medicine Consensus Conference: Definitions for sepsis and organ failure and guidelines for the use of innovative therapies in sepsis. *Crit Care Med* 20:864, 1992.

76. Guidelines Committee: Society of Critical Care Medicine: Guidelines for the care of patients with hemodynamic instability associated with sepsis. *Crit Care Med* 20:1057, 1992.

77. Fiddian-Green RG, Haglund U, Gutierrez G, et al: Goals for the resuscitation of shock. *Crit Care Med* 21:S25, 1993.

78. Silverman HJ, Tuma P: Gastric tonometry in patients with sepsis: Effects of dobutamine infusions and packed red blood cell transfusions. *Chest* 102:184, 1992.

79. Gutierrez G, Clark C, Brown S, et al: The effect of dobutamine on arterial lactate and gastric mucosal pH in septic patients *Am Rev Respir Dis* (in press).

XIII. Neurologic Problems in the Intensive Care Unit

Section Editor
David A. Drachman

182. An Approach to Neurologic Problems in the Intensive Care Unit

David A. Drachman

Neurologic problems present in the intensive care unit (ICU) in two separate modes: (1) primary neurologic problems, usually under the care of a neurologist or neurosurgeon; and (2) secondary neurologic complications, occurring in patients with other medical or surgical disorders. Only a handful of common clinical situations bring neurologists and patients together in the ICU, although they may be caused by myriad disease states [1]. These situations include:

1. Depressed state of consciousness; coma
2. Altered mental function
3. Required support of respirations or other vital functions
4. Monitoring of increased intracranial pressure (ICP), respirations, state of consciousness
5. Determination of brain death
6. Prevention of further damage to the CNS
7. Management of seizures or status epilepticus
8. Evaluation of a neurologic disease that occurs in the course of a severe medical disease
9. Management of a severe medical disease that develops in the course of a neurologic illness

Patients with primary neurologic problems most commonly have conditions with an identified cause, such as myasthenia gravis, Guillain-Barré syndrome, head trauma, or stroke. Such patients are admitted to the ICU for close observation and management of vital functions, such as respiration or control of ICP. These patients represent the minority of neurologic problems seen in the ICU. Far more frequently the neurologist is called on to evaluate the neurologic complications of medical disease: impairment of consciousness in a patient who has undergone cardiopulmonary resuscitation; development of delirium in an elderly patient with a serious infection; or occurrence of focal neurologic deficits in a patient with a ponderous medical record that reveals long-standing diabetes, renal failure, hypertension, and pulmonary disease.

The questions posed to the neurologic consultant are often imperfectly framed. Background observations regarding the origin, onset, and course of the neurologic abnormality may be unavoidably sparse and the history unavailable. The classic neurologic methodology, which involves a comprehensive history and meticulous examination, is rarely possible in patients encumbered with endotracheal tubes, cardiac monitors, and indwelling arterial and venous lines. For these reasons, the neurologist must adopt special strategies to function effectively in the ICU, focusing sharply on the specific question with which he or she is dealing.

Indications for Neurologic Consultation in the ICU

DEPRESSED STATE OF CONSCIOUSNESS. The patient with the most common of ICU neurologic problems—a depressed state of consciousness, ranging from lethargy to coma—raises a host of questions. Does the patient have a focal brainstem lesion or diffuse cerebral involvement? Is there an anatomic lesion or a metabolic disorder? Have vital brainstem functions been impaired? Is intracranial pressure increased?

The most common primary neurologic causes of depressed consciousness include head trauma, intracranial hemorrhage, and, less commonly, inapparent seizures. The secondary conditions seen most often are metabolic, such as anoxia, drug intoxication, or diabetic acidosis. Sometimes the diagnosis is evident, as in head trauma; other times determination of the cause of depressed consciousness may present a diagnostic challenge, demanding a race against the clock to avoid irreversible changes. In every case, it is crucial to establish whether depressed consciousness is due to intrinsic brainstem damage, increased intracranial pressure, toxins, widespread anoxia-ischemia, or some other less common cause. It is particularly important to sort out rapidly the component(s) that may be treatable.

Examination of the patient with depressed consciousness exemplifies some of the difficulties of neurologic care in the ICU. Details of this examination are described elsewhere [2]. Like the standard neurologic examination, however, it includes evaluation of mental status; cranial nerve functions; motor functions and coordination; reflexes; sensation; and vascular integrity. The observations made must be used to answer the questions posed above, supplemented by appropriate laboratory studies when possible.

A detailed evaluation of memory and cognitive function is rarely possible in patients who are lethargic and never possible in those who are stuporous or comatose. Instead, the physician must estimate the patient's responsiveness. Can the patient say any words? Does the patient open his or her eyes? Does the patient groan in response to a painful stimulus or attempt to remove it in a purposeful way? If not, do any vital functions remain? Is the respiratory pattern disturbed?

Cranial nerve evaluations include determination of vision, done by observing how the patient follows a large object or a light, gazes toward right and left visual fields, or blinks to a threat. Pupillary size and responsiveness to light are assessed. Corneal reflexes, cough, and vibrissal (nasal) reflexes are evaluated. "Doll's eyes" responses are determined by rotation of the head from side to side; if absent, ice water caloric testing can be carried out. Facial movements are assessed in response to painful supraorbital stimuli; the gag reflex is tested in the usual fashion.

Motor function is evaluated as completely as possible. All limbs are observed for spontaneous movement and symmetry as well as tremor or other adventitious movements. If no spontaneous movements take place, a pinch or another noxious stimulus may be used to observe purposeful defensive movements. Decerebrate (i.e., four-limb extensor) and decorticate (i.e., upper limbs flexor, lower limbs extensor) rigidity are observed. Tone is assessed passively for spasticity or rigidity. Deep tendon reflexes are checked in the usual way, working around restraints and intravenous tubing. Grasp, suck, snout, and plantar reflexes are evaluated.

Pain is often the only sensory modality that can be tested.

The physician must determine whether withdrawal from pinch or pinprick is appropriately defensive or (in the lower extremities) merely part of an exaggerated extensor-plantar response with "triple flexion" (flexion at hip, knee, and great toe). Finally, the vascular status is evaluated by listening for bruits over the carotid and subclavian arteries, the vertebral arteries, and the orbits.

Such an examination reveals the patient's state of consciousness, the integrity of brainstem reflexes, and the presence or absence of lateralizing or focal neurologic deficits. The value of the systematic (if limited) neurologic examination cannot be overestimated. For example, in a comatose patient the finding of decerebrate rigidity that points to significant damage at the level of the pons may be more valuable than many laboratory studies, and unilateral weakness of limbs will indicate a focal brain disorder rather than a diffuse metabolic problem.

Neurodiagnostic studies are often critical in the analysis of comatose patients in the ICU, but the patient's immobility and dependence on life support systems present special difficulties. A neuroradiology suite that is distant from the ICU presents additional obstacles. It is always difficult to obtain an MRI scan, CT scan, or arteriogram on a patient who is dependent on a respirator. Paradoxically, in the patients with the most urgent problems, it is often least convenient to obtain the maximum amount of neurodiagnostic information. The decision that a patient is "too sick" to have the crucial study performed is often incorrect. In such desperate cases, risks must be taken to obtain lifesaving information.

Management of the patient with depressed consciousness depends largely on the cause. Techniques for eliminating toxins, reducing intracranial pressure, and maintaining vital functions must be applied, depending on the diagnostic context (see Chap. 183).

ALTERED MENTAL FUNCTION. In patients who remain relatively alert, other organic disorders may affect mental function, producing an often perplexing variety of clinical patterns. These include confusion, delirium, aphasia, and isolated memory impairment. The first question for the physician is whether the patient's abnormal mental function represents a recent change that is part of the present illness or is part of a long-standing problem. It is also critical to note whether the change developed abruptly (e.g., after surgery or cardiac arrest) or if there is no known precipitating event, and whether it is improving, worsening, or stable.

Confusion and delirium are commonly reversible and generally result from metabolic and toxic disorders (see Chap. 184). Persistent aphasia and isolated memory impairment suggest focal damage to the brain, and an anatomic lesion should be sought. Dementia cannot be accurately evaluated in patients who have a depressed state of consciousness or the other mental changes indicated above. When dementia occurs de novo in a patient with a clear sensorium, it may indicate either reversible conditions (e.g., drug-induced, depression-related) or irreversible damage (e.g., diffuse anoxia or ischemia) (see Chap. 185).

Any recent change of mental status in a patient in the ICU requires prompt investigation. Whether it signals worsening of the underlying medical disorder or direct involvement of the brain, the change should be assessed by an experienced neurologist as early in its evolution as possible, before it is complicated by the passage of time, advance of disease, and effects of additional treatments.

SUPPORT OF RESPIRATION AND OTHER VITAL FUNCTIONS. Respiratory support is needed for neurologic patients in two circumstances: loss of brainstem reflex control of respiration, and impairment of effective transmission of reflex impulses to functioning respiratory muscles. Ischemia, anoxia, compression, hemorrhage, and toxic depression may alter brainstem control of respirations, producing characteristic respiratory patterns that depend on the site of damage [2], such as central neurogenic hyperventilation, Cheyne-Stokes or periodic breathing, or apnea. The neurologist should be familiar with use of positive end-expiratory pressure (PEEP) and other respiratory regimens, operation of the hospital's respirators, and endotracheal intubation equipment. Further, the neurologist must understand the neurologic significance of different respiratory patterns, which are as much a part of the ICU neurologic examination as is reflex testing.

Effective transmission of respiratory impulses may be impaired at the cervical spinal cord, anterior horn cells, peripheral nerves, neuromuscular junctions, or muscles of respiration. Cervical traumatic injuries, amyotrophic lateral sclerosis (ALS), Guillain-Barré syndrome, myasthenia gravis, and muscular dystrophy may interfere with breathing at the respective levels noted. Some of these conditions are transitory (e.g., Guillain-Barré syndrome) or treatable (e.g., myasthenia gravis), with complete recovery depending largely on the success of maintaining respiration. Even in incurable conditions (e.g., ALS), sustaining respiration during periods of decompensation, such as respiratory infections, can prolong life significantly.

MONITORING OF INTRACRANIAL PRESSURE AND STATE OF CONSCIOUSNESS. In a number of neurologic disorders extremely close observation is needed to avoid the development of dangerous, often irreversible, further damage to the brain. The most common disorder requiring such monitoring is head trauma. The lethargic patient must be carefully observed for evidence of increasing intracranial pressure due to cerebral edema, intracranial (subdural, epidural, intracerebral) hemorrhage, or both [3].

The need for prompt recognition and early treatment of significantly increased intracranial pressure cannot be overemphasized. Once uncal or tonsillar herniation with brainstem compression has occurred, the consequences of this secondary effect of brain injury may far outweigh the initial damage. (The methods for monitoring intracranial pressure with pressure-detecting catheters or bolts and assessing consciousness and brainstem functions with the Glasgow Coma Scale are described in Chap. 175.)

DETERMINATION OF BRAIN DEATH. With the recognition that death of the brain and brainstem is equivalent to death of the patient, even though the heart continues to beat and respirations are sustained by artificial ventilation, the need to ascertain brain death has become more critical. Early identification of brain death has three important justifications: (1) the use of viable donor organs for transplantation, (2) the termination of the hopeless vigil of a distraught family, and (3) the freeing of ICU beds for salvageable patients. When one or more of these conditions prevails, it is important to determine the occurrence of brain death as soon as possible. When none of the conditions is present, there is no urgency in declaring the patient brain-dead.

It should be emphasized that brain death is specifically a determination that the brain *and* the brainstem are *already* dead, not a prediction that useful recovery is unlikely. It is also true that the longer one waits in even marginally uncertain cases, the clearer the evidence of brain death becomes. (The criteria for brain death are discussed extensively in Chap. 197.) The following mnemonic may be useful in recalling the established criteria for brain death: *CADRE*—*C*oma, *A*pnea, *D*ilated, fixed pupils, *R*eflex (brainstem) absence, and *E*EG silence.

PREVENTION OF FURTHER DAMAGE TO THE CENTRAL NERVOUS SYSTEM. A variety of neurologic disorders have the potential to cause further damage to the CNS. Stroke in evolution, for example, demands immediate efforts to arrest the progress of ischemia by anticoagulation; in the foreseeable future, thrombolytic treatment may reverse the underlying ischemic process, and neuroprotective agents may prevent further damage. Spinal cord compression by tumor urgently requires radiation therapy to avoid irreversible complete cord transection. Although much of neurologic practice involves disorders whose progress is measured in months or years, cerebral ischemia, anoxia, hemorrhage, increased ICP, spinal cord compression, and other acute disorders require prompt institution of treatment to avoid extension of the initial process. It is useful to remember that, as a postmitotic structure, the brain is incapable of regeneration and its ability to survive without a continuing supply of nutrients is measured in minutes. Only in the ICU, with its facilities for careful monitoring and adjustment of therapy, can many of these treatments be successfully carried out.

MANAGEMENT OF STATUS EPILEPTICUS. Unlike simple, brief seizures, status epilepticus threatens lasting deficits or death if not controlled (see Chap. 186). Any patient whose sequential seizures cannot be arrested promptly with routine management (e.g., IV phenytoin) must be observed in the ICU, where therapy ranging up to general anesthesia with artificial ventilation may be required.

EVALUATION OF NEUROLOGIC DISEASE ACCOMPANYING SEVERE MEDICAL DISEASE. Many patients admitted to the ICU for myocardial infarction, subacute bacterial endocarditis, cardiac arrhythmia, pneumonia, renal disease, and other similar disorders develop neurologic signs or symptoms while under treatment for the primary medical problem. Numerous questions are raised: Is the neurologic finding a consequence of the underlying disease, or is it coincidental? Does it demand further investigation at once, or can it wait? Should therapy be changed, or should new therapy be started? These issues demand the attention of the neurologist.

MANAGEMENT OF SEVERE MEDICAL DISEASE ACCOMPANYING NEUROLOGIC ILLNESS. Patients in this group most often develop unrelated medical illness in the setting of a chronic neurologic disorder. The demented patient may suffer a myocardial infarct, or the patient with multiple sclerosis (MS) may develop septicemia. Indirect relationships should be sought. Does the demented patient have multiple cerebral emboli from underlying cardiac disease? Is the MS patient septicemic from a bladder infection due to impaired urinary control? Early recognition of a change in the seriousness of the neurologic patient's condition is often difficult, but it may be critical to a successful outcome.

Prognostic and Ethical Considerations

When severe damage involves the brain, either as a separate neurologic condition or as a secondary consequence of other medical disease, both the physician who requested neurologic consultation and the family often need guidance regarding the probable outcome. There are three critical questions: Will the patient survive? Has irreversible brain damage occurred? What is the likely degree of residual disability?

There are few simple rules that can be applied infallibly to determine the prognosis in, for example, comatose patients, especially early in the course. The most important consideration is often whether irreversible damage has affected crucial areas of the brain, rather than the depth of impairment of consciousness. The patient with glutethimide poisoning, for example, may show no evidence of any neurologic function, yet can recover fully if vital functions are maintained. In contrast, the comatose patient with head trauma resulting in pontine hemorrhage and decerebrate rigidity may have a far worse prognosis. The probability of neurologic recovery generally declines with advancing age, size and location of lesion, and duration of deficit. A number of studies have provided statistical guidelines that are of value in gauging the probability of recovery [4].

Early in the course of coma the physician should not be hasty in abandoning hope and vigorous medical efforts, both to maintain survival and to limit neurologic damage. Late in the course it is important to recognize the outer limits of possible recovery, and judiciously continue life support accordingly. The patient's wishes, expressed in a living will or durable power of attorney for health care (DPAHC) and as interpreted by close, responsible family members ("substituted judgment"), should combine with the physician's prognostic judgment to help determine a medical course of action. Although management in the ICU usually entails the unstinting use of every available means of life support and treatment, there must eventually be a transition either to recovery or to a permanent state of dependence, and the nature and extent of continued treatment should be adjusted accordingly. The technical means of maintaining survival almost indefinitely by the use of extraordinary measures is, of course, now available. It is important for both the physician and the patient's family to consider whether, in the case of a patient with irreversible and severe neurologic damage, they are extending life or prolonging the process of dying [5].

It is clear that neurologic problems abound in the ICU. A successful approach to these disorders requires the physician to recognize the nature of the clinical situation prompting neurologic consultation or admission to the ICU. An analysis of which of the nine types of neurologic clinical situations is being encountered will often guide the physician initially in diagnosis and management.

The following chapters discuss some of the more common neurologic problems encountered in the ICU, with specific attention to management in the ICU and a broader view of the neurologic conditions in general.

References

1. Ropper AH (ed.): *Neurological and Neurosurgical Intensive Care.* New York, Raven Press, 1993
2. Plum F, Posner JB: *The Diagnosis of Stupor and Coma.* 3rd ed. Philadelphia, FA Davis, 1982.
3. Jennett B, Teasdale G: *Management of Head Injury.* Philadelphia, FA Davis, 1981.
4. Levy DE, Caronna JJ, Singer BH, et al: Predicting outcome from hypoxic-ischemic coma. *JAMA* 253:1420, 1985.
5. Wanzer SH, Federman DD, Adelstein SJ, et al: The physician's responsibility toward hopelessly ill patients: A second look. *N Engl J Med* 320:844, 1989.

183. Evaluating the Patient with Altered Consciousness in the Intensive Care Unit

Kevin J. Felice, William J. Schwartz, and David A. Drachman

The spectrum of disease that leads to acute impairment of consciousness is broad; the disorders are potentially life-threatening and may be treatable if recognized early. The clinician evaluating the patient with an altered level of consciousness must do so in a systematic and efficient fashion. The approach consists of: (1) rapidly determining the type of mental status change; (2) administering life support measures where urgently needed; (3) obtaining a detailed history and physical examination directed at determining more precisely the cause of the nervous system disorder; (4) selecting appropriate and informative laboratory studies; and (5) initiating more definitive treatment based on this assessment.

As a practical matter, *consciousness* refers to a state of awareness of self and environment that depends on intact *arousal* and *content* [1,2]. Arousal is the level of attentive wakefulness and readiness to respond to relevant sensory information. Alerting stimuli activate the ascending reticular activating system (ARAS), extending from the superior pons to the thalamus and projecting to multiple cortical areas. Diminished arousal implies dysfunction of either the ARAS or both cerebral hemispheres; lesions of the brainstem sparing the ARAS (e.g., of the medulla) or of only one hemisphere do not affect wakefulness. The content of consciousness is the sum of all intellectual and affective mental activity. Some cognitive functions, such as the use of language, can be localized to specific cortical regions, but they cannot be fully assessed if arousal is also impaired.

In this chapter altered states of consciousness are defined, a systematic approach to bedside evaluation of the comatose patient is presented, and definitive therapies for selected neurologic emergencies are discussed.

Altered States of Consciousness

Neurologists are frequently consulted for patients who appear unconscious, confused, or awake and alert but noncommunicative.

THE PATIENT WHO APPEARS UNCONSCIOUS. These patients lie mostly motionless, usually with their eyes closed and seemingly unaware of their environment. The causes of this condition include normal sleep, depressed consciousness, psychogenic coma, locked-in state, and brain death.

Sleep. The normal unconsciousness of sleep is characterized by prompt reversibility on threshold sensory stimulation and maintenance of wakefulness following arousal. The degree of stimulation required depends on the stage of sleep (stage IV non-REM sleep is the deepest) and the sensory stimulation used.

Depressed Consciousness. Consciousness is deemed depressed when suprathreshold sensory stimulation is required

for arousal and wakefulness cannot be maintained unless the stimulation is continuous [1,2]. Responsible specific lesions involve the ARAS and/or cerebral hemispheres bilaterally, the former by brainstem destruction or compression from masses situated in other compartments and the latter by multifocal insults or unilateral lesions with associated mass effect. In addition, a wide array of metabolic derangements, toxic effects, or diffuse injuries may depress consciousness by affecting the ARAS, cerebral hemispheres, or both. The spectrum of depressed states—lethargy, hypersomnolence, obtundation, stupor and coma—is defined by the level of consciousness observed on examination. The etiologies are diverse (Table 183-1), with the degree of depression dependent on the nature of the insult, its duration, and the location and extent of the brain injury.

The first signs of brain dysfunction may be mild and barely noticed. The patient may be described as lethargic or hypersomnolent prior to progressing to a more depressed state. *Hypersomnolent* patients maintain arousal only with vigorous and continuous sensory stimulation; while awake, however, they may be oriented and make appropriate responses. The most common cause of hypersomnolence in the hospital is sleep deprivation, mostly iatrogenic, especially in the around-the-clock care setting of the intensive care unit (ICU). Patients with discrete diencephalic or midbrain tegmentum lesions may also present with hypersomnolence [3,4]. Since these lesions affect the ARAS and spare the cerebral hemispheres, content of consciousness is usually preserved. Rostral extension of a midline lesion may involve thalamic structures (especially the dorsomedial nuclei) and cause difficulties with the ability to store new memories. Other mesencephalic structures may be affected and account for the presence of abnormalities of pupillary function, internuclear ophthalmoplegia, and third nerve dysfunction.

Obtunded patients usually can be aroused by light stimuli but are mentally dulled and unable to maintain wakefulness. *Stuporous* patients can be aroused only with vigorous noxious stimulation. While awake, neither obtunded nor stuporous pa-

Table 183-1. Differential Diagnosis of Depressed Consciousness

I. Depressed consciousness with lateralizing signs of brain disease:
   Brain tumor, cerebral hemorrhage, cerebral thrombosis, cerebral embolism, concussion, subdural or epidural hemorrhage, brain abscess, hypertensive encephalopathy

II. Depressed consciousness with signs of meningeal irritation:
   Meningitis, subarachnoid hemorrhage, leptomeningeal carcinoma or lymphoma

III. Depressed consciousness without lateralizing or meningeal signs:
   Alcohol, barbiturate, or opiate intoxication: carbon monoxide poisoning, anoxia, hypoglycemia, diabetic coma, uremia, hepatic coma, hypercapnia, nonconvulsive status epilepticus

Adapted from RD, Victor M: *Principles of Neurology:* New York, McGraw-Hill, 1989, p 287.

tients demonstrate a normal content of consciousness (if testable), but both may display purposeful movements, as in attempts to ward off painful stimuli or remove intravenous lines.

Patients in *coma* are unarousably unresponsive to suprathreshold sensory stimulation, including noxious stimulation strong enough to arouse a deeply sleeping patient but not so strong as to cause physical injury. Although the patient usually lies motionless, movements such as stereotyped, inappropriate postures (decerebration and decortication) and spinal cord reflexes (triple flexion and Babinski responses) may occur. Whatever the etiology, the duration of coma is typically no longer than 2 to 4 weeks, after which one of three conditions supervenes: arousal to full or partial recovery, persistent vegetative state, or death.

Psychogenic Coma. Patients in psychogenic coma appear comatose but have clinical and laboratory evidence of wakefulness [1]. Psychogenic unresponsiveness is diagnosed by demonstrating that the patient is more aware of the environment than he or she seems. Psychogenic coma may be suggested by active resistance or rapid closure of the eyelids, pupillary constriction to visual threat, fast phase of nystagmus (i.e., a saccade) on oculovestibular or optokinetic testing, and avoidance of self-injury. Electroencephalographic (EEG) alpha waves that attenuate with eye opening are inconsistent with coma or sleep. Psychiatric conditions that may be associated with psychogenic coma are conversion reactions secondary to hysterical personality, severe depression, or acute situational reaction; catatonic schizophrenia; dissociative or "fugue" states; severe psychotic depression; and malingering.

Locked-In State. The locked-in state is a paralysis without loss of consciousness [5]. Since the most common cause of this state is destruction of the base of the pons, the patient is completely paralyzed except for muscles subserved by midbrain structures (i.e., vertical eye movements and blinking). Consciousness is preserved because the ARAS is located in the tegmentum of the pons, dorsal to the damaged area. Less frequent etiologies of the syndrome are acute polyneuropathy (Guillain-Barré syndrome), acute poliomyelitis, toxins that block transmission at the neuromuscular junction, and myasthenia gravis. Some patients who have survived chronically in this state have been taught to communicate by moving their eyes and blinking in Morse code.

Brain Death. Brain death is the irreversible destruction of the brain, with the resulting total absence of all cortical and brainstem function, although spinal cord reflexes may remain [6,7]. It is not to be confused with incomplete brain damage with a poor prognosis or with a vegetative state, conditions in which some function of vital brain centers still remains. In brain death, pupils are midposition and round (not oval), and apnea persists even when arterial carbon dioxide tension (PCO_2) is raised to levels that should stimulate respiration. Table 183-2 summarizes the guidelines used in the United States. The signs of brain death simulated by drug intoxications do not persist longer than 36 hours in most cases. The EEG and blood flow studies (^{99m}Tc scan or arteriography) are not mandatory but may be useful in cases of extensive brainstem destruction. As an example, a patient with absent brainstem function after basilar artery thrombosis may continue to exhibit cortical activity on the EEG and carotid arterial blood flow.

THE PATIENT WHO APPEARS CONFUSED. *Confusion* is a general term used for patients who fail to think with customary speed, clarity, or coherence. The causes of this condition in-

Table 183-2. Criteria for Brain Death

An individual with irreversible cessation of all functions of the entire brain including the brainstem is dead.
1. *Cessation* is recognized when evaluation discloses findings of (a) and (b):
    a. Cerebral functions are absent.
       There must be "cerebral unresponsivity and unreceptivity. . . ."
    b. Brainstem functions are absent.
       These include "pupillary light, corneal, oculocephalic, oculovestibular, oropharyngeal, and respiratory reflexes." Apnea is tested with a nasal cannula delivering oxygen and demonstrating failure of respiratory effort with $PaCO_2$ >60 mm Hg. "Spinal cord reflexes may persist after death. True decerebrate posturing or seizures are inconsistent with the diagnosis of death."
2. *Irreversibility* is recognized when evaluation discloses findings of (a) and (b) and (c):
    a. The cause of coma is established and is sufficient to account for the loss of brain functions.
    b. "The possibility of recovery of any brain function is excluded. . . ."
    c. The cessation of all brain functions persists for an appropriate period of observation or trial of therapy—. . . confirmation of clinical findings by EEG is desirable when objective documentation is needed to substantiate the clinical findings . . . complete cessation of circulation to the normothermic adult brain for more than 10 minutes is incompatible with survival of brain tissue . . . absent cerebral blood flow, in conjunction with the clinical determination of cessation of all brain functions for at least 6 hours, is diagnostic of death. . . ."

Complicating Conditions
A. Drug and metabolic intoxication
   "Drug intoxication is the most serious problem in the determination of death. . . . In cases where there is any likelihood of sedative presence, toxicology screening for all likely drugs is required. If exogenous intoxication is found, death may not be declared until the intoxicant is metabolized or intracranial circulation is tested and found to have ceased . . . before irreversible cessation of brain functions can be determined, metabolic abnormalities should be considered and, if possible, corrected."
B. Hypothermia
   Criteria for reliable recognition of death are not available in the presence of hypothermia (<32.2°C core temperature).
C. Children
   "The brains of infants and young children have increased resistance to damage and may recover substantial functions even after exhibiting unresponsiveness on neurologic examination for longer periods than do adults. Physicians should be particularly cautious in applying neurologic criteria to determine death in children younger than five years. . . .
D. Shock
   "Physicians should also be particularly cautious in applying neurologic criteria to determine death in patients in shock because the reduction in cerebral circulation renders clinical examination and laboratory tests unreliable. . . ."

$PaCO_2$ = arterial carbon dioxide tension; EEG = electroencephalogram.
Source: Reference 7, as adapted from *Defining Death: Medical, Legal, and Ethical Issues in the Determination of Death*. President's Commission for the Study of Ethical Problems in Medicine and Biomedical and Behavioral Research, US Government Printing Office, 1981. With permission.

clude an acute confusional state; dementia; inapparent seizures; and receptive aphasia.

Acute Confusional State. When the cerebral hemispheres are insulted by toxic, metabolic, anoxic, structural, or infectious processes the patient may appear acutely confused [8]. Both poor arousal and an abnormal content of consciousness may contribute to the clinical presentation, and the etiologies are legion (Table 183-3).

Patients with *clouded consciousness* are easily distracted or startled by environmental stimuli. Their processing of information is slow and tedious, arousal fluctuates from drowsiness to hyperexcitability, and poor attention span impairs recall and recent memory. If sensorial clouding becomes more advanced, sensory input is increasingly misinterpreted, daytime drowsiness alternates with nocturnal agitation, disorientation for place and time becomes apparent, and repeated prompting is required for a response to even the simplest commands.

Delirious patients manifest confusion with psychomotor overactivity, agitation, autonomic instability, and often visual hallucinations. Hyperexcitability may alternate with periods of drowsiness or relative lucidity. Signs of autonomic overactivity include pupillary dilatation, diaphoresis, tachycardia, and hypertension. Patients with delirium do not sleep, sometimes for periods of several days; the success of treatment may be judged by the development of normal sleep. Delirium tremens, the most serious consequence of ethanol withdrawal, is perhaps the best known example of this state.

In *beclouded dementia* confusion is superimposed on an underlying subacute or chronic cognitive disorder. The preexisting cerebral dysfunction may be a mental retardation, dementia, or the deficits from a vascular, neoplastic, or demyelinative process. In some cases, the underlying disorder is not diagnosed until the confusion appears secondary to an intercurrent illness (e.g., sepsis, congestive heart failure, surgical procedures, anemia, drug overdose, or intolerance).

Dementia. Patients with dementia have subacute or chronic intellectual dysfunction unaccompanied by a reduction in arousal [9]. The patient exhibits a decline in multiple cognitive functions, including memory, spatial orientation, personality, abstract thinking, and insight. The ability to carry out testing requires relative preservation of attention and language comprehension. The causes of dementia include degenerative processes (Alzheimer's disease, Pick's disease, Huntington's disease), metabolic and nutritional disorders (hypothyroidism, pellagra, vitamin B_{12} deficiency), infectious diseases (subacute spongiform encephalopathy, AIDS dementia, neurosyphilis, chronic meningitis, progressive multifocal leukoencephalopathy), cerebrovascular disorders (multiinfarct dementia, anoxiaischemia), hydrocephalus with normal or increased intracranial pressure, and toxins.

Inapparent Seizures. Patients with nonconvulsive status epilepticus may appear disoriented, episodically unresponsive, or alternately lucid and confused; the EEG shows continuous or frequent epileptiform discharges [10,11,12]. Careful observation may alert the clinician to seizure phenomena, such as episodic staring, eye deviation or nystagmoid jerks, facial or hand clonic activity, and automatisms. The syndrome may be the result of a generalized (absence) status or a complex partial status. Absence seizures are rare in adults and are diagnosed by a characteristic 3 Hz spike and wave activity on an EEG. Complex partial status is the more common form seen in the ICU and may not be preceded by a history of complex partial seizures. The origin of the abnormal focal discharge may be from the temporal, frontal, or occipital lobes, and the EEG pattern during

Table 183-3. Classification of Acute Confusional States (ACS)

I. ACS not associated with focal or lateralizing neurologic signs and normal CSF
  A. Metabolic disorders
    1. Hepatic encephalopathy
    2. Uremia
    3. Hypercapnia
    4. Hypoglycemia
    5. Diabetic ketotic coma
    6. Porphyria
    7. Hypercalcemia
  B. Infectious disorders
    1. *Septicemia
    2. *Pneumonia
    3. *Typhoid fever
    4. *Rheumatic fever
  C. Drug intoxication
    1. Opiates
    2. Barbiturates
    3. Tricyclic antidepressants
    4. Other sedatives
    5. *Amphetamines
    6. *Anticholinergic medications
  D. Abstinence states (i.e., withdrawal states)
    1. *Alcohol (delirium tremens)
    2. *Barbiturates
    3. *Benzodiazepines
  E. States that reduce cerebral blood flow or oxygen content
    1. Hypoxic encephalopathy
    2. Congestive heart failure
    3. Cardiac arrhythmias
  F. Situational psychoses (diagnoses)
    1. *Postoperative psychosis
    2. *Posttraumatic psychosis
    3. *Puerperal psychosis
    4. *ICU psychosis
II. ACS associated with focal or lateralizing neurologic signs and/or abnormal CSF
  A. Cerebrovascular disease or space-occupying lesions (especially of the right parietal, inferofrontal, and temporal lobes)
    1. *Ischemic infarct
    2. *Neoplasm
    3. *Abscess
    4. *Hemorrhage (intraparenchymal, subdural, epidural)
    5. Granuloma
  B. Infectious disorders
    1. *Meningitis
    2. *Encephalitis
  C. *Subarachnoid hemorrhage
  D. *Cerebral contusion and laceration
III. ACS sometimes associated with focal or lateralizing neurologic signs
  A. *Postconvulsive delirium
  B. Acute hydrocephalus
  C. Nonconvulsive status epilepticus
  D. Nonketotic diabetic coma

*The disorders preceded by an asterisk may be associated with signs of psychomotor overactivity or delirium.
ACTH = adrenocorticotropic hormone; CSF = cerebrospinal fluid.
Adapted from Adams RD, Victor M: *Principles of Neurology,* New York, McGraw-Hill, 1989, p 329.

the ictus is variable. A benzodiazepine, such as diazepam or lorazepam, may eliminate the discharge and improve the patient's confusion.

Receptive Aphasia. Patients with receptive aphasia often appear confused because they have a disorder of language comprehension [8]. The patient is awake and alert but unable to comprehend written or verbal commands despite voluminous (fluent) spontaneous speech. Paraphasias may be present (especially when the patient is asked to name objects) and consist of either inappropriately substituted words or nonsensical jargon. The responsible lesions are located in the dominant temporoparietal cortex and are often associated with subtle focal neurologic signs, including mild pronator drift of the right hand, right homonymous hemianopsia or superior quadrantanopsia, and right-sided sensory loss; gross hemiparesis is usually not found. Rarely, a "pure word deafness" (auditory agnosia) prevents comprehension of verbal commands, but reading comprehension and writing or copying are normal.

THE PATIENT WHO APPEARS AWAKE AND ALERT BUT NONCOMMUNICATIVE.

Although sensory stimulation may arouse these patients, they seem unable or unwilling to speak. The causes of this condition include mutism, akinetic mutism, and the persistent vegetative state.

Mutism. Mutism is a manifestation of many clinical conditions, including aphonia, anarthria, oral-lingual apraxia, and aphasia. Only in aphasia, however, is written expression also impaired (i.e., agraphia).

Aphonia due to paralysis of the vocal cords and anarthria due to paralysis of the articulatory muscles are usually evident clinically in patients who are unable to make sounds but who mouth words appropriately. Oral-lingual (facial) apraxia is a disorder of learned mouth movements (e.g., speaking, blowing kisses, sucking through a straw, protruding the tongue to command) seen with isolated and discrete lesions involving the facial area of the dominant motor cortex [13].

Patients with expressive aphasia are unable to communicate normally by verbal or written language [8]. Nonfluent (Broca's) aphasia with diminished "telegraphic" output is usually intensely frustrating to the patient; occasionally, singing his or her words, rather than merely saying them, improves speech. Lesion location differs depending on whether comprehension is also affected or whether comprehension and repetition of words are relatively preserved or lost. At the least, the dominant frontal cortex is involved, and some degree of right hemiparesis is usually present.

Akinetic Mutism. Patients with akinetic mutism appear alert and exhibit sleep-wake cycles, but they show little evidence of cognitive function and do not meaningfully interact with the environment [1]. Brainstem function is intact, and the patient may open his or her eyes to verbal stimuli or track moving objects. There is a paucity of movement even to noxious stimulation, despite little evidence of corticospinal or corticobulbar damage. Akinetic mutism is associated with large bilateral lesions of the basomedial frontal lobes, small lesions of the paramedian reticular formation in the posterior diencephalon and midbrain, and subacute communicating hydrocephalus.

Persistent Vegetative State. Patients in a persistent vegetative state are also akinetic and mute but lack outward manifestations of any significant brain activity other than reflex responses [1,14]. These may include decerebrate or decorticate posturing, deep tendon reflexes, Babinski or triple flexion reflexes, yawning, and so on. The term is usually reserved for the patient who

has recovered only to this extent from coma due to a severe anoxic, metabolic, or traumatic brain injury. Neuropathologic findings may include cortical laminar necrosis, cerebellar Purkinje cell loss, and necrosis of hippocampal cortex, but relative sparing of brainstem structures.

Bedside Evaluation of the Comatose Patient

Coma in the ICU is a medical emergency. The goal of each evaluation is to identify and treat promptly (if applicable) the cause of the comatose state; even if no definitive treatment is available, general and neurologic support are necessary. A neurologic consultation should be obtained early; the practice of obtaining imaging studies prior to a careful and systematic examination is often counterproductive when it delays focused evaluation and treatment. The proper approach requires (1) immediate administration of life support measures, (2) completion of a general physical examination, (3) performance and interpretation of the neurologic examination, (4) selection of ancillary tests, and (5) institution of definitive treatment, based on the above observations.

INITIAL MEASURES. As in all emergencies, vital signs, respiration, and circulation are first stabilized and monitored; the comatose patient usually requires an endotracheal tube for respiratory support and airway protection. A large-bore intravenous line is started and blood is drawn for a complete blood count, glucose, electrolytes (including Ca^{2+}), BUN, creatinine, liver transaminases, and a toxicology screen. Arterial blood is obtained for determination of oxygen tension (PO_2), PCO_2, and pH. If there is any doubt about the etiology of coma, 100 mg of thiamine, 50 mg of glucose, and 0.4 mg of naloxone are administered intravenously.

GENERAL PHYSICAL EXAMINATION. In addition to the usual complete examination, several points deserve special attention [2]. Severe hypothermia (rectal temperature ≤32°C or 89.6°F) may cause coma (as in elderly patients exposed to the cold) or provide clues to other etiologies (e.g., overwhelming sepsis, drug or alcohol intoxication, hypothyroidism, hypoglycemia, Wernicke's encephalopathy) [15]. Severe hyperthermia may result from intracranial causes, including infection and anterior hypothalamic or pontine destruction. Meningeal signs (e.g., nuchal rigidity) may be absent in deeply comatose patients, even in the presence of overwhelming bacterial meningitis. *This sign should never be sought if cervical spine fracture or dislocation is suspected.*

The skin should be thoroughly inspected for signs of trauma. Basilar skull fractures may be signaled by blood behind the ear (Battle's sign), cerebrospinal rhinorrhea, or otorrhea. Orbital fractures may cause bleeding into periorbital tissues ("raccoon eyes").

The breath odor may suggest metabolic derangement or intoxication. The spoiled fruit odor of diabetic coma, the uriniferous odor of uremia, and the musty fetor of hepatic encephalopathy sometimes can be recognized. Although the odor of alcohol is usually noted, its presence does not rule out superimposed structural causes of coma (e.g., subdural hematoma), and its absence does not rule out intoxication with odorless spirits (e.g., vodka).

Respiratory patterns in comatose patients are distinctive [1].

Bilateral hemispheric or diencephalic disturbances as well as systemic disorders may lead to periodic breathing in which increasing and then decreasing breaths (crescendo-decrescendo) alternate with apnea (Cheyne-Stokes respirations). Lesions of the midbrain-pontine tegmentum may give rise to tachypnea and a respiratory alkalosis unresponsive to oxygen (central neurogenic hyperventilation), but this is much less common than hyperpnea due to low PO_2, metabolic acidosis, or a primary respiratory alkalosis (e.g., salicylate poisoning). Lesions of the inferior pons may be associated with 2- to 3-second pauses following full inspiration (apneustic breathing). Compressive or intrinsic lesions of the medulla may cause chaotic breathing of varying rate and depth (Biot breathing). Complete brainstem destruction results in apnea unresponsive to elevated PCO_2.

NEUROLOGIC EXAMINATION. The goal of the neurologic examination in the comatose patient is to determine the location of the lesion (ARAS or bilateral cerebral hemispheres) and its etiology (structural, causing destruction or compression of brain substance; toxic, metabolic, anoxic, or traumatic, affecting the nervous system in a diffuse or multifocal manner; subarachnoid blood or infection; or nonconvulsive status epilepticus). A critical part of this determination is the history, and heroic efforts to locate family members, witnesses, and medication lists are almost always rewarded. For example, truly sudden coma in a healthy person suggests drug intoxication, intracranial hemorrhage, meningoencephalitis, or an unwitnessed seizure.

Neurologic assessment must include a description of the level of consciousness; examination of the pupils; direct ophthalmoscopy; observation of spontaneous and induced ocular movements; elicitation of the corneal reflex; and tests of motor system function (including spontaneous and induced limb movements, asymmetries of tone, deep tendon reflexes, and pathologic reflexes). The importance of repeat examinations to document the temporal course of the patient's condition cannot be overemphasized.

Level of Consciousness. The level of consciousness is determined first by observing the patient undisturbed for several minutes. Any spontaneous (e.g., yawning, sneezing) or responsive (e.g., to ventilator noise) movements or postures are noted. A battery of graduated sensory stimuli is applied (whispered names; shouted names; loud noise; visual threat; noxious stimulation by supraorbital compression, sternal rub, nail bed compression, or medial thigh pinch) and the response recorded (e.g., opens eyes, squeezes eyes shut, blinks symmetrically to visual threat, nods, turns head, groans, grimaces, purposefully withdraws, displays stereotyped posturing). Such careful documentation allows serial assessments of subtle changes over time by multiple examiners.

Pupils. The pupils are examined for size, equality, and reactivity to light. Normal pupils confirm the integrity of a circuit involving the retina, optic nerve, midbrain, third cranial nerve, and pupillary constrictors. A strong flashlight and magnifying glass are usually necessary, and lighting conditions should be noted.

Symmetrically small, light-reactive pupils (miosis) are normally seen in elderly and sleeping patients. Opiates, organophosphates, pilocarpine, phenothiazines, and barbiturates produce small pupils that may appear to be unreactive to light, whereas a large lesion of the pons (i.e., hemorrhage) characteristically produces tiny "pinpoint" pupils. Symmetrically large pupils (mydriasis) that do not react to light suggest midbrain damage, but they may also be seen following resuscitation

when atropine has been used (in this case, the pupils do not constrict to 1% pilocarpine) [16], in cases of anoxia, following pressor doses of dopamine [17], and often in amphetamine or cocaine intoxication. Bilaterally fixed and midposition pupils indicate absent midbrain function, although severe hypothermia [15], hypotension, or intoxication with succinylcholine [18] or glutethimide [19] must be ruled out.

Pupillary asymmetry (anisocoria) suggests neurologic dysfunction if it is of recent onset, the inequality is greater than 1 mm, and the degree of anisocoria changes with ambient lighting [20]. When the *larger* pupil is sluggishly reactive or fixed to light (but the contralateral consensual response is spared), uncal herniation due to an ipsilateral hemispheric mass compressing the third cranial nerve against the petroclinoid ligament must be considered. Unilateral pupillary dilatation may also indicate a mass in the cavernous sinus, aneurysm of the posterior communicating artery, focal seizure, or topical atropine. On the other hand, with Horner's syndrome the affected pupil is *smaller*. In this condition the pupillary asymmetry is increased in darkness and the smaller pupil is associated with partial ptosis of the upper eyelid, straightening of the lower eyelid, and facial anhidrosis. It may be caused by damage to sympathetic fibers from the brainstem to the cervical spinal cord, the thorax or the carotid artery.

Direct Ophthalmoscopy. Direct ophthalmoscopy may be limited by miosis or cataracts, but *the pupils should never be pharmacologically dilated without clear documentation* or if the patient's condition is uncertain or unstable. Obscuration of the disc margins, absent venous pulsations, and flame-shaped hemorrhages suggest early papilledema from an intracranial mass or systemic hypertension [21]. Subhyaloid and vitreous hemorrhages are observed in the patient with subarachnoid hemorrhage or suddenly increased intracranial pressure.

Ocular Movements. Assessment of ocular movements begins by observing for tonic deviation of the eyes at rest [1]. The eyes may deviate toward the side of a lesion in the motor cortex (away from the hemiparetic limbs) but usually can be induced to cross the midline (a gaze preference). The eyes deviate away from the side of a pontine lesion (toward the hemiparetic limbs) and cannot be moved across the midline (a gaze paralysis). A seizure focus in the frontal (area 8) or supplementary motor (area 6) cortex can drive the eyes or cause nystagmoid jerks contralaterally (toward the side of the convulsing limbs) [22]. Tonic upward eye deviation may be seen after anoxia [23], and tonic downward deviation may be seen in thalamic hemorrhage, midbrain compression, and hepatic encephalopathy.

Spontaneous eye movements may have a localizing value. Roving eye movements (slow and random, usually conjugate and horizontal) and periodic alternating ("ping-pong") gaze (cyclic, conjugate excursions to the extremes of lateral gaze every 2–3 seconds) [24] are found in patients with intact brainstem function. Ocular bobbing consists of a rapid conjugate downward jerk followed by a slow upward drift (rate and rhythm are variable) and suggests a lesion in the posterior fossa, especially if horizontal eye movements are impaired [25]. The reverse movement, ocular dipping (slow downward, fast upward) can be seen after anoxia and status epilepticus [26]. Conjugate spasmodic eye movements, rotating the eyes upward for minutes or longer (oculogyric crisis), in some patients may be an untoward effect of neuroleptic medications.

If spontaneous eye movements are absent or restricted to a particular direction, reflex movements should be tested by oculocephalic (doll's eyes) and oculovestibular (caloric) stimulation [1,27]. Full eye movements induced by these maneuvers confirm the integrity of the brainstem tegmentum from the medullary-pontine junction to the midbrain. *Oculocephalic testing is never done in patients with suspected cervical spine fracture or dislocation.* The maneuver is performed by holding the patient's eyelids open and briskly rotating the head from one side to the other (for horizontal eye movements) and from flexion to extension (for vertical eye movements). In comatose patients with an intact brainstem, the eyes deviate to the side opposite the direction of head movement. If the oculocephalic response is not obtained or the movements are limited or asymmetric, the oculovestibular reflex must be tested. *This is never done until the tympanic membrane is examined and seen to be intact.* The patient's head is elevated to 30 degrees above horizontal and up to 120 ml of ice water is instilled slowly in the external auditory meatus with a large syringe and attached Teflon catheter. Each ear is tested separately for horizontal eye movements, with a 5-minute interval between right and left ears. In awake patients (or those in psychogenic coma), nystagmus with the fast phase away from the irrigated ear is induced. In comatose patients with an intact brainstem, a tonic conjugate eye deviation toward the irrigated ear is seen; a defective response implies brainstem failure. Vertical eye movements can be induced by irrigating both ears simultaneously with cold water (eyes deviate downward) and with warm (44°C) water (eyes deviate upward). Absent or deranged responses can be caused, in addition to various brainstem lesions, by previous vestibular (labyrinthine end-organ) lesions, vestibulosuppressant drugs (e.g., benzodiazepines, antihistamines, anticholinergics), hepatic encephalopathy, and neuromuscular blockers (e.g., succinylcholine). An ophthalmoplegia after intravenous phenytoin is well known [28].

Corneal Reflex. The corneal reflex is obtained by lightly touching the limbus of the cornea with a fine material (wisp of cotton, rolled corner of tissue paper). Both eyes should blink to unilateral stimulation, confirming the integrity of a circuit involving the fifth cranial nerve, trigeminal sensory and facial motor nuclei in the pons, and both seventh cranial nerves. An absent blink on the stimulated side with an intact contralateral (consensual) response indicates ipsilateral motor damage.

Motor System. The examination of the motor system identifies whether limb movements are appropriate and purposeful or inappropriate and stereotyped. Left-right asymmetries or worsening of the motor response over time must be carefully noted. Appropriate movements include spontaneous turning in bed, drawing up the sheets, crossing the legs modestly, or rapid withdrawal (especially abduction) from noxious stimulation. Inappropriate movements include spontaneous or induced flexion-internal rotation of the arms with extension of the legs (decortication) or extension-adduction of all limbs (decerebration); whether flexor or extensor postures are induced depends partly on the position of the limbs [29]. These responses may occur occasionally in toxic-metabolic coma [30,31], but are more common with anatomic brainstem lesions. Facial grimaces or groans despite absent motor responses suggest that sensory pathways are grossly intact. Flexion of the leg at the hip, knee, and ankle (triple flexion response) is a spinally mediated exaggerated Babinski reflex that may persist in brain death.

Interpretation of the Neurologic Examination

In general, focal neurologic signs suggest a structural cause of coma. Nevertheless, focal weakness is not unknown in hypo-

glycemia, hyponatremia, and hepatic and uremic encephalopathies, and continuous focal motor seizures (epilepsia partialis continua) may be a presenting sign of the hyperglycemic nonketotic hyperosmolar state [32]. Focal signs due to preexisting deficits may deceive even the ablest clinician. For example, if a patient with an old hemiplegia due to a cerebral infarction develops generalized seizures from a new metabolic imbalance, apparently focal convulsions of the nonplegic limbs might falsely suggest a structural lesion of the intact cerebral hemisphere contralateral to the previously infarcted one. Other "false localizing" signs include sixth nerve palsies (due to transmitted increased intracranial pressure), visual field cuts (due to compression of the posterior cerebral artery), and hemiparesis ipsilateral to a third nerve palsy (due to compression of the contralateral cerebral peduncle against the tentorium [Kernohan's notch]).

Conversely, a nonfocal examination does not invariably indicate toxic-metabolic coma. Symmetric neurologic dysfunction may be caused by meningoencephalitis, subarachnoid hemorrhage, bilateral subdural hematomas, or thrombosis of the superior sagittal sinus. Multifocal seizures, myoclonus, asterixis, or fluctuation of the examination do suggest a toxic or metabolic etiology, although periodic increases in intracranial pressure (plateau waves) and nonconvulsive seizures may lead to a waxing and waning mental status.

A preserved pupillary light reflex—even in deep coma with absent oculovestibular and motor responses—suggests a toxic or metabolic etiology. It is important to note that the pupils may be unreactive to light in severe hypothermia, deep barbiturate coma (the patient is usually apneic and hypotensive if the pupils are fixed), and glutethimide overdose. In addition, an expanding posterior fossa mass (e.g., cerebellar hemorrhage) may present with early signs of pontine compression and small, light-reactive pupils [33].

A useful rule is that toxic-metabolic coma usually has incomplete but symmetric dysfunction of neural systems affecting many levels of the neuraxis simultaneously, while retaining the integrity of other functions at the same levels. Structural coma is characterized by regionally restricted anatomic defects [1]. For example, toxic-metabolic coma might present with intact pupillary reactivity and corneal reflexes but an absence of both horizontal (pontine) and vertical (midbrain) reflex eye movements to oculovestibular testing. Such a presentation would be inconsistent with coma from a structural cause.

Ancillary Tests

A computed tomographic (CT) scan without contrast infusion demonstrates intracranial hemorrhage and hydrocephalus; contrast enhancement may be required for suspected infectious or neoplastic masses. The CT scan does not reliably rule out inflammation, subarachnoid blood, or early ischemia, and of course toxic-metabolic coma and psychogenic unresponsiveness are not diagnosed by imaging. It is not always logistically possible to perform magnetic resonance imaging (MRI) on patients in the ICU, but this technology can demonstrate early ischemia and encephalitis and produces excellent images of the posterior fossa, brainstem, and craniovertebral junction. The cerebrospinal fluid (CSF) must be examined if meningoencephalitis is suspected or if subarachnoid blood is not visualized on the CT scan. Occasionally, a sterile CSF pleocytosis follows status epilepticus [34]. Of all the tests available, only EEG provides a physiologic marker of brain function and may be helpful in nonconvulsive status epilepticus and psychogenic coma and for documenting (but not primarily establishing) brain death by the presence of electrocerebral silence.

Initiation of Emergency Treatment

Definitive treatment of altered consciousness depends on the underlying pathophysiologic process, but urgent therapeutic interventions may be required in life-threatening conditions or to prevent further central nervous system insult. Meticulous nursing care (fluid replacement; oxygenation and prevention of aspiration; nutrition; corneal protection; and conscientious skin, bowel, and bladder care) is essential. Unnecessary sedation should be avoided.

INCREASED INTRACRANIAL PRESSURE. The treatment of increased intracranial pressure secondary to space-occupying masses, hydrocephalus, or edema is discussed in Chapters 9 and 164. Intracranial hypertension is harmful because cerebral arterial perfusion fails and the brain parenchyma shifts (herniates) into adjacent compartments, compressing and damaging the brain further [35]. Medical management includes raising the head of the bed to 45 degrees, ensuring minimal stimulation (visitors, noise, suctioning), fluid restriction, mechanical hyperventilation to a PCO_2 of 25 mm Hg, and osmotic diuresis with mannitol (1 gm/kg of a 20% solution IV over 10–30 minutes followed by $\leq$0.5 gm/kg every 4 hours) to maintain serum osmolarity at 300 to 320 mOsm per kilogram. Corticosteroids (dexamethasone, 10 mg IV followed by 4–6 mg every 6 hours) are usually indicated for the edema associated with primary or metastatic tumors.

STATUS EPILEPTICUS. The treatment of status epilepticus is discussed in Chapter 186. Phenytoin (20 mg/kg IV at a rate of 50 mg/min) is usually effective, but occasionally phenobarbital (up to 20 mg/kg IV) may be required. Diazepam has only a brief anticonvulsant action and may cause respiratory depression or hypotension (especially with barbiturates), but it may be given initially to control seizure activity. Diazepam is not indicated in patients with one or a few isolated seizures.

SUBARACHNOID HEMORRHAGE. The treatment of subarachnoid hemorrhage due to ruptured aneurysm, arteriovenous malformation, or trauma is discussed in Chapter 148. Preoperative complications include rebleeding, vasospasm, hydrocephalus, and mass effect; initial therapy includes mannitol and dexamethasone for increased intracranial pressure, antihypertensive agents if indicated, phenobarbital for sedation and seizure prophylaxis, and stool softeners and volume expansion for vasospasm [36]. The Ca^{2+} channel inhibitor nimodipine (60 mg every 4 hours) may also reduce the incidence and severity of ischemic deficits from vasospasm [37].

INTRACRANIAL INFECTIONS. The treatment of intracranial infections is discussed in Chapter 87. Initial therapy for common bacterial pathogens should include broad-coverage antibiotics and should not be postponed while waiting for a CT scan. We prefer ceftriaxone (1 gm IV every 12 hours) and penicillin G (12–15 million units IV in 4 to 6 divided doses per day for 10–14 days). Gentamicin is added for suspected *Listeria* and Enterobacteriaceae, and a penicillinase-resistant penicillin should be used for suspected *Staphylococcus aureus*. Prompt therapy

of herpes simplex encephalitis (acyclovir 10 mg/kg IV three times per day) may be the deciding factor for the patient's possible recovery to a functionally independent existence [38].

Conclusions

Altered consciousness is common in patients in the ICU. A systematic and efficient approach is required to determine the location of the responsible lesion(s) and cause(s) and to allow institution of definitive therapies.

References

1. Plum F, Posner JB: *The Diagnosis of Stupor and Coma*. Philadelphia, FA Davis, 1982.
2. Fisher CM: The neurological examination of the comatose patient. *Acta Neurol Scand* 45(suppl 36):1, 1969.
3. Caplan LR: "Top of the basilar" syndrome. *Neurology* 30:72, 1980.
4. Bogousslvsky J, Regli F, Uske A: Thalamic infarcts: Clinical syndromes, etiology, and prognosis. *Neurology* 38:837, 1988.
5. Patterson JR, Grabois M: Locked-in syndrome: A review of 139 cases. *Stroke* 17:758, 1986.
6. President's Commission for the Study of Ethical Problems in Medicine and Biomedical and Behavioral Research: *Defining Death: Medical, Legal, and Ethical Issues in the Determination of Death*. Washington, DC, US Government Printing Office, 1981.
7. Black PMcL: Guidelines for the diagnosis of brain death, in Ropper AH, Kennedy SF (eds): *Neurological and Neurosurgical Intensive Care*. 2nd ed. Rockville, MD, Aspen, 1988, p 323.
8. Adams RD, Victor M: *Principles of Neurology*. 4th ed. New York, McGraw-Hill, 1989.
9. Strub RL, Black FW: *Neurobehavioral Disorders: A Clinical Approach*. Philadelphia, FA Davis, 1988.
10. Tomson T, Svangorg E, Wedlund JE: Nonconvulsive status epilepticus: High incidence of complex partial status. *Epilepsia* 27:276, 1986.
11. Simon RP, Aminoff MJ: Electrographic status epilepticus in fatal anoxic coma. *Ann Neurol* 20:351, 1986.
12. Cascino GD: Nonconvulsive status epilepticus in adults and children. *Epilepsia* 34(suppl 1):S21, 1993.
13. Geschwind N: The apraxias: Neural mechanisms of disorders of learned movement. *Am Sci* 63:188, 1975.
14. Jennett B, Plum F: Persistent vegetative state after brain damage. *Lancet* 1:734, 1972.
15. Fischbeck KH, Simon RP: Neurological manifestations of accidental hypothermia. *Ann Neurol* 10:384, 1981.
16. Thompson HS, Newsome DA, Loewenfeld IE: The fixed dilated pupils: Sudden iridoplegia or mydriatic drops? A simple diagnostic test. *Arch Ophthalmol* 86:21, 1971.
17. Ong GL, Bruning HA: Dilated fixed pupils due to administration of high doses of dopamine hydrochloride. *Crit Care Med* 9:658, 1981.
18. Tyson RN: Simulation of cerebral death by succinylcholine sensitivity. *Arch Neurol* 30:409, 1974.
19. Brown DG, Hammill JF: Glutethimide poisoning: Unilateral pupillary abnormalities. *N Engl J Med* 285:806, 1971.
20. Glaser JS: *Neuro-ophthalmology*. Philadelphia, JB Lippincott, 1990.
21. Neetens A, Smets RM: Papilledema. *Neuro-ophthalmology* 9:81, 1989.
22. Wyllie E, Ludes H, Morris HH, et al: The lateralizing significance of versive head and eye movements during epileptic seizures. *Neurology* 36:606, 1986.
23. Keane JR: Sustained upgaze in coma. *Ann Neurol* 9:409, 1981.
24. Stewart JD, Kirkham TH, Mathieson G: Periodic alternating gaze. *Neurology* 29:222, 1979.
25. Mehler MF: The clinical spectrum of ocular bobbing and ocular dipping. *J Neurol Neurosurg Psychiatry* 51:725, 1988.
26. Ropper AH: Ocular dipping in anoxic coma. *Arch Neurol* 28:297, 1981.

27. Leigh RJ, Hanley DF, Munschauer FE, et al: Eye movements induced by head rotation in unresponsive patients. *Ann Neurol* 15:465, 1984.
28. Spector RH, Davidoff RA, Schwartzman RJ: Phenytoin-induced ophthalmoplegia. *Neurology* 26:1031, 1976.
29. Barolet-Romana G, Larson SJ: Influence of stimulus location and limb position on motor responses in the comatose patient. *J Neurosurg* 61:725, 1984.
30. Greenberg DA, Simon RP: Flexor and extensor postures in sedative drug-induced coma. *Neurology* 32:448, 1982.
31. Seibert DG: Reversible decerebrate posturing secondary to hypoglycemia. *Am J Med* 78:1036, 1985.
32. Singh BM, Strobos RJ: Epilepsia partialis continua associated with nonketotic hyperglycemia: Clinical and biochemical profile of 21 patients. *Ann Neurol* 8:155, 1980.
33. Cuneo RA, Caronna JJ, Pitts L, et al: Upward transtentorial herniation. *Arch Neurol* 36:618, 1979.
34. Devinsky O, Nadi NS, Theodore WH, et al: Cerebrospinal fluid pleocytosis following simple, complex partial, and generalized tonic-clonic seizures. *Ann Neurol* 23:402, 1988.
35. Rockoff MA, Kennedy SK: Physiology and clinical aspects of raised intracranial pressure, in Ropper AH, Kennedy SF (eds): *Neurological and Neurosurgical Intensive Care.* 2nd ed. Rockville, MD, Aspen, 1988, p 9.
36. Solomon RA, Fink ME: Current strategies for the management of aneurysmal subarachnoid hemorrhage. *Arch Neurol* 44:769, 1987.
37. Pickard JD, Murray GD, Illingworth R, Effect of oral nimodipine on cerebral infarction and outcome after subarachnoid hemorrhage: British Aneurysm Nimodipine Trial. *Br Med J* 298:636, 1989.
38. Skoldenberg B, Forsgren M, Alestig K, et al: Acyclovir versus vidarabine in herpes simplex encephalitis: Randomized multicenter study in consecutive Swedish patients. *Lancet* 2:707, 1984.

184. Metabolic Encephalopathy

Paula Ravin and Frank Walsh

Metabolic encephalopathy is a general term used to describe any process that affects global cortical function by altering the biochemical function of the brain. It is the most common cause of altered mental status in an ICU setting, either medical or surgical, and is also one of the most treatable. Early recognition of metabolic encephalopathy is, therefore, critical to management of the ICU patient. It should be suspected in any individual who suffers from delirium or decreased alertness, decreased awareness of the surroundings, or cognitive dysfunction (see Chap. 183). Patients with metabolic encephalopathy may progress slowly from a state of delirium to one of depressed consciousness or may develop depressed consciousness initially without any antecedent signs (e.g., in hypoglycemia). In mild cases it is easily mistaken for fatigue or psychogenic depression. More severe cases may develop into stupor or coma and are life-threatening.

The patients most at risk for developing a metabolic encephalopathy are those with single or multiple organ failure, the elderly (older than 60 years), those receiving multiple central nervous system (CNS) toxic agents, and those with severe nutritional deficiencies, such as cancer patients and alcoholics. Other risk factors include infection, temperature disorders (both hypothermia and fever), chronic degenerative neurologic or psychiatric diseases, such as dementia or schizophrenia, and endocrine disorders.

The typical patient with metabolic encephalopathy appears to be asleep, with normal posturing of the limbs and stable vital signs. The respiratory pattern varies depending on the level of cerebral depression, though it is usually slow and regular. Other unusual patterns of respiration are key to specific types of metabolic encephalopathies (see below). Waxing and waning arousal, spontaneous or with external stimuli, is characteristic and occurs over hours, often resulting in conflicting reports regarding the patient's neurologic status. Increased motor activity, including asterixis, myoclonus, tremors, rigidity, and muscle spasms, is also seen with many different types of metabolic encephalopathies. Finally, seizures—either focal or generalized—are a frequent occurrence in acute metabolic encephalopathy and should be recognized as not representing a primary epileptiform disturbance (Table 184-1).

Other disorders that can be confused with metabolic encephalopathy include brain tumors, encephalitis, meningitis, closed head trauma, and brainstem cerebrovascular events. Brain tumors are usually recognizable because they produce focal neurologic deficits, such as hemiplegia or hemianopsia, as do traumatic lesions of the brain and cortical strokes. Hypoglycemic encephalopathy can also present focally (see below). Brainstem stroke due to thrombosis of the basilar artery can be deceptive, because there may be a gradual progression of signs and symptoms over several hours rather than a sudden presentation. Table 184-2 outlines some of the cardinal differences between brainstem stroke and metabolic encephalopathy.

Evaluation

The evaluation of a patient with metabolic encephalopathy is straightforward but should be performed expeditiously to prevent permanent neurologic sequelae.

Table 184-1. Patient Profile in Metabolic Encephalopathy

Gradual onset over hours
Progressive if untreated
Waxing and waning level of consciousness
Patient treated with multiple CNS-acting drugs
Patient with organ failure, postoperative state, electrolyte disturbance, endocrine disease
No evidence of brain tumor or stroke on neurologic exam—usually nonfocal (except hypoglycemia)
Sometimes heralded by seizures—focal or generalized
Increased spontaneous motor activity—restlessness, asterixis, myoclonus, tremors, rigidity, etc.
Abnormal blood chemistries, blood gases, anemia
Usually normal CNS imaging studies
Generalized EEG abnormalities—slowing, triphasic waves
Gradual recovery once treatment is initiated

Table 184-2. Depressed State of Consciousness: Brainstem Stroke Versus Metabolic Encephalopathy

Clinical evaluation	Brainstem CVA	Metabolic disorder
Acute onset of mental status changes (minutes)	+	− ($\overline{x}$ hypoglycemia)
Waxing and waning mental status	+	+
Small, normoactive pupils	+ (pons, medulla)	+
Horner's or unilateral dilated pupil	+	−
Skew deviation of pupils	+	−
Unilateral sensory loss to noxious stimuli	+	−
Periodic respirations	−	+
Apneustic, ataxic breathing	+	−
Hemiplegia or paraplegia	+	− ($\overline{x}$ hypoglycemia)
Nonfocal motor exam	−	+

CVA = cerebrovascular accident

GENERAL EXAMINATION. The general examination should include testing for arousability, observation of the patient's respiratory pattern without stimulation, and measurement of the pulse and blood pressure. Auscultation of the heart to check for arrhythmia and of the carotids to rule out bruits is performed before beginning a detailed neurologic examination.

NEUROLOGIC EXAMINATION. The neurologic examination (see Chap. 158) must begin with careful scrutiny of the patient's mental status; a mild behavior change is the earliest manifestation of metabolic encephalopathy (Table 184-3). Lack of attentiveness to the surroundings and a paucity of spontaneous speech give the patient the appearance of being apathetic or withdrawn. Specific questioning for orientation and simple mental abilities, however, reveals mild confusion and a variable level of alertness. The"mini-mental status exam" is useful for grading the patient'scognitive level sequentially, although in patients with impaired consciousness this is invariably unreliable [1]. The patient's posture may suggest the etiology of the encephalopathy: Decorticate or decerebrate postures are consistent with brainstem lesions due to stroke, tumor, or other causes of increased intracranial pressure. Hemiplegia also suggests a focal lesion, such as a stroke or a mass (i.e., intracerebral hemorrhage or tumor), but may be seen in hypoglycemia as well.

Respiratory Pattern. Changes in the respiratory pattern are the next most important findings for the diagnosis of metabolic encephalopathy and also provide a clue as to its etiology. In the mildly confused patient breathing may be normal, but lethargic or mildly obtunded patients tend to hyperventilate, with brief spells of apnea. This is due to transient lowering of the carbon dioxide tension PCO_2 below 15 mm Hg without the appropriate CNS drive to breathe more rapidly at a lower tidal volume. After 12 to 30 seconds of apnea, the cycle of hyperventilation appears again, resulting in a pattern of periodic respirations [2]. Hypoventilation is usually seen with depressant drug overdoses, chronic pulmonary failure, and metabolic alkalosis of any cause. Cheyne-Stokes respiration, a rhythmic cycle of waxing and waning hyperpnea-apnea, is another pattern occasionally seen in metabolic encephalopathy caused by uremia or hypoxia, but more commonly this indicates bilateral structural lesions of the cortex. Other neurogenic respiratory patterns, such as constant or "central" hyperpnea, cluster breathing, and ataxic breathing, are signs of brainstem dysfunction due to structural damage or suppression by barbiturates. These changes are seen only when the patient is stuporous or comatose.

Pupillary Responses. Pupillary responses are helpful in distinguishing between a metabolic encephalopathy and a structural lesion producing depressed consciousness. As a rule, the pupils are small, symmetric, and responsive to light in metabolic causes of obtundation or coma. Noteworthy exceptions are anticholinergic poisoning (1-methyl-4phenyl-1,2,36 tetrahydropyridine [MPTP], atropine, scopolamine), which produces dilated, sluggish pupils, and glutethimide (Doriden) poisoning, which results in unequal mid-sized to large sluggish or fixed pupils [3].

Ocular Movements. Ocular movements are usually unaffected by metabolic encephalopathy; the eyes are generally at the midline or slightly deviated outward at rest. Doll's eye maneuvers produce conjugate deviation of the eyes opposite to the direction of head rotation. As the level of brainstem suppression progresses to coma, oculocephalic and caloric responses are blunted and may disappear completely, especially with an overdose of sedative drugs. In the face of hyperpnea and decerebrate rigidity, the preservation of ocular responses is a useful sign pointing to a primary metabolic cause of coma.

Increased Motor Activity. Increased motor activity is characteristic of most metabolic encephalopathies and is quite varied in appearance; tremors, myoclonus, asterixis, and rigidity may be seen.

Tremors. Tremors are rhythmic, involuntary oscillatory movements seen in all limbs and often exaggerated during voluntary movement. Tremors occur most often in early hypoglycemic encephalopathy, thyrotoxicosis, acute uremia, chronic dialysis encephalopathy, hypercapnia, and drug intoxication—especially with sympathomimetic agents.

Myoclonus. Myoclonus is multifocal, appearing as brief shocklike contractions of large muscle groups. Synchronous my-

Table 184-3. Evaluation for Metabolic Encephalopathy

Neurologic exam	Mental status
	Pupillary responses
	Oculomotor responses
	Respiratory pattern
	Motor activity, strength
	DTRs, plantar responses
	Sensory exam—pin, light touch
Initial labs	BS, electrolytes, LDH, ALT, AST, ammonia
	BUN, creatinine, WBC/diff, Hgb, Hct, blood gases
EEG	
Neuroimaging	Head CT or MRI
± Lumbar puncture, toxicology screens, serum and urine osmolality, psychiatric exam	

DTR = deep tendon reflexes, BS = blood sugar; LDH = lactate dehydrogenase; BUN = blood urea nitrogen; WBC = white blood cell count; Hgb = hemoglobin; Hct = hematocrit; ALT = alanine aminotransferase; AST = aspartate aminotransferase.

oclonic jerks in all limbs can be seen in any patient who is slipping in and out of a drowsy state—also known as sleep onset myoclonus. This is often seen in patients on large doses of narcotics. Multifocal asynchronous myoclonus, in contrast, is seen in hypoxic-ischemic encephalopathy, chronic hepatic failure of all types, uremia, pulmonary failure, and intoxication with methaqualone and psychedelic agents [4].

Asterixis. Asterixis is a "flapping" movement produced by unsustained muscle contraction against gravity. There is rhythmic extension and flexion of the outstretched limb that disappears at rest. The most common setting for this is in hepatic encephalopathy of any cause, frequently with flapping of the hands, feet, jaw, and tongue. Subacute uremia and pulmonary failure produce asterixis accompanied by myoclonus, which may produce a picture of almost constant muscle twitching.

Rigidity. Rigidity or generalized muscle spasms are states of constant muscle contraction seen when the degree of metabolic encephalopathy is more severe and leads to stupor or coma. This can be the result of end-stage hepatic failure, hypoglycemia (< 25 mg/dl) lasting more than a few minutes, acute renal failure, hyperthermia, and hypothermia below 92°F rectally. Rigidity with dystonic posturing is a clue to amphetamine or phenothiazine poisoning. Choreoathetosis, on the other hand, occurs in chronic hepatic failure, subacute bacterial endocarditis (SBE), posthypoxic insult, Reye's syndrome, chronic dialysis, chronic hypoglycemia, and chronic hypoparathyroidism.

Abnormal Autonomic Responses. Abnormal autonomic responses in metabolic encephalopathy may demand intervention and can cause significant morbidity and mortality. Hypotension, which is unresponsive to volume expansion, points to intoxication with barbiturates or opiates, myxedema, or Addisonian crisis. In this setting, occult sepsis must always be ruled out before treating for specific metabolic derangements. Fever and leukocytosis may be absent in very debilitated patients. Examination of urine, blood counts and coagulation factors, blood and sputum cultures, chest radiograph, and a lumbar puncture are essential to rule out infection. If there remains any doubt about the cause of hypotension, empirical antibiotics, Naloxone for possible opiate overdose, IV glucose (1 ampule), and pressor agents should be added to other supportive measures while the cause is being investigated.

Seizures. Seizures are another significant symptom of metabolic encephalopathy, especially in uremia, hypoglycemia, pancreatic failure, and various types of metabolic acidosis (e.g., ethylene glycol, salicylates). They occur most often at the onset of the metabolic disturbance (e.g., as the BUN is climbing acutely) and as a preterminal expression of severe neuronal injury in a comatose patient. Management of seizures is typically ineffective until the underlying cause is corrected. In renal failure, however, one-third to one-half of the standard loading doses of phenytoin or phenobarbital may be all that is needed to control seizures. The interictal electroencephalogram (EEG) serves as a guideline to the need for continued treatment once the encephalopathy has cleared or has become chronic and stable. A persistent focus of epileptiform activity warrants further investigation and anticonvulsant therapy.

Laboratory Investigation. The laboratory investigation of patients with delirium or coma is crucial in defining the cause of a metabolic encephalopathy. Blood tests for glucose, electrolytes, and blood gases should be drawn immediately, along with a panel of hepatic function tests (ALT, AST, lactate dehydrogenase, ammonium), BUN, and creatinine. Serum and urine osmolality, cerebrospinal fluid (CSF) analysis, serum magnesium and phosphate levels, and specific hormone levels may be needed to define the cause of encephalopathy further. Careful review of all medications taken prior to and during hospitalization may direct attention to specific toxicology screens of blood and urine. The general toxicology screen should be sensitive to opiates, benzodiazepines, caffeine and salicylates, theophylline, barbiturates, and alcohol. Additional drug levels should be ordered if their use is known or suspected (e.g., digoxin, cocaine, phenytoin). If there has been a *sudden* change in mental status, a bolus of 25 gm of glucose should be administered intravenously without hesitation, to avoid prolonged hypoglycemia.

Electroencephalogram. In general, the EEG in metabolic encephalopathy is abnormal; background slowing is the most common pattern found (< 9 Hz). Other patterns can also be useful in identifying or corroborating the cause of encephalopathy. Slow activity prominent frontally, with deep "triphasic" waves (range 2–4 Hz), is characteristic of hepatic encephalopathy but can also be seen in renal failure [5]. Spreading of the slow activity toward the occipital leads is a sign of deepening coma in this setting. Bursts of high-voltage activity amidst normal background frequencies are also a sign of diffuse metabolic disturbance. More important, the EEG in a patient with an acute encephalopathy of unknown cause may reveal subclinical (electrical) status epilepticus, warranting urgent and aggressive treatment. This is particularly common in the case of alcoholics and diabetics who are at risk for multiple CNS insults.

Neuroimaging. Computed tomography (CT) and magnetic resonance imaging (MRI) scans of the brain are often crucial when there is rapid deterioration of mental status without focal signs or an obvious metabolic cause, such as hypoglycemia. Most mass lesions, such as subdural hematomas or brain tumors, are evidenced clinically by a rostrocaudal progression of neurologic signs. The initial picture may be nonfocal with obtundation, but this is followed sequentially by flexor or extensor posturing on one or both sides, then the loss of pupillary or caloric responses. Later, medullary respiratory patterns or bradycardia appear. A noncontrast head CT or MRI scan is definitive in many cases but does not always distinguish a brainstem stroke. When the diagnosis of a metabolic cause of impaired consciousness is not clearly evident, early consultation by a neurologist is necessary.

Lumbar Puncture. A lumbar puncture is also indicated when there is a rapid onset of encephalopathy, especially with a fever, headache, or meningismus. Occult subarachnoid hemorrhage, infection, or elevated intracranial pressure may be found in the absence of funduscopic changes or a clear-cut clinical history. Ideally the lumbar puncture should be performed atraumatically with a small (22-gauge) spinal needle and a simultaneous sample of serum obtained to compare glucose levels in the blood and CSF.

Etiology

HEPATIC FAILURE. The clinical onset of hepatic encephalopathy may be subtle, with a blunting of affect and lethargy, or dramatic (10–20% of patients), with mania or an agitated delirium [6]. It is easy to recognize hepatic encephalopathy in an individual with the obvious stigmata of chronic liver disease, such as ascites, varices, or jaundice. In those with inapparent liver disease, the mental changes may also appear after an additional metabolic demand on the liver. Such stressors are a high-protein meal, gastrointestinal (GI) bleeding with increased blood absorption from the gut, or ingestion of hepatically metabolized drugs [7]. Sedatives and acetazolamide are particularly offensive in this situation.

Asterixis is the next most common clinical sign, appearing in all limbs, jaw, and tongue. As the patient progresses into a coma, this may be replaced by general spasticity and decorticate or decerebrate posturing to stimulation. Plantar responses and gaze-evoked ocular movements are variable at this stage; pupillary responses are always preserved. Oculocephalic and oculovestibular (caloric) responses remain until the patient is moribund. Hyperventilation is another consistent sign of hepatic encephalopathy and results in respiratory alkalosis. The ocular, pupillary, and respiratory patterns above help distinguish severe hepatic encephalopathy from space-occupying lesions of the cortex and brainstem.

The pathophysiology of hepatic coma is not certain, but it is thought to be caused by portacaval shunting of neurotoxic substances. These putative toxins include excess ammonia, "large molecules" normally excluded by the blood-brain barrier [8], increased water, and the "false" neurotransmitter octopamine [9]. Hypoglycemia as a result of decreased glycogen stores in the liver may complicate the CNS picture.

The serum transaminases are usually elevated two- to threefold, and serum ammonia is at least in the high normal range once the patient is lethargic, with a linear correlation thereafter between higher lab values and lower cognitive state. The CSF remains normal until the serum bilirubin exceeds about 5 mg per deciliter, which tints the fluid yellow. The EEG characteristically shows progressive slowing from the frontal to the occipital leads as coma deepens. Triphasic waves are seen in most cases but are not pathognomonic.

Therapy for hepatic encephalopathy is directed toward decreasing the amount of toxic substances being shunted to the brain. Neomycin and lactulose help sterilize and flush the gut. A protein-restricted diet and exclusion of hepatically cleared drugs decrease the metabolic load while intravenous glucose effectively maintains the serum glucose level. Neurologic recovery then depends on the capacity of the liver to regenerate at least 25 percent of its full function. With prolonged or repeated bouts of hepatic coma there may be residual signs of basal ganglia dysfunction evidenced by chorea, postural tremors, or a parkinsonian picture (acquired hepatocerebral degeneration) [10].

REYE'S SYNDROME. This is a unique and quite morbid form of acute hepatic encephalopathy seen in children, usually aged 1 to 10 years. Reye's syndrome occurs in the clinical setting of an acute viral infection, such as chicken pox or influenza A or B, plus aspirin therapy [11]. Approximately 4 to 7 days after the viral symptoms start, the child becomes irritable, with vomiting and sometimes headache or blurred vision. An agitated delirium, combativeness, and progressive obtundation rapidly ensue over hours, followed by hyperventilation, pupillary dilatation, and generalized seizures. Later in the course, decerebrate rigidity, extensor Babinski responses, and papilledema may develop as well.

The pathology of Reye's syndrome includes infiltration of the liver and other visceral organs with small fat droplets, and diffuse cerebral edema. In cases complicated by severe hypoglycemia and seizures, anoxic damage with laminar necrosis of the cerebral cortex is also found. The cause of these changes is presumed to be mitochondrial poisoning, but the pathogenic

agent has not yet been identified. Acetylsalicylic acid has consistently been implicated in this cellular damage. This has led to the standard practice of prescribing acetaminophen instead of aspirin for viral symptoms in children, thereby reducing the incidence of Reye's syndrome [12].

The differential diagnosis relies on measurement of liver function and a high index of suspicion in the appropriate setting. The serum transaminases rise three- to fivefold in the first 48 hours and the serum ammonia is dramatically increased, sometimes to the range of 200 μg per deciliter. Hypoglycemia is also an early sign, aggravating the lactic acidosis and respiratory alkalosis seen later in the course.

Treatment for Reye's syndrome is directed toward diminishing the cerebral edema, controlling seizures, and providing adequate electrolytes and glucose for support while the liver is effectively "shut down" with respect to oxidative metabolism. This is best achieved in an ICU with a standard protocol for Reye's syndrome using intracranial pressure (ICP) monitoring and mannitol or glycerol for reduction of ICP [13].

The prognosis in recent years has improved markedly; mortality and morbidity are now 10 to 20 percent, as opposed to 40 to 50 percent in the 1970s. Factors that contribute to a poor outcome are age less than 1 year, serum ammonia levels greater than five times normal at their peak, and prothrombin time greater than 20 seconds. Other negative prognostic indicators are renal failure and a very rapid progression of liver failure in the first 48 hours. Early intervention is the key to a good outcome neurologically and systemically.

RENAL FAILURE. Uremic encephalopathy may develop acutely, be superimposed on chronic renal insufficiency, or occur as a consequence of chronic dialysis. It is often a complication of systemic diseases that independently affect the CNS—collagen vascular disease, malignant hypertension, drug overdoses, diabetes, or bacterial sepsis. The clinical picture is initially variable and does not correlate directly with measures of renal dysfunction, such as BUN and creatinine.

The first sign of encephalopathy in uremia is delirium or a decrease in level of consciousness; hyperventilation and increased motor activity follow as the patient becomes obtunded. There is also a high frequency of generalized convulsions at the outset and of metabolic acidosis with a low serum bicarbonate. The motor component is prominent in many patients with multifocal myoclonus, hypertonus or asterixis, and tremors together, producing a picture of "twitch-convulsive," as if the patient had fasciculations [14]. While oculomotor function and pupillary responses are normal, deep tendon reflexes may be asymmetric and focal weakness often occurs, with shifting hemipareses during a single period of encephalopathy. The variability of focal motor signs helps rule out a structural lesion but does not obviate the need to look for multifocal seizures in a patient with overt twitching and depressed consciousness.

Studies of the effect of uremia on neuronal function have not been successful in demonstrating a direct correlation between the cognitive state and BUN levels, nor a correlation with any other biochemical or electrolyte markers [15]. The EEG, while becoming slower with higher levels of BUN, also does not correlate with mental status changes, especially in chronic uremia [16]. Hence, the pathophysiology of uremic encephalopathy is not known.

The major diagnostic differential to consider is between a hypertensive crisis and uremic encephalopathy, since malignant hypertension often leads rapidly to renal failure and neurologic signs. Evidence of papilledema, retinal vasospasm, and cortical blindness or aphasia, with a diastolic blood pressure of greater than 120 mm Hg, argues strongly for a hypertensive crisis. In contrast, a sudden rise of BUN alone is most consistent with uremic encephalopathy.

Two variants of this disorder are seen in patients on peritoneal dialysis or hemodialysis. The acute dialysis dysequilibrium syndrome is seen in children more often than in adults undergoing hemodialysis with large exchanges of dialysate. A sudden shift of solutes out of the vascular compartment produces a hyperosmolar state in the brain and subsequent water reabsorption intracerebrally. This results in water intoxication with florid encephalopathy within 30 to 60 minutes. Slower dialysis prevents the problem in general [17].

Dialysis dementia is insidious by comparison and is evidenced by postdialysis lethargy, asterixis, myoclonus, dysphasia, and progressive loss of cognitive abilities over years. This disorder has been linked to increased amounts of aluminum in the dialysate, augmented by aluminum-containing antacids in the diet [18]. While the brains of patients suffering from this disorder do not contain excess aluminum compared to other dialysis patients, elimination of aluminum from these sources helps reverse the symptoms in the early stages. This syndrome is now relatively rare.

PULMONARY FAILURE. A combination of hypoxemia and hypercarbia can produce typical changes of a metabolic encephalopathy in patients with underlying pulmonary failure. Individuals with chronic obstructive pulmonary disease, for example, tolerate a PCO_2 of 50 to 60 mm Hg without mental status changes. However, a sudden increase of PCO_2 up to 65 to 70 mm Hg due to hypoventilation or impaired oxygen exchange can lead to lethargy, headaches, and a rise in intracranial pressure. Associated signs are papilledema or retinal vein congestion, Babinski signs, asterixis, myoclonus, and, often, generalized tremors. Seizures are rarely seen, and pupillary and oculomotor function are preserved unless there is a concomitant hypoxic-ischemic insult [19].

This course of events may be precipitated by systemic infection with fatigue of ventilatory muscles, paralysis of these muscles by neuromuscular disease or Guillain-Barré syndrome, and sedative drugs, with their depressant effect on the medullary respiratory center. In the well-compensated hypercarbic individual, oxygen therapy may be counterproductive by decreasing respiratory drive from the medulla. Rapid correction of hypercarbia by artificial ventilation, on the other hand, worsens the chronic metabolic alkalosis these patients have, possibly resulting in a further depression of mental status plus seizures [20].

The critical factor in the development of pulmonary encephalopathy is a rapid increase in serum PCO_2. This may be complicated by the presence of sedatives, hypoxemia, cardiac failure, and renal hypoperfusion. Treatment is directed toward slow correction of hypercarbia while maintaining an adequate oxygen tension (PO_2) and good cerebral flow. Prognosis for full neurologic recovery is good if the patient is not subjected to cerebral ischemia as well.

HYPOGLYCEMIC ENCEPHALOPATHY. Hypoglycemia can occur as an isolated problem or a complication of liver failure, tumors producing insulin like substances, or urea cycle defects. The most common case is that of a diabetic with an accidental or deliberate overdose of insulin or oral hypoglycemic agents. An initial "insulin reaction" occurs when the serum glucose drops below about 40 mg per deciliter, producing flushing, sweating, faintness, palpitations, nausea, and anxiety. This per-

sists several minutes before the patient becomes confused and either agitated or drowsy [21]. Focal neurologic signs, such as hemiparesis, cortical blindness, or dysphasia, may appear at this point, mimicking an acute stroke [22]. If the serum glucose drops precipitously below 30 mg per deciliter, generalized convulsions may occur in flurries, followed by a postictal coma. Prompt correction of the hypoglycemia at this point leads to reversal of the neurologic deficits, but repeated episodes can result in a subtle dementia evolving over many years [23].

When severe hypoglycemia is sustained for more than 10 minutes, a stepwise progression of neurologic signs occurs. The first step is motor restlessness, with frontal release signs such as sucking, grasping, and a tonic jaw jerk. Diffuse muscle spasms and sometimes myoclonic jerks appear next. Finally, decerebrate rigidity is seen before the so-called medullary phase, a state of deep coma with dilated pupils, bradycardia, hypoventilation, and generalized flaccidity, much like hypoxic-ischemic coma. The pathologic changes associated with bouts of hypoglycemic encephalopathy are also similar to hypoxic-ischemic insults, though the cerebellum is relatively spared [24].

Differentiating hypoglycemic coma from a seizure disorder, cerebrovascular accident, or drug overdose is not possible at the outset unless a stat serum glucose is obtained prior to administering IV fluids. If there is doubt about the cause of a rapidly evolving coma, treatment with a bolus of 50 ml of 50% glucose (1 ampule) should not be delayed, since hypoglycemic encephalopathy can result in permanent neurologic deficits if not reversed in 20 minutes or less. The first bolus of glucose must be followed by close monitoring of blood glucose levels, because most agents leading to symptomatic hypoglycemia are long-acting [25].

HYPERGLYCEMIC ENCEPHALOPATHY. Hyperglycemia that is severe enough to produce mental status changes rarely occurs in isolation from other metabolic disturbances. Hypokalemia and hypophosphatemia, hyperosmolality and ketoacidosis or lactic acidosis often accompany serum glucose levels greater than 300 mg per deciliter. In contrast, acidosis may be absent in nonketotic hyperglycemic hyperosmolar states, while the serum osmolality is often greater than 350 mOsm per kilogram and serum glucose greater than 800 mg per deciliter. The neurologic changes in any case appear to correlate best with abnormalities of serum osmolality and the rate at which it is corrected [26].

In juvenile or "brittle" diabetics, ketoacidosis develops after a dose of insulin is missed or due to an occult infection. The first changes are mild confusion, lethargy, and deep regular inspirations (Kussmaul's breathing) in addition to signs of dehydration. Elderly patients are more prone to nonketotic hyperglycemia, especially when they have an inadequate diet, take medications that interfere with insulin metabolism (e.g., Dilantin, steroids), or take oral hypoglycemic agents [27]. Lactic acidosis may be present, in particular, with phenformin (an oral hypoglycemic currently in disuse). These patients also tend to have focal or generalized seizures and transient or shifting hemiplegia as the level of coma deepens. The preservation of pupillary and oculocephalic responses helps identify the clinical picture in such cases as being metabolic rather than structural.

The hyperosmolality attendant to hyperglycemia of any type causes a shift of water from the intracerebral to intravascular space and, hence, brain shrinkage [28]. How this produces the neurologic changes observed is not known. More importantly, rapid correction of hyperosmolality by IV hydration and insulin results in cerebral water intoxication and signs of increased intracranial pressure. This is exemplified by the patient who begins to awaken from a hyperglycemic coma during IV therapy but later develops a headache and recurrent lethargy and seems to drift back into the previous state. Significant morbidity and mortality follows if these fluctuations are not observed and the IV treatment modified appropriately [29]. Other details of the management of diabetic coma are addressed in Chapter 93.

OTHER ELECTROLYTE DISTURBANCES. Hyponatremia and hypernatremia both cause fluid shifts and critical changes in serum osmolality, with the same effects on cerebral dysfunction as those described above. Mild to moderate hyponatremia (120–130 mEq/L) is evidenced by confusion or delirium, with asterixis and multifocal myoclonus. If the serum sodium drops below 110 mEq per liter or at a rate greater than 5 mEq per liter per hour to 120 mEq per liter and below, seizures and coma are likely to follow. This course of events portends permanent neurologic damage even after careful therapy [30]. Common causes of hyponatremia are the syndrome of inappropriate antidiuretic hormone excretion (SIADH, with a myriad of etiologies), excess volume expansion with hypotonic IV solutions, and renal failure with a decreased glomerular filtration rate [31]. Less common causes include psychogenic polydipsia, severe congestive heart failure, and Addison's disease.

The neurologic signs of hyponatremia are nonspecific, and the general approach to evaluation of an encephalopathy will often identify the problem. Treatment is directed toward the underlying cause, with fluid restriction in mild cases. In moderate cases (i.e., a serum sodium of 105–115 mEq/L), oral sodium supplementation may be needed as well. A serum sodium below 100 mEq per liter is life-threatening. This requires judicious treatment with IV hypertonic saline at a rate calculated to replace about one-half of the total sodium deficit in 3 to 6 hours (or < 0.5–1.0 mg of Na^+ per hour). The remainder of the deficit should be administered in the next 24 to 48 hours [32]. Excessively rapid correction of severe hyponatremia, especially in alcoholic or malnourished individuals, can be associated with central pontine myelinolysis (CPM), another serious neurologic complication [33]. Central pontine myelinolysis starts with a flaccid quadriparesis and inability to chew, swallow, or talk over a period of days. If the patient recovers from the underlying systemic disorder, he or she is left with a spastic quadriparesis and pseudobulbar speech for a number of months or permanently.

Hypernatremia is not seen very often outside the hospital setting, except in children with severe diarrhea and inadequate oral fluid intake. Excess diuretic therapy, hyperosmolar tube feedings, and restricted access to oral fluids are reflected in a serum sodium greater than 155 mEq per liter in institutionalized patients. Clinically progressive confusion and obtundation are seen in subacute cases. With levels of sodium greater than 170 mEq per liter developing acutely, subdural hematomas can occur due to stretching of the dural vessels off the dehydrated cortex. These patients may complain of headache, develop seizures, or simply drift into a stupor. Catastrophic complications such as venous sinus thrombosis and irreversible coma are seen with a serum sodium level greater than 180 mEq per liter, due to the marked hyperosmolality that accompanies it.

The cause of profound hypernatremia is often diabetes insipidus (DI), which may be secondary to head trauma. Impaired thirst mechanisms or depressed consciousness interferes with the polydipsia that is pathognomonic of DI [34].

The treatment of symptomatic hypernatremia depends on its cause: dehydration alone or complicated by additional sodium depletion due to hyperosmolar diuresis or excessive sweating. Fluid replacement is accomplished with D_5W at a rate dependent on the total body water deficit—one-half of the water

needed being administered by IV in the first 12 to 24 hours, and no faster. Saline solutions of one-half normal strength (0.45%) are used in most other cases. The exception is hyperosmolar diabetic coma, in which case both insulin and normal saline are necessary to correct the severe serum hypertonicity.

Metabolic acidosis by itself produces only mild delirium or confusion, but it may be accompanied by organ failure, direct CNS toxicity from drug metabolites, or volume depletion [35]. The first sign of an encephalopathy caused by metabolic acidosis is hyperpnea followed by mental status changes and mild muscular rigidity. Ingestion of toxic doses of poisons such as methanol, ethylene glycol, and salicylates results in encephalopathy along with low serum bicarbonate levels (< 15 mEq/L) [36]. Therapy must be directed toward vigorous correction of the metabolic acidosis while the specific cause is being elucidated.

PANCREATIC FAILURE. Acute pancreatitis rarely leads to mental status changes during the initial bout. When recurrent or chronic, symptoms of encephalopathy may prominently wax and wane [37]. The clinical presentation is abdominal pain followed over 2 to 5 days by hallucinosis, delirium, focal or generalized seizures, and bilateral Babinski responses. As the serum amylase continues to rise, the patient may lapse into a coma as a result of secondary hyperglycemia, hypocalcemia, and hypotension. The prognosis and treatment depend on the underlying cause and severity of the pancreatitis [38].

ENDOCRINE DISORDERS. Adrenal disorders are an important consideration in acute encephalopathy, since both hypo- and hyperadrenalism produce alterations in CNS function.

Addison's disease or secondary adrenocortical deficiency occurs acutely in the setting of septicemia, surgery, and, most frequently, sudden withdrawal of chronically administered steroids. In the latter case, one does not see the stigmata of chronic adrenocorticotropic hormone (ACTH) deficiency, but rather hypotension, a mild hyponatremia, hypoglycemia, and hyperkalemia, together with a delirium or stupor that fluctuates erratically [39]. The electrolyte disturbances in most cases are not severe enough to explain the encephalopathy; other pathologic mechanisms, such as cerebral hypoperfusion or water intoxication, have been suggested. Unlike many metabolic encephalopathies, adrenocortical insufficiency is associated with decreased muscle tone and deep tendon reflexes. Seizures and papilledema may appear when the patient has a profound ACTH deficiency and coma. The neurologic picture does not clear until cortisone replacement is given along with treatment of the electrolyte imbalances. These patients are also particularly sensitive to sedative medications and may lapse into coma with small doses of narcotics or barbiturates [40].

Excess steroids produce different forms of encephalopathy depending on whether the source is endogenous or exogenous. In Cushing's disease, psychomotor depression and lethargy are the norm, while high doses of prednisone usually cause elation, delirium, or frank psychosis [41]. The latter is not uncommon in the ICU setting, due to the administration of stress levels of steroids and multiple other CNS toxins. The behavioral changes are key to recognizing this problem, since there are no specific metabolic markers [42]. Treatment consists of withdrawal of the steroids and sometimes temporary use of tranquilizers or lithium for the psychiatric features. Full neurologic recovery may lag behind the treatment by several days to weeks.

Hypothyroidism is now a rare cause of encephalopathy and coma. It may be confused initially with other causes of hypotension, hypoventilation, and hyponatremia, such as septic shock, brainstem infarcts, or an overdose of sedatives. The diagnosis should be considered in any patient with hypothermia, pretibial edema, pseudomyotonic stretch reflexes (e.g., delayed relaxation of the patellar jerk), and coarse hair or facies. Muscle enzymes, serum cholesterol, and lipids may be elevated along with the thyroid-stimulating hormone (TSH) level [43]. Diagnostic confirmation is often delayed pending results of thyroid function tests, but replacement therapy should be initiated early with IV triiodothyronine or thyroxine. The constitutional symptoms may take several weeks to respond, but the neurologic picture clears promptly with proper treatment.

Thyrotoxicosis is more difficult to recognize, since it can present in an apathetic form, as a "thyroid storm," or in a subacute form (see Chap. 111). Elderly patients are more likely to appear depressed or stuporous and without evidence of hypermetabolism [44]. The key to the diagnosis in such cases is evidence of recent weight loss and atrial fibrillation, often with congestive heart failure and a proximal myopathy. In a thyroid storm the patient with indolent hyperthyroidism may be stressed by an infection or surgery and responds with marked signs of hypermetabolism: tachycardia, fever, profuse sweating, and pulmonary or congestive heart failure. Neurologically the individual becomes acutely agitated, delirious, and then progresses into a stupor [45]. The subacute picture that precedes this is one of mild irritability, nervousness, tremors, and hyperactivity and is often misconstrued as an affective disorder rather than one that is endocrine in origin. Ophthalmologic signs, such as proptosis, chemosis, and periorbital edema, are useful in identifying this form of thyrotoxicosis.

Therapy for thyrotoxic encephalopathy is aimed at ablation of the gland, but supportive care may require beta-blockers, digoxin, diuretics, and sometimes dexamethasone and sedatives for the associated hypermetabolic state.

Encephalopathy is also seen in disorders of the pituitary gland and parathyroid gland, though rarely as a primary process. Hypopituitarism may result from radiation or surgery to the area of the sella and can present as a chronic encephalopathy with features of thyroid and/or adrenal insufficiency. An acute coma due to infarction or hemorrhage of the pituitary gland, known as pituitary apoplexy, can be seen in acromegalics with large adenomas or in patients with postpartum hemorrhage and hypotension (Sheehan's syndrome) [46]. Subarachnoid blood and ocular abnormalities plus signs of increased intracranial pressure help identify the lesion in such cases. Encephalopathy from hyperpituitarism reflects the specific neurohumoral substance that is being released in excess and does not represent a unique syndrome.

Hyperparathyroidism may be manifest neurologically with asthenia, or a vague change in personality. The patient is mildly depressed, lacks energy, and fatigues easily. A serum calcium greater than 12 mg per deciliter and elevated parathormone levels are important diagnostic findings. Occasionally, psychiatric symptoms predominate, starting with delirium and psychosis, or obtundation and coma when the serum calcium exceeds 15 mg per deciliter. Hypercalcemia caused by metastatic bone lesions, paraneoplastic parathyroid hormonelike substances, sarcoidosis, primary bone diseases, and renal failure is associated with a subacute or chronic encephalopathy similar to hyperparathyroidism. Treatment in these cases must be directed toward the underlying disease rather than the hypercalcemia alone. Primary hyperparathyroidism is effectively managed by ablation of the overactive gland. This is not always possible, since often the glands are ectopic and may escape discovery on selective angiography or exploratory surgery.

Hypocalcemia due to hypoparathyroidism produces an encephalopathy that parallels the depression of serum calcium levels. At less than 4.0 mEq per liter of calcium, a blunted affect and seizures are common and may be confused with a dementing process or epilepsy. The motor signs of hypocalcemia (i.e., tetany or neuromuscular irritability) should raise the suspicion of a metabolic disturbance [39]. Another diagnostic dilemma is the occasional presentation of hypocalcemia with papilledema and headache. The opening pressure on lumbar puncture is elevated to the same degree as in pseudotumor cerebri, but a CT scan of the head is likely to show basal ganglia calcifications [47]. Furthermore, the presence of cataracts and mental dullness in a previously normal individual should lead one to check the serum calcium and parathormone levels.

The mechanism by which hypocalcemia and hypoparathyroidism produce these varied neurologic symptoms is not known. Replacement of serum calcium by dietary means is usually inadequate to correct the CNS disorder. Supplementation with vitamin D and calcitriol enhances the absorption and use of oral calcium.

OTHER CAUSES OF ENCEPHALOPATHY. The list of causes of diffuse or metabolic encephalopathies is so lengthy that the problem of diagnosis must be resolved by a process of elimination.

Drugs and Toxins. Drugs and toxins lead all other possible causes, with a frequency of about 50 percent (Chap. 128). Hepatic, renal, or pulmonary failure are causative in another 12 percent of cases, and endocrine or electrolyte disturbances in about 8 percent. Less common etiologies include thiamine deficiency (Wernicke's encephalopathy), cardiac bypass surgery, subacute bacterial endocarditis, and hyperthermia. All of these disorders produce microembolic or microhemorrhagic-petechial lesions in specific areas of the brain.

Wernicke's Encephalopathy. Wernicke's encephalopathy develops acutely in the clinical setting of an alcoholic or malnourished individual, especially when given IV glucose solutions without vitamin supplementation. Since thiamine is a cofactor in the use of cerebral glucose, it is depleted by the IV infusion [48]; confusion, obtundation, and loss of short-term memory rapidly ensue. The hallmark of this entity is a striking impairment of ocular movements, causing an external ophthalmoplegia, nystagmus, and diminished oculocephalic responses. Prompt IV and oral administration of 100 mg of thiamine restores ocular function completely. The cerebral symptoms resolve slowly with the addition of 100 mg of oral thiamine for 3 days or more. Untreated, the patient lapses into a coma due to autonomic failure accompanied by shock and hypothermia, and usually dies. Repeated or untreated episodes of Wernicke's disease may result in a chronic Korsakoff's psychosis with profound memory impairment [49].

Hyperthermia. Hyperthermia due to heat stroke also has a characteristic clinical setting—young individuals suffering from excessive sweating due to overactivity and elderly people on anticholinergics who are exposed to a hot environment [50]. In both cases neurologic changes occur when the core body temperature reaches 42°C (107.6°F). The patient may become agitated and confused, with intermittent generalized seizures, or may immediately lapse into a coma, as if due to a stroke. The presence of tachycardia, hot and dry skin, and diffuse hypertonus along with the appropriate circumstances identifies the likely etiology. Normal pupillary and oculocephalic responses and the absence of focal motor signs also point to a nonstructural lesion. However, if the core body temperature is not lowered early in the course, the patient may be left with sequelae similar to those seen in hypoxic ischemic encephalopathy.

Other causes of temperature greater than 42°C are rare and are not discussed here [51] (see Chap. 73).

Bacterial or Marantic Endocarditis. Up to 20 percent of patients with bacterial or marantic endocarditis can present with a subacute encephalopathy manifested by confusion and hyperpnea with or without fever [52]. It should be suspected in any patient with gram-negative sepsis; ovarian cancer; malignant melanoma; or adenocarcinoma of the lung, breast, prostate, or pancreas; and in anyone with an immunocompromised state. Definitive diagnosis rests on the blood culture results and an echocardiogram showing vegetations. Treatment is directed toward reducing or removing the cardiac source (see Chap. 88).

Conclusions

Metabolic encephalopathy is one of the most frequent neurologic disorders seen in the ICU arena. It is also one of the most diverse in its clinical presentations and requires a systematic approach to define the etiology and institute effective treatment. The features that distinguish most metabolic encephalopathies from structural lesions are: a nonfocal neurologic examination, increased motor activity, intact ocular and pupillary reflexes, and laboratory abnormalities supporting the clinical picture. Additional tests, such as an EEG, head CT, or toxicology screen, are useful in ruling out other possible causes.

One should keep in mind that many patients in the ICU have an underlying chronic encephalopathy due to long-standing illness. Therefore, they are more susceptible to minor metabolic perturbations induced by small doses of drugs, slight shifts of fluid balance, or worsening organ failure. Early recognition and correction of such factors improves the patient's prognosis for a full neurologic recovery. Toward this end, it is prudent to consult the neurologist before the complications of multiple treatments and secondary changes confound the clinical course.

References

1. Folstein MF, Folstein SE, McHugh PR: "Mini-mental state": A practical method for grading the cognitive state of patients for the clinician. *J Psychiatr Res* 12:189, 1975.
2. Plum F, Posner JB: The physiologic pathology of signs and symptoms of coma, in *The Diagnosis of Stupor and Coma.* 3rd ed. Philadelphia, FA Davis, 1980, p 33.
3. Cohen PJ: Signs and stages of anesthesia, in Goodman LS, Gilman A (eds): *The Pharmacological Basis of Therapeutics.* 5th ed. New York, Macmillan, 1975, p 60.
4. Celesia GG, Grigg MM, Ross E: Generalized status myoclonus in acute anoxic and toxic-metabolic encephalopathies. *Arch Neurol* 45:781, 1988.
5. Sheridan PH, Sato S: Triphasic waves of metabolic encephalopathy versus spike-wave stupor. *J Neurol Neurosurg Psychiatry* 49:108, 1986.
6. Fischer JE, Baldessarini RJ: Pathogenesis and therapy of hepatic coma, in Schaeffner F, Popper H (eds): *Progress in Liver Disease.* vol. 5. New York, Grune & Stratton, 1976.
7. Christensen E, Krintel JJ, Hansen SM, et al: Prognosis after the first episode of gastrointestinal bleeding or coma in cirrhosis: Survival and prognostic factors. *Scand J Gastroenterol* 24:999, 1989.
8. Laursen H, Westergaard G: Enhanced permeability to horseradish peroxidase across cerebral vessels in the rat after portacaval anastomosis. *Neuropathol Appl Neurobiol* 3:29, 1979.
9. James JH, Escourroule J, Fisher JE: Blood-brain neutral amino-acid

10. transport activity is increased after portacaval anastomoses. *Science* 200:1395, 1978.
11. Bleasel AF, Waugh RC, McCaughan GW: Development of chronic hepatocerebral degeneration eight years after a distal splenorenal (Warren) shunt. *Gut* 30:1419, 1989.
12. Hurwitz ES: Reye's syndrome. *Epidemiol Rev* 11:249, 1989.
13. Arrowsmith JB, Kennedy DL, et al: National patterns of aspirin use and Reye's syndrome reporting, United States, 1980–1985. *Pediatrics* 79:858, 1987.
14. Fishman RA: Brain edema and disorders of intracranial pressure, in Rowland LP (ed): *Merritts Textbook of Neurology.* 8th ed. Philadelphia, Lea & Febiger, 1989, p 262.
15. Chadwick D, French AT: Uremic myoclonus: An example of reticular reflex myoclonus? *J Neurol Neurosurg Psychiatry* 42:52, 1979.
16. Plum F, Posner JB: Renal encephalopathy, in *The Diagnosis of Stupor and Coma.* 3rd ed. Philadelphia, FA Davis, 1980, p 225.
17. Hagstam KE: EEG frequency content related to clinical blood parameters in chronic uremia. *Scand J Urol Nephrol* 7(suppl):1 1971.
18. Raskin NH, Fishman RA: Neurologic disorders in renal failure. *N Engl J Med* 294:143, 1976.
19. Alfrey AC: Dialysis encephalopathy syndrome. *Ann Rev Med* 29:93, 1978.
20. Glaser G, Pincus JH: Neurologic complications of internal disease, in Baker AB, Baker LH (eds): *Clinical Neurology.* Philadelphia, Harper & Row, 1983, p 17.
21. Rotherman EB, Safar P, Robin ED: CNS disorder during mechanical ventilation in chronic pulmonary disease. *JAMA* 189:993, 1964.
22. Fishbain DA, Rotundo D: Frequency of hypoglycemic delirium in a psychiatric emergency service. *Psychosomatics* 29:346, 1988.
23. Garty BZ, Dinari G, Nitzan M: Transient acute cortical blindness associated with hypoglycemia. *Pediatr Neurol* 3:169, 1987.
24. Malouf R, Brust JCM: Hypoglycemia: Causes, neurological manifestations and outcome. *Ann Neurol* 17:421, 1985.
25. Foster JW, Hart RG: Hypoglycemic hemiplegia: Two cases and a clinical review. *Stroke* 18:944, 1987.
26. Kitabchi EA, Goodman RC: Hypoglycemia, pathophysiology and diagnosis. *Hosp Pract* 22:45, 1987.
27. Wachtel TS, Silliman RA, Lamberton P: Predisposing factors for the diabetic hyperosmolar state. *Arch Intern Med* 147:499, 1987.
28. Arieff AI, Carroll HJ: Cerebral edema and depression of sensorium in nonketotic hyperosmolar coma. *Diabetes* 23:525, 1974.
29. Ryner MM, Fishman RA: Protective adaptation of brain to water intoxication. *Arch Neurol* 28:49, 1973.
30. Plum F, Posner JB: Multifocal, diffuse and metabolic brain diseases causing stupor and coma, in *The Diagnosis of Stupor and Coma.* 3rd ed. Philadelphia, FA Davis, 1980, p 234.
31. Ayus JC, Krothapalli RK, Arieff AI: Treatment of symptomatic hyponatremia and its relation to brain damage: A prospective study. *N Engl J Med* 317:1190, 1987.
32. Streeton DH, Moses AM, Miller M: Disorders of the neurohypophysis, in *Harrison's Principles of Internal Medicine.* 11th ed. New York, McGraw-Hill, 1987, p 1729.
33. Victor M: Neurologic disorders due to alcoholism and malnutrition, in Baker AB, Baker LH (eds): *Clinical Neurology.* Philadelphia, Harper & Row, 1983, p 57.
34. Hattori S, Mochio S, Isogai Y, et al: Central pontine myelinolysis followed by frequent hyperglycemia and hypoglycemia: Report of an autopsy case. *Brain Nerve* 41:795, 1989.
35. Adams RD, Victor M: Hypothalamic pituitary syndromes: Diabetes insipidus, in *Principles of Neurology.* 4th ed. New York, McGraw-Hill, 1989, p 448.
36. Levinsky N: Fluids and electrolytes: Metabolic acidosis, in *Harrison's Textbook of Internal Medicine.* 11th ed. New York, McGraw-Hill, 1987, p 210.
37. Perry S: Substance induced organic mental disorders, in Halis and Yudofsky (eds): *Textbook of Neuropsychiatry.* Washington, DC, American Psychiatry Press, 1987.
38. Sjaastad O, Gjessing L, Ritland S, et al: Chronic relapsing pancreatitis, encephalopathy with disturbance of consciousness and CSF amino acid aberration. *J Neurol* 220:83, 1979.
39. Johnson DA, Tong NT: Pancreatic encephalopathy. *South Med J* 70:165, 1977.
40. Kaminski HJ, Ruff RL: Neurologic complications of endocrine diseases. *Neurol Clin* 7:489, 1989.

40. Plum F, Posner JB: Adrenal insufficiency, in *The Diagnosis of Stupor and Coma*. 3rd ed. Philadelphia, FA Davis, 1980, p 236.
41. Whybrow P, Hurwitz TI: Psychological disturbances associated with endocrine disease and hormone therapy, in Sachar EJ (ed): *Hormones, Behavior and Pathophysiology*. New York, Raven, 1976.
42. Boston Collaborative Drug Surveillance Program: Acute adverse reactions to prednisone in relation to dosage. *Clin Pharmacol Ther* 13:694, 1972.
43. Greene R: The thyroid gland: Its relationship to neurology, in Vinken PJ, Bruyn GW (eds): *The Handbook of Clinical Neurology* Vol 27, part 1. New York, Elsevier North-Holland, 1976, p 253.
44. Thomas TB, Mazzaferri EL, Skillman TG: Apathetic thyrotoxicosis: A distinctive clinical and laboratory entity. *Ann Intern Med* 72:679, 1970.
45. Nemeroff CB: Clinical significance of psychoneuroendocrinology in psychiatry: Focus on the thyroid and adrenal. *J Clin Psychol* 50(Suppl):13, 1989.
46. Tsementzis SA, Loizou LA: Pituitary apoplexy. *Neurochirurgie* 29:90, 1986.
47. Delplace PO, Wery D, Lemort M, et al: A case of multiple brain calcifications associated with hypoparathyroidism. *J Belge Radiol* 72:263, 1989.
48. Goto I, Nagara H, Tateishi J, et al: Thiamine-deficient encephalopathy in rats: Effects of deficiencies of thiamine and magnesium. *Brain Res* 372:31, 1986.
49. Victor M: Neurologic disorders due to alcoholism and malnutrition, in Baker AB, Baker LH (eds): *Clinical Neurology*. Philadelphia, Harper & Row, 1983, p 24.
50. Costrini AM, Pitt HA, Bustafson AB, et al: Cardiovascular and metabolic manifestations of heat stroke and severe heat exhaustion. *Am J Med* 66:296, 1979.
51. Muller PS: Diagnosis and treatment of neuroleptic malignant syndrome: A review. *Neuro View* 3:1, 1987.
52. Terpenning MS, Guggy BP, Kauffman CA: Infective endocarditis: Clinical features in young and elderly patients. *Am J Med* 83:626, 1987.

185. Generalized Anoxia/Ischemia of the Nervous System

Carol F. Lippa

Hypoxic brain injury results from a prolonged period of inadequate oxygen supply to the brain. The clinical picture of patients with this disorder ranges from mild confusion to deep coma with loss of brainstem responses, motor function, and reflexes. Patients with global anoxia constitute a large number of intensive care unit (ICU) admissions. Anoxic damage can be caused by circulatory collapse, respiratory failure, or inadequate hemoglobin binding to oxygen. *Ischemia* is the term used to describe insufficient oxygen delivery to the brain related specifically to hypoperfusion (cardiovascular collapse) [1].

Pathogenesis

The brain is unique because it uses almost exclusively aerobic metabolism of glucose to meet its energy needs. For this reason the cerebral blood flow, which delivers the oxygen, cannot be interrupted if the brain is to function normally. The continuous availability of oxygen is secured by the cerebral vasculature's autoregulatory mechanism [2], which controls the rate of blood flow over a wide range of blood pressures. If blood pressure drops too low for autoregulatory mechanisms to operate, the brain is still protected because oxygen extraction from the blood then increases. When there is a further decline in blood pressure, these compensatory mechanisms fail and oxygen supplies to the brain are insufficient. This results in an arrest of aerobic metabolism.

Intracellularly, oxygen is essential for the operation of the Krebs (tricarboxylic acid) cycle and the electron transport chain. In cardiac arrest, depletion of brain oxygen reserves occurs within 10 seconds, thereby eliminating the major source of neuronal adenosine triphosphate (ATP) and phosphokinase. The immediate result is depolarization of the neuronal membrane, which leads to an influx of fluid and calcium into neurons. The resulting intracellular (cytotoxic) edema is responsible for the increased intracranial pressure that develops. The changeover to anaerobic metabolism results in neuronal catabolism. The increased intraneuronal calcium activates proteases and lipases, which cause further injury to the neuron. When the anoxic insult is due to cardiovascular collapse, loss of venous outflow leads to the extracellular accumulation of lactic acid and pyruvate, the end products of anaerobic metabolism. Buildup of these catabolites potentiates the cellular damage.

Diagnosis

The first question to address when evaluating a comatose patient with a possible hypoxic insult is whether the coma is the result of a metabolic insult or a structural brain lesion. A mass lesion causing coma is usually associated with abnormalities or asymmetries of pupillary size and response to light. Often other obvious focal abnormalities are disclosed on neurologic examination. When the examination shows a focal abnormality, a computed tomography (CT) scan can aid in ruling out subarachnoid or intracerebral hemorrhage, infarction, abscess, tumor, or herpes encephalitis. When the physical examination is nonfocal, a metabolic cause should be suspected. In these cases the CT scan cannot differentiate hypoxic/ischemic encephalopathy from other types of metabolic coma. Similarly, electroencephalographic findings are often nonspecific and therefore of limited diagnostic value in determining which metabolic abnormality is present in a patient whose physical examination is suggestive of metabolic coma.

In cases of anoxic brain injury, the diagnosis is often suggested by the clinical setting (cardiac arrest in patients with arrhythmias or myocardial infarctions, or severe episodes of intraoperative hypotension). When arterial blood gas determination is immediately available it can confirm the diagnosis. A PO_2 of less than 40 mm Hg causes obvious confusion. A PO_2 of less than 30 mm Hg results in coma [1]. Other abnormalities that may potentiate anoxic damage to the brain include anemia, acidosis, an increased PCO_2, and a systolic blood pressure of less than 70 mm Hg. The presence or absence of these factors greatly influences the degree of hypoxemia a given individual can tolerate.

The internist or neurologist is often consulted for the patient who has well-documented cerebral hypoperfusion during surgical operations that require the use of extracorporeal circulation. The physical examination is symmetric and suggestive of global neurologic dysfunction. Because surgical patients with such a history often have preexisting illnesses (vascular disease, borderline renal function, hepatic impairment, diabetes), it is the obligation of the intensive care physician to determine all new deficits due to the anoxic encephalopathy and other treatable conditions secondary to metabolic, infectious, and iatrogenic factors such as sedating medications. Intracerebral hemorrhage and subdural hematomas can occur spontaneously in the perioperative period, especially in patients who have been anticoagulated, and should be sought.

Clinical Course

The symptomatology and clinical outcome of patients who have sustained anoxic injuries depend on the degree and duration of oxygen deprivation to the brain as well as the maintenance of blood flow. Clinical changes observed with lesser degrees of hypoxia include confusion, impaired learning, and short-term memory deficits. These cognitive changes can be apparent when the PO_2 drops below 70 mm Hg, but rapid clinical improvement is seen when the hypoxemia is corrected.

With complete cessation of blood flow to the brain, consciousness is lost after several seconds. If the duration of oxygen deprivation is moderately prolonged, the patient usually wakens but may have residual deficits, such as cognitive impairment, or later sequelae, including extrapyramidal movement disorders or seizures, that may not develop for days to weeks.

With prolonged, severe hypoxia the patient is comatose with loss of brainstem reflexes. Many patients with severe anoxic changes die within 48 hours; others live in vegetative states. In patients who survive, the rate of improvement slows after the first few weeks or months; return of cognitive function late in the clinical course is rare.

An interesting but rare syndrome after hypoxic injury is seen with the following sequence of events. Initially after sustaining an anoxic insult the patient is comatose. Clinical improvement is seen for several days. Three to 30 days after the insult there is a functional decline characterized by irritability, confusion, lethargy, and motor symptoms, including clumsiness and abnormal muscle tone. Many victims deteriorate to coma and die. This rare condition occurs most commonly in cases of carbon monoxide poisoning. Pathologically, widespread demyelination is seen without gray matter changes. The cause is unknown, but it may be due to alteration of enzymatic processes

as normal brain function is reestablished or to edema or damage to small blood vessels [1,3].

Prognosis

The overall prognosis for a meaningful recovery in patients with nontraumatic coma is poor. The longer patients are in coma, the worse the outcome [4,5]. In patients who improve, most improvement occurs within the first 30 days. Comatose patients with anoxic/ischemic events have a better prognosis than those whose coma results from structural brain injuries, such as cerebrovascular disease and subarachnoid hemorrhage, but a poorer prognosis than those with other forms of metabolic coma. A good outcome is seen in 50 percent of patients who wake within 24 hours. Few patients who remain in a vegetative state or coma beyond 1 day return to normal functioning. The occurrence of seizures or myoclonus is not related to ultimate recovery [4]. Other factors that are not predictive include the patient's sex and the reason for cardiac arrest.

If consciousness is maintained during a hypoxic event there is rarely permanent brain damage. Irreversible damage is rarely seen in healthy individuals if the duration of anoxia is less than 4 minutes; however, it may be incurred in individuals with preexisting cerebrovascular disease in shorter periods of time.

In cases of nontraumatic coma, the most valuable prognostic information is obtained from the physical examination. If brainstem reflexes (pupillary light, corneal, and vestibulo-ocular) are present within 48 hours of the anoxic event, the prognosis is more favorable. Conversely, 99 percent of patients who do not regain at least two of these reflexes within 48 hours fail to recover [4]. Another favorable sign is the return of purposeful responses to painful stimuli by 24 hours. The loss of vestibulo-ocular responses at 12 hours and the presence of decerebrate or decorticate posturing at 24 hours also mitigate against a favorable outcome [5,6]. When prognosticating by these criteria one must be careful that no sedative, anesthetic, or anticonvulsant (Dilantin, phenobarbital) is being used, since these agents can suppress brainstem reflexes.

Studies of the effect of age on outcome in cases of hypoxic encephalopathy have generally shown that children have a better prognosis than adults for recovery of neurologic function [7]. Similarly, young adults have a more favorable prognosis than elderly individuals [8].

Maintenance of circulation can affect the degree of brain damage from hypoxia, making the prognosis better in cases where it is due primarily to respiratory dysfunction [9]. Similarly, a low PO_2 in itself does not necessarily convey a bad prognosis in cases of isolated hypoxia [10]; normal neurologic recoveries can be seen after prolonged hypoxia if circulation is carefully maintained [11]. Conversely, the presence of metabolic abnormalities, such as lactic acidosis, worsens prognosis. Patients who were hypothermic at the time of their anoxic event may do better neurologically than would otherwise be expected; drowning victims submerged in cold water up to 40 minutes may return to normal neurologic function [12].

In cases of out-of-hospital cardiac arrest, if the duration of untreated cardiac arrest is less than 6 minutes, prognosis for recovery is related to cardiopulmonary resuscitation (CPR) time; more than half of patients on whom CPR is performed less than 30 minutes make a good neurologic recovery. When CPR time is longer, prognosis for neurologic recovery drops to 3 percent. If untreated arrest time is over 6 minutes, 50 percent of patients recover if CPR time was less than 5 minutes; recovery drops to 19 percent in cases of 6 to 15 minutes of CPR time, and when

CPR time is greater than 15 minutes virtually no patients recover [13]. Similarly, if attempts to resuscitate patients before their arrival in the emergency room fail, recovery is extremely unlikely [14].

Radiologic and other laboratory studies are of limited help in prognostication. The presence of either diffuse edema or watershed infarctions on CT scans often portends a poor prognosis [15]. Prognostication by electroencephalography (EEG) is most reliable when the severity of EEG abnormality is at either extreme—normal or severe [16]. Waiting to obtain a record until 48 hours after an anoxic event improves its predictive value. Serial recordings indicate a good prognosis if there is improvement and a poor prognosis if interval deterioration of the tracing is seen [17].

Short-latency somatosensory tests are noninvasive tests of the sensory system that are absent in brain death but preserved in severe reversible comas, such as barbiturate coma, that can mirror brain death [18,19]. If done in comatose patients 8 hours after cardiorespiratory arrest, patients with unobtainable evoked cortical potentials are not likely to waken. If a short-latency somatosensory potential is elicitable, however, there is a 25 percent chance of significant neurologic recovery [19].

A diagnostic test that may prove useful for prognostication is proton magnetic resonance spectroscopy. If done within 2 days of an anoxic event, patients demonstrating elevated cerebral lactic acid levels do very poorly, whereas individuals without detectable lactic acid levels return to normal neurologic function or have minimal deficits [20].

Cerebrospinal fluid (CSF) lactate levels [21], neuron-specific enolase, and brain-type creatine kinase isoenzyme (CK-BB) levels may have predictive value when obtained 24 hours after cardiac arrest. If CSF neuron-specific enolase is greater than 24 ng per milliliter at 24 hours patients usually die; many patients with lower levels live. A potentially useful laboratory screening test when lumbar puncture is not feasible is the serum neuron-specific enolase level, which has a fair correlation with outcome [22].

After out-of-hospital cardiac arrest the overall probability of awakening is roughly 50 percent [23,24]. Much of this depends on the duration of time patients are in coma. In cases of cardiac arrest, complete recovery occurs in 80 percent of patients in whom the coma resolves within 24 hours [24,25]. Others have shown that 72 hours is the upper limit for recovery of brain function sufficient to permit some degree of speech [25].

Treatment

Treatment approaches for cardiac arrest victims and perioperative hypoxic encephalopathy are similar. Optimal therapy is directed at preventing the recurrence of hypoxia. To ensure that the oxygen-carrying capacity of the blood is restored, excess oxygen administration is suggested for several hours after anoxic events. Blood pressure is maintained at normotensive or mildly elevated levels. Mean arterial pressure should be 90 to 110 mm Hg in patients who are usually normotensive. The PaO_2 should be greater than 100 mm Hg, and to reduce intracranial pressure PCO_2 is kept slightly low (25–35 mm Hg). To optimize cerebral vasoconstriction, pH should be maintained at 7.35 to 7.40. In an attempt to minimize the increase in intracranial pressure, if it is not medically contraindicated, it may be beneficial to keep the patient mildly hypovolemic for several days and to elevate the head of the bed 30 degrees. Vital signs, hematocrit, electrolytes, blood sugar, and serum osmolality should be maintained in the normal range [10]. In cases where

the cause of coma is in doubt or the neurologic examination discloses a focal abnormality, a CT scan should be obtained. In all comatose patients, complete metabolic blood studies should be done to determine other metabolic derangements and to obtain baseline information. When any uncertainties exist, a neurologist should be consulted.

Seizures occur in 25 percent of patients in anoxic coma [4]. They are best treated with loading and then maintenance doses of phenytoin (Dilantin) (loading dose 17 mg/kg in saline, rate not to exceed 50 mg/min, slower in elderly or frail patients; maintenance dose 5 mg/kg/day). Phenobarbital is the drug of second choice. In patients with cardiac conduction abnormalities, phenobarbital is the drug of first choice (loading dose in adults up to 500 mg IV, maintenance dose 2–4 mg/kg/day). Occasionally comatose patients are in status epilepticus without any obvious motor signs following an anoxic event [26,27]. Since status epilepticus or frequent untreated seizures can damage the brain, an EEG should be obtained if there is any question of subclinical epileptiform activity. If seizures are overt and are easily controlled, an EEG obtained after 48 hours will generate more prognostic information [17].

Within the first few weeks of recovery some postanoxic patients develop intention myoclonus. This can be distinguished from seizure activity because the latter is accompanied by an epileptiform discharge on the EEG. In addition, the motor disturbance is frequently more dramatic when true seizures are occurring. Intention myoclonus can be treated with valproic acid.

Steroid administration is of little proved help in cases of postanoxic encephalopathy because the increased intracranial pressure is due to neuronal swelling from loss of normal neuronal osmotic gradients. When this (cytotoxic) edema occurs, damage to the gray matter is so extensive that steroids are unlikely to help. No therapy exists to reverse the neuronal anoxic damage. Steroids, mannitol, and glycerol result in elevated serum glucose blood sugar levels, which increase the brain's production of lactic acid, possibly potentiating preexisting damage.

One experimental therapeutic approach has been the administration of high-dose barbiturates. The rationale is that barbiturates may decrease intracranial pressure, diminishing the requirement for osmotic agents and thus avoiding metabolic abnormalities secondary to rapid diuresis. They also may decrease the brain's oxygen requirements. Barbiturate therapy is ineffectual in global cerebral anoxia because intracranial pressure rises rapidly after withdrawal of the drug. Although individual cases have been reported to improve with high-dose phenobarbital [28], in most individuals this treatment *delays* the deleterious effects of increased intracranial pressure *but does not prevent them* [29]. Similar studies using rapid-acting barbiturate (thiopental) administrations have not proved it to be effective [5]. Other experimental approaches include administration of calcium channel blockers. Although these improve outcome after subarachnoid hemorrhage and possibly strokes, they are ineffective in global anoxic injuries [30].

If the patient wakens, an empiric 7 to 10 days of bed rest may minimize the chance of developing postanoxic encephalopathy, particularly in cases of carbon monoxide poisoning, since these patients are at increased risk for the development of this condition [1,3].

Conclusions

Global anoxic damage occurs when the cerebral blood flow cannot provide enough oxygen to meet the metabolic demands of the brain. The effects of oxygen deprivation depend on many factors. The degree and duration of hypoxia are the most important. In cases of cardiac arrest, brain damage is proportional to the amount of time without perfusion. The patient's age, underlying medical conditions, infection, and other metabolic imbalances also play a role in the body's ability to withstand oxygen deprivation.

Treatment strategies for the acute phase focus on supportive care. Elevation of the head of the bed, maintaining a relatively hypovolemic state, and avoidance of hypotension may be of benefit. A vigorous search should be made for concurrent metabolic abnormalities. Administration of steroids, osmotic agents, and phenobarbital or other anticonvulsants (prophylactically), calcium channel blockers, or anesthetics does not improve outcome and may complicate medical management.

Prognosis is best determined by the early return of brainstem/ cranial nerve function. If it has not reappeared by 48 hours after the event it is unlikely the patient will make a good recovery. Other poor prognostic signs include a brainstem auditory evoked response (BAER) showing no cortical waves 8 hours after the arrest and a CT scan demonstrating diffuse edema or watershed infarcts. An EEG with a relatively preserved background or improvement on serial EEGs conveys a more positive prognosis. For all patients who present in a coma, the overall functional recovery rate is approximately 13 percent. If a patient has not regained consciousness by 6 hours, the chance of survival for 1 year is 10 percent, and many of these survivors remain in a vegetative state.

References

1. Plum F, Posner JB: *The Diagnosis of Stupor and Coma.* Philadelphia, FA Davis, 1982.
2. Kety SS, Schmidt CF: Effects of active and passive hyperventilation and cerebral blood flow, cerebral oxygen consumption, cardiac output and blood pressure of normal young men. *J Clin Invest* 24:839, 1946.
3. Plum F, Posner JB, Hain RF: Delayed neurological deterioration after anoxia. *Arch Intern Med* 110:56, 1962.
4. Levy DE, Bates D, Caronna, JJ, et al: Prognosis in nontraumatic coma. *Ann Intern Med* 94:293, 1981.
5. Snyder BEAD, Ramirez-Lassepas M, Lippert DM: Neurologic status and prognosis after cardiopulmonary arrest. 1. A retrospective study. *Neurology* 27:807, 1977.
6. Caronna JJ, Finkelstein S: Neurologic syndromes after cardiac arrest. *Stroke* 9:517, 1978.
7. Garcia JH: Morphology of cerebral ischemia. *Crit Care Med* 16:979, 1988.
8. Dickey W, Adgey AAJ: Resuscitation: Mortality within hospital after resuscitation from ventricular fibrillation outside hospital. *Br Heart J* 67:334, 1992.
9. Myers RE, DeCourten CM, Yamaguchi S: Failure of marked hypoxia with maintained blood pressure to produce brain injury in cats. *J Neuropathol Exp Neurol* 39:378, 1980.
10. Safar P, Bleyaert A, Nemoto EM, et al: Resuscitation after global brain ischemia-anoxia. *Crit Care Med* 6:215, 1978.
11. Gray FD, Horner GJ: Survival following extreme hypoxia. *JAMA* 211:1815, 1970.
12. Siebke H, Breivik H, Rod T, et al: Survival after forty minutes submersion without cerebral sequelae. *Lancet* 1:1275, 1975.
13. Abramson NS, Safar P, Detre KM: Neurologic recovery after cardiac arrest: Effect of duration of ischemia. *Crit Care Med* 14:930, 1985.
14. Gray WA, Capone RJ Most AS: Unsuccessful emergency medical resuscitation: Are continued efforts in the emergency department justified? *N Engl J Med* 325:1393, 1991.
15. Kjos BO, Brant-Zawadzki, Young RG: Early CT findings of global central nervous system hypoperfusion. *Am J Roentgenol* 141:1227, 1983.
16. Silverman D: *Handbook of Electroencephalography and Clinical Neurophysiology.* vol. 12. Amsterdam, Elsiever, 1975, pp 81–94.
17. Neidermeyer E, Lopes de Silva, F: *Electroencephalography: Basic Principles, Clinical Applications and Related Fields.* Baltimore, Urban & Schwarzenberg, 1987, pp 383–389.
18. Facco E, Liviero MC, Munari M, et al: Short latency evoked potentials: new criteria for brain death? *J Neurol Neurosurg Psychiatry* 3:351, 1990.
19. Brunko E, Zegers de Beyl: Prognostic value of early cortical somatosensory evoked potentials after resuscitation from cardiac arrest. *Electroencephalogr Clin Neurophysiol* 66:15, 1987.
20. Lechleitner P, Felber S, Birbamer G, et al: Proton magnetic resonance spectroscopy of brain after cardiac resuscitation. *Lancet* 340:913, 1992.
21. Risto O, Somer H, Kaste M, et al: Neurologic outcome after out-of-hospital cardiac arrest: Prediction by cerebrospinal fluid enzyme analysis. *Arch Neurol* 46:753, 1989.
22. Edgren E, Hedstrand U, Nordin M, et al: Prediction of outcome after cardiac arrest. *Crit Care Med* 15:820, 1987.
23. Longstreth WT, Inui TS, Cobb LA, et al: Neurologic recovery after out-of-hospital cardiac arrest. *Ann Intern Med* 98:588, 1983.
24. Ernest MP, Yarnell PR, Merrill SL, et al: Long-term survival and neurological status after resuscitation from out-of-hospital cardiac arrest. *Neurology (NY)* 30:1298, 1980.
25. Tweed WA, Thomassen A, Wernberg M: Prognosis after cardiac arrest based on age and duration of coma. *Can Med Assoc J* 126:1058, 1982.
26. Lowenstein DH, Aminoff MJ: Clinical and EEG features of status epilepticus in comatose patients. *Neurology* 42:100, 1992.
27. Simon RP, Aminoff MJ: Electrographic status epilepticus in fatal anoxic coma. *Ann Neurol* 20:351, 1986.
28. Woodcock J, Ropper AH, Kennedy SK: High dose barbiturates in non-traumatic brain swelling: ICP reduction and effect on outcome. *Stroke* 13:785, 1982.
29. Rockoff MA, Marshall LF, Shapiro HM: High-dose barbiturate therapy in humans: A clinical review of 60 patients. *Ann Neurol* 6:194, 1979.
30. Brain Resuscitation Clinical Trial II Study Group: A randomized clinical study of a calcium-entry blocker (lidoflazine) in the treatment of comatose survivors of cardiac arrest. *N Engl J Med* 324:1225, 1991.

186. Status Epilepticus

Catherine A. Phillips and
Andrew M. Blumenfeld

Definition and Classification

Status epilepticus has been defined as "epileptic seizures that are so frequently repeated or so prolonged as to create a fixed and lasting epileptic condition" [1]. Alternatively stated, the definition includes seizures lasting more than 30 minutes or sequential seizures in which there is no return to baseline neurologic status between attacks. Status epilepticus is usually classified into three clinical types: (1) convulsive status epilepticus, in which the patient does not regain consciousness between repeated generalized tonic-clonic attacks; (2) simple partial status epilepticus, characterized by continuous or repetitive focal seizures without loss of consciousness [2]; and (3) nonconvulsive status epilepticus, such as absence or complex partial status, characterized by a prolonged "twilight" state of 30 minutes or more. Accurate assessment of seizure type is crucial, for certain seizures may be sensitive to specific antiepileptic drugs or may suggest a specific etiology.

CONVULSIVE STATUS EPILEPTICUS. Most generalized tonic-clonic status consists of partial seizures that have secondarily generalized; primary generalized status is less common [3,4]. The focal origin of the seizures may not be evident clinically and may be revealed only on an electroencephalogram (EEG). Most patients do not convulse continuously. Instead, seizures of a few minutes' duration may be followed by a prolonged period of unconsciousness that leads to the next seizure. With recurrent seizures, the clonic phase is shortened and the tonic phase lengthened. Status involving only tonic seizures does occur but is uncommon and is usually seen in mentally retarded children with a chronic seizure disorder. During convulsive status, massive autonomic discharge occurs with tachycardia and hypertension. Corneal and pupillary reflexes are lost, and there may be a Babinski response. The EEG shows repetitive spiking at the start of the seizure, which may be generalized (primary generalized epilepsy) or have a focal onset with subsequent generalization (partial epilepsy that secondarily generalizes). As status continues, the seizures may become subclinical without visible convulsive activity and then are evident only on EEG.

Myoclonic status epilepticus is often classified as a form of convulsive status, is rare, and usually occurs in children with chronic epilepsy and mental retardation. It is characterized by repetitive, asynchronous myoclonus with variable clouding of consciousness and may evolve into generalized tonic-clonic status. The EEG shows generalized polyspike and slow wave complexes. In adults, the myoclonic syndromes that occur are almost always secondary to acute or subacute encephalopathies whose origins are either toxic or metabolic (anoxia, liver or kidney failure), infections (Creutzfeldt-Jakob disease), or degenerative (Ramsay Hunt syndrome, neurolipidosis, Unverricht-Lundborg syndrome). Whether or not these syndromes should be considered myoclonic status epilepticus is controversial [5]. In these latter syndromes, the EEG shows the characteristic features of the underlying disorder.

SIMPLE PARTIAL STATUS EPILEPTICUS. This is the second most common form of status, after generalized tonic-clonic status. In *partial motor status,* focal clonic or tonic-clonic activity is localized to the face or an extremity. This activity may spread, corresponding to the somatotopic organization of the motor cortex, known as a *jacksonian march.* Alternatively, partial motor seizures can be multifocal and in this case are often precipitated by metabolic disorders, such as hyperglycemia in the hyperosmolar nonketotic state [6]. *Epilepsia partialis continua* refers to a form of partial motor status characterized by continuous, highly localized seizures that do not secondarily generalize and in which consciousness is maintained. The ictal EEG discharges are variable and may consist of focal spiking or sharp waves, focal slowing, diffuse irregular slowing, or no clear abnormality on scalp recording [7].

NONCONVULSIVE STATUS EPILEPTICUS. This includes absence and complex partial status. Clinically, both may resemble a psychiatric fugue state. Absence status involves a variable level of altered consciousness accompanied by subtle myoclonic movements of the face and occasional automatisms of the face and hands. The EEG is diagnostic and helps distinguish nonconvulsive from myoclonic status epilepticus. Characteristically, the EEG demonstrates continuous or discontinuous generalized 2- to 3-Hz spike and slow wave activity. Complex partial status involves either a series of complex partial seizures with staring, unresponsiveness, and motor automatisms, separated by a twilight state, or a more prolonged state of partial responsiveness and semipurposeful automatisms. The EEG reveals focal rhythmic or semirhythmic slow or sharp activity superimposed on a slow background. In both of these forms of status, the patient is partially or totally amnestic for the episode.

Etiology

Some of the major underlying etiologies and precipitants of status epilepticus are shown in Table 186-1. Precipitants are factors that provoke status where it otherwise would not have occurred, but they are not the underlying cause of the seizure disorder. Symptomatic status, defined as status resulting from an acute or subacute neurologic or metabolic insult, is typically more common than idiopathic status [3]. In most series, at least two-thirds of cases of status are symptomatic [4].

The most common cause of status in known epileptics is a change in antiepileptic drug serum levels. Of interest, the incidence of status has increased over the past century coincident with the introduction of antiepileptic drugs, supporting a connection between the use (or misuse) of these drugs and status epilepticus [3].

In adults without a prior history of epilepsy, the most common causes of status are brain tumors, particularly astrocytomas, and brain trauma, particularly acute open injuries. Lesions

Table 186-1. Etiologies and Precipitants of Status Epilepticus

A. Etiologies
　1. Structural brain lesion　Brain trauma
　　　　　　　　　　　　　　Brain tumors
　　　　　　　　　　　　　　Stroke
　2. CNS infections　　　　　Encephalitis
　　　　　　　　　　　　　　Meningitis
　3. Toxic　　　　　　　　　Drugs, e.g., theophylline, lidocaine,
　　　　　　　　　　　　　　　penicillin
　　　　　　　　　　　　　　Withdrawal states, e.g., alcohol, barbi-
　　　　　　　　　　　　　　　turate
　4. Metabolic　　　　　　　Hypocalcemia
　　　　　　　　　　　　　　Hypomagnesemia
　　　　　　　　　　　　　　Hypoglycemia, hyperglycemia
　　　　　　　　　　　　　　Hyponatremia
　　　　　　　　　　　　　　Hyperosmolar state
　　　　　　　　　　　　　　Anoxia
　　　　　　　　　　　　　　Uremia

B. Precipitants
　1. Changes in anticonvulsant blood levels
　　　Errors in medication
　　　Change in drug regimens
　　　Altered drug absorption
　　　Noncompliance
　2. Intercurrent infection
　　　Fever, e.g., UR or GI infections
　3. Alcohol withdrawal

CNS = central nervous system; UR = upper respiratory; GI = gastrointestinal.

of the frontal lobes are more likely to produce status than lesions at other sites [3]. Viral encephalitis caused by agents such as Epstein-Barr or herpes simplex virus may rarely have an abrupt onset heralded by status epilepticus. Human immunodeficiency virus (HIV) and illicit drug use are increasingly listed as a cause of status in recent series [8].

Prognosis and Sequelae of Status Epilepticus

The prognosis of status epilepticus depends on the etiology, duration of the episode, and secondary physiologic effects. The acute insult triggering status is one of the most important factors influencing mortality. In particular, the presence of a destructive brain lesion has a strong influence on poor outcome [9]. Patients with idiopathic status, where an acute central nervous system (CNS) insult is not a factor, have very low mortality.

The duration of status strongly affects the ultimate prognosis. In one study, the mean duration of convulsive status was 90 minutes in patients who did not have neurologic sequelae, 10 hours in patients with sequelae, and 13 hours for patients who died as a result of their status [10].

Despite improved medical care, in recent years convulsive status has been associated with a 7 to 16 percent acute mortality [11,12]. Other adverse outcomes include intellectual deterioration, permanent neurologic deficits, and chronic epilepsy.

Status epilepticus itself can produce profound neuronal damage. Neuropathologic studies of the brains of children and adults who died shortly after status reveal ischemic neuronal changes in the hippocampus, middle layers of the cerebral cortex, cerebellum (Purkinje cells), basal ganglia, thalamus, and hypothalamus [13]. These changes mimic those of severe hypoxia or hypoglycemia. The degree of hyperthermia during an

episode of status epilepticus has also been shown to correlate closely with the degree of CNS damage [14]. When seizures were artificially induced in paralyzed and mechanically ventilated primates, the neuronal injury still occurred, sparing the cerebellum [15]. This suggests that while the cerebellar damage may be due to hypoxia or hyperpyrexia, additional factors are responsible for the remainder of the neuronal damage.

The mechanism of neuronal damage is probably due to both increases in neuronal metabolic demands and decreases in energy substrates. Neuronal damage resulting from abnormal neuronal activity alone is supported by the presence of permanent neurologic residua following complex partial and partial motor status epilepticus, since in these situations systemic effects such as hypotension, hypoxia, and hyperpyrexia do not occur. Chronic memory impairment may follow complex partial status epilepticus [16,17], and focal neuronal necrosis (and edema) in the region of brain involved with seizure activity has been found following partial motor status [18,19].

Systemic Complications

If convulsive status epilepticus is not terminated promptly, secondary metabolic and medical complications occur (Table 186-2). Cardiac arrhythmias occur due to autonomic overactivity, acidosis, and hyperkalemia. This can be further complicated by shock due to lactic acidosis or pharmacologic intervention. Respiratory dysfunction may be caused by mechanical impairment from tonic muscle contraction, disturbed respiratory center function, massive autonomic discharge producing increased bronchial constriction and secretions, aspiration pneumonia, and neurogenic pulmonary edema. Neurogenic pulmonary edema results from ictal increases in pulmonary circulation with transcapillary fluid flux [14]. Renal impairment is also multifactorial, resulting from a combination of rhabdomyolysis with myoglobinuria and hypotension with poor renal perfusion.

Hyperthermia results from excessive muscle activity and hy-

Table 186-2. Medical Complications of Status Epilepticus

	Early	Late (after 30 min)
1. Cardiovascular system	Tachycardia Hypertension	Bradycardia Cardiac arrest Hypotension Shock
2. Respiratory system	Tachypnea Apnea with CO_2 retention	Apnea Cheyne-Stokes Aspiration pneumonia Neurogenic pulmonary edema
3. Renal system		Uremia Acute tubular necrosis Myoglobinuria
4. Autonomic nervous system	Mydriasis Salivary and tracheobronchial hypersecretion Excessive sweating Bronchial constriction	Hyperpyrexia
5. Metabolic	Lactic acidosis Hyperglycemia Hyperkalemia	Lactic acidosis Hypoglycemia Liver failure Elevated prolactin

pothalamic dysfunction; alternatively, it may be due to an underlying infection that is responsible for the initiation of status epilepticus. The distinction of hyperthermia from an infection or status epilepticus itself can be complicated by the peripheral leukocytosis [14] that occurs with status epilepticus due to demargination. This can result in a white blood cell count in the range of 12,700 to 28,000 cells per cubic millimeter. The differential may be normal or may show lymphocytic or polymorphonuclear predominance, but band forms are rarely present. In addition, a mild cerebral spinal fluid (CSF) pleocytosis can occur with status epilepticus [14]. The maximum cell count is usually less than 80 cells per cubic millimeter, with an initial polymorphonuclear predominance that reverts to a lymphocytic predominance as the pleocytosis resolves over a few days. Mild transient elevations in CSF protein may also occur. Lowering of the CSF glucose level does *not* occur, however, and reduced CSF glucose must immediately suggest an underlying bacterial or fungal infection.

Increased lactate production from maximally exercised muscles results in a metabolic acidosis within minutes after the start of status epilepticus. There is a variable respiratory contribution to the acidosis from carbon dioxide retention. The degree of acidosis does not correlate with the extent of neuropathologic damage [14]. Following cessation of the seizure, lactate is rapidly metabolized, resulting in spontaneous resolution of the acidosis.

Initially, hyperglycemia develops due to catecholamine and glucagon release; later, however, hypoglycemia occurs due to increased plasma insulin, increased cerebral glucose consumption, and excessive muscle activity.

Initial Assessment and Medical Management

Status epilepticus is a medical emergency and must be treated immediately. Ideally, a management protocol should be worked out in advance so the appropriate treatment can be initiated as soon as the diagnosis is made. This discussion concentrates on generalized tonic-clonic status epilepticus, since it is the most common form of status in adults and has the most harmful neurologic sequelae.

The initial step is to confirm the diagnosis. Since patients with generalized tonic-clonic status usually do not convulse continuously, a few minutes of observation may be appropriate to witness recurrence of generalized seizures without subsequent recovery of consciousness. Several seizures, or even a flurry of seizures, separated by a normal level of consciousness does not constitute status epilepticus. In the case of nonconvulsive or focal motor status, the diagnosis should not be made until 30 minutes of continuous clinical (or electrical) seizure activity has been observed. Once the diagnosis is made, treatment must proceed rapidly but deliberately. Table 186-3 outlines a management protocol.

It is important to obtain as much history as possible within the first few minutes of assessment, including any history of a chronic seizure disorder and antiepileptic drug use. The sedating and respiratory depressant effects of some drugs used to treat status may be more pronounced in a patient who already has a significant serum level of phenobarbital. Obtaining information about all medications the patient has used helps the physician anticipate any potential adverse effects.

After appropriate blood samples have been obtained, glucose administration is recommended. Hypoglycemia is a rare but easily reversible cause of status and will result in irreversible

Table 186-3. Management Protocol for Generalized Status Epilepticus in Adults

1. If diagnosis is uncertain, observe recurrence of generalized seizures without subsequent recovery of consciousness.
2. Assess cardiopulmonary status; establish airway.
3. Start intravenous line with normal saline.
4. Draw blood for CBC/diff, glucose, BUN/creatinine, electrolytes, Ca/Mg, antiepileptic drug levels, toxin screen.
5. Give glucose (D_{50}) 50 ml and thiamine 100 mg IV.
6. Monitor respirations, blood pressure, ECG, and, if possible, EEG.
7. Give lorazepam 0.1 mg/kg IV bolus, <2 mg/min, if patient is actively seizing.
8. Immediately start phenytoin 20 mg/kg IV, <50 mg/min, with slower rate if hypotension develops.
9. Give additional boluses of phenytoin (5 mg/kg), to a maximum of 30 mg/kg, if patient is still seizing.
10. If status continues after phenytoin infusion is completed, immediately start phenobarbital 20 mg/kg IV, <100 mg/min. Intubation is necessary either before or during phenobarbital infusion.
11. If status persists, induce coma with short-acting barbiturate:
    a. During induction, continuous EEG to monitor for control of seizures and level of anesthesia is needed.
    b. Pentobarbital: 5 mg/kg IV load, given slowly; give additional 5 mg/kg boluses as necessary to produce burst-suppression pattern.
    c. Maintenance infusion of 0.5–5 mg/kg/hr.
    d. Monitor EEG every 1–2 hr once burst-suppression pattern is present.
    e. Stop pentobarbital at 12 hr; if seizures recur, resume infusion for 24 hr, then stop again. Continue this process as necessary.

CNS damage if left untreated. Since glucose administration may precipitate Wernicke-Korsakoff syndrome in some individuals with marginal nutrition, thiamine should also be given. Subsequent intravenous infusions should consist of saline solution, as some antiepileptic drugs precipitate in glucose solutions.

The patient must be assessed for other metabolic consequences of status. Hyperthermia should be detected and treated using alcohol sponge baths, cooling blankets, or ice packs. Oxygenation must be maintained, but maximal oxygenation is not necessary. The metabolic acidosis that occurs does not adversely affect neurologic outcome and should not be treated with bicarbonate [14]. Blood pressure must be carefully monitored; the systemic hypertension and decreased cerebrovascular resistance of early status provide adequate blood flow for the increased metabolic demand in the brain, but eventually hypotension may occur, making the brain vulnerable to inadequate perfusion. Pharmacologic intervention for the seizures can exacerbate any hypotension.

Maximum effort must be made to determine whether a metabolic disorder is causing the status. In these cases, pharmacologic intervention alone is not effective. Systemic and CNS infections must be excluded, and lumbar puncture is often necessary, even though peripheral leukocytosis, fever, and CSF pleocytosis may be secondary to convulsive status epilepticus itself. Contrast-enhanced head computed tomography (CT) scan may demonstrate a structural cause of status; this procedure should be deferred, however, until the patient has been medically stabilized and the status has terminated.

Pharmacologic Management

A variety of drugs are available to treat status. It is important to understand the pharmacokinetics of these drugs to ensure ef-

Table 186-4. Properties of Drugs Used to Treat Status Epilepticus

	Route	Loading dose	Rate of administration	Time to enter brain	Time to peak brain concentration	Minimum effective plasma concentration (μg/ml)	Side effects
Diazepam	IV, rectal	0.1–0.2 mg/kg up to 20 mg	2 mg/min	IV < 10 sec	8 min	0.2–0.8	Respiratory depression/ apnea (may be abrupt), hypotension, sedation, especially in combination with barbiturates
Lorazepam	IV	0.1 mg/kg	2 mg/min	< 2–3 min	23 min	0.03–0.1	Same as diazepam; amnesia
Phenytoin	IV	20 mg/kg	50 mg/min	1–3 min	3–6 min	15–30	Hypotension and ECG changes during acute administration; sedation at high doses
Phenobarbital	IV	20 mg/kg	100 mg/min	3 min	5–15 min	10–40	Respiratory depression and sedation common with increasing doses, especially when benzodiazepines used; hypotension
Lidocaine	IV	100 mg IV bolus, repeat in 5 min if necessary (2–3 mg/kg)	25–50 mg/ min	< 20 sec	< 1 min	Unknown	Cardiovascular depression, ECG changes, seizures, disorientation; respiratory arrest at high doses

fective use (see Chap. 213). Table 186-4 outlines some of these properties.

If the patient has ongoing continuous seizure activity, therapy with an intravenous benzodiazepine should be initiated. If the seizures have stopped temporarily or if prolonged stuporous periods are present between attacks, intravenous phenytoin should be started immediately and benzodiazepines avoided entirely. Some authorities advocate the use of phenobarbital as initial therapy and believe it may be as safe and effective as the combination of benzodiazepines and phenytoin. However, CNS depression is a major side effect of this therapy [20].

Diazepam is an extremely effective anticonvulsant but has a brief duration of action (10–25 minutes), and some no longer consider it the benzodiazepine of first choice [21,22]. Lorazepam is equally effective in treating generalized status epilepticus and has a much longer duration of action (2 to >24 hours) [23,24,25]. Lorazepam does not have extensive peripheral tissue uptake, unlike diazepam, which distributes rapidly and extensively into fat. Lorazepam has slower and less complete CNS penetration than diazepam, but in clinical practice this difference is rarely significant. The onset of action for lorazepam is usually under 3 minutes, rapid enough to be acceptable in the treatment of status [26].

Both diazepam and lorazepam have significant cardiac, respiratory, and CNS depressant side effects, and the incidence of these side effects has been shown to be essentially the same for the two drugs [23,25]. *Respiratory depression and apnea may occur abruptly with doses as small as 1 mg.* Previous administration of sedative drugs, such as barbiturates, and increasing age potentiate cardiorespiratory side effects. Hypotension, which occasionally occurs, may be partially due to the propylene glycol solvent contained in the intravenous forms of diazepam and lorazepam.

If intravenous access is not available, rectal diazepam is an alternative that has been successful in achieving rapid therapeutic levels and effectively terminating prolonged generalized seizures. The intravenous preparation is administered per rectum, using a 7.5 to 10 mg dose for adults and a 5 to 7.5 mg dose for children younger than 3 years [27,28]. The dose is repeated in 5 minutes if necessary. Significant respiratory depression has not been reported. Intramuscular administration results in delayed peak levels, ranging from 40 to 60 minutes for diazepam and 90 minutes for lorazepam, rendering this route unsuitable for the treatment of status [27,29]. Furthermore, the peak concentration after intramuscular injection is much less than that following intravenous injection for both agents.

Although benzodiazepines stop active seizures, phenytoin is the drug of choice for definitive therapy of status epilepticus. A 20 mg per kilogram load is recommended, given at 50 mg per minute. Intramuscular administration should not be used since it results in precipitation at the injection site and has slow, erratic absorption. Hypotension, electrocardiogram (ECG) changes, and respiratory depression can occur and may be due partly to the propylene glycol diluent [30]. Simultaneous cardiac monitoring should be performed, and slower infusion rates (25 mg/min) should be considered in patients who are elderly or have a history of cardiac arrhythmias, compromised pulmonary function, or hypotension. The most common adverse effect is hypotension, which is age-related and reportedly does not occur in patients younger than 40 years [21].

A loading dose of approximately 20 mg per kilogram of phenytoin results in a plasma level of 25 μg per milliliter when the initial level is zero [21]. The half-life at this level is prolonged to approximately 40 hours because of zero-order kinetics. Maintenance therapy, therefore, need not be started until 18 to 24 hours after the loading dose is given. A full additional phenytoin load in known epileptic patients who already have therapeutic phenytoin plasma levels results in levels of 35 to 40 μg per milliliter [21]. Nystagmus, ataxia, and sedation may be seen with levels in this range but generally do not pose a major problem in this clinical setting. Cardiotoxicity is a concern only at the time of acute administration.

The anticonvulsant effect of phenytoin is maximal within 10 minutes after infusion is completed. Therefore, if status persists after this time, intravenous phenobarbital should be given immediately. Up to 20 mg per kilogram may be necessary, though often an initial dose of 10 mg per kilogram is given and then repeated if seizures continue. Phenobarbital may be administered more rapidly than phenytoin (100 mg/min). *Respiratory depression is a major side effect,* especially if benzodiazepines have been used. It is imperative to monitor respirations and ensure an adequate airway.

If status continues after full loading doses of phenytoin and phenobarbital have been given, then drug-induced coma is indicated. Barbiturates are most commonly used for this. All patients must be intubated by this time. Various agents have been used, including thiopental and methohexital, but pentobarbital has been used most commonly [31,32]. All are extremely effective at suppressing clinical and electrographic seizures. Thiopental has relatively higher fat solubility and slower metabolism because of nonlinear kinetics at high doses and may not be the preferred drug [31]. Phenobarbital is not used for this purpose since it results in a very prolonged coma. Cardiac depression is often produced, and careful hemodynamic monitoring is required. Pressors are frequently needed.

Simultaneous EEG monitoring is mandatory during induction of barbiturate coma. The dose of pentobarbital must be sufficient to produce a burst-suppression EEG pattern, characterized by a flat background punctuated by bursts of mixed-frequency activity. If the bursts contain electrographic seizure activity the coma should be deepened, at times to virtual electrocerebral silence. The goal is to terminate electrical seizure activity, not just to produce a burst-suppression pattern. Maintenance doses of phenytoin and phenobarbital should be continued and the serum levels followed.

Continuous diazepam infusion can be used as an alternative to barbiturate anesthesia. It should not be given to a patient who has received intravenous phenobarbital. A serum level of 0.2 to 0.8 μg per milliliter is recommended and can be maintained by an infusion rate of 0.13 mg per minute (100 mg diazepam in 500 ml D_5W at 40 ml/hr) [33].

Lidocaine may occasionally be effective in controlling status if more conventional therapy has failed [34]. An initial intravenous dose of 100 mg is recommended, followed by a second dose of 100 mg if seizures continue or recur. The efficacy of this drug should be evident within 20 to 30 seconds, and the effect only lasts 20 to 30 minutes. If seizures remit and later recur, a continuous infusion at a rate of 3 to 10 mg/kg/hr may be started. Lidocaine does not cause drowsiness or respiratory depression, but high doses may result in cardiac arrhythmias, hypotension, and convulsions. The dose should be reduced if congestive heart failure or liver disease is present.

Paraldehyde has also been used to treat refractory status but is no longer available in the United States in a form suitable for parenteral use. Rectal administration of paraldehyde can be considered if this is the only route available, other medications have failed, or the patient is allergic to conventional medications [35]. It is well absorbed rectally, though levels do not peak until 2 to 4 hours after administration. The dose is 0.3 ml per kilogram diluted 2:1 in oil. A repeat dose may be given in 15 to 20 minutes [36]. Metabolic acidosis, pulmonary edema, and right heart failure have been reported after parenteral administration. Paraldehyde decomposes to acetaldehyde and acetic acid in the presence of light and air; an outdated drug may therefore result in chemical proctitis when given rectally.

Inhalation anesthetics are used less often for treating status epilepticus. Isoflurane (1.5–2%) has been used successfully, suppressing both clinical and electrographic seizures. Unlike halothane and enflurane, it has few hemodynamic effects and no known toxic metabolites. These agents are cumbersome to administer and may result in increased intracranial pressure [37].

Nonconvulsive status must be treated quickly, although the urgency is not as great as for convulsive status. Diazepam and lorazepam are both effective in treating complex partial, partial motor, and absence status. The response to benzodiazepines may be helpful in confirming the diagnosis if it is in question. The patient should also be started on antiepileptic medication appropriate for long-term management, given as a loading dose if appropriate. Ethosuximide and valproic acid are the drugs of choice for absence status, but neither is available in an intravenous form. Valproic acid is preferable if there is any history of generalized tonic-clonic seizures. The recommended starting dose is 15 mg/kg/day for valproic acid and 500 mg per day for ethosuximide. Complex partial and partial motor status both respond to phenytoin and phenobarbital, though epilepsia partialis continua can be notoriously resistant to treatment. The drug of choice for myoclonic status is valproic acid, but phenytoin and phenobarbital are also effective.

Fosphenytoin, or "phenytoin prodrug," is an investigational agent that is the disodium phosphate ester of phenytoin [38,39]. It is rapidly converted enzymatically to phenytoin. Fosphenytoin has much greater aqueous solubility than phenytoin; therefore propylene glycol is not needed as a diluent. It is nonirritating, whether given intramuscularly or intravenously, and well tolerated. Rapid and complete absorption occurs after intramuscular administration. Time to peak phenytoin levels after intravenous injection of the prodrug is 19 minutes and after intramuscular injection is 180 minutes. In the future, the combination of lorazepam and fosphenytoin may be the method of choice for treating status epilepticus.

Conclusion

Status epilepticus is a true medical emergency and needs to be treated promptly and definitively. In convulsive status, lorazepam is the drug of choice for immediate, short-term termination of ongoing seizure activity. A phenytoin loading dose should be administered simultaneously with the lorazepam; if the patient is not actively seizing, benzodiazepines are not needed. Phenytoin is safe and effective, has a rapid onset of seizure control, and may be used for maintenance therapy. If these drugs are ineffective phenobarbital should be added, and if status still persists barbiturate coma should be induced. Physicians should be familiar with a treatment protocol, since appropriate therapy greatly reduces morbidity and mortality.

References

1. Gastaut H (ed): *Dictionary of Epilepsy I. Definition.* Geneva, Switzerland, World Health Organization, 1973.
2. Treiman DM, Delgado-Escueta AV: Status epilepticus, in Thompson RA, Green JR (eds): *Critical Care of Neurologic and Neurosurgical Emergencies.* New York, Raven, 1980, p 53.
3. Janz D: Etiology of convulsive status epilepticus, in Delgado-Escueta AV, Wasterlain CG, Treiman DM, et al (eds): *Advances in*

Neurology. vol. 34. Status Epilepticus. New York, Raven, 1983, p 47.

4. Hauser WA: Status epilepticus: Frequency, etiology, and neurologic sequelae, in Delgado-Escueta AV, Wasterlain CG, Treiman OH, et al (eds): *Advances in Neurology. vol. 34. Status Epilepticus*. New York, Raven, p 3.

5. Gastaut H: Classification of status epilepticus, in Delgado-Escueta AV, Wasterlain CG, Treiman DM, et al (eds): *Advances in Neurology. vol. 34. Status Epilepticus*. New York, Raven, 1983, p 15.

6. Singh BM, Strobos RJ: Epilepsia partialis continua associated with nonketotic hyperglycemia: Clinical and biochemical profile of 21 patients. *Am Neurol* 8:155, 1980.

7. Thomas JE, Reagan TJ, Klass DW: Epilepsia partialis continua: A review of 32 cases. *Arch Neurol* 34:266, 1977.

8. Holtzman DM, Kaku DA, So YT: New-onset seizures associated with human immunodeficiency virus infection: Causation and clinical features in 100 cases. *Am J Med* 87:173, 1989.

9. Celesia GC: Prognosis in convulsive status epilepticus, in Delgado-Escueta AV, Wasterlain CG, Treiman DM, et al (eds): *Advances in Neurology. vol. 34. Status Epilepticus*. New York, Raven, 1983, p 55.

10. Rowan AJ, Scott DF: Major status epilepticus: A series of 42 patients. *Acta Neurol Scand* 46:573, 1970.

11. Celesia GG: Modern concepts of status epilepticus. *JAMA* 235:1571, 1976.

12. Aminoff MJ, Simon RP: Status epilepticus: Causes, clinical features and consequences in 98 patients. *Am J Med* 69:657, 1980.

13. Corsellis JAN, Bruton CJ: Neuropathology of status epilepticus in humans, in Delgado-Escueta AV, Wasterlain CG, Treiman DM, et al (eds): *Advances in Neurology. vol. 34. Status Epilepticus*. New York, Raven, 1983, p 129.

14. Simon RP: Physiologic consequences of status epilepticus. *Epilepsia* 26:S58, 1985.

15. Meldrum BS, Vigouroux RA, Brierley JB: Systemic factors and epileptic brain damage. *Arch Neurol* 29:82, 1973.

16. Engel J, Ludwig BE, Fettell M: Prolonged partial complex status epilepticus: EEG and behavioral observations. *Neurology* 28:863, 1978.

17. Trieman DM, Delgado-Escueta AV: Complex partial status epilepticus, in Delgado-Escueta AV, Wasterlain CG, Treiman DM, et al (eds): *Advances in Neurology. vol. 34. Status Epilepticus*. New York, Raven, 1983, p 69.

18. Sammaritano M, Andermann F, Melanson D, et al: Prolonged focal cerebral edema associated with partial status epilepticus. *Epilepsia* 26:334, 1985.

19. Soffer D, Melamed E, Assaf Y, et al: Hemispheric brain damage in unilateral status epilepticus. *Ann Neurol* 20:737, 1986.

20. Shaner DM, McCurdy SA, Herring MO, et al: Treatment of status epilepticus: A prospective comparison of diazepam and phenytoin versus phenobarbital and optional phenytoin. *Neurology* 38:202, 1988.

21. Leppik IE: Status epilepticus. *Clin Ther* 7:272, 1985.

22. Treiman DM: Pharmacokinetics and clinical use of benzodiazepines in the management of status epilepticus. *Epilepsia* 30(suppl 2):S4, 1989.

23. Leppik IE, Derivan AT, Homan RW, et al: Double-blind study of lorazepam and diazepam in status epilepticus. *JAMA* 249:1452, 1983.

24. Greenblatt DJ, Divoll M: Diazepam versus lorazepam: Relationship of drug distribution to duration of clinical action, in Delgado-Escueta AV, Wasterlain CG, Treiman DM, et al (eds): *Advances in Neurology. vol. 34. Status Epilepticus*. New York, Raven, 1983, p 487.

25. Levy RJ, Krall RL: Treatment of status epilepticus with lorazepam. *Arch Neurol* 41:605, 1984.

26. Homan RW, Walker JE: Clinical studies of lorazepam in status epilepticus, in Delgado-Escueta AV, Wasterlain CG, Treiman DM, et al (eds): *Advances in Neurology, vol. 34. Status Epilepticus*. New York, Raven, 1983, p 493.

27. Schmidt D: Benzodiazepines: Diazepam, in Levy RH, Dreifuss FE, Mattson RH, et al (eds): *Antiepileptic Drugs*. New York, Raven, 1989, p 735.

28. Graves NM, Kriel RL: Rectal administration of antiepileptic drugs in children. *Pediatr Neurol* 3:321, 1987.

29. Homan RW, Unwin DH: Benzodiazepines: Lorazepam, in Levy RH, Dreifuss FE, Matson RH, et al (eds): *Antiepileptic Drugs*. New York, Raven, 1989, p 841.

30. Uthman BM, Wilder BJ: Emergency management of seizures: An overview. *Epilepsia* 30(suppl 2):533, 1989.

31. Rashkin MC, Young C, Penovich P: Pentobarbital treatment of refractory status epilepticus. *Neurology* 37:500, 1987.

32. Lowenstein DH, Aminoff MJ, Simon RP: Barbiturate anesthesia in the treatment of status epilepticus. *Neurology* 38:395, 1988.

33. Delgado-Escueta AV, Wasterlain C, Treiman DM: Management of status epilepticus. *N Engl J Med* 306:1337, 1982.

34. Pascval J, Sedano MJ, Polo Jose M, et al: Intravenous lidocaine for status epilepticus. *Epilepsia* 29:584, 1988.

35. Browne TR: Status epilepticus, in Browne TR, Feldman RD (eds): *Epilepsy, Diagnosis and Management*. Boston, Little, Brown, 1983, p 341.

36. Lockman LA: Paraldehyde, in Levy RH, Dreifuss FE, Mattson RH, et al (eds): *Antiepileptic Drugs*. New York, Raven, 1989, pp 881–886.

37. Ropper AH, Kofke A, Brumfield EB, et al: Comparison of isoflurane, halothane, and nitrous oxide in status epilepticus. *Ann Neurol* 19:98, 1986.

38. Smith RD, Brown BS, Maher RW, et al: Pharmacology of ACC-9653 (phenytoin prodrug). *Epilepsia* 30(suppl 2):515, 1989.

39. Leppik IE, Boucher R, Wilder BJ, et al: Phenytoin prodrug: Preclinical and clinical studies. *Epilepsia* 30(suppl 2):2, 1989.

187. *Cerebrovascular Disease*

Marc Fisher and John P. Weaver

Cerebrovascular disease encompasses stroke due to thrombotic or embolic ischemia, intracerebral hemorrhage, and subarachnoid hemorrhage. Many patients with cerebrovascular disease require management in the intensive care unit (ICU) because their illness is severe or the treatment is complex. This chapter reviews the basic concepts of pathogenesis, diagnosis, evaluation, and management for patients with each of these types of stroke.

Ischemic Cerebrovascular Disease

Ischemic cerebrovascular disease (ICVD) is the most common neurologic problem that leads to acute hospitalization. It is typically not managed in an ICU except under special circumstances, including impaired consciousness with or without cerebral edema; crescendo transient ischemic attacks; stroke in evolution; major associated illnesses (myocardial infarction [MI], sepsis, pulmonary embolus); or in a patient already in an ICU (ICVD complicates 1–2% of cases of acute MI). It can be anticipated that as therapies directed at preserving ischemic brain tissue and lysis of occluding thrombi in cerebral arteries are developed, many more patients with ICVD will be managed in a general medical ICU or a specialized stroke unit. This change will occur over the next few years. These treatments will require prompt diagnosis and institution of appropriate therapy, and many of them will require careful assessment and titration to improve therapeutic efficacy and avoid side effects.

To ensure accurate diagnosis and appropriate therapy, ICVD is categorized along three axes: degree of completeness, anatomic territory, and underlying mechanism.

DEGREE OF COMPLETENESS OF STROKE. Three degrees of completeness can be recognized: transient ischemic attack (TIA), stroke-in-evolution, and completed stroke [1]. A TIA is an episode of temporary focal cerebral dysfunction occurring on a vascular basis that evolves rapidly. It typically resolves within minutes but may last up to 24 hours.

A stroke-in-evolution, or progressing stroke, is a neurovascular event that worsens over several hours (carotid circulation) to several days (vertebral-basilar system). This type of event is difficult both to define and to recognize clinically, except in retrospect.

A completed stroke is a neurovascular event in which the deficit has been fixed for at least 24 hours in those portions of the brain supplied by the carotid artery and for 72 hours in those portions of the brain supplied by the vertebral-basilar system.

ANATOMIC TERRITORY OF STROKE. Two broad clinical, anatomic categories of ICVD syndromes are recognized, based on division of the vascular supply of the brain into those areas supplied by the carotid system and those supplied by the vertebral-basilar system [2]. Symptoms commonly encountered in carotid system disease include monoparesis or hemiparesis, monoparesthesias or hemiparesthesias, monocular visual loss, homonymous hemianopsia, and various aphasic syndromes. Symptoms seen in vertebral-basilar system disease include binocular visual disturbance, vertigo, diplopia, ataxia, dysarthria, paresis, and paresthesias, frequently with involvement of one side of the face and the contralateral body.

In posterior cerebrovascular ischemia, loss of consciousness rarely occurs without other vertebral-basilar symptoms. Isolated symptoms, such as vertigo, diplopia, amnesia, dysarthria, and light-headedness, cannot by themselves serve as a basis for the diagnosis of a vertebral-basilar event [3]. However, these symptoms together with other brainstem symptoms may support the diagnosis of a vertebral-basilar ischemic event. A small percentage of patients experience symptoms at different times in both the carotid and vertebral-basilar systems. In addition, some cerebrovascular symptoms cannot be adequately localized, even by experienced clinicians.

UNDERLYING MECHANISM OF THE STROKE. Acute ICVD should be categorized into large vessel atherothrombic occlusions, small vessel occlusions, cardioembolic strokes, or "watershed" infarcts.

Large Vessel Atherothrombotic Occlusions. These strokes are due to atherosclerosis in the carotid or vertebral-basilar arteries and are a common cause of acute ICVD. The initial symptoms occur abruptly, and the stroke may evolve in any of

the three patterns noted previously. Many different clinical syndromes relate to the particular vascular territory involved and the adequacy of collateral flow [4].

Small Vessel Occlusions.. These strokes, in which the lenticulostriate arteries or basilar penetrators are occluded by microatheromata or lipohyalinosis, lead to the development of small infarcts called *lacunes* (Fig. 187-1). If a lacune is strategically placed in the internal capsule, thalamus, or basis pontis, substantial neurologic deficits occur. The most common lacunar syndromes are pure motor hemiparesis, pure sensory stroke, ataxic hemiparesis, and clumsy-hand dysarthria syndrome [5]. Similar clinical findings may be caused by mechanisms such as tumors, aneurysms, and large artery infarcts.

Cardioembolic Strokes. As the technology for detecting underlying cardiac sources of emboli has improved, an embolic origin of thrombus has been recognized with increasing frequency. Cardioembolic strokes typically present with maximal deficit at onset, although a small minority may have a stuttering course. Diagnosis may be difficult if the patient has coexistent large arterial lesions; indeed, as many as one-third of patients with a cardiac embolic source have another potential explanation for their strokes [6]. In these cases, it may be difficult to identify a precise etiology. The most common cardiac sources associated with cerebral embolic events are outlined in Table 187-1. Nonvalvular atrial fibrillation is associated with a stroke

Fig. 187-1. Lacunar infarct involving the left internal capsule seen on a CT scan.

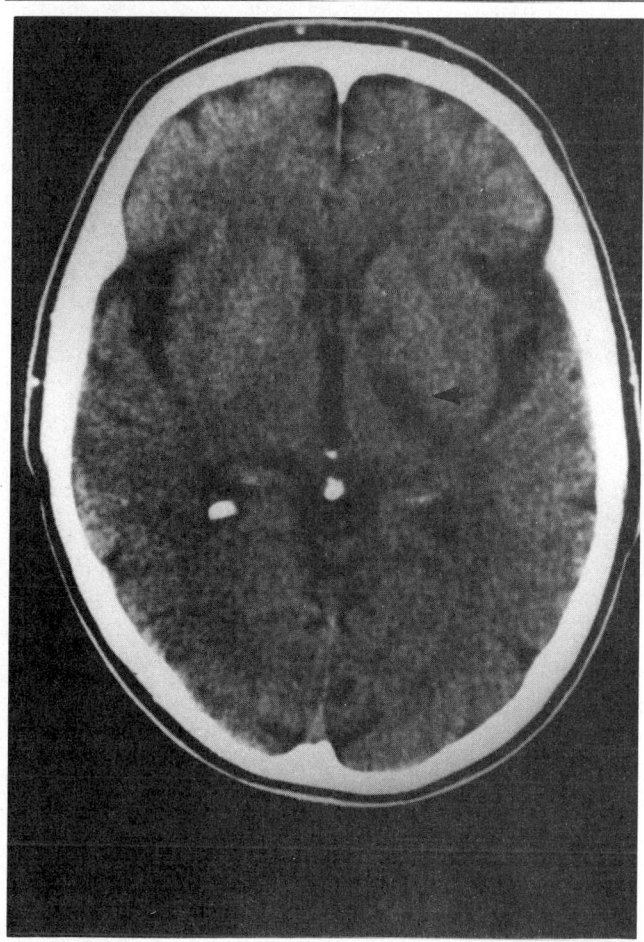

Table 187-1. Cardiac Sources for Cerebral Emboli

Common
    Nonvalvular atrial fibrillation
    Acute anterior wall myocardial infarction
    Ventricular aneurysms and dyskinetic segments
    Rheumatic valvular disease
    Prosthetic cardiac valves
    Right-to-left shunts
    Bacterial endocarditis

Less common
    Mitral valve prolapse
    Cardiomyopathy
    Bicuspid aortic valve
    Atrial myxoma
    Nonbacterial endocarditis
    Mitral annulus calcification
    Idiopathic hypertrophic subaortic stenosis
    Atrial septal aneurysm

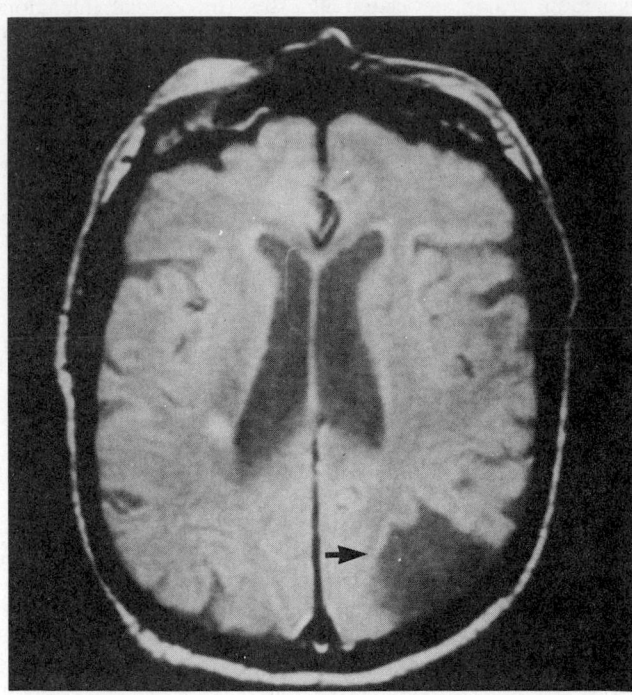

Fig. 187-2. T_1-weighted MRI scan demonstrating a watershed infarction (*arrow*) in the border zone between the middle and posterior cerebral arteries.

risk of 4 to 5 percent per year, increasing with advancing age, the presence of paroxysmal atrial fibrillation, and an enlarged left atrium [7]. Patients with acute transmural myocardial infarctions, especially those with ventricular thrombi noted on echocardiography, have an increased risk for embolic stroke. Cerebral emboli constitute a major complication of mechanical cardiac valves. The risk is higher in patients with coexistent atrial fibrillation and lower in those with bioprosthetic valves. Patent right-to-left cardiac shunts have been recognized with increasing frequency in younger stroke patients by contrast echocardiography [8]. These right-to-left shunts are clearly associated with stroke risk, but the mechanism is uncertain in most cases.

Watershed infarcts are due to globally diminished cerebral blood flow resulting from cardiac arrest or systemic hypotension, with focal infarction and deficits occurring in well-described patterns (Fig. 187-2) [9]. In the carotid circulation, watershed infarcts occur between the distribution of the middle cerebral artery and both the anterior and posterior cerebral arteries. The usual anterior infarction causes contralateral weakness and sensory loss sparing the face; in posterior watershed infarcts homonymous hemianopsia with little or no weakness is most common. Quadriparesis, cortical blindness, or bilateral arm weakness may also be seen in other vascular territory watershed infarcts.

PROGNOSIS. The eventual prognosis of a completed stroke in either the carotid or vertebral basilar distribution cannot be predicted with certainty during the initial phase of the ictus. The overall mortality varies from 3 to 20 percent in both vascular distributions [10]. Patients with an altered level of consciousness or coma have a significantly greater mortality than those who remain alert. A dense hemiplegia and conjugate eye deviation are other early signs that point toward a poorer prognosis in carotid system strokes.

Functional outcome also varies widely, with a favorable outcome observed in 20 to 70 percent of cases [11]. Lacunar syndromes are associated with very low 1-month mortality (approximately 1%) and good functional recovery in 75 to 80 percent of patients 1 to 3 months after stroke. The clinical course varies: one-third of patients with large artery atherothrombotic strokes have a progressive or fluctuating course, whereas less than one-fifth of patients with cardioembolic disease follow a similar pattern [12]. In patients with vertebral-basilar symptoms, more than 40 percent were observed to have a progressive course.

DIFFERENTIAL DIAGNOSIS. The history and neurologic examination usually enable the physician to differentiate among the major subtypes of ICVD: degree of completeness, territory involved, and ischemic mechanism. In some cases, however, this may require further laboratory investigation.

It is especially important to differentiate ICVD patients from those with primary intercerebral hemorrhage. Patients with cerebral hemorrhage typically have a progressive course, with evolution of symptoms over hours [13]. Early obtundation or even coma is much more common in intracerebral hemorrhage than in ICVD because of mass effect on the brainstem reticular arousal system, which occurs rapidly with expanding hematomas. Seizures, headache, and vomiting are also much more common in patients with intracerebral hemorrhage. If this diagnosis is suspected, early imaging with computed tomographic (CT) or magnetic resonance imaging (MRI) scan is imperative.

Other conditions besides cerebral vascular events can occcasionally cause acute focal neurologic deficits and must be considered. Patients with primary or metastatic brain tumors can rapidly develop focal neurologic signs due to hemorrhage into the tumor or other mechanisms (Fig. 187-3). Subdural hematomas may rarely present with the rapid development of focal neurologic deficits and must be considered in elderly patients, even without a history of head trauma. Acute neurologic deficits are occasionally the presenting manifestations of tumors, further supporting the need for an early imaging study. Patients with migraine headaches commonly develop focal neurologic symptoms either before or during the early phase of the head-

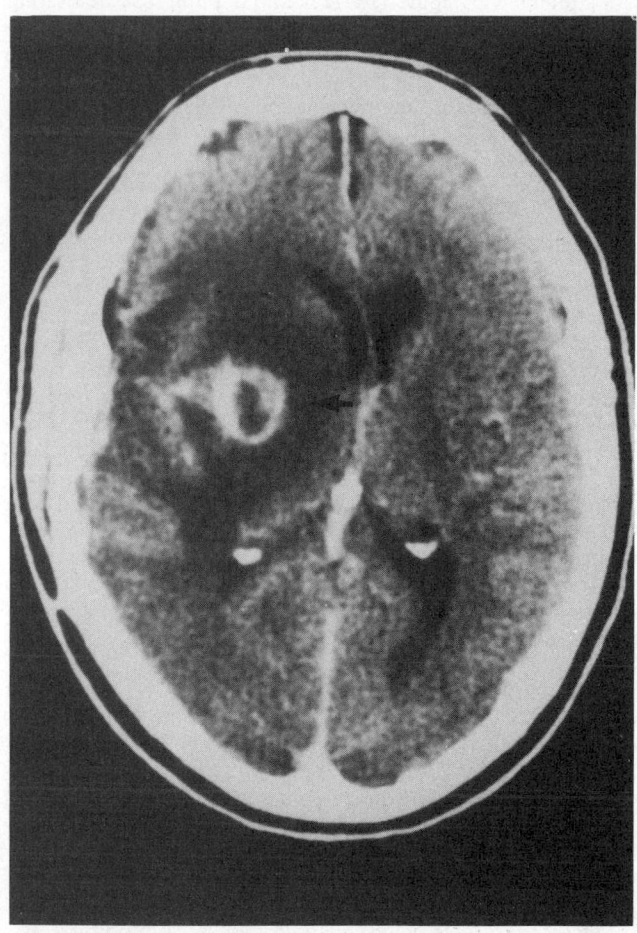

Fig. 187-3. Malignant glioma with associated edema on a CT scan in a patient who abruptly developed a pure motor deficit.

ache. Rarely, these deficits may persist and are associated with frank areas of infarction on imaging studies (migrainous stroke) [14]. Patients with focal seizures may develop sensory and aphasic symptoms that can mimic ICVD, although they are usually stereotyped and transient and march in a different pattern. Occasionally, focal neurologic deficits may follow seizures and persist for 24 hours or longer (Todd's paralysis).

LABORATORY AND RADIOLOGIC EVALUATION. Early imaging in most ICVD patients helps in the differential diagnosis and may determine the need for therapeutic intervention. Both CT and MRI scans are reliable and sensitive means of differentiating between ICVD, hemorrhage, and other mass lesions. Often MRI scans are more sensitive than CT scans for the identification of brain tumors and subdural hematomas and will identify areas of focal ischemic infarction at an earlier stage (within 12–24 hours), but early differentiation of hemorrhage may occasionally be difficult [15]. Newer MRI techniques, such as diffusion weighted imaging and perfusion imaging, are being developed [16]. With diffusion imaging, ischemic lesions can be seen within minutes of onset, and these images can be used to follow therapy in vivo. Perfusion imaging with contrast agents can detail microvascular perfusion and its absence in ischemic regions.

An electrocardiogram (ECG) should be obtained to look for underlying cardiac rhythm disturbances or ischemic changes. Confusion may arise because T wave, S–T segment, or QRS complex changes as well as rhythm disturbances may occur secondary to the cerebral ischemic event. Two-dimensional transthoracic or transesophageal echocardiography and ECG monitoring need not be performed routinely because of their relatively low yield, but they should be considered in younger ICVD patients and those with a significant cardiac history, abnormal cardiac examination, or abnormal baseline ECG (Fig. 187-4). A contrast echocardiogram or transesophageal echocardiogram should be considered in younger stroke patients who do not have an obvious source for their ischemic event. A multiple profile blood chemistry screen, chest radiograph, erythrocyte sedimentation rate, syphilis serology, complete blood count, partial thromboplastin time, prothrombin time, and urinalysis should be obtained in all patients. Other blood studies, including anticardiolipin antibodies, clotting studies, serum viscosity, serum protein electrophoresis, fibrinogen, and lipid studies, may be helpful in some patients. The need for routine lumbar puncture has diminished with the availability of imaging studies that reliably diagnose hemorrhage. A lumbar puncture should be performed if meningitis is suspected or subarachnoid hemorrhage is a consideration, despite a negative result in an imaging study. Electroencephalography may be helpful when associated seizure activity is suspected.

Noninvasive studies of the carotid arteries, such as B-mode and Doppler ultrasound, are a useful and safe method for assessing the extracranial vessels in ICVD patients, especially those with carotid territory infarcts. Even patients with lacunar infarcts or cardiac sources for stroke should have noninvasive vascular studies, because carotid artery atheroma leading to embolus formation may be the source of the stroke, and coexistent carotid disease is not uncommon in patients with cardiac embolic sources. Transcranial Doppler (TCD) ultrasound is becoming available and can provide information about the status of the intracranial vessels, both in the carotid and vertebral-basilar arterial territories [17]. Atherosclerotic narrowing of the middle cerebral or basilar arteries can be identified, as can embolic occlusions. It can also be used to demonstrate intracranial emboli in patients with a cardiac or extracranial arterial source [18]. The information obtained from these techniques

Fig. 187-4. Echocardiogram in a patient with cardioembolic stroke, demonstrating a large thrombus attached to the left mitral valve.

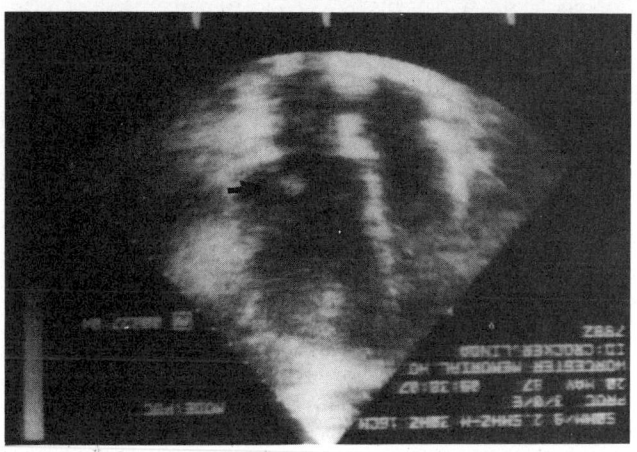

may increase the ability to diagnose more accurately and manage more effectively patients with certain ICVD subtypes.

TREATMENT. The treatment of ICVD can be divided into four major categories: prevention, supportive therapy, standard interventions, and newer experimental approaches.

Prevention. Stroke prevention has improved as risk factors have been identified and treatments developed [19]. The treatment of hypertension, a primary stroke risk factor, clearly reduces ICVD risk. Smoking is another risk factor that can be ameliorated. The treatment of diabetes and hyperlipidemia is less clearly beneficial. Patients with TIA have a substantial risk of stroke, and patients with carotid territory symptoms and greater than 70 percent stenosis of the ipsilateral carotid artery clearly benefit from carotid endarterectomy [20]. In nonsurgical TIA patients, antiplatelet therapy with aspirin or ticlopidine is beneficial. Atrial fibrillation with or without valvular heart disease is associated with a high stroke risk. Several large recent trials demonstrated that warfarin, and perhaps aspirin, reduce primary stroke risk in patients with nonvalvular atrial fibrillation [21].

Supportive Therapy. Supportive therapy for ICVD patients should begin on hospitalization [18]. Elevated blood pressure should be observed at least 4 to 6 hours before antihypertensive therapy is initiated, unless malignant hypertension with focal neurologic signs is present. The blood pressure typically returns to baseline with bed rest; if it remains substantially elevated it should be carefully lowered by no more than 20 percent of the mean arterial pressure. Subcutaneous heparin therapy should be considerd in immobilized ICVD patients to reduce the risk of pulmonary emboli. Indwelling urinary catheters and excessive intravenous (IV) lines should be avoided, as they can promote infection. Aspiration pneumonia can be avoided by delaying oral feedings until swallowing is well performed. Early mobilization and rehabilitation should be attempted.

Standard Interventions. Standard therapies in ICVD patients are directed at treating the neurologic deficit and preventing progression. They include antithrombotic agents and medications to reduce cerebral edema.

Anticoagulants have been employed for many years in ICVD, but definitive proof of their efficacy in many circumstances is lacking. Acute anticoagulation with heparin is considered in patients with cardioembolic stroke to prevent recurrence; in patients with stroke-in-evolution to prevent progression; and in multiple TIA patients to prevent stroke development. Cardioembolic stroke patients have a 4 to 10 percent risk of recurrence within 2 weeks of the initial event. Heparin therapy may reduce this risk and should be considered within 24 to 48 hours of the initial stroke [7]. Patients with large infarcts should not receive heparin, because they have a higher risk of bleeding into the area of infarction [22]. An alternative approach is to begin warfarin as soon as the patient can safely swallow, leading to adequate anticoagulation within 5 to 7 days of stroke onset. Stroke-in-evolution is difficult to define and quantitate, but if it is suspected heparin therapy should be considered [23]. Definitive proof that heparin impedes progression is not available. Heparin therapy is also employed in patients with incomplete or partial deficits, even if they are not actively progressing, to prevent worsening. One recent double-blind, randomized trial of heparin versus placebo in this setting demonstrated no benefit for heparin [24]. A large trial with a heparinoid is in progress and may finally answer this vexing problem. Patients with multiple TIAs may be at higher risk of stroke development

than patients with single TIAs [25], and heparin may be used in these patients despite lack of proof that it is effective. Many authorities do not recommend heparin for patients with single TIAs. Heparin should be initiated as a constant infusion, maintaining the partial thromboplastin time at 1.5 to 2 times control. Aspirin may reduce the risk of stroke after TIA and is widely employed for this indication [26]. Ticlopidine, a new antiplatelet medication, can reduce the risk for recurrent stroke more effectively than aspirin [27], but the rate and severity of side effects is greater than with aspirin. Aspirin or ticlopidine prophylaxis should be considered in patients with ICVD because both can prevent recurrence and are relatively safe.

The development of cerebral edema in ICVD patients is maximal 48 to 72 hours after onset, predominantly due to cytotoxic and vasogenic mechanisms, in contrast to the primarily vasogenic edema associated with brain tumors. This difference in mechanism explains why corticosteroids have not been effective in ICVD [28]. Hyperglycemia associated with corticosteroids may be detrimental as well [29]. Osmotic diuretics such as mannitol are of uncertain value for cerebral edema associated with ICVD, but we consider using pulse doses (1 gm/kg then 0.25 gm/kg every 6 hours) if massive edema begins to develop. Intracranial pressure monitoring to guide therapy should also be considered. Glycerol may be given intravenously if preparations with fructose (to reduce hemolysis) are available.

Experimental Approaches. There is no therapy available that has proved value for improving neurologic outcome or reducing mortality in ICVD patients. Potential therapies and newer therapeutic agents are aimed at either (1) correcting or modifying the cellular consequences of ischemia or (2) restoring impaired blood flow, primarily by dissolving the occluding thrombus.

Intracellular calcium influx is an important cellular consequence of ischemia that can lead to irreversible neuronal injury. A voltage-sensitive calcium channel blocker, nimodipine, has been tried in clinical trials of acute ICVD. Several large trials (all with flawed designs) did not demonstrate effectiveness of nimodipine in acute ICVD. However, a meta-analysis suggests that when nimodipine therapy was initiated within 12 hours of stroke onset, it did improve neurologic outcome [30]. Receptor-mediated calcium channels, primarily activated by excitatory amino acids such as glutamate and aspartate, are probably more important conduits for early intracellular calcium accumulation. Blockers of both the N-methyl-D-aspartate (NMDA) and d-amino-3-hydroxy-5-methyl-4-isoxazole propionate (AMPA) channels were developed and shown to reduce ischemic lesion size substantially in animal stroke models [31,32]. Side effects, such as psychotomimetic effects, hypertension, nausea, vomiting, and sedation, may limit the utility of these agents, but several NMDA antagonists are in early clinical trials.

Free radicals are generated in areas of ischemic brain that are partially perfused or reperfused after clot dissolution. These toxic oxygen metabolites can lead to increased tissue injury. In animal models, therapy with superoxide dismutase and catalase, naturally occurring free radical defense mechanisms, reduces tissue injury and cerebral edema. Lipid peroxidation can be inhibited by the novel corticosteroid derivatives, 21-aminosteroids, and in an animal stroke model these agents (without glucocorticoid or mineralocorticoid side effects) improved outcome and reduced neuronal damage [33]. A clinical trial of Tirilazad is being organized.

Hemodilution therapy has been tried because lowering blood viscosity improves cerebral blood flow and tissue oxygenation. There is currently little enthusiasm for the treatment, after several studies showed negative results [34]. Fibrinolytic therapy with urokinase and streptokinase to remove the offending thrombus was attempted in the past but was discontinued because of excessive hemorrhagic complications. The availability of relative fibrin-specific fibrinolytic molecules, such as tissue plasminogen activator (t-PA), has revived enthusiasm. In animal models, t-PA has been shown to dissolve intracranial cerebral thrombi effectively and safely and to improve neurologic outcome [35]. Human trials have demonstrated that t-PA can be given relatively safely. Efficacy trials are in progress [36].

Other potentially cytoprotective drugs are also being studied. The ganglioside GM-1 was evaluated in a large early treatment trial. Although the overall results were negative, a trend toward benefit was observed in younger patients. Modulation of presynaptic sodium-calcium channels and presynaptic glutamate release is another approach. RS-87476, a drug with these effects, reduces lesion size in animals and is currently being studied in an efficacy trial [37]. Activation of presynaptic kappa-opioid receptors may impede glutamate release. CI-977, a kappa-opioid agonist, has protective effects in animals. Further study of presynaptic modulators may prove interesting.

Summary. An effective treatment to reduce neurologic morbidity of ICVD remains elusive. Stroke treatment requires early intervention (within hours of onset) and careful assessment for favorable responses and side effects. It is probable that a combination of treatments directed at the multiple metabolic and perfusion abnormalities associated with ICVD will be required.

SINUS THROMBOSIS. A variant of ischemic stroke, probably underdiagnosed, is that related to venous sinus thrombosis (ST). The sagittal sinus is the most common venous structure prone to thrombosis [38]. Sinus thrombosis occurs in relationship to a variety of other medical conditions, such as local or systemic infection, head injury, brain and other tumors, coagulation disorders, and dehydration [38]. The majority of postpartum strokes are related to ST [39]. Patients with ST may present with isolated headaches or headache associated with focal neurologic signs and seizures. Head CT scans demonstrate an area of infarction when present, typically parasagittally with a hemorrhagic component. Only a minority of patients have evidence of a vascular occlusion. Standard MRI and magnetic resonance angiography (MRA) are now the imaging technologies of choice in patients with suspected ST. The latter is noninvasive and can reliably document the presence of thrombi in an occluded venous structure (Fig 187-5). Supportive management of ST patients, with fluid replacements, analgesics, and anticonvulsants, is widely employed. The utility of anticoagulant therapy has engendered controversy. Hemorrhagic risks must be balanced with utility to prevent propagation of thrombus. In a small prospective trial of intravenous heparin, active therapy reduced mortality and improved morbidity; this has led to the frequent use of heparin in ST patients [40]. Thrombolytic therapy has also been used in ST, but controlled trials are not available to assess its efficacy and risks.

Nontraumatic Intracranial Hemorrhage

Although occurring less frequently than ischemic cerebrovascular disease, nontraumatic intracranial hemorrhage often requires management in the ICU. The majority of cases are due to spontaneous (primary) intracerebral hemorrhage (ICH) or rupture of saccular aneurysms and arteriovenous malforma-

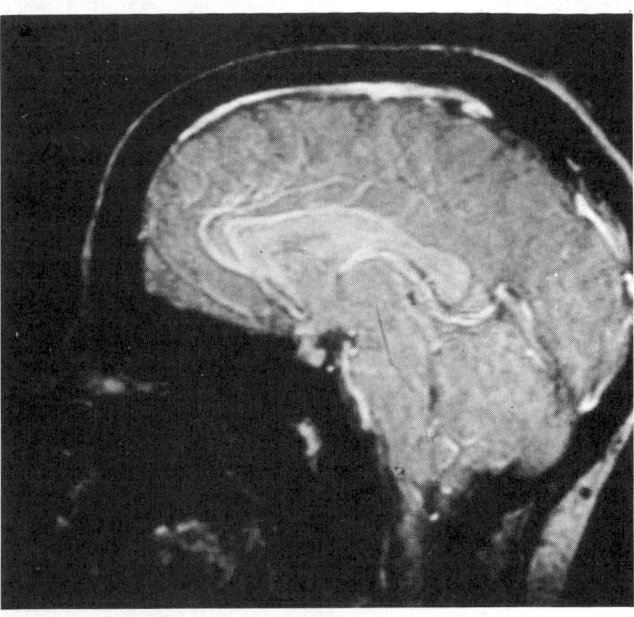

Fig. 187-5. Occluded sagittal sinus on the venous phase of MR angiography.

tions. As the approach to these entities and their management differs considerably, they are discussed separately.

Primary ICH is defined as bleeding within the brain parenchyma without an underlying cause, such as neoplasm, vasculitis, bleeding disorder, prior embolic infarction, aneurysm, vascular malformation, or trauma. One-half of cases of primary ICH result from long-standing hypertension. Due to the aggressive control of hypertension, the incidence of ICH has decreased since the mid-1960s [41]. The ability of CT scanning to identify smaller hemorrhages formerly misdiagnosed as bland infarcts has contributed to a lower apparent fatality rate [42]. Nonetheless, ICH accounts for 4 to 11 percent of all stroke cases in the United States and 16 to 26 percent of all stroke-related deaths [43].

PATHOPHYSIOLOGY. Intracerebral hemorrhage is believed to be due to extravasation of arterial blood from ruptured microaneurysms along the walls of small intracerebral arterioles. Charcot and Bouchard first described these microaneurysms in 1868, and further investigation has confirmed that they tend to form on vessels at the usual sites of ICH. These Charcot-Bouchard miliary aneurysms are 300 to 900 μm in diameter and are outpouchings of vessels 100 to 300 μm in diameter. They develop at sites of vascular branching, where mechanical stress is maximal. The aneurysm wall lacks normal vascular histology; it is composed mainly of connective tissue layers, which represent a weak point in the arterial system. The formation of these aneurysms is favored by the processes of lipohyalinosis and fibrinoid necrosis, which weaken the walls of arterioles, and accelerated by chronic hypertension. Although Charcot-Bouchard aneurysms also appear in the normotensive aging brain, their frequency is notably increased in hypertensive patients. They are commonly observed along the lenticulostriate arteries, thalamoperforant arteries, and paramedian branches of the basilar artery [41]. Although this distribution corresponds to the common sites of ICH, it is impossible to prove that these aneurysms are always the cause of bleeding, and the concept of arteriolar microdissection has been raised as an alternative explanation [44].

Continued extravasation of blood results in the formation of a hematoma, with secondary accumulation of cerebral edema. The lesion may become massive enough to cause midline shift of cerebral structures. This may be followed by transtentorial herniation, which leads to secondary brainstem hemorrhages known as Duret hemorrhages. These linear lesions in the midbrain and upper pons are generally multiple and bilateral. Progression of this process results in brainstem dysfunction and death. Depending on the size and location of the ICH, intraventricular extension can occur and blood may be identified in the subarachnoid space. Some cases of thromboembolic stroke may be misclassified as ICH, because large hematomas may accumulate into areas of infarction. This secondary hemorrhage may be mislabeled if an early imaging study is not performed.

CLINICAL MANIFESTATIONS. The clinical presentation of ICH is distinctive. In most cases the onset is during the waking state when the patient is active; it is unusual for ICH to occur during sleep. The onset is abrupt, and the development of neurologic deficits occurs progressively over minutes to hours. This contrasts with the fluctuating or stepwise progression of deficits commonly seen in atherothrombotic infarcts and with the appearance of maximal deficits at onset in cardioembolic strokes. In addition, prior TIA is rare with ICH and relatively common with ischemic stroke. The average age of onset of ICH, 50 to 70 years, is younger than that of other types of stroke. Patients may complain of lateralized headache, and vomiting is common. Nuchal rigidity may be present. Seizures are seen more frequently at the onset of ICH (17%) than in ischemic cerebrovascular disease and are more likely to occur if the bleeding involves cerebral cortex [45]. Forty-four to 72 percent of patients are comatose when first seen by a physician [31].

The clinical presentation of ICH is monophasic, with active bleeding lasting no more than 2 hours. Subsequent clinical deterioration is due to the effects of cerebral edema [46]. When circulating erythrocytes were labeled with radioactive chromium between 1 and 5 hours after hemorrhage, no radioactivity was found in the primary hematomas at postmortem examination [47]. It was recently suggested that thalamic hemorrhages may bleed further in patients whose hypertension is not adequately controlled [48].

DIAGNOSIS. The diagnosis of ICH can be made by CT scan, which provides accurate information about the size and site of the hematoma as well as the degree of extension, midline shift, and development of cerebral edema. Ordinarily the hemorrhage is hyperintense on CT scan during the acute phase, although in patients who are severely anemic the hematoma may appear isodense due to the reduced concentration of hemoglobin (Fig. 187-6).

The appearance of blood on the MRI scan varies, since signal intensity is related to the state of degradation of the hemoglobin (Fig. 187-7). This state changes with time, therefore MRI is not the study of choice for initial imaging of ICH. In summary, deoxyhemoglobin is found in the first 3 days after ICH and is not well visualized on T_1-weighted images but will appear as an area of reduced signal intensity on T_2-weighted images. From 3 to 10 days after ICH methemoglobin appears as increased signal intensity of T_1-weighted images, but the intracellular portion has reduced signal intensity on T_2-weighted images. In the chronic state the ICH has broken down to hemosiderin, which is poorly visualized on T_1-weighted images

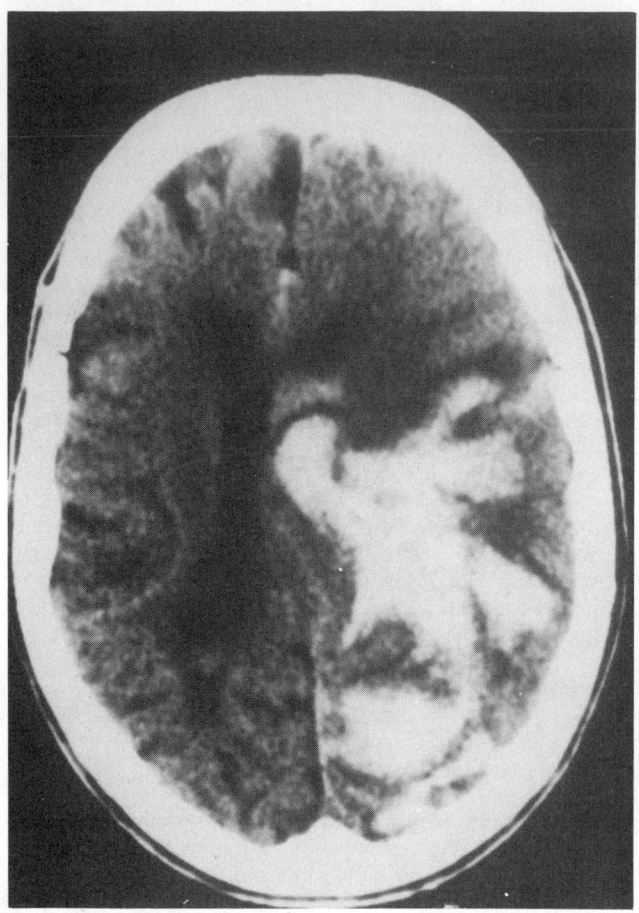

Fig. 187-6. Massive intracerebral hemorrhage with ventricular extension.

but appears as reduced signal intensity on T_2-weighted images. Magnetic resonance angiography should be considered in selected cases, if an underlying aneurysm or arteriovenous malformation is suspected.

Lumbar puncture is contraindicated in ICH because of the risk of herniation from mass effect. Testing on admission for ICH should include coagulation profile and platelet count in all patients, as well as bleeding time if the patient is on aspirin. Prophylaxis against venous thrombosis should be accomplished with pneumatic boots, as subcutaneous heparin is best avoided.

DIFFERENTIAL DIAGNOSIS. Although the majority of ICH is hypertensive in origin, other etiologies should always be considered. Secondary cerebral hemorrhage may occur following embolic infarction. The lodged embolus fragments and ischemic distal vessels may rupture on reperfusion. This is more common in patients with large embolic infarcts, in patients who are anticoagulated, and in patients with poorly controlled hypertension. Intracerebral hemorrhage secondary to reperfusion may also occur following carotid endarterectomy.

Intracerebral hemorrhage accounts for 0.5 to 1.5 percent of all bleeding events related to the use of oral anticoagulants. Oral anticoagulation increases the risk of ICH 8- to 11-fold compared to nonanticoagulated patients. Compared with pa-

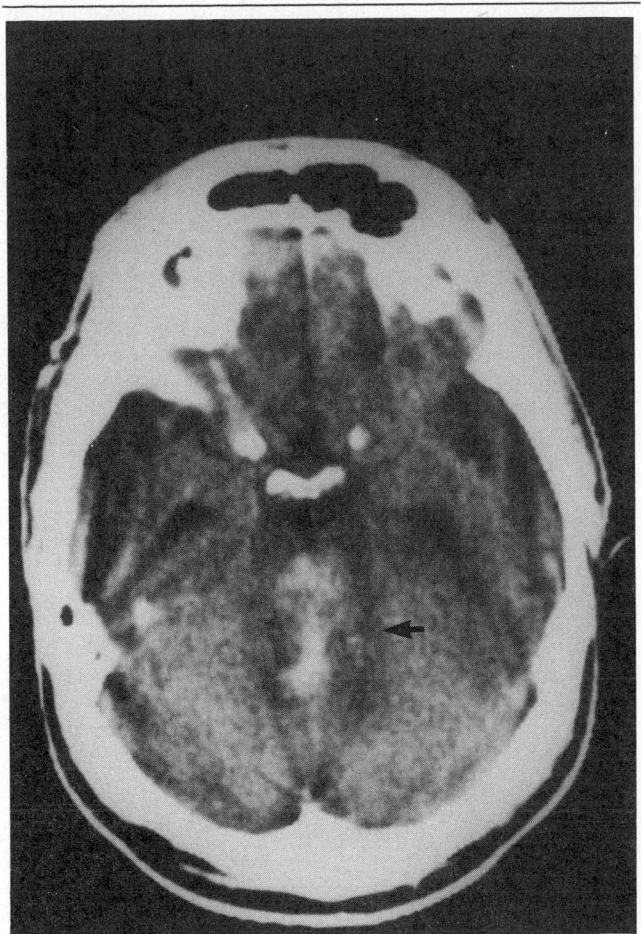

Fig. 187-7. Midline cerebellar hemorrhage (*arrow*) as seen on a head CT scan.

tients with spontaneous ICH, there is a trend toward larger hematomas and a higher mortality rate in patients on anticoagulants [49]. Intracerebral hemorrhage associated with anticoagulants carries a higher mortality, and the incidence of ICH increases with excessive prolongation of prothrombin time. Cerebellar hemorrhage is relatively common in anticoagulated patients, and mortality in these cases may be as high as 65 percent. Therefore, in anticoagulated patients, the onset of focal neurologic signs, even if slowly progressive, necessitates CT scan to rule out ICH [50].

The use of fibrinolytic therapy, such as t-PA, for coronary artery occlusion has also been associated with ICH, especially when concomitant heparin therapy is used. These cases have shown a predilection for the subcortical white matter and lobar areas, generally having a poor prognosis [51]. Surprisingly, the risk for ICH is slightly higher with t-PA than with streptokinase [52].

Intracerebral hemorrhage associated with the presence of primary or secondary brain tumors is infrequent, accounting for only 2 percent of all cases of ICH. Higher-grade malignancies, such as glioblastoma multiforme, are more likely to bleed. The presence of thin-walled vessels in areas of neovascularization is thought to be the underlying reason for these hemorrhages. Metastatic lesions with the tendency to bleed include bronchogenic carcinoma, melanoma, renal cell carcinoma, and choriocarcinoma [41].

Intracerebral hemorrhage is frequent in hematologic disorders such as leukemia and reflects both the underlying thrombocytopenia and disseminated intravascular coagulopathy (DIC). When DIC is due to other organ failures it can also lead to ICH. Intracerebral hemorrhage is noted in 30 percent of hemophiliac deaths and may complicate idiopathic thrombocytopenic purpura [53].

Sympathomimetic drugs, such as methamphetamine, pseudoephedrine, and phenylpropanolamine, have caused ICH in the subcortical white matter. These agents are suspected of inducing a vasculitis. Cocaine, which blocks dopamine and norepinephrine reuptake, has been associated with ICH. Cocaine, especially crack cocaine, appears to incite cerebral vasospasm rather than a vasculitis. The secondary hypertension related to sympathetic stimulation may also cause ICH from any of these agents. This may explain the lack of abnormal angiographic findings in some of these cases [54,55]. Acute elevation of blood pressure in otherwise normotensive people, such as that which may follow migraine, is postulated to result at times in ICH.

SPECIFIC SYNDROMES OF INTRACEREBRAL HEMORRHAGE. Intracerebral hemorrhage tends to occur in stereotyped locations. In order of descending frequency, these locations are the putamen (30–50%), subcortical white matter (15%), thalamus (10%), pons (10%), and cerebellum (10%) [56].

Intracerebral hemorrhage in the putamen is caused by bleeding from a lenticulostriate vessel. Clinically, it is manifested by abrupt development of flaccid hemiplegia, hemisensory disturbances of all primary modalities, homonymous hemianopsia, paralysis of conjugate gaze to the side opposite the lesion, and early alteration in level of consciousness. Subcortical aphasia may occur when a putaminal hemorrhage involves the dominant hemisphere and a hemineglect syndrome when it is on the nondominant side.

Hemorrhages in the subcortical white matter (lobar hemorrhages) are being observed with increasing frequency and are less commonly related to hypertension than is ICH in other locations. The signs and symptoms depend on the location. Lobar ICH occurs at the gray-white junction and is therefore associated with a higher incidence of seizures and headache at onset; it most commonly occurs in the parietal and occipital lobes. Of all ICH locations, lobar hemorrhages have the lowest mortality (about 15%) and carry the best prognosis for a good functional recovery. Lobar ICH is frequently caused by cerebral amyloid angiopathy due to the deposition of amyloid in the walls of the small vessels of the cortex and leptomeninges, typically in the frontal and occipital lobes. The process generally spares vessels of the basal ganglia, deep white matter, brainstem, and cerebellum. The abnormal vessel walls take up Congo red stain, thus the alternative term congophillic angiopathy. Amyloid angiopathy weakens the walls of many arteries and may be associated with recurrent lobar ICH. Five to 10 percent of cases of spontaneous ICH result from amyloid angiopathy, making it second to hypertension as an etiology for ICH [57].

Thalamic ICH is characterized by a unilateral sensorimotor deficit in which sensory findings predominate. There may be a unique downward deviation of the eyes with impairment of vertical gaze and small, sluggish, or unreactive pupils. These ocular findings, collectively known as Parinaud's syndrome, are the result of downward pressure on the vertical gaze center in the midbrain tectum. Depending on the side of the ICH, aphasia or apractagnosia may result. There may be forced conjugate deviation of the eyes, either contralaterally or ipsilaterally. A marked gait disturbance can occur as a consequence of sensory loss. A permanent skew deviation may leave the patient with persistent diplopia. Due to the location, thalamic ICH may rupture into the ventricular system.

Pontine ICH has the highest mortality. Many patients rapidly develop coma. Quadriplegia, brainstem dysfunction, and small unreactive pupils are seen at presentation. Bleeding typically arises from a paramedian branch of the basilar artery and almost always extends into the fourth ventricle. Cases of unilateral pontine ICH have a less dismal outcome [58].

Cerebellar ICH most commonly involves the dentate nucleus. Alteration of consciousness is unusual at onset, but progressive deterioration with drowsiness typically occurs. The majority of patients will initially manifest two of the following: (1) gait, truncal, or limb ataxia; (2) lower motor neuron facial paresis; and (3) an ipsilateral gaze palsy. Other common presenting signs and symptoms are nausea, vomiting, vertigo, nystagmus, and limb ataxia [59]. Early surgical intervention is indicated for lesions greater than 3 cm or in smaller lesions with clinical progression, because cerebellar hemorrhage causes death in up to 60 percent of cases. Surgical mortality is greatly reduced if the patient is still awake before operation; therefore, early intervention is indicated [41].

Approximately 3 percent of cases of ICH are primarily intraventricular in location. These events have minimal focal signs, but generally there is loss of consciousness at onset. Hydrocephalus is a major complication [60].

TREATMENT. The acute medical management of ICH is aimed at correction of any predisposing systemic factors to prevent further clinical deterioration. Control of hypertension is a major management problem in these cases. In response to the acute elevation of intracranial pressure (ICP) caused by the hematoma, systemic blood pressure will rise to maintain adequate cerebral perfusion pressure (CPP). This response, known as Cushing's reflex, serves to protect the brain against ischemia, but autoregulation of cerebral blood flow can be impaired after ICH or infarction. In patients with underlying chronic hypertension the result may be excessively high blood pressure. The best management of this dilemma remains controversial. In chronic hypertension, the lower limit of cerebral autoregulation is shifted toward higher blood pressure; acute lowering of systolic blood pressure is known to result in unfavorable decreases in CPP. Sustained hypertension in the acute phase of ICH, however, can lead to further bleeding or rapid accumulation of cerebral edema [41]. The recommended goal of systolic blood pressure in the acute phase of ICH is between 110 and 160 mm Hg [61]. Some would argue that treatment of hypertension should be avoided unless systolic pressures exceed 200 mm Hg. Blood pressure should be lowered gently, and beta-blockers are the agents of choice. Diuretics may lead to dehydration and electrolyte imbalances, and are second-choice agents. Calcium channel blockers, nipride, and hydralazine should be avoided because as vasodilators they can promote cerebral edema and elevate intracranial pressure [41].

If the hematoma and associated cerebral edema raises ICP, clinical deterioration typically occurs. Acutely, hyperventilation effectively lowers ICP, but only for a matter of hours. Hyperosmolar agents, such as mannitol, sorbitol, and glycerol, provide more sustained reductions in ICP. These drugs reduce the fluid content of the intact brain so the cranial cavity can accommodate cerebral edema. The osmotic diuresis induced by these agents can lead to dehydration, electrolyte imbalances, and pulmonary edema if the patient is not closely monitored. Treatment of ICH with steroids can be detrimental to overall outcome; they are not routinely administered [62]. The value of intracranial pressure monitoring in these situations remains controversial [61]. Elevation of ICP due to hydrocephalus is treated with ventricular shunting.

Anticonvulsants are not routinely used in ICH. If seizures are not present at onset, patients are generally at low risk to develop seizures. Hemorrhage into the cortex, regardless of site of origin, predisposes to seizures, however. Subarachnoid or intraventricular extension of bleeding does not increase the risk of seizures. Seizures have been noted with hemorrhages in the caudate but not with putaminal or thalamic events. Although the incidence of chronic epilepsy from ICH is low (6.5–13%), any seizures usually begin within the first 2 years after the event [45,63].

After the patient is acutely stabilized, angiography may be performed if there is no history of hypertension and the bleeding is in an atypical location. This is particularly true for younger patients, in whom a larger percentage of cases of ICH are due to underlying vascular lesions, such as arteriovenous malformation or aneurysm.

At present, surgery may be indicated for lobar ICH in which the patient continues to deteriorate and for most cerebellar ICH. Emergency ventricular shunting to relieve hydrocephalus should be considered if this condition develops acutely. Surgical intervention for putaminal ICH remains controversial; it is inappropriate for thalamic and pontine hemorrhages [64].

The prognosis for ICH is worse for larger lesions. By location, pontine ICH has the highest mortality, followed by cerebellar and then basal gangliar lesions. Lobar ICH carries the most favorable outlook for survival and functional recovery [49]. Three factors that have accurately predicted 30-day survival in 92 percent of ICH patients reviewed are hemorrhage size, Glasgow coma scale score, and pulse pressure [42].

References

1. Hachinski VC, Norris JW: *The Acute Stroke*. Philadelphia, FA Davis, 1985.
2. Caplan LR, Stein RW: *Stroke: A Clinical Approach*. Boston, Butterworths, 1986.
3. Heyman A, Leviton A, Millikan CH, et al: Transient focal cerebral ischemia: Epidemiological and clinical aspects. *Stroke* 5:271, 1974.
4. Kase CS: Clinicoanatomic correlations, in Woods JH (ed): *Cerebral Blood Flow*. New York, McGraw-Hill, 1987, p 92.
5. Mohr JP: Lacunes. *Stroke* 13:3, 1982.
6. Bogousslavsky J, Hachinski VC, Boughner DR, et al: Cardiac and arterial lesions in carotid transient ischemic attacks. *Arch Neurol* 43:223, 1988.
7. Asinger RW, Dyken ML, Fisher M, et al: Cardiogenic brain embolism. *Arch Neurol* 46:727, 1989.
8. Lechat P, Mas JL, Lascault G, et al: Prevalence of patent foramen ovale in patients with stroke. *N Engl J Med* 318:1148, 1988.
9. Bogousslavsky J, Regli F: Unilateral watershed cerebral infarcts. *Neurology* 36:372, 1988.
10. Chambers BR, Norris JW, Shurvell BL, et al: Prognosis of acute stroke. *Neurology* 27:221, 1987.
11. Bogousslavsky J, Van Melle G, Regli F: The Lausanne stroke registry. *Stroke* 19:1083, 1988.
12. Jones HR, Millikan CM: Temporal profile (clinical course) of acute carotid system cerebral infarction. *Stroke* 7:64, 1976.
13. Mohr JP, Caplan LR, Melski JW, et al: The Harvard cooperative stroke registry. *Neurology* 28:754, 1978.
14. Rothrock JF, Walicke P, Swenson MR, et al: Migrainous stroke. *Arch Neurol* 45:63, 1988.
15. Kertesz A, Black SE, Nicholson L, et al: The sensitivity and specificity of MRI in stroke. *Neurology* 37:1580, 1987.
16. Fisher M, Sotak CH, Minematsu K, Li L: Innovative magnetic resonance technologies for evaluating cerebrovascular disease. *Ann Neurol* 32:115, 1992.
17. Dewitt LD, Wechsler LR: Transcranial Doppler. *Stroke* 19:915, 1988.

18. Tegler CH, Burke GL, Dalley GM, Stump DA: Carotid emboli predict poor outcome in stroke. *Stroke* 24:186, 1993.

19. Dyken ML, Wolf PA, Barnett HJM, et al: Risk factors in stroke. *Stroke* 15:1105, 1984.

20. North American Symptomatic Carotid Endarterectomy Trial Collaborators: Beneficial effects of carotid endarterectomy in symptomatic patients with high grade carotid stenosis. *N Engl J Med* 325:445, 1991.

21. Rothrock JF, Hart RG: Antithrombotic therapy in cerebrovascular disease. *Ann Intern Med* 115:885, 1991.

22. Cerebral Embolism Study Group: Cardiogenic stroke, early anticoagulation and brain hemorrhage. *Arch Intern Med* 147:636, 1987.

23. Gauthier JC: Stroke in progression. *Stroke* 16:729, 1985.

24. Duke RJ, Block RF, Turpie AG, et al: Intravenous heparin for the prevention of stroke in acute partial stable stroke. *Ann Intern Med* 105:821, 1986.

25. Keith DS, Phillips SJ, Whisnant JP, et al: Heparin treatment for recent transient focal cerebral ischemia. *Mayo Clin Proc* 62:1101, 1987.

26. The European Stroke Prevention Study (ESPS): Principal endpoints. *Lancet* 2:1351, 1987.

27. The Canadian-American ticlopidine study in thromboembolic stroke. *Lancet* 1:1215, 1989.

28. Levine SR: Acute cerebral ischemia in a critical care unit. *Arch Intern Med* 149:90, 1989.

29. Woo E, Ma JTC, Robinson JD, et al: Hyperglycemia is a stress response in acute stroke. *Stroke* 19:1359, 1988.

30. The International Nimodipine Study Group: Meta-analysis of nimodipine trials in acute ischemic stroke. *Stroke* 23:148, 1992.

31. Scatton B, Carter C, Benavides J, Giroux C: N-methyl-d-aspartate receptor antagonists. *Cerebrovasc Dis* 1:121, 1991.

32. Smith SE, Meldrum BS: Cerebroprotective effect of a non-N-methyl-d-aspartate antagonist, CYKI 52466, after focal ischemia in the rat. *Stroke* 2:861, 1992.

33. Hall ED, Pazara KE, Braughler JM: 21-Aminosteroid lipid peroxidation inhibitor U74006F protects against cerebral ischemia in gerbils. *Stroke* 19:997, 1988.

34. Italian Acute Stroke Study Group: Hemodilution in acute ischemic stroke: Results of the Italian hemodilution trial. *Lancet* 1:318, 1988.

35. Zivin JA, Fisher M, DeGirolami U: Tissue plasminogen activator reduces neurologic damage after cerebral embolism. *Science* 320:1289, 1985.

36. del Zoppo GJ, Poeck K, Pessin MS, et al: Recombinant tissue plasminogen activator in acute thrombotic and embolic stroke. *Ann Neurol* 32:78, 1992.

37. Kucharczyk J, Mintorovitch J, Moseley ME, et al: Ischemic brain damage: Reduction by sodium-calcium channel modulator, RS 87976. *Radiology* 179:321, 1991.

38. Encvoldson TP, Ross Russell RW: Cerebral venous thrombosis: New causes for an old syndrome. *Q J Med* 284:1255, 1990.

39. Wiebers DO: Ischemic cerebrovascular complications of pregnancy. *Arch Neurol* 42:1106, 1985.

40. Einhaupl KM, Villringer A, Meister W, et al: Heparin treatment in sinus venous thrombosis. *Lancet* 338:597, 1991.

41. Omae T, Ueda K, Ogata J, et al: Parenchymatous hemorrhage: Etiology, pathology and clinical aspects, in Toule JF (ed): *Handbook of Clinical Neurology.* vol 10. New York, Elsevier, 1989, p 287.

42. Tuhrim S, Dambrosia JM, Price TR, et al: Prediction of intracerebral hemorrhage survival. *Ann Neurol* 24:258, 1988.

43. Yatsu FM, Becker C, McLeroy KR, et al: Community hospital-based stroke programs: North Carolina, Oregon, and New York. I. Goals, objectives, and data collection procedures. *Stroke* 17:276, 1986.

44. Fisher CM: Pathological observations in hypertensive cerebral hemorrhage. *J Neuropathol Exp Neurol* 30:536, 1971.

45. Berger AR, Lipton RB, Lesser ML, et al: Early seizures following intracerebral hemorrhage: Implications for therapy. *Neurology* 38:1363, 1988.

46. Fisher CM: Clinical syndromes in cerebral hemorrhage, in Fields WS (ed): *Pathogenesis and Treatment of Cerebrovascular Disease.* Springfield, IL, Charles C. Thomas, 1961, p 318.

47. Herbstein DJ, Schaumberg HH: Hypertensive intracerebral hematoma: An investigation of the initial hemorrhage and rebleeding using chromium Cr 51-labelled erythrocytes. *Arch Neurol* 30:412, 1974.

48. Chen ST, Chen SD, Hsu CY, et al: Progression of hypertensive intracerebral hemorrhage. *Neurology* 39:1509, 1989.

49. Radberg JA, Olson JE, Radberg CT: Prognostic parameters in spontaneous hematomas with special reference to anticoagulation treatment. *Stroke* 22:571, 1991.

50. Kase CS, Robinson RK, Stein RW, et al: Anticoagulant-related intracerebral hemorrhage. *Neurology* 35:943, 1983.

51. Kase CS, O'Neil AM, Fisher M, et al: Intracranial hemorrhage after use of tissue plasminogen activator. *Ann Intern Med* 112:17, 1990.

52. ISIS-3 Collaborative Group: A random trial of streptokinase vs tissue plasminogen activator vs anistreplase. *Lancet* 339:753, 1992.

53. Biggs R: Hemophillia treatment in the United Kingdom from 1969–1974. *Br J Haematol* 35:484, 1977.

54. Wojak JC, Flamm ED: Intracranial hemorrhage and cocaine use. *Stroke* 18:712, 1987.

55. Toffol GJ, Biller J, Adams HP: Nontraumatic intracerebral hemorrhage in young adults. *Arch Neurol* 44:483, 1987.

56. Duff TA, et al: Neurosurgical management of spontaneous intracerebral hematomas. *Barrows Neurol Inst Q* 1:29, 1985.

57. Masferrer R, Zabramski J, Hunt S, et al: Cerebral amyloid angiopathy and recurrent spontaneous intracerebral hematomas. *Barrows Neurol Inst Q* 1:29, 1985.

58. Chung CS, Park CM: Primary pontine hemorrhage: A new CT classification. *Neurology* 42:830, 1992.

59. Ott KH, Kase CS, Ojemann RG, et al: Cerebellar hemorrhage: Diagnosis and treatment—A review of 56 cases. *Arch Neurol* 31:160, 1974.

60. Darby DG, Donnan GA, Saling MA, et al: Primary intraventricular hemorrhage: Clinical and neuropsychological findings in a prospective stroke series. *Neurology* 38:68, 1988.

61. Borges LF: Management of nontraumatic brain hemorrhage, in Ropper AM, Kennedy SF (eds): *Neurological and Neurosurgical Intensive Care.* Rockville, MD, Aspen, 1988, p 209.

62. Poungvarin N, Bhoopat W, Viniarejakul A, et al: Effects of dexamethasone in primary supratentorial intracerebral hemorrhage. *N Engl J Med* 316:1229, 1987.

63. Faught E, Peters D, Bartolucci A, et al: Seizures after primary intracerebral hemorrhage. *Neurology* 39:1089, 1989.

64. Waga S, Miyazaki M, Okada M, et al: Hypertensive putaminal hemorrhage: Analysis of 182 patients. *Surg Neurol* 26:159, 1986.

188. Neurooncologic Problems in the Intensive Care Unit

Massimo S. Fiandaca and
Lawrence D. Recht

While nearly one-fifth of all cancer patients develop direct or indirect neurologic symptoms or signs during the course of their disease, only about 2 percent have primary brain malignancies. Deterioration in neurologic function, however, remains a tremendous hardship on all patients struggling with malignant tumors. Furthermore, despite dismal cure rates, early and appropriate intervention in a large number of these patients can result in prolonged survival with reduced treatment morbidity or mortality.

This chapter addresses situations encountered in the patient harboring a malignancy in which urgent neurologic management is necessary. The first section evaluates emergent complications commonly encountered in brain tumor patients; the second deals with those seen in patients with systemic cancer. For a more general overview of the neurologic complications of systemic cancer, the reader is referred to a number of excellent recent reviews [1,2,3].

Primary Brain Tumors

Primary brain tumors encompass a large and diverse group of neoplasms that arise from the neural or supporting tissues (e.g., glia, leptomeninges) (Table 188-1). Although they are of diverse histologic types, all of these tumors produce clinical symptoms in essentially the same way: by compressing, displacing, and/or infiltrating the normal neural tissues. Before the development of sophisticated neuroimaging modalities such as computed

Table 188-1. Histologic Types of Brain Tumors

	Univ. MD (7/91–3/93)*		Univ. MA (1978–1985)*	
	No.	%	No.	%
Malignant intracranial tumors	138	63.0	86	76.8
Glioblastoma multiforme	33	15.1	45	40.2
Anaplastic astrocytoma	19	8.7	15	13.4
Anaplastic oligo	3	1.4		
Astrocytoma	14	6.4	20	17.9
Mixed glioma	2	—		
Medulloblastoma	6	2.8	4	3.6 (PNET)
Ependymoma	2	—	1	—
Metastasis	48	21.9		
Other malignancies	11	5.0	1	—
Benign intracranial tumors	81	37.0	26	23.2
Meningioma	37	16.9	18	16.0
Pituitary adenoma	25	11.4		
Schwannoma	7	3.2	4	3.6
Other benign tumors	12	5.5	4	3.6

* Operative pathologic specimens obtained during stated period at each institution. Note the increase in metastatic tumor specimens obtained in the more recent series, reflecting a more aggressive approach toward these lesions [31].

tomography (CT) and magnetic resonance imaging (MRI) scanning, clinicians localized these tumors primarily by the symptoms or signs of brain dysfunction that historically have been correlated to specific anatomic locations in the brain. Clinical symptoms and signs alone, however, have occasionally misled the clinician, as increased intracranial pressure (ICP) often associated with these tumors can cause false localizing signs. One of the most common false localizing signs is diplopia, which is due to an abducens nerve palsy and associated with a frontal tumor. Rather than localizing the lesion to the frontal lobe, the cranial nerve dysfunction in this case points falsely to the posterior fossa or cavernous sinus as the site of pathology.

Despite the fact that the majority of these tumors remain incurable, treating physicians strive to optimize patient survival and quality of life and to support the patient's family through these difficult periods. Neurooncology encompasses the surgical, medical, and radiotherapeutic treatment of patients with these various central nervous system (CNS) tumors and, as a medical subspecialty area, is much too broad to cover in one chapter. Therefore, this discussion is limited to the recognition and treatment of the critical situations the physician faces in caring for these patients.

INCREASED INTRACRANIAL PRESSURE AND BRAIN EDEMA. If left untreated, the increased intracranial pressure associated with certain intracranial neoplasms results in major morbidity and death. While slow-growing tumors occasionally grow to large size before causing clinical symptoms, rapidly growing intracranial tumors usually lead to earlier and more serious neurologic deterioration as a result of a decompensation of the brain mechanisms that normally control pressure within the cranium. These latter tumors displace brain structures along paths of least resistance, and from one intracranial compartment to another, in what has been termed herniation syndromes. Without rapid initiation of treatment, this tumor-associated complication is often fatal. It is therefore critical that clinicians recognize and treat ICP and brain edema before neurologic deterioration becomes irreversible.

Pathogenesis. Under normal conditions, brain volume consists of 80 percent interstitial tissue, 10 percent blood volume, and 10 percent cerebrospinal fluid (CSF). Intracranial pressure is regulated by controlling these three major intracranial components. With increases in tissue volume, as is seen in brain tumors, blood volume is initially squeezed out of intracranial venous capacitance vessels in an effort to maintain an overall normal amount of intracranial volume. With further tumor growth, CSF volume decreases and further production is reduced. While these measures temporarily compensate for a growing intracranial mass, continued tumor growth (i.e., increased volume) eventually leads to increased ICP. Although ICP is normally compensated by reductions in intracranial venous blood and CSF volumes, in this situation the brain loses its compliance—the ability to handle positive volume changes

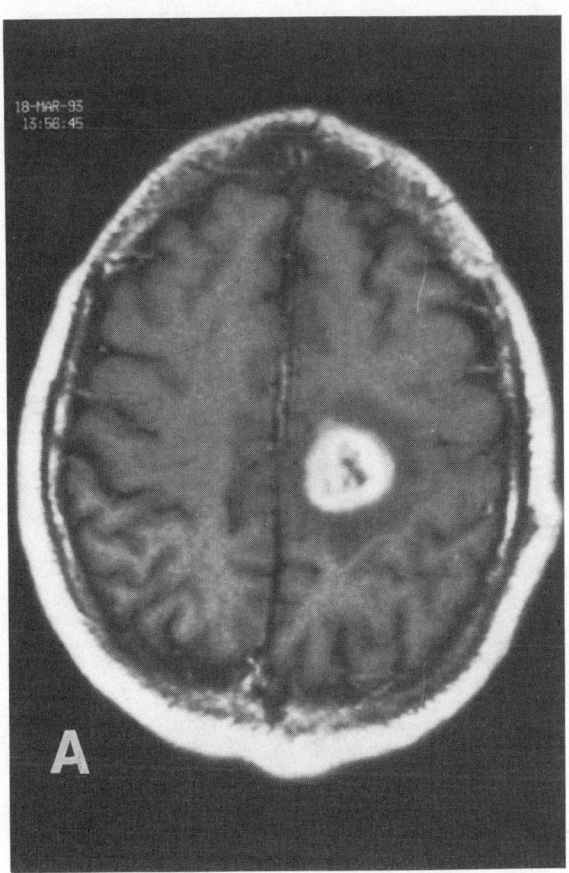 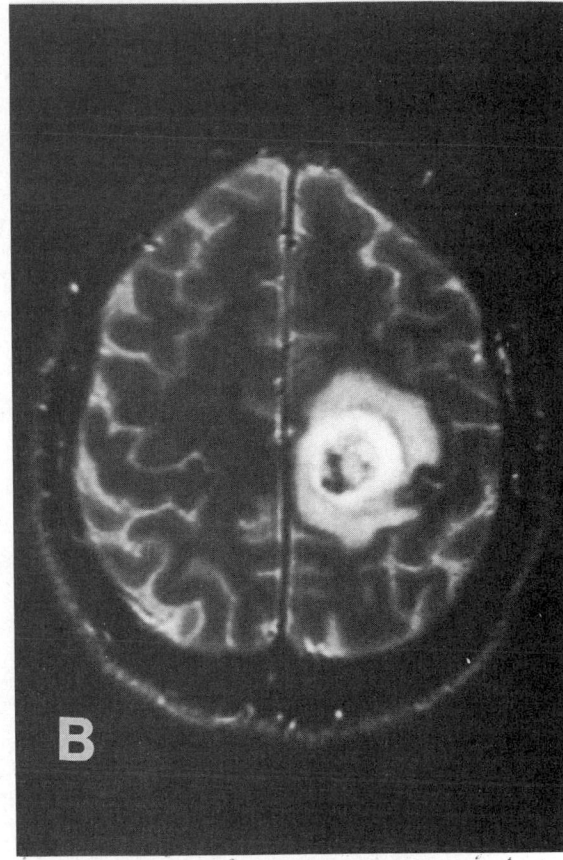

Fig. 188-1. MRI scan of a left frontoparietal glioblastoma multiforme. A. Enhanced axial T_1-weighted image, showing the enhancing tumor and surrounding low-intensity edema. B. Axial T_2-weighted image of the same case, highlighting the hyperintense edema surrounding the tumor.

without increases in ICP. The more rapid the tumor growth, the less time for the compensatory compliance mechanisms to act, and the more likely there will be decompensation of intracranial volume and associated increased ICP. One of the major tumor-associated variables impacting on tissue volume is brain edema.

Brain neoplasms increase in volume through the growth of cellular mass as well as the propensity to increase interstitial *extra*cellular water or *peritumoral edema* [4] (Fig. 188-1). The edema results from either excessive permeability of tumoral or peritumoral vessels, or tumor production of edematogenic substances [5,6]. Since this particular edema is associated with leaky vasculature, it is often designated *vasogenic edema* (as distinguished from edema that results from increased *intra*cellular water, which is usually due to membrane ion pump failure and termed *cytotoxic edema*). Vasogenic edema is very responsive to steroid therapy [7,8].

Diagnosis. The patient with increased ICP may present with headache, diplopia, lethargy, or visual blurring. Often a pre-existing focal neurologic deficit will worsen. Funduscopic examination discloses papilledema (especially in children) in many cases. In its most malignant form, such as in rapidly growing tumors, increased ICP causes one of the herniation syndromes (Table 188-2). The more chronic the tumor growth,

the more gradual the elevation of ICP and the changes in associated clinical findings, such as headaches progressing in severity, evolving encephalopathies, or progressive blindness.

In association with sustained subacute or chronic ICP elevation, rapid deterioration of neurologic function has been correlated with periodic elevations of ICP to levels greater than 50 mm Hg. Visualized with intracranial pressure monitoring, these "plateau" waves [9] last between 5 and 20 minutes and can be associated with acute headache, vomiting, and obtundation. Transient alterations of cerebral autoregulation and reduced CSF absorption are proposed mechanisms for these ICP alterations, but the actual mechanism remains unknown.

Patients suspected of having increased ICP due to tumors should have either a CT or MRI scan to assess the amount of mass effect present. Studies should be performed without and with intravenous contrast to rule out a hemorrhage associated with a tumor. Magnetic resonance imaging is preferable in most circumstances because it allows better anatomic resolution and delineation of the lesion in axial, coronal, and sagittal planes. An MRI scan is especially important for the surgeon planning an operative approach to the lesion (Fig. 188-2).

Treatment. In many instances, relieving increased ICP significantly improves the neurologic status of patients with intracranial tumors. Specific medical therapies can improve headache as well as cognitive and motor deficits. Under specific circumstances, such as with obstructive hydrocephalus or significant lobar mass effect, surgical therapy offers the best chance of providing long-term palliation.

Effective medical treatment of elevated ICP in brain tumor

Table 188-2. Sites of Brain Herniation, Structures Involved, and Resulting Clinical Signs

Site of herniation	Structures involved	Signs
Lateral tentorial (uncal)	Oculomotor nerve	Ptosis, mydriasis, lateral deviation
	Cerebral peduncle	Hemiparesis
	Posterior cerebral artery	Hemianopsia
Posterior tentorial (tectal)	Tectal plate (posterior commissure and superior colliculi)	Bilateral ptosis, failure of upgaze
Central tentorial (axial-brainstem)	Reticular formation	Depression of consciousness
	Corticospinal tracts	Decerebrate rigidity
	Midbrain and pons	Impairment or absence of eye movement reflexes, irregular respirations
	Medulla	Arterial hypertension and bradycardia, irregular respirations, apnea
Foramenal (tonsillar)	Medulla	Apnea
Subfalcine (cingulate)	Cingulate gyrus	Leg weakness
	Anterior cerebral artery	

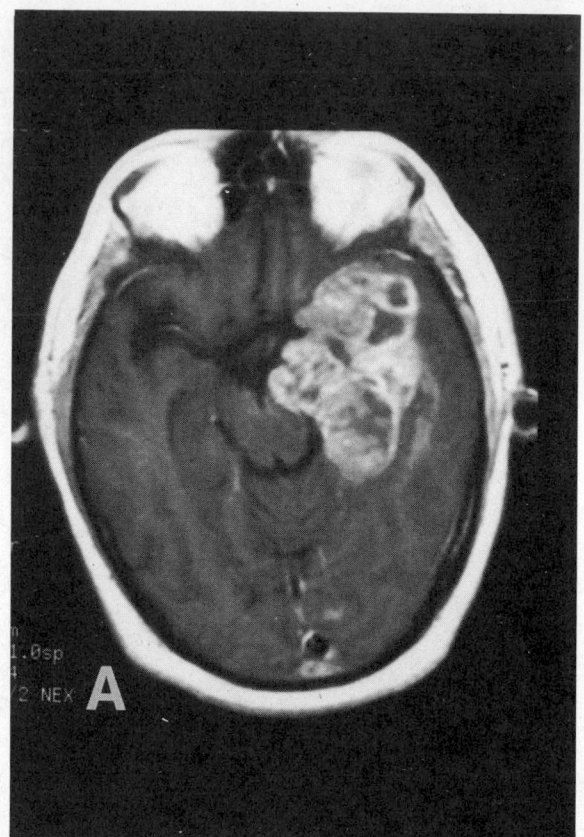

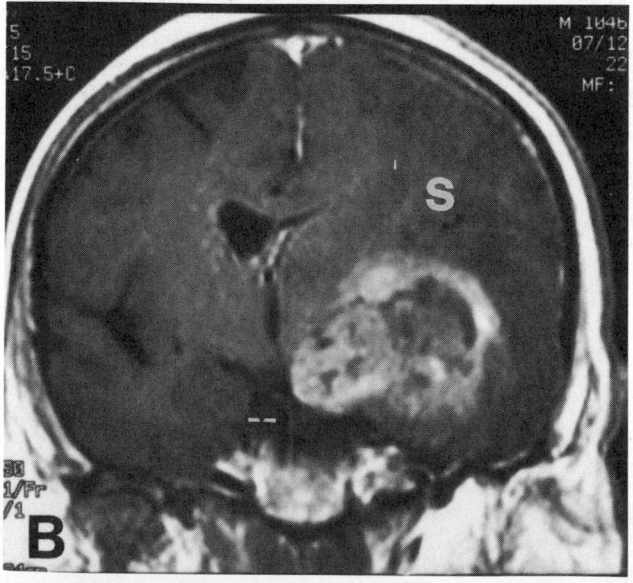

Fig. 188-2. MRI scan of a left temporal glioblastoma multiforme. A. Enhanced axial T_1-weighted image, showing the extent of the tumor within the temporal lobe, cystic and solid components, and associated brainstem compression. B. Enhanced coronal T_1-weighted image, indicating the medial-lateral extent of the tumor within the temporal lobe as well as the relationship to the brainstem and basilar artery (white —) and Sylvian fissure (S).

patients includes controlling ventilation and the judicious use of osmotic diuretic agents and steroids (Fig. 188-3). Hyperventilation is the most rapid medical means of decreasing elevated ICP. As a direct effect on the cerebral vasculature, lowering $PaCO_2$ levels reduces cerebral blood flow (CBF) and ICP almost immediately. Specifically, decreasing the $PaCO_2$ 5 to 10 mm Hg can lower elevated ICP by as much as 25 to 30 percent. This effect is rather short-lived, however, and chronic hyperventilation therapy is not recommended for the management of increased ICP. As a control measure in very acute situations, hyperventilation is most useful as an interim measure until the longer-lasting osmotic diuretic agents and/or steroids express themselves.

Due to the relatively impermeable nature of the blood-brain barrier, intravenous osmotic agents such as mannitol increase the oncotic pressure within the blood and tend to draw water from the edematous brain to the vasculature for clearance. In addition, mannitol improves blood viscosity, which allows better perfusion of ischemic zones of brain adjacent to tumor masses [10] and may cause pial vessel vasoconstriction, thereby decreasing total cerebral blood volume (CBV).

In brain tumor patients with elevated ICP, too rapid an infusion of intravenous mannitol may cause a deterioration in neurologic function by expanding vascular volume and, secondarily, CBV. Under such circumstances, pretreating the patient with 5 to 10 mg of intravenous (IV) furosemide (before mannitol infusion) will lower the starting intravascular volume via its diuretic effect and prevent this significant untoward response. Because the brain needs adequate intravascular volume to maintain proper perfusion, the patient's volume status at the start of these therapeutic interventions must be known and maintained in the euvolemic (rather than hypovolemic or hypervolemic) range. In addition, in patients with ICP monitors

EMERGENCY TREATMENT OF ELEVATED ICP
IN PATIENTS WITH BRAIN TUMORS

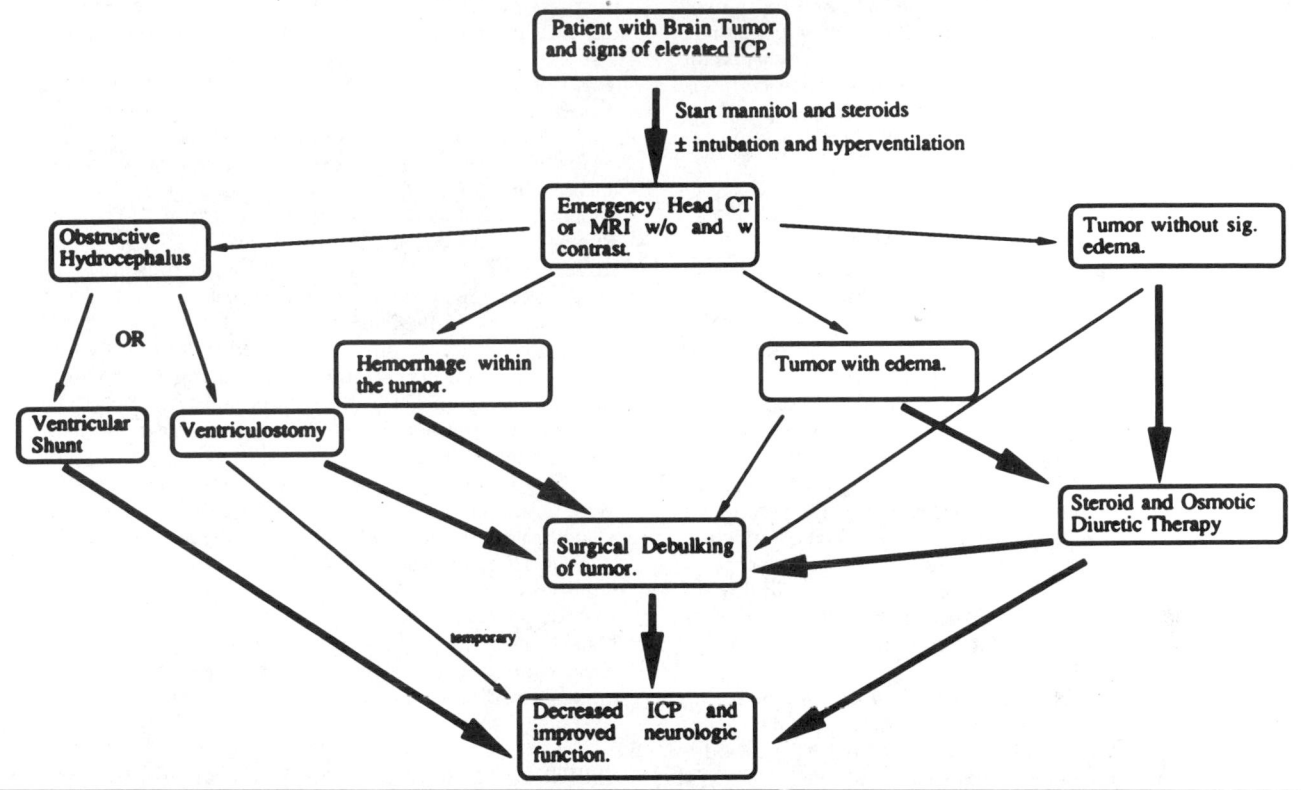

Fig. 188-3. Emergency treatment of elevated ICP in patients with brain tumors.

cerebral perfusion pressure (CPP) may be followed to fine-tune the therapeutic interventions.

Mannitol does not lower ICP as rapidly as hyperventilation. Once the effect takes place, however, mannitol can control elevated ICP over longer periods. Prolonged mannitol therapy remains controversial and may be ill-advised in the management of these patients, since surgical resection of the mass more effectively treats the edematogenic source. Following mannitol therapy (1 gm/kg via IV push), ICP starts to decrease within 20 to 60 minutes; there is also improvement in brain compliance during this interval. Serum osmolality should be maintained in the range of 300 to 310 mOsm per liter for optimum long-term therapy. The standard dose used to maintain this therapeutic range over prolonged periods is 25 gm of mannitol delivered IV every 4 to 6 hours. Overshooting of the serum osmolality to levels greater than 310 mOsm per liter must be avoided, since this alone can lead to neurologic complications (e.g., hyperosmolar coma).

Steroids are the longer-acting agents used to control elevated ICP in brain tumors, and adrenocorticosteroids, such as dexamethasone or solumedrol, are the mainstays of chronic therapy for controlling elevated ICP in brain tumor patients. Steroids ameliorate peritumoral vasogenic edema in both experimental animals and patients; they decrease tumor capillary permeability, favorably alter exchange of sodium and water across endothelial cells, decrease pinocytotic transfer across the blood-brain barrier, and inhibit tumor production of certain edematogenic substances. All of these functions can result in long-term beneficial effects on ICP.

Dexamethasone remains the most commonly used steroid for the treatment of brain tumors. It is one of the most potent glucocorticoids and has minimal mineralocorticoid-associated effects. Compared to the other ICP-lowering agents mentioned above, its onset of action requires a longer interval; other measures, therefore, should be used first in urgent situations. Symptomatic brain tumor patients normally receive 16 to 40 mg of dexamethasone per day in divided doses. Higher doses are given initially, then tapered to an effective lower dose once the patient's clinical status is ameliorated. Intravenous and oral doses are equally effective. Gastrointestinal (GI) side effects (gastritis, upper GI bleeding) are quite common, especially in patients with peptic ulcer disease. Coadministration of medications to prevent gastric irritations is recommended. Prolonged administration of steroids is the norm in many brain tumor patients and has been associated with other deleterious side effects, such as a predisposition to infection, aseptic necrosis of long bones, and myopathy.

Over the long history of brain tumor and elevated ICP treatment, other medical therapies have been used, but none has been very effective. With recent advances in understanding of the biochemistry and mechanisms of brain edema, novel agents are being developed and evaluated for their efficacy in controlling vasogenic edema associated with brain neoplasms. The 21-aminosteroids (Lazeroids), for example, may provide the anti-edema effects of steroids without the associated hyperglucocorticoid side effects [11]. These drugs may provide more effective treatment of vasogenic edema associated with brain tumors with less of the associated morbidity [12].

Course and Prognosis. In the majority of symptomatic patients mentioned above, elevated ICP due to brain edema usually can be managed in the acute phase effectively with medical measures. Medical treatments alone, however, are palliative at best and not recommended over long periods. Surgical intervention, radiation, and/or chemotherapy is usually required for successful long-term management of the majority of brain tumor patients.

TUMOR-ASSOCIATED HYDROCEPHALUS

Pathogenesis. Cerebrospinal fluid is formed continuously in the choroid plexus of the brain's ventricular system by an active transport mechanism. It is circulated via bulk flow from the lateral ventricles, through the brain, to the posterior fossa, where it enters the subarachnoid space. From the posterior fossa, CSF flows cephalad over the cerebral convexities and eventually to the arachnoid granulations, which allow absorption of the CSF into the venous system. Hydrocephalus is an abnormal increase of CSF volume in the intracranial compartment, commonly associated with enlargement of the ventricular system. Hydrocephalus results when there is an overproduction of CSF relative to absorption (very rare, occasionally seen with choroid plexus papillomas) or obstruction of the bulk flow of CSF along its normal route of circulation. In brain tumor patients the latter is clearly the most common mechanism for development of hydrocephalus.

Ventriculomegaly is the resultant finding on neuroimaging studies. Computed tomography scans show ventricular dilatation and hypodensities around the lateral ventricles. These findings are seen in even better detail with MRI (Fig. 188-4). A periventricular low density on CT and periventricular hyperintensity on T_2-weighted (or gradient echo) MRI scans associated with hydrocephalus commonly indicate acute elevations in ICP, with periventricular stasis of extracellular fluid that normally circulates into the ventricles. A tumor can block the flow of CSF either in the ventricles or within the connecting channels (foramina or aqueduct) within the brain, causing *noncommunicating* or *obstructive hydrocephalus,* or in the subarachnoid pathways to or including the arachnoid granulations, causing a *communicating hydrocephalus.* On neuroimaging studies, noncommunicating hydrocephalus is demonstrated by dilatation of the ventricular system proximal to the obstruction with normal-sized pathways distal to the block. For example, a midbrain tumor can cause obstruction at the aqueduct of Sylvius, with dilatation of the lateral and third ventricles but a normal-sized fourth ventricle [13]. In communicating hydrocephalus, however, all four ventricles are enlarged, as occurs commonly with meningeal seeding of CNS tumors. Deep unilateral hemispheric tumors can occasionally obstruct the outflow from the contralateral lateral ventricle by mass effect on the foramen of Monro, resulting in a trapped ventricle [14].

Diagnosis. Patients with brain tumors whose symptoms arise from associated hydrocephalus also present with symptoms and signs of increased intracranial pressure. A decrease in mental status, gait ataxia, incontinence, and obtundation are common clinical findings. Seizures rarely result from hydrocephalus. Papilledema and false localizing signs may be found on examination. If the patient is left untreated cerebral herniation may occur, since the hydrocephalus exacerbates any mass effect or elevation in ICP caused by the tumor.

Both CT and MRI scans are useful in defining the pathologic anatomy leading to the hydrocephalus, with MRI providing the best anatomic details. In children with open fontanelles, cranial ultrasound also can be used to evaluate the hydrocephalus associated with tumors. Whether to treat a patient with a brain tumor-associated hydrocephalus is often a clinical decision and depends primarily on symptomatology and overall prognosis.

Treatment. The ultimate management of tumor-associated hydrocephalus depends on its specific etiology and clinical picture. Ideally, removal of the tumor should relieve the hydrocephalus. In practice, however, this may not be immediately feasible, and a CSF diversion via ventriculostomy may be used initially to stabilize the patient and control ICP. This approach allows for removal of the CSF diversion following definitive surgery, if the hydrocephalus is no longer present. While ventricular shunting procedures once were advocated prior to brain tumor surgery to facilitate resection [15], today many believe the tumor should be directly attacked (with temporary ventriculostomy, if necessary), rather than placing a permanent shunt early in management. If the patient still has symptomatic hydrocephalus after definitive tumor resection, a permanent shunt can then be placed.

Avoidance of a permanent shunt has many advantages in brain tumor patients: there is no chance of clinical deterioration related to hardware obstruction or malfunction; the chance of symptomatic infection is greatly reduced, especially in cases of multiple operations for tumor treatment; and the chance of spreading a CNS tumor systemically via the shunt is eliminated. If a shunt is required, however, the symptomatic spread of CNS tumors rarely leads to death: most patients succumb to their intracranial disease rather than to systemic metastases.

SEIZURES. Seizures are an important cause of morbidity (and occasionally, mortality) in patients with brain tumors. Approximately 40 percent of patients with glioma present with seizure as the earliest manifestation of disease and 55 percent have at least one spell by the time their tumor is diagnosed [16,17].

Pathogenesis. The morbidity normally associated with seizures in patients without intracranial tumors is magnified in tumor patients, due to the lack of brain compliance. With the already elevated ICP associated with most tumors, a seizure causing increased CBF and elevated $PaCO_2$ can precipitate a neurologic emergency. Under these circumstances, brain herniation and death have been reported.

Certain lower-grade glial tumors, such as oligodendrogliomas and certain astrocytomas, are more likely to present with seizures than are glioblastomas [16,17]. The pathologic change of a glial tumor to a more malignant phenotype occasionally may be heralded by an increase in seizure frequency. Status epilepticus is common and may be the only presenting clinical condition. In patients presenting with status epilepticus of unknown etiology, a frontal brain tumor must be sought [18].

Diagnosis. Although classically associated with focal or jacksonian epilepsy, brain tumors can produce virtually any type of epilepsy in the adult. A CT or MRI scan should be performed in all adult patients with new onset seizure.

The usefulness of electroencephalography (EEG) in most patients with seizures secondary to a known tumor is limited. It is most useful when considering resection of a brain tumor for the purpose of controlling seizures. Chronic EEG recordings and electrocorticography can help the surgeon pinpoint the seizure focus in reference to the tumor and/or critical cortical structures and allow optimal treatment.

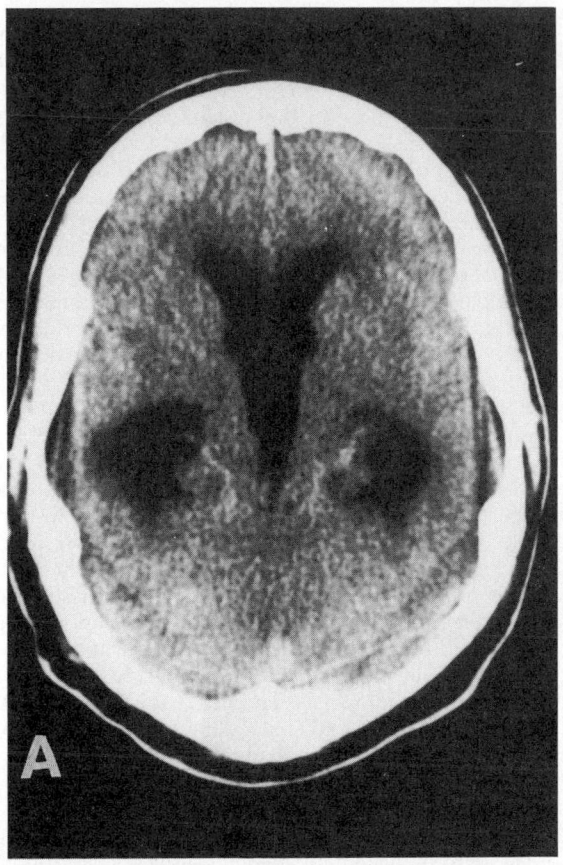
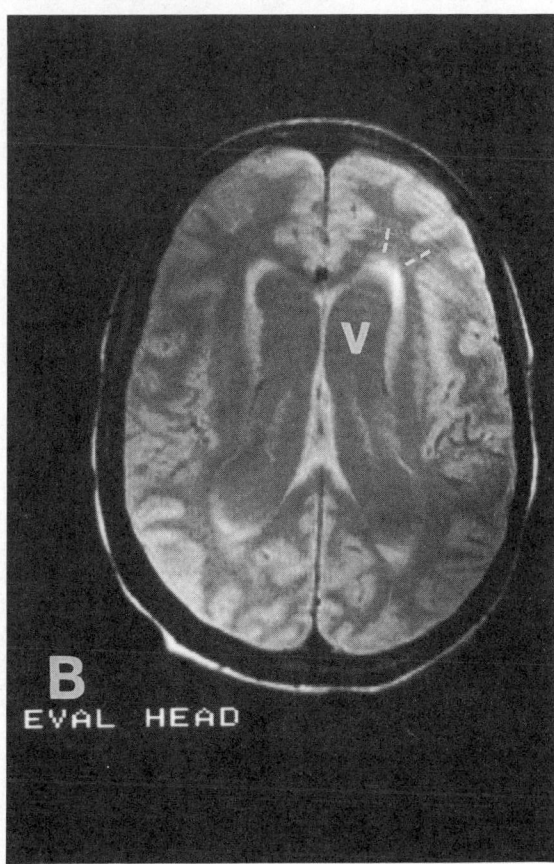

Fig. 188-4. A. Nonenhanced axial CT scan of the brain, showing a typical picture of acute noncommunicating hydrocephalus, with ventriculomegaly and increased periventricular low density. B. Nonenhanced gradient-echo MRI scan of acute hydrocephalus. Note the hyperintense appearing stasis of periventricular fluid (bordered by white —), distinct from the hypointense ventricular fluid (v).

Treatment. For patients with symptomatic seizures due to tumors in the frontal and temporal lobes, surgical resection can provide effective relief, with or without additional pharmacologic therapy.

Pharmacologic therapy for tumors in brain tumor patients is unique in a number of respects. Brain tumor patients are often receiving other medications (e.g., chemotherapy, dexamethasone) that may interact with anticonvulsants. Patients on dexamethasone frequently require higher doses of phenytoin for therapeutic levels and seizure control; conversely, as the steroid is tapered phenytoin levels can increase into the toxic range [19,20]. Brain tumor patients frequently receive cranial irradiation, which predisposes some patients on anticonvulsants to Stevens-Johnson syndrome and erythema multiforme reactions. This is especially true of phenytoin [21]. Finally, these patients often have other neurologic impairments associated with their tumors that can make anticonvulsant side effects much more intolerable. For example, patients with brain tumors treated with phenobarbital are particularly prone to developing shoulder-hand syndrome and diffuse arthralgias. In these specific circumstances, phenobarbital is discontinued and another anticonvulsant used.

Despite the above-mentioned complications, phenytoin remains the first-line drug for seizures in most tumor patients. If complications, breakthrough seizures, or allergic reactions occur, carbamazepine, phenobarbital, or valproate can be substituted. Breakthrough seizures in cases of low-grade glioma occasionally respond to surgical resection.

Occasionally seizures are noted in brain tumor patients following the administration of iodinated contrast agents during CT examinations. This cause of seizure can be diminished by pretreating the patient with 5 mg of intravenous diazepam. The treatment of status epilepticus in brain tumor patients is similar to that of patients with idiopathic epilepsy (see Chap. 186).

Course and Prognosis. Most patients with tumor-associated epilepsy are treated with a single pharmacologic agent (monotherapy). Under certain circumstances, however, some tumor patients may require more than one drug to control their seizures (polytherapy). In cases of refractory seizures despite polytherapy, surgical resection of the seizure focus (and tumor) may be indicated, especially if the tumor is otherwise stable.

Prophylactic anticonvulsants usually are not indicated for patients with brain metastases or primary brain tumors but no clinical seizures [22]. Such patients may be managed temporarily with prophylactic anticonvulsants during the perioperative period (discontinued 7 days after surgery) and during periods of significant ICP elevations, in an effort to prevent acute catastrophic deteriorations. Patients with primary brain tumors are usually treated with anticonvulsants perioperatively; the medication can then be continued for patients who had seizures in their preoperative period.

TREATMENT-RELATED NEUROONCOLOGIC EMERGENCIES.
With the more intensive therapeutic management schemes used in recent years, it is necessary to distinguish between treatment morbidity and tumor progression.

Complications of Neurosurgical Oncologic Procedures.
Modern neurosurgical techniques have greatly reduced operative morbidity and mortality in neurooncologic patients, when practiced with experienced anesthesiologists. While operative mortalities are generally less than 2 percent, medical and neurological morbidity occurs in up to 30 percent, strongly correlating with patient age and neurologic condition [23].

Although most cranial tumor cases are considered "clean," perioperative prophylactic antibiotics reduce infection rates, compared to patients not receiving antibiotics [24]. Meningitis, subdural empyema, and brain abscess all have been associated with brain tumor surgery but are much less frequent today than even 5 to 10 years ago. The majority of infections are related to skin organisms, most commonly *Staphylococcus* species. Careful attention to surgical detail (planning the scalp flap, prevention of subgaleal hematoma, skin closure) and gentle handling of the tissues go a long way in preventing these complications. Patients with high fever, new neurologic deficits, signs of meningeal irritation, CSF leak, and elevated blood leukocyte counts are promptly started on a broad-spectrum antibiotic regimen [25]. With additional objective clinical information and consultation with infectious disease specialists, more specific antibiotics can be prescribed. The patient's symptoms and signs of infection may occasionally be masked by steroid therapy or age. Subdural empyemas, heralded by seizures, focal neurologic deficits, and extraaxial collections on neuroimaging studies, usually should be drained via craniotomy. Further collections require reoperation and drainage. Patients with empyemas and abscesses are followed with serial neuroimaging studies. Brain abscesses can occasionally be treated via freehand or stereotactic aspirations in addition to appropriate antibiotics. Persistent reaccumulations after repeated aspirations, however, may require open craniotomy for abscess resection.

Hemorrhage occurring after open cranial surgery or stereotactic surgery is a readily treatable complication in the postoperative neurooncologic patient. It can usually be prevented by good surgical techniques but may also occur due to other causes. Coagulation studies should be performed to rule out a postoperative coagulopathy. In addition, blood pressure should be maintained in the normal range, preventing hypo- or hypertension. Diagnosis of a hemorrhage in the tumor bed is usually confirmed by neuroimaging studies. If the clot is small and the patient asymptomatic, it usually can be managed without surgery. If the patient is symptomatic and the clot is large, in most cases the clot should probably be evacuated surgically. The dilemma usually occurs in the case of the asymptomatic patient with a fairly large clot. Unless the clot is in a particularly precarious position (i.e., medial temporal lobe, cerebellum), it is best to be conservative.

Another common surgical complication is shunt malfunction [26]. Following a CSF flow obstruction and rise in ICP, a CSF shunt obstruction can mimic signs of tumor progression: decreased mental status, papilledema, and false localizing signs. A CT or MRI scan can assist in the diagnosis, but to evaluate the situation properly the clinician must first suspect the shunt malfunction. Continuity of the shunt system must be confirmed via plain radiographs (head/neck, chest, and abdomen; anteroposterior and lateral) and palpation. Shunt tapping may be necessary to determine the etiology and location of the malfunction (obstruction vs. infection, proximal vs. distal). A radionuclide shunt study may occasionally be necessary to document abnormal flow in the system or a partial obstruction. Malfunctioning shunts are best treated by replacing the malfunctioning portion with a new section of shunt.

Stereotactic radiosurgical procedures in patients with brain tumors rarely cause severe acute complications but may cause late neurologic decompensations. Stereotactic radiosurgery in neurooncology currently involves precise stereotactic delivery of a single high-dose fraction of radiation to a limited volume of tumor in the brain, with rapid radiation dose falloff outside the target. Stereotactic radiosurgery has occasionally produced seizures, nausea, and vomiting around the time of the procedure. In most cases, the seizures are related to acute effects of the single high-dose fraction of radiation on susceptible cortical neurons and are easily prevented or controlled by standard anticonvulsant therapy. The nausea and vomiting probably are related to a transient increase in ICP secondary to the brain's reaction to the large single fraction of radiation and can be treated symptomatically with antiemetics or a short course of steroids. The majority of patients undergoing these procedures are treated prophylactically with anticonvulsants and steroids to decrease the risk of these acute complications. The major delayed complication is focal radiation necrosis, which can behave as an expanding mass and mimic tumor progression clinically and on CT and MRI evaluation. Positron emission tomography (PET) scanning is used to differentiate between radiation necrosis and tumor; a tumor has a markedly elevated metabolic status, whereas necrosis is nearly devoid of metabolic activity. Treatment is symptomatic, with mannitol and steroids or, if refractory to medical management, surgical resection.

Complications are related to the mode of therapeutic delivery with interstitial brachytherapy. As with stereotactic radiosurgery, complications are both acute and delayed. Overall complication rates are significantly higher with the latter treatment modality. Acute complications are related to the percutaneous placement of guide catheters into the tumor bed, usually via stereotactic guidance. These catheters exit from the brain, skull, and skin and are afterloaded with specific radioisotopes. The loaded catheters are left in situ for a specific period (2–3 days), during which time the isotopes deliver their high-dose radiation continuously and intrinsically in the brain tumor. The catheters are then removed percutaneously following treatment. Hemorrhage, brain edema, and infection can result from catheter placement or following catheter removal from the brain and tumor. Because of the percutaneous placement of the catheters the risk of infection is fairly high, despite prophylactic antibiotics, especially if CSF leaks from the wound sites during or after treatment. Hemorrhage and brain edema are treated symptomatically during the acute period, usually with mannitol and steroids. Rarely, these early complications require acute surgical intervention to prevent irreversible neurologic deterioration. Delayed skull and skin flap infections may occur and necessitate debridement and bone flap removal. Radiation necrosis has been another rather frequent, delayed sequela of interstitial brachytherapy for brain tumors [27]. Teatment is similar to that for stereotactic radiosurgery.

Complications of Radiation Therapy.
External beam radiation therapy (RT) is another mainstay of the neurooncologic management of brain tumors. In conventional fractions, RT can result in symptomatic worsening during the course of therapy (acute) or as a delayed effect, occurring weeks (subacute) or

months (chronic) after its completion. The early reactions are primarily related to steroid-responsive brain edema. As with stereotactic radiosurgery and interstitial brachytherapy, delayed effects tend to be more serious and related to the development of radiation necrosis.

Complications of Chemotherapy. The role of chemotherapy and immunotherapy in neurooncology is less restricted today than formerly. Today, the majority of malignant brain neoplasms are aggressively treated with one or more chemotherapeutic agents. Specific agents and modalities are each associated with their own complications, but discussion is beyond the scope of this chapter. The interested reader is referred to the textbook by DeVita et al. [3] and other currently available references.

DEEP VENOUS THROMBOSIS AND PULMONARY EMBOLISM IN THE BRAIN TUMOR PATIENT. Because of the increased incidence of deep vein thrombosis (DVT) and pulmonary embolism (PE) in patients with brain tumors, it is important to discuss these issues as real management possibilities, especially since treatment with anticoagulation may increase morbidity in patients with brain tumors.

Pathogenesis. Because of the increased immobility of neurologically impaired patients, as well as the release of tissue thromboplastins from brain, venous thrombosis is quite common in brain tumor patients. With an incidence as high as 33 percent [28], the clinician should watch for DVT at any time during the disease, although the highest-risk period is within the first 6 weeks following craniotomy. Early recognition and treatment of DVT is the most effective way of preventing PE.

Diagnosis. Since brain tumor patients are at high risk for venous thrombosis, patients with leg pain or increased leg circumference should be screened for DVT with impedance plethysmography or duplex scanning. Sometimes venography is necessary to define the extent of the thrombotic process. Should a patient suddenly develop shortness of breath, chest pain, or encephalopathy of unclear etiology, PE should be ruled out with radionuclide lung scanning. When PE is highly probable or diagnosed, therapy usually is necessary to prevent further complications or death.

Treatment. Prevention is the major goal in this high-risk population. Early ambulation or, if the patient is bedridden, pneumatic compression boots are mandatory. The role of screening with either impedance plethysmography or duplex scanning remains controversial, but eventually it may prove cost-effective in preventing complications related to DVT and PE. Prophylactic subcutaneous heparin is rarely indicated following craniotomy for brain tumors.

Optimal therapy for brain tumor patients with PE remains controversial, especially after recent brain surgery (< 4 weeks), when the potential for neurologic complications due to anticoagulation is increased [29,30]. After the early postoperative period (> 4 weeks), anticoagulation with heparin and warfarin may be necessary and can be carried out with relatively low morbidity in symptomatic patients. For DVT alone, the placement of inferior vena cava filters helps prevent PE. Placement of a filter does not correct the hypercoagulable state, nor does it prevent symptomatic clots from developing above the filter or in the upper extremities (see Chap. 69).

Systemic Cancer Patients

Approximately 15 percent of cancer patients develop neurologic problems during the course of illness. Despite the incurable nature of the disease in many of these patients, proper diagnosis and management of neurologic sequelae can greatly improve the quality of life and survival. Again, complete discussion of neurologic complications related to cancer is beyond the scope of this chapter. This section focuses on the common complications requiring emergent management.

BRAIN METASTASIS. The brain is a relatively common site of involvement for certain systemic cancers. At autopsy, about 25 percent of patients with systemic cancer have brain metastases. More than two-thirds of these patients will have had clinical symptoms attributable to these lesions.

Pathogenesis. Metastatic tumors most commonly spread to the brain via hematogenous routes. There is a correlation between the location of metastatic tumors within the brain and CBF. With the carotid circulation carrying 85 percent of the CBF, metastases to the cerebral hemispheres are much more common than to posterior fossa structures. Within the brain, the gray matter structures have the highest CBF. The cortical gray-white matter junction is a common location for tumor emboli to lodge, due to the rich vascular supply and the rapid change in caliber of the vessels at this location, where pial conductance vessels branch and narrow to form penetrating nutrient arteries. Metastatic lesions may be single or multiple (Fig. 188-5) and cystic or solid and have been reported to occur from almost every type of systemic cancer. The most frequently seen brain metastases are from lung and breast cancers. Melanoma has a particularly high predilection for metastasizing to the brain. Systemic lymphoma also tends to spread to the brain. Certain metastatic brain tumors tend to present as a hemorrhagic mass (or masses), particularly hypernephromas, choriocarcinomas, and melanomas. Infrequently (10–15% of all cases), an extensive preoperative metastatic workup does not reveal the primary site of the cancer, and the histologic diagnosis can be confirmed only at the time of cranial surgery.

Diagnosis. Symptoms and signs associated with brain metastases are quite nonspecific and dependent on lesion location(s) and whether there is an associated increase in ICP. Headaches, seizures, and focal neurologic deficits are common presenting complaints but are also features of primary tumors and other brain pathologies. Twenty percent of patients present with one or more seizures. As part of an ongoing evaluation of cancer patients, clinicians must have a high index of suspicion and a low threshold for performing diagnostic imaging studies, specifically when seeking brain metastases.

Contrast-enhanced MRI imaging is the test of choice for evaluating metastatic brain disease, yielding a correct diagnosis in 95 percent of patients. Computed tomography scans performed without and with contrast are useful options for patients in whom MRI scanning is contraindicated (e.g., those with cardiac pacemakers or metallic ocular implants). When a new mass lesion is found in the brain of a previously undiagnosed patient, a systematic search for the primary lesion is warranted. At a minimum, the diagnostic workup should include a chest CT scan, mammography (in women), stool guaiac, abdominal CT scan, and pelvic CT scan. Additional diagnostic testing can be done but is only rarely useful in defining a primary lesion.

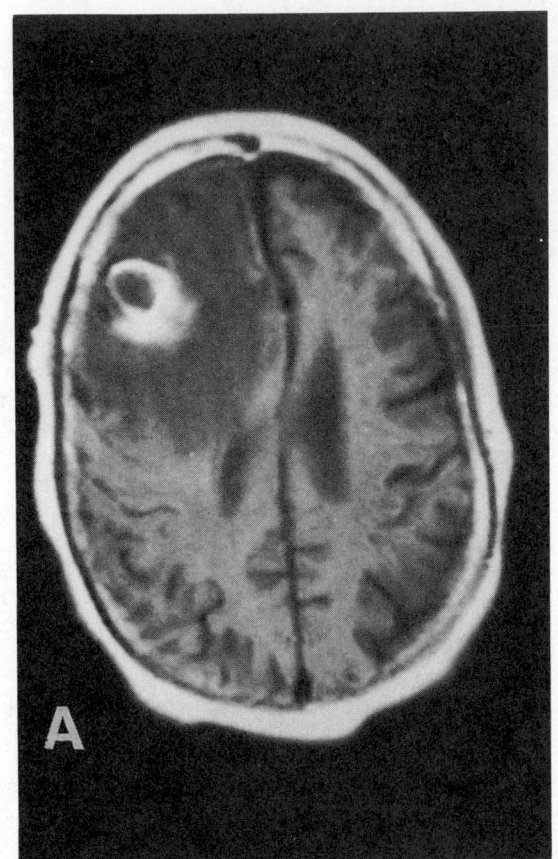

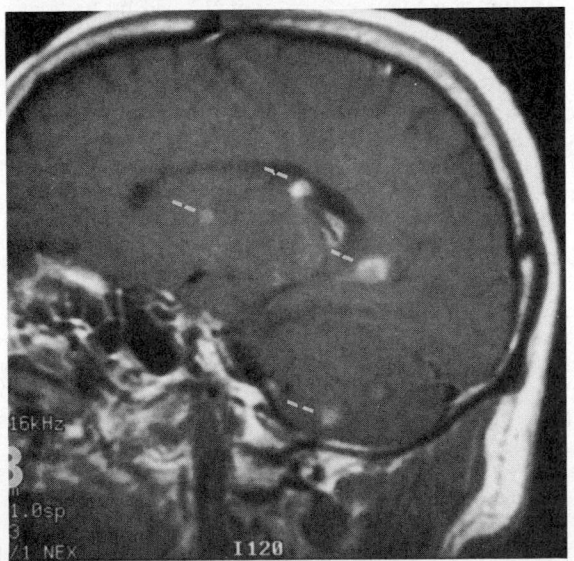

Fig. 188-5. Examples of symptomatic cerebral metastases visualized on MRI scans. A. Axial contrast-enhanced T_1-weighted image of a right frontal single solitary metastasis from a lung primary. Note the significant surrounding edema and mass effect despite the relatively small size of the enhancing lesion. B. Sagittal contrast-enhanced T_1-weighted image, showing multiple supra- and infratentorial metastases (white —) from a cutaneous melanoma primary.

Treatment. When a cerebral metastasis is diagnosed, the initial goal is stabilization of patient and amelioration of the neurologic symptoms and signs. Seizures should be controlled with anticonvulsants. Increased ICP should be managed according to the scheme outlined above (Fig. 188-3). In the majority of patients, headaches and mild neurologic deficits can be greatly improved by treatment with steroids in moderate dosages (i.e., 4 mg dexamethasone four times per day or every six hours). Although they do not impact significantly on long-term outcome, these early measures offer effective early palliation and allow for the planning of additional therapies that can improve long-term outcome.

Once the patient is stabilized, treatment is dependent on one major question: whether there is one lesion or more than one. For long-term control, a single solitary brain metastasis usually is treated aggressively with surgical resection of the lesion, followed by whole brain RT [31]. In the majority of patients single lesions in deep or eloquent brain areas can be removed aggressively using stereotactic microsurgical techniques and cortical brain mapping. Patients with multiple brain metastases are infrequently treated with open craniotomy. An exception is with localized clustering of metastases in a single noneloquent brain area, where the surgeon can intervene in the same manner as for a single lesion. When there is no evidence of a systemic primary tumor, surgical intervention for diagnosis is indicated in the majority of patients. For single lesions, resection is usually indicated; for multiple brain lesions, stereotactic biopsy provides the opportunity for tissue analysis and a definitive diagnosis. In the majority of patients, external beam RT follows surgical intervention [32,33,34]; for a minority of patients chemotherapy is also available.

The role of stereotactic radiosurgery in the treatment of brain metastases is still being defined. Its use has significant theoretic promise. Precisely focused high-dose single-fraction therapy can be applied safely to the intracerebral tumor volume, thereby sparing the surrounding critical brain structures. The precise targeting capabilities of this technology coupled with improved neuroimaging may in the future permit even more aggressive yet lower-risk treatment of brain metastasis (especially multiple metastases).

Course and Prognosis. Therapeutic interventions for cerebral metastases often result in effective CNS palliation. Following optimal surgical intervention more than two-thirds of patients remain stable or improve neurologically for the remainder of the course of their disease. Unfortunately, even with effective control of the CNS pathology, survival is short due to systemic disease, with death occurring within 6 to 12 months. Longer-term survivors are much more common today, with the multimodality treatments available for certain cancers.

EPIDURAL SPINAL CORD COMPRESSION. Epidural spinal cord compression is a frequent neurologic complication of metastatic cancer, found in 5 percent of cancer patients. Back pain in a cancer patient, therefore, is sufficient grounds for immediate evaluation and diagnosis, and makes possible treatment prior to the development of a worsening neurologic picture.

Pathogenesis. Spinal cord compression due to epidural metastatic tumor is most commonly due to breast and lung carcinomas but is also frequently seen with melanoma, lymphoma, and colon cancer [35]. Epidural metastatic tumors usually originate as an extension out of an involved vertebral body. Any vertebral body may be invaded with cancer, and it is not unusual for multiple levels to be involved at once. Most vertebral metastases originate in the vertebral pedicle and extend ventrally to involve varying amounts of the vertebral body. These tumors cause pain by expanding the overlying periosteum and cause neurologic symptoms and signs by compressing the adjacent neural structures. Acute pain and neurologic deterioration are frequently seen in association with bony collapse of the involved vertebra or, occasionally, tumor compression of epidural veins. Some tumors, such as lymphoma, may cause minimal if any bony abnormalities while growing as epidural masses. These tumors tend to grow into the epidural space through the neural foramina from paravertebral masses.

Diagnosis. Back pain remains the most common early symptom of epidural compression and occurs in more than 95 percent of afflicted patients [35]. Associated neurologic symptoms and signs primarily depend on the spinal level of involvement and range from pain alone to a complete loss of function below the involved level.

Early detection and treatment of spinal epidural compression is essential for successful future ambulation, since neurologic function at the time of treatment is the most important determinant of function after treatment. A complaint of back pain in a cancer patient almost always warrants a neurologic examination and radiographic studies to rule out bony spinal metastases. Bone scans are particularly effective in showing the multiplicity of lesions involving the spine. Plain films and CT or MRI scans are more effective for evaluating specific pathology. The chance of finding significant epidural pathology in a patient increases when a myelopathy or radiculopathy is present or when vertebral collapse is documented [36]. Spinal MRI scan is the test of choice for evaluating patients with possible spinal epidural compression due to tumor [37,38] (Fig. 188-6).

Treatment. As with other CNS tumors, steroids provide effective, temporary relief of the symptoms and signs of spinal epidural. Pain relief is particularly gratifying to the patient suffering from this condition. High-dose dexamethasone (50–100 mg IV, followed by 10 mg IV every 6 hours, on a tapering daily schedule) is the treatment of choice in the presence of myelopathy or progressive neurologic deterioration. This therapy is most effective, however, when surgery and/or RT is initiated shortly thereafter. When a stable nonprogressive block is viewed on the MRI or myelogram, lower doses of steroids may be administered [39,40].

Definitive treatments for epidural compression due to metastatic tumor include surgery and RT. In most circumstances, RT is the primary treatment modality. Although metastatic tumors have varying degrees of sensitivity to RT, most patients are effectively palliated by a conventional dosage regimen of 10 fractions of 3 Gy each [35]. Posterior laminectomy is rarely indicated as the only surgical treatment of these lesions but occasionally may be used for primarily dorsolateral lesions or with transpedicular modifications for ventrolateral debulking in the poor-risk patient. More definitive anterior and anterolateral debulking procedures with stabilization and reconstruction are indicated in patients with stable disease and moderate to long expected survival [41].

Course and Prognosis. *The most important prognostic factor in determining ambulation after treatment of an epidural compression is whether the patient is ambulatory at the time of diagnosis and treatment.* Early diagnosis is therefore crucial. By definition, patients with epidural compression due to cancer have advanced disease. Maintaining the ability to ambulate, however, greatly improves the patient's quality of life.

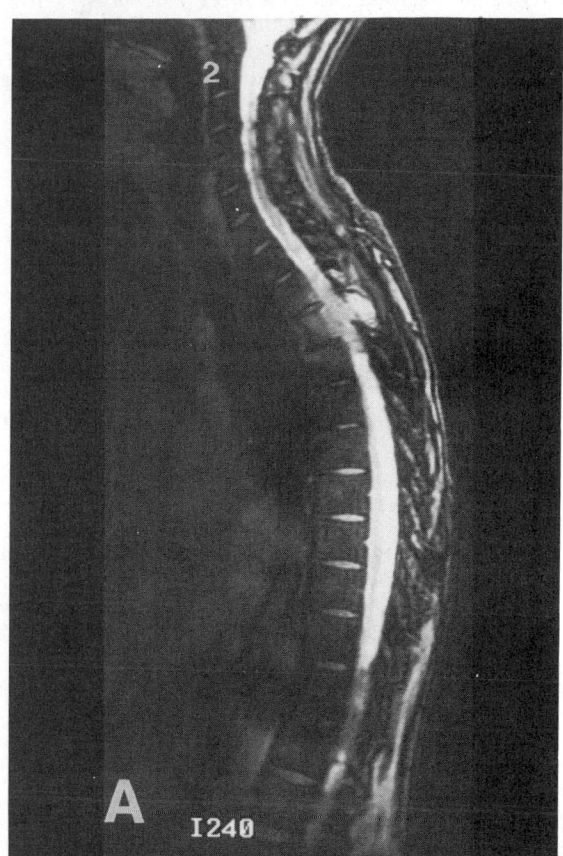

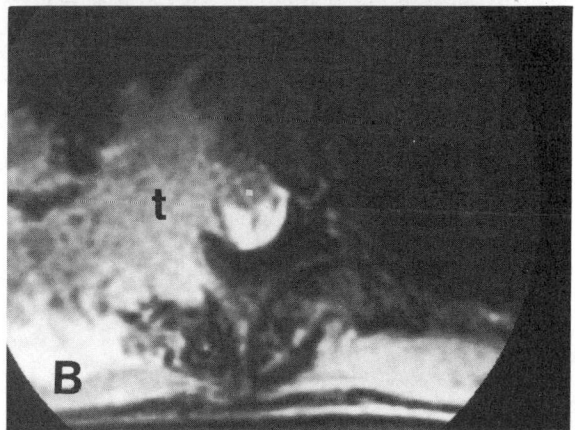

Fig. 188-6. Spinal MRI scan delineating epidural spinal cord compression from a primary lung cancer. A. Midline sagittal T_2-weighted image delineating the focal lesion at T_3 (2 denotes C_2). Note the normal spinal alignment and no other apparent vertebral pathology from C_1 to L_1. B. Axial T_2-weighted image at the T_3 level indicating the primarily right-sided tumor (t) involving the right lamina, pedicle and vertebral body, and paraspinal tissues. The spinal cord (small white square) is only slightly impinged on by the epidural portion of this tumor.

STROKE. Like other individuals, cancer patients can suffer the sudden onset of a neurologic deficit. The differential diagnosis should include thromboembolic stroke, intracranial metastases (especially with intratumoral bleeding), and leptomeningeal carcinomatosis (which may occasionally occlude cerebral arteries). Approximately 15 percent of cancer patients have significant cerebrovascular pathology noted at autopsy [42].

Pathogenesis. At least half of cases of symptomatic strokes in the population have a cause other than primary vascular disease [42]. A unique reason for this is that disseminated intravascular coagulopathies occur in patients with solid tumors. Migratory thrombophlebitis, bleeding, and arterial emboli (Trousseau's syndrome) occur and are often associated with mucin-secreting tumors. In addition, cancer patients receiving certain myelosuppressive agents (particularly patients with lymphoma or leukemia) are especially prone to hemorrhagic events, manifesting at times as intracranial hemorrhages. The approach to stroke in the cancer patient, therefore, should be slightly different than that taken with the general population.

Nonhemorrhagic and Hemorrhagic Stroke Syndromes. Cancer patients have been known to present with at least three types of unique stroke syndromes as a result of a hypercoagulable state: nonbacterial thrombotic endocarditis (NBTE), disseminated intravascular coagulation (DIC), and cerebral vein occlusion.

Pathologically, NBTE in cancer patients, especially those with adenocarcinomas, features sterile vegetations on normal heart valves [43,44]. Typically, stroke due to NBTE is a late manifestation of cancer; rarely is it the initial symptom of an underlying tumor. Most patients present with an acute event, but one-third can present with a progressive neurologic syndrome and no focal neurologic deficits. Echocardiography rarely visualizes the vegetations but is used to rule out other cardiac causes of stroke. Whereas heparin may be useful in preventing further embolization, this effect has not been shown for warfarin. Prognosis in these cases is so poor that, most commonly, no therapy is instituted.

Disseminated intravascular coagulation is a very important complication of cancer, especially the lymphomas and leukemias. It can occlude small vessels and result in neurologic syndromes characterized by focal signs and a fluctuating encephalopathy. A decreasing platelet count and increase in fibrin split products confirm the diagnosis. Anticoagulation with heparin is the treatment of choice but must be used with caution, especially if platelet counts are low or the patient has had recent surgery.

Occlusions of cerebral veins or dural sinuses can occur in cancer patients due to metastatic infiltration or as a nonmetastatic complication. The very common combination of dehydration (due to nausea and vomiting) and chemotherapy, espe-cially with L-asparaginase, predisposes the patient to the formation of a thrombus in the superior sagittal sinus, resulting in headaches and generalized seizures. The diagnosis of a superior sagittal sinus thrombosis can be inferred from the MRI picture and noninvasively confirmed with MRA. Treatment with anticoagulation is controversial, since many patients have hemorrhagic venous infarctions in their cerebral hemispheres parasagittally and generally do well with conservative treatment.

Hemorrhage. As in other patients, spontaneous intracranial hemorrhage occurs in cancer patients, but all too often with fatal consequences. Patients who present with cancer-related hemorrhages most commonly have hematologic malignancies, especially with thrombocytopenia or coagulopathy. Hemor-rhage into metastatic tumors may also occur, especially with melanoma.

CENTRAL NERVOUS SYSTEM INFECTIONS. Due to the immunocompromised condition of many cancer patients, the spectrum and presentation of CNS infections in this population differs significantly from that of the normal population. While the anatomic sites of infection are similar, the offending organisms causing the CNS infections differ.

Pathogenesis. The specific type of organism that infects the immunocompromised patient depends on the specific immune abnormality present, and the type of infectious microorganism depends on whether there is an abnormality in leukocyte function or dysfunction of cell-mediated or humoral immunity. Decreased numbers of neutrophils (e.g., in aplastic anemia or preleukemia) or neutrophil dysfunction can occur with steroid administration or cachexia. Leukocyte abnormalities predispose the patient to infections with gram-negative enteric bacteria or *Staphylococcus.* Abnormalities in cell-mediated (T cell and macrophage) immunity commonly occur in lymphomas and predispose the patient to "exotic" infections, such as fungi *(Cryptococcus* and *Candida),* parasites (toxoplasmosis), and unusual bacteria (especially *Listeria*). Humoral (B cell) immunity is impaired in conditions such as multiple myeloma. Lack of opsonizing antibodies to promote bacterial phagocytosis predisposes patients to infections with encapsulated organisms such as *Streptococcus pneumoniae.*

Diagnosis. Cancer patients with CNS infections may present in a manner identical to similarly infected individuals without cancer. Signs of infection in some patients may be more subtle, however, due to their immunocompromised state. For example, a cancer patient with bacterial meningitis may present with only an alteration in mental status, rather than the more typical high fever and meningeal signs.

Treatment. Treatment of CNS infections is specifically tailored to the isolated organism and is beyond the scope of this chapter. Localized infections, such as epidural abscess, brain abscess, or subdural empyema, require prompt surgical evacuation and intervention, in addition to antibiotic therapy, for the best possible results.

References

1. Henson RA, Urich H: *Cancer and the Nervous System: The Neurological Manifestations of Systemic Malignant Disease.* Oxford, Blackwell 1982.
2. Posner JB: Neurological complications of systemic cancer. *Med Clin North Am* 63:783, 1979.
3. DeVita VT, Hellman S. Rosenberg SA (eds): *Cancer: Principles and Practices of Oncology.* Philadelphia, JB Lippincott, 1989.
4. Bartkowski H: Peritumoral edema. *Prog Exp Tumor Res* 27:179, 1984.
5. Bruce J, Criscuolo G, Merrill M, et al: Vascular permeability induced by protein product of malignant brain tumors: Inhibition by dexamethasone. *J Neurosurg* 67:880, 1987.
6. Black KL, Hoff JT, McGillicuddy JE, Gebarski SS: Increased leukotriene C4 and vasogenic edema surrounding brain tumors in humans. *Ann Neurol* 19:592, 1986.
7. Shapiro WR, Posner JB: Corticosteroid hormones: Effects in an experimental brain tumor. *Arch Neurol* 30:217, 1974.
8. Yamada K, Ushio Y, Hayakawa T, et al: Effects of methylprednisolone on peritumoral brain edema: A quantitative autoradiography study. *J Neurosurg* 59:612, 1983.

9. Rosner MJ, Becker DP: Origin and evolution of plateau waves. *J Neurosurg* 60:312, 1984.

10. Muizelaar J, Wei E, Kontos H, et al: Mannitol causes compensatory cerebral vasoconstriction and vasodilation in response to blood viscosity changes. *J Neurosurg* 59:822, 1983.

11. King WA, Black KL, Ikezaki K, et al: Tumor-associated neurological dysfunction prevented by lazaroids in rats. *J Neurosurg* 74:112, 1991.

12. Joo F, Klatzo I: Role of cerebral endothelium in brain oedema. *Neurol Res* 11:67, 1989.

13. Raimondi A, Tomita T: Hydrocephalus and infratentorial tumors: Incidence, clinical picture and treatment. *J Neurosurg* 55:174, 1981.

14. Weaver D, Winn R, Jane J: Differential intracranial pressure in patients with unilateral mass lesions. *J Neurosurg* 55:660, 1982.

15. Schmid U, Seiler R: Management of obstructive hydrocephalus secondary to posterior fossa tumors by steroids and subcutaneous ventricular catheter reservoir. *J Neurosurg* 65:649, 1986.

16. Ketz E: Brain tumors and epilepsy, in Vinken JPJ, Bruyn GW (eds): *Handbook of Clinical Neurology*. vol. 16. Amsterdam, Elsevier, 1974, p 254.

17. McKeran R, Thomas D: The clinical study of gliomas, in Thomas DGT, Graham DI (eds): *Brain Tumours: Scientific Basis, Clinical Investigation and Current Therapy*. London, Butterworths, 1980, p 194.

18. Oxbury JM, Whitty C: Causes and consequences of status epilepticus in adults: A study of 86 cases. *Brain* 94:733, 1971.

19. Chalk J, Ridgeway K, Brophy T, et al: Phenytoin impairs the bioavailability of dexamethasone in neurological and neurosurgical patients. *J Neurol Neurosurg Psychiatry* 47:1087, 1984.

20. Wong D, Longenecker RG, Liepman M, et al: Phenytoin-dexamethasone: A potential drug interaction. *JAMA* 254:2062, 1985.

21. Delattre J, Safai B, Posner JB: Erythema multiforme and Stevens-Johnson syndrome in patients receiving cranial irradiation and phenytoin. *Neurology* 38:194, 1988.

22. Cohen N, Stauss G, Lew R, et al: Should prophylactic anticonvulsants be administered to patients with newly-diagnosed cerebral metastases? A retrospective analysis. *J Clin Oncol* 6:1621, 1988.

23. Fadul C, Wood J, Thaler H, et al: Morbidity and mortality of craniotomy for excision of supratentorial gliomas. *Neurology* 38:1374, 1988.

24. Haines D: Efficacy of antibiotic prophylaxis in clean neurosurgical operations. *Neurosurgery* 24:401, 1989.

25. Ross D, Rosegay H, Pons V: Differentiations of aseptic and bacterial meningitis in postoperative neurosurgical patients. *J Neurosurg* 69:669, 1988.

26. Sekhar L, Moossy J, Guthkelch N: Malfunctioning ventriculoperitoneal shunts: Clinical and pathological features. *J Neurosurg* 56:411, 1982.

27. Gutin P, Leibel S, Wara W, et al: Recurrent malignant gliomas: Survival following interstitial brachytherapy with high-activity iodine-125 sources. *J Neurosurg* 67:864, 1987.

28. Ruff R, Posner JB: Incidence and treatment of peripheral venous thrombosis in patients with glioma. *Ann Neurol* 13:334, 1983.

29. Swann K, McL Black M: Management of symptomatic deep venous thrombosis and pulmonary embolism on a neurosurgical service. *J Neurosurg* 64:563, 1986.

30. Choucair A, Silver P, Levin V: Risk of intracranial hemorrhage in glioma patients receiving anticoagulant therapy for venous thromboembolism. *J Neurosurg* 66:357, 1987.

31. Patchell RA, Tibbs PA, Walsh JW, et al: A randomized trial of surgery in the treatment of single metastases. *N Engl J Med* 322:494, 1990.

32. Borgelt B, Gelber R, Kramer S, et al: The palliation of brain metastases: Final results of the first two studies by the RTOG. *Int J Radiat Oncol Biol Phys* 6:1, 1980.

33. Cairncross J, Kim J, Posner JB: Radiation therapy for brain metastases. *Ann Neurol* 7:529, 1980.

34. Sheline G, Brady L: Radiation therapy for brain metastases. *J Neurooncol* 4:219, 1987.

35. Gilbert R, Kim J, Posner J: Epidural spinal cord compression from metastatic tumor: Diagnosis and treatment. *Ann Neurol* 3:40, 1978.

36. Rodichok L, Harper G, Ruckdeschel J, et al: Early diagnosis of spinal epidural metastases. *Am J Med* 70:1181, 1981.

37. Godersky J, Smoker W, Knutzon R: Use of magnetic resonance imaging in the evaluation of metastatic spinal disease. *Neurosurgery* 21:676, 1987.

38. Hagenau C, Grosh W, Currie M, et al: Comparison of spinal magnetic resonance imaging and myelography in cancer patients. *J Clin Oncol* 5:1663, 1989.

39. Delattre J, Arbit E, Thaler H, et al: A dose-response study of dexamethasone in a model of spinal cord compression caused by epidural tumor. *J Neurosurg* 70:920, 1989.

40. Slatkin N, Posner JB: Management of spinal epidural metastases. *Clin Neurosurg* 30:698, 1983.

41. Cybulski G: Methods of surgical stabilization for metastatic disease of the spine. *Neurosurgery* 25:240, 1989.

42. Graus F, Rogers L, Posner J: Cerebrovascular complications in patients with cancer. *Medicine* 64:16, 1985.

43. Koolker J, MacLean J, Sumi S: Cerebral embolism caused by marantic endocarditis and cancer. *Arch Neurol* 33:260, 1976.

44. Min K, Gyorkey F, Sata C: Mucin-producing adenocarcinomas and nonbacterial thrombotic endocarditis: Pathogenetic role of tumor mucin. *Cancer* 45:2374, 1980.

189. *The Guillain-Barré Syndrome*

David A. Chad

Introduction

The Guillain-Barré syndrome (GBS) is an acute inflammatory-demyelinating polyradiculoneuropathy—affecting nerve roots and cranial and peripheral nerves—of unknown cause that occurs at all ages. It was described by Guillain, Barré, and Strohl in 1916 [1] as an acute, flaccid paralysis with areflexia and elevated spinal fluid protein without pleocytosis. Today it is the most common cause of rapidly progressive weakness, with an annual incidence of 0.6 to 2.0 cases per 100,000 population [2]. Over the years it has become clear that the condition may be fatal because of respiratory failure and autonomic nervous system abnormalities [3]. It is therefore recognized as a potential medical and neurologic emergency that may require the use of intensive care units experienced in handling the complications of the illness [4].

Pathogenesis

Guillain-Barré syndrome is thought to be produced by immunologically mediated demyelination of the peripheral nervous system [3]. It is likely that both humoral and cellular components of the immune system participate in macrophage-induced peripheral nerve demyelination [2]; however, the exact antigens to which the immune system response is directed have not been identified [3,4]. While P-2 and galactocerebroside—constituents of peripheral nerve myelin—produce an experimental model of GBS-like inflammatory neuropathy in rats and rabbits, only a few GBS patients have detectable antibody to these antigens [5]. In some patients, especially those with severe, acute GBS, there is evidence that the target antigen is a ganglioside [5].

Support for the idea of an immunologic pathogenesis comes from the work of Waksman and Adams in 1959 [6], who described an animal model similar to GBS called experimental allergic neuritis (EAN). They noted that inoculation of rabbits with peripheral nerve antigen and Freund's adjuvant led to symmetric ataxic paralysis of the extremities within about 2 weeks. The disease could be passively transferred with white blood cells (T cells) of affected animals but not with their sera, suggesting a greater role for cell-mediated than for humoral-mediated immunity. Indeed, elevated levels of soluble IL-2 receptors are found in the circulation of GBS patients, providing evidence for T cell activation [7]. Nonetheless, considerable evidence has accrued for an equally important role for the humoral arm of the immune response: Saida et al. [8] demonstrated that intraneural injections of sera from EAN animals produced demyelination; Feasby et al. [9] obtained similar results using sera from GBS patients. Complement-fixing antibodies to peripheral nerve myelin can be detected in the sera of GBS patients when neurologic symptoms first occur, and clearance of these antibodies from the sera correlates well with improvement in clinical status [10]. Last, dramatic improvement in GBS following plasmapheresis further supports a major role for humoral factors [11].

Diagnosis

OVERVIEW. Guillain-Barré syndrome often occurs 2 to 4 weeks after a flulike or diarrheal illness caused by a variety of infectious agents [3], including cytomegalovirus, Epstein-Barr and herpes simplex viruses, mycoplasma, chlamydia, and *Campylobacter jejuni* [12]. It can also be an early manifestation of human immunodeficiency virus (HIV) infection before the development of an immunosuppressed state [13]. Lyme disease may rarely produce a syndrome of polyradiculopathy reminiscent of GBS [14]. Other antecedent events include immunization [3], general surgery [15], and renal transplantation [16]. Guillain-Barré syndrome is also seen in patients with conditions associated with suppression of the immune system, such as Hodgkin's disease [17] and lupus erythematosus [3].

The illness is heralded by the presence of dysesthesias of the feet or hands or both. The major feature is weakness that evolves rapidly (usually over days) and classically has been described as ascending from legs to arms and, in severe cases, to respiratory and bulbar muscles [18]. Approximately 50 percent of patients reach the nadir of their clinical course by 2 weeks into the illness, 80 percent by 3 weeks, and 90 percent by 1 month [19]. In a variant of GBS, weakness progresses beyond 1 month, sometimes for 6 to 8 weeks [19]. An inflammatory demyelinating polyradiculoneuropathy (IDP) progressing beyond 2 months is designated chronic IDP (CIDP), a disorder with a natural history different from GBS. A small percentage of patients (2–5%) have recurrent GBS [20].

The extent and distribution of weakness in GBS are variable. Within a few days a patient can become quadriparetic and respirator-dependent, or the illness can take a benign course and after progression for 3 weeks produce only mild weakness of the face and limbs.

PHYSICAL FINDINGS. In a typical case of moderate severity, the physical examination discloses symmetric weakness in both proximal and distal muscle groups associated with attenuation or loss of deep tendon reflexes. In the early stage of illness, there is no muscle wasting or fasciculation. (If the attack is particularly severe and axons are interrupted, then after a number of months muscles undergo atrophy and scattered fasciculations may be seen [vide infra]). Sensory loss is usually mild, although a variant of GBS is described in which sensory loss (involving large fiber modalities) is widespread, symmetric, and profound [19]. Respiratory muscles are often involved; 10 and 25 percent of patients require ventilator assistance [21] initiated within 18 days (mean of 10 days) after onset [22]. *Need for a ventilator cannot be predicted on the basis of extent of weakness; therefore patients must be followed carefully with serial vital capacity measurements* until weakness has stopped progressing, so the respiratory insufficiency can be anticipated and managed appropriately.

There is often mild to moderate bilateral facial weakness. Mild weakness of tongue muscles and the muscles of deglutition can also develop. Ophthalmoparesis from extraocular motor nerve involvement is unusual in the typical patient with GBS. However, in the Miller Fisher variant [23], there is ophthalmoplegia in combination with ataxia and areflexia, with little limb weakness per se. Pupillary abnormalities have been noted in GBS [24] and in the Miller Fisher variant [25], presumably a consequence of postganglionic parasympathetic and sympathetic nerve involvement. Papilledema (with raised intracranial pressure) is exceedingly rare [26]; it could be related to abnormalities in the absorption of CSF through the arachnoid granulations.

Disturbances of the autonomic nervous system are found in 50 percent of patients and are potentially lethal [3,4]. Autonomic dysfunction takes the form of either excessive or inadequate activity of the sympathetic nervous system or the parasympathetic nervous system, or both [27]. Common findings include cardiac arrhythmias (persistent sinus tachycardia, bradycardia, ventricular tachycardia, atrial flutter, atrial fibrillation, and asystole), orthostatic hypotension, and transient and persistent hypertension. Other changes include transient bladder paralysis, increased or decreased sweating, and paralytic ileus. These changes are not completely understood but may be due to inflammation of the thinly myelinated and unmyelinated axons of the peripheral autonomic nervous system. Young et al. [28] described a neuropathy affecting the peripheral autonomic nervous system exclusively that may have a pathogenesis similar to that of GBS.

LABORATORY FEATURES. The most characteristic laboratory features of GBS are an abnormal CSF profile showing albuminocytologic dissociation (elevated protein without pleocytosis); nerve conduction abnormalities consisting of reduced nerve conduction velocities, prolongation of distal latencies and late responses; and, in the rare instances in which it is obtained, a nerve (sural) biopsy disclosing inflammation-demyelination.

Cerebrospinal fluid examination is most helpful in reaching the diagnosis of GBS. Although the CSF profile is almost always normal within the first 48 hours after onset [19], by 1 week into the illness the CSF protein is elevated in most patients, sometimes to levels as high as 1 gm per deciliter. Rarely, even several weeks after onset of GBS, the CSF protein remains normal and the diagnosis must rest on the presence of otherwise typical clinical features [19]. The cell count may be slightly increased but rarely exceeds 10 cells per cubic millimeter; the cells are mononuclear in nature. When GBS occurs as a manifestation of HIV infection or Lyme disease, the CSF white cell count is generally increased (25–50 cells). Except when there is papilledema, the opening pressure is normal. The CSF glucose is always normal.

Electrodiagnostic studies typically disclose slowing (< 80% of normal) of nerve conduction velocity, most often along proximal nerve segments, with increases in distal motor and sensory latencies [19,29]. The amplitude of the evoked motor response may be reduced (because of axon loss or nerve conduction block), and the response is frequently dispersed because of differential slowing along still-conducting axons [19,29]. At times, because the pathologic process may be maximum and even restricted to spinal nerve roots and proximal nerve segments, routine nerve conduction studies are normal. However, in such cases F responses are usually prolonged because of involvement of the most proximal segments of the motor fibers. Early in the course of GBS, electromyography (EMG) may demonstrate only decreased numbers of motor units firing on voluntary effort because of nerve conduction block. Several weeks later, active denervation changes, such as fibrillation potentials and positive sharp waves, may be seen if there has been axon loss. In some patients with especially severe forms of GBS, both motor and sensory nerves are electrically inexcitable, strongly suggestive of primary axonal degeneration rather than axonal degeneration following demyelination [30]. Another disorder that produces electrodiagnostic studies indicative of an acute motor axonal neuropathy occurs in China during the summer months among children and young adults, most of whom reside in rural areas [31].

Except for a mild increase in the erythrocyte sedimentation rate, hematologic studies are normal. Serum electrolytes may disclose hyponatremia [3], sometimes to a marked degree, because of inappropriate secretion of antidiuretic hormone caused by a disturbance of peripheral volume receptors. There may be evidence of previous viral or *Mycoplasma* infection, such as lymphopenia or atypical lymphocytes. In some cases, evidence of recent viral infection may be sought by measuring antibody (IgM) titers against specific infectious agents, especially cytomegalovirus (CMV) and Epstein-Barr virus. In selected cases, screening for HIV infection should be undertaken.

PATHOLOGY. Pathologic studies of nerves in patients dying with GBS have usually shown infiltration of the endoneurium by mononuclear cells, with a tendency to distribution in a perivenular distribution [32]. The inflammatory process occurs throughout the length of the nerve, from its origin at a root level to the distal ramifications of nerve twigs in the substance of muscle fibers. The brunt of the inflammatory process, however, occurs at more proximal levels (roots, spinal nerves, and major plexuses) and takes the form of discrete foci of inflammation. The pathologic process affecting individual nerve fibers is primarily demyelinating, and electron micrographs show macrophages stripping normal myelin from axons [3]. Axonal degeneration is found, however, in some cases [32]. Patients with axon loss are least likely to recover fully and may be left with functionally significant residual motor weakness.

Differential Diagnosis

A number of well-defined conditions cause an acute or subacute onset of generalized weakness and must be differentiated

Table 189-1. Conditions that May Mimic Guillain-Barré Syndrome

Disorder	Major distinguishing features
Myasthenia gravis	Reflexes are spared Ocular weakness predominates Positive response to edrophonium EMG: decremental motor response
Botulism	Predominant bulbar involvement Autonomic abnormalities EMG: normal velocities, low amplitudes
Tick paralysis	Weakness and prominent sensory loss Tick present
Shellfish poisoning	Rapid onset—face, finger, toe numbness Follows consumption of mussels/clams
Toxic neuropathies	EMG: usually axon loss
Organophosphorus toxicity	Acute cholinergic reaction
Porphyric neuropathy	Mental disturbance Abdominal pain
Diphtheritic neuropathy	Prior pharyngitis Myocarditis
Poliomyelitis	Weakness, pain and tenderness Preserved sensation CSF: protein *and* cell count elevated
Periodic paralysis	Reflexes normal Cranial nerves and respiration spared Abnormal serum [K]
Critical illness neuropathy	Sepsis and multi-organ failure >2 wk EMG: axon loss
Pancuronium-related	Tetraparesis and areflexia Follows prolonged Rx with pancuronium Trauma-associated
Status asthmaticus-related	Clinical and EMG features of myopathy

CSF = cerebrospinal fluid; EMG = electromyelogram

from GBS (Table 189-1). These are disorders of the neuromuscular junction (myasthenia gravis and botulism), disorders of peripheral nerve (tick paralysis, shellfish poisoning, toxic neuropathy, acute intermittent porphyria, and diphtheritic neuropathy), motor neuron disorders (amyotrophic lateral sclerosis and poliomyelitis), and disorders of muscle (periodic paralysis, metabolic myopathies, and inflammatory myopathies). There are a number of less well understood conditions characterized by severe generalized weakness that are defined by the setting in which they are encountered—the ICU. They include critical illness polyneuropathy and the weakness associated with pancuronium and with status asthmaticus—conditions that may be toxic in nature and affect both nerve and muscle (neuromyopathies).

DISORDERS OF THE NEUROMUSCULAR JUNCTION. Although myasthenia gravis can cause limb weakness, it is almost always associated with weakness of cranial nerve-supplied muscles, most notably the ocular muscles (see Chap. 190). In this disorder, limb weakness tends to have a proximal predominance and is usually mild. Muscular fatigability is a hallmark of the disease. Weakness often improves after intravenous administration of a short-acting anticholinesterase (edrophonium). Reflexes are preserved and there is no sensory abnormality. A helpful laboratory clue to diagnosis is the electrodiagnostic finding that the muscle action potential shows a decremental response to repetitive stimulation at low rates (2–3 Hz) [33]. Botulism can also cause acute weakness 6 to 36 hours after ingestion of the toxin formed by *Clostridium botulinum*. The condition is characterized by weakness of cranial nerve-innervated muscles and autonomic abnormalities, such as unreactive pupils and ileus. Weakness may involve respiratory muscles, leading to the need for ventilator assistance. Electrodiagnostic testing shows low motor amplitudes that decline with repetitive stimulation at a slow rate. Some facilitation of muscle response occurs after the muscle has been briefly exercised [33].

DISORDERS OF PERIPHERAL NERVE. Tick paralysis is produced by a toxin contained in the head of the tick *Dermacentor andersoni* or *vanabilis*, which blocks nerve conduction in the fine terminal portions of both motor and sensory nerves. Weakness associated with sensory impairment develops rapidly after the tick has embedded itself in the victim, usually over 1 to 2 days. Shellfish poisoning gives rise to symptoms immediately after contaminated mussels and clams are eaten. Patients complain of face, finger, and toe numbness and then note the development of rapidly progressive descending paralysis, which may involve respiratory muscles. Toxic neuropathies can be caused by a number of heavy metals, including arsenic, thallium, and lead. These and other potential neurotoxins (e.g., the bacteriostatic agent nitrofurantoin) and industrial agents (e.g., the hexocarbons) may produce a rapidly evolving peripheral neuropathy. The majority of acute toxic neuropathies are axon loss neuropathies, but in the case of arsenic poisoning electrodiagnostic features may suggest a demyelinating neuropathy identical to GBS [34]. Organophosphorus insecticide toxicity causes a short-lived acute cholinergic phase marked by miosis, salivation, sweating, and fasciculation followed in 2 to 3 weeks by an acute axon loss polyneuropathy [35]. An intermediate syndrome occurring 24 to 96 hours after the cholinergic phase and characterized by multiple cranial nerve palsies and respiratory failure has also been described [36]. The latter is probably a result of a defect at the neuromuscular junction. Acute intermittent porphyria causes an acute polyneuropathy clinically similar to GBS but differing by its association with mental disturbance and abdominal pain. Attacks of paralysis are precipitated by ingestion of a variety of drugs, including alcohol, barbiturates, estrogens, phenytoin, and sulfonamides. The diagnosis can be established by demonstrating increased levels of porphobilinogen and delta-aminolevulinic acid in the urine. Diphtheritic neuropathy occurs 2 to 8 weeks after a throat infection. During the height of the infection there is numbness of the lips and paralysis of pharyngeal and laryngeal muscles. At the time of the neuropathy, diphtheria organisms may be cultured from the throat. Other clues to the diagnosis are clinical and electrocardiographic features of myocarditis.

DISORDERS OF MOTOR NEURONS. Amyotrophic lateral sclerosis (ALS) is a rare cause of acute weakness. Patients can present with weakness of the bulbar musculature or rapid development of profound respiratory muscle weakness, leading to a need for ventilator assistance. Amyotrophic lateral sclerosis is distinguished from GBS by its usually much slower onset (months) and increased reflex activity, absence of sensory abnormalities, and normal CSF studies. Poliomyelitis is now rare, but it can be associated with weakness of rapid onset and severe muscle pain and tenderness. Respiratory muscles are often involved. Deep tendon reflexes are depressed. The illness is distinguished from GBS by preservation of sensation and an increase of both cells and protein in the CSF. Antibody studies may help identify the illness.

DISORDERS OF MUSCLES. Periodic paralysis (hyperkalemic or hypokalemic) is a disorder of muscle usually inherited in an autosomal dominant fashion. Patients develop generalized weakness over a period of hours. Cranial nerve-supplied muscles are spared, there is generally no respiratory muscle involvement, reflexes are normal, and there is no sensory involvement. Serum potassium measurements aid in the diagnosis. Metabolic myopathies can present with the sudden onset of muscle weakness. Patients with abnormalities of glycogen metabolism (e.g., phosphorylase deficiency and phosphofructokinase deficiency) can develop weakness associated with severe cramps and muscle fiber necrosis; the latter may result in muscle serum enzyme (creatine kinase) elevations and myoglobinuria. Patients with disturbed lipid metabolism (carnitine palmityl transferase deficiency) can develop a similar syndrome. Dermatomyositis, an inflammatory myopathy, can present with the acute onset of proximal muscle (and, rarely, respiratory muscle) weakness. In contrast to GBS, in dermatomyositis reflexes are spared, cranial nerves are rarely involved, and serum creatine kinase is elevated.

ICU-RELATED WEAKNESS. Critical illness polyneuropathy [37] is present in at least 50 percent of patients who have been septic and critically ill with multiorgan system failure longer than 2 weeks. It is characterized by difficulty in weaning from the ventilator, distal greater than proximal muscle weakness, and reduced or absent reflexes. The electrophysiologic findings are distinct from GBS because they show features of axon loss and not of demyelination. Most patients recover over weeks to months after appropriate treatment of the underlying sepsis or critical illness has begun. Pancuronium-associated neuromyopathy is associated with tetraparesis and areflexia after prolonged treatment with pancuronium (>6 days) and a few days of methylprednisolone (50–75 mg/day) [38]. Most patients are trauma victims. In some patients electrodiagnostic studies and muscle biopsies point strongly toward a neurogenic disorder, while in others a myopathic process is evident. The cause is uncertain—prolonged paralysis has been proposed as one possibility, although therapeutic agents toxic to muscle and nerve could be partly responsible. Tumor necrosis factor may also play a role [39]. Status asthmaticus-associated neuromyopathy is characterized by the acute onset of weakness during the treatment of status asthmaticus [40]. Weakness is moderate to severe in degree and often widely distributed, involving the respiratory muscles on occasion. Electrodiagnostic and histologic studies suggest that the disorder is primarily myopathic in nature, but a neuropathic component has been identified in some patients. We believe the combination of high-dose IV corticosteroids, paralytic agents, and drugs such as aminophylline and antibiotics, all used in critically ill asthmatics, exerts a reversible toxic effect on muscle and nerve [40].

Natural History and Prognostic Factors

The natural history of GBS in the moderately to severely affected patient (a patient who is unable to walk or who has severe respiratory muscle weakness requiring a ventilator) is one of gradual improvement. The ability to walk unassisted returns, on average, in about 3 months; in the subset of respirator-dependent patients the average time to recovery is 6 months [41]. Four factors correlate with poor outcome: a mean distal motor amplitude of less than 20 percent of normal; age greater than 60 years; the need for ventilator support; and severe, rapidly progressive disease [42]. Among these factors, the most powerful predictor of poor outcome is severe reduction in mean distal motor amplitude [43].

Management

The three major treatment issues in the GBS are controlling respiration and deciding when to intubate the patient; recognizing and managing autonomic dysfunction; and determining which patients are candidates for plasmapheresis.

Patients with GBS require excellent nursing care, medical management, and emotional support. Respiratory failure is one of the most serious complications of GBS; therefore around-the-clock measurements of maximum inspiratory pressure and forced vital capacity (VC) (Fig. 189-1) are necessary to recognize and manage appropriately respiratory muscle weakness. A normal forced vital capacity is 65 ml per kilogram; a level of 30 ml per kilogram is generally associated with a poor forced cough and requires careful observation and management with

supplemental oxygen and chest physical therapy. At 25 ml per kilogram, the sigh mechanism is compromised and atelectasis occurs, leading to hypoxemia. Ropper and Kehne [44] suggest intubation if any one of the following criteria are met: mechanical ventilatory failure with reduced expiratory VC of 12 to 15 ml per kilogram; oropharyngeal paresis with aspiration; falling VC over 4 to 6 hours; or clinical signs of respiratory fatigue at a VC of 15 ml per kilogram. Intubation should be accomplished with a soft cuff, low-pressure endotracheal tube. A decision to delay tracheostomy for 7 to 10 days is likely to avoid the operation in as many as one-third of patients who improve rapidly and can be extubated after the first few days [44]. Complications of intubation and ventilator assistance are described in other chapters.

The nursing and medical team must also be aware of the many autonomic nervous system disturbances that can occur [27]. Fluctuating blood pressure with transient hypertensive episodes sometimes associated with extreme degrees of agitation may be present. Other manifestations of sympathetic nervous system overactivity include sudden diaphoresis and general vasoconstriction, as well as sinus tachycardia. Evidence of underactivity of the sympathetic nervous system includes presence of marked postural hypotension and heightened sensitivity to dehydration and sedative-hypnotic agents. Excessive parasympathetic nervous system activity is reflected in facial flushing associated with a feeling of generalized warmth and bradycardia. Electrocardiographic changes, consisting of S–T and T wave changes, also occur. Therefore, careful monitoring of blood pressure, fluid status, and cardiac rhythm is absolutely essential to manage the GBS patient. Hypertension may be managed with short-acting alpha-adrenergic blocking agents, hypotension with fluids, and bradyarrhythmias with atropine

Fig. 189-1. Relations between vital capacity (VC), pathophysiology of lung function, and suggested therapy in mechanical ventilatory failure. (From Ropper AH: Guillain-Barré syndrome, in Ropper AH, Kennedy SK, Zervas NT (eds): *Neurological and Neurosurgical Intensive Care.* Baltimore, University Park Press, 1983. With permission.)

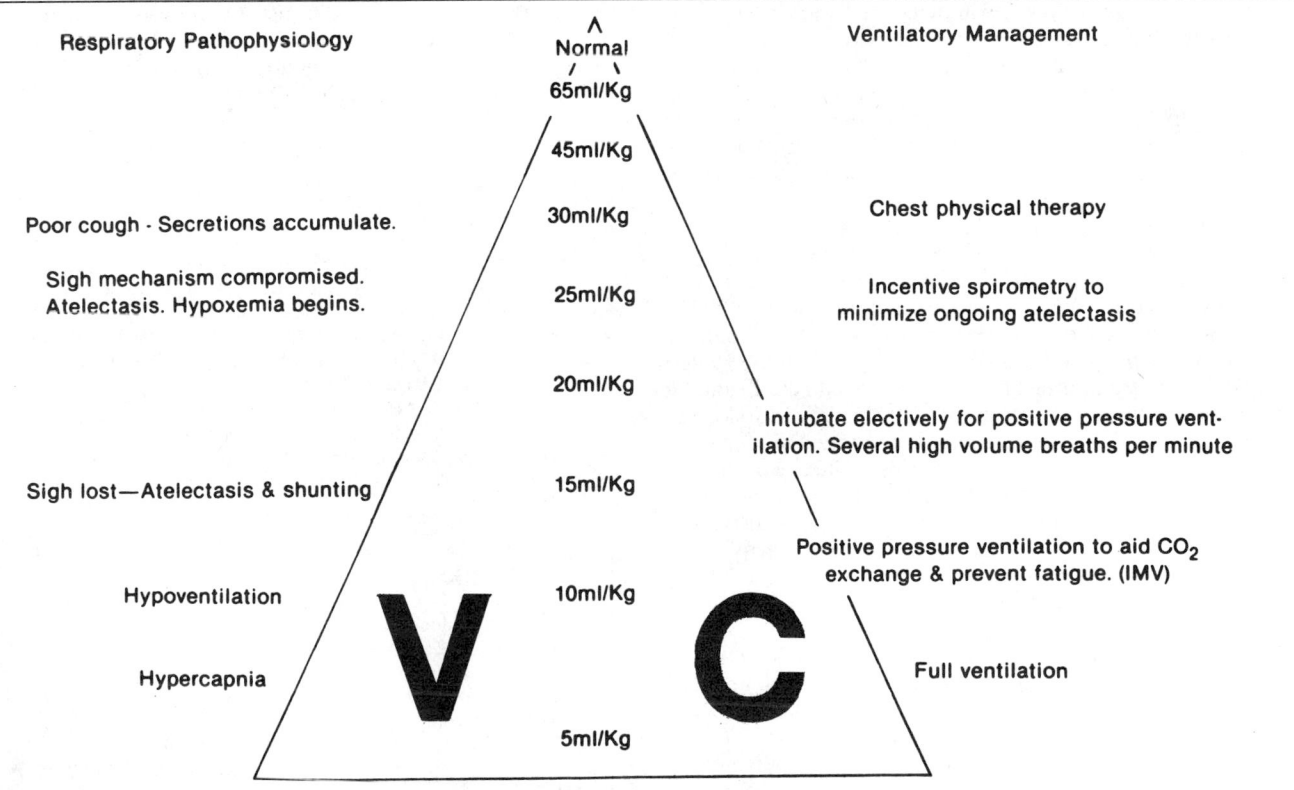

Respiratory Pathophysiology		Ventilatory Management
	∧ Normal ∕ ∖ 65ml/Kg	
	45ml/Kg	
Poor cough - Secretions accumulate.	30ml/Kg	Chest physical therapy
Sigh mechanism compromised. Atelectasis. Hypoxemia begins.	25ml/Kg	Incentive spirometry to minimize ongoing atelectasis
	20ml/Kg	
Sigh lost—Atelectasis & shunting	15ml/Kg	Intubate electively for positive pressure ventilation. Several high volume breaths per minute
Hypoventilation	10ml/Kg	Positive pressure ventilation to aid CO_2 exchange & prevent fatigue. (IMV)
Hypercapnia		Full ventilation
	5ml/Kg	

[27]. As noted earlier, hyponatremia may occur and is probably best managed by fluid restriction.

The bedridden patient needs to be turned frequently to avoid the development of pressure sores. Paralyzed limbs require the attention of the physiotherapist so that passive limb movements can be carried out and contractures prevented. The team needs to be aware of the potential for development of compression neuropathies (most commonly of the ulnar and peroneal nerves), and insulating pads may need to be placed over the usual susceptible sites (the elbow and the head of the fibula). Pain is sometimes severe but may respond to quinine sulfate [45]. When pain is disabling, epidural morphine may be necessary [46]. Deep venous thrombosis and pulmonary embolism are ever-present dangers in the bedridden patient with immobilized limbs; for these patients, in addition to physical therapy, subcutaneous heparin (5000 units twice per day) is recommended.

The use of corticosteroids in the management of GBS has been somewhat controversial (see Hughes et al. [21]); today they have no place in the treatment plan. Ongoing studies may establish a role for these agents in the future.

A number of multicenter studies [11,41,47] have shown that plasmapheresis has a beneficial effect on the course of the illness, even in patients with several poor prognostic signs [42]. Patients treated with plasmapheresis are able to walk, on average, 1 month earlier than untreated patients; respirator-dependent patients so treated walk 3 months sooner than those who do not receive plasma exchange [42]. Plasmapheresis is recommended for patients who reach or are approaching inability to walk unaided, who require intubation or demonstrate a falling vital capacity, and who have weakness of the bulbar musculature leading to dysphagia and aspiration [48]. In a small number of patients (approximately 5%), spontaneous relapse occurs within days to weeks after improvement; a second course of plasmapheresis appears to benefit these patients [49]. Plasmapheresis is safe in pregnant women and children [4]. The GBS study group guidelines recommend exchanging 200 to 250 ml of plasma per kilogram body weight over 7 to 14 days in four to six treatments [41]. Plasmanate or 5% salt-poor albumin is used as replacement fluid (fresh frozen plasma should be avoided). Plasmapheresis is generally not employed in mildly affected patients who are still ambulatory or patients who are no longer progressing 21 days or more after the onset of GBS.

There has been a growing interest in the use of human immune globulin (HIG) for the treatment of GBS. Early studies were promising [50,51], and a large randomized trial performed by Dutch investigators [52] concluded that treatment with HIG was at least as effective as plasmapheresis and might be superior. Following that study, however, two groups in the United States [53,54] presented results of uncontrolled HIG treatment in which more than half of patients (59%) relapsed following therapy, compared to a relapse rate of no more than 5 percent among large numbers of plasmapheresis-treated patients [55]. At present, HIG might be considered for patients in whom IV access is problematic or in settings where plasmapheresis is not possible, but until further studies comparing plasmapheresis and HIG are done plasmapheresis remains the immunotherapy of first choice in the treatment of the severely affected GBS patient.

Finally, it is most important to address the emotional needs of the patient with GBS, who will almost certainly be anxious, fearful, and depressed. We point out the strong likelihood of a good outcome (see below) even in ventilated patients. Sometimes it is helpful for the patient to speak with a person who has recovered from GBS.

Outcome

In most patients recovery occurs over weeks or months, but in some patients muscle strength may take 1.5 to 2 years to reach its best state with an intensive rehabilitation program [2]. Recovery is not always complete, with only about 15 percent of patients resolving with no residual deficits [4]. Another 50 to 65 percent of patients are restored to nearly normal function and can resume their work and leisure activities, although some degree of ankle dorsiflexor weakness or numbness of the feet is commonly encountered. Many patients never regain normal stretch reflexes. Severe residual motor weakness or major proprioceptive loss that seriously impairs walking occurs in about 10 percent of patients. Patients requiring the longest time to recover and those with severe residual motor and sensory deficits tend to have had impressive EMG evidence of axon loss [56]. Inability to walk unassisted at 12 to 18 months after onset of GBS is associated with permanent severe leg weakness [57]. Despite close monitoring in the ICU, deaths from GBS do occur, with mortality in the range of 3 to 8 percent [4]. Causes of fatal outcomes include dysautonomia, sepsis, acute respiratory distress syndrome, and pulmonary emboli [4].

Conclusion

Careful attention to the patient's history and thorough examination usually point to the diagnosis of GBS. A variety of conditions of the motor unit need to be considered in the differential diagnosis, but these can usually be excluded and the diagnosis of GBS established with selected laboratory studies. The challenge is the management of GBS. The mainstay of treatment is excellent nursing and medical care with close attention to respiratory and autonomic function. Most patients with GBS recover nicely, and plasmapheresis can enhance recovery. While we still have much to learn about the pathogenesis of GBS, it stands as an eminently manageable neuropathy with an excellent prognosis for recovery.

References

1. Guillain G, Barré JA, Strohl A: Sur un syndrome de radiculo-nevrite avec hyperalbuminose du liquide cephalo-rachidien sans reaction cellulaire: Remarques sur les characteres cliniques et graphiques des relexes tendineux. *Bull Mem Soc Med Hop Paris* 40:1462, 1916.
2. Ropper AH, Wijdicks EFM, Truax BT: Guillain-Barré syndrome. Philadelphia, FA Davis, 1991.
3. Arnason BGW: Acute inflammatory demyelinating polyradiculoneuropathy, in Dyck PJ, Thomas PK, Griffin JW, et al (eds): *Peripheral Neuropathy.* Philadelphia, WB Saunders, 1993, p 1437.
4. Ropper AH. The Guillain-Barré syndrome. *N Engl J Med* 326:1130, 1992.
5. Yuki N, Yamada M, Sato S, et al: Association of IgG anti-GD1a antibody with severe Guillain-Barré syndrome. *Muscle Nerve* 16:642, 1993.
6. Waksman BH, Adams RD: Allergic neuritis: Experimental disease of rabbits induced by peripheral nervous tissue and adjuvants. *J Exp Med* 102:213, 1955.
7. Hartung HP, Hughes RAC, Taylor WA, et al: T-cell activation in Guillain-Barré syndrome and in MS: Elevated serum levels of soluble IL-2 receptors. *Neurology* 40:215, 1990.
8. Saida T, Saida K, Silberberg DH, et al: Transfer of demyelination by intraneural injection of experimental allergic neuritis serum. *Nature* 272:639, 1978.

9. Feasby TE, Hahn AF, Gilbert JJ: Passive transfer of demyelinating activity in Guillain-Barré polyneuropathy. *Neurology* 30:362, 1980.

10. Koski CL, Gratz E, Sutherland J, Mayer RF: Clinical correlation with anti-peripheral-nerve myelin antibodies in Guillain-Barré syndrome. *Ann Neurol* 19:573, 1986.

11. Dyck PJ, Kurtzke JF: Plasmapheresis in Guillain-Barré syndrome. *Neurology* 35:1105, 1985.

12. Ropper AH: Campylobacter diarrhea and Guillain-Barré syndrome. *Arch Neurol* 45:655, 1988.

13. Cornblath DR, McArthur JC, Kennedy PGE, et al: Inflammatory demyelinating peripheral neuropathies associated with human T-cell lymphotropic virus type III infection. *Ann Neurol* 21:32, 1987.

14. Pachner AR, Steere AC: The triad of neurologic manifestations of Lyme disease: Meningitis, cranial neuritis, and radiculoneuritis. *Neurology* 35:47, 1985.

15. Arnason BG, Asbury AK: Idiopathic polyneuritis after surgery. *Arch Neurol* 18:500, 1968.

16. Drachman DA, Patterson PY, Berlin BS, Roguska I: Immunosuppression and the Guillain-Barré syndrome. *Arch Neurol* 23:385, 1970.

17. Lisak RP, Mitchell M, Zweiman B, et al: Guillain-Barré syndrome and Hodgkin's disease: Three cases with immunological studies. *Ann Neurol* 1:72, 1977.

18. Osler LD, Sidell AD: The Guillain-Barré syndrome: The need for exact diagnostic criteria. *N Engl J Med* 262:964, 1960.

19. Asbury AK, Cornblath DR: Assessment of current diagnostic criteria for Guillain-Barré syndrome. *Ann Neurol* 27(suppl):S21, 1990.

20. Grand'Maison F, Feasby TE, Hahn AF, Koopman WJ: Recurrent Guillain-Barré syndrome: Clinical and laboratory features. *Brain* 115:1093, 1992.

21. Hughes RAC, Radlubowski M, Hufschmidt A: Treatment of acute inflammatory polyneuropathy. *Ann Neurol* 9(suppl):70, 1981.

22. Andersonn T, Siden A: A clinical study of the Guillain-Barré syndrome. *Acta Neurol Scand* 66:316, 1982.

23. Fisher CM: Unusual variant of acute idiopathic polyneuritis (syndrome of ophthalmoplegia, ataxia and areflexia). *N Engl J Med* 255:57, 1956.

24. Williams D, Brust JCM, Abrams G, et al: Landry-Guillain-Barré syndrome with abnormal pupils and normal eye movements: A case report. *Neurology* 29:1033, 1979.

25. Keane JR: Tonic pupils with acute ophthalmoplegic polyneuritis. *Ann Neurol* 2:93, 1977.

26. Sullivan RL, Reeves AG: Normal cerebrospinal fluid proteins, increased intracranial pressure, and the Guillain-Barré syndrome. *Ann Neurol* 1:108, 1977.

27. Lichtenfeld P: Autonomic dysfunction in the Guillain-Barré syndrome. *Am J Med* 50:772, 1971.

28. Young RR, Asbury AK, Corbett JL, Adams RD: Pure pan-dysautonomia with recovery: Description and discussion of diagnostic criteria. *Brain* 98:613, 1975.

29. Albers JW: AAEM Case report #4: Guillain-Barré syndrome. *Muscle Nerve* 12:705, 1989.

30. Feasby TE, Gilbert JJ, Brown WF, et al: An acute axonal form of Guillain-Barré polyneuropathy. *Brain* 109:1115, 1986.

31. McKhann GM, Cornblath DR, Griffin JW, et al: Acute motor axonal neuropathy: A frequent cause of acute flaccid paralysis in China. *Neurology* 33:333, 1993.

32. Asbury AK, Arnason BG, Adams RD: The inflammatory lesion in idiopathic polyneuritis: Its role in pathogenesis. *Medicine* 489:173, 1969.

33. Kimura J: *Electrodiagnosis in Diseases of Nerve and Muscle: Principles and Practice*. Philadelphia, FA Davis, 1983, p 511.

34. Donofrio PD, Wilbourn AJ, Albers JW, et al: Acute arsenic intoxication presenting as Guillain-Barré syndrome. *Muscle Nerve* 10:114, 1987.

35. Senanayake N, Johnson MK: Acute polyneuropathy after poisoning by a new organophosphate insecticide. *N Engl J Med* 306:155, 1982.

36. Senanayake N, Karalliedde L: Neurotoxic effects of organophosphorus insecticides: An intermediate syndrome. *N Engl J Med* 316:761, 1987.

37. Zochodne DW, Bolton CF, Wells GA, et al: Critical illness polyneuropathy: A complication of sepsis and multiple organ failure. *Brain* 110:819, 1987.

38. Op de Coul AAW, Lambregts PC, Koeman J, et al: Neuromuscular complications in patients given Pavulon (pancuronium bromide) during artificial ventilation. *Clin Neurol Neurosurg* 87:17, 1985.

39. Op de Coul AAW, Verheul GA, Leyten ACM, et al: Critical illness polyneuropathy after artificial ventilation. *Clin Neurol Neurosurg* 93:27, 1991.

40. Lacomis D, Smith TW, Chad DA: Acute myopathy and neuropathy in status asthmaticus: Case report and literature review. *Muscle Nerve* 16:84, 1993.

41. The Guillain-Barré Syndrome Study Group: Plasmapheresis and acute Guillain-Barré syndrome. *Neurology* 35:1096, 1985.

42. McKhann GM, Griffin JW, Cornblath DR, et al and the Guillain-Barré Syndrome Study Group: Plasmapheresis and Guillain-Barré syndrome: Analysis of prognostic factors and the effect of plasmapheresis. *Ann Neurol* 23:347, 1988.

43. Cornblath DR, Mellits ED, Griffin JW, et al: Motor conduction studies in Guillain-Barré syndrome: Description and prognostic value. *Ann Neurol* 23:354, 1988.

44. Ropper AH, Kehne SM: Guillain-Barré syndrome: Management of respiratory failure. *Neurology* 35:1662, 1985.

45. Nixon RA: Quinine sulfate for pain in the Guillain-Barré syndrome. *Ann Neurol* 4:386, 1978.

46. Rosenfeld B, Borel C, Henley D: Epidural morphine treatment of pain in the Guillain-Barré syndrome. *Arch Neurol* 43:1194, 1986.

47. French Cooperative Group on Plasma Exchange in Guillain-Barré Syndrome: Efficiency of plasma exchange in Guillain-Barré syndrome: Role of replacement fluids. *Ann Neurol* 22:753, 1987.

48. McKhann GM, Griffin JW: Plasmapheresis and the Guillain-Barré syndrome. *Ann Neurol* 22:762, 1987.

49. Osterman PO, Fagius J, Safwenberg J, et al: Early relapses after plasma exchange in acute inflammatory polyradiculoneuropathy. *Lancet* 2:1161, 1986.

50. Kleyweg RP, van der Meche FGA, Meulstee J: Treatment of Guillain-Barré syndrome with high-dose gamma globulin. *Neurology* 38:1639, 1988.

51. Shahar E, Murphy EG, Roifman CM: Benefit of intravenously administered immune serum globulin in patients with Guillain-Barré syndrome. *J Pediatr* 116:141, 1990.

52. van der Meche FGA, Schmitz PIM, Dutch Guillain-Barré Study Group: A randomized trial comparing intravenous immune globulin and plasma exchange in Guillain-Barré syndrome. *N Engl J Med* 326:1123, 1992.

53. Irani DN, Cornblath DR, Chaudhry V, et al: Relapse in Guillain-Barré syndrome after treatment with human immune globulin. *Neurology* 43:872, 1993.

54. Castro LHM, Ropper AH: Human immune globulin infusion in Guillain-Barré syndrome: Worsening during and after treatment. *Neurology* 43:1034, 1993.

55. Bleck TB: IVIg for GBS: Potential problems in the alphabet soup. *Neurology* 43:857, 1993.

56. Eisen A, Humphreys P: The Guillain-Barré syndrome: A clinical and electrodiagnostic study of 25 cases. *Arch Neurol* 30:438, 1974.

57. Ropper AH: Severe acute Guillain-Barré syndrome. *Neurology* 36:429, 1986.

190. Myasthenia Gravis in the Intensive Care Unit

Randall R. Long

Few physicians have more than a passing acquaintance with myasthenia gravis, although it is by no means rare. The key to handling the emergent problems associated with myasthenia is simply the management of airway and ventilatory support with the same care as in any other instance of respiratory failure (see Chaps. 66 and 67). With respiration under control, the treatment of the underlying disease can be unhurried and orderly, and in the vast majority of patients is successful. This chapter reviews briefly the pathogenesis, clinical spectrum, and diagnosis of myasthenia gravis and focuses on the intensive care setting, including management of the patient in crisis and in the perioperative period.

Pathogenesis

Myasthenia gravis is an autoimmune disorder of neuromuscular transmission [1]. Circulating antibodies react with components of acetylcholine receptors within postsynaptic muscle membrane and may block receptors (i.e., interfere with normal receptor activation by acetylcholine) as well as accelerate receptor degradation. The result is fewer receptors that can be activated at affected neuromuscular junctions, causing weaker muscular contraction. Electrophysiologic study of myasthenic neuromuscular junctions discloses miniature end plate potentials that are normal in number but diminished in amplitude [2]. These observations have been clearly linked to the receptor alterations and an altered postsynaptic response to normal quantal transmitter release from the presynaptic nerve terminal. Understanding of this underlying pathophysiology has, in turn, enabled rational approaches to treatment. Various immunosuppressive therapies and acetylcholinesterase inhibitors are primary therapeutic options in managing myasthenia gravis (see below).

Epidemiology

Myasthenia gravis is not rare: Its prevalence in Western populations is approximately 1 in 20,000 [3]. The overall female-to-male ratio is about 3:2, although there are two distinct sex-specific incidence peaks, the incidence among women peaking in the third decade and that among men in the fifth to sixth decades. A mild familial predisposition has been noted, although Mendelian inheritance does not apply.

Clinical Spectrum

The clinical spectrum of myasthenia gravis is characterized as much by its diversity as it is by its common themes. It may range from a mild and relatively inconsequential disease over a normal lifetime, to a fulminant, incapacitating disorder. The course of given individuals may also vary widely. The clinical hallmarks of the disease are weakness and exaggerated muscle fatigue. The specific muscles involved and the severity of weakness are highly variable, both between individuals and within the same individual over time.

Ocular muscles are most frequently involved: diplopia is common, and various patterns of ophthalmoparesis are seen. Bulbar muscles are also frequently affected, leading to varying combinations of facial paresis, dysarthria, and dysphagia. Ptosis is common, but the pupils are never affected. Limb muscle involvement may vary from very isolated weakness to generalized weakness and fatigability. Respiratory muscle weakness is unfortunately not rare, and respiratory insufficiency as well as the inability to handle oral and upper airway secretions are the critical problems that bring myasthenics to the intensive care setting. Myasthenia should also be considered in any patient who cannot be weaned from ventilator support after an otherwise uncomplicated surgical procedure.

Approximately 15 to 20 percent of myasthenics have only ocular and eyelid involvement. Longitudinal studies indicate that if an individual manifests only oculomotor weakness for more than 2 years, there is little chance of later limb or respiratory weakness. Although several clinical classification schemes have been devised, categorizing myasthenics according to the distribution and severity of their disease, it is preferable to emphasize the fact that myasthenics often fluctuate over time, variability rather than constancy being the norm. Some factors contributing to fluctuations of strength are recognizable (see below); many fluctuations appear to be random occurrences.

Diagnostic Studies

The diagnosis of myasthenia gravis is clinically suggested in patients who present with chronic ocular, bulbar, or appendicular weakness, variable over time, with preservation of normal sensation and reflexes. More restricted presentations require a much broader differential diagnosis. Myasthenia gravis should always be considered in the differential diagnosis of isolated ocular or bulbar weakness. Again, prominent muscular fatigability and temporal fluctuation are key features of the disease. Normal pupils, normal sensation, and normal reflexes are to be expected and are helpful in diagnosing myasthenia gravis when coincident with an acute or subacute paralytic illness.

Once the diagnosis of myasthenia gravis is suggested, confirmation rests on the exclusion of other diseases and supporting clinical and laboratory studies. It is important to stress that, although abnormal tests may be diagnostic, normal test results do not exclude the diagnosis.

TENSILON TEST. Edrophonium hydrochloride (Tensilon) is a fast, short-acting parenteral cholinesterase inhibitor. It reaches peak effect within 1 minute after intravenous injection and persists to some extent for at least 10 minutes. Myasthenic weakness typically improves transiently after administration of 4 to 10 mg (0.4–1.0 cc). The Tensilon test may be blinded, either Tensilon or normal saline being injected. Whether drug or placebo, a 0.2-cc test dose is given to screen for excessive cholinergic side effects, such as cardiac arrhythmia, gastrointestinal hyperactivity, or diaphoresis. A "crash cart" should always be available, and patients with known cardiac disease and elderly patients warrant electrocardiographic monitoring. The remaining 0.8 cc is given after 1 minute. Interpretation of the test depends on identifying and observing a clear muscular deficit.

Ptosis and ophthalmoparesis, if present, are semiquantifiable and well suited; if respiratory compromise is present, monitoring maximum inspiratory pressure or vital capacity is useful. As a general rule, positive responses are dramatic; if there is any doubt about the positivity of the test, it should be considered negative. False positive Tensilon tests are quite rare; false negatives are common. In children, the appropriate test dose is 0.03 mg per kilogram, one fifth of which may be given as a test dose.

Neostigmine is a longer-acting parenteral cholinesterase inhibitor that sometimes effects a more obvious clinical response. It is also typically associated with more obvious autonomic side effects. The 1.5-mg test dose (0.04 mg/kg in children) should therefore be preceded by 0.5 mg of atropine; both may be given subcutaneously.

ANTIACETYLCHOLINE RECEPTOR ANTIBODIES.
Recognition of the immune nature of myasthenia gravis has provided a relatively sensitive and highly specific diagnostic study. Except for purely ocular myasthenia, where antibodies are often absent, approximately 85 percent of myasthenics have detectable serum antibodies, which bind to acetylcholine receptors [4]. The antibodies themselves constitute a heterogeneous group, reacting against various receptor subunits. Although the actual antibody titer is of little significance, correlating poorly with the severity of disease or clinical response to therapy, the presence of antibodies is a strong indication of the disease. A normal test does not exclude the diagnosis, especially in the patient presenting with predominantly ocular symptoms and signs. Myasthenics also have an increased incidence of other autoantibodies, including antithyroid antibodies, antiparietal cell antibodies, and antinuclear antibodies, although routine screening for these is not part of the diagnostic evaluation for suggested myasthenia gravis.

ELECTROMYOGRAPHIC STUDIES.
First described by Johns et al. in 1956 [5], the electromyographic hallmark of myasthenia gravis is a decrement in the amplitude of the muscle potential seen after exercise or slow repetitive nerve stimulation. The decrement should be at least 10 percent and preferably 15 percent or more. Routine motor and sensory conduction studies are normal, as is the conventional needle examination. The more severely affected patient is more likely to evidence a decremental response; responses are most consistently elicited from facial and proximal muscles. If a significant decrement is observed, edrophonium often transiently reverses the decrement. The protocol used is the same as that in conventional Tensilon testing. One can increase the sensitivity of repetitive stimulation with regional curare testing [6], although it is still not highly sensitive. Single-fiber electromyography is relatively sensitive, documenting increased "jitter" [7], variability in the temporal coupling of single fibers within the same motor unit.

Increased jitter, however, is far from specific, most peripheral neurogenic diseases also leading to increased jitter.

MUSCLE BIOPSY.
There are no specific findings on muscle biopsies from myasthenic patients. Muscle biopsy should be considered primarily when the differential diagnosis also includes either neurogenic or inflammatory processes.

MISCELLANEOUS STUDIES.
Myasthenia gravis may be associated with either malignant thymoma or thymic hyperplasia. Once a diagnosis is established, computed tomography of the chest should be obtained. Because there is also a significant association with thyroid and other autoimmune diseases, appropriate screening studies are indicated in the newly diagnosed myasthenic.

Critical Care of the Myasthenic

THE PATIENT IN CRISIS.
Crisis refers to threatened or actual respiratory compromise in a myasthenic patient. It may reflect respiratory muscle insufficiency or inability to handle secretions and oral intake but is typically a combination of the two. With currently available treatments, myasthenic crisis is not common. An occasional patient presents with fulminant disease; crisis management then coincides with initial evaluation and institution of therapy. Otherwise, crisis may be precipitated by other illness, such as influenza or other infections.

GENERAL MEASURES.
The respiratory function of any acutely deteriorating or severely weak myasthenic should be monitored compulsively. When the weakening myasthenic reaches a point at which increased respiratory effort is required, fatigue often prevents the effective use of secondary muscles, and failure rapidly ensues. Arterial blood gas values and even oxygen saturation are poor indicators of incipient failure in the face of respiratory muscle compromise. Forced vital capacity (FVC), maximum inspiratory pressure (MIP), and maximum expiratory pressure (MEP) are better indices and should be serially charted. The FVC should be assessed with the patient both sitting and supine, as diaphragmatic paresis may be accentuated in the supine position. The MIP and MEP measurements require special care if the patient also has significant facial weakness. An FVC less than 20 ml per kilogram, an MIP greater than (i.e., less negative than) −25 cm H_2O, or an MEP less than 40 cm H_2O suggests impending failure and usually warrants intubation. If a downward trend is noted, elective intubation should be considered even sooner, unless there is a realistic expectation of reversal.

Acute deterioration in a myasthenic always warrants consideration of contributing circumstances or concurrent illness that may accentuate the underlying defect in neuromuscular transmission. The major considerations are listed in Table 190-1 and discussed below.

The possibility of cholinergic crisis in patients receiving anticholinesterase drugs (e.g., pyridostigmine), although no longer common, should not be overlooked. The presence of fasciculations, diaphoresis, or diarrhea should alert the clinician to this possibility. Tensilon testing can be helpful: Abrupt deterioration after a conventional 10-mg test dose indicates overdosage with cholinesterase inhibitors. One must be adequately prepared for deterioration as well as increased respi-

Table 190-1. Conditions That May Underlie Interim Deterioration in Myasthenic Patients

Intercurrent infection; occult infection should be excluded
Electrolyte imbalance (Na, K, Ca, P, Mg)
Cholinergic crisis: if any doubt, discontinue cholinesterase inhibitors
Thyrotoxicosis, hypothyroidism
Medication effects (see Table 190-2)

ratory secretions. If there is any doubt, it may simply be assumed that the patient is in true cholinergic crisis, and cholinesterase inhibitors should be withheld for at least 24 hours. This assumes that adequate respiratory monitoring and support are in effect. There is rarely an adverse response to this approach, and a brief "holiday" from cholinesterase inhibition often results in an enhanced response to therapy when reinstituted.

Intercurrent infection is often associated with increased weakness in the myasthenic patient. There should be a compulsive search for systemic infection in the deteriorating patient, particularly the patient receiving immunosuppressive therapy. Any infections should be treated aggressively. Both hypothyroid and hyperthyroid states are often associated with increased weakness. Again, there is an increased association between thyrotoxicosis and myasthenia gravis. The manifestations of electrolyte imbalance may be enhanced in myasthenics. Otherwise insignificant electrolyte effects on transmitter release or muscle membrane excitability may be amplified at the myasthenic neuromuscular junction. Potassium, calcium, phosphate, and magnesium alterations should be corrected. Myasthenia gravis may also impart enhanced sensitivity to a number of medications that have only minimal effects on neuromuscular function in normal individuals. Aminoglycoside antibiotics, beta-blockers, and many antiarrhythmics may have adverse effects. Anticholinergics, respiratory depressants, and sedatives of any kind should be avoided or used only with great caution. *Neuromuscular blocking agents should never be administered to myasthenics in the ICU setting,* as they often have profound and prolonged effects. This increased sensitivity occasionally results in postoperative failure to wean in an undiagnosed mild myasthenic who has undergone surgery for an unrelated problem. Table 190-2 provides a comprehensive listing of medications that may further impair neuromuscular transmission in myasthenic patients.

Some attention should also be given to the general environment in which the myasthenic is managed. The typical noisy, brightly illuminated ICU is not conducive to rest and sleep, which are necessities for the myasthenic patient, in whom fatigue may be critical.

Special consideration must be given to respiratory care of the myasthenic. Incentive spirometry should be avoided, because muscular fatigue outweighs any potential benefit, even in the postoperative patient. Careful attention to respiratory toilet is key and can be complicated by cholinesterase inhibitors, which increase respiratory secretions. Atropine may be used to minimize this effect, but its other autonomic side effects, such as ileus, constipation, and delirium, may limit longer-term use.

THERAPY IN MYASTHENIC CRISIS. Therapeutic agents used in the critical care setting parallel those available to the patient with milder myasthenia gravis. Immunosuppressive therapies are the major considerations. Any myasthenic in crisis, if not already receiving immunosuppressive therapy, will require it. Although the mainstay of therapy in the past, cholinesterase inhibitors are now primarily used on a shorter-term basis, pending response to other modalities. Plasmapheresis, intravenous human immune globulin, corticosteroids, and longer-term immunosuppressants and cholinesterase inhibitors are discussed individually.

Plasmapheresis. Recognition of the role of immunoglobulins in the pathogenesis of myasthenia gravis stimulated clinical trials of plasmapheresis as soon as efficient pheresis technology became available. The results have been quite favorable [8]. Most patients demonstrate a significant clinical response within 48 hours of initiation of plasmapheresis, although the response is short-lived unless therapy is continued on an intermittent basis. Plasmapheresis is too invasive to be used for long-term therapy, but the rapid response can be crucial in the face of crisis, providing a short-term reprieve during which alternative therapy can be initiated or any intercurrent medical problems resolved. About 50 ml per kilogram should be exchanged per session [9], approximating 60 to 70 percent of total plasma volume. Plasma removed is replaced by an equal volume of normal saline and 5% albumin, adjusted to maintain physiologic concentrations of potassium, calcium, and magnesium. The usual course of treatment includes three to seven pheresis sessions at 24- to 48-hour intervals. Many patients develop increased sensitivity to cholinesterase inhibitors after plasmapheresis; dosage should be correspondingly reduced. The

Table 190-2. Medications That May Accentuate Weakness in Myasthenics

Antibiotics	NM blockers and muscle relaxants	Antiarrhythmics and antihypertensives	Antirheumatics	Antipsychotics	Others
Amikacin	Anectine (succinylcholine)	Lidocaine	Chloroquine	Lithium	Opiate analgesics
Clindamycin	Norcuron (vecuronium)	Quinidine	D-penicillamine	Phenothiazines	Oral contraceptives
Colistin	Pavulon (pancuronium)	Procainamide		Antidepressants	Antihistamines
Gentamicin	Tracrium (atacurium)	Beta-blockers			Anticholinergics
Kanamycin	Benzodiazepines	Calcium blockers			
Lincomycin	Curare				
Neomycin	Dantrium (dantrolene)				
Polymyxin B	Flexeril (cyclobenzaprine)				
Streptomycin	Lioresal (baclofen)				
Tobramycin	Robaxin (methocarbamol)				
Tetracyclines	Soma (carisoprodol)				
Trimethoprim/ sulfamethoxazole	Quinamm (quinine sulfate)				

major potential complications of plasmapheresis include hypotension, arrhythmia, and hypercoagulability due to hemoconcentration. Coincident cardiovascular disease is a relative contraindication to plasmapheresis.

Longer-Term Immunosuppression. Intravenous human immune globulin also frequently leads to rapid yet transient improvement in myasthenics [1]. Although its mechanism of action remains unclear, it is a therapeutic option in the event of crisis or in the perioperative period, particularly if the patient's cardiovascular status limits plasmapheresis. The customary dose is 400 mg/kg/day for 5 consecutive days. Maximal improvement occurs by the second week after therapy, and the therapeutic response usually persists for several weeks. Fluid overload is the major practical consideration. Corticosteroids have proved to be an effective long-term therapy for almost all myasthenics whose clinical manifestations cannot be well managed with low doses of cholinesterase inhibitors. Despite potential side effects associated with corticosteroid therapy, a response rate of greater than 80 percent supports its use [10]. Side effects can be minimized with appropriate precautions. Carbohydrate metabolism, electrolytes, blood pressure, and diet should be closely monitored; calcium (250–500 mg three times per day) and vitamin D supplementation (at least 50,000 units twice weekly) are prudent to minimize osteopenia. Screening for tuberculosis exposure with skin testing and chest radiographs should be done before initiation of therapy. Occult infection must be excluded in the deteriorating myasthenic.

Recommendations regarding corticosteroid preparation, dose, and regimen vary, but we prefer to begin with 25 mg of prednisone or its equivalent as a single daily dose, increasing the dose by 5 mg every third day to 60 mg in most patients. Difficulty arises with patients who are severely weak, especially if they have marginal respiratory or bulbar function; if given larger initial doses, many become transiently weaker before they improve. Seybold and Drachman [12] recommended a more gradual introduction of therapy to minimize interim deterioration, although this, in turn, delays therapeutic response. In the critical care setting, concurrent plasmapheresis may offset initial steroid-related deterioration, enabling more rapid institution of therapy.

Once maximal response is obtained, usually within 1 to 2 months, patients may be gradually shifted to alternate-day therapy by concurrently reducing the "off-day" dose and increasing the "on-day" dose, with a 10-mg shift made once each week. Some individuals note a definite off-day adverse effect; this can usually be countered with a 10-mg alternate-day dose. Once stabilized on alternate-day therapy, the on-day dose can be tapered by 5 mg per month. Many patients can be maintained in remission with as little as 20 to 25 mg of prednisone every other day (or alternating with 10 mg). Only rare patients remain in remission if therapy is discontinued, and overenthusiastic tapering of steroids is an all-too-common precipitant of unnecessary disability, or even crisis. Myasthenia sometimes remits spontaneously, and if the patient has undergone thymectomy (see below), the probability of remission increases appreciably, making discontinuation of therapy a more realistic option.

Azathioprine and cyclosporine are alternative agents for longer-term immunosupression [2,3]. Azathioprine is limited by a relatively long delay before its effects are clinically evident, up to 6 months, but its side effect spectrum compares favorably with steroids over a time frame of many years. If a patient tolerates a 50 mg per day test dose, the daily dose can be increased by 50 mg each week up to 2 mg/kg/day. This dose is then gradually adjusted up or down until the white blood count (WBC) is maintained in the range of 3000 to 4000 per cubic millimeter. Azathioprine therapy is often initiated after a patient attains remission on corticosteroids or when corticosteroid side effects become limiting. In such cases, leukocytosis may complicate dose regulation; a total lymphocyte count of 5 to 10 percent of the WBC is then a better target. The gastrointestinal system and liver are the other major sites of toxicity. Nausea may be countered by dividing the dose or giving doses with meals. Hepatic transaminases should be monitored regularly. Initially employed in transplant recipients, cyclosporine has also been shown to be an effective immunosuppressant in myasthenia gravis. Its major limitations are renal toxicity and a relatively high cost. The former can be minimized by divided dosing and gradual introduction of therapy. Five mg/kg/day can be given in two equal and equally spaced doses, followed by adjustments so as to maintain a predose trough level in the range of 100 to 200 ng per milliliter (by radioimmunoassay). Renal function (BUN and creatinine) must be continually monitored. Significant hypertension and preexisting renal disease are contraindications to the use of cyclosporine.

Many variables influence the choice of a longer-term immunosuppressant agent. In the absence of specific contraindications, I favor azathioprine for younger patients. It is introduced after remission is achieved with corticosteroids. The longer-term side effects of corticosteroids are of somewhat lesser concern in older patients. I reserve cyclosporine in most instances, due primarily to the relatively high costs associated with its use.

Cholinesterase Inhibitors. Cholinesterase inhibition was the mainstay of pharmacotherapy for myasthenia gravis before the advent of the immunosuppressive therapies and thymectomy. Many patients are now maintained in remission on corticosteroids or azathioprine, while many others require only low or occasional doses of an oral anticholinesterase drug, such as pyridostigmine (Mestinon). If an acutely deteriorating patient has been taking a cholinesterase inhibitor, cholinergic crisis should be excluded. It is reasonable to discontinue anticholinesterase therapy for 24 hours, managing respiratory status meanwhile. If further anticholinesterase therapy is then deemed necessary, it can be reinstituted by the intravenous route, which assures precise control of drug delivery until the patient stabilizes. Both neostigmine and pyridostigmine preparations are available for continuous intravenous infusion. Therapy should be resumed at about one-half the prior equivalent dosage (Table 190-3), as increased sensitivity often follows a "drug holiday." One milligram of neostigmine given intravenously is roughly equivalent to 120 mg of pyridostigmine taken by mouth. Thus, a patient taking 60 mg of pyridostigmine every 6 hours would receive 1 mg of neostigmine as a continuous intravenous infusion over 24 hours. The infusion rate can be gradually increased or decreased depending on clinical status, side effects, and so on. The dosage equivalents of all anticholinesterase preparations are given in Table 190-3.

Perioperative Management of the Myasthenic Patient

An intercurrent problem requiring surgical intervention was a common source of major morbidity and mortality for myasthenics before the 1960s. Subsequent developments in critical care techniques, especially respiratory care, and in therapy of the underlying disease have dramatically improved this situation. Perioperative management must be compulsive, yet my-

Table 190-3. Cholinesterase Inhibitors and Dosage Equivalents

		Route and dose (mg)	
Agent	Commercial name	Oral	Parenteral
Pyridostigmine bromide	Mestinon	60	2
Neostigmine bromide	Prostigmin	15	—
Neostigmine methylsulfate	Prostigmin	—	0.5

asthenia gravis should rarely preclude surgical treatment that is otherwise indicated.

PREOPERATIVE CONSIDERATIONS. Myasthenia gravis is a major variable in surgical management, whether the surgery is elective or emergent. A neurologist (preferably the neurologist who has been managing the patient) should be considered an integral member of the operative team. If the procedure is elective, the patient's myasthenic status should be optimized before anesthesia and surgery. Pulmonary functions should be reviewed in detail; if respiratory or bulbar muscle function is compromised, therapy adjustments should be undertaken to improve the patient's status. All therapeutic options should be considered, with the possible exception of corticosteroids. If the patient is not receiving steroids, it is prudent to forego or delay this treatment until after surgery, as corticosteroids may increase the risk of infection and retard wound healing. If the patient is already receiving corticosteroids, therapy should be continued, with a short-term increment in dose to compensate for the added stress of anesthesia and surgery. Plasmapheresis or intravenous human immune globulin are often useful in the preoperative setting, providing a transient therapeutic benefit through the preoperative and postoperative periods. Once dose and regimen are optimized, cholinesterase inhibitors may be continued up to the time of surgery. They should then be discontinued, as they will stimulate respiratory secretions.

It is crucial that all physicians involved in perioperative management of the myasthenic be aware of the particular medications that may accentuate the underlying defect in neuromuscular transmission. It is appropriate to post a warning regarding specific medications on the patient's chart, in a manner analogous to that for medication allergies. Neuromuscular blockade should be avoided during surgery unless absolutely essential; if required, the shortest-acting agents should be employed at minimal doses. Accentuated and prolonged effects should be anticipated. Aminoglycoside antibiotics should also be avoided when alternatives are available. There is no clear consensus in favor of any one halogenated anesthetic agent; ether adversely affects neuromuscular transmission. Again, close attention to metabolic homeostasis cannot be overemphasized.

POSTOPERATIVE CARE. Postoperative care of the myasthenic patient should not differ greatly from that of other patients, provided preoperative and intraoperative management have been successful. The patient's status before surgery is often the best indicator of the postoperative course. Intubation and mechanical ventilatory support must be continued until the patient is alert and responsive, and demonstrates and maintains adequate pulmonary function. Serial pulmonary functions indicate when the patient can be extubated. An FVC greater than 20 ml per kilogram and maximum inspiratory pressure less than (i.e., more negative than) -25 cm H_2O are minimum requirements. If needed, cholinesterase inhibitors may be resumed as

a continuous intravenous infusion until bowel function is restored and oral intake allowed. Increased sensitivity to cholinesterase inhibitors is the norm after surgical procedures, especially thymectomy. Resumption at a rate of no more than one-half the preoperative equivalent is often sufficient. Subsequent adjustments should reflect clinical indices. The myasthenic whose neuromuscular function deteriorates during the postoperative period is the exception. In all probability an intercurrent, reversible factor underlies the deterioration. The spectrum of metabolic, infectious, and pharmacologic issues discussed above should be reviewed.

THYMECTOMY. After several decades of controversy, there is a consensus that thymectomy favorably alters the natural history of myasthenia gravis, especially in younger patients, independent of the presence or degree of thymic hyperplasia [12,13]. Thymectomy should be considered early in the course of myasthenia, except in elderly, frail patients. Thymectomy remains an elective procedure, however. The myasthenic with marginal respiratory or bulbar function should be optimally treated before surgery. The perioperative management considerations discussed above apply to prethymectomy and postthymectomy management. Some controversy persists regarding the appropriate thymectomy procedure. Most centers favor the transsternal approach. Although more invasive, this approach facilitates recognition and removal of all thymus tissue and avoids postoperative respiratory compromise. There are some proponents of transcervical, mediastinoscopic thymectomy; in experienced hands this remains an alternative. Thymectomy by conventional thoracotomy has no place in the treatment of myasthenia.

Conclusion

Respiratory failure is no longer the major source of morbidity and mortality in myasthenia gravis. When it does occur, appropriate ventilatory support and airway protection provide time for resolution of any intercurrent problems and therapy of the underlying myasthenia. Plasmapheresis and immunosuppression are usually successful; extended intensive care stays should be rare occurrences.

References

1. Drachman DB, deSilva S, Ramsay D, Pestronk A: Humoral pathogenesis of myasthenia gravis, in Drachman DB (ed): *Myasthenia Gravis: Biology and Treatment.* New York, New York Academy of Sciences, 1987, p 90.
2. Elmqvist D, Hoffman WW, Kugelberg J, Quastel DMJ: An electrophysiological investigation of neuromuscular transmission in myasthenia gravis. *J Physiol* 174:417, 1964.
3. Osserman KE, Genkins G: Studies in myasthenia gravis: A review of a 20 year experience in over 1200 patients. *Mt Sinai J Med* 38:497, 1971.
4. Howard FM Jr, Lennon VA, Finley J, et al: Clinical correlations of antibodies that bind, block, or modulate human acetylcholine receptors in myasthenia gravis, in Drachman DB (ed): *Myasthenia Gravis: Biology and Treatment.* New York, New York Academy of Sciences, 1987, p 526.
5. Johns RJ, Grob D, Harvey AM: Studies in neuromuscular function. 2. Effects of nerve stimulation in normal subjects and in patients with myasthenia gravis. *Bull Johns Hopkins Hosp* 99:125, 1956.
6. Brown JC, Charlton JE: A study of sensitivity to curare in myasthenia

disorders using a regional technique. *J Neurol Neurosurg Psychiatry* 38:27, 1975.

7. Stahlberg E, Ekstedt J, Broman A: Neuromuscular transmission in myasthenia gravis studies with single fiber electromyography. *J Neurol Neurosurg Psychiatry* 37:540, 1974.

8. Asura E: Experience with intravenous immunoglobulin in myasthenia gravis. *Clin Immunol Immunopathol* 53:5170, 1989.

9. Pinching AJ, Peters DK, Newson-Davis J: Remission of myasthenia gravis following plasma exchange. *Lancet* 2:1373, 1976.

10. Perlo VP, Shahani B, Huggins C, et al: Effect of plasmapheresis in myasthenia gravis. *Ann NY Acad Sci* 377:709, 1981.

11. Johns TR: Long-term corticosteroid treatment of myasthenia gravis, in Drachman DB (ed): *Myasthenia Gravis: Biology and Treatment*. New York, New York Academy of Sciences, 1987, p 568.

12. Seybold ME, Drachman DB: Gradually increasing doses of prednisone in myasthenia gravis. *N Engl J Med* 290:81, 1974.

13. Matell G: Immunosuppressive drugs: azathioprine in the treatment of myasthenia gravis. *Ann NY Acad Sci* 505:588, 1987.

14. Tindall RSA, Rollins JA, Phillips JT, et al: Preliminary results in a double-blind, randomized, placebo-controlled trial of cyclosporine in myasthenia gravis. *N Engl J Med* 316:719, 1987.

15. Perlo VP, Arnason B, Poskanzer D, et al: The role of thymectomy in the treatment of myasthenia gravis. *Ann NY Acad Sci* 183:308, 1971.

16. Genkins G, Papatestas AE, Horowitz SH, Kornfeld P: Studies in myasthenia gravis: Early thymectomy. *Am J Med* 58:517, 1975.

191. Miscellaneous Neurologic Problems in the Intensive Care Unit

Nancy M. Fontneau and Ann L. Mitchell

A wide variety of neurologic problems, both primary and those that are secondary to an underlying disorder, may confront the physician in the intensive care unit. While a comprehensive review is beyond the scope of this chapter, we discuss several important disorders for which basic information is not readily available. Suicidal hanging, electrical shock, acute carbon monoxide poisoning, and decompression sickness ordinarily present so blatantly that the initial diagnosis is rarely in question, yet the range of clinical manifestations and their management may be unanticipated. By contrast, cerebral fat embolism and atropinelike poisoning are often not initially suspected if other surgical or medical issues take precedence. Hiccough is an all-too-common secondary problem that not only bedevils patients (and their physicians) but may further weaken the already cachectic individual. Critical illness polyneuropathy is a complication of overwhelming sepsis, which is now seen frequently because of improved survival of these patients. Compression neuropathies may complicate prolonged bed rest. Unexpectedly prolonged action of neuromuscular blocking agents is relatively common in ICU patients.

Suicidal Hanging

Hanging is the third most common means of committing suicide, with a male-to-female predominance ratio of 3:1 [1,2]. Introduced in England in the fifth century by the Angles, Jutes, and Saxons, hanging proceeded to become the official form of execution [3]. Early on there was no exact procedure, and most hangings resulted in slow strangulation [1–6]. Ultimately, an English judiciary committee established official guidelines for the Commonwealth, such that, given the weight of the victim, a force of 1260 ft pounds would be generated [4]. This specification and the use of the hangman's knot in the submental location produced a consistently fatal bilateral axis-pedicle fracture, with complete herniation of the disc and the severance of the ligaments between C_2 and C_3 [1–4,6–9]. This injury causes almost immediate death by destroying the cardiac and respiratory centers, lacerating the carotid artery, and injuring the pharynx [1,2].

Suicidal hangings are rarely so expert, and death usually results from strangulation due to the interruption of cerebral blood flow rather than upper airway obstruction [1,2,5]. A minimal amount of compression occludes the jugular veins, resulting in stagnation of cerebral blood flow [1]. Slightly more force (a pull of 3.5 kg on a ligature around the neck) occludes the carotid arteries, while a much larger force (16.6 kg) is necessary to arrest blood flow in the vertebral arteries [1,2]. Pressure on the jugular veins from the noose results in venous obstruction and stagnation of cerebral blood flow, resulting in hypoxia and loss of consciousness. Cervical muscle tone then decreases, allowing arterial compression and, ultimately, occlusion [2]. In addition, external compression of the carotid bodies or vagal sheath can increase parasympathetic tone, while pressure on the pericarotid area stimulates sympathetic tone; either can result in cardiac arrest [1]. The altered autonomic tone may also affect the respiratory smooth muscle tone, resulting in respiratory acidosis and a further insult to cerebral oxygenation [1,2].

If blood flow is quickly restored, then full recovery can probably be expected. If the blood flow is interrupted more than a few minutes, however, hypoxia causes cell death as well as cytotoxic and vasogenic edema, with increased intracranial pressure. There is a selective vulnerability of the cortex (particularly the third layer), the globus pallidus, thalamus, hippocampus, and Purkinje cells of the cerebellum to anoxia and ischemia. The maximum duration of postanoxic unconsciousness consistent with complete clinical recovery is thought to be 48 hours, but any coma persisting longer than 24 hours in this setting implies a considerable chance of major neurologic dysfunction on recovery of consciousness [5].

DIAGNOSIS. While the diagnosis is rarely in doubt, the patient may show a range of findings, varying from rope burns to coma and/or fracture of the odontoid. In the immediate posthanging period the patient most commonly shows evidence of an altered level of consciousness, ranging from restlessness, delirium, or violence to lethargy, stupor, or coma. Seizures may occur [1,2,5] or hyperthermia [6] may be present because of hypoxic damage to the hypothalamus. Development of the acute respiratory distress syndrome (ARDS) may result from central nervous system (CNS) catecholamine changes that cause constriction of the pulmonary venules [2]. Although infrequent in suicidal hangings, fracture of the odontoid and injury to the spinal cord can occur.

Initial evaluation should include radiographs of the cervical spine, arterial blood gas determination, electrocardiogram (ECG), cardiac monitoring, and frequent monitoring of vital signs and for any evidence of stridor. Careful neurologic examination should be performed, with particular attention to any alterations in the level of consciousness and any evidence of spinal cord injury, such as paraparesis, quadriparesis, or urinary retention.

TREATMENT. The patient may appear dead but still be resuscitable, requiring both artificial respiratory support and external cardiac massage. The goals of treatment are to maintain an adequate level of cerebral oxygenation, to decrease the raised intracranial pressure, and to monitor and treat any cardiac arrhythmias or respiratory distress that may develop. In hangings, the mechanical trauma induced by strangulation can also cause hemorrhage and edema in the paratracheal and laryngeal areas and result in a delayed but significant airway obstruction at any time within the first 24 hours. Endotracheal intubation may be required if there is evidence of hypoxia on the basis of ARDS, airway obstruction, or increased intracranial pressure [2]. The increased intracranial pressure is treated with hyperventilation-induced hypocarbia, with its resultant reflex cerebral vasoconstriction [1]. A fracture of the odontoid requires immediate neurosurgical or orthopaedic intervention to stabilize the cervical spine and protect the cord from injury.

COURSE. Other neurologic sequelae can become manifest either in the immediate posthanging period or after a relatively asymptomatic latent period [1,2,5]. The individual may show evidence of a confusional state, a circumscribed retrograde amnesia, Korsakoff's syndrome, or even progressive dementia. Abnormal movements, motor restlessness, and myoclonic jerks also can characterize this period [5]. Eventually, most patients who survive the initial event recover partially or completely.

Electrical Injuries

Approximately 4000 injuries and 1000 deaths from electrical shock occur annually in the United States. Most fatalities occur in the workplace, but one-third result from contact with household current. A smaller number of individuals die annually from lightning injury [10].

PATHOPHYSIOLOGY. Low-voltage injuries are almost always less serious than high-voltage injuries. Deep tissue injury and mortality are determined by the amperage (I), or current flowing between two potentials, which is equal to the voltage (V) divided by the resistance (R) to current flow (I = V/R). Although it is unknown in most cases, resistance varies by tissue type and is inversely proportional to the water content of the tissue. The nervous system and blood vessels have lower than

expected resistances and are thus more sensitive to electrical injury than would be predicted by their water content. Immediate tissue injury results from the conversion of electrical energy into heat. Delayed injury also occurs, due to vascular occlusion. The extent of injury depends on the path of the current through the victim, the area of contact and current exit, and whether the current is direct or alternating. Alternating current is more dangerous than direct current because it tends to produce tetanic contractions that prevent voluntary release from the current source, and at the usual 60-Hz frequency, alternating current commonly causes cardiac arrhythmias and respiratory arrest [11].

Electrical shocks cause several types of injuries, including burns from direct current or ignition of clothing; muscle necrosis from direct thermal injury or secondary to vascular occlusion; renal failure secondary to myoglobinuria; fractures and other musculoskeletal injuries secondary to tetanic muscular contractions or falls; and premature development of cataracts. Arrhythmia (especially ventricular or atrial fibrillation) and asystole are the most common cardiac manifestations and may be immediate or delayed [12].

Neurologic sequelae occur in more than 25 percent of electrical injuries and affect both central and peripheral nervous systems [13,14,15]. The spinal cord is most commonly involved, due to the frequency of hand-to-hand or hand-to-foot current flow. Acute weakness, ranging from monoparesis to quadriplegia, is a common presentation and usually involves C_4 to C_8. Paresthesias and pain may also be prominent. Acute reversible injuries apparent at presentation usually clear within 24 hours; those that last longer are likely to leave persistent residuals. Permanent spinal cord sequelae are more likely if the contact point is near the spine and if the current is sufficient to produce thermal injury to the cord. Delayed spinal cord injury may develop after a latent period of days to months and progresses slowly. Segmental atrophy is more common after low-voltage injuries and reflects anterior horn cell injury, while delayed myelopathy is more common with exposure to greater than 1000 V. The myelopathy probably results from electrical injury to spinal cord arterioles and is more prominent in patients with preexisting arterial disease.

Electrical contact with the head usually results in unconsciousness. Usually there is rapid return to consciousness, but transient seizures, confusion, sensorimotor dysfunction, deafness, blindness, tinnitus, headache, and retrograde amnesia may occur. In more severe injuries, cerebral edema may result in increased intracranial pressure, but this is usually transient. Subarachnoid hemorrhage and petechial cortical hemorrhages may occur. Acute hypoxic ischemic cerebral injury may also result from cardiac arrhythmias (especially ventricular fibrillation) and central respiratory paralysis, which result from electrical injury. Lightning strikes to the head are fatal in 30 percent of cases.

Delayed cerebral sequelae include encephalopathy, seizures, extrapyramidal syndromes (parkinsonism, chorea), aphasia, hemiparesis, pupillary dysfunction, and dysphagia. Like the delayed effects of electricity on the spinal cord, these injuries are probably the result of changes in the cerebral arteries and arterioles. The electroencephalogram (EEG) may demonstrate focal or generalized slowing or epileptiform discharges. Burns of the scalp and underlying bone may also be present.

Peripheral nerve injuries are usually found at the site of electrical contact or exit. The median nerve is most frequently affected, but all the nerves and plexi of the upper and lower extremities are at risk. The injury probably results from heating of the nerve by the passage of current, and injury to both axon and myelin sheath has been reported. The clinical presentation is of mononeuropathy, mononeuropathy multiplex, plexopathy, or local pain or paresthesias related to burns. Gradual improvement is usually noted.

Vasoconstriction is noted in the limbs after electrical injury and reflects autonomic dysfunction. Delayed reflex sympathetic dystrophy may also occur.

CLINICAL MANIFESTATIONS. After serious electrical injury, patients may be asystolic or in ventricular fibrillation, and apneic. Hypotension may also be present, due to extravasation of fluid into necrotic tissues or through surface burns. Electrical burns range from small areas of thermocoagulation at discrete entrance or exit wounds to more diffuse, spiderlike areas of redness and blistering. Vertebral and other fractures may be present. Muscle necrosis is frequently present and may be progressive and too deep to visualize. Myoglobinuria and renal failure may result. Metabolic acidosis also results from anaerobic metabolism in ischemic tissues. Pulmonary edema, sepsis, and gastrointestinal hemorrhage or necrosis may also complicate serious electrical injuries.

Neurologic examination of the electrically injured patient should begin with assessment of the level of consciousness. Many patients are comatose initially, especially after high-voltage or lightning injury. Coma is usually brief but may be followed by a period of encephalopathy lasting hours to days and characterized by confusion, apathy, and sometimes agitation [13]. Seizures are uncommon. The cranial nerve examination may reveal blindness and papilledema. Pupillary dysfunction may also be present and persistent. Hearing may be reduced or tinnitus may be present, and rupture of the tympanic membranes is common following electrical contact with the head. The motor system is evaluated carefully for signs of weakness and reflex changes indicative of cerebral, spinal cord, or peripheral nerve injury. Cerebral injuries may result in contralateral hemiparesis. Spinal cord injuries are most common in the cervical region and produce paraparesis or quadriparesis. The extent of motor deficit may not be apparent on initial examination, since electrical effects are frequently delayed and may be progressive. Peripheral nerve injuries in the period immediately after injury are usually localized to areas of severe burns. Sensory loss is less frequent than motor deficit and is maximal in burned areas. Hyper- or hyporeflexia may be present.

Laboratory evaluation should include serial determinations of electrolytes, renal function, and hematocrit to ensure adequate fluid replacement and determination of creatine kinase and urinary myoglobin as measures of muscle necrosis. Arterial blood gases may reveal metabolic acidosis. Radiologic examination of the spine, long bones, and skull is indicated when fractures or deep burns are suspected on the basis of history or physical examination. Myelography may be needed to rule out spinal cord compression if delayed signs of myelopathy develop. Cranial computed tomography (CT) scanning is indicated when there is prolonged alteration of consciousness and may reveal evidence of subarachnoid hemorrhage or cerebral edema. Lumbar puncture is not usually indicated, except when infection is suspected. Following electrical injury the cerebrospinal fluid (CSF) protein may be mildly elevated and a minimal increase in the number of white blood cells may be found [13]. When there is subarachnoid hemorrhage or petechial cortical hemorrhages, the CSF red blood cell count is elevated. Nerve conduction studies and electromyography may be useful in localizing and following axonal and demyelinating electrical injuries to the peripheral nerves and plexi but are generally not used in the acute phase of illness. The EEG is useful to rule out status epilepticus when alteration of consciousness is prolonged. In addition, background slowing may be seen even when the mental status has returned to normal.

MANAGEMENT. Initial management consists of safe removal of the victim from the electricity source. Cardiopulmonary resuscitation is frequently required, since asystole and ventricular fibrillation are common and because central respiratory arrest may occur even in the absence of current passage through the brainstem [16]. Even when there is no cardiopulmonary arrest, cardiac monitoring is required because delayed arrhythmias may occur if the current has passed through the thorax.

Fluid and electrolyte management using isosmotic solutions is key for maintaining circulatory volume and preventing renal failure. Although electric shock victims usually have myoglobinuria secondary to burns, their fluid needs are similar to those of patients with crush injuries. Central venous pressure monitoring is usually needed and urine output should be maintained at greater than 50 ml per hour. Alkalinization of the urine and osmotic diuresis with mannitol also help prevent myoglobin nephropathy.

Extensive burns are best treated in specialized burn units. Skin grafts are sometimes required. Debridement of necrotic muscle and fasciotomy are sometimes necessary to prevent secondary ischemia from a compartment syndrome. Amputation is required if there is significant necrosis. In these patients, arteriography may assist in identifying the level of viability [17]. Tetanus prophylaxis and prevention of superinfection are also needed. Spine and long bone fractures require stabilization.

Recurrent seizures are treated with phenytoin (18–20 mg/kg loading dose followed by 5–7 mg/kg/day in divided doses). Since fluid restriction is contraindicated, patients with signs of increased intracranial pressure require osmotic diuresis with mannitol. A loading dose of 0.75 to 1 gm per kilogram is followed by maintenance doses of 0.25 to 0.5 gm per kilogram every 4 to 6 hours as needed to maintain serum osmolarity to 305 to 310 mOsm per liter. Intracranial pressure monitoring is useful. Specific treatment for electrical spinal cord injuries is not available, and early institution of physical therapy is recommended.

Prognosis is difficult to predict for electrical injuries to the nervous system. Patients with deficits at presentation frequently recover fully, while those with delayed onset of neurologic deficits may have syndromes that progress over months to years, or remit, allowing some recovery.

Carbon Monoxide Poisoning

Carbon monoxide is a colorless, tasteless, odorless gas that may give no warning of its presence [18]. It is normally present in the atmosphere in a concentration of less than 0.001%, but a concentration of 0.1% can be lethal [18]. Carbon monoxide is found in automobile exhaust (sometimes offering a mode of suicide), fires, charcoal-burning grills, methylene chloride, volcanic gas, and cigarette smoke. It is also endogenously formed from the degradation of hemoglobin, resulting in a baseline carboxyhemoglobin saturation between 1 and 3 percent [18,19,20]. Smoking more than 40 cigarettes per day can raise the endogenous level to 6 to 7 percent saturation [19]. For further information on the pathogenesis, diagnosis, and treatment of carbon monoxide poisoning, see Chapter 71.

DIAGNOSIS. It is important to consider carbon monoxide in the differential diagnosis of any individual who presents with an altered state of consciousness, particularly in the setting of a long car ride or other exposure to poorly ventilated and incompletely combusted fuel. A carboxyhemoglobin saturation of less than 10 percent can be associated with a mild headache and, in susceptible individuals, dyspnea on exertion [18–22]. A level between 10 and 20 percent is more consistently associated with symptoms of a headache and easy fatigability [18,19,20]. In the range of 20 to 30 percent saturation, the headache becomes pounding and is associated with impaired motor dexterity, blurring of vision, and irritability [18,19,20]. At 30 to 40 percent saturation, symptoms of muscle weakness, nausea, vomiting, and mental confusion or delirium surface [18,19,20]. At greater than 40 percent saturation, tachycardia and cardiac irritability appear, and at greater than 50 percent there can be seizures, respiratory insufficiency, and even coma, at 60 percent. In the range of 60 to 70 percent saturation or higher, coma is routinely present and respiratory failure and death ensue [18,19,20]. In addition, there can be evidence of rhabdomyolysis [23], hepatic damage [18,19,20], flame-shaped superficial retinal hemorrhages [18,19,20,24], and, occasionally, a cherry red discoloration best appreciated in the lips, mucous membranes, and skin [18,19]. The cherry red discoloration is fairly uncommon, appearing only at carboxyhemoglobin levels above 30 to 40 percent, and even then infrequently [19,23]. A CT scan of the brain may be normal early on or show signs of cerebral edema as inferred from narrowed ventricles and effacement of the cerebral sulci. Later in the clinical course, the CT scan may show symmetric bilateral hypodensities of the basal ganglia, particularly of the globus pallidus and substantia nigra [18]. The EEG usually demonstrates diffuse slowing but is generally of little prognostic value.

TREATMENT. The criteria for hospital admission include loss of consciousness at any time; neurologic deficit at any time; any clinical or electrocardiographic signs of cardiac compromise; metabolic acidosis; an abnormal chest radiograph; a carboxyhemoglobin level greater than 25 percent, greater than 15 percent with a history of cardiac disease, or greater than 10 percent in pregnancy; a PO_2 less than 60 mm Hg; and/or any metabolic acidosis on the basis of carbon monoxide poisoning [23].

All patients should be treated with 100% oxygen as soon as the diagnosis of carbon monoxide poisoning is even considered. It should be administered through a tight-fitting, nonrebreathing mask or after endotracheal intubation in severely sensorium-compromised patients. The administration of 100% oxyen can shorten the half-life of carbon monoxide in the blood from 320 minutes to the range of 80 to 90 minutes [18,19]. Therapeutically, the carboxyhemoglobin must be reduced below 5 percent [19]. (See Chaps. 56 and 58 for a discussion of hyperbaric oxygen therapy.)

In addition to the usefulness of the 100% oxygen and, if available, hyperbaric therapy in treating acute cerebral edema, mechanical hyperventilation and monitoring of fluid and electrolyte status are important. Steroids have not been proved effective in cerebral postanoxic states and may increase the risk of oxygen toxicity seizures if hyperbaric therapy is being considered [23].

COURSE. The delayed appearance of neurologic sequelae found in many posthypoxic states occurs with particular frequency and severity after carbon monoxide poisoning [18,19,21–27]. The post-carbon monoxide syndrome begins 7 to 21 days after the initial insult and is characterized by gait disturbances, incontinence, and memory impairment. The initial neurologic effect usually includes impairment of consciousness that evolves into restlessness and confusion with impaired

memory storage. The cerebral edema occasioned by the hypoxia can reach lethal proportions. There may be seizures, cortical blindness, scotomas, and flame-shaped retinal hemorrhages. Korsakoff's psychosis, peripheral neuropathy, irritability, violence, hemiplegia, chorea, and extrapyramidal dysfunction with akinesia, masklike facies, and shuffling gait can also be found. These signs and findings can fluctuate so widely that their evanescent quality falsely suggests hysterical symptoms [24].

Between 10 and 30 percent [23] of patients develop the delayed neurologic signs, and there are no guidelines to indicate which patients are at greatest risk. Although there seems to be a rough correlation between duration of initial unconsciousness and rate of subsequent late relapse [21], even patients with mild toxicity can progress to develop the tardive signs [18,26]. At times, the appearance of the late sequelae appears to be temporally associated with increased patient activity in the early postexposure period.

On average, 75 percent of affected individuals largely recover within a year of the insult, although 20 percent of these individuals continue to show evidence of a mild to moderate impairment of memory and/or extrapyramidal dysfunction [27]. Although the specific cause of the delayed syndrome is unknown, it does correlate temporally with the pathologic findings of cerebral hemisphere white matter demyelination found in the chronic stages of the illness, as opposed to the largely gray matter edema, ischemia, and hemorrhagic necrosis found in the acute stage [21,25]. There is no treatment for the delayed neuropsychiatric syndrome [27].

Decompression Sickness

Decompression sickness ("the bends") occurs when gases dissolved in body fluids come out of solution, forming bubbles in tissues and venous blood (see Chap. 68). Situations in which decompression sickness arise include rapid ascent to the surface by tunnel workers or scuba divers (caisson disease), flying after scuba diving, decompression or rapid ascent in an airplane, and high-altitude flying with inadequate cabin pressurization. In all of these situations, nitrogen and other inert gases that supersaturate the tissues under high pressure are released as bubbles under conditions of decreased pressure. As the bubbles coalesce, they may cause local tissue ischemia due to compression or venous obstruction. The microcirculation is further compromised by activation of platelets, coagulation factors, and complement, capillary endothelial edema, and hemoconcentration due to fluid extravasation [28,29,30].

Symptoms of decompression sickness are variable. In most cases the onset is within 6 hours of decompression and in 97 percent onset occurs within 12 hours [31]. Fulminant cases present early. Any organ system can be affected, and symptoms range from pruritic skin rash ("the creeps"), cough ("the chokes"), and joint pain to paraplegia, vertigo, altered level of consciousness, seizure, shock, and apnea. Joint pain is the most common symptom and most frequently involves the knee, shoulder, or elbow [31]. The pain is probably due to bubble formation within the joint itself [32], thus the colloquial name "the bends."

Almost 80 percent of patients with decompression sickness have neurologic symptoms. The most frequent neurologic presentation is of paresthesias, which may be diffuse or focal and results from gas bubble formation in the skin, joints, peripheral nerves or spinal cord. Weakness, ranging from monoparesis to quadriplegia secondary to spinal cord involvement, may also occur. Cerebral symptoms are infrequent and range from headache and lethargy to vertigo, visual disturbances, paralysis, and unconsciousness [31]. Positron emission tomography (PET) scanning has demonstrated cerebral perfusion deficits in patients with neurologic decompression sickness even without overt cerebral symptoms [33].

Air embolism is a more serious decompression illness and onset is usually within 5 minutes of decompression. Unconsciousness and stupor are the most frequent symptoms. It probably results from tearing of the lung parenchyma secondary to overinflation as the gases in the lungs expand during ascent. The gas escapes into the pulmonary vein and may embolize into large vessels [29]. Gas embolism may also result from paradoxical embolism through a patent foramen ovale [34]. Based on their buoyancy, the emboli often produce neurologic symptoms by floating into and occluding cerebral arterioles. Death from cardiopulmonary arrest may occur, but in a majority of patients (60%) improvement in symptoms accompanies the redistribution of the gas emboli to the venous circulation [29].

Recompression is the definitive treatment for decompression diseases. The patient should be transported to the nearest decompression chamber with minimal delay. Aircraft used in transport should be pressurized to sea level or fly as low as possible [29]. Commercial aircraft are usually pressurized only to the equivalent of 5000 feet [35]. The National Diving Accident Network maintains a 24-hour phone consultation service to assist with diving accidents (Duke University; 919-684-2948 daytime or 919-684-8111 24-hour emergency line).

While awaiting recompression, the patient is placed in a slight Trendelenburg position on the left side, to prevent coalescence of gas bubbles in the left ventricle and subsequent systemic embolization. One hundred percent oxygen administered via tight-fitting mask is given at 10 liters per minute. If a prolonged period prior to recompression is anticipated, air breaks should be planned to avoid the development of pulmonary oxygen toxicity [29]. Tracheal intubation is required for severe pulmonary edema and in patients with poorly compensated respiration that worsens after recompression. Serial arterial blood gas determinations are useful to follow pulmonary function. Chest radiographs are required to rule out pneumothorax, hemopneumothorax, and pneumomediastinum, particularly in patients with suspected air embolism. If present, they should be treated with chest tube drainage, unless a small nonprogressive pneumothorax is present.

Cardiac monitoring is generally required, and arrhythmias and evidence of ischemia may be noted. They should be treated in the usual fashion. Volume expansion with colloid is required to offset fluid loss by extravasation into the extracellular fluid compartment. Serial determinations of hematocrit and electrolytes assist in gauging the adequacy of this therapy. Central pressure monitoring and vasopressors are sometimes required in severe cases. The urinary bladder may become hypotonic if the spinal cord is affected, and bladder catheterization may be needed.

There is no proved role for medications in decompression sickness. Corticosteroids are frequently used to reduce cerebral edema. Intravenous lidocaine may speed neurologic recovery when used in standard doses [29].

Remarkable recovery may occur after recompression. Delay in treatment can limit its effectiveness, but recompression should be attempted even up to 2 weeks after the onset of symptoms. Relapse requiring repeated hyperbaric treatment may occur in as many as 50 percent of patients with decompression sickness and 30 percent of patients with air embolism [29]. Patients with long-term sequelae from decompression ill-

nesses should not be reexposed to conditions that allow their recurrence.

Cerebral Fat Embolism Syndrome

Fat embolism syndrome is characterized by diffuse pulmonary insufficiency with hypoxemia, neurologic dysfunction, pyrexia, tachycardia, tachypnea, and petechiae occurring 12 to 48 hours after trauma [36,37]. At least subclinically, fat embolism is present after all fractures involving the long bones [38,39]. It is clinically recognized in 0.5 to 2 percent of patients with long bone fractures and in 5 to 10 percent of patients who have sustained multiple fractures [38,40]. It has also been recognized in conjunction with extensive burns, rapid decompression syndrome, sickle cell disease, cardiopulmonary bypass, renal transplant, diabetes, and neoplasms [41,42].

PATHOGENESIS. The two main pathogenetic hypotheses to explain fat embolism syndrome are the mechanical and chemical theories. The mechanical theory holds that because of physical disruption to bone and blood vessels at the fracture site, free fat globules from the bone marrow are able to enter venous sinusoids and then embolize to the lungs. The chemical theory posits that a trauma-induced catecholamine surge results in either lipid mobilization from the fat stores or the coalescence of chylomicrons into fat globules [36,41,43]. It has been shown that cerebral fat emboli and ischemia, rather than cerebral anoxia, produce the neurologic damage seen in this condition. The brain is edematous and shows a leptomeningeal inflammatory reaction and cortical surface petechiae. Microscopically there are fat emboli and ball, ring, and perivascular hemorrhages. The fat emboli are more prevalent in the gray matter but the hemorrhages are more common in the centrum semiovale, internal capsule, and cerebral and cerebellar white matter [44].

DIAGNOSIS. Characteristically, there is a symptom-free interval of 12 to 48 hours between trauma and the onset of fat embolism syndrome [36,38,39,41,43]. Sudden onset of fever, tachycardia, and tachypnea often herald onset of the syndrome. Respiratory distress and hypoxemia with an oxygen tension (PO$_2$) less than 60 mm Hg is common and may be either the initial or the only laboratory abnormality in otherwise subclinical fat embolism. The chest radiograph may be unremarkable in half the cases, but fine stippling or hazy infiltrates of both lung fields should be sought, as they are consistent with fat embolism syndrome [43].

Petechiae are present in 50 to 60 percent of clinically recognized cases and are most often found on the lower palpebral conjunctivae, neck, anterior axillary folds, and anterior chest wall [38,40,41]. There is both an associated thrombocytopenia, believed to be caused by the consumption of platelets with their aggregation around the embolic fat droplets, and a progressive anemia with hemoglobin levels commonly less than 9.5 gm per 100 ml [43].

Retinal fat emboli and lipuria are each in evidence in more than 50 percent of patients [43]. The retinal emboli appear as small rosaries of microinfarcts surrounding the macula of both eyes, which over the course of the following 10 to 14 days evolve into yellowish fatty plaques [40,41].

The CNS manifestations range from confusion to coma, and while they almost always accompany respiratory insufficiency they can be the initial and sometimes only symptomatic manifestation of fat embolism syndrome [36,37,38,40]. Impaired consciousness is the earliest recognizable sign. The symptoms can begin with restlessness and confusion and may evolve gradually or abruptly to stupor and coma. Coma, especially if it develops abruptly, portends a poor prognosis [40]. Focal or generalized seizures can occur and may antedate the onset of coma [38]. Decerebrate rigidity is found in 10 to 15 percent of cases and pyramidal signs of hyperreflexia and extensor plantar responses are found in 30 to 70 percent [40]. Focal neurologic signs, such as aphasia and hemiparesis, may be seen in about one-third of patients and are usually restricted to patients with more severe disturbances of consciousness [37,40].

TREATMENT. Rapid immobilization of fractures and their early definitive management decreases the likelihood of the clinical appearance of fat embolism syndrome [43]. Sequential clinical examinations, chest radiographs, and arterial blood gas determinations in patients believed to be at high risk may help identify early on those needing more aggressive care. These patients should have early and expedient replacement of fluids and blood and administration of 40% oxygen by mask [43].

The support of respiration and maintenance of arterial oxygen levels greater than 70 mm Hg sometimes requires intubation and mechanical ventilation. Placement of a central venous pressure line is useful in monitoring the patient for shock. Increased intracranial pressure can be treated with hyperventilation and the resultant hypocarbia-induced vasoconstriction. Steroids have been advocated as treatment to blunt the inflammatory response, to help preserve vascular integrity, and to minimize interstitial edema formation, but there are as yet no controlled trials assessing their benefits [38]. A CT scan of the brain is indicated to assess whether there are any direct cerebral traumatic injuries accounting for neurologic symptoms. The most common finding on head CT in fat embolism syndrome is evidence of diffuse brain edema, as shown by small ventricles and flattened sulci [45]. Areas of decreased attenuation from infarcts appear about 1 week into the course; evidence of cerebral atrophy becomes manifest later [45].

PROGNOSIS. Mortality in fat embolism syndrome can reach 10 to 20 percent; survival for more than 3 or 4 days after the onset of the cerebral fat embolism syndrome portends a good prognosis [40]. Unfortunately, 25 percent of patients experience permanent neurologic deficits [44].

Restoration of normal arterial oxygen levels commonly provides little relief from the CNS signs and symptoms, which usually resolve only 24 to 48 hours after pulmonary manifestations [36,37].

Atropinelike Poisoning

An acute overdose produces a bimodal CNS response of stimulation followed by depression [46]. The hallucinations found in atropine poisoning are usually visual and typically lilliputian but can also be auditory or tactile [47]. Severe overdoses can result in profound CNS depression, with coma, seizures, respiratory failure, and cardiac asystole [46]. Even after ophthalmic administration, clinical manifestations ranging from restlessness, ataxia, and hallucinations to seizures, coma, and death can occur [46,48,49,50]. For further discussion of all aspects of anticholinergic poisoning, including treatment, see Chapter 111.

DIAGNOSIS. Neurologic examination of the patient to determine the level of consciousness should be performed (see Chap. 183), with particular emphasis on the adequacy of respiration and presence of seizures. Dilated pupils, fever, and hot, dry skin in an agitated, confused patient are suggestive of atropinelike poisoning. The differential diagnosis of other toxic and metabolic disorders requires screening with assays of blood determination—glucose, BUN, electrolytes, complete blood count (CBC), and toxicology; an arterial blood gas; and urine for a toxicology screen. Anticholinergic blood level assays are not generally useful in making treatment decisions. Careful monitoring for cardiac arrhythmias, hypertension, and, frequently, hypotension and shock should be carried out.

Hiccough

Hiccough is usually a benign, self-limited condition. Prolonged hiccough can produce fatigue, sleeplessness, weight loss, difficulty in ventilation, and, in postoperative patients, wound dehiscence [51]. In intubated patients, persistent hiccough may result in hyperventilation [52].

PATHOPHYSIOLOGY. Hiccough results from a sudden reflex contraction of the diaphragm that causes forceful inspiration, which is arrested almost immediately by glottic closure, producing the characteristic sound. Afferent pathways include the vagus and phrenic nerves as well as thoracic sympathetic fibers. The efferent pathway includes the phrenic nerve (to the diaphragm), the vagus nerve (to the larynx), and spinal nerves innervating the accessory muscles of inspiration. Central control of this reflex is not well defined but probably involves lower brainstem and possibly upper cervical spinal levels. The central mechanism appears to be separate from the respiratory center [52].

ETIOLOGY. Hiccough most frequently results from irritation of the stomach wall, diaphragm, or phrenic nerve. In nearly one-fourth of cases, surgical therapy of the gastrointestinal or genitourinary tracts, chest, or brain precedes the onset of intractable hiccough. Abdominal disorders causing hiccough include gastric ulceration, gastric distention, hiatus hernia, cholecystitis, peritonitis, subdiaphragmatic abscess, ileus, and bowel obstruction. Thoracic disorders that may precipitate hiccough include esophagitis, pericarditis, myocardial infarction, pneumonia, and neoplasm. Neck masses compressing the phrenic nerve, such as neoplasm and goiter, may also result in hiccough. Brainstem neoplasm or ischemia, multiple sclerosis, and meningoencephalitis are CNS causes. Metabolic disorders, such as uremia, electrolyte disorders, diabetes mellitus, drugs, and toxins, have also been implicated [53]. Some patients have idiopathic or psychogenic hiccoughs.

EVALUATION. A history of gastrointestinal, cardiac, pulmonary, or CNS complaints or surgery may assist in determining the etiology of intractable hiccough. The physical examination should rule out inflammation or neoplasm in the thorax, abdomen, CNS, and neck. Chest and abdominal radiographs should be obtained routinely, and fluoroscopic evaluation of the diaphragm is sometimes needed. Radiographic or endoscopic evaluation of the gastrointestinal tract is sometimes warranted. If the CNS is implicated, cranial CT or magnetic resonance imaging (MRI) may be useful. Computed tomography or

MRI may also be useful if soft tissue lesions of the neck are suspected. Electrocardiography is required. Other investigations include determinations of electrolytes, renal function, glucose, creatine kinase (if myocardial infarction is suspected), and a toxic screen for alcohol and barbiturates. Lumbar puncture is required if there is a suspicion of CNS infection. Electromyography may be useful if surgical therapy for hiccough is contemplated.

MANAGEMENT. Initial management should be directed specifically at treatment of underlying disorders that may cause hiccough, such as inflammation or infection and gastric dilatation. When this is unsuccessful, both pharmacologic and nonpharmacologic treatments are available for intractable hiccough [51,54,55].

Drug therapy should be initiated using chlorpromazine 25 to 50 mg orally or intramuscularly three or four times per day. If this is ineffective in 2 to 3 days, then a slow intravenous infusion of chlorpromazine 25 to 50 mg in 500 to 1000 ml of normal saline is indicated. Although hypotension may result from intravenous administration, chlorpromazine may be most effective by this route [55]. If intravenous chlorpromazine is ineffective, it should be discontinued and 10 mg of metoclopramide given orally four times per day. Other medications used in refractory patients include haloperidol (5 mg three times per day), anticonvulsants (phenytoin, carbamazepine, and valproic acid), lioresal, amitriptyline, nifedipine, and amantadine [54,55].

Nonpharmacologic therapies are directed at altering the reflex arc responsible for hiccough. Mechanical stimulation of the posterior pharynx by the introduction of a red rubber catheter through the nares to a distance of 3 to 4.5 inches, followed by a jerky to-and-fro movement of the catheter, was successful in 84 of 85 patients [51]. Nasogastric intubation and the home remedy, dry granulated sugar taken orally, probably exert their effects by mechanical stimulation of the posterior pharynx as well.

Most patients respond to drug or mechanical therapy. In refractory cases, transcutaneous stimulation of the phrenic nerve [56] or phrenic nerve block or ablation [55] may be useful. However, since there are multiple efferent pathways involved, hiccough may present even after phrenic nerve ablation.

Miscellaneous Neuromuscular Problems in the ICU

CRITICAL ILLNESS POLYNEUROPATHY. A complication of sepsis with multiple organ system failure, critical illness polyneuropathy (CIP) is most commonly seen in patients with sepsis of greater than 2 weeks' duration and is usually suspected when these patients are improving but fail to wean from the ventilator. The incidence may be as high as 50 percent in critically ill septic patients. Clinical features include weakness of respiratory muscles, distal (and, when severe, proximal) limb muscles, reduced or absent deep tendon reflexes, and sensory abnormalities [57]. Mild facial weakness may occur, but other cranial nerve functions are spared. Clinical examination is often difficult because patients with CIP are frequently encephalopathic or sedated. Electrophysiologic studies are remarkable for reduced compound muscle and sensory action potential amplitudes; near normal conduction velocities, distal latencies and F waves; and signs of widespread acute denervation on needle electromyography [58]. The intercostals may also be denervated [57]. The presence of relatively normal conduction velocities

and prominent denervation as well as the normal CSF helps distinguish these patients from those with Guillain-Barré syndrome. Neuromuscular transmission is unaffected. Biopsy and postmortem specimens confirm that the primary pathology is axonal degeneration of motor and sensory nerve fibers with a distal preponderance. Demyelination and inflammation are not seen. Muscle biopsies demonstrate grouped atrophy consistent with denervation [59].

The etiology is unclear. The severity of CIP has not been linked to any particular drug, infectious organism, metabolic derangement (e.g., hypophosphatemia, hypoxemia, renal or liver dysfunction), nutritional deficiency, or use of total parenteral nutrition [60]. Since patients who are most severely ill are most likely to develop CIP, it is probably linked to some other toxic aspect of overwhelming sepsis. Patients who survive their illness recover from CIP over weeks to months [58]. Treatment is aimed at control of the underlying sepsis and supportive treatment of multiple organ failure, maintenance of adequate nutrition, and prevention of compression palsies and contractures through proper nursing technique and early physical therapy.

COMPRESSION NEUROPATHIES. Compression neuropathies are common in the general population. In the ICU population several nerves are particularly at risk, compression of which may result in delayed morbidity. The ulnar nerve may be compressed in the condylar groove posterior to the medial epicondyle when the arms are positioned in a flexed, pronated, or semipronated fashion or when the flexed elbows are used by the patient for repositioning. Ulnar palsy causes weakness of the intrinsic muscles of the hand as well as numbness of the fourth and fifth fingers. The peroneal nerve is also at risk as it courses around the fibular head. The everted immobile position of the leg in severely weak or paralyzed patients contributes to its vulnerability. Proper positioning of the limbs to avoid compression of these nerves between the bed and bony prominences is key to prevention. Other compression neuropathies and brachial plexopathy may result from positions assumed during prolonged coma prior to hospitalization. Hematomas resulting from clotting disorders, anticoagulation, local injection, arterial puncture, or phlebotomy may also compress the peripheral nerves and plexi.

NEUROMUSCULAR BLOCKERS. Neuromuscular blockers are frequently used in the ICU to facilitate intubation and mechanical ventilation. There are two main types: depolarizing agents (succinylcholine) and nondepolarizing competitive blocking agents (curarelike).

Succinylcholine is a short-acting agent that acts like acetylcholine (ACh) by binding to the acetylcholine receptor (ACh-R), resulting in membrane depolarization. This action is more sustained than that caused by ACh due to the prolonged presence of the drug on the ACh-R, since the drug is less rapidly hydrolyzed by plasma cholinesterase than is acetylcholine by acetylcholinesterase. Hydrolysis of succinylcholine may be decreased in patients with atypical plasma cholinesterase and in patients with decreased plasma cholinesterase (liver disease, pregnancy), resulting in prolonged neuromuscular blockade. Membrane depolarization by succinylcholine is accompanied by transient muscle fasciculations and a rise in extracellular potassium [61]. This may result in symptomatic hyperkalemia in patients who have developed an excess of ACh-R due to injury, including those with burns, crush injury, diffuse neuropathy, and spinal cord and other upper motor neuron injuries. Upregulation of the ACh-R may occur within a few days of the

Table 191-1. Characteristics of Neuromuscular Blocking Agents [61]

Drug characteristics	Succinylcholine	d-Tubocurarine	Pancuronium	Vecuronium	Atacurium
Route(s) of excretion	Plasma, cholinesterase	Kidney, liver	Kidney, liver	Liver, kidney	Hydrolysis
Onset (minutes)	1–5	5	3–4	<3	2–3
Duration of action (minutes)	<15	90	90	30–45	30–45
Cardiovascular effects	Bradycardia	Hypotension	Tachycardia, hypertension, increased cardiac output	None	Hypotension, tachycardia
Other	Fasciculations, myalgias, increased K^+	Potent histamine releaser			Histamine releaser

original injury and may persist for years, depending on the type of injury [62]. Succinylcholine also causes malignant hyperthermia in susceptible patients and may cause increased intracranial pressure, increased intraocular pressure, and bradycardia.

The nondepolarizing agents are often used for more sustained neuromuscular blockade in the ICU. These agents act by competitive blockade of the ACh-R and generally produce no CNS effects. The agents should be selected based on drug and patient characteristics and used in sedated patients. Table 191-1 outlines pertinent drug characteristics that aid in their selection. Patient considerations include weight; presence of cardiac, renal or hepatic dysfunction; presence of trauma or nervous system injury; and age. Dosage should be based on lean body weight in obese patients, since the drugs are only slightly lipid-soluble. For patients with significant cardiac problems or renal failure, vecuronium is the drug of choice. In patients with renal and hepatic failure atracurium is the drug of choice, although a metabolite possessing CNS stimulant properties may accumulate in patients with renal failure who are treated more than 24 hours [63]. Patients with burns, trauma, upper or lower motor neuron injuries, chronic anticonvulsant use, or chronic use of nondepolarizing blockers develop increased numbers of ACh-Rs and relative resistance to these medications. In diseases that affect the neuromuscular junction (myasthenia gravis, Lambert-Eaton myasthenic syndrome, organophosphate poisoning) there may be a marked increase in sensitivity to the nondepolarizing blockers. In contrast, myasthenics are resistant to the depolarizing blockers [61]. Neuromuscular blocking agents frequently have a prolonged duration in the elderly, due to their reduced renal and hepatic function. Aminoglycosides and other drugs administered concurrently may also prolong the duration of nondepolarizing blockers.

In ICU patients excessive dose, advanced age, and presence of neuromuscular junction or renal or hepatic dysfunction may result in prolonged neuromuscular blockade. The nondepolarizing blockers can be partially reversed with cholinesterase inhibitors (e.g., pyridostigmine), which may aid in discriminating between prolonged neuromuscular blockade and alternatives such as neuropathies or severe CNS dysfunction.

References

1. McHugh TP, Stout M: Near-hanging injury. *Ann Emerg Med* 12:774, 1983.
2. Campbell W, Cantrill S: Neck injuries, in Rosen P (ed): *Emergency Medicine, Concepts and Clinical Practice.* 2nd ed. St. Louis, CV Mosby, 1988, p 419.
3. Scheider R, Livingston K, Cave A, et al: "Hangman's fracture" of the cervical spine. *J Neurosurg* 22:141, 1965.
4. Garfin S, Rothman R: Traumatic spondylolisthesis of the axis (hangman's fracture), in Bailey R (ed): *The Cervical Spine.* Philadelphia, JB Lippincott, 1983, p 223.
5. Berlyne N, Strachan M: Neuropsychiatric sequelae of attempted hanging. *Br J Psychiatry* 114:411, 1968.
6. Calvanese J, Spohr M, Nevada R: Hyperthermia from a near hanging. *Ann Emerg Med* 113:152, 1982.
7. Levine A, Edwards C: The management of traumatic spondylolisthesis of the axis. *J Bone Joint Surg* 67A:217, 1985.
8. Francis W, Fielding J, Hawkins R, et al: Traumatic spondylolisthesis of the axis. *J Bone Joint Surg* 63B:313, 1981.
9. Eddendi B, Roy D, Cornish B, et al: Fractures of the ring of the axis. *J Bone Joint Surg* 63B:319, 1981.
10. Apfelberg DB, Masters FW, Robinson DW: Pathophysiology and treatment of electrical injuries. *J Trauma* 14:453, 1974.
11. Solem L, Fischer RP, Strate RG: The natural history of electrical injury. *J Trauma* 17:487, 1977.
12. Jensen PJ, Thomsen PEB, Bagger JP, et al: Electrical injury causing ventricular arrhythmias. *Br Heart J* 57:279, 1987.
13. Pause F: Electrical lesions of the nervous system, in Vinken PJ, Bruyn GW (eds): *Handbook of Clinical Neurology.* vol. 7. New York, Elsevier, 1970, p 344.
14. Farrell DF, Starr A: Delayed neurological sequelae of electrical injuries. *Neurology* 18:601, 1968.
15. Silversides J: The neurological sequelae of electrical injury. *Can Med Assoc J* 91:195, 1964.
16. Amy BW, McManus WF, Goodwin CW, et al: Lightning injury with survival in five patients. *JAMA* 253:243, 1985.
17. Hunt JL, McManus WF, Haney WP, et al: Vascular lesions in acute electric injuries. *J Trauma* 14:461, 1974.
18. Bryson P: Carbon monoxide, in Bryson P (ed): *Comprehensive Review of Toxicology.* 2nd ed. Rockville, MD, Aspen, 1989, p 223.
19. Prete MR, Litovitz T: Carbon monoxide, in Edlich R, Spyker D (eds): *Current Emergency Therapy '84.* Norwalk, CT, Appleton-Century-Crofts, 1984, p 706.
20. Goldfrank L, Lewin N, Kirstein R, et al: Carbon monoxide, in Goldfrank L, Flomenbaum N, Lewin N, et al (eds): *Goldfrank's Toxicologic Emergencies.* 3rd ed. Norwalk, CT, Appleton-Century-Crofts, 1986, p 662.
21. Ginsburg R, Romano J: Carbon monoxide encephalopathy: Need for appropriate treatment. *Am J Psychiatry* 133:317, 1976.
22. Gozal D, Ziser A, Shupak A, et al: Accidental carbon monoxide poisoning. *Clin Pediatr* 24:132, 1985.
23. Dinerman N, Huber J: Inhalation injuries, in Rosen P (ed): *Emergency Medicine: Concepts and Clinical Practice.* 2nd ed. St. Louis, CV Mosby, 1988, p 585.
24. Remick R, Miles J: Carbon monoxide poisoning: Neurologic and psychiatric sequelae. *Can Med Assoc J* 117:654, 1977.
25. Garland H, Pearce J: Neurological complications of carbon monoxide poisoning. *Q J Med* 36:445, 1967.
26. Choi I: Delayed neurologic sequelae in carbon monoxide intoxication. *Arch Neurol* 40:433, 1983.
27. Min SK: A brain syndrome associated with delayed neuropsychiatric sequelae following acute carbon monoxide intoxication. *Acta Psychiatr Scand* 73:80, 1986.
28. Hallenbeck JM, Bove AA, Elliott DH: Mechanisms underlying spinal cord damage in decompression sickness. *Neurology* 25:308, 1975.

29. Gorman DF: Decompression sickness and arterial gas embolism in sports scuba divers. *Sports Med* 8:32, 1989.

30. Cockett ATK, Pauley SM, Zehl DN, et al: Pathophysiology of bends and decompression sickness. *Arch Surg* 114:296, 1979.

31. Rivera JC: Decompression sickness among divers: An analysis of 935 cases. *Mil Medicine* 129:314, 1964.

32. Harding RM, Mills FJ: Problems of altitude. II. Decompression sickness and other effects of pressure changes. *Br Med J* 286:1, 1983.

33. Adkisson GH, Hodgson M, Smith F, et al: Cerebral perfusion deficits in dysbaric illness. *Lancet* 2:119, 1989.

34. Wilmshunst PT, Byrne JC, Webb-Peploc MM: Neurological decompression sickness (letter). *Lancet* 1:731, 1989.

35. Schwartz GR: Trauma from environmental pressure alterations (diving and altitude emergencies), in Schwartz GR (ed): *Principles and Practice of Emergency Medicine*. Philadelphia, WB Saunders, 1986, p 1586.

36. Findlay JM, DeMajo W: Cerebral fat embolism. *Can Med Assoc J* 131:755, 1984.

37. Jacobson D, Terrence C, Reinmuth O: The neurologic manifestations of fat embolism. *Neurology* 36:847, 1986.

38. Gossling H, Pellegrini V Jr: Fat embolism syndrome. *Clin Orthop* 165:68, 1982.

39. Schonfeld S, Ploysongsang Y, Diligio R, et al: Fat embolism prophylaxis with corticosteroids. *Ann Intern Med* 99:438, 1983.

40. Thomas J, Ayyar DR: Systemic fat embolism. *Arch Neurol* 26:517, 1972.

41. Oh W, Mital M: Fat embolism: Current concepts of pathogenesis, diagnosis and treatment. *Orthop Clin North Am* 9:769, 1978.

42. Dines D, Burgher L, Okazaki H: The clinical and pathologic correlation of fat embolism syndrome. *Mayo Clin Proc* 50:407, 1975.

43. Peltier L: Fat embolism, in Schwartz G (ed): *Principles and Practice of Emergency Medicine*. Philadelphia, WB Saunders, 1986, p 1589.

44. Kamenar E, Burger P: Cerebral fat embolism: A neuropathological study of a microembolic state. *Stroke* 11:477, 1980.

45. Miller J: Fat embolism: A clinical diagnosis. *Am Fam Physician* 35:129, 1987.

46. Bryson P: Anticholinergic drugs and plant alkaloids, in Bryson P (ed): *Comprehensive Review of Toxicology*. 2nd ed. Rockville, MD, Aspen, 1989, p 75.

47. Goldfrank L, Lewin N, Flomenbaum N, et al: Antidepressants: Tricyclics, tetracyclics, monamine oxidase inhibitors, and other monoxides, in Goldfrank L, Flomenbaum N, Lewin N, et al (eds): *Goldfrank's Toxicologic Emergencies*. 3rd ed. Norwalk, CT, Appleton-Century-Crofts, 1986, p 351.

48. Oderda G: Anticholinergics, in Edlich R, Spyker D (eds): *Current Emergency Therapy '84*. Norwalk, CT, Appleton-Century-Crofts, 1984, p 690.

49. O'Connor P, Mumma J: Atropine toxicity. *Am J Ophthalmol* 99:613, 1985.

50. Epstein F, Eilers M: Poisoning-anticholinergic poisoning, in Rosen P (ed): *Emergency Medicine Concepts and Clinical Practice*. 2nd ed. St. Louis, CV Mosby, 1988, p 350.

51. Salem MR, Baraka A, Rattenborg CC, et al: Treatment of hiccups by pharyngeal stimulation in anesthetized and conscious subjects. *JAMA* 202:126, 1967.

52. Davis JN: An experimental study of hiccup. *Brain* 93:851, 1970.

53. Souadjian JV, Cain JC: Intractable hiccup: Etiologic factors in 220 cases. *Postgrad Med* 43:72, 1968.

54. Lipsky MS: Chronic hiccups. *Am Fam Physician* 34:173, 1986.

55. Williamson BWA, MacIntyre IMC: Management of intractable hiccup. *Br Med J* 2:501, 1977.

56. Aravot DJ, et al: Noninvasive phrenic nerve stimulation for intractable hiccups (letter). *Lancet* 2:1047, 1989.

57. Bolton CF: The peripheral nervous system: Effects of sepsis and critical illness. *Ann R Coll Phys Surg Can* 19:371, 1986.

58. Bolton CF: Electrophysiologic studies of critically ill patients: *Muscle and Nerve* 10:129, 1987.

59. Zochodne DW, Bolton CF, Wells GA, et al: Critical illness polyneuropathy: A complication of sepsis and multiple organ failure. *Brain* 110:819, 1987.

60. Zochodne DW, Bolton CF, Wells GA, et al: Polyneuropathy in critical illness: Analysis of etiologic factors. *Can J Neurol Sci* 12:177, 1985.

61. Larijani GE, Gratz I, Silverberg M, et al: Clinical pharmacology of the neuromuscular blocking agents. *DICP* 25:54, 1991.

62. Martyn JAJ, White DA, Gronert GA, et al: Up-and-down regulation of skeletal muscle acetylcholine receptors. *Anesthesiology* 76:822, 1992.

192. Subarachnoid Hemorrhage

John P. Weaver, Daniel Hanley,
Dimitar Danchev, and Marc Fisher

Introduction

Intracranial hemorrhage secondary to the rupture of saccular aneurysms accounts for 6 to 8 percent of all strokes and is responsible for nearly two-thirds of subarachnoid hemorrhages (SAHs). Intracranial aneurysms are found in approximately 1 percent of the population at autopsy and rupture at a rate of 4 to 10 per 100,000 per year, with a 25 percent mortality during the first 24 hours. Fifty percent of patients die within the first 3 months of the initial event, and 50 percent of the survivors are left with significant neurologic impairment. The mortality and morbidity associated with SAH are significant despite modern medical and surgical management, with extensive disability, lost productivity and expensive rehabilitation and chronic care. Intensive care medical and surgical intervention is necessary in the management of these cases [1–4].

Subarachnoid hemorrhage represents the most treatable form of stroke. Since the mid-1970s substantial changes have occurred in all aspects of the care of this disease. Current acute care management includes early surgery to limit rebleeding, a calcium antagonist to ameliorate cerebral injury secondary to vasospasm, volume replacement, and some form of circulatory manipulation (regional or global).

Extensive efforts at multiple centers have led to improvements in functional outcome. New treatment issues in the areas of cerebral protection, interventional neuroradiology, cerebrospinal fluid (CSF) manipulation, and cardiocirculatory control are reviewed here.

Pathogenesis

Saccular, or berry, aneurysms must be distinguished from other types of intracerebral aneurysms, such as traumatic, dissecting, mycotic, and tumor-related aneurysms. Saccular aneurysms are characterized by a vascular wall lacking the normal muscular media and elastic lamina layers. Normal intracerebral vessels have a prominent muscular media layer, although the external elastic lamina is found only in extracranial vessels [5]. Eighty-five percent of saccular aneurysms are located in the anterior circulation and 15 percent are along the posterior circulation vessels [6]. Common sites for aneurysms are at the junction of the anterior cerebral and anterior communicating arteries, the junction of the posterior communicating and internal carotid arteries, the middle cerebral artery trifurcation, the bifurcation of the internal carotid into middle and anterior cerebral arteries, and at the top of the basilar artery. Some 12 to 31 percent of patients have multiple aneurysms. Nine to 19 percent have aneurysms located at identical sites bilaterally, and multiple aneurysms may occur within families [7]. Systemic diseases, such as polycystic kidney, Marfan's syndrome, Ehlers-Danlos syndrome, pseudoxanthoma elasticum, fibromuscular dysplasia, and coarctation of the aorta, are associated with an increased incidence of intracerebral aneurysms [8].

The pathogenesis of aneurysms and subsequent rupture is uncertain. Central to this controversy are the questions of whether aneurysms are congenital or acquired and to what extent environmental factors are involved. Support for a congenital origin comes from the frequency of multiple aneurysms, familial occurrence of aneurysms, and association of aneurysms with arteriovenous malformations and other systemic inherited disease. Alternatively, the degenerative theory is supported by the increased frequency of aneurysms with age, hypertension, and atherosclerosis. Furthermore, pathologic specimens reveal intimal changes, calcification, and thrombosis within aneurysms. No theory of saccular aneurysm formation and rupture has been uniformly accepted [9].

Symptoms

The signs and symptoms of intracranial aneurysms result from their expansion or rupture. Aneurysmal expansion can lead to localized headache, facial pain, pupillary dilatation from compression of the pupilloconstrictor fibers of the oculomotor nerve, and visual field defects. Aneurysmal rupture typically produces severe headache, back pain, nausea, and vomiting; photophobia and lethargy are also common. At the time of rupture, 45 percent of patients lose consciousness, reflecting the acute rise in intracranial pressure that may transiently equal or exceed mean arterial pressure [10]. The elevation of intracranial pressure may result in an abducens nerve palsy. In some cases, funduscopy demonstrates subhyaloid retinal hemorrhages and papilledema. Other symptoms, such as paresis, paresthesias, aphasia, visual hallucinations, vertigo, and ataxia, may also develop. Following SAH, 26 percent of patients experience seizures, the majority occurring shortly after bleeding. The occurrence of seizures has no relationship to the location of the aneurysm or the patient's prognosis and may reflect an acute rise in intracranial pressure [11,12].

CLINICAL GRADING AND PROGNOSIS. The clinical grading scale developed by Hunt and Hess is useful in correlating the patient's clinical status with prognosis (Table 192-1) [13]. Changes in grade during the clinical course are also helpful in following the patient. Patients who are grade I or II at presentation have a relatively good prognosis, whereas grade IV or V

Table 192-1. Hunt and Hess Subarachnoid Hemorrhage Grading Scale

Grade I	Asymptomatic or minimal headache and slight nuchal rigidity
Grade II	Moderate to severe headache, nuchal rigidity, no neurologic deficit other than cranial nerve palsy
Grade III	Drowsiness, confusion, or mild focal deficit
Grade IV	Stupor, moderate to severe hemiparesis, possibly early decerebrate rigidity and vegetative disturbances
Grade V	Deep coma, decerebrate rigidity, moribund appearance

Serious systemic diseases such as hypertension, diabetes, severe arteriosclerosis, chronic obstructive pulmonary disease, and severe vasospasm result in placement of the patient in the next less favorable category.

patients have a poor prognosis, and grade III patients are intermediate.

Diagnostic Evaluation

The initial investigation if SAH is suspected should be a noncontrast head computed tomography (CT) scan to identify, localize, and quantify the bleeding. A lumbar puncture is indicated if CT scanning is nondiagnostic or unavailable. The estimates of CT scan sensitivity for subarachnoid hemorrhage vary with the series, but it may be negative in as many as 35 percent of patients with a "warning leak" or sentinel hemorrhage [14].

If the CSF is examined at least 2 hours after the initial hemorrhage, it will be xanthochromic; all specimens should be spun down and examined carefully against white paper in comparison to a tube of water. Cell counts remain uniform in all of the tubes of CSF in a true SAH. Protein may be elevated and glucose may be very slightly depressed. Opening pressure at the time of lumbar puncture may reflect the elevation of intracranial pressure.

Repeat CT scanning with contrast enhancement can identify the source of bleeding for aneurysms larger than 5 mm, but this is rarely indicated since cerebral arteriography is necessary to localize the lesion, define the vascular anatomy, and assess the degree of vasospasm. A four-vessel angiogram is essential due to the frequency of multiple aneurysms and should be performed within 24 to 48 hours after admission if early surgery is contemplated. If angiography does not reveal an aneurysm, it may be repeated in 2 to 3 weeks, as vasospasm of the parent vessel or intraluminal thrombus can occasionally interfere with angiographic visualization of aneurysms [15].

General Medical Management

The complications of SAH are fatal in 25 percent of cases [16]. General medical management should include provisions for quiet bed rest with the head of the bed elevated at 30 degrees to improve cerebral venous return. Good pulmonary toilet is essential to avoid atelectasis and pneumonia. Bed rest requires prophylaxis against thrombophlebitis with pneumatic boots. All patients should receive stool softeners. Nausea and vomiting should be controlled with antiemetics, such as hydroxyzine or trimethobenzamide. Pain control is best accomplished with agents such as codeine or meperidine, so as not to mask mental status changes. Systolic blood pressures greater than 180 mm Hg should be lowered gently, but agents that can depress consciousness, such as alphamethyl dopa, should be avoided. Blood pressure is managed with beta-blockers, agents that may also reduce the risk of cardiac arrhythmias.

A manifestation of hypothalamic dysfunction is the syndrome of inappropriate antidiuretic hormone with resultant hyponatremia. After subarachnoid hemorrhage there may be a salt-wasting diuresis due to an increase in circulating atrial natriuretic peptide levels. Accordingly, fluid input and output must be followed closely, along with serum electrolytes and osmolarity [17]. Sedation, if necessary, can be induced with diazepam or low doses (30–60 mg every 8 hours) of phenobarbital, which will also serve as an anticonvulsant. Phenytoin is the preferred anticonvulsant, especially in patients who have suffered a seizure, as it does not alter the level of consciousness. Elevation of intracranial pressure must be treated promptly with agents such as mannitol and furosemide. The utility of dexamethasone in these cases remains controversial, but it is often administered to patients with progressive increases in intracranial pressure and to treat headache due to meningeal irritation.

Cardiac Function After Subarachnoid Hemorrhage

Hypothalamic dysfunction leads to cardiac dysrhythmias due to excessive sympathetic stimulation in 20 percent of SAH cases. The increased levels of circulating catecholamines influence the alpha-receptors of the myocardium and can result in prolonged myofibril contraction, eventually causing myofibrillar degeneration and necrosis. An alternative theory suggests that coronary artery spasm is the mechanism for the myocytolysis. Subarachnoid hemorrhage is the most frequent neurologic cause for electrocardiographic (ECG) changes: large upright T waves and prolonged Q–T intervals (on average about 0.53 seconds). In addition, prominent U waves, inverted T waves, and minor elevation or depression of the S–T segment can occur. Pathologic Q waves are not common and suggest myocardial infarction. Arrhythmias are very common. A prospective study of 120 patients performed using 24-hour Holter monitoring indicated a 90 percent incidence of ventricular and supraventricular arrhythmias in the first 48 hours of hospitalization [18]. These do not appear to account for significant mortality.

The issue of diagnosing ischemic cardiac disease in the SAH victim is complex and would benefit from further study. Most case series suggest a low incidence of ischemia despite ST–T changes [19,20]. These changes do not consistently correlate with elevated cardiac enzymes or focal dyskinetic segments on echocardiography; they seem to correlate more closely with severity of the neurologic insult. A potentially nonbenign subgroup of patients has been reported who may have primary coronary vasospasm; the determinants and mechanism of this phenomenon are not clear [21].

Cardiac complications of SAH therapy do occur and are important to recognize. Congestive heart failure is common when hypervolemic hypertensive therapy is aggressively used. The role the calcium antagonist nimodipine plays in this complication is not clear from the clinical data, but the known negative inotropic action of this class of drugs would argue for an important interaction. Cardiac complications have also been reported by Spetzler and Solomon after hypothermic cardiac arrest [24,53]. The cause of these cardiac and pulmonary complications could be the circulatory arrest or may be additive to the stress response that accompanies the patient's SAH.

Neurologic Complications

Rebleeding from aneurysmal rerupture, cerebral vasospasm with ischemia, and hydrocephalus are the three major neurologic complications following SAH.

Rebleeding is a serious and frequent neurologic complication of SAH. One-third of patients rebleed in the first month and 50 percent within 6 months if the aneurysm is not treated surgically. One-half to two-thirds of patients die at the time of rebleeding. The peak incidence of rebleeding occurs during the first day after SAH; a secondary peak occurs 1 week later. Clinically, rebleeding presents with increasing headache, nausea, vomiting, depressed level of consciousness, and the appearance of new neurologic deficits. Occasionally, seizures occur, but they are the result and not the cause of rebleeding. Rebleeding is postulated to be due to breakdown of the perianeurysmal clot [2].

Clot formation and tissue damage stimulate fibrinolytic activity in the CSF [2]. This process underlies the rationale for the use of antifibrinolytic agents to prevent rebleeding. These agents retard clot lysis by inhibiting the formation of proteolytic enzymes and reduce the concentration of fibrin degradation products in the CSF. The two antifibrinolytic agents currently available are epsilon aminocaproic acid and tranexamic acid. These agents reduce the risk of rebleeding but are associated with an increased risk of deep venous thrombosis, pulmonary embolism, and delayed cerebral ischemia. The use of epsilon aminocaproic acid as a means of preventing secondary hemorrhage is controversial and generally reserved for patients in whom surgery is to be delayed. Antifibrinolytic therapy is not administered to patients undergoing early surgery or those at high risk of vasospasm. In any patient with clinical or angiographic evidence of vasospasm, antifibrinolytic agents should be immediately discontinued. The delayed fibrinolysis of clots surrounding arteries at the base of the brain may account for the increased incidence of vasospasm and stroke associated with the use of these drugs. Attempts to prevent rebleeding by drug-induced hypotension and bed rest have not been successful [22–26].

A major cause of morbidity and mortality in patients recovering from SAH is cerebral vasospasm. This term implies delayed cerebral ischemia, but many patients are asymptomatic despite various degrees of arterial narrowing on the cerebral arteriogram; the role of actual spasm in the pathogenesis of ischemia is debated [23]. Unlike rebleeding, the clinical presentation of vasospasm occurs slowly over hours to days. Although it is noted angiographically in 70 percent of patients, it is symptomatic in only 36 percent [27]. This difference probably reflects the adequacy of collateral circulation in the individual patient as well as the degree of spasm. Delayed cerebral ischemic events are usually first noted on the third day after hemorrhage and peak between days 4 and 12. Unfortunately, the problem may occur as long as 3 weeks after SAH [2,4]. The neurologic deficits are correlated with the areas of brain supplied by the narrowed arteries. Although spasm is currently identified by angiography, it may also be identified noninvasively using transcranial Doppler techniques [28].

The amount of blood in the subarachnoid space and its location predict the degree and location of delayed cerebral ischemic events. In theory, the pathogenesis of spasm is related to local erythrocyte breakdown products that may be spasmogenic. Potential inducers of spasm include oxyhemoglobin, angiotensin, histamine, serotonin, prostaglandin, and catecholamines [4]. Vasospasm may occur because of structural changes in the arterial wall, rather than muscle contraction. The mechanism of arterial wall changes might be an inflammatory response, depression of vessel wall respiration, or damage from prolonged active arterial wall contraction. Other theories include impairment of normal vasodilatation, the mechanical effects of arterial compression by clot, and development of a proliferative vasculopathy. There are secondary disturbances of cerebral autoregulation noted at the microcirculatory level as well. Pathologic specimens of affected vessels demonstrate intimal proliferation and medial necrosis [29]. Thus, the pathogenesis of cerebral vasospasm is a complicated, multifactorial process. Vasospasm occurs more frequently in patients with a poor clinical grade or early cortical enhancement on contrast head CT scans. Patients with thick focal blood clots or a diffuse layer of blood in the subarachnoid space are also at high risk for vasospasm.

Hydrocephalus may develop acutely within the first 24 hours after bleeding, due to blood within the basal cisterns or ventricular system causing obstruction of CSF outflow. Ventricular drainage may be indicated in some cases. Hydrocephalus developing subacutely over a few days following SAH is manifested clinically by the loss of vertical gaze and progressive lethargy. Patients may appear to be abulic. Although treatment is CSF drainage, there is a danger of rebleeding of an untreated aneurysm, which is associated with abrupt decreases in intracranial pressure (ICP). Therefore, diuresis is often attempted before ventricular drainage. A delayed form of hydrocephalus manifested by disorders of gait may be observed several weeks after SAH; in these cases, a ventriculoperitoneal shunt may be indicated [4].

Hyperdynamic Therapy

Circulatory manipulation has for some time been a potential treatment for regional cerebral ischemia; it appears we are now closer to realizing clinical benefit with predictable frequency [30,31]. Although there is no proved treatment for cerebral vasospasm, the current mainstay of therapy is hypervolemic-hypertensive-hemodilution therapy. The aim of this therapy is to augment cerebral perfusion pressure by raising systolic blood pressure, cardiac output, and intravascular volume. Progress in this area has been predominantly in the area of small cohort studies of intermediate variables, cerebral blood flow (CBF), and systemic blood volume. Muizelaar and others have demonstrated that elevation of systemic arterial pressure produces a significant increase in the regional cerebral blood flow [32,33,34]. Typically an elevation of mean arterial pressure (MAP) of 20 to 30 mm Hg produces an increase of CBF from 15 to 25 ml/min/100 gm. Additionally demonstrated is the ability of volume augmentation to prevent the otherwise predictable loss of circulating blood volume in the SAH patient and provide subsequent hemodilution, which leads to improvement in cerebral microcirculation due to decreased viscosity [35]. Inotropic drugs, such as dopamine and dobutamine, are used to keep systolic blood pressures 20 to 40 points over pretreatment levels, and plasma volume is expanded with albumin, hetastarch, or plasmanate. Hematocrit is maintained around 30 percent. This therapy is continued for 48 to 72 hours, then gradually withdrawn under close observation for recurrent

vasospasm. Risks of therapy include myocardial infarction, congestive heart failure, dysrhythmias, hemorrhagic infarcts, rebleeding, hyponatremia, and hemothorax. This treatment is essentially reserved for the postoperative period due to the risks of aneurysmal reruption before surgery [36]. Early surgery and careful cardiac monitoring for congestive heart failure appear to be necessary for the prevention of significant complications. Selection criteria include increasing blood flow velocity signals by transcranial Doppler measurement (TCD), focal deficit, and global impairment of consciousness without hydrocephalus. However, a precise delineation of the selection criteria for blood volume and blood pressure augmentation remains to be tested in an outcome study, and a clinically useful algorithm for blood pressure management in the presence of progressive vasospasm is needed.

Calcium Antagonists

Several controlled studies have shown an important role for the calcium antagonist nimodipine in ameliorating neurologic deficits caused by delayed vasospasm. While the original hypothesis suggested a vascular mechanism, it now appears that the beneficial activity of this drug is in the decrease of neuronal intracellular calcium, which is elevated following injury [37]. Recent investigations revealed that calcium influx plays a major role in the process of neuronal death after ischemia [38,39,40].

The neurologic outcome and mortality rates of SAH victims prophylactically treated with 4 mg/kg/day nimodipine are improved 25 to 50 percent over controls. Fewer infarcts are noted in these patients, although there is no difference in the incidence or extent of arteriographic vasospasm [41]. Adverse drug effects are minimal and include mild transient hypotension lasting less than 1 hour. By contrast, verapamil, nifedipine, and diltiazem have less lipid solubility, are not capable of crossing the blood-brain barrier, and do not produce a cerebral protective effect. Nicardipine has also been tested in studies of SAH, but preliminary reports do not suggest a beneficial effect despite its availability as an intravenous preparation [42]. Whether this apparent differential benefit is a function of inadequate brain tissue levels associated with greater lipid solubility or another factor remains to be demonstrated. Calcium channel blocking agents dilate leptomeningeal vessels and may exert a beneficial effect by improving collateral circulation to ischemic areas, improving erythrocyte deformability or exerting an antiplatelet aggregating effect [24]. Current recommendations are to administer 60 mg of nimodipine orally every 4 hours for a 21-day course beginning at the onset of SAH. The long-term efficacy of this therapy for vasospasm is still to be determined.

Surgical Management

The appropriate timing for surgical intervention is less controversial than just a few years ago. Patients with a grade IV to V presentation are rarely candidates for intracranial clip ligation. In patients of a better grade who are radiographically free of vasospasm, acute or emergent operative intervention is advocated as a means of inhibiting the processes that induce rebleeding and vasospasm [43,44,45]. Following acute angiography, patients with a grade I to III presentation should in most instances undergo microsurgical clip ligation via craniotomy.

Current intracranial management necessitates craniotomy for clip occlusion of the aneurysmal neck, using systemic intraoperative hypotension and microsurgical techniques [46–49]. Unique problems that dictate the use of specialized techniques include vertebral-basilar system aneurysms [47], giant aneurysms (>25 mm), and multiple aneurysms. Aneurysms with sessile or nonpedunculated bases may require external reinforcement techniques [50,51]. Moreover, some giant aneurysms or aneurysms in which the major contributing vessels are not part of the aneurysmal stalk can be isolated from the intracerebral circulation with antecedent superficial temporal artery-middle cerebral artery or other microvascular bypass techniques. Common carotid ligation [27,52] may still be an effective way to reduce intraaneurysmal pressure and reduce the occurrence of subsequent hemorrhage in certain aneurysms (e.g., internal carotid-posterior communicating).

Hypothermia and Intraoperative Cerebral Protection

Hypothermia is a well-known cytoprotective strategy used in cardiac surgery. Recent animal work has demonstrated that moderate drops in brain temperature are associated with decreased concentrations of tissue neurotransmitters that would otherwise promote injury. In addition, the cerebral metabolic rate of oxygen uptake ($CMRO_2$) decreases as temperature falls: below 28°C cerebral electrical activity is minimal, as is further reduction of $CMRO_2$. Lower temperatures may have advantages in protecting other body tissues where the temperature dependence of metabolic rate has a wider range [38]. Because cardiac standstill is helpful for the atraumatic reconstruction of giant aneurysms, the value of hypothermia has been investigated in several groups of these patients.

Spetzler et al. used deep hypothermia (22–18°C) with a short (10–15 minutes) circulatory arrest [53]. This is brought about with femoral arterial/venous exchange transfusion of up to 4 liters of iced saline. Barbiturate anesthesia is also administered. Previous bleeding disorders, predisposition to hemorrhage, and prior cardiopulmonary disease are all relative contraindications to deep hypothermia. Pooled data from recent series suggest that this remains a high-morbidity procedure, with less than 50 percent of patients achieving a good outcome. Reported complications include postoperative hemorrhage, deep vein thrombophlebitis, and pulmonary embolism. The threshold for developing intraoperative ischemia to brain, heart, and kidneys is unclear, as are effective monitoring mechanisms.

Thrombolysis of the Subarachnoid Space

The presence of hemoglobin in the cranial subarachnoid space produces a histologic and arteriographic picture consistent with vasospasm. Furthermore, the severity of spasm/ischemia appears to relate to the amount of blood in the CSF space. Thus, there is significant interest in removing this spasmogen from the pial space. Initial work by Findlay and Weir demonstrated that application of the thrombolytic agent tissue plasminogen activator (t-PA) enhances the clearance of clotted blood from the pial space. An effect of treatment timing was also noted, with the arteriographic spasm syndrome being preventable if the t-PA is administered in the initial 24 hours after bleeding [55]. A drop in resistance to CSF outflow has been noted after experimental treatment with t-PA [54]. Thus, animal experi-

ments strongly suggested that the human vasospasm syndrome might be ameliorated by lysis of clot in the CSF space.

Human phase I studies have demonstrated that similar clearing of the human subpial space can be accomplished. Arteriographic follow-up study suggests that removal of hemoglobin/clot from the CSF space is associated with a decreased incidence of arteriographic vasospasm [56]. To date, the use of t-PA has been reported in 109 patients, with one hemorrhagic death due to an epidural hematoma and four nonfatal cases of epidural and intracerebral hematoma, as well as one extradural hematoma [55,56].

Postoperative Management

If intraoperative angiography was unavailable, then follow-up care includes angiography to assess the position of the clip, confirm the successful occlusion of the aneurysm, and determine the patency of surrounding vessels [57]. The patient is usually discharged from the ICU when the risk of vasospasm has passed, the aneurysm has been surgically obliterated, and other urgent medical problems have been successfully treated. The control of protracted elevation of intracranial pressure may require continuing use of pressure monitoring systems, and the requirements of continuing hypervolemic-hypertensive therapy for postoperative vasospasm dictate the continuing use of central venous pressure monitoring.

Free Radical Scavengers in Subarachnoid Hemorrhage

The large amount of blood deposited in the basal cisterns by subarachnoid hemorrhage undergoes degradation with release of free iron. Because this iron can catalyze free radical reactions, including lipid peroxidation, the role of this process in producing vasospasm and neural injury has been investigated. Animal studies suggest that the 21-aminosteroid inhibition of lipid peroxidation has the benefit of reducing delayed vasospasm [58]. A single human study using another potential free radical scavenging agent, nizofenone, has further promoted this suggestion. Ohta et al. treated 208 patients in a controlled manner and demonstrated improvement based on functional recovery [59], especially in patients with delayed ischemic symptoms, moderate severity of preoperative deficits (grade II or III presentation), and diffuse high-density areas in pre- and postoperative CT scans.

The 21-aminosteroid U74006F-tirilazad mesylate has been shown to inhibit lipid peroxidation and protect cell membranes by scavenging destructive free radicals, similar to vitamin E. A major North American study is underway investigating the combined use of U74006F and nimodipine in prevention of cerebral vasospasm after SAH compared to nimodipine alone [60].

Advances in Neuroradiologic Techniques

The development of interventional neuroradiology has allowed for increasingly accurate descriptions of the human cerebral vasculature and increasingly safe and precise access to the cerebral vasculature. Endovascular balloon occlusion, coil technologies, angioplasty, and intraoperative arteriographic definition of vascular reconstruction represent technical advances that produce improved outcomes.

Angioplasty is a proved technique for management of the coronary circulation. It is not surprising that the former Soviet Union would pioneer the use of this technique for vasospasm in SAH, given their extensive experience with neuroradiologic treatments for cerebral aneurysms. Zubkov et al. reported the first series of SAH patients in whom balloon dilation was technically feasible [61]. Heishima et al. reported the development of a soft silicon balloon that could be navigated into the basilar, posterior cerebral (P1), middle cerebral (M1, M2) and anterior cerebral (A1, A2) arteries and yet provide appropriate pressure to dilate these vascular locations [62].

These balloons deliver 1 to 3 atm of pressure to the vessels via inflation with 0.10 ml of saline. Patient selection criteria are the presence of arteriographic vasospasm without infarction in a patient with a clipped aneurysm. A correlation of symptoms with anatomic vascular lesion is helpful but not always present, since obtundation is often the presenting symptom of vasospasm. Failure of calcium antagonist prophylaxis or complications of hypervolemic hypertensive therapy are appropriate indications for considering this procedure. In two large series totaling 69 patients, the outcome was successful in 71 percent and 10 percent of patients died. Most successful angioplasties have been performed in the first 48 hours after onset of major symptoms. Angioplasty has also been used to treat catheter-induced spasm. Newell et al. described the use of transcranial Doppler study to monitor the effectiveness of angioplasty [63].

Vorkapic and co-workers recently identified the timing and extent of alteration of vessel inelastic elements in the production of vasospasm [64]. In the rabbit SAH model initial vessel narrowing is due to physiologic mechanisms, then anatomic fibrosis increases over the next 5 to 7 days until it accounts for more than 60 percent of the caliber changes. Thus angioplasty, directed at the anatomic fibrotic component of this disorder, should be effective. Recent attempts to address the physiologic component have also been successful. Several groups have reported SAH patients who benefited from intracarotid infusions of papaverine [65].

The technique of endovascular balloon occlusion, pioneered by DeBrun, allows the fluoroscopically directed placement of a detachable silicone occlusive balloon within the aneurysmal sac [66]. It has the advantage of easy access to the vascular defect without craniotomy and the disadvantage of being blind to the extent of the arterial wall defect. Aneurysms of the intracavernous carotid represent the largest group of endovascular lesions accessible with this technique. The ideal treatment preserves the normal course of the vessel but eliminates the wall defect. When this is not possible (often), the aneurysm may be trapped by obstructing flow above and below the site of the defect. Temporary occlusion with neurologic monitoring of the patient's condition, electroencephalogram (EEG), and transcranial Doppler study have been used in this situation. The predictive validity of these tests has not been prospectively demonstrated. Pooled series of 1026 cases of endovascularly trapped aneurysms show a 78 percent success rate with a 15 to 20 percent incidence of ischemia. Rupture, the other major complication, is the most common cause of perioperative death. Other complications include embolic events and incomplete aneurysm obliteration.

Another promising therapy is endovascular aneurysm occlusion achieved by placing detachable platinum coils into the aneurysm sac. A low positive direct electric current transmitted through the guidewire detaches the coil from the stainless steel microcatheter by electrolysis and causes intraaneurysmal elec-

trothrombosis by the attraction of local blood components. Early clinical reports demonstrate a relatively high success rate and low morbidity and mortality in skilled hands [67,68].

Until recently most surgeons obtained postsurgical arteriograms when uncertain about clip placement or if they wished to diagnose vasospasm. The availability of portable digital angiography has made intraoperative angiography quite practical. Barrow et al. recently reported a series of 115 procedures with intraoperative arteriography in which 19 studies resulted in an altered surgical plan, presumably saving reoperation [69]. Selection criteria currently rely on the operative difficulty of clip placement, visualization of clip placement, and surgical judgment. This technique is likely to see greater use.

Transcranial Doppler ultrasound techniques are now widely employed at most cerebral vascular surgical centers. This simple bedside test of arterial blood flow velocity is sensitive to the vasospasm syndrome. Elevated blood velocity is often detected before the occurrence of ischemic complications of vasospasm, making this a very sensitive test (100%), although specificity is lower (56.8%) [70]. Preliminary evaluations of this technology suggest this sensitivity is clinically useful. Furthermore, the use of transcranial Doppler study for large groups of patients has allowed daily charting of the velocity changes that occur with the vasospasm syndrome, The time course of these changes is long, lasting more than 14 days in most cases. Evidence suggests that the onset and remission of spasm are gradual and consistent, making transcranial Doppler study a very good tool with which to stratify patients into risk groups [71].

References

1. Sacco RL, Wolf PA, Bharucha NE, et al: Subarachnoid and intracerebral hemorrhage: Natural history, prognosis, and precursive factors in the Framingham study. *Neurology* 34:847, 1984.
2. Biller J, Godersk JC, Adams HP: Management of aneurysmal subarachnoid hemorrhage. *Stroke* 19:1300, 1988.
3. McCormick WF, Nofziger JD: Saccular intracranial aneurysm: An autopsy study. *J Neurosurg* 21:155, 1965.
4. Heros RC, Kistler JP: Subarachnoid hemorrhage due to a ruptured saccular aneurysm, in Ropper AH, Kennedy SF (eds): *Neurological and Neurosurgical Intensive Care.* Rockville, MD, Aspen, 1988, p 219.
5. Stebbens WE: Ultrastructure of aneurysms. *Arch Neurol* 32:798, 1975.
6. Stebens WE: *Pathology of the Cerebral Blood Vessels.* St. Louis, CV Mosby, 1972, p 351.
7. Wilkins RM: Subarachnoid hemorrhage and saccular intracranial aneurysm: An update. *Surg Neurol* 15:92, 1981.
8. Heros RC, Kistler JP: Intracranial arterial aneurysm: An update. *Stroke* 14:628, 1983.
9. Sekher LN, Neros RC: Origin, growth, and rupture of saccular aneurysms: A review. *Neurosurgery* 8:248, 1981.
10. Fisher CM: Clinical syndromes in cerebral thrombosis, hypertensive hemorrhage and ruptured saccular aneurysms. *Clin Neurosurg* 22:117, 1975.
11. Hart RG, Byer JA, Slaughter JR, et al: Occurrence and implications of seizures in subarachnoid hemorrhage due to ruptured intracranial aneurysms. *Neurosurgery* 8:417, 1981.
12. Sundaram MBM, Chow F: Seizures associated with spontaneous subarachnoid hemorrhage. *Can J Neurol* 13:229, 1986.
13. Hunt WE, Hess RM: Surgical risk as related to time of intervention in the repair of intracranial aneurysms. *J Neurosurg* 28:14, 1968.
14. Leblanc R: The minor leak preceeding subarachnoid hemorrhage. *J Neurosurg* 66:35, 1987.
15. West HH, Mani RI, Eisenberg RL: Normal cerebral arteriography in patients with spontaneous subarachnoid hemorrhage. *Neurology* 27:592, 1972.

16. Kassell NF, Torner JC: The international cooperative study in timing of aneurysm surgery: An update. *Stroke* 15:566, 1984.
17. Norris JW: Effects of cerebrovascular lesions of the heart. *Neurol Clin* 1:87, 1983.
18. Di Pasquale G, Pinelli G, Andreoli A, et al: Holter detection of cardiac arrhythmias in intracranial subarachnoid hemorrhage. *Am J Cardiol* 59:596, 1987.
19. Brouwers PJAM, Wijdicks EFM, Hasan D, et al: Serial electrocardiographic recording in aneurysmal subarachnoid hemorrhage. *Stroke* 20:1162, 1989.
20. Hart GK, Humphrey L, Weiss J: Subarachnoid hemorrhage: Cardiac complications. *Crit Care Rep* 1:88, 1989.
21. Yuki K, Kodama Y, Onda J, et al: Coronary vasospasm following subarachnoid hemorrhage as a cause of stunned myocardium. *J Neurosurg* 75:308, 1991.
22. Kassell NF, Torner JC, Adams HP: Antifibrinolytic therapy in the acute period following aneurysmal subarachnoid hemorrhage: Preliminary observations from the cooperative aneurysm study. *J Neurosurg* 61:225, 1984.
23. Vermeulen M, Lindsay KW, Murray GD, et al: Antifibrinolytic treatment in subarachnoid hemorrhage. *N Engl J Med* 311:432, 1984.
24. Solomon RA, Fink ME: Current strategies for the management of aneurysmal subarachnoid hemorrhage. *Arch Neurol* 44:769, 1987.
25. Nibbelink DW, Henderson WG, Torner JC: Intracranial aneurysms and subarachnoid hemorrhage: Report on a randomized treatment study. IV-A. Regulated bedrest. *Stroke* 8:202, 1977.
26. Nibbelink DW: Cooperative aneurysm study: Antihypertensive and antifibrinolytic therapy following subarachnoid hemorrhage from ruptured intracranial aneurysm, in Whisnant JP, Sandok BA (eds): *Cerebral Vascular Diseases.* New York, Grune & Stratton, 1975, p 155.
27. Tindall GT, Goree JA, Lee JF: Effect of common carotid ligation on size of internal carotid aneurysms and distal intracarotid and retinal artery pressures. *J Neurosurg* 25:503, 1966.
28. Kassell NF, Sasaki T, Colohan ART, et al: Cerebral vasospasm following aneurysmal subarachnoid hemorrhage. *Stroke* 16:562, 1985.
29. Chyatte D, Sundt TM: Cerebral vasospasm after subarachnoid hemorrhage. *Mayo Clin Proc* 59:498, 1984.
30. Kosnik EJ, Hunt WE: Postoperative hypertension in the management of patients with intracranial arterial aneurysms. *J Neurosurg* 45:148, 1976.
31. Hanley DF, Kirsch JR: Cerebral vasospasm: Use of hypervolemic hypertensive therapy. *Crit Care Rep* 1:80, 1989.
32. Muizelaar JP, Becker DP: Induced hypertension for the treatment of cerebral ischemia after subarachnoid hemorrhage: Direct effect on CBF. *Surg Neurol* 25:317, 1986.
33. Yonas H, Sekhar L, Johnson DW, Gur D: Determination of irreversible ischemia by Xenon-enhanced computed tomographic monitoring of CBF in patients with symptomatic vasospasm. *Neurosurgery* 24:368, 1989.
34. Volby B: Pathophysiology of subarachnoid hemorrhage: Experimental and clinical data. *Acta Neurochir Suppl* 45:1, 1988.
35. Diringer MN, Wu KC, Verbalis JG, Hanley DF: Hypervolemic therapy prevents volume contraction but not hyponatremia following subarachnoid hemorrhage. *Ann Neurol* 31:543, 1992.
36. Heros RC, Zervas NT, Varsos V: Cerebral vasospasm after subarachnoid hemorrhage: An update. *Ann Neurol* 14:599, 1983.
37. Wong MCW, Haley EC Jr: Calcium antagonists: Stroke therapy coming of age. *Curr Concepts Cerebrovasc Dis Stroke* 24:31, 1989.
38. Buchan AM, Sharma M: Experimental study of the pathogenesis and treatment of stroke. *Curr Opin Neurol Neurosurg* 4:38, 1991.
39. Heffez DS, Passonneau JV: Effect of Nimodipine on cerebral metabolism during ischemia and recirculation in the mongolian gerbils. *J Cereb Blood Flow Metab* 5:523, 1985.
40. Svendgaard N-Aa, Brismar J, Delgado T, et al: Late cerebral arterial spasm: The cerebrovascular response to hypercapnia, induced hypertension and the effect of Nimodipine on blood flow autoregulation in experimental subarachnoid hemorrhage in primates. *Gen Pharmacol* 14:167, 1983.
41. Petruk KC, West M, Mohr G, et al: Nimodipine treatment in poorgrade aneurysm patients: Results of a multicenter double-blind placebo-controlled trial. *J Neurosurg* 68:505, 1988.
42. Flamm ES, Adams HP Jr, Beck DW, et al: Dose-escalation study of intravenous Nicardipine in patients with aneurysmal subarachnoid hemorrhage. *J Neurosurg* 68:393, 1988.
43. Sano K, Saito I: Timing and indications of surgery for ruptured intracranial aneurysms with regard to cerebral vasospasm. *Acta Neurochir* 41:49, 1978.
44. Suzuki J, Yoshimoto T, Onuma T: Early operations for ruptured intracranial aneurysms: Study of 31 cases operated on within the first four days after ruptured aneurysm. *Neurol Med Chir* 18:82, 1978.
45. Whisnant JP, Phillips LH, Sundt TM: Aneurysmal subarachnoid hemorrhage. *Mayo Clin Proc* 57:471, 1982.
46. Farrar JK, Gamache FW, Ferguson GG: Effects of profound hypotension on cerebral blood flow during surgery for intracranial aneurysms. *J Neurosurg* 55:857, 1982.
47. Drake CD: Management of cerebral aneurysm. *Stroke* 12:273, 1981.
48. Fox JL: Microsurgical exposure of intracranial aneurysms. *J Microsurg* 1:2, 1979.
49. Sundt TM, Whisnant JP: Subarachnoid hemorrhage from intracranial aneurysm. *N Engl J Med* 299:116, 1978.
50. Hayes GJ, Leiser RC: Methyl methacrylate investment of intracranial aneurysms. *J Neurosurg* 25:79, 1966.
51. Todd GM, Shelden CH, Crue BJ: Plastic jackets for certain intracranial aneurysms. *JAMA* 179:935, 1962.
52. Miller JD, Jawad K, Jannett B: Safety of carotid ligation and its role in the management of intracranial aneurysms. *J Neurol Neurosurg Psychiatry* 40:64, 1977.
53. Spetzler RF, Hadley MN, Rigamonti D, et al: Aneurysms of the basilar artery treated with circulatory arrest, hypothermia, and barbiturate cerebral protection. *J Neurosurg* 68:868, 1988.
54. Brinker T, Seifert V, Stolke D: Effect of intrathecal fibrinolysis on cerebrospinal fluid absorption after experimental subarachnoid hemorrhage. *J Neurosurg* 74:789, 1991.
55. Findlay JM, Weir BKA, Kassell NF, et al: Intracisternal recombinant tissue plasminogen activator after aneurysmal subarachnoid hemorrhage. *J Neurosurg* 75:181, 1991.
56. Mizoi K, Yoshimoto T, Fujiwara S, et al: Prevention of vasospasm by clot removal and intrathecal bolus injection of tissue-type plasminogen activator: Preliminary report. *Neurosurgery* 28:807, 1991.
57. Drake CG, Vanderlinden RG: The late consequences of incomplete surgical treatment of cerebral aneurysm. *J Neurosurg* 27:266, 1967.
58. Sakaki S, Ohta S, Nakamura H, Takeda S: Free radical reaction and biological defense mechanism in the pathogenesis of prolonged vasospasm in experimental subarachnoid hemorrhage. *J Cereb Blood Flow Metab* 8:1, 1988.
59. Ohta T, Kikuchi H, Hashi K, Kudo Y: Nizofenone administration in the acute stage following subarachnoid hemorrhage. *J Neurosurg* 64:420, 1986.
60. Kanamaru K, Weir BKA, Simpson I, et al: Effect of 21-aminosteroid U-74006F on lipid peroxidation in subarachnoid clot. *J Neurosurg* 74:454, 1991.
61. Zubkov YN, Nikiforov BM, Shustin VA: Balloon catheter technique for dilatation of constricted cerebral arteries after aneurysmal SAH. *Acta Neurochir* 70:65, 1984.
62. Higashida RT, Halbach VV, Cahan LD, et al: Transluminal angioplasty for treatment of intracranial arterial vasospasm. *J Neurosurg* 71:648, 1989.
63. Newell DW, Eskridge JM, Mayberg MR, et al: Angioplasty for the treatment of symptomatic vasospasm following subarachnoid hemorrhage. *J Neurosurg* 71:654, 1989.
64. Vorkapic P, Bevan RD, Bevan JA: Pharmacologic irreversible narrowing in chronic cerebrovasospasm in rabbits is associated with functional damage. *Stroke* 21:1478, 1990.
65. Weir B: Recent development in cerebral vasospasm. Second World Congress of Stroke, Washington, DC, September 1992.
66. Weil SM, van Loveren HR, Tomisick TA, et al: Management of inoperable cerebral aneurysms by the navigational balloon technique. *Neurosurgery* 21:296, 1987.
67. Guglielmi G, Vinuela F, Sepetka I, et al: Electrothrombosis of saccular aneurysms via endovascular approach. *J Neurosurg* 75:1, 1991.
68. Guglielmi G, Vinuela F, Dion J, et al: Electrothrombosis of saccular aneurysms via endovascular approach. *J Neurosurg* 75:8, 1991.

69. Barrow DL, Boyer KL, Joseph GJ: Intraoperative angiography in the management of neurovascular disorders. *Neurosurgery* 30:153, 1992.

70. Sloan MA, Haley EC Jr, Kassell NF, et al: Sensitivity and specificity of transcranial Doppler ultrasonography in the diagnosis of vasospasm following subarachnoid hemorrhage. *Neurology* 39:1514, 1989.

71. Harders A, Gilsbach J: Hemodynamic effectiveness of Nimodipine on spastic brain vessels after subarachnoid hemorrhage evaluated by the TCD method: A review of clinical studies. *Acta Neurochir Suppl* 45:21, 1988.

XIV. Transplantation

Section Editor
David L. Dunn

193. Transplant Immunology and the Use of Immunosuppressive Agents in Solid Organ Transplantation

Gary L. C. Chan and Daniel M. Canafax

The 1990s will be referred to in future years as the decade of immunosuppressive drug development for transplantation. The immunosuppressive agents in use today have been and are essential for the present high rates of transplant success, but many new drugs are soon to be in widespread clinical use. Although the immune response directed against the allograft diminishes with time, indefinite administration of immunosuppressive agents is necessary to maintain allograft function. These agents act on diverse targets in the immunologic system, have numerous toxicities, and are often used in conjunction with one another for prevention or treatment of rejection. This chapter reviews the pharmacology and clinical use of these agents in solid organ transplantation.

Mechanism of Transplant Rejection

Host immunity presents a barrier to allograft acceptance as an extension of its physiologic role in the defense against foreign antigens. Current evidence underlines the central role portrayed by T-lymphocytes in mediating acute allograft rejection. Understanding the complex immunologic events occurring between alloantigen recognition and cytotoxicity is essential to the optimal use of transplant immunosuppressants.

Allograft rejection is primarily directed against antigens encoded by the major histocompatibility complex (MHC), also known in humans as the human leukocyte antigen (HLA) complex, located on chromosome 6. The HLA complex encodes both class I antigens (HLA-A, -B, and -C), which are expressed by most tissues except erythrocytes, and class II antigens (HLA-DR, -DP, and -DQ), which are limited in distribution to dentritic cells, monocytes, macrocytes, and B-lymphocytes. Initiation of the immune response normally requires presentation of the foreign proteins in the context of self MHC products (MHC-restricted recognition). In comparison, in transplant rejection, the allogenic HLA products may serve as both presenting molecules and foreign peptides [1]. Class I and class II HLA products are recognized by cytotoxic/suppressor (CD8+) and helper/inducer (CD4+) T-cells, respectively.

For the initiation of the rejection process, donor antigens are first digested and processed by intragraft antigen presenting cells such as dentritic leukocytes [2]. Fragments of alloantigens then bind to HLA molecules on the surface of the antigen presenting cell. This complex of HLA molecules and foreign peptide is recognized by direct interaction with the T-cell receptor (TCR) on recipient helper or cytotoxic T-cells [1]. Interaction between TCR and its ligand results in signal transduction through the CD3 complex, a group of transmembrane polypeptides juxtapositioned to the TCR, and subsequent activation of cytoplasmic events [3]. In addition, co-stimulatory signals mediated by other receptors and ligands such as CD4, CD8, CD2, and LFA-3 are necessary for T-cell activation [2] (Fig. 193-1).

The antigen-primed T-helper cell is further activated by the macrophage-derived cytokine, interleukin-1 (IL-1) [1]. In the presence of these signals, helper T-cells produce interleukin-2 (IL-2) as well as IL-2 receptors [1]. Interleukin-2 exerts autocrine function by augmenting its own production, and paracrine function by triggering the activation and proliferation of other helper and cytotoxic T-cells. Activated helper T-cells also produce gamma-interferon (γ-IFN), which further activates macrophages and enhances the expression of intragraft HLA class I and class II molecules [1] Thus expression of IL-2 and γ-IFN provides essential positive feedback for the continued propagation of the allogenic response. Furthermore, helper T-cells elaborate a battery of other lymphokines that result in activation of B-cells and recruitment of polymorphonuclear cells [2]. Recent evidence indicates that T-cell-derived lymphokines also activate vascular endothelium, which expresses proinflammatory products and adhesion molecules essential for the recruitment of new lymphocytes to the rejection process [2].

Damage to the allograft is caused by both specific and nonspecific mechanisms [1]. Cytotoxic T-cells cause lysis of foreign cells by direct contact. In addition, the initial antigen-specific response elicits effector components that result in a nonspecific response. These nonspecific components include expression of thromboxanes, leukotrienes, chemotaxins, and tumor necrosis factor by macrophages; recruitment of polymorphonuclear and natural killer cells; and coagulation activation leading to ischemic damage [1].

Cyclosporine

PHARMACOLOGY AND PHARMACOKINETICS. Cyclosporine (CSA) acts by interrupting the signal transduction essential for cytokine synthesis in antigen-primed T-lymphocytes [4]. Within the cytoplasm, CSA inhibits an enzyme called cytophilin, which possesses peptidyl-prolyl cis-trans isomerase (PPIase) activity [5]. Although the binding of CSA to cyclophilin is required for its immunosuppressive activity, inhibition of the PPIase activity does not seem to be relevant to this process. Current evidence suggests that the CSA-cyclophilin complex binds to and inhibits a Ca^{2+}-dependent phosphatase called calcineurin [5]. Calcineurin is required for the proper assembly of the transcription factor NF-AT, which then binds to the IL-2 gene in the nucleus to initiate IL-2 synthesis [6]. Inhibition of calcineurin by the CSA-cyclophilin complex thus inhibits mRNA transcription for IL-2 and other cytokines. Deprivation of these essential lymphokines disrupts the activation and proliferation of helper and cytotoxic T-cells that is essential for the rejection process [4].

Oral CSA has a mean bioavailability of 30 percent but ade-

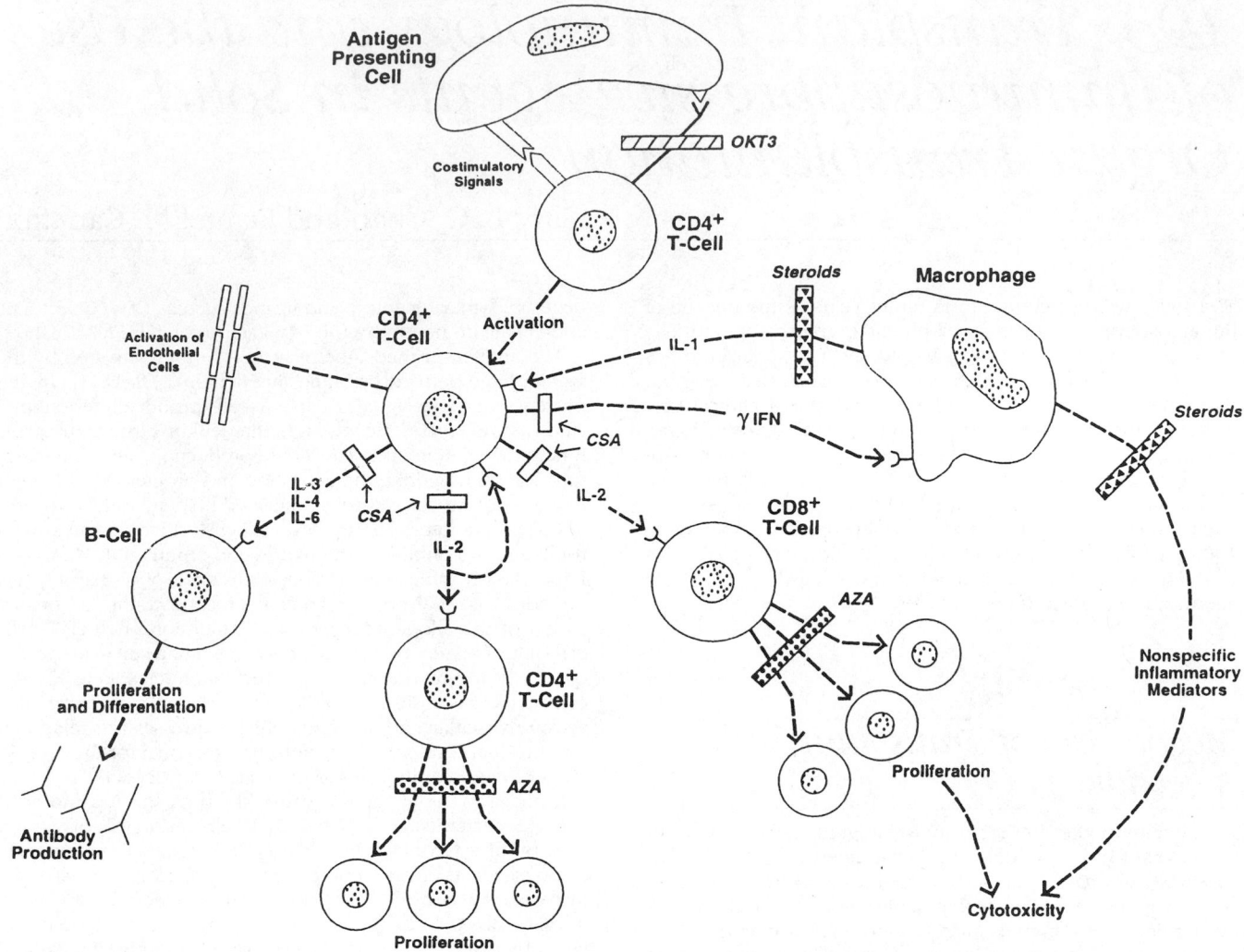

Fig. 193-1. Immunologic cascade of allograft rejection and sites of action of immunosuppressive agents. CSA = cyclosporine; AZA =azathioprine; IL = interleukin.

quate absorption depends on the presence of bile salts [7,8]. In liver transplant patients, bioavailability of CSA in the early post-transplant period is particularly low (<10%), due to biliary diversion from the intestine [7]. Clamping of the T-tube or feeding of bile acids significantly improves the bioavailability of CSA in these patients. Other factors that impair CSA absorption include cholestasis, short bowel, diarrhea, postoperative ileus, and gastroparesis [7]. On the other hand, the bioavailability of CSA increases with time after transplantation, and reduction of CSA dosage is often required to avoid excessive CSA blood levels.

Cyclosporine is primarily metabolized in the liver by the cytochrome P-450IIIA enzyme subfamily. The mean blood clearance is 5 ml/min/kg, and the half-life is approximately 10 hours [7]. Pediatric transplant recipients have significantly higher clearance and require higher CSA dose per kg body weight than adult patients [7]. In the presence of hepatic dysfunction, the clearance of CSA is impaired, and accumulation of both unchanged CSA and metabolites occurs in the blood. Since less than 1 percent of unchanged CSA is excreted into the urine,

dosage adjustment is not required in patients with renal dysfunction. Numerous CSA metabolites have been identified, but the immunosuppressive or toxic activities of these metabolites have not been established [9].

CLINICAL USE

Indication. The use of CSA is one of the most important factors contributing to improved outcome in the field of clinical transplantation during the past decade. In kidney transplantation, allograft survival has improved by 10 to 20 percent, and the use of CSA has been particularly advantageous in high-risk patients such as the elderly, diabetic patients, and patients who undergo retransplantation [10]. The impact of CSA on heart and liver transplantation is even more noticeable. While there has been an almost exponential growth in the number of heart and liver transplants performed over the last 10 years, the greatly improved allograft survival rates also translate into an increased number of lives saved.

Since CSA interferes with the continued activation of T-cells, it is effective for the prevention of rejection. Cyclosporine has also been used to treat steroid-resistant rejections in kidney transplant patients [11] and to prevent progression of mild rejection in heart allografts [12]. Despite these reports of successful rejection reversal, the efficacy of CSA in treating ongoing rejections is probably limited. In clinical practice, CSA is mostly used in combination with other immunosuppressants, such as azathioprine (AZA) and/or prednisone, although some centers have achieved satisfactory results with CSA monotherapy in kidney transplant patients [13].

Cyclosporine is available as soft gelatin capsules and as a liquid preparation for oral administration. The liquid form requires dispersion in beverages such as milk or orange juice before administration and has comparable bioavailability to capsule formulation. Intravenous CSA is formulated in the vehicle Cremophor EL (polyoxyethylated castor oil), which has been associated with rare cases of anaphylactoid reaction and potentiation of CSA-induced nephrotoxicity [14]. Since the high peak concentration of CSA that occurs after an intravenous bolus may be excessively nephrotoxic, CSA should be given by intravenous infusion over 6 hours or as a constant infusion.

Cyclosporine administration is typically initiated prior to transplant surgery as a 6 to 12 mg/kg oral loading dose and the drug is continued postoperatively at 4 to 10 mg/kg/day orally in a once or twice daily regimen. Much higher initial dosage (10–20 mg/kg/day) may be required for liver transplant patients [15]. Some centers administer intravenous CSA during the immediate posttransplant period to ensure therapeutic CSA blood levels, using infusion over 6 hours or constant-rate infusion at 2 to 5 mg/kg/day. This practice is especially important for the care of liver transplant patients, who inevitably have malabsorption of CSA in the early posttransplant period due to ileus and biliary diversion [15]. When gastrointestinal function returns, oral CSA is started and intravenous therapy may be stopped or tapered according to measured blood levels of CSA. In patients who require conversion from oral to intravenous therapy, the same CSA blood levels can be maintained by administering one third the oral dose intravenously.

Therapeutic Drug Monitoring. Since there is substantial variation in CSA blood levels achieved with any given dose [8], monitoring of CSA levels is a common practice. In addition to maintaining CSA levels within a specified therapeutic range, measurement of CSA may help ascertain patient compliance and differentiate allograft dysfunction from drug toxicity.

Several assays are commercially available for measuring CSA levels, such as HPLC, [125]I- or ^{3}H-RIA (Sandoz, Incstar) or polyclonal or monoclonal FPIA (Abbott). These assays measure either only parent CSA levels (specific) or both parent CSA and metabolites levels (nonspecific). In the presence of liver dysfunction, accumulation of CSA metabolites may result in elevated nonspecific CSA levels while specific CSA levels remain unchanged [7]. This is particularly important in liver transplant patients because lowering the CSA dose in response to elevated nonspecific levels may lead to suboptimal immunosuppression and trigger a rejection episode. Cyclosporine levels may be measured in either whole blood or plasma. Since the binding of CSA to red blood cells (RBCs) is temperature-dependent [7], whole blood CSA levels may yield more consistent results. Based on these arguments, specific CSA assay with whole blood as the matrix appears to be the preferred method [8,9].

Cyclosporine level monitoring is most commonly performed as steady-state predose levels. Since the time to peak CSA level after an oral dose is variable, the peak concentration is not usually measured. The desirable therapeutic range varies from center to center, and depends on factors such as assay methodology, assay matrix, immunosuppressive protocol, time after transplant, and type of organ transplant. Typical target CSA levels maintained in the early posttransplant period are 200 to 300 ng/ml, measured in whole blood by specific FPIA. There

is general agreement that lower CSA levels may be maintained after the first 6 months posttransplant without compromising graft outcome. However, the optimal target CSA level that minimizes chronic CSA nephrotoxicity and chronic rejection remains to be defined.

Drug Interaction. Drug interactions that have been reported for CSA and are sustained by controlled studies or clinical experience are summarized in Table 193-1. Drugs that induce P-450IIIA enzymes, such as phenytoin and rifampin, can cause significant decrease in CSA levels, which has been associated with unexpected allograft rejection. On the other hand, drugs that are metabolized by the same enzymes, such as erythromycin, may inhibit CSA biotransformation by competition, and elevated CSA levels have been associated with various toxicities. In addition, P-450IIIA enzymes have been isolated from human intestinal mucosa [16]. Induction and inhibition of these enzymes may impair or enhance oral CSA absorption, respectively. Close monitoring of CSA levels is mandatory when these interacting agents are started or discontinued. Because of the high cost of CSA, inhibitors of CSA metabolism have been used to deliberately decrease CSA dose requirement in transplant patients. For example, ketoconazole [17,18] and diltiazem [19] have been shown to decrease CSA dose requirement by approximately 80 percent and 50 percent, respectively. Moreover, a number of drugs may augment the nephropathy associated with CSA. Use of these agents requires careful balance of the potential benefits against increased toxicity.

ADVERSE EFFECTS. A significant side effect of CSA is nephropathy. The acute form of nephrotoxicity is mediated by altered intrarenal hemodynamics. Cyclosporine enhances the response of glomerular blood vessels to vasoconstrictor hormones by increasing cell membrane permeability to calcium [20]. By a separate mechanism, CSA also inhibits the release of counterbalancing vasodilatory prostacyclin in the glomerulus [20]. Cyclosporine may also enhance the release of vasoconstricting endothelin and inhibit the activity of vasodilators (e.g., nitric oxide) of endothelial origin [20]. This in turn results in decreased renal blood flow and glomerular filtration rate. Sustained vasculopathy may eventually lead to the chronic form of tubulointerstitial damage.

In cadaver renal transplant patients, CSA may aggravate ischemic injury of the allograft and result in increased incidence or severity of delayed graft function. Heart and liver transplant patients who have marginal renal function pretransplant may also be at increased risk of developing acute CSA nephrotoxicity posttransplant. For this reason, some centers administer an antilymphocyte preparation after transplantation for 5 to 14 days and start CSA therapy only after adequate renal function has been established in the patient (sequential therapy). Cy-

Table 193-1. Drug Interactions of Cyclosporine Substantiated by Controlled Studies or Clinical Experience

Increase in cyclosporine level	Decrease in cyclosporine level	Enhanced nephrotoxicity
Verapamil	Rifampin	Aminoglycosides
Diltiazem	Phenytoin	Amphotericin B
Ketoconazole	Phenobarbital	NSAIDs
Erythromycin	Carbamazepine	
Metoclopramide		
Methylprednisolone		

closporine nephrotoxicity may also develop at any time post-transplant as evidenced by a gradual rise in serum creatinine that is often associated with elevated CSA level [4]. Reduction in CSA dose usually leads to decrease in serum creatinine level within 24 to 48 hours.

Long-term administration of CSA has been associated with histological evidence of interstitial fibrosis and tubulointerstitial injury [21]. These initial reports of progressive development of renal failure in heart transplant patients may have been related to the high CSA dosages used in these studies. The prevalence of progressive CSA nephropathy under current protocols of relatively low-dose CSA is unknown. Current data suggest that renal function in heart transplant patients declines initially after exposure to CSA but then stabilizes after 6 months posttransplant without further loss of renal function [22,23]. Similarly, development of renal failure with chronic CSA dosing in liver transplant has been unusual [15]. Stable kidney transplant patients receiving CSA generally maintain higher serum creatinine levels than patients receiving conventional immunosuppression, but progressive decline in renal function has not been a consistent finding [24]. Even when a trend of declining creatinine clearance is demonstrated, the rate of decrease is comparable to that observed with conventional therapy [23,25], suggesting that the decline may be caused by insidious immunologic injury rather than CSA. The optimal care of patients who develop chronic CSA nephrotoxicity is not well established, although reduction of CSA dose with addition of AZA or another immunosuppressive agent to prevent rejection may be beneficial.

Numerous other side effects have been associated with CSA. Hypertension is a common finding in transplant patients receiving CSA. For hypertension associated with renal insufficiency, fluid retention and judicious use of diuretics may be indicated. However, a significant number of CSA-treated patients require antihypertensive medications. Preliminary evidence suggests that calcium channel blockers may help to ameliorate CSA nephrotoxicity [26], decrease kidney allograft rejection [27], and reduce the incidence of cardiac allograft vasculopathy [28]. Consequently, calcium channel blockers may be the drug of choice for managing CSA-induced hypertension. CSA also has been associated with a constellation of neurologic side effects such as tremor, mood changes, anxiety, headache, insomnia, psychosis, encephalopathy, seizures, cortical blindness, hemiplegias, coma, and speech apraxia [15]. Liver transplant patients, and patients with low serum magnesium and cholesterol levels seem to be at greater risk [15]. These neurologic side effects tend to disappear with discontinuation of CSA, although residual disorders may persist in some patients [15]. Elevation of hepatic transaminases and cholestasis also has been associated with high CSA levels and requires careful differentiation from hepatitis caused by viruses and other drugs. Various metabolic disorders have also been reported. These include hyperkalemia, hypomagnesemia, and hyperuricemia. Gingival hypertrophy and hirsutism also have been reported during long-term CSA administration. Hypercholesterolemia associated with CSA therapy is often refractory to treatment, although low-dose HMG CoA reductase inhibitors may provide effective therapy when dietary therapy alone fails.

Azathioprine

PHARMACOLOGY. Azathioprine (AZA) suppresses allograft rejection by inhibiting de novo purine synthesis in lymphocytes.

The immunosuppressive activity of AZA is dependent on formation of active intracellular metabolites, particularly thioinosinic acid and 6-thioguanine nucleotide. Thioinosinic acid inhibits an essential step of de novo purine synthesis, whereas 6-thioguanine nucleotide is incorporated into DNA, resulting in chromosome breaks and nucleic acid malfunction [29].

CLINICAL USE. Since the early 1960s, AZA was the mainstay of transplant immunosuppression until the advent of CSA. The combination of AZA with prednisone, with or without antilymphocyte preparation, is often referred to as conventional therapy. In the CSA era, AZA is mostly used in combination with CSA and prednisone in so-called triple therapy for prophylaxis of allograft rejection. Whether AZA can be safely omitted from an immunosuppressive protocol that incorporates CSA continues to be a subject of controversy.

Azathioprine is available in both an intravenous and an oral form. Oral AZA typically is initiated pretransplant as a 4 to 5 mg/kg loading dose and is continued posttransplant at 1 to 2 mg/kg once daily. Based on the fractional presystemic absorption of 40 to 50 percent [29], patients who require conversion to the intravenous route should receive half of the oral dose intravenously. The dose of AZA should be adjusted according to white blood cell (WBC) and platelet counts because leukopenia and thrombocytopenia are frequent complications. In some heart transplant programs, it has been suggested that the AZA dose should be adjusted to maintain the WBC at 4500 to 6500 cells/mm^3. Azathioprine should be stopped for a WBC count below 2500 cells/mm^3 or a platelet count below 50,000 cells/mm^3. Allopurinol enhances the toxicity of oral AZA by inhibiting xanthine oxidase, which is essential for the degradation of AZA [29]. Therefore, the AZA dose should be reduced by 75 percent in patients receiving allopurinol.

ADVERSE EFFECTS. Reversible myelotoxicity caused by AZA typically develops 7 to 14 days after AZA administration is initiated and frequently manifests itself as leukopenia, although thrombocytopenia, anemia, and pancytopenia can also occur. Leukopenia may exacerbate the patient's susceptibility to infections and must be differentiated from leukopenia caused by cytomegalovirus. Monitoring of liver function tests is mandatory during AZA administration because hepatitis has been associated with AZA therapy. Differentiation of hepatitis caused by AZA from that of viral origin is difficult but often critical, because the management of and prognosis for these two conditions are quite different. Other side effects of AZA include mild pancreatitis, gastrointestinal disturbances, alopecia, and increased incidence of neoplasia such as squamous cell carcinoma.

Corticosteroids

PHARMACOLOGY. Corticosteroids suppress both the alloantigen-specific and nonspecific immune responses that encompass organ transplant rejection. Upon entry into the cell, corticosteroids bind to an intracytoplasmic receptor. The steroid-receptor complex then binds to nuclear DNA, modifying mRNA transcription of various enzymes and cytokines [30]. In particular, corticosteroids inhibit the synthesis of IL-1 by macrophages [31]. Since IL-1 provides an essential signal for the activation of helper T-lymphocytes, steroids interfere with the specific allogenic response at an early stage. In addition, corticosteroids inhibit the chemotaxis of inflammatory cells and the production of proinflammatory molecules such as prostaglandins, which partly mediate the nonspecific cytotoxicity triggered by alloantigens.

CLINICAL USE. The most commonly used steroids for transplant immunosuppression are prednisone, prednisolone, and methylprednisolone. These agents have relatively low mineralocorticoid activity and are less likely to cause sodium or fluid retention than other types of steroids. They also have potent antiinflammatory activity, which complements their specific inhibitory effect on the allogenic response. Prednisone is available only in oral form and is the most commonly used steroid for chronic immunosuppression. Because prednisone must be converted in the liver to prednisolone for activity, some liver transplant programs prefer to use prednisolone rather than prednisone. Prednisolone is available in both intravenous and oral preparations, and the same dose can be used for both routes of administration. Prednisone and prednisolone are equipotent in their adrenocorticoid activity, and successful immunosuppression has been achieved with either agent. Methylprednisolone is also available in both oral and intravenous forms and is used primarily for antirejection therapy as a series of intravenous boluses. Methylprednisolone is 25 percent more potent than prednisone or prednisolone, and an oral dose of methylprednisolone of 4 mg is thus equipotent to 5 mg of prednisone. Occasionally, a patient who cannot tolerate oral prednisone may take oral methylprednisolone instead. However, the high cost of oral methylprednisolone compared with prednisone limits its use for long-term immunosuppression.

The role of corticosteroids in the treatment and prevention of allograft rejection has been firmly established. However, despite extensive clinical experience with the steroids over the past 30 years, the optimal dosage that is associated with maximum efficacy and minimum toxicity is not well established.

For the treatment of ongoing rejections, use of intravenous methylprednisolone remains the gold standard. In kidney and heart transplant patients, 75 to 85 percent of rejection episodes are reversed using intravenous methylprednisolone as first-line therapy [32,33,34]. A variety of methylprednisolone regimens have been used, and daily doses ranging from 250 mg to 1 gm appeared to be equally effective [33]. In current practice, the typical regimen consists of 500 mg to 1 gm of intravenous methylprednisolone administered daily or on alternate days for 3 to 5 doses. This is often followed by an increase of oral prednisone to 1 to 3 mg/kg/day, which is then tapered back to baseline over 7 to 14 days ("recycling" of prednisone). However, a recent study suggests that steroid taper may not be necessary after steroid pulse therapy [35]. Oral prednisone regimens appear to be as effective as intravenous methylprednisolone for reversal of rejection in kidney treatment patients and in treating mild or moderate cardiac allograft rejections without hemodynamic compromise.

Steroids also are used extensively for maintenance immunosuppression. The introduction of CSA has allowed a 50 percent reduction in the concurrent steroid dose compared with AZA-based conventional protocols. Further decrease in the steroid dose has been made feasible by the adoption of triple drug therapy. The typical prophylactic regimen consists of oral prednisone starting at 1 to 2 mg/kg/day, tapered to 0.5 mg/kg/day at 1 month, 0.3 mg/kg/day at 3 months, and 0.1 mg/kg/day at 1 year posttransplant. Methylprednisolone 1 gm also may be given initially intravenously pretransplant. In kidney trans-

plant patients, rapid tapering and early discontinuation of prednisone at 6 to 20 days posttransplant has been associated with a higher incidence of rejection compared to long-term prednisone administration [36]. On the other hand, in patients who receive murine monoclonal antibody OKT3 prophylaxis, the concurrent prednisone dosage can be safely reduced to 0.25 mg/kg/day. At the end of the course of OKT3, prednisone may be increased to 1 mg/kg/day and then tapered back to a lower level over 10 to 14 days. This prednisone taper is designed to suppress the rapid reappearance of peripheral lymphocytes that may occur after OKT3 is discontinued, to prevent the development of rejection [37]. It is interesting to note that this strategy is employed by many heart transplant programs but is rarely used by kidney transplant centers.

ADVERSE EFFECTS. Many of the steroid-induced adverse effects are dependent on the total dose and duration of administration. Particularly in the high dosages used immediately posttransplant, corticosteroids have been associated with infections and poor wound healing. Gastrointestinal complications may be relatively minor (nausea, vomiting, and gastric ulceration) or serious (gastroduodenal or colonic perforation). Gastrointestinal perforation and peritonitis are associated with high mortality rates, because the antiinflammatory activity of steroids may mask the patient's signs and symptoms, resulting in a delay in diagnosis and treatment. Other side effects include the onset of diabetes mellitus, fluid retention, hypertension, hyperlipidemia, osteoporosis, cushingoid habitus, weight gain, acne, glaucoma, and cataracts. In children who have growth retardation induced by steroids, conversion to an alternate day regimen may offer some benefit.

Cyclosphosphamide

PHARMACOLOGY. Cyclophosphamide is a pro-drug and its pharmacologic activity depends on the formation of the active metabolite phosphoramide mustard [38]. Phosphoramide mustard readily undergoes hydrolysis to a reactive aziridium intermediate that alkylates DNA [38]. This results in the formation of intra- and interstrand cross-linkages of DNA, strand breaks, and cell death [38]. On a cellular level, cyclophosphamide is unique in its ability to preferentially suppress B-lymphocytes relative to helper and cytotoxic T-cells.

CLINICAL USE. Early studies of the immunosuppressive activity of cyclophosphamide were inconclusive. With the availability of other potent immunosuppressive agents, cyclophosphamide is not routinely used for transplant immunosuppression in the United States. However, recent studies suggest that cyclophosphamide may be as efficacious as AZA [39,40]. It is occasionally used to replace AZA in cases of severe AZA-induced side effects, such as pancreatitis or hepatitis. It is also used in conjunction with other immunosuppressive measures to suppress B-cell activity in documented vascular rejection [37]. The typical oral dose is 1 to 2 mg/kg/d.

ADVERSE EFFECTS. Leukopenia is a common side effect of cyclophosphamide, and the nadir WBC count usually occurs 7 to 14 days after drug initiation [41]. Less frequently, thrombocytopenia may occur, and nausea, vomiting, and alopecia are also common adverse effects [41]. Hemorrhagic cystitis is a unique toxicity of cyclophosphamide and the associated symptoms include gross hematuria, frequency, dysuria, burning, urgency, and incontinence. Other adverse effects include azospermia, ovarian failure, and teratogenicity [41].

Vincristine

Vincristine inhibits mitosis by binding to the microtubular proteins of the mitotic spindle. In transplantation, vincristine has been used after a course of antilymphocyte preparation to prevent T-cell expansion and development of posttreatment rejection. In a prospective study, heart transplant patients received 6 to 8 doses of 0.015 to 0.025 mg/kg intravenous vincristine over 9 to 12 weeks, beginning 2 days after completion of either OKT3 or ATG [42]. No difference in rejection rate was observed between vincristine-treated patients and control patients. However, subgroup analysis of patients at high risk for rejection (women and patients <55 years of age) indicated that fewer vincristine-treated patients had rejection at 6 months and more were successfully weaned off steroids at 1 year [42]. However, the incidence of side effects was high and 43 percent of the vincristine-treated patients developed peripheral neuropathy [42].

Methotrexate

Methotrexate binds reversibly to dihydrofolate reductase, and inhibits conversion of dihydrofolate to tetrahydrofolate, which normally provides one-carbon fragments for the synthesis of purine nucleotides and thymidylate. This in turn inhibits DNA synthesis and mitosis. In addition, methotrexate suppresses the synthesis of IL-1 and antibody production in response to antigens, thereby inhibiting T- and B-cell activity [43,44].

In preliminary studies in heart transplant patients, methotrexate has been shown to be effective for patients who have persistent or recurrent rejections despite aggressive treatment with intravenous methylprednisolone or antilymphocyte preparations [45–48]. A variety of regimens were used in these studies; they consisted of intravenous or oral methotrexate 2.5 to 50 mg weekly for 1 to 18 weeks [45–48]. Over 90 percent of ongoing rejection episodes were reversed by methotrexate. Rejection reversal is typically delayed by 3 weeks, although resolution also has been observed within 3 days of starting methotrexate [46]. Treatment with methotrexate was also associated with a substantial decrease in the incidence of recurrent rejection in those patients who have demonstrated a high propensity to develop frequent rejections [47,48]. On the other hand, development of leukopenia is common during methotrexate therapy and has resulted in fatal infections in some patients [45,46,48]. The optimal methotrexate dose and duration of treatment are currently unknown and await clarification by prospective controlled studies.

Polyclonal Antilymphocyte Preparations

PHARMACOLOGY. The mechanism of action of polyclonal antilymphocyte preparations has been a subject of much de-

bate. Administration of these products results in rapid clearance of peripheral T-lymphocytes. This may be caused by opsonization of the lymphocytes followed by uptake of the reticuloendothelial system or by complement-mediated lysis [49]. However, lymphopenia does not seem to be essential for the observed immunosuppressive activity [50]. An additional mechanism of action may involve generation of suppressor cells. It has been suggested that the initial immunosuppressive activity may be caused by the depletion of functional T-lymphocytes, whereas inhibition of T-cell proliferation is sustained by suppressor cells after the antilymphocyte preparation is discontinued [49].

CLINICAL USE. Several polyclonal antilymphocyte preparations are currently available in the United States. These include antilymphocyte globulin (ATG) of either horse (Upjohn Atgam) or rabbit origin (Stanford, Virginia, Pittsburgh) and rabbit antithymocyte serum (Nashville ATS). In addition, an equine antilymphoblast globulin (Minnesota ALG) has been used extensively by some transplant centers, but its distribution has recently been halted. These products differ in concentration, potency, route of administration, and dose requirement. The particular product that is used depends largely on local availability. Of these preparations, only Upjohn Atgam is approved for marketing by the Food and Drug Administration.

Polyclonal antilymphocyte products are prepared by immunizing animals with human lymphoid cells, which are either cultured lymphoblasts (ALG) or T-lymphocytes isolated from thymic tissue (ATG, ATS) removed during pediatric cardiothoracic surgery. The animal serum is then harvested and extraneous antibodies against RBCs, platelets, and serum proteins are removed by adsorption. Although the antisera from different animals are pooled to achieve a degree of uniformity in content, batch-to-batch variation is inevitable. The IgG fraction is often separated before release of the product (ATG, ALG), although the unfractionated antiserum is occasionally used (ATS).

Polyclonal antilymphocyte preparations are used for the reversal and prevention of rejections. Due to the longer duration of treatment, the need for hospitalization, and side effects associated with ALG/ATG therapy, these preparations are generally reserved for rejections that fail to respond to high-dose steroids. In patients receiving CSA, success rates for treatment of steroid-resistant rejections with polyclonal antilymphocyte preparations have been reported to be over 80 percent [51]. For preventing rejection, these products have been used immediately posttransplant so that CSA can be avoided until the patient has acquired adequate renal function.

Atgam (Upjohn) is typically administered intravenously at 10 to 20 mg/kg/day for 7 to 14 days for the prevention or treatment of rejection. To detect prior sensitization, it is recommended that a skin test be performed with 0.1 ml of a 1:1000 dilution (total dose 5 μg) administered intradermally before the first Atgam dose. The usefulness of the skin test in screening for anaphylaxis is, however, controversial. Since infusion of Atgam by peripheral vein may cause phlebitis or thrombosis, use of a central vein is recommended. If a central vein is not available, the hemodialysis access may be used, though there is a risk of occluding the dialysis access. The required Atgam dose may be diluted to 4 mg/ml in normal saline or half-normal saline and infused over 6 hours to avoid development of hypotension. Lower final concentrations of 1 to 2 mg/ml are sometimes recommended [50], but the associated fluid load may be excessive for patients with oliguric renal failure. The Atgam dose should be adjusted according to WBC and platelet count. For WBC count below 2500/mm^3 or platelet count below 50,000/mm^3, discontinuation of Atgam should be considered.

ADVERSE EFFECTS. Common side effects associated with polyclonal antilymphocyte products include fever, chills, nausea, vomiting, diarrhea, myalgia, arthralgia, and rash. These symptoms may be mediated by cytokines released during lymphocytolysis and may be alleviated by premedications such as acetaminophen and diphenhydramine. Because these preparations often contain unwanted antibodies directed against other blood elements, leukopenia and thrombocytopenia frequently occur, but tend to respond readily to dose reduction. Development of anti-ALG antibodies in a titer 1:100 or greater has recently been observed in 40 percent of kidney transplant patients and is associated with rapid clearance of ALG from the serum and inferior allograft survival [52]. In a minority of patients, these anti-ALG/ATG antibodies may also precipitate serum sickness. In addition, an increased incidence of infectious complications has been observed in patients receiving polyclonal antilymphocyte preparations.

Orthoclone OKT3

PHARMACOLOGY. OKT3 is an IgG_{2a} antibody produced by fusion of mouse splenocytes with myeloma cells. The resultant hybridoma has the indefinite capability to produce antibodies of a single lineage against a specific antigen. OKT3 binds to the CD3 complex on the lymphocyte surface and causes an initial rapid clearance of the opsonized T-cells by the reticuloendothelial system [53]. Lymphopenia, however, does not seem necessary for immunosuppression because OKT3 is effective in reversing liver allograft rejection, when the reticuloendothelial system is not fully functional. More important, binding of OKT3 to the CD3 complex results in removal of the CD3 and TCR molecules from the cell surface [54]. These T-cells are thus deprived of the essential receptors for alloantigen recognition. OKT3 may also inhibit the activity of T-lymphocytes located within the allograft.

CLINICAL USE

Indications. OKT3 is effective for the treatment of acute cellular rejections. In kidney transplant patients, more rejections were reversed by OKT3 as first-line therapy compared with steroids (94% vs. 75%) [32]. Similarly, in liver transplant patients, use of OKT3 as initial treatment reversed over 70 percent of rejections [55]. In addition, OKT3 appears to be uniquely effective in the treatment of acute vascular rejections [56,57]. In one report, 91 percent of vascular rejection in kidney transplant patients responded to OKT3 [56].

OKT3 has also been used successfully to reverse rejection episodes that are refractory to conventional therapy such as high-dose steroids or ALG/ATG. Approximately 70 to 85 percent of kidney, heart, or liver allograft rejections that failed initial intensified immunosuppression responded to OKT3 treatment [10,58,59,60]. The outcome, however, differs between adults and children, with recurrent and breakthrough rejections occurring more frequently with children [58]. For the treatment of rejection episodes that failed high-dose steroid, OKT3 and polyclonal antilymphocyte preparations appear to be equally effective [61].

OKT3 has also been used in quadruple immunosuppressive protocols for prophylaxis of allograft rejection. However, whether OKT3 induction offers any advantage compared with triple drug therapy alone remains controversial.

OKT3 is typically given as an intravenous bolus of less than 1 minute at 5 mg/day for 7 to 14 days. Recent evidence suggests that the efficacy of OKT3 is not correlated with the administered dose. Similar allograft survival and rejection rates were observed in renal transplant patients who received low-dose (2–2.5 mg/d) or standard-dose (5 mg/d) OKT3 induction [62,63]. Similarly, in patients who are treated with OKT3 for ongoing rejections, both low-dose and standard-dose regimens were associated with comparable reversal rate [64]. However, low-dose OKT3 may be associated with less severe side effects and fewer infections and is less expensive. When the low-dose regimen is used, immunologic monitoring is essential, since one third of the patients may require a dose increase to maintain adequate suppression of circulating CD3+ cells [62].

Immunologic Monitoring. Administration of OKT3 results in rapid depletion of peripheral lymphocytes beginning within minutes [53]. With continued OKT3 therapy, T-lymphocytes reappear in the circulation within 2 to 7 days [53]. However, these T-cells lack the CD3 surface molecule and are thus nonfunctional. Reappearance of CD3+ cells during a course of OKT3 is often due to the formation of anti-OKT3 antibodies and may be associated with treatment failure [65]. However, OKT3 occasionally continues to be effective despite reappearance of CD3 molecules on T-cells due to a lack of expression of TCR molecules [66]. On the other hand, suppression of CD3+ cells does not guarantee treatment success, presumably due to the existence of alternate pathways of allogenic response [37]. In general, CD3+ cells should be maintained below 25 cells/mm^3 during OKT3 therapy to ensure adequate immunosuppressive activity.

The host immune system responds to OKT3, a murine IgG, by producing human anti-mouse antibody (HAMA). This HAMA reaction may partly negate the suppressive effect of OKT3 on CD3+ T-cells and necessitate an increase in OKT3 dose. Moreover, development of high antibody titer of 1:1000 or greater has been associated with retreatment failure [65] and may thus preclude repeat use of OKT3 in the same patient. Recently, development of HAMA reaction has also been linked to the occurrence of vascular rejection in cardiac transplant patients [67]. The incidence of the HAMA reaction and the antibody titer depends on concurrent immunosuppression [68]. With low-dose AZA and prednisone, sensitization has been observed in over 80 percent of patients receiving OKT3. With concurrent low-dose CSA, the sensitization rate was reduced to 11 percent [69]. In addition, the incidence of the HAMA reaction varies strikingly with the specific type of organ transplantion [70]. Positive HAMA reaction and titers of 1:1000 or greater develop most frequently in liver transplant patients, followed by kidney transplant patients, and are least frequent in heart transplant patients [70]. Due to the different assays used at individual centers, there is substantial variation in the reported incidence of sensitization [70].

ADVERSE EFFECTS. The initial dose of OKT3 often is associated with a syndrome characterized by fever, chills, dyspnea, nausea, vomiting, diarrhea, chest tightness, myalgia, and arthralgia. With subsequent OKT3 doses, these symptoms tend to dissipate, but they may persist throughout the entire course of OKT3 treatment. This syndrome is generally considered to be mediated by the release of cytokines such as tumor necrosis factor by lymphocytes activated by OKT3. These distressing symptoms may be partly relieved by the administration of 500 mg intravenous methylprednisolone 1 to 4 hours before the first dose and the use of premedications such as acetaminophen and diphenhydramine before the first and second doses.

More serious adverse reactions also have been associated with OKT3. In heart transplant patients, OKT3 elicits a biphasic hemodynamic response after the first dose [71]. Within 1 to 2 hours postdose, there can be evidence of a hyperdynamic state with increased cardiac index and decreased peripheral resistance, followed in several hours by hypotension, decreased cardiac index consistent with a negative inotropic effect, and increased pulmonary capillary wedge pressure, suggesting a capillary leak syndrome [71]. The hypotension may be severe and may mandate vasopressor or inotropic support. OKT3 may also induce pulmonary edema. Consequently, before OKT3 is initiated, absence of heart failure or fluid overload should be confirmed by chest roentgenogram, and the patient's body weight should not exceed lean body weight by 3 percent. Encephalopathy has also been reported and may manifest as confusion, coma, seizures, blindness, hallucinations, or psychosis [72,73]. Aseptic meningitis is another complication of OKT3, although it may resolve on its own despite continued OKT3 administration. As a potent immunosuppressive agent, OKT3 has been associated with development of opportunistic infections and lymphoproliferative disease.

Immunosuppressive Combinations

TRIPLE THERAPY AND DOUBLE THERAPY. Since CSA, AZA, and prednisone act on different immunologic targets in the allogenic response, these agents are often used together in so-called triple therapy. The purpose of triple combination therapy is to exploit the synergism between CSA and AZA [74], decrease the dose requirement of CSA and prednisone, and thereby further reduce the incidence of drug-related side effects. Excellent clinical results have generally been achieved using triple therapy.

The acceptance of triple therapy in clinical practice was initially prompted by retrospective comparison with historic controls. In cadaver renal transplant patients, the 1-year allograft survival rate in patients receiving triple therapy was 89 percent, which compared favorably with historic controls treated with CSA-prednisone (82%) or AZA-prednisone-ALG (77%) [75]. In heart transplant recipients receiving triple therapy, the Minneapolis group reported a 1-year graft survival of 92 percent, compared to 80 percent achieved with CSA-prednisone in Stanford and Pittsburgh [76]. Similarly, the use of triple therapy has made possible 1-year graft survival of approximately 80 percent in liver transplant patients [77].

More recently, a number of studies have attempted to prospectively compare different combinations of immunosuppressive agents. Overall, these comparisons show that satisfactory allograft survival rates are achieved with CSA-based immunosuppressive regimens regardless of the exact composition of the protocols.

In kidney transplant patients, the aggregate data from several prospective, randomized studies suggest that comparable clinical results are achieved with either triple therapy or CSA-prednisone [78–83]. These studies consistently found that patient and allograft survival, incidence of rejection, and posttransplant renal function were similar between the two regimens. Except for one study [83], the same infection rate was also observed for the two protocols. It should be pointed out that, in these CSA-prednisone protocols, CSA was initiated at 12 to 15 mg/kg/day and higher CSA levels were maintained than in triple therapy. High initial CSA dosages have previously been correlated with development of chronic nephrotoxicity in heart transplant patients [21,84]. Long-term follow-up is required to evaluate whether similar progressive nephrotoxicity is associated with high-dose CSA in a CSA-prednisone protocol in kidney transplant patients.

In heart transplant patients, a comparable outcome has been observed with triple therapy and steroid-free immunosuppression consisting of CSA and AZA. A steroid-free protocol has the advantage of avoiding numerous steroid-related side effects. Prompted by early reports of satisfactory outcome achieved with CSA-AZA [85], several studies have compared triple therapy with CSA-AZA in heart transplant patients. Initial findings suggested that CSA-AZA was associated with more rejections but fewer infectious episodes [86,87]. With longer follow-up, patients receiving triple therapy or CSA-AZA had similar 5-year survival, ventricular function, serum creatinine, and infection rates [88]. More early rejections occurred in the CSA-AZA group, but similar rejection rates were observed beyond 3 months [88]. Patients receiving triple therapy had higher serum cholesterol levels and more severe hypertension, although there was no difference in diabetes, obesity, or bone diseases between the two groups [88]. However, half of patients who began on CSA-AZA required conversion to maintenance steroids, mostly due to development of recurrent rejections [88,89,90]. This suggests that the use of initial CSA-AZA without concurrent steroids may offer suboptimal immunosuppression in half of the patients.

In summary, good allograft survival can be achieved with CSA-prednisone in renal transplant patients or with CSA-AZA in cardiac transplant patients. Nonetheless, neither of these double therapy regimens has been demonstrated to be superior to the CSA-AZA-prednisone combination. In addition, the use of a three-drug combination facilitates individualized patient care by permitting dose adjustment of any of the three agents in response to adverse reactions [91]. Until further evidence is available, triple therapy remains the immunosuppressive protocol of choice in organ transplantation.

SEQUENTIAL THERAPY. The observation of early rejections and renal dysfunction in patients receiving CSA from the day of transplantation has prompted the development of so-called sequential therapy. In this regimen, either polyclonal or monoclonal antilymphocyte preparations are used in conjunction with AZA and prednisone in the immediate posttransplant period. With recovery of postoperative renal function, antilymphocyte preparations are discontinued and CSA is started. Long-term immunosuppression is therefore maintained with CSA-AZA-prednisone. In different reports, this same basic protocol has also been referred to as quadruple or induction therapy. Several objectives are intended for sequential therapy. First, initial withholding of CSA avoids superimposing drug-induced nephrotoxicity on preexisting renal allograft preservation injury and may facilitate recovery of renal function. Second, the immediate onset of the potent immunosuppressive activity of antilymphocyte preparations may curtail the incidence of rejection. Third, induction with cytolytic agents early after alloantigen exposure may establish a state of donor-specific unresponsiveness or tolerance.

Numerous studies have compared sequential therapy with triple therapy to evaluate the benefit of cytolytic induction in various types of organ transplantation. Thus far, sequential therapy has not been conclusively demonstrated to be superior to noninduction regimens, and the aforementioned objectives are only partly fulfilled. A decrease in the incidence or duration of delayed graft function in kidney transplant patients has been seen with sequential ALG protocols [92,93], but has not been uniformly observed with OKT3 [94,95]. Similarly, although OKT3 induction reduced the incidence of early renal dysfunction in liver transplant patients [96,97], renal function at 3 months posttransplant was not affected [98]. Prospective studies in kidney, heart, and liver transplant patients have not demonstrated a consistent decrease in rejection rates [98,99,100], although there is some evidence that the onset of the first rejection may be delayed by the use of potent antilymphocyte preparations early posttransplant [98,101]. This delay in rejection onset may facilitate patient care, but this must be balanced against the risk of infection, lymphoproliferative disease, and the high cost of these antilymphocyte products. Moreover, both regimens are associated with excellent yet equivalent allograft survival, and complete transplant tolerance is not accomplished.

A number of studies have also compared OKT3 with polyclonal antilymphocyte preparations in induction protocols in kidney and heart transplant patients. These studies in general showed that monoclonal and polyclonal antilymphocyte products are equally efficacious for immunosuppressive prophylaxis. In kidney transplant patients, OKT3 was associated with fewer rejection episodes than ALG in an initial, nonrandomized study [102]. Subsequent prospective studies, however, have reported similar patient and graft survivals and incidence of rejection [103–106]. While the use of ALG appears to be associated with more cytomegalovirus infections [103,106], OKT3 induction may result in more side effects [103,104]. Similarly, in heart transplant patients, induction with either OKT3 or polyclonal preparations achieved equivalent allograft survival rates and incidence of infection. The effects on rejection rate and time to first rejection provided conflicting results; a difference between monoclonal and polyclonal products has not been demonstrated conclusively [107–110].

Until further information is available, application of sequential therapy in selective transplant patients seems reasonable. Given the well-known nephrotoxicity of CSA, it may be advisable to avoid early exposure to CSA in kidney transplant patients with delayed graft function or in heart and liver transplant patients with preexisting renal dysfunction. This may help facilitate recovery of renal function and curtail the need for dialysis and associated patient morbidity. In patients at high risk of immunologic graft injury, such as retransplant or highly sensitized patients, there are at least theoretical reasons to maximize immunosuppressive treatment with an induction protocol. Current evidence does not support the routine use of sequential therapy in kidney transplant patients with immediate graft function or in heart or liver transplant patients without preexisting renal dysfunction.

CYCLOSPORINE WITHDRAWAL. While CSA has substantially improved allograft survival compared with AZA-based conventional regimens, much of the benefit is limited to the early posttransplant period. Beyond the first 6 months after kidney transplantation, the survival curves of CSA- and AZA-treated patients declined in parallel, suggesting similar rates of graft loss over time [111,112]. This observation indicates that long-term treatment with CSA may not be necessary for the improved outcome. Discontinuation of CSA may also help prevent the development of progressive nephrotoxicity and reduce the cost of long-term immunosuppression. For these reasons, it has been advocated that CSA may be used initially for engraftment followed by conversion to AZA-prednisone.

A number of studies have attempted to evaluate the impact of CSA withdrawal, but the findings appear inconclusive. Overall, CSA withdrawal in kidney transplant patients has been associated with an increase in the incidence of rejection, especially during the first 6 months after conversion. A recent meta-analysis suggests that the increase in postconversion rejections is not affected by the manner of CSA withdrawal (early or late posttransplant, abruptly or in a tapered schedule) or by whether prednisone is temporarily increased [113]. These rejection episodes tend to respond readily to intravenous steroids

and do not generally result in short-term graft loss. However, with long-term follow-up, some studies have demonstrated late-onset rejections and impaired graft survival [114]. On the other hand, conversion from CSA to AZA-prednisone usually results in improved renal function, particularly in patients who have CSA-induced nephrotoxicity that does not respond to CSA dose reduction [114]. Moreover, nonrenal side effects of CSA such as hypertension, hyperlipidemia, and hyperuricemia are also ameliorated by CSA withdrawal.

Given the increased incidence of rejection after CSA withdrawal, and the possible association with graft loss, this strategy cannot be routinely recommended. This is particularly important in cardiac transplant patients, because fatal rejections after conversion have been reported [115]. In patients who experience CSA-induced nephrotoxicity after long-term administration, an alternative strategy of CSA dose reduction and addition of AZA may be attempted [116,117]. This approach essentially converts the patient to low-dose CSA-AZA-prednisone triple therapy, and has been demonstrated to be effective in managing CSA-related nephrotoxicity. In a minority of patients who develop intractable nephrotoxicity despite CSA dose reduction or who cannot tolerate the nonrenal side effects of CSA, discontinuation of CSA may prove necessary.

STEROID WITHDRAWAL. Since administration of steroids is associated with debilitating side effects, there has been considerable interest in curtailing long-term exposure to steroids. Accumulating evidence in the CSA era suggests that steroids may be withdrawn in selected transplant patients without adversely affecting graft survival.

In kidney transplant patients, steroid withdrawal has consistently led to amelioration of steroid-induced side effects such as hypertension, hyperlipidemia, and cushingoid syndrome [10]. Discontinuation of steroids does not seem to result in increased incidence of rejection in well-matched LRD renal transplant patients, particularly those who demonstrate donor-specific hyporesponsiveness in mixed lymphocyte reaction [118]. In cadaver kidney transplant patients, the result has been less consistent, and unexpected occurrence of rejection has been observed after steroids are discontinued in some studies [10]. In a recent analysis, the success of steroid withdrawal was correlated with the timing of the attempt. When steroid withdrawal was attempted within 6 months posttransplant, only 41 percent of the patients were successfully weaned off steroids, compared with 79 percent success when the attempt was postponed to at least 6 months posttransplant [119].

In heart transplantation, the case for steroid withdrawal is even more controversial. Since allograft failure almost inevitably leads to patient death, the proposed benefits of steroid withdrawal must be carefully balanced against the potentially life-threatening risks of more frequent rejections and cardiac allograft vasculopathy. In fact, in several centers that attempted steroid withdrawal late (>6 months) posttransplant, there was no significant improvement in hypertension, hypercholesterolemia, or patient obesity, despite a success rate of steroid withdrawal of over 80 percent [88,120,121]. This could be because these patients were receiving only low-dose prednisone after the first 6 months, and steroid withdrawal did not offer additional benefits. In comparison, steroid withdrawal early (within 4 months) posttransplant has been shown to reduce the number of major abdominal complications and improve weight, blood pressure, and serum cholesterol control [122,123]. However, 51 percent of patients who attempted early steroid withdrawal developed more than three episodes of allograft rejection and required reinstitution of steroid therapy [122]. It has been pointed out that steroid withdrawal may simply select for the group of patients who have low innate propensity for developing rejections [122]. Attempts to discontinue steroids may be particularly successful in low immunologic responders, such as elderly males with a negative donor-specific crossmatch or patients who have survived for 6 months posttransplant without developing rejections in the past 3 months [120,120].

Alternate Immunosuppressive Strategies

TOTAL LYMPHOID IRRADIATION. Ionizing radiation causes cell death by causing DNA strand breaks and crosslinking. In vivo, total lymphoid irradiation (TLI) changes the proportions of T-lymphocyte subsets, with decreased CD4+ cells and an increase in CD8+ cells. After discontinuation of TLI, a persistent state of donor-specific hyporesponsiveness has been observed [124].

In kidney transplant patients, pretransplant induction has been associated with improved clinical outcome in the pre-CSA era. However, results with TLI and conventional therapy were inferior to that achievable with CSA [125]. Consequently, preoperative TLI is no longer routinely used in kidney transplantation.

In recent years, TLI has been used in heart transplant patients to treat rejections that are refractory to intravenous steroids or antilymphocyte preparations, rejections that recur rapidly after conventional therapy, or severe rejections that occur within 7 days posttransplant [125–128]. The TLI regimen used by the Stanford group consisted of 80 cGy per treatment, two treatments per week, for a goal of 800 cGy [126]. The impact of TLI on the rejection process is delayed and concomitant antirejection therapy may be required to arrest the ongoing episode [128]. The major advantage of TLI appears to be marked reduction in the rejection rate, which may persist for as long as 24 months after treatment [129]. During TLI therapy, development of leukopenia and thrombocytopenia is common and may necessitate frequent adjustment of dose or dosing interval [126,128].

PLASMAPHERESIS. Plasmapheresis has been used for the treatment of vascular rejections because of its ability to remove circulating antibodies. Studies on the antirejection efficacy of plasmapheresis have been inconclusive. Since vascular rejections seldom respond to conventional therapy, plasmapheresis continues to be used as salvage therapy in some centers. Anecdotal success has been reported with plasmapheresis alone or in conjunction with ALG or OKT3 [130,131]. However, the efficacy of plasmapheresis as an antirejection therapy remains to be established.

PHOTOPHERESIS. In photopheresis, patients receive oral 8-methoxypsoralen and then undergo leukapheresis [132,133]. The 8-methoxypsoralen in the separated lymphocytes is activated by extracorporeally administered ultraviolet-A irradiation. Reinfusion of these lymphocytes into the patient triggers an autoimmune response directed against the photomodulated cells. In heart transplant patients, photopheresis has been used successfully to reverse moderate rejections [132]. Comparison between photopheresis and conventional antirejection therapy is not available.

New Immunosuppressive Agents

In recent years, improved understanding of the immune response has accelerated the discovery of new immunosuppressive agents. These include the macrolides (FK506, rapamycin), anti-proliferative agents (brequinar, RS61443, mizoribine), OG 37-325, 15-deoxyspergualin, and various monoclonal antibodies (e.g., OKT4A, anti-Tac, anti-ICAM-1). In particular, FK506 (tacrolimus) and RS61443 (mycophenolate mofetil) are currently undergoing extensive clinical testing. Preliminary evidence suggests that these two agents may be effective for both prophylaxis and salvage therapy of rejections. The exact role of these new immunosuppressive agents in clinical transplantation awaits the final analysis of prospective controlled studies.

CONCLUSION. Over the past decade, substantial progress has been made in the field of transplant immunosuppression. This coincides with and at least partly accounts for the dramatic improvement in transplant outcome. Under CSA-based therapy, however, acute rejections occur frequently and chronic graft attrition continues to occur. The vast array of new immunosuppressive agents on the horizon may help remedy these problems. Together with recent development in tolerance induction and xenotransplantation, these advances promise to further extend the benefit of transplantation to patients with end-stage organ diseases.

References

1. Chandler C, Passaro E: Transplant rejection: Mechanisms and treatment. *Arch Surg* 128:279, 1993.
2. Strom TB: Summation of the biologic aspects of the Congress. *Transplant Proc* 25:1284, 1993.
3. Acuto O, Reinherz EL: The human T-cell receptor: Structure and function. *N Engl J Med* 312:1100, 1985.
4. Kahan BD: Cyclosporine. *N Engl J Med* 321:1725, 1989.
5. Schumacher A, Norheim A: Progress towards a molecular understanding of cyclosporin A—Mediated immunosuppression. *Clin Invest* 70:773, 1992.
6. Schreiber SL, Crabtree GR: The mechanism of action of cyclosporin A and FK 506. *Immunol Today* 13:136, 1992.
7. Ptachcinski RJ, Venkataramanan, R, Burckart GJ: Clinical pharmacokinetics of cyclosporine. *Clin Pharmacokinet* 11:107, 1986.
8. Fahr A: Cyclosporin clinical pharmacokinetics. *Clin Pharmacokinet* 24:472, 1993.
9. Consensus document: Hawk's Cay meeting on therapeutic drug monitoring of cyclosporine. *Transplant Proc* 22:1357, 1990.
10. Chan GLC, Gruber SA, Skjei KL, et al: Principles of immunosuppression. *Crit Care Clin* 6:841, 1990.
11. Margreiter R, Lang A, Koenig P, et al: Cyclosporine in the treatment of acute allograft rejection refractory to high dose methylprednisolone: Results of a prospectively randomized trial. *Transplant Proc* 16:1202, 1984.
12. Kobashigawa J, Stevenson LW, Morguchi J, et al: Randomized study of high dose oral cyclosporine therapy for mild acute cardiac rejection. *J Heart Transplant* 8:53, 1989.
13. Hillebrand G, Schneeberger H, Schleibner S, et al. Ten years' experience with cyclosporine monotherapy after renal transplantation. *Transplant Proc* 25:513, 1993.
14. Abraham JS, Bentley FR, Garrison RN, et al: The influence of the cyclosporine vehicle, Cremophor EL, on renal microvascular blood flow in the rat. *Transplantation* 52:101, 1991.
15. Lake JR, Roberts JP, Ascher NL: Maintenance immunosuppression after liver transplantation. *Semin Liver Dis* 12:73, 1992.
16. Watkins PB, Wrighton SA, Schuetz EG, et al: Identification of glu-

cocorticoid-inducible cytochromes P-450 in the intestinal mucosa of rats and man. *J Clin Invest* 80:1029, 1987.

17. Butman SM, Wild JC, Nolan PE, et al: Prospective study of the safety and financial benefit of ketoconazole as adjunctive therapy to cyclosporine after heart transplantation. *J Heart Lung Transplant* 10:351, 1991.
18. First MR, Schroeder TJ, Michael A, et al: Safety and efficacy of long-term cyclosporine-ketoconazole administration and preliminary results of a randomized trial. *Transplant Proc* 25:591, 1993.
19. Valantine H, Keogh A, McIntosh N, et al: Cost containment: coadministration of diltiazem with cyclosporine after heart transplantation. *J Heart Lung Transplant* 11:1, 1992.
20. Skorecki KL, Rutledge WP: Acute cyclosporine nephrotoxicity—Prototype for a renal membrane signalling disorder. *Kid Int* 42:1, 1992.
21. Moran M, Tomlanovich S, Myers BD, et al: Cyclosporine-induced chronic nephropathy in human recipients of cardiac allografts. *Transplant Proc* 17(suppl 4):185, 1985.
22. Gonwa TA, Mai ML, Pilcher J, et al: Stability of long-term renal function in heart transplant patients treated with induction therapy and low-dose cyclosporine. *J Heart Lung Transplant* 11:926, 1992.
23. Lewis RM, Van Buren CT, Kerman RH, et al: A review of long-term cyclosporine use in renal transplantation. *Clin Transplant* 4:313, 1990.
24. Almond PS, Gillingham KJ, Sibley R, et al. Renal transplant function after ten years of cyclosporine. *Transplantation* 53:316, 1992.
25. Montagnino G, Colturi C, Tarantino A, et al. The impact of azathioprine and cyclosporine on long-term function in a kidney transplantation. *Transplantation* 51:772, 1991.
26. Kirk AJB, Omar I, Dark JH: Long-term improvement in renal function using nifedipine in cyclosporine-associated hypertension. *Transplantation* 50:1061, 1990.
27. Palmer BF, Dawidson I, Sagalowsky A, et al: Improved outcome of cadaveric renal transplantation due to calcium channel blockers. *Transplantation* 52:640, 1991.
28. Schroeder JS, Gao SZ, Alderman EL, et al: A preliminary study of diltiazem in the prevention of coronary artery disease in heart transplant recipients. *N Engl J Med* 328:164, 1993.
29. Chan GLC, Canafax DM, Johnson CA: The therapeutic use of azathioprine in renal transplantation. *Pharmacotherapy* 7:165, 1987.
30. Fauci AS: Mechanisms of the immunosuppressive and anti-inflammatory effects of glucocorticosteroids. *J Immunopharmacol* 1:1, 1978.
31. Snyder DS, Unanue ER: Corticosteroids inhibit immune macrophages' Ia expression and interleukin-1 production. *J Immunol* 129:1803, 1982.
32. Ortho Multicenter Transplant Study Group: A randomized clinical trial of OKT3 monoclonal antibody for acute rejection of cadaveric renal transplants. *N Engl J Med* 313:337, 1985.
33. Wahlers T, Heublein B, Cremer J, et al: Treatment of rejection after heart transplantation: What dosage of pulsed steroids is necessary? *J Heart Lung Transplant* 9:568, 1990.
34. Miller LW: Treatment of cardiac allograft rejection with intravenous corticosteroids. *J Heart Transplant* 9:283, 1990.
35. Lonquest JL, Radovancevic B, Vega JD: Reevaluation of steroid tapering after steroid pulse therapy for heart rejection. *J Heart Lung Transplant* 11:913, 1992.
36. Schulak JA, Mayes JT, Montz CE, et al: A prospective randomized trial of prednisone versus no prednisone maintenance therapy in cyclosporine-treated and azathioprine-treated renal transplant patients. *Transplantation* 49:327, 1990.
37. Woodley SL, Renlund DG, O'Connell JB, et al: Immunosuppression following cardiac transplantation. *Cardiol Clin* 8:83, 1990.
38. Goodman, Gillman (eds): *The Pharmacologic Basis of Therapeutics,* 8th ed. New York, Pergamon Press, 1990, pp 1209–1218.
39. Yadav RVS, Indudhara R, Kamar P, et al: Cyclophosphamide in renal transplantation. *Transplantation* 45:421, 1988.
40. Wagoner LE, Olsen SL, Taylor DO, et al: Cyclophosphamide as an alternative immunosuppressive agent in cardiac transplant recipients with recurrent rejection. *J Heart Lung Transplant* 11:199, 1992.
41. Frasier LH, Kanekal S, Kehrer JP: Cyclophosphamide toxicity. *Drugs* 42:781, 1991.

42. Carandall BG, Gilbert EM, Renlund DG, et al: A randomized trial of the immunosuppressive efficacy of vincristine in cardiac transplantation. *Transplantation* 50:34, 1990.
43. Olsen NJ, Murray L: Antiproliferative effects of methotrexate on peripheral blood mononuclear cells. *Arthritis Rheum* 32:378, 1989.
44. Rosenthal GJ, Weigand GW, Germolec DR: Suppression of B cell function by methotrexate and trimetrexate. *J Immunol* 141:410, 1988.
45. Costanzo-Nordi MR, Grusk BB, Silver MA, et al: Reversal of recalcitrant cardiac allograft rejection with methotrexate. *Circulation* 78(suppl III):45, 1988.
46. Olsen SL, O'Connell JB, Bristow MR, et al: Methotrexate as an adjunct in the treatment of persistent mild cardiac allograft rejection. *Transplantation* 50:773, 1990.
47. Hosenpud JD, Hershberger RE, Ratkovec RR, et al: Methotrexate for the treatment of patients with multiple episodes of acute cardiac allograft rejection. *J Heart Lung Transplant* 11:739, 1992.
48. Bourge RC, Kirklin JK, White-Williams C, et al: Methotrexate pulse therapy in the treatment of recurrent acute heart rejection. *J Heart Lung Transplant* 11:1116, 1992.
49. Carey JA, First WH: Use of polyclonal antilymphocytic preparations for prophylaxis in heart transplantation. *J Heart Lung Transplant* 9:297, 1990.
50. Cosimi AB: Antilymphocyte globulin and monoclonal antibodies, in Morris PJ (ed), *Kidney Transplantation: Principles and Practice,* ed 3. Philadelphia, WB Saunders, 1988.
51. Tellis VA, Matas AJ, Quinn TA, et al: Antilymphoblast globulin treatment of steroid-resistant rejection in cyclosporine immunosuppressed renal transplant recipients. *Transplant Proc* 19:1892, 1987.
52. Filo RS, Book B, Pescovitz MD: Association of sensization to horse antilymphocyte/thymocyte globulin with recipient age and decreased renal allograft survival rates. *Transplant Proc* 25:577, 1993.
53. Todd PA, Brogden RN: Muromonab CD3: A review of its pharmacology and therapeutic potential. *Drugs* 37:871, 1989.
54. Bach J-F, Chatenoud L: Immunologic monitoring of Orthoclone OKT3-treated patients: The problem of anti-monoclonal immune response. *Transplant Proc* 19(suppl 1):17, 1987.
55. Fung JJ, Markus BH, Gordon RD, et al: Impact of orthoclone OKT3 on liver transplantation. *Transplant Proc* 19(suppl 1):37, 1987.
56. Schroeder TJ, Weiss MA, Smithe RD, et al: The use of OKT3 in the treatment of acute vascular rejection. *Transplant Proc* 23:1043, 1991.
57. Delaney VB, Campbell WG, Nasr SA, et al: Efficacy of OKT3 monoclonal antibody therapy in steroid-resistant, predominantly vascular acute rejection. *Transplantation* 45:743, 1988.
58. Woodle ES, Thistlewaite JR, Emond JC, et al: OKT3 therapy for hepatic allograft rejection. *Transplantation* 51:1207, 1991.
59. Solomon H, Gonwa TA, Mor E, et al: OKT3 rescue for steroid-resistant rejection in adult liver transplantation. *Transplantation* 55:87, 1993.
60. Gilbert EM, Dewitt CW, Eiswirth CC, et al: Treatment of refractory cardiac allograft rejection with OKT3 monoclonal antibody. *Am J Med* 82:202, 1987.
61. Deeb GM, Bolling SF, Steimle CN, et al: A randomized prospective comparison of MALG with OKT3 for rescue therapy of acute myocardial rejection. *Transplantation* 51:180, 1991.
62. Alloway RR, Kotb M, Gaber LW, et al: Standard versus low-dose OKT3 induction therapy of cadaveric renal transplantation: Comparison of outcome data versus OKT3 dose and serum levels. *Clin Transplant* 46:468, 1992.
63. Brown M, Korb S, Light JA, et al: Low-dose OKT3 induction therapy following renal transplantation leads to improved graft function and decreased adverse effects. *Transplant Proc* 25:553, 1993.
64. Schweizer RT, Roper L, Hull D, et al: Low-dose OKT3 for cadaveric renal transplantation. *Transplant Proc* 24:2592, 1992.
65. First MR, Schroeder TJ, Hurtubise PE, et al: Immune monitoring during retreatment with OKT3. *Transplant Proc* 21:1753, 1989.
66. Gabel HM, Lebech LL, Jensik SC, et al: Discordant expression of CD3 and T-cell-receptor antigens on lymphocytes from patients treated with OKT3. *Transplant Proc* 21:1745, 1989.
67. Hammond EH, Wittwer CT, Greenwood J, et al: Relationship of OKT3 sensitization and vascular rejection in cardiac transplant

patients receiving OKT3 rejection prophylaxis. *Transplantation* 50:776, 1990.
68. Schroeder TJ, First MR, Mansour ME, et al: Antimurine antibody formation following OKT3 therapy. *Transplantation* 49:48, 1990.
69. Hricik DE, Mayes JT, Schulak JA: Inhibition of anti-OKT3 antibody generation by cyclosporine—results of a prospective randomized trial. *Transplantation* 50:237, 1990.
70. Kimball JA, Normal DJ, Shield CF, et al: OKT3 Antibody Response Study (OARD): A multicenter, comparable study. *Transplant Proc* 25:558, 1993.
71. Breisblatt WM, Schulman DS, Stein K, et al: Hemodynamic response to OKT3 in orthotopic heart transplant recipients: Evidence for reversible myocardial dysfunction. *J Heart Lung Transplant* 10:359, 1991.
72. Chan GL, Weinstein SS, Wright CE, et al: Encephalopathy associated with OKT3 administration. *Transplantation* 52:148, 1991.
73. Marks WH, Perkal M, Bia M, et al: Aseptic encephalitis and blindness complicating OKT3 therapy. *Clin Transplant* 5:435, 1991.
74. Squifflet J-P, Sutherland DER, Field J, et al: Synergistic immunosuppressive effect of cyclosporin-A and azathioprine. *Transplant Proc* 15:520, 1983.
75. Simon RL, Canafax DM, Fryd DS, et al: New immunosuppressive drug combinations for mismatched related and cadaveric renal transplantation. *Transplant Proc* 18(suppl 1):76, 1986.
76. Olivari M-T, Kubo SH, Braunlin EA, et al: Five-year experience with triple-drug immunosuppressive therapy in cardiac transplantation. *Circulation* 82(suppl IV):276, 1990.
77. Ascher NL, Stock PG, Bungardner GL, et al: *Surg Gynecol Obstet* 167:474, 1988.
78. Albrechtsen D, Flatmark A, Brynger H, et al: Dual vs triple immunosuppressive therapy: Equally safe and effective in kidney transplantation? *Transplant Proc* 23:2206, 1991.
79. Bowman JS, Angstadt JD, Waymack JP, et al: A comparison of triple-therapy with double-therapy immunosuppression in cadaveric renal transplantation. *Transplantation* 53:556, 1992.
80. Brinker KR, Dickerman RM, Gonwa TA, et al: A randomized trial comparing double-drug and triple therapy in primary cadaveric renal transplants. *Transplantation* 50:43, 1990.
81. Lindholm A, Albrechtsen D, Tufveson G, et al: A randomized trial of cyclosporine and prednisolone versus cyclosporine, azathioprine and prednisolone in primary cadaveric renal transplantation. *Transplantation* 54:624, 1992.
82. Hardie IR: Optimal combination of immunosuppressive agents for renal transplantation: First report of a multicentre, randomized trial comparing cyclosporine and prednisone with cyclosporine and azathioprine and with triple therapy in cadaveric renal transplantation. *Transplant Proc* 25:583, 1993.
83. Ponticelli C, Tarantino A, Montagnini G, et al: A randomized trial comparing triple-drug and double-drug therapy in renal transplantation. *Transplantation* 45:913, 1988.
84. Greenberg A, Egel JW, Thompson ME, et al: Early and late forms of cyclosporine nephrotoxicity: Studies in cardiac transplant recipients. *Am J Kid Dis* 9:12, 1987.
85. Yacoub M, Alivizatos P, Khaghani A, et al: The use of cyclosporine, azathioprine, and antithymocyte globulin with or without low-dose steroids for immunosuppression of cardiac transplant patients. *Transplant Proc* 17:221, 1985.
86. Esmore DS, Spratt PM, Keogh AM, et al: Cyclosporine and azathioprine immunosuppression without maintenance steroids: A prospective randomized trial. *J Heart Transplant* 8:194, 1989.
87. Katz MR, Barnhart GR, Szentpetery S, et al: Are steroids essential for successful maintenance of immunosuppression in heart transplantation? *J Heart Transplant* 6:293, 1987.
88. Keogh A, MacDonald P, Mundy J, et al: Five-year follow-up of a randomized double-drug versus triple-drug therapy immunosuppressive trial after heart transplantation. *J Heart Lung Transplant* 11:550, 1992.
89. Moore CK, Renlund DG, Rasmussen LG, et al: Long-term morbidity of cyclosporine with corticosteroid-free maintenance immunosuppression in cardiac transplantation. *Transplant Proc* 22(suppl 1):25, 1990.
90. Lee KF, Pierce JD, Hess ML, et al: Cardiac transplantation with corticosteroid-free immunosuppression: Long-term results. *Ann Thorac Surg* 52:211, 1991.
91. Gugenheim J, Samuel D, Saliba F, et al: Use of flexible triple-drug immunosuppressive therapy in liver transplantation. *Transplant Proc* 19:3805, 1987.
92. Sommer BG, Henry M, Ferguson RM: Sequential antilymphoblast globulin and cyclosporine for renal transplantation. *Transplantation* 43:85, 1987.
93. Michael HJ, Fancos GC, Burke JF, et al: A comparison of the effects of cyclosporine versus antilymphocyte globulin on delayed graft function in cadaver renal transplant recipients. *Transplantation* 48:805, 1989.
94. Abramowicz D, Goldman M, De Paw L, et al: The long-term effects of prophylactic OKT3 monoclonal antibody in cadaveric kidney transplantation—A single-center, prospective, randomized study. *Transplantation* 54:433, 1992.
95. Shield CF III: Use of OKT3 as prophylaxis in cadaveric renal transplantation. *Transplant Proc* 21(suppl 2):15, 1989.
96. Cosimi B, Jenkins RL, Rohrer RJ, et al: A randomized clinical trial of prophylactic OKT3 monoclonal antibody in liver allograft recipients. *Arch Surg* 125:781, 1990.
97. Millis JM, McDiarmid SV, Hiatt JR, et al: Randomized prospective trial of OKT3 for early prophylaxis of rejection after liver transplantation. *Transplantation* 47:82, 1989.
98. McDiarmid SV, Busuttil RW, Levy P, et al: The long-term outcome of OKT3 compared with cyclosporine prophylaxis after liver transplantation. *Transplantation* 52:91, 1991.
99. Johnson CP, Slakey DP, Callaluce RD, et al: Prospective randomized comparison of quadruple vs triple therapy for first cadaver transplants with immediate function. *Transplant Proc* 25:585, 1993.
100. Balk AHMM, Weimar W, Mochtar B, et al: Immunosuppression with OKT3 or cyclosporine in heart transplantation. Preliminary report of a controlled trial. *J Heart Transplant* 8:102, 1989.
101. Normal DJ, Kahana L, Stuart FP, et al: A randomized clinical trial of induction therapy with OKT3 in kidney transplantation. *Transplantation* 55:45, 1993.
102. Light JA, Khawand N, Ali A, et al: Comparison of Minnesota antilymphocyte globulin and OKT3 for induction of immunosuppression in renal transplant patients. *Transplant Proc* 21:1738, 1989.
103. Frey DJ, Matas AJ, Gillingham KJ, et al: Sequential therapy—A prospective randomized trial of MALG versus OKT3 for prophylactic immunosuppression in cadaver renal allograft recipients. *Transplantation* 54:50, 1992.
104. Steinmuller DR, Hayes JM, Novick AC, et al: Comparison of OKT3 with ALG for prophylaxis for patients with acute renal failure after cadaveric renal transplantation. *Transplantation* 52:67, 1991.
105. Hanto DW, Jendrisak MD, McCullough CS, et al: A prospective randomized comparison of prophylactic ALG and OKT3 in cadaver kidney allograft recipients. *Transplant Proc* 23:1050, 1991.
106. Broyer M, Gagnadoux MF, Guest G, et al: Prophylactic OKT3 monoclonal antibody versus antilymphocyte globulins: A prospective randomized study in 148 first cadaver kidney grafts. *Transplant Proc* 25:570, 1993.
107. MacDonald PS, Mundy J, Keough AM, et al: A prospective randomized study of prophylactic OKT3 versus equine antithymocyte globulin after heart transplantation—Increased morbidity with OKT3. *Transplantation* 55:110, 1993.
108. Laske A, Gallino A, Schneider J, et al: Prophylactic cytolytic therapy in heart transplantation: Monoclonal versus polyclonal antibody therapy. *J Heart Lung Transplant* 11:557, 1992.
109. Menkis AH, Powell A-M, Novick RJ, et al: A prospective randomized controlled trial of initial immunosuppression with ALG versus OKT3 in recipients of cardiac allograft. *J Heart Lung Transplant* 11:569, 1992.
110. Costanzo-Nordin MR, O'Sullivan EJ, Johnson MR, et al: Prospective randomized trial of OKT3 versus horse antithymocyte globulin-based immunosuppressive prophylaxis in heart transplantation. *J Heart Transplant* 9:306, 1990.
111. Calne RY: Cyclosporin in cadaveric renal transplantation: 5 year follow-up of a multicenter trial. *Lancet* 2:506, 1987.
112. Canadian Multicenter Transplant Study Group: A randomized clinical trial of cyclosporine in cadaveric renal transplantation: Analysis at 3 years. *N Engl J Med* 314:1219, 1986.
113. Kasiske BL, Heim-Duthoy K, Ma JZ: Elective cyclosporine withdrawal after renal transplantation. *JAMA* 269:395, 1993.

114. Flechner SM, Lorber M, Van Buren C, et al: The case against conversion to azathioprine in cyclosporine-treated renal recipients. *Transplant Proc* 17(suppl 1):276, 1985.
115. Stevens L, Halbrook H, Berron K, et al: Conversion from cyclosporine to azathioprine in heart transplant recipients. *J Heart Transplant* 7:119, 1988
116. Perkins JD, Sterioff S, Wiesner RH, et al: Conversion from standard cyclosporine to low-dose cyclosporine and azathioprine therapy as treatment for cyclosporine-related complications in liver transplant patients. *Transplant Proc* 19:2434, 1987.
117. Canafax DM, Marter EJ, Ascher NL, et al: Two methods of managing cyclosporine nephrotoxicity: Conversion to azathioprine, prednisone or cyclosporin, azathioprine, and prednisone. *Transplant Proc* 17:1176, 1985.
118. Flechner SM, Kerman RH, Van Buren CT, et al: The use of cyclosporine-treated living-related renal transplantation. Donor-specific hyporesponsiveness and steroid withdrawal. *Transplantation* 38:685, 1984.
119. Hricik DE, Whalen CC, Lautman J, et al: Withdrawal of steroids after renal transplantation—Clinical predictors of outcome. *Transplantation* 53:41, 1992.
120. Kobashigawa JA, Stevenson LW, Brownfield ED, et al: Initial success of steroid weaning late after heart transplantation. *J Heart Lung Transplant* 11:428, 1992.
121. Miller LW, Wolford T, McBride LR, et al: Successful withdrawal of corticosteroids in heart transplantation. *J Heart Lung Transplant* 11:431, 1992.
122. Price GD, Olsen SL, Taylor DO, et al: Corticosteroid-free maintenance immunosuppression after heart transplantation: Feasibility and beneficial effects. *J Heart Lung Transplant* 11:403, 1992.
123. Pritzker MR, Lake K, Rentzel T, et al: Steroid-free maintenance immunotherapy: Minneapolis Heart Institute experience. *J Heart Lung Transplant* 11:415, 1992.
124. Saper V, Chow ED, Engleman RT, et al: Clinical and immunological studies of cadaveric renal transplant recipients given total lymphoid irradiation and maintained on low dose prednisone. *Transplantation* 45:540, 1988.
125. Levin B, Bohannon L, Warvariv V, et al: Total lymphoid irradiation (TLI) in the cyclosporine era—Use of TLI in resistant cardiac allograft rejection. *Transplant Proc* 21:1793, 1989.
126. Hung SA, Strober S, Hoppe RT, et al: Total lymphoid irradiation for treatment of intractable cardiac allograft rejection. *J Heart Lung Transplant* 10:211, 1991.
127. Frist WH, Winterland AW, Gerherdt EB, et al: Total lymphoid irradiation in heart transplantation: Adjustment treatment for recurrent rejection. *Ann Thorac Surg* 48:863, 1989.
128. Salter MM, Kirklin JK, Bourge RC, et al: Total lymphoid irradiation in the treatment of early or recurrent heart rejection. *J Heart Lung Transplant* 11:902, 1992.
129. Bourge RC, Naftel DC, Geroge JF, et al: Total lymphoid irradiation in cardiac transplantation: Is there a prolonged effect on allograft rejection? *J Heart Lung Transplant* 12:S86, 1993.
130. Haberal M, Sert S, Gulay H, et al: Treatment of steroid-resistant renal allograft rejection with OKT3 and plasmapheresis. *Transplant Proc* 22:1761, 1990.
131. Mehta HJ, Desai JD, Chafekar DS, et al: The therapeutic role of plasma exchange in acute renal allograft rejection. *Transplantation* 50:885, 1990.
132. Costanzo-Nordin MR, Hubbell EA, O'Sullivan EJ, et al: Successful treatment of heart transplant rejection with photopheresis. *Transplantation* 53:808, 1992.
133. Rose EA, Barr ML, Xu H, et al: Photochemotherapy in human heart transplant recipients at high risk for fatal rejection. *J Heart Lung Transplant* 11:746, 1992.

194. Critical Care Problems in Kidney Transplant Recipients

Ranier W. G. Gruessner

Kidney transplantation has emerged as the treatment of choice for end-stage renal failure. A successful transplant, compared with dialysis, offers a better quality of life at an overall lower cost. One-year patient survival rates approach 90 to 95 percent; one-year graft survival rates, 80 to 85 percent. Half-life projected for all cadaver transplant grafts surviving the first year is about 8 years; for living related transplant grafts, 13 to 26 years, depending on HLA match [1]. Despite the improvement in surgical techniques, immunosuppression, and patient and graft survival rates, various problems remain. This chapter discusses complications after kidney transplantation and their implications for critical care.

Pretransplant Evaluation

Successful transplantation depends largely on careful selection and thorough pretransplant evaluation of the recipient. Above all, the evaluation process may reveal absolute contraindica-

tions to transplantation. It may also provide information about the need for perioperative intensive care unit (ICU) monitoring.

The pretransplant workup should assess and document any cardiovascular, gastrointestinal, pulmonary, neurologic, and genitourinary risk factors and disclose any potential sources of infection. Patients with increased risk for coronary artery disease or cardiac dysfunction, especially diabetic candidates, should undergo stress thallium testing. Depending on the results, a coronary angiogram might be indicated. Some patients may require coronary artery bypass or percutaneous coronary artery balloon dilatation pretransplant to decrease cardiac morbidity and mortality posttransplant [2]. Patients with cholelithiasis should undergo cholecystectomy pretransplant. Those with documented colonic disease (e.g., previous episodes of diverticulitis) should undergo colonic surgery. Patients with documented ulcer disease should be treated with H_2 blockers; if ulcers are present on repeat gastroscopies, selective proximal vagotomy may be indicated. If appropriate therapeutic measures are taken pretransplant, many potential complications (sometimes life-threatening) will not become an issue posttransplant. A thorough pretransplant workup will also help identify patients who need posttransplant ICU monitoring.

Pretransplant Preparation

Overall graft and patient survival rates depend in part on proper pretransplant preparation of the recipient. Most patients come to surgery after recent dialysis, so metabolic abnormalities can be present pretransplant. Fluid overload, hyperkalemia, hyperglycemia, and acidosis require correction. A chest x-ray and EKG should be routinely obtained pretransplant to assess recent pulmonary or cardiac abnormalities such as pneumonia, uremic pericarditis, or myocardial infarction. The dialysis access site should be examined to prevent exacerbation of local infection posttransplant. Hypocoagulability due to uremia and recent dialysis may require correction with fresh frozen plasma. Pretransplant central venous line placement allows monitoring of the central venous pressure, which facilitates intraoperative and postoperative fluid management (particularly in high-risk recipients). Arterial line placement is less frequently indicated. Swan-Ganz catheter monitoring occasionally benefits patients with advanced cardiac dysfunction (e.g., ejection fraction <30%).

Intraoperative and Postoperative Care

To decrease the incidence of acute tubular necrosis (ATN) posttransplant, a liberal hydration policy (including crystalloids and blood, in combination with diuretics before revascularization) should be employed intraoperatively. On unclamping, the patient should be well hydrated to prevent hypotension, which would cause poor transplant perfusion due to volume depletion. In patients with initial allograft function, fluid replacement can be regulated by replacing urine volumes hourly; if cardiac dysfunction is not present, urine output can initially be replaced cc for cc. For patients with high-output diuresis (≥500 ml/hr), 1% dextrose with 0.45% normal saline solution is recommended; potassium replacement may also be necessary but should not exceed 0.3 mEq/kg/hr intravenously (otherwise, cardiac monitoring is required). For patients with cardiac dysfunction and high-output diuresis (≥500 ml/hr), the volume of fluid replacement should be smaller than urine output (e.g., 0.5 cc of replacement for 1 cc of urine). In general, 24 hours posttransplant, urine output is appropriate for the patient's weight and renal function; fluid replacement is straight-rated (e.g., at a rate of 125 ml/hr). If urine output is <500 ml/hr, fluid replacement in nondiabetic patients should be with 5% dextrose with 0.45% normal saline solution. Diabetic patients should not be given 5% dextrose solution; instead, they should be placed on 20% dextrose solution at 20 ml/hr and on an insulin infusion pump to closely titrate serum glucose levels. Maintenance fluid replacement is with 1% dextrose with 0.45% normal saline. In patients with low urine output (≤50 ml/hr), urine should be replaced with an equal volume to avoid overreplacement and subsequent congestive heart failure and pulmonary edema. Patients with early dysfunction should, in addition, receive a small amount to account for insensible losses. Hyperkalemia is corrected with rectal administration of ion exchange resin sodium polystyrene sulfonate (Kayexalate), and dialysis may be necessary for patients with ATN.

The patient will spend the first hours posttransplant in the recovery room. This is the time to decide whether the patient can be safely transferred to the regular surgical ward or whether temporary ICU management is required.

In uncomplicated cases, nasogastric decompression is usually discontinued after 24 hours, at which time the patient is started on clear liquids. A Foley catheter is carefully monitored for obstruction and gently irrigated under sterile conditions if occluded (clot). The Foley catheter is discontinued 3 to 4 days posttransplant. Antibiotic ointment is placed around the urethral meatus during that time. Reversal of uremia frequently causes dialysis shunts to clot early posttransplant; no further treatment is usually necessary.

Trimethoprim-sulfamethoxazole (Bactrim; 80/400 mg/day) is given indefinitely for prophylaxis, primarily against *Pneumocystis carinii* and against urinary tract infections. Nystatin or clotrimazole is used as prophylaxis against fungal infections (e.g., monilial esophagitis). Antacids are given to prevent ulcer formation; in patients with documented history of peptic ulcer disease, H_2 blockers are indicated. Stool softeners or mild laxatives are given routinely (e.g., docusate in nondiabetics and bisacodyl in diabetic patients).

Most kidney allograft recipients are treated on a regular surgical ward posttransplant. ICU monitoring may become necessary if complications develop, at any time and at any stage posttransplant. The higher susceptibility of the transplant population to complications is related to immunosuppression. Various complications directly correlate with the intensity and duration of immunosuppression. For that reason, recipients of cadaver kidneys (which entail more induction and maintenance immunosuppression) are more prone to problems than recipients of living related donor kidneys. Moreover, most patients are in a uremic state pretransplant, and uremia itself is associated with less immunocompetence.

Many risk factors directly correlate with the incidence and severity of posttransplant complications. Between 15 and 30 percent of high-risk kidney transplant recipients require specific critical care.

Transplant-Specific Complications

Acute tubular necrosis (ATN) is the most common cause of impaired kidney function immediately posttransplant. While ATN is rare in living related kidney recipients, its incidence averages about 35 percent with cadaver donors. ATN may occur immediately after revascularization or within a few hours in grafts that have diuresed initially. It is less common after an acute rejection episode. Prognostic factors for the development of ATN are ischemic and immunologic [3,4]. Ischemic damage is caused by certain donor factors such as age, underlying disease (e.g., hypertension), and use of vasopressors, as well as by total ischemia time. Immunologic factors that potentially increase the incidence of ATN are a high percentage of antibodies (% PRA), retransplants, and poor matching. ATN not only has an impact on early kidney graft function, but also has a detrimental effect on graft survival and postoperative morbidity [5,6]. Of note, patients with posttransplant ATN have a higher incidence of acute rejection, which ultimately lowers graft survival rates [7]. In patients with ATN, dialysis frequently needs to be reinstituted; after a few days to several weeks, kidney function eventually recovers. These patients require close monitoring. ATN needs to be differentiated from early rejection. Serial ultrasound studies or graft biopsies are helpful in determining the cause of dysfunction.

Despite triple and quadruple immunosuppression—including corticosteroids, azathioprine, cyclosporine, and anti-T-cell preparations—*rejection* has continued to be a major problem [8] (see Chap. 198 for a complete discussion of rejection).

Technical Complications

Hemorrhage from the venous or arterial anastomosis is rare after kidney transplantation. Most posttransplant bleeding results from unligated vessels in the renal hilum; in the case of arterial bleeding, these vessels were very often in spasm at the time of transplant. Reexploration is seldom required in the immediate posttransplant period.

Although the incidence of vascular thrombosis is low (0.7–5%), it is very often associated with graft loss [9–12]. Patients with high-output intraoperative diuresis, who rapidly develop postoperative anuria, need to be monitored for the development of vascular thrombosis.

Causative factors for *renal artery thrombosis* are unidentified intimal flaps, perfusion or preimplantation damage, size discrepancy between donor and recipient vessels, hypotension or hypoperfusion (especially in pediatric donors receiving kidneys from adult donors), and technical difficulties in kidneys with multiple arteries [10]. Early diagnosis is essential. If urine output suddenly ceases, the Foley catheter needs to be gently irrigated to rule out plugging by a clot; if the central venous pressure is low, but the patient does not adequately respond to a fluid flush by an increase in urine output, Doppler studies are needed to rule out thrombosis. Salvage of such kidneys, although theoretically possible, is unlikely; nephrectomy is usually necessary.

Other arterial complications are aneurysm and stenosis. Aneurysms may be anastomotic (pseudoaneurysm) or infected (mycotic). The diagnosis is usually made by arteriogram. Aneurysms require surgical repair. In patients with iliac or renal artery stenosis, percutaneous balloon dilatation is the treatment of choice; if unsuccessful, surgical repair is necessary. Stenotic and aneurysmatic complications are usually not seen in the early posttransplant period.

Causative factors for *venous thrombosis* are kinking of the anastomosis, intimal injury during organ retrieval, pressure on the vein secondary to lymphocele, urinoma, or hematoma, and extension of iliofemoral thrombosis [9,10]. Rejection and some immunosuppressive drugs (e.g., cyclosporine) may also cause graft thrombosis. Renal vein thrombosis usually occurs within the first few days posttransplant. It is characterized by sudden onset of pain and graft swelling and, in the case of iliofemoral thrombosis, a swollen leg [10]. Hematuria with clots and tissue debris is common. The diagnosis is confirmed by Doppler study, which often shows a pulsatile renal artery running into the hilum of an enlarged kidney, possibly surrounded by hematoma. If thrombosis is complete, nephrectomy is necessary, although recovery of function after surgical embolectomy [13] or after intravenous infusion of thrombolytic agents [14] has been reported. When thrombosis is incomplete, the recommendation is immediate thrombectomy (or, alternatively, urokinase and heparin treatment). Vascular complications usually require ICU monitoring.

Urologic complications include hematuria, urinary leakage, and ureteral obstruction. *Hematuria* from the distal ureter or the cystostomy suture line generally ceases within the first 12 to 24 hours after surgery. More extensive bleeding maintained by urokinase release from the bladder may lead to the formation of blood clots and the obstruction of the urinary tract—the most common cause of sudden cessation of diuresis in the immediate postoperative period. If repeated or continuous bladder irrigations do not restore diuresis, cystoscopy may be necessary to evacuate or dissolve the clot. The diagnosis of bladder clots is confirmed by ultrasound. Infarcted papillae are a rare cause of significant hematuria, and nephrectomy usually is necessary. Prompt nephrectomy is also indicated in patients with kidney rupture due to fulminant rejection that causes hematuria and retroperitoneal bleeding. If hematuria is caused by posttransplant biopsy, with subsequent clot formation in the renal pelvis, temporary percutaneous placement of a nephrostomy tube is necessary. Most hematuria-related complications require close urine output monitoring, but rarely ICU admission.

Urinary leakage occurs secondary to technical complications or necrosis of the distal ureter. Percutaneous nephrostomy can initially be done, but reimplantation is generally necessary. Clinical symptoms of urinary leakage in the early posttransplant period are graft swelling and tenderness, fever, wound drainage, and edema of the scrotum, labia, or ipsilateral thigh. Minor urinary leakage may spontaneously resolve by temporary Foley catheter insertion.

Ureteral stenosis manifests itself months posttransplant and occurs secondary to rejection, ischemia, or infection. Percutaneous nephrostomy with balloon dilatation or surgical repair (reimplantation into the bladder or uretero-ureterostomy) is necessary. Urinary leakage and ureteral stenosis usually do not require ICU admission [15].

Lymphoceles or hematomas can cause deep venous thrombosis and impaired graft function, and may require external drainage. Recurrent lymphoceles are treated by either open laparotomy [16] or laparoscopy [17] to create a peritoneal window at the transplant site for drainage.

The incidence of *wound infection* ranges between 1 and 6 percent. This low wound complication rate is due to thorough skin preparation pretransplant and irrigation with an antibiotic solution at the end of the transplant. Intraoperative hemostasis must be meticulous to avoid small hematomas. Because most wound infections are derived from organisms in the recipient bladder, irrigation and instillation of 100 to 250 cc antibiotic solution at the beginning of the transplant procedure are recommended. If wound infection occurs, it is treated according to standard surgical principles of drainage and debridement.

Cardiovascular Complications

The incidence of *cardiac complications* posttransplant depends on the level of renal function and the recipient's underlying disease and cardiac history. Correction of uremia by immediate posttransplant allograft function improves the cardiac index, stroke volume, and ejection fraction. In contrast, patients with ATN experience persistent uremia and, in addition, perioperative fluid overload [18]. They carry a high risk of cardiac dysfunction and may require posttransplant hemodialysis to correct fluid retention and the metabolic state. Patients with diabetes, hypertension, and significant coronary disease are most likely to develop cardiac complications if there is no immediate posttransplant kidney allograft urine output. They may therefore require perioperative ICU monitoring, especially if left ventricular function is poor (ejection fraction <30%). Swan-Ganz catheter placement to optimize hemodynamics might be prudent, especially in diabetic recipients with coronary artery disease.

Myocardial infarction is uncommon in the perioperative period. It is mostly seen in patients with diabetic hypotension or preexisting coronary artery disease. These patients are subject to ICU admission and require close monitoring of their hemodynamic parameters, especially in the case of postoperative ATN. Although rare in the early posttransplant period, myocardial infarction is one of the major causes of death long-term in the transplant population. In diabetic recipients, the duration of this disease and the presence of preexisting coronary artery disease have an impact on the incidence and severity of posttransplant myocardial infarction, which is the main cause of death in this subgroup [19]. Other risk factors, as has been established for the general population, include hyperlipidemia, hypertension, and cigarette smoking.

Pericarditis in the early posttransplant period has in incidence of 1 to 3 percent [20]. It has been attributed to infections (mainly cytomegalovirus [CMV] infection), fluid overload, and medication (e.g., minoxidil). The main factor, however, is uremia. The incidence of pericarditis is significantly higher in patients who experience early posttransplant ATN. Most patients present with episodes of viral or uremic pericarditis during the first 8 weeks posttransplant. In contrast, bacterial pericarditis develops later, often in patients with advanced septic complications. Bacterial pericarditis is less frequent than viral or uremic pericarditis, but usually requires, besides antibiotic treatment, surgical or ultrasound/CT-guided drainage. Pericardiocentesis is mandatory if patients develop cardiac failure, hypertension, or cardiac tamponade. Patients with clinical symptoms of pericarditis require ICU monitoring.

Infective endocarditis is rare. It may be noted in patients with severe septicemia or longstanding immunosuppression [21]. As with all potentially life-threatening infections, the amount of immunosuppression must be reduced and appropriate antibiotics initiated.

Although *hypertension* is a major long-term problem that complicates kidney transplant outcome, it may also require close attention in the immediate posttransplant period. Hypertension can occur in patients with intraoperative hyperhydration (with or without development of ATN posttransplant) or in patients whose antihypertensive drugs were abruptly stopped pretransplant. Monitoring is required in patients with systolic blood pressures >200 mm Hg and diastolic pressures >110 mm Hg. If continuous intravenous infusion is necessary (e.g., titration with sodium nitroprusside), ICU admission should be considered. In most cases, early posttransplant hypertension can be controlled with appropriate medical treatment.

Hypertension is the most common long-term complication after kidney transplantation, with an incidence of up to 50 percent [22]. Children are especially prone to hypertension. It is also an important risk factor with cardiovascular disease and atherosclerosis [23,24]. Hypertension is associated with lower graft survival. Patient survival is also poorer, particularly if the original renal failure was caused by hypertension. Posttransplant hypertension very often has multiple causes, both intrinsic and extrinsic [24].

Intrinsic causes include chronic rejection, and to a lesser extent, acute rejection and recurrent disease. The mechanisms causing hypertension in transplant recipients who experience chronic rejection are similar to those of chronic renal disease in general [23]. Hypertension during acute rejection has been attributed to high-dose steroid treatment and stimulation of the renin-angiotensin system [25]. Angiotensin II is a potent vasoconstrictor, stimulating antidiuretic hormone (ADH) and aldosterone release, which results in sodium retention. Focal glomerulosclerosis is the most common recurrent disease associated with hypertension posttransplant.

Extrinsic factors include renal artery stenosis, native kidney-induced hypertension, and drug (cyclosporine, steroids) induced hypertension. Renal artery stenosis is treated by either percutaneous transluminal dilatation or, if unsuccessful, by sur-

gical repair. Native kidney-induced hypertension requires removal of the native kidneys due to the activation of the renin-angiotensin system. The pathophysiologic relationship of cyclosporine to hypertension is not fully understood, but afferent renal artery vasoconstriction resulting in renal sodium retention and release of potent vasopressor (endothelin) have been discussed [26,27]. In most patients with a longstanding history of hypertension, ICU monitoring is not necessary. Patients are often treated with a combination of calcium channel blockers, angiotensin I-converting-enzyme (ACE) inhibitors, cardioselective beta-adrenergic blockers, vasodilators, and diuretics. Consensus has not been reached on the optimal antihypertensive therapy, since many drugs interfere with kidney function and cyclosporine metabolism; treatment is based on each individual's response.

Hypotension, either intraoperatively or during the immediate posttransplant period, may cause severe damage to the transplanted kidney. Intraoperative hypotension is usually caused by volume depletion or is related to anesthetic agents. Hypovolemia should be corrected rapidly by restoring intravascular volume. It is prudent to monitor central venous pressure before unclamping to avoid poor perfusion of the transplanted kidney. Posttransplant hypovolemia, especially in patients with immediate graft function, is often caused by inadequate fluid replacement and should be treated accordingly. Cardiac dysfunction and bleeding must be ruled out in patients with early posttransplant hypotension. In diabetic patients with orthostatic dysfunction causing pronounced hypotension due to autonomic nephropathy, treatment with fludrocortisone or ephedrine can be successful. *Anaphylactic* reactions causing hypotension due to posttransplant immunosuppression (e.g., methylprednisolone, sodium succinate) are rare [28].

Previously uremic patients are more prone to develop *deep venous thrombosis* (DVT) posttransplant, compared with the general population. DVT has been linked to both high-dose corticosteroid therapy early posttransplant and "rebound" hypercoagulability. The latter is attributed to overcorrection of impaired platelet aggregation and thrombin generation, both associated with uremia [29,30]. Other thrombophilic factors that may occur within the first few weeks posttransplant are decreased fibrinolytic activity and increased plasminogen activation inhibitors [31,32]. Standard therapy is systemic heparinization followed by coumadin administration for 3 to 6 months. If DVT occurs in the immediate postoperative period, when heparinization can cause major bleeding, a vena cava filter is an appropriate alternative [33]. Because the kidney is a "high-flow" organ, DVT usually stops at the level of, or distal to, the renal vein anastomosis. Surgical intervention is indicated only if phlegmasia cerulea dolens develops. Venous thrombectomy (with or without creation of a temporary arteriovenous fistula) and, if necessary, fasciotomy, are the treatments of choice.

The incidence of DVT ranges from 1 to 4 percent [9,34]. The diagnosis is made clinically and confirmed by Doppler studies to assess the extent of DVT and the potential involvement of the kidney graft in the thrombotic event. In about two thirds of cases, DVT occurs on the transplant side. Pulmonary embolism as a result of DVT occurs in less than 1 percent of the transplant population, but, if it does, the mortality rate is about 40 percent [9]. Other factors predisposing to DVT are hematoma and lymphocele formation posttransplant, which diminish the venous return from the leg and may result in stasis and ultimately thrombosis. In contrast, neither transient marked elevation nor moderate sustained elevation of hemoglobin levels per se seems to be directly associated with an increased incidence of thromboembolic complications; DVT rarely occurs during periods of peak hemoglobin elevation [35]. In contrast, high hemoglobin levels (in combination with increased whole blood viscosity, iron deficiency, hypertension), as well as patient age and diabetes contribute to the occurrence of thrombotic events posttransplant. Aggressive therapeutic phlebotomy to maintain the hematocrit <55 percent has been recommended [35].

Pulmonary Complications

Most renal transplant recipients do not require ventilatory support postoperatively and are extubated in the recovery room. Prolonged ventilatory support is indicated in patients with pulmonary dysfunction secondary to intraoperative fluid overload, cardiac dysfunction, or underlying lung disease.

Pulmonary edema usually is the result of fluid overreplacement intraoperatively [36]. Causative factors also include high ventricular filling pressure, pulmonary hypertension, alterations of oncotic hydrostatic gradient, and increased cardiac output. It may occasionally appear in patients with immediate transplant diuresis, especially in those with cardiac dysfunction. In patients with immediate renal dysfunction, fluid restriction and diuresis with intravenously administered diuretics should be implemented. If this approach fails, dialysis is necessary. It is prudent to routinely obtain a chest x-ray in the recovery room to assess fluid status. This is particularly important in transplant recipients who receive monoclonal anti-T-cell treatment with OKT3 for induction or rejection therapy; fluid-overloaded patients can respond to their first dose of OKT3 with pulmonary edema [37,38]. If the interval is short between surgery and posttransplant dialysis, minimal anticoagulation is desirable to avoid bleeding. In patients with unstable hemodynamics, dialysis might be disadvantageous due to the associated decreases in cardiac index, cardiac output, stroke volume, pulmonary artery pressure, and central venous pressure—all of which can aggravate hypotension [39,40]. In these cases, sequential ultrafiltration (i.e., ultrafiltration first, then conventional hemodialysis) or hemofiltration is an alternative. Hemofiltration, in particular, results in stable circulation due to adequate vasoconstriction. Continuous forms of hemofiltration are also well tolerated in patients with hemodynamic instability and allow removal of a greater volume of fluid, compared with hemodialysis.

Pneumonia remains one of the most common posttransplant infections, with an incidence of 10 to 25 percent. It is most frequently observed within the first few months posttransplant, but it can occur at any time, often after treatment of acute rejection [41]. An aggressive approach to diagnosis is required, usually including bronchoscopy to determine the pathogen(s) involved. Most pneumonias are of viral (especially CMV) origin. However, bacterial infections (frequently caused by opportunistic pathogens or gram-negative rods) are not uncommon. Fungal infections occur with increasing frequency in patients who have been extensively treated with immunosuppressive or antibiotic agents; they may also occur as superinfections during treatment of primary pneumonia. Dual infections or superinfections have an associated mortality rate of up to 100 percent [42]. Bacterial pneumonias frequently cause fever and clinical symptoms; viral, fungal, or protozoal infections tend to develop subacutely or chronically over days before they become a clinical entity. Pending culture results, the appearance of the chest x-ray can help differentiate among the forms of pneumonia; CMV and pneumocystis-induced pneumonia cause interstitial infiltrates; bacterial pneumonia (including Legionella species), a lobar or diffuse consolidation; and fungal, mycobacterial, and nocardial infections, nodular infiltrates.

Rapid diagnosis is usually feasible. Fiberoptic bronchoscopy with bronchopulmonary lavage, with or without transbronchial biopsy, is employed. Incipient respiratory failure (PO$_2$ <60 mm Hg) requires oxygen supplementation. If arterial blood gases worsen, temporary ventilation may be necessary. Reduction or even discontinuation of immunosuppression might be indicated.

Pulmonary embolism is rare (<1%) after kidney transplantation. It is, however, more common than in the uremic nontransplanted population. In kidney transplant recipients, especially those who were uremic pretransplant, the hemostatic balance is activated and enhanced during the first week posttransplant [43]. This may explain the overall higher incidence of pulmonary embolism in the transplanted versus the uremic population. In general, quick recovery after kidney transplantation lowers the rate of pulmonary embolism.

Metabolic Complications

Hyperkalemia is frequently noted in the perioperative period, making serial serum potassium determinations necessary. Of note, in recently dialyzed patients, the serum potassium level is not predictive, because of the time lapse needed before equilibration. Surgical trauma, cellulitis, and transfusion of banked blood might cause intraoperative hyperkalemia. This can be corrected intraoperatively by intravenous glucose and insulin infusion, which will drive extracellular potassium into the cells. After transplantation, hyperkalemia can develop in patients with ATN and in patients with poor graft function due to severe acute or chronic rejection. Hyperkalemia can also be a drug-related side effect (e.g., impeded intracellular potassium entry by beta blocker). Therapeutically, a potassium-binding ion exchange resin (e.g., Kayexalate) can be given or, in patients requiring a rapid decrease of serum potassium, intravenous glucose and insulin infusions. Patients with hyperkalemia due to poor graft function may require dialysis.

Copious diuresis (≥500 ml/hr) immediately posttransplant may result in *hypokalemia* and requires appropriate potassium replacement. If potassium is substituted in patients requiring more than a dose of ≥0.3·mEq/kg/hr, they should be placed on a cardiac monitor.

Less frequently, *hypomagnesemia* and *hypophosphatemia* are noted in patients with high-output diuresis initially.

Infectious Complications

Infections are by far the most common posttransplant problem. They contribute substantially to the morbidity and mortality of renal transplant recipients. The incidence has decreased in recent years due to a better understanding of pathophysiology, improvements in prophylaxis and early detection, more aggressive treatment, and development of new drugs. Yet, infections remain the leading cause of death during both the early and the late posttransplant period. About 30 percent of all kidney transplant recipients require hospitalization at least once for treatment of infection [44]. The risk of infection is higher for older individuals, for diabetic patients, and for recipients with (multiple) episodes of antirejection treatment. Infections can be classified by the organism, the organ system involved, and the time of appearance posttransplant [45,46]. They do not occur at random, but frequently according to a timetable. Bacterial infections caused by common pathogens tend to occur early (<4 months), affecting predominantly the urinary and respiratory systems. Opportunistic bacterial infections occur later, correlated with duration and intensity of immunosuppression. Except for herpes simplex virus (HSV) infection, most viral infections (e.g., CMV) tend to occur after the first month posttransplant. Similarly, most fungal infections (e.g., aspergillus, cryptococcus) occur later, correlated to duration and intensity of immunosuppression. In contrast, candidal infections are also noted in the early posttransplant period. Protozoal infections are uncommon in the early posttransplant period. Overall, about 45 percent of all infections are viral, 30 percent bacterial, and 10 percent fungal. In 15 percent of cases, infections are polymicrobial (see Chap. 198).

Bacterial infections are the most common form in the early posttransplant period, predominantly causing wound infections, pneumonia, and urinary tract infections. Frequent organisms are staphylococci, streptococci, and gram-negative rods. These early posttransplant bacterial infections tend to cause septicemia and require prompt identification and treatment. If the causative pathogen or the source of severe bacterial infection is uncertain, antibiotics that provide coverage for gram-positive (e.g., vancomycin) and gram-negative organisms (e.g., a third-generation cephalosporin) should be given until culture and sensitivity results are available. Particularly in older patients with pneumonia requiring intubation and ventilation, as well as in patients with urosepsis, reducing or stopping immunosuppression may be necessary. Total parenteral nutrition is an important tool for critically ill patients to minimize tissue catabolism. More sophisticated treatments have been developed in recent years, including broad spectrum gammaglobulin, hormonal stimulation factors (GCSF, GMCSF), and anti-endotoxin-antibody therapy.

Viral infections are frequent in both the early and the late posttransplant periods. Most are due to organisms of the herpes virus family and include pathogens such as CMV, Epstein-Barr virus (EBV), HSV, and varicella-zoster virus (HZV).

CMV infection with symptomatic disease occurs in 20 to 45 percent of solid organ transplant recipients. It has been associated with chronic allograft rejection and decreased graft and patient survival [47,48]. Some limited success has been achieved in preventing CMV infection with prophylactic acyclovir, anti-CMV immune globulin, and vaccination; the disease itself, with potentially fatal dissemination, has not been eliminated [49,50,51]. Symptoms include fever, malaise, headache, myalgias, and arthralgia; leukopenia occurs in more than 70 percent of patients. CMV infection can present as neuritis, gastritis, or colitis, the latter often causing upper gastrointestinal bleeding. CMV can also cause retinitis, hepatitis, adenopathy, hepatosplenomegaly, and nephritis, frequently during the first 6 months posttransplant. CMV infections occur either as primary infection (e.g., seropositive donor kidney into a seronegative recipient), as reactivation infection (seropositive recipient after inception of immunosuppression), or as CMV superinfection (by separate strains of CMV).

Diagnosis is made by rising antibody titers (>4). Conversion in previously CMV-negative patients occurs frequently (initial titer 0, subsequent titers >4). Blood and urine samples, as well as tissue specimens (obtained at bronchoscopy [with bronchoalveolar lavage] or from kidney or GI biopsies), are examined for cultural evidence of CMV (centrifugation-enhanced shell vial culture rapid antigen [RA] technique). The specimen, after being cultured with fibroblasts, is stained with an immunofluorescent-labeled anti-CMV-specific murine monoclonal antibody and confirmed by immunofluorescence. More advanced technologies, such as complementary DNA (cDNA) probe for CMV or polymerase chain reaction (PCR), have the potential to increase the sensitivity for CMV diagnosis [52].

When the diagnosis of CMV disease is established, treatment is initiated with intravenous ganciclovir (5 mg/kg q 12 hrs if creatinine <1.5 mg/dl, with dose adjustment according to renal function, and 1.2 mg/kg q 48 hrs if patient is on dialysis). Dose reduction or temporary cessation of ganciclovir is indicated if leukopenia (WBC <3000/ml) or thrombocytopenia (platelet count <100,000/ml) occurs. Ganciclovir is usually administered for 14 days. Additional CMV hyperimmune globulin may occasionally be needed. In carefully selected patients with simultaneous occurrence of CMV and acute rejection, simultaneous treatment is feasible: ganciclovir therapy should begin 1 to 3 days before increasing immunosuppression [53]. It should be emphasized, however, that the amount of immunosuppression and the degree of suppression of host defense mechanisms directly correlate with the incidence of CMV disease. Since cell-mediated immunity is markedly impaired in CMV infection, superinfection by other opportunistic pathogens is a risk. Kidney allograft dysfunction (glomerulopathy) during or after active CMV infection has also been described [47,54].

While primary HSV infections are rare, reactivations are frequent. Symptomatic HSV infections are common with orofacial or genital lesions. Occasionally, conjunctivitis or corneal ulceration develops. Topical application of 5% acyclovir ointment accelerates healing and shortens the duration of virus shedding. Oral acyclovir (200 mg 5×/day) is also effective. If disseminated disease occurs (e.g., hepatitis, meningoencephalitis), intravenous acyclovir (5.0 mg/kg q8hrs × 7–14d) is necessary.

Varicella zoster virus (HZV) also requires systemic therapy with acyclovir, usually over a 7-day period.

Epstein-Barr virus infections have been associated with mononucleosis-like symptoms, and with the occurrence of fulminant, widespread lymphoproliferative disease (B-cell lymphoma) posttransplant. Lymphomas usually occur several years posttransplant in heavily immunosuppressed patients. Immunosuppression is then discontinued; conventional lymphoma treatment may be required because many EBV-induced lymphomas do not respond to acyclovir treatment.

Other viruses causing morbidity after successful transplantation are adeno- and influenza-viruses (involving the respiratory tract), papova viruses (progressive multifocal leukoencephalopathy), and hepatitis viruses. For more detailed information, the reader is advised to consult the standard textbooks on infection.

Fungal infections, both local and systemic, occur fairly often in kidney transplant recipients. In the early posttransplant period, oropharyngeal moniliasis is most common. Most fungal infections are prevented with oral nystatin or clotrimazole solutions. Systemic fungal infections are especially noted in patients with excessive immunosuppression; if they occur as superinfections, they are associated with a high mortality rate. Patients with cerebral, pulmonary, or visceral involvement, such as meningitis, pneumonia, or endocarditis (most frequently caused by candida or aspergillus), require reduction or (temporary) cessation of immunosuppression. They also need intravenous amphotericin B and possibly 5-flucytosine. Amphotericin is administered in dosages up to 1.0 mg/kg/day and total dosages of 0.5 to 1 gm, which may result in renal allograft loss due to the nephrotoxic side effects. Nocardia infections are best treated with trimethoprim-sulfamethoxazole. Candida can also cause an uncommon but life-threatening complication: a mycotic pseudoaneurysm. This usually results in allograft nephrectomy, with or without ligation of the external iliac artery, followed by intravenous amphotericin B. Once the infectious course is controlled, arterial revascularization of the lower extremity can be done. Cryptococcus and aspergillus can cause severe pulmonary and cerebral infections requiring systemic amphotericin B.

The most common pathogen of *protozoal infections* is *Pneumocystis carinii* causing interstitial pneumonia, relatively late in the posttransplant course. Since trimethoprim-sulfamethoxazole is given prophylactically posttransplant, the incidence of *Pneumocystis carinii*-induced pneumonia has decreased significantly. This infection is still seen in heavily immunosuppressed patients. Therapy consists of intravenous trimethoprim-sulfamethoxazole (dosage adjusted according to renal function) and, in case of hypersensitivity, pentamidine. *Pneumocystis carinii*-induced pneumonia, like most other severe infections, requires reduction or temporary cessation of immunosuppression.

Gastrointestinal and Pancreaticobiliary Complications

The incidence of posttransplant gastrointestinal (GI) complications is 5 to 25 percent. They are a major cause of morbidity and mortality in the kidney transplant population.

In the *upper GI* tract the most common problem is peptic ulcer disease and its associated complications (bleeding, perforation) [55]. However, the overall incidence of posttransplant upper GI complications after renal transplantation has declined considerably over the last two decades, mainly due to the development of H_2 blockers and routine prophylactic administration of more potent antacids [55]. Severe upper GI bleeding used to occur in more than 10 percent of the transplant population, with a mortality rate of up to 65 percent [56]; most of these bleeding episodes developed in the early postoperative period, half in the first three months [57]. Prophylactic gastric surgery (various forms of vagotomy) became very popular in the 1970s. This surgery was done pretransplant in patients with chronic renal failure, in an attempt to decrease morbidity and mortality of peptic ulcer disease [58]. With the advent of H_2 blockers (cimetidine, ranitidine) and inhibitors of the H + -K + ATPase enzyme system (omeprazole), prophylactic gastric surgery is now subject to treatment with antacids. For those with a documented history of gastric ulcer disease, the use of H_2 receptor antagonists is indicated. If severe upper GI bleeding occurs despite prophylactic treatment, and cannot be controlled by conservative means (including gastroscopy with submucosal injection of Adrenalin), the same surgical options (resection, vagotomy) apply as for nontransplant patients. In renal transplant candidates, the various forms of vagotomy effectively reduce the (mean) basal gastric acid output (BAO) by 70 to 90 percent and the (mean) maximal acid output (MAO) by 49 to 87 percent [59]. Although angiographic embolization for acute hemorrhage has been advocated [56], we have been reluctant to recommend it. Usually it requires embolization of two arteries with the risk of subsequent (gastric) necrosis and infection. Patients with severe upper GI bleeding require ICU monitoring; it is important to stabilize them before they undergo surgery, since gastric emergency procedures in transplant recipients have a high mortality rate [60]. If extensive gastroduodenal surgery is done, immunosuppressive reduction is mandatory and postoperative ICU monitoring recommended.

Peptic ulcer disease secondary to hyperacidity has become less common, due to prophylactic medical treatment, but ulcer disease secondary to viral infections, mainly CMV, has become more common [55]. An unexpectedly high incidence of CMV infection has been observed in apparent peptic ulcers in kidney transplant recipients. Diagnostic and immunohistochemical improvements have made it easier to detect tissue-invasive CMV infection [53]. In these cases, intravenous ganciclovir must be initiated [55].

The impact of hypercalcemia on the pathogenesis of peptic ulcer disease and its therapeutic consequences is controversial. Hypercalcemia due to hyperparathyroidism may aggravate peptic ulcer disease. Immediate and permanent cessation of gastric bleeding has been noted after subtotal parathyroidectomy in renal transplant recipients [56].

The most common *small bowel* complication is intestinal obstruction. Since most renal transplants are done retroperitoneally (except in children), this complication is often related to previous intraabdominal procedures (e.g., native nephrectomies, splenectomy) or infections. The same therapeutic principles apply as for the nontransplanted population.

Complications of the *lower GI tract* after renal transplantation occur at an incidence of 1 to 10 percent [55,61,62,63]. Colon perforation and lower GI hemorrhage are the two most common and frequently fatal (30–70%) lower GI complications.

Perforation can be due to diverticulitis, ischemic colitis, stercoral ulceration, or fecal impaction or to less common or undetermined forms of colitis. About 50 percent of all colon perforations occur within the first 3 months posttransplant [62,64]. Peritoneal signs, the hallmark of hollow organ perforation, are frequently absent in immunosuppressed patients [64].

The presentation and course of *diverticulitis* are different in renal transplant recipients than in the general population. Younger patients are more susceptible to this disease and have more free perforations overall [62,65]. The result is higher morbidity and mortality rates due to perforated diverticulitis. These patients have to deal not only with the insult of peritonitis, but also with the side effects of immunosuppression and the added morbidity of potential graft loss. Steroids are thought to be responsible for the difference between the transplant and the nontransplant population: they mask symptoms and impair the host's ability to localize and contain the perforation. Furthermore, steroids adversely affect colon wall microcirculation and also worsen peritoneal defense mechanisms [65]. The percentage of diverticular disease is highest in patients undergoing renal transplantation for (adult) polycystic kidney disease [66], but these patients do not have a higher predisposition to develop colonic perforation [62]. Patients with diverticulitis require resection of the sigmoid colon, with creation of a colostomy and Hartman's pouch. Broad spectrum antibiotics are given according to sensitivity testing (based on intraoperatively obtained cultures). It is important to test for aerobic and anaerobic pathogens, as well as for fungal organisms, since Candida peritonitis is not uncommon in the transplant population.

Ischemic colitis has been associated with impaired blood flow to the colonic wall, stenosis or occlusion of the inferior mesenteric artery, insufficient vascular collateralization, previous retroperitoneal surgery, immunosuppressive and antibiotic therapy, and diseases such as vasculitis and hypercoagulopathy [67,68]. Other causative factors are (intermittent or temporary) hypotension and irregular blood volume distribution [67]. However, often no explanation is apparent, especially in young patients with normal mesenteric vessels. Ischemic colitis may be segmental or pancolic. Some patients with ischemic colitis have shown, at laparotomy, features suggestive of inflammatory bowel disease, but microscopically without the typical lesions of Crohn's disease [67].

Pseudomembranous colitis caused by *Clostridium difficile* toxin is increasingly recognized. It can result in the development of toxic megacolon. Diagnosis is made from stool or biopsy cultures [62,67]. Patients are usually treated conservatively, with oral vancomycin (125 mg q6h for 10 days) or metronidazole (250 mg qid for 10 days).

Neutropenic enterocolitis causes mucosal ulceration of the bowel wall. It is associated with profound neutropenia and invasion by clostridial organisms (e.g., *Clostridium septicum*). The course of neutropenic enterocolitis is progressive, requiring treatment with metronidazole and possibly surgical intervention [69]. Infectious colitis is frequently due to CMV infection, which often causes lower GI hemorrhage. Infectious colitis can also be due to bacterial (e.g., myobacteria), viral (e.g., herpes), and fungal (e.g., Candida) infections. Diagnosis is from endoscopic biopsy and stool cultures; therapy requires intravenous antimicrobial therapy. Surgical intervention is not desirable due to the increased morbidity and mortality.

Cecal volvulus is a rare complication, but requires prompt surgical intervention [70]. In cases without evidence of gangrene, a cecopexy should be done; if a perforation has taken place, resection and creation of a colostomy are imperative.

The incidence of *acute colonic pseudo-obstruction (Ogilvie's syndrome)* is 1.5 percent in the transplant population [71]; it causes paralytic ileus, particularly with cecal dilatation. This complication is more frequent in patients with delayed onset of graft function. It usually requires nonoperative therapy (colonoscopic decompression). Like fecal impaction and stercoral ulceration, Ogilvie's syndrome can cause colonic perforation, thus necessitating surgical resection.

In general, survival rates in patients with colonic perforation can be improved with early diagnosis and prompt treatment [62,63,67]. With treatment for septicemia and peritonitis, patients may also need to stop immunosuppression and thus risk losing the kidney graft. Of note, rejection in the presence of severe infection is not common. Once the patient's condition improves, immunosuppression should cautiously be restarted.

Lower GI *hemorrhage* is most commonly due to opportunistic colitis. GI lesions thought to be peptic, particularly when associated with upper GI bleeding, are frequently the result of CMV infection [55,72]. Fungal ulceration has also been described as a source of lower GI hemorrhage: H_2 blockers and antacids promote fungal overgrowth due to achlorhydria [72]. Another factor causing lower GI bleeding is the ulcerogenic effect of steroids and their tendency to impair the reparative mechanisms of the bowel wall. In addition, conditions such as uremia and diabetes result in colonic distention and impaction, due to autonomic nephropathy; both contribute to the pathogenesis of colonic ulcers. In cases with lower GI bleeding, colonoscopy must be done urgently so that treatment is not delayed. To prevent fungal superinfection dissemination, prophylactic treatment of the GI tract with antifungal agents (e.g., nystatin or clotrimazole) is helpful.

Successfully managing colonic complications posttransplant requires an aggressive approach. Bacteriologic, radiologic (e.g., CT, gastrografin enema), and endoscopic evaluation must be done on an emergency basis. If necessary, surgical intervention must be rapid. The perioperative treatment of these patients requires close ICU monitoring.

The incidence of *pancreatitis* posttransplant ranges from 1 to 6 percent; its mortality rate, from 30 to 90 percent [73–76]. The mortality appears to be highest if pancreatitis develops after the first 3 months posttransplant [76]. Renal transplant recipients are exposed to many factors known to be associated with pancreatitis: immunosuppression (corticosteroids, azathioprine, cyclosporin A), other pharmacologic agents (e.g., furosemide, thiazide diuretics), hypercalcemia with or without hyperparathyroidism, infections (CMV, herpes), operative procedures (splenectomy, nephrectomy), and uremia, hypertension, hyperlipidemia, and diabetes. Steroids increase the viscosity of pancreatic secretions (theoretically leading to obstruction and dilatation of the pancreatic duct); they can also cause epithelial duct proliferation and peripancreatic fat necrosis [74]. An equally serious side effect of steroids is that they mask abdominal pain during episodes of pancreatitis, thus delaying proper diagnosis. Hypercalcemia secondary to (tertiary) hyperparathyroidism is also considered a major causative factor [77]; exces-

sive ionic calcium accelerates the conversion of trypsinogen, promoting pancreatic autodigestion [74]. Infection, especially CMV, is a well-documented cause of posttransplant pancreatitis [78], but bacterial infections causing pancreatitis have also been reported [74]. The term *rejection pancreatitis* [74,79] arose from speculation that the host forms antibodies that are not only reactive with the graft (vascular rejection), but also with antigens on the surface of pancreas cells (vascular pancreatitis). Biliary tract disease and alcoholism, the most frequent causes of pancreatitis in the nontransplant population, are of minor importance in the kidney transplant group.

Diagnosis of pancreatitis depends mainly on an increase in the serum amylase level. However, hyperamylasemia in uremic patients is not uncommon (30%) due to reduced amylase clearance in light of insufficient renal function [73,75]. The amylase/creatinine clearance ratio appears to be a more sensitive index of pancreatitis in patients without good renal function. The degree of hyperamylasemia is not a prognostic factor [73]. Diagnosis is best confirmed by contrast-enhanced CT scanning; this study is helpful in both staging pancreatitis and distinguishing between edematous and hemorrhagic/necrotic pancreatitis with or without abscess formation [77]. For the edematous form of pancreatitis, conservative treatment is usually successful. Patients with hemorrhagic or necrotic pancreatitis require ICU monitoring, with specific attention to volume replacement and cardiovascular status. In these patients, reduction of immunosuppression, broad spectrum antibiotic coverage, and ICU monitoring are imperative.

The role of early surgical intervention is still controversial. Patients with well-defined abscesses and necroses may benefit from aggressive surgical therapy, including removal of all infected necrotic material and drainage and irrigation of the abdominal cavity. In these cases, regular relaparotomies may be necessary. Since overwhelming sepsis is the most common cause of death, intensive management of infection is essential. Surgical intervention is also required if unresolving pseudocysts develop, although maturation of pseudocysts may take longer in kidney transplant recipients [77]. Pseudocyst complications, such as erosions of adjacent vascular and viscous structures, predispose to early intervention. The mortality rate from complications of posttransplant pancreatitis appears to be higher than from other forms of pancreatitis. A rapid reduction of immunosuppression is necessary to minimize septic complications.

Renal transplant candidates are screened by ultrasonography for the presence of gallstones during their pretransplant workup; and consideration is given at many centers to cholecystectomy if symptoms are or have been present. Yet, *acalculous cholecystitis* has become more common in recipients with a complicated posttransplant course (e.g., septicemia, multiorgan failure). Diagnosis is made clinically and, especially if the patient is intubated and on the ventilator, by ultrasound. A cholecystectomy is desirable. However, CT-guided drainage may also be helpful if the patient is too sick to undergo surgery. Reduction of immunosuppression and adequate antibiotic coverage are imperative.

Neurologic Complications

Up to 30 percent of kidney transplant recipients have neurologic problems posttransplant [80]. The incidence of life-threatening central nervous system (CNS)-related complications in the immediate posttransplant period ranges from 1 to 5 percent. Causative factors are not only the sequelae of the transplant itself, but also the underlying disease (more common in patients with diabetes, hypertension, or soft tissue diseases) and pretransplant conditions (uremic or nonuremic). *Cerebrovascular events* (infarct, TIA, hemorrhage) are the most frequent complications, usually peaking during the first few months posttransplant [80,81]. Hypertension, atherosclerosis, diabetes, hyperlipidemia, hypercoagulability, and advanced age play a major role in the pathogenesis of these complications [81,82,83]. In patients with brain infarctions or TIA, conservative treatment (heparinization, aspirin) is best, although carotid endarterectomy can benefit those with ulcerated carotid lesions or severe but accessible stenosis [81]. The prognosis of intracerebral hemorrhage is poor; posttransplant hypertension is one of the major causative factors.

All CNS *infections* are considered life-threatening. Patients are often left with various degrees of disability. Infections are caused by bacteria (*Listeria monocytogenes,* pseudomonas), viruses (CMV, herpes), fungi (Cryptococcus, Aspergillus, Mucorales), and parasites (Toxoplasma). *Listeria monocytogenes* is the most common and usually causes meningitis. Aspergillus frequently results in brain abscesses. Mucor infection can cause cavernous sinus thrombosis [81,82]. Dissemination of CMV may include the CNS, although the overall incidence is low [84]. Acute polyradiculoneuritis has also been associated with CMV infection [85]. Similarly, dissemination of the varicella-zoster virus can involve the CNS [86]. It is crucial to diagnose and treat these infections early and aggressively. Intrathecal administration of antimicrobial drugs or drainage in patients with brain abscesses may be necessary.

Seizures are usually associated with excessively high cyclosporine (CSA) serum levels. Children are more prone to this complication than adults [87–90]. Treatment consists of CSA dose reduction and anticonvulsants. CSA is highly lipid-soluble and thus crosses the blood–brain barrier. Such seizures have also been related to hypertension and hypomagnesemia [80]. Other CSA-related complications, such as tremor, dysesthesias, ataxia, and psychological disorders, usually do not require ICU monitoring. Another drug-related complication is aseptic meningitis caused by OKT3 [37,38]. Treatment consists of stopping monoclonal antibody therapy and temporarily administering anticonvulsants. In general, seizures can also be related to discontinuation of pretransplant antiseizure medication for apparent metabolic problems due to uremia (electrolyte/fluid imbalances).

Immunosuppression also predisposes to the development of CNS *neoplasms.* The rate of neoplastic complications is significantly higher in kidney transplant recipients. Unlike in the general population, non-Hodgkin's lymphomas predominate [91]. Depending on the aggressiveness of the disease and the treatment, patients may require ICU monitoring and interdisciplinary cooperation among the neurologist, neurosurgeon, and transplant surgeon.

In contrast to CNS-related problems, peripheral neurologic complications do not require ICU monitoring. Compressive *neuropathy* (involving the femoral nerve or the lateral femoral cutaneous nerve) is due to hematoma, ischemia, or retraction injury at the time of transplant. It is always located ipsilateral to the side operated on. This complication has a high degree of reversibility [92].

References

1. Cecka JM, Terasaki PI: The UNOS Scientific Renal Transplant Registry, in Terasaki PI, Cecka JM (eds): *Clinical Transplants 1992,* UCLA Tissue Typing Laboratory, Los Angeles, pp 1–17.

2. Philipson JD, Carpenter BJ, Itzkoff J, et al: Evaluation of cardiovascular risk for renal transplantation in diabetic patients. *Am J Med* 81:630, 1986.

3. Merkus JWS, Hoitsma AJ, Koene RAP: Detrimental effect of acute renal failure on the survival of renal allografts: Influence of total ischemia time and anastomosis time. *Nephrol Dial Transplant* 6:881, 1991.

4. Rocher LL, Landis C, Dafoe DC, et al: The importance of prolonged posttransplant dialysis requirement in cyclosporine-treated renal allograft recipients. *Clin Transplantation* 1:29, 1987.

5. Canafax DM, Torres A, Fryd DS, et al: The effects of delayed function in recipients of cadaver renal allografts. A study of 158 patients randomized to cyclosporine or ALG-azathioprine. *Transplantation* 41:177, 1986.

6. Sanfilippo F, Vaughn WK, Spees EK, et al: The detrimental effects of delayed graft function in cadaver donor renal transplantation. *Transplantation* 38:643, 1984.

7. Troppmann C, Almond PS, Payne WD, et al: Does acute tubular necrosis affect renal transplant outcome? The impact of rejection episodes. *Transplant Proc* 25:905, 1993.

8. Iwaki Y, Terasaki PI: Primary nonfunction in human cadaver kidney transplantation: Evidence for hidden hyperacute rejection. *Clin Transplantation* 1:125, 1987.

9. Louridas G, Botha JR, Meyers AM, et al: Vascular complications in renal transplantation: The Johannesburg experience. *Clin Transplantation* 1:240, 1987.

10. Harmon WE, Stablein D, Alexander SR, et al: Graft thrombosis in pediatric renal transplant recipients. *Transplantation* 51:406, 1991.

11. Goldman MH, Tilney NL, Vineyard GC, et al: A twenty-year survey of arterial complications of renal transplantation. *Surg Gynecol Obstet* 141:758, 1975.

12. Jones RM, Murie JA, Ting A, et al: Renal vascular thrombosis of cadaveric renal allografts in patients receiving cyclosporin, azathioprine and prednisolone triple therapy. *Clin Transplantation* 2:122, 1988.

13. Merion RM, Calne RY: Allograft renal vein thrombosis. *Transplant Proc* 17:1746, 1985.

14. Robinson JM, Cockrell CH, Tisnado J, et al: Selective low-dose streptokinase infusion in the treatment of acute transplant renal vein thrombosis. *Cardiovasc Intervent Radiol* 9:86, 1986.

15. Waltzer WC, Frischer Z, Shabtai M, et al: Early aggressive management for the prevention of renal allograft loss and patient mortality following major urologic complications. *Clin Transplantation* 6:318, 1992.

16. Stephanian E, Matas AJ, Gores P, et al: Retransplantation as a risk factor for lymphocele formation. *Transplantation* 53:676, 1992.

17. McCullough CS, Soper NJ, Clayman RV, et al: Laparoscopic drainage of a posttransplant lymphocele. *Transplantation* 51:725, 1991.

18. Lai KN, Barnden L, Mathew TH: Effect of renal transplantation on left ventricular function in hemodialysis patients. *Clin Nephrol* 18:74, 1982.

19. Basadonna G, Matas AJ, Gillingham K, et al: Kidney transplantation in patients with Type I diabetes: 26 years experience at the University of Minnesota, in Terasaki PI, Cecka JM (eds), *Clinical Transplants 1992.* UCLA Tissue Typing Laboratory, Los Angeles, 1993, pp 227–236.

20. Sever MS, Steinmuller DR, Hayes JM, et al: Pericarditis following renal transplantation. *Transplantation* 51:1229, 1991.

21. Masutani M, Ikeoka K, Sasaki R, et al: Post transplanted infective endocarditis. *Jpn J Med* 30:458, 1991.

22. Van Ypersele de Strihou C, Vereerstaeten P, Wauthier M, et al: Prevalence, etiology, and treatment of late posttransplant hypertension, in Hanburger J, Crosnier J, Grunfield J, et al (eds): *Advances in Nephrology,* Vol. 12. Chicago-London, Year Book Medical, 1983, pp 41–60.

23. Laskow DA, Curtis JJ: Posttransplant hypertension. *Am J Hypertension* 3:721, 1990.

24. Curtis JJ: Distinguishing the causes of posttransplantation hypertension. *Pediatr Nephrol* 5:108, 1990.

25. Gunnels JC, Stickel DL, Robinson RR: Episodic hypertension associated with positive renin assays after renal transplantation. *N Engl J Med* 274:543, 1966.

26. Curtis JJ, Luke RG, Jones PA, et al: Hypertension in cyclosporine-

treated renal transplant patients is sodium dependent. *Am J Med* 85:134, 1988.

27. Lau DCW, Wong K-L, Hwang WS, et al: Cyclosporine toxicity on cultural rat microvascular endothelial cells. *Kidney Int* 35:604, 1989.

28. Peces R, Gorostidi M, Azofra J, et al: Anaphylaxis following intravenous methylprednisolone sodium succinate in a renal transplant recipient. *Nephron* 59:497, 1991.

29. Ozsoylu S, Strauss HS, Diamond LK: Effect of corticosteroids on coagulation of the blood. *Nature* 195:1214, 1962.

30. von Kaulla KN, von Kaulla E, Wasantapruck S, et al: Blood coagulation in uremic patients before and after hemodialysis and transplantation of the kidney. *Arch Surg* 92:184, 1966.

31. Wardle EN, Menon IS, Uldall PR, et al: Proteins and fibrinolysis in recipients of renal allografts. *J Clin Pathol* 24:124, 1971.

32. Blohme I, Brynger H: Malignant disease in renal transplant patients. *Transplantation* 39:23, 1985.

33. Pasquale MD, Abrams JH, Najarian JS, et al: Use of Greenfield filters in renal transplant patients—Are they safe? *Transplantation* 55:439, 1993.

34. Murie JA, Allen RD, Michie CA, et al: Deep venous thrombosis after renal transplantation. *Transplant Proc* 19:2219, 1987.

35. Gruber SA, Simmons RL, Najarian JS, et al: Posttransplant erythrocytosis and the risk of thromboembolic complications: Correlation from a prospective randomized study of cyclosporine versus azathioprine-antilymphocyte globulin. *Clin Transplantation* 2:60, 1988.

36. Boyes R, Pur VK, Toledo L, et al: Pulmonary edema in renal transplant patients. *Am Surgeon* 53:647, 1987.

37. Thislethwaite JR Jr, Stuart JK, Mayes JT, et al: Monitoring and complications of monoclonal therapy. Complications and monitoring of OKT3 therapy. *Am J Kid Dis* 11:112, 1988.

38. Ortho Multicenter Transplant Study Group: A randomized clinical trial of OKT3 monoclonal antibody for acute rejection of cadaveric renal transplants. *N Engl J Med* 313:337, 1985.

39. Hampl J, Paeprer H, Unger V, et al: Hemodynamic changes during hemodialysis, sequential ultrafiltration, and hemofiltration. *Kidney Int* 18:S-83, 1980.

40. Campese VM: Cardiovascular instability during hemodialysis. *Kidney Int* 33(suppl 24):S186, 1988.

41. Briggs WA, Merrill JP, O'Brien TF, et al: Severe pneumonia in renal transplant patients. *Ann Int Med* 75:887, 1971.

42. Ramsey PG, Rubin RH, Tolkoff-Rubin NE, et al: The renal transplant patient with fever and pulmonary infiltrate: Etiology, clinical manifestations and management. *Medicine* 59:206, 1980.

43. Fellstrom B, Siegbahn A, Liljenberg G, et al: Primary haemostasis, plasmatic coagulation and fibrinolysis in renal transplantation. *Thrombosis Research* 59:97, 1990.

44. Peterson PK, Ferguson R, Fryd DS, et al: Infectious diseases in hospitalized renal transplant recipients: A prospective study of a complex and evolving problem. *Medicine* 61:360, 1982.

45. Rubin RH, Wolfson JS, Cosimi AB, et al: Infection in the renal transplant patient. *Am J Med* 70:405, 1981.

46. Cohen J, Hopkin J, Kurtz J: Infectious complications after renal transplantation, in Morris PJ (ed), *Kidney Transplantation: Principles and Practice*. Philadelphia, Saunders 1989, pp 533–574.

47. Peterson PK, Balfour HH, Marker SC, et al: Cytomegalovirus disease in renal allograft recipients: A prospective study of the clinical features, risk factors and impact on renal transplantation. *Medicine* 59:283, 1980.

48. Marker SC, Howard RJ, Simmons RL, et al: Cytomegalovirus infection: A quantitative prospective study of three hundred twenty consecutive renal transplants. *Surgery* 89:660, 1981.

49. Balfour HH, Chage BA, Stapleton JT: A randomized, placebo-controlled trial of oral acyclovir for the prevention of cytomegalovirus disease in recipients of renal allografts. *N Engl J Med* 320:1381, 1989.

50. Snydman DR, Werner BG, Heinze-Lacey B: Use of cytomegalovirus immune globulin to prevent cytomegalovirus disease in renal transplant recipients. *N Engl J Med* 317:1049, 1987.

51. Brayman KL, Dafoe DC, Smythe WR, et al: Prophylaxis of serious cytomegalovirus infection in renal transplant candidates using live human cytomegalovirus vaccine. *Arch Surg* 123:1502, 1988.

52. Demmler GJ, Buffone GJ, Schmbor CM, et al: Detection of cytomegalovirus in urine from newborns by using polymerase chain reaction DNA amplification. *J Infect Dis* 158:1177, 1989.

53. Dunn DL, Mayoral JL, Gillingham KJ, et al: Simultaneous treatment of concurrent rejection and tissue invasive cytomegalovirus disease without detrimental effects upon patient or allograft survival. *Clin Transplantation* 46:413, 1992.

54. Richardson WP, Colvin RB, Cheeseman SH, et al: Glomerulopathy associated with cytomegalovirus viremia in renal allografts. *N Engl J Med* 305:57, 1981.

55. Troppmann C, Papalois BE, Chiou A, et al: Incidence, complications, treatment, and outcome of ulcers of the upper gastrointestinal tract after renal transplantation during the cyclosporine era. *J Am Coll Surg* 180:433, 1995.

56. Sarosdy MF, Cruz AB, Saylor R, et al: Upper gastrointestinal bleeding following renal transplantation. *Urology* 26:347, 1985.

57. Bansky G, Huynh Do U, Largiadèr F, et al: Gastroduodenal complications after renal transplantation: The role of prophylactic gastric surgery in hyperacid kidney allograft recipients. *Clin Transplantation* 1:209, 1987.

58. Uhlschmid G, Largiadèr F: Surgical prophylaxis of gastroduodenal complications associated with renal allotransplantation. *World J Surg* 1:397, 1977.

59. Linder MM, Kösters W, Rethel R: Prophylactic gastric operations in uremic patients prior to renal transplantation. *World J Surg* 3:501, 1979.

60. Cohen EB, Komorowski RA, Kauffman HM Jr, et al: Unexpectedly high incidence of cytomegalovirus infection in apparent peptic ulcers in renal transplant recipients. *Surgery* 97:606, 1985.

61. Flanigan RC, Reckard CR, Lucas BA: Colonic complications of renal transplantation. *J Urol* 139:503, 1988.

62. Lao A, Bach D: Colonic complications in renal transplant recipients. *Dis Colon Rectum* 31:130, 1988.

63. McCune TR, Nylander WA, VanBuren DH, et al: Colonic screening prior to renal transplantation and its impact on posttransplant colonic complications. *Clin Transplantation* 6:91, 1992.

64. Church JM, Braun WE, Novick AC, et al: Perforation of the colon in renal homograft recipients. *Ann Surg* 203:69, 1986.

65. Squiers EC, Pfaff WW, Patton PR, et al: Early posttransplant colon perforation: Does it remain a problem in the cyclosporine era? *Transplant Proc* 23:1782, 1991.

66. Scheff RT, Zuckerman A, Harter H, et al: Diverticular disease in patients with chronic renal failure due to polycystic kidney disease. *Ann Int Med* 92:202, 1980.

67. Indudhara R, Kochhar R, Mehta SK, et al: Acute colitis in renal transplant recipients. *Am J Gastroenterol* 85:964, 1990.

68. Hellström PM, Rubio C, Odar-Cederlöf I, et al: Ischemic colitis of the cecum after renal transplantation masquerading as malignant disease. *Dig Dis Sci* 36:1644, 1991.

69. Frankel AH, Barker F, Williams G, et al: Neutropenic enterocolitis in a renal transplant patient. *Transplantation* 52:913, 1991.

70. Guerra EE, Nghiem DD: Posttransplant cecal volvulus. *Transplantation* 50:721, 1990.

71. Love R, Sterling JR, Sollinger HW, et al: Colonoscopic decompression for acute colonic pseudo-obstruction (Ogilvie's syndrome) in transplant recipients. *Gastrointest Endosc* 34:426, 1988.

72. Stylianos S, Forde KA, Benvenisty AI, et al: Lower gastrointestinal hemorrhage in renal transplant recipients. *Arch Surg* 123:739, 1988.

73. Fernandez JA, Rosenberg JC: Posttransplantation pancreatitis. *Surg Gynecol Obstet* 143:795, 1976.

74. Browning NG, Botha JR: Pancreatitis after renal transplantation: A potentially lethal condition. *Clin Transplantation* 4:93, 1990.

75. Fernandez-Cruz L, Targarona EM, Alcaraz ECA, et al: Acute pancreatitis after renal transplantation. *Br J Surg* 76:1132, 1989.

76. Johnson WC, Nabseth DC: Pancreatitis in renal transplantation. *Ann Surg* 171:309, 1970.

77. Chapman WC, Nylander WA, Williams LF Sr, et al: Pancreatic pseudocyst formation following renal transplantation: A lethal development. *Clin Transplantation* 5:86, 1991.

78. Frick TW, Fryd DS, Sutherland DER, et al: Hypercalcemia associated with pancreatitis and hyperamylasemia in renal transplant recipients: Data from the Minnesota randomized trial of cyclosporine versus antilymphoblast azathioprine. *Am J Surg* 154:487, 1987.

79. Tilney NL, Collins JJ, Wilson RE, et al: Hemorrhagic pancreatitis: A fatal complication of renal transplantation. *N Engl J Med* 274:1051, 1966.

80. Adams HP Jr, Dawson D, Coffman TJ, et al: Stroke in renal transplant recipients. *Arch Neurol* 43:113, 1986.
81. Bruno A, Adams H: Neurologic problems in renal transplant recipients. *Neurol Clin* 6:305, 1988.
82. Kassike BL, Umen AJ: Persistent hyperlipidemia in renal transplant patients. *Medicine* 66:300, 1987.
83. Rao KV, Smith EJ, Alexander JW, et al: Thromboembolic disease in renal allograft recipients. *Arch Surg* 111:1086, 1976.
84. Simmons RL, Matas AJ, Rattazzi LC, et al: Clinical characteristics of the lethal cytomegalovirus infection following renal transplantation. *Surgery* 82:537, 1977.
85. Pouteil-Noble C, Vial C, Moreau T, et al: Acute polyradiculoneuritis associated with cytomegalovirus infection in renal transplantation. *Clin Transplantation* 7:158, 1993.
86. Peterson, LR, Ferguson RM: Fatal central nervous system infection with varicella-zoster virus in renal transplant recipients. *Transplantation* 37:366, 1984.

87. McEnery PT, Nathan J, Bates SR, et al: Convulsions in children undergoing renal transplantation. *J Pediatr* 115:532, 1989.
88. Arora P, Kohli A, Kher V, et al: Complex partial seizure, an unusual complication of cyclosporine in renal transplantation. *Clin Transplantation* 46:458, 1992.
89. Rubin A: Transient cortical blindness and occipital seizures with cyclosporine toxicity. *Transplantation* 47:572, 1989.
90. Thompson CB, June CH, Sullivan KM, et al: Association between cyclosporine neurotoxicity and hypomagnesaemia. *Lancet* 2:1116, 1984.
91. Blohme I, Brynger H: Malignant disease in renal transplant patients. *Transplantation* 39:23, 1985.
92. Kumar A, Dalela D, Bhandari M, et al: Femoral neuropathy—An unusual complication of renal transplantation. *Transplantation* 51:1305, 1991.

195. Specific Critical Care Problems in Heart, Heart-Lung, and Lung Transplant Recipients

Sara J. Shumway

The advent of thoracic organ transplantation has brought new hope to a number of patients previously doomed by end-stage cardiac, pulmonary, or combined cardiopulmonary disease. The first heart transplant was performed on December 3, 1967 [1]. Fourteen years passed before the first successful heart-lung transplant was done on March 9, 1981 [2]. Heart-lung transplantation established lung transplantation as a viable option; the first successful single-lung transplant was performed in 1983 [3].

The indications and limitations of heart transplantation are well-established. Heart-lung transplantation is increasingly limited by the number of status 1 heart recipients who have priority, as well as the usual difficulty in meeting donor criteria for lung donation. Lung transplantation is still undergoing evaluation in terms of the correct operation for a given patient. Much progress has been made, and exciting new developments promise better care for these critically ill patients.

pulmonary vascular disease, that is, either primary or secondary pulmonary hypertension. [4]. Occasionally a patient with septic lung disease has coexistent heart failure such that a heart-lung transplant is required as, for example, in the patient with cystic fibrosis and cardiomyopathy.

Patients with end-stage septic lung disease such as cystic fibrosis or bronchiectasis require bilateral lung transplantation to remove all native lung tissue as a potential source of contamination. [5]. Single-lung transplantation was initially performed for patients with pulmonary fibrosis, and is now also undertaken for those with chronic obstructive pulmonary disease (COPD), including patients with alpha 1 antitrypsin deficiency emphysema. Recently, single-lung transplantation has been used in conjunction with repair of congenital heart defects in patients with secondary pulmonary hypertension [6]. The results have been encouraging.

Indications

Approximately 90 percent of patients with end-stage cardiac disease have some form of cardiomyopathy; half have an idiopathic cardiomyopathy, and the other half have an element of coronary artery disease or an ischemic cardiomyopathy. The remaining 10 percent of heart recipients have either a congenital heart ailment and a smaller number have a more exotic reason for their heart disease, such as an infiltrative cardiomyopathy, Adriamycin-induced cardiotoxicity, Chagas' disease or graft atherosclerosis.

Heart-lung transplants are performed almost exclusively for

Patient Selection

Many of the specific critical care problems seen in thoracic organ recipients can be avoided by careful patient selection. This is underscored by the fact that these patients must have a less than 50 percent chance of living two years. In the compensated patients a week-long outpatient evaluation is performed. Relative contraindications to thoracic organ transplantation are: (1) age greater than 65 years; (2) irreversible hepatic or renal dysfunction, (3) peripheral or cerebral vascular disease, (4) recent pulmonary emboli, (5) systemic disease that could limit survival or rehabilitation, (6) insulin-requiring diabetes mellitus with evidence of end-organ damage, (7) active peptic ulcer disease, (8) active diverticular disease, (9) cachexia, (10) psychiatric illness or history of noncompliance, and (11) poor psychosocial situation [7].

Patients with only end-stage cardiac disease should be evaluated for cardiac transplantation with the above-mentioned criteria being considered.

A specific contraindication to cardiac transplantation is related to the need to rule out severe pulmonary hypertension that could cause right heart failure after the transplant, as well as the presence of serious chronic obstructive pulmonary disease. Previous cardiac or thoracic surgery is a relative contraindication to heart-lung transplantation, as the phrenic nerve pedicles may be difficult to preserve. Bilateral single lung transplantation should be offered to the patient with cystic fibrosis who is young, female, and whose FEV_1 is less than 30 percent predicted [8]. Any patient with cystic fibrosis with increasing difficulty maintaining weight or an increasing number of hospitalizations should also be evaluated.

Donor Criteria

Ideally, a donor heart exhibits a normal echocardiogram and the donor requires minimal inotropic support (i.e., dopamine less than 10 µg/kg/min). A central venous pressure less than 10 mm Hg is also desirable. Nonspecific ST-T wave changes are common ECG findings in a brain dead patient. Any evidence of coronary artery disease is a relative contraindication and cine angiography may be performed in the older donor (age >45 years) to exclude its presence.

Donor criteria for lung donation have been liberalized over the past several years [9]. A small pulmonary contusion is not a contraindication. Bronchoscopy is performed whenever aspiration or serious infection is a possibility. A pO_2 of greater than 100 on an FIO_2 of 40 percent is desirable. Fungal organisms in the sputum or evidence of lobar consolidation remain contraindications. Diuretics and physiologic PEEP (5 cm H_2O) can aid in improving oxygenation. Peak airway pressures should be followed along with serial arterial blood gases.

Operative Techniques

Donor Operation. At the donor operation, the adult heart is protected with a liter of cold cardioplegic solution. Topical cold saline solution is also applied. The lungs are flushed with modified Euro-Collins solution, usually 60 cc/kg, and gently ventilated. The inferior vena cava is divided and a defect created in the left atrial appendage to avoid distention of the heart while the pulmonary flush solution is administered. At some centers Prostaglandin E_1 (500 µg in 50 ml normal saline) is given intravenously to promote pulmonary vasodilatation in the donor [10].

Once the cardioplegia and pulmonary flush solution have been delivered the heart is excised in situ. Care is taken to leave adequate left atrial cuff for each lung. The lung block is then removed and the two lungs are separated on the back table. The lungs are left inflated and transported in cold saline solution; a staple line protects the airway.

HEART TRANSPLANT. At the recipient operation a heart transplant proceeds similar to other cardiac procedures. First, cardiopulmonary bypass is established. Total bypass is achieved, and the aorta then is cross-clamped. The heart is excised along the atrioventricular groove. The great vessels are divided just above their respective semilunar valves. The anastomoses are performed in the usual order: left atrial, right atrial, pulmonary arterial, and aortic [11]. Temporary pacing wires are left on the donor right atrium and right ventricle.

HEART-LUNG TRANSPLANT. At the donor operation care is taken to protect the tissue surrounding the distal trachea and carina. The recipient is placed on cardiopulmonary bypass. The heart is excised first, then each lung is removed. Care is taken to protect the phrenic neurovascular bundles bilaterally [12]. The left recurrent laryngeal nerve is also at risk for damage in the region of the ligamentum arteriosum. For that reason some surgeons leave a portion of the main and left pulmonary artery in situ. The tracheal anastomosis is performed first. Although it can be wrapped with omentum, because the coronary-bronchial collateral circulation is generally excellent it does not need to be. Performance of the right atrial anastomosis is followed by that of the aortic anastomosis. Bleeding from collateral vessels can be a real problem in the patient with secondary pulmonary hypertension.

SINGLE-LUNG TRANSPLANT. The recipient procedure is performed through a standard posterolateral thoracotomy with the ipsilateral groin exposed. If cardiopulmonary bypass is needed the patient may be positioned with the given hemothorax elevated 30 degrees on a roll, and a submammary incision with the extension across the sternum may be used. The recipient's pulmonary artery is occluded briefly to determine its effect on the other lung's pulmonary artery pressure and on systemic blood pressure, and an arterial blood gas is obtained. It is safer to err on the side of cardiopulmonary bypass, as sudden decompensation can be difficult to manage. The bronchial anastomosis is done first, followed by the pulmonary artery, and left atrial anastomosis [13]. A telescoped anastomosis has reduced the need for omental wrapping in this series of patients at the University of Minnesota. However, in pediatric patients, a telescoped anastomosis can lead to significant narrowing of the bronchus. The left atrial anastomosis must join endocardium to endocardium, as thrombosis at this site can have serious consequences. Similarly, care must be taken to avoid a purse-string effect of the pulmonary artery anastomosis.

BILATERAL SINGLE LUNG TRANSPLANT. The bilateral sequential lung, or bilateral single lung, transplant has effectively replaced the double-lung transplant [14]. Double-lung transplantation had an unacceptable number of problems with the healing of the tracheal anastomosis. Bilateral single lung transplantation usually requires cardiopulmonary bypass when performed for a primary pulmonary hypertension or Eisenmenger's complex, but otherwise bypass can be avoided. A double-lumen endotracheal tube should be used in those patients in whom cardiopulmonary bypass is not anticipated.

Perioperative Care

After heart or heart-lung transplantation, cardiac output is sustained by establishing a heart rate of 90 to 110 beats per minute using either temporary epicardial atrial pacing or low-dose isoproterenol (0.01 to 0.02 µg/kg/min). Adequate preload is important in a patient who may have transient right heart failure. This is obtained by filling the heart before discontinuing cardiopulmonary bypass and maintaining the CVP and left atrial pressures at 8 to 15 mm Hg. An oximetric Swan-Ganz catheter to monitor pulmonary artery pressures and measure cardiac outputs is not mandatory but can be helpful.

Postoperatively urine output and arterial blood gases are carefully monitored. Hypotension and a low cardiac output usually respond to an infusion of volume and minor adjustments in inotropic support. In the case of cardiac transplantation, cardiac tamponade should always be considered under the same circumstances it would be for any postoperative cardiac surgery patient.

When the cardiac transplant recipient has an elevated pulmonary vascular resistance, especially above 6 Wood units, then a prostaglandin E1 infusion through the central line can be started with norepinephrine or epinephrine infused through a left atrial catheter. Patients with a transpulmonary gradient in excess of 15, or a fixed pulmonary vascular resistance greater than 6, are not considered good candidates for orthotopic heart transplantation [15].

Serious ventricular failure after cardiac transplantation is unusual and can be related to poor donor organ selection, poor graft preservation, a long ischemia time, or, rarely, hyperacute rejection due to either ABO blood group mismatching or the presence of preformed antibodies. The usual inotropic support and pulmonary vasodilators can be used to manage this situation with the addition of an intra-aortic balloon pump and even ventricular assist devices if the donor graft is expected to recover. In the case of very severe rejection the patient's only option is to be relisted for retransplantation.

One of the major difficulties in lung transplantation has been successful organ preservation and early function of the lung graft. Initial lung changes seen after heart-lung transplantation were referred to as the "reimplantation response" [16]. This was seen during the first few days following transplantation. These changes included pulmonary infiltrates, perihilar flaring, and pleural effusions. More recently, with the routine use of transbronchial biopsy early after transplantation, these changes have been found to be due to acute lung injury associated with the preservation of the graft or the early onset of graft rejection. In patients who undergo single-lung transplantation for pulmonary hypertension, reperfusion edema develops because of the elevated blood flow through the transplanted lung. Blood flow preferentially travels into the lower pulmonary vascular resistance in the transplanted lung so postoperative perfusion scans may show over 80 percent of the blood flow into the transplanted lung. Single-lung transplantation, performed for COPD, may be associated with mismatching of ventilation. The nontransplanted emphysematous lung can cause compression and underventilation of the transplanted lung. This can be especially problematic in the patient with bullous emphysema. One way to avoid this is to perform bilateral sequential lung transplantation [17]. Single-lung transplant for obstructive lung disease can be performed if the recipients are carefully selected. It is helpful if the donor lung is the same size as or larger than the native remaining lung. Careful management of the respiratory tract during mechanical ventilation and immediately following extubation is important. Patients often have to be treated for anxiety during the immediate postextubation period.

Acute failure of a transplanted lung is more commonly seen than acute failure of a heart transplant. The reasons for this are many: poor lung preservation, unrecognized injury or trauma to the donor lung, and reperfusion edema. Lung graft failure can be manifested by hypoxemia, perihilar and parenchymal infiltrates on chest x-ray, and, occasionally, copious secretions when reperfusion edema occurs. These patients require active

diuresis. High levels of PEEP can be used to maintain small airway patency. The patients are kept intubated and paralyzed. Transbronchial biopsy can be performed to rule out rejection when the patient is stable enough. Bronchoalveolar lavage is done to rule out early infection. Extracorporeal membrane oxygenation (ECMO) is used as a last resort and has occasionally been successful.

Pulmonary emboli can be devastating in a patient post-lung transplant. All lung transplant recipients have sequential compression devices placed on both lower extremities in the operating room. Heparin, 5000 units subcutaneous twice a day, is administered until patients are fully ambulatory. In this way embolic phenomena are minimized. If there is any history of deep venous thrombosis, an inferior vena caval filter is inserted before lung transplantation.

Immunosuppression

Thoracic organ transplantation is based on triple-drug immunosuppression: azathioprine, prednisone, and cyclosporine A [18]. The main problem with azathioprine in the immediate postoperative period is that of suppression of the white blood cell count. Occasionally it is necessary to stop the azathioprine, and, even more rarely, it is necessary to give granulocyte colony-stimulating factor. Prednisone is responsible for a wealth of difficulties, primarily hypertension and relative glucose intolerance, as well as obesity and osteoporosis. Cyclosporine acts synergistically with prednisone to cause hypertension. Additionally, it is nephrotoxic and causes neurological problems and hirsutism. The current immunosuppressive regimen used at the University of Minnesota is shown in Table 195-1.

Airway Complications

Airway complications can occur only after heart-lung or lung transplantation. They are rare after heart-lung transplantation because the coronary-bronchial collaterals provide good blood supply to the tracheal anastomosis. Unfortunately, the bronchial anastomosis is at much greater risk for partial dehiscence or airway stenosis, or both [19]. During the first few days after transplantation, regional anastomotic blood flow is established by retrograde collateral flow from pulmonary to bronchial arterial circulation. This flow can be compromised by hypotension, poor lung preservation, rejection, or infection, and so cause ischemic necrosis and poor healing of the airway. This may lead to partial or total dehiscence or chronic narrowing of the bronchus. It is not known whether prolonged mechanical ventilation or PEEP contributes to the development of this necrosis.

Late airway stenosis has been seen in patients whose initial bronchial healing was apparently excellent. Such strictures are thought to be the result of ischemia occurring either at or distal to the anastomosis in an area between the donor organ's retrograde pulmonary artery–bronchial artery circulation and the recipient's antegrade collateral circulation arising from the tracheobronchial region and any omentopexy. Most early complications of the airway have been attributed to the delayed healing caused by steroids.

Postoperative surveillance of the bronchial anastomosis is crucial. In the operating room an intraoperative bronchoscopy is done to establish a baseline appearance of the bronchial anastomosis. Frequent routine bronchoscopy is useful to survey

Table 195-1. Triple-Drug Immunosuppression

Pre-operative	Cyclosporine 6–10 mg/kg by mouth Azathioprine 2.5 mg/kg by mouth	One hour before OR
Intraoperative	Methylprednisolone 500 mg IV	Just before release of aortic cross-clamp or pulmonary artery clamp
Postoperative	Cyclosporine 1–2 mg/hr IV	For 24–48 hr
	Cyclosporine 3–5 mg/kg by mouth	BID
	Azathioprine 2.5 mg/kg by mouth	Daily
	Methylprednisolone 125 mg IV	q 8 hr × 3, then
	Prednisone 1 mg/kg by mouth	In four divided doses for 3 days, then in two divided doses, then taper to BID over 3-week period

the anastomosis for early signs of dehiscence, as well as to monitor for rejection and infection.

Dehiscence usually occurs within three to six weeks after transplantation. Some centers perform routine bronchoscopy on a weekly basis during the first month posttransplant and then every two weeks for the following month. The early signs of anastomotic dehiscence include postoperative pallor, gray or black mucosa at the suture line, loosened sutures or knots within the airway, and herniation of tissue into the airway if a wrap was performed. If the patient is clinically stable and the area of dehiscence is small, conservative management with antibiotics and serial bronchoscopy is appropriate. The development of a bronchopleural or bronchovascular fistula requires operation.

Chronic stenosis may be managed in a variety of ways. When associated with bronchomalacia a metallic stent is usually required to maintain the airway. Granulation tissue may be debrided using laser photocoagulation and repeated dilations of the airway with a rigid bronchoscope. Silastic stents tend to be easily dislodged. Ways to avoid airway complications include: (1) dividing the donor mainstem bronchus within two rings of the lobar bronchus, (2) reinforcing the anastomosis with surrounding vascularized tissue, either pleura, pericardium, or omentum, and (3) using a telescoped anastomosis. In a recent review of patients at the University of Minnesota from June 1989 to July 1993, 75 lung transplants were performed in 73 patients (58 single-lung and 17 bilateral single lung). All airway anastomoses were performed with monofilament nonabsorbable suture material. The first 27 single-lung transplants and the first 4 bilateral single lung transplants had end-to-end anastomoses performed with reinforcement with an omentopexy or the internal mammary artery. The second group of 31 single-lung transplants and 13 bilateral single lung transplants had telescoped bronchial anastomoses without reinforcement. In the first group there were two instances of bronchial dehiscence with stricture formation in four patients. In the second group there was stricture formation in three patients. These airway complications were successfully managed by operative revision in one patient, dilation and laser treatments in five patients, and metallic bronchial stents in three patients. The need for revascularization in the form of an internal mammary artery to bronchial artery anastomosis has not been established [20].

Renal Failure

Renal failure in the perioperative period is almost always the direct result of nephrotoxicity from cyclosporine. Mild impairment of renal function preoperatively is acceptable as long as the risk of severe renal impairment during the postoperative period is recognized as a possible complication. The minimal acceptable level for a creatinine clearance in a potential thoracic organ transplant recipient is 50 ml/min. Two of the 26 heart-lung transplant recipients at the University of Minnesota have undergone successful renal transplantation months after successful heart-lung transplant. In both cases, both sets of grafts continue to function well.

Gastrointestinal Problems

Serious complications of the alimentary tract following heart and heart-lung transplantation have been well documented and remain a major source of morbidity and mortality [21]. For that reason patients with active peptic ulcer disease or diverticular disease are not considered for thoracic organ transplantation, at least until these problems are resolved. A recent review of some 75 patients undergoing lung transplantation at the University of Minnesota revealed 18 had sustained abdominal complications. Four patients had prolonged adynamic ileus, three had a diaphragmatic hernia following omental wrapping of the bronchial anastomosis, two patients had ischemic bowel requiring resection, one patient had colitis with hemorrhage, and one had a splenic injury following colonoscopy. Four patients had colonic perforation, two patients had cholelithiasis and/or choledocholithiasis, and one patient had a mesenteric pseudoaneurysm. These last seven complications occurred more than one month to one year after transplantation. Three patients died from causes directly related to their abdominal complication, and in each case there was a delay between the onset of symptoms and the diagnosis and/or intervention to relieve the complication [22].

Mild liver dysfunction as evidenced by elevation of serum transaminases and hyperbilirubinemia often occurs in patients on high doses of cyclosporine. This is a chemical hepatitis that usually responds to a decrease in the dosage. Other immunosuppressants such as azathioprine have been implicated in a similar process. Hepatitis may also be secondary to hepatitis B, cytomegalovirus, herpes simplex virus, hepatitis A, or hepatitis C [23].

Biliary tract disease is common in the thoracic organ transplant population. In heart transplant recipients an incidence of cholelithiasis ranged from 30 to 39 percent, which is more than twice that expected for age and gender match controls [24]. The primary cause of this problem is thought to be gallbladder stasis and the side effects of specific immunosuppressants.

Rejection

In the case of cardiac rejection the means for diagnosis and treatment are well established (see Chap. 198). Endomyocardial biopsies have been obtained since the mid-1970s, and with the pioneering work of Dr. Margaret Billingham and others, a grading scale for cardiac rejection is now well understood and well distributed [25]. Treatment of cardiac rejection is also well established. Pulse steroids are given intravenously for three days with or without a taper. If that is unsuccessful either a polyclonal preparation such as ATGAM or a monoclonal preparation such as OKT3 is used. Photochemotherapy or photopheresis, in addition to conventional immunosuppression, has been used by the team at Columbia to treat patients who have preexistent high levels of panel reactive antibodies [26]. Of course, when a patient has no other options, retransplantation is necessary to treat chronic, unrelenting rejection. Unfortunately, these patients tend to be quite ill and are not always able to wait until a new donor heart becomes available. It is in this particular instance that patients are placed on ventricular assist devices.

In the field of heart-lung transplantation, it was initially thought that endomyocardial biopsy would be a way of determining when the lung was rejecting at the same time [27]. Unfortunately, the lungs are much more susceptible to rejection and quite often reject despite normal endomyocardial biopsies [28]. The use of the transbronchial biopsy has started to reveal what is occurring in the lungs during the perioperative period, and later when changes are seen on chest x-ray or early changes are noted in pulmonary function studies [29]. While some progress has been made in grading lung rejection it is still unclear to pathologists and clinicians alike whether a single process, such as rejection, is occurring or whether there is an ongoing bronchitis or some form of infection as well. Treatment of recurrent lung rejection consists of the pulse steroids with or without a taper. Most surgeons consider using a polyclonal antithymocyte globulin or antilymphocyte preparation when confronted with a third biopsy still showing rejection. Some believe that there may be a role for methotrexate in the treatment of chronic rejection, and some consideration has been given to photopheresis in patients with chronic rejection.

Infection

Patients who have undergone thoracic organ transplantation are susceptible to bacterial, fungal, and viral infections. The most common source for infection is pulmonary for all thoracic organ transplant recipients. Infection is a particular problem in patients who have undergone lung transplantation [30]. Bacterial infections due to a variety of gram-negative and gram-positive pathology occur, but generally are readily treated. Fungal infections due to Candida and Aspergillus are more serious. As many as 15 to 20 percent of these patients may develop some type of clinically apparent infectious disease process (see Chap. 198). The majority of infections with Aspergillus occur within the first three months after transplantation. This infection is caused by the inhalation of aerosolized fungal spores. In patients with cystic fibrosis, colonization of the paranasal sinuses with Aspergillus can provide an endogenous source for respiratory tract infection. The antibiotic of choice for infection with Aspergillus remains amphotericin B. The goal of treatment is a total cumulative dose of 1.5 to 3 grams, but this often requires a prolonged course of administration because of nephrotoxicity. An every other day schedule may be necessary. The newer, oral antifungal agent, itraconazole is also effective against Aspergillus, but is still being evaluated as a first-line therapy [31].

The most morbid viral infection that occurs in thoracic organ transplant recipients is caused by cytomegalovirus (CMV) [32]. CMV is commonly acquired early in life and persists in a latent state capable of reactivation. Transmission of CMV by a donor organ is very common and for that reason prophylaxis with ganciclovir in all CMV-mismatched lung transplant recipients is performed at the University of Minnesota (see Table 195-2).

Table 195-2. Ganciclovir Therapy for CMV

FOR:	All lung recipients whose donor is seropositive or who are seropositive themselves.
STARTED:	Day 8 posttransplant
DOSAGE:	Ganciclovir 5 mg/kg IV BID × 14 days, then 5 mg/kg IV qd × until postoperative day 90
DURATION:	90 days

Patients who are seronegative at the time of transplantation and receive grafts from seropositive donors sustain the highest rate of infection and exhibit the most severe form of CMV disease. Ganciclovir is the treatment of choice.

Graft Atherosclerosis

The development of graft atherosclerosis can lead to myocardial infarction and sudden death in the cardiac transplant recipient. Routine yearly coronary angiography is performed to permit an accurate assessment of the time of onset and rate of progression of coronary artery disease. Graft atherosclerosis occurs in 30 to 40 percent of transplant recipients at 3 years follow-up and in 40 to 60 percent of patients by 5 year posttransplant [33]. It remains the major obstacle to long-term survival in cardiac transplant recipients. Donor age is the one factor that is suggested as a possible factor in the etiology of graft atherosclerosis [34]. A correlation between CMV infection and accelerated allograft atherosclerosis has also been identified [35]. Immunologically mediated endothelial damage has been proposed as a stimulus for the development of this graft atherosclerosis. Treatment can be temporizing in the form of angioplasty for focal lesions; however, when the disease involves tapering of the distal vessels, only retransplantation will deal with the problem definitively.

Obliterative Bronchiolitis

Obliterative bronchiolitis (OB) occurs with equal frequency in lung and heart-lung transplant recipients. Up to 30 percent of patients develop OB after successful lung or heart-lung transplantation [36]. It usually requires 3 months to manifest itself. Clinically, the patient presents with dyspnea, clear chest radiograph, and obstructive pulmonary function tests. The histologic findings are bronchial and bronchiolar inflammation with organization of the bronchiolar lumen. OB appears to be a manifestation of chronic pulmonary allograft rejection. Its pathogenesis is slowly emerging. It appears that infection can cause OB, especially cytomegalovirus and adenovirus. Basically, it is a fibroproliferative disorder, and after the diagnosis is made therapy is limited primarily to retransplantation [37].

Retransplantation

Most institutions performing heart and lung transplants have had limited experience with retransplantation. The primary indications for retransplantation appear to be early graft failure and the later occurrence of graft atherosclerosis or obliterative bronchiolitis. At the University of Minnesota three patients have undergone retransplantation after heart transplantation. Two of these patients are long-term survivors; the other died of recurrent graft atherosclerosis 14 months after retransplantation. As of August 1992, according to the St. Louis International Lung Transplant Registry, 66 patients had undergone retransplantation [38]. At the University of Minnesota one patient underwent single-lung transplantation for obliterative bronchiolitis after heart-lung transplantation. This patient had an anesthetic complication that led to hypoxic brain injury and death. One patient had a single-lung transplant, had graft failure within one month, and then was retransplanted approximately 2 months post–initial transplant. Retransplantation has been successful in this case. Two patients undergoing single-lung transplantation were converted to bilateral single lung transplants for obliterative bronchiolitis. One patient is alive and well now, more than 2 years post-retransplantation, and the other patient died in the perioperative period of problems related to heart failure.

Conclusions

Heart transplantation has been a clinical entity for 27 years. Lung transplantation reemerged just 12 years ago. Our knowledge about each is relative to the duration of our experimental and clinical experience. Increasingly, patients with primary pulmonary hypertension undergo bilateral single lung transplant, as opposed to a single-lung transplant or even a heart-lung transplant. The patient with extensive bullous emphysema may also require bilateral single lung transplant, and lobar lung transplantation has been considered. It seems certain that new immunosuppressants will improve long-term results in thoracic transplantation and may make graft atherosclerosis and obliterative bronchiolitis less common. As our understanding of lung rejection continues to expand, we can expect increasingly better results as these forms of therapy are employed in patients with end-stage cardiac and/or pulmonary disease.

References

1. Bernard CN: A human cardiac transplant: An interim report of a successful operation performed at Groote Schuur Hospital, Cape Town. *S Afr Med J* 41:1271, 1967.
2. Reitz BA, Wallwork JL, Hunt SA, et al: Heart-lung transplantation: Successful therapy for patients with pulmonary vascular disease. *New Engl J Med* 306:557, 1982.
3. Toronto Lung Transplant Group: Unilateral lung transplantation for pulmonary fibrosis. *New Engl J Med* 314:1140, 1986.
4. Jamieson SW, Stinson EB, Oyer PE, et al: Heart-lung transplantation for irreversible pulmonary hypertension. *Ann Thorac Surg* 38:554, 1984.
5. Patterson GA, Cooper JD, Dark JH, et al: Experimental and clinical double lung transplantation. *J Thorac Cardiovasc Surg* 95:70, 1988.
6. Spray TL, Huddleston CB: Pediatric lung transplantation, in Patterson GA, Cooper JD (eds): *Lung Transplantation, vol 3. Chest Surgery Clinics of North America.* Philadelphia, W. B. Saunders Company, 1993:123–143.
7. Achuff SC: Clinical evaluation of potential heart transplant recipients, in Baumgartner WA, Reitz BA, Achuff SC (eds): *Heart and Heart-Lung Transplantation.* Philadelphia, W. B. Saunders Company, 1990, pp 51–57.
8. Kerem E, Reisman J, Corey M, et al: Prediction of mortality in patients with cystic fibrosis. *N Engl J Med* 326:1187, 1992.
9. Schumway SJ, Hertz MI, Petty MG, eta al: Liberalization of donor criteria in lung and heart-lung transplantation. *Ann Thorac Surg* 57:92, 1994.
10. Calhoon JH, Grover FL, Gibbons WJ, et al: Single lung transplantation—Alternative indications and technique. *J Thorac Cardiovasc Surg* 101:816, 1991.
11. Smith CR: Techniques in cardiac transplantation. *Prog Cardiovasc Dis* 32:383, 1990.
12. Starnes VA: Heart-lung transplantation: An overview. *Cardiol Clin* 8:159, 1990.
13. Kshettry VR, Shumway SJ, Gauthier RL, et al: Technique of single-lung transplantation. *Ann Thorac Surg* 56:520, 1993.
14. Kaiser LR, Pasque MK, Trulock EP, et al: Bilateral sequential lung transplantation: The procedure of choice for double-lung replacement. *Ann Thorac Surg* 52:436, 1991.
15. Kubo SH, Ormaza SM, Francis GS, et al: Trends in patient selection for heart transplantation. *J Am Coll Cardiol* 21:975, 1993.
16. Veith FJ: Lung transplantation. *Surg Clin North Am* 58:357, 1978.
17. Pasque MK, Cooper JD, Kaiser LR, et al: Improved technique for bilateral lung transplantation: Rationale and initial clinical experience. *Ann Thorac Surg* 49:785, 1990.
18. Shumway SJ: Heart and heart-lung immunosuppression: Clinical strategies. *Clin Transplant* 5:554, 1991.
19. Shumway SJ, Hertz MI, Maynard R, et al: Airway complications after lung and heart-lung transplantation. *Transplant Proc* 25:1165, 1993.
20. Patterson GA: Airway revascularization: Is it necessary? *Ann Thorac Surg* 56:807, 1993.
21. Kirklin JK, Holm A, Adrete JS, et al: Gastrointestinal complications after cardiac transplantation. Potential benefit of early diagnosis and prompt surgical intervention. *Ann Surg* 211:538, 1990.
22. Smith P, Slaughter M, Petty M, et al: Abdominal complications following lung transplantation. *J Heart Lung Transplant* 14:44, 1995.
23. Gulbis B, Adler M, Ooms HA, et al: Liver-function studies in heart transplant recipients treated with cyclosporine A. *Clin Chem* 34:1772, 1988.
24. Steck TB, Costanzo-Nordin MR, Keshavarzian A: Prevalence and management of cholelithiasis in heart transplant patients. *J Heart Lung Transplant* 10:1029, 1991.
25. Billingham ME, Cary NRB, Hammond ME, et al: A working formulation for the standardization of nomenclature in the diagnosis of heart and lung rejection: Heart rejection study group. *J Heart Lung Transplant* 9:587, 1990.
26. Rose EA, Barr ML, Xu H, et al: Photochemotherapy in human heart transplant recipients at high risk for fatal rejection. *J Heart Lung Transplant* 11:746, 1992.
27. Glanville AR, Imoto E, Baldwin JC, et al: The role of right ventricular endomyocardial biopsy in the long-term management of heart-lung transplant recipients. *J Heart Transplant* 6:357, 1987.
28. Griffith BP, Hardesty RL, Trento A, et al: Heart-lung transplantation: Lessons learned and future hopes. *Ann Thorac Surg* 43:6, 1987.
29. Starnes VA, Theodore J, Oyer PE, et al: Evaluation of heart-lung transplant recipients with prospective serial transbronchial biopsies and pulmonary function studies. *J Thorac Cardiovasc Surg* 98:683, 1989.
30. Hofflin JM, Potasman I, Baldwin JC, et al: Infectious complications in heart transplant recipients receiving cyclosporine and corticosteroids. *Ann Intern Med* 106:209, 1987.
31. Kramer MR, Marshall SE, Denning DW, et al: Cyclosporine and itraconazole interaction in heart and lung transplant recipients. *Ann Intern Med* 113:327, 1990.
32. Costanzo-Nordin MR, Swinnen LJ, Fisher SG, et al: Cytomegalovirus infections in heart transplant recipients: Relationship to immunosuppression. *J Heart Lung Transplant* 11:837, 1992.
33. Griepp RB, Stinson EB, Bieber CP, et al: Control of graft atherosclerosis in human heart transplant recipients. *Surgery* 81:262, 1977.
34. Gao SZ, Schroeder JS, Alderman EL, et al: Clinical and laboratory correlates of accelerated coronary artery disease in the cardiac transplant patient. *Circulation* 76:V56, 1987.
35. McDonald K, Rector TS, Braunlin EA, et al: Association of coronary artery disease in cardiac transplant recipients with cytomegalovirus infection. *Am J Cardiol* 64:359, 1989.
36. Glanville A, Baldwin J, Burke C, et al: Obliterative bronchiolitis after heart-lung transplantation: Apparent arrest by augmented immunosuppression. *Ann Intern Med* 107:300, 1987.

37. Hertz MI, Henke CA, Nakhleh RE, et al: Obliterative bronchiolitis after lung transplantation: A fibroproliferative disorder associated with platelet-derived growth factor. *Proc Natl Acad Sci USA* 89:10385, 1992.

38. Trulock EP: Recipient selection, in Patterson GA, Cooper JD (eds): *Lung Transplantation.* Chest Surgery Clinics of North America. Vol. 3, 1993:3.

196. Care of the Pancreas Transplant Recipient

Scott A. Gruber and
David E. R. Sutherland

Pancreas transplantation can establish normoglycemia and insulin independence in diabetic recipients by providing functioning beta cells and has the potential to halt the progression of vascular complications that affect the eyes, nerves, kidneys, and other organ systems. No current method of exogenous insulin administration can produce a euglycemic, insulin-independent state over the long term akin to that achievable with a technically successful, immediately vascularized whole pancreas graft. Pancreas transplantation was first performed clinically in 1966 at the University of Minnesota [1]. The frequency of pancreas transplantation has increased as the results have improved, and by the end of 1993, over 5000 pancreas transplants had been performed at more than 160 institutions worldwide and reported to the International Pancreas Transplant Registry (IPTR) [1a]. Fig 196-1 illustrates the number of pancreas transplants worldwide annually and the rapid increase in application since the advent of the United Network for Organ Sharing (UNOS) in 1987. More than 500 have been done every year since 1989 in the United States. Currently 900 patients await pancreas transplantation at about 100 U.S. medical institutions offering the procedure.

Factors responsible for progressive improvement in pancreas transplant outcome include: (1) development of the bladder drainage (BD) technique and use of urinary amylase to monitor graft function; (2) improved techniques of multiorgan procurement and organ preservation with University of Wisconsin (UW) solution; (3) use of cyclosporine (CSA)-based multidrug immunosuppressive protocols, with more potent agents for prophylaxis and treatment of rejection (OKT3); (4) development of better drugs for prophylaxis and treatment of cytomegalovirus (CMV) infection (i.e., ganciclovir); and (5) generalized improvements in the quality of patient care.

In contrast to liver, heart, and lung transplants, pancreas transplants, like renal transplants, are not performed to save a life but to improve the quality of life over that achieved by the alternative treatment (exogenous insulin administration for diabetes and dialysis for renal failure). It is now generally accepted that renal transplantation, with the attendant need for immunosuppression, is a better option than dialysis for most uremic diabetic patients. In fact, it has been demonstrated that diabetics treated with chronic dialysis have a shortened life span when compared with patients who receive a successful kidney transplant [2]. Such agreement does not currently exist with respect to the widespread application of pancreas transplantation to type I diabetes, because the side effects of immunosuppression may exceed the complications of diabetes, which any individual patient is destined to develop. This has

resulted in the preferential performance of pancreas transplants in diabetic patients already obligated to receive immunosuppression to prevent rejection of a simultaneously or previously transplanted kidney in whom organ-specific lesions have already appeared and which may be self-perpetuating. Following this line of reasoning, solitary pancreas transplantation would be appropriate only in the hyperlabile diabetic whose day-to-day quality of life is so poor from a management standpoint that chronic immunosuppression is justified simply to achieve insulin independence. Although multiple studies have examined the effect of successful pancreas transplantation on the already existing metabolic abnormalities and secondary complications of type I diabetes, the potential for pancreas transplantation to *prevent* secondary complications has never been seriously tested and would need to be examined in the context of a randomized, controlled trial [3]. Thus, it is unlikely that pancreas transplantation will be applied early in the course of diabetes until antirejection strategies are available whose potential for causing morbidity is clearly less than the potential morbidities associated with diabetes.

Several surgical techniques have been used to manage pancreas graft exocrine secretions in the recipient, including enteric drainage (ED) into the proximal jejunum [4], synthetic polymer injection of the pancreatic duct [5], and urinary drainage [6–9]. The main advantage of urinary drainage is the ability to detect pancreas rejection episodes early, before hyperglycemia develops, by noting a decrease in serial urine amylase measurements [6]. Draining exocrine secretions into the urinary tract was first described by Gliedman et al. [7] in five patients who underwent pancreatic duct–ureteral anastomosis. BD was introduced in 1982 by Sollinger and colleagues [8], who anastomosed a button of duodenum surrounding the ampulla of Vater to the bladder, and then modified to its current form by Ngheim and Corry [9] to include a segment of duodenum. BD has been associated with lower technical failure rates and higher actuarial graft survival rates than ED or duct injection [10] and has now become the standard technique of establishing exocrine drainage of the pancreatoduodenal allograft.

Recipient Categories and Results

The results of pancreas transplantation must be discussed in light of the three major recipient categories: (1) simultaneous cadaveric pancreas/kidney transplant (SPK); (2) pancreas after

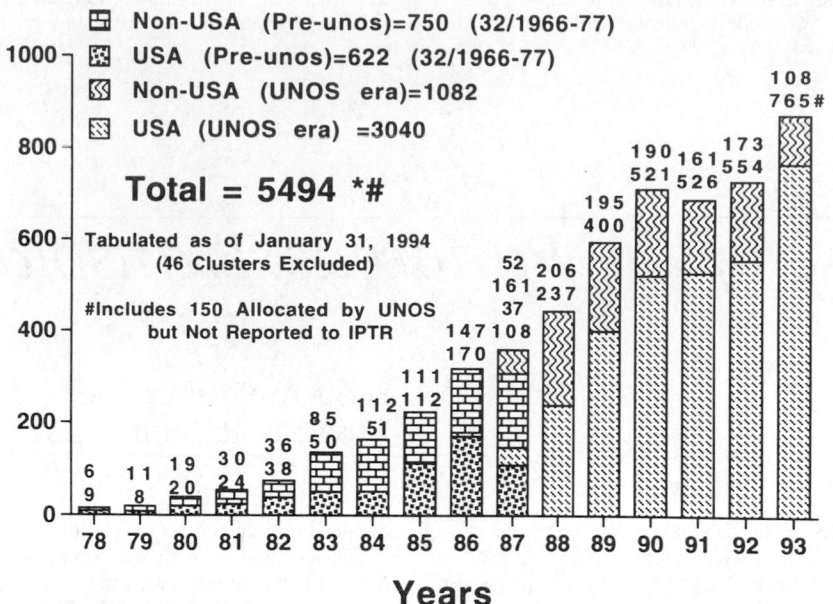

Fig. 196-1. Number of United States and non-US pancreas transplants reported by year to the International Pancreas Transplant Registry (IPTR).

a living-related or cadaveric kidney transplant (PAK); and (3) pancreas transplant alone (PTA). Figs. 196-2 and 196-3 give the actuarial patient and graft survival rates by recipient category for cases performed in the U.S. from October 1987 to November 1993. Graft function is defined by normoglycemia and insulin independence. Only one center, the University of Minnesota, has a large experience with PTA in patients without end-stage diabetic nephropathy.

Most rejection episodes in SPK recipients are heralded first by an increase in serum creatinine, followed by a decrease in urinary amylase, and last, a rise in plasma glucose. Thus, even with BD and the availability of urinary amylase determinations, the functional pancreas survival rate in PAK and PTA patients was initially less than that in SPK recipients [11], in whom the kidney from the same donor serves as an early marker of rejection at a time when the process may be subclinical in the pancreas graft, but nevertheless ongoing. However, with more attention being paid recently to (1) using potent induction immunosuppressive protocols (14 days of antilymphocyte therapy) [12,13]; (2) minimizing HLA mismatches [13,14]; (3) utilizing a smaller decline in urinary amylase (25%) as an indication for rejection treatment; (4) employing transcystoscopic pancreas allograft biopsy for diagnosis of rejection [15]; (5) assuming all rejection episodes are steroid resistant; and (6) liberalizing use of ganciclovir for prophylaxis and treatment of CMV infection, the one-year pancreas graft survival rate in PTA and PAK patients now approaches that of SPK recipients at the University of Minnesota [16–18]. It has been demonstrated that minimizing HLA mismatches is critically important to success in PTA and PAK cases nationwide, but not in SPK cases [11]. Finally, data from the UNOS Registry suggest that preservation up to 30 hours has no detrimental influence on graft functional survival rates and that recipients of 45 years or younger do better [11].

At several of the major pancreas transplant centers in the United States, one-year pancreas graft survival in SPK recipients is in the 80 to 90 percent range and approaches that of renal graft survival, with a similar fall-off over the longer term [19–25]. Data from the University of Wisconsin demonstrate that HLA-DR matching significantly improves long-term graft survival in SPK recipients [26]. Pancreas transplantation results are similar to those of the other solid organ transplants.

Indications for Pancreas Transplantation

In a recent technical review and position statement [27,28], the American Diabetes Association reviewed the safety, efficacy, and indications for pancreas transplantation. It was felt that the main rationale for pancreas transplantation currently is to significantly improve the quality of life of people with diabetes, to eliminate acute complications of the disorder, and not to prevent or retard the development and progression of long-term complications or to prolong life. At the University of Minnesota, all uremic type I diabetics who would be candidates for renal transplantation are also considered potential candidates for pancreas transplantation, with the risks versus the benefits of adding the pancreas evaluated on an individual basis.

There are three transplant options for the diabetic with renal failure: (1) living-related donor (LRD) renal transplant followed by cadaveric pancreas transplant (PAK); (2) simultaneous cadaveric pancreas/kidney transplant (SPK); and (3) LRD or cadaveric kidney transplant alone (KTA). If an LRD kidney is available, we recommend proceeding first with LRD renal transplantation and then subsequently with cadaveric pancreas transplantation (PAK), rather than with SPK. From the standpoint of treatment of uremia, diabetic patients who receive an LRD KTA or LRD renal transplant and then PAK demonstrate significantly better long-term kidney graft survival than those who receive an SPK [29]. Furthermore, patients who receive an LRD kidney may avoid the need for dialysis or a prolonged waiting period on dialysis, and the cadaver kidney can be made available for others—an important consideration in this era of organ shortage. Finally, although pancreas graft survival rates

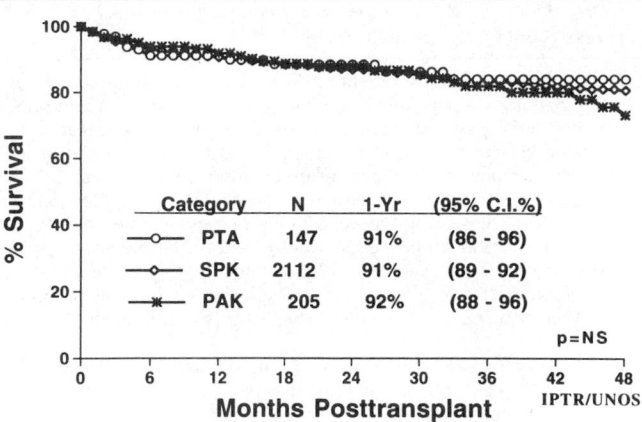

Fig. 196-2. Bladder-drained cadaveric pancreas transplant patient survival in the United States by recipient category for cases reported to the IPTR/UNOS Registry 1987–93.

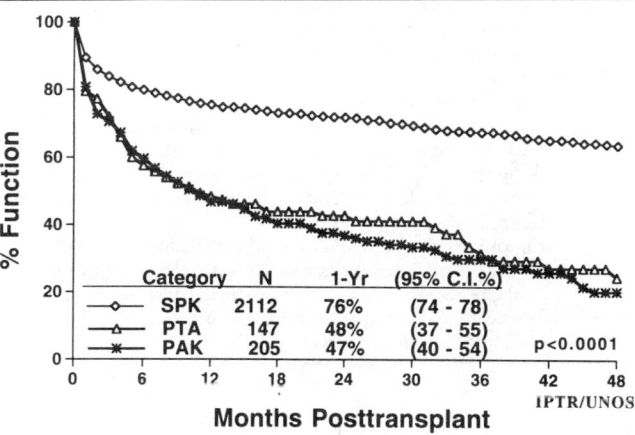

Fig. 196-3. Bladder-drained cadaveric pancreas transplant graft survival in the United States by recipient category for 1987–93.

have been lower in PAK than in SPK recipients, these differences can be minimized by strict attention to the factors discussed earlier. There is no detrimental effect of pancreas transplantation on the function of a previously transplanted kidney at one and two years [30].

If a living-related donor renal transplant is not an option, Table 196-1 summarizes the advantages and disadvantages of SPK, respectively, when compared with KTA in the appropriately chosen uremic diabetic recipient and serves as a guideline for discussion with the patient. For the vast majority of patients, the advantages outweigh the disadvantages, and there is no reason not to make them insulin independent, as well as dialysis-free, by adding a pancreas as long as the surgical risk is low. The degree of immunosuppression currently used to prevent rejection of cadaveric pancreas transplants far exceeds that which has been necessary to prevent autoimmune recurrence of disease in identical twin pancreas transplant cases; therefore, recurrence of disease is not a real consideration [49,50].

The indication for PTA in nonuremic diabetics is twofold and given in Table 196-2. In patients with early diabetic nephropathy, albuminuria indicates disease at a stage where progression is inevitable should the patient remain diabetic [52], but the

Table 196-1. Decision to Perform SPK versus KTA in Appropriately Selected Uremic Diabetic Patients

Advantages
1. Overall actuarial patient survival is the same or higher in SPK patients up to five years posttransplant [19–24,31–34].
2. Overall actuarial kidney graft survival is the same or higher in SPK patients up to five years posttransplant [19–24,31–35].
4. There is no difference in mean serum creatinine levels up to five years posttransplant [19,22,23,33].
5. Improved quality of life from being insulin-independent and euglycemic: freedom from personal, social, and dietary restrictions [31,36–41].
6. Protection from recurrent diabetic nephropathy [42,43].
7. Slowing the process of neuropathy [44–48].

Disadvantages
1. The pancreas is more immunogenic than the kidney and the "antigen load" to the host is greater for two organs, resulting in:
   a. A higher incidence of acute rejection episodes in SPK patients [19,21,22,33].
   b. The need for heavier immunosuppressive therapy for induction (10–14 days versus 7 days of antilymphocyte therapy and higher initial steroid doses) and for treatment of rejection episodes (usually steroid-resistant) in SPK patients.
2. The incidence of wound complications, urologic complications, urinary tract infections, and bacterial and fungal (but not viral) infections is higher in SPK patients [19,21,22,33]. The data are conflicting regarding the incidence of CMV infection.
3. Initial postoperative hospital stay and first-year posttransplant readmission rate are higher in SPK patients, resulting in higher cost [19–23,32]

Table 196-2. Indications for PTA in Nonuremic Diabetic Patients

1. A constellation of diabetic problems *currently* more serious than the potential morbidity from undergoing a major surgical procedure and the side effects of long-term immunosuppression. This includes extremely labile patients with oscillating episodes of ketoacidosis and hypoglycemia with unawareness who need constant attention and cannot live independently, as well as patients with a high glycohemoglobin in the face of proven hypoglycemic episodes with or without oscillating ketoacidosis [51].
2. Early but progressive secondary diabetic complications *predictably* more serious than the potential side effects of chronic immunosuppression with or without day-to-day management problems. Such patients usually have retinopathy and neuropathy, but the main criterion is early nephropathy characterized by [10]:
   a. Albuminuria
   b. Diabetic lesions on kidney biopsy
      Mesangium 20–40% of glomerular volume (<20% is normal; >40% is severe nephropathy)
   c. Creatinine clearance >70 ml/min (CSA will be tolerated)

lesions are early enough so that progression might be halted by a successful pancreas transplant.

Pretransplant Evaluation

In addition to the general preoperative evaluation performed for all potential organ transplant recipients before the initiation of immunosuppressive therapy, all patients considered for pancreas transplantation undergo extensive evaluation of those organ systems predominantly affected by diabetes mellitus (Table 196-3). Examination of the cardiovascular system is most important, because significant coronary artery disease may be present without angina in diabetic recipients with neuropathy. Thus, dipyridamole thallium stress tests and echocardiography are obtained routinely, and coronary angiography follows if the stress test is positive or there is a previous history of angina or myocardial infarction. If significant and correctable lesions are detected on arteriography, candidates should undergo angioplasty or bypass surgery in the pretransplant period. Detailed neurologic, ophthalmologic, renal, psychiatric, joint, and metabolic testing is also performed. An ultrasound of the gallbladder is obtained to permit prophylactic cholecystectomy in patients with cholelithiasis. Because numerous studies have demonstrated that, even with CSA-based immunosuppression, graft survival is significantly better in patients who have been transfused [53–55], we continue to deliberately transfuse pancreas transplant candidates under low-dose azathioprine coverage to prevent sensitization.

Preoperatively, all pancreas transplant recipients receive a mechanical and antibiotic bowel prep and intravenous antimicrobial coverage with imipenem/cilastatin, vancomycin, and fluconazole. Central venous pressure monitoring is performed routinely. Insertion of a pulmonary artery catheter and arterial line with preoperative optimization of end-diastolic volume and systemic vascular resistance is reserved for those patients with decreased cardiac reserve secondary to ischemic or valvular heart disease.

Patients are accepted on the waiting list for SPK as early as it can be determined that the patient will require either transplantation or dialysis support within the foreseeable future. Morbidity and mortality can be reduced if patients have transplantation early in the course of their renal failure, and the majority of patients should be transplanted before the need for dialysis arises. Although a patient may have met the general criteria necessary to be placed on the waiting list for a pancreas or combined pancreas/kidney transplant, the patient's medical condition at the time the organ(s) become available must be reassessed, especially if the waiting time is longer than one year, to prevent transplantation in the setting of infection, as well as other problems.

Donor Selection

The absolute contraindications for cadaver pancreas donation are those applied to organ donation in general (systemic lupus erythematosus and other collagen vascular diseases; congenital and acquired metabolic disorders; sickle cell anemia and related hemoglobinopathies; malignancy other than that confined to low-grade, noninvasive tumors of the skin or central nervous system; generalized viral or bacterial infections; and hepatitis B or HIV carrier state) and a history of diabetes mellitus. Relative contraindications include a history of pancreatic disease or previous duodenal or pancreatic surgery, physiologic age older than 60 years, and amylase levels >100 U/L [56]. Examination of the pancreas at the time of procurement is often the best or only way to confirm suitability of a given organ for donation and transplantation. If sclerotic, calcific, or markedly discolored, the pancreas should not be used. An attempt should be made to maintain plasma glucose levels of the donor within the 100 to 150 mg/dl range, with insulin administration as needed.

With the development of standard techniques for vascular reconstruction of the arterial blood supply to the pancreas graft [57–63], there is currently no question that both the liver and whole-organ pancreas can be procured from the same donor

Table 196-3. Work-up Orders for Potential Pancreas or Pancreas/Kidney Transplant Recipients

1. Consults to: Dental (if patient has not seen a dentist in past year); gynecology—pap smear for all females who have not had one within the past year; radiology—mammography for females over 35 who have not had one in the past year; ophthalmology—refraction visual acuity, applanation tension, dilate OU, fluorescein angiography; neurology—clinical exam, EMG, autonomic studies, temperature test; nephrology—kidney biopsy, renal function studies; endocrinology—24-hour metabolic profile with plasma glucose, serum insulin, and C-peptide levels determined before and 1 and 2 hours after each meal; arginine stimulation test; orthopedics, psychiatry (when indicated).
2. Tests:
    a. Laboratory—CBC with platelets and differential, sed rate, PT/PTT, electrolytes, liver function tests, amylase, serum protein electrophoresis, lipid panel (LDL, HDL, triglycerides, apoprotein A1 and B), glycosylated hemoglobin, hepatitis A, B, and C profile; CMV, EBV, HSV, and VSV titers; pregnancy test; HIV antibody (with consent); urinalysis, culture, and sensitivities, throat and blood cultures; 24-hour urine collection for creatinine clearance, quantitative albumin and protein determination, and amylase and glucose concentrations; fecal occult blood test × 2; peritoneal fluid cell count, Gram stain, and culture for peritoneal dialysis patients; FS blood glucoses at 6 a.m., 11 a.m., 4 p.m., 9 p.m., and as needed for 1 week.
    b. Radiologic/endoscopic—VCUG if history of infection, polycystic kidney disease, congenital anomaly, or hematuria; CXR: PA and lateral; upper GI endoscopy if indicated by past ulcer history, current symptoms, or stool positive for occult blood; gallbladder ultrasound; abdominal ultrasound to rule out abdominal aortic aneurysm in patients over 45 years.
    c. Cardiopulmonary—ECG; dipyridamole-thallium scan (stress test); echocardiogram; cardiac catheterization if indicated by the above or in patients with cardiac history; pulmonary function tests and arterial blood gas if history of asthma, smoking, or pulmonary problems.

with no deleterious effects on the subsequent function of either organ [24,64]. In fact, it is very rare today that the pancreas is procured from a donor in whom the liver is not also removed.

Surgical Techniques

BENCHWORK PREPARATION OF THE DONOR PANCREAS. Our technique of multiorgan procurement has previously been described in detail [65]. The pancreas graft is prepared for implantation either before or simultaneously with the dissection and preparation of the recipient vessels. First, the spleen is removed, and care is taken to avoid injury to the tail of the pancreas. Next, the distal duodenal segment is mobilized to an area approximately 3 cm distal to the ampulla of Vater, and the excess bowel is removed following ligation and division of the blood vessels between pancreas and duodenum to minimize urinary bicarbonate loss. The total length of the remaining duodenal segment is approximately 10 cm. The proximal duodenal staple line is undersewn and then inverted. Last, vascular reconstruction of the splenic artery and superior mesenteric artery (SMA) is performed. Most commonly, a donor iliac artery Y-graft is used, with the internal iliac artery anastomosed end-to-end to the splenic artery and the external iliac artery anastomosed end-to-end to the SMA (Fig. 196-4). The common iliac artery stump is then anastomosed end-to-side to the com-

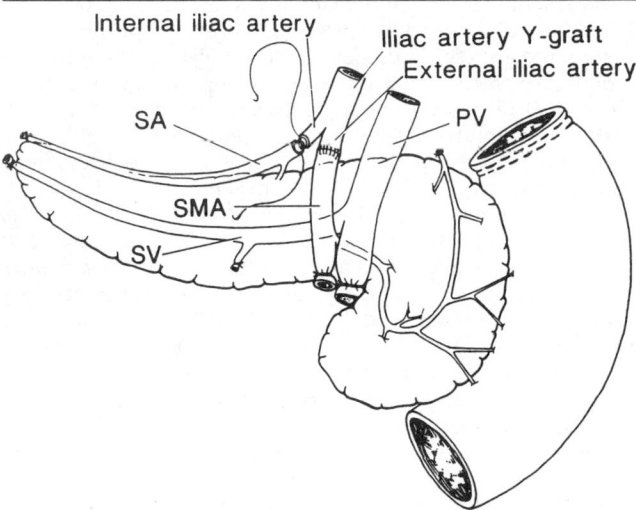

Fig. 196-4. Arterial reconstruction of the donor pancreas utilizing a donor iliac artery Y-graft. SA = splenic artery; PV = portal vein; SMA = superior mesenteric artery; SV = splenic vein.

mon iliac artery of the recipient. Another possibility for vascular reconstruction is end-to-side splenic artery–SMA anastomosis, either directly or through an iliac artery interposition graft. This technique is particularly useful when the donor iliac artery is not usable in whole or in part because of extensive atherosclerotic disease. Finally, in the rare case in which the liver is not procured from a pancreas donor and the celiac axis is allowed to remain with the pancreas graft together with the SMA on a common aortic patch, no vascular reconstruction is necessary.

SIMULTANEOUS PANCREAS/KIDNEY TRANSPLANTA-TION. Vancomycin 1 gm, imipenem-cilastatin 500 mg, fluconazole 200 mg, methylprednisolone 1 mg/kg, and azathioprine 2.5 mg/kg are administered intravenously before induction of anesthesia. Thigh-high TED hose and pneumatic boots are applied. A triple-lumen central venous or Swan-Ganz catheter is inserted through the right internal jugular vein. The abdomen is entered through a midline skin incision extending from midway between the xiphoid process and umbilicus down to the pubis. The lateral attachments of the bladder are freed with the cautery, and the medial umbilical ligaments are ligated and divided so as to completely mobilize the bladder. The lateral peritoneal attachments of the terminal ileum and cecum are divided and the sigmoid colon, small bowel, and cecum are packed away from the area of dissection. The right ureter is mobilized from surrounding tissues and looped so that it will lie medial to the iliac vessels. If necessary, the right gonadal vein and round ligament may be ligated and divided in females to allow the right fallopian tube and ovary to fall into the pelvis to facilitate approximation of the graft duodenum to the bladder. The common, external, and proximal internal iliac arteries are dissected free from surrounding tissues. Larger lymphatic bundles are ligated and divided; smaller lymphatics are cauterized. The common and external iliac veins are dissected free from surrounding tissues. The hypogastric vein, smaller deep external iliac vein branches, and the first lumbar vein, if necessary, are doubly ligated and divided to mobilize the iliac vein well up into the operative field from the vena cava to the inguinal ligament. This mobilization both facilitates the subse-

quent performance of the end-to-side venous anastomosis to the portal vein of the pancreatoduodenal graft, which should be kept short to prevent kinking, and obviates the need for a venous interposition graft. Care is taken not to stricture the main vein when the branches are ligated.

Attention is then turned toward dissection of the left iliac fossa, where the kidney will be implanted. The lateral attachments of the sigmoid colon are divided and the sigmoid mobilized medially. The external iliac artery and vein are dissected free from surrounding tissues so that adequate length is obtained for the end-to-side vascular anastomoses. Because the kidney is generally placed on the left side of the SPK recipient, the left donor kidney (with longer renal vein) is usually selected to be transplanted with the pancreas and the right donor kidney is used for KTA. While the operative field is set up, implantation of the renal allograft is performed first in the standard fashion (unless the preservation time is >18 hours), but the ureteroneocystostomy is not done until after the pancreas transplant is completed. Heparin 70 units/kg is administered intravenously before beginning the vascular anastomoses, and lasix 1 mg/kg and mannitol 12.5 to 25 g are administered intravenously during completion of the arterial anastomosis. Placing the vascular anastomoses lateral to the medially reflected mesentery of the sigmoid colon facilitates percutaneous biopsy of the intraperitoneal kidney by minimizing the interposition of large and small bowel between the kidney and the lateral abdominal wall.

Once the kidney is revascularized, exposure of the right iliac fossa is again obtained for implantation of the pancreatic allograft. The external iliac vein is brought lateral to the external iliac artery. The end-to-side arterial and venous anastomoses are usually made to the recipient common iliac artery and distal common or proximal external iliac vein, respectively. An additional 25 g of mannitol is administered during completion of the arterial anastomosis to reduce reperfusion edema of the graft. The venous clamps are removed first, and if there is no significant bleeding, the arterial clamps are removed in the following order while the graft artery is occluded with a vascular clamp: hypogastric, then common iliac, then external iliac. The graft artery is then released, and bleeding sites on the surface of the gland are controlled with fine suture ligation, taking care not to injure the pancreatic parenchyma. A sample of fluid for Gram stain plus aerobic, anaerobic, and fungal culture is obtained from the duodenum.

Attention is then turned toward performing the duodenocystostomy. Instead of using a hand-sewn, two-layer anastomosis, the circular stapler is usually employed for construction of the stoma [66]. The circular staple line is oversewn and inverted from within the bladder and if necessary, the staple line may also be inverted from the outside. Moreover, the medial umbilical ligaments mobilized at the beginning of the case may be wrapped around the bladder anastomosis for additional reinforcement. Finally, the open duodenum is closed and trimmed using a TA 55 or TA 90 stapler, and the staple line is then inverted with suture. The bladder is thoroughly irrigated with amphotericin B solution (10 mg/L), and the Foley catheter is irrigated to ensure patency. After performing a Leadbetter-Politano ureteroneocystostomy and closing the bladder in three layers, the grafts are inspected for perfusion and hemostasis, and the abdomen is copiously irrigated with triple-antibiotic (kanamycin 250 mg + bacitracin 5000 units + polymyxin B 500,000 units/L of normal saline) and amphotericin B solutions. Fig. 196-5 depicts the location of the pancreas and renal allografts at the completion of the combined procedure. No intraperitoneal or wound drains are placed.

In PTA or PAK recipients, the same technique as that described above for the pancreas is used, with the graft being placed in the right iliac fossa, if possible. In uremic diabetic

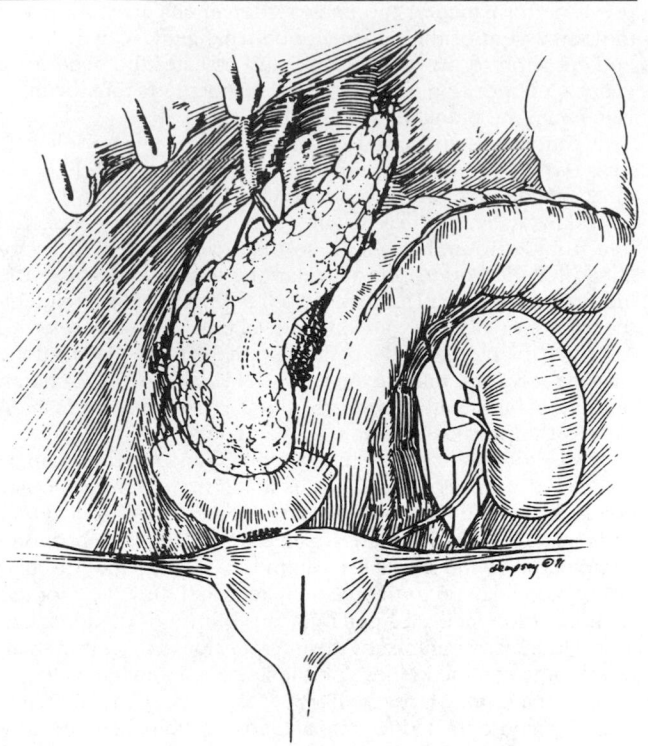

Fig. 196-5. Completed combined pancreas/kidney transplant.

Imipenem/cilastatin and vancomycin are discontinued after 7 days, and oral trimethoprim/sulfamethoxazole prophylaxis is begun; fluconazole is administered for 2 weeks. The immunosuppressive protocol utilized for SPK recipients is given in Table 196-4. In PAK recipients on triple therapy preoperatively, prednisone and antithymocyte globulin (ATGAM) or OKT3 are given as for SPK recipients, azathioprine is continued beginning at 2.5 mg/kg/day, and CSA is administered by continuous IV infusion beginning immediately postoperatively at an initial dose of 3 mg/kg/24 hours, with subsequent conversion to oral dosing and adjustment to maintain whole-blood trough levels by HPLC between 250 and 300 ng/ml. In PTA recipients, azathioprine, prednisone, and ATGAM or OKT3 are given as for SPK recipients, and CSA (14 mg/kg) is given preoperatively and then administered postoperatively as for PAK recipients. Prophylactic CMV therapy consists of acyclovir, 800 mg orally four times per day, until 3 months posttransplant.

Duplex ultrasonography and radionuclide perfusion scans of the pancreas and kidney are performed when clinically indicated. Daily urine amylase levels are monitored by a timed 8-hour collection. Patients are taught to monitor urinary pH because a reduction of the exocrine bicarbonate-rich secretion from the graft is reflected in a decreased pH and may be an early sign of graft rejection. Toward the end of the second postoperative week, patients are given instructions and education for home care, self-medication, and outpatient testing, and additional neurologic, ophthalmologic, and metabolic baseline testing is performed. Pancreatic allograft recipients with an uncomplicated course are generally discharged from the hospital during the third postoperative week.

patients who can receive an LRD renal transplant, the kidney should be placed on the left side, saving the right side for a subsequent cadaveric pancreas transplant. For PAK recipients who already have a functioning renal transplant on the right side, the pancreatoduodenal graft is placed on the left. Care must be taken to leave the transplant ureter undisturbed when mobilizing the bladder in PAK recipients.

Routine Postoperative Care

In general, the pancreas transplant recipient does not require intensive care in the postoperative period, and extubated patients are moved from the recovery room to the transplant nursing unit. Laboratory monitoring during the first postoperative day includes glucose determinations every 2 hours and CBC and electrolytes every 4 hours. Thereafter, plasma glucose is checked every 4 hours, and CBC, electrolytes, and serum amylase are monitored daily. Nasogastric suction and intravenous fluids are continued for the first several days until bowel function returns and oral alimentation can be initiated. In SPK recipients, urine output is replaced hourly on a milliliter per milliliter basis for the first 48 hours, similar to the initial fluid management for renal allograft recipients, and then tapered to maintenance requirements. In the early postoperative period, an infusion of regular insulin is routinely employed to maintain plasma glucose levels less than 150 mg/dl, because it has been demonstrated that chronic hyperglycemia is detrimental to beta cells. Patients who excrete large amounts of bicarbonate from the pancreatic graft, as evidenced by falling serum bicarbonate levels, are begun on oral bicarbonate replacement. The Foley catheter is left in for 10 to 14 days.

Diagnosis and Treatment of Rejection

As mentioned in Recipient Categories and Results and in Chapter 198, rejection episodes in SPK recipients are usually heralded first by an increase in serum creatinine, followed by a decrease in urinary amylase, and last, a rise in plasma glucose. In all patients, a 25 percent decline in urinary amylase from baseline is considered an indication for antirejection treatment. Febrile rejections are common in pancreas transplant recipients, and a rise in serum amylase and a fall in urinary pH may also be early signs of rejection. Antirejection therapy is usually begun before biopsy confirmation is obtained or infection is completely ruled out. In cases where renal transplant biopsy is not possible (PTA recipients) or helpful (PAK recipients or SPK recipients without serum creatinine elevation), transcystoscopic biopsy may be employed for diagnosis of isolated pancreatic rejection [15]; this technique has proved useful in differentiating between rejection and CMV infection. Other tests that may prove useful in monitoring pancreas allograft function and in diagnosing acute rejection include urine cytology [67], serum levels of anodal trypsinogen [68,69], and determination of the glucose disappearance constant [70], particularly in PAK and PTA patients or in patients with ED.

We assume all rejection episodes are steroid resistant and utilize the treatment protocol outlined in Table 196-5. The rationale for this protocol is derived from previous experience at the University of Minnesota, where the majority of acute rejection episodes did not respond to initial use of steroids alone or were followed by early second rejection episodes if anti-T cell therapy was not utilized. The total amount of ATGAM and OKT3 during the first 4 months posttransplant is limited to 21 doses, so if there is a second rejection in this interval, then

Table 196-4. Immunosuppressive Protocol for SPK Recipients

1. *Azathioprine*
   Oral doses listed; if administered IV, one-half oral dose is given:
Day	
0	5 mg/kg pre-op; none post-op
1–2	5 mg/kg/day
3–5	4 mg/kg/day
6–8	3 mg/kg/day
9+	2.5 mg/kg/day and adjust according to WBC count

2. *CSA*
   Begin when creatinine ≤ 3.0 mg/dl, usually day 5, 8 mg/kg/day orally, and adjust to maintain whole-blood trough levels by HPLC between 250 and 300 ng/ml the first six months, 200–250 ng/ml the next six months, and 150–200 ng/ml after the first year.

3. *Prednisone*
Day	
0	1 mg/kg pre-op; 1 mg/kg post-op
1–2	2 mg/kg/d (in 4 divided doses)
3–5	1.75 mg/kg/day
6–8	1.5 mg/kg/day
9–11	1.25 mg/kg/day
12–14	1.0 mg/kg/day
15–17	0.9 mg/kg/day (in 2 divided doses)
18–20	0.8 mg/kg/day
21–24	0.7 mg/kg/day
25–27	0.6 mg/kg/day
Month 2–3	0.5 mg/kg/day
4–5	0.45 mg/kg/day
6–7	0.4 mg/kg/day (single dose daily)
8–9	0.35 mg/kg/day
10–12	0.3 mg/kg/day
13+	0.25 mg/kg/day

4. *Antithymocyte globulin (ATGAM)/OKT3*
   ATGAM: Day 0 0 *or*   OKT3: Day 0 5 mg
   1–14 20 mg/kg/day   1–14 5 mg/day

Table 196-5. Antirejection Treatment Protocol for Pancreas Transplant Recipients

1. *Prednisone*
Day	
0	500 mg IV × 1 dose and 2 mg/kg orally
1	2 mg/kg/day
2–3	1.5 mg/kg/day
4–5	1.0 mg/kg/day
6–7	0.75 mg/kg/day
8–9	0.5 mg/kg/day
10+	Back to original tapered schedule (i.e., pre-rejection dose)

2. *ATGAM/OKT3*
   ATGAM: 20 mg/kg/day for 7 days *or* OKT3: 5 mg for 7 days

steroids only are used with a slow taper. Thereafter OKT3 or ATGAM is used for rejection episodes that occur with intervals of at least 3 months. Acyclovir is administered prophylactically from the initiation of OKT3 or ATGAM treatment for a total of 6 weeks. Chronic rejection is characterized by slowly rising blood glucose levels or increased insulin requirements with a progressive decline in urine amylase and C-peptide concentrations in patients with multiple previous acute rejection episodes and is not treated with more immunosuppression. Rejection remains the most common cause of graft loss.

Surgical Complications

In contrast to other solid organ transplants, the pancreas is susceptible to a unique set of complications because of its exocrine secretions and low blood flow. Overall, the incidence of graft-related complications has decreased significantly in recent years with the introduction of UW preservation solution, use of the "no-touch" technique of donor duodenopancreaticosplenectomy using the spleen and duodenum as handles, intraperitoneal placement of the organ through a midline incision, and use of the duodenal segment technique of BD.

THROMBOSIS. It is often difficult to determine whether pancreatic allograft thrombosis is simply due to a technical problem or is associated with high vascular resistance in the grafts secondary to preservation injury (pancreatitis with edema) or immunologic injury (severe acute rejection). The incidence ranges from 2 to 9 percent in recent single-center reports [19, 20,24,71,72] and is 6 percent in cases reported to the UNOS Registry [11]. The risk of graft thrombosis can be minimized by administering low-dose heparin/antiplatelet agents in the early postoperative period, as well as by keeping the donor portal vein short with full mobilization of the recipient iliac vein to reduce mechanical factors contributing to venous outflow obstruction. Arterial and venous thrombosis most commonly occur within the first several days posttransplant and are heralded by a rise in blood glucose, increased insulin requirement, and a fall in urine amylase. Venous thrombosis is also characteristically accompanied by hematuria and tenderness and swelling of the graft and ipsilateral lower extremity. Treatment is removal of the graft.

HEMORRHAGE. The risk of postoperative bleeding may be minimized at the initial procedure by meticulous control of bleeding sites on the surface of the gland with fine Prolene suture ligatures, tension-free vascular anastomoses, and doubly ligating the mesenteric axis and splenic hilar vessels with individual heavy silk sutures. Although hemorrhage may be exacerbated by anticoagulants/antiplatelet drugs, their benefit seems to outweigh the risk, since bleeding is a much less significant cause of graft loss than is thrombosis (0.9% versus 6%, respectively, in the UNOS Registry [11]). Evidence of significant bleeding is treated by immediate reexploration.

PANCREATITIS. Most cases of early graft pancreatitis are self-limited and due to ischemic/preservation injury. Clinical manifestations may include graft tenderness and fever in addition to hyperamylasemia. Treatment consists of fasting and IV fluid replacement. In some cases, peripancreatic fluid collections may develop, necessitating operative evacuation, debridement of necrotic tissue, initiation of a close suction/irrigation drainage system, and use of total parenteral nutrition. Later episodes of allograft pancreatitis may be caused by reflux or CMV infection, in which case treatment consists of Foley catheter drainage or ganciclovir, respectively. Pancreatitis is responsible for graft loss in approximately 2 percent of patients [11].

UROLOGIC COMPLICATIONS. Hematuria is a not uncommon occurrence in the first several months posttransplant but is usually transient and self-limiting. On occasion, however, it may result in significant blood loss and discomfort from clots and bladder distention. If not responsive to continuous bladder irrigation, persistent hematuria requires cystoscopy, clot evacuation, and cauterization of the bleeding source, which is usually along the duodenocystostomy. Bladder calculi may develop, usually in the setting of recurrent urinary tract infections and exposed staples along the duodenocystostomy, which may serve as a nidus for stone formation. Treatment consists of cystoscopy with removal of the staples and electrohydraulic lithotripsy [20]. Other urinary complications include chronic refractory metabolic acidosis from bicarbonate loss and persistent and recurrent urinary tract infections with severe dysuria, which, in addition to recurrent hematuria, are the major indications for converting exocrine secretions from BD to ED [73].

URINARY LEAKS. Most commonly, these are duodenal segment leaks, related to devascularization during the benchwork or during inversion of the distal duodenal staple line, and typically occur during the first several weeks after transplantation. Small leaks can be successfully managed by prolonged (at least 2 weeks) Foley catheter drainage; larger leaks require surgical intervention. Immediate operative closure of the leak and prolonged Foley catheter decompression are the treatment of choice. Leaks may give rise to pancreatic fistula or peripancreatic abscess. In two recent reports from major pancreas transplant centers, the incidence of duodenal segment leaks requiring surgical correction was 12 percent [24] and 7 percent [71]; however, only 0.4 percent of patients in the UNOS Registry have lost their grafts because of this problem [11].

INFECTION. Besides use of the duodenal segment BD technique and abandonment of extraperitoneal organ placement, the development of wound and peripancreatic infections can be minimized by: (1) irrigation of the duodenum with antibiotic/antifungal solution during the donor procedure; (2) opening the distal duodenum on the back table and thoroughly irrigating out the bowel contents with UW solution; (3) use of an appropriate perioperative antimicrobial regimen for prophylaxis, covering gram-positive and gram-negative bacteria as well as yeast, as the most common pathogens isolated from wound and intraabdominal infections are *Staphylococcus epidermidis*, *Streptococcus faecalis* (enterococcus), Candida albicans, and *Pseudomonas aeruginosa* and other gram-negative aerobic microbes; (4) copious irrigation of the abdominal cavity, bladder, and subcutaneous tissue with antibiotic/antifungal solution during the transplant procedure; and (5) using monofilament suture for fascial closure and not carrying the skin and fascial incision to the pubis [74]. The urinary tract is the most common site of infection; early infections are due to prolonged Foley catheter drainage, and later/persistent infections are due to neurogenic bladder or retained bladder suture or stones. Intraabdominal and peripancreatic infection may occur in association with pancreatitis or urinary leak or without such concurrent problems and are identified on CT scan by the development of fluid collections that prove to be abscesses or, more rarely, infected allograft pseudocysts. Operative exploration and drainage are often required. The incidence of surgical infections requiring operative or invasive radiologic intervention in SPK recipients was 3.6 percent [24] and 5 percent [71] in two recent reports, but close follow-up at the University of Minnesota indicates that approximately 10 percent of patients may develop intraabdominal infection. In the UNOS Registry, infection was responsible for graft loss in 2 percent of pancreas transplant patients [11].

Early Posttransplant Course

At least 10 percent of recipients have a prolonged initial hospitalization due to acute rejection or surgical complications, and more than 50 percent require readmission during their first posttransplant year, the majority of readmissions being for treatment of rejection episodes and opportunistic (e.g., CMV) infections [74]. The majority of readmissions occur within the first 3 months, and hospitalizations after the first year are much less frequent [20,21]. In a representative report from the University of Nebraska [71], the mean number of inpatient days was 38 for SPK recipients during the first posttransplant year, with a mean 2.8 readmissions per patient, 67 percent experiencing at least one rejection episode, and 30 percent requiring reoperation for some reason.

Effect on Quality of Life

Although pancreas transplantation has a relatively high frequency of complications, a successful transplant has several benefits. While the potential for pancreas transplantation to have a favorable effect on secondary complications of diabetes is important, it is the overall impact on quality of life, including that associated with insulin independence *per se,* that should be emphasized. The studies conducted so far are nearly unanimous in finding that patients with successful transplants rate their quality of life to be better after than before the transplant [75–84]. In the largest study to date on solitary pancreas transplant recipients [76,83], 131 patients were analyzed 1 to 10 years posttransplant; half had functioning grafts (n = 65) and half had grafts that ultimately failed (n = 66). Overall, 92 percent stated that managing immunosuppression was easier than managing diabetes [76]. When asked which was more demanding on their families' time and energy, the transplant or diabetes, 63 percent felt that their diabetes was more demanding, 29 percent that the two were equal, and 9 percent that the transplant was more demanding. Of the 65 patients with functioning grafts, 89 percent stated that they were more healthy than before the transplant. Indices of well-being were quantified by standard tests and were significantly higher in patients with functioning grafts than those without [83]. Virtually 100 percent of the patients with continuous graft function and 85 percent whose grafts ultimately failed said they encourage others with similar complications of diabetes to consider pancreas transplantation [76]. In addition, most of the patients with failed grafts desired retransplantation, and those with functioning grafts said they would undergo a retransplant if their current graft failed.

Summary and Conclusion

Currently, pancreas transplantation is most widely applied as an adjunct to kidney transplantation in preuremic, uremic, or posturemic diabetic patients [85]. Application to nonuremic patients, particularly those with hyperlabile diabetes, has increased in recent years [86], but current immunosuppressive regimens have many side effects [87] so the recipients must be carefully selected [88].

Nearly all uremic diabetic candidates for a kidney transplant are also candidates for a pancreas or islet transplant. The best treatment option is to receive a living related donor kidney transplant first, and later a pancreas transplant from either a living related (segmental graft) or cadaver (whole organ or segmental) donor [89,90]. For uremic patients who do not have a living related donor for a kidney, a pancreas transplant can be performed simultaneously with a kidney transplant from a cadaver donor [91–94].

There are several potential surgical complications of pancreas transplants. As for all transplants, immunosuppressive complications also occur. However, patient survival rates are similar to those for kidney transplant recipients, and pancreas graft survival rates are similar for those who receive both organs or a well-matched pancreas alone [1a].

When anti-rejection strategies become available that have fewer consequences than the present regimens, there will be an incentive to use pancreas transplants as a treatment for diabetes before the predisposition to secondary complications declares itself. For now, pancreas transplantation is a routine therapy in renal allograft recipients with Type I diabetes. It is also used to treat selected nonuremic patients with extremely labile diabetes or other diabetic problems that are not well served by other alternatives.

References

1. Kelly WD, Lillehei RC, Merkel FK, et al: Allotransplantation of the pancreas and duodenum along with the kidney in diabetic nephropathy. *Surgery* 61:827, 1967.
1a. Sutherland DER, Moudry-Munns K, Gruessner A: Pancreas transplant results in United Network for Organ Sharing United States of America Registry with a comparison to non-USA data in the International Registry, in Terasaki P (ed): *Clinical Transplantation—1993*, pp 47–69.
2. Vollmer WM, Wahl PW, Blagg CR: Survival with dialysis and transplantation in patients with end-stage renal disease. *N Engl J Med* 308:1553, 1983.
3. Sutherland DER: Commentary on pancreas transplantation. *Diabetes/Metabolism Review* 7:129, 1991.
4. Groth CG, Lundgren G, Klintmalm G, et al: Successful outcome of segmental human pancreatic transplantation with enteric exocrine diversion after modifications in technique. *Lancet* 2:522, 1982.
5. Dubernard JM, Traeger J, Neyra P, et al: A new method of preparation of segmental grafts for transplantation: trials in dogs and in man. *Surgery* 84:633, 1978.
6. Prieto M, Sutherland DER, Fernandez-Cruz L, et al: Experimental and clinical experience with urine amylase monitoring for early diagnosis of rejection in pancreas transplantation. *Transplantation* 43:71, 1987.
7. Gliedman ML, Gold M, Whittaker J, et al: Clinical segmental pancreatic transplantation with ureter-pancreatic duct anastomosis for exocrine drainage. *Surgery* 74:171, 1973.
8. Sollinger HW, Cook K, Kamps D, et al: Clinical and experimental experience with pancreaticocystostomy for exocrine pancreatic drainage in pancreas transplantation. *Transplant Proc* 16:749, 1984.
9. Nghiem DD, Corry RJ: Technique of simultaneous pancreatoduodenal transplantation with urinary drainage of pancreatic secretion. *Am J Surg* 153:405, 1987.
10. Sutherland DER, Moudry-Munns KC: Pancreas transplantation for type I diabetes mellitus. *Adv Endocrinol Met* 2:27, 1991.
11. Sutherland DER, Gruessner A, Moudry-Munns K: Analysis of United Network for Organ Sharing (UNOS) United States of America (USA) pancreas transplant registry data according to multiple variables, in Terasaki P (ed): *Clinical Transplants 1992*. Los Angeles, UCLA Tissue Typing Laboratory, 1993, pp 45–59.
12. Sutherland DER: Immunosuppression for clinical pancreas transplantation. *Clin Transplantation* 5(Spec issue):549, 1991.
13. Brayman KL, Sutherland DER: Factors leading to improved outcome following pancreas transplantation—The influence of immunosuppression and HLA matching. *Transplant Proc* 24(Suppl 2):91, 1992.
14. So SKS, Moudry-Munns KC, Gillingham K, et al: Short-term and long-term effects of HLA matching in cadaveric pancreas transplantation. *Transplant Proc* 23:1634, 1991.
15. Brayman KL, Moss A, Morel P, et al: Exocrine dysfunction evaluation of bladder-drained pancreaticoduodenal transplants using a transcystoscopic biopsy technique. *Transplant Proc* 24:901, 1992.
16. Sutherland DER, Moudry-Munns KC, Gillingham K, et al: Solitary pancreas transplantation: Alone in nonuremic and after a kidney in uremic diabetic patients. *Transplant Proc* 23:1637, 1991.
17. Sutherland DER, Dunn DL, Moudry-Munns KC, et al: Pancreas transplants in nonuremic and posturemic diabetic patients. *Transplant Proc* 24:780, 1992.
18. Sutherland DER, Gruessner R. Gillingham K, et al: A single institution's experience with solitary pancreas transplantation: A multivariate analysis of factors leading to improved outcome, in Terasaki P (ed): *Clinical Transplants 1991*. Los Angeles, UCLA Tissue Typing Laboratory, 1992, pp 141–152.
19. Schulak JA, Mayes JT, Hricik DE: Kidney transplantation in diabetic patients undergoing combined kidney-pancreas or kidney-only transplantation. *Transplantation* 53:685, 1992.
20. Shaffer D, Madras PN, Sahyoun AI, et al: Combined kidney and pancreas transplantation. A 3-year experience. *Arch Surg* 127:574, 1992.
21. Rosen CB, Frohnert PP, Velosa JA, et al: Morbidity of pancreas transplantation during cadaveric renal transplantation. *Transplantation* 51:123, 1991.
22. Cheung AHS, Sutherland DER, Dunn DL, et al: Morbidity following simultaneous pancreas-kidney transplants vs kidney transplants alone in diabetic patients. *Transplant Proc* 24:866, 1992.
23. Stratta RJ, Taylor RJ, Ozaki CF, et al: Combined pancreas-kidney transplantation versus kidney transplantation alone: Analysis of benefit and risk. *Transplant Proc* 25:1298, 1993.
24. Sollinger HW, Knechtle SJ, Reed A, et al: Experience with 100 consecutive simultaneous kidney-pancreas transplants with bladder drainage. *Ann Surg* 214:703, 1991.
25. Sasaki T, Pirsche JD, D'Allesandro AM, et al: Simultaneous pancreas-kidney transplantation at the University of Wisconsin-Madison Hospital, in Terasaki P (ed): *Clinical Transplants 1991*. Los Angeles, UCLA Tissue Typing Laboratory, 1992, pp 135–139.
26. Sasaki T, Pirsch JD, Ploeg RJ, et al: Effects of DR mismatch on long-term graft survival in simultaneous kidney-pancreas transplantation. *Transplant Proc* 25:237, 1993.
27. American Diabetes Association: Technical review: Pancreas transplantation for patients with diabetes mellitus. *Diabetes Care* 15:1668, 1992.
28. American Diabetes Association. Position statement: Pancreas transplantation for patients with diabetes mellitus. *Diabetes Care* 15:1673, 1992.
29. Cheung AHS, Matas AJ, Gruessner RG, et al: Should uremic diabetic patients who want a pancreas transplant receive a simultaneous cadaver kidney-pancreas transplant or a living related donor kidney first followed by cadaver pancreas transplant? *Transplant Proc* 25:1184, 1993.
30. Morel P, Sutherland DER, Almond PS, et al: Assessment of renal function in type I diabetic patients after kidney, pancreas, or combined kidney-pancreas transplantation. *Transplantation* 51:1184, 1991.
31. Secchi A, Di Carlo V, Martinenghi S, et al: Effect of pancreas transplantation on life expectancy, kidney function and quality of life in uraemic type 1 (insulin-dependent) diabetic patients. *Diabetologia* 34(Suppl 1):S141, 1991.
32. USRDS 1992 Annual Data Report: VIII. Simultaneous kidney-pancreas transplantation versus kidney transplantation alone: patient survival, kidney graft survival, and post-transplant hospitalization. *Am J Kid Dis* 20(Suppl 2):61, 1992.
33. Basadonna GP, Arrazola L, Matas AJ, et al: Morbidity, mortality, and long-term allograft function in kidney transplantation alone and simultaneous pancreas-kidney in diabetic patients. *Transplant Proc* 25:1321, 1993.
34. Brekke IB, Holdaas H, Albrechtsen D, et al: Combined pancreatic and renal transplantation: Improved survival of uremic diabetic patients and renal grafts. *Transplant Proc* 22:1580, 1990.
35. Nordén G, Nyberg G, Hedman L, et al: Transplantation in patients with diabetic nephropathy. Outcome of combined pancreas and kidney transplantation compared with kidney transplantation only. *Transplant Int* 3:234, 1990.
36. Zehrer CL, Gross CR: Quality of life of pancreas transplant recipients. *Diabetologia* 34(Suppl 1):S145, 1991.
37. Gross CR, Zehrer CL: Health-related quality of life outcomes of pancreas transplant recipients. *Clin Transplantation* 6:165, 1992.
38. Gross CR, Zehrer CL: Impact of the addition of a pancreas to the quality of life in uremic diabetic recipients of kidney transplants. *Transplant Proc* 25:1293, 1993.

39. Zehr PS, Milde FK, Hart LK, et al: Life quality of pancreatic transplant recipients: A comparison. *Transplant Proc* 24:850, 1992.

40. Voruganti LNP, Sells RA: Quality of life of diabetic patients after combined pancreatic-renal transplantation. *Clin Transplantation* 3:78, 1989.

41. Nakache R, Tydén G, Groth C-G: Quality of life in diabetic patients after combined pancreas-kidney or kidney transplantation. *Diabetes* 38(Suppl 1):40, 1989.

42. Bilous W, Mauer SM, Sutherland DER, et al: The effects of pancreas transplantation on the glomerular structure of renal allografts in patients with insulin-dependent diabetes. *N Engl J Med* 321:80, 1989.

43. Wilczek HE, Jaremko, G, Tydén G, et al: Pancreatic graft protects a simultaneously transplanted kidney from developing diabetic nephropathy: A 1- to 6-year follow-up study. *Transplant Proc* 25:1314, 1993.

44. Solders G, Tydén G, Persson A, et al: Diabetic neuropathy four years after pancreas transplantation. *Transplant Proc* 24:856, 1992.

45. Secchi A, Martinenghi S, Galardi G, et al: Effects of pancreatic transplantation on diabetic polyneuropathy. *Transplant Proc* 23:1658, 1991.

46. Gaber AO, Cardoso S, Pearson S, et al: Improvement in autonomic function following combined pancreas-kidney transplantation. *Transplant Proc* 23:1660, 1991.

47. Hathaway D, Abell T, Cardoso S, et al: Improvement in autonomic function following pancreas-kidney versus kidney-alone transplantation. *Transplant Proc* 25:1306, 1993.

48. Kennedy WR, Navarro X, Goetz FC, et al: Effects of pancreatic transplantation on diabetic neuropathy. *N Engl J Med* 322:1031, 1990.

49. Sutherland DER, Goetz FC, Sibley RK: Recurrence of disease in pancreas transplants. *Diabetes* 38(Suppl 1):85, 1989.

50. Sibley RK, Sutherland DER: Pancreas transplantation: An immunohistologic and histopathologic examination of 100 grafts. *Am J Pathol* 128:151, 1987.

51. Sutherland DER: Is there a need for pancreas transplantation? *Transplant Proc* 25:47, 1993.

52. Viberti GC, Hill RD, Jarre HRJ, et al: Microalbuminuria as a predictor of clinical diabetic nephropathy. *Lancet* 1:1430, 1982.

53. Opelz G: Effect of HLA matching, blood transfusions, and presensitization in cyclosporine treated kidney transplant recipients. *Transplant Proc* 17:2179, 1985.

54. Salvatierra O: The role of blood transfusions in transplantation. In: Cerilli GJ (ed): *Organ Transplantation and Replacement.* Philadelphia, J. B. Lippincott, 1988, pp 151–61.

55. Cecka J: The transfusion effect, in Terasaki P (ed): *Clinical Transplants 1987.* Los Angeles, UCLA Tissue Typing Laboratory, 1987, pp 287–301.

56. Toledo-Pereyra LH, Mittal VK, Gordon DA: Experience of the Mount Carmel Mercy Hospital, Detroit, Michigan, USA, in Dubernard JM, Sutherland DER (eds): *International Handbook of Pancreas Transplantation,* Dordrecht, Kluwer Academic Publishers, 1989, pp 365–370.

57. Bandlien KO, Mittal VK, Toledo-Pereyra LH: Procurement and workbench procedures in preparation of pancreatic allografts. Factors essential for a successful pancreas transplant. *Am Surg* 54:578, 1988.

58. Marsh CL, Perkins JD, Sutherland DER, et al: Combined hepatic and pancreatoduodenal procurement for transplantation. *Surg Gynecol Obstet* 168:254, 1989.

59. Mayes JT, Schulak JA: Pancreas revascularization following combined liver and pancreas procurement. *Transplant Proc* 22:588, 1990.

60. Yang HC, Gifford RRM, Dafoe DC, et al: Arterial reconstruction of the pancreatic allograft for transplantation. *Am J Surg* 162:262, 1991.

61. Fernández-Cruz L, Astudillo E, Sanfey H, et al: Combined whole pancreas and liver retrieval: Comparison between Y-iliac graft and splenomesenteric anastomosis. *Transplant Int* 5:54, 1992.

62. Sanseverino R, Martin X, Dawahra M, et al: Reconstruction of the vascular pedicle of the pancreatic graft after combined harvesting with liver: Comparison among different surgical options. *Transplant Proc* 24:805, 1992.

63. Bechstein WO, Reed AI, Sollinger HW: Alternative technique of pancreas graft arterialization. *Clin Transplant* 6:67, 1992.

64. Dunn DL, Morel P, Schlumpf R, et al: Evidence that combined procurement of pancreas and liver grafts does not affect transplant outcome. *Transplantation* 51:150, 1991.

65. Brayman KL, Najarian JS, Sutherland DER: Transplantation of the pancreas, in Cameron JL (ed): *Current Surgical Therapy—4.* Toronto, B. C. Decker, 1992, pp 458–475.

66. Pescovitz MD, Dunn DL, Sutherland DER: Use of the circular stapler in construction of the duodenoneocystostomy for drainage into the bladder in transplants involving the whole pancreas. *Surg Gynecol Obstet* 169:169, 1989.

67. Radio SJ, Stratta RJ, Taylor RJ, et al: The utility of urine cytology in the diagnosis of allograft rejection after combined pancreas-kidney transplantation. *Transplantation* 55:509, 1993.

68. Perkal M, Marks C, Lorber MI, et al: A three-year experience with serum anodal trypsinogen as a biochemical marker for rejection in pancreatic allografts. *Transplantation* 53:415, 1992.

69. Ploeg RJ, D'Alessandro AM, Groshek M, et al: Clinical efficacy of human anodal trypsinogen (HAT) for detection of pancreatic allograft rejection (abstract). Presented at the Nineteenth Annual Meeting of the American Society of Transplant Surgeons, Houston, 1993.

70. Elmer DS, Hathaway DK, Shokooh-Amiri H, et al: The relationship of glucose disappearance rate (K_G) to acute pancreas allograft rejection. *Transplantation* 57:1400,1994.

71. Ozaki CF, Stratta RJ, Taylor RJ, et al: Surgical complications in solitary pancreas and combined pancreas-kidney transplantations. *Am J Surg* 164:546, 1992.

72. Gruessner A, Gruessner R, Moudry-Munns K, et al: Influence of multiple factors (age, transplant number, recipient category, donor source) on outcome of pancreas transplantation at one institution. *Transplant Proc* 25:1303, 1993.

73. Stephanian E, Gruessner RWG, Brayman KL, et al: Conversion of exocrine secretions from bladder to enteric drainage in recipients of whole pancreaticoduodenal transplants. *Ann Surg* 216:663, 1992.

74. Sutherland DER, Dunn DL, Goetz FC, et al: A 10-year experience with 290 pancreas transplants at a single institution. *Ann Surg* 210:274, 1989.

75. Gross CR, Zehrer CL: Impact of the addition of a pancreas to quality of life in uremic diabetic recipients of kidney transplants. *Transplant Proc* 25:1293, 1993.

76. Zehrer CL, Gross CR: Quality of life of pancreas transplant recipients. *Diabetologia* 34:S145, 1991.

77. Nakache R, Tyden G, Groth CG: Quality of life in diabetic patients after combined pancreas-kidney or kidney transplantation. *Diabetes* 39:802, 1991.

78. Voruganti LNP, Sells RA: Quality of life of diabetic patients after combined pancreatic renal transplantation. *Clin Transplant* 3:78, 1989.

79. Zehr PS, Milde FK, Hart LK, Corry RJ: Pancreas transplantation: Assessing secondary complications and life quality. *Diabetologia* 34:S138, 1991.

80. Nathan DM, Fogel H, Norman D, et al: Long-term metabolic and quality of life results with pancreatic/renal transplantation in insulin-dependent diabetes mellitus. *Transplantation* 52:85, 1991.

81. Secchi AV, Di Carlo S, Martinenghi S, et al: Effect of pancreas transplantation on life expectancy, kidney function and quality of life in uremic type I (insulin-dependent) diabetic patients. *Diabetologia* 34:S141, 1991.

82. Wheeler SJ, Sollinger H, Pirsch JD: Quality of life in diabetics following simultaneous pancreas/kidney and kidney transplants (abstract). Presented at the American Society of Transplant Surgeons and the International Congress of the Transplantation Society, Chicago, 1992.

83. Gross CR, Zehrer CL: Health-related quality of life outcomes of pancreas transplant recipients. *Clin Transplant* 6:165, 1992.

84. Gross CR, Zehrer CL: Impact of the addition of a pancreas to quality of life in uremic diabetic recipients of kidney transplants. *Transplant Proc* 25:1293, 1993.

85. Sutherland DER: Pancreatic transplantation: State of the art. *Transplant Proc* 24:762, 1992.

86. Sutherland DER: Present status of pancreas transplantation alone in nonuremic diabetic patients. *Transplant Proc* 26:379, 1994.

87. Sutherland DER: Immunosuppression for clinical pancreas transplantation. *Clin Transplant* 5:549, 1991.

88. Lebebvre PH: Pancreatic transplantation: Why, when, and who? *Diabetologia* 35:494, 1992.
89. Sutherland DER, Gruessner RWG, Moudry-Munns KC, Cecka M: Tabulation of cases from the International Pancreas Transplant Registry and analysis of United Network for Organ Sharing United States Pancreas Transplant Registry data according to multiple variables. *Transplant Proc* 25:1707, 1993.
90. Sutherland DER, Moudry-Munns KC, Gillingham KJ, et al: Solitary pancreas transplantation: Alone in nonuremic and after a kidney in uremic diabetic patients. *Transplant Proc* 23:1637, 1991.
91. Sollinger H, Stratta RJ, D'Allessandro AM et al: Experience with simultaneous pancreas-kidney transplantation. *Ann Surg* 208:478, 1988.
92. Sutherland DER, Dunn DL, Goetz FC, et al: A 10-year experience with 290 pancreas transplants at a single Institution. *Ann Surg* 210:274, 1989.
93. Garvin PJ, Castaneda M, Carney K: Simultaneous cadaver renal and pancreas transplantation in type I diabetes. *Arch Surg* 122:274, 1987.
94. Stratta RJ, Taylor RJ, Ozaki CF, et al: A comparative analysis of results and morbidity in type I diabetics undergoing preemptive versus post-dialysis combined pancreas-kidney transplantation. *Transplantation* 55:1097, 1993.

197. Management of the Organ Donor

Christoph Troppmann and
David L. Dunn

Introduction

In 1993, approximately 3,000 patients on national organ transplant waiting lists in the United States died before a suitable donor organ became available. These unfortunate individuals represented ~6 percent (1400 patients) of kidney, ~25 percent (n = 650) of liver, and ~33 percent (n = 950) of heart transplant candidates on each waiting list [1]. Almost assuredly, these numbers underestimate the actual magnitude of the problem. Many patients with end-stage organ failure are currently not even considered for transplantation (and consequently are not listed) because of the increasingly strict selection criteria that are being applied as a result of the severe, ongoing organ shortage. The widening gap between available cadaver organs and the number of patients waiting is a result of the explosive, increased use of organ transplantation therapy over the past decade (Tables 197-1 and 197-2) with which the cadaver donor pool has not kept pace (Fig. 197-1).

The single most important factor that has been identified in this equation is the failure to maximize the use of potential cadaver donors, primarily because of the inability to obtain consent for organ retrieval. The rates of consent granted by families of potential cadaver donors range from 0 to 75 percent and appear to vary widely among geographic regions and ethnic groups [14,15]. The national average is only 57 percent [16]. Lack of dissemination and poor presentation of information to the public and misperceptions in the general population regarding the beneficial nature of organ transplantation and the necessity of organ retrieval from brain-dead cadaver donors have led to the stagnation of the organ supply [17].

The role of physicians who care for critically ill patient is crucial [18]. It is their responsibility to perform the preliminary screening tests to ascertain whether donation is possible (Table 197-3), to seek early referral to an organ procurement organization (OPO) should brain death appear imminent, and to coordinate the approach to the family before and after brain death has been declared, thus laying the foundation for obtaining consent. Intensive care and emergency medicine physicians are obligated ethically and morally to provide the best possible outcome for a very ill patient. However, after brain death has been declared they are also obligated to seek the best possible outcome for those patients with end-stage failure of a vital organ waiting for a transplant by attempting to ensure that organ donation occurs.

Current Status of Solid Organ Transplantation

The increased numbers of solid organ transplant procedures performed during the last decade has been paralleled by a significant improvement in outcome with regard to both patient and allograft survival (see Table 197-2). This phenomenon has been attributed to a variety of factors that include: (1) the introduction in the early 1980s of the powerful immunosuppressive agent cyclosporin A (CSA), (2) the availability of antilymphocyte antibody preparations to treat rejection episodes (antilymphocyte globulin [ALG], antithymocyte globulin [ATG], anti-CD3 murine monoclonal antibody [OKT3]), (3) improvements in organ preservation (e.g., use of University of Wisconsin [UW] solution), (4) thorough preoperative patient screening for the presence of existing disease processes, and (5) increasing sophistication in the postoperative intensive care of both normal and high-risk recipients. In addition, the availability of potent, nontoxic antibacterial, antifungal, and antiviral agents [19] has allowed opportunistic infections in immunocompromised transplant patients to be treated more effectively. In combination with refinement of surgical techniques, these factors have led to increasing success of solid organ replacement therapy [20].

Thus, transplantation has become the treatment of choice for many patients with end-stage failure of the kidneys, liver, endocrine pancreas, heart, lungs, and most recently the small bowel. Criteria for potential recipients have been expanded to include infants, children, and individuals thought to be at higher risk for complications (e.g., diabetics, elderly patients) [9,21]. Currently, the only patients who are excluded from undergoing transplantation are those with metastatic malignancies, uncontrolled infections, and diseases with high allograft recurrence rates or those who are unable to withstand major surgery or who have a significantly shortened life expectancy due to disease processes unrelated to their organ dysfunction or failure.

Table 197-1. Number of Solid Organ Transplants from Cadaver Donors per Year in the U.S.A.: 1982 versus 1992*

Organ	1982	1992
Kidney	3681	7698
Liver	62	3024
Pancreas	38	552
Heart	103	2172
Heart-lung	8	48
Lung	0	535

* References: 2, 3, 4

Table 197-2. One-Year Graft Survival Rates (Cadaver Donors): 1982 versus 1992[a]

Organ	1982[b]	1992
Kidney	80%	89%
Liver	35%	69%
Pancreas	23%	71%
Heart	65%	81%
Lung	—[c]	66%

[a] References: 1982: 5–8; 1992: 9–12; [b] results without cyclosporin A based immunosuppression; [c] No lung transplants were performed in 1982.

KIDNEY. Currently, patients undergoing kidney transplants exhibit excellent graft survival rates (89% and 70% at 1 and 5 years, respectively) [9]. Renal replacement therapy serves to improve quality of life and rehabilitates the recipients from a social perspective. Kidney transplants are also less expensive from a socioeconomic standpoint than chronic hemodialysis. For pediatric patients with chronic renal failure, a functioning renal allograft is the only way to preserve normal growth and ensure adequate central nervous, mental, and motor development [21].

LIVER. Patients with end-stage liver failure will die unless they receive a transplant. Liver transplants are an effective treatment for many patients, both pediatric and adult, regardless of the cause of liver failure: congenital (i.e., structural or metabolic defects), acquired (i.e., due to infection, trauma, intoxication), or idiopathic (e.g., cryptogenic cirrhosis, autoimmune hepatitis) [10]. A dramatic improvement in graft survival occurred after the introduction of CSA (see Table 197-2). There is currently no reliable means to substitute, even temporarily, for a failing liver, other than with a transplant. Extracorporeal perfusion, using either animal livers or bioartificial livers (hepatocytes suspended in bioreactors, separated from the perfusate by a membrane), may someday bridge the gap between complete liver failure and a liver transplant, but these therapeutic modalities are still experimental and are far from becoming standard clinical tools. Use of hepatocyte transplants to treat fulminant liver failure and to correct congenital enzyme deficiencies is also in the preliminary stages of study.

SMALL BOWEL. Small bowel transplants are being performed increasingly in patients with congenital or acquired short gut, especially if liver dysfunction occurs due to long-term administration of total parenteral nutrition and if difficulty in establishing or maintaining central venous access occurs. If the liver

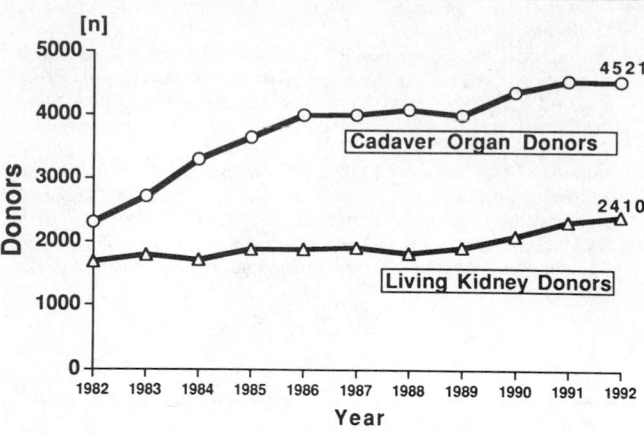

Fig. 197-1. The evolution of the number of cadaver organ donors and living kidney donors between 1982 and 1992 in the United States (references 2, 4, 13).

disease is advanced, a combined liver-small bowel, or in selected cases, a multivisceral transplant (liver, stomach, small bowel, with or without pancreas) has been performed. Early results are encouraging and a significant increase in the number of small bowel and multivisceral transplants is to be expected over the next decade [22].

PANCREAS AND ISLET CELLS. Primary prevention of Type I insulin-dependent diabetes mellitus is still not possible, but transplantation of the entire pancreas or isolated islet cells can correct the endocrine insufficiency once it occurs. Glucose sensor systems that continuously monitor blood sugar levels coupled with real-time command of an insulin delivery system (implantable pump) are not yet available. Development of bioartificial and hybrid biomechanical insulin-secreting devices is in the early experimental stages. Thus, the only effective current option to restore continuous near-physiologic normoglycemia is a pancreas transplant or, possibly in the near future, an islet cell transplant. Recently published evidence demonstrates that good metabolic glycemic control decreases the incidence and severity of secondary diabetic complications (neuropathy, retinopathy, gastropathy, and nephropathy) [23]. Most pancreas transplants are performed simultaneously with a kidney transplant in preuremic patients with significant renal dysfunction or in uremic patients with end-stage diabetic nephropathy. At some centers, nonuremic patients with brittle

Table 197-3. Organ Donor Screening by the Critical Care Physician

Age: 0–80 years
Heart-beating
Near brain death or brain-dead
Contraindications:
    Current untreated severe local bacterial, fungal, or protozoal infection
    Evidence of systemic sepsis syndrome
    Viral encephalitis or severe systemic viral infection
    HIV-positive serology
    Malignancy (except nonmelanoma skin cancers and primary brain tumors with little propensity to disseminate)

Type I diabetes mellitus (with progression of the autonomic neuropathy to the point of hypoglycemic unawareness and repetitive episodes of diabetic ketoacidosis) have undergone a solitary pancreas transplant without a concomitant kidney transplant [24] to improve their quality of life and to prevent the manifestation and progression of secondary diabetic complications. The evidence suggests that a successful pancreatic transplant achieves these goals in both uremic and nonuremic recipients [25]. Islet transplants are undergoing intensive clinical investigation, and recent results of transplanting alloislets from cadaver donors are encouraging [26]. Within the next 5 to 10 years they may become a routine form of therapy.

HEART. Heart transplants are the treatment of choice for patients with end-stage congenital and acquired parenchymal and vascular diseases and are recommended generally after all conventional medical or surgical options have been exhausted. After a spectacular start in 1967, poor results were observed over the ensuing decade. In the 1980's, however, the field of cardiac transplantation experienced dramatic growth (see Table 197-1) because of significant improvements in outcome, probably most directly related to immunosuppressive therapy and to refinements in diagnosis and treatment of rejection episodes [27]. Mechanical pumps, such as ventricular assist devices or the bioartificial heart, serve only to bridge the time between end-stage cardiac failure and a transplant and are by no means a permanent substitute for the transplant itself.

HEART-LUNG AND LUNG. Heart-lung and lung transplants are effective treatment for patients with advanced pulmonary parenchymal or vascular disease, with or without primary or secondary cardiac involvement. This relatively new field has evolved rapidly since the first single-lung transplant with long-term success was performed in 1983 (see Table 197-1). The spectacular increase in lung transplants each year is mainly due to technical improvements resulting in fewer surgical complications, as well as to the extremely limited availability of heart lung donors. Previously, many patients with end-stage pulmonary failure would have waited for an appropriate heart-lung donor. Currently, they undergo a single or a bilateral single-lung transplant instead. Double en bloc lung transplants have been abandoned because of technical difficulties related to the bronchial anastomotic blood supply. Single-lung transplants are most common, which allows one cadaver donor to donate up to three lifesaving thoracic organs. Bilateral single-lung transplants are generally performed in patients with septic lung diseases (e.g., cystic fibrosis, α-1 antitrypsin deficiency) in which the native contralateral lung could cross-contaminate the transplanted lung [28,29]. Mechanical ventilation or extracorporeal membrane oxygenation (ECMO) can be used as a temporary bridge to this type of transplantation, but use of these modalities does not obviate the need for organ replacement therapy.

Current Status of Organ Donation

The once steady increases in most types of organ-transplant procedures have reached a plateau over the last several years. This is due to an insufficient augmentation of the donor pool (see Tables 197-1 and 197-2 and Figure 197-1). The 55 mile per hour speed limit, stricter seat belt and helmet laws, improved trauma care and the AIDS epidemic have all had a significant impact on the number of available brain-dead organ donors [14,30]. In 1991, the three leading causes of death among brain-

dead donors in the United States were motor vehicle accidents, gunshot or stab wounds, and cerebrovascular accidents, followed by head trauma, asphyxiation, and other miscellaneous causes [31].

According to recent estimates, there are 7000 or 8000 *potential* brain-dead donors in the United States per year [13]. In 1992, however, there were 4521 *actual* organ donors in the United States. The single most important reason for lack of organ retrieval from 35 to 45 percent of the potential donor pool is the inability to obtain consent. Several studies have shown that family refusal to provide consent or the inability to identify, locate, or contact family members to obtain consent within an appropriate time frame are the leading causes for the nonuse of many potential donors [14,15,32,33].

The overall consent rate is steadily dropping even today [16]. A recent public opinion survey [17] showed that 69 percent of respondents would be very or somewhat willing to donate their organs, and 93 percent would honor the expressed wishes of a family member. However, only 52 percent of these individuals had communicated their wishes to their family. Moreover, 37 percent of respondents did not comprehend that a brain-dead person should be considered dead and unable to recover, and 59 percent either believed or were unsure whether or not organs can be bought and sold on the "black market." Finally, 42 percent did not realize that organ donation costs the family of the deceased nothing in the United States.

Correcting these misperceptions and attempting to increase awareness of the importance of organ transplant must be the focus of public educational campaigns. Such efforts can be successful, especially among minorities where mistrust and the perception of inequitable access to medical care and organ transplant therapy have led to disappointingly low organ donation and recovery rates [34,35]. It is very important that adequate communication, empathy, and an informative, humane approach to the family of the deceased occur to ensure reasonable consideration of donation. Educational efforts to enhance organ donation must also be directed at health care professionals and medical students, whose views and knowledge of these issues are often inconsistent and limited [36,37]. Physicians, too, need to be better trained to recognize and identify potential organ donors.

Recently, the potential for financial compensation or other rewards (e.g., compensation for funeral expenses) for donor families has been considered as a means to increase organ donation rates. Although the ethical debate that this has engendered is beyond the scope of this discussion, it centers around concerns that any form of reimbursement—direct or indirect—might lead to the commercialization of organ donation with the inherent risk of turning potential donors and transplantable organs into a commodity. Opponents of this concept believe that, rather than serving to enhance organ donation, such a system might alienate the public and further exacerbate the current organ shortage. Moreover, the use of financial compensation or rewards would continue to raise the issue of fairness with regard to access to transplant therapy for those who are disadvantaged and often underrepresented in both the population and transplant programs [38].

Options to Increase Organ Availability

Mechanisms that might serve to increase the number of available organs for transplantation include: (1) optimization and maximal utilization of the current actual donor pool; (2) increasing the number of living donor transplants; (3) use of unconventional and controversial donor sources, such as non–heart-beating cadaver donors, anencephalic donors, and executed prisoners; and (4) performing xenotransplants, using animal organs as a potentially unlimited supply for transplantation into humans. The two first mechanisms are of current practical interest, whereas the last two are likely to be those confronting critical care physicians, nurses, and the lay population over the next years in the form of an ongoing, intense public debate.

OPTIMAL USE OF THE CURRENT DONOR POOL. Required request laws have now been enacted in all states in the United States. They obligate hospitals to notify an OPO of potential donors and to offer the option of donation to the family of brain-dead potential donors. Results of this legislation have not been very encouraging so far: the number of cadaver donors has not significantly increased (see Fig. 197-1). As a result of the ongoing organ shortage, transplant surgeons have attempted to refine procurement techniques so that maximal use of the available donor pool occurs. For example, 76 percent of all brain-dead donors in 1991 were multiple-organ donors (Fig. 197-2) [31]. Simultaneous procurement of thoracic and abdominal organs does not adversely affect outcome, after heart and lung transplant procedures. Similarly, combined procurement of abdominal organs (i.e., liver, pancreas, kidneys) has had no detrimental impact on graft survival [39,40]. Recovery of the liver and pancreas from the same donor, initially touted as impossible because of their shared blood supply [41], has become routine, even in donors with significant splanchnic arterial anatomical abnormalities and variations [42,43]. Extension of the organ presentation time by a variety of techniques, including new preservation solutions, has facilitated allocation of organs to geographically distant transplant centers [44].

Marginal donors—elderly patients, patients with a history of hypertension, poisoning victims, patients with significant complications of brain death (e.g., hypotension, oliguria or anuria, disseminated intravascular coagulation)—are now used not only for recovery of the kidney or pancreas, but also increasingly for vital organs such as the heart and liver [45–48]. Procurement techniques also have been adapted to facilitate use of older donors with significant aortic atherosclerosis [49]. Organs with anatomical abnormalities (e.g., multiple renal arteries or ureters, horseshoe kidney, annular pancreas) also increasingly are being used [50,51]. Improvements in operative technique permit the en bloc transplantation of two kidneys from very young donors that would have been too small to be used separately in one recipient. To maximize the use of livers, adult donor livers can be split and the two size-reduced grafts transplanted into two recipients (e.g., a pediatric and an adult recipient) [52]. A similar principle has also been proposed for the pancreas and has been reported on at least one occasion [53].

The advent of single-lung transplants has made it possible to distribute the heart and lungs of one donor to three recipients. Formerly, transplanting a heart-lung bloc into one recipient was the treatment of choice for end-stage pulmonary disease. If the native heart of a heart-lung recipient is healthy, a "domino transplant" can be performed: the heart-lung recipient donates his or her heart to another patient in need of a heart transplant (31 such cases were reported 1988–1991) [31]. Finally, again in an attempt to optimize utilization of scarce donor resources, the reuse of a transplanted heart has been reported [54].

Unfortunately, these methods allow only for better utilization of organs from the existing donor pool. The cornerstone for an effective *increase* in the number of organ donors remains heightened public awareness and education to improve consent rates. Thus, if the organ shortage problem is to be improved in the near future, the steadily declining consent rates for organ donation must be reversed.

LIVING DONORS. The use of living donors, traditionally limited to kidney transplants, has been expanded to the pancreas, liver, and lung over the past decade [31,55,56]. Most living donors are related to the recipient—siblings, parents, adult children—although more distant relations also have been used. The use of living unrelated kidney donors, who are only emotionally related to the recipient (spouses, close friends), also has increased as a result of the organ shortage.

Compared to the total number of cadaver donor transplants, the proportion of living donor transplants for extrarenal organs is small (<1% for liver, pancreas, and lung). In spite of the overall shortage of kidneys, the increase in living donor transplants has paralleled the slight increase in cadaver donors, keeping the proportion nearly unchanged. Among the 10,108 kidney transplants in 1992 in the United States, 2410 (24%) living donors and 7698 (76%) kidneys from cadaver donors were used (see Table 197-1 and Fig. 197-1). Living donor transplants help alleviate the organ shortage for certain organs (kidneys) and certain recipient subgroups (living related pediatric liver transplant recipients). Overall, however, no significant increases in living donation can be expected.

NON–HEART-BEATING CADAVER DONORS. The use of non–heart-beating cadaver donors has recently been the focus of public discussion. These patients have been declared dead by cardiopulmonary, rather than by the classic brain death, criteria [57]. Certain other countries have experience with the use of non–vital organs from non–heart-beating cadaver donors, but not the United States. One OPO in this country has now preliminarily implemented the use of this donor source, causing considerable debate. Critical care physicians will likely be confronted in the future with the issues surrounding this novel donor source, which potentially could lead to a very significant expansion of the donor pool. Due to practical concerns regarding the cessation of oxygen supply to vital organs after cardiopulmonary death, two main categories of donors are under consideration: (1) non–heart-beating cadaver donors after uncontrolled death (e.g., trauma, sudden cardiovascular event) and (2) non–heart-beating cadaver donors whose time and place of death are controlled.

In the first category, femoral arterial perfusion cannulas must

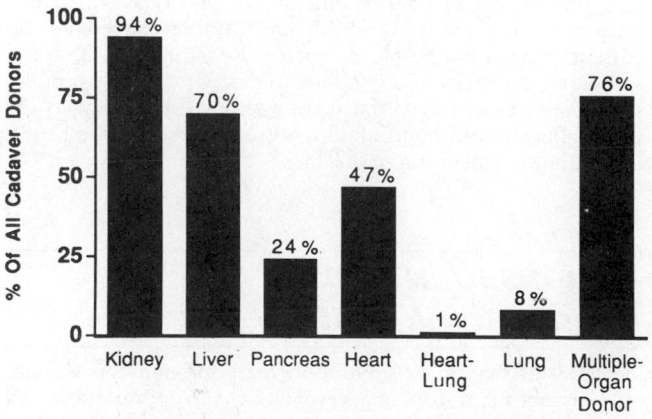

Fig. 197-2. Organ recovery rates from 4532 cadaver donors (100%) in the United States (1991) by organ type (reference 31).

be inserted and advanced into the abdominal aorta immediately after death has been pronounced. The kidneys are flushed and preserved (until surgical removal) by infusion of cold preservation solution through the femoral catheter and by additional topical cooling through percutaneously inserted intraperitoneal cannulas. Family consent for donation has to be obtained immediately after perfusion begins.

In the second category, patients with end-stage chronic cardiorespiratory or degenerative diseases (e.g., amyotrophic lateral sclerosis, multiple sclerosis) may decide, after thorough discussion, to forgo any further life-sustaining treatment (e.g., mechanical ventilation) and to donate their organs. Similarly, families of unconscious patients with severe, irreversible terminal brain injuries who do not fulfill the formal criteria of brain death might decide to forgo any further life-sustaining treatment and to donate the organs. In either scenario, the patient would be brought to the operating room. Life-supporting treatment would be discontinued and organ procurement initiated as soon as death has been pronounced. In this controlled situation, vital and ischemia-sensitive organs such as heart and liver can also be procured.

Ethical problems related to the first category center on when to stop the resuscitation effort, how to avoid hastening death, and whether it is ethical to perform a procedure that presumes consent before actually obtaining it from the family. Issues surrounding the second category include establishing a definition of death after discontinuing life support, the possibility of the patient at least temporarily surviving the withdrawal of support systems, and the conflict between providing optimal care for the patient and promoting suitable organ procurement and maintaining donor organ viability [58]. These concerns must be contrasted with the right of self-determination and the final wishes of a competent patient or family. Extensive debate by the medical community and the general public is crucial to resolving these complex moral and ethical issues [57]. Without such thorough consideration, the brain-dead organ donor concept and donor retrieval system currently in place might be harmed or discredited.

OTHER HUMAN DONOR ORGAN SOURCES. Certain countries use organs from executed prisoners. Use of this group would contribute only very small numbers of donors in the United States and this concept has been rejected by the transplant community here [59]. Likewise, the use of anencephalic babies for solid organ transplantation would not significantly alleviate the organ shortage, because only a few babies fulfill all brain death criteria. Proposals to use organs from executed prisoners or anencephalic babies would engender a very passionate, emotional debate that could have a negative impact on public opinion and thereby decrease the overall organ availability [59,60]. These options are therefore not being actively explored.

XENOTRANSPLANTATION. Xenotransplantation of organs from animals into humans offers a potentially unlimited supply of donors. Several attempts have received significant public attention [61], but numerous problems remain before this procedure will become a clinical routine. Immunologic concerns include hyperacute rejection (mediated by circulating, preformed natural antibodies), which occurs in vascularized solid organ transplantation between virtually all discordant species. Also, the biocompatibility of protein synthesized by an animal liver and the human organism is not fully established, and infectious diseases could be transmitted using nonhuman primates as donors. Genetic engineering of animals before their use as donors to overcome the immunologic barriers is an area

of intensive investigation. Significant experimental progress in this area is to be expected; a breakthrough could fundamentally change the field of organ transplantation. Needless to say, ethical concerns regarding the use of animal organs for transplantation have been raised [62].

PRESUMED CONSENT LAWS. Presumed consent laws have been implemented in many areas of the world, most notably in several countries in Europe. These laws permit organ procurement unless the potential donor has objected explicitly. A permanently and easily accessible registry of objectors is a prerequisite for such a system. Emphasis is placed on an individual's decision while family input is limited. In the United States, presumed consent legislation does not have broad support, and it is uncertain whether the public could be sufficiently informed and able to reach a consensus on this issue. Presumed consent would not alleviate the problem of insufficient donor identification and recognition [63], and no mechanism currently exists to record the decision of individuals who do not wish to participate in such a system.

Almost assuredly the only way to increase donor organ availability in the near future is to increase awareness and insight of the public into the above mentioned issues. Both the public and the medical community need to become more knowledgeable regarding the concepts of brain death and organ donation to enhance patient access to transplantation therapy.

Regulation and Organization of Organ Retrieval and Allocation

In the early 1980s the introduction of new immunosuppressive agents engendered a rise in organ transplant activity. Tissue matching (e.g., living related donor–recipient combinations) became less important at many centers, and the use of brain-dead cadaver donors increased (Fig. 197-1). In the wake of these developments, consolidation and national regulation of the organ sharing and allocation organizations, which had previously functioned mainly at a local and regional level, became necessary.

In the United States, the National Organ Transplant Act of 1984 called for a national system to ensure equitable access to transplant therapy for all patients, a major component of which was fair organ allocation. The federal government commissioned a task force on organ transplantation to define such an allocation system. This task force, whose members were appointed by the U.S. Department of Health and Human Services, resolved that human organs are a "national resource to be used for public good" and recommended the creation of a National Organ Procurement and Transplantation Network (OPTN). In 1986, the U.S. Department of Health and Human Services awarded the OPTN contract to the United Network for Organ Sharing (UNOS). Pursuant to the contract, UNOS was asked to design a network to achieve balance in the goals of equity in organ access and distribution and in optimal medical outcome [64]. In 1986, the Omnibus Budget Reconciliation Act mandated that only hospital members of the OPTN could perform Medicare- and Medicaid-reimbursed transplant procedures. In 1988, the Organ Transplant Amendments reaffirmed the federal interest in equitable organ allocation by locating authority in UNOS as opposed to local transplant organizations.

The national OPTN is operated by the nonprofit UNOS and is accountable to the U.S. Department of Health and Human Services. All patients on waiting lists of a transplant program are registered with UNOS, which maintains a centralized computer system linking all OPOs and transplant centers. The United States has been divided into eleven regions for organ procurement, allocation, and sharing purposes (Fig. 197-3). Organs are registered, shared, and allocated through the central UNOS computer, which generates a list of recipients for each available organ. Patients awaiting cadaveric transplantation are ranked according to UNOS policies, based on medical and scientific criteria such as tissue type, blood type, length of time waiting on the list, age (pediatric versus adult), level of presensitization (percent panel reactivate antibody), and medical status. National sharing of genotypic and phenotypic 6-antigen (A, B, and DR HLA loci) matched kidneys is mandated. In all other cases, and for all other organs, allocation first takes place locally. If no suitable local recipients are available, organs are allocated regionally or nationally [64].

Legal Aspects of Organ Donation and Brain Death

UNIFORM ANATOMICAL GIFT ACT. The Uniform Anatomical Gift Act, adopted in 1968 and in force throughout the United States, allows any adult individual (over age 18) to donate all or part of the body for transplantation, research, or education. Explicit consent, which may be revoked anytime, is required. The act also permits legal next of kin to give consent for donation [65]. Donor cards or driver's licenses, on which individuals indicate their consent to postmortem organ donation, are promoted by many states but serve ultimately as a tool to heighten public awareness [66]. Most hospitals continue to require consent from the next of kin. Therefore, educational efforts must urge potential donors to make their wishes known to their next of kin.

UNIFORM DETERMINATION OF DEATH ACT. Over the past two decades, brain death has legally become equated with death in most developed countries. Brain death means that all brain and brain stem function has irreversibly ceased, while circulatory and ventilatory functions are maintained temporarily. The recognition of brain death became possible only after substantial advances in intensive care medicine (e.g., cardiovascular support, prolonged mechanical ventilation). The first classic description of brain death was published in 1959 in France and termed "coma dépassé" (beyond coma). An ad hoc commission of the Harvard Medical School defined brain death criteria in the United States in 1968 [67]. These criteria were judged by some as being too extensive and too exclusive. In 1981, the President's Commission for the Study of Ethical Problems in Medicine and Biomedical and Behavioral Research formulated the Uniform Determination of Death Act, which established a common ground for statutory and judicial law related to the diagnosis of brain death. The commission stated that "an individual who has sustained . . . irreversible cessation of all functions of the entire brain, including the brain stem, is dead," and left the criteria for diagnosis to be determined by "accepted medical standards."

Those standards were defined in a related report to the President's Commission on the diagnosis of death by 56 medical consultants in 1981. The guidelines in that report have now been accepted as the standard for determining brain death in the United States. They are as follows: "Cessation is recognized when: (1) all cerebral functions and (2) all brain stem functions are absent. The irreversibility is recognized when: (1) the cause of the coma is established and is sufficient to account for the

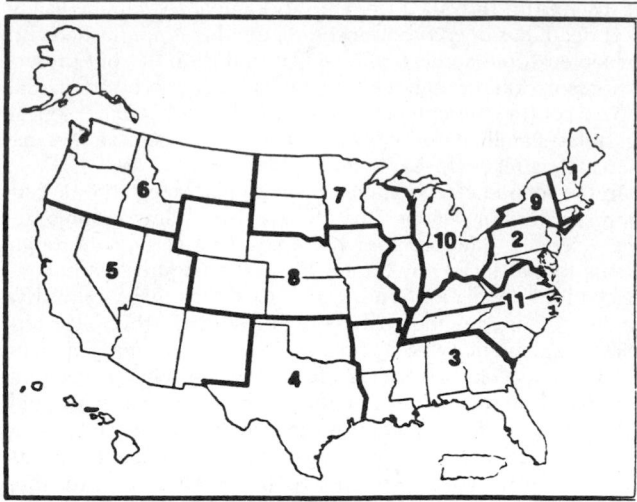

24 hour DONOR REFERRALS: 1-800-24SHARE

Fig. 197-3. United Network for Organ Sharing regions in the United States (24 hour access number: 1-800-24SHARE). The United States has been divided into eleven regions for organ procurement, allocation, and sharing purposes.

loss of brain functions, (2) the possibility of the recovery of any brain functions is excluded, and (3) the cessation of cerebral and brain stem function persists for an appropriate period of observation and/or trial of therapy" [68]. Unfortunately, substantial confusion regarding this well-founded and accepted medicolegal concept of the equivalence of brain death and death of a human being persists among physicians, other health care professionals, and the general public [17,37]. Specifically, in the field of transplantation it should be unequivocally clear to the potential donor's family and anyone involved in the patient's care that the time of death is the time at which the diagnosis of brain death is established and not the time of cardiac arrest during the organ retrieval. Providing education targeted individually at these groups and society at large is of paramount importance to reverse the decline in consent rates.

CLINICAL DIAGNOSIS OF BRAIN DEATH. The clinical diagnosis of brain death rests on three criteria: (1) irreversibility of the neurologic insult, (2) absence of clinical evidence of cerebral function, and, most important, (3) absence of clinical evidence of brain stem function (Table 197-4) [68]. Irreversibility is established if structural disease (e.g., trauma, intracranial hemorrhage) or an irreversible metabolic cause is known to have occurred. Hypothermia, medication side effects, drug overdose, or intoxication need to be ruled out when testing for brain death. Plasma concentrations of sedative or analgesic drugs sometimes correlate poorly with cerebral effects. Residual effects of those drugs can therefore be excluded only by passage of time, if any doubts exist. The observation period (the waiting time between two sequential brain-death examinations) should be at least 6 hours for structural causes and preferably 12 to 24 hours for metabolic causes, drug overdose, or intoxication. Even with potentially reversible metabolic alterations (e.g., hepatic or uremic encephalopathy), recovery has not been described after duration of the brain-death state for more

Table 197-4. Brain Death Criteria and Clinical Diagnoses of Brain Death

1. Irreversible, well-defined etiology of unconsciousness
   a. Structural disease or metabolic cause
   b. Exclusion of hypothermia, hypotension, and drug or substance intoxication
   c. Sufficient observation period (at least 6 hours) between two brain-death examinations
2. No clinical evidence of cerebral function
   a. No spontaneous movement, eye opening, or movement or response after auditory, verbal, or visual commands
   b. No movement elicited by painful simuli to the face and trunk (e.g., sternal rub, pinching of a nipple or finger nail bed), other than spinal cord reflex movements
3. No clinical evidence of brain stem function
   a. *No pupillary reflex:* pupils are fixed and mid position; no change of pupil size in either eye after shining a strong light source in each eye sequentially in a dark room
   b. *No corneal reflex:* no eyelid movements after touching the cornea (not the conjunctiva) with a sterile cotton swab or tissue
   c. *No gag reflex:* no retching or movement of the uvula after touching the back of the pharynx with a tongue depressor or after moving the endotracheal tube
   d. *No cough reflex:* no coughing with deep tracheal irrigation and suctioning
   e. *No oculocephalic reflex (doll's eyes reflex):* no eye movement in response to brisk turning of the head from side to side with the head of the supine patient elevated 30 degrees
   f. *No oculovestibular reflex (caloric reflex):* no eye movements within 3 minutes after removing earwax and irrigating each tympanic membrane (if intact) sequentially with 50 ml of ice water for 30–45 seconds, while the head of the supine patient is elevated 30 degrees
   g. *No integrated motor response to pain:* no localizing or withdrawal response, no extensor or flexor posturing
   h. *No respiratory efforts on apnea testing [PaCO$_2$ >60 mm Hg]:* the patient is oxygenated with an FiO$_2$ of 100% for 10–15 minutes, preferably with an arterial line in place for rapid blood gas measurements, while adjusting ventilatory rate and volume such that the PaCO$_2$ reaches ~40–45 mm Hg. After a baseline arterial blood gas is obtained, and the patient is disconnected from the ventilator, O$_2$ at 6–8 L/min is delivered through a T-piece connected to the endotracheal tube or a cannula advanced 20–30 cm into the endotracheal tube. Continuous pulse oximetry is used for early detection of desaturation, which does not usually occur when using this protocol. In most cases, a PaCO$_2$ >60 mm Hg is achieved within 3–5 minutes after withdrawal of ventilatory support; at this point the patient should be reconnected to the ventilator (or earlier, should hemodynamic instability, desaturation, or spontaneous breathing movements occur). Obtaining an arterial blood gas sample immediately before reinstitution of mechanical ventilation to confirm the PaCO$_2$ rise to >60 mm Hg is recommended but is not mandatory. If there is no evidence of spontaneous respirations before reinstitution of mechanical ventilation in the presence of a PaCO$_2$ of >60 mm Hg, the criteria for a positive apnea test are met.
4. Other points
   a. Spinal reflexes, such as deep tendon reflexes and triple flexion responses, may be preserved and do not exclude the diagnosis of brain death
   b. Shivering, goose bumps, arm movements, reaching of the hands toward the neck, forced exhalation, and thoracic respiratorylike movements are possible after brain death and are likely release phenomena of the spinal cord including the upper cervical cord. All these findings are compatible with the diagnosis of brain death.
   c. Confirmatory tests should be used in cases if the observation period needs to be shortened (e.g., unstable donors) in equivocal situations or if one of the potential pitfalls (see Table 197-5) cannot be ruled out (demonstration of absence of intracranial circulation by angiographic contrast or radioisotopic flow studies or electrocerebral silence documented by an electroencephalogram).

than 12 hours. Clinical testing of cerebral and brain stem function is detailed in Table 197-4 [69,70]. Note that brain-death criteria are more stringent for very young pediatric patients, particularly so for newborns, in whom criteria for brain death also include demonstration of the absence of blood flow on cerebral flow studies.

After brain death, the pupils become fixed in mid position because both sympathetic and parasympathetic input are lost. Decerebrate (abnormal extension) and decorticate (abnormal flexion) responses to painful stimuli imply the presence of some brain stem function and are incompatible with the diagnosis of brain death. In contrast, spinal-cord–mediated tendon reflexes and other spinal-cord–generated movements (which can occur during apnea testing) are compatible with the presence of brain death [71]. The occurrence of these reflex movements can be quite distressing if observed by the next of kin, and it is therefore not advisable that they be present during the apnea test.

Very rarely, ascending acute reversible inflammatory polyneuropathy (Guillain-Barré syndrome) can simulate brain death and inhibit all motor functions, including pupillary reactions and brain stem reflexes. The typical clinical history, coupled with evidence of progressive weakness, yields the correct diagnosis and precludes a diagnosis of brain death being established.

The American Academy of Neurology has stated that special confirmatory tests are not necessary to diagnose brain death in the vast majority of cases. Only in equivocal or questionable circumstances do tests demonstrating absence of intracranial blood flow or the presence of an isoelectric electroencephalogram need to be performed. The most sensitive and specific test for assessing intracranial blood flow is four-vessel cerebral arteriography. All other adjunctive tests are less sensitive (e.g., digital subtraction angiography, transcranial Doppler ultrasonography), are less specific (e.g., brain stem acoustic evoked potentials), measure only hemispheric flow (e.g., radioisotope angiography), or are indirect (e.g., computed tomography, echoencephalography). If either hemispheric neuronal function (electroencephalogram) or hemispheric flow is assessed, reliable clinical testing of the brain stem must be performed to confirm the diagnosis.

Four-vessel cerebral arteriography is indicated in all conditions that can temporarily cause an isoelectric electroencephalogram (e.g., extreme intoxication). If the indication for cerebral arteriography is unclear, the benefits must be weighed against the risks of transporting an unstable patient, of hypotension after contrast injection, and of the nephrotoxic effects of injection of contrast media that potentially may affect early renal allograft function [69,70]. Confirmatory tests may serve to shorten the waiting period between the two brain-death examinations, should donor hemodynamic instability occur. Certain potential pitfalls exist in clinical brain-death testing, and the diagnosis should not be considered to have been estab-

Table 197-5. Pitfalls in Clinical Brain Death Testing and Potential Remedial Measures*

Pitfalls	Remedial Measure
1. Hypotension, shock	Fluid resuscitation, use of pressor agents
2. Hypothermia	Use warmed fluids, ventilatory warmer
3. Intoxication or drug overdose	If measurable, check drug levels and toxicology screens or increase waiting time between brain-death examinations
4. Neuromuscular and sedative drugs, which can interfere with elicitation of motor responses	Discontinue muscle relaxants and mood- or consciousness-altering medications, increase waiting time between brain-death examinations
5. Pupillary fixation, which may be caused by anticholinergic drugs (e.g., atropine given during a cardiac arrest), neuromuscular blocking agents, or preexisting disease	Discontinue anticholinergic medications and muscle relaxants, increase waiting time between brain-death examinations, obtain careful patient history
6. Corneal reflexes absent due to overlooked contact lenses	Remove contact lenses before brain-death examination
7. Oculovestibular reflexes diminished or abolished after prior use of toxic drugs (e.g., aminoglycosides, loop diuretics, vancomycin), or agents with suppressive side effects on the vestibular system (e.g., tricyclic antidepressants, anticonvulsants, barbiturates), or due to preexisting disease	Obtain careful medication history and patient history

* If one of the listed conditions cannot be ruled out, confirmatory testing (cerebral flow studies or electroencephalography) is necessary before declaring brain death.

Table 197-6. Organ Donation Algorithm*

1. Early identification of the potential donor by the critical care physician or health care professional (see Table 197-3).
2. Early contact with the local or regional organ procurement organization (OPO) for medical, legal, and logistic assistance. If the OPO address or phone number is unknown, a 24-hour access number to the United Network for Organ Sharing (UNOS) is available: 1-800-24SHARE.
3. Completion of the preliminary screening by the OPO by obtaining all remaining laboratory and serologic studies, in consultation with the transplant surgeon for decisions regarding marginal donors.
4. Brain death diagnosis and confirmation (see Table 197-4).
5. Family notification and explanation of death and brain death with its legal and medical implications. Sufficient time for acceptance must be allowed.
6. Request for organ donation. Needs to be made in clear temporal separation from step 5, if possible.
7. After consent for organ donation is obtained, the focus switches from treatment of elevated intracranial pressure and brain protection to preservation of organ function and optimization of peripheral oxygen delivery (see Table 197-7).
8. Any further studies and tests required in equivocal situations should be performed at this point (e.g., coronary angiography for older or marginal heart donors).
9. Final organ allocation by the OPO and the United Network for Organ Sharing (UNOS), coordination of the organ recovery operation, and notification of the abdominal and thoracic surgical teams. Modification may become necessary under special circumstances, for example, in hemodynamically unstable donors.
10. Certification of death.
11. Multiple-organ procurement operation.

* Steps 4, 5, and 6 should not involve physicians who are part of the transplant team.

lished until these all have been excluded (Table 197-5). If these cannot be excluded, confirmatory testing is mandatory.

In summary, the diagnosis of brain death can be established by performance of routine neurologic examinations including cold caloric and apnea testing on two separate occasions, coupled with prior establishment of the underlying diagnosis and prognosis in most cases. More sophisticated tests are required in cases in which the diagnosis cannot be unequivocally established. However, brain death must be diagnosed in accordance with state laws. Details on the locally prevailing regulations are available through the state medical board or the local OPO.

The Organ Donation Process

The three key elements leading to successful organ donation are: (1) early donor recognition, (2) a well-coordinated approach in dealing with the donor family to request and obtain consent, and (3) appropriate critical care therapy of the brain-dead donor. The optimal course of events is summarized in Table 197-6.

EARLY DONOR RECOGNITION. The evidence is substantial that brain death eventually leads to cardiac arrest, even when cardiorespiratory support is maintained [72]. Cardiac arrest occurs in 4 to 28 percent of potential donors in the maintenance phase. While approximately 50 percent of all potential donors die within 24 hours without appropriate support, as many as 25 percent are not recognized for 48 hours or longer, identification occurring only at the time of cardiovascular death. Early recognition of the potential donor minimizes the loss of transplantable organs due to unexpected cardiac arrest and death, hemodynamic instability, serious nosocomial infection, or complications related to intensive care. For example, an inverse correlation exists between the duration of mechanical ventilation and the suitability of the donor for lung donation. The previously outlined screening criteria should be used to assess any potential donor after admission to the hospital or intensive care unit (see Table 197-3). Early contact with OPOs is essential, because they provide assistance with the evaluation of any patient who is currently or is anticipated to become brain dead [73].

DONOR EVALUATION

General Guidelines. During the initial contact with the OPO, the physician should provide the potential donor's name, age, sex, height, weight, and blood type. Also needed are the date of admission and diagnosis, the nature and extent of any trauma, a concise medical and social history, and the time of brain death (if applicable). Whether local investigative agencies (e.g., medical examiner, coroner) need to be notified also should be specified. The current medical status including vital signs, urine output, cardiorespiratory status, medications, and culture results must be communicated. If possible, basic laboratory parameters (i.e., arterial blood gases, BUN, creatinine, electrolytes, hemoglobin, hematocrit, white blood cell count, platelet count, serum amylase, total bilirubin, alkaline phosphates, alanine aminotransferase [ALT, SGPT], aspartate aminotransferase [AST, SGOT], coagulation profile [prothrombin time (PT), partial thromboplastin time (PTT), thrombin time (TT)], and urinalysis and urine culture) should be available, along with electrocardiogram and chest radiograph results. In the case of potential lung donors, chest circumference and radiographic thoracic measurements, as well as the results of an oxygenation challenge (PaO$_2$ measurement after ventilation for 10 minutes with an FiO$_2$ of 1.0), will be needed. The OPO will provide further procedural, administrative, legal, and logistic help and begin the organ allocation process immediately after brain death has been declared and consent has been obtained. All further testing (human leukocyte antigen [HLA]-tissue typing; serologic screening for cytomegalovirus [CMV]; hepatitis A, B, and C viruses; human immunodeficiency virus [HIV]; human T-cell lymphotropic virus type I [HTLV-1] and syphilis; blood, sputum, and urine cultures) will then be coordinated through the OPO if the donor passes the preliminary screening tests. If prospective tissue typing is to be done, performing a surgical inguinal lymph node biopsy at the donor hospital may be necessary after brain death is declared but before proceeding with the actual organ recovery several hours later.

The medical status and the life expectancy of the potential recipient without the organ transplant are taken into account when the final decision about transplantation of a specific donor organ is made. The ultimate decision regarding the use of a donor is made by the transplant surgeon. At this point, the transplant center may need to obtain further tests to assess the functional status of one or more organ systems. For example, if the heart is to be retrieved, a cardiac echogram is usually obtained. In the case of donors who demonstrate some degree of cardiac disease, coronary angiography sometimes is performed. Pulmonary status can be further assessed by bronchoscopy after considering the results of the chest radiograph, oxygenation challenge, and sputum cultures.

If concern over the suitability of organs arises, then direct inspection by the transplant surgeon is necessary at the time of the organ procurement operation. In some cases, an open biopsy (e.g., for kidney or liver) and frozen section pathologic analysis will also help in the final decision making. Direct inspection also is important in organ donors declared brain dead after a blunt injury to the head and trunk (e.g., motor vehicle accident). Under these circumstances, intraabdominal organs have been used successfully, despite the presence of small parenchymal tears or subcapsular hematomas in either the liver or kidney.

In summary, each patient who is brain dead or anticipated to progress to brain death should be considered at least initially as a potential donor, regardless of cause of death, history, age, or medical condition [1,46,74]. With few exceptions (*vide infra*) organ donation should never be excluded *a priori* because of the clinical situation, the results of imaging studies, or the magnitude of an injury, without first having contacted an OPO (24-hour access number: 1-800-24SHARE).

Organ-Specific Considerations. The use of kidneys retrieved from older donors (>65 years), donors dying of cardiovascular disease, or donors requiring large doses of inotropic drugs for cardiovascular support entails a higher rate of delayed or diminished graft function and is associated with decreased graft survival [75,76]. Organs from these marginal donors are nevertheless routinely used, given the current prolonged periods of time (>2 years) that some recipients may wait for available organs during which time their medical condition may deteri-

orate. Many investigators believe that organ function is more important than donor biological age In equivocal cases (donors with elevated baseline serum creatinine levels or a history of hypertension) renal biopsies at the time of organ recovery may identify the presence of preexisting donor arteriosclerosis or glomerulosclerosis. If severe disease is present, most transplant surgeons believe that this type of organ should not be used.

Under certain circumstances, liver donors are used despite the presence of an abnormal liver enzyme or coagulation profile [77,78]. Elevated hepatic enzyme levels may reflect transient hepatic ischemia at the time of resuscitation. Abnormal clotting times may be due to disseminated intravascular coagulation (commonly a result of brain injury and not primary hepatic dysfunction). The trends observed in the results of serial laboratory tests may be more important than absolute values. Unfortunately, tests proposed for assessing the biochemical function of the liver (e.g., the formation kinetics of monoethylglycinexylidide [MEGX] after bolus lidocaine administration) have proven unreliable [79]. The decision to use a liver from a marginal donor has to be made on the basis of relatively crude information. Often, only direct inspection with or without a biopsy of the liver at the time of organ recovery provides a final answer and may be the only way to assess a donor with a history of significant ethanol intake. Fatty liver degeneration related to ethanolism is one of the most significant factors predictive of early posttransplant hepatic dysfunction or failure [80].

In general, donors over 55 years should probably not be considered for pancreatic donation. Donors with hyperglycemia or hyperamylasemia are not to be excluded *a priori* from pancreas donation, however, as these factors do not necessarily influence posttransplant outcome [81]. The only absolute contraindications to pancreas donation are a history of impaired glucose tolerance or insulin-dependent diabetes mellitus, direct blunt or penetrating trauma to the pancreas, or the finding of acute or chronic pancreatitis at the time of the donor operation.

Regarding heart donation, the most important criterion appears to be good donor heart ventricular function immediately before retrieval as judged by the cardiac surgeon [74]. No potential heart donor should be excluded solely on the basis of wall motion abnormalities, a borderline or abnormal ejection fraction, inotropic medication requirements or heart murmurs, arrhythmias, or other ECG changes (which often occur in brain-dead individuals in whom no cardiac disease is present).

Risk factors associated with poor outcome after lung transplantation include a history of aspiration, purulent secretions observed during bronchoscopy, an abnormal chest radiograph, or an unsatisfactory oxygenation challenge (PaO$_2$ < 400 mm Hg after 10 minutes of ventilation with FiO$_2$ = 1.0) alone or in combination in lung donors. Lungs obtained from such marginal donors have been successfully transplanted, however, [1]. Bronchoscopy is often performed as a final confirmatory test in the operating room by the transplant surgeon immediately before retrieval. Direct intraoperative inspection of the lungs determines whether significant contusions are present, which would preclude use of the organs.

In conclusion, the traditional donor criteria have been considerably expanded over recent years, for both thoracic and abdominal organs, due to the ongoing, severe donor shortage.

Transmission of Infectious Diseases. Transmission of bacterial or fungal infection through organ transplantation generally is due to contamination of the organ itself during organ procurement or storage [82]. Transmission of these types of pathogens is rare and usually caused by virulent organisms such as *Pseudomonas aeruginosa* [83]. Potential donors who exhibit or develop active bacterial or fungal infection that is unresponsive to adequate source control and antibiotic therapy or evidence of severe systemic sepsis with positive blood cultures (even without a primary source) should be rejected. Similarly, active tuberculosis is a contraindication to organ donation. Positive urine cultures do not preclude renal donation [84]. Donors with serologic evidence of syphilis and no known risk factors for acquiring this disease have been successfully used [85], although this remains controversial.

Absolute contraindications to donation include evidence of significant acute viral infections (e.g., viral encephalitis; systemic herpes simplex virus infections; Guillain-Barré syndrome; acute viral hepatitis A, B, or C; seropositivity for HIV or HTLV-I, or the acquired immunodeficiency syndrome (AIDS). Individuals known to be at high risk for acquiring such diseases (e.g., intravenous drug addicts, prostitutes, homosexuals) are often excluded as well.

The identification of disease due to hepatitis B virus (HBV) precludes organ donation. This includes the presence of serologic evidence of HBV surface antigen (HBsAg); acute active, chronic active, or chronic persistent hepatitis due to HBV; or a history of jaundice with evidence of IgM antibody directed against HBsAg (anti-HBs) or the HBV core particle (anti-HBc). The presence of such positive HBV serologies precludes donation, with two exceptions: (1) donors in whom anti-HBs is the result of previous hepatitis B vaccination or (2) only IgG and not IgM antibodies directed against either HBsAg, HBc, or both are present without evidence of HBsAg or liver enzyme abnormalities. Recipients who receive an organ from a donor with any type of serologic evidence of HBV should undergo HBV vaccination and should receive HBV immunoglobulin (HBIg) at the time of transplant. Ideally, however, all potential organ transplant recipients should receive HBV immunization with the recombinant vaccine during the pretransplant evaluation.

Recently, the use of hepatitis C (HCV)-seropositive donors in certain situations has been advocated and implemented by certain transplant centers [86]. In the absence of a test to detect active hepatitis C viremia and disease coupled with the substantial false positive rate (~6–18%), this issue is very controversial. In essence, exclusion of all HCV-positive donors increases the organ shortage while preventing what would appear to be relatively limited disease transmission. Routine screening ELISA-type tests remain less specific than recombinant immunoblot assay (RIBA)-based tests, but the latter require too long to perform to make them useful in the screening of the brain-dead donor. The final decision must be made on an individual basis by each transplant surgeon [87]. The decision to accept donors from subgroups of individuals at high risk for acquiring either HBV or HCV (IV drug abusers, prostitutes, homosexuals, residents of sub-Saharan Africa) in the absence of any positive viral serologic studies must be individualized [88], and many centers do not retrieve organs from donors with positive HBV and HCV serologies if such a history is obtained.

CMV also may be transmitted by donor tissue, particularly to CMV seronegative patients. Effective prophylaxis and treatment of CMV disease have become a reality with the advent of effective antiviral agents such as ganciclovir [19]. Positive CMV serologies do not preclude organ donation but have been used to identify high-risk donor-recipient combinations (CMV seropositive donor–CMV seronegative recipient) where prophylaxis should be used and careful surveillance for CMV disease is important. Some transplant centers in Canada refrain from transplanting CMV seropositive organs into CMV seronegative recipients. This policy has not been adopted by most transplant centers in the United States for two reasons: (1) this might further constrain access to organs and (2) CMV disease can be effectively treated, with fatality being rare.

Transmission of Malignancy. Transmission of malignancy through donor organs is very rare (<100 cases in over 150,000 transplants) [89]. Donor selection is particularly important in this regard, such that donors with most types of cancer should not be used. The exceptions are those with low-grade skin malignancies, such as basal cell carcinoma and most squamous cell carcinomas; carcinoma *in situ* of the uterine cervix; or primary brain tumors, which rarely spread outside the central nervous system (CNS) (e.g., astrocytomas, meningiomas, and hemangioblastomas but not high-grade glioblastomas). It is important to ensure that a CNS tumor does not represent a focus of metastatic disease from the primary site. Metastases from choriocarcinomas, bronchial or renal malignancies, and malignant melanomas may present as what appears to be a primary brain tumor or may bleed and be mistaken for an intracranial hemorrhage due to an arteriovenous malformation or a ruptured aneurysm. Previous treatment of a neoplasm, menstrual irregularities after a pregnancy or a spontaneous abortion in women of childbearing age (indicative of a choriocarcinoma), or evidence of lesions at other sites in the patient with a purported primary CNS malignancy should preclude organ donation. Donors with primary brain tumors should not be used if they have undergone radiotherapy, chemotherapy, ventriculoperitoneal or ventriculoatrial shunting, or craniotomies, because these treatments either are associated with high-grade malignancies or create potential pathways for the systemic dissemination of tumor cells [89].

If a potential donor has had successful cancer treatment in the past, the transplant surgeon needs to weigh the small potential risk of transmitting micrometastases against discarding a potentially lifesaving organ. In general, patients with a history of malignancy with little propensity to recur after therapy (e.g., small noninvasive lesions treated by complete surgical excision) should be considered as organ donors, particularly if they have remained without evidence of recurrence for over 5 years. Patients who have experienced invasive cancer in which a substantial risk of recurrence exists (e.g., breast cancer, malignant melanoma), particularly if a large lesion was initially present and chemotherapy or radiation therapy was employed, should not be considered for donation.

BRAIN DEATH EXAMINATION AND REQUIRED REQUEST FOR ORGAN DONATION. After the suitability of a potential donor is determined, the next important steps are the brain-death examination and the legally required request for organ donation (see Tables 197-4, 197-5, and 197-6). Those steps should not involve any of the physicians associated with the transplant team, as this would represent a potential conflict of interest. In 1987, federal required request legislation became effective and has since been adopted by every state in the United States. Required request laws mandate that the family of a brain-dead potential organ donor be offered the option of organ donation. The hospital must notify the respective OPO of the presence of a potential organ donor.

It is of utmost importance to ensure that: (1) the family understands and accepts the concept of brain death, including its legal and medical equivalence with death, and (2) the request for organ donation is not made at the same time that brain death is explained (unless the family voiced the wish to consider donation earlier during the hospitalization). Sufficient time must be given to next of kin to begin coping with this information and to accept the loss of the family member. Only then, in clear temporal separation from the explanation of death, should the subject of organ donation be broached and an appropriate request be made. As a case in point, within one region of the United States, consent rates were 18 percent when the discussion of death and the request for donation were combined but rose to 65 percent when these issues were discussed separately [90].

Although driver's license and signed donor cards are considered valid legal documents, the family's wishes are virtually always honored. The Uniform Anatomical Gift Act of 1968 specifies the legal next of kin priority for donors over age 18 in the following order: (1) spouse, (2) adult son or daughter, (3) either parent, (4) adult brother or sister, and (5) legal guardian [65]. Similarly, the order of priority for donors under age 18 is: (1) both parents, (2) one parent (if both parents are not available and no wishes to the contrary of the absent parent are known), (3) the custodial parent (if the parents are divorced or legally separated), and (4) the legal guardian (if there are no parents). Finally, the family must be informed that after declaration of brain death all hospital costs relating to donation will be paid by the OPO.

Critical Care Management of the Brain-Dead Organ Donor

PATHOPHYSIOLOGY OF BRAIN DEATH. The majority of our knowledge of the pathophysiologic changes during and after brain death has been derived from experiments performed using animal models. Hemodynamic instability during the phase of impending brain herniation is the result of autonomic dysregulation secondary to the progressive loss of central neurohumoral regulatory control of vital functions. The continuous increase in intracranial pressure with worsening brain ischemia leads to severe systemic hypertension (Cushing response) and frequently is associated with tachyarrhythmias. This process is mediated by an increase in sympathetic activity and an excess of circulating catecholamines ("autonomic storm") [91]. A brief period of transient bradycardia associated with the hypertensive response can be seen in the early phase of brain herniation (Cushing reflex).

During the phase of increased sympathetic activity, there is evidence that coronary blood flow is significantly impaired, resulting in cardiac microinfarcts. Furthermore, decreased hepatic perfusion due to increased intrahepatic shunting has been demonstrated as a result of the excessive sympathetic activity. Neurogenic pulmonary edema is thought to develop during the autonomic storm phase secondary to the temporary elevation of left atrial pressures over the level of pulmonary arterial and alveolar capillary pressures. This causes massive transudation of fluid from the microvasculature into the alveoli and interstitial hemorrhage [91,92]. Within about 15 minutes after brain herniation and brain death, catecholamines decrease to below baseline values.

The resting vagal tone is abolished because of destruction of the nucleus ambiguus, eliminating all chronotropic effects of atropine administered after brain death. The total CO_2 production after brain death is low, due to the absence of cerebral metabolism and the presence of hypothermia and decreased muscle tone. The subsequent chronic maintenance phase of brain-dead donors is frequently characterized by hypotension, resulting mainly from a complete arterial and venous vasomotor collapse with significant peripheral venous pooling.

ROUTINE CARE AND MONITORING. Regular nursing care must be continued after brain death. Frequent turning for decubitus ulcer prophylaxis, skin care, dressing changes, urinary and intravascular catheter care, and catheter site care must be meticulous to minimize the risk of infection. Other indwelling devices should be removed, if possible (e.g., ventriculostomies and ventriculoatrial or ventriculoperitoneal shunts, which may have been inserted in certain patients for monitoring or treatment of elevated intracranial pressure). Any urinary and intravascular catheters that may have been inserted under suboptimal, emergent conditions without appropriate aseptic technique at the time of original injury should be replaced. A nasogastric tube should always be inserted for gastric decompression and prevention of aspiration.

Arterial lines should be inserted only into peripheral arteries of the upper extremities, because femoral arterial line readings can become inaccurate due to surgical manipulation of the abdominal aorta during organ procurement. Similarly, central venous catheters should not be inserted through the femoral vein as dissection and manipulation of the interior vena cava occurs during organ procurement. In addition, venous catheters inserted through the femoral vein can cause iliac vein thrombosis. This increases the risk of pulmonary embolization, particularly during surgical venous dissection. It can also render the iliac veins unsuitable for use in vascular reconstruction, which may be necessary in some types of abdominal or thoracic organ transplants.

The following parameters need to be determined routinely and frequently for all organ donors using various monitoring devices: core temperature (esophageal, rectal, or indwelling bladder catheter temperature probes), heart rate (continuous electrocardiographic monitoring), systemic blood pressure (arterial catheter), central venous blood pressure (subclavian or internal jugular central venous catheter), arterial oxygen saturation (pulse oximetry), and hourly urine output (Foley catheter). Use of a Swan-Ganz catheter for measurement of pulmonary arterial and left ventricular wedge pressure and central venous oximetry is only rarely necessary; its use should be reserved for unstable donors whose volume status is uncertain or who have persistent acidosis with evidence of tissue hypoperfusion.

Laboratory parameters also need to be checked regularly: arterial blood gases, serum electrolytes, BUN, creatinine, lactate, liver enzymes, total bilirubin, hemoglobin, hematocrit, platelet count, and coagulation tests. Testing is adapted to the individual clinical situation—frequent electrolyte determinations if diabetes insipidus has been diagnosed, lactate monitoring in acidotic donors, and repeated coagulation profiles in the presence of disseminated intravascular coagulation.

If infection is suspected, blood, urine, sputum, cerebrospinal fluid, and wound drainage cultures need to be obtained. Routine surveillance cultures (usually blood and urine cultures) may be required, depending on the protocol of the local OPO and the organ type. Blood cultures should be obtained using peripheral venipuncture, rather than arterial or central venous catheters, to avoid contamination. Prophylactic antibiotics only should be administered immediately prior to the retrieval procedure. Any source of infection should be identified, characterized from a microbiologic standpoint, and treated.

GENERAL MANAGEMENT GOALS. The most important overall goal in the management of brain-dead multiple-organ donors is to optimize organ perfusion and tissue oxygen delivery [93]. Organ viability and function after transplantation are closely correlated with adequacy of resuscitation and hemodynamic stability during the organ donor maintenance phase.

The events associated with the cause of brain death (e.g., hemorrhagic shock, cardiac arrest) can lead to significant physiologic abnormalities. Head injury preceding brain death is known to induce a hypermetabolic response, equivalent to that observed after a second- or third-degree burn involving approximately 40 percent of the total body surface area. Significant metabolic stress and impairment of organ perfusion occur during brain herniation, and both events are related to excessive catecholamine release. Any additional circulatory compromise in the time period afterward potentiates the deleterious consequences of these previous adverse events. Posttransplant organ function can be negatively affected by such episodes of cardiovascular dysregulation, particularly in such ischemia-sensitive organs as the heart and liver. For example, even with optimal heart donor management the recipient often needs inotropic support and may exhibit subendocardial myocyte necrosis on biopsy specimens obtained during the early posttransplant period [94]. Anticipating these changes associated with brain death and providing optimal management should they occur during the organ donor maintenance phase, as well as optimizing organ function, are of utmost importance.

Parameters associated with adequate tissue perfusion in stable donors in the absence of lactic acidosis are listed in Table 197-7. They include: systolic blood pressure 100 to 120 mm Hg, central venous pressure 8 to 10 mm Hg, oxygen saturation of the arterial blood $\geq$ 95 percent, core temperature $\geq$ 35°C, and hematocrit 30 to 35 percent [95], the latter balancing slightly decreased oxygen transport capacity of the red blood cell mass with the beneficial effects of low viscosity on blood flow. Maintaining adequate hemoglobin concentration is also essential in preparation for organ recovery, in which hemodynamic stability throughout the operation is crucial, especially if blood loss occurs.

The use of vasopressors should be minimized if at all possible because of their splanchnic vasoconstrictive effects. Efforts to elevate blood pressure beyond the normal range can adversely affect outcome and should be avoided: high doses of vasopressors can cause arrhythmias and increase myocardial oxygen consumption and pulmonary edema after excessive fluid administration can render lungs unsuitable for transplantation. After the lung, the pancreas is the organ most prone to tissue edema. Normal central venous pressure and low positive end-expiratory pressure (PEEP) help maintain an adequate perfusion gradient across the hepatic microcirculatory bed (i.e., that between the portal vein and hepatic artery on one side and the inferior vena cava and right atrium on the other) [96].

Use of pulmonary artery catheterization needs to be considered in donors who do not respond to routine management and continue to exhibit hypotension or persistent lactic acidosis after adequate volume loading, particularly in those in whom this occurs despite use of moderate doses of dopamine. Determining pulmonary artery and capillary wedge pressures, cardiac output and index, pulmonary and systemic vascular resistive indices, oxygen availability and consumption, and other parameters helps to differentiate the cause of instability. Appropriate therapy can then be administered (e.g., fluid balance correction or PEEP adjustments, additional inotropic support, preload or afterload reduction). Once the hemodynamic instability has resolved, pulmonary artery catheters should be removed promptly to eliminate the inherent risks of infection, induction of arrhythmias, and mechanical endomyocardial damage.

A potential management conflict exists when the lungs are to be procured in combination with other organs from the same donor. Maintaining a central venous pressure of 8 to 10 mm Hg usually represents an acceptable compromise between the need for sufficient hydration to maintain adequate perfusion and good diuresis versus provoking pulmonary edema in potential lung donors.

Overall, optimizing hemodynamic parameters is of paramount importance during the donor maintenance phase. Hypotension must be treated aggressively by proper fluid management, while minimizing the use of vasopressors. Hypertensive crises and tachyarrhythmic episodes require prompt intervention. Last, PEEP exceeding 5 cm H_2O should be used with caution as hypotension may ensue.

CARDIOVASCULAR SUPPORT. Hypotension is the most common hemodynamic abnormality seen in brain-dead organ donors. The usual cause is hypovolemia, due to a combination of vasomotor collapse after brain death and the effects of treatment protocols to decrease intracranial pressure, which require minimizing hydration and use of osmotic diuretics (see Tables 197-8 and 197-9). After brain death is declared, adequate volume resuscitation of the donor can require several liters of fluid. Until a euvolemic state is achieved, dopamine ($\leq$10 μg/kg/min) can be used temporarily; the dose should be titrated to maintain an adequate systolic blood pressure [95]. Dopamine infusions <3 μg/kg/min enhance renal perfusion. Infusion rates >10 μg/kg/min have been associated with increased rates of acute tubular necrosis and decreased renal allograft survival. High infusion rates also lead to decreased perfusion of other organs due to splanchnic vasoconstriction.

Dopamine is also the drug of choice if hemodynamic instability persists after fluid resuscitation and adequate volume loading. Use of isoproterenol and dobutamine should be avoided in this context because of their vasodilatory effects. Drugs with alpha-adrenergic agonist effects such as phenylephrine (IV infusion 0.15–0.75 μg/kg/min) or metaraminol (IV 0.5–7 μg/kg/min) should be added only if hypotension persists in the face of euvolemia and titration of the dopamine infusion up to 15 μg/kg/min. Alpha-adrenergic agonists can cause severe peripheral vasoconstriction and reduce renal and hepatic perfusion, and for this reason they must be used judiciously. Once these drugs are used, the need for their continued use must be frequently reassessed. In those rare cases in which the necessity for use of other inotropic agents in addition to dopamine is established, preference should be given to dobutamine over isoproterenol. Dobutamine increases myocardial oxygen consumption to a lesser extent than isoproterenol. Finally, epinephrine and norepinephrine should not be used because of their marked vasoconstrictive side effects.

Measurement of urine output alone as a means of assessing adequacy of fluid resuscitation is notoriously unreliable in brain-dead donors. The presence of a systolic blood pressure between 100 and 120 mm Hg, a central venous pressure between 8 and 10 mm Hg, and the absence of metabolic acidosis (with or without infusion of a small amount of dopamine) are usually better indirect indicators of donor stability and sufficient oxygen delivery to organs and tissues. It is important to remember, however, that the use of vasoconstrictor or inotropic agents does not serve to replace adequate fluid resuscitation. Thus, proper fluid management remains the cornerstone of successful donor management.

When attempting to determine the etiology of hypotension in an organ donor, underlying cardiac disease (e.g., coronary artery disease, valve defects) and factors related to the cause of brain death (e.g., myocardial infarction, cardiac tamponade, or myocardial contusion) must be included in the differential diagnosis. Electrolyte abnormalities such as hypophosphatemia, hypocalcemia, hypokalemia, and hypomagnesemia are common in brain-dead organ donors. The presence of these entities must also be considered when hemodynamic instability is encountered, and frequent testing and correction of these significant electrolyte imbalances are important. Hypophosphatemia and hypocalcemia can decrease myocardial contractility and

Table 197-7. Maintenance Therapy End Points in the Brain-Dead Organ Donor

Systolic blood pressure	100–120 mm Hg
Central venous pressure	8–10 mm Hg
Urine output	100–300 ml/hr
Core temperature	≥35°C
PaO_2	80–100 mm Hg
Systemic arterial oxygen saturation	95%
pH	7.37–7.45
Hgb	10–12 g/dl
Hematocrit	30–35%

Table 197-8. Differential Diagnosis of Hypotension in the Brain-Dead Organ Donor

Hypovolemia
Hypothermia
Cardiac dysfunction
   Arrhythmia (ischemia, catecholamines, hypokalemia,
      hypomagnesemia)
   Acidosis
   Hypooxygenation
   Excessive positive end-expiratory ventilatory pressure
   Congestive heart failure due to excessive fluid administration
   Hypophosphatemia
   Causes related to the injury leading to brain death (e.g., cardiac
      tamponade, myocardial contusion)
   Myocardial sequelae of autonomic storm
   Preexisting cardiac disease
Drug side effect or overdose (e.g., long-acting β-blocker, calcium
   channel antagonist, antihypertensive agent)
Hypocalcemia

Table 197-9. Differential Diagnosis of Hypovolemia in the Brain-Dead Organ Donor

Arterial and venous vasomotor collapse due to loss of central neuro-
   humoral control
Dehydration (fluid restriction to treat head injury)
Insufficient resuscitation after the injury leading to brain death (e.g.,
   ongoing hemorrhagic shock with coagulopathy after polytrauma)
Polyuria
   Osmotic diuresis (mannitol, hyperglycemia)
   Diabetes insipidus
   Hypothermia
   Administration of other diuretics
Massive third spacing in response to the original injury
Decreased intravascular oncotic pressure after excessive resuscitation
   with crystalloid fluids

provoke hypotension [97]; hypokalemia and hypomagnesemia can impair hemodynamics by causing dysrhythmias.

As a general rule, medications that possess rapid reversibility and a short half-life should be chosen to treat arrhythmias or hypertension. Hemodynamic instability can be pronounced after brain death, with wide swings between the extremes of hypotension and hypertension, rendering the brain-dead donor more susceptible to cardiovascular drug effects. Hypertension can be treated with short-acting vasodilatory agents (e.g., nitroprusside) or a rapidly reversible beta-adrenergic antagonist (e.g., esmolol hydrochloride) as hypertension usually is associated with increased circulating catecholamines. Other drugs, such as calcium channel blockers (e.g., verapamil, nifedipine) or longer-acting beta-blockers (e.g., labetatol, propanolol), should be avoided because of their negative inotropic effects and the inability to titrate them precisely. Bradyarrhythmias during the early phase of brain herniation are part of the Cushing reflex and do not usually require any treatment, unless associated with hypotension and asystole. Because of the lack of chronotropic effects by atropine after brain death, use of either isoproterenol or epinephrine is required to treat hemodynamically significant bradyarrhythmias.

Tachyarrhythmias are associated with the increased catecholamine release that occurs during and immediately after brain herniation. Administration of short-acting beta blockers (e.g., esmolol hydrochloride) serves not only to treat arrhythmias but also to mitigate hypertension during autonomic storm. Use of additional short-acting intravenous antiarrhythmics (e.g., lidocaine) may become necessary if tachyarrhythmias do not resolve after beta blocker therapy. Calcium channel blockers

(e.g., verapamil) must be avoided under these circumstances because of their negative inotropic effects. Cardiac glycosides (e.g., digoxin) also should not be used because they can induce and potentiate bradyarrhythmias and tachyarrhythmias, and they also have splanchnic vasoconstrictive side effects.

Cardiac arrest occurs in about 25 percent of all donors during the maintenance phase after brain death and should be treated by routine measures, with the exception that isoproterenol or epinephrine must be substituted for atropine. No intracardiac injections should be given during cardiopulmonary resuscitation because they can render the heart unsuitable for transplantation.

RESPIRATORY AND ACID–BASE MAINTENANCE. Use of endotracheal suctioning is usually minimized during the treatment of cerebral edema to avoid any unnecessary stimulation that would increase intracranial pressure. In contrast, after brain death is declared, vigorous tracheobronchial toilet is important with frequent suctioning using sterile precautions. Percussion and turning for postural drainage are instituted as well. The lungs must be expanded by manual inflation at regular intervals. Even if the lungs are unsuitable for donation, it is important to minimize the risk of atelectasis and infection. Preventing atelectasis facilitates oxygenation and may obviate the need for detrimental high levels of PEEP. Steroids administered to some patients as part of the treatment for increased intracranial pressure predispose to pulmonary infectious complications. The presence of pneumonia can preclude donation of the lungs as well as other organs, depending on its severity and association with systemic sepsis. Routine respiratory care of all donors also includes use of 5 cm H_2O of PEEP to increase alveolar recruitment and prevent microatelectasis [95].

In potential lung donors the endotracheal tube should not be advanced more than several centimeters into the trachea to prevent damage to areas that may become anastomotic lines. A sample of sputum should be obtained for Gram stain and cultures to exclude the presence of infection. The samples may be obtained using bronchoscopy, a procedure that is often routinely performed before lung donation. Peak airway pressures should be <30 cm H_2O using a tidal volume of 10 to 15 ml/kg. The lowest FIO_2 capable of maintaining a PaO_2 >100 mm Hg should be selected. If oxygenation is insufficient, PEEP should be increased, rather than increasing the FIO_2. High levels of PEEP negatively affect cardiac output, which should be carefully monitored in this setting. If hypotension occurs, PEEP should be reduced. Under these circumstances, use of pulmonary artery catheterization generally is necessary to balance PEEP requirements against those of organ perfusion. In contrast, in non–lung donors an increase in FiO$_2$ is preferred over high levels of PEEP to correct insufficient arterial oxygenation.

The etiology of pulmonary edema in organ donors can be cardiogenic, neurogenic, aspiration induced, or a result of trauma or fluid overload. Neurogenic pulmonary edema usually precludes lung or combined heart-lung donation, but not donation of other organs (e.g., heart, kidney, liver, pancreas). The treatment for pulmonary edema is supportive and should be directed at maintaining adequate arterial oxygenation without using high levels of PEEP. Fluids must be administered carefully to maintain organ perfusion while avoiding exacerbation of the edema. Excessive use of crystalloid fluids during the initial resuscitation after brain death is declared can render the lungs unsuitable for transplantation. If large amounts of fluid are required, colloids (e.g., albumin solutions) or blood transfusions (if the hemoglobin is <10 g/dl) should be considered in addition to the infusion of crystalloid solutions [95].

Brain-dead organ donors can develop respiratory alkalosis secondary to mechanical hyperventilation as part of the treatment protocol for elevated intracranial pressure. After brain death, the arterial pH should be adjusted to normal values, because alkalosis has many undesirable side effects, such as increased cardiac output, systemic vasoconstriction, bronchospasm, and a shift to the left of the oxyhemoglobin dissociation curve [95]. The latter decreases oxygen unloading in the tissues and impairs oxygen delivery.

Lactic metabolic acidosis is frequent in brain-dead donors. it should be treated by compensation with a slight respiratory alkalosis until the underlying abnormality has been corrected (e.g., dehydration, tissue ischemia). Administration of sodium bicarbonate should be contemplated only if the increased minute ventilation necessary to induce respiratory alkalosis leads to a decrease in cardiac output. In either situation, the most important aspect of managing metabolic acidosis is to treat the underlying cause. In certain cases, this may require pulmonary artery catheterization to assess the adequacy of hydration, cardiac output, and tissue oxygen delivery.

RENAL FUNCTION, FLUIDS AND ELECTROLYTE MANAGEMENT. Maintaining adequate systemic perfusion pressure and brisk urine output (1–2 ml/kg/hr), while minimizing use of vasopressors, contributes to good renal allograft function and reduces the rate of acute tubular necrosis posttransplantation. If the urine production is still insufficient (<1 ml/kg/hr) after adequate volume loading, loop diuretics (furosemide, ethacrynic acid, bumetanide) or osmotic diuretics (mannitol) should be used to initiate diuresis. The use of nephrotoxic drugs (e.g., aminoglycosides) and agents that may exert adverse effects on renal perfusion (e.g., nonsteroidal antiinflammatory drugs) should be avoided. Cephalosporins, monobactams, carbapenems, and quinolones are examples of less nephrotoxic but equally effective antibiotics.

Polyuria in brain-dead donors is a frequent finding. It can be due to diabetes insipidus, osmotic diuresis (induced by mannitol administered to decrease elevated intracranial pressures or hyperglycemia), physiologic diuresis due to previous massive fluid administration during resuscitation after the original injury with return of third-space fluid into the intravascular space, or hypothermia.

Diabetes insipidus often heralds brain death in head-injured patients. It is the most frequent cause of polyuria during the organ donor maintenance phase. Found in up to 80 percent [70] of all brain-dead bodies, it is related to insufficient blood levels of antidiuretic hormone (vasopressin), resulting in the production of large quantities of dilute urine. Diabetes insipidus should be suspected when urine volumes exceed 300 ml/hr (or

7 ml/kg/hr) in conjunction with hypernatremia (serum sodium >150 mEq/L), elevated serum osmolality (>310 mOsm/L), and a low urinary sodium concentration. In addition to hypernatremia, other electrolyte abnormalities frequently observed during diabetes insipidus include hypokalemia, hypocalcemia, and hypomagnesemia. The appropriate replacement of these electrolyte losses can be guided by urinary electrolyte determinations, which will easily allow calculation of the amount of the electrolyte to be replaced. Once urine output due to diabetes insipidus exceeds 300 ml/per hour, desmopressin (1-desamino-8-D-arginine vasopressin [dDAVP]), a synthetic analog of vasopressin, should be administered [98]. Desmopressin has a long duration of action and a high antidiuretic/pressor ratio, reducing the undesirable splanchnic vasoconstrictive effects that occur with administration of arginine vasopressin. Doses of 1 to 2 μg dDAVP are administered intravenously every 8 to 12 hours to titrate the urine output to values of 100 to 300 ml per hour [99,100].

Because diabetes insipidus is so common, mannitol administration should be discontinued after brain death is declared. Hyperglycemia (serum glucose >180 mg/dl) also can induce an osmotic diuresis and should be treated with insulin. The physiologic diuresis that occurs during resolution of third-space fluid loss is characterized by the absence of marked serum electrolyte abnormalities with the exception of a moderate degree of hypokalemia, higher urine sodium levels than those usually associated with diabetes insipidus, and an eventual spontaneous decrease in urine output. Intravenous maintenance fluids administered to brain-dead organ donors must always contain glucose, which is important to maintain intrahepatic glycogen stores that appear to be associated with normal liver allograft function in the early posttransplant period.

During the initial resuscitation phase after brain death is declared, infusion solutions with a low sodium content should be used. Subsequently, maintenance fluid should consist of 5% dextrose in 0.45% sodium chloride with 20 mEq of potassium added to each liter, administered at a rate of 2 ml/kg/hr during the maintenance phase if urine output is adequate (>1 to 2 ml/kg/hr). If the urine output is >2ml/kg/hr, intravenous fluids should be administered at the rate equal to the urine output during the previous hour (IV intake = urine output). If the serum sodium concentration exceeds 150 mEq/L, the maintenance fluid should consist of 5% dextrose in 0.2% sodium chloride with 20 mEq of potassium added to each liter. Should the hourly fluid administration rate exceed 500 ml per hour, the dextrose concentration of the maintenance fluid should be decreased to 1% dextrose to avoid excessive hyperglycemia. The sodium content of certain intravenous fluids and plasma expanders (e.g., albumin solutions) also must be taken into consideration in hypernatremic patients.

The use of blood transfusions and other blood products should be minimized in organ donors as in other patients. If transfusion or blood component therapy is necessary, CMV seronegative blood products and/or leukocyte filters should be used whenever possible [95]. All blood must be screened for HIV, HBV, and HCV, and seropositive units should not be used.

ENDOCRINE THERAPY. According to recent studies, pituitary hormone blood levels do not uniformly decrease after brain death. As noted, about 80 percent of brain-dead donors develop diabetes insipidus due to low or absent blood levels of vasopressin [70]. These findings are a direct consequence of brain death, which abolishes both vasopressin production in the hypothalamic nuclei (supraoptic and paraventricular nuclei) and vasopressin storage and release in the posterior pituitary. In contrast, levels of anterior pituitary hormones such as thyroid stimulating hormone (TSH), adrenocorticotropic hormone (ACTH), and growth hormone have been documented to remain normal after brain death [101–104]. Their persistence is probably due to the preservation of small subcapsular areas in the anterior pituitary, whose blood supply is derived from small branches of the inferior hypophyseal artery. The latter arises from the extradural internal cartoid artery, which is relatively protected from increases in intracranial pressure [105].

The principle of pharmacologic replacement therapy for deficient posterior pituitary vasopressin after brain death is well established [98–100]. In contrast, controversy exists regarding the benefits of supplementation with some of the hormones synthesized by organs under anterior pituitary control (triiodothyronine [T_3], thyroxine [T_4], corticosteroids) [106,107,108]. Initially, the presence of low T_3 blood levels was demonstrated after brain death in animal experiments [109]. Administration of exogenous T_3 to donor animals improved a variety of metabolic parameters before and after preservation [110,111,112] as well as organ function after transplantation [113]. These findings suggested the possible positive effects of T_3 in human donors. However, although favorable influences of donor T_3 pretreatment on hemodynamic and metabolic parameters during the donor maintenance phase [72,114,115] and on outcome after heart transplantation [116,117,118] have been demonstrated in a limited number of uncontrolled clinical trials, these findings have not been reproduced by other investigators.

In recent years, evidence has accumulated that the low T_3 levels in human donors do not correlate with the presence of hemodynamic stability [119,120] or outcome after transplantation [121,122,123]. Animal [124] and human [107] studies testing the effect of donor T_3 pretreatment have not demonstrated improved outcome. The typical thyroidal hormonal pattern after brain death consists of decreased T_3, normal or decreased T_4, and normal TSH and is not consistent with acute insufficiency of the hypothalamic-pituitary-thyroid axis or clinically overt hypothyroidism, being similar to changes observed in other groups of critically ill individuals [125]. Thyroid hormone administration to such patient is not only ineffective but potentially detrimental in some cases [125,126]. Therefore, thyroid hormonal supplementation of organ donors should currently be limited to large, controlled clinical trials until its efficacy is proven.

Similarly, routine administration of corticosteroids is not to be recommended. Normal human serum ACTH and cortisol levels have been demonstrated after brain death [101–104]. Only those donors who have been receiving chronic steroid therapy may be at risk for adrenal insufficiency and development of an Addisonian crisis. These individuals probably should receive prophylactic corticosteroids, although this remains somewhat controversial.

Although brain death is not associated with primary pancreatic endocrine dysfunction, hyperglycemia is frequent in brain-dead donors. Hyperglycemia can be caused by increased catecholamine release, altered carbohydrate metabolism, steroid administration for treatment of cerebral edema, infusion of large amounts of dextrose-containing intravenous fluids, or peripheral insulin resistance. Treating hyperglycemia in brain-dead donors appears to be important with regard to pancreatic islet cell function. Experimental evidence suggests that high glucose levels may produce transient or irreversible damage to β-cells in the pancreatic islets, both in vitro and in vivo [127,128]. This glucose toxicity was attenuated during in vivo experiments by correcting hyperglycemia [129]. Clinical studies in pancreas transplant recipients have demonstrated that donor hyperglycemia is a risk factor for decreased graft survival [81]. It was not established in these studies, however, whether donor hyperglycemia was indicative of marginal or insufficient β-cell mass

or whether impaired pancreatic graft function was related to islet cell dysfunction as a result of hyperglycemia.

Finally, hyperglycemia in and of itself is known to cause insulin resistance [130]. Studies in brain-dead donors have suggested that a state of hyperinsulinemia coupled with peripheral insulin resistance exists, as evidenced by elevated C-peptide/glucose molar ratios [131]. For all these reasons, it is prudent to maintain blood glucose levels in donors between 100 and 200 mg/dl. Insulin should be administered as needed according to the blood glucose values to mitigate any potential adverse effects of hyperglycemia on pancreatic islets, which could impair glucose homeostasis posttransplant. If hyperglycemia persists despite initial bolus insulin therapy, then continuous intravenous insulin infusion should be instituted to facilitate titration of glucose levels. Glycemic control also acts to prevent ketoacidosis and osmotic diuresis, both of which can be significant problems in the management of brain-dead donors.

HYPOTHERMIA. After brain death, the body becomes poikilothermic because of the loss of thalamic and hypothalamic central temperature control mechanisms, and hypothermia usually ensues [132]. Systemic vasodilatation causes additional heat loss. Hypothermia can be aggravated by administering room-temperature intravenous fluids and cold blood products. Adverse effects of hypothermia include decreased myocardial contractility, hypotension, cardiac dysrhythmias, cardiac arrest, hepatic and renal dysfunction, and acidosis and coagulopathy [133,134,135]. Donor core temperature therefore must be maintained at 35°C. It is usually sufficient to use humidified, heated ventilator gases; warmed intravenous fluids and blood products; and warming blankets to achieve rewarming and to maintain an adequate body temperature. Rewarming with peritoneal dialysis or bladder irrigations generally should not be performed in organ donors.

COAGULATION SYSTEM. Coagulopathy and disseminated intravascular coagulation are common findings in brain-dead donors, particularly after head injuries [48]. Pathologic activation of the coagulation cascade occurs when brain tissue, which is very rich in tissue thromboplastin, comes in contact with blood after trauma. Massive blood transfusions can produce dilutional thrombocytopenia, and subsequent ongoing hemorrhage, hypothermia, and acidosis are all able to trigger or further aggravate coagulopathy. Clinical findings can include pathologic bleeding, abnormal prothrombin time (PT), thrombocytopenia, hypofibrinogenemia, and increased levels of fibrin/fibrinogen degradation products. Treatment of coagulopathy entails use of blood components such as platelets, fresh frozen plasma, or cryoprecipitate and correction of the underlying pathophysiology (e.g., hypothermia, acidosis, surgical hemorrhage). ε-aminocaproic acid should not be used because of its potential for inducing microvascular thrombosis, thereby rendering organs potentially unsuitable for transplantation.

OTHER ASPECTS. Various attempts to pharmacologically pretreat donors to optimize transplant outcome have been reported. For example, administration of either lidocaine or prostacyclin intravenously before and during organ recovery has been associated with improved renal allograft function in uncontrolled trials [136,137,138]. Similarly, beneficial effects on organ function after administering allopurinol, naloxone, catalase, or superoxide dismutase during hemodynamic instability have been observed in experimental animal models [139,

140,141]. In a small animal model, defibrotide provided favorable effects on cardiac and renal cellular metabolism after procurement and preservation as determined by intracellular nucleotide levels [142]. In another study, a positive impact on experimental liver preservation was attributed to donor pretreatment with chlorpromazine [143]. Finally, calcium channel antagonists have been used experimentally for donor pretreatment to reduce intracellular calcium levels, which increase with ischemia [144]. Verapamil mitigated the adverse impact of elevated cytosolic calcium levels on renal allograft function [145] and on myocardial cellular morphology [146] after donor hemodynamic instability. All these pretreatment methods must be investigated more extensively in controlled clinical trials, however, before they can be applied routinely.

The Multiple-Organ Donor Operation

After consent is obtained, the OPO schedules and organizes the organ recovery operation. Often, several surgical terms from different locations participate; their transportation and the preparation of the recipients in the various hospitals must be meticulously coordinated. After certification of death according to the state laws occurs, the donor is brought to the operating room. Full cardiovascular and ventilatory support is maintained throughout the operation, until the organs are flushed and cooled. The principles of donor management should be reviewed with the anesthesiologist, unless he or she is familiar with the specific clinical aspects of cardiovascular and ventilatory support for brain-dead organ donors. Hemodynamic stability must be maintained during the surgical organ retrieval, which is the equivalent of a combined major abdominal and thoracic operation and can last up to several hours. Transient tachycardia and hypertension may occur while the surgical incision is being made; they most likely reflect spinal reflexes causing vasoconstrictive responses and adrenal stimulation. Subsequently, consideration must be given to the increased heat loss caused by the wide abdominal and thoracic incisions and the duration of the surgery. Vecuronium or pancuronium should be used to inhibit reflex muscular contractions. Tubocurarine should not be used in brain-dead donors because of its association with hypotension as a consequence of histamine release and ganglionic blockade. Maintenance fluid administration throughout the operation needs to take into account the significant intraoperative fluid losses resulting from extensive dissection, transsection of lymphatic channels, and massive third-space fluid loss. All organs to be recovered are completely mobilized and their vascular pedicles are dissected free. At the end of the operation, systemic heparinization occurs and cannulas are inserted (depending on the organs to be procured) into the abdominal aorta, inferior vena cava, portal vein, aortic arch, and pulmonary artery. Only then is circulatory and respiratory support terminated. The organs are flushed in situ with preservation solution to remove blood and to cool the organs to a temperature of 4 to 7°C. Simultaneously, topical external cooling is provided by the application of ice slush. The organs are then individually removed, by dividing the remaining attachments and vascular pedicles, and then packaged. Storage in preservation solution at 4 to 7°C in a cooler surrounded by crushed ice allows maximal preservation times of 4 to 6 hours for heart and lungs, about 30 hours for livers and pancreata, and about 40 hours for kidneys. These preservation constraints are taken into consideration as organs are allocated. Critical care donor management ends when controlled cardiac arrest occurs at the completion of the surgical organ recovery. This finality is ephemeral, however, because it results in the start of a new life after a successful organ transplant.

References

1. Kron IL, Tribble CG, Kern JA, et al: Successful transplantation of marginally acceptable thoracic organs. *Ann Surg* 217:518, 1993.
2. Organ transplantation. Issues and recommendation. *Report of the Task Force on Organ Transplantation, U.S. Department of Health and Human Services,* 1986, p 36.
3. Heffron TG: Organ procurement and management of the multiorgan donor, in Hall JB, Schmidt GA, Wood LDH (eds): *Principles of Critical Care.* New York, 1992, McGraw-Hill, Inc., p 891.
4. UNOS releases 1992 transplant statistics. *UNOS Update* 9:9, 1993.
5. Najarian JS, Strand M, Fryd DS, et al: Comparison of cyclosporine versus azathioprine-antilymphocyte globulin in renal transplantation. *Transplant Proc* 15(Suppl 1):2463, 1983.
6. Starzl TE, Iwatsuki S, Van Thiel DH, et al: Report of Colorado-Pittsburgh liver transplantation studies. *Transplant Proc* 15(Suppl 1):2582, 1983.
7. Sutherland DER: Pancreas transplantation: Overview and current status of cases reported to the registry through 1982. *Transplant Proc* 15(Suppl 1):2597, 1983.
8. Oyer PE, Stinson EB, Jamieson SW, et al: Cyclosporine in cardiac transplantation: a 2-1/2 year follow-up. *Transplant Proc* 15(Suppl 1):2546, 1983.
9. Basadonna G, Matas AJ, Gillingham KJ, et al: Kidney transplantation in patients with type I diabetes: 26-year experience at the University of Minnesota, in Terasaki PI, Cecka JM (eds): *Clinical Transplants 1992.* Los Angeles, UCLA Tissue Typing Laboratory, 1993.
10. Belle SH, Beringer KC, Murphy JB, et al: The Pitt-UNOS liver transplant registry, in Terasaki PI, Cecka JM (eds): *Clinical Transplants 1992.* Los Angeles, UCLA Tissue Typing Laboratory, 1993.
11. Sutherland DER, Gruessner A, Moudry-Munns K: Analysis of united network for organ sharing (UNOS) United States of America (USA) pancreas transplant registry data according to multiple variables, in Terasaki PI, Cecka JM (eds): *Clinical Transplants 1992.* Los Angeles, UCLA Tissue Typing Laboratory, 1993.
12. Breen TJ, Keck B, Hosenpud JD, et al: Thoracic organ transplants in the United States from October 1987 through December 1991: A report from the UNOS scientific registry for organ transplants, in Tersaki PI, Cecka JM (eds): *Clinical Transplants 1992.* Los Angeles, UCLA Tissue Typing Laboratory, 1993.
13. Evans RW, Orians CE, Ascher NL: The potential supply of organ donors. An assessment of the efficiency of organ procurement efforts in the United States. *JAMA* 267:239, 1992.
14. Ivatury RR, Grewal H, Simon RJ, et al: Analysis of organ procurement failure at an urban trauma center and the impact of HIV on organ procurement at a regional transplantation center. *J Trauma* 33:424, 1992.
15. Mackersie RC, Bronsther OL, Shackford SR: Organ procurement in patient with fatal head injuries. *Ann Surg* 213:143, 1991.
16. Rapaport FT: Continuing dilemma of organ procurement for clinical transplantation. *Transplant Proc* 25:2494, 1993.
17. Gallup poll surveys views on organ donation. *Nephrology News & Issues* (May):16, 1993.
18. Tolle SW, Bennett WM, Hickam DH, et al: Responsibilities of primary physicians in organ donation. *Ann Int Med* 106:740, 1987.
19. Dunn DL, Mayoral JL, Gillingham KJ, et al: Treatment of invasive cytomegalovirus disease in solid organ transplant patients with ganciclovir. *Transplantation* 51:98, 1991.
20. Schweitzer EJ, Matas AJ, Gillingham KJ, et al: Causes of renal allograft loss: progress in the 1980s, challenges for the 1990s. *Ann Surg* 214:679, 1991.
21. Najarian JS, Frey DJ, Matas, AJ, et al: Renal transplantation in infants. *Ann Surg* 212:353, 1990.
22. Todo S, Tzakis AG, Abu-Elmagd K, et al: Intestinal transplantation in composite visceral grafts or alone. *Ann Surg* 216:223, 1992.
23. The Diabetes Control and Complications Trial Research Group: The effect of intensive treatment of diabetes on the development

and progression of long-term complications in insulin-dependent diabetes mellitus. *N Engl J Med* 329:977, 1993.

24. Sutherland DER: Indication for pancreas transplantation alone, in Dubernard JM, Sutherland DER (eds): *International Handbook of Pancreas Transplantation.* Dordrecht, The Netherlands, Kluwer Academic, 1989.

25. Sutherland DER: Effect of pancreas transplantation on secondary complications of diabetes, in Dubernard JM, Sutherland DER (eds): *International Handbook of Pancreas Transplantation.* Dordrecht, The Netherlands, Kluwer Academic, 1989.

26. Gores PF, Najarian JS, Stephanian, et al: Insulin dependence in type I diabetes after transplantation of unpurified islets from single donor with 15-deoxyspergualin. *Lancet* 341:19, 1993.

27. Kay MP: The registry of the international society for heart and lung transplantation: tenth official report—1993. *J Heart Lung Transplant* 12:541, 1993.

28. Bolman RM III, Shumway SJ, Estrin JA, et al: Lung and heart-lung transplantation. Evolution and new applications. *Ann Surg* 214:456, 1991.

29. Griffith BP, Hardesty RL, Armitage JM, et al: A decade of lung transplantation. *Ann Surg* 218:310, 1993.

30. Donor pool shrinking? Decreasing vehicular fatalities, increases in AIDS reducing donor pool. *UNOS Update* 9:9, 1993.

31. Ellison MD, Breen TJ, Glascock F, et al: Organ donation in the United States: 1988 through 1991, in Terasaki PI, Cecka JM (eds): *Clinical Transplants 1992.* Los Angeles, UCLA Tissue Typing Laboratory, 1993.

32. Kennedy AP Jr, West JC, Kelley SE, et al: Utilization of trauma-related deaths for organ and tissue harvesting. *J Trauma* 33:516, 1992.

33. Cheung, AHS, Luna GK: Cadaveric organ donor availability: Regional trauma center vs. community hospital. *J Trauma* 30:1366, 1990.

34. Callender CO, Hall LE, Yeager CL, et al: Organ donation and blacks. A critical frontier. *N Engl J Med* 325:442, 1991.

35. Blagg CR, Helgerson S, Warren CW, et al: Awareness and attitudes of Northwest Native Americans regarding organ donation and transplantation. *Clin Transplantation* 46:436, 1992.

36. Pollak R: Medical student education and organ donation—A medical school survey. *Clin Transplantation* 6:372, 1992.

37. Youngner SJ, Landefeld CS, Coulton CJ, et al: Brain death and organ retrieval. A cross-sectional survey of knowledge and concepts among health professionals. *JAMA* 261:2205, 1989.

38. Caplan AL, Van Buren CT, Tilney NL: Financial compensation for cadaver organ donation: Good idea or anathema. *Transplant Proc* 25:2740, 1993.

39. Morel PH, Troppmann C, Almond PS, et al: Multiorgan procurement does not affect the immediate outcome of kidney transplants. *Clin Transplantation* 5:381, 1991.

40. Dunn DL, Morel PH, Schlumpf R, et al: Evidence that combined procurement of pancreas and liver grafts does not affect transplant outcome. *Transplantation* 51:150, 1991.

41. Starzl TE, Hakala TR, Shaw BW, et al: A flexible procedure for multiple cadaveric organ procurement. *Surg Gynecol Obstet* 158:223, 1984.

42. Marsh CL, Perkins JD, Sutherland DER, et al: Combined hepatic and pancreaticoduodenal procurement for transplantation. *Surg Gynecol Obstet* 168:254, 1989.

43. Shaffer D, Lewis WD, Jenkins RL, et al: Combined liver and whole pancreas procurement in donors with a replaced right hepatic artery. *Surg Gynecol Obstet* 175:204, 1992.

44. Todo S, Ner J, Yanaga K, et al: Extended preservation of human liver grafts with UW solution. *JAMA* 261:711, 1989.

45. Troppmann C, Almond PS, Escobar FS, et al: Donor age and cause of death affect cadaver renal allograft outcome. *Transplant Proc* 23:1365, 1991.

46. Alexander JW, Vaughn WK: The use of "marginal" donors for organ transplantation. *Transplantation* 51:135, 1991.

47. Snyder JW, Unkle DW, Nathan HM, et al: Successful donation and transplantation of multiple organs from a victim of cyanide poisoning. *Transplantation* 55:425, 1993.

48. Hefty TR, Cotterell LW, Fraser SC, et al: Disseminated intravascular coagulation in cadaveric organ donors. Incidence and effect on renal transplantation. *Transplantation* 55:442, 1993.

49. Fukuzawa K, Schwartz ME, Katz E, et al: An alternative technique for in situ arterial flushing in elderly liver donors with atherosclerotic occlusive disease. *Transplantation* 55:445, 1993.

50. Rosenberg L, Granke K, Campbell DA, et al: Procurement of kidneys with anomalies. Long-term outcome. *Transplant Proc* 20:768, 1988.

51. Barone GW, Henry ML, Elkhammas EA, et al: Whole organ transplant of an annular pancreas. *Transplantation* 53:492, 1992.

52. Emond JC, Whitington PF, Thistlethwaite JR, et al: Transplantation of two patients with one liver. Analysis of a preliminary experience with 'split liver' grafting. *Ann Surg* 212:14, 1990.

53. Sutherland DER, Morel PH, Gruessner RWG: Transplantation of two diabetic patients with one divided cadaver donor pancreas. *Transplant Proc* 22:585, 1990.

54. Pasic M, Gallino A, Carrel T, et al: Brief report: reuse of a transplanted heart. *N Engl J Med* 328:319, 1993.

55. Broelsch CE, Whitington PF, Emond JC, et al: Liver transplantation in children from living related donors. *Ann Surg* 214:428, 1991.

56. Sutherland DER, Goetz FC, Najarian JS: Pancreas transplants from related donors. *Transplantation* 38:625, 1984.

57. Youngner SJ, Arnold RM: Ethical, psychosocial, and public policy implications of procuring organs from non–heart-beating cadaver donors. *JAMA* 269:2769, 1993.

58. Fox RC: An ignoble form of cannibalism: Reflections on the Pittsburgh protocol for procuring organs from non–heart-beating cadavers. *Kennedy Institute of Ethics Journal* 3:231, 1993.

59. Guttmann RD: On the use of organs from executed prisoners. *Transplantation Reviews* 6:189, 1992.

60. Caplan AL: Ethical issues in the use of anencephalic infants as a source of organs and tissues for transplantation. *Transplant Proc* 20:42, 1988.

61. Starzl TE, Fung J, Tzakis A, et al: Baboon-to-human liver transplantation. *Lancet* 341:65, 1993.

62. Caplan AL: Ethical issues raised by research involving xenografts. *JAMA* 254:3339, 1985.

63. Spital A: The shortage of organs for transplantation. Where do we go from here? *N Engl J Med* 325:1243, 1991.

64. Dennis JM: A review of centralized rule-making in American transplantation. *Transplantation Reviews* 6:130, 1992.

65. Sadler AM Jr, Sadler BL, Stason EB: The uniform anatomical gift act. A model for reform. *JAMA* 206:2501, 1968.

66. Overcast TD, Evans RW, Bowen LE, et al: Problems in the identification of potential organ donors. Misconceptions and fallacies associated with donor cards. *JAMA* 251:1559, 1984.

67. Beecher HK, Adams RD, Barger AC, et al: A definition of irreversible coma. Report of the ad hoc committee of the Harvard medical school to examine the definition of brain death. *JAMA* 205:337, 1968.

68. Guidelines for the determination of death. Report of the medical consultants on the diagnosis of death to the President's Commission for the Study of Ethical Problems in Medicine and Biomedical and Behavioral Research. *JAMA* 246:2184, 1981.

69. Powner DJ: The diagnosis of brain death in the adult patient. *J Intensive Care Med* 2:181, 1987.

70. Darby JM, Stein K, Grenvik A, et al: Approach to management of the heartbeating 'brain dead' organ donor. *JAMA* 261:2222, 1989.

71. Jørgensen EO: Spinal man after brain death. The unilateral extension-pronation reflect of the upper limb as indication of brain death. *Acta Neurochir* 28:259, 1973.

72. Taniguchi S, Kitamura S, Kawachi K, et al: Effects of hormonal supplements on the maintenance of cardiac function in potential donor patients after cerebral death. *Eur J Cardiothorac Surg* 6:96, 1992.

73. Najarian JS: The crucial role of the practicing surgeon in securing permission for organ donation. *Am J Surg* 154:253, 1987.

74. Koerner MM, Posival H, Minami K, et al: Heart transplantation at the Heart Center North Rhine-Westphalia, in Terasaki PI, Cecka JM (eds): *Clinical Transplants 1992.* Los Angeles, UCLA Tissue Typing Laboratory, 1993.

75. Troppmann C, Almond PS, Payne WE, et al: Does acute tubular necrosis affect renal transplant outcome? The impact of rejection episodes. *Transplant Proc* 25:905, 1993.

76. Whelchel JD, Diethelm AG, Phillips MG, et al: The effect of high-dose dopamine in cadaver donor management on delayed graft

function and graft survival following renal transplanataion. *Transplant Proc* 18:523, 1986.

77. Pruim J, Klompmaker IJ, Haagsma EB, et al: Selection criteria for liver donation: a review. *Transpl Int* 6:226, 1993.

78. Mor E, Klintmalm GB, Gonwa TA, et al: The use of marginal donors for liver transplantation. *Transplantation* 53:383, 1992.

79. Reding R, Wallemacq P, De Ville De Goyet J, et al: The unreliability of the lidocaine/monoethylglycinexylidide test for assessment of liver donors. *Transplantation* 56:323, 1993.

80. Ploeg RJ, D'Alessandro AM, Knechtle SJ, et al: Risk factors for primary dysfunction after liver transplantation—A multivariate analysis. *Transplantation* 55:807, 1993.

81. Gores PF, Gillingham KJ, Dunn DL, et al: Donor hyperglycemia as a minor risk factor and immunologic variables as major risk factors for pancreas allograft loss in a multivariate analysis of a single institution's experience. *Ann Surg* 215:217, 1992.

82. Gottesdiener KM: Transplanted infections: Donor-to-host transmission with the allograft. *Ann Intern Med* 110:1001, 1989.

83. Van der Vliet JA, Tidow G. Kootstra G, et al: Transplantation of contaminated organs. *Br J Surg* 67:596, 1980.

84. Harrington JC, Bradley JW, Zalneraitis B, et al: Relevance of urine cultures in the evaluation of potential cadaver kidney donors. *Transplant Proc* 16:29, 1984.

85. Gibel LJ, Sterling W, Hoy W, et al: Is serological evidence of infection with syphilis a contraindication to kidney donation? Case report and review of the literature. *J Urol* 138:1226, 1987.

86. Roth D, Fernandez JA, Babischkin S, et al: Transmission of hepatitis C virus with solid organ transplantation: Incidence and clinical significance. *Transplant Proc* 25:1476, 1993.

87. Pereira BJG, Milford EL, Kirkman RL, et al: Transmission of hepatitis C virus by organ transplantation. *N Engl J Med* 325:454, 1991.

88. Patijn GA, Strengers PFW, Harvey M, et al: Prevention of transmission of HIV by organ and tissue transplantation. HIV testing protocol and a proposal for recommendations concerning donor selection. *Transpl Int* 6:165, 1993.

89. Penn I: Malignancy in transplanted organ. *Transpl Int* 6:1, 1993.

90. Garrison RN, Bentley FR, Raque GH, et al: There is an answer to shortage of organ donors. *Surg Gynecol Obstet* 173:391, 1991.

91. Cooper DKC, Novitzky D, Witcomb WN: The pathophysiological effects of brain death on potential donor organs, with particular reference to the heart. *Ann R Coll Surg Engl* 71:261, 1989.

92. Minnear FL, Barie PS, Malik AB: Effects of transient pulmonary hypertension on pulmonary vascular permeability. *J Appl Physiol: Respirat Environ Exercise Physiol* 55:983, 1983.

93. Wijnen RMH, van der Linden CJ: Donor treatment after pronouncement of brain death: A neglected intensive care problem. *Transplant Int* 4:186, 1991.

94. Frist WH, Fanning WJ: Donor management and matching. *Cardiol Clin* 8:55, 1990.

95. Guidelines for multiorgan donor management and procurement. *UNOS Update* 9:14, 1993.

96. Matuschak GM, Pinsky MR, Rogers RM: Effects of positive end-expiratory pressure on hepatic blood flow and performance. *J Appl Physiol* 62:1377, 1987.

97. Davis SV, Olichwier KK, Chakko SC: Reversible depression of myocardial performance to hypophosphatemia. *Am J Med Sci* 295:183, 1988.

98. Richardson DW, Robinson AG: Desmopressin. *Ann Intern Med* 103:228, 1985.

99. Bodenham A, Park GR: Care of the multiple organ donor. *Intensive Care Med* 15:340, 1989.

100. Grebenik CR, Hinds CJ: Management of the multiple organ donor. *Br J Hosp Med* 38:62, 1987.

101. Hall GM, Mashiter K, Lumley J, et al: Hypothalamic-pituitary function in the "brain-dead" patient. *Lancet* 2:1259, 1980.

102. Gramm H-J, Meinhold H, Bickel U, et al: Acute endocrine failure after brain death. *Transplantation* 54:851, 1992.

103. Howlett TA, Keogh AM, Perry L, et al: Anterior and posterior pituitary function in brain-stem-dead donors. A possible role for hormonal replacement therapy. *Transplantation* 47:828, 1989.

104. Powner DJ, Hendrich A, Lagler RG, et al: Hormonal changes in brain dead patients. *Crit Care Med* 18:702, 1990.

105. Seeger W (ed): *Atlas of Topographical Anatomy of the Brain and Surrounding Structures,* New York, Springer-Verlag, 1978.

106. Pennefather SH, Bullock RE: Triiodothyronine treatment in brain-dead multiorgan donors—A controlled study. *Transplantation* 55:1443, 1993.

107. Randell TT, Höckerstedt KAV: Triiodothyronine treatment in brain-dead multiorgan donors—A controlled study. *Transplantation* 54:736, 1992.

108. Novitzky D, Cooper DKC, Muchmore JS, et al: Pituitary function in brain-dead patients. *Transplantation* 48:1078, 1989.

109. Novitzky D, Wicomb WN, Cooper DKC, et al: Electrocardiographic, hemodynamic and endocrine changes occurring during experimental brain death in the chacma baboon. *J Heart Transplantation* 4:63, 1984.

110. Novitzky D, Cooper DKC, Morrell D, et al: Change from aerobic to anaerobic metabolism after brain death, and reversal following triiodothyronine therapy. *Transplantation* 45:32, 1988.

111. Novitzky D, Wicomb WN, Cooper DKC, et al: Improved cardiac function following hormonal therapy in brain dead pigs: Relevance to organ donation. *Cryobiology* 24:1, 1987.

112. Wicomb WN, Cooper DKC, Novitzky D: Impairment of renal slice function following brain death, with reversibility of injury by hormonal therapy. *Transplantation* 41:29, 1986.

113. Pienaar H, Schwartz I, Roncone A, et al: Function of kidney grafts from brain-dead donor pigs. The influence of dopamine and triiodothyronine. *Transplantation* 50:580, 1990.

114. Washida M, Okamoto R, Manaka D, et al: Beneficial effect of combined 3,5,3′-triiodothyronine and vasopressin administration on hepatic energy status and systemic hemodynamics after brain death. *Transplantation* 54:44, 1992.

115. García-Fages LC, Antolín M, Cabrer C, et al: Effects of substitutive triiodothyronine therapy on intracellular nucleotide levels in donor organs. *Transplant Proc* 23:2495, 1991.

116. Orlowski JP, Spees EK: Improved cardiac transplant survival with thyroxine treatment of hemodynamically unstable donors. 95.2% graft survival at 6 and 30 months. *Transplant Proc* 25:1535, 1993.

117. Novitzky D, Cooper DKC, Reichart B: Hemodynamic and metabolic responses to hormonal therapy in brain-dead potential organ donors. *Transplantation* 43:852, 1987.

118. Novitzky D, Cooper DKC, Chaffin JS, et al: Improved cardiac allograft function following triiodothyronine therapy to both donor and recipient. *Transplantation* 49:311, 1990.

119. Robertson KM, Hramiak IM, Gelb AW: Endocrine changes and haemodynamic stability after brain death. *Transplant Proc* 21:1197, 1989.

120. Koller J, Wieser C, Gottardis M, et al: Thyroid hormones and their impact on the hemodynamic and metabolic stability of organ donors and on kidney graft function after transplantation. *Transplant Proc* 22:355, 1990.

121. Wahlers T, Fieguth HG, Jurmann M, et al: Does hormone depletion of organ donors impair myocardial function after cardiac transplantation? *Transplant Proc* 20:792, 1988.

122. Macoviak JA, McDougall IR, Bayer MG, et al: Significance of thyroid dysfunction in human cardiac allograft procurement. *Transplantation* 43:824, 1987.

123. Gifford RRM, Weaver AS, Burg JE, et al: Thyroid hormone levels in heart and kidney cadaver donors. *J Heart Transplant* 5:249, 1986.

124. Schwartz I, Bird S, Lotz Z, et al: The influence of thyroid hormone replacement in a porcine brain death model. *Transplantation* 55:474, 1993.

125. Hershman JM: Free thyroxine in nonthyroidal illness, in Chopra IJ (moderator): Thyroid function in nonthyroidal illnesses. *Ann Intern Med* 98:947, 1983.

126. Hess ML: Letters to the Editor. *J Heart Transplant* 5:486, 1986.

127. Dohan FC, Lukens FDW: Lesions of the pancreatic islets produced in cats by administration of glucose. *Science* 105:183, 1947.

128. Collier SA, Mandel TE, Carter WM: Detrimental effect of high medium glucose concentration on subsequent endocrine function of transplanted organ-cultured foetal mouse pancreas. *Aust J Exp Biol Med Sci* 60:437, 1982.

129. Clark A, Bown E, King T, et al: Islet changes induced by hyperglycemia in rats. Effects of insulin or chlorpropamide therapy. *Diabetes* 31:319, 1982.

130. Unger RH, Grundy S: Hyperglycemia as an inducer as well as a consequence of impaired islet cell function and insulin resistance:

Implications for the management of diabetes. *Diabetologia* 28:119, 1985.

131. Masson F, Thicoipe M, Gin H, et al: The endocrine pancreas in brain-dead donors. A prospective study in 25 patients. *Transplantation* 56:363, 1993.

132. Powner DJ, Jastremski M, Lagler RG: Continuing care of multiorgan donor patients. *J Intensive Care Med* 4:75, 1989.

133. Swain JA: Hypothermia and blood pH. *Arch Intern Med* 148:1643, 1988.

134. Koncke GM, Nichols RRD, Mendenhall JT, et al: Ectothermic philosophy of acid-base balance to prevent fibrillation during hypothermia. *Arch Surg* 121:303, 1986.

135. Reuler JB: Hypothermia: pathophysiology, clinical settings, and management. *Ann Int Med* 89:519, 1978.

136. Schulak JA, Novick AC, Sharp WV, et al: Donor pretreatment with lidocaine decreases incidence of early renal dysfunction in cadaver kidney transplantation. *Transplant Proc* 22:353, 1990.

137. Walaszewski J, Rowinski W, Pacholczyk M, et al: Multiple risk factor analysis of delayed graft function (ATN) after cadaveric transplantation: Positive effect of lidocaine donor pretreatment. *Transplant Proc* 23:2475, 1991.

138. Mühlbacher F, Sautner T, Schemper M: Improved renal graft function after prostacyclin pretreatment. *Transplant Proc* 14:4162, 1987.

139. Cederna J, Bandlien K, Toledo-Pereyra LH, et al: Effect of allopurinol and/or catalase on hemorrhagic shock and their potential application to multiple organ harvesting. *Transplant Proc* 22:444, 1990.

140. Castillo M, Toledo-Pereyra LH, Shapiro E, et al: Protective effect of allopurinol, catalase, or superoxide dismutase in the ischemic rat liver. *Transplant Proc* 22:490, 1990.

141. Toledo-Pereyra LH, Frantzis P, Prough D, et al: Better renal function with naloxone treatment following hemorrhage and brain death. *Transplant Proc* 22:462, 1990.

142. Ferrero ME, Marni A, Salari PC, et al: Usefulness of defibrotide treatment during organ procurement and preservation in rats. *Transplant Proc* 23:2359, 1991.

143. Sundberg R, Ar'Rajab A, Ahrén B: Improved liver preservation with UW solution by chlorpromazine donor pretreatment. *Transplant Proc* 22:508, 1990.

144. Humes DH: Role of calcium in pathogenesis of acute renal failure. *Am J Physiol* 250:F579, 1986.

145. Korb S, Albornoz G, Brems W, et al: Verapamil pretreatment of hemodynamically unstable donors prevents delayed graft function post-transplant. *Transplant Proc* 21:1236, 1989.

146. Novitzky D, Cooper DKC, Rose AG, et al: Prevention of myocardial injury by pretreatment with verapamil hydrochloride prior to experimental brain death: Efficacy in a baboon model. *Am J Emerg Med* 5:11, 1987.

198. Diagnosis and Treatment of Rejection, Infection, and Malignancy in Transplant Recipients

Timothy P. O'Connor,
M. Francesca Egidi, Patrick J. Brennan,
John E. Tomaszewski, and
Kenneth L. Brayman

The transplantation of solid organs has been carried out with increasing success over the past 30 years. In the 1960s, 1970s, and 1980s, the evolution of techniques to accomplish efficient organ procurement, preservation, and implantation, as well as advances in immunosuppression (cyclosporine), led to dramatic improvements in graft survival. In the 1990s, graft and patient survival rates following organ transplantation continue to improve due in part to improved methods for the diagnosis and treatment of rejection, infection, and malignancy. Cumulative experience obtained over the past 30 years in the management of organ transplant recipients clearly demonstrates that the use of immunosuppressive agents is a double-edged sword. More immunosuppression may prevent or treat rejection, but "over immunosuppression" concomitantly increases the risk of serious infection or certain types of malignancy, conditions that adversely impact on patient and graft survival. This chapter reviews the diagnosis and treatment of rejection following solid organ transplantation, as well as infections and malignancies of special concern to the internist and others involved in the management of immunosuppressed allograft recipients.

Rejection of Solid Organ Allografts

OVERVIEW OF REJECTION. Allograft rejection is a dynamic immunologic process. Essentially, the rejection process is a complex multilevel immunologic response to the presence of non–self antigens. Recognition of non–self (the afferent limb) and generation of an effector response (efferent limb) are both key components of this process. The three broad categories of the rejection response, initially defined histologically and by the temporal relation of the rejection to the time of transplantation, include hyperacute, acute, and chronic rejection.

Hyperacute rejection, initially described following renal transplantation [1] and subsequently applied to other organ allografts, usually occurs within minutes to hours following transplantation. Preformed recipient anti-donor antibodies, usually directed against ABO blood group or human leukocyte antigens (HLA) of the major histocompatibility complex (MHC), rapidly bind to these antigens following reperfusion of the allograft. Antibody binding to vascular endothelial cells initiates a cascade of events including complement activation, which in turn rapidly leads to local endothelial injury with subsequent vasospasm, fibrin and/or platelet deposition, granulocyte infiltration, interstitial hemorrhage, and microvascular thrombosis with rapid loss of graft function. With certain organs, pretransplant screening and donor-recipient crossmatch testing for the presence of preformed anti-donor antibodies helps to select donor-recipient combinations unlikely to result in hyperacute rejection. Peritransplant or posttransplant immunosuppressive agents do not prevent hyperacute rejection [2].

Acute rejection typically occurs within days to weeks following transplantation. This response involves recognition of donor antigens, primarily by T cells, and is characterized by T-cell activation and generation of a cell-mediated immune response. Mismatched HLA groups, the most important antigens involved in acute allograft rejection, seem to be particularly important in this response and include the MHC Class I and Class II antigens, which are coded for by different regions of the genome and expressed on different cell types. Class I antigens are expressed on all nucleated cells, whereas Class II antigens are expressed in a more restricted fashion (primarily on antigen presenting cells, such as monocytes, macrophages, B lymphocytes, dendritic cells, and inducible on others). Mature T cells, classified as either CD8+ or CD4+ (referring to proteins associated with the idiotype-specific T cell receptor [TCR] on the cell surface) specifically recognize peptide antigens presented in the context of Class I and Class II, respectively. Class I or Class II alloantigens are also potent stimulators of T cells either by allo HLA:TCR interactions (direct presentation) or as processed antigens presented by self HLA on self antigen presenting cells (indirect presentation) [3]. In addition to MHC restricted TCR engagement with allo-peptide, costimulation by a second signal is also necessary for T cell activation. This may occur through interaction of adhesion molecules (such as CD28) on the T lymphocyte with its ligand (e.g., B7) on the antigen presenting cell [4].

Once TCR binding, triggering, and simultaneous costimulation occur, a cascade of intracellular events occurs which leads to T cell activation. Tyrosine kinases are activated, which in turn activate several components of T cell activation, including ras and G proteins, phospholipase C-γ1, protein kinases, phosphatidyl inositol-3-kinase, and others (Fig. 198-1). In response to these events, calcium is released from the endoplasmic reticulum, activating calcium-dependent enzymes, including calcineurin which causes NF-AT cytoplasmic factor to translocate to the nucleus and complex with nuclear factors, leading to rapid transcription of mRNA for the cytokine IL-2. IL-2 acts in an autocrine and paracrine fashion to engage its receptor (IL-2R), leading to upregulation of IL-2 and IL-2R production, induction of a number of other cytokines, and clonal expansion of the activated T cell population [5].

The site of the initial T cell–antigen interaction may be within the allograft but also may occur in host (recipient) lymphoid tissue. Subsequent T cell–endothelial interactions involving alternatives in adhesion molecules and permeability changes allow direct interaction of recipient lymphoid cells with donor parenchymal antigens. The immunologic response that follows T cell activation involves specific and nonspecific effectors of inflammation and tissue damage. In many ways, acute rejection resembles a delayed type hypersensitivity response, and a primary lymphocytic infiltrate occurs. Specific effectors in the efferent phase of the response include cytotoxic T cells, and later in the response immunoglobulins play a role. Nonspecific effector cells recruited to and active in graft destruction include macrophages (the main effector), and lesser numbers of eosinophils and neutrophils are involved. Edema and fibrosis occur along with changes in vascular flow during this response.

Commonly used immunosuppressive agents interact with the

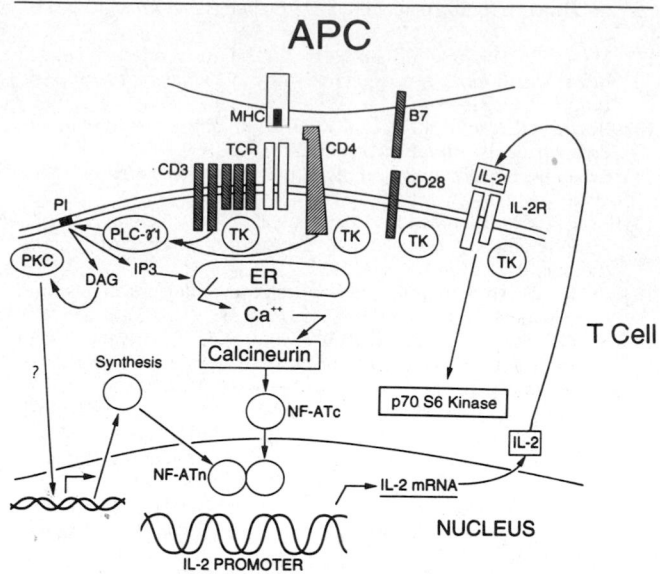

Fig. 198-1. Signal transduction in the T cell, focusing on events that lead to activation of transcription of the IL-2 gene. TK = tyrosine kinase; PLC = phospholipase C; IP3 = phosphatidyl inositol-3-kinase; DAG = diacyl glycerol; PKC = phosphokinase C; ER = endoplasmic reticulum. (Halloran PF, et al: The molecular immunology of acute rejection: An overview. *Trans Immunol* 1:3, 1993.)

immune system at a number of sites to prevent and treat the development of the acute rejection response. Adrenal corticosteroids (prednisone, methylprednisone) bind to a steroid receptor to form a complex that then migrates to the nucleus to downregulate specific mRNA production [6]. IL-2 production is severely impaired by corticosteroids. Lymphocyte-directed signals are also blocked by corticosteroids. Cyclosporine and FK506 each bind to separate binding proteins, which then bind to calcineurin to interfere with IL-2 mRNA production and T cell activation [7]. Azathioprine, an antimetabolite, interferes with nucleic acid synthesis, particularly of rapidly replicating cells such as lymphocytes [8]. Mycophenolate mofetil, a semisynthetic derivative of mycophenolic acid currently being evaluated in clinical trials, causes specific inhibition of de novo purine synthesis, blocking proliferation of both T and B cells, which lack a "salvage" pathway of purine synthesis present in other cells [9]. The murine anti-human monoclonal antibody OKT3 (Ortho-Biotech) binds to the CD3 molecule, which is associated with the TCR/CD3 complex. OKT3 binding to CD3 leads to downregulation of T cell activity through mechanisms that include cell lysis by opsonization and inactivation by antigenic modulation of the CD3 molecule on the surface of T cells [10]. Importantly, the capacity of this agent to inhibit the activity of established effector cytotoxic T cells makes it useful in the therapy of ongoing rejection. Polyclonal anti-T cell agents (antilymphocyte globulin preparations) act on similar cell populations as OKT3 but also bind to a wider array of target antigens [11], a phenomenon that augments their effectiveness and potency.

The cellular mechanisms responsible for chronic rejection are less well understood from an immunologic perspective and are the subject of intense investigation. Chronic rejection usually occurs months or years after transplantation and is a gradual process characterized by progressive functional deterioration. Histologically, vascular changes occur, the most prominent of which is concentric fibrointimal thickening of blood vessels and interstitial fibrosis. The histologic changes of chronic rejection have been seen to occur following all types of organ allografts. Both immunologic and nonimmunologic mechanisms are postulated to be involved pathologically, and it is hypothesized that chronic rejection may be a consequence of tissue-destructive mechanisms activated or sustained by repetitive episodes of acute rejection or from smaller foci of rejection that resolve spontaneously without clinical detection [12]. Late graft loss secondary to chronic rejection remains a formidable problem and challenge for organ transplantation in the 1990s.

REJECTION OF THE RENAL ALLOGRAFT. Hyperacute rejection due to binding of recipient preformed antidonor antibodies is a dramatic phenomenon that occurs minutes to hours after reperfusion of the renal allograft (see Chap. 194). The perfused renal allograft suddenly becomes blue and mottled, and urine output ceases. Microscopically, vascular thrombosis with slight neutrophil infiltrate is observed. Fortunately, pretransplant crossmatching to detect antidonor antibodies in the serum of the recipient has nearly eliminated hyperacute rejection of kidneys (and pancreata) today. Immediate hyperacute rejection is irreversible and transplant nephrectomy is always required [13].

More than half of renal transplant recipients experience at least one episode of acute rejection in the first 6 months posttransplantation [14]. In those patients who experience acute rejection, 1-year graft survival is decreased [15]. The diagnosis of acute rejection is based on clinical, biochemical, and histologic features [16]. Since the introduction of cyclosporine as the backbone of maintenance immunosuppressant drug therapy, the clinical signs of acute rejection, such as graft tenderness and swelling, have become more subtle. A rise in serum creatinine and blood urea nitrogen values with a concomitant fall in urine output may be related to the presence of rejection, but the differential diagnosis should also always include other possible causes of graft dysfunction, such as acute tubular necrosis (delayed graft function), ureteral obstruction or urinary leak, and cyclosporine nephrotoxicity and causes unrelated to the allograft, such as dehydration leading to prerenal azotemia.

A variety of noninvasive radiologic procedures have been employed in attempts to confirm the diagnosis of acute rejection of the renal allograft [17,18]. Ultrasound examination can provide information about the dimensions and volume of the allograft, which during acute rejection episodes increase in size. Sonographic signs commonly associated with acute rejection include a decrease in renal sinus echogenicity, an increase in cortical thickness, and enlargement of the renal pyramids. Color duplex sonography can also be useful in assessing blood flow to the transplanted kidney. The duplex Doppler is employed to measure quality and characteristics of the blood flow in the major renal vessels. In the case of acute rejection, the diastolic blood flow in the renal artery also may be reduced [19].

Radionuclide scintigraphy with ^{99m}Tc DPTA or ^{131}I Hippuran (renal scan) may demonstrate a poor uptake of radioactivity in the renal transplant with active rejection, but this abnormal scintigraphic pattern may not differentiate acute allograft rejection from other causes of renal dysfunction [17]. The renal scan also may permit a diagnosis of obstruction or urinary leak to be made. Magnetic resonance imaging may be useful to evaluate the differentiation between the cortex medulla in the kidney graft during rejection; however, the observed changes are not specific, and similar changes may occur at ATN [20]. At the present time, no single noninvasive radiologic imaging technique has been unequivocally demonstrated to yield a certain diagnosis of rejection.

Renal biopsy and histologic analysis of transplanted tissue remains the gold standard in the diagnosis of rejection. Percutaneous core needle biopsy of the renal allograft can be performed under ultrasound guidance to better localize the graft, although localization with ultrasound is often not required for the experienced operator. Though serious risks are rare, the renal biopsy should be used in those cases where noninvasive techniques have failed to establish the diagnosis of rejection and the need for histologic confirmation is mandatory. The complications of percutaneous core biopsy include bleeding, hematuria, perirenal hematoma, and arteriovenous fistula [21].

Acute rejection of the renal allograft may take one of two morphologic forms. *Acute cellular rejection* is characterized by a cellular infiltrate in the interstitium, tubules, vessels, and glomeruli. The intensity, cell composition, and distribution of the infiltrate vary with the severity of the cellular rejection process. This type of rejection is primarily mediated by T cells. *Acute vascular rejection* is characterized by endothelial cell swelling, intravascular coagulation, and fibrinoid necrosis of vessels. This latter form of acute rejection is often seen in patients with previously high levels of cytotoxic anticlass I antibodies (panel reactive antibodies [PRA]) that subsequently decreased before transplantation [5,22,23]. Renal function may abruptly decline several days following transplantation. The mechanism thought to be responsible for this is a secondary antibody response leading to the above described morphologic changes. Thrombotic microangiopathy, associated with cytomegalovirus (CMV) infection or cyclosporine, may show features similar to acute vascular rejection but through different mechanisms. An international standardization scheme for the histologic diagnosis of renal allograft rejection has been developed [24].

Chronic rejection is characterized by a gradual deterioration in graft function and/or proteinuria occurring several months to years after renal transplantation. In addition to obliterative fibrosis of the small vessels, progressive interstitial fibrosis and tubular atrophy are seen. Retrospective studies [25,26] have shown that an acute rejection episode significantly increases the risk of developing biopsy-proven chronic rejection. This risk may be even higher in patients with more than one acute rejection episode and in those whose rejection episode occurred in the first 60 days after transplantation.

Fine needle aspiration biopsy (FNAB) is a cytologic approach to confirm kidney transplant rejection or other causes of graft dysfunction, such as ATN and cyclosporine nephrotoxicity [27,28,29]. FNAB is a safe technique that is easily performed. Results are usually available in 1 to 2 hours in experienced centers. Since the risks of the procedure are low (lower than the core biopsy), a major advantage of FNAB is that transplanted patients can be monitored sequentially during rejection episodes. The presence of immunocompetent cells (lymphoblasts, plasma cells, macrophages, etc.) in the aspirates permits the diagnosis of "acute cellular rejection," with good correlation to the histologic findings of core-biopsy when both are performed simultaneously. During ATN and cyclosporin A toxicity episodes, the tubular and endothelial cells demonstrate characteristic features on FNAB. In particular, cyclosporin A may induce isometric vacuolization with cytoplasmic inclusions (erythrophagocytosis); these lesions are dose-related and reversible in most cases with appropriate cyclosporine dosage reduction. Because FNAB cannot evaluate structural abnormalities, conditions such as acute vascular rejection and chronic rejection are more difficult to evaluate with this technique.

Treatment of acute renal allograft rejection is usually initiated with high dose steroid boluses (500–1000 mg of intravenous methylprednisolone daily, for 3–6 days). If stabilization and/or reversal of rejection has not occurred following treatment with steroids, monoclonal OKT3 (Ortho) antibody treatment (5 mg/

day IV) or polyclonal antithymocyte globulin (ATGAM [Up-john], 15 mg/kg/day) is administered for 7–14 days. It is important that the renal transplant recipient not be overly hydrated when OKT3 treatment is started, because massive cytokine release that occurs following T cell lysis with the initial dose of OKT3 may increase pulmonary endothelial permeability and precipitate pulmonary edema and respiratory failure [30].

Treatment of chronic rejection with increased immunosuppression has been virtually ineffective. Baseline immunosuppression should be maintained and retransplantation considered when recurrence of end-stage renal failure occurs. Once all allograft function is lost immunosuppression can be stopped after drug dosage reduction takes place. Rapid withdrawal of immunosuppression may lead to the development of perigraft pain and hematuria secondary to accelerated rejection of the remaining parenchyma. Nephrectomy may be required if this occurs but is not necessary for cases where the drugs are stopped and symptoms related to rejection do not occur.

REJECTION OF THE PANCREAS ALLOGRAFT. Historically, documentation of acute rejection following pancreatic transplantation has presented a difficult problem because of the lack of a specific and sensitive marker for diagnosing early reversible rejection episodes (see Chap. 196). Clinical symptoms such as fever, graft tenderness, and biochemical alterations including elevated serum amylase may be related not only to rejection but also to several types of pancreatitis with different etiologies (manipulation of the pancreas during surgery, partial venous thrombosis, bacterial and viral infection). Hyperglycemia is a late manifestation of pancreas allograft rejection. When the exocrine drainage of the pancreas allograft is directed into the recipient's bladder by duodenal cystostomy, a decrease in urine amylase has been determined to be the most accurate parameter signaling acute rejection of the pancreas allograft [31,32]. Because most pancreas transplants have been performed simultaneous with a kidney transplant and the organs are from the same cadaver donor, rejection of the kidney, which is readily diagnosed by elevations in serum creatinine, has resulted in initiation of anti-rejection treatment for both organs since acute rejection commonly manifests simultaneously in both sites. Obviously, rejection of the renal allograft cannot occur when the pancreas is transplanted alone or in pancreas after kidney transplantation where the renal and the pancreas allograft are derived from different donors. In the latter situation, rejection of the pancreas can occur independently from that of the kidney. Hyperglycemia is not a reliable marker of early acute rejection because an elevated fasting blood glucose may be due to a steroid treatment of rejection or other drugs that cause altered glucose metabolism, (e.g., thiazide diuretics or beta-blocking agents). Hyperglycemia is a late manifestation of rejection and occurs only after approximately 90 percent of the beta cell islet mass is destroyed or rendered dysfunctional. Treatment of acute rejection after hyperglycemia occurs does not usually result in return of significant endocrine function, although isolated cases of short-term graft salvage have been described [33].

Percutaneous biopsy of the pancreas allograft has been reported [34]. The potential risks of pancreas core biopsy include bleeding, pancreatitis, and fistula formation. These are uncommon following percutaneous [34] or transcystoscopic transduodenal pancreas biopsy [35,36]. Histologically, pancreas rejection does not affect all components of the gland in its earliest stages [37]. Characteristic findings of acute pancreas rejection include diffuse mononuclear cell infiltrates in the pancreatic parenchyma with ductitis, vasculitis, and necrosis. Insulitis and selective loss of beta cells from islets are more typical of recurrent autoimmune type I diabetes than is graft rejection.

Serum anodal trypsinogen has recently been shown to be useful in the diagnosis of pancreas rejection [38] as have urine and serum measurements of IL-2 [39]. Theoretically, fine needle aspiration biopsy of the pancreas should be less hazardous than core biopsy, because the needle used in the procedure is much smaller (25 gauge) than that required for core biopsy (18 gauge). Therefore, interest in FNAB of the pancreas allograft recently has increased [40]. In Europe, pancreatic juice, temporarily drained to the exterior by means of a pancreatic duct catheter left in at the time of surgery, makes possible daily determinations of amylase output and studies of pancreatic cytology; however, this technique is not employed widely in the United States to monitor the pancreas allograft for the development of rejection.

Radionuclide scanning is usually not sensitive enough to be a reliable indication of pancreatic allograft rejection. The lack of flow to the pancreas graft in this study may signal complete graft dysfunction (especially if obtained early following transplantation and the urinary amylase has dropped suddenly or the urine has become hemorrhagic), or it may represent artifact due to lower blood flow to the pancreas relative to other organs. A confirmatory angiogram is required to rule out mechanical problems such as torsion of the vessels or graft thrombosis if the nuclear scan is suggestive. More recently, magnetic resonance imaging has been used as an adjunct to aid in the diagnosis of acute rejection of the pancreas allograft. An increase in inhomogeneity from a baseline study or the failure of the pancreas graft to enhance following gadolinium injection suggests acute rejection [41,42].

The treatment of acute rejection in simultaneous pancreas-kidney or pancreas alone transplantation allografts is similar to that for renal allografts. It has been observed that most recipients of pancreas grafts undergo rejection episodes (> 75%), and these rejection episodes are often resistant to steroid treatment and require OKT3 for control. To delay or decrease the severity of pancreas rejection, a prophylactic 7- to 10-day course of monoclonal or polyclonal anti-T cell agents is commonly administered immediately peritransplant. The routine use of induction therapy seems to diminish the severity of acute rejection of pancreas allografts.

REJECTION OF THE LIVER ALLOGRAFT. Acute rejection of the liver allograft differs from acute rejection of other commonly transplanted organs in several ways. Hyperacute rejection of the liver allograft is uncommon, even in highly sensitized patients. Thus, performing a pretransplant crossmatch is not a requirement for liver transplantation. The histologic picture of acute rejection may appear to resolve in some instances with no changes in immunosuppression. Chronic rejection can sometimes be treated successfully. Also, occasional patients retain good graft function after cessation of all immunosuppression, implying that a state of tolerance has been achieved [43].

ABO compatibility, graft size, and quality are the main parameters considered in assessing the quality of a donor liver for transplantation. Characteristics of the liver graft believed to abrogate the effect of circulating anti-donor antibody include the release of soluble MHC antigens, which may bind antidonor antibody; the presence of a sinusoidal network coated with Kupffer cells, which may also absorb antidonor antibody; and dual afferent blood supply to the liver (portal vein, hepatic artery), which may limit ischemic injury from vascular rejection [44]. The success of combined liver-kidney transplantation in sensitized patients attests to the ability of the liver to abrogate the effect of circulating antidonor antibodies.

The waiting time for organ transplants of all types grows longer as the recipient list expands. Patients *in extremis* and near death from liver failure may receive an ABO-incompatible liver allograft when an ABO-matched graft is not immediately available. Early graft failure from rejection and vascular complications is much higher in this situation and is attributed to the presence of high titer circulating anti-donor ABO antibodies and the frequency of the target ABO antigen [45]. Patients receiving an ABO-incompatible liver allograft may experience graft dysfunction within hours, and liver enzymes may rise steeply for several days. Occasionally, the liver may never produce coagulation factors (primary nonfunction). An arteriogram may be necessary to rule out thrombosis. Liver biopsy may reveal areas of coagulation necrosis, red cell congestion, parenchymal hemorrhage, fibrin deposits, and neutrophilic exudate [46]. Hepatic artery thrombosis is common in this situation. Retransplantation is always necessary for primary nonfunction.

Acute rejection following ABO-compatible liver transplantation occurs in 50 to 70 percent of liver allografts and 90 percent of these episodes occur within the first three months following transplantation [47,48]. Liver enzymes become elevated and a cholestatic picture is commonly seen, but neither the pattern nor the amplitude of enzyme and bilirubin elevation is specific [46,49]. Vascular thrombosis, biliary obstruction or leak, infection, and preservation injury must be included in the differential diagnosis of hepatocellular enzyme elevation in the early posttransplant period. A core liver biopsy, T-tube cholangiogram, and color duplex ultrasound or arteriogram should be obtained to ascertain the cause of liver dysfunction. The diagnosis of acute rejection is based on correlation of clinical course, liver test abnormalities, and histopathologic evaluation. The histologic features of acute rejection include activated mononuclear cell infiltrates in the portal spaces along with bile ductular damage and venulitis. The most specific feature of rejection, when present, is endothelitis of the portal venules and hepatic arterioles. Grading of acute rejection is based on the degree of inflammation, the degree of tissue damage, and the presence of arteritis and/or ischemic necrosis (see Table 198-1) [46].

Fine needle aspiration biopsy has been shown to correlate with histologic assessment of rejection by core liver biopsy and, in conjunction with cytoimmunologic monitoring of peripheral blood, can differentiate between intragraft activation from CMV infection and acute rejection [50]. However, to date, the routine use of fine needle aspiration biopsy has been limited to protocol studies and has not achieved widespread use for the diagnosis of acute rejection. Cytologic monitoring of bile for inflammatory cells is not specific for rejection but may be an indicator of persistent rejection [51].

Table 198-1. Histopathologic Grading System of Acute Cellular Rejection in Liver Transplantation

Mild	Mild predominantly mononuclear portal tract infiltrate with evidence of bile duct damage, with subendothelial inflammation
Moderate	Portal expansion secondary to predominantly mononuclear inflammation with duct damage and "spillover" into the lobule with or without periportal hepatocyte necrosis; no evidence of arteritis or central or bridging necrosis (rejection-related ischemia)
Severe	Usually marked but variable portal inflammation with evidence of arteritis and/or rejection-related ischemic damage in addition to duct damage

Source: Demetrius AJ: The pathology of liver transplantation, in *Progress in Liver Diseases.* 9:687, 1990.

Corticosteroids are the first-line agent in the treatment of acute hepatic rejection, but the total dose administered and required is usually less than that for other organ transplants. Typically 500 to 1000 mg methylprednisolone is given intravenously, followed by a steroid taper over 1 week ("steroid recycle"), with daily monitoring of liver enzymes and bilirubin. A repeat liver biopsy may be obtained at the completion of treatment to assess the impact of therapy on the persistence of rejection. A poor or incomplete histologic and enzyme response to steroids necessitates treatment with an additional agent, either OKT3 or ATGAM, usually for 7 to 14 days. Conversion from cyclosporin A to FK506 has also been effective for treating persistent acute rejection that is not responsive to initial treatment with steroids, an antilymphocyte agent, and a second course of steroids [52]. Early graft failure from acute rejection is uncommon following liver transplantation, except when neoplasm or infection prevents use of increased immunosuppression. Histopathologic evidence of mild or moderate rejection in a liver biopsy with or without hepatic dysfunction may, in some cases, resolve with no change in immunosuppression [46,53,54].

Late acute rejection (>6 months posttransplant) is more likely to be resistant to treatment, possibly because of a longer time to diagnosis. This is frequently associated with low cyclosporine levels, often because of patient noncompliance. Biliary obstruction or cholangitis may increase liver immunogenicity by upregulating expression of MHC antigens on biliary epithelium and thus precipitating rejection. Late rejection that occurs in the absence of other causes should prompt a biliary evaluation by percutaneous transhepatic cholangiography or endoscopic retrograde cholangiography [55].

Chronic rejection occurs in 10 to 20 percent of liver allograft recipients [56]. Reported risk factors for development of chronic rejection include acute rejection, CMV infection, positive crossmatch, and HLA mismatch. Chronic rejection is a syndrome characterized clinically by an indolent but progressive increase in a cholestatic picture. Impairment of synthetic function is a late manifestation of chronic rejection. Time to occurrence and rate of progression are variable and may ultimately result in graft failure; in one series only 20 percent of patients recovered [57]. The histologic diagnosis is based on a loss of small bile ducts and portal venules or arterial intimal thickening and hyalinization. Also, cholestasis and a paucity of portal inflammation may be present [46]. FK506 may be useful in treatment of chronic rejection. In a nonrandomized trial, conversion from cyclosporin A to FK506 was successful in 73 percent of treated patients with histologic diagnosis of chronic rejection [58].

REJECTION OF THE CARDIAC ALLOGRAFT. Cardiac rejection, as with rejection of other allografts, may be classified as hyperacute, acute, or chronic (see Chap. 195). Hyperacute or accelerated rejection, due to the presence of preformed anti-donor antibodies, may occur within minutes or a few days postoperatively. Hemodynamic support by inotropic or mechanical means may be necessary for several days. If ventricular dysfunction does not resolve, retransplantation may be required. Plasmapheresis to remove preformed antibodies and substitution of cyclophosphamide for azathioprine have been advocated, but, in general, treatment of hyperacute cardiac rejection has not been successful [59]. To reduce the incidence of hyperacute rejection, candidates for cardiac transplantation are assessed pretransplant for the presence of preformed antibodies to HLA Class I specificities using a microcytotoxicity assay. A PRA result of reactivity to greater than 10 to 15 percent of wells in the panel indicates that the prospective recipient is significantly sensitized and at risk for hyperacute rejection, and a pretransplant crossmatch is then routinely performed using lymphocytes from the cardiac donor. This is not done if the PRA is lower (0 to 15 percent). Pretransplant crossmatching is difficult to perform routinely in cardiac transplantation, largely for logistical reasons. The cold preservation time of a donor heart must be quite short (4–6 hours) to optimize posttransplant function. Cardiac transplant recipients with donor-specific crossmatches that were performed retrospectively and demonstrated to be incompatible ("positive") should be observed closely for early rejection and treated aggressively.

Acute cardiac rejection, similar to acute rejection of other solid organs, is a T cell mediated event. It occurs most frequently within the first 3 months, but may also take place later. Before the development of endomyocardial biopsy and the use of cyclosporine, the diagnosis of acute cardiac rejection was based primarily on physical signs of congestive heart failure or electrocardiographic findings of diminished voltage or arrhythmia [60]. Percutaneous transvenous right ventricular endomyocardial biopsy, now performed routinely, allows for effective screening and early treatment of rejection episodes [61]. Cyclosporine has also changed the character of rejection episodes; clinical and electrocardiographic signs are much subtler and frequently absent, in part because rejection in cyclosporine-treated patients is associated with less edema. Clinical signs of acute rejection may include fever, fatigue, malaise, dyspnea, and other signs of cardiac dysfunction.

Endomyocardial biopsy remains the gold standard for diagnosis of acute cardiac rejection. It has high specificity and sensitivity and a good safety profile and can be performed on an outpatient basis. Biopsy schedules vary, but generally biopsies are performed frequently during the first 3 months, with much less frequent surveillance biopsies performed indefinitely thereafter. Diagnosis and grading of acute cardiac rejection is based on the presence and degree of perivascular or interstitial mononuclear infiltrate, myocyte necrosis, edema, and interstitial hemorrhage [62]. A number of histologic grading systems have been developed. The widely used International Grading System is described here (see Table 198-2) [63].

Several noninvasive methods have been investigated as possible screening and diagnostic modalities in recipients at risk for the development of acute cardiac rejection, but to date none have achieved sufficient sensitivity [64]. However, several of these techniques may be useful as adjuncts to guide the timely use of biopsy and to monitor overall cardiac function. Electrocardiographic frequency analysis by fast Fourier transformation and the use of power spectral analysis of respiratory sinus arrhythmia are being investigated. Echocardiography and magnetic resonance imaging can provide information about rejection as well as cardiac function. Nuclear scintigraphy techniques may also be useful [65]. Determination of lymphocyte activation by cytoimmunologic monitoring levels of IL-2 receptors, beta-2 microglobulin [66], lymphocyte transferrin receptors, neopterin levels, and other immunologic markers are currently not sensitive or specific enough to replace endomyocardial biopsy; differentiation of infection from rejection is the main obstacle to success using these latter techniques.

Treatment of acute cardiac rejection depends on its severity, the presence or absence of hemodynamic compromise, and the patient's current maintenance immunosuppressive regimen [59]. A histologic picture of mild rejection in a patient not receiving chronic corticosteroid therapy may be treated with an oral prednisone pulse and taper, with follow-up biopsy. Moderate rejection without hemodynamic compromise is treated with pulse intravenous methylprednisolone (1 gm daily for 3 days), followed by oral steroid taper, with follow-up biopsies. If evidence of hemodynamic compromise is present (by echocardiography, elevated jugular venous pressure, new S3 gallop

Table 198-2. The International Grading System for Cardiac Rejection

Grade 0	No rejection
Grade 1	A = Focal (perivascular or interstitial) infiltrate without necrosis
	B = Diffuse but sparse infiltrate without necrosis
Grade 2	One focus only with aggressive infiltration and/or focal myocyte damage
Grade 3	A = Multifocal aggressive infiltrates and/or myocyte damage
	B = Diffuse inflammatory process with necrosis
Grade 4	Diffuse aggressive polymorphous ± infiltrate, ± edema, ± hemorrhage, ± vasculitis, with necrosis

Source: Billingham ME, et al: A working formulation for the standardization of nomenclature in the diagnosis of heart and lung rejection: Heart Rejection Study Group. *J Heart Transplant* 9:587, 1990.

or other signs), or if rejection persists after steroid treatment, a monoclonal or polyclonal anti-T cell antibody agent is added. Very few early acute rejection episodes are resistant to treatment such that retransplantation is required. Nevertheless, 15 to 20 percent of cardiac allograft failure is due to recurrent episodes of acute rejection [67].

Accelerated coronary artery atherosclerosis in the cardiac allograft is a major cause of mortality 2 years posttransplantation, affecting up to 50 percent of patients by 5 years after transplantation [68,69,70]. This condition may represent a form of chronic rejection, but thus far a mechanism has not been elucidated. The coronary arteries are affected by concentric intimal proliferation along the entire length, including the epicardial and intramyocardial regions [61,63,71]. This diffuse vasculopathy affects all coronary vessels, and collaterals do not develop. Risk factors for the development of graft atherosclerosis include the type of immunosuppression administered and the presence of CMV infection but etiologic factors have not been consistently identified in all cases. Diltiazem may prevent or slow the reduction in coronary artery diameter seen in this syndrome [72]. Congestive heart failure, ventricular arrhythmias, or myocardial infarction may be a consequence of this progressive vasculopathy. Angina pectoris does not occur because the cardiac allograft is denervated, and sudden death may be the first manifestation of this problem in heart transplant recipients. Routine annual coronary arteriography may identify this lesion prior to ischemic graft injury, but due to its diffuse nature, the lesion is usually not amenable to angioplasty or coronary bypass grafting. Retransplantation should be considered when the severity of the disease becomes life-threatening.

REJECTION OF THE LUNG ALLOGRAFT. Acute rejection occurs in nearly all recipients of lung allografts [73,74] (see Chap. 175). Prompt diagnosis and treatment are important because, in the absence of definitive therapy, rejection may rapidly lead to respiratory insufficiency. Moreover, the later development of obliterative bronchiolitis has been associated with the number and severity of rejection episodes following lung transplantation [75]. The principal challenge in the diagnosis of acute rejection of the lung allograft is the differentiation of this process from opportunistic or other pulmonary infections. Bronchoalveolar lavage (BAL) is an accurate and sensitive means for diagnosing opportunistic infections of the lung; its usefulness in diagnosing rejection is an area of active investigation. Transbronchial lung biopsy with 3 to 5 samples per lung can provide adequate tissue for histologic diagnosis [76,77].

Recipients of combined heart-lung transplants have pulmonary rejection episodes more frequently than rejection of a cardiac allograft alone. Thus, endomyocardial biopsies have not been useful in monitoring for rejection of the lung following combined heart-lung transplantation.

Symptoms of acute rejection may include breathlessness, chest tightness, and cough as patients perceive changes in their lung function. Clinical signs include low-grade fever and decreases in PaO_2, FEV_1, VC, TLC, and DLCO. The chest radiograph may reveal a fluffy hilar infiltrate, but this occurs later than other signs [78]. Single lung transplant recipients usually have a decrease in percent of total blood flow to the transplanted lung by radionuclide perfusion scan during rejection episodes, a sensitive but not specific finding [79]. Bronchoscopy may reveal erythema of the bronchus distal to the anastomosis as well.

Histologically, acute rejection is diagnosed by the presence of perivascular, interstitial, and vascular lymphocytic infiltrates often associated with similar infiltration of the bronchial mucosa. The working formulation for the diagnosis of lung resection [80], proposed in 1990, recognizes four grades (Table 198-3). These changes can be distinguished from those occurring with infection,which include pneumonialike changes with an extensive alveolitis [81,82,83]. Concurrent infection and rejection, often in different lobes, may occur in over one quarter of rejection episodes; thus, biopsy and BAL are performed in each lobe of a lung [77].

In the absence of risk factors for opportunistic infections, the diagnosis of acute rejection may be made on clinical grounds alone and treatment initiated. A favorable response to a steroid pulse helps confirm the diagnosis. A second episode of acute rejection commonly occurs in the second or third week following the first episode, and a biopsy diagnosis is more appropriate at that time to ascertain whether infection, rejection, or both are occurring. After the first month posttransplant, acute rejection is much less common.

Treatment of acute rejection depends on the immunosuppressive regimen used. An initial steroid-free regimen following lung transplantation has been advocated to facilitate bronchial anastomotic healing. In such cases, rejection is treated with pulse steroid therapy and the episode is usually responsive. Improvement should be noted within 24 hours [74]. A lack of improvement should prompt further evaluation including bronchoalveolar lavage and transbronchial biopsy. Steroid-resistant rejection may require a monoclonal or polyclonal anti-T cell agent [84,85].

Obliterative bronchiolitis, a manifestation of chronic rejection in the lung recipient, affects about 50 percent of heart-lung recipients and somewhat fewer lung-only recipients. This condition causes submucosal fibrosis and results in obliteration of the airways, leading to loss of lung function [77]. The severity and persistence of early acute rejection episodes, and the occurrence of CMV or *Pneumocystis carinii* pneumonia, correlate with subsequent development of obliterative bronchiolitis [75,86,87]. Initial manifestations of the syndrome include a dry cough, dyspnea, occasional sputum production, and an obstructive picture on pulmonary function tests. Chest radiographs may be unremarkable. Transbronchial or open-lung biopsy confirms the diagnosis. Treatment of coexisting acute rejection may be helpful, but retransplantation may need to be considered because obliterative bronchiolitis is not reversible once the pathologic changes supervene.

Table 198-3. Working Formulation for Classification and Grading of Pulmonary Rejection

A. Acute Rejection
  0. Grade 0—No significant abnormality
  1. Grade 1—Minimal acute rejection
    a. With evidence of bronchiolar inflammation
    b. Without evidence of bronchiolar inflammation
    c. With large airway inflammation
    d. No bronchioles are present
  2. Grade 2—Mild acute rejection
    a. With evidence of bronchiolar inflammation
    b. Without evidence of bronchiolar inflammation
    c. With large airway inflammation
    d. No bronchioles to evaluate
  3. Grade 3—Moderate acute rejection
    a. With evidence of bronchiolar inflammation
    b. Without evidence of bronchiolar inflammation
    c. With large airway inflammation
    d. No bronchioles to evaluate
  4. Grade 4 - Severe acute rejection
    a. With evidence of bronchiolar inflammation
    b. Without evidence of bronchiolar inflammation
    c. With large airway inflammation
    d. No bronchioles to evaluate
B. Active airway damage without scarring
  1. Lymphocytic bronchitis
  2. Lymphocytic bronchiolitis
C. Chronic airway rejection
  1. Bronchiolitis obliterans—subtotal
    a. Active
    b. Inactive
  2. Bronchiolitis obliterans—total
    a. Active
    b. Inactive
D. Chronic vascular rejection
E. Vasculitis

Infection Following Solid Organ Transplantation

Infection remains a major cause of morbidity and mortality following solid organ transplantation despite significant improvements in prevention and treatment. Refinements in patient selection, surgical technique, immunosuppression, and antibiotic prophylaxis have all had favorable impact on the incidence of posttransplant infections [88]. Infectious complications following transplantation have been described since the earliest series of kidney and liver transplantations [89,90,91]. These early series noted the association of intensification of immunosuppression as a risk factor for infection, as well as the propensity for infection to result from microbial flora endogenous to the recipient. Posttransplant infections often occur at the site of graft implantation. Forty-one percent of infections in kidney transplant recipients occur in the urinary tract, 38 percent occur in the thorax in heart recipients, and 35 percent in the abdomen of liver recipients [92].

Despite advances in immunosuppression, it is not yet possible to selectively suppress the immune system and completely maintain intact host defenses against infection [73]. Pharmacologic immunosuppression, the use of medical devices during hospitalization, and conditions such as diabetes mellitus, hepatitis, leukopenia, splenectomy, persistent uremia, cadaveric (versus living donor) allografts, and treatment of persistent or recurrent rejection episodes are associated with diminution in host immunity [94]. In the early postoperative period, infection is most likely to be the result of a quiescent infection that was undetected at the time of transplant (e.g., hepatitis B, tuberculosis) or the effect of a hospital-related event (e.g., surgery, catheterization, mechanical ventilation). Infections following the initial hospitalization are more likely to be caused by opportunistic pathogens. The donor organ and the organ procurement process are potential vehicles for transmission of pathogenic microbes to the recipient. Human immunodeficiency virus, the Herpesvirus family and hepatitis B, C, and D have been clearly documented to be transmitted to the recipient by the donor organ vector [95,96,97]. Bacteria, including tuberculosis, fungi, and parasites, have also been spread in this fashion.

The diagnosis of infection in the transplant recipient presents special challenges. Immunosuppression may blunt some of the standard clinical signs of infection such as fever, erythema, purulence, and nuchal rigidity. The early posttransplant period is the most likely time for rejection or infection, either of which may present with fever, malaise, pain, and organ dysfunction. Thus, the clinician must entertain the possibility of infection when investigating most such symptoms in the transplant recipient.

BACTERIAL INFECTIONS. Bacterial infections occur primarily in the first few weeks posttransplant, a time when opportunistic (i.e., fungal, viral, and protozoal) infections are uncommon. The major sites of bacterial infection during this period are the wound, respiratory tract, urinary tract, and bacteremias. Nosocomial infections are the result of the surgical procedure, underlying diseases, and medical device use. At our institution, the risk of nosocomial infection after transplantation varies by organ and severity of illness. Kidney recipients experience a 3.2 percent annual nosocomial infection rate, whereas the rate for liver recipients is 16.2 percent. Kidney-pancreas and heart recipients experience levels of risk intermediate to these two extremes [97a].

Wound infections have been found to be significantly decreased in renal transplant recipients by the use of perioperative systemic antibiotics administration [90,91], and this strategy has been applied to extrarenal organ transplantation as well. The most important factors in wound infection are technical in nature [92]. Purulent wound drainage should prompt local wound exploration, and superficial wound infections should be treated with drainage, open packing of the wound, and appropriate antibiotics.

Urinary tract infections are markedly reduced posttransplantation by daily administration of one double-strength trimethoprim-sulfamethoxazole tablet [100,101]. Additionally, trimethoprim-sulfamethoxazole provides protection against Listeria, Nocardia, Legionella, and Pneumocystis when continued for at least 6 months [102,103,104]. Urinary tract infections in the early postoperative period should be treated with the appropriate intravenous antibiotics.

Liver transplant recipients have a reported incidence of nonviral infections between 38 and 83 percent, most of which are bacterial [105–110] being caused by aerobic gram-positive organisms [105,106]. Intraabdominal infections predominate in this group and also in pancreas transplant patients [105,110]. Selective bowel decontamination to decrease gram-negative gut flora has been advocated to decrease the infection rate [110–113]. Prophylactic antibiotics are recommended before any biliary manipulation or liver biopsy in patients with a choledochojejunostomy [114].

Bacterial infections occur commonly following lung transplantation. Antibiotic prophylaxis may be individualized based on pretransplant surveillance sputum cultures in the transplant candidate and from the cadaver donor. Bacterial pneumonia occurs commonly in lung transplant recipients. Most episodes occur in the transplanted lung between 4 and 8 weeks posttransplant. Most are caused by gram-negative rods with *Pseudomonas aeruginosa, Serratia marcescens,* and *Enterobacter* predominating [114,115]. Pleural space infection may occur as a result of pneumonia, mediastinitis from a bronchial anastomotic leak, prolonged chest tube drainage, or a surgical procedure. A new or enlarging pleural effusion in an asymptomatic patient should be aspirated for diagnosis [115]. Early posttransplant pleural effusions that progress to infection are often the result of the lung transplant operation or pneumonia and are usually bacterial in origin. Empyema should be treated with antibiotics and drainage. Tube thoracostomy is usually adequate, but if infected material cannot be drained, the cavity does not decrease in size, or sepsis persists, open drainage is required. Bacterial bronchitis constitutes 25 percent of bacterial infections; predisposing factors to recurrent bouts of bronchitis include obliterative bronchiolitis, Silastic endobronchial stents, and concurrent sinusitis (especially in cystic fibrosis patients) [115]. Mediastinitis may occur from direct spillage of infected respiratory secretions at transplantation, airway anastomotic dehiscence, or sternal osteomyelitis. Fever, chest pain, and dyspnea may occur. Diagnostic work-up should include bronchoscopy and computed tomography of the chest. Debridement, drainage, and antibiotics are the mainstay of treatment.

VIRAL INFECTIONS. Certain viral infections are particularly common following organ transplantation. Herpesviruses, papovavirus, hepatitis viruses (especially B and C), and occasionally adenovirus can cause infection with increased frequency following transplantation [117]. Among the herpesvirus group, herpes simplex 1 and 2 frequently reactivate and the mucocutaneous lesions are treated with acyclovir [118]. Invasive herpetic infections are also occasionally seen. Varicella zoster virus reactivation causing shingles should also be treated with intravenous acyclovir [119]. CMV is clinically the most significant member of the herpesvirus group and is discussed below. Hepatitis C infection and liver dysfunction following organ transplantation of all types are more common than previously appreciated. Unfortunately, no definitive therapy for hepatitis C infection is available although alpha-interferon treatment has been attempted. Papovaviruses, including human papilloma virus, may cause numerous warts and also predispose the immunosuppressed host to certain malignancies. Primary adenovirus infection occurs in 10 percent of pediatric liver transplant recipients but is uncommon in adults [120,121]. Human immunodeficiency virus (HIV) infection has been transmitted with transplanted organs [122], but the risk for this is now minimal given the routine use of highly specific and sensitive screening assays, which are performed in all donors. HIV-infected transplant recipients progress more rapidly to AIDS defining illness. Progression to AIDS occurred on average 32 months after infection, whereas in nontransplant patients, AIDS-related illness occurs, on average, 9 years after infection.

CYTOMEGALOVIRUS. CMV, like other members of the herpesvirus family, establishes latent infection in its host and persists throughout life. Subclinical reactivation of CMV infection cause shedding of virus in saliva and urine. The presence of CMV-reactive antibodies is caused by prior infection, but they do not imply immunity to either reactivation of latent infection or reinfection (superinfection) by another strain. While CMV infection is subclinical in most normal individuals, it is an important source of morbidity and mortality in immunosuppressed allograft recipients, who can experience an incidence of CMV infection as high as a 75 percent following transplantation, especially in groups at high risk for the development of primary infection (e.g., CMV seropositive donor, CMV seronegative recipient) [123].

Clinical CMV infection may occur as a result of (1) primary viral infection in a CMV seronegative recipient receiving an allograft from a CMV seropositive donor, (2) reactivation of endogenous latent virus in a patient who was seropositive for CMV antibody pretransplantation, or (3) superinfection in a seropositive recipient due to a different CMV strain derived from a seropositive donor. Blood products as well as all types of allografts are capable of transmitting CMV [124]. The incidence, timing, and many disease manifestations of CMV infection are similar for all types of allografts. Those patients at risk for primary infection have the highest incidence of CMV disease, followed by those at risk for reactivation and superinfection; seronegative recipients of grafts from seronegative donors have the lowest risk. The severity of the clinical manifestation of CMV infection has been correlated with the overall degree of immunosuppression. CMV infection usually occurs 4 to 12 weeks following transplantation or treatment of rejection [117,125], especially when monoclonal or polyclonal anti-T cell antibody agents are used. OKT3 treatment increases the incidence and severity of disease in seropositive patients, but it does not increase the already high incidence of disease in patients at risk of primary diseases [126].

A wide spectrum of disease manifestations may be seen during CMV infection in organ transplant recipients. Some CMV infections may be subclinical, but most often, CMV infection causes a febrile mononucleosislike syndrome that may manifest one or more of the following: leukopenia, atypical lymphocytosis, hepatosplenomegaly, myalgia, arthralgia, pneumonia, and mild transaminase elevation [117]. Interstitial pneumonitis is less common than the mononucleosis syndrome but has higher morbidity and mortality. Chest radiographs usually show an interstitial pattern. Dyspnea, hypoxia, and respiratory failure can result. *Pneumocystis carinii* is a frequent copathogen at centers that do not use trimethoprim-sulfamethoxazole prophylaxis [127]. CMV hepatitis with elevation of liver enzymes and bilirubin is of special importance in liver transplantation, and pancreatitis also can occur [128]. Central nervous system involvement, which is seen with CMV infection in a number of immunosuppressed states, is uncommon following organ transplantation [113].

Expeditious diagnosis of CMV infection is advantageous because early treatment may limit or decrease the severity of disease manifestations. Detection of virus in blood or body fluids by inoculation of fibroblast cultures and identification of a cytopathic effect requires 3 days to 2 weeks, depending on the concentration of virus in the specimen [129]. CMV in blood and urine is coated with beta-2 microglobulin, a nonpolymorphous component of HLA Class I, hampering immunologic recognition in vivo and in vitro. Therefore, methods have been developed for identification of viral antigens, DNA, or specific mRNA transcripts. Immunocytochemical detection of CMV immediate early (IE) antigens in blood leukocytes, tissue specimens, or body fluids can be determined within hours using the CMV rapid antigen (shell vial) assay. In this test, the relevant specimen is cocultured with a layer of fibroblasts for 18 hours, the monolayer is washed, and the presence of CMV antigens in the monolayer is detected immunocytochemically. High IE antigenemia levels (>100 positive cells per 50,000 leukocytes) have a significant correlation with CMV-related clinical manifestations in heart recipients [130]. Patients with lower levels are less likely to subsequently develop a symptomatic infection. The sensitivity and specificity of this assay for the diagnosis of active CMV infection are 90 percent or greater, and sensitivity is near 100 percent in asymptomatic patients [131]. In renal transplantation, a cutoff level of 10 positive cells per 50,000

leukocytes may differentiate between significant and clinically unimportant infections in renal transplant recipients [132]. Polymerase chain reaction (PCR) detection of CMV-specific viral DNA is also very sensitive but has not been useful as a marker of symptomatic CMV disease [133]. During active infection, CMV replicates in peripheral blood leukocytes; thus, identification of specific mRNA transcripts may become a method to detect patients at high risk of symptomatic infection [134].

CMV disease also may be identified by histologic analysis of biopsy specimens to identify the characteristic changes associated with CMV. This technique is useful in identifying CMV as a cause of esophagitis, pneumonitis, liver dysfunction, or gastrointestinal ulceration after transplantation. Identification of large giant cells with intranuclear inclusion bodies is characteristic of CMV infection. A neutrophilic infiltrate surrounding infected hepatocytes is seen in CMV hepatitis. Less well defined cytoplasmic inclusions may help distinguish CMV from other herpesviruses infections [135]. In situ hybridization and culture can also identify CMV in a biopsy specimen.

Treatment of CMV infection in organ transplant recipients depends on the severity of the disease (e.g., pulmonary or liver involvement) and the overall degree of immunosuppression (both current and cumulative). An infection detected by screening in an asymptomatic patient who has no signs or laboratory abnormalities suggestive of disease may usually be observed without treatment. CMV tissue invasion or symptomatic disease is generally treated with intravenous ganciclovir and a reduction in immunosuppression [136]. CMV hyperimmune globulin is often added to ganciclovir in the hope of controlling severe CMV infections, although an additive effect has not been proved [137]. The transplant recipient with laboratory evidence of CMV and minimal symptoms such as solely fever may resolve the infection without treatment or may progress. Both treatment and observation have been proposed, with proponents for each strategy. The ongoing debate as to whether or not to treat underscores the need to further refine strategies to identify and define early, clinically significant CMV disease or factors likely to define disease progression. In general, when fever and leukopenia occur, it is recommended to treat with ganciclovir because the therapy is usually benign but disease progression can be life-threatening.

Ganciclovir, a nucleoside antiviral, is effective in suppressing CMV replication and also possesses activity against herpes simplex 1 and 2. The usual dose, 5 mg/kg/every 12 hours, should be adjusted if renal impairment is present. Neutropenia and thrombocytopenia are common side effects of ganciclovir use. Paradoxically, the leukopenia associated with CMV infection almost always improves during ganciclovir therapy. Duration of treatment can vary from 7 to 21 days or more depending on the severity of disease and the response to treatment. Ganciclovir resistance of the CMV strain may develop with prolonged treatment courses [138,139]; in these cases, foscarnet has been used successfully [140].

Pharmacologic immunosuppression is usually temporarily reduced during CMV infection for two reasons. First, this allows for a more effective immune response to the virus. Second, CMV infection increases the net state of immunosuppression through a poorly understood mechanism and predisposes the host to concurrent opportunistic infections, with Nocardia, Aspergillus and Pneumocystis occurring among others [110]. In patients receiving multidrug immunosuppression, azathioprine is often temporarily discontinued. In the face of overwhelming infection, the dose of cyclosporine may also be reduced. Many patients with severe CMV infection can be maintained on as little as 10 mg prednisone daily. As the life-threatening manifestations of the infection subside, cyclosporine and azathioprine can be added back to the daily immunosuppressive maintenance regimen.

Over the last 15 years, several agents have been used in attempts to decrease the risk for developing CMV infection or disease using a prophylactic strategy [141]. CMV disease in renal transplant recipients at risk for primary infection, reactivation, or superinfection can be decreased with prophylactic high-dose oral acyclovir (800 mg/four times per day) for 6 to 12 weeks [142] or with CMV hyperimmune globulin administered in several doses over a 4-month period [123]. Antilymphocyte antibody treatment of transplant recipients, for either prevention or treatment of allograft rejection, increases the incidence of CMV disease in at-risk patients and decreases the efficacy of prophylactic measures to prevent CMV disease [143].

Prophylaxis with ganciclovir plus hyperimmune globulin for 1 week immediately posttransplant has been attempted and appears to be less effective than long-term treatment with acyclovir, confirming that CMV transmission or reactivation does not occur solely within the first few weeks posttransplant [144,145]. In liver, heart, and lung transplant recipients, various prophylactic regimens have not demonstrated a decreased incidence of primary infection, but decreases in the incidence of reactivation infection or superinfection have been described [110]. Merigan has reported decreased rates of CMV disease in seropositive but not seronegative heart transplant recipients receiving ganciclovir prophylactically [146]. The Towne vaccine, a live attenuated virus vaccine, has been proved efficacious in preventing severe CMV disease in seronegative recipients of seropositive kidneys [147]. This vaccine is currently not available, but, theoretically, a recombinant vaccine should allow for the same or better protection than the Towne vaccine. Although the optimal regimen for CMV prophylaxis has yet to be determined in terms of agent, dose, route, duration, and cost, most centers have gravitated toward the use of prophylactic acyclovir as originally described by the Minnesota group [142].

FUNGAL INFECTIONS. Fungal infections in transplant recipients are most commonly caused by Candida species; Aspergillus accounts for a much smaller percentage, as do fungi responsible for regional mycoses (Trichosporon, Histoplasma, Coccidioides, and others). The incidence of fungal infection following liver transplantation is higher than following renal, heart, or lung transplantation, reflecting the increased overall susceptibility to infection in recipients with end-stage liver disease. Candidal overgrowth of the oropharynx and gastrointestinal tract in the early posttransplant period or during other periods of heavy immunosuppression is common with all types of allografts. Topical nystatin (mycostatin 5 ml PO tid and qhs) or clotrimazole (50×10^5 U PO qid) may prevent thrush and candidal esophagitis [92]. Invasive mycoses most often occur in patients already compromised by other infections, intensive treatment for rejection, or early posttransplant surgical complications (e.g., anastomotic leak, wound infection).

Aspergillus species infection in immunosuppressed patients may be limited to pulmonary involvement, but commonly this fungus has a tendency to invade blood vessels, leading to infarction, necrosis, and widespread hematogenous dissemination [148]. Invasive aspergillosis should be treated with amphotericin B but has a much higher mortality than invasive Candida infections. Amphotericin B, along with overall reduction of immunosuppression, has been the gold standard for treatment of posttransplant fungal infections. Renal dysfunction frequently occurs with amphotericin use and is exacerbated by concurrent cyclosporine use; hepatotoxicity is also seen. As an alternative, fluconazole is less toxic than amphotericin B and has been

demonstrated to be effective in the treatment of oropharyngeal, esophageal, and systemic candidiasis as well as cryptococcal meningitis. It should be noted that fluconazole is ineffective against Aspergillus and *Candida krusei*, its dose should be reduced in renal insufficiency, and it may increase cyclosporine levels. Itraconazole has recently been approved by the Food and Drug Administration of the United States for oral treatment of histoplasmosis and blastomycosis. Itraconazole may also have a place in the treatment of Aspergillus in patients unable to tolerate conventional amphotericin B therapy or in those patients who require prolonged treatment [136,149,150,151]. In most life-threatening infections with fungi in organ transplant recipients, treatment is carried out with amphotericin B despite its toxicity.

Asymptomatic candiduria may occur following transplantation, especially in diabetic renal transplant recipients. Preemptive treatment with 2 weeks of fluconazole, or low dose amphotericin B (10 mg/day) plus flucytosine has been advocated [110]. Amphotericin bladder irrigation may also be used. Fungus balls may develop in patients with abnormal bladder emptying, causing signs and symptoms of obstruction. Although rare, the diagnosis can be made with cystoscopy or during a cystogram.

The reported incidence of fungal infections in liver transplant patients is variable, ranging from 7 to 92 percent [108, 109,152,153]. Mortality due to fungal infections accounts for nearly a quarter of all deaths following liver transplantation. Risk factors for fungal infection include retransplantation, prolonged operating time, high intraoperative transfusion requirement, urgent status on transplant waiting list, number of steroid boluses, vascular complications, prolonged antibiotic use, and Roux-en-y choledochojejunostomy [152]. End-stage liver patients have a very high rate of gastrointestinal colonization by Candida. A 10- to 14-day course of intravenous amphotericin B in the early postoperative period has been advocated in liver recipients at risk for the disease [111], and prophylactic fluconazole is being studied to assess its benefit on fungal infections in this setting.

Infection with *Cryptococcus neoformans* is an important cause of central nervous system infection following organ transplantation [154]. Infection is first established as a subclinical infection in most cases, with subsequent dissemination and seeding of the meninges. Dissemination occasionally manifests as skin nodules. New skin lesions in a transplant recipient may be evidence of a systemic fungal infection and should be biopsied and cultured. First-line therapy for cryptococcal infection is amphotericin B, although fluconazole may be effective in less severely ill patients.

PROTOZOAL INFECTIONS. *Pneumocystis carinii* pneumonia (PCP) is a rare but potentially fatal posttransplant infection. In transplant recipients receiving oral trimethoprim-sulfamethoxazole (one single-strength tablet daily) or inhaled pentamidine prophylaxis, PCP is extremely uncommon but occurs in 3 to 15 percent of patients who do not receive prophylaxis [109,127,155]. Eighty percent of PCP infections occur in the first 6 months posttransplant, and the incidence of PCP infection is higher in patients receiving OKT3 and in patients with cytomegalovirus infection. Patients typically have symptoms of dyspnea and dry cough that progress over several days, with or without fever. A diffuse interstitial infiltrate is eventually present on chest radiograph, but this is a late finding. Diagnosis of PCP in transplant recipients generally requires bronchoalveolar lavage, and a positive methenamine silver stain of a cytospin smear of lavage fluid is diagnostic. Sputum induction is a noninvasive technique for obtaining deep respiratory specimens for the diagnosis of PCP in HIV-infected persons. The utility of this technique in transplant patients is not known, but transplant patients typically have a much smaller cyst burden than HIV-infected persons, and the sensitivity is likely to be decreased. Intravenous trimethoprim-sulfamethoxazole is generally administered for 2 weeks as definitive treatment for PCP. Defervescence can occur within 2 days, but improvement in respiratory symptoms may not be seen for 3 to 5 days [114]. Pentamidine can be added in patients who do not respond to initial therapy. In patients with delayed response to treatment, a reduction in maintenance immunosuppression and a search for concurrent viral (especially CMV) infections should be undertaken.

Toxoplasmosis is of particular concern following heart transplantation. *Toxoplasma gondii* cysts may reside in the donor heart and give rise to disease in the immunosuppressed recipient. Transplantation of a heart from a seropositive donor to a seronegative recipient warrants 3 to 6 months of prophylaxis with pyrimethamine and sulfadiazine. Clinical manifestations of toxoplasmosis in this population can include lymphadenopathy and fatigue without fever, pneumonitis, myocarditis, maculopapular rash, or encephalitis. Diagnosis is usually based on elevated IgG or IgM antibody titers. Toxoplasmosis in an immunosuppressed patient is treated with pyrimethamine and sulfadiazine for at least 4 to 6 weeks after resolution of symptoms [156].

Malignancy

Organ transplant recipients have an increased risk for developing certain types of malignancies following transplantation and institution of immunosuppressive therapy. Malignancies that occur after transplantation may be divided into three categories: de novo cancers, recurrence of preexisting tumors of recipient origin, and neoplasms of donor origin. Particularly important in the first group are B cell lymphoproliferative diseases. Possible mechanisms to account for the increased risk for developing malignancy include impaired immunosurveillance, reactivation of latent oncogenic viruses, chronic alloantigenic stimulation, direct oncogenic effects of immunosuppressive agents [157], and transmission of malignant cells. De novo malignancies noted to be increased in incidence include nonmelanomatous skin cancers, lymphoproliferative disease, gynecologic and urologic cancers, and Kaposi's sarcoma. Other malignancies have not consistently been noted to occur in increased incidence in transplant recipients. Overall rates of cancer development are not markedly different between kidney, liver, and heart allograft recipients.

SKIN CANCER. Skin cancers are the most common malignancies in transplant patients and may occur at any time following transplantation. The reported incidence in renal transplant recipients in the Netherlands is 40 percent at 20 years, and in Australia and New Zealand 66 percent at 24 years [158]. These cancers tend to be located on sun-exposed areas (head, neck, lower lip, and upper extremities), on the same body sites as warts, and are often associated with numerous keratoses, Bowen's disease, and keratoacanthomas. Squamous cell carcinomas account for more than half of these skin cancers (in contrast to the general population, in which the basal cell to squamous cell carcinoma ratio is 7:1), tend to be multiple, and have an increased predilection for metastasis (5–7 percent). A mortality rate for skin cancer in transplant recipients of 6 percent has been reported [159] and has accounted for 2.4 percent of all deaths in one transplant series [160]. Human papilloma virus

(HPV) DNA has been detected in half of premalignant lesions and squamous cell carcinomas, suggesting that immunosuppression may have a permissive effect for HPV proliferation [161]. Routine patient and physician surveillance of areas with warts or premalignant lesions is important. Diagnosis is based on skin examinations and biopsy of suspicious lesions. Treatment is the same as for the general population, and may involve local excision, cryosurgery, radiotherapy, or topical 5-fluorouracil cream. Reduction of immunosuppressive medications has not been shown to affect the occurrence or progression of these lesions [157].

POSTTRANSPLANT LYMPHOPROLIFERATIVE DISEASE. Lymphomas constitute the largest group of noncutaneous neoplasms that occur in organ transplant recipients. The vast majority of these (86%) consist of a spectrum of Epstein Barr virus (EBV)-associated B cell proliferation disorders known collectively as posttransplant lymphoproliferative disease (PTLD). Overall, PTLD occurs in 1 to 2 percent of renal transplant recipients, 2.5 percent of liver recipients [162,163,164], 7 to 9 percent of pediatric liver recipients [165,166], 1 to 5.5 percent of heart recipients, and 2 to 7 percent of lung recipients. Risk factors include overall degree of immunosuppression, use of OKT3 or polyclonal anti-T cell antibody agents [166,167], and primary EBV infection posttransplant [168,169].

EBV, a herpesvirus, is nearly ubiquitous in the adult population, with 90 percent of adults showing serologic evidence of prior infection [170,171]. Primary infection involves invasion, viral replication, and lysis of epithelial cells, primarily of the oropharynx and parotid duct, causing pharyngitis and viral deposition in saliva [172]. EBV may then invade B cells (via the C3B receptor) passing through oropharyngeal lymphoid tissue and entering the circulation; cell proliferation (rather than lysis) is stimulated and little, if any, viral proliferation occurs. Viremia has not been demonstrated [170,173]. Most primary infections occur at an early age and are subclinical. Classic infectious mononucleosis involves primary EBV infection and a vigorous T cell-mediated immune response to proliferating B cells that infiltrate the liver, bone marrow, spleen, and brain. Following primary infection, EBV may be detected in saliva throughout life and at a fairly constant rate that can be directly correlated with the numbers of circulating infected B cells [174].

The oropharynx and parotid appear to be the main reservoirs of infection throughout life. Renal transplant recipients have increased shedding from the pharynx [175], which is assumed to be due to a dampening of immunosurveillance mechanisms. Proliferating EBV-infected B cells unchecked by an adequate T cell immune response can lead to lymphoma. PTLD has been categorized into three groups [176], which may represent sequential progression of the disease from a benign to truly malignant process. In the first group, patients present with an infectious mononucleosislike disease (fever, sore throat, generalized lymphadenopathy) and, histologically, a polymorphic diffuse B cell hyperplasia is seen. In the second group, a polymorphic, polyclonal B cell proliferation occurs with large, malignant-appearing atypical immunoblasts having early malignant transformation. This may progress to the third group, monoclonal B cell proliferation with cytogenetic abnormalities, which constitutes true malignancy. Recipient B lymphocytes are believed to be the cells of origin in the majority of these lymphomas. However, in several cases, donor tissue has been shown to be the source [174,175,176].

Transplant patients undergoing primary, rather than reactivation, EBV infection are at increased risk for PTLD, explaining the higher incidence of PTLD in pediatric transplant patients. Profound inhibition of T cell activation also increases the risk of PTLD. A number of reports have documented an increased risk of PTLD in patients receiving OKT3, with a markedly greater risk at higher total doses and short intervals between separate courses of therapy. This has also been reported with polyclonal antithymocyte or antilymphocyte globulin administration. Time to onset of PTLD is much less when these agents are used.

A wide variety of clinical manifestations may be seen with PTLD, depending on location, clonality, and extent of disease [163,176]. Symptoms may be systemic and include fever, fatigue, weight loss, or progressive encephalopathy. Lymphadenopathy may be localized, diffuse, or absent and may cause airway obstruction in children [180]. PTLD occurring late after transplantation has a tendency to present with asymptomatic localized lymphadenopathy and has a monoclonal, malignant histology. Intrathoracic PTLD may have several radiologic manifestations; multiple, well-circumscribed pulmonary nodules with or without mediastinal adenopathy are highly suggestive of PTLD [181]. Abdominal pain, rectal bleeding, or bowel perforation may occur with visceral involvement. Allograft involvement may occur and cause organ dysfunction, particularly in kidney or liver grafts undergoing treatment for rejection. EBV hepatitis, similar to infectious mononucleosis, may be seen in liver allografts. CNS involvement, either isolated or part of a multifocal disease, is much more frequent than in nontransplant lymphomas.

Diagnosis is confirmed by histologic examination of tissue specimens. The lesion may be classified into one of the above categories based on histologic appearance, determination of clonality, and extent of disease. Adjunctive studies in the workup of recipients with suspected PTLD should include imaging of the head, thorax, abdomen, and allograft biopsy. In situ hybridization for EBV in tissue sections may be helpful in confirming the diagnosis [182].

Treatment measures include reduction of immunosuppression, intravenous antiherpesviral agents such as acyclovir and ganciclovir, and surgical extirpative therapy. A reduction in immunosuppression may improve T cell-mediated immunity against EBV-infected proliferating B cells. Acyclovir blocks EBV replication by inhibiting DNA polymerase activity and thus stops oropharyngeal shedding of EBV during the treatment period, but it has no effect in the in vitro proliferation of latently infected B cells. B cells within the PTLD lesion may not be sites of significant viral replication; thus, the effectiveness of acyclovir in inducing remission implies that viral replication in pharyngeal epithelial cells, with secondary infection of B cells, may be a necessary link in the progression of disease. A local effect of acyclovir within the lesion has also been proposed [183]. Remissions with no treatment, or with acyclovir alone, have been reported. Some form of surgical treatment has been involved in 35 percent of cases [164].

Diffuse B cell hyperplasia of EBV hepatitis usually is responsive to a combination of reduction of immunosuppression and intravenous acyclovir (800 mg/m^2/8h); either one alone has also been reported to be effective. Polymorphic, polyclonal lymphoma with early malignant transformation requires more aggressive treatment. Immunosuppression should be stopped if the organ is not vital (kidney or pancreas) and decreased by at least 50 percent for other grafts. Some patients with liver grafts will tolerate dramatic decreases in, or cessation of, immunosuppression. If rejection occurs it should not be treated immediately [163,176,184]. Intravenous acyclovir should be administered. Graft nephrectomy may be necessary for nonvital organs. In contrast, monoclonal B cell PTLD has undergone true malignant transformation and is not usually responsive to reduction of immunosuppression or acyclovir. Conventional

lymphoma treatment involving chemotherapy, radiotherapy, and/or surgery should be administered [163,176].

Other treatment modalities that have been used with some success include anti-B cell monoclonal antibodies and alpha interferon plus gamma globulin. Fischer et al reported 26 patients with monoclonal PTLD or disease unresponsive to immunosuppression reduction and acyclovir who were given anti-B cell monoclonal antibodies (CD21-specific and CD24-specific). Eleven patients were alive and disease free at median follow-up of 35 months [185]. Shapiro et al have observed dramatic responses in 5 patients with monoclonal or polyclonal PTLD treated with alpha interferon and intravenous gamma globulin [186].

OTHER DE NOVO NEOPLASMS. Gynecologic cancers are the third most frequent type of de novo cancer after organ transplantation. The risk of cervical carcinoma in situ is increased as high as 14-fold. HPV, which has been linked to the development of cervical neoplasia, is found at twofold higher prevalence in renal transplant recipients [187,188]. Thus, routine pelvic examinations and Pap smears are especially important for female transplant recipients. Routine colposcopic examinations have also been advocated. Treatment is the same for immunosuppressed patients. Squamous cell carcinoma of the vulva, vagina, perineum, and anus is also more common.

Kaposi's sarcoma has been reported in 0.4 percent of renal transplant patients in North America. A 4 percent incidence has been seen in transplant recipients in Saudi Arabia [189]. Most patients present with skin lesions, characteristically multiple, irregular, bluish dermal plaques or nodules; gingival or intraabdominal lesions may also occur. About two thirds are benign, and complete remissions are frequently achieved by reduction of immunosuppression, with or without chemotherapy or radiotherapy. The malignant type is often fatal despite aggressive treatment.

Other malignancies have an increased incidence in transplant recipients. Conventional treatment is appropriate for most malignancies after transplantation. Chemotherapy has not been shown to induce rejection [190]. To date, the adjunctive use of granulocyte-colony stimulating factor (G-CSF) in combination with marrow suppressive chemotherapy agents for prevention of neutropenia has not been found to cause allograft rejection. G-CSF stimulates proliferation of granulocytes but not cells involved in antigen presentation or immune activation lineages.

RECURRENCE OF PREEXISTING TUMORS. Of 855 patients with malignancies treated before or at the time of transplantation reported to the Cincinnati Transplant Tumor Registry (CTTR), 191 (22%) had recurrences; half of these occurred in patients treated within 2 years or less pretransplantation [191]. Tumors with an intermediate recurrence rate (11–25%) were uterine, Wilms', colon, breast, and prostate cancers. A feature favoring absence of recurrence of these tumors was a long time interval between treatment of the cancer and transplantation. Tumors with a high recurrence rate (>26%) after transplantation included bladder carcinoma, sarcoma, malignant melanoma, and symptomatic renal carcinoma. Tumors with a low recurrence rate (0–10%) included incidental renal neoplasms, testicular tumors, cervical carcinoma (in situ), thyroid carcinoma, and Hodgkin's or non-Hodgkin's lymphoma. Of 82 patients with preexisting tumors first treated after transplant, 35 percent had persistent or recurrent tumors, whereas 65 percent had no recurrence at a mean follow-up of 49 months.

The Cincinnati Transplant Tumor Registry has also reported

recurrences in 637 patients undergoing liver transplantation for primary or metastatic hepatic malignancies [192]. Forty percent of tumors recurred, and 81 percent of deaths from recurrence occurred in the first two years posttransplantation. Tumors with favorable recurrence rates and 5 year survival greater than 50 percent were incidental hepatoma, fibrolamellar hepatoma, hepatoblastoma, epithelioid hemangioendothelioma, and metastatic endocrine tumors. Clinical trials using pretransplant and posttransplant adjunctive therapy are currently under way. In general, results of transplantation for recurrence of liver tumors have been poor, and palliative measures should be considered.

TRANSPLANTED MALIGNANCY. Organs procured from donors harboring a malignancy may transmit the malignancy to the transplant recipient. In the largest collected series of 91 patients receiving organs from donors with neoplasia, 37 (41%) developed malignancy [157]. These consisted of primary renal tumors in 12 and disseminated bronchial carcinoma, breast carcinoma, or melanoma in the other 25 recipients. In 5 recipients developing extrarenal metastases, graft nephrectomy and cessation of immunosuppression led to regression of the transplanted malignancy. Ideally, one should avoid transplantation of organs from donors with cancer or a recent history of cancer. Donors with low-grade skin cancers or primary brain neoplasms with very low risk of extracranial spread may be acceptable. However, there have been reports of medulloblastoma and glioblastoma, which have higher risk of extracranial spread than other CNS lesions, transmitted from donor to recipient [193].

Current heart-beating cadaver donor management and organ procurement protocols should minimize the risk of transplanting a malignancy. A good history and survey of laboratory and other test results are important. A head CT of the prospective donor is essential if a primary CNS process is suspected. The abdomen and possibly the thorax should be explored during organ recovery, especially in elderly donors. Procured organs should be carefully inspected for the presence of tumor. This is especially true for kidneys, in which a nephroma may lurk beneath Gerota's fascia. Biopsy and frozen section examination of any suspicious lesion (including brain biopsy, if an unidentified lesion is present) should be obtained before transplantation of the organ(s). The increasing utilization of organs from elderly donors warrants a special vigilance in identifying tumors present at the time of procurement. Following diagnosis of a transplanted malignancy, immunosuppression should be reduced and the graft removed, if possible. This may be curative if the tumor is limited to the allograft.

Summary

The results of solid organ transplantation continue to improve and an ever-expanding population of potential recipients is being considered for organ replacement therapy. Rejection, infection, and malignancy remain formidable problems following transplantation and continue to hamper overall long-term success as manifested by decreased patient and graft survival. The prevention, diagnosis, and timely treatment of rejection, infection, and malignancy in organ transplant recipients remain key to improved graft and patient survival. In an era of ever-lengthening waiting time and focus on cost effectiveness of organ replacement, the limited organ supply and proper management of rejection, infection, and malignancy will weigh heavily in the overall equation of the appropriateness of organ transplantation in the 1990s and beyond.

References

1. Porter KA: Rejection in treated renal allografts. *J Clin Pathol* 20:518, 1967.
2. Auchincloss HA, Sachs DH: Transplantation and graft rejection, in *Fundamental Immunology*, Second Edition. New York, Raven Press Ltd, 1989, pp 899–922.
3. Benichow G, Takizawa PA, Olson CA, et al: Donor major histocompatibility complex (MHC) peptides are presented by recipient MHC molecules during graft rejection. *J Exp Med* 175:305, 1992.
4. Jane CH, Ledbetter JA, Linsley PS, et al: Role of the CD28 receptor in T-cell activation. *Immunol Today* 11:211, 1990.
5. Halloran PF, Broski AL, Batuik TD, et al: The molecular biology of acute rejection: An overview. *Trans Immunol* 1:3, 1993.
6. Kirkham BW, Panayi GS: Steroids, in, Rugstad HE, et al (eds): *Immunopharmacology in Autoimmune Disease and Transplantation.* New York, Plenum Press, 1992, pp 103–121.
7. Schreiber SL, Crabtree GR: The mechanism of action of cyclosporin A and FK506. *Immunol Today* 13:136, 1992.
8. Bach JF: Mode of action of thiopurines: Azathioprine and 6-mercaptopurine, in Rugstad HE, et al (eds): *Immunopharmacology in Autoimmune Disease and Transplantation.* New York, Plenum Press, 1992.
9. Franklin TJ, Cook JM: The inhibition of nucleic acid synthesis by mycophenolic acid. *Biochem J* 113:515, 1992.
10. Goldstein G: Overview of the development of orthoclone OKT3: Monoclonal antibody for therapeutic use in transplantation. *Transplant Proc* 19(2 Suppl 1):1, 1987.
11. ATGAM Product Information. *Physicians Desk Reference* 47th Edition, Medical Economics Data, Montvale, NJ, 1993, pp. 2433–2434.
12. Paul LC, Bendiktsson H: Chronic transplant rejection: Magnitude of the problem and pathogenic mechanisms. *Trans Review* 7:96, 1993.
13. Halloran PF, Srinivasa NS, Soley K, et al: The role of the antibody in clinical rejection syndromes, in Burdick JF, Racusen LC, Soley K, et al. (eds): *Kidney Transplant Rejection: Diagnosis and Treatment.* New York, Marcel Dekker, 1992, pp 359–372.
14. Keown PA: Annual Review of Transplantation, in Terasaki D (ed): *Clinical Transplants 1991.* Los Angeles, UCLA Press, 1991, pp 205–224.
15. Cecka JM, Terasaki PI: Early rejection episodes, in *Clinical Transplants 1989.* Los Angeles, UCLA Tissue Typing Laboratory, 1989, pp 425–434.
16. Saluman JR: Monitoring in renal transplantation. *Immunol Letter* 29:139, 1991.
17. Abecassis MM, Kirduer PT, Hunsicker LT, et al: Diagnostic radiology of kidney transplantation, in Makowka L (ed): *The Handbook of Transplantation Management.* Austin, TX, 1991, pp 541–561.
18. Meyer M, Paushter S, Steinmuller DR: The use of duplex Doppler ultrasonography to evaluate renal allograft dysfunction. *Transplantation* 50:974, 1990.
19. Saarinen I, Shonen J, Isoniami H, et al: Acute rejection in kidney grafts with delayed onset of graft function: A Duplex–Doppler study. *Transplant Int* 5:159, 1992.
20. Grist TM, Charles HC, Sostman HD: Renal transplant rejection: Diagnosis with ^{31}P MR spectroscopy. *Am J Radiol* 156:105, 1991.
21. Wilczek HE: Percutaneous needle biopsy of the renal allograft. A clinical safety evaluation of 1129 biopsies. *Transplantation* 50:790, 1990.
22. Halloran PF, Wadgyman A, Ritchie S, et al: The significance of the anti-class I antibody response. I: Clinical and pathologic features of anti-class I mediated rejection. *Transplantation* 49:85, 1990.
23. Halloran PF, Schlart J, Soley K, et al: The significance of the anti-class I response. II: Clinical and pathologic features of renal transplants with anti-class I-like antibody. *Transplantation* 53:550, 1992.

24. Solez K, Axelsen RA, Benediktsson H, et al: International standardization of criteria for the histologic diagnosis of renal allograft rejection: The Banff working classification of kidney transplant pathology. *Kidney Int* 44:411, 1993.

25. Basadonna G, Matas AJ, Gillingham KT, et al: Early versus late acute renal allograft rejection: Impact on chronic rejection. *Transplantation* 55:993, 1993.

26. Reinsmoen NL, Matas AJ: Improved late renal transplant outcome correlates with the development of in vitro donor antigen-specific hyporesponsiveness. *Transplantation* 55:1017, 1993.

27. Hayry P, von Willebrand E: Practical guidelines for fine needle aspiration biopsy of human renal allografts. *Ann Clin Res* 13:288, 1981.

28. Egidi F: Fine needle aspiration biopsy. *Contr Nephrol* 69:81, 1989.

29. Egidi F: Fine needle aspiration biopsy in renal transplantation. *Diag Cytopathol* 6:330, 1990.

30. Cosimi AB: OKT3: First dose safety and success. *Nephron* 46(Suppl 1):12, 1987.

31. Ngheim D, Gonwa TA, Corry RJ: Metabolic monitoring in renal-pancreatic transplants with urinary pancreatic exocrine drainage. *Transplant Proc* 19:2350, 1987.

32. Prieto M, Collins W, Scott MH, et al: Method for home monitoring of urinary amylase after pancreas transplantation. *Diabetes* 38(Suppl. 1):68, 1989.

33. McMaster P: The diagnosis and treatment of pancreatic rejection, in Dubenard JM, Sutherland DER (eds): *International Handbook of Pancreas Transplantation.* Boston, Kluwer Academic Publishers, 1989, pp 187–202.

34. Allen RDM, Wilson TG, Grierson JM, et al: Percutaneous biopsy of bladder drained pancreas transplants. *Transplantation* 51:1213, 1991.

35. Pekins JD, Munn SR, Narsh CL, et al: Safety and efficacy of cystoscopically directed biopsy in pancreatic transplantation. *Trans Proc* 22:665, 1990.

36. Brayman KL, Moss A, Morel P, et al: Exocrine dysfunction evaluation of bladder-drained pancreaticoduodenal transplants using a transcystoscopic biopsy technique. *Transplant Proc* 24:901, 1992.

37. Nakhleh RE, Gruesner RW, Swanson PE, et al: Pancreas transplant pathology. A morphologic, immunohistochemical, and electron microscope comparison of allogeneic grafts with rejection, syngeneic grafts and chronic pancreatitis. *Am J Surg Pathol* 15:246, 1991.

38. Perkel M, Marks W, Lorber M, et al: A three year experience with serum anodal trypsinogen as a biochemical marker for rejection in pancreatic allografts. *Transplantation* 53:415, 1992.

39. Georgi BA, Dempsey RA, Corry RJ: Interleukin-2 assay in serum and urine as a means of monitoring pancreatic allograft rejection. *Transplant Proc* 21:2784, 1989.

40. Allen RDM, Wilson TG, Grierson JM, et al: Percutaneous pancreas transplant fine needle aspiration and needle core biopsies are useful and safe. *Transplant Proc* 22:663, 1990.

41. Yuh WTC, Wiese JA, Slur-Yousef MM, et al: Pancreatic transplant imagery. *Radiology* 167:679, 1988.

42. Contis J, O'Connor T, Holland G, et al: Noninvasive evaluation of bladder drained whole pancreaticoduodenal transplants with magnetic resonance angiography. *Transplant Proc* 1993. (In Press).

43. Reyes J, Tzakis A, Zeevi A, et al: Chimerism and the frequent achievement of a drug free state after orthotopic liver transplantation. (abstract) American Society of Transplant Surgeons. I-5, p 39, 1993.

44. Mor E, Solomon H, Gibbs JF, et al: Acute cellular rejection following liver transplantation: Clinical pathologic features and effect on outcome. *Sem Liver Dis* 12:28, 1992.

45. Demetris AJ, Jaffe R, Tzakis A, et al: Antibody mediated rejection of human orthotopic liver allografts: A study of liver transplantation across ABO blood group barrier. *Am J Pathol* 132:489, 1988.

46. Demetris AJ: The pathology of liver transplantation, in: *Progress in Liver Diseases,* 9:687, 1990.

47. Adams DH, Neuberger JM: Treatment of acute rejection. *Sem Liver Dis* 12:80, 1992.

48. Klintinalm GB, Nevy JR, Husberg BS, et al: Rejection in liver transplantation. *Hepatology* 10:978, 1989.

49. Colina F, Mollejo M, Moreno E, et al: Effectiveness of histopathological diagnoses in dysfunction of hepatic transplantation. *Arch Pathol Lab Med* 115:998, 1991.

50. Schlitt HJ, Nashan B, Ringe B, et al: Differentiation of liver graft dysfunction by transplant aspiration cytology. *Transplantation* 51:786, 1991.

51. Roberti I, Lieberman KV, Manzarbeitia C, et al: Evidence that the systemic analysis of bile cytology permits monitoring of hepatic allograft rejection. *Transplantation* 54:471, 1992.

52. United States Multicenter FK506 Liver Study Group: Use of Prograf (FK506) as rescue therapy for refractory rejection after liver transplantation. *Transplant Proc* 25:679, 1993.

53. Dousset B, Hubscher SG, Padbury RTA, et al: Acute liver allograft rejection—Is treatment always necessary? *Transplantation* 55:529, 1993.

54. Schlitt HJ, Nashan B, Krick P, et al: Intragraft immune events after human liver transplantation. *Transplantation* 54:273, 1992.

55. Mor E, Gonwa TA, Husberg BS, et al: Late-onset acute rejection in orthotopic liver transplantation—Associated risk factors and outcome. *Transplantation* 54:821, 1992.

56. Freese DK, Snover DC, Sharp HL, et al: Chronic rejection after liver transplantation: A study of clinical, histopathological and immunological features. *Hepatology* 13:882, 1991.

57. Van Hoek B, Wiesner RH, Krom RAF, et al: Severe ductopenic rejection following liver transplantation: Incidence, time of onset, risk factors, treatment and outcome. *Sem Liver Dis* 12:41, 1992.

58. United States Multicenter FK506 Liver Study Group: Prognostic factors for successful conversion from cyclosporine to FK506-based immunosuppressive therapy for refractory rejection after liver transplantation. *Transplant Proc* 25:641, 1993.

59. O'Connell JB, Renlund DG: Diagnosis and treatment of cardiac allograft rejection, in ME Thompson (ed): *Cardiac Transplantation.* Philadelphia, F.A. Davis Company, 1990, pp. 147–162.

60. Slater AD, Klein JB, Gray LA, et al: Clinical orthotopic cardiac transplantation. *Am J Surg* 153:582, 1987.

61. Caves PK, Stinson EB, Billingham ME, et al: Percutaneous transvenous endomyocardial biopsy in human heart recipients. *Am J Thorac Surg* 16:325, 1973.

62. Billingham ME: Pathology of the transplanted heart and lung. *Cardiovascular Clinics* 20:71, 1990.

63. Billingham ME, et al: A working formulation for the standardization of nomenclature in the diagnosis of heart and lung rejection: Heart Rejection Study Group. 9:587, 1990

64. Kobashiagawa, J, Stevenson LW: Noninvasive detection of acute cardiac allograft rejection, in Kapoor AS, et al (eds): *Cardiomyopathies and Heart-Lung Transplantation.* McGraw Hill, 1991, pp 293–303.

65. Iturralde MP: Radionuclide imaging procedures in the evaluation of heart transplant recipients, in Kapoor AS, et al (eds): *Cardiomyopathies and Heart-Lung Transplantation.* McGraw Hill, 1991, pp 305–323.

66. Teufelsbauer H, Prischl FC, Havel M, et al: β-Microglobulin: A reliable parameter for differentiating between graft rejection and severe infection after cardiac transplantation. *Circulation* 80:1681, 1989.

67. Nielsen H, Sorensen FB, Nielsen B, et al: Reproducibility of the acute rejection diagnosis in human cardiac allografts. The Stamford Classification and the International Grading System. *J Heart Lung Trans* 12:239, 1993.

68. Gao SZ, Schroeder JS, Alderman EL, et al: Clinical and laboratory correlates of accelerated coronary artery disease in cardiac transplant recipients. *Circulation* 76:(Suppl V)56, 1987.

69. Uretsky BF, Murali S, Reddy PS, et al: Development of coronary artery disease in cardiac transplant recipients receiving immunosuppressive therapy with cyclosporine and prednisone. *Circulation* 76:827, 1987.

70. Gao SZ, Schroeder JS, Alderman EL, et al: Prevalence of accelerated coronary artery disease in heart transplant survivors: Comparison of cyclosporine and azathioprine. *Circulation* 80:(Suppl. 3)100, 1989.

71. Kottke-Marchant K, Ratliff NB: Endomyocardial biopsy: Pathologic findings in cardiac transplant recipients. *Pathology Annual* 25:211, 1990.

72. Schroeder JS, Gao SZ, Alderman EL, et al: A preliminary study of diltiazem in the prevention of coronary artery disease in heart transplant recipients. *N Engl J Med* 328:164, 1993.

73. Griffith BP, Hardesty RL, Armitage JM, et al: Acute rejection of lung allografts with various immunosuppressive protocols. *Ann Thorac Surg* 54:846, 1992.

74. Kaiser LR, Cooper JD: The current status of lung transplantation. *Adv Surg* 25:259, 1992.

75. Youssem SA, Dauber JA, Kennan R, et al: Does histologic acute rejection in lung allografts predict the development of bronchiolitis obliterans? *Transplantation* 52:306, 1991.

76. Higenbottam T, Stewart S, Penketh A, et al: Transbronchial lung biopsy for the diagnosis of rejection in heart-lung transplant patients. *Transplantation* 46:532, 1988.

77. Higenbottam T, Clelland C: Lung rejection after transplantation. *Transplant Review* 5:1, 1991.

78. Herman SJ: Radiologic assessment after lung transplantation. *Clin Chest Med* 11:333, 1990.

79. The Toronto Lung Transplant Group. Unilateral lung transplantation for pulmonary fibrosis. *N Engl J Med* 314:1140, 1986.

80. The International Society of Heart Transplantation: A working formulation for the standardization of nomenclature in the diagnosis of heart and lung rejection: Lung Rejection Study Group. *J Heart Trans* 9:594, 1990.

81. Nakhleh RE, Bolman RM, Henke CA, et al: Lung transplant pathology: A comparative study of pulmonary acute rejection and cytomegaloviral infection. *Am J Surg Pathol* 15:1197, 1991.

82. Sibley RK, Berry GJ, Tazelaar HD, et al: The role of transbronchial biopsies in the management of lung transplant recipients. *J Heart Lung Trans* 12:308, 1993.

83. Paradis IL, Duncan SR, Dauber JH, et al: Distinguishing between infection, rejection, and the adult respiratory distress syndrome after human lung transplantation. *J Heart Lung Transplant* 11:232, 1992.

84. Lawrence EC: Diagnosis and management of lung allograft rejection. *Clin Chest Med* 11:269, 1990.

85. Kirby TJ, Mehta A, Rice TW, et al: Diagnosis and management of acute and chronic lung rejection. *Thorac Card Surg* 4:126, 1992.

86. Scott JP, Higenbottom TW, Clellan C, et al: The natural history of obliterative bronchiolitis. *J Heart Transplant* 9:150, 1990.

87. Youssem SA, Paradis IL, Dauber JH, et al: Pulmonary atherosclerosis in long term human heart-lung transplant recipients. *Transplantation* 47:564, 1989.

88. Brayman KL, Stephanian E, Matas J, et al: Analysis of infectious complications occurring after solid-organ transplantation. *Arch Surg* 127:38, 1992.

89. Hume DM, Merrill JP, Miller BF, et al: Experiences with renal homotransplantation in the human: Report of nine cases. *Science* 34:327, 1955.

90. Rifkind D, Marchioro TL, Waddell WR, et al: Infectious disease associated with renal homotransplantation: I. Incidence, types, and predisposing factors. *JAMA* 189:87, 1964.

91. Fulginiti VA, Scribner R, Groth CG, et al: Infections in recipients of liver homografts. *N Engl J Med* 279:619, 1968.

92. Ho M, Wajszczuk CP, Hardy A, et al: Infections in kidney, heart, and liver transplant recipients on cyclosporine. *Transplant Proc* 15:2768, 1983.

93. Green M, Tzakis A, Scantlebury V, et al: Infectious complications of pediatric liver transplantation under FK506. Abstract of the 1990 ICAAC. p 169.

94. Dunn DL, Najarian JS: Infectious complications in transplant surgery in *Principles and Management of Surgical Infection.* Philadelphia, J.B. Lippincott, 1990, pp 425–464.

95. Gottesdiener KM: Transplanted infections: Donor-to-host transmission with the allograft. *Ann Intern Med* 110:1001,

96. Pereira BJG, Milford EL, Kirkman RL, et al: Prevalence of hepatitis C virus RNA in organ donors positive for hepatitis C antibody and in the recipients of their organs. *N Engl J Med* 327:910, 1992.

97. Roth D, Fernandez JA, Babischkin S, et al: Detection of hepatitis C virus infection among cadaver organ donors: Evidence for low transmission of disease. *Ann Intern Med* 117:470, 1992.

97a. Brennan PJ: unpublished data.

98. Tilney NL, Strom TB, Vineyard GC, et al: Factors attributing to the declining mortality rate in renal transplantation. *N Engl J Med* 299:1321, 1978.

99. Tillegard A: Renal transplant wound infection: The value of prophylactic antibiotic treatment. *Scand J Urol Nephrol* 18:215, 1984.

100. Tolkoff-Rubin NE, Cosimi AB, et al: A controlled study of trimethoprim-sulfamethoxazole prophylaxis of urinary tract infection in renal transplant recipients. *Rev Infect Dis* 4:614, 1982.

101. Fox BC, Sollinger HW, Belzer FO, et al: A prospective, randomized, double-blind study of trimethoprim-sulfamethoxazole for prophylaxis of infection in renal transplantation: Clinical efficacy, absorption of trimethoprim-sulfamethoxazole, effects on the microflora, and the cost-benefit of prophylaxis. *Am J Surg* 89:255, 1990.

102. Higgins RM, Bloom SL, Hopkin JM, et al: The risks and benefits of low-dose cotrimoxazole prophylaxis for *Pneumocystis* pneumonia in renal transplantation. *Transplantation* 47:558, 1989.

103. Peters C, Peterson P, Marabella P, et al: Continuous sulfa prophylaxis for urinary tract infection in renal transplant recipients. *Am J Med* 146:589, 1983.

104. Peterson PK, Gerfuson R, Fyrd DS, et al: Infectious disease in hospitalized renal transplant recipients: A prospective study of a complex and evolving problem. *Medicine* 61:360, 1982.

105. Paya CV, Hermans PE, Washington JA, et al: Incidence, distribution, and outcome of episodes of infection in 100 orthotopic liver transplantations. *Mayo Clin Proc* 64:555, 1989.

106. Cuervas-Mons V, Barrios C, Garrido A, et al: Bacterial infections in liver transplant patients under selective decontamination with norfloxacin. *Transplant Proc* 21:3558, 1989.

107. Pirsch JD, Armbrust MJ, Stratta RJ, et al: Perioperative infection in liver transplant recipients under a quadruple immunosuppressive protocol. *Transplant Proc* 21:3559, 1989.

108. Colonna JO, Winston DJ, Brill JE, et al: Infectious complications in liver transplantation. *Arch Surg* 123:360, 1988.

109. Kusne S, Dummer JS, Singh H, et al: Infections after liver transplantation. An analysis of 101 consecutive cases. *Medicine* 67:132, 1988.

110. Rubin RH, Tolkoff-Rubin NE: Antimicrobial strategies in the care of organ transplant recipients. *Antimicrobial Agents and Chemotherapy* 37:619, 1993.

111. Mora NP, Klintmalm G, Solomon H, et al: Selective amphotericin B prophylaxis in the reduction of fungal infections after liver transplant. *Transplant Proc* 24:154, 1992.

112. Wiesner RH: The incidence of gram-negative bacterial and fungal infections in liver transplant patients treated with selective decontamination. *Infection* 18(Suppl. 1):S19, 1990.

113. Wiesner RH, Hermans PE, Rakela J, et al: Selective bowel decontamination to decrease gram-negative aerobic bacterial and candida colonization and prevent infection after orthotopic liver transplantation. *Transplantation* 45:570, 1988.

114. Dummer JS, Montero CG, Griffith BP, et al: Infections in heart-lung transplant recipients. *Transplantation* 41:725, 1986.

115. DeHoyos A, Maurer JR: Complications following lung transplantation. *Sem Thorac Cardiovasc Surg* 4:132, 1992.

116. Bubak ME, Porayko MK, Krom RAF, et al: Complications of liver biopsy in liver transplant patients: Increased sepsis associated with choledochojejunostomy. *Hepatology* 14:1063, 1991.

117. Ho M: Human cytomegalovirus infections in immunocompromised patients, in *Cytomegalovirus: Biology and Infection.* 2nd Ed. New York, Plenum Medical Book Co., 1991, pp 249–300.

118. Meyers JD, Wade JC, Mitchell CD, et al: Multicenter collaborative trial of intravenous acyclovir for treatment of mucocutaneous herpes simplex virus infection in the immunocompromised host. *Am J Med* 73:229, 1982.

119. Balfour HH, Bean B, Laskin OL, et al: Acyclovir halts progression of herpes zoster in immunocompromised patients. *N Engl J Med* 308:1448, 1983.

120. Michaels M, Green M, Wald E, et al: Adenovirus infection in pediatric orthotopic liver transplant recipients. *J Infect Dis* 165:170, 1992.

121. Koneru B, Jaffe R, Esquivel CO, et al: Adenoviral infections in pediatric liver transplant recipients. *JAMA* 258:489, 1987.

122. Erice A, Aleja, Rhone FS, et al: Human immunodeficiency virus infection in patients with solid organ transplants: Report of five cases and review. *J Infect Dis* 13:537, 1991.

123. Snydman: Cytomegalovirus infection in solid organ transplantation. *Transplant Rev* 4:59, 1990.

124. Weir HR, Henry ML, Blackmore M, et al: Incidence and morbidity of cytomegalovirus disease associated with a seronegative recipient receiving seropositive donor specific transfusion and living related donor transplantation. *Transplantation* 45:111, 1988.

125. Rubin RH: Impact of cytomegalovirus infection on organ transplant recipients. *Rev Infect Dis* 12(Suppl. 7):S754, 1990.

126. Hibberd PL, Tolkoff-Rubin NE, Cosimi AB, et al: Symptomatic cytomegalovirus disease in the cytomegalovirus antibody seropositive renal transplant recipient treated with OKT3. *Transplantation* 53:68, 1992.

127. Hardy AM, Wajszczuk CP, Suffredini AF: *Pneumocystis carinii* pneumonia in renal-transplant recipients treated with cyclosporine and steroids. *J Infect Dis* 149:143, 1984.

128. Paya CV, Hermans PE, Wiesner RH, et al: Cytomegalovirus hepatitis in liver transplantation: Prospective analysis of 93 consecutive orthotopic liver transplantations. *J Infect Dis* 160:752, 1989.

129. Ho M: Virological diagnosis and infections in cells and tissues, in *Cytomegalovirus: Biology and Infection*. 2nd Ed. New York, Plenum Medical Book Co., 1991, pp 75–100.

130. Koskinen PK, Nieminen MS, Matlila SP, et al: The correlation between symptomatic CMV infection and CMV antigenemia in heart allograft recipients. *Transplantation* 55:547, 1993.

131. The TH, van der Big W, van der Berg AP: Cytomegalovirus antigenemia. *Rev Infect Dis* 12(Suppl.7):S737, 1990.

132. van der Berg AP, van der Big W, van Son WJ, et al: Cytomegalovirus antigenemia as a useful marker of symptomatic cytomegalovirus infection after renal transplantation—A report of 130 consecutive patients. *Transplantation* 48:991, 1989.

133. Delgado R, Lumbreras C, Alba C, et al: Low predictive value of polymerase chain reaction for diagnosis of cytomegalovirus disease in liver transplant recipients. *J Clin Microbiol* 30:1876, 1992.

134. Bitsch A, Kirchner H, Dupke R: Cytomegalovirus transcripts in peripheral blood leukocytes of actively infected transplant patients detected by reverse transcription-polymerase chain reaction. *J Infect Dis* 167:740, 1993.

135. Ho M: Pathology of cytomegalovirus infection, in *Cytomegalovirus: Biology and Infection*. 2nd Ed. New York, Plenum Medical Book Co., 1991, pp 189–204.

136. Dupont B: Itraconazole therapy in aspergillosis: Study in 4 patients. *J Am Acad Dermatol* 23:607, 1990.

137. Lautenschlager I, Abonen J, Eklund B, et al: Hyperimmune globulin therapy of clinical cytomegalovirus infection in renal allograft recipients. *Scand J Infec Dis* 21:139, 1989.

138. Erise A, Chou S, Byron KK, et al: Progressive disease due to ganciclovir-resistant cytomegalovirus in immunocompromised patients. *N Engl J Med* 320:289, 1989.

139. Drew WL, Miner RC, et al: Prevalence of resistance in patients receiving ganciclovir for serious cytomegalovirus infection. *J Infect Dis* 163:716, 1991.

140. Jacobsen MA, Drew WF, Feinberg J, et al: Foscarnet therapy for ganciclovir-resistant cytomegalovirus retinitis in AIDS. *J Infect Dis* 163:1348, 1991.

141. Balfour HH: Options for prevention of cytomegalovirus disease. *Ann Intern Med* 114:598, 1991.

142. Balfour HH, Chace BA, Stapleton JT, et al: A randomized, placebo-controlled trial of oral acyclovir for the prevention of cytomegalovirus disease in recipients of renal allografts. *N Engl J Med* 320:1381, 1989.

143. Martin M: Cytomegalovirus prophylaxis in solid organ transplantation. *Transplant Sci* 2:83, 1992.

144. Dunn DL, Mayoral JL, Gillingham KJ, et al: Treatment of invasive cytomegalovirus disease in solid organ transplant patients with ganciclovir. *Transplantation* 51:98, 1991.

145. Dunn DL, Gillingham KJ, Kramer MA, et al: A prospective randomized study of acyclovir versus ganciclovir plus human immune globulin prophylaxis of CMV infection after solid organ transplantation. *Transplantation* (Submitted).

146. Mericon TC, et al: A controlled trial of ganciclovir to prevent CMV disease after heart transplantation. *N Engl J Med* 326:1182, 1992.

147. Plotkin, SA, Starr SE, Friedman HM, et al: Effect of Towne live virus vaccine on cytomegalovirus disease after renal transplantation. *Ann Intern Med* 114:525, 1991.

148. Dar MA, Ahmed M, Weinstein AJ, et al: Thoracic aspergillosis. *Clev Clin Q* 51:615, 1984.

149. Burno-Murtha L, Sugar AM: Emerging agents of the treatment of invasive fungal-infections in transplant patients: An outlook for the future. *Transplant Sci* 100, 1992.

150. Denning DW, Tucker RM, Hanson LG, et al: Treatment of invasive aspergillosis with itraconazole. *Am J Med* 86:791, 1989.

151. van't Wout JW, Novakova I, Verhagen CA, et al: The efficacy of itraconazole against systemic fungal infections in neutropenic patients: A randomized comparative study with amphotericin B. *J Inf* 22:45, 1991.

152. Castaldo P, Stratta RJ, Wood RP, et al: Clinical spectrum of fungal infections after orthotopic liver transplantation. *Arch Surg* 126:149, 1991.

153. Wajszccyuk CP, Dummer JS, Ho M, et al: Fungal infections in liver transplant recipients. *Transplantation* 40:347, 1985.

154. Hooper DC, Pruitt AA, Rubin RH: Central nervous system infection in the chronically immunosuppressed. *Medicine* 61:166, 1982.

155. Hofflin JM, Potasman I, Baldwin JC, et al: Infectious complications in heart transplant recipients receiving cyclosporine and corticosteroids. *Ann Intern Med* 106:209, 1987.

156. Wilson CB, Remington JS: Toxoplasmosis, in Feigin RD, Cheng JD (eds): *Textbook of Pediatric Infectious Diseases*. 3rd Ed. Philadelphia, W.B. Saunders, 1992, pp 2057–2069.

157. Hanto DW, Shelton MW, and Simmons RL: Malignancies after organ transplantation, in Paul LC, Solez K (eds): *Organ Transplantation Long Term Results*. New York, Marcel Dekker, 1992, pp 319–351.

158. Shiel AGR, Disney APS, Matthew TH, et al: De novo malignancy emerges as a major cause of morbidity and late failure in renal transplantation. *Transplant Proc* 25:1383, 1993.

159. Penn, I: Risk of cancer in the transplant patient, in Flye MW (ed): *Principles of Organ Transplantation*. Philadelphia, W.B. Saunders, 1989, pp 634–643.

160. Hardie IR, Strong RW, Hartley CCJ, et al: Skin cancer in caucasian renal allograft recipients living in a subtropical climate. *Surgery* 87:177, 1980.

161. Euvrard S, Chardonnet Y, Pouteil-Noble CP, et al: Skin malignancies and human papillomavirus in renal transplant recipients. *Transplant Proc* 25:1392, 1993.

162. McAlister V, Grant D, Roy A, et al: Posttransplant lymphoproliferative disorders in liver recipients treated with OKT3 or ALG induction immunosuppression. *Transplant Proc* 25:1400, 1993.

163. Starzl TE: The diagnosis and treatment of posttransplant lymphoproliferative disorders. *Current Prob Surg* 25:371, 1988.

164. Stieber AC, Boillot C, Scotti-Foglieni C, et al: The surgical implications of the posttransplant lymphoproliferative disorders. *Transplant Proc* 23:1477, 1991.

165. Malatack JJ, Gartner JC, Urbach AH, et al: Orthotopic liver transplantation, Epstein-Barr virus, cyclosporine, and lymphoproliferative disease: A growing concern. *J Pediatr* 118:667, 1991.

166. Renard TH, Andrews WS, Foster ME: Relationship between OKT3 administration, EBV seroconversion and the lymphoproliferative syndrome in pediatric liver transplant recipients. *Transplant Proc* 23:1473, 1991.

167. Solomon H, Gonwa TA, Mor E, et al: OKT3 rescue for steroid resistant rejection in adult liver transplantation. *Transplantation* 55:87, 1993.

168. Ho M, Jaffe R, Miller G, et al: The frequency of Epstein-Barr virus infection and associated lymphoproliferative syndrome after transplantation and its manifestations in children. *Transplantation* 45:719, 1988.

169. Sheil AGR, Disney APS, Matthew TH, et al: De novo malignancy emerges as a major cause of morbidity and late failure in renal transplantation. *Transplant Proc* 25:1383, 1993.

170. Allday MJ, Crawford DH: Role of epithelium in EBV persistence and pathogenesis of B-cell tumors. *Lancet* 855, 1988.

171. Ho M: Infection and organ transplantation, in Gelman S (ed): *Anesthesia and Organ Transplantation*. Philadelphia, W.B. Saunders, 1987, pp 49–60.

172. Sixberg JW, Nedrud JG, Raab-Traub N, et al: Epstein-Barr virus replication in oropharyngeal epithelial cells. *N Engl J Med* 310:1225, 1984.

173. Rickinson AB, Epstein MA, Crawford DH: Absence of Epstein-Barr virus in blood in acute infectious mononucleosis. *Nature* 258:236, 1975.

174. Yao QY, Rickinson AB, Epstein MA: A re-examination of the Epstein-Barr virus carrier state in healthy seropositive individuals. *Int J Cancer* 35:35, 1985.

175. Cheeseman, SH, Henle W, Rubin RH, et al: Epstein-Barr virus infection in renal transplant recipients. *Ann Intern Med* 93:39, 1980.

176. Hanto DW, Frizzera G, Gaji-Peczalska KJ, et al: Epstein-Barr virus, immunodeficiency, and B cell lymphoproliferation. *Transplantation* 39:461, 1985.

177. Spiro IJ, Yandell DW, Li C, et al: Brief report: Lymphoma of donor origin occurring in the porta hepatis of a transplanted liver. *N Engl J Med* 329:27, 1993.

178. Hjelle B, Evans-Holm M, Yen TSB, et al: A poorly differentiated lymphoma of donor origin in a renal allograft recipient. *Transplantation* 47:945, 1989.

179. Medure G, Fromenti L, Vieilleford A, et al: Donor-related non-Hodgkin's lymphoma in a renal allograft recipient. *Transplant Proc* 23:2649, 1991.

180. Sculerati N, Arriaga M: Otolaryngologic management of posttransplant lymphoproliferative disease in children. *Ann Otol Rhinol Laryngol* 99:445, 1990.

181. Dodd GD, Ledesma-Mediver J, Baron RL: Posttransplant lymphoproliferative disorder: Intrathoracic manifestations. *Radiology* 11184:65, 1992.

182. Montone KT, Friedman H, Hodinka RL, et al: In situ hybridization for Epstein-Barr virus not I repeats in posttransplant lymphoproliferative disorder. *Mod Pathol* 5:292, 1992.

183. Katz BZ, Raab-Traub N, Miller G: Latent and replicating forms of Epstein-Barr virus DNA in lymphomas and lymphoproliferative diseases. *J Infec Dis* 160:589, 1989.

184. Hanto DW, Frizzera G, Gajl-Peczalska, KL, et al: Acyclovir therapy of Epstein-Barr virus-induced posttransplant lymphoproliferative diseases. *Transplant Proc* 17:89, 1985.

185. Fischer A, Blanche S, LeBidois J, et al: Anti-B cell monoclonal antibodies in the treatment of severe B-cell lymphoproliferative syndrome following bone marrow and organ transplantation. *N Engl J Med* 324:1451, 1991.

186. Shapiro R, Chauvenet A, McGuire W, et al: Treatment of B-cell lymphoproliferative disorders with interferon alfa and intravenous gamma globulin. *N Engl J Med* 318:1334, 1988.

187. Busnach G, Civati G, Brando B, et al: Viral and neoplastic changes of the lower genital tract in women with renal allografts. *Transplant Proc* 25:1389, 1993.

188. Alloub MI, Barr BBB, McLaren KM, et al: Papillomavirus infection and cervical intraepithelial neoplasia in women with renal allografts. *Br Med J* 298:153, 1989.

189. Qunibi WY, Barri Y, Alfurayh O, et al: Kaposi's sarcoma in renal transplant recipients: A report on 26 cases from a single institution. *Transplant Proc* 25:1402, 1993.

190. Horn M, Phebus C, Blatt J: Cancer chemotherapy after solid organ transplantation. *Cancer* 66:1468, 1990.

191. Penn I: Effect of immunosuppression on preexisting cancers. *Transplant Proc* 25:1380, 1993.

192. Penn I: Hepatic transplantation for primary metastatic cancers of the liver. *Surgery* 110:726, 1991.

193. Colquhoun S, Shaked A, Rosenthol T, et al: Transmission of CNS malignancy by organ transplantation (abstract). 111-9:101, 1993.

XV. Metabolism and Nutrition

Section Editor
Frank B. Cerra

199. The Multiple Organ Dysfunction Syndrome

Stephen O. Heard, Mitchell P. Fink, and Frank B. Cerra

The past two decades have witnessed dramatic improvements in the initial resuscitation and subsequent management of critically ill patients. These therapeutic advances have substantially decreased the incidence of early death due to cardiovascular collapse or the acute respiratory distress syndrome (ARDS) in patients with sepsis, massive hemorrhage, major trauma, necrotizing pancreatitis, and other acute, serious medical and surgical conditions. Nevertheless, patients sustaining a variety of acute insults often develop a syndrome characterized by progressive deterioration in the function of multiple organ systems, a phenomenon that has been termed the "multiple organ dysfunction syndrome" (MODS) [1,2,3]. MODS is the leading cause of mortality among patients requiring care in a surgical intensive care unit (ICU) [1]. The financial costs attributable to MODS are enormous. The mean length of ICU stay for patients with MODS is 21 days [1]. For survivors, total hospital and rehabilitation costs average $385,000 [1]. The emotional costs for patients and families are incalculable.

Attention was first drawn to MODS by Skillman et al. [4], who described the concurrence of respiratory failure, sepsis, and jaundice in ICU patients following hemorrhage due to erosive gastritis. Tilney et al. [5] noted that sequential organ system failure was a common occurrence after apparently successful repair of ruptured abdominal aortic aneurysms. Although several subsequent reports stressed the relationship between "uncontrolled" sepsis and remote organ system dysfunction [6–9], it is currently apparent that infection is only one of several factors underlying the development of MODS (see following).

Epidemiology and Prognostication

The pattern for the evolution of MODS is apparently independent of the initiating insult. Respiratory failure (i.e., ventilator-dependence and widened alveolar–arterial PO_2 gradient) is almost always present initially, whereas the timing of the onset of dysfunction of other organ systems is variable [10,11]. Not all organ systems are necessarily involved, and, for organs that are dysfunctional, the magnitude of physiologic derangement is variable. In addition to respiratory failure, common clinical manifestations of MODS include azotemia, hyperbilirubinemia, ileus, thrombocytopenia, and altered mental status (Table 199-1) [10–14].

Although the development of MODS is usually preceded by a period of hemodynamic instability, the precise risk factors for the development of the syndrome remain poorly defined. Factors known to increase the risk of MODS include the degree of initial physiologic derangement, age 65 years or more, and presence of a "nonoperative diagnosis" (e.g., sepsis or cardiac arrest) [13,14]. Risk factors for the development of ARDS (an important component of MODS) include sepsis, aspiration of gastric contents, multiple blood transfusions, and pulmonary contusion [15,16]. Other factors that may predict the development of MODS are calculated oxygen debt (see following) [17]

and circulating levels of several substances, including neopterin (a macrophage product) [18], elastase-alpha$_1$ protease complex [19], C5a [20], and lipopolysaccharide (LPS) [21,22,23].

The derangements in organ function observed during MODS are a continuum rather than discrete events signalling the failure of a particular organ. However, research evaluating patient outcome during MODS has focused on organ failure rather than dysfunction. Thus, outcome in MODS has been found to be determined both by the number of failed organ systems and the duration of organ system failure [13]. In one study, the death rate was 22 percent for patients with single organ system failure lasting less than 24 hours, but after 7 days of single organ failure, the death rate increased to 41 percent [13]. The death rate was 80 percent when three or more organs were dysfunctional for less than 24 hours and increased to 100 percent when three or more organs were dysfunctional for over 4 days.

Pathophysiology

The development of MODS tends to occur in patients with a constellation of signs, symptoms, and laboratory abnormalities that are indicative of a generalized inflammatory response. This systemic inflammatory response syndrome (SIRS) [3] commonly occurs as a result of infection, although other conditions, such as necrotizing pancreatitis, severe trauma, or even salicylate toxicity [24] also can lead to systemic manifestations of poorly controlled inflammation. According to the parlance recently adopted by the American College of Chest Physicians and the Society of Critical Care Medicine, SIRS due to infection is referred to as "sepsis" [3]. Although documented infection is not a prerequisite for the development of MODS, SIRS, sepsis, and MODS appear to be closely related phenomena. Hence, a coherent discussion of the pathophysiology of MODS demands that all these syndromes be considered together.

DERANGEMENTS IN OXYGEN DELIVERY AND CONSUMPTION; UNCOUPLING OF OXIDATIVE PHOSPHORYLATION; AEROBIC GLYCOLYSIS; DETERMINANTS OF BLOOD LACTATE CONCENTRATION. In many tissues, O_2 consumption (VO_2) is determined by metabolic demand rather than O_2 delivery (DO_2). When DO_2 is reduced by a moderate amount, VO_2 is maintained by increased O_2 extraction. VO_2 becomes "supply-dependent" when DO_2 is reduced to such an extent that extraction is maximized (Fig. 199-1). The point at which VO_2 becomes supply-dependent is called the critical DO_2. In anesthetized humans, the critical DO_2 is approximately 330 ml per minute per square meter [25,26].

Tissues (or species) that manifest a biphasic relationship between DO_2 and VO_2, such as the one depicted in Figure 199-1, have been called "oxygen regulators" [27]. In some tissues, such as skeletal muscle [28,29], VO_2 is determined by oxygen availability over a wide range of values for the latter parameter. Such

Table 199-1. Definitions of Individual Organ System Failure (OSF)

If the patient has one or more of the following during a 24-hour period (regardless of other values), OSF exists on that day.

I. Cardiovascular failure (presence of one or more of the following):
   A. Heart rate ≤ 54/min
   B. Mean arterial blood pressure ≤ 49 mm Hg
   C. Occurrence of ventricular tachycardia and/or ventricular fibrillation
   D. Serum pH ≤ 7.24 with a $PaCO_2$ of ≤ 49 mm Hg

II. Respiratory failure (presence of one or more of the following):
   A. Respiratory rate ≤ 5/min or ≥ 49/min
   B. $PaCO_2$ ≥ 50 mm Hg
   C. $AaDO_2$ ≥ 350 mm Hg; $AaDO_2 = (713 \cdot FiO_2) - PaCO_2 - PaO_2$
   D. Dependent on ventilator on the fourth day of OSF (i.e., not applicable for the initial 72 hr of OSF)

III. Renal failure (presence of one or more of the following):
   A. Urine output ≤ 479 ml/24 hr or ≤ 159 ml/8 hr
   B. Serum BUN ≥ 100 mg/100 ml
   C. Serum creatinine ≥ 3.5 mg/100 ml

IV. Hematologic failure (presence of one or more of the following):
   A. WBC ≤ 1000 mm³
   B. Platelets ≤ 20,000 mm³
   C. Hematocrit ≤ 20%

V. Neurologic failure
   Glasgow Coma Score ≤ 6 (in absence of sedation at any one point in day)

VI. Liver failure
   A. Prothrombin time > 4 seconds over control (in absence of systemic anticoagulation)
   B. Bilirubin > 6 mg%

Source: From Knaus WA, Wagner DP: Multiple systems organ failure: Epidemiology and prognosis. *Crit Care Clin* 5:221, 1989, with permission.

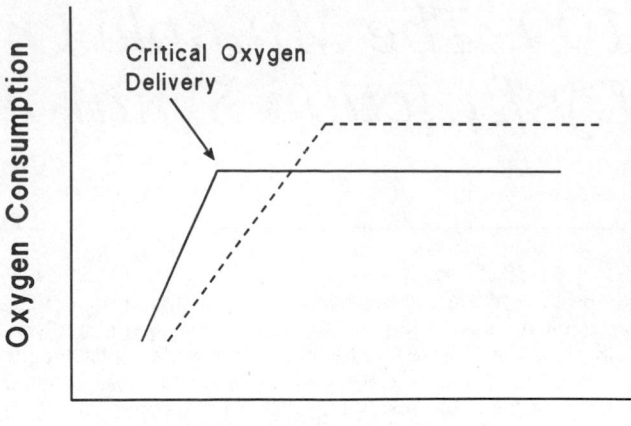

Oxygen Delivery

Fig. 199-1. Oxygen consumption as a function of oxygen delivery. Normally oxygen consumption (solid line) is independent of delivery. The point where O_2 consumption becomes dependent upon O_2 delivery is termed the critical O_2 delivery. The slope of the dependent portion of the curve is equal to the O_2 extraction ratio. In some septic patients (dashed line), oxygen consumption is supply dependent over a wide range of O_2 delivery, and the O_2 extraction ratio is reduced. The supply independent area of the curve is hypothetical and has not been demonstrated in patients with pathologic O_2 supply dependency.

tissues have been termed "oxygen conformers" [27]. Liver expresses an intermediate pattern, such that oxygen regulation is apparent at high rates of DO_2, but oxygen conformation occurs when oxygen availability is limited by only a modest degree [30].

In many patients with sepsis or ARDS, VO_2 is apparently supply-dependent over a wide range of DO_2 values (see Fig. 199-1) [31–48]. Since the relationship between oxygen transport and consumption in critically ill patients *without* sepsis or ARDS is typically one of regulation [41,42], the apparent coupling of these two parameters in patients with sepsis or ARDS has been termed "pathologic supply-dependency" [49].

Despite the large number of studies showing evidence of "pathologic supply-dependency" in patients with sepsis or ARDS, the validity of this concept has been challenged. Recent studies suggest that this phenomenon may be more artifactual than real. In most studies, VO_2 has not been measured directly but has been calculated according to the Fick principle as the product of cardiac output times the difference in oxygen contents between arterial and mixed venous blood. Similarly, DO_2 has been calculated as the product of cardiac output times arterial oxygen content. Thus, relatively small errors in the measurement of either or both of the shared parameters (i.e., arterial oxygen content and cardiac output) will lead to artifactual correlation of VO_2 and DO_2. This methodologic problem, called mathematical coupling [50,51], can be obviated by measuring systemic VO_2 by a method, such as analysis of respiratory gases with a "metabolic cart," which is independent from the means used to calculate systemic DO_2. Using this approach, several studies have found that systemic VO_2 is independent of systemic DO_2 in patients with sepsis or ARDS [52–57] (Fig. 199-2). Indeed, several carefully perfomed studies using the Fick

equation to calculate systemic VO_2 also have failed to find evidence of "pathologic supply-dependency" in patients with sepsis or ARDS [58,59]. Conversely, if mathematical coupling were to account for supply-dependency, it should always be present. Several studies have observed differences in the DO_2–VO_2 relationship between surviving and nonsurviving patients [44]. Further study is needed to clarify the effect that mathematical coupling has on DO_2–VO_2 relationships.

In addition to mathematical coupling, two other methodologic problems have contributed to confusion regarding the issue of "pathologic supply-dependency" of VO_2 in sepsis and ARDS. First, many investigators have performed regression analyses of VO_2 as a function of DO_2 using data pooled from individual experiments in multiple subjects. Analyzing the data in this way ignores the contribution of variability among (rather than within) patients and can lead to overestimation of the dependency of VO_2 on DO_2 [60]. Second, many studies have failed to control adequately for the fact that DO_2 normally tracks VO_2. Spontaneous changes in metabolic demand due, for example, to variations in the degree of sedation of patients can lead to the appearance that VO_2 is "pathologically" dependent on DO_2 when, in actuality, the relationship between these two parameters is physiologic [61,62,63].

In addition to the results obtained from clinical studies, conflicting data regarding the existence of "pathologic" supply dependency in sepsis also have been obtained in studies using animal models of bacteremia or endotoxemia. On the one hand, Shumacker and colleagues have reported that critical DO_2 is increased and maximal oxygen extraction is decreased in septic dogs [49,64,65]. On the other hand, several groups have determined that oxygen extraction is unimpaired in models of sepsis in rats, rabbits, dogs, and pigs [66–69]. Thus, even in animal models, the existence of "pathologic" supply-dependency of oxygen uptake in sepsis remains an open question.

The presence of pathologic supply-dependency has been interpreted as meaning that an oxygen deficit exists at the cel-

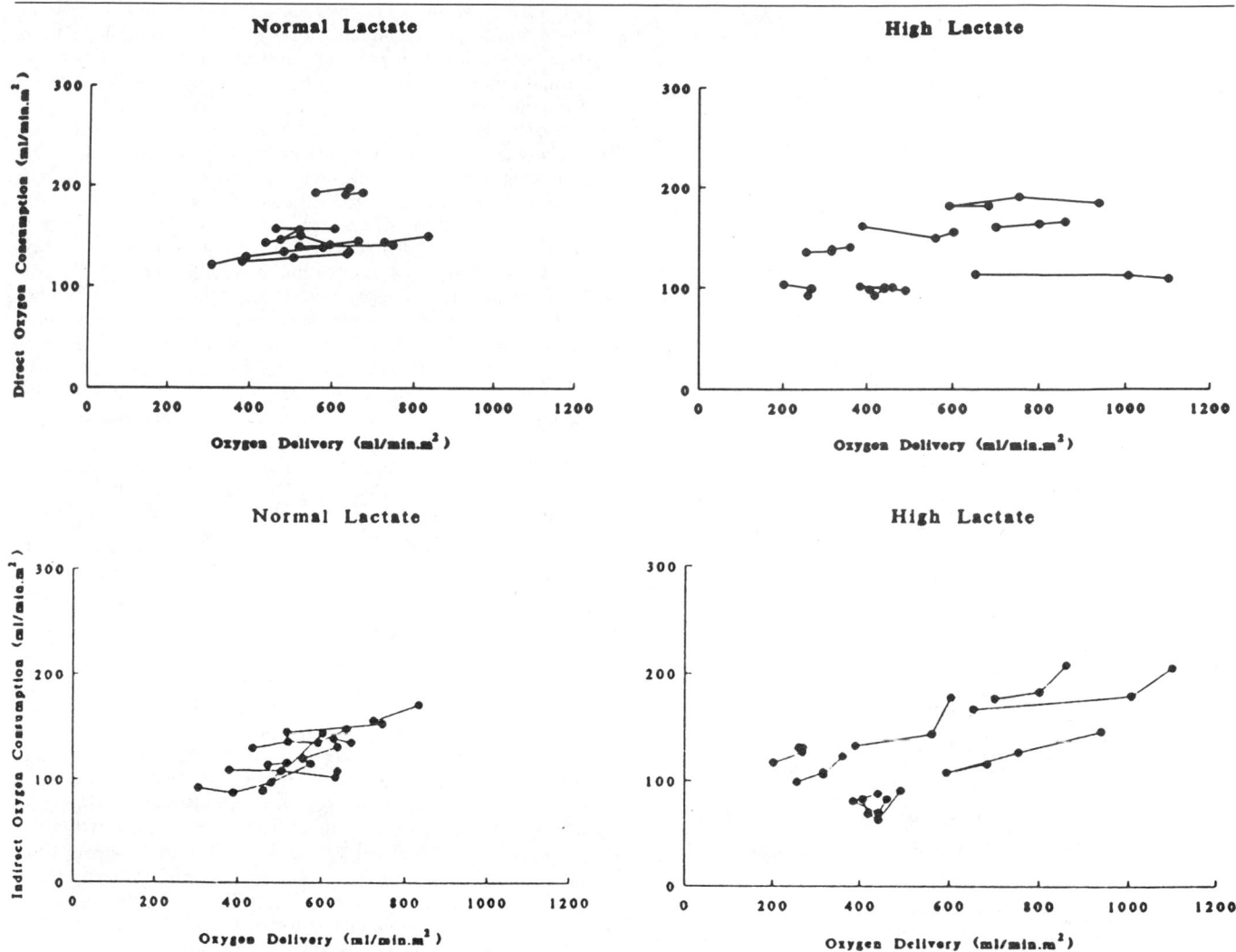

Fig. 199-2. Oxygen consumption as a function of oxygen delivery in critically ill patients with normal or elevated lactate levels. Oxygen consumption in the upper graphs was measured directly with a metabolic chart. No supply dependency is observed in those patients with either normal or elevated lactate concentrations. In contrast, oxygen consumption, measured at the same time using the Fick method, is supply dependent (the lower graphs) irrespective of the lactate levels. (From: Ronco JJ, Fenwick JC, Wiggs BR, et al: Oxygen consumption is independent of increases in oxygen delivery by dobutamine in septic patients who have normal or increased plasma lactate. *Am Rev Resp Dis* 147:25-31, 1993. Reproduced with permission.)

lular level. This notion is supported by studies that indicate that only septic or ARDS patients with elevated blood lactate levels manifest evidence of supply-dependency of VO_2 [35–38]. To the extent that elevated blood lactate levels are indicative of anaerobic metabolism (see following), these data indicate that, in patients with sepsis or MODS, VO_2 is often less than the amount necessary to meet metabolic demand, even when DO_2 is normal or even supranormal. In other words, in sepsis and MODS, some tissues may be relatively ischemic even when global perfusion is preserved. According to this hypothesis, inadequate production of adenosine triphosphate (ATP) (or other high-energy phosphates) at the cellular level may be an important factor leading to organ failure in MODS.

Interestingly, some studies have found that pathologic sup-

ply-dependency of VO_2 occurs only in those septic patients with normal lactate levels [39] or in septic patients irrespective of blood lactate concentration [40]. In addition, metabolic data from studies of sepsis and SIRS following resuscitation are not consistent with the presence of significant anaerobic glycolysis. The observed stoichiometric presence and release of alanine, lactate, and pyruvate and increased oxidation of amino acids and fatty acids indicate a "hyperfunctioning" Krebs cycle, a process referred to as aerobic glycolysis [1,70]. Thus, the relationship between supply-dependency of VO_2 and the presence of (occult) anaerobic metabolism remains uncertain.

One or more of several mechanisms could account for "pathologic" supply-dependency in sepsis and MODS (if it exists). These mechanisms include (1) alterations in vasomotor responsiveness [71–83], leading to derangements in the regulation of regional blood flow, such that some vascular beds are underperfused whereas others are hyperperfused; (2) plugging of capillaries by activated leukocytes and platelets leading to regions of ischemia [84,85]; and (3) deranged microvascular perfusion due to decreased erythrocyte deformability [86,87].

In addition to pathologic supply-dependency of VO_2, uncoupling of mitochondrial oxidative phosphorylation is another factor that may lead to energy starvation at the cellular level in sepsis and MODS. Uncoupling means that ADP is not esterified

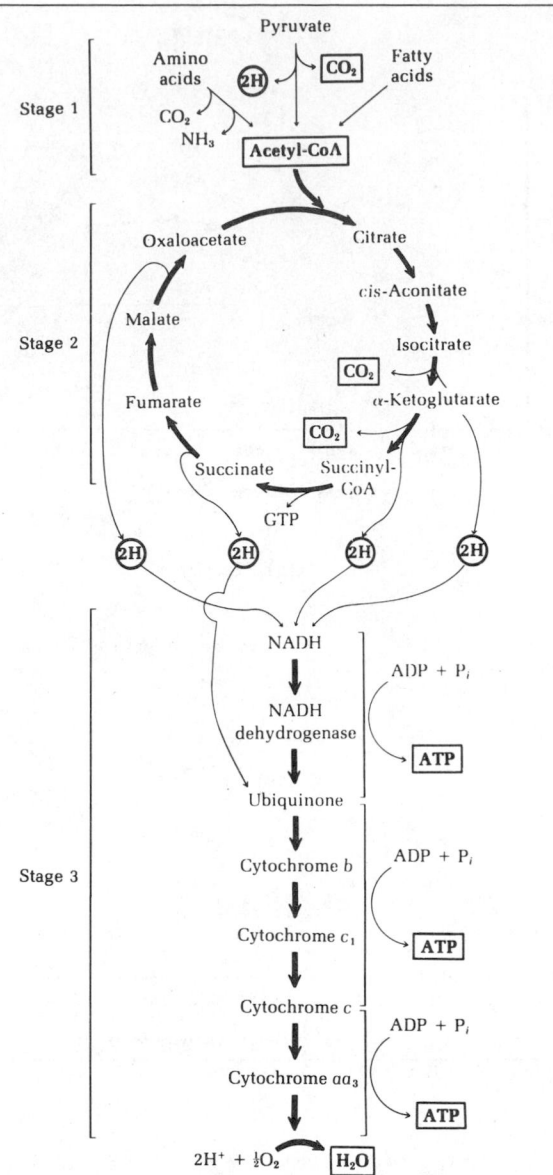

Fig. 199-3. Stages in cell respiration. Stage 1 is the formation of acetyl-CoA from glucose, fatty acids, and amino acids. Stage 2 is the citric acid or Krebs cycle. Stage 3 is electron transport and oxidative phosphorylation. (From Lehninger AL: *Principles of Biochemistry.* New York, Worth Publishers, Inc., 1982, with permission.)

to ATP as normally occurs in mitochondria, although oxygen continues to function as the final electron acceptor for the reducing equivalents (nicotinamide adenine dinucleotide [NADH] and flavin adenine dinucleotide [FADH]) generated by the Krebs cycle (Fig. 199-3). Thus, uncoupling can lead to cellular depletion of ATP despite normal (or typically supranormal) rates of oxygen consumption and can cause tremendous heat production. The existence of this phenomenon in animal or in vitro models of sepsis or endotoxicosis is quite controversial. Some experimental studies have provided evidence of uncoupling of oxidative phosphorylation [88–91], whereas others have not [92–95]. It is unknown whether uncoupling of oxidative phosphorylation occurs in patients with sepsis or MODS. However, the data on energetics during SIRS and MODS following

resuscitation show (1) normal intracellular lactate/pyruvate ratio without excess lactate and a normal stoichiometric relationship between lactate/pyruvate and alanine; (2) a reasonably normal mitochondrial redox state as reflected in the beta-hydroxybutyrate/acetoacetate ratio; (3) increased energy expenditure (by using isotopes and measuring oxidation directly); (4) a relative decrease in glucose oxidation via pyruvate dehydrogenase and proportionate increases in the oxidation of fatty acids and amino acids in the Krebs cycle; and (5) an overactive Cori cycle, which produces much less heat than does uncoupling. These data suggest that uncoupling of oxidative phosphorylation is not present in the patient with SIRS or MODS who has been adequately resuscitated [96].

When oxygen delivery is inadequate to support mitochondrial oxidative phosphorylation, some measure of metabolic compensation is provided by increased anaerobic metabolism through the glycolytic (Embden-Meyerhof) pathway (Fig. 199-4). The end product of this pathway is pyruvate. In addition to generating pyruvate, the flow of glucose through the Embden-Meyerhof pathway generates NADH, which must be oxidized to NAD^+ for reuse in glycolysis. During anaerobic metabolism, pyruvate is converted to lactate, the former serving as a (temporary) electron acceptor (in place of oxygen) for the oxidation of NADH:

$$NADH + pyruvate \rightarrow NAD^+ + lactate$$

During aerobic metabolism of glucose through the Krebs cycle, pyruvate enters the mitochondria and undergoes conversion to acetyl coenzyme A (acetyl-CoA). This reaction is catalyzed by an enzyme complex called pyruvate dehydrogenase (PDH). Since this reaction is the first irreversible step in the mitochondrial oxidative pathway for pyruvate, PDH represents a major control point in carbohydrate metabolism. PDH is capable of existing in either an active (dephosphorylated) or an inactive (phosphorylated) form. Ordinarily the proportion of PDH in the active form is under tight metabolic control. In sepsis, however, there is evidence that an increased proportion of PDH is converted to the inactive form, effectively shunting an increased fraction of pyruvate into lactate formation, even when oxidative metabolism is adequate [97,98,99]. Predictable consequences of this metabolic derangement are increased glucose cycling and elevated blood lactate levels, findings that are often observed in patients with SIRS [100]. Thus, elevated blood lactate levels in sepsis may be indicative of relative tissue ischemia, derangements in carbohydrate metabolism in the absence of ischemia, or both. It is important to remember, however, that elevated lactate levels are not necessarily indicative of anaerobic metabolism. Other causes for increased concentrations of blood lactate include decreased hepatic lactate clearance, increased protein catabolism, increased lactate production by red blood cells, and increased *aerobic* glycolysis [70].

Even if VO_2 is not "pathologically" dependent on DO_2 in patients with ARDS, data exist to support the view that inadequate oxygen utilization is a major factor contributing to the development of MODS in certain high-risk populations. In patients who have suffered major trauma [101], it appears that a systemic VO_2 less than 150 ml per min-M^2 and a blood lactate concentration greater than 2.5 mM per liter at 12 hours following admission are significant independent predictors for the subsequent development of MODS. In high-risk surgical patients, estimated perioperative cumulative oxygen deficits correlate with the development of MODS and death [17]. Thus, an early period of hypoperfusion may be an important factor contributing to the development of MODS, at least in surgical patients. This idea derives further support from two recent studies that suggest the risk of MODS is markedly increased if patients sustain two successive "hits," namely an early episode of severe

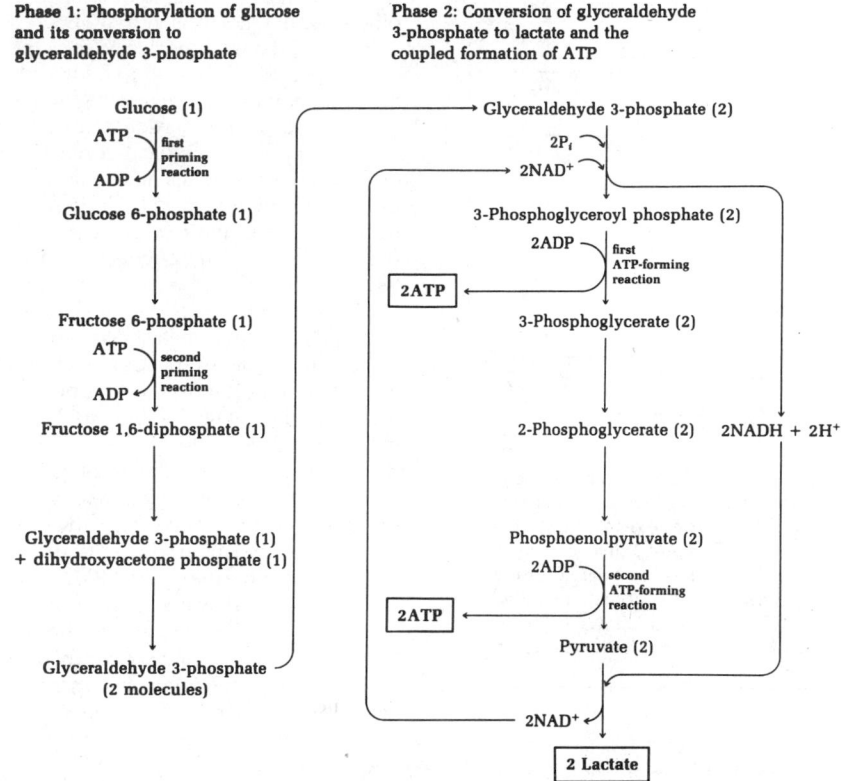

Phase 1: Phosphorylation of glucose and its conversion to glyceraldehyde 3-phosphate

Phase 2: Conversion of glyceraldehyde 3-phosphate to lactate and the coupled formation of ATP

Fig. 199-4. A schematic diagram depicting anaerobic glycolysis. (From Lehninger AL: *Principles of Biochemistry.* New York, Worth Publishers, Inc., 1982, with permission.)

global hypoperfusion (i.e., hemorrhagic or hypovolemic shock) followed by an infectious challenge [102,103].

ROLE OF INFLAMMATORY AND VASOACTIVE MEDIATORS.

As noted previously, early descriptions of MODS stressed the etiologic importance of uncontrolled infection [6–9]. Subsequent clinical series have substantiated the notion that sepsis is a key risk factor for MODS. Nevertheless, it is apparent that MODS complicates the course of many critically ill patients without documented infections. For example, one retrospective study determined that only 33 percent of trauma patients with MODS had evidence of infection [10]. Another study found that infection was absent in 8 percent of patients with ARDS and MODS [12]. It has been proposed that extensive tissue injury (as in trauma or pancreatitis) *and* sepsis are both capable of triggering the systemic release of inflammatory mediators that lead to further tissue injury and MODS [10,104,105,106].

Inflammatory mediators that may be involved in the pathogenesis of MODS include complement-derived peptides, activated neutrophils (and products secreted by them), reactive oxygen species, kinins, vasoactive lipids (e.g., thromboxane A_2, leukotrienes, and platelet-activating factor), cytokines (e.g., tumor necrosis factor and interleukin-1), opioid peptides, and nitric oxide.

Complement, Neutrophils, and Reactive Oxygen Metabolites.

The complement cascade is activated through the classical pathway by antibody-coated targets or antigen–antibody complexes. The complement system also can be activated through the alternative pathway by aggregated immunoglobulins, products of tissue trauma, lipopolysaccharide (LPS), and other complex polysaccharides (e.g., zymosan). C5a, a polypeptide generated as a result of complement activation, causes neutrophil activation and margination [107]. Activated polymorphonuclear leukocytes (PMNLs) are capable of plugging capillaries and damaging endothelium by releasing lysozomal enzymes (e.g., elastase) and toxic oxygen radicals (Table 199-2). The adherence of PMNLs to vascular endothelium requires the participation of a variety of adhesion molecules on both PMNLs and endothelial cells. These receptors include the CD11b/CD18 integrin on PMNLs (also called MAC-1 and CRIII), ICAM-1 on endothelial cells, and several proteins, called selectins, which bind to lectin-like carbohydrate domains on target cells [108,109]. Endotoxin, inflammatory mediators such as tumor necrosis factor-α, and toxic oxygen metabolites induce increased expression of these adhesion molecules and thereby enhance the sequestration of PMNLs in tissues [110–119] (Fig. 199-5).

Considerable data support the notion that complement-mediated activation of neutrophils is important in the pathophysiology of MODS [120,121]. Most studies, whether

Table 199-2. Neutrophil Enzymes and Oxygen Radical Metabolites Capable of Causing Tissue Damage

Myeloperoxidase	Superoxide anion
Lactoferrin	Hydroxyl radical
Lysozyme	Hydrogen peroxide
Elastase	Hypochlorite anion
Collagenase	
Cathepsins B,D,G	

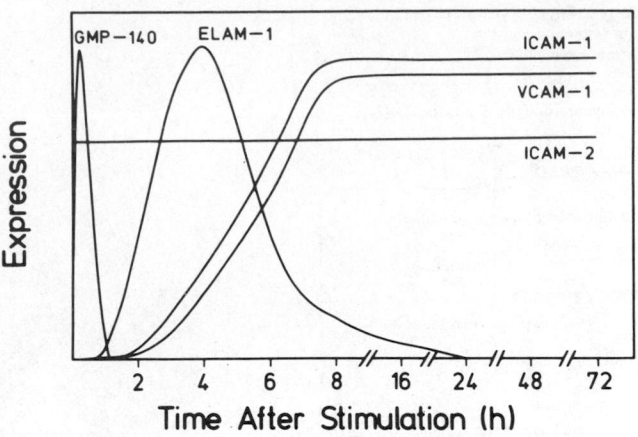

Fig. 199-5. Time course of activation of adhesion molecules on endothelial surfaces by inflammatory mediators such as endotoxin and TNF-α. GMP-140 = granule membrane protein 140; ELAM-1 = endothelial leukocyte adhesion molecule 1; ICAM-1 and -2 = intercellular adhesion molecules 1 and 2; VCAM-1 = vascular cell adhesion molecule 1. (From McEver RP: Role of the endothelium in the inflammatory response, in Taylor RW, Shoemaker WC (eds): *Critical Care: State of the Art.* The Society of Critical Care Medicine (Fullerton, CA), 1991. Reproduced with permission.)

clinical or experimental, have focused on the ARDS component of MODS; this topic is briefly reviewed here, but a more thorough discussion is presented in Chapter 55. Several studies have provided evidence of complement activation in patients with ARDS [20,120–124], and products of complement activation are clearly capable of eliciting an ARDS-like syndrome in experimental animals [125,126,127]. The idea that C5a plays a key role in the pathophysiology of sepsis-induced ARDS is supported by data showing that sepsis-induced acute lung injury is ameliorated in nonhuman primates treated with anti-C5a antibodies [128] and is lessened in mice with a genetic deficiency of C5 [129].

Although ARDS clearly can occur in patients with few circulating neutrophils [130,131], data from numerous clinical studies implicate the PMNL as an important etiologic factor in many cases of acute lung injury [132]. Activation of neutrophils (as evidenced by an increased number of cell surface complement receptors) occurs in burn patients with elevated plasma levels of C3a desArg, a cleavage fragment of C3 [133], and in trauma patients developing ARDS [134]. Scans using intravenous gallium-67 citrate or PMNL labeled with indium-111 suggest that neutrophils accumulate in the lungs of at least some patients with ARDS [135,136]. Furthermore, bronchoalveolar lavage (BAL) fluid from patients with ARDS contains increased numbers of PMNLs as well as elevated levels of several markers of complement or neutrophil activation, including C3a desArg, lactoferrin, and elastase-alpha$_1$-protease inhibitor complexes [124,137–142]. Circulating levels of lactoferrin are also increased in patients with ARDS [143].

These clinical data are supported by results from numerous studies using animal models of ARDS that indicate that neutrophils are important in the pathogenesis of the syndrome [111,115,118,144,145,146]. Nevertheless, the role of the neutrophil in the pathogenesis of ARDS is brought into question by other studies using animal models of acute lung injury that show that neutrophil depletion is without effect [147,148]. Thus, it seems probable that activated neutrophils are only one of several mediators capable of injuring the lung (and presumably other organs) in sepsis and MODS.

Reactive oxygen species (e.g., superoxide radical [O$^-$], hydrogen peroxide [H$_2$O$_2$], and hydroxyl radical [OH$^-$] result from the reduction of molecular oxygen in single electron steps (Fig. 199-6). Hydrogen peroxide can be generated from two molecules of superoxide radical, a reaction that is catalyzed by the enzyme superoxide dismutase. Another enzyme, catalase, promotes the conversion of hydrogen peroxide to water and molecular oxygen. Hydroxyl radical can be generated from superoxide radical and hydrogen peroxide, a process that requires the presence of certain transition metal (especially iron) ions, and is often referred to as the Haber-Weiss reaction.

Reactive oxygen metabolites are capable of injuring tissues by damaging DNA ("nicking"), cross-linking cellular proteins, and, most importantly, causing peroxidation of membrane lipids (see Fig. 199-6) [149]. Lipid peroxidation can diminish membrane fluidity and increase membrane permeability with disastrous effects on cellular integrity and function.

Although reactive oxygen species are generated by a variety of intracellular reactions (e.g., the reaction catalyzed by cyclooxygenase), two main sources of these mediators are implicated in the pathophysiology of MODS: activated PMNLs and xanthine oxidase. Activated PMNLs are capable of generating reactive oxygen species through the reaction catalyzed by nicotinamide adenine dinucleotide phosphate (NADPH) oxidase. In addition, PMNLs contain an enzyme (myeloperoxidase) that catalyzes the reaction of hydrogen peroxide plus chloride anion

Fig. 199-6. The top figure depicts the sequential reduction of molecular oxygen. The bottom figure details the lipid peroxidation reactions initiated by the hydroxyl-radical (PUFA = polyunsaturated fatty acids). (From Southern PA, Powis G: Free radicals in medicine. I. Chemical nature and biologic reactions. *Mayo Clin Proc* 63:381, 1989, with permission.)

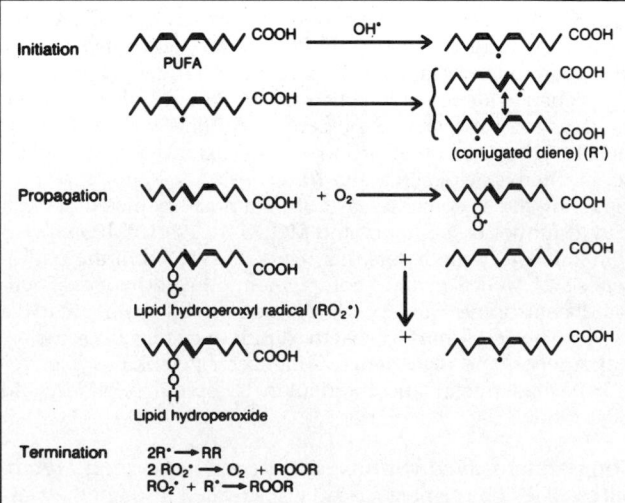

to form hypochlorous acid and water. Hypochlorous acid, the active ingredient in laundry bleach, is a potent oxidizing and chlorinating agent with great potential to damage vital cellular constituents [149]. Under normal conditions, xanthine oxidase exists as a purine dehydrogenase that does not generate free radicals. In ischemic tissues, however, the dehydrogenase form is converted to the oxidase form. The principal substrates for xanthine oxidase are hypoxanthine and xanthine, molecules that are present in high concentration after ischemia as a result of the metabolism of ATP. During *reperfusion,* the delivery of molecular oxygen permits the reactions catalyzed by xanthine oxidase to proceed and leads to the production of reactive oxygen species. Xanthine oxidase is present in a wide variety of tissues, including endothelial cells [150].

Accumulating data from clinical and laboratory studies strongly implicate toxic oxygen metabolites as important pathophysiologic mediators of ARDS. In humans with ARDS, plasma levels of lipid peroxides are elevated [151]. Furthermore, patients with ARDS have reduced levels in plasma or bronchoalveolar lavage fluid of important naturally occurring oxidant scavengers, including vitamin E and reduced glutathione [151,152]. These findings represent circumstantial evidence that ARDS patients have been subjected to "oxidant stress." Interestingly, levels of certain naturally occurring antioxidant substances, including ceruloplasmin, transferrin, catalase, and superoxide dismutase, are increased in plasma or bronchoalveolar lavage fluid from patients with ARDS [153,154,155], possibly reflecting an effort by the body to control the effects of the excessive release of oxidant species.

There is biochemical evidence of lipid peroxidation in plasma and lung in various animal models of acute pulmonary injury [156,157,158]. Moreover, the degree of lipid peroxidation and lung injury can be ameliorated by treatment with various antioxidants, including catalase, flurbiprofen, ibuprofen, or *N*-acetylcysteine [159–164]. Also, beta-agonists, such as dobutamine, can diminish LPS-induced lung lipid peroxidation in sheep, an effect that may be related to the effect of these agents on intracellular levels of cyclic adenosine monophosphate [165]. Despite these promising results in animals, there is a lack of data demonstrating that antioxidant strategies improve outcome in humans with ARDS. Indeed, in a recent randomized, prospective trial, no improvement in key clinical parameters, such as the ratio of PaO_2 to inspired fraction of oxygen, was observed in 32 ARDS patients treated with intravenous *N*-acetylcysteine as compared to 34 patients treated with placebo [166].

Catalase, but not superoxide dismutase or hydroxyl radical scavengers, ameliorates lung injury during ovine endotoxicosis [167,168]. Therefore, it seems likely that acute respiratory dysfunction in this model is mediated, at least in part, by hydrogen peroxide rather than other reactive oxygen species. Additional support for the idea that hydrogen peroxide is a key mediator in acute lung injury derives from recent clinical studies showing that levels of this compound are elevated in the expiratory condensate of mechanically ventilated patients with ARDS [169,170,171].

The role of reactive oxygen species in sepsis and MODS is more controversial than it is in ARDS. Some data suggest that systemic oxidant injury is a key feature of experimental sepsis and endotoxicosis [172–178], hemorrhage [179,180,181], and burn trauma [182,183]. Other data from experimental studies fail to support the notion that oxidant injury is pathophysiologically important in experimental models of MODS caused by sterile peritonitis, sepsis, or endotoxicosis [184,185,186]. There are conflicting clinical data regarding the role of reactive oxygen metabolites in sepsis or MODS per se (as distinguished from

ARDS). In one study, plasma levels of lipid peroxides were elevated and vitamin E was decreased in critically ill patients [187] whereas in another study, there was no evidence of oxidant-induced membrane damage within 2 to 6 hours after injury in a cohort of 43 victims of major blunt trauma [188]. In a recent, prospective, randomized trial, recombinant human superoxide dismutase (rhSOD), administered as a constant infusion for 5 days in patients with multiple trauma, attenuated multiple organ dysfunction, reduced length of ICU stay, and curtailed the release of inflammatory mediators [189]. These encouraging results will need to be confirmed in a larger clinical series.

The Kallikrein-Kinin System. The kallikrein-kinin system is part of the contact system (complement, coagulation, and kallikrein-kinins). LPS, tissue injury, or activated complement activates (Hageman) Factor XII of the intrinsic coagulation pathway. Activated Hageman factor is capable of converting prekallikrein to kallikrein. The latter protein is a proteolytic enzyme that acts on high molecular weight kininogen (HMWK) to form the small, vasoactive peptide, bradykinin (BK). Other proteolytic enzymes (e.g., plasmin) are also capable of catalyzing the formation of BK. Effects of BK include vasodilation and increased microvascular permeability.

A considerable body of evidence suggests that the kallikrein-kinin system participates in the pathophysiology of sepsis and MODS. Circulating BK levels are elevated in endotoxic monkeys [190,191], septic patients [192], and healthy volunteers injected with LPS [193], and correlate with the development of hypotension [190,191,192]. Circulating levels of Hageman factor, prekallikrein, HMWK, and endogenous kallikrein inhibitors decrease in endotoxic dogs [194] and patients with septic shock [195–198]. Use of a monoclonal antibody to Factor XII in a baboon model of gram-negative bacteremia prevents activation of HMWK, limits the degree of hypotension, and prolongs survival [199].

Despite these data, the role of the kallikrein-kinin system in the pathophysiology of sepsis and MODS is far from established with certainty, in part because BK is labile and difficult to assay accurately. Decreased plasma levels of BK precursors may represent consumption and activation of the kallikrein-kinin pathway, but also may reflect redistribution of plasma proteins into other fluid compartments or decreased synthesis. Indeed, results from two recent studies failed to support the idea that BK is an important mediator in experimental endotoxicosis [200,201]. A trial of a BK receptor antagonist for the adjuvant therapy of sepsis in humans is currently in progress.

Prostaglandins. Prostaglandins (PG) and related compounds (collectively referred to as prostanoids) are inflammatory mediators derived from arachidonic acid through the enzyme cyclooxygenase. Arachidonic acid, in turn, is derived from membrane phospholipids through the enzyme phospholipase A_2 (PLA_2). Among the prostanoids are thromboxane (Tx) A_2 and prostacyclin (PGI_2). TxA_2 causes platelet and neutrophil activation and aggregation, vasoconstriction, bronchoconstriction, and increased capillary permeability, whereas PGI_2 causes platelet disaggregation and vasodilation [202].

An extensive literature supports the idea that prostanoids are key pathophysiologic mediators in experimental endotoxicosis, sepsis, and ARDS [202,203]. These findings can be summarized briefly as follows: (1) concentrations of 6-keto-$PGF_{1\alpha}$ (PGI_2 metabolite) and TxB_2 (TxA_2 metabolite) are elevated in plasma and pulmonary lymph in animal models of sepsis, endotoxicosis, and ARDS [204–207]; (2) survival and hemodynamics are improved in experimental endotoxic or septic shock when prostanoid synthesis is inhibited pharmacologically [205,208–

211] or nonpharmacologically (by inducing a state of essential fatty acid deficiency) [212]; (3) pulmonary hypertension, a characteristic feature of experimental endotoxicosis, sepsis, and ARDS, is abrogated by inhibitors of TxA_2 synthesis or TxA_2 receptor antagonists [213,214,215]; (4) cyclooxygenase inhibitors attenuate acute lung injury in porcine *Pseudomonas* bacteremia [216,217]; (5) inhibiting cyclooxygenase improves oxygenation in experimental pneumonia [206].

At present, support for the notion that prostanoids are important mediators of MODS and sepsis in humans is somewhat tenuous. Data favoring this view include the following observations: (1) previous treatment with ibuprofen prevents some of the manifestations of sepsis (e.g., tachycardia, fever, elevated plasma levels of "stress" hormones) that are elicited when human volunteers are injected with tiny doses of LPS [218]; (2) plasma and urinary concentrations of prostanoids are variably elevated in selected patients with sepsis, septic shock, or ARDS [219–225]; (3) plasma PLA_2 levels are elevated in patients with septic shock, pancreatitis, or salicylate-induced MODS and correlate with the degree of hypotension [226,228]; (4) indomethacin has been shown to improve oxygenation in a small group of critically ill patients with pneumonia [229]; (5) in a randomized, placebo-controlled prospective trial that enrolled 30 patients with sepsis, treatment with ibuprofen (800 mg given by retention enema every 4 hours for three doses) significantly decreased heart rate and temperature and tended to increase the likelihood for the normalization of blood pressure among patients with arterial hypotension at the time of entry into the study [225].

In contrast to these observations, there are data that call into question the role of prostanoids in human sepsis and ARDS. Ibuprofen fails to prevent the hyperdynamic cardiovascular response to LPS in human volunteers [230]. In two small studies, dazoxiben, an inhibitor of TxA_2 synthesis, was shown to have no effect in patients with established ARDS [231,232], and in another preliminary study, administering ibuprofen to patients with sepsis did not affect hemodynamics, respiratory function, or outcome [233].

Leukotrienes. The leukotrienes (LT) are another group of lipid mediators derived from arachidonic acid [234,235]. The sulfidopeptide LT (C_4, D_4, and E_4) cause vasoconstriction, bronchoconstriction, and increased microvascular permeability; these compounds represent the slow-reacting substance of anaphylaxis. LTB_4 is a potent chemoattractant.

Accumulating data suggest that LTs are important mediators in experimental sepsis, other shock states, and ARDS. Biliary excretion of LT metabolites is increased in rats subjected to one of several different stresses that are relevant to the problem of MODS (specifically endotoxicosis, burn injury, and extensive soft-tissue trauma) [236,237].

Treatment with sulfidopeptide LT receptor antagonists improves survival in experimental shock due to hemorrhage [238], trauma [239], gut ischemia [240], and endotoxicosis [241]. In experimental models of LPS-induced shock and/or ARDS, sulfidopeptide LT receptor antagonists improve regional perfusion [242,243,244], ameliorate gut mucosal acidosis [242], improve pulmonary function [243,245], and increase survival [246]. Recent data indicate that treatment with an LTB_4 receptor antagonist (LY255283) prevents lung injury and arterial hypoxemia in a porcine model of endotoxic shock and ARDS, possibly by blocking the recruitment of PMNLs into alveoli [247,248]. Other recent studies call into question the importance of the 5-lipoxygenase products of arachidonic acid metabolism in experimental models of sepsis [249,250].

Clinical studies have implicated the sulfidopeptide LTs and LTB_4 in the pathogenesis of ARDS. Immunoreactive LTD_4 levels are higher in pulmonary edema fluid from patients with ARDS compared with edema fluid from patients with congestive heart failure [251]. Urinary or bronchoalveolar lavage fluid concentrations of sulfidopeptide LTs are elevated in patients with ARDS or at risk for the development of ARDS [252,253]. Plasma concentrations of immunoreactive LTC_4 are higher in multiple trauma patients with ARDS compared with similar patients without ARDS [254]. Furthermore, bronchoalveolar lavage fluid levels of LTC_4 and LTE_4 correlate with the onset of ARDS in trauma patients [254]. Evidence of increased production of LTB_4 also has been obtained in patients with ARDS [255,256].

Platelet-Activating Factor. Platelet-activating factor (PAF), another potent lipid mediator that may be important in the pathophysiology of sepsis and MODS, is synthesized and released by platelets, neutrophils, monocytes, macrophages, endothelial cells, and other cell types (Fig. 199-7) [257]. PAF has a variety of biologic actions, including aggregaton of platelets, activation of neutrophils, bronchoconstriction, enhancement of microvascular permeability, and coronary artery vasoconstriction. In endotoxic rats, PAF levels are elevated and inversely correlated with blood pressure and cardiac output [258]. PAF levels are also elevated in the peritoneal fluid of rats subjected to extensive soft-tissue trauma [259]. Pretreatment with one of several PAF-receptor antagonists improves survival in endotoxic rats or guinea pigs [258,260,261]. In experimental animals of several species, PAF-receptor antagonists ameliorate several adverse effects of LPS, including hypotension [258,260–263], intestinal epithelial necrosis [264], acute lung injury [258,265,266,267], myocardial depression [268], and acute renal failure [269].

The release and actions of PAF are closely interrelated with several other mediators, including the prostanoids, LT, and reactive oxygen metabolites [270]. For example, pharmacologic blockade of PAF receptors blunts LPS-induced prostanoid release in experimental endotoxicosis [265], and hydrogen peroxide stimulates PAF release by cultured endothelial cells [271].

Limited data suggest that PAF participates in the pathophys-

Fig. 199-7. Metabolic pathway of platelet activating factor (alkyl acyl GPC = 1-0-alkyl-2 acetyl-su-glyceryl-3-phosphorylcholine. (From Braquet P, Touqui L, Shen TY, et al: Perspectives in platelet-activating factor research. *Pharmacol Rev* 39:97, 1987, with permission.)

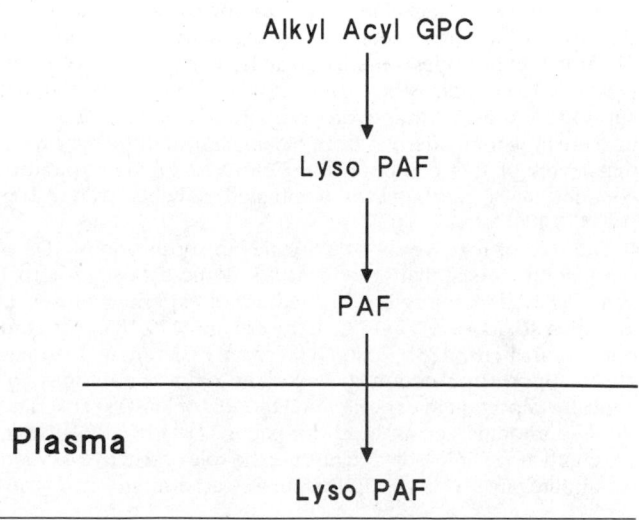

iology of human sepsis or MODS. Elevated levels of PAF have been measured in empyema fluid [272]. Indirect evidence of PAF release in human sepsis was obtained in a study showing that platelets from septic patients manifest increased occupancy of PAF receptors and contain high levels of cell-associated PAF [273]. More recently, elevated plasma concentrations of PAF and depressed levels of lyso-PAF (the precursor to PAF) have been assayed in septic patients [274,275]. PAF also has been implicated in the pathogenesis of ARDS [276].

Cytokines. Cytokines are small proteins with autocrine, paracrine, or endocrine activity that are secreted by immune cells. Several cytokines, namely tumor necrosis factor alpha (TNF-α), interleukin-1 (IL-1), interleukin-6 (IL-6), and interleukin-8 (IL-8), are currently the focus of intense investigation as potential key mediators of sepsis and MODS.

TNF-α, IL-1, and IL-6 have unique and overlapping biologic activities; as such, these cytokines appear to represent an inflammatory mediator system. Moreover, many of the phenomena mediated by these cytokines appear to be triggered or elaborated by other mediator systems, including the prostanoids, the complement cascade, activated neutrophils, and catecholamines.

TNF-α has a wide range of biologic effects, among which are the activation of PMNLs and the promotion of the adherence of these cells to endothelium [277,278,279]. These are effects that seem particularly noteworthy in view of the apparent importance of neutrophil-mediated endothelial damage in the pathophysiology of sepsis and MODS (see above). TNF-α also is capable of affecting the physiology of endothelial cells directly (i.e., in the absence of PMNLs) [280,281].

The notion of a cytokine *system* is supported by the observation that TNF-α can stimulate the synthesis and release of other cytokines [280–283]. Furthermore, many of the actions of TNF-α are enhanced by the simultaneous presence of LPS or IL-1 [284–287] and modified by other mediators such as PAF, prostanoids, other interleukins, and hormones (cortisol and catecholamines).

The concept that TNF-α is a mediator of septic shock was initially advanced by Beutler et al. [288,289]. In the first study, antibodies to TNF-α were shown to prevent LPS-induced mortality in mice [288]. In the second, injecting rats with recombinant human TNF-α was shown to reproduce many of the pathologic features (including death) elicited by a lethal dose of LPS [289]. Anti-TNF-α antibodies were subsequently shown to improve survival in baboons rendered bacteremic by an intravenous infusion of viable *Escherichia coli* or *Staphylococcus aureus* bacteria [290,291,292]. This last finding, in addition to providing support for the TNF-sepsis hypothesis, has profound implications for the adjuvant treatment of sepsis and MODS in humans and represents a particularly exciting avenue of investigation.

Numerous recent studies using experimental animals have further delineated the importance of TNF-α in the pathophysiology of sepsis and MODS. In guinea pigs, administration of recombinant human TNF-α leads to histologic evidence of damage to multiple organs and physiologic evidence of widespread increases in microvascular permeability to proteins (i.e., "capillary leak" syndrome) [293]. Interestingly, these phenomena are abrogated by previous depletion of PMNLs, suggesting that the effects of TNF-α in this model of MODS are mediated through activation of neutrophils. Infusing rats for 24 hours with recombinant human TNF-α leads to pulmonary edema and decreased pulmonary compliance, key features of ARDS in humans [294]. Recombinant human TNF-α also produces an ARDS-like syndrome in sheep [295,296]. Reversible myocardial depression, an important feature of sepsis in humans (see Chap.

197), is elicited in dogs and guinea pigs infused with recombinant human TNF-α [297,298,299]. TNF-α depresses myocardial adrenergic responsiveness in vitro [300]. Low calculated systemic vascular resistance (SVR) is a characteristic feature of sepsis in patients; this same hemodynamic derangement is elicited by TNF-α in a variety of species [296–302]. In vitro, incubation of vascular rings with TNF-α has been shown to diminish vascular smooth muscle contractility [303].

TNF-α also might be responsible for another of the characteristic features of sepsis and MODS, namely impaired oxygen extraction (see above). Recent data have documented that TNF-α inhibits mitochondrial oxygen utilization by digitonin-permeabilized rat hepatocytes [304].

Results from an increasing number of clinical studies clearly suggest that TNF-α plays an important role in the pathogenesis of human sepsis, septic shock, and MODS. When tiny doses of LPS are injected into human volunteers, TNF-α levels in plasma increase [305,306]. Plasma TNF-α levels in these studies correlate with circulating levels of acute-phase reactants and also correspond to the development of clinical features of sepsis, such as fever and tachycardia. When humans are injected with authentic recombinant human TNF-α, metabolic and cardiovascular changes are elicited that are similar to those observed in compensated sepsis: energy expenditure, cardiac output, glycerol turnover, and free fatty acid turnover increase and SVR decreases [307,308,309].

Two studies in septic pediatric patients suggest that elevated plasma TNF-α levels correlate with mortality [310,311]. Other studies also have documented elevated circulating TNF-α levels in selected critically ill patients, particularly those with arterial hypotension secondary to sepsis [312–317]; nevertheless, high plasma TNF-α concentrations are not a consistent finding in human sepsis [318]. Thus, it seems probable that massive TNF-α release is an early and transient event in septic shock. Support for this notion comes from a recent case report describing early, transient elevations in TNF-α following the self-administration of 1 mg of *Salmonella minnesota* endotoxin [319]. Down-regulation of TNF-α production or synthesis of TNF-α inhibitors may also explain this phenomenon [320,321]. Alternatively, lower levels of TNF-α may be secreted during the subacute phases of sepsis and MODS and may act in an autocrine or paracrine fashion to affect tissue and organ system function. This thesis is supported by a recent study demonstrating high bronchoalveolar lavage concentrations of TNF-α but near-normal plasma TNF-α levels in patients with early ARDS [322].

Several studies of adjuvant therapy with either anti-TNF-α antibodies or recombinant soluble TNF-α receptors have been completed. Although some of these studies have enrolled large numbers of patients, only preliminary data have been reported at the time of this writing [323,324].

Like TNF-α, IL-1 has a wide variety of biologic actions (Fig. 199-8) [325,326,327]. IL-1 is released by numerous cell types, including monocytes, macrophages, endothelial cells, B lymphocytes, astrocytes, and microglial cells in the central nervous system, keratinocytes, and renal mesangial cells. IL-1 is an important mediator of the acute-phase response [326,328]. Thus, actions of IL-1 include the induction of fever and the stimulation of hepatic synthesis of acute-phase reactants (e.g., serum amyloid A protein, C-reactive protein, and the complement component C3). LPS, C5a, and TNF-α are all capable of triggering the release of IL-1. This emphasizes the close interrelationship among these various mediators.

The potential role of IL-1 in MODS and sepsis is illustrated by studies showing that this cytokine elicits a hyperdynamic state when infused into rabbits or dogs [329,330]. The role of IL-1 as a mediator of the hyperdynamic, low SVR state charac-

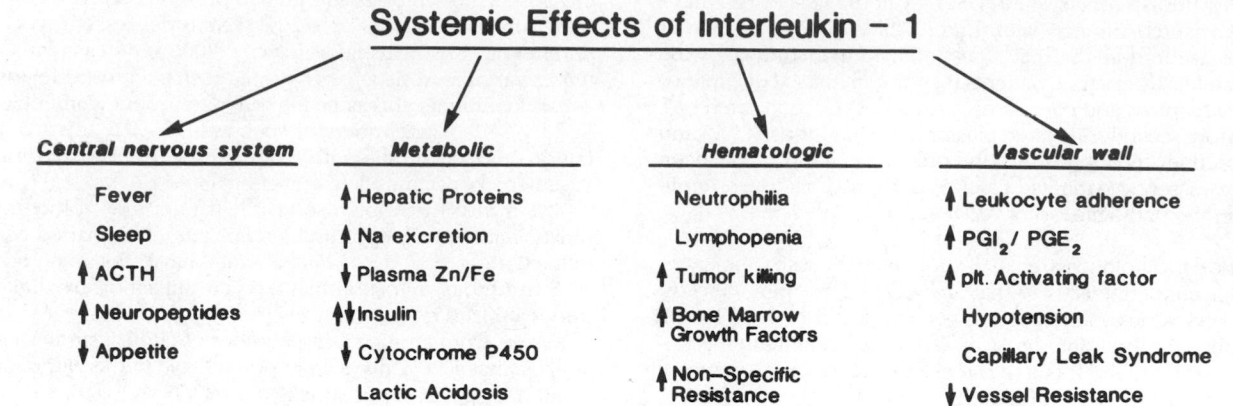

Fig. 199-8. Systemic effect of interleukin 1. (From Dinarello CA: Biology of Interleukin-1. *FASEB J* 2:108, 1988, with permission.)

teristic of the sepsis syndrome is further supported by in vitro studies showing that this cytokine depresses the contractility of vascular smooth muscle [331,332], perhaps by a process involving nitric oxide (see following) [333]. In addition, endotoxic shock is prevented in rabbits and mortality is reduced in mice subjected to cecal ligation and puncture if these animals are pretreated with a specific IL-1 receptor anatgonist (IL1-RA) [334,335]. Two human trials of a recombinant IL-1RA for the adjuvant therapy of septic shock have been completed; however, results have been reported only in abstract form.

As already noted, many of the in vivo effects of IL-1 or TNF-α are enhanced if both cytokines are infused together. This apparent synergy between IL-1 and TNF-α is exemplified by data obtained in rabbits showing that bolus administration of either cytokine alone has no effect on plasma levels of lactate, glucose, or triglycerides [286]. Metabolic derangements reminiscent of sepsis in humans (i.e., hyperglycemia, hypertriglyceridemia, and lactic acidosis) occur when IL-1 and TNF-α are administered together, however. Coadministration of IL-1 and TNF-α also diminishes the activity of PDH in hepatic mitochondria [286], a finding that is of considerable interest in view of the apparent importance of alterations in the activity of this enzyme complex in sepsis (see above). Coadministration of IL-1 and TNF-α also amplifies the hemodynamic effects of the former [329].

Muscle wasting or "autocannibalism" [336] is a key feature of the sepsis syndrome in humans. This phenomenon is apparently due, at least in part, to the actions of circulating peptides, one of which may be a cleavage product of IL-1 [337,338]. In human cancer patients, administration of recombinant human TNF-α increases the efflux of amino acids from the forearm musculature, suggesting that TNF-α also may be one of the factors promoting catabolism of skeletal muscle in sepsis [307]. Indeed, trace amounts of TNF-α may be necessary for elaboration of the muscle wasting effects of IL-1 or its cleavage products, since in rabbits [287] and rats [339] recombinant human TNF-α promotes muscle catabolism, whereas recombinant human IL-1 does not [287]. Recombinant human IL-1, however, is synergistic with TNF-α in this animal model of the metabolic response to sepsis.

Many of the effects of IL-1 are secondarily mediated by prostanoids. Fever is one key example [340]. Another PG-mediated effect of IL-1 (or perhaps TNF-α plus IL-1) is increased protein degradation in skeletal muscle [341]. Some of the hemodynamic effects of IL-1 and TNF-α also may be mediated by PG, since

purified human IL-1 induces PGI_2 synthesis by endothelial cells [342] and the low systemic vascular resistance state induced by these cytokines in rabbits is abrogated by ibuprofen [329].

In two studies, circulating IL-1 levels have been shown to be inversely correlated with survival in critically ill patients [317,343,344,345]. In contrast, in some studies, septic patients who died had higher plasma levels of IL-1 than did survivors [311]. Yet, in still more investigations, IL-1 levels have been undetectable in critically ill patients, including those with septic shock [316,346,347]. Moreover, a recent study suggests that false positives may occur when IL-1β is measured in biologic samples by enzyme-linked immunosorbent assay (ELISA) [348]. Thus, it is unclear whether the actions of IL-1 in sepsis are predominantly beneficial or harmful.

IL-6 and IL-8 are additional cytokines that appear to be important mediators of sepsis and MODS. IL-6 has a broad range of biologic actions, many of which (e.g., induction of fever) overlap those of TNF-α and IL-1 [349,350]. IL-1 and IL-6 act synergistically to enhance the synthesis of acute-phase proteins by hepatocytes. In patients with major burns, serum IL-6 levels are strongly correlated with body temperature and circulating levels of C-reactive protein [351]. Plasma levels of IL-6 are elevated in patients with sepsis and are directly correlated with mortality [316,352]. IL-8 is produced by a variety of cells in response to LPS, TNF-α, and IL-1. In baboons during lethal septic shock and sublethal endotoxemia, IL-8 plasma levels are elevated [353,354]. A major action of IL-8 appears to be the inducement of adhesion moclecule expression, thereby aiding in neutrophil venular transmigration [355]. Elevated circulating levels of IL-8 have been shown to correlate with mortality in patients with bacteremia [356]. IL-8 levels in bronchoalveolar lavage fluid are elevated in patients with ARDS, and very high concentrations of this cytokine in the airspaces of patients with ARDS are associated with mortality [357].

Opioid Peptides. The opioid peptides have been implicated as being important mediators in shock states (see Chaps. 195 and 197). The role of these compounds in MODS is not as well delineated.

Nitric Oxide. Nitric oxide (NO), an inorganic free radical gas, is derived in biologic systems from one of the terminal gaunidino nitrogens of L-arginine. The five-electron reaction is catalyzed by a group of enzymes called NO synthases. Two general classes of NO synthases have been described: constitutive (calcium-dependent) NO synthases and inducible (calcium-independent) NO synthases. NO is released by a variety of cells and tissues, including endothelium, vascular smooth muscle, neutrophils, and mononuclear, glial, mast, hepatic, and adrenal medullary cells [358,359,360].

One of the prominent physiologic actions of NO is vasorelaxation. Accumulating data suggest that NO may play a significant role in the pathophysiology of sepsis and MODS. Some data indicate that endotoxin and cytokines such as TNF-α increase the production of NO in both cultured endothelial cells and vascular rings via the calcium-independent NO synthase [361,362,363], although other data suggest that endothelial synthesis of NO is actually decreased by LPS or cytokines [364,365]. In animal models of septic shock, hypotension can be reversed by the administration of NO synthase inhibitors, although such treatment can cause liver injury and actually increase mortality [366,367,368]. In addition to its vascular effects, NO may play a role in sepsis-related myocardial dysfunction, since recent data suggest that LPS- or cytokine-induced myocardial dysfunction in vitro can be reversed by treatment with NO synthase inhibitors [369,370].

Currently, the clinical data implicating NO as a mediator in sepsis and/or MODS are quite limited. Anecdotally, it has been shown that pharmacologic inhibition of NO synthase can increase arterial blood pressure in some people with septic shock [371]. In septic patients, there is increased urinary excretion of nitrite and nitrate, two end products of NO metabolism [372]. Moreover, the excretion of nitrite and nitrate is inversely correlated with systemic vascular resistance, suggesting that NO is a mediator of the loss of vascular tone in sepsis [372]. The excretion of nitrate also has been shown to increase dramatically following administration of a cytokine, IL-2, which, when infused in humans, can induce a syndrome reminiscent of MODS [373].

NO appears to be an important component in macrophage function against various pathogens [374]. Therefore, treatment directed against NO-induced hypotension may have an adverse effect on the host response to infection. A recent report also indicates that the use of NO synthase inhibitors may worsen hepatic damage during murine endotoxemia [375]. Thus, although NO may be a factor contributing to the development of hypotension and organ dysfunction in patients with sepsis and/or MODS, the implications of inhibiting the production of this potent mediator remain to be elucidated.

DERANGEMENTS IN THE BARRIER FUNCTION OF THE INTESTINAL MUCOSA. Derangements in gut mucosal barrier function may contribute to the pathophysiology of MODS. Normally, the mucosa and lymphoid tissue of the gastrointestinal (GI) tract represent an effective barrier that prevents the systemic absorption of intraluminal microbes and microbial products (including LPS). This barrier consists of the tight junctions between mucosal epithelial cells, the mucous layer secreted by the epithelium, secretory IgA, and local cell-mediated immune mechanisms [376]. It has been hypothesized that derangements in the gut's barrier function permit the systemic absorption of gut-derived microbes (a process termed "translocation") and microbial products.

During critical illnesses, the gut mucosal barrier can be damaged. An extensive literature supports the notion that the gut is a major target organ in hypodynamic (i.e., low cardiac output) shock states (see also Chaps. 187 and 171). In experimental endotoxic shock, however, gut perfusion decreases dramatically, even when total cardiac output is well maintained [377]. Thus, it seems likely that absolute or relative mesenteric ischemia is a common occurrence in most forms of shock, including those, like septic shock, characterized by low SVR and normal or elevated cardiac output.

The tips of the intestinal villi are particularly susceptible to

ischemia because their nutrient vessels form a counter-current arrangement, and hence oxygen tensions at the apex of the loop are normally low [378]. In addition, the nutrient arteries supplying the villi take off from their parent vessels at right angles, an arrangement that may promote "plasma skimming," further diminishing oxygenation of the mucosal epithelium [379].

Shock is not the only factor that can adversely affect the integrity of GI tract mucosa. Nutritional factors may be important as well. Glutamine is a major energy substrate for the small intestine, and under conditions of stress, glutamine consumption across the mesenteric bed increases markedly [380]. The influence of glutamine on the ecology of the gut mucosa is dramatized by studies showing that experimental animals develop diarrhea, villous atrophy, mucosal ulcerations, and intestinal necrosis when they are deprived of glutamine by being infused with glutaminase [381]. The importance of glutamine is further supported by numerous studies showing that glutamine supplementation preserves gut mucosal integrity and function in a variety of experimental models of critical illness [382,383]. Because glutamine is labile (and was formerly considered an unessential amino acid), current total parenteral nutrition formulations do not contain glutamine. Thus, it is possible that glutamine deficiency contributes to deranged mucosal function in critically ill patients.

The role of altered GI barrier function in the pathogenesis of MODS in humans remains poorly defined. Nevertheless, several observations from both animal and clinical studies provide circumstantial evidence to support the idea that the gut is the "motor" of MODS [384]. The following are some of these observations:

1. Bacterial translocation to mesenteric lymph nodes occurs in patients with simple mechanical bowel obstruction, a finding that bolsters the idea that translocation occurs in humans [385].
2. A large proportion of patients with hemorrhagic shock have positive blood cultures [386].
3. The most common microbial species isolated from cultures of the proximal GI tract in critically ill surgical patients (i.e., *Candida albicans*, coagulase-negative *Staphylococcus*, and *Pseudomonas*) are also the most common species causing invasive infection in these patients [387].
4. Administration of LPS to human volunteers increases intestinal permeability [388].
5. Total parenteral nutrition and bowel rest (factors that have been shown to impair barrier function in animals and that are commonly present in critically ill patients) augment the acute-phase, endocrine, and cytokine responses to LPS in human volunteers [389].
6. Survival after hemorrhagic shock is improved in germ-free animals [390] or after the oral administration of nonabsorbable antibiotics active against gram-negative bacteria [391].
7. The permeability of the intestinal mucosa to various hydrophilic solutes, such as lactulose or polyethylene glycol, increases in human volunteers injected with LPS [392] and in patients with sepsis [393] or thermal trauma [394,395]. In victims of burn injury, the degree of gut mucosal hyperpermeability correlates with the extent of injury [395].

Other data fail to support the notion that increased translocation of microbes or increased permeability of the gut to hydrophilic solutes is a key feature contributing to MODS in critically ill patients [396]. In one investigation of 20 victims of major torso trauma, endotoxin was not detected in portal venous or systemic blood samples obtained over the first five days of hospitalization [397]. Although nine of 242 systemic and portal venous blood cultures were positive, virtually all of the isolates were probably contaminants. Another investigation in patients with major torso trauma failed to demonstrate positive mesenteric lymph node culture despite 40 percent of the patients developing major complications, including ARDS and gram-negative bacteremia [398]. Gut mucosal permeability to hydrophilic solutes is increased in many critically ill patients, but the increase in permeability does not correlate with APACHE II score, sepsis score, or survival [399].

GENETIC REGULATION OF CELLULAR FUNCTION. Recent data suggest that altered gene expression may have a profound effect on cellular and host responses during sepsis and shock. Apoptosis (programmed cell death) may occur when accumulated injuries reach a threshold [400]. Stress genes, including acute-phase and heat-shock genes, are expressed in a variety of disease states. The acute-phase proteins protect the *host* from the effects of inflammation, whereas heat-shock proteins appear to be necessary for survival of the *cell* [401]. Both can be induced individually, and induction is mutually exclusive [401]. Accumulating evidence indicates that heat-shock genes are expressed preferentially over the acute-phase genes in stress and shock states. Such a priority of gene expression may lead to organ dysfunction [401,402,403].

Prevention and Treatment of Multiple Organ Dysfunction Syndrome

From the foregoing discussion, it is apparent that our understanding of the pathophysiology of MODS remains sketchy, although rapid progress is being made in the search for the mechanisms involved. Thus, the prevention and treatment of MODS are nonspecific, and the goals are to maintain adequate tissue oxygenation, to find and treat infection, to provide adequate nutritional support, and, when necessary, to provide artificial support, such as dialysis, for dysfunctional organ systems.

RESUSCITATION. The most common events antedating the development of MODS are episodes of circulatory shock (see Chap. 171). Thus, timely and adequate restoration of DO_2 (see above) is of paramount importance in preventing (or ameliorating) MODS in high-risk patients. Controversy exists regarding the optimal fluid for resuscitation; this topic is discussed in depth in Chapters 171 and 172. Controversy also exists regarding the optimal circulating hemoglobin concentration; high hemoglobin concentrations increase blood viscosity and potentially adversely affect microvascular perfusion [404], whereas low hemoglobin concentrations can impair O_2 extraction by tissues [379,405]. Our practice is to maintain a blood hemoglobin concentration of 10 to 12 gm per deciliter in high-risk patients.

Assessing the adequacy of tissue oxygenation is difficult given the current state of the art. Commonly used clinical parameters include arterial blood pressure, skin color and temperature, urine flow, mixed venous O_2 saturation, and blood lactate concentration. Shoemaker et al. [406] have suggested that systemic DO_2, systemic VO_2, and cardiac output may be particularly valuable indices of the adequacy of resuscitation. In a randomized, prospective study of surgical patients considered

to be at high risk for MODS and death, these authors showed that survival was significantly improved if predetermined levels of DO_2 (>600 ml/min-M²), VO_2 (>170 ml/min-M²) and cardiac index (>4.5 L/min-M²) were maintained in the early period after major operations or trauma [407]. Other studies that have evaluated similar therapeutic endpoints in patients with septic shock or suffering from trauma support such a strategy [408,409,410] (Fig. 199-9). Taken together, the results from these trials have been interpreted as indicating that resuscitation to supranormal levels of cardiac output, DO_2, and VO_2 improves outcome in a wide variety of critically ill patients.

Despite these data, a few words of caution are in order. First, pushing cardiac output to supranormal levels (by infusing large volumes of fluid or chronotropic and inotropic drugs) carries its own risks, such as exacerbation of pulmonary edema or precipitation of myocardial ischemia [411]. Indeed, two recent studies have suggested that minimizing the volume of infused fluid improves outcome in critically ill patients [412,413]. Second, while it seems quite clear that patients at high risk for MODS do better if high levels of oxygen transport are maintained, it remains to be established unequivocally whether supranormal indices of oxygen metabolism are a causative factor leading to improved survival or whether the ability to achieve a high cardiac output and DO_2 is merely a marker of good "physiologic reserve" that portends a good outcome. Third, this approach assumes that oxygen is the limiting "nutrient."

Other approaches that may be of value for assessing the adequacy of tissue oxygenation remain largely experimental and include measurement of intramyocardial pH during cardiac surgical procedures [414]; tonometric determination of subcutaneous tissue PO_2 [415,416]; monitoring of conjunctival PO_2 [417]; use of near infrared spectroscopy to assess the oxidation state of cerebral cytochrome aa3 [418]; and tonometric estimation of GI mucosal pH [419,420]. The last method, discussed in greater detail in Chapter 187, is simple and minimally invasive.

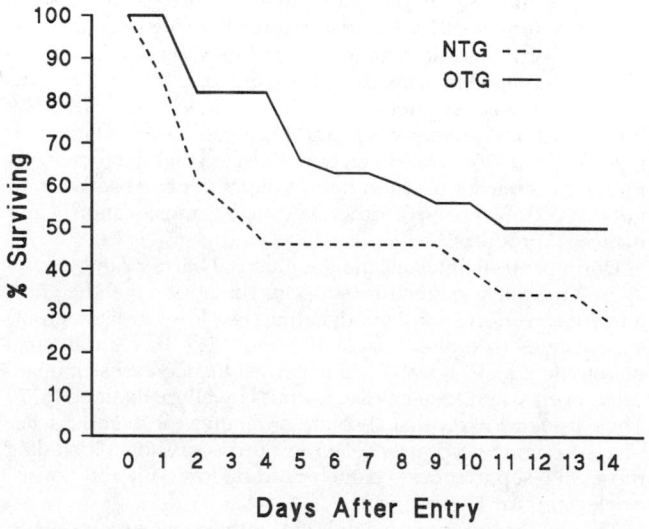

Fig. 199-9. Life table analysis of patients with septic shock randomized to be resuscitated to a cardiac index of 3.0 liters/min-M² (normal treatment group, NTG) or 6.0 liters/min-M² (optimal treatment group, OTG). There is a trend favoring optimal treatment (p = 0.14). (From Tuchschmidt J, Fried J, Astiz M, Rackow E: Elevation of cardiac output and oxygen delivery improves outcome in septic shock. *Chest* 102:216-220, 1992. Reproduced with permission.)

Tonometric evidence of gastric mucosal acidosis has been shown to correlate with both short- and long-term mortality in critically ill patients [420,421,422] and the development of complications after cardiac surgical procedures [419]. In addition, prevention of gastric intramucosal acidosis by using aggressive fluid resuscitation and inotropic therapy may reduce mortality [423]. However, recent data suggest that easily obtained clinical data such as base deficit are as accurate as tonometric estimation of gastric intramucosal pH in predicting outcome [424]. Additional research is needed before gastric tonometry becomes a routine clinical tool.

DEBRIDEMENT OF DEAD TISSUE AND FRACTURE STABILIZATION. The presence of devitalized tissue seems to be a major risk factor for the development of MODS, and hence careful debridement of dead tissue is an important element in the prevention of the syndrome. Early surgical stabilization of major lower extremity fractures has been shown to decrease the incidence of ARDS and pneumonia [425,426,427], and this practice should be considered the standard of care in the management of trauma patients.

INFECTION. Sepsis is an important cause (or correlate) of MODS. In critically ill patients with signs of deteriorating organ system function, the onus is on the physician to exclude untreated or inadequately treated infection. Although truly prophylactic antibiotics should be avoided, empiric administration of broad-spectrum antibiotics is often indicated in febrile patients with impending or established MODS, pending the results of further diagnostic studies [428]. In patients with normal liver function tests, the prophylactic administration of ketoconazole (200 mg/day by mouth or gavage) has been shown to reduce the incidence of both ARDS [429] and systemic fungal infections [430]. Although these results need to be confirmed in other studies before the practice of prophylactically administering ketoconazole can be advocated, the use of this agent warrants consideration and further investigation.

Intraabdominal Sepsis. Early and adequate treatment of intraabdominal sepsis (see Chap. 223) is important to prevent the development of MODS; unfortunately, it is unclear whether drainage of infected peritoneal collections improves outcome once MODS is established [431]. In an effort to improve outcome in high-risk cases of intraabdominal sepsis or necrotizing pancreatitis, several centers, including our own, advocate the use of multiple planned reoperations [432,433] or open packing (marsupialization) of the peritoneal cavity [434–437]. Although anecdotal results support the use of open management in selected cases of intraabdominal sepsis, the lack of data from a well-controlled randomized trial renders it impossible to advocate this approach strongly. It seems likely that in the absence of supportive clinical or radiographic evidence, however, repeat celiotomy for sepsis or MODS does not clearly alter outcome [438,439].

Pulmonary Sepsis. Nosocomial pneumonia is a major problem in the management of critically ill patients and can play a role in the development and course of MODS. This topic is discussed in greater detail elsewhere (see Chaps. 92 and 103). Accumulating data suggest that the pathogenesis of pneumonia in intubated patients is related, at least in part, to the colonization of the proximal GI tract and oropharynx with gram-negative bacteria and the subsequent aspiration of these organisms around the cuff of the endotracheal tube. Early studies suggested that treatment with H-2 blockers or antacids to prevent erosive gastritis may contribute to the development of pneumonia by raising gastric pH and thus promoting the overgrowth of gram-negative bacteria [440,441,442]. More recent studies have shown that the use of H-2 blockers is not associated with increased risk of nosocomial pneumonia, indicating that it is the combination of high gastric pH *and* high gastric volume associated with the use of antacids that is most likely important in the development of nosocomial pneumonia [443,444]. Sucralfate seems to be as effective as gastric alkalinization in preventing bleeding from erosive gastritis, and use of this agent may lessen the risk of nosocomial pneumonia [441].

Data, mostly from investigators in Europe, suggest that oropharyngeal and gut "decontamination" with topical nonabsorbable antibacterial and antifungal agents (plus a short course of systemic antibiotics) may lessen the incidence of nosocomial pneumonia in high-risk patients [445–449]. Recent trials of "selective digestive decontamination" have yielded conflicting results, with some studies indicating that this strategy improves outcome [450,451,452], but others suggesting that outcome is unaffected [453,454]. One study indicates that selective decontamination tends to improve outcome, but only in selected subpopulations of patients [455]. At least as practiced in North America, selective digestive decontamination is expensive. Furthermore, this strategy carries the risk of selecting multidrug-resistant strains of gram-negative organisms or enterococci [456].

It has been known for many years that early ambulation decreases the incidence of respiratory complications after surgical procedures. It is noteworthy, therefore, that postural oscillation with a rotating bed has been shown to decrease the incidence of nosocomial respiratory tract infections in high-risk patients [457,458].

Adherence of bacteria to endotracheal tubes in a biomatrix may be another factor contributing to the development of pneumonia in intubated patients [459], although one study found no correlation between the presence of the matrix and the development of nosocomial pulmonary infections [460].

Catheter-Related Sepsis (CRS). CRS can be a contributing factor in the development of MODS, and diligent efforts should be made to decrease the incidence of this problem (see Chap. 104). Strict aseptic technique (including cap, gown, and gloves for central venous and pulmonary artery catheters) is required for the insertion of intravascular catheters. Catheters that are placed with suboptimal attention to asepsis during emergency situations should be removed or replaced as soon as possible. Catheters should be left in place no longer than absolutely necessary. In the past, it was common to replace or exchange central venous, pulmonary artery, or arterial catheters if catheterization extended beyond 72 to 96 hours [461–466]. However, recent randomized studies demonstrated that such a routine practice is unnecessary and indeed may have adverse consequences for the patient [467,468]. If catheter infection is suspected and guide wire exchange is performed, the intradermal segment should be cultured semiquantitatively [469]. If cultures reveal evidence of significant colonization (15 or more colony-forming units), then the (new) catheter should be removed and another catheter inserted, this time using a different site.

A silver-impregnated collagen cuff that fits around the catheter in subcutaneous tissue has become commercially available. Several studies have suggested that use of this device reduces the density of bacterial growth on intravascular catheters, but the sample sizes of these studies were too small to permit definitive conclusions regarding the efficacy of the silver-impregnated cuff in reducing the incidence of CRS [471,472]. Another strategy to reduce the incidence of catheter infection utilizes a catheter with an antiseptic (silver sulfadiazine and chlorhexidine) surface [473]. Preliminary data indicate the use of such a catheter reduces the incidence of significant bacterial colonization and catheter-related bacteremia.

The Gut as a Source of Sepsis. If alterations in intestinal permeability leading to systemic absorption of gut-derived microbes and microbial products are important in the pathophysiology of sepsis and MODS, then selective bowel decontamination regimens may be of benefit (see above). Although the role of this strategy in unselected ICU patients remains controversial, it seems likely that gut decontamination, at the very least, is useful for controlling outbreaks of infection due to multiply-resistant gram-negative bacilli [474].

The use of the gut for nutritional support may be a key maneuver to help preserve the integrity of the mucosal barrier. This topic is discussed below and in Chapter 201.

Other approaches for limiting the development of what Border calls the "gut origin septic state" [475] are experimental and include intraluminal administration of agents that bind LPS (e.g., activated charcoal, bentonite, or polymyxin B) [476,477]; gut lavage (as performed for mechanical bowel preparation before colon surgery or colonoscopy); and systemic administration of polyclonal or monoclonal antibodies against LPS to high-risk patients [478].

Other Sources of Sepsis. Other sources of infection in critically ill patients include purulent sinusitis [479,480], suppurative thrombophlebitis, otitis media, perirectal abscess, epididymitis, prostatitis, calculous or acalculous cholecystitis, meningitis or brain abscess (particularly after instrumentation of the central nervous system), prosthetic intravascular graft infection, lower or upper urinary tract infection, and endocarditis. These conditions should be excluded on the basis of history, physical examination, laboratory studies (including cultures of relevant body fluids), and appropriate radiographic studies.

NUTRITIONAL SUPPORT. Malnutrition can contribute to morbidity and death rate in sepsis and MODS [7] (see also Chaps. 200 and 201). Proteolysis is a key feature of sepsis, and although it is not suppressed by infusing amino acids, positive nitrogen balance can be achieved by aggressive nutritional support. Early and aggressive nutritional support seems to prevent septic complications after thermal injury or multiple trauma [481,482,484]. Supplementation of amino acid formulas with branched chain amino acids improves nitrogen retention [485–489] and immune function in critical illness [489] but has not been shown to improve mortality in septic patients [490].

Accumulating data suggest that enteral feeding is preferable to parenteral feeding. In rats with bacterial peritonitis fed the same solution either enterally or parenterally, mortality is significantly lower when nutrition is provided by the enteral route [491]. Compared with isocaloric and isonitrogenous enteral feeding, total parenteral nutrition (TPN) increases cecal bacterial colony counts, reduces secretory IgA concentrations in bile, and enhances bacterial translocation [492]. In a randomized, prospective study of nutritional support in trauma patients, Moore et al. [483] showed that enteral feeding through needle-catheter jejunostomy (beginning within 12 hours of operation) is associated with significantly fewer septic complications than is a regimen of TPN that achieved comparable nitrogen balance. Remarkably similar results were recently reported by Kudsk et al., who also compared early enteral to early parenteral nutrition in a prospective, randomized fashion in trauma patients [484]. In contrast to these data, Cerra et al. [493] have been unable to document the superiority of enteral compared with parenteral nutrition in septic, hypermetabolic patients.

Regardless of route, overfeeding should be avoided. In a guinea pig model of peritonitis, caloric intake greater than 150 kcal per kilogram per day increased mortality [494]. Excess administration of carbohydrate results in the conversion of glucose to fat, increases the respiratory quotient and CO_2 production, and can delay weaning from mechanical ventilation [495,496]. Administration of an excessive caloric load, irrespective of the relative proportion of carbohydrates, has been shown to increase CO_2 production [497]. Excess administration of carbohydrate can also affect hepatic metabolic functions and alter drug clearance []. Current guidelines for support of hypermetabolic patients with sepsis or MODS include a total nonprotein caloric intake of 25 to 35 kcal per kilogram per day (3–5 gm/kg/day of glucose plus 0.5–1.0 gm/kg/day of fat) and 1.5 to 2.0 gm per kilogram per day of protein [499,500]. The number of calories needed for a given patient can be estimated using the Harris-Benedict equation [500], indirect calorimetry, or data obtained with a pulmonary artery catheter [501].

THERAPEUTIC ADJUNCTS OF UNPROVED BENEFIT

Corticosteroids and Prostaglandin E_1. In view of the data suggesting that mediators of inflammation play a key role in the pathophysiology of sepsis and MODS, one might expect that antiinflammatory drugs would play a major role in the management of these problems. Currently available data, however, do not strongly support this view.

Results from several recent randomized, prospective trials indicate that a short course of corticosteroids is without value in septic shock, SIRS, or ARDS (Fig. 199-10) [502–506]. Some data suggest that administering high doses of methylprednisolone can actually worsen outcome for selected subpopulations of these patients [503,506]. Despite these negative data, recent anecdotal data suggest that prolonged administration of glucocorticoids can hasten resolution of established ARDS in patients with evidence of pulmonary inflammation by gallium citrate scanning [136] or high pulmonary microvascular permeability as assessed by [113m]In-transferrin lung extravascular uptake [507]. Randomized, prospective studies will be required to determine the effectiveness of prolonged steroid therapy in the treatment of established ARDS.

Fig. 199-10. Cumulative mortality rates in patients with sepsis treated with placebo or methylprednisolone. (From The Veterans Administration Systemic Sepsis Cooperative Study Group: Effect of high-dose glucocorticoid therapy on mortality in patients with clinical signs of systemic sepsis. *N Engl J Med* 317:659, 1987, with permission.)

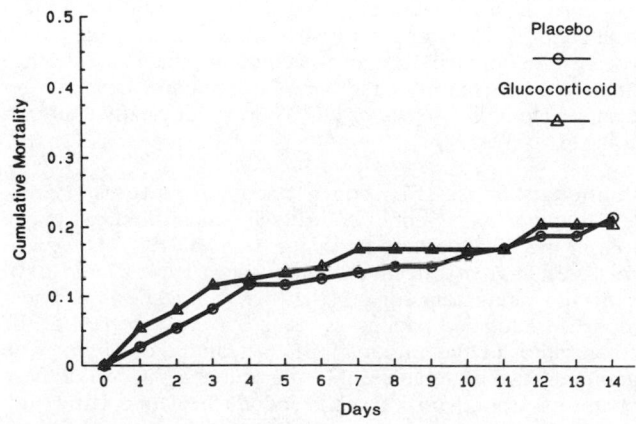

Prostaglandin E₁ possesses potent antiinflammatory activity. In a single-center, randomized, prospective trial, infusion of PGE₁ was shown to decrease the 30-day death rate but not the overall death rate in patients with ARDS [508]. Unfortunately, these encouraging findings were not confirmed in susequent trials [509,510]. Although some data suggest that PGE₁ improves oxygen transport in patients with ARDS [509], other studies fail to support this idea [511].

Immunotherapy. Endotoxemia is correlated with the development of ARDS [21,512] and gram-negative sepsis (Fig. 199-11) [513]. Injection of small doses of LPS into human volunteers reproduces key features of SIRS [308,514]. In view of the apparent importance of LPS as an early trigger of the cascade of events leading to MODS, there has been considerable interest in passive immunization against so-called core determinants shared by the endotoxins of a variety of species and strains of gram-negative bacteria [478,515]. Three recent randomized, prospective, placebo-controlled trials using either polyclonal or monoclonal antibodies directed against the core determinant of LPS have yielded either negative or conflicting results [516,517,518]. As yet, there is no immunotherapeutic modality that has been approved by the Food and Drug Admininstration. Other potential immunotherapeutic agents include anti-C5a antibody [128], anti-TNF-α antibody [290,323,324], antibodies directed against adhesion molecules, soluble TNF-α receptors, IL-I receptor antagonist, bacterial permeability–increasing protein (a white cell product that binds LPS), anti-TNF-α receptor antibody, granulocyte colony-stimulating factor, and antiidiotopic monoclonal antibodies specific for monoclonal antibodies directed against the core determinants of LPS [519–522].

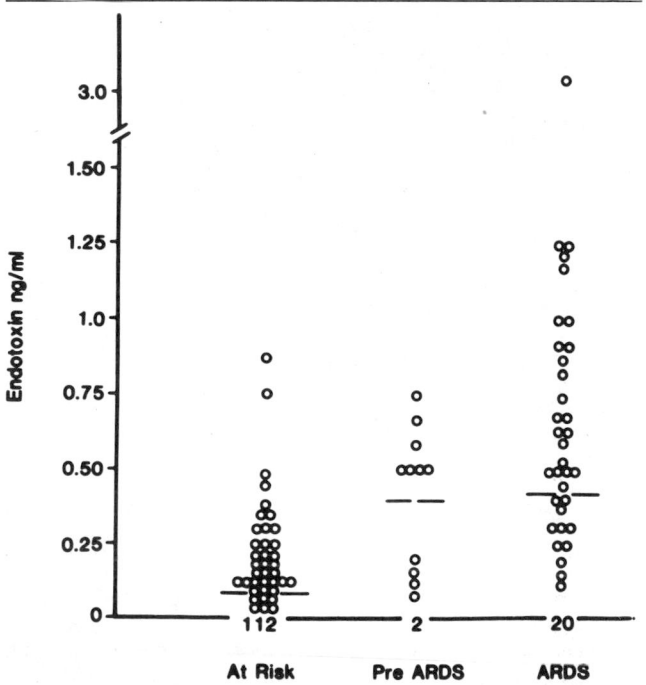

Fig. 199-11. Endotoxin levels (ng/ml) in patients (1) at risk for the development of ARDS, (2) eventually developing ARDS, and (3) with ARDS. (From Parsons PE, Worthen JS, Moore EE, et al: The association of circulating endotoxin with the development of the adult respiratory distress syndrome. *Am Rev Respir Dis* 144:294, 1989, with permission.)

Fibronectin. Fibronectin is a complex glycoprotein important in the normal functioning of the phagocytic cell ("reticuloendothelial") system (see Chap. 171). Circulating levels of fibronectin are depressed in patients with trauma and correlate directly with the likelihood of survival [523]. These and other data have prompted considerable interest in using fibronectin as an adjunctive agent in the management of patients with sepsis, trauma, and MODS. Early, uncontrolled trials suggested that therapy with cryoprecipitate, a rich source of fibronectin, improves organ system function in patients with sepsis or trauma [524]. Unfortunately, these findings were not confirmed in a large, prospective, controlled trial [525].

Extracorporeal Hemofiltration and Hemoperfusion. With the advent of continuous arteriovenous hemofiltration (CAVH) as a form of artificial renal support, interest has focused on this modality as a means for removing or reducing the concentration of circulating mediators associated with sepsis and MODS. Anecdotal results from a small study of patients with MODS caused by sepsis suggest that plasmapheresis and CAVH may be beneficial in reducing mortality [526]. Many of the inflammatory mediators that have been implicated in the etiology of sepsis and MODS (e.g., TNF-α) have molecular weights greater than 10,000 daltons. Thus, for CAVH to be effective, the filter must be able to remove molecules larger than 10,000 daltons, a capability not all CAVH filters possess. Extracorporeal hemoperfusion through columns containing materials capable of binding LPS is currently undergoing evaluation using animal or in vitro models [527,528].

Miscellaneous Agents of Unproved Benefit. An extensive literature supports the notion that nonsteroidal antiinflammatory agents, such as ibuprofen, improve survival and organ function in experimental models of septic shock, ARDS, and acute endotoxicosis [202,203]. A multicenter, randomized trial of ibuprofen as adjunctive therapy for the sepsis syndrome is currently underway.

Other agents that are attracting attention as potential adjuncts for the care of patients with MODS (or at risk of developing the syndrome) include pentoxyphylline [529,530,531] and a variety of agents with antioxidant activity [532].

Another agent that offers promise as an adjunct to the therapy of MODS and sepsis is human recombinant TNF-α. Although implicated as an important mediator of sepsis, exogenous administration of low doses of this cytokine, alone or in combination with IL-1, reduces mortality in experimental sepsis [533,534].

Summary

Although some progress may be made in the therapy of established MODS, greater strides are likely if patients at high risk for developing the syndrome can be identified so that measures to prevent MODS can be instituted. Since the pathophysiology of MODS clearly involves numerous mediators, it is doubtful that all patients can be adequately treated with a single agent or mode of therapy. Rather, combination therapy will probably be employed in the future. For now, the keys to preventing MODS seem to be aggressive early resuscitation so that prolonged periods of hypoperfusion are avoided; prevention of sepsis by careful attention to aseptic technique, and possibly other adjunctive measures; aggressive debridement of devitalized tissue; and aggressive medical and surgical treatment of sepsis when it is present.

References

1. Barton R, Cerra FB: The hypermetabolism multiple organ failure syndrome. *Chest* 96:1153, 1989.
2. DeCamp MM, Demling RH: Posttraumatic multisystem organ failure. *JAMA* 260:530, 1988.
3. American College of Chest Physicians/Society of Critical Care Medicine Consensus Conference: Definitions for sepsis and organ failure and guidelines for the use of innovative therapies in sepsis. *Crit Care Med* 20:864, 1992.
4. Skillman JJ, Bushnell LS, Goldman H, et al: Respiratory failure, hypotension, sepsis and jaundice. *Am J Surg* 117:523, 1969.
5. Tilney NL, Bailey GL, Morgan AP: Sequential system failure after rupture of abdominal aortic aneurysms: An unsolved problem in postoperative care. *Ann Surg* 178:117, 1973.
6. Churchill ED: Multiple, progressive, or sequential systems failure: A syndrome of the 1970's. *Arch Surg* 110:779, 1975.
7. Polk HC, Shields C: Remote organ failure: A valid sign of occult intra-abdominal infection. *Surgery* 81:310, 1977.
8. Fry DE, Pearlstein L, Fulton R, et al: Multiple system failure: The role of uncontrolled infection. *Arch Surg* 115:136, 1980.
9. Ferraris VA: Exploratory laparotomy for potential abdominal sepsis in patients with multiple-organ failure. *Arch Surg* 118:1130, 1983.
10. Goris RJ, Boekhorst TPA, Nuytinck JKS, et al: Multiple-organ failure—Generalized autodestructive inflammation? *Arch Surg* 120:1109, 1985.
11. Bone RC, Balk R, Slotman G, et al: Adult respiratory distress syndrome. Sequence and importance of development of multiple organ failure. *Crit Care Med* 101:320, 1992.
12. Bell RC, Coalson JJ, Smith JD, et al: Multiple organ system failure and infection in adult respiratory distress syndrome. *Ann Intern Med* 99:293, 1983.
13. Knaus WA, Draper EA, Wagner DP, et al: Prognosis in acute organ system failure. *Ann Surg* 202:685, 1985.
14. Knaus WA, Wagner DP: Multiple systems organ failure with epidemiology and prognosis. *Crit Care Clin* 5:221, 1989.
15. Pepe PE, Potkin RT, Holtman D, et al: Clinical predictors of the adult respiratory distress syndrome. *Am J Surg* 144:124, 1982.
16. Pepe PE, Thomas RG, Stager MA, et al: Early prediction of the adult respiratory distress syndrome by a simple scoring method. *Ann Emerg Med* 12:749, 1983.
17. Shoemaker WC, Appel P, Kram HB: Tissue oxygen debt as a determinant of lethal and nonlethal postoperative organ failure. *Crit Care Med* 16:1117, 1988.
18. Pacher R, Redl H, Frass M, et al: Relationship between neopterin and granulocyte elastase plasma levels and the severity of multiple organ failure. *Crit Care Med* 17:221, 1989.
19. Redl H, Paul E, Goris RJA, et al: Plasma levels of elastase 1 protease inhibitor complex in the monitoring of ARDS and multi-organ failure—A summary of three clinical trials. *Adv Exp Med Biol* 240:457, 1988.
20. Hammerschmidt DE, Weaver LJ, Hudson LD, et al: Association of complement activation and elevated plasma-C5a with adult respiratory distress syndrome. *Lancet* 1:947, 1980.
21. Brandtzaeg P, Kierulf P, Gaustad P, et al: Plasma endotoxin as a predictor of multiple organ failure and death in systemic meningococcal disease. *J Infect Dis* 159:195, 1989.
22. Danner RL, Elin RJ, Hosseini JM, et al: Endotoxemia in human septic shock: *Chest* 99:169, 1991.
23. Vijaykumar E, Raziuddin S, Wardle EN: Plasma endotoxin in patients with trauma, sepsis and severe hemorrhage. *Clin Intensive Care* 2:4, 1991.
24. Leatherman JW, Schmitz PG: Fever, hyperdynamic shock, and multiple system organ failure: A pseudo-sepsis syndrome associated with chronic salicylate intoxication. *Chest* 100:1391, 1991.
25. Shibutani K, Komatsu T, Kubal K, et al: Critical level of oxygen delivery in anesthetized man. *Crit Care Med* 11:640, 1983.
26. Komatsu T, Shibutani K, Okamoto K, et al: Critical level of oxygen delivery after cardiopulmonary bypass. *Crit Care Med* 15:194, 1987.
27. Hochachka PW: Metabolic suppression and oxygen availability. *Can J Zool* 66:152, 1987.

28. Gutierrez G, Pohil RJ, Strong R: Skeletal muscle oxygen consumption and energy metabolism during hypoxemia. *J Appl Physiol* 66:2117, 1989.
29. Duran WN, Renkin EM: Oxygen consumption and blood flow in resting mammalian skeletal muscle. *Am J Physiol* 226:173, 1974.
30. Edelstone DI, Paulone ME, Holzman IR: Hepatic oxygenation during arterial hypoxemia in neonatal lambs. *Am J Obstet Gynecol* 150:513, 1984.
31. Powers SR, Mannal R, Neclerio M, et al: Physiologic consequences of positive end-expiratory pressure (PEEP) ventilation. *Ann Surg* 178:265, 1973.
32. Danek SJ, Lynch JP, Weg JG, et al: The dependence of oxygen uptake on oxygen delivery in the adult respiratory distress syndrome. *Am Rev Respir Dis* 122:387, 1980.
33. Kaufman BS, Rackow EC, Falk JL: The relationship between oxygen delivery and consumption during fluid resuscitation of hypovolemic and septic shock. *Chest* 85:336, 1984.
34. Kariman K, Burns SR: Regulation of tissue oxygen extraction is disturbed in adult respiratory distress syndrome. *Am Rev Respir Dis* 132:109, 1985.
35. Haupt MT, Gilbert EM, Carlson RW: Fluid loading increases oxygen consumption in septic patients with lactic acidosis. *Am Rev Respir Dis* 131:912, 1985.
36. Kruse JA, Haupt MT, Puri VK, Carlson RW: Lactate levels as predictors of the relationship between oxygen delivery and consumption in ARDS. *Chest* 98:959, 1990.
37. Fenwick JC, Dodek PM, Ronco JJ, et al: Increased concentrations of plasma lactate predict pathological dependence of oxygen consumption on oxygen delivery in patients with adult respiratory distress syndrome. *J Crit Care* 5:81, 1990.
38. Vincent JL, Roman A, DeBacker D, Kahn RJ: Oxygen uptake/supply dependency: Effects of short-term dobutamine infusion. *Am Rev Respir Dis* 142:2, 1990.
39. Steffes CP, Bender JS, Levison MA: Blood transfusion and oxygen consumption in surgical sepsis. *Crit Care Med* 19:512, 1991.
40. Bakker J, Coffernils M, Leon M, et al: Blood lactate levels are superior to oxygen-derived variables in predicting outcome in human sepsis. *Chest* 99:956, 1991.
41. Gutierrez G, Pohil RJ: Oxygen consumption is linearly related to O_2 supply in critically ill patients. *J Crit Care* 1:45, 1986.
42. Wolf YG, Cotev S, Perel A, et al: Dependence of oxygen consumption on cardiac output in sepsis. *Crit Care Med* 15:198, 1987.
43. Astiz ME, Rackow EC, Falk JL, et al: Oxygen delivery and consumption in patients with hyperdynamic septic shock. *Crit Care Med* 15:26, 1987.
44. Bihari D, Smithies M, Gimson A, et al: The effects of vasodilation with prostacyclin on oxygen delivery and uptake in critically ill patients. *N Engl J Med* 317:397, 1987.
45. Astiz ME, Rackow EC, Kaufman B, et al: Relationship of oxygen delivery and mixed venous oxygenation to lactic acidosis in patients with sepsis and acute myocardial infarction. *Crit Care Med* 16:655, 1988.
46. Clarke C, Edwards JD, Nightingale P, et al: Persistence of supply dependency of oxygen uptake at high levels of delivery in adult respiratory distress syndrome. *Crit Care Med* 19:497, 1991.
47. Lorente JA, Renes E, Gomez-Aquinaga MA, et al: Oxygen delivery-dependent oxygen consumption in acute respiratory failure. *Crit Care Med* 19:770, 1991.
48. Ronco JJ, Montaner JSG, Fenwick JC, et al: Pathologic dependence of oxygen consumption on oxygen delivery in acute respiratory failure secondary to AIDS-related *Pneumocystis carinii* pneumonia. *Chest* 98:1463, 1990.
49. Nelson DP, Beyer C, Samsel RW, et al: Pathological supply dependence of O_2 uptake during bacteremia in dogs. *J Appl Physiol* 63:1487, 1991.
50. Archie JP, Jr.: Mathematic coupling of data: A common source of error. *Ann Surg* 193:296, 1981.
51. Stratton HH, Feustel PJ, Newell JC. Regression of calculated variables in presence of shared measurement error. *J Appl Physiol* 62:2083, 1987.
52. Vermeij CG, Feenstra BWA, Adrichem WJ, Bruining HA: Independent oxygen uptake and oxygen delivery in septic and postoperative patients. *Chest* 99:1438, 1991.

53. Ronco JJ, Fenwick JC, Wiggs BR, et al: Oxygen consumption is independent of increases in oxygen delivery by dobutamine in septic patients who have normal or increased plasma lactate. *Am Rev Respir Dis* 147:25, 1993.

54. Ronco JJ, Phang PT, Walley KR, et al: Oxygen consumption is independent of changes in oxygen delivery in severe adult respiratory distress syndrome. *Am Rev Respir Dis* 143:1267, 1991.

55. Carlile PV, Gray BA: Effect of opposite changes in cardiac output and arterial PO$_2$ on the relationship between mixed venous PO$_2$ and oxygen transport. *Am Rev Respir Dis* 140:891, 1989.

56. Vermeij CG, Feenstra BWA, Bruining HA: Oxygen delivery and oxygen uptake in postoperative and septic patients. *Chest* 98:415, 1990.

57. Marik PE, Sibbald WJ: Effect of stored-blood transfusion on oxygen delivery in patients with sepsis. *JAMA* 269:3024, 1993.

58. Dietrich KA, Conrad SA, Hebert CA, et al: Cardiovascular and metabolic response to red blood cell transfusion in critically ill volume-resuscitated nonsurgical patients. *Crit Care Med* 18:940, 1990.

59. Mink RB, Pollack MM: Effect of blood transfusion of oxygen consumption in pediatric septic shock. *Crit Care Med* 18:1087, 1990.

60. Feldman HA: Families of lines: Random effects in linear regression analysis. *J Appl Physiol* 64:1721, 1988.

61. Weissman C, Kemper M: The oxygen uptake-delivery relationship during ICU interventions. *Chest* 99:430, 1991.

62. Villar J, Slutsky AS, Hew E, Aberman A: Oxygen transport and oxygen consumption in critically ill patients. *Chest* 98:687, 1990.

63. Boyd O, Grounds M, Bennett D: The dependency of oxygen consumption on oxygen delivery in critically ill postoperative patients is mimicked by variations in sedation. *Chest* 101:1619, 1992.

64. Nelson DP, Samsel RW, Wood LDH, Schumacker PT: Pathological supply dependence of systemic and intestinal O$_2$ uptake during endotoxemia. *J Appl Physiol* 64:2410, 1988.

65. Samsel RW, Nelson DP, Sanders WM, et al: Effect of endotoxin on systemic and skeletal muscle O$_2$ extraction. *J Appl Physiol* 65:1377, 1988.

66. Heard SO, Baum TD, Wang H, et al: Systemic and mesenteric O$_2$ metabolism in endotoxic pigs: Effect of graded hemorrhage. *Circ Shock* 35:44, 1991.

67. Rackow EC, Astiz ME, Weil MH: Increases in oxygen extraction during rapidly fatal septic shock in rats. *J Lab Clin Med* 109:660, 1987.

68. Hurtado FJ, Gutierrez AM, Silva N, et al: Role of tissue hypoxia as the mechanism of lactic acidosis during *E. coli* endotoxemia. *J Appl Physiol* 72:1895, 1992.

69. Hirschl RB, Heiss KF, Cilley RE, et al: Oxygen kinetics in experimental sepsis. *Surgery* 112:37, 1992.

70. Hotchkiss RS, Karl IE: Reevaluation of the role of cellular hypoxia and bioenergetic failure in sepsis. *JAMA* 267:1503, 1992.

71. Zweifach BW, Thomas L: The relationship between the vascular manifestations of shock produced by endotoxin, trauma, and hemorrhage. *J Exp Med* 106:385, 1957.

72. Fink MP, Homer L, Fletcher JR: Diminished pressor response to exogenous norepinephrine and angiotensin II in septic, unanesthetized rats: Evidence for a prostaglandin-mediated effect. *J Surg Res* 38:335, 1985.

73. McKenna M, Martin FM, Chernow B, et al: Vascular endothelium contributes to decreased aortic contractility in experimental sepsis. *Circ Shock* 19:267, 1986.

74. McKenna M, Martin FM, Chernow B, et al: Enhanced vascular effect of cyclic GMP in septic rat aorta. *Am J Physiol* 254:R436, 1988.

75. Lubbe AS, Garrison RN, Cryer HM, et al: EDRF as a possible mediator of sepsis-induced arteriolar dilation in skeletal muscle. *Am J Physiol* 262:H880, 1992.

76. Baker CH, Sutton ET: Arterial endothelium-dependent vasodilation occurs during endotoxic shock. *Am J Physiol* 264:H1118, 1993.

77. Nelson S, Steward RH, Traber L, Traber D: Endotoxin-induced alterations in contractility of isolated blood vessels from sheep. *Am J Physiol* 260:H1790, 1991.

78. Szabo C, Mitchell JA, Gross SS, et al: Nifedipine inhibits the induction of nitric oxide synthase by bacterial lipopolysaccharide. *J Pharmacol Exp Ther* 265:674, 1993.

79. Fleming I, Gray GA, Stoclet J-C: Influence of endothelium on induction of the L-arginine-nitric oxide pathway in rat aortas. *Am J Physiol* 264:H1200, 1993.

80. Ochoa JB, Udekwu AO, Billiar TR, et al: Nitrogen oxide levels in patients after trauma and during sepsis. *Ann Surg* 214:621, 1991.

81. Myers PR, Wright TF, Tanner MA, Adams HR: EDRF and nitric oxide production in cultured endothelial cells: Direct inhibition by *E. coli* endotoxin. *Am J Physiol* 262:H710, 1992.

82. Wylam ME, Samsel RW, Umans JG, et al: Endotoxin *in vivo* impairs endothelium-dependent relaxation of canine arteries *in vitro*. *Am Rev Respir Dis* 142:1263, 1990.

83. Landry DW, Oliver JA: The ATP-sensitive K$^+$ channel mediates hypotension in endotoxemia and hypoxic lactic acidosis in dogs. *J Clin Invest* 89:2071, 1992.

84. Barroso-Aranda J, Schmid-Schonbein GW, Zweifach BW, et al: Granulocytes and no-reflow phenomenon in irreversible hemorrhagic shock. *Circ Res* 63:437, 1988.

85. Barroso-Aranda J, Schmid-Schonbein GW: Transformation of neutrophils as indicator of irreversibility in hemorrhagic shock. *Am J Physiol* 257:H846, 1989.

86. Hurd TC, Dasmahapatra KS, Rush BF Jr, et al: Red blood cell deformability in human and experimental sepsis. *Arch Surg* 123:217, 1988.

87. Machiedo GW, Towell RJ, Rush BF Jr, et al: The incidence of decreased red blood cell deformability in sepsis and the association with oxygen free radical damage and multiple-system organ failure. *Arch Surg* 124:1386, 1989.

88. Mela L, Bacalzo LD, Miller LD: Defective oxidative metabolism of rat liver mitochondria in hemorrhagic and endotoxin shock. *Am J Physiol* 220:571, 1971.

89. Greer GG, Milazzo FH: *Pseudomonas aeruginosa* lipopolysaccharide: An uncoupler of mitochondrial oxidative phosphorylation. *Can J Microbiol* 21:877, 1975.

90. Tavakoli H, Mela-Riker LM: Alterations of mitochondrial metabolism and protein concentration in subacute septicemia. *Infect Immunol* 78:536, 1982.

91. Stadler J, Bentz BG, Harbrecht BG, et al: Tumor necrosis factor alpha inhibits hepatocyte mitochondrial respiration. *Ann Surg* 216:539, 1992.

92. Geller ER, Jankauskas S, Kirkpatrick J: Mitochondrial death in sepsis: A failed concept. *J Surg Res* 40:514, 1986.

93. Fry DE, Silva BB, Rink RD, et al: Hepatic cellular hypoxia in murine peritonitis. *Surgery* 85:652, 1979.

94. Decker GA, Daniel AM, Blevings S, et al: Effect of peritonitis on mitochondrial respiration. *J Surg Res* 11:528, 1971.

95. Mela-Riker L, Bartos D, Viessis AA, et al: Chronic hyperdynamic sepsis in the rat. II. Characterization of liver and muscle energy metabolism. *Circ Shock* 36:83, 1992.

96. Cerra FB: Multiple organ failure syndrome. *Dis Mon* 38:843, 1992.

97. Vary TC, Siegel JH, Nakatani T, et al: Effect of sepsis on activity of pyruvate dehydrogenase complex in skeletal muscle and liver. *Am J Physiol* 250:E634, 1986.

98. Kilpatrick-Smith L, Erecinska M: Cellular effect of endotoxin in vitro: I. Effect of endotoxin on mitochondrial substrate metabolism and intracellular calcium. *Circ Shock* 11:85, 1983.

99. Vary TC, Martin LF: Potentiation of decreased pyruvate dehydrogenase activity by inflammatory stimuli in sepsis. *Circ Shock* 39:299, 1993.

100. Shaw JHF, Klein S, Wolfe RR: Assessment of alanine, urea, and glucose interrelationships in normal subjects and in patients with sepsis with stable isotope tracers. *Surgery* 97:557, 1985.

101. Moore FA, Haenel JB, Moore EM, Whitehill TA: Incommensurate oxygen consumption in response to maximal oxygen availability predicts postinjury multiple organ failure. *J Trauma* 33:58, 1992.

102. Moore FA, Moore EE, Poggetti RS, Read RA: Postinjury shock and early bacteremia: A lethal combination. *Arch Surg* 127:893, 1992.

103. Henao FJ, Daes JE, Dennis RJ: Risk factors for multiorgan failure: A case-control study. *J Trauma* 31:74, 1991.

104. Goris RJA, Boekholtz WKS, van Bebber IPT, et al: Multiple-organ failure and sepsis without bacteria: An experimental model. *Arch Surg* 121:897, 1986.

105. Nuytinck HKS, Offermans XJMW, Kubat K: Whole-body inflammation in trauma patients: An autopsy study. *Arch Surg* 123:1519, 1988.

106. Steinberg S, Flynn W, Kelley K, et al: Development of a bacteria-

independent model of the multiple organ failure syndrome. *Arch Surg* 124:1390, 1989.

107. Jacob HS, Craddock PR, Hammerschmidt DE, et al: Complement-induced granulocyte aggregation: An unsuspected mechanism of disease. *N Engl J Med* 302:789, 1980.

108. Ruoslahti E: Integrins. *J Clin Invest* 87:1, 1991.

109. Bevilacqua MP, Nelson RM: Selectins. *J Clin Invest* 91:379, 1993.

110. Wright SD, Ramos RA, Hermanowski-Vosatka A, et al: Activation of the adhesive capacity of CR3 on neutrophils by endotoxin: Dependence on lipopolysaccharide binding protein and CD14. *J Exp Med* 173:1281, 1991.

111. Lo SK, Everitt J, Gu J, Malik AB: Tumor necrosis factor mediates experimental pulmonary edema by ICAM-1 and CD18-dependent mechanisms. *J Clin Invest* 89:981, 1992.

112. Gasic AC, McGuire G, Krater S, et al: Hydrogen peroxide pretreatment of perfused canine vessels induces ICAM-1 and CD18-dependent neutrophil adherence. *Circulation* 84:2154, 1991.

113. Argenbright LW, Barton RW: Interactions of leukocyte intregrins with intercellular adhesion molecule 1 in the production of inflammatory vascular injury in vivo. The Shwartzman reaction revisited. *J Clin Invest* 89:259, 1992.

114. Ruoslahti E: Integrins. *J Clin Invest.* 87:1, 1991.

115. Walsh CJ, Carey PD, Cook DJ, et al: Anti-CD18 antibody attenuates neutropenia and alveolar capillary-membrane injury during gram-negative sepsis. *Surgery* 110:205, 1991.

116. L-selectin function is required for β_2-integrin-mediated neutrophil adhesion at physiologic shear rates in vivo. *Am J Physiol* 263:H1034, 1992.

117. Worthen GS, Avdi N, Vukajlovich S, Tobias PS: Neutrophil adherence induced by lipopolysaccharide in vitro: Role of plasma component interaction with lipopolysaccharide. *J Clin Invest* 90:2526, 1992.

118. Mulligan MS, Polley MJ, Bayer RJ, et al: Neutrophil-dependent acute lung injury: Requirement for P-selectin (GMP-140). *J Clin Invest* 90:1600, 1992.

119. Windsor ACJ, Walsh CJ, Mullen PG, et al: Tumor necrosis factor-α blockade prevents neutrophil CD18 receptor upregulation and attenuates acute lung injury in porcine sepsis without inhibition of neutrophil oxygen radical generation. *J Clin Invest* 91:1459, 1993.

120. Robbins RA, Russ WD, Rasmussen JK, et al: Activation of the complement system in the adult respiratory distress syndrome. *Am Rev Respir Dis* 135:651, 1987.

121. Dofferhoff ASM, De Jong HJ, Bom VJJ, et al: Complement activation and the production of inflammatory mediators during the treatment of severe sepsis in humans. *Scand J Infect Dis* 24:197, 1992.

122. Duchateau J, Haas M, Schreyen H, et al: Complement activation in patients at risk of developing the adult respiratory distress syndrome. *Am Rev Respir Dis* 130:1058, 1984.

123. Ketai LH, Grum CM: C3a and adult respiratory distress syndrome after massive transfusion. *Crit Care Med* 14:1001, 1986.

124. Fowler AA, Hyers TM, Fisher BJ, et al: The adult respiratory distress syndrome: Cell populations and soluble mediators in the air spaces of patients at high risk. *Am Rev Respir Dis* 136:1225, 1987.

125. Gee MH, Perkowski SZ, Tahamont MV, et al: Thromboxane as a mediator of pulmonary dysfunction during intravascular complement activation in sheep. *Am Rev Respir Dis* 133:269, 1986.

126. Till GO, Ward PA: Systemic complement activation and acute lung injury. *Fed Proc* 45:13, 1986.

127. Johnson A, Cooper JA, Malik AB: Effect of complement activation with cobra venom factor on pulmonary vascular permeability. *J Appl Physiol* 61:2202, 1986.

128. Stevens JH, O'Hanley P, Shapiro JM, et al: Effects of anti-C5a antibodies on the adult respiratory distress syndrome in septic primates. *J Clin Invest* 77:1812, 1986.

129. Olson LM, Moss GS, Baukus O, et al: The role of C5 in septic lung injury. *Ann Surg* 202:771, 1985.

130. Ognibene FP, Martin SE, Parker MM, et al: Adult respiratory distress syndrome in patients with severe neutropenia. *N Engl J Med* 315:547, 1986.

131. Maunder RJ, Hackman RC, Riff E, et al: Occurrence of the adult respiratory distress syndrome in neutropenic patients. *Am Rev Respir Dis* 133:313, 1986.

132. Repine JE, Beehler CJ: Neutrophils and adult respiratory distress syndrome: Two interlocking perspectives in 1991. *Am Rev Respir Dis* 144:251, 1991.

133. Moore FD, Davis C, Rodrick M, et al: Neutrophil activation in thermal injury as assessed by increased expression of complement receptors. *N Engl J Med* 314:948, 1986.

134. Simms HH, D'Amico R: Increased PMN CD11b/CD18 expression following post-traumatic ARDS. *J Surg Res* 50:362, 1991.

135. Powe JE, Short A, Sibbald WJ, et al: Pulmonary accumulation of polymorphonuclear leukocytes in the adult respiratory distress syndrome. *Crit Care Med* 10:712, 1982.

136. Hooper RG, Kearl RA: Established ARDS treated with a sustained course of adrenocortical steroids. *Chest* 97:138, 1990.

137. Lee CT, Fein AM, Lippmann M, et al: Elastolytic activity in pulmonary lavage fluid from patients with adult respiratory distress syndrome. *N Engl J Med* 304:192, 1981.

138. Weiland JE, Davis WB, Holter JF, et al: Lung neutrophils in the adult respiratory distress syndrome: Clinical and pathophysiologic significance. *Am Rev Respir Dis* 133:218, 1986.

139. Modig J, Samulesson T, Hallgreen R: The predictive and discriminative value of biologically active products of eosinophils, neutrophils and complement in bronchoalveolar lavage and blood in patients with adult respiratory distress syndrome. *Resuscitation* 14:121, 1986.

140. Hallgren R, Samulesson T, Modig J: Complement activation and increased alveolar-capillary permeability after major surgery and in adult respiratory distress syndrome. *Crit Care Med* 15:189, 1987.

141. Zheutlin LM, Thonar E, Lemley-Gillespie S, et al: C3a DES ARG and elastase-alpha 1-protease inhibitor levels in lavage fluid from patients with adult respiratory distress syndrome. *J Crit Care* 2:86, 1987.

142. Zilow G, Joka T, Obertacke U, et al: Generation of anaphylatoxin C3a in plasma and bronchoalveolar lavage fluid in trauma patients at risk for the adult respiratory distress syndrome. *Crit Care Med* 20:468, 1992.

143. Hallgren R, Borg T, Venge P, et al: Signs of neutrophil and eosinophil activation in adult respiratory distress syndrome. *Crit Care Med* 12:14, 1984.

144. Patterson CE, Barnard JW, Lafuze JE, et al: The role of activation of neutrophils and microvascular pressure in acute pulmonary edema. *Am Rev Respir Dis* 140:1052, 1989.

145. Barie PS, Tahamont MV, Malik AB: Prevention of increased pulmonary vascular permeability after pancreatitis by granulocyte depletion in sheep. *Am Rev Respir Dis* 126:904, 1982.

146. Basadre JO, Sugi K, Traber DL, et al: The effect of leukocyte depletion on smoke inhalation injury in sheep. *Surgery* 104:208, 1988.

147. Winn R, Maunder R, Chi E, et al: Neutrophil depletion does not prevent lung edema after endotoxin infusion in goats. *J Appl Physiol* 62:116, 1987.

148. Basadre JO, Singh H, Herndon DN, et al: Effect of antibody-mediated neutropenia on the cardiopulmonary response to endotoxemia. *J Surg Res* 45:266, 1988.

149. Carden DL, Smith JK, Zimmerman BJ, et al: Reperfusion injury following circulatory collapse: The role of reactive oxygen metabolites. *J Crit Care* 4:294, 1989.

150. Friedl HP, Till GO, Ryan US, et al: Mediator-induced activation of xanthine oxidase in endothelial cells. *FASEB J* 3:2512, 1989.

151. Richard C, Lemonnier F, Thibault M, et al: Vitamin E deficiency and lipoperoxidation during adult respiratory distress syndrome. *Crit Care Med* 18:4, 1990.

152. Pacht ER, Timerman AP, Lykens MG, Merola AJ: Deficiency of alveolar fluid glutathione in patients with sepsis and the adult respiratory distress syndrome. *Chest* 100:1397, 1991.

153. Leff JA, Parsons PE, Day CE, et al: Increased serum catalase activity in septic patients with the adult respiratory distress syndrome. *Am Rev Respir Dis* 146:985, 1992.

154. Krsek-Staples JA, Kew RR, Webster RO: Ceruloplasmin and transferrin levels are altered in serum and bronchoalveolar lavage fluid of patients with the adult respiratory distress syndrome. *Am Rev Respir Dis* 145:1009, 1992.

155. Leff JA, Parson PE, Day CE, et al: Serum antioxidants as predictors of adult respiratory distress syndrome in patients with sepsis. *Lancet* 341:777, 1993.

156. Demling RH, LaLonde C, Ryan P, et al: Endotoxemia produces an increase in arterial but not venous lipid peroxides in sheep. *J Appl Physiol* 64:592, 1988.

157. Demling RH, LaLonde C, Jin LJ, et al: Endotoxemia causes increased lung tissue lipid peroxidation in unanesthetized sheep. *J Appl Physiol* 60:2094, 1986.

158. Demling RH, LaLonde C, Daryani R, et al: Relationship between the lung and systemic response to endotoxin: Comparison of physiologic change and the degree of lipid peroxidation. *Circ Shock* 34:364, 1991.

159. Seekamp A, LaLonde C, Zhu D, et al: Catalase prevents prostanoid release and lung lipid peroxidation after endotoxemia in sheep. *J Appl Physiol* 65:1210, 1988.

160. Demling R, LaLonde C, Seekamp A, et al: Endotoxin causes hydrogen peroxide-induced lung lipid peroxidation and prostanoid production. *Arch Surg* 123:1337, 1988.

161. Milligan SA, Hoeffel JM, Goldstein IM, et al: Effect of catalase on endotoxin-induced acute lung injury in unanesthetized sheep. *Am Rev Respir Dis* 137:420, 1988.

162. LaLonde C, Knox J, Daryani R, Zhu D, Demling RH: Topical flurbiprofen decreases burn wound-induced hypermetabolism and systemic lipid peroxidation. *Surgery* 109:645, 1991.

163. Kennedy TP, Rao NV, Noah W, et al: Ibuprofen prevents oxidant injury and in vitro lipid peroxidation by chelating iron. *J Clin Invest* 86:1565, 1990.

164. Bernard GR, Lucht WD, Niedermeyer ME, et al: Effect of N-acetylcysteine on the pulmonary response to endotoxin in the awake sheep and upon granulocyte function. *J Clin Invest* 73:1772, 1984.

165. Demling RH, Knox J, Youn Y-K, et al: Effect of dobutamine infusion on endotoxin-induced lipid peroxidation in awake sheep. *Surgery* 111:79, 1992.

166. Jepsen S, Herlevsen P, Knudsen P, et al: Antioxidant treatment witn N-acetycysteine during adult respiratory distress syndrome: A prospective, randomized, placebo-controlled study. *Crit Care Med* 20:918, 1992.

167. Traber DL, Adams T, Sziebert L, et al: Potentiation of lung vascular response to endotoxin by superoxide dismutase. *J Appl Physiol* 58:1005, 1985.

168. Wong C, Fox R, Demling RH: Effect of hydroxyl radical scavenging on endotoxin-induced lung injury. *Surgery* 97:300, 1985.

169. Baldwin SR, Grum CM, Boxer LA, et al: Oxidant activity in expired breath of patients with adult respiratory distress syndrome. *Lancet* 1:11, 1986.

170. Sznajder JI, Fraiman A, Hall JB, et al: Increased hydrogen peroxide in the expired breath of patients with acute hypoxemic respiratory failure. *Chest* 96:606, 1989.

171. Kietzmann D, Kahl R, Muller M, et al: Hydrogen peroxide in expired breath condensate of patients with acute respiratory failure and with ARDS. *Intensive Care Med* 19:78, 1993.

172. McKechnie K, Furman BL, Parratt JR: Modification by oxygen free radical scavengers of the metabolic and cardiovascular effects of endotoxin infusion in conscious rats. *Circ Shock* 19:429, 1986.

173. Morgan RA, Manning PB, Coran AG, et al: Oxygen free radical activity during live *E. coli* septic shock in the dog. *Circ Shock* 25:319, 1988.

174. Broner CW, Shenep JL, Stidham GL, et al: Effect of scavengers of oxygen-derived free radicals on mortality in endotoxin-challenged mice. *Crit Care Med* 16:848, 1988.

175. Pearce RA, Finley RJ, Mustard RA Jr, et al: 2,3-dihydroxybenzoic acid: Effect on mortality rate in a septic rat model. *Arch Surg* 120:937, 1985.

176. Takeda K, Shimada Y, Okada T, et al: Lipid peroxidation in experimental septic rats. *Crit Care Med* 14:719, 1986.

177. Novelli GP: Oxygen radicals in experimental shock: Effects of spin-trapping nitrones in ameliorating shock pathophysiology. *Crit Care Med* 20:499, 1992.

178. Pogrebniak HW, Merino MJ, Hahn SM, et al: Spin trap salvage from endotoxemia: The role of cytokine down-regulation. *Surgery* 112:130, 1992.

179. Crowell JW, Jones CE, Smith EE: Effect of allopurinol on hemorrhagic shock. *Am J Physiol* 216:744, 1969.

180. Allan G, Cambridge D, Tsang-Tan LL, et al: The protective action of allopurinol in an experimental model of hemorrhagic shock and reperfusion. *J Pharmacol* 89:149, 1986.

181. Jacobs DM, Julsrud JM, Bubrick MP: Iron chelation with a deferoxamine conjugate in hemorrhagic shock. *J Surg Res* 51:484, 1991.

182. Demling RH, LaLonde C, Liu Y, et al: The lung inflammatory response to thermal injury: Relationship between physiologic and histologic changes. *Surgery* 106:52, 1989.

183. Demling RH, LaLonde C: Early postburn lipid peroxidation: Effect of ibuprofen and allopurinol. *Surgery* 107:85, 1990.

184. Novotny MJ, Laughlin MH, Adams HR: Evidence for lack of importance of oxygen free radicals in *Escherichia coli* endotoxemia in dogs. *Am J Physiol* 254:H954, 1988.

185. Broner CW, Shenep JL, Stidham GL, et al: Effect of antioxidants in experimental *Escherichia coli* septicemia. *Circ Shock* 29:77, 1989.

186. van Bebber IPT, Lieners CFJ, Kodewijn EL, et al: Superoxide dismutase and catalase in an experimental model of multiple organ failure. *J Surg Res* 52:265, 1992.

187. Takeda K, Shimada Y, Amano M, et al: Plasma lipid peroxide and alpha-tocopherol in critically ill patients. *Crit Care Med* 12:957, 1984.

188. Girotti MJ, Khan N, McLellan BA: Early measurement of systemic lipid peroxidation products in the plasma of major blunt trauma patients. *J Trauma* 31:32, 1991.

189. Marzi I, Buhren V, Shuttler A, Trentz O: Value of superoxide dismutase for prevention of multiple organ failure after multiple trauma. *J Trauma* 35:110, 1993.

190. Nies AS, Forsyth RP, Williams HE, et al: Contribution of kinins to endotoxin shock in unanesthetized rhesus monkeys. *Circ Res* 22:155, 1968.

191. Reichgott MJ, Melmon KL, Forsyth RP, et al: Cardiovascular and metabolic effects of whole or fractionated gram-negative bacterial endotoxin in the unanesthetized rhesus monkey. *Circ Res* 33:346, 1973.

192. O'Donnell TF, Clowes GHA, Talamo RC, et al: Kinin activation in the blood of patients with sepsis. *Surg Gynecol Obstet* 143:539, 1976.

193. Kimball HR, Melmon KL, Wolff SH: Endotoxin-induced kinin production in man. *Exp Biol Med* 139:1078, 1972.

194. Gallimore MJ, Aasen AO, Lyngaas KHN, et al: Falls in plasma levels of prekallikrein, high molecular weight kininogen, and kallikrein inhibitors during lethal endotoxin shock in dogs. *Thromb Res* 12:307, 1978.

195. Mason JW, Kleeberg U, Dolan P, et al: Plasma kallikrein and Hageman factor in gram-negative bacteremia. *Ann Intern Med* 73:545, 1970.

196. Hirsch EF, Nakajima T, Oshima G, et al: Kinin system responses in sepsis after trauma in man. *J Surg Res* 17:147, 1974.

197. Aasen AO, Smith-Erichsen N, Amundsen E: Plasma kallikrein-kinin system in septicemia. *Arch Surg* 118:343, 1983.

198. Robinson JA, Klodnycky ML, Loeb HS, et al: Endotoxin, prekallikrein, complement and systemic vascular resistance: Sequential measurements in man. *Am J Med* 59:61, 1975.

199. Pixley RA, De La Cadena R, Page JD, et al: The contact system contributes to hypotension but not disseminated intravascular coagulation in lethal bacteremia. In vivo use of a monoclonal anti-factor XII antibody to block contact activation in baboons. *J Clin Invest* 91:61, 1993.

200. Janssen HF, Pugh JL, Lange DL: Bradykinin does not contribute to hypotension in early canine endotoxemia. *Circ Shock* 23:197, 1987.

201. Mann R, Woodson LC, Traber LD, et al: The role of bradykinin in ovine endotoxemia. *Circ Shock* (*in press*).

202. Ball HA, Cook JA, Wise WC, et al: Role of thromboxane, prostaglandins and leukotrienes in endotoxic and septic shock. *Intensive Care Med* 12:116, 1986.

203. Fink MP: Role of prostaglandins and related compounds in the pathophysiology of endotoxic and septic shock. *Semin Respir Med* 7:17, 1985.

204. Fink MP, Gardiner WM, Roethel R, et al: Plasma levels of 6-keto-PGF, but not TxB_2 increase in rats with peritonitis due to cecal ligation. *Circ Shock* 16:297, 1985.

205. Fink MP, Rothschild HR, Deniz YF, et al: Systemic and mesenteric O_2 metabolism in endotoxic pigs: Effect of ibuprofen and meclofenamate. *J Appl Physiol* 67:1950, 1989.

206. Hanly PJ, Sienko A, Light RB: Role of prostacyclin and thrombox-

ane in the circulatory changes in acute bacteremic *Pseudomonas* pneumonia in dogs. *Am Rev Respir Dis* 137:700, 1988.

207. Demling RH, Smith M, Gunther R, et al: Pulmonary injury and prostaglandin production during endotoxemia in conscious sheep. *Am J Physiol* 240:H348, 1981.

208. Wise WC, Cook JA, Eller T, et al: Ibuprofen improves survival from endotoxic shock in the rat. *J Pharmacol Exp Ther* 215:160, 1980.

209. Tempel GE, Cook JA, Wise WC, et al: Improvement in organ blood flow by inhibition of thromboxane synthetase during experimental endotoxic shock in the rat. *J Cardiovasc Pharmacol* 8:514, 1986.

210. Halushka PV, Cook JA, Wise WC: Beneficial effects of UK 37248, a thromboxane synthetase inhibitor, in experimental endotoxic shock in the rat. *Br J Clin Pharmacol* 15:133S, 1983.

211. Jacobs ER, Bone RC, Balk R, et al: Increased survival in bacteremic sheep treated with ibuprofen. *J Crit Care* 1:142, 1986.

212. Cook JA, Wise WC, Halushka PV: Elevated thromboxane levels in the rat during endotoxic shock: Protective effect of imidazole, 13-azaprostanoic acid, or essential fatty acid deficiency. *J Clin Invest* 65:227, 1980.

213. Casey LC, Fletcher JR, Zmudka MI, et al: Prevention of endotoxin-induced pulmonary hypertension in primates by the use of a selective thromboxane synthetase inhibitor, OKY 1581. *J Pharmacol Exp Ther* 222:441, 1982.

214. Kuhl PG, Bolds JM, Loyd JE, et al: Thromboxane receptor-mediated bronchial and hemodynamic responses in ovine endotoxemia. *Am J Physiol* 254:R310, 1988.

215. Svartholm E, Berguvist D, Hedner U, et al: Thromboxane A₂-receptor blockade and prostacyclin in porcine *Escherichia coli* shock. *Arch Surg* 124:669, 1989.

216. Lee CC, Surgerman HJ, Tatum JL, et al: Effects of ibuprofen on a pig *Pseudomonas* ARDS model. *J Surg Res* 40:438, 1986.

217. Steinberg SM, Dehring DJ, Martin DT, et al: Amelioration of pulmonary pathophysiology of adult respiratory distress syndrome by sulindac, a cyclooxygenase inhibitor. *J Trauma* 27:1323, 1987.

218. Revhaug A, Michie HR, Manson JM, et al: Inhibition of cyclooxygenase attenuates the metabolic response to endotoxin in humans. *Arch Surg* 123:162, 1988.

219. Halushka PV, Reines HD, Barrow SE, et al: Elevated plasma 6-keto-prostaglandin F₁ in patients in septic shock. *Crit Care Med* 13:451, 1985.

220. Oettinger WKE, Walter GO, Jensen UM, et al: Endogenous prostaglandin F₂ in the hyperdynamic state of severe sepsis in man. *Br J Surg* 70:237, 1983.

221. Oettinger W, Berger D, Berger HG: The clinical significance of prostaglandins and thromboxane as mediators of septic shock. *Klin Wochenschr* 65:61, 1987.

222. Slotman GJ: Interaction of prostaglandins, activated complement, and granulocytes in clinical sepsis and hypotension. *Surgery* 99:744, 1986.

223. Reines HD, Cook JA, Halushka PV, et al: Plasma thromboxane concentrations are raised in patients dying with septic shock. *Lancet* 2:174, 1982.

224. Deby-Dupont G, Braun M, Lamy M, et al: Thromboxane and prostacyclin release in adult respiratory distress syndrome. *Intensive Care Med* 13:167, 1987.

225. Bernard GR, Reines HD, Halushka PV, et al: Prostacyclin and thromboxane A₂ formation is increased in human sepsis syndrome: effects of cyclooxygenase inhibition. *Am Rev Respir Dis* 144:1095, 1991.

226. Vadas P, Pruzanski W, Stefanski E, et al: Pathogenesis of hypotension in septic shock: Correlation of circulating phospholipase A₂ levels with circulatory collapse. *Crit Care Med* 16:1, 1988.

227. Vadas P, Scott K, Smith G, et al: Serum phospholipase A₂ enzyme activity and immunoreactivity in a prospective analysis of patients with septic shock. *Life Sci* 50:807, 1992.

228. Vadas P, Schouten BD, Stefanski E, et al: The association of hyperphospholipasemia A₂ with multisystem organ dysfunction due to salicylate intoxication. *Crit Care Med* (*in press*).

229. Hanly PJ, Roberts D, Dobson K, et al: Effect of indomethacin on arterial oxygenation in critically ill patients with severe bacterial pneumonia. *Lancet* 1:351, 1987.

230. Martich GD, Parker MM, Cunnion RE, Suffredini AF: Effects of ibuprofen and pentoxifylline on the cardiovascular response of normal humans to endotoxin. *J Appl Physiol* 73:925, 1992.

231. Leeman M, Boeynaems JM, Degaute JP, et al: Administration of dazoxiben, a selective thromboxane synthetase inhibitor, in the adult respiratory distress syndrome. *Chest* 87:726, 1985.

232. Reines HD, Halushka PV, Olanoff LS, et al: Dazoxiben in human sepsis and adult respiratory distress syndrome. *Clin Pharmacol Ther* 37:391, 1985.

233. Haupt MT, Jastremski MS, Clemmer TP, et al: Effect of ibuprofen in patients with severe sepsis: A randomized, double-blind, multicenter study. *Crit Care Med* 19:1339, 1991.

234. Garcia JGN, Noonan TC, Jubiz W, et al: Leukotrienes and the pulmonary microcirculation. *Am Rev Respir Dis* 136:161, 1987.

235. Sprague RS, Stephenson AH, Dahms TE, et al: Proposed role for leukotrienes in the pathophysiology of multiple systems organ failure. *Crit Care Clin* 5:315, 1989.

236. Keppler D, Hagmann W, Rapp S: Role of leukotrienes in endotoxin action in vivo. *Rev Infect Dis* 9:580S, 1987.

237. Denzingler C, Rapp S, Hagmann W, et al: Leukotrienes as mediators in tissue trauma. *Science* 230:330, 1985.

238. Bitterman H, Smith BA, Lefer AM: Beneficial actions of antagonism of peptide leukotrienes in hemorrhagic shock. *Circ Shock* 24:159, 1988.

239. Hock CE, Loprest L, Lefer AM: Inhibitors of lipoxygenase products improves survival in traumatic shock. *Prostaglandins* 28:557, 1984.

240. Bitterman H, Lefer AM: Use of a novel peptide leukotriene receptor antagonist, LY-163443, in splanchnic artery occlusion shock. *Prostaglandins Leukot Essent Fatty Acids* 32:63, 1988.

241. Keppler D, Hagmann W, Denzlinger C: Leukotrienes as mediators in endotoxin shock and tissue trauma. *Prog Clin Biol Res* 236A:301, 1987.

242. Cohn SM, Kruithoff KL, Rothschild HR, et al: LY 171883 preserves mesenteric perfusion in porcine endotoxin shock. *J Surg Res* 49:37, 1990.

243. Cohn SM, Fink MP, Lee PC, et al: LY203647 selective leukotriene (LT C₄-D₄) antagonist, improves pulmonary function and mesenteric perfusion in a porcine model of septic shock and ARDS. *Surg Forum* 15:105, 1989.

244. Etemadi AR, Temple GE, Farah BA, et al: Beneficial effects of a leukotriene antagonist on endotoxin-induced acute hemodynamic alterations. *Circ Shock* 22:5, 1987.

245. Gross D, Dahan JB, Landau EH: Effect of leukotriene inhibitor LY-171883 on the pulmonary response to *Escherichia coli* endotoxemia. *Crit Care Med* 18:190, 1990.

246. Turner CR, Lackey MN, Quinlan MF, et al: Therapeutic intervention in a rat model of adult respiratory distress syndrome: II. Lipoxygenase pathway inhibition. *Circ Shock* 34:263, 1991.

247. Wollert PS, Menconi MJ, O'Sullivan BP, et al: LY255283, a novel leukotriene B₄ receptor antagonist, limits activation of neutrophils and prevents acute lung injury induced by endotoxin in pigs. *Surgery* (*in press*).

248. Fink MP, O'Sullivan BP, Menconi MJ, et al: LY255283, a novel leukotriene B₄ receptor antagonist, ameliorates hypoxemia and abrogates pulmonary edema in a porcine model of circulatory shock and acute lung injury caused by lipopolysaccharide. *Crit Care Med* (*in press*).

249. Miller RF, Lefferts PL, Snapper JR: Effect of sulfidopeptide leukotriene receptor antagonists on endotoxin-induced pulmonary dysfunction in awake sheep. *Am Rev Respir Dis* 146:997, 1992.

250. Kuratomi Y, Lefferts PL, Christman BW, et al: Effect of a 5-lipoxygenase inhibitor on endotoxin-induced pulmonary dysfunction in awake sheep. *J Appl Physiol* 74:596, 1993.

251. Matthay MA, Eschenbacher WL, Goetzl EJ: Elevated concentrations of leukotriene D₄ in pulmonary edema fluid of patients with adult respiratory distress syndrome. *J Clin Immunol* 4:479, 1984.

252. Bernard GR, Korley V, Chee P, et al: Persistent generation of peptido leukotrienes in patients with the adult respiratory distress syndrome. *Am Rev Respir Dis* 144:263, 1991.

253. Stephenson AH, Lonigro AJ, Hyers TM, et al: Increased concentrations of leukotrienes in bronchoalveolar lavage fluid of patients with ARDS or at risk for ARDS. *Am Rev Respir Dis* 138:714, 1988.

254. Knoller J, Schonfeld W, Joka T, et al: Generation of leukotrienes in polytraumatic patients with adult respiratory distress syndrome (ARDS). *Prog Clin Biol Res* 236A:311, 1987.

255. Antonelli M, Bufi M, DeBlasi RA, et al: Detection of leukotrienes B₄, C₄ and of their isomers in arterial, mixed venous blood and

bronchoalveolar lavage fluid from ARDS patients. *Intensive Care Med* 15:296, 1989.

256. Davis JM, Meyer JD, Barie PS, et al: Elevated production of neutrophil leukotriene B$_4$ precedes pulmonary failure in critically ill surgical patients. *Surg Gynecol Obstet* 170:495, 1990.

257. Braquet P, Touqui L, Shen TY, et al: Perspectives in platelet-activating factor research. *Pharmacol Rev* 39:97, 1987.

258. Chang SW, Feddersen CO, Henson PM, et al: Platelet-activating factor mediates hemodynamic changes and lung injury in endotoxin-treated rats. *J Clin Invest* 79:1, 1987.

259. Lefer AL: Induction of tissue injury and altered cardiovascular performance by platelet-activating factor: Relevance to multiple systems organ failure. *Crit Care Clin* 5:331, 1989.

260. Doebber TW, Wu MS, Robbins JC, et al: Platelet activating factor (PAF) involvement in endotoxin-induced hypotension in rats, studies with PAF-receptor antagonist kadsurenone. *Biochem Biophys Res Commun* 127:799, 1985.

261. Terashita Z, Imura Y, Nishikawa K, et al: Is platelet activating factor (PAF) a mediator of endotoxin shock? *Eur J Pharmacol* 109:257, 1985.

262. Adnot S, Lefort J, Lagente V, et al: Interference of BN 52021, a PAF-acether antagonist, with endotoxin-induced hypotension in the guinea pig. *Pharmacol Res Commun* 18:197, 1986.

263. Handley DA, Van Valen RG, Tomesch JC, et al: Biological properties of the antagonist SRI 63-441 in the PAF and endotoxin models of hypotension in the rat and dog. *Immunopharmacology* 13:125, 1987.

264. Caplan MS, Kelly A, Hsueh W: Endotoxin and hypoxia-induced intestinal epithelial necrosis in rats: The role of platelet activating factor. *Pediatr Res* 31:428, 1992.

265. Sessler CN, Glauser FL, Davis D, et al: Effects of platelet-activating factor antagonist SRI 63-441 on endotoxemia in sheep. *J Appl Physiol* 65:2624, 1988.

266. Byrne K, Surgerman HJ, Tatum JL, et al: Successful use of an anti-platelet-activating factor agent in the porcine *Pseudomonas* ARDS model. *Surg Forum* 39:61, 1988.

267. Siebeck M, Weiprt J, Keser C, et al: A trazolodiazepine platelet activating factor receptor antagonist (WEB 2086) reduces pulmonary dysfunction during endotoxin shock in swine. *J Trauma* 31:942, 1991.

268. Baum TD, Heard SO, Feldman HS, et al: Endotoxin-induced myocardial depression in rats: Effect of ibuprofen and SDZ 64-688, a platelet activating factor receptor antagonist. *J Surg Res* 48:629, 1990.

269. Tollins JP, Vercellotti DM, Wilkowske M, et al: Role of platelet activating factor in endotoxemic acute renal failure in the male rat. *J Lab Clin Med* 113:316, 1989.

270. Lefer AM: Significance of lipid mediators in shock states. *Circ Shock* 27:3, 1989.

271. Lewis MS, Whatley RE, Cain P, et al: Hydrogen peroxide stimulates the synthesis of platelet-activating factor by endothelium and induces endothelial cell-dependent neutrophil adhesion. *J Clin Invest* 82:2045, 1988.

272. Oda M, Satouchi K, Ikeda I, et al: The presence of platelet-activating factor associated with eosinophil and/or neutrophil accumulations in the pleural fluids. *Am Rev Respir Dis* 141:1469, 1990.

273. Diez FL, Nieto ML, Fernandez-Gallardo S, et al: Occupancy of platelet receptors for platelet-activating factor in patients with septicemia. *J Clin Invest* 83:1733, 1989.

274. Bussolino F, Porcellini MG, Varese L, Bosia A: Intravascular release of platelet-activating factor in children with sepsis. *Thromb Res* 48:619, 1987.

275. Leonelli FM, Leong LL, Strum MJ, et al: Plasma levels of the lyso-derivative of platelet-activating factor in acute severe systemic illness. *Clin Sci* 77:561, 1989.

276. Fink A, Geva D, Zung A, et al: Adult respiratory distress syndrome: Roles of leukotriene C$_4$ and platelet activating factor. *Crit Care Med* 18:905, 1990.

277. Larrick JW, Graham D, Toy K, et al: Recombinant tumor necrosis factor causes activation of human granulocytes. *Blood* 69:640, 1987.

278. Pohlman TH, Stanness KA, Beatty PG, et al: An endothelial cell surface factor induced *in vitro* by lipopolysaccharide, interleukin 1, and tumor necrosis factor-alpha increases neutrophil adherence

by a CDw18-dependent mechanism. *J Immunol* 136:4548, 1986.

279. Gamble JR, Harlan JM, Klebanoff SJ, et al: Stimulation of the adherence of neutrophils to umbilical vein endothelium by human recombinant tumor necrosis factor. *Proc Natl Acad Sci USA* 82:8667, 1985.

280. Le J, Vilcek J: Tumor necrosis factor and interleukin 1: Cytokines with multiple overlapping biological activities. *Lab Invest* 56:234, 1987.

281. Strieter RM, Kunkle SL, Showell HJ, et al: Endothelial cell gene expression of a neutrophil chemotactic factor by TNF-alpha, LPS, or IL-1-beta. *Science* 243:1467, 1989.

282. Dinarello CA, Cannon JG, Wolff SM, et al: Tumor necrosis factor (cachectin) is an endogenous pyrogen and induces production of interleukin-1. *J Exp Med* 163:1433, 1986.

283. Bachwich PR, Chensue SW, Larrick GW, et al: Tumor necrosis factor stimulates interleukin-1 and prostaglandin E$_2$ production in resting macrophages. *Biochem Biophys Res Commun* 136:94, 1986.

284. Rothstein JL, Schreiber H: Synergy between tumor necrosis factor and bacterial products causes hemorrhagic necrosis and lethal shock in normal mice. *Proc Natl Acad Sci USA* 85:607, 1988.

285. Elias JA, Gustilo K, Freundlich B: Human alveolar macrophage and blood monocyte inhibition of fibroblast proliferation: Evidence for synergy between interleukin-1 and tumor necrosis factor. *Am Rev Respir Dis* 138:1595, 1988.

286. Tredget EE, Yu YM, Zhong S, et al: Role of interleukin 1 and tumor necrosis factor on energy metabolism in rabbits. *Am J Physiol* 255:E760, 1988.

287. Flores EA, Bistrian BR, Pomposelli JJ, et al: Infusion of tumor necrosis factor/cachectin promotes muscle catabolism in the rat: A synergistic effect with interleukin 1. *J Clin Invest* 83:1614, 1989.

288. Beutler B, Milsark IW, Cerami AC: Passive immunization against cachectin/tumor necrosis factor protects mice and lethal effect of endotoxin. *Science* 229:869, 1985.

289. Tracey KJ, Beutler B, Lowry S, et al: Shock and tissue injury induced by recombinant human cachectin. *Science* 234:470, 1986.

290. Tracey KJ, Fong Y, Hesse DG, et al: Anti-cachectin/TNF monoclonal antibodies prevent septic shock during lethal bacteremia. *Nature* 330:662, 1987.

291. Hinshaw LB, Tekamp-Olson P, Chang ACK, et al: Survival of primates in LD$_{100}$ septic shock following therapy with antibody to tumor necrosis factor (TNFa). *Circ Shock* 30:279, 1990.

292. Hinshaw LB, Emerson TE Jr, Taylor FB Jr, et al: Lethal *Staphylococcus aureus*-induced shock primates: prevention of death with anti-TNF antibody. *J Trauma* 33:568, 1992.

293. Mallick AA, Ishizaka A, Stephens KE, et al: Multiple organ damage caused by tumor necrosis factor and prevented by prior neutrophil depletion. *Chest* 95:1114, 1989.

294. Ferrari-Daliviera E, Mealy K, Smith RJ, et al: Tumor necrosis factor induces adult respiratory distress syndrome in rats. *Arch Surg* 124:1400, 1989.

295. Johnson J, Meyrick B, Jesmok G, et al: Human recombinant tumor necrosis factor alpha infusion mimics endotoxemia in awake sheep. *J Appl Physiol* 66:1448, 1989.

296. Krcil EA, Greene E, Fitzgibbon C, et al: Effect of recombinant human tumor necrosis factor alpha, lymphotoxin, and *Escherichia coli* lipopolysaccharide on hemodynamics, lung, microvascular permeability, and eicosanoid synthesis in anesthetized sheep. *Circ Res* 65:502, 1989.

297. Natanson C, Eichenholz PW, Danner RL, et al: Endotoxin and tumor necrosis factor challenges in dogs simulate the cardiovascular profile of human septic shock. *J Exp Med* 169:823, 1989.

298. Pagani FD, Baker LS, Hsi C, et al: Left ventricular systolic and diastolic dysfunction after infusion of tumor necrosis factor-alpha in conscious dogs. *J Clin Invest* 90:389, 1992.

299. Heard SO, Perkins MW, Fink MP: Tumor necrosis factor-α causes reversible myocardial depression in guinea pigs. *Crit Care Med* 20:523, 1992.

300. Gulick T, Chung MK, Pieper SJ, et al: Interleukin 1 and tumor necrosis factor inhibits cardiac myocyte beta-adrenergic responsiveness. *Proc Natl Acad Sci USA* 86:6753, 1989.

301. Schirmer WJ, Schirmer JM, Fry DE: Recombinant human tumor necrosis factor produces hemodynamic changes characteristic of sepsis and endotoxemia. *Arch Surg* 124:445, 1989.

302. Pagani FD, Baker LS, Knox MA, et al: Load-insensitive assessment of myocardial performance after tumor necrosis factor alpha in dogs. *Surgery* 111:683, 1992.

303. Hollenberg SM, Cunnion RE, Parrillo JE: The effect of tumor necrosis factor on vascular smooth muscle: *In vitro* studies using rat aortic rings. *Chest* 100:1133, 1991.

304. Stadler J, Bentz BG, Harbrecht BG, et al: Tumor necrosis factor alpha inhibits hepatocyte mitochondrial respiration. *Ann Surg* 216:539, 1992.

305. Hesse DG, Tracey KJ, Fong Y, et al: Cytokine appearance in human endotoxemia and primate bacteremia. *Surg Gynecol Obstet* 166:147, 1988.

306. Michie HR, Manogue KR, Spriggs DR, et al: Detection of circulating tumor necrosis factor after endotoxin administration. *N Engl J Med* 318:1481, 1988.

307. Starnes HF, Warren RS, Jeevanandam M, et al: Tumor necrosis factor and the acute metabolic response to tissue injury in man. *J Clin Invest* 82:1321, 1988.

308. Michie HR, Spriggs DR, Manogue KR, et al: Tumor necrosis factor and endotoxin induce similar metabolic responses in human beings. *Surgery* 104:280, 1988.

309. Kimura K, Taguchi T, Urushizaki I, et al: Phase I study of recombinant human tumor necrosis factor. *Cancer Chemother Pharmacol* 20:223, 1987.

310. Girardin E, Grau GE, Dayer JM, et al: Tumor necrosis factor and interleukin-1 in the serum of children with severe infectious purpura. *N Engl J Med* 319:397, 1988.

311. Sullivan JS, Kilpatrick L, Costarino AT, et al: Correlation of plasma cytokine elevations with mortality rate in children with sepsis. *J Pediatr* 120:510, 1992.

312. Debets JM, Kampmeijer R, van der Linden MP, et al: Plasma tumor necrosis factor and mortality in critically ill septic patients. *Crit Care Med* 17:489, 1989.

313. Damas P, Reuter A, Gysen P, et al: Tumor necrosis factor and interleukin-1 serum levels during severe sepsis in humans. *Crit Care Med* 17:975, 1989.

314. Dofferhoff ASM, Bom VJJ, De Vries-Hospers HG, et al: Patterns of cytokines, plasma endotoxin, plasminogen activator inhibitor, and acute-phase proteins during the treatment of severe sepsis in humans. *Crit Care Med* 20:185, 1992.

315. Endo S, Inada K, Inoue Y, et al: Two types of septic shock classified by the plasma levels of cytokines and endotoxin. *Circ Shock* 38:264, 1992.

316. Damas P, Ledoux D, Nys M, et al: Cytokine serum level during severe sepsis in humans: IL-6 as a marker of severity. *Ann Surg* 215:356, 1992.

317. Cannon JG, Friedberg JS, Gelfand JA, et al: Circulating interleukin-1β and tumor necrosis factor-α concentrations after burn trauma in humans. *Crit Care Med* 20:1414, 1992.

318. de Groote MA, Martin MA, Densen P, et al: Plasma tumor necrosis factor levels in patients with presumed sepsis. Results in those treated with antilipid A antibody vs placebo. *JAMA* 262:249, 1989.

319. Taveira da Silva AM, Kaulbach HC, Chuidian FS, et al: Brief report: Shock and multiple organ dysfunction after self-administration of *Salmonella* endotoxin. *N Engl J Med* 328:1457, 1993.

320. Munoz C, Carlet J, Fitting C, et al: Dysregulation of in vitro cytokine production by monocytes during sepsis. *J Clin Invest* 88:1747, 1991.

321. Cavaillon JM, Munoz C, Fitting C, et al: Circulating cytokines: The tip of the iceberg? *Circ Shock* 38:145, 1992.

322. Suter PM, Suter S, Girardin E, et al: High bronchoalveolar levels of tumor-necrosis factor and its inhibitors, interleukin-1, interferon, and elastase in patients with the adult respiratory distress syndrome after trauma, shock, or sepsis. *Am Rev Respir Dis* 145:1016, 1992.

323. Fisher CJ Jr, Opal SM, Dhainaut J-F, et al: Influence of an antitumor necrosis factor monoclonal antibody on cytokine levels in patients with sepsis. *Crit Care Med* 21:318, 1993.

324. Vincent J-L, Bakker J, Marecaux G, et al: Administration of anti-TNF antibody improves left ventricular function in septic shock patients: Results of a pilot study. *Chest* 101:810, 1992.

325. Kaplan E, Dinarello CA, Gelfand JA: Interleukin-1 and the response to injury. *Immunol Res* 8:118, 1989.

326. Dinarello CA: Biology of interleukin 1. *FASEB J* 2:108, 1988.

327. Mizel SB: Interleukins. *FASEB J* 3:2379, 1989.

328. Dinarello CA: Interleukin-1 and the pathogenesis of the acute-phase response. *N Engl J Med* 311:1413, 1984.

329. Okusawa S, Gelfand JA, Ikejima T, et al: Interleukin 1 induces a shock-like state in rabbits. *J Clin Invest* 81:1162, 1988.

330. Fukushima R, Saito H, Taniwaka K, et al: Different roles of IL-1 and TNF on hemodynamics and interorgan amino acid metabolism in awake dogs. *Am J Physiol* 262:E275, 1992.

331. McKenna TM, Reusch DW, Simpkins CO: Macrophage-conditioned medium and interleukin 1 suppress vascular contractility. *Circ Shock* 25:187, 1988.

332. Beasley D, Cohen RA, Levinsky NG: Interleukin 1 inhibits contraction of vascular smooth muscle. *J Clin Invest* 83:331, 1989.

333. Beasley D, Schwartz JH, Brenner BM: Interleukin 1 induces prolonged L-arginine-dependent cyclic guanosine monophosphate and nitrite production in rat vascular smooth muscle cells. *J Clin Invest* 87:602, 1991.

334. Wakabayashi G, Gelfand JA, Burke JF, et al: A specific receptor antagonist for interleukin 1 prevents *Escherichia coli*-induced shock in rabbits. *FASEB J* 5:338, 1991.

335. Alexander HR, Doherty GM, Fraker DL, et al: Human recombinant interleukin-1α protection against the lethality of endotoxin and experimental sepsis in mice. *J Surg Res* 50:421, 1991.

336. Cerra FB, Siegel JH, Coleman B, et al: Septic autocannibalism: A failure of exogenous nutritional support. *Ann Surg* 192:570, 1980.

337. Clowes GHA, George BC, Villef CA, et al: Muscle proteolysis induced by a circulating peptide in patients with sepsis or trauma. *N Engl J Med* 308:545, 1983.

338. Clowes GHA, Hirsch E, George BC, et al: The significance of altered protein metabolism regulated by proteolysis inducing factor, the circulating cleavage product of interleukin-1. *Ann Surg* 202:446, 1985.

339. Zamir O, Hasslegran PO, Kunkel SL, et al: Evidence that tumor necrosis factor participates in the regulation of muscle proteolysis during sepsis. *Arch Surg* 127:170, 1992.

340. Dinarello CA, Bernheim HA: Ability of human leukocytic pyrogen to stimulate brain prostaglandin synthesis *in vitro*. *J Neurochem* 37:702, 1981.

341. Baracos V, Rodemann P, Dinarello CA, et al: Stimulation of muscle protein degradation and prostaglandin E₂ release by leukocytic pyrogen (interleukin-1): A mechanism for the increased degradation of muscle proteins during fever. *N Engl J Med* 308:553, 1983.

342. Rossi V, Breviario F, Ghezzi P, et al: Prostacyclin synthesis induced in vascular cell by interleukin-1. *Science* 229:174, 1985.

343. Lugar A, Graf H, Schwarts HP, et al: Decreased serum interleukin 1 activity and monocyte interleukin 1 production in patients with fatal sepsis. *Crit Care Med* 14:458, 1986.

344. Cannon JG, Tompkins RG, Gelfand JA, et al: Circulating interleukin-1β and tumor necrosis factor in septic shock and experimental endotoxin fever. *J Infect Dis* 161:79, 1990.

345. Munoz C, Carlet J, Fitting C, et al: Dysregulation of *in vitro* cytokine production by monocytes during sepsis. *J Clin Invest* 88:1747, 1991.

346. Hoch RC, Rodriquez R, Manning T, et al: Effects of accidental trauma on cytokine and endotoxin production. *Crit Care Med* 21:839, 1993.

347. Pinsky MR, Vincent J-L, Deviere J, et al: Serum cytokine levels in human septic shock: Relation to multiple-system organ failure and mortality. *Chest* 103:565, 1993.

348. Herzyk DJ, Wewers MD: ELISA detection of IL-1β in human sera needs independent confirmation. *Am Rev Respir Dis* 147:139, 1993.

349. Helle M, Brakenhoff JPJ, De Groot ER, et al: Interleukin-6 is involved in interleukin-1 induced activity. *Eur J Immunol* 18:957, 1988.

350. Moshage HJ, Roelofs HMJ, van Pelt JF, et al: The effect of interleukin-1, interleukin-6 and its interrelationship on the synthesis of serum amyloid A and C-reactive protein in primary cultures of adult human hepatocytes. *Biochem Biophys Res Commun* 155:112, 1988.

351. Nijsten MWN, De Groot ER, ten Duis HJ, et al: Serum levels of interleukin-6 and acute phase responses. *Lancet* 2:921, 1987.

352. Hack EE, De Groot ER, Felt-Bersma JF, et al: Increased plasma levels of interleukin-6 in sepsis. *Blood* 74:1704, 1989.

353. Van Zee KJ, DeForge LE, Fischer E, et al: IL-8 in septic shock, endotoxemia, and after IL-1 administration. *J Immunol* 146:3478, 1991.

354. Redl H, Schlag G, Bahrami S, et al: Plasma neutrophil-activating peptide-1/interleukin-8 and neutrophil elastase in a primate bacteremia model. *J Infect Dis* 164:383, 1991.

355. Huber AR, Kunkul SL, Todd RF, Weiss SJ: Regulation of transendothelial neutrophil migration by endogenous interleukin-8. *Science* 254:99, 1991.

356. Hack CE, Hart M, Strack RJM, et al: Interleukin-8 in sepsis: Relation to shock and inflammatory mediators. *Infect Immunol* 60:2835, 1992.

357. Miller EJ, Cohen AB, Nagao S, et al: Elevated levels of NAP-1/interleukin-8 are present in the airspaces of patients with the adult respiratory distress syndrome and are associated with increased mortality. *Am Rev Respir Dis* 146:427, 1992.

358. Vane JR, Anggard EE, Botting RM: Regulatory functions of the vascular endothelium. *N Engl J Med* 323:27, 1990.

359. Moncada S, Palmer RMJ, Higgs EA: Nitric oxide: Physiology, pathophysiology, and pharmacology. *Pharmacol Rev* 43:109, 1991.

360. Palmer RMJ: The discovery of nitric oxide in the vessel wall: A unifying concept in the pathogenesis of sepsis. *Arch Surg* 128:396, 1993.

361. Salvemini D, Korbut R, Anggard E, Vane J: Lipopolysaccharide increases release of nitric oxide-like factor from endothelial cells. *Eur J Pharmacol* 17:135, 1989.

362. Fleming I, Gray GA, Stoclet J-C: Influence of endothelium on induction of the L-arginine pathway in rat aortas. *Am J Physiol* 264:H1200, 1993.

363. Fleming I, Gray GA, Julou-Schaeffer G, et al: Incubation with endotoxin activates the L-arginine pathway in vascular tissue. *Biochem Biophys Res Commun* 171:562, 1990.

364. Myers PR, Wright TF, Tanner MA, Adams HR: EDRF and nitric oxide production in cultured endothelial cells: Direct inhibition by *E. coli* endotoxin. *Am J Physiol* 262:H710, 1992.

365. Aoki N, Siegfried M, Lefer A: Anti-EDRF effect of tumor necrosis factor in isolated, perfused cat carotid arteries. *Am J Physiol* 256:H1509, 1989.

366. Kilbourn RG, Jubran A, Gross SS, et al: Reversal of endotoxin-mediated shock by N^G-methyl-L-arginine, an inhibitor of nitric oxide synthesis. *Biochem Biophys Res Commun* 172:1132, 1990.

367. Cobb JP, Natanson C, Hoffman WD, et al: N^w-amino-L-arginine, an inhibitor of nitric oxide synthase, raises vascular resistance but increases mortality rates in awake canines challenged with endotoxin. *J Exp Med* 176:1176, 1992.

368. Lorente JA, Landin L, Renes E, et al: Role of nitric oxide in the hemodynamic changes of sepsis. *Crit Care Med* 21:759, 1993.

369. Finkel MS, Addis CV, Jacob TD, et al: Negative inotropic effects of cytokines on the heart mediated by nitric oxide. *Science* 257:387, 1992.

370. Brady AJB, Poole-Wilson PA, Harding SE, Warren JB: Nitric oxide production within cardiac myocytes reduces their contractility in endotoxemia. *Am J Physiol* 263:H1963, 1992.

371. Petros A, Bennett D, Vallance P: Effect of nitric oxide synthase inhibition on hypotension in patients with septic shock. *Lancet* 338:1557, 1991.

372. Ochoa JB, Udekwu AO, Billiar TR, et al: Nitrogen oxide levels in patients after trauma and during sepsis. *Ann Surg* 214:621, 1991.

373. Hibbs JB, Westenfelder C, Taintor R, et al: Evidence for cytokine-inducible nitric oxide synthesis from L-arginine in patients receiving interleukin-2 therapy. *J Clin Invest* 89:867, 1992.

374. Malawista SE, Montgomery RR, Van Blaricom G: Evidence for reactive nitrogen intermediates in killing of staphylococci by human neutrophil cytoplasts. A new microbicidal pathway for polymorphonuclear leukocytes. *J Clin Invest* 90:621, 1992.

375. Harbrecht BG, Billiar TR, Stadler J, et al: Nitric oxide synthesis serves to reduce hepatic damage during acute murine endotoxemia. *Crit Care Med* 20:1568, 1992.

376. Jones AL: The intestinal immune system: A time for the reaper. *Gastroenterology* 87:234, 1984.

377. Fink MP, Cohn SM, Lee PC, et al: Effect of lipopolysaccharide on intestinal intramucosal hydrogen ion concentration in pigs: Evidence of gut ischemia in a normodynamic model of septic shock. *Crit Care Med* 17:641, 1989.

378. Hallback DA, Hulten L, Jodal M, et al: Evidence for the existence of a countercurrent exchanger in the small intestine in man. *Gastroenterology* 74:683, 1978.

379. Kiel JW, Riedel GL, Shephard AP: Effects of hemodilution on gastric and intestinal oxygenation. *Am J Physiol* 256:H171, 1989.

380. Souba WW, Smith RJ, Wilmore DW: Glutamine metabolism by the intestinal tract. *J Parenteral Enteral Nutr* 9:608, 1985.

381. Baskerville A, Hambleton P, Benbough JE: Pathologic features of glutaminase toxicity. *Br J Exp Pathol* 61:132, 1980.

382. Fox AD, Kripke SA, Berman JR, et al: Reduction of the severity of enterocolitis by glutamine-supplemented enteral diets. *Surg Forum* 38:43, 1987.

383. Fox AD, DePaula JA, Kripke SA: Glutamine-supplemented elemental diets reduced endotoxemia in a lethal model of enterocolitis. *Surg Forum* 29:46, 1988.

384. Carrico CJ, Meakins JL, Marshall JC, et al: Multiple-organ-failure syndrome. *Arch Surg* 121:196, 1986.

385. Deitch EA: Simple intestinal obstruction causes bacterial translocation in man. *Arch Surg* 124:699, 1989.

386. Rush BF Jr, Sori AJ, Murphy TF, et al: Endotoxemia and bacteremia during hemorrhagic shock: The link between trauma and sepsis? *Ann Surg* 207:549, 1988.

387. Marshall JC, Christou NV, Horn R, et al: The microbiology of multiple organ failure: The proximal gastrointestinal tract as occult reservoir of pathogen. *Arch Surg* 123:309, 1988.

388. O'Dwyer SD, Michie HR, Ziegler TR, et al: A single dose of endotoxin increases intestinal permeability in healthy humans. *Arch Surg* 123:1459, 1988.

389. Fong Y, Marano MA, Barber A, et al: Total parenteral nutrition and bowel rest modify the metabolic response to endotoxin in humans. *Ann Surg* 210:449, 1989.

390. Rush BF Jr, Redan JA, Flanagan JJ Jr, et al: Does the bacteremia observed in hemorrhagic shock have clinical significance? A study in germ-free animals. *Ann Surg* 210:342, 1989.

391. Frank HA, Jacob SW, Schweinburg FD, et al: Traumatic shock. XXI: Effectiveness of an antibiotic in experimental hemorrhagic shock. *Am J Physiol* 168:430, 1952.

392. O'Dwyer S, Michie HR, Ziegler TR, et al: A single dose of endotoxin increases intestinal permeability in healthy humans. *Arch Surg* 123:1459, 1988.

393. Ziegler TR, Smith RJ, O'Dwyer ST, et al: Increased intestinal permeability associated with infection in burn patients. *Arch Surg* 123:1313, 1988.

394. Deitch EA: Intestinal permeability in burn patients shortly after injury. *Surgery* 107:411, 1990.

395. Ryan CM, Yarmush ML, Burke JF, Tompkins RG: Increased gut permeability early after burns correlates with the extent of burn injury. *Crit Care Med* 20:1508, 1992.

396. Fink MP: The importance of the gut as a central organ in the pathogenesis of the multiple organ dysfunction syndrome (MODS). In: Vincent J-L, ed. *Update in Intensive Care and Emergency Medicine.* Berlin: Springer-Verlag (in press).

397. Moore FA, Moore EE, Poggetti R, et al: Gut bacterial translocation via the portal vein: A clinical perspective with major torso trauma. *J Trauma* 31:629, 1991.

398. Peitzman AB, Udekwu AO, Ochoa J, Smith S: Bacterial translocation in trauma patients. *J Trauma* 31:1083, 1991.

399. Harris CE, Griffiths RD, Freestone N, et al: Intestinal permeability in the critically ill. *Intensive Care Med* 18:38, 1992.

400. Cipolle MD, Pasquale MD, Cerra FB: Secondary organ dysfunction. From clinical perspectives to molecular mediators. *Crit Care Clin* 9:261, 1993.

401. Schoeniger LO, Reilly PM, Bulkley GB, Buchman TG: Heat-shock gene expression excludes hepatic gene expression after resuscitation from hemorrhagic shock. *Surgery* 112:355, 1992.

402. Cabin DE, Buchman TG: Molecular biology of circulatory shock. Part III. Human hepatoblastoma (HepG2) cells demonstrate two patterns of shock-induced gene expression that are independent, exclusive, and prioritized. *Surgery* 108:902, 1990.

403. Barke RA, Brady PS, Brady LJ: The effect of peritoneal sepsis on the hepatic gene expression and hepatic mitochondrial long-chain fatty acid oxidation in rats. *Surg Forum* 42:62, 1991.

404. Snyder JV: Oxygen transport: The model and reality, in Snyder JV, Pinsky MR, eds: *Oxygen Transport in the Critically Ill.* Chicago, Year Book Medical Publishers, 1987, p 3.

405. Bredle DL, Bradley WE, Chapler CK, et al: Muscle perfusion and oxygenation during local hyperoxia. *J Appl Physiol* 65:2057, 1988.

406. Shoemaker WC, Czer LSC: Evaluation of the biologic importance

of various hemodynamic and oxygen transport variables: Which variables should be monitored in postoperative shock? *Crit Care Med* 7:424, 1979.

407. Shoemaker WC, Appel PL, Kram HB, et al: Prospective trial of supranormal values of survivors as therapeutic goals in high-risk surgical patients. *Chest* 94:1176, 1988.

408. Tuchschmidt J, Fried J, Astiz M, Rackow F: Elevation of cardiac output and oxygen delivery improves outcome in septic shock. *Chest* 102:216, 1992.

409. Fleming A, Bishop M, Shoemaker W, et al: Prospective trial of supranormal values as goals of reuscitation in severe trauma. *Arch Surg* 127:1175, 1992.

410. Yu M, Levy MM, Smith P, et al: Effect of maximizing oxygen delivery on morbidity and mortality rates in critically ill patients: A prospective, randomized, controlled study. *Crit Care Med* 21:830, 1993.

411. Hayes MA, Yau EHS, Timmins AC, et al: Response of critically ill patients to treatment aimed at achieving supranormal oxygen delivery and consumption. Relationship to outcome. *Chest* 103:886, 1993.

412. Humphrey H, Hall J, Sznajder I, et al: Improved survival in ARDS patients associated with a reduction in pulmonary capillary wedge pressure. *Chest* 97:1176, 1990.

413. Mitchell JP, Schuller D, Calandrino FS, Schuster DP: Improved outcome based on fluid management in critically ill patients requiring pulmonary artery catheterization. *Am Rev Respir Dis* 145:990, 1992.

414. Khuri SF, Josa M, Marston W, et al: First report of intramyocardial pH in man: II. Assessment of adequacy of myocardial preservation. *J Thorac Cardiovasc Surg* 86:667, 1983.

415. Gottrup F, Gellett S, Kirkegaard L, et al: Continuous monitoring of tissue oxygen tension during hyperoxia and hypoxia: Relation of subcutaneous, transcutaneous, and conjunctival oxygen tension to hemodynamic variables. *Crit Care Med* 16:1229, 1988.

416. Jensen JA, Goodson WH, O'Machi RS, et al: Subcutaneous tissue oxygen tension falls during hemodialysis. *Surgery* 101:416, 1987.

417. Abraham E, Oye RK, Smith M: Detection of blood volume deficits through conjunctival oxygen tension monitoring. *Crit Care Med* 12:931, 1984.

418. Piantadosi CA: Near infrared spectroscopy: Principles and application to noninvasive assessment of tissue oxygenation. *J Crit Care* 4:308, 1989.

419. Fiddian-Green RG, Baker S: Predictive value of the stomach wall pH for complications after cardiac operations: Comparison with other monitoring. *Crit Care Med* 15:153, 1987.

420. Gys T, Hubens A, Neels H, et al: Prognostic value of gastric intramural pH in surgical intensive care patients. *Crit Care Med* 12:1222, 1988.

421. Doglio GR, Pusalo JF, Egurrola MA, et al: Gastric mucosal pH as a prognostic index of mortality in critically ill patients. *Crit Care Med* 19:1037, 1991.

422. Marik PE: Gastric intramucosal pH: A better predictor of multiorgan dysfunction syndrome and death than oxygen-derived variables in patients with sepsis. *Chest* 104:225, 1993.

423. Gutierrez G, Palizas F, Doglio G, et al: Gastric intramucosal pH as a therapeutic index of tissue oxygenation in critically ill patients. *Lancet* 339:19, 1992.

424. Boyd O, Mackay CJ, Lamb G, et al: Comparison of clinical information gained from routine blood-gas analysis and gastric tonometry for intramural pH. *Lancet* 341:142, 1993.

425. Goris RJA: Prevention of ARDS and MOF by prophylactic mechanical ventilation and early fracture stabilization. *Prog Clin Biol Res* 236B:163, 1987.

426. Lozman J, Deno DC, Feustel PJ, et al: Pulmonary and cardiovascular consequences of immediate fixation or conservative management of long-bone fractures. *Arch Surg* 121:992, 1986.

427. Johnson KD, Cadambi A, Siebert GB: Incidence of adult respiratory distress syndrome in patients with multiple musculoskeletal injuries: Effect of early operative stabilization of fractures. *J Trauma* 25:375, 1985.

428. Macho JR, Luce JM: Rational approach to the management of multiple systems organ failure. *Crit Care Clin* 5:379, 1989.

429. Slotman GJ, Burchard KW, D'Arezzo A, et al: Ketoconazole prevents acute respiratory failure in critically ill surgical patients. *J Trauma* 28:648, 1988.

430. Slotman GJ, Burchard KW: Ketoconazole prevents candida sepsis in critically ill surgical patients. *Arch Surg* 122:147, 1987.

431. Norton LW: Does drainage of intraabdominal pus reverse multiple organ failure? *Am J Surg* 149:347, 1985.

432. Teichmann W, Wittmann DH, Andreone PA: Scheduled reoperations (etappenlavage) for diffuse peritonitis. *Arch Surg* 121:147, 1986.

433. Garcia-Sabrido JL, Taado JM, Christou NV, et al: Treatment of severe intra-abdominal sepsis and/or necrotic foci by an "open-abdomen" approach: Zipper and zipper-mesh techniques. *Arch Surg* 123:152, 1988.

434. Anderson ED, Mandelbaum DM, Ellison EC, et al: Open packing of the peritoneal cavity in generalized bacterial peritonitis. *Am J Surg* 145:131, 1983.

435. Davidson ED, Bradley EL III: "Marsupialization" in the treatment of pancreatic abscess. *Surgery* 89:252, 1981.

436. Ivatury RR, Nallathambi, Rao PM, et al: Open management of the septic abdomen: Therapeutic and prognostic considerations based on APACHE II. *Crit Care Med* 17:511, 1989.

437. Wertheimer MD, Norris CS: Surgical management of necrotizing pancreatitis. *Arch Surg* 121:484, 1986.

438. Bunt TJ: Urgent relaparotomy: The high-risk, no-choice operation. *Surgery* 98:555, 1985.

439. Bunt TJ: Non-directed relaparotomy for intra-abdominal sepsis: A futile procedure. *Am Surg* 52:294, 1986.

440. du Moulin GC, Paterson DG, Hedley-Whyte J, et al: Aspiration of gastric bacteria in antacid-treated patients: A frequent cause of postoperative colonization of the airway. *Lancet* 1:242, 1982.

441. Driks MR, Craven DE, Bartolome RC, et al: Nosocomial pneumonia in intubated patients given sucralfate as compared with antacids or histamine type 2 blockers. *N Engl J Med* 317:1376, 1987.

442. Garvery BM, McCambley JA, Tuxen D: Effects of gastric alkalization on bacterial colonization in critically ill patients. *Crit Care Med* 17:211, 1989.

443. Martin LF, McL Booth FV, Karlstadt RG, et al: Continuous intravenous cimetidine decreases stress-related upper gastrointestinal hemorrhage without promoting pneumonia. *Crit Care Med* 21:19, 1993.

444. Fabian TC, Boucher BA, Croce MA, et al: Pneumonia and stress ulceration in severely injured patients. A prospective evaluation of the effects of stress ulcer prophylaxis. *Arch Surg* 128:185, 1993.

445. van Uffelen R, Rommes JH, van Saene HDF: Preventing lower airway colonization and infection in mechanically ventilated patients. *Crit Care Med* 15:99, 1987.

446. Stoutenbeek CP, van Saene HDF, Miranda DR, et al: The effect of oropharyngeal decontamination using topical nonabsorbable antibiotics on the incidence of nosocomial respiratory tract infections in multiple trauma patients. *J Trauma* 27:357, 1987.

447. Unertl K, Ruckdeschel G, Selbmann HD, et al: Prevention of colonization and respiratory infections in long-term ventilated patients by local antimicrobial prophylaxis. *Intensive Care Med* 13:106, 1987.

448. Johanson WG, Seidenfeld JJ, de Los Santos R, et al: Prevention of nosocomial pneumonia using topical and parenteral antimicrobial agents. *Am Rev Respir Dis* 137:265, 1988.

449. Ledingham IM, Eastway AT, McKay IC, et al: Triple regimen of selective decontamination of the digestive tract, systemic cefotaxime, and microbiological surveillance for prevention of acquired infection in intensive care. *Lancet* 1:785, 1988.

450. Cockerill FR, Muller SR, Anhalt JP, et al: Prevention of infection in critically ill patients by selective decontamination of the digestive tract. *Ann Intern Med* 117:545, 1992.

451. Kerver AJH, Rommes JH, Mevissen-Verhage EAE: Prevention of colonization and infection in critically ill patients: A prospective randomized study. *Crit Care Med* 1087, 1988.

452. Pugin J, Auckenthaler R, Lew DP, Suter PM: Oropharyngeal decontamination decreases incidence of ventilator-associated pneumonia. A randomized, placebo-controlled, double-blind clinical trial. *JAMA* 265:2704, 1991.

453. Hammond JMJ, Potgieter PD, Saunders GL, Forder AA: Double-blind study of selective decontamination of the digestive tract in intensive care. *Lancet* 340:5, 1992.

454. Gastinne H, Wolff M, Delatour F: A controlled trial in intensive care units of selective decontamination of the digestive tract with nonabsorbable antibiotics. *N Engl J Med* 326:594, 1992.

455. Blair P, Rowlands BJ, Lowry K, et al: Selective decontamination of the digestive tract: A stratified, randomized, prospective study in a mixed intensive care unit. *Surgery* 110:303, 1991.

456. Fink MP: Selective digestive decontamination: A gut issue for the nineties. *Crit Care Med* 20:559, 1992.

457. Gentilello L, Thompson DA, Tonnesen AS, et al: Effect of a rotating bed on the incidence of pulmonary complications in critically ill patients. *Crit Care Med* 17:783, 1988.

458. Fink MP, Helsmoortel CM, Stein KL, et al: The efficacy of an oscillating bed in the prevention of lower respiratory tract infection in critically ill victims of blunt trauma. *Chest* 97:132, 1990.

459. Sottile FD, Marrie TJ, Prough DS, et al: Nosocomial pulmonary infection: Possible etiologic significance of bacterial adhesion to endotracheal tubes. *Crit Care Med* 14:265, 1986.

460. Diaz-Blanco J, Clawson RC, Roberson SM, et al: Electron microscopic evaluation of bacterial adherence to polyvinyl endotracheal tubes used in neonates. *Crit Care Med* 17:1335, 1989.

461. Pinilla JC, Ross DF, Martin T, et al: Study of the incidence of intravascular catheter infection and associated septicemia in critically ill patients. *Crit Care Med* 11:21, 1983.

462. Sitzmann JV, Townsend TR, Siler MC: Septic and technical complications of central venous catheterization. *Ann Surg* 202:766, 1985.

463. Hudson-Civetta JA, Civetta JM, Martinez OV, et al: Risk and detection of pulmonary artery catheter-related infection in septic surgical patients. *Crit Care Med* 15:29, 1987.

464. Heard SO, Davis RF, Sherertz RJ, et al: Influence of sterile protective sleeves on the sterility of pulmonary artery catheters. *Crit Care Med* 15:499, 1987.

465. Pettigrew RA, Lang SDR, Haydock DA, et al: Catheter related sepsis in patients on intravenous nutrition: A prospective study of quantitative catheter cultures and guidewire changes for suspected sepsis. *Br J Surg* 72:52, 1985.

466. Plit ML, Liman J, Eidelman J, et al: Catheter related infection: A plea for consensus with review and guidelines. *Intensive Care Med* 14:503, 1988.

467. Cobb DK, High KP, Sawyer RG, et al: A controlled trial of scheduled replacement of central venous and pulmonary-artery catheters. *N Engl J Med* 327:1062, 1992.

468. Eyer S, Brummitt C, Crossley K, et al: Catheter-related sepsis: Prospective, randomized study of three methods of long-term catheter maintenance. *Crit Care Med* 18:1073, 1990.

469. Maki DG, Weise CE, Sarafini HW: A semi-quantitative culture method for identifying intravenous-catheter-related infection. *N Engl J Med* 296:1305, 1977.

470. Kotilainen HR, Curley FJ, Fink MP, et al: A program to reduce line associated bacteremia. *Antimicrob Agents Chemother* 1081, 1989 (Abstr).

471. Maki DG, Cobb L, Garman JK, et al: An attachable silver-impregnated cuff for prevention of infection with central venous catheters: A prospective randomized multicenter trial. *Am J Med* 85:307, 1988.

472. Flowers RH, Schwenzer KJ, Kopel RF: Efficacy of an attachable subcutaneous cuff for the prevention of intravascular catheter-related infection: A randomized, controlled trial. *JAMA* 261:878, 1989.

473. Maki DG, Wheeler SJ, Stolz SM: Study of a novel antiseptic-coated central venous catheter. *Crit Care Med* 19:S99, 1991.

474. Brun-Buisson C, Legrand P, Rauss A, et al: Intestinal decontamination for control of nosocomial multiresistant gram-negative bacilli. *Ann Intern Med* 110:873, 1989.

475. Border JR, Hassett J, LaDuca J, et al: The gut origin septic state in blunt multiple trauma: ISS +40 in the ICU. *Ann Surg* 206:427, 1987.

476. From AHL, Fong JSC, Good RA: Polymyxin B sulphate modification of bacterial endotoxin: Effects on the development of endotoxin shock in dogs. *Infect Immunol* 23:660, 1979.

477. Ditter B, Urbaschek R, Urbaschek B: Ability of various absorbents to bind endotoxins *in vitro* and to prevent orally induced endotoxemia in mice. *Gastroenterology* 84:1547, 1983.

478. Baumgartner JD, Glauser MP, McCutchan JA, et al: Prevention of gram-negative shock and death in surgical patients by antibody to endotoxin core glycolipid. *Lancet* 2:59, 1985.

479. Grindlinger GA, Niehoff J, Hughes L, et al: Acute paranasal sinusitis related to nasotracheal intubation of head-injured patients. *Crit Care Med* 15:214, 1987.

480. Fassoulaki A, Pamouktsoglou P: Prolonged nasotracheal intubation and its association with inflammation of paranasal sinuses. *Anesth Analg* 69:50, 1989.

481. Alexander JW, MacMillan BG, Stinnett JD, et al: Beneficial effects of aggressive protein feeding in severely burned children. *Ann Surg* 192:505, 1980.

482. Moore EE, Jones TN: Benefits of immediate jejunostomy feeding after major abdominal trauma—A prospective, randomized study. *J Trauma* 26:874, 1986.

483. Moore FA, Moore EE, Jones TN: TEN versus TPN following major abdominal trauma-reduced septic morbidity. *J Trauma* 29:916, 1989.

484. Kudsk KA, Croce MA, Fabian TC, et al: Enteral versus parenteral feeding: Effects on septic morbidity after blunt and penetrating abdominal trauma. *Ann Surg* 215:503, 1992.

485. Cerra FB, Mazuski J, Teasley K, et al: Nitrogen retention in critically ill patients is proportional to the branched chain amino acid load. *Crit Care Med* 11:775, 1983.

486. Eyer SD, Micon LT, Konstantinides FN, et al: Early enteral feeding does not attenuate metabolic response after blunt trauma. *J Trauma* 34:639, 1993.

487. Mizock BA: Branched-chain amino acids in sepsis and hepatic failure. *Arch Intern Med* 145:1284, 1985.

488. Cerra F, Hirsch J, Mullen K, et al: The effect of stress level, amino acid formula, and nitrogen dose on nitrogen retention in traumatic and septic stress. *Ann Surg* 205:282, 1987.

489. Cerra FB, Mazuski JE, Shute E, et al: Branched chain metabolic support: A prospective, randomized, double-blind trial in surgical stress. *Ann Surg* 199:286, 1984.

490. Bower RH, Muggia-Sullam M, Vallgren S, et al: Branched chain amino acid-enriched solutions in the septic patient. *Ann Surg* 203:13, 1986.

491. Kudsk KA, Stone JM, Carpenter G, et al: Enteral and parenteral feeding influences mortality after hemoglobin-*E. coli* peritonitis in normal rats. *J Trauma* 23:605, 1983.

492. Alverdy JC, Aoys E, Moss GS: Total parenteral nutrition promotes bacterial translocation from the gut. *Surgery* 104:185, 1988.

493. Cerra FB, McPherson JP, Konstantinides FN, et al: Enteral nutrition does not prevent multiple organ failure syndrome (MOFS) after sepsis. *Surgery* 104:727, 1988.

494. Alexander JW, Gonce SJ, Miskell W, et al: A new model for studying nutrition in peritonitis: The adverse effect of overfeeding. *Ann Surg* 209:334, 1989.

495. Herve P, Simonneau G, Girard P, et al: Hypercapnic acidosis induced by nutrition in mechanically ventilated patients: Glucose versus fat. *Crit Care Med* 13:537, 1985.

496. Delafosse B, Bouffard Y, Viale JP, et al: Respiratory changes induced by parenteral nutrition in postoperative patients undergoing inspiratory pressure support ventilation. *Anesthesiology* 66:393, 1987.

497. Talpers SS, Romberger DJ, Bunce SB, Pingleton SK: Nutritionally associated increased carbon dioxide production. Excess total calories vs high proportion of carbohydrate calories. *Chest* 102:551, 1992.

498. Pantuck E, Pantuck CB, Weissman C, et al: Effects of parenteral nutritional regimens on oxidative drug metabolism. *Anesthesiology* 60:534, 1984.

499. Cerra F: Hypermetabolism-organ failure syndrome: A metabolic response to injury. *Crit Care Clin* 5:289, 1989.

500. Berger R, Adams L: Nutritional support in the critical care setting (part 1). *Chest* 96:139, 1989.

501. Liggett SB, St. John RE, Lefrak SS: Determination of resting energy expenditure utilizing the thermodilution pulmonary artery catheter. *Chest* 91:562, 1987.

502. Sprung CL, Caralis PV, Marcial EH, et al: The effects of high dose corticosteroids in patients with septic shock. *N Engl J Med* 311:1137, 1984.

503. Bone RC, Fisher CJ, Clemmer TP, et al: A controlled clinical trial of high-dose methylprednisolone in the treatment of severe sepsis and septic shock. *N Engl J Med* 317:653, 1987.

504. Hinshaw L, Peduzzi P, Young E, et al: Effect of high-dose glucocorticoid therapy on mortality with clinical signs of systemic sepsis. *N Engl J Med* 317:659, 1987.

505. Bernard G, Luce JM, Sprung CL, et al: High-dose corticosteroids in patients with adult respiratory distress syndrome. *N Engl J Med* 317:1565, 1987.

506. Bone RC, Fisher CJ Jr, Clemmer TP, et al: Early methylprednisolone treatment for septic syndrome and the adult respiratory distress syndrome. *Chest* 92:1032, 1987.

507. Braude S, Haslam P, Hughes D, et al: Chronic adult respiratory distress syndrome—a role for corticosteroids? *Crit Care Med* 20:1187, 1992.

508. Holcroft JW: Prostaglandin E$_1$ and survival in patients with the adult respiratory distress syndrome. *Ann Surg* 203:371, 1986.

509. Bone RC, Maunder R, Silverman H: Randomized double-blind, multicenter study of prostaglandin E$_1$ in patients with the adult respiratory syndrome. *Chest* 96:114, 1989.

510. Vassar MJ, Fletcher MP, Perry CA, Holcroft JW: Evaluation of prostaglandin E$_1$ for prevention of respiratory failure in high risk trauma patients: A prospective clinical trial and correlation with plasma suppressive factors for neutrophil activation. *Prostaglandins Leukot Essent Fatty Acids* 44:223, 1991.

511. Russell JA, Ronco JJ, Bodek PM: Physiologic effects and side effects of prostaglandin E$_1$ in the adult respiratory distress syndrome. *Chest* 97:684, 1990.

512. Parsons PE, Worthen GS, Moore EE, et al: The association of circulating endotoxin with the development of the adult respiratory distress syndrome. *Am Rev Respir Dis* 140:294, 1989.

513. van Deventer SJH, Buller HR, ten Cate JW, et al: Endotoxaemia: An early predictor of septicaemia in febrile patients. *Lancet* 1:605, 1988.

514. Suffredini AF, Fromm RE, Parker MM: The cardiovascular response of normal humans to the administration of endotoxin. *N Engl J Med* 321:280, 1989.

515. Ziegler EJ, McCutchan A, Fierer J, et al: Treatment of gram-negative bacteremia and shock with human antiserum to a mutant *Escherichia coli. N Engl J Med* 307:1225, 1982.

516. J5 Study Group: Treatment of severe infectious purpura in children with human plasma from donors immunized with *Escherichia coli* J5: A prospective double-blind study. *J Infect Dis* 165:695, 1992.

517. Ziegler EJ, Fisher CJ, Sprung CL, et al: Treatment of gram-negative bacteremia and septic shock with HA-1A human monoclonal antibody directed against endotoxin. A randomized, double-blind, placebo-controlled trial. *N Engl J Med* 324:429, 1991.

518. Greenman RL, Schein RMH, Martin MA, et al: A controlled clinical trial of E5 murine monoclonal IgM antibody to endotoxin in the treatment of gram-negative sepsis. *JAMA* 266:1097, 1991.

519. St. John R, Dorinsky PM: Immunologic therapy for ARDS, septic shock and multiple organ failure. *Chest* 103:932, 1993.

520. Cunnion RE: Clinical trials of immunotherpy for sepsis. *Crit Care Med* 20:721, 1992.

521. O'Reilly M, Silver GM, Greenhalgh DG, et al: Treatment of intra-abdominal infection with granulocyte colony-stimulating factor. *J Trauma* 33:679, 1992.

522. Su S, Ward MM, Apicella MA, Ward RE: A nontoxic, idiotope vaccine against gram-negative bacterial infections. *J Immunol* 148:234, 1992.

523. Saba TM: Plasma fibronectin (opsonic glycoprotein): Its synthesis by vascular endothelial cells and role in cardiopulmonary integrity after trauma as related to reticuloendothelial function. *Am J Med* 68:577, 1980.

524. Annest SJ, Scovill WA, Blumenstock FA, et al: Increased creatinine clearance following cryoprecipitate infusion in trauma and surgical patients with decreased renal function. *J Trauma* 20:726, 1980.

525. Hesselvik F, Brodin B, Carlsson C, et al: Cryoprecipitate infusion fails to improve organ function in septic shock. *Crit Care Med* 15:475, 1987.

526. Barzilay E, Kessler D, Berlot G, et al: Use of extracorporeal supportive techniques as additional treatment for septic-induced multiple organ failure patients. *Crit Care Med* 17:634, 1989.

527. Bende S, Bertok L: Elimination of endotoxin from the blood by extracorporeal activated charcoal hemoperfusion in experimental canine endotoxin shock. *Circ Shock* 19:239, 1986.

528. Bysani GK, Shenep JL, Hildner WK, et al: Detoxification of plasma containing lipopolysaccharide by adsorption. *Crit Care Med* 18:67, 1990.

529. Lilly CM, Sandhu JS, Ishizaka A, et al: Pentoxifylline prevents tumor necrosis factor-induced lung injury. *Am Rev Respir Dis* 139:1371, 1989.

530. Harada H, Ishizaka A, Yonemaru M, et al: The effects of aminophylline and pentoxifylline on multiple organ damage after *Escherichia coli* sepsis. *Am Rev Respir Dis* 140:974, 1989.

531. Tighe B, Moss R, Hynd J, et al: Pretreatment with pentoxifylline improves the hemodynamic and histologic changes and decreases neutrophil adhesiveness in a pig cecal peritonitis model. *Crit Care Med* 18:184, 1990.

532. Heffner JE, Repine JE: Pulmonary strategies of antioxidant defense. *Am Rev Respir Dis* 140:531, 1989.

533. Sheppard BC, Fraker DL, Norton JA: Prevention and treatment of endotoxin and sepsis lethality with recombinant human tumor necrosis factor. *Surgery* 106:156, 1989.

534. Cross AS, Sadoff JC, Kelly N, et al: Pretreatment with recombinant murine tumor necrosis factor alpha/cachectin and murine interleukin 1 alpha protects mice for lethal bacterial infection. *J Exp Med* 169:2021, 1989.

200. Total Parenteral Nutrition

Nancy J. Evans and James L. Mullen

Nutritional metabolic support is an increasingly important modality in the care of the critically ill patient. With the advances and increases in many therapeutic technologies, we are able to sustain critically ill patients much longer after medical catastrophes than has previously been possible. During illnesses of long duration, the quantity and quality of the nutrient supply to the patient may actually become an increasingly important determinant in his or her outcome. The severe metabolic alterations that occur during periods of critical illness present a unique challenge to the clinician providing nutritional metabolic support and rightfully demand attention to detail, extensive education and training, and meticulous critical care expertise that is not present in the average clinician. The disturbances in the macronutrient and micronutrient metabolism create an environment where providing such nutritional support without in-depth expertise and a comprehensive understanding of metabolic changes can be extremely detrimental to the patient and adversely impact on his or her outcome. The patient's existence is often fragile and may hinge on accumulation of multiple small improvements. Parenteral nutrition is clearly a life-sustaining therapy for the critically ill patient whose gastrointestinal tract is not functioning efficiently to fully support the patient's metabolic demands. Without such nutrient supply, the longevity of the critically ill patient in the intensive care unit (ICU) is measured in days and weeks, not months and years.

Total parenteral nutrition (TPN) initially evolved in the ICU of the University of Pennsylvania Medical Center, and we have actively participated in its development during the past 25 years. The use of parenteral nutrition in our medical center has undergone substantial changes (Fig. 200-1). Although the inpatient average daily TPN census has remained relatively constant, the type of patient receiving TPN has changed. Because the less critically ill patients are receiving their TPN at home, their place has been taken by an ever-increasing use of TPN in the critical care arena. During a 12-month period the severity index of the average TPN patient increased 40 percent. We hope our 25-year perspective can enhance TPN application in critical care medicine.

The Problem

Metabolic alterations in critical illness will quickly lead to the demise of the patient if untreated or if treated improperly. Severe critical illness results in a well-orchestrated set of events that can be summarized as hypermetabolism and hypercatabolism: the increased expenditure of energy and the increased destruction of existing tissues. The neuroendocrine response orchestrates to the disruption of normal metabolic balance where synthesis and catabolism are usually equal. When decreased nutrient intake and decreased synthetic production are coupled with increased tissue catabolism, the net tissue balance is severely negative, leading to a rapid depletion of body tissue stores and critical elements such as functional protein. Skeletal muscle and fat stores are rapidly depleted to provide fuel and substrates for more vital organs as nutrients are redistributed internally in response to the insult. This is adaptive and protective initially, but without enhancement of the synthetic side of the equation, the body cell mass, including functional host defenses, will be rapidly depleted, significantly reducing the patient's chance of survival. A reasonable hope for the future is the ability to modulate such catabolic events by altering their messages or the effects of these messages. Such interventions need to be approached with caution so that all effects are assessed to clearly establish that the net benefit is positive. The goal of nutritional metabolic support in these critically ill patients is to minimize the net negative protein and energy daily balances, which accumulate into net negative tissue protein and fat store balances over time, by providing substrate to at least partially offset the obligatory catabolic losses and to provide fuel for oxidative purposes. Such interventions probably translate into decreased mortality and morbidity as well as enhanced functional capacity.

Why Bother?

One could not legitimately support an intensive nutritional metabolic intervention with its concomitant cost and adverse im-

Fig. 200-1. Average daily census for TPN from the Hospital of the University of Pennsylvania from 1979 to 1993. Inpt = inpatient.

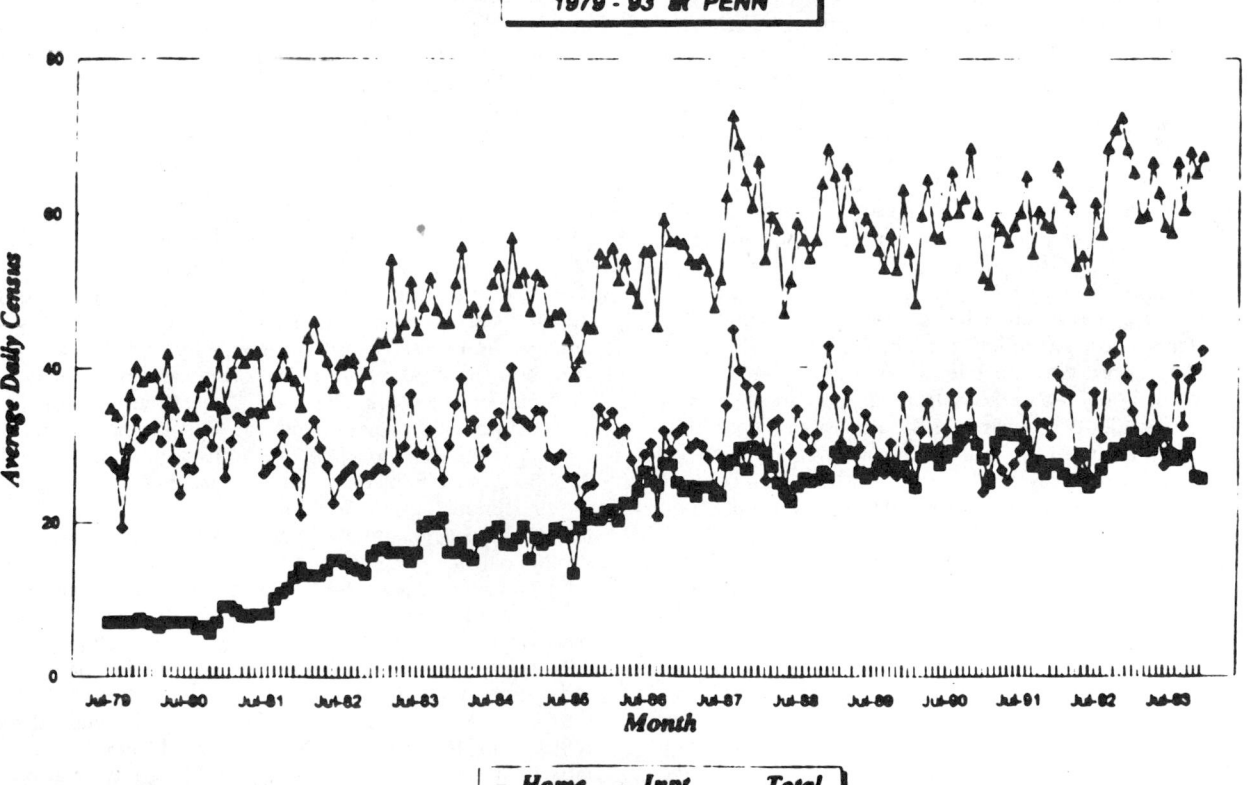

pacts on the care of other disorders in the critically ill patient unless there is some rational basis to conclude or suspect that improved clinical outcome can be achieved. One could speculate that the increase in use of nutritional metabolic support in the ICU is a result of the cumulative wisdom of critical care intensivists as to the beneficial effects of such support. This supposition may be correct but somewhat dangerous in that it is difficult to link specific outcomes with any one of a multitude of interventions employed in the care of a very complicated critically ill patient. Nevertheless, it is important to examine any evidence that intervention will bring about measurable improvements in clinical outcomes. The increased severity of patient illness and the frequency of change in other interventions have limited our ability to perform controlled intervention studies in the rapidly changing environment of the ICU. This challenge has been met with attempts to look at outcome in a number of ways, and the cumulative effect of these studies supports the aggressive use of nutritional metabolic intervention in the ICU.

TPN was developed to improve patient outcome. Initially, the obvious desired outcome was survival, and TPN was able to sustain patients with a chronic nonfunctional gastrointestinal system who would not have otherwise survived. As the therapy advanced and clinicians became more familiar with administration techniques, applications of TPN broadened to include many other patient populations. TPN, with seemingly few adverse side effects, became a widely prescribed therapy for many surgical patients, preoperatively to "beef them up" and postoperatively when gastrointestinal function was significantly delayed. TPN therapy not only held the promise of increasing survival in postsurgical care, it also carried the potential for prospectively changing the nutritional status of patients in the hopes of improving outcome. To more closely evaluate the role of TPN, clinicians began to critically evaluate the efficacy of TPN, because complications such as catheter infection, pneumothorax, and electrolyte imbalances were sometimes not inconsequential. Many of the initial investigations were conducted using surgical patients. Early studies sought to define specific outcome measures, such as infectious complications, wound healing, and mortality, that could be influenced by the implementation of TPN. In several investigations, preoperative TPN has been shown to reduce mortality and morbidity in a select group of surgical patients, being most effective in the severely malnourished patient [1,2]. These findings were based on well-defined objective criteria so clinicians could prospectively identify those malnourished patients who may benefit from the administration of TPN.

We developed a predictive index mostly based on serum proteins. This predictive index was applied and validated in various populations to prospectively identify risks. Patients with the highest risk benefited the most from TPN; the most severely malnourished patients receiving TPN had a significant reduction in postoperative mortality and morbidity. Those patients not malnourished or only mildly malnourished did not demonstrate significant reduction in postoperative morbidity/mortality. TPN was ineffective if the patient was not severely malnourished. This was examined in our multi-institutional clinical trial conducted by the Veteran's Administration TPN Cooperative Study Group [3]. The degree of malnutrition was rated by a nutritional risk index score composed of weight loss and serum albumin level, and subjective global assessment. The final sample included 395 patients who were randomly assigned to TPN or no TPN. TPN was administered 7 to 15 days before major intracavitary surgery and at least 3 days postoperatively. Complication rates were monitored for 90 days and included such things as major and minor infectious complica-

tions, major and minor noninfectious complications, catheter-related complications, and 90-day mortality rate. Severely malnourished patients who received TPN had significantly fewer noninfectious complications (p=0.03). An interesting unexpected finding was an increase in infectious complications in the well-nourished group receiving TPN. Preoperative TPN (the therapy) should be administered only to those patients who have severe malnutrition.

The benefits of parenteral nutrition may be evident in less clinically obvious measures such as changes in body composition. Hill and coworkers administered a 14-day course of TPN to surgical patients with gastrointestinal disease [4]. Patients initially presenting with moderate to severe protein depletion gained total body protein. This gain was somewhat diminished when the measured resting energy expenditure (REE) was elevated in the sicker subset. Patients with moderate to severe protein depletion had a significant increase in their serum pre-albumin and transferrin levels.

Extrapolation of much of the clinical outcome data to the critically ill should be viewed with considerable caution. Few limited studies examine efficacy of TPN specifically in the critically ill population. This is most likely related to limitations encountered in studying a complex heterogenous sample such as critically ill patients with nutritional diagnostic difficulties and rapidly changing interventions. Traditional outcome variables such as morbidity and mortality are influenced by a multitude of other factors occurring in the intensive care setting. For example, the timing of intervention was studied by one group of investigators by randomizing 67 patients with severe acute pancreatitis to either TPN within 72 hours or TPN after 72 hours; early intervention led to fewer complications [5].

The critically ill patient is at risk for severe unchecked losses in total body protein because of the hypercatabolism. It is important to understand what impact nutritional metabolic support has on the accelerated destruction of body protein. One would hope that providing exogenous amino acids could ameliorate the unrelenting catabolism.

Streat and associates measured body composition in 8 septic postoperative patients supported on mechanical ventilation [6]. Body composition was measured at baseline, before the initiation of TPN, and after 10 days of TPN. Mean energy intake was 2750 nonprotein calories, and mean protein intake was 1.8 gm protein/kg body weight/day. Baseline measurements of body composition indicated that patients were not totally depleted of body protein but after 10 days lost a mean of 1.5 kg of protein, or 12.2 percent of total body protein. They did demonstrate a significant gain in energy and fat stores but were unable to significantly increase protein stores. Others have examined the excessive protein losses through kinetic studies, concluding that net protein catabolism can be cut by no more than 50 percent using TPN [7,8]. These investigators demonstrated increased protein synthesis in septic and severely injured patients receiving TPN. It is important to understand that TPN does not significantly alter the protein catabolism; providing exogenous nutrients will benefit the patient by increasing the synthesis side of the equation and thus increasing the net protein balance.

Ziegler administered TPN to patients undergoing allogenic bone marrow transplants [9]. TPN was provided at 1.5 times basal energy requirements, with 1.5 gm of protein/kg/day, and one group had a TPN solution enriched with glutamine. The glutamine-enriched formula resulted in significantly improved nitrogen retention; nitrogen balance was significantly more negative in the non-glutamine group. Still other investigators have manipulated both the type and quantity of protein to improve nitrogen retention [10,11].

Many of the outcome data in the field of nutritional metabolic reports relate to the degree of preexisting protein energy of malnutrition and examine how correcting existing protein energy malnutrition (PEM) or reducing the potential development can impact on outcome. In many clinical settings the delivery of TPN can effectively prevent the occurrence of PEM. Windsor correctly suggests that the clinical importance of energy malnutrition is overemphasized [12]. Emphasis should be directed toward the loss of body protein and how this affects physiologic functions such as respiratory function, wound healing, and the immune system and the core organs such as skeletal muscles.

The role of nutritional metabolic support in altering patient outcome during periods of critical illness will be more clearly defined as research extends our knowledge of the response to severe insult. In many cases where the gastrointestinal tract is not functional and the patient's period of critical illness is prolonged, TPN clearly contributes to improving survival. In terms of improving outcome, studies suggest that, at best, net protein catabolism can be reduced by 50 percent. The future of nutrition support will in large part be identifying specific substrates that target clearly defined functional deficits.

Which Critically Ill Patient Should Receive TPN and When?

The use of TPN in the critical care unit is somewhat dependent on one's philosophy of patient care. We view TPN as a relatively inexpensive ICU therapy whose side effects are many, but often not serious and easily treated. As such, we err on the side of using TPN in the hope of avoiding the consequences of not using it in a single patient who may benefit. If TPN were overly expensive or fraught with untreatable lethal complications, we would be much more reluctant to take on such an approach.

The criteria for starting TPN in the critically ill patient are somewhat subjective, but experience guides us that a rational first criterion to begin TPN would be if the gastrointestinal tract were nonfunctional either due to dysmotility, disrupted continuity, or ischemia.

Dysmotility has a multifactorial etiology and can be noted from excessive proximal gastrointestinal drainage via intestinal tubes and vomiting. The inability to obtain enteral access below the point of dysmotility precludes the use of enteral feeding. Dysmotility can also present as excessive diarrhea of greater than 1500 ml over 24 hours. Obviously the enteral route is not feasible if the gastrointestinal tract is not intact due to a fistula, coupled with inability to get enteral access distal to the fistula. Intestinal ischemia is a common reason for a nonfunctional gastrointestinal tract in the critically ill patient, and the enteral route should not be used with cardiovascular instability since this sets the stage for intestinal ischemia and gangrene.

The second criterion is the anticipation that the patient will not have an adequate oral intake for at least 3 to 5 days if he or she is well nourished at the onset of the critical illness. If the patient has significant malnutrition at the onset of the critical illness, a delay in achieving an oral intake of only 1 to 3 days should be allowed before starting TPN.

The current nutritional status of the patient is the third criterion, since patients with chronic disease are often suboptimally nourished. Various degrees and types of malnutrition existing prior to the onset of critical illness may well have a profound impact on patients' ability to withstand a particular stress. The difficulty we face in evaluating the nutritional status of patients during a period of critical illness is that many of the traditional "nutritional assessment" parameters are unreliable. Nutritional assessment is a snapshot look at the static tissue reserves of the body, focusing very little on functional capacity, although that view is changing with time. We receive few clues from the patient history since patients are often uncommunicative and determining the adequacy of prior nutrient intake from the family is not very reliable. The body weight changes must be cautiously evaluated since critical illness distorts the normal distribution of body fluid, changing the composition of various compartments, and affects the interpretation of weight. Current weight should be compared to the patient's usual and ideal weight, with particular attention paid to estimating the dry weight of the patient. If there is a period of significant (greater than 10%) weight loss prior to the onset of critical illness, this should alert the clinician that the patient will more quickly deplete stores to dangerously low levels. Weight, as compared to ideal body weight, can be used very effectively as a marker in a gross way to identify how the patient's fat stores compare with normal. This is particularly useful in nutrient prescription; most critically ill patients do not suffer from a deficiency of caloric stores, which are readily utilizable during the hypermetabolic period. Serum proteins, usually important nutritional assessment parameters, are often distorted because of the aforementioned fluid shifts. Serum albumin, transferrin, and prealbumin, which normally give a balanced composite view of the patient's serum protein status, are not particularly useful in this postresuscitation setting. In addition, the reprioritization of the liver synthetic pathways and the increased catabolism of certain of these proteins make them much more an indicator of severe illness than a measure of the liver's synthetic ability. Serum proteins still have a considerable prognostic value, but certainly they are less reflective of static serum protein stores. Serum albumin continues to be a very good prognostic outcome factor despite all the factors that should make it a bad predictor. During critical illness, the body mass of albumin is redistributed, with a tendency to move from the intravascular space to the extravascular space. Increases in extracellular fluid further contribute to the decreased serum level of albumin and to an increased catabolic rate and decreased synthetic rate. Despite the many reasons why the serum level is distorted, it seems to retain its ability to predict bad outcomes quite well.

The fourth major factor in deciding which patients should receive support is the anticipated clinical course of the illness. Obviously, a self-limited, acute, single-organ illness does not scream for TPN the way a catastrophic multiorgan failure situation does.

Goal Definition

To adequately treat an individual with a particular technology one needs to be very clear in defining realistic goals, which will not be the same for all patients. Once the goals are defined, the specific nutrient requirements to achieve these goals can be outlined in the nutrient prescription designed. The general goals of TPN in the critically ill patient are to reduce the overall net negative protein balance and to provide maintenance levels of substrates within the constraints of the organ disposal mechanisms. Hopefully these metabolic goals will be coupled with a reduction in mortality and morbidity and a maintenance of vital organ structure and function. In usual circumstances, it is unrealistic to have goals of fat repletion and muscle building during periods of critical illness.

How Much?

Once realistic goals are defined, how much of what should the patient receive in the TPN? Once the requirements are defined, nutrient prescription is straightforward.

Total energy expenditure (TEE) is the amount of calories burned in a 24-hour period, which can be measured directly by heat loss or indirectly by gas exchange involving oxygen consumption and carbon dioxide production. A patient's total energy expenditure is the sum of resting energy expenditure, dietary-induced and cold thermogenesis, and activity energy expenditure. Each of these components may change under varying circumstances, which will influence the total caloric expenditure of the patient and thus the caloric requirements. To make a rational caloric prescription, one needs to know the individual patient's TEE. Energy balance in a patient would be achieved if sufficient exogenous calories were supplied in an amount equal to the TEE. Over a period of time, a patient in energy balance should not suffer substantial changes in body caloric stores, overwhelmingly predominated by fat stores. Negative energy balance occurs when the exogenous caloric supply is less than the TEE; this results in a net fat tissue loss over time as the patient's fat calorie stores are gradually utilized to meet energy demands not being met by exogenous supply. Positive energy balance occurs when exogenous caloric supply exceeds total energy expenditure and results in a net increased storage of calories, predominantly as fat. Daily energy balance multiplied by time results in tissue store changes.

The most variable portion of TEE is the REE. This changes dramatically in sick people for a variety of reasons. The sicker the patient, the more variable the individual REE, as compared to that of a normal individual with a normal body composition. Critically ill patients have a marked reduction in exogenous intake, and REE trends are downward in starvation, both on a whole patient basis and on a per kilogram of tissue basis [13,14]. In the opposite direction, the REE in critical illness changes in an upward direction often directly related to the severity of illness or injury [13,15,16,17]. In general, the energy expenditure data reported in the past have been overly high due to technical and procedural difficulties and the changes that occur with a critical illness are increasingly being seen as more modest. The elevations in REE with acute illness occur in most critical illnesses and exceed those seen with the most ambitious surgical procedures, where REE increases only 5 to 10 percent in the immediate postoperative period and often returns to normal within several days if no complications ensue [18]. Head trauma patients have documented REE measures 125 percent predicted but can be normalized or driven below predicted measures during barbiturate therapy [19]. Patients who become critically ill with a complication or with the cancer cachexia syndrome demonstrate a great deal of variability in their measured energy expenditure, as has been found in heterogeneous groups [20], between tumor types [21], and between stages in a given tumor type [22]. Interestingly, the abnormalities in REEs in cancer patients are ablated by the curative removal of the tumor, whereas a limited palliative operative approach often aggravates the hypermetabolism of these patients [23].

Dietary-induced and cold thermogenesis probably have only minor influences on the TEE in critically ill patients. This probably occurs only when the exogenous caloric supply rate exceeds the energy expenditure rate. With increasing diligence, intensivists must continue to focus on avoiding overfeeding of the critically ill patient because of the untoward effects that ensue, such as fluid overload, increased CO_2 production, increased O_2 consumption, and hepatic steatosis.

Another moderate component of the TEE of the critically ill patient is the activity energy expenditure (AEE). Although TEE is sometimes twice REE in normal adults, due to the large AEE, this is not true in sick patients. The sicker the patient, the less AEE occurs and the more TEE approaches REE. Routine intensive care procedures do contribute to AEE, accounting for as much as 10 percent of the TEE [24,25]. For non-ICU hospitalized patients, TEE can often be estimated as 130 percent of the directly measured REE. As one approaches a more homogeneous intensive care group, TEE approaches between 100 and 120% of REE.

How can TEE be determined? The TEE can be determined directly by measuring heat exchange with a direct calorimeter or with continuous 24-hour indirect calorimetry. Although these are technologically possible, they are clinically impractical and substitute approaches have been developed. The simplest approach is to estimate a patient's REE from a variety of predictive equations and add stress and activity factors to this calculation to estimate the patient's TEE. Unfortunately, the predictive equations for REE have been developed in normal individuals with normal body composition, which has little relationship with the sick patients with distorted body composition in our intensive care unit. In addition, stress and activity factors are averages that have a great deal of variability among patients, and their applicability in an individual patient is very suspect. A number of studies have examined this issue, and most active investigators have settled on the approach of measuring the REE of the patient and adding a small increment from 10 to 30 percent to determine the TEE. The effects of disease, its treatment, and nutrient intake will be considered in the measured REE. The magnitude of the added factor is determined by the degree of illness of the patient; the sicker the patient, the less is added to REE, reflecting less estimated AEE.

When should the ICU patient's REE be determined? It certainly should be determined at the outset to determine the severity of the hypermetabolism, on a weekly basis thereafter, and on a more frequent ad hoc basis when there have been significant changes in clinical course. The REE can be measured any time during the day with maximum repeatability using the modern indirect calorimetry that has been developed over the past 15 years.

The purpose of determining TEE is to acquire a measure of severity of hypermetabolism that has predictive benefits but allows you to provide a rational nutrient prescription purely based on your therapeutic goals for the patient. If the desire is to replenish the patient's depleted caloric fat stores, one would have to supply more exogenous calories than the TEE. In most cases, this represents a caloric prescription of 130 to 150 percent of REE or 110 to 120 percent of TEE. This modest "overfeeding" will slowly replete the fat stores, but should be abandoned at the first sign of difficulties with hepatic, renal, or respiratory excretory pathways of the body. If one's goal is to maintain the patient's current fat stores, one would have to supply exogenous calories equivalent to the patient's TEE. If, as in many patients, the caloric fat stores are excessive, as defined by a weight far greater than 120 percent of ideal body weight, then one would supply calories at a rate significantly below the TEE. A practical approach is to supply 800 glucose calories and 2 gm protein/kg/day to such patients.

In critical care, particular attention is paid to disorders that lead to cerebral dysfunction. Hypoxia is the most common example, and considerable effort is devoted to avoiding this problem. If the brain is deprived of fuel, as in hypoglycemia, the outcome is similar, yet far less attention is paid to maintaining an adequate and appropriate long-term fuel supply.

In the early days of TPN, patients were provided 12.6 to 20.9 millijoules (MJ) (3000–5000 kcal) per day with the "thought" that "hyper" alimentation was good. Energy requirements of sick patients were ill defined and "guess work" at best. Energy prescription often consisted of "three bottles per day" and such input often exceeded the capacity of the body's disposal systems. Unfortunately, serious adverse events accompanied overfeeding: hyperglycemia, hyperosmolar states, steatosis, excessive carbon dioxide production, increased norepinephrine secretion, and fluid overload. When any or all these events occurred, the temptation for the clinician was to abandon forced feeding and blame TPN. However, only misuse of TPN is to blame. We must approach energy prescription much as we approach medication prescriptions, with precision based on objective scientific information.

Indirect calorimetry measures gas exchange in contrast to the heat exchange measurements of direct calorimetry. Multiple studies have validated their comparable results in varying settings. Although the mouthpiece or mask is still used occasionally, the canopy technique is preferred for clinical studies. Clinically useful indirect calorimeters must have portability, automated calibration, limited sensor drift, the ability to collect gas exchange measurements under a variety of circumstances, flexibility in their computer software, and a minimal warm-up time. A calibration checklist must be followed, and the system must be checked for any leaks to maintain stable inspired oxygen concentration as well as sufficient desiccant to remove excess humidity. Should the indirect calorimetry measurements be continuous over 24 hours to measure a patient's TEE, or can a "snapshot" measurement of REE be performed and extrapolated to an estimate of TEE? We measure a spot REE and extrapolate, controlling physical activity and nutrient intake; others have favored random multiple "snapshots" of nonresting measurements for more accurate extrapolation. REE test conditions include 0.5-hour rest in bed, no nutrient intake within 2 hours before the test, and a thermoneutral environment. Gas-exchange results must demonstrate a steady state such that five consecutive 1-minute measurements have a coefficient variation of less than 5 percent. Using this rigid approach, we can be confident that our "snapshot" REE measurements are truly representative. If the measured REE is greater than 120 percent or less than 80 percent of that expected, if the minute ventilation is less than 5 liters or greater than 10 liters, or if the respiratory quotient (RQ) is greater than 1.00, we review the raw data to confirm an accurate collection. We have a 2 percent coefficient of variation in REE measured multiple times during the same day. Rumpler and coworkers showed that the coefficient of variation of REE measured on five consecutive days was 2 percent and only 3 percent when the REE was measured weekly for 1 month in the same subject [26]. Furthermore when TEE was measured for 24 hours, the daily measurements had a coefficient of variation of 3 percent and only 5 percent when done weekly. The lack of nitrogen excretion data has little influence on REE calculations and can essentially be ignored, as shown by other investigators [27].

Whether one need measure REE in sick patients should no longer be debated. Multiple studies have adequately shown that the variability of measured REE compared with predictions for individuals is substantial: measured REE ranges from 50 to 150 percent of the expected metabolic rate in different study populations [28]. Such wide variability compared with that expected precludes the use of a predictive formula to clinically define energy requirements, since the risk of substantial underfeeding or overfeeding is unacceptably high. The degree of variability is closely linked to disease severity and is due to distorted body composition, abnormal metabolic activity per unit of tissue, and multiple thermogenic and thermodepressive clinical interventions. In a study conducted by Cox, quadriplegics had an REE 30 percent below the expected value and paraplegics had one 10 percent below the expected value [29]. Sepsis, operations,

trauma, and respiratory failure all generate elevated energy expenditure in some, but not all, sick patients. The concept of attributing a certain degree of elevation of TEE to a given disease and extrapolating this to all patients with that disease, regardless of severity and time course, is a serious error. In many patients an initial hypermetabolism often slowly declines over time.

The whole body protein catabolic rate can be measured, using urinary nitrogen excretion over a defined period of time, usually 24 hours. These data result in a calculated catabolic index [30] as well as a urea generation rate [31]. The formula for the nitrogen balance is:

N intake − (urinary N + change BUN + 4)
change in BUN (g) = $(0.6 \times \text{weight})(\text{SUN}f − \text{SUN}i)$

where i and f are the initial and final values in the measurement period, SUN is serum urea nitrogen (g/L), and weight is body weight in kilograms. With the rapidity of changing clinical status in the intensive care unit, repeat measurements of both the metabolic rate and catabolic rate should be done with significant changing clinical status or at least weekly. One must caution that changes in blood urea levels need to be accounted for in the calculations of nitrogen balance since urea is distributed throughout total body water and this is metabolically "outside" the body, and should be included on the output side of the nitrogen balance equation. Cumulative energy balance is synonymous with tissue fat balance, and if energy supply to the patient exceeds the TEE, fat stores will increase. If the exogenous energy supply is less than TEE, body fat stores will decline over time.

Having determined TEE, our energy prescription is based on our goal for the patient's fat stores. If the patient's current weight is less than 90 percent of ideal weight, the patient's fat stores are subnormal and we prescribe an energy supply to replete those fat stores (energy supply >TEE). How much greater depends on how rapidly we want to restore fat stores and the ability of the patient's liver to convert and export the energy overload to peripheral fat stores. If the patient's current weight is between 90 and 120 percent of ideal body weight, the fat stores are normal and our energy goal is to maintain these fat stores at their current size (energy supply = TEE). If the patient's dry current body weight is greater than 120 percent of idea body weight, the fat stores are excessive and we would not be unhappy if they were partially depleted over the hospital course. We supply energy at a rate less than the patient's TEE, driving the cannibalization of endogenous fat stores. This approach has worked well and has brought rationality to the energy prescription process.

We have explored the hypothesis that one may simultaneously create a positive clinical outcome, positive nitrogen balance, and negative energy or fat balance in sick patients. Our study population consisted of morbidly obese patients with over 1674 MJ (400 000 kcal) of fat stores who had an intraabdominal abscess and enterocutaneous fistula and were "sick" with these potentially lethal postoperative complications [32]. It made no sense to provide sufficient energy to maintain or expand the fat stores in patients who already had an excessive amount, so energy was supplied at only 30 percent of their TEE. By design the other energy source would be their endogenous fat stores, so these fat stores and body weight would gradually decline. We provided protein at a rate of 2 gm protein per kilogram of ideal body weight. The patients lost 1.5 kg weight per week, primarily as fat, as evidenced by their RQ of 0.75. For the clinician, the results were dramatic. All fistulas healed, and patients were in slightly positive nitrogen balance at +2 gm per day, and their serum proteins gradually returned to normal. Once positive N balance was achieved, closure of wounds and enterocutaneous fistulas occurred.

Our overall philosophy of energy prescription in the critically ill patient emphasizes a balanced approach with a provision of energy at the lowest level possible to achieve maximal benefit. We must be cognizant of the limitations of the respiratory, renal, and hepatic disposal systems. There is no obvious benefit in creating or maintaining obesity and no indication as to why we should "fatten-up" the patient. Endogenous fat can provide energy needs, and with this rational approach to energy prescription there is a great reduction in the number of complications of excessive energy delivery.

How To Deliver

The two main caloric sources are carbohydrate and fat. Glucose is the primary source of carbohydrate and necessary fuel for brain, bone marrow cells, and certain other tissues. One could view minimum requirement as 200 gm per day, particularly in a patient with major extensive surgical wounds [33]. Although there is a protein-sparing effect of glucose in the unstressed starving patient, it diminishes in importance as the individual becomes "sick" [34,35]. The limitations on the exogenous supply of glucose are really related to the limitations of glucose oxidation. During severe critical illness, there is no deficit in available glucose as glucose production is enhanced and glucose oxidation is relatively unimpaired [36]. Enhanced gluconeogenesis is nonsuppressible by exogenous supplies of glucose. The maximum rate of glucose oxidation is probably in the range of 7 gm/kg/day. The fate of glucose supplied above the oxidation rate is important to understand. Long and co-workers studied several groups, including cancer patients, septic patients, and trauma patients receiving glucose infusions of 5 to 6 mg/kg/min, and found oxidation of glucose contributed 60 percent to the CO_2 production (ml/min or ml/μ^2) [37]. Glucagon production is enhanced, as are fat synthesis and storage. The cost of converting excess glucose to the storage forms of glucagon and fat is about 10 percent of the energy value [38] of the stored fuel as glucagon, and once glucagon supplies are repleted this cost is closer to the 20 to 30 percent range [39] when lipid storage is involved. This cost of storing oversupplied exogenous calories contributes to the hypermetabolism when there is overfeeding. This is obviously greatly enhanced if the exogenous fuels are supplied at an accelerated rate for only part of the day rather than the same quantity spread out in a continuous infusion over 24 hours. There are clearly consequences to glucose overfeeding, which have been well defined in the literature and are really an indictment of the prescribing habits of clinicians. Complications of fluid overload, hepatic steatosis, excessive CO_2 production, respiratory failure, and the increased energy expenditure related to the storage cost certainly have caused great concerns about the use of TPN and in reality should be a concern about the prescribing habits of the practitioners. We rarely see "hepatic dysfunction" since our energy prescription is in tune with the concepts elucidated above.

Supplemental insulin may provide mild improvement in nitrogen utilization, probably related to the insulin effect on the skeletal muscle. This is not a major rationale for using insulin, which should be primarily directed at maintaining a reasonable serum glucose level. Glucose solutions are available in concentrations ranging from 2.5 percent up to 70 percent; solutions above 10 percent must be delivered via a central vein.

The other major caloric source of fuel is fat, which is the preferred fuel in the critically ill patient. Fatty acid mobilization from peripheral fat stores is increased in this patient population and is not suppressed by glucose infusion [40]. Fatty acid oxidation is also increased. However, they are not directly linked, and one cannot extrapolate from one to the other. As in carbohydrate metabolism, a recycling occurs in fat metabolism, with fatty acids being recycled and transported back to the adipose tissue for storage [40,41]. Fat is a calorically dense, effectively utilized fuel source, and use of exogenous fat in sick patients can obviate the negative effects of excessive carbohydrate infusion [42]. Most practitioners supply 30 to 50 percent of the daily caloric requirement as fat and limit total dose to 2.5 gm/fat/kg/day. Although alternative carbohydrate sources are available, more is known and promising in the use of different lipid preparations. The most common type of lipid used as a caloric source in TPN is long-chain triglycerides (LCT) in a lipid emulsion derived from soybean or safflower oil. These triglycerides are 16 to 18 carbons long, and the predominant fatty acid is linoleic acid. Some reported disadvantages of long-chain triglycerides (LCTs) are their immunosuppressive effects on neutrophil function and macrophage phagocytosis and a general impairment in the function of the reticuloendothelial system [43]. LCTs are not cleared by lipoprotein lipase as efficiently as one would hope and they are dependent on a carnitine-controlled oxidative pathway, which is impaired in sepsis. The medium-chain triglycerides (MCTs), derived from palm and coconut oils and composed of mainly 8 to 10 carbon fatty acids, are alternatives to LCTs. MCTs are more rapidly and efficiently oxidized by carnitine-independent pathways and have less uptake in the reticuloendothelial system and may result in improved nitrogen retention [44,45,46]. MCT infusions have been shown to increase oxygen demand and change minute ventilation if infused too quickly [47] and are not as well stored in adipose tissue. A number of experimental admixtures of MCT and LCT are currently being evaluated, with the goal of producing a product with minimized host defense impairments and maximized oxidative capacity.

Can lipid infusions be used with the patient in sepsis? Sepsis is a very common occurrence in the critically ill patient, and the answer is certainly yes. Although lipid particles are trapped particularly in the reticuloendothelial cells and partially disrupt the function of these cells, there are no overwhelming studies that convince us that such infusions seriously alter the host defense capabilities in a clinically relevant way [48]. In fact, lipid supplementation of omega-3 fatty acids may have benefits in reducing the severity of septic shock. Lipid emulsions should be given slowly, optimally over 24 hours, to reduce the release of vasoactive thromboxanes, which can impair pulmonary function [49] or minimize metabolic complications [50]. The rate should be less than 3 mg/kg/min to avoid this effect. The use of lipid emulsions during episodes of acute pancreatitis should not be restricted since there is no evidence suggesting they exacerbate the primary disease process [51]. The only exception would be when clearance of lipids is impaired in the patient due to acute pancreatitis or any other disorder.

Should the glucose-amino acid standard mixture be combined with lipid emulsion or infused separately? Although this issue has been studied in less sick patients, the conclusions are probably applicable. Mixed fuel systems such as those used in total nutrient admixture are certainly well tolerated and can achieve acceptable or better nitrogen balance results [8,52, 53,54].

Protein Requirements

During critical illness, protein is redistributed and mobilized from various sources, such as the intestinal tract, skeletal muscle, albumin mass, and the skin, to provide precursors for the body protein synthesis. The losses that occur in the critically ill patient are often staggering. Most of this protein is utilized for precursor to synthesize higher priority needs. Some is oxidized for energy, with a proportion ranging from a normal amount of 15 to 20 percent to sometimes as high as 30 percent [55]. During critical illness urinary nitrogen losses can exceed 50 gm per day. One must remember that 33 gm of urinary nitrogen represents a loss of 1 kg of lean tissue in the body. Losses between 30 and 50 gm of urinary nitrogen are not infrequent in the multiply injured patient, septic patient, and bone marrow transplant patient. We must be cognizant of the fact that if a patient is losing 4 gm protein per day, it is unlikely that nitrogen balance will improve by exogenously providing only 1 gm protein per day. A rational approach would suggest starting these patients on 2 gm protein per day, assuming the hepatic and renal disposal systems are functioning in a normal fashion. The protein content of the TPN prescription in the critically ill patient should be 2 gm/kg/current body weight. If current body weight is greater than 130 percent of ideal body weight, one should use 130 percent of the ideal body weight as the denominator. This avoids oversupply of amino acids to significantly obese patients. The adequacy of the protein intake can be assessed over time using nitrogen balance techniques. Limitations in protein may be imposed because of the inadequacies of the patient's disposal systems, particularly the liver and kidney. If these disposal pathways are impaired and accumulation occurs, there is no great advantage to continue a high intake. Protein intake can be adjusted early both in quantity and quality as defined by the amino acid profile; variations of formulations will be discussed later. The normal way to supply protein is with the synthetic crystalline amino acid solutions, available in concentrations ranging from 1 to 15 percent, a mix of essential and nonessential amino acids. Decades of amino acid research have produced specialty amino acid solutions specific for certain disease states, and this exciting area of research continues as we search for any advantages in the treatment of the critically ill patients. Most studies have shown nutritional metabolic improvements in the patient, but it has been difficult to demonstrate clinical effectiveness, given the complexity of the milieu and environment in which these products are delivered.

Glutamine is a conditionally essential amino acid that is required because of its increased utilization during severe stress. It is normally synthesized and stored in skeletal muscle and is a major fuel for the intestine and host-defense–replicating cells. During critical illness, skeletal muscle releases large amounts of glutamine, causing blood and tissue levels to fall in concert with the severity of illness. The skeletal muscle is the primary organ releasing glutamine, with the lungs contributing to a modest degree. Alteration in glutamine metabolism is evident following surgery as well as episodes of sepsis. Increased glutamine utilization is mediated by cytokines, glucocorticoids, and hormones and is very likely directed to lymphocyte and macrophagic activity for cell proliferation [56]. When the increased release is not countered by increased uptake, a negative balance ensues. Glutamine supplementation can potentially help replete these depleted storehouses. Several clinical studies seem to provide evidence that there are clinical benefits in certain postoperative patients and in the bone marrow transplant group [9,57,58]. Glutamine may also have an important clinical role in maintaining the integrity of intestinal mucosa, and several studies demonstrate a beneficial effect of glutamine in preventing mucosal atrophy [59,60]. The role of glutamine in preventing the intestinal mucosal atrophy that develops during TPN is still being investigated but may in fact be a relatively simple intervention with few side effects. Since glutamine is utilized by rapidly replicating cells, there is some concern that

glutamine supplementation in a tumor-bearing host may accelerate unwanted tumor growth. The concern is probably not warranted in view of studies where glutamine's effect on tumor growth and host tissue was marginal and did not increase tumor size, DNA content, or tumor glutamine metabolism [61]. Despite all the promising effects of glutamine supplementation, its routine administration has been limited because it is not standardly included in commercially available parenteral solutions. The stability issue relates to the increased rapid breakdown of glutamine to ammonia and glutamate, which can be toxic. However, more recent data indicate that parenteral glutamine preparations are stable for prolonged periods of time and have limited toxic side effects [62,63], and thus preparation should no longer limit appropriate administration.

The second amino acid that has received considerable attention is arginine. Increased plasma levels of arginine stimulate secretion of insulin, glucagon, growth hormone, prolactin, and adrenal catecolamines. Arginine is important in wound healing, and deficiencies may certainly lead to impairment of wound healing [64,65]. Most major attention has been focused on its role in the immune system and its necessity for effective T-cell function. Immunomodulation with arginine has been studied extensively, and evidence is accumulating that it is important in maintaining or enhancing the host defense capabilities as well as having a secondary positive effect on overall body nitrogen balance [66–69].

Vitamins and Trace Elements

The requirement of vitamins and trace elements during periods of critical illness is not completely understood. During acute periods of stress and accelerated metabolic demand there may in fact be an increased need for vitamins and trace elements. However, this has not been clearly defined, partly because of the difficulty in accurately measuring the total body stores of vitamins and trace elements. Specifically, serum measures are costly and may have little clinical yield in the setting of critical illness. If stores are depleted from a prolonged chronic illness prior to the onset of acute illness, deficiencies may exist even if serum levels appear normal. Table 200-1 outlines current recommendations for daily parenteral vitamin supplementation that have been defined by the Nutrition Advisory Group (NAG)

Table 200-1. Multivitamin Formulation for Adults*

Vitamin	Intravenous dose (NAG† guidelines)
A$_1$ (IU)	3300
D (IU)	200
E (IU)	200
Ascorbic acid (mg)	100–200
Folate (μg)	400–600
Niacin (mg)	40
Thiamine (mg)	3
Riboflavin (mg)	3.6
Pyridoxine (mg)	4.0–6.0
Cyanocobalamin (mg)	5.0
Pantothenic acid (mg)	15
Biotin (mg)	60

* Data from Baumgartner TG (ed): *Clinical Guide to Parenteral Micronutrition,* 2nd ed. Deerfield, IL, Fujisawa USA, Inc., 1991, pp 343–590.
† NAG = Nutrition Advisory Group of the American Medical Association.

[70]. One milligram of vitamin K is added daily to TPN solution to provide maintenance needs. Additional vitamin K, required because of suspected deficiency or because of clotting abnormalities, can be delivered in intermittent intramuscular injection. Repletion doses of vitamin K should be administered parenterally secondary to the potential for anaphylactic reaction when administered too rapidly. Maintenance parenteral iron is generally not recommended during periods of critical illness. Iron stores in men are up to 1000 mg and in women are up to 500 mg, which could provide iron for at least one year in the absence of bleeding [71]. Furthermore, during periods of acute bleeding in which transfusions are required, each unit of packed red blood cells provides significant amounts of iron. Parenteral iron dextran is not compatible with lipids and therefore cannot be added to lipid-containing TPN solutions. Iron overload is a potential danger if the parenteral dose is not carefully calculated and closely monitored. Vitamins should be deleted from intradialytic TPN since the multivitamins are lost in the course of the dialysis treatment.

Trace elements are required during periods of increased metabolic demands. However, like vitamins, there is little evidence of specific needs during periods of acute illness, but previously depleted patients may be at risk for trace element deficiencies. Increased demand for zinc is seen in the adult with acute catabolic stress, and deficiencies can contribute to poor wound healing [72]. Therefore, an additional 2 mg over the maintenance dose is recommended. Furthermore, addition of 12.2 mg for each liter of small intestinal fluid and an additional 17.1 mg for each liter of ileostomy or stool output is recommended to maintain normal serum levels. Chromium losses may be increased during acute periods of stress, and deficiency can result in difficulty with glucose control [73]. Trace element requirements can be delivered to the critically ill patient by daily addition as outlined in Table 200-2. Further research is needed to define additional demands during periods of critical illness.

Fluid and Electrolyte Requirements

A multitude of factors contribute to a patient's fluid and electrolyte homeostasis during periods of critical illness. Significant losses in various body compartments can occur from massive blood loss, excessive gastrointestinal losses, large nasogastric outputs, high-volume enteric or pancreatic fistulas, or high-volume diarrhea. Increased insensible losses are associated with persistent fever, with the presence of tracheostomy requiring frequent suctioning, and with burn injuries.

Assessing the fluid and electrolyte status of a critically ill patient is challenging given the potential for massive shifts of fluids and electrolytes between body compartments. Ordinarily intracellular fluid, which accounts for 50 to 55 percent of total body water, is the storage for almost all the body potassium. Total body potassium is approximately 3200 mg, and all but about 60 mg is located intracellularly. Extracellular fluid is mainly composed of sodium chloride, and 85 percent of the sodium is located extracellularly and accounts for approximately 1500 mEq, with total body chloride reaching about 2300 mEq [74]. A variety of clinical situations can alter fluid and electrolyte distribution among body compartments and impact on the parenteral prescription. For example, starvation results in increased extracellular fluid, decreased total body potassium, decreased total body magnesium, and decreased total body phosphate. During acute injury there may be an initial period where there is sodium and water retention. During periods of hemodynamic instability, patients may be resuscitated with large volumes of exogenous fluid or blood products, which has an impact on total body fluid status and serum measures of various electrolytes.

When carefully prescribed, parenteral nutrition is an excellent vehicle for fluid and electrolyte administration. Most standard TPN solutions that contain maintenance doses of electrolytes range anywhere from one-fourth to one-half normal saline. For example, 1 liter of normal saline contains 164 mEq of sodium. A typical TPN regimen provided in 2 liters of fluid containing maintenance doses of sodium chloride (80 mEq) is approximately one-fourth normal saline. Many factors affect the electrolyte recommendations during periods of critical illness, and fluid and electrolyte requirements can change on an hourly or daily basis. Table 200-3 outlines typical electrolyte requirements and factors that can affect these requirements during periods of critical illness. Disruption of normal renal function usually requires limitation of several electrolytes. Synthesis of new tissue can result in rapid depletion of serum levels of potassium, magnesium, and phosphate, as all of these are driven into the cell for synthesis. Persistent excessive gastrointestinal losses contribute largely to depletion of electrolytes and total body water.

Careful attention to the fluid and electrolyte needs in the critically ill adult is necessary to achieve successful administration of parenteral nutrition. Maximally concentrating all solutions in the critically ill patient avoids premature discontinuation of TPN when fluid status quickly changes and patients no longer tolerate the same fluid prescription. Additional fluids needed as requirements increase are easily provided through simultaneous infusions of other parenteral fluid. To facilitate consistent delivery of nutrient regimens, the TPN should be

Table 200-2. Trace Element Recommendations in Critical Illness*

Trace element	Recommended daily needs for adult patients on TPN[†]	MTE-5[‡]	Special needs during critical illness
Zinc (as sulfate)	2.5–4.0 mg	5 mg	Add 2 mg/day for acute catabolic stress (may need to be reduced with renal insufficiency)
Copper (as sulfate)	0.5–1.5 mg	1 mg	Reduced need with biliary obstruction
Manganese (as sulfate)	0.15–0.8 mg	0.5 mg	Reduced need with biliary obstruction
Chromium (as chloride)	10–15 μg	10 μg	Reduced need with renal failure or insufficiency
Selenium	40–80 μg	60 μg	Increased losses in burns and in gastrointestinal diseases

* From Frankel WL, Evans NJ, Rombeau JL: Scientific rationale and clinical application of parenteral nutrition in critically ill patients, in Rombeau JL, Caldwell MD (eds): *Parenteral Nutrition.* Philadelphia, WB Saunders, 1993, p 606.
[†] TPN = total parenteral nutrition.
[‡] LyphoMed.

Table 200-3. Electrolyte Requirements for Critically Ill Patients

Electrolyte	Daily requirement (mEq/day)	Causes of increased requirements	Causes of decreased requirements
Na	70–100	Administration of loop diuretics	Hypertension Fluid overload
K	70–100	Early nutritional repletion Postobstructive diuresis Diuretic therapy ↑ Gastrointestinal losses	Renal failure
Mg	15–20	Early nutritional repletion Diuretic therapy ↑ Gastrointestinal losses	Renal failure
Ca	10–20	Multiple blood transfusions	—
PO_4	20–30 mmol/day	Early nutritional repletion	Renal failure
Cl	80–120	Prolonged gastric losses	—
Acetate	0–60	Metabolic acidosis Excessive diarrhea Drug therapy—PO_4 binders	Metabolic alkalosis

From Frankel WL, Evans NJ, Rombeau JL: Scientific rationale and clinical application of parenteral nutrition in critically ill patients, in Rombeau JL, Caldwell MD (eds): *Parenteral Nutrition.* Philadelphia, WB Saunders, 1993, p 605.

ordered each day. Daily evaluation of laboratory values and patient status will prevent overestimation or underestimation of fluid and electrolyte requirements.

Acid-base balance is of critical importance during periods of severe illness. Acid-base balance is disrupted for many reasons, including gastrointestinal losses, sepsis, and renal failure. Although primary intervention should fix the underlying problem, the parenteral nutrition solution can contribute to the correction of acid-base balance. Acetate can be provided in the form of the sodium or potassium salt. The TPN solution itself can contribute, very minimally, to the disruption of the patient's acid-base balance, but it is easily correctable with the addition of acetate. TPN solutions designed for central administration generally have a pH in the range of 4 to 5, which increases with the addition of lipids.

Blood sugar control is particularly labile during periods of severe illness. The use of a mixed fuel system that delivers a combination of lipid and dextrose calories will generally ease the demand for exogenous insulin. However, in the event of persistent hyperglycemia, insulin can be added to the parenteral nutrition. There is no question of the availability of insulin in the parenteral nutrition solution, given the evidence provided by investigators who examined the recovery of Humulin-R insulin from ethylene vinyl acetate plastic bags and found that at least 90 percent of the insulin was recovered [75]. One consideration when adding insulin to the TPN solution is the precipitous changes in blood glucose that often accompany periods of critical illness. For example, the hyperglycemia associated with an episode of sepsis may quickly resolve once the septic focus is eliminated. Therefore, for short-term management, insulin can be delivered outside the TPN solution until the total daily insulin requirement is defined. In this way the insulin-containing TPN is not acutely stopped and discarded if the patient's glucose suddenly normalizes.

Delivery Considerations: Infection Control

Infusate contamination is a rare but preventable complication of TPN administration. Meticulous aseptic technique is imper-

ative to ensure that TPN is given with minimal complications. Infusate contamination can occur at the time of TPN compounding, while attaching administration sets, or during any incorrect manipulation of the TPN solution. Strict quality control measures instituted over the past 10 to 15 years have essentially eliminated the infusate as a source of contamination by dedicating specially trained personnel responsible for daily solution preparation under a laminar flow hood and providing for proper storage after preparation. Routine surveillance of solution sterility has been abandoned.

Clinicians are often misinformed that current TPN solutions are good growth media for bacteria and fungi. Early TPN solutions (protein hydrolysates) did support growth of bacteria and fungi better than current amino acid sources (synthesized crystalline amino acids) [76,77]. Current formulations using crystalline amino acids are hypertonic and have a very low pH, which renders them a poor growth media [78,79,80]. The addition of albumin increases the support of bacterial proliferation [81]. Isolated lipid emulsions support growth of bacteria and fungi more than dextrose amino acid mixtures because of the increased pH of lipid emulsions, generating debate regarding safe hang time [82,83,84]. Several investigators have identified microbial growth in lipid solutions in concentrations greater than 10^3 colony-forming units/ml/24 hours [84,85]. The Centers for Disease Control and Prevention (CDC) recommend that such separate lipid infusions be completed within 12 hours [86,87]. However, other investigators found no significant difference in microbial growth when lipids were infused at less than or at greater than 12 hours [88]. Total nutrient admixtures (TNA) or 3-in-1 solutions have lipid emulsions combined with more bacteriostatic dextrose and amino acid solutions. The TNA has a slightly higher pH, allowing better growth than dextrose-amino acid solutions alone, but far less than isolated lipid emulsion [89,90].

To prevent proliferation of bacteria or fungi if the solution is contaminated, it is imperative that recommendations for storage and administration are followed. All compounded parenteral solutions should be stored at 5°C. Solutions must be used within 24 hours of warming to room temperature. The use of in-line filters to trap contaminants is controversial. Filters must be 0.22 μm in order to remove bacteria, fungi, and particulate matter; the 0.22-μm filter is too small to be used with the total nutrient admixture solution. A 1.2-μm filter, acceptable for 3-in-1 solutions, can remove *Candida;* however, *Escherichia coli* and *Staphylococcus epidermidis* pass through these filters. Increased manipulation of the filters and administration sets may actually increase line contamination.

CENTRAL VENOUS ACCESS. Central venous access is mandatory to safely and efficiently deliver the macronutrient and micronutrient requirements during critical illness. Solutions that are calorically dense and contain large amounts of nitrogen must often be prepared in a minimal volume. Central venous access is required to deliver any solution with an osmolarity greater than 900 mOsm. TPN solutions prepared with 70% dextrose and maximally concentrated amino acid solutions well exceed 900 mOsm and are typically in the range of 1400 to 1800 mOsm. Peripheral parenteral nutrition is not a practical option in most critically ill patients.

Percutaneous central venous catheters (CVC) have been used increasingly for three decades. Historically, TPN was delivered through protected lines placed only for TPN, but there is no logical reason for this approach if previously used catheters have been properly maintained. The proper setting for placement of a CVC in the critically ill patient includes hemodynamic stability, no coagulation abnormalities, and no anatomic or physiologic limitations. The large superior central venous system is used for central venous access. The use of the inferior central venous system carries an increased infection risk and increased morbidity if a venous thrombosis occurs (see Chap. 2).

Since the 1980s, central access catheters with multiple lumens have been used increasingly to deliver the variety of lifesaving medications required during periods of critical illness. Several investigators have evaluated the infection rates between single lumen and multiple lumen catheters [91,92,93,94]. Definitive conclusions are elusive; much of the data are retrospective and uncontrolled and lack consistent definition of catheter-related sepsis. Catheter infection rates should be defined as the number of infectious episodes per catheter-day at risk. Multiple-lumen catheters have increased infection rates (per catheter but not per lumen) as compared to the single-lumen catheters [95]. Reducing the number of catheter lumens is neither a practical nor realistic approach in the intensive care setting. Other catheters that are used during periods of critical illness include hemodynamic monitoring lines, such as pulmonary artery (PA) catheters. Although it is safe to infuse TPN through such monitoring catheters, it should be administered only through a proximal port because infusions via distal ports may increase the risk of artery inflammation [96,97]. TPN should not be infused through side ports of introducer sheaths.

It is important to understand the etiology of the catheter sepsis and avoid implicating TPN. Sick immunocompromised patients often require TPN, and such patients are prone to catheter infections. TPN is a good marker for a sick patient but is not an independent variable in the generation of catheter sepsis. The predominant etiology for catheter-related sepsis is the migration of skin flora down the subcutaneous tract [98]. TPN itself does not cause catheter-related bacteremia or sepsis. Confusion occurs because TPN is often a common therapeutic modality in a critically ill immunocompromised patient who is a prime candidate for catheter-related sepsis. To minimize catheter-related sepsis it is important to follow strict protocols for CVC insertion and maintenance. The evidence is inconclusive regarding the most effective dressing protocol that will reduce infection rates. A variety of antimicrobial cleansing agents are available. The most commonly used agents are alcohol and povidone-iodine. Chlorhexidine, which is not a new agent, is being used increasingly in the care of CVCs. It has the advantage

of a longer-acting antibacterial effect and has been shown to reduce the incidence of catheter-related infection [99]. Although CVC dressing protocols have been extensively studied over the years, neither gauze nor transparent semipermeable film predominates [100–103]. Regardless of the type of dressing protocol used, it is important that the dressing remains sealed and intact and is applied using a well-defined protocol. A variety of new catheter designs purport to decrease the risk of catheter-related sepsis. Commercially available devices include antibiotic bonded CVCs as well as those with a subcutaneous implantable cuff that acts as a mechanical and chemical barrier to migration of bacteria down the tract.

Impaired Disposal Systems

The disposal systems of the body handle the end products of metabolism. When such systems are impaired, the exogenous nutrient supply must be adjusted. Impairments in the functional capacity of the kidney, liver, and respiratory system are common in the critically ill.

RENAL FAILURE. Renal failure commonly occurs during critical illness as a result of preexisting insufficiency, severe hemodynamic instability, or nephrotoxic agents. Decreased renal function impairs the ability to excrete the end products of metabolism. The characteristic rise in blood urea nitrogen (BUN), creatinine, and electrolytes alerts the clinician to worsening function.

Energy expenditure and caloric requirements during acute renal failure are often increased, but the largest contributor to this elevation is usually an underlying acute event, such as sepsis. Glucose calories must be administered carefully because of the glucose intolerance that occurs with sepsis. Fat calories can be delivered, but hypertriglyceridemia can occur due to the reduced activity of plasma and tissue lipoprotein lipase.

Limiting exogenous nutrient supply, as may be indicated in the critically ill hypermetabolic patient to prevent or delay dialytic therapy, is unwise and will result in severe cumulative deficits in both energy and nitrogen balance. The concept of limiting or withholding nutrients to prevent the need for dialysis is shortsighted since urea generation still continues as skeletal muscle is catabolized, despite limiting exogenous nutrient provision. Dialysis therapy contributes to protein losses nearing 10 gm per day and even higher in acute renal patients receiving peritoneal dialysis [104]. On the other hand, peritoneal dialysis and continuous arteriovenous hemofiltration dialysis contribute significantly to the exogenous nonprotein caloric supply. Sixty percent of the glucose calories in peritoneal dialysis are absorbed [105]. For example, a patient receiving hourly exchanges of 1500 ml of 1.5% dialysate alternating with 2.5% dialysate will absorb approximately 1400 nonprotein kcal per day. It is essential that the TPN nutrient prescription account for the contribution such therapies make toward energy goals in order to avoid overfeeding. TPN protein prescription in renal failure has generated debate both in terms of the amount and the type of protein. Patients with impaired renal function who are effectively dialyzed can tolerate protein prescriptions ranging from 1.2 to 2 gm/kg/day [106,107]. Protein prescription must be frequently reevaluated since changes in effectiveness of dialysis as well as the intrinsic renal function may vary. Reducing the protein prescription may be necessary if the BUN is consistently over 100 mg per deciliter despite maximal dialytic therapy. The role of essential amino acids in the care of the patient with renal failure is controversial. Theoretically, providing only essential amino acids is thought to slow the rise of BUN because of reduced urea synthesis or recycling of urea to make nonessential amino acids. Only limited studies support the effectiveness of this approach, and we use a mix of nonessential and essential amino acids in the setting of renal failure. A disadvantage of the essential amino acid solutions is their limited concentration, which may be less well tolerated in these patients who are often fluid restricted.

Fluid and electrolyte homeostasis is a unique challenge in the patient with renal failure. Accumulation of free water and hyponatremia are common [108]. Maximally concentrating nutrient solutions in order to minimize fluid volume necessary to provide nutrient substrates is an effective approach to the care of the patient with renal failure. Electrolytes such as magnesium, potassium, and phosphate should be deleted and reintroduced at half the daily requirements when serum levels are low. Acid-base balance is often disrupted in renal failure because of the decreased ability to excrete acid by-products. Acetate in the form of sodium or potassium salt can be added to the TPN solution as needed. Vitamin and trace element requirements are similar to those in other critically ill patients, but water-soluble vitamins are often lost in the dialysis process and therefore should not be provided during intradialytic TPN. Excretion of fat-soluble vitamins is decreased, although accumulation during acute episodes of short duration is unlikely. Zinc and chromium are excreted in the urine and sometimes deleted from nutrient regimens. A practical clinical approach with acute renal failure patients within the setting of increased catabolism, often of short duration, is to provide maintenance levels of vitamins and trace elements in daily TPN prescriptions.

Maximizing the successful delivery of TPN in the setting of renal failure requires careful attention to all aspects of nutrient prescriptions. The most optimal way to provide nutritional and metabolic support is through daily infusions. Intradialytic TPN is usually of limited use, since intermittent TPN infusions will never meet the metabolic demands of critical illness. Furthermore, 4-hour infusions impose limits on the quantity of both nutrient and fluid delivery. Renal failure patients requiring TPN often have limited vascular access; hemodialysis access catheters should be utilized for TPN administration off dialysis.

HEPATIC FAILURE. Impairment in hepatic function can result from a variety of causes and becomes clinically most apparent when there is greater than a 70 percent loss in hepatocyte mass. Injury can be imparted to the liver as a result of cell destruction, cell impairment, limitation in blood supply, or metabolic impairment [109.] Hepatic failure in the setting of critical illness is associated with a poor clinical outcome. Structural and functional changes in the injured liver include formation of scar tissue from cell death and regeneration, which subsequently impedes normal blood perfusion. The end result of this is portal-systemic venous shunting, which inevitably deprives hepatic tissue of the nutrient-rich portal blood. Hepatic failure results in several alterations in metabolism, but the albumin synthesis rate is usually maintained despite chronic or acute impairment [110]. Naturally, during periods of superimposed acute illness, albumin synthesis rates may decline secondary to the production of acute-phase reactants. Depletion in serum protein measures is generally a reflection of the overall fluid status and of the presence of ascites. Furthermore, decreased intake often accompanying chronic liver failure largely contributes to the depletion in overall protein status. Alteration in glucose metabolism is clinically evidenced by glucose intolerance. End-stage liver failure can result in hypoglycemia if damage is severe enough to impair gluconeogenesis. The liver produces approx-

imately 150 gm per day of glucose, so the baseline requirement for glucose is 6 gm per hour, which is equivalent to 480 glucose calories per day [111]. Alterations in lipid metabolism accompanying liver failure may be the result of increased levels of plasma-free fatty acids, which can occur because of a decrease in the activity of lipoprotein lipase as well as impaired clearance.

Vitamin and trace element metabolism can be impaired as liver function continues to deteriorate. Decreased retention of water-soluble vitamins may occur in liver failure. Furthermore, decreases in vitamin A and vitamin B_{12} are notable since the liver is a primary storage place for these vitamins. Decreased synthesis of retinol-binding protein results in a decreased plasma level of vitamin A. Additionally, impairment occurs in converting vitamin D to its active form, thus risking progressive bone disease. Decreased hepatic synthesis of vitamin K contributes to abnormalities in clotting function that may already result from decreased synthesis of essential clotting factors. Forty percent of intravascular zinc is transported bound to albumin, and therefore deficiencies in zinc can result from increased excretion and decreased intestinal absorption [111]. The most common vitamin deficiencies accompanying alcohol abuse and cirrhosis include thiamine deficiency, which is thought to be a result of a defect in the phosphorylation of thiamine; impaired formation and excretion of folic acid; and increased breakdown of vitamin B_6.

The goals of therapy are to support the regeneration of hepatic tissue as well as protein synthesis while minimizing metabolic complications. The energy prescription must provide at least 150 gm of glucose per day, matching daily liver production in order to prevent hypoglycemia. Providing a mixed-fuel system is recommended since glucose intolerance is common. Several studies have supported the safety of providing up to 30 percent of the total calories as lipid [112,113]. The protein prescription during periods of impaired liver function is widely debated. The traditional approach to protein prescription has included strict limitations to prevent encephalopathy. This approach further contributes to protein depletion and negative nitrogen balance. Patients with liver dysfunction will usually tolerate an initial protein load of 1.5 gm protein/kg/day if moderately catabolic. However, during periods of severe catabolism it is recommended that protein be increased to 2.0 gm protein/kg/day. It is imperative that the nitrogen metabolism be assessed with nitrogen balance data. Protein prescription should be restricted only if encephalopathy occurs or worsens and is not due to other factors such as gastrointestinal bleeding, sepsis, and shock.

The role of modified amino acids in the setting of impaired liver function is somewhat controversial. In liver failure there is an increase in plasma levels of aromatic amino acids and a decrease in branched-chain amino acids. Hepatic failure solutions are low in aromatic amino acids and high in branched-chain amino acids. The empiric goal of such formulas is to normalize this abnormal plasma amino acid profile. Early studies demonstrated an ability to correct this amino acid profile with solutions high in branched-chain amino acids and to improve the patient's mental status [114,115]. However, other studies have been unable to demonstrate significant differences in reversing encephalopathy [116,117]. A meta-analysis by Naylor includes five randomized controlled studies and concludes that there is significant improvement in mental recovery but no difference in overall survival [118]. A practical clinical approach is to begin with a standard amino acid profile and closely monitor nitrogen balance and mental status. Only in the setting of uncontrolled encephalopathy should the hepatic failure solutions be tried.

The role of nutritional and metabolic support after liver transplantation is still evolving. There is increasing evidence that pre-transplant nutritional status is important. Malnutrition was found to correlate with patient survival in a retrospective review of 160 adult transplant patients [119]. Nutrient requirements are often increased during the immediate post-transplant period. Documented hypermetabolism up to 30 percent above predicted has been shown using indirect calorimetry [120]. Accelerated nitrogen loss has also been documented and is accelerated by steroid use. Investigators have documented increased nitrogen losses after liver transplantation approaching 22 gm per day early after transplantation and continuing at 12.5 gm per day throughout postoperative day 7 [120,121,122]. One outcome study evaluated 28 transplant patients randomized to receive standard TPN, TPN with high branched-chain amino acid solutions, or nothing and found that both TPN groups were off mechanical ventilation sooner, out of the ICU sooner, and, most importantly, had a less negative cumulative nitrogen balance [122]. The use of postoperative TPN in the uncomplicated liver transplant patient is still debated. Certainly when transplantation is accompanied by serious complications, postoperative TPN is important. Early transition to enteral support is an especially important goal.

RESPIRATORY FAILURE. Respiratory failure can result from an acute process such as acute respiratory distress syndrome or from superimposed illness that worsens long-standing chronic pulmonary disease. Preexisting malnutrition is often associated with chronic pulmonary disease and reduces available reserves needed to survive periods of acute stress. Respiratory function can be impaired by malnutrition and acute catabolic processes. Acute catabolic processes that result in the mobilization of body protein deplete respiratory skeletal muscle, including the diaphragm and intercostal muscles. Chronic malnutrition can result in a loss of diaphragm muscle mass parallel to the body weight loss [123,124]. Pathophysiologic changes that accompany this depletion include decreased vital capacity, decreased muscle strength, decreased endurance, decreased ventilatory response to hypoxemia, and impairment in pulmonary defense mechanisms. The clinically relevant functional outcomes that occur as a result of such physiologic changes can be significant [125]. The risk of bacterial colonization and potential for nosocomial lung infections result from impaired function of alveolar macrophage and impaired phagocyte activity. Protein and energy deficits are of particular concern in the critically ill since theoretically they can result in the inability to successfully wean a patient from mechanical ventilation. Kelly and colleagues documented improvement in respiratory muscle strength in 21 of 29 critically ill patients receiving TPN for two weeks [126]. However, not a great deal of quality data exist to assure us that optimizing nutritional status is a large contributor to the success of extubating patients. However, it would be prudent to provide TPN when one expects a prolonged period of illness rather than risk further depletion.

In this population it is particularly important that energy expenditure be measured and not calculated since overfeeding can quickly exceed the ability of compromised lungs to handle the excess carbon dioxide. Patients with pulmonary impairment may not be able to respond to the increase in carbon dioxide produced by adjusting their minute ventilation. We have extensively studied this problem and reached several conclusions: (1) providing no exogenous calories minimizes carbon dioxide production at extreme cost to the patient; (2) providing exogenous calories at or below metabolic rate only increases carbon dioxide production marginally (10%); (3) providing exogenous calories above metabolic rate (overfeeding) greatly accelerates

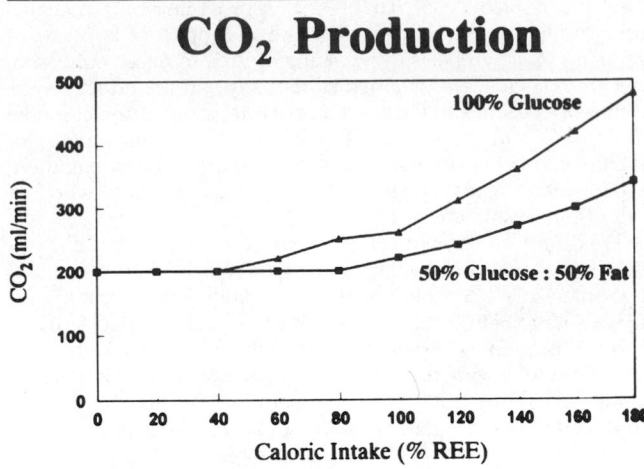

CO$_2$ Production

200-2. CO$_2$ production (ml/min) with different caloric sources (100% dextrose or 50% glucose: 50% fat) and varying caloric supply expressed as a percentage of metabolic rate.

carbon dioxide production (Fig. 200-2); (4) the type of calorie is far less important (glucose vs. fat); and (5) the degree of hypermetabolism influences the carbon dioxide production response to caloric supply; the hypermetabolic patient generates more carbon dioxide in response to a given caloric supply, particularly in the "overfeeding" range (Fig. 200-3) [127]. Talpers and colleagues administered a variety of nutrient regimens to stable mechanically ventilated patients, comparing carbon dioxide production [128]. They also concluded that the total caloric intake contributed more to excessive carbon dioxide production than the ratio of glucose to fat. The concept of reducing or eliminating exogenous caloric intake to facilitate weaning from the ventilator is of questionable utility.

Fig. 200-3. CO$_2$ production with varying caloric intake stratified by metabolic group.

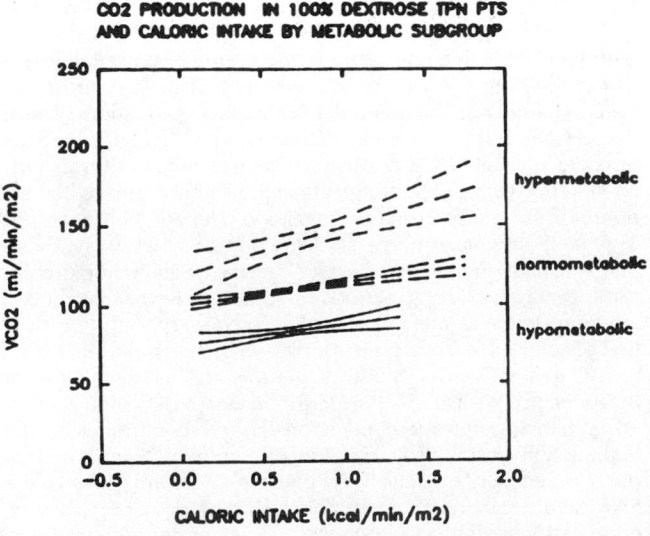

CO2 PRODUCTION IN 100% DEXTROSE TPN PTS AND CALORIC INTAKE BY METABOLIC SUBGROUP

Measuring Goal Achievement: How Did We Do?

It is important to thoughtfully consider whether we have achieved our goals in the delivery of nutritional metabolic support. This should obviously reflect the goals that are set at the time of the initial patient evaluation. The energy prescription must reflect the goals for overall weight and fat stores. Serial monitoring should include body weights. During brief acute illness, body weight will reflect fluid shifts rather than any tissue gains or losses in fat stores. Over time (weeks), accurate body weight changes more accurately reflect tissue accretion or depletion and are an important measure of goal achievement. It is important to obtain serial measures of energy expenditure to determine whether the energy prescription reflects the changing metabolic state of the patient. Certainly this measure is useful not only to assess the caloric prescription but also to provide information for the respiratory failure patient, regarding the level of carbon dioxide production. Considerable attention is directed to offset the ongoing total body nitrogen losses from catabolism through high nitrogen prescription. It is important to serially assess measures of nitrogen and protein stores. A realistic nitrogen balance goal is not necessarily to achieve a positive nitrogen balance, but rather to reduce the net negativity. One is hopeful that the majority of exogenous protein is utilized for synthesis rather than oxidation for fuel. Serial serum proteins such as albumin, transferrin, and prealbumin reflect changes in the visceral protein compartment over time, which has considerable prognostic significance. Maintenance or repletion of the skeletal muscle protein pool will not occur in the critically ill patient given the effects of disuse and severe catabolic pathways. During periods of critical illness the weight loss is two-thirds lean tissue and one-third fat mass. During repletion, we have the ability to define the composition of replaced tissue. Using a low-protein, high-calorie approach we will generate weight gain of two-thirds fat mass and one-third lean body mass. Using a high-protein, low-calorie approach we can put on weight predominated by lean tissue [129].

The overall goal of nutritional metabolic support is to improve survival and decrease morbidity and mortality by improving the organ function of critically ill patients. Improved survival is obvious and evident in the ability to sustain patients who have inadequate functioning of the gastrointestinal tract. The monitoring of morbidity includes wound healing and a multitude of complications of both the primary disease and the treatment. Monitoring specific functional outcomes includes examining the response of acute phase reactants during periods of critical illness, the recovery of respiratory muscles and subsequent ability to get off the ventilator, and improved physical therapy performance.

The incidence and seriousness of complications of total parenteral nutrition in the critically ill patient are much less onerous than the consequences of not feeding. One must make every effort to minimize both the occurrence and severity of the complications, which are inevitable accompaniments of the technique. It is no longer acceptable to withhold forced feeding in these patients because of an irrational exaggerated fear of the complications of parenteral nutrition. Parenteral nutrition has acquired a multitude of myths surrounding its use, many of which are poorly, if at all, supported by data and facts.

The complications of TPN can be divided into three major categories: mechanical complications, metabolic complications, and infectious complications. Much has been written about TPN complications, and they are probably more frequent in the literature than they are in actual occurrence. With effective monitoring strategies, early detection, and immediate intervention, most TPN complications are easily treated and pale in comparison to the devastating effects on clinical outcome when patients are not fed.

Most mechanical complications center around the insertion of the central venous line into the patient. Although many have been described, the most common complication is pneumothorax. This can be kept at a reasonable rate (1%) by a credentialing process and an active educational process that would allow physicians of all specialties to insert this line. This approach works well, and there are no significant differences in frequency of complications among different specialties.

The metabolic complications of TPN are usually related to the oversupply or undersupply of the various nutrients in TPN (Fig. 200-4). The aberrations induced by critical illness are substantial. They can be effectively minimized with an aggressive monitoring program and immediate interventions to correct adverse trends—a major contribution of the nutrition support team. Since critically ill patients receive frequent phlebotomies, the monitoring solely for TPN can be done on a weekly basis, provided there is coordination between TPN and non-TPN blood monitoring. Abnormal serum electrolyte measures can be easily managed by adjusting the TPN prescription on a daily basis. When TPN infusions are intermittent, the need to taper these infusions or to use a hypertonic 10% glucose infusion before coming off TPN is questionable. The field of home TPN has shown us that such tapering and the use of 10% glucose solutions are really unnecessary. Ordering TPN in the critically ill more than a day in advance is not rational. The most onerous complication of TPN is caloric overfeeding. Excessive caloric supply has plagued the therapy from its inception and has generated complications such as hepatic steatosis, excessive carbon dioxide production and respiratory insufficiency, and fluid overload, as well as contribution to the hypermetabolic state in critically ill patients. If a patient is "overfed" with energy, the excess is stored as fat. This occurs mainly in the liver, and hepatic steatosis and "dysfunction" are not uncommon complications of TPN when excessive energy content is used. In our institution, we have rarely seen abnormal liver function tests since we started providing energy based on the actual measurement of energy expenditure. This is an important advance because the development of "hepatic dysfunction" often leads the non-expert clinician to conclude that forced feeding is bad and to stop feeding the patient. The problem is the poor prescription and not the technology.

Foster and associates reviewed the guidelines for energy requirements published in the literature [18]. They used 100 malnourished TPN patients who were fed for more than 7 days. In their study the measured EE had the usual variability in that only 48 percent had a measured EE within 90 to 110 percent of the expected rate. We compared energy prescription based on their actual measured TEE with the energy prescription based on all available applicable recommendations in the literature. The published guidelines recommended supplying 2.1 to 8.4 MJ (500–2000 kcal) per day more than the recommendation based on actual measured TEE. Blindly following such published guidelines would lead to considerable overfeeding and all its adverse clinical events, as well as economic disadvantages. In our institution in one year, using a measured TEE-based energy prescription methodology, we reduced the total volume of TPN from 33,000 liters per year to 26,000 liters per year; this reduction in TPN of over 7000 liters per year is not inconsequential. Caloric supply must be tailored to the fat stores in individual patients and their metabolic rate. The demise of few patients occurs because they run out of calories; their fat stores often still have plenty of available calories.

The third category of complications consists of infections of the central line that are almost never initiated at the time of

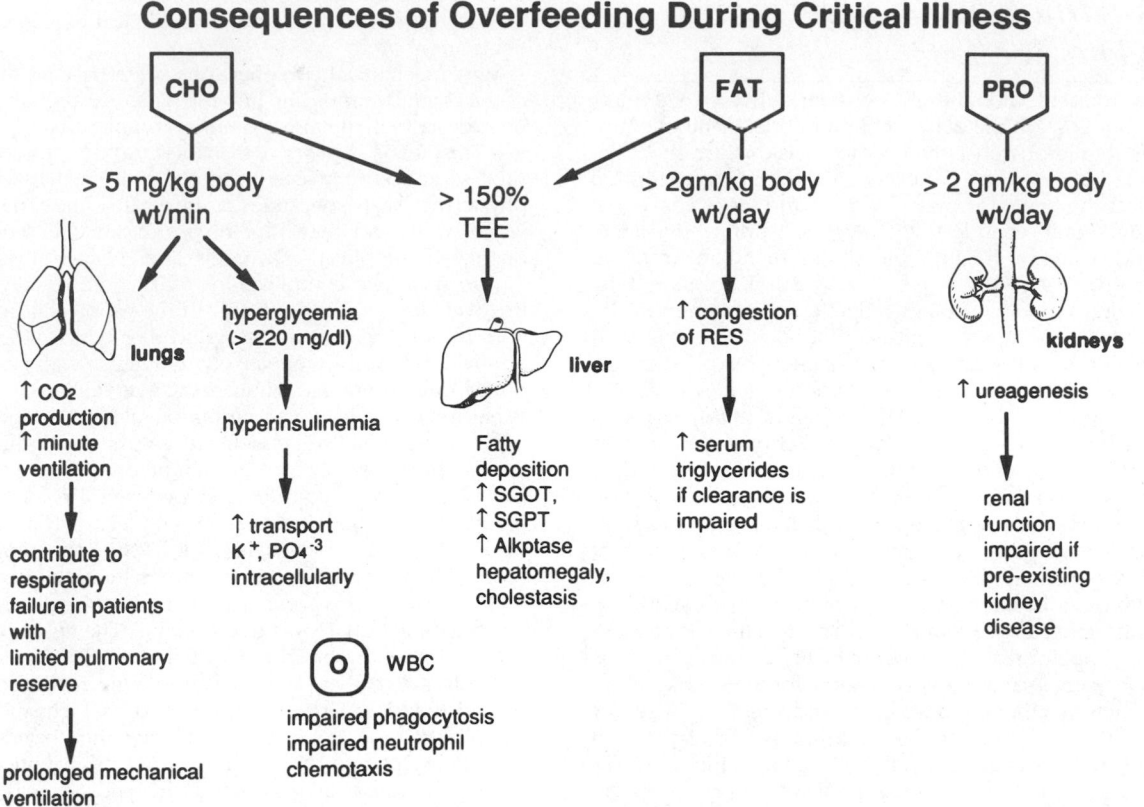

Consequences of Overfeeding During Critical Illness

Fig. 200-4. Metabolic consequences of protein-calorie overfeeding in the critically ill adult. CHO = carbohydrate; PRO = protein; TEE = total energy expenditure; RES = reticuloendothelial system; SGOT = serum glutamic oxaloacetic transaminase; SGPT = serum glutamic pyruvic transaminase; WBC = white blood cells. (From Frankel WL, Evans NJ, Rombeau JL: Scientific rational and clinical application of parenteral nutrition in critically ill patients, in Rombeau JL, Caldwell MD [eds]: *Clinical Nutrition: Parenteral Nutrition.* Philadelphia, Saunders, 1993, reproduced with permission.)

insertion of the catheter or from contamination of infusates flowing through the catheter. Although these two etiologies may have been frequent in the early developmental days of TPN, they are infrequent or nonexistent at this time. There is an inevitable level of catheter infection that will occur, but this should be minimized with protocols enforcing strict aseptic techniques. Over the years, fungi have become more prevalent as the invader, and suspicion of a fungal infection should be maintained at a high level. When a fever occurs in a patient with a temporary central line, this line can be changed over a wire and cultured and blood withdrawn through the catheter. If the patient shows clinical signs of sepsis, the catheter should be removed and not changed over a wire. If the catheter tip culture from a guidewire change becomes positive, the newly inserted replacement line needs to be removed. If the patient has a tunneled central line, bacterial infection can be eradicated one-half to two-thirds of the time with adequate antimicrobial therapy.

Proper maintenance of the central venous access is crucial to minimizing the risk of infectious complications in TPN patients. Several investigators confirm that prophylactic change of the CVC will not reduce the incidence of catheter-related infections and will increase the number of mechanical insertion complications [130,131,132]. Eyer and coworkers prospectively randomized ICU patients with triple-lumen catheters, PA catheters, or arterial catheters to one of the following groups: (1) new placement every seven days using a new site; (2) no weekly changes unless indicated by clinical situation; and (3) guidewire change using the same site every seven days [131]. They found no significant difference in catheter sepsis rate or bacteremia rate comparing all regimens. A second controlled trial in an adult ICU population assigned patients to one of four regimens: (1) catheter replacement every three days using a new site, (2) replacement by guidewire exchange every 3 days, (3) replacement when clinically indicated using a new site, or (4) guidewire change only when clinically indicated [132]. The incidence of catheter-related infections, defined per 1000 catheter days, was not significantly different between regimens.

One should view the inability to deliver the prescribed nutrients as a complication of therapy that should be assessed periodically. A multitude of factors thwart complete delivery of the prescribed nutrients. Most can be corrected with a very proactive approach and meticulous attention to detail. One must always be conscious that the efficacy of one's clinical service might be limited by how well one can deliver the energy prescribed. We reviewed 758 forced feeding days in the surgical ICU, evaluating the achievement of the calorie and protein goals; average daily mean intake was 70 to 75 percent [133]. Parenteral versus enteral route was not a factor. The main reasons for nondelivery were logistical problems (e.g., no available access, fluid restrictions, or decreased clearance through disposal systems). Interestingly, electrolyte abnormalities did not impede TPN delivery, reflecting the benefits of monitoring and writing daily TPN orders. If one can only deliver 70 percent of the prescribed energy, it makes little sense to expend considerable resources to precisely define unachievable energy goals.

Once the macronutrient quantities are defined for an individual, decisions on how to deliver the substrate need to be made. Underachievement of nutrient goals is preventable if a very aggressive approach is employed to monitoring the administration of parenteral therapies and encouraging timely intervention.

Summary

TPN remains an essential tool in critical care for those patients without a functioning accessible gastrointestinal tract. TPN can be administered safely and should be initiated early rather than late in a rational selective approach. Its contents should be minimized to a level that achieves the maximal effects without impairing the body's hepatic, renal, and respiratory disposal systems. The future holds increasing hope of disease-specific approaches with defined clinical benefits.

References

1. Mullen JL, Buzby GP, Matthews DC, et al: Reduction of operative morbidity and mortality by combined preoperative and postoperative nutritional support. *Ann Surg* 192:604, 1980.
2. Muller JM, Keller HN, Brenner U, et al: Indicators and effects of preoperative parenteral nutrition. *World J Surg* 10:53, 1986.
3. VA Cooperative Study: Perioperative total parenteral nutrition in surgical patients. *N Engl J Med* 325:525, 1991.
4. Hill GL, Witney GB, Christie PN, et al: Protein status and metabolic expenditure determine the response to intravenous nutrition—a new classification of surgical malnutrition. *Br J Surg* 78:109, 1991.
5. Kalfarentozos FE, Karavias DD, Karatzas TM, et al: Total parenteral nutrition in severe acute pancreatitis. *J Am Coll Nutr* 10:156, 1991.
6. Streat J, Beddoe AH, Hill GL: Aggressive nutritional support does not prevent protein loss despite fat gain in septic intensive care patients. *J Trauma* 27:262, 1987.
7. Shaw JHF, Wildbore M, Wolfe PR: Whole body protein kinetics in severely septic patients. *Ann Surg* 205:288, 1987.
8. Shaw JH, Wolfe RR: An integrated analysis of glucose, fat, and protein metabolism in severely traumatized patients: Studies in the basal state and the response to TPN. *Ann Surg* 209:63, 1989.
9. Zeigler TR, Young LS, Benfell K, et al: Clinical and metabolic efficacy of glutamine-supplemented parenteral nutrition after bone marrow transplantation. *Ann Intern Med* 116:821, 1992.
10. Wolfe RR, Goodenough RD, Burke JF, et al: Response of protein and urea kinetics in burn patients to different levels of protein intake. *Ann Surg* 197:163, 1983.
11. Cerra FB, Blackburn G, Hirsch et al: The effect of stress level, amino acid formula, and nitrogen dose on nitrogen retention in traumatic and septic stress. *Ann Surg* 205:282, 1987.
12. Windsor JA: Underweight patients and the risks of major surgery. *World J Surg* 17:165, 1993.
13. Shaw-Delanty SN, Elwyn DH, Askanazi J, et al: Resting energy expenditure in injured, septic, and malnourished adult patients on intravenous diets. *Clin Nutr* 9:305, 1990.
14. Keys A, Brozek J, Henschel A, et al: *The Biology of Human Starvation* (Vol I), Minneapolis, The University of Minnesota Press, 1950.
15. Kinney JM, Duke JH, Long CL, et al: Tissue fuel and weight loss after injury. *J Clin Pathology* 23(Suppl 4):65, 1970.
16. Dickerson RN, Guenter PA, Gennarelli TA, et al: Increased contribution of protein oxidation to energy expenditure in head injured patients. *J Am Coll Nutr* 9:86, 1990.
17. Bouffard YH, Delafosse BX, Annat GJ, et al: Energy expenditure during severe acute pancreatitis. *J Parenteral Enteral Nutr* 13:26, 1989.
18. Foster GD, Knox LS, Dempsey DT, et al: Caloric requirements in total parenteral nutrition. *J Am Coll Nutr* 6:231, 1987.
19. Dempsey DT, Guenter P, Mullen JL, et al: Energy expenditure in acute head trauma with and without barbiturate therapy. *Surg Gynecol Obstet* 170:128, 1985.
20. Knox LS, Crosby LO, Feurer ID, et al: Energy expenditure in malnourished cancer patients. *Ann Surg* 197:30, 1983.
21. Dempsey DT, Feurer ID, Crosby LO, et al: Energy expenditure in malnourished gastrointestinal cancer patients. *Cancer* 53:1265, 1984.
22. Dempsey DT, Knox LS, Mullen JL, et al: Energy expenditure in malnourished patients with colorectal cancer. *Arch Surg* 121:789, 1986.
23. Luketich JD, Mullen JL, Feurer ID, et al: Ablation of abnormal energy expenditure by curative tumor resection. *Arch Surg* 125:337, 1990.
24. Weissman C, Kemper M, Damask MC, et al: Effect of routine intensive care interactions on metabolic rate. *Chest* 86:815, 1984.
25. Swinamer DL, Phang PT, Jones RL: Twenty-four hour energy expenditure in critically ill patients. *Crit Care Med* 15:637, 1987.
26. Rumpler WV, Seale JL, Conway JM, et al: Repeatability of 24-hr energy expenditure measurements in humans by indirect calorimetry. *Am J Clin Nutr* 51:147, 1990.
27. Bursztein S, Saphar P, Singer P, et al: A mathematical analysis of indirect calorimetry measurements in acutely ill patients. *Am J Clin Nutr* 50:227, 1989.
28. Feurer ID, Crosby LO, Mullen JL: Measured and predicted resting energy expenditure in clinically stable patients. *Clin Nutr* 3:27, 1984.
29. Cox AR, Weiss S, Posuniak RA, et al: Energy expenditure after spinal cord injury: An evaluation of stable rehabilitating patients. *J Trauma* 25:419, 1985.
30. Blackburn GL, Bistrian BR, Maini BS, et al: Nutritional and metabolic assessment of the hospitalized patient. *J Parenteral Enteral Nutr* 1:11, 1977.
31. Bistrian BR: A simple technique to estimate the severity of stress. *Surg Gynecol Obstet* 148:675, 1979.
32. Dickerson RN, Rosato EF, Mullen JL: Net protein anabolism with hypocaloric parenteral nutrition in obese stressed patients. *Am J Clin Nutr* 44:747, 1986.
33. Frankel WL, Evans NJ, Rombeau JL: Scientific rationale and clinical application of parenteral nutrition in critically ill patients, in Rombeau JL, Caldwell MD (eds): *Clinical Nutrition: Parenteral Nutrition,* Philadelphia, WB Saunders, 1993.
34. Shaw JHF, Klein S, Wolfe RR: Assessment of alanine, urea and glucose interrelationships in normal subjects and in patients with sepsis with stable isotopic tracers. *Surgery* 97:557, 1985.
35. Wolfe BM, Culebras JM, Sim AJW, et al: Substrate interaction in intravenous feeding: Comparative effects of carbohydrate and fat on amino acid utilization in fasting man. *Ann Surg* 186:518, 1977.
36. Wolfe RR, Jahoor F, Herndon DN, et al: Isotopic evaluation of the metabolism of puruvate and related substrates in normal adult volunteers and severely burned children: Effect of dichloroacetate and glucose infusion. *Surgery* 110:54, 1991.
37. Long CL, Nelson KM, Akin JM, et al: A physiologic basis for provision of fuel mixtures in normal and stressed patients. *J Trauma* 30:1088, 1990.
38. Himms-Hagan J: Cellular thermogenesis. *Annu Rev Physiol* 38.315, 1976.
39. Askanazi J, Carpenter YA, Elwyn DH, et al: Influence of total parenteral nutrition on fuel utilization in injury and sepsis. *Ann Surg* 191:40, 1980.
40. Goodenough RD, Wolfe RR: Effect of total parenteral nutrition on free fatty acid metabolism in burned patients. *J Parenteral Enteral Nutr* 8:357, 1984.
41. Wolfe RR, Shaw JHF, Durkot MJ: Effect of sepsis on VLDL kinetics: Response in basal state and during glucose infusion. *Am J Physiol* 248:E732, 1985.
42. Nordenstrom, J, Carpentier YA, Askanazi J, et al: Free fatty acid mobilization and oxidation during total parenteral nutrition in trauma and infection. *Ann Surg* 198:725, 1983.
43. Carpentier YA, Van Gossum A, Dubois DY, et al: Lipid metabolism in parenteral nutrition, in Rombeau JL, Caldwell MD (eds): *Clinical Nutrition: Parenteral Nutrition,* Philadelphia, WB Saunders, 1993.
44. Babineau TJ, Pomposelli J, Forse RA, et al: Lipids, in Zaloga GP (ed): *Nutrition in Critical Care.* St Louis, CV Mosby, 1994.
45. Bach AC, Storck D, Meraihi Z: Medium-chain triglyceride-based

fat emulsions: An alternative energy supply in stress and sepsis. *J Parenteral Enteral Nutr* 12:82S, 1988.

46. Jiang Z-M, Zhang S-Y, Wang X-R, et al: A comparison of medium-chain and long-chain triglycerides in surgical patients. *Ann Surg* 217:175, 1993.

47. Chassard D, Guiraud M, Gauthier J, et al: Effects of intravenous medium-chain triglycerides or pulmonary gas exchanges in mechanically ventilated patients. *Crit Care Med* 22:248, 1994.

48. Palmblad J: Intravenous lipid emulsions and host defense a critical. *Clin Nutr* 10:303, 1991.

49. Huang T-L, Huang S-I, Chen M-F: Effects of intravenous fat emulsion on respiratory failure. *Chest* 97:934, 1990.

50. MacFie J, Courtney DF, Brennan TG: Continuous versus intermittent infusion of fat emulsions during total parenteral nutrition: A clinical trial. *Nutrition* 7:99, 1991.

51. Robin AP, Campbell R, Colathur K, et al: Total parenteral nutrition during acute pancreatitis: Clinical experience with 156 patients. *World J Surg* 14:572, 1990.

52. Jeejeebhoy KN, Anderson GH, Nakhooda AT, et al: Metabolic studies in total parenteral nutrition with lipid in man. *J Clin Invest* 57:125, 1976.

53. Nordenstrom J, Askanazi J, Elwyn DH, et al: Nitrogen balance during total parenteral nutrition. *Ann Surg* 187:27, 1983.

54. Shaw JHF, Holdaway CM: Protein sparing effect of substrate infusion in surgical patients is governed by the clinical state, and not by the individual substrate infused. *J Parenteral Enteral Nutr* 12:433, 1988.

55. Long JM, Long CL: Fuel Metabolism, in Zaloga GP (ed): *Nutrition in Critical Care*, St. Louis, CV Mosby, 1994.

56. Souba WW, Austgen TR: Interorgan glutamine flow following surgery and infection. *J Parenteral Enteral Nutr* 14(Supp):90, 1990.

57. Stehle P, Zander J, Mertes N, et al: Effect of parenteral glutamine peptide supplements on muscle glutamine loss and nitrogen balance after major surgery. *Lancet* 1:231, 1989.

58. Hammarqvist F, Wernerman J, Ali R, et al: Addition of glutamine to total parenteral nutrition after elective abdominal surgery spares free glutamine in muscle, counteracts the fall in muscle protein synthesis, and improves nitrogen balance. *Ann Surg* 209:455, 1989.

59. Tamanda H, Nazu R, Imamura I, et al: The dipeptide alanyl-glutamine prevents intestinal mucosal atrophy in parenterally fed rats. *J Parenteral Enteral Nutr* 16:110, 1992.

60. Van Der Hulst RWJ, Van Kreel NK, Von Meyenfeldt MF, et al: Glutamine and the preservation of gut integrity. *Lancet* 341:1363, 1993.

61. Austgen TR, Dudrick PS, Sitren H, et al: The effects of glutamine-enriched total parenteral nutrition on tumor growth and host tissues. *Ann Surg* 215:107, 1992.

62. Khan K, Hardy B, Elia M: The stability of l-glutamine in total parenteral nutrition solutions. *Clin Nutr* 10:193, 1991.

63. Lowe DK, Benfell K, Smith RJ, et al: Safety of glutamine-enriched parenteral nutrition solutions in humans. *Am J Clin Nutr* 52:1101, 1990.

64. Barbul A, Fishel RS, Shimazus, et al: Intravenous hyperalimentation with high arginine levels improves wound healing and immune function. *J Surg Res* 38:328, 1985.

65. Barbul A, Lazarou S, Efron DT, et al: Arginine enhances wound healing in humans. *Surgery* 108:331, 1990.

66. Daly J, Reynolds J, Thom A, et al: Immune and metabolic effects of arginine in the surgical patient. *Ann Surg* 208:512, 1988.

67. Barbul A, Sisto A, Wasserkrug HL, et al: Metabolic and immune effect of arginine in post-injury hyperalimentation. *J Trauma* 21:970, 1981.

68. Gonce SJ, Peck MD, Alexander JW, et al: The effect of supplemental arginine on recovery from peritonitis in guinea pigs. *J Parenteral Enteral Nutr* 14:237, 1990.

69. Saito H, Trocki O, Wang S, et al: Metabolic and immune effects of dietary arginine supplementation after burn. *Arch Surg* 122:784, 1987.

70. Multivitamin preparations for parenteral use: A statement by the Nutrition Advisory Group. *J Parenteral Enteral Nutr* 3:258, 1979.

71. Solomons NW: Trace elements, in Rombeau JL, Caldwell MD (eds): *Clinical Nutrition: Parenteral Nutrition*. Philadelphia, WB Saunders, 1993.

72. Fleming R: Trace element metabolism in adult patients requiring total parenteral nutrition. *Am J Clin Nutr* 49:573, 1989.

73. Herr DL: Trace elements, in Zaloga GP (ed): *Nutrition in Critical Care*. St Louis, CV Mosby, 1994.

74. Albina JE, Melink G: Fluids, electrolytes, and body composition, in Rombeau JL, Caldwell MD (eds): *Clinical Nutrition: Parenteral Nutrition*. Philadelphia, WB Saunders, 1993.

75. Marcuard SP, Dunham B, Hobbs, et al: Availability of insulin from total parenteral nutrition solutions. *J Parenteral Enteral Nutr* 14:262, 1990.

76. Goldman DA, Martin WT, Worthington JW: Growth of bacteria and fungi in total parenteral nutrition solutions. *Am J Surg* 126:314, 1973.

77. Rowlands DA, Wilkinson WR, Yoshimura N: Storage ability of mixed hyperalimentation solutions. *Am J Hosp Pharm* 30:436, 1973.

78. Mershon J, Nogami W, Williams JM, et al: Bacterial/fungal growth in a combined parenteral nutrition solution. *J Parenteral Enteral Nutr* 10:498, 1986.

79. D'Angio R, Quercia RA, Treiber NK, et al: The growth of microorganisms in total parenteral nutrition admixtures. *J Parenteral Enteral Nutr* 11:394, 1987.

80. Maki DG: Pathogenesis, prevention, and management of infections due to intravascular devices used for infusion therapy, in Bisno AL, Waldrogel FA (eds): *Infections Associated with Indwelling Medical Devices*. Washington, DC, American Society for Microbiology, 1989.

81. Mirtallo JM, Caryer K, Schneider PJ, et al: Growth of bacteria and fungi in parenteral nutrition solutions containing albumin. *Am J Hosp Pharm* 38:1907, 1981.

82. Melly MA, Meng HC, Schaffner W: Microbial growth in lipid emulsions used in parenteral nutrition. *Arch Surg* 110:1479, 1975.

83. Kim CH, Lewis DE, Kumar A: Bacterial and fungal growth of intravenous fat emulsions. *Am J Hosp Pharm* 40:2159, 1983.

84. Keammerer D, Mayhall CG, Hall GO, et al: Microbial growth pattern in intravenous fat emulsions. *Am J Hosp Pharm* 40:1650, 1983.

85. Crocker KS, Naga R, Filibeck DJ, et al: Microbial growth comparisons of five commercial parenteral lipid emulsions. *J Parenter Enteral Nutr* 8:391, 1984.

86. Williams WW: Infection control during parenteral nutrition therapy. *J Parenteral Enteral Nutr* 9:735, 1985.

87. Simmons BP, Holton TM, Wong ES, et al: CDC Guidelines for prevention of intravascular infections. *Infect Control* 3:52, 1982.

88. Ebbert ML, Farraj M, Hwang LT: The incidence and clinical significance of intravenous fat emulsion contamination during infusion. *J Parenteral Enteral Nutr* 11:42, 1987.

89. Gilbert M, Gallagher SC, Eads M, et al: Microbial growth patterns in total parenteral nutrition formulation containing lipid emulsion. *J Parenteral Enteral Nutr* 10:494, 1986.

90. Rowe CE, Fukuyama TT, Martinoff JT: Growth of microorganisms in total nutrient admixtures. *Drug Intell Clin Pharm* 21:633, 1987.

91. Gil RT, Kruse JA, Thaill-Baharozian MC, et al: Triple- vs single-lumen central venous catheters. *Arch Intern Med* 149:1139, 1989.

92. Lee RB, Buckner M, Sharp KW: Do multi-lumen catheters increase central venous catheter sepsis compared to single-lumen catheters? *J Trauma* 28:1472, 1988.

93. Rose SG, Pitsch RJ, Karrer FW, et al: Subclavian catheter infections. *J Parenteral Enteral Nutr* 12:511, 1986.

94. Pemberton LB, Lyman B, Lander V, et al: Sepsis from triple- vs single-lumen catheters during total parenteral nutrition in surgical or critically ill patients. *Arch Surg* 121:591, 1986.

95. Clark-Christoff N, Watters VA, Sparks W, et al: Use of triple-lumen subclavian catheters for administration of total parenteral nutrition. *J Parenteral Enteral Nutr* 16:403, 1992.

96. Schlichtig R, Ayres SM, eds: *Nutritional Support of the Critically Ill*. Chicago, Year Book Medical Publishers, 1988.

97. Horowitz HW, Dworkin DM, Savino JA, et al: Central catheter-related infections: Comparison of pulmonary artery catheters and triple lumen catheters for the delivery of hyperalimentation in a critical care setting. *J Parenteral Enteral Nutr* 14:588, 1990.

98. Maki DG: Infections due to infusion therapy, in Bennett JV, Brachman PS (eds): *Hospital Infections*. Boston, Little, Brown & Co, 1992.

99. Maki DG, Ringer M, Alvarado CJ: Prospective randomized trial of

povidone-iodine, alcohol, and chlorhexidine for prevention of infection associated with central venous and arterial catheters. *Lancet* 338:339, 1991.

100. Young GP, Alexeyeff M, Russell D, et al: Catheter sepsis during parenteral nutrition: The safety of long-term Opsite dressings. *J Parenteral Enteral Nutr* 12:365, 1988.

101. Powell C, Regan C, Fabri PJ, et al: Evaluation of Opsite dressing. *J Parenteral Enteral Nutr* 12:365, 1988.

102. Conly JM, Greives K, Peter B: A prospective, randomized study comparing transparent and dry gauze dressings for central venous catheters. *J Infect Dis* 59:310, 1989.

103. Hoffman KK, Weber DJ, Samsa GP, et al: Transparent polyurethane film as an intravenous catheter dressing: A meta-analysis of the infection risks. *JAMA* 267:2072, 1992.

104. Alvestrand A, Bergstrom J: Renal diseases, in Kinney JM, Jeejeebhoy KN, Hill GL, Owen OE (eds): *Nutrition and Metabolism in Patient Care.* Philadelphia, WB Saunders, 1988.

105. Grodstein GP, Blumenkrantz MJ, Kopple JD, et al: Glucose absorption during continuous ambulatory peritoneal dialysis. *Kidney Int* 19:564, 1981.

106. Shuler CL, Wolfson M: Nutrition in acute renal failure, in Rombeau JL, Caldwell MD (eds): *Clinical Nutrition: Parenteral Nutrition.* Phildelphia, WB Saunders, 1993.

107. Compher C, Mullen JL, Barker CF: Nutritional support in renal failure. *Surg Clin North Am* 71:597, 1991.

108. Li S: Acute renal failure, in Fischer JE (ed): *Total Parenteral Nutrition.* Boston, Little, Brown & Co, 1991, pp 191–202.

109. Hiyama DT, Fischer JE: Nutritional support in hepatic failure: The current role of disease-specific therapy, in Fischer JE (ed): *Total Parenteral Nutrition.* Boston, Little, Brown & Co, 1991.

110. O'Keefe SJD, Ogden J, Rund J: The use of ^{14}C phenylalanine to trace deranged aromatic amino acid metabolism in liver failure: A functional indicator with prognostic potential. *Gastroenterology* 96:A641, 1989.

111. O'Keefe SJD: Parenteral nutrition and liver disease, in Rombeau JL, Caldwell MD (eds): *Clinical Nutrition: Parenteral Nutrition.* Philadelphia, WB Saunders, 1993.

112. Muscaritoli M, Cangiano C, Cascino A, et al: Exogenous lipid clearance in compensated liver cirrhosis. *J Parent Enteral Nutr* 10:599, 1986.

113. Nagayama M, Takai T, Okuno M, et al: Fat emulsion in surgical patients with liver disorders. *J Surg Res* 47:59, 1989.

114. Fischer JE, Rosen HM, Ebeid AM, et al: The effect of normalization of plasma amino acids on hepatic encephalopathy in man. *Surgery* 80:77, 1976.

115. Cerra FB, Cheung NK, Fischer JE, et al: Disease-specific amino acid infusion (F080) in hepatic encephalopathy: A prospective, randomized, double-blind, controlled trial. *J Parenteral Enteral Nutr* 9:288, 1985.

116. Wahren JJ, Denis J, Desurmont P, et al: Is intravenous administra-

tion of branched chain amino acids effective in the treatment of hepatic encephalopathy? A multicenter study. *Hepatology* 4:475, 1983.

117. Michel H, Pomier-Layrogues G, Duhamel O, et al: Intravenous infusion of ordinary and modified amino acid solutions in the measurement of hepatic encephalopathy (controlled study, 30 patients). *Gastroenterology* 79:1038, 1980.

118. Naylor CD, O'Rourke K, Detsky AS, et al: Parenteral nutrition with branched chain amino acids in hepatic encephalopathy: A meta-analysis. *Gastroenterology* 97:1033, 1989.

119. Shaw BW, Wood RP, Gordon RD, et al: Influence of selected patient variables and operative blood loss on 6 month survival following liver transplantation. *Semin Liver Dig* 5:385, 1985.

120. Delafosse JL, Faure Y, Boufferd JP, et al: Liver transplantation-energy expenditure, nitrogen loss and substrate oxidation rate in the first two postoperative days. *Transplant Proc* 21:2453, 1989.

121. O'Keefe SJD, William R: "Catabolic" loss of body protein after human liver transplantation. *BMJ* 280:1107, 1980.

122. Reilley J, Metha R, Teperman L, et al: Nutritional support after liver transplantation: A randomized prospective study. *J Parenteral Enteral Nutr* 14:386, 1990.

123. Arora NS, Rochester DF: Effect of body weight and muscularity on human diaphragm muscle mass, thickness and area. *J Appl Physiol* 52:64, 1982.

124. Lewis MI, Sieck GC: Effect of acute nutritional deprivation on diaphragm structure and function. *J Appl Physiol* 68:1933, 1990.

125. Gaare JM, Manner T, Wiese S, et al: Nutrition in pulmonary diseases, in Rombeau JL, Caldwell MD (eds): *Clinical Nutrition: Parenteral Nutrition.* Philadelphia, WB Saunders, 1993.

126. Kelly SM, Rosa A, Field S, et al: Inspiratory muscle strength and body composition in patients receiving total parenteral nutrition therapy. *Am Rev Respir Dis* 130:33, 1984.

127. Compher CW, Mullen JL: Parenteral caloric supply and CO_2 production. *Clin Nutr* 9:29, 1990.

128. Talpers SS, Romberger DJ, Bunce SB, et al: Nutritionally associated increased carbon dioxide production. Excess total calories vs high protein of carbohydrate calories. *Chest* 102:551, 1992.

129. Elwyn DH, Gump PE, Munro HN, et al: Changes in nitrogen balance of depleted patients with increasing infusions of glucose. *Am J Clin Nutr* 32:1597, 1979.

130. Powell C, Kudsk KA, Kulich PA, et al: Effect of frequent guide wire changes on triple-lumen catheter sepsis. *N Engl J Med* 12:464, 1988.

131. Fyer S, Brummit C, Crossley K, et al: Catheter-related sepsis: Prospective, randomized study of three methods of long-term catheter maintenance. *Crit Care Med* 18:1810, 1990.

132. Cobb K, High KP, Sawyer G, et al: A controlled trial of scheduled replacement of central venous and pulmonary-artery catheters. *J Parenteral Enteral Nutr* 327:10628, 1992.

133. Evans NJ, Sorouri BB, Feurer ID: Constraints of nutrient supply in the intensive care unit. *J Parenteral Enteral Nutr* 15:34S, 1991.

201. Enteral Nutrition

William T. Adamson and
John L. Rombeau

The critically ill patient presents complex nutritional and metabolic challenges to the critical care team. The demands of the stressed state create hypermetabolic imbalances that can lead to an adverse clinical outcome. When these stresses become overwhelming, a progressive catabolic cascade culminates in the systemic inflammatory response syndrome. Recent investigations of the critically ill patient have significantly increased understanding of the hemodynamic, septic, inflammatory, and other components of this multisystem response [1,2]. Moreover, these studies demonstrate that therapy directed toward restoring homeostasis improves the success in caring for these patients. Integral to reestablishing homeostasis is the arrest of catabolism and the provision of specific nutrient fuels to potentiate anabolism.

As discussed in previous chapters, nutrient requirements are greatly increased for the intensive care unit (ICU) patient. To meet these increased needs, the critically ill patient is force-fed by several routes. While parenteral nutrition can provide a balanced nutrient supply to help correct nitrogen losses and reverse catabolism, simply replenishing the nutrients does not fully replace gut function. With increasing understanding of the importance of the endocrine and immune systems in critical illness, it has become evident that the gut performs greater and more complex functions than simply digesting and absorbing nutrients. For example, impairment of the barrier function of the gut has been proposed as a central factor in the development of sepsis in the severely ill patients who go on to develop systemic inflammatory response syndrome (SIRS) [3]. Restoring gut function with enteral nutrition helps reestablish immune competence and may reduce sepsis due to disrupted gut barrier function [4,5]. Thus, enteral nutrition offers several therapeutic advantages to the critically ill patient. Moreover, multiple centers have shown in prospective, randomized, controlled clinical trials that enteral feeding is safe and efficacious in the critically ill patient [6,7]. This chapter discusses the rationale, delivery, and formulation of enteral nutrition in the critically ill patient.

The Catabolic State: Hypermetabolism in the Critically Ill

The critically ill patient faces multiple metabolic stresses, which place markedly increased energy demands on an already compromised system. A global acceleration of metabolism occurs in patients recovering from major trauma, major surgery, burns, and other critical illness. After injury, the body's response to illness undergoes an initial metabolic dormancy and then accelerates, reaching a hypermetabolic peak at approximately 72 to 96 hours after onset of stress [8]. This catabolic response is characterized by increased oxygen consumption and carbon dioxide production, increased cardiac output, decreased systemic vascular resistance, and an overall increase in resting energy expenditure. Increased metabolic demand leads to a catabolic state wherein energy stores are mobilized to provide the glucose and other fuels needed to mount the stress response. Normal amino acid metabolism is greatly altered. Approximately 30 percent of energy needs are met by the breakdown of amino acids, primarily mobilized from skeletal muscle [8]. Metabolically, this protein breakdown is exemplified by net increases in urea nitrogen [9]. In the liver, altered hepatic metabolism generates needed glucose to meet increased demands and produces a net buildup of less useful aromatic amino acids and toxins [10]. Branched-chain amino acids, which are associated with enhanced nitrogen retention and restoration of muscle mass, are reduced in serum due to enhanced oxidation in peripheral tissues [11]. Provision of exogenous nutrients meets these increased needs and helps reverse catabolism.

Nutritional support, including parenteral and enteral feeding, is a mandatory component of the critical care plan. Aggressive nutritional support with standard diets alone, however, does not prevent proteolysis of skeletal muscle in the severely ill [12,13,14]. Specific fuels such as glutamine and branched-chain amino acids may be required to blunt the catabolic process and help restore metabolic balance [11,15].

Increased energy needs are only part of the stress response. Upregulation of metabolism in the stressed patient is at least partly regulated by hormonal and inflammatory mediators. Inadequate insulin levels and elevated glucagon, glucocorticoids, and catecholamines generate glucose at the expense of nitro-

gen stores [16]. Hyperglycemia and glucose resistance follow [17]. The hypothalamic-pituitary axis is stimulated in response to illness and injury [18]. Growth hormone, perhaps through insulin-like growth factor 1, augments insulin response to glucose mobilization and use of fat stores and improves nitrogen balance during both normal and hypocaloric dietary intakes [19–22]. Critically ill surgical patients given growth hormone in a randomized trial significantly improved uptake of amino acids and maintained lean body mass [23]. Growth hormone also enhances wound healing [24].

In addition to altered hormonal response, multiple inflammatory mediators including cytokines such as TN-F, IL-1, IL-2, IL-6, and IL-8 promote hypermetabolism [25]. Restoration of a normal milieu of these hormonal and other regulators would seem to complement a provision of nutrients to support the catabolic patient.

Systemic Inflammatory Response Syndrome

Critical illness can progress to SIRS with its concomitant mortality of 35 percent [2]. A predictable cascade of pulmonary failure with infection followed by hepatic and renal failure, metabolic imbalance, gastrointestinal bleeding, and sepsis characterizes this overwhelming process. Alterations of the immune system are intrinsic to this systemic response and appear to be mediated through multiple inflammatory cytokines including interleukins, prostaglandins, catecholamines, and oxygen radicals [25,26]. Additionally, the endogenous inflammatory response can provoke a cytotoxic neutrophil response causing tissue injury, which may progress to necrosis, sepsis, and organ failure [27].

The gut has been proposed as a primary contributor to sepsis seen in SIRS. In critical illness, the gut undergoes characteristic changes in villous structure and barrier function. This is discussed in the following section.

THE GUT IN CRITICAL ILLNESS. The gastrointestinal tract undergoes characteristic changes during critical illness, including disruptions of motility, villous architecture, and nutrient processing. Paralytic ileus often occurs, impeding normal motility and nutrient delivery to the villi [28]. Starvation models in animals predict the gut function seen in critically ill patients. Levels of insulin, a primary anabolic hormone, are decreased. Glycogenolysis and gluconeogenesis produce increased levels of hepatic glucose. Lipolysis with mobilization of free fatty acids from adipose tissue and catabolic breakdown of skeletal muscle provide necessary energy sources [29].

Starvation alters the structural integrity of the gut. Atrophy is manifested by decreased villous height, crypt cell depth, and cellular mass in the absence of enteral nutrition [30,31]. Normal cellular migration patterns from crypt to villi are disrupted and retarded. Starvation decreases mitotic indices in the mucosa and depresses the rate of cell differentiation [32].

Starvation induces specific changes at the luminal interface as well. Brush border activity is generally decreased. In early stages of starvation, elevated levels of aminopeptidases and lactase are detected within the brush border as the gut attempts to conserve protein [33]. Maintenance and regulation of the brush border are dependent on nutrient delivery. Direct contact with nutrient fuels is vital to villous integrity. Nutrient provision by parenteral nutrition alone does not reverse starvation-induced changes in villous height, cellular mass, and brush border activity [30].

Nutrient processing is also altered in starvation. Carrier-mediated transport of amino acids within the cells is disrupted. Vitamin absorption is decreased, chylomicron transport is depressed, and fatty acid uptake is altered, resulting in steatorrhea. Similarly, the carbohydrate malabsorption that is often present is compounded by a lack of disaccharidases and other glucose transport proteins [32].

Specific fuels are trophic for the enterocytes within the gut. Glutamine, in preference to glucose or ketone bodies, is the primary oxidizable fuel source for small bowel enterocytes [34,35]. Circulating levels of glutamine, the most abundant free amino acid in healthy patients, are markedly decreased in stressed patients [12]. Glutamine supports fibroblasts and other rapidly proliferating tissue [36]. Additionally, glutamine serves as an energy source for immunologically active tissue through oxidation, providing carbon and nitrogen precursors for biosynthetic processes that may be upregulated in stressed patients [15]. In postoperative patients, glutamine increases skeletal muscle ribosomes [37]. Short-chain fatty acids (SCFA) are a primary fuel for the colonocytes. When administered enterally or parenterally, SCFAs maintain mucosal mass and DNA content [38,39]. The provision of specialized fuels may improve clinical outcome in the critically ill patient.

BARRIER FUNCTION.

In addition to processing enteral nutrients, the gut also provides vital barrier function against enteric pathogens. Enteric bacteria translocated across the gut barrier are thought to contribute to sepsis and damage to peripheral organs by provoking an inflammatory immune response. Damage to mucosa may provide a route of entry for enteric organisms. Histologically, stress-induced mucosal lesions progress downward from the apices of the villi, even separating the epithelium from the lamina propria [40]. Local hypoxia is thought to correlate with exfoliation by increasing mucosal permeability and decreasing mucus production [41]. Endotoxin produced by enteric bacteria and transmigrated into mesenteric tissues may mediate this response. Animals given lethal doses of bacterial toxin have disruption of intracellular tight junctions [42].

Translocation of bacteria from within the gut lumen into mesenteric tissues is associated with decreased immune competence and increased bacterial load in mesenteric and systemic tissues [43]. Macrophage secretion of cytokines is increased and neutrophil proteases stimulate tissue oxidation [44,45]. Widespread use of antibiotics in the ICU kills normal enteric flora, allowing bacterial overgrowth by potential pathogens. Bacterial overgrowth has been implicated in gut dysfunction and can be measured clinically by monitoring breath H_2 levels, urine lactulose, and fecal alpha-1-antitrypsin.

In protein-deficient burn patients, translocated bacteria are associated with significant morbidity [43]. A prospective study of burn patients with ICU-acquired infection found that 30 of 33 patients concomitantly cultured the same pathogen from the upper gastrointestinal tract [3,46]. This concurrence of isolation of a clinically significant pathogen with gut colonization correlated with increased mortality.

Studies defining a mechanism for bacterial translocation have been equivocal. In an animal model combining burn injury with partial mesenteric ischemia, bacteria cultured from mesenteric lymph nodes correlated with bacteria cultured from the gastrointestinal lumen 24 hours previously [47]. A randomized sampling of portal blood in trauma patients for 5 days post-injury failed to culture clinical pathogens, despite the later development of multiple organ failure in 30 percent of these patients.

It is concluded that the relationship between compromised gut integrity and translocation of enteric bacteria in the evolution of systemic inflammatory response syndrome is unclear.

RATIONALE FOR ENTERAL NUTRITION.

Restoring intestinal integrity and preserving barrier functions of the gut, then, provide a rationale for prescribing enteral nutrition early in critical illness. Enteral nutrition reduces gut atrophy in animal models of stress. Enteral nutrition improves gut structure by maintaining mucosal mass [48]. Animals given balanced oral nutrition had increased gut weight and mucosal thickness, higher epithelial cell proliferation and DNA content, increased mucosal protein levels, and greater disaccharidase activity [49]. Direct contact with nutrients preserves enteral growth and the ability of rapidly dividing enteric tissue to undergo trophic adaptation after bowel resection [50,51,52]. In an animal model of bacterial peritonitis, enteral repletion of malnourished animals enhanced survival over animals repleted parenterally [53]. Feedings correct the pH balance of the gut and help to reduce bacterial overgrowth [53]. Enteral feedings significantly reduce the incidence of gastrointestinal bleeding in ICU patients [54]. Early feeding enhances motility by minimizing the delay in gastric emptying often seen in these patients [8].

Multiple randomized trials report that early enteral feeding administered by tube into the gastrointestinal tract is safe, efficacious, cost-effective, and associated with improved outcome [4,6,7,55,56,57]. Immediate enteral feeding of burn patients was associated with decreased gut atrophy, decreased resting energy expenditure, and decreased catabolic hormone production [58,59]. Compared with similar patients who received adequate nutrition parenterally, these patients lost less weight and had improved nitrogen balance. An increased balance of constitutive proteins versus acute-phase proteins was noted in enterally fed patients [60].

Maintenance of mucosal integrity and function with enteral nutrition directly correlates with improved outcome in the critically ill. Early enteral feeding in major trauma patients resulted in fewer septic complications compared to total parenteral nutrition (TPN) alone [6]. Some of the changes within the gut in critical illness and the potential changes from nutrition are described in Figure 201-1. A meta-analysis of published series of trauma and blunt trauma patients noted a reduction of sepsis in 18 to 35 percent of patients [7]. In summary, enteral nutrition provides the nutrients to enhance recovery and avoid catabolism while maintaining gut structural and functional competence and avoiding the complications associated with gut atrophy.

Enteral Delivery

ASSESSMENT.

While the role for enteral nutrition in the most severely ill trauma patients is well defined, not all patients require forced enteral feeding. Selection of patients to receive nutritional supplementation is based on premorbid nutritional status, the expected duration of illness, and the severity of injury. Assessment of nutritional status is discussed in detail in Chapter 200.

A patient's premorbid nutritional status should be determined. History and physical examination of the patient provide height and weight indices as well as a baseline control for that patient. Patients with weight loss of 10 percent or more of usual body weight are arbitrarily defined as severely malnourished and should receive nutritional support. Serum levels of albu-

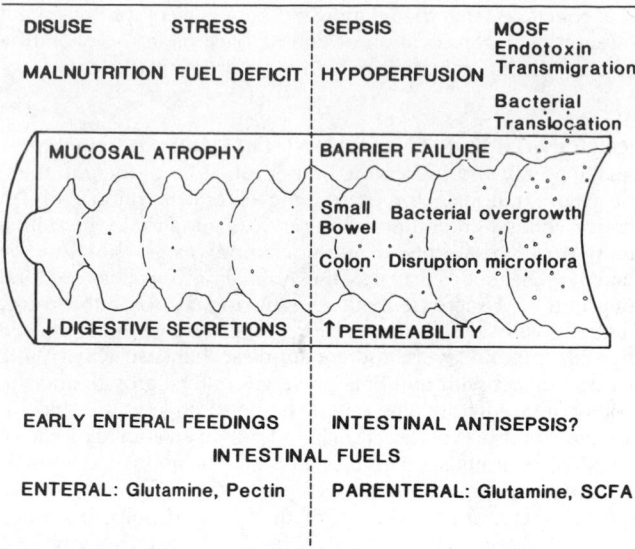

Fig. 201-1. Schematic representation of changes within the gastrointestinal tract in response to critical illness and possible sites of benefit of nutrition. (From Rolandelli RH, Rombeau JL: Enteral nutrition in critically ill patients. *Perspect Crit Care* 2:1, 1989.)

Table 201-1. Indications for Enteral Nutrition in Critically Ill Patients

Hypermetabolism
  Trauma
  Burns
  Sepsis
  Following major surgery
  Preoperative malnutrition
Gastrointestinal disease
  Esophageal obstruction
  Mild or resolving pancreatitis
  Pancreaticobiliary surgery
  Major upper gastrointestinal surgery
  Inflammatory bowel disease
  Short bowel syndrome
  Fistula—low output
Organ system failure
  Prolonged ventilatory dependence
  Cardiac cachexia
  Closed head injury
  Head and neck surgery
  Renal insufficiency
  Hepatic failure

Modified from Rolandelli RH, Koruda MJ, Guenter P, et al: Enteral nutrition: Advantages, limitations, and formula selection. *J Crit Illness* 3(10):93, 1988.

min, transferrin, prealbumin, retinol-binding protein, and other serum transport proteins have been included in nutritional assessment [61,62]. Only serum albumin has been proved to have predictive value. Serum albumin levels of less than 2.5 gm per deciliter correctly identified 93 percent of survivors of critical illness [62]. Estimates of nitrogen balance reflect the degree of protein catabolism. The creatinine-height index estimates the severity of protein depletion in hospitalized patients [63]. Nitrogen excretion over 24 hours can be measured directly. 3-Methyl histidine, a by-product of the catabolism of skeletal muscle, can also be measured but requires normal renal function. A handgrip test to measure adductor pollicis fatigue can monitor muscle strength [64,65].

This clinical assessment can be used to determine which patients are appropriate for forced feeding. The American Society of Parenteral and Enteral Nutrition (ASPEN) has established guidelines for initiating forced feedings [66]. Enteral or parenteral forced feeding should be administered in severely malnourished patients who have not eaten for 1 to 3 days or in previously well-nourished or mildly malnourished patients who have not eaten for 5 to 7 days. Additionally, those patients not expecting to eat for 7 to 10 days or anticipating a prolonged inability to eat will benefit from forced feedings. A subset of patients preparing to undergo major surgery will benefit from preoperative nutritional supplementation. Preoperative TPN correlated with a reduction in major complications in those patients who were severely malnourished prior to undergoing major surgery [67].

Table 201-1 lists some of the indications for enteral nutrition in patients in whom it would be efficacious. In the critical care setting, enteral nutrition is particularly useful in those patients who are obtunded or paralyzed. Patients recovering from neurologic injury and sedated ventilator-dependent patients should receive post-pyloric enteral feeding. Patients with proximal gastrointestinal obstruction, including nasopharyngeal or esophageal disorders, are also ideal candidates for enteral feeding. Enteral nutrition is particularly useful in patients susceptible to stress gastritis, such as burn patients.

Some patients are not candidates for enteral feeding. Restoration of gut function with enteral feedings is not possible in hemodynamically unstable patients. Priority must be given to optimization of cardiopulmonary function, tissue oxygenation, and acid-base and electrolyte balances. For example, care of ventilator-dependent patients must include concern for the potential increase in carbon dioxide production that may accompany enteral feeding. Absolute contraindications to enteral feedings include distal intestinal obstruction or new distal gastrointestinal anastomosis, massive upper gastrointestinal bleeding, intestinal ischemia, and high gastric output. Vomiting and/or increased risk of aspiration of gastrointestinal contents precludes gastric feeding in some patients. Diarrhea, greater than three loose stools per day, is a relative contraindication to enteral feeding. Table 201-2 lists some of the contraindications to enteral feeding.

ACCESS. Once a decision has been made to give enteral nutrition, access to the gastrointestinal tract must be established. Delivery of enteral formulas is most often through Silastic or similar flexible tubes. Several decisions must be considered when placing a feeding tube. Tubes are placed in either gastric or post-pyloric, most often jejunal, position. Feedings are given

Table 201-2. Contraindications to Enteral Feeding

Absolute contraindications
  Severe enteritis or peritonitis
  Distal gastrointestinal obstruction
  Severe diarrhea
  Upper gastrointestinal bleeding
  Severe pancreatitis
Relative contraindications
  Ileus
  Vomiting
  High risk of aspiration pneumonia
  Enterocutaneous fistula (>500 ml/day)

by bolus into the stomach or continuously into the small intestine. Tube placement is performed either at the bedside or in the operating room or endoscopy suite. Each of these options has advantages and disadvantages that must be tailored to the individual patient.

Gastric feedings most fully reestablish the normal enteral pathway. Nasogastric tubes are easily placed at the bedside and are inexpensive. Feeding is given by bolus, with frequent monitoring of the gastric residual. Risk of aspiration is greatest in patients fed via nasogastric tube versus other routes, although clinical significance of this risk has been debated. Incidence of aspiration with nasogastric feedings has been documented as high as 95 percent, with one-third of these associated with morbidity [68]. Other studies have shown that nasogastric feedings can be given safely if the head of the patient's bed is elevated at a 30-degree angle and if residuals are frequently checked [69]. If residuals are large (150 to 200 ml) gastric feedings should be discontinued. Gastroparesis is common in critically ill patients and may preclude gastric feedings.

Since nasogastric tubes are frequently dislodged and are uncomfortable for the patient, a permanent gastric feeding route can be established through a tube placed directly into the stomach. Gastric tubes offer an ideal route for the awake, alert patient who tolerates intermittent bolus feeds. Percutaneous endoscopic placement of gastric tubes can be placed in cooperative patients under local anesthesia, as depicted in Figure 201-2. Patients must be able to tolerate upper gastrointestinal endoscopy. Risk of injury to neighboring organs, including transverse colon, is small but real. Gastric tubes are also placed operatively, but this requires a general anesthetic in most cases.

Tubes placed into the jejunum offer several advantages for the critically ill patient. Ileus from operation or illness in the small bowel often resolves more quickly than gastroparesis, so patients can be fed earlier into the jejunum [70]. Feedings are given as a continuous infusion. Continuous feeds require an infusion pump and supervision but offer better nutrient utilization and patient tolerance. Jejunal feeds are associated with decreased stool frequency, an important consideration in these patients for whom diarrhea can be a major problem [71]. One study documented a higher percentage of daily nutrient goal delivered, a greater increase in serum prealbumin levels, and a lower incidence of pneumonia in patients who were fed in the jejunum as opposed to the stomach [72].

Nasojejunal tubes are placed at the bedside, with passage of the tube through the nasopharynx past the pylorus into the proximal jejunum. Success rates of this procedure range from 15 to 61 percent, with greatest success in patients given metoclopramide and monitored with serial radiographs [69,73]. Nasoenteric tubes are uncomfortable and frequently dislodged; therefore, patients requiring forced feeding for greater than 1 month should receive a permanent tube. Jejunostomy can be established directly by operative placement of a tube into a loop of jejunum secured to the anterior abdominal wall. A gastrostomy can be converted to a gastrojejunostomy by distal placement of the tube in the small intestine under fluoroscopic or endoscopic guidance. Newer methods of jejunostomy placement through laparoscopy and endoscopy offer potentially less invasive access than traditional laparotomy.

Enteral Formulas

CALCULATION OF NUTRIENT NEEDS. Once enteral access has been gained, the specific nutrient needs of the patient are determined. Multiple formulas are commercially available to meet specific patient requirements. Careful consideration of the patient's nutritional status as well as his or her protein calorie and carbohydrate calorie needs will help select the appropriate formula.

As a first approximation, basal nonprotein caloric need is roughly 20 to 25 kcal/kg/day in the resting volunteer [74]. A normal adult may need approximately 0.4 gm of N_2/kg/day and up to 2 gm N_2/kg/day to maintain positive nitrogen balance. A useful value for basal energy expenditure can be derived from the Harris-Benedict equation (discussed in Chapter 200), which predicts nonprotein caloric requirements based on weight, height, gender, and age of the patient [75]. This estimate of basal energy expenditure (BEE) can then be adjusted for the patient's illness state. For example, malnourished patients may need 135 percent of BEE to avoid catabolism. Severe injury may require 130 percent of BEE, while the catabolic states of sepsis and burn injury may demand 160 percent and 200 percent, respectively. Protein needs in critical illness are similarly increased. Once a formulation has been ordered, frequent monitoring is required to ensure that the ordered formulation is being delivered fully and that desired clinical goals are met.

AVAILABLE FORMULAS. Enteral formulas exist in two general categories: balanced (polymeric) and modified. Formulas are generally isotonic and lactose-free. Balanced, polymeric formulas provide a natural protein source, usually soy or egg, and include a mixture of simple and complex carbohydrates, which require some digestion by the gut. Balanced formulas provide 100 percent of RDA and are the least expensive category of formula. Modified or elemental formulas are composed of crystalline amino acids or oligopeptides and medium-chain triglycerides rather than long-chain triglycerides. These simple molecules require minimal digestion and provide low residue in the colon. Modified diets, however, are hyperosmolar and more expensive than balanced polymeric diets.

Most formulas contain 1 calorie per milliliter, but concentra-

Fig. 201-2. Placement of gastric feeding tube via endoscopically guided percutaneous method. Needle placement of wire is performed under direct endoscopic vision, then feeding tube is pulled through in direction of arrow. (From Rombeau JL, Rolandelli RH, Wilmore DW: Nutritional support. Care of the Surgical Patient, Section II, Subsection 10. © 1988 Scientific American, Inc. All rights reserved.)

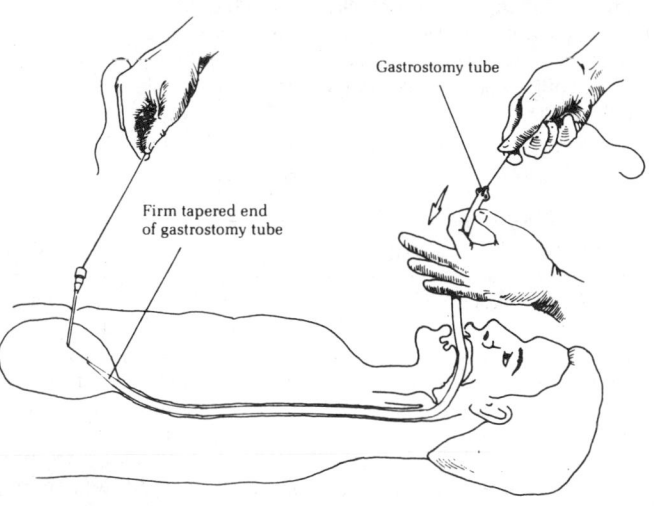

Gastrostomy tube

Firm tapered end
of gastrostomy tube

tions of 0.6 kcal per milliliter, 1.5 kcal per milliliter, and 2 kcal per milliliter are available. Protein is usually provided in a ratio of 1 gm of nitrogen (1 gm $N_2 = 6.25$ gm of protein) for every 150 nonprotein calories. In recognition of the increased protein needs in the critically ill, formulas modified for stress provide protein in a ratio of 1:80 or 1:100 gm N_2 per kilocalorie (nonprotein). These formulas are hyperosmolar and expensive. A protein supplement can be added to standard formulation as powder or liquid. Some stress formulas also provide specific amino acids, which are thought to be most needed in hypermetabolism. Branched-chain amino acids (BCAA) are catabolized from skeletal muscle under hormonal control in response to stress. Balanced formulas deliver approximately 25 to 30 percent of protein as BCAA. Some stress formulas deliver 44 to 50 percent of amino acids as BCAA based on the rationale that provision of exogenous BCAA will arrest muscle breakdown. Formulas enriched with BCAA enhance nitrogen retention, visceral protein mass, and indices of survival [11,76].

Simple sugars and lipids provide the source of nonprotein calories. While glucose is the body's primary fuel source, the addition of lipid more completely serves the body's broad range of metabolic needs. Lipid has a lower oxygen content than does glucose for a given amount of calories and thus, when metabolized, produces less carbon dioxide [77,78]. Lower CO_2 production may be clinically important in patients with pulmonary compromise [79,80]. While incorporation of lipid into the diet may reduce net CO_2 production, increasing lipid content in enteral feeds has the metabolic cost of increased diarrhea. Lipid utilization has been shown to be increased in trauma patients [81].

Lipids are also important in the inflammatory response. Omega-3 fatty acids, primarily eicosapentaenoic acid found in fish oil, are structured lipids that replace and avoid the immune suppression of omega-6 fatty acids, found in balanced diets [82,83]. Omega-6 fatty acids are precursors in the inflammatory cascade that produce toxic cytokines PGE_2 and PGI_2 [84,85]. Processing of omega-3 fatty acids, however, provides biologically less inflammatory cytokine competitors to PGE_2. Omega-3 fatty acids stimulate the gut immune system and help maintain mucosal integrity [5] and are efficacious in burn patients [86,87].

Lipid is provided primarily as long-chain triglycerides (LCTs) in balanced formulas. Some studies using a higher proportion of LCTs have failed to show a benefit in stressed animals [88,89]. LCTs are processed intracellularly via a carnitine-dependent transport into mitochondria. Carnitine may be limited in stress states [90]. Medium-chain triglycerides (MCTs), which enter mitochondria by passive diffusion, have been advocated by some investigators as a more easily utilized fuel than LCTs. MCT emulsions were more efficacious over a standard LCT formula in one burn model [91].

Lipid building blocks, the short-chain fatty acids (SCFAs), appear to play a fundamental role in gut metabolism. SCFAs, primarily butyrate, are the primary fuel source of colonocytes and are associated with enhanced colonic proliferation, mucosal blood flow, and mucosal growth [38,92]. SCFAs are generated from the colonic fermentation of dietary polysaccharides, which are provided primarily as dietary fiber and undigested starch. In experimental models of colitis, one source of fiber, fruit pectin, has been associated with a decreased degree of bowel injury in rats [93,94].

Recent work has focused on the addition of specific amino acids to nutrient formulations. As discussed earlier, glutamine serves as a primary fuel source for the gut [34,95]. The addition of glutamine to parenteral nutrition is associated with decreased gut atrophy and stimulation of brush border activity [96]. Given to catabolic critical care patients, glutamine improves nitrogen balance and counteracts the decrease in muscle protein synthesis by sparing glutamine stores in skeletal muscle [97].

Arginine enhances recovery of nitrogen balance and weight loss in malnourished and post-traumatic animals [98,99]. Addition of arginine to nutrient formulas is associated with increased survival in septic animals and is postulated to exert an immune-enhancing effect through stimulation of the hormonal response to stress [100,101,102]. Both glutamine and arginine are now components of some commercially available enteral formulas. Other specialty formulas are available in renal and hepatic failure. These are discussed in other chapters.

Complications of Enteral Nutrition

Approximately 10 to 15 percent of patients encounter some complication that disrupts enteral feeding [103]. Most problems are easily recognized and corrected. Mechanical problems can occur from the tube leaking or becoming clogged. Patients may suffer from excoriation of the skin by acidic gastrointestinal contents at the tube exit site. Diarrhea is by far the most frequent gastrointestinal complication, accounting for significant morbidity in 10 to 20 percent of patients [104]. Diarrhea can be defined as greater than 600 ml of stool per day [28] or more than three large stools in a day [8]. If adjustment of the feeding schedule or formula composition does not eliminate this problem, kaolin-pectin can be given [105]. Bacteria cultured from enteral feeding bags have been implicated as a contributor to diarrhea in these patients [106–109].

Delayed gastric emptying, vomiting, and gastrointestinal bleeding have also been attributed to enteral nutrition in a few patients. In general, the presence of food in the gut lumen is protective of intestinal mucosa and facilitates gastric emptying by restoring gut competence. Nausea and vomiting occur in 10 to 20 percent of patients on enteral feeds [104]. Formula odor, fat content, lactose, high osmolarity, and delayed gastric emptying are thought to contribute to this problem.

By far the most serious complication of enteral nutrition is aspiration pneumonia, which occurs in 1 to 44 percent of patients on enteral feeding [68,103,110,111]. Patients receiving gastric feedings are particularly at risk. Keeping the head of the patient's bed elevated 30 degrees, frequently checking the gastric residuals, and keeping endotracheal tube cuffs inflated can help reduce this risk [110]. With the exception of the risk of aspiration pneumonia, the risks of enteral feedings are minimal. In many patients, enteral feedings avoid the complications from providing nutrition by the parenteral route. In particular, line sepsis can be avoided in patients fed enterally. Some of the complications of enteral and parenteral feedings are compared in Table 201-3.

Clinical Trials

Findings from recent clinical trials of enterally fed patients have confirmed current understanding of the benefits of enteral feeding on gut atrophy, immunocompetence, and nitrogen balance observed in stress models. The value of postinjury nutritional support was demonstrated in 75 consecutive trauma patients who were given either no supplemental nutrition or fed elemental diets via jejunostomy during the first 5 days [6]. Enterally fed patients improved nitrogen balance and had fewer septic complications than controls.

Table 201-3. Complications of Enteral Feeding

Infectious
  Aspiration pneumonia
Gastrointestinal
  Diarrhea
  Delayed gastric emptying
  Nausea and vomiting
  Gastrointestinal bleeding
Mechanical problems
  Obstruction
  Tube leakage
  Tube clogging
  Excoriation of skin at tube exit site

Enteral feeding has also compared favorably with parenteral feeding of critically ill patients. Forty-six multiple trauma patients who underwent laparotomy were randomized to central venous parenteral nutrition or enteral nutrition by jejunostomy [55]. No differences were found in injury severity, estimated caloric needs, average daily caloric intake, nitrogen balance, and complication rates. A similar randomized, prospective study in 20 patients undergoing major upper gastrointestinal or pancreaticobiliary surgery demonstrated adequate nutritional support in both enterally and parenterally fed groups [56].

Septic complications were examined in a series of 75 patients who underwent laparotomy to feeding via parenteral catheter or by jejunostomy [4]. Caloric and nitrogen delivery and nitrogen balance were equivalent in both groups. Traditional serum protein markers were improved in the enteral group. Septic morbidity in the parenteral group (20%) was much higher than in the enteral group (3%). These results were reinforced in another study of 98 patients randomized to enteral or parenteral nutrition at laparotomy for trauma [57]. Significantly lower septic morbidity was seen in blunt and penetrating trauma patients fed enterally. Another study depicted in Figure 201-3 demonstrated a lower incidence of sepsis in enterally fed patients as duration of ICU days increased.

Fig. 201-3. Enteral nutrition and sepsis. Duration of ICU stay is associated with a lower incidence of sepsis in enterally fed patients. (Data from Border JR, Hassett J, LaDuca J, et al: The gut origin septic states in blunt multiple trauma (ISS = 40) in the ICU. *Ann Surg* 206(4):427, 1987.)

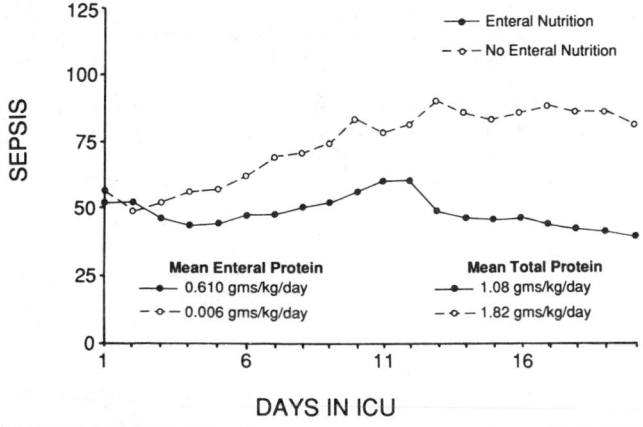

ENTERAL NUTRITION AND SEPSIS

A meta-analysis of eight prospective, randomized trials in 194 high-risk surgical patients compared early enteral feeding (within 48 hours postoperative) to parenteral feeding [7]. Both groups demonstrated improved nutritional markers, although baseline and final nitrogen intake, nitrogen balance, and net weight gain were significantly lower in the enteral group. Enterally fed patients also experienced greater abdominal discomfort and diarrhea. Complications, however, both septic and nonseptic, were significantly lower in enterally fed groups. Even with exclusion of catheter sepsis, a significant reduction in the rate of septic complications was still seen in the enterally fed patients. These differences were particularly noted in blunt trauma patients. Enteral nutrition is not indicated in all critically ill patients; however, clinical and experimental data now confirm that early enteral nutrition is safe and efficacious and has profound effects on patient nutritional indices and rate of complications.

Future Directions

A role for enteral nutrition in the critical care setting is now clear. Investigations on the interaction of specific nutrients with the digestive, immune, and other organ systems in the critical care setting will further define this role. The interplay between nutrition and hormonal mediators of the stress response, such as the growth factors, with enteral feeding is now opening exciting areas for further clinical applications. Glutamine- and arginine-enriched formulas are just two examples of the type of nutritional modulation that will be seen as our understanding of the role of the gut in critical illness unfolds. Enteral nutrition will continue to be an important adjuvant therapy in the critical care setting.

References

1. Carrico CJ: The elusive pathophysiology of multiple organ failure syndrome. *Ann Surg* 218(2):109, 1993.
2. Carrico CJ, Meakins JM, Marshall JC, et al: Multiple-organ-failure syndrome. *Arch Surg* 121:196, 1986.
3. Marshall JC, Christou NV, Meakins JL: The gastrointestinal tract: The "undrained abscess" of multiple organ failure. *Ann Surg* 218(2):111, 1993.
4. Moore FA, Moore EE, Jones TN, et al: TEN versus TPN following major abdominal trauma—reduced septic morbidity. *J Trauma* 29(7):916, 1989.
5. McClave SA, Lowen CC, Snider HL: Immunonutrition and enteral hyperalimentation of critically ill patients. *Dig Dis Sci* 37:1153, 1992.
6. Moore EE, Jones TN: Benefits of immediate jejunostomy feeding after major abdominal trauma—a prospective, randomized study. *J Trauma* 26(10):874, 1986.
7. Moore FA, Feliciano DV, Andrassy RJ, et al: Early enteral feeding, compared with parenteral, reduces postoperative septic complications, the results of a meta-analysis. *Ann Surg* 216(2):172, 1992.
8. Bower RH: Nutritional and metabolic support of critically ill patients. *J Parenter Enter Nutr* 14(5):257S, 1990.
9. Cuthbertson DP: Observations on disturbance of metabolism produced by injury to limbs. *Q J Med* 25:233, 1932.
10. Gump FE, Long CL, Killian P, et al: Studies of glucose intolerance in septic injured patients. *J Trauma* 14:378, 1974.
11. Cerra FB, Shronts EP, Konstantinides NN, et al: Enteral feeding in sepsis: A prospective, randomized, double-blind trial. *Surgery* 98(4):632, 1985.
12. Wilmore DW: Catabolic illness: Strategies for enhancing recovery. *N Engl J Med* 325:695, 1991.

13. Loder PB, Smith RC, Kee AJ, et al: What rate of infusion of intravenous nutrition solution is required to stimulate uptake of amino acids by peripheral tissues in depleted patients? *Ann Surg* 211:360, 1990.

14. Kinney JM, Elwyn DH: Protein metabolism in the traumatized patient. *Acta Chir Scand Suppl* 522:45, 1985.

15. Newsholme EA, Newsholme P, Curi R, et al: A role for muscle in the immune system and its importance in surgery, trauma, sepsis, and burns. *Nutrition* 4:261, 1988.

16. Baracos V, Rodemann HP, Dinarello CA: Stimulation of muscle protein degradation and prostaglandin E2 release by leukocytic pyrogen (interleukin-1). *N Engl J Med* 308:553, 1983.

17. Inamura M, Clowes GH, Blackburn G: Liver metabolism and gluconeogenesis in trauma and sepsis. *Surgery* 77:868, 1975.

18. Wilmore DW: Hormonal responses and their effects on metabolism. *Surg Clin North Am* 56:999, 1976.

19. Manson JM, Wilmore DW: Positive nitrogen balance with human growth hormone and hypocaloric intravenous feedings. *Surgery* 100:188, 1986.

20. Ziegler TR, Young LS, Manson JM, et al: Metabolic effects of recombinant human growth hormone in patients receiving parenteral nutrition. *Ann Surg* 208:6, 1988.

21. Clemmons DR, Snyder DK, Williams R, et al: Growth hormone administration conserves lean body mass during dietary restriction in obese subjects. *J Clin Endocrinol Metab* 64:878, 1987.

22. Ziegler TR, Young LS, Ferrari-Baliviera E, et al: Use of human growth hormone combined with nutritional support in a critical care unit. *J Parenter Enter Nutr* 14:574, 1990.

23. Weir JB deV: New methods for calculating metabolic rate with special reference to protein metabolism. *J Physiol* 109:1, 1949.

24. Wilmore DW: *The Metabolic Management of the Critically Ill.* New York, Plenum, 1977.

25. Tracey KJ, Vlassara H, Cerami A: Cachectin/tumour necrosis factor. *Lancet* 1:1122, 1989.

26. Fry DE: Multiple system organ failure. *Surg Clin North Am* 68(1):107, 1988.

27. Anderson BO, Harken AH: Multiple organ failure: Inflammatory priming and activation sequences promote autologous tissue injury. *J Trauma* 30(12):S44, 1990.

28. Koruda MJ, Guenter P, Rombeau JL: Enteral nutrition in the critically ill. *Crit Care Clin* 3(1):133, 1987.

29. Baker JP, Lemoyne M: Nutritional support in the critically ill patient: If, when, how, and what. *Crit Care Clin* 3(1):97, 1987.

30. Wilmore D, Smith R, O'Dwyer S, et al: The gut: A central organ in sepsis. *Surgery* 104:917, 1988.

31. Altmann GG: Influence of starvation and refeeding on mucosal size and epithelial renewal in the rat small intestine. *Am J Anat* 133:391, 1972.

32. Brunser O: Effects of malnutrition on intestinal structure and function in children. *Clin Gastroenterol* 6:341, 1977.

33. Raul F, Noriega R, Doffoel M, et al: Modifications of brush border enzyme activities during starvation in the jejunum and ileum of adult rats. *Enzyme* 28:328, 1982.

34. Windmueller HG: Glutamine utilization by the small intestine. *Adv Enzymol Relat Areas Mol Biol* 53:201, 1982.

35. Ardawi MSM, Newsholme EA: Fuel utilization in colonocytes of the rat. *Biochem J* 231:713, 1985.

36. Caldwell MD: Local glutamine metabolism in wounds and inflammation. *Metabolism* 38(Suppl 1):34, 1989.

37. Hammarqvist F, Wernerman J, Ali R, et al: Addition of glutamine to total parenteral nutrition after elective abdominal surgery spared free glutamine in muscle, counteracts the fall in muscle protein synthesis, and improves nitrogen balance. *Ann Surg* 209:455, 1989.

38. Sakata T: Stimulatory effect of short chain fatty acids on epithelial proliferation in the rat intestine: A possible explanation for trophic effects of fermentable fibre, gut microbes and luminal trophic factors. *Br J Nutr* 58:95, 1987.

39. Roediger WEW: Utilization of nutrients by isolated epithelial cells of the rat colon. *Gastroenterology* 83:424, 1982.

40. Saadia R, Schein M, MacFarlane C, et al: Gut barrier function and the surgeon. *Br J Surg* 77:487, 1990.

41. Jones WG, Minei JP, Barber AE, et al: Splanchnic vasoconstriction and bacterial translocation after thermal injury. *Am J Physiol* 261:H1190, 1991.

42. Dietch EA, Berg R, Specian R: Endotoxin promotes the translocation of bacteria from the gut. *Arch Surg* 122:185, 1987.

43. Deitch EA: Bacterial translocation of the gut flora. *J Trauma* 30:S184, 1992.

44. Dietch EA: Multiple organ failure: Pathophysiology and potential future therapy. *Ann Surg* 216:117, 1992.

45. Zhi-Yong S, Yuan-Lin D, Xiao-Hong W: Bacterial translocation and multiple system organ failure in bowel ischemia and reperfusion. *J Trauma* 32:148, 1992.

46. Marshall JC, Christou NV, Horn R, et al: The microbiology of multiple organ failure: The proximal gastrointestinal tract as an occult reservoir of pathogens. *Arch Surg* 123:309, 1988.

47. Saydjari R, Beerthuizen GIJM, Townsend C, et al: Bacterial translocation and its relationship to visceral blood flow, gut mucosal ornithine decarboxylase activity, and DNA in pigs. *J Trauma* 31(5):639, 1991.

48. Lowry SF: The route of feeding influences injury responses. *J Trauma* 30:S10, 1990.

49. Levine GM, Deren JJ, Steiger ET, et al: Role of oral intake in maintenance of gut mass and disaccharide activity. *Gastroenterology* 67:975, 1974.

50. Feldman EJ, Dowling RH, et al: Effects of oral versus intravenous nutrition on intestinal adaptation after small bowel resection in the dog. *Gastroenterology* 70:712, 1976.

51. Reinken EO, Menge H: Nutritive effects of food constituents on the structure and function of the intestine. *Acta Hepatogastroenterol* 24:388, 1977.

52. Ryan GP, Dudrick SJ, et al: Effects of various diets on colonic growth in rats. *Gastroenterology* 77:658, 1979.

53. Petersen SR, Kudsk KA, Carpentier G, et al: Malnutrition and immunocompetence: Increased mortality following an infectious challenge during hyperalimentation. *J Trauma* 21:528, 1984.

54. Pingleton SK, Hadzima SK: Enteral alimentation and gastrointestinal bleeding in mechanically ventilated patients. *Crit Care Med* 11(1):13, 1983.

55. Adams S, Dellinger EP, Wertz MJ, et al: Enteral versus parenteral nutritional support following laparotomy for trauma: A randomized prospective trial. *J Trauma* 26(10):882, 1986.

56. Bower RH, Talamini MA, Sax HC, et al: Postoperative enteral vs parenteral nutrition: A randomized controlled trial. *Arch Surg* 121:1040, 1986.

57. Kudsk KA, Croce MA, Fabian TC, et al: Enteral *vs.* parenteral feeding: Effects on septic morbidity after blunt and penetrating abdominal trauma. *Ann Surg* 215(5):503, 1992.

58. Mochizucki H, Trocki O, Dominioni L, et al: Mechanism of prevention of postburn hypermetabolism and catabolism by early enteral feeding. *Ann Surg* 200:297, 1984.

59. Saito H, Trocki O, Alexander JW, et al: The effect of route of nutrient administration on the nutritional state, catabolic hormone secretion, and gut mucosal integrity after burn injury. *J Parenter Enter Nutr* 11:1, 1987.

60. Moore EE, Moore FA: Immediate enteral nutrition following multisystem trauma: A decade perspective. *J Am Coll Nutr* 10(6):633, 1991.

61. Foley EF, Borlase BC, Dzik WH, et al: Albumin supplementation in the critically ill: A prospective, randomized trial. *Arch Surg* 125:739, 1990.

62. Apelgren KN, Rombeau JL, Twomey PL, et al: Comparison of nutritional indices and outcome in critically ill patients. *Crit Care Med* 10(5):305, 1982.

63. Bistrian BR, Blackburn GL, Sherman M, et al: Therapeutic index of nutritional depletion in hospitalized patients. *Surg Gynecol Obstet* 141:512, 1975.

64. Merton PA: Voluntary strength and fatigue. *J Physiol* 123:533, 1954.

65. Edwards RHT: Physiological analysis of skeletal muscle weakness and fatigue. *Clin Sci Mol Med* 54:463, 1978.

66. American Society for Parenteral and Enteral Nutrition Board of Directors: Guidelines for use of parenteral and enteral nutrition in the adult and pediatric patients. *J Parenter Enter Nutr* 17(4):8SA, 1993.

67. The Veterans Affairs Total Parenteral Nutrition Cooperative Study Group: Perioperative total parenteral nutrition in surgical patients. *N Engl J Med* 325(8):525, 1991.

68. Winterbauer RH, Durning RB, Barron E, et al: Aspirated nasogastric

feeding solution detected by glucose strips. *Ann Intern Med* 95:67, 1981.

69. Marian M, Rappaport W, Cunningham D, et al: The failure of conventional methods to promote spontaneous transpyloric feeding tube passage and the safety of intragastric feeding in the critically ill ventilated patient. *Surg Gynecol Obstet* 176:475, 1993.

70. Rothie NG, Harper RAK, Catchpole BN: Early postoperative gastrointestinal activity. *Lancet* 2:64, 1963.

71. Moore FA, Moore EE, Poggetti R, et al: Gut bacterial translocation via the portal vein: A clinical perspective with major torso trauma. *J Trauma* 31(5):629, 1991.

72. Montecalvo MA, Steger KA, Farber HW, et al: Nutritional outcome and pneumonia in critical care patients randomized to gastric versus jejunal tube feedings. *Crit Care Med* 20(10):1377, 1992.

73. Grant JP, Curtas MS, Kelvin FM: Fluoroscopic placement of nasojejunal feeding tubes with immediate feeding using a nonelemental diet. *J Parenter Enter Nutr* 7:299, 1983.

74. Borlase BC, Babineau TJ, Forse RA, et al: Enteral nutrition support, in Rippe et al (eds): *Intensive Care Medicine*. Boston, Little, Brown & Co, 1991.

75. Van Way CW: Variability of the Harris-Benedict equation in recently published textbooks. *J Parenter Enter Nutr* 16(6):566, 1992.

76. Cerra FB, Upson D, Angelico R, et al: Branched chain amino acids support postoperative protein synthesis. *Surgery* 92:192, 1982.

77. Askanazi J, Carpenter VA, Elwyn DH, et al: Influence of total parenteral nutrition of fuel utilization in injury and sepsis. *Ann Surg* 191:40, 1980.

78. Askanazi J, Elwyn DH, Silverberg PA, et al: Respiratory distress secondary to a high carbohydrate load of TPN: A case report. *Surgery* 87:596, 1980.

79. Collins JP, Oxby CB, Hill GL: Intravenous amino acids and intravenous hyperalimentation as protein sparing therapy after major surgery. A controlled clinical trial. *Lancet* 1:788, 1978.

80. Larca L, Greenbaum DM: Effectiveness of intensive nutritional regimens in patients who fail to wean from mechanical ventilation. *Crit Care Med* 10:297, 1982.

81. Oparo O, Burch W, Akwari OE: Enhancement of endocrine pancreatic secretions by essential fatty acids. *J Surg Res* 48:329, 1990.

82. Gottschlich M, Alexander J: Fat kinetics and recommended dietary intake in burns. *J Parenter Enter Nutr* 11:80, 1987.

83. Heird W, Grundy S, Hubbard V: Structured lipids and their use in clinical nutrition. *Am J Clin Nutr* 43:320, 1986.

84. Endres S, Ghorbani R, Kelley VE, et al: The effect of dietary supplementation with W-3 polyunsaturated fatty acids on the synthesis of interleukin-1 and tumor necrosis factor by mononuclear cells. *N Engl J Med* 320:265, 1989.

85. Lee TH, Hoover RL, Williams JD, et al: Effect of dietary enrichment with eicosapentaenoic and docohexanenoic acids on in vitro neutrophil and monocyte leukotriene generation and neutrophil function. *N Engl J Med* 312:1217, 1985.

86. Alexander JW, Saito H, Trocki O, et al: The importance of lipid type in the diet after burn injury. *Ann Surg* 204:1, 1986.

87. Mochizuki H, Trocki O, Dominioni L, et al: Optimal lipid content for enteral diets following thermal injury. *J Parenter Enter Nutr* 8:638, 1984.

88. Nordenstrom JA, Carpentier YA, Askanazi JH, et al: Free fatty acid mobilization and oxidation during total parenteral nutrition in trauma and infection. *Ann Surg* 198:725, 1983.

89. Stein TP, Fried RC, Leskiw MJ, et al: The effect of calorie source (glucose, LCT, MCT) on protein metabolism in septic rat. *Am J Physiol* 250:E312, 1986.

90. Fritz IB: The role of acylcarnitine esters and carnitine palmityltransferase in the transport of fatty acyl groups across mitochondrial membranes. *Proc Natl Acad Sci (USA)* 54:1226, 1965.

91. Mok KT, Maiz A, Yamazaki A, et al: Structured medium- and long-chain triglyceride emulsions are superior to physical mixtures in sparing body protein in the burned rat. *Metabolism* 33:901, 1984.

92. Sakata T, Yajima T: Influence of short chain fatty acids on the epithelial cell division of the digestive tract. *Q J Exp Physiol* 69:639, 1984.

93. Rolandelli RH, Saul SH, Settle RG, et al: Comparison of parenteral nutrition and enteral feeding with pectin in experimental colitis in the rat. *Am J Clin Nutr* 47:715, 1988.

94. Koruda MJ, Rolandelli RH, Settle RG, et al: Small bowel disaccharidase activity in the rat as affected by intestinal resection and pectin feeding. *Am J Clin Nutr* 47:448, 1988.

95. Souba WW, Herskowitz K, Austgen TR, et al: Glutamine nutrition: Theoretical considerations and therapeutic impact. *J Parenter Enter Nutr* 14: 237S, 1990.

96. Grant J, Snyder PJ: Use of L-glutamine in total parenteral nutrition. *J Surg Res* 44:506, 1988.

97. Stehle P, Zander J, Mertes N, et al: Effect of parenteral glutamine peptide supplements on muscle glutamine loss and nitrogen balance after major surgery. *Lancet* 1(8632):231, 1989.

98. Steffee CH, Wissler RW, Humphreys EM, et al: Studies in amino acid utilization. V: The determination of minimum daily essential amino acid requirements in protein depleted adult male albino rats. *J Nutr* 40:483, 1950.

99. Chyun JH, Griminger P: Improvement of nitrogen retention by arginine and glycine supplementation and its relation to collagen synthesis in traumatized mature and aged rats. *J Nutr* 144:1687, 1984.

100. Madden HP, Breslin RJ, Wasserkrug HL, et al: Stimulation of T cell immunity enhances survival in peritonitis. *J Surg Res* 44:658, 1988.

101. Saito H, Trocki O, Wang S, et al: Metabolic and immune effects of dietary arginine supplementation after burn. *Arch Surg* 122:784, 1987.

102. Daly JM, Lieberman MD, Goldfine J, et al: Enteral nutrition with supplemental arginine, RNA, and omega-3 fatty acids in patients after operation: Immunologic, metabolic, and clinical outcome. *Surgery* 112(1):56, 1992.

103. Cataldi-Belcher EL, Seltzer MH, Slocum BA, et al: Complications occurring during enteral nutrition support: A prospective study. *J Parenter Enter Nutr* 7:546, 1983.

104. Heymsfield SB, Bethel RA, Ansley JD, et al: Enteral hyperalimentation: An alternative to central venous hyperalimentation. *Ann Intern Med* 90:63, 1979.

105. Jones BJM, Payne S, Silk DBA: Indications for pump-assisted enteral feeding. *Lancet* 1:1057, 1980.

106. Hosteller C, Lipman TO, Geraghty M, et al: Bacterial safety of reconstituted continuous drip tube feeding. *J Parenter Enter Nutr* 6:232, 1982.

107. Scheimer RL, Fitzer H, Gfell MA, et al: Environmental contamination of continuous drip feedings. *Pediatrics* 63:232, 1979.

108. Schroeder P, Fisher D, Volz M, et al: Microbial contamination of enteral feeding solutions in a community. *J Parenter Enter Nutr* 7:364, 1983.

109. White WT, Acuff TE, Sykes TR, et al: Bacterial contamination of enteral nutrient solution: A preliminary report. *J Parenter Enter Nutr* 3:459, 1979.

110. Taylor T: Comparison of two methods of nasogastric tube feeding. *Neurol Nurs* 14:49, 1982.

111. Toews A, de la Rocha AG, et al: Oropharyngeal sepsis with endothoracic spread. *Can J Surg* 23:265, 1980.

202. Disease-Specific Nutrition

Todd W. Mattox, Judy Fish, and
Eva P. Shronts

The benefits of specialized nutrition support in patients unable to consume adequate nutrients by mouth have been well documented. While patients with stable, uncomplicated malnutrition appear to respond well to parenteral or enteral nutrition, the data are less clear in critically ill patients with mild or moderate malnutrition [1]. Technologic advances over the past two decades have facilitated intense study of critically ill patients and the metabolic consequences associated with injury or underlying disease states. This body of information has fueled a marked growth in the number of commercially available parenteral and enteral products designed for use in patients with specific metabolic abnormalities and nutrient requirements. A clear understanding of the biochemical and physiologic basis for development of these formulas is necessary for appropriate evaluation of the scientific literature and subsequent clinical application in patients. This chapter reviews parenteral and enteral formulas designed for use in patients with specific organ dysfunction and metabolic stress. The rationale and clinical role of these solutions are discussed as well.

"Standard" versus "Disease-Specific" Nutrition Regimens

Disease-specific nutrition regimens differ from "standard" regimens in several aspects. Standard total parenteral nutrition (TPN) regimens are generally composed of dextrose; a standard crystalline amino acid solution containing a balanced profile of essential, semiessential, and nonessential L-amino acids; and, in some instances, lipid emulsion. Appropriate electrolytes and recommended daily allowances of vitamins and trace elements are also added. Standard formulas for enteral nutrition support (ENS) are usually lactose-free and contain carbohydrate, protein, and fat in a high molecular form that requires normal absorption and digestion. These formulas usually provide carbohydrate as glucose oligosaccharides, protein as lactalbumin, casein or whey, and fat as long-chain triglycerides (LCTs) from corn, soy, safflower, sunflower, or canola oils. Some formulas may contain a combination of LCTs and medium-chain triglycerides (MCTs). These formulas provide recommended daily allowances of both macronutrients and micronutrients and are generally intended for use in non–critically ill patients with a relatively normal absorptive and digestive capacity. Some may be used as an oral supplement. These formulas are isosmolar to moderately hyperosmolar.

Both parenteral and enteral regimens designed for use in altered medical conditions differ from conventional or standard regimens by specific modifications in the type or concentrations of both micronutrients and macronutrients. Sources of carbohydrate, protein, and fat tend to be similar for TPN and enteral formulas, respectively, although concentrations of each nutrient may be altered to better meet demands caused by metabolic abnormalities. For example, disease-specific TPN regimens usually differ in the dose of protein infused, or the profile of the amino acid solution may be modified to meet altered amino acid requirements. In addition, carbohydrate and fat concentra-

tions may be altered to modify the non–protein calorie-to-nitrogen ratio (NPC:N). Disease-specific enteral formulas may provide protein in a simpler, hydrolyzed form such as smaller peptide fragments or free amino acids. Some products may contain combinations of larger proteins and hydrolyzed proteins. Fat is usually provided as LCTs and MCTs or as combinations of omega-6 and omega-3 fatty acids. Specialty parenteral amino acid solutions used for disease-specific TPN and enteral formulas tend to be more expensive than their standard counterparts. In general, the rationale for the use and clinical role of disease-specific regimens is controversial.

Hypermetabolism

Critically ill patients present with a wide spectrum of metabolic abnormalities that change as an individual patient's medical condition changes. The characteristic metabolic alterations that accompany the response to injury or infection have been well described in a variety of patients [2–6]. In general, patients frequently demonstrate a measured energy expenditure that is greater than predicted during metabolic stress states such as major surgery, trauma, sepsis, and burns [2]. Other metabolic changes in carbohydrate, fat, and protein substrates not normally seen in simple starvation have been described in patients with metabolic stress. Increased glucocorticoid and glucagon levels stimulate gluconeogenesis at the expense of lean body tissue, predominantly skeletal muscle. Protein synthesis is increased although the rate of catabolism is accelerated [7]. This net protein loss is manifested by large urinary nitrogen losses and low serum visceral protein concentrations. Ineffective peripheral utilization of glucose occurs, manifested by elevated plasma glucose despite normal or elevated levels of insulin [8]. Fatty acids are increasingly utilized for fuel. The degree of these abnormalities is directly proportional to the extent of injury [4]. Multiple investigations have studied the biochemical basis for these metabolic derangements in an attempt to facilitate provision of more efficiently utilized nutrient substrates and to prevent further metabolic complications associated with nutrition support.

Many studies have focused on altered protein metabolism. Investigations in critically ill patients have demonstrated decreased plasma levels of the branched-chain amino acids (BCAAs) leucine, isoleucine, and valine, presumably due to their preferential utilization for energy [9]. This phenomenon has been hypothesized to occur in septic patients because of a peripheral energy deficit of unknown etiology, which promotes BCAA consumption by skeletal muscle for energy production [10]. However, this theory has been challenged [11]. Other studies have investigated the use of alternative energy fuels, such as glycerol and MCTs. Glycerol is oxidized independently of insulin, and MCTs are more readily absorbed from the gastrointestinal tract [12,13]. MCTs also do not require carnitine for oxidation and are more rapidly cleared when given intravenously. More recent investigations suggest that the etiology of these metabolic abnormalities is associated with an inflammatory response that is caused by a complex series of interactions

Table 202-1. Hypermetabolism Amino Acid Product Comparison

	Branch Amin 4%[a] (Clintec Nutrition Co.)	Branch Amin 4%[b] with Travasol 10% (Clintec Nutrition)	FreAmine HBC (McGaw Labs)	Aminosyn HBC (Abbott Labs)
Protein concentration	4%	7%	6.9%	7%
Nitrogen (gm/100 ml)	.44	1.05	.97	1.12
Essential amino acids (mg/100 ml)				
Histidine	-	240	160	154
Isoleucine	1380	990	760	789
Leucine	1380	1055	1370	1576
Lysine	-	290	410	265
Methionine	-	200	250	206
Phenylalanine	-	280	320	228
Threonine	-	210	200	272
Tryptophan	-	90	90	88
Valine	1240	910	880	789
Nonessential amino acids (mg/100 ml)				
Alanine	-	1035	400	660
Arginine	-	240	580	507
Proline	-	340	630	448
Serine	-	250	330	221
Tyrosine	-	515	330	660
Glycine	-	20	-	33
Electrolytes (mEq/L)				
Sodium	-	-	10	7
Chloride	-	40	<3	≤40
Acetate	-	-	57	72
Amino acid composition	100% BCAA[c] 100% EAA	42% BCAA 61% EAA	45% BCAA 66% EAA	46% BCAA 63% EAA

[a] Provides increased BCAA when added to a standard amino acid solution.
[b] 1:1 ratio BranchAmin to Travasol 10%.
[c] BCAA, branched chain amino acid; EAA, essential amino acid.

between hormones, cytokines, and lipid mediators [6]. Several nutrient substrates have been investigated for their potential as a more efficiently utilized fuel and for their ability to modulate the inflammatory response [14,15].

PARENTERAL AND ENTERAL FORMULATIONS. Parenteral formulations designed for use in hypermetabolic patients are generally restricted to the type of amino acids provided and manipulation of the NPC:N, using LCT-based lipid emulsion and dextrose. Specialty amino acid solutions marketed for use in patients with severe metabolic stress are listed in Table 202-1. The products contain essential, semiessential, and nonessential amino acids with higher concentrations of BCAAs. These solutions are available as a premixed solution or as an additive solution of 100 percent BCAAs, which is mixed with a standard amino acid solution. Other parenteral amino acid modifications currently under investigation include high-dose arginine and glutamine. Arginine is provided in currently available standard amino acid products in amounts lower than doses that have demonstrated immunomodulating properties [15]. Because glutamine has limited solubility and stability in solution, it is not available in standard amino acid solutions. However, it is available as a supplement to standard amino acid solutions or an essential amino acid solution usually marketed for use in renal failure. Glutamine must be added to the TPN solution as a separate additive at the time of compounding.

A variety of enteral products have been introduced for use in patients with metabolic stress (Table 202-2). In general, these products are nutritionally complete formulas with a low NPC:N. Enteral formulas designed for use in hypermetabolic patients contain high concentrations of BCAAs. While both standard formulas and other formulas targeted for use in critically ill patients usually contain 15 to 20 percent of BCAAs, BCAA-enriched formulas should generally contain greater than 40 percent of BCAAs. Because of the limited stability of these formulas, BCAA-enriched enteral products are available in powder form and must be reconstituted prior to use. Other unique enteral formulas have been introduced for use in critically ill patients. Elemental formulas (Table 202-3) containing free amino acids and peptide-containing formulas were developed for use in patients with marginally functioning gastrointestinal (GI) tracts. Elemental formulas contain very little fat and therefore provide a large percentage of total calories as carbohydrate. This may contribute to the development of essential fatty acid deficiency and difficult blood glucose control in critically ill patients. Peptide-based formulas (Table 202-3) provide protein as small-molecular-weight peptides or a mixture of peptides and free amino acids. Most peptide-based formulas contain fat as a mixture of LCTs and MCTs. Fiber has also been added to several formulas. The most recent formulas introduced for use in hypermetabolic patients are solutions containing glutamine, arginine, omega-3 fatty acids, and nucleotides, as single agents or in combination.

CLINICAL STUDIES. Multiple investigations of parenteral and enteral products have been conducted in an effort to define the therapeutic effectiveness and clinical role of solutions designed for use in critically ill patients. BCAA solutions have received considerable attention in the past. Many clinical investigations have been performed to evaluate the effectiveness of high BCAA solutions as compared to standard amino acid solutions, and most have utilized parenteral nutrition. Early studies of high

Table 202-2. High Nitrogen Enteral Formula Product Comparison

	Protein						Fat				Carbohydrate	
	gm/1000 kcal	% kcal	Sources	Glutamine (gm/1000 kcal)/(H)	Arginine (gm/1000 kcal)	% BCAA protein	gm/1000 kcal	% kcal	Sources n-6:n-3	gm/1000 kcal	% kcal
Alitraq (A)	52.5	21	Soy and lactalbumin hydrolysates, whey, free amino acids	14.2	4.5	18.2	15.5	13	MCT, Safflower oil 4.29:1	164	66
Immun-Aid (G)	80	32	Lactalbumin, free amino acids	9	14	20	22	20	Canola: MCT 1:1	120	48
Perative (B)	51.23	20.5	Partially hydrolyzed sodium caseinate, lactalbumin hydrolysate, L-arginine	0	6.19	8.0	28.76	25	Canola, MCT, corn oils 4.8:1	136.3	54.5
Stresstein (F)	58	23	Free amino acids	0	4	44	23	21	MCT, soybean oil 7.2:1	142	56
Vivonex Plus (F)	45	18	Free amino acids	10	6.2	30	6.7	6	Soybean oil 7:1	190	76
Crucial (A)	62.6	25	Hydrolyzed casein	4.8	10	17.6	45	39	MCT, Fish oil, soy oil, lecithin 2:1	90	36
Impact (F) or Impact w/guar	56	22	Sodium and calcium caseinates, L-arginine	0	12.5	17.1	28	25	Structured lipid from palm kernel oil and sunflower menhaden oil. 1.3:1	132	53
Protain XL (C)	55	22	Sodium and calcium caseinates	0	1.76	21	30	27	MCT, corn oil 27.9:1	138	51
TraumaCal (E)	55	22	Calcium and sodium caseinates	0	2.2	23	45	40	Soy oil, MCT 6.2:1	95	38
Isotein HN (F)	57	23	Lactalbumin	5	1.6	22	29	25	Partially hydrogenated, soybean oil, MCT, 31.5:1	133	52
Nitrolan (D)	60	19.1	Sodium and calcium caseinates	0	0	12.3	32	29	Corn oil, MCT 27:1	129	52
Promote (A)	62.4	25	Sodium and calcium caseinates, soy protein isolates	0	2.4	20.23	26	23	Safflower oil, Canola oil, MCT oil 6.8:1	133	52
Replete (A) unflavored	62.5	25	Casein	5.6	2.4	16	34	30	Canola oil, MCT 3:1	113	45
Sustacal (E)	61	24	Casein, soy	0	2.6	21	23	21	Partially hydrogenated corn oil, 20.5:1	140	55

BCAA parenteral nutrition solutions in small numbers of catabolic patients have reported improvements in nitrogen retention, visceral protein status, measurements of immune function, and normalization of plasma amino acid profiles [16,17]. However, these results have not been reproduced in other investigations [18,19]. Results of larger trials disagree as well. A randomized, double-blind, multicenter study of postsurgical patients at varying levels of stress reported better nitrogen retention as measured by nitrogen balance in patients receiving TPN regimens, including high BCAA formulas [20]. Thirty-four patients were randomized to receive a TPN regimen of standard amino acids and glucose in a fixed ratio of 114 glucose calories per gram of nitrogen. Fifty-three patients received the same regimen except the amino acid source contained a final concentration of 50 percent of BCAA. No lipid emulsion was given to either group during the 7-day study period. Both regimens were isocaloric and isonitrogenous. The authors confirmed the findings of an earlier investigation with a similar study design. They reported a proportionate response to the dose of high BCAA protein administered and the extent of nitrogen retention [21]. The effect was also proportional to the level of metabolic stress. The authors did not report effects on morbidity or mortality. In a clinical trial of similar design, Okada et al. studied

173 patients who underwent either total or subtotal gastrectomy for 7 days [22]. Data were reported for 163 patients, and patient data were stratified according to type of surgery. Forty total gastrectomy patients and 39 subtotal gastrectomy patients received a TPN regimen containing standard amino acids (26% BCAAs) providing 40 kcal/kg/day and 1.5 gm/kg/day protein by day 2 after initiating nutrition support. Forty total gastrectomy patients and 41 subtotal gastrectomy patients received the same regimen, although the amino acid source provided 36 percent BCAAs. The authors reported no significant difference in cumulative nitrogen balance, cumulative urinary 3-methylhistidine excretion, or concentrations of visceral protein markers (total protein, albumin, retinol-binding protein, prealbumin, and transferrin) between treatment groups in either the total or subtotal gastrectomy subsets. The authors reported no morbidity or mortality results. Von Meyenfeldt et al. conducted a prospective randomized, double-blind controlled study of 101 septic and traumatized patients for 7 days [23]. Fifty-two patients received a TPN regimen containing standard amino acids (15.6% BCAAs) with non–protein calories provided as glucose and lipid emulsion. Forty-nine patients received a similar regimen; however, the amino acid source provided 50.2 percent BCAAs. Both patient groups received approximately 30 to 35

Sources	NPC:N	Calorie density (kcal/ml)	Fiber (gm)	Ultra Trace Elements	Cartinine (gm)	Taurine (gm)	Per 1000 kcal Vitamin A β-carotene (mg)	Vitamin C (mg)	Zinc (mg)	Nucleic acids
Sucrose, fructose, hydrolyzed corn starch	94:1	1.0	0	Yes	.1	.2	3998 IU Vitamin A	200	17.7	0
Malto dexins	53:1	1.0	0	Yes	.1	.2	2665 IU	60	25	1.0
Hydrolyzed corn starch	97:1	1.3	0	Yes	.10	.10	6666 IU	200	15	0
Hydrolyzed corn starch	97:1	1.21	0	Yes	0	0	2100 IU	25	6.3	0
Maltodextrin modified starch	115:1	1.0	0	Yes	.200	.100	4170 IU	62	12.5	0
Maltodextrin, starch	67:1	1.5	0	Yes	.1	.1	10,000 IU 60% β-carotene	667	24	0
Hydrolyzed corn starch	71:1	1.0	0 or 10	Yes	0	0	6680 IU (1/2 β-carotene, 1/2 vitamin A palmitate)	80	15	1.3
Maltodextrin	89:1	1.0	8	Yes	0	0	Vitamin A IU 6000 1/2 β-carotene	240	36	0
Corn syrup, sugar	91:1	1.5	0	No	0	0	1552 IU	98	9.8	0
Hydrolyzed corn starch, fructose	86:1	1.19	0	Yes	0	0	2400 IU	43	7.1	0
Maltodextrin	104:1	1.24	0	Yes	0	0	3226 IU	116	9.7	0
Hydrolyzed corn starch, sucrose	75:1	1.0	0	Yes	.12	.12	Vitamin A 4000 IU	240	18	0
Maltodextrin, corn syrup solids	75:1	1.0	0 or 14	Yes	.100	.100	4000 IU Vitamin A 3332 IU β-carotene	340	24	0
Corn syrup, sucrose	79:1	1.0	0 or 8	No	0	0	4700 IU	56	14.1	0

(A) = Clintec, Nutrition Co., (B) = Ross Labs, (C) = Sherwood Medical, (D) = Elan Pharma, (E) = Mead Johnson, (F) = Sandoz Nutrition, (G) = McGaw Labs, (H) = represents added free glutamine

kcal/kg/day provided as 85 percent glucose calories and 15 percent fat calories, and 0.17 gm/kg/day nitrogen (approximately 1.0–1.1 gm/kg/day protein). The authors reported no significant differences in nitrogen balance or urinary 3-methylhistidine excretion. They also reported no difference in morbidity as measured by an organ function scoring system, and there was no significant difference in overall mortality. Jimenez-Jimenez et al. studied 80 septic, postoperative patients in a randomized controlled trial for 15 days [24]. Forty patients received TPN containing a standard amino acid solution (22.5% BCAAs) at a dose of approximately 1.4 gm/kg/day. Sixty percent of the non-protein calories were provided as glucose, and 40 percent were provided as lipid emulsion. The NPC:N was 150:1. Forty patients in the study group received the same regimen although the amino acid source provided 45 percent BCAAs. The authors reported a more positive nitrogen balance in the study group at day 7, with no significant difference between groups at day 15. Urinary 3-methylhistidine declined significantly from baseline in the study group at day 7 and day 15 when compared to controls. There was no significant difference in mortality between groups.

Patients who reportedly responded to high BCAA parenteral solutions met criteria for stress level equal to or greater than 2 and were provided BCAA at a dose of ≥ 0.5 gm/kg/day [16,21]. While the trials reviewed above used a variety of stress stratification systems, the patients would appear to meet such criteria described by Cerra et al. [14]. However, these large trials have demonstrated inconsistent improvement in certain metabolic and nutritional markers in highly stressed, critically ill patients with no clear difference in morbidity or mortality.

Enteral formulas containing high BCAA concentrations have received relatively little study. However, much like the studies of high BCAA TPN, studies of high BCAA enteral formulas also disagree. Cerra et al. compared a standard enteral formula containing 28 percent BCAAs and a modified enteral formula containing 44 percent BCAA in a prospective, randomized, double-blind study of septic surgical patients [25]. The formulas were isocaloric and isonitrogenous. Patients were fed nasoduodenally with 5 gm/kg/day nitrogen (approximately 2 gm/kg/day protein) for 7 days. The study group achieved a significantly more positive nitrogen balance by day 7. When the data were adjusted for 2 patients who received suboptimal nitrogen

Table 202-3. High Nitrogen Peptide and Amino Acid Enteral Formula Product Comparison

	ACCUPEP HPF (Sherwood Medical)	ALITRAQ (Ross Labs)	PEPTAMEN (Clintec Nutrition)	PERATIVE (Ross Labs)	REABILAN HN (Elan Pharma)	STRESSTEIN (Sandoz Nutrition)	VITAL HN (Ross Labs)	VIVONEX PLUS (Sandoz Nutrition)	CRUCIAL (Clintec Nutrition)
Carbohydrate									
gm/1000 kcal	188.8	164	127	177.2	119	142	185	190	90
% kcal	75.5	66	51	54.5	47.5	57	74	76	36
source	Maltodextrin	Hydrolyzed corn starch, sucrose, fructose	Maltodextrin starch	Hydrolyzed cornstarch	Maltodextrin tapioca starch	Hydrolyzed cornstarch	Hydrolyzed cornstarch, sucrose, lactose	Maltodextrin modified starch	Maltodextrin, starch
Protein									
gm/1000 kcal	40	52.5	40	66	44	58	41.7	45	62.6
% kcal	16	21	16	20.5	17.5	23	17	18	25
source	Hydrolyzed lactalbumin	Hydrolyzed soy and lactalbumin, whey, free amino acids, 1-arginine, glutamine	Enzymatically hydrolyzed whey	Partially hydrolyzed sodium caseinate lactalbumin, 1-arginine	Hydrolyzed whey, casein	Free amino acids	Partially hydrolyzed whey, meat and soy free essential amino acids	Free amino acids, 1-arginine, glutamine	Hydrolyzed casein, 1-arginine, glutamine
Fat									
gm/1000 kcal	10	15.5	39	37.4	39	23	10	6.7	45
% kcal	8.5	13	33	25	35	21	9.5	6	39
source	MCT, corn oils	MCT, safflower oils	MCT, sunflower oils	Canola, MCT, corn oils	MCT, soy oneothera biennis oils	MCT, soybean oils	Safflower MCT	Soybean oil	MCT, fish, soy, lecithin
Caloric density									
kcal/ml	1.0	1.0	1.0	1.3	1.0	1.0	1.33	1.0	1.5
NPC:N	134:1	94:1	131:1	97:1	117:1	97:1	125:1	115:1	67:1
Osmolality	490	575	270	385	490	910	500	650	490
Packaging	Powder	Powdered, vanilla flavored	Ready to feed, flavored	Ready to feed, flavored	Ready to feed	Powder	Powder, vanilla flavored	Powder, flavor packets	Ready to feed

amounts for 2 study days, the study group achieved significantly more positive nitrogen balance by day 3. In the study group, the authors also reported a higher percentage of patients who had a rise in transferrin greater than 20 mg per deciliter and more than 500 lymphocytes per square millimeter after the 7-day study period. They did not report if the difference between the groups was statistically significant. Patient mortality or morbidity was not reported. The results of this investigation disagree with the findings of a more recent study in burn patients. Yong-Ming et al. compared an egg protein formulation containing approximately 20 percent BCAAs and a high BCAA formulation containing approximately 44 percent BCAAs in a prospective, cross-over study of 12 burn patients with an average burn surface area of 36 percent [26]. Patients were studied while receiving each formula over 2 to 4 days. Choice of which formula patients received first was by random selection. Studies were conducted at an average of 25 days following burn. Patients in both groups received approximately 40 kcal/kg/day, with the egg diet group receiving 0.26 gm/kg/day nitrogen and those in the BCAA group receiving 0.24 gm/kg/day nitrogen. The enteral formulations differed in the type of protein and source of fat. The authors reported no statistical difference in nitrogen balance between the two study periods. Visceral protein measurements were not reported, nor were rates of morbidity or mortality. Although the patients in both of these trials no doubt suffered from metabolic stress, one might argue that burn injury may not elicit the same degree or type of metabolic stress as sepsis. This may account for the differences in results. Use of high BCAA solutions remains controversial because of considerable disagreement in results from several clinical trials as well as the relative expense of these specialty solutions. In general, several large investigations of patients receiving high BCAA nutrition support have demonstrated that these regimens may be responsible for facilitating improvement in certain biochemical markers (hepatic transport proteins, nitrogen retention, lymphocytes) in a specific group of critically ill patients. Although the improvements were statistically significant, to date no effect has been demonsrated on morbidity or mortality [27,28].

Several other enteral formulas have been developed and targeted for use in hypermetabolic patients (see Table 202-2). Although many critically ill patients maintain reasonably normal gut absorptive capacity and are able to tolerate the macronutrient mix of most isotonic standard formulas, others may develop symptoms of impaired absorption [29]. In an attempt to maximize benefits of enteral alimentation, multiple investigations have focused on the study of macronutrients in a form that patients may assimilate and physically tolerate more effectively. Early investigations identified amino acids as the most efficiently absorbed form of protein utilized by the gut [30]. Elemental formulas containing free amino acids were developed from these studies. However, more recent investigations suggest that protein in the form of small dipeptides and tripeptides appears to be absorbed more efficiently in the intestine than free amino acids or intact proteins [31,32]. Enhanced assimilation of these smaller proteins is thought to occur due to non-competitive transport of peptides into the intestinal mucosa. Subsequent to these reports, formulas designed to provide protein as peptides or mixtures of peptides and free amino acids were developed. These formulas also contain fat, usually as mixtures of LCT and MCT, and are generally marketed for use in patients who are considered to have marginally functional GI tracts (Table 202-3). Some recent reports have supported the use of peptide-based formulas in critically ill, hypoalbuminemic patients [33]. Hypoalbuminemia is associated with increased incidence of diarrhea in critically ill patients receiving enteral support [34]. Decreased serum albumin is the-

orized to promote increased permeability of the GI tract and development of secretory diarrhea as a result of decreased oncotic pressure [35]. Peptide formulas may allow for improved nitrogen absorption, resulting in reduced stool output and increased serum albumin. However, the extent of preferred peptide absorption in critically ill patients has been challenged [36]. In addition, the proposed clinical advantage of better nitrogen absorption with decreased diarrhea is controversial. Mowatt-Larrsen et al. compared a peptide enteral formula with a standard enteral formula in a prospective, randomized study of 41 acutely injured, hypoalbuminemic patients [37]. Twenty-one patients who received the peptide enteral formula and 20 patients who received a standard enteral formula were studied for a minimum of 5 days and a maximum of 10 days. The authors reported no difference in prevalence of diarrhea or elevated gastric residuals between the groups. They also reported no difference in prealbumin, transferrin, or albumin. While nitrogen balance increased significantly from baseline in both groups on both study days, the increase was significantly higher at day 10 in the group fed the peptide formula. The results of this investigation agree with the findings of a study evaluating the influence of serum albumin concentration on enteral feeding tolerance. Patterson et al. retrospectively reviewed the clinical response of 88 hypoalbuminemic patients who received a standard isotonic formula for a minimum of 48 hours [38]. The formula contained intact protein and had a caloric concentration of 1 kcal per milliliter. The first 10 days of enteral support were designated as the study period. The authors reported no statistical difference in the enteral feeding tolerance defined as more than 3 stools per day for more than 48 hours, or gastric residuals greater than twice the infusion rate for more than 48 hours.

Comparison of results from investigations utilizing different peptide formulas is difficult. Currently available peptide-based formulas may vary in the proportion of total peptides, peptide-chain composition, and molecular weights [39]. Beneficial effects of peptides are associated with shorter chain length (3–5 amino acids) and molecular weights less than 1000. However, physiologic effects of peptides with similar molecular weights may differ with chain amino acid composition. In addition, type of fat and carbohydrate used in the formula may also alter peptide absorption.

Other investigations of enteral feedings in critically ill patients have studied the potential clinical utility of fiber-containing formulas. Soluble fiber is associated with beneficial effects in treating hypercholesterolemia and in blood glucose control, while insoluble fiber is associated with improvement in bowel function [40]. Initially, dietary fiber was added to enteral formulas to normalize bowel function. Dietary fiber is usually promoted as a preventive treatment for constipation in normal individuals as it increases fecal bulk. However, in hospitalized patients, fiber is generally used as a preventive measure for treatment of diarrhea or diarrhea associated with enteral feedings. Although the mechanism is not clear in humans, experimental models have demonstrated generation of short-chain fatty acids by colonic bacterial fermentation of fiber, which facilitates absorption of fluid and electrolytes by the gut lumen [41,42]. The effect of fiber-containing formulas on diarrhea associated with enteral feeding is controversial [42]. Studies of hospitalized patients with varying degrees of critical illness have reported no difference in stool frequency when comparing patients who received fiber-containing formulas with patients who received lower residue formulas [43,44]. Numerous enteral products with added soluble fiber are currently available, including selected formulas designed for use in critically ill patients. Although guidelines exist for a recommended dietary intake of fiber for healthy individuals, there is no consensus for the optimal dose of fiber to promote better bowel function and gut regeneration in critically ill patients.

Recent studies of nutritional intervention in critically ill patients have investigated the clinical effects of certain nutrients considered semiessential or conditionally essential, such as glutamine. Other nutrients that have received attention for their apparent immunomodulating properties when given in pharmacologic doses include arginine, RNA, and omega-3 fatty acids. In general, these nutrients have received little study as individual immunomodulating agents in humans. However, several formulas are now commercially available that contain a variety of mixtures of these nutrients (see Table 202-2).

RECOMMENDATIONS. Nutritional goals in critically ill patients include detection and correction of preexisting malnutrition, prevention of progressive protein-calorie malnutrition, optimization of patients' metabolic status including fluid and electrolyte management, and reduction of morbidity and subsequent duration of recovery [45]. The optimal dose range for protein appears to be approximately 1.5 to 2 gm/kg/day. However, an accurate urine collection for nitrogen excretion may be helpful in guiding the clinician to determine a more individualized dose [46,47,48]. In most patients the use of a standard mix of essential, semiessential, and nonessential amino acids is indicated. Until further evidence of greater clinical benefit is demonstrated, routine use of high BCAA formulas cannot be recommended [27,28]. The optimal caloric range appears to be approximately 25 to 30 kcal/kg/day, or 120 to 140 percent of basal energy expenditure as calculated by the Harris-Benedict equation. Carbohydrate should be provided at a rate not to exceed 4 to 7 mg/kg/min. The dose of lipid emulsion in critically ill patients is controversial because of results from earlier studies that reported decreased immunocompetence associated with long-chain fatty acids from commercially available lipid emulsion [3,47,49]. However, provision of approximately 1 gm/kg/day, not to exceed 30 percent of total calories, appears to be a reasonable compromise in view of the lack of clear data concerning effects on morbidity and mortality in human models and the clinical utility of lipid emulsion as a noncarbohydrate source for hyperglycemic patients and possibly those with carbon dioxide–retaining ventilator dependency [49,50]. The route of nutrition support in critically ill patients has been shown to be a major determining factor in clinical outcome [51,52]. Critically ill patients who receive early enteral feedings appear to have lower septic complications. Choice of which enteral formulation to use is difficult and dependent on an individual patient's clinical condition. Characteristics of an optimal enteral formula in this patient population include a low NPC:N (~ 100:1), with 20 to 30 percent of total calories as fat. The optimal source of nitrogen remains controversial. Based on current data, peptide formulas should not be routinely used in stable, critically ill patients with or without hypoalbuminemia who require enteral nutrition. These solutions may be most useful in patients who have failed therapy with standard formulas and selected patients with functionally or anatomically compromised small bowel function. There are no data to support the concept that fiber-containing formulas offer any advantage to critically ill hypermetabolic patients from the standpoint of diarrhea. These formulas may be most effective in stable patients receiving long-term enteral feeding for management of constipation or diarrhea. Further study of enteral formulas containing high concentrations of semiessential or immunomodulating nutrients is needed before routine use of these solutions can be recommended.

Liver Failure

Liver failure may be caused by a number of insults, such as trauma, sepsis, viral infection, hypoperfusion, or hepatotoxic agents [53]. In all cases there is some degree of cellular compromise. If tissue death occurs, the liver may eventually begin a cellular regeneration and form fibrotic tissue. Depending on the course of the disease, the patient may either recover with few residual effects, develop stable chronic disease, or even die. Development of chronic liver dysfunction and the characteristic pathologic events that follow are usually referred to as *cirrhosis*. Eventually, the underlying disease begins to worsen the condition of the vasculature and parenchymal tissue, resulting in a reduction of functional hepatocytes. As this process continues, resistance to hepatic blood flow increases, causing portal hypertension, which may lead to development of collateral vessels, esophageal varices, and GI bleeding. Clinical signs and symptoms of these pathologic changes may include ascites, jaundice, central nervous system (CNS) changes, and encephalopathy. Liver failure that occurs more acutely may be referred to as fulminant hepatic failure (FHF). FHF is defined as hepatic failure with development of encephalopathy within 8 weeks of the first symptoms of illness without preexisting liver disease. Late-onset hepatic failure (LOHF) occurs in patients without preexisting disease who develop encephalopathic liver failure within 8 weeks to 6 months of the first symptoms of illness [54]. Because the liver is the central organ for nutrient metabolism, patients with hepatic failure may present with multiple abnormalities in carbohydrate, fat, and protein metabolism [55]. Although glucagon and insulin levels are elevated, the insulin:glucagon ratio is decreased, favoring sustained gluconeogenesis and glucose intolerance [55,56]. Decreased hepatic degradation of cortisol and epinepherine contributes to increased catabolism and glucose intolerance. However, patients with FHF may experience hypoglycemia [57]. These patients appear to develop depletion of glycogen stores in the setting of impaired gluconeogenesis and decreased insulin clearance. Fat utilization may be impaired secondary to poor liver metabolism and impaired lipoprotein lipase activity. Long-chain fatty acids are incompletely metabolized, causing an accumulation of short-chain fatty acids. Protein metabolism is also abnormally affected by liver failure [57,58]. Increased gluconeogenesis results in the accelerated use of the body's protein stores. Muscle use of BCAAs for energy is increased, resulting in decreased plasma concentrations. Other amino acids usually metabolized by the liver, such as methionine, glutamine, and the aromatic amino acids (AAAs) tryptophan, phenylalanine, and tyrosine, begin to accumulate. In addition, ammonia levels are usually elevated secondary to ineffective detoxification of ammonia to urea.

Patients with advanced liver disease have demonstrated neurologic and behavioral changes that may range from confusion to bizarre behavior and coma. These changes are collectively referred to as hepatic encephalopathy [59]. Multiple metabolic derangements, such as fluid and electrolyte imbalances, perfusion abnormalities, or infection, may contribute to the development of encephalopathy. However, several hypotheses have been proposed to explain the etiology of CNS changes that are characteristic of liver failure [59,60]. Elevated ammonia concentrations have been suggested as a causative agent. The specific mechanism is not known, but it has been shown that plasma levels correlate poorly with the degree of encephalopathy [59]. Interestingly, studies have demonstrated improvement in mental status by bowel cleansing with lactulose and bowel sterilization with neomycin [59]. Elevated concentrations of mercaptans and short-chain fatty acids have been hypothesized to act synergistically with ammonia. Another hypothesis was proposed by Fischer and Baldessarini [61]. According to this hypothesis, during liver failure the imbalance of BCAAs and AAAs in the plasma and alterations in the blood-brain barrier (BBB) work together to promote influx of increased concentrations of AAAs, methionine, and tryptophan into the CNS. Increased cerebral spinal fluid (CSF) levels of AAAs may result in the formation of weakly stimulatory, or "false," neurotransmitters that compete with normal neurotransmitters for binding sites. In addition, tryptophan is converted to the inhibitory neurotransmitter serotonin. The unified theory of hepatic encephalopathy bridges the ammonia and false neurotransmitter theories [62]. This hypothesis maintains that increased plasma ammonia concentrations worsen the encephalopathic process by crossing the BBB and forming glutamine in the CNS. Glutamine shares an exchange carrier at the BBB with the AAAs. As glutamine efflux increases, AAA influx into the CNS increases. Recently, another hypothesis has been proposed. Data suggest that increased activity of the inhibitory neurotransmitter gamma-aminobutyric acid (GABA) may also contribute to development of hepatic encephalopathy [63].

PARENTERAL AND ENTERAL FORMULATIONS. Formulas for use in patients with liver failure have been developed based on the Fischer and Baldessarini hypothesis of encephalopathy. Hepatamine (McGaw) (Table 202-4) is the only intravenous solution commercially available in the United States that contains high concentrations of BCAAs and low concentrations of AAAs and methionine. Two commercial enteral solutions have been developed based on previous studies of plasma amino acid derangements (Table 202-5). Both parenteral and enteral modified amino acid solutions are designed to normalize plasma amino acid concentrations in an attempt to improve encephalopathy. Hepatic Aid II (McGaw) contains essentially no electrolytes or vitamins and should be supplemented with appropriate amounts of each when used as the patient's primary source of nutrient intake. NutriHep (Clintec) is a newer formula, which replaces Travasorb Hepatic (Clintec). Unlike the Travasorb Hepatic, NutriHep is ready to use and provides 100 percent of the recommended daily allowances for vitamins and minerals.

CLINICAL STUDIES. The role of specialized nutrition intervention in the overall supportive care of patients with liver failure is controversial. Multiple investigations of patients with varying degrees of liver failure and hepatic encephalopathy have reported conflicting results. Several publications have reviewed these investigations [59,64–69]. The use of parenteral

Table 202-4. Hepatic and Renal Failure Parenteral Amino Acid Product Comparison

	Renal failure			Liver failure
	NephrAmine (McGaw Labs)	Aminosyn-RF (Abbott Labs)	RenAmin (Clintec Nutrition)	Hepatamine (McGaw Labs)
Protein concentration	5.4%	5.2%	6.5%	8.0%
Nitrogen (gm/100 ml)	.64	.79	1	1.2
Amino acids (mg/100 ml)				
Histidine	250	429	420	240
Isoleucine	560	462	500	900
Leucine	880	726	600	1100
Lysine	640	535	450	610
Methionine	880	726	500	100
Phenylalanine	880	726	490	100
Threonine	400	330	380	450
Tryptophan	200	165	160	66
Valine	640	528	820	840
Nonessential amino acids (mg/100 ml)				
Alanine	—	—	560	770
Arginine	—	600	630	600
Proline	—	—	350	800
Serine	—	—	300	500
Tyrosine	—	—	40	—
Glycine	—	—	300	900
Cysteine	<20	<20	—	<20
Glutamic acid	—	—	—	—
Electrolytes (mEq/L)				
Sodium	5	—	—	10
Chloride	<3	—	31	<3
Acetate	44	105	60	62
Potassium	—	5.4	—	—
Phosphate (mmol/liter)	—	—	—	10
Amino acid composition	39% BCAA	33% BCAA	30% BCAA	36% BCAA
	20% aromatic amino acids	22% aromatic amino acids	11% aromatic amino acids	3% aromatic amino acids
	99% essential amino acids	89% essential amino acids	67% essential amino acids	56% essential amino acids

Table 202-5. Liver Failure Enteral Formula Product Comparison

	NutriHep (Clintec Nutrition Co.)		Hepatic Aid II (McGaw Labs)	
	Source	per 1000 kcal	Source	per 1000 kcal
Carbohydrate	Maltodextrin modified cornstarch	193 gm	Maltodextrins Sucrose	143 gm
Amino acids	L-amino acids Whey protein 50% BCAA 2.4% aromatic amino acids	26.7 gm protein 31 gm amino acids	L-amino acids 46% BCAA 1.87% aromatic amino acids	33.4 gm protein 37.5 gm amino acids
Fat	MCT (66%) Canola Soy lecithin Corn oil	14 gm	Soybean oil Lecithin Monoglycerides and diglycerides	30.8 gm
Sodium		213.3 mg 9.3 mEq		<288 mg <12.5 mEq
Potassium		880 mg 22.6 mEq		<196 mg <5 mEq
Caloric density (kcal/ml)	1.5		1.2	
Packaging	Ready to feed Flavoring available		Powdered flavored	

and enteral modified amino acid solutions in encephalopathic patients has normalized plasma amino profiles, which correlated with improved encephalopathy in some studies. A recent meta-analysis of the benefits of parenteral modified amino acids reported a significant and beneficial effect on mental recovery from hepatic encephalopathy [68]. However, the discrepancy in other clinical outcomes among the 9 trials selected for the analysis was large enough for the authors to question the benefits of parenteral modified amino acids on mortality. When homogeneous subsets of the trials were analyzed, there appeared to be a trend toward a positive effect on mortality in patients who received modified amino acid solutions. The importance of nutritional intervention in patients with liver failure has been demonstrated in a study by Cerra et al. [69]. Hospitalized patients with chronic alcoholic cirrhosis were prospectively randomized to receive either a modified amino acid TPN regimen without lipid emulsion or concentrated dextrose and neomycin. Forty patients received TPN, and 35 patients received concentrated dextrose and neomycin for up to 14 days. The TPN group demonstrated a statistically significant improvement in encephalopathy while achieving a mean positive nitrogen balance by days 3 to 4. Survival was statistically greater in the TPN group.

RECOMMENDATIONS. Nutrition support of patients with liver failure generally depends on the degree of liver dysfunction and associated metabolic abnormalities [66,70]. Stable patients with cirrhosis but without encephalopathy should receive amounts of standard amino acids and calories appropriate for the level of metabolic stress and degree of malnutrition. A low-fat diet supplemented with MCT should be considered in those patients with steatorrhea. Sodium and fluids should be restricted in patients with ascites, and recommended daily allowances of vitamins and minerals should be provided. Patients with cirrhosis and mild encephalopathy should initially receive standard amino acids in doses of 0.7 gm/kg/day, advancing this dose as tolerated. If the clinical status of the patient progresses to stage 2 encephalopathy at minimum doses of standard pro-

tein, a modified amino acid nutrition support regimen should be considered. Patients with uncomplicated, acute hepatitis should receive 30 to 35 kcal/kg/day or approximately 130 percent of calculated basal energy expenditure and protein doses of at least 1 gm/kg/day. The role of modified amino acid solutions in patients with FHF is not clear. These patients demonstrate amino acid profiles not consistent with cirrhosis and chronic liver failure [58]. However, current data tend to support the judicious use of high-BCAA, low-AAA formulas in encephalopathic patients who present with acute liver decompensation superimposed on a history of cirrhosis [71].

Renal Failure

Although dialysis has increased survival in critically ill patients with acute renal failure (ARF) following surgery or trauma, their mortality is still 50 to 70 percent [45]. Those patients greater than 60 years of age have an 80 percent or higher mortality [72]. Critically ill patients with renal failure tend to be both catabolic and hypermetabolic in a setting of fluid and protein restriction. Despite the limitations in providing nutrition support, sufficient nutrients may assist in recovery of kidney function and will avoid complications associated with malnutrition.

Hypotension and hypovolemia are the usual causes of acute renal failure. Many other factors can play a role in deteriorating renal function, such as hemorrhage, sepsis, loss of GI fluids, anesthetic agents, antibiotics, and blood transfusions [72]. Patients with chronic renal failure (CRF) and critical illness will have similar metabolic derangements as patients with ARF, but they will also have many other long-term nutritional disadvantages. Long-term dialysis can increase risk of malnutrition from poor dietary intake and catabolism. These patients may also have metabolic bone disease, hypertriglyceridemia, and individual vitamin or mineral deficiencies from their long-term disease and the losses and demands of dialysis. Nutrition support can be provided effectively to both ARF and CRF patients in the ICU, but close monitoring is necessary to avoid harmful effects of excess nutrients or underfeeding.

The metabolic alterations in ARF are a combination of hypermetabolism in response to injury, coupled with the metabolic disorders associated with ARF. Catabolism causes increased release of phosphate, sulfate, potassium, magnesium, and other ions from muscle tissue. Hyperphosphatemia develops from decreased renal excretion, which in turn causes decreased serum calcium concentrations, increased parathyroid hormone secretion, and depression of 1,25-dihydroxycholecalciferol. Accumulation of trace elements may also occur because of poor excretion. Carnitine deficiency is associated with dialysis therapy, long-term enteral or parenteral nutrition support, and increased urinary carnitine losses following surgery or with sepsis. Many critically ill patients with renal failure have a combination of these factors. Edema, hyponatremia, and metabolic acidosis are often present, making fluid and electrolyte management challenging. Energy requirements appear to be influenced mostly by the primary disease rather than by the renal failure. Therefore, energy provision should be similar to that provided for other critically ill patients. Unfortunately, renal failure is often accompanied by alterations in carbohydrate and fat metabolism, making provision of adequate energy difficult. Increased glycogenolysis and decreased glycogen synthesis result in less glycogen available as a short-term energy source. Insulin levels may be elevated because of poor clearance by the kidney, but glucose is poorly tolerated secondary to insulin resistance. ARF patients often present with a Type IV hyperlipoproteinemia due to increased hepatic triglyceride production and altered very low density lipoprotein catabolism [72]. For these reasons, energy is best provided with mixed substrates.

Nitrogen metabolism in renal failure has been the area of greatest interest and controversy. Both quantity and quality of protein must be considered. Animal data suggest that dietary protein restriction slows the rate of progression of CRF. However, any level of stress can induce catabolism and lead to negative nitrogen balance. Patients requiring hemodialysis or peritoneal dialysis have increased catabolism and loss of protein into the dialysate. Therefore, a protein restriction is not appropriate. The metabolism of several amino acids, such as histidine, taurine, and arginine, is altered in CRF. Provision of essential amino acids combined with a high energy intake has been suggested in an attempt to neutralize urea nitrogen for synthesis of nonessential amino acids and reduce blood urea nitrogen (BUN) levels. BCAAs have also been suggested for nutrition in patients with hypermetabolism and ARF. BCAAs are a principal source of energy for muscle during stress or following injury. Supplemental BCAAs may provide a more efficient source of nitrogen to patients who are highly catabolic. In oliguric patients with ARF, early and frequent dialysis is acceptable to control uremia and fluid overload. This allows lesser fluid and protein restrictions and, therefore, more complete nutritional supplementation. In patients with severe fluid intolerance, ultrafiltration may also be necessary. Although dialysis can improve fluid and protein management, there are several disadvantages. Dialysis can increase catabolism and alter the metabolism of other nutrients. Significant losses of protein and amino acids in hemodialysis and peritoneal dialysis have been documented. Losses during peritoneal dialysis appear to be greatest.

Vitamins can also be affected by renal failure. Water-soluble vitamins can be lost in dialysate. Fat-soluble vitamins may accumulate in patients with renal failure. The conversion of vitamin D to the active form is reduced in patients with end-stage renal disease, and such patients may require supplementation if serum calcium is reduced.

PARENTERAL AND ENTERAL FORMULATIONS. As with all patients, enteral nutrition support is the preferred route in ARF. There are several types of enteral formulas specifically designed for renal failure patients (Table 202-6). Some products contain only essential amino acids and histidine, with little to no vitamins, minerals, or electrolytes. These formulas are designed for short-term use when dialysis is not possible. Other products have reduced protein (standard essential amino acids and nonessential amino acids), potassium, phosphorus, vitamin A, and vitamin D and are enriched in vitamin B_6 and folate. Many of the newer formulas also have added histidine, arginine, taurine, and carnitine. Non–protein calorie to nitrogen ratios vary and can be applied to patients with or without dialysis. A ratio of approximately 400:1 meets most predialysis patient needs. A ratio of approximately 150:1 is preferable for those patients receiving dialysis. All renal failure formulas are calorically concentrated for better fluid management. Most of these formulas are palatable as oral supplements or may be fed via a feeding tube.

Enteral nutrition is often not possible in renal failure because of ileus, nausea, vomiting, or gastric bleeding. Under these circumstances, parenteral nutrition is appropriate. Several parenteral amino acid solutions designed for renal failure have been developed (see Table 202-4). Those containing only essential amino acids have limited use for short-term situations when dialysis is not possible. Amino acid solutions with 35 to 40 percent of BCAAs have been designed for hypermetabolic patients and may help reduce rising BUN. A 100 percent BCAA supplement is also available that may be added to standard amino acid formulas [73]. This may be most useful when concentrated solutions are needed. Utilizing concentrated stock amino acid solutions (15%), dextrose (70%), and lipid (20%) will assist in restricting fluid. Standard parenteral vitamins are recommended.

CLINICAL STUDIES. Research involving nutrition support of renal failure patients began in 1963 when Giordano reported that a diet containing only essential amino acids (EAAs) as a nitrogen source plus adequate calories fed to uremic patients lowered BUN levels, decreased catabolism, and maintained nitrogen balance [74]. Giovannetti and Maggiore had similar findings [75]. The benefits of using only EAAs were proposed based on the theory that urea nitrogen is recycled to synthesize nonessential amino acids (NEAAs). Further studies were carried out using parenteral nutrition support. Abel et al. [76] compared uremic patients receiving intravenous EAAs and dextrose to intravenous dextrose without nitrogen. They reported stabilization of BUN; decreased serum magnesium, phosphorus, and potassium; and more rapid return of renal function in the group receiving EAA.

A later study done by Feinstein et al. [77] compared 30 uremic patients receiving IV EAA with dextrose to EAA and non-essential amino acids (NEAA) with dextrose. A third group received glucose alone. They found a similar benefit in the EAA solution in that there was a lower rate of urea nitrogen appearance. Two studies [78,79] performed in the early 1980s had designs similar to Feinstein's study but showed no benefit to the EAA solution versus EAA and NEAA solution. The control groups showed similar survival, recovery of renal failure, and serum BUN, phosphorus, and magnesium to that of the EAA group. Many of these conflicting results can be attributed to variability in renal function, disease state, and quantity and quality of amino acids infused. Several clinical studies have indicated that nitrogen from urea plays a minimal role in protein synthesis and is most likely recycled for synthesis of urea [80]. Varcol et al. reported that only a small amount of urea nitrogen is incorporated into

Table 202-6. Calorically Dense and Renal Failure Enteral Formula Comparison

	AminAid (McGaw Labs)	Deliver 2.0 (Mead Johnson)	Magnacal (Sherwood Nutrition)	Nepro (Ross Labs)	Nutren 2.0 (Clintec Nutrition Co.)	Suplena (Ross Labs)	Travasorb Renal (Clintec Nutrition Co.)	Two Cal HN (Ross Labs)
Carbohydrate								
gm/1000 kcal	187	100	125	107.6	98	128	200	109
% kcal	74.8	47	50	43	39	51	81.1	43.2
Source	Maltodextrins Sucrose	Corn syrup	Maltodextrins Sucrose	Hydrolyzed cornstarch, sucrose	Corn syrup solids Maltodextrins Sucrose	Hydrolyzed cornstarch, sucrose	Glucose Oligosaccharides sucrose	Hydrolyzed cornstarch, sucrose
Protein								
gm/1000 kcal	10	38	35	34.9	40	15	17	42
% kcal	4	15	14	14	16	6	6	16.7
Source	Essential amino acids plus histidine	Sodium and calcium caseinate	Sodium, calcium caseinates	Calcium, magnesium, and Sodium caseinates	Casein	Sodium and calcium caseinates	Essential amino acids Select nonessential amino acids	Sodium and calcium caseinates
Fat								
gm/1000 kcal	24	51	40	47.8	63	48	13	45
% kcal	21.2	45	36	43	45	43	12	40.1
Source	Partially hydrogenated soybean oil, lecithin, Monoglycerides and diglycerides	Soy oil MCT	Soy oil	Safflower oil Soy oil	MCT Canola oil Lecithin	Safflower oil Soy Oil	MCT Sunflower Oil	Corn and MCT oils
NPC:N	800:1	145:1	157:1	154:1	131:1	393:1	339:1	125:1
Caloric density	2.0	2.0	2.0	2.0	2.0	2.0	1.35	2.0
Sodium								
mg/1000 kcal	<173 mg	400	500	415	500	391	0	655
mEq/1000 kcal	<7.5 mEq	17.4	21.8	18.1	21.8	17.0	0	28.4
Potassium								
mg/1000 kcal	<118 mg	850	625	528	1250	558	0	122.1
mEq/1000 kcal	<3 mEq	22	16	13.5	32.1	14.3	0	31.2
Calcium								
mg/1000 kcal	0	500	500	686	700	692	0	526
Magnesium								
mg/1000 kcal	0	200	200	105	340	105	0	210
Phosphorus								
mg/1000 kcal	0	500	500	343	700	364	0	526
Water-soluble vitamins	No	Yes	Yes	Yes	Yes	Yes	Yes	Yes
Fat-soluble vitamins	No	Yes	Yes	Yes	Yes	Yes	No	Yes

albumin [81]. These studies seem to imply that EAAs alone may not support protein synthesis.

Few studies have been performed comparing enteral formulas in renal failure. Sofio et al. [82] gave an EAA enteral formula as a sole nitrogen source or as a supplement to a low-protein diet to patients with ARF or CRF. They found a slower rise in BUN, stabilized serum potassium and phosphorus, and positive or improved nitrogen balance in all groups.

RECOMMENDATIONS. Although some of the research in renal failure remains controversial, there are many sound recommendations of nutrition support based on clinical experience. Overall, it is agreed that adequate calorie provision is essential to avoid excessive catabolism in critically ill patients with ARF. In general, 25 kcal per kilogram will meet most patient needs, but indirect calorimetry is helpful when estimates seem inadequate. Fluid restriction can limit the actual amount of calories provided. A common guideline for fluid allowance is 500 ml plus 24-hour urine losses. Concentrated enteral formulas (2 kcal/ml) and concentrated parenteral stock solutions can provide maximum calories in a limited volume. Carbohydrate and fat intolerance can occur, so a mix of substrates is recommended (20–50% of total calories as carbohydrate and 30–40% as fat). Patients receiving peritoneal dialysis may absorb up to 500 to 800 calories in dextrose from the dialysate. These calories should be considered when planning nutrition support. To calculate kilocalories (kcal) from dialysate, the following equation can be used [83]:

Kcal from dialysate = glucose concentration (gm/L) × 3.4 kcal/gm × 0.8 × volume (L)

Monitoring serum glucose daily and triglycerides weekly is necessary to evaluate substrate tolerance. Insulin may be required to achieve normal serum blood glucose levels, but smaller amounts may be necessary in renal failure. Protein requirements vary largely with disease process and dialysis. Critically ill patients require 1.5 to 2.0 gm of protein per kilogram of body weight, but in the setting of renal failure, this is usually decreased to 0.5 to 1.0 gm per kilogram. When dialysis is utilized, protein can be increased to 1.2 gm per kilogram in hemodialysis and 1.5 gm per kilogram for peritoneal dialysis. In most ARF patients, standard amino acid mixtures are tolerated. Solutions or formulas with only EAAs are reserved for those patients who cannot receive dialysis and have progressive renal deterioration. Clinical trials comparing EAAs alone to a mixture of NEAAs and EAAs have had conflicting results. Excessive (greater than 40 gm) EAAs may cause hyperammonemia. NEAAs (arginine, ornithine, and citrulline) are necessary for ammonia detoxification via the urea cycle, and without these amino acids there may be increased serum ammonia levels [45]. For these reasons, EAAs and glucose should be limited to short-term use and to patients in whom renal replacement therapy cannot be instituted. Serum ammonia levels should be closely monitored when only EAAs are provided [45]. BCAA parenteral solutions may be useful in patients with severe stress or sepsis. The beneficial effects of BCAAs have not been clearly shown in clinical trials, although a decreased rate of urea generation has been documented [73]. Formulas higher in BCAAs may be useful in patients with hypercatabolic renal failure who have a BUN greater than 100 mg per deciliter while receiving 40 to 70 gm of a standard amino acid mixture [72]. Minerals and electrolytes can require frequent adjustments and should be monitored daily. Most ARF patients require phosphorus, magnesium, and potassium restriction. Supplemental calcium may be recommended to treat decreased serum calcium. Vitamin requirements for ARF are derived from data for CRF. Water-soluble vitamins are lost in dialysate, but losses appear no greater than in the urine of normal healthy persons. Supplementation may be necessary for patients with high output receiving dialysis. Serum vitamin A tends to be above normal in patients with renal failure, so supplementation should be avoided. Serum values for vitamin D and calcium will dictate whether vitamin D supplementation is necessary. Trace elements are excreted via the kidney, and the current standard of practice is to provide them only three times per week in the parenteral solution and in reduced amounts in enteral formulas, although no substantial data exist to support this practice. Iron is usually supplemented in renal failure patients but should be avoided during sepsis.

There are many limitations in providing nutrition to renal failure patients, but with careful monitoring and early intervention, adequate nutrition can be provided.

Respiratory Failure

Malnutrition in patients with respiratory disease has been well recognized. Several researchers have documented decreased weight and other anthropometric measures as well as a decline in visceral proteins in approximately 25 percent of patients with chronic obstructive pulmonary disease (COPD) [84,85,86]. These studies also found that malnutrition correlated with severity of disease. Those patients with nutrition compromise had lower arterial oxygen pressure (PO_2) and higher carbon dioxide pressure (PCO_2). Nutritional status appears to have an effect on pulmonary function. Autopsies comparing diaphragmatic muscle mass in depleted patients and normal healthy subjects have shown 43 percent less muscle in the depleted patients [87]. Several researchers have shown decreased respiratory function in malnourished patients compared with healthy subjects [88]. Whittaker et al. reported improved maximum expiratory pressure and mean sustained inspiratory pressure in COPD patients receiving 1000 calories daily via tube feeding [89]. While others have shown that patients who are starved are more likely to develop pneumonia [88], Keys et al. measured respiratory function in healthy men after 12 weeks of semistarvation and during refeeding. They observed a decrease in respiratory efficiency over 24 weeks of semistarvation and return of function with refeeding [90]. These data seem to imply that nutritional status corresponds with disease state in respiratory disease and that nutrition support may improve respiratory function.

Although nutrition support can be helpful in treating respiratory disease, overfeeding can be equally detrimental. When calories provided exceed energy requirements, lipogenesis occurs, causing a rise in carbon dioxide (CO_2) production. In a normal individual, an increased CO_2 will result in increased minute ventilation to expire the excess gas. However, in patients with respiratory compromise, this adaptive mechanism is inefficient. When macronutrients (carbohydrate, protein, and fat) are metabolized, oxygen is consumed (VO_2) and carbon dioxide is produced (VCO_2). These gases can be measured and represented in a ratio (VCO_2:VO_2) called the respiratory quotient (RQ). Oxidation of macronutrients results in specific RQ values: carbohydrate 1.0, protein 0.8, fat 0.7, and mixed substrate 0.85. RQ values greater than 1.0 are thought to represent fat synthesis.

Many patients with COPD tend to have elevated resting energy expenditures. Schols et al. reported a lack of a hypometabolic adaptive response to caloric restriction in COPD patients [91].

Protein requirements also tend to be increased in patients with respiratory failure. Protein has been shown to increase minute ventilation, oxygen consumption, ventilatory response to hypoxia, and hypercapnia [92]. BCAAs have been proposed as a stimulator to ventilatory drive via alterations of neurotransmitters. Studies of the effect of BCAAs on respiratory function have been performed in healthy subjects; therefore, the effect of BCAAs on patients with respiratory disease is still unclear [92]. In patients with acute respiratory compromise, high levels of protein may further fatigue the patient, and protein may need to be temporarily reduced. Carbohydrate and fat content of nutrition support has been well studied. When amounts of carbohydrate administered exceed maximum oxidation (4–7 mg/kg/min), lipogenesis and increased CO_2 production occur. Askanazi et al. compared provision of dextrose and fat versus dextrose alone in critically ill patients [93]. They reported VCO_2 and RQ levels significantly increased with dextrose administration. Based on data of carbohydrate intolerance in this patient population, higher fat solutions have been suggested for provision of adequate calories. Tolerance of enteral and parenteral fat can also be a concern. Patients who are hypermetabolic from stress or sepsis may have reduced metabolism of triglycerides. Excess lipid infusion has been shown to interfere with the function of the reticuloendothelial system and pulmonary diffusion capacity [94].

In patients with pulmonary edema or acute respiratory distress syndrome (ARDS), fluid restriction to produce slight hypovolemia is often desirable. Phosphorus plays an important role in respiratory function and oxidation. Hypophosphatemia can develop from decreased renal reabsorption secondary to theophylline, stress, and refeeding. Reduced phosphorus can cause decreased 2,3-diphosphoglycerate levels in red blood cells, which deliver oxygen to tissues and decrease contractility of respiratory muscles. Gravelyn et al. showed improved inspiratory and expiratory pressures with repletion of serum phosphorus [95]. Providing supplemental phosphorus in malnourished patients and monitoring serum phosphorus levels should be routine in patients with respiratory failure. Other essential nutrients (e.g., potassium, calcium, and magnesium) should be provided in adequate amounts to maintain respiratory muscle function [93].

Parenteral and Enteral Formulations. Designing an appropriate nutrition support regimen begins with an accurate assessment of caloric requirements. Indirect calorimetry is helpful whenever stress or body weight makes estimates difficult. Patients with FIO_2 greater than 60 percent will have increased error in measurement of resting energy expenditure. In general, 35 kcal per kilogram will maintain body weight and avoid overfeeding. Fluid restriction can sometimes limit caloric provision; therefore, calorically dense enteral formulas (Table 202-7) and concentrated parenteral stock solutions should be utilized. When patients have excess CO_2 production or are unable to be weaned from a ventilator, nutrient composition should be adjusted to 40 to 50 percent of calories as fat and 30 to 40 percent of calories as carbohydrate. Enteral fat is usually well tolerated, but diarrhea can develop with higher fat formulas that contain small amounts of medium-chain triglycerides (MCTs). Omega-6 fatty acids are thought to be more immunosuppressive than omega-3 fatty acids. Current IV lipid emulsions have high omega-6/omega-3 polyunsaturated fatty acid ratios, and many enteral products high in fat are being redesigned to provide more MCTs and omega-3 fatty acids. Weekly monitoring of serum triglycerides will help evaluate fat tolerance. Protein requirements are usually estimated as 1.5 to 2.0 gm per kilogram in critically ill patients. If respiratory distress is exacerbated, protein can be decreased to 1.0 to 1.5 gm per kilogram. Supplemental phosphorus can be provided enterally or parenterally. A total of 30 to 40 mM of phosphorus can be provided in most parenteral solutions, but smaller volumes may limit phosphorus provision. Enteral solutions can be supplemented with additional phosphate such as Neutra-Phos, 1 to 2 capsules dissolved in 75 to 150 ml of enteral formula 2 to 4 times daily. Some enteral products for respiratory failure have additional phosphorus already incorporated. Monitoring serum phosphorus once or twice weekly is recommended.

CLINICAL STUDIES. Research on the effects of carbohydrate and fat on respiratory function began with parenteral solutions. Askanazi et al. [96] compared parenteral nutrition with dextrose as a sole non–protein calorie source, versus a mixed substrate containing 50 percent of non–protein calories as dextrose and 50% as fat. They also made this comparison in five nutritionally depleted patients versus 12 critically ill patients. The depleted patients were crossed over from dextrose only to dextrose and fat. The dextrose alone caused a 20 percent increase in CO_2 and a 15 percent increase in RQ. When the acutely ill group was crossed over in a similar fashion, there was a rise in VCO_2 but the RQ remained less than 1. This suggests that critically ill patients have continued fat oxidation even with sufficient calories [88]. A similar study compared mechanically ventilated patients without chronic lung disease to mechanically ventilated patients with COPD. They also found increased VCO_2 and RQ when patients received dextrose as the sole non–protein calorie source. Only a few studies have been performed involving enteral nutrition in patients with respiratory failure. Angelillo et al. [97] compared a low-, medium-, and high-fat diet in ambulatory patients with COPD, in a randomized, prospective double-blind design. Patients who received the high-fat, low-carbohydrate diet had lower VCO_2 and RQ values. Al-Saady et al. [98] compared two calorically dense enteral products (standard carbohydrate and fat versus high fat) in stable ventilated patients. They reported less CO_2 production and less average time on the ventilator with the high-fat formula, but it is unclear if the calories provided were equal between groups. Other researchers [99] have found the level of calories to have a greater effect than the level of carbohydrate. Currently, there are no published studies comparing enteral formulas designed for respiratory failure, so decisions on enteral formulas should be based on formula composition.

RECOMMENDATIONS. Overall recommendations for nutrition support in the care of respiratory failure are straightforward. Most importantly, early intervention may prevent further complications from nutritional depletion. The benefits of enteral feeding warrant aggressive attempts to feed using the GI tract, taking precautions against aspiration. Fluid may need to be restricted to 1 to 1.5 liters daily. Protein can be provided as 1.5 to 2.0 gm per kilogram and decreased to 1.2 gm per kilogram when fatigue is a concern. Electrolytes and minerals, particularly phosphorus, should be monitored and supplemented when necessary. Finally, overfeeding must be avoided by measuring energy requirements and monitoring weight. Indirect calorimetry should be performed to estimate calorie requirements when providing nutrition support to patients in acute respiratory failure. To avoid overfeeding and excessive CO_2 production, calories should provide for maintenance during respiratory failure, and for repletion only when respiratory function is stable. If VCO_2 continues to be excessive, a trial of a higher-fat formula may be worthwhile. When using higher fat in nutrition support regimens, serum triglycerides and overall tolerance

Table 202-7. Respiratory Failure Enteral Formula Product Comparison

	High-fat low-carbohydrate				Calorically dense			
	Pulmocare (Ross Labs)	Respalor (Mead Johnson)	Nutrivent (Clintec Nutrition Co.)	Glucerna (Ross Labs)	Deliver 2.0 (Mead Johnson)	TwoCal HN (Ross Labs)	Magnacal (Sherwood Nutrition)	Nutren 2.0 (Clintec Nutrition Co.)
Carbohydrate								
gm/1000 kcal	70.5	97	67	93.7	100	108.6	125	98
% kcal	28	39	27	33	40	43.2	50	38
Protein								
gm/1000 kcal	4.17	50	45	41.8	38	41.8	35	40
% kcal	17	20	18	17	15	17	14	16
Fat								
gm/1000 kcal	62.2	46.7	63	55.7	51	45.4	40	53
% kcal	55	41	55	50	45	40.1	36	45
Source	55% canola 20% MCT 14% corn oil 7% safflower	30% MCT 70% canola	40% MCT 43% canola 13% corn	85% safflower oil 15% soybean oil	70% soy oil 30% MCT	80% corn oil 20% MCT	Soy oil	Canola, MCT
Omega 6:Omega 3	4:1	2.4:1	4:1	17.8:1	6.72:1	N/A	7.6:1	4:1
Caloric density	1.5	1.52	1.5	1.0	2.0	2.0	2.0	2.0
Sodium								
mg/1000 kcal	873	835	500	930	400	655	500	500
mEq/1000 kcal	38	36	22	40.4	17.5	28.4	21.8	21.7
Phosphorus								
mg/1000 kcal	704	467	800	704	500	526	500	700

should be monitored. All of these recommendations can be achieved with parenteral and/or enteral solutions. Like all critically ill patients, respiratory failure patients should receive parenteral nutrition only when the GI tract is dysfunctional or enteral nutrition has failed. Enteral nutrition support is the most preferable route for nutrition support, and feeding into the small bowel rather than into the stomach may help to avoid the risk of aspiration. Specialty enteral formulas can be selected or modular components can be added to a standard formula to achieve the desired macronutrient profile.

References

1. Fischer JE: Metabolism in surgical patients: Protein, carbohydrate and fat utilization by oral and parenteral routes, in Sabiston DC, Jr (ed): *Textbook of Surgery: The Biological Basis of Modern Surgical Practice.* 14th ed. Philadelphia, WB Saunders, pp 103–140.
2. Bessy PQ: Parenteral nutrition and trauma, in Rombeau JL, Caldwell MD (eds): *Parenteral Nutrition.* 2nd ed. Philadelphia, WB Saunders, 1993, pp 538–565.
3. Mattox TW, Teasley-Strausburg KM: Overview of biochemical markers used for nutrition support. *Ann Pharmacother* 25:265, 1991.
4. Long CL, Schaffel N, Geiger JW, et al. Metabolic response to injury and illness: Estimation of energy and protein needs from indirect calorimetry and nitrogen balance. *J Parenter Enteral Nutr* 3:452, 1979.
5. Dietch EA: Multiple organ failure: Pathophysiology and potential future therapy. *Ann Surg* 216:117, 1992.
6. Wilmore DW: Catabolic illness: Strategies for enhancing recovery. *N Engl J Med* 325:695, 1991.
7. Shaw JHF, Wolfe RR: An integrated analysis of glucose, fat, and protein metabolism in severely traumatized patients: Studies in the basal state and the response to total parenteral nutrition. *Ann Surg* 209:63, 1989.
8. Black PR, Brooks DC, Bessey PQ, et al: Mechanisms of insulin resistance following injury. *Ann Surg* 196:420, 1982.
9. Skeie B, Kvetan V, Gil KM, et al: Branched-chain amino acids: Their metabolism and clinical utility. *Crit Care Med* 18:549, 1990.
10. Cerra FB, Caprioli J, Siegel JH, et al: Proline metabolism in sepsis, cirrhosis and general surgery. *Ann Surg* 190:577, 1979.
11. Jahoor F, Shangraw RE, Miyoshi H, et al: Role of insulin and glucose oxidation in mediating the protein metabolism of burns and sepsis. *Am J Physiol* 257 (Endocrinol Metab 20):E323, 1989.
12. Singer P, Burszstein S, Kirvela O, et al: Hypercaloric glycerol in injured patients. Surgery 112:509, 1992.
13. Bell SJ, Mascioli EA, Bistrian BR, et al: Alternative lipid sources for enteral and parenteral nutrition: Long- and medium-chain triglycerides, structured triglycerides and fish oils. *J Am Diet Assoc* 91:74, 1991.
14. Cerra FB, Holman RT, Bankey PE, Mazuski JE: Nutritional pharmacology: Its role in the hypermetabolism-organ failure syndrome. *Crit Care Med* 18:S155, 1990.
15. Daly JM, Reynolds J, Sigal RK, et al: Effect of dietary protein and amino acids on immune function. *Crit Care Med* 18:S86, 1990.
16. Cerra FB, Upson D, Angelico R, et al: Branched chains support postoperative protein synthesis. *Surgery* 92:192, 1982.
17. Cerra FB, Mazuski JE, Chute E, et al: Branched chain metabolic support: A prospective, randomized double blind trial in surgical stress. *Ann Surg* 199:286, 1984.
18. Oki JL, Cuddy PG: Branched-chain amino acid support of stressed patients. *Ann Pharmacother* 23:399, 1989.
19. Melnik G: Parenteral nutrition products, in Zaloga GP (ed): *Nutrition in Critical Care.* St Louis, Mosby-Year Book, 1994.
20. Cerra FB, Blackburn G, Hirsch J, et al: The effect of stress level, amino acid formula, and nitrogen dose on nitrogen retention in traumatic and septic stress. *Ann Surg* 205:282, 1987.
21. Cerra FB, Mazuski J, Teasley K, et al: Nitrogen retention in critically-ill patients is proportional to the branched chain amino acid load. *Crit Care Med* 11:775, 1983.
22. Okada A, Mori S, Totsuka M, et al: Branched-chain amino acids metabolic support in surgical patients: A randomized, controlled trial in patients with subtotal or total gastrectomy in 16 Japanese institutions. *J Parenter Enteral Nutr* 12:332, 1988.
23. Von Meyenfeldt MF, Soeters PB, Vente JP, et al: Effect of branched chain amino acid enrichment of total parenteral nutrition on nitrogen sparing and clinical outcome of sepsis and trauma: A prospective, randomized, double-blind trial. *Br J Surg* 77:924, 1990.
24. Jimenez-Jimenez FJ, Ortiz Leyba C, Morales Menez S, et al: Prospective study on the efficacy of branched-chain amino acids in septic patients. *J Parenter Enteral Nutr* 15:252, 1991.
25. Cerra FB, Shronts EP, Konstantinides NN, et al: Enteral feeding in sepsis: A prospective, randomized, double-blind trial. *Surgery* 98:632, 1985.
26. Yu Y-M, Wagner DA, Walesrewski JL, et al: A kinetic study of leucine metabolism in severely burned patients: A comparison between a conventional and branched-chain amino acid-enriched nutritional therapy. *Ann Surg* 207:421, 1988.
27. Brennan MF, Cerra F, Daly JM, et al: Report of a research workshop: Branched-chain amino acids in stress and injury. *J Parenter Enteral Nutr* 10:446, 1986.
28. Bessey PQ: Invited commentary. *World J Surg* 15:133, 1991.
29. Rolandelli RH, DePaula JA, Guenter P, Rombeau JL: Critical illness and sepsis, in Rombeau JL, Caldwell MD (eds): *Enteral and Tube Feeding.* 2nd ed. Philadelphia, WB Saunders, 1990, pp 288–305.
30. Koretz RL, Meyer JH: Elemental diets—facts and fantasies. *Gastroenterology* 78:393, 1980.
31. Keohane PP, Silk DBA: Peptides and free amino acids, in Rombeau JL, Caldwell MD (eds): *Enteral and Tube Feeding.* Philadelphia, WB Saunders, 1984, pp 44–59.
32. Silk DA, Fairclough PD, Clark ML, et al: Use of peptide rather than amino acid nitrogen source in chemically defined "elemental" diets. *J Parenter Enteral Nutr* 4:548, 1980.
33. Brinson RR, Pitts WM: Enteral nutrition in the critically ill patient: Role of hypoalbuminemia. *Crit Care Med* 17:367, 1989.
34. Brinson RR, Kolts BE: Hypoalbuminemia as an indicator of diarrheal incidence in critically ill patients. *Crit Care Med* 15:506, 1987.
35. Kaminsky MV, Williams SD: Review of the rapid normalization of serum albumin with modified total parenteral nutrition solutions. *Crit Care Med* 18:327, 1990.
36. Heimburger DC: Peptides in clinical perspective. *Nutr Clin Prac* 5:225, 1990.
37. Mowatt-Larrsen CA, Brown RO, Wojtysiak SL, Kudsk KA: Comparison of tolerance and nutritional outcome between a peptide and a standard enteral formula in critically-ill, hypoalbuminemic patients. *J Parenter Enteral Nutr* 16:20, 1992.
38. Patterson ML, Dominguez JM, Lyman B, et al: Enteral feeding in the hypoalbuminemic patient. *J Parenter Enteral Nutr* 14:362, 1990.
39. Shronts EP, Havala T: Enteral nutrition I: Formulas, in Teasley-Strausburg KT, et al (eds): *Nutrition Support Handbook. A Compendium of Products with Guidelines for Usage.* Cincinnati, Harvey Whitney Publishers, 1992, pp 147–186.
40. Slavin J: Commercially available enteral formulas with fiber and bowel function measures. *Nutr Clin Prac* 5:247, 1990.
41. Palacio JL, Rolandelli RH, Settle RG, Rombeau JL: Dietary fibers physiologic effects and potential applications to enteral nutrition, in Rombeau JL, Caldwell MD (eds): *Enteral and Tube Feeding.* 2nd ed. Philadelphia, WB Saunders, 1990, pp 556–574.
42. Silk DBA: Fibre and enteral nutrition. *Gut* 30:246, 1989.
43. Heymsfield SB, Roongspisuthipong C, Evert M, et al: Fiber supplementation of enteral formulas: Effects on the bioavailability of major nutrients and gastrointestinal tolerance. *J Parenter Enteral Nutr* 12:265, 1988.
44. Frankenfield DC, Beyer PL: Soy polysaccharide fiber: Effect on diarrhea in tube fed, head-injured patients. *Am J Clin Nutr* 50:533, 1989.
45. A.S.P.E.N. Board of Directors: Guidelines for the use of parenteral and enteral nutrition in adult and pediatric patients. *J Parenter Enteral Nutr* 17:20SA, 1993.
46. Konstantinides FN: Nitrogen balance studies in clinical nutrition. *Nutr Clin Prac* 7:231-238, 1992.
47. Shronts EP, Lacy J: Metabolic support, in Gottschlich MM, Materese LE, Shronts EP (eds): *Nutrition Support Dietetics, Core Curriculum.* 2nd ed. Silver Spring, MD, ASPEN, 1993, pp 351–365.

48. Fish J, Shronts EP: A case for nitrogen balance vs caloric balance in critically ill patients. *Nutrition and Immunology Digest* 2(1):1, 1993.

49. Hamawy KJ, Moldawer LL, Georgieff M, et al: The effect of lipid emulsion on reticuloendothelial system function in the injured animal. *J Parenter Enteral Nutr* 9:559, 1985.

50. Frankel WL, Evans NJ, Rombeau JL: Scientific rationale and clinical application of parenteral nutrition in critically ill patients, in Rombeau JL, Caldwell MD (eds): *Parenteral Nutrition.* 2nd ed. Philadelphia, WB Saunders, 1993, pp 597–616.

51. Moore FA, Feliciano DV, Andrassy RJ, et al: Early enteral feeding compared with parenteral, reduces post-operative septic complications: The results of a meta-analysis. *Ann Surg* 216:172, 1992.

52. Kudsk KA, Croce MA, Fabian TC, et al: Enteral versus parenteral feeding: Effects on septic morbidity after blunt and penetrating abdominal trauma. *Ann Surg* 215:503, 1992.

53. Conn HO, Atterbury CE: Cirrhosis, in Schiff L, Schiff ER (eds): *Diseases of the Liver.* 7th ed. Philadelphia, JB Lippincott, 1993, pp 875–934.

54. Gimson AES, O'Grady J, Roland J, et al: Late onset hepatic failure: Clinical, serological and histologic features. *Hepatology* 6:288, 1986.

55. Soeters PB, Fischer JE: Insulin, glucagon, amino acid imbalances and hepatic encephalopathy. *Lancet* 2:880, 1976.

56. Blei AT, Robbins DC, Drobny E, et al: Insulin resistance and insulin receptors in hepatic cirrhosis. *Gastroenterology* 83:1191, 1982.

57. Riegler JL, Lake JR: Fulminant hepatic failure. *Med Clin North Am* 77:1057, 1993.

58. Fischer JE, Rosen HM, Ebeid AM, et al: The effect of normalization of plasma amino acids on hepatic encephalopathy in man. *Surgery* 80:77, 1976.

59. Conn HO: Hepatic encephalopathy, in Schiff L, Schiff ER (eds): *Diseases of the Liver.* 7th ed. Philadelphia, JB Lippincott, 1993, pp 1036–1060.

60. Record CO: Neurochemistry of hepatic encephalopathy. *Gut* 32:1261, 1991.

61. Fischer JE, Baldessarini RJ: Pathogenesis and therapy of hepatic coma, in Popper H, Schaffner F (eds): *Progress in Liver Disease.* vol V. New York, Grune & Stratton, 1976, pp 363–397.

62. Hoyumpa AM, Schneker S: Perspectives in hepatic encephalopathy. *J Lab Clin Med* 100:477, 1982.

63. Basile AS, Hughes RD, Harrison PM, et al: Elevated brain concentrations of 1,4-benzodiazepines in fulminant hepatic necrosis. *N Engl J Med* 325:473, 1991.

64. Marsano L, McCalin CJ: Nutrition and alcoholic liver disease. *J Parenter Enteral Nutr* 15:337, 1991.

65. Eriksson LS, Conn HO: Branched-chain amino acids in the management of hepatic encephalopathy: An analysis of variants. *Hepatology* 10:228, 1989.

66. Talbot JM: Medical foods for specific diseases and disorders, in Guidelines for the scientific review of enteral food products for special medical purposes. *J Parenter Enteral Nutr* 15:115S, 1991.

67. Mattox TW, Brown RO: Use of modified amino acid formulas in the enteral nutrition support of patients with portosystemic encephalopathy: A review. *Nutrition* 4:7, 1988.

68. Naylor CP, O'Rourke K, Detsky AS, et al: Parenteral nutrition with branched-chain amino acids in hepatic encephalopathy: A meta-analysis. *Gastroenterology* 97:1033, 1989.

69. Cerra FB, Cheung NK, Fischer JE, et al: Disease specific amino acid infusion (F080) in hepatic encephalopathy: A prospective, randomized, double-blind, controlled trial. *J Parenter Enteral Nutr* 9:288, 1985.

70. Shronts EP, Fish J: Hepatic failure, in Gottschlich MM, Matarese LE, Shronts EP (eds): *Nutrition Support Dietetics, Core Curriculum.* 2nd ed. Silver Spring, MD, ASPEN, 1993, pp 311–326.

71. Fischer JE: Branched-chain enriched amino acid solutions in patients with liver failure: An early example of nutritional pharmacology. *J Parenter Enter Nutr* 14(5):249S, 1990.

72. Freund HR: Renal failure, in Lang CE (ed): *Nutritional Support in Critical Care.* Rockville, MD, Aspen Publishers, 1987, pp 315–328.

73. Maliakkal RJ, Bistrian BR: Nutritional support of ICU patients with acute renal failure: Steps to foster protein synthesis, reverse catabolism, reduce mortality. *J Crit Illness* 7(8):1261, 1992.

74. Giordano C: Use of exogenous and endogenous urea for protein synthesis in normal and uremic subjects. *J Lab Clin Med* 62:231, 1963.

75. Giovannetti S, Maggiore Q: A low nitrogen diet with protein of high biological value for severe chronic uremia. *Lancet* 1:1000, 1964.

76. Abel RM, Abbott WM, Fisher JE: Acute renal failure: Treatment without dialysis by total parenteral nutrition. *Arch Surg* 103:512, 1971.

77. Feinstein EL, Bumenkrantz MJ, Healy M, et al: Clinical and metabolic responses to parenteral nutrition in acute renal failure. *Medicine* 60:124, 1981.

78. Pelosi G, Proietti R, Areagneli A, et al: Total parenteral nutrition infusate: An approach to its optimal composition in post-trauma acute renal failure. *Resuscitations* 9:45, 1981.

79. Mirtallo JM, Schneider PJ, Mavko K, et al: A comparison of essential and general amino acid infusion in the nutritional support of patients with compromised renal function. *J Parenter Enteral Nutr* 6:109, 1982.

80. Nakasaki H, Katavama T, Yokoyama S: Complication of parenteral nutrition composed of essential amino acids and histidine in adults with renal failure. *J Parenter Enteral Nutr* 17:86, 1993.

81. Varcol AR, Halliday D, Carson ER, et al: Oral essential amino acids in the management of acute and chronic renal failure. *Am J Clin Nutr* 31:1601, 1978.

82. Sofio CA, Nicora RW, Osborn TW, et al: Oral essential amino acids in the management of acute and chronic renal failure. *J Parenter Enteral Nutr* 3:506, 1979 (Abstract).

83. Pemberton CM, Moxness KM, German MJ, et al: *Mayo Clinic Diet Manual.* 6th ed. Philadelphia, B.C. Decker, 1988, p 225.

84. Wilson DO, Rogers RM, Wright EC, et al: Body weight in chronic obstructive pulmonary disease: The National Institutes of Health intermittent positive-pressure breathing trial. *Am Rev Respir Dis* 139:1435, 1989.

85. Openbrier DR, Irwin MN, Rogers RM, et al: Nutritional status and lung function in patients with emphysema and chronic bronchitis. *Chest* 83:17, 1983.

86. Schols A, Mostert R, Soeters P, et al: Inventory of nutritional status in patients with COPD. *Chest* 96:247, 1989.

87. Arora NS, Rochester DF: Effect of body weight and muscularity on human diaphragm muscle mass, thickness and area. *J Appl Physiol* 52:64, 1982.

88. Mowatt-Larssen CA, Brown RO: Therapy review: Specialized nutritional support in respiratory disease. *Clin Pharm* 12(4):276, 1993.

89. Whittaker JC, Ryan CF, Buckley PA, et al: The effects of refeeding on peripheral and respiratory muscle function in malnourished chronic obstructive pulmonary disease patients. *Am Rev Respir Dis* 142:283, 1990.

90. Keys A, Brozek J, Hesnschel A, et al: *Biology of Human Starvation.* Minneapolis, University of Minnesota Press, 1950.

91. Schols AM, Fredrix EW, Soeters PB, et al: Resting energy expenditure in patients with chronic obstructive pulmonary disease. *Am J Clin Nutr* 54:983, 1991.

92. Takala J: Branch chain amino acids and respiratory function in man, in Kinney JM, Brown PR (eds): *Perspectives in Clinical Nutrition.* Baltimore, Urban & Schwarzenberg, 1989.

93. Askanazi J, Rosenbaum SH, Hylman AL, et al: Respiratory changes induced by large glucose loads of total parenteral nutrition. *JAMA* 243:1444, 1980.

94. A.S.P.E.N. Board of Directors: Guidelines for the Use of Parenteral and Enteral Nutrition in Adult and Pediatric Patients. *J Parenter Enteral Nutr* 17(4)(Suppl):17SA, 1993.

95. Gravelyn TR, Brophy N, Siegert C, et al: Hypophosphatemia-associated respiratory muscle weakness in general inpatient population. *Am J Med* 84:870, 1988.

96. Askanazi J, Nordenstrum J, Rosenbaum SH, et al: Nutrition for the patient with respiratory failure: Glucose vs fat. *Anesthesiology* 54:373, 1981.

97. Angelillo VA, Bedi S, Durfee D, et al: Effects of low and high carbohydrate feedings in ambulatory patients with chronic obstructive pulmonary disease and chronic hypercapnia. *Ann Intern Med* 103:883, 1985.

98. Al-Saady N, Blackmore C, Bennet ED: High fat, low carbohydrate enteral feedings reduce $PaCO_2$ and the period of ventilation in ventilated patients. *Chest* 94(Suppl):49S, 1989.

99. Talpers SS, Romberger DJ, Bunce SB, Pingleton SK: Nutritionally associated increased carbon dioxide production excess total calories vs high proportion of carbohydrate calories. *Chest* 102:551, 1992.

203. Modulating the Inflammatory Response and Its Associated Immune Dysfunction

Frank B. Cerra

The characterization of the systemic inflammatory response and multiple organ dysfunction (SIRS-MODS) and its associated physiology and metabolism have been presented in earlier chapters in this section. A summary of some of their manifestations is presented in Tables 203-1 and 203-2.

Immune Dysfunction as a Manifestation of the Inflammatory Response

Dysfunction of the specific and nonspecific immune systems is a major feature of SIRS-MODS, one manifestation of which is nosocomial infections. The specific antigen response system is complex and has a number of potential areas where dysfunction could occur (Fig. 203-1). Hemorrhage, tissue injury, and bacterial products can produce alterations in T-cell function [1,2,3]. The ability of CD4 and CD8 cells to respond to specific antigens is diminished. There is reduced release by CD4 Th1 cells of TNF, IL-2, and interferon, and an increased release by CD4 Th2 cells of IL-4, IL-5, and IL-10. In addition, there are excessive amounts of prostaglandin E_2 in the cell-cell interaction milieu [4]. The net result of this altered signaling may be a reduced capacity of antigen processing and presentation functions and reduced proliferative responses by the T-cell system [1–5]. Thus, the dysfunction in the immune system is most likely a reflection of the inflammatory process itself.

Nosocomial infections are typical of SIRS-MODS and usually begin 7 to 10 days following injury. The major sites are sinuses, lower respiratory tract, invasive lines or prosthetic devices, and urinary tract. The organisms involved tend to be those harbored in the gut. Within a few days of injury, the enteral flora will have colonized the skin, upper gut, and respiratory tract in up to 80 percent of patients. Within 7 to 10 days of injury, up to 80 percent of those colonized will manifest a nosocomial infection. Organisms that are characteristic of these infections include *Pseudomonas* species, *Enterobacter* or *Klebsiella* species, *Candida* species, and *Staphylococcus epidermis*. These pathogens are frequently found in aspirates of gastric contents, sinuses, line infections, and in pneumonias.

There are two mechanisms hypothesized through which this colonization could occur, both originating from a failure of the gut barrier functions. In one, the organisms move up the gut from colon to small bowel to stomach to respiratory tract [6]. In the other, the organisms move through the wall of the gut and into regional lymph drainage and then systemically [7,8]. The organisms that move are primarily the gut aerobic flora that reside in the lumen, and not the anaerobic flora that reside in the crypts. The precise mechanisms responsible for these phenomena are not clear. Generally, the mechanisms are felt to include ischemia-reperfusion injury during shock and resuscitation, mucosal atrophy resulting from bowel rest, reduced function of the nonspecific immune system such as decreased IgA production, and the inflammatory response itself within the gut. It is also hypothesized that the gut may be another source of increased systemic inflammatory mediator release. Whether the upward migration of bacteria in the gut lumen is enhanced by gastric pH modulation in the prevention of stress ulceration remains controversial [9,10]. Attempts to suppress the gut flora with selective decontamination regimens are associated with reduced nosocomial colonization and infection rates, but no demonstrable improvement in patient outcomes [11].

Table 203-1. Characteristics of the Inflammatory Response

Physiologic response	Mediators
Vasodilatation	Hageman factor, bradykinin, lactate, acidosis, nitric oxide, prostacyclin
Vasoconstriction	Thromboxane, leukotriene B4,C5a
Vascular permeability	PgE2, C3a, C5a, leukotriene C and D, Hageman factor, bradykinin, prostacyclin
PMN chemotaxis, adherence, phagocytosis	Interleukin1, C3a, C5a, PAF, TNF, fibrinectin, heparan, collagen fragments, leukotriene, laminin
Fever	TNF, interleukin, PgE2
Pain	PgE2

Table 203-2. Characteristics of the Systemic Inflammatory Response*

Characteristic	Starvation	Systemic inflammation
Oxygen consumption	−	+ +
Cardiac output	−	+ +
Systemic vascular resistance	NC	− −
Gluconeogenesis	−	+ + +
Ketonemia	+ + +	−
Proteolysis	+	+ + +
Ureagenesis	+	+ +
Total nitrogen excretion	+	+ + +
Net catabolism	+	+ + +
Lipolysis	+	+ +
Acute phase protein synthesis	+	+ +
Rate of malnutrition developing	+	+ + +
Neuroendocrine activation	−	+ +
Cytokine production	−	+ +

* − = decreased; + = increased; NC = no change.

IMMUNEDYSFUNCTION: SPECIFIC ANTIGEN RESPONSE

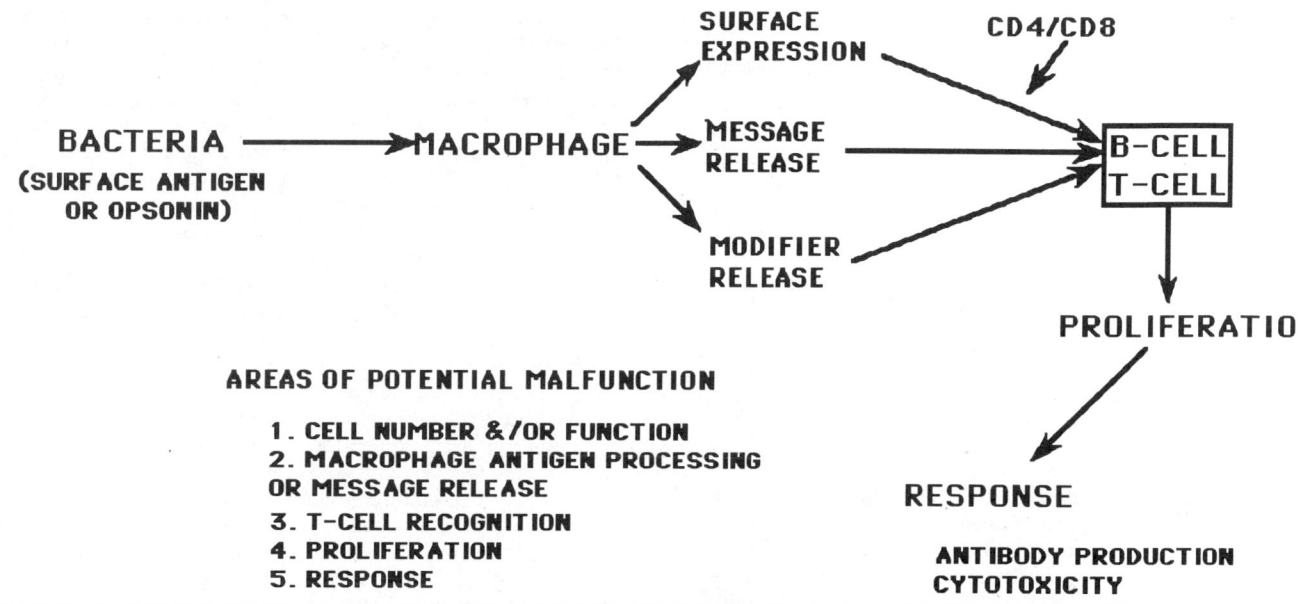

Fig. 203-1. Immune dysfunction: Specific antigen response.

General Nutrition Support of the Inflammatory Response

The metabolic response to injury increases nutrient requirements, and deficiency states can develop rapidly in the absence of the provision of adequate amounts of nutrients. This relates in part to the increased metabolic needs, in part to the inaccessibility of body stores during the inflammatory response, and in part to increased losses in stool, urine, wounds and body fluids. Examples of such deficiency states are presented in Table 203-3. Thus, one of the major therapeutic modalities in supporting immune function is adequate general nutrition support. This approach is presented in the Chapters 201 and 202 on enteral and parenteral nutrition in this section.

Recent research has focused on the route and timing of nutrient administration as a therapeutic mechanism for preserving or restoring gut barrier function and reducing nosocomial infection rates. This is quite a different approach from that of parenteral nutrition. The effect of current parenteral nutrition on immune function appears to be in the prevention of nutrient deficiencies and in the treatment of moderate to severe malnutrition, frequently not present until several days after injury. The effect of enteral nutrition on immune function appears to be directly on gut barrier and immune functions as well as that of providing general nutrition support. The clinical studies most illustrative of this point were performed in patients who sustained abdominal trauma [12,13,14]. An abdominal trauma index of 15 or greater was required for admission to these randomized, prospective studies with feeding started 12 to 24 hours following injury. The first study evaluated 98 trauma patients with the primary outcome being infectious complications

over a 15-day study period [12]. A significant reduction in infectious complications was observed in the enterally fed group. The septic complications included pneumonia, abdominal abscess formation, line sepsis, empyema, fasciitis, and wound dehiscence.

The second study evaluated 75 patients who had sustained abdominal trauma [13]. The primary outcome analysis was septic complications. Feedings were adjusted to achieve maximum nitrogen retention. A substantial early elevation in visceral proteins and a reduction in infectious complications from 37 percent to 17 percent was observed in the enterally fed group. The third study was a meta-analysis of eight prospective, randomized clinical trials performed in different institutions where the same enteral and parenteral formulas were used in all studies and feedings were begun within 30 hours of injury [13]. Four studies were performed exclusively in trauma patients with an abdominal trauma index of 15 or greater and four studies were performed in trauma/general surgery patients. A total of 118 patients received enteral nutrition, with 26 dropouts; and a total of 112 patients received total parenteral nutrition (TPN), with 10 dropouts. The first analysis excluded all dropouts and demonstrated a difference in infectious complications of 17 percent (18% enteral and 35% TPN). The second analysis included all patients (intent to treat) and confirmed the first analysis.

Since these studies all provided early nutrition support, the consideration of another study is necessary to evaluate the issue of the timing of initiation of nutrition support relative to the injury event and the onset of the inflammatory response. This study evaluated patient outcome when either enteral nutrition or parenteral nutrition was begun after the systemic inflammatory response was established [15]. The study was performed in 66 general surgery intensive care unit (ICU) patients who were randomized to receive either enteral or parenteral nutrition after the systemic inflammatory response was established.

Table 203-3. Specific Nutrient Deficiencies

Amino acid	
BcAA LYS METH	
ARG	More bacterial infections
	T-cell and macrophage functions decreased
	Lymphoproliferative responses suppressed
METH	Decreased complement levels (C3)
PHE/TYR	Decreased phagocyte function
Vitamins	
C	Reduced chemotaxis and random migration
A	Lymphoid atrophy, decreased T and B function, decreased phagocytosis
E	Antioxidant
	High doses suppressant and low doses stimulant to immune function
Trace elements	
Iron	Decreased phagocytic bactericidal activity
Zinc	Lymphoid atrophy; T and B cell dysfunction; impaired phagocytosis and impaired wound healing
Selenium	Impaired antibody production; cardiomyopathy
Magnesium	Arrhythmias, particularly ventricular

Nutrition intake was adjusted to achieve maximum nitrogen retention. There were no demonstrable effects of the route of nutrition administration on nutrition outcomes or on such patient outcomes as the incidence of organ failure or mortality.

Thus, there appears to be a window within which the enteral route can improve patient outcome in those patients in whom enteral nutrition can be performed. This window appears to be the initiation of enteral nutrition sometime between the injury event and the establishment of the systemic inflammatory response. The patient outcome where there was benefit was a reduced incidence of infectious complications in the enterally fed group when the nutrition support was initiated within the first 1 or 2 days after injury. This reduction in infection rate appears to be for both line sepsis and for infections other than line sepsis. Presumably, this beneficial outcome effect represents an effect of the enteral nutrients on gut barrier and immune functions.

Nutrients as Modulators of the Inflammatory Response

The concept has evolved that the inflammatory response itself can become a pathogenic mechanism for the organ dysfunctions and may be a major contributing factor to the morbidity, mortality, and cost associated with SIRS-MODS. Thus, therapies are being directed at modulating the inflammatory response. These therapies are both specific and nonspecific. Specific therapy is targeted against a defined mediator, such as endotoxin, IL-1 receptors, or TNF (Fig. 203-2). One of the best studied specific therapies is the monoclonal antibody directed against endotoxin [16]. When this antibody was administered to new ICU admissions who had infection with sepsis and gram-negative bacteremia, a reduction in mortality was observed. Unfortunately, this beneficial effect did not hold up in further clinical studies. Currently, a number of monoclonal antibodies targeted against various mechanisms involved in the pathogenesis of the inflammatory response are either in testing or going into testing. They include antibodies designed to interfere with PMN adher-

ence (anti CD 18 or CD 11), IL-1 receptors, or to bind TNF. To date, the results are disappointing. Testing is continuing, and it is fully anticipated that combination therapy with multiple agents administered together or at various timing intervals will also be undertaken.

The other approach to modulating the inflammatory response and its associated immune dysfunction does not focus on specific mediators. Rather, this approach focuses on the cells producing mediators and the target cells for these mediators (Fig. 203-3). These nonspecific therapies are targeted at general response mechanisms such as second messenger generation, eicosanoid release from cell membranes, and the molecular regulation of metabolism. Specific nutrients constitute the agents under investigation. These nutrients are designed to effect specific cell functions. Thus, the approach is often referred to as *nutrient pharmacology.* The best studied targeted nutrients are those whose use is designed to suppress the overactive macrophage and reduce the output of interleukin, TNF, and eicosanoids such as PgE_2 and LTb_4, and whose use is designed to stimulate lymphocyte proliferation in response to specific antigen stimulation. The former would include w-3 PUFA such as eicosapentanoic acid (EPA) and docasahexanoic acid (DHA); and the latter would include arginine, uracil or ribonucleic acid (RNA), and omega-3 polyunsaturated fatty acids.

Arginine is a potent endocrinologic secretagogue that can stimulate the release of growth hormone, prolactin, insulin, and glucagon. In cell culture systems it is essential for growth but not viability or release of cytokine. Arginine is an essential component in polyamine and nucleic acid synthesis and thus is necessary for mitotic responses [17–20]. Arginine is also a major source of nitric oxide [21]. Nitric oxide is an important mediator of vascular dilatation, of protein synthesis in hepatocytes, and of electron transport in hepatocyte mitochondria. A number of immune effects have also been observed with the administration of arginine, including increased survival in septic animals; increased survival of tumor-bearing animals; an increase in the number of T cells and delayed hypersensitivity responses in athymic nude mice; increased thymic and peripheral blood lymphocyte responses to mitogen-induced blastogenesis; and increased allograft rejection in rodents [22]. Clinical data suggest that arginine supplementation may be associated with reduced length of stay following major cancer surgery [23].

Purines and pyrimidines are precursors of deoxyribonucleic acid (DNA) and ribonucleic acid (RNA). Restriction of dietary nucleotides results in suppression of cellular immune responses and prolongation of allograft survival in rodents [24–27]. Uracil administration in mice can restore delayed-type hypersensitivity responses to various foreign antigens, stimulate T-cell antigenic proliferative responses in T cells, and reduce abscess formation to gram-positive organisms. Dietary nucleotides may also be effective in promoting macrophage activation of the T helper/inducer populations. Uracil has also been reported to reverse the immunosuppression associated with blood transfusion in experimental settings [27].

The polyunsaturated fatty acids (PUFA) are a major component of the cell membrane. They are responsible for the structural integrity of membranes, eicosanoid production and release, and signal transduction through the phospholipid-dependent second messenger pathways. The major PUFA constituents of membranes are of the n-6 family. There are very low levels of the n-3 family, which are major constituents of fish oils. The incorporation of n-3 PUFA, such as 20:5n-3 (EPA) and 22:5n-3 (DHA), into macrophages occurs within 3 to 6 hours in cell culture and is stabilized within a few days in vivo [28]. Once incorporated, fluidity increases, inositol phosphate production and dienoic eicosanoid release are reduced, and interleukin release and tumor necrosis factor release in re-

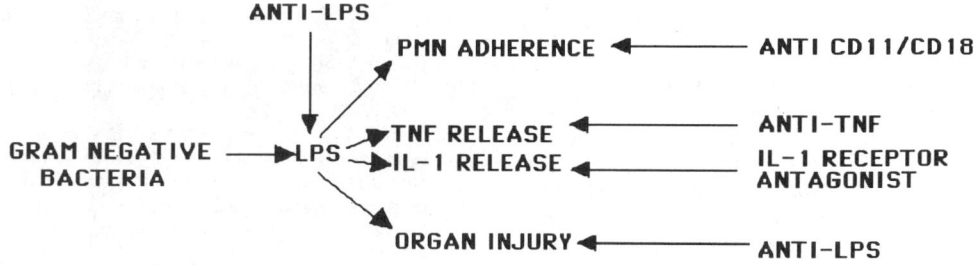

MULTIPLE(SEQUENTIAL) HIGHLY SPECIFIC ANTI-INFLAMMATORY THERAPY FOR SEPSIS-MOF

Fig. 203-2. Multiple (sequential) highly specific antiinflammatory therapy for sepsis-MOF.

sponse to lipopolysaccharide are altered [28,29]. The release of dienoic eicosanoids and TNF and IL1 release by the macrophage are related to the n-6:n-3 ratio and n-3 and n-6 total PUFA content of the cell membrane [28,29,30]. The prostanoid products of eicosapentanoic acid (20:5 n-3) are less inflammatory than those of linoleic acid (18:2 n-6). A relative excess of linoleic acid substrate stimulates PGE$_2$ production, which decreases the ability of cytokines to stimulate IL-2 synthesis by endothelial cells and suppresses T-cell proliferative responses to lectin and specific antigen stimulation [28,29,30]. In rat models of bacterial peritonitis, n-3 PUFA in the diet was associated with a reduction in mortality [31].

These three nutrients have been combined and provided in studies of enteral nutrition support. Since all these nutrients were present in the enteral formulas, an evaluation of the effects of the components is not possible. One study was performed in patients sustaining burn injury [32]. The study diet consisted of a modular tube feeding formula of whey protein enriched with arginine, cysteine, and histidine; low in total fat and re-stricted in linoleic acid; and enriched with omega-3 PUFA. The two control diets were high in n-6 PUFA, with a low and high nonprotein calorie-to-nitrogen ratio. Fifty patients normalized for burn size and severity were studied for a 3- to 4-week period. The experimental formula was associated with significant reductions in wound infection and length of stay adjusted for percent burn. Another series of studies evaluated an enteral formula fortified with menhaden oil, arginine, and ribonucleic acid. The first study evaluated the effects of this formula on in vitro tests of immune function in surgical ICU patients [33]. The experimental formula consistently enhanced these in vitro tests. Another study evaluated these same formulas in 88 patients undergoing upper gastrointestinal surgery for malignancy [34]. The results of this study confirmed the observations made with the in vitro tests of immune function and also observed a significant reduction in length of stay and in infectious complications in patients who received the enhanced formula. The last study was a multicenter trial in which the primary outcome variable was length of stay [35]. The dominant patient group was patients who sustained multiple trauma. A significant reduction in length of stay and in infectious complications was observed, and formula composition functioned as an independent variable. There were no observed differences in mor-

Fig. 203-3. Nonspecific modulation of inflammatory and immune function.

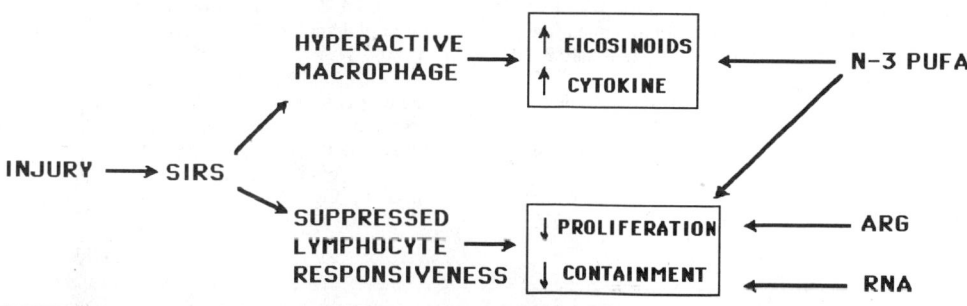

NONSPECIFIC MODULATION OF INFLAMMATORY AND IMMUNE FUNCTION

tality. The mortality observed was much less than that predicted by the APACHE II score or TISS score, perhaps reflecting the use of early enteral feeding. The experimental formula appeared to help those patients who were going to survive to survive more rapidly. Reductions in length of stay and infectious complications and the incidence of organ failures have been observed in other recent studies that have employed immune-enhancing enteral formulas [35–38].

Summary and Conclusions

Alterations in immune function with an increased incidence of acquired infections appear to be one of the consequences of the inflammatory response following injury. Nutrition support can modulate this effect of the inflammatory response on immune responsiveness with an associated reduction in acquired infections and, in some studies, significant reductions in length of stay. These beneficial patient outcomes are related to the route and timing of nutrient administration and the composition of the formula administered. Enteral nutrition that is initiated as soon as possible after resuscitation has been achieved following tissue injury and that utilizes formula compositions that can enhance immune function appears to be associated with the beneficial outcome effects. These effects are observed when appropriate general nutrition is provided so that generalized and single nutrient deficiencies are effectively treated or prevented.

References

1. Munster AM, Winchurch RA, Birmingham WJ, et al: Longitudinal assay of lymphocyte responsiveness in patients with major burns. *Ann Surg* 192:772, 1980.
2. Abraham E, Chang Y-H: The effects of hemorrhage on mitogen-induced lymphocyte proliferation. *Circ Shock* 15:171, 1985.
3. Abraham E, Regan RF: The effects of hemorrhage and trauma on interleukin 2 production. *Arch Surg* 120:1341, 1985.
4. Meyer JD, Yurt RW, Duhaney R, et al: Tumor necrosis factor-enhanced leukotriene B4 generation and chemotaxis in human neutrophils. *Arch Surg* 123(12):1454, 1988.
5. Kinsella J, Lakesh B, Boughton S: Dietary PUFA and eicosanoids potential effects on the modulation of inflammation and immune cells. *Nutrition* 6:24, 1
6. Atherton ST, White DJ: Stomach as a source of bacteria colonising respiratory tract during artificial ventilation. *Lancet* 2:968, 1983.
7. Deitch EA, Maejima K, Berg R: Effect of oral antibiotics and bacterial overgrowth on the translocation of the GI-tract microflora in burned rats. *J Trauma* 25:385, 1985.
8. Wells CL, Maddaus MA, Simmons RL: Proposed mechanism for the translocation of enteric bacteria. *Rev Infect Dis* 10:958, 1988.
9. Driks M, Craven DE, Bartolome R, et al: Nosocomial pneumonia in intubated patients given sucralfate as compared with antacids or histamine type 2 blockers. *N Engl J Med* 317:1376, 1987.
10. Ryan P, Dawson J, Teres D, et al: Continuous infusion of cimetidine vs sucralfate: Incidence of pneumonia and bleeding compared. *J Crit Care Med* 18(4):S253, 1990.
11. Blair PHB, Rowlands K, Lowry H, et al: A stratified randomized prospective study in a mixed ICU. *Surgery* (in press).
12. Kudsk KA, Croce MA, Fabian TC, et al: Enteral vs parenteral feeding. *Ann Surg* 215:503, 1992.
13. Moore FA, Moore EE, Jonew TN, et al: TEN vs TPN following major abdominal trauma-reduced septic morbidity. *J Trauma* 29:916, 1989.
14. Moore FA, Feliciano DV, Andrassy RJ, et al: Early enteral feeding, compared with parenteral, reduces postoperative septic complications. *Ann Surg* 216:172, 1992.
15. Cerra FB, McPherson J, Konstantinides FN, et al: Enteral nutrition does not prevent multiple organ failure syndrome after sepsis. *Surgery* 104(4):727, 1988.
16. Ziegler EJ, et al: Treatment of gram-negative bacteremia and septic shock with HA-1A human monoclonal antibody against endotoxin. *N Engl J Med* 324:429, 1991.
17. Barbul A: Arginine and immune function. *Nutrition* 6:53, 1990.
18. Rose WC: The nutritional significance of amino acids and certain related comounds. *Science* 86:298, 1937.
19. Barbul A, Sisto DA, Wasserkrug HL, et al. Metabolic and immune effects of arginine in post-injury hyperalimentation. *J Trauma* 21:970, 1981.
20. Barbul A, Wasserkrug HL, Sisto DA, et al: Thymic and immune stimulatory actions of arginine. *J Parenter Enteral Nutr* 4:446, 1980.
21. Stuehr D, Gross S, Sakuma I, et al: Activated murine macrophages secrete a metabolite of arginine with the bioactivity of endothelium-derived relaxing factor and the chemical reactivity of nitric oxide. *J Exp Med* 169:1011, 1989.
22. Barbul A, Sisto DA, Wasserkrug HL, et al: Arginine stimulates lymphocyte immune response in healthy humans. *Surgery* 90:244, 1981.
23. Reynolds JV, Thom AK, Zhang SM, et al: Arginine, protein calorie malnutrition and cancer. *J Surg Res* 45:513, 1988.
24. Kulkarni SS, Bhateley DC, Zander AR, et al: Functional impairment of T lymphocytes in mouse radiation chimeras by a nucleotide-free diet. *Exp Hematol* 12:694, 1984.
25. Van Buren CT, Kulkarni AD, Rudolph F: Synergistic effect of a nucleotide-free diet and cyclosporine on allograft survival. *Transplant Proc* Suppl 1-2:2967, 1983.
26. Kulkarni AD, Fanslow WC, Rudolph FB, et al: Effect of dietary nucleotides on response to bacterial infections. *J Parenter Enteral Nutr* 10:169, 1986.
27. Rudolph FB, Kulkarni AD, Fanslow WC, et al: Role of RNA as a dietary source of pyrimidines and purines in immune function. *Nutrition* 6:45, 1990.
28. Kinsella J, Lokesh B, Boughton S, et al: Dietary PUFA and eicosanoids: Potential effects on the modulation of inflammatory and immune cells: An overview. *Nutrition* 6:24, 1990.
29. Holman RT: Control of polyunsaturated acids in tissue lipids. *J Am Coll Nutr* 5:236, 1986.
30. Billiar TR, Bankey PE, Svingen BA, et al: Fatty acid intake and Kupffer cell function: Fish oil alters eicosanoid and monokine production to endotoxin stimulation. *Surgery* 104:343, 1988.
31. Cerra FB, Alden PA, Negro F, et al: Clinical sepsis, endogenous and exogenous lipid modulation. *J Parenter Enteral Nutr* 12:63, 1988.
32. Alexander JW, Saito H, Trocki O, et al: The importance of lipid type in the diet after burn injury. *Ann Surg* 204:1, 1986.
33. Cerra FB, Lehman S, Konstantinides N, et al: Effect of enteral nutrient on in vitro tests of immune function in ICU patients: A preliminary report. *Nutrition* 6:84, 1990.
34. Daly JM, Lieberman D, Goldfine MS, et al: Enteral nutrition with supplemental arginine, RNA, and omega 3 fatty acids in patients after operation: Immunologic, metabolic, and clinical outcome. *Surgery* 112:56, 1992.
35. Bower RH, Cerra FB, Bershadsky B, et al: Early enteral feeding of a formula supplemented with arginine, nucleotides, and fish oil in intensive care unit patients; results of a multicenter, prospective, randomized clinical trial. *Crit Care Med* 23:436, 1995.
36. Moore FA, Moore EE, Kudsk KA, et al: Clinical benefits of an immune-enhancing diet for early postinjury enteral feeding. *J Trauma* 37:607, 1994.
37. Kamen M, Senkal M, Homann H-H, et al: Early postoperative enteral feeding with arginine, n-3 fatty acids and RNA-supplemented diet versus placebo in cancer patients: An immunologic evaluation of impact. *Crit Care Med* 23:652, 1995.
38. Daly J, Weintraub FN, Shou J, et al: Early nutrition during multimodality therapy in upper gastrointestinal cancer patients. *Ann Surg* 221:327, 1995.

204. Transitioning

Joan Mandt Shopbell

Nutritional support has become an essential component of the overall metabolic and supportive therapies utilized in the care of critically ill patients. As changes in the clinical status of these patients occur, the optimal route for delivery of nutrients may change as well.

Transitional feeding occurs when one route of feeding delivery is being changed to another (e.g., parenteral nutrition [PN] to enteral nutrition [EN], enteral to oral nutrition [PO], or any combination of these). The goal is for a smooth transition from one feeding modality to the next without causing a significant disruption in total nutrient intake during the process. Transitional feeding is an important element of total patient care.

This chapter will focus on assessment of the optimal route for feeding delivery and evaluation of nutritional goals. Key concepts in transitioning from parenteral to enteral feeding, parenteral to oral feeding, enteral to oral feeding, and enteral to parenteral feeding will be reviewed. Suggested guidelines for monitoring and case examples are also included.

Assessment of Gastrointestinal Tract Function

Optimal nutrition support requires careful evaluation of the patient's gastrointestinal tract function to determine the most appropriate route for nutrient delivery. Evidence strongly suggests that patients should be fed enterally whenever possible [1]. The guideline to follow is "if the gut works, use it."

Enteral feedings provide several benefits to the patient. Luminal stimulation increases mesenteric blood flow and maintains gut digestive and absorptive functions [1,2,3]. In addition, enteral nutrition has been shown to maintain gut barrier function and decrease the risk for bacterial translocation from the gut. As a result, morbidity and septic complications may be decreased. Enteral feedings are also less costly than total parenteral nutrition (TPN), and the complications related to central venous catheter use may be avoided [1,2,3].

In assessing the readiness of the patient for transition from one feeding modality to another, a number of factors must be considered. Age, disease, surgery, and medical treatments may negatively affect a patient's gastrointestinal tract function [4]. Use of antibiotics, radiation, or chemotherapy will greatly influence a patient's tolerance to enteral nutrients. The length of time the gastrointestinal tract has not been used and the actual gastrointestinal tract surface area available for digestion and absorption also need to be carefully evaluated. Patients with short bowel syndrome, Crohn's disease, radiation enteritis, or severe malnutrition may require the use of modified feeding formulations for optimal tolerance.

Assessment of Nutritional Status

Assessment of the patient's current nutritional status is essential in determining goals for the next phase of nutritional management. This includes assessment of visceral protein nutriture, weight status, weight changes over time, nitrogen balance, fluid status, oral intake, vitamin and mineral nutriture, and medication-related nutrient-drug interactions [2]. Results of this assessment will establish goals for maintenance or repletion of nutritional status. It will then be necessary to estimate nutrient requirements, including energy, protein, fluid, electrolytes, minerals, vitamins, and trace elements. Optimal distribution of carbohydrate, protein, and fat substrates should be based on disease state and clinical status. The nutritional assessment will guide the clinician in choosing an appropriate enteral or parenteral formulation.

The patient's prognosis and anticipated length of therapy will ultimately influence both the route of feeding and the overall goals for nutritional therapy.

Feeding Transitions: Parenteral to Enteral Feeding

As soon as adequate gastrointestinal tract function is present, enteral feedings should be initiated. Assessment of current clinical and nutritional status will enable determination of appropriate goals for caloric and protein intake. Access for enteral feeding must be established using a small-bore nasointestinal feeding tube, gastrostomy, jejunostomy, percutaneous endoscopic gastrostomy (PEG), or percutaneous endoscopic jejunostomy (PEJ), based on the functional capacity of the gastrointestinal tract and anticipated length of therapy.

An appropriate enteral formula must be selected based on nutritional assessment and goals for therapy, as well as gastrointestinal function. Modified nutrient formulas may be indicated in the presence of gastrointestinal disease, intestinal resection, or enteritis.

Generally, enteral feedings may be initiated full strength at a rate of 20 to 50 ml per hour. Gastrointestinal function and length of time the patient has been without oral intake (NPO) should be considered when the initial rate of feedings is determined. Enteral feedings can generally be advanced every 8 to 12 hours, as tolerated, in increments of 20 to 50 ml to goal rate. If intolerance to formula administration develops (i.e., bloating, abdominal distention, diarrhea, cramping), the rate of infusion should be decreased to the previously tolerated level of administration. If intolerance persists, dilution of hyperosmolar formulas may be necessary with a gradual readvancement to full strength and goal rate.

As the enteral feeding is advanced to goal rate of administration, the TPN can be tapered. Ideally, calorie and protein intake should be kept relatively constant during the transition. If protein or fluid restrictions are in place, care must be taken to balance both enteral and parenteral infusions to keep levels of both relatively constant.

As most enteral formulas provide a source of essential fatty acids, the parenteral lipid infusion can generally be discontinued with the initiation of tube feedings. When the patient demonstrates tolerance to the enteral formula at one-third to one-half the goal volume, the parenteral infusion may be decreased by half. Parenteral nutrition may be discontinued when the patient demonstrates tolerance to the enteral feeding at the goal rate established to meet estimated nutritional requirements. A step-by-step summary of the transition from parenteral to enteral feeding is provided in Table 204-1.

CASE EXAMPLE 1: PARENTERAL TO ENTERAL FEEDING.

H.O. is a 72-year-old woman with a history of chronic pulmonary disease and aortic valvular insufficiency with an ascending aortic arch aneurysm. An aortic valve replacement with ascending aortic graft was performed. On postoperative day 1, H.O. was returned to the operating room after developing a mediastinal blood clot.

The gastrointestinal examination revealed a firm, distended abdomen, lack of bowel sounds, and suspected small bowel ileus. At this time, the patient was started on TPN for nutritional support. The formula provided 73 gm of protein (1.5 gm/kg) and 1420 calories per day (130% estimated basal energy expenditure).

On postoperative day 6, the patient's abdomen no longer appeared distended, with resolution of small bowel ileus, and a nasoduodenal feeding tube was placed for transition to enteral feedings. A high-nitrogen, polymeric tube feeding was initiated using full-strength formula at a rate of 20 ml. The IV lipid infusion was discontinued at this time, and the parenteral nutrition infusion was decreased to 50 percent of the previous rate. The enteral feeding was advanced to goal rate 24 hours later. No symptoms of intolerance to the enteral formula infusion were apparent, and the parenteral nutrition infusion was discontinued.

The total nutrient intake during the feeding transition is as follows:

DAY	TPN	ENTERAL FEEDING	TOTAL
1	1420 kcal, 73 gm protein	None	1420 kcal, 73 gm protein
2	950 kcal, 45 gm protein	480 kcal, 27 gm protein	1430 kcal, 72 gm protein
3	514 kcal, 37 gm protein	800 kcal, 45 gm protein	1314 kcal, 82 gm protein
4	Discontinued	1440 kcal, 81 gm protein	1440 kcal, 81 gm protein

Feeding Transitions: Parenteral to Oral Feeding

In transitioning to oral intake from total parenteral nutrition, several factors should be considered. Functional capacity of the gastrointestinal tract should be evaluated on an ongoing basis. As soon as adequate function is confirmed, oral nutrition should be initiated. The patient must be willing and able to eat orally without risk of aspiration. Appropriate goals for calorie and protein intake should be determined based on current clinical and nutritional assessment.

A speech pathology assessment of the patient's functional ability to swallow may be indicated if neurologic or physical deficits are present. This is often helpful in cases involving prolonged use of an endotracheal tube or presence of a tracheostomy. Oral feeding should be initiated using small volumes of a liquid diet of appropriate consistency, and advanced to solid foods according to patient tolerance and physical ability.

Prolonged disuse of the gastrointestinal tract may predispose patients to lactose and fat intolerance and other functional changes [5]. Low-lactose and low-fat foods may be better tol-

Table 204-1. Parenteral to Enteral Feeding

1. Assess adequacy of gastrointestinal function.
2. Determine appropriate goals for calorie and protein intake.
3. Establish appropriate enteral feeding access.
4. Choose an appropriate enteral formula.
5. Initiate formula at a rate of 25–50 ml full strength.
6. Advance the formula every 8–12 hours as tolerated to goal rate.
7. Discontinue the lipid infusion with initiation of enteral feeding.
8. When the patient demonstrates tolerance to the enteral formula at one-third to one-half of the desired volume, the TPN may be decreased to one-half the total volume.
9. TPN may be discontinued when the patient demonstrates tolerance to the enteral formula at a rate adequate to meet estimated nutritional requirements.
10. If restrictions on protein or fluid intake are necessary, care must be taken to balance both enteral and parenteral infusions to keep protein and/or fluid provision relatively constant.

erated initially with a gradual reintroduction of lactose- and fat-containing food to the diet as adaptation occurs. Oral intake should be monitored using calorie and protein counts. Smaller, more frequent meals may also be helpful to reduce stomach distention and feelings of fullness.

Although controversial, some literature exists suggesting that continuous infusion of parenteral nutrition may be associated with suppression of appetite [6]. For this reason, a night-time cyclic schedule for TPN administration may be of benefit. Infusion of nutrients over an 8- to 16-hour period will allow "time off" and may improve appetite during the day.

When daily calorie intake reaches approximately 500 calories, the IV lipid infusion can be discontinued. If protein consumption is near half of estimated requirements to meet goals for nutritional therapy, the parenteral nutrition infusion can be decreased to one-half the volume. When oral intake reaches two-thirds to three-fourths of nutritional needs, parenteral nutrition may be discontinued.

Abrupt discontinuation of parenteral nutrition should be avoided to safeguard against sudden hypoglycemia. The rate should be lowered by 50 percent the first hour, then by 50 percent the second hour, and then discontinued [7].

Monitoring calorie and protein intake should be continued to ensure adequate nutrition. Use of supplements may be necessary to meet nutritional goals. If the patient is unable to continue to meet two-thirds of requirements orally after three to five days, enteral tube feedings should be considered. Table 204-2 summarizes the steps involved in a transition from parenteral nutrition to oral feeding.

CASE EXAMPLE 2: PARENTERAL TO ORAL FEEDING.

L.M., a 27-year-old woman with myelodysplastic syndrome, was admitted for a bone marrow transplant. She underwent two courses of chemotherapy prior to admission. She then received a combination of chemotherapy and radiation therapy in preparation for bone marrow transplant.

L.M. developed radiation enteritis with mucositis and was unable to ingest adequate nutrition orally. As a result of severe mucositis, placement of a feeding tube was contraindicated and TPN was initiated for nutritional support. The formula provided an average of 1750 calories (~ 130% estimated BEE) and 110 gm of protein (1.75 gm/kg). The TPN was continued for 5 weeks. At this time, L.M. was able to resume some oral intake, and calorie counts were initiated. A goal of 1600 to 1800 calories with 60 to 70 gm of protein was set for oral intake.

Table 204-2. TPN to Oral Feeding

1. Assess adequacy of gastrointestinal function.
2. Assess patient's willingness and ability to eat without aspirating.
3. Determine appropriate goals for calorie and protein intake.
4. Begin with small volumes of a clear liquid diet.
5. Advance diet to solid foods as tolerated. Consider the possibility of lactose and fat intolerance and the need for modified food consistencies.
6. Monitor oral intake with calorie and protein counts.
7. A nocturnal cyclic administration for TPN may be considered.
8. When calorie intake reaches approximately 500 calories per day, lipid infusion may be discontinued and the parenteral nutrition infusion decreased to one-half.
9. When oral intake reaches two-thirds to three-fourths of nutritional needs, parenteral nutrition may be discontinued.
10. Avoid abrupt discontinuation of parenteral nutrition infusion. Instead, lower rate by 50% the first hour, then by 50% the second hour, then discontinue infusion.
11. Use of oral nutritional supplements may be necessary to ensure adequate oral intake.
12. If patient is unable to consume two-thirds of requirements orally, enteral tube feeding should be considered.

After several days, L.M. was eating approximately 375 calories and 10 gm of protein. At this time, the IV lipid infusion was discontinued. The parenteral nutrition infusion was continued until oral intake improved.

Five days later, L.M.'s oral intake reached 850 calories and 35 gm of protein, and the parenteral nutrition infusion was decreased to 50 percent of the previous volume. Several days later, L.M.'s oral intake was 1200 calories and 50 gm of protein, and the parenteral nutrition infusion was discontinued. L.M. continued to maintain adequate nutritional intake orally with the addition of enteral supplements.

Feeding Transitions: Enteral to Oral Feeding

It is important to evaluate the ability of a patient to eat orally on an ongoing basis while the patient is receiving enteral feedings. Barring any physical impairments that prevent oral intake, as clinical status improves, oral feedings may gradually be reintroduced. The patient must be alert and willing to eat orally. Assessment of the patient's ability to swallow safely is also very important. Evaluation by a speech pathologist may be indicated prior to initiation of oral intake if there is a question of any deficits in this area. Once the speech pathologist's assessment is complete, an appropriate oral diet may be initiated and advanced as tolerated. Oral intake should be monitored using calorie and protein counts.

As a continuous infusion of enteral nutrients often contributes to a feeling of fullness, a night-time cycle for tube feeding administration may result in an improved appetite during the day. The feeding may be infused over an 8- to 16-hour time period based on patient tolerance and the volume of formula required. Formula volume should be decreased as oral intake improves, resulting in a shorter night-time infusion schedule.

When the patient consumes two-thirds to three-fourths of estimated nutritional requirements orally for two to three days, the tube feeding can be discontinued. Calorie and protein counts should be continued, and if the patient is unable to

achieve and maintain two-thirds to three-fourths of required intake, oral nutritional supplements should be provided. If inadequate oral intake persists and enteral feedings need to be continued indefinitely, education for home enteral nutrition may be required. Teaching for home tube feeding should be provided to the patient, family, or caregivers as appropriate, and ideally prior to discharge from the hospital. Table 204-3 summarizes the steps involved in transition from enteral tube feedings to an oral diet.

CASE EXAMPLE 3: ENTERAL TO ORAL FEEDING. C.O., a 36-year-old woman, was admitted to the medical intensive care unit with severe acute respiratory distress syndrome of unclear etiology. She was intubated and maintained on enteral tube feedings throughout much of her 3-month intensive care unit stay. The enteral feedings provided an average of 1850 calories and 100 gm of protein per day.

A tracheostomy had been placed several weeks after admission. Ten weeks following intubation, C.O.'s clinical and neurologic status had improved sufficiently to allow a trial of oral nutrition. Evaluation by the speech pathologist confirmed adequate swallow function, and a low-fat, low-lactose liquid diet was initiated. Oral intake progressed and the diet was advanced to solid foods as the patient tolerated.

C.O. consumed 575 calories and 20 gm of protein by day 3 and was complaining of a constant feeling of fullness. The tube feeding was then transitioned to a nocturnal infusion providing a total of 1300 calories and 75 gm of protein over 14 hours.

C.O.'s oral intake increased progressively to 1200 calories and 50 gm of protein by day 7, using small, frequent meals and liquid nutritional supplements. The feeding cycle was shortened to 8 hours, with a subsequent increase in oral intake. On day 10 of oral intake, C.O. was consuming a regular diet, 1900 calories, and 84 gm of protein, and the tube feeding was discontinued.

Situations may arise that necessitate a change from enteral tube feedings to parenteral nutrition. Examples may include temporary loss of enteral access, small bowel ileus, bowel obstruction, high-output enteric fistulas, severe intolerance to enteral feedings (i.e., intractable diarrhea, severe abdominal distention, and cramping), or an insult resulting in loss of small bowel function.

In the majority of situations, enteral feedings may already have been discontinued and parenteral nutrition initiated. If abrupt cessation of tube feeding is unnecessary, a gradual decrease in feeding rate should take place as the parenteral nutrition infusion is advanced to the desired goal rate.

Care should be taken to avoid extremes in the level of nutrients provided to guard against hyperglycemia/hypoglycemia

Table 204-3. Enteral Tube Feeding to Oral Intake

1. Assess the patient's willingness and ability to eat and swallow safely.
2. Determine appropriate goals for calorie and protein intake.
3. Begin appropriate oral diet, advancing as tolerated.
4. Monitor oral intake with calorie and protein counts.
5. A nocturnal cycle for tube feeding may improve the patient's appetite during the day.
6. Formula volume should be decreased as oral intake improves.
7. When the patient consumes two-thirds to three-fourths of nutritional requirements by mouth, tube feeding can be discontinued.
8. Oral supplements and calorie/protein counts should be continued as needed.

Table 204-4. Suggested Guidelines for Monitoring

	Parenteral nutrition	Enteral nutrition
Weight	Daily	Daily
Fluid intake/output	Daily	Daily
Bowel function	Daily	Daily
Glucose	Daily to 3×/week	Daily to 2×/week
Electrolytes	Daily to 3×/week	Daily to 2×/week
BUN/creatinine	Daily to 3×/week	Daily to 2×/week
Phosphorus, magnesium	Day 1, then 2×/week	Day 1, then once/week
Calcium, transferrin	Day 1, then once/week	Day 1, then once/week
Albumin, zinc	Day 1, then as indicated	Day 1, then as indicated
Liver function tests, triglycerides	Day 1, then once/week	As needed
Nitrogen balance	Weekly	Weekly

and protein and/or fluid overload. Enteral nutrition should be resumed as soon as gastrointestinal function allows.

Monitoring

Total calorie and protein intake should be monitored carefully during transitional feedings. Adequate nutrient intake is necessary to avoid a decline in nutritional status, and additional nutrient supplementation may be required. On the other hand, it is desirable to avoid excessive calorie and protein intake for a prolonged period during the transition as this can result in complications related to overfeeding [2].

A number of complications can occur as a result of excessive nutrient infusion. For example, hyperglycemia can lead to osmotic diuresis and resulting hyperosmolar nonketotic coma. Sudden discontinuation of an excessive infusion of glucose may result in rebound hypoglycemia. Infusion of excessive carbohydrate or total calories may lead to respiratory insufficiency as a result of increased CO_2 production. Hepatic steatosis and cholestasis have also been associated with excessive parenteral infusions over a prolonged period of time, especially of glucose [8]. Records of parenteral and enteral fluid intake, along with total calorie and protein consumption by the oral route, need to be assessed.

Biochemical assessment should include markers of visceral protein status such as albumin, transferrin, or prealbumin levels. Nitrogen balance studies also assess adequacy of protein intake. Serum electrolytes, blood urea nitrogen, creatinine, glucose, triglycerides, and liver function tests should also be monitored as clinically indicated. Vitamin and mineral status should be assessed if clinical deficiency symptoms are apparent on clinical examination or suspected as a result of clinical status. Table 204-4 summarizes suggested monitoring guidelines.

References

1. Zaloga GP, MacGregor DA: What to consider when choosing enteral or parenteral nutrition. *J Crit Illness* 5(11):1180, 1990.
2. Zibrida JM, Carlson SJ: Transitional feeding, in Gottschlich MM, Matarese LE, Shronts EP (eds): *Nutrition Support Dietetics Core Curriculum.* 2nd ed. Silver Spring, MD, A.S.P.E.N., 1993, pp 459–465.
3. Hasse J, Suneson J: A practical guide to adult nutrition support. Baylor University Medical Center, *Clinical Nutrition Services,* 1990, pp 69–71.
4. Wade J: Parenteral and enteral transition techniques, in Krey SH, Murray RL (eds): *Dynamics of Nutrition Support.* Norwalk, CT, Appleton-Century-Crofts, 1986, pp 489–496.
5. Krey S, Murray R: Modular and transitional feedings, in Rombeau J, Caldwell M (eds): *Clinical Nutrition, Enteral and Tube Feeding.* 2nd ed. Philadelphia, WB Saunders, 1990, pp 140–148.
6. Gil KM, Skeie B, Kvetan V, et al: Parenteral nutrition and oral intake: Effect of glucose and fat infusion. *J Parenter Enteral Nutr* 15:426, 1991.
7. Wagman LD, Miller KB, Thomas RB, et al: The effect of acute discontinuation of total parenteral nutrition. *Ann Surg* 204(5):524, 1986.
8. Freund HR: Abnormalities of liver function and hepatic damage associated with total parenteral nutrition. *Nutrition* 7:1, 1991.
9. Havala T, Shronts EP, Refeeding the chronically malnourished patient. *Nutr Clin Pract* 5(1):23, 1990.

XVI. Pharmacokinetics and Pharmacodynamics

Section Editor
Darwin Zaske

205. Applied Pharmacokinetics: Specific Application for the ICU

Paula L. Townsend, John R. Reynolds, and Darwin E. Zaske

Introduction

In intensive care medicine, the physician frequently encounters patients who exhibit extreme changes in physiologic parameters secondary to injury, sepsis, and/or underlying disease. The magnitude of change can be further altered by therapeutic interventions commonly used by the intensivist to improve oxygen delivery or cardiac output, including fluid therapy, ventilation, and concurrent medications. These critically ill patients require aggressive therapy, and the margin for error is small. The condition of critically ill patients is dynamic, and pharmacokinetic parameters change as therapy progresses and the patient improves.

Recommended dosage regimens are generally based on studies from normal volunteers or a limited number of patients who have minimal disease. Their physiologic and metabolic parameters are obviously much more homogeneous, and they are representative only of the normal population. Patients in the intensive care unit (ICU) have serious or life-threatening medical conditions or injuries. Their physiologic and metabolic parameters are substantially altered from baseline, which directly affects drug disposition and dosage requirements. Many of these changes may not be anticipated by monitoring estimates of renal function (i.e., serum creatinine). The routine use of conventional dosage regimens may expose a substantial portion of the ICU patient population to high risk of treatment failure or drug toxicity. Careful titration of the ICU patient's dosage regimen becomes imperative to ensure the ideal outcome. Serum drug concentration monitoring and pharmacokinetic concepts become clinically important tools to assist in making appropriate dosage adjustments.

This chapter acquaints the clinician with applied pharmacokinetic principles that can be used as a basis for evaluating serum drug concentrations and designing and adjusting drug dosage regimens. Knowledge of the patient's clinical status and functional status of vital organ systems (e.g., cardiovascular system) can be qualitatively used to anticipate which patients require more intensive monitoring of drug regimens. The pharmacokinetic approaches presented here are simplified to increase their clinical utility for ICU patients. For an in-depth understanding of the pharmacokinetic concepts, the reader is referred to one of the many excellent clinical pharmacokinetic textbooks [1,2,3].

Definition

Pharmacokinetics is the study of the relationships between the dose of a drug, the resulting concentration of the drug in the body fluids, and time. Pharmacokinetic mathematical relationships describe the movement of drugs into, throughout, and out of the body. Pharmacodynamics is a more specific study of the relationships between drug concentration and the intensity and time course of the pharmacologic response. Applied pharmacokinetics is the process of using measured drug concentrations, pharmacokinetic principles, and pharmacodynamic information to optimize drug therapy for individual patients. Applied pharmacokinetics thereby becomes a clinical tool that enables the clinician to become more quantitative when adjusting a patient's dosage regimen. The clinician must actively assess the patient's clinical status, define therapeutic endpoints, continually monitor the patient's response, and make appropriate adjustments in the dosage regimen to ensure a satisfactory outcome. Applied pharmacokinetics has become a useful clinical tool prospectively to minimize the effect of the heterogenicity in the ICU population and improve outcome of patient treatment.

Processes Affecting Drug Disposition

Drug disposition is a very dynamic process influenced by several pharmacokinetic processes (Fig. 205-1). The change in drug concentration over time is related to the rate of drug absorption/administration, amount of drug administered, volume of distribution, rate of drug distribution from the central compartment to the tissue compartment, and rate of drug elimination. Agents administered orally or intramuscularly are absorbed into the central compartment from the gastrointestinal (GI) tract or site of injection. Less common methods of administration include transdermal, pulmonary inhalation, buccal, and intraocular. The drug is administered directly into the central compartment when given intravenously. Within the central compartment, most drugs are transported by means of systemic circulation to their site of action, which is generally within the tissue compartment. Drug binding to circulating plasma proteins (e.g., albumin or alpha-1-acid glycoprotein) occurs mainly in the central compartment. Drug distribution from the central compartment to the tissue compartment may be rapid enough that the central compartment and tissue compartment appear to be contiguous. If the drug equilibrates more slowly from the central compartment to the tissue compartment, the serum concentrations may be better characterized by more complex modeling (i.e., two-compartment modeling) (Fig. 205-2). The rate of drug administration, elimination rate, and time for equilibrium collectively determine whether the drug's concentrations are more accurately characterized by one-compartment behavior or multiple-compartment phenomena. The agent is then eliminated from the body via the kidney unchanged or metabolized by the liver or other organs. The metabolites are eliminated via the kidney. Drug elimination can also be via fecal, skin, and pulmonary routes.

Absorption of the drug is required for all methods of drug administration, except intravascular administration. Figure 205-3 illustrates serum drug concentration versus time curves for an identical drug administered in three ways: intravascularly as a bolus, orally as a rapid-release product, and orally as a sus-

One-Compartment Model

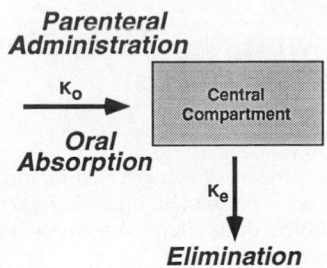

Fig. 205-1. In a one-compartment model, drug absorption/administration occurs at rate K_o, followed by immediate distribution. The drug is further eliminated from the body at rate K_e.

Two-Compartment Model

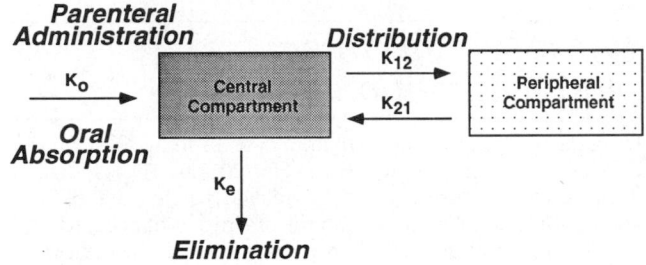

Fig. 205-2. In a two-compartment model, drug absorption/administration occurs at rate K_o, followed by distribution from the central compartment to the peripheral compartment. The drug distributes from the central compartment to the peripheral compartment (K_{12}) and from the peripheral compartment to the central compartment (K_{21}). The drug is further eliminated from the body at K_e.

tained-release product. In intensive care patients, absorption may be altered after oral and intramuscular administration, and serum concentration-time profiles may be further altered. The initial upward slope of the serum drug concentration versus time curve signifies that absorption predominates. During this initial phase, the rate of absorption is greater than the rate of elimination, thus the concentration in serum increases. The highest serum concentration on the curve, "peak," occurs at the time when the rate of entry into the circulation is equal to the rate of elimination from the circulation. Thus, the time to peak depends on the relative rates of absorption and elimination. Elimination of any drug begins as soon as it enters the systemic circulation. Following the peak serum drug concentration, elimination predominates and the slope turns downward.

Drug Administration/Absorption

The complexity of drug administration for the intensive care patient has increased steadily in the last several years and will likely continue. A larger number of drug entities is now needed to manage these patients. In some of the more critically ill patients, 80 to 100 different dosage administrations may be necessary daily. Administration of these medications needs to be carefully designed and scheduled to achieve the desired patient response. This includes the method of drug administration (bolus injections, continuous infusions, and intermittent infusions) and determination of which drugs are added to specific solutions, so as to minimize or prevent drug incompatibilities and ensure the desired pharmacologic response. Application of pharmacokinetic concepts and principles is essential to optimize the treatment regimen.

The rate of drug absorption or administration is clinically important because it influences or determines the time required to achieve therapeutic serum concentrations. For most patients in the ICU, the pharmacologic response must be achieved as quickly as possible. In ICU patients, drug absorption from the GI tract and from intramuscular administration is frequently not reliable and consistent. Blood supply to the GI tract or capillary flow within the muscle may be altered by sepsis or underlying medical disease and further affect drug absorption. Oral or intramuscular administration of medications should be approached cautiously and used only for select drugs in patients in whom the rate of absorption may not be as critical for achieving the drug's response. Intravenous administration is certainly the most reliable method of drug administration in the ICU.

After intravenous administration, the resultant serum concentrations are influenced by the dose, rate of administration, and length of infusion. If the intravenous dose is the same, the serum concentration-time curve differs for the common methods of intravenous administration, but the area under the serum concentration-time curve is similar for most drugs. This applies to all drugs that follow linear pharmacokinetic behavior, meaning a proportional increase in serum concentrations or area under the serum concentration-time curve occurs as increasing doses are administered. Common drugs that do not follow linear pharmacokinetic principles include alcohol, theophylline, and phenytoin.

Three common methods of intravenous drug administration for ICU patients are intravenous bolus, intermittent infusion, and continuous administration. Retrograde infusions (direct injection into the intravenous catheter via a Y site) are also frequently used in pediatric patients, and the resulting serum concentration-time curve generally mimics that of an intermittent infusion. These methods of intravenous administration produce different serum concentration time profiles and can therefore result in different dose-response effects. Many of these untoward responses can be anticipated and prevented by using a different method of administration. Careful selection of the method of administration maximizes the drug's effectiveness and minimizes the risks of adverse reactions.

A bolus infusion is a dose administered intravenously directly into the vascular compartment via a vein or artery. A bolus infusion is closely approximated by injecting the drug solution at the distal end of the catheter prior to insertion in the vein or artery. The catheter must be clamped proximal to the injection site or retrograding of the drug will rapidly occur in the catheter proximal to the injection site. Advantages of this route of administration include rapid delivery of drug to the site of activity, which enhances the time of drug responsiveness. This route is advantageous for the pressor and inotropes used in hypotensive patients but may be problematic for some drugs with a rapid respiratory depressant effect, central nervous system effect, or cardiovascular effect. Examples of drugs that have these effects are the narcotic analgesics, lidocaine, and propylene glycol. The latter is used as a solubilizing vehicle in many con-

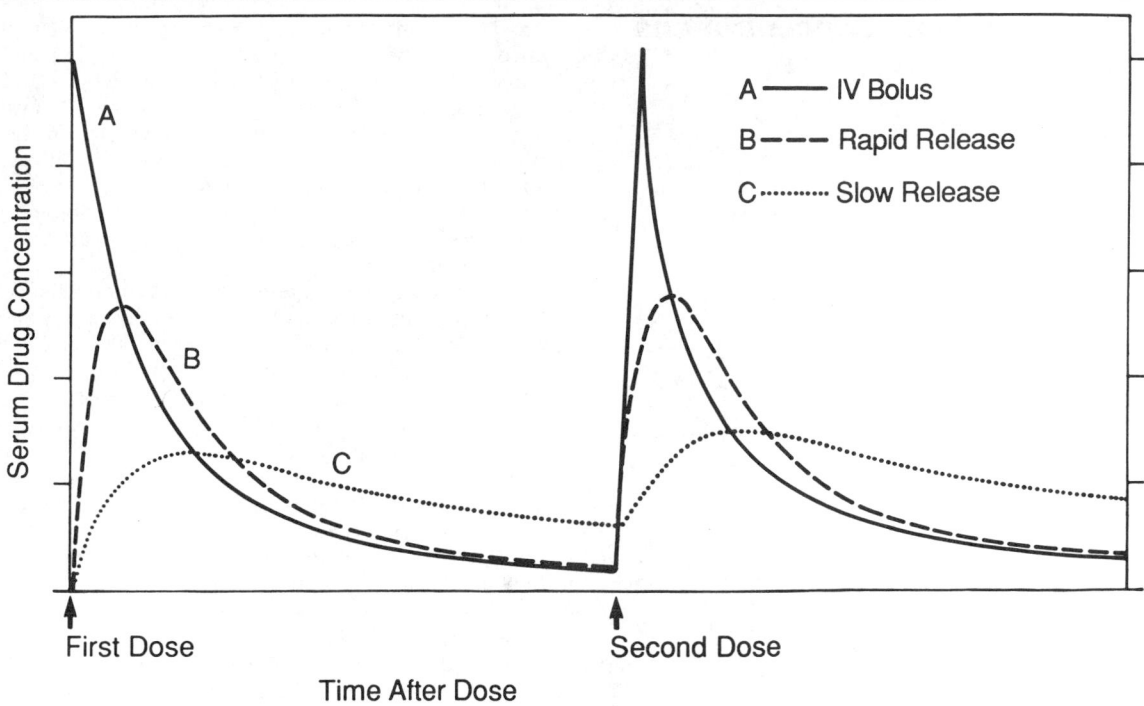

Fig. 205-3. Serum drug concentration versus time curves for drugs with different rates of absorption or administration.

centrated parenteral drug products, such as phenytoin and many benzodiazepines.

An intermittent infusion is intravenous administration of a dose, generally at a fixed rate for a defined period of time. The drug and accompanying solution are administered at a continuous rate over a fixed period of time and repeated at desired intervals (e.g., 100 mg of drug X in 100 ml of D_5W administered at 100 ml/hr over 60 minutes and repeated every 6 hours). It is important to emphasize that the drug and the solution might be administered into the patient's IV line as ordered, but because considerable mixing occurs in the line the patient receives an infusion rate that is substantially different [4]. Drug mixing occurs in the line with solution already in the line and with the drug retrogrades in the line after completion of the infusion. With an intermittent infusion (using the previous example), the actual infusion realized is considerably affected by the fluid mixing dynamics within the line. In the above example, the rate of drug administration into the IV line is 100 mg per hour, but the rate of drug received by the patient at the IV site is much lower and the infusion will actually persist longer than the 60 minutes. Drug mixing in-line is most likely accomplished by brownian movement of molecules within the IV line. Factors such as fluid currents and solution tunneling within the line and drug/solution adherence to the catheter may also contribute to the mixing of solutions and drugs within the line. In-line mixing of drug can be decreased by using faster rates of drug administration, smaller-bore catheter lines, catheter sets with less dead space, and solutions with similar osmolarity. Obviously, dedicated lines or multiluminal catheters also reduce or eliminate the problem. This is especially important for the administration of drugs with a high risk of chemical or physical incompatibility (e.g., phenytoin) or when serum samples are measured for drug dose adjustments.

A drug administered as a continuous infusion is infused at the same rate over a prolonged period. After five elimination half-lives of the drug, the serum concentrations are assumed to have reached steady-state values after continuous or intermittent infusion (Fig. 205-4). The delay in attaining therapeutic values may be a disadvantage with continuous infusions. Therapeutic serum concentrations can be achieved more quickly with the use of a bolus injection or a more rapid rate of infusion when initiating therapy. This approach is specifically useful when initiating lidocaine or phenytoin. Infusion pumps are generally used for continuous infusion. Altered infusion rates can cause a change in responsiveness to a dosage regimen. If more than one drug is being continuously infused on the same IV catheter set with a Y connector, the infusion rates of the second pump can be inadvertently altered by changing the rate of the first pump. This rate change persists until the solution mixing ratio reaches a new equilibrium. The use of dedicated lines or multiluminal catheters may be necessary to ensure the desired rate of drug administration, especially of inotropes, pressors, and antiarrhythmics.

Drug administration with IV pumps also can be inadvertently interrupted and alter the patient's response, especially to vasoreactive drugs. This occurs only at low infusion rates and is caused by the "dead space" in the pump's cycle. This is the point in the cycle when the pump refills with solution before resuming its pumping action. At normal infusion rates, this period is minute compared to the pumping period and therefore the dead space is not important clinically. At low infusion rates, however, the dead space becomes a larger fraction of the total pumping cycle and noticeably interrupts the continuous administration of drug. Pumps specifically designed for lower pumping rates should be used, especially for administration of vasoactive agents or inotropes.

If the same dose is administered intravenously by the three different methods, serum concentrations are highest after a bolus infusion. However, these measured values are from the central compartment and may not be indicative of concentrations in the tissue compartment, which is generally the effect compartment for the pharmacologic or toxic response. Some

Time to Steady State Concentrations

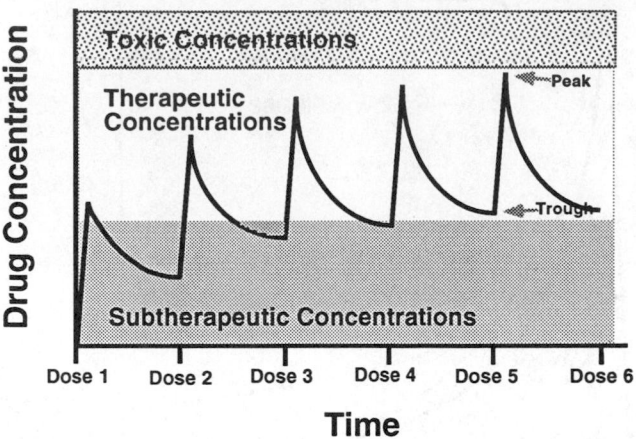

Fig. 205-4. A gradual increase in serum drug concentrations occurs until steady-state conditions are achieved. This is assumed to occur after five half-lives of the drug. The method of drug administration is not a factor in attaining steady state.

drugs appear to have different effect compartments, each of which appears to reach equilibrium more rapidly with the central compartment, such as lidocaine. The central nervous system effects (e.g., seizures) of lidocaine may be more quickly evident before the cardiovascular effects (e.g., antiarrhythmic activity) are present. Therefore, bolus injections should be used only when the pharmacologic effect is needed immediately (e.g., pressors and inotropes) and the drug effect can be achieved safely. With lidocaine, for example, therapeutic serum concentrations can be initially obtained with a bolus and then the effective concentrations maintained by continuous infusion.

For drugs administered intramuscularly (IM) or subcutaneously (SC), the extent of absorption usually approaches about 100 percent, but the rate of absorption varies greatly, depending on the formulation, chemical properties of the drug, and physiologic factors, such as tissue composition, temperature, blood pH, and blood perfusion at the site of administration. Because tissue perfusion can be dramatically altered in ICU patients, drug absorption after IM or SC administration is often delayed and variable. If the patient experiences an adverse reaction the effect is more prolonged than generally observed after IV administration, because of continued absorption with IM or SC administration. For these reasons, IM and SC administration are generally avoided in critically ill patients.

The rate of absorption is important for drugs critical to the treatment of acute conditions such as seizures. The relative need to achieve therapeutic serum concentrations quickly determines the product or route of administration chosen. For example, oral phenytoin is absorbed slowly, with a half-life for absorption of approximately 8 hours; therefore it is administered initially intravenously to attain effective serum concentrations. Once effective concentrations have been attained, it may be administered by a different route, such as orally via nasogastric feeding tube.

Bioavailability refers to both the amount of drug absorbed and the rate at which it becomes available. Systemically, several factors influence a drug's bioavailability, and some of these are especially important for ICU patients. The first factor is the fraction of active drug in a product formulation. Drugs are often provided in salt conjugate forms to maintain solubility or influence in vivo ionization. For example, aminophylline is 84 to 87 percent anhydrous theophylline, the active drug, and about 15 percent ethylenediamine, the salt conjugate. Bioavailability is also influenced by the rate of product dissolution, the chemical properties of the dissolved drug (lipophilicity, pKa, molecular size), GI motility, blood flow to the GI tract, blood pH, surface area available for absorption, and the physiology of the absorptive surface. Disease, drugs, and surgery are known to alter these factors.

Intravenously administered drugs are generally assumed to be 100 percent bioavailable. An exception is parenteral drugs administered as prodrugs. Chloramphenicol succinate, for example, is inactive until it undergoes hydrolysis by the liver to yield the active drug, chloramphenicol. Bioavailability is dependent on the efficiency of kidney to eliminate the unchanging prodrug, chloramphenicol succinate, before it can be hydrolyzed to the active form. For this agent, bioavailability is assumed to be 60 to 90 percent [5,6]. Intravenously administered drugs may also be bound to the plastic in the catheter sets (e.g., nitroglycerin and nifedipine) or may be inactivated by the ultraviolet light (e.g., amphotericin). Generally, these drugs must be administered with special precautions.

For absorption of a drug administered orally it must first undergo dissolution, which is often the rate-limiting step. Dissolution depends on the chemical properties of the drug, the formulation, and physiologic factors such as GI pH. In cases of oral drug overdose, the dissolution rate may be dependent on the amount of drug ingested [7]. If the drug has a slow dissolution rate or is administered as a sustained-release product and the patient has increased GI motility (i.e., short transit time) or a short bowel, the drug may not dissolve completely, hence bioavailability will be decreased and less drug will be absorbed. Similarly, diarrhea can decrease absorption of some drugs due to shortened transit time. Drugs may be administered already dissolved in solution to bypass the dissolution step and effect more rapid absorption.

Most oral drugs are absorbed primarily by passive diffusion in the small bowel. Absorption from the stomach is usually minimal, regardless of the pKa of the drug. Thus, gastric emptying time is often the rate-limiting step following dissolution. Many drugs alter gastric motility and the rate at which other orally administered drugs are absorbed. Commonly encountered drugs that slow gastric emptying include anticholinergic agents (e.g., atropine, tricyclic antidepressants), phenothiazines, narcotics, antacids, and anesthetics (e.g., ganglionic blocking drugs) [8,9]. In one study volunteers consumed 400 ml of juice containing 20 mg per kilogram of acetaminophen together with a nonabsorbable isotopic marker for measuring the rate of gastric emptying. Administration of meperidine (150 mg) prolonged the mean time of 50 percent gastric emptying from 12 to 90 minutes. As would be expected, the resulting peak serum drug concentrations were significantly decreased [10]. A commonly used drug that increases gastric emptying rate is metoclopramide.

Many disease states alter gastric emptying. Diabetic gastriparesis is associated with significantly delayed gastric emptying [8]. In Crohn's disease, drug absorption may be increased or decreased, depending on the drug and individual pathology [11]. Most acute illnesses seen in the ICU have the potential to decrease gastric motility and influence drug absorption [8]. As patients improve, drug absorption and, hence, serum drug concentrations may increase. In these patients, follow-up monitoring of serum concentrations and/or dosage adjustments may be necessary to prevent toxicity.

Gastrointestinal surgery alters the anatomy and physiology

of the GI tract, and can thus alter both the rate and extent of drug absorption. Venho et al. studied the effect of four gastrostomy procedures on the absorption rate of quinidine (a base), ethambutol (a neutral drug), and sulfafurazole (an acid) [12]. After antrectomy with gastroduodenostomy plus selective vagotomy, gastric emptying and the rate of absorption of all the drugs were significantly decreased. After antrectomy and gastroduodenostomy without vagotomy, no change was identified. Small bowel resection or ileojejunal bypass also affects drug bioavailability. In a study that compared absorption of a 200-mg test dose of phenytoin in seven obese patients with ileojejunal bypass with absorption in nine healthy controls, the relative bioavailability in the bypass patients was only 30 percent that in the controls [13].

Administration of food or tube-feeding solutions can significantly decrease the bioavailability and rate of absorption of many drugs. Adsorption of drug onto food components may be an important mechanism of this interaction. One of the most important examples in the ICU is the dramatic decrease in phenytoin serum drug concentrations observed in patients who receive enteral tube feeding when the drug is changed from IV to nasogastric (NG) administration using the suspension formulation [14].

Drugs absorbed distal to the oropharynx enter the portal system and are delivered to the liver before reaching the systemic circulation. For drugs that are hepatically metabolized, bioavailability may be decreased. This is referred to as the first-pass effect. The fraction of the drug dose metabolized during one pass through the liver is termed the hepatic extraction ratio (E).

$$A = \frac{C_{in} - C_{out}}{C_{in}} \tag{1}$$

where C_{in} is the concentration of drug entering the liver and C_{out} is the concentration existing in the liver; E ranges from 0 to 1.

For example, if 100 mg of drug A is administered orally and 90 mg is absorbed and 20 mg is extracted by the liver before reaching the systemic circulation, then:

$$E = \frac{90 \text{ mg} - 7 \text{ mg}}{90 \text{ mg}} = 0.22$$

and overall bioavailability (F) = 0.78.

In practice, bioavailability is calculated by comparing the areas under the serum drug concentration versus time curve (AUC) resulting from the oral dose with that of the intravascular dose, where bioavailability of the latter is assumed to be 100 percent. The first-pass effect is taken into account when calculating the "normal dosage" for a drug. Increased bioavailability after oral administration is seen when the metabolic capacity of the liver is impaired by disease and the drug has a large first-pass effect. In patients who have cirrhosis, the enzymatic capacity of the liver is diminished and, in addition, blood is shunted around the liver through collateral channels, increasing bioavailability. In patients with cirrhosis and portal hypertension who have undergone various portal venous shunting procedures for variceal bleeding, the bioavailability of orally administered drugs with large hepatic extraction values (e.g., propranolol, verapamil, meperidine) can be markedly increased and doses need to be adjusted accordingly.

Hepatic metabolism can be saturable, leading to dose-dependent bioavailability. For example, propranolol has a very high extraction ratio (0.7–0.9) and is extensively metabolized. Bioavailability of propranolol is lowest when the concentration is low (i.e., with small doses) or the rate of administration is slow. Increasing the dose results in decreased first-pass clearance and increased bioavailability [15,16].

Distribution

After reaching the systemic circulation, drug is available for transport into various peripheral tissue compartments. The rate and extent of distribution depend on the chemical properties of the drug (e.g., lipid solubility, affinity for active transport pumps, affinity for tissue and plasma protein binding sites) and physiologic status of the patient (e.g., body tissue composition, age, hydration, blood pH, tissue perfusion, organ function) The drug's distribution profile has important clinical implications. For example, an antibiotic chosen to treat meningitis must cross the blood-brain barrier, and the dose selected must achieve adequate cerebrospinal fluid (CSF) drug concentrations.

The apparent volume of distribution (V_d) is a proportionality constant that relates the total amount of drug in the body to the resulting serum drug concentrations. It may simply be defined as the size of the bucket within which the drug distributes. It is the calculation of the theoretical volume into which a drug would have to distribute after an instantaneous injection if the measured concentration were uniform throughout the body. This volume is termed "apparent" because it is generally not a true physiologic or anatomic volume. The V_d is determined, in part, by where a drug distributes. A simplified mathematical version of V_d is:

$$V_d = \frac{Dose}{C_p} \tag{2}$$

where the serum drug concentration (C_p) is the result of a single instantaneously administered dose. This formula is based on several assumptions: the initial serum drug concentration is zero; the drug is administered instantaneously by means of the intravascular route; distribution is uniform and occurs instantaneously; and there is no elimination of the drug. Given these conditions, the dose in the body is equal to the dose administered. According to this equation, the lower the serum drug concentrations relative to a dose, the larger the volume of distribution, and vice versa (Fig. 205-5). Factors that decrease the serum drug concentrations, such as high lipid solubility, high tissue binding, or low serum protein binding, tend to increase volume of distribution.

Because elimination begins as soon as a drug enters the systemic circulation, an accurate calculation of V_d is more complex. One method of calculation is:

$$V_d = \frac{Dose}{AUC \times Ke} \tag{3}$$

where AUC is the area under the serum drug concentration versus time curve and K_e is the elimination rate constant. It is important to remember that V_d is a function of the patient's physiology and the drug's chemistry and is independent of the drug's clearance.

These examples assume there is instantaneous and uniform drug distribution consistent with a one-compartment model (Fig. 205-1). In reality, the distribution of most drugs occurs over a measurable time period. Drugs do not distribute homogeneously in the body, because some are concentrated in the fat, others in extracellular fluid, and others with proteins. In a two-compartment model (Fig. 205-2), the drug distributes initially into a "central compartment" consisting of blood and highly perfused tissues. Later the drug is distributed to tissues

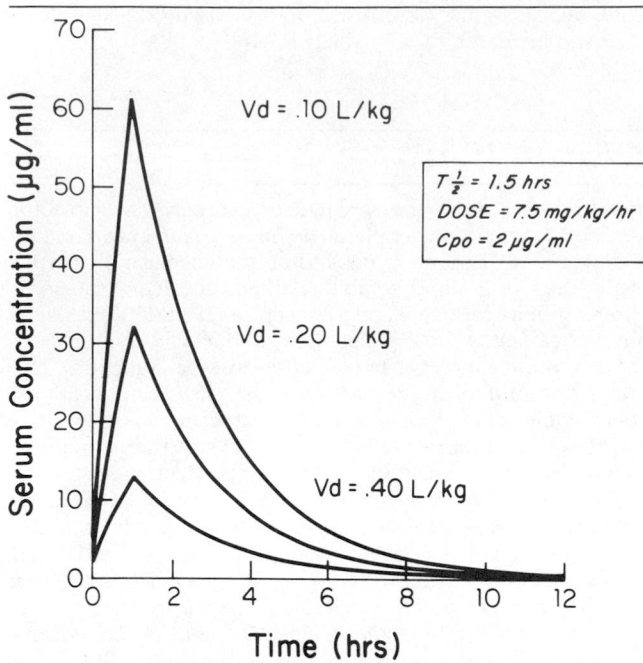

Fig. 205-5. The effects of different distribution volumes (V_d) on serum concentrations under similar conditions: serum concentration-time curve for three hypothetical patients after receiving the same dose over 1 hour and having the same half-life and initial serum concentration. The patients with lower drug volumes have higher peak levels and those with higher volumes have lower peak levels.

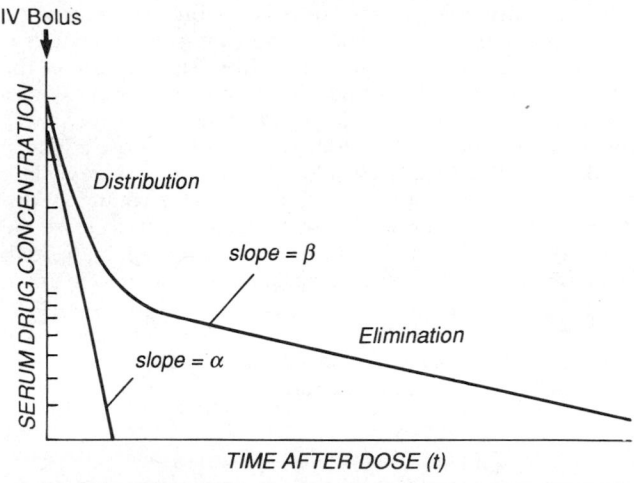

Fig. 205-6. Log of the serum drug concentration versus time curve for a drug following two-compartment behavior. Slopes of the distribution (α) and elimination (β) processes are expressed as natural logarithms.

that are less well perfused ("peripheral compartment"). Distribution between the central and peripheral compartments is described by the rate constants K_{12} and K_{21}. A serum drug concentration obtained immediately after administration of an initial IV bolus dose reflects the volume of the central compartment (V_{d_c}).

$$V_{d_c} = \frac{\text{Dose}}{C_{P0}} \tag{4}$$

where C_{P0} is the drug concentration immediately after an instantaneous dose. As distribution takes place, the serum drug concentration rapidly decreases (Fig. 205-6). The rate of decline reflects both distribution and elimination. When distribution is complete, the slope of the decline decreases, reflecting only elimination.

Drug distribution is usually a first-order process and is associated with the distribution rate constant alpha α. Using this constant, distribution half-life can be calculated as follows:

$$t_{1/2\alpha} = \frac{0.693}{\alpha} \tag{5}$$

where $t_{1/2\alpha}$ is the time required for distribution to be 50 percent complete. Distribution is 96.9 percent complete after five distribution half-lives. Most drugs have a $t_{1/2\alpha}$ value between 5 and 30 minutes.

Similarly, when elimination is a first-order process, the elimination phase is associated with an elimination rate constant (K_e) or beta (β). K_e and β are commonly used abbreviations, used interchangeably in this text. Using this constant, the elimination half-life can be calculated as follows:

$$t_{1/2} = \frac{0.693}{K_e} \tag{6}$$

where $t_{1/2}$ (also referred to as elimination $t_{1/2}$) is the time required for the serum drug concentration to decline by 50 percent. Elimination is 96.9 percent complete after five elimination half-lives.

When a drug has a large volume of distribution, the difference in volume of the central compartment (V_{dc}) and volume of distribution (V_d) is large, and a distinct biphasic decay pattern is observed with serial serum drug concentrations. Volume of the central compartment and α determine the rate at which many drugs can be administered without attaining extremely high serum concentrations. For example, the total loading dose of a drug is calculated using the apparent (postdistribution) volume of distribution and desired serum concentration. If the entire dose is administered as an IV bolus, the initial (predistribution) serum drug concentrations is high. The importance of this high serum drug concentration is determined by the pharmacodynamics of the drug. If a drug's pharmacologic or toxic response correlates with concentration in the central compartment, the predistribution value becomes important and determines the safe maximal rate of administration. A slower rate of administration will decrease the peak concentration in the central compartment. If the response is correlated only with postdistribution serum drug concentrations, the initial level is irrelevant. For example, with lidocaine, seizures are associated with high initial concentrations and may be avoided by splitting the total loading dose into several smaller bolus doses to reduce predistribution serum drug concentrations. The initially toxic serum drug concentrations can also be eliminated by administering the loading dose in the form of a slow infusion, as is done with procainamide and quinidine. Conversely, the pharmacologic effects of digoxin are correlated with postdistribution serum drug concentration; initial predistribution concentrations are usually irrelevant.

Some drugs have responses associated with both predistribution and postdistribution serum drug concentrations. The bronchodilatory response to theophylline correlates with postdistribution serum drug concentrations, and administration of the drug at a rate faster than it can be distributed does not lead to a faster onset of effect. However, tachycardia tends to correlate with high initial serum drug concentrations, and slowing the rate of administration (and thus lowering the initial serum drug concentrations) may prevent or limit the development of tachycardia. In summary, volume of distribution determines the size of the dose necessary to obtain desired serum drug concentrations, and volume of distribution for the central compartment can influence the rate of administration.

Although volume of distribution is not a true physiologic entity, it can be used as a rough indicator of where the drug distributes. In general, a small volume of distribution suggests that tissue distribution is minimal. Volume of distribution generally correlates well with body weight and is often expressed in units of liters per kilogram of total body weight; this value corresponds to plasma volume. A volume of distribution of 0.25 liter per kilogram of total body weight is associated with distribution primarily in extracellular fluid. A volume of distribution of 0.65 liter per kilogram with a drug that is highly water-soluble suggests distribution to total body water. A large volume of distribution (>1 L/kg) suggests extensive tissue distribution and peripheral concentration.

Another commonly encountered drug distribution volume is volume of distribution at steady state (V_{dss}). V_{dss} relates the amount of drug in the body to the serum drug concentrations at steady state. Calculation of V_{dss} is beyond the scope of this discussion, but V_{dss} values are usually about 10 percent less than volume of distribution. V_{dss} and V_d can be used interchangeably in the simplified calculations presented here.

Protein Binding

Many drugs associate, or bind to plasma proteins. Two plasma proteins, albumin and alpha-1-acid glycoprotein (AAG), are responsible for about 95 percent of all drug binding. Most of this binding is readily reversible, and an equilibrium between bound and free drug is established such that the free fraction remains relatively constant for any given protein concentration. Only the free drug is pharmacologically active. In most cases, protein binding capacity is much larger than necessary and the fraction of free drug is independent of the total serum drug concentrations. With a few drugs, notably valproic acid [17] and salicylates [18], binding sites can be saturated with usual therapeutic doses. If saturation occurs, the total serum drug concentrations can be within the normal range, but the free fraction and, hence, the pharmacologic effect, can be increased. In overdose, saturation of protein binding sites becomes clinically more important.

Anionic drugs and weak acids usually bind to albumin. Examples are phenytoin, warfarin, and salicylates. Albumin is synthesized in the liver and normally constitutes about 60 percent of total plasma protein, or about 4 gm per deciliter. Many disease states are associated with significant decreases in plasma albumin concentrations. In the ICU, the most common are malnutrition, burns, sepsis, renal disease, and liver disease [19,20]. If the albumin concentration is decreased, binding sites are proportionally decreased and the percentage of free drug increases:

$$f = \frac{C_{pfree}}{C_{ptotal}} \tag{7}$$

where f is the fraction of free drug in blood, C_{pfree} is the concentration of free drug, and C_{ptotal} is the free serum drug concentration plus the concentration of bound drug.

If the free fraction (f) is greater than 0.5, less than one-half of the drug is bound, and changes in albumin concentrations usually have an insignificant effect on free serum drug concentrations. For example, for a drug with f of 0.5, decreasing albumin concentration by 25 percent increases the free drug concentration from 50 percent to 62.5 percent of the total drug. In contrast, if f is 0.1, a 25 percent decrease in albumin concentration increases free serum drug concentration from 10 percent to 33 percent of the total drug, more than a threefold increase. The therapeutic range for phenytoin, which is about 90 percent bound to albumin, is 10 to 20 µg per milliliter (total serum drug concentrations). Because f is 0.1 for this drug, the equivalent free drug therapeutic range is 1 to 2 µg per milliliter. In hypoalbuminemic patients who have an altered free fraction, measured total serum drug concentrations can be used to estimate the total serum drug concentrations that would have been measured if the serum albumin level and hence the number of available binding sites were normal ($C_{ptotal\text{-}adjusted}$). For example, if it is assumed the free fraction is proportional to measured albumin (the affinity constant does not change), the patient's albumin is 2.0 gm per deciliter, and the measured total serum drug concentration is 7 µg per milliliter, then:

$$C_{ptotal\text{-}adjusted} = \frac{f_{normal}}{f_{patient}} \times \text{Measured } C_{ptotal} \tag{8}$$

$$
\begin{aligned}
C_{ptotal\text{-}adjusted} &= \frac{\text{Normal albumin}}{\text{Patient albumin}} \times \text{Measured } C_{ptotal} \\
&= \frac{4.0 \text{ gm/dl}}{2.0 \text{ gm/dl}} \times 7 \text{ µg/ml} \\
&= 14 \text{ µg/ml}
\end{aligned}
\tag{9}
$$

Therefore, a serum drug concentration of 7 µg per milliliter in this patient is approximately equal to a serum drug concentration of 14 µg per milliliter in a patient with an albumin of 4.0 gm per deciliter.

Most clinical drug assay procedures measure total drug concentration. Some laboratories can measure free drug concentrations for drugs that are highly protein-bound. This procedure is expensive and time-consuming but can be helpful in the management of patients whose plasma protein binding is likely to be altered. If available, the physician should use the free and total serum drug concentrations to calculate the patient's f value. Using the phenytoin example, if the free serum drug concentration is 1.5 µg per milliliter and the total serum drug concentration is 7 µg per milliliter, then f is 0.21. The patient's individualized therapeutic range in terms of total serum drug concentrations can be calculated as follows:

$$
\begin{aligned}
\text{Individual therapeutic range} &= \frac{f_{normal}}{f_{patient}} \times \text{Usual therapeutic range} \\
&= \frac{0.1}{0.21} \times 10 \text{ µg/ml} \\
&= 4.8 \text{ µg/ml}
\end{aligned}
$$

and

$$
\begin{aligned}
&= \frac{0.1}{0.21} \times 20 \text{ ug/ml} \\
&= 9.5 \text{ ug/ml}
\end{aligned}
\tag{10}
$$

In this patient, the therapeutic range for phenytoin is 4.8 to 9.5 μg per milliliter. With this information the physician can continue to use the total serum drug concentration information and will need to recheck the free serum drug concentrations only when the serum albumin concentration changes significantly.

Cationic drugs and weak bases usually bind to globulins, specifically AAG. Examples are methadone, quinidine, propranolol, clindamycin, and lidocaine. Alpha-1-acid glycoprotein is an acute phase reactant synthesized by the liver, with a normal serum concentration of 80 mg per deciliter. Trauma, surgery, burns, psychiatric conditions, acute inflammation, and myocardial infarction are associated with large increases in AAG (up to 500–600 mg/dl) and consequent decreases in circulating concentrations of free drug [20]. The increases in AAG may render some drugs thought to be unbound into highly bound in specific patients. A good example is clindamycin, which was previously thought to be unbound but is now considered to be bound up to 98 percent in trauma patients.

Another phenomenon that can affect the serum free drug concentration is the displacement of drugs from their binding sites by endogenous ligands. For example, in patients with either acute or chronic uremia, free drug concentrations of both diazepam and phenytoin are greatly increased [21]. The exact ligand involved has not been identified, but binding site displacement is thought to be the mechanism.

Drug protein binding is usually nonspecific, so that one drug can displace another on a binding site. The drug with higher binding affinity displaces the one with lower affinity. Many drug interactions result from displacement reactions at the binding protein. Free drug distributes in the plasma and tissue compartments. The smaller the volume of distribution of the drug, the greater the significance of changes in free ratio. Drugs that are highly protein-bound tend to have small volumes of distribution.

Clearance

Elimination of drugs from the body depends on the chemical properties of the drug (molecular size, structure, pKa, lipophilicity), the route of elimination, and the patient's physiologic status. In humans, the primary routes of elimination are the liver, kidneys, and lungs.

Lipophilic drugs usually must undergo metabolism to more polar (hydrophilic) compounds to be eliminated. Phase I metabolism (nonsynthetic reactions, such as oxidation, reduction, and hydrolysis) transform lipophilic drugs into relatively polar substances. Oxidation reactions generally occur in the hepatic microsomal enzyme system. Hydrolysis often takes place in the plasma, and reduction often occurs in the GI tract. Phase II metabolism (synthetic reactions) combines relatively polar compound with other lipophilic substances, rendering the latter hydrophilic. The most common conjugation reaction is glucuronidation, which generally takes place in the hepatic microsomal enzyme system. Metabolites formed in the liver can be excreted into the intestinal tract via bile and eliminated in the feces or reabsorbed into the blood. The latter process is referred to as enterohepatic reabsorption or recirculation. Some active lipophilic drugs also undergo enterohepatic recirculation. Hydrophilic drugs and metabolites are often excreted by the kidneys via the urine. Volatile anesthetics are the only major pharmacologic agents that undergo primarily pulmonary excretion.

Clearance refers to the volume of blood, plasma, or serum from which a drug is completely removed (or cleared) per unit time. Clearance is expressed in units of volume per time (L/hr

Drug Clearance

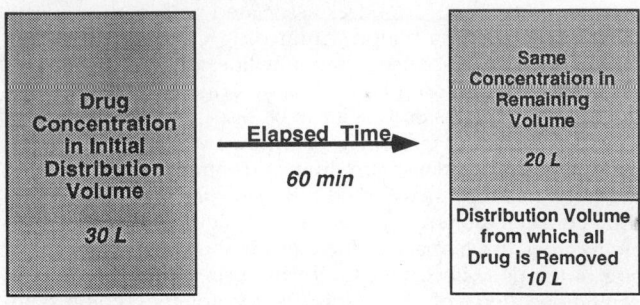

Fig. 205-7. Drug clearance is the volume from which the drug is removed over time. In this illustration, the volume is 30 liters, and 10 liters is cleared over 60 minutes. The clearance is 10 L/60 min.

or ml/min). This volume is theoretical; no single liter of blood necessarily has all of its drug removed during one pass through the clearance organ. Rather, a fraction of drug is removed from each of the many liters perfusing an organ. This fraction is expressed as though it were derived by completely clearing a smaller volume of blood of all of its drug. Figure 205-7 illustrates this concept. Clearance is a measure of the intrinsic ability of the body to eliminate the drug.

Clearance usually involves more than one organ. Total body clearance (Cl) is the sum of all the individual organ clearances, as shown in the equation:

$$Cl = Cl_H + Cl_R + Cl_{other} \qquad (11)$$

where Cl_H is hepatic clearance, Cl_R is renal clearance, and Cl_{other} resents the sum of all other routes of drug elimination.

Consider a single well-perfused organ that eliminates a drug:

$$\begin{array}{ll} C_{in} & C_{out} \\ Q \rightarrow & Organ \rightarrow \end{array}$$

where Q is blood flow through the organ, C_{in} is the concentration of drug entering the organ, and C_{out} is the concentration existing the organ. If drug is eliminated by the organ, C_{in} is greater than C_{out}. As previously described, the fraction of drug eliminated during one pass through the organ is termed the extraction ratio (E). The amount of drug available for elimination is dependent on blood flow to the organ. It follows that:

$$Cl = Q \times \frac{C_{in} - C_{out}}{C_{in}} = Q \times E \qquad (12)$$

If drug elimination is a first-order process, then clearance can also be expressed as the proportionality constant that relates the drug's elimination rate to its concentration:

$$Cl = \frac{Rate\ of\ elimination\ (amount/time)}{C_p}$$

In first-order drug elimination, Cl is independent of the serum drug concentration. For example, if the elimination rate of a drug is 10 mg per hour and the serum drug concentration is 1 mg per liter, then Cl is 10 per hour. While clearance remains constant, the elimination rate and the serum drug concentration change proportionately.

RENAL CLEARANCE. Measurement of renal clearance using Equation 12 requires very invasive methods, so it is usually calculated using Equation 13:

$$Cl_R = \frac{\text{Rate of elimination in urine}}{C_{pmid}} \qquad (13)$$

where C_{pmid} is the serum drug concentration at the midpoint of the urine collection interval. It follows that:

$$Cl_R = \frac{Q_{urine} \times C_{urine}}{C_{pmid}} \qquad (14)$$

where Q_{urine} is urine flow and C_{urine} is the drug concentration in the urine.

When a drug is freely filtered and neither secreted nor reabsorbed, renal clearance is equivalent to glomerular filtration rate. Only unbound free drug can be filtered. Thus:

$$Cl_R = C_{pfree} \times GFR \qquad (15)$$

where GFR is glomerular filtration rate.

Knowledge of the mechanism of drug clearance is important in anticipating the influence of disease or altered physiology on serum drug concentrations and dosing regimen. The need for adjustments in dosing regimens in patients who have altered renal function is determined by the therapeutic indices of the drugs or consequences of drug accumulation. In general, if renal clearance accounts for 50 percent or more of total clearance, the dosing regimen in patients with renal dysfunction should be adjusted to maintain serum drug concentrations in the same range as in patients with normal kidneys.

Factors that determine renal clearance include glomerular filtration, active tubular secretion, and passive reabsorption. For a drug that is freely filtered by the glomerulus and neither secreted nor reabsorbed, renal clearance is equivalent to glomerular filtration rate. Inulin, an example of such an agent, is often used to measure GFR. Renal secretion involves a carrier-mediated system that is capacity-limited and saturable. Reabsorption, which can be active or passive, occurs after filtration. Drugs that undergo significant tubular secretion have renal clearance values greater than the GFR, whereas drugs that are filtered and then reabsorbed have renal clearance values less than the GFR even when the drug is actively secreted. Thus, for renally eliminated drugs, dosage adjustments are based on estimates of the fractional reduction in GFR.

Creatinine, an endogenous product of muscle metabolism, is normally released from muscle at a constant rate. It may also be absorbed from the GI tract following ingestion of protein. The concentration of creatinine in the serum (SCr) is determined by both the rate of production and its subsequent elimination by the kidneys. Creatinine clearance (CrCl) is a close approximation of GFR. For a given GFR, the relationship between SCr and GFR is largely dependent on muscle mass. When renal function is stable, CrCl and SCr are highly correlated; thus, SCr is often used to estimate CrCl and thus glomerular filtration rate. Creatinine clearance can be estimated as follows:

$$CrCl(ml/min) = \frac{(140 - \text{Age}) \times \text{Lean body weight}}{72 \times SCr} \qquad (16)$$

This result is multiplied by 0.85 for women [22]. This equation takes into consideration the effects of weight, age, and gender on muscle mass and, thus, on creatinine production.

Serum creatinine is highly correlated with GFR only if several important conditions are satisfied. First, GFR must be stable and the concentration of creatinine must be constant. Following a change in GFR, SCr changes over time and is not useful for predicting CrCl until SCr is again stable. Second, creatinine production must be constant. Many pathologic states seen in ICU patients are associated with altered creatinine production, including sepsis, malnutrition, systemic muscular diseases, and prolonged immobilization. Elderly or morbidly obese patients also have significant alterations in creatinine production, leading to poor correlation between SCr and GFR. In addition, when SCr is very high, extrarenal routes can account for 16 to 66 percent of creatinine elimination and SCr will be much lower than expected for a given GFR [23]. Because creatinine is cleared by dialysis, SCr in dialysis patients is not a good predictor of GFR.

In the ICU, drug dosage adjustments in patients with renal failure should never be based solely on SCr. The CrCl can be estimated by performing the calculation presented in Equation 16, although this method can lead to erroneous values. If possible, the actual CrCl should be measured and used as a guide for dosing when the therapeutic index is low and serum drug concentrations cannot be easily measured by a clinical laboratory. The 24-hour CrCl can be estimated using an 8-hour urine collection with about a 20 percent error [24]. If the patient is receiving a drug that is eliminated solely by glomerular filtration, and serum drug concentrations are obtained from which renal clearance can be calculated, renal clearance can be considered to be equal to GFR and used to adjust the doses of other drugs the patient is receiving. Thus, if the patient is receiving an aminoglycoside antibiotic, the total clearance for the aminoglycoside can be considered to be equal to GFR and can then be used to guide adjustments in the dose of other renally excreted drugs he or she is receiving. Recently it was found that the extraction ratio of aminoglycosides appears to change during severe sepsis and to be quite dynamic. The relationship of renal clearance of aminoglycosides with creatinine clearance also appears to change rapidly during a patient's course of treatment. Hence, the use of renal clearance for one drug to estimate the renal clearance of another renally cleared drug should be approached cautiously.

HEPATIC CLEARANCE. Hepatic clearance depends on blood flow to the liver (Q), the intrinsic activity of hepatic enzymes involved in removing the drug from blood (Cl_{int}), and the fraction of drug that is unbound and free to interact with these enzymes (f).

$$Cl_H = Q \times E = Q \times \frac{f \times Cl_{int}}{Q + (f \times Cl_{int})} \qquad (17)$$

Normal hepatic blood flow is approximately 1 to 2 liters per minute. Maximal hepatic clearance equals hepatic blood flow. Changes in blood flow change the rate of drug delivery and alter hepatic clearance. The magnitude of this effect depends on the liver's ability to extract the drug. This is represented by the value of extraction ratio (E). If a drug has a high intrinsic clearance ($E_1 > 0.6$), then hepatic clearance is dependent on blood flow; that is, hepatic clearance is flow-limited. Alterations in hepatic blood flow (caused by other drugs, surgical procedures, or disease) cause significant changes in the rate of elimination of flow-limited drugs. Disease states common in the ICU patient that decrease hepatic blood flow include shock and heart failure. Drugs that decrease hepatic blood flow include propranolol and norepinephrine; drugs that increase hepatic blood flow include dopamine, glucagon, and isoproterenol [25]. Examples of flow-limited drugs are listed in Table 205-1.

Table 205-1. "Flow-Limited" Agents Frequently Used in the ICU

Gentamicin	Ceftazidime
Tobramycin	Lidocaine
Amikacin	Aztreonam
Cefazolin	Netilmicin
Piperacillin	Vancomycin
Ranitidine	Meperidine
Ampicillin	Imipenem

Table 205-2. "Capacity-Limited" Agents Frequently Used in the ICU

Drug	Binding sensitive	Binding insensitive	Unknown
Phenytoin	Yes		
Clindamycin	Yes		
Lorazepam			Yes
Theophylline		Yes	
Midazolam	Yes		
Cimetidine		Yes	
Diazepam			Yes

For drugs with low intrinsic clearances (E < 0.3) the amount of drug removed per unit time is dependent on the enzyme system itself and is relatively independent of hepatic blood flow. Enzyme induction or inhibition can significantly alter the Cl_H of drugs with a low extraction efficiency (E). Changes in the percentage of protein binding can also affect clearance of these drugs. If the free fraction is less than 0.5, then binding is not a significant factor determining clearance and hepatic clearance is most affected by changes in enzymatic activity. Agents of this sort are referred to as capacity-limited, binding-insensitive drugs (Table 205-1). If the free fraction is less than 0.2, hepatic clearance may be sensitive to changes in protein binding, because the fraction of drug available for enzymatic processing changes significantly with alterations in protein binding. These drugs are described as capacity-limited, binding-insensitive (Table 205-2). Clearance of drugs with intermediate extraction ratios (0.3–0.6) can be affected by changes in both blood flow and intrinsic clearance (Cl_{int}). Thus, changes in hepatic clearance because of pathophysiologic alterations can be difficult to predict. These drugs are considered to be flow/capacity-sensitive. With advancing age, hepatic blood flow decreases, thus hepatic clearance for flow-limited drugs (e.g., lidocaine) decreases. In addition, elderly patients can exhibit a decrease in maximal enzyme activity and a corresponding decrease in hepatic clearance [26].

Hepatic disease usually results in reduced liver blood flow. In addition, there is often extensive portosystemic shunting of blood, causing marked reduction in the hepatic clearance of flow-limited drugs. For capacity-limited agents, liver disease causes a greater reduction in the elimination of drugs undergoing phase I reactions. The hepatic clearance of drugs that undergo phase II (conjugative) metabolism is less likely to be altered.

It is difficult to predict which patients with hepatic dysfunction will have significantly decreased drug clearance. This is partially the result of the large variability in drug clearance in normal individuals and the lack of homogeneity among patients with "liver disease." The problem is further complicated by the effects of concurrent medications, activity level, or environmental factors (e.g., smoking, diet) that modify rates of hepatic metabolism and hepatic blood flow. Antipyrine is extensively metabolized in the liver, and its hepatic clearance is independent of hepatic blood flow. The elimination half-life of antipyrine is used as an indicator of hepatic enzyme capacity. In one study, the prolonged antipyrine elimination half-life correlated with the presence of encephalopathy, ascites, and a prolonged prothrombin time [27]. Resolution of these manifestations of hepatic disease was associated with a decrease in antipyrine elimination half-life. Although elevated serum albumin and bilirubin concentrations were weakly correlated with a prolonged antipyrine elimination half-life, there was considerable overlap between normal subjects and patients with hepatic dysfunction. Aspartate aminotransferase or glutamyltranspeptidase levels do not correlate well with antipyrine elimination half-life. Alterations in antipyrine half-life may not correlate well with the clearance of drugs that are flow-limited or highly protein-bound.

References

1. Gibaldi M, Perrier D (eds): *Pharmacokinetics*. New York, Marcel Dekker, 1982.
2. Evans W, Schentag J, Jusko W (eds): *Applied Pharmacokinetics: Principles of Therapeutic Drug Monitoring*. Vancouver, WA, Applied Therapeutics, 1990.
3. Shargel L, Yu A (eds): *Applied Biopharmaceutics and Pharmacokinetics*. Norwalk, CT, Appleton-Century-Crofts, 1985.
4. Leissing N, Story K, Zaske D: Inline fluid dynamics in piggyback and manifold drug delivery systems. *Am J Hosp Pharm* 46:89, 1989.
5. Nahata M, Powell D: Bioavailability and clearance of chloramphenicol after intravenous chloramphenicol succinate. *Clin Pharmacol Ther* 30:368, 1981.
6. Nahata M, Powell D: Comparative bioavailability and pharmacokinetics of chloramphenicol after intravenous chloramphenicol succinate in premature infants and older patients. *Dev Pharmacol Ther* 6:23, 1983.
7. Jung D, Powell J, Walson P, et al: Effect of dose on phenytoin absorption. *Clin Pharmacol Ther* 28:479, 1980.
8. Nimmo W: Drugs, diseases and altered gastric emptying. *Clin Pharmacother* 1:189, 1976.
9. Welling P: Interactions affecting drug absorption. *Clin Pharmacokinet* 9:404, 1984.
10. Nimmo W, Heading R, Wilson J, et al: Inhibition of gastric emptying and drug absorption by narcotic analgesics. *Br J Clin Pharmacol* 2:509, 1975.
11. Gubbins P, Bertch K: Drug absorption in gastrointestinal disease and surgery. *Pharmacotherapy* 9:285, 1989.
12. Venho V, Aukee S, Jussila J, et al: Effect of gastric surgery on the gastrointestinal drug absorption in man. *Scand J Gastroenterol* 10:43, 1975.
13. Kennedy M, Wade D: Phenytoin absorption in patients with iliojejunal bypass. *Br J Clin Pharmacol* 7:515, 1979.
14. Bauer L: Interference of oral phenytoin absorption by continuous nasogastric feedings. *Neurology* 32:570, 1982.
15. Walle T, Conradi E, Walle U, et al: 4-Hydroxypropranolol and its glucuronide after single and long-term doses of propranolol. *Clin Pharmacol Ther* 27:22, 1980.
16. Walle T, Fagan T, Walle U, et al: Food-induced increase in propranolol bioavailability: Relationship to protein and effects on metabolites. *Clin Pharmacol Ther* 30:790, 1981.
17. Yu H: Clinical implications of serum protein binding in epileptic children during sodium calproate maintenance therapy. *Ther Drug Monit* 6:414, 1984.
18. Ekstrand R, Alvan G, Borga O: Concentration dependent plasma protein binding of salicylate in rheumatoid patients. *Clin Pharmacokinet* 4:137, 1979.
19. Tillement J, Lhoste F, Giudicelli J: Diseases and drug protein binding. *Clin Pharmacokinet* 3:144, 1978.
20. Svensson C, Woodruff M, Baxter J, et al: Free drug concentration monitoring in clinical practice: Rationale and current status. *Clin Pharmacokinet* 11:450, 1986.
21. Tiula E, Neuvonen P: Effect of total drug concentration on the free fraction in uremic sera. *Ther Drug Monit* 8:27, 1986.
22. Cockroft D, Gault M: Prediction of creatinine clearance from serum creatinine. *Nephron* 16:31, 1976.

23. Jones J, Burnett P: Creatinine metabolism in humans with decreased renal function: Creatinine deficit. *Clin Chem* 20:1204, 1974.

24. Baumann T, Staddon J, Horst H, et al: Minimum urine collection periods for accurate determination of creatinine clearance in critically ill patients. *Clin Pharm* 6:393, 1987.

25. Richardson P, Withrington P: Liver blood flow. II. Effects of drugs and hormones on liver blood flow. *Gastroenterology* 81:356, 1981.

26. Mayersohn M (ed): Special pharmacokinetic considerations in the elderly. Vancouver, WA, Applied Therapeutics, 1986.

27. Farrell G, Cooksley W, Hart P, et al: Identification of patients with impaired hepatic drug metabolism. *Gastroenterology* 75:580, 1978.

Suggested Readings

Evans WE, Schentag JJ, Jusko WJ (eds): *Applied Pharmacokinetics: Principles of Therapeutic Drug Monitoring*. 3rd ed. Vancouver, WA, Applied Therapeutics, 1990.

Extensive discussions on general aspects of pharmacokinetics (e.g., protein binding, renal clearance) and in-depth discussions on the pharmacokinetics and dose/response data of various commonly monitored drugs.

Taylor WJ, Caviness MHD (eds): *A Textbook for the Clinical Application of Therapeutic Drug Monitoring*. Irving, TX, Abbott Laboratories, Diagnostics Division, 1986.

A brief introduction to principles of therapeutic drug monitoring, followed by individual chapters on a large number of drugs.

Winter ME: Koda-Kimble MA, Young LY (eds): *Basic Clinical Pharmacokinetics*, 2nd ed. Vancouver, WA, Applied Therapeutics, 1988. *Simplified explanations of pharmacokinetic concepts and chapters on the calculation of doses for commonly monitored drugs, with multiple examples.*

206. Physiologic Clearance and Pharmacokinetic Parameters to Individualize and Monitor Dosage Regimens of ICU Patients

Darwin E. Zaske

Introduction

Intensive care patients have a broad array of underlying diseases and medical complications. They become one of the most heterogeneous group of patients requiring the most assertive interventions and technology to maintain life. Drug disposition in these patients also demonstrates the most dynamic characteristics of any patient group [1–74]. The extremes of rapid or slow drug elimination rates are readily apparent for many drugs used in this group. These alterations are driven by the major changes known to occur in the patient's physiologic parameters, such as cardiac output, oxygen consumption and delivery, rate of metabolism, organ blood flow, serum protein changes, fluid balance, and organ function, especially liver and kidney [39,40,51,55,56,60,68,75–113]. These physiologic changes are secondary to underlying disease, sepsis, or injury.

The alteration in drug disposition can directly affect the patient's response to pharmacotherapy [1,4,114–117]. Disregarding these dynamic changes in the patient's drug disposition results in greater variation in drug response and leads to a higher risk of treatment failure or serious drug-induced toxicity. Many patients on the intensive care unit (ICU), even patients of select subgroups, demonstrate substantial variation in dosage requirements [70,71,74]. This variation is not readily identifiable by common organ function tests, such as serum creatinine or liver function tests [13,26,31,32,36,53,55,56,70,71,118–123] and

thus often is independent of concurrent changes noted in organ function, such as kidney or liver [55,56,61].

The magnitude of patient variation in physiologic response to injury and medical complications can also change substantially over time within the same patient [55,56,61]. Successful treatment of an infection in a ICU patient will likely change the magnitude of the stimuli previously driving the dynamic changes in metabolic and physiologic response. When patient demands for oxygen delivery decrease over time as the patient's injury resolves, cardiac output and blood flow to vital organs decrease in a parallel manner. Medical conditions that compromise cardiac output (i.e., congestive heart failure) can be successfully treated and blood flow to vital organs may improve [80,85–88,98,101]. Dosage requirements of many agents also demonstrate a substantial intrapatient variation over time that parallels the change in many physiologic parameters [55,56,61]. This intrapatient variation can be substantial and often is not apparent if common parameters of renal and hepatic function are used solely [55,56,61].

The number of pharmacologic agents used in treating complications in the ICU patients is substantial as they frequently require complex and multiple drug therapies [99,100]. These agents include antibiotics, analgesics, pressors, inotropes, H_2 antagonists, anticonvulsants, beta-blockers, neuromuscular blockers, and benzodiazepines. Many of these agents are used to treat life-threatening complications, and the margin of error for ensuring efficacious therapy is small. The costs of these therapies have recently become a focus of review and concern, and the need to institute the most efficacious treatment quickly is emphasized [124,125]. These patients also may be predisposed to a higher risk of serious toxicity due to serious underlying disease [126]. There is an obvious clinical need to approach treatment in a quantitative manner. This includes anticipating physiologic changes and making appropriate alterations in a timely manner, preferably prospectively [55,56,61].

Many of the pharmacokinetic and pharmacodynamic alterations in ICU patients can be anticipated by knowing the patient's physiologic response to underlying disease(s), trauma, complications, sepsis, and concurrent treatment interventions [25,32,55,56,61,93,127,128]. The technology used to monitor intensive care patients frequently can provide estimates of cardiac output and oxygen delivery and clearance [75,82,83]; subsequent pharmacokinetic changes for many pharmacologic agents can be predicted and appropriate alterations in drug therapy can be instituted. The magnitude of the physiologic changes is generally known to the clinician. The reported relationship of these changes to drug disposition [55,56,61] can assist the clinician in planning the therapeutic regimen or identifying patients at a higher risk of treatment failure or toxicity. These patients may require more intensive monitoring of serum concentration measurements.

This chapter describes the relationships of physiologic alterations and pharmacokinetic parameters describing drug disposition in ICU patients, which are useful in anticipating and describing the wide interpatient and intrapatient variation in drug disposition. The concepts of physiologic clearance and applied pharmacokinetics are important clinical tools to optimize treatment and improve outcome.

Physiologic Response to Underlying Disease, Injury, and Complications

The physiologic and metabolic changes secondary to underlying disease, trauma, sepsis, and their related complications are substantial   [40,48,75,76,78,80–88,91,92,103,104,106,107,108, 124,129–135]. The mechanisms and steps involved in activating and mediating the injury-related responses are controversial and unclear. Many current studies may further delineate the pathways of injury-related responses and mechanisms involved [78,80,95,96,97,103,104,112,113,130,134,136,137].   End-organ responses are better understood and meaningful if the patient is hypermetabolic or hypometabolic. In hypermetabolic patients drug disposition and dosage requirements may be affected and dosages may need adjustment to optimize therapy. The dosage regimen may need further adjustment as the clinical course improves and the physiologic response lessens. Assessment of the patient's physiologic response can help determine whether a dosage adjustment is needed and what dosage adjustment is appropriate.

The end-organ responses to injury associated with changes in drug disposition include oxygen clearance, cardiac output, serum proteins, vascular volume, extracellular fluid volume, metabolic rate, urinary urea nitrogen, urinary catecholamines, regional shunting in blood flow, amino acid utilization, and organ blood flow [40,75,77,80–86,88,101,130,133]. The magnitude of the physiologic response demonstrates considerable heterogeneity among a group of hyperdynamic or hypodynamic patients. Many other physiologic or metabolic changes have been identified but may not be associated with changes

in physiologic parameters describing drug disposition. These variables are not included in the following discussion.

The increased oxygen requirements in the hyperdynamic patient are mainly achieved by increased cardiac output via increased heart rate and stroke volume. Changes in the cardiac output can be substantial (>100% increase), especially in the younger trauma patient [75,81,83,133,138]. This increase in cardiac output progressively increases over the first 6 to 9 days after injury (Fig. 206-1). The increased cardiac output further increases blood flow to other organs, including the liver and kidney. Liver blood flow may increase 50 to 70 percent over baseline by 3 to 5 days after injury [138]. The liver also receives a larger fraction of the cardiac output over the first 6 to 9 days after injury, indicating a redistribution of blood flow following hypermetabolic stimuli [107,109,129,132,139]. The fraction of cardiac output received by the liver may increase by 50 percent over baseline. The organs principally responsible for drug clearance can thus receive more blood volume per unit time during the period following hypermetabolic stimuli. This hyperdynamic phase may be further stimulated by medical complications such as sepsis [80,87,88,92]. In patients improving clinically, this hypermetabolic phase resolves as the patient recovers from the injury or complications.

Organ blood flow is also altered during the perioperative period in patients undergoing elective surgery [107,109, 127,128,129,132,139]. In a group of patients undergoing appendectomy, liver blood flow decreased from 1600 ml per minute at baseline to 750 ml per minute during the surgery. Many factors could explain the decreased organ blood flow during surgery, including analgesics, anesthetics, regional shunting of blood flow, decreased body temperature, and the injury. Many of the same factors are found in victims of motor vehicle accidents, especially when there is substantial blood loss from a major fracture and an external or internal bleed. Blood flow to vital organs can be further altered and the energy-dependent processes, such as drug metabolism, affected.

Drug metabolizing systems appear to be affected by the physiologic changes secondary to injury in humans and animal models [3,47,58,89,118,132,140,141]. Boucher and others [3,142] systematically studied oxidizing enzyme systems and conjugative systems in head-injured patients. Their model utilized lorazepam, antipyrine, and indocyanine green as markers of hepatic glucuronidation, oxidation, and hepatic blood flow, respectively. Antipyrine clearance was significantly increased on study days 4, 7, and 14 when compared to baseline [3]. The increases at day 14 were 14 to 207 percent over baseline. Lorazepam clearance was significantly increased on day 14, with values ranging from 9 to 130 percent higher than baseline. Indocyanine green clearance did not change longitudinally; this was unexpected based on other data. These data indicate that the metabolic systems responsible for hepatic oxidation and glucuronidation are stimulated in the head-injured patient. Drugs metabolized by these enzyme systems should be closely monitored in the hypermetabolic patient, and dosage adjustments may be needed to achieve the desired pharmacologic response.

Changes in drug metabolizing systems have also been verified in animal models [118,140,141]. In a bilateral fracture model using the rat, the cytochrome P-450 system was affected by injury [118]. The content and activity of the cytochrome P-450 system were decreased by 25 to 35 percent within 24 hours of injury (Fig. 206-2) and returned to baseline within 48 to 72 hours after injury. In an abdominal aorta ligation model of the rat, the activity of the cytochrome P-450 system decreased by 50 percent and the content of cytochrome P-450 remained the same [140,141]. These data suggest a heterogeneity of responses from

Physiologic Changes Post-trauma

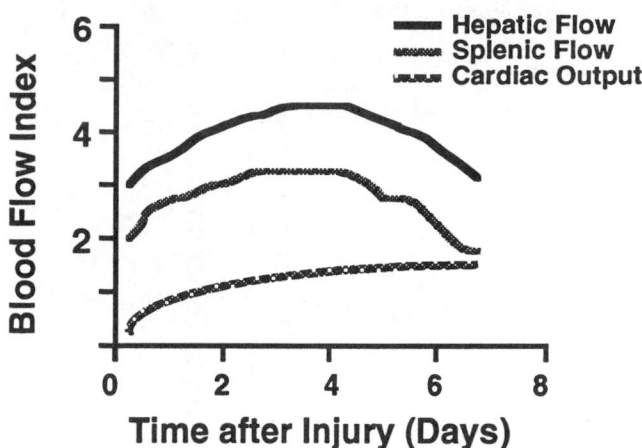

Fig. 206-1. Physiologic changes after trauma. The hepatic blood flow and cardiac output rise substantially in the immediate days after trauma. This end organ response is reflective of the hyperdynamic state that many posttraumatic patients experience [138].

Effect of Abdominal Aorta Ligation on Cytochrome P-450

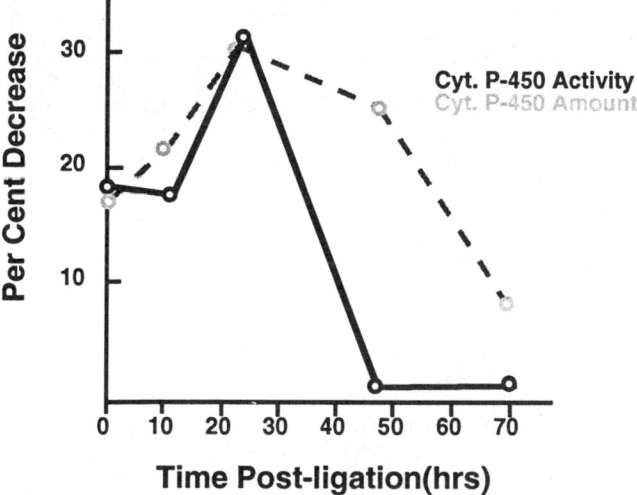

Fig. 206-2. Effect of abdominal aorta ligation on cytochrome P-450. A substantial decrease in the activity and content was noted in the rat model within the first 24 hours after aorta ligation. These data indicate that oxidative enzyme systems conducted via the cytochrome P-450 system are impacted by trauma [140,141].

the same or similar stimuli studied in human or animal models. Some enzyme systems appear to be upregulated by the same stimuli that downregulate other enzyme systems. Physiologic stimuli from medical disease or trauma may have a less predictable response on the major systems responsible for metabolizing drugs.

The vascular and extracellular fluid volumes are known to be altered in postinjury patients and those with underlying medical disease, such as congestive heart failure. [138,143,144]. Fluid shifts between physiologic spaces can occur and may affect the distribution of drugs to tissue compartments and the volume of distribution for many agents. The vascular volume increases by 10 to 20 percent in the first 6 to 9 days after trauma. The extracellular fluid volume and vascular volume can be further increased by direct intervention to maximize cardiac output and oxygen delivery. A decrease in fluid volumes can occur rapidly with administration of rapid-acting diuretics and diuresis. Changes in fluid volumes can be quite dynamic from patient to patient or in the same patient over time. Fluid changes and their effect on drug disposition can be anticipated.

Serum proteins can demonstrate substantial changes secondary to underlying disease or after injury [1,2,10,14,15,22, 32,45,58,68,76,90,110,132,145–149]. Serum albumin concentrations can decrease by 50 percent in the first days after injury. Albumin concentrations can also be affected by many medical conditions, including liver disease, ascites, kidney disease, and malignancies. Stress proteins, such as alpha-1-acid glycoprotein, are released into vascular circulation in patients following a myocardial infarction, trauma, and psychosis. The concentrations of alpha-1-acid glycoprotein can increase to values four to five times baseline (Fig. 206-3). Peak values occur 9 to 12 days after injury or myocardial infarction. These values return to normal as the patient's medical condition resolves.

Changes in protein concentration and total amount can alter the binding of drugs that are acids (e.g., phenytoin) [3,7,9–12, 15, 19, 21, 24, 29, 30, 33, 36, 37, 42, 45, 51–54, 62, 64, 73, 114, 137,145,147,149–161] or bases (e.g., lidocaine) [1,5,8,11,14, 16,22,26,27,34,38,41,46,60,62,64,66,72,73,145,146,147,152, 162–165]. Basic drugs bind to alpha-1-acid glycoprotein and the acidic agents to albumin. In the postmyocardial infarction or trauma patient, stress proteins (e.g., alpha-1-acid glycoprotein) are increased; acidic drugs are more highly bound and the free

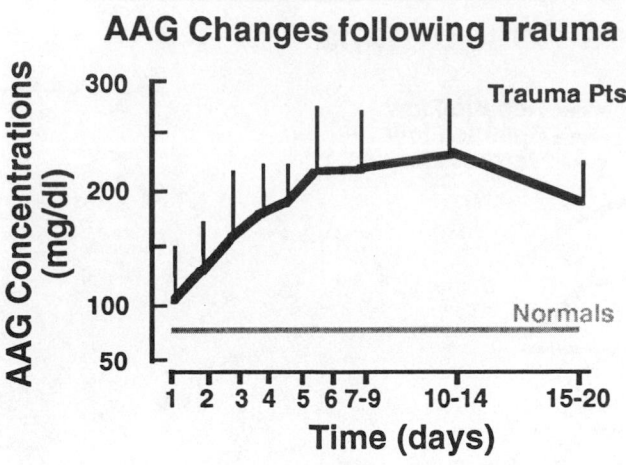

Fig. 206-3. Alpha-1-acid glycoprotein (AAG) changes following trauma. The normal concentration of AAG is approximately 80 mg/dl. In the traumatized patient, AAG concentrations increase by 10–14 days by as much as five- to sixfold over baseline values. This increase can substantially impact the protein binding of specific drugs [146].

fraction is decreased. Also in these patients, serum albumin concentration and total amounts are decreased; the basic drugs thus have higher free fractions, and more of the total concentration is available for the agent's pharmacologic effect.

The magnitude of the physiologic response to injury parallels the severity of injury, within the limits of aerobic metabolism the patient can maintain (Fig. 206-4) [77,82,85,86,87,98, 101,102,105,108,112,113,166]. More severe patient injuries (e.g., burns and multiple fractures) result in more exaggerated changes in physiologic parameters, including oxygen demand, cardiac output, energy requirements, and blood flow to the kidney or liver. Complications such as sepsis increase the physiologic stress and end-organ responses are elevated further. The magnitude of the physiologic responses continues to increase until the patient can no longer deliver enough oxygen to the tissues to maintain aerobic metabolism [105,106,108,131, 166,167]. When anaerobic metabolism begins (multiple organ system failure), as indicated by rising lactate values and so on, the functional level or efficacy of vital organs diminishes markedly. Indices of end-organ function demonstrate marked decreases in functionality. The disposition of many drugs follows the changes in organ function, especially those agents that are dependent on organ blood flow for clearance.

Physiologic Clearance

The qualitative pharmacokinetic changes, for many of the pharmacologic agents used in the ICU patient, can be anticipated knowing the patient's response to underlying diseases, fluid balance, injury, sepsis, and the drug's physiologic clearance properties. It is essential to identify the clinical parameters that describe the patient's hyperdynamic or hypodynamic state (including cardiac output and oxygen clearance) in order to assess the patient's physiologic or metabolic response. Classifying a patient as generally hypermetabolic or hypometabolic is useful to anticipate decreased or increased dosage requirements.

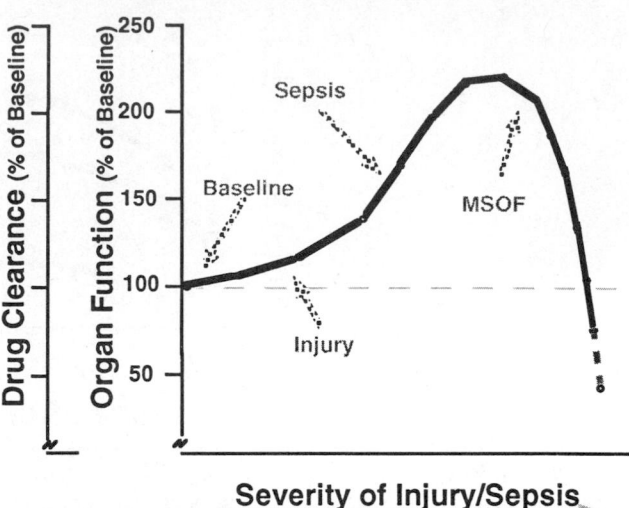

Fig. 206-4. Organ function and drug clearance with increasing severity of injury/sepsis. End-organ functions, such as cardiac output, liver blood flow, and oxygen clearance, markedly increase as the severity of injury increases or metabolic complications such as sepsis develop in traumatized patients. Multiple system organ failure (MSOF) begins to develop when aerobic conditions cannot be maintained and organ effectiveness begins to deteriorate. This qualitative relationship parallels the clearance observed for many drugs cleared by the liver or kidney.

HYPERMETABOLIC STATE. A patient with high cardiac output, oxygen clearance, or metabolic rate can be described as being hypermetabolic, a state that is secondary to injury-related changes and complications such as sepsis [39,61,75,76, 77,82,84,98,101,102,112,133,136,166,168]. Physiologic parameters, such as oxygen clearance, cardiac output, energy requirements, and blood flow to the kidney and liver, increase. As blood flow to the organ increases, drug clearance may also increase.

HYPOMETABOLIC STATE. The patient who develops severe congestive heart failure or multiple system organ failure may have substantial decreases in organ function, such as cardiac output and organ blood flow [105,106,108,131,166,167]. The functional capacity of the kidney or liver in removing drugs decreases markedly with the onset of changes in blood chemistry and clinical indicators of organ failure. The change in drug disposition may occur before the change in blood chemistry or other physiologic markers are evident. Drug elimination or clearance is frequently reduced to values unexpectedly low compared to estimates from volunteers or adjusted for renal or hepatic function.

PHYSIOLOGIC CLEARANCE MODEL. Physiologic clearance concepts are useful in predicting and anticipating pharmacokinetic changes in the intensive care patients. For many patients, the clinician may order interventions aimed at expanding the vascular volume to maximize cardiac output and oxygen delivery, maximizing cardiac output (i.e., inotropes) and increasing oxygen delivery, or altering the underlying dynamic state of the patient. In addition, any medical complication or drug toxicity that compromises the function of the kidney or liver may change the organ's ability to eliminate drug, thereby altering the drug's clearance and dosage requirements. Clinical assessment of the patient's medical condition can identify physiologic parameters that are directly applicable to the intrinsic clearance model and can be useful in anticipating changes in drug disposition and dosage requirements.

Systemic clearance or total clearance of a drug can be defined as the sum of clearances from all organs responsible for the drug's elimination. The drug clearance of an individual organ (e.g., liver) is dependent on the blood flow to the organ (Q) and the extraction ratio (E):

$$Cl = Q \times E \qquad (1)$$

The extraction ratio (E) is further defined as the difference between arterial concentration (C_a) and venous concentration (C_v) across an organ.

$$E = \frac{C_a - C_v}{C_a} \qquad (2)$$

A physiologic approach to clearance can be derived by explaining extraction ratio (Equation 1) in terms of blood flow, the fraction free in perfused blood (f_B), and the free intrinsic clearance of the organ (Cl_{int}):

$$Cl = \frac{Q \times f_B \times Cl_{int}}{Q + (f_B \times Cl_{int})} \qquad (3)$$

Pharmacologic agents can be divided into three classes according to their physiologic clearance characteristics, described by blood flow (Q), protein binding (f_B), and intrinsic clearance (Cl_{int}). These classes are flow-limited agents, capacity-limited binding-insensitive agents, and capacity-limited binding-sensitive agents (Fig. 206-5). These categories of agents behave in a predictable manner, and this information can be of assistance in qualitatively assessing changes in a patient's dosage requirements. Specific agents that fall between flow-limited and capacity-limited characteristic or between binding-sensitive or binding-insensitive can change when the patient becomes either hyperdynamic or hypodynamic.

Flow-Limited Agents. The clearance of "flow-limited" agents is principally dependent on the blood flow to the organ (Q) and extraction efficiency (E), as described in Equation 1. In hypermetabolic states, blood flow increases secondary to the elevated cardiac output values and increased blood supply. The agents eliminated by the kidney via glomerular filtration and/or active secretion follow flow-limited characteristics. This group includes most of the penicillins, cephalosporins, aminoglycosides, and H_2 antagonists (see Table 205-1). These agents generally follow linear principles of pharmacokinetic behavior, which greatly simplifies the mathematical approach to clinically adjusting dosage requirements. Most agents used in the ICU are classified as flow-limited.

Capacity-Limited Binding-Insensitive. The clearance of capacity-limited binding-insensitive agents is dependent on the intrinsic clearance of the organ responsible for the drug's elimination. The primary organ is the liver, but the gut, respiratory tract, and other organs can be important contributors to the total clearance of specific agents. The drug metabolizing activity of the liver has several important enzyme systems that can be

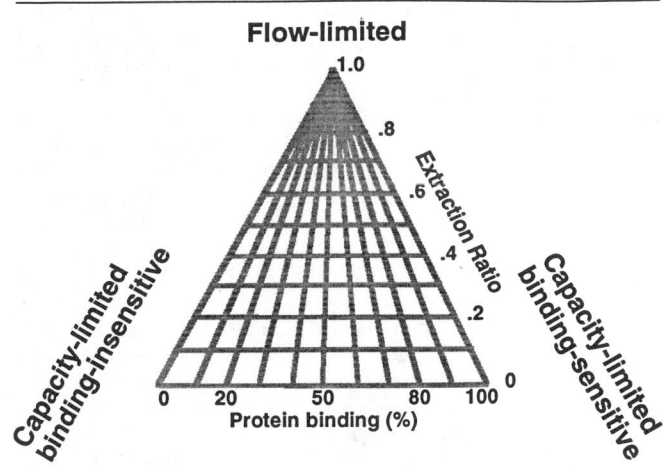

Fig. 206-5. Physiologic clearance model. The clearance of drugs can generally be divided into two groups, depending on the extraction ratio. If the extraction ratio is high, the drug will follow flow-limited characteristics. If the extraction ratio is low, the drug will following capacity-limited characteristics. Clearance can also be impacted by the degree of protein binding. For capacity-limited drugs, the clearance is impacted by protein binding if values exceed 70–80%. The clearance for these agents closely follows capacity as long as it has binding-sensitive characteristics. For agents not extensively bound to proteins, clearance follows capacity-limited, binding-insensitive characteristics.

influenced differently by the same stimuli. Different enzyme systems can be upregulated and others downregulated by the same stimuli (e.g., catecholamines). The different enzyme systems responsible for phase I or phase II reactions may also behave differently under the same stimuli. Clearance of these agents is dependent on the capacity of the enzyme systems responsible for their elimination or the drug's intrinsic clearance (Cl_{int}). These agents are not extensively bound to serum proteins ($f_B > 0.7$) (see Table 205-2). Chloramphenicol and theophylline are examples of agents that follow capacity-limited binding-insensitive characteristics. This group of agents can exhibit nonlinear characteristics and should be considered in making dosage adjustments.

Capacity-Limited Binding-Sensitive. The clearance of these agents is dependent on the drug's intrinsic clearance (Cl_{int}) and the free fraction(f_B). Changes in blood flow rates (cardiac output) should not influence the drug's clearance characteristics unless the same stimuli affecting the cardiac output also affect the enzyme system responsible for the drug's elimination. The drug's protein binding characteristics become an important factor influencing its clearance if the free fraction (f_B) is less than 0.7 (see Table 205-2). Agents binding to alpha-1-acid glycoprotein, such as clindamycin and the narcotic analgesics, may demonstrate substantial change in the degree of protein binding over the course of a patient's hospitalization. These dynamic changes can also occur with agents that bind to albumin (i.e., phenytoin), especially in ICU patients, who may also have dramatic changes in serum albumin concentrations.

Clinical Application of Physiologic Clearance. Physiologic drug clearance can be explained in terms of three physiologic variables that the clinician can use to make qualitative assessments and inferences regarding a drug's disposition characteristics. These include the patient's cardiac output, serum proteins (i.e., albumin or alpha-1-acid glycoprotein), and organ function. Much of this information is available for patients in the ICU. The physiologic clearance concepts are a useful tool to identify patients who need more intensive monitoring assessments and who may require changes in dosing regimens.

Drugs eliminated via the kidney by glomerular filtration generally appear to follow flow-limited characteristics. Those agents actively secreted by the kidney may have a saturation point, but within the amounts administered clinically their clearance seem to follow flow-limited characteristics. The clearance of flow-limited drugs directly parallels changes in blood flow to the primary organ responsible for the drug's elimination. In the hypermetabolic patient, drug clearance generally increases in parallel with the change in blood flow as long as the intrinsic function of the organ is not altered by medical complications (e.g., shock), altered renal function, altered hepatic function, or drugs (e.g., aminoglycosides).

Drugs metabolized by various enzyme systems are generally more complex and less predictable than the flow-limited agents. Their clearance characteristics are categorized as capacity-limited, meaning clearance is not primarily dependent on blood flow to the organ, but rather on the intrinsic clearance capacity of the drug's enzyme system. These enzyme systems respond differently to the common mediators of injury-related stress. For example, some enzyme systems can be upregulated by catecholamines and some can be downregulated. Various enzyme systems have been studies in vitro or in animal models. Although the results cannot be extrapolated to the patient with assurance, the data indicate that changes in the rate of drug metabolism occur after injury. The mechanisms responsible for regulating these enzyme systems have received considerable study, and the results may contribute to understanding of drug metabolism in critical care patients.

Several drugs are known to be capacity-limited; for example, phenytoin has an elevated clearance rate. These agents have higher dosage requirements in hypermetabolic patients and lower dosage requirements in hypometabolic patients. This is likely explained by the dichotomy in response of different enzyme systems to the same stimuli in the posttraumatic patient. Specific enzyme systems may be upregulated by the mediators of the injury-related response and others may be downregulated by the same stimuli. Further study is required to predict the qualitative response of different enzyme systems.

The clearance of the capacity-limited agents can be affected further by protein binding characteristics of the drug if it is highly protein-bound (>90%). The binding characteristics of acidic and basic drugs can be affected by changes in protein concentration (i.e., amount of albumin or stress proteins, such as alpha-1-acid glycoprotein). The concentration and amount of albumin decrease in hypermetabolic patients. Acidic drugs (e.g., phenytoin) are highly bound to albumin in hypermetabolic patients; generally less of these drugs bind to the albumin. Because more of the drug exists in the free unbound form, a higher percentage of the total drug is pharmacologically active. The free fraction describes the amount or concentration of a drug that is related to the drug's pharmacologic effect and also the amount of drug available for elimination via metabolism. Basic drugs (e.g., clindamycin and morphine) bind to alpha-1-acid glycoprotein (Fig. 206-6). The free fraction may be decreased by 300 to 500 percent over baseline values in the hypermetabolic patient. Capacity-limited agents that are highly bound (>90%) to either albumin or alpha-1-acid glycoprotein are referred to as capacity-limited binding-sensitive. Changes in amount or concentration of albumin directly affect the binding of basic drugs, and changes in the amount or concentration of alpha-1-acid glycoprotein directly affect the binding of acidic drugs.

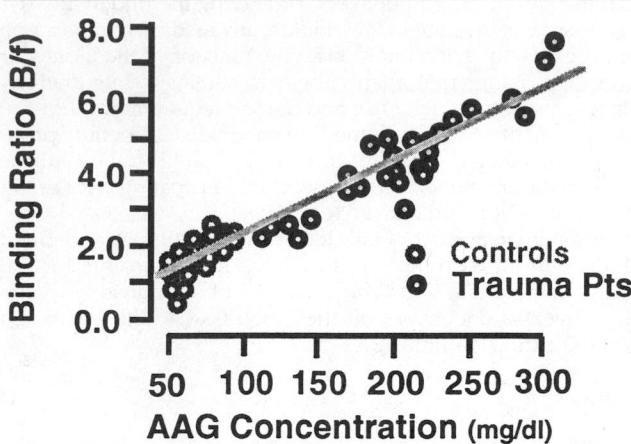

Fig. 206-6. Lidocaine binding. As the concentration of alpha-1-acid glycoprotein (AAG) increases in patients immediately after trauma or myocardial infarction, the binding of specific drugs can be impacted substantially. For example, the ratio of bound lidocaine to free lidocaine is changed substantially as the concentration of AAG increases. The amount of free lidocaine available from pharmacologic activity is markedly reduced [146].

Pharmacokinetic Principles Used to Individualize a Patient's Dosage Regimen

Pharmacokinetic parameters for a specific drug for an individual patient can be determined from the serum concentration versus time and used to calculate dosage regimens to attain desired serum concentrations. The patient's pharmacokinetic parameters are an important clinical tool to calculate the dosage regimen quickly and inexpensively. The clinician must define serum concentration endpoints that balance the risks of treatment failure with the risks of toxicity. These endpoints have been defined for some drugs, and guidelines exist to facilitate decision-making.

Dosage regimens should be designed to maximize the therapeutic benefits against the risks of toxicity. In selected patients, some drugs (e.g., lidocaine) should be administered initially as a loading dose to achieve the desired pharmacologic effect quickly; other drugs may be effectively administered as a maintenance dose initially. The following discussion describes methods to determine a patient's pharmacokinetic parameters, and loading dose and maintenance dose requirements to achieve desired concentration endpoints.

PHARMACOKINETIC MODEL SELECTION. The pharmacokinetic model is selected to maximize the mathematical fit of serum concentration-time data, thereby minimizing the error or biases realized in using a less appropriate model. The ultimate goal is to use the model with the highest predictive performance in estimating dosage regimens in a cost-effective manner. For most drugs used in the ICU, a simple one-compartment model that assumes linear behavior between serum concentrations and dose can be used. The mathematical fit of the data can generally be improved with additional serum concentration values, but the predictive performance may not be improved; therefore it is not necessary to incur the excessive costs of many

Fitting Amikacin Concentrations with a One Compartment Model

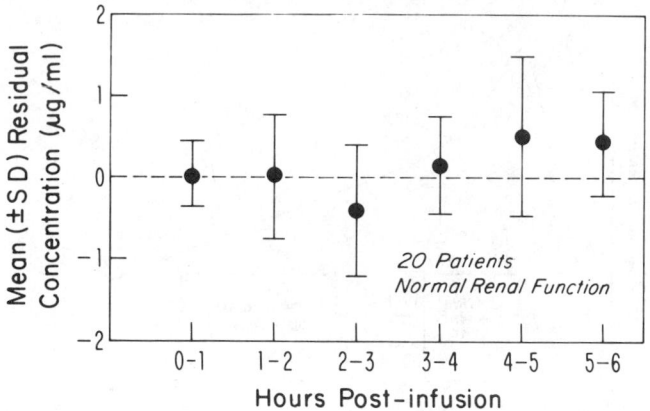

Fig. 206-7. Fitting amikacin concentrations. Postinfusion serum concentration-time data were fitted by nonlinear least squares regression analysis assuming a monoexponential decay. The differences between measured and fitted concentrations were grouped and summed for each 1-hour interval. For each time period, the mean and standard deviation of the residual concentrations are illustrated. The use of the one-compartment model demonstrated minimal bias after administering the drug as a 1-hour infusion.

serum drug concentrations (Fig. 206-7) [49,50,70,71]. Most drugs used in the ICU follow linear pharmacokinetic principles, meaning the change in serum concentration or the area under the serum concentration-time curve produced by a change in the patient's dosage regimen is directly proportional. These drugs include most antibiotics and analgesics. A notable exception is phenytoin, which follows nonlinear principles in epileptic patients but may follow linear principles in many hyperdynamic trauma patients and within the dosages used or serum concentrations attained in these patients. This is due to alteration of the capacity of different enzyme systems in hyperdynamic patients.

ONE-COMPARTMENT LINEAR MODEL. The least expensive model is the one-compartment model that assumes linear behavior [49,50]. Of the various models it requires the least samples and is therefore most cost-effective. Pharmacokinetic parameters can be calculated from the first dose or from steady-state conditions. This model can be used to estimate dosage requirements prospectively, to monitor a course of treatment, and to modify dosage regimens as clinical conditions change. Imprecision or model biases are the major criticism of this model, which may be justifiable when it is used as a clinical research tool [71].

The elimination rate of a drug is described by its half-life or elimination rate constant. The half-life ($t_{1/2}$) is the time required for the serum concentration to decrease to 50 percent of its initial value. The elimination rate constant (K_d) is the negative slope of the log of serum concentration versus time, or the ln of 2 divided by the half-life:

$$t_{1/2} = \frac{\ln 2}{K_d} = \frac{0.693}{K_d} \tag{4}$$

$$K_d = \frac{0.693}{t_{1/2}}$$

The volume of distribution (V_d) is the size of the space within which the drug distributes. It can be further defined by the change in serum concentration (ΔC_p) produced by a known dose (D) of drug administered by an instantaneous intravenous bolus. This relationship can be further modified to resemble clinical conditions in the ICU, where the drug may not be administered by bolus. Equation 6 considers the amount of drug eliminated during the infusion period to estimate more accurately the volume of distribution. The infusion rate (K_o), defined as the amount per time, and the infusion period (t') must be known. The volume of distribution can be standardized to body weight to reduce some of the interpatient variation in a patient sample [49,50].

$$V_d = \frac{\Delta C_p}{D} = \frac{C_{p post} - C_{p pre}}{D} \tag{5}$$

$$V_d = \frac{K_o}{K_d} \times \frac{(1 - e^{-K_{d0}'})}{(C_{p post} - C_{p pre}\, e^{-K_{dt}'})} \tag{6}$$

The drug's clearance (Cl) is the volume of drug cleared from the body per unit time. It can be standardized by weight to reduce some of the interpatient variation. It can be determined by dividing the dose by the area under the serum concentration-time curve (AUC).

$$Cl = \frac{D}{AUC} \tag{7}$$

$$Cl = K_d \times V_d \tag{8}$$

In many ICU patients, the relationship of the drug's half-life with the distribution volume (V_d) and clearance (Cl) is apparent. This relationship becomes quite useful clinically in monitoring the patient's dosage regimen over time where the extracellular fluid volume is intentionally changed to maximize cardiac output or where excess fluid is diuresed with rapid-acting loop diuretics (e.g., furosemide). The volume of distribution for the penicillins and aminoglycosides closely resembles the extracellular fluid volume and is altered clinically by changes in the patient's state of hydration. The half-life is directly proportional to the volume of distribution and inversely related to clearance (Cl).

$$t_{1/2} = \frac{V_d \times 0.693}{Cl} \tag{9}$$

Since the clearance of a flow-limited drug by an organ (Cl) is related to the blood flow to the organ (Q) and the extraction efficiency (E), the relationship of half-life in Equation 6 can be rewritten to be more useful for monitoring dosage regimens:

$$Cl = Q \times E \tag{10}$$

$$t_{1/2} = \frac{V_d \times 0.693}{Q \times E} \tag{11}$$

The half-life is directly related to the volume of distribution and inversely related to the blood flow to the organ and extraction efficiency. This relationship (Equation 11) is a useful tool to anticipate changes in drug disposition and estimate dosage regimens when qualitative changes in the volume of distribution and blood flow are known. For example, if a patient has clinical signs of edema and a rapid-acting diuretic is used to remove the excess fluid, the volume of distribution will decrease for drugs primarily distributed in the extracellular fluid volume (e.g., aminoglycosides and beta-lactams). The half-life of the drug will also become shorter as the excess fluid is diuresed and may further change the dosage regimen needed to maintain the same peak and trough serum concentrations.

Dosage regimens can be estimated using general assumptions of pharmacokinetic parameters for a drug with a wide margin of safety (e.g., a beta lactam), or calculated estimates of the patient's half-life and volume of distribution for a drug with a narrow therapeutic index (e.g., an aminoglycoside). The patient's dosage regimen (D), administered as a continuous infusion, can be estimated using the desired serum concentration (C_p) and the clearance (Cl):

$$D = C_p \times Cl \tag{12}$$

For drugs administered as intermittent infusions, the infusion rate (K_o) is determined using the drug's elimination rate constant (K_d), distribution volume (V_d), desired peak serum concentration (C_{pmax}), dosing interval (π), and infusion period (t') [49,50]:

$$K_o = K_d V_d C_{pmax} \frac{(1 - e^{-K_d\pi})}{(1 - e^{-K_d t'})} \tag{13}$$

The dose is equal to the infusion rate (K_o) times the infusion period (t'). The dosage interval (π) necessary to achieve targeted peak serum concentrations (C_{pmax}) and desired trough serum concentration (C_{pmin}) can be calculated for a specific patient using the elimination rate constant (k_d) and infusion period (t') [49,50].

$$\pi = \frac{-1}{K_d} \ln \frac{C_{pmin}}{C_{pmax}} + t' \tag{14}$$

TWO-COMPARTMENT LINEAR MODELS. After intravenous infusions, the drug reaches equilibrium between the vascular compartment and the tissue compartment. With certain drugs, the serum concentration-time curve will appear biphasic (Fig. 206-8). The first phase is actually the combination of drug diffusing into the tissue compartment and that being eliminated from the body. The second phase is attributed to the drug being eliminated from the body. The interpatient variation of the pharmacokinetic parameters describing the two-compartment characteristics of drugs is substantial. It is further attenuated by changes made in fluid therapy and state of hydration.

Determining serum sampling intervals necessary to describe the two-compartment phenomena of a specific drug is difficult [169]. At least six concentration-time pairs are needed. The practical limitations of this model make it more useful as a research tool. Errors incurred by applying a one-compartment model to a drug displaying two-compartment phenomena can be minimized by obtaining serum samples on the elimination phase of the serum concentration time curve, using longer infusion periods to decrease the infusion rate, and monitoring the patient carefully during therapy and making appropriate changes in the dosage regimen. Generally, one-compartment models can be used to estimate the pharmacokinetic parameters of drugs displaying two-compartment phenomena, providing the necessary precautions are implemented to prevent underestimating drug accumulation.

NONLINEAR PHARMACOKINETIC MODEL. The pharmacokinetic behavior of a limited number of agents used in the ICU cannot be adequately characterized by linear models [170]. Nonlinearity is generally limited to agents that are metabolized. The enzyme system becomes saturated with substrate and reaches its maximal rate of converting parent compound to

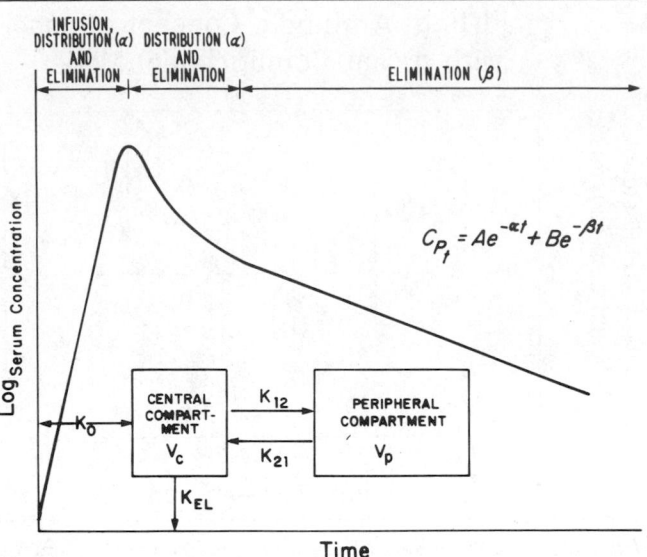

Fig. 206-8. Two-compartment pharmacokinetic behavior will likely be observed for pharmacologic agents that diffuse slowly into the peripheral compartment, those that are infused at more rapid rates, and those that are eliminated slowly. The elimination portion of the curve can generally be anticipated, and serum sampling conducted or devise the capture of that specific portion of the curve within the patient care setting.

metabolite. For these agents (e.g., phenytoin) Michaelis-Menten kinetics are generally used to assist in quantitatively determining dosage regimens. The pharmacokinetic parameters can be determined only while the patient is at steady state (requiring several days) and requires two to three dosage adjustments with measured serum concentrations after each. This method is generally not useful in the ICU because the time required to achieve steady state for each dosage increment is too long. Dosages of these drugs need to be increased cautiously at smaller incremental steps to avoid serious risks of adverse reactions. Serum concentrations may need to be monitored after steady state has been achieved to avoid serious toxicity and to attain therapeutic values quickly.

A nonlinear serum drug concentration versus time curve on both coordinate and semilogarithmic plots can result from a variety of mechanisms. Drugs with a capacity-limited or saturable clearance pathway are said to demonstrate nonlinear pharmacokinetics. As the serum drug concentration increases, clearance decreases, saturation occurs, and elimination approaches zero-order. As saturation occurs, disproportionate increases in serum drug concentrations are observed with increasing drug doses. The Michaelis-Menten function can be used to describe the rate of elimination and clearance of these drugs as follows:

$$\text{Elimination rate} = \frac{V_{max} \times C_{ps}}{K_m + C_{ps}} \tag{15}$$

where V_{max} is the maximum rate of elimination in units of amount/time, K_m is the Michaelis-Menten constant (i.e., the serum drug concentration at which elimination is half maximal), and C_{ps} is the serum drug concentration at steady state. For drugs with saturable elimination:

$$Cl = \frac{V_{max}}{K_m + C_{ps}} \tag{16}$$

When the usual therapeutic drug concentrations for a drug are much smaller than its K_m, clearance is independent of serum drug concentration and the drug exhibits first-order elimination. With most hepatically eliminated drugs, serum concentrations can be increased to points at which the capacity of the liver to metabolize the drug is exceeded, thus these agents exhibit nonlinear pharmacokinetics. Nonlinear elimination is frequently observed in overdose, where the primary route of elimination of many drugs depends on metabolism. With a few drugs, most notably phenytoin and salicylates, saturation occurs at serum concentrations in the usual therapeutic range.

LOADING DOSE. Loading doses (LD) can be determined by rearranging Equation 2 and using a population-based volume of distribution (V_d). Loading doses are calculated by:

$$LD = \frac{(C_{pdesired} - C_{pobs}) \times V_d}{F} \tag{17}$$

where the difference in desired serum drug concentration ($C_{pdesired}$) and the current serum drug concentration (C_{pobs}) is multiplied by the volume of distribution. If the patient has not received any drug yet, then current serum drug concentration equals zero.

MAINTENANCE DOSE. Pharmacokinetic principles are useful to anticipate the dynamic parameters describing drug disposition and calculate maintenance dosage regimens. These parameters can further be used as a clinical tool to adjust dosage regimens in the ICU patient. The following discussion describes the principles and concepts to determine maintenance dosage regimens. Maintenance dosage regimens can be either continuous or intermittent infusions.

The patient's dosage regimen (D), administered as a continuous infusion, can be established by using the desired average serum concentration (C_p) and the clearance (Cl).

$$D = C_p \times Cl \tag{18}$$

Estimates of average serum concentration (C_p) over the entire dosing interval may also be used to determine intermittent dosage regimens.

For drugs administered as intermittent infusions, the infusion rate (K_o) is determined using the drug's elimination rate constant (K_d), distribution volume (V_d), desired peak serum concentration (C_{pmax}), dosing interval (π), and infusion period (t') [49,50].

$$K_o = K_d V_d C_{pmax} \frac{(1 - e^{-K_d\pi})}{(1 - e^{-K_dt'})} \tag{13}$$

The dose is equal to the infusion rate (K_o) times the infusion period (t').

$$D = K_o t' \tag{19}$$

The dosage interval (π) necessary to achieve targeted peak serum concentrations (C_{pmax}) and desired trough serum concentration (C_{pmin}) can be calculated for a specific patient knowing the elimination rate constant (K_d) and infusion period (t'): [49,50]

$$\pi = \frac{-1}{K_d} \ln \frac{C_{pmin}}{C_{pmax}} + t' \tag{14}$$

The dosage regimens determined using these equations should be used as a guideline. The clinician should always consider other commonly used methods of estimating dosage requirements. Also, these dosages should be implemented gradually in steps (e.g., theophylline, phenytoin), if clinically possible, and the response and need for higher dosage regimens reassessed. Necessary adjustments in dosage should be made to minimize risk of toxicity or treatment failure.

Monitoring the Patient's Dosage Regimen

After successfully implementing a patient's dosage regimen, the clinician should continually assess the response and changes in the patient's pharmacokinetic parameters. The response will indicate whether treatment is successful and dosage regimens can be decreased or whether the treatment is failing and other therapies should be considered. In addition, the patient's pharmacokinetic parameters may change during therapy and may necessitate changes in dosage. These changes can be determined by periodically checking serum concentrations during treatment or by anticipating changing physiologic parameters that may further affect dosage requirements.

ANTICIPATING PHARMACOKINETIC CHANGES BASED ON PHYSIOLOGIC CHANGES. Many physiologic changes observed between ICU patients and within the same patient have predictable consequences on the drug's pharmacokinetic parameters and on dosage requirements [55,56,61]. These include a change in fluid status to maximize cardiac output or a rapid diuresis (affects the volume of distribution for many antibiotics), altered physiologic stimuli from the injury and/or complications (affects organ clearance, drug-inactivating enzyme systems, and protein binding), and damage to the organ responsible for drug elimination (affects intrinsic clearance) (Figs. 206-9 and 206-10). This clinical information and assessment combined with pharmacologic and pharmacokinetic information make qualitative estimates of drug disposition clinically feasible and useful in adjusting dosage regimens or determining the appropriate time to obtain serum samples.

CHANGING FLUID STATUS. The extracellular and intravascular fluid volumes are frequently expanded in ICU patients to ensure optimal perfusion or due to underlying medical complications [55,56,61]. Hyperdynamic patients generally have an adequate cardiovascular reserve and respond to the increased vascular volume with increased ventricular filling pressures and increased cardiac output. This directly affects the volume of distribution of water-soluble drugs (e.g., the beta-lactams and aminoglycosides). The distribution volume expands in parallel to the volume of the extracellular fluid space, further changing the dynamics of drug disposition. The drug's half-life increases in parallel with the change in the volume of distribution if the clearance is not altered by the volume (Equation 11). This change can alter the serum concentration-time relationship (Fig. 206-6). The peak serum concentration is inversely related and trough values are directly related to the volume of distribution.

For drugs with a narrow therapeutic index (e.g., aminoglycosides), the altered serum concentration-time relationship may necessitate a change in dosage regimen to ensure an optimal response [6,35,63,70,71,74,122,171–173]. Drug clearance in patients with changing fluid dynamics does generally not change

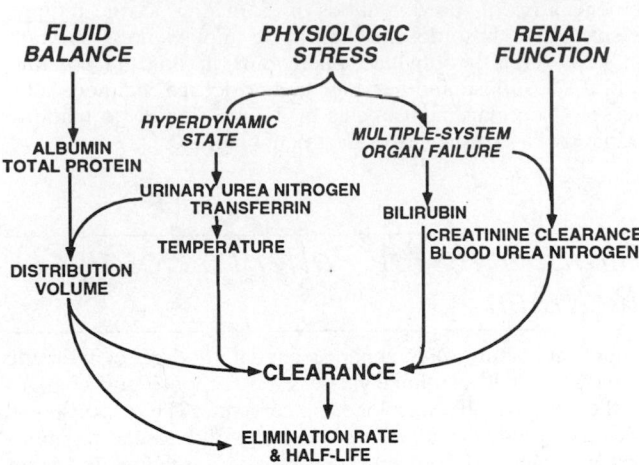

Fig. 206-9. Variables altering aminoglycoside clearance. In traumatized patients, factors associated with aminoglycoside clearance can be grouped into three categories: factors or variables associated with the state of hydration or extracellular fluid compartment, those associated with kidney function, and those that may be indicative of the hyperdynamic or hypodynamic state. The factors identified for each group were statistically related to either the drug's distribution volume or the drug's clearance. The statistical relationships indicate that variables descriptive of the magnitude of stress describe the most variance in drug clearance within this group of patients [61].

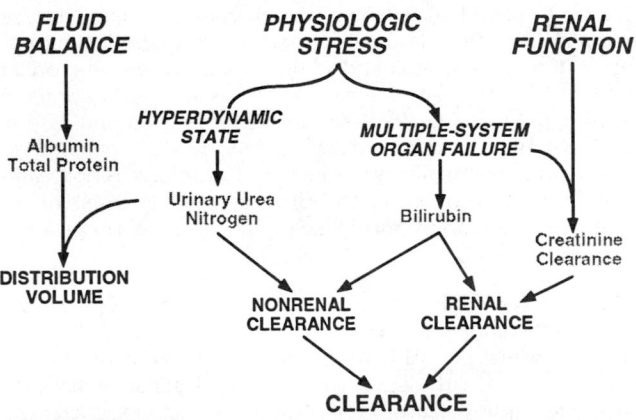

Fig. 206-10. The factors associated with piperacillin clearance can be categorized into factors influencing the extracellular fluid compartment, those associated with renal function, and those associated with the physiologic stress secondary to trauma. These factors are statistically related to the drug's volume of distribution or clearance as shown here [55,56].

unless cardiac output or the enzyme system for the drug's elimination is affected. The volume of distribution of water-soluble agents is affected to a greater magnitude than that of the lipid-soluble agents. The increased volume of distribution requires a larger dose (Equation 13), but the dosing interval needs to be prolonged (longer half-life; Equation 15) to attain the same peak and trough serum concentrations. The total daily dose may actually remain constant while the patient's volumes are changing. The distribution volumes can change rapidly from day to day, but generally this change is obvious by examining the patient or monitoring the amount of fluid administered. The volumes of distribution for water-soluble drugs generally decrease over time and as the patient clinically improves.

HYPERDYNAMIC/HYPODYNAMIC STATES

Flow-Limited Agents. The physiologic effects and effects on drug disposition of the hypermetabolic state are predictable for the flow-limited agents. The change in drug clearance is directly proportional to the change in blood flow rates or other markers of the hyperdynamic state while aerobic metabolism is maintained (Equation 10). The dosage requirements of flow-limited agents are increased in the hyperdynamic state. The magnitude of the increase may be five to six times the standard dosage. If oxygen delivery cannot be maintained to achieve aerobic conditions as observed in hyperdynamic patients, the clearance of flow-limited agents appears to be quite sensitive; marked decreases in drug clearance and dosage requirements are quickly observed. There is also substantial intrapatient variation as the patient's underlying trauma and medical complications resolve [55,56,61]. This change occurs over 10 to 14 days, sometimes longer, depending on the clinical response.

Capacity-Limited Agents. The patient's hyperdynamic effects on capacity-limited agents become specific to the drug and the enzyme system responsible for its degradation. Some of these agents appear to have increased clearance rates in hyperdynamic patients and others appear to have decreased clearance values. This might be explained by the same mediator of the physiologic change secondary to trauma having opposite effects on different enzyme systems. This is supported by animal studies and the limited data derived from ICU patients.

The protein binding characteristics of the capacity-limited binding-sensitive agents can change markedly during the patient's hospital stay [10,14,15,22,42,45,46,60,62,64,152, 155,165,174,175]. The amount of serum albumin and alpha-1-acid glycoprotein is very dynamic in the ICU patient. The amount of albumin decreases as the magnitude of posttrauma physiologic response increases. The amount of acute phase reactants (e.g., alpha-1-acid glycoprotein) increases as the magnitude of physiologic response increases. The amount of intrapatient fluctuation in serum albumin and alpha-1-acid glycoprotein is substantial during an ICU stay. A five- to sixfold variation in alpha-1-acid glycoprotein can be observed. Parenteral administration of albumin to increase osmotic pressure likely complicates drug disposition parameters for the binding-sensitive agents. Attainment of steady state pharmacokinetic parameters with capacity-limited binding-sensitive drugs is not a very dependable assumption to make but is done frequently. Serious errors can be minimized by increasing dosage regimens of the binding-sensitive agents slowly and continually reassessing the patient's response.

COMPROMISED RENAL FUNCTION. Dosage regimens of drugs primarily eliminated by the kidney must be adjusted frequently in ICU patients [47,121,123,171]. Several approaches

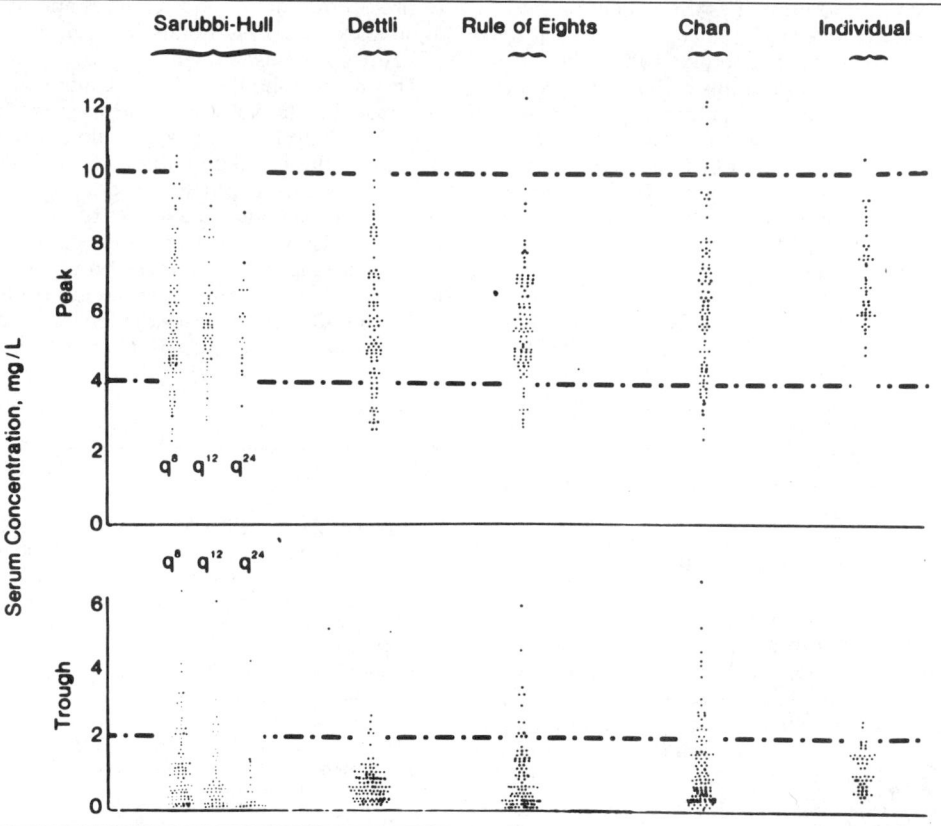

Fig. 206-11. Serum concentrations from four predictive dosing methods (calculated) and measured for the individual [49,50] are compared. Individualized method produced peak concentrations of 4–10 mg/L and troughs of 2 mg/L or less in significantly more patients (94%) than all predictive methods (p<0.01) [176].

are available; the choice of method depends on the drug's therapeutic index, the severity of the patient's clinical condition, and the risks or consequences of an adverse reaction. The risks of treatment failure and toxicity must be weighed against the costs of the method of dosage adjustment.

The use of serum concentrations may be expensive. Quantitative approaches using serum drug measurements to calculate dosage regimens necessary to attain desired serum concentrations have been evaluated in clinical settings and have improved patient survival rates or significantly decreased ICU stay [115,116,117]. Frequently these are the most cost-effective methods to maximize dosage regimens of aminoglycosides, theophylline, digoxin, vancomycin, and the anticonvulsants [176]. These approaches are highly recommended for situations, such as in the ICU, where there is substantial interpatient and intrapatient variation in pharmacokinetic parameters and dosage requirements.

Measurements of the patient's pharmacologic response or pharmacodynamic endpoints are useful for many other agents used in the ICU, including heparin, H_2 antagonists, beta-blockers, lidocaine, calcium channel blocking agents, inotropes, pressors, and narcotic analgesics. The therapeutic response is useful for determining the dosage regimen and making necessary adjustments.

Nomograms have been frequently recommended to adjust dosage regimens in patients with renal or liver impairment. Several assumptions are made, which can lead to substantial

error in individual patients [176]. These approaches can be recommended only for drugs with a wide therapeutic index, including the penicillins, cephalosporins, and H_2 antagonists. The assumptions that lead to substantial error in estimating dosage requirements for the ICU patient (Fig. 206-11) include the following.

1. Good correlation exists between measured and estimated creatinine clearances in the ICU patient.
2. Good correlation exists between measured or estimated creatinine clearances and drug clearance.
3. The volume of distribution remains constant for the patient.
4. The unrecognized patient response to trauma and/or sepsis leads to the hyperdynamic state.

The use of these nomograms frequently leads to substantial errors in estimating dosage requirements of aminoglycosides, theophylline, digoxin, vancomycin, and anticonvulsants. Nomograms are not recommended for estimating dosage requirements of these agents other than the initial dose. The use of serum concentration measurements is highly recommended when using these agents, especially for ICU patients.

CHANGING SERUM PROTEIN CONCENTRATIONS. The serum protein concentrations profile changes substantially in trauma patients and those who have serious underlying disease. Serum albumin concentrations and intravascular amounts of albumin frequently decrease by 50 percent or more [2, 159]. Acute phase reactant proteins (alpha-1-acid glycoprotein) may increase in certain patients, reaching peak values in 7 to 10 days [58]. These changes in albumin and alpha-1-acid glycoprotein concentrations return to normal as the patient reaches the convalescent stages of recovery.

The changes in serum protein concentrations affect the protein binding characteristics of several drugs commonly used in the ICU and may be important factors determining patient response. Acidic drugs bind to albumin (e.g., phenytoin) and basic agents to alpha-1-acid glycoprotein (e.g., meperidine, morphine, methadone, lidocaine, clindamycin, and propranolol). The free fraction of acidic drugs such as phenytoin is higher for the same total serum concentration measured in these patients. The basic drugs have lower free fractions and thus less of the total drug available for the pharmacologic activity. For example, methadone's free fraction changes from 92 percent to 8.8 percent when the alpha-1-acid glycoprotein concentration changes from 0.05 to 2 gm per liter [14,46].

The free fraction of the drug is both pharmacologically active and available for elimination. The net effect on the patient is difficult to anticipate because the drug's clearance increases as the free fraction increases and pharmacologic activity increases as the free fraction increases. Frequently, free serum concentrations are required to monitor the drug's pharmacologic response. Changes in protein concentrations thus affect protein binding of specific agents used in the ICU and are a factor in the wide interpatient variation in response.

The concentrations of albumin and alpha-1-acid glycoprotein demonstrate substantial variation in the initial 2 to 3 weeks after trauma or onset of underlying disease [2,14,27,32,33,39,45, 58,90,93,102,145,152]. The protein binding characteristics of acidic and basic drugs are quite dynamic during this period. The patient's pharmacologic response and dosage requirements can also vary substantially during the hospital course [1,2,10,19,26–29, 41–43, 45, 52, 99, 120, 122, 150, 151, 156, 158, 159, 163, 177, 178]. Due to the dynamic nature of protein concentrations, many ICU patients are never at steady state while recovering from their injury or sepsis. This observation can explain some of the intrapatient variation.

Computerized Pharmacokinetics

With recent advances in computer technology and the development of commercially available pharmacokinetic software, clinicians are better equipped to provide accurate serum drug concentration evaluations without the tedious mathematical tasks commonly associated with clinical pharmacokinetics. Commercially available software programs employ a variety of dosing and analysis functions, ranging from simple population-based dosing methods to sophisticated Bayesian feedback curve-fitting functions.

The initial segments of most programs are used to categorize physiologic, pathophysiologic, and pharmacologic factors contributing to variability in volume of distribution and clearance. Some programs automatically adjust pharmacokinetic parameters if the magnitude of the reported variability is great. For example, the population-based estimate of volume of distribution for gentamicin would be increased in an edematous patient.

Many programs provide dosing recommendations and a graphic display of predicted versus observed serum drug concentrations, providing the user with an estimate of the value of the simulation in predicting serum drug concentrations (i.e., predictive performance). Using a series of curve-fitting techniques, the user can attempt to reconcile the predicted and actual serum drug concentrations to improve predictive performance and thereby increase the potential for achieving the desired serum drug concentrations and associated pharmacologic responses. Easy storage and retrieval of data are features of many programs.

The novice should exercise caution in the application of pharmacokinetic software. The user is presumed to have a strong background in the application of pharmacokinetic principles and their clinical application. With the continued development of on-screen help functions and tutorials, and further progress in computerized access of medication administration records and laboratory data, the effectiveness of these programs is likely to improve. Still, these programs are only an aid or a tool in decision-making, and do not substitute for good clinical judgment. Always, clinical judgment must supersede computer-generated recommendations that seem unreasonable.

References

1. Bodenham A, Shelley MP, Park GR: The altered pharmacokinetics and pharmacodynamics of drugs commonly used in critically ill patients. *Clin Pharm* 14:347, 1988.
2. Boucher BA, Rodman JH, Jaresko GS, et al: Phenytoin pharmacokinetics in critically ill trauma patients. *Clin Pharmacol Ther* 44:675, 1988.
3. Boucher BA, Kuhl DA, Fabian TC, Robertson JT: Effect of neurotrauma on hepatic drug clearance. *Clin Pharmacol Ther* 50:487, 1991.
4. Beller JP, Pottecher T, Lugnier A, et al: Prolonged sedation with propofol in ICU patients: Recovery and blood concentration changes during periodic interruptions in infusion. *Br J Anaesth* 61:583, 1988.
5. Beemer GH, Bjorksten AR, Crankshaw DP: Pharmacokinetics of atracurium during continuous infusion. *Br J Anaesth* 65:668, 1990.
6. Dasta JF, Armstrong DK: Variability in aminoglycoside pharmacokinetics in critically ill surgical patients. *Crit Care Med* 16:327, 1988.
7. Dirksen MSC, Vree TB, Driessen JJ: Midazolam in the intensive care unit (letter). *DICP* 20:805, 1986.
8. Donati F: Atracurium, pharmacokinetics and metabolites. *Can J Anaesth* 36:257, 1989.
9. Dirksen MSC, Vree TB, Driessen JJ: Clinical pharmacokinetics of long-term infusion of midazolam in critically ill patients: Preliminary results. *Anaesth Intens Care* 15:440, 1987.
10. Griebel ML, Kearns GL, Fiser DH, et al: Phenytoin protein binding in pediatric patients with acute traumatic injury. *Crit Care Med* 18:385, 1990.
11. Fruncillo RJ, Digregorio GJ: Pharmacokinetics of pentobarbital, quinidine, lidocaine, and theophylline in the thermally injured rat. *J Pharm Sci* 73:1117, 1984.
12. Friedrich LV, White RL, Kays MB, et al: Aztreonam pharmacokinetics in burn patients. *Antimicrob Agents Chemother* 35:57, 1991.
13. Hickling KG, Begg EJ, Perry RE, et al: Serum aminoglycoside clearance is predicted as poorly by renal aminoglycoside clearance as by creatinine clearance in critically ill patients. *Crit Care Med* 19:1041, 1991.
14. Julius HC, Levine HL, Williams WD: Meperidine binding to isolated alpha 1-acid glycoprotein and albumin. *DICP* 23:568, 1989.
15. Kangas L, Kanto J, Forsstrom J, Iisalo E: The protein binding of diazepam and N-demethyldiazepam in patients with poor renal function. *Clin Nephrol* 5:114, 1976.
16. Larijani GE, Gratz I, Silverberg M, Jacobi AG: Clinical pharmacology of the neuromuscular blocking agents. *DICP Ann Pharmacother* 25:54, 1991.
17. Langley MS, Heel RC: Propofol: A review of its pharmacodynamic and pharmacokinetic properties and use as an intravenous anaesthetic. *Drugs* 35:334, 1988.
18. Kushimo OT, Darowski MJ, Morris P, et al: Dose requirements of atracurium in paediatric intensive care patients. *Br J Anaesth* 67:781, 1991.

19. Kohler TR, Dellinger EP, Simonowitz DA, et al: Cimetidine pharmacokinetics in trauma patients. *Surg Forum* 30:12, 1979.

20. Kanto J, Gept E: Pharmacokinetic implications for the clinical use of propofol. *Clin Pharmacokinet* 17:308, 1989.

21. Kanto JH: Midazolam: The first water-soluble benzodiazepine—Pharmacology, pharmacokinetics, and efficacy in insomnia and anesthesia. *Pharmacotherapy* 5:138, 1985.

22. Macnab MSP, Macrae DJ, Guy E, et al: Profound reduction in morphine clearance and liver blood flow in shock. *Intensive Care Med* 12:366, 1986.

23. Majerus TC: Predicting serum gentamicin levels in adult trauma patients. *Clin Ther* 3:316, 1980.

24. Mandema JW, Tuk B, van Steveninck AL, et al: Pharmacokinetic-pharmacodynamic modeling of the central nervous system effects of midazolam and its main metabolite alpha-hydroxymidazolam in healthy volunteers. *Clin Pharmacol Ther* 51:715, 1992.

25. Mann HJ, Fuhs DW, Cerra FB: Pharmacokinetics and pharmacodynamics in critically ill patients. *World J Surg* 11:210, 1987.

26. Mann H, Townsend R, Fuhs D, Cerra F: Decreased hepatic clearance of clindamycin in critically ill patients with sepsis. *Clin Pharm* 6:154, 1987.

27. Markowsky S, Skaar D, Shikuma L, Zaske D: Pharmacokinetics of clindamycin in surgical intensive care patients. (In review.)

28. Martyn JAJ, Liu LMP, Szyfelbein SK, et al: The neuromuscular effects of pancuronium in burned children. *Anesthesiology* 59:561, 1983.

29. Martyn JAJ, Greenblatt DJ, and Quinby WC: Diazepam kinetics in patients with severe burns. *Anesth Analg* 62:293, 1983.

30. Martyn J, Greenblatt DJ: Lorazepam conjugation is unimpaired in burn trauma. *Clin Pharmacol Ther* 43:250, 1988.

31. Martyn JAJ, Bishop AL, Oliveri MF: Pharmacokinetics and pharmacodynamics of ranitidine after burn injury. *Clin Pharmacol Ther* 51:408, 1992.

32. McLean AJ, Morgan, DJ: Clinical pharmacokinetics in patients with liver disease. *Clin Pharmacokinet* 21:42, 1991.

33. Muschitto LJ, Greenblatt DJ: Concentration-independent plasma protein binding of benzodiazepines. *J Pharm Pharmacol* 35:179, 1983.

34. Neill EAM, Chapple DJ, Thompson CW: Metabolism and kinetics of atracurium: an overview. *Br J Anaesth* 55:23S, 1983.

35. Niemiec PW, Allo MD, Miller CF: Effect of altered volume of distribution on aminoglycoside levels in patients in surgical intensive care. *Arch Surg* 122:207, 1987.

36. Oldenhof H, de Jong M, Steenhock A, Janknegt R: Clinical pharmacokinetics of midazolam in intensive care patients: A wide interpatient variability? *Clin Pharmacol Ther* 43:263, 1988.

37. Park GR, Manara AR, Dawling S: Extra-hepatic metabolism of midazolam. *Br J Clin Pharmacol* 27:634, 1989.

38. Parker CJR, Jones JE, Hunter JM: Disposition of infusions of atracurium and its metabolite, laudanosine, in patients in renal and respiratory failure in an ITU. *Br J Anaesth* 61:531, 1988.

39. Pentel P, Benowitz, N: Pharmacokinetic and pharmacodynamic considerations in drug therapy of cardiac emergencies. *Clin Pharmacokinet* 9:273, 1984.

40. Perkins MW, Dasta JF, DeHaven, B: Physiologic implications of mechanical ventilation on pharmacokinetics. *DICP* 23:316, 1989.

41. Perry S, Inturrisi CE: Analgesia and morphine disposition in burn patients. *J Burn Care Rehab* 4:276, 1983.

42. Perucca E: Plasma protein binding of phenytoin in health and disease: Relevance to therapeutic drug monitoring. *Ther Drug Monit* 2:331, 1980.

43. Peter JV, Awni WM: Quantifying hepatic function in the presence of liver disease with phenazone (antipyrine) and its metabolites. *Clin Pharmacokinet* 20:50, 1991.

44. Plaisance K, Drusano G, Forrest A, et al: Pharmacokinetic evaluation of two dosage regimens of clindamycin phosphate. *Antimicrob Agents Chemother* 33:618, 1989.

45. Pugh CB: Phenytoin and phenobarbital protein binding alterations in a uremic burn patient. *Drug Intell Clin Pharm* 21:264, 1987.

46. Romach M, Piafsky K, Abel J, et al: Methadone binding to orosomucoid (alpha 1 acid glycoprotein): Determinant of free fraction in plasma. *Clin Pharmacol Ther* 29:211, 1981.

47. Runciman WB, Myburgh JA, N UR: Pharmacokinetics and pharmacodynamics in the critically ill. *Baillieres Clin Anaesthesiol* 4:271, 1990.

48. Sarfeh I, Balint J: Hepatic dysfunction following trauma: Experimental studies. *J Surg Res* 22:370, 1977.

49. Sawchuk R, Zaske D: Pharmacokinetics of dosing regimens which utilize multiple intravenous infusion: Gentamicin in burn patients. *Pharmacokinet Biopharma* 4:183, 1976.

50. Sawchuk R, Zaske D, Cipolle R, et al: Application of a kinetic model for gentamicin dosing using individual patient parameters. *Clin Pharmacol Ther* 21:362, 1977.

51. Segal JL, Brunnemann SR: Clinical pharmacokinetics in patients with spinal cord injuries. *Clin Pharmacokinet* 17:109, 1989.

52. Segal JL, Brunnemann SR, Eltorai IM, Vulpe M: Decreased systemic clearance of lorazepam in humans with spinal cord injury. *J Clin Pharmacol* 31:651, 1991.

53. Shelly MP, Mendel L, Park GR: Failure of critically ill patients to metabolize midazolam. *Anaesthesia* 42:619, 1987.

54. Shelly MP, Sultan MA, Bodenham A, Park GR: Midazolam infusions in critically ill patients. *Eur J Anaesth* 8:21, 1991.

55. Shikuma L, Ackerman B, Weaver R, et al: Thermal injury effects on drug disposition: A prospective study with piperacillin. *J Clin Pharmacol* 30:632, 1990.

56. Shikuma LR, Ackerman BH, Weaver RH, et al: Effects of treatment and the metabolic response to injury on drug clearance: A prospective study with piperacillin. *Crit Care Med* 18:37, 1990.

57. Sjovall S, Kanto J, Himberg JJ, et al: CSF penetration and pharmacokinetics of midazolam. *Eur J Clin Pharmacol* 25:247, 1983.

58. Slaughter RL, Hassett JM: Hepatic drug clearance following traumatic injury. *Drug Intell Clin Pharm* 19:799, 1985.

59. Somogyi A, Gugler R: Clinical pharmacokinetics of cimetidine. *Clin Pharmacokinet* 8:463, 1983.

60. Tatman AJ, Wrigley SR, Jones RM: Resistance to atracurium in a patient with an increase in plasma alpha-1 globulins. *Br J Anaesth* 67:623, 1991.

61. Tholl D, Shikuma L, Miller T, et al: The physiologic response of stress and aminoglycoside clearance in critically ill patients. *Crit Care Med* 21:248, 1993.

62. Thomson PD, Melmon KL, Richardson JA, et al: Lidocaine pharmacokinetics in advanced heart failure, liver disease, and renal failure in humans. *Ann Intern Med* 78:488, 1973.

63. Townsend PL, Fink MP, Stein KL: Aminoglycoside pharmacokinetics: Dosage requirements and nephrotoxicity in trauma patients. *Crit Care Med* 17:154, 1989.

64. van Dalen R, Vree TB, Baars IM: Influence of protein binding and severity of illness on renal elimination of four cephalosporin drugs in intensive-care patients. *Weekblad* 9:98, 1987.

65. van Dalen R, Vree TB: Pharmacokinetics of antibiotics in critically ill patients. *Intensive Care Med* 16(suppl 3):S235, 1990.

66. Vandenbrom RHG, Mark J, Wierda KH, Agoston S: Pharmacokinetics and neuromuscular blocking effects of atracurium besylate and two of its metabolites in patients with normal and impaired renal function. *Clin Pharmacokinet* 19:230, 1990.

67. Wermeling DP, Blouin RA, Porter WH, et al: Pentobarbital pharmacokinetics in patients with severe head injury. *Drug Intell Clin Pharm* 21:459, 1987.

68. Xia Z-F, Coolbaugh MI, He F, et al: The effects of burn injury on the acute phase response. *J Trauma* 32:245, 1992.

69. Yuen GJ, Drusano GL, Plaisance K, et al: Ciprofloxacin pharmacokinetics in critically ill trauma patients. *Am J Med* 87(suppl 5A):70S, 1989.

70. Zaske D, Cipolle R, Rotschafer J, et al: Gentamicin pharmacokinetics in 1640 patients: A method to control serum concentrations. *Antimicrob Agents Chemother* 21:407, 1982.

71. Zaske D, Strate R, Kohls P: Amikacin pharmacokinetics: Wide interpatient variation in 98 patients. *J Clin Pharmacol* 31:158, 1991.

72. Ziemniak JA, Watson WA, Saffle JR, et al: Cimetidine kinetics during resuscitation from burn shock. *Clin Pharmacol Ther* 36:228, 1984.

73. Zokufa HZ, Solem LD, Rodvold KA, et al: The influence of serum albumin and alpha-1 acid glycoprotein on vancomycin protein binding in patients with burn injuries. *J Burn Care Rehabil* 10:425, 1989.

74. Zaske D, Chin T, Kohls P, et al: Initial dosage regimens of gentamicin in patients with burns. *J Burn Care & Rehabil* 12:46, 1991.

75. Siegel JH, Cerra FB, Coleman B, et al: Physiological and metabolic correlations in human sepsis. *Surgery* 86:163, 1979.

76. Stahl WM: Acute phase protein response to tissue injury. *Crit Care Med* 15:545, 1987.

77. Stoner HB: Interpretation of the metabolic effects of trauma and sepsis. *J Clin Pathol* 40:1108, 1987.

78. Suffredini AF: Endotoxin administration to normal humans, in *Septic Shock in Humans: Advances in the Understanding of Pathogenesis, Cardiac Dysfunction, and Therapy. Ann Intern Med* 113:227, 1990.

79. Trunkey DD: Trauma. *Sci Am* 249:28, 1983.

80. Tuchsmidt J, Fried J, Swinney R, Sharma OP: Early hemodynamic correlates of survival in patients with septic shock. *Crit Care Med* 17:719, 1989.

81. Villar J, Slutsky AS, Hew E, Aberman A: Oxygen transport and oxygen consumption in critically ill patients. *Chest* 98:687, 1990.

82. Shoemaker WC, Appel PL, Kram HB: Incidence, physiologic description, compensatory mechanisms, and therapeutic implications of monitored events. *Crit Care Med* 17:1277, 1989.

83. Shoemaker WC, Appel PL, Kram HB: Tissue oxygen debt as a determinant of lethal and nonlethal postoperative organ failure. *Crit Care Med* 16:1117, 1988.

84. Shoemaker WC: Circulatory mechanisms of shock and their mediators. *Crit Care Med* 15:787, 1987.

85. Parrillo JE: Cardiovascular pattern during septic shock, in *Septic Shock in Humans: Advances in the Understanding of Pathogenesis, Cardiovascular Dysfunction, and Therapy. Ann Intern Med* 113:227, 1990.

86. Parker MM: Cardiac dysfunction in human septic shock, in *Septic Shock in Humans: Advances in the Understanding of Pathogenesis, Cardiovascular Dysfunction, and Therapy. Ann Intern Med* 113:227, 1990.

87. Ognibene FP: Management of septic shock, in *Septic Shock in Humans: Advances in the Understanding of Pathogenesis, Cardiovascular Dysfunction, and Therapy. Ann Intern Med* 113:227, 1990.

88. Natanson C: A canine model of septic shock, in *Septic Shock in Humans: Advances in the Understanding of the Pathogenesis, Cardiovascular Dysfunction, and Therapy. Ann Intern Med* 113:227, 1990.

89. Murray M: P450 enzymes. *Clin Pharmacokinet* 23:132, 1992.

90. Morgan DJ, Smallwood RA: Clinical significance of pharmacokinetic models of hepatic elimination. *Clin Pharmacokinet* 18:61, 1990.

91. Michie HR, Majzoub JA, O'Dwyer ST, et al: Both cyclooxygenase-dependent and cyclooxygenase-independent pathways mediate the neuroendocrine response in humans. *Surgery* 108:254, 1990.

92. Matuschak G, Rinaldo J: Organ interactions in the adult respiratory distress syndrome during sepsis: Role of the liver in host defense. *Chest* 94:400, 1988.

93. Klotz U: Pathophysiological and disease-induced changes in drug disposition volume: Pharmacokinetic implications. *Clin Pharmacokinet* 1:204, 1976.

94. Johnston RB: Current concepts: Immunology monocytes and macrophages. *N Engl J Med* 318:747, 1988.

95. Heinemeyer G, Roots I, Lestau P, et al: D-Glucaric acid excretion in critical care patients: Comparison with 6β-hydroxycortisol excretion and serum glutamyltranspeptidase activity and relation to multiple drug therapy. *Br J Clin Pharmacol* 21:9, 1986.

96. Hartl WH, Herndon DN, Wolfe RR: Kinin/prostaglandin system: Its therapeutic value in surgical stress. *Crit Care Med* 18:1167, 1990.

97. Fischer JE, Hasselgren P-O: Cytokines and glucocorticoids in the regulation of the "hepato-skeletal muscle axis" in sepsis. *Am J Surg* 161:266, 1991.

98. Feustel PJ, Fortune JB, Stratton H, Newell JC: Oxygen delivery and consumption in head-injured and multiple trauma patients. 30:1259, 1990.

99. Farina ML, Bonati M, Iapichino G, et al: Clinical pharmacological and therapeutic considerations in general intensive care: A review. *Drugs* 34:662, 1987.

100. Farina M, Levati A, Tognon G: A multicenter study of ICU drug utilization. *Intensive Care Med* 7:125, 1981.

101. Edwards JD: Practical application of oxygen transport principles. *Crit Care Med* 18:S45, 1990.

102. Douglas RG, Shaw JHF: Metabolic response to sepsis and trauma. *Br J Surg* 76:115, 1989.

103. Dinarello CA, Mier JW: Current concepts: Lymphokines. *N Engl J Med* 317:940, 1987.

104. Danner RL: Mediators and endotoxin inhibitors, in *Septic Shock in Humans: Advances in the Understanding of Pathogenesis, Cardiovascular Dysfunction, and Therapy. Ann Intern Med* 113:227, 1990.

105. Cerra FB, Holman RT, Bankey PE, Mazuski JE: Nutritional pharmacology: Its role in the hypermetabolism-organ failure syndrome. *Crit Care Med* 18:S154, 1990.

106. Carrico CJ, Meakins JL, Marshall JC, et al: Multiple-organ-failure syndrome. *Arch Surg* 121:196, 1986.

107. Bryan-Brown, CW: Blood flow to organs: Parameters for function and survival in critical illness. *Crit Care Med* 16:170, 1988.

108. Brown KA, Sheagren JN: Recognition and emergent treatment of septic shock/multiple organ systems failure syndrome. *IM* 11:3, 1990.

109. Brosen K: Recent developments in hepatic drug oxidation: Implications for clinical pharmacokinetics. *Clin Pharmacokinet* 18:220, 1990.

110. Bonate P: Pathophysiology and pharmacokinetics following burn injury. *Clin Pharmacokinet* 18:118, 1990.

111. Bihari D, Smithies M, Gimson A, Tinker J: The effects of vasodilatation with prostacyclin on oxygen delivery and uptake in critically ill patients. *N Engl J Med* 317:397, 1987.

112. Becker W, Konstantinides F, Eyer S, et al: Plasma amino acid clearance as an indicator of hepatic function and high-energy phosphate in hepatic ischemia. *Surgery* 102:777, 1987.

113. Abraham E: Host defense abnormalities after hemorrhage, trauma, and burns. *Crit Care Med* 17:934, 1989.

114. Albanese J, Martin C, Lacarelle B, et al: Pharmacokinetics of long-term propofol infusion used for sedation in ICU patients. *Anesthesiology* 73:214, 1990.

115. Whipple J, Ausman R, Franson T, Quebbeman E: Effect of individualized pharmacokinetic dosing on patient outcome. *Crit Care Med* 19:1480, 1991.

116. Zaske D, Bootman J, Solem L, Strate R: Increased burn patient survival with individualized dosages of gentamicin. *Surgery* 91:142, 1982.

117. Solem L, Zaske D, Strate R: Ecthyma gangrenosum: Survival with individualized antibiotic therapy. *Arch Surg* 114:580, 1979.

118. Rauckman EJ, Rosen GM, Post SE, Gillogly SD: Effect of model traumatic injury on hepatic drug metabolizing enzymes. *J Trauma* 20:884, 1980.

119. Robert S. Zarowitz B: Is there a reliable index of glomerular filtration rate in critically ill patients. *DICP* 25:169, 1991.

120. Martyn JJA, Greenblatt DJ, Abernethy DR: Increased cimetidine clearance in burn patients. *JAMA* 253:1288, 1985

121. Lott R, Uden D, Strate R, Zaske D: Correlation of predicted versus measured creatinine clearance values in burn patients. *J Am Hosp Pharm* 35:717, 1977.

122. Martin C, Alaya M, Bras J, et al: Assessment of creatinine clearance in intensive care patients. *Crit Care Med* 18:1224, 1990.

123. Freysz M, Lafleur P, Dupont G, et al: Comparison of creatinine and inulin clearances in multiple trauma. *Biomed Pharmacother* 44:175, 1990.

124. Madoff RD, Sharpe SM, Fath JJ, et al: Prolonged surgical intensive care. *Arch Surg* 120:696, 1985.

125. Jacobs P, Noseworthy T: National estimates of intensive care utilization and costs: Canada and the United States. *Crit Care Med* 18:1282, 1990.

126. French MA, Cerra FB, Plaut ME, Schentag JJ: Amikacin and gentamicin accumulation pharmacokinetics and nephrotoxicity in critically ill patients. *Antimicrob Agents Chemother* 19:147, 1981.

127. Miller KW, Chan KKH, McCoy HG, et al: Cephalothin kinetics: Before, during, and after cardiopulmonary bypass surgery. *Clin Pharmacol Ther* 26:54, 1979.

128. Miller KW, McCoy HG, Chan KKH, et al: Effect of cardiopulmonary bypass on cefazolin disposition. *Clin Pharmacol Ther* 27:550, 1980.

129. Woodhouse KW, Wynee HA: Age-related changes in liver size and hepatic blood flow: The influence on drug metabolism in the elderly. *Clin Pharmacokinet* 15:287, 1988.

130. Stames NF, Warren RS, Jeevandam M, et al: Tumor necrosis factor and the acute metabolic response to tissue injury in man. *J Clin Invest* 82:1321, 1988.
131. Sarfeh IJ, Balint JA: The clinical significance of hyperbilirubinemia following trauma. *J Trauma* 18:58, 1978.
132. Sarfeh IJ, Balint JA: Hepatic dysfunction following trauma: Experimental studies. *J Surg Res* 22:370, 1977.
133. Naylor-Shepherd MF, Fuhs DW, Angaran DM: Oxygen homeostasis: Theory, measurement, and therapeutic implications *DICP* 24:1195, 1990.
134. Damas P, Reuter A, Gysen P, et al: Tumor necrosis factor and interleukin-1 serum levels during severe sepsis in humans. *Crit Care Med* 17:975, 1989.
135. Dahn MS, Lange P, Lobdell K, et et al: Splanchnic and total body oxygen consumption differences in septic and injured patients. *Surgery* 101:69, 1987.
136. Spitzer JA: Altered Ca^{2+} homeostasis and functional correlates in hepatocytes and adipocytes in endotoxemia and sepsis. *J Trauma* 30:S192, 1990.
137. Boosalis MG, Ott L, Levine AS, et al: Relationship of visceral protein to nutritional status in chronic and acute stress. *Crit Care Med* 17:741, 1989.
138. Gottlieb ME, Sarfeh IJ, Stratton H, et al: Hepatic perfusion and splanchnic oxygen consumption in patients postinjury. *J Trauma* 23:836, 1983.
139. Wang P, Ba ZF, Chaudry IH: Hepatic extraction of indocyanine green is depressed early in sepsis despite increased hepatic blood flow and cardiac output. *Arch Surg* 126:219, 1991.
140. Griffeth LK, Rosen GM, Rauckman EJ: Effects of model traumatic injury on hepatic drug metabolism in the rat. II. In vivo metabolism on hexobarbital and zoxazolamine. *Drug Metab Dispos* 12:582, 1984.
141. Griffeth LK, Rosen GM, Tschanz C, Raukman EJ: Effects of model traumatic injury on hepatic drug metabolism in the rat. I. In vivo antipyrine metabolism. *Drug Metab Dispos* 11:517, 1983.
142. Crom WR, Webster SL, Bobo L, et al: Simultaneous administration of multiple model substrates to assess hepatic drug clearance. *Clin Pharmacol Ther* 41:645, 1987.
143. Goodwin CW, Aulick LH, Becker RA, Wilmore DW: Increased renal perfusion and kidney size in convalescent burn patients. *JAMA* 244:1588, 1980.
144. Gottlieb ME, Stratton HH, Newell JC, Shah DM: Indocyanine green: Its use as an early indicator of hepatic dysfunction following injury in man. *Arch Surg* 119:264, 1984.
145. Bloedow DC, Hansbrough JF, Hardin T, Simons M: Postburn serum drug binding and serum protein concentration. *J Clin Pharmacol* 26:147, 1986.
146. Edwards DJ, Lalka D, Cerra F, Slaughter RL: Alpha 1-acid glycoprotein concentration and protein binding in trauma. *Clin Pharmacol Ther* 31:62, 1982.
147. Edwards DJ, Axelson JE, Slaughter RL, et al: Factors affecting quinidine protein binding in man. *Clin Pharmacokinet* (9S):96, 1984.
148. Fruncillo RJ, DiGregorio GJ: The effect of thermal injury on drug metabolism in the rat. *J Trauma* 23:523, 1983.
149. Vree TB, Shimoda M, Driessen JJ, et al: Decreased plasma albumin concentration results in increased volume of distribution and decreased elimination of midazolam in intensive care patients. *Clin Pharmacol Ther* 46:537, 1989.
150. Morrison G, Chiang ST, Koephe HH, Walker BR: Effect of renal impairment and hemodialysis on lorazepam kinetics. *Clin Pharmacol Ther* 35:646, 1984.
151. Martyn J, Goldhill DR, Goudsouzian NG: Clinical pharmacology of muscle relaxants in patients with burns. *J Clin Pharmacol* 26:680, 1986.
152. Martyn JAJ, Abernethy DR, Greenblatt DJ: Plasma protein binding of drugs after severe burn injury. *Clin Pharmacol Ther* 35:535, 1984.
153. Harris CE, Grounds RM, Murray AM, et al: Propofol for long-term sedation in the intensive care unit. *Anaesthesia* 45:366, 1990.
154. Guthrie RD, Hines C, Jr: Use of intravenous albumin in the critically ill patient. *Am J Gastroenterol* 86:255, 1991.
155. Greenblatt DJ, Ehrenberg BL, Gunderman J, et al: Kinetic and dynamic study of intravenous lorazepam: Comparison with intravenous diazepam. *J Pharmacol Exp Ther* 250:134, 1989.
156. Dundee JW, Collier PS, Carlisle RJT, Harper KW: Prolonged midazolam elimination half-life. *Br J Clin Pharmacol* 21:425, 1986.
157. Cloyd J: Pharmacokinetic pitfalls of present anticpileptic medications. *Epilepsia* 32:(suppl 5):S53, 1991.
158. Bowdles TA, Neal GD, Levy RH, Heimbach DM: Phenytoin pharmacokinetics in burned rats and plasma protein binding of phenytoin in burned patients. *J Pharmacol Exp Ther* 213:97, 1980.
159. Bauer LA, Edwards WAD, Dellinger EP, et al: Importance of unbound phenytoin serum levels in head trauma patients. *J Trauma* 23:1058, 1983.
160. Bailie GR, Cockshott ID, Douglas EJ, Bowles BJM: Pharmacokinetics of propofol during and after long term continuous infusion for maintenance of sedation in ICU patients. *Br J Anaesthesia* 68:486, 1992.
161. Allonen H, Ziegler G, Klotz U: Midazolam kinetics. *Clin Pharmacol Ther* 30:653, 1981.
162. Ball M, Moore RA, Fisher A, et al: Renal failure and the use of morphine in intensive care. *Lancet* April 6:784, 1985.
163. Durbin CGJ: Neuromuscular blocking agents and sedative drugs: Clinical uses and toxic effects in the critical care unit. *Crit Care Clin* 7:489, 1991.
164. Flaherty J, Rodondi L, Guglielmo J, et al: Comparative pharmacokinetics and serum inhibitory activity of clindamycin in different dosing regimens. *Antimicrob Agents Chemother* 32:1825, 1988.
165. Kemner JM, Snodgrass WR, Worley SE, et al: Interaction of oxygen-carrying resuscitation fluids and morphine. *J Lab Clin Med* 104:433, 1984.
166. Astiz ME, Rackow EC, Kaufman B, et al: Relationship of oxygen delivery and mixed venous oxygenation to lactic acidosis in patients with sepsis and acute myocardial infarction. *Crit Care Med* 16:655, 1988.
167. Cerra F, Negro F, Abrams J: APACHE II score does not predict multiple organ failure or mortality in postoperative surgical patients. *Arch Surg* 125:519, 1990.
168. Long C, Lowry S: Hormonal regulation of protein metabolism. 14:55, 1990.
169. Yuen GJ, Drusano GL, Forrest A, et al: Prospective use of optimal sampling theory: Steady-state ciprofloxacin pharmacokinetics in critically ill trauma patients. *Clin Pharmacol Ther* 46:451, 1989.
170. Ludden TM: Nonlinear pharmacokinetics: Clinical implications. *Clin Pharmacokinet* 20:429, 1991.
171. Reed R, Wu A, Miller-Crotchett P, et al: Pharmacokinetic monitoring of nephrotoxic antibiotics in surgical intensive care patients. *J Trauma* 29:1462, 1989.
172. Reed LR, Ericsson CD, Wu A, et al: The pharmacokinetics of prophylactic antibiotics in trauma. *J Trauma* 32:21, 1992.
173. Cipolle R, Seifert R, Zaske D, Strate R: Hospital acquired Gram-negative pneumonias: Response rate and dosage requirements with individualized tobramycin therapy. *Ther Drug Monit* 2:359, 1980.
174. Shanks CA: Pharmacokinetics of the non-depolarizing neuromuscular relaxants applied to calculation of bolus and infusion dosage regimens. *Anesthesiology* 64:72, 1986.
175. Michalk S, Moncorge C, Fichelle A, et al: Midazolam infusion for basal sedation in intensive care: Absence of accumulation. *Intensive Care Med* 15:37, 1988.
176. Lesar, T, Rotschafer J, Strand L, et al: Gentamicin dosing errors with four commonly used nomograms. *JAMA* 248:1190, 1982.
177. Follath F: Problems of drug elimination in intensive care patients. *Resuscitation* 16(suppl):S63, 1988.
178. Shafer A, Doze VA, White PF: Pharmacokinetic variability of midazolam infusions in critically ill patients. *Crit Care Med* 18:1039, 1990.

207. Antiarrhythmic Agents

Robert J. Straka, Shawn Hansen,
Eric Wittbrodt, and Henry J. Mann

Overview

Issues relevant to the pharmacokinetics and pharmacodynamics of antiarrhythmic agents in the critically ill patient are discussed in this chapter. We focus primarily on the pharmacokinetics of antiarrhythmic agents, specifically in the context of the hypodynamic and hyperdynamic patient. Unfortunately, there is a general lack of good clinical studies describing the use of antiarrhythmic agents in critically ill patients. Nonetheless, knowledge of the basic principles of drug disposition (absorption, distribution, and elimination) and of some commonly observed physiologic changes in critically ill patients allows the intensivist to make reasonable decisions regarding antiarrhythmic drug dosing in critically ill patients.

Antiarrhythmic drugs represent a relatively diverse class of pharmacologic agents. For this reason, many clinicians use the Vaughn-Williams classification to categorize individual agents in terms of their fundamental and predominant electrophysiologic effects. This classification scheme is summarized in Table 207-1. Although this classification scheme has its faults, it does represent a venue by which clinicians can attempt to organize these agents in a practical way.

Table 207-1. Vaughn-Williams Classification of Antiarrhythmic Drugs

Class	Action	Drugs
I	Sodium channel blockers	
IA	Moderate phase 0 depression Moderate conduction slowing Prolongs repolarization	Quinidine Procainamide Disopyramide
IB	Minimal phase 0 depression Shortens repolarization	Lidocaine (IV) Tocainide Mexiletine
IC	Marked phase 0 depression Marked conduction slowing Slight effect on repolarization	Flecainide Encainide Propafenone[b]
I[a]	Sodium channel blockers–mechanism not clearly defined	Moricizine[a] Recainam
II	Beta-blockers	Propranolol Acebutolol
III	Prolong repolarization	Bretylium Amiodarone[b] Sotalol[b]
IV	Calcium channel blockers	Verapamil Diltiazem
	Purine nucleosides Digitalis glycosides	Adenosine Digoxin Digitoxin

[a] Also has type Ia activity (decreases conduction velocity more than most Class Ib agents)
[b] Also has type II (beta-blocking) activity

Quinidine

Quinidine is a class IA antiarrhythmic agent employed in the conversion of atrial tachyarrhythmias and for control of many ventricular arrhythmias.

PHARMACOLOGY [1]. Suppression of transcellular sodium ion transport results in decreased conduction velocity and increased ERP in the atria and ventricles. Ventricular automaticity is decreased, but quinidine does not appreciably affect atrial automaticity. On electrocardiogram (ECG), QRS complex widening and P–R interval lengthening are commonly observed. Quinidine causes blockade of alpha-adrenergic receptors, which manifests clinically as a decrease in peripheral vascular resistance and hypotension.

THERAPEUTIC RANGE. The accepted therapeutic range for quinidine is approximately 2 to 5 μg per milliliter. Toxicity is likely with serum concentrations greater than 10 μg per milliliter.

PREPARATIONS. Quinidine is available as gluconate, sulfate, and polygalacturonate salts.

Gluconate salt extended-release (Quinaglute Dura-tabs, Quinalan, Duraquin, generic)	324-mg, 330-mg
Sulfate salt immediate-release (Cin-Quin, Quinova, generic)	200-mg, 300-mg capsules 100-mg, 200-mg, 300-mg tablets
Sulfate salt extended-release (Quinidex Extentabs)	300-mg tablets
Polygalacturonate salt immediate-release (Cardioquin)	275-mg
Sulfate parenteral (generic)	80 mg/ml
Glucanate parenteral (generic)	275 mg/ml

PHARMACOKINETICS. Table 207-2 summarizes the pharmacokinetic properties of quinidine.

Absorption. Oral quinidine is approximately 70 percent bioavailable, with wide variability. Since absorption from the gastrointestinal (GI) tract is nearly complete, a significant amount of quinidine is metabolized by the liver before it reaches the systemic circulation. Absorption after intramuscular administration is erratic and incomplete and therefore not recommended.

Distribution. Quinidine is rapidly distributed into all body tissues except the central nervous system (CNS). It concentrates in the heart, liver, kidneys, and skeletal muscle and also distributes into erythrocytes. Protein binding is significant, with about 70 to 90 percent bound to both albumin and alpha-1-acid glycoprotein (AAG).

Table 207-2. Pharmacokinetic Properties of Antiarrhythmic Agents [2,3,4]

Drug	Protein binding (%)	Percent excreted unchanged	Half-life (hr)	V_{dss} (L/kg)	V_d in CHF (L/kg)	Bioavailability (%)	Therapeutic range
Quinidine	80	19.5 (7.77)	6.50 (1.67)	2.61 (1.10)	1.8 (.5)	60—sulfate 40—gluconate & polygalactate	2–5 µg/ml
Procainamide	15	52 (11)	3.3 (0.64)	2.0 (0.42)	1.5	72—tabs and caps	4–10 µg/ml
NAPA		88.5 (4)	6.2 (0.67)	2.0 (0.42)	1.4		15–25 µg/ml
Lidocaine	70		1.6 (0.18) 3.66 CHF 4.22 AMI	1.08 (0.12)	0.9		2–6 µg/ml
Mexiletine	70	10–20	6–12	5–12		90	0.5–2 µg/ml
Moricizine	95	<1	2–4	>4	—	38	?
Flecainide	37–50	25–40	14(7)	8–10		90–100	0.2–1.0 µg/ml
Propafenone	90	1	5.5 EM 17.2 PM	3.6	—	5–12 (dose-dependent)	Not clear: An EM needs less, a PM needs more
Amiodarone	96	<1	10–50 days (25)	60	—	42	1–2.5 µg/ml
Sotalol	0	75	13 (5)	1.6–2.4		~100	1–4 µg/ml
Digoxin	25	72 (8) IV 54 PO	36 (8)	6.7 (1.4) 4.5 (renal patients)		75 - tabs 95 - caps 80 - elixir 100 - IV	0.5–2 ng/ml

Items inside parentheses indicate standard deviation
EM = extensive metabolizers; PM = poor metabolizers; NAPA = N-acetylprocainamide; AMI = acute myocardial infarction; CHF = congestive heart failure.

Elimination. The liver is primarily responsible for clearance of quinidine, with about 10 to 20 percent renally excreted as unchanged drug. The major metabolites, 3-hydroxyquinidine and 2-quinidinone, are produced by hydroxylation and possess an unknown degree of antiarrhythmic activity. Urinary excretion of the parent drug and its metabolites is via filtration and is reduced in the presence of an elevated urine pH.

PHYSIOLOGIC CLEARANCE

Hypodynamic. The rate but not the extent of absorption of quinidine is diminished in congestive heart failure (CHF) after oral administration, because of alterations in mucosal blood flow [5,6]. Reduced renal function does not affect quinidine excretion. Reductions in serum proteins may increase the amount of circulating unbound quinidine, predisposing certain patients to its toxic effects. Physiologic states that reduce liver blood flow may impair metabolism of the parent compound. Few studies have been done to ascertain the disposition of quinidine in hypodynamic patients.

Hyperdynamic. There is little information about quinidine pharmacokinetics in this population.

DOSING GUIDELINES

Loading Dose. Intravenous loading of quinidine may be instituted with the gluconate (800 mg) or sulfate salt (600 mg) diluted in D_5W and infused at 1 ml per minute. Close observation of ECG and blood pressure is necessary to avoid adverse cardiovascular effects. For oral loading, quinidine sulfate (200–300 mg) is given every 2 to 3 hours until the arrhythmia is controlled.

Maintenance Dose. Quinidine sulfate (200–300 mg three to four times daily) is administered for maintenance therapy. In the gluconate form, 324 to 660 mg every 6 hours is administered. When extended-release quinidine is used for chronic suppression of arrhythmias, the regimen is 300 to 600 mg of quinidine sulfate every 8 to 12 hours or 324 to 660 mg of quinidine glucaronate every 6 to 12 hours.

DRUG INTERACTIONS. Table 207-3 summarizes the important drug interactions with quinidine.

COMMON PITFALLS
1. Obtain trough concentrations to monitoring risk of quinidine toxicity.
2. Different dosages are required, depending on the choice of quinidine salt.

Procainamide

Procainamide is a class IA (membrane stabilizing) antiarrhythmic agent used for the prophylaxis and treatment of ventricular and supraventricular arrhythmias.

Table 207-3. Important Drug Interactions with Quinidine [7]

Drug	Effect	Mechanism
Antacids (maalox); urinary alkalinizers ($NaHCO_3$)	Increased serum quinidine concentrations	pH-related decrease in urinary excretion of quinidine; increased tubular reabsorption of un-ionized drug
Barbiturates	Decreased quinidine serum concentrations and elimination half-life	Probably enhanced metabolic clearance of quinidine
Cimetidine	Increased quinidine serum concentrations and enhanced pharmacologic and toxicologic effects of quinidine	Increased quinidine absorption, decreased quinidine metabolism, or both
Phenytoin	Decreased quinidine serum concentrations and potential loss of therapeutic effect of quinidine	Increased quinidine metabolism due to stimulation of hepatic microsomal enzyme system by phenytoin
Rifampin	Decreased quinidine serum concentrations and potential loss of therapeutic effect of quinidine	Increased quinidine metabolism due to stimulation of hepatic microsomal enzyme system by rifampin
Anticoagulants	Hypoprothrombinemia and potential bleeding	Quinidine may itself inhibit hepatically synthesized clotting factors
Digoxin	2–3-fold increase in serum digoxin concentration and potential digoxin toxicity	Increased bioavailability and decreased volume of distribution and clearance of digoxin
Amiodarone	Increase in serum quinidine concentration and potentially fatal cardiac dysrhythmias	Unknown
Propafenone	Serum propafenone concentration may double and serum 5-hydroxypropafenone concentration may be cut in half in extensive metabolizers, with no apparent change in pharmacologic activity of propafenone	Quinidine is a specific and potential inhibitor of the enzyme P-450 IID6, which is responsible for the hepatic hydroxylation of propafenone
Verapamil	Potentiation of pharmacologic activity of quinidine; possible hypotension, bradycarida, ventricular tachycardia, A-V block, and pulmonary edema	Verapamil interferes with the clearance of quinidine
Neuromuscular blockers	Potentiation or prolongation of blockade	Postsynaptic blockade of acetylcholine receptors

PHARMACOLOGY [1]. Direct effects on the heart include a decrease in automaticity and lengthening of the action potential duration. Lengthening of the refractory potential and slowing of conduction in the atrium, atrioventricular (AV) node, and ventricle also occur. On ECG, prolongation of the QRS complex is most common, although at high doses P–R interval prolongation or heart block may be seen. Extracardiac effects primarily involve peripheral vasodilatation, resulting in hypotension.

THERAPEUTIC RANGE. Table 207-4 summarizes the concentration effect relationship of procainamide.

PREPARATIONS

Procainamide immediate-release (Pronestyl, Promine, generic)	250-mg, 375-mg, 500-mg tablets
Procainamide sustained-release (Procan SR)	250-mg, 500-mg, 750-mg, 1000-mg tablets
Procainamide injection (Pronestyl, generic)	100 mg/ml, 500 mg/ml

PHARMACOKINETICS. Table 207-2 summarizes the pharmacokinetic properties of procainamide.

Absorption. Procainamide is rapidly absorbed after IM administration and variably absorbed when given orally (50–95%), depending on the formulation. Absorption of procainamide from the IM route may be erratic in critically ill patients; the IV route may be preferred in such patients. The bioavailability of an immediate-release formulation has been reported as 85 percent, while that of an extended-release formulation was 68 percent [10]. Absorption may be delayed immediately following acute myocardial infarction (MI), presumably due to impaired mucosal blood flow.

Distribution. On reaching the bloodstream, procainamide rapidly distributes into all major organs, including the CNS, heart, liver, and kidneys. Volume of distribution has been estimated as 2 liters per kilogram [11]. At therapeutic concentrations in the plasma, approximately 14 to 23 percent of the drug is bound to plasma proteins.

Elimination. Procainamide is acetylated in the liver to *N*-acetylprocainamide (NAPA). The rate of acetylation is genetically determined and varies between patients. In vitro studies suggest production of a hydroxylamine metabolite by hepatic microsomes [11,12]. This metabolite has been implicated in the pathogenesis of procainamide-induced lupus syndrome. Forty to 70 percent of procainamide is excreted in the urine as unchanged drug and the rest as metabolites, depending on acetylator phenotype.

PHYSIOLOGIC CLEARANCE

Hypodynamic. As a flow-limited drug, procainamide is cleared from the body less efficiently in hypodynamic low flow states. Decreased renal function (<60 ml/min) and increased age (>60 years) have been shown to reduce significantly clearance of procainamide and the NAPA-procainamide concentration ratio. Conflicting data for CHF patients have been reported. One study reported significantly reduced clearance in patients with CHF as compared with controls [13]. However, no significant effect on clearance of procainamide was detected in post-

Table 207-4. Concentration-Effect Relationship of Procainamide [8,9]

Concentration (μg/ml)	Effect
4–10 (P only)	Accepted therapeutic range
>10 (P only)	Increased risk of toxicity
25–30 (P + NAPA)	Increased risk of toxicity

P = procainamide; NAPA = N-acetylprocainamide

MI or CHF patients in two other studies [14,15]. Changes in protein status do not appreciably affect procainamide pharmacokinetics, since it is not extensively protein-bound.

Hyperdynamic. Little is known about procainamide pharmacokinetics in this population. Pediatric patients have demonstrated increased dosage requirements. One study reported that five children receiving therapy with procainamide had rapid clearance and a short half-life ($t_{1/2}$) [16]. The effect of clearance may necessitate continuous-infusion procainamide in this age group.

DOSING GUIDELINES

Loading Dose. Although a loading dose of procainamide is not always necessary, it can be achieved using either intravenous or oral drug. For immediate suppression of an arrhythmia an intravenous load is preferred, at a dose of 17 mg per kilogram IBW of procainamide HCl infused at a rate not to exceed 50 mg per minute. Alternatively, a bolus injection of 100 mg of procainamide HCl may be administered over 2 minutes and repeated every 5 minutes until the arrhythmia is controlled or a cumulative dose of 17 mg per kilogram IBW is reached. For oral loading with procainamide the immediate-release preparation should be used, given as a single dose of 17 mg per kilogram IBW or in divided doses given every 2 hours for rapid absorption and onset. The loading dose should be reduced to 12 mg per kilogram IBW in patients with severe renal impairment or reduced cardiac output.

Maintenance Dose. Maintenance therapy with procainamide can be achieved by using oral immediate-release, oral sustained-release, or IV continuous infusion of procainamide HCl. Intravenous procainamide is generally reserved for situations in which oral therapy is not feasible. Oral maintenance therapy can be initiated empirically with a dose of 50 mg per kilogram IBW per day in divided doses of the immediate-release preparation given every 3 to 4 hours or the sustained-release preparation given every 6 to 8 hours. Intravenous maintenance therapy, which is often required in the ICU, is initiated as a continuous infusion of procainamide HCl at a rate of 2 to 4 mg per minute. Reduced maintenance doses may be required in patients with renal insufficiency and in the elderly. No specific information regarding dosing of hypodynamic or hyperdynamic patients is available. However, in hypodynamic patients, procainamide and NAPA clearances are likely to be reduced, necessitating cautious dosing in this group. Dosage adjustment during maintenance therapy is guided by arrhythmia control and steady-state serum concentrations.

DRUG INTERACTIONS. Cimetidine [17] and trimethoprim [18] can decrease the renal clearance of procainamide by about one third, probably through competitive inhibition of secretion

of the parent drug and NAPA. Amiodarone can significantly increase procainamide and NAPA serum concentrations through an unknown mechanism and produce additive effects on a number of electrophysiologic parameters, necessitating close monitoring of serum procainamide and NAPA concentrations and a decrease in procainamide dose in a number of patients [19,20].

COMMON PITFALLS
1. Monitor serum trough concentrations immediately prior to the next dose.
2. Monitor ECG to assess clinical effectiveness of the procainamide dose.
3. Evaluate procainamide and NAPA concentrations individually. Accumulation of NAPA is likely in renal failure, and accumulation of procainamide is possible in renal or hepatic failure.

Disopyramide

Disopyramide is a class IA antiarrhythmic indicated for the suppression of ventricular arrhythmias.

PHARMACOLOGY [1]. Decreased conduction velocity and lengthening of the effective refractory period is caused by a reduction in excitability of the atria and ventricles. Disopyramide may also decrease automaticity of the atria and ventricles. On ECG, the effects of disopyramide manifest as milder versions of quinidine or procainamide effects. Disopyramide possesses slight anticholinergic properties.

THERAPEUTIC RANGE. The putative therapeutic range for disopyramide is 2 to 5 μg per milliliter. No clear relationship has been established between total plasma concentration of disopyramide and an increased risk of myocardial depression [21].

PREPARATIONS

Disopyramide immediate-release (Norpace)	100-mg, 150-mg capsules
Disopyramide extended-release (Norpace CR)	100-mg, 150-mg, 250-mg capsules

PHARMACOKINETICS
Absorption. Disopyramide is about 85 percent bioavailable, and absorption from the GI tract is rapid after an oral dose.

Distribution. Disopyramide concentrates in the extracellular fluid and is not tissue-bound to a great extent. Concentrations of disopyramide in the heart are reportedly double that in the plasma. Protein binding is variable and concentration-dependent, such that in the upper therapeutic range protein binding decreases. Therefore, at higher concentrations, more free drug is available to exert a therapeutic effect at the myocardium or result in toxicity. Disopyramide has a three times greater affinity for AAG than for albumin. Approximately 50 to 65 percent of disopyramide is protein-bound at therapeutic concentrations.

Elimination. Disopyramide is metabolized in the liver to an N-monodealkylated moiety (15–25%). Between 40 and 60 percent is excreted in urine as unchanged drug, 10 percent is excreted as unidentified metabolites, and 10 percent is excreted in feces as unchanged drug.

PHYSIOLOGIC CLEARANCE

Hypodynamic. The effects of myocardial infarction on disopyramide disposition have been studied [22]. Lowered plasma concentrations of disopyramide were noted, supposedly because absorption of orally administered disopyramide was diminished after acute MI. Elimination rate, body clearance, degree of protein binding, and volume of distribution did not differ between the acute MI and recovery phases. A study of disopyramide pharmacokinetics in renal transplant and dialysis patients revealed widely variable plasma drug concentrations and decreased unbound fraction, indicating that in this population, interpatient protein binding changes are magnified [23]. In patients with moderate to severe renal impairment, disopyramide dosing intervals should be modified (see Dosing Guidelines).

Hyperdynamic. Since AAG is released in the acute phase of injury or stress, an increase in this protein may decrease the fraction of unbound drug.

DOSING GUIDELINES

Loading Dose. Disopyramide (300 mg) is administered orally. If necessary, 200 mg every 6 hours may be given for a maximum of 48 hours or until control of the arrhythmia has been achieved.

Maintenance Dose. Disopyramide (150 mg every 6 hours) is administered orally. The usual maximum dose is 800 mg per day. Dosage intervals (CrCl) should be adjusted for patients with renal insufficiency as follows: 30 to 40 ml per minute every 8 hours; 15 to 30 ml per minute every 12 hours; less than 15 ml per minute every 24 hours.

DRUG INTERACTIONS.

Concomitant use of drugs with negative inotropic effects, such as beta-blockers or verapamil, may result in additive depression of myocardial function.

COMMON PITFALLS

1. Avoid use of other drugs with negative inotropic effects, such as beta-blockers or verapamil, concomitantly with disopyramide.
2. Avoid use of anticholinergic drugs with disopyramide, which may result in increased anticholinergic effects, especially in patients being treated for atrial fibrillation or flutter.

Lidocaine

Lidocaine is perhaps the most important parenteral antiarrhythmic agent used by practicing intensivists. Although quite complex in terms of its clinical pharmacokinetics and pharmacodynamics in the intensive care patient, it enjoys wide recognition as a safe and effective therapy for acute management of ventricular arrhythmias. Lidocaine, which is the prototype IB antiarrhythmic agent, has structure and pharmacology similar to those of mexiletine and tocainide. Subtle modifications to the original lidocaine molecule allow for improved bioavailability and hence more practical oral routes of administration for mexiletine and tocainide compared to lidocaine. Available for IV use only, lidocaine is a highly protein-bound, high-clearance drug that requires dosage modification in the hypo- and hyperdynamic patient. Failure to consider dosage modification of lidocaine in certain intensive care patients can result in potentially significant toxicities or lack of efficacy [24].

PHARMACOLOGY.

The pharmacology of all of the class IB antiarrhythmic agents is similar. The basic cellular electrophysiologic effects on automaticity include little if any effect of the sinus node in the absence of preexisting disease, decreases in the slope of phase 4 depolarization in Purkinje fibers, and abolishment of triggered activity due to digitalis-induced delayed afterdepolarizations [25,26]. Relative to other Vaughn Williams classes of antiarrhythmics, lidocaine and other class IB agents have no effect on conduction velocity in normal tissues [27]. They cause little change in the duration of action potential for atrial fibers, in contrast to decreases in action potential duration for Purkinje fibers, ventricular muscle, and portions of the His-Purkinje system [28,29]. These minimal effects on atrial tissue translate into a minimal effectiveness compared to class IA agents in the treatment of atrial flutter or atrial fibrillation for either conversion or rate reduction. Furthermore, lidocaine's effects tend to reduce the spatial dispersion of refractoriness. This translates into a minimal effect of these agents observed on the surface ECG at typical therapeutic concentrations [27].

THERAPEUTIC RANGE.

As with other class IB antiarrhythmic agents, there is substantial interpatient variability in the ratio of therapeutic to toxic plasma concentrations of lidocaine. The therapeutic endpoint was established via observed suppression of ventricular ectopy, namely suppression of PVCs [2]. The earliest reports to determine a therapeutic range based on efficacy [30–35] tended to identify ranges approximating the currently reported range of 2 to 6 μg per milliliter [2]. Similarly, early and late reports of the relationship between concentration and toxicity [24,30,35–40] tended to implicate levels in excess of 6 μg per milliliter as more commonly associated with toxicities than lower levels.

The contribution of active lidocaine metabolites (monoethylglycinexylidide [MEGX] and glycinexylidide [GX]) to the toxicity of lidocaine is unclear. The antiarrhythmic potency of MEGX and GX is approximately 80 to 90 percent and 10 to 26 percent that of lidocaine, respectively, based on animal models of arrhythmia [41,42]. The two metabolites have been identified in the blood of patients receiving lidocaine infusions. In cardiac patients, the ratio of serum concentrations of MEGX to lidocaine has ranged from 0.11 to 0.36, while that of GX to lidocaine has ranged from 0.5 to 0.11 [43,44]. Reports of lidocaine toxicity in patients with total lidocaine concentrations within the therapeutic range may be explained by accumulation of the metabolites [41,43,45] or alterations in protein binding [2]. This latter point may be particularly relevant in the intensive care patient, where trauma, burns, and so on may cause substantial alterations in the protein binding and hence free concentrations of lidocaine in the blood. A therapeutic range of free (unbound) lidocaine of 0.5 to 2.0 μg per milliliter has been suggested based on concentration-dependent binding [2].

The clinical use of lidocaine for suppression of ventricular tachycardia should be guided by the ECG response and total lidocaine blood (or serum or plasma) concentrations of 2 to 6 μg per milliliter. A serum lidocaine concentration exceeding 2 μg per milliliter is generally necessary in the treatment of ventricular tachycardia or fibrillation [2].

PREPARATIONS. Lidocaine is available as a parenteral formulation only. Typical availability in an institutionalized setting includes either prepared bags containing 2-, 4-, or 8-mg per milliliter solutions in 5% dextrose ready for infusion or 4%, 10%, or 20% additive syringes or single-dose vials for IV admixtures. Additional forms are available for direct IV and IM administration. These include a 1% and 2% single-dose disposable syringe (without preservatives) and various IM injections forms (10% solution in 5 ml amps and a 300 mg/3 ml automatic injection device).

PHARMACOKINETICS. Table 207-2 summarizes the pharmacokinetic properties of lidocaine.

Absorption. Although lidocaine is rapidly and extensively absorbed after oral administration, this route is not used due to reported abdominal discomfort and massive first-pass hepatic extraction, resulting in extremely poor systemic bioavailability [46], ranging from 18 to 46 percent in noncirrhotic subjects [47]. Rectal administration of an aqueous solution of lidocaine (HCl has been investigated as a means to avoid the portal circulation and thereby improve systemic availability. Only partial avoidance of first-pass hepatic extraction was observed using this route [48]. Intramuscular administration, which avoids presystemic elimination, has been studied extensively; considerable efficacy was demonstrated using doses of 200 to 400 mg [31,32,33,49–52]. Although lidocaine concentrations were influenced by the site of IM administration, concentrations in excess of 1.0 μg per milliliter persisted over 2 hours, suggesting that IM administration is a viable alternative in patients in whom the IV route is not possible.

Of potential importance to the intensive care patient is the risk of systemic absorption following use of lidocaine as a local anesthetic. Clinically significant serum concentrations of lidocaine have been reported following lidocaine use as a local anesthetic for electrophysiologic studies, catheterization procedures, and bronchoscopy [53–56].

Distribution. Lidocaine distribution follows a two-compartment open pharmacokinetic model, partitioning initially into the central compartment, including high perfused tissues such as the lungs, heart, and kidneys, and then extensively into remaining body tissues. Lidocaine binds extensively (70%) to serum proteins, including AAG (50%) and albumin (20%) [57]. The extent of lidocaine protein binding can be significantly altered by disease-inducing changes in plasma protein concentrations, especially AAG. The degree of protein binding tends to increase with age from birth through adulthood [58]. The volume of distribution of lidocaine is relatively large and is influenced by several factors, including gender and various disease states. In young, healthy volunteers, the volume of distribution for the central compartment after a single bolus is approximately 0.5 liter per kilogram, while that at steady state is about 1 liter per kilogram [59]. Females appear to have 33 percent greater volume of distribution of lidocaine than males [60,61]. The volume of distribution in patients with CHF is reduced in the central compartment (0.3 L/kg) and at steady state [62,63] while in patients with acute viral hepatitis it is significantly larger in the central compartment (1 L/kg) and at steady

state (3.1 L/kg) [64]. The volume of distribution of lidocaine does not appear to be influenced by renal disease [62] or age [60].

Elimination. Lidocaine is primarily metabolized in the liver by the cytochrome P-450 system to two active metabolites (MEGX and GX) and several inactive metabolites, all of which are excreted almost entirely in the urine. Less than 5 percent of lidocaine is excreted as unchanged drug in the urine [44,65]. Lidocaine clearance is influenced by many factors, including gender, age, and various disease states. In healthy male volunteers, the systemic clearance and half-life of lidocaine after a single IV bolus is approximately 16 ml/min/kg at 1.6 hours [2]. Females appear to have an increased clearance and half-life of lidocaine [60,61]. Increased age [60,66] and various conditions, such as congestive heart failure, [62,67,68,69], acute myocardial infarction [68,70,71,72], chronic liver disease [62,73], and hypotension [74], are associated with a significant reduction in lidocaine clearance and increase in half-life.

PHYSIOLOGIC CLEARANCE. The disposition of lidocaine after bolus administration and during continuous infusion is extremely susceptible to changes in the patient's physiologic state. Due to rapid and extensive metabolism by hepatic microsomal enzymes, lidocaine clearance is largely determined by hepatic blood flow and thus, indirectly, by cardiac output. Physiologic alterations in critically ill patients producing high-flow or low-flow states may, therefore, have a profound effect on lidocaine disposition. Furthermore, since lidocaine is extensively protein-bound in serum and tissues, the volume of distribution and half-life can be altered by disease-induced changes in serum protein concentrations and due to displacement of lidocaine from protein binding sites. Thus, changes in hepatic blood flow and drug binding are major determinants of lidocaine half-life.

Given the complexity of lidocaine pharmacokinetics and prevalence of physiologic alterations in critically ill patients, lidocaine therapy must be individualized and carefully monitored in the ICU. Elderly patients and those with CHF, acute myocardial infarction (AMI), and hypotension all tend to have reduced hepatic blood flow associated with decreased cardiac output and are therefore susceptible to lidocaine accumulation and toxicity. Elderly men and women demonstrate a reduced clearance and prolonged half-life [60,66], suggesting that lidocaine infusion rates should be reduced by 20 to 30 percent to achieve drug concentrations comparable to those in young patients [2]. In patients with CHF, lidocaine clearance is reduced by 35 percent and the half-life is increased more than twofold [62,66,67,68]. After AMI, lidocaine clearance is reduced by 40 percent and the half-life is increased two- to threefold [68,70,71,72]. An increase in serum AAG concentrations of approximately 20 percent occurring within 36 hours after AMI [75] may result in a reduced free fraction of lidocaine in the serum [76]. Therefore, the increase in half-life after AMI is likely due to an increase in the volume of distribution of lidocaine, increased protein binding, and a decrease in lidocaine clearance secondary to reduced hepatic blood flow [2].

Patients with AMI and CHF are especially susceptible to lidocaine accumulation, with a half-life of nearly five times normal [68,71,77]. Postsurgical and other stressed patients may also undergo acute changes liver blood flow and serum AAG concentrations, resulting in significant changes in lidocaine pharmacokinetics. Changes in lidocaine binding that increase or decrease the free fraction of drug may not be detected through routine monitoring of total serum lidocaine levels. Chronic liver disease, such as chronic active hepatitis [64] and cirrhosis [62,73], has been associated with various degrees of reduced hepatic clearance of lidocaine, possibly due to reduced hepatic blood flow or impaired metabolism [2]. The disposition of lidocaine is relatively unchanged in patients with renal dysfunction [62,78].

DOSING GUIDELINES. The multicompartment pharmacokinetics of lidocaine dictate that optimal serum concentrations and antiarrhythmic efficacy be attained through the administration of several intravenous bolus doses followed by a continuous infusion. The initial IV bolus dose distributes rapidly from the blood into the central compartment, resulting in rapidly declining serum concentrations. A second IV bolus dose is required to maintain therapeutic serum concentrations while drug accumulates from the continuous infusion. Several dosing regimens have been proposed to achieve rapidly and maintain therapeutic lidocaine concentrations for the duration of lidocaine therapy [63,79–83]. A well-accepted and relatively simple method is described below.

Loading Dose. Lidocaine therapy is generally indicated with an IV bolus injection of 1.0 to 1.5 mg/kg, followed by one or more IV bolus injections of 0.5 to 1.5 mg per kilogram every 5 to 15 minutes to a total loading dose of 3 mg per kilogram. Reduction of premature ventricular contractions and suppression of ventricular arrhythmias may aid in determining the size and number of bolus injections administered. Due to the relatively high lipophilicity of lidocaine and observed increase in volume of distribution in obese subjects [61], initial loading doses may be based on total body weight.

Maintenance Dose. Maintenance therapy with lidocaine is generally initiated at a dose of 1 to 4 mg per minute, beginning immediately after completion of the first bolus dose. Initial selection of a maintenance infusion rate may be best guided by use of mean population clearance values. Table 207-5 summarizes the mean systemic clearance and recommended infusion rates for selected patient populations. However, because these are mean clearance values, some patients may be somewhat under- or overtreated at these infusion rates. Since the mean half-life of lidocaine in normal volunteers is 1 to 2 hours, steady-state concentrations are normally achieved within 10 hours. In contrast, critically ill patients with reduced hepatic blood flow and/or alterations in drug binding may not achieve steady-state concentration for up to 24 hours or longer. Therefore, dose adjustment during maintenance therapy is best guided by serum concentration monitoring and clinical observation, including suppression of arrhythmia and signs of lidocaine toxicity (CNS side effects). It should be remembered, however, that lidocaine disposition can change rapidly in critically ill patients and thereby continually complicate the design of dosage regimens.

DRUG INTERACTIONS
Beta-Adrenergic Antagonists. Beta-blockers and other drugs that reduce cardiac output and hepatic blood flow can result in higher lidocaine levels and toxicity. The interaction is most significant with propranolol, since it also directly inhibits hepatic metabolism of lidocaine [2]. Propranolol [84,85] and metoprolol [84] can reduce lidocaine clearance by 40 to 50 percent and 30 percent, respectively.

Cimetidine. Cimetidine can reduce the systemic clearance of lidocaine by 15 to 45 percent [2,86], resulting in lidocaine tox-

icity [87]. Cimetidine reduces lidocaine intrinsic clearance by competing for hepatic microsomal enzymes. The effect of ranitidine appears to be negligible.

Antiarrhythmics. Many drugs can alter serum AAG concentrations and displace lidocaine from binding sites. Quinidine and disopyramide displace lidocaine from protein binding sites, increasing the free fraction of lidocaine by 34 percent and 21 percent, respectively [88].

COMMON PITFALLS
1. Failure to administer the second bolus within 15 to 30 minutes of the initial bolus dose of lidocaine results in subtherapeutic serum concentrations, due to rapid of lidocaine from the central compartment.
2. Failure to reduce the dose of lidocaine in elderly patients and those in low flow states (CHF, AMI, hypotension) can rapidly result in lidocaine toxicity.
3. The CNS signs and symptoms of lidocaine toxicity (confusion, paresthesias, tremor, ataxia, seizures, psychosis) must be recognized.

Mexiletine

Mexiletine is a class IB antiarrhythmic agent. It is indicated for the treatment of documented life-threatening ventricular arrhythmias. Mexiletine also has local anesthetic and anticonvulsant properties.

PHARMACOLOGY. Mexiletine is a primary amine with close structural similarities to lidocaine. It appears to produce a rate-dependent blocking of the sodium channel with minimal in vivo effects on sinus node discharge rate and atrial refractory note [89]. Despite increases in the relative and effective refractory periods in the His-Purkinje system, serious A-V conduction disturbances are unusual in the absence of overdose situations. Class IB agents are notable in general for their minimal effects on hemodynamic variables. Although occasional hypotension has been observed, mexiletine rarely adversely affects cardiac output [90].

THERAPEUTIC RANGE. Therapeutic plasma concentrations of mexiletine range from 0.5 to 2 μg per milliliter [89]. Plasma concentrations correlate well with adverse effects. As with other class IB agents, there is considerable interpatient variability in the ratio of toxic to therapeutic plasma concentrations of mexiletine.

PREPARATIONS

Mexiletine immediate-release	100-mg, 150-mg, 250-mg capsules
Mexiletine sustained-release	360-mg capsules

PHARMACOKINETICS. The pharmacokinetic properties of mexiletine are summarized in Table 207-2.

Absorption. Mexiletine is extensively (~90%) absorbed from the upper portion of the small intestine, achieving peak plasma concentrations within 2 to 3 hours in normal subjects [91]. Of

Table 207-5. Mean Systemic Clearance and Recommended Infusion Rates for Selected Patient Population [2]

Population	Mean (± SD) systemic clearance (ml/min/kg)	Infusion rate to achieve 3 µg/ml (mg/min/70 kg)	
		Mean	Range
Normal	15.6 ± 4.6	3.3	2.3–4.3
CHF	5.5 ± 1.7	1.2	0.8–1.5
AMI	9.1 ± 2.0	1.9	1.5–2.3
CHF and AMI	6.3 ± 1.4	1.3	1.1–1.6
Chronic liver disease	6.0 ± 3.2	1.3	0.6–1.9
Renal disease	13.2 ± 3.2	2.8	2.1–3.4
Propranolol coadministered	9.4 ± 3.1	2.0	1.3–2.7

AMI = acute myocardial infarction; CHF = congestive heart failure.

interest, in patients with AMI delayed gastric emptying has resulted in a significant delay in attainment of peak plasma concentrations [92,93]. Other clinical situations in which gastric emptying time is reduced also delay absorption of mexiletine. The extensive absorption of mexiletine combined with minimal first-pass hepatic extraction results in excellent systemic bioavailability, approaching 90 percent [93].

Distribution. Mexiletine distributes in a biphasic manner, initially partitioning rapidly into a central compartment and then slowly and extensively into peripheral tissues. Substantial tissue uptake of mexiletine results in a large but variable volume of distribution of 5 to 7 liters per kilogram [93,94]. Plasma protein binding is moderate, at 50 to 60 percent.

Elimination. Mexiletine is primarily metabolized in the liver to mostly inactive metabolites, except for N-methylmexiletine, which is less than 20 percent as potent as mexiletine [3,95,96]. Renal clearance of mexiletine can be substantial depending on urine pH, ranging from 35 percent of total clearance if the urine is acidic to 1 percent of total clearance if the urine is alkaline [97]. However, the clinical importance of this phenomenon is probably minimal, since renal insufficiency does not appear to prolong significantly the elimination half-life of mexiletine [98,99], which in normal subjects varies from 8 to 10 hours. It is somewhat longer (up to 14 hours) in patients with arrhythmias or AMI [92]. Hepatic impairment can significantly prolong the elimination half-life, to 25 hours or longer. Smoking, for unknown reasons, enhances mexiletine elimination, reducing the half-life by 35 percent compared to nonsmokers [100].

PHYSIOLOGIC CLEARANCE. Information is lacking regarding the disposition of mexiletine in the hypodynamic or hyperdynamic patient. Renal insufficiency does not significantly alter the elimination of mexiletine. Patients with chronic liver disease, such as hepatic cirrhosis, undergo a marked reduction in the hepatic metabolism of mexiletine [101].

DOSING GUIDELINES
Loading Dose. An initial dose of 400 mg may be used when rapid control of ventricular arrhythmias is essential.

Maintenance Dose. Most patients can be adequately treated with 200 to 300 mg every 8 hours. An initial dose of 200 mg every 8 hours may be gradually increased at 3-day intervals to 250 mg and then 300 mg every 8 hours, if necessary. If 300 mg

every 8 hours is tolerated but ineffective, the dosage may be increased to a maximum of 400 mg every 8 hours. Dosage titration is best guided by the development of adverse CNS effects and suppression of ventricular ectopic beats and ventricular arrhythmias, as documented by programmed electrical stimulation or ambulatory electrocardiographic monitoring.

DRUG INTERACTIONS. Phenytoin, rifampin, and phenobarbital induce hepatic enzymes and thereby lower mexiletine plasma concentrations. Antacid therapy, cimetidine, and narcotic analgesics can slow the absorption of mexiletine [89].

COMMON PITFALLS
1. A relatively high incidence (~70%) of minor adverse effects, such as tremor, diplopia, nausea, and vomiting, can result in poor patient compliance.

Moricizine

Moricizine is a class I antiarrhythmic with properties of IA, IB, and IC subclasses. It was approved by the FDA in 1990 to treat documented life-threatening ventricular arrhythmias.

PHARMACOLOGY. Moricizine is a phenothiazine derivative that is chemically unrelated to any currently approved antiarrythmic drug. As for all class I antiarrhythmic agents, moricizine reduces the fast inward sodium current of the action potential. Excitability, conduction velocity, and automaticity are diminished through slowing of A-V nodal and His-Purkinje conduction, resulting in decreased duration of the action potential and the effective refractory period [102,103]. In humans, a dose-related increase in the P–R, QRS, and corrected Q–T intervals is seen [104,105].

THERAPEUTIC RANGE. Plasma concentrations of moricizine and its metabolites do not appear to predict antiarrhythmic efficacy or toxicity [106].

PREPARATIONS

Moricizine (Ethmozine)   200-mg, 250-mg, 300-mg tablets

PHARMACOKINETICS [103,107]. Table 207-2 summarizes the pharmacokinetic properties of moricizine.

Absorption. Moricizine is readily absorbed from the GI tract. Systemic bioavailability is reduced to 30 to 40 percent due to significant first-pass metabolism in the liver [106]. Peak plasma concentrations are achieved within 1 to 2 hours after a single oral dose [108]. Giving the drug with food delays the time to peak plasma concentration but affects the absolute peak plasma concentration [106].

Distribution. Moricizine is widely distributed in peripheral tissue and is highly protein-bound (95%) to AAG and albumin [106].

Elimination. Moricizine is almost completely biotransformed in the liver by several processes. Approximately 40 metabolites have been isolated, although their antiarrhythmic potencies are unknown. Less than 1 percent of moricizine is excreted unchanged in the urine [106]. Approximately 39 percent of the parent compound and its metabolites is eliminated in the urine, and 56 percent is excreted by the fecal route. The mean terminal elimination half-life is 3 to 4 hours in normal subjects [109] and 6 to 13 hours in patients with arrhythmias [110].

PHYSIOLOGIC CLEARANCE. Few data exist regarding the use of moricizine in critically ill patients or patients with renal or hepatic insufficiency. Given the extensive metabolism of moricizine, prolonged elimination in patients with compromised renal function is not expected and has not been demonstrated [111]. Critically ill patients and other patients under physiologic stress with increased serum concentrations of AAG may have a reduced free fraction of moricizine in serum, although the clinical significance of this is unknown.

DOSING GUIDELINES
Loading Dose. A loading does has not been proposed for moricizine.

Maintenance Dose. Moricizine doses required to produce antiarrhythmic effects are variable. Most patients can be adequately treated with 200 to 300 mg every 8 hours. An initial dose of 200 mg every 8 hours may be gradually increased at 3-day intervals to 250 mg and then 300 mg every 8 hours [112,113]. A linear relationship exists between the dose of moricizine and the suppression of PVCs [112]. Therefore, in the absence of established concentration-effect relationships, dosage titration is best guided by suppression of ventricular ectopic beats and ventricular arrhythmias, as documented through programmed electrical stimulation or ambulatory electrocardiographic monitoring [105,106,114].

DRUG INTERACTIONS. The effects of moricizine and other drugs that affect cardiac conduction may be additive. Cimetidine (300 mg four times per day) can reduce moricizine clearance by nearly 50 percent and prolong the elimination half-life by 35 percent [109]. Ranitidine does not alter moricizine disposition. Moricizine increases plasma concentrations of theophylline by 46 to 68 percent and prolongs the elimination half-life by 20 to 34 percent [115].

COMMON PITFALLS
1. Moricizine may worsen cardiac performance in patients with preexisting left ventricular dysfunction or a history of CHF [116,117,118].
2. Moricizine has the potential to exacerbate ventricular arrhythmias; its use must be critically evaluated in the context of potential risks and lack of proven benefit in the CAST I and II trials.

Flecainide

Flecainide is a class IC antiarrhythmic indicated for the suppression of life-threatening ventricular arrhythmias and prevention of paroxysmal supraventricular tachycardia and paroxysmal atrial flutter and fibrillation.

PHARMACOLOGY [1]. Flecainide slows electrical conduction through the atria, ventricles, and A-V node, which decreases the automaticity of these tissues and lengthens the effective refractory period. The His-Purkinje system is most profoundly affected by the electrophysiologic properties of flecainide. It is, to a small degree, a negative inotrope.

THERAPEUTIC RANGE. The reported therapeutic range for flecainide is 0.3 to 2.5 μg per milliliter [119].

PREPARATIONS

Flecainide (Tambocor)	50-mg, 100-mg, 150-mg tablets

PHARMACOKINETICS. Table 207-2 summarizes the pharmocokinetic properties of flecainide.

Absorption. Absorption of flecainide from the GI tract is rapid and virtually complete. First-pass metabolism through the liver is negligible and minimally affects bioavailability, which is approximately 85 to 90 percent.

Distribution. Rapid and extensive distribution follows parenteral administration of flecainide, as documented in studies of healthy human volunteers. In vitro studies suggest that flecainide is 40 to 50 percent protein-bound, mostly to AAG.

Elimination. Flecainide is hepatically metabolized (dealkylated and oxidized) to two major metabolites, *m-O*-dealkylated flecainide and *M-O*-dealkylated lactam derivative, which possess 20 to 50 percent and 10 percent of the antiarrhythmic activity of the parent compound, respectively. Both metabolites are further conjugated. Elimination of unchanged drug and its metabolites is via the urine.

PHYSIOLOGIC CLEARANCE
Hypodynamic. In patients with diminished renal function, the elimination of flecainide and its metabolites decreases as the creatinine clearance decreases [120–122]. In patients with ventricular arrhythmias, flecainide has been shown to exhibit nonlinear elimination, which may affect predictability of plasma concentrations and drug response [123]. A reduction in the plasma clearance of flecainide was reported in patients with cirrhosis, probably because of impaired hepatic function [124].

Congestive heart failure may also decrease flecainide clearance, resulting in prolonged elimination half-life [125].

Hyperdynamic. A study in 63 pediatric patients aged 0 to 12 years with ventricular arrhythmias was performed to determine the pharmacokinetics of flecainide. The half-life of flecainide in patients aged 1 to 12 years was approximately 8 hours, one-third less than that of adult patients [126]. Infants (< 1 year) were found to have a flecainide half-life of 11 to 12 hours, about the same as adults. Administration of flecainide every 12 hours, however, suppressed arrhythmia activity in 80 percent of patients aged 1 to 12 years.

DOSING GUIDELINES

Loading Dose. Due to the proarrhythmic risks associated with early peak concentrations of flecainide, loading doses are not recommended.

Maintenance Dose. For suppression of life-threatening ventricular arrhythmias, flecainide is initiated at 100 mg orally every 12 hours. The dosage may be increased by 50 mg per dose every 4 days to a maximum of 150 mg every 12 hours, if necessary. In patients with severe renal insufficiency (creatinine clearance <35 ml/min/1.73 m^2), flecainide is started at a dose of 50 mg every 12 hours.

DRUG INTERACTIONS. Amiodarone has reportedly doubled the serum concentrations of flecainide when the two drugs are concomitantly administered. A reduction in the flecainide dose by 50 percent is suggested when this combination is used.

COMMON PITFALLS

1. Serum concentrations of flecainide may be useful as an indicator of toxicity. Trough plasma concentrations greater than 1 μg per milliliter have been associated with increased cardiac toxicity, such as bradycardia.
2. Reserve flecainide for suppression of life-threatening ventricular arrhythmias in patients for whom no suitable alternative therapy exists.
3. Loading doses of flecainide are not recommended.

Propafenone

Propafenone is a class IC antiarrhythmic agent indicated for the suppression of life-threatening ventricular arrhythmias.

PHARMACOLOGY. Propafenone slows electrical conduction through the AV node, ventricles, and the His-Purkinje system, which decreases the automaticity of these tissues and lengthens the effective refractory period. The His-Purkinje system is most profoundly affected by the electrophysiologic properties of propafenone. These effects are more pronounced in ischemic tissue than in normal myocardium.

THERAPEUTIC RANGE. No consistent range for therapeutic concentrations for propafenone has been defined [127]. The wide interpatient variability of propafenone concentrations and the nonlinearity of propafenone elimination have hampered efforts at elucidation of its therapeutic range.

PREPARATIONS

Propafenone (Rythmol)   150-mg, 300-mg tablets

PHARMACOKINETICS. Table 207-2 summarizes the pharmacokinetic properties of propafenone.

Absorption. Propafenone is rapidly and completely (90%) absorbed. However, due to significant first-pass metabolism through the liver, the absolute bioavailability of propafenone ranges from 5 to 50 percent, depending on the patient's genetically determined capacity to metabolize the drug extensively. Giving propafenone with food may significantly increase the systemic bioavailability in extensive metabolizers by diminishing the first-pass extraction of the drug [128].

Distribution. The steady-state volume of distribution is large, reportedly between 1.9 and 3.0 liters per kilogram [129]. Distribution is rapid and extensive into tissues including the heart, lungs, and liver. The major metabolite of propafenone, 5-hydroxypropafenone, and the parent compound are equally distributed between the atria and ventricles. Propafenone is highly protein-bound (>95%), predominantly to AAG. The protein binding characteristics of the metabolites of propafenone remain unclear.

Elimination. Through first-pass hepatic metabolism, propafenone is converted into several metabolites, including 5-hydroxypropafenone, which possesses a degree of antiarrhythmic activity similar to that of the parent compound. The metabolism of propafenone has been characterized as a polymorphic, saturable system [130]. The extent of propafenone metabolism is genetically determined based on phenotype. Approximately 90 percent of patients extensively metabolize of propafenone, resulting in serum 5-hydroxypropafenone concentrations between 60 and 100 percent of those of propafenone. The remaining 10 percent are poor metabolizers, and 5-hydroxypropafenone concentrations are approximately 35 percent of those of propafenone [131]. Elimination is by both renal and fecal routes. Less than 1 percent of propafenone is eliminated through the kidneys as unchanged drug, and the metabolites are 38 percent renally excreted and 53 percent fecally excreted.

PHYSIOLOGIC CLEARANCE

Hypodynamic. Liver disease appears to have a profound effect on the disposition of propafenone because of impaired biotransformation of the parent compound and decreased albumin production [132]. Significantly enhanced systemic bioavailability, reduced clearance, and decreased protein binding of propafenone have been observed in this population. Renal insufficiency has not been shown to have any effect on the pharmacokinetics of propafenone [133].

Hyperdynamic. Since AAG is released in the acute phase of injury or stress, an increase in this protein may decrease the fraction of unbound propafenone.

DOSING GUIDELINES

Loading Dose. No guidelines for loading doses of propafenone have been proposed.

Maintenance Dose. Recommended initial oral dosing of propafenone is 150 mg every 8 hours. Dosing may be increased to 225 mg every 8 hours after 4 days. After that, the dose may be further increased to 300 mg every 8 hours if adequate control of ventricular arrhythmia has not been achieved.

DRUG INTERACTIONS

Digoxin. Digoxin serum concentrations may be increased 35 to 85 percent due to impairment of nonrenal clearance of digoxin.

Quinidine. Quinidine is a specific and potent inhibitor of the enzyme P450IID6, which is responsible for the hepatic hydroxylation of propafenone. The serum propafenone concentration may double and serum 5-hydroxypropafenone concentration may be cut in half in extensive metabolizers of propafenone. However, there is no apparent change in the pharmacologic activity of propafenone [134].

Warfarin. An increased prothrombin time of 25 percent may occur. The mechanism is unclear.

COMMON PITFALLS

1. Do not use serum concentrations of propafenone to guide therapy, as an indicator of either efficacy or toxicity.
2. Loading doses of propafenone are not suggested.

Amiodarone

Amiodarone is a class III antiarrhythmic agent used in the chronic management of ventricular arrhythmias.

PHARMACOLOGY [1]. Amiodarone affects cardiac electrical conduction in several ways. Primarily, the action potential duration and the effective refractory period are prolonged in the atria and ventricles. In addition, the automaticity of the sinoatrial node is diminished. On ECG, lengthening of the P–R and Q–T intervals and widening of the QRS complex are commonly observed. Vascular tone is dampened in both the systemic and coronary vessels as a result of alpha- and beta-adrenergic receptor blockage.

THERAPEUTIC RANGE. A therapeutic range of 1.0 to 2.5 μg per milliliter has been reported; however serum concentration monitoring is controversial [135,136]. The efficacy and toxicity of amiodarone are determined more by tissue deposition than by serum concentration. Moreover, accumulation of the active metabolite desethylamiodarone may further confuse the situation. Therefore, the use of serum drug level monitoring with amiodarone is generally not recommended.

PREPARATIONS

Amiodarone (Cordarone)   200-mg scored tablets

PHARMACOKINETICS. Table 207-2 summarizes the pharmacokinetic properties of amiodarone.

Absorption. After oral administration, amiodarone is slowly absorbed from the GI tract. Variability in absorption ranges from 22 to 86 percent, with an average bioavailability of about 50 percent.

Distribution. Amiodarone widely distributes into body tissues, and the tissue concentration generally exceeds that in the plasma. It is highly lipophilic and has an extremely long elimination half-life of 53 days. The half-life of the major metabolite of amiodarone, N-desethylamiodarone, is about 57 to 61 days. It is 96 percent bound to plasma proteins, mainly to albumin and, to a lesser extent, a high-density lipoprotein (probably beta-lipoprotein).

Elimination. Metabolism occurs in the liver and possibly in the GI tract. The major metabolite, N-desethylamiodarone, may possess antiarrhythmic activity. Amiodarone is excreted in the feces as unchanged drug or metabolites.

PHYSIOLOGIC CLEARANCE

Hypodynamic. The disposition of amiodarone was examined in a study of 21 surgical patients, 12 of whom had received short-term therapy (<4 weeks) and 9 of whom had received long-term therapy (>4 weeks) [137]. Blood and atrial tissue samples were assayed for amiodarone concentration. Drug plasma concentrations did not differ significantly between short- and long-term treatment groups, but mean desethylamiodarone metabolite concentrations were significantly higher in the long-term treatment group. Average atrial tissue concentrations of both amiodarone and desethylamiodarone were significantly greater in the long-term treatment group. Amiodarone concentrations were four to five times higher than those of the metabolite in pericardial fat tissue in both treatment groups. The time course for equilibration of amiodarone concentrations between the atria and the plasma (at least 4 weeks) is a potential reason for its delayed onset of activity. The parent compound appears to have a higher affinity for adipose tissue, where it accumulates during long-term treatment.

Hyperdynamic. There is little information about amiodarone pharmacokinetics in this population.

DOSING GUIDELINES

Loading Dose. The recommended loading dose of amiodarone is 800 to 1600 mg administered orally for 1 to 3 weeks. The dose may be divided if the total daily dose is greater than 1000 mg or if GI upset occurs. A lower dose of 600 to 800 mg orally is administered for at least 1 week for the management of supraventricular tachycardia.

Maintenance Dose. The lowest possible dose that prevents arrhythmia recurrence is the goal. Typical oral maintenance doses for suppression of ventricular or supraventricular arrhythmias is 200 to 400 mg daily.

DRUG INTERACTIONS

Anticoagulants. Potentiation of the anticoagulant effect through inhibition of warfarin metabolism can occur.

Digoxin. Up to a 70 to 100 percent increase in digoxin serum concentration can occur. Digoxin renal and nonrenal clearance is reduced.

Phenytoin. A two- to three-fold increase in phenytoin serum concentrations can occur. The mechanism is unclear.

COMMON PITFALLS

1. Serum concentration monitoring of amiodarone must be considered in light of its limitations. Improvement in symp-

toms and ECG parameters and monitoring for long-term adverse effects are more useful monitoring tools.

2. Therapy needs to be continued for at least 1 to 3 weeks for an adequate trial of amiodarone. Tissue concentrations of amiodarone in the myocardium may not be sufficient to produce a therapeutic response for several weeks, due to the extensive distribution and high lipophilicity of amiodarone. This contributes to a delayed onset of action in most patients.

Bretylium

Bretylium is a class III antiarrhythmic agent used in the management of ventricular arrhythmias refractory to initial therapy.

PHARMACOLOGY

[1]. As a quaternary ammonium compound, bretylium exhibits ganglionic blocking activity in adrenergic neurons. Release of norepinephrine is impeded by bretylium at the synaptic junction. Bretylium increases the action potential duration and lengthens the effective refractory period in the atria, ventricles, and A-V node. The effect of bretylium on automaticity is negligible. On ECG, bretylium lengthens the P–R and Q–T intervals.

THERAPEUTIC RANGE.

The reported therapeutic range is 0.5 to 2.0 μg per milliliter [138]. Plasma concentrations greater than 3 μg per milliliter have been associated with transiently increased vascular tone. Serum concentrations of bretylium are useful to gauge the likelihood of toxicity, which may lead to nausea, vomiting, and hypotension.

PREPARATIONS

Bretylium parenteral (Bretylol, generic)	50 mg/ml, 100 mg/ml

PHARMACOKINETICS

Absorption. Bretylium is well absorbed after IM administration, which may be a consideration in critically ill patients in whom vascular access is limited.

Distribution. Bretylium concentrates in tissues rich in adrenergic innervation, such as the spleen. Protein binding of bretylium is 1 to 10 percent.

Elimination. Bretylium is completely eliminated by the kidneys, with an elimination half-life of approximately 5 to 10 hours [138].

PHYSIOLOGIC CLEARANCE

Hypodynamic. Clearance of bretylium correlates well with creatinine clearance [139]. Elimination by the renal route is significantly reduced in patients with creatinine clearances less than 30 ml per minute. Decreased blood flow to the renal bed or acute renal failure is likely to decrease total body clearance of bretylium. Changes in protein status do not affect bretylium pharmacokinetics, since it is negligibly protein-bound.

Hyperdynamic. Little is known about bretylium pharmacokinetics in this population.

DOSING GUIDELINES

Loading Dose. For treatment of ventricular fibrillation, bretylium is administered in undiluted form as an intravenous injection. The usual regimen is 5 mg per kilogram followed by 10 mg per kilogram every 15 to 30 minutes until the arrhythmia is controlled or until a total dose of 30 mg per kilogram has been administered. In the management of all other ventricular arrhythmias, 5 to 10 mg per kilogram is diluted in a proper medium (500 mg in at least 50 ml of diluent) and given every 1 to 2 hours until the arrhythmia is controlled or a total dose of 40 mg per kilogram has been reached.

Maintenance Dose. Bretylium is intended for short-term use and should be stopped after 3 to 5 days, with subsequent conversion of the patient to an oral antiarrhythmic, if necessary. Intermittent infusion of 5 to 10 mg per kilogram every 6 to 8 hours or a continuous infusion of 1 to 2 mg per minute are common regimens. Intramuscular bretylium is administered in undiluted form at 5 to 10 mg per kilogram every 6 to 8 hours for temporary maintenance of stable ventricular arrhythmias.

DRUG INTERACTIONS

[24]. Initial release of norepinephrine from sympathetic ganglia caused by bretylium may potentiate digoxin toxicity when the two are given together. This dose-dependent phenomenon occurs when the sudden surge in circulating norepinephrine aggravates ventricular arrhythmias due to digoxin toxicity. Bretylium is contraindicated in patients with arrhythmias, due to cardiac glycoside toxicity, and should be used cautiously in all other patients receiving digoxin. Bretylium should be used cautiously in hypotensive patients, since exogenous catecholamines administered as vasopressors may be rendered ineffective by the prevention of norepinephrine release from nerve terminals.

COMMON PITFALLS

1. Bretylium is relegated to a second-line agent for the management of ventricular arrhythmias due to its propensity to cause hypotension and contraindication in patients with arrhythmias caused by digoxin toxicity.
2. Expect nausea and vomiting after bretylium administration.

Sotalol

Sotalol hydrochloride is an antiarrhythmic agent with unique electrophysiologic properties. It is indicated for the treatment of life-threatening ventricular arrhythmias, such as sustained ventricular tachycardia or ventricular fibrillation. It has also demonstrated benefit in the treatment of supraventricular arrhythmias, hypertension, angina, and acute myocardial infarction, although it lacks an official indication for such uses.

PHARMACOLOGY.

Sotalol was originally evaluated in 1965 as a specific beta-adrenergic blocking drug [140]. By 1970 it was recognized as possessing unique electrophysiologic properties [141], which have recently been shown to confer significant broad-spectrum antiarrhythmic activity [142,143]. It is now clear that sotalol possesses two distinct properties, a combination of class II and class III antiarrhythmic activity, that distinguish it from other antiarrhythmic agents. The antiarrhythmic activity of sotalol in patients with life-threatening ventricular arrhythmias, however, is attributed largely to its class III activity. Like all beta-adrenoreceptor antagonists, sotalol contains a chiral center. It is commercially available as the racemic mixture of its stereoisomers, the additive properties of which account for its dual mechanism of antiarrhythmic action. The dextrorotatory isomer, d-sotalol, is currently being evaluated in clinical trials. The electrophysiologic properties of sotalol are summarized in Table 207-6.

The class II activity of sotalol is characterized by competitive antagonism of beta-adrenergic receptors [140,145,146] with an in vivo potency of one-fourth to one-third that of propranolol [147,148]. Beta blockade with sotalol, as measured by reduction in heart rate during exercise, is dose- and concentration-dependent [149]. As a beta-blocker, sotalol is noncardioselective and lacks intrinsic sympathomimetic activity (except at very high doses), membrane-stabilizing activity, and local anesthetic effects [141,147,150]. Beta blockade is primarily due to the levoisomer, which has 50 times the beta-blocking activity of the dextroisomer [151]. D-sotalol is essentially devoid of beta-blocking activity [48,140,152,153,154] and has been used successfully in experimental situations where a beta-blocker is contraindicated [155].

The class III activity of sotalol is characterized by selective lengthening of the action potential duration and effective refractory period in all cardiac tissues [141,145,156] and is independent of its beta-blocking properties [151,153,156,157]. Sotalol prolongs the monophasic action potential in the atria and ventricles [151,158,159,160] and lengthens the intranodal conduction time and effective refractory period in atrial and ventricular muscle, the A-V node, and bypass tracts in both the antegrade and retrograde directions [142,143,161,162,163]. Sotalol selectively alters repolarization, as opposed to depolarization, as evidenced by a lack of effect on the upstroke velocity of phase 0 of the action potential and relatively unaltered sinoatrial conduction [150,164]. Sotalol's effect on repolarization manifests as lengthening of the Q–Tc interval on the surface of ECG and is dose- and concentration-dependent [141,145,150, 151,157,165]. Data in healthy volunteers indicate that the effect of sotalol on Q–Tc prolongation at steady state can be reliably predicted based on the degree of Q–Tc prolongation 3 hours after a single 320-mg oral dose [165]. His-Purkinje conduction and QRS duration are unaltered. Like most of the newer class III agents, sotalol demonstrates "reverse use-dependence" or rate-dependent effects on repolarization, producing greater Q–Tc prolongation at slower heart rates [143]. The proposed mechanism by which sotalol prolongs repolarization involves a substantial inhibition of the outward potassium current (delayed rectifier current) in association with a small decrease in the background current (inward rectifier current) [156]. In contrast to the beta-blocking activity of sotalol, for which the levoisomer is solely responsible, the levoisomer, dextroisomer, and racemate are equipotent in their effects on repolarization [48,151,166].

Table 207-6. Electrophysiologic Properties of Sotalol [141]

Class II	Slows heart rate
	Lowers cardiac output
	Lowers systolic blood pressure
	Increases systemic vascular resistance
Class III	Prolongs action potential duration in atria and ventricles
	Increases effective refractory period in atria, ventricles, A-V node, A-V accessory pathways
	Lengthens intranodal conduction time
	Prolongs Q–T interval
	Minimal change in QRS duration

The hemodynamic effects of sotalol are unique, especially in terms of the apparent lack of substantial myocardial depressant effects [146,162,167,168]. Sotalol produces a proportionate reduction in heart rate and cardiac output at rest and during exercise without a change in stroke volume and increase in systemic vascular resistance while producing little or no increase in left ventricular end-diastolic pressure [169,170,171]. The negative chronotropic effects of sotalol are primarily due to beta blockade by the levoisomer. D-sotalol, however, can also lower heart rate during exercise through a beta-receptor-independent mechanism, probably through prolongation of the action potential duration in the sinus node [154]. The myocardial depressant effect of sotalol from its beta-blocking activity may be offset by an increase in contractility resulting from its effects on action potential duration, thus distinguishing it from conventional beta-blockers. An intrinsic positive inotropic effect has been clearly demonstrated in vitro [147,151,162,172, 173] and is probably due to lengthening of the action potential duration and subsequent delay in inactivation of the slow calcium channel, allowing a net increase in intracellular calcium per beat [157,174]. In patients with heart failure, sotalol has been reported to lack significant depressant effects on systemic hemodynamics [168]; however, worsening heart failure in small numbers of patients has been observed [142,143,175]. If D-sotalol is given alone, presumably a net increase in contractility would be observed. Studies in anesthetized animals have indicated that sotalol has significantly less myocardial depressant effects than conventional beta-blockers [146,162,167,173]. Thus, the net hemodynamic effect of the racemic mixture in humans may be no depressant effect or possibly even an augmentation of myocardial contractility.

THERAPEUTIC RANGE. Routine measurement of racemic sotalol as well as enantiospecific measurement of D-sotalol and I-sotalol concentrations in plasma is available using high-performance liquid chromatography [176]. A wide range of serum sotalol concentrations has been observed in patients effectively treated with the drug. The suggested therapeutic range is 1 to 4 μg per milliliter [177]. Several investigators have demonstrated a linear relationship between serum sotalol concentration and the drug's effect on heart rate [178,179] and repolarization, as measured by Q–Tc interval duration [160,165,179,180,181]. The concentration at which each of these effects occurs, however, may be very different. Minimal beta-blocking activity (50%) with sotalol has been reported to occur at drug concentrations much lower than those generally required to produce significant Q–Tc prolongation (804 ng/ml and 2550 ng/ml, respectively) [181]. This finding has been disputed by others, however, who contend that use of a more accurate formula for calculating Q–Tc indicates that the plasma concentrations of sotalol required to produce minimal beta blockade and Q–Tc prolongation are similar, occurring at 840 ng per milliliter and 680 ng per milliliter, respectively [179]. Nevertheless, the suggested therapeutic range of 1 to 4 μg per milliliter is considered broad enough to forego monitoring in most situations [177].

PREPARATIONS

Sotalol (Betapace)	80-mg, 160-mg, 240-mg scored tablets
Sotalol IV	Not available in the United States

PHARMACOKINETICS. Table 207-2 summarizes the pharmacokinetic properties of sotalol. The disposition of sotalol can be described by an open, linear, two-compartment model that follows first-order kinetics [182]. While many beta-blockers undergo enantioselective disposition, sotalol enantiomers have nearly identical pharmacokinetics [151,176,183,184]. Chronic therapy with sotalol does not significantly alter its pharmacokinetics [185]. However, the Q–Tc interval reportedly lengthens to a greater degree following long-term administration than after acute intravenous administration [144].

Absorption. Sotalol is rapidly (2–3 hours) and completely (>90%) absorbed from the GI tract with an oral bioavailability of nearly 100 percent. The bioavailability is unaffected by age [186] and pregnancy [187]. Food, especially milk and milk products, reduces absorption by 20 percent [187]. Peak plasma concentrations [165] and peak beta-blocking effects [148] occur within 2 to 3 hours. Steady-state concentrations are reached in 2 to 3 days and demonstrate little intersubject variability.

Distribution. The volume of distribution of sotalol ranges from 1.6 to 2.4 liters per kilogram, although it may be decreased in the elderly [185]. Sotalol demonstrates no plasma protein binding and, due to its low lipophilicity, crosses the blood-brain barrier poorly. Sotalol is an extremely hydrophilic compound with slow entry into the CSF, a low brain-plasma ratio [188,189], and little or no CNS activity [190].

Elimination. Sotalol is eliminated primarily by glomerular filtration [188]. Approximately 75 percent of a single dose is detected as unchanged drug in the urine within 72 hours [191]. Renal clearance values of 1.5 times creatinine clearance have been observed for sotalol enantiomers, indicating the additional likelihood of active tubular secretion [183]. Sotalol is not metabolized in the liver, and no metabolites have been detected [192]. Plasma half-lives ranging from 7 to 18 hours have been reported for patients with normal renal function and vary linearly with creatinine clearance [193–197]. Berglund et al. reported an elimination half-life of about 8 hours in patients with normal renal function (CrCl>39 ml/min), 24 hours in patients with moderate renal dysfunction (CrCl 8–38 ml/min), and 34 hours in patients on dialysis [195]. Hemodialysis effectively reduces the half-life to approximately 6 hours and the plasma concentrations by 35 to 75 percent [195]. The plasma half-life is reportedly unaffected by pregnancy [186] but may increase in the elderly due to the effects of age on glomerular filtration. In contrast, the manufacturer maintains that sotalol clearance increases by 60 percent during pregnancy due to increases in renal plasma flow and glomerular filtration rate. Plasma clearance of sotalol may be reduced by drinking alcohol [197].

PHYSIOLOGIC CLEARANCE. Certain physiologic changes that may occur in critically ill patients may have an impact on the distribution and clearance of sotalol. Physiologic changes in serum protein concentrations, hepatic blood flow, and metabolic activity are not expected to alter sotalol elimination due to the drug's lack of protein binding and metabolism. However, physiologic changes in total body water or renal blood flow may have an impact on the volume of distribution and renal elimination, respectively. Because sotalol is hydrophilic and primarily distributed into extracellular fluid, the volume of distribution is likely to increase in volume-overloaded patients.

Hypodynamic. The hypodynamic patient may experience a reduction in sotalol clearance and an increase in elimination half-life in response to reduced renal blood flow. Due to the high degree of glomerular filtration, sotalol clearance decreases in proportion to renal blood flow.

Hyperdynamic. The hyperdynamic patient may experience an increase in sotalol clearance and a decreased half-life in response to increased renal blood flow. Supraphysiologic rates of glomerular filtration result in enhanced elimination of sotalol.

DOSING GUIDELINES

Loading Dose. With the oral form of sotalol, no loading dose is necessary; therapy should begin with 80 mg twice daily. With the intravenous form, doses ranging from 0.2 to 1.5 mg per kilogram administered slowly over 5 minutes have been shown to be well-tolerated. The intravenous form should be administered under ECG and blood pressure control.

Maintenance Dose. Maintenance therapy with sotalol is initiated with 80 mg twice daily and adjusted every 2 to 3 days as needed to allow attainment of steady-state serum concentrations. For maximum absorption, sotalol should be taken on an empty stomach. Beta blockade with sotalol is evident at doses as low as 25 mg per day; it reaches half-maximum at 80 mg per day and maximum between 320 and 640 mg per day. Prolongation of the action potential duration is evident at doses of 160 mg and greater. The lowest single dose shown to have antiarrhythmic activity is 80 mg; however, most patients require maintenance doses of 240 to 320 mg per day. Occasionally, patients with refractory arrhythmias require doses as high as 480 to 640 mg per day. The maximum dose should not exceed 640 mg per day and the dose must be adjusted for renal impairment (Table 207-7). In patients with a CrCl less than 25 ml per minute sotalol should be used cautiously, with careful monitoring of the Q–Tc interval and serum concentrations (if available).

DRUG INTERACTIONS. The unique and favorable pharmacokinetic profile of sotalol, including rapid and complete absorption and lack of protein binding and metabolism, render it free of many potential drug interactions. However, many drugs have the potential to prolong refractoriness, and their concomitant use with sotalol is generally not recommended. Such drugs include class IA antiarrhythmics (quinidine, procainamide, disopyramide), other class III drugs (amiodarone), certain antihistamines (terfenadine, astemizole), phenothiazines, and tricyclic antidepressants. The interacting drug should be withdrawn a minimum of 2 to 3 half-lives before sotalol therapy is begun. When these combinations are necessary, sotalol plasma concentrations and the Q–T interval should be carefully monitored. Successful combinations of sotalol with class IA drugs (procainamide and quinidine), class IB drugs (mexiletine and tocainide), and class IC drugs (flecainide, propafenone) have been reported in small numbers of patients [198]. Due to the class II activity of sotalol, concomitant beta-blocker therapy should be avoided. Hyperglycemia may occur with sotalol, requiring adjustment of insulin or oral hypoglycemic agents. Rebound hypertension sometimes observed with clinidine withdrawal may be exacerbated due to the beta-blocking activity of sotalol. Beta-agonists may need to be administered in higher dosages if used concurrently with sotalol.

Table 207-7. Sotalol Dosing in Renal Impairment

Creatinine clearance (ml/min)	Dosing interval (hr)
>60	12
30–60	24
10–30	36–48
<10	Individualized

COMMON PITFALLS

1. Sotalol should be used with caution in patients with marginal cardiac compensation, as deterioration in cardiac performance may occur. Premarketing studies demonstrated a 3.3 percent incidence of new or worsened CHF, which led to discontinuation of sotalol in 1 percent of patients [174].
2. Sotalol-induced Q–Tc prolongation can be associated with *Torsades de pointes,* especially under conditions of hypokalemia [188], bradycardia, high serum drug concentrations (potentially induced by renal failure), and preexisting lengthening of the Q–Tc interval. Rarely, in the absence of these risk factors, *Torsades de pointes* may occur with serum drug concentrations in the normal range [189].

Verapamil

Verapamil is the prototype calcium channel blocker of the phenylalkylamine type and is designated a class IV antiarrhythmic agent in the Singh-Vaughan-Williams classification scheme. It is widely used and indicated for the treatment of supraventricular tachyarrhythmias, including atrial fibrillation and flutter. For more information on the pharmacology, pharmacokinetics, and dosing of verapamil, the reader is referred to Chapter 210.

PHARMACOLOGY. Verapamil binds to slow calcium channels in the sinoatrial and A-V nodes and inhibits the transmembrane influx of calcium across myocardial cell membranes. By inhibiting calcium entry into the cell, verapamil slows conduction, prolongs refractoriness, and decreases automaticity of the sinoatrial and A-V nodes. Prolongation of the P–R interval, but not the Q–T interval, is usually seen on the ECG. The A–V nodal effects of verapamil are greater than those of diltiazem and substantially greater than those of nifedipine.

THERAPEUTIC RANGE. Plasma verapamil concentrations, while not routinely measured, correlate reasonably well with P–R interval prolongation and antiarrhythmic effect. Plasma concentrations greater than 100 ng per milliliter are required to achieve the acute antiarrhythmic effect of verapamil. Considerable interindividual and intraindividual variation in plasma concentration is seen with oral verapamil. Oral doses of 120 mg every 6 hours using conventional tablets result in mean steady-state plasma concentrations of 125 to 400 ng per milliliter. A single 240-mg dose of an extended-release verapamil capsule or tablet produced peak plasma concentrations of 77 and 150 to 165 ng per milliliter, respectively. A single IV injection of 10 mg of verapamil produced peak plasma concentrations ranging from 10 to 1500 ng per milliliter.

PREPARATIONS

Verapamil immediate-release	40-mg, 80-mg, 120-mg tablets
Verapamil extended-release	180-mg, 240-mg tablets
Verapamil extended-release	120-mg, 240-mg capsules
Verapamil injectable	2.5 mg/ml

PHARMACOKINETICS. Verpamil is administered clinically as a racemic mixture of optically active stereoisomers, which exhibit different pharmacokinetic and pharmacodynamic properties, including differential first-pass hepatic extraction after oral administration, protein binding, and A-V nodal effects [199]. These differences may contribute to inter- and intraindividual variability in patient response, especially after oral administration, given potential variability in the composition of commercially available verapamil.

Absorption. Although approximately 90 percent of oral verapamil is rapidly absorbed from the GI tract, it subsequently undergoes extensive first-pass hepatic elimination, resulting in a low systemic oral bioavailability of 20 to 35 percent. Peak plasma concentrations are reached within 1 to 2 hours after oral administration of conventional tablets, while extended-release tablets and capsules produce peak plasma concentrations within 4 to 8 hours and 7 to 9 hours, respectively. Food decreases the rate and extent of absorption of extended-release tablets but has little or no effect on the absorption of conventional tablets or extended-release capsules.

Distribution. The volume of distribution of verapamil ranges from 1.5 to 7.0 liters per kilogram in healthy adults. Verapamil is highly bound (95–99%) to plasma proteins. It distributes into the CNS, placenta, and breast milk.

Elimination. Verapamil is eliminated in a biphasic manner, with an elimination half-life of 4 to 12 hours. The half-life appears to increase with chronic dosing, due to saturation of hepatic enzymes [200]. Verapamil is almost completely metabolized in the liver to at least 12 metabolites, one of which (norverapamil) is the active metabolite. Norverapamil has approximately 20 percent of the cardiovascular activity of verapamil. Since only 3 to 4 percent of verapamil is excreted in the urine as unchanged drug, dose adjustment is unnecessary in renal dysfunction, but severe liver dysfunction may result in reduced clearance. Verapamil clearance is also decreased in the elderly, resulting in prolongation of the elimination half-life [199].

PHYSIOLOGIC CLEARANCE. Verapamil is considered a high-clearance drug that is highly protein-bound. Hepatic enzymes have a large capacity to metabolize verapamil. Its disposition after oral or IV administration is extremely susceptible to changes in the patient's physiologic state, especially of organ blood flow. Physiologic alterations in liver blood flow and serum protein concentrations can significantly alter the bioavailability and clearance of verapamil. Due to extensive first-pass hepatic elimination, the systemic bioavailability of oral verapamil is sensitive to alterations in hepatic blood flow, increasing in low flow states and decreasing in high flow states. Regardless of the route of administration, verapamil clearance is sensitive to these changes.

Hypodynamic. Patients with reduced hepatic blood flow may have reduce clearance of verapamil due to lower amounts of the drug reaching the liver. In addition, reduced serum protein concentrations and/or displacement of verapamil from serum binding sites can increase the fraction of pharmacologically active drug in the serum.

Hyperdynamic. Patients with increased hepatic blood flow may have enhanced clearance of verapamil due to increased amounts of drug reaching the liver.

DOSING GUIDELINES

Loading Dose. Verapamil is generally administered intravenously for the acute management of supraventricular tachyarrhythmias, especially for those associated with symptoms. Five to 10 mg (0.075–0.15 mg/kg) is given by slow IV push over no less than 2 minutes, preferably over 3 to 5 minutes. If the patient does not respond to the first dose, a second dose of 10 mg may be given 15 to 30 minutes after the initial dose.

Maintenance Dose. Oral maintenance doses of 240 to 480 mg per day are generally required to control ventricular response rate in patients with atrial flutter and/or fibrillation and for the prevention of paroxysmal supraventricular tachycardia. The daily dose is given in 3 to 4 divided doses for regular-release tablets or as a single daily dose for sustained-release tablets or capsules. Daily doses as low as 120 to 180 mg may be adequate for some patients. Continuous verapamil infusions at doses of approximately 1 to 5 μg/kg/min have been used successfully in the management of refractory supraventricular tachyarrhythmias [201,202,203].

DRUG INTERACTIONS

Antiarrhythmic Drugs. Quinidine, procainamide, and disopyramide should be avoided or used with extreme caution in combination with verapamil, due to additive effects on the cardiac conduction system. Furthermore, a pharmacokinetic interaction exists between verapamil and quinidine. Although the exact mechanism is unknown, verapamil appears to inhibit the clearance and prolong the half-life of quinidine [204]. Hypotension, pulmonary edema, ventricular tachycardia, bradycardia, and A-V block have been reported with this combination [205].

Digoxin. Verapamil can increase serum digoxin concentrations by 50 to 75 percent within the first week of combined therapy, primarily by decreasing the total body clearance of digoxin. The degree of interaction is dose-dependent up to 240 mg per day of verapamil [206]. Digoxin serum concentrations should be monitored and the dose adjusted accordingly.

Rifampin. Rifampin, a potent inducer of hepatic enzymes, has been shown significantly to enhance the first-pass hepatic extraction of oral verapamil, resulting in a 90 percent reduction in systemic bioavailability and loss of effectiveness of verapamil [207]. In this situation, oral verapamil should be replaced with IV verapamil or another agent.

Carbamazepine. Verapamil appears to impair the hepatic metabolism of carbamazepine, resulting in significantly increased carbamazepine levels [208].

COMMON PITFALLS

1. Exercise caution when using IV verapamil in elderly subjects, as they are often more susceptible to the hypotensive effects of the drug. Pretreatment with IV calcium has been shown to counteract the peripheral vascular effects of verapamil without inhibiting its A-V nodal effects [203,209].
2. Patients with heart failure may decompensate when given verapamil.

Diltiazem

Diltiazem is the prototype calcium channel antagonist of the benzothiazepine type and, like verapamil, is designated a class IV antiarrhythmic agent in the Singh-Vaughan-Williams classification scheme. It is similar to verapamil in that it has significant inhibitory effects on the cardiac conduction system and is therefore useful in the treatment of supraventricular tachyarrhythmias when administered intravenously. This section focuses primarily on the use of IV diltiazem in the acute management of supraventricular arrhythmias. For additional information on the pharmacology, pharmacokinetics, and dosing of oral diltiazem, the reader is referred to Chapter 210.

PHARMACOLOGY. Diltiazem share the pharmacologic actions of verapamil described previously. Ditiazem slows A-V nodal conduction and prolongs A-V nodal refractoriness when conduction through the A-V node is rapid.

THERAPEUTIC RANGE. Routine monitoring of diltiazem serum concentrations is not recommended. Mean steady-state plasma concentrations achieved during continuous infusions of 10 and 15 mg per hour in 32 patients with atrial fibrillation or flutter were approximately 242 and 470 ng per milliliter, respectively [210]. Plasma concentrations of diltiazem correlated well with percent reduction in heart rate in most patients, with the maximum mean percent reduction in heart rate seen at 294.4 ng per milliliter.

PREPARATIONS

Diltiazem immediate-release	30-mg, 60-mg, 90-mg, 120-mg tablets
Diltiazem sustained-release	60-mg, 90-mg, 120-mg capsules (twice daily)
	120-mg, 180-mg, 240-mg, 300-mg capsules (once daily)
Diltiazem injectable	5 mg/ml

PHARMACOKINETICS

Absorption. Intravenous diltiazem is 100 percent bioavailable, and peak effects on heart rate occur within 5 minutes in most cases. Approximately 80 percent of an oral dose of diltiazem is absorbed, but due to extensive first-pass metabolism in the liver only 40 percent of the dose reaches the systemic circulation. However, the systemic bioavailability of oral diltiazem increases disproportionately with increasing doses, due to saturation of hepatic enzymes.

Distribution. Approximately 75 to 80 percent of diltiazem is bound to plasma proteins, half of which are albumin. Diltiazem distributes into milk at concentrations equal to those in maternal serum.

Elimination. Diltiazem obeys first-order elimination, with a half-life of approximately 3.5 to 9 hours. Diltiazem is almost entirely metabolized in the liver by rapid deacetylation, N-demethylation, and O-demethylation to form one active and at least five inactive metabolites. The two principal metabolites are deacetydiltiazem, which has approximately 25 to 50 percent of the coronary vasodilating activity of diltiazem, and N-desmethydiltiazem, which is inactive. Only 2 to 4 percent of diltiazem is excreted as unchanged drug in the urine, so no adjustment for renal dysfunction is necessary.

Diltiazem exhibits nonlinear disposition during continuous IV infusion. In a study of 32 patients with atrial fibrillation and flutter, a higher maintenance dose (15 mg/hr vs. 10 mg/hr) resulted in a lower mean systemic clearance, a lower mean volume of distribution, and a disproportionately higher mean steady-state serum concentration [210]. However, the mean apparent elimination half-lives of diltiazem were similar for each infusion rate.

PHYSIOLOGIC CLEARANCE. Unlike verapamil, diltiazem is not a high-clearance drug and is only moderately bound to plasma proteins. Diltiazem clearance is only moderately dependent on liver blood flow and on the intrinsic metabolic capacity of the liver. Physiologic alterations in liver blood flow or hepatic function that may occur in the hyperdynamic and hypodynamic patient are not likely to affect diltiazem clearance unless these functions are severely depressed. Furthermore, due to only moderate protein binding, changes in the serum concentration of unbound diltiazem are not likely to be clinically significant.

DOSING GUIDELINES. Only intravenous diltiazem is indicated for the acute management of supraventricular tachycardias, although maintenance therapy with oral diltiazem may be useful for the prevention of recurrent paroxysmal supraventricular tachycardia. For more information regarding oral maintenance dosing of diltiazem, the reader is referred to Chapter 210.

Loading Dose. Diltiazem is initially given as a 0.25 mg/kg IV bolus administered over 2 minutes. If a response is not achieved, a second IV bolus of 0.35 mg/kg is given. Response rates have reached 75 percent after the first bolus and 90 percent after the second bolus.

Maintenance Dose. After the initial loading dose(s), a continuous infusion of 10 to 15 mg per hour is indicated for up to 24 hours.

DRUG INTERACTIONS. Since diltiazem is not a high-clearance drug and exhibits only moderate protein binding, few drug interactions have been identified.

Antiarrhythmics. Concurrent use of diltiazem and other drugs with additive effects on the cardiac conduction system, such as procainamide, quinidine, disopyramide, and other antiarrhythmic agents, should be considered a relative contraindication.

Cimetidine. Cimetidine may inhibit the clearance of diltiazem and its active metabolite, desacetyldiltiazem [211]; it has been recommended that the diltiazem dose be reduced by one-third when using this combination [212].

COMMON PITFALLS
1. Exercise caution when using IV diltiazem in elderly subjects, as they are often more susceptible to the hypotensive effects of the drug.
2. Patients with heart failure may decompensate when given diltiazem.

Adenosine

Adenosine is a synthetic form of a naturally occurring nucleoside compound indicated for the emergency management of paroxysmal supraventricular tachycardia involving the A-V node. Adenosine was approved for this indication by the FDA in 1989. Due to its superior safety profile, adenosine has become an attractive alternative to verapamil in the acute management of paroxysmal supraventricular tachycardia, including that associated with accessory bypass tracts, such as Wolff-Parkinson-White syndrome, for which calcium antagonists are contraindicated [213]. Adenosine has also been used extensively in the diagnosis of broad-complex tachycardias [214,215] and appears to be safe and effective for use in infants and children [216,217].

PHARMACOLOGY. Adenosine is an endogenous purine nucleoside compound normally present in all cells of the human body. It is produced intracellularly and extracellularly by degradation of adenine nucleotides and is released from cells under physiologic and pathophysiologic conditions [218,219,220]. Accordingly, this ubiquitous substance has a wide spectrum of biologic activity. The cardiovascular effects of adenosine are of particular interest in the clinical setting and perhaps the best studied in humans.

The degree of activity of adenosine depends on its concentration in the extracellular space, its functional compartment. Adenosine binds to extracellular purine receptors, whereupon most of its physiologic effects are mediated through cyclic adenosine monophosphate (cyclic AMP)-dependent and independent modulation of ionic movement through cell membranes [221]. The inhibitory effects of adenosine on the sinus and A-V nodes are mediated through cyclic AMP-independent activation of outward cellular potassium currents, resulting in hyperpolarization of the cell membrane and slowing or block of spontaneous activity [222,223].

When administered by rapid IV bolus, adenosine exerts a potent but transient negative dromotropic and chronotropic effect in humans, usually within 20 to 30 seconds [224]. Under these circumstances, adenosine directly slows electrical conduction through the A-V node and depresses automaticity of cardiac pacemakers. This activity accounts for its effectiveness in terminating reentry circuits that often perpetuate supraventricular tachycardia. Ventricular pacemakers are most sensitive to suppression by adenosine, followed by junctional pacemakers and then sinus pacemakers [225]. Depression of sinoatrial node automaticity results in transient sinus bradycardia (~10 seconds), followed by sinus tachycardia (~20 sec) [226,227], the latter of which may be due to adenosine-induced sympathetic activation [228].

THERAPEUTIC RANGE. Physiologic concentrations of adenosine range from 0.1 to 1 μM per liter [229]. Therapeutic plasma concentrations have not been established, due to the rapid disappearance of adenosine from the blood.

PREPARATIONS

Adenosine (Adenocard) injection   6-mg/2 ml flip-top vials

PHARMACOKINETICS

Absorption. Exogenously administered adenosine is not absorbed orally, but only after intravenous administration.

Distribution. During IV administration, adenosine is rapidly and widely distributed into cellular and extracellular fluid as well as into interstitial vascular space, where it is transported into and out of most cell types by a nucleoside transport system

[225]. Transport into the cell is necessary for subsequent enzymatic degradation. The actual volume of distribution of adenosine has not been characterized, due to its rapid disposition after intravenous administration.

Elimination. Adenosine is rapidly metabolized in the blood, with a reported half-life of less than 10 seconds [218,230]. Total clearance from the plasma occurs in less than 30 seconds [226]. At physiologic concentrations, adenosine is phosphorylated by adenosine kinase to form adenosine monophosphate (AMP) within erythrocytes, but after exogenous administration resulting in supraphysiologic concentrations adenosine is preferentially metabolized intracellularly by adenosine deaminase [229,231]. Deamination of adenosine forms inosine, which is then further broken down to hypoxanthine, xanthine, and, ultimately, uric acid, all of which are excreted by the kidneys [218,230].

PHYSIOLOGIC CLEARANCE. The actual clearance of adenosine is unknown due to its short half-life. Changes in the physiologic state of the patient are unlikely to affect the clearance of adenosine, due to the drug's lack of protein binding and lack of dependence on renal or hepatic mechanisms of elimination. No dosing adjustments are required for renal or hepatic dysfunction. Patients in a hyperdynamic or hypodynamic state, however, may undergo changes in circulation time that could affect the distribution of adenosine to its site of action in the heart. Therefore, site and technique of IV administration are critical to the drug's effectiveness in these situations.

DOSING GUIDELINES. The minimum effective dose of adenosine in terminating paroxysmal supraventricular tachycardia has been shown to vary up to 10-fold between patients, possibly due to variability in the site and technique of administration, circulation time, and level of adrenergic or vagal tone, which may antagonize or enhance the effects of adenosine [214]. Therefore, site and technique of administration are critical. Under these circumstances, adenosine should be administered as a rapid IV bolus over 1 to 2 seconds directly into a central or peripheral vein or into the most proximal site of an IV catheter or infusion line. Administration into a central vein as opposed to a peripheral vein has been shown more rapidly to terminate the tachycardia [232]. However, lower doses may be required with central administration, due to the decreased circulation time before the bolus reaches the heart [214]. To maximize the amount of drug reaching the systemic circulation and thus cardiac adenosine receptors, all connecting lines should be clamped to avoid retrograde flow of the solution and the line should be immediately flushed with at least 5 ml of saline.

Loading Dose. Initially, a 6-mg bolus of adenosine is administered intravenously over 1 to 2 seconds. If the tachycardia remains after 1 to 2 minutes, a second dose of 12 mg should be administered, followed by a third dose of 12 mg, if needed. Single doses exceeding 12 mg are not recommended by the manufacturer.

Maintenance Dose. There are no recommendations for maintenance therapy with adenosine in the treatment of supraventricular tachycardia. Adenosine infusions have been used experimentally in situations other than paroxysmal supraventricular tachycardia [233,234]. However, depending on the dose and route of administration, the cardiovascular effects of adenosine may vary. After a typical IV bolus of adenosine, A-V nodal

and cardiac pacemaker effects predominate, whereas during low-dose continuous infusion, vascular effects predominate. Adenosine infusions are associated with a lack of inhibition of A-V nodal conduction and a dose-dependent sinus tachycardia, presumably due to low concentrations of adenosine at the A-V node and reflex sympathetic activation due to systemic vasodilation, respectively [235,236]. Therefore, this method of administration would presumably be ineffective in the management of paroxysmal supraventricular tachycardia.

DRUG INTERACTIONS. The A-V nodal effects of adenosine are potentiated by dipyridamole, which inhibits the adenosine transport system, thereby slowing its uptake into cells and subsequent degradation [237,238]. It has been suggested that the adenosine dose be decreased to one-fourth the usual dose in patients taking dipyridamole [239].

Methylxanthines, such as caffeine and theophylline, are competitive antagonists of adenosine. These agents may completely block the electrophysiologic effects of the drug by competitively binding to adenosine receptors [214].

COMMON PITFALLS
1. Adenosine administered by rapid intravenous bolus may result in transient A-V block, sinus tachycardia or bradycardia, and/or various dysrhythmias such as ventricular tachycardia and atrial fibrillation [213,214,240].
2. Adenosine should not be used in patients with atrial fibrillation-flutter, as it is ineffective and may shorten the atrial action potential duration and accelerate the tachycardia [225,226].
3. Adenosine should be used with caution in patients with reactive airway disease, due to its potential bronchoconstrictor effects [214]. Although bronchoconstriction has been reported after inhalation of adenosine [247] but not during continuous intravenous infusion [242], the potential exists for such an effect to occur during rapid IV bolus administration and may underlie the dyspnea experienced in up to 20 percent of patients receiving the drug in this fashion [214].

Digoxin

Digoxin is a cardiac glycoside used in the treatment of congestive heart failure and atrial tachyarrhythmias.

PHARMACOLOGY [1]. Most notably, digoxin exerts a positive inotropic effect, thereby enhancing the force of myocardial contraction. The mechanism has not been fully elucidated, but an alteration in the intracellular concentrations of sodium and potassium in the myocardial cell appears to be the most likely explanation. Also, an increase in intracellular calcium ion appears to be important for the facilitation of increased myocardial work. Direct effects of digoxin include prolongation of the effective refractory period (ERP) in the atria and the A-V node, which diminishes the conduction velocity through those regions. A reduction in the ERP is experienced by the ventricles, with a subsequent increase in automaticity. Indirectly, vagal tone is enhanced, causing a decreased ERP in the atria. On ECG, an increased P–R interval and decreased Q–T interval are observed. Depression of the T wave and S–T segment are occasionally seen.

Table 207-8. Concentration-Effect Relationships for Digoxin [243–246]

Concentration (ng/ml)	Effect
0.8–1.5	Enhanced myocardial contraction
1.0–2.0	Control of atrial arrhythmias
>2.0	Increased risk of cardiac toxicity

THERAPEUTIC RANGE. Table 207-8 summarizes the concentration-effect relationships for digoxin. The generally accepted therapeutic range is 0.8 to 2.0 ng per milliliter. Higher concentrations (1.5–2.0 ng/ml) are often needed for control of ventricular response in atrial arrhythmias than for inotropic support in patients with left ventricular dysfunction (0.8–1.5 ng/ml).

PREPARATIONS

Digoxin tablets (Lanoxin)	0.125-mg, 0.25-mg, 0.5-mg
Digoxin liquid-filled capsules (Lanoxicaps)	0.05-mg, 0.1-mg, 0.2-mg
Digoxin elixir (Lanoxin Pediatric)	0.05 mg/ml
Digoxin injectable	0.1 mg/ml, 0.25 mg/ml

PHARMACOKINETICS. Table 207-2 summarizes the pharmocokinetic properties of digoxin.

Absorption. Digoxin is passively absorbed from the GI tract after an oral dose. The bioavailability of the parenteral form is 20 to 25 percent greater than of oral forms, with the exception of the liquid-filled capsules, which are nearly 100 percent bioavailable. The clinician should be mindful of the differences in the bioavailability of the different formulations when switching patients from one route to another.

Distribution. Over time, digoxin is widely distributed into body tissues, especially the heart, kidneys, liver, and skeletal muscle. Therapeutic effect is usually noted within 6 hours of administration. Digoxin is protein-bound to a modest extent (20–30%), primarily to albumin.

Elimination. The kidneys are responsible for most of the elimination of digoxin from the body. Elimination half-life is approximately 36 hours in patients with normal renal function. The role of the liver in digoxin elimination is unclear, but 20 to 25 percent of the drug may be metabolized, with some biliary excretion of the metabolites.

PHYSIOLOGIC CLEARANCE

Hypodynamic. Since digoxin is primarily renally eliminated, patients with hypodynamic low flow states should be monitored for renal function. Clearance of digoxin is reduced in renal failure, which results in increased serum concentrations. In the presence of decreased renal clearance, extrarenal elimination of digoxin accounts for a larger share of drug clearance. Changes in protein status do not appreciably affect digoxin pharmacokinetics, since it is not extensively protein-bound.

Hyperdynamic. Digoxin is highly tissue-bound, and it is unlikely the pharmacokinetics of the drug would be appreciably altered in hyperdynamic patients. However, if renal blood flow, and thus digoxin clearance, is increased in a hyperdynamic patient, then digoxin clearance would be enhanced.

DOSING GUIDELINES

Loading Dose. Digoxin loading is generally reserved for the treatment of acute atrial arrhythmias associated with a rapid ventricular response rate. If desired, rapid digitalization can be achieved by giving 10 to 15 μg per kilogram IBW of digoxin IV in divided doses. Usually, 50 percent of the total loading dose is administered immediately, followed by 25 percent 6 hours later and 25 percent 6 hours after that. In less acute situations, such as when initiating digoxin for congestive heart failure, the patient can be loaded in the same manner using oral digoxin or simply started on maintenance therapy without a loading dose.

Table 207-9. Important Drug Interactions with Digoxin [7]

Drug	Effect	Mechanism
Amiodarone	Approximate doubling of digoxin level	Multifactorial; reduced V_d and renal and nonrenal clearance; possible displacement of digoxin from tissue binding sites
Bepridil	Serum digoxin concentration may be elevated; additive negative chronotropic effects	Unknown
Cholestyramine	Decreased bioavailability of digoxin	Impaired absorption and Colestipol enterohepatic recycling of digoxin
Cyclosporine	Increased digoxin serum concentrations and severe toxicity, including arrhythmias	Significant decrease in V_d and clearance of digoxin
Oral antibiotics (erythromycin, neomycin, tetracycline)	Increased serum concentrations in approximately 10% of patients	Inhibition of gut flora responsible for digoxin metabolism in certain patients
Metoclopramide	Decreased absorption and bioavailability of digoxin	Increased gut motility
Propafenone	Increased serum digoxin level and possible digoxin toxicity	Possible reduction in V_d and renal and nonrenal clearance of digoxin
Quinidine	Doubling of digoxin serum level	Decreased V_d and clearance of digoxin
Verapamil	50–75% increase in digoxin level	Reduced clearance of digoxin

Maintenance Dose. For maintenance therapy 0.125 to 0.25 mg of digoxin is administered once daily as tablets, capsules, or solution, or an injection is given as a single daily dose. One commonly used method (Jelliffe method) for the individualization of maintenance digoxin dosing incorporates an estimate of the patient's renal function using the formula shown below [247].

$$MD_{iv} = LD \times \frac{(14 + CrCl/5)}{100} \qquad MD_{po} = MD_{iv}/0.72$$

MD_{iv} = maintenance dose of IV digoxin
MD_{po} = maintenance dose of oral digoxin, accounting for oral bioavailability
LD = loading dose
CrCl = creatinine clearance in ml/min as estimated by various formulae [248–252]
$\frac{14 + CrCl/5}{100}$ represents the percent daily loss of digoxin

DRUG INTERACTIONS. Table 207-9 summarizes important drug interactions with digoxin.

COMMON PITFALLS

1. Digoxin serum concentrations should not be obtained within 6 hours after a dose, due to the slow distribution of the drug. Erroneously high serum concentrations may otherwise result. In many ICUs maintenance doses of digoxin are administered between noon and 4 P.M. so that a digoxin serum trough concentration may be drawn with routine laboratory tests the following morning.
2. Consider serum digoxin concentrations in the context of monitoring for *clinical* toxicity.
3. Steady-state serum concentrations are not reached for 5 to 7 days. It is reasonable to obtain a trough concentration before the fourth maintenance dose, at which time the concentration should be approximately 60 percent of the steady-state concentration.
4. The presence of a digoxinlike immunoreactive substance (DLIS) has been detected in patients with renal failure [253,254], hepatorenal failure [255], and during pregnancy [256], none of whom were receiving digoxin. This substance interferes with the assay for digoxin in the serum, and concentrations of digoxin may be falsely increased in these patient groups. Interpretation of such concentrations should be approached with caution.

References

1. Jacob LS: *Pharmacology (National Medical Series for Independent Study)*. New York, Wiley, 1987.
2. Evans WE, Schentag JJ, Jusko WJ: Applied Pharmacokinetics, Spokane Applied Therapeutics, 1992.
3. Olin B: *Drug Facts and Comparisons*. Philadelphia, JB Lippincott, 1993.
4. McEvoy GK: *American Hospital Formulary Service Drug Information*. Bethesda, MD, 1993.
5. Crouthamel WG: The effect of congestive heart failure on quinidine pharmacokinetics. *Am Heart J* 90:335, 1975.
6. Ueda CT, Dzindzio BS: Bioavailability of quinidine in congestive heart failure. *Br J Clin Pharmacol* 11:571, 1981.
7. Tatro D: *Drug Interaction Fact*. St. Louis, Facts & Comparisons, 1992.
8. Koch-Weser J: Clinical application of the pharmacokinetics of procainamide. *Cardiovasc Clin* 6:63, 1974.
9. Koch-Weser J: Serum procainamide levels as therapeutic guides. *Clin Pharmacokinet* 2:389, 1977.
10. Grasela TH, Sheiner LB: Population pharmacokinetics of procainamide from routine clinical data. *Clin Pharmacokinet* 9:545, 1984.
11. Uetrecht JP, Sweetman BJ, Woosley RL, et al: Metabolism of procainamide to a hydroxylamine by rat and human hepatic microsomes. *Drug Metab Dispos Biol Fate Chem* 12:77, 1984.
12. Budinsky RA, Roberts SM, Coats EA, et al: The formation of procainamide hydroxylamine by rat and human liver microsomes. *Drug Metab Dispos Biol Fate Chem* 15:37, 1987.
13. Bauer LA, Black D, Gensler A, et al: Influence of age, renal function, and heart failure on procainamide clearance and n-acetylprocainamide serum concentrations. *Int J Clin Pharmacol Ther Toxicol* 27:213, 1989.
14. Wyman MG, Goldreyer BN, Cannom DS, et al: Factors influencing procainamide total body clearance in the immediate postmyocardial infarction period. *J Clin Pharmacol* 21:20, 1981.
15. Kessler KM, Kayden DS, Estes DM, et al: Procainamide pharmacokinetics in patients with acute myocardial infarction or congestive heart failure. *J Am Coll Cardiol* 7:1131, 1986.
16. Singh S, Gelband H, Mehta AV, et al: Procainamide elimination kinetics in pediatric patients. *Clin Pharmacol Ther* 32:607, 1982.
17. Christian CD, Meredith CG, Speeg KV: Cimetidine inhibits renal procainamide clearance. *Clin Pharmacol Ther* 36:221, 1984.
18. Vlasses PH, Kosoglou T, Chase SL, et al: Trimethoprim inhibition of the renal clearance of procainamide and n-acetylprocainamide. *Arch Intern Med* 149:1350, 1989.
19. Saal A: *Am J Cardiol* 53:1264, 1984.
20. Marchlinski F: *Circulation* 78:583, 1988.
21. Morady F, Scheinman MM, Desai J: Disopyramide. *Ann Intern Med* 96:337, 1982.
22. Pentkainen PJ, Huikuri H, Jounela AJ, et al: Disopyramide pharmacokinetics in patients with acute myocardial infarction. *Eur J Clin Pharmacol* 28:45, 1985.
23. Haughey DB, Kraft CJ, Matzke GR, et al: Protein binding of disopyramide and elevated alpha-1-acid glycoprotein concentrations in serum obtained from dialysis patients and renal transplant recipients. *Am J Nephrol* 5:35, 1985.
24. Deglin SM, et al: Rapid serum lidocaine determination in the coronary care unit. *JAMA* 244:571, 1980.
25. Rosen M, Danilo PJ, Alonso M, et al: Effects of therapeutic concentrations of diphenylhydantoin on transmembrane potentials of normal and depressed Purkinje fibers. *J Pharmacol Exp Ther* 197:594, 1976.
26. Peon J, Ferrier G, Moe G: The relationship of excitability to conduction velocity in canine Purkinje tissue. *Circ Res* 43:125, 1978.
27. Gilman AG, Ral T, Nies A, et al: *The Pharmacological Basis of Therapeutics*. New York, Macmillan, 1990.
28. Colaatsky T: Mechanisms of action of lidocaine and quinidine on action potential duration in rabbit cardiac Purkinje fibers: An effect on steady state sodium currents? *Circ Res* 50:17, 1982.
29. Wittig J, Harrison L, Wallace A: Electrophysiological effects of lidocaine on distal Purkinje fibers of canine heart. *Am Heart J* 86:69, 1973.
30. Gianelly R, et al: Effect of lidocaine on ventricular arrhythmias in patients with coronary heart disease. *N Engl J Med* 277:1215, 1967.
31. Bellet S, et al: Intramuscular lidocaine in the therapy of ventricular arrhythmias. 27:291, 1971.
32. Fehmers M, Dunning A: Intramuscularly and orally administered lidocaine in the treatment of ventricular arrhythmias in acute myocardial infarction. *Am J Cardiol* 29:514, 1972.
33. Schwartz M, et al: Antiarrhythmic effectiveness of intramuscular lidocaine. Influence of different injection sites. *J Clin Pharmacol* 15:77, 1974.
34. Sheridan DJ, et al: Antiarrhythmic action of lidocaine in early myocardial infarction. *Lancet* 1:824, 1977.
35. Lie KI, et al: Lidocaine in the prevention of primary ventricular fibrillation. *N Engl J Med* 291:571, 1974.
36. Foldes FF, et al: Comparison of toxicity of intravenously given local anesthetic agents in man. *JAMA* 172:1493, 1972.
37. Buckman K, et al: Lidocaine efficacy and toxicity assessed by a new rapid method. *Clin Pharmacol Ther* 28:177, 1980.
38. Pfeifer HJ, et al: Clinical use and toxicity of intravenous lidocaine: A report from the Boston Collaborative Drug Surveillance Program. *Am Heart J* 92:168, 1976.
39. Aiderman E, et al: Evaluation of lidocaine resistance in man using

intermittent large-dose infusion techniques. *Am J Cardiol* 34:342, 1974.

40. Wyman MG, et al: Multiple bolus technique for lidocaine in acute ischemic heart disease. II. Treatment of refractory ventricular arrhythmias and the pharmacokinetic significance of severe left ventricular failure. *J Am Coll Cardiol* 2:764, 1983.

41. Strong JM, et al: Pharmacologic activity, metabolism and pharmacokinetics of glycinexylidide. *Clin Pharmacol Ther* 17:184, 1975.

42. Burney R, et al: Antiarrhythmic effects of lidocaine metabolites. *Am Heart J* 88:765, 1974.

43. Halkin H, et al: Influence of congestive heart failure on blood levels of lidocaine and its active monodeethylated metabolite. *Clin Pharmacol Ther* 17:669, 1975.

44. Drayer DE, et al: Plasma levels, protein binding and elimination data of lidocaine and active metabolites in cardiac patients of various ages. *Clin Pharmacol Ther* 34:14, 1983.

45. Wing L, et al: Lidocaine disposition: Sex differences and effects of cimetidine. *Clin Pharmacol Ther* 35:695, 1984.

46. Keenaghan JB, Boyes RN: The tissue distribution, metabolism and excretion of lidocaine in rats, guinea pigs, dogs, and man. *J Pharmacol Exp Ther* 180:454, 1972.

47. Bennett PN, et al: Pharmacokinetics of lidocaine and its deethylated metabolite. dose and time dependency studies in man. *J Pharmacokinet Biopharm* 10:265, 1982.

48. Johnston GD, Finch MB, McNeill JA, et al: A comparison of the cardiovascular effects of (+)-sotalol and (±)-sotalol following intravenous administration in normal volunteers. *Br J Clin Pharmacol* 20:507, 1985.

49. Ryden L, et al: Comparison between effectiveness of intramuscular and intravenous lidocaine on ventricular arrhythmia complicating acute myocardial infarction. *Br Heart J* 35:1124, 1973.

50. Perucca E, Richens E: Reduction of oral bioavailability of lidocaine by induction of first pass metabolism in epileptic patients. *Br J Clin Pharmacol* 8:21, 1979.

51. Cohen LS, et al: Plasma levels of lidocaine after intramuscular administration. *Am J Cardiol* 29:520, 1972.

52. Ryden L, et al: Blood levels of lidocaine after intramuscular administration to patients with proven or suspected acute myocardial infarction. *Br Heart J* 34:1012, 1972.

53. Nattel, et al: Therapeutic blood lidocaine concentrations after local anesthesia for cardiac electrophysiologic studies. *N Engl J Med* 301:418, 1979.

54. Schwartz ML, et al: Blood levels of lidocaine following subcutaneous administration prior to cardiac catheterization. *Am Heart J* 88:721, 1974.

55. Estes NAM, et al: Therapeutic serum lidocaine and metabolite concentrations in patients undergoing electrophysiologic study after discontinuation of intravenous lidocaine infusion. *Am Heart J* 117:1060, 1989.

56. Jones D, et al: Plasma concentrations of lignocaine and its metabolites during fiberoptic bronchoscopy. *Br J Anaesth* 54:853, 1982.

57. Routledge PA, et al: Lidocaine plasma protein binding. *Clin Pharmacol Ther* 27:247, 1980.

58. Lerman J, et al: Effects of age on the serum concentration of alpha-1-acid glycoprotein and the binding of lidocaine in pediatric patients. *Clin Pharmacol Ther* 91:219, 1989.

59. Rowland M, et al: Disposition kinetics of lidocaine in normal subjects. *Ann NY Acad Sci* 179:383, 1971.

60. Abernathy DR, Greenblatt DJ: Impairment of lidocaine clearance in elderly male subjects. *J Cardiovasc Pharmacol* 5:1093, 1983.

61. Abernathy DA, Greenblatt DJ: Lidocaine disposition in obesity. *Am J Cardiol* 53:1183, 1984.

62. Thomson PD, et al: Lidocaine pharmacokinetics in advanced heart failure, liver disease and renal disease in humans. *Ann Intern Med* 78:499, 1973.

63. Wyman M, et al: Multiple bolus technique for lidocaine administration during the first hours of a myocardial infarction. *Am J Cardiol* 41:313, 1978.

64. Williams RL, et al: Influence of aviral hepatitis on the disposition of two compounds with high hepatic clearance: Lidocaine and indocyanine green. *Clin Pharmacol Ther* 20:290, 1976.

65. Beckett AH, et al: The metabolism and excretion of lidocaine in man. *J Pharm Pharmacol* 18:765, 1966.

66. Nation RL, et al: Lidocaine kinetics in cardiac patients and aged subjects. *Br J Clin Pharmacol* 4:439, 1977.

67. Zito RA, Reid PA: Lidocaine pharmacokinetics predicted by indocyanine green clearance. *N Engl J Med* 298:1160, 1978.

68. Sawyer DR, et al: Continuous infusion of lidocaine in patients with cardiac arrhythmias: Unpredictability of plasma concentrations. *Arch Intern Med* 141:43, 1981.

69. Huet M, et al: Bioavailability of lidocaine in normal volunteers and cirrhotic patients. *Clin Pharmacol Ther* 25:230, 1979.

70. Lelorier J, et al: Pharmacokinetics of lidocaine after prolonged intravenous infusions in uncomplicated myocardial infarction. *Ann Intern Med* 87:700, 1977.

71. Prescott LF, et al: Impaired lidocaine metabolism in patients with myocardial infarction. *Br Med J* 1:939, 1976.

72. Bax NDS, et al: Lidocaine and indocyanine green kinetics in patients following myocardial infarction. *Br J Clin Pharmacol* 10:353, 1980.

73. Forrest JA, et al: Antipyrine, paracetamol and lidocaine elimination in chronic liver disease. *Br Med J* 1:1384, 1977.

74. Feely J, et al: Effect of hypotension on liver blood flow and lidocaine disposition. *N Engl J Med* 307:866, 1982.

75. Johansson BG, et al: Sequential changes of plasma proteins after myocardial infarction. *Scand J Clin Lab Invest* 29:117, 1972.

76. Routledge PA, et al: Relationship between alpha-1-acid glycoprotein and lidocaine disposition in myocardial infarction. *Clin Pharmacol Ther* 30:154, 1981.

77. Lalka D, et al: Lidocaine pharmacokinetics and metabolism in acute myocardial infarction patients. *Clin Res* 28:329A, 1980.

78. Collinsworth KA, et al: Pharmacokinetics and metabolism of lidocaine in patients with renal failure. *Clin Pharmacol Ther* 18:59, 1975.

79. Rodman JH, et al: Clinical studies with computer assisted initial lidocaine therapy. *Arch Intern Med* 144:703, 1984.

80. Aps C, et al: Logical approach to lidocaine therapy. *Br Med J* 1:13, 1975.

81. Ridell JG, et al: A new method for constant plasma drug concentrations: Applications to lidocaine. *Ann Intern Med* 100:25, 1984.

82. Salzer LB, et al: A comparison of methods of lidocaine administration in patients. *Clin Pharmacol Ther* 29:617, 1981.

83. Sebaldt RJ, et al: Lidocaine therapy with an exponentially declining infusion. *Ann Intern Med* 101:632, 1984.

84. Conrad KA, et al: Lidocaine elimination: Effects of metoprolol and of propranolol. *Clin Pharmacol Ther* 33:133, 1983.

85. Ochs HR, et al: Reduction in lidocaine clearance during continuous infusion and by co-administration of propranolol. *N Engl J Med* 303:373, 1980.

86. Thomson AH, et al: Changes in lidocaine disposition during long-term infusion in patients with acute ventricular arrhythmias. *Ther Drug Monit* 9:283, 1987.

87. Knapp A, Maguire W, Keren G, et al: The cimetidine-lidocaine interaction. *Ann Intern Med* 98:174, 1983.

88. McNamara PJ, et al: Factors influencing the serum free fraction of lidocaine in man. *Clin Pharmacol Ther* 27:271, 1980.

89. Campbell RWF: Mexiletine. *N Engl J Med* 316:29, 1987.

90. Stein J, Podrid P, Lown B: Effects of oral mexiletine on left and right ventricular function. *Am J Cardiol* 54:575, 1984.

91. Woosley R, Wang T, Stone W, et al: Pharmacology, electrophysiology, and pharmacokinetics of mexiletine. *Am Heart J* 107:1058, 1984.

92. Pentikainen P, Halinen M, Helin M: Pharmacokinetics of oral mexiletine in patients with acute myocardial infarction. *Eur J Clin Pharmacol* 25:773, 1983.

93. Pottage A, Campbell R, Achuff S, et al: The absorption of oral mexiletine in coronary care patients. *Eur J Clin Pharmacol* 13:393, 1978.

94. Vozeh S, Katz G, Steiner V, et al: Population pharmacokinetic parameters in patients treated with oral mexiletine. *Eur J Clin Pharmacol* 23:445, 1982.

95. Beckett A, Chidomere E: The distribution, metabolism and excretion of mexiletine in man. *Postgrad Med* 53(suppl 1):60, 1977.

96. Brown J, Shand D. Therapeutic drug monitoring of antiarrhythmic agents. *Clin Pharmacokinet* 7:125, 1982.

97. Upward J, Holt D, Jackson G: A study to compare the efficacy,

plasma concentration profile and tolerability of conventional mexiletine and slow-release mexiletine. *Eur Heart J* 5:247, 1984.

98. El Allaf D, Henrard L, Crochelet L, et al: Pharmacokinetics of mexiletine in renal insufficiency. *Br J Clin Pharmacol* 14:431, 1982.

99. Wang T, Wuellner D, Woosley R, et al: Pharmacokinetics of mexiletine in renal failure. *Clin Pharmacol Ther* 37:649, 1985.

100. Grech-Belanger O, Gilbert M, Turgeon J, et al: Effect of cigarette smoking on mexiletine kinetics. *Clin Pharmacol Ther* 37:638, 1985.

101. Nitsch J, Steinbeck G, Luderitz B: Increase of mexiletine plasma levels due to delayed hepatic metabolism in patients with chronic liver disease. *Eur Heart J* 4:810, 1983.

102. Bigger JT, Hoffman BF: *Antiarrhythmic Drugs.* Elmsford, NY, Pergamon, 1990.

103. Clyne CA, Estes NAM, Wang PJ: Moricizine. *N Engl J Med* 327:255, 1992.

104. Salerno DM, Ettinger A, Hodges M: The electrocardiographic effects of encainide, flecainide, and moricizine in a subgroup of the Cardiac Arrhythmic Suppression Trial. *J Am Coll Cardiol* 17 (suppl 56A), 1991.

105. Smetnev AS, Shugushev KK, Rosenshtraukh LV: Clinical, electrophysiologic and antiarrhythmic efficacy of moricizine HCl. *Am J Cardiol* 60:40F, 1987.

106. Woosley RL, Morganroth J, Fogoros RN, et al: Pharmacokinetics of moricizine HCl. *Am J Cardiol* 60:35F, 1987.

107. Mann HJ: Moricizine: A new class I antiarrhythmic. *Clin Pharmacol* 9:842, 1990.

108. Howrie DL, Pieniazek HJ, Forgoros RN, et al: Disposition of moracizine (ethmozine) in healthy subjects after oral administration of rediolabeled drug. *Eur J Clin Pharmacol* 32:607, 1987.

109. Biollaz J, Shaheen O, Wood AJJ: Cimetidine inhibition of ethmozine metabolism. *Clin Pharmacol Ther* 37:665, 1983.

110. Shand DG: Alpha-1-acid glycoprotein and plasma lidocaine binding. *Clin Pharmacokinet* 9 (suppl): 27, 1984.

111. Pieniaszek HJ, McEntegart, Mayersohn M, et al: Moricizine pharmacokinetics in renal insufficiency: Reevaluation of elimination half-life. *J Clin Pharmacol* 32:412, 1992.

112. Morganroth J: Dose effect of moricizine on suppression of ventricular arrhythmias. *Am J Cardiol* 65:26D, 1990.

113. Podrid PJ, Lyakishev A, Lown B, et al: Ethmozin, a new arrhythmic drug for suppressing ventricular premature complexes. *Circulation* 61:450, 1980.

114. Morganroth J, Pratt CM, Kennedy HL, et al: Efficacy and tolerance of ethmozine (moricizine HCl) in placebo-controlled trials. *Am J Cardiol* 50:48F, 1987.

115. Siddoway LA, Schwartz SL, Barbey JT, et al: Clinical pharmacokinetics of moricizine. *Am J Cardiol* 65:21D, 1990.

116. CAPS: The cardiac arrhythmia pilot study. *Am J Cardiol* 57:91, 1986.

117. Podrid PJ, Beau SL: Antiarrhythmic drug therapy for congestive heart failure with focus on moricizine. *Am J Cardiol* 65:56D, 1990.

118. Greene HL, Richardson DW, Hallstrom AP, et al: Congestive heart failure after acute myocardial infarction in patients receiving antiarrhythmic agents for ventricular premature complexes (Cardiac Arrhythmic Pilot Study). *Am J Cardiol* 63:393, 1989.

119. Roden DM, Woosley RL: Drug therapy: Flecainide. *N Engl J Med* 315:36, 1986.

120. Forland SC, Cutler RE, McQuinn RL, et al: Flecainide pharmocokinetics after multiple dosing in patients with impaired renal function. *J Clin Pharmacol* 28:727, 1988.

121. Braun J, Kollert JR, Becker JU: Pharmacokinetics of flecainide in patients with mild and moderate renal failure compared with patients with normal renal function. *J Clin Pharmacol* 31:711, 1987.

122. Williams AJ, McQuinn RL, Walls J: Pharmacokinetics of flecainide acetate in patients with severe renal impairment. *Clin Pharmacol Ther* 43:449, 1988.

123. Boriani G, Strocchi E, Capucci A, et al: Flecainide: Evidence of non-linear kinetics. *Eur J Clin Pharmacol* 41:57, 1991.

124. McQuinn RL, Pentkainen PJ, Chang SF, et al: Pharmacokinetics of flecainide in patients with cirrhosis of the liver. *Clin Pharmacol Ther* 44:566, 1988.

125. Cavalli A, Maggioni AP, Marchi S, et al: Flecainide half-life prolon-

gation in 2 patients with congestive heart failure and complex ventricular arrhythmias. *Clin Pharmacokinet* 14:187, 1988.

126. Perry JC, McQuinn RL, Smith RT, et al: Flecainide acetate for resistant arrhythmias in the young: Efficacy and pharmacokinetics. *J Am Coll Cardiol* 14:185, 1989.

127. Frabetti L, Marchesini B, Capucci A, et al: Antiarrhythmic efficacy of propafenone: Evaluation of effective plasma levels following single and multiple doses. *Eur J Clin Pharmacol* 30:665, 1986.

128. Axelson J: *Br J Clin Pharmacol* 23:735, 1987.

129. Seipel L, Breithardt G: Propafenone: A new antiarrhythymic drug. *Eur Heart J* 1:309, 1980.

130. Siddoway LA, Thompson KA, McAllister CB, et al: Polymorphism of propafenone metabolism and disposition in man: Clinical and pharmacokinetic consequences. *Circulation* 75:785, 1987.

131. Hii JTY, Duff HJ, Burgess ED: Clinical pharmacokinetics of propafenone. *Clin Pharmacokinet* 21:1, 1991.

132. Lee JT, Yee YG, Dorian P, et al: Influence of hepatic dysfunction on the pharmacokinetics of propafenone. *J Clin Pharmacol* 27:384, 1987.

133. Burgess E, Duff H, Wilkes P: Propafenone disposition in renal insufficiency and renal failure. *J Clin Pharmacol* 29:112, 1989.

134. Funck-Brentano C: *Br J Clin Pharmacol* 27:435, 1989.

135. Zipes DP, Prystowsky EN, Heger JJ: Amiodarone: Electrophysiologic actions, pharmacokinetics and clinical effects. *J Am Coll Cardiol* 3:1059, 1984.

136. Holt DW, Tucker GT, Jackson PR, et al: Amiodarone pharmacokinetics. *Am Heart J* 106:840, 1983.

137. Barbieri E, Conti F, Zampieri P, et al: Amiodarone and desethylamiodarone distribution in the atrium and adipose tissue of patients undergoing short- and long-term treatment with amiodarone. *J Am Coll Cardiol* 8:210, 1986.

138. Anderson JL, Patterson E, Wagner JG, et al: Oral and intravenous bretylium disposition. *Clin Pharmacol Ther* 28:468, 1980.

139. Josselson J, Narang PK, Adir J, et al: Bretylium kinetics in renal insufficiency. *Clin Pharmacol Ther* 33:144, 1983.

140. Lish PM, Weikel JH, Dungan KW: Pharmacological and toxicological properties of two new beta-adrenergic receptor antagonists. *J Pharmacol Exp Ther* 149:161, 1965.

141. Singh BN, Vaughan-Williams EM: A third class of anti-arrhythmic action: Effects on atrial and ventricular intracellular potentials, and other pharmacologic actions on cardiac muscle of MJ 1999 and AH 3474. *Br J Pharmacol* 39:675, 1970.

142. Nadamanee K, Feld G, Hendrickson J, et al: Electrophysiologic and antiarrhythmic effects of sotalol in patients with life-threatening ventricular tachyarrhythmias. *Circulation* 72:555, 1985.

143. Senges J, Lengfelder W, Jauernig R, et al: Electrophysiologic testing of therapy with sotalol for sustained ventricular tachycardia. *Circulation* 69:577, 1984.

144. Singh BN, Deedwania P, Nadamanee K, et al: Sotalol: A review of its pharmacodynamic and pharmacokinetic properties, and therapeutic use. *Drugs* 34:311, 1987.

145. Strauss HC, Bigger JT, Hoffman BF: Electrophysiological and beta-receptor blocking effects of MJ 1999 on dog and rabbit cardiac tissue. *Circ Res* 26:661, 1970.

146. Goldstein RE, Hall CA, Epstein SE: Comparison of relative inotropic and chronotropic effects of propranolol, practolol and sotalol. *Chest* 64:619, 1973.

147. Aberg G, Dzedin T, Lundholm L, et al: A comparative study of some cardiovascular effects of sotalol (MJ 1999) and propranolol. *Life Sci* 8:353, 1969.

148. Lewis MJ, Grey AC, Henderson AH: Inotropic beta-blocking potency (pA2) and partial against activity of propranolol, practolol, sotalol and acebutolol. *Eur J Pharmacol* 86:71, 1983.

149. Johansson SR, McCall M, Wilhelmsson C, et al: Duration of action of beta-blockers. *Clin Pharmacol Ther* 27:593, 1980.

150. Nakaya H, Kimura S, Nakao Y, et al: Effects of nipradilol (K-351) on the electrophysiologic properties of canine cardiac tissues: Comparison with propranolol and sotalol. *Eur J Pharmacol* 104:335, 1984.

151. Kato R, Ikeda N, Yabek S, et al: Electrophysiologic and antiarrhythmic effects of sotalol in patients with life-threatening ventricular tachyarrhythmias. *Circulation* 72:555, 1986.

152. Somani P, Watson DL: Antiarrhythmic activity of the dextro- and

levo-rotatory isomers of 4-(2-isopropylamino-1-hydroxyethyl) methanesulfonanalide (MJ1999). *J Pharmacol Exp Ther* 164:317, 1968.

153. Funck-Bretano C: A mechanism of D-(+) sotalol effects on heart rate not related to beta-adrenoreceptor antagonism. *Br J Clin Pharmacol* 30:195, 1990.

154. Yasuda SU, Barbey JT, Funck-Brentano C, et al: d-Sotalol reduces heart rate in vivo through a beta-adrenergic receptor-independent mechanism. *Clin Pharmacol Ther* 53:436, 1993.

155. Kuntz RE, Ruskin JN, Weinberger S, et al: The advantage of D-sotalol over Dl-sotalol in a patient with ventricular arrhythmias and comorbid bronchospasm. *Chest* 102:1627, 1992.

156. Carmeliet E: Electrophysiologic and voltage clamp analysis of sotalol effects in cardiac muscle and Purkinje fibers. *J Pharmacol Exp Ther* 232:817, 1985.

157. Prakash R, Parmley WW, Allen HN, et al: Effects of sotalol on clinical arrhythmias. *Am J Cardiol* 29:397, 1972.

158. Edvardsson N, Hirsch I, Emanuelsson H, et al: Sotalol-induced delayed ventricular repolarization in man. *Eur Heart J* 1:335, 1980.

159. Edvardsson N, Olsson SB: Effects of acute and chronic beta-receptor blockade on ventricular repolarization in man. *Br Heart J* 45:628, 1981.

160. Echt DS, Bert LE, Clusin WT, et al: Prolongation of the human cardiac monophasic action potential by sotalol. *Am J Cardiol* 50:1082, 1982.

161. Ward DE, Camm AJ, Spurrel RAJ: The acute cardiac electrophysiological effects of intravenous sotalol hydrochloride. *Clin Cardiol* 2:185, 1979.

162. Nathan AW, Hellestrand KJ, Bextan RS, et al: Electrophysiological effects of sotalol: Just another beta-blocker? *Br Heart J* 47:515, 1982.

163. Toubol P, Atullah G, Kirkonian G, et al: Clinical electrophysiology of intravenous sotalol, a beta-blocking drug with class III antiarrhythmic properties. *Am Heart J* 107:888, 1984.

164. Shimatori M, Kobayashi M, Chiba S: Comparative study of five beta-adrenoreceptor blocking agents in sino-atrial conduction time in isolated blood-perfused canine atria. *Arch Int Pharmacodyn Ther* 274:240, 1985.

165. LeCoz F, Funck-Brentano C, Poirier JM, et al: Prediction of sotalol-induced maximum steady-state QTc prolongation from single-dose administration in healthy volunteers. *Clin Pharmacol Ther* 52:417, 1992.

166. Lynch JJ, Coskey LA, Montgomery DG, et al: Prevention of ventricular fibrillation by dextrorotatory sotalol in a conscious canine model of sudden coronary death. *Am Heart J* 109:949, 1985.

167. Hoffmann RP, Grupp G: The effects of sotalol and propranolol on contractile force and atrioventricular conduction time of the dog heart in situ. *Chest* 55:229, 1969.

168. Brooks H, Banas J, Meister S, et al: Sotalol-induced beta-blockade in cardiac patients. *Circulation* 42:99, 1970.

169. Thumala A, Hammermeister KE, Campbell WB, et al: Hemodynamic studies with sotalol in man, performed at rest, during exercise, and during right ventricular pacing. *Am Heart J* 82:439, 1971.

170. Hutton I, Lorimer AR, Hillis WS, et al: Haemodynamics and myocardial infarction after sotalol. *Br Heart J* 34:787, 1972.

171. Taylor SH: General review of the hemodynamic effects of beta-adrenoreceptor blocking drugs. *Curr Ther Res* 28:83S, 1980.

172. Kaumann AJ, Olson CB: Temporal relationship between long-lasting aftercontractions and action potentials in cat papillary muscles. *Science* 163:293, 1968.

173. Gomoll AW, Braunwald E: Comparative effects of sotalol and propranolol on myocardial contractility. *Arch Int Pharmacodyn Ther* 205:338, 1973.

174. Singh BN, Nademanee K: Control of cardiac arrhythmias by selected lengthening of repolarization: Theoretic considerations and clinical observations. *Am Heart J* 109:421, 1985.

175. Soyka LF, Wirz C, Spangenburg RB: Clinical safety profile of sotalol in patients with arrhythmias. *Am J Cardiol* 65:74A, 1990.

176. Sallustio BC, Morris RG: High-performance liquid chromatographic determination of sotalol in plasma. I. Application to the disposition of sotalol enantiomers in humans. *J Chromatogr* 576:321, 1992.

177. Follath F: The utility of serum drug level monitoring during therapy with class III antiarrhythmic agents. *J Cardiovasc Pharmacol* 20 (suppl 2): S41, 1992.

178. Harron DWG, Balnave K, Kinney CD, et al: Effects of exercise tachycardia during forty-eight hours of a series of doses of atenolol, sotalol, and metoprolol. *Clin Pharmacol Ther* 29:295, 1981.

179. Funck-Bretano C, Kibleur Y, LeCoz F, et al: Rate dependence of sotalol-induced prolongation of ventricular repolarization during exercise in humans. *Circulation* 83:536, 1991.

180. Neuvonen PJ, Elonen E, Tanskanen A, et al: Sotalol and prolonged QTc interval. *Lancet* 2:426, 1981.

181. Wang T, Bergstrand RH, Thompson KA, et al: Concentration-dependent pharmacologic properties of sotalol. *Am J Cardiol* 57:1160, 1986.

182. Ritschel WA: Compilation of pharmacokinetic parameters of beta-adrenergic blocking agents. *Drug Intell Clin Pharm* 14:746, 1980.

183. Poirier JM, Jaillon P, Lecocq B, et al: The pharmocokinetics of d-sotalol and d,1 sotalol in healthy volunteers. *Eur J Clin Pharmacol* 38:579, 1990.

184. Carr RA, Foster RT, Lewanczuk RZ, et al: Pharmacokinetics of sotalol enantiomers in humans. *J Clin Pharmacol* 32:1105, 1992.

185. McDevitt DG, Shanks RG: Evaluation of once daily sotalol administration in man. *Br J Clin Pharmacol* 4:153, 1977.

186. Ishizaki T, Hirayama H, Tawara K, et al: Pharmacokinetics and pharmacodynamics in young normal and elderly hypertensive subjects: A study using sotalol as a model drug. *J Pharmacol Exp Ther* 212:173, 1980.

187. O'Hare MF, Leahey W, Murnaghan GA, et al: Pharmacokinetics of sotalol during pregnancy. *Eur J Clin Pharmacol* 24:521, 1983.

188. McKibbin JK, Pocock WA, Barlow JB, et al: Sotalol, hypokalemia, syncope, and torsade de pointes. *Br Heart J* 51:157, 1984.

189. Krapf R, Gertsch M: Torsade de pointes induced by sotalol despite therapeutic plasma sotalol concentrations. *Br Med J* 290:1784, 1985.

199. Abernethy D, Schwartz J, Todd E, et al: Verapamil pharmacodynamics and disposition in young and elderly hypertensive patients. *Ann Intern Med* 105:329, 1986.

200. Schwartz J, Keefe D, Kirsten E, et al: Prolongation of verapamil elimination kinetics during chronic oral administration. *Am Heart J* 104:198, 1982.

201. Iberti T, Benjamin E, Paluch T, et al: Use of constant-infusion verapamil for the treatment of postoperative supraventricular tachycardia. *Crit Care Med* 14:283, 1986.

202. Barbarash R, Bauman J, Lukazewski A, et al: Verapamil infusions in the treatment of atrial tachy-arrhythmias. *Crit Care Med* 14:886, 1986.

203. Barnett J, Touchon R: Short-term control of supraventricular tachycardia with verapamil infusion and calcium pretreatment. *Chest* 97:1106, 1990.

204. Edwards D, Lavoie R, Beckman H, et al: The effect of coadministration of verapamil on the pharmacokinetics and metabolism of quinidine. *Clin Pharmacol Ther* 41:68, 1987.

205. Epstein S, Rosing D: Verapamil: Its potential for causing serious complications in patients with hypertrophic cardiomyopathy. *Circulation* 64:437, 1981.

206. Klein H, Lang R, Weiss E, et al: The influence of verapamil on serum digoxin concentration. *Circulation* 65:998, 1982.

207. Barbarash R, Bauman J, Fischer J, et al: Near-total reduction in verapamil bioavailability by rifampin: Electrocardiographic correlates. *Chest* 94:954, 1988.

208. Macphee G, McInnes G, Thompson G, et al: Verapamil potentiates carbamazepine neurotoxicity: A clinically important inhibitory interaction. *Lancet* 1:700, 1986.

209. Salerno D, Anderson B, Sharkey P, et al: Intravenous verapamil for treatment of multifocal atrial tachycardia with and without calcium pretreatment. *Ann Intern Med* 107:623, 1987.

210. Dias V, Weir S, Ellenbogen K: Pharmacokinetics and pharmacodynamics of intravenous diltiazem in patients with atrial fibrillation or atrial flutter. *Circulation* 86:1421, 1992.

211. Winship L, McKenney J, Wright J, et al: The effect of ranitidine and cimetidine on single-dose diltiazem pharmacokinetics. *Pharmacotherapy* 5:16, 1985.

212. Piepho R, Culbertson V, Rhodes R: Drug interactions with calcium-entry blockers. *Circulation* 75(suppl V):181, 1987.

213. Rankin A, Brooks R, Ruskin J, et al: Adenosine and the treatment of supraventricular tachycardia. *Am J Med* 92:655, 1992.

214. DiMarco J, Sellers T, Lerman B, et al: Diagnostic and therapeutic use of adenosine in patients with supraventricular arrhythmias. *J Am Coll Cardiol* 6:417, 1985.
215. Griffith M, Linker N, Ward D, et al: Adenosine in the diagnosis of broad complex tachycardias. *Lancet* 1:672, 1988.
216. Clarke B, Till J, Rowland E, et al: Rapid and safe termination of supraventricular tachycardia in children by adenosine. *Lancet* 1:299, 1987.
217. Overholt E, Rheuban K, Gutgesell H, et al: Usefulness of adenosine for arrhythmias in infants and children. *Am J Cardiol* 61:336, 1988.
218. Berne R, DiMarco J, Belardinelli L: Dromotropic effects of adenosine and adenosine triphosphate in the treatment of cardiac arrhythmias involving the atrioventricular node. *Circulation* 69:1195, 1984.
219. Sparks H, Bardenheuer H: Regulation of adenosine formation by the heart. *Circ Res* 58:193, 1987.
220. Camm A, Garrat C: Adenosine and supraventricular tachycardia. *N Engl J Med* 325:1621, 1991.
221. Mosqueda-Garcia R: Adenosine as a therapeutic agent. *Clin Invest Med* 15:445, 1992.
222. West G, Belardinelli L: Correlation of sinus slowing and hyperpolarization caused by adenosine in sinus node. *Pflugers Arch* 403:75, 1985.
223. Belardinelli L, Giles W, West A: Ionic mechanisms of adenosine actions in pacemaker cells from rabbit heart. *J Physiol* (Lond) 405:615, 1988.
224. Drury A, Szent-Gyorgi A: The physiological activity of adenine compounds with special reference to their action upon mammalian heart. *J Physiol* 68:214, 1929.
225. Pelleg A, Porter S: The pharmacology of adenosine. *Pharmacotherapy* 10:157, 1990.
226. DiMarco J, Sellers T, Berne R, et al: Adenosine: Electrophysiologic effects and therapeutic use for terminating paroxysmal supraventricular tachycardia. *Circulation* 68:1254, 1983.
227. Watt A, Routledge P: Transient bradycardia and subsequent sinus tachycardia produced by intravenous adenosine in healthy adult subjects. *Br J Clin Pharmacol* 21:533, 1986.
228. Biaggioni I, Killian T, Mosqueda-Garcia R, et al: Adenosine increases sympathetic nerve traffic in humans. *Circulation* 83:1668, 1991.
229. Moser G, Schrader J, Deussen A: Turnover of adenosine in plasma of human and dog blood. *Am J Physiol* 256:C799, 1989.
230. Ontyd J, Schrader J: Measurement of adenosine, inosine and hypoxanthine in human plasma. *J Chromatogr* 307:404, 1984.
231. Ohisalo J: Regulatory functions of adenosine. *Med Biol* 65:181, 1987.
232. Belhassen B, Pelleg A: Adenosine triphosphate and adenosine: Perspectives in the acute management of paroxysmal supraventricular tachycardia. *Clin Cardiol* 8:460, 1985.
233. Abreu A, Mahmarian J, Nishimura S, et al: Tolerance and safety of pharmacologic coronary vasodilation with adenosine in association with thallium-201 scintigraphy in patients with suspected coronary artery disease. *J Am Coll Cardiol* 18:730, 1991.
234. Sollevi A, Lagerkranser M, Irestedt L, et al: Controlled hypotension with adenosine in cerebral aneurysm surgery. *Anesthesiology* 61:400, 1984.
235. Biaggioni I, Olafsson B, Robertson R, et al: Cardiovascular and respiratory effects of adenosine in conscious man: Evidence for chemoreceptor activation. *Circ Res* 61:779, 1987.
236. Conradson T, Dixon C, Clark B, et al: Cardiovascular effects of infused adenosine in man: Potentiation by dipyridamole. *Acta Physiol Scand* 129:387, 1987.
237. Klabunde R: Dipyridamole inhibition of adenosine metabolism in human blood. *Eur J Pharmacol* 93:21, 1983.
238. Watt A, Bernard M, Webster J: Intravenous adenosine in the treatment of supraventricular tachycardia: A dose-ranging study and interaction with dipyridamole. *Br J Clin Pharmacol* 21:227, 1986.
239. Lerman B, Belardinelli L: Cardiac electrophysiology of adenosine: Basic and clinical concepts. *Circulation* 83:1499, 1991.
240. Wesley R, Belardinelli L: Role of adenosine on ventricular overdrive suppression in isolated guinea pig hearts and Purkinje fibers. *Circ Res* 57:517, 1985.
241. Cushley M, Tattersfield A, Holgate S: Inhaled adenosine and guanosine on airway resistance in normal and asthmatic subjects. *Br J Clin Pharmacol* 15:161, 1985.
242. Larsson K, Sollevi A: Influence of infused adenosine on bronchial tone and bronchial reactivity in asthma. *Chest* 93:280, 1988.
243. Goldman S, Probst P, Selzer A, et al: Inefficacy of "therapeutic" serum levels of digoxin in controlling the ventricular rate in atrial fibrillation. *Am J Cardiol* 35:651, 1975.
244. Hoeschen RJ, Cuddy TE: Dose-response relation between therapeutic levels of serum digoxin and systolic time intervals. *Am J Cardiol* 35:469, 1975.
245. Redfors A: Plasma digoxin concentration: Its relation to digoxin dosage and clinical effects in patients with atrial fibrillation. *Br Heart J* 34:383, 1971.
246. Beller GA, Smith TW, Abelmann WH, et al: Digitalis intoxication: A prospective clinical study with serum level correlations. *N Engl J Med* 284:989, 1971.
247. Jelliffe RW: Factors to consider in planning digoxin therapy. *J Chron Dis* 24:407, 1971.
248. Cockcroft DW, Gault MH: Prediction of creatinine clearance from serum creatinine. *Nephron* 16:31, 1976.
249. Jelliffe RW: Creatinine clearance: Bedside estimate. *Ann Intern Med* 79:604, 1973.
250. Hallynck T, Soep HH, Thomis J, et al: Prediction of creatinine clearance from serum creatinine concentration based on lean body mass. *Clin Pharmacol Ther* 30:414, 1981.
251. Kampmann J, Siersbek-Nielsen K, Kristensen M, et al: Rapid evaluation of creatinine clearance. *Acta Med Scand* 196:517, 1974.
252. Siersbaek-Nielsen K, Hansen JM, Kampmann J, et al: Rapid evaluation of creatinine clearance. *Lancet* 1:1133, 1971.
253. Craver JL, Valdes R: Anomalous serum digoxin concentrations in uremia. *Ann Intern Med* 98:483, 1983.
254. Heazlewood VJ, Heazlewood RL, Jellett LB: An endogenous digoxin-like substance and renal failure. *Ann Intern Med* 100:618, 1984.
255. Gault MH, Vasdev SC, Longerich LL: Endogenous digoxin-like substance(s) and combined hepatic and renal failure. *Ann Intern Med* 101:567, 1984.
256. Barbarash RA: Serum digoxin measurements during pregnancy. *Eur J Clin Pharmacol* 27:125, 1984.

208. Neuromuscular Blocking Agents

Tanyia L. Abel and Philip R. Kohls

Neuromuscular blocking agents (NMBAs) are used in the intensive care unit (ICU) to immobilize patients for selected procedures, such as intubation for airway control, to decrease oxygen consumption requirements, and to improve patient compliance with mechanical ventilator therapies refractory to sedative-hypnotics. They are classified as either nondepolarizing (competitive) or depolarizing agents and are subdivided by duration of action. Extensive research for use in intensive care patients does not exist, therefore methods of administration and drug selection vary between clinicians, based on clinical experience. This chapter focuses on the pharmacodynamics and pharmacokinetics of nondepolarizing neuromuscular blocking agents and their use in mechanically ventilated critically ill patients.

Pharmacology

NEUROMUSCULAR TRANSMISSION. At the neuromuscular junction the neurotransmitter, acetylcholine, is released from vesicles in the end terminal into the synaptic cleft. Released acetylcholine binds with postsynaptic receptors in the motor end plate, causing ion channels to open, thus permitting a sudden influx of sodium. Exchange of sodium and potassium ions results in depolarization of the nerve and triggers a local action potential stimulating skeletal muscle fibers to contract. Within milliseconds of its liberation into the synaptic cleft, remaining acetylcholine is hydrolyzed by acetylcholinesterase to inactive choline and acetic acid. The cell membrane then pumps sodium from the cell and replaces it with potassium, regaining impermeability to sodium, resulting in repolarization of the motor end plate and muscle fiber. Plasma cholinesterases are synthesized in the liver and have a half-life of 3 to 5 minutes. Acetylcholine's action on the motor end plate may be prolonged in situations where concentrations of the enzymes are reduced, such as liver disease, pregnancy, and renal dialysis. Pharmacologic interference with the physiology of the neuromuscular transmission will interrupt nerve impulses arriving at the end plate [1,2].

Neuromuscular blockade can occur via different mechanisms: interference with the synthesis and/or transmission of acetylcholine (calcium deficiency, magnesium excess, aminoglycosides, local anesthetics), competitive blockade (pancuronium, vecuronium, atracurium, etc.), depolarizing blockade (succinylcholine), or desensitization blockade, in which the motor end plate is insensitive to drugs or acetylcholine (repeated doses of succinylcholine) [1,2].

DEPOLARIZING NEUROMUSCULAR BLOCKING AGENTS. The depolarizing NMBA in widespread use today is succinylcholine. Primarily used in surgery to facilitate general anesthesia and intubation, this drug has limited use in ICUs due to its potentially adverse effects. Succinylcholine is less suitable for prolonged use because an unpredictable duration of neuromuscular blockade (phase II block) may develop.

Initially, succinylcholine mimics the effects of acetylcholine on the postsynaptic acetylcholine receptor. However, while acetylcholine is unbound and hydrolyzed within a few milli-seconds by plasma cholinesterases, succinylcholine's effect is terminated when it diffuses away from the neuromuscular junction motor end plate. This mechanism causes a more sustained depolarization of the muscle fiber. Therefore, succinylcholine stimulates with a brief period of excitation and transient fasciculation and then causes a blockade of neuromuscular transmission and flaccid paralysis. Succinylcholine offers the most rapid onset of action (60–90 seconds) of the neuromuscular blockers and is rapidly hydrolyzed by plasma cholinesterases. The half-life is 2 minutes, with a duration of action of 6 to 10 minutes.

COMPETITIVE NEUROMUSCULAR BLOCKING AGENTS. Competitive (nondepolarizing) NMBAs compete with acetylcholine at its receptor sites on the motor end plate to prevent depolarization and contraction of skeletal muscle fibers (Table 208-1). They also block presynaptic receptors, thereby possibly preventing positive feedback on presynaptic receptors by decreasing the production of acetylcholine, which is evident by tetanic fade and train-of-four fade responses to nerve stimulation [3,4]. Because only a single molecule of the antagonist is required to prevent acetylcholine binding and two acetylcholine molecules are required to produce a muscle contraction, the competitive inhibition is biased in favor of the antagonist [5].

Therapeutic Range/Monitoring

Clinical monitoring of a patient's neuromuscular function is used as the pharmacodynamic endpoint for neuromuscular blocker titration. Data for dose-effect responses are primarily from studies of patients undergoing general anesthesia, using American Society of Anesthesia (ASA) scores I to III. Neuromuscular blockade after surgery can be evaluated clinically on the basis of hand grip strength, vital capacity, positive inspiratory pressure, head lift, or spontaneous movement. The use of peripheral nerve stimulators has become standard in anesthesia, where they are used to observe skeletal muscle responses after stimulation to prevent overdosage. Their use in ICUs to monitor patients receiving neuromuscular blockers is increasing. However, in critically ill patients neuromuscular blockade serves different needs, and clinical assessment as well as nerve stimulation is needed to evaluate completely the depth of blockade. To avoid prolonged neuromuscular blockade, many clinicians recommend the combination of clinical monitoring and peripheral nerve stimulators [6,7,8].

The different methods of nerve stimulation used to study the effects of NMBAs include single twitch, tetanic stimulus, post-tetanic stimulation, double-burst stimulation, and train-of-four (TOF) stimulation [9]. Most studies comparing methods of stimulation have observed sensitivities in detecting residual neuromuscular block of postsurgical patients in recovery phases. Train-of-four sensitivity has been shown to be more sensitive than single twitch or tetanic stimulation, especially for monitoring nondepolarizing neuromuscular blockade [10]. Double-burst stimulation is more sensitive than TOF in detecting fade for residual block [11]. However, double-burst stimulation and tetanic stimulation are more painful than TOF, and the current

Table 208-1. Structural Characteristics of Competitive Neuromuscular Blocking Agents [2]

Steroidal structure
  Pancuronium
  Vecuronium
  Pipecuronium
Bezylisoquinolines
  d-tubocurarine
  Atracurium
  Doxacurium
  Mivacurium

Table 208-2. Procedure for Train-of-Four [10,21,110]

1. Prepare skin by cleaning with alcohol swabs.
2. Place two electrodes on volar surface of wrists
  a. First, on radial side of flexor carpi ulnaris muscle about 1 cm from wrist crease.
  b. Second, 2–3 cm proximal to first electrode.
3. Attach alligator clips of peripheral nerve stimulator to electrode (black clip closest to fingers).
4. Abduct patient's thumb with two fingers.
5. Press TOF touchpad on peripheral nerve stimulator and feel for number of twitches in thumb ignoring movement in fingers, start power at 25 mA.
6. If no response increase milliamperage of nerve stimulator and re-check response. If still no response repeat procedure at different site, for example, the ankle or elbow.

recommendation is to monitor function with TOF [10,12,13]. Routine use of peripheral nerve stimulators with TOF may make it possible to individualize dosages and prevent overdose during prolonged and repeated administration [10,14].

Train-of-four stimulation delivers four stimuli of 2 Hz every 0.5 seconds and can be repeated every 12 seconds. Because muscle stimulation follows an "all-or-none" response, if the stimulus intensity exceeds a certain threshold there will be maximal muscle contraction; therefore, a normal response to TOF stimulation is four contractions of equal force. After neuromuscular blockade, the force of muscle contraction is reduced and the measured reduction in the contraction force is an expression of the degree of neuromuscular blockade [10]. The force of contraction is graded from 0 to 100 percent, and TOF response begins to decrease when more than 70 to 75 percent of receptors are blocked as the force of muscle contraction decreases [10,15]. In the presence of NMBAs the force of contraction response to TOF fades with each stimulation. To assess the muscle response to TOF stimulation, one can measure or count the tactile/visual muscle movements. A TOF ratio is calculated to measure the stimulus response; this ratio is the height of the first twitch divided by the height of the fourth twitch. The need for recording devices and measurement of control height makes this method less attractive for the ICU. Tactile and visual assessment by counting the number of twitches present after stimulation with TOF is currently recommended for monitoring in the ICU [16,17,18].

The most accessible nerve to follow TOF is the ulnar nerve, which, when stimulated, results in adduction of the thumb [5,9]. Sensitivity of the ulnar nerve correlates well with the blockade and recovery of neuromuscular function of the diaphragm in the presence of NMBAs [19]. Other monitoring sites include the posterior tibial nerve, which causes plantar flexion of the foot; the lateral popliteal nerve, which causes dorsiflexion of the foot; and the temporal branch of the facial nerve, which causes elevation of the eyebrow. The facial nerve recovers TOF responses more rapidly than the diaphragm from redosing and residual NMBA effects [20]. For monitoring the depth of neuromuscular block, the ulnar nerve is the site of choice. If there is no response, repositioning or choosing another site for TOF must be considered before changing the doses of NMBA agents. A condensed description of the procedure for TOF nerve stimulation is shown in Table 208-2 [10].

The intensity of a stimulus (supermaximal or submaximal) required for an adequate response from TOF nerve stimulation has been studied. By comparing the error of monitoring with submaximal and supramaximal stimulation, Helbo-Hanson and associates concluded that the accuracy of TOF is unacceptable at currents less than 25 mA [21]. Kopman and Lawson also concluded that supramaximal stimulation is mandatory and that some patients require up to 50 to 60 mA to elicit a response and patients with increased wrist circumferences may need stimulation in excess of 50 mA [22]. This is clinically important, because inadequate stimulation may lead to overestimation of

the degree of neuromuscular blockade and result in inappropriate dosing.

Because TOF monitoring involves counting the number of twitches in response to a stimuli, there is still a subjective component [13]. Viby-Mogenson et al. evaluated clinicians' ability to detect TOF fade. They found that it frequently went undetected (14 to 37 observations) and concluded that complete recovery was very difficult to estimate, visually or manually, with TOF. However, the lower depth of neuromuscular blockade required in mechanically ventilated patients was detected in 100 percent of cases [23]. While it is difficult to evaluate residual TOF fade, the number of responses evoked is a relatively reliable assessment. The degree of neuromuscular suppression can be estimated by counting the number of twitches, with four twitches indicating less than 75 percent of clinically relevant muscle relaxation and no twitches indicating more than 90 percent maximal relaxation. Op de Coul et al. recommend monitoring TOF every 15 to 30 minutes if a patient is receiving intermittent boluses. Repeated doses of NMBAs should not be administered until at least a single twitch reappears. If a patient is receiving a continuous infusion, administration rates should be titrated to the detection of one or two twitches [24]. This is because complete blockade is rarely necessary in intensive care patients.

Train-of-four assessment can be influenced by stimulus strength, location of electrodes, electrode type, tissue and electrode impedance, and interpatient receptor sensitivity. Understanding these variables improves the assessment of a patient's response [25]. Although still controversial, use of peripheral nerve stimulators can help achieve more precise neuromuscular blockade and possibly prevent adverse effects from overdosing and accumulation. This may possibly lower drug dosages and associated costs.

Many other factors may influence the titration of NMBAs. First, there is a great variability in patient response to these agents, which is probably more pronounced in the critically ill. Coadministered drugs, such as sedatives and analgesics, can also affect the dosages required, but the extent of these interactions is currently unknown. The severity of illness may further alter the pharmacokinetics and pharmacodynamics, influencing dosage titration. The potential effect of pathophysiology on NMBAs is discussed later in the chapter.

Preparations

Neuromuscular blockers are available for intravenous administration only. Intramuscular injections are not recommended, due to a slow onset of action and erratic absorption. Pancuronium is available for injection in vials of 1 or 2 mg per milliliter. Atracurium is available in a vial of 10 mg per milliliter. Both of these products must be refrigerated for storage. Vecuronium is available as a 10-mg vial that requires reconstitution prior to administration. Vecuronium does not need to be refrigerated until it is reconstituted.

Pharmacokinetics

The pharmacokinetics of NMBAs are intricately related to their pharmacodynamics, which are illustrated by a sigmoid E_{max} model describing the relationship of receptor occupancy and concentration to effect [26,27,28]. Time to onset of paralysis has a clinically relevant pharmacokinetic relationship and is determined by dose, distribution/redistribution kinetics, time lag from serum concentrations to site of effect concentrations, and receptor sensitivity [29]. Large doses correlate with high serum concentrations and increased drug concentrations at the site of effect soon after IV administration [27]. This concept is illustrated by a faster time to maximum blockade with a more rapid bolus of vecuronium [30]. Alterations in volumes of distribution affect peak concentrations and the time of onset of maximum paralysis. Changes in volume of distribution due to different disease states are discussed in the following section.

The duration of neuromuscular blockade is related to the time interval required for plasma concentration to decline below the concomitant effective concentration. This concentration threshold may occur during distribution or elimination phases. For example, after small doses, plasma concentrations fall below the effective concentration during the distribution phase. After large or repeated doses, plasma concentrations fall below the effective concentration during the terminal elimination phase; this may result in greater than double the duration of action [28,31,32]. Feldman described a variable dosing technique for vecuronium, in which increasing single-bolus doses of 100, 150, 200, and 250 μg per kilogram resulted in increases in the duration of action to 28.4, 40.9, 54.2, and 72.4 minutes, respectively [33]. The effect after repeated doses follows a similar pattern. Fisher and Rosen found that increased or repeated dosing techniques affected the duration for pancuronium and vecuronium but not atracurium [31]. Recovery from atracurium should generally correlate with the elimination phase, due to its unique metabolism. Atracurium may exhibit a change in duration in proportion to the dose administered, although some investigators have not observed this [28,29,34]. Variations in intensity and duration of neuromuscular blockade vary from patient to patient due to altered pharmacokinetics and pharmacodynamic responses, despite similar plasma concentrations and dosing techniques [28,29]. The combined pharmacokinetic/dynamic model provides insight into details of dose-response relationship for neuromuscular blockade. Further applications of the model in settings of pathophysiology may help with proper dosing in different patient populations [29].

All NMBAs share important physiochemical properties. They contain quaternary ammonium groups in large bulky molecules, which are highly ionized regardless of pH, limiting their absorption and distribution to extracellular water [35]. Onset of action varies between the different agents, but in general occurs within 3 to 5 minutes. Duration depends on the method of administration and specific drug used [14]. Elimination of NMBAs varies by route of metabolism and excretion. The different pharmacokinetics of these agents influences their use for different clinical goals. Pancuronium, vecuronium, and atracurium are discussed in detail in the following sections. Pharma-

cokinetic parameters of depolarizing and competitive NMBAs are summarized in Table 208-3.

ABSORPTION. Because all NMBAs contain one to three quaternary ammonium groups, they are poorly absorbed from the gastrointestinal tract and must be administered by intravenous injection [3]. Intramuscular administration is not recommended due to a slower onset of action and less predictable absorption, however intramuscular injection of vecuronium is being investigated for use in extreme situations [36].

DISTRIBUTION. Because these agents contain quaternary ammonium groups, following intravenous administration they are distributed into extracellular fluid. The volumes of distribution in adults range from 0.17 to 0.35 liter per kilogram [3,35]. Distribution accounts for termination of muscle relaxation during single doses, but after multiple doses and continuous infusions, metabolism and excretion play a larger role in determining the duration of action [14]. Because the agents are primarily ionized, there is negligible cerebrospinal fluid (CSF) penetration. There is variable binding (30–90%) to plasma proteins between different agents, mostly to albumin and gamma globulin [37,38]. Patients with physiologic stress (e.g., trauma) may have a decreased free fraction due to increase in concentrations of alpha-1-acid glycoprotein and thereby display increased binding capacities. This could be responsible for increased dosage requirements of NMBAs, such as tubocurarine and atracurium [39,40]. Differences in ultracentrifugation methods, drug concentrations, or methods for determining drug loss may account for the variations in protein binding [41]. More study is needed to determine the extent of protein binding and its clinical significance [3].

EXCRETION/METABOLISM

Pancuronium. Up to 60 percent of the parent drug pancuronium is eliminated by the kidney as unchanged drug, and 30 to 40 percent is converted by hepatic oxidative enzymes [42]. The 3-OH deacetylated metabolite exhibits 50 percent the activity of pancuronium and is eliminated by the kidney. This metabolite may accumulate to a significant degree in renal failure, prolonging the duration of action after repeated doses or during continuous infusion [43]. Biliary elimination accounts for 11 percent of unchanged drug and metabolites [14,42,44].

Vecuronium. The main route of excretion for vecuronium is hepatobiliary clearance. This drug undergoes spontaneous deacetylation to 3-hydroxy, 17-hydroxy, and 3,17-hydroxy compounds. The 3-hydroxy metabolite appears to exhibit at least 50 percent of the neuromuscular activity of the parent compound and may become clinically significant in severe renal dysfunction [4]. Biliary excretion accounts for 30 to 50 percent of unchanged drug and another 30 percent of 3-hydroxy metabolite. Up to 10 percent of the dose is excreted in the urine unchanged, and most urinary excretion occurs within 4 to 6 hours after single doses.

Khuenl-Brady et al. studied the effects of vecuronium's metabolites on its pharmacodynamic effect. They found that vecuronium in combination with the 3-desacetyl metabolite had additive effects, but low concentrations of vecuronium in combination with the 3,17-desacetyl metabolite exhibited antagonistic activity. Given the interpatient variability in the critically ill and specific changes in biotransformation and elimination, these metabolites may play a role in the development of resis-

Table 208-3. Summary of Kinetic Parameters for Depolarizing and Nondepolarizing Neuromuscular Blockers

Drug	Onset	Duration	Metabolism	Elimination	Half-life	Cum*	Ref
Depolarizing							
Succinylcholine	0.5–1 min	4–6 min	Plasma cholinesterases	10% unchanged in urine	30 sec	+	16
Nondepolarizing							
Long-acting							
Pancuronium	2–3 min	30–60 min	30–40% by the liver, active metabolite (3-OH pancuronium)	60% unchanged drug and metabolites in urine, 11% in bile	120 min	+ + +	3,16,42
Doxacurium	5–10 min	100–160 min	Negligible	Unchanged drug in bile and urine	70–99 min	NA	35,127
Pipecuronium	5 min	60–120 min	20% metabolized by liver by deacetylation	Unchanged drug and metabolites in urine	98 min	NA	35
Tubocurarine	2–5 min	25–95 min	1% metabolized by N-demethylation	33–75% unchanged drug and metabolites in urine, 11% in bile	170 min	NA	3,125
Intermediate-acting:							
Vecuronium	2–5 min	20–40 min	Spontaneous deacetylation and liver metabolism, active metabolites (3-OH vecuronium and 3-desacetyl vecuronium)	20% unchanged drug in urine, 45% unchanged drug and 25% metabolites in bile	30–80 min	+ +	3
Atracurium	3–5 min	20–35 min	Ester hydrolysis and Hofman elimination in plasma	Unchanged drug and metabolites in urine and bile	20 min	+	3
Short-acting							
Mivacurium	3–5 min	15–30 min	Ester hydrolysis by plasma cholinesterase in plasma	Unchanged drug and metabolites in urine and bile	2 min	NA	16,124

* The drug's potential to accumulate.

tance in some patients [45]. One case report describes a patient who was resistant to vecuronium and responded to normal doses of pancuronium. High concentrations of the metabolite 17-hydroxy vecuronium were the only corresponding alteration [46].

Atracurium. The majority of atracurium undergoes spontaneous decomposition, at physiologic pH and normal body temperatures, by a base-catalyzed reaction called Hofman elimination. This reaction causes a breakage of the link between a quaternary nitrogen and carbonyl in the central chain, thereby forming laudanosine and monoquaternary methacrylate. The remainder of atracurium is hydrolyzed by non-specific plasma cholinesterases, yielding a quaternary alcohol and quaternary acid. These by-products have not exhibited neuromuscular activity in humans. Hofman elimination is not dependent on blood flow or organ enzymes for metabolism. However, Parker et al. compared elimination of atracurium in the elderly and in a younger population and found a reduced clearance and longer elimination half-life with advancing age [47].

Hofman elimination may be affected by certain physiologic pH and temperature changes [48–52]. This may necessitate clinical dosage adjustments, but more clinical studies are required to establish guidelines.

Laudanosine formation and possible accumulation is of concern in critically ill patients [50,53,54]. The threat of toxicity during-long term infusions is still controversial. Laudanosine is a central nervous stimulant that has caused seizures in dogs after very large intravenous doses [55]. Because of its high lipophilicity and large volume of distribution, accumulation in CNS tissue is possible. However, significant CSF levels would require prolonged continuous infusions [56]. There is no clinical evidence of drug-related convulsive behavior [49,57]. The risk of serious side effects from laudanosine is still of concern, especially in patients with renal dysfunction [58,59,60].

Physiologic Clearance Characteristics

HYPODYNAMIC PATIENTS

Pancuronium. Hypodynamic patients are in various stages of decreased organ function, which may decrease pancuronium's clearance. This drug's clearance is mostly affected by renal insufficiency but also by hepatic failure. In chronic renal failure the terminal half-life increases from an average of 1 to 2 hours to an average of 8 to 10 hours and total body clearance decreases from 60 to 80 ml per minute to 18 to 22 ml per minute [61]. The disparate changes between clearance and half-life indicate an increase in distribution volume in renal failure that could require a larger loading dose.

Hepatobiliary disease affects pancuronium clearance by changes in both biliary clearance and metabolism by the P-450 mixed oxidase system. In patients with cirrhosis, plasma clearance was decreased by 22 percent compared to control [62]. This study also found a 50 percent increase in distribution volume, which would partially explain reports of drug resistance in such patients. These results should be contrasted with patients having primarily biliary obstruction, who demonstrated a 50 percent decrease in total clearance compared to a control group. The recovery time was twice as long as in the control group, with serum concentrations for recovery in both groups at 20 to 25 μg per milliliter [44].

Peritoneal dialysis does not seem to affect the clearance of pancuronium in renal failure patients. Data for hemodialysis or hemofiltration are not available.

Vecuronium. Vecuronium's predominantly hepatobiliary clearance has been investigated in patients with both renal and hepatic dysfunction. Single-dose studies in patients with renal dysfunction have found no change in clearance. Patients in end-stage renal failure after repetitive dosing, however, have manifested a prolonged recovery time [63,64,65]. An active metabolite, 3-desacetylvecuronium, was recently implicated in prolonging neuromuscular recovery by accumulating in critically ill patients with renal failure [6]. These patients had been on varying doses of vecuronium infusions for longer than 6 days.

Studies in patients with alcoholic cirrhosis and viral hepatitis have shown little change in clearance with single 0.1-mg per kilogram doses. Clearance and volume of distribution were not altered compared to healthy controls [66,67]. Because the recovery time doubled in studies using larger (0.2-mg/kg) doses in cirrhotic patients versus healthier controls, saturation of the elimination system might be a more likely cause of prolonged recovery time in cirrhotic patients.

In patients with cholestasis, vecuronium clearance is reduced by approximately 50 percent. The recovery time also doubled in these patients. Control patients and cholestatic patients achieved 75 percent recovery at 200 to 300 ng per milliliter, indicating a predominately pharmacokinetic change to explain the prolonged recovery. Similar increases in duration of action and half-life have been seen in patients with stable cirrhosis [68,69,70].

Atracurium. Atracurium clearance is not impaired in renal failure [58,71,72]. A study of patients with acute hepatic and renal failure showed no difference in clearance after a single dose [73]. When the drug was administered as an infusion (<48 hours) in critically ill patients with and without renal failure, there was no difference in total clearance [59,74].

Hepatobiliary dysfunction has little effect on atracurium's clearance whether it is administered as single doses or short-term infusions [75,76].

HYPERDYNAMIC PATIENTS

Pancuronium and Vecuronium. Data for pancuronium and vecuronium in physiologically stressed patients come primarily from investigations with burn patients. These investigations indicate a need for an increase in dosing requirements due to pharmacodynamic drug resistance. Mean serum concentrations for 50 percent maximal effect are two to three times those in control patients. This may be due to the proliferation of extrajunctional nicotinic receptors, which occupy the drug.

There is good correlation between increased burn size and the need for increased doses of steroid NMBAs. In a study of pancuronium in pediatric patients with approximately 50 percent total body surface area burns, the patients were studied at 34.2 ± 7.9 days after their injury [77]. Vecuronium was studied by the same group in pediatric patients at 6 to 35 days after burn injury [78]. Both studies were conducted on induction of general anesthesia, and in both the pharmacokinetics were not significantly different between control and burn patients. Therefore, the explanation for increased dosing needs in this patient population is either a decrease in sensitivity to NMBAs or a change in pharmacodynamics.

Atracurium. Atracurium in hyperdynamic patients may require increases in dosages over 2 to 3 days after onset of injury or sepsis. An investigation involving mostly surgical/trauma patients receiving atracurium for 36 to 219 hours noted a 50 to 100 percent increase in dosing requirements in 14 to 15 patients in the first 72 hours [49]. A report of two young trauma patients receiving infusions for 22 and 106 hours recorded required doses of 1 and 1.38 mg/kg/hr [79]. This increase in drug requirement could be attributed partially to increased alpha-acid glycoprotein binding and hence decreased free concentrations, increased clearance, or acquired pharmacodynamic resistance.

Atracurium continues the trend of resistance to competitive neuromuscular blockers in burn patients. A single-dose study showed no difference in pharmacokinetics compared to controls [80]. However, serum concentrations for 50 percent of effect were approximately threefold higher in patients with burns on greater than 33 percent of total body surface area and greater than 1 week after injury [81]. This effective resistance may continue up to 3 months after injury but eventually returns to normal [82].

Dosing Guidelines

Most NMBA dosing guidelines are derived from data in surgical patients under general anesthesia. General anesthetics, more commonly inhaled anesthetics, are known to potentiate the blockade of NMBAs and reduce the dose required [83–86]. Because in ICUs patients usually are not under the influence of anesthetics, NMBA dosing requirements may be greater than those described in the anesthesiology literature. Conversely, the degree of neuromuscular blockade required to facilitate mechanical ventilation may be less than what is required for surgery.

Dosing of competitive NMBAs should be individualized and based on patient mass. The appropriate effect can be improved and interpatient variability decreased by basing the dose on lean body weight [87]. This is because competitive NMBAs distribute mainly in the extracellular fluid compartment [3]. Initial recommendations for intermittent doses, loading doses, and continuous infusions are summarized in Table 208-4. Subsequent titration of each dosage regimen should be based on clinical goals and patient response.

INTERMITTENT DOSING. Traditionally, long-acting NMBAs have been administered in ICUs by intermittent bolus as needed to achieve the clinical goals. Pancuronium and vecuronium can be useful when administered as intermittent boluses, with the pharmacokinetic and pharmacodynamic parameters determining the onset of action and duration of blockade as discussed above. After an intravenous bolus of 0.1 to 0.15 mg per kilogram of pancuronium, intubating conditions should be adequate 90 to 120 seconds after the dose, and duration of action is about 60 minutes [17]. After the initial bolus, repeated doses of 0.1 to 0.2 mg per kilogram can be administered every 1 to 3 hours as needed based on clinical signs [3]. This regimen theoretically reduces significant accumulation, but it may not

Table 208-4. Initial Dosing Guidelines for ICU Patients[a][3,15,16,110]

Drug	Intermittent dose	Continuous infusion	
		Loading dose[b]	Maintenance dose
Pancuronium	0.1–0.2 mg/kg every 1–3 hr	0.03–0.1 mg/kg	0.06–0.1 mg/kg/hr
Vecuronium	0.1–0.2 mg/kg every 1 hr	0.1 mg/kg	0.05–0.1 mg/kg/hr
Atracurium	—	0.5 mg/kg	0.4–1.0 mg/kg/hr

[a] Dosing recommendations for patients with no underlying organ dysfunction
[b] Loading doses usually administered over 5–10 minutes.

provide continuous blockade for synchronous mechanical ventilation.

Vecuronium can also be administered by intermittent intravenous bolus. Following a dose of 0.1 to 0.2 mg per kilogram, adequate intubating conditions occur in 60 seconds [3,88]. To decrease the time to maximal effect a high-dose vecuronium regimen of 0.4 to 0.5 mg per kilogram has been suggested as an alternative to depolarizing NMBAs [89]. However, patients are likely to exhibit a prolonged duration of action, due to pharmacokinetic and pharmacodynamic differences with larger doses. There are reports that the time of onset may decrease proportionately with doses up to 0.3 mg per kilogram and higher doses will simply increase the duration of action [32].

Atracurium given in doses of 0.5 mg per kilogram for intubation can achieve maximal effect within 2 to 2.5 minutes. For patients at increased risk of histamine release and reactions (e.g., asthmatics), initial doses should be reduced and administration time prolonged. At higher doses atracurium's duration of action may be prolonged, but because its usual duration is short (20 minutes) intermittent bolus therapy is impractical for intensive care use.

CONTINUOUS INFUSION. Continuous infusion, a common method of administration in ICUs for prolonged, complex mechanical ventilation, may reduce required daily dosages compared to intermittent bolus therapy. Suggested loading doses provide profound muscle relaxation in healthy patients. Maintenance infusion doses are intended as initial guidelines. Because of differing goals, adjuvant drugs, and varying patient response to neuromuscular agents, subsequent infusion rates should be titrated based on individual response.

Pancuronium requires a loading dose of 0.03 to 0.1 mg per kilogram, with a maintenance infusion of 0.06 to 0.1 mg/kg/hr titrated to the patient's response [3,17,90]. A loading dose of vecuronium of 0.1 mg per kilogram should be followed within 20 to 40 minutes by a maintenance infusion of 0.05 to 0.1 mg/kg/hr [3,91]. Atracurium's initial loading dose is 0.5 mg per kilogram and the initial maintenance infusion starts at 0.4 to 1.0 mg per hour [3,87].

DOSING IN HYPODYNAMIC PATIENTS. Guidelines for dosing in patients with decreased organ function start with drug selection, considering the elimination pathways of the different agents. For example, in patients with renal dysfunction pancuronium dosing would have great variability due to its 60 percent renal elimination. However, with appropriate decreases in dosage based on accurate monitoring it may be a cost-effective agent for intensive care patients.

There have been conflicting results in investigations of pharmacokinetics and pharmacodynamics of neuromuscular blockers in the elderly. Bell et al. studied differences in dose-response curves of atracurium, vecuronium, and pancuronium after single doses in elderly versus young surgical patients. They found no significant difference in dose-response curves or potencies [67]. There was also no change in pharmacokinetic effects of atracurium in elderly surgical patients after initial bolus and short-term infusions [92].

On the other hand, vecuronium was found to have a significantly longer time for recovery after single doses in elderly patients [93]. Surgical elderly patients after single bolus doses of vecuronium also exhibited significantly longer half-lives [94]. Both studies determined the differences to be due to pharmacokinetic changes in the elderly population. McLeod et al. looked at pharmacokinetic differences of pancuronium in elderly patients undergoing surgery with no evidence of major organ dysfunction; they found the elderly had a decrease in

rate of decline of plasma concentration and increase in recovery time [95]. Patients with changing renal and hepatic function due to the aging process and alterations in body composition may require smaller daily doses of NMBAs.

Guidelines for NMBA dosage reduction for hypodynamic patients with renal and hepatic dysfunction have not been reported. Due to pancuronium's primarily renal clearance, reductions in dosing up to 50 percent may be required for patients with renal dysfunction [61] and patients with primary biliary obstruction [44]. Loading doses of pancuronium remain the same in most situations, unless the volume of distribution has changed as discussed previously. Vecuronium is cleared predominantly via hepatobiliary excretion; therefore in patients with cholestasis and hepatic dysfunction maintenance infusions may need to be reduced by 50 percent [68,96]. Loading doses of vecuronium remain the same. Studies have indicated that dose reduction of atracurium in patients with renal and hepatic dysfunction is not required [59,73,74,76].

DOSING IN HYPERDYNAMIC PATIENTS. Burn patients have been most studied when comparing NMBA dosing in hyperdynamic and nonhypermetabolic patient populations. Hyperdynamic patients exhibit a decreased sensitivity to competitive neuromuscular blockers, which can start as early as 1 week after injury, peak at 15 to 40 days after injury, and last many months [80]. Because of their increased resistance to these agents, patients with major burns have dose requirements 2.5 to 5.0 times the normal dose [77,78,80,81,97,98]. Hypermetabolic states gradually decrease with burn wound healing, but NMBA resistance may outlast the hypermetabolic state of the burn injury [98]. Initial doses of pancuronium and atracurium in patients with more than 40 percent total body surface area burn are 0.13 and 2.0 mg per kilogram, respectively, compared to 0.05 and 0.25 mg per kilogram in patients without burns. Patients with intermediate-sized burns (15–40% total body surface area) require more standard dosing. Recovery from high-dose neuromuscular blockade is not significantly impaired in burn patients with normal renal and hepatic function [98].

Increases in dosage requirements have also been described for critically ill patients receiving prolonged continuous infusions. Coursin et al. described two cases of critically ill patients whose vecuronium requirements increased up to sixfold. Both received infusions for 12 weeks, and the authors could not identify any physiologic parameter that was clearly associated with the increased requirements [99]. One possible explanation is the proliferation of extrajunctional receptors secondary to prolonged competitive blockade. Changes in the neuromuscular junction may be a mechanism causing resistance after prolonged paralysis with NMBAs lasting days to months [99,100]. Chapple et al. investigated the mechanism of increased resistance to atracurium in dogs and found that resistance was probably due to prolonged immobility, not to atracurium [101]. Prolonged immobility may result in an upregulation of extrajunctional acetylcholine receptors and an increased sensitivity to acetylcholine, which may cause an increased requirement of drug to induce neuromuscular block [100,101]. The mechanism of resistance in critically ill patients from weeks of neuromuscular blockade is still being investigated.

Drug Interactions

Many drugs used in ICUs may influence the degree and duration of neuromuscular blockade (Table 208-5). Clinical significance of these reactions can only be related to individual situ-

Tables 208-5. Drug Interactions

Drug	Interaction	References
Antibiotics		103
Aminoglycosides	Potentiation of blockade by decreasing amount of acetylcholine release	102
Tetracyclines	Potentiation of blockade	103
Clindamycin, lincomycin	Potentiation of blockade	103
Vancomycin	Potentiation of blockade	103,123
Sedative/anesthetics	May potentiate blockade	
Cardiovascular agents		
Furosemide	Potentiate blockade at low doses, antagonize blockade at high doses	121,122
Beta-blockers	Potentiate blockade	3
Procainamide	Potentiate blockade	3
Quinidine	Potentiate blockade	3
Calcium channel blockers	Potentiate blockade	120
Methylxanthines (theophylline)	Antagonize blockade	119
Antiepileptic drugs		
Phenytoin	Resistance to blockade from chronic use	104,105,106,118
	Potentiation after acute administration	107
Carbamazepine	Resistance to blockade	117
Ranitidine	Antagonize blockade	115, 116
Lithium	Mild potentiation of blockade	114
Immunosuppressive agents		
Azathioprine	Mild antagonism by inhibiting phosphodiesterase in the motor terminal	113
Cyclosporine	Potentiate blockade	111
Corticosteroids	May potentiate steroid myopathy	8
Local anesthetics	Potentiate blockade	11

Adapted from [3].

ations. For example, patients with significant burn injury have similar increases in requirements despite being on aminoglycosides; therefore there is no clinical significance [98]. The following drug interactions should be considered when using NMBAs.

Several classes of antibiotics can influence neuromuscular blockade and paralysis via prejunctional, postjunctional, and synaptic cleft effects. Aminoglycosides are known to prolong NMBA effects by decreasing the amount of acetylcholine liberated by nerve impulses and stabilizing postjunctional membranes. Calcium can antagonize this effect by restoring the amount of acetylcholine released to control levels [102]. Clindamycin has a complex mechanism of action; it has a local anesthetic effect on myelinated nerves, stimulates nerve terminals, and blocks postsynaptic cholinergic receptors [103].

Chronic anticonvulsant use may cause an increased resistance to neuromuscular blocking effects. This mechanism of action in neurosurgical patients may be manifested by decreased sensitivity of acetylcholine at receptor sites, increased metabolism of NMBAs, and/or increased number of receptors secondary to intracranial pathology [104]. Hickey et al. and Tempelhoff et al. described an increased resistance to NMBAs in neurosurgical patients chronically treated with phenytoin and carbamazepine. They suspect the mechanism may involve hepatic enzyme induction, which increases the metabolism of NMBAs. Other proposed mechanisms include decreased sensitivity of acetylcholine at receptor sites, increased receptor density, increased end plate anticholinesterase activity, and reduced acetylcholine secretion in response to action potentials [100,105,106]. Careful monitoring of NMBA requirements is recommended in neurosurgical patients on anticonvulsants. The acute administration of phenytoin with neuromuscular blockade may potentiate the effects of NMBAs by a different mechanism [107].

Recently, many reports of prolonged paralysis or acute generalized neuromyopathy have been published. A common factor of some reports includes continuous NMBA infusions for greater than 5 days. Other reports involve patients with renal failure and those treated concomitantly with corticosteroids [108]. Myopathy occurring after long-term paralysis in critically ill asthmatics may be caused by the combined effects of corticosteroids and muscle relaxants on the muscle cell [8]. Loss of myosin filaments has been observed in muscle biopsies from asthmatic patients who have remained quadriplegic after treatment with methylprednisolone and vecuronium [109]. Most case reports have involved pancuronium and vecuronium and not atracurium, but this may reflect the limited experience with prolonged infusions of atracurium. Atracurium does differ in chemical structure and elimination pathways and may be less likely to cause or exacerbate steroid myopathy. Risk factors for developing persistent weakness/paresis include renal failure, concomitant treatment with corticosteroids, and continuous infusions longer than 5 days. Clinicians have recommended limiting continuous infusions whenever possible, avoiding overdosing by clinical monitoring with peripheral nerve stimulator or allowing patient movement every 24 hours, avoiding or limiting corticosteroid administration, and being aware of potential for severe muscle weakness in recovering patients [108].

Common Pitfalls in Management

1. Failure to use adequate sedation and analgesia. There is a persisting misconception that administration of nondepolarizing NMBAs also provides sedation and analgesia. Appropriate pain and sedation management renders the patient less aware of surroundings and physical state, and therefore less anxious and more comfortable. Adequate sedation is often difficult to assess, but unexplained tachycardia and hypertension may be indications of awareness. Pain is also

difficult to assess. Similar clinical signs should be monitored while manipulating catheters, caring for wounds, or applying daily hygiene. The experiences of nurses and physicians as patients in ICUs have illustrated the lack of adequate sedation and pain relief. Both sedation and analgesia must be administered for the duration of neuromuscular blockade [3,16].

2. Failure to monitor depth of blockade consistently or to reassess with improved clinical status. Peripheral nerve stimulators, when properly applied, may assist greatly in preventing excessive blockade.

3. Failure to consider drug selection and dosage changes for patients with underlying renal or hepatic dysfunction.

References

1. Feldman S: Neuromuscular transmission and block, in Scurr C, Feldman S, Soni N. (eds): *Scientific Foundations of Anaesthesia: The Basis of Intensive Care.* 4th ed. Chicago, Year Book, 1990, pp 497–505.

2. Taylor P: Agents acting at the neuromuscular junction and autonomic ganglia, in Goodman A, Gilman R, Rall TW, Nies AS, Taylor P (eds): *Goodman and Gilman's The Pharmacological Basis of Therapeutics.* 8th ed. New York, Pergamon, 1990, pp 167–178.

3. Buck ML, Reed MD: Use of nondepolarizing neuromuscular blocking agents in mechanically ventilated patients. *Clin Pharm* 10:32, 1991.

4. Torda TA: The 'new' relaxants: A review of the clinical pharmacology of atracurium and vecuronium. *Anaesth Intensive Care* 15:72, 1987.

5. Larijani GE, Gratz I, Silverberg M, et al: Clinical pharmacology of the neuromuscular blocking agents. *DICP* 25:54, 1991.

6. Segredo V, Caldwell JE, Matthay MA, et al: Persistent paralysis in critically ill patients after long-term administration of vecuronium. *N Engl J Med* 327:524, 1992.

7. Gooch JL, Suchyta MR, Balbierz JM, et al: Prolonged paralysis after treatment with neuromuscular junction blocking agents. *Crit Care Med* 19:1125, 1991.

8. Griffin D, Fairman N, Coursin D, et al: Acute myopathy during treatment of status asthmaticus with corticosteroids and steroidal muscle relaxants. *Chest* 102:510, 1992.

9. Ali HH, Savarese JJ: Monitoring of neuromuscular function. *Anesthesiology* 45:216, 1976.

10. Viby-Mogensen J: Clinical assessment of neuromuscular transmission. *Br J Anaesth* 54:209, 1982.

11. Drenck NE, Ueda N, Olsen NV, et al: Manual evaluation of residual curarization using double burst stimulation: A comparison with train-of-four. *Anesthesiology* 70:578, 1989.

12. Connelly NR, Silverman DG, Z OT, et al: Subjective response to train-of-four and double burst stimulation in awake patients. *Anesth Analg* 70:650, 1990.

13. Bevan DR: Monitoring, new drugs, and reversal of neuromuscular blocking drugs. *Can J Anaesth* 38:R89, 1991.

14. Durbin CG: Neuromuscular blocking agents and sedative drugs: Clinical uses and toxic effects in the critical care unit. *Crit Care Clin* 7:489, 1991.

15. Willatts SM: Paralysis for ventilated patients? Yes or no? *Intensive Care Med* 11:2, 1985.

16. Isenstein DA, Venner DS, Duggan J: Neuromuscular blockade in the intensive care unit. *Chest* 102:1258, 1992.

17. Sharpe MD: The use of muscle relaxants in the intensive care unit. *Can J Anaesth* 39:949, 1992.

18. Fiamengo SA, Savarese JJ: Use of muscle relaxants in intensive care units. *Crit Care Med* 19:1457, 1991.

19. Donati F, Antzaka C, Bevan D: Potency of pancuronium at the diaphragm and the adductor pollicis muscle in humans. *Anesthesiology* 64:1, 1986.

20. Caffrey RR, Warren ML, Becker KE Jr: Neuromuscular blockade monitoring comparing the orbicularis oculi and adductor pollicis muscles. *Anesthesiology* 65:95, 1986.

21. Helbo-Hansen HS, Bang U, Nielsen HK, et al: The accuracy of train-of-four monitoring at varying stimulating currents. *Anesthesiology* 76:199, 1992.

22. Kopman AF, Lawson D: Milliamperage requirements for supramaximal stimulation of the ulnar nerve with surface electrodes. *Anesthesiology* 61:83, 1984.

23. Viby-Mogensen J, Jensen NH, Engbraek J, et al: Tactile and visual evaluation of the response to train-of-four nerve stimulation. *Anesthesiology* 63:440, 1985.

24. Op de Coul A, Lambrects P, Koeman T: Neuromuscular complications in patients given pavulon during artificial ventilation. *Clin Neurol Neurosurg* 87:17, 1985.

25. Mylrea K, Hameroff S, Calkins J, et al: Evaluation of peripheral nerve stimulators and relationship to possible errors in assessing neuromuscular blockade. *Anesthesiology* 60:464, 1984.

26. Donati F, Meistelman C: A kinetic-dynamic model to explain the relationship between high potency and slow onset time for neuromuscular blocking drugs. *J Pharmacokinet Biopharm* 19:537, 1991.

27. Hennis PJ, Stanski DR: Pharmacokinetic and pharmacodynamic factors that govern the clinical use of muscle relaxants. *Semin Anesth* 4:21, 1985.

28. Shanks CA: Kinetic-dynamic modelling of neuromuscular blockade, in van Boxtel CJ, Holford NHG, Danhof M (eds): *The in vivo study of drug action.* Amsterdam, Elsevier, 1992, pp 205–217.

29. Swerdlow BN, Holley FO: Intravenous anaesthetic agents: Pharmacokinetic-pharmacodynamic relationships. *Clin Pharmacokinet* 12:79, 1987.

30. Feldman SA, Soni N, Kraayenbrink MA: Effect of rate of injection on the neuromuscular block produced by vecuronium. *Anesth Analg* 69:624, 1989.

31. Fisher DM, Rosen JI: A pharmacokinetic explanation for increasing recovery time following larger or repeated doses of nondepolarizing muscle relaxants. *Anesthesiology* 65:286, 1986.

32. Kaufman JA, Dubois MY, Chen JC, et al: Pharmacodynamic effects of vecuronium: A dose response study. *J Clin Anesth* 1:434, 1989.

33. Feldman SA: Vecuronium—A variable dose technique. *Anaesthesia* 42:199, 1987.

34. Ward S, Neill A, Weatherley B, et al: Pharmacokinetics of atracurium besylate in healthy patients (after a single I.V. bolus dose). *Br J Anaesth* 55:113–118, 1983.

35. Agoston S, Vanderbrom RH, Wierda JMK: Clinical pharmacokinetics of neuromuscular blocking drugs. *Clin Pharmacokinet* 22:94, 1992.

36. Alpert CC, Bailey MK, Brahen NH, et al: Intramuscular use of vecuronium bromide. *J Cardiothorac Vasc Anesth* 6:265, 1992.

37. Duvaldestin P, Henzel D: Binding of tubocurarine, fazadinium, pancuronium and ORG NC 45 to serum proteins in normal man and in patients with cirrhosis. *Br J Anaesth* 54:513, 1982.

38. Foldes F, Deery A: Protein binding of atracurium and other short-acting neuromuscular blocking agents and their interaction with human cholinesterases. *Br J Anaesth* 55(suppl1):31S, 1983.

39. Tatman A, Wrigley S, Jones R: Resistance to atracurium in a patient with an increase in plasma alpha1 globulins. *Br J Anaesth* 67:623, 1991.

40. Thompson DF: Neuromuscular blocking agents in burn patients. *DICP* 23:1006, 1989.

41. Ramzan MJ, Somogyi AA, Walker JS, et al: Clinical pharmacokinetics of the non-depolarising muscle relaxants. *Clin Pharmacokinet* 6:25, 1981.

42. Agoston S, Vermeer GA, Kersten UW, et al: The fate of pancuronium bromide in man. *Acta Anaesthesiol Scand* 17:267, 1973.

43. Vandenbrom RHG, Wierda JMKH: Pancuronium bromide in the intensive care unit: A case of overdose. *Anesthesiology* 69:996, 1988.

44. Somogyi AA, Shanks CA, Triggs EJ: Disposition kinetics of pancuronium bromide in patients with total biliary obstruction. *Br J Anaesth* 49:1103, 1977.

45. Khuenl-Brady KS, Mair P, Koller J: Antagonism of vecuronium by one of its metabolites in vitro. *Eur J Pharmacol* 222:153, 1992.

46. Cozanitis D: Probable resistance to vecuronium involving the 17-hydroxy metabolite. *Br J Anaesth* 69:110, 1992.

47. Parker CJR, Hunter JM, Snowdon SL: Effect of age, sex and anaes-

thetic technique on the pharmacokinetics of atracurium. *Br J Anaesth* 69:439, 1992.

48. Neill EAM, Chapple DJ: Metabolic studies in the cat with atracurium: A neuromuscular blocking agent designed for non-enzymatic inactivation at physiological pH. *Xenobiotica* 12:203, 1982.

49. Yate PM, Flynn PJ, Arnold RW, et al: Clinical experience and plasma laudanosine concentrations during the infusion of atracurium in the intensive therapy unit. *Br J Anaesth* 59:211, 1987.

50. Nigrovic V, Banoub M: Pharmacokinetic modeling of a parent drug and its metabolite: Atracurium and laudanosine. *Clin Pharmacokinet* 22:396, 1992.

51. Platt M, Hayward A, Cooper A, et al: Effect of arterial carbon dioxide tension on the duration of action of atracurium. *Br J Anaesth* 66:45, 1991.

52. Denny NM, Kneeshaw JD: Vecuronium and atracurium infusions during hypothermic cardiopulmonary bypass. *Anaesthesia* 41:919, 1986.

53. Nigrovic V, Fox JL: Atracurium decay and the formation of laudanosine in humans. *Anesthesiology* 74:446, 1991.

54. Nigrovic V, Smith S: Involvement of nucleophiles in the inactivation of atracurium. *Br J Anaesth* 59:617, 1987.

55. Hennis PJ, Fahey MR, Canfell PC, et al: Pharmacology of laudanosine in dogs. *Anesthesiology* 65:56, 1986.

56. Fahey MR, Hosobuchi Y, Canfell C, et al: Cerebrospinal fluid concentrations of laudanosine in man. *Anesthesiology* 63:A312, 1986.

57. Wadon AJ, Dogra S, Anand S: Atracurium infusion in the intensive care unit. *Br J Anaesth* 58:64S, 1986.

58. Vandenbrom RHG, Wierda JMKH, Agoston S: Pharmacokinetics and neuromuscular blocking effects of atracurium besylate and two of its metabolites in patients with normal and impaired renal function. *Clin Pharmacokinet* 19:230, 1990.

59. Parker CJR, Jones JE, Hunter JM: Disposition of infusions of atracurium and its metabolite, laudanosine, in patients in renal and respiratory failure in an ITU. *Br J Anaesth* 61:531, 1988.

60. Kent AP, Parker CJR, Hunter JM: Pharmacokinetics of atracurium and laudanosine in the elderly. *Br J Anaesth* 63:661, 1989.

61. McLeod K, Watson MJ, Rawlins MD: Pharmacokinetics of pancuronium in patients with normal and impaired renal function. *Br J Anaesth* 48:341, 1976.

62. Duvaldestin P, Agoston S, Henzel D, et al: Pancuronium pharmacokinetics in patients with liver cirrhosis. *Br J Anaesth* 50:1131, 1978.

63. Starsnic MA, Goldberg ME, Ritter DE, et al: Does vecuronium accumulate in the renal transplant patient? *Can J Anaesth* 36:35, 1989.

64. Smith CL, Hunter JM, Jones RS: Vecuronium infusions in patients with renal failure in an ITU. *Anaesthesia* 42:387, 1987.

65. Bevan DR, Donati F, Gyasi H, et al: Vecuronium in renal failure. *Can Anaesth Soc J* 31:491, 1984.

66. Arden JR, Lynam DP, Castagnoli KP, et al: Vecuronium in alcoholic liver disease: A pharmacokinetic and pharmacodynamic analysis. *Anesthesiology* 68:771, 1988.

67. Bell PF, Mirakhur RK, Clarke RSJ: Dose-response studies of atracurium, vecuronium and pancuronium in the elderly. *Anaesthesia* 44:925, 1989.

68. Lebrault C, Duvaldestin D, Henzel D, et al: Pharmacokinetics and pharmacodynamics of vecuronium in patients with cholestasis. *Br J Anaesth* 58:983, 1986.

69. Hilgenberg JC: Comparison of the pharmacology of vecuronium and atracurium with that of other currently available muscle relaxants. *Anesth Analg* 62:524, 1983.

70. Bencini AF, Mol WEM, Scaf AHJ, et al: Uptake and excretion of vecuronium bromide and pancuronium bromide in the isolated perfused rat liver. *Anesthesiology* 69:487, 1988.

71. Fahey MR, Rupp SM, Fisher DM, et al: The pharmacokinetics and pharmacodynamics of atracurium in patients with and without renal failure. *Anesthesiology* 61:699, 1984.

72. Ward S, Boheimer B, Weatherley BC, et al: Pharmacokinetics of atracurium and its metabolites in patients with normal renal function, and in patients with renal failure. *Br J Anaesth* 59:697, 1987.

73. Ward S, Neill E: Pharmacokinetics of atracurium in acute hepatic failure (with acute renal failure). *Br J Anaesth* 55:1169, 1983.

74. Griffiths RB, Hunter JM, Jones RS: Atracurium infusions in patients with renal failure on an ITU. *Anaesthesia* 41:375, 1986.

75. Lawhead RG, Matsumi M, Peters R, et al: Plasma laudanosine levels in patients given atracurium during liver transplantation. *Anesth Analg* 76:569, 1993.

76. Parker C, Hunter J: Pharmacokinetics of atracurium and laudanosine in patients with hepatic cirrhosis. *Br J Anaesth* 62:177, 1989.

77. Martyn JAJ, Liu LMP, Szyfelbein SK, et al: The neuromuscular effects of pancuronium in burned children. *Anesthesiology* 59:561, 1983.

78. Mills AK, Martyn JAJ: Neuromuscular blockade with vecuronium in paediatric patients with burn injury. *Br J Clin Pharmac* 28:155, 1989.

79. Gwinnutt CL, Eddleston JM, Edwards D, et al: Concentrations of atracurium and laudanosine in cerebrospinal fluid and plasma in three intensive care patients. *Br J Anaesth* 65:829, 1990.

80. Dwersteg JF, Pavlin EG, Heimbach DM: Patients with burns are resistant to atracurium. *Anesthesiology* 65:517, 1986.

81. Marathe PH, Dwersteg JR, Pavlin EG, et al: Effect of thermal injury on the pharmacokinetics and pharmacodynamics of atracurium in humans. *Anesthesiology* 70:752, 1989.

82. Pavlin EG, Haschke RH, Marathe P, et al: Resistance to atracurium in thermally injured rats. *Anesthesiology* 69:696, 1988.

83. Shanks CA, Avram MJ, Fragen RJ, et al: Pharmacokinetics and pharmacodynamics of vecuronium administered by bolus and infusion during halothane or balanced anesthesia. *Clin Pharmacol Ther* 42:459, 1987.

84. Beattie WS, Buckley DN, Forrest JB: Continuous infusions of atracurium and vecuronium, compared with intermittent boluses of pancuronium: Dose requirements and reversal. *Can J Anaesth* 39:925, 1992.

85. Miller RD, Way WL, Dolan WM, et al: The dependence of pancuronium and d-tubocurarine induced neuromuscular blockades on alveolar concentrations of halothane and forane. *Anesthesiology* 37:573, 1972.

86. Stanski DR, Ham J, Miller RD, et al: Pharmacokinetics and pharmacodynamics of d-tubocurarine during nitrous-oxide and halothane anesthesia in man. *Anesthesiology* 51:235, 1979.

87. Beemer GH, Bjorksten AR, Crankshaw DP: Pharmacokinetics of atracurium during continuous infusion. *Br J Anaesth* 65:668, 1990.

88. Culling RD, Middaugh RE, Menk EJ: Rapid tracheal intubation with vecuronium: The timing principle. *J Clin Anesth* 1:422, 1989.

89. Ginsberg B, Glass PS, Quill T, et al: Onset and duration of neuromuscular blockade following high-dose vecuronium administration. *Anesthesiology* 71:201, 1989.

90. Clyburn PA, Marshall RD: Control of ventilation by continuous infusion of pancuronium bromide. *Anaesthesia* 36:860, 1981.

91. Fitzpatrick KTJ, Black GW, Crean PM, et al: Continuous vecuronium infusion for prolonged muscle relaxation in children. *Can J Anaesth* 38:169, 1991.

92. Rowlands DE: Atracurium in the elderly. *Br J Anaesth* 58:39S, 1986.

93. McCarthy G, Elliott P, Mirakhur RK, et al: Onset and duration of action of vecuronium in the elderly: Comparison with adults. *Acta Anaesthesiol Scand* 36:383, 1992.

94. Lien CA, Matteo RS, Ornstein E, et al: Distribution, elimination, and action of vecuronium in the elderly. *Anesth Analg* 73:39, 1991.

95. McLeod K, Hull C, Watson M: Effects of aging on the pharmacokinetics of pancuronium. *Br J Anaesth* 51:435, 1979.

96. Hunter JM, Parker CJR, Bell CF, et al: The use of different doses of vecuronium in patients with liver dysfunction. *Br J Anaesth* 57:758, 1985.

97. Martyn JAJ, Szyfelbein SK, Ali HH, et al: Increased d-tubocurarine requirement following major thermal injury. *Anesthesiology* 52:352, 1980.

98. Martyn J, Goldhill DR, Goudsouzian NG: Clinical pharmacology of muscle relaxants in patients with burns. *J Clin Pharmacol* 26:680, 1986.

99. Coursin DB, Klasek G, Goelzer SL: Increased requirements for continuously infused vecuronium in critically ill patients. *Anesth Analg* 69:518, 1989.

100. Martyn JAJ, White DA, Gronert GA, et al: Up-and-down regulation of skeletal muscle acetylcholine receptors: Effects on neuromuscular blockers. *Anesthesiology* 76:822, 1992.

101. Chapple D, Dodd P, Macleod D: Requirements for blocking agents during prolonged anesthesia in the anesthetized dog. *Br J Anaesth* 59:1321, 1987.

102. Brazil OV, Prado-Franceschi J: The nature of neuromuscular block

produced by neomycin and gentamicin. *Arch Int Pharmacodyn* 179:78, 1969.

103. Sokoll MD, Gergis SD: Antibiotics and neuromuscular function. *Anesthesiology* 55:148, 1981.

104. Chen J, Kim YD, Dubois M, et al: The increased requirement of pancuronium in neurosurgical patients receiving dilantin chronically. *Anesthesiology* 59:A288, 1983.

105. Hickey DR, Sangwan S, Bevan JC: Phenytoin-induced resistance to pancuronium. *Anaesthesia* 43:757, 1988.

106. Tempelhoff R, Modica PA, Jellish WS, et al: Resistance to atracurium-induced neuromuscular blockade in patients with intractable seizure disorders treated with anticonvulsants. *Anesth Analg* 71:665, 1990.

107. Gray HSJ, Slater RM, Pollard BJ: The effect of acutely administered phenytoin on vecuronium-induced neuromuscular blockade. *Anaesthesia* 44:379, 1989.

108. Hansen-Flaschen J, Cowen J, Raps EC: Neuromuscular blockade in the intensive care unit: More than we bargained for. *Am Rev Respir Dis* 147:234, 1993.

109. Danon MJ, Carpenter S: Myopathy with thick filament (myosin) loss following prolonged paralysis with vecuronium during steroid treatment. *Muscle Nerve* 14:1131, 1991.

110. Topulos GP: Neuromuscular blockade in adult intensive care. *New Horizons* 1:447, 1993.

111. Matsuo S, Rao DBS, Chaudry I, et al: Interaction of muscle relaxants and local anesthetics at the neuromuscular junction. *Anesth Analg* 57:580, 1978.

112. Wood GG: Cyclosporine-vecuronium interaction. *Can J Anaesth* 36:358, 1989.

113. Dretchen KL, Morgenroth VH III, Standaert FG, et al: Azathioprine: Effects on neuromuscular transmission. *Anesthesiology* 45:604, 1976.

114. Waud BE, Farrell L, Waud DR: Lithium and neuromuscular transmission. *Anesth Analg* 61:399, 1982.

115. Law SC, Ramzan IM, Brandom BW, et. al: Intravenous ranitidine antagonizes intense atracurium-induced neuromuscular blockade in rats. *Anesth Analg* 69:611, 1989.

116. McCarthy G, Mirakhur RK, Elliott P, et al: Effect of H2-receptor antagonist pretreatment on vecuronium and atracurium induced neuromuscular block. *Br J Anaesth* 66:713, 1991.

117. Roth S, Ebrahim ZY: Resistance to pancuronium in patients receiving carbamazepine. *Anesthesiology* 65:691, 1987.

118. Ornstein E, Matteo RS, Schwartz AE, et al: The effect of phenytoin on the magnitude and duration of neuromuscular block following atracurium or vecuronium. *Anesthesiology* 67:191, 1987.

119. Doll DC, Rosenberg H: Antagonism of neuromuscular blockage by theophylline. *Anesth Analg* 58:139, 1979.

120. Durant NN, Nguyen N, Katz RL: Potentiation of neuromuscular blockade by verapamil. *Anesthesiology* 60:298, 1984.

121. Azar I, Cottrell J, Gupta B, et al: Furosemide facilitates recovery of evoked twitch response after pancuronium. *Anesth Analg* 59:55, 1980.

122. Scappaticci KA, Ham JA, Sohn YJ, et al: Effects of furosemide on the neuromuscular junction. *Anesthesiology* 57:381, 1982.

123. Huang KC, Heise A, Shrader AK, et al: Vancomycin enhances the neuromuscular blockade of vecuronium. *Anesth Analg* 71:194, 1990.

124. Savarese JJ, Ali HH, Basta SJ, et al: The clinical neuromuscular pharmacology of mivacurium chloride (BW B1090U). *Anesthesiology* 68:723, 1988.

125. Matteo RS, Backus WW, McDaniel DD, et al: Pharmacokinetics and pharmacodynamics of *d*-tubocurarine and metocurine in the elderly. *Anesth Analg* 64:23, 1985.

126. Caldwell JE, Castagnoli KP, Canfell PC, et al: Pipecuronium and pancuronium: Comparison of pharmacokinetics and duration of action. *Br J Anaesth* 61:693, 1988.

127. Faulds D, Clissold SP: Doxacurium: A review of its pharmacology and clinical potential in anaesthesia. *Drugs* 42:673, 1991.

209. Sedative Agents

Lori L. Hoey, Avi Nahum, and Kyle Vance-Bryan

Introduction

Most mechanically ventilated intensive care unit (ICU) patients and many nonventilated patients require sedation to control anxiety, minimize distress during uncomfortable procedures, and attenuate the physiologic responses to stress, such as tachycardia and hypertension. Severely agitated and/or delirious patients pose a significant risk of self-harm by interruption of medical care (i.e., self-extubation, dislodgement of cardiac pacing wires or intravascular catheters). In addition, agitation may result in hemodynamic alterations associated with angina, heart failure, and cardiac arrhythmias by increasing myocardial work and oxygen consumption. Sedation is a vital component of the treatment plan for the critically ill patient experiencing agitation or difficulty with mechanical ventilation.

In the past, heavy or complete sedation was common to facilitate different aspects of mechanical ventilation. Today, depth of sedation for the mechanically ventilated patient is titrated to achieve a clinical endpoint that may allow some degree of spontaneous breathing. Complete sedation has several disadvantages over partial sedation, including respiratory muscle atrophy and prolonged weaning secondary to sedation.

All of the potential complications of coma (i.e., deep venous thrombosis, compression injuries to peripheral nerves, and infection) are more likely to occur with complete sedation [1]. Titration to the level of sedation that optimizes alertness and responsiveness should minimize the incidence of such adverse effects.

Drugs used for ICU sedation have changed over the years from barbiturates to benzodiazepines and several new agents. Benzodiazepines quickly gained popularity for the treatment of agitation in the ICU due to their efficacy and more favorable safety profile compared to the barbiturates. Several benzodiazepines commonly used in the ICU are diazepam, lorazepam, and midazolam. Originally diazepam was most commonly employed, but because of its prolonged terminal elimination half-life($t_{1/2}$) and the presence of active metabolites, newer agents with shorter half-lives, such as lorazepam, are more commonly used today. Lorazepam is unique because it is metabolized to inactive metabolites and has an intermediate half-life. Midazolam offers the advantages of a rapid onset of action, enhanced water solubility, and a very short half-life; a disadvantage is that it may accumulate with long-term use.

An example of the nonbenzodiazepine agents used for sedation in the ICU is propofol, a short-acting intravenous anesthetic with rapid onset and offset sedative properties. Isoflurane is an anesthetic agent that in preliminary studies has shown sedative effects equivalent to those of midazolam and propofol. Several adjunctive agents are used to optimize sedation of the critically ill patient. Haloperidol is used primarily when delirium is a significant component of agitation. Flumazenil is a benzodiazepine antagonist used to reverse undesired sedation associated with prior benzodiazepine administration. Finally, since pain is not uncommon in the ICU patient, analgesic agents with sedative properties can be used to provide or enhance sedation associated with concurrently administered sedative agents. Morphine and fentanyl are the primary analgesic agents used for sedation in the ICU. The pharmacokinetics/pharmacodynamics of analgesic agents are covered elsewhere in this text.

This chapter addresses the relevant drug administration and pharmacokinetic aspects of sedative agents currently used to manage the ICU patient. No single sedative regimen is suitable for all ICU patients. The pharmacokinetic disposition of these drugs may be markedly altered in hypermetabolic and hypometabolic patients; therefore individualization of dosing is required. A knowledge of the basic principles influencing sedative drug disposition in critically ill patients enables the development of an optimal therapeutic plan.

Benzodiazepines

Benzodiazepines are well suited to the ICU because of their hypnotic, anxiolytic, and amnestic properties. They do not have any analgesic properties but may reduce the intensity of painful stimuli by decreasing apprehension. These agents are frequently used for prolonged sedation because they have minor effects on the respiratory and cardiovascular system, elimination of concomitant drugs, and adrenocortical function. Several benzodiazepines are available, each with distinct pharmacokinetic parameters. Differences between the agents include terminal half-life route of hepatic metabolism (oxidation versus glucuronidation), presence or absence of metabolites, and extent of protein binding. A particular agent may be more advantageous in the presence of a hyperdynamic or hypodynamic state.

Here we focus on selected agents most commonly used in the ICU (Table 209-1). Diazepam is the widely used prototype benzodiazepine, but it may have disadvantages in the ICU due to a long half-life and metabolism of the parent compound resulting in production of active metabolites. These metabolites may accumulate with long-term use and predispose the patient to undesirable periods of prolonged sedation. Chlordiazepoxide is another benzodiazepine with a long elimination half-life and active metabolites; it is used primarily as a sedative for the management of alcohol withdrawal. In contrast to diazepam and chlordiazepoxide, lorazepam may offer an advantage in the ICU because it has a shorter half-life and no active metabolites. Lorazepam's pharmacokinetics are not affected by age or hepatic failure, unlike the longer-acting agents; therefore it may be a good choice in the critically ill patient. Midazolam has gained much popularity in the ICU because it has a very short half-life and is water-soluble, in contrast to the benzodiazepines mentioned above. Midazolam may be useful when rapid recovery from sedation is needed, as in patients requiring frequent neurologic evaluation, patients being weaned from mechanical ventilation, or during brief invasive procedures.

Table 209-1. Benzodiazepines Most Commonly Used in the ICU

	Chlordiazepoxide	Diazepam	Lorazepam	Midazolam
Bioavailability	100%	100%	90%	N/A
Time to effect				
PO	1–3 hr	1–3 hr	1–3 hr	N/A
IV	1–5 min	1–5 min	1–5 min	1–5 min
Protein binding	96%	98%	85%	95–100%
V_d	0.25–0.5 L/kg	1–2 L/kg	1–3 L/kg	0.5–1.5 L/kg
Clearance	0.25–0.5 ml/min/kg	25–40 ml/min	1 ml/min/kg	6–8 ml/min/kg
Hemodialysis	Not dialyzed	Not dialyzed	Not dialyzed	Not dialyzed
Elimination half-life	5–30 hr	20–50 hr	10–20 hr	3–26 hr
Metabolic pathway	Oxidation	Oxidation	Conjugation	Oxidation
Clinically significant metabolites	Demoxepam, desmethyl-chlordiazepoxide	Desmethyldiazepam	None	1-hydroxymethyl-midazolam
Physiologic parameters	Low intrinsic clearance	Low intrinsic clearance	Enhanced lorazepam clearance in burn patients; increased half-life in hepatic dysfunction	Metabolic clearance dependent on hepatic blood flow and intrinsic clearance; circadian effect may result in increased midazolam levels
Factors influencing pharmacokinetics	Increased V_d & half-life with age and liver disease; females have increased V_d	Increased V_d & half-life in cirrhotics & elderly; increased V_d in females	Gender, age, or renal dysfunction do not influence pharmacokinetics	Increased half-life in elderly, hepatic, and renal dysfunction
Equivalent dose (approx)	10 mg	4 mg	1 mg	1 mg

N/A = not available

PHARMACOLOGY. Benzodiazepines have anxiolytic, hypnotic, anticonvulsant, muscle relaxant, and antegrade amnestic properties. The exact sites and mode of action of the benzodiazepines are unknown; however, they appear to act at the limbic, thalamic, and hypothalamic levels of the central nervous system (CNS). The clinical effects of benzodiazepines may be mediated through the inhibitory neurotransmitter gamma-aminobutyric acid (GABA).

Anxiolytic effects are thought to occur through an increase of the glycine inhibitory neurotransmitter [2]. After several days of benzodiazepine therapy, a decrease in rapid eye movement (REM), stage 3, and stage 4 sleep occurs. An REM rebound does not occur when benzodiazepines are discontinued. The hypnotic effect of benzodiazepines is believed to be related to GABA accumulation and occupation of a benzodiazepine receptor.

Benzodiazepine receptors are mainly in the CNS, which may explain the relative absence of non-CNS effects [3]. It is thought that separate benzodiazepine and GABA receptors coupled to a common ionophore (chloride) channel become simultaneously occupied and produce membrane hyperpolarization and neuronal inhibition. The result is interference with GABA reuptake and thus accumulation of GABA, which causes hypnosis.

The skeletal muscle relaxation associated with benzodiazepine therapy appears to occur through inhibition of spinal polysynaptic afferent pathways but may also involve inhibition of monosynaptic afferent pathways. This is postulated to occur through inhibition of the neuronal transmitters or excitatory synaptic transmission. Direct depression of motor nerve and muscle function may also occur with benzodiazepines, mediated through glycine receptors in the spinal cord [2].

Anticonvulsant activity in animals has been shown to occur through augmentation of presynaptic inhibition. Enhancement of GABA's action on the motor circuits of the brain may explain the anticonvulsant properties [2]. Benzodiazepines suppress the spread of seizure activity but do not abolish the abnormal discharge from an epileptic focus. Benzodiazepines affect electroencephalograph (EEG) readings and in low doses result in decreases in the percentage of alpha activity and increases in the prevalence of beta waves over 18 Hz [4]. After administration of higher doses of benzodiazepines, theta and delta activity predominate. These EEG effects are characteristic for anxiolytic sedatives [5].

LORAZEPAM. Lorazepam (Ativan) has a moderately long half-life and is commonly used as a sedative in the ICU. Because lorazepam is metabolized via glucuronidation to an inactive metabolite, it may offer advantages over some of the benzodiazepines that are metabolized via oxidation (e.g., diazepam), as in critically ill patients requiring extended sedation and the elderly population. Because hepatic dysfunction generally affects oxidation much sooner than glucuronidation, lorazepam may be a better choice in patients with evidence of mild hepatic dysfunction.

Therapeutic Range. There are very few data evaluating the use of lorazepam in the ICU. The only published study was done in a respiratory ICU and evaluated the safety and efficacy of the drug after intermittent intravenous administration of 4 mg every 4 to 6 hours [6]. Clinically, the sedative effects of lorazepam have a linear correlation with serum concentration [7]. The duration and frequency of anterograde amnesia are also influenced by lorazepam dose, but the dosage requirements for amnesia do not necessarily correlate with those providing sedation [8–11]. The peak concentrations obtained after

doses of 2 mg and 4 mg are approximately 20 to 30 and 40 to 50 mg per milliliter, respectively [12,13].

Preparations. Lorazepam is available as oral tablets in strengths of 0.5 mg, 1 mg, and 2 mg as well as a 2 mg per milliliter oral concentration solution that contains polyethylene glycol and propylene glycol as additives. A parenteral formulation is available for intramuscular or intermittent intravenous administration. The parenteral injection is available as a 2 or 4 mg per milliliter formulation that contains 2% benzyl alcohol, polyethylene glycol 400, and propylene glycol to solubilize the lorazepam. Although lorazepam may be administered as a large volume parenteral by continuous intravenous infusion, few published data support the safety and efficacy of this route.

Pharmacokinetics

ABSORPTION. Although lorazepam undergoes significant enterohepatic recirculation when administered orally [14], the absolute bioavailability is approximately 90 percent. Peak plasma concentrations occur within 2 hours after an oral dose is administered [12,15,16]. The rate of lorazepam absorption after intramuscular administration depends on blood flow to the injection site. The deltoid muscles receive relatively high blood flow; therefore peak plasma levels generally occur 1.5 hours following injection [12]. Injection into areas of lower blood flow results in a longer time to achieve peak plasma levels [17]. After intramuscular administration mean absorption half-life values are 20 minutes or less, with mean systemic availability of greater than 90 percent [18]. Intravenous lorazepam has a rapid onset of sedative-hypnotic activity (1–2 minutes) [19] with maximum plasma concentrations and activity generally attained in 30 minutes [20].

The rate of uptake of the various benzodiazepine derivatives into the cerebrospinal fluid (CSF) may determine the clinical response [21,22]. The rates of onset for clinical effects are as follows: diazepam, midazolam > chlordiazepoxide > lorazepam. The slightly longer onset of action for lorazepam compared to other benzodiazepines may be explained by a slow penetration through the blood-brain barrier [23–28]. Very low levels of unconjugated CSF lorazepam compared to its serum protein binding support a slow and incomplete penetration through the blood-CSF barrier [23]. On the contrary, others have reported that lorazepam peak brain tissue concentrations occur 10 minutes after serum peak concentrations [29,30,31]. In Greenblatt and co-workers' study, although peak plasma concentrations were obtained immediately after IV administration of both low- and high-dose (0.025 and 0.045 mg/kg, respectively), EEG effects were not maximal until 30 minutes after initiation of the infusion [27].

DISTRIBUTION. Lorazepam is widely distributed into body tissues, including the CNS. Lorazepam is extensively bound to albumin, with a free fraction of 8 to 12 percent. The volume of distribution (V_d) in healthy volunteers is 1.0 to 1.3 liters per kilogram [32].

ELIMINATION. Lorazepam is primarily eliminated via hepatic biotransformation to lorazepam glucuronide, an inactive, nontoxic metabolite eliminated by the kidney [12,16,24,33]. Less than 1 percent of lorazepam is excreted unchanged in the urine [24,34]. Lorazepam elimination after a single intravenous dose is a biphasic process. Initially, a rapid decline in plasma levels occurs as a drug is distributed into the peripheral tissues. Following distribution, the plasma concentration curve enters a slower phase representing elimination [15].

The mean elimination half-life of lorazepam is approximately 21 hours (range 9–32 hours) in healthy individuals [12,16,18,

35,36]. The values for accumulation half-life for lorazepam are essentially unchanged between single and multiple dosage [35,37]. Mean total clearance of lorazepam is approximately 1.0 ml/min/kg [15]. The elimination half-life of lorazepam after ingestion of large doses is essentially unchanged from that for usual therapeutic doses. The biotransformation of lorazepam to the active glucuronide metabolite after administration of large doses does not appear to be a saturable process [38].

Physiologic Clearance Characteristics. As a parent compound lorazepam is almost completely biotransformed to the conjugated metabolite 3-glucuronide; systemic clearance reflects the overall metabolic activity in the involved organs (i.e., total intrinsic clearance) [7,39,40,41]. Plasma binding and free intrinsic clearance approximate the clearance from tissue water [42]. Lorazepam has a low hepatic extraction ratio, therefore, due to first-pass metabolism, only a fraction (7–10%) of an orally administered dose fails to reach the systemic circulation [43].

HYPERDYNAMIC PATIENTS. Benzodiazepine metabolism via oxidation (e.g., diazepam) is significantly impaired in the burn patient population [44,45]. In contrast, the degradation of lorazepam, which undergoes mainly hepatic glucuronidation, is not impaired and may even be enhanced in burn patients. On days 8 through 28 after injury, burn patients with mean percent body surface area burn of 42.6 have increased V_d and clearance of lorazepam, with significant reductions in elimination half-life [46]. Although the free fraction of lorazepam is increased in burn patients, they usually have decreased serum and total protein concentration and altered drug binding. This suggests that the enhanced lorazepam clearance in burn patients is not an artifact of an increased free drug fraction [46].

HYPODYNAMIC PATIENTS. Multiple system organ failure may alter lorazepam disposition, depending on the organ systems involved. Lorazepam elimination is not altered by age or renal disease [36,39]. Although there are reports of renal failure patients with a prolonged lorazepam elimination half-life, the alterations are in distribution rather than elimination rate, since clearance is not reduced in these patients [47]. As renal function decreases. clearance does not change while the lorazepam V_d increases [48]. In contrast, the pharmacokinetics of the glucuronide metabolite are markedly affected by renal dysfunction. Because the glucuronide is pharmacologically inactive and nontoxic, accumulation in renal dysfunction appears to be clinically unimportant [36,48]. Hemodialysis has minimal effects on the systemic clearance of lorazepam [36,48].

Although the glucuronidation pathway is less sensitive to hepatic diseases than oxidation, lorazepam may be affected by significant hepatic dysfunction. Hepatic diseases may also result in changes in plasma protein binding, which, depending on the extent of change, may affect systemic clearance and distribution of total lorazepam [15,39,49]. Cirrhosis has been associated with a prolonged lorazepam elimination half-life, attributed to an increase in free lorazepam. Acute viral hepatitis may result in similar findings, but additional study is necessary to confirm this [39].

Although lorazepam may have a slightly smaller V_d in the elderly (aged >60 years), elimination half-life is not influenced by age [16]. Clinically, lorazepam's effects appear unaltered in the elderly [39,50]. In addition, gender does not appear to alter lorazepam kinetics [51].

Dosing Guidelines. Little information is available in regard to the appropriate dosing of lorazepam in the critically ill patient. Sedative doses have ranged from 0.03 to 0.07 mg per kilogram or 2 to 4 mg every 4 to 6 hours by intermittent intravenous injection [6,11]. Initial loading and maintenance doses may be safely initiated in this range. Because lorazepam has an intermediate half-life it is most often administered by intermittent intravenous injection. A potential advantage of this route is that it allows assessment of the need for further sedation prior to administration of the next dose. Continuous infusion has also been used, but this method of administration is not approved by the FDA and data in support of this method from clinical trials with critically ill patients have not been reported.

Drug Interaction. Few drug interactions occur with lorazepam because, unlike most benzodiazepines, it bypasses the hepatic oxidation step. For example, there is no interaction between lorazepam and cimetidine; this is in contrast to many of the benzodiazepines that undergo hepatic oxidation [18,52]. Lorazepam produces additive pharmacodynamic effects on the CNS when used in combination with other CNS depressants, such as narcotic analgesics and anticonvulsants.

Pitfalls of Management. Failure to correlate anticipated pharmacodynamic effect with administration time may result in over- or underdosing. Sedation (fatigue, drowsiness, lethargy), dizziness, ataxia, muscle weakness, and impaired mental function are dose-related adverse effects [53]. Paradoxical stimulation, confusion, and blurred vision have also been reported [15]. As a benzodiazepine, lorazepam has the potential to produce chemical dependence [15], but this is unlikely to occur during the short duration of use in the ICU. Prolonged administration (several weeks) may require tapering rather than abrupt discontinuation to avoid withdrawal seizures.

Problems may arise if one fails to consider the pharmaceutical excipients in the commercial preparation of lorazepam, because it contains propylene glycol as a vehicle. Propylene glycol may result in hypotension on infusion. Since propylene glycol is metabolized to lactic acid, at high doses acidosis may develop [54]. In addition, IM injection of lorazepam may produce discomfort, muscle irritation, and, occasionally, phlebitis due to the propylene glycol [15].

MIDAZOLAM. Midazolam (Versed) is a short-acting, water-soluble benzodiazepine. Indications for midazolam include use as an intramuscular premedicant, an intravenous induction agent for general anesthesia, and an intravenous agent for conscious sedation prior to short diagnostic or endoscopic procedures. In the ICU, continuous intravenous infusion of midazolam is used to provide relief from anxiety and agitation as well as to provide amnesia. Midazolam may offer an advantage over longer acting benzodiazepines (i.e., diazepam, chlordiazepoxide, lorazepam) when a prolonged sedative effect is undesirable.

Therapeutic Range. After short-term infusion, the clinical effect of midazolam, as measured by a sedation index, can be correlated with plasma concentrations (r = 0.73–0.97) [55]. This is despite large interpatient variability in midazolam steady-state serum concentrations. Concentrations of 40 ng per milliliter appear to be the threshold for efficacy. Hypnotic activity is present at concentrations above 80 ng per milliliter, and at concentrations above 100 ng per milliliter patients are drowsy but arousable. After long-term infusions, plasma levels producing a sedative effect are much higher, at times ranging greater than 1000 ng per milliliter [56,57]. Considerable interpatient variation exists even when plasma concentrations and free fractions of midazolam are similar. One explanation may involve variable penetration into the CSF and/or the number or affinity of the benzodiazepine receptors in the brain [58,59]. Serum levels of midazolam and metabolites during infusion provide limited clinically useful information. While no correlation has been defined between plasma midazolam concentrations and time of awakening following infusion, some data suggest that plasma concentrations of 1-hydroxy midazolam (1-OH mida- zolam), an active midazolam metabolite, in the range of 20 to 40 ng per milliliter are associated with awakening [60].

In critically ill patients, midazolam's EEG effects show a rel- atively fast (alpha or beta) frequency activity superimposed on delta slowing, alpha frequency coma pattern, transient burst suppression pattern, and spindle coma, effects similar to those seen with other benzodiazepines [61,62]. Electroencephalo- graphic measurements of the effects of the hydroxy metabolite suggest it has potent activity and may contribute significantly to the effects of midazolam [63].

Attempts have been made to correlate plasma midazolam concentration with EEG wake activity [64,65]. High-dose mid- azolam results in burst suppression and some spindle coma patterns consistent with CNS depression [66].

Preparations. Midazolam is water-soluble and available in a parenteral formulation for intramuscular or slow intravenous injection. Continuous intravenous infusion for ICU sedation is not FDA-approved but is commonly used. Intraarterial injection or extravasation of midazolam should be avoided. Midazolam maleate is an oral dosage form currently not available in the United States. Each milliliter of the parenteral formulation con- tains midazolam hydrochloride equivalent to 1 or 5 mg of mid- azolam compounded with 0.8% sodium chloride and 0.01% disodium acetate, and 1% benzyl alcohol as preservative; the pH is adjusted to 3 with hydrochloric acid. If administered intramuscularly, midazolam should be injected deep into the muscle. For intravenous administration midazolam may be di- luted with 0.9% sodium chloride injection or 5% dextrose injec- tion. Intravenous boluses should be administered slowly over at least 2 minutes. Intravenous boluses do not require dilution prior to administration. Midazolam doses and rate of adminis- tration should be reduced in patients who are older or debili- tated, those with chronic diseases (e.g., congestive heart fail- ure), and those with reduced pulmonary reserve. Depression of respiration may occur with midazolam injection, especially at higher doses (0.1–0.15 mg/kg), and may result in hypoven- tilation or apnea.

Pharmacokinetics

ABSORPTION. Midazolam is 80 to 100 percent absorbed after an intramuscular injection [20]. Due to midazolam's lipophilic properties, it is rapidly absorbed from the deltoid muscle, with mean peak plasma concentrations occurring within 0.38 to 0.69 hour [67]. Intramuscular peak concentrations of midazolam generally are one-half those seen with equivalent intravenous doses. The rapid response to midazolam cannot be explained by rapid passage into the human lumbar CSF [59]; this is in contrast to benzodiazepines such as diazepam and lorazepam [23,68] for which CSF penetration has been correlated with onset of effect.

DISTRIBUTION. Midazolam's V_d is approximately 0.5 to 1.5 liter per kilogram [55,69–72]. The V_d varies highly with plasma al- bumin concentrations in the critically ill patient [73] and may increase 1.5- to 3.0-fold in patients with chronic renal failure or congestive heart failure [74]. The V_d is larger in women than in men, in obese than in nonobese patients, in supine than in ambulant patients, and in elderly than in young patients [70,75,76,77].

Midazolam is highly protein-bound to albumin (95–100%) [55,70]. Subsequently, the drug is found in low concentrations in the CSF [59,78]. The free fraction of midazolam is higher in

patients with liver cirrhosis and patients with chronic renal failure, which leads to larger V_d values and higher clearance rates when total drug (bound and free) is evaluated [79].

ELIMINATION. Midazolam is hepatically metabolized by the cy- tochrome P-450 III A4 enzymes via hydroxylation and subse- quent conjugation with glucuronic acid [55,80]. Extrahepatic metabolism of midazolam has been demonstrated in patients undergoing liver transplantation during the anhepatic period [81]. 1-OH midazolam, the principal metabolite, is active but shows much less activity than the parent drug and has a shorter elimination half-life (45 minutes) [69,82,83]. 1-OH midazolam usually does not contribute to the clinical activity of midazolam because it is rapidly conjugated with a glucuronide and ex- creted as an inactive compound by the kidney [69,83]. Very small amounts of two other metabolites, 4-hydroxymidazolam and alpha 4-dihydroxymidazolam, are also excreted in the urine (3% and 1%, respectively) [69]. Excretion of unchanged mida- zolam in the urine is negligible (< 1%) [19,84,85].

Midazolam has a short half-life (range 1–4 hours) and is rap- idly cleared (6–8 ml/min/kg) after single-dose administration and after discontinuation of continuous intravenous infusion in normal volunteers without evidence of altered renal, hepatic, or tissue binding changes [58,70,71,72,86]. The elimination half- life varies in critically ill patients. In those without evidence of organ dysfunction or protein binding changes, elimination half- life may be as short as 4 to 12 hours with continuous infusion with no prolonged sedation after discontinuation [87]. With pro- longed administration of midazolam, the elimination half-life may vary between 3 and 26 hours [56,69,79,86]. Impaired mid- azolam elimination in critically ill patients has been attributed to a larger V_d [88]. However, a variety of other reasons, such as decreased hepatic perfusion and metabolic capacity, fluid shifts, altered protein binding, pharmacogenetic abnormalities, and the effects of concomitant medication, may contribute as well [79,89]. Altered pharmacokinetics may lead to unwanted cu- mulative effects, although the development of tolerance to the central effects of benzodiazepines during continuous infusion may counteract these effects [78].

A large interindividual variation in midazolam pharmaco- kinetics exists in the critically ill patient as judged by the ratio of midazolam to total 1-OH midazolam [57,87]. After long-term infusion of midazolam to patients with kidney dysfunction, ac- cumulation of the hydroxymetabolites may alter the plasma ratio of midazolam and 1-OH-midazolam. When the renal ex- cretion of 1-OH-midazolam is inhibited, deglucuronization is more apparent, with increasing plasma concentrations of 1-OH- midazolam. The sedative effects of midazolam may be more pronounced if 1-OH-midazolam accumulates.

Midazolam may accumulate after repeated dosages [60]. The intra- and interindividual variations in midazolam pharmaco- kinetics make it difficult to predict which critically ill patients will accumulate midazolam. For some patients the sedative ef- fects may persist several days after discontinuation [89]. Be- cause it is uncertain which patients will have longer elimination half-lives, it is difficult to predict which patients will accumulate the drug [56,57,69,79,86]. Although some studies have reported a lack of accumulation when midazolam is administered by continuous intravenous infusion, these studies did not include patients with altered hepatic, renal, cardiac, or neurologic func- tion [90,91]. The prolonged effects of midazolam in some criti- cally ill patients may be due to altered hepatic blood flow or impaired metabolic capacity of the P-450-CYP3A4 hepatic en- zyme system [89,92,93].

Consideration of the attributes of specific subpopulations may predict some of the variations in midazolam pharmacoki- netics. These alterations may result from changes in midazolam half-life and/or V_d. Midazolam's elimination half-life is prolonged in older patients and those undergoing major operations [76,92]. The pharmacologically active metabolite, 1-OH midazolam, has a prolonged elimination half-life in elderly men and women [67]. With short-term use, midazolam pharmacokinetics are essentially unchanged between younger and older women [67,75]; small increases in V_d may occur in older women without a change in elimination half-life [67,75]. There are significant age-related differences in the elimination and clearance of midazolam in men [70]. The age-related and gender differences in midazolam have been reported for other benzodiazepines metabolized by the hepatic microsomal oxidation system [94]. The elderly have more extensive and rapid distribution of midazolam, which may explain the greater pharmacologic effects often seen in this group [70,95]. Obesity may result in a significant prolongation of midazolam half-life due to an increase in V_d [27].

Organ dysfunction may also alter the pharmacokinetics of midazolam. Patients with chronic renal failure (CRF) have significantly higher V_d and clearance of midazolam compared to normal subjects [72]. Protein binding is reduced, with significantly higher free fractions in CRF patients (6.5%) compared to healthy patients (3.9%). Correction for protein binding differences reveals no difference between V_d and clearance for unbound drug. Changes in hepatic function may influence midazolam pharmacokinetics as well [96,97].

Posture and circadian rhythm are important variables affecting blood flow-dependent hepatic elimination of midazolam [77]. Midazolam total blood clearance is relatively high at approximately 500 ml per minute (mean extraction ratio 0.34) or one-third of hepatic blood flow; therefore the major determinants for midazolam disposition are the rate of delivery of drug to the liver and the capacity of drug metabolizing systems [55]. Positional changes may influence hepatic blood flow significantly (40–60%); thus hepatic elimination of high clearance drugs such as midazolam may be altered.

Hypovolemia may reduce hepatic blood flow, thus decreasing drug clearance and prolonging pharmacologic action of midazolam [71]. The hypotensive and sedative effects of midazolam may be potentiated by volume depletion.

Physiologic Clearance Characteristics. Midazolam has a hepatic extraction ratio in the intermediate range of 30 to 70 percent; therefore metabolic clearance is determined by hepatic blood flow as well as intrinsic clearance [55,69,96,98,99]. Midazolam is highly protein-bound (>95%); like other benzodiazepines, however, but in contrast to diazepam, hepatic clearance is nonrestrictive, since the extraction ratio is higher than the free fraction [55]. This implies that bound and unbound drug may be degraded by the liver enzymes. Midazolam blood clearance averages 502 ml per minute [55], which represents approximately one-third of liver blood flow (Q = 1500 ml/min). This suggests that the hepatic extraction ratio (E) is high (0.34), even higher than the measured free fraction (0.06).

It is possible that some individuals may experience a circadian rhythm effect on the clearance of midazolam, resulting in higher plasma concentrations at night [58]. Fluctuations do not appear to be related to changes in protein binding but perhaps are a result of altered hepatic blood flow.

Dosing Guidelines. Midazolam dosing guidelines are quite variable due to the wide range of variability in pharmacokinetics among patients, particularly in the ICU patient. In studies evaluating critically ill patients, loading doses employed range from 0.05 to 0.5 mg per kilogram [57,90,100,101]. A conservative approach would be a loading dose of 0.05 to 0.1 mg per kilogram, which may be repeated if the desired effect is not obtained within a few minutes. Maintenance doses are highly variable, ranging from 0.025 to 0.212 mg/kg/hr [57,100,101]. A reasonable starting maintenance dose is 0.05 to 0.1 mg/kg/hr, depending on the patient's individual pharmacokinetic parameters and the severity of agitation. Therapy is initiated at a low infusion rate and titrated up to the desired effect, if necessary. Lower dosing should be used in the elderly, those with altered protein binding, and those with low cardiopulmonary reserve. In greater than 74 percent of critically ill patients a loading dose of 0.1 mg per kilogram followed by a maintenance dose of 0.1 to 0.2 mg/kg/hr provides adequate sedation [102]. If intermittent intramuscular dosing is used, it is important to consider absorption characteristics. After an intramuscular midazolam injection, the onset of effect may not appear for 15 minutes, with the peak effect usually occurring 30 to 60 minutes after injection.

Drug Interactions. Midazolam produces additive pharmacodynamic effects on the CNS when used in combination with other CNS depressants, such as narcotic analgesics and anticonvulsants. Midazolam may interact with cimetidine, resulting in increased midazolam pharmacologic effect.

Common Pitfalls. Failure to titrate midazolam to specific clinical endpoints may result in dose-dependent adverse effects, such as ataxia, dizziness, nystagmus, slurred speech, and amnesia. The effects on respiratory function are similar for all benzodiazepines, with a decrease in tidal volume, decrease in ventilation rate, and reduction in the ventilatory response to hypoxia.

Midazolam also has vasodilating properties [103]. Administration of small doses (0.05 mg/kg) or continuous intravenous infusions to patients with coronary artery disease does not, however, result in significant depression of the cardiovascular system [100,104]. Administration of anesthesia induction doses of midazolam (0.3 mg/kg) to patients undergoing coronary artery bypass surgery results in increased heart rate and decreased systemic arterial pressure and pulmonary artery pressure. The magnitude of these changes is not clinically significant [105]. During the postperfusion period of cardiopulmonary bypass surgery, midazolam's half-life increases (4.5 hours vs. 2 hours) while V_d remains unchanged. This suggests a slower metabolism of midazolam during the postperfusion period [106].

Benzodiazepine tolerance may develop even with short-term use of midazolam. This results in the need for progressively larger doses to achieve the same clinical endpoint. Increasing midazolam requirements to achieve the same degree of sedation signals the need to evaluate for the presence of tolerance [97]. Emergence of withdrawal symptoms after prolonged administration may complicate benzodiazepine tolerance [97]. Patients who have developed tolerance require longer periods of benzodiazepine taper to avoid withdrawal symptoms.

In critically ill patients, accumulation of midazolam prolongs time to awakening following cessation of a midazolam infusion. Accumulation may result in prolonged ventilation or difficulty in assessment of neurologic function. A benzodiazepine antagonist, such as flumazenil, may alleviate some of these problems. However, flumazenil administration may induce seizures in patients who have been on benzodiazepines chronically or in those undergoing treatment with other drugs that decrease the seizure threshold (e.g., tricyclic antidepressants).

PROPOFOL. Propofol (Diprivan) is an intravenous agent, originally approved for induction and maintenance of anesthesia, that was recently approved for ICU sedation. Propofol is useful for severely agitated patients. Its rapid onset and offset are advantages when neurologic assessment or rapid weaning from sedation is essential.

Pharmacology. Propofol is a 2,6-diisopropylphenol with sedative-hypnotic properties suitable for use in induction and maintenance of anesthesia or sedation. In rats, propofol induces EEG changes similar to those produced by rapid-acting barbiturates [107]. Burst suppression is produced at approximately the median hypnotic dose. Anticonvulsant activity has been documented in both animals and humans [108,109]. Controversy exists over the incidence of convulsive activity of propofol. There are more than 100 reports of seizurelike activity following propofol administration [110,111] and withdrawal seizures following discontinuation of propofol have also been reported [112]. In contrast, other studies report the successful use of propofol for the treatment of status epilepticus [113].

Therapeutic Range. A linear relationship exists between propofol blood concentration and duration of sleep [114,115]. A variation in response seen among individuals is most likely a result of interindividual variation in the distribution phase [115]. The anesthesia literature reports that propofol blood concentrations of 2 to 4 μg per milliliter provide adequate sedation for anesthesia, while at 1 μg per milliliter or less patients awaken [114–119]. For sedation of intensive care patients on mechanical ventilators the range of effective propofol concentrations is approximately 0.1 to 2.0 μg per milliliter [120].

Blood propofol concentrations have also been correlated with other effects. Systolic and diastolic blood pressures decrease with increasing blood propofol concentrations [117]. There may be a wide variability in patient specific blood pressure changes, with a 10 to 20 percent reduction in blood pressure not uncommon. Heart rate often remains unchanged and may be due to a resetting of the baroreceptor reflex setpoint by propofol [121]. Propofol blood concentrations also are correlated with EEG activity [122].

Preparations. Propofol exists as an oil at room temperature and is formulated as an emulsion to enable intravenous administration. It was originally formulated as a 2% solution containing 16% polyoxyethylated castor oil (Cremophor EL) and 8.66% ethyl alcohol. However, because this formulation was painful on injection and Cremophor EL was associated with anaphylactoid reactions, an alternative formulation of propofol in a 1% solution with 10% soybean oil, 2.25% glycerol, and 1.2% purified egg phosphatide is now available. The new formulation, in contrast to the old, has not been associated with histamine release [118,123,124]. Propofol should not be administered to patients with a known hypersensitivity to soybean oil, egg lecithin, or glycerol.

As is true with any emulsion, propofol must not be administered through filters with a pore size less than 5 μM. Propofol for injection is available in ready-to-use 20-ml ampules and 50-ml infusion vials containing 10 mg per milliliter of propofol. Again due to the emulsion formulation, extreme caution must be used when considering the compatibility of propofol with other products. Propofol has been shown to be compatible with the following intravenous fluids when administered into a running intravenous catheter: 5% dextrose (D), lactated Ringer's solution (LR), LR and 5% D, 5% D and 0.45% sodium chloride (SC), and 5% D and 0.2% SC.

Strict aseptic technique must be used when handling propofol because it does not contain antimicrobial preservatives.

Because vehicle can support rapid growth of microorganisms, propofol has a 6-hour expiration period after opening [125].

Pharmacokinetics

ABSORPTION. Propofol has a very rapid onset (within minutes) and a short duration of action after intravenous injection. Blood and brain concentrations of propofol decline rapidly after a single dose, due to extensive distribution and rapid elimination.

DISTRIBUTION. Propofol pharmacokinetic modeling studies have suggested a blood-brain equilibration half-life of approximately 2 minutes and a distribution half-life of 2 to 4 minutes [126,127]. The volume of the central compartment is between 22 and 55 liters and the V_d is 171 to 329 liters, indicating extensive distribution to the tissues [119,128,129]. Volumes of distribution during the terminal phase are two to three times those during the steady state, indicating that a small proportion of the dose is eliminated very slowly [130].

Propofol is highly plasma protein-bound (97–99%) and the extent of protein binding is similar in young and elderly patients [130]. Propofol crosses the placenta, achieving increasing concentrations in the fetus in a time-dependent fashion [122].

ELIMINATION/METABOLISM. Propofol undergoes extensive metabolism in the liver to produce inactive, water-soluble glucuronide and sulfate conjugates. After a single dose, unchanged propofol is recovered in less than 0.3 percent of the urine and less than 2 percent of the feces [131]. Clearance values equal or exceed hepatic blood flow, which suggests that extrahepatic metabolism and/or extrarenal elimination (i.e., via the lungs) may occur [126].

Propofol's elimination is best characterized using a three-compartment kinetic model, but two-compartment models have been used by some investigators [127,128,129,131–134]. When the three-compartment model is used, the first exponential phase (half-life 2–3 minutes) mirrors the rapid onset of action and the second half-life (34–56 minutes) that of the high metabolic clearance. The long third exponential phase (half-life 184–480 minutes) describes the slow elimination of a small amount of the drug remaining in poorly perfused tissues [122, 128,129,134].

Some investigators have suggested that propofol's long terminal elimination half-life may result in accumulation with long-term infusion [126,127]. Clinical experience with long-term propofol infusion, however, is still limited: Most studies have used continuous infusions for less than 24 hours [120,135]. Albanese et al. evaluated propofol for ICU sedation for 72 hours [136] and found that the termination half-life correlated strongly with the length of the sampling period [137]. They concluded that with long-term infusion the half-life is prolonged and the V_d is increased. However, other investigators have not substantiated these findings. In several studies, the pharmacokinetics in ICU patients during long-term sedation with continuous infusions of propofol have been similar to those seen with single-dose studies [103,139,140,141]. Propofol may produce dose-dependent reductions in systolic, diastolic, and mean arterial blood pressure of 15 to 30 percent [126]. This effect may be accentuated if it is used in combination with an opioid analgesic, in the elderly, in hypovolemic patients, or in those with impaired left ventricular function. At higher doses, propofol has been shown to decrease stroke volume, cardiac index, left ventricular stroke work index, and systemic vascular resistance. Decreases in myocardial blood flow and myocardial oxygen consumption have occurred, as has increased myocardial lactate production, in those with coronary artery disease.

Dosing Guidelines. For ICU sedation, propofol may be initiated at an infusion rate of 5 $\mu g/kg/min$. This rate may be increased by increments of 5 to 10 μg/kg/min every 5 to 10 minutes until the desired level of sedation is achieved. If desired, an initial bolus of 10 to 20 mg may be administered. Most adult patients require maintenance propofol infusion rates of 5 to 50 μg/kg/min to achieve adequate levels of sedation [102,116,120,135,136,138,139,140]. Patient monitoring should include vital signs, cardiac output, and pulmonary capillary wedge pressure when available. The infusion rate of propofol should be decreased if mild hypotension develops. For severe hypotension and/or cardiovascular depression, propofol should be discontinued. Wake-up assessments should be performed every 24 hours to ensure the minimal effective propofol infusion rate is employed. Abrupt discontinuation of propofol should be avoided; rather, the drug should be decreased by increments of 5 to 10 μg/kg/min every 10 to 15 minutes. Due to its rapid offset, propofol may be discontinued 15 minutes prior to extubation.

Pitfalls of Management. Green and red-brown urine color occurs during propofol infusion due to the quinol metabolites of propofol. The color is darkened with alkalinization of the urine [141].

Propofol infusions elevate triglyceride concentrations. Even with the lower infusion rates used for ICU sedation compared to anesthesia, problems may occur due to the emulsion lipid load and supplementation of a considerable amount of calories (1 cal/ml). A dosage range of 1 to 3 mg/kg/hr corresponds to approximately 300 to 500 ml of a 10% fat emulsion. Most patients can easily tolerate this amount, but when designing a nutrition regimen consideration of the lipid contribution of propofol is important. Serum cholesterol and triglyceride concentrations progressively increase as the duration of infusion and dosage increase [142]. Monitoring of serum triglyceride concentration is important to avoid the complications of fat overload. In addition, because propofol can support bacterial growth at the same rate as Intralipid 10%, aseptic technique should be used in preparation [125].

The possibility of tolerance development to propofol must be considered when increasing infusion rates are required over time [143]. High infusion rates may be problematic due to the volume of lipid necessary to achieve a therapeutic effect as well as the high cost of the drug.

HALOPERIDOL. Agitation associated with delirium frequently occurs in the intensive care patient. Rapid, effective treatment is usually necessary to facilitate the diagnosis and treatment of underlying medical problems and to prevent unnecessary morbidity. Disconnection of catheters, self-extubation, or difficulty in ventilating the patient may all contribute to morbidity [144]. Delirium is not adequately treated by administration of commonly used sedative agents; therefore, adjunctive use of haloperidol in these instances is beneficial.

Pharmacology. Haloperidol (Haldol) is a butyrophenone-derivative antipsychotic agent. The mechanism of antipsychotic action is unknown but may be a result of CNS depression at the subcortical level of the brain, midbrain, and brainstem reticular formation. Haloperidol may also inhibit the ascending reticular activating system of the brainstem, which interrupts the impulse between the diencephalon and the cortex. The drug may antagonize the actions of glutamic acid within the extrapyramidal system. Haloperidol may also inhibit catecholamine receptors and inhibit the reuptake of neurotransmitters in the brain. The drug has strong central antidopaminergic and weak central anticholinergic activity. It produces a ganglionic blockade and reduces affective responses. It also directly affects

the chemoreceptor trigger zone, which may be the mechanism of its antiemetic activity.

Therapeutic Range. There is no established therapeutic range for haloperidol used to treat delirium in an ICU patient. Serum concentrations of 3 to 20 ng per milliliter have been reported as therapeutic in several studies assessing antipsychotic activity [145]. Intravenous injection of 0.125 mg per kilogram produces peak serum concentrations of 15 to 50 ng per milliliter with marked sedation [146]. Haloperidol concentrations are detectable in the serum for several weeks after administration of a single dose.

Preparations. Available oral haloperidol preparations are solution containing 2 mg per milliliter, scored tablets containing 0.5, 1, 2, 5, 10, and 20 mg, and film-coated tablets in 0.5, 1, 2, and 5 mg. The oral solution or crushed tablets can be administered via a nasogastric tube.

Haloperidol for intramuscular administration is available in two formulations. Haloperiodol lactate contains 5 mg per milliliter and is available in preservative and preservative-free formulations. Haloperidol deconoate contains 50 mg per milliliter and is available in a sesame oil formulation, which allows slow release of the drug in a depot fashion. The deconoate formulation should be used only for patients requiring long-term antipsychotic therapy. Haloperidol lactate may be administered intramuscularly for acute treatment of delirium in the ICU patient.

Intravenous administration is not FDA approved, but there is substantial literature to support its safety and efficacy [147–158]. Haloperidol lactate containing 5 mg per milliliter may be administered intravenously. Haloperidol deconoate should not be administered intravenously.

Pharmacokinetics

ABSORPTION. After oral administration, haloperidol appears in the serum within 60 to 90 minutes, followed by peak serum concentrations in 2 to 6 hours. Oral haloperidol may undergo enterohepatic recirculation and immediate deactivation by the liver during initial transport from the portal system to the systemic circulation. This results in interindividual differences in bioavailability and effectiveness. The bioavailability of oral haloperidol is approximately 60 percent; therefore parenteral doses should be one-half to two-thirds the oral dose.

Following intramuscular administration of haloperidol lactate, rapid and complete absorption results in peak serum concentrations of haloperidol within 10 to 20 minutes and peak pharmacologic action within 30 to 45 minutes. Intravenous administration of haloperidol lactate results in immediate peak serum concentrations of haloperidol. Intravenous administration therefore allows rapid and titratable delivery without the problems associated with oral and intramuscular administration, such as unpredictable absorption of the drug due to impaired peripheral tissue perfusion and gastrointestinal dysfunction.

DISTRIBUTION. Haloperidol distribution into human body tissues and fluids has not been fully elucidated. In animal models, the drug is distributed mainly into the liver, with smaller concentrations reaching the brain, lungs, kidneys, spleen, and heart. Haloperidol is 92 percent bound to plasma proteins.

ELIMINATION. Haloperidol is principally metabolized in the liver via oxidative N-dealkylation and reduction. The reduced metabolite, hydroxyhaloperidol, may have some limited activity, but the other metabolites are inactive. Haloperidol and its metabolites are excreted into the urine and feces. Approximately 40 percent of a single oral dose is excreted in the urine and 15 percent in the feces within 5 days; small amounts of haloperidol continue to be excreted for approximately 28 days after a single dose. Dosages must be decreased in patients with significant hepatic dysfunction. No adjustment is necessary in patients with renal dysfunction.

Serum half-life averages 16 hours (range 12–22 hours), regardless of the route of administration (excluding the deconoate formulation). However, there does not appear to be a correlation between half-life and effect evidenced by the frequent dosing (i.e., every 2–4 hours) required by the delirious ICU patient.

Dosage and Administration. There is a large interindividual variability in dose response to haloperidol. An initial dose of 1 to 5 mg, given no faster than 5 mg per minute, is appropriate. The smaller doses may be initially used in elderly patients or those with hepatic dysfunction. Repeat doses may be administered every 20 to 30 minutes, with dosage adjusted according to the initial response. If agitation persists after administration, doubling each previous dose every 20 minutes has been recommended. Once the patient's agitation has been controlled, the dose that controlled the patient may be used in subsequent doses [159,160,161].

Intravenous administration of haloperidol lactate has been used without evidence of cardiovascular or respiratory difficulties even, at high doses (>100 mg/day) [147,162,163,164]. Both oral and intramuscular haloperidol have also been used without cardiovascular side effects in patients with cardiac dysrhythmias or cardiogenic shock [154,163]. Haloperidol, unlike the benzodiazepines and barbiturates, does not depress the medullary respiratory center and has no well-documented evidence of respiratory depression. Bedell and colleagues attempted to correlate a 2-mg intramuscular dose of haloperidol with the respiratory arrest of an 80-year-old woman, but others believed the arrest was more likely the result of undersedation [165,166].

Drug Interactions. Haloperidol may potentiate the sedative effects of CNS depressants, such as opiates, or other analgesics, barbiturates, or other sedatives. Concomitant administration of benzodiazepine and haloperidol may result in hypotension, particularly if the patient is hypovolemic before treatment [158]. Concomitant administration of lithium may result in an intoxication syndrome characterized by extrapyramidal side effects, decreased sensorium, hyperthermia, and permanent neurologic sequelae. Haloperidol blocks guanethidine's access to the presynaptic reuptake pump; therefore blood pressure may increase.

Pitfalls of Management. Autonomic effects (dry mouth, blurred vision, urinary retention, sedation, orthostatic hypotension) may be associated with haloperidol, although less so than with low-potency neuroleptics. Hypotension may occasionally occur, but haloperidol has been safely used in high doses in cardiovascular patients. Some neuroleptics decrease the seizure threshold, but there is little clinical evidence that haloperidol causes such an effect [159]. Other potential side effects include tardive dyskinesia with long-term use, catonia, and neuroleptic malignant syndrome.

Haloperidol is a dopamine receptor antagonist; therefore extrapyramidal reactions may occur. This is more likely in patients with a prior history of extrapyramidal side effects or a family history of Parkinson's disease. Most clinicians have reported a low incidence of extrapyramidal symptoms with the use of intravenous haloperidol [156,157,167]. In fact, intravenous administration has been reported to cause less extrapyramidal symptoms than oral or intramuscular administration [147,156, 157,168–175], although some have questioned this [146]. Even higher doses of intravenous haloperidol (530 mg over 24 hours)

have rarely resulted in extrapyramidal symptoms [157, 158,162,172,176,177,178]. While several studies have evaluated the extrapyramidal effects associated with haloperidol the study populations have been relatively small in most cases; therefore further study is needed to determine the risk associated with haloperidol use in critically ill patients.

Opioids

While opioids are useful for pain management in the ICU, the high dose needed to provide sedation when used as a single agent makes opioids inappropriate for this use. The high doses required may result in accumulation of the parent drug or metabolites in a critically ill patient with renal or hepatic dysfunction [102,179,180]. Adverse effects commonly associated with the opioids include nausea and vomiting, decreased gut motility, depressed ventilation in spontaneously breathing patients, induction of miosis, hypotension, and dose-related immune depressant effects [102,181]. Morphine is the opioid most frequently used in the ICU. It is extensively taken up by the tissues, is not very lipid-soluble, has slow blood-brain barrier penetration, and may be problematic in severe hepatic and/or renal failure. Alternative opioids include alfentanil, a short-acting agent currently being studied in ICU patients as a sedative [183,184,185]. No cumulative effects have been noted with alfentanil, although clearance may be decreased in critically ill and cirrhotic patients [182,183]. Opioids are very effective sedative agents when used in combination with other CNS depressants. Nevertheless, the major use of opioids in the ICU is as analgesic agents. When opioids are used in combination with a benzodiazepine and/or haloperidol the clinically effective dose of each agent is usually lower.

Barbiturates

Although barbiturates were originally employed for sedation, today there is little use for this class of agents in the ICU for sedation, as many other agents with better side-effect profiles are available. Barbiturates are used mainly to sedate patients with head injuries, because they can lower intracranial pressure. Accumulation of barbiturates may hinder neurologic assessment [184]. Barbiturates also depress respiration, circulation, thermogenesis, bowel movement, and immune function. Because they may cause induction or inhibition of hepatic enzymes, the potential for a large number of drug interactions also exists.

Isoflurane

Various anesthetics have been evaluated for their efficacy as sedative agents. Nitrous oxide was used as an ICU sedative until concern over bone marrow suppression restricted its use [185]. Use of halothane, enflurane, and isoflurane for sedation is limited due to concern about cardiovascular depression, arrhythmias, and hepatic effects. Recently isoflurane, a volatile fluorinated anaesthetic agent, was studied for use as a sedative in the ICU due to its favorable physicochemical properties. It has a low solubility in blood that facilitates control of anesthetic concentrations, enabling rapid titration and recovery. Isoflurane is a particularly attractive alternative for the critically ill patient because its elimination is independent of renal and hepatic function. The few studies that have compared isoflurane to other sedatives have found isoflurane to be a viable alternative to continuous infusion midazolam [186,187] and propofol [188]. Further study is needed to assess the use of isoflurane beyond 24 hours for efficacy and toxicity. Concern has been raised about the potential for fluoride accumulation in the setting of renal dysfunction [189]. Another limiting factor is the expensive scavenging equipment necessary for administration of isoflurane. The high cost of isoflurane may also prohibit its routine use as a sedative agent in the ICU. Isoflurane may prove to be a valuable option for sedation in the critically ill patient, but further evaluation is necessary before it can be routinely used in clinical practice.

Flumazenil

Occasionally administration of benzodiazepines, including short-acting agents such as midazolam, may cause prolonged sedation of the critically ill patient [60,89]. Flumazenil is a benzodiazepine antagonist that rapidly reverses benzodiazepine effects [190]. Pepperman showed that patients who received flumazenil after the discontinuation of midazolam administered by continuous infusion for greater than 12 hours were less sedated, able to obey commands, and extubated significantly faster than those receiving placebo [191]. Flumazenil has been used in critically ill trauma patients for periodic reversal of benzodiazepine sedation to assess neurologic status [192,193]. Although flumazenil consistently reverses the CNS effects of benzodiazepines, its ability to reverse respiratory depression is not completely established. It reverses some components of benzodiazepine-induced ventilatory depression (e.g., minute ventilation at end-tidal CO_2 tension and tidal volume), but does not affect others (i.e., the slope of the CO_2 response) [194].

Based on animal studies that support the use of flumazenil to reverse subsensitivity to GABA induced by chronic benzodiazepine therapy [195,196,197], flumazenil is being evaluated for its efficacy in humans for preventing as well as reversing benzodiazepine tolerance. If supported by further study, intermittent administration of flumazenil to selected patients during prolonged continuous infusions of benzodiazepines may allow better periodic neurologic evaluation. Theoretically, the administration of flumazenil in this manner may precipitate withdrawal seizures. Of interest, flumazenil has some anticonvulsant activity [198] at less than 60 percent receptor occupancy, suggesting it might be possible to reverse tolerance with little risk of provoking withdrawal seizures [199]. The rationale behind this theory is that partial receptor occupancy would still allow benzodiazepines to bind to the receptors and exert anticonvulsant activity. Flumazenil exhibits dose-dependent effects, with doses of 1 to 2 mg producing 50 percent receptor occupation in the brain, whereas doses of 15 mg produce almost 100 percent receptor occupation [199,200]. Benzodiazepine occupancy of all available receptors is not needed for efficacy; for example, clonazepam administered in therapeutic doses occupies only 37 percent of the benzodiazepine receptors [201]. Further investigation is necessary to determine the value of intermittent flumazenil for preventing or reversing tolerance to benzodiazepine agonists. Because flumazenil has a shorter half-life (90 minutes) than most benzodiazepines, residual sedation may be problematic in a large percentage of patients unless repeat doses or continuous infusion is administered.

Flumazenil is available as an intravenous preparation in a 0.1

mg per milliliter concentration. It may be administered intermittently as 0.2- to 0.5-mg boluses or as a continuous infusion initiated at 0.1 to 0.5 mg per hour [202]. After intravenous administration, flumazenil plasma concentrations follow linear pharmacokinetics, with a short elimination half-life (0.7–1.3 hours) and a high total body clearance (54–67 L/hr) [203]. Peak plasma concentrations are proportional to the administered dose; generally those between 10 and 20 μ per liter effectively reverse benzodiazepine-induced CNS depression and may be achieved after an IV bolus of 2.5 mg [204,205]. Maximum concentrations are attained in the CNS within 5 to 8 minutes after administration. The effects of protein binding are minimal, with 40 to 50 percent bound to albumin. The volume of distribution is 77 to 96 liters. Flumazenil is rapidly metabolized to an inactive free carboxylic acid, which is then bound to a glucuronide and excreted with less than 0.2 percent unchanged in the urine. Patients with hepatic dysfunction may experience prolonged effects from flumazenil [206].

Adverse effects of flumazenil have been reported in a subgroup of patients. Flumazenil should not be used to reverse benzodiazepine effect in patients with severe head injury with unstable intracranial pressure (ICP), as it has been shown to increase ICP significantly in this population [207]. Flumazenil may provoke acute anxiety reactions in predisposed individuals [208], but in normal volunteers there is no evidence of acute anxiety or stress [209]. Food given during flumazenil administration increases clearance 50 percent, most likely due to an increase in hepatic blood flow. Additional adverse effects associated with flumazenil include precipitation of benzodiazepine withdrawal symptoms, seizures, and arrhythmias. The use of flumazenil has been associated with seizures, most frequently in patients who have been on long-term benzodiazepines or in tricyclic antidepressant overdose.

References

1. Ritz R: Benzodiazepine sedation in adult ICU patients. *Intensive Care Med* 17:S11, 1991.
2. Richter J: Current theories about the mechanisms of benzodiazepines and neuroleptic drugs. *Anesthesiology* 54:66, 1981.
3. Study R, Barker J: Cellular mechanisms of benzodiazepine action. *JAMA* 247:2147, 1982.
4. Fink M: Cerebral electrometry-quantitative EEG applied to human psychopharmacology, in Dolce G, Kunkel (eds): *Computerized EEG Analysis*. Stuttgart, Gustave Fischer Verlag, 1975, pp 271–288.
5. Mandema J, Danhof M: Electroencephalogram effect measures and relationships between pharmacokinetics and pharmacodynamics of centrally acting drugs. *Clin Pharmacokinet* 23:191, 1992.
6. Dundee J, Johnston H, Gray R: Lorazepam as a sedative-amnesic in an intensive care unit. *Curr Med Res Opin* 4:290, 1976.
7. Greenblatt D, Schillings R, Kyriakopoulos A, et al: Clinical pharmacokinetics of lorazepam. *Clin Pharmacol Ther* 20:329, 1976.
8. Blitt C, Petty W, Wright W, et al: Clinical evaluation of injectable lorazepam as a premedicant: The effect on recall. *Anesth Analg* 55:522, 1976.
9. Pandit S, Heisterkamp D, Cohen P: Further studies of the anti-recall effect of lorazepam: A dose time-effect relationship. *Anesthesiology* 45:495, 1976.
10. Dundee J, George K: The amnesic action of diazepam, flunitrazepam and lorazepam in man. *Acta Anaesthesiol Belg* 27 (suppl):3, 1976.
11. Camu F: Clinical use of lorazepam in postoperative intensive care. *Acta Anaesthesiol Belg* 29:191, 1978.
12. Greenblatt D, Shader R, Franke K: Pharmacokinetics and bioavailability of intravenous, intramuscular, and oral lorazepam in humans. *J Pharm Sci* 68:57, 1979.
13. Dundee J, Lilburn J, Toner W, et al: Plasma lorazepam levels. *Anaesthesia* 33:15, 1978.

14. Herman R, Duc Van Pham J, Szakacs C: Disposition of lorazepam in human beings: Enterohepatic recirculation and first-pass effect. *Clin Pharmacol Ther* 46:18, 1989.

15. Ameer B, Greenblatt D: Lorazepam: A review of its clinical pharmacological properties and therapeutic uses. *Drugs* 21:161, 1981.

16. Greenblatt D, et al: Lorazepam kinetics in the elderly. *Clin Pharmacol Ther* 26:103, 1979.

17. Evans E, Proctor J, Fratkin M, et al: Blood flow in muscle groups and drug absorption. *Clin Pharmacol Ther* 17:44, 1975.

18. Greenblatt D: Clinical pharmacokinetics of oxazepam and lorazepam. *Clin Pharmacokinet* 6:89, 1981.

19. Smith M, Eadie M, O'Rourke Brophy T: The pharmacokinetics of midazolam in man. *Eur J Clin Pharmacol* 19:271, 1981.

20. Crevoisier C, Ziegler W, Eckert M, et al: Relationship between plasma concentration and effect of midazolam after oral and intravenous administration. *Br J Clin Pharmacol* 16:51S, 1983.

21. Bliding A: Effects of different rates of absorption of two benzodiazepines on subjective and objective parameters. *Eur J Clin Pharmacol* 7:201, 1974.

22. Bonati M, Kanto J, Tognoni G: Clinical pharmacokinetics of CSF. *Clin Pharmacokinet* 7:312, 1982.

23. Aaltonen L, Kanto J, Salo M: Cerebrospinal fluid concentrations and serum protein binding of lorazepam and its conjugate. *Acta Pharmacol Toxicol* 46:156, 1980.

24. Elliott H: Metabolism of lorazepam. *Br J Anaesth* 48:1017, 1976.

25. George K, Dundee J: Relative amnestic actions of diazepam, flunitrazepam and lorazepam in man. *Br J Clin Pharmacol* 4:45, 1977.

26. Conner J, Katz R, Bellville J, et al: Diazepam and lorazepam for intravenous surgical premedication. *J Clin Pharmacol* 18:285, 1978.

27. Greenblatt D, Ehrenberg B, Gunderman J, et al: Kinetic and dynamic study of intravenous lorazepam: Comparison with intravenous diazepam. *J Pharmacol Exp Ther* 250:134, 1989.

28. Tedeschi G, Smith A, Dhillon S, et al: Rate of entrance of benzodiazepines into the brain determined by eye movement recording. *Br J Clin Pharmacol* 15:103, 1983.

29. Walton N, Treiman D: Lorazepam treatment of experimental status epilepticus in the rat: Relevance to clinical practice. *Neurology* 40:990, 1990.

30. Miller L, Greenblatt D, Paul S, et al: Benzodiazepine receptor occupancy in vivo: Correlation with brain concentrations and pharmacodynamic actions. *J Pharmacol Exp Ther* 240:516, 1987.

31. Arendt R, Greenblatt D, deJong R, et al: In vitro correlates of benzodiazepine cerebrospinal fluid uptake, pharmacodynamic action, and peripheral distribution. *J Pharmacol Exp Ther* 227:95, 1983.

32. Greenblatt D: Clinical pharmacokinetics of oxazepam and lorazepam. *Clin Pharmacokinet* 6:89, 1981.

33. Greenblatt D, Schillings R, Kyriakopoulos A, et al: Absorption and disposition of oral C-lorazepam. *Clin Pharmacol Ther* 20:329, 1976.

34. Verbeeck R, Tjandramaga T, Verberckmoes R, et al: Biotransformation and excretion of lorazepam in patients with chronic renal failure. *Br J Clin Pharmacol* 3:1033, 1976.

35. Greenblatt D, Allen M, MacLaughlin D, et al: Single- and multiple-dose kinetics of oral lorazepam in human: The predictability of accumulation. *J Pharmacokinet Biopharm* 7:159, 1979.

36. Verbeeck R, Tjandramaga T, Verberckmoes R, et al: Biotransformation and excretion of lorazepam in patients with chronic renal failure. *Br J Clin Pharmacol* 3:1033, 1976.

37. Greenblatt D, Allen M, MacLaughlin D, et al: The predictability of accumulation. *J Pharmacokinet Biopharm* 7:159, 1979.

38. Allen M, Greenblatt D, Lacasse Y, et al: Pharmacokinetic study of lorazepam overdosage. *Am J Psychiatry* 137:1414, 1980.

39. Kraus J, Desmond P, Marshall J, et al: Effects of aging and liver disease on disposition of lorazepam. *Clin Pharmacol Ther* 24:411, 1978.

40. Schillings R, Schrader S, Ruelius H: Urinary metabolites of lorazepam in humans and four animal species. *Arzneimittelforschung* 21:1059, 1971.

41. Knowles J, Comer W, Ruelis H: Disposition of lorazepam in humans. *Arzneimittelforschung* 21:1055, 1971.

42. Wilkinson G, Shand D: A physiological approach to hepatic drug clearance. *Clin Pharmacol Ther* 18:377, 1975.

43. Wilkinson G, Shand D: A physiological approach to hepatic drug clearance. *Clin Pharmacol Ther* 18:377, 1975.

44. Martyn J, Greenblatt D, Quinby W: Diazepam kinetics in patients with severe burns. *Anesth Analg* 62:293, 1983.

45. Ciaccio E, Fruncillo R: Urinary excretion of D-glucaric acid by severely burned patients. *Clin Pharmacol Ther* 25:340, 1979.

46. Martyn J, Greenblatt D: Lorazepam conjugation is unimpaired in burn trauma. *Clin Pharmacol Ther* 43:250, 1987.

47. Verbeeck R, Tjandramaga T, DeSchepper P, et al: Impaired elimination of lorazepam following subchronic administration in two patients with renal failure. *Br J Clin Pharmacol* 12:749, 1981.

48. Morrison G, Chiang S, Koepke H, et al: Effect of renal impairment and hemodialysis on lorazepam kinetics. *Clin Pharmacol Ther* 35:646, 1984.

49. Kraus J, Marshall J, Johnson R, et al: Lorazepam elimination in liver disease. *Gastroenterology* 73:1288, 1977.

50. Aaltonen L, Kanto J, Arola M, et al: Effect of age and cardiopulmonary bypass on the pharmacokinetics of lorazepam. *Acta Pharmacol Toxicol* 51:126, 1982.

51. Greenblatt D, Allen M, Locniskar A, et al: Lorazepam kinetics in the elderly. *Clin Pharmacol Ther* 26:103, 1979.

52. Greenblatt D, Abernethy D, Koepke H, et al: Interaction of cimetidine with oxazepam, lorazepam, and flurazepam. *J Clin Pharmacol* 24:187, 1984.

53. Richards D: Clinical profile of lorazepam, a new benzodiazepine tranquilizer. *J Clin Psychiatry* 39:58, 1978.

54. D'Ambrosio J, Borchardt-Phelps P, Nolen J, et al: Propylene glycol-induced lactic acidosis secondary to a continuous infusion of lorazepam. *Pharmacotherapy* 13:274, 1992.

55. Allonen H, Ziegler G, Klotz U: Midazolam kinetics. *Clin Pharmacol Ther* 30:654, 1981.

56. Dirksen M, Vree T, Driessen J: Midazolam in the intensive care unit. *Drug Intel Clin Pharm* 20:805, 1986.

57. Oldenhof H, de Jong M, Steenhoek A, et al: Clinical pharmacokinetics of midazolam in intensive care patients: A wide interpatient variability? *Clin Pharmacol Ther* 43:263, 1988.

58. Klotz U, Reimann I: Chronopharmacokinetic study with prolonged infusion of midazolam. *Clin Pharmacokinet* 9:469, 1984.

59. Sjovall S, Kanto J, Himberg J, et al: CSF penetration and pharmacokinetics of midazolam. *Eur J Clin Pharmacol* 25:247, 1983.

60. Shelly M, Mendel L, Park G: Failure of critically ill patients to metabolise midazolam. *Anaesthesia* 42:619, 1987.

61. Herkes G, Wszolek Z, Westmoreland B, et al: Effects of midazolam on electroencephalograms of seriously ill patients. *Mayo Clin Proc* 67:334, 1992.

62. Brown C, Sarnquist F, Canup C, et al: Clinical, electroencephalographic, and pharmacokinetic studies of a water-soluble benzodiazepine, midazolam maleate. *Anesthesiology* 50:467, 1979.

63. Mandema J, Tuk B, van Steveninck A, et al: Pharmacokinetic-pharmacodynamic modeling of the central nervous system effects of midazolam and its main metabolite alpha-hydroxymidazolam in healthy volunteers. *Clin Pharmacol Ther* 51:715, 1992.

64. Koopmans R, Dingemanse J, Danhof M, et al: Pharmacokinetic-pharmacodynamic modeling of midazolam effects on the human central nervous system. *Clin Pharmacol Ther* 44:14, 1988.

65. Greenblatt D, Ehrenberg B, Gunderman J, et al: Pharmacokinetic and electroencephalographic study of intravenous diazepam, midazolam, and placebo. *Clin Pharmacol Ther* 45:356, 1989.

66. Herkes G, Wszolek A, Westmoreland B, et al: Effects of midazolam on EEG's of seriously ill patients. *Mayo Clin Proc* 67:334, 1992.

67. Holazo A, Winkler M, Patel I: Effects of age, gender and oral contraceptives on intramuscular midazolam pharmacokinetics. *J Clin Pharmacol* 28:1040, 1988.

68. Kanto J, Kangas L. Siirtola T: Cerebrospinal fluid concentrations of diazepam and its metabolites in man. *Acta Pharmacol Toxicol* 36:328, 1975.

69. Heizmann P, Eckert M, Ziegler W: Pharmacokinetics and bioavailability of midazolam in man. *Br J Clin Pharmacol* 16:43S, 1983.

70. Greenblatt D, Abernethy D, Lockniskar A, et al: Effect of age, gender, and obesity on midazolam kinetics. *Anesthesiology* 61:27, 1984.

71. Adams P, Gelman S, Reves J, et al: Midazolam pharmacodynamics

and pharmacokinetics during acute hypovolemia. *Anesthesiology* 63:140, 1985.

72. Vinik H, Reves J, Greenblatt D, et al: The pharmacokinetics of midazolam in chronic renal failure patients. *Anesthesiology* 59:390, 1983.

73. Vree T, Shimoda M, Driessen J, et al: Decreased plasma albumin concentration results in increased volume of distribution and decreased elimination of midazolam in intensive care patients. *Clin Pharmacol Ther* 46:537, 1989.

74. Versed PI. 1993;.

75. Avram M, Fragen R, Caldwell N: Midazolam kinetics in women of two age groups. *Clin Pharmacol Ther* 34:505, 1983.

76. Collier P, Kawar P, Gamble J, et al: Influence of age on pharmacokinetics of midazolam. *Br J Clin Pharmacol* 13:602P, 1982.

77. Klotz U, Ziegler G: Physiologic and temporal variation in hepatic elimination of midazolam. *Clin Pharmacol Ther* 32:108, 1982.

78. Kroboth P, Smith R, Erb R: Tolerance to alprazolam after intravenous bolus and continuous infusion: Psychomotor and EEG effects. *Clin Pharmacol Ther* 43:270, 1988.

79. Shafer A, Doze V, White P: Pharmacokinetic variability of midazolam infusions in critically ill patients. *Crit Care Med* 18:1039, 1990.

80. Dundee J, Halliday N, Harper K, et al: Midazolam: A review of its pharmacological properties and therapeutic use. *Drugs* 28:519, 1984.

81. Park G, Manara A, Dawling S: Extra-hepatic metabolism of midazolam. *Br J Clin Pharmacol* 27:634, 1989.

82. Kronbach T, Mathys D, Umeno M, et al: Oxidation of midazolam and triazolam by human liver cytochrome P450 III A4. *Mol Pharmacol* 36:89, 1989.

83. Ziegler W, Schalch E, Leishman B, et al: Comparison of the effects of intravenously administered midazolam, triazolam and their hydroxy metabolites. *Br J Clin Pharmacol* 16:63S, 1983.

84. Dundee J, Collier P, Carlisle R, et al: Prolonged midazolam elimination half-life. *Br J Clin Pharmacol* 21:425, 1986.

85. Puglisi C, Meyer J, D'Arconte L, et al: Determination of water-soluble imidazo-1, 4-benzodiazepines in blood by electroncapture gas-liquid chromatography and in urine by differential pulse polarography. *J Chromatogr* 145:81, 1978.

86. Dundee J, Samuel I, Toner W, et al: Midazolam: A water-soluble benzodiazepine. *Anaesthesia* 35:454, 1980.

87. Dirksen M, Vree T, Driessen J: Clinical pharmacokinetics of long-term infusion of midazolam in critically ill patients: Preliminary results. *Anaesth Intensive Care* 15:440, 1987.

88. Malacrida R, Fritz M, Suter P, et al: Pharmacokinetics of midazolam administered by continuous intravenous infusion to intensive care patients. *Crit Care Med* 20:1123, 1992.

89. Byatt C, Lewis L, Dawling S, et al: Accumulation of midazolam after repeated dosage in patients receiving mechanical ventilation in an intensive care unit. *Br Med J* 289:799, 1984.

90. Michalk S, Moncorge C, Fichelle A, et al: Midazolam infusion for basal sedation in intensive care: Absence of accumulation. *Intensive Care Med* 15:37, 1988.

91. Lowry K, Dundee J, McClean E, et al: Pharmacokinetics of diazepam and midazolam when used for sedation following cardiopulmonary bypass. *Br J Anaesth* 57:883, 1985.

92. Harper K, Collier P, Dundee J, et al: Age and nature of operation influence the pharmacokinetics of midazolam. *Br J Anaesth* 57:866, 1985.

93. Murray M: P450 enzymes. *Clin Pharmacokinet* 23:132, 1992.

94. Greenblatt D, Allen M, Harmatz J, et al: Diazepam disposition determinants. *Clin Pharmacol Ther* 27:301, 1980.

95. Collier P, Kawar P, Gamble J, et al: Influence of age on pharmacokinetics of midazolam. *Proc BPS* December:602P, 1981.

96. Macgilchrist A, Birnie G, Cook A, et al: Pharmacokinetics and pharmacodynamics of intravenous midazolam in patients with severe alcoholic cirrhosis. *Gut* 27:190, 1986.

97. Shelly M, Sultan M, Bodenham A, et al: Midazolam infusions in critically ill patients. *Eur J Anaesthesiol* 8:21, 1991.

98. Kanto J: Midazolam: The first water-soluble benzodiazepine. *Pharmacotherapy* 5:138, 1985.

99. Bodenham A, Shelly M, Park G: The altered pharmacokinetics and pharmacodynamics of drugs commonly used in critically ill patients. *Clin Pharmacokinet* 14:347, 1988.

100. Shapiro J, Westphal L, White P, et al: Midazolam infusion for sedation in the intensive care unit: Effect on adrenal function. *Anesthesiology* 64:394, 1986.

101. Mikhail M, Thangathurai D: Sedating patients in ICU's. *West J Med* 157:566, 1992.

102. Aitkenhead A, Pepperman M, Willatts S, et al: Comparison of propofol and midazolam for sedation in critically ill patients. *Lancet* Sept 23:704, 1989.

103. Forster A, Gardez J, Suter P, et al: I.V. midazolam as an induction agent for anesthesia: A study in volunteers. *Br J Anaesth* 52:907, 1980.

104. Fragen R, Meyers S, Barresi V, et al: Hemodynamic effects of midazolam in cardiac patients. *Anesthesiology* 51:S103, 1979.

105. Kawar P, Carson I, Clarke R, et al: Hemodynamic changes during induction of anaesthesia with midazolam and diazepam (Valium) in patients undergoing coronary artery bypass surgery. *Anaesthesia* 40:767, 1985.

106. Kanto J, Himberg J, Heikkila H, et al: Midazolam kinetics before, during and after cardiopulmonary bypass surgery. *Int J Clin Pharm Res* 2:123, 1985.

107. Glen J: Animal studies of the anaesthetic activity of ICI 35 868. *Br J Anaesth* 52:731, 1980.

108. Bone M, Wilkins C, Lew J: A comparison of propofol and methohexitone as anaesthetic agents for electroconvulsive therapy. *Eur J Anaesthesiol* 8:141, 1988.

109. Simpson K, Halsall P, Carr C, et al: Propofol reduces seizure duration in patients having anaesthesia for electroconvulsive therapy. *Br J Anaesth* 61:343, 1988.

110. Shearer E: Convulsions and propofol. *Anaesthesia* 45:255, 1990.

111. Collier C, Kelly K: Propofol and convulsions: The evidence mounts. *Anaesth Intensive Care* 19:573, 1991.

112. Au J, Walker W, Scott D: Withdrawal syndrome after propofol infusion. *Anaesthesia* 45:741, 1990.

113. Mackenzie J, Kapadia F, Grant I: Propofol infusion for control of status epilepticus. *Anaesthesia* 45:1043, 1990.

114. Kay N, Stephenson D: Dose-response relationship for disoprofol: Comparison with methohexitone. *Anaesthesia* 36:863, 1981.

115. Adam H. Kay B, Douglas E: Blood disoprofol levels in anaesthetised patients: Correlation of concentrations after single or repeated doses with hypnotic activity. *Anaesthesia* 37:536, 1982.

116. Beller J, Pottecher T, Lugnier A, et al: Prolonged sedation with propofol in ICU patients: Recovery and blood concentration changes during periodic interruptions in infusion. *Br J Anaesth* 61;583, 1988.

117. Vuyk J, Engbers F, Lemmens H, et al: Pharmacodynamics of propofol in female patients. *Anesthesiology* 77:3, 1992.

118. Shafer A, Doze V, Shafer S, et al: Pharmacokinetics and pharmacodynamics of propofol infusions during general anesthesia. *Anesthesiology* 69:348, 1988.

119. Cockshott I, Briggs L, Douglas E, et al: Pharmacokinetics of propofol in female patients: Studies using single bolus injections. *Br J Anaesth* 59:1103, 1987.

120. Newman L, McDonald J, Wallace P, et al: Propofol infusion for sedation in intensive care. *Anaesthesia* 42:929, 1987.

121. Cullen P, Turtle M, Prys-Roberts C, et al: Effect of propofol anesthesia on baroreflex activity in humans. *Anesth Analg* 66:1115, 1987.

122. Kanto J, Gepts E: Pharmacokinetic implications for the clinical use of propofol. *Clin Pharmacokinet* 17:308, 1989.

123. Withington D: Basophil histamine release studies in the evaluation of a new anesthetic agent. *Agents Actions* 23:337, 1988.

124. Kay B: Propofol and alfentanil infusion. *Anaesthesia* 41:589, 1986.

125. Tessler M, Dascal A, Gioseffini S, et al: Growth curves of *Staphylococcus aureus, Candida albicans,* and *Moraxella osloensis* in propofol and other media. *Can J Anaesth* 39:509, 1992.

126. White P: Propofol: Pharmacokinetics and pharmacodynamics. *Semin Anesth* 7(Suppl 1):4, 1988.

127. Cockshott I: Propofol pharmacokinetics and metabolism: An overview. *Postgrad Med J* 61:45, 1985.

128. Kay N, Sear J, Uppington J, et al: Disposition of propofol in patients undergoing surgery. *Br J Anaesth* 58:1075, 1986.

129. Schuttler J, Stoeckel H, Schwilden H: Pharmacokinetic and pharmacodynamic modeling of propofol in volunteers and surgical patients. *Postgrad Med J* 61:53, 1985.

130. Kirkpatrick T, Cockshott I, Douglas E, et al: Pharmacokinetics of propofol in elderly patients. *Br J Anaesth* 60:146, 1988.

131. Simons P, Cockshott I, Douglas E, et al: Blood concentrations, metabolism and elimination after a subanesthetic intravenous dose of 14-C-propofol to male volunteers (abstract). *Postgrad Med J* 61:64, 1985.

132. Briggs L, White M, Cockshott I, et al: The pharmacokinetics of propofol in female patients. *Postgrad Med J* 61(Suppl 3):58, 1985.

133. Gepts E, Claeys M, Camu F: Pharmacokinetics of propofol administered by continuous intravenous infusion in man: A preliminary report. *Postgrad Med J* 61:51, 1985.

134. Gepts E, Camu F, Cockshott I, et al: Disposition of propofol administered as constant-rate infusions. *Anesth Analg* 66:1256, 1987.

135. Grounds R, Lalor J, Lumley J, et al: Propofol infusion for sedation in the intensive care unit: a preliminary report. *Br Med J* 294:929, 1987.

136. Albanese J, Martin C, Lacarelle B, et al: Pharmacokinetics of long-term propofol infusion used for sedation in ICU patients. *Anesthesiology* 73:214, 1990.

137. Campbell G, Morgan D, Kumar K, et al: Extended blood collection period required to define distribution and elimination kinetics of propofol. *Br J Clin Pharmacol* 26:187, 1988.

138. Harris C, Grounds R, Murray A, et al: Propofol for long-term sedation in the intensive care unit. *Anaesthesia* 45:366, 1990.

139. Bailie G, Cockshott I, Douglas E, et al: Pharmacokinetics of propofol during and after long term continuous infusion for maintenance of sedation in ICU patients. *Br J Anaesth* 68:486, 1992.

140. Albanese J, Auffray J, Lacarelle B, et al: Pharmacokinetics of propofol administered by continuous intravenous infusion in man. *Anesthesiology* 67:A667, 1987.

141. Simons P, Cockshott I, Douglas E, et al: Blood concentrations, metabolism and elimination after a subanesthetic intravenous dose of 14 C-propofol to male volunteers. *Postgrad Med J* 61(Suppl 3):64, 1985.

142. Cook S, Palma O: Propofol as a sole agent for prolonged infusion in the intensive care. *J Drug Dev* 2(Suppl 2):65, 1989.

143. Harper J, Buckley P, Carr K: A study of the utility of continuous infusions of propofol and alfentanil in ventilated intensive care patients. *J Drug Dev* 2(Suppl 2):75, 1989.

144. Sanders K, Minnema A, Murray G: Low incidence of extrapyramidal symptoms in treatment of delirium with intravenous haloperidol and lorazepam in the intensive care unit. *J Intensive Care Med* 4:201, 1989.

145. Perry. *Psychotropic Drug Handbook.* 5th ed., 1988.

146. Magliozzi J, Gillespie H, Lombrozo L, et al: Mood alteration following oral and intravenous haloperidol and relationship to drug concentration in normal subjects. *J Clin Pharmacol* 25:285, 1985.

147. Settle E, Ayd F: Haloperidol: A quarter century of experience. *J Clin Psychiatry* 44:440, 1983.

148. Ayd F: Haloperidol update: 1975. *Proc R Soc Med* 69:14, 1976.

149. Ayd FJ: Intravenous haloperidol therapy. *Int Drug Ther News* 13:20, 1978.

150. Giacobini E, Lassenius B: Haloperidol in the treatment of delirium tremens. *Svenska Lakartidningen* 58:1429, 1961.

151. Gomez J, Daily P: Intravenous tranquilization with ECT. *Br J Psychiatry* 127:604, 1975.

152. Dudley D, Rowlett D, Loebel P: Emergency use of intravenous haloperidol. *Gen Hosp Psychiatry* 1:240, 1979.

153. Moeller H, Kissling W, Doerr P, et al: Studies on the effects and side effects of haloperidol after I.V. and oral administration. *Arzneimittelforschung* 30:1201, 1980.

154. Pratt I: Twilight sleep after infarction. *Br Med J* 3:475, 1971.

155. Lichko A, Marchenko B, Prakhow V, et al: Reactions to intravenous introduction of haloperidol. *Zh Nevropatol Psikhiatr* 71:443, 1971.

156. Sos J, Cassem N: Managing postoperative agitation. *Drug Ther* 10:103, 1980.

157. Tesar G, Murray G, Cassem N: Use of high-dose intravenous haloperidol in the treatment of agitated cardiac patients. *J Clin Psychopharmacol* 5:344, 1985.

158. Adams F: Neuropsychiatric evaluation and treatment of delirium in the critically ill cancer patient. *Cancer Bull* 35:156, 1980.

159. Settle E, Ayd F: Haloperidol: A quarter century of experience. *J Clin Psychiatry* 44:440, 1983.

160. Tesar G, Stern T: Rapid tranquilization of the agitated intensive care unit patient. *J Intensive Care Med* 3:195, 1988.

161. Moore D: Rapid treatment of delirium in critically ill patients. *Am J Psychiatry* 134:1431, 1977.

162. Tesar G, Murray G, Cassem N: Use of high-dose intravenous haloperidol in the treatment of agitated cardiac patients. *J Clin Psychopharmacol* 5:344, 1985.

163. Cameron O: Safe use of haloperidol in a patient with cardiac dysrhythmia. *Am J Psychiatry* 135:1244, 1978.

164. Donlon P, Hopkin J, Schaffer C: Cardiovascular safety of rapid treatment with intramuscular haloperidol. *Am J Psychiatry* 136:233, 1979.

165. Glinkman L: Haloperidol: Did it cause the respiratory arrest? *JAMA* 267:54, 1992.

166. Bedell S, Deitz D, O'Leeman D: Incidence and characteristics of preventable iatrogenic cardiac arrests. *JAMA* 265:2815, 1991.

167. Menza M, Murray G, Holmes V, et al: Controlled study of extrapyramidal reactions in the management of delirious, medically ill patients: Intravenous haloperidol versus intravenous haloperidol plus benzodiazepines. *Heart Lung* 17:238, 1988.

168. Menza M, Murray G, Holmes V, et al: Decreased extrapyramidal symptoms with intravenous haloperidol. *J Clin Psychiatry* 48:278, 1987.

169. Lawson J, McGowan S: Haloperidol in obstetrics. *Lancet* 1:1205, 1962.

170. Dyrberg V: Haloperidol in the prevention of postoperative nausea and vomiting. *Acta Anesthesiol Scand* 6:37, 1962.

171. Danik J, Goverdham M: Haloperidol in the treatment of 120 psychotic patients. *Am J Psychiatry* 120:389, 1963.

172. Lerner Y, Lwow E, Levitin A: Acute high-dose parenteral haloperidol treatment of psychosis. *Am J Psychiatry* 136:1061, 1979.

173. Kulenkampff C: Acute psychotic states. *Med Welt* 22:802, 1971.

174. Forsman A: Individual variability in response to haloperidol. *Proc R Soc Med* 69(suppl 1):9, 1976.

175. Denker S: High-dose treatment with neuroleptics in the acute phase of mental disorder. *Proc R Soc Med* 69(suppl 1):32, 1976.

176. Dudley D, Rowlett D, Pierre J: Emergency use of intravenous haloperidol. *Gen Hosp Psychiatry* 240, 1979.

177. Cassem N: Critical care psychiatry: State of the art, in Shoemaker WC, Thompson WL (eds): Society of Critical Care Medicine, 1983, pp 1–31.

178. Adams F, Fernandez F, Anderson B: Emergency pharmacotherapy of delirium in the critically ill cancer patient. *Psychosomatics* 27(suppl):33, 1986.

179. Osborne R, Joel S, Slevin M: Morphine intoxication in renal failure: The role of morphine-6-glucuronide. *Br Med J* 292:1548, 1986.

180. Shelly M, Cory E, Park G: Pharmacokinetics of morphine in two children before and after liver transplantation. *Br J Anaesth* 58:1218, 1986.

181. Prys-Roberts C, Kelman G: The influence of drugs used in neuroleptic analgesia on cardiovascular and respiratory function. *Br J Anaesth* 39:134, 1967.

182. Yate P, Thomas D, Short S, et al: Comparison of infusions of alfentanil or pethidine for sedation of ventilated patients on the ITU. *Br J Am* 58:1091, 1986.

183. Ferrier C, Marty J, Bottard Y, et al: Alfentanil pharmacokinetics in cirrhosis. *Anesthesiology* 62:480, 1985.

184. Carlon G, Kahn R, Goldiner P, et al: Long-term infusion of sodium thiopental: Hemodynamic and respiratory effects. *Crit Care Med* 6:311, 1978.

185. Amos R, Amess J, Hinds C, et al: Incidence and pathogenesis of acute megaloblastic bone-marrow change in patients receiving intensive care. *Lancet* 2:835, 1982.

186. Spencer E, Willatts S: Isoflurane for prolonged sedation in the intensive care unit: Efficacy and safety. *Intensive Care Med* 18:415, 1992.

187. Kong K, Tyler J, Willatts S, et al: Isoflurane sedation for patients undergoing mechanical ventilation: Metabolism to inorganic fluoride and renal effects. *Br J Anaesth* 64:159, 1990.

188. Millane T, Bennett E, Grounds R: Isoflurane and propofol for long-term sedation in the intensive care unit. *Anesthesiology* 47:768, 1992.

189. Park G, Burns A: Isoflurane compared with midazolam in the ICU.

190. Bodenham A, Brownlie G, Dixon J, et al: Reversal of sedation by prolonged infusion of flumazenil. *Anaesthesia* 43:376, 1988.

191. Pepperman M: Double-blind study of the reversal of midazolam-induced sedation in the ICU with flumazenil: Effect on weaning from ventilation. *Anaesth Intensive Care* 18:38, 1990.

192. Geller E, Halperri P, Leykin Y, et al: Midazolam infusion and

benzodiazepine antagonist for sedation in ICU. *Anesthesiology* 65:A65, 1986.

193. Chiolero R, Ravussin P, Anderes J, et al: The effects of midazolam reversal by RO 15-1788 on cerebral perfusion pressure in patients with severe head injury. *Intensive Care Med* 14:196, 1988.
194. Gross J, Weller R, Conard P: Flumazenil antagonism of midazolam-induced ventilatory depression. *Anesthesiology* 75:179, 1991.
195. Gonsalves S, Gallager D: Spontaneous and Ro 15-1788 induced reversal of subsensitivity to GABA following chronic benzodiazepines. *Eur J Pharmacol* 110:163, 1985.
196. Nutt D, Costello M: Rapid induction of lorazepam dependence and reversal with flumazenil. *Life Sci* 43:1045, 1984.
197. Gallager D, Lakoski J, Gonsalves S, et al: Chronic benzodiazepine treatment decreases postsynaptic GABA sensitivity. *Nature* 308:74, 1984.
198. Hart Y, Meinardi H, Sander J, et al: The effect of intravenous flumazenil on interictal EEG epileptic activity: Results of a placebo-controlled study. *J Neurol Neurosurg Psychiatry* 54:305, 1991.
199. Savic I, Widen L, Stone-Elander S: Feasibility of reversing benzodiazepine tolerance with flumazenil. *Lancet* 337:133, 1991.
200. Persson S, Pauli S, Halldin C, et al: Saturation analysis of specific (11)C-Ro 15—1788 binding to human neocortex using PET. *Hum Psychopharm* 4:21, 1989.
201. Shinitoh H, Ivo M, Yamada T: Detection of benzodiazepine receptor occupancy in the human brain by positron emission tomography. *Psychopharmacology* 99:202, 1989.
202. Hojer J, Baehrendtz S, Magnusson A, et al: A placebo-controlled trial of flumazenil given by continuous infusion in severe benzodiazepine overdosage. *Acta Anaesthesiol Scand* 35:584, 1991.
203. Brogden R, Goa K: Flumazenil: A reappraisal of its pharmacological properties and therapeutic efficacy as a benzodiazepine antagonist. *Drugs* 42:1061, 1991.
204. Klotz U, Ziegler G, Reimann I: Pharmacokinetics of the selective benzodiazepine antagonist Ro 15-1788 in man. *Eur J Clin Pharmacol* 27:115, 1984.
205. Klotz U, Ziegler G. Ludwig L, et al: Pharmacodynamic interaction between midazolam and a specific benzodiazepine antagonist in humans. *J Clin Pharmacol* 25:400, 1985.
206. Park G: Plasma concentrations of flumazenil during liver transplantation. *Anaesthesia* 47:887, 1992.
207. Chilero R, Ravussin P, Anderes J, et al: The effects of midazolam reversal by Ro 15-1788 oncerebral perfusion pressure in patients with severe head injury. *Intensive Care Med* 14:196, 1988.
208. Ricou B, Forster A, Bruckner A, et al: Clinical evaluation of a specific benzodiazepine antagonist. *Br J Anaesth* 58:1005, 1986.
209. White P, Shafer A, Boyle W, et al: Benzodiazepine antagonism does not provoke a stress response. *Anesthesiology* 70:636, 1989.

210. Antihypertensive Agents

Robert J. Straka, Bruce Lohr, Pamela Borchardt-Phelps, and Shawn Hansen

Overview

Numerous agents can be used to manage elevated blood pressure in the intensive care patient. This chapter summarizes the salient pharmacokinetic features of the more widely used or clinically relevant antihypertensive agents, with the perspective of the intensivist in mind.

Beta-Adrenergic Antagonists

Beta-adrenergic receptor antagonists are an important group of agents with varied pharmacokinetics and pharmacologic properties. As a class, they are similar in general mechanism of action—competitive beta-adrenergic receptor blockade—yet are dissimilar in pharmacologic properties such as relative cardioselectivity, intrinsic sympathomimetic activity, and alpha-receptor blocking activity. Use of beta-blockers in the management of hypertension, angina, and dysrrhythmias is based largely on the pharmacologic actions, available routes of administration, and pharmacokinetic profiles of the individual agents. Major differences between specific agents in terms of protein binding, bioavailability, and major route of elimination may have clinical consequences in the intensive care setting.

All of the beta-adrenergic antagonists are included in this section, but only propranolol, metoprolol, labetalol, atenolol, nadolol, and esmolol are discussed in depth.

PHARMACOLOGY. Table 210-1 summarizes the pertinent pharmacologic properties of the beta-adrenergic antagonists. As a class, beta-blockers exert their pharmacologic action by competitive blockade of the beta-receptors of the autonomic nervous system. They may be nonselective, such as propranolol, or selective, such as atenolol. Selective beta-receptor antagonists have a concentration-dependent specificity for blockade of beta$_1$-receptors over beta$_2$-receptors. This cardioselectivity can have clinical relevance when targeting cardiac beta$_1$-receptor antagonism while attempting to preserve beta$_2$-receptor stimulation by endogenous catecholamines. This may be the goal in a patient in whom a beta-blocker is the optimal treatment for a specific condition but who has a relative contraindication to its use, such as a questionable history of mild reactive airway disease. A cautious trial of a cardioselective beta-blocker may be in order.

Beta-adrenergic receptor blocking agents compete with beta-adrenergic agonists for available beta-receptor sites. Propranolol, nadolol, timolol, penbutolol, carteolol, sotalol, and pindolol inhibit both the beta$_1$ receptors (located chiefly in cardiac muscle) and beta$_2$ receptors (located chiefly in the bronchial and vascular musculature), inhibiting the chronotropic, inotropic, and vasodilator responses to beta-adrenergic stimulation. Metoprolol, acebutolol, bisoprolol, esmolol, betaxolol, and atenolol are cardioselective and preferentially inhibit beta$_1$ receptors.

Intrinsic sympathomimetic activity (ISA) refers to the property possessed by some beta-blockers that act as partial agonists while occupying the receptor in such a way as to behave simultaneously as an antagonist. The predominance of agonist/

Table 210-1. Pharmacologic and Pharmacokinetic Properties of Beta-Adrenergic Blocking Agents [4,75,182]

	Adrenergic receptor blocking activity	Intrinsic sympatho-mimetic activity	Lipid solubility	Extent of absorption (%)	Absolute oral bio-availability (%)	Half-life (hr)	Protein binding (%)	Clearance (ml/min)	Metabolism/excretion
Acebutolol	$\beta_1{}^a$	+	Low	90	20–60	3–4	26	615	Hepatic, renal excretion 30–40%, non-renal excretion 50–60% (bile, intestinal wall)
Atenolol	$\beta_1{}^a$	0	Low	50	50–60	6–9	6–16	130	≈ 50% excreted unchanged in feces
Betaxolol	$\beta_1{}^a$	0	Low	≈ 100	89	14–22	≈ 50	NA	Hepatic; > 80% recovered in urine, 15% unchanged
Bisoprolol	$\beta_1{}^a$	0	Low	≥ 90	80	9–12	≈ 30	NA	≈ 50% excreted unchanged in urine, remainder as inactive metabolites; < 2% excreted in feces
Esmolol	$\beta_1{}^a$	0	Low	na	na	0.15	55	170 ml/min/kg	Rapid metabolism by esterases in cytosol of red blood cells
Metoprolol, long-acting	$\beta_1{}^a$	0	Moderate	95	40–50 77	3–7	12	1100	Hepatic, renal excretion, < 5% unchanged
Carteolol	β_1, β_2	+ +	Low	80	85	6	23–30	NA	50–70% excreted unchanged in urine
Nadolol	β_1, β_2	0	Low	30	30–50	20–24	30	200	Urine, unchanged
Penbutolol	β_1, β_2	+	High	≈ 100	≈ 100	5	80–98	NA	Hepatic (conjugation and oxidation); renal excretion of metabolites (17% as conjugate)
Pindolol	β_1, β_2	+ + +	Moderate	95	≈ 100	3–4^b	40	400	Urinary excretion of metabolites (60–75%) and unchanged drug (35–40%)
Propranolol, long-acting	β_1, β_2	0	High	90	30 9–18	3–5 8–11	90	1000	Hepatic; < 1% excreted unchanged in urine
Sotalol	β_1, β_2	0	Low	ND	90–100	12	0	150	Not metabolized; excreted unchanged in urine
Timolol	β_1, β_2	0	Low to moderate	90	75	4	10	660	Hepatic; urinary excretion of metabolities and unchanged drug
Labetalol	$\beta_1, \beta_2,$ alpha$_1$	0	Moderate	100	30–40	5–5.8	50	2700	55–60% excreted in urine as conjugates or unchanged drug

^{a} Inhibits β_2 receptors (bronchial and vascular) at higher doses.
^{b} In elderly hypertensive patients with normal renal function, $t_{1/2}$ is variable (7–15 hr)
NA = not applicable (available IV only); ND = no data
0 = none; + = low; + + = moderate; + + + = high

antagonist activity is largely thought to be a function of relative circulating catecholamines. At higher levels of circulating catecholamines (e.g., in a patient with congestive heart failure), these agents behave similar to beta-blockers without ISA. On the other hand, in a patient with a low circulating catecholamine level with borderline bradycardia, a beta-blocker with ISA may be preferable to one without ISA to preserve an otherwise modest resting heart rate.

Local anesthetic activity is one property of beta-blockers of little known practical significance. This will not be discussed in detail other than to point out its possible link to the antiarrhythmic mechanism of action for some beta-blockers.

One aspect of the pharmacology of beta-blockers is their stereochemistry. With the exception of timolol and practolol, all commercially available beta-blockers are available as racemic mixtures of the dextrorotary (d) and levorotary (l) enantiomer. It is the l-enantiomer that is largely responsible for the beta-blocking effects of this class of agents. Stereoselective clearance, variability in enantiomeric protein binding, and volume of distribution can result in variable concentrations of the active/inactive forms of racemic mixtures. Their concentrations may be affected more in hyperdynamic than in nonstressed patients because the enantiomers are affected differently by altered hepatic or renal perfusion.

THERAPEUTIC RANGE. Therapeutic ranges associated with beta-blockers are of little clinical significance. This is largely due to the substantial interpatient variability in drug concentrations relative to dose and the accessibility of heart rate and blood pressure as monitoring tools. Serum concentration monitoring of beta-blockers is therefore generally not recommended.

PREPARATIONS. Table 210-2 summarizes the available preparations of beta-adrenergic antagonists.

PHARMACOKINETICS. Table 210-1 summarizes the pharmacokinetic properties of the beta-adrenergic antagonists. Specific pharmacokinetic information is provided below for selected agents.

Propranolol. Propranolol, available as a racemic mixture of the d- and l-enantiomers, enjoys extensive use for the treatment of numerous FDA-approved and unapproved indications. The l-enantiomer is the more potent of the two enantiomers and is responsible for the majority of the beta-receptor blocking action of the drug. Several important aspects of the pharmacokinetics of propranolol may have clinical implications for its use in hyperdynamic or hypodynamic patients. These include high first-pass metabolism, protein binding, and aspects of its stereopharmacology that relate to these factors.

ABSORPTION. Propranolol's absorption is virtually 100 percent due to its high degree of lipid solubility. The formulation of oral propranolol has a profound effect on absorption. Immediate-release propranolol is very rapidly absorbed from the gastrointenstinal tract, with peak plasma concentrations occurring within 1 to 2 hours, compared with 4 to 6 hours for the long-acting formulation [1].

The systemic availability of propranolol is compromised substantially by its high degree of first-pass metabolism, for several reasons. The dosage formulation and hence rate of presentation of drug to the metabolizing enzymes of the liver once absorbed influences bioavailability. Absolute oral bioavailability is highly variable but is considered in most subjects to be approximately

36 percent [2] of that of the intravenous formulation at steady state [3]. The absolute bioavailability of the sustained-release formulation has been reported to be approximately 9 to 18 percent [4]. Under similar conditions, in normal volunteers, the relative bioavailability of the long-acting form compared to equal doses of the immediate-release form is approximately 50 percent [5]. This demonstrates the saturability of the enzymes responsible for removal of the drug following oral absorption. The same phenomenon may explain the sensitivity of propranolol's bioavailability to dosage rate. Silber et al. [6] demonstrated the nonlinearity of propranolol's bioavailability with increasing dosages ranging from 40 to 320 mg of propranolol at steady state. There was a 56 ± 20 percent reduction in intrinsic clearance and a 175 percent increase in half-life over these dosages.

As with many high-clearance drugs, propranolol's apparent oral clearance decreases with chronic dosing. Wood et al. [3] demonstrated an increase in bioavailability from 22 percent following single doses to 34 percent after steady-state dosing with corresponding increases in the area under the curve (AUC). A small but statistically insignificant reduction in systemic clearance and concomitant increase in half-life was also observed of interest, the degree of accumulation or increase in AUC following steady-state dosing compared to single-dose studies appears not to differ between immediate-release (49%) and sustained-release (68%) formulations. Furthermore, the accumulation observed after total steady-state dosing and single doses of d- and l-enantiomer AUC appears to occur to a similar degree for each enantiomer. Lalonde et al. [7] demonstrated the l/d accumulation ratio to be 1.52 after single doses compared to 1.32 after steady-state dosing.

DISTRIBUTION. The overall volume of distribution of propranolol is quite large. Values of approximately 200 liters [8] indicate extensive distribution throughout the body and substantial tissue accumulation [9]. High tissue levels in the central nervous system (CNS) produce CNS side effects. Serum protein binding is significant. Straka et al. [10] report binding to be in excess of 90 percent. However, like other weak bases, propranolol's binding to acute-phase reactant proteins such as alpha-1-acid glycoprotein (AAG) may be clinically significant [11,12]. Given propranolol's variability in other pharmacokinetic properties [8] and in the relationship between free concentrations and pharmacodynamic effect [1], the clinical relevance of binding to AAG may be limited to subtle differences in stereoselective binding to AAG [13]. Walle et al. noted that the unbound l:d propranolol ratio decreased from 0.93 to 0.81 as overall protein binding of propranolol increased [13]. It was suggested that this may result in a decrease in cardioactive l-enantiomer in settings where AAG levels are temporally elevated beyond normal values [14]. This may be the case in extreme stress, as is commonly encountered in intensive care patients.

ELIMINATION. Propranolol's elimination is largely based on its extensive metabolism by the liver. Walle et al. [15] reported that less than 1 percent of an administered dose is recovered unchanged in the urine. The bulk of the total recovery of propranolol within 24 hours is in the forms of propranolol glucuronide (17%), naphthoxylactic acid (21%), 4-hydroxypropranolol sulfate (22%), and 4-hydroxypropranolol glucuronide (12%). Although there is evidence of accumulation of propranolol's metabolites in renal dysfunction, there appears to be no need to adjust the dose in this patient population.

The metabolism of few drugs have been as extensively studied as that of propranolol. The metabolism of propranolol is largely by the P-450 mixed function oxidase system. The saturability of enzymes responsible for propranolol's metabolism was already discussed (see Absorption). The dependence of propranolol's metabolism on hepatic blood flow and intrinsic clearance following intravenous administration make these im-

Table 210-2. Preparations and Dosing Guidelines for Beta-Adrenergic Antagonists [4,33]

Agent	Available preparations	Starting dose	Usual maintenance dose	Maximum dose
Acebutolol	200, 400 mg tablets	400 mg/day	400–800 mg/day	1200 mg/day
Atenolol	25, 50, 100 mg tablets 5 mg/10 ml injection	po: 50 mg qd IV (post-MI): 5 mg over 5 min, then 5 mg in 10 min	50–100 mg/day	200 mg/day
Betaxolol	10, 20 mg tablets	10 mg qd	10–20 mg/day	40 mg/day
Bisoprolol	5, 10 mg tablets	5 mg qd	10 mg/day	20 mg/day
Carteolol	2.5, 5 mg tablets	2.5 mg qd	5–10 mg/day	10 mg/day
Esmolol	10, 250 mg/ml injection	500 μg/kg	50 μg/kg/min, increase by 50 μg/kg/min with a 500 μg/kg bolus prior	Maximum rate 300 μg/kg/min
Labetalol	100, 200, 300 mg tablets 5 mg/ml injection	po: 100 mg bid IV: 20 mg over 2 min; may repeat 40–80 mg q10min	po: 200–400 mg bid	po: 2.4 g/day IV: 300 mg
Metoprolol	50, 100 mg IR tablets 50, 100, 200 mg XR tablets 1 mg/ml injection	po IR: 50 mg bid po XR: 100 mg qd IV (post-mI): 5 mg q2 min × 3	po: 100–450 mg/day	po: 450 mg/day
Nadolol	20, 40, 80, 120, 160 mg tablets	40 mg bid	40–80 mg/day	240 mg/day
Penbutolol	20 mg tablet	20 mg qd	20 mg/day	40 mg/day
Pindolol	5-mg, 10-mg tablets	5 mg bid	20–40 mg/day	60 mg/day
Propranolol	10, 20, 40, 60, 80, 90 mg tablets 60, 80, 120, 160 mg SR capsules 4, 8, 80 mg/ml oral solution 1 mg/ml injection	po: 40 mg bid po SR: 80 mg qd IV: 1–3 mg; may repeat × 1 in 2 minutes	po: 120–240 mg/day po SR: 120–160 mg	640 mg/day
Sotalol	80, 160, 240 mg tablets	80 mg bid	240–360 mg/day	480–640 mg day
Timolol	5, 10, 20 mg tablets	10 mg bid	20–40 mg/day	60 mg/day

IR = immediate release; XR = extended release; SR = sustained release

portant considerations in the intensive care patient. Numerous factors may affect liver blood flow and intrinsic clearance (e.g., interacting drugs, hypo/hyperdynamic states) and consequently may contribute to altered metabolism of propranolol.

The elimination half-life of propranolol at steady state varies but has been reported to average approximately 4 hours [2,3]. The half-life may be dose dependent due to saturability of the enzymes responsible for propanolol's metabolism [16]. The clinical significance of the variability in half-life is limited due to the dissociation between the pharmacokinetic half-life and pharmacodynamic response. Although the pharmacodynamic half-life is variable based on the parameter being monitored, the pharmacodynamic half-life for blood pressure control can be longer than propanolol's pharmacokinetic half-life [1]. This argument has been used to justify once or twice daily dosing of regular-release propranolol formulation for hypertension [17,18]. In spite of rapidly falling drug concentrations due to propanolol's short half-life, the minimum concentration needed to lower blood pressure is maintained for an extended period of time.

More than 22 metabolites were identified by Walle et al. [15]. The major routes of metabolism following an oral dose include ring oxidation (accounting for approximately 31%), side chain oxidation (approximately 22%) and glucuronide formation of propranolol itself (approximately 15%) and its metabolic prod-

ucts [19]. The 4-hydroxypropranolol metabolite, though active, probably has little clinical significance.

Metoprolol

ABSORPTION. Absorption of oral metoprolol is complete, with a reported bioavailability of 40 to 50 percent. Metoprolol undergoes extensive first-pass metabolism, resulting in substantial intersubject variability in oral bioavailability [20,21]. Food may increase oral bioavailability, but the clinical importance of this is probably limited [20].

DISTRIBUTION. Metoprolol is considered a lipophilic drug, although it is considerably less lipophilic than propranolol. It is substantially less protein-bound than propranolol, reportedly as low as 12 percent [22].

ELIMINATION. Like propranolol, metoprolol is extensively metabolized in the liver. Only 10 percent of the dose is recovered in the urine as unchanged drug, with the remainder metabolized to alpha-hydroxymetoprolol (10%) or an amphoteric metabolite [23] by demethylation and secondary oxidation. Two unique aspects of metoprolol's metabolism are the polymorphic nature of the metabolism and the stereopharmacokinetic differences in metabolism of its enantiomers. Metoprolol cosegregates with the P-450IID6, or debrisoquine, pathway. Six to 9 percent of the North American Caucasian population are deficient in this enzyme. These individuals have longer half-lifes and reduced clearance of metoprolol [24,25]. This pharmacogenetically based variability in pharmacokinetics, discussed at length elsewhere [26], has two consequences for intensive care patients. First, if it is unknown whether an individual has a P-450IID6 isozyme deficiency, metoprolol dosing should proceed slowly and drug accumulation (due to reduced clearance) and duration of response (due to increased half-life) should be monitored. Poor metabolizers (those lacking P-450IID6) may have a greater than sixfold increase in AUC and a half-life up to 2.5 times longer than that in extensive metabolizers (those possessing P-450IID6) [24]. Consequently, it may take longer to achieve steady state in poor metabolizers than in extensive metabolizers. The second consideration is potential drug-drug interactions. Extensive metabolizers behave as poor metabolizers (who are deficient for P-450IID6) when the enzyme is inhibited. Drugs such as quinidine and the selective serotonin reuptake inhibitors (e.g., fluoxitine, paroxitine and sertraline) inhibit this enzyme, thus effectively converting an extensive metabolizer to a poor metabolizer. Coadministration of these agents may therefore have profound consequenses. This is particularly true if, for example, metoprolol is titrated to a goal heart rate or blood pressure in an extensive metabolizer and an inhibitor is added or removed at some point. There are numerous reports of decompensation of patients under these conditions [27]. Addition of these inhibitors to a poor metabolizer's drug regimen has no effect.

The issue of stereopharmacology is less clinically important. Like many other beta-blockers metoprolol is administered as a racemic mixture of the active l- and inactive d-enantiomers. The ratio of these enantiomers is deferent between extensive and poor metabolizers (extensive metabolizers having a higher l-AUC:d-AUC ratio), but this is of little clinical significance.

As a result of the polymorphic nature of metoprolol's metabolism and its stereopharmacology, reported half-life and clearance must to be qualified. Table 210-3 depicts the differences in half-lives (expressed as elimination rate constants) between extensive and poor metabolizers of P-450IID6 system. Overall, half-lives of approximately 3 hours for extensive metabolizers and 6 hours or more for poor metabolizers are most likely to be seen.

Labetolol. Labetalol, a nonselective beta-antagonist, is unique in that it also possesses alpha$_1$-adrenergic antagonistic activity. It is therefore the only beta-blocking agent that tends to decrease peripheral vascular resistance while lowering blood pressure. It is also unique in that, having two chiral (asymmetric) centers, it is actually a mixture of four separate enantiomers, each of which has slightly different pharmacologic activity.

Atenolol and Nadolol

ABSORPTION. As hydrophilic drugs, these agents have modest absorption, resulting in bioavailabilities of approximately 50 percent following oral administration [28,29].

DISTRIBUTION. Both atenolol and nadolol are distributed more slowly and to a lesser extent than their lipophilic counterparts.

Table 210-3. Pharmacokinetic Differences Between Extensive and Poor Metabolizers of Metoprolol [25]

Parameter	Extensive metabolizers	Poor metabolizers
Number of subjects	7	4
AUC (−) metoprolol (Ng × hr/ml)	767	2549
k (elimination rate constant) (hr-1)	0.245	0.115
AUC (−enantiomer/+enantiomer)	1.33	0.9

AUC = area under concentration-time curve

Time to maximum response within a dosing interval is therefore typically longer for these agents than for propranolol or metoprolol. Furthermore, their hydrophilicity can be argued to limit their likely penetratability into the CNS and hence elicit likely CNS side effects attributed to more lipophilic beta-blockers.

ELIMINATION. The elimination of both atenolol and nadolol depends substantially on renal function. Both drugs accumulate in patients with compromised renal function. Given that approximately 18 percent of nadolol and up to 45 percent of atenolol is excreted unchanged in the urine, dosages must be adjusted in patients with renal dysfunction. Reported serum half-lives are 6 to 9 hours for atenolol and 20 to 24 hours for nadolol in patients with normal renal function (Table 210-1), compared with greater than 50 hours for either drug in patients with severely compromised (GFR < 10 ml/min) renal function [30,31].

Esmolol.

Esmolol is an ultra-short-acting beta-adrenergic blocking agent. It is cardioselective, with no intrinsic sympathomimetic or alpha-blocking activity. It is FDA-approved for treatment of paroxysmal supraventricular tachycardia (PSVT) but is often used as an antihypertensive agent.

ABSORPTION. Esmolol is available for intravenous use only. It is administered as a bolus and continuous infusion. Additional boluses may sometimes be required, but due to its extremely short half-life, this is often not necessary.

DISTRIBUTION. The volume of distribution of esmolol is approximately 3.43 ± 1.42 liter per kilogram [32].

ELIMINATION. Elimination of esmolol is unlike that of other beta-blockers in that the parent drug is rapidly metabolized in blood to an acid metabolite with a reported half-life of 3.7 hours [32]. This metabolite is eliminated renally. The elimination of esmolol is unaffected by hepatic or renal insufficiency. This is in contrast to most other beta-blockers, for which compromised renal or hepatic function may result in accumulation of the parent or its metabolite.

PHYSIOLOGIC CLEARANCE.

The physiologic clearance characteristics for selected agents are described below.

Propranolol

HYPODYNAMIC. Because propranolol's elimination is dependent on liver blood flow, the decreased liver blood flow in hypodynamic patients is likely to cause a decrease in systemic clearance of the parent compound. The result may be negative chronotropism and inotropism or exaggerated hypotensive effects. This agent should therefore be used with caution in hypodynamic patients with close monitoring of the patient's hemodynamics.

The effects of propranolol in this patient population depend largely on the magnitude of decline in liver blood flow and (as a consequence) of altered intrinsic clearance. However, since propranolol's effects may be related to free (unbound) concentrations and patients in a hypodynamic state may respond with the creation and liberation of acute phase reactants, such as AAG, the anticipated exaggerated effects may be somewhat attenuated.

HYPERDYNAMIC. Patients with substantially increased hepatic blood flow (due to stress, etc.) may experience a diminished response to typical doses of propranolol. This may be a consequence of both an increased capacity to mctabolize the drug (as a result of increase in blood flow) and a need for higher concentrations of the drug to offset heightened competition for beta-blockade at the receptor level, given higher circulating catacholamines and a likely increase in protein binding to AAG. Consequently, propranolol may be used more aggressively, but cautiously. Hemodynamic endpoints such as blood pressure and heart rate may require adjustment, depending on the indication for the drug. Alternatively, selection of another beta-blocker may simplify the predictability of response in the hyper- or hypodynamic patient.

Metoprolol and Labetolol

HYPODYNAMIC. Metoprolol's elimination in the hypodynamic patient is likely to be affected to a limited degree. Although difficult to predict because of its relative dependence on hepatic blood flow, its elimination is likely to be reduced in the modestly perfused hypodynamic patient. The magnitude of difference in elimination and hence pharmacologic effect is likely to be less profound than that seen in the hypodynamic patient on propranolol.

HYPERDYNAMIC. A hyperdynamic patient given metoprolol is likely to have a somewhat increased clearance and hence possibly shorter half-life. In both hypodynamic and hyperdynamic cases, metoprolol's hemodynamic effect should be carefully monitored.

Atenolol and Nadolol

HYPODYNAMIC. In the hypodynamic state, the risk of compromised renal function and hence renal elimination of nadolol and atenolol exists. The consequences of this physiologic effect may necessitate a decrease in dose or, more likely, the frequency of administration. Alternatively, given the lack of a clear relationship between pharmacologic response and pharmacokinetic alterations of beta-blockers, careful monitoring of the response may suffice.

HYPERDYNAMIC. Significant consequences due to increased perfusion of eliminating organs are unlikely. Although some change in renal function may result, it is unlikely to necessitate major dosage adjustments.

Esmolol. Because this agent is cleared by esterases in red blood cells, no dosage adjustment is necessary in hypodynamic and hyperdynamic patients with physiologic alterations in organ blood flow.

DOSING GUIDELINES. Table 210-2 summarizes the dosing guidelines for the beta-adrenergic antagonists. Additional dosing information for esmolol is provided below.

Esmolol

LOADING DOSE. Because of its extremely short half-life, a loading dose is recommended to achieve concentrations that approximate those at steady state. Usually a dose of 0.5 mg per kilogram over 1 minute is given. This may be administered from an IV bag, diluted to 10 mg per milliliter, or a 10-mg per milliliter ampule may be used. The maintenance infusion should be started immediately after the first bolus is given. Additional boluses (0.5 mg/kg for 1 minute) may be administered but are often not necessary and may result in a precipitous drop in blood pressure and, perhaps, heart rate.

MAINTENANCE DOSE. Usually, a maintenance infusion of one-tenth the loading dose or 0.05 mg/kg/min (or 50 μg/kg/min) is started after the loading dose is given. The maintenance infusion may be increased by 50 μg/kg/min every 10 to 15 minutes as needed to control heart rate or blood pressure.

DRUG INTERACTIONS. Calcium channel blocking agents when combined with beta-blockers can potentiate the phar-

macologic effects of beta-blockers. When combination therapy is used, careful monitoring of cardiac function (heart rate, blood pressure, cardiac output, etc.) is prudent.

Flecainide when combined with beta-blockers can increase the bioavailability of the beta-blocker, possibly increasing pharmacologic effects.

H2 antagonists when combined with beta-blockers may inhibit metabolism of the beta-blocker. This is most likely to occur with cimetidine but can occur with other agents. The magnitude and consistency of this interaction is variable.

Hydralazine may interact with certain beta-blockers (e.g., propranolol and metoprolol) that tend to increase serum levels and hence pharmacologic effect. This is a bi-directional interaction: beta-blockers may also cause increased hydralazine serum levels.

Propafenone when combined with certain beta-blockers (e.g., metoprolol) may increase serum levels due to enzyme (P-450IID6) inhibition and combined beta-blocking effects of both propafenone and the coadministered beta-blocker.

Quinidine when combined with beta-blockers may increase serum levels due to its ability to inhibit P-450IID6 and thus convert extensive metabolizers into poor metabolizers (see Elimination).

Quinolones such as ciprofloxacin may increase the bioavailability of beta-blockers due to inhibition of cytochrome P-450 metabolism.

Thyroid hormones when coadministered with beta-blockers to convert a hypothyroid patient to a euthyroid state, may decrease the pharmacologic effects of beta-blockers.

Anticoagulants may have their effect exaggerated when coadministered with beta-blockers (e.g., propranolol with warfarin).

Clonidine when abruptly withdrawn either in combination with beta-blockers or alone has been reported to cause life-threatening increases in blood pressure response.

Lidocaine levels may increase when coadministered with beta-blockers.

The hypoglycemic effects of sulfonylureas may be attenuated when coadministered with beta-blockers.

Theophylline elimination may be reduced by coadministering certain beta-blockers. In addition, there is pharmacological antagonism when co-administering theophylline and a beta-blocker to a patient with reactive airway disease (regardless of cardioselectivity).

COMMON PITFALLS

1. Beta$_1$-receptor cardioselectivity of beta-blocking agents is a relative property. At higher doses and in select patients at relatively low doses, agents possessing cardioselectivity may behave as both beta$_1$- and beta$_2$-antagonists. Even cardioselective beta-antagonists should be used with caution in patients with a contraindication to beta$_2$-antagonism.

2. Intensive care patients may exhibit physiologically appropriate tachycardia and hypertension. Use of beta-blocking agents to lower heart rate and mitigate elevated blood pressure should be evaluated in the context of physiologic need for the observed tachycardia and hypertension.

3. An approach to the use of beta-blockers in hyper- and hypodynamic patients requires consideration of the specific agent's properties. No one approach may apply to all beta-blockers. The time course and complexity of the interplay of elevations of acute phase reactant protein production secondary to stress or hyper- or hypodynamic states and their effects on drug metabolism and elimination should be continuously reevaluated.

Loop Diuretics

INTRODUCTION. So named because they act primarily on the thick ascending limb of Henle's loop, the loop diuretics are the most potent diuretics in clinical use. Furosemide, the prototype loop diuretic, was introduced in 1966. The other two loop diuretics available in the United States are bumetanide and ethacrynic acid. Despite their different chemical structures, the three loop diuretics have similar actions. They are used primarily for their diuretic action in the treatment of edema associated with congestive heart failure, hepatic cirrhosis, and renal disease, including nephrotic syndrome. They are generally not used as first-line agents in the treatment of hypertension because they do not modify arteriolar tone to the same degree as the thiazide diuretics. Furthermore, because the loop diuretics are shorter-acting they must be given more frequently than the thiazides. Thus, the loop diuretics are generally reserved for hypertensive patients with significantly impaired renal function who no longer respond to thiazides. Ethacrynic acid is the only nonsulfonamide diuretic, except for the potassium-sparing agents. It is useful in patients who cannot tolerate sulfonamide compounds [33].

PHARMACOLOGY. The loop diuretics are actively secreted via the nonspecific organic acid transport system into the lumen of the thick ascending limb of Henle's loop. There they inhibit the coupled transport of sodium and chloride from the lumen into the cell. Normally this nephron segment reabsorbs 20 to 30 percent of the filtered load of sodium chloride. The natriuretic effect of the loop diuretics also depends on a prostaglandin-mediated increase in renal blood flow that serves to decrease the interstitial concentration of solutes. As a result of inhibition of coupled transport and increased renal blood flow, medullary hypertonicity is decreased and the kidney's ability to reabsorb water is diminished. Excretion of sodium, chloride, potassium, hydrogen ion, calcium, magnesium, ammonium, bicarbonate, and possibly phosphate is enhanced. All loop diuretics also produce an acute increase in venous capacitance by venodilation of the large veins, particularly within the thorax. This effect is noted within minutes of intravenous administration and is independent of diuretic effect. Loop diuretics can produce rapid improvement in pulmonary edema via this effect [33,34,35].

THERAPEUTIC RANGE. No therapeutic range has been established for the loop diuretics.

PREPARATIONS

Furosemide	20-mg, 40-mg, 80-mg oral tablets; 8-mg/ml and 10-mg/ml oral solution; 10-mg/ml IM, IV injection [33]
Bumetanide	0.5-mg, 1-mg, 2-mg oral tablets; 0.25-mg/ml IM, IV injection [33]
Ethacrynic Acid	25-mg and 50-mg oral tablets; 50-mg powder for IM, IV injection [33]

PHARMACOKINETICS. The pharmacokinetic properties of the loop diuretics are summarized in Table 210-4.

PHYSIOLOGIC CLEARANCE

Hypodynamic. The loop diuretics are flow-dependent drugs, as blood flow to the kidney and liver are the primary determinants of clearance. All of these agents have elimination half-lives of approximately 1 hour in normal subjects. Although elimination is reduced in patients with renal failure, these patients require, rather than a reduction in dosage, higher doses, because of reduced efficacy. This reduced efficacy is due to two factors. First, the nephron mass available to respond to the diuretic is reduced. Second, the proximal tubular organic acid transport system that actively delivers loop diuretics into the lumen of the nephron is competitively inhibited by organic acids that accumulate in chronic renal failure, thereby reducing drug delivery to its site of action within the nephron. Patients with congestive heart failure, nephrotic syndrome, and liver cirrhosis may also require larger, rather than reduced, doses of loop diuretics because of altered pharmacokinetics. The full oral absorption of furosemide is delayed due to edema in the gut wall. This does not appear to affect bumetanide oral absorption. Congestive heart failure is also associated with reduced blood flow to the kidney, resulting in decreased delivery of loop diuretics to the tubule. The hypoalbuminemia seen in patients with nephrotic syndrome and liver cirrhosis results in a reduction in protein binding of the loop diuretics (normally 90% protein-bound), increasing the unbound fraction. However, the unbound drug diffuses into the tissues, thereby in-

Table 210-4. Pharmacokinetic Parameters of the Loop Diuretics [4,33,34]

	Furosemide oral	Vumetanide oral	Ethacrynic acid oral
Bioavailability	40–70%	72–96%	95–100%
Onset of diuresis	0.5–1 hr	0.5–1 hr	0.5 hr
Peak diuresis	1–2 hr	1–2 hr	2 hr
Duration of Diuresis	6–8 hr	4–6 hr	6–8 hr
V_{dss}	0.091–0.174 L/kg	9.45–19.7 L	—
Protein binding	96–99%	92–96%	> 90%
Elimination half-life (healthy adults)	0.5–2 hr[a]	1–1.5 hr[a]	1 hr[a]
Metabolism	Liver	Liver	Liver
Active metabolites	—	No	Yes
Excretion	Renal + biliary/fecal[b]	Renal + biliary/fecal[c]	Renal + biliary/fecal[d]

[a] The terminal half-life is prolonged in patients with renal and/or hepatic dysfunction.
[b] 60–70% excreted renally (20–55% as parent drug)
[c] 81% excreted renally (45% as parent drug)
[d] 65% excreted renally (20% as parent drug)

creasing the volume of distribution and reducing the amount of drug delivered to the peritubular sites of loop diuretic transport in the kidney [4,33,34,35].

Hyperdynamic. Little is known about the pharmacokinetics of the loop diuretics in the hyperdynamic population. Theoretically, hyperdynamic patients with normal serum albumin levels would have increased physiologic clearance of loop diuretics because of increased blood flow to the kidney and liver. They may require more frequent dosing due to a shorter duration of diuretic effect. Hyperdynamic patients with reduced serum albumin levels may require higher doses of loop diuretics, because protein binding to albumin is necessary for delivery to the peritubular sites of loop diuretic transport into the lumen of the nephron.

DOSING GUIDELINES. Table 210-5 summarizes the dosing guidelines for the loop diuretics.

DRUG INTERACTIONS

Aminoglycosides. Auditory toxicity resulting from parenteral aminoglycoside antibiotics appears to be increased when coadministered with loop diuretics. Experimental data suggest a synergistic ototoxicity when the agents are combined that appears to be related to dose and serum concentration of the two drugs. The risk of ototoxicity is increased further in patients with renal insufficiency. Hearing loss of varying degree may occur, and irreversible hearing loss has occurred. Excessive doses of each agent should be avoided in patients with impaired renal function. Periodic monitoring of hearing acuity may be useful [36,37].

Digitalis Glycosides. Loop diuretic-induced electrolyte disturbances may predispose to digitalis-induced arrhythmias, especially in patients with preexisting cardiac abnormalities. Plasma levels of potassium and magnesium should be monitored when these drugs are used in combination and patients with low electrolyte levels should receive supplements. Further electrolyte disturbances can be prevented with dietary sodium restriction or the addition of potassium- and magnesium-sparing diuretics [38,39].

Cisplatin. Coadministration of loop diuretics and cisplatin may increase the potential for ototoxicity far greater than expected from either agent alone. This combination should be avoided, if possible. If it is necessary to use this combination of agents, hearing tests should be performed for early detection of hearing loss [40,41].

Nonsteroidal Antiinflammatory Drugs. Coadministration of nonsteroidal antiinflammatory drugs (NSAIDs) and loop diuretics may reduce the natriuretic and antihypertensive effects of the loop diuretics due to inhibition of prostaglandin synthesis. A higher dose of loop diuretic may be required or a different antiinflammatory drug may be used. The interaction has been reported most often with indomethacin, ibuprofen, and sulindac [42,43,44].

Warfarin. Ethacrynic acid may increase the hypoprothrombinemic effect of warfarin. Furosemide and bumetanide do not appear to interact. Patients receiving this combination should be monitored for enhanced anticoagulant effect and the warfarin dose adjusted accordingly [33].

Lithium. Loop diuretics may increase the therapeutic and toxic effects (e.g., gastrointestinal symptoms, polyuria, muscular weakness, lethargy, tremor) of lithium. Lithium levels should be monitored and the dose lowered if necessary [33].

COMMON PITFALLS

1. Acute hypotensive episodes have occasionally occurred within several hours of initial doses of angiotensin-converting enzyme (ACE) inhibitors in patients receiving loop diuretics. Hypovolemia due to diuretic therapy appears to be a predisposing factor. Therapy with ACE inhibitors should be undertaken with caution. It may be desirable to withdraw the diuretic temporarily prior to starting the ACE inhibitor. If this is not possible, lower initial doses of the ACE inhibitor should be used [45,46].
2. Excessive potassium loss may result from concomitant administration of corticosteroids and loop diuretics. This is more likely to occur with corticosteroids possessing significant mineral corticoid effects, such as hydrocortisone, cortisone, and, to a lesser extent, prednisone, prednisolone, and methylprednisolone. Special attention should be given to serum potassium levels when corticosteroids are given to patients receiving loop diuretics. Corticosteroids such as dexamethasone and triamcinolone have minimal potassium wasting activity [47].
3. Hepatic encephalopathy and/or coma has been precipitated in patients with hepatic cirrhosis and ascites due to sudden alterations in fluid and electrolyte balance from the use of loop diuretics. Loop diuretics should be initiated at low doses in a hospital setting, with careful monitoring of fluid and electrolyte balance and clinical status. Supplemental therapy with potassium chloride or potassium-sparing diuretics may be used to prevent hypokalemia and metabolic alkalosis in these patients [33].

Table 210-5. Dosing Guidelines for Loop Diuretics in the Treatment of Hypertension [4,33]

	Furosemide[a,b,c]	Bumetanide[a,b,c]	Ethacrynic acid[a,b]
Starting dose	10–20 mg po bid	0.5 mg po qd	25–50 mg po qd
Usual maintenance dose	20–40 mg po bid	1–2 mg po qd	25–50 mg po bid
Maximum dose	160–240 mg po bid	5 mg po bid	100 mg po bid

[a] The hypotensive effect of antihypertensive agents may be enhanced during concomitant loop diuretic administration. The dosage of the antihypertensive agent should be reduced when a loop diuretic is added to an existing antihypertensive regimen.
[b] The loop diuretics are contraindicated in patients with anuria.
[c] No specific information regarding dosing of hyperdynamic patients is available. Patients with renal disease and liver disease may require higher doses of the loop diuretics.

Thiazides and Related Diuretics

INTRODUCTION. The thiazide class of sulfonamide diuretics includes a large number of compounds with similar chemical structures. Also in this group are a number of sulfonamide diuretics that differ chemically from the thiazides but have pharmacologic activity that is indistinguishable from that of the thiazides. These include chlorthalidone, quinethazone, metolazone, and indapamide.

The thiazides and related diuretics are the most frequently used antihypertensive agents in the United States. They are first-line agents in the pharmacologic management of hypertension and have been used as monotherapy or in combination with other classes of antihypertensives. A reduction in morbidity and mortality has been demonstrated with these agents in clinical studies. All of the thiazide and related diuretics are equally effective in lowering blood pressure. The major differences between them are potency, elimination half-life, and duration of diuretic effect. However, these differences may not be clinically relevant, as the elimination half-life does not correlate with the duration of hypotensive effect [33,34].

PHARMACOLOGY. The thiazides and related diuretics enhance the renal excretion of sodium, chloride, and water by interfering with the transport of sodium ions across the renal tubular epithelium in the cortical diluting segment of the nephron. They also increase potassium, magnesium, and bicarbonate excretion. Calcium and uric acid excretion are decreased [33,34].

The exact mechanism of action for the antihypertensive effect of the thiazides and related diuretics is unknown. Acutely, they lower blood pressure by causing a diuresis with a resultant reduction in plasma volume and cardiac output. After several weeks of therapy the plasma and extracellular fluid volumes approach but remain slightly below normal. Peripheral vascular resistance falls below pretreatment baseline. It is the reduction in peripheral vascular resistance that is responsible for the an-

tihypertensive effect of chronic thiazide therapy. It is postulated that this reduction is due in part to a direct arteriolar dilation effect, as well as mobilization of sodium and water from arteriolar walls [33,34].

Thiazides can induce hyperglycemia, exacerbate preexisting diabetes mellitus, or precipitate diabetes in prediabetic patients. The mechanism for this effect of thiazides is not known [33,34].

THERAPEUTIC RANGE. No therapeutic range has been established for the thiazide and related diuretics.

PREPARATIONS. Table 210-6 summarizes the available thiazide and related diuretic preparations.

PHARMACOKINETICS. Table 210-7 summarizes the pharmacokinetic parameters for the thiazide and related diuretics.

PHYSIOLOGIC CLEARANCE

Hypometabolic. The clearance for most of these agents is primarily via glomerular filtration and secretion as unchanged drug. Clearance is decreased in patients with renal dysfunction and congestive heart failure. Patients with mild to moderate renal insufficiency generally require no dosage adjustments. The thiazides and related drugs (except metolazone and indapamide) become ineffective when the glomerular filtration rate drops below 25 ml per minute. Thus, their use is not recommended in severe renal failure [33].

Indapamide is extensively metabolized in the liver to glucoronide and sulfate conjugates. Excessive accumulation does not occur in patients with decreased or no renal function. Liver dysfunction probably results in reduced clearance of indapamide, therefore the drug should be used with caution in this population. Hepatic dysfunction should not affect the clearance of the other thiazides, as they are primarily excreted by the kidneys unchanged. They may, however, induce hepatic en-

Table 210-6. Preparations and the Oral Dosing Guidelines for the Thiazide and Related Diuretics for the Treatment of Hypertension [33]

Diuretic*	Preparations	Starting dose	Maintenance dose	Maximum dose
Chlorothiazide	250, 500 mg tablets, 250 mg/5 ml oral suspension	250–500 mg/day	250–1000 mg/day	1000 mg/day
Hydrochlorothiazide	25, 50, 100 mg tablets 50 mg/5 ml, 100 mg/ml oral solution	50–100 mg/day	25–100 mg/day	200 mg/day
Bendroflumethiazide	5, 10 mg tablets	5–20 mg/day	2.5–15 mg/day	20 mg/day
Cyclothiazide	2 mg tablets	2 mg/day	2–4 mg/day	6 mg/day
Methyclothiazide	2.5, 5 mg tablets	2.5–5 mg/day	2.5–5 mg/day	5 mg/day
Benzthiazide	50 mg tablets	25–50 mg bid	25–50 mg bid	200 mg/day
Hydroflumethiazide	50 mg tablets	50 mg bid	50–100 mg/day	200 mg/day
Trichlormethiazide	2, 4 mg tablets	2 mg/day	2–4 mg/day	4 mg/day
Polythiazide	1, 2, 4 mg tablets	2 mg/day	1–4 mg/day	4 mg/day
Quinethazone	50-mg tablets	50–100 mg/day	50–100 mg/day	200 mg/day
Metolazone	2.5, 5, 10 mg extended-release tablets	2.5–5 mg/day	2.5–5 mg/day	10 mg/day
Metolazone	0.5 mg prompt tablets	0.5 mg/day	0.5–1 mg/day	1 mg/day
Chlorthalidone	25, 50, 100 mg tabs	25 mg/day	25–50 mg/day	100 mg/day
Indapamide	2.5 mg tablets	2.5 mg/day	2.5–5 mg/day	5 mg/day

* No specific information regarding dosing of hypodynamic or hyperdynamic patients is available.

Table 210-7. Pharmacokinetic Parameters of the Thiazide and Related Diuretics [4,33,34,35]

	Bioavailability	V_{dss}	Protein binding	Elimination half-life[a]	Metabolism	Excretion
Chlorothiazide	10–21%	—	20–80%	1–2 hr	None	Renal (unchanged)
Hydrochlorothiazide	65–75%	3L/kg	40%	6–15 hr	None	Renal (unchanged)
Bendroflumethiazide	95–100%	—	94%	8–9 hr	None	Renal (unchanged)
Cyclothiazide	—	—	—	—	—	Renal
Methyclothiazide	—	—	—	—	—	Renal
Benzthiazide	—	—	—	—	None	Renal (unchanged)
Hydroflumethiazide	50%	—	74%	17 hr	—	Renal
Trichlormethizide	—	—	—	—	—	Renal
Polythiazide	—	—	84%	—	Liver	Renal + biliary/fecal
Quinethazone	—	—	—	—	—	Renal
Metolazone	64%[b]	113 L	50–70%	8–14 hr	Liver	Renal + biliary/fecal[c]
Chlorthalidone	64%	—	75%	40 hr	—	Renal[d]
Indapamide	90%	60–110 L	75–80%	14–18 hr	Liver	Renal + biliary/fecal[e]

[a] In patients with uncompensated congestive heart failure or impaired renal function, excretion may be delayed.
[b] Bioavailability of the extended-release formulation. The prompt formulation (MyKrox) is more rapidly and completely absorbed.
[c] 70–90% excreted renally unchanged.
[d] 30–60% excreted renally unchanged.
[e] 60–70% excreted renally (7% as parent drug); approximately 16–23% excreted in feces via biliary elimination.

cephalopathy in this population and should be used with caution.

Hypermetabolic. No information is available on the clearance of these agents in hypermetabolic patients. Theoretically, clearance should be increased via enhanced renal blood flow, but this greater clearance is probably not clinically significant.

DOSING GUIDELINES. Table 210-6 summarizes the dosing guidelines for the thiazide and related diuretics.

DRUG INTERACTIONS
Digitalis Glycosides. A dose-dependent reduction in serum potassium and magnesium by thiazide diuretics may predispose patients to digitalis-induced arrhythmias. Plasma levels of potassium and magnesium should be monitored when administering digitalis glycosides concurrently; patients with low electrolyte levels should receive supplements. Further losses should be prevented with dietary sodium restriction and/or potassium-sparing diuretics [48,49].

Sulfonylureas. Thiazides increase fasting blood glucose and may decrease the hypoglycemic effect of concomitantly administered sulfonylureas. These effects may occur within days or months of initiation of therapy. Blood glucose should be closely monitored. If hyperglycemia develops, it may possibly respond to a higher dose of sulfonylurea. Hyponatremia has occurred with concurrent chlorpropamide and thiazide therapy [50,51].

Lithium. The thiazide and related diuretics may increase the therapeutic and toxic effects of lithium (e.g., gastrointestinal symptoms, polyuria, muscular weakness, lethargy, tremor) by decreasing its renal clearance. Despite this interaction, lithium and thiazides have been used together. Plasma lithium levels should be monitored and the patient observed for symptoms of toxicity. A reduction in lithium dose may be necessary [52,53,54].

Cholestyramine and Colestipol. The anion-exchange resins cholestyramine and colestipol bind thiazide diuretics and decrease their absorption. The actions of the oral thiazides may be reduced. Administration of cholestyramine and colestipol should be separated from thiazide administration by at least 2 hours, longer if possible. An increased dose of thiazide may still be necessary [33,55].

Nonsteroidal Anti-inflammatory Agents. The thiazide and related diuretics may increase the risk of NSAID-induced renal failure. Inhibition of renal prostaglandins by NSAIDs appears to be the mechanism leading to decreased renal blood flow and renal failure. In addition, NSAIDs may interfere with the diuretic and antihypertensive effects of the thiazides and related diuretics. Patients receiving the drugs concomitantly should be monitored for declining renal function and/or attenuation of thiazide-induced therapeutic effects [33].

COMMON PITFALLS
1. To avoid the possibility of severe hypotension when a thiazide diuretic is added to the antihypertensive regimen of a patient, the dosage of the other hypotensive agent(s) should initially be reduced.
2. Metolazone and indapamide are the only thiazide and thiazidelike diuretics that are effective as diuretics in patients with a GFR less than 15 to 25 ml per minute.
3. Patients receiving thiazide therapy who develop serum potassium levels less than 3.0 mEq per liter may not respond to potassium supplements, as they rarely correct hypokalemia of this severity. The concurrent use of a potassium-sparing diuretic may be effective [13].
4. The thiazides and related diuretics should be used with caution in patients with severe renal disease, because these drugs decrease the GFR and may precipitate azotemia. They should also be used with caution in patients with impaired hepatic function or progressive liver disease, as these drugs may precipitate hepatic coma as a result of alterations in electrolyte balance, particularly hypokalemia [33].

Potassium-Sparing Diuretics

INTRODUCTION. The three currently available potassium-sparing diuretics are spironolactone, triamterene, and amiloride. Although they act by different mechanisms, they interfere with sodium reabsorption at the distal tubule of the kidney, thus decreasing potassium excretion. They exert mild to moderate antihypertensive and diuretic effect when used alone. Their major use is to enhance the antihypertensive and diuretic effects of the thiazides and loop diuretics and to counteract their kaliuretic action [33].

PHARMACOLOGY

Spironolactone. Spironolactone is a specific aldosterone antagonist that acts from the interstitial side of the distal tubular epithelium to block reabsorption of sodium and secretion of potassium and hydrogen ions. This produces a mild diuresis with sodium, chloride, and calcium excretion with retention of potassium and magnesium. The antihypertensive activity of spironolactone is equivalent to that of the thiazides for the treatment of mild to moderate hypertension [56,57].

Triamterene and Amiloride. These two agents act directly at the luminal surface of the cortical collecting duct of the distal tubule. They inhibit the reabsorption of sodium ions in exchange for potassium and hydrogen ions, producing a mild diuresis that is independent of aldosterone levels. Sodium, chloride, calcium, and possibly bicarbonate excretion are increased, while potassium and possibly magnesium excretion are decreased. Their antihypertensive activity is inconsistent and weaker than that of spironolactone or the thiazides [56,58].

THERAPEUTIC RANGE. No therapeutic range has been established for spironolactone, triamterene, and amiloride.

PREPARATIONS

Spirolactone	25-mg, 50-mg, 100-mg oral tablets
Triamterene	50-mg and 100-mg oral capsules
Amiloride	5-mg oral tablet

PHARMACOKINETICS. Table 210-8 summarizes the pharmacokinetic parameters of the potassium-sparing diuretics.

PHYSIOLOGIC CLEARANCE

Spironolactone

HYPOMETABOLIC. Spironolactone is rapidly and extensively metabolized in the liver to 7-alpha-thiomethyl-spirolactone (major metabolite), canrenóne, and other sulfur-containing metabolites that contribute to the pharmacologic activity of the drug. The metabolites are eliminated primarily renally. Although the clearance of spironolactone's metabolites is reduced in renal failure, dosage adjustment is not necessary in mild to moderate failure. Lower doses should be used in severe renal failure and with caution because of the potential for hyperkalemia. Clearance is expected to be reduced in liver dysfunction, but high doses are generally tolerated. Downward dosage adjustment is not necessary [33,56,59].

HYPERMETABOLIC. No information is available on the clearance of spironolactone in this population. Theoretically, clearance should be increased and higher doses required to produce the desired response.

Table 210-8. Pharmacokinetic Parameters of the Potassium-Sparing Diuretics in Normal Subjects [57,58,60,183]

	Spironolactone	Triamterene	Amiloride
Bioavailability (%)	90	30–70	15–25
Onset (hr)	24–48	2–4	2
Peak (hr)	48–72	6–8	6–10
Duration (hr)	48–72	12–16	24
V_{dss}	—	—	—
Protein binding (%)	98	50–67	23
Elimination half-life (hr)	1–2	2–4	6–12
Metabolism	Liver	Liver	None
Active metabolites	Yes	Yes	No
Excretion	Metabolites renally + biliary/fecal[a]	Parent + metabolites excreted renally + biliary/fecal, 15% excreted unchanged	Renal + fecal[b]

[a] Less than 10% excreted renally unchanged
[b] Approximately 50% excreted renally (unchanged) and 40% fecal (unchanged)

Triamterene

HYPOMETABOLIC. Triamterene is rapidly metabolized in the liver by hydroxylation, followed by immediate conjugation with active sulfate to form p-hydroxy-triamterene sulfuric acid ester. This metabolite possesses the same activity as triamterene. Both the parent compound and the sulfate conjugate are excreted renally by filtration and secretion. Clearance of triamterene and metabolite is reduced in renal failure patients. However, dosage adjustment is not necessary in mild to moderate failure. Patients with severe renal dysfunction should not receive the drug because of the risk of hyperkalemia. Because triamterene is extensively metabolized in the liver, its clearance is markedly decreased in patients with severe liver disease. Bioavailability is also enhanced in liver failure because of a significant first-pass effect. The drug should be used cautiously, if at all, in this population [33,56,60].

HYPERMETABOLIC. No information is available on the clearance of triamterene in this population. Enhanced liver and renal blood flow would theoretically increase the clearance of the parent drug and active metabolite. Higher doses may be necessary to achieve the desired response.

Amiloride

HYPOMETABOLIC. Amiloride is cleared mainly by urinary excretion of unmetabolized drug. Clearance is markedly reduced in renal dysfunction. In individuals with renal impairment, the elimination half-life (creatinine clearance 5–46 ml/ml) of the drug ranged from 21 to 144 hours (normal 6–12 hours). In patients with mild to moderate renal failure, the dose of amiloride should be decreased by 50 percent. Patients with severe renal dysfunction should not receive the drug because of the risk of hyperkalemia. In patients with mild to moderate liver disease, clearance is not expected to change. However, in patients with severe liver disease, amiloride should be used cautiously, if at all, because of the risk of producing hepatic encephalopathy [33,56,61].

HYPERMETABOLIC. Although information is not available on the clearance of amiloride in hypermetabolic patients, it should not be changed significantly, as its predominant route to clearance is renal.

DOSING GUIDELINES.
Table 210-9 summarizes the dosing guidelines for the potassium sparing diuretics.

DRUG INTERACTIONS
Spironolactone, Triamterene, and Amiloride
ANGIOTENSIN CONVERTING ENZYME INHIBITORS. Concurrent administration of ACE inhibitors with potassium-sparing diuretics may result in elevated serum potassium concentrations in some patients. Patients receiving concomitant therapy with these agents should have regular measurements of serum potassium concentrations [62,63].

POTASSIUM SUPPLEMENTS. Coadministration with potassium-sparing diuretics may result in hyperkalemia and possibly subsequent cardiac arrhythmias or cardiac arrest. Coadministration of these agents should be avoided, especially in patients with renal dysfunction. If this combination is required, serum potassium concentrations should be monitored closely [64,65].

Spironolactone
DIGOXIN. Spironolactone increases the elimination half-life of digoxin by reducing renal and possibly nonrenal clearance. This may result in increased serum digoxin levels and subsequent digoxin toxicity. The digoxin maintenance dose may need to be reduced when spironolactone is initiated [66]. In addition, the negative inotropic effect of spironolactone may attenuate the positive inotropic effect of digoxin [67].

SALICYLATES. Spironolactone-induced natriuresis but not the antihypertensive effect may be blocked by salicylates. Canrenone, the principal unconjugated metabolite of spironolactone, appears to have its renal tubular secretion inhibited by aspirin. Blood pressure and serum sodium should be monitored in patients receiving spironolactone and salicylates. The effects of the interaction may be reversed by increasing the dose of spironolactone [68,69].

Triamterene
AMANTADINE. Triamterene may decrease the renal clearance of amantadine, with subsequent toxic effects such as ataxia and agitation. Approaches to management of this interaction include discontinuation of triamterene, lowering the dose of amantadine, or discontinuing amantadine and substituting another drug [70].

INDOMETHACIN. Concomitant triamterene administration may possibly produce acute renal failure. It is thought that indo-

Table 210-9. Dosing Guidelines for the Potassium-Sparing Diuretics [33]

	Spironolactone[a,b]	Triamterene[a,b]	Amiloride[a,b]
Starting dose	25–100 mg po qd	50–100 mg po bid	5 mg po qd
Usual maintenance dose	50–100 mg po qd	50–100 mg po qd-bid	5–10 mg po qd
Maximum dose	200 mg po qd	150 mg po bid	20 mg po qd

[a] Should be taken with food
[b] When used in conjunction with other diuretics, reducing the doses of these agents may be required.
[c] No specific information regarding dosing in hypodynamic or hyperdynamic patients is available.

methacin blocks the triamterene-induced increases in prostaglandins E and F that normally protect the kidney from triamterene toxicity. This combination should be used only when it is clearly needed, and the patient should be monitored for acute renal failure. If renal failure occurs both drugs should be discontinued [71,72].

Amiloride
DIGOXIN. The pharmacologic effects of digoxin may be reduced by concurrent administration of amiloride. Possible mechanisms for a decrease in digoxin's inotropic effect include inhibition of sarcolemmal cation exchange. Patients on this combination need to be monitored for reduced pharmacologic effects of digoxin. The effects appear to be independent of digoxin serum levels [73,74].

COMMON PITFALLS.
The potassium-sparing diuretics should not be used in patients with anuria, acute or chronic renal insufficiency, or evidence of diabetic neuropathy, because potassium retention is accentuated and may result in rapid development of hyperkalemia [33].

Calcium Channel Antagonists

INTRODUCTION.
Calcium channel antagonists are a large group of drugs used to treat hypertension, angina, and, in some cases, arrhythmias. The following discussion is limited to the pharmacology and use of calcium channel blockers with respect to the management of hypertension only. The use of verapamil and diltiazem for the management of arrhythmias is discussed in Chapter 207.

Like the beta-antagonists, calcium channel antagonists are composed of a collection of agents that differ in terms of predominant pharmacologic effects, pharmacokinetic parameters, and electrophysiologic activity. They also differ in terms of the predominance of effect on myocardial vascular smooth muscle and on the conduction system. The following refers to these differences in the context of their use in the critical care patient.

PHARMACOLOGY.
The calcium antagonists are made up of three structurally different classes, the phenylalkylamines, benzothiazepines, and dihydropyridines. The prototype agents for these classes are verapamil, diltiazem, and nifedipine, respectively. Recent additions to the calcium channel antagonist class are the so-called "second-generation" dihydropyridines, including such drugs as amlodipine, felodipine, isradipine, nicardipine, and nimodipine. In general, the second-generation dihydropyridines differ by having greater vascular selectivity and less cardiac effects compared to nifedipine. However, the clinical benefits of these agents over nifedipine are questionable. Overall, the second-generation dihydropyridines tend to have longer half-lives and differ somewhat in dosing and pharmacokinetics. These features and cost may make these agents more attractive for a given intensive care patient.

When extracellular calcium enters arterial smooth muscle cell, it results in the contraction of myocytes and relaxation of smooth muscle. Calcium channel antagonists exert their effects by inhibiting this influx of calcium across the membranes, resulting in the negative inotropic and/or hypotensive effects of this class of agents. The electrophysiologic effects of calcium channel antagonists are more complex and vary between the subtypes of agents. Basically, calcium channel antagonists act to depress conduction velocity and depolarization through the atrioventricular (A-V) node. These effects are particularly associated with phenylalkylamines, such as verapamil, and to some extent the benzothiazepine diltiazem. In vivo, the effects on conduction through the A-V node are less clinically relevant for the dihydropyridine class of calcium channel antagonists, such as nifedipine. This may be due to a reflex increase in catecholamines secondary to the more profound vasodilatory effect of the dihydropyridines. This increase in catecholamines may offset the A-V node blocking effects. The reader is referred to Chapter 207 for further discussion on the electrophysiologic effects of these agents. Intercellular calcium is regulated by several types of calcium channels controlled by a complex series of gating mechanisms. There are basically three sites for calcium ion influx: voltage-dependent channels, the major site of action of calcium channel antagonists; receptor-operated channels; and sodium-calcium exchange gating mechanisms. Each gating mechanism plays a role in the modulation of calcium ion influx, resulting in the hemodynamic and vascular effects of these agents.

The overall effects of calcium channel blockade are to lower blood pressure, alter A-V conduction, and create negative inotropism. In the case of hypertension, calcium is the link between various types of stimuli involved in smooth muscle contraction. Calcium is involved in the final common pathway, where the calcium-calmodulan complex activates myosin light chain kinase, which then activates myosin, promoting the interaction between actin and myosin [75]. The ultimate effect is contraction of smooth muscle. When this pathway is inhibited by calcium channel antagonists, the ultimate effect is relaxation of smooth muscle, resulting in a lower of systolic and diastolic blood pressure.

Although these agents resemble one another in terms of their effects on the slow calcium channel, they differ in the degree of selectivity on the various tissues they tend to affect. Their effects on vascular smooth muscle, myocardial muscle, and specialized conduction or pacemaker tissues differ [75]. Generally, verapamil has the most profound effect on myocardial contractility, with diltiazem having less effect, and nifedipine and the second-generation dihydropyridines having the least effect. Similarly, verapamil and diltiazem are thought to have the most significant effects on A-V conduction, hence their use for supraventricular arrhythmias. Nifedipine and the second-generation dihydropyridines have the potential for a reflex increase in heart rate due to their vascular selectivity. Finally, coronary artery selectivity is thought to be most significant for the dihyropyridine class, although each of the classes has positive hemodynamic effects for anginal patients. This heterogeneity in calcium channel blockers influences the selection of an appropriate agent for a particular patient.

Table 210-10 compares the myocardial and vascular effects of selected calcium channel antagonists.

The following describes overall pharmacokinetics and clinically important information pertaining to these agents, with the exception of bepridil and nimodipine. Bepridil, although a calcium channel antagonist, differs substantially in its pharmacologic effect, which is mainly related to its antiarrhythmic properties. In addition to being a calcium channel antagonist, it is also a sodium channel blocker and is approved for use in ventricular tachyarrhythmias. Nimodipine is unique because it selectively vasodilates the cerebral vasculature and is therefore indicated for the treatment of subarachnoid hemorrhage. Neither agent is discussed in detail in this chapter.

THERAPEUTIC RANGE. Although occasionally referred to in the scientific literature, the therapeutic range for the antihypertensive or antiarrhythmic properties of calcium channel antag-

Table 210-10. Comparative Myocardial and Vascular Effects of Selected Calcium Channel Antagonists

	Verapamil	Diltiazem	Nifedipine	Second-generation dihydropyridines
Myocardial contractility	Moderate decrease	Moderate to slight decrease	Slight decrease	Minimal to no effect
Arterial selectivity	Minimal	Moderate	Moderate	Pronounced
A-V nodal conduction	Moderate decrease	Slight decrease	No effect	No effect
Heart rate	Slight increase or decrease	No change or slight decrease	Increase (reflex)	Increase (reflex)

onists does not correlate well with efficacy or toxicity. The pharmacologic effects of clinically administered doses are best monitored by observing for the predominant effect associated with the class of calcium channel antagonist being used. Specifically, blood pressure, heart rate, cardiac function (negative inotropicity), or conduction (ECG) should be monitored. See Table 210-11 for suggested therapeutic ranges.

PREPARATIONS. Table 210-12 summarizes the available preparations of calcium channel antagonists. For more information regarding the use of intravenous calcium channel antagonists, the reader is referred to Chapter 207.

PHARMACOKINETICS. Table 210-11 summarizes the pharmacokinetic properties of the calcium channel antagonists..

Amlodipine. This second-generation dihydropyridine has an extremely long half-life (approximately 30–50 hours). Consequently, there is a delayed peak onset of action of about 6 to 12 hours after the dose and substantial delay in offset of action on discontinuation. The peak onset of action is not substantially affected by food. The bioavailability ranges from 64 to 90 percent, which is clinically unaffected by food. Unlike some of the other second-generation agents, amlodipine has only a few select drug-drug interactions.

Felodipine. Felodipine has a half-life of approximately 10 hours, but the product is formulated as an extended-release preparation, permitting once daily dosing. Felodipine's bioavailability is not affected by food, with the exception of grapefruit juice, which, when ingested in large amounts is reported to increase bioavailability. Bailey et al. described an increase of up to a 206 percent in plasma AUC following ingestion of 200 ml of grapefruit juice in nine healthy men [76]. The mechanism of this interaction is believed to be related to inhibition of metabolism of felodipine by a component of grapefruit juice.

Isradipine. Approved for the treatment of hypertension, isradipine is typically administered twice daily. Its bioavailability is an extremely low 15 to 24 percent, with some risk of food delaying time to peak concentration but not AUC.

Nicardipine. Nicardipine is indicated for the treatment of chronic stable angina and essential hypertension. It is available as a sustained-release formulation that can be dosed twice daily.

Table 210-11. Pharmacokinetic Properties of Oral Calcium Channel Antagonists [4]

	Extent of absorption (%)	Absolute oral bio-availability (%)	Onset of action (min)	Time to peak plasma levels (hr)	Therapeutic range (ng/ml)	Metabolite formation	Half-life (hr)
Nifedipine (XL form)	90	45–70	20	0.5 (6)	25–100	Acid or lactone[a]	2–5
Verapamil	90	20–35	300	1–2	80–300	Norverapamil[b]	3–7
Diltiazem (SR form)	80–90	40–65	30–60	2–3 (6–11)	30–60	Desacetyldiltiazem[c]	3.5–6 (5–7)
Nicardipine	~ 100	35	20	0.5–2	28–50	Glucuronide conjugates	2–4
Nimodipine	ND	13	ND	≤1	ND	Unknown[a]	1–2
Isradipine	90–95	15–24	120	1.5	ND	Monoacids and cyclic lactone[d]	8
Bepridil	~ 100	59	60	2–3	1–2	4-OH-N-phenylbepridil	24
Felodipine	~ 100	20	120–300	2.5–5	ND	Six unidentified[a]	11–16
Amlodipine	ND	64–90	ND	6–12	ND	90% converted to inactive	30–50

ND = no data; XL = extended release; SR = sustained release
[a] Inactive
[b] Pharmacologic activity 20% of verapamil
[c] Pharmacologic activity 25–50% of diltiazem; plasma levels 10–20% of parent drug
[d] Of 6 metabolites identified, account for >75%

PHYSIOLOGIC CLEARANCE

Hypodynamic. In the hypodynamic patient, there are two concerns. First, many of the calcium channel blocking agents, have extensive first-pass elimination (Table 210-11). Although the majority of these agents are well absorbed, verapamil, nicardipine, nimodipine, isradipine, and felodipine undergo extensive metabolism. As relatively high-clearance drugs, these agents are subject to some alteration in pharmacokinetic and possibly pharmacodynamic response as a result of altered hepatic blood flow in the hypodynamic patient. The lack of perfusion to the liver may result in a greater bioavailability and a possible exaggeration of pharmacodynamic response.

Second, verapamil and diltiazem have active metabolites. Although the clinical significance is doubtful, accumulation of the active metabolites may have some clinical consequence in select patients experiencing profound reductions in ability to clear these renally eliminated agents. In both cases, prudent judgment in assessment of the hemodynamic effects of these agents in the hypodynamic patient should be exercised.

Hyperdynamic. The hyperdynamic patient may have an increased capacity to eliminate agents cleared mainly by hepatic metabolism, particularly verapamil, nicardipine, isradipine, and felodipine. Enhanced liver blood flow for extended periods may increase the ability to metabolize these agents.

DRUG INTERACTIONS [4,33].

The calcium channel blocking agents differ from one another somewhat in potential drug-drug interactions. Generally, all calcium channel blocking agents inhibit P-450 enzyme systems and affect digoxin clearance. Amlodipine, however, has minimal drug interactions with agents that typically interact with other calcium channel blocking agents, such as theophylline, digoxin, and H2 blockers. This is in contrast to the known interactions between diltiazem and verapamil with digoxin and carbamazepine. Diltiazem and ver-

apamil also interact with several other drugs, including antiepileptic drugs.

H2 Blockers. Although there is no effect when coadministered with amlodipine, H2 blockers can increase diltiazem, felodipine, nicardipine, nifedipine, and verapamil concentrations. Since these drugs are often coadministered, prospective dosage adjustment or, more practically, careful evaluation of altered hemodynamics and heart rate is prudent. This effect has been seen with both ranitidine and cimetidine, but is not usually clinically important.

Antiepileptic Drugs. Diltiazem and verapamil increase carbamazepine levels. Downward adjustment in the carbamazepine dosage may be necessary. No information is available for amlodipine or isradipine, and nifedipine does not appear to interact. Plasma levels of felodipine may decrease when coadministered with carbamazepine.

Cyclosporine. Diltiazem, nicardipine, and verapamil have all been reported to increase cyclosporine levels; nifedipine has no effect. There are no reports on amlodipine, isradipine and felodipine. This interaction may be used to some benefit when these agents are used to minimize the cyclosporine needs of posttransplant patients.

Digoxin. Digoxin levels tend to increase after initiation of verapamil, diltiazem, nifedipine, and felodipine. Verapamil may increase digoxin levels by up to 75 percent, whereas more modest increases in dioxin levels have been observed from coadministration of diltiazem and nifedipine. Amlodipine, isradipine, and nicardipine seem not to be affected.

Beta-Blockers. Combinations with beta-blockers may have pharmacodynamic consequences as a result of the common negative inotropic and chronotropic effects, independent of

Table 210-12. Preparations and Dosing Guidelines for Calcium Channle Antagonists

Agent	Available preparations	Starting dose	Usual maintenance dose	Maximum dose
Amlodipine	2.5, 5, 10 mg tablets	5 mg qd	5 mg/day	10 mg/day
Bepridil	200, 300, 400 mg tablets	200 mg/day	300 mg/day	400 mg/day
Diltiazem IR	30, 60, 90, 120 mg tablets	30 mg 4 times/day	160–360 mg/day	360 mg/day
Diltiazem SR	60, 90, 120 mg capsules	60 mg bid	240–360 mg/day	360 mg/day
Diltiazem CD, XR	120, 180, 240, 300 mg capsules	180 mg qd	180–360 mg/day	360 mg/day
Isradipine	2.5, 5 mg capsules	2.5 mg bid	10 mg/day	20 mg/day
Felodipine	5, 10 mg tablet	5 mg qd	5–10 mg/day	20 mg/day
Nicardipine IR	20, 30 mg capsules	20 mg tid	20–40 mg tid	ND
Nicardipine SR	30, 45, 60 mg capsules	30 mg bid	30–60 mg bid	ND
Nifedipine IR	10, 20 mg capsules	10 mg tid	10–20 mg tid	120 mg/day
Nifedipine XL, CC	30, 60, 90 mg tablets	30 mg qd	60–90 mg/day	120 mg/day
Verapamil IR	40, 80, 120 mg tablets	80 mg tid	240–360 mg/day	480 mg/day
Verapamil SR	120, 180, 240 mg tablets	240 mg qd	360 mg/day	480 mg/day

IR = immediate release; SR, XL, CD, XR, CC = sustained release; ND = no data

potential pharmacokinetic consequences. Diltiazem, verapamil, and isradipine have been shown to increase the beta-blocker area under serum concentration-time curves. The combination of beta-blockers and calcium channel antagonists should always be approached with caution in the intensive care patient.

Theophylline. Nifedipine, verapamil, and diltiazem have been shown to enhance the activity of theophylline, presumably through a reduction in theophylline clearance secondary to enzyme inhibition. Information on other agents is limited.

Erythromycin. Pharmacologic effects of felodipine may be exaggerated when it is co-administered with erythromycin, due to enzyme inhibition.

COMMON PITFALLS

1. The negative inotropism of verapamil and perhaps other calcium channel blocking agents should not go unrecognized. This may be particularly relevant to the hypodynamic patient with underlying compromised cardiac output. Although less of a concern with the second-generation dihydropyridines, for optimal antihypertensive activity this should always be considered when selecting a calcium channel antagonist.
2. The interaction between digoxin and verapamil (or other calcium channel antagonists) can dramatically influence the clinical interpretation of serum digoxin levels. Serum digoxin level should be closely monitored after recent addition, removal, or alteration in dosage of calcium channel antagonists. Some calcium channel antagonists do not have this interaction and thus may be optimal agents in select patients.
3. Many of the calcium channel antagonists have long half-lives inherently (isradipine, amlodipine, felodipine) or as a result of sustained-release formulation (verapamil SR, Dilacor XR, Cardizem CD, Procardia XL, Adalat CC). For rapid hemody-

namic effects, agents with quick onset of action (short time to peak plasma levels) should be selected. For drugs formulated as sustained-release products, their integrity should not be compromised by crushing or chewing. This has been reported to result in a bolus effect, precipitating angina or even myocardial infarction.

Angiotensin Converting Enzyme Inhibitors

INTRODUCTION. The ACE inhibitors include benazepril, captopril, enalapril, fosinopril, lisinopril, quinapril, ramipril, and enalaprilat. Enalaprilat is currently the only ACE inhibitor available as an injection. The ACE inhibitors are indicated for treatment of hypertension. Captopril, enalapril, benazepril, lisinopril, and quinapril are also indicated for treatment of congestive heart failure.

PHARMACOLOGY. The ACE inhibitors act on the renin-angiotensin-aldosterone system by preventing conversion of angiotensin I to angiotensin II, a potent vasoconstrictor that stimulates aldosterone secretion from the adrenal cortex. Inhibition of ACE results in decreased angiotensin II concentrations. The net result is vasodilation, reduction in blood pressure, reduction in aldosterone secretion, and sodium and fluid loss. The hypotensive effect lasts longer than ACE inhibition in the blood. Other proposed mechanisms of ACE inhibitor hypotensive effect include a longer inhibition of ACE in vascular epithelium than in blood (a local effect), vasodilation secondary to an accumulation of bradykinin, or an increase in prostaglandin synthesis or release [77].

In hypertensive patients, ACE inhibitors reduce blood pressure by decreasing total peripheral resistance, with no effect on heart rate, cardiac output, or cerebral blood flow [77]. They cause both arterial and venous vasodilation. Pulmonary vascular resistance is unchanged. An increase in renal blood flow, characterized by preferential vasodilation of the efferent arterioles of the glomeruli, can occur in patients receiving ACE inhibitors. Increases in BUN and creatinine are seen in patients with preexisting renal disease or with renovascular hypotension. In ICU patients it is common to see a rise in BUN and creatinine on initiation of ACE inhibitor therapy, particularly when combined with diuretics. It is thought that sodium depletion secondary to diuretic therapy may increase the dependency of the GFR on a functioning renin-angiotensin system, potentiating the renal failure effects of ACE inhibitors [78,79]. Onset of effect of ACE inhibitors ranges from 15 minutes to 1 hour. There can be a precipitous fall in blood pressure on initiation of therapy, called the first dose effect. Care should be taken on initiation of therapy, particularly in volume-depleted patients and those receiving concomitant diuretic therapy [80]. In patients with renal artery stenosis, angiotensin II may be vital to maintaining adequate filtration pressure to the glomeruli by constricting the efferent arterioles. Impairment of renal function can be seen on initiation of ACE inhibitors in these patients but is usually reversible after withdrawal of the ACE inhibitor [77].

THERAPEUTIC RANGE. Although therapeutic ranges have been identified for many ACE inhibitors, routine serum concentration monitoring is not recommended. The ACE inhibitors are usually dosed to antihypertensive effect.

PHARMACOKINETICS AND PHYSIOLOGIC CLEARANCE. Table 210-13 summarizes the pharmacokinetic properties of the ACE inhibitors.

Captopril. Captopril is well absorbed. Peak serum concentrations occur within 1 hour, and the drug is cleared rapidly, almost entirely in the urine. Thus, elimination is dependent on blood flow to the kidney (flow-limited). Forty percent is eliminated as unchanged drug and the remainder is eliminated as disulfide metabolites [77]. About 30 percent of captopril is protein-bound to albumin. Limited data are available on the effect of the hypodynamic or hyperdynamic state on captopril pharmacokinetics. In the hypodynamic state, the elimination half-life of captopril is increased in proportion to the degree of diminished renal function [81]. The drug may be more extensively metabolized to its disulfide metabolites in the presence of renal failure [82]. There is evidence that both captopril and its metabolites accumulate in renal failure, but they can undergo reversible metabolic interconversions resulting in accumulation not only of the active drug but also of disulfide metabolites, with the potential of conversion back to active drug [83]. The effect of hepatic failure on captopril's pharmacokinetics is unknown. In patients with liver cirrhosis, the reactivity of the renin-angiotensin-aldosterone system is intact, and blood pressure effects are seen [84]. In a hyperdynamic state, the drug metabolism and excretion may be increased, requiring larger doses to achieve the antihypertensive effect. Since protein binding of captopril is low, displacement from protein binding sites should not result in a significant change in clinical effect.

Table 210-13. Pharmacokinetic Properties of ACE Inhibitors [4,33,86,184]

Agent	Available strengths	Absorption	Time to onset (hr)/ peak effect	Duration of effect (hr)	Prodrug	Mode of elimination	Half-life (hr)	Dialyzed
Benazepril (Lotensin)	5, 10, 20, 40 mg tablets	37%	0.5/2–4	24 +	Yes	Renal	22	Yes
Captopril (Capoten)	12.5, 25, 50, 100 mg tabs	60–75%	0.25/1–1.5	2–6 increase with increasing doses	No	Renal	1.7	Yes
Enalapril (Vasotec)	2.5, 5, 10, 20 mg tabs	60%	1/4–6	24	Yes	Renal	1.3	Yes
Enalaprilat (Vasotec IV)	1.25 mg/ml, 1 and 2 ml vials for injection	NA	0.25/1	6	No	Renal	11	Yes
Fosinopril (Monopril)	10, 20 mg tablets	36%	1/2–6	24	Yes	Hepatic, biliary, renal	12	No
Lisinopril (Prinivil, Zestril)	5, 10, 20, 40 mg tabs	25%	1/6	24	No	Renal	12.6	Yes
Quinapril (Accupril)	5, 10, 20, 40 mg tabs	60%	1/2–4	24 +	Yes	Renal 60%, biliary 30%	2	No
Ramipril (Altace)	1.25, 2.5, 5, 10 mg caps	50–60%	1–2/3–6	24 +	Yes	Renal 60%, biliary 40%	13–17	

NA = not available

Enalapril and Enalaprilat. Enalapril itself is an inactive prodrug; after absorption it is metabolized to the active drug enalaprilat by ester hydrolysis. Since both enalapril and enalaprilat are renally eliminated, they exhibit flow-dependent renal elimination characteristics. Enalapril is also dependent on liver metabolism to the active drug enalaprilat and may exhibit capacity-limited pharmacokinetic characteristics. Since protein binding of enalaprilat is less than 50 percent, changes in protein binding should not produce a significant change in clinical effect.

No data are available on the effect of the hypodynamic or hyperdynamic states on the elimination of enalapril or analaprilat. One would expect that a flow-dependent, capacity-limited drug could be affected by these conditions. In the hypodynamic state, flow to both the kidney and the liver are expected to be diminished. In fact, enalaprilat can accumulate in renal failure, leading to dose-related side effects such as hypotension or hyperkalemia [85,86]. Liver failure may affect the pharmacokinetics of enalapril by diminishing the conversion of enalapril to the active drug, enalaprilat [87]. Dosage modification is necessary in patients in the hypodynamic state. In a hyperdynamic state, the renal elimination of enalaprilat may be increased, requiring increasing doses. Whether the conversion of enalapril to enalaprilat is altered in the hyperdynamic state is unknown. In any case, larger doses may be needed, and enalapril should be dosed to antihypertensive effects.

Lisinopril. Lisinopril is a lysine analog of enalaprilat and is an active substance, not a prodrug. The elimination of lisinopril is primarily renal and it therefore exhibits flow-dependent elimination. Protein binding is minimal, so displacement from protein binding sites should not produce a significant clinical effect. Data on the effects of the hyperdynamic and hypodynamic state on lisinopril pharmacokinetics and pharmacodynamics are lacking. It is clear that elimination of the drug declines with declining renal function [87,88,89]. Increases in AUC and maximum concentrations of lisinopril, indicating accumulation in renal failure, are more pronounced with lisinopril than with enalapril [85]. In a hypodynamic state, it is expected that elimination of lisinopril would be reduced and dosage modification required. Likewise, the elimination of lisinopril may be increased in the hyperdynamic state, requiring larger than usual doses. In both cases, the dosing of lisinopril should be titrated to effect.

Fosinopril. Fosinopril is a prodrug that is hydrolyzed by hepatic esterases to its active form, fosinoprilat. Fosinopril is a unique ACE inhibitor because it exhibits dual hepatic and renal elimination. Urinary excretion accounts for 44 percent of elimination, while hepatobiliary excretion accounts for 46 percent [90]. Negligible amounts of the prodrug are detected in the urine or plasma. Data regarding administration in the hypodynamic or hyperdynamic states are lacking. In declining renal function, renal elimination of fosinoprilat is reduced, but this does not result in a significant accumulation of fosinoprilat. This may be explained by a compensatory shift to nonrenal clearance in the presence of renal failure [85]. While no dosage adjustment is advised for patients in renal failure, there is considerable interpatient variability in the accumulation of fosinoprilat in renal failure [85]. Therefore, caution is advised. The effect of hepatic failure on the pharmacokinetics of fosinopril or fosinoprilat is unknown. The conversion of fosinopril to fosinoprilat may be slowed. If biliary excretion mechanisms are impaired, accumulation of fosinoprilat may occur. Despite the advantages of the dual elimination of fosinopril, caution is advised when using it in the presence of renal and hepatic dysfunction. Conversely, elimination may be more rapid in a hyperdynamic state. Fosinopril should be dosed to antihypertensive effect.

Quinapril. Quinapril is converted by hydrolysis to the active drug quinaprilat. At least 60 percent of quinapril is renally eliminated as quinaprilat and other metabolites. About one-third of quinapril appears in the feces. Quinaprilat is eliminated primarily through tubular secretion in the kidneys [91]. The effect of the hypodynamic and hyperdynamic states on quinapril's disposition is unknown. In hepatic and renal dysfunction, the conversion of quinapril to quinaprilat may be impaired [91]. The renal elimination of quinapril is slowed in a hypodynamic patient with renal dysfunction [92]. Quinaprilat is 97 percent protein-bound. The effects in renal failure of protein binding displacement or competition with organic acids for tubular secretion on the elimination of quinaprilat are unknown. In the hyperdynamic state, quinapril may be more rapidly hydrolyzed and secreted, resulting in a need for higher doses.

Ramipril. Ramipril is converted by hydrolysis to the active drug ramiprilat. The active metabolite is excreted primarily through the kidneys [93]. In renal failure, the parent compound does not accumulate but the elimination of ramiprilat is reduced in proportion to the extent of renal function [94]. In a hypodynamic patient with renal dysfunction or hepatic dysfunction, an accumulation of the active metabolite would be expected, and dosages should be adjusted downward [95]. In a hyperdynamic patient it possible that elimination of both ramipril and ramiprilat would be accelerated, resulting in a need for higher doses. In either case, the drug should be titrated to effect.

Benazepril. Benazepril is hydrolyzed in the liver to the active metabolite benazeprilat. While benazeprilat is primarily excreted through the kidneys, nonrenal mechanisms contribute approximately 12 percent to the elimination of benazeprilat [96,97]. In a hyperdynamic patient with renal failure, the half-life of benazeprilat is expected to the prolonged. While the non-renal mechanisms of elimination can partially compensate for the reduction in renal excretion, dosage modification is still necessary. In hepatic failure the pharmacokinetics of benazepril are not significantly changed, therefore dosage modification is not necessary [97]. In a hyperdynamic patient, it is possible an increase in elimination can occur and higher than usual doses may be needed. Dosages in hyperdynamic patients should be titrated to effect.

DOSING GUIDELINES. Tables 210-14 and 210-15 summarize the dosing guidelines for the ACE inhibitors.

DRUG INTERACTIONS

Thiazide Diuretics. Concomitant administration of thiazide diuretics and ACE inhibitors may result in an increased hypotensive response to the ACE inhibitor and an increased risk of renal failure.

Antacids. Concomitant administration of ACE inhibitors and antacids may result in a decreased bioavailability of the ACE inhibitor.

Potassium-Sparing Diuretics and Potassium Supplements. There is an increased risk of hyperkalemia when these agents are given with an ACE inhibitor.

Nonsteroidal Antiinflammatory Agents. Concomitant administration of NSAIDs and ACE inhibitors may reduce the blood pressure response to ACE inhibitors, probably by inhibiting prostaglandins.

Table 210-14. Dosing Guidelines for the ACE Inhibitors [4,33]

Drug	Initial dose	Maintenance dose	Hypodynamic	Hyperdynamic
Benazepril	10 mg qd	20–80 mg qd	Reduce doses—see Table 210-15	10 mg qd, titrate upward, divide bid if response diminished at end of dosing interval
Captopril	12.5–25 mg bid–tid	25–150 mg/day divided bid or tid	Reduce doses—see Table 210-15	25 mg tid, titrate upward to response
Enalapril	5 mg qd	10–40 mg/day divided qd or bid	Reduce doses—see Table 210-15	5 mg qd, titrate upward, divide bid if response diminished at end of dosing interval
Enalaprilat	1.25 mg IV q6h	2.5 mg IV q6h	Begin 0.625 mg IV q6h, however, a q8h dosing interval may be required in some cases	1.25 mg IV q6h, titrate upward to response
Fosinopril	10 mg qd	20–80 mg qd	No change	10 mg qd, titrate to response, divide bid if response diminished at end of dosing interval
Lisinopril	10 mg qd	20–40 mg qd	Reduce doses—see Table 210-15	10 mg qd, titrate to response
Quinapril	10 mg qd	20–80 mg/day divided qd or bid	Reduce doses—see Table 210-15	10 mg qd, titrate to response divide bid if response is diminished at end of dosing interval
Ramipril	2.5 mg qd	2.5–20 mg/day divided qd or bid	Reduce doses—see Table 210-15	2.5 mg qd, titrate to response, divide bid if response is diminished at end of dosing interval

Insulin. The ACE inhibitors may increase insulin sensitivity in diabetic patients. The risk of hypoglycemia should be considered.

Lithium. Increased lithium serum concentrations and lithium toxicity can occur.

Phenothiazines. An increase in the pharmacologic effect of ACE inhibitors may be seen when they are given concomitantly with phenothiazines.

Rifampin. The pharmacologic effects of enalapril may be decreased in patients receiving rifampin.

Table 210-15. Initial Dosing Guidelines for ACE Inhibitors in Renal Dysfunction [4,33]

	Creatinine clearance (ml/min)		
	30–50	10–30	< 10
Benazepril	10 mg qd	5 mg qd	5 mg qd*
Captopril	25 mg tid	25 mg bid	12.5–25 mg qd–bid*
Enalapril	5 mg qd	2.5 mg qd	2.5 mg qd*
Enalaprilat	1.25 mg IV q6h	0.625 mg IV q6h	0.625 mg IV q6h*
Fosinopril	10 mg qd	No change	No change
Lisinopril	10 mg qd	5 mg qd	2.5 mg qd*
Quinapril	5 mg qd	2.5 mg qd	2.5 mg qd
Ramipril	2.5 mg qd	1.25 mg qd	1.25 mg qd

* Supplemental doses needed after hemodialysis

COMMON PITFALLS

1. Patients receiving a diuretic are at a higher risk of increased hypotensive effect. Initial doses should be reduced or the diuretic discontinued 2 days prior to ACE inhibitor initiation.
2. Patients receiving diuretics are at increased risk of renal failure due to ACE inhibitors. Diuretics should be discontinued if possible before starting ACE inhibitors.
3. Failure to monitor potassium levels closely can lead to hyperkalemia, especially if the patient is also receiving a potassium supplement or potassium-sparing diuretic.
4. First-dose effect (excessive hypotension) can occur, especially if the patient is receiving diuretics concomitantly.
5. Patients on high doses of ACE inhibitors should have their WBC and platelets monitored.

Centrally Acting Antiadrenergic Agents

INTRODUCTION. In this antihypertensive category are the four agents methyldopa, clonidine, guanabenz, and guanfacine. It is thought that all four agents have as their mechanism of action the stimulation of central alpha$_2$-adrenergic receptors in the central nervous system (CNS). These agents have been used as monotherapy in the treatment of mild to moderate hypertension but are generally used as step agents in conjunction with a diuretic [33].

PHARMACOLOGY. These agents stimulate postsynaptic alpha$_2$-adrenergic receptors in the CNS, which activate inhibitory neurons to produce a decrease in sympathetic outflow. These actions result in a reduction in peripheral vascular resistance, renal vascular resistance, heart rate, and blood pressure. There is also a reduction in renin release by inhibitory adrenergic input to the juxtaglomerular apparatus in the kidney. These agents can decrease diastolic blood pressures by an average of 10 mm Hg when used as monotherapy [33,98,99,100].

THERAPEUTIC RANGE. No therapeutic range has been established for methyldopa, guanabenz, and guanfacine. A therapeutic range of 0.2 to 2 μg/per milliliter (0.9–9 nM/L) has been suggested for clonidine, although routine serum concentrations are not recommended [101].

PREPARATIONS

Clonidine	0.1-mg, 0.2-mg, 0.3-mg oral tablets and 0.1-mg/24 hr, 0.2-mg/24 hr, 0.3-mg/24 hr transdermal topical patches
Methyldopa	125-mg, 250-mg, 500-mg oral tablets
Methyldopate	250-mg/5-ml injection for intravenous administration
Guanabenz	4-mg, 8-mg oral tablets
Guanfacine	1-mg oral tablet

PHARMACOKINETICS. Table 210-16 summarizes the pharmacokinetic properties of the alpha$_2$-receptor agonists.

PHYSIOLOGIC CLEARANCE

Clonidine

HYPODYNAMIC. Clonidine is a flow-dependent drug, and its clearance is determined by renal and hepatic blood flow. The normal half-life of 6 to 20 hours is increased to 42 hours in end-stage renal failure. The dose of clonidine should be reduced by 50 to 75 percent in patients with a GFR less than 10 ml per minute. Patients with moderate to severe liver dysfunction should receive the lowest possible dose of clonidine, with final dosage adjustment titrated to hemodynamic effect [33,101].

HYPERDYNAMIC. Little is known about the pharmacokinetics of clonidine in this population. Theoretically, hyperdynamic patients would require higher doses because of increased clearance due to enhanced renal and liver blood flow.

Methyldopa

HYPODYNAMIC. Methyldopa is extensively metabolized to active and inactive metabolites, probably in the gastrointestinal tract and the liver. Methyldopa and metabolites are then excreted via the kidney. In patients with renal failure, urinary elimination of methyldopa and the O-sulfate conjugate metabolite is decreased. They accumulate and may cause increased hypotensive effect. Moderate to severe liver dysfunction may increase the oral bioavailability of methyldopa significantly due to decreased first-pass effect. Final dose adjustments in liver failure patients should be based on hemodynamic response and patient tolerance [33,102].

HYPERDYNAMIC. Little is known about the pharmacokinetics of methyldopa in this population. Theoretically, hyperdynamic patients would require higher doses because of enhanced liver metabolism and renal clearance.

Guanabenz

HYPODYNAMIC. Guanabenz is metabolized extensively in the liver to several metabolites that are then excreted predominately by the kidney. Only 1 to 2 percent of guanabenz is excreted renally as the parent compound. Therefore, the clearance of guanabenz is not greatly affected by renal dysfunction. However, as with other sympatholytic drugs, enhanced hypotensive action may be seen and a slower rate of increase in dosage is recommended during initiation of therapy. Hepatic impairment substantially reduces the clearance of guanabenz, therefore the lowest possible dose is recommended [33,98].

HYPERDYNAMIC. Little is known about the pharmacokinetics of guanabenz in this population. Theoretically, hyperdynamic patients would require higher maintenance doses because of enhanced physiologic clearance secondary to increased hepatic blood flow.

Guanfacine

HYPOMETABOLIC. The physiologic clearance of guanfacine is flow-dependent. Blood flow to the liver and kidney are the primary determinants of clearance. Following hepatic biotransformation into inactive metabolites, guanfacine and metabolites are excreted mainly by the kidney, with approximately 50 percent of a dose as parent drug. Guanfacine clearance is reduced in patients with renal dysfunction. However, drug plasma levels are only slightly increased and dosage adjustment is usually not necessary. No information is available on the kinetics of guanfacine in patients with hepatic dysfunction, but 50 percent of a

Table 210-16. Pharmacokinetic Parameters of the Alpha$_2$-Receptor Agonists [33,98,99,100, 102]

	Oral clonidine	Oral methyldopa	Oral guanabenz	Oral guanfacine
Bioavailability (%)	75–95	25–50	75	80
Onset (hr)	0.5–1.0	2	1	1–2
Peak (hr)	1–3	4–6	3	1–4
Duration (hr)	6–8	24–48	6–12	24
V_{dss} (L/kg)	2.1 ± 0.4	0.37	93–147	6.3
Protein binding (%)	20–40	10–15	90	70
Elimination half-life (hr)	6–24	1–2	6	10–30
Metabolism	Liver	Liver	Liver	Liver
Active metabolites	No	Yes	No	No
Excretion	65% renal[a], 20% feces	Renal[b]	Renal[c] + feces	Renal

[a] 40–50% excreted renally as clonidine
[b] 18% excreted renally as methyldopa
[c] 1.4% excreted renally as guanabenz
[d] 30–50% excreted renally as guanfacine

dose is liver metabolized. No clinically significant first-pass effect occurs. It is recommended that the lowest possible dose be used in liver failure patients [33,99].

HYPERMETABOLIC. Little is known about the physiologic clearance of guanfacine in hypermetabolic patients. Younger patients tend to have shorter elimination half-lives (13–14 hours) than older patients (20–30 hours). Theoretically, hypermetabolic patients may require higher maintenance doses because of enhanced physiologic clearance [99].

DOSING GUIDELINES. Table 210-17 summarizes the dosing guidelines for the alpha$_2$-receptor agonists.

DRUG INTERACTIONS
Clonidine

BETA-BLOCKERS. The severity of withdrawal hypertension caused by abrupt discontinuation of clonidine may be greater in patients taking beta-blockers. This is possibly due to unopposed alpha-adrenergic stimulation. Also, the combination of clonidine and beta-blockers has uncommonly caused paradoxical hypertension. Blood pressure should be closely monitored after initiation or discontinuation of clonidine or a beta-blocker especially when they are used concurrently. Both agents should be discontinued gradually (over several days), removing the beta-blocker first, when both are used [103,104].

TRICYCLIC ANTIDEPRESSANTS. The antihypertensive effect of clonidine may be blocked by tricyclic antidepressants with resultant loss of blood pressure control and possibly life-threatening elevations in blood pressure. Inhibition of central alpha$_2$ adrenergic receptors has been postulated. The combination of clonidine and tricyclic antidepressants should be avoided; other antihypertensive agents or nontricyclic antidepressants should be used [105,106].

Methyldopa

SYMPATHOMIMETICS. The coadministration of methyldopa and sympathomimetics may result in an increased pressor response, possibly resulting in hypertension. The mechanism of the interaction is unknown. Blood pressure should be monitored during coadministration of methyldopa and sympathomimetic agents [107,108].

COMMON PITFALLS
1. Abrupt discontinuation of the alpha$_2$-adrenergic agonists may occasionally lead to rebound hypertension or overshoot hypertension. A compensatory increase in norepinephrine release following discontinuation of presynaptic alpha$_2$-receptor stimulation is thought to occur. This reaction is most commonly reported with previous administration of high oral doses (more than 1.2 mg/day) of clonidine or with concomitant beta-blocker therapy (unopposed alpha-receptor stimulation). Alpha$_2$-agonists should be gradually withdrawn over several days [33,109].
2. Therapeutic plasma levels of clonidine are not achieved until 2 to 3 days after the initial application of the clonidine transdermal delivery system. Concomitant antihypertensive therapy with oral clonidine or other agents may be necessary for several days to maintain blood pressure control [33].
3. Tolerance to methyldopa therapy may occur, usually during the second or third month of therapy. Adding a diuretic or increasing the dosage of methyldopa usually restores blood pressure control. A thiazide diuretic is recommended if therapy was not initiated with a thiazide or if effective blood pressure cannot be maintained on 2 gm of methyldopa daily [33].

Postganglionic Sympathetic Inhibitors

INTRODUCTION. Guanethidine and guanadrel are postganglionic adrenergic blocking agents that produce a selective block of efferent, peripheral sympathetic pathways. Because of their potential to cause orthostatic hypotension and syncope, impotence, and explosive diarrhea, these agents are usually restricted to use in patients with hypertension refractory to other antihypertensive drugs. They are seldom used [33].

PHARMACOLOGY. Guanethidine and guanadrel lower blood pressure by depleting norepinephrine from postganglionic sympathetic nerve terminals and inhibiting the release of norepinephrine in response to sympathetic nerve stimulation. This results in a reduction in cardiac output, peripheral vascular resistance, and systolic blood pressure more than diastolic pressure. The hypotensive effect of these agents is much greater in upright posture, and postural hypotension is common because reflex-mediated vasoconstriction is blocked. Guanadrel has a faster onset and shorter duration of action than guanethidine [33,110].

Table 210-17. Dosing Guidelines for the Alpha$_2$-Receptor Agonists [33]

	Oral clonidine[a,b,c]	Transdermal clonidine[a,b,c]	Oral methyldopa[a,b,c]	Injectable methyldopa[a,b,c]	Oral guanabenz[a,b,c]	Oral guadfacine[b]
Starting dose	0.1 mg bid	One #1 patch weekly	250 mg bid	250 mg–1 gm IV q6h	4 mg bid	1 mg at bedtime
Usual maintenance dose	0.3 mg bid	One #1–#3 patch weekly	500 mg–2 gm/day in 2–4 doses	250 mg–1 gm IV q6h	16 mg bid	1–3 mg qd
Maximum dose	2.4 mg/day	Two #3 patches weekly	2 gm/day	250 mg–1 gm IV q6h	32 mg bid	3 mg qd

[a] Dosage adjustment necessary in patients with severe renal dysfunction
[b] Dosage adjustment may be necessary in patients with severe hepatic failure
[c] No specific information available regarding dosing of hypodynamic and hyperdynamic patients

THERAPEUTIC RANGE. Adrenergic blockade occurs at 8 μg per milliliter (40 nM/L) or greater for guanethidine [111].

PREPARATIONS

Guanethidine   10-mg and 25-mg oral tablets
Guanadrel   10-mg and 25-mg oral tablets

PHARMACOKINETICS. Table 210-18 summarizes the pharmacokinetic properties of guanethidine and guanadrel.

PHYSIOLOGIC CLEARANCE

Guanethidine

HYPOMETABOLIC. Guanethidine is extensively metabolized in the liver to metabolites that have less than 10 percent of the hypotensive activity of the parent compound. The drug and its metabolites are excreted predominately by the kidney. Patients with severe renal dysfunction require reduced doses because of reduced clearance and enhanced hypotensive action similar to that of other sympatholytic drugs in renal failure. No information is available with regard to the clearance of guanethidine in liver failure patients. Final dose adjustments should be based on hemodynamic response and patient tolerance [33,112].

HYPERMETABOLIC. No information is available concerning the pharmacokinetics of guanethidine in this population. It could be postulated that clearance would be increased because of increased liver blood flow.

Guanadrel

HYPOMETABOLIC. The liver metabolizes approximately 40 to 50 percent of a dose of guanadrel to several metabolites. The hypotensive activity of the metabolites is unknown. Renal excretion is the primary route of elimination for the metabolites and parent drug. Forty to 50 percent of a dose is excreted as guanadrel. The total body clearance of guanadrel is significantly reduced by renal insufficiency. It is recommended that the dosing interval be extended from daily in patients with normal renal function to every 2 to 3 days and every 5 days in patients with moderate and severe renal insufficiency, respectively. No information on the clearance of guanadrel in liver dysfunction is available. It could be assumed that clearance would be reduced and a reduction in dosage would be appropriate. Final

dosage should be based on hemodynamic response and patient tolerance [33,113].

HYPERMETABOLIC. Although no information is available on the clearance of guanadrel in this population, one could conclude that clearance would be increased secondary to increased liver metabolism and renal excretion. These patients may require higher doses of the drug.

DOSING GUIDELINES. Table 210-19 summarizes the dosing guidelines for guanethidine and guanadrel.

DRUG INTERACTIONS

Direct-Acting Sympathomimetics. Guanethidine and guanadrel potentiate the effect of the direct-acting sympathomimetics (epinephrine, norepinephrine, phenylephrine, metaraminol, methoxamine) by making the receptors more sensitive to these agents. An increase in pressor response and arrhythomogenic potential may occur. This combination of drugs should be avoided [114,115].

Tricyclic Antidepressants. The hypotensive action of guanethidine and guanadrel may be inhibited by concurrent tricyclic antidepressant administration. The uptake of guanethidine and guanadrel into their site of action at the nerve terminal is inhibited. Blood pressure should be monitored and alternative antihypertensive therapy used if necessary for blood pressure control [116].

Amphetamines, Methylphenidate. The hypotensive effects of guanethidine and guanadrel can be reversed by concurrent amphetamine or methylphenidate administration. The mechanism of the interaction is unknown. If there is loss of blood pressure control the amphetamine or methylphenidate should be discontinued, or an alternative hypotensive therapy instituted [117].

Monoamine Oxidase Inhibitors. The hypotensive effect of guanethidine and guanadrel may be inhibited by monoamine oxidase inhibitors. Their concurrent use is generally contraindicated. The monoamine oxidase inhibitor should be discontinued at least 1 week before guanethidine or guanadrel is started [33,118].

Phenothiazines, Thioxanthenes, Haloperidol. The hypotensive action of guanethidine and guanadrel may be inhibited by the concurrent administration of these agents. Inhibition of the uptake of guanethidine and guanadrel into its site of action in the nerve endings is thought to occur. This interaction is

Table 210-18. Pharmacokinetic Parameters for Guanethidine and Guanadrel in Healthy Subjects [33,112,113]

	Guanethidine	Guanadrel
Bioavailability	3–50%	90–100%
Onset	Several days	30–120 min
Peak	1–3 wk	4–6 hr
Duration	1–3 wk	14 hr
V_{dss}	—	—
Protein binding	—	< 20%
Elimination half-life	4–8 days	4–12 hr
Metabolism	Liver	Liver
Active metabolites	Yes	?
Excretion	Kidney[a]	Kidney[b]

[a] Approximately 6% of a dose is excreted renally as parent drug
[b] Approximately 85% of the drug is eliminated in the urine with about 40–50% of a dose as parent drug

Table 210-19. Dosing Guidelines for the Postganglionic Inhibitors [33]

	Guanethidine[a,b]	Guanadrel[b,c]
Starting dose	10 mg po qd	5 mg po bid
Usual maintenance dose	10–100 mg/day po	20–75 mg/day po
Maximum dose	300 mg/day po	150 mg/day po

[a] May need to adjust dosage in patients with creatinine clearance less than 10 ml/min
[b] No specific information available regarding dosing of hypodynamic or hyperdynamic patients
[c] Dosage adjustment necessary in renal dysfunction patients

most commonly reported with chlorpromazine. An alternative antihypertensive therapy should be used if guanethidine or guanadrel is no longer effective and continued antipsychotic therapy is necessary [119,120].

Rauwolfia Derivatives/Reserpine. Concurrent use of guanethidine and guanadrel with rauwolfia derivatives or reserpine may cause excessive postural hypotension, bradycardia, and mental depression due to additive effects [4].

Digitalis Glycosides. Guanethidine and guanadrel in combination with digitalis glycosides may result in excessive slowing of heart rate. Patients should be monitored for changes in heart rate [4].

COMMON PITFALLS

1. The maximum hypotensive response to guanethidine may not occur for up to 1 to 3 weeks after initiation or changes in dosage. Frequent dosage increment changes should be avoided to prevent excessive hypotension.
2. Clinicians should have a thorough knowledge of potential drug interactions associated with this class of antihypertensive agents before using these drugs in combination with other agents.

Nitroglycerin

INTRODUCTION. Nitroglycerin is generally not used as a first-line antihypertensive agent. However, an intravenous infusion can be a useful alternative agent, particularly in patients with concurrent myocardial ischemia or infarction. The drug has been used to control blood pressure in perioperative hypertension, especially hypertension associated with cardiovascular procedures, and to control severe hypertension or hypertensive emergencies [33,121].

PHARMACOLOGY. Nitroglycerin relaxes vascular smooth muscle via increases in cyclic GMP [122]. The venous side of the vasculature is affected to a greater degree than the arterial side, which explains why nitroglycerin is less effective as an antihypertensive than an agent such as nitroprusside, which predominantly dilates the arterial blood vessels. The drug has a quick onset of action (2–5 minutes), and offset is nearly the same when the infusion is stopped. Nitroglycerin also lowers pulmonary vascular resistance and maintains or improves collateral coronary circulation [33,121].

THERAPEUTIC RANGE. No therapeutic range has been established for nitroglycerin.

PREPARATIONS. Intravenous nitroglycerin is available as a 5 mg per milliliter concentrate injection containing 70% alcohol. The injection must be diluted in 5% dextrose or 0.9% sodium chloride prior to administration.

PHARMACOKINETICS [33]

Absorption. The onset of antihypertensive effect of nitroglycerin is approximately 2 to 5 minutes with a duration of effect of 10 to 20 minutes on discontinuation.

Distribution. Nitroglycerin is widely distributed in the body. The drug has an apparent volume of distribution of 3.3 ± 1.2 liters per kilogram. The drug is 87 ± 1 percent plasma protein-bound.

Elimination. The plasma elimination half-life of nitroglycerin is about 1 to 4 minutes. The drug is metabolized in the liver to less active dinitro and inactive mononitro metabolites.

PHYSIOLOGIC CLEARANCE

Hypodynamic. The clearance of intravenous nitroglycerin is predominantly dependent on liver metabolism. Therefore, clearance is not expected to be altered in renal failure patients. The use of intravenous nitroglycerin in severe liver failure should proceed with caution because of possible reduced liver clearance. Hemodynamic response and patient tolerance should guide dosage adjustments [33].

Hyperdynamic. Information on the clearance of nitroglycerin in this population is not available. Theoretically, clearance may be increased and higher infusion rates required to achieve the desired hemodynamic response.

DOSING GUIDELINES

Loading Dose. Initial loading doses are not necessary, as the drug has a very quick onset; steady state at a given infusion rate is achieved in approximately 5 minutes.

Maintenance Dose. A continuous intravenous infusion is initiated at a rate of 5 to 10 μg per minute using an infusion pump. Dosage must be titrated to the individual patient's response. The dosage can be increased by 5 to 10 μg per minute every 5 to 10 minutes until a response is noted. If no response occurs at 20 μg per minute, increments of 10 to 20 μg/min can be used. Once partial blood pressure response occurs, incremental increases should be decreased and intervals increased. For control of hypertension or in hypertensive emergencies, doses of up to 150 to 200 μg per minute or higher may be needed [2]. No specific information regarding dosing of hypodynamic or hyperdynamic patients is available.

DRUG INTERACTIONS. Nitroglycerin infusions have been reported to inhibit the anticoagulant effect of heparin, but this has not been a consistent finding. The mechanism of this possible interaction has not been determined. During coadministration of intravenous nitroglycerin and heparin, coagulation status should be monitored and the heparin dose adjusted accordingly. Patients may have an increase in their aPTT when the nitroglycerin infusion is stopped [123,124].

COMMON PITFALLS

1. Because nitroglycerin readily migrates into many plastics, the type of intravenous administration set used (polyvinyl chloride [PVC] or non-PVC [polyethylene]) must be considered in initial dosage estimations. Dosages commonly used in published studies are based on the use of PVC administration sets and are too high when non-PVC sets are used. An initial dose of 5 to 10 μg per minute should be used when using non-PVC sets [33].
2. The principal toxic effect of nitroglycerin is hypotension, which may exacerbate myocardial ischemia. Nitrate-induced hypotension responds readily to fluid replacement therapy. Other potential complications of intravenous nitroglycerin

include tachycardia, paradoxical bradycardia, hypoxemia caused by increased pulmonary ventilation-perfusion mismatch, methemoglobinemia, and headache. In general, the drug is well tolerated [33].

Nitroprusside

INTRODUCTION. Nitroprusside is an injectable, fast-acting vasodilator that relaxes the smooth muscle of both arteriolar and venous vascular beds. It is indicated for the treatment of hypertensive crisis and to produce controlled hypotension to reduce bleeding during surgery. It is commonly used in the ICU during hypertensive emergency, acute valvular insufficiency, low cardiac output states, and congestive myocardial failure.

PHARMACOLOGY. Nitroprusside produces a hypotensive effect by inducing vascular smooth muscle relaxation, possibly via an increase in intracellular cyclic GMP [125]. Both arteriolar and venous vasodilation are produced. Onset of action occurs within seconds of administration, and duration of action is 3 to 5 minutes. In addition to reducing blood pressure, nitroprusside produces an increase in heart rate and a reduction in systemic vascular resistance, pulmonary capillary wedge pressure, and mean arterial pressure [126]. It has a variable effect on cardiac output. While it usually has no effect on renal blood flow and GFR, nitroprusside-induced azotemia has been reported [4,127].

THERAPEUTIC RANGE. There is no identified therapeutic range for nitroprusside serum concentrations. Cyanide-induced toxicity begins to appear at red cell cyanide concentrations of 0.5 to 1.0 mg per liter. Thiocyanate toxicity begins to appear at serum thiocyanate levels of 10 mg per deciliter [128].

PREPARATIONS. Nitroprusside is available as a powder for injection. A 50-mg vial should be dissolved with 2 to 3 ml of dextrose in water. The solution is then further diluted in 250 to 1000 ml of 5% dextrose injection. A usual concentration is 50 to 400 mg nitroprusside diluted in 250 ml of D5W. The solution should be protected from light.

PHARMACOKINETICS. Sodium nitroprusside contains 44% cyanide. Each molecule of nitroprusside contains five cyanide moieties [128]. Nitroprusside distributes mainly in the plasma volume, with a distribution volume approximately the same as the extracellular space. Nitroprusside is broken down in the plasma through a reaction with sulfhydryl groups to release cyanide. Thiosulfate then donates a sulfur to cyanide to convert it to thiocyanate. This reaction is catalyzed by the enzyme rhodanese as well as other enzymes [128,129]. Thiocyanate is eliminated through the kidneys, with a half-life of about 3 days [130].

PHYSIOLOGIC CLEARANCE. Nitroprusside exhibits capacity-limited pharmacokinetics. The metabolism of cyanide is dependent on the availability of thiosulfate. Thiosulfate stores are limited, which results in saturable elimination pharmacokinetics for cyanide. This is particularly dangerous when thiosulfate stores are depleted in patients with poor nutrition, chronic disease, recent surgery, or chronic diuretic use [128]. Thiosulfate

stores are depleted at nitroprusside infusion rates as low as 1 to 2 μg/kg/min. Theoretically, the depletion of thiosulfate could cause cyanide concentrations to rise indefinitely, as long as nitroprusside continues to be infused. Red cell cyanide concentrations rise in proportion to the infusion rate [130]. Cyanide toxicity occurs when red cell cyanide concentrations reach 1.0 mg per liter. Whole blood concentrations of 0.5 to 1.0 μg per milliliter are associated with tachycardia and flushing, 1 to 2.5 μg per milliliter with decreased level of consciousness, 2.5 to 3.0 μg per milliliter with coma, and concentrations greater than 3.0 μg per milliliter with death [131]. Cyanide bonds to cytochrome oxidase, preventing oxidative phosphorylation and oxygen consumption. Symptoms of cyanide toxicity include agitation, lethargy, disorientation, seizures, coma, tachypnea, and hypotension. Signs of cyanide toxicity include cardiac arrhythmias, lactic acidosis, increased anion gap, and a narrowed arteriovenous oxygen difference. Cyanosis and death are late-occurring signs of cyanide toxicity. An increasing dosage requirement for nitroprusside to maintain blood pressure and a lactic acidosis are the earliest signs of cyanide toxicity [132].

Data regarding the effect of a hypometabolic or hypermetabolic state on the fate of nitroprusside are lacking. Known risk factors for the development of cyanide toxicity include malnutrition, recent surgery, diuretic use, hepatic impairment, hypoalbuminemia, tobacco smoking, hypothermia, and cardiopulmonary bypass surgery [128,132]. The most important factor, however, is the dose of nitroprusside administered [130,132]. In a hypometabolic state, liver and renal function are likely less than optimal. Liver dysfunction may prevent nitroprusside's metabolism. Conversely, some authors suggest that the presence of rhodanese throughout the body allows peripheral metabolism of nitroprusside, even in patients with cirrhosis [132]. Renal dysfunction is certainly a risk factor for the development of thiocyanate toxicity, since it is eliminated renally [133]; toxicity is usually not a concern if nitroprusside infusions are limited to 6 to 7 days. Thiocyanate toxicity as a result of nitroprusside infusions is usually characterized by CNS dysfunction (agitation, delusions, disorientation, tremor, nervousness). In severe cases, this can progress to convulsions, coma, and death. Thiocyanate can also compete with iodine for thyroidal uptake, producing hypothyroidism. Although fatigue can occur with thiocyanate concentrations of 80 mg per liter, thiocyanate toxicity usually requires concentrations of 100 mg per liter. The treatment is discontinuation of the infusion and hemodialysis. While data are lacking, it is possible that hyperdynamic patients may metabolize nitroprusside more quickly, leading to a more rapid depletion of thiosulfate stores. This, in theory, could lead to a greater potential for the development of cyanide toxicity. It is difficult to state whether the presence of cysteine or cystine sulfur donors in parenteral nutrition have a protective effect.

DOSING GUIDELINES. Dosing of nitroprusside is the same regardless of the patient's "dynamic" condition: the lowest possible dose to obtain an adequate blood pressure response should be used. Recent FDA guidelines call for an initial dose of 0.3 μg/kg/min and titration to a maximum dose of 10 μg/kg/min. Infusions of 10 μg/kg/min should never last more than 10 minutes [134]. An adequate blood pressure response can usually be obtained at infusion rates of 2 μg/kg/min or less. Cyanide toxicity can be completely avoided by adding sodium thiosulfate to a nitroprusside infusion at a concentration of 1 gm per 100 mg of nitroprusside [132,135]. This does not, however, prevent the accumulation of thiocyanate in the presence of renal dysfunction. Suspected cyanide poisoning can be treated with the Lilly Cyanide Antidote Kit. Treatment guidelines include the inhalation of amyl nitrite for 15 to 30 seconds every

1 to 3 minutes while sodium nitrite is being prepared. Then 300 mg of sodium nitrite is immediately infused over 3 to 5 minutes. Immediately thereafter, 12.5 gm of sodium thiosulfate is infused. The sulfur donor present converts cyanide to thiocyanate. Additional doses of one-half the original amount may be given [136].

DRUG INTERACTIONS [33,137]

Clonidine. Severe hypotensive reactions with the combined use of clonidine and nitroprusside have been reported. The possibility exists that this interaction may occur with guanabenz and guanfacine as well.

Diltiazem administration reduces the dose of nitroprusside required to produce hypotension and may enhance nitroprusside-induced hypotension. Data on other calcium channel blockers are lacking.

The hypotensive effects of nitroprusside are additive when used concomitantly with ganglionic blocking agents, negative inotropic agents, and general anesthetics.

COMMON PITFALLS

1. Failure to begin nitroprusside dosing at the lowest possible dose
2. Failure to administer nitroprusside infusions with thiosulfate
3. Failure to recognize early warning signs of cyanide toxicity (increasing dosage requirement of nitroprusside, metabolic acidosis, and CNS changes)
4. Utilization of thiocyanate levels to assess the presence of cyanide toxicity or utilization of cyanide levels to assess the presence of thiocyanate toxicity
5. Failure to monitor for symptoms of thiocyanate toxicity in patients with renal failure

Alpha₁ Postsynaptic Adrenergic Blockers

INTRODUCTION. Prazosin, terazosin, and doxazosin are selective alpha₁-receptor blockers; they do not elicit the reflex tachycardia that is associated with nonselective alpha-blockers. The nonselective alpha-blockers phentolamine and phenyoxybenzamine block both postsynaptic alpha₁- and presynaptic alpha₂-receptors. In low doses, the selective alpha-blockers may be used as monotherapy in the treatment of mild to moderate hypertension. They are generally used as step two agents [33].

PHARMACOLOGY. The postsynaptic alpha₁-receptor blockers produce arterial and venous dilation and a reduction in total peripheral resistance. These agents cross the blood-brain barrier and may cause CNS side effects such as lassitude, vivid dreams, and depression. An important side effect of alpha₁-blockers is the so-called first-dose phenomenon, characterized by transient dizziness, palpitations, and possibly syncope, which occurs within 1 to 3 hours of the first dose. It may also occur during rapid upward dosage titration or when adding an another antihypertensive agent [138,139].

THERAPEUTIC RANGE. There is no established correlation between plasma levels and clinical effect for the alpha₁-blockers.

PREPARATIONS

Prazosin	1-mg, 2-mg, 5-mg oral capsules
Terazosin	1-mg, 2-mg, 5-mg 10-mg oral tablets
Doxazosin	1-mg, 2-mg, 4-mg, 8-mg oral tablets

PHARMACOKINETICS. Table 210-20 summarizes the pharmacokinetic parameters of the alpha₁-adrenergic blockers.

PHYSIOLOGIC CLEARANCE

Prazosin

HYPOMETABOLIC. Prazosin is extensively metabolized in the liver by demethylation and conjugation. Ninety percent is excreted in feces and the rest by the kidney. The elimination half-life of the drug is longer in congestive heart failure, the elderly, and pregnancy. The pharmacokinetics of prazosin may be altered in chronic renal failure because of decreased protein binding, resulting in elevated peak serum concentrations. This population may require smaller doses. Because prazosin is subject to significant first-pass metabolism, moderate to severe hepatocellular dysfunction may be expected to increase bioavailability and reduce systemic clearance. Final dose adjustments should be made based on hemodynamic response and patient tolerance [33,140].

HYPERMETABOLIC. No information is available on the clearance of prazosin in this population. Enhanced first-pass metabolism and liver metabolism would be expected to increase physiologic clearance and possibly dosage requirements.

Terazosin

HYPOMETABOLIC. Terazosin is extensively metabolized in the liver, with the major route of excretion through the biliary tract. It undergoes minimal hepatic first-pass metabolism. Plasma clearance is 80 ml per minute, but renal clearance is only 10 ml per minute. The clearance of terazosin is decreased slightly in the elderly, but drug dosage adjustments have not been necessary. Moderate to severe renal dysfunction does not alter

Table 210-20. Pharmacokinetic Parameters of the Alpha₁-Adrenergic Blockers [140,141,142]

	Prazosin	Terazosin	Doxazosin
Bioavailability (%)	50–70	80–90	60–70
Onset (hr)	1–2	1–2	1–2
Peak (hr)	1–3	1–2	6
Duration (hr)	8–10	18+	18–36
V_{dss} (L/kg)	0.6–0.8	0.2–0.4	1.0–1.5
Protein binding (%)	96–98	90–94	98
Elimination half-life (hr)	2–3	9–12	17–22
Metabolism	Liver	Liver	Liver
Active metabolites	Yes	No	No
Excretion	Feces + kidney[a]	Biliary/feces + kidney[b]	Feces + kidney[c]

[a] 90% excreted in feces and 10% renally with 3–4% as prazosin in the urine
[b] 60% excreted in feces and 40% in urine; approximately 10% of an oral dose excreted as parent drug in the urine and approximately 20% as parent drug in the feces
[c] 65% excreted in feces and 9% in urine with 1–5% of unchanged drug in urine and 5% in feces

clearance significantly, but greater effects may be seen in these patients. Clearance remains unchanged in congestive heart failure. No information is available regarding clearance in chronic liver failure. Doses should be titrated to the desired effect in this population [33,141].

HYPERDYNAMIC. Information on the clearance of terazosin in this population is not available. Although clearance may be increased, it is unlikely to be clinically significant.

Doxazosin

HYPOMETABOLIC. Doxazosin is extensively metabolized in the liver, mainly by 0-demethylation or hydroxylation. Because its clearance is by nonrenal metabolism and no evidence suggests there are active metabolites, there is no need for dose adjustments in patients with renal failure. As is true with other antihypertensive agents, greater effects may be seen in end-stage renal disease. No information is available regarding clearance in hepatic dysfunction. Doses should be titrated to the desired effect in this population [33,142].

HYPERDYNAMIC. Information on the clearance of doxazosin in this population is not available. Clearance may be enhanced due to increased liver metabolism.

DOSING GUIDELINES. Table 210-21 summarizes the dosing guidelines for the alpha$_1$-adrenergic blockers.

DRUG INTERACTIONS

Verapamil. The addition of verapamil to prazosin therapy appears to increase prazosin concentrations and may increase sensitivity to prazosin-induced postural hypotension. The mechanism of this interaction is unknown. The patient should take precautions regarding postural hypotension when these drugs are used in combination [143].

Beta-Adrenergic Blockers. Acute postural hypotension following the initiation of prazosin therapy may be enhanced by concurrent beta-blocker therapy. Patients who require both drugs should be advised that symptomatic hypotension may occur. Terazosin and doxazosin have been combined with beta-blockers with no adverse reaction [144].

COMMON PITFALLS. The first-dose phenomenon may be minimized by limiting the initial dose to 1 mg of prazosin or terazosin (given at bedtime) or doxazosin. The dosage should be increased slowly, with increases in dose every 2 weeks.

Table 210-21. Dosing Guidelines for the Alpah$_1$-Adrenergic Blockers [33]

	Prazosin[a,b,c,d]	Terazosin[c,d]	Doxazosin[c,d]
Starting dose	1 mg bid–tid	1 mg/day	1 mg/day
Usual maintenance dose	2–20 mg/day (divided doses)	1–20 mg/day	1–16 mg/day
Maximum dose	20–40 mg/day (divided doses)	20 mg/day	16 mg/day

[a] First dose at bedtime
[b] Patients with renal failure may require smaller doses.
[c] Dosage adjustments may be necessary in patients with severe liver failure.
[d] No specific information available regarding dosing of hypodynamic or hyperdynamic patients

Additional antihypertensives should be given with caution. Patients should avoid situations where injury could result should syncope occur during initiation of therapy or dosage titration.

Vasodilators

INTRODUCTION. Hydralazine and minoxidil cause direct arteriolar smooth muscle relaxation and therefore vasodilation. They have minimal effect on venous circulation. This class of antihypertensive agents is not appropriate as initial monotherapy of hypertension in most patients because of reflex sympathetic stimulation and activation of the renin-angiotensin system. They are usually reserved for patients with severe and moderately severe hypertension who do not respond to two or three antihypertensives [33].

PHARMACOLOGY. The direct arteriolar smooth muscle relaxation of hydralazine and minoxidil is via mechanisms that increase the intracellular concentration of cyclic guanosine monophosphate. The resultant reduction in peripheral vascular resistance lowers blood pressure and afterload. Acutely, they substantially lower blood pressure. If used alone, their antihypertensive effect is attenuated by 75 to 80 percent because of activation of baroreceptor reflexes, which results in an increase in sympathetic outflow from the vasomotor center in the CNS. This leads to an increase in heart rate, cardiac output, and renin release. Consequently, the antihypertensive effect diminishes in time unless a sympathetic inhibitor and a diuretic are used concurrently to counteract the compensatory responses brought about by baroreceptor reflexes. Elderly patients with mild hypertension may be treated with low doses of hydralazine monotherapy without causing reflex tachycardia because of blunted baroreflexes. However, sodium and fluid retention may still be a problem [33,145–152].

THERAPEUTIC RANGE. No therapeutic or toxic ranges have been established for hydralazine or minoxidil.

PREPARATIONS

Hydralazine	10-mg, 25-mg, 50-mg, 100-mg oral tablets
Minoxidil	2.5-mg and 10-mg oral tablets

PHARMACOKINETICS. Table 210-22 summarizes the pharmacokinetic parameters of hydralazine and minoxidil.

PHYSIOLOGIC CLEARANCE
Hydralazine

HYPODYNAMIC. Hydralazine is metabolized extensively in the gastrointestinal mucosa during absorption and in the liver by acetylation, hydroxylation, and conjugation with gluconic acid. The drug is then rapidly excreted in the urine, mainly as metabolites. First-pass acetylation in the gastrointestinal mucosa and liver is related to genetic acetylator phenotype. Slow acetylators generally have higher plasma levels of hydralazine than fast acetylators and require lower doses to maintain control of blood pressure. Hydralazine clearance is reduced in renal failure. In mild to moderate renal dysfunction, the dosing interval should be increased from 6 hours to 8 hours. In severe renal

Table 210-22. Pharmacokinetic Parameters of Hydralazine and Minoxidil [153,154,185]

	Hydralazine	Minoxidil
Bioavailability (%)	30–50	90–95
Onset (hr)	1	0.5
Peak (hr)	1–2	2–3
Duration (hr)	6–8	75
V_{dss} (L/kg)	0.46–7.7	2.7
Protein binding (%)	87	Negligible
Elimination half-life (hr)	1–6	3–4
Metabolism	Liver	Liver
Active metabolites	?	Yes
Excretion	Renal + feces[a]	Renal[b]

[a] 86% excreted in urine (12–14% as hydralazine) and 11% in feces as metabolites
[b] At least 90% of a dose metabolized and excreted in urine along with unchanged drug

Table 210-23. Dosing Guidelines for Hydralazine and Minoxidil

	Hydralazine[a,b,c,d]	Minoxidil[c,d]
Starting dose	10 mg qid po	5 mg qd po
Usual maintenance dose	10–50 mg qid po	10–40 mg/day po
Maximum dose	300 mg/day po	100 mg/day po

[a] Should be taken with meals (food enhances bioavailability)
[b] Dosage adjustments necessary in patients with moderate to severe renal dysfunction
[c] Dosage adjustments may be necessary in patients with severe hepatic failure.
[d] No specific information available regarding dosing of hypodynamic or hyperdynamic patients

failure, dosing intervals of 8 to 16 hours for fast acetylators and 12 to 24 hours for slow acetylators are recommended [153,154].

No information is available about the clearance of hydralazine in liver failure. Theoretically the bioavailability of orally administered hydralazine would be increased in these patients and therefore a reduction in dosage may be necessary.

HYPERMETABOLIC. The clearance of hydralazine in hypermetabolic patients is unknown. It could be speculated that higher doses may be necessary in these patients because of enhanced gastrointestinal and liver metabolism and renal excretion.

Minoxidil

HYPODYNAMIC. Minoxidil is extensively metabolized in the liver to a glucuronide conjugate and also by conversion to more polar metabolites. The metabolites are considerably less active than the parent drug. The drug and its metabolites are excreted by the kidney by glomerular filtration. No change in minoxidil clearance has been reported in renal failure. However, greater hypotensive effects may be produced in this patient population. No information is available concerning the clearance of minoxidil in hepatic failure. Dosage adjustment may be necessary in patients with severe liver failure [4,33].

HYPERDYNAMIC. There is no information on the clearance of minoxidil in hyperdynamic patients. Hypothetically, clearance should be increased secondary to increased liver and renal blood. These patients may require higher maintenance doses.

DOSING GUIDELINES. Table 210-23 summarizes the dosing guidelines for hydralazine and minoxidil.

DRUG INTERACTIONS. Concomitant therapy with minoxidil and guanethidine can result in profound orthostatic hypotension. Guanethidine should be discontinued 1 to 3 weeks before initiation of minoxidil therapy or minoxidil therapy should be initiated in the hospital [4].

COMMON PITFALLS
1. To prevent fluid retention, minoxidil must usually be administered with a diuretic, and almost always a loop diuretic is required.
2. Hydralazine and minoxidil can precipitate angina or ECG evidence of myocardial ischemia in patients with underlying coronary artery disease unless the baroreceptor reflex mech-

anism is blocked. For minoxidil, this usually requires the use of a beta-adrenergic blocker, as other sympathetic inhibitors are inadequate.
3. Doses of hydralazine of 200 mg or more per day have been associated with a higher risk of a syndrome similar to systemic lupus erythematosus. Symptoms include joint pain and skin rash and only rarely cerebritis and nephritis. Daily dosage of hydralazine affects the frequency, with no cases reported at 50 mg per day, 5.4 percent of patients at 100 mg per day, and 10.4 percent at 200 mg per day. Women have a higher incidence of this syndrome (11.6% for women vs. 2.8% for men). Women taking 200 mg per day had an incidence of 19.4 percent. Slow acetylator phenotype may also increase the risk for the syndrome. This syndrome is reversible on discontinuation of the drug [155].

Diazoxide

INTRODUCTION. Diazoxide is a parenteral nondiuretic antihypertensive that is structurally related to the thiazide diuretics. It may be used in the acute treatment of severe hypertension. The newer parenteral antihypertensives have replaced diazoxide as first-line agents for treating severe hypertension [156].

PHARMACOLOGY. Diazoxide reduces total peripheral vascular resistance and blood pressure via a direct relaxation of arteriolar smooth muscle. An increase in heart rate and cardiac output occurs as blood pressure is reduced. Coronary blood flow is maintained. The drug causes transient hyperglycemia in the majority of patients by inhibiting insulin release and peripheral utilization of glucose [156].

THERAPEUTIC RANGE. Plasma concentrations of 35 μg per milliliter (152 μM/L) produce a 25 percent reduction in mean arterial pressure [157].

PREPARATIONS. Diazoxide is available as a 15 mg per milliliter injection for intravenous administration.

PHARMACOKINETICS
Absorption. Although diazoxide is well absorbed following oral administration (86–96%), it must be administered intravenously to be an effective antihypertensive [33]. The onset of antihypertensive effect is within 1 to 2 minutes, with a peak

effect at 2 to 5 minutes and a duration of effect of 3 to 15 hours [33].

Distribution. Diazoxide is extensively bound to serum proteins (> 90%) and may displace other highly protein-bound drugs. The volume of distribution is 0.21 ± 0.02 liter per kilogram in patients with normal renal function [157,158].

Elimination. Diazoxide is partially metabolized in the liver by oxidation and sulfate conjugation and excreted slowly in the urine as unchanged drug (about 20%) and metabolites. It has an elimination half-life of 28 ± 8.3 hours, which can be prolonged in renal failure in proportion to creatinine clearance [33].

PHYSIOLOGIC CLEARANCE
Hypodynamic. The clearance of diazoxide is determined by liver and renal clearance (flow-dependent). In patients with renal impairment, the half-life of diazoxide is prolonged in proportion to decreases in creatinine clearance. No information is available concerning the clearance of the drug in patients with hepatic dysfunction. In this patient population, the dosing should be based on hemodynamic response and patient tolerance [138,156].

Hyperdynamic. Information concerning the clearance of diazoxide in this population is not available. It could be speculated that clearance may be increased in this population and dosage requirements may be higher.

DOSING GUIDELINES
Loading Dose. A slow intravenous infusion administered at a rate of 15 to 30 mg per minute is given via a peripheral vein to a total dosage of 5 mg per kilogram or until adequate blood pressure reduction is achieved. This dosing method may avoid the excessive reduction in blood pressure that may occur with rapid intravenous push administration. Alternatively, intravenous push doses of 1 to 3 mg per kilogram may be administered every 5 to 15 minutes until adequate blood pressure response is achieved [159,160].

Maintenance Dose. Doses may be repeated every 4 to 24 hours as needed to maintain blood pressure control. The drug should not be used longer than 10 days. No specific information regarding dosing of hypodynamic or hyperdynamic patients is available.

DRUG INTERACTIONS
Thiazide Diuretics. The coadministration of diazoxide with thiazide diuretics potentiates hyperglycemia. This may become a particular problem if diazoxide therapy is continued for several days. Symptoms similar to frank diabetes may occur. If possible, this combination of drugs should be avoided or blood and urine glucose levels monitored frequently. Thiazides may also potentiate the antihypertensive and hyperuricemic effects of diazoxide [161,162].

Sulfonylureas. Diazoxide appears to inhibit insulin release from pancreatic islet cells and may antagonize the effect of the oral sulfonylureas, resulting in hyperglycemia. Blood glucose should be carefully monitored and the dosage of each drug adjusted as needed. The dosage of the sulfonylurea may need to be increased to maintain the blood glucose within the desired range [163,164].

Phenytoin. Several days of continuous diazoxide therapy may result in increased hepatic metabolism of phenytoin, with a possible decrease in anticonvulsant effect and subtherapeutic phenytoin levels. Patients receiving concomitant phenytoin and diazoxide should be monitored for signs of decreased phenytoin levels [165].

COMMON PITFALLS
1. Repeated administration of diazoxide can lead to sodium and water retention. A diuretic may be necessary for maximal blood pressure reduction and to avoid congestive failure [33].
2. Diazoxide should not be administered intramuscularly or subcutaneously. The drug solution's alkalinity is irritating to tissue; extravasation should be avoided. Subcutaneous administration has produced inflammation and pain without subsequent necrosis. If extravasation occurs, it should be treated with warm compresses and rest [33].

Reserpine

INTRODUCTION. Reserpine lowers blood pressure via several different mechanisms that result in sympathetic inhibition. The drug was used in conjunction with other antihypertensive agents in many early clinical trials that documented benefit in treating hypertension [166–169]. Reserpine is one of the least expensive agents available for the treatment of hypertension [170].

PHARMACOLOGY. Reserpine depletes norepinephrine from postganglionic adrenergic neurons and blocks the transport of norepinephrine into the storage granules of the neuron. Thus, less norepinephrine is released into the synapse when the nerve is stimulated. This leads to a diminution in sympathetic tone with a resulting decrease in peripheral vascular resistance and blood pressure. It has only mild antihypertensive activity and is only effective as monotherapy in mild hypertension. It is most effective when used in combination with a diuretic or other antihypertensive agents, which permits the use of lower dosages of each drug and possibly minimizes side effects [33].

THERAPEUTIC RANGE. No therapeutic range has been established for reserpine. The onset and duration of the pharmacologic effects do not appear to be related to concentration in the blood.

PREPARATIONS. Reserpine is available as 0.1-mg, 0.25-mg, and 1-mg oral tablets.

PHARMACOKINETICS
Absorption. Reserpine is incompletely absorbed and has a bioavailability of approximately 40 to 50 percent following oral administration. Peak plasma levels of 0.15 to 0.3 ng per milliliter were reported 1 to 3 hours after an oral dose of 0.25 mg [33].

Distribution. Reserpine appears to be widely distributed in the tissues, especially adipose tissue. The drug crosses the blood-brain barrier and the placenta. It is extensively bound (96%) to plasma proteins [33].

Elimination. Reserpine is extensively metabolized in the liver, with more than 90 percent excreted in metabolized form. Approximately 1 percent is recovered in the urine unchanged and 11 percent as metabolites. Reserpine and metabolites are also excreted in the feces. The drug has an elimination half-life of 50 to 100 hours [33].

PHYSIOLOGIC CLEARANCE

Hypodynamic. Reserpine is extensively metabolized in the liver, with a large portion of a dose excreted in feces. Renal dysfunction probably does not change total clearance significantly. However, as with other sympatholytics, renal dysfunction patients may require lower maintenance doses of reserpine because of enhanced hypotensive response. Although no information is available, it can be deduced that patients with severe hepatic failure will require lower doses of reserpine due to reduced clearance [33].

Hyperdynamic. No information is available on the clearance of reserpine in hyperdynamic patients.

DOSING GUIDELINES

Loading Dose. The initial dosage for reserpine is 0.5 mg per day orally for 1 to 2 weeks.

Maintenance Dose. The maintenance dose for reserpine is 0.1 to 0.25 mg orally per day. No specific information regarding dosing of hypodynamic or hyperdynamic patients is available. The full effects of fixed oral doses of the drug are usually delayed for 2 to 3 weeks. Cardiovascular and CNS effects may persist several days to several weeks following discontinuation of chronic therapy.

Drug Interactions. Reserpine may increase receptor sensitivity to the direct-acting sympathomimetics, such as epinephrine, norepinephrine, and phenylephrine, resulting in an enhanced pressor response to these agents, which may result in hypertension. The pressor response to the indirect acting sympathomimetics, such as ephedrine, may be antagonized in patients receiving reserpine. If direct or indirect sympathomimetic agents and reserpine must be used together, blood pressure should be monitored. Depending on the type of sympathomimetic used, the dose may need to be increased or decreased [171,172,173].

COMMON PITFALLS. The incidence of reserpine-induced depression can be minimized by using doses of 0.25 mg per day or less. However, the drug should be avoided in patients with a known or suspected history of mental depression [174].

Trimethaphan Camsylate

INTRODUCTION. Trimethaphan is a nonselective, nondepolarizing ganglionic blocking agent. It is administered as a continuous intravenous infusion for short-term acute control of blood pressure in hypertensive emergencies, for controlled hypotension during surgery, and in emergency treatment of pulmonary edema in patients with pulmonary hypertension associated with systemic hypertension. Many clinicians consider the drug the agent of choice for the management of blood pressure

and the rate of left ventricular pressure rise in patients with acute dissection of the aorta. Trimethaphan's adverse parasympatholytic effects limit its usefulness; therefore, other parenteral antihypertensive agents are usually preferred as first-line agents and trimethaphan is now rarely used [33,175,176].

PHARMACOLOGY. Trimethaphan blocks the transmission of impulses at sympathetic and parasympathetic ganglia. It occupies ganglion receptors and stabilizes postsynaptic membranes against the action of acetylcholine liberated from presynaptic nerve endings. Through blockade of sympathetic ganglia, trimethaphan causes vasodilation and decreased blood pressure. The drug may also have a direct peripheral vasodilation effect. Tachyphylaxis develops within 24 to 72 hours, making transition to other antihypertensive agents mandatory [33].

THERAPEUTIC RANGE. No therapeutic range has been established for trimethaphan.

PREPARATIONS. Trimethaphan is available as a intravenous injection of 500 mg per 10 ml amp. The injection must be diluted prior to administration. Intravenous infusions are usually prepared by adding 500 mg of trimethaphan to 500 ml of 5% dextrose injection.

PHARMACOKINETICS. Intravenous infusion of trimethaphan produces almost immediate reduction in blood pressure. Blood pressure begins to rise when the infusion is slowed or stopped and usually returns to pretreatment levels within 10 to 15 minutes. The drug may be metabolized by pseudocholinesterase but is predominately eliminated renally by filtration and secretion, mostly unchanged [33].

PHYSIOLOGIC CLEARANCE

Hypometabolic. Trimethaphan is primarily eliminated renally as the parent compound. No information is available on clearance in renal dysfunction, however it should be decreased. Patients with renal dysfunction should respond to lower doses. Mild to moderate liver dysfunction should have little effect on clearance. The drug should be used with caution in patients with severe liver failure.

Hypermetabolic. No information is available on the clearance of trimethaphan in this population. Theoretically, hypermetabolism should not change its clearance significantly as clearance is primarily renal.

DOSING GUIDELINES

Loading Dose. Loading doses of trimethaphan are not necessary, as the drug has a quick onset of action and steady-state plasma levels are attained within minutes of starting a continuous intravenous infusion.

Maintenance Dose. A continuous intravenous infusion of trimethaphan is initiated at a rate of 0.5 to 1 mg per minute using an infusion pump. Subsequent titration to the desired blood pressure can be made in increments of 0.5 to 1mg per minute every 3 to 5 minutes. A marked variation in individual responses to the drug occurs. The usual dosage response is in the range of 0.3 to 6 mg per minute. No specific information regarding dosing of hypodynamic or hyperdynamic patients is available. However, geriatric patients generally require smaller doses than do young patients [33,175,177].

DRUG INTERACTIONS

Succinylcholine. Trimethaphan is a potent noncompetitive inhibitor of pseudocholinesterase. Concurrent administration of these two drugs may result in a decreased rate of succinylcholine metabolism and prolong neuromuscular blockade. Trimethaphan may also directly decrease the sensitivity of the respiratory center, contributing to prolongation of apnea. This drug combination should be avoided if possible. Nitroprusside would be an appropriate alternative to trimethaphan [178,179].

Nondepolarizing Neuromuscular Blockers. Trimethaphan may potentiate the neuromuscular blocking action of the nondepolarizing muscle relaxants, probably due to a curarelike effect of trimethaphan. This combination of drugs should be avoided if possible. Nitroprusside would be an appropriate alternative agent [180,181].

COMMON PITFALLS

1. Animal studies indicate that aggressive dosing of trimethaphan may result in respiratory arrest. Rare cases of respiratory arrest have occurred in humans, although a causal relationship has not been established. Respiratory status should be closely monitored.
2. Trimethaphan can cause pupillary dilation. Therefore, mydriasis does not necessarily indicate anoxia or reflect the depth of anesthesia [33].
3. Trimethaphan should be avoided during pregnancy because it crosses the placenta and can cause decreased fetal gastrointestinal motility and resulting meconium ileus. In addition, trimethaphan-induced hypotension may have other serious adverse effects on the fetus [33].

References

1. Lalonde RL, et al: Propranolol pharmacodynamic modeling using unbound and total concentrations in healthy volunteers. *J Pharmacokinet Biopharm* 15:569, 1987.
2. Kornhauser DM, et al: Biological determinants of propranolol disposition in man. *Clin Pharmacol Ther* 23:165, 1978.
3. Wood AJJ, et al: Direct measurement of propranolol bioavailability during accumulation to steady-state. *Br J Clin Pharmacol Ther* 6:345, 1978.
4. Olin BR, Hebel SK (eds): *Drug Facts and Comparisons.* St. Louis, Facts and Comparisons, Inc., 1993.
5. Lalonde RL, et al: Propranolol pharmacokinetics and pharmcodynamics after single doses and at steady-state. *Eur J Clin Pharmacol* 32:315, 1987.
6. Silber BM, et al: Dose-dependent elimination of propranolol and its major metabolites in humans. *J Pharm Sci* 72:725, 1983.
7. Lalonde R, et al: Nonlinear accumulation of propranolol enantiomers. *Br J Clin Pharmacol* 26:100, 1988.
8. Routledge PA, Shand D: Clinical pharmacokinetics of propranolol. *Clin Pharmacokinet* 4:73, 1979.
9. Bianchetti G, et al: Kinetics of distribution of dl-propranolol in various organs and discrete brain areas of the rat. *J Pharmacol Exp Ther* 214:682, 1980.
10. Straka R, Lalonde R, Pieper J, et al: Nonlinear pharmacokinetics of unbound propranolol after oral administration. *J Pharm Sci* 76:521, 1987.
11. Piafsky KM, Borga O: Plasma protein binding of basic drugs. II. Importance of alpha-1-acid glycoprotein for interindividual variation. *Clin Pharmacol Ther* 22:545, 1977.
12. Routledge PA, et al: Increased plasma propranolol binding in myocardial infarction. *Br J Clin Pharmacol* 9:438, 1980.
13. Walle UK, et al: Stereoselective binding of propranolol to human plasma, alpha-1-acid glycoprotein, and albumin. *Clin Pharmacol Ther* 34:718, 1983.
14. Evans WE, Schentag JJ, Jusko WJ (eds): *Applied Pharmacokinetics.* Spokane, Applied Therapeutics, 1992.
15. Walle T, et al: Quantitative account of propranolol metabolism in urine of normal man. *Drug Metab Dispos Biol Fate Chem* 13:204, 1985.
16. Walle T, et al: The predictable relationship between plasma levels and dose during chronic propranolol therapy. *Clin Pharmacol Ther* 24:688, 1978.
17. Wilson M, et al: The effect on blood pressure of beta-adrenoceptor blocking drugs administered once daily and their duration of action when therapy is ceased. *Br J Clin Pharmacol* 3:857, 1976.
18. Wilcox EG: Randomized study of six beta blockers and a thiazide diuretic in essential hypertension. *Br Med J* 2:383, 1978.
19. Walle T, et al: Stereoselective ring oxidation of propranolol in man. *Br J Clin Pharmacol* 18:741, 1984.
20. Melander A, et al: Enhancement of the bioavailability of propranolol and metoprolol by food. *Clin Pharmacol Ther* 22:108, 1977.
21. Johnsson G, et al: Combined pharmacokinetic and pharmacodynamic studies in man of the adrenergic beta-1 receptor antagonist metoprolol. *Acta Pharmacol Toxicol* 36:31, 1975.
22. Johnsson G, Regardh C-G: Clinical pharmacokinetics of beta-adrenoreceptor blocking drugs. *Clin Pharmacokinet* 1:233, 1976.
23. Borg K, Carlsson E, Hoffmann K, et al: Metabolism of metoprolol-(3-H) in man, the dog and the rat. *Acta Pharmacol Toxicol* 36(suppl 5):125, 1975.
24. Lennard M, Silas J, Freestone S, et al: Defective metabolism of metoprolol in poor hydroxylators of debrisoquine. *Br J Clin Pharmacol* 14:301, 1982.
25. Straka R, Johnson K, Gross C, et al: Pharmacodynamic modeling of metoprolol enantiomers in poor and extensive metabolizers of debrisoquine (abstract). *Clin Pharmacol Ther* 49:157, 1991.
26. Lennard M, Tucker G, Woods H: The polymorphic oxidation of beta adrenergic antagonists: Clinical pharmacokinetic considerations. *Clin Pharmacokinet* 11:1, 1986.
27. Eichelbaum M, Gross A: The genetic polymorphism of debrisoquine/sparteine metabolism: Clinical aspects. *Pharmacol Ther* 46:377, 1990.
28. Mason W, et al: Kinetics and absolute bioavailability of atenolol. *Clin Pharmacol Ther* 25:408, 1979.
29. Dreyfuss J, et al: Pharamcokinetics of nadolol, a beta receptor antagonist: Administration of therapeutic single and multiple-dosage regimens to hypertensive patients. *J Clin Pharmacol* 19:712, 1979.
30. Reeves PR, et al: Metabolism of atenolol in man. *Xenobiotica* 8:313, 1978.
31. Flouvar B, et al: Pharmacokinetics of atenolol in patients with terminal renal failure and influence of hemodialysis. *Br J Clin Pharmacol* 9:379, 1980.
32. Sum CY, et al: Kinetics of esmolol, an ultra-short-acting beta-blocker, and of its major metabolite. *Clin Pharmacol Ther* 34:427, 1983.
33. McEvoy GK (ed): *American Hospital Formulary Service Drug Information.* Bethesda, MD, American Society of Hospital Pharmacists, 1993.
34. Boles Ponto LL, Schoenwald RD: Furosemide (frusemide): A pharmacokinetic pharmacodynamic review (two parts). *Clin Pharmacokinet* 18:381, 460, 1990.
35. Olsen UB: The pharmacology of bumetanide. *Acta Pharmacol Toxicol* 41:1, 1977.
36. Brummett RE, Bendrick T, Himes D: Comparative ototoxicity of bumetanide and furosemide when used in combination with kanamycin. *J Clin Pharm* 21:628, 1981.
37. Kaka JS, Lyman C, Kilarski D: Tobramycin-furosemide interaction. *Drug Intell Clin Pharm* 18:235, 1984.
38. Cohen L, Kitzes R: Magnesium sulfate and digitalis-toxic arrhythmias. *JAMA* 249:2808, 1983.
39. Multiple Risk Factor Intervention Trial Research Group: Multiple risk factor intervention trial: Risk factor changes and mortality results. *JAMA* 248:351, 1982.

40. Brummett RE: Ototoxicity resulting from the combined administration of potent diuretics and other agents. *Scand Audiol* 14:215, 1981.

41. Komune S, Snow JB: Potentiating effects of cisplatin and ethacrynic acid in ototoxicity. *Otolaryngology* 107:594, 1981.

42. Brater DC: Effect of indomethacin on salt and water homeostasis. *Clin Pharmacol Ther* 25:322, 1979.

43. Skinner MH, Mutterperl R, Zeitz HJ: Sulindac inhibits bumetanide-induced sodium and water excretion. *Clin Pharmacol Ther* 42:542, 1987.

44. Laiwah ACY, Mactier RA: Antagonistic effect of non-steroidal anti-inflammatory drugs on frusemide-induced diuresis in cardiac failure. *Br Med J* 283:714, 1981.

45. Atkinson AB, Brown JJ, Leckie B, et al: Captopril in a hyponatremic hypertensive: Need for caution in initiating therapy. *Lancet* 1:557, 1979.

46. Vlasses PH, Ferguson RK, Chatterjee K: Clinical pharmacology and benefit-to-risk ratio in hypertension and congestive heart failure. *Pharmacotherapy* 2:1, 1982.

47. Thorn GW: Clinical consideration in the use of corticosteroids. *N Engl J Med* 274:775, 1966.

48. Seller RH, Cangiano J, Kim K, et al: Digitalis toxicity and hypomagnesemia. *Am Heart J* 79:57, 1970.

49. Steiness E, Olesen KH: Cardiac arrhythmias induced by hypokalemia and potassium loss during maintenance digoxin therapy. *Br Heart J* 38:167, 1976.

50. Goldner MG, Zarowitz H, Akgun S: Hyperglycemia and glycosiuria due to thiazide derivatives administered in diabetes mellitus. *N Engl J Med* 262:403, 1960.

51. Frishman WH: Pharmacology of the nitrates in angina pectoris. *Am J Cardiol* 56:81, 1985.

52. Solomon JG: Lithium toxicity precipitated by a diuretic. *Psychosomatics* 21:425, 1980.

53. Nurnberger JI: Diuretic-induced lithium toxicity presenting as mania. *J Nerv Ment Dis* 173:316, 1985.

54. Levy ST, Forrest JN, Heninger GR: Lithium-induced diabetes insipidus: Manic symptoms, brain and electrolyte correlates, and chlorothiazide treatment. *Am J Psychiatry* 130:1014, 1973.

55. Hunninghake DB, King S: Effect of cholestyramine and colestipol on the absorption of methyldopa and hydrochlorothiazide. *Pharmacologist* 20:220, 1978.

56. Lant A: Clinical pharmacology and therapeutic use. *Drugs* 29:57, 162, 1985.

57. Skluth HA, Gums JG: Spironolactone: A re-examination. *Drug Intell Clin Pharm* 24:52, 1990.

58. Macfie HL, Colvin CL, Anderson PO: Amiloride. *Drug Intell Clin Pharm* 15:94, 1981.

59. Welling PG: Pharmacokinetics of the thiazide diuretics. *Biopharm Drug Dispos* 7:501, 1986.

60. Sorgel F, Hasegawa J, Lin E, et al: Oral triamterene disposition. *Clin Pharmacol Ther* 38:306, 1985.

61. Beerman B, Groschinsky-Grind M: Clinical pharmacokinetics of diuretics. *Clin Pharmacokinet* 5:221, 1980.

62. Atlas SA, Case DB, Sealey JE, et al: Interruption of the renin-angiotensin system in hypertensive patients by captopril induces sustained reduction in aldosterone secretion, potassium retention and natriuresis. *Hypertension* 1:274, 1979.

63. Maslowski AH, Ikram H, Nicholls MG, et al: Haemodynamic, hormonal, and electrolyte responses to captopril in resistant heart failure. *Lancet* 1:71, 1981.

64. Shapiro S, Slone D, Lewis GP, et al: Fatal drug reactions among medical inpatients. *JAMA* 216:467, 1971.

65. Greenblatt DJ, Koch-Weser J: Adverse reactions to spironolactone. *JAMA* 225:40, 1973.

66. Steiness E: Renal tubular secretion of digoxin. *Circulation* 50:103, 1974.

67. Waldorff S, Berning J, Buch J, et al: Systolic time intervals during spironolactone treatment of digitalized and non-digitalized patients with ischemic heart disease. *Eur J Clin Pharmacol* 21:269, 1981.

68. Elliott HC: Reduced adrenocortical steroid excretion rates in man following aspirin administration. *Metabolism* 11:1015, 1962.

69. Ramsey LE, Harrison IR, Shelton JR, et al: Influence of acetylsalicyclic acid on the renal handling of a spironolactone metabolite in healthy subjects. *Eur J Clin Pharmacol* 10:43, 1976.

70. Wilson TW, Rajput AH: Amantadine-dyazide interaction. *Can Med Assoc J* 129:974, 1983.

71. Lynn KL, Bailey RR, Swainson CP, et al: Renal failure with potassium sparing diuretics. *N Z Med J* 98:629, 1985.

72. Faure L, Glasson PH, Riondel A, et al: Interaction of diuretics and non-steroidal anti-inflammatory drugs in man. *Clin Sci* 64:407, 1983.

73. Waldorff S, Hansen PB, Kjaergard H, et al: Amloride-induced changes in digoxin dynamics and kinetics: Abolition of digoxin-induced inotropism with amiloride. *Clin Pharmacol Ther* 30:172, 1981.

74. Kennedy RH, Akera T, Brody TM: Suppression of positive inotropic and toxic effects of cardiac glycosides by amiloride. *Eur J Pharmacol* 115:199, 1985.

75. Gilman AG, Ral T, Nies A, et al: *The Pharmacological Basis of Therapeutics.* New York, MacMillan, 1990.

76. Bailey DG, Arnold MO, Munoz C, et al: Grapefruit juice-felodipine interaction: Mechanism, predictability, and effect of naringin. *Clin Pharmacol Ther* 53:637, 1993.

77. Brunner HR, Waeber B, Nussberger J: Angiotensin converting enzyme inhibitors in arterial hypertension. *Wiener Mediziniche Wochenshrift* 140:22, 1990.

78. Bridoux F, Hazzan M, Pallot JL, et al: Acute renal failure after the use of angiotensin converting enzyme inhibitors in patients without renal artery stenosis. *Nephrol Dial Transplant* 7:100, 1992.

79. Lee HC, Dettinger WH: Diuretics potentiate the angiotensin converting enzyme inhibitor-associated acute renal dysfunction (letter). *Clin Nephrol* 38:236, 1992.

80. Advisory Committee ADR: ACE inhibitor first dose effect. *Med J Aust* 158:208, 1993.

81. Duchin KL, Pierides AM, Heald A, et al: Intravenous captopril in patients with renal failure. *Kidney Int* 25:942, 1984.

82. Drummer OH, Workman BJ, Miach PJ, et al: The pharmacokinetics of captopril and captopril disulfide conjugates in uremic patients on maintenance dialysis: Comparison in patients with normal renal function. *Eur J Clin Pharmacol* 32:267, 1987.

83. Feinfeld DA, Frishman WH: Renal considerations in cardiovascular therapy. *Cardiol Clin* 5:675, 1987.

84. Belz GG, Kirch W, Kleinbloesen CH: Angiotensin converting enzyme inhibitors: Relationship between pharmacodynamics and pharmacokinetics. *Clin Pharmacokinet* 15:295, 1988.

85. Sica DA, Cutler RE, Parmer RJ, et al: Comparison of the steady-state pharmacokinetics of fosinopril, lisinopril, and enalapril in patients with chronic renal insufficiency. *Clin Pharmacokinet* 20:420, 1991.

86. Kelly JG, Doyle GD, Carmody M, et al: Pharmacokinetics of lisinopril, enalapril and enalaprilat in renal failure: Effects of hemodialysis. *Br J Clin Pharmacol* 26:781, 1988.

87. Gautam DC, Vargas E, Lye M: Pharmacokinetics of lisinopril in healthy young and elderly subjects and in elderly patients with cardiac failure. *J Pharm Pharmacol* 39:929, 1987.

88. Jackson B, Cubela RB, Conway EL, et al: Lisinopril pharmacokinetics in chronic renal failure. *Br J Pharmacol* 25:719, 1988.

89. Thomson AH, Kelly JG, Whiting B: Lisinopril population pharmacokinetics in elderly and renal disease patients with hypertension. *Br J Clin Pharmacol* 27:57, 1989.

90. Singhvi SM, Duchin KL, Morrison RA, et al: Disposition of fosinopril sodium in healthy subjects. *Br J Clin Pharmacol* 25:9, 1988.

91. Olson S, Horvath A, Michniewicz B, et al: The clinical pharmacokinetics of quinapril. *Angiology* 40:351, 1989.

92. Begg EJ, Robcon RA, Bailey RR, et al: The pharmacokinetics and pharmacodynamics of quinapril and quinaprilat in renal impairment. *Br J Clin Pharmacol* 30:213, 1990.

93. Witte PV, Irmisch R, Hajdu P, et al: Pharmacokinetics and pharmacodynamics of a novel orally active angiotensin converting enzyme inhibitor in healthy subjects. *Eur J Clin Pharmacol* 27:577, 1984.

94. Schunkert H, Knoller J, Gassmann M, et al: Steady-state kinetics of ramipril in renal failure. *J Cardiovasc Pharmacol* 13:552, 1989.

95. Kindler J, Schunkert H, Gassmann M, et al: Therapeutic efficacy and tolerance of ramipril in hypertensive patients with renal failure. *J Cardiovasc Pharmacol* 13:555, 1989.

96. Bell J: Benazepril: A new ACE inhibitor. *ANNA J* 20:187, 1993.

97. Kaiser G, Ackermann R, Sioufi A: Pharmacokinetics of a new angiotensin converting enzyme inhibitor: Benazepril hydrochloride in special populations. *Am Heart J* 117:746, 1989.

98. Holmes B, Brogden RN, Hael RC, et al: Guanabenz: A review of its pharmacodynamic properties and therapeutic efficacy in hypertension. *Drugs* 26:212, 1983.

99. Sorkin EM, Heel RC: Guanfacine: A review of its pharmacodynamic and pharmacokinetic properties and therapeutic efficacy in the treatment of hypertension. *Drugs* 31:301, 1986.

100. Van Zwieten PA: Pharmacology of centrally acting hypotensive drugs. *Br J Clin Pharmacol* 10:13S, 1980.

101. Lowentahl DT, Matzek KM, MacGregor TR: Clinical pharmacokinetics of clonidine. *Clin Pharmacokinet* 14:287, 1988.

102. Myhre E, Rugstad HE, Hansen T: Clinical pharmacokinetics of methyldopa. *Clin Pharmacokinet* 7:221, 1982.

103. Bailey RR, Meale TJ: Rapid clonidine withdrawal with blood pressure overshoot exaggerated by beta blockade. *Br Med J* 1:942, 1976.

104. Strauss FG, Stanley SF, Lewin AJ, et al: Withdrawal of antihypertensive therapy. *JAMA* 238:1734, 1977.

105. Briant RH, Reid JL, Dollery CT: Interaction between clonidine and desipramine in man. *Br Med J* 1:522, 1973.

106. Hui KK: Hypertensive crisis induced by interaction of clonidine with imipramine. *Geriatr Soc* 31:164, 1983.

107. Pettinger W, Horwitz D, Spector S, et al: Enhancement of methyldopa of tyramine sensitivity in man. *Nature* 200:1107, 1963.

108. Dollery CT, Harington M, Hodge JV: Haemodynamic studies with methyldopa: Effect on cardiac output and response to pressor amines. *Br Heart J* 25:670, 1963.

109. Reid JL, Campbell BC, Hamilton CA: Withdrawal reactions following cessation of central alpha-adrenergic receptor agonists. *Hypertension* 6:71-II, 1984.

110. Palmer JD, Nugent CA: Guanadrel sulfate: A postganglionic sympathetic inhibitor for the treatment of mild to moderate hypertension. *Pharmacotherapy* 3:220, 1983.

111. Walter IE, Khandelwal J, Falkner F, et al: The relationship of plasma guanethidine levels to adrenergic blockade. *Clin Pharmacol Ther* 18:571, 1975.

112. Hengstmann JH, Falkner FC: Disposition of guanethidine during chronic oral therapy. *Eur J Clin Pharmacol* 15:121, 1979.

113. Finnerty FA, Brogden RN: Guanadrel: A review of its pharmacodynamic and pharmacokinetic properties and therapeutic use in hypertension. *Drugs* 30:22, 1985.

114. Laurence DR: The effects of bretylium and guanethidine on the pressor responses to noradrenaline and angiotensin. *Br J Pharmacol* 21:403, 1963.

115. Muelheims GH, Entrup RW, Paiewonsky D, et al: Increased sensitivity of the heart to catecholamine-induced arrhythmias following guanethidine. *Clin Pharmacol Ther* 6:757, 1965.

116. Poe TE, Edwards JL, Taylor RB: Hypertensive crisis possibly due to drug interaction. *Postgrad Med* 66:235, 1979.

117. Ober KF, Wang RI: Drug interactions with guanethidine. *Clin Pharmacol Ther* 14:190, 1973.

118. Gulati OD, Dave BT, Gokhale SE, et al: Antagonism of adrenergic neuron blockade in hypertensive subjects. *Clin Pharmacol Ther* 7:510, 1966.

119. Janowsky DS, El-Yousef MK, Davis JM, et al: Antagonism of guanethidine by chlorpromazine. *Am J Psychiatry* 130:808, 1973.

120. Gilder DA, Fain W, Simpson LL: A comparison of the abilities of chlorpromazine and molindone to interact adversely with guanethidine. *J Pharmacol Exp Ther* 198:255, 1976.

121. Chiariello M, Gold HK, Leinbach RC, et al: Comparison between the effects of nitroprusside and nitroglycerin on ischemic injury during acute myocardial infarction. *Circulation* 54:766, 1976.

122. Mason DT: Symposium on vasodilator and inotropic therapy of heart failure. *Am J Med* 65:101, 1978.

123. Habbab MA, Haft JL: Intravenous nitroglycerin and heparin resistance. *Ann Intern Med* 105:305, 1986.

124. Habbab MA, Haft JL: Heparin resistance induced by intravenous nitroglycerin. *Arch Intern Med* 147:857, 1987.

125. Murphy J, Lavie C, Breshahan D (eds): *Nitroprusside.* Philadelphia, WB Saunders, 1990.

126. Borchardt-Phelps PK, Lohr BC (eds): *Optimization of Drug Doses.* St. Louis, Quality Medical Publishing, 1993.

127. Reid GM, Muther RS: Nitroprusside-induced acute azotemia. *Am J Nephrol* 7:313, 1987.

128. Curry SC, Arnold-Capell P: Nitroprusside, nitroglycerin, and angiotensin-converting enzyme inhibitors. *Crit Care Clin* 7:555, 1991.

129. Ivankovich A, Miletich D, Tinker J: Sodium nitroprusside: Metabolism and general considerations. *Int Anesthesiol Clin* 16:4, 1978.

130. Schulz V: Clinical pharmacokinetics of nitroprusside, cyanide, thiosulphate, and thuocyanate. *Clin Pharmacokinet* 9:239, 1984.

131. Hall A, Rumack B: Clinical toxicology of cyanide. *Ann Emerg Med* 15:1067, 1986.

132. Rindone J, Sloane E: Cyanide toxicity from sodium nitroprusside: Risks and management. *Ann Pharmacother* 26:515, 1992.

133. Schulz V, Bonn R, Kindler J: Kinetics of elimination of thuocyonate in 7 healthy subjects and in 8 subjects with renal failure. *Klin Wochenschr* 57:243, 1979.

134. *FDA Medical Bulletin*, March 1991.

135. Schulz V, Gross R, Pasch T, et al: Cyanide toxicity of sodium nitroprusside in therapeutic use with and without sodium thuosulfate. *Klin Wochenschr* 6:1393, 1982.

136. Holland M, Kozlowski L: Clinical features and management of cyanide poisoning. *Clin Pharm* 5:737, 1986.

137. Hansten P, Horn J (eds): *Drug Interactions and Updates.* Vancouver, WA, Applied Therapeutics, 1993.

138. Ram VS, Kaplan NM: Individual titration of diazoxide dosage in the treatment of severe hypertension. *Am J Cardiol* 43:627, 1979.

139. Reid JL: Alpha-adrenergic receptors and blood pressure control. *Am J Cardiol* 57:6E, 1986.

140. Vincent J, Meredith PA, Reid JL, et al: Clinical pharmacokinetics of prazosin. *Clin Pharmacokinet* 10:144, 1985.

141. Patterson SE: Terazosin kinetics after oral and intravenous doses. *Clin Pharmacol Ther* 38:423, 1985.

142. Young RA, Brogden RN: Doxazosin: A review of its pharmacodynamic and pharmacokinetic properties and therapeutic efficacy in mild or moderate hypertension. *Drugs* 35:525, 1988.

143. Elliott HL, Meredith PA, Campbell L, et al: The combination of prazosin and verapamil in the treatment of essential hypertension. *Clin Pharmacol Ther* 43:554, 1988.

144. Elliott HL, McLean K, Sumner DJ, et al: Immediate cardiovascular response to oral prazosin: Effects of concurrent beta-blockers. *Clin Pharmacol Ther* 29:303, 1981.

145. Caris TN (ed): *A Clinical Guide to Hypertension.* Littleton, MA, PSG, 1985.

146. Kaplan NM (ed): *Clinical Hypertension.* 4th ed. Baltimore, Williams & Wilkins, 1986.

147. Genest J, Kuchel O, Hamet P, et al (eds): *Hypertension, Physiopathology and Treatment.* 2nd ed. New York, McGraw-Hill, 1983.

148. Kincaid-Smith PS, Whitworth JA (eds): *Hypertension: Mechanisms and Management.* New York, ADIS Health Science Press, 1980.

149. Meyer P (ed): *Hypertension Mechanisms and Clinical and Therapeutic Aspects.* Oxford, Oxford University Press, 1980.

150. McCarron DA: Management of hypertension: Pathophysiologic and therapeutic perspectives. *J Cardiovasc Pharmacol* 6:464, 1984.

151. Chobanian AV: Hypertension. *Clin Symp* 34:3, 1982.

152. McMahon FG (ed): *Management of Essential Hypertension: The New Low-dose Era.* 2nd ed. Mount Kisco, NY, Futura, 1984.

153. Lacourciere Y, Poirier L, Dion D, et al: Antihypertensive effect of irsadipine administered once or twice daily on ambulatory blood pressure. *Am J Cardiol* 65:467, 1990.

154. Ludden TM, McNay JL, Shepherd AMM: Clinical pharmacokinetics of hydralazine. *Clin Pharmacokinet* 7:185, 1982.

155. Cameron HA, Ramsay LE: The lupus syndrome induced by hydralazine: A common complication with low-dose treatment. *Br Med J* 289:410, 1984.

156. Speight TM: Diazoxide: A review of its pharmacological properties and therapeutic use in hypertensive crisis. *Drugs* 2:78, 1971.

157. Ogilvie RI, Nadeau JH, Sitar DS: Diazoxide concentration-response relation in hypertension. *Hypertension* 4:167, 1982.

158. Pearson RM, Breckenridge AM: Renal function, protein binding and pharmacological response to diazoxide. *Br J Clin Pharmacol* 3:169, 1976.

159. Andreasen F, Botker HE, Christenson JH, et al: The biological relevance of protein binding of diazoxide. *Acta Pharmacol Toxicol* 57:30, 1985.

160. Joint National Committee (Fifth Report): Hypertension: Steps forward and steps backward. *Arch Intern Med* 153:149, 1993.

161. Dollery CT, Pentecost BL, Samaan NA, et al: Drug-induced diabetes. *Lancet* 2:735, 1962.

162. Okun R, Russell RP, Wilson WR: Use of diazoxide with trichlor-methiazide for hypertension. *Arch Intern Med* 112:882, 1963.
163. Graber AL, Porte D, Williams RH: Clinical use of diazoxide and mechanisms for its hyperglycemic effects. *Diabetes* 15:143, 1966.
164. Wales JK, Grant AM, Wolff FW: Reversal of diazoxide effects by tolbutamide. *Lancet* 1:1137, 1967.
165. Roe TF, Podosin RL, Blaskovics ME, et al: Drug interaction: Diazoxide and diphenylhydantoin. *J Pediatr* 87:480, 1975.
166. VACSAA: Effects of treatment on morbidity in hypertension: Results in patients with diastolic pressures averaging 115-129 mmHg. *JAMA* 202:1028, 1967.
167. VACSAA: Effects of treatment on morbidity in hypertension. II. Results in patients with diastolic blood pressure averaging 90-114 mmHg. *JAMA* 213:1143, 1970.
168. Hypertension DaF-UPCG: Five year findings of the hypertension, detection and follow-up program. I. Reduction in mortality of persons with high blood pressure, including mild hypertension. *JAMA* 242:2562, 1979.
169. Moser M: Cost containment and hypertension. *Ann Intern Med* 108:148, 1988.
170. Moser G, Schrader J, Deussen A: Turnover of adenosine in plasma of human and dog blood. *Am J Physiol* 256:C799, 1989.
171. Eger EI, Hamilton WK: The effect of reserpine on the action of various vasopressors. *Anesthesiology* 20:641, 1959.
172. Ziegler CH, Lovette JB: Operative complications after therapy with reserpine and reserpine compounds. *JAMA* 176:916, 1961.
173. Sneddon JM, Turner P: Ephedrine mydriasis in hypertension and the response to treatment. *Clin Pharmacol Ther* 10:64, 1969.
174. Borreson RE: The case for reserpine in hypertension. *Hosp Formul* 20:719, 1985.
175. Becker CE, Benowitz NL: Hypertensive emergencies. *Med Clin North Am* 63:127, 1979.
176. Palmer RF, Lasseter NL: Nitroprusside and aortic dissecting aneurysm. *N Engl J Med* 294:1976.
177. Gifford RW (ed): *Management and Treatment of Essential Hypertension, Including Malignant Hypertension and Emergencies.* 2nd ed. New York, McGraw-Hill, 1983.
178. Tewfik GI: Its effect on the pseudo-cholinesterase level of man. *Anaesthesia* 12:326, 1957.
179. Sklar GS, Lanks KW: Effects of trimethaphan and sodium nitroprusside on hydrolysis of succinylcholine in vitro. *Anesthesiology* 47:31, 1977.
180. Deacock AR, Davies TDW: The influence of certain ganglionic blocking agents on neuromuscular transmission. *Br J Anaesth* 30:217, 1958.
181. Dale RC, Schroeder ET: Respiratory paralysis during treatment of hypertension with trimethaphan camsylate. *Arch Intern Med* 136:816, 1976.
182. Singh BN, Deedwania P, Nadamanee K, et al: Sotalol: A review of its pharmacodynamic and pharmacokinetic properties, and therapeutic use. *Drugs* 34:311, 1987.
183. Gardiner P, Schrode K, Quinlan D, et al: Spironolactone metabolism: Steady-state serum levels of the sulfur-containing metabolites. *J Clin Pharmacol* 29:342, 1989.
184. Knoben JE, Anderson PO (eds): *Handbook of Clinical Drug Data.* Hamilton, IL, Drug Intelligence Publications, 1993.
185. Fleishaker JC, Andreadis NA, Welshman IR, et al: The pharmacokinetics of 2.5 to 10 mg oral doses of minoxidil in healthy volunteers. *J Clin Pharmacol* 29:162, 1989.

211. Theophylline

Philip R. Kohls and Susan J. Markowsky

Theophylline (1,3-dimethylxanthine) is a smooth muscle relaxant and bronchodilator used in the prevention and treatment of hyperreactive airway disease. In the intensive care unit (ICU), its primary indication is in the treatment of bronchospasm. It is occasionally used as an aid in liberating patients from the ventilator [1,2].

Pharmacology

Theophylline is a direct-acting smooth muscle relaxant with a bronchodilatory mechanism of action that is still unclear. Proposed mechanisms include inhibition of cyclic adenosine monophosphate (cyclic AMP) phosphodiesterase; inhibition of cellular calcium translocation; inhibition of leukotriene production; reduction in the uptake or metabolism of catecholamines; and blockade of adenosine receptors [3]. Only the last two mechanisms appear likely to occur at clinically obtainable theophylline concentrations. Enprofylline, a related xanthine, is a potent bronchodilator but is not an adenosine receptor antagonist; thus, this mechanism of action is also open to question.

Theophylline has many physiologic effects, which are briefly summarized in Table 211-1.

Therapeutic Range and Toxicity

The accepted therapeutic range for theophylline is 10 to 20 mg per liter. In an early study of nine hospitalized but otherwise healthy asthma patients who were recovering from an acute exacerbation of their disease, peak expiratory flow rate, or forced expiratory volume in 1 second divided by forced vital capacity (FEV_1/FVC), increased in proportion to the log of the serum theophylline concentration (STC) over a range of 5 to 20 mg per liter [4,5]. Measurable improvement was observed at 5 mg per liter, although optimal bronchodilator effects are often described at concentrations greater than 10 mg per liter [6]. The degree of airway obstruction in an individual patient tends to determine the degree of improvement in pulmonary function and the steepness of the dose-response curve over the range of 5 to 20 mg per liter. An STC between 5 and 10 mg per liter may be appropriate for some individuals, especially children with mild asthma. Although additional bronchodilation can be induced by increasing the STC to greater than 20 mg per liter, the high frequency of adverse effects at these drug concentrations makes them generally prohibitive. The beneficial effects of theophylline on diaphragmatic strength are demonstrable at concentrations of approximately 14 mg per liter [1,2,7].

Signs and symptoms of theophylline toxicity are an extension of the pharmacologic properties of the drug and correlate with

Table 211-1. Physiologic Effects of Theophylline

Central nervous system
    Stimulation of cortical centers
    Stimulation of medullary respiratory center
    Nausea and emesis
    Cerebral vasoconstriction (suggested)
    Decreased cerebral blood flow
Cardiovascular
    Positive inotropic and chronotropic effects
    Vascular smooth muscle relaxation
Pulmonary
    Bronchial smooth muscle relaxation
    Increased ventilation
    Stimulation of diaphragmatic and intercostal muscles
Gastrointestinal
    Increased gastric acid and pepsin secretion
    Relaxation of cardioesophageal smooth muscle, possible reflux
Renal
    Increased blood flow and glomerular filtration rate
    Increased diuresis (<48 hr)
Endocrine
    Increased plasma catecholamines
    Augmented dopamine beta-hydroxylase and renin
Metabolic
    Lipolysis
    Gluconeogenesis and glycogenolysis
Musculoskeletal
    Augmented contractility
    Disturbances in depolarization (e.g., tremor)

the STC (see Chap. 148). Sinus tachycardia frequently occurs within the therapeutic range [8]. Nausea, vomiting, diarrhea, tremor, and central nervous system (CNS) excitation (anxiety, agitation) are usually observed at STCs greater than 20 mg per liter [9,10]. In patients receiving chronic theophylline therapy (>24 hours), hypotension, serious arrhythmias, and seizures are usually observed with an STC above 35 mg per liter. In acute poisoning, serious side effects (e.g., seizures, arrhythmias) are usually not observed unless the STC is 70 mg per liter or greater [11,12]. Cases of serious toxicity occasionally have been reported in individuals with STCs lower than these guidelines, especially in patients with underlying CNS or cardiovascular pathology. Common theophylline-induced arrhythmias include supraventricular tachyarrhythmias and ventricular irritability, leading to ventricular tachycardia or fibrillation. Seizures are usually of the tonic-clonic type, are often relatively resistant to therapy, and are associated with a high rate of morbidity and mortality. No consistent warning signs or symptoms predict subsequent development of serious arrhythmias or seizures. Elevated STCs may be the only warning of impending serious toxicity. In excess of 30 to 35 mg per liter, STCs are not predictive of the risk of life-threatening toxicity [13,14].

Preparations

Theophylline for IV administration is available primarily as aminophylline, the ethylenediamine salt of theophylline. Ethylenediamine is added to increase the water solubility of theophylline but may have some respiratory stimulant activity of its own [15]. Ethylenediamine can cause hypersensitivity reactions, most commonly rashes ranging from maculopapular eruptions to exfoliative dermatitis and urticaria [16,17]. Aminophylline for injection is 80% to 85% anhydrous theophylline,

depending on the product chosen. It has a pH of 8.6 to 9.0 and should not be administered through IV catheters used to administer alkali-sensitive drugs (e.g., epinephrine, norepinephrine, isoproterenol, penicillin, cephalosporins). Premixed theophylline (without ethylenediamine) in D_5W recently became available for IV administration. This product has a pH of 3.5 to 6.5. In its most concentrated form, this preparation contains only 4 mg per milliliter of theophylline, which may limit its usefulness in fluid-restricted patients. Rapid administration of theophylline or aminophylline can cause flushing, palpitations, profound bradycardia, hypotension, and cardiopulmonary arrest. The maximum rate of administration should be 25 mg per minute [18,19].

Intramuscular injection can cause intense local pain, precipitation of drug at the injection site, and delayed absorption and is not recommended.

Oral theophylline preparations are available in different salt forms (Table 211-2), and confusion about the exact dose of theophylline being administered is common. Many of the salt forms of theophylline were originally developed to increase the pH and water solubility of the drug and, hence, its absorption. However, absorption is determined by the lipophilic character of the drug and the absorption of these preparations is no faster or more complete than is the case for anhydrous theophylline. The different oral products should be ordered based on the dose of anhydrous theophylline.

Oral formulations are available as liquids, rapid-release tablets, sustained-release tablets, and sustained-release capsules. Many of the solutions contain 5% to 20% ethanol. Theophylline solutions are generally dilute, necessitating the administration of relatively large volumes in adults, leading to ingestion of substantial amounts of alcohol, unless an ethanol-free product is specifically chosen. In patients with nasogastric (NG) tubes, more concentrated aminophylline solutions may be appropriate. Sustained-release tablets should not be crushed and administered via an NG tube.

Pharmacokinetics

Table 211-3 summarizes the pharmacokinetic parameters of theophylline.

ABSORPTION. Absorption of theophylline depends on the formulation [20,21]. Plain uncoated tablets and oral solutions are rapidly and completely absorbed, with peak serum levels observed in approximately 1 to 2 hours. Enteric-coated formulations demonstrate incomplete or erratic delays in absorption. The rate and extent of absorption vary among the different sustained-release formulations of theophylline, although the bioavailability is 90 to 100 percent. The peak STC typically occurs approximately 4 hours after ingestion of theophylline formulated as a sustained-release product.

Table 211-2. Amount of Theophylline in Various Salts

Salt	Theophylline (%)
Aminophylline anhydrous (theophylline ethylenediamine)	84–86
Aminophylline hydrous	78–82
Sodium glycinate	50
Oxtriphylline (choline theophyllinate)	65

Table 211-3. Theophylline Pharmacokinetic Parameters

Bioavailability	90–100%
Protein binding	40%
V_d central	0.3 L/kg (range 0.2–0.4)
V_d steady-state	0.45 L/kg (0.3–0.6)
Distribution half-life	6–10 min
Elimination half-life (adult, nonsmoking, good organ function)	6–8 hr
Clearance	
Hepatic	85–95%
Renal	10–15%
Peritoneal dialysis	0.027 L/kg/hr
Hemodialysis	0.024–0.072 L/kg/hr
Hemoperfusion	0.14–0.24 L/kg/hr

The range of STCs observed over a given dosage interval depends on rate of absorption, dosing interval, and clearance. The STC can vary over a wide range between peak and trough concentrations [22]. In smokers or patients receiving enzyme-inducing drugs, STC fluctuations are exaggerated by increased clearance of the drug. The fluctuation in serum levels can be decreased by using a product with slower absorption or shortening the dosing interval but keeping the daily dose the same. In patients with high theophylline clearance, most sustained-release products must be administered every 8 hours to decrease STC fluctuations to less than 100 percent. Products designed for once-daily administration often depend on "normal" gastrointestinal (GI) pH for dissolution or absorption and may exhibit erratic, incomplete, or too rapid absorption ("dose dumping") [23]. These products are not recommended for seriously ill patients.

DISTRIBUTION. The apparent volume of distribution (V_d) of theophylline averages 0.45 liter per kilogram (range 0.3–0.6 L/kg) [24]. A V_d of 0.5 per kilogram should be used to calculate doses. Theophylline pharmacokinetics are best characterized using a two-compartment open model with a distribution half-life of approximately 6 to 10 minutes and completion of distribution within 30 to 60 minutes [25]. The heart responds to theophylline as if it were in the central compartment. Cardiac arrhythmias and hypotension can occur following bolus doses of theophylline. A 30- to 60-minute infusion is recommended when loading doses are administered. This method results in lower central compartment concentrations and reduces the risk of infusion-related toxicity.

Approximately 40 percent of the theophylline dose is bound to plasma albumin. Free drug is distributed into extracellular body water [26]. Alterations in protein binding are not clinically significant.

Whether V_d is best related to ideal or actual body weight (IBW or ABW) in obese patients (defined as > 150% of lean body weight) is controversial [27,28,29]. Initial doses should be based on IBW.

CLEARANCE. Eighty-five to 95 percent of theophylline is metabolized by the liver via the cytochrome P-450 component of the mixed-function oxidase system [30]. In adults, theophylline undergoes N-demethylation and hydroxylation to form three primary metabolites, only one of which (3-methylxanthine) is active. Metabolites are eliminated in the urine at a rate greater than that at which they are produced and therefore exert no pharmacologic activity. Less than 15 percent of administered theophylline is eliminated as unchanged drug in the urine [31].

Although theophylline is often characterized as exhibiting overall first-order elimination, all the metabolic pathways are capacity-limited. Depending on the K_m and V_{max} values for each pathway in a given patient, clearance can decrease with increasing STCs, thus changes in dosage can result in disproportionate changes in STC [30,32]. Pooled estimates of V_{max} and K_m for theophylline from one study are 1960 mg per day and 24.1 mg per liter, respectively [33]. Nonlinear elimination of theophylline is observed most frequently with high STCs due to overdosage.

The average theophylline clearance in adult nonsmokers is 0.044 L/kg/hr. There are conflicting data regarding the effect of age in adults on theophylline clearance [33,34].

Smoking (>20 cigarettes/day) induces the cytochrome P-450 enzyme system, resulting in increased theophylline clearance [35]. This effect persists in elderly patients (>60 years) [36]. Smokers require about 1.5 to 2 times the daily dose of theophylline required by nonsmokers. This effect decreases to about 30 percent over normal within 1 week after cessation of smoking, but increased clearance can persist up to 2 months [35,37]. Smoking marijuana increases metabolism of theophylline to a similar degree [38]. High-protein diets, especially with charcoal-broiled foods, can increase theophylline clearance [39].

In the average adult nonsmoker, the serum half-life ($t_{1/2}$) of theophylline is 6 to 8 hours. In elderly patients, it is prolonged to 8 to 12 hours. Smoking decreases the half-life to about 3 to 4 hours. In patients with cirrhosis, it may be prolonged to as long as 60 hours [41] and in patients with acute hepatitis or cholestasis to 15 to 20 hours [40].

HYPODYNAMIC PATIENTS. Clearance is decreased as much as 50 percent in patients with congestive heart failure (cardiac index <2 L/min/m²), cor pulmonale, hepatic cirrhosis, acute hepatitis, and possibly cholestasis [40–44]. Patients with acute viral illnesses may also manifest decreased theophylline clearance [45]. Renal disease has little effect on theophylline clearance [46,47].

HYPERDYNAMIC PATIENTS. Theophylline clearance in patients with surgical sepsis or major trauma has not been studied extensively. Two studies in multiple organ failure have shown decreased, increased, and no change in clearance [48,49]. The possibility of significantly increased clearance with capacity-limited drugs such as theophylline in septic surgical patients is based on two studies. An investigation in 22 patients used hexobarbital to demonstrate increased drug clearance by 87 percent to 143 percent at 1 to 3 weeks, compared to the first few days of intensive care stay [50]. Hexobarbital is a capacity-limited drug primarily metabolized by the IIC9 isoenzyme of the P-450 system. A recent study in 10 neurotrauma patients demonstrated increase in antipyrine clearance by 14 to 207 percent over 2 weeks in intensive care [51]. Antipyrine is a marker drug for the capacity of the CYP1A2 isoenzyme in the P-450 system to metabolize drugs, such as theophylline.

Dosage and Administration

The parenteral loading dose of theophylline for patients with no recent theophylline ingestion (i.e., within the last 24 hours) is 5 mg per kilogram (i.e., 6 mg/kg of aminophylline), based on the following calculations:

$$\text{Loading Dose} = V_d \times \text{desired STC}$$
$$= 0.5 \text{ L/kg} \times 10 \text{ mg/L theophylline}$$
$$= 5 \text{ mg/kg theophylline (6 mg/kg of aminophylline)}$$

A desired STC at the low end of the therapeutic range is used to estimate this dose because of the variability in V_d. If the patient has a very small V_d (0.3 L/kg) the STC resulting from this loading dose will be approximately 16 μg per milliliter, still well within the therapeutic range. If the patient has a history of recent theophylline ingestion, a partial loading dose of 2.5 mg per kilogram (3 mg/kg aminophylline) can be administered to increase the STC by approximately 5 μg per milliliter. Each increment (mg/kg) of theophylline administered should result in an increase in the STC of approximately 2 mg per liter:

$$\text{Change in STC} = \text{Dose}/V_d$$

$$= \frac{1 \text{ mg/kg}}{0.5 \text{ L/kg}}$$

$$= 2 \text{ mg/L}$$

Further dosing should be based on STC determinations.

Loading doses should be administered over 30 to 60 minutes to decrease the risk of toxic effects due to high predistribution STCs. If tachycardia or nausea occurs, the rate of administration should be decreased.

Theophylline STCs should be obtained 30 to 60 minutes after the loading dose is completed. This STC can be used to estimate the individual patient's V_d (Dose/STC = V_d). This individualized value can then be used when calculating any further bolus doses. If the postloading STC is low (e.g., <10 μg/ml), another dose can be administered to increase the level to the target STC using this V_d value. With this baseline STC, it is not necessary to wait until a steady state is achieved to ensure that the doses are in the therapeutic range. In addition, this STC will serve as a baseline to aid in evaluating the maintenance infusion.

Following the loading dose, a maintenance infusion is calculated based on a population-derived estimate of the patient's clearance (Table 211-4). These IV maintenance dose (MD) guidelines are designed to achieve STCs of 10 μg per milliliter at steady state. The maintenance dose (mg/hr) can be calculated, using the average expected clearance (Cl) for the patient:

$$MD = Cl \times \text{STC at steady state}$$

$$= 0.044 \text{ L/kg/hr} \times 10 \text{ mg/L}$$

$$= 0.44 \text{ mg/kg/hr of theophylline (0.5 mg/kg/hr of aminophylline)}$$

Again because the guidelines are conservative, based on a desired STC of 10 μg per milliliter, patients with clearance values above the reported mean will have subtherapeutic STC. If a loading dose is not administered, it takes approximately five times the serum half-life of the drug (about 24 hours) to reach steady state.

A second STC should be obtained approximately 8 to 12

Table 211-4. Intravenous Infusion Rates for Theophylline (STC goal of 10 μg/ml)

Disease state	Age (yr)	Infusion rate (mg/kg/hr)	Clearance rate (mg/kg/hr)
Smoker	12–16	0.7	0.084–0.096
Nonsmoker	12–16	0.5	0.054–0.084
Smoker	17–50	0.7	0.066–0.108
Nonsmoker	17–50	0.4	0.040–0.052
Cardiac index <2 L/min/m²		0.2	0.018–0.027
Cor pulmonale, cirrhosis, or liver failure		0.2	0.018–0.027

hours after beginning the maintenance dose. This second STC should be compared with the initial (postloading) STC to determine whether the maintenance dose is resulting in rising, falling, or steady STCs. If the two STCs are approximately equal, the initial infusion rate chosen can be continued. If the second STC is significantly higher than the baseline, the drug is accumulating and levels should be closely followed or the rate decreased to prevent toxicity. If the second STC is significantly lower than the baseline, the patient's clearance is greater than the rate of administration, and the infusion should be increased.

Clearance (Cl) can be estimated using these two non-steady state levels:

$$Cl = \frac{2 \times \text{rate of infusion (mg/hr)}}{STC_1 + STC_2} + \frac{2 V_d (STC_1 - STC_2)}{(STC_1 + STC_2)(t_2 - t_1)}$$

where STC_1 is the postloading STC, STC_2 is the 8-hour STC, V_d is the estimated V_d in liters, and t_1 and t_2 are the times in hours when STC_1 and STC_2 were measured [46]. This estimate of clearance can be used to calculate the infusion rate necessary to obtain a desired STC at steady state:

$$MD = \text{STC at steady state} \times Cl$$

If the first two STCs suggested are not obtained, an STC level should be obtained within 24 hours of beginning theophylline therapy. In patients in whom drug half-lives are less than 6 hours, this 24-hour STC will reflect steady state.

The above equation can be used to aid in dosage adjustments at steady state. This method, however, assumes that a steady state has been established. Thus, if it is used early in therapy and the elimination half-life for the drug is very long, leading to slow accumulation, this method may result in an overestimate of clearance and the appropriate dose. If two STCs have been obtained 24 hours apart on the same dose and are relatively equivalent, steady state can be assumed. For example, if a patient has a STC of 10 μg per milliliter at steady state on 35 mg per hour of aminophylline and the physician wants to increase the STC to 15 μg per ml, the appropriate dose can be calculated:

$$35 \text{ mg/hr aminophylline} = 30 \text{ mg/hr theophylline}$$

$$30 \text{ mg/hr theophylline} = 10 \text{ mg/L} \times Cl$$

$$Cl = 3 \text{ L/hr}$$

$$\text{New MD} = 15 \text{ mg/L} \times 3 \text{ L/hr}$$

$$\text{New MD} = 45 \text{ mg/hr theophylline or 56 mg/hr of aminophylline}$$

In a 60- to 70-kg patient with a normal clearance of 0.044 liter/kg/hr, a change in the aminophylline infusion rate of 5 mg per hour should increase the theophylline STC by only 1 to 1.5 mg per liter. Before making large dosing adjustments, the physician should ensure that errors in mixing aminophylline, setting infusion pumps, and obtaining STCs have not occurred and that the estimated clearance makes sense clinically.

In critically ill patients, STCs should be assessed daily until dosage and STCs are stable. Thereafter, STCs should be obtained twice weekly while the patient is in the ICU. In addition, STCs should be obtained when starting or stopping other interacting drugs or if the patient's hemodynamic or metabolic status changes significantly.

When the patient is able to take medications via the GI tract, IV theophylline can be stopped just before the first oral dose is given. It is not necessary to overlap the IV with the oral product. The total daily IV theophylline dose is calculated and divided into the number of doses appropriate to the product chosen.

Oral solutions to be administered via the NG tube should be divided into six daily doses, administered every 4 hours. This regimen minimizes fluctuations between peak and trough levels. The NG tube should be flushed with 30 to 60 ml of saline or water to ensure complete delivery of the drug. In patients receiving rapid-release theophylline products STCs should be obtained just before the next dose is given (i.e., as a trough level) to ensure meaningful day-to-day comparisons between STCs, doses, and clearances. In patients with high clearance values and high peak-to-trough fluctuations, trough STCs should be specifically ordered, even when administering sustained-release products. If a patient exhibits signs or symptoms of toxicity early in the dosing interval, peak and trough levels may be obtained to assess the extent of fluctuation in STCs.

Drug Interactions

There are numerous clinically significant interactions between theophylline and other drugs [52,53]. Food and antacids containing aluminum hydroxide or magnesium hydroxide can decrease the rate at which theophylline is absorbed from rapid-release formulations but not the extent of absorption. The effect of food on the pharmacokinetics of extended-release products varies depending on the product. Potentially toxic amounts of theophylline are released from once-daily formulations in the presence of food, so these products should be avoided. Continuous NG feedings can significantly decrease absorption of oral theophylline (liquid and sustained-release tablets) [54].

Because theophylline is extensively metabolized by the hepatic cytochrome P-450 enzyme system, drugs that induce these enzymes can significantly increase theophylline clearance and significantly decrease STCs. The effects of inducing drugs are usually seen within 2 to 14 days after their initiation and may take several weeks to dissipate after the inducing agent is discontinued. Drugs that increase theophylline clearance include carbamazepine (60%), phenobarbital (25%), pentobarbital (25%), phenytoin (50%), and rifampin (80%) [52,53].

Drugs that inhibit hepatic microsomal enzymes decrease clearance and increase STCs. The decrease in clearance can be observed 2 to 10 days after starting concomitant administration of the inhibiting agent. The administration of cimetidine is associated with decreases in clearance of 25 to 100 percent. The effect of ranitidine is less predictable. Other drugs that can decrease clearance include enoxacin (50%), other fluoroquinolones with varying effect [55,56], and erythromycin (25%) [52]. Beta-blockers, especially nonselective agents, can inhibit the metabolism of theophylline and decrease clearance. In one study, 120 and 720 mg of propranolol decreased theophylline clearance by 30 and 52 percent, respectively [57]. Verapamil inhibits the metabolism of theophylline and can increase STCs by 100 percent. Other calcium channel blockers are less likely to cause this effect [53]. Chronic administration of isoniazid can decrease theophylline clearance. Contrary to the expected effect, ketaconazole does not appear to inhibit theophylline metabolism [53].

Theophylline metabolism is increased in hyperthyroid patients and decreased in hypothyroid patients. Initiation of thyroid hormone replacement tends to reduce STCs [52].

All of these interactions have been studied in noncritically ill patients. Major physiologic changes associated with critical illness can negate or exaggerate the effect of these interacting drugs. Therefore, when any of the above agents is administered concomitantly with theophylline, STCs should be carefully monitored.

Common Pitfalls in Management

1. Failure to check STCs on a frequent basis in ICU patients receiving theophylline.
2. Failure to order *trough* theophylline levels when using rapid-release products.
3. Failure to increase the aminophylline infusion by an amount large enough to increase the STC. Increases of 5 mg per hour usually do not significantly alter STCs.
4. Failure to consider drug interactions and check STCs at appropriate times when starting and stopping other medications.

References

1. Murciano D, Aubier M, Lecocquic Y, et al: Effects of theophylline on diaphragmatic strength and fatigue in patients with chronic obstructive pulmonary disease. *N Engl J Med* 311:349, 1984.
2. Matthay RA, Berger HJ, Lake J, et al: Effects of aminophylline upon right and left ventricular performance in chronic obstructive pulmonary disease: Noninvasive assessment of radionuclide angiocardiography. *Am J Med* 65:903, 1978.
3. Rall TW: Central nervous system stimulants: The methylxanthines, in Gilman AG, Goodman LS, Rall TW, et al (eds): *Goodman and Gilman's The Pharmacological Basis of Therapeutics.* 7th ed. New York, Macmillan, 1985, p 589.
4. Mitenko PA, Ogilvie RI: Rational intravenous doses of theophylline. *N Engl J Med* 289:600, 1973.
5. Vozeh S, Kewitz G, Perruchoud A, et al: Theophylline serum concentrations and therapeutic effect in severe acute bronchial obstruction: The optimal use of intravenously administered aminophylline. *Am Rev Respir Dis* 125:181, 1982.
6. Weinberger M, Bronsky E: Evaluation of oral bronchodilator therapy in asthmatic children. *J Pediatr* 84:421, 1974.
7. Vires N, Aubier M, Murciano D, et al: Effects of aminophylline on diaphragmatic fatigue during acute respiratory failure. *Am Rev Respir Dis* 129:396, 1984.
8. Ogilvie R, Fernandez P, Winsberg F: Cardiovascular response to increasing theophylline concentrations. *Eur J Clin Pharmacol* 12:409, 1977.
9. Hendeles L, Bighley L, Richardson R, et al: Frequent toxicity from IV aminophylline infusion in critically ill patients. *Drug Intell Clin Pharm* 11:12, 1977.
10. Jacobs MH, Senior RM, Kessler G: Clinical experience with theophylline: Relationships between dosage, serum concentrations and toxicity. *JAMA* 235:1983, 1976.
11. Zwillich CW, Sutton FD, Neff TA, et al: Theophylline induced seizures in adults: Correlation with serum concentrations. *Ann Intern Med* 82:784, 1975.
12. Paloucek FP, Rodvold KA: Evaluation of theophylline overdoses and toxicities. *Ann Emerg Med* 17:135, 1988.
13. Shannon M, Lovejoy FH: Life-threatening events after theophylline intoxication: A prospective analysis of 144 cases. *Ann Emerg Med* 18:446, 1989.
14. Aitken ML, Martin TR: Life-threatening theophylline toxicity is not predictable by serum levels. *Chest* 91:10, 1987.
15. Marais OAS, McMichael J: Theophylline-ethylenediamine in Cheyne-Stokes respiration. *Lancet* 2:437, 1937.
16. Allergy to aminophylline (editorial). *Lancet* 2:1192, 1984.
17. Elias J, Levinson A: Hypersensitivity reactions to ethylenediamine and aminophylline. *Am Rev Respir Dis* 123:550, 1981.
18. Gult JE: A fatal reaction to aminophylline given intravenously. *Med J Aust* 51:148, 1964.
19. Camarata SJ, Weil MH, Hanashiro PK, et al: Cardiac arrest in the critically ill. 1. A study of predisposing causes in 132 patients. *Circulation* 44:688, 1971.
20. Hendeles L, Weinberger M, Bighley L: Absolute bioavailability of oral theophylline. *Am J Hosp Pharm* 34:525, 1977.

21. Weinberger M, Hendeles L, Bighley L: The relation of product formulation to absorption of oral theophylline. *N Engl J Med* 299:852, 1978.

22. Hendeles L, Iafrate P, Weinberger M: A clinical and pharmacokinetic basis of the selection and use of slow-release theophylline products. *Clin Pharmacokinet* 9:95, 1984.

23. Hendeles L, Weinberger M, Milavetz G, et al: Food induced dumping from "once a day" theophylline product as a cause of toxicity. *Chest* 87:758, 1985.

24. Hendeles L. Weinberger M, Bighley L: Disposition of theophylline after a single intravenous infusion of aminophylline. *Am Rev Respir Dis* 118:97, 1978.

25. Mitenko PA, Ogilvie RI: Pharmacokinetics of intravenous theophylline. *Clin Pharmacol Ther* 14:509, 1973.

26. Shaw LM, Fields L, Mayock R: Factors influencing theophylline serum protein binding. *Clin Pharmacol Ther* 32:490, 1982.

27. Gal P, Jusko WJ, Yurchak AM, et al: Theophylline disposition in obesity. *Clin Pharmacol Ther* 23:438, 1978.

28. Shum L, Jusko WJ: Theophylline disposition in obese rats. *J Pharmacol Exp Ther* 228:380, 1984.

29. Blouin RA, Elgert JF, Bauer LA: Theophylline clearance: Effect of marked obesity. *Clin Pharmacol Ther* 28:619, 1980.

30. Tang Liu DS, Williams RL, Riegelman S: Non-linear theophylline elimination. *Clin Pharmacol Ther* 31:358, 1982.

31. Levy G, Koysooko R: Renal clearance of theophylline in man. *J Clin Pharmacol* 16:329, 1976.

32. Lesko LJ: Dose dependent elimination kinetics of theophylline. *Clin Pharmacokinet* 4:449, 1979.

33. Wagner JG: Theophylline: Pooled Michaelis-Menten parameters (V_{max} and Km) and implications. *Clin Pharmacokinet* 10:432, 1985.

34. Fox RW, Samoan S, Bukantz SC, et al: Theophylline kinetics in a geriatric group. *Clin Pharmacol Ther* 34:60, 1983.

35. Jusko WJ, Schentag JJ, Clark JH, et al: Enhanced biotransformation of theophylline in marijuana and tobacco smokers. *Clin Pharmacol Ther* 24:406, 1978.

36. Lusak B, Kelly JG, Lavan J, et al: Theophylline kinetics in relation to age: The importance of smoking. *Br J Clin Pharmacol* 10:109, 1980.

37. Lee BL, Benowitz NL, Jacob P: Cigarette abstinence, nicotine gum and theophylline disposition. *Ann Intern Med* 106:553, 1987.

38. Jusko W, Schentag J, Clark J, et al: Enhanced biotransformation of theophylline in marijuana and tobacco smokers. *Clin Pharmacol Ther* 24:405, 1978.

39. Kappas A, Anderson K, Conney A, et al: Influence of dietary protein and carbohydrate on antipyrine and theophylline metabolism in man. *Clin Pharmacol Ther* 20:643, 1976.

40. Mangione A, Imhoff TE, Lee RV, et al: Pharmacokinetics of theophylline in hepatic disease. *Chest* 73:616, 1978.

41. Piafsky KM, Sitar DS, Rangno RE, et al: Theophylline disposition in patients with hepatic cirrhosis. *N Engl J Med* 296:1495, 1977.

42. Staib AH, Schuppan D, Lissner R, et al: Pharmacokinetics and metabolism of theophylline in patients with liver disease. *Int J Clin Pharmacol Ther Toxicol* 18:500, 1980.

43. Piafsky KM, Sitar DS, Rangno RE, et al: Theophylline kinetics in acute pulmonary edema. *Clin Pharmacol Ther* 21:310, 1977.

44. Powell JR, Vozeh S, Hopewell P, et al: Theophylline disposition in acutely ill hospitalized patients: The effects of smoking, heart failure, severe airway obstruction, and pneumonia. *Am Rev Respir Dis* 118:229, 1978.

45. Chang K, Lauer B, Bell T, et al: Altered theophylline pharmacokinetics during acute respiratory viral illness. *Lancet* 1:1132, 1978.

46. Kraan J, Jonkman JGH, Koeter GH, et al: The pharmacokinetics of theophylline and enprofylline in patients with liver cirrhosis and in patients with chronic renal disease. *Eur J Clin Pharmacol* 35:357, 1988.

47. Bauer LA, Bauer SP, Blouin RA: The effect of acute and chronic renal failure on theophylline clearance. *J Clin Pharmacol* 1982:65, 1982.

48. Schregel W, Kuntz H-D, Vitt M: Hepatic disposition in multiple organ failure. *Acta Anaesthesiol Scand* 32:638, 1988.

49. Toft P, Heslet L, Hansen M, et al: Theophylline and ethylenediamine pharmacokinetics following administration of aminophylline to septic patients with multi organ failure. *Intensive Care Med* 17:465, 1991.

50. Rietbrock I, Lazarus G, Richter E, et al: Hexobarbitone disposition at different stages of intensive care treatment. *Br J Anaesth* 53:283, 1981.

51. Boucher BA, Kuhl DA, Fabian TC, et al: Effect of neurotrauma on hepatic drug clearance. *Clin Pharmacol Ther* 50:487, 1991.

52. Edwards DJ, Zarowitz BJ, Slaughter RL: Theophylline, in Evans WF, Schentag JJ, Jusko WJ (eds): *Applied Pharmacokinetics: Principles of Therapeutic Drug Monitoring.* 3rd ed. Vancouver, WA, 1992.

53. Hendeles L, Weinberger M: Theophylline: A "state of the art" review. *Pharmacotherapy* 3:2, 1983.

54. Gal P, Layson R: Interference with oral theophylline absorption of continuous nasogastric feedings. *Ther Drug Monit* 8:421, 1986.

55. Edwards DJ, Bowles SK, Svensson CK, et al: Inhibition of drug metabolism by quinolone antibiotics. *Clin Pharmacokinet* 15:194, 1988.

56. Fuhr U, Anders E-M, Mahr G: Inhibitory potency of quinolone antibacterial agents against cytocrome P450IA2 activity in vivo and in vitro. *Antimicrob Agents Chemother* 36:942, 1992.

57. Miners JO, Wing LM, Lillywhite KJ, et al: Selectivity in dose-dependency of the inhibitory effect of propranolol on theophylline. *Br J Clin Pharmacol* 20:219, 1985.

212. Antimicrobial Agents

John C. Rotschafer, Karla J. Walker, and Karl J. Madaras-Kelly

Success or failure of antimicrobial treatment in the eradication or prevention of bacterial infection is predicated on situation recognition and prompt and appropriate clinical intervention. Clinical attempts to alter the infectious process focus primarily on the use of surgery and/or antibiotic therapy. Surgical intervention can be used to alter environmental oxygen tension, pH, and the infectious milieu of localized bacterial infections through debridement and drainage [1]. Prophylactic or adjunctive antibiotic intervention with local or systemic therapy can

also dramatically reduce the bacterial burden and often proves crucial to a successful clinical outcome [2–6].

Another factor to consider in the treatment of bacterial infection is the release of toxins or bacterial cell wall components (e.g., peptidoglycan, teichoic acid, and lipopolysaccharide), which may be induced by the action of certain antimicrobials [7,8]. These mediators in turn stimulate the release of cellular cytokines, such as tumor necrosis factor (TNF), various interleukins (IL-1, -2, -6 and -8), prostaglandins, platelet-activating factor, and others, thereby initiating a sequential activation of the septic cascade. Ultimately, the full sequence of events can lead to multisystem organ failure and death. Parrillo recently described the pathogenesis of septic shock and the resultant sequelae [9]. While current understanding of the exact sequence and nature of these events is incomplete, substantial research efforts are being directed toward the development of immunologic and pharmacologic interventions that may alter the effects of these cytokine mediators and the activation of the septic cascade leading to septic shock [9].

Successful antibiotic therapy depends on appropriate selection, dosage, and method of administration. Antibiotic selection is governed by the likelihood that certain bacterial pathogens are present and the clinician's comfort with a single agent or preference for a combination of antibiotics for possible additive or synergistic effects. Historically, antibiotic dosage is an empirically derived, fixed regimen for most patients. Unless there exists some abnormality in renal function, hepatic function, or body size, the "usual" antibiotic regimen is prescribed. With the introduction of studies characterizing antibiotic pharmacokinetic parameters in specific patient populations, the "usual" or "normal" antibiotic dosage has in many situations proved to be inadequate or potentially toxic [10–19]. Pharmacodynamic studies that characterize antibiotic performance in killing bacterial pathogens as concentration-dependent or concentration-independent have challenged traditional concepts of antibiotic administration and dosing [1]. These data may have significant therapeutic implications, especially for the critically ill, in whom the ability to eliminate antibiotic can vary hour-to-hour and where there is a heavier dependence on the antibiotic to sterilize the infected site. Ultimately, appropriate alterations in dose and method of antibiotic administration may optimize antibiotic effect on bacterial pathogens and clinical outcome [1].

This chapter focuses on vancomycin, imipenem, clindamycin, and the aminoglycosides gentamicin, tobramycin, and amikacin. These antibiotics are commonly used in critically ill patients where a hypo- or hypermetabolic state may exist for at least a portion of the intensive care hospitalization and are representative of the broader classes of antibiotics currently available for use in this environment.

Vancomycin

At present vancomycin is the only licensed glycopeptide antibiotic available in the United States. The antimicrobial spectrum of vancomycin is primarily limited to gram-positive organisms and select anaerobes [20,21,22]. The drug is effective for penicillin-sensitive, penicillin-resistant, and methicillin-resistant strains of *Staphylococcus aureus* and *S. epidermidis* as well as enterococci, streptococci, *Clostridium difficile,* and diphtheroids [20–23]. Vancomycin generally produces a postantibiotic effect of 2 hours or greater for *S. aureus* [24]. With the exception of limited reports of vancomycin-resistant *S. haemolyticus* and *S. epidermidis,* clinically significant resistance has not been reported with vancomycin despite its availability for more than 35 years [25]. Except for enterococci and some tolerant (MBC/MIC >32) strains of staphylococci, vancomycin is a bactericidal (MBC/MIC ≤4) antibacterial agent [20,21,22,26]. Some investigators have questioned whether vancomycin is as effective as penicillinase-resistant penicillins in killing *S. aureus* [27–29].

Vancomycin is commonly used in combination with other antibiotics. For tolerant staphylococci, some investigators have suggested the addition of rifampin for possible additive or synergistic effects or to eliminate intracellular carriage of staphy-

lococcal pathogens [30]. Other investigators have suggested little or no benefit associated with this combination of antimicrobial agents [31,32]. Vancomycin must be combined with either gentamicin or streptomycin in the treatment of serious enterococcal infections to overcome bacterial tolerance. There are concerning reports of vancomycin-resistant enterococci, which may limit the use of this drug in the future [33–37]. Leclercq et al. reported vancomycin and teicoplanin resistance to be plasmid-mediated [38].

As staphylococci are facultative organisms, knowledge of antibiotic performance under both aerobic and anaerobic conditions could be an important factor. Unfortunately, anaerobic MICs are not routinely performed. Knowles et al. reported that both vancomycin and teicoplanin are not significantly affected by aerobic versus anaerobic conditions in killing *S. aureus;* however, this effect was dependent on the type of media used in testing [39].

PHARMACOLOGY. Vancomycin is a unique antimicrobial agent in that the antibiotic has three different sites of action [40,41,42]. Most notably, vancomycin has an effect on cell wall synthesis at a site different than that affected by beta-lactam compounds. Vancomycin also has an effect on the cytoplasmic membrane and inhibits RNA synthesis. These three distinct effects on bacterial pathogens provide a likely explanation for the very limited extent of bacterial resistance seen with this compound.

THERAPEUTIC RANGE. Geraci proposed that the therapeutic range for vancomycin is 30 to 40 mg per liter for peak concentrations and 5 to 10 mg per liter for trough concentrations [43]. While serum concentration monitoring practices for vancomycin (especially "peak" determinations) have significant geographic variability, most institutions do attempt to monitor vancomycin concentrations [44]. Controversies surrounding therapeutic drug monitoring of vancomycin have been extensively debated [19,45,46]. To date, there are very few rigorous clinical data on clinical efficacy or toxicity to support the recommended ranges for either peak or trough vancomycin concentrations [45–48].

Vancomycin has been reported to be a concentration-independent killer of gram-positive pathogens at concentrations used clinically, and most gram-positive pathogens have an MIC of 1.5 mg per liter or less [21,49,50]. Thus, maintaining a trough concentration at or above 5 mg per liter (approximately 3 times the MIC) will likely optimize the clinical response to vancomycin. Trough concentrations maintained above 10 mg per liter may be associated with a higher incidence of nephrotoxicity [51,52,53]. Because of the rapid alpha (distribution) phase, the peak concentration is maintained for only a short time; the clinical relevance of this value is unknown. Geraci et al. reported that auditory toxicity has been associated with serum levels of 80 to 95 mg per liter [54]. This report is often misrepresented by referring to these values as "peak" concentrations; however, the vancomycin levels were obtained at 3 and 6 hours after infusion [54]. A variety of risk factors that were also present in this patient complicate the interpretation of this report. Traber et al. reported vancomycin ototoxicity in a patient with normal renal function who had 1-hour postinfusion vancomycin concentrations of 50 mg per liter [55]. However, because the investigators did not take into account the multi-compartmental nature of the vancomycin serum concentration time curve, the true peak concentration (end of infusion) was likely much higher [56].

Given currently available information regarding vancomycin

toxicity and the relationship to vancomycin serum concentrations, patients would appear to be safely treated by adhering to the original recommendations of Geraci [57]. Whether to monitor peak and/or trough concentrations and whether to monitor vancomycin levels at all remain unanswered questions. Given the concentration-independent nature of vancomycin bacterial killing, the large distribution volume, and the low extent of vancomycin protein binding, there does not appear to be a reason to exceed Geraci's original recommendations [46].

PREPARATIONS. The commercially available vancomycin in the United States has undergone many significant improvements since the late 1950s [40,58,59]. The factor B (vancomycin) content of the current Eli Lilly product approximates 93%, while various generic products have approximately 85% factor B content [40,58,59,60]. There appears to be no clinically significant difference between these products, based on MIC or MBC determinations [61]. However, there are very few peer reviewed data regarding the purity, efficacy, or toxicity of generic vancomycin products.

Depending on the manufacturer, vancomycin is available as 125-mg and 250-mg pulvule and various ampules containing lyophilized powder, suitable for intravenous administration when reconstituted. Vancomycin can be administered orally (pulvules and suspension) or intravenously. It should not be administered intramuscularly, due to extreme pain and discomfort at the injection site.

PHARMACOKINETICS. The serum concentration time profile and pharmacokinetic parameters of vancomycin are heavily dependent on the intensity of serum sampling, the times at which samples are obtained, and the modeling approach utilized. The serum concentration time curve cannot be adequately described using a one-compartment model and is probably best represented using a two- or three-compartment model [62,63].

During intravenous administration, distribution and elimination occur simultaneously. When infusion of drug ends, the true peak concentration is obtained [19]. The distribution, or alpha, phase immediately follows the peak concentration during which distribution and elimination occur simultaneously. Approximately 3 hours after infusion the distribution of vancomycin is complete; from this point on in the serum concentration time curve a log-linear elimination or beta-phase is observed [63].

Absorption. When given intravenously, vancomycin is completely bioavailable. While it has been used orally to treat pseudomembranous colitis and staphylococcal enterocolitis successfully, very little drug is systemically absorbed, even in anephric patients; therefore, oral administration is not appropriate for treatment of systemic infections [64]. Some investigators have reported clinically significant serum vancomycin concentrations following oral administration in a limited number of patients treated for pseudomembranous colitis [65,66].

Distribution. Vancomycin is best characterized using a pharmacokinetic model incorporating a central and peripheral [62,63]. Drug is introduced to the central compartment (approximately 0.2 L/kg) through intravenous infusion and from there is distributed to the peripheral compartment. This transport is governed by two transfer constants: one (K_{12}) governs distribution from the central to the peripheral compartment and the other K_{21} regulates transport from the peripheral to the central compartment [21]. Overall, vancomycin has a relatively large distribution volume ($V_{d\beta}$ approximately 0.7 L/kg) [21]. This appears to be most directly correlated with total body weight [67,68].

The rate of intravenous infusion of vancomycin has been associated with so-called red man or red neck syndrome. Vancomycin infusions of 1 gm or more (>15 mg/kg/hr) over 1 hour or less may precipitate this adverse reaction of rash, vasoflushing, nausea, facial edema, and hypotension [69]. For unexplained reasons this reaction seems to be much more common in healthy volunteers given rapid infusions of vancomycin than in patients [69]. Polk proposed that the underlying mechanism is vancomycin-induced release of histamine stores [69]. Maintaining vancomycin infusion rates at less than 15 mg/kg/hr or premedicating patients with diphenhydramine may prevent this reaction [62].

Vancomycin appears to distribute well throughout the body and does not usually require direct injection into the central nervous system. Some authors suggest consideration of intraventricular administration bacterial meningitis, but only if the patient does not respond clinically to intravenous administration. Congeni et al. suggested a daily 5 mg intraventricular dose in addition to continued intravenous administration in this situation [70]. This recommendation has been supported by other investigators [71]. The clinician should appreciate that the pharmacokinetics of vancomycin outside and within the central nervous system are likely to differ and the dose and frequency of administration may have to be altered. The critical factor is not how the amount of vancomycin in the central nervous system compares to serum concentration, but the relationship between the amount of vancomycin present in the central nervous system and the susceptibility of the infecting bacterial pathogen. When the ratio between the concentration of antibiotic in the central nervous system and the MIC-90 of the likely bacterial pathogens exceeds 10, there is reason to expect a satisfactory clinical outcome.

While early investigators reported vancomycin to be negligibly protein-bound [72], recent studies have demonstrated protein binding to be on the magnitude of 40 to 50 percent in healthy volunteers and 30 to 40 percent in patients [73–79]. Current data would suggest the primary protein involved is albumin. Investigations into the contribution of the reactive protein, alpha-1-acid glycoprotein, to the overall binding of vancomycin have concluded that this protein has little to no effect on the overall magnitude of vancomycin protein binding [76,77]. Sun et al. reported substantial binding of vancomycin to the immunoglobulin IgA but not IgG or IgM [77].

Elimination. The vast majority of vancomycin clearance occurs through glomerular filtration. Rodvold and colleagues also reported a limited degree of tubular secretion [63]. Nonrenal clearance of vancomycin is thought to occur primarily through hepatic elimination [62,80]. Vancomycin elimination has been reported to correlate strongly with age [74,81–85] and renal function [62,63,86]. Select patient populations, such as intravenous drug abusers with right-sided endocarditis and burn patients, have been identified as having high rates of vancomycin elimination [87,88,89].

PHYSIOLOGIC CLEARANCE CHARACTERISTICS. Because the primary route of elimination is glomerular filtration, vancomycin clearance is predictively sensitive to renal blood flow. Thus, any alterations in heart rate or stroke volume resulting in changes in cardiac output ultimately affect renal blood flow and vancomycin clearance. The kidney's ability to eliminate vancomycin is directly related to the number of functioning nephrons.

While nonrenal clearance of vancomycin is usually quite small, the presence of renal dysfunction presents a larger vancomycin fraction to the liver for elimination. Most patients in total renal shutdown require only weekly doses of vancomycin. However, some individuals in renal failure require much more frequent dosing of vancomycin, possibly due to increased nonrenal clearance.

Standard hemodialysis with cellulose acetate or cuprophane membranes and peritoneal dialysis have a negligible effect on vancomycin serum concentrations [90–94]. Hemodialysis with polyacrylonitrile or polysulfone membranes has a more dramatic affect on vancomycin clearance than with cellulose acetate or cuprophane membranes [90,91]. The usual weekly dosage interval is shortened if patients are regularly hemodialyzed using these newer membranes, but in most situations immediate replacement of vancomycin following 3 to 4 hours of hemodialysis is not required.

Continuous or intermittent hemofiltration has become a popular method to treat critically ill patients with end-stage renal disease. Hemofiltration has been shown to increase vancomycin clearance significantly [95,96].

When monitoring patients in renal failure, careful consideration should be given to the assay method. Morse et al. reported that vancomycin degradation products may be measured as vancomycin when a fluorescence polarization immunoassay (TDx, Abbott Laboratories) is used [97]. Thus, fluorescence polarization immunoassay would be expected to overpredict vancomycin concentrations in patients with end-stage renal disease [98].

Orally administered activated charcoal has been reported to speed the clearance of vancomycin in an overdose when combined with exchange transfusion [99]. Davis et al. reported virtually no change in clearance parameters with and without activated charcoal in a population of healthy volunteers with usual serum concentrations of vancomycin [100].

Overall, vancomycin offers a favorable pharmacokinetic profile from a variety of perspectives. The average half-life in adult patients with normal renal function is 6 to 8 hours, which eliminates the need for frequent or continuous infusion. Vancomycin has a relatively large distribution volume (0.7 L/kg), which eliminates the need to produce unusually high serum concentrations in an attempt to drive the drug to a distant site of infection. Because vancomycin is not extensively protein-bound, a large portion of the drug is unbound and free to distribute throughout the body and to interact with bacterial pathogens. Finally, vancomycin is a concentration-independent killer of bacteria. As such, increases in serum concentration to many times the MIC do not improve the efficacy with which vancomycin kills bacteria. As most staphylococci and streptococci have minimum inhibiting concentrations (≤1.5 mg/L) clinical outcome is unlikely to improve by producing vancomycin concentrations above the accepted range for peak (30–40 mg/L) and trough (5–10 mg/L) concentrations.

DOSING GUIDELINES. A variety of methods have been suggested for appropriate dosing of vancomycin. Empiric or fixed doses (1 gm every 12 hours or 500 mg every 6 hours) have been traditionally suggested for adult patients with normal renal function. Dosage based on body weight and underlying disease state has also been suggested [21]. Daily dosages have ranged up to 60 mg/kg/day in young burn patients or patients with gram-positive bacterial meningitis [21]. Rapid intravenous administration of vancomycin has been associated with red man or red neck syndrome [69,101]. Though some investigators have suggested that the syndrome is caused by a vancomycin-induced release of histamine, others question this finding [69,101].

Limiting the rate of infusion to 12 mg/kg/hr or less usually prevents this syndrome. Premedicating the patient with an antihistamine, such as diphenhydramine, has also been suggested as a mechanism for preventing the syndrome.

A variety of nomograms have also appeared in the literature. Nielsen, Matzke, Moellering, and Lake suggested different methods for adjusting the dose of vancomycin [86,102,103,104]. Zokufa et al. evaluated these dosage regimens in 37 patients and found that the Matzke method produced peak concentrations in excess of 40 mg per liter in 97 percent of patients studied and that trough concentrations were less than 5 mg per liter in 40 percent of the patient population [10]. The Nielsen and Moellering methods produced peak concentrations less than 30 mg per liter in 64 percent and 51 percent of the patient population and trough concentrations less than 5 mg per liter in 46 percent and 35 percent of the patient population, respectively. The Lake method produced peak concentrations above 40 mg per liter and less than 30 mg per liter in 32 percent and 32 percent of the patient population, respectively; trough concentrations were below 5 mg per liter in 22 percent of the patient population [10]. Both peak (30–40 mg/l) and trough (5–10 mg/l) concentrations were within the previously defined range in 30 percent, 8 percent, 3 percent, and 16 percent of the patient population for the Matzke, Nielsen, Moellering, and Lake methods, respectively [10]. In a separate evaluation of vancomycin dosing methods, Pryka et al. concluded that the Moellering and Lake methods offered the least biased and most precise predictions of vancomycin dosage [48].

DRUG INTERACTIONS. Parenteral vancomycin is associated with few if any clinically significant drug-drug interactions. There have been reports suggesting a pharmacodynamic interaction between the parenteral use of vancomycin in combination with aminoglycosides in potentiating nephrotoxicity [51,52].

The combination of oral vancomycin with resin binding agents such as cholestyramine can reduce the functional concentration of vancomycin and alter the desired effect in the treatment of pseudomembranous colitis.

COMMON PITFALLS. The most frequently seen problems with vancomycin include attempting to characterize vancomycin with a one-compartment model and obtaining the "peak" concentration at some time after the intravenous infusion. This practice results in mythical pharmacokinetic parameters: The "peak" is not the real peak, the "half-life" is not the real terminal half-life, and the "distribution volume" is not the real volume when monoexponential interpretation is used. Not only do these parameters have no factual derivation, there is no established range of normal values to apply to their interpretation.

Careful documentation of infusion times and the time of serum sampling represent significant problems in attempting to monitor vancomycin therapy.

Occasionally, inexperienced clinicians, not realizing that vancomycin is not absorbed from the gastrointestinal tract, attempt to convert a patient receiving intravenous vancomycin for a systemic infection over to oral vancomycin therapy.

Imipenem

Structurally, imipenem is a carbapenem antibiotic and the only product of this class currently marketed in the United States.

Imipenem has the broadest spectrum of activity for any commercially available antibiotic, and many clinical trials have shown it to be a valuable agent for the treatment of polymicrobial and monomicrobial infections encountered in the intensive care unit. In the treatment of abdominal infections, comparisons of imipenem to combinations of aminoglycosides, penicillins, and clindamycin or metronidazole have revealed that imipenem is at least equal to and perhaps superior to double or triple antibiotic regimens [105–109]. In addition, imipenem is an effective therapy for nosocomially acquired pneumonia, urinary tract infections, skin and soft tissue infections, and osteomyelitis [105,106].

PHARMACOLOGY. Imipenem is the N-formimidoyl derivative of thienamycin, a carbapenem antibiotic produced by the fungal species *Streptomyces cattleya*. Carbapenems are structural analogues of beta-lactam antibiotics; a carbon atom is substituted for a sulfur atom and a double bond is added to the five-membered ring of penicillin [110].

Commercially, imipenem is combined with cilastatin, which prevents hydrolysis of imipenem by inhibition of dehydropeptidase-1, resulting in increased 6-hour urinary recovery of imipenem. Animal studies have shown that the coadministration of cilastatin prevents the formation of hydrolytic metabolites, which are nephrotoxic [105,106].

The primary mechanism of action of imipenem is similar to that of beta-lactam antibiotics. Imipenem inhibits cell wall synthesis by covalently binding to penicillin binding proteins (PBPs), which results in a bactericidal effect and cell death. The affinity of imipenem for PBPs in gram-negative bacteria is greatest for PBPs 1a, 1b, and 2a and least for PBP 3 [105,111]. Against *S. aureus* and *Bacteroides fragilis,* imipenem has been shown to have a high affinity for PBPs 1 to 4 [105].

The antimicrobial spectrum of imipenem encompasses a wide variety of community- and hospital-acquired organisms. Imipenem exhibits bactericidal activity against most *Streptococcus* spp, *Staphylococcus* spp (except methicillin-resistant *Staphylococcus*), Enterobacteriaceae (including *Enterobacter* spp, *Serratia* spp, *Citrobacter* spp), and *Pseudomonas aeruginosa.* Imipenem is also effective against many enteric and oropharyngeal anaerobes, including *Bacteroides fragilis* and nonfragilis *Bacteroides* spp.

The major mechanism of resistance to imipenem is thought to be due to an alteration in outer membrane proteins [105,112,113]. Decreased permeability has been documented as a mechanism of resistance primarily in *P. aeruginosa* and has also been observed in *Enterobacter* spp and *Acinetobacter* spp [105]. Mechanisms of resistance to imipenem are generally not associated with hydrolysis by beta-lactamases. The hydroxyethyl side chain of imipenem is in the *trans* configuration, opposite that of conventional beta-lactam antibiotics. This structural difference makes imipenem resistant to most beta-lactamases [110]. However, most strains of *Xanthomonas maltophilia* produce carbapenem hydrolases that can inactivate imipenem [105,106,110]. Some strains of *Enterococcus faecium,* methicillin-resistant *Staphylococcus, Pseudomonas cepacia, P. aeruginosa, Serratia marcescens, B. fragilis,* and *Enterobacter* spp have also been reported to produce carbapenem hydrolases [105,106,110].

THERAPEUTIC RANGE. There is no established therapeutic range for imipenem. Several investigators have suggested that beta-lactam antibiotics should be dosed to maintain concentrations above the bacterial MIC for the entire dosing interval [114,115]. In vitro studies suggest that beta-lactam antibiotics in general are no more effective when dosed to achieve concentrations many times the MIC than when dosed to achieve concentrations only several times greater than the MIC [114,115,116]. Further, improved bacterial eradication is seen when beta-lactam concentrations are above the MIC for the entire dosing interval [114,115,116]. Many bacterial species have MIC-90-values for imipenem less than 2 mg per liter, but certain strains of *Pseudomonas* or Enterobacteriaceae may exhibit higher MICs. Indirectly, these data would suggest that concentrations should be maintained at least at 2 to 4 mg per liter for the entire dosing interval, and possibly higher for more resistant pathogens.

PREPARATIONS. There are two currently available imipenem preparations: an intravenous preparation that contains equal portions of cilastatin and anhydrous imipenem with 20 mg of sodium bicarbonate, and a preparation for intramuscular injection that contains equal portions of cilastatin and anhydrous imipenem. Use of the IM preparation should be reserved for mild to moderate infections; the IM preparation should be reconstituted with 1% lidocaine [117].

PHARMACOKINETICS

Asorption. Imipenem is not absorbed appreciably after oral administration and must be administered by intravenous injection or deep intramuscular injection. Imipenem is incompletely absorbed following intramuscular administration of the commercially available intramuscular preparation [105].

Distribution. The volume of distribution for imipenem approximates that of extracellular body fluids; total apparent volume of distribution has been reported to range from 0.23 to 0.35 liter per kilogram in adult patients [105,106,118]. A two-compartment model best fits the pharmacokinetics of imipenem and cilastatin, with alpha distribution reaching completion within 15 to 30 minutes of the end of administration [106]. Imipenem is 10 to 20 percent bound to albumin [106]. Imipenem distributes into human body tissues within 30 minutes to 1 hour after administration; concentrations in peritoneum, abdominal organs, meninges, sputum, prostate, bone, and renal tissue are in excess of most aerobic bacterial MICs [105,106, 118,119,120].

Elimination. Imipenem, imipenem metabolites, and cilistatin are cleared predominantly through the kidney. Glomerular filtration is the primary elimination mechanism, but 20 to 30 percent of the renal excretion of imipenem occurs by tubular secretion [121]. Nonrenal hydrolysis of the carbapenem ring accounts for formation of approximately 20 to 30 percent of the metabolite [121]. Negligible amounts of imipenem are excreted via the hepatobiliary tract, with 1 to 2 percent of imipenem being recovered in the feces [110,117].

The average elimination half-life of imipenem in patients with normal renal function has been reported to be 0.8 to 1.3 hours. Cilistatin has an elimination half-life of slightly less than 1 hour in patients with normal renal function. When imipenem is administered alone, approximately 20 percent of the parent compound is excreted unchanged in the urine. When it is administered with equal concentrations of cilastatin, approximately 70 percent of imipenem is excreted unchanged in the urine, and approximately 29 percent is excreted as the inactive open lactam metabolite [110,117,122].

PHYSIOLOGIC CLEARANCE CHARACTERISTICS. Patients who experience trauma, sepsis, or burns may experience physiologic changes that can affect the pharmacokinetics of imipenem. Almost all beta-lactam antibiotics are eliminated by the kidney and therefore exhibit flow-limited characteristics. The elimination of imipenem should parallel changes in blood flow to the kidneys, provided the kidneys are not physiologically deficient. Several authors have shown a correlation between both increased and decreased creatinine and imipenem clearance [118,122,123,124]. However, some intensive care patients may experience changes in renal drug clearance that are not reflected by changes in creatinine clearance.

No published studies have specifically studied the clearance of imipenem in hypodynamic intensive care patients. Theoretically, however, certain patients, such those who develop low cardiac output and multisystem organ failure, may exhibit decreases in flow dependent imipenem clearance. Eventually, changes in serum creatinine reflect decreases in renal function; however, clearance of flow-dependent antibiotics such as imipenem may be decreased prior to changed in renal function indicators. In patients who exhibit hypodynamic characteristics, the potential for decreased imipenem clearance and cumulative toxicity should be considered.

Recent data suggest that patients in acute renal failure have a significantly greater degree of nonrenal imipenem elimination than chronic renal failure patients (95 ml/min vs. 51 ml/min), and therefore have greater total clearance [125]. Intensive care patients who exhibit a temporary decrease in renal function without a corresponding decrease in other organ system function may be able to tolerate larger doses of imipenem than end-stage renal failure or multisystem organ failure patients [125].

Several studies have investigated the pharmacokinetics of imipenem in intensive care patients, but no studies have specifically investigated the pharmacokinetics of imipenem in hyperdynamic patients. In general, pharmacokinetic parameters in intensive care patients are similar to those in healthy individuals, and 500 to 1000 mg administered every 6 hours provide plasma imipenem concentrations above the MIC for most pathogens for the duration of the dosing interval [118,124,126]. However, it is difficult to interpret these data with regard to hypermetabolism. In all studies, selection of patients for pharmacokinetic study was not based on hypermetabolic considerations, and mean creatinine clearances were not appreciably different from those in studies investigating healthy volunteers. In addition, plasma imipenem concentrations were reported as mean values and subgroup analysis of hypermetabolic patients was not performed.

Theoretically, the use of standard dosing regimens and routes of administration could produce subtherapeutic imipenem concentrations in patients with increased cardiac output and corresponding increased flow-dependent glomerular filtration and tubular secretion. In these patients, more frequent dosing of imipenem may be required to maintain concentrations above bacterial MICs.

Boucher et al. studied the pharmacokinetics of 500 mg of imipenem, every 6 hours in 11 adult patients at least 5 days after experiencing severe burns [124]. The pharmacokinetic parameters in this population were not statistically different from previously reported parameters in normal healthy volunteers; however, substantial variability existed between individual patients. Creatinine clearances (CrCl) ranged from 17 to 218 ml per minute, and imipenem elimination was significantly related to creatinine clearance. Pharmacokinetic data obtained from two patients with measured CrCl greater than 150 ml/min/1.73m^2 revealed that a regimen of 500 mg every 6 hours did not provide sustained concentration of imipenem throughout the entire dosing interval. Multidose simulations of 500 mg every 4 hours provided imipenem concentrations in excess of most imipenem MICs (1 mg/L) for the entire dosing interval, whereas doses of 1000 mg every 6 hours did not. These results suggest that while 500 mg dosed every 6 hours may be adequate for many patients, hyperdynamic patients who exhibit increased measured creatinine clearances may exhibit a corresponding increase in imipenem clearance. In any patient receiving imipenem who exhibits hypermetabolic characteristics, an increase in the frequency of imipenem administration should be considered.

DOSING GUIDELINES. Microbial susceptibility of the causative organisms should be considered when dosing imipenem. In general, the MIC-90 for most Enterobacteriaceae, *Pseudomonas* spp, anaerobes, and gram-positive aerobes is quite low in relation to achievable serum and tissue concentrations of imipenem. However, development of pseudomonal resistance to imipenem during treatment has been reported frequently. Some investigators have reported resistance rates as high as 16 to 60 percent for *P. aeruginosa* [127,128,129]. If MIC values of any isolated organism indicate only moderate susceptibility (MIC $\geq$4 mg/L) or if the likelihood of *P. aeruginosa* as a causative organism is high, imipenem dosages such as 1 gm every 6 hours or the addition of an aminoglycoside may be advantageous.

For most patients, the manufacturer's suggested guidelines of 500 mg every 6 hours administered intravenously for moderately severe infections caused by susceptible microorganisms or 1000 mg every 6 to 8 hours for severe infections caused by moderately susceptible organisms should be adequate. However, hypodynamic or hyperdynamic patients with impaired renal function may require alternative dosing strategies.

The primary pharmacokinetic consideration of imipenem dosing in the hypodynamic patient is renal function. In all patients who have creatinine clearances of less than 70 ml/min/1.73 m^2 the dosage of imipenem should be reduced [105]. The manufacturer's guidelines suggest that patients with creatinine clearances between 30 and 70 ml/min/1.73 m^2 should receive 500 mg every 6 to 8 hours. Patients with creatinine clearances between 20 and 30 ml/min/1.73 m^2 should receive 500 mg every 8 to 12 hours, and patients with creatinine clearances less than 20 ml/min/1.73 m^2 should receive 250 to 500 mg of imipenem every 12 hours. Patients with acute renal compromise deserve special consideration. These patients may require 500 mg every 8 hours or 750 mg every 12 hours, due to increased extrarenal metabolism [125]. The potential for adverse central nervous system effects must be weighed against the severity of infection when aggressive therapy is desired. Administration of excessive doses of imipenem is not without consequence: The incidence of seizures increases dramatically in patients with reduced renal function who receive large doses of imipenem.

The optimal dosing of imipenem in the hypermetabolic patient is speculative, due to limited pharmacokinetic data. Patients who exhibit increased cardiac output resulting in increased renal blood flow may benefit from more frequent dosing, such as 500 mg every 4 hours. Measured creatinine clearance (>150 ml/min/1.73 m^2) may help determine which patients may benefit from 4-hour dosing [124]. Alternatively, patients with normal or slightly increased renal function and the potential for infections caused by pathogens with MICs greater than 4 mg per liter may benefit from 1 gm or more every 6 hours [124,130]. Shortened dosage intervals or larger imipenem doses should be selected on a case-by-case basis, taking into consideration the potential for dose-related adverse effects and the patient's pharmacokinetic characteristics. In addition, the microbial etiology of the infection and susceptibility of the microorganisms must be considered when dosing imipenem.

DRUG INTERACTIONS. The concurrent use of imipenem with other antimicrobials has been studied in detail. When traditional synergy testing methods (e.g., checkerboard testing) are employed, additivity has been frequently reported when imipenem is combined with aminoglycosides [105,106]. However, synergy has been reported, with the degree of synergy varying from strain to strain against *P. aeruginosa* and Enterobacteriaceae [105,106]. When imipenem was combined with aminoglycosides against *E. faecalis,* the majority of strains tested (36–100%) showed synergy [105,106].

The concurrent use of imipenem with other beta-lactam antibiotics has been reported to be antagonistic [105,106,131]. Imipenem has been reported to antagonize the effects of aztreonam, ureidocillins, and second- and third-generation cephalosporins against *P. aeruginosa* and Enterobacteriaceae [105,106]. The mechanism of antagonism is thought to be the induction of beta-lactamase production. Imipenem is a strong inducer of Sykes class 1 cephalosporinase; therefore, antimicrobial therapy should not include the concurrent use of imipenem with other beta-lactam antibiotics [105,106,131]. Against *P. aeruginosa* and Enterobacteriaceae, both synergy and additivity have been reported when imipenem was combined with Ag; however, strain to strain variation is common [105,106].

COMMON PITFALLS. The use of imipenem has been associated with superinfection and colonization. The overall incidence of colonization has been reported to be 16 percent (11% *Candida* spp, 1.0% other fungi, and 3.5% resistant bacteria) [105,106]. The incidence of colonization with imipenem therapy is considered to be similar to that of cephalosporin antibiotics. Superinfection occurred in 5.5 percent (1.5% *Candida* spp, 2.4% imipenem-susceptible bacteria, and 1.6% imipenem-resistant bacteria) [105,106]. Microbes commonly associated with superinfection include *Enterococcus* spp, *Pseudomonas* spp, and coagulase-negative *Staphylococcus* [105,106].

The most commonly reported adverse effects in patients receiving imipenem include nausea, vomiting, and diarrhea (3.2–4.2%) [105,106,132,133]. The potential for nausea can be reduced by increasing the duration of infusion to at least 30 minutes for a 500-mg dose and 1 hour for a 1-gm dose.

The most serious sequelae reported with imipenem use are central nervous system effects such as seizures, myoclonus, or convulsions. The mechanism is thought to be binding of imipenem to GABA receptors [134]. The overall incidence of seizures during imipenem therapy is comparable to that seen with beta-lactam antibiotics (1.5–3%). However, in certain patient populations (elderly; patients with renal failure, seizure history, or treated with large doses of imipenem) the risk of seizures during imipenem therapy increases substantially [132–135]. The risk of imipenem-induced seizures is associated primarily with excessive dose and renal dysfunction [135]. Patients with renal insufficiency who are administered dosages in excess of the manufacturer's recommended guidelines exhibit a higher frequency of seizures (11.8% vs. 2.6%) than patients with renal insufficiency who receive adjusted dosages [135]. Patients with a history of central nervous system disorders are at increased risk of developing seizures when administered imipenem doses in excess of manufacturer's guidelines, compared with patients with central nervous system disorders who are administered standard dosages (24.4% vs. 11.3%) [135]. Patients with a history

of both central nervous system disorders and renal insufficiency who receive excessive dosages of imipenem are at greatest risk of developing seizures. The incidence of seizures is 32.1 percent for these patients versus 20 percent for patients with the same underlying central nervous system disorders and renal insufficiency who receive correct dosages [135].

Due to the increased risk of adverse central nervous system effects, patients with renal insufficiency should receive imipenem only when dosages are adjusted for renal failure. The importance of central nervous system lesions is difficult to interpret due to the variables associated with seizure activity; however, lesions in combination with either excessive dosage or renal dysfunction increase the risk of seizures, and these patients should not receive imipenem unless the doses are adjusted for renal failure [135]. Patients with central nervous system disorders and no other risk factors do not need dosage reduction [135].

Methods of treatment for imipenem-induced seizures have shown variable results [135]. In general, seizures due to beta-lactam antibiotic administration are considered refractory to phenytoin therapy [105,106], but in some cases seizure activity has been eliminated with phenytoin [105,106,133,135]. Favorable response to benzodiazepine administration has been reported in other cases of antibiotic-related seizures [135]. The treatment of imipenem-induced seizures and concomitant use of imipenem should be evaluated for risk versus benefit on an individualized basis.

Clindamycin

Clindamycin is a semisynthetic derivative of lincomycin, a natural compound that was isolated from the fermentation products of *Streptomyces lincolnensis* [136,137,138]. The 7-chloro substitution of the 7-hydroxyl group of the natural compound resulted in improved oral absorption, decreased toxicity, and increased activity [137,138,139].

Clindamycin is widely used in the treatment of serious pulmonary, intraabdominal, and pelvic anaerobic infections and, in combination with an aminoglycoside, is regarded by many as standard therapy for mixed aerobic-anaerobic infections [138,140,141]. Clindamycin is particularly useful in the treatment of surgical and gynecologic infections [134,140].

PHARMACOLOGY. Clindamycin exerts a bacteriostatic effect through inhibition of bacterial protein synthesis. The drug binds exclusively to the 50S subunit of bacterial ribosomes and may inhibit either the binding of aminoacyl-tRNA to the ribosomes or the translocation that follows binding of the amino acid [138].

Clindamycin is active against most aerobic gram-positive bacteria, with the notable exceptions of enterococci and methicillin-resistant staphylococci [138,139,142]. Both gram-positive and gram-negative anaerobic bacteria, including *Bacteroides fragilis* and *Actinomyces* spp, are typically susceptible [138, 139,140,142–145]. A substantial postantibiotic effect (2–5 hours) against *B. fragilis* has been demonstrated [146,147].

Subinhibitory concentrations of clindamycin have a positive effect on the function of polymorphonuclear cells (PMNs), both in vitro and in vivo [148,149,150]. This effect is lost or reversed at higher concentrations [148]. Clindamycin is liposoluble and actively penetrates PMNs via the nucleotide transport mechanism; however, the mechanism for the potentiating effect is unknown [151,152]. In addition to the effect on PMNs, subinhibitory concentrations of clindamycin exert a direct effect on the susceptibility of various bacteria to opsonization, phago-cytosis, and intracellular killing [153,154,155].

THERAPEUTIC RANGE.

A therapeutic range has not been established for clindamycin. Presumably, efficacy depends in part on the achievement of inhibitory concentrations of unbound antibiotic at the site of the infection.

PREPARATIONS.

Clindamycin is available as capsules (75 mg and 150 mg, clindamycin hydrochloride), a pediatric suspension (75 mg/5 ml, clindamycin palmitate hydrochloride), and for injection (150 mg/ml, clindamycin phosphate). Clindamycin palmitate and clindamycin phosphate are both rapidly hydrolyzed in vivo to the active base [156].

PHARMACOKINETICS.

Pharmacokinetic data for clindamycin are limited, primarily because most of the early studies used microbiologic assay techniques that are unable to differentiate between clindamycin and active metabolites. Pharmacokinetic studies using chromatography techniques have not been performed in large numbers of patients.

Absorption. Clindamycin, as both the hydrochloride and palmitate ester, is rapidly and virtually completely absorbed from the gastrointestinal tract; absorption is not decreased by food [138,157].

Distribution. Peak serum concentrations of clindamycin are achieved within 45 to 60 minutes after oral administration and 1 to 3 hours after intramuscular injection [156,157]. Clindamycin phosphate is rapidly hydrolyzed in vivo to the active base; peak serum concentrations of the base occur at the end of intravenous infusions [156]. Reported peak values after intravenous infusion vary widely and increase linearly, but not proportionally, with increases in dosage (peak concentrations 10–20 mg/L for 600–1200-mg doses in normal volunteers) [138,141,156]. In general, higher peak levels have been seen in acutely ill patients than in normal volunteers [138,158].

The distribution volume of clindamycin in healthy volunteers averages 0.9 to 1.1 liters per kilogram and tends to increase as the dose increases [141]. Clindamycin is widely distributed in many body tissues and fluids; significant concentrations are attained in saliva, sputum, respiratory tissues, pleural fluid, soft tissues, prostate, semen, bones and joints, and fetal blood and tissues [137,156,159–166]. Significant concentrations are not achieved in cerebrospinal fluid or brain tissue [137,167].

Clindamycin is extensively protein-bound (60–95%) to alpha-1-acid glycoprotein (AAG) [168,169,170]. Protein binding is dependent on the serum concentrations of both AAG and clindamycin; the degree of protein binding increases with increased AAG concentrations and decreased clindamycin concentrations [168].

Elimination. The elimination of clindamycin occurs primarily (approximately 85%) through hepatic metabolism to N-demethylclindamycin and clindamycin sulfoxide. The N-demethyl metabolite is several times more active than the parent compound; the sulfoxide metabolite is less active [156]. Both metabolites are excreted in the urine and bile [138,164,165]. Urinary excretion of unchanged clindamycin is minimal (5–10%), and only small quantities are found in the feces [137,138]. Reported elimination half-lives for clindamycin in normal volunteers range between 1.5 and 4.0 hours [137,141,156, 157,171,172,173]. The elimination half-life is unchanged in pa-

tients with chronic renal failure; blood levels are not affected by hemodialysis [171]. Prolonged elimination half-lives and elevated serum concentrations have been demonstrated in patients with hepatic failure; however, these changes were modest and were not associated with drug accumulation or toxicity [138,172,174–178]. In one study, the elimination half-life of clindamycin was strongly associated with total bilirubin (r = 0.86) and indirect bilirubin (r = 0.925); the elimination half-life could be estimated by the following equation: $t_{1/2}$ (hr) = (3.2 × Indirect bilirubin) + 0.48 [176].

More rapid elimination and greater urinary excretion of clindamycin has been shown for infants and children as compared to adults [157,179]. Elderly patients, however, presumably metabolize the drug more slowly, as prolonged half-lives (>4 hours) have been demonstrated in this patient population [180].

PHYSIOLOGIC CLEARANCE CHARACTERISTICS.

Clindamycin is highly protein-bound and has a low extraction ratio, placing it in the general pharmacokinetic category of capacity-limited, binding-sensitive drugs [168,169,170,181,182,183]. Clindamycin is primarily bound to AAG, an acute phase reactant. In response to trauma and stress, AAG can be increased in critically ill patients to several times normal concentrations [184]. Increased protein binding of clindamycin in these patients should result in decreased drug clearance. In addition, clindamycin clearance may be decreased in patients with hepatic dysfunction.

The mean total body clearance of clindamycin in a group of critically ill patients with sepsis was less than half that of healthy volunteers (0.166 vs. 0.37 L/hr/kg) [158]. However, a reduction in clindamycin clearance did not occur in all patients; linear regression analysis failed to demonstrate strong correlations between pharmacokinetic parameters and patient physiologic, laboratory, or outcome variables [158].

Protein binding of clindamycin in critically ill patients remains an important consideration. Although increased binding may lead to decreased clearance, the unbound concentration of drug may not change significantly. It is likely that increased protein binding alone would have little negative effect on the pharmacodynamics of clindamycin.

DOSING GUIDELINES.

In patients with serious infections, clindamycin phosphate is generally administered intravenously in doses of 1.2 to 2.7 gm per day in two to four divided doses. Doses of up to 4.8 gm per day have been administered for very serious life-threatening infections. Dosage adjustments are unnecessary in patients with renal failure. Patients with hepatic failure will likely tolerate standard doses of clindamycin without accumulation; however, caution should be used in patients with severe hepatic disease. Critically ill patients may have decreased clearance of clindamycin; however, no discriminating variables for decreased clearance have been identified. Given that there are no known concentration-related toxicities, routine dosage adjustment for these patients is not recommended.

DRUG INTERACTIONS.

Clindamycin has neuromuscular blocking properties that may enhance the action of other neuromuscular blocking agents; caution should be used in patients receiving concomitant therapy. In vitro antagonism has been demonstrated between clindamycin and erythromycin.

COMMON PITFALLS.

Clindamycin has been associated with the development of severe and possibly fatal pseudomembranous colitis, characterized by diarrhea, abdominal pain, fever, and mucus and blood in the stool [138]. A toxin produced by *C. difficile* is responsible for this syndrome. The development of significant diarrhea warrants discontinuation of clindamycin. If the colitis is severe or does not respond to discontinuation of the drug, oral vancomycin or metronidazole therapy may be necessary.

Diarrhea is reported in approximately 8 percent of patients receiving clindamycin, and 10 percent develop skin rashes. Other adverse reactions, which are uncommon, include Stevens-Johnson syndrome, itching, urticaria, drug fever, granulocytopenia, thrombocytopenia, hepatotoxicity, and anaphylactic reactions [138,185,186,187].

Aminoglycosides

Despite the introduction of expanded-spectrum beta-lactam and fluoroquinolone antibiotics, aminoglycosides remain first-line therapy in the management of gram-negative sepsis [188,189]. Gentamicin, kanamycin, netilmicin, tobramycin, streptomycin, and amikacin are the parenteral aminoglycosides commercially available in the United States. Gentamicin and tobramycin are available as generic products and are relatively inexpensive. While the aminoglycosides have proved to be very clinically efficacious the adverse reactions of nephrotoxicity and ototoxicity limit usage and universal endorsement [188–192].

PHARMACOLOGY. Aminoglycosides interfere with the 30S and 50S ribosomes, ultimately resulting in inhibition of protein synthesis [188]. The antimicrobial action of aminoglycosides has been reported to be concentration-dependent [1]. Thus, higher aminoglycoside serum concentrations will kill susceptible bacteria with increased efficiency, kill a larger fraction of the bacterial population, and theoretically extend the postantibiotic effect [1].

The antimicrobial action of the aminoglycoside is bactericidal, meaning the ratio between the bacterial MBC and MIC is usually four or less [188]. However, this factor is directly dependent on the specific aminoglycoside and bacterial pathogen in question. The antimicrobial activity of aminoglycosides can be dramatically altered by changes in pH, the presence of divalent cations, and the absence of oxygen [188]. These drugs tend to be much more active in an alkaline rather than an acid environment. Unlike many antibiotics, aminoglycosides have an antibacterial effect in both exponential and stationary growth [188]. They are also reported to have a postantibiotic effect of several hours for gram-negative pathogens but only a modest effect against gram-positive pathogens [1,24].

Aminoglycosides are used primarily in the management of Enterobacteriaceae and pseudomonal infections. On the basis of MICs, tobramycin tends to be a more effective aminoglycoside than gentamicin in the management of *P. aeruginosa*, while gentamicin tends to be more active than tobramycin in the management of *S. marcescens* infections [188]. Current data would suggest that maximizing the ratio between achievable antibiotic concentration and the MIC of the infecting pathogen will improve antibiotic performance [191].

The use of streptomycin has been limited to the treatment of enterococcal infections and management of *Mycobacterium tuberculosis*. In both situations, streptomycin must be combined with other antibiotics to effect a successful outcome. Classically, enterococci are tolerant to the action of penicillins and vancomycin, and for this reason these antibiotics must be combined with either streptomycin or gentamicin for successful treatment of systemic infections.

Resistance to aminoglycosides is primarily enzymatically mediated through adenylation, acetylation, or phosphorylation. Adenylation represents the most common method for aminoglycoside inactivation and is capable of destroying both gentamicin and tobramycin but not amikacin [188]. Amikacin and netilmicin are inactivated by acetylating enzymes but not adenylating enzymes. Most gram-negative bacterial pathogens, however, do not possess both capabilities, and in many situations amikacin can be successfully used to manage gentamicin- and tobramycin-resistant gram-negative pathogens.

THERAPEUTIC RANGE. Despite the acceptance of therapeutic drug monitoring of aminoglycoside therapy for over 50 years, the therapeutic range for these drugs remains ill defined [193–199]. Generally, peak concentrations of 6 to 8 μg per milliliter for gentamicin and tobramycin and 25 to 32 μg per milliliter for amikacin have been considered acceptable ranges [188]. Trough concentrations of less than 2 μg per milliliter for gentamicin and tobramycin between 5 and 8 μg per milliliter for amikacin are generally accepted [188].

Noone et al. and Jackson and Riff were among the first investigators to establish that unsuccessful clinical outcomes resulted when subtherapeutic peak concentrations of aminoglycoside were achieved in infected patients [196,197]. Following this work, other investigators have continued to report such relationships and have established the need to determine patient-specific pharmacokinetic parameters, especially in unique patient settings [11–16,193,199–213]. The definition of a "peak concentration" varies substantially from investigator to investigator. In many well-known clinical trials, the "peak" concentration is actually a 30- or 60-minute postinfusion concentration [189,190,191,206,214–219]. In these situations, the actual peak concentration is actually higher than the value reported [214]. The difference between the actual peak and the defined peak depends on the patient's half-life, distribution volume, and duration of intravenous infusion. Rigorous means must be also employed to document accurately infusion start times, infusion stop times, and the time at which serum concentrations are actually collected and to document that the patient is truly at steady state when trough and peak aminoglycoside studies are performed. Without such rigor, the value of the data must be called into question.

Clinical studies that helped define the therapeutic range for aminoglycosides utilized older (microbiologic, radioenzymatic, or radioimmunoassays) technologies. Over the last 20 years, quantitative drug assay technology has become increasingly more sophisticated. However, whether the aminoglycoside therapeutic range needs to be redefined in view of this new technology has not been addressed. Rotschafer et al. and Bleske et al. have demonstrated assay performance bias between different assay technologies that resulted in the generation of significantly different pharmacokinetic parameters and aminoglycoside dosage regimens from serum-concentration-time data [194,198,199].

The demonstration that single daily dose aminoglycoside therapy (6 mg/kg/day for gentamicin, netilmicin, and tobramycin) can be administered to patients with at least equal rates of toxicity and efficacy as compared to conventional dosing creates a new variable in defining the therapeutic range of aminoglycosides. Rotschafer et al. reported that dosages of this magnitude will produce serum concentrations well beyond the conventionally defined range for aminoglycoside peak and trough concentrations when large patient populations with varying pharmacokinetic parameters are treated in this fashion [1].

At present there are three major philosophies regarding aminoglycoside therapeutic drug monitoring. The first is that there are insufficient data to demonstrate conclusively a benefit of adjusting aminoglycoside therapy to obtain predefined concentration ranges. The second group believes very strongly in therapeutic drug monitoring of aminoglycosides and utilizes conventional peak and trough concentrations in patients monitoring. The third group advocates the use of a single daily dose of aminoglycosides. While there may exist some question as to definition of the therapeutic range for aminoglycosides, pharmacokinetic (Sawchuk-Zaske) or bayesian methods have been established as clearly superior to conventional dosing strategies at achieving desired serum concentrations [192,220].

PREPARATIONS. The various aminoglycoside preparations are too numerous to mention and beyond the scope of this chapter. The drugs are available as topical creams and ointments, ophthalmic, and otic dosage forms. Preservative-free forms of gentamicin and tobramycin are available for intrathecal or intraventricular injection. Available pediatric and adult products for intramuscular or intravenous administration differ only in concentration.

Unlike tobramycin, amikacin, and netilmicin, which are pure antibiotic entities, gentamicin is actually a mixture of three components: C1, C1A, and C2. From manufacturer to manufacturer and lot to lot there are likely to be differences in the C1, C1A, and C2 content of gentamicin. There are, however, tolerance specifications for these components in the production and certification of gentamicin. Nahata et al. reported significant interlot variability between the labeled concentration and the actual measured concentration of both gentamicin and tobramycin available from various manufacturers [221]. These investigators report that an 80-mg dose of gentamicin may actually contain 107 mg of drug and an 80-mg dose tobramycin may actually provide 98 mg of drug. For obvious reasons such variability may significantly complicate attempts to monitor aminoglycoside therapy pharmacokinetically.

PHARMACOKINETICS

Absorption. Oral and rectal administration are not viable routes of aminoglycoside therapy for systemic infections, as aminoglycosides are virtually nonabsorbable. For selective gut decontamination or treatment of intestinal parasitic infections, clinicans can capitalize on the poor systemic absorption of the aminoglycoside; treatment is accomplished without exposing the patient to the systemic adverse effects of the aminoglycoside.

Systemic infections must be managed with intramuscular or intravenous administration. Aminoglycoside bioavailability is 100 percent for intravenous administration and very close to 100 percent when these drugs are administered intramuscularly. As with all agents administered intramuscularly, absorption is dependent on muscle mass at the site of injection as well as regional blood flow. Erratic absorption can be seen in patients with peripheral vascular disease or diabetes or in patients who are obese or emaciated. Generally, peak aminoglycoside concentrations are achieved within 60 minutes following intramuscular injection.

Distribution. Generally, aminoglycosides have a relatively small distribution volume (approximately 10–20 liters; 0.25–0.35 L/kg when standardized to body weight). This "normal" range of values may have to be adjusted based on the assay technology used at a particular institution [194,198,199]. Because of the relatively small size of the distribution volume, this compartment can be greatly influenced by dehydration or overhydration and is likely to vary throughout the course of hospitalization, especially in critically ill patients.

When distribution volume is standardized to actual body weight (L/kg) and when there is a large difference between actual and lean body weight, a different range of normal values should be used. A typical distribution volume in a patient at or near lean body weight would be 0.25 to 0.35 liter per kilogram actual body weight, whereas in an obese patient of identical body stature the normal value might be 0.10 to 0.15 liter per kilogram actual body weight. Adipose tissue does contribute to overall distribution volume, but to a lesser degree than lean tissue. If actual body weight is used to calculate the distribution volume (in L/kg) the denominator is disproportionately high in obese patients; therefore the distribution volume is lower. Sketris et al. documented the effect of obesity on overall distribution volume [222].

While aminoglycosides are distributed from the blood to a variety of body tissues, there are some notable exceptions. Aminoglycosides do not distribute well to the central nervous system or into the eye [188]. When aminoglycosides are intended as treatment for infections of these tissues or fluids, the drug must be directly injected at the site of infection. Variable concentrations can be seen in the bile and in lung tissue. If the infecting pathogen has a low minimum inhibiting concentration (≤0.5 mg/L), even small amounts of aminoglycoside may be sufficient to eradicate the infection. However, when the MIC of the infecting pathogen is higher and the absolute amount of aminoglycoside distributing to the site of infection is small, a satisfactory clinical outcome may not be seen. In these circumstances, higher serum concentrations of aminoglycoside or the addition of a second antibiotic, such as a beta-lactam compound, may be necessary.

Limited data suggest that aminoglycoside distribution to the inner ear and to the kidney may be a saturable phenomenon [208,223,224]. As a result, administration of the aminoglycoside in divided doses may result in more tissue accumulation and therefore toxicity than administration of the entire dose at one time. This observation has been offered in part as rationale for single daily dosing of aminoglycosides.

Elimination. Aminoglycosides are primarily excreted unchanged by the kidney. Glomerular filtration plays the predominant role in the elimination of aminoglycosides, but there is limited information suggesting a small contribution from tubular secretion [188]. For this reason, aminoglycoside elimination is heavily dependent on cardiac output and ultimately renal blood flow. Alterations in renal perfusion or the number of functioning nephrons impact on aminoglycoside elimination and contribute to the variability often seen in aminoglycoside clearance over the course of hospitalization. Clinical interventions to alter heart rate or stroke volume resulting in changes in cardiac output ultimately affect renal blood flow and, therefore, aminoglycoside clearance.

Aminoglycosides are readily removed by hemodialysis. While the effect of hemodialysis on aminoglycoside clearance is dependent on the rate of blood flow, the dialysis membrane material used, the aminoglycoside being dialyzed, and the duration of the procedure, a typical 3-hour hemodialysis procedure will remove approximately 25 percent of the aminoglycoside present prior to the start of hemodialysis. Usually these patients have an aminoglycoside half-life of 30 to 70 hours off hemodialysis and approximately 7 hours on hemodialysis. Following hemodialysis, patients experience a modest increase in serum aminoglycoside concentrations (a rebound effect). Peritoneal dialysis also affects the clearance of aminoglycosides.

Aminoglycoside that is added to the peritoneal dialysate can also be expected to cross over to the systemic circulation.

PHYSIOLOGIC CLEARANCE CHARACTERISTICS. Zaske and colleagues have over the years reported substantial inter-patient and intrapatient variability in distribution volume and the rate of aminoglycoside clearance among a wide range of patients [11–16,201,204,220,225,226]. Initially, reports of extraordinary dosage requirements in burn patients by Zaske and others prompted many clinicians to consider pharmacokinetics in this patient population as a unique exception to the usual aminoglycoside pharmacokinetics [11,16,201,204]. The underlying principles contributing to the changes in distribution volume and clearance of aminoglycoside seen in burn patients also apply to the critically ill. A young traumatized patient with a high cardiac output clears aminoglycosides at a much faster rate during the hypermetabolic state compared to the normal state. Dehydrated or overhydrated patients obviously require less or more drug, respectively, to achieve targeted concentrations for aminoglycoside serum concentration. Extremely hypotensive patients and patients in renal shutdown do not require aminoglycoside with the same frequency as a hypermetabolic patient. Thus the patient's underlying condition or any attempts to alter preload, afterload, stroke volume, heart rate, or any alterations in distribution volume affect aminoglycoside dosage requirements.

DOSING GUIDELINES

Loading Dose. In most situations, an aminoglycoside loading dose is not required. Patients with normal serum half-lives (2–3 hours) or those with very short half-lives (<2 hours) will reach 87 percent of steady state after three half-lives and 97 percent of steady state after five half-lives. Thus, in most patients steady-state aminoglycoside concentrations are achieved after only one or two doses of drug. If a loading dose is to be used, there is usually only a modest difference between the loading and maintenance dose. For gentamicin and tobramycin, a typical loading dose would be 1.75 to 2 mg per kilogram, while the maintenance dose would approximate 1.5 mg per kilogram. For amikacin, a typical loading dose would be 7.5 mg per kilogram, whereas the maintenance dose would approximate 5 mg per kilogram.

Maintenance Dose. Appropriate dosing of aminoglycosides is directly linked to renal function. A variety of nomograms have been developed in an attempt to incorporate some measure of renal function into the determination of aminoglycoside dose; however, most nomograms continue to promote 8-hour dosing. Lesar et al. [220] compared the dosing methods of Dettli [213], Sarubbi and Hull [227], and Chan et al. [211] and the manufacturer's dosage recommendations [228] to an individualized pharmacokinetic approach [225] in establishing appropriate peak and trough aminoglycoside serum concentrations. This work clearly established the superiority of an individualized approach over nomogram dosing of aminoglycosides at achieving a targeted range of aminoglycoside concentrations. This work has been confirmed by others [192].

While dependence on population data for establishing aminoglycoside dosage throughout the course of therapy is inappropriate, population data can be used to establish an initial aminoglycoside dose and interval that can later be refined with the use of actual serum-concentration-time data. In attempting to perform these calculations, several patient-specific parameters need to be determined or calculated [229]. Actual body weight (ABW) needs to be determined and lean body weight

(LBW) needs to be calculated (LBW-male = 50 + 2.3 (no. of inches > 5 ft in height); LBW-female = 45 + 2.3 (no. of inches > 5 ft in height)). If there is a large difference between ABW and LBW, many clinicians prefer to use dosing body weight (DBW), which is calculated as LBW plus 40 percent of the difference between ABW and LBW (DBW = LBW + 0.40 (ABW − LBW)).

After determining LBW, the patient's age and serum creatinine need to be determined. From these data, creatinine clearance (CrCl) can be calculated using the method of Cockroft and Gault [230]. An estimated elimination rate constant can then be calculated using the method of Dettli (K_d = 0.0024 (CrCl) + 0.01) [213]. An estimated half-life can then be determined by dividing the natural logarithm of 2 by the calculated elimination rate constant ($t_{1/2} = Ln_2/K_d = 0.693/K_d$) [229].

If desired, a loading dose of 1.75 to 2 mg per kilogram of gentamicin or tobramycin or 7.5 mg per kilogram of amikacin can be administered. The loading dose and maintenance dose for these drugs should be based either on LBW or, if there is a large discrepancy between LBW and ABW, on DBW. Initial maintenance doses of gentamicin and tobramycin should be 1.5 mg per kilogram and for amikacin 5 mg per kilogram.

Dosage intervals can be estimated by multiplying the calculated half-life by a factor of 2 to 3 and adding the time for the aminoglycoside infusion. This value can then be rounded to a convenient interval of 6, 8, 12, or 24 hours.

Assuming the patient's fluid status and renal function remain stable, actual trough and peak aminoglycoside concentration can be determined after the patient has received the drug for three to five half-lives (87–97% of steady state). For this determination there cannot be significant variance from scheduled administration times and actual time of infusion. Once these data are available, a new dose and dosage interval can be determined using the method of Sawchuk et al. [225]. Using this method, patient-specific values for the elimination rate constant and distribution volume are used to individualize the patient's dose and dosage interval to obtain desired peak and trough concentrations.

Single Daily Dose Therapy. Over the past few years, once daily or single daily dosing of aminoglycosides has become popular among some clinicians [208]. The rationale behind this dosing strategy is multifactorial. Because aminoglycosides are concentration-dependent killers of bacteria, increased concentrations of aminoglycoside would theoretically increase the rate and extent of bacterial killing [1,208]. With a longer than traditional dosage interval (24 hours vs. 8 hours), aminoglycoside accumulation, and hence drug-related adverse effects, are theoretically reduced. There is also evidence to suggest that transport of aminoglycoside into the inner ear and kidneys may be a saturable process [208,224]. Thus, administering the daily dose of aminoglycoside as a single dose may result in lower tissue concentrations than if the same dose were divided and administered several times over the course of 24 hours. Finally, long dosage intervals that promote an aminoglycoside washout or a relatively aminoglycoside-free period during the dosage interval may overcome bacterial adaptive resistance mechanisms reported for aminoglycosides [1,208,223,224,231]. Adaptive resistance may also be overcome by combining the aminoglycoside with a beta-lactam antibiotic [123].

Rotschafer et al. reported that routine use of a 6 mg/kg/day dose of gentamicin or tobramycin in a large patient population would in some cases result in extremely high peak and trough concentrations and in other patients produce conventional levels of aminoglycoside [1]. These authors suggest that a combination of patient-specific pharmacokinetic parameters, relative susceptibility data of bacterial pathogens to aminoglycosides, and the pharmacodynamic principles associated with single daily dose therapy would likely result in a more favorable clinical outcome. They caution that in patients with long aminoglycoside half-lives ($\geq$ 4 hours) or in patients with resilient bacterial pathogens (gentamicin or tobramycin MICs $\geq$ 4 mg/L), single daily dose therapy may not be appropriate. Other patients with extremely sensitive pathogens (MIC $\leq$ 0.5 mg/L) may respond optimally to conventional levels (6–8 mg/L gentamicin or tobramycin) of aminoglycoside depending on the site of infection [1].

DRUG INTERACTIONS. Aminoglycosides are seldom used as single agents for the treatment of gram-negative infections. This is especially true with pseudomonal infections, for which aminoglycosides are generally combined with an antipseudomonal penicillin or an antipseudomonal cephalosporin. In some institutions the antipseudomonal penicillin is mixed in the same intravenous piggyback container with the aminoglycoside, in an attempt to reduce the cost of parenteral antibiotic administration. This combination is unstable, however, in that the antipseudomonal penicillin inactivates the aminoglycoside [232–237].

This chemical reaction is governed by the molar quantities of the antipseudomonal penicillin, molar quantities of aminoglycosides, the generation of penicillin intermediates, temperature, and the period of time over which the reaction is allowed to progress [232–235]. Of the antipseudomonal penicillins, carbenicillin is the most problematic in this reaction [236,237]. Of the aminoglycosides, gentamicin and tobramycin were more likely to be inactivated, while amikacin was more stable to inactivation [234,235]. As a result of these studies, the practice of mixing antipseudomonal penicillins with aminoglycosides has been abandoned.

From a clinical perspective, this chemical reaction could still be a problem when aminoglycoside serum concentrations are measured in the presence of beta-lactam antibiotics. The laboratory should have in place a procedure (sera separated and refrigerated or frozen) where blood samples obtained for aminoglycoside analysis are rapidly processed, especially during evening, weekend, and holiday hours. The crucial link in this process is the rapid transportation of the blood sample from the patient's bedside to the laboratory for appropriate processing.

Schentag et al. suggested chemical complexation between the aminoglycoside and either ticarcillin or carbenicillin as an alternative to hemodialysis in reducing elevated serum levels of aminoglycoside [238]. Complexation could be used in situations where there may be an extended delay in implementing hemodialysis. The procedure would undoubtedly be less expensive when compared to hemodialysis and possibly associated with less toxicity. While these authors clearly demonstrate that the use of ticarcillin or carbenicillin can lower aminoglycoside serum concentrations, few data are available regarding the potential toxicity of the chemical complex. This strategy is obviously of considerably less value for amikacin than for gentamicin or tobramycin.

COMMON PITFALLS. Perhaps the greatest difficulty in monitoring aminoglycoside therapy is the evaluation of serum concentration-time data. Documentation of the exact start time and stop time of the intravenous infusion and the exact times that serum samples are obtained are crucial to any meaningful interpretation of the serum concentration-time data. These data should be permanently recorded in the patient's medical record.

The aminoglycoside concentration obtained following antibiotic administration, the so-called "peak concentration," must be evaluated in a proper spatial relationship to the end of intravenous infusion. The dose of aminoglycoside must be evenly administered during the infusion period, with a tubing flush during infusion. This is especially critical in pediatric or neonate patients, in whom the period of intravenous infusion may only deposit the aminoglycoside into the intravenous infusion set but not deliver the entire dose or even a high percentage of the dose to the patient. If another medication is to be administered using the same intravenous line following administration of the aminoglycoside, the remaining aminoglycoside present in the infusion set will be delivered to the patient, further corrupting the pharmacokinetic study.

Distribution volume is a dose-sensitive parameter that can be significantly altered when the patient receives more aminoglycoside or less aminoglycoside than what is assumed to be the correct dose. Any situation where the patient receives less drug than what is assumed will result in an overestimate of distribution volume. Conversely, any situation where the patient receives more drug than what is assumed will result in an underestimate of distribution volume.

A number of clinical situations can affect the calculation of the distribution volume [229]. Intravenous infiltration or incomplete administration that results in the patient receiving only a fraction of the assumed dose will result in an overestimate in distribution volume. Aminoglycosides must be administered at an even rate throughout the period of intravenous administration if an accurate determination of distribution volume is to be made. Errors in preparation and/or administration of the drug such that the patient receives less aminoglycoside than the assumed correct dose will result in an overestimate of distribution volume. Another artifact that can alter the determination of distribution volume is aminoglycoside inactivation. As previously discussed, this can result from mixing the beta-lactam antibiotic with the aminoglycoside in the same container or through improper handling and processing of aminoglycoside serum samples that contain beta-lactam antibiotic. Calculating distribution volume from trough and peak determinations not performed under steady-state conditions will also misrepresent the true distribution volume [206]. Artifact from aminoglycoside quantitative assay methods can affect the distribution volume determination especially if the same patient is studied at different times using different assay methods [194,198,199]. As previously discussed, there are differences in what constitutes a normal range of values for distribution volume (L/kg) in a patient at or near their LBW compared to obese patients. A distribution volume of 0.30 liter per kilogram in an obese patient may be the equivalent of 0.60 liter per kilogram in a patient at LBW. This "normal" distribution volume can be easily overlooked in the obese patient and potentially result in an overdose, whereas the abnormal volume of 0.60 liter per kilogram in a patient at or near LBW is much less likely to be overlooked.

There are physiologic situations in which distribution volume may be quite large. Anasarca, ascites, pleural effusion, active profuse bleeding, and the presence of a surgical drain that results in removal of large quantities of fluid containing aminoglycoside are situations in which the distribution volume is larger than normal. Infusion of large quantities of intravenous fluids and/or blood products over short periods to maintain homeostasis can have a dilutional effect on aminoglycoside concentrations, making the volume appear larger than it actually is.

Any situation that results in the patient receiving more drug than what is assumed to be the correct dose will result in an underestimate of distribution volume. The most common physiologic reason for a reduced distribution is dehydration. When distribution volume is expressed in liter per kilogram of ABW, the value for body weight should be checked for accuracy and possible transcription error.

Whenever distribution volume appears outside the "normal" range, the clinician should seek biologic explanations. The lack of such explanation dictates the need for timely follow-up studies to confirm the original pharmacokinetic data and dosage recommendations. Clinical experience would suggest that artifact is responsible for the vast majority of abnormal distribution volumes. Only when the original pharmacokinetic parameters are confirmed with follow-up data should the clinician accept an explanation of the patient being a statistical outlier.

Conclusion

The critically ill patient represents a unique challenge to the clinician in terms of appropriate antibiotic selection and dosage. Current data suggest that empiric or fixed doses of antibiotic are in many cases not likely to accommodate the physiologic changes seen in hypermetabolic or hypometabolic critically ill patients. Because most antibiotics are cleared renally, appropriate dosage is extremely sensitive to the interventions attempted clinically to alter cardiac output and support blood pressure. Because of the variation seen among patients and within the same patient with regard to antibiotic pharmacokinetic parameters and dosage requirements, objective serum-concentration-time data may represent the only practical means of appropriately adjusting dose and dosage interval. Obviously, more data are required to establish the value of a large dose but infrequent administration of antibiotics that demonstrate concentration-dependent antibacterial activity or continuous administration of antibiotics that demonstrate concentration-independent antibacterial activity.

References

1. Rotschafer JC, Zabinski RA, Walker KJ: Pharmacodynamic factors of antibiotic efficacy. *Pharmacotherapy* 12:S64, 1992.
2. Classen DC, Evans RS, Pestotnik SL, et al: The timing of prophylactic administration of antibiotics and the risk of surgical-wound infection. *N Engl J Med* 326:281, 1992.
3. Ericsson CD, Fischer RP, Rowlands BJ, et al: Prophylactic antibiotics in trauma: The hazards of underdosing. *J Trauma* 29:1356, 1989.
4. Page CP, Bohnen JMA, Fletcher R, et al: Antimicrobial prophylaxis for surgical wounds: Guidelines for clinical care. *Arch Surg* 128:79, 1993.
5. Reed RL, Ericsson CD, Wu A, et al: The pharmacokinetics of prophylactic antibiotics in trauma. *J Trauma* 32:21, 1992.
6. Reed RL: Antibiotic choices in surgical intensive care unit patients. *Surg Clin North Am* 71:765, 1991.
7. Dofferhoff ASM, Nijland JH, deVries-Hospers HG, et al: Effects of different types and combinations of antimicrobial agents on endotoxin release from gram-negative bacteria. *Scand J Infect Dis* 23:745, 1991.
8. Hurley JC, Louis WJ, Tosolini FA, et al: Antibiotic-induced release of endotoxin in chronically bacteriuric patients. *Antimicrob Agents Chemother* 35:2388, 1991.
9. Parrillo JE: Pathogenetic mechanisms of septic shock. *N Engl J Med* 328:1471, 1993.
10. Zokufa HZ, Rodvold KA, Blum RA, et al: Simulation of vancomycin peak and trough concentrations using five dosing methods in 37 patients. *Pharmacotherapy* 9:10, 1989.
11. Zaske DE, Chin T, Kohls PR, et al: Initial dosage regimens of gentamicin in patients with burns. *J Burn Care Rehabil* 12:46, 1991.
12. Zaske DE, Strate RG, Kohls PR: Amikacin pharmacokinetics: Wide interpatient variation in 98 patients. *J Pharmacol* 31:158, 1991.
13. Zaske DE, Cipolle RJ, Rotschafer JC, et al: Gentamicin pharmacokinetics in 1,640 patients: Method for control of serum concentrations. *Antimicrob Agents Chemother* 21:407, 1982.
14. Zaske DE, Irvine P, Strand LM, et al: Wide interpatient variations in gentamicin dose requirements for geriatric patients. *JAMA* 248:3122, 1982.
15. Zaske DE, Cipolle RJ, Strate RJ: Gentamicin dosage requirements: Wide interpatient variations in 242 surgery patients with normal renal function. *Surgery* 87:164, 1980.
16. Zaske DE, Sawchuk RJ, Gerding DN, et al: Increased dosage requirements of gentamicin in burn patients. *J Trauma* 16:824, 1976.
17. Shikuma LR, Ackerman BW, Weaver RH, et al: Effects of treatment and the metabolic response to injury on drug clearance: A prospective study with piperacillin. *Crit Care Med* 18:37, 1990.
18. Shikuma LR, Ackerman BW, Weaver RH, et al: Thermal injury effects on drug disposition: A prospective study with piperacillin *J Clin Pharmacol* 30:632, 1990.
19. Rodvold KA, Zokufa H, Rotschafer JC: Routine monitoring of serum vancomycin concentrations: Can waiting be justified? *Clin Pharm* 6:655, 1987.
20. Rotschafer JC, Garrison MW, Rodvold KA: Therapeutic update on glycopeptide and lipopeptide antibiotics *Pharmacotherapy* 8:211, 1988.
21. Rotschafer JC: *Vancomycin.* Irving, TX, Abbott Laboratories, 1986.
22. Matzke GR: *Vancomycin.* 3rd ed. Vancouver, WA, Edwards Brothers, 1992.
23. Fekety R, Silva J, Armstrong J: Treatment of antibiotic associated enterocolitis with vancomycin. *Rev Infect Dis* 3:S273, 1981.
24. Craig WA: *The Postantibiotic Effect.* Baltimore, Williams & Wilkins, 1986.
25. Schwalbe RS, Stapleton JT, Gilligan PH: Emergence of vancomycin resistance in coagulase-negative staphylococci. *N Engl J Med* 316:927, 1987.
26. Sabath LD, Wheeler N: A new type of penicillin resistance of *Staphylococcus aureus. Lancet* 1:443, 1977.
27. Chambers HF, Miller RT, Newman MD: Right-sided *Staphylococcus aureus* endocarditis in intravenous drug abusers: Two week combination therapy. *Ann Intern Med* 109:619, 1988.
28. Small PM, Chambers HF: Vancomycin for *Staphylococcus aureus* endocarditis in intravenous drug users. *Antimicrob Agents Chemother* 34:1227, 1990.
29. Karchmer AW: *Staphylococcus aureus* and vancomycin: The sequel. *Ann Intern Med* 115:739, 1991.
30. Faville RJ, Zaske DE, Kaplan EL, et al: *Staphylococcus aureus* endocarditis: Combined therapy with vancomycin and rifampin. *JAMA* 240:1963, 1978.
31. Levine DP, Fromm BS, Reddy BR: Slow response to vancomycin or vancomycin plus rifampin in methicillin-resistant *Staphylococcus aureus* endocarditis. *Ann Intern Med* 115:674, 1991.
32. Tofte RW, Solliday J, Rotschafer J, et al: *Staphylococcus aureus* infection of dialysis shunt: Absence of synergy with vancomycin and rifampin. *South Med J* 74:612, 1981.
33. Murray BE: New aspects of antimicrobial resistance and the resulting therapeutic dilemmas. *J Infect Dis* 163:1185, 1991.
34. Murray BE: The life and times of the *Enterococcus. Clin Microbiol* 3:46, 1990.
35. Noble WC, Virani Z, Cree RGA: Co-transfer of vancomycin and other resistance genes from *Enterococcus faecalis* NCTC 12201 to *Staphylococcus aureus. FEMS Microbiology Letters* 93:195, 1992.
36. Caron F, Carbon C, Gutmann L: Triple-combination penicillin-vancomycin-gentamicin for experimental endocarditis caused by a moderately penicillin- and highly glycopeptide resistant isolate of *Enterococcus faecium. J Infect Dis* 164:888, 1991.
37. Herman DJ, Gerding DN: Antimicrobial resistance among enterococci. *Antimicrob Agents Chemother* 35:1, 1991.
38. Leclercq R, Derlot E, Duval J, et al: Plasmid-mediated resistance to vancomycin and teicoplanin in *Enterococcus faecium. Med Intell* 319:157, 1988.
39. Knowles D, Good V, Autie M, et al: Antistaphylococcal activity of vancomycin and teicoplanin under anaerobic conditions. *Antimicrob Agents Chemother* 31:323, 1993.
40. Cooper GL, Given DB: *Vancomycin: A Comprehensive Review of*

30 Years of Clinical Experience. New York, Park Row Publishers, 1986.

41. Pfeiffer RR: Structural features of vancomycin. *Rev Infect Dis* 3:S205, 1981.
42. Watanakunakorn C: The antibacterial action of vancomycin. *Rev Infect Dis* 3:S210, 1981.
43. Geraci JE: Vancomycin. *Mayo Clin Proc* 52:631, 1977.
44. Fitzsimmons WE, Postelnick MJ, Tortorice PV: Survey of vancomycin monitoring guidelines in Illinois hospitals. *Drug Intell Clin Pharm* 22:598, 1988.
45. Edwards DJ, Pancorbo S: Routine monitoring of serum vancomycin concentrations: Waiting for proof of its value. *Clin Pharm* 6:652, 1987.
46. Freeman CD, Quintiliani R, Nightingale CH: Vancomycin therapeutic drug monitoring: Is it necessary? *Ann Pharmacother* 27:594, 1993.
47. Pryka RD, Rodvold KA, Garrison M, et al: Individualizing vancomycin dosage regimens: One- versus two-compartment bayesian models. *Ther Drug Monit* 11:450, 1989.
48. Pryka RD, Rodvold KA, Erdman SM: An updated comparison of drug dosing methods. IV. Vancomycin. *Clin Pharmacokinet* 20:463, 1991.
49. Ackerman BH, Vannier AM, Eudy EB: Analysis of vancomycin time kill studies with *Staphylococcus* species by using a curve stripping program to describe the relationship between concentration and pharmacodynamic response. *Antimicrob Agents Chemother* 36:1766, 1992.
50. Peetermans WE, Hoogeterp JJ, Hazekamp-van Dokkum AM, et al: Antistaphylococcal activities of teicoplanin and vancomycin in vitro and in an experimental infection. *Antimicrob Agents Chemother* 34:1869, 1990.
51. Farber BF, Moellering RC: Retrospective study of the toxicity of preparations of vancomycin from 1974 to 1981. *Antimicrob Agents Chemother* 23:138, 1983.
52. Rybak MJ, Albrecht LM, Boike SC, et al: Nephrotoxicity of vancomycin, alone and with an aminoglycoside. *J Antimicrob Chemother* 25:679, 1990.
53. Cimino MA, Rotstein C, Slaughter RL, et al: Relationship of serum antibiotic concentrations to nephrotoxicity in cancer patients receiving concurrent aminoglycoside and vancomycin therapy. *Am J Med* 83:1091, 1987.
54. Geraci JE, Heilman FR, Nichols DR, et al: Antibiotic therapy of bacterial endocarditis. VII. Vancomycin for acute micrococcal endocarditis. *Staff Meet Mayo Clin* 33:172, 1958.
55. Traber PG, Levine DP: Vancomycin ototoxicity in a patient with normal renal function. *Ann Intern Med* 95:458, 1981.
56. Lackner TE: Relationship of vancomycin concentrations of ototoxicity. *Arch Intern Med* 144:419, 1984.
57. Bailie GR, Neal D: Vancomycin ototoxicity and nephrotoxicity: A review. *Med Toxicol* 3:376, 1988.
58. Alexander MR: A review of vancomycin after 15 years of use. *Drug Intell Clin Pharm* 8:520, 1974.
59. Griffith RS: Introduction to vancomycin. *Rev Infect Dis* 3:S200, 1981.
60. New preparations of vancomycin. *Med Lett* 28:121, 1986.
61. Conte JE: Comparative antibacterial activity of vancocin and generic vancomycin. *Antimicrob Agents Chemother* 31:333, 1987.
62. Rotschafer JC, Crossley K, Zaske DE, et al: Pharmacokinetics of vancomycin: Observations in 28 patients and dosage recommendations. *Antimicrob Agents Chemother* 22:391, 1982.
63. Rodvold KA, Blum RA, Fischer JH, et al: Vancomycin pharmacokinetics in patients with various degrees of renal function. *Antimicrob Agents Chemother* 32:848, 1988.
64. Bryan CS, White WL: Safety of oral vancomycin in functionally anephric patients. *Antimicrob Agents Chemother* 14:634, 1978.
65. Dudley MN, Quintiliani R, Nightingale CH, et al: Absorption of vancomycin. *Ann Intern Med* 101:144, 1984.
66. Spitzer PG, Eliopoulos GM: Systemic absorption of enteral vancomycin in a patient with pseudomembranous colitis. *Ann Intern Med* 100:533, 1984.
67. Vance-Bryan K, Guay DR, Gilliland SS, et al: Effect of obesity on vancomycin pharmacokinetic parameters as determined by using a bayesian forecasting technique. *Antimicrob Agents Chemother* 37:436, 1993.
68. Blouin RA, Bauer LA, Miller DD, et al: Vancomycin pharmacoki-

netics in normal and morbidly obese subjects. *Antimicrob Agents Chemother* 21:575, 1982.
69. Polk RE: Anaphylactoid reactions to glycopeptide antibiotics. *J Antimicrob Chemother* 27:17, 1991.
70. Congeni B, Tan J, Salstrom SJ: Kinetics of vancomycin after intraventricular and intravenous administration (abstract 799). *Pediatr Res* 13:459, 1979.
71. Luer MS, Hatton J: Vancomycin administration into the cerebrospinal fluid: A review. *Ann Pharmacother* 27:912, 1993.
72. Lindholm DD, Murray JS: Persistence of vancomycin in the blood during renal failure and its treatment by hemodialysis. *N Engl J Med* 274:1047, 1966.
73. Krogstad DJ, Moellering RC, Greenblatt DJ: Single dose kinetics of intravenous vancomycin. *J Clin Pharmacol* 20:197, 1980.
74. Cutler NR, Narang PK, Lesko LJ, et al: Vancomycin disposition: The importance of age. *Clin Pharmacol Ther* 36:803, 1984.
75. Ackerman BH, Taylor EH, Olsen KM, et al: Vancomycin serum protein binding determination by ultrafiltration. *Drug Intell Clin Pharm* 22:300, 1988.
76. Zokufa HZ, Solem LD, Rodvold KA, et al: The influence of serum albumin and alpha-1-acid glycoprotein on vancomycin protein binding in patients with burn injuries. *J Burn Care Rehabil* 10:425, 1989.
77. Sun H, Maderazo EG, Krusell AR: Serum protein-binding characteristics of vancomycin. *Antimicrob Agents Chemother* 37:1132, 1993.
78. Wittendorf RW, Swagzdis JE, Gifford R, et al: Protein binding of glycopeptide antibiotics with diverse physical-chemical properties in mouse, rat, and human serum. *J Pharmacokinet Biopharm* 15:5, 1987.
79. Albrecht LM, Rybak MJ, Warbasse LH, et al: Vancomycin protein binding in patients with infections caused by *Staphylococcus aureus.* *Ann Pharmacother* 25:713, 1991.
80. Brown N, Ho DHW, Fong KL, et al: Effects of hepatic function on vancomycin clinical pharmacology. *Antimicrob Agents Chemother* 23:603, 1983.
81. Alpert G, Campos JM, Harris MC, et al: Vancomycin dosage in pediatrics reconsidered. *Am J Dis Child* 138:20, 1984.
82. Gross JR, Kaplan SL, Kramer WG, et al: Vancomycin pharmacokinetics in premature infants. *Pediatr Pharmacol* 5:17, 1985.
83. James A, Koren G, Milliken J, et al: Vancomycin pharmacokinetics and dose recommendations for preterm infants. *Antimicrob Agents Chemother* 31:52, 1987.
84. Naqvi SH, Keenan WJ, Reichley RM, et al: Vancomycin pharmacokinetics in small, seriously ill infants. *Am J Dis Child* 140:107, 1986.
85. Schaad UB, McCracken GH, Nelson JD: Clinical pharmacology and efficacy of vancomycin in pediatric patients. *J Pediatr* 96:119, 1980.
86. Moellering RC, Krogstad DJ, Greenblatt DJ: Pharmacokinetics of vancomycin in normal subjects and in patients with reduced renal function. *Rev Infect Dis* 3:S230, 1981.
87. Bailie GR, Ackerman BH, Fischer J, et al: Increased vancomycin dosage requirements in young patients. *J Burn Care Rehabil* 5:376, 1984.
88. Garrelts JC, Peterie JD: Altered vancomycin dose vs serum concentration relationship in burn patients. *Clin Pharmacol Ther* 44:9, 1988.
89. Rybak MJ, Albrecht LM, Berman JR, et al: Vancomycin pharmacokinetics in burn patients and intravenous drug abusers. *Antimicrob Agents Chemother* 34:792, 1990.
90. Lanese DM, Alfrey PS, Molitoris BA: Markedly increased clearance of vancomycin during hemodialysis using polysulfone dialyzers. *Kidney Int* 35:1409, 1989.
91. Torras J, Cao C, Rivas MC, et al: Pharmacokinetics of vancomycin in patients undergoing hemodialysis with polyacrylonitrile. *Clin Nephrol* 36:35, 1991.
92. Blevins RD, Halstenson CE, Salem NG, et al: Pharmacokinetics of vancomycin in patients undergoing continuous ambulatory peritoneal dialysis. *Antimicrob Agents Chemother* 25:603, 1984.
93. Morse GD, Farolino DF, Apicella MA, et al: Comparative study of intraperitoneal and intravenous vancomycin pharmacokinetics during continuous ambulatory peritoneal dialysis. *Antimicrob Agents Chemother* 31:173, 1987.
94. Magera BE, Arroyo JC, Rosansky SJ, et al: Vancomycin pharma-

cokinetics in patients with peritonitis on peritoneal dialysis. *Antimicrob Agents Chemother* 23:710, 1983.

95. Slugg PH, Haug MT, Bosworth C, et al (eds): *Comparative Vancomycin Kinetics in Intensive Care Unit Patients with Acute Renal Failure: Intermittent Hemodialysis versus Continuous Hemofiltration Hemodialysis.* Basel, Karger, 1991.

96. Matzke GR, O'Connell MB, Collins AJ, et al: Disposition of vancomycin during hemofiltration. *Clin Pharmacol Ther* 40:425, 1986.

97. Morse GD, Nairn DK, Bertino JS, et al: Overestimation of vancomycin concentrations utilizing fluorescence polarization immunoassay in patients on peritoneal dialysis. *Ther Drug Monit* 9:212, 1987.

98. Perino LM, Mueller BA: Accuracy of vancomycin serum concentrations in patients with renal failure. *Ann Pharmacother* 27:892, 1993.

99. Burkhart KK, Metcalf S, Shurnas E, et al: Exchange transfusion and multidose activated charcoal following vancomycin overdose. *Clin Toxicol* 30:285, 1992.

100. Davis RL, Roon RA, Koup JA, et al: Effect of orally administered activated charcoal on vancomycin clearance. *Antimicrob Agents Chemother* 31:720, 1987.

101. Polk RE, Healy DP, Schwartz LB, et al: Vancomycin and the redman syndrome: Pharmacodynamics of histamine release. *J Infect Dis* 157:502, 1988.

102. Matzke GR, McGory RW, Halstenson CE, et al: Pharmacokinetics of vancomycin in patients with various degrees of renal function. *Antimicrob Agents Chemother* 25:433, 1984.

103. Nielsen HE, Hansen HE, Korsager B, et al: Renal excretion of vancomycin in kidney disease. *Acta Med Scand* 197:261, 1975.

104. Lake KD, Peterson CD: A simplified dosing method for initiating vancomycin therapy. *Pharmacotherapy* 5:340, 1985.

105. Buckley MM, Brogden RN, Barradell LB, et al: Imipenem/cilastatin: A reappraisal of its antibacterial activity, pharmacokinetic properties and therapeutic efficacy. *Drugs* 44:408, 1992.

106. Clissold SP, Todd PA, Campoli-Richards DM: Imipenem/cilastatin. *Drugs* 33:183, 1987.

107. Danziger LH, Creger RJ, Shwed JA, et al: Randomized trial of imipenem-cilastatin versus gentamicin plus clindamycin in the treatment of polymicrobial infections. *Pharmacotherapy* 8:315, 1988.

108. Jaresko GS, Barriere SL: Imipenem monotherapy versus combination therapy in the management of mixed bacterial infection: A critical appraisal. *Pharmacotherapy* 8:324, 1988.

109. Solomkin JS, Dellinger EP, Christou NV, et al: Results of a multicenter trial comparing imipenem/cilastatin to tobramycin/clindamycin for Intra-abdominal infections. *Ann Surg* 212:581, 1990.

110. Hellinger WC, Brewer NS: Imipenem. *Mayo Clin Proc* 66:1074, 1991.

111. Sobel JD: Imipenem and aztreonam. *Infect Dis Clin North Am* 3:613, 1989.

112. Quinn JP, Studemeister AE, DiVincenzo CA, et al: Resistance to imipenem in *Pseudomonas aeruginosa*: Clinical experience and biochemical mechanisms. *Rev Infect Dis* 10:892, 1988.

113. Livermore DM: Interplay of impermeability and chromosomal b-lactamase activity in imipenem-resistant *Pseudomonas aeruginosa*. *Antimicrob Agents Chemother* 36:2046, 1992.

114. Craig WA, Ebert SC: Continuous infusion of b-lactam antibiotics. *Antimicrob Agents Chemother* 36:2577, 1992.

115. Drusano GL: Human pharmacodynamics of beta-lactams, aminoglycosides and their combinations. *Scand J Infect Dis* 74:235, 1991.

116. Vogelman B, Gudmundsson S, Leggett J, et al: Correlation of antimicrobial pharmacokinetic parameters with therapeutic efficacy in an animal model. *J Infect Dis* 158:831, 1988.

117. *Imipenem and Cilastatin Sodium.* Bethesda, MD, American Society of Hospital Pharmacists, 1993.

118. MacGregor RR, Gibson GA, Bland JA: Imipenem pharmacokinetics and body fluid concentrations in patients receiving high-dose treatment for serious infections. *Antimicrob Agents Chemother* 29:188, 1986.

119. Wise R, Donovan IA, Lockley MR, et al: The pharmacokinetics and tissue penetration of imipenem. *J Antimicrob Chemother*. 18:93, 1986.

120. Erttmann M, Krause U, Ullmann U: Pharmacokinetics of imipenem in patients undergoing major colon surgery. *Infection* 18:367, 1990.

121. Norrby SR, Alestig K, Bjornegard B, et al: Urinary recovery of n-formimidoyl thienamycin (MK0787) as affected by coadministra-

tion of n-formimidoyl thienamycin dehydropeptidase inhibitors. *Antimicrob Agents Chemother* 23:300, 1983.

122. Verpooten GA, Verbist L, Buntinx AP, et al: The pharmacokinetics of imipenem (thienamycin-foramidine) and the renal dihydropeptidase inhibitor cilastatin sodium in normal subjects and patients with renal failure. *Br J Clin Pharmacol* 18:183, 1984.

123. Toon S, Hopkins KJ, Garstang FM, et al: Pharmacokinetics of imipenem and cilastatin after their simultaneous administration to the elderly. *Br J Clin Pharmacol* 23:143, 1987.

124. Boucher AB, Hickerson WL, Kuhl DA, et al: Imipenem pharmacokinetics in patients with burns. *Clin Pharmacol Ther* 48:130, 1990.

125. Mueller BA, Scarim SK, Macias WL: Comparison of imipenem pharmacokinetics in patients with acute or chronic renal failure treated with continuous hemofiltration. *Am J Kidney Dis* 21:172, 1993.

126. Zajac BA, Fisher MA, Gibson GA, et al: Safety and efficacy of high-dose treatment with imipenem-cilastatin in seriously ill patients. *Antimicrob Agents Chemother* 27:745, 1985.

127. Acar JF: Therapy for lower respiratory tract infections with imipenem/cilastatin. *Rev Infect Dis* 7:S513, 1985.

128. Eron LJ: Imipenem/cilastatin therapy of bacteremia. *Am J Med* 78:95, 1985.

129. Salata RA, Gebhart RL, Palmer DL, et al: Pneumonia treated with imipenem/cilastatin. *Am J Med* 78:104, 1985.

130. King JH, Kailath EJ, Hardy DB: Successful use of higher than recommended dosage of imipenem in *Pseudomonas aeruginosa* endocarditis. *Ann Pharmacother* 26:639, 1992.

131. Tausk F, Evans ME, Patterson LS, et al: Imipenem-induced resistance to antipseudomonal β-lactams in *Pseudomonas aeruginosa*. *Antimicrob Agents Chemother* 28:41, 1985.

132. Calandra GB, Wang C, Aziz M, et al: The safety profile of imipenem/cilastatin: Worldwide clinical experience based on 3470 patients. *J Antimicrob Chemother* 18:193, 1986.

133. Calandra GB, Brown KR, Grad CL, et al: Review of adverse experiences and tolerability in the first 2,516 patients treated with imipenem/cilastatin. *Am J Med* 78:73, 1985.

134. Eng RHK, Munsif AN, Yangco BG, et al: Seizure propensity with imipenem. *Arch Intern Med* 149:1881, 1989.

135. Calandra GB, Lydick E, Carrigan J, et al: Factors predisposing to seizures in seriously ill infected patients receiving antibiotics: Experience with imipenem/cilastatin. *Am J Med* 84:911, 1988.

136. Soper DE: Clindamycin. *Obstet Gynecol Clin North Am* 19:483, 1992.

137. Rimmer D, Sales JEL: Lincomycin and clindamycin. *Antibiot Chemother* 23:204, 1978.

138. LeFrock JL, Molavi A, Prince RA: Clindamycin. *Med Clin North Am* 66:103, 1982.

139. Geddes AM, Bridgwater FAJ, Williams DN, et al: Clinical and bacteriological studies with clindamycin. *Br Med J* 2:703, 1970.

140. Bartlett JG, Sutter VL, Finegold SM: Treatment of anaerobic infections with lincomycin and clindamycin. *N Engl J Med* 16:1006, 1972.

141. Flaherty JF, Rodondi LC, Guglielmo BJ, et al: Comparative pharmacokinetics and serum inhibitory activity of clindamycin in different dosing regimens. *Antimicrob Agents Chemother* 32:1825, 1988.

142. Phillips I, Fernandes R, Warren C: In-vitro comparison of erythromycin, lincomycin, and clindamycin. *Br Med J* 2:89, 1970.

143. Pien FD, Thompson RL, Martin WJ: Clinical and bacteriologic studies of anaerobic gram-positive cocci. *Mayo Clin Proc* 47:251, 1972.

144. Lerner PI: Susceptibility of actinomyces species to lincomycin and its 7-halogenated analogues. *Antimicrob Agents Chemother* 461, 1968.

145. Nastro LJ, Finegold SM: Bactericidal activity of five antimicrobial agents against *Bacteroides fragilis*. *J Infect Dis* 126:104, 1972.

146. Craig W, Mattie H (eds): *Postantibiotic Effect (PAE) with Bacteroides Fragilis.* Abstracts of the 1986 ICAAC, 147, 1986.

147. Yagi BH, Schaadt RD, Zurenko GE: The bactericidal activity and postantibiotic effect of trospectomycin. *Diagn Microbiol Infect Dis* 15:417, 1992.

148. Santos JI, Arbo A, Pavia N: In vitro and In vivo effects of clindamycin on polymorphonuclear leukocyte function. *Clin Ther* 14:578, 1992.

149. Arbo A, Santos JI: The in vitro effects of clindamycin on polymorphonuclear leukocyte function: A reassessment. *Drug Invest* 2:235, 1990.

150. Noess A, Hauge B, Solberg CO: Effects of clindamycin and cefuroxime on leukocyte membrane receptors and function. *Chemotherapy* 35:193, 1989.

151. Klempner MS, Styrt B: Clindamycin uptake by human neutrophils. *J Infect Dis* 144:472, 1981.

152. Hand WL, King-Thompson NL: Membrane transport of clindamycin in alveolar macrophages. *Antimicrob Agents Chemother* 21:241, 1982.

153. Howard RJ, Soucy DM: Potentiation of phagocytosis of bacteroides fragilis following incubation with clindamycin. *J Antimicrob Chemother* 12:63, 1983.

154. Lianou PE, Bassaris HP, Votta EG, et al: Interaction of subminimal inhibitory concentrations of clindamycin and gram-negative aerobic organisms: Effects on adhesion and polymorphonuclear leukocyte function. *J Antimicrob Chemother* 15:481, 1985.

155. Gemmell CG, Peterson PK, Schmeling D, et al: Potentiation of opsonization and phagocytosis of *Streptococcus pyogenes* following growth in the presence of clindamycin. *J Clin Invest* 67:1249, 1981.

156. DeHaan RM, Metzler CM, Schellenberg D, et al: Pharmacokinetic studies of clindamycin phosphate. *J Clin Pharmacol* 190, 1973.

157. DeHaan RM, Metzler CM, Schellenberg D, et al: Pharmacokinetic studies of clindamycin hydrochloride in humans. *Int J Clin Pharmacol Ther Toxicol* 6:105, 1972.

158. Mann HJ, Townsend RJ, Fuhs DW, et al: Decreased hepatic clearance of clindamycin in critically ill patients with sepsis. *Clin Pharm* 6:154, 1987.

159. Panzer JD, Brown DC, Epstein WL, et al: Clindamycin levels in various body tissues and fluids. *J Clin Pharmacol* 259, 1972.

160. Plott MA, Roth H: Penetration of clindamycin into synovial fluid. *Clin Pharmacol Ther* 11:577, 1970.

161. Vacek V, Hejzlar M, Slavik M, et al: Penetration of clindamycin into bone in man. *Chemotherapy* 17:22, 1972.

162. Nicholas P, Meyers BR, Levy RN, et al: Concentration of clindamycin in human bone. *Antimicrob Agents Chemother* 8:220, 1975.

163. Alexander JW, Alexander NS: The influence of route of administration on wound fluid concentration of prophylactic antibiotics. *J Trauma* 16:489, 1976.

164. Brown RB, Martyak SN, Barza M, et al: Penetration of clindamycin phosphate into the abnormal human biliary tract. *Ann Intern Med* 84:168, 1976.

165. Sales JEL, Sutcliffe M, O'Grady F: Excretion of clindamycin in the bile of patients with biliary tract disease. *Chemotherapy.* 19:11, 1973.

166. Philipson A, Sabath LD, Charles D: Transplacental passage of erythromycin and clindamycin. *Med Intell* 288:1219, 1973.

167. Picardi JL, Lewis HP, Tan JS, et al: Clindamycin concentrations in the central nervous system of primates before and after head trauma. *J Neurosurg* 43:717, 1975.

168. Kays MB, White RL, Gatti G, et al: Ex vivo protein binding of clindamycin in sera with normal and elevated alpha-1-acid glycoprotein concentrations. *Pharmacotherapy* 12:50, 1992.

169. Suh B, Craig WA, England AC, et al: Effect of free fatty acids on protein binding of antimicrobial agents. *J Infect Dis* 143:609, 1981.

170. Gordon RC, Regamey C, Kirby WMM: Serum protein binding of erythromycin, lincomycin, and clindamycin. *J Pharm Sci* 62:1074, 1973.

171. Eastwood JB, Gower PE: A study of the pharmacokinetics of clindamycin in normal subjects and patients with chronic renal failure. *Postgrad Med J* 50.710, 1974.

172. Avant GR, Schenker S, Alford RH: The effect of cirrhosis on the disposition and elimination of clindamycin. *Dig Dis* 20:223, 1975.

173. Metzler CM, DeHaan R, Schellenberg D, et al: Clindamycin dose-availability relationships. *J Pharm Sci* 62:591, 1973.

174. Lesar TS, Zaske DE: Antibiotics and hepatic disease. *Med Clin North Am* 66:257, 1982.

175. Williams DN, Crossley K, Hoffman C, et al: Parenteral clindamycin phosphate: pharmacology with normal and abnormal liver function and effect on nasal staphylococci. *Antimicrob Agents Chemother* 7:153, 1975.

176. Eng RHK, Gorski S, Person A, et al: Clindamycin elimination in patients with liver disease. *J Antimicrob Chemother* 8:277, 1981.

177. Brandl R. Arkenau C, Simon C, et al: Zur Pharmakokinetik von Clindamycin bei gestorter leber- und nierenfunktoin. *Med Wschr* 97:1057, 1972.

178. Hinthorn DR, Baker LH, Romig DA, et al: Use of clindamycin in patients with liver disease. *Antimicrob Agents Chemother* 9:498, 1976.

179. Bongiorno JR, Alcasid ML, Chiaramonte LT: Treatment of pneumonia in children with cleocin palmitate. *Curr Ther Res* 13:667, 1971.

180. Campbell IW, Hossack DJN, Munro JF: Absorption and urinary excretion of clindamycin palmitate in the elderly. *Curr Med Res Opin* 1:369, 1973.

181. Williams RL, Mamelok RD: Hepatic disease and drug pharmacokinetics. *Clin Pharmacokinet* 5:528, 1980.

182. Wilkinson GR, Shand DG: A physiological approach to hepatic drug clearance. *Clin Pharmacol Ther* 18:377, 1975.

183. Blaschke TF: Protein binding and kinetics of drugs in liver diseases. *Clin Pharmacokinet* 2:32, 1977.

184. Edwards DJ, Lalka D, Cerra F, et al: Alpha-1-acid glycoprotein concentration and protein binding in trauma. *Clin Pharmacol Ther* 31:62, 1982.

185. Pisciotta AV: Agranulocytosis during antibiotic therapy: Drug sensitivity or sepsis? *Am J Hematol* 42:132, 1993.

186. Hinthorn DR, Baker LH, Romig DA, et al: Endocarditis treated with clindamycin: Relapse and liver dysfunction. *South Med J* 70:823, 1977.

187. Elmore M, Rissing JP, Rink L, et al: Clindamycin-associated hepatotoxicity. *Am J Med* 57:627, 1974.

188. Zaske DE: *Aminoglycosides.* 3rd ed. Vancouver, WA, Edwards Brothers, 1992.

189. Moore RD, Smith CR, Lietman PS: The association of aminoglycoside plasma levels with mortality in patients with gram-negative bacteremia. *J Infect Dis* 149:443, 1984.

190. Moore RD, Smith CR, Lipsky JJ, et al: Risk factors for nephrotoxicity in patients treated with aminoglycosides. *Ann Intern Med* 100:352, 1984.

191. Moore RD, Lietman PS, Smith CR: Clinical response to aminoglycoside therapy: Importance of the ratio of peak concentration to minimal inhibitory concentration. *J Infect Dis* 155:93, 1987.

192. Erdman SM, Rodvold KA, Pryka RD: An updated comparison of drug dosing methods. III. Aminoglycoside antibiotics. *Clin Pharmacokinet* 20:374, 1991.

193. Dahlgren JG, Anderson ET, Hewitt WL: Gentamicin blood levels: A guide to nephrotoxicity. *Antimicrob Agents Chemother* 8:58, 1974.

194. Bleske BE, Larson TA, Rotschafer JC: Observed differences in amikacin pharmacokinetic parameters and dosage recommendations determined by enzyme immunoassay and fluorescence polarization immunoassay. *Ther Drug Monit* 9:48, 1987.

195. McConnell JS, Cohen J: Release of endotoxin from *Escherichia coli* by quinolones. *J Antimicrob Chemother* 18:765, 1986.

196. Jackson GG, Riff LJ: Pseudomonas bacteremia: Pharmacologic and other bases for failure of treatment with gentamicin. *J Infect Dis* 124:185, 1971.

197. Noone P, Parsons TMC, Pattison JR, et al: Experience in monitoring gentamicin therapy during treatment of serious gram-negative sepsis. *Br Med J* 16:475, 1974.

198. Rotschafer JC, Morlock C, Strand L, et al: Comparison of radioimmunoassay and immunoassay methods in determining gentamicin pharmacokinetic parameters and dosages. *Antimicrob Agents Chemother* 22:648, 1982.

199. Rotschafer JC, Berg HG, Nelson RB, et al: Observed differences in gentamicin pharmacokinetic parameters and dosage recommendations determined by fluorescent polarization immunoassay and radioimmunoassay methods. *Ther Drug Monit* 5:443, 1983.

200. Zaske DE, Cipolle RJ, Rotschafer JC, et al: Individualizing amikacin regimens: accurate method to achieve therapeutic concentrations. *Ther Drug Monit* 13:502, 1991.

201. Zaske DE, Bootman JL, Solem LB, et al: Increased burn patient survival with individualized dosages of gentamicin. *Surgery* 91:142, 1982.

202. Triginer C, Izquierdo I, Fernandez R, et al: Gentamicin volume of distribution in critically ill septic patients. *Intensive Care Med* 16:30, 1990.

203. Tholl DA, Shikuma LR, Miller TQ, et al: Physiologic response of stress and aminoglycoside clearance in critically ill patients. *Crit Care Med* 21:248, 1993.

204. Solem LD, Zaske D, Strate RG: Ecthyma gangrenosum: Survival with individualized antibiotic therapy. *Arch Surg* 114:580, 1979.

205. Rodvold KA, Pryka RD, Kuehl PG, et al: Bayesian forecasting of serum gentamicin concentrations in intensive care patients. *Clin Pharmacokinet* 18:409, 1990.

206. Rodvold KA, Zokufa H, Rotschafer JC: Aminoglycoside pharmacokinetic monitoring: An integral part of patient care? *Clin Pharm* 7:608, 1988.

207. Gill MA, Kern JW: Altered gentamicin distribution in ascitic patients. *Am J Hosp Pharm* 36:1704, 1979.

208. Gilbert DN: Once-daily aminoglycoside therapy. *Antimicrob Agents Chemother* 35:399, 1991.

209. Garrison MW, Zaske DE, Rotschafer JC: Aminoglycosides: Another perspective. *Ann Pharmacother* 24:267, 1990.

210. Destache CJ, Meyer SK, Bittner MJ, et al: Impact of a clinical pharmacokinetic service on patients treated with aminoglycosides: A cost-benefit analysis. *Ther Drug Monit* 12:419, 1990.

211. Chan RA, Benner EJ, Hoeprich RD: Gentamicin therapy in renal failure: A nomogram for dosage. *Ann Intern Med* 76:775, 1978.

212. Bootman JL, Wertheimer AI, Zaske D, et al: Individualizing gentamicin dosage regimens in burn patients with gram-negative septicemia: A cost-benefit analysis. *J Pharm Sci* 68:267, 1979.

213. Dettli LC: Drug dosage in patients with renal disease. *Clin Pharmacol Ther* 16:274, 1974.

214. Zaske DE, Crossley KB, Strate RJ: Aminoglycoside toxicity (Letter.) *N Engl J Med* 303:1002, 1980.

215. Smith CR, Baughman KL, Edwards CQ, et al: Controlled comparison of amikacin and gentamicin. *N Engl J Med* 296:349, 1977.

216. Smith CR, Lipsky JJ, Laskin L, et al: Double-blind comparison of the nephrotoxicity and auditory toxicity of gentamicin and tobramycin. *N Engl J Med* 302:1106, 1980.

217. Smith CR, Lipsky JJ, Lietman PS: Relationship between aminoglycoside-induced nephrotoxicity and auditory toxicity. *Antimicrob Agents Chemother* 15:780, 1979.

218. Flint LM, Gott J, Short L, et al: Serum level monitoring of aminoglycoside antibiotics: Limitations in intensive care unit-related bacterial pneumonia. *Arch Surg* 120:99, 1985.

219. Arroyo JC, Milligan WL, Davis J, et al: Impact of aminoglycoside serum assays on clinical decisions and renal toxicity. *South Med J* 79:272, 1986.

220. Lesar TS, Rotschafer JC, Strand LM, et al: Gentamicin dosing errors with four commonly used nomograms. *JAMA* 248:1190, 1982.

221. Nahata MC, Hipple TF, Clotz M: Interlot variability in gentamicin and tobramycin concentration and its possible significance. *Ther Drug Monit* 8:256, 1986.

222. Sketris I, Lesar T, Zaske DE, et al: Effect of obesity on gentamicin pharmacokinetics. *J Clin Pharmacol* 21:288, 1981.

223. Daikos GL, Jackson GG, Lolans VT, et al: Adaptive resistance to aminoglycoside antibiotics from first-exposure down-regulation. *J Infect Dis* 162:414, 1990.

224. Daikos GL, Lolans VT, Jackson GG: First-exposure adaptive resistance to aminoglycoside antibiotics in vivo with meaning for optimal clinical use. *Antimicrob Agents Chemother* 35:117, 1991.

225. Sawchuk RJ, Zaske DE, Cipolle RJ, et al: Kinetic model for gentamicin dosing with the use of individual patient parameters. *Clin Pharmacol Ther* 21:362, 1977.

226. Cipolle RJ, Siefert RD, Zaske DE, et al: Hospital acquired gramnegative pneumonias: Response rate and dosage requirements with individualized tobramycin therapy. *Ther Drug Monit* 2:359, 1980.

227. Sarubbi FA, Hull JH: Amikacin serum concentrations: Prediction of levels and dosage guidelines. *Ann Intern Med* 89:612, 1978.

228. *Garamycin sulfate.* Oradell, NJ, Medical Economics, 1981.

229. Rotschafer JC, Steinberg I: A rational approach to aminoglycoside therapy. *Minn Pharm* 6, 1985.

230. Cockroft DW, Gault MH: Prediction of creatinine clearance from serum creatinine. *Nephron* 16:31, 1976.

231. Jackson GG, Lolans VT, Daikos GL: The inductive role of ionic binding in the bacterial and postexposure effects of aminoglycoside antibiotics with implications for dosing. *J Infect Dis* 162:408, 1990.

232. Lackner TE, Rotschafer JC, Crossley K, et al: Assay specificity for biologically active gentamicin in serum. *Am J Hosp Pharm* 39:647, 1982.

233. Gensmantel NP, Page MI: The aminolysis of penicillin derivatives: Rate constants for the formation and breakdown of the tetrahedeal addition intermediate. *Chem Soc London* 2:137, 1979.

234. Glew RH, Pavuk RA: Stability of gentamicin, tobramycin, and amikacin in combination with four beta-lactam antibiotics. *Antimicrob Agents Chemother* 24:474, 1983.

235. Blair DC, Duggan DO, Schroeder ET: Inactivation of amikacin and gentamicin by carbenicillin in patients with end-stage renal failure. *Antimicrob Agents Chemother* 22:376, 1982.

236. Konishi H, Goto M, Nakamoto Y, et al: Tobramycin inactivation by carbenicillin, ticarcillin, and piperacillin. *Antimicrob Agents Chemother* 23:653, 1983.

237. Thompson MIB, Russo ME, Saxon BJ, et al: Gentamicin inactivation by piperacillin or carbenicillin in patients with end-stage renal disease. *Antimicrob Agents Chemother* 21:268, 1982.

238. Schentag JJ, Simons GW, Schultz RW, et al: Complexation versus hemodialysis to reduce elevated aminoglycoside serum concentrations. *Pharmacotherapy* 4:374, 1984.

213. Anticonvulsant Drugs

Susan J. Markowsky and Philip R. Kohls

Phenytoin

Phenytoin is an anticonvulsant indicated for the treatment of status epilepticus, tonic-clonic seizures, and partial seizures with complex symptomatology. It is also used for prophylaxis of seizures following trauma or neurosurgical procedures. Its value as an antiarrhythmic agent remains limited to the treatment of digitalis-induced arrhythmias.

PHARMACOLOGY. Phenytoin limits seizure development by selectively suppressing rapid, sustained, neuronal firing and ectopic burst generation. The probable mechanism involves blockade of sodium channels in excitatory pathways and prevention of increases in extracellular potassium concentrations and decreases in calcium concentrations. Limiting those perturbations inhibits neuronal depolarizations [1].

Phenytoin is also a class IB antiarrhythmic agent similar to lidocaine. Rapid infusion of phenytoin can precipitate arrhythmias. Hypotension also can result from the pharmacologic effects of the cosolvent, propylene glycol [2].

---

* For newer anticonvulsants, the authors recommend refernces 132, 133, 134 and 135 for information and applying the principles from this chapter.

THERAPEUTIC RANGE. The accepted therapeutic range for total serum phenytoin concentration (SPC) is 10 to 20 mg per liter, although levels as high as 25 to 30 mg per liter may be optimal in selected patients, especially those in status epilepticus. Based on an unbound (free) fraction of 10 percent, the therapeutic free concentration range is 1 to 2 mg per liter.

A 3-year prospective study of 32 patients demonstrated a significant decrease in seizure activity when SPCs were controlled to greater than 10 mg per liter [3]; when SPCs were increased to greater than 10 mg/L and later to greater than 14 mg/L, seizure frequency decreased by 30 percent and 70 percent, respectively. Results were similar for tonic-clonic and partial seizures. In another prospective study of the efficacy of SPCs, the mean (± SD) SPC required to maintain 100 percent seizure control for at least 1 year was 14 ± 9 mg per liter in patients with tonic-clonic seizures and 23 ± 9 mg per liter in patients with partial seizures [4]. In this study, 68 percent of patients were treated with phenytoin as a single agent.

Early signs of phenytoin toxicity include nystagmus, ataxia, and/or cognitive difficulty. At SPCs greater than 20 mg per liter, the most common adverse effect is nystagmus. With levels greater than 30 mg per liter, ataxia frequently occurs. If SPCs are greater than 40 mg per liter, lethargy or decreased cognition is likely [5]. The elderly seem to be more susceptible to these adverse effects. Increased seizure activity has been reported at concentrations greater than 40 mg per liter, but this adverse phenomenon is more probable when levels are greater than 80 mg per liter [6].

PREPARATIONS. Phenytoin is available for intravenous (IV) and oral administration. The most commonly used dosage forms (i.e., IV solutions and capsules) contain phenytoin sodium, which is 92% phenytoin. Chewable tablets and suspensions contain 100% phenytoin acid.

Solid dosage forms include 50-mg chewable tablets, prompt-release capsules (30 and 100 mg), and extended-release capsules (30 and 100 mg). The extended-release form is commonly known by the trade name Dilantin (Parke Davis, Morris Plains, NJ). Pediatric and adult formulations of Dilantin suspension contain 30 mg per 5 ml and 125 mg per 5 ml, respectively.

The parenteral formulation for intravenous administration contains 50 mg per milliliter of solution in 40% propylene glycol and 10% ethanol and has a pH of 10 to 12. Parenteral phenytoin is most compatible with normal saline at concentrations of 8 to 20 mg per milliliter [7]. Parenteral phenytoin should not be administered intramuscularly (IM).

A prodrug of phenytoin is currently undergoing clinical trials [8]. This drug is soluble in aqueous solutions without the need for a propylene glycol plus ethanol cosolvent system. This formulation may decrease the incidence of adverse cardiac effects and phlebitis due to intravascular precipitation of phenytoin. This new agent is rapidly converted to phenytoin by blood phosphatases and is more suitable than the commercially available phenytoin formulation for IM administration.

PHARMACOKINETICS. Table 213-1 summarizes phenytoin's pharmacokinetic parameters.

Absorption. Oral forms are 90 to 100 percent bioavailable. Absorption rates vary for different products (brands); therefore, it is advisable to use a product from one manufacturer consistently. Phenytoin absorption is slow due to the poor dissolution of phenytoin in acidic aqueous fluids. Peak SPCs occur 3 to 12 hours after an oral dose. Due to phenytoin's long elimination half-life, oral maintenance doses can usually be administered

Table 213-1. Summary of Phenytoin Pharmacokinetic Parameters

Bioavailability	
Capsules	92%
Chewable tablets	100%
Protein binding	90% (85–95%)
V_{dss}	0.8 L/kg
Clearance	Varies with concentration
	Capacity-limited metabolism
	V_{max} 5–7 mg/kg/day
	K_m 5–6 mg/L
	Hepatic >95%
	Renal <5%
Peritoneal dialysis	Negligible
Hemodialysis	Negligible
Hemoperfusion	Significant removal
Elimination half-life	Varies with phenytoin concentration

once daily, except in patients who rapidly metabolize phenytoin.

The absorption rate is dose-dependent, which means the rate of absorption decreases at higher doses [9,10,11]. For example, peak SPCs occur approximately 1 to 2 hours after a 200-mg oral dose. In contrast, the peak SPC is observed approximately 18 hours after an 800-mg dose. The concept of prolonged absorption with higher doses is important when administering loading doses and in overdose situations. Oral loading doses of phenytoin should be administered in divided doses of no more than 400 mg per dose every 2 to 4 hours.

The suspension should be used when phenytoin is administered via a nasogastric (NG) or feeding tube. The tube should be flushed before and after the dose with at least 30 ml of normal saline solution or water. Diluting the suspension enhances passage through the NG tube [12]. Continuous NG enteral feedings interfere with phenytoin absorption and lower serum phenytoin concentrations by up to 80 percent in trauma patients [13]. There are conflicting data in the literature regarding this problem [14].

Distribution. Distribution of phenytoin is complete in approximately 30 to 60 minutes [15]. Brain and cerebrospinal fluid concentrations are equal to plasma concentrations 10 to 20 minutes following infusion of a loading dose [16,17]. An IV infusion of phenytoin yields pharmacokinetic data best described by a one-compartment model with a mean V_{dss} of 0.75 liter per kilogram (range 0.6-1.0 L/kg) [15,18].

Phenytoin is extensively bound to serum albumin. The free fraction is normally about 10 percent of total drug [19]. Only free phenytoin is pharmacologically active. Phenytoin protein binding is decreased (i.e., the free fraction is increased) in hypoalbuminemic states and renal failure. Altered protein binding in renal failure may be explained by altered albumin conformation or the presence of an endogenous substance that displaces phenytoin from binding sites [20]. This displacing agent appears to be an endogenous peptide [21]. In addition to a decreased albumin concentration, patients with hepatic failure may have high serum bilirubin concentrations, which can displace phenytoin from binding sites on circulating proteins and increase the free fraction [22,23].

Hypoalbuminemic states with potential for an increased phenytoin free fraction include major trauma, burns, nephrotic syndrome, malnutrition, and surgery. In addition, elderly and chronically debilitated patients often have decreased serum albumin concentrations [23]. An increased free fraction occurs whenever albumin binding sites are decreased significantly relative to total drug concentrations. At therapeutic concentrations of phenytoin, a significant alteration of protein binding is most likely to occur when serum albumin concentrations are 2.5 gm per deciliter or less.

Due to competition for binding sites, the free fraction of phenytoin can be increased by other drugs with a high binding affinity for albumin. Such drugs include warfarin, sulfonamides, valproic acid, salicylates, and phenylbutazone [24].

Elimination/Metabolism. Phenytoin is 95 percent metabolized by the hepatic cytochrome P-450 system to inactive metabolites. The primary metabolite, 5-(p-hydroxyphenyl)-5-phenylhydantoin, is subsequently glucuronidated and renally excreted [25]. The Michaelis-Menten function can be used to describe the rate of elimination and clearance of phenytoin [26]. Thus,

$$\text{Rate of elimination} = \frac{V_{max} \times SPC_{ss}}{K_m SPC_{ss}}$$

where V_{max} is the maximum rate of elimination (velocity) in units of amount/time, K_m is the Michaelis-Menten constant, and SPC_{ss} is the steady-state phenytoin serum concentration (see Chap. 176).

The average values for V_{max} and K_m in adult epileptic patients are 6 to 8 mg per kilogram per day and 5 to 6 mg per liter, respectively [27,28]. However, these parameters exhibit wide variability. Since V_{max} and K_m occur at commonly used doses and concentrations, nonlinear pharmacokinetics are clinically observed and small changes in dosage can result in large changes in SPCs. When the dose administered and concentration obtained are lower than the patient's V_{max} and K_m values, linear pharmacokinetics will be observed. Aging is associated with decreasing V_{max} and lower phenytoin dosage requirements [29,30].

Clearance and elimination half-life ($t_{1/2}$) are concentration- and dose-dependent terms, which change during the dosing interval as concentration changes and thus are not commonly used when describing phenytoin elimination.

Extracorporeal clearance by peritoneal dialysis or hemodialysis is not clinically significant and extra doses after dialysis are not necessary [31].

PHYSIOLOGIC CLEARANCE CHARACTERISTICS.

Based on the physiologic models of hepatic drug clearance, phenytoin is classified as a capacity-limited, binding-sensitive drug [32,33]. It has a low hepatic extraction ratio (E = 0.03) associated with a low hepatic intrinsic clearance. Phenytoin is also highly protein-bound, with an unbound fraction of approximately 10 percent (f = 0.1). In addition, phenytoin exhibits nonlinear pharmacokinetics due to saturable metabolism [26,33]. Hepatic drug clearance is dependent on three factors: hepatic blood flow, drug metabolizing enzyme activity (hepatic intrinsic clearance), and protein binding [33]. Based on the physiologic model of hepatic metabolism, total hepatic clearance of capacity-limited, binding-sensitive drugs depends primarily on two of these factors: drug metabolizing enzyme activity and protein binding. Metabolism of low extraction drugs is independent of liver blood flow [33].

Hypodynamic States. If sustained, shock states may result in hepatic dysfunction characterized by jaundice, hyperbilirubinemia, or morphologic hepatic changes including cholestasis, centrilobular congestion, and hepatic necrosis [34–39]. Impaired hepatic function would be expected to reduce liver drug metabolizing activity by cytochrome enzymes. Since hepatic

clearance of phenytoin is independent of liver blood flow [33], hypodynamic states may theoretically lead to decreased hepatic total and unbound clearance due to decreased microsomal enzyme capacity. Frequent SPC monitoring is indicated to guide dosage adjustments. Coexisting conditions such as hypoalbuminemia and acute renal failure may increase phenytoin total clearance secondary to an increased unbound fraction (see Distribution).

Liver disease reduces clearance (Cl) of phenytoin and increases free concentrations of the drug [32]. Decreases in protein binding, which may occur secondary to hypoalbuminemia or drug displacement, also increase the free fraction of phenytoin. Free phenytoin is cleared faster than the bound drug. The net result may be lower total SPCs, a higher free fraction, unaltered dosage requirements, and an equivalent amount of free active drug in the serum. In this situation, monitoring of free SPCs is advised, if this assay is available.

Hyperdynamic States. Although not well studied, the hyperdynamic states observed following acute neurotrauma, major surgery, burn injuries, and brain hemorrhage may be associated with altered hepatic drug clearance. Due to dynamic fluctuations in the physiologic status of intensive care unit (ICU) patients, true steady-state conditions for drug elimination may not be achieved. Boucher et al. reported evidence suggesting that metabolism of phenytoin may be increased over time during the first 2 weeks following head trauma [40]. The mean V_{max} increased to 1348 mg per day (range 372–474 mg/day) during the first 2 weeks of therapy in patients with head injury. The median K_m value was 4.8 mg per liter (range 2.6–20 mg/L). Total phenytoin concentrations often drop well below the expected therapeutic range of 10 to 20 mg per liter within days following the initial IV loading doses and parenteral maintenance doses of 5 to 7.5 mg/kg/day in head trauma patients. The time-dependency and nonlinearity of phenytoin's pharmacokinetics in ICU patients make SPCs difficult to predict and steady-state conditions unlikely.

Hyperdynamic patients may have altered phenytoin protein binding due to hypoalbuminemia accompanying the hypermetabolic state [41,42]. Bauer et al. investigated the relationship between total and unbound phenytoin concentrations in 10 comatose head trauma patients [41]. They reported a higher fraction of free phenytoin in head trauma patients (21 + 3.2%) than in 10 otherwise healthy patients with epilepsy (10 + 1.3%, p < 0.0002). Hypoalbuminemia may result in increased total phenytoin hepatic clearance and decreased total phenytoin concentration due to an increase in the phenytoin free fraction [42].

DOSING GUIDELINES

Loading Dose. The recommended loading dose is 15 to 18 mg per kilogram [43]. A 15-mg per kilogram dose produces a postdistribution SPC of approximately 20 mg per liter. Thus,

$$\begin{aligned} \text{Dose} &= SPC \text{ desired} \times V_{dss} \\ &= 20 \text{ mg/L} \times 0.75 \text{ L/kg} \\ &= 15 \text{ mg/kg} \end{aligned}$$

This loading dose is usually adequate for seizure prophylaxis following head trauma or neurosurgical procedures. A loading dose of 18 to 20 mg per kilogram is recommended for status epilepticus. This dose produces initial postdistribution SPCs of 20 to 30 mg per liter [43].

Phenytoin should be diluted in 0.45% or 0.9% sodium chloride solution to a concentration of 8 to 20 mg per liter [7,44]. Further dilution markedly lowers the pH and concentration of propylene glycol (stabilizer), resulting in precipitation. A solution containing 10 mg per milliliter is recommended for peripheral infusion to decrease the incidence of phlebitis and discomfort [45]. The loading dose should be administered via a rate-controlling pump at a maximum rate of 50 mg per minute. Intravenous doses given faster than 50 mg per minute can cause hypotension and ventricular arrhythmias. These effects are probably due to the propylene glycol solvent [46]. For patients older than 70 years and those with atherosclerotic cardiovascular disease or hemodynamic instability, the maximum rate should be 25 mg per minute [45,47]. Due to potential hemodynamic instability, severe sepsis and therapeutic pentobarbital coma are other possible risk factors for phenytoin hypotension [48]. If hypotension or arrhythmias occur, the rate should be slowed by 50 percent and the patient should be reevaluated and other potential causes for the cardiac complications excluded [49].

An SPC can be obtained 1 to 2 hours after the loading dose has been completely infused to ensure that therapeutic drug levels have been achieved. This postloading SPC also can be used to calculate the patient-specific V_d, which can be used to individualize future bolus doses. In addition, this level acts as a baseline for evaluating the maintenance dose.

Maintenance Dose. The initial maintenance dose should be determined using population-based pharmacokinetic values. The first maintenance dose should be given approximately 12 hours after the loading dose. Table 213-2 provides recommendations for initial maintenance doses. Steady-state conditions for phenytoin clearance are not predictable in ICU patients; therefore dosing methods that utilize dosing nomograms or equations [29] should not be used in this patient population.

For young adult epileptic patients with normal liver function, the usual maintenance dose is 5 to 6 mg/kg/day administered in one to two daily doses to achieve accepted therapeutic total and unbound phenytoin concentrations of 10 to 20 and 1 to 2 mg per liter, respectively. In the majority of epileptic patients, daily doses of 5 to 6 mg/kg/day result in the accepted therapeutic range of phenytoin concentrations [30].

• Elderly patients and patients with significant hepatic dysfunction (e.g., cirrhosis and hepatic encephalopathy) require lower doses, frequent monitoring of SPCs, and physical examination for signs of phenytoin toxicity.

Hypodynamic ICU patients with sustained shock or multiple organ dysfunction syndrome secondary to sepsis may also require lower maintenance doses, but the supporting evidence is anecdotal and wide intrapatient and interpatient variability exists.

For hyperdynamic patients following trauma or central nervous system hemorrhage, 6 to 7.5 mg/kg/day can be administered in two to three divided doses. Patients with acute brain injury may require an increase in phenytoin dosage over time

to maintain therapeutic concentrations, possibly due to the hypermetabolic state [50]. In occasional patients with large dosage requirements (10–15 mg/kg/day), dosing intervals of IV phenytoin should be 6 to 8 hours to minimize peak-to-trough SPC fluctuations. Because oral formulations are absorbed slowly, they can be administered once or twice daily in most patients.

To ensure therapeutic drug levels, a trough SPC (i.e., a sample collected within 1 hour before the next dose) should be obtained 3 days after initiating the maintenance dose and twice weekly thereafter while the patient is in the ICU. Phenytoin clearance frequently increases in hyperdynamic surgical, burn, trauma, and neurosurgical patients during ICU care; however, during convalescence reversal of phenytoin hypermetabolism may be observed, resulting in multiple dosage adjustments. Medical and neurologic ICU patients (e.g., stroke, status epilepticus, metabolic disorders) typically require less frequent monitoring (once weekly) after the first week, if the seizure disorder is well controlled.

If a postloading SPC was obtained, it can be used as a baseline to evaluate the adequacy of the maintenance dose. If a postloading SPC was not obtained, an SPC drawn prior to the next morning dose can be used as a baseline or the postloading SPC can be estimated using the following equation:

$$SPC \text{ achieved} = SPC \text{ observed} + \frac{Dose}{V_d}$$

For example, if the morning SPC observed is 5 mg per liter, and a 600-mg phenytoin partial loading dose is administered intravenously to a 70-kg patient, then the estimated postloading SPC achieved is calculated as follows:

$$SPC \text{ achieved} = 5 + \frac{600 \text{ mg}}{(0.75 \text{ L/kg} \times 70 \text{ kg}}$$
$$= 5 + 11.4$$
$$= 16.4 \text{ mg/L}$$

If the trough level obtained on the third or fourth day of the maintenance dosage regimen decreases by 50 percent or more from the baseline or the SPC drops below 10 mg per liter, the patient should receive a partial loading dose to increase the SPC to approximately 15 to 20 mg per liter, followed by an increase in the maintenance dosage as described below. This method of reloading and monitoring SPCs circumvents the requirement that SPCs be obtained during steady-state conditions. Due to frequent changes in drug clearance in ICU patients, the condition of steady state cannot be assumed. Partial loading doses can be calculated using the following equation:

$$Dose = (SPC \text{ desired} - SPC \text{ observed}) \times V_d$$

Table 213-2. Phenytoin Initial Maintenance Dose Recommendations

Age	Disease state	Initial dose	Dose requirement range
Young adult	Epilepsy Mild head trauma Brain tumor	5–6 mg/kg/day	4–7 mg/kg/day
Adult	Severe head trauma Subarachnoid hemorrhage	6–7.5 mg/kg/day	7–15 mg/kg/day
Age > 70 yr	Epilepsy Stroke	4–5 mg/kg/day	3–6 mg/kg/day
Any age	Hepatic encephalopathy Cirrhosis	1–3 mg/kg/day	Reduced requirements Variable

For example, if the trough SPC is 7 mg per liter in a 70-kg patient, and the desired SPC is 15 mg per liter, then the estimated additional loading dose is calculated as follows:

$$\text{Dose} = (15 \text{ mg/L} - 7 \text{ mg/L}) \times (0.75 \text{ L/kg} \times 70 \text{ kg})$$
$$= 420 \text{ mg (which can be rounded off to 400 mg)}$$

If a postloading SPC is available, an estimate of the patient's V_d could be used in place of the population estimate (V_d = loading dose/observed SPC). Following the partial loading dose, the maintenance dose should be increased. Maintenance dose adjustments based on SPCs for ICU patients are summarized in Table 213-3.

The estimated therapeutic range of 10 to 20 mg per liter can be individualized as patient-specific experience is gained. If the patient has seizures or unexpected neurologic changes during therapy, an SPC obtained before an additional dose is administered can provide useful information regarding the patient-specific concentration-response relationship. A seizing patient can be given 50 percent of the initial loading dose in an effort to terminate the convulsion.

Measurements of free phenytoin concentrations may be of value in adjusting dosages in critically ill patients with hypoalbuminemia and is indicated when the albumin concentration is 2.5 gm per deciliter or less. If renal failure develops or drugs that displace phenytoin are added to the medication regimen, clinically significant changes in the free fraction can occur and free and total SPCs should be monitored more frequently.

When changing from IV to oral therapy, an equivalent dose of phenytoin should be administered. Since the suspension and tablet forms have 8 percent more phenytoin acid, consideration should be given to decreasing the dose slightly in patients well stabilized on the IV dosage form.

To decrease the effect of continuous enteral feedings on phenytoin absorption, tube feedings can be withheld for 1 hour before and after each phenytoin dose. Some patients receiving tube feedings require a significant increase in phenytoin dosage due to decreased availability. If the dose has been well-titrated in the presence of continuous enteral feedings, it is important to remember to decrease or withhold the dose if tube feedings are withheld for any reason. Because phenytoin exhibits nonlinear pharmacokinetics, a large change in absorption associated with discontinuing tube feedings can result in very high SPCs.

Following stabilization of head trauma patients, phenytoin clearance and dosage requirements decrease, often within the

Table 213-3. Phenytoin Maintenance Dosage Adjustment in ICU Patients

If the total phenytoin concentration is <10 μg/ml (free <15%) *or* the free phenytoin concentration is <1.0 μg/ml, then
1. Give partial loading dose to achieve total of 15 μg/ml
2. Increase maintenance dose by 0.5–1.0 mg/kg/day (for medical/neurologic patients) or 1.5–2 mg/kg/day (for patients with severe brain injury)

If the total phenytoin concentration is 10–20 μg/ml *or* the free phenytoin concentration is 1.0–2.0 μg/ml, then no change is necessary; unless seizures are uncontrolled

If the total phenytoin concentration is >20 μg/ml *or* the free phenytoin concentration is >2.0 μg/ml, then
 Suspend administration of the drug until the SPC is <20 μg/ml, and then
 Decrease the maintenance dose by 0.5–1.0 mg/kg/day (for medical/neurologic patients) or 1.5–2.0 mg/kg/day (for patients with severe brain injury)

first 3 months following the initial injury. Thus, doses that produced appropriate SPCs in the ICU can lead to toxic SPCs during convalescence. Phenytoin toxicity will most likely occur within the first month after transfer from the ICU. Weekly SPC determinations should be obtained and patients closely monitored for signs of toxicity during this period.

DRUG INTERACTIONS. A complete review of potential drug interactions with phenytoin is beyond the scope of this text; the reader is referred to references 51 and 52 for a complete listing. Interactions common in the ICU are discussed briefly here. Phenytoin is metabolized by the cytochrome P-450 enzyme system. It can enhance the metabolism of other drugs metabolized by this system; conversely, other drugs can enhance or inhibit the metabolism of phenytoin. Generally, the effects of enzyme induction are observed within 2 days to 2 weeks after starting the inducing agent. The effects of induction can last for weeks after the inducing agent is discontinued. Inhibition reactions generally occur quickly (within 1–2 days). When the drug that causes the inhibition reaction is stopped, the effects generally dissipate as soon as the drug is cleared from the system.

Trimethoprim can inhibit the clearance of phenytoin by as much as 50 percent, leading to increased SPCs [53]. The metabolism of phenytoin is also inhibited by erythromycin [52], cimetidine [54], chloramphenicol [36], amiodarone [55], omeprazole [56], isoniazid [52], ketaconazole [52], fluconazole [57], and possibly fluoxitene [58]. Valproic acid is capable of inhibiting the metabolism of phenytoin and also displaces phenytoin from binding sites on albumin, thereby increasing the free drug fraction. Since free drug is cleared faster than bound drug, the net effect of SPCs is difficult to predict [51]. Phenytoin can enhance the metabolism of valproic acid and decrease valproate serum concentrations [52]. In general, free concentrations of phenytoin should be monitored when valproic acid is administered concomitantly.

Ethanol induces the enzyme system responsible for the metabolism of phenytoin, and chronic alcoholics often require larger than normal doses. The effect of this interaction is difficult to predict in alcoholics with cirrhosis, since hepatic dysfunction decreases phenytoin clearance [59].

Carbamazepine induces the metabolism of phenytoin and can decrease SPCs [51]. Normal doses of phenobarbital can induce hepatic metabolism of phenytoin, leading to decreased SPCs. However, higher doses of phenobarbital can competitively inhibit phenytoin metabolism, resulting in increased SPCs. A complete review of this complex interaction is presented in reference 60.

Phenytoin increases the metabolism of theophylline, quinidine, disopyramide, corticosteroids, dexamethasone, warfarin, chloramphenicol, cyclosporine, and carbamazepine [51,52].

COMMON PITFALLS IN MANAGEMENT
1. Failure to obtain SPCs as a trough when administering IV formulations.
2. Failure to obtain or estimate a baseline postloading SPC with which to compare later SPCs when evaluating maintenance dose regimens. Without a baseline, an evaluation of whether the SPC is increasing or decreasing on the chosen dose cannot be made.
3. Failure to change the phenytoin dose or monitor SPCs when enteral tube feedings are discontinued or suspended.
4. Failure to monitor SPCs frequently during ICU stay and when patients are initially discharged from the ICU. This is especially important in head injury patients with high dosage

requirements in the ICU, whose clearance is expected to change dramatically over time.

5. Failure to monitor SPCs following hospital discharge. Follow-up clinic visits may be necessary to monitor SPCs as drug clearance may change and, due to nonlinearity, may result in SPCs outside the therapeutic window.

6. Failure to monitor SPCs when adding drugs enzyme inhibitors such as fluconazole and cimetidine or inducers such as phenobarbital or pentobarbital.

Phenobarbital

Phenobarbital is a long-acting barbiturate with sedative-hypnotic and anticonvulsant activity. In the ICU, phenobarbital is primarily used in the treatment of generalized tonic-clonic seizures or epilepsia partialis continua or in patients who cannot tolerate phenytoin or in whom phenytoin is ineffective. Phenobarbital is also an effective alternative in the prophylaxis of posttraumatic seizures. Phenobarbital is a secondary agent for the treatment of alcohol withdrawal.

PHARMACOLOGY. Barbiturates probably act by potentiating the actions of the neurotransmitter gamma aminobutyric acid (GABA) at neuronal synapses [61]. Noradrenergic activity also may be depressed by barbiturates. Phenobarbital limits the spread of seizure activity and elevates the seizure threshold. Barbiturates probably augment the inhibitory effects of GABA at postsynaptic GABA receptors in the brain or presynaptic receptors in the spinal cord. Barbiturates also enhance the binding of benzodiazepines to GABA receptors [61]. The relationship between the biochemical and electrophysiologic effects of barbiturates is not clearly understood.

Phenobarbital causes dose-dependent depression of most central nervous system (CNS) activities, except the reaction to pain. The drug depresses the neurogenic component of the respiratory drive with doses of 5 to 10 mg per kilogram [61]. Anesthetic doses of phenobarbital inhibit smooth, skeletal, and cardiac muscle, leading to hypotonia, vasodilation, hypotension, decreased cardiac contractility, decreased gastric motility, and ileus. Partial inhibition of ganglionic transmission contributes to hypotension, especially in patients with congestive heart failure or hypovolemic shock.

Therapeutic Range. The accepted therapeutic range for phenobarbital is 10 to 40 mg per liter [4]. This range was originally based on data from 11 patients hospitalized for frequent seizures [62]. Paroxysmal activity on the electroencephalogram (EEG) decreased by 90 percent at 4 mg per liter for 3 patients, at 8 to 15 mg per liter for 7, and at approximately 22 mg per liter for 1. The average serum concentration required for this response was 10 mg per liter. In another study, the therapeutic range was based on the concentration at which seizures were recorded following phenobarbital withdrawal [63]. The occurrence of seizures coincided with an average phenobarbital serum concentration of 9.9 mg per liter. Pooled data from three retrospective trials and one prospective trial, representing 568 patients, yielded the following results [63]. In 84 percent of patients, seizure control was obtained with serum phenobarbital concentrations (SPbCs) ranging from 10 to 14 mg per liter. A minimal increase in efficacy was observed when SPbCs exceeded 40 mg per liter. Ataxia, sedation, and nystagmus are generally absent at concentrations lower than 30 mg per liter. Serum phenobarbital concentrations greater than 50 mg per liter

are associated with clinically significant neurologic and respiratory depression. Serum concentrations greater than 80 mg per liter can be lethal in the absence of ventilatory and cardiovascular support. True pharmacodynamic tolerance to sedation occurs with phenobarbital; thus, naive patients experience some sedation even when SPbCs are within the low therapeutic range. Tolerance to sedation usually develops after 1 to 2 weeks of appropriate treatment [64], although this response is variable and cognitive deficits may persist when drug levels are within the therapeutic range. Dysarthrias, incoordination, ataxia, and nystagmus usually appear when SPbCs exceed 40 mg per liter [62,65]. Elderly patients with cognitive deficits are more likely to become agitated at SPbCs tolerated by others. The degree of CNS depression is greater in patients receiving benzodiazepines. Symptoms usually disappear with reduction in dose or discontinuation of the drug. Due to tolerance to phenobarbital after prolonged periods, abrupt discontinuation can cause withdrawal syndromes, which may not be manifested for several days.

Although SPbCs of 10 to 40 mg per liter should be the initial therapeutic goal, some patients may require higher or lower SPbCs for optimal benefit. Once experience is obtained in an individual patient, patient-specific therapeutic goals can be established to guide dosing.

Preparations Available. Phenobarbital is available for IV, IM, and oral administration. The parenteral formulation contains 68.8% propylene glycol. If this diluent is administered too rapidly, hypotension can occur. The maximum administration rate for IV infusions of phenobarbital is 60 mg per minute. Inadvertent intraarterial injection can cause distal gangrene.

Intramuscular injection should be deep into a large muscle. Injection into or near peripheral nerves can result in a permanent neurologic deficit.

Phenobarbital is available for oral administration in tablets and as an elixir. The elixir should be used for administration via an NG tube.

PHARMACOKINETICS. Table 213-4 summarizes phenobarbital's pharmacokinetic parameters.

Absorption. In adults, oral phenobarbital is 90 to 100 percent bioavailable. Peak serum concentrations occur 0.5 to 4 hours after an oral dose [66]. The ileum is the primary site of absorption. Oral absorption may be slowed because of decreased gastric motility after high doses of phenobarbital. In cases of

Table 213-4. Summary of Phenobarbital Pharmacokinetic Parameters

Bioavailability	90–100%
Protein binding	50% (40–60%)
V_{dc}	0.3 L/kg
V_{dss}	0.7 L/kg (0.5–1.0 L/kg)
Clearance	2.1–4.1 ml/kg/hr
Hepatic	65%
Renal	35% pH-dependent
Peritoneal dialysis	Not significant
Hemodialysis*	60–75 ml/min
Hemoperfusion*	100–300 ml/min
Distribution half-life	12 min (3–24 min)
Elimination half-life	96 hours (50–120 hr)

* Clearance is dependent on equipment used and serum concentration of the drug. May require dose supplementation.

phenobarbital poisoning, absorption may be delayed up to 12 hours. If ileus occurs secondary to intoxication, phenobarbital absorption may resume with recovery of gut motility, resulting in increasing SPbCs. Phenobarbital is completely absorbed from IM injection sites.

Distribution. The pharmacokinetics of phenobarbital are characterized by a two-compartment model with a mean distribution half-life of 12 minutes (range 3–24 minutes). In adults, V_{dc} and V_{dss} are approximately 0.3 liter per kilogram and 0.5 to 1.0 liter per kilogram, respectively [67,68]. Because of the large difference in V_{dc} and V_{dss}, phenobarbital infusions should be administered slowly to avoid high concentrations in the central compartment, which can lead to respiratory or cardiovascular toxicity.

Phenobarbital distributes to the brain and cerebrospinal fluid. The peak brain/plasma concentration ratio occurs at 20 to 40 minutes [17]. The steady-state brain/plasma concentration ratio ranges from 0.59 to 0.82 [16]. Phenobarbital is 40 to 60 percent bound to plasma proteins, primarily albumin [69].

Phenobarbital is a weak acid with a pKa of 7.2. When the physiologic pH equals the pKa, 50 percent of the drug is ionized. Both the value of V_d and the sites to which phenobarbital distributes are pH-dependent. Only the un-ionized drug crosses the blood-brain barrier. Acidosis increases the concentration of the un-ionized drug and thus increases the pharmacologic effect of phenobarbital. Alkalosis increases trapping of the drug in the serum, resulting in higher SPbCs for a given dose, decreased calculated V_d, and decreased pharmacologic effect (despite the higher SPbCs).

Elimination/Metabolism. Approximately 65 to 70 percent of a phenobarbital dose is metabolized by hydroxylation and parahydroxylation via the cytochrome P-450 system in the hepatic endoplasmic reticulum [70,71,72]. Twenty to 25 percent (up to 40%) of a dose is excreted by the kidneys as unchanged drug.

The average elimination half-life of phenobarbital is 96 hours (4 days; range 50–140 hours) [70,71]. Steady-state levels are achieved in about 3 weeks in patients with stable clearance on a stable dose.

PHYSIOLOGIC CLEARANCE CHARACTERISTICS. Phenobarbital is a capacity-limited, binding-insensitive drug [32] eliminated primarily by hepatic metabolism; however, filtration by the kidney is significant. Phenobarbital is a low-clearance drug (E < 0.3), indicating that hepatic clearance is dependent on enzyme capacity and is not affected by changes in hepatic blood flow. Since phenobarbital is not highly protein-bound (F > 0.2), alterations in serum albumin concentrations are unlikely to cause significant changes in free phenobarbital concentrations.

Total body clearance ranges from 2.1 to 4.1 ml/kg/hr (0.05–0.1 L/kg/day) [66,67]. Clearance is decreased in patients with cirrhosis and patients with severe renal failure (CrCl <10 ml/min). In addition, clearance is usually low in patients older than 70 years; therefore the daily dose requirements is typically about 30 percent lower in older patients. The renal clearance of phenobarbital is enhanced by alkalizing the urine (pH >7.5) and increasing urine flow [73]. Hemodialysis significantly removes phenobarbital, and supplemental doses are indicated.

Hypodynamic States. Theoretical considerations of the effects of hypodynamic states on hepatic clearance of capacity-limited or low extraction drugs is discussed in the section on phenytoin (Physiologic Clearance Characteristics). The impact on phenobarbital metabolism is unknown.

Hyperdynamic States. Theoretical considerations for hyperdynamic patients receiving low extraction drugs was discussed previously (see Phenytoin), but phenobarbital metabolism has not been studied in this patient population.

DOSE AND ADMINISTRATION

Loading Dose. A loading dose of 15 mg per kilogram achieves a postdistribution SPbC of approximately 20 mg per liter. Loading doses greater than 10 mg per kilogram can transiently depress respiratory drive. Therefore, in the absence of mechanical ventilation, a dose of 10 mg per kilogram should be administered initially, followed after approximately 30 to 60 minutes by an additional 5 mg per kilogram. For mechanically ventilated patients, 15 mg per kilogram can be administered as the initial dose. Thus,

$$SPbC = \frac{Dose}{V_d}$$

$$= \frac{15 \text{ mg/kg}}{0.7 \text{ L/kg}}$$

$$= 21 \text{ mg/L}$$

The loading dose should be diluted in 5% dextrose in water or 0.9% normal saline and infused slowly over 30 to 60 minutes. Although the maximum rate of administration is listed as 60 mg per minute, loading doses administered at this rate are likely to cause hypotension. Blood pressure should be monitored during the loading infusion; if hypotension occurs the infusion rate should be reduced by 50 percent. If seizures are not controlled with the initial loading dose, an extra 5 to 10 mg per kilogram can be administered. Total loading doses greater than 25 mg per kilogram are not likely to increase efficacy; if seizures persist another drug should be considered. A postdistribution SPbC can be obtained 1 to 2 hours after completion of the loading infusion to assess adequacy of the dose. This SPbC can be used to estimate the patient's V_d, which can be used to calculate the amount of additional partial loading dose doses, if required. This SPbC also serves as a baseline for evaluating the adequacy of the chosen maintenance dose.

Maintenance Dose. The first maintenance dose should be administered approximately 24 hours after the loading dose. The initial maintenance dose for adults based on an estimated clearance of 0.1 liter/kg/day is 1.0 to 3.0 mg/kg/day to achieve a steady-state SPbC of 10 to 30 mg per liter. Thus,

$$Dose = Cl \times SPbC \text{ desired}$$

$$= 0.1 \text{ L/kg/day} \times 20 \text{ mg/L}$$

$$= 2 \text{ mg/kg}$$

In general, each increment of 1 mg/kg/day results in an incremental increase in the steady-state SPbC of about 10 mg per liter. In elderly patients or patients with significant liver dysfunction or severe renal failure, the initial clearance estimate, and thus the dose, should be lower.

Following the initiation of the maintenance dose, an SPbC should be obtained as a trough in 6 to 8 days, depending on the patient's clinical status. Hyperdynamic trauma and surgery patients in the ICU may have time-dependent alterations in drug clearance, and the SPbC should be obtained 3 to 4 days following initiation of the maintenance dose. Hypodynamic patients or patients with acid-base disturbances should also have their SPbC checked earlier to determine whether levels of the drug are accumulating, decreasing, or remaining relatively constant.

If the SPbC is within the therapeutic range, seizures are controlled, and the SPbC is similar to the postloading concentration, then dosage adjustments are not required. If the SPbC has increased by 25 to 50 percent, it should be closely followed or the maintenance dose decreased to prevent development of toxicity. If the SPbC is decreasing, then clearance is greater than anticipated and the maintenance dose should be increased. It is not necessary to wait until a steady state is achieved to make adjustments in dosage to maintain the patient within the therapeutic range. It must be recognized, however, that further adjustments may be necessary when steady-state concentrations are achieved. If seizures recur, or if toxicity is suspected, an SPbC should be obtained to help establish the patient-specific dose-response relationship.

Subsequent SPbC should be obtained weekly in ICU patients whose seizures are well controlled. A true steady state will not be achieved for 2 to 4 weeks (5 half-lives). It can be assumed that a steady state has been achieved when similar SPbCs are measured approximately 3 weeks apart in stable convalescing patients.

Due to the excellent bioavailability of phenobarbital, its IM and oral dosage forms are equivalent to the IV form. Due to its long elimination half-life, the maintenance dose can be administered once or twice daily. In patients with high clearance values who require relatively large doses, a twice daily regimen is most appropriate. During chronic therapy, phenobarbital can be administered once daily in the evening to decrease daytime sedation [74]. Supplemental doses may be required after hemodialysis.

DRUG INTERACTIONS. A complete review of drug interactions involving phenobarbital is beyond the scope of this chapter; the reader is referred to references 51, 52, and 75 for a complete listing. Interactions that commonly occur in the ICU are presented here.

Phenobarbital is metabolized by the cytochrome P-450 enzyme system and can induce the metabolism of many other drugs metabolized by this system. The effects of phenobarbital enzyme induction generally take longer than 1 week to become apparent. Phenobarbital increases the clearance of carbamazepine, which is additive to the autoinduction of metabolism observed with this drug [76]. The anticoagulant effect of warfarin is decreased, corresponding to a decreased serum concentration [75,77]. Phenobarbital also increases the clearance of chloramphenicol, clonazepam, dexamethasone, digoxin, tricyclic antidepressants, beta-adrenergic blockers metabolized by the liver, disopyramide, quinidine, theophylline, and corticosteroids [52,77]. Phenobarbital can increase the clearance of verapamil by four to five times when verapamil is administered orally and by two times when administered IV [78]. The clearance of nifedipine can be doubled [79].

Phenytoin and phenobarbital compete for the same metabolic pathway, thus phenytoin clearance may be increased, decreased, or unchanged when phenobarbital is added to the medication regimen [80,81].

Valproic acid, which inhibits phenobarbital metabolism and decreases drug clearance, results in increased SPbCs. When valproic acid is added to the phenobarbital regimen, the phenobarbital dose should be reduced by 50 percent [82]. Serum phenobarbital concentrations should be checked before and 3 to 4 days after instituting valproic acid therapy. Thereafter, SPbCs should be obtained weekly while the patient is hospitalized. In addition, because phenobarbital can increase the metabolism of valproic acid, serum concentrations of this drug should be monitored.

COMMON PITFALLS IN MANAGEMENT

1. Failure to administer an adequate loading dose of phenobarbital. In a 70-kg patient, a loading dose of 15 mg per kilogram is approximately 1 gm of phenobarbital and will result in a SPbC of approximately 20 mg per liter.
2. Failure to administer IV phenobarbital slowly. A slow infusion of phenobarbital (25 mg/min) is less likely to cause hypotension than multiple IV bolus doses.
3. Failure to consider the effects of phenobarbital administration on the metabolism and dosage requirements of other hepatically metabolized medications.
4. Failure to obtain follow-up steady-state SPbCs on the chosen dose. Because the elimination half-life of phenobarbital is long and steady state is not achieved for several weeks after the patient stabilizes, the patient is often transferred to another chronic care service where SPbCs are not closely followed.
5. Failure to reduce the dose of phenobarbital when valproic acid is added to the regimen, to avoid phenobarbital accumulation and toxicity.

Pentobarbital

Pentobarbital is a barbiturate used as a sedative-hypnotic and anticonvulsant. In the ICU, pentobarbital is sometimes used to reduce intracranial pressure (ICP) in patients with head trauma, cerebral aneurysms, or Reyes syndrome after conservative therapy has failed [83,84]. It is also used as a tertiary agent to control status epilepticus or acute seizures in patients with meningitis, alcohol withdrawal, tetanus, chorea, poisoning, or eclampsia [85,86]. Intravenous pentobarbital can be used for general and regional anesthesia or for intubation. Oral pentobarbital has been used in withdrawal therapy for barbiturate addiction.

PHARMACOLOGY. The pharmacologic effects of pentobarbital include dose-dependent CNS depression ranging from mild sedation to death. The anticonvulsant mechanisms are probably similar to those postulated for phenobarbital. The proposed mechanisms for pentobarbital-induced cerebral protection and ICP reduction include decreased cerebral oxygen utilization, decreased cerebral blood flow, and free radical scavenging [61,83].

Respiratory rate and depth are always suppressed to some extent with pentobarbital. However, this effect is most prominent when the hypnotic dosage range is exceeded; therefore, assisted ventilation is required during high-dose therapy [61].

Rapid IV administration can induce arrhythmias and hypotension [87,88]. Therapeutic pentobarbital-induced coma frequently results in adverse cardiovascular effects, including vasodilation of capacitance vessels, decreased ventricular filling pressures and cardiac output, and loss of baroreceptor reflexes [61]. Hypotension can result in inadequate cerebral perfusion pressure (CPP) [61,83,88]. It is unclear whether pentobarbital is a direct myocardial depressant or if reduced cardiac output occurs only as a result of peripheral vasodilation and diminished ventricular filling.

THERAPEUTIC RANGE. Serum concentrations of 1 to 5 mg per liter generally produce sedation, and concentrations of 5 to 10 mg per liter produce sleep in most patients. The accepted therapeutic range for barbiturate-induced coma is 20 to 50 mg per liter. In the treatment of increased ICP, the therapeutic goal is an induced coma state characterized by absent brainstem reflexes, suppression of the EEG, and reduced cerebral oxygen utilization and blood flow. Electroencephalogram burst suppression following anesthetic doses of pentobarbital is accompanied by a significant reduction in cerebral blood flow and oxygen utilization [83,89]. Electroencephalogram burst suppression is reported to occur at pentobarbital concentrations ranging from 20 to 50 mg per liter [83,89]. The clinical endpoint is decreased ICP.

The optimal therapeutic range for the use of pentobarbital in status epilepticus is not established [90]. Anesthetic doses are usually required for anticonvulsant activity [61]. The therapeutic endpoint is seizure control, with EEG monitoring indicating suppression of aberrant electrical activity.

PREPARATIONS. Pentobarbital is available for IV, IM, and oral administration. The injectable formulation contains 40% propylene glycol and 10% ethanol, adjusted to a pH of approximately 9.5. Oral formulations include an elixir suitable for administration via NG tube and capsules.

PHARMACOKINETICS. The pharmacokinetic parameters of pentobarbital are summarized in Table 213-5.

Absorption. Absorption of oral pentobarbital is approximately 100 percent. The onset of action occurs in approximately 15 to 60 minutes [61,91]. Similar to the other barbiturates, ileus and delayed absorption can occur following pentobarbital poisoning. As serum concentrations decline and gut motility improves, cyclic coma can result from absorption of residual pentobarbital present in gastric fluid.

Distribution. Pentobarbital pharmacokinetics are best characterized by a two-compartment model, with a distribution half-life of 10 to 60 minutes. In adults, V_{dc} and V_{dss} are approximately 0.5 liter per kilogram and 1 liter per kilogram, respectively [90,91,92]. Due to the small V_{dc}, the initial concentrations following IV bolus administration or rapid infusions are high and can result in significant hypotension or cardiac arrhythmias.

Pentobarbital is 40 to 60 percent bound to albumin. Pentobarbital is widely distributed in the body, including the cerebrospinal fluid and brain. It has a greater affinity for fat than does phenobarbital, and it crosses the blood-brain barrier quickly, resulting in a rapid onset of anesthesia.

Elimination/Metabolism. Pentobarbital is almost completely metabolized (99%) to inactive metabolites by the cytochrome P-450 enzyme system in the liver. The elimination half-life of pentobarbital in normal volunteers is 22.3 ± 4 hours [91]. In

two studies of patients with head trauma, the elimination half-life of pentobarbital was 15.6 ± 31 3.9 hours [92] and 19.1 ± 10.9 hours [93].

PHYSIOLOGIC CLEARANCE CHARACTERISTICS. Pentobarbital is a capacity-limited, binding-insensitive drug eliminated primarily by hepatic clearance. Pentobarbital is a low clearance drug (E < 0.3), indicating that elimination depends on enzyme capacity and is not affected by changes in hepatic blood flow. Pentobarbital clearance is not significantly influenced by changes in protein binding.

Hypodynamic States. Although data are limited, pentobarbital is expected to follow a pattern similar to that for phenytoin (see above). Liver diseases or hepatic dysfunction subsequent to shock or sepsis would be expected to impair pentobarbital clearance and result in lower dosage requirements.

Hyperdynamic States. Hypermetabolic states are expected to increase pentobarbital clearance, as discussed for phenytoin. Limited data and clinical observations support increased clearance and dosage requirements in critically ill trauma and neurosurgery patients. Total body clearance is approximately 0.53 ml/kg/min in normal volunteers [91] and approximately 0.4 to 1.2 ml/kg/min in patients with severe head injury [92,93,94]. As for phenytoin, pentobarbital clearance may be time-dependent and can increase within several days in ICU patients [94].

DOSE AND ADMINISTRATION. The doses of pentobarbital recommended for ICP control (Table 213-6) and reported by other investigators [89,95] are based on the pharmacokinetic

Table 213-6. High-Dose Pentobarbital Protocol for Increased Intracranial Pressure

Loading infusion
  1. Administer 20 mg/kg infusion IV over 2 hr. (Dilute in 0.9% or 0.45% saline to 5–20 mg/ml.)
  2. If SBP drops 10–20 mm Hg, decrease rate of infusion by 50%.
  3. If SBP drops > 20 mm Hg, discontinue infusion until SBP stabilizes.
  4. If ICP increases significantly, administer an additional 10 mg/kg loading infusion over 1 hr.
Maintenance infusion
  1. Initiate infusion at 1.0 mg/kg/hr (diluted in saline to 4–10 mg/ml).
  2. Adjust (± 0.5–1.0 mg/kg/hr) based on assessment of serum pentobarbital concentrations and physiologic monitoring parameters.
  3. Expected dose requirements range from 0.5–3.5 mg/kg/hr.
Physiologic monitoring parameters and therapeutics goals
  1. Mechanical ventilation
  2. Absence of brain stem reflexes
  3. ICP < 20 mm Hg; CPP > 60 mm Hg (CPP = MAP − ICP)
  4. SBP < 170–180 mm Hg; MAP adequate to maintain CPP
  5. EEG burst suppression pattern
  6. Normal sinus rhythm
  7. Adequate urine output, CVP, PCWP, and cardiac index
Pentobarbital serum concentration monitoring
  1. Therapeutic range 20–50 μg/ml
  2. Peak serum concentration (1–2 hr following loading infusion)
  3. Daily serum concentrations

SBP = systolic blood pressure; ICP = intracranial pressure; CPP = cerebral perfusion pressure; MAP = mean arterial pressure; CVP = central venous pressure; PCWP = pulmonary capillary wedge pressure

Table 213-5. Summary of Pentobarbital Pharmacokinetic Parameters

Bioavailability	100% (capsules)
Protein binding	40–60%
V_{dc}	0.5 L/kg
V_{dss}	1.0 L/kg
Clearance	0.53 ml/kg/min
Hepatic	99%
Renal	Negligible
Peritoneal dialysis	Negligible
Hemodialysis	Negligible
Distribution half-life	10–30 min
Elimination half-life	24 (15–72) hr

parameters of the drug. They are designed to attain therapeutic serum pentobarbital concentrations (approximately 20 mg/L) rapidly with minimal adverse cardiovascular effects.

Loading Dose. The recommended loading dose for ICP control is 20 mg per kilogram administered over 2 hours. This dose results in a serum pentobarbital concentration of approximately 20 mg per liter. Thus,

$$\text{Serum pentobarbital concentration} = \frac{\text{Dose}}{V_{dss}}$$
$$= \frac{20 \text{ mg/kg}}{1 \text{L/kg}}$$
$$= 20 \text{ mg/L}$$

This dose should be diluted in 0.45% or 0.9% sodium chloride at a concentration of 5 to 20 mg per milliliter and delivered using a rate-control device. A 2-hour infusion time minimizes the risk of adverse cardiovascular effects due to high predistribution serum concentrations. If hypotension or tachycardia occurs, the infusion can be slowed by 50 percent.

A serum concentration should be determined 1 to 2 hours after infusion of the loading dose to determine whether a therapeutic concentration (20–50 mg/L) has been achieved. The V_d can be calculated using this level and used to determine the size of further loading doses, if required, since:

$$V_d \text{ for the individual patient} = \frac{\text{Dose}}{\text{Resulting drug concentration}}$$

If the systolic blood pressure (SBP) drops by 10 to 20 mm Hg, the infusion rate should be decreased by 50 percent. If the SBP drops by 20 mm Hg or is below the therapeutic goals for the individual patient, the infusion should be discontinued to allow the blood pressure to stabilize. Then the loading infusion can be restarted at 50 percent of the initial rate. Intravascular volume loading may be required to counter decreased ventricular filling pressures resulting from pentobarbital-induced peripheral vasodilation. If hypotension persists, the infusion should be discontinued or, if further therapy is warranted, vasopressor support with dopamine initiated to increase mean arterial blood pressure and, hence, CPP. If clinically significant arrhythmias occur, the drug should be discontinued.

If intracranial hypertension or status epilepticus is not controlled or EEG burst suppression not achieved after the loading infusion, a serum pentobarbital concentration should be obtained before further loading doses are administered. The size of further doses can be calculated based on the individualized V_d. Alternatively, 10 mg per kilogram can be administered over 1 hour. This dose should increase the serum pentobarbital concentration by about 10 mg per liter. If intracranial hypertension, seizure, or EEG burst suppression goals still are not achieved, further loading doses should be administered only if serum pentobarbital levels are lower than 50 mg per liter and the patient is expected to tolerate the potential adverse effects on arterial blood pressure.

For control of seizures, a smaller loading dose of pentobarbital (5–10 mg/kg) should be employed initially. This dose can be repeated as necessary to a maximum cumulative dose of 30 mg per kilogram. Additional loading doses beyond this point should be guided by serum pentobarbital concentrations. These doses should be administered as a slow infusion, with monitoring similar to that recommended in the discussion of ICP control.

Maintenance Dose. The initial maintenance dose for ICP control is 1 to 2 mg/kg/hr administered as a continuous infusion. The drug should be diluted in 0.45% or 0.9% sodium chloride to a concentration of 4 to 10 mg per milliliter. An initial maintenance infusion of 2 mg/kg/hr is designed to attain a steady-state serum concentration of approximately 30 mg per liter based on a clearance estimate of 0.53 ml/kg/min (0.032 L/kg/hour). Thus,

$$\text{Steady-state concentration} = \frac{\text{Dose/dosing interval}}{\text{Cl}}$$
$$= \frac{1.0 \text{ mg/kg/hr}}{0.032 \text{ L/kg/hr}}$$
$$= 31 \text{ mg/L}$$

This clearance estimate is based on data from normal volunteers [91]. Our experience suggests that this value is an underestimate, since measured serum concentrations are generally lower than predicted. In addition, higher clearance values and time-dependent changes in clearance have been reported in hypermetabolic trauma patients [92,93,94]. Thus, in hyperdynamic ICU patients, reloading infusions may be required and the maintenance dose may need to be increased up to 3 to 4 mg/kg/hr over time; this should be based on measured drug concentrations.

A serum pentobarbital concentration obtained 24 hours after beginning the maintenance infusion does not reflect the true steady-state value but nevertheless can be used to adjust the dose. If the 24-hour concentration reflects a change in concentration from the postloading level of 33 to 50 percent and is less than 20 mg per liter or greater than 50 mg per liter, the rate of infusion should be increased or decreased by 0.5 to 1.0 mg/kg/hr, respectively. Daily serum pentobarbital concentrations should be obtained to assess changes in clearance and thus dose requirements.

If ICP increases during the maintenance infusion, serum pentobarbital concentration should be obtained and a reloading infusion of 5 to 10 mg per kilogram administered. The maintenance infusion can be increased by 0.5 to 1.0 mg/kg/hr. The typical mean maintenance dose requirement is 2.0 mg/kg/hr (range 0.5–4) mg/kg/hr.

The following parameters are reasonable therapeutic endpoints: mean arterial pressure (MAP) 70 to 80 mm Hg, CPP greater than 60 mm Hg, and ICP lower than 20 mm Hg. If the EEG is used as a monitoring tool, it should show a 30- to 60-second burst suppression pattern. The neurologic examination should show absence of muscular movement and brainstem reflexes.

Pentobarbital therapy should be discontinued after 72 hours of ICP control or if there is deterioration of cardiovascular status. The pentobarbital infusion should be tapered over 48 to 72 hours by reducing the infusion rate by 25 percent every 12 hours. The patient should be monitored for increasing ICP or seizures following pentobarbital withdrawal. Once pentobarbital is discontinued, the elimination half-life can be estimated from two concentrations obtained 12 hours apart. Thus,

$$K_e = \frac{\ln SDC_2 - \ln SDC_1}{\text{Time between concentrations (hr)}}$$

where K_e is the elimination rate constant and SDC_1 and SDC_2 are the serum drug concentrations obtained at times 1 and 2.

$$t_{1/2} = \frac{0.693}{K_e}$$

Half-life can be used to estimate the time required before pentobarbital serum concentrations decline below a desired serum concentration (e.g., 5 mg/L). Thus,

$$\text{Projected SDC} = \text{SDC}_2 \times e^{-K_e \times t}$$

where SDC_2 is the last measured serum drug concentration and t is the time in hours following the SDC_2 at which one wishes to know the projected SDC. If the initial concentration is 20 mg per liter and half-life is 15 hours, it will take about 30 hours for the concentration to decrease to 5.0 mg per liter.

For control of status epilepticus, we recommend an initial continuous infusion rate of 0.5 to 1.0 mg/kg/hr, which can be increased as necessary in increments of 0.5 mg/kg/hr. Serum pentobarbital concentrations should be obtained daily to assess changes in clearance.

DRUG INTERACTIONS. Pentobarbital is a potent inducer of the hepatic cytochrome P-450 enzyme system. Enzyme induction typically occurs during the first 5 to 10 days of therapy and, can generally be expected to increase hepatic clearance of susceptible drugs by 50 to 100 percent. Drug interactions with pentobarbital have been documented for many hepatically metabolized drugs, including theophylline, warfarin, corticosteroids, phenytoin, quinidine, and tricyclic antidepressants, resulting in increased clearance and decreased concentrations [52,96].

Occasionally, pentobarbital competitively inhibits the metabolism of other drugs (particularly phenytoin and tricyclic antidepressants), resulting in increased serum drug concentrations and pharmacologic effects [52].

Serum concentrations of drugs with a narrow therapeutic range should be monitored frequently after initiating pentobarbital therapy. Drugs that have shorter elimination half-lives are more rapidly affected than drugs with long half-lives.

COMMON PITFALLS IN MANAGEMENT
1. Failure to administer IV pentobarbital slowly. A continuous infusion is less likely to cause adverse hemodynamic effects than multiple bolus doses.
2. Failure to load IV pentobarbital adequately to achieve therapeutic serum concentrations in the initial hours of therapy.
3. Failure to maintain pentobarbital serum concentrations in the therapeutic range. Prolonged infusion of high maintenance doses eventually leads to overshooting the therapeutic range and delayed pentobarbital coma once therapy is discontinued due to the long elimination half-life.
4. Failure to consider the elimination half-life of pentobarbital when obtaining serial concentrations to determine when the drug has been eliminated. Following discontinuation of the drug, an estimation of the patient's half-life using two serum pentobarbital concentrations can be used to predict when this level will drop below any desired value. A confirmatory level can be obtained at the time the drug is predicted to be eliminated. This approach will significantly decrease the number of level determinations necessary.

Carbamazepine

Carbamazepine is an anticonvulsant drug indicated for the treatment of generalized tonic-clonic, simple, and complex partial seizures [1]. It is an alternative for seizure control or prophylaxis in neurotrauma patients, especially during rehabilitation [97]. Carbamazepine is used to treat trigeminal and glossopharyngeal neuralgias and posttraumatic paresthesias [1,98]. This agent is gaining acceptance in psychiatry for the treatment of bipolar disorders [99].

PHARMACOLOGY. Carbamazepine is an iminostilbene derivative, similar in structure to imipramine. Pharmacologically, carbamazepine is similar to phenytoin. The mechanism of action has not been clearly delineated.

In animals, carbamazepine is more effective than phenytoin in reducing electrical discharge and blocking pentylenetetrazol-induced seizures [1]. An antidiuretic effect can occur, which is sometimes associated with reduced vasopressin levels; thus, carbamazepine has been used to treat diabetes insipidus. In high doses, carbamazepine has anticholinergic activity, particularly in overdose. In trigeminal neuralgias, it may decrease synaptic transmission in the spinal trigeminal nucleus [1]. Carbamazepine may be effective in treating manic-depressive patients, including some who are resistant to lithium.

THERAPEUTIC RANGE. The generally accepted therapeutic range is 4 to 12 mg per liter. The imprecision in the estimate for the therapeutic range is probably due to variabilities in seizure types and severity, concomitant use of other anticonvulsant drugs, variations in protein binding, and differences in the coexisting concentrations of carbamazepine's active metabolite, carbamazepine-10, 11-epoxide. The therapeutic threshold for seizure control in most patients is 4 mg per liter. The upper half of the range (8–12 mg/L) is often required for monotherapy, whereas the lower half (4–8 mg/L) may be sufficient for patients simultaneously receiving other anticonvulsant drugs. Most patients experience neurotoxicity at serum carbamazepine concentrations greater than 12 mg per liter. Neurotoxic symptoms include gait disturbances, dysdiadochokinesia, diplopia, dizziness, and/or loss of accommodation [100–105]. At serum concentrations of 15 to 25 mg per liter, patients can be combative or hallucinatory or have choreiform movements [105]. When serum concentrations exceed 25 mg per liter, seizures or significant CNS depression can be observed [105]. Ventricular arrhythmias and various degrees of heart block have been reported following overdose.

One study suggests that carbamazepine-induced neurotoxicity correlates with free serum carbamazepine concentrations greater than 1.7 mg per liter [106]. Further studies are needed to define the therapeutic range of carbamazepine in terms of free drug concentrations. Similarly, the concentration-response relationship for the active metabolite carbamazepine-10, 11-epoxide has not been adequately studied. Carbamazepine has many adverse reactions that are not concentration-related.

PREPARATIONS. Carbamazepine is available only for oral administration. In addition to tablets, a suspension is available that can be administered via NG tube. A 1:1 dilution of the suspension can be administered rectally [107].

PHARMACOKINETICS. Table 213-7 summarizes the pharmacokinetic parameters of carbamazepine.

Absorption. Absorption studies are confounded by the lack of an IV dosage form, since bioavailability is usually determined by comparing the areas under the serum concentration-time curves for oral and IV administration. Using radioisotope stud-

Table 213-7. Summary of Carbamazepine Pharmacokinetic Parameters

Bioavailability	80–90%
Protein binding	75%
V_{dss}	0.8–2.2 L/kg
Clearance	
Initial monotherapy	0.01–0.03 L/kg/hr
Chronic monotherapy	0.05–0.07 L/kg/hr
Polytherapy	0.08–0.17 L/kg/hr
Hepatic	95%
Renal	Negligible
Peritoneal dialysis	Negligible
Hemodialysis	Negligible
Hemoperfusion	0.09 L/kg/hr
Elimination half-life	
Initial monotherapy	18–30 hr
Chronic monotherapy	12–18 hr
Polytherapy	6–12 hr

ies, however, bioavailability has been estimated to be 75 to 85 percent, with the tablet and suspension being equivalent [108,109,110]. Carbamazepine is highly lipophilic; thus, the rate-limiting step in absorption is dissolution. Peak serum drug concentrations following a single dose are usually observed in 4 to 8 hours. With chronic dosing, peak serum concentrations are observed earlier (1–3 hours) due to autoinduction and higher carbamazepine clearance [111]. The rate of absorption is dose-dependent. Because the rate of absorption is reduced at high doses (10–20 mg/kg/day) [111,112], the daily dose is administered in three to four divided doses. The dose-related decrease in absorption rate is especially important in overdose [105]. Enteral feedings can decrease the rate, but not the extent, of absorption [113].

Distribution. The accurate calculation of V_d is hampered by the lack of a parenteral product. Assuming bioavailability of 100 percent, the apparent V_d is estimated to be 0.8 to 2.2 liters per kilogram, reflecting the high lipophilicity of this drug [114,115]. The brain-to-plasma concentration ratio is 0.8 to 1.6 for carbamazepine and 0.6 to 1.5 for its epoxide metabolite [116,117]. Carbamazepine is approximately 75 percent bound to albumin and alpha-(1)-acid glycoprotein (AAG), whereas its epoxide metabolite is approximately 50 percent bound to albumin [114,118]. Salivary concentrations appear to correlate with free carbamazepine concentrations.

Elimination/Metabolism. Carbamazepine is completely metabolized by the liver [119]. The most important pathway is epoxidation by hepatic monooxygenases to the active metabolite, carbamazepine-10,11-epoxide. The epoxide is hydrolyzed, glucuronidated, and excreted in the urine [119,120,121]. When used as the sole anticonvulsant (monotherapy), 25 percent of the carbamazepine dose is metabolized via this pathway. When used in combination with other anticonvulsants, such as phenytoin or phenobarbital, 40 to 50 percent is metabolized via this pathway.

Carbamazepine induces its own metabolism (autoinduction), resulting in time-dependent changes in clearance. The onset of autoinduction can be observed during the first few days of therapy, with the peak effect occurring after 3 to 4 weeks [111,122,123]. The initial clearance of carbamazepine is approximately 0.01 to 0.03 L/kg/hr [111]. Following autoinduction, clearance is about 0.05 to 0.07 L/kg/hr [124]. Administration of other anticonvulsants further increases the clearance of carbamazepine to 0.8 to 0.17 L/kg/hr [125].

The elimination half-life of carbamazepine following single doses is 18 to 30 hours [126]. With chronic dosing and autoinduction, it decreases to 12 to 18 hours [124]. Polytherapy with other anticonvulsant drugs results in a half-life of 6 to 12 hours [125]. The epoxide metabolite has an elimination half-life of approximately 5 to 8 hours [126].

PHYSIOLOGIC CLEARANCE CHARACTERISTICS. Carbamazepine is a capacity-limited, binding-sensitive drug. The effects of hypodynamic or hyperdynamic states on carbamazepine hepatic clearance is unknown. Carbamazepine is approximately 75 percent bound to albumin and AAG, whereas its epoxide metabolite is approximately 50 percent bound to albumin [114,118]. There is considerable interpatient variability in protein binding. Significant increases in serum AAG concentrations following trauma, burns, major surgery, and myocardial infarction can contribute to a decreased free fraction of carbamazepine, although the clinical significance of this effect has not been adequately studied. Theoretically, for this low extraction (E < 0.3) drug, increases in protein binding would be expected to reduce clearance, increase total drug concentration, and have no effect on free drug concentration. Thus the dose-response relationship would be maintained, although the dose-measured concentration relationship would be altered.

Peritoneal dialysis and hemodialysis do not substantially affect carbamazepine clearance due to the large V_d, and extra doses are not necessary after dialysis.

DOSING GUIDELINES. Since high peak serum carbamazepine concentrations are associated with a high frequency of neurotoxicity and high doses are associated with increased gastrointestinal side effects, a loading dose is not recommended. Instead, this drug is started at a low dose that is gradually increased as clearance increases. Because clearance changes with time, changes in the dosing regimen are carried out empirically. The initial dose is 5 mg/kg/day, divided into two daily doses. After the first week of therapy, the dose can usually be increased to 7 to 10 mg/kg/day. By the third week of therapy, an increase to 15 mg/kg/day may be required. All dosage increases should be guided by trough serum carbamazepine concentrations and clinical evaluation. After autoinduction, the usual adult dosage requirement during monotherapy is 7 to 15 mg/kg/day to achieve a trough serum carbamazepine concentration of approximately 6.0 mg per liter. Higher doses are often required in patients receiving other anticonvulsant drugs, and reported dosage requirements are as high as 17 to 25 mg/kg/day. The optimal dosing frequency is two to three times daily during carbamazepine monotherapy and three to four times daily during combination therapy. If a patient has a relatively low trough serum carbamazepine concentration but experiences mild neurotoxicity several hours after a dose, the dosing interval can be shortened (same daily dose) to decrease fluctuation in serum concentrations. This adjustment may obviate the necessity of decreasing the dose.

Weekly trough serum carbamazepine concentration measurements are necessary to assess clearance changes and establish a patient-specific therapeutic range based on seizure event records and adverse effects. The frequency of serum concentration determinations can be decreased after the patient is stabilized on a dose and several concentration determinations are consistent (i.e., there is evidence that steady state has been achieved). If toxicity or seizures occur, a serum concentration should be obtained. Since carbamazepine can itself cause seizures at high levels, poisoning must be ruled out before increasing the dose further. Serum carbamazepine concentrations must be obtained when initiating or discontinuing other medications that affect the hepatic microsomal enzyme system.

DRUG INTERACTIONS. Carbamazepine is a potent hepatic microsomal enzyme-inducing drug and therefore affects the metabolism of many other drugs metabolized via this system. Reported interactions usually involve medications for which a clinical assay procedure is readily available, but the potential to alter the clearance of other medications should be remembered. Carbamazepine can increase the clearance of theophylline, valproic acid, corticosteroids, alprazolam, tricyclic antidepressants, cyclosporine, and haloperidol [1,52,127,128].

The metabolism of phenytoin can be competitively inhibited by carbamazepine, and carbamazepine can induce the metabolism of phenytoin [129,130]. The net result is variable and difficult to predict. In addition, phenytoin can induce the metabolism of carbamazepine. Concentrations of both medications should be monitored.

As previously mentioned, the metabolism of carbamazepine can be induced by other anticonvulsant drugs [52,128]. Drugs that induce metabolism of carbamazepine also increase the concentration of carbamazepine-10, 11-epoxide. Carbamazepine clearance can be decreased by valproic acid, erythromycin, cimetidine, propoxyphene, diltiazem, and isoniazid, resulting in increased serum carbamazepine concentrations [52,128, 131,132]. Clinical observations suggest that carbamazepine metabolism is decreased by fluconazole, as documented for phenytoin.

COMMON PITFALLS IN MANAGEMENT

1. Failure to obtain serum carbamazepine concentrations as a trough.
2. Failure to recognize the potential for drug interactions with any medication metabolized via the microsomal enzyme system.
3. Failure to split the total daily dose into three to four divided doses when administering large doses.
4. Failure to closely monitor serum carbamazepine concentrations until the effects of autoinduction are complete and a true steady state has been achieved.

References

1. Rall TW, Scheifer LS: Drugs effective in the therapy of the epilepsies, in Gilman AG, Goodman LS, Rall TW, et al (eds): *Goodman and Gilman's The Pharmacological Basis of Therapeutics.* 7th ed. New York, Macmillan, 1985, p 450.
2. Reynolds EH: Phenytoin toxicity, in Levy R, Dreifuss FE, Mattson R, et al (eds): *Antiepileptic Drugs.* 3rd ed. New York, Raven, 1989, p 241.
3. Lund L: Anticonvulsant effect of diphenylhydantoin relative to plasma levels: A prospective three-year study in ambulant patients with generalized epileptic seizures. *Arch Neurol* 31:289, 1974.
4. Schmidt D, Einicke I, Haenel F: The influence of seizure type on the efficacy of plasma concentrations of phenytoin, phenobarbital and carbamazepine. *Arch Neurol* 43:263, 1986.
5. Kutt H, Winters W, Kokenge R, McDowell R: Diphenylhydantoin metabolism, blood levels and toxicity. *Arch Neurol* 11:642, 1964.
6. Osorio I, Burnstine TH, Remler B, et al: Phenytoin-induced seizures: A paradoxical effect at toxic concentrations in epileptic patients. *Epilepsia* 30:230, 1989.
7. Markowsky SJ, Kohls PR, Ehresman D, Leppik IE: Compatibility and pH variability of four injectable phenytoin sodium products. *Am J Hosp Pharm* 48:510, 1991.
8. Leppik IE, Boucher BR, Wilder BJ, et al: Phenytoin prodrug: Preclinical and clinical studies. *Epilepsia* 39(suppl 2):S22, 1989.
9. Jusko WJ, Koup JR, Alvan G: Non-linear assessment of phenytoin bioavailability. *J Pharmacokinet Biopharm* 4:327, 1976.
10. Jung D, Powell JR, Walson P, Perrier D: Effect of dose on phenytoin absorption. *Clin Pharmacol Ther* 28:479, 1980.
11. Osborn HA, Zisfein J, Sparano R: Single dose phenytoin loading. *Ann Emerg Med* 16:407, 1987.
12. Cacek AT, DeVito J, Koonce JR: In vitro evaluation of nasogastric administration methods for phenytoin. *Am J Hosp Pharm* 43:689, 1986.
13. Bauer LA: Interference of oral phenytoin absorption by continuous nasogastric feedings. *Neurology* 32:570, 1982.
14. Krueger KA, Garnett WR, Comstock TJ, et al: Effect of two administration schedules of an enteral nutrient formula on phenytoin bioavailability. *Epilepsia* 28:706, 1987.
15. Suzuki T, Saitoh Y, Nishihara K: Kinetics of diphenylhydantoin disposition in man. *Chem Pharm Bull* 18:405, 1970.
16. Ramsey RE, Hammond EJ, Perchalski RJ, Wilder BJ: Brain uptake of phenytoin, phenobarbital and diazepam. *Arch Neurol* 36:535, 1979.
17. Paulson OB, Gyory A, Hentz MM: Blood-brain barrier transfer and cerebral uptake of antiepileptic drugs. *Clin Pharmacol Ther* 32:466, 1982.
18. Browne TR, Evans JE, Szabo GK, et al: Studies with stable isotopes I: Changes in phenytoin pharmacokinetics and biotransformation during monotherapy. *J Clin Pharmacol* 25:43, 1985.
19. Hooper WD, Bochner F, Eadie MJ, Tyrer JH: Plasma protein binding of diphenylhydantoin: Effects of sex hormones, renal and hepatic disease. *Clin Pharmacol Ther* 15:276, 1974.
20. Olsen GD, Bennett WM, Porter GA: Morphine and phenytoin binding to plasma proteins in renal and hepatic failure. *Clin Pharmacol Ther* 17:677, 1975.
21. Kinniburgh DW, Boyd ND: Isolation of peptides from uremic plasma that inhibit phenytoin binding to normal plasma proteins. *Clin Pharmacol Ther* 30:276, 1981.
22. Bloedow DC, Hansbrough JF, Hardin TH, Simons M: Postburn serum drug binding and serum protein concentrations. *J Clin Pharmacol* 26:147, 1986.
23. Svensson CK, Woodruff MN, Lalka D: Influence of protein binding and use of unbound drug concentrations, in Jusko WS, Schentag JJ, Evans WF (eds): *Applied Pharmacokinetics: Principles of Therapeutic Drug Monitoring.* 2nd ed. Spokane, Applied Therapeutics 1986, p 187.
24. Lunde PKM, Rane A, Yaffe Si, et al: Plasma protein binding of diphenylhydantoin in man: Interaction with other drugs and effect of temperature and plasma dilution. *Clin Pharmacol Ther* 11:846, 1970.
25. Glasko AJ, Chang T, Baukema J, et al: Metabolic disposition of diphenylhydantoin in human subjects following intravenous administration. *Clin Pharmacol Ther* 10:498, 1969.
26. Martin E, Tozer TN, Sheiner LB, et al: The clinical pharmacokinetics of phenytoin. *J Pharmacokinet Biopharm* 5:579, 1977.
27. Bauer LA, Blouin RA: Phenytoin Michaelis-Menten pharmacokinetics in Caucasian paediatric patients. *Clin Pharmacokinet* 8:545, 1983.
28. Bauer LA, Blouin RA: Age and phenytoin kinetics in adult epileptics. *Clin Pharmacol Ther* 31:301, 1982.
29. Winter ME, Tozer TN: Phenytoin, in Evans WE, Schentag JJ, Jusko WJ (eds): *Applied Pharmacokinetics: Principles of Therapeutic Drug Monitoring.* 2nd ed. Spokane, Applied Therapeutics, 1986, p 494.
30. Leppik IE: Metabolism of antiepileptic medication: Newborn to elderly. *Epilepsia* 33(suppl 4):S32, 1992.
31. Martin E, Gambertoglio JG, Alder DS, et al.: Removal of phenytoin by hemodialysis in uremic patients. *JAMA* 238:1750, 1977.
32. Blaschke TF: Protein binding and kinetics of drugs in liver diseases. *Clin Pharmacokinetics* 2:32, 1977.
33. Wilkinson GR, Shand DG: A physiological approach to hepatic drug clearance. *Clin Pharmacol Ther* 18:377, 1975.
34. Sarfeh IJ, Balint JA: Hepatic dysfunction following trauma: Experimental studies. *J Surg Res* 22:370, 1977.
35. Sarfeh IJ, Balint JA: The clinical significance of hyperbilirubinemia following trauma. *J Trauma* 18:58, 1978.

36. Nunes G, Blaisdell W, Margaretten W: Mechanism of hepatic dysfunction following shock and trauma. *Arch Surg* 100:546, 1970.

37. Schmid M, Hefti ML, Galtiker R, et al.: Benign postoperative intrahepatic cholestasis. *N Engl J Med* 272:545, 1965.

38. Shoemaker WC, Szanto PB, Fitch LB, Brill NR: Hepatic physiologic and morphologic alterations in hemorrhagic shock. *Surg Gynecol Obstet* 118:828, 1964.

39. Gottlieb ME, Stratton HH, Newell JC, Shah DM: Indocyanine green: Its use as an early indicator of hepatic dysfunction in man. *Arch Surg* 119:264, 1984.

40. Boucher BA, Rodman JH, Jaresko GS, et al.: Phenytoin pharmacokinetics in critically ill trauma patients. *Clin Pharmacol Ther* 44:675, 1988.

41. Bauer LA, Edwards WAD, Dellinger ED, et al.: Importance of unbound phenytoin serum levels in head trauma patients. *J Trauma* 23:1058, 1983.

42. Rapp RP, Young B, Twyman D, et al: The favorable effect of early parenteral feeding on survival in head-injured patients. *J Neurosurg* 58:906, 1983.

43. Cloyd JC, Gumnit RJ, McLain W: Status epilepticus: The role of intravenous phenytoin. *JAMA* 244:1479, 1980.

44. Cloyd JD, Bosch DE, Sawchuk RJ: Concentration-time profile of phenytoin after admixture with small volumes of intravenous fluids. *Am J Hosp Pharm* 35:45, 1978.

45. Earnest ED, Marx JA, Drury LA: Complications of I.V. phenytoin for acute treatment of seizures: Recommendations for usage. *JAMA* 249:762, 1983.

46. Louis S, Kutt H, McDowell E: The cardiac circulatory changes caused by intravenous dilantin and its solvent. *Am Heart J* 74:523, 1967.

47. Donovan PJ, Cline D: Phenytoin administration by constant intravenous infusion: Selective rates of administration. *Ann Emerg Med* 20:139, 1991.

48. Isenstein D, Nasraway SA: Hypotension during slow phenytoin infusion in severe sepsis. *Crit Care Med* 18:1036, 1990.

49. York RC, Coleridge ST: Cardiopulmonary arrest following intravenous phenytoin loading. *Am J Emerg Med* 6:255, 1988.

50. Temkin NR, Dikmen SS, Wilensky AJ, et al: A randomized, double-blind study of phenytoin for the prevention of post-traumatic seizures. *N Engl J Med* 323:497, 1990.

51. Kutt H: Phenytoin: Interactions with other drugs, in Levy R, Dreifuss FE, Mattson R, et al (eds): *Antiepileptic Drugs*. 3rd ed. New York, Macmillan, 1989, p 339.

52. Hansten PD, Horn JR: *Drug Interactions and Updates*. Vancouver, WA, Applied Therapeutics, 1990.

53. Hanson JM, Kampmann JP, Siersbalk-Nielsen K, et al: The effect of different sulfonamides on phenytoin metabolism in man. *Acta Med Scand* 624(suppl):106, 1979.

54. Philips P, Hansky J: Phenytoin toxicity secondary to cimetidine administration. *Med J Aust* 141:602, 1984.

55. Nolan PE, Marcus FI, Hoyer GL, et al: Pharmacokinetic interaction between intravenous phenytoin and amiodarone in healthy volunteers. *Clin Pharmacol Ther* 46:43, 1989.

56. Prichard DJ, Walt RP, Kitchingman GK, et al: Oral phenytoin pharmacokinetics during omeprazole therapy. *Br J Clin Pharmacol* 24:543, 1987.

57. Mitchell AS, Holland JT: Fluconazole and phenytoin: A predictable interaction. *Br Med J* 398:1315, 1989.

58. Jalil P: Toxic reaction following the combined administration of fluoxetine and phenytoin: Two case reports. *J Neurol Neurosurg Psychiatry* 55:412, 1992.

59. Katen RM, Roggin G, Robon F, et al: Increased rate of clearance of drugs from the circulation of alcoholics. *Am J Med Sci* 258:35, 1969.

60. Hansten PD: Interactions between anticonvulsant drugs: Primidone, diphenylhydantoin and phenobarbital. *Northwest Med J* 1:17, 1974.

61. Harvey SC: Hypnotics and sedatives, in Gilman AG, Goodman LS, Rall TW, Murad F (eds): *Goodman and Gilman's The Pharmacological Basis of Therapeutics*. 7th ed. New York, Macmillan, 1985.

62. Buchthal F, Svensmark O, Simonson H: Relation of EEG and seizures to phenobarbital in serum. *Arch Neurol* 19:567, 1968.

63. Booker HE: Phenobarbital: Relationship of plasma concentrations to seizure control, in Woodbury DM, Penry JK, Pippinger CE (eds): *Antiepileptic Drugs*. New York, Raven, 1982.

64. Butler TC, Mahafee C, Waddell WJ: Phenobarbital: Studies of elimination, accumulation, tolerance, and disease schedules. *J Pharmacol Exp Ther* 111:425, 1954.

65. Mattson R, Cramer J, Collins J, et al: Comparison of carbamazepine, phenobarbital, phenytoin, and primidone in partial and secondarily generalized tonic-clonic seizures. *N Engl J Med* 313:145, 1985.

66. Nelson E, Powell JR, Conrad K, et al: Phenobarbital pharmacokinetics and bioavailability in adults. *J Clin Pharmacol* 23:87, 1982.

67. Browne TR, Evans JE, Szabo GK, et al: Studies with stable isotopes. II. Phenobarbital pharmacokinetics during monotherapy. *J Clin Pharmacol* 25:51, 1985.

68. Welinsky, AJ, Friel PN, Levy RH, et al: Kinetics of phenobarbital in normal subjects and epileptic patients. *Eur J Clin Pharmacol* 23:87, 1982.

69. Jusko W, Gretch M: Plasma and tissue binding of drugs in pharmacokinetics. *Drug Metab Rev* 5:43, 1979.

70. Maynert EW, Van Dyke HB: The metabolism of barbiturates. *Pharmacol Rev* 1:217, 1949.

71. Waddell WJ, Butler TC: The distribution and excretion of phenobarbital. *J Clin Invest* 36:1217, 1957.

72. Alvin J, McHorse T, Hoyumpa A, et al: The effect of liver disease in man on the disposition of phenobarbital. *J Pharmacol Exp Ther* 192:224, 1975.

73. Henderson LW, Merrill JP: Treatment of barbiturate intoxication. *Ann Intern Med* 64:876, 1966.

74. Wroblewski BA, Garvin WH: Once daily administration of phenobarbital in adults: Clinical efficacy and benefit. *Arch Neurol* 42:699, 1985.

75. Eadie MJ: Anticonvulsant drugs: An update. *Drugs* 27:328, 1984.

76. Eichelbaum M, Kothe KW, Hoffman F, von Unruh GE: Kinetics and metabolism of carbamazepine during combined antiepileptic drug therapy. *Clin Pharmacol Ther* 26:366, 1979.

77. Perucca E: Clinical implications of hepatic microsomal enzyme induction by antiepileptic drugs. *Pharmacol Ther* 33:139, 1987.

78. Rutledge DR, Pieper JA, Mirvis DM: Effects of chronic phenobarbital on verapamil disposition in humans. *J Pharmacol Exp Ther* 246:7, 1988.

79. Schilleno JHM, Vander Wart JH, Brugman M, Briermer DD: Influence of enzyme induction and inhibition on the oxidation of nifedipine, sparteine, mephenytoin, and antipyrine in humans as assessed by a cocktail study design. *J Pharmacol Exp Ther* 249:638, 1989.

80. Browne TR, Szabo GK, Evans J, et al: Phenobarbital does not alter phenytoin steady-state serum concentration or pharmacokinetics. *Neurology* 38:639, 1988.

81. Eadie MJ, Lander CM, Hooper WD, Tyrer JH: Factors influencing plasma phenobarbital levels in epileptic patients. *Br J Clin Pharmacol* 4:541, 1977.

82. Kapetanovic IM, Kupeferberg HJ, Porter R, et al: Mechanism of valproate-phenobarbital interaction in epileptic patients. *Clin Pharmacol Ther* 29:480, 1981.

83. Piatt JH, Schiff Si: High dose barbiturate therapy in neurosurgery and intensive care. *Neurosurgery* 15:427, 1984.

84. Belopavlovic M, Buchthal A, Beks JWF: Barbiturates for cerebral aneurysm surgery: A review of preliminary results. *Acta Neurochir* 76:73, 1985.

85. Delgado-Escueta AV, Wasterlain C, Treiman DM, et al: Current concepts in neurology: Management of status epilepticus. *N Engl J Med* 306:1337, 1982.

86. Osorio I, Reed RC: Treatment of refractory generalized tonic-clonic status epilepticus with pentobarbital anesthesia after high dose phenytoin. *Epilepsia* 30:464, 1989.

87. Traeger SM, Henning RJ, Dubkin W, et al: Hemodynamic effects of pentobarbital therapy for intracranial hypertension. *Crit Care Med* 11:697, 1983.

88. Todd MM, Drummond JC, Hoi Sang U: Hemodynamic effects of high dose pentobarbital: Studies in elective neurosurgical patients. *Neurosurgery* 20:559, 1987.

89. Kassell NF, Peerless SJ, Drake CG: Treatment of ischemic deficits from cerebral vasospasm with high dose barbiturate therapy. *Neurosurgery* 7:593, 1980.

90. Lowenstein DH, Aminoff MJ, Simon RP: Barbiturate anesthesia in the treatment of status epilepticus: Clinical experience with 14 patients. *Neurology* 38:395, 1988.

91. Ehrnebo M: Pharmacokinetics and distribution properties of pen-

tobarbital in humans following oral and intravenous administration. *J Pharm Sci* 63:1114, 1974.

92. Bayliff CD, Schwartz ML, Hardy GB: Pharmacokinetics of high-dose pentobarbital in severe head trauma. *Clin Pharmacol Ther* 38:457, 1985.

93. Wermeling DP, Blouin RA, Porter WH, et al: Pentobarbital pharmacokinetics in patients with severe head injury. *Drug Intell Clin Pharm* 21:459, 1987.

94. Heinemeyer G, Roots I, Dennhardt R: Monitoring of pentobarbital plasma levels in critical care patients suffering from increased intracranial pressure. *Ther Drug Monit* 8:145, 1986.

95. Eisenberg HM, Frankowski RJ, Contant CF, et al: High-dose barbiturate control of elevated intracranial pressure in patients with severe head injury. *J Neurosurg* 69:15, 1988.

96. Dahlquist R, Steiner E, Koike Y, et al: Induction of theophylline metabolism by pentobarbital. *Ther Drug Monit* 11:408, 1989.

97. Wroblewski BA, Glenn MD, Whyte J, Singer WD: Carbamazepine replacement of phenytoin, phenobarbital and primidone in a rehabilitation setting: Effects on seizure control. *Brain Inj* 3:149, 1989.

98. Patterson JF: Carbamazepine in the treatment of phantom limb pain. *South Med J* 81:1100, 1988.

99. Ballenger JC: The use of anticonvulsants in manic-depressive illness. *J Clin Psychiatry* 49(suppl):21, 1988.

100. Riva R, Albani F, Ambrosetto G, et al: Diurnal fluctuations in free and total steady-state plasma levels of carbamazepine and correlation with intermittent side effects. *Epilepsia* 25:476, 1984.

101. Callaghan N, O'Callaghan M, Duggan B, Feely M: Carbamazepine as a single drug in the treatment of epilepsy: A prospective study of serum level and seizure control. *J Neurol Neurosurg Psychiatry* 41:907, 1978.

102. Troupin AS, Ojeman LM, Halpern L, et al: Carbamazepine: A double blind comparison with phenytoin. *Neurology* 27:511, 1977.

103. Strandjord RE, Johannessen SI: Single drug therapy with carbamazepine in patients with epilepsy: Serum levels and clinical effect. *Epilepsia* 21:655, 1980.

104. Reynolds EH: Neurotoxicity of carbamazepine. *Adv Neurol* 11:345, 1975.

105. Weaver DF, Camfield P, Fraser A: Massive carbamazepine overdose: Clinical and pharmacologic observations in five episodes. *Neurology* 38:755, 1988.

106. Perucca E: Free level monitoring of antiepileptic drugs. *Clin Pharmacokinet* 9(suppl 1):71, 1984.

107. Graves NM, Kriel RL, Jones-Saete C, Cloyd JC: Relative bioavailability of rectally administered carbamazepine suspension in humans. *Epilepsia* 26:429, 1985.

108. Cotter LAR, Eadie LS, Hooper WD: The pharmacokinetics of carbamazepine. *Eur J Clin Pharmacol* 12:451, 1977.

109. Neuvonen PJ, Tokola O: Bioavailability of rectally administered carbamazepine mixture. *Br J Clin Pharmacol* 24:839, 1987.

110. Morselli PL, Monaco F, Gerna M: Bioavailability of two carbamazepine preparations during chronic administration to epileptic patients. *Epilepsia* 16:259, 1975.

111. Bertillson L, Tomson T: Clinical pharmacokinetics and pharmacological effects of carbamazepine 10,11 epoxide: An update. *Clin Pharmacokinet* 11:177, 1986.

112. Levy RH, Pitlick WH, Troupin AS, et al: Pharmacokinetics of carbamazepine in normal man. *Clin Pharmacol Ther* 17:657, 1975.

113. Bass J, Miles MV, Tennison MD, et al: Effects of enteral tube feedings on the absorption and pharmacokinetic profile of carbamazepine suspension. *Epilepsia* 30:364, 1989.

114. Westenberg HGM, van der Klejn E, Oeitt de, Zeeuw RA: Kinetics of carbamazepine and carbamazepine 10,11 epoxide determined by use of plasma and saliva. *Clin Pharmacol Ther* 23:320, 1978.

115. Eichelbaum M, Kothe KW, Hoffman F, et al: Use of stable labeled carbamazepine to study its kinetics during chronic carbamazepine treatment. *Eur J Clin Pharmacol* 23:241, 1982.

116. Frits ML, Christiansen J, Hvidberg EF: Brain concentration of carbamazepine and carbamazepine 10,11 epoxide in epileptic patients. *Eur J Clin Pharmacol* 14:47, 1978.

117. Morselli PL, Barruzzi A, Gerna M, et al: Carbamazepine and carbamazepine 10,11 epoxide concentrations in human brain. *Br J Clin Pharmacol* 4:535, 1977.

118. Hooper WD, Dubetz DK, Bochner F, et al: Plasma protein binding of carbamazepine. *Clin Pharmacol Ther* 17:433, 1975.

119. Lertratananykoon K, Horning MG: Metabolism of carbamazepine. *Drug Metab Dispos* 10:1, 1981.

120. Bourgeois BFD, Wad N: Individual and combined antiepileptic and neurotoxic activity of carbamazepine and carbamazepine 10,11 epoxide in mice. *J Pharmacol Exp Ther* 231:411, 1984.

121. Tomson T, Bertilsson L: Potent therapeutic effect of carbamazepine 10,11 epoxide in trigeminal neuralgia. *Arch Neurol* 41:598, 1984.

122. McNamara PJ, Colburn WA, Gilbaldi M: Time course of carbamazepine self-induction. *J Pharmacokinet Biopharm* 7:63, 1979.

123. Makati MA, Browne TR, Collins JF: Time course of carbamazepine autoinduction. *Neurology* 39:592, 1989.

124. Eichelbaum M, Tomson T, Tybring G, Bertilsson L: Carbamazepine metabolism in man: Induction and pharmacogenetic aspects. *Clin Pharmcokinet* 10:80, 1985.

125. Eichelbaum M, Kothe KW, Hoffman F, et al: Kinetics and metabolism of carbamazepine during combined anti-epileptic drug therapy. *Clin Pharmacol Ther* 26:366, 1979.

126. Tomson T, Tybring G, Bertilsson L: Single dose kinetics and metabolism of carbamazepine-10,11-epoxide. *Clin Pharmacol Ther* 33:58, 1983.

127. Bowdle TA, Levy RH, Cutler RE: Effects of carbamazepine on valproic acid in normal man. *Clin Pharmacol Ther* 26:629, 1979.

128. Baciewicz AM: Carbamazepine drug interactions. *Ther Drug Monit* 8:305, 1986.

129. Browne TR, Szabo GK, Evans JH, et al: Carbamazepine increases phenytoin serum concentrations and reduces phenytoin clearance. *Neurology* 38:1146, 1988.

130. Zielinski JJ, Haedukewych D, Leketa BJ: Carbamazepine-phenytoin interaction: Elevation of plasma phenytoin concentrations due to carbamazepine comedication. *Ther Drug Monit* 7:51, 1985.

131. Wong JYY, Ludden TM, Bell RD: Effect of erythromycin on carbamazepine kinetics. *Clin Pharmacol Ther* 33:460, 1983.

131. Oles KS, Mivza W, Penry JK: Catastrophic neurologic signs due to drug interaction: Tegretol and Darvon. *Surg Neurol* 32:144, 1989.

132. Bebin M, Bleck TP: New anticonvulsant drugs. Focus on flunarizine, fosphenytoin, midazolam and stirpentol. *Drugs* 48:153, 1994.

133. Walker MC, Sander JW: Developments in antiepileptic drug therapy. *Curr Opin Neurol* 7:131, 1994.

134. Davis R, Peters, DH, McTavish D: Valproic acid: A reappraisal of its pharmacologic properties and clinical efficacy in epilepsy. *Drugs* 47:332, 1994.

135. Levy RH, Mattson, RH, Meldrun, et al: *Antiepileptic Drugs*. 4th ed. New York, Raven Press, 1995.

214. Cyclosporine

David I. Min and Daniel M. Canafax

Introduction

The indications for cyclosporine are prevention of allograft rejection [1], graft-versus-host disease in bone marrow transplant recipients [2], and treatment of autoimmune diseases, such as uveitis [3], diabetes [4], and myasthenia gravis [5]. Allograft survival rates for renal, cardiac, hepatic, and pancreatic transplant recipients have significantly improved since cyclosporine became available for clinical use in 1983 [1].

Pharmacology

Cyclosporine blocks cytokine synthesis and receptor expression needed for T-lymphocyte activation by interrupting the signal transduction [6]. Cyclosporine binds cyclophilin and the cyclosporine-cyclophilin complex binds to and inhibits the Ca^{2+}-dependent phosphatase calcineurin [7]. Calcineurin is required for the proper assembly of a transcription factor, which then binds to the IL-2 gene and initiates IL-2 synthesis [8]. A lack of cytokine disrupts the activation and proliferation of helper and cytotoxic T cells that are essential for the rejection process [6].

The mechanism of cyclosporine-induced nephrotoxicity appears to involve interference with prostaglandin synthesis in renal cortical tissue that increases thromboxane A_2 concentrations, causing intrarenal vasoconstriction [6]. These effects produce a decrease of renal blood flow and glomerular filtration rate, usually without morphologic changes, although chronic effects may progress to interstitial fibrosis.

Therapeutic Range

Table 214-1 summarizes the therapeutic ranges for the various analytic methods and blood matrices in clinical use. A precise cyclosporine concentration versus response relationship for both therapeutic and toxic effects has been difficult to define as a result of the many confounding patient factors, such as use of other immunosuppressants, and different analytic methods. Cyclosporine concentrations do, however, help identify patients with low or high values, who might benefit from dosage changes.

The two analytical methods used for clinical monitoring of cyclosporine concentrations produce differing results. The high-performance liquid chromatographic (HPLC) method, a monoclonal radioimmunoassay (MRIA), and a monoclonal fluorescence polarization immunoassay (M-FPIA) technique are specific for cyclosporine, whereas the polyclonal radioimmunoassay (P-RIA) and the polyclonal fluorescence polarization immunoassay (P-FPIA) methods are nonspecific, cross-reacting with cyclosporine metabolites. Results from nonspecific assay methods must be interpreted with caution in patients with reduced hepatic function, since accumulation of metabolites occurs. Whole blood concentrations are usually two times greater than serum concentrations, since cyclosporine distributes into erythrocytes. This distribution is temperature-dependent, with plasma concentration decreasing by 50 percent if the blood sample is separated at room temperature versus at 37°C. It has been recommended that whole blood be the standard analytical matrix and a specific assay method used for analysis [9]. Assay accuracy is poor at concentrations less than 50 ng per milliliter, which becomes important at low doses of cyclosporine.

Adverse reactions associated with high cyclosporine concentrations include renal dysfunction, tremor, hypertension, and hepatotoxicity. Nephrotoxicity, the most common adverse effect, is dose-related and decreasing the cyclosporine dose usually decreases the creatinine level. In renal allograft recipients, it is often difficult to differentiate between cyclosporine renal effects and acute rejection episodes. Measurement of cyclosporine concentrations may be helpful in this situation; high levels are more likely associated with cyclosporine effects and low levels with rejection [10].

Twelve- or 24-hour trough cyclosporine concentrations (depending on the dosing frequency) are used for monitoring therapy. When using PRIA or P-FPIA to analyze serum concentrations, a range of 100 to 250 ng per milliliter is a reasonable target for immunosuppressive activity [11]. Cyclosporine-induced nephrotoxicity can be minimized by keeping concentrations (HPLC, whole blood) between 150 to 250 ng per milliliter during the first 4 months and 100 to 200 ng per milliliter thereafter [12].

Table 214-1. Cyclosporine 12-Hour Trough Concentration Ranges for Various Analytic Methods

Transplant	Sample matrix	Analytic method[a]	Target range (ng/ml)
Kidney	Blood	HPLC	150–250 (day 0–day 120) 100–200 (after day 120)
	Blood	P-FPIA or P-RIA[b]	200–800
	Blood	M-RIA of M-FPIA	150–400
	Serum/ plasma	P-FPIA	100–250
Liver	Blood	HPLC	150–300
		M-RIA or M-FPIA	150–400
		P-FPIA	400–800
Heart	Blood	HPLC	150–300
		M-RIA or M-FPIA	150–400
Bone marrow	Serum/ plasma	P-FPIA or P-RIA[b]	100–250

[a] HPLC: high performance liquid chromatography, M-RIA: monoclonal radioimmunoassay, M-FPIA: monoclonal fluorecence polarization immunoassay, P-FPIA: polyclonal fluorescence polarization immunoassay, P-RIA: polyclonal radioimmunoassay
[b] no longer available

Preparations

Cyclosporine for IV administration is available in 5-ml sterile ampules, with each milliliter containing 50 mg of cyclosporine, 650 mg of polyoxyethylated castor oil (Cremophor EL), and 32.9% alcohol. Cyclosporine for IV use must be diluted before administration. The diluents can cause acute toxic effects, including flushing, shortness of breath, tachycardia, and hypotension. Intramuscular injection is not recommended because of low bioavailability.

Two oral cyclosporine preparations are available: 50-ml bottles of an olive oil solution that contains 100 mg per milliliter and gelatin capsules that contain 25 or 100 mg. Cyclosporine capsules and solution are bioequivalent [13]. The oral solution can be administered by nasogastric tube. To make the oral solution more palatable, it can be diluted with chocolate milk or juice.

Pharmacokinetics

Table 214-2 summarizes cyclosporine's pharmacokinetic parameters.

ABSORPTION. Cyclosporine is only partially absorbed after an oral dose, with a mean bioavailability of 30 percent, (range 7–92%) [14,15]. Because of low fractional absorption and significant first-pass metabolism, oral cyclosporine doses are three times larger than IV doses, to achieve equivalent circulating concentrations. The absorption of cyclosporine is influenced by factors such as the type of organ transplanted, time since transplantation, presence of external biliary drainage, liver function, intestinal dysfunction, and use of drugs that alter gastrointestinal motility. Other factors that may be responsible for reduced cyclosporine absorption include carrier-controlled absorption, reduced bile production, and intestinal wall metabolism. It appears that cyclosporine absorption is dose-dependent [16].

Some patients achieve adequate cyclosporine concentrations before transplant but using the same dose have markedly reduced concentrations immediately after transplant. These patients need higher oral doses or IV therapy for a short period. Poor absorption of cyclosporine in the early postoperative period has been attributed to prolonged postoperative ileus. Bile salts are necessary for oral cyclosporine absorption, which may account for the slow and incomplete absorption seen in liver transplant patients with external bile drainage. There can also be a significant increase in cyclosporine concentrations after T tube clamping in these patients. A new oral formulation of cyclosporine (Neoral) is in clinical trials, and it is expected to be available soon in the United States. This oral formulation incorporates drug in a microemulsion preconcentrate. According to the preliminary data, its absorption in the gastrointestinal tract appears to be bile or food independent. It showed a significantly reduced inter- and intrasubject variability in cyclosporine absorption compared with the current formulation [37].

Any factor affecting gastric emptying time and intestine transit time may influence the rate and extent of cyclosporine absorption in the gut. Metoclopramide increases the rate and amount of cyclosporine absorption, whereas severe diarrhea can cause decreased absorption, resulting in low trough concentrations.

Oral cyclosporine bioavailability gradually improves for several weeks after transplant. The time to peak cyclosporine concentrations is 3 to 5 hours after oral administration. After single high doses of 17.5 mg per kilogram given once daily, peak

Table 214-2. Summary of Cyclosporine Pharmacokinetic Parameters [1,4,11][a]

Parameter	Population average ($\pm$ SD)
Bioavailability (oral)	$30.6 \pm 12.7\%$
Protein binding	98%
CL (ml/min/kg)	12.62 ± 5.7
Tmax (hr)	4.0 ± 1.8
C_{max} (ng/ml)[b]	1103 ± 570
V_{dc} (L/kg)	0.8 ± 0.2
V_{dss} (L/kg)	4.24 ± 2.7
Distribution half-life	1.1 ± 0.3 hr
Elimination half-life	9.6 ± 5.8 hr
Hemodialysis	No effect ($<1\%$)
Peritoneal Dialysis	No data
Hemoperfusion	No effect

[a] All parameters based on whole-blood samples and HPLC assay.
[b] This C_{max} is based on a dose of 10 mg/kg.

serum concentrations ranged from 1800 to 3300 ng per milliliter (P-RIA, serum) in renal transplant patients [11]. Patients with cyclosporine bioavailability of less than 25 percent have an increased risk of renal allograft loss (63% vs. 83%) [15].

DISTRIBUTION. The distribution half-life of cyclosporine is about 1.1 hours [17]. Cyclosporine is lipophilic and distributes widely throughout body tissues, concentrating in organs such as liver, pancreas, lungs, kidneys, and, especially, fat, producing higher cyclosporine concentrations than in the serum. For example, the ratio of cyclosporine concentrations in renal tissue to whole blood is 5.5:1 [18]. Cyclosporine is not bound to albumin, but is highly bound to lipoproteins, which comprise 10 to 15 percent of all plasma proteins. Among the blood fractions, 10 to 20 percent of cyclosporine concentrations are found in the leukocytes, 40 to 50 percent in the erythrocytes, and 30 to 40 percent in the plasma [19]. Whole blood cyclosporine concentrations are two to three times higher than serum or plasma concentrations. Cyclosporine persists in body tissue for weeks to months after therapy is discontinued. Cyclosporine does not readily penetrate the blood-brain barrier, but cyclosporine-induced neurotoxicity occurs most frequently at very high blood concentrations, low cholesterol levels, during hypomagnesemia, and in liver transplant recipients [20,21]. Cyclosporine crosses the placental barrier and can be found in amniotic fluid during pregnancy [22]. Cyclosporine was detected in an infant's blood up to 48 hours after birth and was detectable in the breast milk of women receiving the drug. The volume of distribution (V_2) for cyclosporine does not appear to increase in obese patients; however, because obese patients have higher blood concentrations than normal patients, cyclosporine doses should be based on lean body weight [23]. The V_d is not altered in patients with hepatic or renal failure.

CLEARANCE. Cyclosporine is extensively metabolized by the liver, with more than 90 percent of a dose excreted as metabolites into the bile and eliminated in the feces. Renal excretion of unchanged cyclosporine accounts for less than 1 percent of a dose and urinary excretion of metabolites for less than 6 percent [24]. Cyclosporine is primarily metabolized by the hepatic oxidase cytochrome P-450 IIIA enzyme system. There are 17 suspected metabolites, the structures of 9 of which have been identified. Of these metabolites 17, 1, and 21 are the most common. The cyclosporine metabolites identified to date maintain the cyclic oligopeptide structure of the parent drug, with minor oxidative changes on the amino acid side chains. The immunosuppressive properties of these metabolites appear to be minimal [25]. There is no evidence that any of these metabolites have renal effects.

Various factors can alter the rate of cyclosporine metabolism, such as hepatic function, patient age, and interactions with other drugs. Cyclosporine clearance in pediatric renal and liver transplant recipients is significantly faster than in adults. Systemic clearance of cyclosporine is about 50 percent less in patients with moderate hyperbilirubinemia (bilirubin level > 2.0 mg/dl). Hemodialysis and hemoperfusion do not remove cyclosporine from the body.

HALF-LIFE. The mean elimination half-life varies from 7 to 24 hours, depending on the type of transplant and concurrent disease states [9,14]. In adult renal transplant recipients with near normal renal function, the mean half-life of cyclosporine is about 10 hours. Patients with liver failure have relatively long cyclosporine elimination half-lives, averaging 20 hours (range 10–48 hours) [9]. Cyclosporine doses should be decreased in most patients with hepatic failure. Cyclosporine trough levels can double a few months after transplant from increased hematocrit and lipoproteins [26].

Dosage and Administration

Initial oral cyclosporine doses are usually about 10 mg/kg/day. For living donor kidney recipients, cyclosporine is given 1 to 2 days before transplantation to achieve therapeutic concentrations at the time of transplantation [27]. This dose is divided twice daily and adjusted to maintain the desired cyclosporine concentrations. Dosage adjustment is empirical as a result of extreme intrapatient variability in absorption and clearance. Antilymphoblast globulin or OKT3 is often used in the early post-transplant period for cadaver kidney recipients to allow holding cyclosporine until serum creatinine concentrations are less than 3 mg per deciliter, in an attempt to avoid adverse renal effects of cyclosporine [28].

Oral administration of cyclosporine is usually preferred. However, for patients who cannot tolerate oral therapy or whose cyclosporine absorption is poor, IV doses of 3 to 6 mg/kg/day can be given. Hepatic, heart-lung, and pancreatic allograft recipients usually require IV cyclosporine in the first few weeks after transplant. Loading doses are not used when beginning cyclosporine therapy, since side effects would likely occur. Before use, IV cyclosporine solution should be diluted in 20 ml to 100 ml of normal saline or D_5W for injection and given as a slow IV infusion over 2 to 6 hours. The IV cyclosporine dose can be given by a continuous 24-hour infusion, which may reduce the renal effects of the drug. The IV dose is adjusted using trough levels. Blood samples for cyclosporine analysis should not be drawn from the IV lines used for administration, to avoid spuriously high levels. Patients receiving IV cyclosporine can be changed to oral therapy by giving two to three times the IV dose and measuring cyclosporine concentrations. To ensure cyclosporine absorption and assess the adequacy of the dose, a trough level should be taken within the first 2 or 3 days after starting therapy. Because absorption and clearance change during the first weeks of therapy, levels should be obtained at least two or three times weekly. After

discharge from the hospital, levels should be obtained at least twice per week until stable, usually within 1 or 2 months. Chronic cyclosporine dosing is guided by weekly and then monthly blood concentrations and serum creatinine levels, with most patients requiring approximately 5 to 6 mg per kilogram of cyclosporine daily.

Drug Interactions

Numerous reported interactions between cyclosporine and other drugs can produce troublesome clinical effects [29,30,31].

Food appears to increase cyclosporine levels by increasing the amount absorbed. It is not known whether antacids can decrease cyclosporine absorption, but there appears to be no effect. No effects were seen from cholestyramine given 1 hour before or 4 hours after a cyclosporine dose. Metoclopramide increases cyclosporine levels, and severe diarrhea can decrease cyclosporine levels [32].

Since cyclosporine is extensively metabolized by the hepatic cytochrome P-450 IIIA enzyme system, various drugs that induce or inhibit these enzymes usually have significant effects on cyclosporine concentrations. The antiepileptic drugs, such as phenytoin, phenobarbital, and carbamazepine, induce these enzymes and decrease the concentrations of cyclosporine. Phenytoin effects on cyclosporine metabolism last at least 2 weeks after discontinuation and usually require two to three times higher cyclosporine doses [31]. A good alternative antiepileptic drug might be valproic acid, which has fewer effects on cyclosporine concentrations. The antitubercular drugs, rifampin, and isoniazid are also potent inducers of the P-450 IIIA enzymes and reduce cyclosporine concentrations [29,33].

Drugs that inhibit the hepatic microsomal enzymes increase cyclosporine concentrations. For example, ketoconazole caused 10-fold increases in cyclosporine concentrations with subsequent increases in serum creatinine levels [34]. Fluconazole can slightly increase cyclosporine concentrations after 2 weeks of therapy [35]. Giving erythromycin to a patient on cyclosporine typically causes cyclosporine concentrations to increase fivefold 2 to 5 days after initiation of therapy [36].

Calcium channel blockers, such as diltiazem and nicardipine, can slightly increase cyclosporine concentrations, but nifedipine appears to have no effect [31]. Hormones such as danazol, norethisterone, and methyltestosterone have been reported to increase cyclosporine concentrations, but the clinical significance of this interaction remains unclear. Cimetidine likely increases cyclosporine concentrations but ranitidine and famotidine appear to have no effects [31].

Drugs such as amphotericin B, aminoglycosides, trimethoprim-sulfamethoxazole, melphalan, furosemide, mannitol, and indomethacin and the cephalosporins increase the incidence of adverse renal effects when given with cyclosporine. Drugs that decrease cyclosporine-induced renal effects include spironolactone, enalapril, prazosin, thromboxane synthetase inhibitors, and some prostaglandins.

The combination of cyclosporine and lovastatin has been reported to cause a myalgia and rhabdomyolysis syndrome at high doses of cyclosporine [29,30]. Patients on cyclosporine are prone to gingival hyperplasia, which can be worsened by other drugs such as phenytoin and nifedipine.

References

1. Canafax DM, Sutherland DER: Recent advances in solid organ transplantation. *Pharmacotherapy* 7:S20, 1987.

2. Storb R, Deeg HJ, Thomas EL, et al: Preliminary results of prospective randomized trials comparing methotrexate and cyclosporine for prophylaxis of graft-versus-host disease after HLA-identical marrow transplantation. *Transplant Proc* 15:2620, 1983.

3. Nussenblatt RB, Palestine AG, Rook AH, et al: Treatment of intraocular inflammatory disease with cyclosporin A. *Lancet* 2:235, 1982.

4. Stiller C, Depre JP, Gent M, et al: Effects of cyclosporine immunosuppression in insulin-dependent diabetes of recent onset. *Science* 223:1362, 1984.

5. Tindall RFA, Rolands JA, Phillips JT, et al: Preliminary results of a double blind randomized placebo controlled trial of cyclosporine in myasthenia gravis. *N Engl J Med* 316:719, 1987.

6. Kahan BD: Cyclosporine. *N Engl J Med* 321:1725, 1989.

7. Schumacher A, Norheim A: Progress towards a molecular understanding of cyclosporin A-mediated immunosuppression. *Clin Invest* 70:773, 1992.

8. Schreiber SL, Crabtree GR: The mechanism of action of cyclosporin A and FK 506. *Immunol Today* 13:136, 1992.

9. Shaw LM, Bowers LD, Demers L, et al: Critical issues in cyclosporine monitoring: Report of the task force on cyclosporine monitoring. *Clin Chem* 33:1269, 1987.

10. Ferguson RM, Canafax DM, Sawchuk RT, Simmons RS: Cyclosporine blood level monitoring: The early posttransplant period. *Transplant Proc* 18(suppl 2):113, 1986.

11. Keown PA, Stiller CR, Ulan RA, et al: Immunological and pharmacological monitoring in clinical use of cyclosporin A. *Lancet* 1:686, 1981.

12. Moyer TP, Gregory RP, Sterioff S, et al: Cyclosporine nephrotoxicity is minimized by adjusting dosage on the basis of drug concentration in blood. *Mayo Clin Proc* 63:241, 1988.

13. Min DL, Hwang GC, Bergstom S, et al: Bioavailability and patient acceptance of cyclosporine soft gelatin capsules in renal allograft recipients. *Ann Pharmacother* 26:175, 1992.

14. Ptachcinski RJ, Venkataramanan R, Burckart GJ, et al: Clinical pharmacokinetics of cyclosporine. *Clin Pharmacokinet* 11:107, 1986.

15. Lindholm A, Kahan B: Influence of cyclosporine pharmacokinetic parameters, trough concentrations, and AUC monitoring on outcome after renal transplantation. *Clin Pharmacol Ther* 54:205, 1993.

16. Reymond JP, Steimer JL, Niederberger W: On the dose dependency of cyclosporin A absorption and disposition in healthy volunteers. *J Pharmacokinet Biopharm* 16:331, 1988.

17. Follath F, Wenk M, Vozeh S, et al: Intravenous cyclosporine kinetics in renal failure. *Clin Pharmacol Ther* 34:638, 1983.

18. Atkinson K, Boland J, Britton K, et al: Blood and tissue distribution of cyclosporine in humans and mice. *Transplant Proc* 15:2434, 1983.

19. Lemaire M, Tillement JP: Role of lipoproteins and erythrocytes in the in vitro binding and distribution of cyclosporin A in the blood. *J Pharm Pharmacol* 34:715, 1982.

20. Thomson CB, June CH, Sullivan KM, et al: Association between cyclosporine neurotoxicity and hypomagnesaemia. *Lancet* 2:1116, 1984.

21. de Groen PC, Aksamit AJ, Rakela J, et al: Central nervous system toxicity after liver transplantation: The role of cyclosporine and cholesterol. *N Engl J Med* 317:861, 1987.

22. Flechner SM, Katz AR, Rogers AJ, et al: The presence of cyclosporine in body tissue and fluids during pregnancy. *Am J Kidney Dis* 5:60, 1985.

23. Flechner SM, Kolbeinsson ME, Tam J, et al: The impact of body weight on cyclosporine pharmacokinetics in renal transplant recipients. *Transplantation* 47:806, 1989.

24. Mauer G, Loosli HR, Schreier E, et al: Disposition of cyclosporine in several animal species and man. *Drug Metab Dispos* 12:120, 1984.

25. Rosano TG, Freed BM, Cerilli J, et al: Immunosuppressive metabolites of cyclosporine in the blood of renal allograft recipients. *Transplantation* 42:262, 1986.

26. Kasiske BL, Awni WM, Heim-Duthoy KL, et al: Alterations in cyclosporine pharmacokinetics after renal transplantation are like to rapid increases in hematocrit, lipoproteins, and serum protein. *Transplant Proc* 20:485, 1988.

27. Chan GLC, Canafax DM, Ascher NL, et al: HLA-identical renal transplantation: No rejections with a cyclosporine-azathioprine-prednisone protocol. *Clin Transpl* 2:9, 1988.

28. Canafax DM, Min DI, Gruber SA, et al: Immunosuppression for cadaveric renal allograft recipients: A risk-factor matched comparison of the Minnesota randomized trial with an antilymphoblast globulin, azathioprine, cyclosporine and prednisone protocol. *Clin Transpl* 3:110, 1989.

29. Baciewicz AM, Baciewicz FA: Cyclosporine pharmacokinetic drug interactions. *Am J Surg* 157:264, 1989.

30. Lake KD: Cyclosporine drug interactions: A review. *Cardiac Surg* 2:617, 1988.

31. Hansten PD, Horn JR: *Drug Interactions.* 6th ed. Philadelphia, Lea & Febiger, 1989.

32. Wadhwa NK, Schroeder TJ, O'Flaherty E, et al: The effects of oral metoclopramide on the absorption of cyclosporine. *Transplantation* 43:211, 1987.

33. Langhoff E, Madsen S: Rapid metabolism of cyclosporine and prednisolone in kidney transplant patients receiving tuberculostatic treatment. *Lancet* 2:1031, 1983.

34. Ferguson RM, Sutherland DER, Simmons RL, et al: Ketaconazole, cyclosporine metabolism in renal transplantation. *Lancet* 2:822, 1982.

35. Canafax DM, Graves NM, Hilligoss DM, et al: Interaction between cyclosporine and fluconazole in renal transplant recipients. *Transplantation* 51:1014, 1991.

36. Ptachcinski RJ, Carpenter BJ, Burckart GJ, et al: Effect of erythromycin on cyclosporine levels. *N Engl J Med* 313:1416, 1985.

37. Kahan BD, Dunn J, Fitts C, et al: Reduced inter- and intrasubject variability in cyclosporine pharmacokinetics in renal transplant recipients treated with a microemulsion formulation in conjunction with fasting, low-fat meals, or high-fat meals. *Transplantation* 59:505, 1995.

215. *Analgesics*

David R. P. Guay

Opioids

INTRODUCTION. Opioids (also known as narcotic analgesics) are among the most commonly used medications in the intensive care setting. Although most frequently used for analgesia, these agents may be used to alleviate psychologic discomfort, produce sedation, or depress respiratory drive or coughing. Clinicians specializing in critical care need to know not only primary and secondary pharmacological actions of these agents but also their pharmacokinetics, pharmacodynamics, and optimal modes of administration.

PHARMACOLOGY. [1–8]. Sixteen opioid analgesics and two opioid antagonists are currently available in the United States (Table 215-1).

Although five types of opioid receptors have been isolated,

Table 215-1. Chemical Classification and Receptor Specificities of Narcotic Analgesics [1]

	Receptor types		
	Mu	Kappa	Sigma
Opioid agonists			
Morphine	Ag	Ag	—
Hydromorphone (Dilaudid)	Ag	Ag	—
Oxycodone (Percodan, Percocet)	Ag	Ag	—
Codeine	Ag	Ag	—
Meperidine (Demerol)	Ag	Ag	—
Fentanyl (Sublimaze)	Ag	Ag	—
Levorphanol (Levo-Dromoran)	Ag	Ag	—
Oxymorphone (Numorphan)	Ag	Ag	—
Sufentanil (Sufenta)	Ag	Ag	—
Alfentanil (Alfenta)	Ag	Ag	—
Methadone (Dolophine)	Ag	Ag	—
Buprenorphine (Buprenex)	pAg	Ant*	—
Dezocine (Dalgan)	pAg	Ag	—
Opioid agonist antagonists			
Pentazocine (Talwin)	Ant	Ag	Ag
Nalbuphine (Nubain)	Ant	Ag	—
Butorphanol (Stadol)	—	Ag	Ag
Opioid antagonists			
Naloxone	Ant	Ant	Ant
Naltrexone	Ant	Ant	Ant

Ag = agonist; pAg = partial agonist; Ant = competitive antagonist;
* Not yet fully studied

only three (mu, kappa, sigma) are thought to have relevance in humans. Stimulation of mu receptors is thought to be associated with supraspinal analgesia, respiratory depression, euphoria, depressed gastrointestinal (GI) motility, urinary retention, sedation, nausea, vomiting, bradycardia, constipation, pruritus, and tolerance/dependence. Stimulation of kappa receptors is thought to be associated with spinal analgesia and sedation, while sigma receptor stimulation is thought to be associated with respiratory and vasomotor stimulation and dysphoria/hallucinations/delirium. Table 215-1 illustrates the receptor specificities of available opioids and underscores the fact that none of these agents exhibits an ideal profile of receptor stimulation properties.

A variety of central nervous system (CNS) pharmacodynamic effects are associated with opioids. These include narcosis, respiratory depression (depressed rate, minute volume, tidal exchange, response to CO_2), cough suppression, tolerance/dependence, seizures (true seizures with meperidine and nonepileptic clonus with large doses of fentanyl and sufentanil) and muscle rigidity with rapid intravenous (IV) bolus administration of fentanyl, sufentanil, and alfentanil. From a cardiovascular standpoint, these agents may cause hypotension secondary to vasodilatation (due to decreased sympathetic tone and histamine release) and/or bradycardia (due to increased vagal tone). This may be especially problematic in hypovolemic individuals. In contrast, the opioid agonist/antagonists may increase pulmonary vascular resistance and cause systemic hypertension. Fentanyl, sufentanil, and alfentanil appear to have minimal adverse cardiovascular effects.

Direct respiratory effects may include bronchospasm secondary to histamine release and chest wall rigidity (especially in elderly patients or those with renal impairment). Histamine release appears to be greatest for meperidine, codeine, and morphine and absent with fentanyl and its congeners [1,9]. Urinary retention, due to increased sphincter pressure and decreased detrusor tone, is especially problematic with epidural/intrathecal opioid use. Opioids can suppress appetite, cause nausea and vomiting secondary to chemoreceptor trigger zone stimulation and gastric stasis, increase sphincter of Oddi tone, suppress GI motility, and aggravate postsurgical ileus. Although controversial, meperidine and the agonist/antagonists may cause less spasm of the sphincter of Oddi [1,10,11]. Itching and formication may be problematic, especially with epidural/intrathecal agents. IgE-medicated anaphylaxis due to opioids is extremely rare but evidence exists to suggest that cross-reactivity between fentanyl, alfentanil, sufentanil, and meperidine is likely.

THERAPEUTIC RANGE. Few data exist that document therapeutic plasma, serum, or blood concentrations for opioid analgesia. Although a therapeutic range for morphine of 10 to 100 ng per milliliter with a minimal effective concentration of 15 to 65 ng per milliliter has been cited [12], this has been disputed [10,13]. Similarly, therapeutic ranges for fentanyl, alfentanil, and meperidine of 1 to 3 ng/per milliliter, greater than 20 to 25 ng per milliliter, and more than 0.7 μg per milliliter, respectively, have been proposed [14,15,16]. In light of these data, together with the lack of routinely available assays for these compounds in biologic specimens, it appears that the use of therapeutic drug concentration monitoring is of little routine clinical value.

PREPARATIONS. The opioid analgesic and antagonist preparations available in the United States are listed in Table 215-2. Multiple routes of administration, including oral, rectal, parenteral, epidural/intrathecal, and transdermal, are available.

PHARMACOKINETICS. Table 215-3 illustrates the pharmacodynamic and pharmacokinetic parameters for available opioids in adults. Oral bioavailability of opioids is less than quantitative, probably secondary to a substantial degree of presystemic metabolism. Similar reductions in bioavailability after rectal administration have been noted, probably due to both reduced absorption (related to formulation vehicle) and presystemic metabolism.

Most opioids are bound moderately to extensively to plasma proteins (60–95%), both albumin and alpha-1-acid glycoprotein (AAG), and binding may be altered in a variety of circumstances. For example, morphine plasma protein binding is significantly reduced in the presence of renal and hepatic disease, while that of meperidine is reduced in the elderly and increased in postsurgical and burn patients (in the latter probably due to elevated AAG). In addition, alfentanil binding is reduced in the presence of hepatic disease.

Extensive tissue distribution is evidenced by the large terminal phase or steady-state volume of distribution values noted in a variety of populations (1–6 L/kg). All opioids are virtually entirely dependent on hepatic metabolism for elimination, either through oxidative phase I or synthetic phase II (glucuronidation) reactions. The isozymes of cytochrome P-450 requisite for opioid metabolism and the possibility of phenotypic differences in opioid metabolism have not been explored.

Although renal elimination of parent compound constitutes only a small proportion of the clearance mechanism of most opioids, the clearance of active metabolites such as normeperidine, morphine-6-glucuronide (M-6-G), normorphine, and norpropoxyphene may be exquisitely sensitive to renal function. In patients with renal dysfunction, these metabolites may accumulate substantially, leading to either prolonged narcosis (M-6-G) or CNS excitation, including tremors, clonus, and seizures (normeperidine, normorphine [?], norpropoxyphene).

Table 215-2. Narcotic Analgesic Preparations Available in the United States

Drug	Preparation	Drug	Preparation
Codeine	30 or 60 mg with ASA 325 mg tablets	Sufentanil	50 µg/ml × 1, 2, 5 ml ampules
	30 mg with acetaminophen 325 mg (+ caffeine, butalbital) capsules	Dihydrocodeine	16 mg with ASA 356 mg (+ caffeine) capsules
		Dezocine	5, 10, 15 mg/ml × 2 ml vials
	30 mg with ASA 325 mg (+ caffeine, butalbital) capsules		10 mg/ml × 10 ml vials
		Propoxyphene	50 mg with acetaminophen 325 mg tablets
	15, 30, or 60 mg with acetaminophen 300, 325, 650 mg capsules, tablets		65 mg with acetaminophen 650 mg tablets
	12 mg with acetaminophen 120 mg/5 ml elixir		100 mg with acetaminophen 650 mg tablets
Buprenorphine	0.3 mg ampules		50 mg/5 ml oral suspension
Nalbuphine	10 and 20 mg ampules, syringes		65 mg capsules
	10 and 20 mg/ml × 10 ml vials		65 mg with ASA 389 mg (+ caffeine) capsules
Butorphanol	1 mg/ml × 1 ml vials	Meperidine	25, 50, 75, 100 mg/ml × 1 ml syringes
	2 mg/ml × 1 or 2 ml vials		50 mg/ml × 0.5, 1, 1.5, 2 ml ampules
	2 mg/ml × 10 ml vials		50 mg/ml × 30 ml vials
	10 mg/ml nasal solution		100 mg/ml × 20 ml vials
Pentazocine	25 mg with acetaminophen 650 mg tablets		50, 100 mg tablets
	12.5 mg with ASA 325 mg tablets		50 mg/5 ml oral syrup
	50 mg with naloxone 0.5 mg tablets	Alfentanil	0.5 mg/ml × 2, 5, 10, 20 ml ampules
	30 mg/ml × 1, 1.5, 2 ml ampules, syringes	Hydrocodone	2.5, 5, 7.5 mg with acetaminophen 500 mg capsules, tablets
	30 mg/ml × 10 ml vials		
Hydromorphone	1, 2, 4 mg/ml × 1 ml ampules		7.5, 10 mg with acetaminophen 650 mg tablets
	10 mg/ml ampules, vials		5 mg with ASA 500 mg
	2 mg/mL × 20 mL vials	Morphine	0.5 and 1.0 mg/ml × 2, 10 ml ampules (preservative-free)
	1, 2, 3, 4 mg tablets		
	3 mg rectal suppositories		0.5 and 1.0 mg/ml × 10 ml vials
Methadone	10 mg/ml × 1 ml ampules		10, 25 mg/ml × 20 ml ampules
	10 mg/ml × 20 ml vials		10, 20, 100 mg/5 ml oral solution
	5, 10 mg tablets		30 mg/1.5 ml oral solution
	5, 10 mg/5 ml oral solution		20 mg/1 ml oral solution
Fentanyl	2.5, 5, 7.5, 10 mg transdermal patches		15, 30 mg immediate-release tablets
	50 µg/ml × 2, 5, 10, 20 ml ampules		15, 30, 60, 100 mg controlled-release tablets
Levorphanol	2 mg/ml × 1 ml ampules	Naloxone	0.4 mg/ml × 1 ml syringes, ampules
	2 mg/ml × 10 ml vials		0.4 mg/ml × 10 ml vials
	2 mg tablets		1.0 mg/ml × 1, 2 ml syringes, ampules
Oxymorphone	1, 1.5 mg/mL × 1 ml ampules		1.0 mg/ml × 10 ml vials
	5 mg rectal suppositories		0.02 mg/ml × 2 ml ampules
Oxycodone	2.25 or 4.5 mg with ASA 325 mg tablets	Naltrexone	50 mg tablets
	5 mg with acetaminophen 325, 500 mg tablets, capsules		
	5 mg with acetaminophen 325 mg/5 ml oral solution		
	5 mg tablets		
	5 mg/5 ml oral solution		
	20 mg/ml oral solution		

ASA = acetylsalicylic acid

PHYSIOLOGIC CLEARANCE. The clearance of many opioids is high; in general these agents are flow-limited rather than capacity-limited. This is by no means a ubiquitous finding, as data suggest the metabolism of morphine (extraction ratio [E]=0.75), propoxyphene (E>0.90), and pentazocine are flow-limited; meperidine (E=0.50) and alfentanil (E=0.3-0.6) are flow- and capacity-limited; and methadone is capacity-limited, binding-sensitive. Hence, the extraction or metabolism of these agents is dependent on both hepatic blood flow and intrinsic enzymatic metabolic capacity of the liver to variable degrees, depending on the opioid under question.

The effects of critical illness and concomitant pathophysiologic states on opioid pharmacokinetics have been the subject of a number of recent studies [36,37,60–65]. Cardiopulmonary bypass has been associated with the following effects: increased half-life of alfentanil (due to decreased volume of distribution [V_d]) and fentanyl (due to decreased total body clearance [TBC] and increased V_d), depressed fentanyl metabolism due to hypothermia, sequestration of fentanyl and sufentanil in the lungs during the procedure, and adsorption of fentanyl to the bypass

apparatus [60]. In the presence of respiratory acidosis, morphine V_d was decreased, serum and brain concentrations were increased, and half-life in brain was increased more than 50 percent [37]. In respiratory alkalosis due to hyperventilation, fentanyl TBC was decreased [62] while sufentanil half-life and V_d were increased with no change in TBC [63]. In the critically ill, fentanyl half-life and V_d were increased with no change in TBC, as compared to surgical patients. Interindividual variability in fentanyl pharmacokinetic parameters was great [61]. In the presence of septic shock, morphine half-life was increased, TBC was decreased, and V_d was unchanged compared to previous data obtained in surgical patients and normal volunteers. In this study, reduced hepatic blood flow was documented (ICG clearance) [64]. In trauma patients early in the posttrauma period without hepatic or renal dysfunction, meperidine TBC was similar to that noted in previous studies in surgical patients and slightly decreased compared to that noted in previous studies in normal volunteers [36]. Tissue distribution of alfentanil has been determined to be highly dependent on cardiac output [65].

The tremendous variability in opioid pharmacokinetic parameters even in relatively homogenous groups makes dosing recommendations problematic in the critically ill.

DOSING. Opioid dosing recommendations for adults are illustrated in Table 215-4. Unless otherwise noted, these regimens are for patients without significant organ dysfunction and reflect package insert ranges.

Several factors require modification of the usual dosing recommendations noted in Table 215-4 for ICU patients. Because of the unpredictability of pharmacokinetic parameters in ICU patients, medication should be administered to the desired effect. Intravenous administration obviates the unpredictable absorption of these agents attendant on oral, intramuscular, subcutaneous, rectal, or transdermal administration. The following initial dosing regimens in adult ICU patients may be suggested: morphine 2 to 4 mg per hour IV, meperidine 25 to 50 mg every 2 to 3 hours IV, fentanyl 50 to 200 μg per hour (2–5 μg/kg/hr) IV, alfentanil 0.4 to 0.6 μg/kg/h IV, and sufentanil 1 μg/kg/h IV [10]. Pediatric ICU dosing regimens are provided in Table 215-5. Initial slow bolus IV loading dose administration prior to initiation of continuous IV infusion is recommended to hasten achievement of steady-state conditions. In any case, dose titration to patient response is mandatory. It should be remembered that dose requirements may change daily based on the quantity of pain the patient experiences as well as changes in pharmacokinetics. Careful dosing adjustment may be necessary in the elderly and those with hepatic and/or renal dysfunction. In patients with hepatic disease, the following recommendations for dosage adjustment have been made: decrease the oral dose of meperidine and propoxyphene by 50 percent, decrease the oral dose of pentazocine by 67 percent, decrease or do not change the dose of methadone (controversial), and do not change the morphine dose but avoid it in severe hepatic disease. In the presence of renal disease, it is best to avoid meperidine and propoxyphene use and to monitor the patient carefully when morphine is used (due to potential accumulation of M-6-G).

DRUG INTERACTIONS. Opioid therapy may be associated with the development of pharmacokinetic, pharmacodynamic, or combination pharmacokinetic/pharmacodynamic drug interactions (Table 215-6). Numerous physicochemical admixture or Y site administration incompatibilities for parenteral opioids and potential concomitant parenteral agents have been recently reviewed [71]. Potential interacting agents commonly used in the ICU setting include aminophylline, amobarbital, pentobarbital, secobarbital, sodium bicarbonate, glycopyrrolate, heparin, nafcillin, furosemide, dimenhydrinate, perphenazine, ranitidine, diazepam, promethazine, thiethylperazine, chlorothiazide, floxacillin, phenobarbital, phenytoin, thiopental, prochlorperazine, acyclovir, minocycline, tetracycline, cefoperazone, imipenem-cilastatin, mezlocillin, and sargramostim.

COMMON PITFALLS
1. Agonist/antagonist opioids should not be frequently used in the ICU setting due to deleterious CNS (dysphoria/hallucinations/delirium) and hemodynamic (increased pulmonary vascular resistance, systemic hypertension) effects [10]. In addition, these agents exhibit a ceiling effect on analgesia and hence are useful only in mild to moderate degrees of pain. An exception is that buprenorphine is effective in severe pain [31], but buprenorphine is characterized by a slow

onset of effect due to receptor binding characteristics, and reversal of its effects by naloxone may be difficult [13,37]. In addition, all of these agents can precipitate withdrawal in opioid-dependent individuals [6].
2. Intramuscular, SC, PO, PR, and transdermal routes of administration should be avoided in the acutely ill due to the potential for unpredictable absorption.
3. To reverse physical dependence due to long-term opioid administration, oral clonidine or a tapering schedule with methadone should be used [47].
4. Prolonged use of meperidine should be avoided, even in the absence of organ dysfunction, due to the potential for normeperidine accumulation and toxicity. Meperidine and propoxyphene should be avoided in patients with renal dysfunction due to the potential for metabolite accumulation.
5. Extreme caution should be used when reversing opioid effects with naloxone, as extreme agitation, severe hypertension, dysrhythmias, cardiac failure, and cardiac arrest may occur. If naloxone is to be used, small incremental doses of 20 to 40 μg (0.002 mg/kg) should be given and titrated to effect [10, 66].
6. Methadone may be difficult to use due to the danger of drug accumulation attendant upon its long half-life and short duration of action [6].

Local Anesthetics

INTRODUCTION. Local anesthetics applied in appropriate concentrations reversibly depress conduction in nervous tissue. Due to the extensive record of efficacy and safety in providing discrete local analgesia, these agents are administered in perhaps more ways than any other class of therapeutic agents. As all electrically excitable tissues are susceptible to local anesthetic blockade, these agents are also used systemically as antiarrhythmic agents (see Chap. 207) and as adjuncts to general anesthesia.

Local anesthetics have enjoyed more widespread use recently in the management of acute pain, especially in the postoperative setting. These agents may be employed in single injection (to allow for effective onset of the analgesia of systemic agents, such as the opioids) or continuous block techniques. Blocks may be central, thoracic, or peripheral in nature. This section focuses on the nonparenteral and nonsubcutaneous uses of local anesthetics in the management of postoperative or postprocedural pain, common in the ICU. Agents marketed in the United States are listed in Table 215-7.

PHARMACOLOGY. All local anesthetics inhibit nerve conduction by interfering with transit of sodium (Na^+) ions into the nerve cell. This action is thought to involve direct activity of these agents on Na^+ channels [72]. Local anesthetics are thought to bind directly to the Na^+ channel, possibly within the channel pore itself, and disrupt the normal cycling process during an action potential. As local anesthetics are heterogeneous in structure, the channel binding site is not thought to be a true stereospecific drug receptor. However, some structural limitations are placed on local anesthetics, location of the binding site, or the pore structure itself.

Typical local anesthetics are amphipathic, with a lipophilic aromatic ring structure at one end of the molecule and a hydrophilic amino group at the other end. An intermediate amide, ester, or ether linkage combined with a short allyl chain separates the ends an appropriate distance (7–9 Å). Dissociation constants (pKa) range from 7.5 to 9.0, allowing the coexistence

Table 215-3. Pharmacodynamic and Pharmacokinetic Parameters of Narcotic Analgesics in Adults

Drug	Pharmacodynamics			Pharmacokinetics			
	Onset of Effect (min)	Duration of effect (min)	Equivalent doses (mg)	Absorption characteristics	Distribution characteristics	Metabolism/elimination characteristics	References
Morphine	30–60 (IM) 60–90 (PO)	180–300 (IM, PO)	10 (SC)	T_{max} = 0.25–0.33 hr (IM, SC) = 0.5–1.5 hr (PO) F = 22–24% (PO) = 100% (IM) = 30–90% (PR)	V_d = 1–6 L/kg 20–36% PB ↓ PB in renal and hepatic disease	Metabolism via N-demethylation, O-methylation, N-oxidation, glucuronidation (primarily hepatic) M-3-G inactive M-6-G active $t_{1/2}$ = 2–3 hr TBC = 11–33 ml/min/kg Renal disease—M-6-G accumulation → prolonged narcosis, no change for morphine Hepatic disease—↑ $t_{1/2}$, ↓ TBC, ↑ oral F Elderly—↑ C_{max}, ↓ V_d, ↓ TBC Surgery—no effect Burns—no effect	10, 12, 17–30
Meperidine	30–45 (IM) 60–90 (PO)	120–240 (IM, SC) 240–300 (PO)	80–100 (SC)		V_d = 3.7 L/kg 60–70% PB (albumin, AAG) ↓ PB in elderly ↑ PB in burns, postsurgery (AAG) ↔ PB in hepatic disease	Metabolism to normeperidine, meperidinic acid, normeperidinic acid; normeperidine active (toxic) $t_{1/2}$ = 3–6.5 hr (meperidine) = 15–40 hr (normeperidine) TBC = 1020 ml/min Renal disease—normeperidine accumulates → seizures, tremors Hepatic disease—↓ TBC, ↑ $t_{1/2}$, ↑ oral F Elderly—↓ V_d, ↓ TBC	1, 6, 10, 18, 24, 31–41
Hydromorphone	15–30 (IM) 30–45 (PO)	240–300 (IM/SC)	1.5 (SC)	F = 36% (PR) = 50% (PO)		Metabolism to hydroxy metabolites, glucuronidation $t_{1/2}$ = 3–4 hr	1, 6, 18, 19
Codeine	30–60 (IM) 60–90 (PO)	180–360 (IM/SC)	120 (PO)			Metabolism via glucuronidation. Morphine is active metabolite $t_{1/2}$ = 3–4 hr ESRD—↑ $t_{1/2}$, AF	1, 6, 18, 42, 43
Oxycodone	15–30 (IM/PO)	240–300 (IM/SC)	10–15 (SC)			Metabolism to noroxycodone oxymorphone (active), conjugates. $t_{1/2}$ = 3–4 hr	1, 6, 18
Levorphanol	30–60 (IM) 60–90 (PO)	240–300 (IM/SC)	2 (SC)			$t_{1/2}$ = 11–16 hr	1, 18
Methadone	20–60 (PO) 30–45 (IM)	180–300 (IM/SC)	8–10 (SC)	F = 79% (PO) = 67–90% (PR, relative to oral solution)	V_d = 4 L/kg	Metabolism via N-methylation, cyclization $t_{1/2}$ = 20–60 hr TBC = 150 ml/min Hepatic disease—↑ $t_{1/2}$, ↑ V_d, ↔ TBC	1, 18, 19, 27, 44
Propoxyphene			250 (PO)		PB unchanged in hepatic disease	Metabolism to norpropoxyphene (active and toxic) $t_{1/2}$ = 3.5–15 hr (propoxyphene) = 23–37 hr (norpropoxyphene) Renal disease—norpropoxyphene accumulation → seizures, tremors Hepatic disease—↑ $t_{1/2}$, ↓ TBC	6, 44, 45

Table 215-3. (continued)

| Drug | Pharmacodynamics | | | Pharmacokinetics | | | References |
	Onset of Effect (min)	Duration of effect (min)	Equivalent doses (mg)	Absorption characteristics	Distribution characteristics	Metabolism/elimination characteristics	
Dihydrocodeine					V_d = 1.15 L/kg	$t_{1/2}$ = 3.9 hr Renal disease—↑ C_{max}, ↑ AUC, ↔ $t_{1/2}$	44

Fentanyl	60–90 (IV)		0.1 (SC)		V_c = 10–60 L (volunteers)
					    = 3–25 L (surgical patients)
					V_m = 55–335 L (volunteers)
					    = 30–118 L (surgical patients)
					79–87% PB (albumin)
						$t_{1/2}$ = 100–219 minutes (volunteers)
						    = 85–945 minutes (surgical patients)
						TBC = 0.4–1.53 L/min (volunteers)
						    = 0.24–0.99 L/min (surgical patients)
						Elderly—↓ TBC, ↑ $t_{1/2}$, ↑ CNS sensitivity
						Hepatic disease—no effect
							10, 14, 31–33, 37, 46–50

Alfentanil					V_c = 11–12 L (volunteers)
					    = 5.4–12.3 L (surgical patients)
					V_m = 32–47 L (volunteers)
					    = 27–57 L (surgical patients)
					85–92% PB (AAG)
					↓ PB in hepatic disease
						Metabolism via N- and O-dealkylation
						$t_{1/2}$ = 70–103 min (volunteers)
						$t_{1/2}$ = 70–204 min (surgical patients)
						TBC = 0.24–0.34 L/min (volunteers)
						$t_{1/2}$ = 0.18–0.56 L/min (surgical patients)
						Elderly—↓ TBC, ↑ $t_{1/2}$, ↑ CNS sensitivity
						Renal disease—↓ V_c ↓ $t_{1/2}$, ↓ V_m, ↔ TBC
						Hepatic disease—↓ TBC, $t_{1/2}$, ↓ unbound V_d and TBC
							14, 31, 32, 37, 46, 47, 50–57

Sufentanil					V_c = 0.26 L/kg V_m = 1.7–8.7 L/kg 93% PB	$t_{1/2}$ = 2–3 hr (volunteers) $t_{1/2}$ = 8–12 hr (surgical patients) TBC = 12–19 ml/min/kg Renal disease—no effect	1, 14, 37, 46, 58, 59
Pentazocine	30–45 (IM) 30–60 (PO)	120–240 (IM/SC)	30 (SC)			$t_{1/2}$ = 2–5 hr Hepatic disease—↑ $t_{1/2}$, ↔ V_d, ↓ TBC, ↓ oral F ↓ oral F	1, 6, 17, 41
Nalbuphine	30–45 (IM) 30–60 (PO)	240–300 (IM/SC)	10–20 (SC)			$t_{1/2}$ = 3.5–5 hr	1, 6, 17, 37
Butorphanol	30–45 (IM)	120–130 (IM/SC)	2–3 (SC)			$t_{1/2}$ = 3 hr	1, 6, 17
Buprenorphine	10–20 (IM)	240–480 (IM/SC)	0.4 (SC)		V_d = 188 L	Metabolism to N-demethylated metabolite and 3-glucuronide $t_{1/2}$ = 2–4.5 hr TBC = 1275 ml/min Renal disease—no effect	6, 17, 31, 37, 45

Abbreviations: IM = intramuscular; PO = oral; SC = subcutaneous; T_{max} = time to peak plasma concentration; F = systemic bioavailability; V_d = volume of distribution; PB = protein binding; $t_{1/2}$ = terminal disposition half-life; TBC = total body clearance; C_{max} = peak plasma concentration; AAG = alpha-acid glycoprotein; PR = rectal; ESRD = endstage renal disease; AF = accumulation factor (on multiple dosing); AUC = area under the plasma concentration-time curve; V_c = volume of the central compartment; IV = intravenous; V_{ss} steady-state volume of distribution; CNS = central nervous system; ↑ = increased, ↓ = decreased, ↔ = no change.

Table 215-4. Narcotic Analgesic Dosing in Adults*

Drug	Regimen
Codeine-ASA/acetaminophen combination products	1–2 tabs/caps q4h PO prn
Buprenorphine	0.3–0.6 mg up to Q6H IM/IV prn
Nalbuphine	10–20 mg q3–6h IM/SC/IV prn
Butorphanol	0.5–2 mg q3–4h IV prn
	1–4 mg q3–4h IM prn
	1–2 sprays q3–4h intranasally prn
Pentazocine	(With acetaminophen) 1 tab q4h PO prn
	(With ASA) 2 tabs tid–qid PO
	(With naloxone) 1–2 tabs q3–4h PO prn
	30–60 mg q3–4h IM/IV/SC prn
Alfentanil	No FDA-approved analgesia guidelines
Hydrocodone	(With acetaminophen 500 mg) 1–2 tabs q4–6h PO prn
	(With acetaminophen 650 mg) 1 tab q4–6h PO prn
	(With ASA 500 mg) 1–2 tabs q4–6h PO prn
Dezocine	5–20 mg q3–4h IM prn
	2.5–10 mg q2–4h IV prn
Morphine	5–30 ng q4h PO (immediate-release)
Oxymorphone	1–1.5 mg q4–6h SC/IM prn
	0.5–1 mg q4–6h IV prn
	5 mg q4–6h PR prn
Oxycodone	(With ASA/acetaminophen) 1–2 tabs q6h PO prn
	5 mg q6h PO prn
Meperidine	50–150 mg q3–4h IM/SC/PO prn
Hydromorphone	1–2 mg q4–6h IM/SC prn
	2–4 mg q4–6h PO prn
	3 mg q6–8h PR prn
Methadone	2.5–10 mg q3–4h IM/SC/PO prn
Fentanyl	50–100 µg q1–2h IM
Sufentanil	No FDA-approved analgesia guidelines
Levorphanol	2–3 mg per dose SC/PO
Dihydrocodeine	(With ASA) 2 caps q4h PO prn

PO = oral; IM = intramuscular; IV = intravenous; SC = subcutaneous; tid = thrice daily; qid = four times daily; ASA = aspirin; PR = rectal; prn = as needed
* Package insert data

Table 215-5. Narcotic Analgesic Dosing in Pediatric ICU Patients [66]

Drug	Regimen[a]
Morphine	0.08–0.1 mg/kg q2h IV[b]
	0.05–0.06 mg/kg/hr IV[c]
	0.1–0.15 mg/kg q3–4h IM
	0.3 mg/kg q4h PO
Meperidine	0.8–1 mg/kg q2h IV[b]
	0.5–0.6 mg/kg/hr IV[c]
	1–1.5 mg/kg q3–4h IM
	1–2 mg/kg q3–4h PO
Fentanyl	1–2 µg/kg q15–30 min during procedure IV[b]
	1–2 µg/kg/hr IV[c]
Methadone	0.1 mg/kg q2h × 2 doses IV then 0.03–0.08 mg/kg q4–8h IV[b,d]
	0.1–0.15 mg/kg q4–8h PO[d]
Codeine	0.5–1 mg/kg q4h PO

IV = intravenous; IM = intramuscular; PO = oral
[a] Doses should be reduced in patients under 3 months of age, nonintubated patients, those predisposed to respiratory depresssion.
[b] Administer IV boluses slowly over 15–20 min in nonintubated patients.
[c] Loading dose may be necessary prior to initiation of continuous infusion to ensure therapeutic plasma concentrations achieved.
[d] Longer dosing interval (q8–12h) or dose reduction may be necessary if somnolence occurs.

of neutral and charged forms at tissue pH. Size constraints restrict these agents to molecular weights ranging from 200 to 300 d. A summary of the pharmacology of these agents is provided in Table 215-8.

A number of variables influence the degree and type of blockade observed clinically with these agents. These include drug concentration and dose, intrinsic potency, nerve fiber size and length, amount of impulse flow through the nerve, physiologic state of the nerve, and degree of inflammation present (probably related to tissue pH) [73].

An additional factor influencing degree and type of blockade is the enantiomeric form of the agent. Mepivacaine, bupivacaine, prilocaine, and etidocaine are chiral drugs, existing as both R and S stereoisomers (ropivacaine, an investigational agent, is available as the S isomer only). It has been demonstrated that the S forms of prilocaine, bupivacaine, ropivacaine, and mepivacaine are longer-acting than the R forms. This is generally thought to be due to the vasoconstrictive activity of the S forms [76,77,78].

Low systemic concentrations of local anesthetics result in generally benign effects, such as analgesia, anticonvulsant activity, mild sedation, antiarrhythmic activity, and mild increases

in blood pressure, cardiac output, and peripheral vascular resistance [79,80]. In general, the quality and duration of analgesia do not differ between agents when administered in equipotent doses, although this has been disputed. However, if absorbed sufficiently into the systemic circulation, local anesthetics may be associated with a constellation of adverse systemic effects, including those in the CNS (confusion, somnolence, respiratory depression, dysphoria, motor hyperactivity, hallucinations, seizures), cardiovascular system (hypertension or hypotension, arrhythmias, myocardial depression, collapse), and miscellaneous effects (augmentation of neuromuscular blockade, myotoxicity on direct IM injection, dose-dependent bronchoconstriction at low and bronchodilation at high concentrations, methemoglobinemia with prilocaine and possibly lidocaine, and hypersensitivity, especially to ester anesthetics and preservatives) [81–85]. Rather unique side effects associated with 2-chloroprocaine include severe backache on epidural administration (due to ethylenediaminetetraacetic acid [EDTA], drug, or both) and thrombophlebitis (due to solution pH = 3.7).

THERAPEUTIC RANGE. No data exist regarding therapeutic ranges for the efficacy of local anesthetics, due to an inability to sample biologic fluids at the site of action. Data do exist, however, assessing serum, plasma, or whole blood local anesthetic concentration-toxicity relationships. Such relationships need to be interpreted keeping in mind the following factors: plasma or serum versus whole blood drug concentrations (ratio varies between agents [vide infra]), total versus free or unbound serum drug concentrations (protein binding varies between agents and within agents with changing physiologic states [vide infra]), changes in degree of drug ionization (with changes in brain tissue pH), stereochemistry (R vs. S enantiomers), contribution of metabolites (e.g., monoethylglycinexylidide from lidocaine), and arterial versus venous drug concentrations (former may be more relevant vis-à-vis vital organ exposure) [86].

Lidocaine toxicity most frequently occurs with total serum drug concentrations in excess of 5 mg per liter, usually with a gradation in toxicity severity in increments of 5 to 10 mg per liter (dizziness, drowsiness, tinnitus, perioral paresthesias), 10

Table 215-6. Narcotic Analgestic Drug-Drug Interactions [12,31,67–70]

Narcotic	Other Drug	Effect	Comment
Pharmacokinetic interactions			
General	H$_2$ blockers	↓ metabolism of meperidine and fetanyl by cimetidine No effect of cimetidine on morphine metabolism or ranitidine on meperidine metabolism	Use morphine Avoid cimetidine ? Clinical relevance
Alfentanil	Erythromycin	↓ TBC, ↑ t$_{1/2}$ of alfentanil with prolonged narcosis	Decrease alfentanil dose Monitor for prolonged effect Use alternative opioid
Meperidine Methadone Morphine	Hydantoins Barbiturates Rifampin	↑ metabolism of meperidine to normeperidine, ↑ morphine and methadone metabolism, ? ↓ therapeutic effect	May need to ↑ dose for therapeutic effect Monitor for CNS excitation (meperidine)
Morphine	Tricyclic antidepressants	↑ oral morphine bioavailability	May need dose reduction
Propoxyphene	Barbiturates	↑ barbiturate concentrations due to ? ↓ metabolism	? Clinical relevance
	Benzodiazepines	↓ TBC, ↑ t$_{1/2}$ of alprazolam (no effect on diazepam or lorazepam)	Avoid alprazolam
	Carbamazepine	↑ carbamazepine concentrations due to ? ↓ metabolism	Follow carbamazepine serum concentrations and monitor for toxicity Use alternative opioid
	Doxepin	↓ metabolism of doxepin with ↑ CNS depression	Avoid combination
Pharmacodynamic interactions			
General	Barbiturates	↑ sedation	Monitor
General	Hydroxyzine	↑ sedation and respiratory depression	Avoid combination
Alfentanil	Ethanol	Induced tolerance to alfentanil	May need to ↑ alfentanil dose in habitual users
Meperidine	Phenothiazines	↑ sedation and hypotension	Avoid chlorpromazine
Interactions with unknown mechanisms			
Meperidine	Isoniazid	CNS depression and hypotension	Caution with combination Monitor BP frequently
Meperidine	MAOI Furazolidone	Agitation, seizures, diaphoresis, fever → coma, apnea, death	Avoid meperidine up to several weeks postcessation of MAOI Use morphine
Propoxyphene	Warfarin	↑ anticoagulant effect of warfarin	Monitor prothrombin time frequently May need to ↓ warfarin dose
Fentanyl	Diazepam	Hypotension due to ↓ SVR	Avoid combination Otherwise monitor BP closely
Fentanyl	Scopolamine + Pancuronium	Severe tachycardia and myocardial ischemia	Avoid combination
Sufentanil	Succinylcholine Vecuronium β or Ca blocker	Severe bradycardia	Monitor heart rate closely with combination

MAOI = monoamine oxidase inhibitor; TBC = total body clearance; t$_{1/2}$ = terminal disposition half-life; CNS = central nervous system; SVR = systemic vascular resistance

Table 215-7. Systemic Local Anesthetics Available in the United States

Esters
   Chloroprocaine (Nesacaine)
   Procaine (Novocaine)
   Tetracaine (Pontocaine)
Amides
   Mepivacaine (Carbocaine)
   Etidocaine (Duranest)
   Bupivacaine (Marcaine, Sensorcaine)
   Lidocaine (Xylocaine)

to 20 mg/per liter (disorientation, delirium, coma, convulsions), and greater than 20 mg per liter (cardiorespiratory arrest) [75,81]. Although the threshold total serum bupivacaine concentration for toxicity has been quoted as 4 mg per liter [87,88,89] many cases of toxicity, including seizures, have been reported with total serum drug concentrations ranging from 1.5 to 4 mg/per liter [75,90,91,92]. Toxic ranges for procaine, mepivacaine, etidocaine, and prilocaine of 21 to 81, 5 to 6, 2 or greater and 7 to 9 mg per liter, respectively, have also been reported [75,92].

Few data have been published examining the relationship of free or unbound serum drug concentration and toxicity. Two studies have suggested that bupivacaine toxicity is more likely when free drug concentration is 0.24 mg/per liter or greater [93,94]. Of interest, in one of these studies total serum drug concentrations did not distinguish between patients with or without toxicity, while free serum drug concentrations did [93]. With the ready availability of rapid, simple methods to determine free serum drug concentrations in most laboratories, further work in this area is warranted.

The role of therapeutic drug monitoring (TDM) of local anesthetics used for analgesia in routine patient care is controversial. The lack of ready availability of local anesthetic assays (except for lidocaine) in most laboratories seriously compromises TDM. In addition, the multiple factors that may affect drug concentration interpretation alluded to previously and the lack of formally established toxic concentration ranges compromise TDM at present. Therapeutic drug monitoring may be warranted (when assay capabilities exist) in patients receiving long-term infusions of these agents for analgesia (vide infra). However, the caveats for concentration interpretation discussed previously need to be kept in mind and concentration determinations should be interpreted in the context of clinical signs and symptoms.

PREPARATIONS. The systemic local anesthetic preparations available in the United States are listed in Table 215-9.

PHARMACOKINETICS. The absorption, distribution, metabolism, and excretion profiles of local anesthetics are important to consider due to their influence on potential adverse systemic effects following administration for local effect.

Absorption. A major impetus to examine the magnitude of peak and time to peak systemic local anesthetic concentrations after regional anesthesia has been the establishment of ceilings of dosage for each procedure by relating these concentrations to those associated with toxicity (see Therapeutic Range). Systemic uptake of these agents is influenced by factors such as tissue affinity, tissue blood flow, local anesthetic effects on local microcirculation, site of injection, dosage (concentration and volume) injected, and effects of coadministered vasoconstrictors, such as epinephrine (see Drug Interactions) (Table 215-10).

Few data are available regarding the absolute bioavailability to the systemic circulation after nonparenteral administration of local anesthetics. However, the absolute systemic bioavailabilities of lidocaine and bupivacaine after subarachnoid injection were 103 and 96 percent, respectively, while those after epidural injection were 96 and 91 percent, respectively [86,96]. A number of generalizations can be made using the data from Table 215-10. The net systemic absorption of the long-acting, more lipophilic agents is slower (probably due to local tissue binding rather than alterations in vascular activity). Absorption rate decreases in the following order: intercostal block > interpleural block > caudal block > peridural block > brachial plexus block > sciatic and femoral nerve block. Intraperitoneal administration is accompanied by low peak drug concentrations, probably due to extensive first-pass metabolism following absorption into the portal circulation. Increasing the concentration of the local anesthetic injection increases the absorption rate. Plasma concentrations of local anesthetics during regional anesthesia are poorly correlated with age and weight.

Table 215-8. Pharmacologic Properties of Systemic Local Anesthetics [73,74,75]

Drug	pKa	o/w PC	Molecular weight	Relative rate of onset	Relative duration of action	Relative potency	Principal uses
Esters							
Procaine	8.9	3	236	Slow	Short	1	Infiltration
2-Chloroprocaine	8.7	3	271	Fast	Short	1	Most block techniques, obstetric block
Tetracaine	8.4	541	264	Slow	Long	8	Spinal
Amides							
Lidocaine	7.8	110	234	Fast	Intermediate	2	All block techniques
Mepivacaine	7.6	0.8	285	Fast	Intermediate	2	All block techniques
Bupivacaine	8.1	560	288	Intermediate	Long	8	All block techniques
Prilocaine	7.9	18		Fast	Intermediate	2	IV regional, single-dose nerve block
Etidocaine	7.7	287	313	Fast	Long	4	Surgical blocks

o/w PC = oil/water partition coefficient; IV = intravenous.

Table 215-9. Systemic Local Anesthetic Preparations Available in the United States

Drug	Preparation
Chloroprocaine	1% (10 mg/ml) in 30 ml vials
	2% (20 mg/ml) in 30 ml vials
	3% (30 mg/ml) in 30 ml vials
	(1,2% with/2,3% without preservatives)
Procaine	1% (10 mg/ml) in 2, 6 ml ampules and 30 ml vials
	2% (20 mg/ml) in 30 ml vials
	10% (100 mg/ml) in 2 ml ampules
Tetracaine	20 mg ampules
	1% (10 mg/ml) in 2 ml ampules
Mepivacaine	1% (10 mg/ml) in 30, 50 ml vials
	1.5% (15 mg/ml) lin 30 ml vials
	2% (20 mg/ml) in 20, 50 ml vials
Etidocaine	1% (10 mg/ml) in 30 ml vials (with/without epinephrine)
	1.5% (15 mg/ml) in 20 ml vials (with epinephrine)
Bupivacaine	0.25% (2.5 mg/ml) in 10, 30, 50 mL vials/ampules (with/without epinephrine)
	0.5% (5 mg/mL) in 3, 5 ml ampules (with epinephrine)
	in 10, 30, 50 ml vials/ampules (with/without epineprhine)
	0.75% (7.5 mg/ml) in 10, 30 ml vials/ampules (with/without epinephrine)
	15 mg (2 ml) ampule (spinal anesthesia)
	(all above with/without preservatives)
Lidocaine	0.5% (5 mg/ml) in 50 ml vials
	1% (10 mg/ml) in 2, 5, 30 ml ampules
	in 2, 5, 10, 20, 30, 50 ml vials
	1.5% (15 mg/ml) in 5, 20, 30 ml ampules
	in 5, 10, 20 30 ml vials
	2% (20 mg/ml) in 2, 10, 20 ml ampules
	in 2, 5, 10, 20 50 ml vials
	(all above with/without epinephrine)

Distribution. After distribution into the systemic circulation, local anesthetics are reversibly bound to plasma proteins, principally AAG and to a lesser extent albumin [97]. Red blood cell partitioning also occurs. Plasma protein binding appears to be related to the oil-water partition coefficient (i.e., balance between lipophilicity and hydrophilicity), with highly lipophilic agents such as etidocaine and bupivacaine exhibiting greater degrees of binding than less lipophilic agents such as lidocaine and prilocaine (Table 215-11). The blood-plasma distribution follows the opposite relationship (Table 215-12).

The influence of a number of factors on local anesthetic plasma protein binding has been examined. Increasing age was not demonstrated to influence bupivacaine protein binding [112]. Phenytoin, quinidine, meperidine, and desipramine were demonstrated to displace bupivacaine from its plasma protein binding sites in vitro, but only when toxic concentrations of the former agents were present [113]. Thus, it does not appear that significant protein binding displacement interactions occur with local anesthetics. In conditions associated with elevated plasma concentrations of AAG (postoperative, pregnancy), the degree of plasma protein binding of bupivacaine significantly increased [114,115]. The effect of pH and temperature on the in vitro plasma protein binding of prilocaine has been assessed. With decreasing pH, the free or unbound fraction significantly increased (67% at pH 7.40 and 79% at pH 7.00), while the converse was true with increasing pH (47% at pH 8.00). While hyperthermia did not affect protein binding, hypothermia significantly increased the free fraction (56% at 37°C and 68% at

25°C) [116]. This may have ramifications in the critically ill septic patient (vide infra).

In the absence of intravascular injection, the rate of distribution exceeds that of absorption into the systemic circulation such that usually even transiently toxic organ-specific concentrations are not attained. However, sequential distribution occurs following intravascular injection: lung uptake followed by uptake into brain, heart, liver, kidneys, and spleen followed by redistribution into muscle and fat. Local anesthetic uptake into the CNS from the systemic circulation appears to occur by a process of simple diffusion, independent of molecular weight and lipid solubility [117].

Numerous studies have examined the distribution of local anesthetics after subarachnoid, epidural, paravertebral, intercostal, and interpleural administration. The most important factors influencing distribution of local anesthetic solutions after subarachnoid administration include basicity of the solution, position of the patient during injection, dose, and site of injection (i.e., above vs. below the second lumbar vertebrae). Less important factors include patient age, height, spinal cord anatomic configuration, direction of spinal needle during injection, and volume of cerebrospinal fluid (CSF) in the subarachnoid segment. Controversial factors include volume and temperature of local anesthetic solution, vertebral length, changes in posture after injection of nonisobaric solutions, and speed of injection [118]. Systemic fentanyl may increase the spread of lidocaine spinal anesthesia [119]. Warming the local anesthetic to 36 to 37°C prior to epidural injection has been demonstrated to reduce the latent period of onset for bupivacaine and lidocaine [120,121].

In a study of distribution after paravertebral injection of 5 ml volumes, injectate was confined to the paravertebral area after only 18 percent of injections while varying degrees of epidural spread occurred after 70 percent of injections, exclusive epidural spread occurred after 31 percent of injections, and combined paraverebral/epidural spread occurred after 39 percent of injections [122]. Conflicting results of spread after intercostal injection have been reported, including confinement to the intercostal space, spread to the paravertebral space, spread to the epidural space, and spread subpleurally cephalad and caudal. Spread after intercostal injection is probably volume- and/or position-dependent [123]. After interpleural administration, solution spreads to the roots of the intercostal nerves, splanchnic nerves, and sympathetic chain [124].

Metabolism/Excretion. Chemical structure, in general, dictates the metabolic fate of these agents. Ester derivatives of para-aminobenzoic acid (e.g., procaine, tetracaine, benzocaine) are predominantly hydrolyzed by plasma pseudocholinesterase, while hepatic esterases are more important with other ester-type agents [82]. As a result, in vitro disposition half-lives in normal adults are less than 1 minute for procaine and chloroprocaine and slightly longer for tetracaine [125,126]. In turn, circulating concentrations of these agents after regional anesthesia are very low.

Amide anesthetics undergo a more complex pattern of biotransformation, predominantly in the liver (except prilocaine, for which the lungs and/or kidneys play a role in drug metabolism). N-dealkylation of tertiary amine agents such as lidocaine and bupivacaine occurs, producing secondary amines that often retain significant activity. In turn, a second dealkylation or hydrolysis by hepatic amidases occurs. Hydroxylation of the aromatic ring and conjugation with glucuronic acid also occur. Very little amide local anesthetic is excreted renally as unchanged parent compound (1–5% at normal urine pH values) [91,102,127]. Renal impairment does not alter the pharmacoki-

(Text continues on page 2371.)

Table 215-10. Systemic Uptake of Local Anesthetics after Administration for Regional Anesthesia

Drug	Route	Dose (mg)	Concentration (%)	Epinephrine	No. of subjects	Sampling site	Maximum concentration[a] (μg/ml)	Peak time[a] (min)
Lidocaine	PCB	200	1	−	10	VP	2.08±0.09[b]	10
	BP	6.2/kg	1.5	+	7	VP	2.5±0.5	30 (20–60)
	BP	400[c]	2	−	5	VP	≈3.4	25
		400[c]	2	+	5		≈2.4	25
	BP[d]	450	2	−	5	VP	4.51	15
		450	2	+	5		3.62	20
	Pudend[c,1]	1/kg	1	−	6	VS	0.36±0.08	27±18
	ON	200	2	−	6	AP	2.28±0.29	26±7
		300	2	−	6		3.75±0.79	20±6
	IPer	400	0.5	−	7	VS	4.32±1.77	20±16
		400	0.5[c]	+	8		2.30±0.98	58±22
		400	0.5[f]	+	7		1.89±0.69	72±21
	IT	100	5	+	16	VB	0.14±0.03	60
		100	5	−	16		0.28±0.02	120
	IC	400	1	−	8	VP	6.8±0.32	≈15
		400	1	+[g]	12		5.28±0.36	≈20
		400	1	+[h]	10		4.87±0.24	≈10
		400	2	−	11		6.48±0.38	≈15
	IC	400	4	−	13	VP	8.42±0.26	≈15
	IC	3/kg	1.5	+	20	AS	2.0±0.7	9±3
		1/kg/h[i]	1	−	20		4.8±1.0	1800–3240
	Perid	300–500	2	−	15	VB	1.7–9.4	5–35
		300–680	2	+	12		1.0–4.4	12–40
	Perid	5.5/kg	1.5	+	4	VP	3.1±0.7	20–30
	Perid	600	2	+	?	VB	2.72±1.26	30[j]
	Perid	200	2	−	11	VP	3.30±0.07	≈15
		400	2	−	23		4.27±0.24	≈20
		400	2	+[g]	15		2.95±0.29	≈15
		400	2	±[h]	13		3.09±0.38	≈30
		600	2	−	10		7.34±0.37	≈15
		600	3	−	8		6.31±0.26	≈15
	Perid	700	2	−	9	VP	7.43±0.23	≈15
	Perid	300[k]	2	−	6	VP	3.5	25
		300[k]	2	+	8		≈2.6	25
	Perid	400	2	−	5	AP	3.7±0.5	12±3
		400	2	+	5		2.1±0.4	25±4
	Perid	75/hr[i,k]	0.75	−	12	VS	3.2±1.5	720
	Perid	400	2	±	29	VS	1.49–1.87	33–52
		400	2	−	10		2.02±0.21	42±7
	Caud[l]	5/kg	1	−	11	VP	2.05±0.08	28±3
j	Caud[l,m]	11/kg	1.5	+	10	VB	2.20±0.26	45
	Caud	6.6/kg	1.5	+	4	VP	1.8±0.5	40(10–60)
	MT	260	2.0	−	18	VB	1.1	90
Prilocaine	BP[d]	450	1.5	−	5	VP	2.3	30
		450	1.5	+	5		1.2	30
	BP[d]	525	1.5	−	10	VP	3.61 (0.44–10.94)	≈25
	SF	300–450 +250–350	1.5 +1	−	11	VP	2.37 (1.27–3.75)	30
	IC	400	1	−	9	VP	5.09±0.25	≈15
		400	2	−	13		4.46±0.27	≈15
		400	2	+[g]	16		3.63±0.21	≈20
		400	2	+[g]	10		2.79±0.22	≈15
	Perid	600	2	−	?	VB	3.68±2.05	20[c]
		600	2	+	?		1.75±0.84	20[c]
		900	3	−	?		5.23±2.57	20[c]
		900	3	+	?		3.25±1.40	20[c]
	Perid	200	2	−	8	VP	1.69±0.21	≈15
		400	2	−	31		2.67±0.15	≈15
		400	2	+[g]	27		2.21±0.10	≈20
		400	2	+[h]	36		2.23±0.13	≈20
		600	2	−	9		4.47±0.15	≈20
		600	3	−	12		4.90±0.25	≈20
Mepivacaine	PCB	200	1	−	5	VP	1.86 (1.4–2.4)	30[j]
		400	2	−	6		4.47 (2.1–5.6)	30[j]
	Periton	2/kg	0.5	+	7	VB	1.09±0.30	10[j]
	BP	6/kg	2	−	10	VB	2.07±0.73	15[j]
		6/kg	2	+	10		1.49±0.37	30[j]

Table 215-10. (continued)

Drug	Route	Dose (mg)	Concentration (%)	Epinephrine	No. of subjects	Sampling site	Maximum concentration[a] (μg/ml)	Peak time[a] (min)
	BP	5/kg	2	−	15	VB	1.99 ± 0.18[b]	45
		5/kg	2	+	16		1.61 ± 0.13[b]	45
	BP	500	1	−	5	AP	3.68 ± 0.83	24 (15–30)
		500	1	+	5		2.96 ± 0.77	47 (15–129)
	SF	300–450 +250–350	1.5 +1	−	9	VP	5.1 (3.7–7.2)	20
	SF	500	1	−	5	AP	3.59 ± 1.25	31 (25–45)
		500	1	+	5		3.06 ± 1.34	55 (20–110)
	PC/S	731	1.33	+	10	AP	R(+)[n] 1.54 ± 0.34 S(−)[n] 2.34 ± 0.51	40 ± 8 44 ± 12
	IC	500	2	−	5	AP	8.06 ± 1.62	9 (5–15)
		500	2	+	5		3.94 ± 0.69	19 (5–15)
		500	1	−	5		5.91 ± 1.58	11 (5–15)
		500	1	+	5		3.69 ± 0.68	37 (10–60)
	Perid	600	2	−	?	VB	5.56	20[j]
		600	2	+	?		4.00	20[j]
	Perid	6/kg	2	−	6	VB	1.31 ± 0.39	30[j]
		6/kg	2	+	4		1.27 ± 0.20	60[j]
	Perid	500	2	−	5	AP	4.95 ± 0.86	16 (10–20)
		500	2	+	5		3.19 ± 0.60	26 (15–45)
	Perid	200/h[i,o]	2	+	10	VB	$4.65 + 0.55$	300
	Caud	500	2	−	5	AP	5.49 ± 1.52	13 (10–15)
		500	2	+	5		4.60 ± 1.48	40 (25–60)
		500	1	−	5		4.57 ± 1.65	25 (10–60)
		500	1	+	5		2.38 ± 0.45	72 (30–120)
Bupivacaine	Caud[l,m]	11/kg	1.5	+	10	VB	$2.53 + 0.31$	45
	PCB	100	0.5	+	10	VP	0.2 (0.16–1.25)	25 (10–60)
	PCB	100	0.5	−	11	VP	0.8 (0.30–1.87)	15 (5–30)
	PCB	50	0.25	−	8	VP	1.07 ± 0.145[b]	≈15
		50	0.25	+	8		0.53 ± 0.05[b]	≈10
	PCB	50	0.5	−	10	VP	0.9 (0.8–3.2)	5[p] (2–15)
	Pudend[l]	25	0.25	+	11	VP	0.31 (0.11–0.54)	≈20
	Pudend[l]	0.5/kg	0.25	−	6	VS	0.27 ± 0.09	23 ± 5
	BP	300	0.5	+	10	AP	1.71 (1.05–2.40)	30–35
						VP	1.55 (0.94–2.25)	30–35
	BP	150[q]	0.75	−	5	VP	≈1.0	≈25
		150[q]	0.75	+	5		≈0.5	≈30
		150[c]	0.75	−	4		≈0.7	≈30
		150[c]	0.75	+	5		≈0.5	≈30
	BP[d]	150	0.5	−	5	VP	2.16	15
		150	0.5	+	5		1.19	20
	BP	150–210	0.75	+	12	VP	1.63 ± 0.55	30
		0.25/kg/hr[i]	0.25	−	12		1.08 ± 0.35	1440
	BP	150	0.5	−	10	VP	1.57 ± 0.78	45[p] (30–60)
	SF	400	0.5	+	10	AP	1.89 (1.0–3.16)	15
						VP	1.60 (0.84–2.73)	15
	SF	169	0.375	+	11	VP	0.98	60–120
		169	0.375	−	11		1.66	30
	SF	3/kg	0.5	+	11	VP	0.79 ± 0.14	63 ± 7
		3/kg	0.5	−	11		0.70 ± 0.09	60 ± 7
	IC	400	0.5	+	10	AP	3.29 (1.72–4.0)	10–20
						VP	2.52 (1.4–3.45)	10–20
	IC	70	0.5	+	19	AB	0.38	5–10
						VB	0.26	5–10
	IC	105	0.5	+	12	AP/VP	1.36 ± 0.48/ 1.21 ± 0.48	9/13
	IC[l]	2/kg	0.5	+	5	AB	0.77 ± 0.25	5–15
		3/kg	0.5	+	4		1.37 ± 0.23	5–30
		4/kg	0.5	+	11		1.87 ± 0.53	<5–15
	IC	100	0.5	−	12	VP	1.45 ± 0.32	25[p] (10–60)
		0.5/kg/hr[i]	0.5	−	12		4.92 ± 0.70	2880 (300–5760)
	IC	120	0.5	+	8	AB	0.68 ± 0.21	9.1 ± 9.1
		120	0.5	−	7		1.32 ± 0.41	4.2 ± 3.1

Table 215-10. (continued)

Drug	Route	Dose (mg)	Concentration (%)	Epinephrine	No. of subjects	Sampling site	Maximum concentration[a] (μg/ml)	Peak time[a] (min)
	IC[r]	100	0.5	+	9	AP	Dose 1 0.5 ± 0.1	10–20
							Dose 2 0.6 ± 0.1	10–20
							Dose 3 0.9 ± 0.1	10–20
							Dose 4 1.2 ± 0.2	10–20
	IC	100	0.5	−	10	AP	1.5–1.7	3–15
	IT	22.5	0.5	+	10	AP	0.22 ± 0.10	59 ± 31
		22.5	0.5	−	9		0.23 ± 0.11	41 ± 34
	IPer	100	0.125	+	6	VP	0.92 ± 0.33	52 ± 24
	Caud[l,m]	3/kg	0.25	−	45	AP	1.55–1.57	15–20
	Caud[m]	2.5/kg	0.5	−	13	VS	0.97 ± 0.42	28 ± 13
	Caud[l]	2.5/kg	0.25	−	6	VP	1.25 ± 0.09	29 ± 3
	Caud[l]	3.7/kg	0.5	+	10	VB	0.67 ± 0.08	45
	Perid	100	0.5	+	21	AP	0.77 ± 0.32	30[j]
						VP	0.92 ± 0.23	30[j]
	Perid	150	0.5	+	12	VP	1.14	20
		150	0.5	−	5		1.26	20
		225	0.75	+	6		2.33	20
	Perid	70–100	0.5	+	10	VB	0.33 ± 0.04[b]	≈30
	Perid	1.5/kg	0.5	−	8	VB	≈0.5	16[j]
		1.5/kg	0.5	+	8		≈0.4	28[j]
		1.5/kg	0.5	−[s]	8		≈0.58	16[j]
	Perid	150	0.5	+	?	VP	1.14 ± 0.17[b]	≈20
		225	0.75	+	?		2.33 ± 0.41[b]	≈20
	Perid	1.58/kg	0.5	+	8	AP	1.01 ± 0.33[b]	20[j]
						VP	0.82 ± 0.36[b]	30[j]
	Perid	25	0.25	+	27	VP	0.16 ± 0.08	20[j]
	Perid	0.25–0.5/ kg/hr[i]	0.125 or 0.25	−	8	AP	1.67 ± 0.79	1440
							2.16 ± 0.93	2880
	Perid	7.5/hr[i]	0.25	−	10	AP	0.1–0.2	240
	Perid[l]	0.2/kg/ hr[i,t]	0.25	−	6	VP	0.58 ± 0.20	1440–2880
	Perid	100	0.5	−	9	VP	0.79 ± 0.10[b]	5[j]
		100	0.5	+	8		0.74 ± 0.09[b]	15[j]
	Perid	150	0.75	+	10	AP	1.46 (1.13–2.32)	15–20
						VP	1.19 (0.71–1.73)	15–20
		225	0.75	+	10	AP	1.49 (1.12–2.15)	15–30
						VP	1.25 (0.78–1.70)	15–30
	Perid	150	0.75	+	5	AP	1.35 ± 0.63	20 ± 4
	Perid	112.5[q]	0.75	−	6	VP	1.0	25
		112.5[q]	0.75	+	8		0.8	25
		112.5[c]	0.75	−	8		1.0	25
		112.5[c]	0.75	+	7		0.5	25
	Perid	66	0.5	+	22	VP	0.7 ± 0.1	20
	Perid	22.5/hr[i,u]	0.375	−	8	VP	1.86 ± 0.58	1080
		22.5/hr[i,u]	0.375	+	8		1.12 ± 0.38	1080
	Perid	6.25–12.5/ hr[i,v]	0.125	−	10	AP	0.60 ± 0.28	3900
	Perid	15–45/ hr[i,w]	0.125	−	9	VP	3.04 ± 1.20	2640
	IP	50	0.25	+	5	VP	0.76 ± 0.17	20–30
		100	0.50	+	9		0.83 ± 0.18	20–30
	IP	75–100	0.5	−	14	?P	0.82 ± 0.59	30
		12.5–25/ hr[i]	0.25	−	14		1.64 ± 1.04/ 2.29 ± 1.12	1st PO AM/ 2nd PO Am[x]
	IP	150	0.5	+	10	VP	2.07 ± 0.58	21
	IP	22.5/hr[i,y]	0.375	+	39	VP	1.13	1080
	IP	100	0.5	+	8	AP	1.90 ± 0.36	21.6 ± 9.6
						VP	1.65 ± 0.48	25.2 ± 10.2
	IP	105	0.5	+	12	AP/VP	2.07 ± 0.53/ 1.86 ± 0.45	16/20
	IP	100	0.5	+	7	AB	0.29 ± 0.12	3
		100[z]	0.5	+	7		0.21 ± 0.07	5
		100[z]	0.5	−	6		0.79 ± 0.25	6
	IP	0.31/kg/ hr[i]	0.25	−	13	VS	1.8 ± 0.2	1440
		2/kg[r]	0.50	+	12		1.8 ± 0.2/ 3.2 ± 0.4[aa]	

Table 215-10. (continued)

Drug	Route	Dose (mg)	Concentration (%)	Epinephrine	No. of subjects	Sampling site	Maximum concentration[a] (µg/ml)	Peak time[a] (min)
	IP	25[bb]	0.25	+	14	VS	0.21 ± 0.08/ 0.35 ± 0.12[cc]	108/50[cc]
	IP	25/hr[i,dd]	0.25	−	10	AP	0.5	240
	IP	50	0.25	+	8	AP	0.57[p]	10–20
		75	0.375	+	7		0.73[p]	10–20
		100	0.5	+	7		1.18[p]	10–20
	IP[l,m]	1.25–2.5/ kg/hr[i]	0.25	+	14	?A	3.36 ± 0.49	1440
	IP	100	0.5	+	2	AP	0.35	5–15
		100	0.5	−	4		1.68 ± 1.29	30–120
	IP	100	0.5	+	5		0.32 ± 0.02	53 ± 27
		100	0.5	−	6		1.28 ± 0.48	10 ± 2
	IP	50	0.25	+	10	AP	0.62 ± 0.25	15
		75	0.375	+	10		0.82 ± 0.40	15
		100	0.5	+	10		1.20 ± 0.44	15
	IP	1.5/kg	0.5	−	5	AP	2.14 ± 1.23	46 ± 19
	IP	25[ee]	0.25	+	10	VP	0.49 ± 0.09[ff]	15[ff]
	IP	100[gg]	0.5	+	10	VP	3.03[hh]	10–30[hh]
	IA	100	0.25	−	11	VP	0.48 ± 0.20	43 ± 23
	IA	50	0.25	−	7	VP	0.15 ± 0.03	30
		100	0.50	−	7		0.31 ± 0.07	30
		150	0.75	−	7		0.82 ± 0.12	30
	IA	75	0.25	−	7	VP	0.223 ± 0.166	20–30
		150	0.50	−	11		0.625 ± 0.225	20
	MT	225	0.75	−	10	VB	0.50	30
Etidocaine	BP	150	0.5	+	13	VP	0.64 ± 0.12[b]	≈20
	BP[d]	150	0.5	−	5	VP	1.31	15
		150	0.5	+	5		0.86	10
	IC	150	0.25	+	10	AP	1.15 ± 0.23[b]	10–15
		150	0.5	+	10		1.30 ± 0.23[b]	5–10
		200	1	−	8		1.53 ± 0.11[b]	5–20
		200	1	+	10		1.27 ± 0.09[b]	10–15
		300	0.5	+	10		2.39 ± 0.26[b]	5–15
	IC	140	1	+	20	AB	0.52	5–10
						VB	0.46	5–10
	IC	100	0.5	−	5	P	0.8	15
		100	0.5	+	5		0.6	30
	Perid	128	1	+	19	VP	0.8 ± 0.1	20
	Perid	200	1	+	5	AP	0.92 ± 0.19	16 ± 9
		200	1	−	5		1.07 ± 0.16	15 ± 5
	Perid	300	1.5	+	19	VP	1.51	16
	Perid	50	0.25	+	5	AP	0.30 ± 0.40[b]	2–20
		100	0.5	+	8		0.53 ± 0.02[b]	2–15
		150	0.75	+	10		0.68 ± 0.03[b]	5–20
		200	1	+	10		1.27 ± 0.09[b]	10–15
		300	1.5	−	5		2.70 ± 0.31[b]	5–15
		300	1.5	+	5		1.56 ± 0.22[b]	5–20
	Perid	100	0.5	+	?	VP	0.58 ± 0.10	20
		150	0.5	+	6		0.60 ± 0.11[b]	20
		150	0.75	+	?		0.66 ± 0.05[b]	20
		300	1	−	?		1.31 ± 0.09[b]	20
		300	1	+	?		1.18 ± 0.09[b]	20
		300	1.5	+	?		1.69 ± 0.21[b]	20
		450	1.5	+	?		2.44 ± 0.37[b]	20
	Perid	100	0.5	−	9	VP	0.86 ± 0.12[b]	15[j]
		200	1	−	9		0.97 ± 0.10[b]	20[j]
		200	1	+	9		0.69 ± 0.06[b]	10[j]
	Perid	200	1	−	5	AP	1.07 ± 0.16	15 ± 5
		200	1	+	5		0.92 ± 0.19	16 ± 9
	Perid	300	1.5	+	5	AP	1.52 ± 0.64	14 ± 2
	Perid	250	1	−	?	VP	1.33 ± 0.36	
		250	1	+	?		1.26 ± 0.26	
	Caud	150	0.5	+	6	VP	1.33 ± 0.3[b]	≈10

Table 215-10. (continued)

Drug	Route	Dose (mg)	Concentration (%)	Epinephrine	No. of subjects	Sampling site	Maximum concentration[a] (µg/ml)	Peak time[a] (min)
Ropivacaine	Perid	100	0.5	−	5	VS	0.53 ± 0.19	96
		150	0.75	−	5		1.07 ± 0.57	40
		200	1.0	−	5		1.53 ± 0.60	39
	Perid	100	0.5	−	5	VP	0.65 ± 0.15	24 ± 21
		150	0.75	−	5		1.23 ± 0.42	17 ± 8
		200	1.0	−	5		1.30 ± 0.43	44 ± 14

PCB = paracervical block; V = venous; P = plasma; BP = brachial plexus block; ON = obturator nerve block; A = arterial; IPer = intraperitoneal cavity; S = serum; IT = intrathecal; B = whole blood; IC = intercostal block; Perid = peridual (epidural) block; Caud = caudal block; MT = midtarsal block; SF = sciatic/femoral block; Periton = peritonsillar block; PC/S = psoas compartment/sciatic block; Pudend = pudendal block; IP = interpleural block; IA = intraarticular (knee) block
[a] Mean SD
[b] SEM
[c] With bupivacaine
[d] Interscalene approach
[e] With epinephrine 1:320,000
[f] With epinephrine 1:800,000
[g] With epinephrine 1:200,000
[h] With epinephrine 1:80,000
[i] Continuous infusion
[j] Time of mean maximum concentration
[k] After loading dose = 150 mg
[l] Children
[m] Infants
[n] R(+), S(−) enantiomers of chiral drug
[o] After loading dose = 200–300 mg
[p] Median
[q] With chloroprocaine
[r] q6h × 4 doses
[s] Carbonated solution
[t] After loading dose = 1.25 mg/kg
[u] After loading dose = 75 mg
[v] After loading dose = 25–50 mg
[w] After mean loading dose = 65 mg
[x] First postop morning/second postop morning
[y] After loading dose = 75 mg
[z] Two intercostal catheters
[aa] Predose 4/30 minutes postdose 4
[bb] q8h × 12 doses
[cc] First dose/12th dose
[dd] After loading dose = 100 mg
[ee] q8h × 12 doses
[ff] Day 4
[gg] q4h × 6 doses
[hh] Postdose 6
Adapted from Tucker GT, Mather LE: Clinical pharmacokinetics of local anesthetics. Clin Pharmacokinet 4:241, 1979.

Table 215-11. Pharmacokinetic Parameters of Amide-Type Local Anesthetics after Intravenous to Healthy Adult Volunteers

Drug	V (L)	Vd$_{ss}$ (L)	t$_{1/2}$ (hr)	Cl (L/min)	E	f$_B$	References
Lidocaine	8.3 ± 1.6	91 ± 15 157 ± 35	1.6 ± 0.3	0.95 ± 0.21	0.65	0.36	98–101
Mepivacaine	8.1 ± 1.6	84 ± 35	1.9 ± 0.8 2.08 ± 0.53 3.17	0.78 ± 0.25 0.70 ± 0.41 0.40 0.76	0.52	0.22	98,99,102
Bupivacaine	14 ± 8	73 ± 26 34 ± 9	2.7 ± 1.3 1.27 ± 0.93	0.58 ± 0.23	0.38	0.07	98,99,100,103
Etidocaine	12 ± 4	133 ± 75 62 ± 45	2.7 ± 1.1 0.95 ± 0.26	1.11 ± 0.34	0.74	0.09	98,99,100,103
Prilocaine			1.6 ± 0.6	2.84 ± 0.41		0.45	104
Ropivacaine		59 ± 7	1.85 ± 1.03	0.72 ± 0.16		0.06	105

V = apparent initial dilution volume; Vd$_{ss}$ = apparent volume of distribution at steady state; t$_{1/2}$ = terminal disposition half-life; Cl = total body clearance; E = estimated hepatic extraction ratio; f$_B$ = free fraction in blood.

Table 215-12. Blood/Plasma Distribution (B/P) of Amide Local Anaesthetics[a]

Agent	B/P	References
Lidocaine	0.84 ± 0.08[b]	98,99
	0.81 ± 0.05[b]	106
	1.09 ± 0.10[c]	106
Mepivacaine	0.92 ± 0.04[b]	98,99
	1.03 ± 0.05[b]	106
	1.15 ± 0.12[c]	106
	0.80[d]	107
	0.95[c]	107
Bupivacaine	0.73 ± 0.05[b]	98,99
	0.59 ± 0.02[d]	108
	0.62 ± 0.11[c]	108
Etidocaine	0.61 ± 0.06[b]	98,99
	0.55 ± 0.03[e]	109,110
	0.64 ± 0.08[e]	109
	0.72 ± 0.10[d]	109
	1.24 ± 0.64[c]	111
Prilocaine	1.12[d]	107
	1.16[c]	107
Ropivacaine	0.69 ± 0.06[b]	105

[a] Data expressed as mean $\pm$ SD
[b] Normal adult males
[c] Neonate
[d] Pregnant at delivery
[e] Normal adult female

netics or pharmacodynamics of bupivacaine after brachial plexus block [128].

Little is known about the biologic activity of the metabolites of local anesthetics with two notable exceptions. First, metabolism of high-dose prilocaine (> 600 mg epidurally) to 0-toluidine and hydroxy-0-toluidine may cause methemoglobinemia. As premature and full-term infants have decreased levels of methemoglobin reductase and fetal hemoglobin is more easily oxidized than adult hemoglobin, newborns are especially susceptible to developing methemoglobinemia. Thus, prilocaine cannot be recommended for use in neonates. Second, the metabolism of some ester local anesthetics to para-aminobenzoic acid may be responsible for the allergic phenomena noted with this class of agents.

The pharmacokinetics of both ester and amide local anesthetics may be profoundly influenced by physiologic factors unique to neonates and infants [106,129]. Clearance of ester agents may be reduced and hence the effects of these agents enhanced by the relative deficiency of plasma cholinesterase in neonates and infants younger than 6 months. Neonates and infants younger than 3 months also exhibit reduced hepatic blood flow, immature metabolic degradation pathways, and lower levels of AAG and albumin. These physiologic alterations may lead to unpredictable alterations in amide agent pharmacokinetics. For example, premature neonates exhibited a significantly longer terminal disposition half-life, higher renal clearance, lower total body and metabolic clearances, and altered metabolite profiles as compared to adults after IV administration of mepivacaine [106].

Few studies have examined the stereoselective disposition parameters of local anesthetic enantiomers in humans. Those data available suggest that there may be significant differences in enantiomer disposition, at least for bupivacaine and mepivacaine. For example, the plasma concentration versus time profiles for R- and S-bupivacaine were significantly different after administration of racemic bupivacaine as a constant rate intercostal infusion (0.5 mg/kg/hr for 120 hours) to 12 patients

after thoracotomy [130]. In another study, the pharmacokinetic parameters of area-under-the-curve, steady-state volume of distribution, and total body clearance were significantly different between enantiomers after injection of 731 mg of racemic mepivacaine for psoas compartment/sciatic block in 10 male patients. S-enantiomer plasma concentrations were much higher due to the reduced volume of distribution and total body clearance as compared to the R-enantiomer [131].

PHYSIOLOGIC CLEARANCE. For etidocaine, lidocaine, and mepivacaine, hepatic drug clearance approaches 75 percent of hepatic blood flow. These highly extracted agents exhibit flow-dependent pharmacokinetics, thus changes in hepatic blood flow would be expected to play a significant role in systemic drug disposition. For example, reductions in hepatic blood flow secondary to cirrhosis, congestive heart failure (CHF), myocardial infarction even in the absence of CHF, hypotension, beta-blockers, and sympathetic blockade would be expected to reduce systemic clearance, while enhancement of flow secondary to intake of a high-protein meal would be expected to enhance clearance. Little information is available regarding the effect of norepinephrine, epinephrine, dopamine, and dobutamine on hepatic blood flow in humans and hence the kinetics of these highly extracted drugs.

For agents with a lower extraction ratio (i.e., poorly extracted drugs), such as bupivacaine, hepatic metabolism (i.e., intrinsic clearance) plays a more important role in systemic clearance. Some of the factors cited previously that affect hepatic blood flow can affect functioning liver mass and hence the systemic clearance of these agents (decreased perfusion, hypoxia, passive congestion).

Another complicating factor in the critically ill patient is the role of fluctuating levels of AAG (vide supra). Increased serum levels of AAG lead to increased serum protein binding and hence an increase in total serum drug concentration for poorly extracted drugs. However, the unbound or free serum drug concentration remains unchanged, toxicity risk is not altered, and dosage adjustment is not necessary. In contrast, for highly extracted drugs, changes in protein binding lead to little change in total drug clearance (total drug concentration remains unchanged), but free drug concentration rises, increasing the toxicity risk and necessitating dosage adjustment. This again argues for the establishment of free or unbound toxic serum concentration ranges for local anesthetics.

One study specifically examined the pharmacokinetics of lidocaine in four multiple organ failure (MOF) patients ($\geq$ grade 2 Goris [132] MOF score) after epidural drug administration (200 mg loading dose followed by 10–12 mg/kg/hr). All patients suffered from chest wall trauma or had undergone major upper abdominal surgery. Mean total arterial plasma lidocaine concentrations at 8, 12, 24, and 48 hours into therapy were 3.4, 3.8, 3.9, and 4.0 mg per liter, respectively, in the MOF group with corresponding values of 0.8, 0.8, 0.9, and 0.8 mg/per liter in the control non-MOF group (N=4). The MOF patients had adequate volume replacement and positive inotropic support if needed, and cardiac index was maintained at greater than 3.5 liters per minute. Most of the subjects were mildly acidotic during the study. The results suggest that MOF may have pronounced effects on lidocaine disposition, even when attention is paid to maintenance of hepatic blood flow [133].

Other studies have examined specific factors that may impact on local anesthetic disposition in the intensive care patient. Intravenous epinephrine was demonstrated to reduce plasma bupivacaine concentrations after epidural administration of 187.5 mg as compared to IV phenylephrine, possibly secondary to increased cardiac output (unlikely, as bupivacaine is poorly extracted), decreased absorption from the epidural space, or increased distribution to the periphery secondary to increased cardiac output and skeletal muscle blood flow [134]. Orthotopic liver transplantation was shown to have no significant effect of bupivacaine disposition after intercostal block [135]. Hypercarbia and acidosis have been demonstrated in animal studies to decrease the convulsive threshold of local anesthetics and increase total plasma and tissue concentrations of bupivacaine [136,137]. Acidosis has resulted in increased free fractions of lidocaine and bupivacaine [138,139,140]. Acute hypovolemia in dogs slows systemic lidocaine absorption after peridural injection in dogs and prolongs anesthesia in patients undergoing thoracotomy with regional blockade [141,142]. The hyperkinetic circulation of renal disease has been hypothesized to result in significantly decreased duration of brachial plexus block in chronic renal failure patients [143].

Various factors have been assessed for their contribution to augmented risk for local anesthetic toxicity, predominantly for lidocaine. In general, weight, gender, race, parturition status, and renal disease have a minor impact. Cardiovascular disease (CHF, orthostatic hypotension, status postcardiopulmonary resuscitation) is associated with reduced drug clearance (Cl) and volume of distribution (V_d), while cirrhosis is associated with reduced clearance and increased V_d and terminal disposition half-life (t1/2). Neonates exhibit an unchanged or reduced clearance and increased V_d and half-life. Drug interactions may play a significant role (vide infra). The effect of increased age on local anesthetic kinetics and dynamics is controversial, with some studies demonstrating reduced clearance, increased half-life, and faster systemic absorption after epidural and subarachnoid administration of bupivacaine in the elderly and others demonstrating no effect of advanced age on the kinetics or dynamics of epidural bupivacaine or lidocaine in the elderly.

DOSING. Dosing recommendations for FDA-approved and nonapproved indications for local anesthetics are provided in Table 215-13. Pediatric-specific data are included where available. It is prudent to avoid exceeding suggested continuous epidural anesthesia dosing limits in pediatric patients, as these patients do not appear to be more resistant to local anesthetic toxicity than adults and may lack the premonitory signs of impending major CNS toxicity. Should analgesia be inadequate at the upper limit of the suggested dosing range, addition of epinephrine or a systemic opioid, testing of the catheter, or abandonment of the technique should be considered. In pediatric upper abdominal or thoracic surgery, a thoracic epidural approach should be utilized in lieu of caudal or low-placed lumber catheters. Infusion rates should be reduced in pediatric patients at risk for seizures (i.e., past history of febrile convulsions, hypomagnesemia, hyponatremia) [144].

Attempts to avoid toxicity by individualizing nonparenteral local anesthetic dosing based on an individualized pharmacokinetic approach have been described, utilizing repeated one-point and two-point methods [145,146]. Although these techniques accurately predict systemic concentrations after continuous epidural or perineural (lumbar chain, brachial plexus) administration, their utility is compromised by the lack of availability of local anesthetic assays (except for lidocaine) in most patient care settings.

DRUG INTERACTIONS. Drug interactions involving local anesthetics and vasoconstrictors are illustrated in Table 215-14.

COMMON PITFALLS.
1. Use of epidural local anesthetics in anticoagulated patients (exogenous or endogenous) is controversial.
2. Lack of readily available assays for therapeutic drug monitoring for all local anesthetics but lidocaine (despite the plethora of published high-performance liquid and gas chromatographic assays) hampers use of these agents for extended periods in pain control in the critically ill.
3. Combinations of two or more local anesthetics are not superior to single agents used in appropriate doses. Combination therapy may predispose to toxicity by synergistic protein binding displacement interactions, leading to higher-than-expected free serum concentrations of both agents.
4. Interpretation of "toxic" serum drug concentrations in the literature is difficult, as they are based on total and not free drug concentrations and free fraction may be altered with disease.

Nonsteroidal Antiinflammatory Drugs

INTRODUCTION. The nonsteroidal antiinflammatory drugs (NSAIDs) are very commonly prescribed, due in part to the high prevalence of collagen vascular disease and other painful conditions. Despite the modest role these agents may have been previously perceived to have in the ICU, the availability of ketorolac tromethamine, the first parenteral NSAID, has rekindled interest in this analgesic class in the critically ill. In addition, the use of more traditional NSAIDs as adjuvants to opioids in the management of postoperative pain, especially in Europe, lends support to the need for a review of the pharmacologic properties of these agents.

PHARMACOLOGY. Eighteen NSAIDs are currently available in the United States, derived from a variety of chemical classes (Table 215-15). As a group, these agents exhibit antiinflammatory, analgesic, antipyretic, and antiplatelet actions. Although these agents differ chemically, pharmacokinetically, and to some extent pharmacodynamically, the clinical relevance attributable to these differences should be questioned.

From a physicochemical viewpoint, the majority of these agents are weak acids with ionization constants (pKa) ranging from 3 to 5. The pH dependence of NSAID ionization is a major determinant of distribution into tissue, with acidic NSAIDs becoming preferentially sequestered in inflamed tissue such as the synovium. Some NSAIDs, such as sulindac, are prodrugs, with the active moiety being generated in vivo. It has been suggested that because this agent does not seem to affect renal prostaglandin synthesis, it should be preferred in patients with renal disease or threatened renal hypoperfusion. However, this is controversial, as several investigators have failed to demonstrate any such advantage for this agent. These conflicting results may be explained by interindividual variability in the capacity for renal oxidation of sulindac sulfide to inactive metabolites.

The NSAIDs are thought to exert their analgesic, antiinflammatory, antipyretic, and antiplatelet effects principally by local inhibition of cyclo oxygenase, the enzyme responsible for the conversion of arachidonic acid to prostaglandin endoperoxides [149–152]. However, other mechanisms of action have been suggested as well, including inhibition of lipoxygenase, cell

(Text continues on page 2378.)

Table 215-13. Local Anesthetic Dosing Recommendations for FDA-Approved and Nonapproved Indications

Drug	Concentration (%)	Volume (ml)	Total dose (mg)
Chloroprocaine			
Approved			
Mandibular	2	2–3	40–60
Infraorbital	2	0.5–1	10–20
Brachial plexus	2	30–40	600–800
Digital	1	3–4	30–40
Pudendal	2	10/each side	400
Paracervical	1	3/each of 4 sites	≤ 120
Nonapproved			
IVRA[a] upper limb	0.5	40	200
IVRA[a] lower limb	0.5	60	300
Epidural	3	5/increment to T_4 block	150/increment
		20–30/hr[b]	600–900/hr[b]
Tetracaine			
Approved			
Spinal	1	0.5–1.5	5–15
Nonapproved			
Brachial plexus	0.25	4	10
Sciatic/femoral	0.25	4	10
Intercostal	0.25	4	10
	0.1–0.25	0.5–1.5/space	0.5–3.75/space
Caudal	0.25	15–20	37.5–50
			2/kg[c]
Epidural	0.25	6–14	15–35
	0.5	3–10	15–50
Mepivacaine			
Approved			
Cervical, brachial, intercostal,	1	5–40	50–400
pudendal	2	5–20	100–400
		0.4/kg[c]	8/kg[c]
Transvaginal (paracervical + pudendal)	1	≤ 30 (both sides)	≤ 300 (both sides)
Paracervical	1	≤ 20 (both sides)	≤ 200 (both sides)
Caudal and epidural	1	15–30	150–300
	1.5	10–25	150–375
		0.73/kg[c]	11/kg[c]
		10–20	200–400
Therapeutic (pain)	2	1–5	10–50
	2	1–5	20–100
Nonapproved			
Epidural	2	10/hr[b]	200/hr[b]
Etidocaine			
Approved			
Peripheral nerve	1	5–40	50–400
Peridural	1	10–30	100–300
	1.5	10–20	150–300
Caudal	1	10–30	100–300
Retrobulbar	1	2–4	20–40
	1.5	2–4	30–60
Maxillary	1.5	1–5	15–75
Nonapproved			
Intercostal	0.5	30–60	150–300
	1	3/space	30/space
Thoracic epidural	1.5	4/hr[b]	60/hr[b]
Brachial plexus	0.5	20–30	100–150
	0.75	20–30	150–225
Celiac plexus	0.25	40	100
Prilocaine			
Nonapproved			
IVRA[a] upper limb	0.5	40	200
	1	20–40	300–400
Epidural	2	20	400
Brachial plexus	1.5	30	450
Sciatic/femoral	1	25–35	250–350
	1.5	20–30	300–450
Peripheral nerve			5–7/kg[c,d]

Table 215-13. (continued)

Drug	Concentration (%)	Volume (ml)	Total dose (mg)
Lidocaine			
Approved			
IVRA[a]	0.5	10–60	50–300
Brachial plexus	1.5	15–20	225–300
Intercostal	1	3/space	30/space
Paravertebral	1	3–5	30–50
Pudendal (each side)	1	10	100
Paracervical (each side)	1	10	100
Cervical	1	5	50
Lumbar	1	5–10	50–100
Epidural (thoracic)	1	20–30	200–300
(lumbar)	1	25–30	250–300
Caudal (obstetrical)	1	20–30	200–300
(surgical)	1.5	15–20	225–300
Nonapproved			
Interpleural			2.1/min[b]
Intercostal	2	5/space	100/space
	1.5/1[b,e]	0.2/kg/0.1/kg/hr[b,e]	3 per kg/1 per kg per h[b,e]
Epidural	1.5	5/increment to T_4 block	75/increment
	2	15–20	300–400
	2/0.4[b,e]	8–15/0.5–1/min[b,e]	160–300/2–4/min[b,e]
	1.5/0.75[b,e]	10/10/hr[b,e]	150/75/hr[b,e]
Caudal			5–7/kg[c]
	1.5[c]	0.73/kg[c]	11/kg[c]
Brachial plexus	1[c]	10[c]	100[c]
Intraarticular	0.5	20	100
Spinal	2	2.5–3	
			1.2/in of body height 100
	1	1/0.5–1 increment to block	10/5–10 increment to block
Sciatic/femoral	1[c]	1/yr of age[c]	10/yr of age[c]
Bupivacaine			
Approved			
Epidural	0.75	10–20	75–150
	0.5	10–20	50–100
	0.25	10–20	25–50
Caudal	0.5	15–30	75–150
	0.25	15–30	37.5–75
Peripheral nerve	0.5	5 to max 80	25 to max 400
	0.25	5 to max 160	12.5 to max 400
Retrobulbar	0.75	2–4	15–30
Sympathetic	0.25	20–50	50–125
Intraarticular	0.25	20–40	50–100
	0.5	20–30	100–150
	0.75	20	150
Nonapproved			
Caudal	0.75	0.3/kg	2.2/kg
	0.25[c]	1.2/kg[c]	3/kg[c]
	0.5[c]	0.75/kg[c]	3.7/kg[c]
			1.5–2.5/kg[c]
	0.125	1/kg	1.25/kg
Sciatic/femoral	0.25[c]	5–10[c]	12.5–25[c]
	0.25/0.125[b,e]	30/6/hr[b,e]	75/7.5/hr[b,e]
	0.5	0.6/kg	3/kg
	0.375	45	169
	0.25–0.5/0.25–0.5[b,e]	10–20/2–4/hr[b,e]	25–100/5–20/hr[b,e]
	0.25/0.25[b,e]	10/7/hr[b,e]	25/17.5/per hr[b,e]
Peripheral nerve			1.5–2.5/kg[e]
Intercostal	0.25	3/hr[b]	7.5/hr[b]
	0.5/0.5[b,e]	10/5–7/hr[b,e]	50/25–35/hr[b,e]
	0.75/0.25[b,e]	20–28/5–9/hr[b,e]	150–210/12.5–22.5/hr[b,e]
	0.5	12 q8h	60 q8h
	0.5/0.5[b,e]	20/0.1/kg/hr[b,e]	100/0.5/kg/hr[b,e]
	0.5/0.5[b,e]	30/3/hr[b,e]	150/15/hr[b,e]
	0.5/0.5[b,e]	20/5–10/hr[b,e]	100/25–50/hr[b,e]

Table 215-13. (continued)

Drug	Concentration (%)	Volume (ml)	Total dose (mg)
Brachial plexus	0.25[c]	10[c]	25[c]
	0.25–0.5/0.25–0.5[b,e]	10–20/2–4/hr[b,e]	25–100/5–20/hr[b,e]
Lumbar plexus	0.5/0.25[b,c]	0.4/0.14/hr[b,e]	2/kg/0.35/kg/hr[b,e]
Spinal	0.125	6–10	7.5–12.5
	0.5	4	20
	0.5	2.5	12.5
	0.25/0.125[b,e]	1.5/1.5/hr[b,e]	3.75/1.875/hr[b,e]
	0.25	0.5	1.25
Epidural	0.25–0.375/NA[b,e,f]	0.5–1/0.5–1/hr[b,e]	1.25–3.75/1.25–3.75/hr[b,e]
	0.25/0.25 or 0.125[b,e]	12–15/7 or 12/hr[b,e]	30–37.5/15–17.5/hr[b,e]
	0.166[b]	1–6/hr[b]	1.66–9.96/hr[b]
	0.125[b]	10/hr[b]	12.5/hr[b]
	0.25/0.25[b,c,e]	0.5/kg/0.08/kg/hr[b,c,e]	1.25/kg/0.2/kg/hr[b,c,e]
	0.5/0.5[b,c]	20–25/8/hr[b,c]	100–125/40/hr[b,c]
	0.1–0.5[b]	4–18/hr[b]	0.4–90/hr[b]
	0.5	0.5/kg[c]	2.5/kg[c]
			2–2.5/kg/0.4-0.5/kg/hr[c,g]
			2–2.5/kg/0.2–0.25/kg/hr[c,h]
	0.75/0.75/0.25[b,e]	7/4/hr/4/hr[b,e]	52.5/30/hr/10/hr[b,e]
	0.25/0.125[b,e]	10/10/hr[b,e]	25/12.5/hr[b,e]
	0.2/0.2[b,e]	5/3–5/hr/[b,e]	10/6–10/hr[b,e]
	0.25/0.125[b,e]	10/7/hr[b,e]	25/8.75/hr[b,e]
	0.5/0.5[b,e]	20–30/8/hr[b,e]	100–150/40/hr[b,e]
	0.975	16	156
	0.5/0.5[b,c,e]	0.2/kg/0.2/kg/hr[b,c,e]	1/kg/1/kg/hr[b,c,e]
	0.25/0.25[b,c,e]	0.05/kg/segment/0.1/kg/hr[b,c,e]	0.125/kg/segment/0.25/kg/hr[b,c,e]
	0.125[c]	0.75/kg[c]	0.9375/kg[c]
	0.125–0.25[b]	0.1–0.4/kg/hr[b]	0.25–0.5/kg/hr[b]
	0.5/0.25[b,e]	6/3/hr[b,e]	30/7.5/hr[b,e]
	0.125[b]	5/hr[b]	6.25/hr[b]
	0.5/0.125[b,e]	8/7.5/hr[b,e]	40/9.375/hr[b,e]
	0.1[b]	3–6/hr[b]	3–6/hr[b]
	0.25/0.25[b,e]	10–20/7/hr[b,e]	25–50/17.5/hr[b,e]
	0.1/0.1[b,e]	5/5/hr[b,e]	5/5/hr[b,e]
	0.5/0.08[b,e]	6/15/hr[b,e]	30/12/hr[b,e]
	0.5/0.5[b,e]	9/5/hr[b,e]	45/25/hr[b,e]
	0.25/0.25[b,e]	10/3–10/hr[b,e]	25/7.5–25/hr[b,e]
	0.5/0.125[b,e]	10/15/hr[b,e]	50/18.75/hr[b,e]
Interpleural	0.25[b]	5/hr[b]	12.5/hr[b]
			1.5/kg
	0.25[b,c]	0.5/kg/hr[b,c]	1.25/kg/hr[b,c]
	0.25	10–20	25–50
	0.5	20	100
	0.5/0.25[b,e]	20/8/hr[b,e]	100/20/hr[b,e]
	0.5/0.25[b,e]	15–20/5–10/hr[b,e]	75–100/12.5–25/hr[b,e]
	0.375/0.375[b,e]	20/6/hr[b,e]	75/22.5/hr[b,e]
	0.375	20 q4h	75 q4h
	0.25	20–40	50-100
	0.5	20–30	100–150
	0.5	21	105
	0.25[b]	0.125/kg/hr[b]	0.3125/kg/hr[b]
	0.5	0.4/kg q6h	2/kg q6h
	0.25	20 q4h	50 q4h
	0.5	20 q4h	100 q4h
	0.5[b]	10/hr[b]	50/hr[b]
	0.5/0.25[b,e]	20/10/hr[b,e]	100/25/hr[b,e]
	0.25	10 q8h	25 q8h
	0.375	20 q6h	75 q6h
	0.375	20	75
			150
	0.25[b,e]	0.5–1/kg/hr[b,e]	1.25–2.5/kr/hr[b,e]

Table 215-13. (continued)

Drug	Concentration (%)	Volume (ml)	Total dose (mg)
Ropivacaine			
Nonapproved			
Epidural	0.5	15–20	75–100
	0.75	15–20	112.5–150
	1	15–20	150–200
Brachial plexus	0.25	45	112.5
	0.5	30–38	150–190

[a] Intravenous regional anesthesia
[b] Continuous infusion
[c] Pediatric dose
[d] Maximum dose = 600 mg, not recommended ≤ 6 months of age
[e] Loading dose/maintenance dose
[f] NA = not available
[g] Older infants, toddlers, children
[h] Neonates

Table 215-14. Drug Interactions Involving Local Anesthetics and Vasoconstrictors [73,147,148]

Drug	Interacting drug	Effect	Recommendation
Local anesthetics (general)	Alcohol, CNS depressants, parenteral $MgSO_4$	CNS and respiratory depression	Caution in simultaneous use
	Antiarrhythmics (e.g., quinidine)	cardiodepression	Caution in simultaneous use
	Antimyasthenics (e.g., neostigmine)	Antagonism of effect of antimyasthenics on muscle	Caution in simultaneous use
	Carrier molecules (lipids such as iophenyldylate, polymers, liposomes)	duration of action, especially with epidural, spinal, sciatic blocks	Investigational use only
	Clonidine	Prolongs duration of anesthesia and analgesia when admixed with local anesthetic in brachial plexus, femoral, spinal, epidural blocks and administered orally with spinal blocks. No effect on epidural lido or spinal bupiv kinetics	
	Dextran	Controversial; prolongs duration of anesthesia in some studies but not in others. Slows systemic local anesthetic absorption, perhaps by complexation	
	Opioids	Controversial; potentiation of caudal/epidural bupiv by caudal/epidural fentanyl, sufentanil, alfentanil, morphine, butorphanol, meperidine, diamorphine; epidural lido by epidural butorphanol, fentanyl, sufentanil; intraarticular bupiv by intraarticular morphine, IVRA lido by fentanyl; intrathecal bupiv by intrathecal meperidine. No potentiation of epidural chloropro by epidural fentanyl, nalbuphine; epidural bupiv by epidural fentanyl, morphine, sufentanil; epidural lido by epidural nalbuphine; IVRA prilo by IVRA fentanyl; intraarticular bupiv by intraarticular morphine; IVRA lido by IVRA fetanyl	On balance, it appears opioids are useful adjunctive agents to local anesthetics for pain control in patients with suboptimal response to local anesthetics alone
	Phenylephrine	Improves analgesia/anesthesia of spinal tetra and lido but not bupiv when admixed with local anesthetic	

Table 215-14. (continued)

Drug	Interacting drug	Effect	Recommendation
	Epinephrine	Controversial; kinetics (see also Table 215–10): ↓ plasma concentrations of epidural lido, bupiv, prilo; intraperitoneal lido; intercostal lido, prilo, bupiv; brachial plexus mepiv; interpleural bupiv; sciatic/femoral bupiv; intraarticular bupiv; spinal lido No effect on plasma concentrations of epidural lido, etid, mepiv; intercostal etid, bupiv; spinal bupiv; interpleural bupiv; sciatic/femoral bupiv Dynamics: potentiates epidural lido, bupiv, bupiv + fentanyl; caudal mepiv; spinal tetra, lido ↓ plasma potassium (epidural mepiv) No effect on sciatic/femoral bupiv; ulnar bupiv; epidural bupiv, etid; intercostal etid; interpleural bupiv; brachial plexus ropiv	
	Sodium bicarbonate	Controversial; speeds onset of epidural block, no effect on epidural block, speeds onset of brachial plexus block, no effect on brachial plexus block, speeds onset of sciatic nerve block, no effect in intercostal block, speeds onset of IVRA with prilo, no effect on systemic absorption of mepiv or lido	Use only freshly prepared solution (shelf-life unknown at neutral pH) although buffered lido is active for at least 1 wk (room temp) or 2 wk (refrigerated)
Local anesthetics (esters)	Anticholinesterases (e.g., neostigmine), insecticides (e.g., parathion), amide local anesthetics (e.g., bupiv), atypical pseudocholinesterase activity (pregnant women, infants < 3 mo, hepatic disease, familial deficiency)	↓ ester metabolism	Caution in simultaneous use
	Sulfonamides	Inhibition of sulfonamide activity	Caution in simultaneous use
Local anesthetics (amides)	H₂ blockers	Cimetidine: ↑ plasma lido, no effect on plasma bupiv Ranitidine: no effect on plasma lido, controversial effect on plasma bupiv Famotidine: no effect on plasma lido	Caution in simultaneous use
	Benzodiazepines	Midazolam: no kinetic effect on mepiv, bupiv but ↓ AUC for lido, synergistic ↓ in resting ventilation (spinal lido)	Caution in simultaneous use, especially with lidocaine
		Diazepam: ↑ C_{max} and AUC of caudal bupiv but not lido	Caution in simultaneous use, especially with bupivacaine
	Hyaluronidase	Improves regional ophthalmic anesthesia with bupiv, bupiv + lido, etid ↓ duration of anesthesia in brachial plexus block (bupiv)	
Vasoconstrictors	Inhalational anesthetics (e.g., halothane)	↑ cardiac arrhythmias	
	Tricyclic antidepressants	↑ sympathomimetic effects	Use epinephrine cautiously, avoid levonordefrin and norepinephrine.
	β-blockers, adrenergic neuron blockers	Hypertensive and/or cardic reactions.	Caution in simultaneous use
	Neuroleptics	↓ vasoconstrictor activity	Caution in simultaneous use
	Monoamine oxidase inhibitors	↑ sympathomimetic effects	Avoid phenylephrine, use others cautiously
	Local anesthetics (amides)	↑ systemic absorption of epinephrine	Caution in simultaneous use
Meperidine	Prilocaine	Enhanced systemic bioavailability of intrathecal meperidine	Caution in simultaneous use

CNS = central nervous system; lido = lidocaine; bupiv = bupivacaine; IVRA = intravenous regional anesthesia; chloroproc = 2-chloroprocaine; prilo = prilocaine; tetra = tetracaine; mepiv = mepivacaine; etid = etidocaine; ropiv = ropivacaine; AUC = area under the curve; C_{max} = peak concentration.

Table 215-15. Chemical Classification of NSAIDs

Fenamates
  Meclofenamate sodium (Meclomen)
  Mefenamic acid (Ponstel)
Indoles
  Indomethacin (Indocin)
  Sulindac (Clinoril)
  Tolmetin sodium (Tolectin)
Naphthylkanone
  Nabumetone (Relafen)
Oxicam
  Piroxicam (Feldene)
Salicylates
  Acetylsalicylic acid (aspirin)
  Diflunisal (Dolobid)
Phenylacetic acid
  Diclofenac (Voltaren)
Propionic acids
  Fenoprofen calcium (Nalfon)
  Flurbiprofen (Ansaid)
  Ibuprofen (Motrin)
  Ketoprofen (Orudis)
  Naproxen (Naprosyn)
  Oxaprozin (Daypro)
Pyranocarboxylic acid
  Etodolac (Lodine)
Pyrrolopyrrole
  Ketorolac tromethamine (Toradol)

membrane-associated processes (NADPH oxidase, phospholipase C), neutrophil function (cell-cell aggregation, H_2O_2 generation), lymphocyte function, proteoglycan synthesis, and transmembrane ion fluxes [151–157]. More recent data suggest that NSAIDs may exert more central analgesic effects as well [158,159]. Although classified as an NSAID, ketorolac has not shown substantial antiinflammatory activity in animal models at analgesic doses, and pilot clinical trials have demonstrated only marginal efficacy for rheumatic conditions [160].

In general, NSAIDs inhibit platelet aggregation either irreversibly (aspirin) or reversibly (all others). They generally do not exert appreciable effects on the CNS, cardiovascular system (mean arterial pressure, heart rate, stroke volume), respiratory system (pCO_2, response to CO_2), GI transit, or biliary tree dynamics.

The analgesic dose of most NSAIDs is about one-half the antiinflammatory dose, for reasons that are not well understood. For some NSAIDs, such as aspirin, ibuprofen, and fenoprofen, the gap between the small dose required for analgesia and the larger dose required for antiinflammatory activity is considerable, while for others, such as sulindac and piroxicam, the gap is much smaller [161].

THERAPEUTIC RANGE. Few database assessed dose-response or concentration-response relationships for NSAIDs, and those that exist have examined principally the antiinflammatory concentration-response relationships, not those for analgesia. Some investigators have found that NSAIDs exhibit linear antiinflammatory actions that depend on the dose or total or unbound plasma drug concentration in rheumatoid or osteoarthritis patients, while others have not. The relationship between plasma drug concentration and antiinflammatory effect does not explain all of the variability in response, suggesting that some of the variability in response is pharmacodynamic in origin [162,163]. Preliminary data suggest that the analgesic potency of NSAIDs such as ibuprofen, independent of rheumatoid disease, may also be a function of serum drug concentration [164].

Relationships between plasma NSAID concentrations or dosage and toxicity have been noted for ototoxicity due to salicylates and upper GI bleeding and a variety of NSAIDs [165,166,167]. Of interest, the suggested differing pharmacokinetics (vis-à-vis plasma concentrations) of NSAIDs in responders versus nonresponders has not been supported by existing data.

In light of the above data, it appears that, perhaps with the exception of salicylate, the use of therapeutic drug concentration monitoring of NSAIDs is of little routine clinical value [163].

PREPARATIONS. The NSAID preparations available in the United States are listed in Table 215-16. These preparations are predominantly designed for oral administration, although rectal and parenteral routes are available for some agents.

PHARMACOKINETICS. In general, NSAIDs are well-absorbed after oral administration, exhibit low non-flow-dependent hepatic clearance and low to nonexistent first-pass metabolism, are highly plasma protein-bound (principally to albumin), and have small distribution volumes.

Of interest, the disposition of some NSAIDs is complicated by their availability as racemic mixtures of two optical isomers or enantiomers. In most cases, the R enantiomer is inactive as an antiinflammatory agent while the S enantiomer is active (e.g., ibuprofen, ketoprofen, flurbiprofen). Conversion from one enantiomer to the other may occur in vivo, depending on the drug and individual patient [168,169,170]. However, the R enantiomers of some NSAIDs, such as flurbiprofen, may be active as analgesics but devoid of antiinflammatory, gastrotoxic, and peripheral prostaglandin synthesis inhibition effects [168].

Table 215-16. NSAID Preparations Available in the United States

Drug	Preparation
Meclofenamate sodium	50 and 100 mg oral capsules
Mefenamic acid	250 mg oral capsules
Indomethacin	25 and 50 mg oral capsules
	25 mg/5 ml oral suspension
	75 mg sustained-release oral capsule
	50 mg rectal suppositories
Sulindac	150 and 200 mg oral tablets
Tolmetin sodium	200 and 600 mg oral tablets
	400 mg oral capsules
Nabumetone	500 and 750 mg oral tablets
Piroxicam	10 and 20 mg oral capsules
Acetylsalicylic acid	Multiple oral and rectal suppository formulations
Diflunisal	250 and 500 mg oral tablets
Diclofenac	25, 50, and 75 mg oral enteric-coated tablets
Fenoprofen calcium	200 and 300 mg oral capsules
	600 mg oral tablets
Flurbiprofen	50 and 100 mg oral tablets
Ibuprofen	Multiple oral tablet and suspension formulations
Ketoprofen	25, 50, and 75 mg oral capsules
Naproxen	250, 375, and 500 mg oral tablets
	25 mg/ml oral suspension
	275 and 550 mg oral tablets (sodium)
Oxaprozin	600 mg oral tablet
Etodolac	200 and 300 mg oral capsules
Ketorolac tromethamine	15 and 30 mg/ml × 1 ml syringe
	30 mg/ml × 2 ml syringe
	10 mg oral tablets

It should be noted that much of the data presented herein (vide infra, Tables 215-17 and 215-18) may be inaccurate and misleading due to a lack of assessment of unbound pharmacologically active drug concentrations, as opposed to total drug concentrations, and lack of assessment of stereospecific drug disposition for those compounds administered as racemates (vide supra).

Absorption. It is generally believed that the oral absorption of NSAIDs is complete, despite the fact that this hypothesis has been confirmed for only a few of these agents. Oral bioavailabilities of 65, 60, 81, and 38 percent have been reported for aspirin, diclofenac, ketorolac, and nabumetone, respectively.

The oral bioavailabilities of aspirin, diclofenac, and nabumetone are relatively low due to substantial first-pass metabolism, which in the case of nabumetone results in the generation of the active moiety 6-methoxy-naphthylacetic acid (6-MNA) [178].

Distribution. Most NSAIDs are bound extensively ($\geq$ 95%) to albumin, and the drug free fraction may be increased in patients with hypoalbuminemia. Protein binding is saturable in the usual dose range for some NSAIDs (salicylate, naproxen, phenylbutazone, ibuprofen), so that increasing daily doses lead to a less-than-proportional increase in steady-state trough concentrations; in contrast, free drug concentrations increase proportionally with dose.

Several factors have been assessed for their effect on NSAID plasma protein binding. Female gender has been linked to a decrease in naproxen plasma protein binding [185]. Increasing age has been associated with variable effects on NSAID plasma protein binding: decreased binding for diflunisal, salicylate, phenylbutazone, ketorolac; no change for etodolac, ibuprofen, oxaprozin; and conflicting data for piroxicam and naproxen [175,185]. Hepatic and renal disease may be associated with reduced NSAID protein binding as well, in the latter case primarily due to the presence of small-molecular-weight endogenous binding inhibitors [186,187]. The plasma protein binding of salicylate, diflunisal, naproxen, oxaprozin, sulindac (+ metabolites), and phenylbutazone are reduced in patients with renal disease.

The high degree of NSAID plasma protein binding is reflected in the small volumes of distribution, which are approximately 15 percent of body weight.

Metabolism/Excretion. All NSAIDs except indomethacin and oxaprozin are virtually entirely dependent on hepatic metabolism for elimination, either through oxidation or glucuronidation. The isozymes of cytochrome P-450 requisite for NSAID metabolism and the possibility of phenotypic differences in NSAID metabolism have not been explored.

Limited data are available regarding enterohepatic circulation of NSAIDs, but they suggest that there is a potential for this to occur with indomethacin and sulindac due to their extensive degree of biliary excretion.

The renal elimination of parent compound constitutes only a small proportion of the clearance mechanism of most NSAIDs. The clearance of agents such as ketoprofen, fenoprofen, naproxen, indomethacin, and carprofen may be decreased to a variable degree in patients with renal impairment or in those taking probenecid concurrently, due to the retention of unstable acyl-glucuronide metabolites that may hydrolyze to reform the parent compound [188]. This recycling is one reason for caution in the use of these agents in patients with renal impairment [189]. Urine pH plays a major role in the elimination of salicylate when urine pH exceeds 6.5, as renal clearance increases markedly in this urine pH range [186].

PHYSIOLOGIC CLEARANCE. The clearance of most NSAIDs is low, and these drugs are generally capacity-limited rather than flow-limited. The extraction or metabolism of most of these agents is thus dependent on the intrinsic metabolic capacity of the liver. For example, an extraction ratio of 0.002 to 0.09 has been estimated for ketorolac [172]. Clearance of total drug is thus determined by the unbound drug concentration and unbound clearance [190]. Thus, the degree of plasma protein binding plays a potentially key role in the disposition of most NSAIDs, and studies assessing their disposition should be conducted with this in mind. In general, though, displacement of an NSAID from its binding site leads to an increase in clearance and a decrease in total plasma concentration but not the concentration of unbound drug after re-equilibration. Hence, the pharmacologic effect of the drug should remain unchanged.

The effects of hypometabolism and hypermetabolism on the disposition of these agents should follow the physiologic clearance characteristics of a capacity-limited, binding-sensitive agent. However, data from the critically ill patient population have not been systematically obtained.

DOSING. Dosing recommendations for analgesia and antiinflammatory activity for adults and children are illustrated in Table 215-19. Unless otherwise noted, these regimens are for patients without significant organ dysfunction and reflect package insert ranges. Dosage recommendations for hypometabolic and hypermetabolic patients cannot be made at present due to a lack of pharmacokinetic and pharmacodynamic data in these patient populations.

DRUG INTERACTIONS. Therapy with NSAIDs may be associated with the development of pharmacokinetic, pharmacodynamic, or combination pharmacokinetic/pharmacodynamic drug interactions. A summary of NSAID drug-drug interactions is provided in Table 215-20, with an emphasis on those of particular clinical relevance (reviews are available in references 190 to 194). The breadth of these interactions may complicate the use of these agents in the critically ill, who may already be concurrently receiving multiple drugs and have multiple disease entities.

Physicochemical admixture incompatibilities for parenteral ketorolac tromethamine with selected potential concomitant parenteral agents were assessed in a recent study. Ketorolac tromethamine should not be mixed in the same syringe as morphine sulfate, meperidine hydrochloride, promethazine hydrochloride, hydroxyzine hydrochloride, prochlorperazine edisylate, nalbuphine hydrochloride, or diazepam, due to physicochemical incompatibility [195].

COMMON PITFALLS. Use of NSAIDs in the critically ill patient may be problematic due to the frequency and intensity of adverse events secondary to their use. Up to 25 percent of all adverse reactions may be due to NSAIDs, and the spectrum of reactions is broad, including GI, renal, dermatologic, and CNS reactions (in descending order of frequency) [196,197].

Gastrointestinal reactions, including erosions, ulceration, and hemorrhage, may be devastating in critically ill patients already at high risk for stress gastritis. There is no good evidence that differentiates roughly equipotent antiinflammatory doses of one NSAID from another with respect to risk of serious gastrointestinal reactions, with the exception of aspirin [166]. Avoidance of these agents in those at high risk of stress ulcer disease is prudent.

(Text continues on page 2384).

Table 215-17. Pharmacokinetic Parameters of NSAIDs in Adults [167,171–181]

Drug	Absorption characteristics	Distribution characteristics	Metabolism/elimination characteristics
ASA	Presystemic hydrolysis (> 30% dose) Food ↓ C_{max} but no effect on F	V_d = 0.15 L/kg	$t_{1/2}$ = 0.25 hr TBC = 650 ml/min F_e < 2% of dose Salicylate is active metabolite
Salicylate	T_{max} = 2 hr	V_d = 0.17 L/kg (dose-dependent) 80–90% PB (albumin) PB is saturable	$t_{1/2}$ = 2–30 hr (dose-dependent) TBC = 10–60 ml/min (concentration-dependent) F_e = 2–30% of dose (pH-dependent) Dose-dependent kinetics (capacity-limited metabolism) ↑ $t_{1/2}$, ↓ V_d, ↓ TBC in elderly Renal disease— ↓ PB Hepatic disease— ↓ PB, ↓ TBC
Diflunisal	T_{max} = 1–2 hr Food has no effect on F	V_d = 0.10 L/kg > 99% PB (albumin)	$t_{1/2}$ ↑ = 5–20 hr (dose-dependent) TBC = 8 ml/min F_e ≤ 5% of dose Dose-dependent kinetics Renal disease— ↓ TBC, ↓ PB, ↑ V_d ↓ PB in elderly
Phenylbutazone	T_{max} = 2 hr	V_d = 0.17 L/kg 98–99% PB (albumin)	$t_{1/2}$ ↑ = 50–100 hr F_e = 1% dose Active metabolites Dose-dependent kinetics Renal disease— ↓ PB, ↑ V_d, ↑ $t_{1/2}$ Hepatic disease— ↓ PB, ? ↑ TBC, ? ↑ V_d ↓ PB in elderly
Oxyphenbutazone		98–99% PB (albumin)	$t_{1/2}$ = 27–64 hr F_e < 2% of dose Active metabolite of phenylbutazone
Indomethacin	T_{max} = 1–2 hr Food ↓ rate but not extent of F	V_d = 0.15–0.20 L/kg > 90% PB (albumin) but variable	$t_{1/2}$ = 6 hr TBC = 70–140 ml/min F_e < 15% of dose Enterohepatic recirculation
Sulindac	T_{max} = 1–2 hr (sulindac) 2 hr (active metabolite) Food ↓ rate and extent of F	93.1% PB (sulindac) 95.4% PB (active metabolite)	$t_{1/2}$ = 7 (sulindac), 16 (active metabolite) hr F_e = 7% of dose Active metabolite (sulfide) Sulindac ↔ sulfide interconvertible Enterohepatic recirculation
Tolmetin	T_{max} = 0.5–1 hr	V_d = 0.10–0.14 L/kg > 99% PB (albumin)	$t_{1/2}$ = 1–6 hr TBC = 125 ml/min F_e = 15% of dose
Naproxen	T_{max} = 1–2 hr Food no effect on rate or extent of F	V_d = 0.10 L/kg Concentration-dependent PB (97.4 → 99.6%) (albumin)	$t_{1/2}$ = 12–15 hr TBC = 5 ml/min F_e < 10% of dose ↑ renal clearance at high plasma concentrations due to saturable protein binding Renal disease— ↑ TBC, ↑ V_d, ↓ PB ↔ or ↓ PB, ↓ TBC of free drug in elderly
Fenoprofen	T_{max} = 1–2 hr Food ↓ rate and extent of F	V_d = 0.08–0.10 L/kg > 99% PB (albumin)	$t_{1/2}$ = 2–3 hr TBC = 40–90 ml/min F_e = 2–5% of dose
Ketoprofen	T_{max} = 0.5–2 hr	V_d = 0.11 L/kg 98.7% PB (albumin)	$t_{1/2}$ = 1.5 hr TBC = 87 ml/min F_e < 1% of dose ↑ $t_{1/2}$, ↓ TBC in elderly
Flurbiprofen	T_{max} = 1.5–3 hr Food no effect on extent of F	V_d = 0.10–0.16 L/kg ≥ 99% PB (albumin)	$t_{1/2}$ = 3–4 hr TBC = 22 ml/min F_e < 15% of dose
Ibuprofen	T_{max} = 0.5–1.5 hr Food ↓ rate but not extent of F	99% PB (albumin)	$t_{1/2}$ = 1.6–2.5 hr F_e = 1% of dose ↑ $t_{1/2}$, ↓ TBC in elderly males
Diclofenac	T_{max} = 1–3 hr Presystemic elimination (F = 60%) Food ↓ rate but not extent of F	V_d = 0.12 L/kg > 99% PB (albumin)	$t_{1/2}$ = 1–2 hr TBC = 260 ml/min (IV) F_e < 1% of dose

Table 215-17. (continued)

Drug	Absorption characteristics	Distribution characteristics	Metabolism/elimination characteristics
Mefenamic acid	T_{max} = 1–3 hr Food no effect on rate or extent of F		$t_{1/2}$ = 3–4 hr F_e < 6% of dose
Meclofenamic acid	T_{max} = 0.5–2 hr	V_d = 23.3 L 99.8% PB (albumin)	$t_{1/2}$ = 0.8–2.1 hr TBC = 206 ml/min F_e = 2–4% of dose Active hydroxymethyl metabolite Enterohepatic recirculation
Piroxicam	T_{max} = 2–3 hr Food ↓ rate but not extent of F	V_d = 0.12–0.15 L/kg > 99% PB (albumin)	$t_{1/2}$ = 31–57 hr TBC = 2–3 ml/min F_e = 10% of dose Enterohepatic recirculation Renal disease— ↓ $t_{1/2}$, ↑ V_d ↔ or ↓ PB in elderly
Ketorolac	T_{max} = 0.3–1 hr (PO + IM) Food ↓ rate but not extent of F Absolute bioavailability of PO = 80–100% IM = 100%	V_d = 0.1–0.3 L/kg > 99% PB (albumin) Saturable protein binding at high plasma concentrations	TBC = 24–33 mL/min (IV/IM) F_e = 5–10% of dose ↓ TBC, ↑ T_{max} ↓ PB in elderly Renal disease— ↓ TBC, ↓ $t_{1/2}$, ↑ T_{max}
Etodolac	T_{max} = 1–2 hr Food ↓ rate but not extent of F	V_d = 0.41 L/kg > 99% PB (albumin)	$t_{1/2}$ = 6–7 hr Liver disease— ↓ T_{max}
Oxaprozin	T_{max} = 3–6 hr Food no effect on rate or extent of F	V_d = 0.15–0.25 L/kg ≥ 99.5% PB (albumin)	$t_{1/2}$ = 59 hr TBC = 1.3–2.0 ml/min F_e ≥ 90% of dose ↓ V_d, ↓ TBC in elderly Renal disease— ↓ unbound fraction, ↓ TBC of free drug Hepatic disease— ↑ unbound fraction CHF— ↑ V_d, ↓ C_{max}, ↑ unbound fraction, ↑ TBC
Nabumetone	T_{max} (6-MNA) = 3–6 hr Extensive presystemic metabolism to 6-MNA Food ↑ rate but not extent of F	V_d = 7.5 L > 99% PB (6-MNA, albumin)	$t_{1/2}$ (6-MNA) = 21–27 hr TBC (6-MNA) = 3–5 ml/min Active metabolite (6-MNA) ↑ $t_{1/2}$, ↑ C_{max} in elderly Hepatic disease— ↑ T_{max}

C_{max} = peak plasma or serum concentration; F = bioavailability; T_{max} = time to C_{max}, V_d = volume of distribution; $t_{1/2}$ = elimination half-life; TBC = total body clearance; F_e = fraction of the dose excreted in unchanged form in the urine; PB = protein binding; 6 MNA = 6-methoxy-naphthylacetic acid; CHF = congestive heart failure

Table 215-18. Pharmacokinetic Parameters of NSAIDs in Children [164,167,182–184]

Drug	Absorption characteristics	Distribution characteristics	Metabolism/elimination characteristics
ASA		V_d = 0.15 L/kg	
Salicylate		V_d = 0.15 L/kg (dose-dependent) 80–98% PB (albumin) PB is saturable	
Naproxen	T_{max} = 3–4 hr		$t_{1/2}$ = 11–14 hr
Ibuprofen	T_{max} = 0.5–2 hr	V_d = 0.18–0.22 L/kg	$t_{1/2}$ = 1–2 hr TBC = 1.2 ml/kg/min F_e < 10% of dose
Fenoprofen	T_{max} = 1–2 hr	V_d = 0.08–0.11 L/kg	$t_{1/2}$ = 2–4 hr
Ketoprofen	T_{max} = 0.5–6 hr		
Flurbiprofen	T_{max} = 1 hr	V_d = 2.4–6.6 L > 99% PB (albumin)	$t_{1/2}$ = 2.7–3.2 hr
Diclofenac	T_{max} = 0.5–2 hr Presystemic elimination (F = 60%)	V_d = 0.12–0.17 L/kg > 99% PB (albumin)	$t_{1/2}$ = 1.2–1.8 hr F_e = 5–10% of dose
Indomethacin	T_{max} = 1–3 hr	V_d = 0.5–1.5 L/kg (PO) = 0.2–0.5 L/kg (IV)	
Ketorolac (IV)		V_d = 0.26 L/kg	$t_{1/2}$ = 6.1 hr (range 3.5–10 hr) TBC = 4.2 ml/min

ASA = Acetylsalicylic acid; T_{max} = time to peak plasma or serum concentration; F = bioavailability; V_d = volume of distribution; PB = protein binding; $t_{1/2}$ = elimination half-life; TBC = total body clearance; F_e = fraction of the dose exreted in unchanged form in the urine; IV = intravenous; PO = oral.

Table 215-19. NSAID Dosing

Drug	Adults Analgesic	Adults Antiinflammatory	Children Analgesic	Children Antiinflammatory
Meclofenamate sodium	50–100 mg q4–6h	200–400 mg/day (tid or qid)	—	3–7.5 mg/kg/day
Mefenamic acid	500 mg stat, 250 mg q6h	—	—	—
Indomethacin	—	150–200 mg/day (bid or tid)	—	1–2.5 mg/kg/day (max 150 mg/d)
Sulindac	—	150–200 mg bid	—	2–4 mg/kg/day (max 200 mg/day)
Tolmetin sodium	—	600–1800 mg/day (tid)	—	15–30 mg/kg/day (tid or qid)
Nabumetone	—	1000–2000 mg/day (qd or bid)	—	—
Piroxicam	—	10–20 mg/day (qd)	—	0.33 mg/kg/day (qd)
Diflunisal	1000 mg stat, 500 mg q8–12h	500–1500 mg/day (bid)	—	—
Diclofenac	—	100–200 mg/day (bid–qid)	—	2–3 mg/kg/day (bid)
Fenoprofen calcium	200 mg q4–6h	900–3200 mg/day (tid or qid)	—	900–1800 mg/m²/day (qid)
Flurbiprofen	—	200–300 mg/day (bid–qid)	—	4 mg/kg/day (bid–qid)
Ibuprofen	400 mg q4–6h	1200–3200 mg/day (tid or qid)	—	30–40 mg/kg/day (tid or qid)
Ketoprofen	25–50 mg q6–8h	150–300 mg/day (tid or qid)	—	100–200 mg/m²/day (qid) (max 320 mg/day)
Naproxen	500 mg stat, 250 mg q6–8h (max 1250 mg/day)	250–750 mg bid	—	10–20 mg/kg/day (bid)
Oxaprozin	600–1200 mg qd	600–1200 mg qd	—	10–20 mg/kg/day
Etodolac	200–400 mg q6–8h (max 1200 mg/day)	800–1200 mg/day (bid–qid)	—	—
Ketorolac tromethamine	30–60 mg stat, 10–30 mg IV/IM q4–6h (max 150 mg day 1, 120 mg days 2 →) $\quad$ 10 mg PO q4–6h (max 40 mg/day)	—	0.2–0.5 mg/kg IV/IM q4–6h	—

Dosing guidelines refer to package insert and peer-reviewed literature. Analgesic doses are on an as needed basis.
qd = once daily, bid = twice daily, tid = thrice daily, qid = four times daily.

Table 215-20. NSAID Drug-Drug Interactions

Drug affected	NSAID	Effect	Comment
Pharmacokinetic interactions			
Oral anticoagulants	Phenylbutazone and congeners Meclofenamic acid and mefenamic acid	↓ S-warfarin clearance → ↑ anticoagulant effect	Avoid simultaneous therapy; monitor PT otherwise
Oral hypoglycemics	Phenylbutazone and congeners	↓ sulfonylurea clearance → ↑ risk of hypoglycemia	Avoid simultaneous therapy; monitor serum glucose otherwise
	Salicylates	Protein binding displacement, ↓ renal tubular secretion of hypoglycemic → ↑{ risk of hypoglycemia	
Lithium	Indomethacin, diclofenac, piroxicam, phenylbutazone	↓ renal lithium clearance → ↑ plasma lithium concentraton	Monitor plasma concentrations; use ASA or possibly sulindac if NSAID needed
	Sulindac	↑ clearance → ↓ plasma lithium concentration	
Phenytoin	ASA, others	Protein binding displacement	Caution in interpretation of total serum concentration (measure free concentration)
	Phenylbutazone and congeners	↓ clearance → ↑ plasma phenytoin concentration	Avoid simultaneous therapy; monitor serum concentrations otherwise
Methotrexate Antineoplastic dose Antirheumatic dose	Indomethacin, ketoprofen Naproxen, azapropazone, ASA, ibuprofen	↓ renal clearance (? competition for tubular secretion vs. ↓ GFR) → ↑ plasma MTX concentration	Avoid simultaneous therapy, if possible; monitor plasma MTX otherwise (esp. with antineoplastic regimens)
Valproic acid	ASA	↓ valproate clearance → ↑ plasma valproate concentration	Avoid ASA; monitor plasma valproate concentrations

Table 215-20. NSAID Drug-Drug Interactions

Drug affected	NSAID	Effect	Comment
Digoxin	All	↓ GFR → ↑ plasma digoxin concentrations	Avoid simultaneous therapy; monitor plasma creatinine and drug concentrations otherwise
Aminoglycosides	All	↓ GFR → ↑ plasma aminoglycoside concentrations	Avoid simultaneous therapy; monitor plasma creatinine and drug concentrations otherwise
Acetazolamide	ASA	↓ protein binding and renal tubular secretion of acetazolamide	Avoid simultaneous therapy
Other drugs affecting NSAIDs			
Barbiturates	Phenylbutazone, fenoprofen	↑ clearance of NSAID	? ↑ dose or use alternative NSAID
Probenecid	Indomethacin, carprofen, naproxen, ketoprofen documented (probably all)	↓ metabolism and renal clearance of parent compound and glucuronide metabolities (latter hydrolyzed back to parent compound)	
Antacids	ASA	↓ serum salicylate concentration (↑ urine pH, Mg/AlOH),	Monitor serum salicylate concentrations
	Naproxen, diflunisal	AlOH ↓ diflunisal, naproxen absorption	Monitor response to naproxen and diflunisal and ↑ dose if needed
Caffeine	ASA	↑ rate and extent of absorption	
Bile acid binding resins	Piroxicam, naproxen (probably all)	↓ rate and possibly extent of absorption of NSAID	Separate dosing times, may need ↑ NSAID dose
		↓ enterohepatic recycling (piroxicam)	Avoid piroxicam
Metoclopramide	ASA (probably all)	↑ rate and extent of absorption (at least in migrainous patients)	
Corticosteroids	ASA	↑ clearance, ↓ ↓ serum concentrations of ASA	Monitor serum salicylate concentrations and adjust dose
Oral contraceptive steroids	ASA, diflunisal	↑ clearance, ↓ serum concentrations of NSAID	Monitor serum salicylate concentrations and response; adjust dose
Pharmacodynamic interactions			
Diuretics	Indomethacin, others (?except sulindac)	↓ natriuretic/diuretic effect, ↓ hypotensive effect (antiprostaglandin effect)	Avoid NSAID use (use sulindac if NSAID needed); monitor BP and fluid status.
ACE inhibitors (ACEI)	Indomethacin, others (?except sulindac)	↓ hypotensive effect, ↑ risk hemodynamic renal failure and hyperkalemia	Avoid NSAID use (use sulindac or naproxen if NSAID needed); monitor BP and pulse
Beta-blockers	Indomethacin	↓ hypotensive effect	Avoid NSAID use (use sulindac or naproxen if NSAID needed); monitor BP and pulse
Anticoagulants	All	↑ risk of GI bleeding (GI mucosal damage + antiplatelet effect)	Avoid NSAID use, if possible
Hypoglycemics	ASA (high dose)	↑ hypoglycemic effect (unknown mechanism)	Avoid simultaneous therapy; monitor serum glucose otherwise
Combination with enhanced toxicity risk			
Diuretics	All	General— ↑ risk hemodynamic renal failure	Avoid simultaneous therapy; monitor plasma creatinine otherwise
		Triamterene + indomethacin— potentiation of nephrotoxicity	Avoid simultaneous therapy; monitor serum creatinine otherwise
		K-sparing—K retention and ↑ serum K	Avoid simultaneous therapy; monitor serum K concentration otherwise
Zidovudine	Probably all (including acetaminophen)	↑ hematologic toxicity of zidovudine	Monitor blood counts
		↑ bleeding tendency in hemophiliacs	

ASA = acetylsalicylic acid; GFR = glomerular filtration rate; MTX = methotrexate

Prostaglandin inhibition by NSAIDs may cause a spectrum of adverse renal events, including reversible impairment of glomerular filtration, acute renal failure, edema, interstitial nephritis, papillary necrosis, chronic renal failure, and hyperkalemia [198,199]. These events are especially likely to occur in patients with hypovolemic states (salt depletion, hypoalbuminemia) or preexisting renal impairment (age, atherosclerosis, hypertensive renal disease, other intrinsic renal disease). No NSAID is absolutely safe with respect to adverse renal effects; avoidance of these agents in at-risk patients is prudent.

References

1. Teeple E Jr: Pharmacology and physiology of narcotics. *Crit Care Clin* 6:255, 1990.
2. Murkin JM: Central analgesic mechanisms: A review of opioid receptor physiopharmacology and related antinociceptive systems. *J Cardiothorac Vasc Anesth* 5:268, 1991.
3. Pasternak GW: Pharmacological mechanisms of opioid analgesics. *Clin Neuropharmacol* 16:1, 1993.
4. Dickenson AH: Mechanisms of the analgesic actions of opiates and opioids. *Br Med Bull* 47:690, 1991.
5. Sabbe MB, Yaksh TL: Pharmacology of spinal opioids. *J Pain Symptom Manage* 5:191, 1990.
6. Hare BD: The opioid analgesics: Rational selection of agents for acute and chronic pain. *Hosp Formul* 21:64, 1986.
7. Schug SA, Zech D, Grand S: Adverse effects of systemic opioid analgesics. *Drug Safety* 7:200, 1992.
8. Fisher MM, Harle DG, Baldo BA: Anaphylactoid reactions to narcotic analgesics. *Clin Rev Allergy* 9:309, 1991.
9. Flacke JW, Flacke WE, Bloor BC, et al: Histamine release by four narcotics: A double-blind study in humans. *Anesth Analg* 66:723, 1987.
10. Coyle JP: Sedation, pain relief, and neuromuscular blockade in the postoperative cardiac surgical patient. *Semin Thorac Cardiovasc Surg* 3:81, 1991.
11. Thune A, Baker RA, Saccone GTP, et al: Differing effects of pethidine and morphine on human sphincter of Oddi manometry. *Br J Surg* 77:992, 1990.
12. Glare PA, Walsh TD: Clinical pharmacokinetics of morphine. *Ther Drug Monitor* 13:1, 1991.
13. Schug SA, Merry AF, Acland RH: Treatment principles for the use of opioids in pain of nonmalignant origin. *Drugs* 42:228, 1991.
14. Mather LE: Clinical pharmacokinetics of fentanyl and its newer derivatives. *Clin Pharmacokinet* 8:422, 1983.
15. Hill HF, Chapman CR, Saeger LS, et al: Steady-state infusions of opioids in human. II. Concentration-effect relationships and therapeutic margins. *Pain* 43:69, 1990.
16. Austin KL, Stapleton, JV, Mather LE: Relationship between blood meperidine concentrations and analgesic response. *Anesthesiology* 53:460, 1980.
17. McQuay HJ: Opioid clinical pharmacology and routes of administration. *Br Med Bull* 47:703, 1991.
18. Stanski DR, Greenblatt DJ, Lowenstein E: Kinetics of intravenous and intramuscular morphine. *Clin Pharmacol Ther* 24:52, 1978.
19. von Hoogdalen EJ, deBoer AG, Breimer DD: Pharmacokinetics of rectal drug administration. General considerations and clinical applications of centrally acting drugs. *Clin Pharmacokinet* 21:11, 1991.
20. Persson MP, Wiklund L, Hartvig P, et al: Potential pulmonary uptake and clearance of morphine in post-operative patients. *Eur J Clin Pharmacol* 30:567, 1986.
21. Finck AD, Berkowitz BA, Hempstead J, et al: Pharmacokinetics of morphine: Effects of hypercarbia on serum and brain morphine concentrations in the dog. *Anesthesiology* 47:407, 1977.
22. Olsen GD: Morphine binding to human plasma proteins. *Clin Pharmacol Ther* 17:31, 1975.
23. Klotz U: Pathophysiological and disease-induced changes in drug distribution volume: pharmacokinetic implications. *Clin Pharmacokinet* 1:204, 1976.
24. Piafsky KM: Disease-induced changes in the plasma binding of basic drugs. *Clin Pharmacokinet* 5:246, 1980.
25. Bodenham A, Quinn K, Park GR: Extrahepatic morphine metabolism in man during the anhepatic phase of orthotopic liver transplantation. *Br J Anaesth* 63:380, 1989.
26. Moore RA, Baldwin D, Allen MC, et al: Sensitive and specific morphine radioimmunoassay with iodine label: Pharmacokinetics of morphine in man after intravenous administration. *Ann Clin Biochem* 21,318, 1984.
27. Mather LE, Cousins MJ: The pharmacological relief of pain-contemporary issues. *Med J Aust* 156:796, 1992.
28. Milne RW, Nation RL, Somogyi AA, et al: The influence of renal function on the renal clearance of morphine and its glucuronide metabolites in intensive-care patients. *Br J Clin Pharmacol* 34:53, 1992.
29. Owen JA, Sitar DS, Berger L, et al: Age-related morphine kinetics. *Clin Pharmacol Ther* 34:364, 1983.
30. Perry S, Inturrisi CE: Analgesia and morphine disposition in burn patients. *J Burn Clin Res* 4:276, 1983.
31. Mitchell RWD, Smith G: The control of acute post-operative pain. *Br J Anaesth* 63:147, 1989.
32. Burns AM, Shelly MP, Park GR: The use of sedative agents in critically ill patients. *Drugs* 43:507, 1992.
33. Roerig DL, Kotrly KJ, Vucins EJ, et al: First pass uptake of fentanyl, meperidine, and morphine in the human lung. *Anesthesiology* 67:466, 1987.
34. Klotz U, McHorse TS, Wilkinson GR, et al: The effect of cirrhosis on the disposition and elimination of meperidine in man. *Clin Pharmacol Ther* 16:667, 1974.
35. Mather LE, Tucker GT, Pflug AE, et al: Meperidine kinetics in man: Intravenous injection in surgical patients and volunteers. *Clin Pharmacol Ther* 17:21, 1975.
36. Kirkwood CF, Edwards DJ, Lalka D, et al: The pharmacokinetics of meperidine in acute trauma patients. *J Trauma* 26:1090, 1986.
37. Aidkenhead AR: Analgesia and sedation in intensive care. *Br J Anaesth* 63:196, 1989.
38. Szeto, HH, Inturrisi CE, Houde R, et al: Accumulation of normeperidine, an active metabolite of meperidine, in patients with renal failure or cancer. *Ann Intern Med* 86:738, 1977.
39. McHorse TS, Wilkinson GR, Johnson RF, et al: Effect of acute viral hepatitis in man on the disposition and elimination of meperidine. *Gastroenterology* 68:775, 1975.
40. Pond SM, Tong T, Benowitz NL, et al: Presystemic metabolism of meperidine to normeperidine in normal and cirrhotic subjects. *Clin Pharmacol Ther* 30:183, 1981.
41. Neal EA, Meffin PJ, Gregory PB, et al: Enhanced bioavailability and decreased clearance of analgesics in patients with cirrhosis. *Gastroenterology* 77, 96, 1979.
42. Guay DRP, Awni WM, Findlay JWA, et al: Pharmacokinetics and pharmacodynamics of codeine in endstage renal disease. *Clin Pharmacol Ther* 43:63, 1988.
43. Findlay JWA, Jones EC, Butz RF, et al: Plasma codeine and morphine concentrations after therapeutic oral doses of codeine-containing analgesics. *Clin Pharmacol Ther* 24:60, 1978.
44. Chan GLC, Matzke GR: Effects of renal insufficiency on the pharmacokinetics and pharmacodynamics of opioid analgesics. *Drug Intell Clin Pharm* 21:773, 1987.
45. Fitzgerald J: Narcotic analgesics in renal failure. *Conn Med* 55:701, 1991.
46. Shafer SI, Vawel JR: Pharmacokinetics, pharmacodynamics, and rational opioid selection. *Anesthesiology* 74:53, 1991.
47. Dobb GJ, Murphy DF: Sedation and analgesia during intensive care. *Clin Anesthesiol* 3:1055, 1985.
48. Bentley JB, Borel, JD, Nenad RE Jr, et al: Age and fentanyl pharmacokinetics. *Anesth Analg* 61:968, 1982.
49. Haberer JP, Schoeffler P, Couderc E, et al: Fentanyl pharmacokinetics in anaesthetized patients with cirrhosis. *Br J Anaesth* 54:1267, 1982.
50. Scott JC, Stanski DR: Decreased fentanyl/alfentanil dose requirements with increasing age: A pharmacodynamic basis. *Anesthesiology* 63:A374, 1985.
51. Yate PM, Thomas D, Short SM, et al: Comparison of infusions of alfentanil or pethidine for sedation of ventilated patients on the ICU. *Br J Anaesth* 58:1091, 1986.

52. Helmers H, VanPeer A, Woestenborghs R, et al: Alfentanil kinetics in the elderly. *Clin Pharmacol Ther* 36:239, 1984.

53. Bower S, Hull CJ: Comparative pharmacokinetics of fentanyl and alfentanil. *Br J Anaesth* 54:871, 1982.

54. Lemmens HJM, Burm AGL, Bovill JG, et al: Pharmacodynamics of alfentanil: The role of plasma protein binding. *Anesthesiology* 76:65, 1992.

55. Maitre PO, Ausems ME, Vozeh S, et al: Evaluating the accuracy of using population pharmacokinetic data to predict plasma concentrations of alfentanil. *Anesthesiology* 68:59, 1988.

56. VanPeer A. Vercauteren M, Noordiun H, et al: Alfentanil kinetics in renal insufficiency. *Eur J Clin Pharmacol* 30:245, 1986.

57. Ferrier C, Marty J, Bouffard Y, et al: Alfentanil pharmacokinetics in patients with cirrhosis. *Anesthesiology* 62:480, 1985.

58. Sear JW: Sufentanil disposition in patients undergoing renal transplantation: influence of choice of kinetic models. *Br J Anaesth* 63:60, 1989.

59. Hudson RJ, Bergstrom RG, Thomson IR, et al: Pharmacokinetics of sufentanil in patients undergoing abdominal aortic surgery. *Anesthesiology* 70:426, 1989.

60. Hall R: The pharmacokinetic behavior of opioids administered during cardiac surgery. *Can J Anaesth* 38:747, 1991.

61. Alazia M, Levron JC, Guidon C, et al: Pharmacokinetics of fentanyl (F) during continuous infusion in critically ill patients. *Anesthesiology* 67:A665, 1987.

62. Singleton MA, Rosen JI, Fisher DM: Pharmacokinetics of fantanyl in the elderly. *Br J Anaesth* 60:619, 1988.

63. Schwartz AE, Matteo RS, Ornstein E, et al: Pharmacokinetics of sufentanil in neurosurgical patients undergoing hyperventilation. *Br J Anaesth* 63:385, 1989.

64. Macnab MSP, Macrae DJ, Guy E, et al: Profound reduction in morphine clearance and liver blood flow in shock. *Intensive Care Med* 12:366, 1986.

65. Henthron TK, Krejcie TC, Avram MJ: The relationship between alfentanil distribution kinetics and cardiac output. *Clin Pharmacol Ther* 52:190, 1992.

66. Brill JE: Control of pain. *Crit Care Clin* 8:203, 1992.

67. Tomicheck RC, Rosow CE, Philbin DM, et al: Diazepam-fentanyl interaction-hemodynamic and hormonal effects in coronary artery surgery. *Anesth Analg* 62:881, 1983.

68. Richter PA, Burk MP: The potentiation of narcotic analgesics with phenothiazines. *J Foot Surg* 31:378, 1992.

69. Thomson IR, MacAdams CL, Hudson RJ, et al: Drug interactions with sufentanil: Hemodynamic effects of premedication and muscle relaxants. *Anesthesiology* 76:922, 1992.

70. Glazier HS: Potentiation of pain relief with hydroxyzine: A therapeutic myth? *DICP Ann Pharmacother* 24:484, 1990.

71. Trissel LA: *Handbook on Injectable Drugs.* 7th ed. Bethesda, MD, American Society of Hospital Pharmacists, 1992.

72. Butterworth FJ IV, Strichartz GR: Molecular mechanisms of local anesthesia: A review. *Anesthesiology* 72:711, 1990.

73. Yagiela JA: Local Anesthetics. *Anesth Prog* 38:128, 1991.

74. Curran MJA: Options for labor analgesia: techniques of eipdural and spinal analgesia. *Semin Perinatol* 15:348, 1991.

75. Mather LE, Cousins MJ: Local anesthetics and their current clinical use. *Drugs* 18:185, 1979.

76. Aps C, Reynolds F: An intradermal study of the local anaesthetic and vascular effects of the isomers of bupivacaine. *Br J Clin Pharmacol* 6:63, 1978.

77. Fairley JW, Reynolds F: An intradermal study of the local anaesthetic and vascular effects of the isomers of mepivacaine. *Br J Anaesth* 53:1211, 1981.

78. Aberg G: Toxicological and local anaesthetic effects of optically active isomers of two local anaesthetic compounds. *Acta Pharmacol Toxicol* 31:273, 1972.

79. Koppanyi T: The sedative, central analgesic, and anticonvulsant actions of local anesthesia. *Am J Med Sci* 244:646, 1962.

80. DeGiorgio CM, Altman K, Hamilton-Byrd E, et al: Lidocaine in refractory status epilepticus: Confirmation of efficacy with continuous EEG monitoring. *Epilepsia* 33:913, 1992.

81. Gianelly R, von der Groeben JO, Spivack AP, et al: Effect of lidocaine on ventricular arrhythmias in patients with coronary heart disease. *N Engl J Med* 277:1215, 1967.

82. Foldes FF, Davidson GM, Duncalf D, et al: The intravenous toxicity of local anesthetic agents in man. *Clin Pharmacol Ther* 6:328, 1965.

83. McCaughey W: Adverse effects of local anesthetics. *Drug Safety* 7:178, 1992.

84. Glinert RJ, Zachary CB: Local anesthetic allergy: Its recognition and avoidance. *J Dermatol Surg Oncol* 17:491, 1991.

85. Sindel LJ, deShazo RD: Accidents resulting from local anesthetics: True or false? *Clin Rev Allergy* 9:379, 1991.

86. Tucker GT: Pharmacokinetics of local anesthetics. *Br J Anaesth* 58:717, 1986.

87. Dunne NM, Kox WJ: Neurological complications following the use of continuous extradural analgesia with bupivacaine. *Br J Anaesth* 66:617, 1991.

88. Agarwal R, Gutlove DP, Lockhart CH: Seizures occurring in pediatric patients receiving continuous infusion of bupivacaine. *Anesth Analg* 75:284, 1992.

89. McCloskey JJ, Haun SE, Deshpande JK: Bupivacaine toxicity secondary to continuous caudal epidural infusion in children. *Anesth Analg* 75:287, 1992.

90. Yamashiro H: Bupivacaine-induced seizure after accidental intravenous injection: A complication of epidural anesthesia. *Anesthesiology* 47:472, 1977.

91. Mather LE, Long GJ, Thomas J: The intravenous toxicity and clearance of bupivacaine in man. *Clin Pharmacol Ther* 12:935, 1971.

92. Scott DB: Evaluation of the toxicity of local anaesthetic agents in man. *Br J Anaesth* 47:56, 1975.

93. Denson DD, Myers JA, Hartrick CT, et al: The relationship between free bupivacaine concentrations and central nervous system toxicity. *Anesthesiology* 61:A211, 1984.

94. DuPen SL, Kharasch ED, Williams A, et al: Chronic epidural bupivacaine: Opioid infusion in intractable cancer pain. *Pain* 49:293, 1992.

95. Tucker GT, Mather LE: Clinical pharmacokinetics of local anesthetics. *Clin Pharmacokinet* 4:241, 1979.

96. Veering BT, Burm AGL, Vletter AA, et al: The effect of age on systemic absorption and systemic disposition of bupivacaone after subarachnoid administration. *Anesthesiology* 74:250, 1991.

97. Piafsky KM, Knoppert D: Binding of local anesthetics to α_1 acid glycoprotein. *Clin Res* 26:836A, 1978.

98. Tucker GT, Mather LE: Pharmacokinetics of local anaesthetic agents. *Br J Anaesth* 47:213, 1975.

99. Tucker GT, Wiklund L, Berlin-Wahlen A, et al: Hepatic clearance of local anesthetics in man. *J Pharmacokinet Biopharm* 51:111, 1977.

100. Scott DB: Evaluation of clinical tolerance of local anaesthetic agents. *Br J Anaesth* 47:328, 1975.

101. Boyes RN, Scott DB, Jebson PJR, et al: Pharmacokinetics of lidocaine in man. *Clin Pharmacol Ther* 12:105, 1971.

103. Scott DB, Jebson PJR, Boyes RN: Pharmacokinetic study of the local anesthetics bupivacaine (Marcaine) and etidocaine (Duranset) in man. *Br J Anaesth* 45:1010, 1973.

104. Arthur GR, Scott DHT, Boyes RN, et al: Pharmacokinetic and clinical pharmacological studies with mepivacaine and prilocaine. *Br J Anaesth* 51:481, 1979.

105. Lee A, Fagan D, Lamont M et al: Disposition kinetics of ropivacaine in humans. *Anesth Analg* 69:736, 1989.

106. Moore RG, Thomas J, Triggs EJ, et al: The pharmacokinetics and metabolism of the anilide local anesthetics in neonates. III. Mepivacaine. *Eur J Clin Pharmacol* 14:203, 1978.

107. ook R, Greenberg RA, Hehre FW: Continuous lumbar peridural anesthesia in obstetrics. VII. Distribution of local anesthetic agents in maternal and fetal blood. *Anesth Analg* 50:693, 1971.

108. Tucker GT, Boyes RN, Bridenbaugh PO, et al: Binding of anilide-type local anesthetics in human plasma. II. Implications in vivo with special reference to transplacental disposition. *Anesthesiology* 33:304, 1970.

109. Morgan DH, Cousins MJ, McQuillan D, et al: Disposition and placental transfer of etidocaine in pregnancy. *Eur J Clin Pharmacol* 12:359, 1977.

110. Cousins MJ, Augustus JA, Gleason M, et al: Epidural block for abdominal surgery: Aspects of the clinical pharmacology of etidocaine. *Anaesth Intens Care* 6:105, 1978.

111. Morgan DH, McQuillan D, Thomas J: Pharmacokinetics and me-

tabolism of the anilide local anesthetics in neonates. II. Etidocaine. *Eur J Clin Pharmacol* 13:365, 1978.

112. Veering B Th, Burm AGL, Gladines MPRR, et al: Age does not influence the serum protein binding of bupivacaine. *Br J Clin Pharmacol* 32:501, 1991.

113. Ghoneim MM, Pandya H: Plasma protein binding of bupivacaine and its interaction with other drugs in man. *Br J Anaesth* 46:435, 1974.

114. Rosenberg PH, Pere P, Hekali R, et al: Plasma concentrations of bupivacaine and two of its metabolites during continuous interscalene brachial plexus block. *Br J Anaesth* 66:25, 1991.

115. Wulf H, Munstedt P, Maier Ch: Plasma protein binding of bupivacaine in pregnant women at term. *Acta Anaesthesiol Scand* 35:129, 1991.

116. Bachmann B, Biscoping J, Sinning E, et al: Protein binding of prilocaine in human plasma: Influence of concentration, pH, and temperature. *Acta Anaesthesiol Scand* 34:311, 1990.

117. McEllistrem RF, Bennington RG, Roth SH: In vitro determination of human dura mater permeability to opioids and local anesthetics. *Can J Anaesth* 40:165, 1993.

118. Stienstra R, Greene NM: Factors affecting the subarachnoid spread of local anesthetic solutions. *Reg Anesth* 16:1, 1991.

119. Fassoulaki A, Sarantopoulos C, Chondrelli S: Systemic fentanyl enhances the spread of spinal analgesia produced by lignocaine. *Br J Anaesth* 67:437, 1991.

120. Lim ETM, Chong KY, Singh B, et al: Use of warm local anaesthetic solution for caudal blocks. *Anaesth Intensive Care* 20:453, 1992.

121. Mehta PM, Theriot E, Mehrotra D, et al: A simple technique to make bupivacaine a rapid-acting epidural anaesthetic. *Reg Anesth* 12:135, 1987.

122. Purcell-Jones G, Pither CE, Justins DM: Paravertebral somatic nerve block: A clinical, radiographic, and computed tomographic study in chronic pain patients. *Anesth Analg* 68:32, 1989.

123. Moorthy SS, Dierdorf SF, Yaw PB: Influence of volume on the spread of local anesthetic-methylene blue solution after injection for intercostal block. *Anesth Analg* 75:389, 1992.

124. Stromskag KE, Hauge O, Steen PA: Distribution of local anesthetics injected into the interpleural space: Studied by computerized tomography. *Acta Anaesthesiol Scand* 34:323, 1990.

125. Reidenberg MM, James M, Dring LG: The rate of procaine hydrolysis in serum of normal subjects and diseased patients. *Clin Pharmacol Ther* 13:279, 1972.

126. duSoich P, Erill P: Altered metabolism of procainamide and procaine in patients with pulmonary and cardiac diseases. *Clin Pharmacol Ther* 21:101, 1977.

127. Thomas J, Morgan D, Vine J: Metabolism of etidocaine in man. *Zenobiotica* 6:39, 1976.

128. Rice ASC, Pither CE, Tucker GT: Plasma concentrations of bupivacaine after supraclavicular brachial plexus blockade in patients with chronic renal failure. *Anaesthesia* 46:354, 1991.

129. Yaster M, Maxwell LG, Nicholas EJ: Local anesthetics in the management of acute pain in clindren: A primer for the non-anesthesiologist. *Comp Ther* 17:27, 1991.

130. Berrisford RG, Sabanathan S, Mearns AJ, et al: Plasma concentrations of bupivacaine and its enantiomers during continuous extrapleural intercostal nerbe block. *Br J Anaesth* 70:201, 1993.

131. Vree TB, Beumer EMC, Lagerwerf AJ, et al: Clinical pharmacokinetics of R(+)- and S(−)-mepivacaine after high doses of racemic mepivacaine with epinephrine in the combined psoas compartment/sciatic nerve block. *Anesth Analg* 75:75, 1992.

132. Goris RJA, teBoekhorst TPA, Nuytinck JKS, et al: Multiple-organ failure: Generalized autodestructive inflammation? *Arch Surg* 120:1109, 1985.

133. Putensen C, Lingnau W, Putensen-Himmer G, et al: Plasma lignocaine concentrations associated with extradural analgesia in patients with and without multiple organ failure. *Br J Anaesth* 69:513, 1992.

134. Sharrock NE, Go G, Mineo R: Effect of IV low-dose adrenaline and phenylephrine infusions on plasma concentrations of bupivacaine after lumbar extradural anaesthesia in elderly patients. *Br J Anaesth* 67:694, 1991.

135. Bodenham A, Park GR: Plasma concentrations of bupivacaine after intercostal nerve block in patients after orthotopic liver transplantation. *Br J Anaesth* 64:436, 1990.

136. Englesson S: The influence of acid-base changes on central nervous system toxicity of local anaesthetic agents. I. *Acta Anaesthesiol Scand* 18:79, 1974.

137. Englesson S, Grevsten S: The influence of acid-base changes on central nervous system toxicity of local anaesthetic agents. II. *Acta Anaesthesiol Scand* 18:88, 1974.

138. Burney RG, DiFazio CA: Hepatic clearance of lidocaine during N_2O anesthesia in dogs. *Anesth Analg* 55:322, 1976.

139. Denson DD, Coyle DE, Thompson GA, et al: Bupivacaine protein binding in the term parturient: Effects of lactic acidosis. *Clin Pharmacol Ther* 35:702, 1984.

140. Denson D, Coyle D, Thompson G, et al: Alpha$_1$-acid glycoprotein and albumin in human serum bupivacaine binding. *Clin Pharmacol Ther* 35:409, 1984.

141. Morikawa KI, Bonica JJ, Tucker GT, et al: Effects of acute hypovolemia on lignocaine absorption and cardiovascular response following epidural block in dogs. *Br J Anaesth* 46:631, 1974.

142. Quimby CW Jr: Influence of blood loss on the duration of regional anesthesia. *Anesth Analg* 44:387, 1965.

143. Bromage PR, Gertel M: Brachial plexus anesthesia in chronic renal failure. *Anesthesiology* 36:488, 1972.

144. Berde CB: Convulsions associated with pediatric regional anesthesia. *Anesth Analg* 75:164, 1992.

145. Chan K: Predicting plasma concentrations of bupivacaine after epidural administration in obstetric analgesia. *Ther Drug Monit* 11:567, 1989.

146. Denson DD, Thompson GA, Raj PP, et al: Continuous perineural infusions of bupivacaine for prolonged analgesia: A rapid two-point method for estimating individual pharmacokinetic parameters. *Int J Clin Pharmacol Ther Toxicol* 22:552, 1984.

147. Alston TA: Antagonism of sulfonamides by benzocaine and chloroprocaine. *Anesthesiology* 76:475, 1992.

148. Goulet J-P, Perusse R, Turcotte J-Y: Contraindications to vasoconstrictors in dentistry. III. *Oral Surg Oral Med Oral Pathol* 74:692, 1992.

149. Vane JR: Inhibition of prostaglandin synthesis as a mechanism of action for the aspirin-like drugs. *Nature* 231:232, 1971.

150. Vane JR, Botting RM: The mode of action of anti-inflammatory drugs. *Postgrad Med J* 66(suppl):S2, 1990.

151. Abramson SB, Weissman G: The mechanisms of action of non-steroidal anti-inflammatory drugs. *Arthritis Rheum* 32:1, 1989.

152. Forrest M, Brooks PM: Mechanism of action of non-steroidal antirheumatic drugs. *Clin Rheumatol* 2:275, 1988.

153. Kitchen EA, Dawson W, Rainsford KD, et al: Inflammation and possible modes of action of anti-inflammatory drugs, in Rainsford KD (ed): *Anti-inflammatory and Anti-rheumatic Drugs: Inflammation Mechanisms and Actions of Traditional Drugs*. vol. 1. Boca Raton, FL, CRC Press, 1985.

154. Biemond P, Swaak AJ, Penders JM, et al: Superoxide production by polymorphonuclear leucocytes in rheumatoid arthritis and osteoarthritis: In vivo inhibition by antirheumatic drug piroxicam due to interference with activation of the NADPH-oxidase. *Ann Rheum Dis* 45:249, 1986.

155. Bomalaski JS, Hirata F, Clark MA: Aspirin inhibits phospholipase C. *Biochem Biophys Res Commun* 139:115, 1986.

156. Herman JH, Appel AM, Khosla RC, et al: Cytokine modulation of chondrocyte metabolism: In vivo and in vitro effects of piroxicam. *Inflammation* 8(suppl):S125, 1984.

157. Altman RD: Neutrophil activation: An alternative to prostaglandin inhibition as the mechanism of action for NSAIDs. *Semin Arthritis Rheum* 19(suppl 2):1, 1990.

158. Willer JC, DeBroucker T, Bussel B, et al: Central analgesic effect of ketoprofen in humans: Electrophysiological evidence for a supraspinal mechanism in a double-blind and cross-over study. *Pain* 38:1, 1989.

159. Bannwarth B, Demotes-Mainard F, Schaeverbeke T, et al: Where are peripheral analgesics acting? *Ann Rheum Dis* 52:1, 1993.

160. Rooks WH II, Maloney PJ, Shott LD, et al: The analgesic and anti-inflammatory profile of ketorolac and its tromethamine salt. *Drugs Exp Clin Res* 11:479, 1985.

161. Jungnickel PW: Selection of non-steroidal anti-inflammatory drugs. *Fam Pract Res J* 6:33, 1984.

162. Day RO, Furst DE, Dromgoole SH, et al: Relationship of serum

naproxen concentration to efficacy in rheumatoid arthritis. *Clin Pharmacol Ther* 31:733, 1982.

163. Orme ML: The relationship between plasma concentration of non-steroidal anti-inflammatory drugs and their therapeutic effects. *Agents Actions* 17(suppl):151, 1988.

164. Laska EM, Sunshine A, Martero I, et al: The correlation between blood levels of ibuprofen and clinical analgesic response. *Clin Pharmacol Ther* 40:1, 1986.

165. Day RO, Graham GG, Bieri D, et al: Concentration-response relationships for salicylate-induced ototoxicity in normal volunteers. *Br J Clin Pharmacol* 28:695, 1989.

166. Carson JL, Strom BL, Morse ML, et al: The relative gastrointestinal toxicity of non-steroidal anti-inflammatory drugs. *Arch Intern Med* 147:1054, 1987.

167. Needs CJ, Brooks PM: Clinical pharmacokinetics of the salicylates. *Clin Pharmacokinet* 10:164, 1985.

168. Brune K, Geisslinger G, Menzel-Soglowek S: Pure enantiomers of 2-arylpropionic acids: tools in pain research and improved drugs in rheumatology. *J Clin Pharmacol* 32:944, 1992.

169. Jamali F: Pharmacokinetics of enantiomers of chiral non-steroidal anti-inflammatory drugs. *Eur J Drug Metab Pharmacokinet* 13:1, 1988.

170. Evans AM: Enantioselective pharmacodynamics and pharmacokinetics of chiral non-steroidal anti-inflammatory drugs. *Eur J Clin Pharmacol* 42:237, 1992.

171. Verbeeck RK, Blackburn JL, Loewen GR: Clinical pharmacokinetics of non-steroidal anti-inflammatory drugs. *Clin Pharmacokinet* 8:297, 1983.

172. Brocks DR, Jamali F: Clinical pharmacokinetics of ketorolac tromethamine. *Clin Pharmacokinet* 23:415, 1992.

173. Balfour JA, Buckley MMT: Etodolac: A reappraisal of its pharmacology and therapeutic use in rheumatic diseases and pain states. *Drugs* 42:274, 1991.

174. Miller LG: Oxaprozin: A once daily nonsteroidal anti-inflammatory drug. *Clin Pharm* 11:591, 1992.

175. Wallace SM, Verbeeck RK: Plasma protein binding of drugs in the elderly. *Clin Pharmacokinet* 12:41, 1987.

176. Brater DC, Lasseter KC: Profile of etodolac: Pharmacokinetic evaluation in special populations. *Clin Rheumatol* 8(suppl):1, 1989.

177. Conroy MC, Randinitis EJ, Turner JL: Pharmacology, pharmacokinetics, and therapeutic use of meclofenamate sodium. *Clin J Pain* 7(suppl 1):S44, 1991.

178. Roth SH: Nabumetone: A new NSAID for rheumatoid arthritis and osteoarthritis. *Orthop Rev* 21:223, 1992.

179. Friedel HA, Langtry HD, Buckley MM: Nabumetone: A reappraisal of its pharmacology and therapeutic use in rheumatic diseases. *Drugs* 45:131, 1993.

180. Woodhouse KW, Wynne H: The pharmacokinetics of non-steroidal anti-inflammatory drugs in the elderly. *Clin Pharmacokinet* 12:111, 1987.

181. Verbeeck RK, Richardson CJ, Blocka KLN: Clinical pharmacokinetics of piroxicam. *J Rheumatol* 13:789, 1986.

182. Brewer EJ, Arroyo I: Use of non-steroidal anti-inflammatory drugs in children. *Pediatr Ann* 15:575, 1986.

183. Walson PD, Mortensen ME: Pharmacokinetics of common analgesics, anti-inflammatories, and antipyretics in children. *Clin Pharmacokinet* 17(suppl 1):116, 1989.

184. Olkkola KT, Maunuksela E-L: The pharmacokinetics of post-operative intravenous kelorolac tromethamine in children. *Br J Clin Pharmacol* 31:182, 1991.

185. Hundal O, Rugstad HE, Husby G: Naproxen free plasma concentrations and unbound fractions in patients with osteoarthritis: Relation to age, sex, efficacy, and adverse events. *Ther Drug Monit* 13:478, 1991.

186. Day RO, Graham GG, Williams KM: Pharmacokinetics of non-steroidal anti-inflammatory drugs. *Baillieres Clin Rheumatol* 2:363, 1988.

187. Lin JH, Cocchetto DM, Duggan DE: Protein binding as a primary determinant of the clinical pharmacokinetic properties of non-steroidal anti-inflammatory drugs. *Clin Pharmacokinet* 12:402, 1987.

188. Meffin PJ: The effects of renal dysfunction on the disposition of non-steroidal anti-inflammatory drugs forming acyl-glucuronides. *Agents Actions* 17(suppl):85, 1985.

189. Dunn MJ, Patrono C (eds): Renal effects of non-steroidal anti-inflammatory drugs. *Am J Med* 81(suppl 2B):1, 1986.

190. Wilkinson GR: Clearance approaches in pharmacology. *Pharmacol Rev* 39:1, 1987.

191. Tonkin AL, Wing LMH: Interactions of non-steroidal anti-inflammatory drugs. *Clin Rheumatol* 2:455, 1988.

192. Miners JO: Drug interactions involving aspirin (acetylsalicylic acid) and salicylic acid. *Clin Pharmacokinet* 17:327, 1989.

193. Furst DE: Clinically important interactions of non-steroidal anti-inflammatory drugs with other medications. *J Rheumatol* 15(suppl 17):58, 1988.

194. Verbeeck RK: Pharmacokinetic drug interactions with non-steroidal anti-inflammatory drugs. *Clin Pharmacokinet* 19:44, 1990.

195. Knapp AJ, Mauro VF, Alexander KS: Incompatibility of ketorolac tromethamine with selected postoperative drugs. *Am J Hosp Pharm* 49:2960, 1992.

196. O'Brien WM, Bagby GF: Rare adverse reactions to non-steroidal anti-inflammatory drugs. *J Rheumatol* 12:13, 1985.

197. Brooks PM: Side effects of non-steroidal anti-inflammatory drugs. *Med J Aust* 148:248, 1988.

198. Clive DM, Stoff JS: Renal syndromes associated with non-steroidal anti-inflammatory drugs. *N Engl J Med* 310:563, 1984.

199. Stillman MT, Napier J, Blackshear JL: Adverse effects of non-steroidal anti-inflammatory drugs on the kidney. *Med Clin North Am* 68:371, 1984.

XVII. Dermatologic, Rheumatologic, and Immunologic Problems in the Intensive Care Unit

Section Editor
David F. Giansiracusa

216. Rheumatic Diseases in the Intensive Care Unit

Katherine S. Upchurch and
David F. Giansiracusa

Introduction

In the absence of organ system failure (e.g., renal, pulmonary, cardiac), a rheumatologic disease is rarely the primary cause of a patient's admission to an intensive care unit (ICU). However, three groups of patients commonly encountered in the intensive care setting present problems of special concern to the rheumatologist and internist. These include (1) patients with underlying rheumatologic diseases that may pose certain problems in the planning and execution of particular critical care procedures, such as endotracheal intubation, (2) patients who develop acute rheumatologic syndromes while hospitalized for other medical or surgical reasons, and (3) patients who are subject to the complications of prolonged immobilization.

Rheumatic Diseases Complicating Intensive Care Procedures

Difficult endotracheal intubations may be encountered in patients with rheumatoid arthritis (RA), juvenile rheumatoid arthritis (JRA), ankylosing spondylitis (AS), or progressive systemic sclerosis (PSS). The involvement of the cervical spine may limit neck mobility in RA [1], JRA [2], and AS [3], thus preventing proper positioning of the neck for intubation. This condition may be caused in RA by osteochondral destruction with marked pain on motion of the discovertebral joints [4] and ankylosis of the costovertebral joints [2]; in JRA most commonly by ankylosis of the apophyseal joints [5]; and in AS by ossification of the posterior longitudinal ligaments and annulus fibrosis with concomitant syndesmophyte formation and apophyseal joint ankylosis [6]. In each of these instances, a tracheostomy may be required for satisfactory endotracheal intubation (see Chap. 16), although in some patients the use of fiberoptic intubation, laryngoscopy, or blind nasotracheal intubation may suffice (see Chap. 1) [7].

Because of the potential for neurologic sequelae, of more serious consequence is a subluxation of the first and second cervical vertebral bodies (atlantoaxial subluxation) or a staircase cervical subluxation that involves many cervical vertebrae. Both of these complications are frequently found in cases of advanced RA with cervical spine involvement [4] and occur more rarely in certain subgroups of patients with JRA [8]. Although the majority of patients with cervical spine involvement are asymptomatic [9], a forced manipulation of the neck (e.g., during intubation, endotracheal suctioning, or nasogastric tube placement) may precipitate symptoms and signs of spinal cord compression.

Patients at risk should be identified with lateral cervical spine radiographs in the flexed position that should reveal no more than 3 mm of separation between the odontoid process and the arch of the atlantis [10]. If this distance is exceeded, care should be taken to avoid sudden or forced neck flexion during any intensive care procedure, which may be facilitated through the use of a soft cervical collar to maintain the neck in slight extension. If neurologic symptoms that are suggestive of spinal cord compression develop in a patient with either atlantoaxial or staircase subluxation, computerized tomography may be useful to confirm the diagnosis [11].

In addition to cervical spine disease, patients with JRA or, more rarely, RA may have temporomandibular joint disease with a resultant limitation of the motion of the lower jaw and decreased access to the oropharynx. In advanced cases of PSS, soft tissue fibrosis and atrophy may reduce the oral aperture [8] and make orotracheal intubation impossible. This problem may be circumvented in the event of planned or emergency endotracheal intubation by early identification of the patient at risk through careful physical examination and by anticipation of the need for nasotracheal intubation in all patients with limited oral apertures.

Finally, as many as 30 percent of patients with RA or JRA may have involvement of the cricoarytenoid joints at some time during the disease course [12]. These joints rotate during vocal cord adduction and abduction. Prolonged inflammation of the cricoarytenoid joints may restrict joint motion and thereby immobilize the cords in the midline position. The attempted passage of an endotracheal tube through the vocal cords in this situation may produce cord trauma and severe laryngospasm. Thus, in patients with RA or JRA in whom a history of hoarseness is elicited, indirect laryngoscopy to evaluate mobility of the vocal cords and integrity of the cricoarytenoid joints is advisable. If the cords are immobile due to cricoarytenoid joint disease, inhaled corticosteroid preparations may be useful, but preparations should be made for cricothyroidotomy or tracheostomy, should the need arise for establishing an emergency airway [13].

Acute Rheumatic Diseases in an Intensive Care Setting

Several rheumatologic syndromes have been observed to occur with increased frequency in selected populations of hospitalized patients, including those in the ICU. These include gouty arthritis, other microcrystalline arthropathies (calcium hydroxyapatite, calcium oxalate, calcium pyrophosphate), septic arthritis (as a complication of bacteremia), hemarthrosis (as a complication of anticoagulation therapy), and reflex sympathetic dystrophy (as a complication of myocardial infarction).

GOUT

Pathogenesis. Gout is a disorder characterized by one or more attacks of mono- or polyarticular arthritis in the setting of prolonged hyperuricemia, which may occur intermittently or constantly over time. The acute gouty paroxysm is triggered by precipitation of monosodium urate crystals in the joint space or nearby tissues [14–16], provoking an intense inflammatory reaction [17,18]. Regardless of a primary or secondary etiology of hyperuricemia [19], marked fluxes in serum urate [20] increase the risk of acute gout.

Although the specific inciting event that triggers an isolated attack may be difficult to define, the factors that are known to cause fluxes in serum urate and thus an increased incidence of secondary gout are common in patients in an ICU (Table 216-1). (The inborn errors of metabolism that cause primary hyperuricemia are discussed by Wyngaarden and Kelley [20].)

Of the conditions listed in Table 216-1, those that result in decreased renal excretion of uric acid deserve special comment. A reduction in the glomerular filtration rate that is secondary either to intrinsic renal disease or to decreased effective arteriolar blood volume results in a decreased filtered load of uric acid, hyperuricemia, and an increased risk of gout. In cases of decreased effective arteriolar blood volume, there is, additionally, enhanced tubular reabsorption of uric acid. Any condition that causes an accumulation of organic acids (e.g., lactic acid, betahydroxybutyric acid, and acetoacetic acid) may competitively inhibit the renal tubular secretion of uric acid, also leading to hyperuricemia. Possible mechanisms of hyperlactacidemia in the critically ill patient are multiple (see Chap. 115).

Drug-induced hyperuricemia represents one of the most frequently identifiable etiologies of gout in both hospitalized and nonhospitalized patients. Diuretic therapy decreases effective arteriolar blood volume and also may directly inhibit secretion of uric acid. Although thiazide diuretics were the first to be implicated as causes of hyperuricemia and gout [21,22], hyperuricemia has been reported as a side effect of furosemide [23,24], acetazolamide [25], ethacrynic acid [26,27], and diazoxide [28]. Furosemide and diazoxide may induce hyperlactacidemia as well.

In addition to diuretics, some other drugs that may predispose to hyperuricemia include low-dose salicylates (< 2.0 gm/day) [29], pyrazinamide [30], levodopa [31], and alpha-methyldopa [32]. Because of the uricosuric effect of radiocontrast media, a dye study may also precipitate an attack of acute gout. Finally, a hospitalized patient with hyperuricemia who undergoes a surgical procedure is at risk from postoperative gout [33]. The underlying factors that lead to gout are not well defined but may include some of those listed in Table 216-1.

Clinical Features. Gout is generally an easily identifiable and treatable clinical entity. A knowledge of the predisposing factors and the typical clinical features of the disease may aid in early diagnosis and appropriate management. Characteristically, the patient with acute gout will complain of the sudden onset of an exquisitely painful arthritis that (1) may involve one or more joints, (2) is asymmetrical, and (3) may be accompanied by fever, particularly in the case of a polyarticular presentation [34]. The great toe will be involved in over 50 percent of the initial acute attacks [35] and in 90 percent of acute attacks at some time in the course of the disease. The other common sites of involvement in order of observed frequency include insteps, ankles, knees, wrists, fingers, and elbows. Typically the involved area is erythematous, swollen, warm, and painful on motion.

The diagnosis of gout is confirmed when synovial fluid analysis by polarized light microscopy reveals the causative needle-shaped, negatively birefringent monosodium urate crystals located within polymorphonuclear leukocytes (Fig. 216-1). Monosodium urate crystals are yellow when parallel to the plane of the polarized light and are blue when perpendicular. Other characteristic findings of the synovial fluid in gouty ar-

Table 216-1. Factors That Increase Likelihood of Hyperuricemia and Acute Gout in the Critically Ill Patient

A. Conditions associated with increased production of uric acid
  1. Myeloproliferative disorders
  2. Lymphoproliferative disorders
  3. Chronic hemolytic anemias
  4. Multiple myeloma
  5. Severe psoriasis
B. Conditions associated with decreased renal excretion of uric acid
  1. Chronic renal disease (decreased renal functional mass)
  2. Lead nephropathy (decreased fractional excretion of uric acid)
  3. Decreased effective arteriolar blood volume
    a. Congestive heart failure
    b. Sodium depletion
    c. Dehydration
    d. Diabetes insipidus
    e. Drug-induced (diuretics)
  4. Hyperlactic acidemia
    a. Hypoxemia
    b. Sepsis
    c. Shock
    d. Toxemia of pregnancy
    e. Acute alcohol intoxication
  5. Increased levels of beta-hydroxybutyrate and acetoacetate
    a. Starvation
    b. Diabetic ketoacidosis
  6. Drug administration
    a. Pyrazinamide
    b. Diuretics
    c. Salicylates (low dose)
    d. Ethambutol
    e. Levodopa, alpha-methyldopa
C. Radiocontrast dye studies
D. Surgery

thritis are leukocytosis (generally > 2000 leukocytes/mm^3 and occasionally as high as 100,000/mm^3) with a polymorphonuclear leukocyte predominance. Since septic arthritis and gout may rarely be coexistent [36], aspirated fluid should be stained for microorganisms and cultured; both tests will be negative in the case of gout alone.

Hyperuricemia during an acute gouty episode is a variable finding. Other laboratory abnormalities associated with, but not always present in, acute gouty arthritis include a peripheral leukocytosis with an increased polymorphonuclear leukocyte count and an elevated sedimentation rate. These are nonspecific abnormalities, however, and the failure of these parameters to normalize with appropriate therapy and resolution of the acute attack should raise the suspicion of other underlying causes. An infection of both the true joint and the surrounding structures is another important entity to exclude.

Since overlying erythema and edema of a gouty joint may extend beyond the joint capsule, gout may be confused with cellulitis, a condition commonly encountered in an intensive care setting. A carefully performed physical examination of the patient may reveal lymphangitis or lymphadenopathy, and a careful examination of joint motion may reveal little limitation if cellulitis is present because the joint itself is not involved. If there is a small suspicion of joint inflammation, diagnostic arthrocentesis should be avoided until a therapeutic trial of appropriate antibiotics for cellulitis has been completed. Otherwise, there may be a risk of introducing organisms into a sterile joint. If there is marked pain or restriction on joint motion, or radiologic evaluation of the joint suggests an effusion, a diagnostic arthrocentesis should be performed prior to the institution of any therapy.

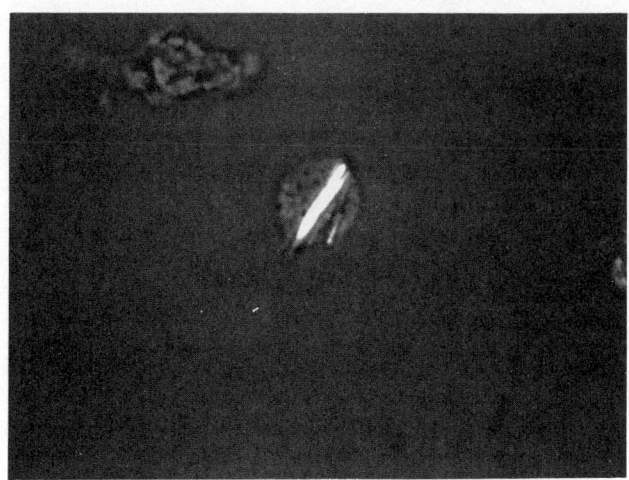

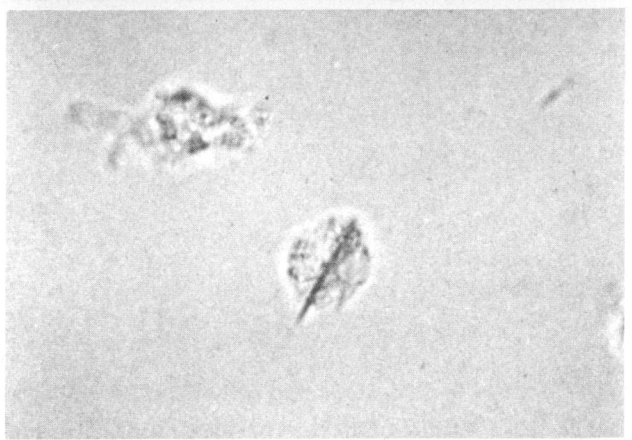

Fig. 216-1. Monosodium urate crystals phagocytosed by a synovial fluid polymorphonuclear leukocyte. In the top section, compensated polarized light clearly demonstrates two longer crystals and one shorter crystal. The bottom section shows the same field under ordinary light. Comparison of the two views demonstrates the superiority of compensated light over ordinary light microscopy when evaluating joint fluid for crystals. (From the Arthritis Foundation Clinical Slide Collection on the Rheumatic Diseases, copyright 1972. Slide 86, with permission of the Arthritis Foundation.)

Therapy. Once the diagnosis of acute gouty arthritis is established, the immediate aim of therapy is to terminate the attack by interruption of the inflammatory response to monosodium urate microcrystals. Several pharmacologic agents are useful, including adrenocorticotropic hormone (ACTH), colchicine, phenylbutazaone, indomethacin, and other newer nonsteroidal antiinflammatory drugs (NSAIDs). In certain settings, corticosteroids (either injected locally into the involved joint or administered parenterally) may be indicated as well. These options are summarized in Table 216-2.

Long-term goals (e.g., prevention of recurrent attacks, sequelae of tophaceous disease or renal stones) need not be considered in the acute setting. In fact, the initiation or discontinuation of any drug that may cause acute fluxes in the serum uric acid, such as allopurinol, probenecid, or salicylates, may prolong an acute attack. Hyperuricemia without clinical gout need not be treated.

ADRENOCORTICOTROPIC HORMONE. ACTH has been used in the treatment of acute gout for many years [37]. Though the mech-

anism of action is unknown, the beneficial response of ACTH is likely due to the release of endogenous adrenocorticosteroids. Recently, it has been shown in a nonblinded study to produce pain relief more rapidly when administered intramuscularly (40 IU) than indomethacin with a mean time to complete pain relief of 3 hours [38]. Of 36 patients receiving ACTH, none experienced side effects [38], an observation that, when coupled with the rapid action of the drug, makes ACTH treatment the therapy of choice for acute gout in the critically ill patient. In an anticoagulated patient, ACTH may be administered subcutaneously or intravenously to avoid possible bleeding associated with intramuscular injection. ACTH should be given for 3 consecutive days, 40 IU/day.

COLCHICINE. Colchicine is a drug that inhibits microtubular formation from subunit protein precursors and inhibits the production and the release from polymorphonuclear neutrophil leukocytes (PMN) of PMN chemotactic factor [39,40]. It may be administered to the patient either orally or intravenously in the doses shown in Table 216-2. The efficacy of this drug is related to the duration of the acute attack prior to its administration. More than 90 percent of patients will report improvement in symptoms if the acute attack has only lasted for a few hours, whereas only 75 percent of patients will respond favorably after 12 to 48 hours of untreated gouty arthritis [41].

A response to oral or intravenous colchicine is not completely diagnostic of gout, since other noninfectious inflammatory arthropathies may also respond to this drug [42]. The major disadvantage of the oral route of administration of colchicine is that 50 to 80 percent of patients will experience significant gastrointestinal toxicity, including abdominal pain, nausea, diarrhea, or vomiting [43].

Because intravenous access is routinely available in a critically ill patient, the intravenous route of colchicine administration is the preferred route in this setting. When used as described in Table 216-2, the incidence of adverse gastrointestinal side effects is markedly lowered, while the therapeutic efficacy is maintained [44]. The complications of intravenous colchicine include severe soft tissue toxicity if extravasation occurs and bone marrow suppression [45]. (Neutropenia is a relative contraindication to the use of intravenous colchicine.)

Renal failure necessitates an increase in the oral or intravenous dose interval of administration (a twofold increase in the case of the anephric patient and a proportional fraction increase in lesser degrees of renal insufficiency [46]). In addition, patients with hepatic insufficiency or those who have recently taken chronic oral colchicine should receive lower doses than those shown in Table 216-2 [47]. Colchicine may be useful in a gouty patient who has been refractory to, or relapsed after, a course of ACTH.

NONSTEROIDAL ANTIINFLAMMATORY DRUGS. Most NSAIDs are useful in the treatment of acute gout, although potential toxicity and, in most cases, the necessity for oral administration make their use less desirable in critically ill patients than parenteral ACTH or colchicine. Though phenylbutazone was one of the first NSAIDs to be used with great success to treat gouty arthritis [48], concern about bone marrow aplasia [49] and profound sodium and water retention [50] has limited its use. Indomethacin and most other NSAIDs are effective as either primary or adjunctive therapy. In general, NSAIDs with short half-lives are preferable to longer-acting agents due to the frequency with which peak serum levels are achieved in the course of therapy. Salicylates should be avoided due to unpredictable effects on urate excretion. For details concerning the use of NSAIDs, see Simon and Mills [51] and Chap. 215.

The potential toxicity of all NSAIDs should be considered, since they are either absolutely or relatively contraindicated in

Table 216-2. Treatment Options in Acute Gout

Medication	Route of administration	Dose	Side effects	Contraindications
Colchicine	Oral	0.6 mg q1h until either symptomatic relief, development of gastrointestinal symptoms, or a total of 10 doses[a]	Nausea, vomiting, diarrhea, abdominal pain	Serious gastrointestinal disease
	Intravenous (diluted in 20 cc saline)	2 mg initially; 1 mg q6h until total dose of 4 mg[a]	Gastrointestinal toxicity rare, bone marrow suppression	Leukopenia, thrombocytopenia, poor intravenous access
NSAIDs				
Indomethacin	Oral	50–75 mg initially; 50 mg q8h until symptoms improve, then 25 mg q8h until resolution	Nausea, abdominal pain, gastrointestinal bleeding, peptic ulceration, headaches, confusion, seizures, renal failure, potentiation of congestive heart failure, platelet dysfunction	Active ulcer disease, gastrointestinal bleeding, inflammatory bowel disease; abnormal mental status; renal insufficiency; congestive heart failure, decreased intravascular or effective arteriolar blood volume from any cause, bleeding disorders
Phenylbutazone	Oral	200–600 mg initially; 100–200 mg q6–8h for 1 day (maximum, 600 mg/day), 100 mg q6h for 2 days, then 100 mg q8h for 4–5 more days	Nausea, vomiting, epigastric pain, diarrhea, peptic ulcer disease, bone marrow suppression,[b] sodium retention[b]	Serious gastrointestinal disease, leukopenia, thrombocytopenia, congestive heart failure, cirrhosis
Other NSAIDs	See reference [50]			
Adrenocorticosteroids				
ACTH	Intramuscular	40–60 IU/day for 3 days	Same as for oral prednisone	Should not be used in anticoagulated patients
	Intravenous	Same as for intramuscular ACTH	Same as for intramuscular ACTH	Same as for intramuscular ACTH
Prednisone	Oral (rarely necessary)	30 mg/day for 2 days, 20 mg/day for 2 days, 10 mg/day for 2 days	Sodium retention, hypokalemia, opportunistic infection, masking of signs of infection; no adrenal suppression within 1 wk	Congestive heart failure, underlying infection
Methylprednisolone	Intravenous	Same as for oral prednisone	Same as for oral prednisone	Same as for oral prednisone
Methylprednisolone acetate or triamcinolone hexacetonide	Intraarticular	20–40 mg (depends on size of affected joint)	Superimposed infection (rare)	Should not be used in anticoagulated patients

[a]Dose of colchicine needs to be modified in renal and hepatic insufficiency. No colchicine should be given for next 7 days.
[b]These two complications have significantly limited the use of phenylbutazone.
NSAIDs = nonsteroidal antiinflammatory drugs; ACTH = adrenocorticotropic hormone.

many critically ill patients (see Chap. 154). Because of myriad gastrointestinal toxicities associated with these agents [52,53], most active gastrointestinal diseases represent absolute contraindications to their use. Diffuse gastritis, duodenitis, active peptic ulcer disease, or lower gastrointestinal bleeding may be induced through the local erosive effects of these drugs or through their inhibition of prostaglandin-mediated gastric cytoprotection. Thus, NSAIDs are absolutely contraindicated in patients with active peptic ulcer disease or gastrointestinal bleeding of any etiology, including "stress ulcers." Inflammatory bowel disease is a relative contraindication because of a reported incidence of bowel perforation in this setting [54,55]. Sucralfate or cytoprotective prostaglandin analogs may reduce the risks of gastric ulcerations when used concomitantly with NSAIDs [52].

Renal toxicity from NSAIDs may occur from a variety of mechanisms [56–62]. Patients with diminished effective arteriolar blood volume from any cause (e.g., congestive heart failure, cirrhosis, intravascular volume depletion) are at risk of developing renal failure after NSAID ingestion due to the inhibition of compensatory prostaglandin-induced renal arteriolar vasodilatation [56,57]. Thus any condition that produces an altered hemodynamic status, such as those listed above, represents either a relative or an absolute contraindication to the use of any NSAID, depending on the degree of hemodynamic compromise and the severity of underlying renal dysfunction.

NSAIDs may cause deterioration of renal function by several other mechanisms as well, including acute intrinsic renal failure, acute allergic interstitial nephritis, and papillary necrosis with chronic interstitial nephritis [58,59]. Other renal side effects of NSAIDs, which have been described, include sodium retention, hyponatremia, hyperkalemia, and aggravation of preexisting hypertension [56,57,60]. As in the case of phenylbutazone, sodium retention in a patient with underlying cardiac disease may have profound deleterious hemodynamic consequences. Thus, any NSAID must be used with extreme caution in this group of patients. Preliminary studies suggest that sulindac may be a potential renal function–sparing NSAID and thus may prove useful in situations in which other more nephrotoxic NSAIDs may be contraindicated [61].

Because of reversible inhibition of platelet function [51], NSAIDs may enhance bleeding tendencies in any patient. A recent history of a bleeding diathesis of any etiology, abnormal clotting studies, or thrombocytopenia therefore represents a relative contraindication to NSAID therapy. Many NSAIDs compete with warfarin for protein-binding sites and may increase the serum concentration of this medication [51]. In patients who are anticoagulated with this drug, NSAID therapy should be administered cautiously, if at all, and clotting parameters as well as possible bleeding sites should be carefully monitored.

CORTICOSTEROIDS. A last option in the management of acute gouty arthritis is the use of corticosteroids. Local corticosteroid injections into involved gouty joints are more useful in an intensive care setting, particularly in the setting of mono- or oligoarthritis. In patients in whom colchicine and NSAIDs are contraindicated, a single injection of a sustained-release corticosteroid preparation into a troublesome joint may provide relief as well as obviate the need for systemically administered medication. Moreover, when all other modes of therapy have been unsuccessful, a rapidly tapered course of systemic corticosteroids may be indicated. This situation is rarely encountered, however, and systemic corticosteroid therapy should be undertaken only after rheumatologic consultation.

OTHER MICROCRYSTALLINE ARTHROPATHIES. Although gout is the best-defined and most frequently occurring microcrystalline arthropathy, several other crystalline-induced syndromes may mimic gout and cause potential diagnostic confusion. These include arthritides due to deposition of calcium pyrophosphate dihydrate (CPPD) [62,63], calcium hydroxyapatite [64,65], or calcium oxalate [66] crystals.

Pathogenesis. The pathophysiology of these entities appears to be similar to that of gouty arthritis, involving a complex series of biochemical reactions that lead to the inflammatory response within the involved joint [67,68]. Like gout, each of these disorders may be more common in certain groups of patients in an ICU.

The acute self-limited form of CPPD deposition (which most closely simulates acute gout and thus is also known by the eponym *pseudogout*) may be precipitated by surgery of any type [69] and may be related to downward fluxes in serum calcium levels that lead to "crystal shedding into intraarticular spaces" [70]. Postsurgical attacks most commonly occur 3 days postoperatively [69] and most frequently involve the knee joint. Severe medical illnesses, such as ischemic heart disease, cerebral infarction, and thrombophlebitis, may also provoke attacks of CPPD deposition [69].

Patients who are undergoing chronic intermittent peritoneal dialysis have recently been described as having a high incidence of acute arthritis that is thought to be associated with either CPPD or calcium hydroxyapatite deposition in articular cartilage [71]. Furthermore, patients who are maintained on chronic hemodialysis have been shown to be at risk of developing arthritis due to calcium oxalate crystals [66].

Clinical Features. Clinically, each of the above entities may be indistinguishable from acute gout. The diagnosis of CPPD deposition is suggested by radiographically demonstrated cartilaginous calcification of the involved joint (articular chondrocalcinosis) and is established with certainty by aspirating the joint and visualizing under polarized microscopy weakly positively birefringent, rhomboid-shaped crystals within synovial fluid PMNs (Fig. 216-2). These crystals are blue when parallel to the plane of polarized light and yellow when perpendicular.

Calcium oxalate crystals, likewise, are positively birefringent, but they are pleomorphic and bipyramidal or rod-like in shape. Smaller hydroxyapatite crystals may be visualized only by examining the synovial fluid with electron microscopy. A diagnosis of acute arthritis due to the smaller crystal may thus be clinically presumed in the proper setting and when other diagnoses have been excluded.

Therapy. Therapeutic options in the crystalline arthropathies are identical to those in acute gout. Of some interest is the fact that patients with pseudogout may respond dramatically on some occasions to colchicine [72], since this response was initially considered to be diagnostic of gout.

SEPTIC ARTHRITIS. Joint infection by a bacterial or fungal pathogen is the most critical diagnosis that must be established rapidly and treated appropriately in any patient who develops acute arthritis of either one or, less commonly, multiple joints. A delay in the diagnosis and treatment of this condition may lead to the destruction of articular cartilage and the loss of joint function [73]. Furthermore, a diagnosis of septic arthritis may lead to early identification of, and therapy for, the source of the septicemia, such as endocarditis (see Chap. 88).

Pathogenesis. A variety of debilitating illnesses predispose to septic arthritis, including diabetes mellitus [74], alcoholism [75], malignancies [76,77], renal failure [75], systemic lupus erythematosus (see Chap. 219) [78], and rheumatoid arthritis (see Chap. 219) [79]. Immunosuppressive therapy, for any reason, increases the risk of infectious complications, including septic arthritis [76,80]. In either the presence or the absence of these predisposing factors, acute infectious arthritis may result from hematogenous spread from another site of infection, direct inoculation (e.g., from a puncture wound), or local extension (e.g., from adjacent soft tissue or bone). Septicemia is especially likely to result in infection of prosthetic joints [81]. Once an infection is established within a joint, a complex cascade of physiologic responses occurs that can lead to cartilage destruction [82], a process whose progression depends on the virulence of the organism.

Clinical Features. Clinically, septic arthritis may be indistinguishable from the acute arthritis of other causes, such as CPPD and the other microcrystalline arthropathies. Typically, septic arthritis is acute in onset; is monoarticular; and produces swelling, tenderness, overlying erythema, warmth, and limitation of motion (due to pain) of the involved joint. Septic arthritis of multiple joints is well described [83]; thus polyarticular arthritis should not preclude consideration of infection as an etiology. Accompanying fever is a variable finding. When it is present, it may be low grade.

Clinical suspicion remains the key to the diagnosis of septic arthritis. Because of the nature of the patients in an ICU, the frequency of invasive procedures can lead to bacteremia and a large number of portals for the entry of organisms (e.g., indwelling catheters, intravenous lines). Any patient in this setting who develops an acutely swollen, painful joint should undergo diagnostic arthrocentesis to exclude infection unless examination of the joint indicates that the underlying process is not intraarticular (e.g., cellulitis).

Diagnosis is confirmed by seeing organisms on Gram stain [83] or positive cultures. Cultures should be planted at the bedside if possible or immediately thereafter in the laboratory. They

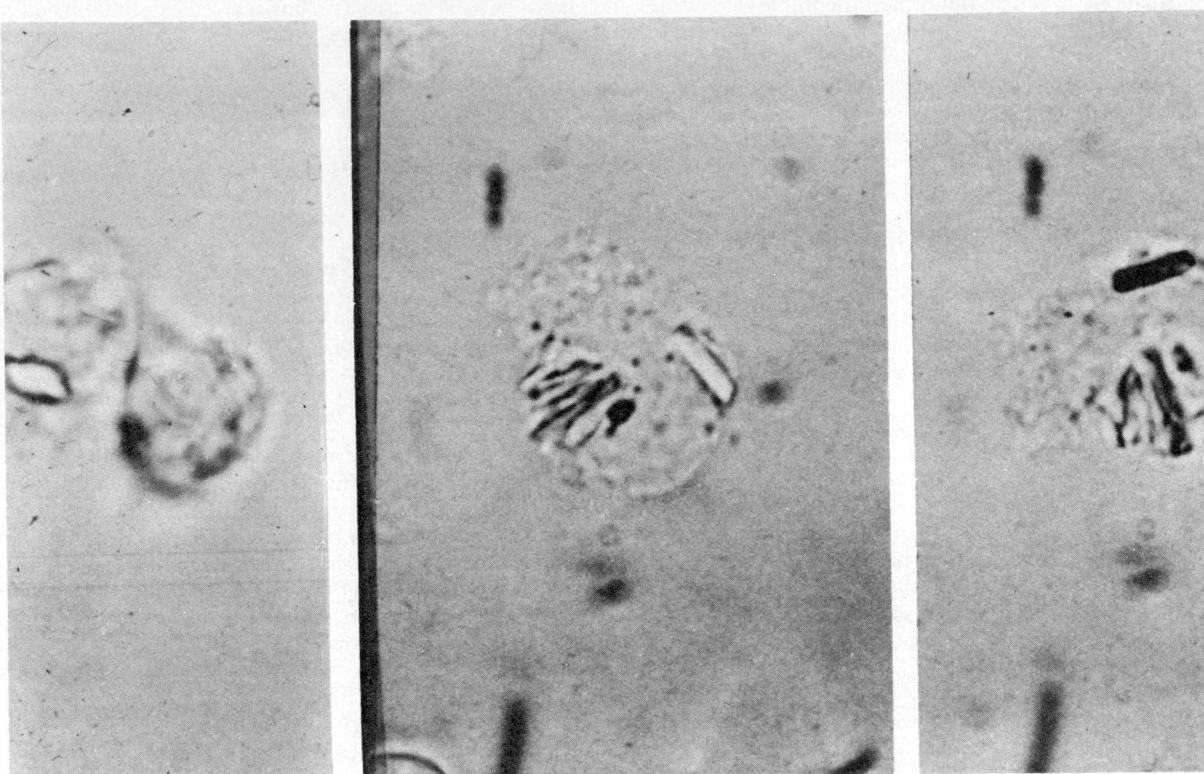

Fig. 216-2. Calcium pyrophosphate crystals phagocytosed by polymorphonuclear leukocytes in synovial fluid. Demonstrated are their rectangular or rhomboid shapes. (From the Arthritis Foundation Clinical Slide Collection on the Rheumatic Diseases, copyright 1972. Slide 91, with permission of the Arthritis Foundation.)

should be performed both anaerobically and aerobically with special requests for fungal cultures and cultures of organisms that require a special medium for growth (e.g., *Neisseria gonorrhoeae*) if indicated. In addition to cultures, synovial fluid should be analyzed for cell count, glucose, and mucin clot formation, which may support a diagnosis of infection.

Although leukocyte counts as low as 5000 per cubic millimeter may occasionally be present in septic arthritis [84], the counts generally exceed 50,000 per cubic millimeter and on occasion may be as high as 200,000 per cubic millimeter, with a marked PMN predominance. Synovial fluid glucose may be low (serum glucose exceeding synovial fluid glucose by 40–50 mg/dl or more) [83,85], and mucin clot formation is poor [83]. Unfortunately, synovial fluid leukocyte count, glucose, and mucin clot are deranged in a similar fashion in RA, making the diagnosis more difficult in this circumstance.

In addition to Gram stain, bacteriologic studies, and routine synovial fluid analysis, several techniques have recently been suggested as aids in the early diagnosis of bacterial joint infections. These include counterimmunoelectrophoresis [86], nitroblue tetrazolium testing [87], and lactic acid determinations on synovial fluid [88–90]. Of these techniques, the last appears to be the most promising, except in cases of *N. gonorrhoeae* infections. However, this test is not yet routinely available for clinical use.

Although radiographs of an infected joint will often be normal early in the course of the infection, they should be obtained as a baseline for future studies, which may show juxtaarticular osteopenia, joint-space narrowing, or subchondral bone loss in later stages, particularly if diagnosis and treatment have been delayed.

Therapy. If the diagnosis of septic arthritis is either strongly suspected on clinical grounds or documented by positive Gram stain or culture, the therapeutic approach involves several steps. First, appropriate antibiotic therapy should be instituted for the presumptive or proved pathogen. In the noncompromised patient, *Staphylococcus aureus* is the most common nongonococcal offender, followed by nonpneumococcal streptococci and *Streptococcus pneumoniae* [80]. In the case of a prosthetic joint infection, *Staphylococcus epidermidis* is usually the causative organism, most commonly followed by *Staphylococcus aureus* and *Streptococcus faecalis* [81]. In the critically ill patient exposed to the multiple organisms that may be found in an ICU, however, broad-spectrum antibiotic coverage should be instituted pending the results of cultures. Tables 216-3 and 216-4 summarize antibiotic therapy for septic arthritis in situations where the organism is known and those in which it is unknown. In most cases, antibiotic therapy should be continued intravenously for at least 3 weeks.

Most fungal arthritis is subacute or chronic and thus is not likely to represent an emergent problem in a critically ill patient. Acute arthritis has been reported to be caused by *Candida* organisms [77,91]. These organisms, however, can be diagnosed by their typical appearance on synovial fluid analysis, and treatment can be initiated while awaiting culture results. Treatment consists of amphotericin B administered alone, intravenously, or in concert with intraarticular instillation (see Chap. 85). Other agents, although potentially less toxic, have not proved to be as efficacious in this setting.

Two other aspects of therapy of an infected joint are (1) immobilization to eliminate painful motion of the joint and (2) repeated (often daily) aspirations of synovial fluid [92] to re-

Table 216-3. Antibiotic Therapy of Acute Bacterial Arthritis in the Critically Ill Adult (Known Pathogen)

Organism	Antibiotic choice	Alternatives
Staphylococcus aureus	Nafcillin 9–12 gm/day (q4h) or oxacillin 9–12 gm/day (q4h)	Cefazolin 4.5–6 gm/day (q8h) or vancomycin 2 gm/day (q12h)
Staphylococcus aureus, methicillin-resistant	Vancomycin 2 gm/day (q12h)	None
Streptococcus pyogenes, Streptococcus pneumoniae	Penicillin G, 12–18 million units/day (q4h)	Cefazolin or vancomycin or clindamycin 1.8 gm/day (q8h)
Nesiseria gonorrhoeae	Ceftriaxone 1–2 gm/day (q12h) Cefotaxine 3–gm/day (q8h)	Penicillin G (tetracycline, aztreonam, or ciprofloxacin)
Pseudomonas aeruginosa	Piperacillin 12 gm/day (q4h) plus tobramycin 4–5 mg/kg/day (q8h)	Ceftazidime 6 gm/day (q8h) or imipenem 2 gm/day or aztreonom 6 gm/day plus tobramycin or gentamicin or ciprofloxacin 400 mg IV (q12h)
Enterobacteriaceae	Third generation cephalosporin [plus gentamicin 4–5 mg/kg/day (q8h)]	Aztreonam 3 gm/day (q8h) plus gentamicin or amikacin

Table 216-4. Antibiotic Therapy of Acute Bacterial Arthritis in the Critically Ill Adult (Known Pathogen)

Gram stain	Presumed organism(s)	Antibiotic(s)
Positive		
Gram-positive cocci	*Staphylococcus aureus*	Oxacillin or nafcillin
Gram-positive cocci (prosthetic joint)	*Staphylococcus epidermidis*	Vancomycin
Gram-negative cocci	*Neisseria gonorrhoeae*	Ceftriaxone or cefotaxime
Gram-negative bacilli	*Escherichia coli, Serratia marcescens* other enterobacteriaceae	Third generation cephalosporin or imipenem or aztreonam or ciprofloxacin
Gram-negative bacilli (thin)	*Pseudomonas aeruginosa*	Ceftazidime (or piperacillin, imipenem, or aztreonam) plus tobramycin or ciprofloxacin
Negative		
Noncompromised host	*Staphylococcus aureus,*[a] enterobacteriaceae	Third generation cephalosporin (ceftriaxone or cefotaxime) plus vancomycin
Compromised host	*Pseudomonas aeruginosa*	Imipenem (or ceftazidime, piperacillin, or aztreonam) plus tobramycin or ciprofloxacin

[a]Treatment for both gram-positive and gram-negative pathogens must be continued until cultures return.

move lysosomal enzymes, which may potentiate joint destruction. If arthrocentesis cannot be frequently and adequately performed to drain the accumulation of synovial fluid, surgical drainage or arthroscopic lavage is indicated.

Finally, since most articular infections occur as a result of hematogenous spread of an organism from another site of primary infection, any patient with septic arthritis without an obvious site of local inoculation should be evaluated for a primary source. Evaluation should include complete cultures from possible portals as well as blood cultures (prior to the institution of antibiotics) and other tests, such as echocardiogram and computerized tomographic or gallium scanning, to exclude valvular vegetations or other sites of infection.

HEMARTHROSIS. In the absence of an underlying inherited disorder of coagulation, hemarthrosis in an intensive care setting is most likely a complication of anticoagulation therapy. It is most frequently described in patients who are receiving oral anticoagulant therapy (sodium warfarin) [93,94], but hemarthrosis may also complicate intravenous heparin therapy [95]. Although an uncommon complication of anticoagulation, hemarthrosis constitutes as much as one-third of major hemorrhagic events in patients who are receiving oral anticoagulants [94]. Hemarthrosis may also constitute the reason for ICU admission in a patient with hemophilia.

Because hemarthrosis may be spontaneous, a history of trauma may not be elicited from patients with this diagnosis. Clinically, hemarthrosis is uniformly monoarticular and presents as a painful, swollen, and warm joint with a tense effusion on examination. A prolongation of coagulation parameters (often beyond the therapeutic range [94]) suggests the diagnosis, but diagnostic arthrocentesis is essential to confirm the diagnosis of hemarthrosis and to exclude the possibility of septic arthritis. When performed aseptically and carefully, arthrocentesis is safe and free of significant long-term morbidity.

A precise definition of hemarthrosis has not been established, but it is suggested by the presence of the synovial fluid hematocrit exceeding 3 percent [94]. The causes of hemarthrosis include trauma (especially with fracture), blood dyscrasias, neuroarthropathy, synovial tumors (primary or metastatic), myeloproliferative disease, sickle cell trait or disease, and joint prosthesis [96].

Despite the fact that repeated hemarthrosis such as in patients with hemophilia may have profound pathophysiologic consequences on joint structure and function [97], spontaneous hemarthrosis has a benign prognosis. Therapy consists of arthrocentesis and the withholding of anticoagulants to improve clotting parameters with or without the addition of vitamin K. The temporary discomfort of hemarthrosis is often less than the risk of inducing a hypercoagulable state by the administration of vitamin K, although in the most severe cases this may be indicated [94]. Some patients who recover from one hemarthrosis will experience another if anticoagulation is resumed. A close monitoring of coagulation parameters and the maintaining of values within the therapeutic range minimize the chance of recurrence.

REFLEX SYMPATHETIC DYSTROPHY SYNDROME. The reflex sympathetic dystrophy syndrome (RSDS), which follows myocardial infarction and other illnesses, is a symptom complex that is occasionally encountered in patients by the intensivist. This syndrome is characterized by (1) pain and swelling in an extremity, with prominent distal articular involvement; (2) trophic skin changes in the extremity, including atrophy, nail changes, hypertrichosis, and hyperhidrosis; (3) vasomotor instability; (4) pain and/or decreased motion in the ipsilateral shoulder; and (5) a precipitating event or illness [98]. The term *shoulder-hand syndrome* (SHS) may be used in the case of upper-extremity involvement.

The pathogenesis of the syndrome remains poorly understood, although recent studies have documented increased blood flow and increased venous oxygen saturation in the affected extremity, suggesting that symptoms may be due to local sympathetic dysfunction with resultant vasodilatation [98].

The precipitating illnesses that have been associated with RSDS and that are typically managed in the ICU are myocardial infarction [98–100], trauma [99,100], and a variety of other diseases, including cerebral infarction, malignancy, thrombophlebitis, polyarteritis nodosa, and other vasculitic syndromes. The older literature suggests that RSDS can be seen as often as 20 to 30 percent of the time following myocardial infarction [101,102], being confined to the SHS variant with onset 3 to 16 weeks after the acute infarction [99].

Although the incidence of SHS following infarction is undoubtedly much lower than this at the present time (possibly because of early mobilization in the periinfarction period), it is important to be alert to this diagnosis for two reasons: (1) the shoulder pain of SHS may antedate other symptoms [100] and may be confused with the referred pain of cardiac origin, and (2) early identification and appropriate intervention may prevent long-term disability [101].

Shoulder pain from SHS may be distinguished from referred cardiac pain by the fact that joint motion is painful and/or limited in SHS, which it is not in the pain of cardiac origin. Further, intrinsic disease of the shoulder will produce pain in the deltoid region (upper outer aspect of the arm), whereas pain from a cardiac source typically involves the pectoral and ulnar regions (upper inner aspect of the arm). Frequently, SHS is bilateral, although involvement is greater on one side than the other [98,103]. The presence of bilateral symptoms, however, does *not* preclude an alternative diagnosis of referred cardiac pain. Other differential diagnostic considerations of SHS include thrombophlebitis, cellulitis, RA, periarthritis, and acute gouty arthritis.

In the early stages of SHS, the diagnosis is clinical. Few supportive ancillary diagnostic tools are available except a perfusion scan, which may reveal increased blood flow in the limb's affected portion. In later stages of disease, bone scintigraphy may reveal a juxtaarticular increase in uptake of nuclide. Radiographs may show patchy demineralization of the involved extremity [103].

If left untreated, SHS may progress to a chronic stage that is characterized by muscular atrophy, flexion contractures (particularly the digits), and dystrophic skin changes. The principles of therapy include (1) early diagnosis, (2) pain management with analgesics or NSAIDs, (3) aggressive physical therapy with emphasis on preservation of joint motion and muscle strengthening, and (4) stellate ganglion (sympathetic) blocks if pain or vasomotor symptoms are incapacitating. Systemic corticosteroid therapy has been advocated by some authors [98,100,104], but early recognition and the preceding measures may obviate the need for this medication and its many associated complications. However, if conservative measures fail, a 4- to 6-week course of corticosteroids may be efficacious.

VASCULITIS. Vasculitis is discussed in Chapters. 165 and 220.

Complications of Immobilization

Critically ill patients may remain immobilized for extended periods of time and thus may be subject to several complications of immobilization. These include muscle weakening, restricted range of joint motion, decubitus ulcers, and diffuse osteoporosis [105] as well as other derangements in bone metabolism in selected patients, such as those with Paget's disease.

MUSCLE WEAKENING. The complete rest of a single muscle will result in a 10 to 15 percent decrement per week of muscle strength [106], leading to atrophy, generalized weakness, and lack of stamina. Furthermore, muscle disease may contribute to joint contractures with a resultant marked limitation of motion. The pathophysiology of this process is not well understood, but it is possibly related to collagen deposition around muscle fibers, a reduction in their normal stretching capacity, and, ultimately, a shortened resting-muscle length [107].

JOINT CONTRACTURES. The restricted range of motion of a joint may develop as early as 4 days after the joint is placed at complete rest [108]. Shortened muscle length is a contributing factor in this process. Other soft tissue supportive joint structures, such as ligaments and tendons, may be similarly affected.

Joint contractures often reflect improper attention to positioning patients who are immobile. The joints that are particularly vulnerable to this problem include the ankles, knees, hips, and shoulders. In particular, the common practice of maintaining the knees in a flexed position through manipulating the hospital bed or placing pillows in the popliteal fossae greatly enhances the development of flexion contractures, while the failure to use a foot board may result in contractures of the Achilles tendons.

DECUBITUS ULCERS. Decubitus ulcers represent one of the most potentially troublesome aspects of immobilization and may contribute significantly to the morbidity of critical illness (see Chaps. 166 and 220). The particularly vulnerable areas of tissue breakdown are those over the bony prominences: anterior superior iliac spines, patellae, humeral tuberosities, trochanters, lateral malleoli, scapulae, sacrum, and calcanei [108]. Positioning methods and preventive skin care are predominantly the province of the skilled critical care nurse and are reviewed in detail by Stryker [109].

DISUSE OSTEOPOROSIS AND OTHER DERANGEMENTS OF BONE METABOLISM. Because bone remodeling is an active, ongoing process in which bone formation is tightly coupled in normal circumstances to bone reabsorption, total bone mass is dependent on factors that modulate either of these parameters. Bone formation is stimulated by exercise and, conversely, markedly diminished by rest. Bone disuse results, therefore, in reduced bone formation due to the reduced activity of the major bone-forming cells (the osteoblasts) and increased bone reabsorption due to the increased activity of the major bone-resorbing cells (the osteoclasts) [110]. This process may occur rapidly in the immobilized patient and result in dramatic decrements in bone density, which predispose the patient to pathologic fractures when normal activity is resumed.

Patients with Paget's disease may be subject to an exaggeration of the above process. In this disease, there is increased osteoclastic and osteoblastic activity, compared to that of normal individuals, and a resultant markedly increased rate of bone turnover. With prolonged complete immobilization and inhibition of osteoblastic function, osteoclastic function proceeds unopposed and may result in hypercalciuria, which occasionally engenders the formation of calcium-containing renal stones and even severe hypercalcemia [111]. Thus it is essential to mobilize patients with Paget's disease early, to monitor closely both serum and urinary calcium levels, and to intervene with appropriate calcium-lowering therapy if indicated.

PREVENTIVE AND THERAPEUTIC APPROACHES. Each of the complications of immobilization discussed here should be addressed from the first day a patient is admitted to an ICU. Both passive and active range-of-motion exercises should be performed routinely on each extremity daily unless contraindicated by underlying medical problems. In this manner, muscle tone will be maintained, and joint contractures will be minimized. Care should be taken to avoid improper positioning that may facilitate the development of flexion contractures. Position changes of the immobile patient should be performed frequently to avoid skin breakdown.

Early mobilization is the key to the prevention of disuse osteoporosis, although in certain patients this may not be feasible. Range-of-motion exercises, patient positioning, skin care, and mobilization are appropriate functions of critical care nurses and ancillary personnel, but they are also the direct responsibility of the attending physician. Appropriate emphasis on these aspects of care of the immobilized patient may facilitate rehabilitation and the return to optimal function after hospitalization.

References

1. Gray TC, Utting JE, Nunn JF (eds): *General Anaesthesia,* ed 4. London, Butterworth, 1980, p 894.
2. Gschwend N: *Surgical Treatment of Rheumatoid Arthritis.* Philadelphia, W.B. Saunders, 1980, p 1.
3. Wright V, Moll JMH: Ankylosing spondylitis. *Br J Hosp Med* 9:331, 1973.
4. Bland JH: Rheumatoid arthritis of the cervical spine. *J Rheumatol* 1:319, 1974.
5. Martel W, Holt JF, Cassidy JT: Roentgenologic manifestations of juvenile rheumatoid arthritis. *Am J Roentgenol* 88:400, 1962.
6. Kelley WN, Harris ED Jr, Ruddy S, et al: (eds): *Textbook of Rheumatology.* Philadelphia, W.B. Saunders, 1981, p 611.
7. Salem MR, Mathrubhutham M, Bennett EJ: Current concepts. Difficult intubation. *N Engl J Med* 295:879, 1976.
8. Arnett FC, Bias WB, Stevens MB: Juvenile-onset chronic arthritis. Clinical and roentgenographic features of a unique HLA-B27 subset. *Am J Med* 69:369, 1980.
9. Smith PH, Benn RT, Sharp J: Natural history of rheumatoid cervical luxations. *Ann Rheum Dis* 31:431, 1972.
10. Martel W: The occipito-atlanto-axial joints in rheumatoid arthritis and ankylosing spondylitis. *Am J Roentgenol* 86:223, 1961.
11. Rosenthal DI, Mankin HJ, Bauman RA: Musculoskeletal applications for computed tomography. *Bull Rheum Dis* 33:1, 1983.
12. Lofgren RH, Montgomery WW: Incidence of laryngeal involvement in rheumatoid arthritis. *N Engl J Med* 267:193, 1962.
13. Vassallo CL: Rheumatoid arthritis of the cricoarytenoid joints. *Arch Intern Med* 117:273, 1966.
14. Garrod AB: *The Nature and Treatment of Gout and Rheumatic Gout.* London, Walton and Maberly, 1859.
15. Zvaifler NJ, Pekin TJ: Significance of urate crystals in synovial fluids. *Arch Intern Med* 111:99, 1963.
16. Seegmiller JE, Laster L, Howell RR: Biochemistery of uric acid and its relation to gout. *N Engl J Med* 268:712, 1963.
17. Faires JS, McCarty DJ Jr: Acute synovitis in normal joints of man and dog produced by injections of microcrystalline sodium urate, calcium oxalate, and corticosteroid esters, abstract. *Arthritis Rheum* 5:295, 1962.
18. Seegmiller JE, Howell RR, Malawista SE: The inflammatory reaction to sodium urate. Its possible relationship to the genesis of acute gouty arthritis. *JAMA* 180:469, 1962.
19. Hall AP, Burry PE, Dawber TR, et al: Epidemiology of gout and hyperuricemia. A long-term population study. *Am J Med* 42:27, 1967.
20. Wyngaarden JB, Kelley WN: *Gout and Hyperuricemia.* New York, Grune & Stratton, 1976, p 215.
21. Aronoff A: Acute gouty arthritis precipitated by chlorothiazide. *N Engl J Med* 262:767, 1960.
22. Warshaw LJ: Acute attacks of gout precipitated by chlorothiazide-induced diuresis. *JAMA* 172:802, 1960.
23. Steele TH: Evidence for altered renal urate reabsorption during changes in volume of the extracellular fluid. *J Lab Clin Med* 74:288, 1969.
24. Steele TH, Oppenheimer S: Factors affecting urate excretion following diuretic administration in man. *Am J Med* 47:564, 1969.
25. Ayvazian JH, Ayvazian LF: A study of the hyperuricemia induced by hydrochlorothiazide and acetazolamide separately and in combination. *J Clin Invest* 40:1961, 1961.
26. Cannon PJ, Heinemann HO, Stason WB, et al: Ethacrynic acid. Effectiveness and mode of diuretic action in man. *Circulation* 31:5, 1965.
27. Bourke E, Ledingham JGG, Stokes GS: Effects of intravenous ethacrynic acid on the renal handling of citrate and urate in man. *Clin Sci* 31:231, 1966.
28. Wyngaarden JB, Kelley WM: *Gout and Hyperuricemia.* New York, Grune & Stratton, 1976, p 370.
29. Klempcrcr F, Bauer W: Influence of aspirin on urate excretion. *J Clin Invest* 23:950, 1944.
30. Shapiro M, Hyde L: Hyperuricemia due to pyrazinamide. *Am J Med* 23:596, 1957.
31. Al-Hujaj M, Schonthal H, Johannes-Krankenhaus E: Hyperuricemia and levodopa. *N Engl J Med* 285:859, 1971.
32. Wyngaarden JB, Kelley WN: *Gout and Hyperuricemia.* New York, Grune & Stratton, 1976, p 373.
33. Linton RR, Talbott JH: Surgical treatment of topaceous gout. *Ann Surg* 117:161, 1943.
34. Hadler NM, Franck WA, Bress NM, et al: Acute polyarticular gout. *Am J Med* 56:715, 1974.
35. Wyngaarden JB, Kelley WN: *Gout and Hyperuricemia.* New York, Grune & Stratton, 1976, p 214.
36. Smith JR, Phelps P: Septic arthritis, gout, pseudogout and osteoarthritis in the knee of a patient with multiple myeloma. *Arthritis Rheum* 15:89, 1972.
37. Axelrod D, Preston S: Comparison of parenteral adrenocorticotropic hormone with oral indomethacin in the treatment of acute gout. *Arthritis Rheum* 31:803, 1988.
38. Wolfson WQ, Cohn C, Levine R: Rapid treatment of acute gouty arthritis by concurrent administration of pituitary adrenocorticotropic hormone (ACTH) and colchicine. *J Lab Clin Med* 34:1766, 1949.
39. Borisy GG, Taylor EW: The mechanism of action of colchicine. Binding of colchicine $<$sup -3$>$H to cellular protein. *J Cell Biol* 34:525, 1967.
40. Spilberg I, Mandell B, Mehta J, et al: Mechanism of action of colchicine in acute urate crystal-induced arthritis. *J Clin Invest* 64:775, 1979.
41. Wallace SL, Bernstein D, Diamond H: Diagnostic value of the colchicine therapeutic trial. *JAMA* 199:525, 1967.

42. Wallace SL: Colchicine. *Semin Arthritis Rheum* 3:369, 1974.
43. Carr AA: Colchicine toxicity. *Arch Intern Med* 115:29, 1965.
44. Davis JS Jr, Bartfield H: The effect of intravenous colchicine on acute gout. *Am J Med* 16:218, 1954.
45. Dixon WE, Malden W: Colchicine with special reference to its mode of action on bone marrow. *J Physiol* 37:50, 1908.
46. Brenner BM, Rector PC: *The Kidney,* ed 2. Philadelphia, W.B. Saunders, 1981, p 2680.
47. Kelley WN, Harris ED, Ruddy S, et al (eds): *Textbook of Rheumatology.* Philadelphia, W.B. Saunders, 1981, p 1421.
48. Johnson HP Jr, Engleman EP, Forsham PH, et al: Effects of phenylbutazone in gout. *N Engl J Med* 250:665, 1954.
49. Mauer EF: The toxic effects of phenylbutazone (butazolidin): Review of the literature and report of the twenty-third death following its use. *N Engl J Med* 253:404, 1955.
50. Gilman AG, Goodman LS, Gilman A (eds): *Goodman and Gilman's The Pharmacological Basis of Therapeutics,* ed 6. New York, Macmillan, 1980, p 700.
51. Simon LS, Mills JA: Nonsteroidal antiinflammatory drugs. *N Engl J Med* 302:1179, 1237, 1980.
52. Schoen RT, Vender RJ: Mechanisms of nonsteroidal antiinflammatory drug-induced gastric damage. *Am J Med* 86:449, 1989.
53. Roth SH: NSAID and gastropathy. *J Rheumatol* 15:912, 1988.
54. Shack ME: Drug-induced ulceration and perforation of the small intestine. *Arizona Med* 23:517, 1966.
55. O'Brien WM: Indomethacin: A survey of clinical trials. *Clin Pharmacol Ther* 9:94, 1968.
56. Dunn JJ, Zambraski EJ: Renal effects of drugs that inhibit prostaglandin synthesis. *Kidney Int* 18:609, 1980.
57. Clive DM, Stoff JS: Renal syndromes associated with nonsteroidal antiinflammatory drugs. *N Engl J Med* 310:563, 1984.
58. Brezin JH, Katz SM, Schwartz AB, Chinitz JL: Reversible renal failure and nephrotic syndrome associated with nonsteroidal antiinflammatory drugs. *N Engl J Med* 301:1271, 1979.
59. Garella S, Matarese RA: Renal effects of prostaglandins and clinical adverse effects of nonsteroidal antiinflammatory agents. *Medicine* 63:165, 1984.
60. Adams DH, Michael J, Bacon PA, et al: Nonsteroidal antiinflammatory drugs and renal failure. *Lancet* 1:57, 1986.
61. Bunning RD, Barth WF: Sulindac. A potentially renal-sparing nonsteroidal anti-inflammatory drug. *JAMA* 248:2864, 1982.
62. McCarty DJ, Kohn NN, Faires JS: The significance of calcium phosphate crystals in the synovial fluid of arthritic patients: The "pseudo gout syndrome": I. Clinical aspects. *Ann Intern Med* 56:711, 1962.
63. Schumacher HR: Pathogenesis of crystal-induced synovitis. *Clin Rheum Dis* 3:105, 1977.
64. Dieppe PA, Crocker P, Huskisson EC, et al: Apatite deposition disease. A new arthropathy. *Lancet* 1:266, 1976.
65. Schumacher HR, Smolyo AP, Tse RL, et al: Arthritis associated with apatite crystals. *Ann Intern Med* 87:411, 1977.
66. Hoffman G, Schumacher HR, Paul H, et al: Calcium oxalate microcrystalline associated arthritis in end stage renal disease. *Ann Intern Med* 97:36, 1982.
67. Caswell A, Guilland-Cumming DF, Hearn PR, et al: Pathogenesis of chondrocalcinosis and pseudogout. Metabolism of inorganic pyrophosphate and production of calcium pyrophosphate dehydrate crystals. *Ann Rheum Dis* (Suppl) 42:27, 1983.
68. Schumacher HR, Tse R, Reginato AJ, et al: Hydroxyapatite-like crystals in synovial fluid and cell vacuoles: A suspected new cause for crystal-induced arthritis. *Arthritis Rheum* 19:821, 1976.
69. O'Duffy JD: Clinical studies of acute pseudogout attacks. Comments on prevalence, predispositions and treatment. *Arthritis Rheum* 19:349, 1976.
70. McCarty DJ: Calcium pyrophosphate dihydrate crystal deposition disease 1975. *Arthritis Rheum* 19:275, 1975.
71. Chalmers A, Reynolds WJ, Oreopoulos DG, et al: The arthropathy of maintenance intermittent peritoneal dialysis. *Can Med Assoc J* 123:635, 1980.
72. Kelley WN, Harris ED, Ruddy S, et al (eds): *Textbook of Rheumatology.* Philadelphia, W.B. Saunders, 1981, p 1452.
73. Ho G Jr, Su EY: Therapy for septic arthritis. *JAMA* 247:797, 1982.
74. Argen RJ, Wilson CH, Wood P: Suppurative arthritis. Clinical features of 42 cases. *Arch Intern Med* 117:661, 1966.

75. Willkens RF, Healey LA, Decker JL: Acute infectious arthritis in the aged and chronically ill. *Arch Intern Med* 106:354, 1960.
76. Douglas GW, Levin RH, Sokoloff L: Infectious arthritis complicating neoplastic disease. *N Engl J Med* 270:299, 1964.
77. Fainstein V, Gilmore C, Hopfer RL, et al: Septic arthritis due to *Candida* species in patients with cancer: Report of five cases and review of the literature. *Rev Infect Dis* 4:78, 1982.
78. Myers AR, Mills JA, Ropes MW: The problem of infection in systemic lupus erythematosus. *Arthritis Rheum* 10:300, 1967.
79. Myers AR, Miller LM, Pinals RS: Pyarthrosis complicating rheumatoid arthritis. *Lancet* 2:714, 1960.
80. Vincenti F, Amend WJ, Feduska NJ, et al: Septic arthritis following renal transplantation. *Nephron* 30:253, 1982.
81. Inman RD, Gallegos KV, Barry BD, et al: Clinical and microbial features of prosthetic joint infection. *Am J Med* 77:47, 1984.
82. Curtess PH Jr: The pathophysiology of joint infections. *Clin Orthop* 96:129, 1973.
83. Goldenberg DL, Cohen AS: Acute infectious arthritis. A review of patients with nongonococcal joint infections (with emphasis on therapy and prognosis). *Am J Med* 60:369, 1976.
84. Newman JH: Review of septic arthritis throughout the antibiotic era. *Ann Rheum Dis* 35:198, 1976.
85. Ward J, Cohen AS, Bauer W: The diagnosis and therapy of acute suppurative arthritis. *Arthritis Rheum* 3:522, 1960.
86. Rytel MW: Microbial antigen detection in infectious arthritis. *Clin Rheum Dis* 4:83, 1978.
87. Gupta RC, Steigerwald JC: Nitroblue tetrazolium test in the diagnosis of pyogenic arthritis. *Ann Intern Med* 80:723, 1974.
88. Riley TV: Synovial fluid lactic acid levels in septic arthritis. *Pathology* 12:69, 1981.
89. Behn AR, Matthews JA, Phillips I: Lactate UV-system: A rapid method for diagnosis of septic arthritis. *Ann Rheum Dis* 40:489, 1981.
90. Riordan T, Doyle D, Tabaqchali S: Synovial fluid lactic acid measurement in the diagnosis and management of septic arthritis. *J Clin Pathol* 35:390, 1982.
91. Noyes FR, McCabe JD, Fekety FR: Acute *Candida* arthritis. *J Bone Joint Surg* [Am] 55:169, 1973.
92. Schmid FR, Parker RH: Ongoing assessment of therapy in septic arthritis. *Arthritis Rheum* 12:529, 1969.
93. McGlaughlin GE, McCarty DJ Jr, Segal BL: Hemarthrosis complicating anticoagulant therapy. Report of three cases. *JAMA* 196:1020, 1966.
94. Wild JH, Zvaifler NJ: Hemarthrosis associated with sodium warfarin therapy. *Arthritis Rheum* 19:98, 1976.
95. Hasselbacher P, Schimmer BM, Weinberger A: Hemarthrosis with sodium warfarin and heparin, (letter). *Arthritis Rheum* 21:740, 1978.
96. McCarty DJ: Synovial fluid, in McCarty DJ (ed): *Arthritis and Allied Conditions,* ed 9. Philadelphia, Lea & Febiger, 1979, p 51.
97. Upchurch KS, Levine PH: Hemophiliac arthropathy, in Kelley WN, Harris ED Jr, Ruddy S, Sledge C (eds): *Textbook of Rheumatology.* Philadelphia, W.B. Saunders, 1989, p 1629.
98. Kozin F, McCarty DJ, Sims J, et al: The reflux sympathetic dystrophy syndrome: I. Clinical and histologic studies: Evidence for bilaterality, response to corticosteroids and articular involvement. *Am J Med* 60:321, 1976.
99. Johnson AC: Disabling changes in the hands resembling sclerodactylia following myocardial infarction. *Ann Intern Med* 19:433, 1943.
100. Steinbrocker O, Spitzer N, Friedman HH: Shoulder-hand syndrome in reflex dystrophy of the upper extremity. *Ann Intern Med* 29:22, 1947.
101. Rosen PS, Graham W: The shoulder-hand syndrome. Historical review with observations on seventy-three patients. *Can Med Assoc J* 77:86, 1957.
102. Steinbrocker O, Argyros TG: The shoulder-hand syndrome: Present status as a diagnostic and therapeutic entity. *Med Clin North Am* 42:1533, 1958.
103. Kozin F, Genant HK, Bekerman C, et al: The reflex sympathetic dystrophy syndrome: II. Roentgenographic and scintigraphic evidence of bilaterality and of periarticular accentuation. *Am J Med* 60:332, 1976.
104. Kozin F, Ryan LM, Carerra GF, et al: The reflex sympathetic dys-

trophy syndrome (RSDS): III. Scintigraphic studies, further evidence for the therapeutic efficacy of systemic corticosteroids, and proposed diagnostic criteria. *Am J Med* 70:23, 1981.

105. Holloway NM: *Nursing the Critically Ill Adult.* Menlo Park, Calif, Addison-Wesley, 1979, p 455.
106. Kottke FJ: Deterioration of the bedfast patient: Causes and effects. *Public Health Rep* 80:437, 1965.
107. Kelley WN, Harris ED, Ruddy S, et al (eds): *Textbook of Rheumatology.* Philadelphia, W.B. Saunders, 1981, p 406.
108. Kottke F: Therapeutic exercise, in Knisen F, Kottke F, Ellwood P

(eds): *Handbook of Physiology and Rehabilitation.* Philadelphia, J.B. Lippincott, 1971, p 365.
109. Stryker RP: *Rehabilitative Aspects of Acute and Chronic Nursing Care.* Philadelphia, W.B. Saunders, 1972, p 127.
110. Meunier P, Courpron P, Edouard C, et al: Physiological senile involution and pathological rarefraction of bone. *Clin Endocrinol Metab* 2:239, 1973.
111. Nagant de Deauxchaisnes C, Krane SM: Paget's disease of bone: Clinical and metabolic observations. *Medicine* 43:233, 1964.

217. Anaphylaxis

Helen M. Hollingsworth,
David F. Giansiracusa,
and Katherine S. Upchurch

Introduction

Anaphylaxis is the most severe and potentially fatal form of the immediate hypersensitivity reactions. The term *anaphylaxis* (antiphylaxis) is derived from the Greek and means *"against protection"* [1]. It describes the shocklike state that is caused by contact with a substance and contrasts with the term *prophylaxis,* which denotes a beneficial or protective state that results from contact with a substance [2].

The clinical features of the anaphylactic reactions are the physiologic sequelae of release of chemical mediators from tissue-based mast cells and circulating basophils and include a potential for life-threatening vascular collapse and respiratory obstruction [3–5]. A clinically and physiologically indistinguishable hypersensitivity reaction, which is called an *anaphylactoid reaction,* differs from anaphylactic reactions only because the chemical mediators are released by nonimmunologic mechanisms. Since the clinical features are indistinguishable, both will be referred to collectively as *anaphylactic reactions* [6].

Pathophysiology of Anaphylactic Reactions

MECHANISMS OF RELEASE OF CHEMICAL MEDIATORS. In humans, anaphylaxis involves a series of steps that result in the release of chemical mediators from tissue-based mast cells and circulating basophils. First, contact with an antigen stimulates the generation of antibodies of the immunoglobulin E (IgE) class (Fig. 217-1). Specific Fab binding sites on the IgE molecules recognize the antigen. Next, the IgE molecules bind by way of their Fc receptor to a glycoprotein receptor on the cell-surface membrane of tissue mast cells and blood-borne basophils that are called *target cells,* and as such, the IgE molecules are called *cytotropic antibodies* [4,7].

As many as 7000 to 100,000 IgE molecules will normally bind to a single target cell, and up to 100,000 to 500,000 in atopic individuals [8,9]. This binding may remain for weeks to months

[9]. When two IgE molecules with the same Fab binding specificity are in close proximity on the surface of mast cells and basophils, the cells are termed *sensitized.* In contrast to this process of active sensitization, an individual's mast cells and basophils may be passively sensitized by the transfusion of IgE that is reactive to a specific antigen [10].

Mast cells and basophils share many characteristics including high-affinity receptors for IgE, certain cell-staining properties, and many of the same chemical mediators. However, it is likely that mast cells and basophils are derived from different bone marrow progenitor cells, as evidenced by the presence of major basic protein and lysophospholipase in basophils and eosinophils but not in mast cells.

In order for a subsequent exposure to the antigen to stimulate the release of mediators from mast cells and basophils, the antigen must bind to the Fab portion of two IgE molecules fixed to the surface of the target cell [7,8,11,12]. This bridging of two IgE molecules initiates a series of biochemical modifications called the *activation-secretion response* (Fig. 217-2). This sequence activates secretion of preformed primary mediators of anaphylaxis from cytoplasmic granules in target cells, including histamine, serotonin, eosinophil chemotactic factor of anaphylaxis (ECF-A), heparin, neutrophil chemotactic factor, and proteolytic enzymes that include tryptase (Table 217-1) [13].

The activation-secretion response also stimulates synthesis of kallikrein [14,15] and newly generated, secondary lipid mediators, which include platelet-activating factor (PAF) [12]; prostaglandin D_2 (PGD_2), a product of the cyclooxygenase pathway of arachidonic acid metabolism [16,17]; and leukotrienes C_4, D_4, and E_4 (LTC_4, LTD_4 and LTE_4), products of the lipoxygenase pathway of arachidonic acid metabolism [8]. LTC_4, LTD_4, and LTE_4 are chemically identical to slow-reacting substance of anaphylaxis (SRS-A) [8,18]. Several cytokines are also released after activation, including interleukins (IL-1, IL-2, IL-3, IL-4, IL-5, and IL-6), tumor necrosis factor, endothelin-1, and granulocyte-macrophage colony stimulating factor [18a].

The release of mediators from mast cells and basophils is modulated by cyclic adenosine monophosphate (cyclic AMP), which suppresses mediator release, and cyclic guanosine monophosphate (cyclic GMP), which enhances mediator release [19]. The substances that elevate intracellular levels of cyclic

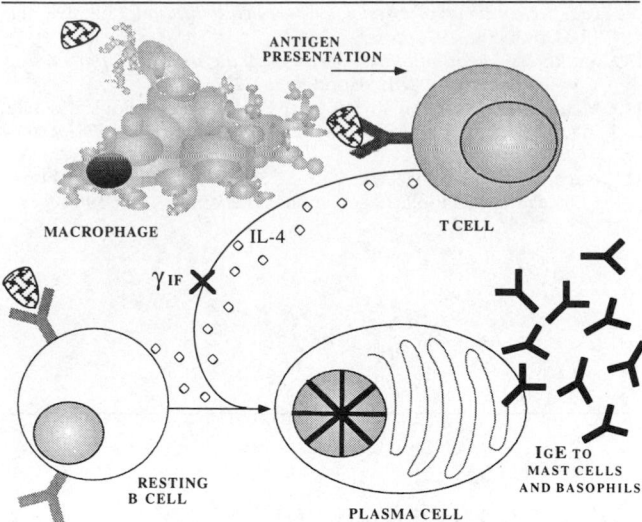

Fig. 217-1. Immunoglobulin E (IgE) production. The sensitization process that results in production of antigen-specific IgE antibody begins with antigen processing by the antigen presenting cell (APC), usually a macrophage, and subsequent display of the antigenic determinants to T lymphocytes. The T lymphocytes then secrete interleukin-4 (IL-4) and probably other cytokines that cause precursor B cells to mature into plasma cells that are able to secrete antigen-specific IgE antibodies. These antibodies attach to receptors on the surface of mast cells and circulating basophils. Interferon-γ can inhibit the switch to E heavy chain and favor the selection of other isotypes. Other cytokines, such as IgE-potentiating factor and IgE-suppressive factor, may influence the maturation process.

AMP, such as beta-adrenergic agonists (epinephrine) and prostaglandins of the E series, will inhibit mediator release, while the substances that increase intracellular cyclic GMP levels, such as adenosine, cholinergic agents, and possibly alpha-adrenergic agonists, will augment mediator release [12,20,21]. A variety of substances may induce IgE antibody formation and, on subsequent challenge, provoke anaphylactic reactions (Table 217-2) [22]. The most common substances are drugs, insect venoms, foods, and allergen extracts used in hyposensitization therapy [4,23].

Anaphylactic reactions have also been reported as a result of treatment with suxamethonium [29,30], alcuronium [31], hydrocortisone [32], thiopentone [33], and thiopental sodium [34] and have occurred after coitus due to contact with semen [35] and as a result of physical stress, such as immersion in cold water [36] or vigorous exercise [37].

Clinically significant examples of non-IgE-mediated anaphylaxis include those associated with blood product transfusion in IgA-deficient individuals, cuprophane membrane exposure during dialysis, nonsteroidal antiinflammatory drugs (NSAIDs), narcotics, and intravascular radiographic contrast media (Table 217-3). Administration of blood, serum, or immunoglobulins to patients who are IgA-deficient can result in immune complex formation between donor IgA and recipient IgG anti-IgA antibodies [6,38]. These immune complexes can then fix complement, causing activation of the complement cascade with release of the C3a and C5a complement fragments. C3a and C5a are *anaphylatoxins* and can directly activate mast cells and basophils. It is presumed that polysaccharide in the cuprophane membrane activates complement with release of anaphylatoxins [6,39].

In addition to stimulating mediator release from target cells,

Table 217-1. Mediators of Human Mast Cells and Basophils

	Mast cell	Basophil
Preformed		
Histamine	+	+
Neutrophil chemotactic factor	+	+
Eosinophil chemotactic factor	+	+
Lysosomal hydrolases (e.g. hexosaminidase, glucuronidase, arylsulfatase)	+	+
Newly generated		
Sulfidopeptides LTC$_4$, LTD$_4$, LTE$_4$, LTB$_4$	+	+
Prostaglandins (mainly PGD$_2$)	+	−
Thromboxane A$_2$	+	?
Monohydroxyeicosatetranoic acids	+	?
PAF	+	?
Adenosine	+	?
Free oxygen radicals	+	?
Granule matrix constituents		
Heparin	+	−
Chondroitin sulfate	−	+
Tryptase, chymotryptic proteinase	+	−
Kallikrein	+	+

LTC$_4$, LTD$_4$, LTE$_4$, and LTB$_4$ = leukotrienes C$_4$, D$_4$, E$_4$, and B$_4$; PGD$_2$ = prostaglandin D$_2$; PAF = platelet-activating factor; + = mediator present; − = mediator absent.
Source: Adapted from Alam R. Role of mast cells and basophils in human disease. Insights into Allergy 2:1–5, 1987.

Table 217-2. Cause of IgE-Mediated Anaphylaxis

Type	Agent	Example
Proteins	Allergen extracts	Pollen, dust mite, mold
	Enzymes	Chymopapain, streptokinase, L-asparginase
	Food	Egg white, legumes, milk, nuts, celery, shellfish, psyllium
	Heterologous serum	Tetanus antitoxin [23], antithymocyte globulin, snake antivenom
	Hormones	Insulin [24], ACTH, TSH [23], insulin, progesterone, salmon calcitonin
	Vaccines	Influenza
	Venoms	Hymenoptera
	Others	Heparin, latex [25], thiobarbiturates, seminal fluid
Haptens	Antibiotics	Beta-lactams [27], ethambutol, nitrofurantoin sulfonamides [28], streptomycin, vancomycin [28]
	Disinfectants	Ethylene oxide
	Local anesthetics [28]*	Benzocaine, tetracaine, xylocaine, mepivicaine
	Others	Aminopyrine, sulfobromophthalein

ACTH = adrenocorticotropic hormone; TSH = thyroid-stimulating hormone.
*Precise mechanism not established.

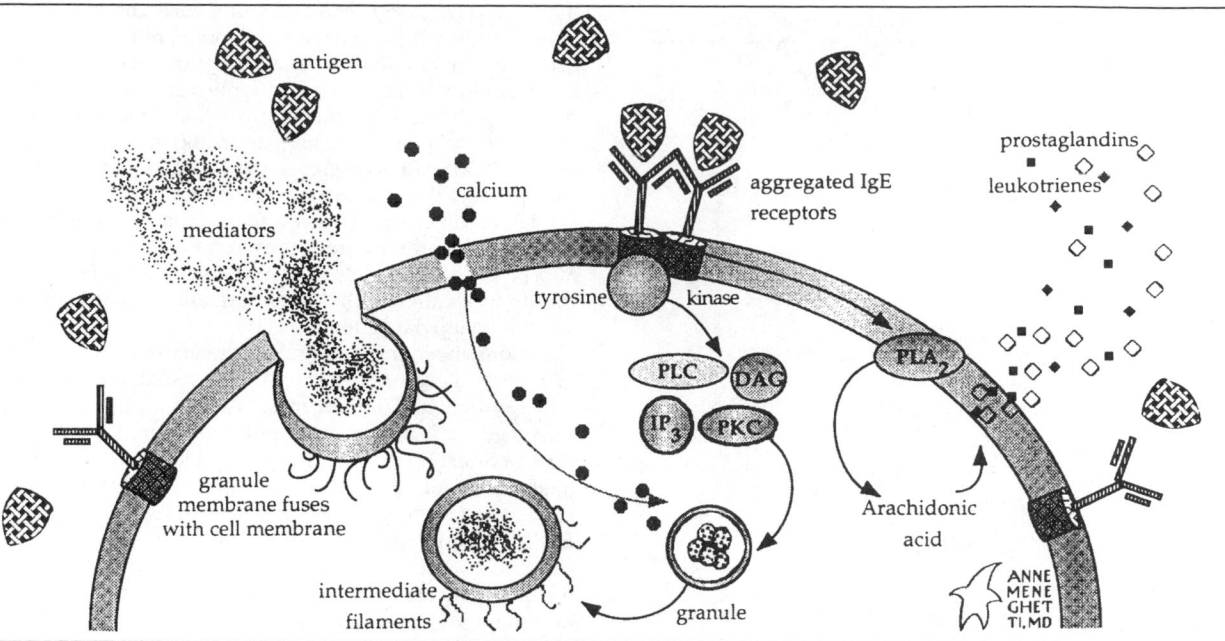

Fig. 217-2. Chemical mediator release. When two immunoglobulin E (IgE) molecules are bridged by an antigen that is specifically recognized by those IgE molecules, a cascade of transmembrane and then intracellular events is triggered. The end result is the extrusion of granule contents (mediators) into the extracellular space and elaboration of other, newly formed mediators. The intricate details of this process are not completely understood. Tyrosine kinase appears to be an important intramembrane messenger that initiates the intracellular cascades. At least one cascade involves phospholipase C (PLC), which mediates calcium influx into the cell and catalyzes hydrolysis of phosphatidylinositol into the secondary messengers 1, 4, 5-triphosphate (IP3) and 1,2-diacylglycerol (DAG). IP3 plays a role in calcium mobilization; DAG mediates production of arachidonic acid metabolites and activates protein kinase C (PKC). PKC, in turn, participates in fusion of granules with the cell membrane. Phospholipase A2 (PLA2) mediates the conversion of membrane phospholipid into arachidonic acid, resulting in elaboration of prostaglandins and leukotrienes.

C5a is also chemotactic for neutrophils and immunocytes [40]. Neutrophils may contribute to anaphylactic reactions by releasing mediators during ingestion of immune complexes [41]. Mononuclear cells may similarly liberate chemical mediators during cellular hypersensitivity reactions [23].

Medications, such as NSAIDs and narcotics, and diagnostic agents, such as radiographic contrast media, are clinically important agents that may precipitate anaphylactic reactions by causing direct mast cell activation with release of chemical mediators [28,40–54] or by causing generation of leukotrienes (Table 217-4) [55–60]. Anaphylaxis may also be idiopathic [61,62].

PHYSIOLOGIC PROPERTIES OF THE CHEMICAL MEDIATORS OF ANAPHYLAXIS.
The most important chemical mediators of anaphylaxis are histamine, leukotrienes LTC_4, LTD_4 and LTE_4, PAF, and bradykinin. Physiologically, these substances act to increase arteriolar vasodilatation, to enhance capillary permeability, and to precipitate bronchiolar constriction [5,63].

Histamine, a bioactive amine, is released as a preformed substance from mast cell and basophil granules by the process of exocytosis [64]. Histamine acts to (1) increase capillary permeability by stimulating terminal arteriolar dilatation and contraction of endothelial cells in postcapillary venules, which opens intercellular gaps [21,65] and, as a result, causes the development of urticaria and angioedema [57]; (2) increase secretion from nasal and bronchial mucous glands [4]; (3) stimulate contraction of smooth muscle [7,12]; (4) enhance prostaglandin synthesis; (5) chemotactically modulate eosinophil migration; and (6) regulate parasympathetic afferent nerve stimulation (a process blocked by atropine), which increases airway resistance and decreases lung compliance [66].

Studies of histamine infusion in normal human volunteers suggest that vasodilatation is mediated by both H_1 and H_2 receptors, whereas bronchoconstriction and tachycardia are mediated by H_1 receptors alone [67].

As noted previously, SRS-A is now recognized as a group of acidic lipopeptides, specifically LTC_4, LTD_4, and LTE_4 [68,69]. Unlike histamine, which exists preformed in the intracellular granules, LTC_4, LTD_4, and LTE_4 are synthesized at the cell membrane, following activation of the mast cell or basophil by either IgE- or non-IgE-mediated mechanisms [70–72]. Once activation of mast cells or basophils occurs, membrane phospholipids are methylated by methyltransferases, which results in opening of membrane calcium channels and in an increase in intracellular calcium. This then activates the calcium-dependent enzyme phospholipase A2, which releases arachidonic acid from the membrane phospholipids. Arachidonic acid is then oxygenated by either cyclooxygenase to form prostaglandins or by lipoxygenase to form leukotrienes. Although our understanding of the myriad SRS-A activities is incomplete, in anaphylaxis these activities are believed to (1) induce a prolonged constrictive effect preferentially on bronchial smooth muscle, which affects the peripheral more than the central airways [73], (2) increase vascular permeability, and (3) act as chemotactic agents for other inflammatory cells [74].

Two additional modulators of anaphylaxis are bradykinin, which appears to be activated by mast cell kallikrein, and PAF. Bradykinin is a nine-amino-acid peptide that stimulates pain

Table 217-3. Causes of Non-IgE-mediated Anaphylaxis

Complement activation
    Blood product transfusion in IgA-deficient patient [41A]
    Hemodialysis with cuprophane membrane
Direct release of chemical mediators of anaphylaxis
    Protamine [42,43]*
    Radiographic contrast media [44,45]
    Dextran [46–49]*
    Hydroxyethyl starch [49]
    Muscle relaxants [50,51]
    Ketamine [52]
    Local anesthetics [28]*
    Codeine and other opiate narcotics [53,54]
    Highly charged antibiotics, including amphotericin B [28]
Generation of leukotrienes
    Nonsteroidal anti-inflammatory drugs [55]
    Indomethacin [56]
    Acetylsalicylic acid [57]
    Mefenamic acid [56]
    Sulindac [58]
    Zomepirac sodium [54]
    Tolmetin sodium [60]
Other
    Antineoplastic agents
    Sulfiting agents
    Exercise [37]
    Idiopathic recurrent anaphylaxis [61,62]

*Precise mechanism not established.

Table 217-4. Pathologic Events in Anaphylaxis

Bronchial muscle contraction	Histamine (H₁ response), leukotrienes C₄, D₄, E₄, acetylcholine, bradykinin
Mucosal edema	Histamine (H₁ response), leukotrienes C₄, D₄, E₄, prostaglandin E₂
Eosinophil infiltrate	Histamine (H₂ response), ECF-A, PAF
Neutrophil infiltration	NCF-A, granule-derived inflammatory factors of anaphylaxis
Mucus secretion	Histamine (H₂ response), acetylcholine, alpha-adrenergic agonists, prostaglandins, PAF
Desquamation	Hydrogen peroxide (H₂O₂), hydroxyl groups (OH), proteolytic enzymes
Basement membrane thickening	O₂⁻, proteolytic enzymes

ECF-A = eosinophil chemotactic factor of anaphylaxis; NCF-A = neutrophil chemotactic factor of anaphylaxis.
Source: Adapted from Mathews KP: Respiratory atopic disease. *JAMA* 248:2587, 1982.

fibers and a slow, sustained contraction of bronchial and vascular smooth muscles while increasing vascular permeability and secretion from mucous glands [4]. PAF contributes to the pulmonary and cardiovascular manifestations of anaphylaxis [75] by inducing platelet aggregation with release of serotonin, adenosine triphosphate, and lysosomal enzymes from preformed granules [76,77]. In vitro studies have shown that platelets are an essential ingredient in PAF-induced bronchoconstriction. It is not known whether this is due to the role of platelet-derived thromboxane A₂, serotonin, or a lipoxygenase product [72]. In addition, PAF is a potent chemotactic factor for eosinophils and can directly increase vascular permeability [72].

Thus, the physiologic consequences of chemical-mediator release in anaphylaxis are (1) an increased vascular permeability; (2) an increased secretion from nasal and bronchiolar mucous glands; (3) smooth-muscle contraction in the blood vessels, the bronchioles, the gastrointestinal tract, and the uterus; (4) migration-attraction of eosinophils and neutrophils; (5) bradykinin generation stimulated by kallikrein substances; and (6) induction of platelet aggregation and degranulation. These events coordinate to increase the vascular permeability that in turn permits the access of a variety of plasma proteins (antibodies, complement, kinins, and coagulation proteins) to tissue sites, which further contributes to the observed inflammation. Substances such as PAF and Hageman factor potentially contribute to local coagulation abnormalities, which may also be seen in anaphylactic reactions [5].

Various mechanisms regulate the activity of these chemical mediators. Recall that cyclic AMP is capable of inhibiting the release of chemical mediators. Thus, in a process termed *negative feedback,* histamine stimulates generation of cyclic AMP, down-regulating further mediator release. A second control mechanism relates to the digestion of mediators by enzymes released from eosinophils that are attracted to target sites by ECF-A [78] and PAF released by mast cells. Eosinophils synthesize and release several products, including (1) arylsulfatase B, which inactivates SRS-A [79]; (2) histaminase, which digests histamine [80]; and (3) phospholipase D, which destroys the activity of PAF [81].

Clinical and Laboratory Features

Urticaria, angioedema, respiratory obstruction, and vascular collapse are the major clinical features of anaphylaxis. These signs and symptoms are due to the direct effects of the chemical mediators released in anaphylaxis on target tissues (see Table 217-4). One marker that correlates well with the severity and duration of anaphylactic reactions is plasma histamine activity [82].

Mast cells are concentrated in the skin, in the mucous membranes of the respiratory and gastrointestinal tracts, and in the perivenular tissue, while basophils are located in the bloodstream. Thus, these target cells are in proximity to sites of exposure to offending antigens (e.g., drugs, diagnostic agents), which may precipitate anaphylactic reactions [17]. Because mast cells are found predominantly in skin and mucous membranes, these organ systems are commonly affected by anaphylactic reactions. Although the respiratory tract and the skin are the most commonly involved target organs in humans, other organ systems, such as the heart, blood vessels, gastrointestinal tract, and genitourinary system, or other structures rich in tissue-fixed mast cells, may be involved [83]. Table 217-5 lists the clinical manifestations of anaphylactic reactions.

Urticarial eruptions are the most common manifestation of anaphylaxis in humans [5]. Other clinical manifestations may include (1) a sense of fright or impending doom, (2) weakness, (3) sweating, (4) sneezing, (5) rhinorrhea, (6) conjunctivitis, (7) generalized pruritus and swelling, (8) cough, (9) wheezing or breathlessness, (10) choking, (11) dysphagia, (12) vomiting, (13) abdominal pain, (14) incontinence, and (15) loss of consciousness [1,18]. Profound hypotension and shock may develop as a result of significant arteriolar vasodilatation, increased vascular permeability, cardiac arrhythmias [84,85], or irreversible cardiac failure [86], even in the absence of respiratory or other symptoms [5,77,87]. Furthermore, transient or sustained hypotension may result in local tissue ischemia, stroke, myocardial infarction, or death [77,87]. Uterine cramps [4] and intravascular coagulation, evidenced by a fall in the levels of

Table 217-5. Clinical Manifestations of Anaphylactic Reactions

System	Reaction	Symptoms	Signs
Respiratory tract	Rhinitis	Nasal congestion and itching	Mucosal edema
	Laryngeal edema	Dyspnea	Laryngeal stridor, edema of vocal cords
	Bronchospasm	Cough, wheezing, sensation of chest tightness	Crackles, respiratory distress, tachypnea, wheezes
Cardiovascular	Hypotension	Syncope, feeling of faintness	Hypotension, tachycardia
	Arrhythmias	Palpitations	ECG changes: nonspecific S–T segment and T-wave changes, nodal rhythm, atrial fibrillation
Skin	Urticaria	Pruritus, hives	Urticarial lesions
	Angioedema	Nonpruritic swelling of extremity or peri-oral or periorbital region	Nonpruritic, frequently asymmetric swelling of extremity, perioral or periorbital region
Gastrointestinal tract	Smooth muscle contraction Mucosal edema	Nausea, vomiting, abdominal pain, diarrhea	Abdominal tenderness, distention
Eye	Conjunctivitis	Ocular itching, lacrimation	Conjunctival inflammation

Source: Adapted from Kelly JF, Patterson R: Anaphylaxis: Course, mechanisms and treatment. *JAMA* 227:1431, 1974.

factors V, VIII, fibrinogen, kininogen, and complement components, have also been described [82].

Anaphylacsis-induced fatalities most often result from involvement of the respiratory tract [77]. The structures throughout the respiratory tract may be affected, but respiratory failure is generally the result of (1) upper respiratory tract obstruction due to laryngeal edema, or (2) obstruction of small airways due to bronchospasm, mucosal edema, and hypersecretion of mucus [77,88]. An intraalveolar hemorrhage may occur that is associated with pulmonary infiltrates [89]. Anaphylaxis may even present as the shock-lung syndrome [90]. The less severe respiratory symptoms include nasal congestion, profuse rhinorrhea, hypopharyngeal edema, and intense pruritus [4].

The physical examination of a patient with anaphylactic shock often reveals a rapid, weak, irregular, or unobtainable pulse; tachypnea, respiratory distress, cyanosis, hoarseness, stridor, or dysphagia secondary to laryngeal edema; diminished breath sounds, crackles, cough, wheezes, and hyperinflated lungs due to severe bronchoconstriction; urticaria; angioedema or conjunctival edema (see Table 217-5) [83]. Any individual patient, though, may manifest only a subset of these findings, perhaps only cardiovascular collapse or only stridor and breathlessness.

Laboratory findings in anaphylaxis include a variety of electrocardiographic abnormalities such as disturbances in rate, rhythm, repolarization, and ectopy [84,85,91,92]. Biochemical abnormalities in anaphylaxis include elevation of blood histamine levels, depression of serum complement components, and decreased levels of high-molecular-weight kininogen [87].

Clinical Course of Anaphylactic Reactions

The characteristic features of anaphylactic reactions are (1) the rapid onset of clinical manifestations that follow the administration of, or the contact with, antigen (or other provocative substances) and (2) the rapid progression of symptoms to a severe and sometimes fatal outcome. Recognition of the early signs and symptoms of anaphylaxis and prompt treatment may prevent progression to irreversible shock and death [93].

The development of clinical symptoms as well as their severity and duration is variable but will depend to some extent on the mode of antigen exposure. Anaphylaxis may occur within seconds following parenteral introduction of antigen [82,94] and usually occurs within 30 minutes. In contrast, anaphylaxis that follows oral administration of an antigen may develop within minutes to several hours [83]. Generally, the more rapid the onset of symptoms, the more severe will be the reaction [1]. Mild systemic reactions often last for several hours, rarely more than 24 hours. Severe manifestations, such as laryngeal edema, bronchoconstriction, and hypotension, if not fatal, may persist or recur for several days. Surprisingly, however, even severe manifestations may resolve within minutes of treatment [83].

Pathologic examinations of patients with fatal anaphylactic reactions due to respiratory compromise have revealed upper airway edema, peribronchial congestion, submucosal edema, air trapping, bronchiole luminal secretions, and eosinophilic infiltration of the hypopharynx, the trachea, and the pulmonary interstitium [77,88]. Postmortem examinations performed on individuals who died of nonrespiratory manifestations of anaphylaxis have demonstrated marked congestion of visceral structures [5].

Diagnosis and Differential Diagnosis of Anaphylaxis

The development of the characteristic clinical features (see Table 217-5) shortly after exposure to an antigen or other inciting agent usually establishes the diagnosis of an anaphylactic reaction. The setting is often suggestive as well: a patient who has just received an antibiotic injection or radiographic contrast media infusion or who presents to the emergency room after a yellow jacket sting.

The clinical disorders that may be confused with anaphylaxis are (1) sudden, acute bronchoconstriction in an asthmatic, (2) vasovagal syncope, (3) tension pneumothorax, (4) mechanical airway obstruction, (5) pulmonary edema, (6) cardiac arrhythmias, (7) myocardial infarction with cardiogenic shock, (8) aspiration of a food bolus, (9) pulmonary embolism, (10) seizures, (11) acute drug toxicity, (12) hereditary angioedema, (13) cold or idiopathic urticaria, (14) septic shock, and (15) toxic shock [4].

Initial laboratory testing is often not helpful. Serum obtained during the acute episode can be assayed subsequently for tryptase and histamine. The presence of these mediators would support a diagnosis of anaphylaxis. Retrospectively, specific skin tests may define the allergic sensitivity, but they must be done in a carefully controlled setting due to the risk of provoking another severe reaction. The measurement of specific IgE antibodies by a radioallergosorbent test (RAST) may indicate sensitization [95].

Treatment of Anaphylaxis

The treatment of anaphylaxis consists primarily of preventive measures, specifically, the avoidance of known precipitants. Once symptoms ensue, however, measures to support cardiopulmonary function are critical, including the aggressive use of pressors, fluid replacement, and medications to counteract the effects of released chemical mediators [96]. Injectable epinephrine, tourniquets, intravenous infusion materials and fluids, antihistamines, intubation equipment, a tracheostomy set, and individuals trained to use these materials should be available. Since symptoms of a systemic anaphylactic reaction may be followed by potentially fatal manifestations, patients must be serially monitored [83]. Many therapeutic and diagnostic agents frequently employed in intensive care settings may induce anaphylactic reactions. Thus, the anticipation and the preparedness to deal with these potential reactions are very important.

EMERGENCY MEASURES. The evaluation of individuals who are suspected of having anaphylaxis must be performed rapidly. The cause and mechanism of antigen exposure should be ascertained in order to accurately assess how long the inciting antigen has been present and, when possible, to limit further absorption. The more immediate the reaction after antigen exposure, the more severe the reaction is likely to be. A history of prior allergic reactions and former treatment may help to guide immediate therapy, obviating the need to try previously failed regimens in a life-threatening situation [36].

Supportive Cardiopulmonary Measures. Particular attention to the respiratory and cardiovascular systems is paramount and must include watching for the development of laryngeal edema and bronchoconstriction as well as monitoring the arterial blood gases, blood pressure, and cardiac rhythm [36]. Close electrocardiographic monitoring is essential because both the sequelae of anaphylaxis and its therapy are potentially arrhythmogenic [91]. For example, hypotension, acidosis, hypoxia, pressors, and bronchodilators may all increase the risk of cardiac arrhythmias (see Chap. 49).

The maintenance of an adequate airway and ventilation are essential. Supplemental oxygen should be administered. Intubation and assisted ventilation may be necessary in cases of severe bronchospasm (see Chap. 1). Although intubation is usually feasible, edema of the tongue, larynx, or vocal cords may obstruct the upper airway and preclude oropharyngeal or nasopharyngeal intubation. To ensure a patent airway in such instances, cricothyroidotomy or tracheotomy may be necessary (see Chap. 16) [18,97]. Cricothyroidotomy is preferred to tracheotomy when performed in an emergent situation, as the former is easier to perform and usually safer [98–101]. Contraindications to cricothyroidotomy include a suspected neck frac-

ture or a serious injury to the larynx or cricoid cartilage (see Chap. 16).

Pharmacologic Therapy. The guidelines for pharmacologic therapy of anaphylaxis are listed in Table 217-6 [83,96]. Beta-adrenergic agonists, such as epinephrine hydrochloride and isoproterenol hydrochloride, act by increasing the intracellular levels of cyclic AMP and thereby inhibiting the activation of tissue-based mast cells and circulating basophils [102–105]. In addition, epinephrine acts on bronchial and cardiac beta-receptors, causing bronchial dilatation and both chronotropic and inotropic cardiac stimulation. An equally important effect of epinephrine is stimulation of alpha-adrenergic receptors on blood vessels, which causes vasoconstriction. This is important in reversing anaphylaxis-induced hypotension and in delaying antigen absorption when infiltrated locally into an injection or sting site [36]. In contrast, isoproterenol has not been found to be efficacious in reversing anaphylactic shock, although it can prevent anaphylaxis in animals if given before antigen exposure [106]. Inhaled beta-adrenergic agents, such as metaproterenol sulfate or albuterol sulfate, may also be helpful in reversing bronchoconstriction and in reducing bronchial mucus secretion. Methylxanthines, such as aminophylline, are also bronchodilators, although the exact mechanism of action is not well-defined.

H_1-receptor-blocking antihistamines may be helpful in reversing the histamine-induced cardiopulmonary effects of vasodilatation, tachycardia, and bronchoconstriction, as well as bothersome cutaneous manifestations, such as flushing, pruritis, and urticaria [67]. However, antihistamines are more effective in prevention than in treatment of full-blown anaphylaxis and should never be used as the primary therapy for anaphylactic shock. H_2-receptor-blocking antihistamines prevent the fall in diastolic blood pressure induced by experimental histamine infusion [67] and the H_2-blocker cimetidine has been reported to reverse refractory systemic anaphylaxis [108,109].

Corticosteroids, although not immediately active in anaphylactic shock, are effective pharmacologic agents that are capable of increasing tissue response to beta-adrenergic agonists as well as inhibiting basophil activation and phospholipase- mediated generation of LTC_4, LTD_4, and LTE_4 [7,110].

Epinephrine should be tried first to treat all initial manifestations of anaphylaxis [36,83,111]. Alone, it may reverse rhinitis, urticaria, bronchoconstriction, and hypotension. The failure to administer epinephrine or a delay in its administration may be fatal [83]. The dose is 0.2 to 0.5 ml of a 1:1000 dilution (0.2–0.5 mg) and is given subcutaneously and repeated every 15 minutes, usually not more than 3 times [36,83]. Absorption of parenterally introduced antigens may be retarded by infiltrating the site with approximately one-half this dose of epinephrine [36]. Tourniquet application proximal to the site of antigen administration that is sufficient to occlude venous and lymphatic returns without interfering with arterial blood flow may also retard absorption of the antigen [111]. The tourniquet should be loosened for approximately 15 to 30 seconds every 10 to 15 minutes. If symptoms are not immediately reversed with subcutaneous epinephrine, H_1 and H_2 antihistamine therapy should be added. The H_1-receptor-blocker diphenhydramine (50 mg for an adult) should be infused intravenously over 3 minutes [111]. The H_2-receptor-blocker cimetidine (300 mg for an adult) can be infused intravenously over 3 to 5 minutes [108,109,112].

If shock develops, subcutaneous epinephrine is unlikely to be absorbed. In this setting, epinephrine should be given intravenously: 1 mg (1 ml of a 1:1000 solution or 10 ml of a 1:10,000 solution) diluted in 500 ml of normal saline and infused at a rate of 0.5 to 2.0 ml/min (1–4 µg/min) with continuous electro-

Table 217-6. Treatment of Anaphylaxis in Adults

Mandatory and immediate

General measures:

  Aqueous epinephrine (1:1000), 0.2 to 0.5 ml SQ or IM; up to 3
    doses at 1- to 5-min intervals
  Tourniquet proximal to antigen injection or sting site
  Aqueous epinephrine (1:1000), 0.1 to 0.3 ml infiltrated into antigen
    injection or sting site

For laryngeal obstruction or respiratory arrest:

  Establish airway: endotracheal intubation, cricothyroidotomy or tra-
    cheotomy
  Supplemental oxygen
  Mechanical ventilation

After clinical appraisal

General measures:

  Diphenhydramine, 1.25 mg/kg to maximum of 50 mg, IV or IM
  Aqueous hydrocortisone, 200 mg, or methylprednisolone, 50 mg,
    IV every 6 hr for 24–48 hr
  Cimetidine, 300 mg, IV over 3–5 min

For hypotension:

  Aqueous epinephrine (1:1000), 1 ml in 500 ml of saline at 0.5–2.0
    ml/min, or 1–4 µg/min, via a central venous line
  Normal saline, lactated Ringer's, or colloid volume expansion
  Levarterenol bitartrate, 4 mg in 1000 ml of D5W at 2–12 µg/min IV
  Glucagon, if patient is receiving β-blocker therapy, 1 mg/ml IV bo-
    lus or infusion of 1 mg/liter of D5W at a rate of 5–15 ml/min

For bronchoconstriction:

  Supplemental oxygen
  Aminophylline, only if patient *not* in shock, 5 mg/kg to maximum
    of 500 mg IV over 20 min, then 0.3–0.8 mg/kg/hr IV
  Metaproterenol (5%), 0.3 ml in 2.5 ml of saline, or albuteral (0.5%),
    0.5 ml in 2.5 ml of saline, by nebulizer
  Isoproterenol, if patient is refractory to other measures, 0.0375 µg/
    kg/min IV, increased slowly to 0.225 µg/kg/min, or 2–20 µg/min

cardiographic monitoring [3]. Intravenous support with normal saline or colloid is also important. If hypotension persists, pressors, such as levarterenol bitartrate (Levophed), dopamine (Inotropin), or metaraminol bitartrate (Aramine), should be administered (see Chap. 147) [113]. If no response to pressors occurs, the central venous pressure (CVP) should be measured. A CVP between 0 and 12 cm H$_2$O suggests that more intravenous fluids should be given, whereas a CVP greater than 12 cm H$_2$O suggests that the hypotension may be based on myocardial failure. For refractory hypotension, pulmonary artery catheterization (see Chap. 4) can help guide further fluid, inotropic, and vasopressor therapy, as outlined in Chap. 171.

If bronchoconstriction does not respond to epinephrine, methylxanthines may be given: 250 to 500 mg of aminophylline may be infused over 20 minutes (see Chap. 56). Since methylxanthines may worsen hypotension and cause unpredictable cardiovascular toxicity, these drugs are not recommended in hypotensive patients [36,83]. In addition, inhaled, nebulized metaproterenol (0.3 ml of 5% solution diluted in 2.5 ml of normal saline) or albuteral (0.5 ml of 0.5% solution diluted in 3 ml of normal saline) is recommended. Alternatively, isoproterenol has been suggested for the hypotensive patient with bronchospasm [83]. Isoproterenol increases myocardial oxygen consumption and should be used with caution in patients with coexisting coronary artery disease. It also is highly arrhythmogenic, and ventricular irritability is a relative contraindication.

Preexisting beta-adrenergic blockade with noncardioselective or cardioselective agents significantly increases the difficulty of treating anaphylactic shock [22,114]. In the presence of beta-blockade, anaphylaxis is characterized by bradycardia with or without atrioventricular nodal delay (in contrast to the usual tachycardia), profound and refractory hypotension, urticaria, and angioedema [114]. Beta-blockade appears to increase anaphylactic mediator synthesis and release, as well as altering end-organ responsiveness. Whether beta-blockade truly increases the chance of developing anaphylaxis or just the severity is not known. Although alpha-adrenergic agents may increase in vitro release of mast cell mediators in the presence of beta-blockade [115,116], the drug of first choice for treating anaphylaxis in the presence of beta-blockade remains epinephrine [114]. Dopamine, which has combined alpha, beta, and dopaminergic activities may be useful for shock refractory to epinephrine. The dose of beta-agonists will likely have to be greater than usual to overcome the beta-blockade. Several case reports note success with glucagon in treating refractory shock. Glucagon appears to increase cardiac cyclic AMP independent of beta-receptors and to increase heart rate despite beta-blockade [114,117].

It has been suggested that although glucocorticosteroids are not of immediate clinical benefit, they often help to reduce bronchospasm and laryngeal edema and to provide blood pressure support when used in high doses and for prolonged attacks [6,83,113]. The generally recommended initial dose of aqueous hydrocortisone is 5 mg/kg to a maximum of 200 mg given intravenously, followed by 2.5 mg/kg to 200 mg given intravenously every 4 to 6 hours [6,83,113] for 24 to 48 hours.

Despite the general sense that glucocorticosteroids prevent late recurrences of anaphylaxis, biphasic anaphylaxis has been reported [118] to occur in 20 percent of anaphylactic reactions in spite of glucocorticosteroid therapy. In this report [118], after an initial response to therapy, life-threatening symptoms recurred up to 8 hours later. Whether glucocorticoid therapy helped prevent recurrences after 8 hours is not known. Because of the possibility of a late recurrence, patients should be monitored in an intensive care setting for 8 to 12 hours after resolution of symptoms. Roughly 30 percent of anaphylaxis cases [118] may have protracted symptoms for 5 to 32 hours despite vigorous therapy including glucocorticosteroids. One characteristic of patients with biphasic or protracted anaphylaxis is oral ingestion of the offending antigen. On this basis, it would be reasonable to include enteral activated charcoal and sorbitol in the therapy of such patients to reduce the absorption and duration of exposure to the antigen (see Chap. 109 on drug overdose).

PREVENTION OF ANAPHYLACTIC REACTIONS. In view of the potential morbidity and mortality from anaphylactic reactions, prevention is of primary importance. Prevention includes obtaining a careful history to identify possible precipitants of anaphylaxis. Allergen skin testing or RAST may be helpful in predicting allergy to beta-lactam antibiotics, stinging insect venoms, local anesthetics, insulin, chymopapain, and foods (see specific sections below). Because of the possibility of a life-threatening reaction to skin testing of food extracts, skin testing should be avoided, or undertaken with caution, in patients who have had a severe anaphylactic event. Skin testing of drugs other than those mentioned may not always be a reliable way to evaluate hypersensitivity, because of the possibility of local irritant reactions [95].

Individuals with a history of anaphylaxis should be encouraged to wear Medic-Alert bracelets, which detail the offending precipitant(s). Physicians should be aware of cross-reacting agents in these sensitized individuals.

Genetic make-up, exogenous factors (e.g., frequency of specific antigen exposure) and concomitant diseases and medications may also influence the risk of developing an anaphylactic reaction. For example, some evidence suggests that atopic persons are not any more susceptible to allergic emergencies than nonatopic persons [36]. Other studies indicate that individuals with personal and/or family histories of allergy and positive intradermal skin reactions are at greater risk of developing an anaphylactic reaction than their healthy counterparts [5].

In IgE-mediated anaphylaxis, prior exposure to an antigen is required for elaboration of IgE antibodies, so the risk of anaphylaxis would be expected to increase with recurrent exposure. On the other hand, amnestic IgE responses may wane with time, so the time interval between exposures may also be important.

Beta-blocking medication may increase the risk of developing an anaphylactic reaction and makes these reactions more refractory to treatment [114]. Thus, patients at risk for recurrent anaphylaxis should not receive beta-blocking medication, unless no reasonable alternative exists. Similarly, allergen skin testing, immunotherapy, and desensitization should not be undertaken in patients on beta-blocking medication until the drug has been discontinued and beta-adrenergic responsiveness recovers [114].

Prevention of anaphylaxis also depends on a heightened awareness of possible cross-sensitizing drugs and situations that have previously been associated with a relatively high risk of anaphylaxis. For example, approximately 15 percent of aspirin-sensitive asthmatics are also sensitive to the agent tartrazine, which is used as a yellow coloring (FD&C #5) for foods and drugs [119]. Other preservatives, such as metabisulfite, ethylenediamine, and methylparabens, have been associated with anaphylactic reactions, so it is helpful to review the inactive ingredients contained in medications temporally associated with anaphylaxis [120].

MANAGEMENT OF ANAPHYLAXIS TO SPECIFIC AGENTS AND PRECIPITANTS

Beta-lactam antibiotic anaphylaxis. The most common cause of anaphylaxis in the United States is penicillin. Systemic reactions complicate approximately 1 to 2 percent of penicillin courses. Approximately 10 percent of the population will have positive skin tests to penicillin. Thus, a substantial portion of the population is at risk for developing anaphylactic reactions to the drug. About 10 percent of these reactions are life-threatening because of induced laryngeal edema, bronchospasm, or shock; 2 to 10 percent of these are fatal [23]. Seventy-five percent of the patients who die of penicillin anaphylaxis have experienced previous allergic reactions to the drug. As with other medications, the risk of a severe reaction is greater with parenteral administration than with oral [23,83].

Skin testing for penicillin hypersensitivity with penicilloyl-polylysine (Pre-Pen), penicillin G, and penicilloic acid is highly efficient in detecting IgE-mediated sensitivity and thereby identifying individuals at risk for developing acute allergic reactions to penicillin [23]. The negative predictive value of skin testing when both major and minor determinants of penicillin are used is excellent for immediate hypersensitivity reactions [121]. This testing does not evaluate other types of sensitivity, such as serum sickness reactions, morbilliform rashes, and interstitial nephritis. Unfortunately, the minor determinants (benzylpenicillin, benzylpenicilloate, and benzylpenicilloyl-N-propanolamine) are not commercially available yet. Therefore, Anderson has described an alternative protocol using penicilloylpolylysine (Pre-Pen; Schwarz Pharma, Kremers Urban Company, Milwaukee, WI), which is the major determinant, and freshly prepared penicillin G potassium, which contains one of the minor determinants [122]. With this method, 3 percent of patients with negative skin tests may have an IgE-mediated reaction when treated with penicillin. If no alternative antibiotic is effective,

and penicillin is absolutely necessary, individuals can be desensitized: a rapid desensitization protocol has been found to be safe [123] (Table 217-7) and might be of benefit in critically ill patients. Otherwise, a slower protocol can be used (see protocol in Patterson and Anderson [23], p 2644).

Patients with a history of penicillin allergy have been reported to have allergic reactions to cephalosporins at a rate of 5.4 to 16.5 percent, compared with patients with a negative history, whose reaction rate was 1 to 2 percent [124,125]. However, not all of these reactions reflect true cross-reactivity, as only 15 to 40 percent of patients with a positive history react to penicillin on subsequent testing [124]. Unfortunately, skin testing with cephalosporin derivatives is not reliable, as severe allergic reactions have occurred in patients with negative cephalosporin skin tests. On the other hand, patients with negative penicillin skin tests have no greater risk of allergic reaction to cephalosporins than the general population [125].

Monobactams (e.g., aztreonam) do not show cross-reactivity with penicillin, but do show some cross-reactivity with the cephalosporins [125]. Carbapenems (e.g., imipenem), in comparison, show a high degree of in vivo cross-reactivity with penicillin and should only be given to patients with a history of penicillin allergy if no reasonable alternative exists and with the same precautions as if giving the patient penicillin [125].

STINGING INSECT VENOM ANAPHYLAXIS. Venom extracts for yellow jacket, white-faced hornet, yellow-faced hornet, wasp, honey bee, and fire ant are available for skin testing to confirm specific IgE mediation and for desensitization [126]. Results with venom desensitization suggest greater than 95 percent protection against anaphylaxis on subsequent stings [126]. The duration of desensitization therapy necessary for long-term protection after discontinuation remains investigational, but likely exceeds 5 years [127,128].

FOOD ANAPHYLAXIS. Food allergy occurs in approximately 8 percent of children and 1 to 2 percent of adults [129]; however, fatal anaphylactic reactions are much less common. A recent review of fatal and severe nonfatal anaphylactic reactions [130] to foods revealed several important features of the fatal anaphylactic reactions: all occurred in patients with asthma, all were in a public setting rather than in the home, and all were associated with delayed administration of epinephrine. The foods that caused these severe reactions were peanuts, cashews, milk, filberts, walnuts, and eggs. In another review of causes of anaphylaxis [131], the five most common foods were pine nuts, peanuts, soy, shellfish, and other nuts. A methodical approach to the diagnosis and treatment of food hypersensitivity has been outlined by Sampson [129].

Processed foods may contain significant amounts of milk products, despite a lack of mention of this on the label ingredient lists [132]. This is important to remember in patients with milk allergy who appear to experience a cryptogenic anaphylactic episode. As noted above, other food additives, such as preservatives, have been implicated as causes of anaphylaxis [126].

LOCAL ANESTHETIC ANAPHYLAXIS. Immediate hypersensitivity reactions to local anesthetics are rare, despite being one of the most commonly used groups of drugs in medicine. Cell-mediated reactions that manifest as contact dermatitis are more common. Local anesthetics are divided into two classes: group I (paraminobenzoic acid ester) consists of benzocaine, tetracaine, and procaine; group II (non-ester-containing) consists of

Table 217-7. Desensitization Schedule for Beta-Lactam Antibiotics

Dose No.	Concentration of stock solution (mg/ml)*	Concentration of infused solution (mg/ml)**
1	0.0005	0.00001
2	0.005	0.0001
3	0.05	0.001
4	0.5	0.01
5	5	0.1
6	50	1
7	500	10

*Stock solution is prepared by solubilizing the antibiotic with nonbacteriostatic saline to a final concentration of 500 mg/ml. Dilutions of 1 ml of each preceding antibiotic dilution to 9 ml of diluent.
**One milliliter of stock solution is further diluted into 50 ml of saline and infused during 20 minutes.
Source: From Borish L, Tamir R, Rosenwasser L: Intravenous desensitization to beta-lactam antibiotics. *J Allergy Clin Immunol* 80:314.

xylocaine, mepivicaine, dibucaine, and cyclomethycaine. Cross-reactivity between the two groups is very rare [133,134]. Skin testing can be helpful to determine whether sensitivity exists and which drugs are likely to be safe in the future.

RADIOCONTRAST MEDIA ANAPHYLAXIS. Because radiocontrast dye studies arc frequently necessary in critically ill patients, it is important to know when a reaction is likely to occur and how to prevent it. Unfortunately, the likelihood of an anaphylactic reaction to radiocontrast dye cannot be predicted by pretesting with oral, conjunctival, or intradermal skin tests [135]. In patients with a history of a previous anaphylactic reaction, the repeat reaction rate is reported to be 35 to 60 percent [136]. Patients with a general history of allergies, whether to inhalant allergens, foods, or medications, have an increased reaction rate compared with nonallergic individuals [136,137].

Pretreatment protocols have been developed for patients with a history of a prior anaphylactic reaction who require additional intravascular dye studies [135–137]. In one study of 192 procedures in patients with previous anaphylactic reactions to contrast media, pretreatment with prednisone, 50 mg orally at 13, 7, and 1 hour before the procedure; diphenhydramine, 50 mg orally or intramuscularly at 1 hour before; and ephedrine, 25 mg orally at 1 hour before resulted in a reaction rate of 3.1 percent [136]. A multicenter study of nonselected patients receiving intravenous contrast media reported a reaction rate of 5.4 percent in 2513 patients given oral methylprednisolone, 32 mg at 12 hours and again at 2 hours before the procedure [137]. In this same study, a single dose of methylprednisolone, 32 mg 2 hours before the procedure was no better than placebo, with a reaction rate of 9.4 percent in 1759 patients. This finding raises the question of how to manage patients with a prior history of anaphylaxis who require an urgent radiocontrast study. In a small study, nine such patients were treated with hydrocortisone, 200 mg intravenously immediately and every 4 hours until the procedure was completed, and diphenhydramine, 50 mg intravenously 1 hour before the procedure [138]. Roughly half of the patients received one dose of hydrocortisone, and half received two doses. No reactions occurred in these patients. Given that this study evaluated only nine patients, it remains unknown whether additional therapy with ephedrine or an H_2-receptor blocking agent, or both, would provide better protection.

The newer, nonionic radiocontrast agents are useful but expensive alternatives to conventional ionic contrast media, especially in high-risk patients who need an emergent contrast study [139]. Clinical trials comparing nonionic and ionic contrast media have shown a significant decrease in the overall adverse reaction rate (i.e., heat sensation, pain, cardiovascular changes) when nonionic contrast is used, but studies have not shown a reduction in nephrotoxicity, life-threatening reactions, or death [140–142]. Whether allergic reactions in particular would be reduced has not yet been elucidated [140,142]. Thus, because of the expense of nonionic media, it is not clear whether universal use of nonionic media would be cost effective. However, preliminary studies suggest that patients with a prior history of contrast media reactions may have a lower recurrence rate when nonionic media are used than when ionic media are combined with corticosteroid pretreatment [142]. This remains an important area for further research. Currently, in patients who have had a prior anaphylactic reaction to contrast media and who require a contrast study, the use of low ionic contrast should be considered in addition to pretreatment with corticosteroids, diphenhydramine and ephedrine or corticosteroids and diphenhydramine, without ephedrine [143].

LATEX-INDUCED ANAPHYLAXIS. Latex allergy can take several forms: contact dermatitis, urticaria, asthma, and anaphylaxis. Perioperative anaphylaxis caused by latex exposure has been described in several children with spina bifida or a history of multiple surgical procedures [144]. In addition, latex allergy has become a more common occupational hazard in the health professions since the institution of universal precautions. Latex is found in a wide spectrum of products, including balloons, elastic thread, rubber bands, condoms, household rubber gloves, surgical gloves, Foley catheters, enema bags, rubber stoppers on medication vials and intravenous line tubing, as well as some surgical drapes and gowns [25,145,146]. Sensitivity seems to be increased in atopic individuals with frequent exposure to latex.

Evaluation with skin testing has been recommended for patients at high risk, although skin test extracts are not yet commercially available [145–147]. Another alternative is a commercial latex RAST (Pharmacia, Uppsala, Sweden or DACI Reference Laboratory at Johns Hopkins University, Baltimore, MD) [25,145,147]. Because the latex extracts used for skin testing are made by individual allergists, the specificity and sensitivity of the skin tests may vary. However, latex skin testing appears to have greater sensitivity than the RAST [145,146].

The most important step in prevention of future anaphylactic reactions to latex is careful patient education. Verbal and written information should be given about the various sources of latex exposure, the importance of alerting health care professionals who may care for the patient in the future, wearing a Medic-Alert bracelet and carrying an Epi-Pen kit, as well as sources of latex-free gloves for patients to take to dentist and doctor visits.

EXERCISE-INDUCED ANAPHYLAXIS. This syndrome has been shown to be distinct from cold and cholinergic urticaria and exercise-induced asthma and usually occurs in individuals who engage in vigorous exercise [37]. A subgroup of these patients are allergic to a specific food, such as shrimp or celery, which acts as a cofactor: manifestations of anaphylaxis only occur if ingestion of the specific food is accompanied by exercise [6,37]. Otherwise, these patients can either ingest the food or perform the exercise without adverse effect. Anaphylaxis can be prevented by delaying exercise at least 2 and preferably

4 hours after eating (48 hours after ingesting a food cofactor) and stopping exercise at the onset of pruritis. Exercising with someone who is capable of administering epinephrine is also recommended. Antihistamines are occasionally of benefit in prevention.

IDIOPATHIC ANAPHYLAXIS. A group of patients has been described who experience recurrent anaphylaxis without an identifiable precipitant, so-called idiopathic anaphylaxis [61]. In these patients, a careful review of all foods, preservatives, and drugs ingested prior to the episodes, as well as physical factors such as exercise, fails to reveal a cause for recurrent life-threatening anaphylaxis. Maintenance therapy with antihistamines, oral corticosteroids, and sympathomimetics has been shown to reduce the frequency and severity of episodes of idiopathic anaphylaxis [62].

ANGIOTENSIN-CONVERTING ENZYME INHIBITOR ANGIOEDEMA. Severe, potentially life-threatening facial and oropharyngeal angioedema may occur in individuals with hypersensitivity to angiotensin-converting enzyme (ACE) inhibitors [148–150]. Onset of angioedema usually starts within the first several hours or up to a week after beginning therapy, but angioedema can develop after months to years of asymptomatic usage [148,149]. Subsequent episodes may occur after days to weeks of continued usage. A late onset of symptoms, 12 to 24 hours after the last dose, has been reported with the long-acting ACE inhibitors lisinopril and enalapril [150]. Cross-reactivity does pertain among the different ACE inhibitors. The mechanism is unknown but is suspected to be related to an alteration in bradykinin metabolism or, possibly, an interaction with components of the complement cascade (e.g., complement 1-esterase inhibitor) [148,149].

MISCELLANEOUS CAUSES OF ANAPHYLAXIS. Insulin therapy has been associated with an increased risk of anaphylaxis, particularly when a patient on insulin therapy has a history of local wheal-and-flare reactions at the site of insulin injections and interrupts insulin therapy for more than 48 hours and then resumes it [23].

The injection of heterologous serum carries a significant risk of anaphylaxis. Human serum should be used whenever available [83]. If heterologous serum must be used (antitoxin for snake bites and clostridia infections and antilymphocytic serum for organ transplantation), the patient should be tested for cutaneous sensitivity by first performing a scratch test with antitoxin or normal horse serum. If there is no reaction, 0.02 ml of a 1:10 serum dilution can be injected intradermally. As with all skin testing, the physician must be prepared to treat any systemic reactions that arise [95].

Patients with mastocytosis appear to be at greater risk for developing anaphylaxis from Hymenoptera stings (even in the absence of IgE mediation) and from mast cell–degranulating agents (see Table 217-2). These patients should carry a bee-sting kit during Hymenoptera season. Administrations of diagnostic and therapeutic agents that might cause mast cell activation should be avoided in these patients [151].

References

1. Weiszer I: Allergic emergencies, in Patterson R (ed): *Allergic Diseases: Diagnosis and Management*. Philadelphia, Lippincott, 1980, p 374.
2. Lichtenstein LM: Anaphylaxis, in Wyngaarden JB, Smith LH (eds): *Cecil Textbook of Medicine*. Philadelphia, Saunders, 1982, p 1803.
3. Parker CW: Systemic anaphylaxis, in Parker CW (ed): *Clinical Immunology*. Philadelphia, Saunders, 1980, p 1215.
4. Frick OL: Immediate hypersensitivity, in Fudenberg HH, Stites DP, Caldwell JL, et al (eds): *Basic and Clinical Immunology*. Los Altos, Calif, Lange Medical Publications, 1980, p 274.
5. Austen KF: Current concepts. Systemic anaphylaxis in the human being. *N Engl J Med* 291:661, 1974.
6. Sheffer AL: Anaphylaxis. *J Allergy Clin Immunol* 75:227, 1985.
7. Austen KF: Tissue mast cell in immediate hypersensitivity. *Hosp Pract* November 1982, p 98.
8. Mathews KP: Respiratory atopic disease. *JAMA* 248:2587, 1982.
9. Manuel PV, Bahna SL: Clinical aspects of serum total IgE level. *Immunol Allergy Pract* 7:212, 1983.
10. Routledge RC, DeKretser DMH, Wadsworth LD: Severe anaphylaxis due to passive sensitization by donor blood. *Br Med J* 1:434, 1976.
11. Ishizaka T, Ishizaka K, Orange RP, et al: The capacity of human immunoglobin E to mediate the release of histamine and slow reacting substance of anaphylaxis (SRS-A) from monkey lung. *J Immunol* 104:335, 1970.
12. Weiszer I: Allergic emergencies, in Patterson R (ed): *Allergic Diseases: Diagnosis and Management*. Philadelphia, Lippincott, 1980, p 381.
13. Sullivan TJ, Kulczycki A: Immediate hypersensitivity responses, in Parker CW (ed): *Clinical Immunology*. Philadelphia, Saunders, 1980, p 131.
14. Newball HH, Talamo RC, Lichtenstein LM: Anaphylactic release of a basophil kallikrein-like activity: II. A mediator of immediate hypersensitivity reactions. *J Clin Invest* 64:466, 1979.
15. Newball HH, Berninger RW, Talamo RC, et al: Anaphylactic release of a basophil kallikrein-like activity: I. Purification and characterization. *J. Clin Invest* 64:457, 1979.
16. Hamberg M, Svensson J, Hedqvist P, et al: Involvement of endoperoxides and thromboxanes in anaphylactic reactions. *Adv Prostaglandin Thromboxane Res* 1:495, 1976.
17. Roberts LJ, Lewis RA, Lawson JA, et al: Arachidonic acid metabolism by rat mast cells. *Prostaglandins* 15:717, 1978.
18. Chatton MJ: General symptoms, in Krupp MA, Chatton MJ (eds): *Current Medical Diagnosis and Treatment*. Los Altos, Calif, Lange Medical Publications, 1982, p 14.
18a. Kaliner M, Lemanske R: Rhinitis and Asthma. *JAMA* 268:2807, 1992.
19. Kaliner M, Austen KF: A sequence of biochemical events in antigen-induced release of chemical mediators from sensitized human lung tissue. *J. Exp Med* 138:1077, 1973.
20. Lichtenstein LM, Margolis S: Histamine release in vitro. Inhibition by catecholamines and methylxanthines. *Science* 161:902, 1968.
21. Kazimierczak W, Diamant B: Mechanisms of histamine release in anaphylactic and anaphylactoid reactions. *Prog Allergy* 24:295, 1978.
22. Austen KF: Systemic anaphylaxis in man. *JAMA* 192.108, 1965.
23. Patterson R, Anderson J: Allergic reactions to drugs and biologic agents. *JAMA* 248:2637, 1982.
24. Lieberman P, Patterson R, Metz R, et al: Allergic reactions to insulin. *JAMA* 215:1106, 1971.
25. Jaeger D, Kleinhans D, Czuppon, Baur X: Latex-specific proteins causing immediate-type cutaneous, nasal, bronchial, and systemic reactions. *J Allergy Clin Immunol* 89:759, 1992.
26. Zipf RE Jr: Fatal anaphylaxis after intravenous iron dextran. *J Forensic Sci* 20:326, 1975.
27. Saleh Y, Tischler E: Severe anaphylactic reaction to intravenous cephaloridine in a pregnant patient. *Med J Aust* 2:490, 1974.
28. Van Arsdel PP: Adverse drug reactions, in Middleton E Jr, Reed CE, Ellis EF (eds): *Allergy: Principles and Practice*. St. Louis, Mosby, 1978, p 1139.
29. Royston D, Wilkes RG: True anaphylaxis to suxamethonium chloride. A case report. *Br J Anaesth* 50:611, 1978.
30. Matthews MD, Ceglarski JZ, Pabari M: Anaphylaxis to suxamethonium. A case report. *Anaesth Intensive Care* 5:235, 1977.
31. Fisher MM, Hallowes RC, Wilson RM: Anaphylaxis to alcuronium. *Anaesth Intensive Care* 6:125, 1978.
32. Hayhurst M, Braude A, Benatar SR: Anaphylactic-like reaction to hydrocortisone. *S Afr Med J* 53:259, 1978.

33. Chung DCW: Anaphylaxis to thiopentone: A case report. *Can Anaesth Soc J* 23:319, 1976.

34. Dolovich J, Evans S, Rosenbloom D, et al: Anaphylaxis due to thiopental sodium anesthesia. *Can Med Assoc J* 124:292, 1982.

35. Levine BB, Siraganian RP, Schenkein I: Allergy to human seminal plasma. *N Engl J Med* 288:894, 1973.

36. Patterson R, Valentine M: Anaphylaxis and related allergic emergencies including reactions due to insect stings. *JAMA* 248:2632, 1982.

37. Sheffer AL, Austen KF: Exercise-induced anaphylaxis. *J Allergy Clin Immunol* 66:106, 1980.

38. Vyas GN, Perkins HA, Fundenberg H: Anaphylactoid transfusion reactions associated with anti-igA. *Lancet* 2:312, 1968.

39. Craddock PR, Fehr J, Brigham KL, et al: Complement and leukocyte mediated pulmonary dysfunction in hemodialysis. *N Engl J Med* 296:769, 1977.

40. Frank MM, Atkinson JP: Complement in clinical medicine. *DM* January 1975, p 1.

41. Cochrane CG, Koffler D: Immune complex disease in experimental animals and man. *Adv Immunol* 16:185, 1973.

41a. Ellis EF, Henney CS: Adverse reactions following administration of human gamma globulin. *J Allergy* 43:45, 1969.

42. Nordstrom L, Fletcher R, Pavek K: Shock of anaphylactoid type induced by protamine: A continuous cardiorespiratory record. *Acta Anaesthesiol Scand* 22:195, 1978.

43. Olinger GN, Becker RM, Bonchek LI: Noncardiogenic pulmonary edema and peripheral vascular collapse following cardiopulmonary bypass: Rare protamine reaction. *Ann Thorac Surg* 29:20, 1980.

44. Fischer HW, Daust VL: An evaluation of pretesting in the problem of serious and fatal reactions to excretory urography. *Radiology* 103:497, 1972.

45. Lieberman P, Siegle RI, Taylor WW: Anaphylactoid reactions to iodinated contrast material. *J Allergy Clin Immunol* 62:174, 1978.

46. Fanous LH, Gray A, Felmingham J: Severe anaphylactoid reactions to dextran 70. *Br Med J* 2:1189, 1977.

47. Adar R, Schneiderman J: Severe anaphylaxis in cirrhotic patients receiving dextran 40. *JAMA* 237:119, 1977.

48. Hedin H, Richter W: Pathomechanisms of dextran-induced anaphylactoid/anaphylactic reactions in man. *Int Arch Allergy Appl Immunol* 68:122, 1982.

49. Ring J, Messmer K: Incidence and severity of anaphylactoid reactions to colloid volume substitutes. *Lancet* 1:466, 1977.

50. Fisher MM: Severe histamine mediated reactions to intravenous drugs used in anesthesia. *Anaesth Intensive Care* 3:180, 1975.

51. Comroe JE Dupps RD: Histamine-like action of curare acid tubocurarine injected intramuscularly and intra-arterially in man. *Anesthesiology* 7:260, 1946.

52. Mathieu A, Goudsouzian N, Snider MT: Reaction to ketamine: Anaphylactoid or anaphylactic? *Br J Anaesth* 47:624, 1975.

53. Lecomte J: Liberation of endogenous histamine in man. *J Allergy* 28:102, 1957.

54. Schoenfeld MR: Acute allergic reactions to morphine, codeine, meperidine, hydrochloride, and opium alkaloids. *NY State J Med* 60:2591, 1960.

55. Friedlaender S: Adverse reactions to aspirin and nonsteroidal antiinflammatory drugs. *Immunol Allergy Pract* 2:73, 1980.

56. Vane JR: Inhibition of prostaglandin synthesis as a mechanism of action of aspirin-like drugs. *Nature [New Biol]* 231:232, 1971.

57. Samter M, Beers RF Jr: Intolerance to aspirin: Clinical studies and consideration of its pathogenesis. *Ann Intern Med* 68:975, 1968.

58. Burrish GF, Kaatz BL: Sulindac-induced anaphylaxis. *Ann Emerg Med* 10:154, 1981.

59. Corre KA, Rothstein RJ: Anaphylactic reaction to zomepirac. *Ann Allergy* 48:299, 1982.

60. Moore ME, Goldsmith DP: Nonsteroidal anti-inflammatory intolerance. An anaphylactic reaction to tolmetin. *Arch Intern Med* 140:1105, 1980.

61. Wong S, Dykewicz MS, Patterson R: Idiopathic anaphylaxis. *Arch Intern Med* 150:1323, 1990.

62. Wong S, Yarnold PR, Yango C, et al: Outcome of prophylactic therapy for idiopathic anaphylaxis. *Ann Intern Med* 114:133, 1991.

63. Lichtenstein LM: Mediators and the mechanism of their release. *Chest* 73:919, 1978.

64. Herson PM, Betz SJ: Low molecular weight mediators of inflammation: Histamine, serotonin, SRS, PAF, and ECF, in Kelley WN, Harris ED, Ruddy S, et al (eds): *Textbook of Rheumatology.* Philadelphia, Saunders, 1981, p 72.

65. Majno G, Shea SM, Leventhal M: Endothelial contraction induced by histamine-type mediators. An electron microscopic study. *J Cell Biol* 42:647, 1969.

66. Nadel JA: Neurophysiologic aspects of asthma, in Austen KF, Lichtenstein L (eds): *Asthma: Physiology, Immunopharmacology and Treatment.* New York, Academic, 1973, p 32.

67. Kaliner M, Sigler R, Summers R, et al: Effects of infused histamine: Analysis of the effects of H-1 and H-2 histamine receptor antagonists on cardiovascular and pulmonary responses. *J Allergy Clin Immunol* 61:365, 1981.

68. Bach MK, Brashler JR, Gorman RR: On the structure of slow reacting substance of anaphylaxis: Evidence of biosynthesis from arachidonic acid. *Prostaglandins* 14:21, 1977.

69. Jakschik BA, Falkenhein S, Parker CW: Precursor role of arachidonic acid in release of slow reacting substance from rat basophilic leukemia cells. *Proc Natl Acad Sci USA* 74:4577, 1977.

70. Brocklehurst WE: The release of histamine and formation of a slow-reacting substance (SRS-A) during anaphylactic shock. *J Physiol* 151:416, 1960.

71. Lewis RA, Wasserman SI, Goetzl EJ, et al: Formation of slow reacting substance of anaphylaxis in human lung tissue and cells before release. *J Exp Med* 140:1133, 1974.

72. Townley RG, Hopp RJ, Agrawal DK, et al: Platelet-activating factor and airway reactivity. *J Allergy Clin Immunol* 83:997, 1989.

73. Brocklehurst WE: Slow reacting substance and related compounds. *Prog Allergy* 6:539, 1962.

74. Orange RP, Austen KF: Slow reacting substance of anaphylaxis. *Adv Immunol* 10:105, 1969.

75. Pinckard RN, Halonen M, Palmer JD, et al: Intravascular aggregation and pulmonary sequestration of platelets during IgE-induced systemic anaphylaxis in the rabbit. Abrogation of lethal anaphylactic shock by platelet depletion. *J Immunol* 119:2185, 1977.

76. Henson PM, Gould D, Becker EL: Activation of stimulus-specific serine esterases (proteases) in the initiation of platelet secretion: I. Demonstration with organophosphorus inhibitors. *J Exp Med* 144:1657, 1976.

77. James LP Jr, Austen KF: Fatal systemic anaphylaxis in man. *N Engl J Med* 270:597, 1964.

78. Kay AB, Austen KF: The IgE-mediated release of an eosinophil leukocyte chemotactic factor from human lung. *J Immunol* 107:899, 1971.

79. Wasserman SI, Austen KF: Arylsulfatase B of human lung: Isolation, characterization, and interaction with slow reacting substance of anaphylaxis. *J Clin Invest* 57:738, 1976.

80. Austen KF: Structure and function of chemical mediators received after activation of mast cells, in Lichtenstein LM, Austin KF (eds): *Asthma: Physiology, Immunopharmacology and Treatment.* New York, Academic, 1977, p 113.

81. Kater LA, Goetzl EJ, Austen KF: Isolation of human eosinophil phospholipase D. *J Clin Invest* 57:1173, 1976.

82. Smith PL, Kagey-Sobotka A, Bleecker ER, et al: Physiologic manifestations of human anaphylaxis. *J Clin Invest* 66:1072, 1980.

83. Kelly JF, Patterson R: Anaphylaxis: Course, mechanisms and treatment. *JAMA* 227:1431, 1974.

84. Bernreiter M: Electrocardiogram of patient in anaphylactic shock. *JAMA* 170:1628, 1959.

85. Levine HD: Acute myocardial infarction following wasp sting. *Am Heart J* 91:365, 1976.

86. Delage C, Mullick FG, Irey NS: Myocardial lesions in anaphylaxis. *Arch Pathol* 95:185, 1973.

87. Hanashiro PK, Weil MH: Anaphylactic shock in man. *Arch Intern Med* 119:129, 1967.

88. Barnard JH: Allergic and pathologic findings in fifty insect sting fatalities. *J Allergy* 40:107, 1967.

89. Delage C, Irey NS: Anaphylactic deaths. A clinicopathologic study of 43 cases. *J Forensic Sci* 17:525, 1972.

90. Edde RR, Burtis BB: Lung injury in anaphylactoid shock. *Chest* 63:636, 1973.

91. Booth BH, Patterson R: Electrocardiographic changes during human anaphylaxis. *JAMA* 211:627, 1970.

92. Petsas AA, Kotler MN: Electrocardiographic changes associated with penicillin anaphylaxis. *Chest* 64:66, 1973.

93. Weiszer I: Allergic emergencies, in Patterson R (ed): *Allergic Diseases: Diagnosis and Management*. Philadelphia, Lippincott, 1980, p 380.

94. Lowell FC, Franklin W, Schiller IW: Acute allergic reactions induced in subjects with hay fever and asthma by the intravenous administration of allergens with observation on blood clot lysis. *J Allergy* 27:369, 1956.

95. Weiszer I: Allergic emergencies, in Patterson R (ed): *Allergic Diseases: Diagnosis and Management*. Philadelphia, Lippincott, 1980, p 389.

96. Weiszer I: Allergic emergencies, in Patterson R (ed): *Allergic Diseases: Diagnosis and Management*. Philadelphia, Lippincott, 1980, p 388.

97. Kleid JJ, Hickman B: *Handbook of Medical Emergencies*. Flushing, NY, Medical Examination Publishing, 1970, p 13.

98. Simon RR, Brenner BE: *Procedures and Techniques in Emergency Medicine*. Baltimore, Williams & Wilkins, 1982, p 67.

99. Boyd AD, Romita MC, Conlan AA, et al: A clinical evaluation of cricothyroidotomy. *Surg Gynecol Obstet* 149:365, 1979.

100. Nicholas TM, Rumer GF: Emergency airway. A plan of action. *JAMA* 174:1930, 1960.

101. Oppenheimer RP: Airway . . . instantly. *JAMA* 230:76, 1974.

102. Ishizaka T, Ishizaka K, Orange RP, et al: Pharmacologic inhibiton of the antigen-induced release of histamine and slow reacting substance of anaphylaxis (SRS-A) from monkey lung tissue mediated by human IgE. *J Immunol* 106:1267, 1971.

103. Orange RP, Austen WG, Austen KF: Immunological release of histamine and slow reacting substance of anaphylaxis from human lung: I. Modulation by agents influencing cellular levels of cyclic 3′,5′ adenosine monophosphate. *J Exp Med* 134:136, 1971.

104. Kaliner M, Austen KF: Cyclic AMP, ATP and reversed anaphylactic histamine release from rat mast cells. *J Immunol* 112:664, 1974.

105. Sutherland EW, Robison GA: Metabolic effects of catecholamines: A. The role of cyclic 3′,5′-AMP in response to catecholamines and other hormones. *Pharmacol Rev* 18:145, 1966.

106. Silverman HJ, Taylor WR, Smith PL, et al: Prevention of canine anaphylaxis with isoproterenol. *Am Rev Respir Dis* 134:243, 1986.

107. Lichtenstein LM, Margolis S: Histamine release in vitro: Inhibition by catecholamines and methylxanthines. *Science* 161:902, 1968.

108. Kambam Jr, Merrill WH, Smith BE: Histamine 2 receptor blocker in the treatment of protamine related anaphylactoid reactions: two case reports. *Can J Anaesth* 36:463, 1989.

109. Yarbrough JA, Moffitt JE, Brown DA, et al: Cimetidine in the treatment of refractory anaphylaxis. *Ann Allergy* 63:235, 1989.

110. Sullivan JJ, Kulczycki A: Immediate hypersensitivity responses, in Parker CW (ed): *Clinical Immunology*. Philadelphia, Saunders, 1980, p 130.

111. Weiszer I: Allergic emergencies, in Patterson R (ed): *Allergic Diseases: Diagnosis and Management*. Philadelphia, Lippincott, 1980, p 386.

112. Kaliner MA: Anaphylaxis. *N Engl Allergy Proc* 5:324, 1984.

113. Weiszer I: Allergic emergencies, in Patterson R (ed): *Allergic Diseases: Diagnosis and Management*. Philadelphia, Lippincott, 1980, p 387.

114. Toogood JH: Risk of anaphylaxis in patients receiving beta-blocker drugs. *J Allergy Clin Immunol* 81:1, 1988.

115. Jacobs RL, Rake GW, Fournier DC, et al: Potentiated anaphylaxis in patients with drug-induced beta-adrenergic blockade. *J Allergy Clin Immunol* 68:125, 1981.

116. Kaliner M, Orange RP, Austen KF: Immunological release of histamine and slow-reacting substance of anaphylaxis from human lung: IV. Enhancement by cholinergic and alpha adrenergic stimulation. *J Exp Med* 136:556, 1972.

117. Zaloga GP, DeLacey W, Holmboe E, et al: Glucagon reversal of hypotension in a case of anaphylactoid shock. *Ann Intern Med* 105:65, 1986.

118. Stark BJ, Sullivan T. Biphasic and protracted anaphylaxis. *J Allergy Clin Immunol* 78:76, 1986.

119. Stevenson DD, Simon RA, Matheson DA: Aspirin-sensitive asthma: Tolerance to aspirin after positive oral aspirin challenge. *J Allergy Clin Immunol* 66:82, 1980.

120. Twarog FJ, Leung DYM: Anaphylaxis to a component of isoetharine (sodium bisulfite). *JAMA* 248:2030, 1982.

121. Sogn DD, Evans R, Shepard GM et al: Results of the National Institutes of Allergy and Infectious Diseases Collaborative Clinical Trial to test the predictive value of skin testing with major and minor penicillin derivatives in hospitalized adults. *Arch Intern Med* 152:1025, 1992.

122. Anderson JA: Allergic reactions to drugs and biological agents. *JAMA* 269:2845, 1992.

123. Borish L, Tamir R, Rosenwasser LJ: Intravenous desensitization to beta-lactam antibiotics. *J Allergy Clin Immunol* 80:314, 1987.

124. Anderson JA: Cross-sensitivity to cephalosporins in patients allergic to penicillin. *Pediatr Infect Dis* 5:557, 1986.

125. Saxon A, Beall GN, Rohr AS, et al: Immediate hypersensitivity reactions to beta-lactam antibiotics. *Ann Intern Med* 107:204, 1987.

126. Valentine MD: Insect venom allergy: Diagnosis and treatment. *J Allergy Clin Immunol* 73:299, 1984.

127. Reisman RE, Lantner R: Further observations of stopping venom immunotherapy: Comparison of patients stopped because of a fall in serum venom-specific IgE to insignificant levels with patients stopped prematurely by self choice. *J Allergy Clin Immunol* 83:1049, 1989.

128. Golden DBK, Addison BI, Gadde J, et al: Prospective observations on stopping prolonged venom immunotherapy. *J Allergy Clin Immunol* 84:162, 1989.

129. Sampson HA: IgE-mediated food intolerance. *J Allergy Clin Immunol* 81:495, 1988.

130. Sampson HA, Mendelson L. Rosen JP: Fatal and near-fatal anaphylactic reactions to food in children and adolescents. *N Engl J Med* 327:380, 1992.

131. Wiggins CA: Characateristics and etiology of 30 patients with anaphylaxis. *Immunol Allergy Prac* 13:313, 1991.

132. Gern JE, Yang E, Evrard HM, Sampson HA: Allergic reactions to milk-contaminated 'nondairy' products. *N Engl J Med* 324:976, 1991.

133. Incaudo G, Schatz M, Patterson R, et al: Administration of local anesthetics to patients with a history of prior adverse reaction. *J Allergy Clin Immunol* 61:339, 1978.

134. de Shazo RD, Nelson HS: An approach to the patient with a history of local anesthetic hypersensitivity: Experience with 90 patients. *J Allergy Clin Immunol* 63:387, 1979.

135. Shehadi WH: Adverse reactions to intravascularly administered contrast media. A comprehensive study based on a prospective survey. *Am J Roentgenol* 124:145, 1975.

136. Greenberger PA: Contrast media reactions. *J Allergy Clin Immunol* 74:600, 1984.

137. Lasser EC, Berry CC, Talner LB, et al: Pretreatment with corticosteroids to alleviate reactions to intravenous contrast material. *N Engl J Med* 317:845, 1987.

138. Greenberger PA, Halwig JM, Patterson R, et al: Emergency administration of radiographic contrast media in high-risk patients. *J Allergy Clin Immunol* 77:630, 1986.

139. Rapoport S, Bookstein JJ, Higgins CB, et al: Experience with metrizamide in patients with previous severe anaphylactoid reactions to ionic contrast agents. *Radiology* 143:321, 1982.

140. Wolf GL, Arenson RL, Cross AP: A prospective trial of ionic vs. nonionic contrast agents in routine clinical practice: comparison of adverse effects. *Am J Roentgenol* 152:939, 1989.

141. Lasser EC, Berry CC: Nonionic vs. ionic contrast media: what do the data tell us? *Am J Roentgenol* 152:945, 1989.

142. McLennan BL: Ionic and nonionic iodinated contrast media: evolution and strategies for use. *Am J Roentgenol* 155:225, 1990.

143. Greenberger PA, Patterson R: The prevention of immediate generalized reactions to radiocontrast media in high-risk patients. *J Allergy Clin Immunol* 87:867, 1991.

144. Blaiss MS: Latex allergy in children: A review. *Pediatric Asthma, Allergy Immunol* 6:71:1992.

145. Fuchs T, Wahl R: Immediate reactions to rubber products. *Allergy Proc* 13:61, 1992.

146. Sussman GL: Latex allergy: Its importance in clinical practice. *Allergy Proc* 13:67, 1992.

147. Ber DV, Davidson AE, Klein DE, et al: Latex hypersensitivity: Two case reports: *Allergy Proc* 13:71, 1992.

148. Roberts JR, Wuerz RC: Clinical characteristics of angiotensin-converting enzyme inhibitor-induced angioedema. *Ann Emerg Med* 20:555, 1991.

149. Israili ZH, Hall WD: Cough and angioneurotic edema associated with angiotensin-converting enzyme inhibitor therapy. *Ann Intern Med* 117:234, 1992.

150. Bielory L, Lee SS, Holland CL, Jaker M: Long-acting ACE-inhibitor-induced angioedema. *Allergy Proc* 13:85, 1992.

151. Lewis RA: Mastocytosis. *J Allergy Clinic Immunol* 74:755, 1984.

218. *Dermatologic Problems in the Intensive Care Unit*

Dianne L. Silvestri and
Thomas G. Cropley

Overview

The cutaneous disorders that are found among patients hospitalized in the intensive care unit (ICU) may be divided into four categories (Table 218-1). The first category consists of the skin diseases that are severe enough to produce life-threatening complications. The second category consists of the serious systemic diseases that have prominent cutaneous involvement. A third group consists of subtle skin abnormalities that may be seen in systemic disorders whose course is often punctuated by sequelae that require critical monitoring. These skin manifestations may be neglected or unrecognized clues to the underlying disease. Finally, there are the skin disorders that are observed frequently in the ICU because of environmental, nutritional, immunologic, or pharmacologic risk factors common among these patients.

Skin Diseases With Life-Threatening Complications

ERYTHEMA MULTIFORME. Erythema multiforme (EM) is a self-limited, episodic, acute inflammatory cutaneous or mucocutaneous disorder. It is characterized by variety among the cutaneous lesions, often including a typical targetlike papule, by a tendency to recur, and by a distinctive histopathology [1,2]. The clinical severity ranges from EM minor, in which skin lesions may be accompanied by mild mucosal involvement, to severe EM major (in the past referred to as Stevens-Johnson syndrome) [3,4], which is characterized by constitutional symptoms and severe affliction of at least two mucosal surfaces, as well as occasional visceral involvement [2]. Many authors now consider toxic epidermal necrolysis (TEN) (see Toxic Epidermal Necrolysis), a disease in which large areas of skin are sloughed, to be an extremely severe form of EM [2,5,6], although they may represent two distinct but similar responses to similar inciting agents [7,8]. Rarely, a case has seemed to progress from EM major to TEN [9] or to resemble both [7,8,10]; in fact, an outbreak of both disorders has been reported following sulfonamide administration during an epidemic of meningitis [11].

It is most likely that EM represents a hypersensitivity state precipitated by any of a variety of antigenic stimuli (Table 218-2). The best documented associations are with herpes simplex virus (HSV) and mycoplasmal infections and with drugs [1,2,12–14]. Recurrent herpes simplex labialis and genitalis infections are a frequent cause of EM minor [15,16]. Even silent herpetic infections may lead to EM [12,16]. Although the exact mechanism of the production of EM is not known, HSV antigens have been detected in circulating immune complexes in patients with EM [17] and in EM skin lesions examined by indirect immunofluorescence [16]. Furthermore, several studies have suggested a possible genetic predisposition related to HLA-B15 and HLA-DQw3, especially in individuals with postherpetic and recurrent EM [18]. In contrast, *Mycoplasma pneumoniae* infection is usually associated with EM major [2,12], but circulating immune complexes to the antigen have not been found. The organism has, however, been cultured from bullous lesions in two patients [2]. Numerous other infectious agents have been reported in cases of EM (see Table 184-2) including the recent occurrence with human parvovirus B19 infection [19].

Of the many drugs implicated as causative factors in EM, the most frequently described are sulfonamides, penicillins, phenytoin, nitrofurantoin, phenobarbital, valproic acid, phenolphthalein, phenylbutazone, and nonsteroidal antiinflammatory agents [2,12,20,21,22].

Histologic examination of skin lesions supports an immunologic etiology for EM, with the presence in early lesions of a lymphohistiocytic perivascular infiltrate in the superficial dermis and along the dermal-epidermal junction [23]. Direct immunofluorescence frequently shows IgM or C3 in dermal vessels and C3 along the dermal-epidermal junction [13,24,25]. Epidermal damage is characteristic, with necrotic epidermal cells and vacuolar degeneration of the basal cells. Edema may lead to subepidermal blister formation [2]. A leukocytoclastic vasculitis is not present.

EM is primarily a disorder of young adults 20 to 40 years of age. Although it occasionally occurs in children and adolescents, it is rarely seen in individuals older than 50. The eruption usually appears within 1 to 3 weeks after the inciting event. Nonspecific prodromal symptoms, such as fever, headache, malaise, and upper respiratory symptoms, precede the skin eruption for at least 1 week in approximately one-third of patients, especially with EM major. Often it is unclear if these

Table 218-1. Dermatologic Problems in the Intensive Care Unit

1. Skin diseases with life-threatening complications
   a. Erythema multiforme (EM)
   b. Toxic epidermal necrolysis (TEN)
   c. Exfoliative erythroderma
   d. Pustular psoriasis of Von Zumbusch
   e. Pemphigus vulgaris
   f. Disseminated cutaneous herpes simplex virus infection
2. Life-threatening systemic diseases with prominent skin involvement
   a. Purpura fulminans
   b. Rocky Mountain spotted fever
   c. Graft-versus-host disease
   d. Toxic shock syndrome
   e. Sepsis
   f. Lyme disease
   g. Brown recluse spider bite (loxoscelism)
   h. Angioedema and anaphylaxis (see Chap. 98)
   i. Acquired immunodeficiency syndrome
   j. Systemic lupus erythematosus
3. Life-threatening systemic diseases with subtle skin manifestations
   a. Hereditary hemorrhagic telangiectasia (Osler-Weber-Rendu)
   b. Pseudoxanthoma elasticum
   c. Ehlers-Danlos syndrome
   d. Malignant atrophic papulosis (Degos' disease)
4. Skin diseases acquired during course of serious systemic illness
   a. Drug eruptions
   b. Moniliasis
   c. Seborrheic dermatitis
   d. Pressure sores
   e. Recurrent herpes simplex virus infection
   f. Contact dermatitis

symptoms are due to an infectious agent or are themselves early components of the EM [2]. In EM minor, skin lesions appear in successive crops over 3 to 5 days, receding after 1 to 3 weeks. There is usually the acute onset of symmetrically distributed acral erythematous macules, which progress to wheals. Central fading may produce rings, and coalescence yields polycyclic and arcuate configurations. Blister formation may ensue. Concentric alterations in color may produce the characteristic "target" lesion, which may have a dusky, papular, blistered, or necrotic center (Plate II-1). In EM major, mucosal lesions are more prominent, although skin lesions may also be present, even generalized [1,12,13]. Oral lesions evolve rapidly from macules through bullae to confluent erosions covered by a pseudomembrane of necrotic epithelium and inflammatory cells. The lips often become denuded with a typical hemorrhagic crust. Ocular involvement is also severe with bilateral palpebral edema and catarrhal conjunctivitis. Erosions of the glans penis may occur, and vulvovaginitis and anal ulcers sometimes occur. The course of EM major may extend 2 to 7 weeks.

No specific laboratory abnormalities occur in EM. Leukocytosis, elevated sedimentation rate, albuminuria, and, rarely, hematuria are seen [1]. Appropriate laboratory tests to identify infectious etiologic agents may be helpful. If the clinical diagnosis is in doubt, a skin biopsy should be performed.

EM must be differentiated from urticaria, lesions of sepsis, and leukocytoclastic vasculitis. It may mimic other blistering diseases, including bullous pemphigoid, pemphigus vulgaris, herpes gestationis, bullous impetigo, dermatitis herpetiformis, staphylococcal scalded skin syndrome, and toxic epidermal necrolysis. The differential diagnosis also includes mucocutaneous disorders, including Reiter's syndrome, Behçet's syndrome, and primary herpetic stomatitis. The clinical picture, a skin biopsy, and appropriate cultures should distinguish among these diseases. Direct immunofluorescence, although not diagnostic in EM, may be necessary to differentiate it from other bullous diseases.

Complications are common, especially in EM major. Ten percent of patients with ocular involvement suffer permanent impairment, some with blindness [12,26]. Gastrointestinal (GI) complications including esophagitis, stricture, hemorrhage, and diarrhea are less common [27,28]. Respiratory mucosa may be involved, resulting in tracheitis or bronchitis; as many as 30 percent of patients with EM major may have pneumonitis, due to either mycoplasma or EM, and pneumothorax and mediastinal emphysema have been reported [2,12,29]. Rarely, acute glomerulonephritis, acute tubular necrosis [30], arrhythmias, or pericarditis [31] may be seen. Vaginal stenosis may ultimately require surgical correction [32]. Most deaths in EM major occur in the elderly or in patients with chronic underlying disease. The mortality rate is from 2 to 25 percent [2,12], but if TEN ensues, it may rise to 65 percent [2].

Patients with EM should be treated according to the etiology and severity of the illness. It is clearly important to remove, treat, or prevent the suspected cause. All nonessential drugs should be discontinued. In recurrent EM minor suspected or verified to be of herpetic origin, prophylactic oral acyclovir may be very effective in preventing future EM [33,34]. Antihistamines and antipyretics may reduce minor symptoms. For minimal skin blistering, wet dressings (e.g., sterile saline or Burow's solution) or baths (e.g., oilated oatmeal) may help dry and debride erosions and prevent secondary infection. If skin cultures document secondary infection, antibiotic therapy may be required. Oral erosions should be cleansed frequently with a 3 percent hydrogen peroxide solution or frequent water or saline irrigation. For mouth pain, local anesthetics (e.g., viscous xylocaine, dyclonine, or mixtures of kaolin with pectin in equal parts of diphenhydramine) may give relief.

Cases of extensive EM major require hospitalization for management of fluid and electrolytes and prevention of desiccation necrosis, frictional trauma, and bacterial overgrowth. Burn unit treatment has improved the outcome in severe cases [35]. Early debridement, topical antibacterial ointments or dressings, and homograft or heterograft applications can reduce morbidity and mortality [35,36]. Prophylactic systemic antibiotics should probably be avoided even in the face of transient leukopenia [35]. An ophthalmologist should always be consulted early and frequently for evaluation and therapy in cases of eye involvement with special attention to removal of synechiae [36a].

There has been growing condemnation of the use of high-dose systemic corticosteroids in EM. In EM minor, many clinicians believe that, in fact, they may prolong recovery [15,37]. In EM major, several patient series have suggested that corticosteroid use may prolong hospitalization, delay skin healing, and increase mortality [35-43a]. Recent anecdotal reports describing the use of cyclosporine-A for treatment of severe erythema multiforme need to be confirmed with controlled studies before that drug can be recommended [43b].

TOXIC EPIDERMAL NECROLYSIS. TEN is an acute, fulminating, life-threatening illness that produces extensive epidermal necrosis, leading to widespread sloughing of skin. As previously discussed, TEN may represent an extremely severe manifestation of EM (see Erythema Multiforme) [44,45].

The specific pathogenesis of TEN remains unknown, although both immunologic mechanisms, such as drug-dependent antiepidermal antibodies, and direct drug-related toxins have been proposed [44,46,47]. TEN most commonly occurs accompanying drug ingestion, and nearly all drugs have been

Table 218-2. Causative Factors Associated with Erythema Multiforme in the Medical Literature

A. Infections
  1. Viral
      a. Herpes simplex*
      b. Infectious mononucleosis*
      c. Vaccinia*
      d. Orf
      e. Milker's nodules
      f. Mumps
      g. Measles
      h. Influenza
      i. Psittacosis
      j. Varicella-zoster
      k. Lymphogranuloma venereum
      l. Enterovirus infections
      m. Adenovirus infections
      n. Hepatitis B
      o. Human parvovirus B19
  2. Bacterial
      a. *Streptococcus*
      b. Typhoid fever
      c. *Pseudomonas*
      d. *Proteus*
      e. Tularemia
      f. *Vibrio parahemolyticus*
      g. Dental infections
      h. Vincent's angina
      i. Pneumococcus
      j. *Yersinia* infections*
      k. Legionnaire's disease
  3. Mycobacterial
      a. Tuberculosis*
      b. Bacillus Calmette-Guérin
  4. Spirochetal: syphilis
  5. Mycoplasmal: *Mycoplasma pneumoniae*
  6. Protozoan: *Trichomonas*
  7. Fungal
      a. Histoplasmosis*
      b. Coccidioidomycosis
      c. Dermatophyte infections
B. Immunizations or hyposensitization
  1. Horse serum
  2. Diphtheria-pertussis
  3. Polio vaccine
  4. Typhoid vaccine
  5. Pollen hyposensitization
  6. Poison ivy hyposensitization
  7. Measles vaccine
C. Systemic drugs*
  1. Sulfonamides
  2. Penicillins
  3. Diphenylhydantoin
  4. Phenylbutazone
  5. Chlorpropamide
  6. Barbiturates
  7. Phenolphthalein
  8. Tetracycline
  9. Acetylsalicylic acid
  10. Alkylating agents
  11. Estrogens
  12. Arsenic
  13. Ethanol
  14. Carbamazepine
  15. Thiouracil
  16. Codeine
  17. Trimethadione
  18. Chloramphenicol
  19. Thiacetazone
  20. Meprobamate
  21. Glutethimide
  22. Quinine
  23. Isoniazid
  24. Furosemide
  25. Rifampin
  26. Glucocorticoids
  27. Zomepirac
  28. Cimetidine
  29. Clindamycin
  30. Methotrexate
  31. Thiabendazole
  32. Ibuprofen
  33. Ethosuximide
  34. Benoxaprofen
  35. Fenoprofen
  36. Minoxidil
  37. Sulindac
  38. Methaqualone
  39. Dapsone
  40. Glucagon
D. Topical agents (chemicals and drugs)
  1. 9-Bromofluorene
  2. Sulfonamides
  3. Anticholinergic eye drops
  4. Primula antigen
  5. Tropical woods
  6. Fire sponge
E. Neoplasms
  1. Leukemia
  2. Lymphoma
  3. Pelvic tumors
  4. Leiomyoma
F. Connective tissue disease: lupus erythematosus
G. Physical agents
  1. Sunlight
  2. X-irradiation of tumors*
H. Food: margarine (emulsifying agent)
I. Inhalants: methylparathion
J. Other diseases or conditions
  1. Inflammatory bowel disease
  2. Sarcoidosis
  3. Pregnancy
  4. Menstruation

*Well-documented precipitating factor(s).
Source: From Huff JC, Weston WL, Tonnesen MG: Erythema multiforme: A critical review of characteristics, diagnostic criteria and causes. *J Am Acad Dermatol* 8:771, 1983, with permission.

implicated. The most commonly cited agents are sulfonamides, barbiturates, allopurinol, antibiotics, carbamazepine, and nonsteroidal antiinflammatory agents, especially butazones and oxicams [22,48–50a]. Recently, pyrimethamine-sulfadoxine malaria prophylaxis has been associated with TEN [51]. Other possible causes include infections [52], vaccinations [53], neoplasms [54], graft-versus-host disease [47,55], beverages [56], and toxins [57]. A particularly severe form of TEN has been described in HIV-infected individuals [57a,57b]. Some cases remain idiopathic (Table 218-3) [52,58].

Histopathologically, there are vacuolar changes in the basal cell layer of the epidermis resulting in subepidermal cleavage and extensive necrosis of the epidermis. Only sparse lymphocytes and histiocytes are present perivascularly in the superficial dermis.

TEN generally affects adults at least 40 years of age, although it has been reported sometimes in children [59–62]. Initially patients may experience a burning sensation of the skin and conjunctivae, with fever, malaise, and arthralgias. Shortly thereafter tender erythema develops on the face and extremities, becoming confluent over a few hours to days. Within 1 to 3 days flaccid multiloculated bullae form, which peel off in sheets to leave painful denuded areas (Plate II-2). Pressure with torsion on an area of erythema produces new areas of cleavage of the skin (Nikolsky's sign). Usually the oral, genital, urethral, and anal mucosae as well as conjunctivae are severely involved with inflammation and erosions. Fingernails, toenails, and hair may be shed, although the palms and soles may be spared.

There are no specific laboratory abnormalities in TEN. There may be transaminase, blood urea nitrogen, and creatinine elevation, thrombocytopenia, albuminuria, and fluid and electrolyte derangement [52]. Granulocytopenia that fails to improve within 1 week has been associated with a grave prognosis [45,63].

TEN clinically resembles a disease of infants and young children called staphylococcal scalded skin syndrome (SSSS), which in the past was described under the name TEN. The two are, however, quite distinct from one another [45]. In SSSS, a superficial cleavage through the granular layer high in the epidermis is caused by a staphylococcal-phage group II exotoxin. The healthy mature kidney is probably capable of excreting this toxin [64,65]. Antibodies may also play a role in the pathogenesis of SSSS [66]. Prompt treatment with antistaphylococcal antibiotics gives children with this disorder an excellent prognosis. SSSS occasionally strikes adults who have renal failure, immunosuppression, immunodeficiency, or overwhelming staphylococcal sepsis, in which case the prognosis is poorer [66–72]. Other conditions to be distinguished from TEN include chemical burns, erythema multiforme, toxic shock syndrome [73], and some bullous diseases of the skin [46,48]. Appropriate bacterial stains and cultures, a frozen section of the roof of a blister, and routine skin biopsy can help in the differentiation.

Systemic involvement in TEN may include acute renal failure due to either acute tubular necrosis or immune-mediated glomerulonephritis [74,75]. Erosions of the GI and respiratory tracts resemble the skin changes histologically, and lead to hemorrhage, tracheitis, and pneumonia [76]. Sepsis, fluid and electrolyte imbalance, and GI hemorrhage are the major complications that have led to death in 20 to 50 percent of patients [12,45,52].

Therapy should begin with the removal of all possible causative drugs. Careful monitoring of fluid balance is essential to avoid pulmonary edema [77]. Frequent cultures of the blood, skin, and mucosal surfaces should be taken to allow prompt appropriate antibiotic administration for documented infection or signs of sepsis [35,77]. Although TEN patients have been likened to patients with second-degree burns, they differ by

Table 218-3. Some Causes of Toxic Epidermal Necrolysis

I. Drugs
  A. Sulfonamides
  B. Barbiturates
  C. Hydantoins
  D. Allopurinol
  E. Antibiotics
  F. Carbamazepine
  G. Nonsteroidal antiinflammatory agents
II. Infectious agents
  A. Viral
    1. Measles
    2. Varicella
    3. Herpes zoster
    4. Herpes simplex
  B. Bacterial
    1. *Escherichia coli*
    2. *Pseudomonas*
    3. *Klebsiella*
  C. Fungal
    1. *Aspergillus*
III. Vaccinations
  A. Measles
  B. Poliomyelitis
  C. Tetanus
  D. Diphtheria
  E. Smallpox
  F. BCG
IV. Neoplasms
  A. Lymphoma
  B. Leukemia
V. Graft-versus-host disease
VI. Connective tissue disease
  A. Systemic lupus erythematosus
VII. Beverages
  A. Quinine
VIII. Toxins
  A. Fumigants (acryl nitrate)
  B. Carbon monoxide
IX. Idiopathic

often having preexisting dehydration due to oral lesions antedating skin injury, usually displaying generalized cutaneous involvement that limits venous access, occasionally suffering visceral involvement, and always retaining an undamaged dermis. Nevertheless, many investigators have found that burn unit management facilitates care while reducing morbidity and mortality [77,78,79]. Controversies persist over the desirable extent of debridement [77,78], the use of allografts, xenografts, or synthetic dressings [77,78,80,81], and the application of topical antibiotics [35,77,78,79]. Systemic corticosteroids should probably be avoided, although frequently recommended in the past [77,78,82]. Controlled studies will be required to know if anecdotal success using plasmapheresis [77,83] or cyclosporine [84] can be confirmed.

Mucous membranes need special attention. Early ophthalmologic intervention may help prevent scarring, keratinization, and late sicca syndrome [45,77,78,85,86]. Oral care similar to that described for EM major (see Erythema Multiforme) may be beneficial. Vaginal lesions may be treated with topical anesthetics and hydrocortisone suppositories. Topical steroids may be used for involvement of the urethral meatus, and urologic consultation may be helpful for therapeutic suggestions to prevent late stricture or phimosis [45,48].

EXFOLIATIVE ERYTHRODERMA. An exfoliative erythroderma is a generalized or near total indurated erythema of the skin accompanied by scaling (exfoliation). It is characterized by an increase in epidermal cell turnover, dermal inflammation, and marked circulatory shunting to the skin [87]. Most commonly, this condition results from the exacerbation of an underlying dermatosis; some cases are due to the administration of a drug (Table 218-4) or the presence of a malignancy; the cause in many cases remains unknown (Table 218-5).

Although erythroderma can occur even at birth, the highest incidence appears to be in individuals over age 45 [88,89]. Men predominate (around 70%) [88,89,90]. The onset may be gradual or sudden. Common complaints include pruritus, which may be severe [91], and chills, probably due to uncontrolled convection and radiant heat losses through the skin [89,92]. There may also be symptoms of congestive heart failure or orthostatic hypotension [93].

Physical findings in addition to the erythroderma often include ectropion, excoriations, fissures, and crusts (Plate II-3) [92,94]. The palms and soles as well as the scalp may be involved with erythema and scaling [92,95]. Ankle edema is common [91,96]. In long-standing cases, alopecia and nail dystrophy may be present [89,91,92,94,97,98]. Mucous membranes are spared [95]. Hypothermia is common and may be life-threatening in itself, or it may conceal the fever of sepsis [99]. Fever may be present with or without evidence of infection [88,93], and may indicate a drug reaction [88,98]. Because of increased transepidermal water loss, hypovolemia is common. Lymphadenopathy is often present [89,92], demonstrating only reactive dermatopathic changes on histopathologic examination unless an underlying lymphoma is present [88,93,94,98,99]. Hepatomegaly is often seen [88,91,98,99]. Splenomegaly, if present, may indicate an underlying lymphoreticular neoplasm [88,92,95,99].

Common abnormalities in laboratory tests include mild anemia and marked elevation of the white blood cell count [89,90,95–98]. Eosinophilia is present in as many as half the patients [88,89] and may be more common in those with underlying atopic dermatitis or drug allergy [89,95,98]. Large numbers of circulating T cells with convoluted nuclei, known as Sézary cells, may help establish the diagnosis of Sezary syndrome, an erythrodermic form of cutaneous T cell lymphoma [95]. Serum protein electrophoresis often shows nondiagnostic irregularities, with hypoalbuminemia in chronic cases [88,91,93]. The skin biopsy demonstrates nonspecific changes or may even be misleading as to cause, except in patients with cutaneous T-cell lymphoma or leukemia, in whom the biopsy may reveal the primary diagnosis [88,92,95,99,100].

Exfoliative erythroderma is distinguished from the toxic erythemas associated with various bacterial and viral infections by its continuous scaling and longer duration. In the newborn, it may mimic widespread candidal infection and some forms of ichthyosis.

The management of exfoliative erythroderma requires elimination of the underlying cause when possible. Any potentially offending systemic or topical drug must be discontinued, and underlying malignancy should be treated [101]. A history of underlying skin disease, such as psoriasis, should not deter the investigation of other possible causes, such as drugs or malignancy [93]. Rarely, even scabies or dermatophytes may produce erythroderma [91,93,102]. Body temperature should be closely monitored and environmental temperature modulated accordingly. Areas of the skin that are fissured or crusted should be compressed after bacterial cultures have been obtained. Bland emollients and oral antihistamines often provide symptomatic relief of pruritus [94]. Topical agents, however, that contain

antibiotics, fragrances, or preservatives known to sensitize should be avoided [89]. Mild or moderate strength corticosteroid ointments with or without occlusion are indicated despite their significant percutaneous absorption. In severe cases not associated with psoriasis, systemic steroids (prednisone up to 60 mg daily tapered over 2 to 4 weeks) may be necessary [98,103,104]. When psoriasis is the underlying cause, systemic steroids should be avoided [103,105]; topical tars and oral antimalarials may also worsen psoriatic erythroderma [88,103,105]. On the other hand, methotrexate [106], ultraviolet light therapy [99,107,108,109], and etretinate [99,104,110], are often beneficial. Erythroderma due to cutaneous T-cell lymphoma has been successfully treated with alpha-interferon

Table 218-4. Drugs Frequently Responsible for Erythroderma

Allopurinol
Antimalarials
Arsenicals
Barbiturates
Gold
Iodides
Isoniazid
Mercurials
Para-amino salicylic acid
Penicillins
Phenylbutazone
Phenytoin
Quinidine
Streptomycin
Sulfonamides
Thiazides

Table 218-5. Summary of 1038 Cases from 11 Reviews of Erythroderma

Cause	No.	%
Underlying dermatosis		
Atopic and other eczema	182	18
Psoriasis	191	18
Contact dermatitis	76	7
Seborrheic dermatitis	38	4
Stasis dermatitis	14	1
Pityriasis rubra pilaris	12	1
Other	35	3
Total	548	52
Drug ingestion or injection		
Penicillin	18	2
Sulfonamide	16	1
Antituberculous agents	17	2
Anticonvulsants	14	1
Antimalarials	10	1
Gold	6	1
Other	91	9
Total	172	17
Malignancy		
Cutaneous T-cell lymphoma	46	4
Other lymphoma	28	3
Solid neoplasm	13	1
Leukemia	12	1
Total	99	10
Unknown	218	21

and, more recently, with extracorporeal photopheresis [110a,110b]. Although erythroderma is often tolerated well for long periods [88,94,103], death has resulted from hypothermia [94,111], congestive heart failure, myocardial infarction, pneumonia, septicemia, and associated malignancy [88,92,94,95, 97,98,100,103].

PUSTULAR PSORIASIS OF VON ZUMBUSCH. Pustular psoriasis of von Zumbusch is a potentially fatal form of psoriasis characterized by the acute onset of generalized pustules, high fever, leukocytosis, and malaise [112,113]. Although the pathogenesis of this disease remains unknown, its victims comprise two distinct groups. In the first are patients who have had stable typical psoriasis vulgaris since early in life and who suddenly develop a flare with widespread pustulation. Usually the episode is triggered by some factor, such as withdrawal of systemic or potent topical steroids [112,113,114], use of nonsteroidal antiinflammatory agents [112] or lithium [115], pregnancy [112,113], sunburn [112,116], infection [112,113,114], alcohol [105,112], emotional factors [105,117], or hypocalcemia [118]. The second group of affected individuals are those who develop psoriasis later in life (41 to 60 years old), often with an atypical distribution (such as flexural or acral) or morphology (especially annular) [112,114]. Their onset is followed shortly by the generalized pustular involvement with no obvious precipitant [112,114]. Recent investigations into the mechanism of this disease have focused on leukotrienes chemotactic for neutrophils [119].

Often an episode of pustular psoriasis is heralded by a mild fever, granulocytosis, and skin hyperesthesia [112]. Mild erythema and edema of the skin are followed by rapidly spreading crops of shallow, sterile pustules that coalesce atop fiery red skin (Plate II-4) [112,113]. Fever reaches 104°F (40°C) and white blood cell counts may be over 30,000. Waves of recurrent pustulation sometimes continue for several weeks with periods of remission [112]. Pustules may form under the nails, resulting in onycholysis. Mucosal lesions include geographic and fissured tongue [120]. As many as one-third of patients eventually develop acute or chronic arthritis, often with distal interphalangeal and sacroiliac involvement [112]. Purulent sterile conjunctivitis or more severe eye problems may occur [112].

Hypoalbuminemia and hypocalcemia are the most common laboratory abnormalities during the acute attacks [112,113, 118,121]. Elevated liver enzymes may be due to drugs, heart failure, or pericholangitis, which has been found on liver biopsy [112,122]. Renal dysfunction has also been reported, and anemia is common [112].

The differential diagnosis of this disease includes infections, such as folliculitis, impetigo, and candidiasis. The marked erythema and edema may suggest cellulitis or thrombophlebitis. Pemphigus foliaceus, subcorneal pustular dermatosis, pustular miliaria, pustular drug eruptions, and Sweet's syndrome may also need to be considered. The diagnosis can be confirmed by finding the characteristic spongiform pustule of Kogoj, a pustule located high in the epidermis, on a biopsy from the skin in pustular psoriasis [123].

The treatment of von Zumbusch's psoriasis is difficult; 26 of 155 patients in one series died from either the disease or the treatment [114]. Hospitalization with bed rest, compresses or baths, and bland emollients is recommended [112]. The patient should be carefully monitored for fluid and electrolyte status, secondary infection, hypocalcemia, and renal and hepatic dysfunction. Systemic steroid administration has been associated with higher morbidity and mortality [112,114,124]. Methotrexate therapy, despite careful monitoring, may cause fatal complications [112,114,124]. Hydroxyurea, which has induced remissions in some patients, has significant bone marrow toxicity [112]. Etretinate, a new aromatic retinoid, is presently the drug of choice for patients with severe disease, often producing rapid improvement [112,125,126,127]. The initial oral dose recommended varies from 0.5 to 2.0 mg per kilogram in a divided daily dose [112,127]. In some instances, methotrexate has been given in combination with etretinate with good results [128,129]. Some cases have cleared on cyclosporin [130], isotretinoin [131], calcipotriol [131a], or photochemotherapy with psoralen and long wave ultraviolet light (PUVA) [132]. Relapses are common in patients whose generalized pustular psoriasis has occurred late in life without a known provocative factor, and maintenance therapy may be required.

PEMPHIGUS VULGARIS. Pemphigus vulgaris is a rare but serious disease characterized by superficial flaccid bullae, which leave large weeping erosions on the skin and mucous membranes when they rupture. The blisters result from the loss of normal adhesion between epidermal cells (acantholysis) [133,134]. Immunopathologic studies reveal IgG and often complement components in the intercellular spaces in the epidermis [133]. Circulating antibody directed against the epidermal cell surface and capable of causing in vitro acantholysis is also found in these patients [133,134]. An autoimmune basis for the disease is further supported by its occasional association with other autoimmune disorders, including thymoma, myasthenia gravis, and systemic lupus erythematosus [133,135]. The occasional occurrence in families, as well as the increased frequency of HLA-A10 and HLA-DR4, suggests a genetic link.

Pemphigus vulgaris affects both men and women of any age [133]. It is more common among people of Jewish or Mediterranean ancestry [133,136]. Over half the patients develop oral lesions weeks to months before the appearance of skin involvement [133,134,136]. Cutaneous blisters measure a centimeter or more and may arise on normal or erythematous skin [133,134]. Their intraepidermal location causes them to rupture easily, producing glistening erosions (Plate II-5). Sites of predilection include the face, axillae, groin, trunk, and areas of trauma [133,136]. In fact, lateral pressure applied to normal appearing skin will often create a new separation of the epidermis (Nikolsky's sign) [133,137]. The entire oral cavity may be involved, as well as the esophagus [138,139], duodenum, colon [140], urethra, vulva, larynx, and conjunctiva [133]. Lesions heal without scarring but occasionally with temporary hyperpigmentation.

Laboratory abnormalities are seldom reported in patients with pemphigus vulgaris, although peripheral eosinophilia may be present in 45 percent [133]. A skin biopsy is the most helpful laboratory test to establish the diagnosis. It demonstrates characteristic cleft formation above the basal cell layer of the epidermis; individual keratinocytes lie free within the cavity [133,134]. A Tzanck smear, a quick cytologic preparation performed by scraping the base of a blister, may show free-lying epidermal cells with pyknotic nuclei [133,141]. Immunofluorescent microscopy of the skin will reveal IgG deposition in the intercellular spaces of the epidermis [133–136]. Eighty to 90 percent of patients also manifest pemphigus IgG antibodies circulating in the serum (visualized by indirect immunofluorescence), the titer of which usually correlates with disease activity [133,134].

The differential diagnosis of pemphigus vulgaris includes other causes of extensive bullae and erosions, such as TEN and EM major (see Toxic Epidermal Necrolysis and Erythema Multiforme), bullous impetigo, and bullous pemphigoid. In the latter disease, which has a much lower morbidity and mortality than pemphigus vulgaris, subepidermal separation produces tense bullae. Polymorphonuclear leukocytes and eosinophils may be present on Tzanck smear, but acantholytic keratinocytes are not. Immunofluorescence in bullous pemphigoid shows immunoglobulins (especially IgG) and complement deposited at the dermal-epidermal junction. In bullous impetigo, a Gram's stain of blister fluid will demonstrate gram-positive cocci and a culture should yield *Staphylococcus aureus* or streptococci.

The management of patients with pemphigus vulgaris is a medical and nursing challenge. Before the advent of antibiotics and corticosteroids, 90 to 100 percent of affected patients died within the first 2 years of diagnosis [142]. Mortality rates continue to be high among those patients who acquire the disease over the age of 50 years and in those whose disease is severe enough to require daily doses of prednisone greater than 180 mg [143,144]. Opportunistic infections may complicate therapy. Pneumonia and sepsis, especially with *S. aureus*, are common causes of death, as are pulmonary embolus, myocardial infarction, and GI hemorrhage [142,144].

In pemphigus vulgaris, prompt institution of therapy is vital [136,142]. For patients with extensive or advancing lesions, corticosteroids should be started at a dosage equivalent to at least 80 to 120 mg of prednisone daily [133,142,145]. If new blister formation is not suppressed within 5 days, the dosage should be incrementally increased [142,145]. Although there is little evidence verifying their clear benefit, various immunosuppressive agents (especially cyclophosphamide, azathioprine, and methotrexate), as well as gold, plasmapheresis, and dapsone have been added to the therapy in an effort to control difficult cases or facilitate steroid tapering after most lesions have healed [133,145,146]. Pulse intravenous corticosteroids given intermittently may reduce long-term sequelae of steroid therapy, although the risk of acute effects such as hyperglycemia, pulmonary edema, and sepsis necessitate in-hospital monitoring [146a]. Plasmapheresis, although attractive theoretically as a means of reducing circulating autoantibodies, may promote sepsis [147], must be performed frequently, and requires the concommitant administration of a cytotoxic drug or high dose of steroid to prevent rebound antibody production [147, 148,149].

Throughout therapy, skin hygiene must be meticulous. Local skin care may include compresses, silver sulfadiazine cream, or semipermeable dressings [150]. Oral ulcers may benefit from topical steroids in a gel or suspension form. Oral irrigation with saline or dilute hydrogen peroxide, as well as frequent rinses with antibacterial and antiyeast suspensions may reduce halitosis and secondary infection.

DISSEMINATED CUTANEOUS HERPES SIMPLEX VIRUS INFECTION. Widespread skin infection with HSV is an uncommon event that rarely is associated with fatal visceral involvement. Primary infection with herpes simplex usually produces localized oral or genital lesions; recrudescence of the virus generally causes a small number of rapidly healing grouped vesicles recurrently at one site. In two principal settings, however, either primary or recurrent infection with HSV can lead to numerous extensive cutaneous lesions: (1) in certain skin disorders (see Table 218-6), the most common being atopic dermatitis, in which the widespread infection is known as eczema herpeticum or Kaposi's varicelliform eruption, and (2) in immunosuppression, especially from lymphoreticular malignancies [151–159]. Either type 1 or type 2 *Herpesvirus hominis* may be responsible [159], and similar eruptions can also result from vaccinia [154,160] or Coxsackie A16 [161]. The exact nature of the immunologic problem that allows dissemination has not been defined [152,162]. Although herpetic lesions may localize to the areas of active dermatitis in patients suffering from atopic dermatitis [162], cutaneous dissemination can occur both in

Table 218-6. Underlying Conditions in Which Cutaneous Dissemination of Herpes Simplex Virus Infection Has Occurred

A. Skin disorder
  1. Atopic dermatitis
  2. Wiskott-Aldrich syndrome
  3. Pemphigus vulgaris
  4. Keratosis follicularis (Darier's disease)
  5. Burns
  6. Pemphigus foliaceus
  7. Seborrheic dermatitis
  8. Ichthyosiform erythroderma (epidermolytic hyperkeratosis)
  9. Ichthyosis vulgaris
  10. Erythroderma
B. Immunocompromised host
  1. Cutaneous T-cell lymphoma (mycosis fungoides)
  2. Other lymphomas
  3. Leukemias
  4. Acquired immunodeficiency syndrome
  5. Systemic lupus erythematosus
  6. Renal transplant
  7. Thymic dysplasia
  8. Pregnancy
  9. Newborn
C. Other
  1. Chronic renal failure, postoperative nephrectomy, and splenectomy
  2. Healthy adult

these patients [151,160,163] and in those suffering from Darier's disease [154] when the skin appears to be normal.

Disseminated cutaneous herpes simplex virus infection is most common in children and young adults [151,152,155]. Lesions begin as crops of 2- to 5-mm umbilicated vesicles or pustules on an erythematous base, appearing over 3 to 7 days (Plate II-6). The usual sites involved are the head, neck, and upper trunk, and sometimes the extremities [151,152,155]. Affected areas may be painful or pruritic with prominent edema and regional lymphadenopathy. Low-grade fever, myalgia, headache, anorexia, and malaise are not uncommon [151,152,154]. The lesions evolve into "punched-out" tiny, round ulcers, which remain discrete or coalesce into large ulcers with scalloped margins. Crusts may be present on earlier lesions at the same time new vesicles continue to appear. Healing may leave hypopigmentation or slight scarring [152]. In patients with underlying skin disorders, the lesions resolve in an average of 16 days [155]. In immunosuppressed individuals, however, new lesions may continue to form over many months, and extensive erosions may be slow to heal [152,155,159].

The diagnosis of HSV infection can be strongly suspected if a Tzanck preparation made by scraping a vesicle demonstrates multinucleated giant keratinocytes, which are only seen in varicella-zoster and HSV infections (Plate II-7) [164]. A viral culture, most sensitive if fresh vesicles are swabbed, may be positive within 24 hours [165]. Even long-standing ulcers in the immunosuppressed patient, however, may yield the virus [166]. Other techniques that may confirm the presence of HSV include fluorescent antibody, polymerase chain reaction, (equivalent in sensitivity to fluorescent antibody) and immunoperoxidase staining of blister cells or tissue [165,167,167a]. The virus has also been recovered from the buffy coat of one patient with a varicelliform eruption [156].

The differential diagnosis of the disseminated eruption of HSV includes infection with varicella or Coxsackie virus, EM (see Erythema Multiforme), impetigo, and other blistering diseases. The characteristic clustering of new vesicles around the first lesion as it crusts may be a clue to the herpetic etiology.

Routine histopathologic examination of a skin biopsy and Tzanck cytology will not distinguish herpes simplex from varicella infection, although viral culture and other tests mentioned previously can. In EM, the vesicles are usually larger. Impetigo should demonstrate streptococci or staphylococci on lesional Gram's stain and culture.

Occasionally herpes virus infections may be mistaken for exacerbations of eczema in atopic individuals. Sometimes recurrences of disseminated HSV infection also occur as well [151,161,162,163]. Clues that the process is not merely dermatitis are (1) the new onset of pain or pruritus; (2) an umbilication of the vesicles; (3) a vesicular diameter as large as 3 to 5 mm; (4) the appearance of new discrete vesicles; and (5) absolutely round ulcers, distinct from the linear, triangular, and irregular erosions produced by excoriations [154,162]. Additionally, most atopic patients who develop disseminated herpes or vaccinia infection have a history of recent exposure to the virus or the vaccination, respectively.

The most common complications of disseminated cutaneous HSV infection are secondary bacterial infection and ocular involvement. Fatalities, although rare, have been reported to result from bacterial superinfection, fluid or electrolyte imbalance, and visceral spread of the virus [151]. Organs of predilection include the lungs, liver, GI tract, adrenal glands, and central nervous system (CNS). Visceral dissemination is rare in individuals who are not immunosuppressed [155], but when it does occur, viral lesions of the mucosa are more often present than is a generalized cutaneous eruption [168–171]. Often, however, visceral infection in the form of hepatitis [171,172], esophagitis [173], or encephalitis [174] develops with no mucosal or skin lesions apparent. In the immunosuppressed patient with widespread cutaneous HSV infection, although the mortality may be as high as 38 percent [155], visceral viral dissemination is seldom documented to be the cause of death [159]. In patients dying of visceral infection, the diagnosis of herpes is rarely made before their death [170,173].

No controlled trials have been reported to investigate the therapy of disseminated cutaneous HSV infection. Although intravenous (IV) adenine arabinoside has been used in the past [151,175], more recently IV followed by oral acyclovir has been reported to promote healing [151,176–179]. Compresses may afford symptomatic relief, and the use of topical antibacterial preparations may reduce secondary infection. The prompt institution of appropriate isolation procedures with strict use of rubber gloves is essential to protect medical personnel from inoculation during routine care of the patient [180].

Life-Threatening Systemic Diseases With Prominent Skin Involvement

PURPURA FULMINANS. Purpura fulminans is a rare but devastating disorder characterized by extensive and rapidly progressive ecchymosis of the skin, fever, hypotension, and disseminated intravascular coagulation (DIC). Histopathology reveals thrombosis of the superficial capillaries and venules of involved skin. The mechanism seems to involve either primary congenital or secondary acquired deficiency of proteins C and S, which are vitamin K–dependent anticoagulant and fibrinolytic proteins [181,182,183]. DIC probably precedes the hemorrhage into the skin [181,184].

Purpura fulminans usually appears in one of three settings. It is most common in children in whom there is a history of recent infection, such as viral-induced upper respiratory illness, gastroenteritis, scarlet fever, scarlatina, varicella, meningococ-

cemia, staphylococcal bacteremia, rubella, roseola, streptococcal pharyngitis, hemophilus meningitis, Rocky Mountain spotted fever, or leptospirosis [181,184,185,186]. In a second group of patients, the purpura accompanies DIC in a serious systemic illness. The third presentation is in those neonates who inherit a homozygous deficiency of protein C [181].

Neonates with protein C deficiency usually develop purpura soon after birth [181]. For the other groups, the latent period from the premonitory event to the onset of purpura varies from 1 day to 3 weeks. The cutaneous changes appear abruptly. Large irregular areas of purpura develop symmetrically (Plate II-8), usually affecting the lower extremities first [184,185,186]. The purpura may extend to the abdomen and upper extremities, but the face, chest, and genitalia are seldom involved [186]. The ecchymotic areas evolve into hemorrhagic and necrotic bullae, and subsequently, hard eschars. Compartment syndromes may occur due to circumferential involvement and edema, and major amputations are common in survivors [184,185,186]. Fever and hypotension are usually present [184,185]. Seizures may accompany the syndrome in one-third of cases [186], and visceral thrombosis may produce hemorrhagic infarction of the bowel or bladder [181]. The disease sometimes progresses in waves, with disease activity for up to 2 weeks [181,184].

Laboratory abnormalities include an elevated white blood cell count with a left shift and anemia. Coagulation studies demonstrate a variable but low platelet count, positive plasma protamine test, reduced fibrinogen level, and increased fibrin degradation products [184].

The differential diagnosis of purpura fulminans includes many other causes of extensive ecchymosis, hemorrhagic bullae, and cutaneous necrosis (Table 218-7). Severe thrombocytopenia on any basis may cause widespread acral or dependent purpura. Cryoglobulinemia, TEN (see Toxic Epidermal Necrolysis), and allergic rheumatologic or septic vasculitis can lead to hemorrhagic bullae. Coumarin or heparin necrosis (see Drug Eruptions), phlegmasia cerulea dolens, necrotizing fasciitis, and many forms of necrotizing cellulitis and ischemia may mimic the necrotic stage.

Complications in patients with purpura fulminans are common due to shock and DIC. Acute respiratory, hepatic, and renal failure occur, as do GI bleeding and cardiomyopathy [186,187]. In patients with sepsis, the mortality is 40 percent, while only 17 percent of children who acquire the syndrome in a postviral setting die [187].

Initial therapy is aimed at prompt reversal of any identifiable cause of underlying DIC. Shock should be treated with fluid and blood replacement and cardiotonic drugs, avoiding peripheral vasconstrictors that may enhance thrombus formation [186,187]. Heparin is recommended in large doses by continuous infusion (100 to 150 U/kg q6h) to arrest further thrombosis [184,188]. Fresh frozen plasma, factor IX concentrate, antithrombin III, and cryoprecipitate can restore protein C or protein S levels and have been recommended by some authors [181,183,184,184a]. Dextran, hyperbaric oxygen, and streptokinase have not been proven beneficial, and corticosteroid use is controversial [184,186]. Surgical intervention must be prompt for fasciotomies, debridement of eschars, amputation, and grafting [184–187]. Burn unit management may be helpful for patients with extensive full-thickness skin loss [187] (see Chap. 179).

ROCKY MOUNTAIN SPOTTED FEVER. Rocky Mountain spotted fever (RMSF), an acute, sometimes fatal, tick-borne rickettsial infection, is discussed in detail in Chapter 142. The incubation period for RMSF ranges from 1 to 14 days, with an

Table 218-7. Some Causes of Purpuric or Necrotic Lesions

I. Within the bloodstream
   A. Platelet disorders (see Chaps. 118 and 120)
      1. Thrombocytopenia
      2. Functional disturbance
      3. Thrombocytosis
   B. Coagulation disorders (see Chaps. 119 and 121)
      1. Factor deficiency
      2. Anticoagulation
      3. Hyperviscosity
   C. Embolization
      1. Atheromatous
      2. Thromboembolic
      3. Myxomatous
      4. Marantic
      5. Fat
      6. Gas
      7. Tumor
   D. Infection
      1. Bacterial
         a. Gram-positive cocci (e.g., *Staphylococcus aureus,* microaerophilic streptococci)
         b. Gram-positive rods (e.g., *Bacillus anthracis, Corynebacterium diphtheriae*)
         c. Gram-negative diplococci (e.g., *Neisseria meningitidis* and *Neisseria gonorrhoeae*)
         d. Gram-negative rods (e.g., *Pseudomonas aeruginosa* and *Pseudomonas cepacia, Serratia marcescens, Campylobacter fetus, Proteus mirabilis, Escherichia coli, Citrobacter freundii, Aeromonas hydrophila, Klebsiella pneumoniae, Salmonella enteritidis,* and *Salmonella typhimurium*)
         e. Acid-fast bacilli (e.g., *Mycobacterium tuberculosis, Mycobacterium leprae,* and *Mycobacterium ulcerans*)
         f. Fusospirochetes
         g. Treponema (e.g., *Treponema pallidum*)
      2. Viral
         a. Herpes simplex
         b. Vaccinia
         c. Varicella-zoster
         d. Rubeola
      3. Rickettsial
         a. Rocky Mountain spotted fever
         b. Typhus
      4. Protozoan
         a. Amebiasis cutis
         b. Schistosomiasis cutis
      5. Fungal
         a. Phycomycosis
         b. Nocardiosis
         c. Actinomycosis
         d. Sporotrichosis
         e. Histoplasmosis
         f. Cryptococcosis
         g. North American blastomycosis
         h. South American blastomycosis
         i. Aspergillosis
      6. Systemic candidiasis
II. Within the vessel walls
   A. Necrotizing vasculitis
      1. Leukocytoclastic vasculitis
         a. Infections
         b. Drugs
         c. Foreign proteins
         d. Chemicals and ingestants
         e. Underlying systemic diseases
         f. Familial C2 deficiency
         g. Urticarial vasculitis
         h. Henoch-Schönlein purpura
      2. Rheumatoid vasculitis
         a. Systemic lupus erythematosus
         b. Mixed connective tissue disease
         c. Sjögren's syndrome
         d. Rheumatoid arthritis
         e. Dermatomyositis
         f. Progressive systemic sclerosis
      3. Granulomatous vasculitis
         a. Allergic granulomatous angiitis (Churg-Strauss syndrome)
         b. Wegener's granulomatosis
         c. Lymphomatoid granulomatosis
      4. Polyarteritis nodosa
      5. Giant cell arteritis (temporal arteritis)
      6. Pyoderma gangrenosum
   B. Altered vessel integrity
      1. Hereditary hemorrhagic telangiectasia
      2. Amyloidosis
      3. Scurvy
      4. Ehlers-Danlos syndrome
      5. Pseudoxanthoma elasticum
      6. Steroid purpura
      7. Senile purpura
      8. Stasis dermatitis
      9. Benign capillaritis (Schamberg's)
   C. Ischemia
      1. Occlusion
         a. Arteriosclerosis
         b. Thromboangiitis obliterans
      2. Vasospasm
         a. Raynaud's syndrome
         b. Vasopressor infusion
         c. Ergotism
         d. Accidental intraarterial infusion
         e. Hypertensive ischemic ulcer
III. Outside the vessel wall
   A. Physical agents
      1. Temperature extremes (e.g., frostbite, thermal burn)
      2. Trauma
      3. Pressure
      4. Radiant energy
      5. Electrical energy
   B. Chemical agents
      1. Topical vesicants and escharotics
      2. Extravasated medications (e.g., daunorubicin hydrochloride, norepinephrine bitartrate, sulfobromophthalein)
      3. Factitious injections
      4. Venoms of snakes, spiders, marine life
   C. Tumor necrosis
   D. Gangrenous cellulitis
      1. Necrotizing fasciitis
      2. Progressive bacterial synergistic gangrene
      3. Clostridial myonecrosis
      4. Synergistic necrotizing cellulitis

average of 4 to 8 days [189,190]. Fever of abrupt onset to 40°C and headache, both refractory to common treatments, are usually present and may precede other signs by a week or more [191]. Other manifestations include malaise, photophobia, myalgia, arthralgia, anorexia, nausea, vomiting, abdominal pain, and diarrhea. The characteristic rash may be absent or overlooked in up to 20 percent of cases [191–193]. It usually occurs by the fifth day of illness, although it may appear as early as the first day of fever or as late as the eighth day [191]. Blanchable irregular 2- to 6-mm macules are noted first on the ankles or wrists (Plate II-9), spreading within hours to the hands and feet, including palms and soles, and finally to the trunk and head [189,190,191]. The macules may become papules, and with advancing disease become petechial and purpuric, often coalescing into large areas of necrosis [189]. Within 4 days of the onset of the rash, periorbital edema and nonpitting, nondependent edema of the face and extremities often develops. Common ocular findings include conjunctivitis, petechiae, and photophobia.

Immunofluorescence or immunoperoxidase stains of a biopsy taken from the rash may show evidence of rickettsiae within the first week of illness, but the technique is not available in many institutions and antibiotic treatment may cause negative results [189,190,191,191a]. Identification of the organism in monocytes has allowed early confirmation but is also not widely used [190].

GRAFT-VERSUS-HOST DISEASE. Graft-versus-host disease (GVHD) can occur whenever lymphoid cells from an immunocompetent donor are introduced into an immunosuppressed histoincompatible recipient. In its acute form GVHD appears in 50 to 60 percent of bone marrow recipients, and it produces chronic changes in 30 percent of all long-term bone marrow transplant survivors [195]. Significant mortality is associated with the disease [195,196]. Methods to prevent GVHD include the use of immunosuppressive agents and the elimination of donor T lymphocytes [196].

Acute GVHD usually occurs by day 60 after transplantation and affects the skin, liver, and GI tract [197,198]. It is probably produced by donor cytotoxic T cells. Most often a somewhat pruritic macular exanthem begins on the palms, soles, and cheeks. It may spread over the extremities and trunk in an evanescent form, or progress to a bullous exfoliative erythroderma or TEN (see Toxic Epidermal Necrolysis) (see Plate II-2) [197,198,199]. Fever, jaundice, and diarrhea are often present. Although the cutaneous eruption may be mimicked by a drug eruption or an infectious exanthem, skin biopsy usually confirms the diagnosis [195,198]. Corticosteroids (topical and parenteral), methotrexate, antihuman antithymocyte globulin, and cyclosporin, as well as other agents, have been used for therapy [196,197,197a].

Chronic GVHD need not be preceded by acute GVHD and may occur months to years after bone marrow transplantation. The liver, intestinal tract, eyes, respiratory tract, oral and genital mucosae, and skin are frequent targets [197]. A localized area of skin may become hyperpigmented and indurated, and subsequently sclerotic. A more generalized eruption may also be seen that resembles lichen planus, with violaceous flat-topped papules and white lacy mucosal lesions [197]. Scaly plaques, desquamation, periungual erythema, and scarring alopecia [195] also may be present. Later in the course of chronic GVHD, a sclerodermalike thickening may ensue, often accompanied by dyspigmentation, telangiectasia, and atrophy (a combination of clinical findings known as *poikiloderma*). In chronic GVHD, the clinical features, laboratory abnormalities such as circulating autoantibodies and increased eosinophils, and pathologic findings of plasmacytosis of viscera and lymph nodes often mimic

Sjögren's syndrome, lupus erythematosus, dermatomyositis, and other autoimmune disorders [199]. Contractures and ulcerations, dry eyes and mouth, pulmonary insufficiency, and weight loss cause major morbidity [200]. Those patients with localized chronic GVHD do well without treatment [195]. For generalized chronic GVHD, prednisone together with either azathioprine or cyclophosphamide has been used [197,200]. PUVA photochemotherapy and particularly extracorporeal photopheresis have been used experimentally for treatment of chronic GVHD and hold much promise [200a,200b,200c].

TOXIC SHOCK SYNDROME. Toxic shock syndrome (TSS) is an acute illness characterized by high fever, diffuse cutaneous erythema, hypotension, and vomiting or diarrhea [201–206]. A detailed discussion of TSS and its treatment appears in Chapter 91.

Usually the illness presents with a precipitous fever of at least 38.9°C (102°F), chills, myalgias, headache, hypotension (systolic blood pressure of 90 mm Hg or less), vomiting or diarrhea, and a widespread rash. The diffuse sunburnlike nontender, blanchable, macular erythema may be prominent or so mild as to be overlooked or attributed to the fever [201,207]. This erythema may evolve into discrete macules [203] and may be localized rather than generalized, for example, to involve only the inguinal area or extremities [201]. Commonly there is brawny nonpitting edema of the face, eyelids, palms, and soles at presentation [201,208]. Mucosal involvement, including pharyngeal redness, palatal petechiae, conjunctival suffusion, tender vulvar hyperemia, and strawberry tongue are variably present [202,208]. Between days 5 and 12, the face, trunk, and extremities show a fine desquamation, which is followed by peeling of the palms and soles. Healing occurs without scarring. Histopathology of the skin rash demonstrates only a nonspecific mild lymphohistiocytic infiltrate around the blood vessels of the upper and middle dermis [207].

The differential diagnosis of TSS includes a variety of diseases that affect multiple organ systems. The cutaneous findings may suggest early SSSS, in which shock and multisystem involvement are not present. Streptococcal scarlet fever usually produces a "sandpapery," granular-feeling exanthem, and evidence of group A streptococci can be found. Mucocutaneous lymph node syndrome (Kawasaki's disease) has many similarities but generally occurs before the age of 5 years and lacks the severe myalgias, abdominal pain, and hypotension. Furthermore, the presence of lymphadenopathy, prolonged fever, and thrombocytosis rather than thrombocytopenia also help differentiate it. In the stage of discrete macules, the cutaneous eruption of TSS may resemble a drug eruption, a viral exanthem, atypical measles, early RMSF, and leptospirosis. In some patients a diagnosis of systemic lupus erythematosus, septic shock, erythema multiforme major, or tick-borne typhus may be entertained.

SEPSIS. Cutaneous lesions may be very important in sepsis. First they may mark the onset of septicemia (Plate II-10) [209–214] or disseminated intravascular coagulation or (DIC) [215]. They may also provide a prognostic indicator [210,215]. Additionally, the lesions may yield the responsible organism [210,211,214,216,217], even when blood cultures are negative [218–221].

The exact pathogenesis of the various skin lesions seen in sepsis is unknown. The major factors that are likely to be responsible are the organisms themselves, endotoxins or other bacterial products, antigen-antibody complexes, and embolized vegetations [218,222].

Table 218-8. Types of Skin Lesions That May Occur with Sepsis

Macules	Vesicles and bullae
Blanchable	Serous
Petechial	Hemorrhagic
Patches	Pustular
Ecchymotic	Necrotic
Gangrenous	Ulcers
Papules	Ruptured vesicles
Blanched center	Necrotic
Erythematous	Nodules
Purpuric	Erythematous
Plaques	Purpuric
Cellulitic	Necrotic
Necrotic	Thrombophlebitic
	Fluctuant

A host of morphologically different cutaneous abnormalities has been associated with sepsis from bacteria, yeast, and fungi (Table 218-8) [209,223]. None of the particular types of lesions is pathognomonic for sepsis or for a particular causative organism. Disseminated purpuric papules and plaques, for example, have been described from causes as diverse as leptospirosis and fungemia to staphylococcal sepsis in an immunocompromised host [218,224]. Splinter hemorrhages, Osler's nodes, and Janeway lesions, once common hallmarks of endocarditis, are now neither common nor specific to that diagnosis [210,214]. Cellulitis, with accompanying sepsis, may be caused by a variety of organisms other than staphylococci, including *Haemophilus influenzae* [225], *Vibrio* species [212,222], and other gram-negative organisms [222] and fungi [209].

Erysipelaslike plaques are usually caused by group A beta-hemolytic streptococci, but similar lesions have also been reported from other streptococci [226,227,228], *Pseudomonas aeruginosa* [210,221], and other organisms [222]. Bacterial causes of large bullae include *Neisseria meningitidis* [210], *Citrobacter freundii* [214], *Vibrio vulnificus* [229], and *Yersinia enterocolitica* [230]. Ecthyma gangrenosum begins as a painless, round erythematous macule, which rapidly becomes indurated, then bullous or pustular centrally, finally sloughing to yield a gangrenous ulcer or black eschar surrounded by a halo of erythema [210,218,231]. Although it was originally thought to occur only with *P. aeruginosa* sepsis, ecthyma gangrenosum has now been reported frequently from *Aeromonas* species and other gram-negative bacilli [210,218], *S. aureus* [210,232], yeast [209,210,218,220], and fungi [209,210]. Furthermore, identical lesions may be produced by vasculitis or malignancy in the absence of sepsis (see Table 218-7) [210]. Similarly, the red-based necrotic pustules associated with disseminated gonococcemia [210,233] may be mimicked by sepsis with staphylococci and nontyphoidal *Salmonella* species [234], as well as by vasculitis and viral infections. A unique central pallor is seen in some papules and nodules of disseminated candidiasis, but not in all [209] (See Moniliasis).

In sepsis, skin lesions may be single or multiple and are frequently acral (Plate II-11) [210]. If numerous, they may be monomorphic [224], or several different types of lesions may be present simultaneously or serially in the same patient [214,221]. Lesions that occur in the thrombocytopenic patient tend to become purpuric.

A Gram's stain and potassium hydroxide preparation performed on vesicle fluid [209,210,211,218,219,229] or skin biopsy tissue [209,210,220,224] may reveal organisms. Identification of the underlying pathogen may be made by culturing an aspirate of the skin lesion [209,211,214,216,219,221,229] or culturing tissue obtained by biopsy [209,210,218,223,232,233]. A touch preparation of the biopsied cutaneous tissue may be useful for obtaining a rapid diagnosis [217]. In disseminated gonococcemia, Gram's stain and culture of skin lesions are usually negative for *Neisseria gonorrhoeae,* but fluorescent antibody staining of the skin biopsy will identify the organism in over half the patients [233].

In sepsis the therapy is directed specifically toward the offending organism(s) and organ(s) involved (see Chap. 173). Occasionally surgical intervention may be required for debridement, drainage of abscesses, amputation, or grafting. It is important to remember that catheters and prosthetic devices may need to be removed in some instances to eradicate infection completely [222].

LYME DISEASE. Lyme disease, named after Lyme, Connecticut, where the original cluster of cases occurred [235], is a multisystem illness that affects primarily the skin, nervous system, heart, and joints. The disease is caused by a tick-transmitted spirochete *Borrelia burgdorferi* [235]. Infection is usually acquired between May and July as nymphal ticks feed [235]. People of all ages and both sexes are affected. Lyme disease, or Lyme borreliosis, has been recognized around the world. The implicated vectors are *Ixodes dammini* ticks in the northeastern and midwestern United States, *I. pacificus* in the western states, *I. racinis* in Europe, and *I. persulcatus* in Asia [235].

Lyme disease occurs in three different clinical stages, each of which may have exacerbations and remissions. A patient may have one or all the stages, and may pass through the first stage with no symptoms. Early infection, which occurs within a month of the tick bite, becomes manifest with a skin eruption. The second stage, which follows in days or weeks corresponds with disseminated infection. Finally, late infection, or stage 3, persistent infection, usually begins a year or more after the onset of infection [235].

In early infection (stage 1) local spread of the spirochetes in the skin from the site of inoculation results in erythema migrans in 60 to 80 percent of patients. The cutaneous findings may be accompanied by fever, regional lymphadenopathy, or mild constitutional symptoms. A typical erythematous macule or papule slowly enlarges surrounding the site of the bite to produce a large single or multiple smaller rings (Plate II-12). Spirochetes have been cultured from skin biopsies taken from the advancing margin [235,236]. The same site may demonstrate the etiologic agent in more than half the biopsies if processed with Gram's monoclonal antibody, Warthin-Starry, or modified Dieterle silver stain [236]. The eruption most frequently appears on the trunk or the proximal extremities, especially the thigh, buttock, and axilla. The lesions usually resolve within 3 or 4 weeks, although rarely they may persist more than a year or recur [235].

Erythema migrans is a characteristic eruption. It may, however, be confused with figurate erythemas, urticaria, serum sickness, erythema multiforme, erythema marginatum, cellulitis, erysipelas, erysipeloid, tinea, and tularemia.

Within days or weeks following injection, the spirochete may spread hematogeneously to various sites, including skin, neurologic and musculoskeletal systems, eyes, heart, liver, spleen, lymph nodes, testes, and respiratory system. Secondary skin lesions appear in about half these patients, resembling the primary lesion of erythema migrans, although usually smaller and less migratory [237]. A malar rash may be seen. Myositis, bone pains, panniculitis, conjunctivitis, hepatitis, lymphadenopathy, splenomegaly, orchitis, cough, pharyngitis, and respiratory distress syndrome may occur in this stage. Malaise and fatigue are often severe [235]. Transplacental transmission of the blood-borne spirochete has been reported [238,239].

Neurologic involvement is manifested in about 15 to 20 percent of patients, most frequently as the triad of meningitis, peripheral radiculoneuropathy, and cranial neuropathy, especially Bell's palsy [235,240]. If meningitis is present, the cerebrospinal fluid usually shows a lymphocytic pleocytosis, normal glucose, and elevated protein. The spirochete has been cultured from spinal fluid.

Cardiac involvement is seen in stage 2 in 4 to 8 percent of patients. The chief abnormality is fluctuating degrees of atrioventricular block [235,241]. More serious cardiac sequelae include acute myopericarditis, left ventricular dysfunction, cardiomegaly, and pancarditis [235,241]. Cardiac abnormalities usually reverse after 3 days to 6 weeks.

In the third stage or that of persistent infection, the affected individual has continuation of previously brief attacks of asymmetric oligoarticular arthritis of the large joints, especially the knee [235,242]. This complication develops in over half the patients in this country. Synovial fluid of affected joints shows white cell counts from 500 to 110,000/ml, predominantly polymorphonuclear leukocytes [235,242]. Borrelia has been cultured infrequently from joint fluid.

Because culture of the spirochete is difficult and its visualization in specimens often unsuccessful [236], serologic studies are currently the most reliable aid in diagnosis. Indirect immunofluorescence or the more sensitive and specific enzyme-linked immunosorbent assay (ELISA) is used to determine antibody response to B. burgdorferi. Antibody titers generally begin to rise several weeks after infection, although unless the special capture IgM ELISA is used, many patients will test negative in the acute phase of illness [235]. Falsely positive serologic results are even more common, especially in patients with autoimmune disorders, RMSF, syphilis, and some neurologic disorders [235]. In addition, test results often vary within and between laboratories [236,243]. Polymerase chain reaction may prove to be a more sensitive and specific test in the future [243a].

The present recommended treatment for early Lyme disease (localized stage 1 or disseminated stage 2) in adults is oral tetracycline 250 mg qid or doxycycline 100 mg bid for 10 to 30 days depending on clinical response [235,244]. Amoxicillin may be given as an alternate choice for adults (500 mg qid) or for children. Penicillin-allergic children may be given erythromycin, 30 mg/kg/day in divided doses [235,244]. Despite antibiotic therapy, about 50 percent of patients experience minor symptoms, including headache, musculoskeletal pain, and lethargy, which correlate with the severity of the initial illness [235].

IV therapy, generally ceftriaxone, 2 gm once daily for at least 2 weeks, is recommended for all patients with objective neurologic abnormalities other than Bell's palsy [235,244]. Alternatives include IV penicillin G (20 million units daily in 6 divided doses) or, for those allergic to ceftriaxone and penicillin G, oral doxycycline, 100 mg bid for 30 days [235,244]. IV ceftriaxone or penicillin should be chosen for patients with high degree atrioventricular block [235,244]. If response is not prompt, prednisone (40 to 60 mg daily) may be indicated [235]. Late arthritis may improve with 3 to 4 weeks of doxycycline, amoxicillin, ceftriaxone, or penicillin G, but studies are inconclusive. Intraarticular steroid use may have a role in refractory cases [235]. The best treatment for Lyme disease in pregnancy is not yet known.

BROWN RECLUSE SPIDER BITE (LOXOSCELISM).

The clinical response to envenomation by the brown recluse spider, known as loxoscelism, varies from an insignificant skin lesion to death [245]. The course of the reaction seems to depend on (1) the amount of venom inoculated, (2) the immune status and age of the victim (younger and older people are at greatest risk), and (3) the site of the bite [245,246] (see Chap. 142 for a complete discussion of loxoscelism).

Bites are reported most frequently between April and October, with the most common sites being the arm, leg, trunk, and hand [247]. Often the initial bite goes unnoticed or the agent is not identified. Two to 6 hours later pain, tingling, or itching, induration, and erythema occur at the site. A halo of pallor may envelop the area [245]. In more severe cases the erythema becomes violaceous or gray over 24 hours and develops bullae [245,248]. Ischemia follows, leading to necrosis, which may progress to an enlarging area of full-thickness necrosis over the subsequent 24 to 48 hours. An eschar forms, followed by ulceration in 2 weeks, which may take months to heal. Histologically there is endothelial swelling in the dermis with degeneration of the vessel walls, fibrin thrombi, hemorrhage, and a massive infiltrate of polymorphonuclear cells [245]. The damage is probably caused at least in part by numerous enzymes in the venom, such as esterase, hyaluronidase, protease, and sphingomyelinase D [245,248].

In addition to the local symptoms, malaise, chills, and sweats are common on presentation [248]. There may be a cellulitislike reaction on the extremity or a fine macular eruption over the entire body [247,249]. Generalized urticaria has also been described and may suggest severe envenomation [250].

Systemic envenomations may be life-threatening. Fever, petechiae, and constitutional symptoms occur within 3 days of the bite and may precede the reaction at the bite site. The systemic reaction is not necessarily proportional to the cutaneous response [245,248,251].

The differential diagnosis of loxoscelism includes a wide range of disorders, depending on the presentation and severity of the case. Notable causes of necrotic skin lesions for consideration are outlined in Table 218-7 (Plate II-13). Treatment for loxoscelism remains controversial (see Chap. 142) [245–248, 252, 253].

ACQUIRED IMMUNODEFICIENCY SYNDROME.

A variety of cutaneous lesions have been reported in individuals with acquired immunodeficiency syndrome (AIDS) (Table 218-9) (see Chap. 93). Although some of these conditions are seen as well in the general population and may be merely coincidental, others are quite rare [255] or, although common, may be more explosive, extensive, severe, or recalcitrant to therapy in AIDS patients [256,257].

Probably the most widely publicized skin abnormality associated with AIDS is Kaposi's sarcoma. Although it is seen primarily in homosexual men, its incidence among those patients at the time of their initial diagnosis of AIDS has steadily fallen (44% in 1981 to 20% in 1987) since it was initially identified as a marker of disease [255]. It has remained uncommon among heterosexual men with AIDS acquired through IV drug use and transfusion-related cases [255]. It has been found at autopsy, however, in more than 90 percent of patients in a variety of risk groups, usually present in the lymph nodes and spleen [258]. Cutaneous involvement is characterized by oval or fusiform macules, papules, plaques, or nodules that vary from brown to blue-violet [255]. Lesions are common on the head, upper trunk, and oropharyngeal mucosa [255]. They may develop rapidly, producing a disseminated bilaterally symmetrical eruption over the trunk and extremities. Lymph node involvement is often present at the time of diagnosis. Although the tumor often causes disability and severe disfigurement by its relentless growth and spread, it is seldom the cause of death.

Table 218-9. Cutaneous Lesions Seen with HIV Infection

Skin infections and infestations	Other
Acanthamoeba	Alopecia
Bacillary angiomatosis	Bullous pemphigoid
Botryomycosis	Drug eruption
Candida	Eosinophilic pustular folliculitis
Cytomegalovirus	Erythema elevatum diutinum
Dermatophyte	Granuloma annulare
Folliculitis	Ichthyosis
Gangrenous stomatitis	Long eyelashes
Hairy leukoplakia	Nail changes
Herpes simplex virus	Papular urticaria
Herpes zoster	Pityriasis rosea
Impetigo	Porphyria cutanea tarda
Molluscum contagiosum	Premature graying of hair
Mycobacteria	Pseudothrombophlebitis
Papilloma virus	Psoriasis
Scabies, Norwegian	Reiter's syndrome
Systemic infections	Seborrheic dermatitis
Coccidioidomycosis	Vasculitis
Cryptococcosis	
Histoplasmosis	
Pneumocystis	
Sporotrichosis	
Syphilis	
Malignancies	
Basal cell epithelioma	
Kaposi's sarcoma	
Lymphoma	
Malignant melanoma	
Mycosis fungoides	
Squamous cell carcinoma	

When circumstances require local treatment, radiotherapy, surgical excision, cryotherapy, and intralesional vinblastine or bleomycin have been used [255]. A biopsy diagnosis of Kaposi's sarcoma may help to establish the diagnosis of AIDS. In some reports the sarcoma tissue has also revealed atypical mycobacteria [259] and undifferentiated lymphoma [260], as well as cytomegalovirus [261,262], which has long been considered a possible causative agent in the malignancy.

Cutaneous reactions to drugs are very common in AIDS and AIDS-related complex (ARC) patients [254,263]. As many as 60 to 70 percent of those receiving trimethoprim-sulfamethoxazole, which is widely used for prophylaxis or therapy of *Pneumocystis carinii* pneumonia, will develop a widespread pruritic erythematous macular, papular, or urticarial eruption from the drug [254,263]. The rash usually appears between 8 and 12 days after beginning therapy, may be accompanied by a drug fever [254] and often persists for many weeks after discontinuation of the drug [263]. The histology of the rash may be similar to that seen in non-AIDS patients with drug eruptions [264], or it may display more severe damage to the epidermis [254]. Exaggerated hypersensitivity in the form of anaphylactoid reactions to ciprofloxacin and rifampicin has also been reported in HIV-infected individuals [265].

Also common among HIV patients is seborrheic dermatitis, which has been reported in over 80 percent of those having AIDS and in approximately 40 percent of those with ARC [254,257]. It is characterized by waxy scale overlying orange-pink or red plaques, which are symmetrically distributed over the face, scalp, chest, and upper trunk [254,257,263]. It is occasionally pruritic on the scalp, but primarily presents a cosmetic problem. It may be the first sign of HIV infection [254,263]. Although the usual modalities used to manage seborrheic dermatitis, such as sulfur, salicylic acid, or tar-containing shampoos, topical ketoconazole, and mild topical steroid preparations may be useful, the disorder is often recurrent and resistant [254,257].

Just as stress or immunodeficiency may predispose to florid seborrheic dermatitis [254], so also it may account for the severe extensive psoriasis, Reiter's syndrome, eczema, and ichthyosis, which have been described in some AIDS patients [254,263]. A generalized pruritic acnelike eruption of pink papules each with a central pustule has been reported with increasing frequency among HIV-infected patients. These pustules are distinguished histologically by the presence of clusters of eosinophils in the superficial portion of the hair follicle [263,266]. This eosinophilic pustular folliculitis may respond to topical acne remedies, oral antihistamines, or ultraviolet B light therapy [263].

Many of the mucosal and cutaneous abnormalities present in HIV-infected patients are manifestations of infection. Candidiasis occurs in 80 to 90 percent of AIDS and ARC patients and is the most frequent opportunistic infection in AIDS patients [254]. In addition to oral manifestations of thrush, monilial diaper rash is common in the pediatric AIDS population [267]. Generally a potassium hydroxide or Gram's stain preparation of a scraping from the beefy red erosion or the easily removed white pseudomembranous exudate will reveal numerous pseudohyphae and budding yeasts [263]. Esophageal spread from oral lesions may produce dysphagia and retrosternal pain or be asymptomatic [254]. Topical nystatin or clotrimazole may be beneficial, but oral ketoconazole is sometimes necessary. Other superficial fungi also often produce intertriginous, palmar, plantar, and nail infections that are difficult to treat [263].

Systemic fungal infections, especially with cryptococcosis or histoplasmosis, may produce umbilicated (molluscumlike) papules, acneform pustules, erosions, or cellulitic plaques [254,263]. Tissue biopsy is essential to confirm the diagnosis. Bacterial skin infections commonly seen include staphylococcal and pneumococcal pustular folliculitis, crusted impetigo, and syphilis in its various manifestations [263]. *Mycobacterium tuberculosis* and *M. avium-intracellulare* may also be revealed by biopsy to be the source of some pustules, nodules, or plaques [263]. Recently a gram-negative bacillus visualized with Warthin-Starry stain has been isolated from an unusual proliferative vascular process of friable domed red papules that has been named epithelioid or bacillary angiomatosis [263,268]. Lesions resolve with erythromycin therapy [268]. Another unique finding termed hairy leukoplakia is probably due to the Epstein-Barr virus [254,263]. It appears as white corrugations or papules usually on the lateral tongue and buccal surface, but sometimes covering the dorsal tongue, palate, and floor of the mouth [254,263]. The eruption may clear on acyclovir in doses of 800 mg qid for 2 weeks [263].

The cytomegalovirus may also affect the skin if resulting thrombocytopenia produces petechiae, or less commonly by producing a generalized morbilliform eruption or localized vesicles and ulcers that mimic herpes simplex–induced lesions [263]. Skin biopsy may demonstrate the intranuclear inclusions characteristic of this virus [263,269]. Recurrent HSV infections often plague the AIDS patient with their pain, extensiveness, and persistence despite acyclovir, and occasionally with dissemination of lesions (see Disseminated Cutaneous Herpes Simplex Virus Infection) [254,263,270]. Chronic extensive anogenital erosions may also be complicated by secondary bacterial infection [254,263]. The incidence of herpes zoster is higher in AIDS patients than in immunocompetent patients of the same age [254], and dissemination of vesicles beyond the affected dermatome is also common [254,263,270,271]. A cytologic examination of scrapings from the base of a vesicle will reveal multinucleated giant keratinocytes in both herpes simplex and zoster [264], but fluorescent antibody staining can differentiate the two causative agents. IV acyclovir may be required in the case of dissemination of lesions of either virus [254]. Dome-shaped pearly 3- to 6-mm papules with depressed centers are typical of infection with the molluscum contagiosum pox virus. AIDS patients may develop hundreds of lesions that may grow quite large, leading to confusion with basal cell carcinomas [254,263,269]. They may be refractory to conventional therapy with liquid nitrogen, curettage, or topical acids. Similarly, human papillomavirus–induced warts are often large, widespread, and refractory to therapy [254,263,270]. Infestations with the scabies mite are also often overwhelming, producing the crusted and hyperkeratotic lesions of so-called Norwegian scabies [263]. Protozoan infections rarely produce cutaneous lesions, but cutaneous *Pneumocystis* nodules of the ear [272,273] and a skin papule due to *Acanthamoeba* [269] have been reported.

Other less common skin findings in HIV-infected patients are listed in Table 218-9 [254,255,256,263,268,269,272–284].

SYSTEMIC LUPUS ERYTHEMATOSUS. Lupus erythematosus is an autoimmune disorder with a widely variable presentation. For detailed discussion of systemic lupus erythematosus (SLE), see Chapter 219.

Cutaneous lesions, often distinctive enough to aid in diagnosis, are very common in lupus (Table 218-10) [285]. In fact, 4 of the 11 criteria for establishing the diagnosis of SLE are skin and mucosal findings [286]. First is the poorly demarcated erythema that usually affects all or part of the malar eminences and the bridge of the nose in a "butterfly" pattern [286]. Second are the chronic scarring "discoid" lesions, usually on sun-exposed sites, which are sharply marginated violaceous plaques with adherent scale and plugged hair follicles [286]. Older scarring lesions have an atrophic epidermis with telangiectasias and hyperpigmentation or hypopigmentation [285]. Photosensitivity and shallow oral or nasopharyngeal ulcers are two additional findings that may support a diagnosis of lupus.

Beyond these common manifestations many other skin changes are also frequently seen (see Table 218-10). Subacute cutaneous lupus, a recently defined subset of lupus [285,287], usually exhibits nonscarring arcuate macules or psoriasislike plaques. Alopecia in lupus may be due to scarring discoid lesions, or it may be diffuse with no scarring. Additionally, a frontal pattern of short broken-off hairs is said to be characteristic [288]. Lesions of panniculitis present as subcutaneous nodules, often with mild erythema or no overlying skin changes. These persistent and relatively nontender masses occur primarily on the cheeks, buttocks, and upper arms, and often develop following trauma or exposure to cold [289]. Tense bullae as a manifestation of lupus may be difficult to distinguish from bullous pemphigoid, dermatitis herpetiformis, and lichen planus [290]. Oral lesions include hemorrhage, ulcerations, and gingivitis [288]. Raynaud's phenomenon occurs in lupus but is more often associated with other autoimmune disorders [286]. Vasculitis in its protean manifestations is seen in approximately 20 percent of patients with lupus. Although the lesions are not in themselves diagnostic of lupus, their presence should suggest a serologic evaluation for the disease.

Laboratory findings in lupus include an array of autoantibodies [286]. Antinuclear antibodies are rarely found in patients with chronic cutaneous scarring lesions except in the 5 percent who eventually develop SLE. More than 60 percent of individuals who have subacute cutaneous lupus have antinuclear and anticytoplasmic antibodies present. Antinuclear antibodies are absent in only approximately 15 percent of patients with SLE; many of these patients are found to have a relatively benign photosensitive disorder with cytoplasmic Ro (SS-A) antibodies present [285,286,287,291,291a]. Recently a relationship has been suggested between recurrent thrombotic events and the presence of antibodies to the phospholipid cardiolipin [289a,292,293].

Histologic features of discoid skin lesions include vacuolar changes of the epidermal basal cell layer, epidermal atrophy, and a dense mononuclear cell infiltrate surrounding the vessels and skin appendages in the superficial and deep dermis. In subacute cutaneous lesions the cellular infiltrate is more superficial, and in the acute cutaneous indurated erythema of SLE, only a sparse mononuclear cell infiltrate is present along with edema of the upper dermis. Immunofluorescent examination usually reveals immunoglobulin and complement deposition along the dermal-epidermal junction in most skin lesions of chronic cutaneous and systemic lupus, as well as in 85 to 90 percent of biopsies of nonlesional deltoid skin of patients with SLE [285]. The presence of this immunofluorescent "lupus band" in normal non-sun-exposed skin of lupus patients may correlate with the presence of antibodies to double-stranded deoxyribonucleic acid, hypocomplementemia, and renal disease [285].

The management of the cutaneous lesions of lupus varies according to the type and severity of the lesion and the activity of the systemic disease. Sunscreens should be recommended [294,295]. Topical, intralesional, and systemic corticosteroids, as well as antimalarials, may be indicated in individual cases [294].

Life-Threatening Systemic Diseases With Subtle Skin Manifestations

This third group of skin disorders consists of subtle abnormalities that are often ignored by the inexperienced examiner. These signs, however, may provide key clues to diagnosing the systemic disease responsible for the major critical care problem.

HEREDITARY HEMORRHAGIC TELANGIECTASIA. Hereditary hemorrhagic telangiectasia (Osler-Weber-Rendu disease) is a mucocutaneous and visceral fibrovascular dysplasia characterized by telangiectasias, aneurysms, and arteriovenous malformations. Although 6 to 20 percent of patients have no known family history of the disease, usually it is inherited in an autosomal dominant mode [296,297].

The characteristic lesion is a macular telangiectasia, dotlike or linear, found on the face, lips, nares, tongue, ears, hands, chest, or feet (Plate II-14) [297]. Many of these telangiectasias usually appear before the age of 30 and increase in size and number with age [296,297]. They may become spiderlike over time but lack the central arterial pulsation of spider angiomata. They are difficult to distinguish from the telangiectasias seen in the CREST (calcinosis, Raynaud's, esophageal dysmotility, sclerodactyly, telangiectasias) variant of scleroderma. Other typical clinical features and the presence of anticentromere antibodies help to differentiate CREST patients [297,298].

The earliest symptom of hereditary hemorrhagic telangiectasia is usually recurrent epistaxis, which may begin in childhood [296,297]. Painless hemorrhage also occurs from the GI mucosa, or less commonly is pulmonary, genitourinary, or intracerebral [297]. An array of different vascular malformations may be present in the celiac and mesenteric vessels, usually not producing bleeding until the fourth or fifth decade [297]. Chronic, recurrent hemorrhage tends to be progressive, and the acute source may elude both endoscopic and angiographic examination [297]. Congestive heart failure from arteriovenous fistulas may also produce the initial symptoms of the disease

Table 218-10. Cutaneous Abnormalities in Lupus Erythematosus (LE)

Histopathology diagnostic of LE	Histopathology not diagnostic of LE
Acute "butterfly blush"	Vasculitis
Subacute psoriasiform patches and plaques	Purpuric papules
	Hemorrhagic bullae
Chronic scarring "discoid" plaques	Stellate infarcts
	Digital gangrene
Lupus (profundus) panniculitis	Digital nodules
Bullous lupus	Ulcers
Hyperkeratotic palmoplantar papules	Recurrent superficial and deep thrombophlebitis
Mucosal ulcerations	Livedo reticularis
Alopecia, scarring	Alopecia, nonscarring
	Photosensitivity
	Periungual erythema
	Raynaud's phenomenon
	Sclerodactyly
	Splinter hemorrhages
	Hyperpigmentation, diffuse
	Depigmentation, focal
	Erythermalgia
	Calcinosis cutis
	Chilblains
	Clubbing
	Rheumatoid nodules
	Urticaria
	Angioedema
	Erythema multiforme
	Pyoderma gangrenosum-like ulcers

[299]. Hereditary hemorrhagic telangiectasia is the most common cause of arteriovenous fistulas of the respiratory tract [300], which affect approximately 15 percent of patients [297] and may be solitary or multiple. The pulmonary involvement may lead to dyspnea, cyanosis, and clubbing. Chest roentgenography, fluoroscopy, and angiography can confirm the diagnosis [297,300]. Neurologic symptoms may result from spinal cord hemorrhage or from pulmonary involvement leading to polycythemia, paradoxic or air embolism, or abscess [297,301,302]. Hepatic arteriovenous fistulas may cause hepatomegaly, pain, hyperdynamic circulatory state, and portal hypertension [297]. Conjunctival and retinal vascular lesions are rare [297,303].

Despite repeated hemorrhage and other problems, life expectancy is not inevitably reduced. In fewer than 10 percent of those affected can death be attributed to complications of the disease. Treatment depends on the site and degree of involvement. Nearly all patients require iron supplementation, and often folate as well. Immunization against hepatitis B should be offered in view of the anticipated frequent blood transfusions [297]. Local measures for epistaxis often fail, necessitating oral estrogen therapy or septal dermoplasty [297]. GI bleeding may require endoscopic coagulation, laser, or segmental bowel resection, although recurrent hemorrhage is likely from remaining sites [297,304]. Pulmonary fistulas have been managed with ligation, resection, or embolization [297,300,300a]. Similar measures for hepatic fistulas may be required to manage high output congestive heart failure [297]. CNS vascular or septic lesions frequently coexist with pulmonary fistulas and should be considered. Cutaneous telangiectasias may respond to laser treatment [305].

PSEUDOXANTHOMA ELASTICUM. Pseudoxanthoma elasticum is a rare disorder of elastic tissue that affects both the skin and the viscera, resulting in hemorrhage and accelerated atherosclerosis. It can be inherited as an autosomal dominant or recessive condition. Similar skin changes, without typical visceral disease, have been described in the L-tryptophan-induced eosinophilia myalgia syndrome [305a,305b] and as a result of D-penicillamine therapy [305c]. Its pathogenesis is poorly understood, but the disease is characterized by fragmented, thickened, and calcified elastic fibers [306,307].

The characteristic cutaneous change appears in adolescence with the asymptomatic onset of coalescent 2- to 5-mm chamois-colored papules most frequently beginning on the nape or lateral neck but also seen symmetrically in the axillae, groin, antecubital and popliteal fossae, and face [307,308]. Slowly these pebbly xanthomalike lesions assume a "peau d'orange" or rippled plaque appearance (Plate II-15). One-third of individuals may later develop yellow cobblestoning inside the lower lip [307]. Skin biopsy is useful to demonstrate the pathognomonic elastic degeneration and differentiate from solar elastosis and cutis laxa [307,308]. Other changes that may be present but are not specific to this disorder are angioid streaks, which represent breaks in the retinal elastic basement membrane (Bruch's) seen in 85 percent of patients [308], and elastosis perforans serpiginosa, which appears as plugged brownish papules arranged in arcuate or serpiginous clusters usually on the neck, cheeks, or extremities [309].

The most common complication requiring critical care is GI hemorrhage secondary to destruction of the elastic fibers in the submucosal vessels. This bleeding usually occurs between the ages of 20 and 30 and is often recurrent [310]. Subarachnoid, pulmonary, and genitourinary hemorrhage are less common [310]. Hypertension due to renal artery involvement occurs in 25 percent of patients [311], often beginning in the teenage years. Mitral valve prolapse is a frequent finding [312]. Premature atherosclerotic disease affects the cerebral, coronary, mesenteric, and peripheral arteries [307,308]. By age 30, most affected individuals have markedly diminished or absent pulses in the extremities and radiographically apparent arterial calcifications [312]. Retinal hemorrhage and neovascularization lead to visual deterioration, and early laser coagulation therapy may be helpful [307,308,313].

At present, there is no specific cure for this disease. Early and regular eye care is critical, together with avoidance of head trauma and heavy straining, which might precipitate retinal hemorrhage [307]. Dietary calcium restriction in childhood and adolescence may be beneficial [307,313]. Pregnancy is known to accelerate the natural course of the disease [307]. Avoidance of cardiovascular risk factors, such as smoking and hypercholesterolemia is advisable [307]. Control of hypertension and gastric acidity with agents that do not promote hypercalcemia is also useful [307]. Pentoxifylline may improve symptoms of intermittent claudication.

EHLERS-DANLOS SYNDROME. Ehlers-Danlos syndrome is a heterogeneous group of heritable disorders of collagen, many of which are characterized by joint hypermobility, skin hyperextensibility, easy bruisability, and atrophic scarring. Of the ten described variants, type I or "gravis," and type IV or "ecchymotic," are especially prone to rupture of the great vessels and GI perforation.

The skin in these patients is velvety, translucent, and fragile. Wounds heal slowly and leave broad flaccid scars [314,315]. In those individuals with hyperelasticity of the skin, loss of recoil in later life may leave loose, overlapping folds. Easy bruising and spontaneous hematomas are hallmarks of the collagen defect in type IV, in which there is minimal joint hypermobility and no excessive skin stretchability [316,317].

Death often occurs in the first two decades of life in patients with severe types [318]. Aneurysm and rupture of large arteries [315,319] and spontaneous GI perforation are the primary causes of death. GI complications in addition to hemorrhage and rupture of viscera include intestinal diverticulae, rectal prolapse, eventration of the diaphragm, and umbilical, hiatal, and inguinal hernias [317]. Pneumothorax may occur spontaneously [320] or may be induced by artificial ventilation. Mitral valve prolapse [312], varicosities, and joint dislocations [315] are common. High risk accompanies angiography [321] and endoscopy [316], as well as the passage of nasogastric tubes and the performance of digital rectal examination [322].

Surgery should be performed with caution because of the risks of profuse bleeding and wound dehiscence [315]. Complications of pregnancy range in severity from premature labor and postpartum hemorrhage to exsanguination from rupture of a major vessel [323,323a].

Currently, the treatment of Ehlers-Danlos syndrome is limited to prevention and supportive care of the unfortunate sequelae. Pharmacologic doses of vitamin C may be beneficial in some forms of the disease [324].

MALIGNANT ATROPHIC PAPULOSIS. Malignant atrophic papulosis, also known as Degos' disease, is a rare, often lethal multisystem disease afflicting young adults and manifested by pathognomonic porcelain white skin lesions. Histologically small vessel lumina are narrowed by endarteritis and occluded by thrombi. The etiology is unknown, although an endothelial defect or anticardiolipin antibodies may play a role [325,326]. A few familial cases have been reported [327,328,329].

Skin lesions are asymptomatic and may be visible months to years before visceral involvement [329]. Crops of pink, gray, or yellow papules arise, then evolve into atrophic white macules bounded by a well-defined elevated erythematous or telangiectatic border (Plate II-16) [329,330,331]. Some lesions may coalesce to form "clover-leaf" patterns. The papules predominate on the trunk and upper arms. Occasionally skin lesions of systemic lupus erythematosus may resemble malignant atrophic papulosis [332].

Additional clinical manifestations result from involvement of other organs with infarctive lesions similar to those in the skin. Most frequently, the GI tract [333,334], CNS (in about 20%) [333,334], and eye [333,335] are affected. GI perforation leading to peritonitis is a common cause of death, as is cerebral infarction [334]. Other organs that may be involved are the heart, lung, kidney, bladder, and gallbladder [334]. Recently, patients with a more benign and chronic course have been described [328,329,333].

Surgical closure of bowel perforations rather than resection is recommended. Various therapies, including cyclophosphamide, steroids, antibiotics, phenformin with ethylestrenol, aspirin with dipyridamole, and ticlopidine have been used without consistent success [325]. Pentoxifylline or heparin administered early may reduce infarction.

Skin Diseases Acquired During the Course of Serious Systemic Illness

DRUG ERUPTIONS. Skin eruptions are the most common form of adverse reaction to drugs [336]. These cutaneous responses vary from mild pruritus to life-threatening anaphylaxis, TEN, or erythroderma. One survey of 464 drug eruptions in Finland found that 46 percent were macular, papular, or morbilliform exanthems; 23 percent were urticarial; 10 percent were fixed drug eruptions; and 5 percent were EM; other forms accounted for less than 5 percent each [337].

The pathogenesis of drug eruptions varies. Eruptions that result from immunologic reactions are appropriately termed drug allergies. Drug reactions that do not involve the immune system may also occur, for example, via nonimmunologic activation of effector pathways, overdosage, cumulative toxicity, side effects, ecologic disturbances, and drug interactions [338]. The exact mechanism of most drug reactions, however, remains undefined.

Often it is difficult to determine which drug is responsible for an adverse reaction. Additionally, nearly all types of drug-related cutaneous reactions, in fact, may also be produced by other agents [339]. Once a drug eruption is considered, any drug should be suspect. Certain clues, however, may help identify the offending agent. First, most drug eruptions are caused by medications that have recently been administered. Morbilliform rashes (Plate II-17) usually develop within 1 week of starting therapy, even when the drug is taken for the first time. Reactions to a few drugs, especially penicillins, may not appear until after 2 weeks of commencing therapy, and may *even begin as late as 2 weeks after therapy has ceased* [338].

The only known risk factor for developing a drug eruption is a history of prior reaction to the drug [340]. The frequency with which various drugs cause skin reactions in hospitalized patients, however, may help determine which drug is most highly suspect in a patient who is receiving multiple drugs. Agents that cause reactions most frequently are antibiotics, especially amoxicillin, trimethoprim-sulfamethoxazole, ampicillin, cephalosporins, erythromycin, and penicillin, and blood products [336]. A recently gathered list of cutaneous reaction rates to many frequently used drugs appears in Table 218-11. Some commonly used drugs that seldom produce skin reactions are listed in Table 218-12 [341].

Furthermore, to decide which of several drugs may be the inciting agent, it may be helpful to know that a certain drug has been implicated in causing a distinct type of eruption, for example EM. Table 218-13 lists some drugs frequently administered in the intensive care unit (ICU) and the common or distinctive eruptions with which they have been associated. Cutaneous side effects of cancer chemotherapeutic agents are summarized in Table 218-14 [342]. Adverse reactions in the skin caused by cardiovascular drugs have recently been reviewed [342a].

As mentioned previously, a variety of cutaneous reaction patterns may be produced by drugs. Urticaria, transient wheals, may occur alone or in conjunction with anaphylaxis, angioedema, or serum sickness (see Chap. 217) [343]. Exanthems, consisting of macular, papular, morbilliform, or scarlatiniform eruptions, are especially common (Plate II-17). Pruritus and eosinophilia may or may not accompany them, and they may be indistinguishable from viral exanthems [338]. Leukocytoclastic vasculitis is usually manifested as crops of purpuric papules, which appear primarily on the lower extremities (Plate II-18) (see Chap. 220). This palpable purpura, however, has a host of possible etiologies other than drugs (Table 218-15) [344]. A fixed drug eruption consists of a cutaneous or mucosal macule, plaque, or bulla—usually pink, red, brown, or gray—that recurs in the same site(s) each time a particular drug is readministered. A photoeruption may result when a patient taking one of certain drugs, such as thiazides or sulfonylureas, is exposed to ultraviolet light. Allergic contact dermatitis may develop in response to a variety of topical therapies (see Contact Dermatitis). In addition, dermatitislike plaques have been reported to occur at sites of subcutaneous heparin injection [345,346]. Certain

Table 218-11. Allergic Skin Reaction Rates to Drugs Commonly Used in the Critically Ill

Drug	Reaction rate per 1000 recipients
Acetylcysteine[b]	8.8
Allopurinol[b]	7.7
Amoxicillin[a]	51.4
Ampicillin[a]	33.2
Atropine sulfate[a]	1.6
Barbiturates[b]	4.0
Blood[a]	21.6
Bromhexine hydrochloride[b]	6.4
Carbocysteine[c]	6.8
Cephalosporins[c]	21.1
Cimetidine[c]	12.8
Cyanocobalamin[c]	17.9
Cyclophosphamide[c]	4.8
Diazepam[a]	0.4
Dihydralazine hydrochloride[c]	19.1
Doxycycline[c]	4.7
Erythromycin[c]	20.4
Furosemide[a]	0.5
Gentamicin sulfate[b]	4.5
Glyburide[c]	2.1
Heparin sodium[b]	1.1
Hydralazine hydrochloride[c]	8.3
Hyoscine butylbromide[c]	13.2
Indomethacin[c]	2.1
Ipodate[c]	27.8
Isoniazid[c]	5.6
Metoclopramide hydrochloride[b]	3.2
Nitrazepam[a]	1.5
Penicillin G[b]	18.5
Penicillin, semisynthetic[b]	20.7
Phenazopyridine hydrochloride[b]	4.5
Pentazopyridine hydrochloride[c]	8.8
Phenylbutazone[c]	11.6
Potassium chloride[a]	0.3
Quinidine[c]	13.4
Trimethoprim-sulfamethoxazole[a]	33.8
Vincristine sulfate[c]	6.3

[a] Drug received by at least 1000 patients.
[b] Drug received by 500 to 999 patients.
[c] Drug received by 100 to 499 patients.
Source: Adapted from Bigby M, Jick S, Jick H, et al: Drug-induced cutaneous reactions. A report from the Boston Collaborative Drug surveillance program on 15438 consecutive inpatients, 1975 to 1982. *JAMA* 256:3358, 1986.

Table 218-12. Drugs Frequently Used in the Intensive Care Unit that Rarely Cause Allergic Skin Reactions

Acetaminophen	Laxatives
Adrenergic agents	Lidocaine
Aminophylline	Methyldopa
Antacids	Multivitamin
Antihistamines	Nitroglycerin
Aspirin	Opiates
Digitalis glycosides	Prednisolone, prednisone
Diphenhydramine	Propranolol hydrochloride
Ferrous sulfate	Tetracycline
Flurazepam hydrochloride	Theophylline
Folic acid	Thyroid hormones
Ganglionic-blocking agents	Tubocurarine
Isosorbide dinitrate	Warfarin

or breasts (Plate II-20) [348]. Recent evidence suggests that individuals deficient in protein C may be at an increased risk of developing coumadin necrosis [348].

Laboratory findings in drug eruptions are generally not helpful. Drug-induced exanthems and contact dermatitis are sometimes accompanied by eosinophilia. Antinuclear antibodies appear in drug-related lupus erythematosus. In leukocytoclastic vasculitis, erythrocyte sedimentation rate is often elevated, and hematuria and proteinuria or occult blood in the stool may demonstrate renal or GI involvement, respectively. The platelet count may fall in heparin necrosis. Skin biopsy often shows distinctive findings in EM, TEN, erythema nodosum, fixed drug eruption, leukocytoclastic vasculitis, coma bullae, and anticoagulant necrosis. Nonspecific histologic changes occur in most other types of drug reactions.

If a drug has caused an eruption, it should be discontinued and not reinstated unless there is no alternative therapy and the need for the medication is critical [338]. Although the drug eruption may appear benign, continuation of the medication, in rare cases, may cause severe sequelae, including death [340]. If the patient is taking several medicines, all those that are not absolutely necessary should be discontinued. Unrelated agents, if available, may be substituted, or those drugs that are not likely to provoke reactions may be reintroduced individually after the eruption has resolved. It is useful but not always safe or practical to attempt to confirm the drug-reaction connection [336,339]. Provocation testing was used to verify the relationship in 62 percent of cases in one study [344], whereas skin testing and lymphocyte toxicity assay prove helpful only occasionally [336,339].

Treatment of drug exanthems is usually supportive with oral antihistamines, topical antipruritic lotions containing menthol and phenol, or topical steroids as necessary. Baths or compresses may be helpful if blisters or oozing lesions are present. Severe reactions, such as anaphylaxis [343] (see Chap. 217), erythroderma (see Exfoliative Erythroderma), and toxic epidermal necrolysis (see Toxic Epidermal Necrolysis), of course, may require prompt specific intervention. For coumarin necrosis, both heparin [348] and prostacyclin [349] have been reported to be useful.

MONILIASIS. Skin eruptions that are common in the general population, such as moniliasis, are also common in the critically ill. Obesity, diabetes, pregnancy, incontinence, and the use of corticosteroids, antibiotics, and oral contraceptives all predispose to the development of *Candida* skin infection [384].

drugs, such as hydralazine and procainamide, can produce a SLE-like syndrome with positive antinuclear antibodies [340,350]. Medications also may give rise to exfoliative dermatitis (see Exfoliative Erythroderma), pigmentary changes, and erythema nodosum. Lichenoid eruptions and exacerbations of psoriasis are seen during the use of beta-blocking agents as well as some other drugs [347]. Monomorphous acneform lesions may follow parenteral steroid administration. During coma from certain narcotics, barbiturates, antidepressants, or carbon monoxide poisoning, characteristic blisters may develop on areas of pressure (Plate II-19). Both coumarin and heparin may produce paradoxic thrombotic purpuric and necrotic lesions usually present on the thighs, buttocks, abdomen,

Table 218-13. Some Cutaneous Reactions to Agents Frequently Used in Critically Ill Patients

Agent	Dermatologic reaction	Reference	Agent	Dermatologic reaction	Reference
Diuretics			Anticoagulants		
Thiazides	Photodermatitis	350	Heparin	Cutaneous necrosis	348
	Urticaria	338		Alopecia	351
	Morbilliform exanthem	338		Eczematous plaque	345,346
	Leukocytoclastic vasculitis	350	Coumarin	Cutaneous necrosis	348
	Lichen planuslike eruption	350		Alopecia	351
Furosemide	Bullous eruption	350	Vasoconstrictors		
	Erythema multiforme	2	Dopamine	Peripheral gangrene	367
	Leukocytoclastic vasculitis	340,344	Vasopressin	Cutaneous necrosis	368
Peripheral vasodilators			Antibiotics		
Hydralazine	Lupus erythematosus eruption	340,350		Morbilliform exanthem	340
	Urticaria	340		Erythema multiforme	2,340
	Vasculitis	344		Toxic epidermal necrolysis	49,340
	Serum sickness	340		Leukocytoclastic vasculitis	340,344
Nitroglycerin paste	Contact dermatitis	427		Exfoliative erythroderma	99,340,369
Antiarrhythmics				Urticaria	340
Digitalis	Rare urticaria	350		Anaphylaxis	340
	Rare exanthem	350		Serum sickness	340
Quinidine	Rare morbilliform exanthem	350		Fixed-drug eruption	340,370
	Urticaria	340	Anticonvulsants		
	Exfoliative erythroderma	350	Phenytoin	Hypertrophy gums, pigmentation	351
	Lichenoid eruption	350		Morbilliform exanthem	371
	Photodermatitis	351,352		Erythema multiforme	2
	Rare acne	353		Toxic epidermal necrolysis	340
	Exacerbation psoriasis	354		Leukocytoclastic vasculitis	340
Procainamide	Lupus erythematosus eruption	340,350		Exfoliative erythroderma	340
Amiodarone	Photosensitivity	355		Hypersensitivity syndrome[a]	372
	Gray violet pigmentation of exposed skin	355,356		Pseudolymphoma syndrome[b]	373
Antihypertensives				Lupus erythematosus eruption	340
Beta-blockers	Rare exanthem	347,350		Urticaria	340
	Lichenoid eruption	347	Barbiturates	Morbilliform exanthem	351
	Psoriasiform dermatitis	347		Erythema multiforme	2
	Eczematous dermatitis	347		Exfoliative erythroderma	340
Captopril	Pityriasis rosealike eruption	357		Urticaria	340
	Morbilliform or urticarial eruption	357		Fixed-drug eruption	340,370
	Pemphiguslike eruption	358	Miscellaneous		
	Vasculitis	359	Aminophylline	Exfoliative erythroderma	340
	Psoriasislike eruption	360	Allopurinol	Hypersensitivity syndrome[c]	374
	Exfoliative dermatitis	361		Leukocytoclastic vasculitis	340
	Mycosis fungoideslike eruption	362		Toxic epidermal necrolysis	340
Enalapril	Mycosis fungoideslike eruption	362		Morbilliform exanthem	351
Diazoxide	Hypertrichosis	363	Blood products	Morbilliform exanthem	340
Minoxidil	Erythema multiforme	2		Urticaria	340
	Hypertrichosis	364		Anaphylactoid reaction	340
Calcium channel blockers				Serum sickness	340
Nifedipine	Exfoliative dermatitis	365	Cimetidine	Rare exanthem	375
	Erythema multiforme	366		Leukocytoclastic vasculitis	340,344
Verapamil	Exfoliative dermatitis	366		Xerosis	376
	Erythema multiforme	366			
Diltiazem	Exfoliative dermatitis	366			
	Erythema multiforme	366			
	Toxic epidermal necrolysis	366			

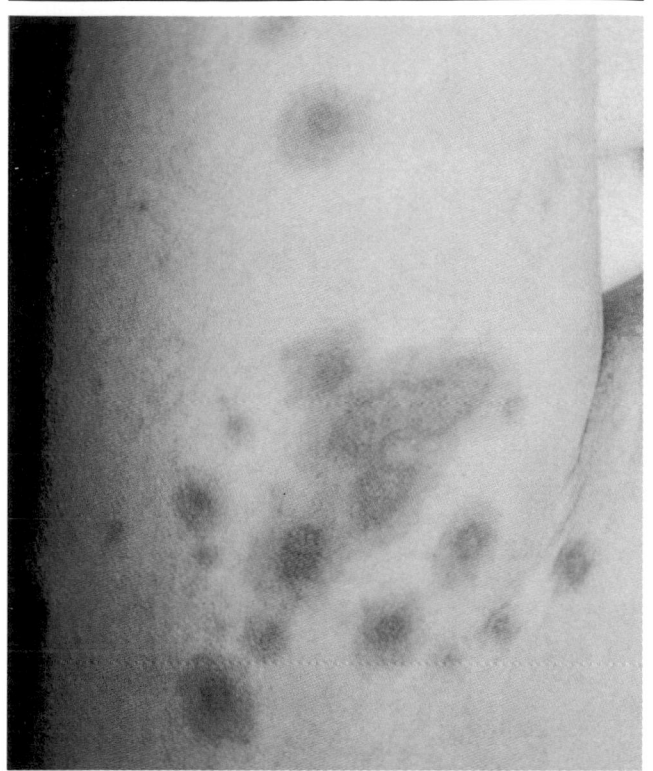

Plate II-1. Typical target lesions of erythema multiforme.

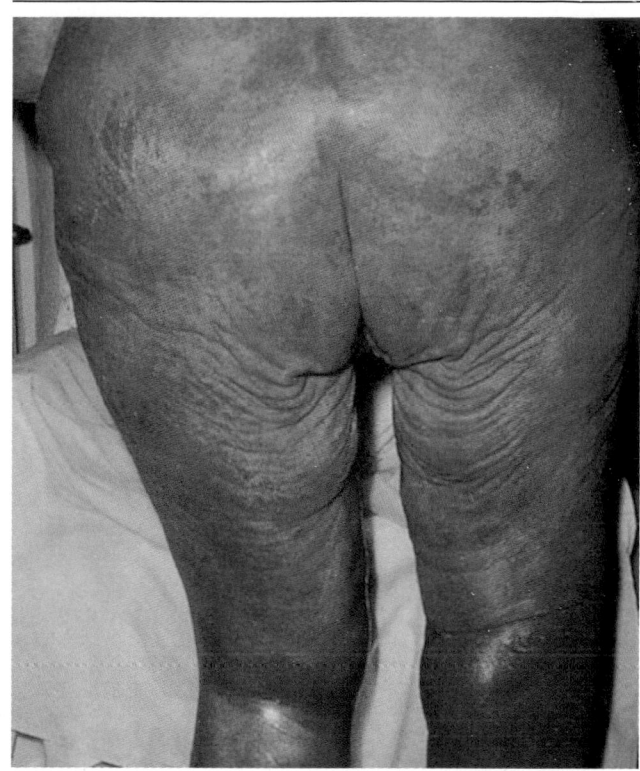

Plate II-3. Generalized erythroderma in patient with psoriasis.

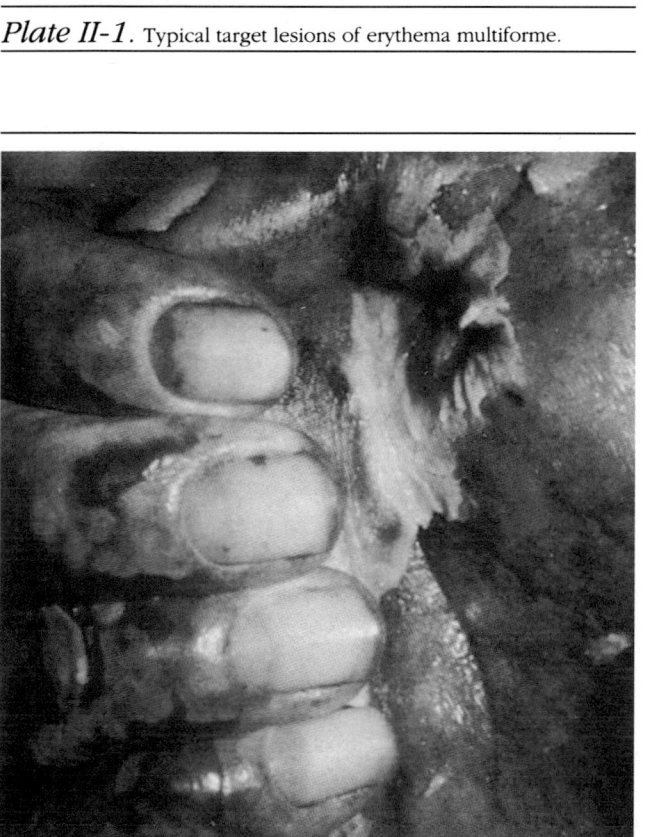

Plate II-2. Toxic epidermal necrolysis in patient with graft-versus-host disease following a bone marrow transplant for aplastic anemia.

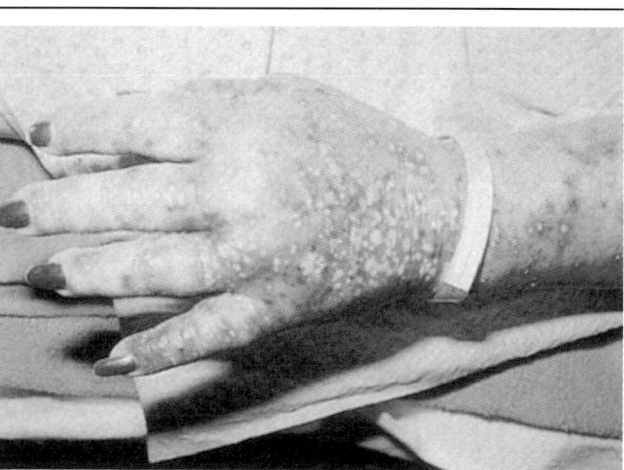

Plate II-4. Lakes of pustules seen in pustular psoriasis of von Zumbusch.

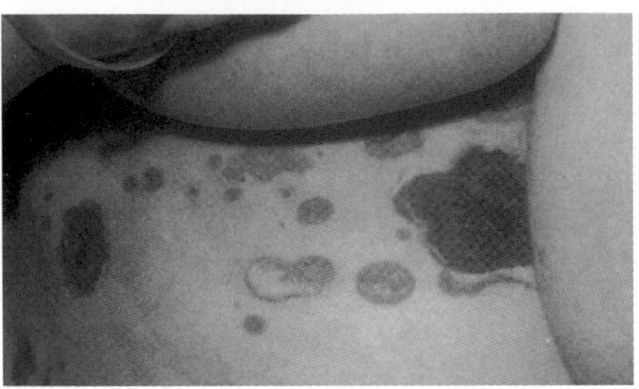

Plate II-5. Flaccid bullae and erosions of pemphigus vulgaris. (Courtesy of Samuel Moschella, M.D.)

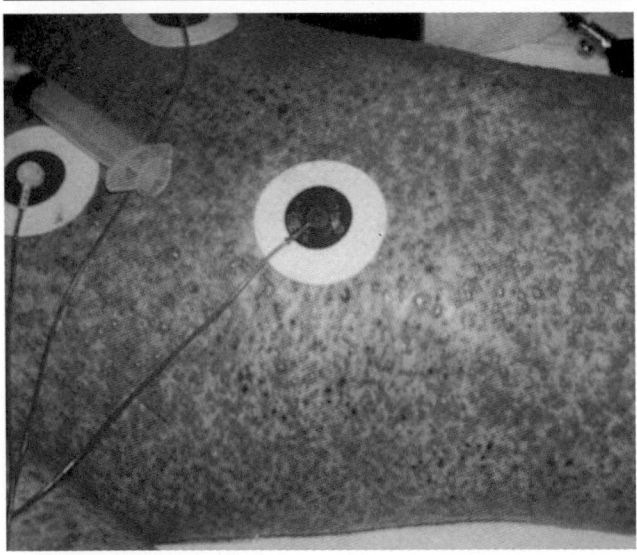

Plate II-6. Disseminated herpes simplex virus infection in patient with Hodgkin's disease.

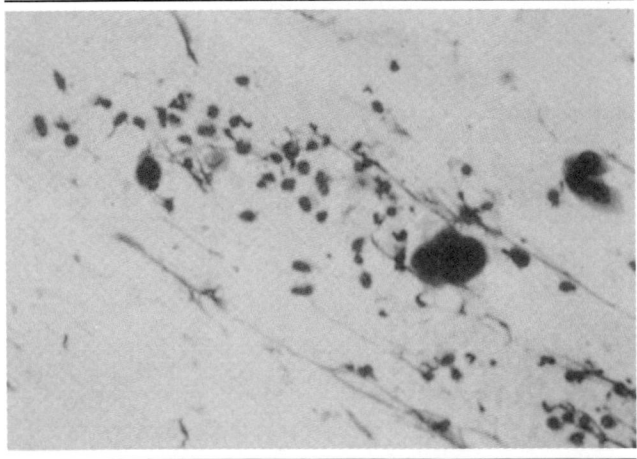

Plate II-7. Tzanck smear showing multinucleated giant keratinocytes seen only in herpes simplex or varicella-zoster virus infections.

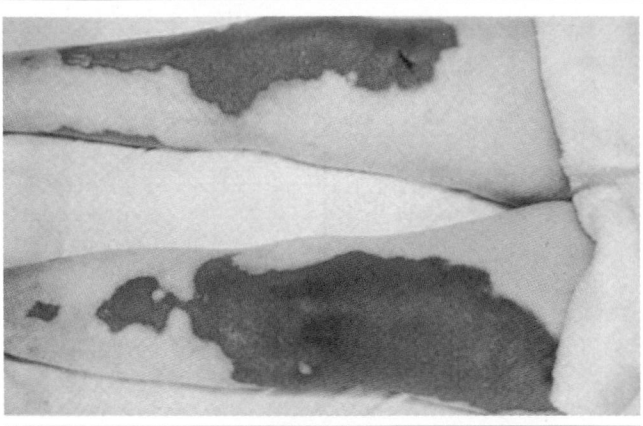

Plate II-8. Large areas of purpura seen in purpura fulminans.

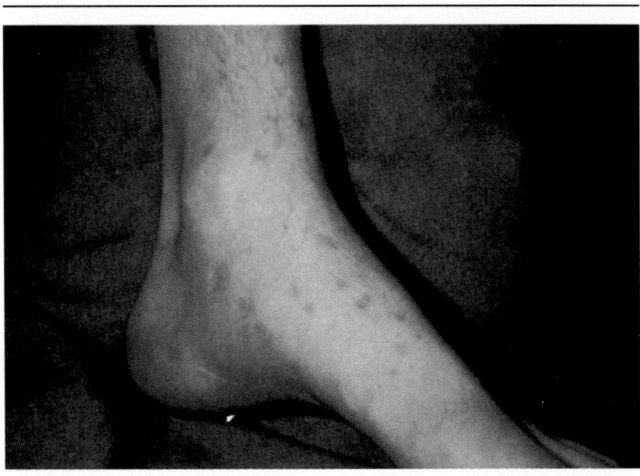

Plate II-9. Nonpurpuric macular and papular lesions of the ankle and foot found early in the course of Rocky Mountain spotted fever. (Courtesy of Gregory Bishop, M.D.)

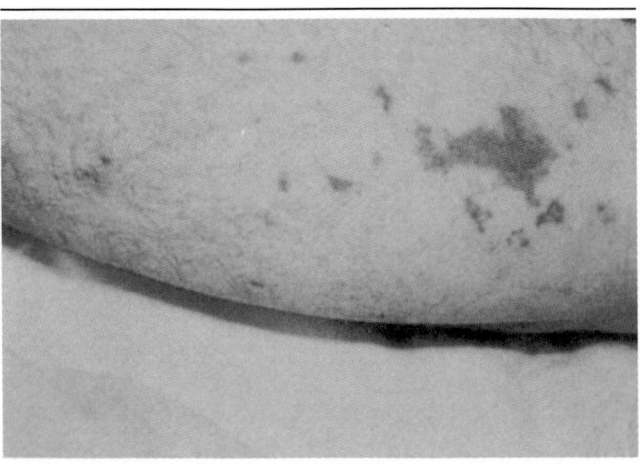

Plate II-10. Purpuric lesions in meningococcemia with characteristic "gun-metal" gray color centrally.

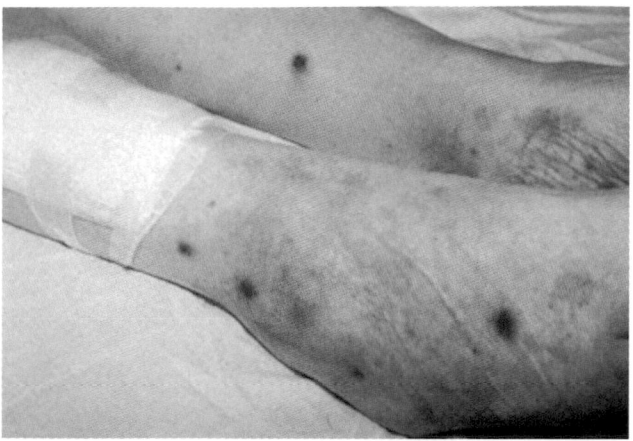

Plate II-11. Purpuric nodules of *Candida* sepsis. (Courtesy of Samuel Moschella, M.D.)

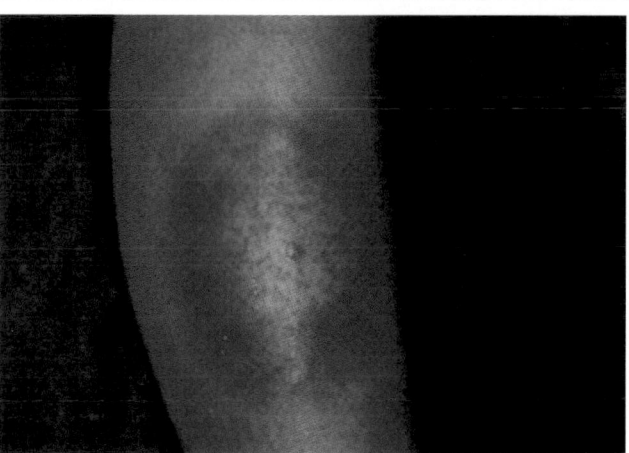

Plate II-12. Annular lesion of erythema chronicum migrans seen in Lyme disease, with central papule at the site of the tick bite. (Courtesy of Gregory Bishop, M.D.)

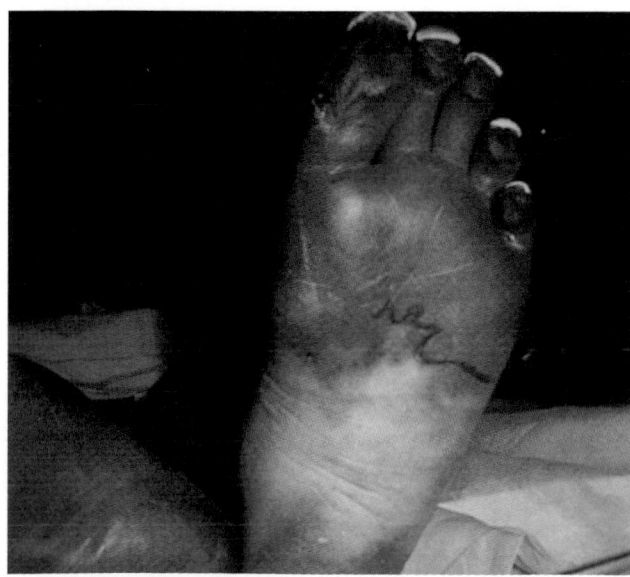

Plate II-13. Purpuric and necrotic lesions produced by "marantic emboli" in patient with carcinoma of the lung.

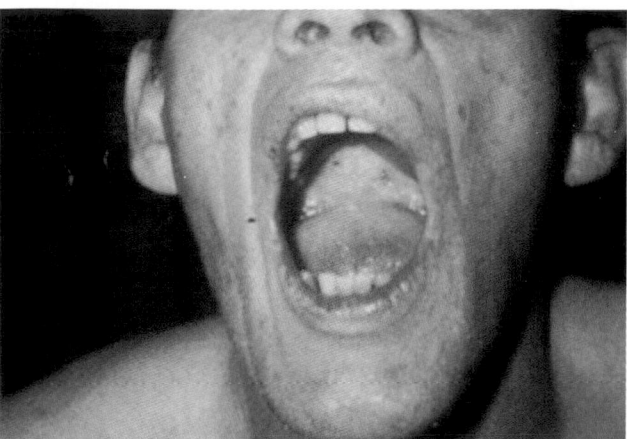

Plate II-14. Telangiectasias of the skin and mucosa seen in hereditary hemorrhagic telangiectasia (Osler-Weber-Rendu).

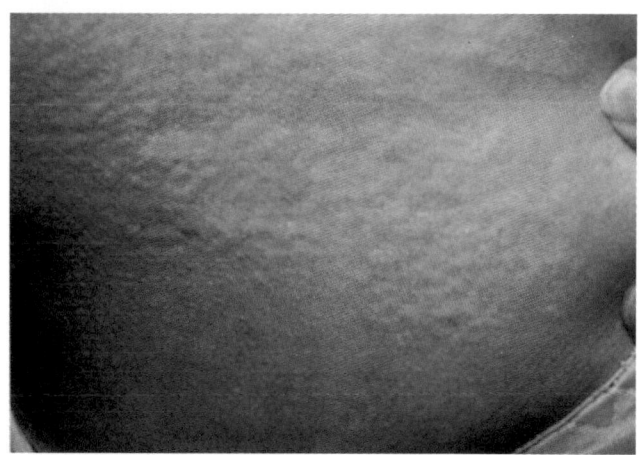

Plate II-15. "Peau d'orange" plaques seen in pseudoxanthoma elasticum. (Courtesy of Samuel Moschella, M.D.)

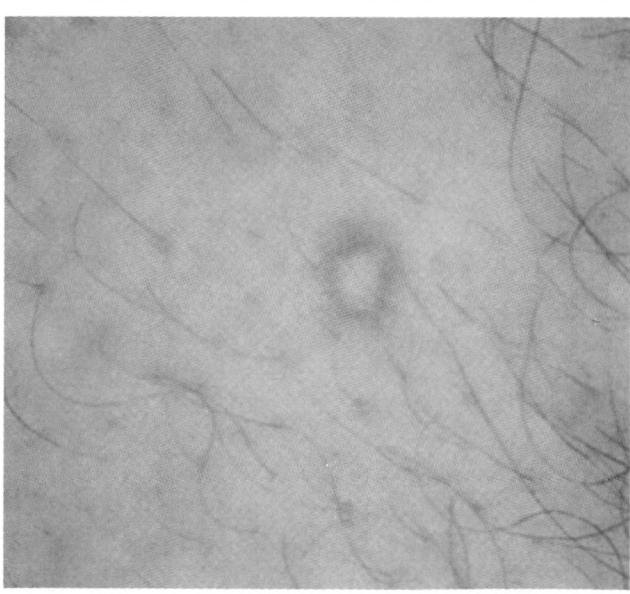

Plate II-16. Characteristic porcelain white skin lesions with erythematous border seen in malignant atrophic papulosis (Degos' disease). (Courtesy of Jessica Fewkes, M.D.)

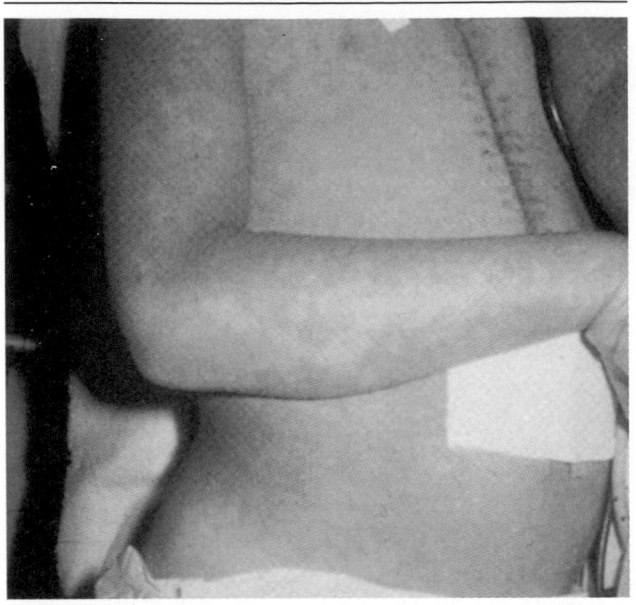

Plate II-17. Morbilliform exanthem caused by a drug.

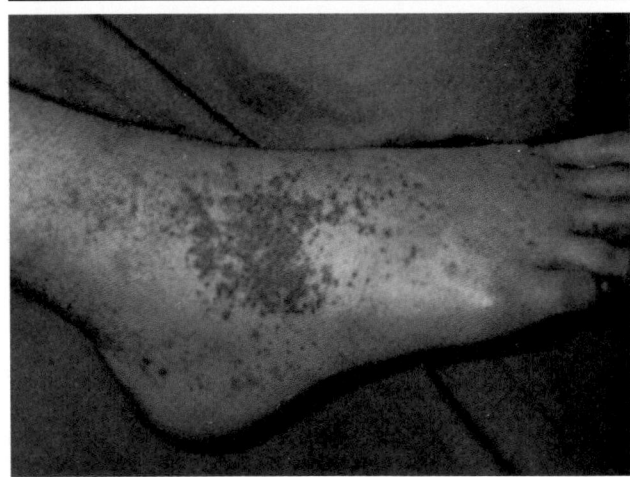

Plate II-18. Palpable purpuric lesions on the foot seen in leuko-cytoclastic vasculitis. (Courtesy of Gregory Bishop, M.D.)

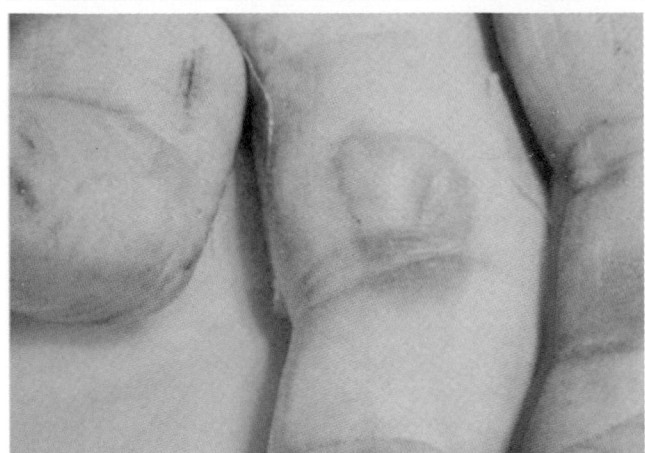

Plate II-19. Blister seen in barbiturate-induced coma.

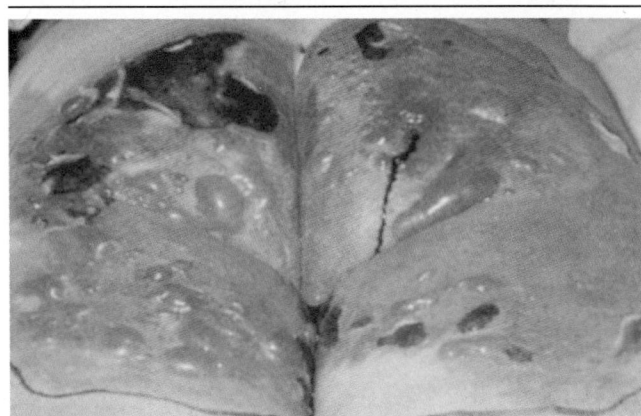

Plate II-20. Extensive area of necrosis with bullae and erosions caused by intravenous heparin.

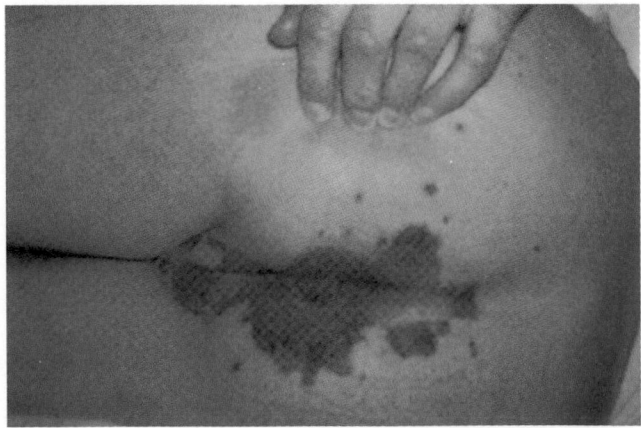

Plate II-21. Acral and periorificial scaly erythematous plaques of acquired acrodermatitis enteropathica seen in patient on zinc-poor parenteral nutrition.

Table 218-15. Some Causes of Leukocytoclastic Vasculitis

1. Drugs
   a. Allopurinol
   b. Amphetamines
   c. Aspirin
   d. Barbiturates
   e. Cimetidine
   f. Coumadin
   g. Furosemide
   h. Gold
   i. Hydantoins
   j. Hydralazine
   k. Iodides
   l. Penicillins
   m. Phenacetin
   n. Phenothiazines
   o. Procainamide
   p. Sulfonamides
   q. Thiazides
   r. Thiouracils
2. Infectious agents
   a. Group A beta-hemolytic streptococci
   b. Hepatitis B virus
   c. Influenza virus
   d. *Mycobacterium leprae*
3. Ingestants and chemicals
   a. Food colorings
   b. Food preservatives
   c. Insecticides
   d. Petroleum products
   e. Weed killers
4. Foreign proteins
   a. Serum
   b. Hyposensitization antigens
   c. Snake antivenom
5. Associated diseases
   a. Complement component deficiency (familial)
   b. Cryoglobulinemia
   c. Dermatomyositis
   d. Henoch-Schönlein purpura
   e. Hyperglobulinemic (Waldenström's) purpura
   f. Inflammatory bowel disease
   g. Intestinal bypass surgery
   h. Malignancy
   i. Mixed connective tissue disease
   j. Rheumatoid arthritis
   k. Sjögren's syndrome
   l. Systemic lupus erythematosus
   m. Urticarial vasculitis

parkinsonian side effects have also been reported to cause seborrheic dermatitislike eruptions [393,396].

The symptoms and signs of seborrheic dermatitis wax and wane. Men are more often affected than women, and the disorder may worsen in the winter [393]. It produces widespread or patchy scalp desquamation with or without pruritus and erythema. Additionally, there are often patches of waxy scale in the medial eyebrows, external ear canals, nasolabial creases, sideburns, beard, and presternal and interscapular areas [393,397]. A marginal blepharitis is common [393]. Body folds may also be involved; the axillary, intergluteal, inframammary, umbilical, and inguinal creases may demonstrate well-defined orange to pink patches with or without a greasy scale. Malodor or oozing and crust formation imply concurrent secondary bacterial infection [397]. The histopathologic changes are nonspecific [393,397].

The skin findings in seborrheic dermatitis may be mistaken for psoriasis or contact dermatitis, which can usually be distinguished by history and distribution. Dermatophytosis and moniliasis can be differentiated by the demonstration of hyphae or pseudohyphae, respectively, on a potassium hydroxide preparation; erythrasma can be recognized by its coral-red fluorescence under a Wood's lamp. Infrequently, rare disorders such as pemphigus erythematosus, acrodermatitis enteropathica (see Acquired Zinc Deficiency), and lupus erythematosus (see Systemic Lupus Erythematosus) may mimic seborrheic dermatitis.

Treatment of the scalp often requires daily use of a shampoo containing sulfur, salicylic acid, selenium sulfide, tar, zinc pyrithione, or chloroxine [393,397]. Recently propylene glycol [394] and ketoconazole [401,402] in topical preparations have also been shown to be effective. Occasionally a short course of a nonfluorinated topical steroid cream, such as hydrocortisone or desonide, may be necessary to clear the glabrous skin [393].

PRESSURE SORES. Pressure sores or decubitus ulcers, are a common complication of immobility, developing in 3 to 11 percent of patients in acute care hospitals [403,404,405]. They are even more common among spinal cord injury victims and geriatric patients in chronic care facilities. These ulcerations usually occur when a setting of immobility leads to sustained pressure, either of low magnitude for a long duration or of high degree for a brief period [405,406]. Additional factors that predispose to skin breakdown include shearing forces, friction, and moisture, including that from perspiration as well as fecal and urinary soilage [403,404,405]. Hypoalbuminemia, presence of a fracture, vitamin C deficiency, other nutritional and health factors, and aging changes of the skin may also predispose to ulceration [403,404] (see Chap. 166).

The histopathology demonstrates initially dilation of the capillaries and venules in the superficial dermis with endothelial cell swelling. Later, edema and hemorrhage appear in the upper dermis. The eccrine glands and subcutaneous fat, and eventually the follicular structures and epidermis as well, become necrotic [407].

A pressure sore may be mistaken for a vasculitic or neurotropic ulcer or an early ischial-rectal abscess. The presence of an everted edge suggests a biopsy should be performed to exclude the presence of an underlying or secondary neoplasm. Peripheral pustules help to differentiate the ulcers associated with deep mycotic infections [405]. Pressure ulcers must also be distinguished from pyoderma gangrenosum, radiation injury, and stasis and ischemic ulcers [403].

The prevention of pressure sores is far preferable to current methods available for their treatment [403,404,405] (see Chap. 166). General measures in treatment include correction of anemia, hypoalbuminemia, diabetes, edema, and incontinence [404]. Early clean ulcerations may be treated with damp compresses [403] or, alternatively, vapor-permeable, polyurethane film or hydrocolloid occlusive dressings left in place for several days [403,404]. Deeper draining ulcers may benefit from hydrophilic substances, such as dextranomer polymer beads, gelatin sponge (Gelfoam), granulated sugar, or calcium alginate [403,404,407a]. The use of topical antibiotics such as silver sulfadiazine and gentamicin is controversial [404] but may be helpful if used temporarily to lower bacterial counts in superficially infected ulcers [403]; topical iodine and other cytotoxic antiseptic solutions should be avoided [403]. Topical or oral metronidazole may help eliminate overgrowth of anaerobes [404]. Enzyme preparations, such as streptokinase-streptodornase and collagenase, fibrinolysin, and deoxyribonuclease (Elase) may facilitate debridement of necrotic tissue [403]. The need for surgical debridement should not be overlooked if necrotic tissue remains [403,404,405]. Bridging with pillows may facilitate pressure relief in some patients. Air-fluidized beds and low-air-loss beds are expensive, but are often beneficial for rehabilitating patients with large ulcers [403,406]. Correction of zinc deficiency is helpful [404]. Ascorbic acid, 500 mg bid, has been shown to reduce ulcer surface area [403]. Topical benzoyl peroxide, heavy metal ions, and karaya powder, hyperbaric oxygen, and laser therapy have been reported to hasten healing in some patients [404] but remain controversial [403]. Systemic antibiotics should be given only if there is evidence of sepsis, cellulitis, or osteomyelitis [403,404,408]. Primary surgical closure, split-thickness skin grafts, or myocutaneous flaps afford definitive ulcer therapy appropriate in some settings [403]. Recurrence is, however, not uncommon if the patient remains immobile.

RECURRENT HERPES SIMPLEX LABIALIS. Recurrent herpes simplex virus-induced lesions of the perioral area occur in 20 to 40 percent of the general population [409]. Factors reported to precipitate symptomatic recurrences include fever [410], severe emotional stress [410], surgery on the trigeminal ganglion [411], and immunosuppression, including renal [412] or bone marrow [413,414] transplantation, chemotherapy of hematologic malignancies [415], and AIDS (see Acquired Immunodeficiency Syndrome). The virus is transiently shed even in the saliva of asymptomatic individuals [416], and it is often present for prolonged periods in the deep chronic ulcers that may develop in immunocompromised patients [417].

Lesions typically appear at the mucocutaneous junction of the lip but may affect the entire perioral area, including the nose and cheeks, and occasionally the oral or pharyngeal mucosa. Vesicles or pustules, from 2 to 5 mm in diameter, may appear early and evolve rapidly into punctate erosions and crusts. The confluence of clustered lesions may create large ulcers or eschars. In immunosuppressed individuals, lesions may arise in atypical sites, become very deep and extensive, develop satellite involvement, and persist for months before healing [415].

Optimally, confirmation of the presence of the virus requires viral culture. A Tzanck cytologic preparation, immunoperoxidase tissue stain, or immunofluorescent labeling of scrapings may also be helpful in identifying the viral source of the lesions [417].

In critically ill patients, lesions of recurrent herpes simplex virus infection may be overlooked. They are often mistakenly accredited to trauma from tape or from nasogastric or endotracheal tubes. They may mimic lesions of impetigo, EM, or drug-induced mucositis. Severe involvement may resemble lesions of histoplasmosis or malignant infiltrate.

Therapy of immunocompetent individuals is palliative. Analgesics, antipyretics, and antipruritics may reduce symptoms. Lesions should be kept clean to avoid secondary bacterial infection. Hospital personnel must wear rubber gloves to avoid contact with the lesions. In immunocompromised patients IV, oral, and topical forms of acyclovir have been shown to reduce the duration of viral shedding, alleviate symptoms, and hasten healing [417].

CONTACT DERMATITIS. Contact dermatitis is a superficial inflammatory pruritic condition of the skin that may be induced by a variety of topical agents, several of which are used in the ICU. The inciting products may be primary irritants or, less commonly, sensitizing allergens that elicit a cell-mediated immunologic response after repeated exposure. Irritant contact dermatitis, a nonallergic skin reaction, can be produced from exposure to a chemical substance in sufficient concentration and duration. Irritants are commonly contacted in soaps, detergents, starch, and solvents. Dermatitis is produced within minutes to hours after exposure to the irritant. Allergic contact dermatitis is elicited when a previously sensitized individual is exposed to the offending allergen or a related cross-reactive chemical. Although the initial sensitization can occur within 7 to 10 days after first contact with the allergen, usually the response is seen after repeated or prolonged exposure. Once contact allergy is acquired, dermatitis develops within 24 to 48 hours following reexposure to the sensitizing agent [418].

Adhesive tapes and gauze bandages are a common cause of dermatitis in the ICU. Most reactions are either secondary to mechanical trauma or a result of occlusion of the eccrine and follicular ostia. This traumatic or irritant reaction usually remains confined to the site of contact. Alternatively, allergic contact dermatitis tends to spread beyond the margins of the tape application. It may represent allergy to the rubber accelerator, antioxidant, or resin in the older adhesive tapes or rarely to the acrylate polymer or monomer in the newer paper tapes [419].

Electrocardiography may produce allergic contact dermatitis. Gels or pastes used in this procedure, rubber-strap fasteners, nickel-plated electrodes, and alcohol sponges have all been implicated [419a]. Nasal cannulas may cause an allergic skin eruption if they contain epoxy resin [419].

Many topical medications have the potential of being sensitizing agents. Neomycin is among the ten most common allergens in North America [420], yet remains widely available in topical antibiotic creams and ointments. A widespread "systemic allergic contact dermatitis" may occur in a previously sensitized individual when the allergenic agent or a similar cross-reacting drug is administered parenterally. Just such an erythroderma has been reported in a neomycin-sensitive patient given systemic gentamicin, which is a closely related chemical [421]. Similarly, individuals who have become sensitized to ethylenediamine, a preservative found in the original Mycolog Cream and in numerous otic, nasal, and ophthalmic solutions, may develop a widespread dermatitis when given systemic aminophylline (theophylline plus ethylenediamine) or ethylenediamine antihistamines, such as hydroxyzine, tripelennamine, or piperazines [422].

Many other topical substances used in the ICU can produce contact dermatitis. Bacitracin [423] and povidone-iodine [424] have only rarely been reported to cause allergic contact dermatitis. Topical nitroglycerin ointment and transdermal discs have been implicated in many cases of contact dermatitis; usually the contact allergy does not preclude sublingual use [425]. The topical anesthetic benzocaine is a frequent and potent sensitizer, yet is still commonly available in numerous over-the-counter preparations. Propylene glycol, which is a widely used vehicle for cosmetics, some topical steroids and otic preparations, K-Y Jelly, and many other products, can also produce allergic as well as irritant cutaneous reactions [426]. The parabens, ubiquitous preservatives in topical antimicrobials, steroids, anesthetics, emollients, vaginal jellies and suppositories, rectal suspensions, ulcer bandages, and eye, ear, and nose drops, are frequent sensitizers.

The hallmark of an allergic contact dermatitis is pruritus, whereas in irritant dermatitis, stiffness and dryness are more common. Either reaction may show erythema, papules, plaques, and blisters evolving into oozing erosions. Often, the eruption will have "artificial borders" coinciding with the boundaries of the agent that was applied to the skin.

For management, avoidance or discontinuation of the irritant or allergen is the best approach. Antihistamines may be effective for pruritus. Compresses with drying agents such as aluminum acetate (Burow's solution) should be used for weeping areas. Moderate strength to strong topical corticosteroids should be applied to the skin. Systemic corticosteroids should be reserved for severely edematous or widespread reactions. Secondary infection, usually manifested by honey-colored exudate and crusting, should be treated with appropriate antibiotics after culture confirmation.

ACQUIRED ZINC DEFICIENCY. Acquired zinc deficiency has been reported in association with a variety of nutritional insults, many of which may be seen in critically ill patients. The prototype of zinc deficiency is the congenital form of acrodermatitis enteropathica, whose manifestations from infancy are thought to result from a defect in intestinal zinc absorption. Similar clinical states, however, have been reported in adults as early as 3 weeks after the start of zinc-poor total parenteral nutrition [427]. Additional cases have been described in adult alcoholic cirrhotics with poor diets [428] in young cachectic women with a diet solely of alcohol [429], in a child with cystic fibrosis [430], and in patients with malabsorption [431].

The usual cutaneous manifestation of acquired acrodermatitis enteropathica consists of sharply demarcated erythematous plaques, often with superficial pustules or erosions. The common sites are the distal extremities, the body folds, and around the orifices (Plate II-21) [431,432]. Paronychia, scalp alopecia, and atrophy of the papillae of the tongue often occur. Reversible personality changes including apathy, lethargy, and irritability have been reported [428]. Diarrhea, fever, and dysgeusia may also occur [427]. In zinc deficiency many steps in both cell-mediated and antibody-mediated immunity are impaired [433].

Because the histologic findings in this eruption are nonspecific, a skin biopsy is generally not helpful [428]. Documentation of a low-serum zinc level and reversal of symptoms and signs within 2 to 10 days of adequate zinc supplementation are diagnostic [429,434]. The laboratory should be consulted regarding proper collection and processing of serum specimens in order to avoid zinc contamination.

Lesions of acrodermatitis enteropathica frequently resemble seborrheic dermatitis, psoriasis, or moniliasis. The skin changes may also be confused with those of essential fatty acid deficiency, which produces a dry, usually asymptomatic ichthyosislike desquamation that begins in body folds [435]. It may develop after 4 to 6 months of IV nutrition lacking in lipid supplementation. Necrolytic migratory erythema, which occurs in the presence of a glucagon-secreting tumor of the pancreas, is also similar to acrodermatitis enteropathica in both its morphology and distribution. Hyperglycemia, anemia, weight loss, cutaneous histopathology, and, in most cases, an elevated serum glucagon help to differentiate this disorder.

References

1. Tonnesen MG, Soter NA: Erythema multiforme. *J Am Acad Dermatol* 1:357, 1979.
2. Huff JC, Weston WI, Tonneson MG: Erythema multiforme: A critical review of characteristics, diagnostic criteria, and causes. *J Am Acad Dermatol* 8:763, 1983.
3. Stevens AM, Johnson FC: A new eruptive fever associated with stomatitis and ophthalmia. *Am J Dis Child* 24:526, 1922.
4. Thomas BA: The so-called Stevens-Johnson syndrome. *Br Med J* 1:1393, 1950.
5. Lyell A: Toxic epidermal necrolysis (the scalded skin syndrome): A reappraisal. *Br J Dermatol* 100:69, 1979.
6. Lever WF, Schaumburg-Lever G: *Histopathology Of The Skin.* Philadelphia, Lippincott, 1983, p 122.
7. Braverman IM: *Skin Signs of Systemic Disease.* Philadelphia, Saunders, 1981, p 484.
8. Chan HL: Observations of drug induced toxic epidermal necrolysis in Singapore. *J Am Acad Dermatol* 10:973, 1984.
9. Assaad D, From L, Ricciatti D, et al: Toxic epidermal necrolysis in Stevens-Johnson syndrome. *Can Med Assoc J* 118:154, 1978.
10. Breathnach SM, Dutt MK, Black MM: A severe bullous eruption occurring in a patient with chronic active hepatitis and glomerulonephritis. *Arch Dermatol* 116:1061, 1980.
11. Bergoend H, Loffler A, Amar R, et al: Reactions cutanees survenues au cours de la prophylaxie de masse la meningite cerebro-spinale par un sulfamide long-retard. *Ann Dermatol Syphiligr* 95:481, 1968.
12. St. Clair K, Duvic M: Erythema multiforme. *IM* 8:113, 1987.
13. Howland WW, Golitz LE, Weston WL, et al: Erythema multiforme: Clinical, histopathologic and immunologic study. *J Am Acad Dermatol* 10:438, 1984.
14. Chan HL, Stern RS, Arndt KA, et al: The incidence of erythema multiforme, Stevens-Johnson syndrome, and toxic epidermal necrolysis. *Arch Dermatol* 126:43, 1990.
15. Edmond BJ, Huff JC, Weston WL: Erythema multiforme. *Pediatr Clin North Am* 30:631, 1983.
16. Huff JC, Weston WL: Recurrent erythema multiforme. *Medicine* 68:133, 1989.
17. Kazmierowski JA, Peizner DS, Wuepper KD: Herpes simplex antigen in immune complexes of patients with erythema multiforme. *JAMA* 247:2547, 1982.
18. Kampgen E, Burg G, Wank R: Association of herpes simplex virus-induced erythema multiforme with the human leukocyte antigen DQw3. *Arch Dermatol* 124:1372, 1988.
19. Lobkowicz F, Ring J, Schwarz TF, et al: Erythema multiforme in a patient with acute human parvovirus B19 infection. *J Am Acad Dermatol* 20:849, 1989.
20. Bianchine JR, Macarage TV, Lasagn AL, et al: Drugs as etiologic factors in the Stevens-Johnson syndrome. *Am J Med* 44:390, 1968.
21. Stran J: Aetiology of febrile mucocutaneous syndromes with special reference to the provocative role of infections and drugs. *Acta Med Scand* 201:131, 1977.
22. Bigby M, Stern R: Cutaneous reactions to nonsteroidal inflammatory drugs. *J Am Acad Dermatol* 12:866, 1985.
23. Ackerman AB, Penneys NS, Clark WH: Erythema multiforme exudativum: Distinctive pathological process. *Br J Dermatol* 84:554, 1971.
24. Bushkell LL, Mackel SE, Jordan RE: Erythema multiforme: Direct immunofluorescence studies and detection of circulating immune complexes. *J Invest Dermatol* 74:372, 1980.
25. Huff JC, Weston WL: Clinical and laboratory features of recurrent erythema multiforme. *Clin Res* 29:599, 1981.
26. Howard GM: The Stevens-Johnson syndrome. Ocular prognosis and treatment. *Am J Ophthalmol* 55:893, 1963.
27. Beck MH, Portnoy B: Severe erythema multiforme complicated by fatal gastrointestinal involvement following co-trimoxazole therapy. *Clin Exp Dermatol* 4:201, 1979.
28. Zweiban B, Cohen H, Chandrasoma P: Gastrointestinal involvement complicating Stevens-Johnson syndrome. *Gastroenterology* 91:469, 1986.
29. Virant FS, Reading GJ, Novack AH: Multiple pulmonary complications in a patient with Stevens-Johnson syndrome. *Clin Pediatr* 23:412, 1984.
30. Comaish JS, Karr DN: Erythema multiforme nephritis. *Br Med J* 2:84, 1961.
31. Schartum F: Stevens-Johnson syndrome with cardiac involvement. *Acta Med Scand* 179:729, 1966.
32. Wilson EE, Malinak LR: Vulvovaginal sequelae of Stevens-Johnson syndrome and their management. *Obstet Gynecol* 71:478, 1988.
33. Green JA, Spruance SL, Wenerstrom G, et al: Postherpetic erythema multiforme prevented with prophylactic oral acyclovir. *Ann Intern Med* 102:632, 1985.
34. Molin L: Oral acyclovir prevents herpes simplex virus-associated erythema multiforme. *Br J Dermatol* 116:109, 1987.
35. Halebian PH, Shires GT: Burn unit treatment of acute, severe exfoliating disorders. *Ann Rev Med* 40:137, 1989.
36. Marvin JA, Heimbach DM, Engrav LH, et al: Improved treatment of the Stevens-Johnson syndrome. *Arch Surg* 119:601, 1984.
36a. Wilkins J, Morrison L, White CR Jr.: Oculocutaneous manifestations of the erythema multiforme/Stevens-Johnson syndrome/

toxic epdermal necrolysis spectrum. *Dermatol Clin* 10:571, 1992.

37. Ting HC, Adam BA: Erythema multiforme–response to corticosteroid. *Dermatologica* 169:175, 1984.

38. Kim PS, Goldfarb JW, Galsford JC, et al: Stevens-Johnson syndrome and toxic epidermal necrolysis: A pathophysiologic review with the recommendations for a treatment protocol. *J Burn Care Rehabil* 4:91, 1983.

39. Rasmussen JE: Erythema multiforme in children: Response to treatment with systemic corticosteroids. *Br J Dermatol* 95:181, 1976.

40. Shum S: Stevens-Johnson syndrome: A pediatric experience. *J La State Med Soc* 128:331, 1976.

41. Ginsburg CM: Stevens-Johnson syndrome in children. *Pediatr Infect Dis* 1:155, 1982.

42. Ting HC, Adam BA: Stevens-Johnson syndrome: A review of 34 cases. *Int J Dermatol* 169:175, 1985.

43. Nethercott JR, Choi BCK: Erythema multiforme (Stevens-Johnson syndrome)—chart review of 123 hospitalized patients. *Dermatologica* 171:383, 1985.

43a. Renfro L, Grant-Kels JM, Feder HM Jr, Daman LA: Controversy: Are systemic steroids indicated in the treatment of erythema multiforme? *Pediatr Dermatol* 6:43, 1989.

43b. Wilkel CS, McDonald CJ: Cyclosporine therapy for bullous erythema multiforme (letter). *Arch Dermatol* 126:397, 1990.

44. Goldstein SM, Wintroub BW, Elias PM: Toxic epidermal necrolysis. Unmuddying the waters. *Arch Dermatol* 123:1153, 1987.

45. Revuz J, Pensco D, Roujeau JC, et al: Toxic epidermal necrolysis. Clinical findings and prognosis factors in 87 patients. *Arch Dermatol* 123:1160, 1987.

46. Reinhoff HY Jr: Toxic epidermal necrolysis. *Johns Hopkins Med J* 151:326, 1982.

47. Merot Y, Savrat JH: Clues to the pathogenesis of toxic epidermal necrolysis. *Int J Dermatol* 24:165, 1985.

48. Lyell A: Toxic epidermal necrolysis (the scalded skin syndrome): A reappraisal. *Br J Dermatol* 100:69, 1979.

49. Guillaume JC, Roujeau JC, Revuz J, et al: The culprit drugs in 87 cases of toxic epidermal necrolysis (Lyell's syndrome). *Arch Dermatol* 123:1166, 1987.

50. Heng MCY: Drug-induced toxic epidermal necrolysis. *Br J Dermatol* 113:597, 1985.

50a. Roujeau JC, Guillaume JC, et al: Toxic epidermal necrolysis (Lyell syndrome): Incidence and drug etiology in France (1981–1985). *Arch Dermatol* 126:37 1990.

51. Olsen VV, Loft S, Christensen KD: Serious reactions during malaria prophylaxis with pyrimethamine-sulfadoxine. *Lancet* 2:994, 1982.

52. Fritsch PO, Elias PM: Toxic epidermal necrolysis. In: Fitzpatrick TB, et al, (eds) *Dermatology In General Medicine*. New York, McGraw-Hill, 1987, p 563.

53. Shoss RG, Rayhanzadeh S: Toxic epidermal necrolysis following measles vaccination. *Arch Dermatol* 110:766, 1974.

54. Lyell A: Toxic epidermal necrolysis: An eruption resembling scalding of the skin. *Br J Dermatol* 68:355, 1956.

55. Peck GL, Herzig GP, Elias PM: Toxic epidermal necrolysis in a patient with graft-versus-host reaction. *Arch Dermatol* 105:562, 1972.

56. Callaway JL, Tate WE: Toxic epidermal necrolysis caused by gin and tonic. *Arch Dermatol* 109:909, 1974.

57. Radimer GF, Davis JH, Ackerman AB: Fumigant-induced toxic epidermal necrolysis. *Arch Dermatol* 110:103, 1974.

57a. Saiag P, Caumes E, Chosidow O, et al: Drug-induced toxic epidermal necrolysis (Lyell syndrome) in patients infected with the human immunodeficiency virus. *J Am Acad Dermatol* 26(4):567, 1992.

57b. Porteous DM, Berger TG: Severe cutaneous drug reactions (Stevens-Johnson syndrome and toxic epidermal necrolysis) in human immunodeficiency virus infection (letter). *Arch Dermatol* 127:740, 1991.

58. Greer KE: Toxic epidermal necrolysis. *Cutis* 24:565, 1979.

59. Jones WG, Halebian P, Madden M, et al: Drug-induced toxic epidermal necrolysis in children. *J Pediatr Surg* 24:167, 1989.

60. Manzella JP, Hall CB, Green JL, et al: Toxic epidermal necrolysis in childhood: Differentiation from staphylococcal scalded skin syndrome. *Pediatrics* 66:291, 1980.

61. Hawk RJ, Storer JS, Daum RS: Toxic epidermal necrolysis in a six week old infant. *Pediatr Dermatol* 2:197, 1985.

62. Adzick NS, Kim SH, Bondoc CC, et al: Management of toxic epidermal necrolysis in a pediatric burn center. *Am J Dis Child* 139:499, 1985.

63. Westly ED, Wechsler HL: Toxic epidermal necrolysis. Granulocytic leukopenia as a prognostic indicator. *Arch Dermatol* 120:721, 1984.

64. Elias PM, Fritsch P, Epstein EH: Staphylococcal scalded skin syndrome: Clinical features, pathogenesis, and recent microbiological and biochemical developments. *Arch Dermatol* 133:207, 1977.

65. Fritsch P, Elias PM, Varga J: The fate of staphylococcal exfoliatin in newborn and adult mice. *Br J Dermatol* 95:275, 1976.

66. Fine JD, Harrist TJ, Radford MJ, et al: Adult scalded skin syndrome fatally complicated by mixed gram-negative sepsis and cellulitis. *Cutis* 27:162, 1981.

67. Elias PM, Fritsch P, Dahl MV, et al: Staphylococcal exfoliative toxin: Pathogenesis and subcellular site of action. *J Invest Dermatol* 65:501, 1975.

68. Sturman SW, Malkinson FD: Staphylococcal scalded skin syndrome in an adult and a child. *Arch Dermatol* 112:1275, 1976.

69. Levine G, Norden CW: Staphylococcal scalded skin syndrome in an adult. *N Engl J Med* 287:1339, 1972.

70. Reid LH, Weston WL, Humbert JR: Staphylococcal scalded skin syndrome: Adult onset in the patient with deficient cell-mediated immunity. *Arch Dermatol* 109:239, 1974.

71. Borchers SL, Gomez EC, Isseroff RR: Generalized staphylococcal scalded skin syndrome in an anephric boy undergoing hemodialysis. *Arch Dermatol* 120:912, 1984.

72. Ridgway HB, Lowe NJ: Staphlylococcal scalded skin syndrome in an adult with Hodgkin's disease. *Arch Dermatol* 115:589, 1979.

73. Hurwitz RM, Rivera HP, Gooch MH, et al: Toxic shock syndrome or toxic epidermal necrolysis? Case reports showing clinical similarity and histologic separation. *J Am Acad Dermatol* 7:246, 1982.

74. Hunter JAA, Davison AM: Toxic epidermal necrolysis associated with pentazocine therapy and severe reversible renal failure. *Br J Dermatol* 88:287, 1973.

75. Krumlovsky FA, DelGreco F, Herdson PB, et al: Renal disease associated with toxic epidermal necrolysis (Lyell's disease). *Am J Med* 57:817, 1974.

76. Roupe G, Ahlmén M, Fagerberg B, et al: Toxic epidermal necrolysis with extensive mucosal erosions of the gastrointestinal and respiratory tracts. *Int Arch Allergy Appl Immunol* 80:145, 1986.

77. Revuz J, Roujeau JC, Guillaume JC, et al: Treatment of toxic epidermal necrolysis. Creteil's experience. *Arch Dermatol* 123:1156, 1987.

78. Heimbach DM, Engrav LH, Marvin JA: Toxic epidermal necrolysis. A step forward in treatment. *JAMA* 257:2171, 1987.

79. Jones WG, Halebian M, Finkelstein J, et al: Drug-induced toxic epidermal necrolysis in children. *J Pediatr Surg* 24:167, 1989.

80. Birchall N, Langdon R, Cuono C: Toxic epidermal necrolysis: An approach to management using cryopreserved allograft skin. *J Am Acad Dermatol* 16:368, 1987.

81. Macfarlane AW, Curley RK: Management of toxic epidermal necrolysis with a hydrogel dressing and fluidized-bead bed: Report of three cases. *Clin Exp Dermatol* 12:354, 1987.

82. Halebian PH, Corder VJ, Madden MR, et al: Improved burn center survival of patients with toxic epidermal necrolysis managed without corticosteroids. *Ann Surg* 204:503, 1986.

83. Kamanabroo D, Schmitz-Landgraf W, Czarnetzki BM: Plasmapheresis in severe drug-induced toxic epidermal necrolysis. *Arch Dermatol* 121:1548, 1985.

84. Renfro L, Grant-Kels JM, Daman LA: Drug-induced toxic epidermal necrolysis treated with cyclosporin. *Int J Dermatol* 28:441, 1989.

85. deFelice GP, Caroli R, Autelitano A: Long-term complications of

toxic epidermal necrolysis (Lyell's disease). Clinical and histopathologic study. *Ophthalmologica* 195:1, 1987.

86. Arstikaitis MJ: Ocular aftermath of Stevens-Johnson syndrome. *Arch Ophthalmol* 90:376, 1973.

87. Smith GB, Shribman AJ: Anaesthesia and severe skin disease. *Anaesthesia* 39:443, 1984.

88. Abrahams I, McCarthy JT, Sanders SL: 101 cases of exfoliative dermatitis. *Arch Dermatol* 87:136, 1963.

89. Hasan T, Jansen CT: Erythroderma: A follow-up of fifty cases. *J Am Acad Dermatol* 8:836, 1983.

90. Gentele H, Lodin A, Skog E: Dermatitis exfoliativa. Cases admitted in the decade 1948-1957 to the Dermatological Clinic, Karolinska Sjukhuset, Stockholm, Sweden. *Acta Derm Venereol (Stockh)* 38:296, 1958.

91. Sehgal VN, Srivastava G: Exfoliative dermatitis. *Dermatologica* 173:278, 1986.

92. Adam JE: Exfoliative dermatitis. *Can Med Assoc J* 99:661, 1968.

93. Adam JE: Exfoliative dermatitis (erythroderma). *Curr Probl Dermatol* 4:1, 1972.

94. Anderson PC, Loeffel ED: Erythrodermatitis. A review of 40 cases. *Mo Med* 67:252, 1970.

95. King LE Jr, Dufresne RG Jr, Lovett GL, et al: Erythroderma: Review of 82 cases. *South Med J* 79:1210, 1986.

96. Wong KS, Wong SN, Tham SN: Generalized exfoliative dermatitis—A clinical study of 108 patients. *Ann Acad Med Singapore* 17:520, 1988.

97. Wilson HTH: Exfoliative dermatitis. Its etiology and prognosis. *Arch Dermatol Syph* 69:577, 1954.

98. Nicolis GD, Helwig EB: Exfoliative dermatitis. A clinicopathologic study of 135 cases. *Arch Dermatol* 108:788, 1973.

99. Marks JM: Erythroderma. *Semin Dermatol* 5:27, 1986.

100. Thestrup-Pedersen K, Halkier-Sorensen L, Sogaard H, et al: The red man syndrome. Exfoliative dermatitis of unknown etiology: A description and follow-up of 38 patients. *J Am Acad Dermatol* 18:1307, 1988.

101. Harper TG, Latuska RF, Sperling HV: An unusual association between erythroderma and an occult gastric carcinoma. *Am J Gastroenterol* 79:921, 1984.

102. Shelley ED, Shelley WB, Schafer RL: Generalized *Trichophyton rubrum* infection in congenital ichthyosiform erythroderma. *J Am Acad Dermatol* 20:1133, 1989.

103. Marks J: Erythroderma and its management. *Clin Exp Dermatol* 7:415, 1982.

104. Mogavero HS Jr: Exfoliative dermatitis, in Provost TT, Farmer ER (eds): *Current Therapy In Dermatology-2*. Philadelphia, BC Decker, 1988, p 20.

105. Boyd AS, Menter A: Erythrodermic psoriasis. Precipitating factors, course, and prognosis in 50 patients. *J Am Acad Dermatol* 21:985, 1989.

106. Roenigk HH Jr, Auerbach R, Maibach HI, et al: Methotrexate guidelines—revised. *J Am Acad Dermatol* 6:145, 1982.

107. Shelley WB, Shelley ED: *Advanced Dermatologic Therapy*. Philadelphia, W.B. Saunders, 1987, p 420.

108. Morison WL, Momtaz KT, Parrish JA, et al: Combined methotrexate-PUVA therapy in the treatment of psoriasis. *J Am Acad Dermatol* 6:46, 1982.

109. Paul BS, Momtaz KT, Stern RS, et al: Combined methotrexate-ultraviolet B therapy in the treatment of psoriasis. *J Am Acad Dermatol* 7:758, 1982.

110. Kingston TP, Matt LH, Lowe NJ: Etretin therapy for severe psoriasis. Evaluation of initial clinical responses. *Arch Dermatol* 123:55, 1987.

110a. Bunn PA Jr, Norris DA: The therapeutic role of interferons and monoclonal antibodies in cutaneous T-cell lymphomas. *J Invest Dermatol* 95:209S, 1990.

110b. Edelson RL: Photopheresis: Present and future aspects. *J Photochemistry & Photobiology* 10:165, 1991.

111. Reuler JB, Jones SR, Girard DE: Hypothermia in the erythroderma syndrome. *West J Med* 127:243, 1977.

112. Lyons JH III: Generalized pustular psoriasis. *Int J Dermatol* 26:409, 1987.

113. Baker H, Ryan TJ: Generalized pustular psoriasis: A clinical and epidemiological study of 104 cases. *Br J Dermatol* 80:771, 1968.

114. Ryan TJ, Baker H: The prognosis of generalized pustular psoriasis. *Br J Dermatol* 85:407, 1971.

115. Lowe NL, Ridgway HB: Generalized pustular psoriasis precipitated by lithium carbonate. *Arch Dermatol* 114:1788, 1978.

116. Landry M, Murrel SA: Generalized pustular psoriasis: Observations on the course of the disease in a familial occurrence. *Arch Dermatol* 105:711, 1972.

117. Tolman MM, Moschella SL: Pustular psoriasis (Zumbusch). *Arch Dermatol* 81:400, 1960.

118. Stewart AF, Battaglini-Sabetta J, Milstone L: Hypocalcemia-induced pustular psoriasis of von Zumbusch. New experience with an old syndrome. *Ann Intern Med* 100:677, 1984.

119. Goldyne ME: Leukotrienes: Clinical significance. *J Am Acad Dermatol* 10:659, 1984.

120. Hubler WR Jr: Lingual lesions of generalized pustular psoriasis: Report of five cases and a review of the literature. *J Am Acad Dermatol* 11:1069, 1984.

121. Braverman IM, Cohen I, O'Keefe E: Metabolic and ultrastructural studies in a patient with pustular psoriasis (von Zumbusch). *Arch Dermatol* 105:189, 1972.

122. Shelley WB: Generalized pustular psoriasis induced by potassium iodide. *JAMA* 201:1009, 1967.

123. Lever WF, Schaumburg-Lever G: *Histopathology Of The Skin*. Philadelphia, Lippincott, 1983, p 145.

124. Ryan TJ, Baker H: Systemic corticosteroids and folic acid antagonists in the treatment of generalized pustular psoriasis. Evaluation and prognosis based on the study of 104 cases. *Br J Dermatol* 81:134, 1969.

125. Wolska H, Jablonska S, Bounameaux Y: Etretinate in severe psoriasis. Results of double blind study and maintenance therapy in pustular psoriasis. *J Am Acad Dermatol* 9:883, 1983.

126. Rubin MG, Hanno R: Short term etretinate for pustular psoriasis. *J Am Acad Dermatol* 12:896, 1985.

127. Lowe NJ, Lazarus V, Matt L: Systemic retinoid therapy for psoriasis. *J Am Acad Dermatol* 19:186, 1988.

128. Rosenbaum MM, Roenigk HH Jr: Treatment of generalized pustular psoriasis with etretinate (Ro 10-9359) and methotrexate. *J Am Acad Dermatol* 10:357, 1984.

129. Tuyp E, MacKie RM: Combination therapy for psoriasis with methotrexate and etretinate. *J Am Acad Dermatol* 14:70, 1986.

130. Meinardi MMHM, Westerhof W, Bos JD: Generalized pustular psoriasis (von Zumbusch) responding to cyclosporin A. *Br J Dermatol* 116:269, 1987.

131. Sofen H, Moy R, Lowe N: Treatment of generalized pustular psoriasis with isotretinoin. *Lancet* 1:40, 1984.

131a. Berth-Jones J, Bourke J, Bailey K, et al: Generalized pustular psoriasis: response to topical calcipotriol. *Br Med J* 305:868, 1992.

132. Honigsmann H, Gschnait F, Konrad K, et al: Photochemotherapy for pustular psoriasis (von Zumbusch). *Br J Dermatol* 97:119, 1977.

133. Korman N: Pemphigus. *J Am Acad Dermatol* 18:1219, 1988.

134. Koulu L, Stanley JR: Clinical, histologic, and immunopathologic comparison of pemphigus vulgaris and pemphigus foliaceus. *Semin Dermatol* 7:82, 1988.

135. Lever WF: Pemphigus and pemphigoid: A review of the advances made since 1964. *J Am Acad Dermatol* 1:2, 1979.

136. Ahmed AR, Graham J, Jordan RE, et al: Pemphigus: Current concepts. *Ann Intern Med* 92:396, 1980.

137. Eaglstein WH, Pariser DM: *Office techniques for diagnosing skin disease*. Chicago, Year Book, 1978, p 65.

138. Kaneko F, Mori M, Tsukinaga I, et al: Pemphigus vulgaris of esophageal mucosa. *Arch Dermatol* 121:272, 1985.

139. Barnes LM, Clark ML, Estes SA, et al: Pemphigus vulgaris involving the esophagus. A case report and review of the literature. *Dig Dis Sci* 32:655, 1987.

140. Schwermann M, Lechner W, Elsner C, et al: Pemphigus vulgaris involving duodenum and colon. *Z Hautkr* 63:101, 1988.

141. Eaglstein WH, Pariser DM: *Office techniques for diagnosing skin disease*. Chicago, Year Book, 1978, p. 23.

142. Seidenbaum M, David M, Sandbank M: The course and prognosis of pemphigus. A review of 115 patients. *Int J Dermatol* 27:580, 1988.

143. Savin JA: Some factors affecting prognosis in pemphigus vulgaris and pemphigoid. *Br J Dermatol* 104:415, 1981.

144. Ahmed AR, Moy R: Death in pemphigus. *J Am Acad Dermatol* 7:221, 1982.

145. Bystryn JC: Adjuvant therapy of pemphigus. *Arch Dermatol* 120:941, 1984.

146. Fine JD, Appell ML, Green LK, et al: Pemphigus vulgaris. Combined treatment with intravenous corticosteroid pulse therapy, plasmapheresis, and azathioprine. *Arch Dermatol* 124:236, 1988.

146a. Pandya AG, Sontheimer RD: Treatment of pemphigus vulgaris with pulse intravenous cyclophosphamide. *Arch Dermatol* 128:1626, 1992.

147. Guillaume JC, Roujeau JC, Morel P, et al: Controlled study of plasma exchange in pemphigus. *Arch Dermatol* 124:1659, 1988.

148. Bystryn JC: Plasmapheresis therapy of pemphigus. *Arch Dermatol* 124:1702, 1988.

149. Blaszczyk M, Chorzelski TP, Jablonska S, et al: Indications for future studies on the treatment of pemphigus with plasmapheresis. *Arch Dermatol* 125:843, 1989.

150. Anhalt GJ: Pemphigus, in Provost TT, Farmer ER (eds): *Current Therapy In Dermatology-2*. Philadelphia, BC Decker, 1988, p 55.

151. Bork K, Bräuninger W: Increasing incidence of eczema herpeticum: Analysis of seventy-five cases. *J Am Acad Dermatol* 19:1024, 1988.

152. Long JC, Wheeler CE Jr, Briggaman RA: Varicella-like infection due to herpes simplex. *Arch Dermatol* 114:406, 1978.

153. Nishimura M, Maekawa M, Hino Y, et al: Kaposi's varicelliform eruption: Development in a patient with a healing second-degree burn. *Arch Dermatol* 120:799, 1984.

154. Toole JWP, Hofstader SL, Ramsay CA: Darier's disease and Kaposi's varicelliform eruption. *J Am Acad Dermatol* 1:321, 1979.

155. Cesario T, Fife LT, Rayhan S, et al: Cutaneous dissemination of herpes simplex virus in individuals fifteen years of age and older. *Am J Med Sci* 273:345, 1977.

156. Naraqi S, Jackson GG, Jonasson OM: Viremia with herpes simplex type 1 in adults: Four nonfatal cases, one with features of chicken pox. *Ann Intern Med* 85:165, 1976.

157. Lagrew DC Jr, Furlow TG, Hager D, et al: Disseminated herpes simplex virus infection in pregnancy: Successful treatment with acyclovir. *JAMA* 252:2058, 1984.

158. Masessa JM, Grossman ME, Knobler EH, et al: Kaposi's varicelliform eruption in cutaneous T cell lymphoma. *J Am Acad Dermatol* 21:133, 1989.

159. Muller SA, Herrmann EC Jr, Winkelmann RK: Herpes simplex infections in hematologic malignancies. *Am J Med* 52:102, 1972.

160. Copeman PWM, Wallace HJ: Eczema vaccinatum. *Br Med J* 2:906, 1964.

161. Higgins PG, Crow KD: Recurrent Kaposi's varicelliform eruption in Darier's disease. *Br J Dermatol* 88:391, 1973.

162. Leyden JJ, Baker DA: Localized herpes simplex infections in atopic dermatitis. *Arch Dermatol* 115:311, 1979.

163. Mailman CJ, Miranda JL, Spock A: Recurrent eczema herpeticum: Widespread cutaneous herpes simplex in atopic patient without active dermatitis. *Arch Dermatol* 89:815, 1964.

164. Solomon AR, Rasmussen JE, Varani J, et al: The Tzanck smear in the diagnosis of cutaneous herpes simplex. *JAMA* 251:663, 1984.

165. Wong KK, Hirsch MS: Herpes virus infections in patients with neoplastic disease: Diagnosis and therapy. *Am J Med* 76:464, 1984.

166. Burkhart CG: Persistent cutaneous herpes simplex infection. *Int J Dermatol* 20:552, 1981.

167. Cao M, Xiao X, Egbert B, et al: Rapid detection of cutaneous herpes simplex virus infection with the polymerase chain reaction. *J Invest Dermatol* 92:391, 1989.

167a. Nahass GT, Goldstein BA, Zhu WY, et al: Comparison of Tzanck smear, viral culture, and DNA diagnostic methods in detection of herpes simplex and varicella-zoster infection. *JAMA* 268:2541, 1992.

168. Jaworski MA, Moffatt MEK, Ahronheim GA: Disseminated herpes simplex associated with *H. influenzae* infection in a previously healthy child. *J Pediatr* 96:426, 1980.

169. Becker WB, Kipps A, McKenzie D: Disseminated herpes simplex virus infection: Its pathogenesis based on virological and pathological studies in 33 cases. *Am J Dis Child* 115:1, 1968.

170. Raga J, Chrystal V, Coovadia HM: Usefulness of clinical features and liver biopsy in diagnosis of disseminated herpes simplex infection. *Arch Dis Child* 59:820, 1984.

171. Auch Moedy JL, Lerman SJ, White RJ: Fatal disseminated herpes simplex virus infection in a healthy child. *Am J Dis Child* 135:45, 1981.

172. Connor RW, Lorts G, Gilbert DN: Lethal herpes simplex virus type 1 hepatitis in a normal adult. *Gastroenterology* 76:590, 1979.

173. Buss DH, Scharyj M: Herpesvirus infection of the esophagus and other visceral organs in adults: Incidence and clinical significance. *Am J Med* 66:457, 1979.

174. Whitley RJ, Soong SJ, Linneman C Jr, et al: Herpes simplex encephalitis. Clinical assessment. *JAMA* 247:317, 1982.

175. Braunstein BL, Greer KL: Treatment of eczema herpeticum with vidarabine. *Arch Dermatol* 118:597, 1982.

176. Parham DM, Gawkrodger DJ, Vestey JP, et al: Disseminated herpes simplex infection complicating Darier's disease: Successful treatment with oral acyclovir. *J Infect* 10:77, 1985.

177. Swart RNJ, Vermeer BJ, van Der Meer JWM, et al: Treatment of eczema herpeticum with acyclovir. *Arch Dermatol* 119:13, 1983.

178. Robinson GE, Underhill GS, Forster GE, et al: Treatment with acyclovir of genital herpes simplex virus infection complicated by eczema herpeticum. *Br J Ven Dis* 60:241, 1984.

179. Jawitz CJ, Hines HC, Moshell AN: Treatment of eczema herpeticum with systemic acyclovir. *Arch Dermatol* 121:274, 1985.

180. Greaves WL, Kaiser AB, Alford RH, et al: The problem of herpetic whitlow among hospital personnel. *Infect Control* 1:381, 1980.

181. Auletta MJ, Headington JT: Purpura fulminans. A cutaneous manifestation of severe protein C deficiency. *Arch Dermatol* 124:1387, 1988.

182. Dominey A, Kettler A, Yiannias J, et al: Purpura fulminans and transient protein C and S deficiency. *Arch Dermatol* 124:1442, 1988.

183. Powars DR, Rogers ZR, Patch MJ, et al: Purpura fulminans in meningococcemia: Association with acquired deficiencies of proteins C and S. *N Engl J Med* 317:571, 1987.

184. Seagle MB, Bingham HG: Purpura fulminans. *Ann Plast Surg* 20:576, 1988.

184a. Fourrier F, Lestavel P, Chopin C, et al: Meningococcemia and purpura fulminans in adults: Acute deficiencies of proteins C and S and early treatment with antithrombin III concentrates. *Intens Care Med* 16(2):121, 1990.

185. Spicer TE, Rau JM: Purpura fulminans. *Am J Med* 61:566, 1976.

186. Silbart S, Oppenheim W: Purpura fulminans. Medical, surgical, and rehabilitative considerations. *Clin Orthop* 193:206, 1985.

187. Chu DZJ, Blaisdell FW. Purpura fulminans. *Am J Surg* 143:356, 1982.

188. Chenaille PJ, Horowitz ME: Purpura fulminans. A case for heparin therapy. *Clin Pediatr* 28:95, 1989.

189. McCalmont C, Zanolli MD: Rickettsial diseases. *Dermatol Clin* 7:591, 1989.

190. Riley HD: Rickettsial diseases. *Curr Probl Pediatr* 11:1, 1981.

191. Kamper CA, Chessman KH, Phelps SJ: Rocky Mountain spotted fever. *Clin Pharm* 7:109, 1988.

191a. Dumler JS, Gage WR, Pettis GL, et al: Rapid immunoperoxidase demonstration of *Rickettsia rickettsii* in fixed cutaneous specimens from patients with Rocky Mountain spotted fever. *Am J Clin Path* 93:410, 1990.

192. MMWR: Rocky Mountain spotted fever—United States, 1988. *Arch Dermatol* 125:1323, 1989.

193. Kelsey DS: Rocky Mountain spotted fever. *Pediatr Clin North Am* 26:367, 1979.

194. Woodward TE: Rocky Mountain spotted fever: Epidemiological and early clinical signs and keys to treatment and reduced mortality. *J Infect Dis* 150:465, 1984.

195. James WD, Odom RB: Graft-vs-host disease. *Arch Dermatol* 119:683, 1983.

196. Breathnach SM: Current understanding of the aetiology and clinical implications of cutaneous graft-versus-host disease. *Br J Dermatol* 114:139, 1986.

197. Mauduit G, Claudy A: Cutaneous expression of graft-v-host disease in man. *Semin Dermatol* 7:149, 1988.

197a. Markus PM, Cai X, Ming W, et al: FK 506 reverses acute graft-versus-host disease after allogeneic bone marrow transplantation in rats. *Surg* 110:357, 1991.

198. Ferrara JLM: Syngeneic graft-vs-host disease. *Arch Dermatol* 123:741, 1987.

199. Harper JI: Cutaneous graft versus host disease. *Br Med J* 295:401, 1987.

200. Shulman HM, Sullivan KM, Weiden PL, et al: Chronic graft-versus-host syndrome in man. A long-term clinicopathologic study of 20 Seattle patients. *Am J Med* 69:204, 1980.

200a. Kapoor N, Pelligrini AE, Copelan EA, et al: Psoralen plus ultraviolet A (PUVA) in the treatment of chronic graft versus host disease: preliminary experience in standard treatment resistant patients. *Semin Hematol* 29:108, 1992.

200b. Jampel RM, Farmer ER, Vogelsang GB, et al: PUVA therapy for chronic cutaneous graft-vs-host disease. *Arch Dermatol* 127:1673, 1991.

200c. McCann S, Solomon R: Chronic graft-versus host disease: Dermatological manifestations, nursing management, and research with extracorporeal chemophotopheresis. *Dermatol Nursing* 3:221, 1991.

201. Wright SW, Trott AT: Toxic shock syndrome: A review. *Ann Emerg Med* 17:268, 1988.

202. Center for Disease Control: Toxic-shock syndrome, United States, 1970–1982. *MMWR* 31:201, 1982.

203. Wager GP: Toxic shock syndrome: A review. *Am J Obstet Gynecol* 146:93, 1983.

204. Reingold AL: Nonmenstrual toxic shock syndrome: The growing picture. *JAMA* 249:932, 1983.

205. Bartlett P, Reingold AL, Graham DR, et al: Toxic shock syndrome associated with surgical wound infections. *JAMA* 247:1448, 1982.

206. Buchdahl R, Levin M, Wilkins B, et al: Toxic shock syndrome. *Arch Dis Child* 60:563, 1985.

207. Findlay RF, Odom RB: Toxic shock syndrome. *Int J Dermatol* 21:117, 1982.

208. Bach MC: Dermatologic signs in toxic shock syndrome—clues to diagnosis. *J Am Acad Dermatol* 8:343, 1983.

209. Radentz WH: Opportunistic fungal infections in immunocompromised hosts. *J Am Acad Dermatol* 20:989, 1989.

210. Spencer LV, Callen JP: Cutaneous manifestations of bacterial infections. *Dermatol Clin* 7:579, 1989.

211. Bagel J, Grossman ME: Hemorrhagic bullae associated with *Morganella morganii* septicemia. *J Am Acad Dermatol* 12:575, 1985.

212. Wickboldt LG, Sanders CV: *Vibrio vulnificus* infection: Case report and update since 1970. *J Am Acad Dermatol* 9:243, 1983.

213. Myskowski PL, Brown AE, Dinsmore R, et al: Mucormycosis following bone marrow transplantation. *J Am Acad Dermatol* 9:111, 1983.

214. Schlossberg D, Ricci JA, Fugate JS: Dermatologic manifestations of *Citrobacter* septicemia. *J Am Acad Dermatol* 5:613, 1981.

215. Robboy SJ, Mihm MC, Colman RW, et al: The skin in disseminated intravascular coagulation: Prospective analysis of thirty-six cases. *Br J Dermatol* 88:221, 1973.

216. Wolinsky S, Grossman ME, Walther RR, et al: Hemorrhagic bullae associated with salmonella septicemia. *NY State J Med* 81:1639, 1981.

217. Held JL, Berkowitz RK, Grossman ME: Use of touch preparation for rapid diagnosis of disseminated candidiasis. *J Am Acad Dermatol* 19:1063, 1988.

218. Kingston ME, Mackey D: Skin clues in the diagnosis of life-threatening infections. *Rev Infect Dis* 8:1, 1986.

219. Shapiro PE, Grossman ME: Disseminated *Nocardia asteroides* with pustules. *J Am Acad Dermatol* 20:889, 1989.

220. Fine JD, Miller JA, Harrist TJ, et al: Cutaneous lesions in disseminated candidiasis mimicking ecthyma gangrenosum. *Am J Med* 70:1133, 1981.

221. Roberts R, Tarpay MM, Marks MI, et al: Erysipelas-like lesions and hyperesthesia as manifestations of *Pseudomonas aeruginosa* sepsis. *JAMA* 248:2156, 1982.

222. Harris RL, Musher DM, Bloom K, et al: Manifestations of sepsis. *Arch Intern Med* 147:1895, 1987.

223. Wolfson JS, Sober AJ, Rubin RH: Dermatologic manifestations of infections in immunocompromised patients. *Medicine (Baltimore)* 64:115, 1985.

224. Shelley WB, Zolin WD: Disseminate intradermal bacterial colonization presenting as palpable purpura in lymphoblastic leukemia. *J Am Acad Dermatol* 8:714, 1983.

225. Goldgeier MK: The microbial evaluation of acute cellulitis. *Cutis* 31:649, 1983.

226. Varghese R, Melo JC, Chun C, et al: Erysipelas-like syndrome caused by *Streptococcus pneumoniae*. *South Med J* 72:757, 1979.

227. Binnick AN, Klein RB, Baughman RD: Recurrent erysipelas caused by group B streptococcus organisms. *Arch Dermatol* 116:798, 1980.

228. Shama S, Calandra GB: A typical erysipelas caused by group G streptococci in a patient with cured Hodgkin's disease. *Arch Dermatol* 118:934, 1982.

229. Nip-Sakamoto CJ, Pien FD: *Vibrio vulnificus* infection in Hawaii. *Int J Dermatol* 28:313, 1989.

230. Olbrych TG, Zarconi J, File TM Jr, et al: Bullous skin lesions associated with *Yersinia enterocolitica* septicemia. *Am J Med Sci* 287:38, 1984.

231. Greene SL, Su WPD, Muller SA: Ecthyma gangrenosum: Report of clinical, histopathologic, and bacteriologic aspects of eight cases. *J Am Acad Dermatol* 11:781, 1984.

232. Turnbull D, Parry MF: Ecthyma-like skin lesions causes by *Staphylococcus aureus*. *Arch Intern Med* 141:689, 1981.

233. Hook EW III, Holmes KK: Gonococcal infections. *Ann Intern Med* 102:229, 1985.

234. Black PH, Kunz LJ, Swartz MN: Salmonellosis—a review of some unusual aspects. *N Engl J Med* 262:921, 1960.

235. Steere AC: Lyme disease. *N Engl J Med* 321:586, 1989.

236. Barbour AG: The diagnosis of Lyme disease: Rewards and perils. *Ann Intern Med* 110:501, 1989.

237. Berger BW: Erythema chronicum migrans of Lyme disease. *Arch Dermatol* 120:1017, 1984.

238. Editor: Update: Lyme disease and cases occurring during pregnancy. *JAMA* 254:736, 1985.

239. Schlesinger PA, Duray PH, Burke BA: Maternal-fetal transmission of the Lyme disease spirochete, *Borrelia burgdorferi*. *Ann Intern Med* 103:67, 1985.

240. Pachner AR, Steere AC: The triad of neurologic manifestations of Lyme disease: Meningitis, cranial neuritis, and radiculoneuritis. *Neurology* 35:47, 1985.

241. Steere AC, Batsford WP, Weinberg M, et al: Lyme carditis: Cardiac abnormalities of Lyme disease. *Ann Intern Med* 93:8, 1980.

242. Steere AC, Schoen RT, Taylor E: The clinical evolution of Lyme arthritis. *Ann Intern Med* 107:725, 1987.

243. Schwartz BS, Golstein MD, Ribeiro JMC, et al: Antibody testing in Lyme disease. A comparison of results in four laboratories. *JAMA* 262:3431, 1989.

243a. Marconi RT, Garon CF: Development of polymerase chain reaction primer sets for diagnosis of Lyme disease and for species-specific identification of Lyme disease isolates by 16S rRNA signature nucleotide analysis. *J Clin Microbiology* 30:2830, 1992.

244. Abramowicz M, et al (eds): Treatment of Lyme disease. *Med Lett Drugs Ther* 31:57, 1989.

245. Young VL, Pin P: The brown recluse spider bite. *Ann Plast Surg* 20:447, 1988.

246. Wasserman GS, Andersen PC: Loxoscelism and necrotic arachnidism. *J Toxicol Clin Toxicol* 21:451, 1983.

247. Rees R, Campbell D, Rieger E, et al: The diagnosis and treatment of brown recluse spider bites. *Ann Emerg Med* 16:945, 1987.

248. Binder LS: Acute arthropod envenomation. Incidence, clinical features and management. *Med Toxicol Adverse Drug Exp* 4:163, 1989.

249. Anderson PC: Necrotizing spider bites. *Am Fam Phys* 26:198, 1982.

250. Hagen MD: Urticaria in loxoscelism. *South Med J* 74:1427, 1981.

251. Sauer G: Transverse myelitis and paralysis from a brown recluse spider bite. *Mo Med* 72:603, 1975.

252. King LE Jr, Rees RS: Treatment of brown recluse spider bites. *J Am Acad Dermatol* 14:691, 1986.

253. Wille RC, Morrow JD: Case report: Dapsone hypersensitivity syndrome associated with treatment of the bite of a brown recluse spider. *Am J Med Sci* 296:270, 1988.

254. Weismann K, Petersen CS, Sondergaard J, et al: *Skin Signs in AIDS*. Copenhagen, Munksgaard, 1988, p 1.

255. Friedman-Kien AE, Ostreicher R, Saltzman B: Clinical manifestations of classical, endemic African, and epidemic AIDS associated

Kaposi's sarcoma, in Friedman-Kien AE (ed): *Color Atlas of AIDS*. Philadelphia, W.B. Saunders, 1989, p 11.

256. Hatcher VA: Mucocutaneous infections in acquired immune deficiency syndrome. In Friedman-Kien AE, Laubenstein LJ (eds): *AIDS: The Epidemic Of Kaposi's Sarcoma And Opportunistic Infections*. New York, Masson, 1984, p 245.

257. Mathes BM, Douglass MC. Seborrheic dermatitis in patients with acquired immunodeficiency syndrome. *J Am Acad Dermatol* 13:947, 1985.

258. Moskowitz LB, Hensley GT, Gould EW, et al. Frequency and anatomic distribution of lymphadenopathic Kaposi's sarcoma in the acquired immunodeficiency syndrome: an autopsy series. *Hum Pathol* 116:447, 1985.

259. Croxson TS, Ebanks D, Mildvan D. Atypical mycobacteria and Kaposi's sarcoma in the same biopsy specimens. *N Engl J Med* 308:1476, 1983.

260. Lind SE, Gross PL, Andiman WA, et al. Malignant lymphoma presenting as Kaposi's sarcoma in a homosexual man with the acquired immunodeficiency syndrome. *Ann Intern Med* 102:338, 1985.

261. Burkes RL, Gal AA, Stewart ML, et al: Simultaneous occurrence of *Pneumocystis carinii* pneumonia, cytomegalovirus infection, Kaposi's sarcoma, and B-immunoblastic sarcoma in a homosexual man. *JAMA* 253:3425, 1985.

262. Gross DJ, Safai B: Kaposi's sarcoma/AIDS cofactors. *Int J Dermatol* 28:571, 1989.

263. Cockerell CJ: Cutaneous signs of AIDS other than Kaposi's sarcoma, in Friedman-Kien AE (ed): *Color Atlas of AIDS*. Philadelphia, Saunders, 1989, p 93.

264. Cockerell CJ: The dermatopathology of AIDS: Cutaneous diseases other than Kaposi's sarcoma. *Semin Dermatol* 5:316, 1986.

265. Wurtz RM, Abrams D, Becker S, et al: Anaphylactoid drug reactions to ciprofloxacin and rifampicin in HIV-infected patients. *Lancet* 1:955, 1989.

266. Frentz G, Niordson AM, Thomsen K: Eosinophilic pustular dermatosis: An early skin marker of infection with human immunodeficiency virus? *Br J Dermatol* 121:271, 1989.

267. Prose NS, Mendez H, Menikoff H, et al: Pediatric human immunodeficiency virus infection and its cutaneous manifestations. *Pediatr Dermatol* 4:67, 1987.

268. Cockerell CJ, LeBoit PE: Bacillary angiomatosis: A newly characterized, pseudoneoplastic, infectious, cutaneous vascular disorder. *J Am Acad Dermatol* 22:501, 1990.

269. Penneys NS, Hicks B: Unusual cutaneous lesions associated with acquired immunodeficiency syndrome. *J Am Acad Dermatol* 13:845, 1985.

270. Goodman DS, Teplitz ED, Wishner A, et al: Prevalence of cutaneous disease in patients with acquired immunodeficiency syndrome (AIDS) or AIDS-related complex. *J Am Acad Dermatol* 17:210, 1987.

271. Cohen PR, Grossman ME: Clinical features of human immunodeficiency virus–associated disseminated herpes zoster virus infection—a review of the literature. *Clin Exp Dematol* 14:273, 1989.

272. Coulman C, Greene I, Archibald RWR: Cutaneous pneumocystosis. *Ann Intern Med* 106:396, 1987.

273. Schinella RA, Breda SD, Hammerschlag PE: Otic infection due to *Pneumocystis carinii* in an apparently healthy man with antibody to the human immunodeficiency virus. *Ann Intern Med* 106:399, 1987.

274. Bakos L, Kronfeld M, Hampe S, et al: Disseminated paracoccidioidomycosis with skin lesions in a patient with acquired immunodeficiency syndrome. *J Am Acad Dermatol* 20:854, 1989.

275. Yeager BA, Hoxie J, Weisman RA, et al: Actinomycosis in the acquired immunodeficiency syndrome–related complex. *Arch Otolaryngol Head Neck Surg* 112:1293, 1986.

276. Toth IR, Kazal HL: Botryomycosis in acquired immunodeficiency syndrome. *Arch Pathol Lab Med* 111:246, 1987.

277. Shaw JC, Levinson W, Montanaro A: Sporotrichosis in the acquired immunodeficiency syndrome. *J Am Acad Dermatol* 21:1145, 1989.

278. Fitzpatrick JE, Eubanks S: Acquired immunodeficiency syndrome presenting as disseminated cutaneous sporotrichosis. *Int J Dermatol* 27:406, 1988.

279. Sitz KV, Keppen M, Johnson DF: Metastatic basal cell carcinoma in acquired immunodeficiency syndrome–related complex. *JAMA* 257:340, 1987.

280. Milburn PB, Brandsma JL, Goldsman CI, et al: Disseminated warts and evolving squamous cell carcinoma in a patient with acquired immunodeficiency syndrome. *J Am Acad Dermatol* 19:401, 1988.

281. Tindall B, Finlayson R, Mutimer K, et al: Malignant melanoma associated with human immunodeficiency virus infection in three homosexual men. *J Am Acad Dermatol* 20:587, 1989.

282. Chren MM, Silverman RA, Sorensen RU, et al: Leukocytoclastic vasculitis in a patient infected with human immunodeficiency virus. *J Am Acad Dematol* 21:1161, 1989.

283. Ghadially R, Sibbald RG, Walter JB, et al: Granuloma annulare in patients with human immunodeficiency virus infections. *J Am Acad Dermatol* 20:232, 1989.

284. Hogan D, Card RT, Ghadially R, et al: Human immunodeficiency virus infection and porphyria cutanea tarda. *J Am Acad Dermatol* 20:17, 1989.

285. Hymes SR, Jordan RE, Arnett FC. Lupus erythematosus. *Dermatol Clin* 4:267, 1986.

286. Condemi JJ: The autoimmune diseases. *JAMA* 258:2920, 1987.

287. Sontheimer RD: Subacute cutaneous lupus erythematosus: a decade's perspective. *Med Clin North Am* 73:1073, 1989.

288. Tuffanelli DL. Lupus erythematosus. *J Am Acad Dermatol* 4:127, 1981.

289. Izumi AK, Takiguchi P. Lupus erythematosus panniculitis. *Arch Dermatol* 119:61, 1983.

289a. Hughes GR: Systemic lupus erythematosus. *Postgrad Med J* 64:517, 1988.

290. Camisa C, Sharma HM. Vesiculobullous systemic lupus erythematosus. Report of two cases and a review of the literature. *J Am Acad Dermatol* 9:924, 1983.

291. Provost TT, Talal N, Harley JB, et al: The relationship between anti-Ro (SS-A) antibody positive lupus erythematosus. *Arch Dermatol* 124:63, 1988.

291a. Sontheimer RD, McCauliffe DP: Pathogenesis of anti-Ro/SS-A autoantibody-associated cutaneous lupus erythematosus. *Dermatol Clin* 8:751, 1990.

292. Sontheimer RD: The anticardiolipin syndrome. A new way to slice an old pie, or a new pie to slice? *Arch Dermatol* 123:590, 1987.

293. Alegre VA, Winkelmann RK: Histopathology and immunofluorescence study of skin lesions associated with circulating lupus anticoagulant. *J Am Acad Dermatol* 19:117, 1988.

294. Connolly SM: Management of the cutaneous manifestations of lupus erythematosus. *Semin Dermatol* 4:82, 1985.

295. Taylor CR, Stern RS, Leyden JJ: Photoaging/photodamage and photoprotection. *J Am Acad Dermatol* 22:1, 1990.

296. Plauchu H, de Chadarevian JP, Bideau A, et al: Age-related clinical profile of hereditary hemorrhagic telangiectasia in an epidemiologically recruited population. *Am J Med Genet* 32:291, 1989.

297. Peery WH: Clinical spectrum of hereditary hemorrhagic telangiectasia (Osler-Weber-Rendu disease). *Am J Med* 82:989, 1987.

298. Fritzler MJ, Arlette JP, Behn AR, et al: Hereditary hemorrhagic telangiectasia vs. CREST syndrome: Can serology aid diagnosis? *J Am Acad Dermatol* 10:192, 1984.

299. Baranda MM, Perez M, DeAndres J, et al: High output congestive heart failure as first manifestation of Osler-Weber-Rendu disease. *J Vasc Dis* 35:568, 1984.

300. Burke CM, Safai C, Nelson DP, et al: Pulmonary arteriovenous malformations: A critical update. *Am Rev Resp Dis* 134:334, 1986.

300a. Whiting JH Jr, Morton KA, Datz FL, et al: Embolization of hepatic arteriovenous malformations using radiolabeled and nonradiolabeled ployvinyl alcohol sponge in a patient with hereditary hemorrhagic telangiectasia: case report. *J Nuclear Med* 33:260, 1992.

301. Reagan TJ, Bloom WH: The brain in hereditary hemorrhagic telangiectasia. *Stroke* 2:361, 1971.

302. Press OW, Ramsey PG: Central nervous system infections associated with hereditary hemorrhagic telangiectasia. *Am J Med* 77:86, 1984.

303. Brant AM, Schachat AP, White RI: Ocular manifestations in hereditary hemorrhagic telangiectasia (Rendu-Osler-Weber disease). *Am J Ophthal* 107:642, 1989.

304. Mathus-Vliegen EMH: Laser treatment of intestinal vascular abnormalities. *Int J Colorect Dis* 4:20, 1989.

305. Parkin JL, Dickson JA: Argon laser treatment of head and neck vascular lesions. *Otolaryngol Head Neck Surg* 93:211, 1985.

305a. Mainetti C, Schmied E, Masouye I, et al: L-tryptophan-induced eosinophilia-myalgia syndrome. Report of two cases with pseudoxanthoma-elasticum-like skin changes. *Dermatologica* 183:57, 1991.

305b. Mainetti C, Masouye I, Saurat JH: Pseudoxanthoma elasticum-like lesions in the L-tryptophan-induced eosinophilia-myalgia syndrome. *J Am Acad Dermatol* 24:657, 1991.

305c. Bolognia JL, Braverman I: Pseudoxanthoma-elasticum-like skin changes induced by penicillamine. *Dermatology* 184(1):12, 1992.

306. Walker ER, Frederickson RG, Mayes MD: The mineralization of elastic fibers and alterations of extracellular matrix in pseudoxanthoma elasticum. Ultrastructure, immunocytochemistry, and X-ray analysis. *Arch Dermatol* 125:70, 1989.

307. Neldner KH: Pseudoxanthoma elasticum. *Clin Dermatol* 6:1, 1988.

308. Viljoen D: Pseudoxanthoma elasticum (Grönblad-Strandberg syndrome). *J Med Genet* 25:488, 1988.

309. Patterson JW: The perforating disorders. *J Am Acad Dermatol* 10:561, 1984.

310. McCreedy CA, Zimmerman TJ, Webster SF: Management of upper gastrointestinal hemorrhage in patients with pseudoxanthoma elasticum. *Surgery* 105:170, 1989.

311. Przybojewski JZ, Maritz F, Tiedt FAC, et al: Pseudoxanthoma elasticum with cardiac involvement: A case report and review of the literature. *S Afr Med J* 59:268, 1981.

312. Pyeritz RE: Cardiovascular manifestations of heritable disorders of connective tissue. *Prog Med Genet* 5:191, 1983.

313. Neldner KH: Pseudoxanthoma elasticum. *Int J Dermatol* 27:98, 1988.

314. Holzerg M, Hewan-Lowe KO, Olansky AJ: The Ehlers-Danlos syndrome: Recognition, characterization, and importance of a milder variant of the classic form. *J Am Acad Dermatol* 19:656, 1988.

315. Serry C, Agomouh OS, Goldin MD: Review of Ehlers-Danlos syndrome. Successful repair of rupture and dissection of abdominal aorta. *J Cardiovasc Surg* 29:530, 1988.

316. Sykes EM Jr: Colon perforation in Ehlers-Danlos syndrome: Report of two cases and review of the literature. *Am J Surg* 147:410, 1984.

317. Spiro MJ, Janiak BD: Spontaneous rupture of the sigmoid colon in a patient with Ehlers-Danlos syndrome. *Ann Emerg Med* 13:960, 1984.

318. Krieg T, Ihme A, Weber L, et al: Molecular defects of collagen metabolism in Ehlers-Danlos syndrome. *Int J Dermatol* 20:415, 1981.

319. Harris SC, Slater DN, Austin CA: Fatal splenic rupture in Ehlers-Danlos syndrome. *Postgrad Med J* 61:259, 1985.

320. Graf CJ: Spontaneous carotid-cavernous fistula: Ehlers-Danlos syndrome and related conditions. *Arch Neurol* 13:662, 1965.

321. Sheiner N, Miller N, Lachance C: Arterial complications of Ehlers-Danlos syndrome. *J Cardiovasc Surg* 26:291, 1985.

322. Nardone DA, Reuler JB, Girard DE: Gastrointestinal complications of Ehlers-Danlos syndrome. *N Engl J Med* 300:863, 1979.

323. Snyder RR, Gilstrap LC, Hauth JC: Ehlers-Danlos syndrome and pregnancy. *Obstet Gynecol* 61:649, 1983.

323a. Kulkarni S, LaGrenade L: Ehlers-Danlos syndrome in pregnancy. *W Indian Med J* 41:86, 1992.

324. Elsas LJ, Miller RL, Pinnell SR: Inherited human collagen lysyl hydroxylase deficiency: Ascorbic acid response. *J Pediatr* 92:378, 1978.

325. Tribble K, Archer E, Jorizzo JL: Malignant atrophic papulosis: Absence of circulating immune complexes or vasculitis. *J Am Acad Dermatol* 15:365, 1986.

326. Englert HJ, Hawkes CH, Boey ML, et al: Degos' disease: Association with anticardiolipin antibodies and the lupus anticoagulant. *Br Med J* 289:576, 1984.

327. Newton JA, Black MM: Familial malignant atrophic papulosis. *Clin Exp Dermatol* 9:298, 1984.

328. Habbema L, Kisch LS, Starink TM: Familial malignant atrophic papulosis (Degos' disease)—Additional evidence for heredity and a benign course. *Br J Dermatol* 114:134, 1986.

329. Plantin P, Labouche F, Sassolas B, et al: Degos' disease: A 10-year follow-up of a patient without visceral involvement. *J Am Acad Dermatol* 21:136, 1989.

330. Degos R: Malignant atrophic papulosis. *Br J Dermatol* 100:21, 1979.

331. Black MM: Malignant atrophic papulosis (Degos' disease). *Int J Dermatol* 15:405, 1976.

332. Doutre MS, Beylot C, Bioulac P, et al: Skin lesion resembling malignant atrophic papulosis in lupus erythematosus. *Dermatologica* 175:45, 1987.

333. Su WP, Schroeder AL, Lee VA, et al: Clinical and histologic findings in Degos' syndrome (malignant atrophic papulosis). *Cutis* 35:131, 1985.

334. Barlow RJ, Heyl T, Simson IW, et al: Malignant atrophic papulosis (Degos' disease)—Diffuse involvement of brain and bowel in an African patient. *Br J Dermatol* 118:117, 1988.

335. Lee DA, Su WP, Liesegane TJ: Ophthalmic changes of Degos' disease (malignant atrophic papulosis). *Ophthalmology* 91:295, 1984.

336. Anderson JA, Adkinson NF: Allergic reactions to drugs and biologic agents. *JAMA* 258:2891, 1987.

337. Kuokkanen K: Drug eruptions: A series of 464 cases in the Department of Dermatology, University of Turku, Finland, during 1966–1967. *Acta Allergol* 27:407, 1972.

338. Wintroub BU, Stern R: Cutaneous drug reactions: Pathogenesis and clinical classification. *J Am Acad Dermatol* 13:167, 1985.

339. Shear NH: Diagnosing cutaneous adverse reactions to drugs. *Arch Dermatol* 126:94, 1990.

340. Van Arsdel PP Jr: Allergy and adverse drug reactions. *J Am Acad Dermatol* 6:833, 1982.

341. Bigby M, Jick S, Jick H, et al: Drug-induced cutaneous reactions. A report from the Boston Collaborative Drug surveillance program on 15,438 consecutive inpatients, 1975 to 1982. *JAMA* 256:3358, 1986.

342. Kerker BJ, Hood AF: Chemotherapy-induced cutaneous reactions. *Semin Dermatol* 8:173, 1989.

342a. Reiner DM, Frishman WH, Luftschein S, Grossman M: Adverse cutaneous reactions from cardiovascular drug therapy. *NY State J Med* 92:137, 1992.

343. Sussman FL, Dolovich J: Prevention of anaphylaxis. *Semin Dermatol* 8:158, 1989.

344. Sams WM: Hypersensitivity angiitis. *J Invest Dermatol* 93:78S, 1989.

345. Klein GF, Kofler H, Wolf H, et al: Eczema-like, erythematous infiltrated plaques: A common side effect of subcutaneous heparin therapy. *J Am Acad Dermatol* 21:703, 1989.

346. Guillet G, Delaire P, Plantin P, et al: Eczema as a complication of heparin therapy. *J Am Acad Dermatol* 20:1130, 1989.

347. Gold MH, Holy AK, Roenigk HH Jr: Beta-blocking drugs and psoriasis. A review of cutaneous side effects and retrospective analysis of their effects on psoriasis. *J Am Acad Dermatol* 19:837, 1988.

348. Cole MS, Minifee PK, Wolma FJ: Coumarin necrosis—A review of the literature. *Surgery* 103:271, 1988.

349. Norris PG: Warfarin skin necrosis treated with prostacyclin. *Clin Exp Dermatol* 12:370, 1987.

350. Almeyda J, Levantine A: Cutaneous reactions to cardiovascular drugs. *Br J Dermatol* 83:313, 1973.

351. Swinyer LJ: Determining the cause of drug eruptions. *Dermatol Clin* 1:417, 1983.

352. Berger TG, Sesody ST: Quinidine-induced lichenoid photodermatitis. *Cutis* 29:595, 1982.

353. Burkhart CG: Quinidine-induced acne. *Arch Dermatol* 117:603, 1981.

354. Harwell WB: Quinidine-induced psoriasis. *J Am Acad Dermatol* 9:278, 1983.

355. Harris L, McKenna WJ, Rowland E, et al: Side effects of long-term amiodarone therapy. *Circulation* 67:45, 1983.

356. Trimble JW, Mendelson DS, Fetter BF, et al: Cutaneous pigmentation secondary to amiodarone therapy. *Arch Dermatol* 119:914, 1983.

357. Wilkin JK, Kirkendall WM: Pityriasis rosea-like rash from captopril. *Arch Dermatol* 118:186, 1982.

358. Katz RA, Hood AF, Anhalt GJ: Pemphigus-like eruption from captopril. *Arch Dermatol* 123:20, 1987.

359. Miralles R, Pedro-Botet J, Farre M, et al: Captopril and vasculitis. *Ann Intern Med* 109:514, 1988.

360. Wolf R, Dorfman B, Krakowski A: Psoriasiform eruption induced by captopril and chlorthalidone. *Cutis* 40:162, 1987.

361. O'Neill PG, Rajan N, Charlat ML, et al: Captopril-related exfoliative dermatitis. *Texas Medicine* 85:40, 1989.

362. Furness PN, Goodfield MJ, MacLennan KA, et al: Severe cutaneous reactions to captopril and enalapril; Histological study and comparison with early mycosis fungoides. *J Clin Pathol* 39:902, 1986.

363. Burton JL, Schutt WH, Caldwell IW: Hypertrichosis due to diazoxide. *Br J Dermatol* 93:707, 1975.

364. Burton JL, Marshall A: Hypertrichosis due to minoxidil. *Br J Dermatol* 70:593, 1979.

365. Reynolds NJ, Jones SK, Crossley J, et al: Exfoliative dermatitis due to nifedipine. *Br J Dermatol* 121:401, 1989.

366. Stern R, Khalsa JH: Cutaneous adverse reactions associated with calcium channel blockers. *Arch Intern Med* 149:829, 1989.

367. Golbranson FL, Lurie L, Vance RM, et al: Multiple extremity amputations in hypotensive patients treated with dopamine. *JAMA* 243:1145, 1980.

368. Wormer GP, Kornblee LV, Gottfried EB: Cutaneous necrosis following peripheral intravenous vasopressin therapy. *Cutis* 29:249, 1982.

369. Kannangara DW, Smith B, Cohen K: Exfoliative dermatitis during cefoxitin therapy. *Arch Intern Med* 142:1031, 1982.

370. Kauppinen K, Stubb S: Fixed eruptions: Causative drugs and challenge tests. *Br J Dermatol* 112:575, 1985.

371. Dunagin WG, Millikan LE: Drug eruptions. *Med Clin North Am* 64:983, 1980.

372. Stanley J, Fallon-Pellicci V: Phenytoin hypersensitivity reaction. *Arch Dermatol* 114:1350, 1978.

373. Charlesworth EN: Phenytoin induced pseudolymphoma syndrome. *Arch Dermatol* 133:477, 1977.

374. Lupton GP, Odom RB: The allopurinol hypersensitivity syndrome. *J Am Acad Dermatol* 1:365, 1979.

375. Ivey KJ: H$_2$-receptor antagonists. *Int J Dermatol* 19:175, 1980.

376. Greist MC, Epinette WW: Cimetidine-induced xerosis and asteatotic dermatitis. *Arch Dermatol* 118:253, 1982.

377. Herschthal D, Robinson MJ: Blisters of the skin in coma induced by amitriptyline and clorazepate dipotassium. Report of a case with underlying sweat gland necrosis. *Arch Dermatol* 115:499, 1979.

378. Heng MCY: Lithium carbonate toxicity: Acneform eruption and other manifestations. *Arch Dermatol* 118:246, 1982.

379. Bakris GL, Smith DW, Timari S: Dermatologic manifestations of lithium: A review. *Int J Psychiatry Med* 10:327, 1980.

380. Schlappner OLA, Shelley WB, Ruberg RL, et al: Acute papulopustular acne associated with prolonged intravenous hyperalimentation. *JAMA* 219:877, 1972.

381. Bigby M: Nonsteroidal anti-inflammatory drug reactions. *Semin Dermatol* 8:182, 1989.

382. McCall CY, Cooper JW: Tolmetin anaphylactoid reaction. *JAMA* 243:1263, 1980.

383. Burrish GF, Katz BL: Sulindac-induced anaphylaxis. *Ann Emerg Med* 19:154, 1981.

384. Montes LF, Wilborn WH: Fungus-host relationship in candidiasis: A brief review. *Arch Dermatol* 121:119, 1985.

385. Jorizzo JL: The spectrum of mucosal and cutaneous candidosis. *Dermatol Clin* 2:19, 1984.

386. Ray TL: Oral candidiasis. *Dermatol Clin* 5:651, 1987.

386a. Patel AS, DeRidder PH, Alexander TJ, et al: Candida cellulitis: A complication of percutaneous endoscopic gastrostomy. *Gastrointest Endosc* 35:571, 1989.

386b. Galimberti RL, Flores V, Gonzalez Ramos MC, Villalba LI: Cutaneous ulcers due to *Candida albicans* in an immunocompromised patient: Response to therapy with itraconazole. *Clin Exp Dermatol* 14:295, 1989.

387. Head E: Laboratory diagnosis of the superficial fungal infections. *Dermatol Clin* 2:93, 1984.

388. Smith EB: Topical antifungal agents. *Dermatol Clin* 2:109, 1984.

389. Abramowicz M, et al, eds: Naftidine for fungal skin infections. *Med Lett Drugs Ther* 30:98, 1988.

390. Lesher JL, Smith JG Jr: Antifungal agents in dermatology. *J Am Acad Dermatol* 17:383, 1987.

391. Sobel JD: *Candida* infections in the intensive care unit. *Crit Care Clin* 4:325, 1988.

391a. Edwards JE Jr., Filler SG: Current strategies for treating invasive candidiasis: Emphasis on infections in nonneutropenic patients. *Clin Infect Dis* 14:S106, 1992.

392. Grossman ME, Silvers DN, Walther RR: Cutaneous manifestations of disseminated candidiasis. *J Am Acad Dermatol* 2:111, 1980.

393. Fox BJ, Odom RB: Papulosquamous diseases: A review. *J Am Acad Dermatol* 12:597, 1985.

394. Faergemann J: Short-term treatment of dandruff with a combination of propylene glycol solution and shampoo. *Cutis* 42:146, 1988.

395. Shuster S: The aetiology of dandruff and the mode of action of therapeutic agents. *Br J Dermatol* 111:235, 1984.

396. Binder RL, Jonelis FJ: Seborrheic dermatitis: A newly reported side effect of neuroleptics. *J Clin Psychiatry* 45:125, 1984.

397. Kligman AM, Leyden JJ: Seborrheic dermatitis. *Semin Dermatol* 2:57, 1983.

398. Tager A, Berlin C, Schen RJ: Seborrheic dermatitis in acute cardiac disease. *Br J Dermatol* 76:367, 1964.

399. Smith LL, Conerly SL: Ataxia-telangiectasia or Louis-Bar syndrome. *J Am Acad Dermatol* 12:681, 1985.

400. Reed WB, Pidgeon J, Becker SW: Patients with spinal cord injury. Clinical cutaneous studies. *Arch Dermatol* 83:379, 1961.

401. Carr MM, Pryce DM, Ive FA: Treatment of seborrhoeic dermatitis with ketoconazole: I. Response of seborrhoeic dermatitis of the scalp to topical ketoconazole. *Br J Dermatol* 116:213, 1987.

402. Green CA, Farr PM, Shuster S: Treatment of seborrhoeic dermatitis with ketoconazole: II. Response of seborrhoeic dermatitis of the face, scalp and trunk to topical ketoconazole. *Br J Dermatol* 116:217, 1987.

403. Allman RM: Pressure ulcers among the elderly. *N Engl J Med* 320:850, 1989.

404. Knight AL: Medical management of pressure sores. *J Fam Pract* 27:95, 1988.

405. Reuler JB, Cooney TG: The pressure sore: Pathophysiology and principles of management. *Ann Intern Med* 94:661, 1981.

406. Klein L, Gilroy K: Evaluating mattress overlays and pressure relieving systems: A question of perception or reality? *J Enterostom Ther* 16:58, 1989.

407. Witkowski JA, Parish LC: Histopathology of the decubitus ulcer. *J Am Acad Dermatol* 6:1014, 1982.

407a. Fowler E, Papen JC: Evaluation of an alginate dressing for pressure ulcers. *Decubitus* 4:47, 1991.

408. Sugarman B: Pressure sores and underlying bone infection. *Arch Intern Med* 147:553, 1987.

409. Spruance SL, Overall JC Jr, Kern ER, et al: The natural history of recurrent herpes simplex labialis. Implications for antiviral therapy. *N Engl J Med* 297:69, 1977.

410. Nahmias AJ, Roizman B: Infection with herpes-simplex viruses 1 and 2. *N Engl J Med* 289:719, 1973.

411. Pazin GJ, Armstrong JA, Lam MT, et al: Prevention of reactivated herpes simplex infection by human leukocyte interferon after operation on the trigeminal root. *N Engl J Med* 301:225, 1979.

412. Cheeseman SH, Rubin RH, Stewart JA, et al: Controlled clinical trial of prophylactic human-leukocyte interferon in renal transplantation. Effects on cytomegalovius and herpes simplex virus infections. *N Engl J Med* 300:1345, 1979.

413. Saral R, Burns WH, Laskin OL, et al: Acyclovir prophylaxis of herpes-simplex-virus infections: A randomized double-blind, controlled trial in bone-marrow-transplant recipients. *N Engl J Med* 305:63, 1981.

414. Gluckman E, Lotsburg J, Devergie A, et al: Prophylaxis of herpes infections after bone-marrow transplantation by oral acyclovir. *Lancet* 2:706, 1983.
415. Burgoyne M, Burke W: Atypical herpes simplex infection in patients with acute myelogenous leukemia recovering from chemotherapy. *J Am Acad Dermatol* 20:1125, 1989.
416. Lindgren KM, Douglas RG Jr, Couch RB: Significance of herpesvirus hominis in respiratory secretions of man. *N Engl J Med* 278:517, 1968.
417. Straus SE, Rooney JF, Sever JL: Herpes simplex virus infection: Biology, treatment, and prevention. *Ann Intern Med* 103:404, 1985.
418. Kaplan AP, Buckley RH, Mathews KP: Allergic skin disorders. *JAMA* 258:2900, 1987.
419. Fisher AA: *Contact dermatitis*. Philadelphia, Lea and Febiger, 1986, p 362.
419a. Ibid. p 352.
420. Storrs FJ, Rosenthal LE, Adams RM: Prevalence and relevance of allergic reactions in patients patch tested in North America—1984 to 1985. *J Am Acad Dermatol* 20:1038, 1989.
421. Guin JD, Phillips D: Erythroderma from systemic contact dermatitis: A complication of systemic gentamicin in a patient with contact allergy to neomycin. *Cutis* 43:564, 1989.
422. Fisher AA, op cit: p 212.
423. Held JL, Kalb RE, Ruszkowski AM, et al: Allergic contact dermatitis from bacitracin. *J Am Acad Dermatol* 17:592, 1987.
424. Marks JG: Allergic contact dermatitis to povidone-iodine. *J Am Acad Dermatol* 6:473, 1982.
425. Fisher AA, op cit: p 154.
426. Ibid. p 245.
427. Bernstein B, Leyden JJ: Zinc deficiency and acrodermatitis after intravenous hyperalimentation. *Arch Dermatol* 114:1070, 1978.
428. Ecker RI, Schroeter AL: Acrodermatitis and acquired zinc deficiency. *Arch Dermatol* 114:937, 1978.
429. West BL, Anderson PC: Alcohol and acquired acrodermatitis enteropathica. *J Am Acad Dermatol* 15:1305, 1986.
430. Hansen RC, Lemen R, Revsin B: Cystic fibrosis manifesting with acrodermatitis enteropathica-like eruption. Association with essential fatty acid and zinc deficiencies. *Arch Dermatol* 119:51, 1983.
431. Ferrandiz C, Henkes J, Peyri J, et al: Acquired zinc deficiency syndrome during total parenteral alimentation. Clinical histopathological findings. *Dermatologica* 163:255, 1981.
432. Brazin SA, Johnson WT, Abramson LJ: The acrodermatitis enteropathica-like syndrome. *Arch Dermatol* 115:597, 1979.
433. Norris D: Zinc and cutaneous inflammation. *Arch Dermatol* 121:985, 1985.
434. Strobel CT, Byrne WJ, Abramovits W, et al: A zinc-deficiency dermatitis in patients on total parenteral nutrition. *Int J Dermatol* 17:575, 1978.
435. Skolnick P, Eaglstein WH, Ziboh VA: Human essential fatty acid deficiency. *Arch Dermatol* 113:939, 1977.

219. *Collagen Vascular Diseases in the Intensive Care Unit*

Nancy Y. N. Liu, David F. Giansiracusa, and Steven L. Strongwater

Rheumatoid Arthritis

Rheumatoid arthritis is a chronic, inflammatory disorder of unknown etiology that affects synovial joints and extraarticular structures. The patient with rheumatoid arthritis may require admission to the intensive care unit (ICU) because of a complication of joint disease such as joint sepsis; airway obstruction due to cricoarytenoid arthritis; severe extraarticular disease such as pulmonary function impairment due to pleural effusions and interstitial disease; cardiac dysfunction due to pericardial, myocardial, or endocardial rheumatoid involvement; necrotizing rheumatoid vasculitis; and neurologic dysfunction due to atlantoaxial subluxation. The physician caring for the rheumatoid arthritis patient in the ICU must be mindful of the effects of both the rheumatic disease as well as of the medications used to treat rheumatoid arthritis, specifically nonsteroidal antiinflammatory drugs, corticosteroids, and cytotoxic agents.

PATHOGENESIS. The inflammation and tissue destruction characteristic of rheumatoid arthritis appear to occur because of humoral and cellular mediated immunologic processes. Humoral interactions between antigens, immunoglobulins, or other tissue constituents such as collagen, cartilage, nuclear material, and antibodies cause tissue injury [1,1a]. Cellular immunity mediated by lymphocytes and macrophages results in tissue damage by the production of cytokines, which stimulate the humoral response, the release of collagenases and proteases, and osteoclastic bone resorption [2].

JOINT INFECTIONS SEPSIS COMPLICATING RHEUMATOID ARTHRITIS. One of the indications for admission of the rheumatoid arthritis patient to an ICU is sepsis, particularly involving joints. Rheumatoid arthritis patients are susceptible to developing bacterial infection of involved joints. Joint infections are more frequently polyarticular and more severe than in patients without rheumatoid arthritis [3–6]. A variety of factors including immunosuppressive drugs, general debility, immobility, and cutaneous ulcers predispose the rheumatoid patient to developing bacterial infections of the skin and respiratory and urinary tracts. These organisms may hematogenously seed inflamed rheumatoid joints [7]. Once bacteria have invaded a rheumatoid joint, a number of pathophysiologic processes interfere with the normal protective mechanisms, including (1) decreased polymorphonuclear (PNM) leukocyte bacterial killing, (2) decreased PMN chemotaxis, and (3) decreased complement and serum bactericidal activity against organisms [8,9,10].

Tables 219A-1 to 219A-9 are found on pages 2649–2651.

Although joint sepsis after intraarticular steroid injection and arthrocentesis is a rare complication, infection has been reported in this context and may be more resistant to treatment [11,12].

A delay in diagnosing joint sepsis in the rheumatoid arthritis patient may also contribute to increased morbidity and mortality [13]. In the rheumatoid arthritis patient, a variety of factors may contribute to a delay in the diagnosis of a joint infection including (1) reduction of the joint pain and inflammation by nonsteroidal antiinflammatory drugs, corticosteroids, and immunosuppressive agents; (2) generalized debility and malnutrition; and (3) the physician and the patient attributing the joint inflammation to the underlying rheumatoid arthritis [14,15]. Failure to recognize septic arthritis complicating rheumatoid arthritis may have disastrous effects [16]. Whenever a single joint or a few joints are more inflamed than others in a patient with rheumatoid arthritis, joint sepsis should be excluded by arthrocentesis, Gram's stain, and cultures of synovial fluid and blood, as well as by other appropriate cultures, particularly if the patient has any systemic signs and symptoms of bacterial infection. Inspection of the skin for a possible portal of bacterial entry and a thorough general examination are of utmost importance.

The microbiology of septic arthritis complicating rheumatoid arthritis consists of a wide range of organisms, but in approximately 80 percent of cases, the organism is *Staphylococcus aureus* [13,17]. Streptococcal species are also common pathogens. Gram-negative organisms, including *Pseudomonas aeruginosa, Escherichia coli, Proteus mirabilis,* anaerobes, fungi, mycobacterium, and polymicrobial infection have all been reported as causes of septic arthritis in the rheumatoid joint [17,18].

Management of septic arthritis, including antibiotic therapy, joint drainage, and joint rest, is discussed in Chapter 216 [19]. As compared to the septic, nonrheumatoid joint, the septic rheumatoid joint more frequently fails to respond to percutaneous needle aspiration. Due to increased tendency for development of loculations and more proliferative synovitis, early open surgical drainage with synovectomy may be the preferred treatment [20].

Septic Arthritis in the Prosthetic Joint. Although rates of infection of artificial joint replacements are generally quite low (0.5–4.0% for hips and knees), rheumatoid arthritis patients have an increased risk of developing infected prosthetic joints [21–24]. Diagnosis of prosthetic joint infection may be difficult. Clinical features include localized pain, fever in one-fourth to one-half of patients, elevation of the erythrocyte sedimentation rate (ESR), a positive gallium scan, and positive cultures on aspirations in only 75 percent of the patients [25,26,27]. Approximately 10 percent of prosthetic joint infections are due to gram-negative organisms in which painful loosening is present, often without systemic symptoms of infection [28]. As such, treatment of suspected prosthetic joint infection before results of cultures and antibiotic sensitivities are available from the microbiology laboratory should include coverage of both gram-negative and gram-positive organisms with a regimen such as vancomycin and an aminoglycoside.

Although in the past, infected prosthetic joints were treated with antibiotics and removal of the prosthesis, if loosening of the prosthesis is not present, cases are being successfully treated with debridement and prolonged antibiotics [24]. After removal of the implant, antibiotics are generally given for 4 to 6 weeks before placement of another prosthesis [27]. One-stage procedures of treating with antibiotics and then removing the infected prosthesis and implanting another prosthesis have met with some success, as has the use of antibiotic-impregnated implants [25,29].

RESPIRATORY TRACT INVOLVEMENT IN RHEUMATOID ARTHRITIS. The respiratory system in the patient with rheumatoid arthritis may be involved in a variety of ways, including upper airway obstruction due to arthritis of the cricoarytenoid joints, pleuritis and pleural thickening, rheumatoid pulmonary nodules, interstitial lung disease, bronchiolitis obliterans, pulmonary vasculitis, pulmonary hypertension, and pulmonary infections, particularly in the patient with poor mucociliary clearance and ineffective cough, on immunosuppressive therapy, or with associated Sjögren's syndrome [30,31,32]. Table 219-1 summarizes respiratory tract involvement in rheumatoid arthritis. Patients with rheumatoid arthritis may also develop respiratory tract disease due to medications, most commonly angioedema and bronchospasm induced or aggravated by aspirin or other nonsteroidal antiinflammatory drugs and interstitial disease as a result of treatment with gold and methotrexate [33–36]. Penicillamine may cause Goodpasture's syndrome and bronchiolitis [37,38].

Cricoarytenoid Arthritis. The cricoarytenoid joints are true synovial joints that allow adduction and abduction of the vocal cords. Inflammation of these joints may cause throat pain, a sense of a foreign object stuck in the throat, odynophagia, dysphagia, hoarseness, shortness of breath, and stridor. During acute inflammation or more insidiously as a result of chronic inflammation, the vocal cords may become fixed in a position of adduction, resulting in upper airway obstruction and respiratory failure [39]. The diagnosis may be made and distinguished from recurrent laryngeal nerve paralysis, tumor, and thyroiditis by visualizing the vocal cords either by indirect laryngoscopy or fiberoptic nasopharyngoscopy. These procedures are also helpful to evaluate for rheumatoid nodules. In the patient with chronic laryngeal inflammation with airway narrowing due to restricted motion of the cricoarytenoid joints, a superimposed insult such as an upper respiratory tract infection or trauma such as intubation may cause sufficient soft tissue swelling to obstruct the airway.

Treatment of life-threatening airway obstruction includes es-

Table 219-1. Respiratory Involvement in Rheumatoid Arthritis

Disease related
Upper airway involvement
  Cricoarytenoid arthritis
  Laryngeal nodules
Bronchial tree
  Bronchitis
  Bronchiolitis
  Bronchial nodules
Parenchyma
  Alveolitis
  Interstitial fibrosis
  Rheumatoid nodules ± cavitation
  Vasculitis
  Infection
  Aspiration
Pleura
  Pleuritis
  Pleural effusions
  Pleural thickening
Respiratory muscle disease—myositis

tablishing an airway by cricothyroidotomy or tracheostomy, high-dose systemic corticosteroids, systemic antirheumatic therapy, and topical aerosolized corticosteroids [40,41].

Micrognathia. Another rheumatoid manifestation that may cause upper respiratory tract obstruction and sleep apnea as well as complicate intubation (as may occur with rheumatoid cervical spine involvement) is micrognathia due to severe involvement of the temporomandibular joints, which occurs more commonly in patients with juvenile rheumatoid arthritis [42].

Pleural Disease. Pleuritis is the most common pulmonary manifestation of rheumatoid arthritis, occurring in approximately 40 percent of individuals studied by ultrasound or at autopsy [43]. Although involvement may be asymptomatic, acute febrile pleurisy or large pleural effusions impairing respiratory function may occur. The differential diagnoses of the pleural effusions include malignancy, pulmonary infarction, viral or bacterial infection, tuberculosis, and empyema. Empyemas occur with increased frequency in patients with preexisting rheumatoid pleural effusions and should be suspected in debilitated, anemic, or hypoproteinemic patients who have been treated with corticosteroids and have persistent fever and pleural effusions [44,45].

Examination of pleural fluid is essential to evaluate for differential possibilities. Rheumatoid pleural effusions are sterile exudates with elevated lactic dehydrogenase levels and often low glucose (< 40 mg/dl) and pH levels. Other characteristics of the effusions include a color that may vary from clear yellow to green-yellow, white cell count of 100 to 7000 cells/ul (predominantly lymphocytes), reduced complement levels, cholesterol crystals, and immune complexes [46].

Symptomatic pleural effusions are managed with nonsteroidal antiinflammatory drugs, aspiration, and in some cases surgical decortication. High-dose corticosteroid therapy may not be effective and carries an increased risk of an empyema [47]. Intrapleural corticosteroids may improve recalcitrant effusions [47a] (see Chap. 65).

Lung Disease. Interstitial rheumatoid lung disease occurs in approximately 20 to 40 percent of rheumatoid patients and is characterized pathologically as alveolar wall thickening; cellular infiltrates of lymphocytes, fibroblasts, and plasma cells; macroscopic honeycombing; and, rarely, peribronchiolar fibrosis [48]. Symptoms include dyspnea on exertion, cough, and chest discomfort, with clubbing of fingers and toes apparent as a late manifestation. Chest radiographs reveal a fine, reticular appearance predominantly involving the lower lobes, associated with restrictive physiology and a decreased diffusion capacity [48,49].

Treatment of rheumatoid interstitial lung disease is generally unsatisfactory. Although approximately 50 percent may improve with corticosteroid treatment, the improvement is often temporary. Reports of small numbers of patients treated with immunosuppressants have appeared, but no controlled studies have demonstrated sustained benefit [48].

Rheumatoid pleural effusions and interstitial lung disease may not be the reason for admission to the ICU, but these respiratory diseases may complicate other respiratory insults such as pulmonary embolism, congestive heart failure, and pulmonary infection. Bacterial pulmonary infection is a particularly frequent and serious form of lung disease in the rheumatoid patient. It has been reported to be the major cause of death in approximately a quarter of rheumatoid patients [50].

Several less common manifestations of rheumatoid lung involvement, which include pulmonary vasculitis, obliterative bronchiolitis, spontaneous pneumothorax, and antirheumatic

drug-related pulmonary disease, may actually require treatment in the ICU. Rarely, chronic vasculitis may involve pulmonary and bronchial arterioles and result in pulmonary hypertension and cor pulmonale [51]. Therapy consists of corticosteroids, generally in combination with cytotoxic agents (see Chap. 220).

Bronchiolitis obliterans has been associated with rheumatoid arthritis. It is often characterized by the abrupt onset of dyspnea and a dry cough with inspiratory crackles, sometimes with a "midinspiratory squeak," a clear chest radiograph or finding of hyperinflation, irreversible airflow obstruction at low volumes on pulmonary function testing, mild to moderate arterial hypoxemia with a respiratory alkalosis, and progressive obliteration of airways 1 to 6 mm in diameter with constrictive bronchiolitis [32,38]. The prognosis is generally poor with a fairly rapid rate of progressive airflow obstruction. Although high-dose corticosteroids with or without cytotoxic agents may be helpful in some cases, progression to death in 2 years is not uncommon [43,52]. Penicillamine has been reported to be associated with the development of obliterative bronchiolitis [53].

Antirheumatic Drug-Induced Pulmonary Complications. These are listed in Table 219-2.

RHEUMATOID CARDIAC INVOLVEMENT. Rheumatoid arthritis may involve all structures of the heart as the result of granulomatous proliferation or vasculitis to cause (1) pericarditis, (2) myocarditis, (3) endocarditis (valvulitis), (4) coronary arteritis, (5) aortitis, and (6) cardiac conduction abnormalities [50,68–71]. Cardiac involvement may be the principal reason for intensive care hospitalization or it may complicate the course of the rheumatoid patient hospitalized in the ICU for other medical or surgical problems.

Pericarditis, the most common of the rheumatoid cardiac manifestations, with an incidence of approximately 50 percent by autopsy studies, rarely causes impairment of left ventricular function [72,73]. However, constrictive pericarditis or a large pericardial effusion may cause cardiac tamponade, requiring pericardial aspiration and pericardiectomy [74]. The pericardial fluid has the same characteristics as pleural fluid (see Respiratory Tract Involvement in Rheumatoid Arthritis).

Pericardial effusions generally respond to administration of 30 to 40 mg prednisone/day over a several week period. Peri-

Table 219-2. Pulmonary Complications of Antirheumatic Drugs

Noncardiogenic Pulmonary Edema [54,55]
  Salicylates
Bronchospasm [33,34]
  Nonsteroidal antiinflammatory drugs (excluding nonacetylated salicylates)
Pulmonary Infiltrates [56]
  Naproxen
Interstitial Pneumonitis [32,35,38,57,58,59]
  Intramuscular gold
  D-penicillamine
Hypersensitivity Interstitial Pneumonitis [36,60,61]
  Methotrexate
Interstitial Fibrosis [62,63]
  Methotrexate
Opportunistic Pulmonary Infection [64,65,66]
  Methotrexate
Rarely Interstitial Pneumonia and Alveolar Cell Atypia [67]
  Cyclophosphamide

cardiocentesis should be performed early if tamponade is suspected (see Chap. 34) or if there is a question of septic or suppurative pericarditis [75].

In contrast to pericardial effusions, steroid treatment of cardiac tamponade is generally unsuccessful. Aspiration of pericardial fluid may temporarily improve cardiac function, but often the viscosity of the fluid, loculations, and thickness of the pericardium necessitate pericardiectomy [74,75a]. In cases of constrictive pericarditis, pericardiectomy is the only effective therapy [74].

The myocardium may be affected by granulomatous inflammation and by vasculitis. Cardiac conduction abnormalities, including complete heart block, may develop because of subcutaneous nodules [76,77]. A mononuclear cell infiltrate may also affect the myocardium in a diffuse manner, generally without clinical significance [78].

Arteritis in the rheumatoid patient may affect the coronary arteries and the aorta. Although coronary arteritis has been found to be present in as many as 20 percent of rheumatoid arthritis patients at autopsy, it is generally subclinical, but in patients with active systemic vasculitis, coronary arteritis may be the cause of myocardial infarction [78,79]. Involvement of the aorta, either by rheumatoid granulomata or inflammation of the aortic vasa vasorum, may result in dilatation of the aortic root and aortic valvular insufficiency [80,81,82,82a].

RHEUMATOID VASCULITIS. The vasculitis that complicates rheumatoid arthritis pathologically is a panarteritis with mononuclear cells, infiltrates of all layers of the involved blood vessels, fibrinoid necrosis in active lesions, and thrombosis associated with intimal proliferation. Rheumatoid vasculitis tends to occur in patients with severe, deforming rheumatoid arthritis, subcutaneous nodules, and high-titer rheumatoid factors and in patients with Felty's syndrome. The clinical features of rheumatoid vasculitis are variable and include (1) palpable purpura, (2) cutaneous ulceration including pyoderma gangrenosum, (3) distal arteritis ranging from fingernail fold infarcts and splinter hemorrhages to digital gangrene, and (4) arteritis of major organs including the bowel, kidneys, heart, lungs, liver, spleen, pancreas, and components of the nervous system in a manner similar to polyarteritis nodosa [83–87,87a]. Severe necrotizing forms of rheumatoid vasculitis, manifested as digital gangrene, intestinal bleeding or perforation, myocardial or renal infarction, and mononeuritis multiplex are associated with a poor prognosis and are treated aggressively in a manner similar to polyarteritis and Wegener's granulomatosis (see Chapter 220) with high-dose corticosteroids, cytotoxic agents, and occasionally pheresis [88,89,90].

NEUROLOGIC COMPLICATIONS OF RHEUMATOID ARTHRITIS. All components of the nervous system may be affected by rheumatoid arthritis. The brain and meninges, spinal cord, peripheral nerves, and muscles may be involved with granulomatous inflammation in the form of rheumatoid nodules or by vasculitis; the spinal cord and cranial and peripheral nerves may also be compressed by skeletal and soft tissue structures, and the nervous system may be affected by hyperviscosity syndrome and medications [91–95].

Spinal cord compression due to cervical instability is one of the most common neurologic complications in patients with rheumatoid arthritis [96–102]. It is particularly pertinent in the ICU due to the vulnerability of the cervical spine during procedures such as bronchoscopy, gastroscopy, and endotracheal intubation. Cervical instability and dislocations most commonly occur at the atlantoaxial (first and second cervical vertebrae)

junction due to erosion of the transverse ligament. This may allow the odontoid (superior peg of the second cervical vertebra) to protrude posteriorly, particularly during neck flexion, and compress the spinal cord and lower medulla or vertebrobasilar arteries [103–105]. Fracture or erosive destruction of the odontoid may allow the atlas (first cervical vertebra) to slide posteriorly on the second cervical vertebra, termed posterior atlantoaxial subluxation. Destruction of the lateral atlantoaxial joints and of the bones of the foramen magnum may allow the axis to sublux upward, so-called vertical subluxation [96,97].

Manifestations of spinal cord compression in the setting of cervical subluxation that require intervention include the sensation of anterior instability of the head during neck flexion, "drop" attacks, loss of urinary bladder and anal sphincter control, dysphagia, vertigo, hemiplegia, dysarthria, nystagmus, changes in level of consciousness, and peripheral paresthesias without evidence of a peripheral cause [106]. Although rheumatoid arthritis patients may have radiographic evidence of cervical subluxations without symptoms, once signs of cord compression become apparent, myelopathy may rapidly progress [107,108]. For patients with manifestations of spinal cord and brainstem compression, surgical reconstruction of normal alignment and stabilization are treatments of choice. For the nonsurgical candidate, a firm collar should be worn to immobilize the neck and prevent further subluxation. Prior to procedures such as intubation, rheumatoid arthritis patients who are at risk for cervical subluxation should be identified by lateral flexion and extension neck radiographs after plain lateral and open-mouth posteroanterior views have excluded odontoid fracture and severe subluxation. During the procedure (intubation, endoscopy, bronchoscopy) the neck should be stabilized and motion minimized by techniques as nasotracheal rather than orotracheal intubation.

Cervical subluxation in the rheumatoid arthritis patient may also occur at levels below C_1 and C_2 and cause cervical myelopathy. Myelography or myelography combined with CT scan is generally indicated to evaluate to level or levels of cord compression [98,109,110].

Systemic Lupus Erythematosus

Systemic lupus erythematosus (SLE) is an autoimmune disease characterized by excessive immune complex deposition in multiple organ systems. The etiology, however, remains to be fully elucidated. Currently experts believe that multiple factors in varying degrees contribute to the development of SLE in any individual [111]. A genetic susceptibility is supported by the increased incidence in females, certain racial groups, and familial aggregates. In addition, individuals with certain human leukocyte antigen (HLA) haplotypes or complement deficiencies are more susceptible to the disease. Environmental factors are also important because SLE has incomplete penetrance in identical twins and family studies. These factors result in immune abnormalities characterized by (1) polyclonal B-cell activation with resultant excessive overproduction of autoantibodies [111] and (2) T-cell abnormalities including impaired T-cell helper and suppressor functions [112,113].

The clinical result of these multiple abnormalities is a disease with a tremendous variation in signs and symptoms that range from arthralgias, rash, and fatigue to life-threatening renal, central nervous system, cardiac, and hematologic manifestations. In the ICU, most patients will have had a diagnosis of SLE based on the clinical criteria set forth by the American College of Rheumatology (Table 219A-1) [114]. In evaluating these patients, utmost care is needed to distinguish active SLE-related problems from secondary conditions that are a result of SLE or complications of therapy. Klippel referred to the latter as "pseudoactive" lupus; [115] examples include infections, drug-induced lupus, nonsteroidal antiinflammatory drug-induced renal dysfunction and aseptic meningitis, and corticosteroid-induced psychosis. Associated diseases include avascular necrosis, hypertensive encephalopathy, pseudotumor cerebri, amyloidosis, myasthenia gravis, and thrombotic thrombocytopenic purpura. Furthermore, SLE should be considered in the differential diagnosis in patients who present to the ICU with acute renal failure, seizures, myocarditis, acute pulmonary deterioration, hemolytic anemias, or thrombocytopenia.

RENAL DISEASE. Renal involvement in SLE has the worst prognosis and is one of the major causes of mortality in SLE patients. The frequency of renal involvement ranges from 38 to nearly 80 percent depending on definition, but clinical lupus nephritis involves approximately 50 percent of the patients [116]. Since the advent of improved diagnostic and therapeutic modalities, 10-year survival of SLE patients with nephritis increased from 65 percent in the 1950s to 93 percent in the late 1980s [117]. However, glomerulonephritis and progressive renal failure remain a major source of morbidity and mortality. Lupus nephritis constitutes approximately 3 percent of all end-stage renal failure in patients on dialysis or requiring transplantation [118]. Of those patients who have transplants, overall graft survival rate has reached 70 percent [118a.]

The pathogenesis of renal disease is complex but is best characterized by the deposition of immune complexes of native DNA and anti-DNA in the glomerular basement membrane and in situ formation of immune complexes in the kidney. These complexes activate the complement cascade and attract inflammatory cells, which may further damage the interstitium, tubules, and possibly the glomeruli.

Classification of lupus-induced glomerulonephritis is based on histopathologic, immunofluorescent, and electron microscopic changes based on the World Health Organization (WHO) classification (Table 219A-2). The classification includes mesangial glomerulonephritis, focal proliferative glomerulonephritis, diffuse proliferative glomerulonephritis, and membranous nephropathy. The renal lesions are commonly pleiomorphic and may even vary from one glomerulus to another. Repeat biopsies have revealed transition of one class to another over time [119]. In addition to the WHO classification, semiquantitative scoring is recommended for assessing potentially reversible lesions characterized by glomerular hypercellularity, karyorrhexis, leukocyte exudation, fibrinoid necrosis, cellular crescents, interstitial inflammation, and hyaline deposits. Irreversible lesions include glomerular sclerosis, fibrous crescents, tubular atrophy, and interstitial fibrosis. Thus, these activity and chronicity indices, respectively, may provide information on prognosis and guidelines for therapeutic options. In particular, the presence of proliferative lesions and chronic lesions is associated with greater mortality.

The clinical manifestations of renal involvement vary tremendously, but rapidly progressive renal failure with attendant fluid overload, congestive heart failure, and hypertension are the most likely events to precipitate an ICU admission. A sudden deterioration in renal function should warrant careful consideration of other causes of acute renal insufficiency (see Chap. 81) before attributing the patient's renal deterioration to active SLE. In particular, hypovolemia, drug-induced interstitial nephritis or renal insufficiency, renal vein thrombosis, and contrast-induced acute tubular necrosis must be excluded. The physical examination may reveal evidence of SLE activity of the dermatologic, musculoskeletal, cardiovascular, pulmonary, hematologic, or nervous systems. Laboratory studies should include the routine ones to assess renal status and fluid balance as well as immunologic studies including double-stranded DNA (dsDNA), total hemolytic complement (CH_{50}), third (C_3), and fourth (C_4) complement levels, and ESR. The latter serologies, dsDNA, C_3, and C_4, may provide evidence of SLE activity if values are abnormal, but normal values do not completely rule out active disease.

Management of lupus nephritis depends on the renal histologic and functional parameters. Thus, a patient with mesangial glomerulonephritis with normal creatinine clearance may require no specific therapy, whereas a patient with increasing azotemia, active urinary sediment, and impaired clearance will require aggressive therapy. Although high-dose corticosteroids (40–50 mg/m²/day or 1.0–1.5/mg/kg/day) have been the accepted therapy for lupus nephritis, there are few randomized studies that have proved this approach is appropriate [117,120].

Other investigations have shown that in severe lupus nephritis (WHO Class III or IV), the combination of prednisone with cytotoxic agents stabilized renal function [121,122.] A National Institute of Health (NIH) study started in 1968 enrolled 111 SLE patients with lupus nephritis into five treatment groups (high-dose prednisone alone, oral azathioprine, oral cyclophosphamide, combined oral azathioprine and cyclophosphamide, and monthly intravenous cyclophosphamide) [122,123]. Recently, analysis of outcome data at 10 years after treatment of all patients reveal that cyclphosphamide, whether oral, intravenous, or in combination with azathioprine, delayed or prevented end-stage renal disease [124]. Toxicities from these regimens are discussed in detail in the section on immunosuppressive therapy in this chapter.

The dosage recommendation for pulse cyclophosphamide is 0.5 to 1.0 g/m² monthly for 3 months [122] and then once every 3 months. Although this regimen was considered less toxic than oral daily corticosteroids, complications included major severe infections and development of secondary amenorrhea.

McCune and associates [125] also noted significant improvement of nephritis with monthly pulse cyclophosphamide as measured by decreased proteinuria, increased creatinine clearance, decreased titer of dsDNA, and improved C_3, C_4, and CH_{50} levels. The dosage protocol is outlined as follows. Patients received 0.50 g/m² of cyclophosphamide as an initial dose. If the white blood cell count remained above 2000 to 3000 cells/μl on day 7 to 14 after treatment, then each subsequent monthly dose was increased by a maximum of 25 percent. No patient received more than 2.5 g of cyclophosphamide at each dose. When the monthly dosage was greater than 1 gm/m², the increments were reduced to 10 percent. If the white blood cell count decreased below 2000 at day 7 to 14 after therapy, the dose was reduced by 25 percent. Toxicities at 6-month follow-up included granulocytopenia, non-life-threatening infections, diarrhea, alopecia, and menstrual irregularities.

In membranous glomerulonephritis (WHO Class V), the optimal therapy is controversial. Progressive renal failure is less frequent. Most authors recommend high-dose steroids for 6–12 weeks, and if proteinuria does not diminish, steroids are discontinued [125a.] Angiotensin converting enzyme inhibitors have been used to reduce proteinuria successfully [125b.]

Plasmapheresis in combination with high-dose daily steroids and cytotoxic agents has been used to treat severe lupus nephritis [125c.] However, a collaborative study of 86 lupus nephritis patients revealed no difference in creatinine or disease manifestations after 2–3 years of follow-up between groups receiving low-dose cyclophosphamide/initial high-dose steroids versus a group receiving the oral regimens with the addition of plasmapheresis [125d.]

CENTRAL NERVOUS SYSTEM DISEASE. Neuropsychiatric involvement occurs in between 25 and 80 percent of SLE patients. Although the central nervous system (CNS) involvement was considered a poor prognostic indicator in the older literature, a retrospective study of 1103 patients by Ginzler and colleagues found little influence of neuropsychiatric lupus in survival rates [126]. Active CNS disease contributed primarily or secondarily to death in 11 percent of the patients [127]. This group, however, made up only 2 percent of the 1,103 patients.

McCune and Globus have categorized CNS disease into nonfocal cerebral dysfunction, seizures, focal deficits, peripheral neuropathy, movement disorders, and others (Table 219A-3) [128]. However divided, an individual SLE patient may have more than one manifestation. Organic brain syndrome, characterized by impaired cognitive function, memory deficits, agitation, or delirium may be accompanied by functional abnormalities such as depression, affective disorders, or other psychiatric illness. Frank psychosis has been estimated to occur in 25 percent of the patients [129]. Often, it is difficult to separate active lupus psychosis from other causes of psychosis [116], but functional disorders, uremia, illicit drugs, metabolic disturbances, medications, and infections must be considered.

Seizures occur in 15 to 35 percent of SLE patients [128] and can antedate the onset of SLE or may develop during the disease course. Grand mal seizures are the most common, but essentially all types have been reported [130,131]. Secondary causes of seizures must be sought as in patients with psychosis. In several prospective studies of SLE patients with neurologic events, 50 to 75 percent of the seizures were due to associated infection, uremia, hypertension, and metabolic abnormalities [132,132a].

Other neurologic abnormalities include cranial neuropathies (10–35%), usually involving eye function [128]. Asymmetric peripheral neuropathies (10–15%) may also include an ascending motor paralysis similar to Guillain-Barré [128]. Cerebrovascular accidents (5–10%) include infarctions secondary to intracranial hemorrhage or arteritis, thrombosis secondary to hypercoagulable states associated with the lupus anticoagulant or antiphospholipid antibody, or embolism from Libman-Sacks endocarditis [133]. Movement disorders include chorea, ataxia, and hemiballismus. Transverse myelitis is a rare but devastating complication of SLE. It is characterized by acute or subacute paraplegia or quadraplegia associated with sensory deficit level and loss of sphincter control. Ischemic spinal cord necrosis secondary to microvascular injury from immune complex mediated vasculitis or hypercoagulability from phospholipid antibodies are postulated [128.] Cerebrospinal fluid (CSF) analysis reveals pleocytosis, low CSF glucose, and high CSF protein [134]. T_2-weighted magnetic resonance imaging (MRI) images usually demonstrate increased signal intensity and cord edema.

Meningitis, usually infectious, may develop in SLE patients. However, aseptic meningitis can be idiopathic or secondary to drug effects of ibuprofen or azathioprine [135,136,137].

The pathogenesis of neuropsychiatric lupus remains unknown. Although immune complex–mediated vasculitis in the CNS would be an attractive hypothesis, fewer than 10 percent of patients from two autopsy series have true vasculitis [130,131]. More common findings were hemorrhage (33–42%), microinfarcts (35–83%), and noninflammatory changes of intimal thickening and proliferation. Some researchers have postulated that these bland changes may be associated with antiphospholipid antibodies directed against endothelial membranes [138]. However, often the clinical manifestations did not correlate with the pathologic lesions. Bluestein and associates have reported antineuronal antibodies of the IgG class in the CSF of patients with organic brain syndromes, seizures, or psychosis [139]. In several animal models, injection of various antibodies to brain, gangliosides, or synaptosomal plasma membranes has produced seizure activity, memory changes, and demyelination [140,141,142]. This has led others to speculate that antineuronal antibodies can cross the CNS blood-brain barrier via immune complex–mediated vascular injury and then interfere with the ability of the neuron to function normally. An autoantibody to ribosomal-phosphoprotein has been reported to be present in 90 percent of SLE patients with lupus psychosis. Whether this antibody has a direct role in pathogenesis remains to be elucidated, but it may be a useful marker of lupus psychosis [143].

The diagnosis of neuropsychiatric lupus from other CNS processes is difficult and remains a process of elimination. Often CNS disease may be active in the setting of inactive SLE in other organ systems. Serologies that are commonly helpful in evaluating other manifestations of active SLE are often *not* helpful in patients with isolated CNS abnormalities. CSF studies are variable and may be normal. However, infectious etiologies should be carefully excluded if pleocytosis and low glucose are present. The presence of immune complexes and oligoclonal bands, depressed levels of complement, and elevated IgG, IgA, or IgM immunoglobulins have been reported in active CNS SLE, but these findings are *not* specific or diagnostic [144,145,146]. Electroencephalography will generally reveal diffuse brain wave slowing, but this may be focal in patients with seizures. Imaging studies such as CT and MRI are helpful to document hemorrhage, infarcts, parenchymal disease, paracranial tumors, or abscesses. MRIs have been able to distinguish diffuse cerebral disease from focal vascular lesions. The former is associated with increased signal intensity in subcortical white matter, which may reverse with treatment. The focal lesions were along the distribution of major vessels and are permanent [147]. Angiography results are positive in only 10 percent of patients with active CNS lupus [128]. The utility of single photon–emission computed tomography (SPECT) scan remains to be clarified.

Management of SLE patients with neuropsychiatric manifestations should focus on specific neurologic symptoms. Causes of non-SLE CNS dysfunction, including infections, uremia, hypertension, metabolic disturbances, hypoxia, or drug toxicities must be identified and appropriately treated. If steroid psychosis is suspected, McCune recommends doubling the steroid dose for 3 days to rule out the possibility of lupus cerebritis. If no improvement or evidence of active lupus is noted, the steroid therapy should be tapered [128]. Appropriate anticonvulsant medications should be instituted if recurrent seizures are present. Status epilepticus should be treated with both anticonvulsants and high-dose steroids. Psychotic patients should receive antipsychotic agents. High-dose steroids have been recommended for neuropsychiatric lupus; dosages have ranged from doubling of the baseline corticosteroid dose to high-dose steroids (prednisone 1.0–1.5 mg/kg/day or its equivalent). In severe cases, pulse intravenous (IV) methylprednisolone in a dose of 1.0–1.5 g/day for 3 days has been recommended [148,149]. As immunosuppressive agents, few prospective studies in the treatment of CNS disease have been performed. In one study of treating severe SLE with pulse monthly IV cyclophosphamide, three patients with active CNS and renal disease improved [125]. Transverse myelitis has been also successfully treated with pulse methylprednisolone and pulse cyclophosphamide [149a]. Plasmapheresis has been used in lupus nephritis, but only two reports described improvement of CNS symptoms [150,151]. Further studies must be done before recommendations can be made.

PULMONARY DISEASE. The pulmonary manifestations of SLE are multiple and variable. Although pulmonary disease in SLE was formerly considered uncommon, more recent reviews (clinical assessment or pathologic examination) have estimated a prevalence of 39 to 88 percent [152,153,154].

The most common clinical symptoms include dyspnea on exertion (49–80%), breathlessness at rest (37%), chest pain (25–35%), and cough (12–44%) [153,154,155]. Physical findings depended on the specific pulmonary syndromes, but only 12 percent of patients in an unselected ambulatory SLE population had pulmonary findings [154]. However, specific entities such as pulmonary hemorrhage (see Chap. 61) or interstitial lung disease have a better correlation with physical findings.

Pulmonary function testing has been the most sensitive indicator of pulmonary involvement. It most often reveals findings of restrictive lung volume patterns and decreased diffusing capacity [154,156].

Pleuritis with or without effusions has been reported in 30 to 60 percent of patients with SLE, depending on the method of study (i.e., clinical history, x-ray findings, or autopsy findings) [157]. Pleural effusions are usually small and bilateral, but massive collections can occur. Thoracentesis is indicated when the etiology of the fluid is uncertain or if respiratory compromise is present. Pleural fluid is characteristically exudative with high protein, pH greater than 7.35 [158], glucose normal or slightly decreased [159], and leukocyte count that is variable, usually less than 10,000 cells/μl. The presence of immune complexes and depressed complement levels in pleural fluid can be seen in SLE patients, but this does not differentiate it from rheumatoid arthritis [159]. The presence of lupus erythematosus (LE) cells is infrequent. Antinuclear antibodies (ANAs) are frequently present in pleural fluids, usually in the context of ANAs in serum, which raises the possibility of diffusion of antibodies from the serum into pleural space [157,160]. Mild pleuritis usually responds to nonsteroidal antiinflammatory drugs (NSAIDs) or low-dose corticosteroids (0.5 mg/kg/day of prednisone or its equivalent). The latter is used only after infectious causes have been excluded (see Chap. 65).

Acute lupus pneumonitis is characterized by parenchymal infiltrates, which are patchy and basilar in location [161]. There are no specific characteristics to differentiate lupus pneumonitis from other forms of bronchopneumonia and thus infectious etiologies have to be ruled out by appropriate studies. Clinically, patients present with fever, severe dyspnea, tachypnea, and hypoxemia [161]. Chest x-ray films reveal alveolar infiltrates, usually basilar in location. In the 12 patients described by Matthay and associates, all received corticosteroids and oxygen; azathioprine was added in seven cases. Mortality remained high at 50 percent—six out of 12 patients [161]. Of the six patients who recovered, three developed chronic restrictive lung disease with decreased diffusing capacity [161]. Pathologically, no distinguishing characteristics were evident. Alveolar wall injury, hemorrhage, edema, and hyaline membrane formation were typical findings [161]. Vasculitis in the lung has been rarely reported. Reports of immunoglobulin or complement staining within pulmonary tissue suggest a role for these humoral agents in pathogenesis [162,163]. Transbronchial biopsies may help distinguish infections from acute immunologically mediated pneumonitis.

Pulmonary hemorrhage is a rare but potentially fatal complication. In case reports patients characteristically present with acute dyspnea, tachycardia, severe hypoxemia, rales, a sudden drop in hematocrit, and hemoptysis [164]. Of note, several patients did not present with hemoptysis and, thus, hemorrhage was not clinically recognized [165]. Pathologic findings include intraalveolar hemorrhage sometimes associated with interstitial

pneumonitis; capillaritis may also be seen. Immunopathologic studies may reveal granular deposition of IgG in alveolar septal walls and pulmonary vessels, thus suggesting a possible immune complex–mediated process [165,166]. Therapy is generally aggressive and includes high-dose steroids (pulse methylprednisolone) and cytotoxic therapy in conjunction with plasmapheresis [167,168], but mortality remains high at 80 percent despite such treatment. See Chapter 61 for an indepth discussion of intrapulmonary hemorrhage and pulmonary-renal bleeding syndromes.

Diffuse interstitial lung disease in SLE patients may represent the end spectrum of acute pneumonitis, and thus some authors have labeled this as chronic lupus pneumonitis. Several large series have not noted this complication in SLE patients, but in 1973, Eisenberg and colleagues reported 18 SLE patients with interstitial lung disease without other identifiable causes [169]. They cited a prevalence of less than 3 percent in their population. Patients usually presented with dyspnea on exertion (DOE) (100%), productive cough (69%), pleuritis (66%), and rales (66%). Pulmonary function tests were consistent with restriction and marked reduction in diffusing capacity. Obstructive abnormalities were not noted. Histology revealed nonspecific interstitial fibrosis in three-fourths of patients. Pulmonary immunohistology done by Eisenberg and colleagues revealed evidence of immunoglobulin and complement in a diffuse or focal pattern in the interstitium of patients with SLE and rheumatoid arthritis not seen in other forms of diffuse interstitial fibrosis (DIF) [170].

Treatment for interstitial fibrosis is not well documented in the literature. Corticosteroids may be beneficial in the prefibrotic stage with active inflammatory lesions [169]. This stage may be detected by gallium scanning or transbronchial biopsy. It is unclear whether bronchoalveolar lavage (BAL) is useful in distinguishing SLE from other causes of chronic interstitial fibrosis [171]. If biopsy reveals little evidence of acute inflammation, it is unlikely that corticosteroids will be of great benefit [172].

Pulmonary hypertension (PH) may be either a primary or secondary entity in SLE and is recognized more in the recent literature, with pathologic studies indicating evidence of pulmonary hypertension in 17 to 40 percent of cases of unselected SLE patients [172,173]. Pathologically, changes of intimal thickening and fibrosis, medial hypertrophy, altered elastic laminae, and periadventitial fibrosis have been similar to changes seen in idiopathic PH [173]. A few cases have reported necrotizing arteritis. Patients usually present with severe dyspnea on exertion and fatigue. There is a greater frequency of Raynaud's phenomenon in patients with PH [174,175,176]. Asherson and colleagues have reported the presence of antiphospholipid antibodies (APLA) in five of six patients with PH. Whether a hypercoagulable state contributes to development of PH remains to be further elucidated [175] (see Chap. 64).

Therapy for PH in lupus patients is limited. Corticosteroids have not been demonstrated to be helpful unless PH results from arteritis, which is quite uncommon. Vasodilators have been variably successful and may be most effective in the early reversible lesions. If APLAs are present, anticoagulation may be potentially useful [177,178].

Dyspnea in SLE may also be secondary to diaphragmatic dysfunction. This is felt to be secondary to a myopathy of the diaphragm, resulting in "sluggish diaphragm" [179] or the entity of "shrinking lungs" [180].

Pulmonary embolism and peripheral vasoocclusive disease are well-known risks in SLE (see Chap. 60). The frequency of deep vein thrombophlebitis (DVT) in a prospective study was approximately 12 percent and pulmonary embolism (PE) was documented at 9 percent [181]. The association of thrombosis with the lupus anticoagulant (LAC) is well known, and more recently the association of venous and arterial occlusions with APLA has also been well characterized [177]. (See Antiphospholipid Antibody Syndrome).

CARDIAC DISEASE. Cardiovascular involvement in SLE has been reported to range from 29 to 66 percent [182]. This tremendous range reflects whether data were based on clinical parameters or pathologic findings at autopsy. Often, the latter studies will document significant findings in the heart without much clinical correlation.

Pericardial disease is by far the most common cardiac manifestation of SLE (see Chap. 34). Subclinical pericarditis is often documented only at autopsy. Pericarditis usually presents during the course of the disease rather than as an initial manifestation of SLE [183,184]. In addition, it occurs usually in association with disease activity in other organ systems rather than during quiescent phases of illness [185].

Patients usually develop anterior or substernal chest pain that is characteristically pleuritic and relieved by leaning forward. The pain may be associated with dyspnea or arrhythmias, ranging from sinus tachycardia to atrial arrhythmias. A pericardial friction rub may be heard on auscultation; chest x-ray film may reveal an enlarging cardiac silhouette; transient ECG changes may be seen (ST segment elevation). Echocardiography, one of the most sensitive tests for the detection of pericardial disease, may reveal pericardial effusion or thickening.

Life-threatening complications of pericarditis include cardiac tamponade and constriction. Both of these entities are rare; tamponade occurs in less than 4 to 7 percent [186] of lupus patients with pericarditis, and constriction has been described in case reports. Because hemodynamically significant pericarditis is rare, only a few patients have required pericardiocentesis. Thus, data regarding pericardial fluid are limited. Typically, pericardial fluid is exudative with high protein and normal to low glucose, compared with serum. The total white blood cell counts from various reports have ranged from 544 to 199,600 cells/μl (a mean of 29,790) [182], with predominantly polymorphonuclear cells. Thus, suppurative pericarditis becomes a significant and important differential in SLE patients with pericarditis. Pericardial fluid complement levels have been reported to be low or undetectable [182,187], while lupus LE cells have been routinely found on smears. Pericardial ANA titers may be positive. However, none of the laboratory findings can differentiate infectious from lupus pericarditis [182].

Constrictive pericarditis may develop after successful treatment of pericarditis with or without corticosteroids. One necropsy report of 36 patients suggested that corticosteroid therapy may have converted the typical fibrinous pericarditis of the presteroid era to adhesive pericarditis in the poststeroid era [188].

Once other causes of pericarditis, including uremia, drugs, or viral infections, have been eliminated, hemodynamically stable and symptomatic pericarditis can be successfully treated with NSAIDs such as indomethacin 50 mg tid and, occasionally, oral corticosteroids at low dosages (15–30 mg/day). If fever is present and the etiology of the pericardial effusion is not clear, a diagnostic pericardiocentesis may be necessary to rule out bacterial or opportunistic infection. Hemodynamically compromising effusions require pericardial aspiration and high-dose intravenous corticosteroids (e.g., equivalent of 1 mg/kg/day of prednisone). If effusions recur despite high-dose steroids, repeat drainage, a pericardial window, or even pericardial stripping may be required [185,186].

Myocardial involvement in SLE is the least frequent manifes-

tation of cardiac disease and should be categorized as primary or secondary. Primary myocarditis is rare, clinically occurring in 2.1 to 14.0 percent of SLE patients [189,190]. Pathologic abnormalities of the myocardium, however, have been reported in as high as approximately 40 percent of patients in the precorticosteroid era [182]. Studies from that era usually reveal mild perivascular infiltrates with inflammatory cells and patchy fibrosis [188]; immunoglobulin deposition is diffuse throughout the myocardium [184]. Clinically, myocarditis has been defined as unexplained tachycardia, congestive heart failure, ventricular arrhythmias, conduction defects, ST-T wave changes, or cardiomegaly without evidence of valvular or pericardial disease [190]. Congestive heart failure from myocarditis is rare and is estimated to occur in 4 percent of cases of myocarditis [183]. One report suggested a clinical correlation of myocarditis with peripheral skeletal myositis [190]. Most studies have evaluated cardiac function by echocardiography [191,192], thallium stress tests [193], and, in one report, invasive hemodynamic studies [194]. Each method has revealed that some SLE patients have elements of reversible myocardial dysfunction or perfusion abnormalities suggestive of functional or obliterative small vessel disease. Of interest, some of these patients did not have cardiac symptoms.

Secondary myocardial dysfunctions in SLE include systemic hypertension, valvular disease, pulmonary disease, coronary artery ischemia (see following discussion), drug toxicity, and amyloidosis. These secondary causes are often more important than true lupus myocarditis.

Therapeutic management of patients with evidence of carditis rests on distinguishing primary from secondary disorders. The latter require treatment of the underlying problems rather than initiation or acceleration of antiinflammatory or immunosupressive therapies directed against SLE. Corticosteroids may exacerbate hypertension, salt and water balance problems, and even accelerate atherosclerosis. However, in the rare patient who does have myocarditis from SLE, high-dose corticosteroids are indicated. Data regarding use of immunosuppressive agents are scarce.

Coronary artery involvement in SLE includes embolic events, thromboses, or a true vasculitis of the vessels as opposed to secondary changes of premature atherosclerosis. Coronary arteritis is rare [195,196]. It may be difficult to distinguish coronary arteritis from atherosclerosis on arteriographic studies unless repetitive studies are performed. In a prospective study of 100 SLE patients, 5 percent of the patients with clinical ischemic symptoms responded to increases in steroid dosage, suggesting active arteritis [192]. This can occur in the absence of extracardiac SLE activity [195].

Myocardial infarctions can occur in young SLE patients and contribute to 3 percent of deaths in SLE patients [126]. Rubin and colleagues [197] noted that the majority of late deaths in SLE patients were attributed to atherosclerotic cardiovascular disease in the absence of active SLE. Gladman and associate [198] reported an incidence of atherosclerosis of 9 percent (45 of 507 patients) in a lupus population followed prospectively. The mean age of these patients was 48 years and overall disease activity was quiescent at the time of angina or myocardial infarction. Pathologically, atherosclerosis is the major cause of coronary artery disease [188,199]. Risk factors for vascular disease include hyperlipidemia, hypertension, antiphospholipids, and corticosteroid use.

Emboli from Libman-Sacks endocarditis or possibly thrombosis associated with APLAs may contribute to myocardial ischemia. More recently, APLAs and the lupus anticoagulant have been reported in young SLE or SLE-like patients presenting with myocardial infarctions [200,201]. Coronary arteriograms in two of four patients revealed no evidence of atherosclerosis. The

APLA has been associated with recurrent arteriovenous thrombosis, possibly via platelet activation, vascular endothelial cell proliferation [202] or interference with prostacyclin production by endothelial cells [203] (see Antiphospholipid Antibody Syndrome).

The management of SLE patients with acute myocardial ischemia should initially be similar to patients with atherosclerotic coronary artery disease. However, the etiology of the ischemia must be determined (see Chap. 50). Because the management of coronary arteritis would differ from and may be countereffective to management of atherosclerotic disease, data must be collected on a clinical basis to guide management. Evidence of extracardiac SLE activity may be helpful. Laboratory tests including ANA, anti-dsDNA, complement levels, complete blood count with differential, and platelet counts may provide some indicators of SLE activity. Lupus anticoagulant and APLAs should be checked. The ECG, echocardiogram, and thallium stress test will not distinguish arteritis from atherosclerosis. A coronary arteriogram may be helpful to separate thrombosis and vasculitis from atherosclerosis. However, arteriographic distinction of the latter two may be difficult. Mandell [182] recommended that, in rare cases in which arteriograms cannot be safely performed, empiric therapy with moderate to high-dose steroids along with antianginal medications be instituted. Once the patient is stabilized, the steroids are tapered. If cardiac symptoms recur, a presumptive diagnosis of coronary arteritis is made. If arteriography reveals thrombosis without evident atherosclerosis and the presence of APLAs is documented, therapy should consist of anticoagulation and antiplatelet medications.

The most characteristic cardiac manifestation of SLE is nonbacterial verrucous endocarditis, first described by Libman and Sacks in 1924 [204]. At autopsy, 15 to 60 percent of SLE patients will have these lesions, which are commonly found on the ventricular surface of the mitral valve, often involving the ventricular endocardium, chordae tendineae, and papillary muscle. Histologically, these lesions have been characterized by proliferating endothelial cells and myocytes with chronic inflammatory cell infiltrates [188]. Immunoglobulins and complement are also found [205]. In addition, a necrotizing valvulitis has also been described secondary to vasculitis of the smaller vessels supplying the valve.

Clinically, the presence of these Libman-Sacks (LS) lesions does not correlate with murmurs. Literature from the presteroid era states that the LS lesions rarely produced significant valvular dysfunction. However, Doherty and Siegel summarized over 50 cases of hemodynamically significant aortic and mitral insufficiency [186]. Some investigators postulate that steroids may contribute to the valvular dysfunction by promoting healing of the verrucous lesions, which results in scarring and retraction [188]. Valve replacements may be required, but the associated mortality has been as high as 25 percent [206].

Rarely, lesional material of LS endocarditis may dislodge and embolize. Case reports have associated cerebral embolic events with the presence of LS endocarditis [207]. Secondary bacterial endocarditis occurs at an incidence of 1 to 7 percent [182,208].

Recently, investigators have noted an association of cardiac valvular disease with the presence of APLA in SLE and SLE-like disease [209,210,211]. Although these lesions were similar echocardiographically and histologically to the lesions of LS endocarditis, there was a much higher incidence of aortic valve involvement [212]. The data are too limited at this time for comment whether these lesions are different pathologically from LS endocarditis. In addition, the pathophysiologic relationship between valvulitis, thrombosis, and APLA remains unclear.

Conduction abnormalities and arrhythmias due to SLE are not usually clinically significant. Although conduction disease has been reported in adult SLE patients, the reports have not detailed contributory variables such as hypertension, ischemia, or drugs. The incidence of AV nodal block is estimated at 5 percent [182], and autopsy studies have demonstrated fibrosis of nodal and conduction tissue [213]. Sinus tachycardia without underlying pathology (fever, dehydration, congestive heart failure, thyroid disease, drug abuse) has been noted by several authors [182,183]. Some have postulated that this may be a subtle manifestation of lupus activity [182].

Recently, neonatal lupus associated with complete heart block has been described. This syndrome in infants is characterized by conduction system abnormalities, rash, and arthritis and is believed to develop as a result from anti-Ro antibodies, which are passively transferred in utero from their mothers. Some of these mothers had SLE or developed Sjögren's syndrome, but over 60 percent of the mothers did not meet clinical criteria for SLE or Sjogren's syndrome [214]. It is believed that anti-Ro antibodies prevent the development of conduction fibers [215].

Conduction abnormalities in SLE patients are more likely to be associated with other processes such as congestive heart failure or ischemia than with lupus activity and should be managed the same as patients without SLE. If acute conduction disease is clinically suspected to be secondary to myocarditis or arteritis, a short trial of corticosteroids could be initiated in the hemodynamically compromised patient [182].

HEMATOLOGIC DISEASE. Hematologic abnormalities constitute one of the criteria for classification of SLE. These include hemolytic anemia, thrombocytopenia, leukopenia, and lymphopenia. Hematologic aberrations vary in SLE subsets. Hemolytic anemia predominates in pediatric populations (73%) [216], circulating anticoagulant in adult populations (55%) [217], and nonhemolytic anemia, lymphopenia, and hypergammaglobulinemia in SLE patients over 60 years old [218].

Anemia is present in 57 to 78 percent of SLE patients [184,219]. Anemia of chronic disease is most common. However, autoimmune hemolytic anemia (AIHA) occurs in 40 percent of lupus patients sometime during the course of their disease [220]. From 18 to 65 percent of SLE patients will have a positive direct Coombs assay, but significant hemolytic anemia will develop in only 10 percent [216]. The presence of both "warm" IgG autoantibodies and complement on the red cell surface is characteristic of SLE AIHA [220]. Clinically, the AIHA is accompanied by an elevated reticulocyte count and indirect bilirubin and decreased haptoglobin levels. Despite the variable degree of severity, AIHA in SLE does not signify a poor prognosis [220].

Seventy-five percent of patients with AIHA will respond to high-dose corticosteroids (60–100 mg/day of prednisone in divided doses) [221]. Response is usually rapid, and prednisone can be slowly tapered after 3 weeks, based on laboratory results. If active hemolysis persists after 3 weeks, other therapeutic modalities include danazol, immunosuppressive agents, and splenectomy; however, splenectomy induces permanent remission in less than 50 percent of patients [222]. Ahn and associates recommended the use of high-dose steroids and danazol, 200 mg three to four times a day, as the initial treatment of severe AIHA, with subsequent gradual tapering of corticosteroids [223]. Danazol was also effective in patients who had failed to respond to other modalities. Uncontrolled trials with azathioprine or cyclophosphamide have shown therapeutic response [222,224]. Plasmapheresis was effective in another study [225].

Other mechanisms of anemia in SLE patients include pure

red cell aplasia, which is presumed to be immune mediated, characterized by bone marrow erythroid hypoplasia. Occult gastrointestinal blood loss as a result of medications, particularly NSAIDs, or peptic ulcer disease should be considered in patients with hypochromic/microcytic indices or an unexplained drop in hemoglobin. Myelosuppression is common with azathioprine and cyclophosphamide. Phenylbutazone has been associated with aplastic anemia and agranulocytosis.

Leukopenia, defined as a total white blood cell count of less than 4500/μl, occurs in 50 to 60 percent of SLE patients [184]; however, associated infections and complications are rare [226]. Lymphopenia, defined as lymphocyte counts lower than 1500/μl, is associated with 84 percent of SLE patients during disease activity [218,220].

Thrombocytopenia, or platelet counts lower than 100,000/μ is observed in 20 to 40 percent of SLE patients and is severe (<50,000/μl) in 10 percent of the patients [227]. Idiopathic thrombocytopenia pupura (ITP) may be the initial presentation of SLE. In evaluating patients with thrombocytopenia, five major causes are outlined by Laurence and Nachman [220]: (1) decreased production from megakaryocyte defects or drug toxicities; (2) ineffective thrombopoiesis; (3) abnormal platelet distribution as in congestive splenomegaly; (4) dilutional effects; and (5) abnormal platelet destruction by disseminated intravascular coagulation, thrombotic thrombocytopenic purpura, hemolytic uremic syndrome, vasculitis, drug-induced infection, or hematologic malignancies. The pathologic mechanism of thrombocytopenia is usually antiplatelet antibodies with resultant splenic sequestration and decreased platelet life span. A bone marrow biopsy is helpful in distinguishing various forms of thrombocytopenia. SLE-associated ITP is characterized by an increased number of megakaryocytes.

Therapy of severe SLE-associated ITP (<50,000/μl) is similar to that of idiopathic autoimmune thrombocytopenia. Corticosteroid therapy at 30 to 50 mg/m²/day is the recommended initial therapy [120]. Subsequent tapering is guided by platelet counts. If corticosteroids are not effective, intravenous gammaglobulin may increase platelet counts rapidly. Recommended doses range from 0.4 g–1 g/d or 6–15 mg/kg/d for 4–7 days. Success at maintaining platelet counts were variable [234,235.]

If either steroids or immunoglobulin fails, splenectomy may be considered. Although most studies report sustained remission in 50 percent of patients following splenectomy, others have questioned its long-term benefit [228,229]. For those patients whose disease has failed to respond to both regimens, danazol 200 mg four times a day alone or in conjunction with corticosteroids has been effective in several studies [230,231]. Immunosuppressive agents include various combinations of vincristine [232] or vinca-loaded platelets, cyclophosphamide [233], and azathioprine [221]. Plasmapheresis may also be beneficial [235a].

The lupus anticoagulant (LAC), which interferes with the activation of prothrombin activator complex (factors Xa and V, Ca²⁺, and phospholipid), affects both the intrinsic and extrinsic pathways. The laboratory findings are markedly prolonged partial thromboplastin time (PTT) and normal or mildly prolonged prothrombin time (PT) that cannot be corrected with mixing normal plasma. Clinically, however, this anticoagulant is associated with arterial and venous thrombosis rather than with bleeding. More recently, antiphospholipid antibodies directed at the phospholipid in the prothrombin activator complex and LACs have also been associated with various clinical syndromes of arterial and venous thrombotic events, recurrent fetal loss, chorea, and valvular heart disease [177]. Although many SLE patients have both the LAC and anticardiolipin antibodies, there are subsets of patients with only one or the other antibody. (See Antiphospholipid Antibody Syndrome.)

GASTROINTESTINAL DISEASE. The gastrointestinal (GI) involvement in SLE is not frequently considered because many GI symptoms can be attributed to complications of drug therapy, particularly salicylates, NSAIDs, corticosteroids, hydroxychloroquine, and azathioprine. GI disease directly caused by SLE has been reported in a range of 1 to 27 percent of lupus patients [236]. Several distinct clinical entities, however, may present acutely and require ICU admission.

The most serious GI complication of SLE is small vessel vasculitis (or mesenteric vasculitis) of the large or small intestine. The severity and extent of involvement vary and can range from segmental edema or ulcerations to perforations [236]. Histologically, specimens reveal small vessel vasculitis [237], although large vessel involvement has been reported [238]. In one retrospective review of all reported cases up to 1980, two-thirds of the patients died when vasculitis was complicated by infarct or perforation of a viscus [239]. Zizic and associates, however, noted that 57 percent of those patients with abdominal vasculitis also had cutaneous vasculitis compared with the 27 percent of controls who did not have cutaneous vasculitis [237]. Other associations with abdominal vasculitis included CNS involvement, thrombocytopenia, and circulating rheumatoid factor. Often, because patients were on chronic steroids, the classical abdominal findings were obscured.

Evaluation should include plain films, paracentesis of ascitic fluid (to rule out perforation or bacterial peritonitis), and barium studies. Mesenteric arteritis has been radiologically characterized by pseudo-obstruction, thumb-printing, or mucosal abnormalities [240]. Arteriography may be helpful, but its role is not as well delineated as in polyarteritis [241]. Direct visualization with endoscopy or colonoscopy may also provide useful information.

Pneumatosis intestinalis, or intramural air, has been associated with bowel infarction in one case report, but others have noted it to be benign [242,243].

Lupus peritonitis is less devastating but often quite dramatic in presentation [244]. The etiology of the serositis is presumed to be secondary to immune complex deposition in mesenteric vessels. Ascites may be present and, on paracentesis, the fluid is exudative and sterile with a low white cell count [245]. Other causes of ascites must be ruled out, including constrictive pericarditis, nephrotic syndrome, and spontaneous bacterial peritonitis.

Recently, protein-losing enteropathy has been described in SLE patients [244a,b] Other GI manifestations, including acute GI bleeding, pancreatitis, and esophageal disease, may be seen in SLE patients, but evidence directly linking these disorders to SLE is variable. Thus, evaluation should screen for other etiologies, and, most importantly, drugs should be considered primary offenders. (See the sections on antirheumatic drugs in this chapter.)

Management of the SLE patient with abdominal pain does not differ significantly from that for non-SLE patients. Hoffman and colleagues suggested that in patients with mild to moderate pain with a chronic course, medications and intercurrent disease should be considered as the cause of the pain first [239]. If no etiology is found, lupus vasculitis or peritonitis should be considered and treated with a moderate increase in steroids. In patients who present acutely, general management should be started and appropriate studies performed. Paracentesis should be obtained to rule out perforation of viscus or infection. A therapeutic trial of high-dose steroids can then be instituted. Rapid (12–48 hours) response usually is consistent with vasculitis or peritonitis; if a patient deteriorates clinically, exploratory laparotomy may be necessary [239].

Drug-induced Lupus

The syndrome of drug-induced lupus should be considered in ICU patients if systemic symptoms of fever, arthralgias, arthritis, and pleuropericarditis develop. Because many ICU patients are on medications that potentially induce SLE (Table 219-3), the diagnosis must be excluded. However, some of the medications, particularly procainamide and hydralazine, produce positive ANA tests, but this does not necessarily imply drug-induced lupus is present [246]. Symptoms typically develop several months after the institution of the medication. CNS, hematologic, and renal manifestations are rare. Males and females are equally susceptible. Laboratory values reveal an elevated ESR, mild leukopenia or thrombocytopenia, and positive LE prep and ANA; antihistone antibodies are present in 90 percent of patients [116]; specific antibodies to dsDNA and Smith (Sm) antigen are absent. Discontinuation of the offending medication results in gradual diminution of symptoms. NSAIDs or low-dose steroids may control the symptoms [247].

As for patients with idiopathic SLE who may require hydralazine, procainamide, isoniazid, phenytoin, beta-blockers, or other medication that can potentially induce lupus, most rheumatologists feel that these medications can be used. However, it is advisable to document the clinical and serologic status of the patient before starting the medication [247].

Antiphospholipid Antibody Syndrome

The antiphospholipid antibody (APLA) syndrome refers to an illness in patients who (1) have SLE, a "lupus-like" disorder, or another connective tissue disease; (2) have antibodies to phospholipids indicated by anticardiolipin antibodies, the lupus anticoagulant, and false positive reactions in the test for syphilis; and (3) manifest venous thrombosis (recurrent deep vein thrombosis, retinal vein thrombosis, Budd-Chiari syndrome), arterial thrombosis (cerebrovascular accidents, coronary thrombosis, retinal artery thrombosis), recurrent fetal loss due to thrombosis and infarction of the placenta, leg ulcers, livedo reticularis, pulmonary hypertension, migraine headaches, chorea, endocardial disease, lupoid sclerosis, thrombocytopenia, and Coombs positive hemolytic anemia [248,249,249a,249b, 249c,249d]. The complex of clinical and laboratory features in patients with no underlying disorder has been referred to as the primary antiphospholipid syndrome [249-255].

The lupus anticoagulant (LAC) and anticardiolipin antibodies (ACLA) are two APLAs, which bind negatively charged phospholipids and most strongly correlate with the development of thromboses. (See Systemic Lupus Erythematosus for a discussion of LAC.) The presence of one of these antibodies is usually associated with the presence of the other, but there is a one-third discordance of positive results in any individual. The most reliable anticardiolipin determination is a solid-phase, enzyme-linked anticardiolipin assay (ELISA), which utilizes bovine heart extract as the substrate.

Two theories for the prothrombotic effects of APLAs have

Table 219-3. Medications Associated with Drug-Related Lupus

Type	Definite	Possible	Unlikely or rare
Antihypertensives/cardiac drugs	Methyldopa Hydralazine Procainamide	Atenolol Acebutolol Propranolol Labetalol Metoprolol Practolol Oxprenolol Captopril Quinidine	Reserpine Minoxidil Chlorthalidone Timolol* Pindolol* Lovastatin*
Anticonvulsant or other neurologic medications		Phenytoin Primidone Carbamazepine Ethosuximide Levadopa Trimethadione	
Psychiatric	Chlorpromazine	Lithium carbonate	
Antibiotics	Isoniazid	Sulfonamides Nitrofurantoin	Streptomycin Tetracycline Penicillin
Endocrine	—	Methimazole Propylthiouracil Methylthiouracil	
Rheumatic		Penicillamine Phenylbutazone Ibuprofen*	Sulfasalazine Gold salts p-Aminosalicylic acid Allopurinol
Others			Oral contraceptives*

Source: Adapted from Schur PH: Clinical Features of SLE, in Kelly WN (ed): *Textbook of Rheumatology,* 3rd ed. Philadelphia, WB Saunders, 1989; and Solinger AM: Drug related lupus: Clinical and etiological considerations. *Rheum Dis Clin North Am* 14:187, 1988.

been advanced: (1) the APLAs, by binding to phospholipid moieties within endothelial cells, prevent arachidonic acid release and prostacyclin formation, which would normally inhibit platelet aggregation and thrombus formation [256,257,258, 258a]; and (2) APLAs, by binding to phospholipid components of platelets, render the platelets more likely to aggregate and form thromboses [177,259,260]. Other possible thrombogenic mechanismsinclude interference with release of plasminogen-activating factor [202,261,262], inhibition of thrombomodulin-induced activation of protein C [263,264,264a], and deficiency of protein S [264b].

Although the clinical manifestations of the vasculopathy associated with antiphospholipid syndromes may resemble vasculitis [249,265–272], occlusive vascular lesions typically appear to be due to thromboses and emboli [249d,272a]. As reported by Alarcon-Segovia and colleagues, however, rarely have these been associated with vasculitis. These authors describe three young patients with antiphospholipid antibodies who developed arterial occlusive lesions of limbs and whose biopsies of skin and muscle revealed leukocytoclastic vasculitis. Biopsies from two of the three individuals displayed mononuclear cell infiltrate in large arteries [273]. Another report described a patient with a lupus anticoagulant who required progressive right lower extremity amputations for ischemia associated with inflammatory vasculitis in multiple arteries and high titers of a cardiolipin antibodies. High-dose corticosteroid therapy reversed the ischemic process [273a].

Thromboses and emboli associated with antiphospholipid antibodies may occur in retinal, mesenteric, coronary, pulmonary, intracranial, and peripheral arteries as well as in superficial and deep leg veins and veins of the liver, kidney, brain, retina, and placenta, thus causing a variety of clinical manifestations. Transient ischemic attacks, ischemic infarctions, multiinfarct dementia, cerebral venous thromboses [274–277,177a], retinal artery and venous occlusion [278], ischemic optic neuropathy, vertebrobasilar artery insufficiency, spontaneous abortions [279–283,283a], and livedo reticularis are clinical components of the syndrome. APLAs are also believed to play a pathogenic role in thrombocytopenia, cardiac valvular lesions (nonbacterial thrombotic endocarditis Libman-Sacks lesions) [210,211,253], aortic and mitral valve insufficiency [209,284], chorea [285], migraine headache, and pulmonary hypertension [285a].

The manifestations of the antiphospholipid syndrome that most likely require ICU admission are cerebrovascular disease [274], venous thrombosis with pulmonary embolism [286], pulmonary hypertension [287], major abdominal or extremity arterial or venous thrombosis, cardiac disease including myocardial infarction in a young individual [201,288,289], recurrent myocardial infarctions [290], possibly some cases of coronary artery bypass graft occlusions [291], severe valvular disease (insufficiency or thrombotic valvular vegetations), and intracardiac thrombosis. Adrenal insufficiency associated with antiphospholipids may complicate the presentation and management of such patients [291a]. The percentage of these disorders caused by thromboses associated with the presence of APLAs is not yet known.

Although treatment of patients with recurrent thromboses in the setting of elevated phospholipid antibodies consists primarily of antiplatelet medications and anticoagulants, optimal therapy has not been established. A study by Rosove and colleagues indicates that intermediate to high-intensity warfarin therapy may provide better protection against recurrent thrombosis than low-intensity warfarin therapy or aspirin [291b]. In patients with superficial and nonthreatening venous thromboses, treatment with antiplatelet therapy in the form of aspirin may be sufficient. Patients with deep venous thrombosis should

be anticoagulated with intravenous heparin then oral warfarin. Most authorities recommend lifelong anticoagulation for serious venous thromboembolic disease associated with APLAs. Management of serious venous thromboses also includes evaluating for predisposing conditions other than APLAs such as venous insufficiency, venous obstruction, nephrosis, and deficiencies of protein C, protein S, and antithrombin III [264b,291c,291d].

For patients with arterial thromboses, a search for causes including cocaine use, valvular heart disease, atrial myxoma, and arterial stenosis should be performed. Treatment consists of intravenous heparin then long-term oral warfarin anticoagulation. There is little experience with thrombectomy and thrombolysis, but in cases that have been so treated, rethrombosis tends to occur [291c]. For arterial thromboses, some recommend either high-dose warfarin (adjusting the protime to 20–25 seconds or the international normalization ratio [INR], to 2.0 to 3.0) or adding aspirin to warfarin, but these measures increase the risk of hemorrhage and are controversial with regard to the balance of risks and benefits [291c]. Several studies document recurrent thrombotic episodes after anticoagulation has been discontinued, and thus emphasize the need for long-term anticoagulation [292,293]. Anticoagulation is not recommended for individuals who possess APLAs but have no evidence of thrombosis.

Studies are now examining the efficacy of low-dose aspirin in pregnant women with APLAs and histories of repetitive spontaneous abortions [294]. It appears that for women with high titers of APLAs and previous fetal losses, the best therapy is low-dose aspirin for gestational weeks 0–12, subcutaneous heparin 10,000–12,000 units bid for weeks 13–32, and aspirin thereafter until delivery [291c]. Low-dose aspirin also appears to decrease the risk of preeclampsia and reduces intrauterine growth retardation [294a]. Combined corticosteroids and aspirin [295,296], subcutaneous heparin [296a], and high-dose intravenous gamma globulin [297,298,299] are other therapeutic modalities which have been used.

Systemic Sclerosis

Systemic sclerosis (SSc), or scleroderma, is a multisystem disease characterized by fibrosis and degeneration of various organs, including the skin, heart, lungs, kidneys, and GI tract. Although the classification of SSc and scleroderma-like disorders is large, only classic SSc will be discussed here. For a complete discussion, refer to the review by Rocco and Hurd [300] and to references 301–317.

Although SSc involves many organ systems, the ICU team generally will manage those patients with severe pulmonary, cardiac, or renal involvement. The following discussion will be accordingly limited to these areas.

PULMONARY DISEASE. Pulmonary involvement in SSc is now the primary cause of mortality. The prevalence ranges from 50 to 92 percent [318]. This tremendous range is due to the subtle aspects of pulmonary disease that may be apparent on biopsy but correlate poorly with either clinical symptoms, laboratory tests, or functional testing [319]. Interstitial fibrosis is the major pulmonary manifestation of SSc. Dyspnea, cough, and basilar crackles are the predominant clinical features. Radiographs may reveal pulmonary fibrosis in 18 to 78 percent of cases [318] with a characteristic reticulonodular pattern at the bases, or honeycombing. Pulmonary function tests may reveal abnormalities even before there are radiographic or clinical findings. The classic pattern is restrictive with decreased total lung capacity and vital capacity. These findings correlate with fibrosis of the chest wall, diaphragm, and pleura [300]. A decrease in diffusing capacity (DC) is often the earliest abnormal parameter. The etiology of the decreased DC was previously attributed to fibrosis of alveolar septa [318]. More recently, because decreased DC was not associated with pathologic changes, some researchers have proposed that ventilation-perfusion mismatch, possibly due to small airway disease, may be the actual mechanism [320,321,322]. Other investigators have also noted the additive detrimental effects of smoking on SSc lung disease [320,323]. Although some investigators have suggested that esophageal dysmotility with resultant aspiration is the pathologic mechanism of pulmonary fibrosis [324,325], other studies have noted pulmonary disease without esophageal involvement [320,326]. Pathologically, fibrotic replacement of alveolar septa with or without varying degrees of inflammation are present. Vascular lesions, described in the following section, are also present.

Although secondary pulmonary arterial hypertension (PAH) from chronic interstitial lung disease may develop, the degree of PAH is disproportionate to the severity of interstitial lung disease [327]. Ungerer and colleagues, in studying 49 patients with SSc, found a 33 percent prevalence of PAH; however, in the subset of CREST patients, a much higher percentage (50%) of PAH was present [328] but without significant interstitial lung disease. This observation has been confirmed by other investigators [329,329a]. Pathologically, intimal hyperplasia, medial hypertrophy, and luminal occlusion by fibromyxoid collagen in the muscular arterioles are noted. Some researchers have postulated a role for Raynaud's phenomenon initiating the vascular lesions in the pulmonary vascular tree [330,331]. However, others have not been able to support this hypothesis [320,332]. The most sensitive tests for predicting PAH are decreased DC to less than 43 percent, chest radiographic changes, and ECG changes [328]. More subtle disease, however, cannot be predicted.

Diagnosis of pulmonary disease in SSc is based on clinical symptoms, abnormal radiographs, and physiologic testing. PAH may be subtle, and right heart catheterization with pressure readings may be necessary. Although gallium scans have been used to assess inflammation, they are less sensitive in SSc than in sarcoidosis or idiopathic pulmonary fibrosis [333,334]. High-resolution computed tomographic (HRCT) scans have documented interstitial disease in 88 percent of SSc patients compared with only 59 percent abnormal chest radiographs in 17 patients tested [335]. Bronchoalveolar lavage has also been advocated in assessing scleroderma lung [336,337]. Inflammatory cells in the washings are variable but 50 percent of SSc patients had neutrophilic alveolitis with also increased numbers of macrophages and eosinophils [338]. Given these bronchoalveolar lavage abnormalities, some researchers have proposed that a more acute, inflammatory stage exists in scleroderma interstitial lung disease and have treated patients with this stage of neutrophilic alveolitis with corticosteroids and cyclophosphamide [338].

Treatment of pulmonary disease is limited and lacks efficacy. Steen and associates in a retrospective study noted improvement of DC from 76 to 87 percent in 44 patients treated with D-penicillamine, while in the 48 patients who were untreated, DC did not change significantly [339]. PAH has been equally difficult to treat, and various vasodilators (nifedipine, prazosin, high-flow oxygen) have had variable success. Corticosteroids and other immunosuppressive agents may have a role in early, inflammatory stages of interstitial lung disease, but data currently are limited. Thus, most of the management remains supportive, with care directed at prevention of infections, especially if patients have esophageal reflux that results in aspiration. Prompt treatment of infection, use of bronchodilators and supplemental oxygen when necessary are other measures.

The contribution of pulmonary disease to mortality varies from 0 to 27 percent [340,341]. The rapidity of pulmonary disease progression also varies, but factors such as Raynaud's phenomenon, interstitial changes on chest radiograph, or smoking may indicate worse prognosis [320,342].

CARDIAC DISEASE. Cardiac involvement in SSc may be a primary process within the heart or secondary to other major organ involvement (i.e., pulmonary, renal, vascular, or thyroid). Primary cardiac disease in SSc was first noted by Weiss and associates [343] and includes pericardial disease, myocardial disease, conduction abnormalities, and arrhythmias. Because the most common symptoms are dyspnea, orthopnea, atypical chest pain, palpitations, easy fatigue, and dizziness, the clinical manifestations of cardiac disease can be confused with other organ systemic involvement.

Pericardial disease is the most common clinical manifestation of scleroderma heart disease. Like SLE, asymptomatic pericardial disease based on autopsy series or recent echocardiographic data has much higher prevalence than symptomatic disease (33–71% versus 7–20%) [344,345,346]. Pericardial effusions are usually small and do not influence prognosis. Larger effusions (>200 ml), however, are associated with poor prognosis. One prospective study reported death in three of four patients with large pericardial effusions [346]. Pericardial tamponade with hemodynamic compromise is rare.

McWhorter and colleagues in a retrospective review described two clinical presentations of pericarditis in SSc patients [345]. One group of patients had chronic pericarditis and presented with dyspnea, congestive heart failure, peripheral edema, and cardiomegaly. Six of eleven patients subsequently developed renal failure within 6 months and died. The second group presented with acute symptoms of fever, dyspnea, chest pain, and auscultable friction rub. Two of the four patients in this group had sudden death. Thus, this study pointed to a poor prognosis in patients with symptomatic pericarditis.

Diagnosis of pericardial disease is based on clinical symptoms, physical findings, ECG or radiographic changes, and echocardiographic findings (see Chap. 34). Pericardiocentesis is rarely required unless the patient is hemodynamically compromised or febrile and an infectious etiology must be ruled out. Pericardial fluid tends to be serous with a wide range of leukocytosis [347]. Complements and immunoglobulins are normal in the pericardial fluid.

Valvular heart disease in SSc appears to be rare. There are case reports of isolated aortic regurgitation without evidence of prior rheumatic heart disease [348]. The prevalence of valvular abnormalities at autopsy, however, does not significantly differ from age-matched control groups [308].

Myocardial involvement is the most common cardiac finding in patients with SSc at autopsy, ranging from 12 to 89 percent [344]; however, symptomatic disease occurs less frequently than pericarditis. Pathologically, the most common findings are focal myocardial fibrosis that is equally distributed throughout the three layers of the heart as well as in both right and left ventricles. Contraction band necrosis is characterized histologically by transverse, dense, eosinophilic bands of contractile elements and subsequent replacement of myocardium with fibrosis. These lesions are usually associated with transient vessel occlusion followed by reperfusion and not with complete occlusion of extramural arteries. Bulkley and colleagues [349] reviewed

23 autopsies of SSc patients with myocardial fibrosis and found no evidence of extramural coronary artery occlusions. Others have noted increased small vessel abnormalities compared to controls at autopsy [308]. This has led to the hypothesis that small vessel vasospasm and fixed structural abnormalities may result in contraction band necrosis and subsequent myocardial fibrosis [349,350]. Alexander and associates demonstrated myocardial abnormalities by thallium perfusion scan, and echocardiography when peripheral vasoconstriction was induced in SSc patients [351]. This could not be reproduced in control subjects. Others have demonstrated improved myocardial perfusion on thallium scanning or echocardiography after pretreatment with calcium channel blockers [352,353]. This again seems to suggest a role of small vessel vasospasm in patients with SSc.

Clinically, myocardial disease may result in cardiomyopathy, congestive heart failure, angina, conduction abnormalities, or malignant arrhythmias. It has been well documented that from 2 to 60 percent of SSc patients will have resting ECG abnormalities [344]. Clements noted that 80 percent of SSc patients without cardiac symptoms had abnormalities in their resting ECG, chest radiograph, Holter monitor, or echocardiogram [354]. Electrophysiologic studies have revealed a high incidence of reentrant supraventricular tachyarrhythmias as well as atrioventricular conduction delays [355]. Ventricular tachycardia may occur in 10 to 13 percent of the patients and may be the etiology of sudden death in SSc [344,356]. Pathologically, advanced myocardial fibrosis rather than selective fibrosis of the conduction system appears to be responsible for conduction abnormalities and arrhythmias.

Evaluation of acutely ill SSc patients for suspected heart disease should include a routine ECG and chest radiograph. Echocardiography provides information regarding the pericardium, valvular function, ventricular systolic and diastolic function, chamber size, and wall thickness. Nuclear scanning may pick up subclinical myocardial disease; arteriography usually will be unremarkable unless the patient has risk factors for arteriosclerosis. Endomyocardial biopsies usually are not helpful if negative, because the pathologic process tends to be patchy. Electrophysiologic studies are helpful for patients who have sustained ventricular tachycardia, sudden cardiac arrest, or syncope of unclear etiology.

Treatment of SSc cardiac disease is tailored to the specific syndrome. Pericarditis can be treated with NSAIDs or low-dose corticosteroids. More aggressive therapy is reserved for the hemodynamically compromised patient. Diuresis should be pursued with caution in patients with large pericardial effusions. Renal failure has been reported in patients after vigorous diuresis, presumably secondary to hypovolemia superimposed on low cardiac output that resulted in decreased renal cortical blood flow [345]. Congestive heart failure symptoms are treated as outlined in Chapter 42. However, if echocardiography reveals evidence of diastolic dysfunction, angiotensin-converting enzyme (ACE) inhibitors or calcium channel blockers may be more appropriate than inotropic agents. As for prevention of progressive myocardial fibrosis, little is known about the efficacy of calcium channel blockers in preventing vasospastic changes or about the use of ACE inhibitors. Furthermore, the results of treatment with D-penicillamine or other agents for cardiac disease in SSc remains unknown.

RENAL DISEASE. In addition to cardiac and pulmonary involvement in diffuse scleroderma, significant morbidity and mortality result from renal disease. The onset of accelerated to malignant hypertension accompanied by signs of microangiopathic hemolytic anemia, hyperreninemia, and rapidly progressive renal failure describes a syndrome referred to as "sclero-

derma renal crisis" (SRC). Up to 15 percent of diffuse scleroderma patients may develop SRC [357]. SRC typically occurs early in the course of disease in patients with diffuse scleroderma, more commonly in the winter months and during the phase of illness accompanied by rapid progression of skin involvement.

Although the pathophysiology of SRC is unknown, several factors contribute to its evolution. Important factors include a change in the effective intravascular volume due to drug therapy (diuretics, calcium channel blockers, etc.), bleeding, or other intrinsic illness (diarrhea and subsequent dehydration); Raynaud's phenomenon affecting renal cortical blood flow; circulating humeral substances that may damage renal epithelium or affect intrarenal hemodynamics; structural or functional changes in the interlobular or arcuate arteries (endothelial cell proliferation, swelling, collagen deposition leading to luminal occlusion); and elevation of plasma renin activity [335]. The role of glucocorticoids in initiating this syndrome has been inconclusively debated. Current theory suggests that a reduction of blood flow to the renal cortex due in part to functional (Raynaud's phenomenon) or structural vascular changes leads to increased renin release, elevation of circulating and perhaps intrarenal angiotensin II (A II), exaggerated renal vasoconstriction, further reductions in renal cortical blood flow, and ultimately sustained hypertension and renal failure [300]. The potent vasoconstrictor A II increases peripheral vascular resistance, contributing to the development of systemic malignant hypertension, and also has intrarenal targets including the mesangial cells and afferent and efferent arterioles. Angiotensin II or similar substances have been implicated in the development of fixed structural lesions such as myointimal cell hypertrophy or hyperplasia, hyalinization of vessel wall media, or fibrinoid necrosis, findings observed in SRC. The compromised endothelium and vessel lumens are postulated to contribute to the development of a microangiopathic hemolytic anemia and thrombocytopenia characterized by elevation of fibrin degradation products, normal fibrinogen levels, reticulocytosis, and the presence of urinary hemosiderin. The urinary sediment is also frequently abnormal, containing small amounts of protein (1–2+ on dipstick evaluation) but typically no red blood cell casts. Without therapy, patients become progressively anuric and develop the systemic complications of sustained or malignant hypertension, including renal failure.

The diagnosis of SRC should be strongly considered in the scleroderma patient with accelerated hypertension, particularly in the ICU setting. Subtle early signs of scleroderma such as sclerodactyly, pitting in the pulp or pad of the digits, proximal scleroderma, or skin thickening above the level of the metacarpophalangeal joints should suggest the diagnosis. Examination of peripheral blood smears may help to rapidly confirm the syndrome of SRC, which in the context of hypertension reveals a microangiopathic process. Virtually all patients with SRC have elevated plasma renin activity, although serial tests of renin levels in patients with scleroderma are not predictive of the onset of this syndrome [358].

In the past, accelerated uncontrollable hypertension in patients with SRC has led to the suggestion that bilateral nephrectomy might be lifesaving. Since the discovery of ACE inhibitors, however, there is evidence to suggest that conservation of and improvement in renal function are possible. Case reports have documented reversal of dialysis-dependent renal failure and return to near-normal kidney function [359]. It is now clear that this class of drugs should be employed as the standard of care in SRC. There are three available ACE inhibitors in the United States including enalapril, captopril, and lisinopril. These agents work by inhibition of ACE with a resultant fall in vascular resistance and blood pressure. Kininase II, responsible in part for the metabolism of bradykinin, is also inhibited by these agents. The combination of a calcium channel blocker (nifedipine) and an ACE inhibitor may provide improved blood pressure control potentially by blunting the peripheral effect of A II on vascular smooth muscle [359]. In many patients treated with ACE inhibitors there may be a transient reduction in glomerular filtration rate and a rise in serum creatinine. Continuation of therapy with ACE inhibitors and calcium channel blockers is recommended as recovery of renal function may take months. The prognosis of patients with SRC has not been well defined, although survival has vastly improved with the availability of more refined and potent pharmacologic agents for blood pressure control.

GASTROINTESTINAL DISEASE. Gastrointestinal involvement is common in SSc with various studies reporting 50 to 80 percent of patients affected [359a]. The most common physiological abnormalities, esophageal dysmotility and decreased lower esophageal sphincter pressure, are manifested by symptoms of dysphagia and heartburn respectively. Pathologically, impaired microvascular perfusion initially alters myoelectrical function of the smooth muscle layer [359b]. In later stages, the persistent decreased perfusion results in fibrosis replacing the muscularis, submucosa, and lamina propria of the esophagus. Although most of the symptoms can be symptomatically treated, serious complications include erosive gastritis with upper gastrointestinal bleeding, Barrett's esophagus, and strictures. Gastric involvement is less common but can include gastric atony with symptomatic outlet obstruction. Telangectasias may rarely bleed.

Patients with small intestinal involvement may present with malabsorption symptoms of bloating, cramping, and intermittent or severe diarrhea. Hypomotility due to progressive smooth muscle atrophy and fibrosis results in bacterial overgrowth. In addition, adynamic ileus or pseudoobstruction may occur. Rarely, complication include volvulus, perforation, or pneumatosis intestinalis cystoides (ruptured cysts resulting in pneumoperitoneum) [359c].

Colonic involvement usually occurs in conjunction with small bowel abnormalities. Although barium studies reveal widemouth sacculations or diverticulae on the antimesenteric border, most patients have relatively few symptoms. Rare complications include obstruction due to fecal impaction, megacolon, and volvulus of the transverse colon [300].

Treatment of esophageal disease includes various antireflux measures, antacids, sulcrafate at bedtime, and H2 blockers for documented peptic esophagitis. Recently cisapride, a prokinetic agent [359d] and intravenous erythromycin have been reported to be useful in treatment of upper GI disease. Intestinal involvement has been treated with antibiotics, low-residue diets, medium-chain triglycerides, and total parenteral nutrition. Soudah reported improvement in bacterial overgrowth and abdominal symptoms with octreotide in a small group of SSc patients with intestinal disease [359e].

Polymyositis and Dermatomyositis

Polymyositis (PM) is a progressive inflammatory disease of muscle that presents with limb girdle weakness. Inflammatory myositis associated with skin disease is termed dermatomyositis (DM). A number of syndromes are recognized under the broad heading of polymyositis. Classification schemes based on clinical symptoms or disease associations have been developed that classify patients into (1) idiopathic PM, (2) idiopathic DM (myositis and characteristic rash), (3) myositis with symptoms of other connective tissue diseases (overlap group), (4) PM/DM of childhood, and (5) myositis associated with malignancy [360]. Another group has been suggested that consists of several less commonly encountered forms of myopathy (Table 219A-4) [361,362,363]. Other forms of inflammatory myopathy are associated with the use of certain drugs (Table 219A-5), infections (Table 219A-6), or other immunological or connective tissue disorders (Table 219A-7).

PM and DM are primarily disorders of skeletal muscle, but it is now clear that visceral organs may be affected. Disease can involve the pulmonary, cardiac, articular, GI, or vascular systems leading to catastrophic illness requiring support in an ICU. Moreover, organ dysfunction may occur in patients without "overlap syndromes." Respiratory failure, cardiac abnormalities, renal insuffficiency, or comorbidity related to immunosuppression are the most common reasons for ICU admission. Because a complete discussion of the presentation, diagnosis, management, and differential diagnosis is beyond the scope of this chapter, please refer to references 364–392.

PULMONARY INVOLVEMENT. Dickey and Myers retrospectively reviewed the pulmonary manifestations of PM/DM in 42 patients. Interstitial lung disease (10%), respiratory insufficiency due to muscle weakness (7%) (intercostal or diaphragmatic muscles), aspiration pneumonia (14%), opportunistic pneumonia (5%), pneumonia from neither aspiration nor opportunistic infection (10%), and concurrent diseases (10%) were described [371]. In other series, pulmonary vasculitis, pulmonary edema, primary pulmonary malignancy, diffuse alveolar damage, fibrinous pleuritis, pulmonary emboli, and diaphragmatic atrophy have been reported. Dyspnea, cough, and chest pain are among the clinical complaints described. Interstitial lung disease is postulated to be immunologically mediated. It presents clinically as progressive dyspnea with or without a nonproductive cough, bibasilar rales, bibasilar reticulonodular infiltrates that may lead to a ground-glass appearance on chest roentgenogram, shrinking lung volumes, and a reduced diffusing capacity on pulmonary function testing. Recent reports have described the association of interstitial lung disease with the antibody Jo-1. Patients with the Jo-1 antibody also have a high prevalence of arthritis, sicca syndrome, Raynaud's phenomenon, and sclerodactyly. Frequently, their disease course is dominated by respiratory insufficiency. Interstitial lung disease is managed primarily with respiratory support and immunosuppression (see Immunosuppressive Therapy) [372].

Bronchopneumonia occurs in PM/DM due to a combination of pharyngeal incompetence leading to poor protection of the airway and subsequent aspiration pneumonitis, iatrogenic immunosuppression, and often a weakened cough. Microbiologic studies reveal a broad range of etiologic agents including virulent bacteria and opportunistic organisms (Table 219A-8). The recognition that AIDs may manifest as PM/DM enlarges the possible spectrum of infectious agents that may be seen [373,374,375]. Hence, respiratory symptoms should be evaluated aggressively with chest roentgenograms and routine and specialized microbiologic techniques (culture for bacteria, mycobacteria, fungi, etc., and smears for *Pneumocystis carinii*).

Respiratory failure from intercostal muscle weakness or diaphragmatic dysfunction has been reported but is unusual in PM and DM. In patients with respiratory symptoms, however, pulmonary mechanics should be evaluated (spirometry, inspiratory force). Serial measurements are often predictive of impending respiratory failure that might necessitate intubation and mechanical ventilation. The management of respiratory failure resulting from muscle weakness should be both supportive (oxygen, mechanical ventilation) and accompanied by therapy directed at the underlying myositis. (See Chap. 58 on extrapulmonary causes of respiratory failure.)

MYOCARDIAL INVOLVEMENT. Cardiac involvement in PM/DM has been recognized since 1899 and is now thought to be the third leading cause of death, following sepsis and malignancy [362,365]. As many as 76 percent of patients studied prospectively have a definable cardiac abnormality (on electrocardiography, phonocardiography, echocardiography, or nuclear medicine evaluation; Table 219A-9) [376]. Accumulated evidence suggests that myocardial inflammation is part of the PM/DM syndrome. The extent to which any abnormality is iatrogenic or arises as a complication of the disease is unclear. For example, steroid therapy results in accelerated atherosclerosis, hypertension, diabetes mellitus, and electrolyte disturbances and, when administered chronically, may decrease cardiac contractility, thereby contributing to the development of myocardial infarction, arrhythmias, or a congestive cardiomyopathy. Similarly, hypoxia from pulmonary involvement contributes to arrhythmias, axis shifts, and strain patterns on electrocardiography. Inflammatory myocardial injury leads to focal myonecrosis, interstitial edema, round cell infiltration, and patchy fibrosis of both the myocardium and conducting tissue. Progression of a normal electrocardiogram to complete heart block over a 4-year period has been reported [377]. The most common site of fibrous replacement of the conducting tissue is the distal His bundle and its branches. Valvular abnormalities are largely confined to the mitral valve. The presence of a cardiomyopathy presents difficult diagnostic and therapeutic challenges and may require transthoracic right-sided endomyocardial biopsy for appropriate diagnosis. Although atypical, myocardial disease may be present and may progress when there is little evidence of active skeletal muscle inflammation. The presence of significant elevations of the isoenzyme creatine kinase CK MB fraction should signify the possibility of ongoing myocardial inflammation due to PM/DM and prompt a careful evaluation including electrocardiography, echocardiography, and other studies as clinically indicated (e.g., extended monitoring for arrhythmias, thallium scanning). The antibody Ro (anti SS-A) has been identified as a marker for underlying cardiac disease in PM/DM, reported in as many as 69 percent of patients [378]. Therapy must be tailored to each patient's problem(s) in concert with immunosuppression for the underlying PM/DM.

RENAL INVOLVEMENT. Renal failure and its attendant metabolic abnormalities are the result of rhabdomyolysis, myoglobinemia, subsequent myoglobinuria, and renal insufficiency [372]. Myoglobinuric renal failure is rare but tends to occur in patients with acute or hyperacute presentations, as a result of widespread muscle necrosis and release of sarcoplasmic materials including myoglobin. Therapy is directed toward the underlying muscle disease while maintaining an adequate urinary output.

ARTICULAR INVOLVEMENT. The presence of arthritis in a febrile ICU patient with PM/DM should raise concern for infection either within the joint or as a peripheral manifestation of endocarditis or of hepatitis. Despite this it is important to recognize that arthralgia or arthritis occurs in 17 to 68 percent of patients. Arthritis is typically symmetrical and nonerosive, affecting the proximal interphalangeal, metacarpophalangeal wrist, and knee joints [379,380]. Carpal tunnel syndrome occurs in some patients with wrist involvement [380]. Synovial fluid analysis reveals leukocyte counts ranging from 650 to 5280 cells/μl, which are predominantly small lymphocytes. Joint subluxation and periarticular calcifications in association with synovitis have also been described. The latter is postulated to result from calcium hydroxyapatite deposition [380].

MALIGNANCY. The relationship of PM/DM to malignancy is controversial. Historically, the risk of developing an associated malignancy has been considered high. More recent studies suggest it has been overstated (380a,380b). In Scandinavia, the relative risk for malignancy was 1.8 for men and 1.7 for women with PM and 2.4 for men and 3.4 for women with DM (380b). The presence of a low CK or a rash, particularly vasculitis, confers a higher risk while patients with overlap syndromes are not as often affected. Despite the appreciation of an increased risk of malignancy, a thorough physical examination and routine health screening is recommended rather than widespread undirected evaluations. Special attention should be paid to the head and neck and testis in young men; breast and gynecological areas in young women. Note that Orientals have a higher incidence of nasopharyngeal cancer.

Eosinophilia Myalgia Syndrome

In 1989, a disorder, eosinophilia myalgia syndrome (EMS) characterized by the development of intense myalgias, various skin rashes, edema, dyspnea, constitutional symptoms and high levels of blood eosinophils (>1000/μl) was described in patients taking large amounts of tryptophan, an oral amino acid supplement used to treat insomnia, premenstrual syndrome, depression, and chronic pain disorders (392a). Many patients developed pulmonary symptoms including dyspnea, hemoptysis, and cough; cardiac symptoms such as chest pain and palpitations; GI symptoms such as nausea, vomiting, abdominal pain, and hematochezia; sclerodermatous skin changes; neurologic abnormalities including proximal myopathy, carpal tunnel syndrome and distal neuropathies; vasculopathy and vasculitis; and articular abnormalities including arthralgia and arthritis. The majority of affected individuals were white females (96% white, 85% female). Careful epidemiologic and biochemical studies point to a contaminant, not tryptophan, as the etiologic agent for EMS. Drug lots that produced this disorder consistently demonstrated the presence of a single peak, peak E, on high-performance liquid chromatography, subsequently determined to be 1,1'-ethylidenebis (tryptophan).

The immune system is activated in EMS, resulting in the release of cytokines, which stimulate the eosinophil (IL-5), activate T cells (increases in circulating CD4+), and stimulate fibroblast collagen production (TGF beta). Eosinophil contents, such as eosinophil basic protein and eosinophil-derived neurotoxin (damages myelinated neurons), and leukotriene C4 (a potent vasoconstrictor) may all be important in disease pathogenesis. Quinolinic acid, a neurotoxic metabolite, and 5-hydroxytryptamine, both products of tryptophan metabolism, may also play a role in EMS.

Blood tests are nondiagnostic, other than detecting eosinophilia. A significant population of patients will have positive antinuclear antibodies, making it important to exclude SLE diagnostically.

Treatment of EMS has been difficult. In the early phase of disease, corticosteroids have been effective in reducing edema and eosinophilia; however, other multisystemic manifestations, such as cutaneous and neurologic aspects of disease, often progress without a known cure.

Nonsteroidal Antiinflammatory Drugs

Nonsteroidal antiinflammatory drugs (NSAIDs) are the cornerstone of therapy in patients with rheumatic diseases. Numerous NSAIDs are currently available, and a rational approach to their use is indicated. Please refer to Chapters 154 and 215 for complete discussion of NSAIDs.

Corticosteroid Therapy

Although nonsteroidal antiinflammatory medications are drugs of choice in the initial treatment of nonseptic inflammatory joint disease, corticosteroids are more effective for the vasculitides and in inflammatory, multisystem autoimmune diseases such as SLE. The physiology and mechanism of action of corticosteroids are beyond the scope of this chapter.

Exogenous corticosteroids at an equivalent dose of prednisone 5.0–7.5 mg/day will inhibit the hypothalamic-pituitary-adrenal (HPA) axis. Thus, patients who are on corticosteroids chronically will require increased "stress" doses when situations such as surgery, sepsis, trauma, or other serious medical complications occur. Pharmacologically, various preparations of corticosteroids are available, which differ in potency, half-life, and mineralocorticoid activity. In the ICU, typical corticosteroids employed are hydrocortisone, methylprednisolone, and prednisone. There are few indications to use the long-acting corticosteroids, such as dexamethasone, in the rheumatic patient. Corticosteroids are primarily bound by transcortin. Once supraphysiologic doses are given, however, most of the binding will be by albumin. If a patient has hypoalbuminemia, a greater percentage of steroid will be free, thus increasing both the antiinflammatory effects and toxicities. Because corticosteroids are metabolized by the liver, the concomitant administration of drugs that increase hepatic microsomal enzyme activity (phenytoin, barbiturates, etc.) will also accelerate corticosteroid metabolism.

Corticosteroids are both antiinflammatory and immunosuppressive. These effects are dependent on the dose and frequency of administration. For example, 20 mg of prednisone tid is a more potent immunosuppressive than one 60 mg/day dose. Some toxicities are also dose dependent. Most patients are very conscious of the physical changes produced by corticosteroids, particularly a cushingoid appearance, acne, hirsutism, and easy bruising. However, the metabolic, psychiatric, immunologic, ophthalmologic, gastrointestinal, and musculoskeletal changes are more concerning and contribute to morbidity and mortality. Some of these complications do not develop for several years. In particular, avascular necrosis often occurs at a time remote from the initiation of corticosteroids. Although some patients (SLE, obese, alcoholic) are more susceptible to avascular necrosis, it is difficult to determine if the duration and dose of corticosteroid is the more important risk factor. Thus, physicians must weigh carefully the potential risks and benefits before initiating corticosteroid therapy.

The dosage and mode of administration of corticosteroids depend on the clinical situation. In rheumatoid patients without evidence of vasculitis, joint symptoms may be controlled with less than 10 mg/day of prednisone. In contrast, a patient with newly diagnosed dermatomyositis will require high-dose prednisone (1.0 mg/kg/day) generally in three divided doses. The more usual situation in the ICU is the patient with multisystem involvement from SLE or vasculitis. High-dose parenteral methylprednisolone may be initiated at 50–100 mg/day [393].

If patients fail conventional high-dose steroids (i.e., 1.0–1.5 mg/kg/day), pulse intravenous methylprednisolone at 1–2 g/day has been advocated [394,395]. This regimen requires infusion over 30 minutes and is repeated daily for 3 consecutive days. Pulse intravenous methylprednisolone may produce minor side effects such as metallic taste, facial flushing, transient hypertension, and hyperglycemia. More significant (but rare) toxicities include seizures, anaphylaxis, intractable hiccoughs, arrhythmias, hemiplegia, psychosis, and sudden death [396,397,398]. In four reported deaths, patients were receiving furosemide concurrently. Theories on the mechanism of death include an electrolyte imbalance resulting in cardiac arrhythmias, cardiovascular collapse due to hypovolemia and vasodilation, and anaphylaxis [399]. Data are limited on the actual mechanism of action by pulse methylprednisolone in suppressing SLE or vasculitis activity. In addition, the long-term toxicities are unknown. Thus, these factors must be weighed against the patient's clinical status.

High-dose divided daily corticosteroids should be tapered to daily doses within 4–6 weeks. If disease activity remains controlled, further tapering to 30 mg/day should be attempted. Switching to alternate-day steroids will reduce or prevent Cushing's syndrome and reduce hypothalamic-pituitary-adrenal axis suppression. This regimen, however, does not prevent steroid-induced osteopenia. If the patient fails to improve with high-dose or pulse corticosteroids, the addition of other immunosuppressive agents must be considered.

Immunosuppressive Therapy

Immunosuppressive agents were initially used in rheumatic diseases as steroid-sparing agents. More recently, there is convincing evidence that these agents can produce dramatic improvement or induce remission in many patients [125,400]. Although various agents have been studied, the most common drugs employed include cyclophosphamide, azathioprine, and methotrexate.

All the immunosuppressive agents interfere with the cell cycle. Cytotoxic effects occur through the inhibition of cell division. Azathioprine, a purine analogue, prevents the biosynthesis of the purine bases, adenine and guanine. Methotrexate inhibits dihydrofolate reductase, an enzyme that forms tetrahydrofolate. By preventing the formation of tetrahydrofolate, thymidilic and inosinic acid are not available for DNA synthesis. Cyclophosphamide is an alkylating agent that binds to DNA and thus prevents cell replication. It is presumed that in the autoimmune diseases, pathogenic cells are inhibited along with those of the bone marrow, skin, mucosal surfaces, and hair follicles. However, McCune and Fox recently described selective rather than global inhibition of T-cell function by high-dose intravenous pulse cyclophosphamide in SLE patients [401]. In addition, autoantibody production is suppressed.

Azathioprine is absorbed from the GI tract and metabolized by the liver to 6-mercaptopurine and subsequently to active and inactive metabolites. The latter are excreted in the urine, but it is unclear whether accumulation of these metabolites in renal insufficiency or failure increases toxicities. Cyclophosphamide is also metabolized by the liver to several active and

Table 219-4. Frequency of Toxicity of Cytotoxic Drugs (When Used in the Dosages Commonly Used in the Rheumatic Diseases

Toxicity	Azathioprine	Cyclophosphamide	Chlorambucil	Methotrexate
Toxicity common to all cytotoxic agents				
Dose-related marrow suppression				
Leukopenia	+ +	+ + to + + +	+ + to + + +	+ to + +
Thrombocytopenia	+ to + +	+	+ +	+ to + +
Susceptibility to infection	+	+	+ +	+ to + +
GI tolerance	+ +	+ +	+	+ +
Rash	+	+ +	+ +	+
Toxicity not shared by all drugs				
Hepatic damage	+	0	0	+ to + + (M)
Oral ulcers	0	0	0	+ +
Hair loss	0	+ + +	+ to + +	+ to + +
Azospermia	0	+ + +	+ +	Uncertain
Anovulation	0	+ + +	+ +	Uncertain
Cystitis (hemorrhagic, fibrotic)	0	+ + (M)	0	0
Teratogenesis	0	+ (M)	+ (M)	+ + + (M)
Neoplasia	Uncertain	Probable (M)	Probable (M)	0
Pneumonitis pulmonary fibrosis	±	±	±	±

Abbreviations: 0, considered not to occur; ± may occur but very rarely; +, occurs but usually in <5% of patients; + +, occurs in >5% of patients; + + +, occurs very frequently (>30–40%); (M), adverse experience of major concern.
Source: From Clements PJ, Davis J: Cytotoxic drugs: Their clinical application to rheumatic diseases. *Semin Arthritis Rheum* 15:231, 1986, with permission.

inactive compounds that are also excreted in the urine. Reports have varied on the effects of hepatic or renal insufficiency on toxicity [402].

Toxicities common to all immunosuppressive agents include bone marrow suppression with leukopenia, especially granulocytopenia (Table 219-4). Anemia and thrombocytopenia usually occur in conjunction with leukopenia but rarely alone. The nadir of the white blood cell (WBC) counts occurs usually 7–14 days after a single dose; recovery occurs within 21–25 days [403]. Infections secondary to immunosuppression may occur with any drug but may not necessarily correlate with the degree of leukopenia, duration of drug therapy, or concomitant corticosteroid therapy [404]. Gastrointestinal irritation and skin rashes may occur with any of the agents.

More specific toxicities of azathioprine include hypersensitivity hepatitis characterized by elevated transaminases and cholestasis. These abnormalities usually resolve after drug discontinuation. Irreversible damage, however, has been reported [405]. Pancreatitis has also been associated with azathioprine. Azoospermia, anovulation, and teratogenesis are unusual. It is uncertain whether neoplasia occurs at a greater incidence in rheumatic patients treated with azathioprine as compared with cancer patients who received azathioprine [406,407]. However, follow-up of the 111 SLE patients followed at the NIH for lupus nephritis on various cytotoxic regimens revealed malignancies in three of the 19 patients who received azathioprine [124].

Cyclophosphamide has much greater potential for toxicities than azathioprine. Although hepatotoxicity is rare, nausea and vomiting with intravenous cyclophosphamide are common. Both oral and intravenous regimens produce gonadal dysfunction in men and women due to injury to germinal epithelium [408]. Azoospermia in males [409] and amenorrhea in premenopausal women [410] may be permanent with periods of cyclophosphamide therapy of a year or longer. Sperm banking for men should be considered before initiating cyclophosphamide therapy. Teratogenesis is well documented in the literature [411]. Malignancy is a significant complication of oral cyclophosphamide therapy. In the previously mentioned NIH study, three of the 18 patients who received oral cyclophosphamide developed malignancies. Other studies have reported a malignancy rate of 25 percent in patients who received cyclophos-

phamide when compared with control group rates of 5 to 13 percent [412,413].

Hemorrhagic cystitis occurs in 20 to 30 percent of patients receiving oral cyclophosphamide [403]. The mechanism is believed to be due to acrolein, a metabolite of cyclophosphamide, or other metabolites. Bladder carcinoma occurs in 10 percent of patients who receive long-term cyclophosphamide therapy [414]. Intravenous bolus cyclophosphamide may have fewer bladder complications than the oral regimen. In the NIH study on treatment of lupus nephritis, none of the 20 patients who received intravenous cyclophosphamide developed acute bladder complications [124]. The intravenous route may reduce the development of hemorrhage cystitis by inactivating the oxazophosphorine metabolite of cyclosphosphamide that irritates the bladder mucosa [415]. One mesna regimen is 0.5 mg of intravenous mesna for every 1 mg of intravenous cyclophosphamide just before the cyclophosphamide infusion and then 0.5 mg of intravenous mesna for every 1 mg of IV cyclophosphamide 2 hr after the cyclophosphamide infusion [416]. Another regimen is to give mesna in a dose of 20 to 40 percent in milligrams of the milligram dose of cyclophosphamide 15 minutes before then every 3 hours for 3 to 4 doses after the cyclophosphamide infusion [417].

Other toxicities of cyclophosphamide include cardiomyopathy at dosages greater than 100 mg/kg during 48 hours [402], pulmonary fibrosis [418], and hepatotoxicity [419]. *Pneumocystis carinii* pneumonia has also occurred in patients with autoimmune diseases who have been treated with cyclophosphamide and steroids in the setting of lymphopenia but adequate granulocytes [420].

Cytotoxic drugs should be initiated in patients with life-threatening or potentially crippling diseases that have failed to respond to conventional therapy. In addition, the patient should have reversible lesions in contrast to end-stage renal failure or class IV rheumatoid arthritis. There should be no evidence of active infection at the start of cytotoxic therapy. A PPD should be placed to evaluate for infection with mycobacteria. If it is positive, some physicians advocate treating with isoniazid, whereas others follow with serial chest radiographs. Once therapy is initiated, laboratory studies need to be monitored carefully.

Low-dose, weekly methotrexate has become established therapy for rheumatoid arthritis and in 1988 was approved by the Food and Drug Administration (US) for this indication. Methotrexate interferes with DNA synthesis by inactivating dihydrofolate reductose and thereby inhibiting the synthesis of thymidylate, but the mechanism of action of low-dose methotrexate in rheumatoid arthritis is unknown. Methotrexate and its metabolites are excreted by the kidney. The dosages generally used to treat rheumatoid arthritis range from 7.5–20 mg weekly given as a single intramuscular injection or oral dose or oral dose divided and taken over 24 hours [421].

The most common adverse reactions are nausea, vomiting, anorexia, diarrhea, and weight loss [422]. Stomatitis may occur and may vary in severity. Alopecia, sensitivity to ultraviolet light result in erythema, urticaria, and cutaneous vasculitis may occur [422].

Major toxicities of methotrexate involve the hematologic system, lungs, and liver. Leukopenia, thrombocytopenia, megaloblastic anemia, and pancytopenia rarely occur. Predisposing factors for hematologic toxicity includes concomitant use of trimethoprim/sulfamethoxazole [423,424], renal insufficiency, viral infections, folic acid deficiency, and concurrent use of probenacid. For a methotrexate overdose or elevation of the mean corpuscular volume (which may indicate methotrexate toxicity), folinic acid, leucovocin, in a dose equal to the methotrexate dose q4–6 h should be given until the serum methotrexate level is no longer detectable [421].

Pulmonary toxicity of methotrexate generally is manifested by dyspnea, fever, nonproductive cough associated with headaches and malaise and bilateral interestitial infiltrates. Pathology consists of inflammatory infiltrates of mononuclear cells, grant cells, granuloma formation, bronchiolitis, and fibrosis which may progress [425,426]. Treatment consists of respiratory support, discontinuation of methotrexate, and corticosteroids.

Opportunistic infections including *Pneumocystis carinii* pneumonia, cryptococcosis, and disseminated herpes zoster have also occurred with low-dose, weekly methotrexate therapy for rheumatoid arthritis [427,428,429]. Methotrexate appears also to increase the risk of postoperative infectious complications [430]. A potential long-term toxicity of methotrexate is hepatic fibrosis [421].

The use of oral and intravenous cyclophosphamide has already been discussed in the sections on rheumatoid arthritis, Wegener's granulomatosis, and lupus nephritis. Azathioprine is usually administered at 1–3 mg/kg/day orally. A hematologic profile is obtained every week to every other week for the first 2 months. If the total leukocyte count is lower than 3500 and the platelet count is lower than 100,000, azathioprine should be held until counts are above the cut-off levels. Once the counts normalize, azathioprine can be restarted at 50 to 75 percent of the original dose, and subsequent adjustments are made within the parameters given. Liver function tests should be obtained at regular intervals of 1–2 months. If a patient develops renal failure, the dose should be reduced by 50 percent [403]. The effects of azathioprine are markedly potentiated by allopurinol therapy requiring a reduction in dosage by approximately 75 percent. Careful monitoring can prevent significant morbidity and even mortality.

References

1. Zvaifler NJ: The immunopathology of joint inflammation in rheumatoid arthritis. *Adv Immunol* 16:265, 1973.
1a. Goronzy JJ, Weyand CM. Interplay of T lymphocytes and HLA-DR molecules in rheumatoid arthritis. *Curr Opin Rheumatol* 51:169, 1993.

2. Harris ED: Pathogenesis of rheumatoid arthritis, in Kelly WM, Harris ED, Ruddy S, Sledge CB, (eds): *Textbook of Rheumatology,* 3rd ed. Philadelphia, Saunders, 1989, p 905.
3. Goldenberg DL: Infectious arthritis complicating rheumatoid arthritis and other chronic rheumatic disorders. *Arthritis Rheum* 32:496, 1989.
4. Goldenberg DL, Reed JI: Bacterial arthritis. *N Engl J Med* 312:764, 1985.
5. Myers AR, Miller LM, Pinals RS: Pyarthrosis complicating rheumatoid arthritis. *Lancet* 2:714, 1969.
6. Karten I: Septic arthritis complicating rheumatoid arthritis. *Ann Intern Med* 70:1147, 1969.
7. Huskisson EC, Hart FD: Severe, unusual and recurrent infections in rheumatoid arthritis. *Ann Rheum Dis* 31:118, 1972.
8. Turner RA, Schumacher R, Meyers AR: Phagocytic function of polymorphonuclear leukocytes in rheumatic diseases. *J Clin Invest* 52:1632, 1973.
9. Mowat AG, Baum J: Chemotaxis of polymorphonuclear leukocytes from patients with rheumatoid arthritis. *J Clin Invest* 50:2541, 1971.
10. Pruzanski W, Leers WD, Wardlaw AC: Bacteriolytic and bactericidal activity of sera and synovial fluids in rheumatoid arthritis and osteoarthritis. *Arthritis Rheum* 17:207, 1974.
11. Hollander JL: Intrasynovial corticosteroid therapy in arthritis. *Md State Med J* 19:62, 1970.
12. Gowans JD, Graieri PA: Septic arthritis: Its relation to intra-articular injections of hydrocortisone acetate. *N Engl J Med* 261:502, 1959.
13. Goldenberg DL, Cohen AS: Acute infectious arthritis: A review of patients with non-gonococcal joint infections (with emphasis on therapy and prognosis). *Am J Med* 60:369, 1976.
14. Kelly PJ, Martin WJ, Coventry MB: Bacterial (suppurative) arthritis in the Adult. *J Bone Joint Surg* 52A:1595, 1970.
15. Newman JH: Review of septic arthritis throughout the antibiotic era. *Ann Rheum Dis* 35:198, 1976.
16. Kraft SM, Panush RS, Longley S: Unrecognized staphylococcal pyarthrosis with rheumatoid arthritis. *Semin Arthritis Rheum* 14:196, 1985.
17. Keroack MA, Weinstein L: Infectious disease emergencies in rheumatoid arthritis, in Blau SP (ed): *Emergencies in Rheumatoid Arthritis*. Mount Kisco, NY, Futura, 1986, p 37.
18. Bayer AS, Chow AW, Louie JS, et al: Gram negative bacillary septic arthritis: Clinical, radiographic, therapeutic, and prognostic features. *Semin Arthritis Rheum* 7:123, 1977.
19. Goldenberg DL, Brandt KD, Cohen AS, et al: Treatment of septic arthritis: Comparison of needle aspiration and surgery as initial modes of joint drainage. *Arthritis Rheum* 18:83, 1975.
20. Gristina AG, Rovere GD, Shoji H: Spontaneous septic arthritis complicating rheumatoid arthritis. *J Bone Joint Surg* 56A:1180, 1984.
21. Gristina AG, Kolkin J: Current concept review: Total joint replacement and sepsis. *J Bone Joint Surg* 65A:128, 1983.
22. Rand JA, Morrey BF, Bryan RS: Management of the infected total joint arthroplasty. *Orthop Clin North Am* 15:491, 1984.
23. Andrews HJ, Arden GP, Hart GM, Owen JW: Deep infection after total hip replacement. *J Bone Joint Surg* 63B:53, 1981.
24. Poss R, Thornhill TS, Ewald FC, et al: Factors influencing the incidence and outcome of infection following total joint arthroplasty. *Clin Orthop* 182:117, 1984.
25. Milney GB, Scheller AD, Turner RH: Medical and surgical treatment of the septic hip with one-stage revision arthroplasty. *Clin Orthop* 170:76, 1982.
26. Rosenthall L, Lisbona R, Hernandez M, Hadjipavlou A: 99mTc-PP and 67 Ga imaging following insertion of orthopedic devices. *Radiology* 133:717, 1979.
27. Fitzgerald RH, Nolan DR, Ilstrup DM, et al: Deep wound sepsis following total hip arthroplasty. *J Bone Joint Surg* 59A:847, 1977.
28. Inman RD, Gallegos KV, Brause BD, et al: Clinical and microbial features of prosthetic joint infections. *Am J Med* 77:47, 1984.
29. Carlsson AS, Josefsson G, Lindberg L: Revision with gentamicin-impregnated cement for deep infection in total hip arthroplasties. *J Bone Joint Surg* 60A:1059, 1978.
30. Walker WC, Wright V: Pulmonary lesions and rheumatoid arthritis. *Medicine* (Baltimore) 47:501, 1968.

31. Hunningshake GW, Fauci AS: Pulmonary involvement in the collagen vascular disease. *Am Rev Respir Dis* 119:471, 1979.

32. Geddes DM, Corrin B, Brewerton DA, et al: Progressive airway obliteration in adults and its association with rheumatoid disease. *Q J Med* 46:427, 1977.

33. Giraldo B, Blumenthal MN, Spink WW: Aspirin intolerance and asthma. A clinical and immunologic study. *Ann Intern Med* 71:479, 1969.

34. Szczeklik A, Gryglewski RJ, Czerniawska-Mysik G, et al: Asthmatic attacks induced in aspirin-sensitive patients by diclofenac and naproxen. *Br Med J* 2:231, 1977.

35. Levinson ML, Lynch JP, Bower JS: Reversal of progressive, life-threatening gold hypersensitivity pneumonitis by corticosteroids. *Am J Med* 71:908, 1981.

36. Sostman HD, Matthay RA, Putnam CE, et al: Methotrexate-induced pneumonitis. *Medicine* (Baltimore) 55:371, 1976.

37. Gibson T, Burry HC, Ogg C: Letter: Goodpasture syndrome and D-penicillamine. *Ann Intern Med* 84:100, 1976.

38. Penny WJ, Knight RK, Rees AM, et al: Obliterative bronchiolitis in rheumatoid arthritis. *Ann Rheum Dis* 41:469, 1982.

39. Chalmers A, Traynor JA: Cricoarytenoid arthritis as a cause of acute upper airway obstruction. *J Rheumatol* 6:541, 1979.

40. Tozman EC, Gottlieb NL: Respiratory emergencies and rheumatoid arthritis, in Blau SP (ed): *Emergencies in Rheumatoid Arthritis*. Mount Kisco, NY, Futura, 1986, p 252.

41. Sladek GD, Vasey FB, Saraceno C., et al: Letter: Beclomethasone dipropionate in the treatment of rheumatoid larynx. *J Rheumatol* 10:518, 1983.

42. Davis SF, Iber D: Obstructive sleep apnea associated with adult-acquired micrognathia from rheumatoid arthritis. *Am Rev Respir Dis* 127:245, 1983.

43. Shiel WC Jr, Prete PE: Pleuropulmonary manifestations of rheumatoid arthritis. *Semin Arthritis Rheum* 13:235, 1984.

44. Jones FL Jr, Blodgett RC Jr: Letter: Empyema and rheumatoid pleuropulmonary disease. *Ann Intern Med* 89:139, 1978.

45. Jones FL, Blodgett RC Jr: Empyema in rheumatoid pleuropulmonary disease. *Ann Intern Med* 74:665, 1971.

46. Shiel SAR, Hunder GG, McDuffie FC, Hepper NG: Pleural fluid complement in systemic lupus erythematosus and rheumatoid arthritis. *Ann Intern Med* 76:357, 1972.

47. Brunk JR, Drash EC, Swindford O Jr: Rheumatoid pleuritis successfully treated with decortication. Report of a case and review of the literature. *Am J Med Sci* 251:545, 1966.

47a. Chapman PT, O'Donnell JL, Moller PW: Rheumatoid pleural effusion: Response to intrapleural corticosteroid. *J Rheumatol* 19:478, 1992.

48. Roschman RA, Rothenberg RJ: Pulmonary fibrosis in rheumatoid arthritis: A review of the clinical features and therapy. *Semin Arthritis Rheum* 16:174, 1987.

49. Frank ST, Weg JG, Harkleroad LE, et al: Pulmonary dysfunction in rheumatoid disease. *Chest* 63:27, 1973.

50. Hollingsworth JW, Saykaly RJ: Systemic complications of rheumatoid arthritis. *Med Clin North Am* 61:217, 1977.

51. Kay JM, Banik S: Unexplained pulmonary hypertension with pulmonary arteritis in rheumatoid disease. *Br J Dis Chest* 71:53, 1977.

52. King TE Jr: Bronchiolitis obliterans: Keys to diagnosis and management. *Immunol Allergy Pract* 11:17, 1989.

53. Veys EM, Gabriel PA, Coigne E, et al: Rheumatoid factor and serum IgG, IgM and IgA levels in rheumatoid arthritis with vasculitis. *Scand J Rheumatol* 5:1, 1976.

54. Brigham KL: Salicylate-induced pulmonary edema. *Pract Cardiol* 8:71, 1982.

55. Heffner JE, Sahn SA: Salicylate-induced pulmonary edema. Clinical features and prognosis. *Ann Intern Med* 95:405, 1981.

56. Buscaglia AJ, Cowden FE, Brill H: Pulmonary infiltrates associated with naproxen. *JAMA* 251:65, 1984.

57. Winterbauer RH, Wilske KR, Wheelis RF: Diffuse pulmonary injury associated with gold treatment. *N Engl J Med* 294:919, 1976.

58. Evans RB, Ettensohn DB, Fawaz-Estrup F, et al: Gold lung: Recent developments in pathogenesis, diagnosis, and therapy. *Semin Arthritis Rheum* 16:196, 1987.

59. Camus P, Degat OR, Justrabo E, et al: D-Penicillamine-induced severe pneumonitis. *Chest* 81:376, 1982.

60. Carson CW, Cannon GW, Egger MJ, et al: Pulmonary disease during treatment of rheumatoid arthritis with low dose pulse methotrexate. *Semin Arthritis Rheum* 16:186, 1987.

61. Searles G, McKendry RJ: Methotrexate pneumonitis in rheumatoid arthritis: Potential risk factors. Four case reports and a review of the literature. *J Rheumatol* 14:1164, 1987.

62. Kaplan RL, Waite DJ: Progressive interstitial lung disease from prolonged methotrexate therapy. *Arch Dermatol* 114:1800, 1978.

63. Bedrossian CW, Miller WC, Luna MA: Methotrexate-induced diffuse interstitial pulmonary fibrosis. *South Med J* 72:313, 1979.

64. Perruquet JL, Harrington TM, Davis DE: Letter: *Pneumocystis carinii* pneumonia following methotrexate therapy for rheumatoid arthritis. *Arthritis Rheum* 26:1291, 1983.

65. Wallis PJ, Ryatt KS, Constable TJ: *Pneumocystis carinii* pneumonia complicating low dose methotrexate treatment for psoriatic arthropathy. *Ann Rheum Dis* 48:247, 1989.

66. Altz-Smith M, Kendall LG Jr, Stamm AM: Cryptococcosis associated with low-dose methotrexate for arthritis. *Am J Med* 83:179, 1987.

67. Sostman HD, Matthay RA, Putnam CE: Cytotoxic drug-induced lung disease. *Am J Med* 62:608, 1977.

68. Hurd ER: Extraarticular manifestations of rheumatoid arthritis. *Semin Arthritis Rheum* 8:151, 1979.

69. Turner R, Collins R, Nomeir AM: Extraarticular manifestations of rheumatoid arthritis. *Bull Rheum Dis* 29:986, 1978–1979.

70. Gordon DA, Stein JL, Broder I: The extraarticular features of rheumatoid arthritis: A systemic analysis of 127 cases. *Am J Med* 54:445, 1973.

71. Harris ED Jr: The clinical features of rheumatoid arthritis, in Kelley WN, Harris ED Jr, Ruddy S, Sledge CS (eds): *Textbook of Rheumatology*, 3rd ed. Philadelphia, Saunders, 1989.

72. Bonfiglio T, Atwater EC: Heart disease in patients with seropositive rheumatoid arthritis: A controlled autopsy study and review. *Arch Intern Med* 127:714, 1969.

73. MacDonald WJ Jr, Crawford MH, Klippel JH, et al: Echocardiographic assessment of cardiac structure and function in patients with rheumatoid arthritis. *Am J Med* 63:890, 1977.

74. Thadini VU, Iveson JM, Wright V: Cardiac tamponade, constrictive pericarditis and pericardial resection in rheumatoid arthritis. *Medicine* (Baltimore) 54:261, 1975.

75. Franco AE, Levine HD, Hall AP: Rheumatoid pericarditis: Report of 17 cases diagnosed clinically. *Ann Intern Med* 77:837, 1972.

75a. Kennedy WP, Partridge RE, Matthews MB: Rheumatoid pericarditis with cardiac failure treated by pericardiectomy. *Br Heart J* 28:602, 1966.

76. Lev M, Bharati S, Hoffman FG, et al: The conduction system in rheumatoid arthritis with complete atrioventricular block. *Am Heart J* 90:78, 1975.

77. Ahern M, Lever JV, Cosh J: Complete heart block in rheumatoid arthritis. *Ann Rheum Dis* 42:389, 1983.

78. Lebowitz WB: The heart in rheumatoid arthritis (rheumatoid disease): A clinical and pathological study of sixty-two cases. *Ann Intern Med* 58:102, 1963.

79. Swezey RL: Myocardial infarction due to rheumatoid arteritis: An antemortem diagnosis. *JAMA* 199:855, 1967.

80. Zvaifler NJ, Weintraub AM: Aortitis and aortic insufficiency in the chronic rheumatic disorders—a reappraisal. *Arthritis Rheum* 6:241, 1963.

81. Reimer KA, Rodgers RF, Oyasu R: Rheumatoid arthritis with rheumatoid heart disease and granulomatous aortitis. *JAMA* 235:2510, 1976.

82. Iveson JM, Thadini U, Ionescu M, et al: Aortic valve incompetence and replacement in rheumatoid arthritis. *Ann Rheum Dis* 34:312, 1975.

82a. Gravallese EM, Corson JM, Coblyn JS, et al: Rheumatoid aortitis: A rarely recognized but clinically significant entity. *Medicine* 68:95, 1989.

83. Soter NA, Mihm MC Jr, Gigli I, et al: Two distinct cellular patterns in cutaneous necrotizing angiitis. *J Invest Dermatol* 66:344, 1976.

84. Fischer M, Mielke H, Glaefke S, Deicher H: Generalized vasculopathy and finger blood flow abnormalities in rheumatoid arthritis. *J Rheumatol* 11:33, 1984.

85. Geirsson AJ, Sturfelt G, Truedsson L: Clinical and serological fea-

tures of severe vasculitis in rheumatoid arthritis: Prognostic implications. *Ann Rheum Dis* 46:727, 1987.

86. Schneider HA, Yonker RA, Katz P, et al: Rheumatoid vasculitis: Experience with 13 patients and review of the literature. *Semin Arthritis Rheum* 14:280, 1985.

87. Scott DGI: Systemic rheumatoid vasculitis: A clinical and laboratory study of 50 cases. *Medicine* 60:288, 1981.

87a. Vollertsen RS, Conn DL, Ballard DJ, et al: Rheumatoid vasculitis: Survival and associated risk factors. *Medicine* (Baltimore) 65:365, 1986.

88. Scott DG, Bacon PA, Elliot PJ, et al: Systemic vasculitis in a district general hospital 1972–80: Clinical and laboratory features, classification, and prognosis of 80 cases. *Q J Med* 51:292, 1982.

89. Naschitz JE, Yeshurun D, Scharf Y, et al: Recurrent massive alveolar hemorrhage, crescentic glomerulonephritis, and necrotizing vasculitis in a patient with rheumatoid arthritis. *Arch Intern Med* 149:406, 1989.

90. Scott DG, Bacon PA: Intravenous cyclophosphamide plus methylprednisolone in treatment of systemic rheumatoid vasculitis. *Am J Med* 76:377, 1984.

91. Louis S, Gerard G: Neurological complications of rheumatoid arthritis, in Blau SP (ed): *Emergencies in Rheumatoid Arthritis*. Mount Kisco, NY, Futura, 1986, p 127.

92. Nakano KK: Neurologic complications of rheumatoid arthritis. *Orthop Clin North Am* 6:861, 1975.

93. Reza MJ, Verity MA: Neuromuscular manifestations of rheumatoid arthritis: A clinical and histomorphological analysis. *Clin Rheum Dis* 3:565, 1977.

94. Nakano KK: The entrapment neuropathies of rheumatoid arthritis. *Orthop Clin North Am* 6:837, 1975.

95. Bathon JM, Moreland LW, DiBartolomeo AG: Inflammatory central nervous system involvement in rheumatoid arthritis. *Semin Arthritis Rheum* 18:258, 1989.

96. Stevens JC, Cartlidge NE, Saunders M, et al: Atlanto-axial subluxation and cervical myelopathy in rheumatoid arthritis. *Q J Med* 40:391, 1971.

97. Weiner S, Bassett L, Spiegel T: Superior, posterior, and lateral displacement of C1 in rheumatoid arthritis. *Arthritis Rheum* 25:1378, 1982.

98. Nakano KK, Schoene WC, Baker RA, Dawson DM: The cervical myelopathy associated with rheumatoid arthritis: Analysis of patients, with 2 postmortem cases. *Ann Neurol* 3:144, 1978.

99. Christophidis N, Huiskisson EC: Misleading symptoms and signs of cervical spine subluxation in rheumatoid arthritis. *Br Med J* 285:364, 1982.

100. Martel W: The occipito-atlanto-axial joints in rheumatoid arthritis and ankylosing spondylitis. *AJR* 86:223, 1961.

101. Raskin RJ, Schnapf DJ, Wolf CR, et al: Computerized tomography in evaluation of atlantoaxial subluxation in rheumatoid arthritis. *J Rheumatol* 10:33, 1983.

102. Breedveld FC, Algra PR, Veilvoye CJ, Cats A: Magnetic resonance imaging in the evaluation of patients with rheumatoid arthritis and subluxations of the cervical spine. *Arthritis Rheum* 30:624, 1987.

103. Smith HP, Challa VR, Alexander E Jr: Odontoid compression of the brain stem in a patient with rheumatoid arthritis. Case report. *J Neurosurg* 53:841, 1980.

104. Marks JS, Sharp J: Rheumatoid cervical myelopathy. *Q J Med* 50:307, 1981.

105. Jacobs B: Cervical spine complications in rheumatoid arthritis, in Blau SP (ed): *Emergencies in Rheumatoid Arthritis*. Mount Kisco, NY, Futura, 1986, p 157.

106. Mayer JW, Messner RP, Kaplan RJ: Brain stem compression in rheumatoid arthritis. *JAMA* 236:2094, 1976.

107. Meyers KAE, Cats A, Kremer HPH, et al: Cervical myelopathy in rheumatoid arthritis. *Clin Exp Rheumatol* 2:239, 1984.

108. Davidson RC, Horn JR, Herndon JH, et al: Brainstem compression in rheumatoid arthritis. *JAMA* 238:2633, 1977.

109. Manz HJ, Luessenhop AJ, Robertson DM: Cervical myelopathy due to atlantoaxial and subaxial subluxation in rheumatoid arthritis. *Arch Pathol Lab Med* 107:94, 1983.

110. Kataoka O, Hirohata K, Kurihara A: The surgical treatment of myelopathy secondary to rheumatoid arthritis of the lower cervical spine. *Int Orthop* 3:103, 1979.

111. Steinberg AD, Klinman DM: Pathogenesis of systemic lupus erythematosus. *Rheum Dis Clin North Am* 14:25, 1988.

112. Smolen JS, Chused TM, Leiserson WM, et al: Heterogenecity of immunoregulatory T cell subset in systemic lupus erythematosus: Correlation with clinical features. *Am J Med* 72:783, 1982.

113. Smolen JS, Morimoto C, Steinberg AD, et al: Systemic lupus erythematosus: Delineation of subpopulations by clinical, serologic and T cell marker analysis. *Am J Med* 289:139, 1985.

114. Tan EM, Cohen AS, Fries JF, et al: The 1982 revised criteria for classification of systemic lupus erythematosus. *Arthritis Rheum* 25:1271, 1982.

115. Klippel JH: Management of the seriously ill systemic lupus erythematosus patient. *Postgrad Adv Rheumatol* II:VII, 1987.

116. Schur PH: Clinical features in systemic lupus erythematosus, in Kelly WM, Harris ED, Ruddy S, Sledge CB (eds): *Textbook of Rheumatology*, 4th ed. Philadelphia, Saunders, 1993, p 1017.

117. Pistiner M, Wallace DJ, Nessim S, et al: Lupus erythematosus in the 1980's: A survey of 570 patients. *Sem Arth Rheum* 21:55, 1991.

118. Balow JE, Austin HA: Renal disease in systemic lupus erythematosus. *Rheum Dis Clin North Am* 16:117, 1988.

118a. Bumgardener GL, Mauer SM, Ascher NL, et al: Longterm outcome of renal transplantation in patients with systemic lupus erythematosus. *Transplant. Proc.* 21:2031, 1989.

119. Hill GS, Hinglais N, Tron F, Bach JF: Systemic lupus erythematosus: Morphological correlations with immunologic and clinical data at time of biopsy. *Am J Med* 64:61, 1978.

119a. McLaughlin J, Gladman DD, Urowitz MB, Bombardier CB, Cole E: Renal biopsy in systemic lupus erythematosus. II. Survival analysis according to biopsy rsults. *Arthritis Rheum*, In press.

120. Steinberg AD: Management of systemic lupus erythematosus, in Kelly WM, Harris ED, Ruddy S, Sledge CB (eds): *Textbook of Rheumatology*, 3rd ed. Philadelphia, Saunders, 1989, p 1130.

121. Donadio JV, Holley KE, Ferguson RH, et al: Treatment of diffuse proliferative lupus nephritis with prednisone and combined prednisone and cyclophosphamide. *N Engl J Med* 299:1151, 1978.

122. Austin HA, Klippel JH, Balow JE, et al: Therapy of lupus nephritis. *N Engl J Med* 314:491, 1986.

123. Balow JE: Therapeutic studies in humans, In: Balow JE (moderator): Lupus nephritis. *Ann Intern Med* 06:79, 1987.

124. Steinberg AD, Steinberg SC: Longterm preservation of renal function in patients with lupus nephritis receiving treatment that includes cyclophosphamide versus those treated with prednisone only. *Arth. Rheum* 34:945, 1991.

125. McCune WJ, Globus J, Zeldes W, et al: Clinical and immunological effects of monthly administration of intravenous cyclophosphamide in severe lupus erythematosus. *N Engl J Med* 318:1423, 1988.

125a. Hahn BH: Management of systemic lupus erythematosus. In: Kelly WM, Harris ED, Ruddy S, Sledge CB (eds): Textbook of Rheumatology, 4th ed. Philadelphia, Saunders, 1993, p 1043.

125b. Shapira Y, Mor F, Friedler A, et al: Antiproteinuric effect of captopril in a patient with lupus nephritis and intractable nephrotic syndrome. *Ann Rheum Dis* 49:725, 1990.

125c. Schroeder JO, Euler HH, Loffler H: Synchronization of plasmapheresis and pulse cyclophosphamide in severe systemic lupus erythematosus. *Ann Int Med* 107:344, 1987.

125d. Lewis EJ, Hunsicker LG, Lan SP, et al: A controlled trial of plasmapheresis therapy in severe lupus nephritis. *N Engl J Med* 326:373, 1992.

126. Ginzler EN, Diamond HS, Weiner M, et al: A multicenter study of outcome in systemic lupus erythematosus: I. Entry variables as predictor of prognosis. *Arthritis Rheum* 25:601, 1982.

127. Rosner S, Ginzler EM, Diamond HS, et al: A multicenter study of outcome in systemic lupus erythematosus: II. Causes of death. *Arthritis Rheum* 25:612, 1982.

128. McCune JW, Globus J: Neuropsychiatric lupus. *Rheum Dis Clin North Am* 14:149, 1988.

129. Rogers M: Psychiatric aspects, in Schur P (ed): *The Clinical Management of Systemic Lupus*. New York, Grune & Stratton, 1983.

130. Ellis SG, Verity MA: Central nervous system involvement in systemic lupus erythematosus: A review of neuropathologic findings in 57 cases 1955–1977. *Semin Arthritis Rheum* 8:212, 1979.

131. Johnson RT, Richardson EP: Neurologic manifestations of systemic lupus erythematosus. *Medicine* (Baltimore) 47:337, 1968.

132. Kaell AT, Shetty M, Lee BC, et al: The diversity of neurologic events in systemic lupus erythematosus. Prospective clinical and CT classification of 82 events in 71 patients. *Arch Neurol* 43:273, 1986.

132a. Wong KL, Woo EKW, Yu YL, Wong RWS: Neurologic manifestations of systemic lupus erythematosus: a prospective study. *Q J Med* 81:857, 1991.

133. Fox IS, Spence AM, Wheelas RF, et al: Cerebral embolism in Libman-Sacks endocarditis. *Neurology* 30:487, 1980.

133a. Boumpas DT, Patronas NJ, Dalakas MC, et al: Acute transverse myelitis in systemic lupus erythematosus: magnetic resonance imaging and a review of the literature. *J Rheum* 17:89, 1990.

134. Andrianakos AA, Duffy J, Suzuki M, et al: Transverse myelopathy in systemic lupus erythematosus. Report of 3 cases and review of the literature. *Ann Intern Med* 83:616, 1975.

135. Welsby P, Smith C: Recurrent sterile meningitis as manifestation of systemic lupus erythematosus. *Scand J Infect Dis* 2:149, 1977.

136. Wasner CC: Ibuprofen meningitis and systemic lupus erythematosus. *J Rheumatol* 5:162, 1978.

137. Lockshin MD, Kagen LJ: Meningitis reaction after azathioprine. *N Engl J Med* 286:1321, 1972.

138. Woods VL, Zvaifler NJ: Pathogenesis of systemic lupus erythematosus, in Kelly WN, Harris ED, Ruddy S, Sledge CB (eds): *Textbook of Rheumatology,* 3rd ed. Philadelphia, Saunders, 1989.

139. Bluestein HG, Williams GN, Steinberg AD: Cerebrospinal fluid antibodies to antineuronal cells: Association with neuropsychiatric manifestations of systemic lupus erythematosus. *Am J Med* 70:240, 1981.

140. Karpiak SE, Graf L, Rappoport MM: Antiserum to brain ganglioside produces recurrent epileptiform activity. *Science* 194:735, 1976.

141. Kobiler D, Fuchs S, Samuel D: The effect of antisynatosomal plasma membrane antibodies on memory. *Brain Res* 15:129, 1976.

142. Simon J, Simon O: Effect of passive transfer of anti-brain antibody to normal recipient. *Exp Neurol* 477:523, 1975.

143. Elkon K, Weissbach H, Brot N: Central nervous system function in systemic lupus erythematosus. *Neurochem Res* 15:401, 1990.

144. Hirohata S, Hirose S, Miyamoto T: Cerebrospinal fluid IgM, IgA, IgG indexes in systemic lupus erythematosus: Their use as estimates of central nervous system disease activity. *Arch Intern Med* 145:1843, 1985.

145. Seibold JR, Buckingham RB, Medsger TA, et al: Cerebrospinal fluid immune complexes in systemic lupus erythematosus involving the central nervous system. *Semin Arthritis Rheum* 12:68, 1982.

146. Ernerudh J, Olsson T, Lindstrom F, et al: Cerebrospinal fluid immunoglobulin abnormalities in systemic lupus erythematosus. *J Neurol Neurosurg Psychiatry* 40:807, 1983.

147. Bell CL, Partington C, Robbins M, et al: Magnetic resonance imaging of central nervous system lesions in patients with systemic lupus erythematosus. Correlation with clinical remission and antineuronal and anticardiolipin antibody titers. *Arth Rheum* 34:432, 1991.

148. Fessel WJ: Megadose corticosteroid therapy in systemic lupus erythematosus. *J Rheumatol* 7:486, 1980.

149. Isenberg DA, Morrow MJ, Snaith ML: Methylprednisolone pulse therapy in treatment of systemic lupus erythematosus. *Ann Rheum Dis* 41:347, 1982.

149a. Barile L, Lavalle C: Transverse myelitis in systemic lupus erythematosus: the effects of IV methylprednisolone and cyclophosphamide. *J Rheum* 19:370, 1992.

150. Fruchter L, Gauthein B, Marino F: Letter: The use of plasmapheresis in a patient with systemic lupus erythematosus and necrotizing cutaneous ulcers. *J Rheumatol* 10:341, 1983.

151. Schena FP, Manno C, Carabellese S, et al: Plasma exchange in systemic lupus erythematosus. *Int J Artif Organs* 6:29, 1983.

152. Pines A, Kaplinsky N, Olchovsky D, et al: Pleuro-pulmonary manifestations of systemic lupus erythematosus: Clinical features and its subgroups. *Chest* 88:129, 1985.

153. Alarcon-Sergovia D, Alarcon DG: Pleural-pulmonary manifestations of systemic lupus erythematosus. *Dis Chest* 39:7, 1961.

154. Silberstein SL, Barland P, Grayzel AL, et al: Pulmonary dysfunction in systemic lupus erythematosus—prevalence, classification, and correlation with other organ involvement. *J Rheumatol* 7:187, 1980.

155. Holgate ST, Glass DDN, Haslam P, et al: Respiratory involvement in systemic lupus erythematosus: A clinical and immunological study. *Clin Exp Immunol* 24:385, 1976.

156. Huang CT, Hennigar GR, Lyons HA: Pulmonary dysfunction in systemic lupus erythematosus. *N Engl J Med* 272:288, 1965.

157. Segal A, Calabrase LH, Ahmad M, et al: The pulmonary manifestations of systemic lupus erythematosus. *Semin Arthritis Rheum* 14:202, 1985.

158. Potts DE, Wilcox MA, Good JT, et al: The acidosis of low glucose pleural effusions. *Am Rev Respir Dis* 117:665, 1978.

159. Halla JT, Schrohenloher RE, Volanakis JE: Immune complex and other laboratory features of pleural effusions—a comparison of rheumatoid arthritis, systemic lupus erythematosus, and other diseases. *Ann Intern Med* 92:748, 1980.

160. Leechawengwong W, Berger HW, Sukumaran M: Diagnostic significance of antinuclear antibodies in pleural effusions. *Mt Sinai J Med* 46:137, 1979.

161. Matthay RA, Schwartz MI, Petty TL: Pulmonary manifestations of systemic lupus erythematosus. Review of twelve cases of acute lupus pneumonitis. *Medicine* (Baltimore) 54:397, 1974.

162. Pertschuk LP, Moccia LF, Rosen Y, et al: Acute pulmonary complications in systemic lupus erythematosus: Immunofluorescent and light microscopy study. *Am J Clin Pathol* 68:553, 1977.

163. Inaue T, Kanayama Y, Ohe A, et al: Immunopathologic studies in pneumonitis of systemic lupus erythematosus. *Ann Intern Med* 91:30, 1979.

164. Mintz G, Galindo LF, Fernandez-Diaz J, et al: Acute massive pulmonary hemorrhage in systemic lupus erythematosus. *J Rheumatol* 5:39, 1978.

165. Eagan JW, Memoli VA, Roberts JL, et al: Pulmonary hemorrhage in systemic lupus erythematosus. *Medicine* (Baltimore) 57:545, 1978.

166. Marino CT, Pertshuk LP: Pulmonary hemorrhage in systemic lupus erythematosus. *Arch Intern Med* 141:201, 1981.

167. Millman RP, Cohen TB, Levenson AL, et al: Systemic lupus erythematosus complicated by acute pulmonary hemorrhage: Recovery following plasmapheresis and cytotoxic drugs. *J Rheumatol* 8:1021, 1981.

168. Isbistar JP, Ralston M, Hayes JM, et al: Fulminant lupus pneumonitis in renal failure and RBC aplasia: Successful management with plasmapheresis and immunosuppression. *Arch Intern Med* 141:1081, 1981.

169. Eisenberg H, Dubois EL, Sherman RP, et al: Diffuse interstitial lung disease in systemic lupus erythematosus. *Ann Intern Med* 19:37, 1973.

170. Eisenberg H, Simmons DH, Barnett EV: Diffuse interstitial pulmonary disease: An immunological study. *Chest* 75:262, 1979.

171. Lawrence EC: Systemic lupus erythematosus and the lung, in Lahita RG (ed): *Systemic Lupus Erythematosus.* New York, Churchill-Livingstone, 1987.

172. Baehr G, Klemperer P, Schifrin A: A diffuse disease of peripheral circulation usually associated with lupus erythematosus and endocarditis. *Trans Assoc Am Physicians* 50:139, 1935.

173. Fayemi AO: Pulmonary vascular disease in systemic lupus erythematosus. *Am J Clin Pathol* 65:284, 1976.

174. Asherson RA, Oakly CM: Pulmonary hypertension and systemic lupus erythematosus. *J Rheumatol* 13:1, 1986.

175. Asherson RA, Higenbottam TW, Xuan ATD, et al: Pulmonary HTN in lupus clinic experience with twenty-four patients. *J Rheum* 17:1292, 1990.

176. Perez HD, Kramer N: Pulmonary hypertension in systemic lupus erythematosus: Report of 4 cases and review of the literature. *Semin Arthritis Rheum* 11:177, 1981.

177. Harris EN, Gharavi AE, Hughes GRV: Antiphospholipid antibodies. *Clin Rheum Dis* 11:591, 1985.

178. Mandell BF: Cardiovascular involvement in SLE. *Semin Arthritis Rheum* 17:126, 1987.

179. Gibson GJ, Edmonds JP, Hughes GR: Diaphragm function and lung involvement in systemic lupus erythematosus. *Am J Med* 63:926, 1977.

180. Rubin LA, Urowitz MB: Shrinking lung syndrome in systemic lupus erythematosus—a clinical pathologic study. *J Rheumatol* 10:973, 1983.

181. Gladman DD, Urowitz MB: Venous syndromes and pulmonary embolism in systemic lupus erythematosus. *Ann Rheum Dis* 51:340, 1980.
182. Mandell B: Cardiovascular involvement in systemic lupus erythematosus. *Semin Arthritis Rheum* 17:126, 1987.
183. Hejtmancik MR, Wright JL, Quint R, et al: The cardiovascular manifestations of systemic lupus erythematosus. *Am Heart J* 68:119, 1964.
184. Estes D, Christian CL: The natural history of systemic lupus erythematosus by prospective analysis. *Medicine* (Baltimore) 50:85, 1971.
185. Carette S: Cardiopulmonary manifestations of SLE. *Rheum Dis Clin North Am* 14:135, 1988.
186. Doherty NE, Siegal RJ: Cardiovascular disease in systemic lupus erythematosus. *Am Heart J* 110:1257, 1985.
187. Hunder GG, Mullen BJ, McDuffie FC: Complement in pericardial fluid of lupus erythematosus. *Ann Intern Med* 80:453, 1974.
188. Bulkley BH, Roberts WC: The heart in systemic lupus erythematosus and changes induced in it by corticosteroids. *Am J Med* 58:243, 1975.
189. Stevens MB: Editorial. *N Engl J Med* 319:861, 1988.
190. Borenstein DG, Fye WB, Arnett FC, et al: The myocarditis of systemic lupus erythematosus. *Ann Intern Med* 89:619, 1978.
191. Baduie E, Garcia-Rubi D, Robles E, et al: The cardiovascular manifestations in systemic lupus erythematosus: Prospective study of 100 patients. *Angiology* 36:431, 1985.
192. Murai K, Oku H, Takeuchi K, et al: Alteration in myocardial systolic and diastolic function in patients with active systemic lupus erythematosus. *Am Heart J* 113:966, 1987.
193. Hosenpud JD, Montanaro A, Hart MV, et al: Myocardial perfusion abnormalities in asymptomatic patients with systemic lupus erythematosus. *Am J Med* 77:286, 1984.
194. Strauer BE, Brune I, Schenk H, et al: Lupus cardiomyopathy: Cardiac mechanics, hemodynamics, and coronary artery blood flow in uncomplicated systemic lupus erythematosus. *Am Heart J* 92:715, 1976.
195. Heibel RH, O'Toole J, Curtiss B, et al: Coronary arteritis in systemic lupus erythematosus. *Chest* 69:700, 1976.
196. Korbet SM, Schwartz MM, Lewis EJ: Immune complex deposition and coronary vasculitis in systemic lupus erythematosus. *Am J Med* 77:141, 1984.
197. Rubin LA, Urowitz MB, Gladman DD: Mortality in systemic lupus erythematosus   the bimodal pattern revisited. *QJ Med* 55:87, 1985.
198. Gladman DD, Urowitz MB: Morbidity in systemic lupus erythematosus. *J Rheumatol* (Suppl 13) 14:223, 1987.
199. Haider YS, Roberts WC: Coronary artery disease in systemic lupus erythematosus—quantification of degree of narrowing in 20 necropsy patients. *Am J Med* 70:775, 1981.
200. MacGregor AJ, Dhillon VB, Binder A, et al: Fasting lipids and anticardiolipin antibodies as risk factors for vascular disease in SLE. *Ann Rheum Dis* 51:152, 1992.
201. Asherson R, Harris N, Gharavi A, et al: Myocardial infarction in systemic lupus erythematosus and "lupus-like" disease. *Arthritis Rheum* 29:1292, 1986.
202. Elias M, Eldor A: Thromboembolism in patients with the lupus type circulating anticoagulant. *Arch Intern Med* 144:510, 1984.
203. Carreros LO, Machin SJ, Denman R, et al: Arterial thrombosis, intrauterine death and "lupus" anticoagulant: Detection of immunoglobulin interfering with prostacyclin formation. *Lancet* 1:244, 1981.
204. Libman E, Sacks B: A hitherto underdescribed form of valvular and mural endocarditis. *Arch Intern Med* 33:705, 1924.
205. Bidani AK, Roberts JL, Schwartz MA, et al: Immunopathology of cardiac lesions in fatal systemic lupus erythematosus. *Am J Med* 69:849, 1980.
206. Dajee H, Hurley EJ, Szarnicki RJ: Cardiac valve replacement in systemic lupus erythematosus. A review. *J Thorac Cardiovasc Surg* 85:718, 1983.
207. Fox IS, Spence AM, Wheelis RF, et al: Cerebral embolism in Libman-Sacks endocarditis. *Neurology* 30:487, 1980.
208. Dubois EL: Causes of death in SLE, in Dubois EL (ed): *Lupus Erythematosus,* 2nd ed. Los Angeles, University of Southern California Press, 1970, p 633.
209. Chartash E, Lans D, Paget S, et al: Aortic insufficiency and mitral regurgitation in patients with SLE and the antiphospholipid syndrome. *Am J Med* 86:407, 1989.
210. Ford PM, Ford SE, Lillicrap DP: Association of lupus anticoagulant with severe valvular heart disease in systemic lupus erythematosus. *J Rheumatol* 15:597, 1988.
211. Asherson RA, Lubbe WF: Cerebral and valve lesions in systemic lupus erythematosus: Association with antiphospholipid antibodies. *J Rheumatol* 15:539, 1988.
212. Galve E, Candell-Riera J, Pigrau C, et al: Prevalence, morphological types and evolution of cardiovascular disease in systemic lupus erythematosus. *N Engl J Med* 319:817, 1988.
213. James TN, Rope CD, Monto RW: Pathology of cardiac conduction system in systemic lupus erythematosus. *Ann Intern Med* 63:402, 1965.
214. Kephart DC, Hood AF, Provost TT: Neonatal lupus erythematosus: New serologic findings. *J Invest Dwermatol* 77:331, 1981.
215. Lockshin MD, Gibofsky A, Peebles CL, et al: Neonatal lupus erythematosus with heart block: Family study of a patient with anti-SSA and SSB autoantibodies. *Arthritis Rheum* 26:210, 1983.
216. Fish AJ, Blau EB, Westberg NG, et al: Systemic lupus erythematosus within the first two decades of life. *Am J Med* 62:99, 1977.
217. Harvey AM, Schulman LE, Tumulty PA, et al: Systemic lupus erythematosus with review of literature and clinical analysis of 138 cases. *Medicine* (Baltimore) 33:291, 1954.
218. Baker SB, Rovira JR, Campion EW, et al: Late onset systemic lupus erythematosus. *Am J Med* 66:727, 1979.
219. Bridman DR, Steinberg AD: Hematologic aspects of systemic lupus erythematosus: Current concepts. *Ann Intern Med* 86:220, 1977.
220. Laurence J, Nachman R: Hematologic aspects of systemic lupus erythematosus, in Lahita RG (ed): *Systemic Lupus Erythematosus.* New York, Churchill-Livingstone, 1987.
221. Eyster ME, Jenkins DE Jr: Erythrocyte coating substances in patients with positive direct antiglobulin reaction. *Am J Med* 46:360, 1969.
222. Dacie JV: *The Haemolytic Anemias, Congenital and Acquired: II. The Autoimmune Hemolytic Anemias,* 2nd ed. New York, Grune & Stratton, 1962.
223. Ahn YS, Harrington WJ, Ravindra PL, et al: Danazol therapy for autoimmune hemolytic anemias. *Ann Intern Med* 102:298, 1985.
224. Corley CC Jr, Lessner HE, Larsen WE: Azathioprine therapy of "autoimmune diseases." *Am J Med* 41:404, 1966.
225. Bernstein MC, Schneider BK, Naimen JL: Plasma exchange in refractory acute autoimmune hemolytic anemia. *J Pediatr* 98:774, 1981.
226. Ginzler E, Diamond H, Kaplan D, et al: Computer analysis of factors influencing frequency of infections in systemic lupus erythematosus. *Arthritis Rheum* 21:37, 1978.
227. Wallace DJ, Dubois EL (eds): *Dubois' Lupus Erythematosus,* 3rd ed. Philadelphia, Lea & Febiger, 1987.
228. Hall S, McCormick JL, Greipp PR, et al: Splenectomy does not cure thrombocytopenia of systemic lupus erythematosus. *Ann Intern Med* 102:325, 1985.
229. Gruenberg JC, VanSlyck EJ, Abraham JP: Splenectomy in systemic lupus erythematosus. *Am Surg* 52:366, 1986.
230. Ahn YS, Harrington WJ, Simon SR, et al: Danazol for the treatment of idiopathic thrombocytopenic purpura. *N Engl J Med* 308:1396, 1983.
231. West SG, Johnson SC: Danazol for treatment of refractory autoimmune thrombocytopenia in SLE. *Ann Intern Med* 108:703, 1988.
232. Ahn YS, Rocha R, Mylvaganam R, et al: Longterm danazol therapy in autoimmune thrombocytopenic purpura: Unmaintained remission and age dependent response in women. *Ann Intern Med* 111:723, 1989.
233. Boumpas DT, Barez S, Klippel JH, Balow JE: Intermittent cyclophosphamide for treatment of autoimmune thrombocytopenia in systemic lupus erythematosus. *Ann Int Med* 112:674, 1990.
234. Gordon DS: Intravenous immunoglobulin therapy. New directions and unanswered questions. *Am J Med* 83 (Suppl 4A):52, 1987.
235. Jacobs P, Wood L: The comparison of gammaglobulin to steroids in treating adult immune thrombocytopenia. An interim analysis. *Blut* 59:92, 1989.
235a. Wall BA, Weinblatt ME, Aguedelo CA: Plasmapherisis in the treat-

ment of resistant thrombocytopenia in systematic lupus erythematosus. *South Med J* 9:305, 1982.

236. Meyer LF: Gastrointestinal manifestations of SLE, in Lahita RG (ed): *Systemic Lupus Erythematosus*. New York, Churchill-Livingstone, 1987, p 709.

237. Zizic TM, Schulman LE, Stevens MB: Colonic perforation in systemic lupus erythematosus. *Medicine* (Baltimore) 54:411, 1975.

238. Pollack VE, Grove WJ, Kank RM, et al: Systemic lupus erythematosus simulating acute surgical condition of the abdomen. *N Engl J Med* 259:258, 1958.

239. Hoffman B, Katz W: The gastrointestinal manifestations of systemic lupus erythematosus: A review of the literature. *Semin Arthritis Rheum* 9:237, 1980.

240. Shapeero LG, Myers A, Oberkircher PE, et al: Acute reversible lupus vasculitis of gastrointestinal tract. *Radiology* 112:569, 1974.

241. Phillips JC, Howland WJ: Mesenteric arteritis in systemic lupus erythematosus. *JAMA* 206:1569, 1968.

242. Freiman D, Chon H, Bilaniu KH: Pneumotosis intestinalis in systemic lupus erythematosus. *Radiology* 116:563, 1975.

243. Kleinman P, Mayers MA, Abbott G, et al: Necrotizing enterocolitis associated with systemic lupus erythematosus and polyarteritis. *Radiology* 121:595, 1976.

244. Ropes MW: *Systemic Lupus Erythematosus*. Boston, Harvard University Press, 1976, p 40.

244a. Perednia DA, Curosh NA: Lupus-associated protein-losing enteropathy. *Arch Int Med* 150:1806, 1990.

244b. Tsutsumi A, Sugiyama T, Matsumura R, et al: Protein losing enteropathy associated with collagen vascular disease. *Ann Rheum Dis* 50:178, 1991.

245. Musher DR: SLE: A cause of medical peritonitis. *Am J Surg* 124:368, 1978.

246. Blomgren SE, Condemi JJ, Bignell MC, et al: Antinuclear antibody induced by procainamide. A prospective study. *N Engl J Med* 281:64, 1969.

247. Solinger AM: Drug related lupus: Clinical and etiological considerations. *Rheum Dis Clin North Am* 14:187, 1988.

248. Hughes GR, Harris NN, Gharavi AE: The anticardiolipin syndrome. *J Rheumatol* 13:486, 1986.

249. Lockshin MD: Lupus anticoagulant-related conditions. *Curr Opin Rheumatol* 1:339, 1989.

249a. Bowles CA: Vasculopathy associated with the antiphospholipid antibody syndrome. *Rheum Dis N Amer* 16:471, 1990.

249b. Sugai S.: Antiphospholipid antibody and antiphospholipid antibody syndrome. *Curr Opin Rheumatol* 4:666, 1992.

249c. McNeil HP, Chesterman CN, Krills ST: Immunology and clinical importance of antiphospholipid antibodies, in Dixon F (ed): *Advances in Immunology*. Duluth, Academic,1991, p 193.

249d. Lockshin MD: Antiphospholipid antibody and antiphospholipid antibody syndrome. *Curr Opin Rheumatol* 3:797, 1991.

250. Alarcon-Segovia D, Sanchez-Guerrero J: Primary antiphospholipid syndrome. (Published erratum appears in *J Rheumatol* 16:1014, 1988). *J Rheumatol* 16:482, 1989.

251. Mackworth-Young CG, Loizou S, Walport MJ: Primary antiphospholipid syndrome: Features of patients with raised anticardiolipin antibodies and no other disorder. *Ann Rheum Dis* 48:362, 1989.

252. Harris EN, Hughes GRV, Gharavi AE: Antiphospholipid antibodies: An elderly statesman dons new garments. *J Rheumatol* 14(Suppl 13):208, 1987.

253. Giansiracusa DF, Stafford-Brady F: A 35-year-old woman with recurrent strokes, and intracardiac lesions, anemia, and thrombocytopenia. Case 37-1988. *N Engl J Med* 319:699, 1988.

254. Hughes GRV, Asherman RA, Khamashta MA: Antiphospholipid syndrome: Linking many specialties. *Ann Rheum Dis* 48:355, 1989.

255. Recker DP, Leff RL: The broad clinical reach of antiphospholipid antibodies. *Contemporary Medicine* Nov/Dec:30, 1989.

256. Rustin MHA, Bull HA, Machin SJ, et al: Effects of the lupus anticoagulant in patients with systemic lupus erythematosus on endothelial cell prostacyclin release and procoagulant activity. *J Invest Dermatol* 90:744, 1988.

257. Carreras LO, Vermylen JG: "Lupus" anticoagulant and thrombosis-possible role of inhibition of prostacyclin formation. *Thromb Haemost* 48:38, 1982.

258. Boey ML, Colaco CB, Gharavi AE, et al: Thrombosis in systemic lupus erythematosus: Striking association with the presence or circulating lupus anticoagulant. *Br Med J* 287:1021, 1983.

258a. Westerman EM, Miles JM, Backonja M, Sundstrom WR: Neuropathic findings in multi-infarct dementia associated with anticardiolipin antibody: Evidence for endothelial injury as the primary event. *Arthritis Rheum* 35:1038, 1992.

259. Khamashta MA, Harris EN, Gharavi AE, et al: Immune mediated mechanism for thrombosis: Antiphospholipid antibody binding to platelet membranes. *Ann Rheum Dis* 47:849, 1988.

260. Howard MA, Firkin BG: Investigations of the lupus-like inhibitor bypassing activity of platelets. *Thromb Haemost* 50:775, 1983.

261. Byron MA, Allington MJ, Chapel HM, et al: Indications of vascular endothelial cell dysfunction in systemic lupus erythematosus. *Ann Rheum Dis* 46:741, 1987.

262. Sanfellippo MJ, Drayna CJ: Prekallikrein inhibition associated with the lupus anticoagulant: A mechanism of thrombosis. *Am J Clin Pathol* 77:275, 1982.

263. Freyssinet JM, Wiesel ML, Gauchy J, et al: An IgM lupus anticoagulant that neutralizes the enhancing effect of phospholipid on purified endothelial thrombomodulin activity—a mechanism for thrombosis. *Thromb Haemost* 55:309, 1986.

264. Esmon CT: The regulation of natural anticoagulant pathways. *Science* 235:1348, 1987.

264a. Malia RG, Kitchen S, Greaves M, Preston FE: Inhibition of activated protein C and its cofactor protein S by antiphospholipid antibodies. *Br J Haematol* 76:101, 1990.

264b. Ruiz-Arguelles GJ, Ruiz-Arguelles A, Alarcan-Segovia D, et al: National anticoagulants in systemic lupus erythematosus: Deficiency of protein S bound to C4bp associates with recent history of venous thrombosis, antiphospholipid antibodies and the antiphospholipid syndrome. *J Rheumatol* 10:552, 1991.

265. Jindal BK, Martin MF, Gayner A: Gangrene developing after minor surgery in a patient with undiagnosed systemic lupus erythematosus and lupus anticoagulation. *Ann Rheum Dis* 42:347, 1983.

266. Ferrante FM, Myerson GE, Goldman JA: Subclavian artery thrombosis mimicking the aortic arch syndrome in systemic lupus erythematosus. *Arthritis Rheum* 25:1501, 1982.

267. Bird AG, Lendrum R, Asherson RA, et al: Disseminated intravascular coagulation, antiphospholipid antibodies, and ischaemic necrosis of extremities. *Ann Rheum Dis* 46:251, 1987.

268. Drew P, Asherson RA, Zuk RJ, et al: Aortic occlusion in systemic lupus erythematosus associated with antiphospholipid antibodies. *Ann Rheum Dis* 46:612, 1987.

269. Mor F, Beigel Y, Inbal A, et al: Hepatic infarction in a patient with the lupus anticoagulant. *Arthritis Rheum* 32:491, 1989.

270. Asherson RA, Derksen RH, Harris EN, et al: Large vessel occlusion and gangrene in systemic lupus erythematosus and "lupus-like" disease: A report of six cases. *J Rheumatol* 13:740, 1986.

271. Ingram SB, Goodnight SH, Bennett RM: An unusual syndrome of devastating noninflammatory vasculopathy associated with anticardiolipin antibodies. Report of two cases. *Arthritis Rheum* 30:1167; 1987.

272. Asherson RA, Baguley E, Khamashta MA, et al: Multiple small-vessel occlusions in systemic lupus erythematosus. *Stroke* 20:127, 1989.

272a. Greisman SG, Thayaparan RS, Godwin TA, Lockshin MD: Occlusive vasculopathy in systemic lupus erythematosus: association with anticardiolipin antibody. *Arch Intern Med* 151:389, 1991.

273. Alarcon-Segovia D, Cardiel MH, Reyes E: Antiphospholipid arterial vasculopathy. *J Rheumatol* 16:762, 1989.

273a. Goldberger E, Elder RC, Schwartz RA, Phillips PE: Vasculitis in the antiphospholipid syndrome: A cause of ischemia responding to corticosteroids. *Arthritis Rheum* 35:569, 1992.

274. Levine SR, Welch KM: The spectrum of neurologic disease associated with antiphospholipid antibodies, lupus anticoagulants and anticardiolipin antibodies. *Arch Neurol* 44:876, 1987.

275. Asherson RA, Mercey D, Phillips G, et al: Recurrent stroke and multi-infarct dementia in systemic lupus erythematosus: Association with antiphospholipid antibodies. *Ann Rheum Dis* 46:605, 1987.

276. Asherson RA, Khamashta MA, Gil A, et al: Cerebrovascular disease and antiphospholipid antibodies in systemic lupus erythe-

matosus, lupus-like disease, and the primary antiphospholipid syndrome. *Am J Med* 86:391, 1989.

277. Harris EN, Gharavi AE, Asherson RA, et al: Cerebral infarction in systemic lupus: Association with anticardiolipin antibodies. *Clin Exp Rheumatol* 2:47, 1984.

277a. Pope JM, Canny CB, Bell DA: Cerebral ischemic events associated with endocarditis, renal vascular disease, and lupus anticoagulant. *Am J Med* 90:299, 1991.

278. Asherson RA, Merry P, Acheson JF, et al: Antiphospholipid antibodies: A risk factor for occlusive ocular vascular disease in systemic lupus erythematosus and the "primary" antiphospholipid syndrome. *Ann Rheum Dis* 48:358, 1989.

279. Hughes GRV: Thrombosis, abortion, cerebral disease and the lupus anticoagulant (editorial). *Br Med J* 287:1088, 1983.

280. Deleze M, Alarcon-Segovia D, Valdes-Macho D, et al: Relationship between antiphospholipid antibodies and recurrent fetal loss in patients with systemic lupus erythematosus and apparently healthy women. *J Rheumatol* 16:768, 1989.

281. Ordi J, Barquinero J, Vilardell M, et al: Fetal loss treatment in patients with antiphospholipid antibodies. *Ann Rheum Dis* 48:798, 1989.

282. Derue GJ, Englert HJ, Harris EN, et al: Fetal loss in systemic lupus: Assocaition with anticardiolipin antibodies. *J Obstet Gynecol* 5:207, 1985.

283. Asherson RA, Hughes GRV: Recurrent deep vein thrombosis and Addison's disease in primary antiphospholipid syndrome. *J Rheumatol* 16:378, 1989.

283a. Out HJ, Kooijman CD, Bruinse HW, Derksen RHWM: Histopathological findings in placentae from patients with intra-uterine fetal death and antiphospholipid antibodies. *Eur J Obstet Gynecol Reprod Biol* 41:719, 1991.

284. Asherson RA, Gibson DG, Evans DW, et al: Diagnostic and therapeutic problems in two patients with antiphospholipid antibodies, heart valve lesions, and transient ischaemic attacks. *Ann Rheum Dis* 47:947, 1988.

285. Khamashta MA, Gil A, Anciones B, et al: Chorea in systemic lupus erythematosus: Association with antiphospholipid antibodies. *Ann Rheum Dis* 47:681, 1988.

285a. Luchi ME, Asherson RA, Lahita RG: Primary idiopathic pulmonary hypertension complicated by pulmonary arterial thrombosis—association with antiphospholipid antibodies. *Arthritis Rheum* 35:700, 1992.

286. Asherson RA, Zulman J, Hughes GRV: Pulmonary thromboembolism associated with procainamide induced lupus syndrome and anticardiolipin antibodies. *Ann Rheum Dis* 48:232, 1989.

287. Anderson NE, Ali MR: The lupus anticoagulant, pulmonary thromboembolism, and fatal pulmonary hypertension. *Ann Rheum Dis* 43:760, 1984.

288. Asherson RA, Mackay IR, Harris EN: Myocardial infarction in a young man with systemic lupus erythematosus, deep vein thrombosis, and antibodies to phospholipid. *Br Heart J* 56:190, 1986.

289. Gharavi Y, Raz E, Gilon D, et al: Cerebrovascular accident and myocardial infarction associated with anticardiolipin antibodies in a young woman with systemic lupus erythematosus. *Ann Rheum Dis* 48:853, 1989.

290. Hamstem A, Bjorkholm M, Norberg R, et al: Antibodies to cardiolipin in young survivors of myocardial infarction: An association with recurrent cardiovascular events. *Lancet* 1:113, 1986.

291. Morton KE, Gavaghan TP, Krilis SA, et al: Coronary artery bypass graft failure—an autoimmune phenomenon? *Lancet* 2:1353, 1986.

291a. Levy EN, Ramsey-Goldman R, Kahl LE: Adrenal insufficiency in two women with anticardiolipin antibodies: cause and effect. *Arthritis Rheum* 33:1842, 1990.

291b. Rosove MH, Brewer PMC: Antiphosopholipid thrombosis: clinical course after the first thrombotic event in 70 patients. *Ann Intern Med* 117:303, 1992.

291c. Lockshin MD: Which patients with antiphospholipid antibody should be treated and how? *Rheum Dis Clin* 119:235, 1993.

291d. Lo SC, Salem HH, Howard MA, et al: Studies of natural anticoagulant proteins and anticardiolipin antibodies in patients with the lupus anticoagulants. *Br J Haemotol* 76:380, 1990.

292. Williams H, Laurent R, Gibston T: The lupus coagulation inhibitor and venous thrombosis: A report of four cases. *Clin Lab Haematol* 2:139, 1980.

293. Asherson RA, Chan JK, Harris EN, et al: Anticardiolipin antibody, recurrent thrombosis and warfarin withdrawal. *Ann Rheum Dis* 44:823, 1985.

294. Lockshin MD: Anticardiolipin antibody. *Arthritis Rheum* 30:471, 1987.

294a. Lindheimer MD, Katz AI: I: Preclampsia: Pathophysiology, diagnosis, and management. *Ann Rev Med* 169:439, 1989.

295. Lubbe WF, Butler WS, Palmer SJ, et al: Lupus anticoagulant in pregnancy. *Br J Obstet Gynaecol* 91:357, 1984.

296. Branch DW, Scott JR, Kochenour NK, et al: Obstetric complications association with the lupus anticoagulant. *N Engl J Med* 313:1322, 1985.

296a. Rosove MY, Tabsh K, Wasserstrum N, et al: Heparin therapy for prevention of pregnancy in women with lupus anticoagulants or anticardiolipin antibodies. *Obstet Gynecol* 75:630, 1990.

297. Francois FA, Freund M, Daffos F, et al: Repeated fetal losses and the lupus anticoagulant (letter). *Ann Intern Med* 109:993, 1988.

298. Parke A, Maier D, Wilson D, et al: Intravenous gamma-globulin, antiphospholipid antibodies, and pregnancy (letter). *Ann Intern Med* 110:495, 1989.

299. Walport MJ: Pregnancy and antibodies to phospholipids. *Ann Rheum Dis* 48:795, 1989.

300. Rocco VK, Hurd ER: Scleroderma and scleroderma-like disorders. *Semin Arthritis Rheum* 16:22, 1986.

301. Subcommittee for Scleroderma Criteria of the American Rheumatism Association Diagnostic and Therapeutic Criteria Committee: Preliminary criteria for classification of systemic sclerosis. *Arthritis Rheum* 23:581, 1980.

302. Medsger TA, Masi AT: Epidemiology of progressive systemic sclerosis. *Clin Rheum Dis* 5:15, 1979.

303. Abraham D, Lupoli S, McWhirter A, et al: Expression and function of surface antigens on scleroderma fibroblasts. *Arthritis Rheum* 34:1164, 1991.

304. Umehara H, Kumagai S, Ishida H et al: Enhanced production of interleukin-2 in patients with progressive systemic sclerosis: hyperactivity of CD-4 positive T cells? *Arthritis Rheum* 31:401, 1988.

305. Khaleh MB: Vascular disease in scleroderma. Endothelial T lymphocyte-fibroblast interactions. *Rheum Dis Clin N Amer* 16(1):53, 1990.

306. Needleman BW: Immunologic aspects of scleroderma. *Curr Opinion Rheum* 4:862, 1992.

307. Gruschwitz MS, Moormann S, Kromer G, et al: Phenotypic analysis of skin infiltrates in comparison with peripheral blood lymphocytes, spleen cells and thymocytes in early avian scleroderma. *J Autoimmun* 4:577, 1991.

308. D'Angelo WA, Fries JF, Masi AT, et al: Pathological observations in systemic sclerosis (scleroderma). *Am J Med* 46:428, 1969.

309. Tuffanelli DL, Winkleman RK: Systemic sclerosis (a clinical study of 727 cases). *Arch Dermatol* 84:359, 1969.

310. Westerman MO, Martinez R, Medsger T, et al: Anemia and scleroderma. Frequency, causes and marrow findings. *Arch Intern Med* 122:39, 1968.

311. Sumithran E: Progressive systemic sclerosis and autoimmune hemolytic anemia. *Postgrad Med J* 52:173, 1971.

312. Rosenthal DS, Sack B: Autoimmune hemolytic anemia in scleroderma. *JAMA* 216:2011, 1971.

313. Tan EM, Rodnan GP: Profiles of antinuclear antibodies in progressive systemic sclerosis. *Arthritis Rheum* 18:430, 1975.

314. Catoggio LJ, Bernstein AM, Black CM, et al: Serological markers of progressive systemic sclerosis: Clinical correlations. *Ann Rheum Dis* 42:23, 1983.

315. Fritzler MJ, Kinsella TD, Garbutt E: The CREST syndrome: A distinct serological entity with anticentromere antibodies. *Am J Med* 69:520, 1980.

316. Jarzabek-Chorzelska M, Blaszczyk M, Jablanska S, et al: Scl 70 antibody—a specific marker of systemic sclerosis. *Br J Dermatol* 115:393, 1986.

317. Maul GG, French BT, van Venrooij WJ, et al: Topoisomerase I identified by scleroderma 70 antisera: Enrichment of topoisomerase at centromere in mouse mitotic cells before anaphase. *Proc Natl Acad Sci USA* 83:5145, 1986.

318. Alton E, Turner-Warwick M: Lung Involvement in scleroderma, in Jayson MV, Black CM (eds): *Systemic Sclerosis: Scleroderma*. Chichester, Wiley, 1988.

319. Cosio M, Ghezzo H, Hogg JC, et al: The relations between struc-

tural changes in small airways and pulmonary function testing. *N Engl J Med* 298:1277, 1978.

320. McCarthy DS, Baragar FD, Dhinga S, et al: The lung in systemic sclerosis (scleroderma): A review and new information. *Semin Arthritis Rheum* 17:271, 1988.

321. Godfrey S, Bluestone R, Higgs BE: Lung function and response to exercise in systemic sclerosis. *Thorax* 24:427, 1969.

322. Guttadauria M, Ellman H, Emmanuel G, et al: Pulmonary function in scleroderma. *Arthritis Rheum* 20:1071, 1977.

323. Steen VD, Owen GR, Fino GJ, et al: Pulmonary involvement in systemic sclerosis (scleroderma). *Arthritis Rheum* 28:882, 1985.

324. Smitham JH: Discussion. *Proc Ro Soc Med* 46:521, 1953.

325. Opie LH: The pulmonary manifestations of generalized scleroderma (progressive systemic sclerosis). *Dis Chest* 28:665, 1955.

326. Orringer MB, Dabich L, Zasabonetis CJ, et al: Gastroesophageal reflux in esophageal scleroderma. Diagnosis and implication. *Ann Thorac Surg* 22:120, 1976.

327. Steckel RJ, Bein ME, Kelley PM: Pulmonary arterial hypertension in progressive systemic sclerosis. *Am J Roentgenol Rad Ther Nucl Med* 124:461, 1975.

328. Ungerer RG, Tashkin DP, Frust D, et al: Prevalence and clinical correlates of pulmonary arterial hypertension in progressive systemic sclerosis. *Am J Med* 75:65, 1983.

329. Salerni R, Rodnan GP, Leon DF, Shaver JA: Pulmonary hypertension in the CREST syndrome variant of progressive systemic sclerosis (scleroderma). *Ann Intern Med* 86:394, 1977.

329a. Yousem SA: The pulmonary pathological manifestations of CREST syndrome. *Human Pathol* 21:467, 1990.

330. Rozkovec A, Bernstein R, Asherson RA, et al: Vascular reactivity and pulmonary hypertension in systemic sclerosis. *Arthritis Rheum* 26:1037, 1983.

331. Sfikakis PP, Kyriakidis M, Vergo C: Diffusing capacity of the lung and nifedipine in systemic sclerosis. *Arth Rheum* 33:1634, 1990.

332. Thurm CA, Wigley FM, Dole WP, Wise RA: Failure of vasodilator infusion to alter pulmonary diffusing capacity in systemic sclerosis. *Am J Med* 90:547, 1991.

333. Baron M, Feiglin D, Hyalin R, et al: Gallium scan in progressive systemic sclerosis. *Arthritis Rheum* 26:969, 1983.

334. Siebolt JR: Scleroderma, in Kelly WN, Harris ED, Ruddy S, Sledge CB (eds): *Textbook of Rheumatology.* Philadelphia, Saunders, 1989.

335. Warrick JH, Bhalla M, Schabel SI, Silver RM: High resolution computed tomography in early scleroderma lung disease. *J Rheum* 18:1520, 1991.

336. Edelson JD, Hyland RH, Ramsden M, et al: Lung inflammation in scleroderma: Clinical, radiological, physiological and cytopathological features. *J Rheumatol* 12:957, 1985.

337. Silver RM, Metcalf JF, LeRoy EC: Interstitial lung disease in scleroderma: Immune complexes in sera and bronchoalveolar lavage fluid. *Arthritis Rheum* 29:525, 1986.

338. Silver RM, Miller KS, Kinsella MB, et al: Evaluation and management of scleroderma lung disease using bronchoalveolar lavage. *Am J Med* 88:470, 1990.

339. Steen VD, Owens GR, Redmond C, et al: The effects of D-penicillamine on pulmonary findings in systemic sclerosis. *Arthritis Rheum* 28:882, 1985.

340. Rodnan GP: The natural history of progressive systemic sclerosis (diffuse scleroderma). *Bull Rheum Dis* 13:301, 1963.

341. Lally EV, Jimenez SA, Kaplan SR: Progressive systemic sclerosis: Mode of presentation, rapidly progressive disease course, and mortality based on analysis of 91 patients. *Semin Arthritis Rheum* 18:1, 1988.

342. Peters-Golden M, Wise RA, Hochberg MD, et al: Carbon monoxide diffusing capacity as a predictor of outcome in systemic sclerosis. *Am J Med* 77:1027, 1984.

343. Weiss O, Stead E, Warren J, et al: Scleroderma heart disease. *Arch Intern Med* 71:749, 1943.

344. Janosik D, Osborn T, Moore T, et al: Heart disease in systemic sclerosis. *Semin Arthritis Rheum* 19:191, 1989.

345. McWhorter JE, LeRoy EC: Pericardial disease in scleroderma (SSc). *Am J Med* 57:566, 1974.

346. Smith JW, Clements PJ, Levisman J, et al: Echocardiographic features of progressive systemic sclerosis. Correlations with hemodynamic and post-mortem studies. *Am J Med* 66:28, 1979.

347. Gladman DD, Gordon DA, Urowitz MB, et al: Pericardial fluid analysis in scleroderma (systemic sclerosis). *Am J Med* 60:1064, 1976.

348. Yunis MB, Radford CM, Masi AT, et al: Aortic regurgitation in scleroderma. *J Rheumatol* 11:384, 1984.

349. Bulkley BH, Ridolfi RL, Salger WR, et al: Myocardial lesions of progressive systemic sclerosis: A cause of cardiac dysfunction. *Circulation* 53:483, 1976.

350. Follansbee WP, Miller TR, Curtiss EI, et al: A controlled clinicopathologic study of myocardial fibrosis in systemic sclerosis (scleroderma). *J Rheum* 17:650, 1990.

351. Alexander EL, Firestein GS, Weiss JL, et al: Reversible cold-induced abnormalities in myocardial perfusion and function in systemic sclerosis. *Ann Intern Med* 105:661, 1986.

352. Kahan A, Devaux J, Amor B, et al: Nifedipine and thallium 201 myocardial perfusion in progressive systemic sclerosis. *N Engl J Med* 314:1397, 1986.

353. Ellis WW, Baer AN, Robertson RM, et al: Left ventricular dysfunction induced by cold exposure in patients with systemic sclerosis. *Am J Med* 80:385, 1986.

354. Clements PJ, Furst DE, Cabeen WR, et al: The relationship of arrhythmias and conduction disturbances to other manifestations of cardiopulmonary disease in progressive systemic sclerosis. *Am J Med* 71:38, 1981.

355. Roberts NK, Cabeen WR, Moss J, et al: The prevalence of conduction defects and cardiac arrhythmias in progressive systemic sclerosis. *Ann Intern Med* 94:38, 1981.

356. Bulkley BH, Klarsman PG, Hutchins GM: Angina pectoris, myocardial infarction, and sudden cardiac death with normal coronary arteries: A clinicopathologic study of nine patients with progressive systemic sclerosis. *Am Heart J* 95:563, 1978.

357. *Primer in the Rheumatic Diseases.* Atlanta, Arthritis Foundation, 1988.

358. Gavras H, Gavras I, Cannon PJ, et al: Is elevated plasma renin activity of prognostic importance in progressive systemic sclerosis? *Arch Intern Med* 137:1554, 1977.

359. Strongwater SL, Galvanek EG, Stoff JS: Control of hypertension and reversal of renal failure in undifferentiated connective tissue disease by enalopril. *Arch Intern Med* 149:582, 1989.

359a. Cohen S, Laufer I, Snape W, et al: The gastrointestinal manifestation of scleroderma: Pathogenesis and management. *Gastroenterology* 79:155, 1980.

359b. Lally EV, Jimenez SA, Kaplan SR: Progressive systemic sclerosis: Mode of presentation, rapidly progressive disease course, and mortality based on an analysis of 91 patients. *Sem Arth Rheum* 18:1, 1988.

359c. Seibold JR: Scleroderma, in Kelly WN, Harris ED, Ruddy S, et al (eds): *Textbook in Rheumatology.* Philadelphia, Saunders Co., 1993, p. 1113.

359d. Kahan A, Chaussade S, Gaudric M: The effect of cisapride on gastroesophageal dysfunction in systemic sclerosis: A controlled manometric study. *Br J Clin Pharm* 31:683, 1991.

359e. Soudah H, Hasler W, Owyang C: Effect of octreotide on intestinal motility and bacterial overgrowth in scleroderma. *N Engl J Med* 325:1461, 1991.

360. Bohan A, Peter JB: Polymyositis and dermatomyositis. Part I and Part II. *N Engl J Med* 292:334, 403, 1975.

361. Rose AL, Walton JN: Polymyositis: A survey of 89 cases with particular reference to treatment and prognosis. *Brain* 89:747, 1966.

362. Devere R, Bradley WG: Polymyositis: Its presentation, morbidity and mortality. *Brain* 98:637, 1975.

363. Henriksson KG, Sandstedt P: Polymyositis—treatment and prognosis. A study of 107 patients. *Acta Neurol Scand* 65:280, 1982.

364. Currie S: Polymyositis and related disorders. Part I, in Walton SJ (ed): *Disorders of Voluntary Muscle,* 4th ed. Edinburgh, Churchill-Livingstone, 1981, p 525.

365. Whitaker JN: Inflammatory myopathy: A review of etiologic and pathogenetic factors. *Muscle Nerve* 5:573, 1982.

366. Benbassat J, Gefel D, Larholt K, et al: Prognostic factors in polymyositis/dermatomyositis: A computer assisted analysis of 92 cases. *Arthritis Rheum* 28:249, 1985.

367. Keil H: The manifestations in the skin and mucous membranes in dermatomyositis with specific reference to the differential di-

agnosis from systemic lupus erythematosus. *Ann Intern Med* 16:828, 1942.

368. Maricq HR, Spencer-Green G, LeRoy EC: Skin capillary abnormalities as indicators of organ involvement in scleroderma (systemic sclerosis), Raynaud's syndrome and dermatomyositis. *Am J Med* 61:862, 1976.

369. Mills JA: Dermatomyositis, in Fitzpatrick TB, Eisen AZ, Wolf K, et al (eds): *Dermatology in General Medicine*. New York, McGraw-Hill, 1979, p 1298.

370. Feldman D, Hochberg MC, Zizic TM, Stevens MB: Cutaneous vasculitis in adult polymyositis/dermatomyositis. *J Rheumatol* 10:85, 1982.

371. Dickey BF, Myers AR: Pulmonary disease in polymyositis/dermatomyositis. *Semin Arthritis Rheum* 14:60, 1984.

372. Bradley WG: Inflammatory diseases of muscle, in Kelley WN, Harris ED, Ruddy S, Sledge CB (eds): *Textbook of Rheumatology*, 2nd ed. Philadelphia, Saunders, 1989, p 1263.

373. Dalakas MC, London WT, Gravell M, Sever JL: Polymyositis in an immunodeficiency disease in monkeys induced by a type D retrovirus. *Neurology* 36:569, 1986.

374. Dalakas MC, Pezeshkpour GH, Gravell M, Sever JL: Polymyositis associated with AIDS retrovirus. *JAMA* 256:2381, 1986.

375. Bohan A, Peter JB, Bowman RL, Pearson CM: A computer assisted analysis of 153 patients with polymyositis and dermatomyositis. *Medicine* (Baltimore) 56:255, 1977.

376. Strongwater SL, Annesley T, Schnitzer TJ: Myocardial involvement in polymyositis. *J Rheumatol* 10:459, 1983.

377. Kehoe R, Bauernfeind R, Tommasco C, et al: Cardiac conduction defects in polymyositis. *Ann Intern Med* 94:141, 1981.

378. Behan WM, Behan PO, Gairns J: Cardiac damage in polymyositis associated with antibodies to ribonuclear proteins. *Br Heart J* 57:176, 1987.

379. Bunch TW, Duffy JD, McLeod RA: Deforming arthritis of the hands in polymyositis. *Arthritis Rheum* 19:243, 1976.

380. Schumacher HR, Schimmer B, Gordon GV, et al: Articular manifestations of polymyositis and dermatomyositis. *Am J Med* 67:287, 1979.

380a. Hidano A, Kaneko K, Arai Y, et al: Survey of the prognosis for dermatomysitis with special reference to its association with malignancy and pulmonary fibrosis. *J Dermatol* 13:233, 1986.

380b. Sigurgeirsson B, Lindelof B, Edhag O, Allander E: Risk of cancer in patients with dermatomyositis or polymyositis. A population based study. *N Eng J Med* 326:363, 1992.

381. Ogasahara S, Takahashi M, Kang J, et al: Serum mitochondrial aspartate aminotransferase in patients with polymyositis. *Ann Neurol* 13:100, 1983.

382. Reichlin M, Arnett FC Jr: Multiplicity of antibodies in myositis sera. *Arthritis Rheum* 27:1150, 1984.

383. Hoffman GS, Franck WA, Raddatz DA, Stallones L: Presentation, treatment and prognosis of idiopathic muscle disease in a rural hospital. *Am J Med* 75:433, 1983.

384. Hochberg MC, Feldman D, Stevens MB: Adult onset polymyositis/dermatomyositis: An analysis of clinical and laboratory features and survival in 76 patients with a review of the literature. *Semin Arthritis Rheum* 15:168, 1986.

385. Tymms KE, Webb J: Dermatopolymyositis and other connective tissue diseases: A review of 105 cases. *J Rheumatol* 12:1140, 1985.

386. Payan J: Electromyography in polymyositis and some related disorders. *Clin Rheum Dis* 10:75, 1984.

387. Warmolts JR: Electrodiagnosis in neuromuscular disease. *Ann Intern Med* 95:599, 1981.

387a. Miller F, Leitman SF, Cronin ME, et al: Controlled trial of plasma exchange and leukapheresis in polymyositis and dermatomyositis. *New Eng J Med* 326:1380, 11992.

387b. Cherin P, Herson S, Wechsler B, et al: Efficacy of intravenous gammaglobulin therapy in chronic refractory polymyositis and dermatomyositis: An open study with 20 adult patients. *Am J Med* 91:162, 1991.

388. McKeran R, Slavin G, Ward P, et al: Hypothyroid myopathy: A clinical and pathological study. *J Pathol* 132:35, 1980.

389. Calabrese LH, Mitsumoto H, Chou SM: Inclusion body myositis presenting as treatment resistant polymyositis. *Arthritis Rheum* 30:397, 1987.

390. Eisen A, Berry K, Gibson G: Inclusion body myositis (IBM) myopathy or neuropathy? *Neurology* (Cleveland) 33:1109, 1983.

391. Centers for Disease Control: Eosinophilia myalgia syndrome—New Mexico. *MMWR* 38:765, 1989.

392. Askari A, Vignos P, Moskowitz RW: Steroid myopathy in connective tissue disease. *Am J Med* 61:485, 1976.

392a. Varga J, Uitto J, Jimenez SA: The cause and pathogenesis of the Eosinophilia-myalgia syndrome. *Ann Int Med* 116:140, 1992.

393. Steinberg AD: Principals in the use of immunosuppressive agents, in Schumacher HR (ed): *Primer in the Rheumatic Diseases*. Atlanta, Arthritis Foundation Publication, 1988.

394. Isenberg DA, Morrow MJW, Snaith ML: Methylprednisolone pulse therapy in treatment of systemic lupus erythematosus. *Ann Rheum Dis* 41:347, 1982.

395. Mackworth Young CG, Morgan SH, Hughes GRV: Intravenous methylprednisolone in treatment of systemic lupus erythematosus. *Scand J Rheumatol Suppl* 54:16, 1984.

396. Ayoub WT, Hale RC, Harrington TM, et al: Adverse effects methylprednisolone pulse therapy in systemic lupus erythematosus. *Arthritis Rheum* 26:S34, 1983.

397. Moses RE, McCormick A, Nickey W: Fatal arrhythmias after pulse methylprednisolone therapy. *Ann Intern Med* 95:781, 1981.

398. Bocanegia TS, Casteneda MO, Espinoza LR, et al: Sudden death after methylprednisolone pulse therapy. *Ann Intern Med* 95:122, 1981.

399. Stubbs SS, Morrell RM: Intravenous methylprednisolone sodium succinate: Adverse reactions reported in association with immunosuppressive therapy. *Transplant Proc* 5:1145, 1973.

400. Fauci AS, Haynes BF, Katz P: The spectrum of vasculitis: Clinical, pathological, immunologic, and therapeutic considerations. *Ann Intern Med* 89:660, 1978.

401. McCune WJ, Fox D: Intravenous cyclophosphamide therapy of severe SLE. *Rheum Dis Clin North Am* 15:455, 1989.

402. Kovarsky J: Clinical pharmacology and toxicity of cyclophosphamide: Emphasis on use in rheumatic diseases. *Semin Arthritis Rheum* 12:359, 1983.

403. Clements J, Davis J: Cytotoxic drugs: Their clinical application to the rheumatic diseases. *Semin Arthritis Rheum* 15:231, 1986.

404. Bradley JD, Brandt KD, Katz BP: Infectious complications of cyclophosphamide treatment for vasculitis. *Arthritis Rheum* 32:45, 1989.

405. Zarday Z, Veith FJ, Gliedman ML, et al: Irreversible liver damage after azathioprine. *JAMA* 222:660, 1972.

406. Kirsner AB, Farber SJ, Sheom RP, et al: The incidence of malignant disease in patients receiving cytotoxic therapy for rheumatoid arthritis. *Ann Rheum Dis* 41(suppl):32, 1982.

407. Kinlen LJ, Scheil AGR, Peto J, et al: Collaborative United Kingdom–Australian study of cancer in patients treated with immunosuppressive drugs. *Br Med J* 2:1461, 1979.

408. Schilsky RL, Lewis BJ, Slerins RJ, Young RC: Gonodal dysfunction in patients receiving chemotherapy for cancer. *Ann Intern Med* 92:019, 1980.

409. Trompeter RS, Evans PR, Barratt JM: Gonadal function in boys with steroid-responsive nephrotic syndrome treated with cyclophosphomide for short periods. *Lancet* 1:1177, 1981.

410. Worne GL, Fairley KF, Hobbs JB, Martin FIR. Cyclophosphomide-induced ovarian failure. *N Engl J Med* 289:1139, 1973.

411. Kirshon B, Wasserstrum N, Willis R: Teratogenic effects of first trimester cyclophosphamide therapy. *Obstet Gynecol* 72:462, 1988.

412. Baker GL, Kahl LE, Zee BC, et al: Malignancy following treatment of rheumatoid arthritis with cyclophosphamide. *Am J Med* 83:1, 1987.

413. Baltus JA, Boersma JW, Hartman AP, et al: The occurrence of malignancies in patients with rheumatoid arthritis treated with cyclophosphamide: A controlled retrospective follow-up. *Ann Rheum Dis* 42:368, 1983.

414. Pedersen-Bjergaard J, Ersboll J, Sorenson HM, et al: Carcinoma of the urinary bladder after treatment with cyclophosphamide for non-Hodgkin's lymphoma. *N Engl J Med* 318:1028, 1988.

415. deVries CR, Freiha ES: Hemorrhagic cystitis. A review. *J Urol* 143:1, 1990.

416. Hahn B: Systemic lupus erythematosus and related syndromes, in WN Kelley, ED Harris Jr, S Ruddy, CB Sledge (eds): *Textbook of Rheumatology*, Philadelphia, Saunders, 4th ed. 1993, p 1050.

417. Wofsy D: Difficult lupus nephritis prognosis and management,

Oct. 15, 1992. American College of Rheumatology National Meetings.

418. Patel AR, Shah PC, Rhee HL: Cyclophosphamide therapy and interstitial pulmonary fibrosis. *Cancer* 38:1542, 1976.

419. Goldberg JW, Lidsky MD: Cyclophosphamide-associated hepatotoxicity. *South Med J* 78:222, 1985.

420. Sen RP, Walsh TE, Fisher W, Brock N. Pulmonary complications of combination therapy with cyclophosphomide and prednisone. *Chest* 99:143, 1991.

421. Weinblatt ME: Methotrexate. In WN Kelley, ED Harris, S Ruddy, CB Sledge (eds): *Textbook of Rheumatology,* 4th edition. Philadelphia, Saunders, 1993, p 767.

422. Weinblatt ME. Toxicity of low dose methotrexate in rheumatoid arthritis. *J Rheumatol* (Suppl.), 12:35, 1985.

423. Maricic M, Davis M, Gale EP: Megaloblastic paneytopenia in a patient receiving concurrent methotrexate and timethoprim-sulfame thoxayole treatment. *Arthritis Rheum* 29:133, 1986.

424. MacKinnon SK, Starkebaum G, Willkens RF: Paneytopenia associated with low dose pulse methotrexate in the treatment of rheumatoid arthritis. *Semin Arthritis Rheum* 15:119, 1985.

425. Searles G, McKendry RJ: Methotrexate pneumonitis in rheumatoid arthritis: Potential risk factors. Four case reports and a review of the literature. *J Rheumatol* 14:1164, 1987.

426. Kaplan RL, Waite DH: Progressive interstitial lung disease from prolonged methotrexate therapy. *Arch Dermatol* 114:1800, 1978.

427. Perruquet JL, Harrington TM, Davis DE: Pneumocystis carinii pneumonia following methotrexate therapy for rheumatoid arthritis (letter). *Arthritis Rheum* 26:1291, 1983.

428. Alty-Smith M, Kendall LG, Stamm AM: Cryptococcosis associated with low dose methotrexate for arthritis. *Am J Med* 83:179, 1987.

429. Shiroky JB, Frost A, Skelton JD, et al: Complications of immunosuppression associated with weekly low dose methotrexate. *J Rheumatol* 18:1172, 1991.

430. Bridges SL Jr, Lopey-Mendez A, Harn KH, et al: Should methotrexate be discontinued before elective orthopedic surgery in patients with rheumatoid arthritis? *J Rheumatol* 18:984, 1991.

220. Vasculitis in the Intensive Care Unit

Nancy Y. N. Liu, David F. Giansiracusa, and Steven L. Strongwater

Overview

The vasculitides are a group of clinicopathologic disorders in which inflammation and necrosis of blood vessel walls result in organ system abnormalities due to thrombosis and hemorrhage [1–4]. The possibility of a systemic vasculitis should be considered in the patient with systemic complaints (Table 220-1) and dysfunction of any and often multiple organ systems (Table 220-2), frequently in the context of severe constitutional symptoms such as fever, malaise, and weight loss. Patients hospitalized in the intensive care unit (ICU) may develop vasculitis as a consequence of an infection, due to a drug reaction, as a consequence of emboli of atheromatous material or from thrombosis during a hypercoagulable state.

Disorders not discussed herein but which may simulate the presentation of vasculitis include endocarditis embolism, cardiac myxoma, hypercoagulable states, hyperviscosity syndromes, chronic ergotism, radiation arteriopathy, and less commonly Ehler's-Danlos syndrome, neurofibromatosis, Sweet's syndrome, pseudoxanthoma elasticum, and Kohlmeier-Danlos diseases [4a,4b].

This chapter addresses several forms of necrotizing vasculitis including polyarteritis, drug-induced vasculitis, vasculitis associated with human immunodeficiency virus (HIV), Wegener's granulomatosis, isolated cerebral angiitis, and cholesterol embolism. Arterial thromboses associated with antiphospholipid antibodies are discussed in Chapter 219. For a more general discussion of vasculitis other references are available [1–4].

Polyarteritis Nodosa

Polyarteritis nodosa (PAN) is a systemic necrotizing arteritis involving the small and medium-size muscular arteries. Vasculitic lesions characteristically occur at the bifurcations or branches of vessels and are often segmental. Almost any organ can be involved but the skin, kidney, peripheral nerves, GI tract, and joints are the principal organs affected. The prevalence of polyarteritis is 6.3 per 100,000 population with an incidence of 0.7–1.8/100,000 [5]. Men are more likely to be affected than women in a ratio of 2 : 1. The mean age of onset is 45 years [6].

The pathogenesis of polyarteritis is unknown. Although immune complex-mediated mechanisms have been proposed, immune deposits are not often found [7]. Hepatitis B surface antigen (HBsAg) has been found in approximately 30 percent of patients with polyarteritis. The presence of circulating immune complexes of HBsAg and antibody in vessel walls has suggested that immune mechanisms may play a role in some forms of polyarteritis [8]. However, other infectious agents can be associated with vasculitis including streptococcal and staphylococcal organisms as well as cytomegalovirus [9], parvovirus [10], human T-cell leukemia virus I (HTLV-I) [11], HTLV-III [12], adenovirus, and herpes zoster [13].

Recently, hepatitis C virus (HCV) has been reported in association with polyarteritis. A study of 56 patients with classic PAN revealed antibodies to HCV in 20 percent of the patients. More specific antibodies to HCV antigens, as detected by recombinant immunoblot assay (RIBA II) and polymerase chain reaction (PCR) to HCV RNA was only positive in 5 percent of all patients (13a). Thus, only a small fraction of PAN patients had documented infection with HCV. In contrast, there is a strong association of the presence of HCV infection in patients with mixed cryoglobulinema type II (13b,13c).

Polyarteritis can be associated with other collagen vascular diseases such as rheumatoid arthritis, systemic lupus erythematosus (SLE), and Sjögren's syndrome (see Chap. 219). In addition, polyarteritis has been associated with malignancies including carcinomas, lymphomas, and other myeloproliferative disorders. Hairy cell leukemia with associated polyarteritis is rare, but some have postulated that cross-reacting antibodies against hairy cell and endothelial cell determinants result in vasculitis [14].

Table 220-1. Complaints of Patients with Systemic Vasculitis

Fever	Chest pain
Weight loss	Weakness
Cough	Numbness and paresthesias
Malaise	Extremity pain
Myalgia	Arthritis and arthralgia
Nausea and vomiting	Skin rashes
Abdominal pain	

Table 220-2. Organ Dysfunction Occurring in Systemic Necrotizing Vasculitis

Renal	*GI*
Hypertension	Cholecystitis
Renal infarction	Bleeding
Glomerulonephritis	Hepatic dysfunction
Interstitial nephritis	Bowel infarction
	Bowel perforation
Skin	*Cardiac*
Rash, purpura	Myocardial infarction
Nodules	Congestive heart failure
Livedo reticularis	Pericarditis
Ulcers	
Nervous System	*Musculoskeletal*
Cerebral vascular accidents	Arthralgias
Altered mental status	Arthritis
Seizures	Myalgias
Peripheral neuro-infarction	Muscle infarction
Mononeuritis multiplex	
Peripheral neuropathy	
Pulmonary	
Pleuritis	
Pneumonitis	
Interstitial lung disease	
Cavitary lesion	

Pathologically, fibrinoid necrosis, predominantly with polymorphonuclear leukocyte infiltrates, involves the entire wall of small and medium-size muscular arteries (Fig. 220-1). Thromboses and aneurysms can be found in lesions. In autopsy series, the kidneys and heart are the most common organs involved (70%), followed by peripheral nerves (50%), liver (50%), and the GI tract (44%) [6]. Less commonly, muscle, pancreas, testes, CNS, and skin are involved [6].

Clinical manifestations vary from mild localized disease to multisystem failure. Patients generally complain of malaise, weight loss, fevers, abdominal or lower extremity pain, and myalgias or arthralgias. Clinical parameters (Table 220-3) include renal involvement with vasculitis (45%), hypertension (54%), and glomerulonephritis (25%) [6]. Abnormal laboratory findings include proteinuria, active urinary sediment, or progressive renal insufficiency. Renal disease, a major cause of mortality, is estimated to range from 45 to 65 percent [6,15]. Peripheral neuropathy occurs in 50 to 70 percent of cases and patterns usually include mixed sensorimotor and mononeuritis multiplex [16]. Sudden-onset paresthesias associated with motor deficits are common manifestations. CNS involvement, including seizures, focal events, and altered mental status is much less common (23%) [6]. Musculoskeletal symptoms occur in 50 percent of patients [6]. Approximately 20 percent of patients will have episodic, polyarthritis that is nondeforming. Vasculitis of skeletal muscles may cause severe myalgias. Abdominal pain may have a variety of causes including intestinal angina, mesenteric thrombosis, or localized gallbladder or liver disease.

Acute GI bleeding, perforation, and infarction are rare but are associated with a high mortality if the diagnosis is not established promptly. Cardiac involvement, observed in nearly 60 percent of autopsy series, is often clinically silent [17]. Congestive heart failure, pericarditis, myocardial infarctions, and conduction abnormalities are the common manifestations. Cutaneous lesions include nonspecific maculopapular rash, livedo reticularis, tender nodular lesions, and ulcers. Arteries of the eye, testes, and lungs, as well as involvement of the temporal arteries, may also develop.

The diagnosis of polyarteritis should be considered when a patient presents with multisystem involvement associated with systemic complaints of malaise, weight loss, and fever. Associated laboratory studies include anemia, leukocytosis, thrombocytosis, elevated erythrocyte sedimentation rates (ESRs), and proteinuria. HBsAg, cryoglobulins, and low serum complements may be present. To establish the diagnosis, histologic documentation of necrotizing vasculitis is usually required. The most accessible tissues include skin, muscle, sural nerve, and kidney. Blind muscle biopsies may reveal arteritis in 30 to 50 percent of cases [18,19]. Renal biopsies usually reveal necrotizing glomerulonephritis but do not help differentiate various forms of vasculitides [20]. If electromyography or nerve conduction studies reveal abnormalities of the sural nerve, biopsies of the sural nerve and muscle often yield tissue evidence of vasculitis [21].

In 80 percent of patients with polyarteritis, the diagnosis is established by arteriograms [6]. Arteriography usually reveals saccular or fusiform aneurysms at multiple sites [22]. The renal arteries are most commonly involved but hepatic, mesenteric, cerebral, splenic, hypogastric, gastroduodenal, intercostal, and pulmonary arteries can also be affected. The differential diagnosis of arterial aneurysms occurring in conjunction with polyarteritis includes SLE, Kawasaki disease, atrial myxomas, endocarditis, drug abuse, HIV infection, Wegener's granulomatosis, thrombotic thrombocytopenia purpura, and fibromuscular dysplasia [6].

Patients with untreated polyarteritis have only a 13 percent 5-year survival rate [17,23]. More recently, survival has improved to 50 to 60 percent with the use of glucocorticoids; the addition of cyclophosphamide may result in even higher survival rates [24]. Whether the use of high-dose corticosteroids alone is adequate or the combination of corticosteroids with an immunosuppressive agent is needed as initial therapy is debated. Cupps and Fauci [6] and Fauci and co-workers [25] recommend cyclophosphamide, 2 mg/kg/day, together with prednisone, 1 mg/kg/day, for severe, progressive systemic necrotizing vasculitis. Conn and Hunder recommend high-dose prednisone (60–100 mg) in divided doses for patients with less severe involvement (e.g., minimal visceral involvement) [24]. If the patient's disease progresses or remains unimproved, then cytotoxic agents or pulse-dose corticosteroids should be given [26].

A recent prospective study demonstrated that the combination of steroids, cyclophosphamide, and plasma exchange can provide improved disease control overall and fewer relapse rate than steroids and plasma exchange alone. However, 10 year survival was similar in the two groups (72% versus 75%) [26].

A subsequent study that tried to delineate optimal initial therapy revealed no benefit of plasma exchange with high-dose steroids from high-dose steroids alone. However, both groups experienced high rate of relapse, which required institution of cytotoxic drugs [26a]. Thus, the final optimal therapy with steroids alone or steroids with cyclophosphamide remains unanswered.

A variety of drugs may cause a necrotizing angiitis that is indistinguishable from polyarteritis including amphetamines,

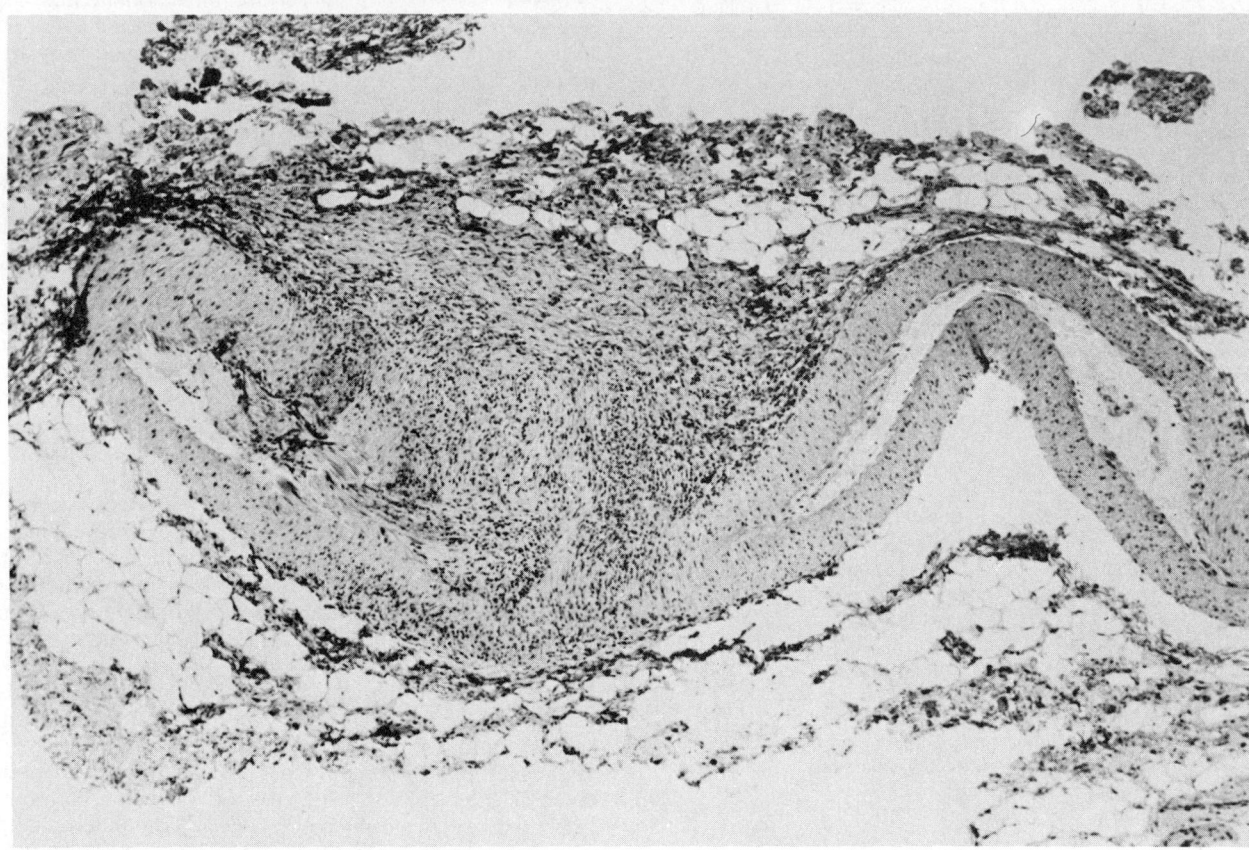

Fig. 220-1. Microscopic section of necrotizing arteritis (polyarteritis nodosa) involving a muscular artery. The process is characteristically focal. The lesion is composed of a transmural acute inflammatory infiltrate with muscle necrosis and luminal occlusion (hematoxylin and eosin stain, low power). (Courtesy of Carolyn Compton, M.D., Department of Pathology, University of Massachusetts Medical Center, Worcester, MA)

ergotamine derivatives, cocaine, phenylpropanolamine, pseudoephedrine, and lysergic acid diethylamide (LSD) [26b].

Drug-Induced Vasculitis

Drug-induced vasculitis is categorized by Fauci and co-workers in the heterogeneous group of hypersensitivity vasculitis [2]. Distinctive features of this group include small vessel involvement that on histologic tissue examination is leukoclastic vasculitis. The pathogenesis of these disorders is a hypersensitive reaction to offending drugs, microorganisms, tumor antigens, or other unidentified antigens resulting in immune complex deposition in the wall of postcapillary venules, particularly of the dermis and other organs. Pathologically, endothelial cells are swollen and necrotic; polymorphonuclear leukocytes (PMNs) infiltrate the vessel wall; leukocytoclasis, evidenced by breakdown of PMNs with visible nuclear debris, fibrinoid necrosis, and red blood cell extravasation are seen [27].

Clinically, drug-induced vasculitis occurs within 7–10 days of exposure to the offending drug. The drugs most commonly causing vasculitis include penicillin, sulfonamides, quinidine, and procainamide, but virtually any drug can produce hypersensitivity vasculitis. Table 220-4 lists some of the drugs that frequently cause hypersensitivity vasculitis. Development of the syndrome is not related to a specific dose [28].

The appearance of palpable purpura on the lower extremities, back, or buttock regions may be accompanied by systemic features of fever, arthralgias, and malaise. The lesions appear in crops. Vesicles and bullae may develop and may become more severe after standing and activity. On healing they may leave areas of hyperpigmentation and in more severe cases, scars. Although 33 percent of patients have no symptoms associated with the lesions, 40 percent complain of burning or pain [29].

Other organs commonly involved with drug-induced vasculitis include the GI tract, kidneys, and nervous system. Small vessel vasculitis of bowel wall may cause abdominal pain, nausea, vomiting, but more severe symptoms of GI bleeding, intussusception, perforation, or infarction can occur. Renal involvement may cause a spectrum of disease from mild proteinuria and hematuria to nephrotic syndrome and renal failure. Neurologic symptoms include headache and diplopia, and less commonly, polyneuropathy or hemiparesis.

Drug-induced vasculitis is usually a self-limited disease that resolves 2–4 weeks after the offending agent is eliminated. If a patient is acutely symptomatic or has evidence of significant organ involvement other than the skin, corticosteroids may be prescribed in a dose of 20–60 mg/day, depending on the severity of disease. Once symptoms improve, corticosteroids should be tapered. Rarely, drug-induced vasculitis recurs despite discontinuation of the offending agent. Repeated courses of corticosteroids may be required. The role of immunosuppressive agents in the treatment of hypersensitivity vasculitis remains unclear [30].

Table 220-3. Clinical Parameters in Patients with Classic PAN

Clinical parameter	Finding	Number of patients
General Considerations		
Age (mean)	45 years	198
Sex ratio (male to female)	2.5 : 1	314
	Percent	
Fever	71	460
Weight loss	54	405
Organ System Involvement		
Kidney renal	70	375
Musculoskeletal system	64	301
Arthritis and arthralgia	53	301
Myalgias	31	238
Hypertension	54	356
Peripheral neuropathy	51	495
GI tract	44	507
Abdominal pain	43	122
Nausea and vomiting	40	30
Cholescystitis	17	64
Bleeding	6	205
Bowel perforation	5	64
Bowel infarction	1.4	140
Skin	43	476
Rash and purpura	30	259
Nodules	15	369
Livedo reticularis	4	194
Cardiac	36	413
Congestive heart failure	12	204
Myocardial infarct	6	64
Pericarditis	4	204
Central nervous system	23	184
Cerebral vascular accident	11	90
Altered mental status	10	90
Seizure	4	90

PAN = polyarteritis nodosa.
Source: From Cupps TR, Fauci AS: Systemic necrotizing vasculitis of the polyarteritis nodosa group, in *The Vasculitides.* Philadelphia, rs Co., 1981, with permission.

Table 220-4. Drugs Associated with Hypersensitivity Vasculitis

Antibiotics	*Anticonvulsants*	*Antiarrhythmics*
Penicillin	Phenobarbital	Quinidine
Sulfonamides	Phenytoin	Procainamide
Tetracycline		
Streptomycin		
Rheumatic Drugs	*Others*	
Aspirin	Phenothiazines	
Levamisole	Iodides	
Allopurinol	Griseofulvin	
Gold	Propylthiouracil	
Phenylbutazone		

Cutaneous lesions that on biopsy reveal leukocytoclastic vasculitis of small vessels are not limited to drug-induced vasculitis. In fact, only 13 percent of all cutaneous vasculitis is related to drug hypersensitivity [30a]. Thus, the differential is broadened after drugs are excluded to include infections (*Streptococcus, Staphylococcus, Salmonella, Yersinia,* mycobacterium, varicella zoster, hepatitis B, cytomegalovirus [CMV], influenza), malignancy, granulomatous vasculitis, rheumatoid arthritis, PAN, SLE, Sjögren's syndrome, cryoglobulinemia, idiopathic (which includes Henoch Schönlein purpura), and urticarial vasculitis.

Vasculitis Associated with Human Immunodeficiency Virus

Infection with HIV has broad immunologic and clinical manifestations (see Chap. 93). Rheumatic manifestations of HIV infections have been recently reviewed in the rheumatology and general literature [31,32,33]. These manifestations include Reiter's syndrome or reactive arthritis, psoriatic arthritis, septic arthritis, polymyositis, Sjögren's syndrome, lupuslike syndrome, and vasculitis. The following discussion is limited to vasculitis.

Calabrese reviewed cases of necrotizing vasculitis from the literature [34]. Clinically, eight cases had medium-size vessel vasculitis involving the skin, nerve, and muscle similar to polyarteritis nodosa with documented fibrinoid necrosis of vessel walls. He emphasized the difficulty in assigning causal relationship of particular vasculitis syndromes to HIV infection. Most cases were case reports and lacked detailed evaluations to exclude other viral infections (such as Epstein-Barr virus [EBV], CMV, hepatitis B), which have been associated with vasculitis.

Eight patients developed medium-size vessel vasculitis involving nerve, muscle, and skin, which was pathologically similar to PAN. Hypersensitivity vasculitis has also been reported. Lymphomatoid granulomatosis, a rare T-cell lymphoproliferative disorder, has been reported in six patients. Although the lungs are the major target organ involved, CNS, peripheral nerves, and kidneys can be involved. Even more intriguing was the development of primary angiitis of the CNS [35,36,37]. Six of the 108 cases in the literature were associated with HIV infection. Causal relationship again was difficult to prove, but one patient who had no evidence of immunodeficiency and was seronegative, died from granulomatous angiitis of CNS. However, HIV was isolated from the cerebrospinal fluid and brain tissue [35].

The pathogenesis of HIV vasculitis may be as heterogeneous as that of other viral-induced vasculitides. Direct invasion of HIV into vessel walls may be a mechanism, given that evidence for this invasion exists in other viral-induced vasculitides [38]. Alternatively, HIV infection may stimulate a humoral or cellular immune response. The support for the former hypothesis is the finding of immune complexes within the vessel wall of one patient with PNA-like vasculitis [39]. Cellular immunity may have a role in the cases involving lymphomatoid granulomatosis; Calabrese postulates that an angiocentric lymphoproliferative disorder may exist in these patients [31].

Treatment of these patients is complicated by their immunocompromised state. In the various case reports, prednisone was used with variable success [40]. One patient received both high-dose prednisone and cyclophosphamide before his HIV infection was documented. This patient died of infectious complications [35]. Thus, therapy in each individual patient must be based on risk-benefit analysis. Calabrese recommends aggressive antimicrobial prophylaxis in patients who require combination chemotherapy [34].

Wegener's Granulomatosis

Wegener's granulomatosis is a disease of unknown etiology characterized by granulomatous vasculitis of the upper and lower respiratory tract, segmental necrotizing glomerulonephritis, and systemic vasculitis of small blood vessels [41]. Although involvement of only the respiratory tract has been described and reported as "limited Wegener's granulomatosis" [42], it is likely that these cases have mild or subclinical renal involvement [43]. Although the disease may affect individuals

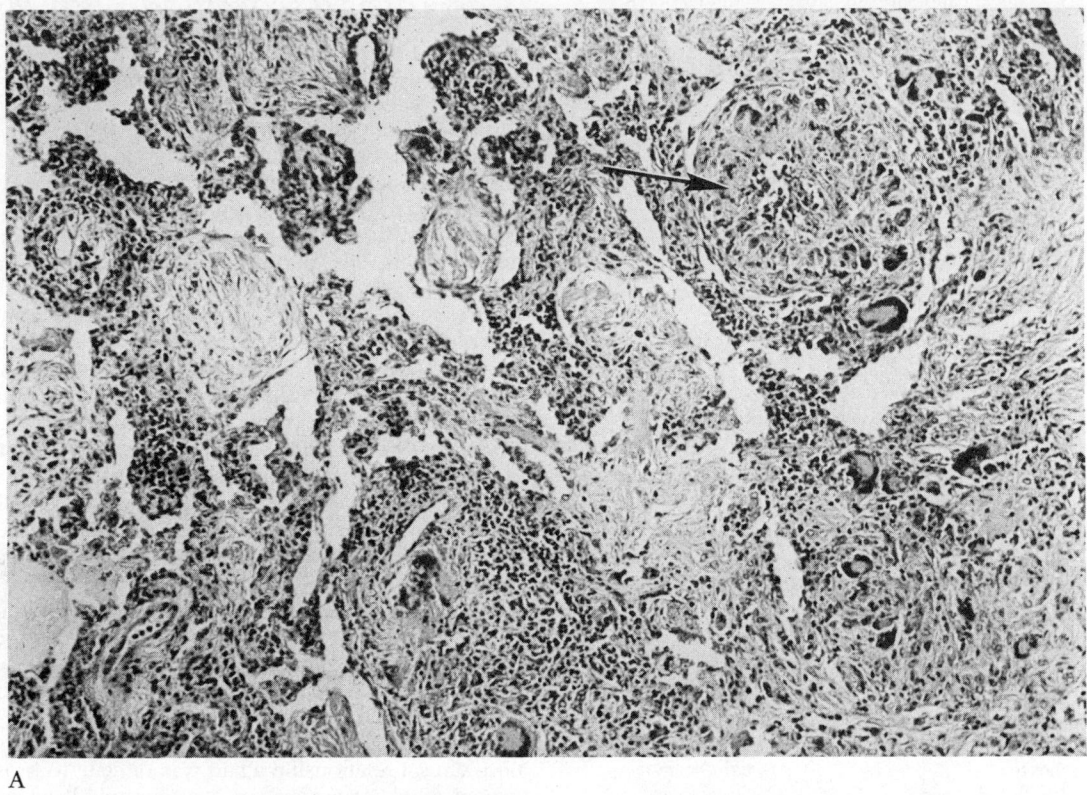

A

Fig. 220-2. Wegener's granulomatosis. A. The characteristic necrotizing granulomatous inflammation with severe vasculitis is seen (involved vessel at arrow). B. This hematoxylin and eosin stain shows transmural inflammation and focal necrosis of an arterial vessel (arrow). C. An affected vessel is more easily recognized in an elastic tissue stain. Disruption of the elastic externa (stained black) is seen where a granuloma with numerous giant cells appears in the arterial wall (arrows).

of a wide range of ages, the disease most commonly affects persons in their fourth or fifth decades of life with a slight predominance of men over women [43,44]. Wegener's granulomatosis is relatively rare with approximately three to four new cases seen per year at major medical centers. Patients most frequently require intensive care treatment for severe pneumonitis, glomerulonephritis, stroke, myocardial infarction, multiorgan system dysfunction secondary to necrotizing vasculitis, and infection due to immunosuppression and anatomic abnormalities secondary to the granulomatous inflammation.

Although the etiology of Wegener's granulomatosis is unknown, involvement of the respiratory tract with necrotizing, granulomatous inflammation raises the possibility of a reaction to an inhaled pathogenic agent. The presence of antibodies to cytoplasmic antigens in PMNs has, over the past several years, been described as a marker for Wegener's granulomatosis and is useful to support the diagnosis and to monitor disease activity [45].

Pathologically, the vessels involved in Wegener's granulomatosis include both small arteries and veins; these vessels are often adjacent to granuloma. The pathology of vasculitis includes fibrinoid necrosis with inflammatory mononuclear cell infiltrates of vessel walls, focal destruction of the elastic lamina, and narrowing or obliteration of vessel lumens. Granulomatous lesions are characterized by areas of central necrosis surrounded by epithelial fibroblasts and scattered multinucleated

giant cells (Fig. 220-2) [46]. Granulomatous vasculitis may involve the lung, skin, CNS, peripheral nerves, heart, and other organs.

CLINICAL FEATURES. The symptoms and findings associated with Wegener's granulomatosis depend on the location and severity of granulomata and of granulomatous vasculitis. Types of organ system involvement in patients with Wegener's granulomatosis are listed in Table 220-5.

The great majority of patients (approximately 85–90%) present with symptoms referable to the upper respiratory tract, including sinusitis, nasal obstruction, rhinitis, otitis, hearing loss, ear pain, gingival inflammation, epistaxis, sore throat, laryngitis, and nasal septal deformity. Fever, in addition to being caused by the underlying disease, may be due to suppurative otitis or Staphylococcus aureus sinusitis [47]. Granulomatous vasculitis of the upper respiratory tract may lead to damage of nasal cartilage resulting in the "saddle-nose" deformity, sore throat, and oral and nasal mucosal ulcers [43,48]. In addition, chondritis of the nose or ear may develop [49]. Laryngeal involvement may result in severe narrowing of the upper respiratory tract [50,51]. Approximately 10 percent of patients present with only nonspecific constitutional symptoms such as arthralgias, myalgias, fever, and weight loss. Unusual manifestations of Wegener's granulomatosis include distinctive "punched out" ulcerative skin lesions appearing as pyodermic gangrenosum [52], and painless subcutaneous nodules occurring in approximately 2 to 5 percent [41].

Although only one-third of patients present with symptomatic lung involvement (including cough, sputum production, dyspnea, chest pain, hemoptysis, and even life-threatening pulmonary hemorrhage), lower respiratory tract disease is found in almost all patients after evaluation (see Chap. 61 on Man-

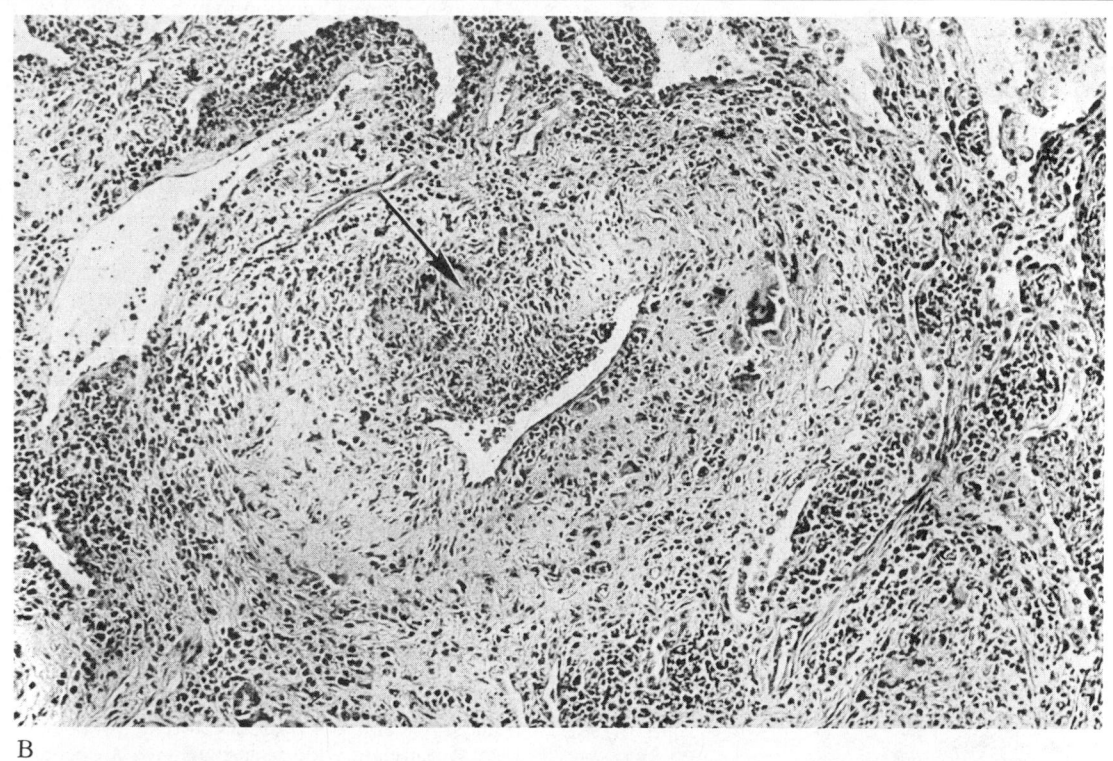

B

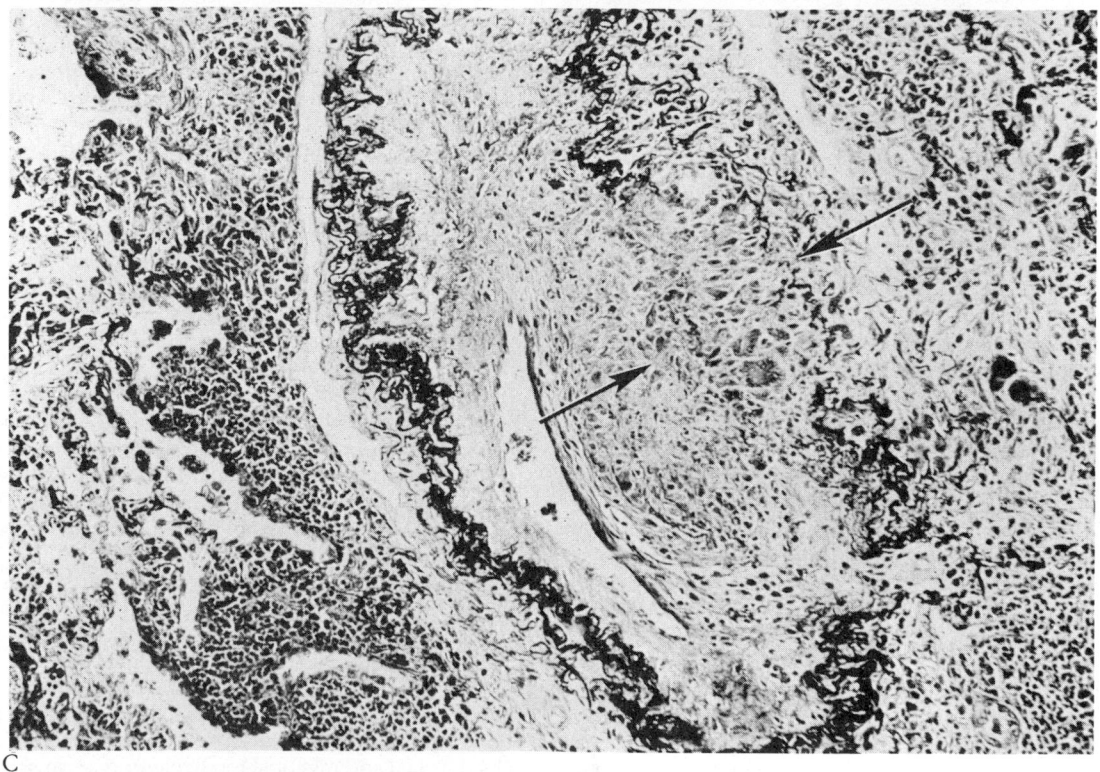

C

aging Hemoptysis). Frequently chest radiographs are abnormal even in the absence of symptoms. The characteristic chest radiographic findings are multiple, nodular, bilateral cavitary infiltrates, but infiltrates without sharp margins occur more frequently than distinct nodules. Cavitation may occur in both distinct nodules as well as in infiltrates with less defined borders. Nodules may have either thick or thin walls. Infiltrates may involve either the lower or upper lobes. In approximately 50 percent of patients, the infiltrates are bilateral. Infiltrates may be transient [43,53]. Less common chest radiographic abnor-

Table 220-5. Organ System Involvement in Wegener's Granulomatosis

Respiratory Tract

Upper	*Lower*
Sinusitis	Pleurisy
Otitis	Pulmonitis
Epistaxis	Cavitary lesions
Laryngitis	
Nasal cartilage erosion	
Nasal or oral mucosal inflammation	

Urinary Tract
Segment, necrotizing glomerulonephritis
Perinephritic hematoma
Ureteral vasculitis with obstruction
Rarely hypertension

Cardiac
Pericarditis
Myocardial infarction
Congestive heart failure
Endomyocarditis
Arrhythmias

Eye
Proptosis
Conjunctivitis, episcleritis, scleritis, uveitis, corneoscleral ulcer
Optic nerve vasculitis
Nasolacrimal duct obstruction

Musculoskeletal
Arthralgias
Arthritis

Skin
Ulcers
Papules
Petechiae
Subcutaneous nodules
Nonhealing surgical wounds

Nervous System
Mononeuritis multplex
Polyneuritis
Cranial nerve, meningeal inflammation from paranasal sinus involvement
Subarachnoid hemorrhage
Intracerebral hemorrhage

malities include paratracheal masses, large cavitary lesions, a miliary pattern, massive pleural effusion, calcified nodule, and masses between the trachea and esophagus [54]. CT scan of the chest may reveal pulmonary lesions not well demonstrated on plain x-ray films.

Although renal manifestations are often asymptomatic, urinalysis reveals renal involvement in approximately 80 percent of patients at presentation [44]. The typical renal lesion is segmental, necrotizing glomerulonephritis [55,56]. Even in patients thought to have disease limited to the respiratory tract, kidney biopsy has revealed involvement in 50 percent. Functional renal impairment may progress rapidly if appropriate therapy is not instituted promptly [43].

The vasculitis of Wegener's granulomatosis may cause a variety of other clinical manifestations including arthralgias and less commonly arthritis, most frequently affecting the knees [57,58], perinephric hematoma, renal artery aneurysms, ureteral obstruction [59], a variety of cutaneous lesions including ulcers, papules, vesicles, and subcutaneous nodules [53], episcleritis, conjunctivitis, scleritis, uveitis, optic nerve vasculitis [60], mononeuritis multiplex or polyneuritis, cranial nerve dysfunction [61], meningitis [62,63], cerebral infarction [64], subarachnoid hemorrhage [61], abdominal pain, intestinal perforation, and diarrhea [65]. CNS as well as ocular, musculoskeletal, and cutaneous manifestations are listed in Table 186-5.

Intensive care admission may be required for patients with cardiac involvement and resultant myocardial infarction secondary to coronary arteritis [66,67,68], pericarditis with tamponade, congestive heart failure due to endocarditis with valvular involvement [67,68], heart block [69], cardiac arrhythmias [70], or pancarditis.

In addition to involving the paranasal sinuses, invasion of other tissue by contiguous granulomatous inflammation may cause cranial nerve palsies, proptosis, eustachian tube obstruction, and diabetes insipidus [43,47].

Laboratory features of Wegener's granulomatosis include normochromic, normocytic anemia, mild to moderate leukocytosis without eosinophilia, thrombocytosis, elevation of the erythrocyte sedimentation rate and C-reactive protein levels, hypergammaglobulinemia, abnormalities on urinalysis including hematuria and red blood cell casts, signs of renal function and impairment, and paranasal sinus and chest radiographic abnormalities [47].

Serum immunoglobulin G autoantibodies against cytoplasmic components of PMNs have recently been reported to be involved in as many as 95 percent of Wegener's patients, particularly those with renal involvement [45,71,72]. The cytoplasmic antineutrophil cytoplasmic antibodies (C-ANCA) are directed against proteinase 3, in contrast to the peripheral antineutrophil cytoplasmic antibody (P-ANCA) which are antibodies to myeloperoxidase or elastase [72a,72b,72c]. In addition to the diagnostic value of the antineutrophil cytoplasmic antibodies (ANCAs), the presence and titer of these antibodies appear to correlate with disease activity. A decrease in titers and reversion to negative results occur during periods of remission. Intercurrent diseases and complications of therapy such as infections have not been associated with increases in titers [73,74]. The presence of ANCAs has also been reported in patients with microscopic polyarteritis [71] and in patients with rapidly progressive glomerulonephritis without Wegener's granulomatosis, idiopathic necrotizing glomerulonephritis [74a], suggesting a possible pathogenic role of the antibody [75,75a]. A number of studies support the concept that antibodies to proteinase 3, C-ANCA, play a pathogenetic role in Wegener's granulomatosis [75b,75c,75d].

The differential diagnosis of Wegener's granulomatosis includes a number of disease entities including granulomatous diseases (tuberculosis, histoplasmosis, sarcoidosis, berylliosis), neoplasmic processes (lymphoma, metastatic carcinoma, lymphomatoid granulomatosis), pulmonary-renal syndromes (Goodpasture's syndrome, Churg-Strauss syndrome, and streptococcal pneumonia complicated by glomerulonephritis), and collagen vascular diseases such as SLE [76]. Churg-Strauss syndrome (allergic angiitis and granulomatosis) is distinguished from Wegener's by a history of bronchial asthma, eosinophilia, and tissue infiltration of eosinophils [43].

The diagnosis of Wegener's granulomatosis is established by the recognition of appropriate clinical and laboratory features and the findings of the classic histopathologic triad of (1) necrotizing granulomatous lesions of the upper or lower respiratory tract, (2) glomerulonephritis, and (3) generalized necrotizing vasculitis of arteries and veins. Granulomatous lesions must be extensively studied with special stains and cultures to exclude fungal and mycobacterial microorganisms that may cause granulomatous vasculitis [76,77]. The detection of anticytoplasmic antibodies supports the diagnosis of Wegener's granulomatosis (see laboratory section, preceding), while the finding of antiglomerular basement membrane antibodies supports a diagnosis of Goodpasture's syndrome [78]. Lymphomatoid granulomatosis (polymorphic reticulosis) is distinguished from Wegener's granulomatosis by absence of glomerulonephritis and by the pathologic features of infiltration around and in blood vessels (angiocentric) of atypical lymphocytes and plasma cells [79,80,81]. Midline granuloma is more erosive than Wegener's granulomatosis and causes destructive lesions of the hard palate and skin of nose and face. In contrast to Wegener's, lymphomatoid granulomatosis localized to the lung and midline granuloma are responsive to radiation therapy [82,83].

A histologic diagnosis of Wegener's granulomatosis is critical and is typically made by lung biopsy, although adequate sampling generally requires limited thoracotomy [44]. Biopsy of involved nasal mucosa or other tissue of the upper respiratory tract may yield diagnostic material, but the sample must be of adequate size to avoid finding only necrotic tissue [51]. Although the renal biopsy findings of focal, segmental glomerulonephritis are not specific for Wegener's granulomatosis, needle biopsy of the kidney may (1) reveal changes consistent with the diagnosis, (2) help define the extent of the disease, (3) exclude other diseases in the differential diagnosis, and (4) provide useful prognostic information, because patients with renal function impairment due to active inflammatory lesions are more likely to experience improvement with treatment than are patients with significant glomerular sclerosis and renal scarring [41].

Treatment of Wegener's granulomatosis has markedly improved the outcome of the disease. Whereas the mortality rate for patients untreated at 2 years had been 90 percent, there is now a 93 percent complete remission rate, as shown by a prospective trial of oral cyclophosphamide (1–2 mg/kg/day) in 85 patients [47]. Although relapses recurred in 25 patients after discontinuation of cyclophosphamide, reinstitution controlled the disease in all but one. Azathioprine has not been as effective in inducing remissions, but may be helpful in maintaining the cyclophosphamide-induced remission in patients unable to continue cyclophosphamide. Cyclophosphamide is generally given in doses of 1–2 mg/kg/day by mouth or in cases of rapidly progressive renal disease, as 2–4 mg/kg/day IV for the first several days. The dose of the medication is then adjusted to maintain a total white blood cell count above 3000 cells/μl or a PMN count above 1500 cells/μl. Complete blood counts and platelet counts should be monitored closely (every few days) until stabilization, then every 1 or 2 weeks, with the knowledge that the nadir of white blood cell counts occurs 7 to 10 days after administration of the drug. Urinalysis should be done every few weeks for hematuria, which may reflect cyclophosphamide-induced hemorrhagic cystitis. Persistent hematuria necessitates cystoscopy and urine cytology studies to evaluate for carcinoma of the bladder [84]. Cyclophosphamide treatment is continued for at least 12 months after all reversible disease is controlled, then tapered by approximately 25 mg every 1 to 3 months. In a recently reported analysis of 158 patients followed for 6 months to 24 years (1229 patient years) [84a], a subset of patients, approximately 8 percent, who were not diagnosed for 5 to 16 years, appeared to have indolent disease generally without renal involvement. Whether this group should be treated less aggressively remains unanswered. One hundred and thirty-three (84%) of the 158 patients were treated with a "standard therapy," glucocorticosteroids and cyclophosphamide. Marked improvement occurred in 91 percent, and remission was achieved in 75 percent after a mean of 12 months of therapy, with range of 1–2 months to 4 or more years [84a]. Of those achieving remission, 50 percent relapsed. Monitoring for reactivation of disease activity should continue in this period [85]. In Hoffman's recent study [84a], 20 percent of 158 patients died, 13 percent directly related to the Wegener's granulomatosis or complications of therapy. Of the 158 patients, many suffered permanent morbidity of the disease or therapy including infertility (57%), chronic sinus disease (47%), cyclophosphamide-induced cystitis (43%), chronic renal insufficiency

(42%), hearing loss (35%), nasal deformity (28%), pulmonary insufficiency (17%), tracheal stenosis (13%), osteoporotic fractures (11%), malignancies (10% of those treated with a cytotoxic agent), visual loss (8%), aseptic necrosis of bone (3%), bladder cancer (4.2%), and myelodysphasia (2%) [84a].

Corticosteroids used alone have not significantly improved the prognosis of Wegener's granulomatosis, but they may be helpful, particularly for the control of constitutional symptoms, pericarditis, arthritis, and vasculitic skin rash when used for a short course in combination with long-term cytotoxic therapy. Severe pulmonary, renal, or skin disease may require long-term steroid therapy in combination with cyclophosphamide treatment. Patients with acute renal failure, fulminant vasculitis, or pulmonary hemorrhage are a subset of patients with poor prognosis [86].

Complications of cyclophosphamide, including increased susceptibility to infection [86a], induction of malignancy, particularly solid tumors, lympho- and myeloproliferative malignancies, and bladder cancer are major concerns. Hemorrhagic cystitis, hepatotoxicity, gonadal dysfunction, ovarian fibrosis, and pulmonary fibrosis are other potential adverse effects [39, 50,84a]. To preserve male fertility, sperm banking may be a consideration if the course of the disease allows postponing cyclophosphamide therapy. Hemorrhagic cystitis associated with pulse intravenous cyclophosphamide may be reduced with concurrent intravenous mesna which binds oxazaphosphorine. One intravenous (IV) mesna regimen is to give one-half of the total IV cyclophosphamide dose in milligrams of mesna before the cyclophosphamide infusion and the remaining half 2 hours after the infusion [84a]. In the treatment of SLE, pulse IV cyclophosphamide has appeared to be associated with lower rates of hemorrhagic cystitis than has daily cyclophosphamide [87].

Several studies using pulse, monthly IV cyclophosphamide for treatment of Wegener's granulomatosis have been performed. Intravenous therapy in a dose of 0.5–1.0 gm/m^2/month resulted in response in two of five patients [87a]. An NIH study of intravenous pulse cyclophosphamide to treat Wegener's granulomatosis resulted in a good initial response, but many beneficial responses were not maintained [87b]. In a study of seven patients who were initially treated with prednisone and daily oral cyclophosphamide but developed toxicities, switching to monthly intravenous cyclophosphamide induced remission in four and partial remission in three patients [47].

Infectious complications such as bacterial sinusitis and pulmonary infection may simulate and even exacerbate the underlying Wegener's [88]. Thorough evaluation of the clinical presentation, measurement of ANCA levels, and obtaining appropriate samples for stains and cultures including bronchoalveolar lavage, transbronchial brushings and biopsies, and even open lung biopsies may be required to distinguish activity of the Wegener's granulomatosis from infectious complications. Pneumocystis pneumonia has been reported in patients with autoimmune diseases treated with cyclophosphamide [88a].

Recently, treatment with trimethoprim-sulfamethoxazole has been noted to favorably affect the course of Wegener's granulomatosis [89]. The use of trimethoprim-sulfamethoxazole for the treatment of mild upper respiratory tract disease and mild exacerbations has been reported [90] and is being studied further at the National Institutes of Health but its role remains controversial [84a].

Alternative therapies for Wegener's granulomatosis are under study. In a pilot study of 29 patients who did not have life-threatening disease, weekly methotrexate in conjunction with glucocorticosteroids resulted in improvement in 76 percent, remission in 69 percent, and progression of disease in 17 percent [90a,90b]. High-dose IV immunoglobulin has also been reported to be beneficial in a total of seven patients with ANCA-positive systemic vasculitis [90c]. This has led to the concept that antiidiotypic antibodies to ANCA may be responsible for the beneficial effect of IV immunoglobulin therapy [90d].

Microscopic polyarteritis, an overlap syndrome between Wegener's granulomatosis and PAN, is a systemic necrotizing small vessel vasculitis. Clinically, it resembles Wegener's in its pulmonary and renal involvement. Thirty per cent of the patients will have pulmonary hemorrhage from capillaritis, and nearly all have necrotizing segmental glomerulonephritis. Skin, eyes, mucous membranes, and peripheral and central nervous systems may also be involved. In addition, there is strong correlation with presence of ANCA. However, the lack of upper respiratory involvement and more frequent involvement of the GI tract is more reminiscent of PAN. Pathologically, the vessels involved are similar to Wegener's but lack granulomata formation or venous involvement. Treatment with prednisone, cyclophosphamide, azathioprine, and plasmapheresis resulted in a 5-year survival rate of 65 percent. The relapse rate, however, was high.

Central Nervous System Vasculitis

A variety of primary and secondary forms of vasculitis affect the CNS [91,92,93]. The clinical manifestation of these disorders varies depending on the size and location of the blood vessels affected. Primary forms of CNS vasculitis, systemic necrotizing vasculitides that also involve the CNS, and a number of rheumatologic disorders, such as systemic lupus erythematosus SLE, cause CNS symptoms. This section reviews the CNS manifestations of selected disorders including granulomatous angiitis of the CNS (isolated CNS vasculitis), temporal arteritis, Takayasu's arteritis, Wegener's granulomatosis, lymphomatoid granulomatosis, and classic polyarteritis nodosa. Secondary causes of CNS vasculitis and syndromes mimicking CNS vasculitis result from drug use, a variety of infections, arterio- and venocclusive diseases, malignancies (metastases, paraneoplastic syndromes including vasculitis), coagulopathies involving subarachnoid, intraparenchymal, or subdural hemorrhage, hypertensive crisis, irradiation, multiple sclerosis, and congenital vascular malformations (Table 220-6). These secondary causes are not discussed here, except to underscore their importance in establishing a differential diagnosis for central neurologic lesions.

The neurologic manifestations of CNS vasculitis are broad and include subacute memory loss, acute encephalopathy, other cognitive and behavioral changes, seizures, cranial nerve abnormalities, focal deficits (cerebrum, cerebellum, and brainstem), spinal cord lesions, meningismus, headache, auditory and vestibular disturbances, intracranial or subarachnoid hemorrhage, and reduced visual acuity or blindness due to retinal vasculitis and optic nerve infarction, respectively. Frequently, patients have hypertension that aggravates their underlying disease or raises questions about their primary diagnosis. Disease manifestations may develop precipitously or gradually over several days or weeks, depending on the disorder.

The diagnostic approach to CNS vasculitis must be aggressive and includes a rapid evaluation with both noninvasive and invasive modalities, where appropriate. A careful, frequently repeated, neurologic examination is critical. Noninvasive studies might include CT scanning, brain scanning (including oxygen-15 positron emission tomographic scanning), electroencephalography, and MRI. Currently, the most expedient approach is an MRI, where available. More invasive studies such as a spinal tap, angiography, and infrequently leptomeningeal and brain biopsy (isolated granulomatous angiitis of the CNS) may also be indicated. Study of serologic markers, as outlined above, including the ANCA, cryoglobulins, ANA, and complement studies facilitates diagnosis and therapeutic planning.

The frequent involvement of the CNS by a variety of connective tissue disorders, particularly SLE, should be appreciated. Fifty-nine percent of 150 patients with SLE reviewed by Estes and Christian had neuropsychiatric manifestations including psychosis, seizures, and paralysis, as well as cranial nerve abnormalities [94]. Unlike other forms of CNS vasculitis, in which pathology develops from direct vascular injury, antineuronal and cross-reactive brain antilymphocytotoxic antibodies may be important. Scleroderma, by causing nerve entrapment, may result in a trigeminal neuropathy. Rheumatoid arthritis, Sjögren's syndrome, Behçet's syndrome, and undifferentiated connective tissue diseases may also cause CNS vasculitis.

Granulomatous angiitis of the CNS, also referred to as isolated angiitis of the CNS, is a disorder largely confined to blood vessels within the CNS [95]. Segmental inflammation and necrosis of small leptomeningeal and parenchymal vessels lead to widespread neurologic symptoms in virtually all patients. Headache, intellectual deterioration, visual disturbances, seizures, ataxia, cranial neuropathy, and transverse myelopathy have all been described (Table 220-7). If untreated the disorder is fatal. The diagnosis is made in the setting of an appropriate history, neurologic deficits associated with angiographic, MRI, or CT abnormalities, and confirmed by histologic examination of leptomeningeal biopsies. All biopsy specimens must be cultured and evaluated for infectious agents. The cerebrospinal fluid is usually abnormal with an elevated opening pressure, elevated protein levels, and a lymphocytosis. Treatment with cyclophosphamide and prednisone is recommended, although long-term studies confirming their efficacy are unavailable.

Two forms of giant cell arteritis cause neurologic symptoms: temporal arteritis and Takayasu's arteritis (see Table 220-7). The most common CNS complaint in temporal arteritis is headache, present in almost all patients [91,92,93]. Headache may be either unilateral or bilateral and has been variably described as lancinating, throbbing, and dull. Visual disturbances occur in 36 to 58 percent of patients, most often due to ischemic optic neuritis; ischemic retrobulbar neuritis and central retinal artery occlusion also occur. Diplopia occurs in approximately 12 percent of patients as a result of ischemia to the extraocular muscles of their cranial nerves [96]. Intracranial lesions are uncommon in temporal arteritis, because pathology is typically confined to blood vessels containing a high content of elastin. Although extracranial vessel elastin content is high, it drops rapidly (within millimeters) after piercing the dura, thereby sparing intracranial structures. However, syncope, stroke, hearing loss, confusion, visual hallucinations, and ataxia have been reported [96].

Neurologic symptoms are usually a late manifestation of Takayasu's arteritis and develop because the branches arising from the aortic arch are compromised [91,92,93]. Transient ischemic attacks, which may progress to completed stroke, and visual disturbances that occur with neck extension are complications of ischemia involving components of the eye and may cause cataracts, atrophy of the iris, and optic nerve atrophy. Brainstem ischemia leading to dysphagia, vertigo, hearing deficits, and facial weakness, as well as a speech deficit due to a subclavian steal syndrome, have all been reported. Stroke is most often referable to the distribution of the middle and anterior cerebral arteries. Eighty to 90 percent of patients have nonspecific complaints of headache and vertigo; focal symptoms (paresis, sensory loss, aphasia) occur in only 36 percent of patients; syn-

Table 220-6. Central Nervous System Vasculitis

1. Primary CNS Vasculitis Syndromes
   a. Granulomatous angiitis of the CNS
   b. Cogan's syndrome
   c. Eales' disease
   d. Isolated spinal cord vasculitis
2. Systemic Necrotizing Vasculitis That May Involve the CNS
   a. PAN (classic PAN; allergic granulomatosis and angiitis of Churg-Strauss; drug abuse–associated vasculitis; hepatitis B—associated vasculitis; overlap group of vasculitis)
   b. Giant cell arteritis (temporal arteritis; Takayasu's arteritis)
   c. Wegener's granulomatosis
   d. Lymphomatoid granulomatosis
   e. Henoch-Schönlein purpura
   f. Cryoglobulinemia
3. Rheumatologic Disorders Affecting the CNS
   a. SLE
   b. Undifferentiated and/or mixed connective tissue disease
   c. Progressive systemic sclerosis
   d. Sjögren's syndrome
   e. Rheumatoid arthritis
   f. Behçet's syndrome
   g. Antiphospholipid or anticardiolipin antibody syndrome
   h. Sarcoidosis
4. Disorders That Mimic or Cause CNS Vasculitis
   a. Atypical migraine (hemiplegia)
   b. Fibromuscular hyperplasia
   c. Myomoya (multiple progressive intracranial arterial occlusion, diffuse meningeal angiomatosis)
   d. Fabry's disease
   e. Malignant atrophic papulosis
   f. Postirradiation hypertensive crisis
   g. Malignancies (particularly Hodgkin's disease)
   h. Left atrial myxoma
   i. Atheroemboli
5. Drugs That Cause CNS Syndromes
   a. Methamphetamines
   b. Ergotamine derivatives
   c. Phenylpropanolamine
   d. Cocaine
   e. Pseudoephedrine
   f. LSD
   g. Birth control pills
   h. Alcohol
6. Infections That Mimic or Cause CNS Vasculitis (Selected List)
   a. HIV (AIDS)
   b. Cytomegalovirus
   c. Mononucleosis
   d. Hepatitis B (cryoglobulinemic vasculitis)
   e. Herpes zoster (ophthalmicus)
   f. Acute or subacute bacterial endocarditis
   g. Tuberculosis
   h. Lyme disease and other spirochetal infections
   i. Rickettsial infection

PAN = polyarteritis nodosa; SLE = systemic lupus erythematosus; AIDS = acquired immunodeficiency syndrome.
Data from: Sigal LH: The neurologic presentation of vasculitis and rheumatologic syndromes. A review. *Medicine (Baltimore)* 66:157, 1987; Moore PM, Cupps TR: Neurological complications of vasculitis. *Ann Neurol* 14:155, 1983; Cohen SB, Hurd ER: Neurological complications of connective tissue and other "collagen vascular" diseases. *Semin Arthritis Rheum* 11:190, 1981.

cope, due in part to a hypersensitive carotid sinus, occurs in approximately 70 percent of patients.

Wegener's granulomatosis affects the CNS by direct granulomatous invasion, by causing other granulomatous lesions, or by affecting the vascular supply via vasculitic lesions. Drachman found that 45 percent of all neurologic lesions were caused by direct invasion by granuloma, 7 percent by discreet granulomatous lesions, and 49 percent by vasculitis [61]. Mononeuritis multiplex and cranial nerve and ocular lesions are also

common. Ocular pathology includes episcleritis, scleritis, uveitis, optic nerve disease, proptosis, ocular muscle weakness, and retinal artery occlusion. Diabetes insipidus, cortical vein thrombosis, aseptic meningitis, mild alterations in cognitive function, seizures, strokes, and encephalopathy have also been described [91,92,93].

Neurologic dysfunction in lymphomatoid granulomatosis has been reported as a presenting manifestation in approximately 20 percent of patients and had an occurrence of 30 percent among patients in different stages of the illness. CNS findings occurred in 30 percent, cranial neuropathy in 11 percent, and peripheral neuropathy in 7 percent of 152 cases reviewed by Katzenstein and coworkers [97]. Because the disease is multifocal, CNS manifestations are diverse, ranging from confusion to paresis (see Table 220-7). Unlike in Wegener's granulomatosis, ocular involvement is unusual.

Involvement of the CNS by PAN occurs in approximately 20 to 40 percent of patients [91,92,93]. It is generally not an isolated manifestation of polyarteritis but part of an overall systemic process. As noted in other multifocal forms of vasculitis, clinical manifestations are varied (see Table 220-7). In one study hemiplegia, aphasia or constructional apraxia, subarachnoid haemorrhagia due to ruptured aneurysms, nonsteroid induced psychosis, drowsiness, and confusion were reported [98]. CNS involvement occurs later than the peripheral neuropathies (mononeuritis multiplex, sensorineuropathy) observed in PAN. Many of the reported abnormalities are irreversible and hence require prompt diagnosis and therapy.

Cholesterol Embolism

Cholesterol (athero-) embolism may produce a variety of multisystemic manifestations and laboratory abnormalities that may resemble connective tissue disease, necrotizing vasculitis, emboli of cardiac origin (subacute bacterial endocarditis, mural thrombi, and atrial myxoma), cryoglobulinemia, and macroglobulinemia [99,100,101]. Awareness of atheroembolism and histologic documentation of cholesterol crystals obstructing arterioles and small arteries allows the clinician to establish the diagnosis and avoid the potentially toxic therapy that might otherwise be prescribed to treat what was incorrectly thought to be a necrotizing vasculitis or connective tissue disease.

Atheromatous material may embolize to the lower extremities as well as to organs throughout the body. Because the most common sources of atheroemboli are atherosclerotic lesions in the aorta, iliac, and femoral arteries, the most susceptible regions are the abdominal viscera, the kidneys, and the lower extremities [102].

The pathologic features of atheromatous emboli in small arteries and arterioles include endothelial and fibroblastic proliferation, foreign body giant cell response to the cholesterol crystals, and lymphocytic perivascular infiltration [103]. Examination of tissue from humans with atheromatous emboli has revealed emboli lodged in interlobar, arcuate, and intralobular renal arteries, as well as in larger arteries [104]. Occasionally, necrotizing angiitis of small arteries occurs and is characterized by polymorphonuclear infiltration of the vessel and fibrinoid necrosis of vessel walls [105,106].

The clinical settings in which atheroemboli most commonly occur are (1) in the presence of an aortic aneurysm, (2) after surgical manipulation of an atheromatous aorta [104,107,108], (3) following blunt abdominal trauma [109], (4) during and after angiography and intraarterial catheterization [4b,104,110–114, 114a], (5) spontaneously [115], and (6) as a complication of warfarin therapy [99,116,117].

Table 220-7. CNS Manifestations of Selected Disorders

Isolated CNS vasculitis	Temporal arteritis	Takayasu's arteritis	Wegener's granulomatosis	Lymphomatoid granulomatosis	PAN
Headache (diffuse or focal)	Headache	Headache	Headache	Confusion	Headache
Confusion	Visual disturbances	Vertigo	Aphasia	Cranial neuropathy	Cerebrovascular syndromes
Intellectual deterioration	Diplopia	Syncope	Subarachnoid hemorrhage	Blindness	Subarachnoid hemorrhage
Hallucinations	Blindness	Paresis	Cranial neuropathy	Cerebrovascular syndromes	Altered mental status
Visual disturbance	Decreased visual acuity	Aphasia	Hypertensive encephalopathy	Aphasia	Seizures
Aphasia	Syncope	Bulbar signs	Hearing loss	Dysarthria	Hemiparesis
Seizures	Dementia	Transient ischemic attacks	Diabetes insipidus	Ataxia	Brain stem lesions
Ataxia	Stroke	Hearing deficits		Seizures	Dysphagia
Cranial neuropathy	Hearing loss	Stroke		Hemiparesis	Cranial neuropathy
Transverse myelopathy	Ataxia	Blindness			
	Visual hallucinations	Hemiparesis and paraparesis			
		Cerebellar symptoms			
		Seizures			
		Memory deficits			

PAN = polyarteritis nodosa.

The clinical features of multiple cholesterol emboli depend on the size and number of emboli and on the organ(s) of the arteries involved. Cyanotic, severely painful toes, which often have bluish patches and hemorrhagic areas due to occlusion of digital arterioles, the so-called blue or purple toe syndrome [4b,118], are often accompanied by ulceration and gangrene, even in the presence of normal pedal arterial pulses [102,119]. Livedo reticularis, a prominent local mottling with a blotchy or netlike (reticular) reddish blue appearance of the skin, commonly involves the lower extremities and occasionally the trunk, due to occlusion of arterioles of the skin [120–123]. Emboli to the kidneys, the most frequently affected visceral organ [124], are manifested by impairment of renal function [114,125], hypertension [125,126,127], and microscopic hematuria, leukocyturia, and proteinuria [125].

The chronology of impaired renal function following angiography may help distinguish radiocontrast dye-induced renal failure from renal failure due to atheromatous microemboli. Renal failure caused by radiocontrast dye tends to appear soon after the study, reaches maximal severity within 7 to 10 days, and then improves, with renal function returning to baseline over several weeks. In contrast, renal failure due to atheromatous microemboli to the kidney generally develops over 1 to 4 weeks or even over several months following the angiographic procedure, and may not be reversible [112].

Multiplicity of organ system involvement and laboratory abnormalities may simulate a systemic vasculitis and systemic connective tissue disease. The following conditions may simulate polyarteritis: skin involvement including livedo reticularis, purpura, nodules, ulcers, and gangrene; clinical evidence of renal involvement; symptoms and signs of nervous system disease including transient ischemic attacks, cerebrovascular accidents, amaurosis fugax, confusion, and mononeuritis [110,115,123,128,129,130]; GI involvement such as abdominal pain, nausea, emesis, melena, hematochezia, gastric ulcers, bowel infarction [114], and pancreatitis [131]; and cardiac manifestations such as angina pectoris and myocardial infarctions [115]. Myalgias, muscle tenderness, severe myopathy with weakness, elevated muscle enzymes, and myopathic features on electromyography simulate polymyositis [132,133].

Laboratory features of cholesterol (atheromatous) embolism are often nonspecific but may also be suggestive of a systemic vasculitis or connective tissue disease. The erythrocyte sedimentation rate is often elevated. Transient or persistent eosinophilia in the setting of multiorgan system disease may suggest Churg-Strauss angiitis (allergic angiitis and granulomatosis) and polyarteritis. Polyarteritis may also be incorrectly suggested by arteriographic findings of multiple stenoses and microaneurysms of medium and small arteries [99,134]. The findings of hypocomplementemia, antinuclear antibodies (ANAs), and rheumatoid factors may occur in the setting of multiple cholesterol emboli and suggest the diagnosis of SLE [99,135], while peripheral gangrene and arterial occlusions of other organs suggest the diagnosis of the antiphospholipid or lupuslike antibody syndrome [136] (see Chap. 219) or of other hypercoagulable states. Findings of vascular inflammation and fibrinoid necrosis of vessel walls on histologic studies of specimens involved with cholesterol emboli may further incorrectly support the diagnosis of a primary vasculitis if cholesterol crystals are not seen [99,105,106].

To establish the diagnosis of atheromatous emboli, one must have a high degree of suspicion based on the clinical presentation, history, physical findings, and laboratory results. The diagnosis is confirmed by the demonstration on histologic samples of biopsied skin, muscle, and kidney or amputated tissue of the characteristic biconvex needle-shaped clefts representing the "ghosts" of the cholesterol crystals within arteries and arterioles that are dissolved during routine histologic preparation (Fig. 220-3) [4b,137–140]. With special histologic preparation, the cholesterol crystals display birefringence when viewed with a polarized light microscope [141].

An important aspect of treatment of atheromatous embolism is prevention. Increased awareness of the risks of atheromatous embolism associated with surgical manipulation and angiographic studies of atheromatous arteries, minimizing intraarterial procedures in atherosclerotic aortas and femoral arteries, use of brachial rather than femoral artery approaches for cardiac catheterization in patients with atheromatous disease of the aorta and iliac arteries, minimizing catheter manipulation, and the use of softer, more flexible catheters may help reduce the incidence and severity of atheromatous embolization [112].

Treatment of atheromatous emboli consists of controlling pain and blood pressure and measures to increase local blood flow with topical glyceryl trinitrate (2% Nitrol) ointment, sym-

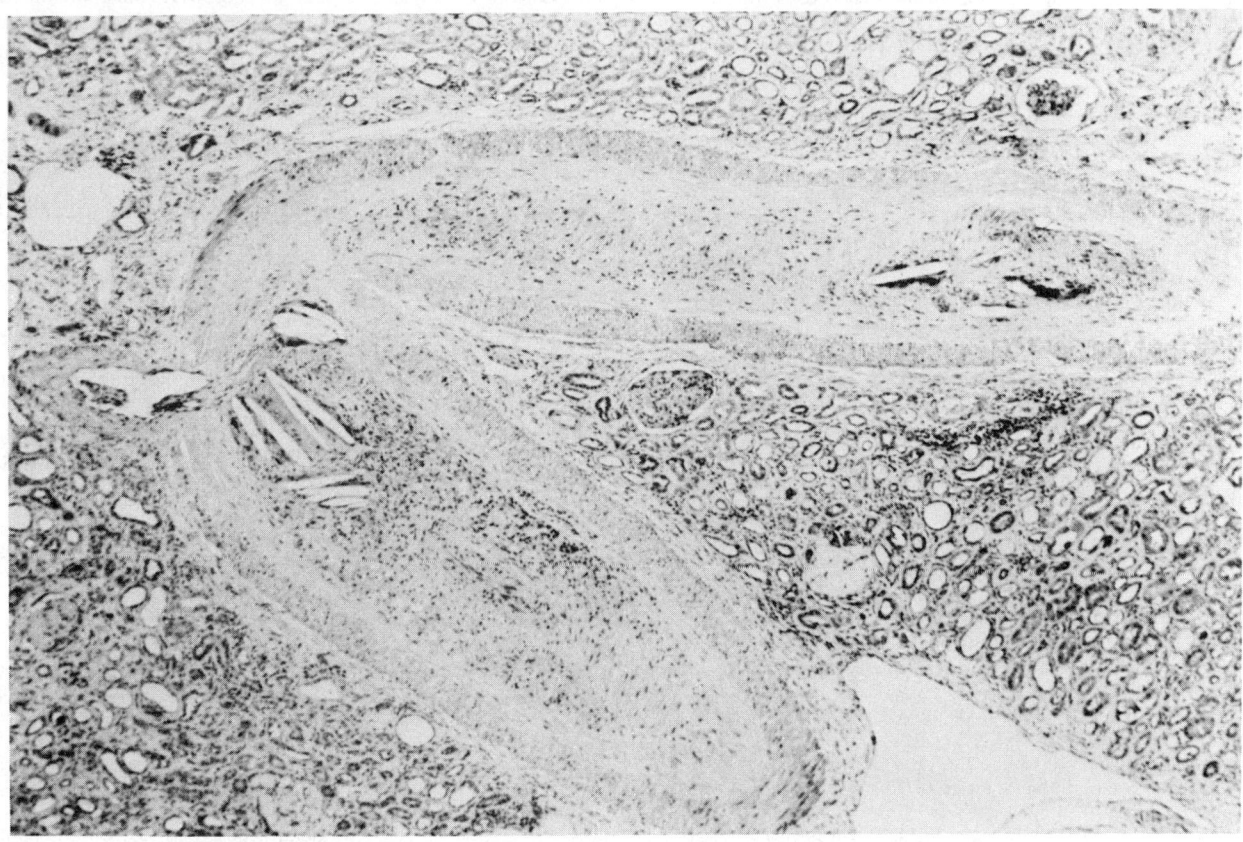

Fig. 220-3. "Ghostlike" appearance of needle-shaped cholesterol crystals in a renal artery, the size of an interlobular vessel, surrounded by occlusive intimal proliferation and fibrous tissue (hematoxylin and eosin stain). (Courtesy of Carolyn Compton, M.D., Department of Pathology, University of Massachusetts Medical Center, Worcester, MA).

pathetic blockade, calcium channel blockers to reduce vasospasm, and perhaps pentoxifylline to improve the rheostatic properties of red blood cells [142,143]. Definitive treatment involves identification and surgical resection of the arterial source of the atheromatous emboli. (For discussion of surgical treatment including embolectomy see Chap. 165). In the case of severe renal function impairment, dialysis may allow time for renal function to improve [122,125].

A number of modalities are ineffective for the treatment of atheromatous emboli, including the use of antiplatelet drugs and low-molecular-weight dextan. Although corticosteroids may theoretically be helpful, evidence of benefit is lacking [144,145].

The use of heparin and warfarin is controversial. The general consensus, however, is that these drugs are contraindicated, because by preventing the formation of an organized thrombus over ulcerated atheromatous plaques, anticoagulants may allow continued breakdown and embolization of material [116, 146,147].

References

1. Cupps TR, Fauci AS: *The Vasculitides.* Philadelphia, Saunders, 1981, p vii.
2. Fauci AS, Haynes BF, Katz P: The spectrum of vasculitis. *Ann Intern Med* 89:660, 1978.
3. Fan PT, Davis JA, Somer T, et al: A clinical approach to systemic vasculitis. *Semin Arthritis Rheum* 9:248, 1980.
4. Conn DL: Update on systemic necrotizing vasculitis. *Mayo Clin Proc* 64:535, 1989.
4a. Lie JT: Vasculitis simulators and vasculitis look-alikes. *Curr Opin in Rheumatol* 4:47, 1992.
4b. O'Keefe ST, Woods B O'B, Breslin DJ, Tsapatasaris NP: Blue toe syndrome. Causes and management. *Arch Intern Med* 152:2197, 1992.
5. Kurland LT, Chuang TY, Hunder GG: The epidemiology of systemic arteritis, in Laurence RE, Schulman (eds): *Current Topics in Rheumatology: Epidemiology of Rheumatic Diseases.* New York, Gower, 1984, p 196.
6. Cupps TR,. Fauci AS: Systemic necrotizing vasculitis of the polyarteritis nodosa group, in *The Vasculitides.* Philadelphia, Saunders, 1981, p 26.
7. Ronco P, Verroust P, Mignon F, et al: Immunopathological studies of polyarteritis nodosa and Wegener's granulomatosis: A report of 43 patients with 51 renal biopsies. *Q J Med* 52:212, 1983.
8. Gocke DJ, Hsu K, Morgan C, et al: Association between polyarteritis and Australian antigen. *Lancet* 2:1149, 1970.
9. Doherty M, Bradfield JW: Polyarteritis nodosa associated with acute cytomegalovirus infection. *Ann. Rheum Dis* 40:419, 1981.
10. Li Loong TC, Coyle PV, Anderson MJ, et al: Human serum parvovirus associated vasculitis. *Postgrad Med J* 62:493, 1986.
11. Haynes BF, Miller SE, Palker TJ, et al: Identification of human T cell leukemia virus in a Japanese patient with adult T cell leukemia and cutaneous lymphomatous vasculitis. *Proc Natl Acad Sci U S A* 80:2054, 1983.
12. Yankner BA, Skolnik PR, Shoukimas GM, et al: Cerebral granulomatous angiitis associated with isolation of human T-lymphotrophic virus type III from the central nervous system. *Ann Neurol* 20:362, 1986.
13. Doyle PW, Gibson G, Dolman CL: Herpes zoster ophthalmicus

with contralateral hemiplegia: Identification of cause. *Ann Neurol* 14:84, 1985.

13a. Carson LW, Conn DL, Czaja AJ, et al: Frequency and significance of antibodies to hepatitis C virus in polyarteritis nodosa. *J Rheum* 20:304, 11993.

13b. Ferri C, Greco F, Longombardo G, et al: Antibodies in hepatitis C virus in patients with mixed cryoglobulinemia. *Arth Rheum* 34:1606, 1991.

13c. Agnello V, Chung RT, Kaplar LU, et al: A role for hepatitis C virus infection in type II cryoglobulinemia. *N Engl J Med* 327:1490, 1992.

14. Posnett DN, Marboe CC, Knowles DM II, et al: A membrane antigen (HC1) selectively present on hairy cell leukemia cells, endothelial cells, and epidermal basal cells. *J Immunol* 132:2700, 1984.

15. Rose GA: The natural history of polyarteritis. *Br Med J* 2:1148, 1957.

16. Chang RW, Bell CL, Hallett M: Clinical characteristics and prognosis of vasculitic mononeuropathy multiplex. *Arch Neurol* 41:618, 1984.

17. Holsinger DR, Osmundson PJ, Edwards JE: The heart in periarteritis nodosa. *Circulation* 25:610, 1962.

18. Maxeiner SR, McDonald JR, Kirklin JW: Muscle biopsy in diagnosis of periarteritis nodosa: An evaluation. *Surg Clin North Am* August 32:1225, 1952.

19. Sack M, Cassidy JT, Bole GG: Prognostic factors in polyarteritis. *J Rheumatol* 2:411, 1975.

20. Weiss MA, Crissman JD: Segmental necrotizing glomerulonephritis: Diagnostic, prognostic and therapeutic significance. *Am J Kidney Dis* 6:199, 1985.

21. Wees SJ, Sunwoo IN, Oh SJ: Sural nerve biopsy in systemic necrotizing vasculitis. *Am J Med* 71:525, 1981.

22. Travers RL, Allison DJ, Brettle RP, et al: Polyarteritis nodosa: A clinical and angiographic analysis of 17 cases. *Semin Arthritis Rheum* 8:184, 1979.

23. Cohen RD, Conn DL, Ilstrup DM: Clinical features, prognosis and response to treatment of polyarteritis. *Mayo Clin Proc* 55:146, 1980.

24. Conn DL, Hunder GG: Vasculitis and related disorders, in Kelley WN, Harris ED, Ruddy S, et al (eds): *Textbook of Rheumatology.* Philadelphia, Saunders, 1989, p 1167.

25. Fauci AS, Katz P, Haynes BF, et al: Cyclophosphamide therapy of severe systemic necrotizing vasculitis. *N Engl J Med* 301:235, 1979.

26. Guillevin L, Jarroussa B, Lok C, et al: A long term follow-up after treatment of polyarteritis nodosa and Churg-Strauss angitis with comparison of steroids, plasma exchange and cyclophosphamide to steroids and plasma exchange. *J Rheum* 18:567, 1992.

26a. Guillevin L, Olivier F, Lhote F, et al: Lack of superiority of steroids plus plasma exchange to steroids alone in the treatment of polyarteritis nodosa and Churg-Strauss syndrome: a prospective randomized trial of 78 patients. *Arth Rheum* 35:108, 1992.

26b. Citron BP, Halpern M, McCarron M, et al: Necrotizing angitis associated with drug abuse. *N Engl J Med* 283:1003, 1970.

27. Wenkleman RK, Ditto WB: Cutaneous and visceral syndromes of necrotizing or "allergic" angiitis. A study of 38 cases. *Medicine* 43:59, 1964.

28. Mullick, FG, McAllister HA Jr, Wagner BM, et al: Drug related vasculitis: Clinicopathologic correlations in 30 patients. *Hum Pathol* 10:313, 1979.

29. Katz P: Vasculitic purpura: Differential diagnosis and therapy. *Semin Thrombosis Hemostasis* 10:202, 1984.

30. Conn DL, Hunder GG: Vasculitis and related disorders, in Kelly WH, Harris ED, Ruddy S, et al (eds): *Textbook of Rheumatology,* 3rd ed. Philadelphia, Saunders, 1989.

30a. Gibson LE, Su WP: Cutaneous vasculitis. *Rheum Dis Clin N Amer* 16:309, 1990.

31. Calabrese LH: The rheumatic manifestations of infection with the human immunodeficiency virus. *Semin Arthritis Rheum* 18:225, 1989.

32. Kaye BR: Rheumatologic manifestations of infection with human immunodeficiency virus. *Ann Intern Med* 111:158, 1989.

33. Winchester R (ed): AIDS and Rheumatic Diseases. *Rheum Dis Clin N Amer* 17:1, 1991.

34. Calabrese LH: Vasculitis and infection with human immunodeficiency virus. *Rheum Dis Clin N Am* 17:131, 1991.

35. Yankner BA, Skolnik PR, Shoukimas GM, et al: Cerebral granulomatous angiitis associated with isolation of human T-lymphotrophic virus type III from the central nervous system. *Ann Neurol* 20:362, 1986.

36. Frank Y, Lim W, Kahn E, et al: Multiple ischemic infarcts in a child with AIDS, varicella zoster, and cerebral vasculitis (abstr). *Ped Neurol* 5:64, 1989.

37. Andar KH, Latta H, Chang BS, et al: Lymphomatoid granulomatosis and malignant lymphoma of the central nervous system in AIDS. *Hum Pathol* 20:326, 1989.

38. Sergent J: Vasculitis associated with viral infection. *Clin Rheum Dis* 6:339, 1980.

39. Bardin T, Gaudauer C, Kuntz D, et al: Necrotizing vasculitis in HIV infection. *Arthritis Rheum* 30:S105, 1987.

40. Schwartz ND, So YT, Hollander H, et al: Eosinophilic vasculitis leading to amaurosis fugax in a patient with acquired immunodeficiency syndrome. *Arch Intern Med* 146:2059, 1986.

41. Cupps TR, Fauci AS: Wegener's granulomatosis, in *The Vasculitides.* Philadelphia, Saunders, 1981, p 72.

42. Carrington CB, Liebo A: Limited forms of angiitis and granulomatosis of Wegener's type. *Am J Med* 41:497, 1966.

43. Fauci AS, Wolff SM: Wegener's granulomatosis: Studies in eighteen patients and a review of the literature. *Medicine (Baltimore)* 52:535, 1973.

44. Wolff SM, Fauci AS, Horn RG, et al: Wegener's granulomatosis. *Ann Intern Med* 81:513, 1974.

45. Van der Woude FJ, Rasmussen N, Lobatto S, et al: Autoantibodies against neutrophils and monocytes: A tool for the diagnosis and marker of disease activity of Wegener's granulomatosis. *Lancet* 1:425, 1985.

46. Godman GC, Churg J: Wegener's granulomatosis: Pathology and review of literature, A.M.A. *Arch Pathol* 58:533, 1954.

47. Fauci AS, Haynes BF, Katz P,. et al: Wegener's granulomatosis: Prospective clinical and therapeutic experience with 85 patients for 21 years. *Ann Intern Med* 98:76, 1983.

48. Schramm VL Jr, Myers EN, Rogerson DR: The masquerade of vasculitis: Head and neck diagnosis and management. *Laryngoscope* 88:1922, 1978.

49. Goldenberg DL, Goodman ML: Case 26-1985. Case records of the Massachusetts General Hospital: Weekly clinicopathological exercises. *N Engl J Med* 312:1695, 1985.

50. Harrington JT, McCluskey RT: Case 24-1979. Case records of the Massachusetts General Hospital: Weekly clinicopathological exercises. *N Engl J Med* 300:1378, 1979.

51. McDonald TJ, DeRemee RA: Wegener's granulomatosis. *Laryngoscope* 93:220, 1983.

52. Bernhard JD, Mark EJ: Case 17-1986. Case records of the Massachusetts General Hospital: Weekly clinicopathological exercises. *N Engl J Med* 314:1170, 1986.

53. McGregor MG, Sandler G: Wegener's granulomatosis. A clinical and radiological survey. *Br J Radiol* 37:430, 1964.

54. Maguire R, Fauci AS, Doppmann JL, et al: Unusual radiographic features of Wegener's granulomatosis. *Am J Rheumatol* 130:233, 1978.

55. Weiss MA, Crissman JD: Renal biopsy findings in Wegener's granulomatosis: Segmental necrotizing glomerulonephritis with glomerular thrombosis. *Hum Pathol* 15:943, 1984.

56. Horn RG, Fauci AS, Rosenthal AS, et al: Renal biopsy pathology in Wegener's granulomatosis. *Am J Pathol* 74:423, 1974.

57. Pritchard MH: Wegener's granulomatosis presenting as rheumatoid arthritis (two cases). *Proc R Soc Med* 69:501, 1976.

58. Rothschild BM, Calabro JJ, Staley H, et al: The arthritis of Wegener's granulomatosis. *Clin Rheumatol in Prac* Jan/Feb, 1984, p 29.

59. Baker SB, Robinson DR: Unusual renal manifestations of Wegener's granulomatosis. Report of two cases. *Am J Med* 64:883, 1978.

60. Haynes BF, Fishman ML, Fauci AS, et al: The ocular manifestations of Wegener's granulomatosis. Fifteen years experience and review of the literature. *Am J Med* 63:131, 1977.

61. Drachman DA: Neurological complications of Wegener's granulomatosis. *Arch Neurol* 8:145, 1963.

62. Parker SW, Sobel RA: Case 12-1988. Case records of the Massachusetts General Hospital: Weekly clinicopathological exercises. *N Engl J Med* 318:760, 1988.

63. Atcheson SG, Van Horn G: Subacute meningitis heralding a diffuse granulomatous angiitis: (Wegener's granulomatosis?). *Neurology (Minneapolis)* 27:262, 1977.

64. Satoh J, Miyasaka N, Yamada T, et al: Extensive cerebral infarction due to involvement of both anterior cerebral arteries by Wegener's granulomatosis. *Ann Rheum Dis* 47:606, 1988.

65. Camilleri M, Pusey CD, Chadwick VS, et al: Gastrointestinal manifestations of systemic vasculitis. *Q J Med* 52:141, 1983.

66. Fauci AS, Walton EW: Giant cell granuloma of the respiratory tract (Wegener's granulomatosis). *Br Med J* 2:265, 1958.

67. McCrea PC, Childers RW: Two unusual cases of giant cell myocarditis associated with mitral stenosis and with Wegener's syndrome. *Br Heart J* 26:490, 1964.

68. Levine H, Madden TJ: Wegener's granulomatosis. Report of a case. *Am Heart J* 53:632, 1957.

69. Allen DC, Doherty CC, O'Reilly DP: Pathology of the heart and the cardiac conduction system in Wegener's granulomatosis. *Br Heart J* 52:674, 1984.

70. Forstot JZ, Overlie PA, Neufeld GK, et al: Cardiac complications of Wegener's granulomatosis: A case report of complete heart block and review of the literature. *Semin Arthritis Rheum* 10:148, 1980.

71. Savage CO, Winearls CG, Jones S, et al: Prospective study of radioimmunoassay for antibodies against neutrophil cytoplasm in diagnosis of systemic vasculitis. *Lancet* 1:1389, 1987.

72. Gross WL, Ludemann G, Kiefer G, et al: Anticytoplasmic antibodies in Wegener's granulomatosis. *Lancet* 1:806, 1986.

72a. Ludemann J, Csernok E, Ulner M, et al: Antineutrophil cytoplasma antibodies in Wegener's granulomatosis: immunodiagnostic value, monoclonal antibodies, and characterization of the target antigen. *Neth J Med* 36:157, 1990.

72b. Hagen EC, Ballieux BEPB, Daha MR, et al: Fundamental and clinical aspects of antineutrophil lytoplasmic antibodies. *Autoimmunity* 11:199, 1992.

72c. Niles JL: Value of tests for antineutrophil cytoplasmic autoantibodies in the diagnosis and treatment of vasculitis. *Curr Opin Rheumatol* 5:18, 1993.

73. Specks U, Wheatley CL, McDonald TJ, et al: Anticytoplasmic autoantibodies in the diagnosis and follow-up of Wegener's granulomatosis. *Mayo Clinic Proc* 64:28, 1989.

74. Nolle, B, Speck U, Ludemann J, et al: Anticytoplasmic antoantibodies: Their immunodiagnostic value in Wegener's granulomatosis. *Ann Intern Med* 111:28, 1989.

74a. Ulner M, Rautmann A, Gross WL: Immunodiagnostic aspects of autoantibodies against myeloperoxidase. *Clin Nephrol* 37:161, 1992.

75. Falk RJ, Jennette JC: Anti-neutrophil cytoplasmic autoantibodies with specificity for myeloperoxidase in patients with systemic vasculitis and idiopathic necrotizing and crescentic glomerulonephritis. *N Engl J Med* 318:1651, 1988.

75a. Falk RJ, Hogan S, Carey TS, et al: Clinical course of neutrophil cytoplasmic autoantibody-associated glomerulonephritis and systemic vasculitis. *Ann Intern Med* 113:656, 1990.

75b. Hoffman GS, Sechler JMG, Gallin JI, et al: Bronchoalveolar lavage analysis in Wegener's granulomatosus. *Am Rev Resp Dis* 143:401, 1991.

75c. Baltaro RJ, Hoffman GS, Sechler JMG, et al: Immunoglobulin G antineutrophil cytoplasmic antibodies are produced in the respiratory tract of patients with Wegener's granulomatosis. *Am Rev Resp Dis* 143:275, 1991.

75d. Savage COS, Pottinger BE, Gaskin G, et al: Vascular damage in Wegener's granulomatosis and microscopic poly presence of anti-endothelial cell antibodies and their relation to anti-neutrophil cytoplasm antibodies. *Clin Exp Immunol* 85:14, 1991.

76. Lynch JP, Matteson E, McCune WJ: Wegener's granulomatosis: Evolving concepts. *Medical Rounds* 2:67, 1989.

77. Smith LR, Heaton CL: Actinomycosis presenting as Wegener's granulomatosis. *JAMA* 240:247, 1978.

78. Bowman C, Lockwood CM: Clinical application of a radioimmunoassay for auto-antibodies to glomerular basement membrane. *J Clin Lab Immunol* 17:197, 1985.

79. DeRemee RA, Weiland LH, McDonald TJ: Polymorphic reticulosis, lymphomatoid granulomatosis. Two diseases in one? *Mayo Clin Proc* 53:634, 1978.

80. Petras RE, Tubbs RR, Gephardt GN, et al: T lymphocyte proliferation in lymphomatoid granulomatosis. *Cleve Clin Q* 52:137, 1985.

81. Fauci AS, Haynes BF, Costa J, et al: Lymphomatoid granulomatosis. Prospective clinical and therapeutic experience over 10 years. *N Engl J Med* 306:68, 1982.

82. Schechter SL, Bole GG, Walker SE: Midline granuloma and Wegener's granulomatosis: Clinical and therapeutic considerations. *J Rheumatol* 3:241, 1976.

83. Fauci AS, Johnson RE, Wolff SM: Radiation therapy of midline granuloma. *Ann Intern Med* 84:140, 1976.

84. Stillwell TJ, Benson RC Jr, DeRemee RA, et al: Cyclophosphamide-induced bladder toxicity in Wegener's granulomatosis. *Arthritis Rheum* 31:465, 1988.

84a. Hoffman GS, Kerr GS, Leavitt RY, et al: Wegener's granulomatosis: an analysis of 158 patients. *Ann Intern Med* 116:488, 1992.

84b. Hahn B: Systemic Lupus Erythematosus and Related Syndromes. In: *Textbook of Rheumatology*, p 1050,

85. Reza MJ, Dornfeld L, Goldberg LS, et al: Wegener's granulomatosis. Long term followup of patients treated with cyclophosphamide. *Arthritis Rheum* 18:501, 1975.

86. Cupps TR, Fauci AS: Management and treatment, in *The Vasculitides*. Philadelphia, Saunders, 1981, p 162.

86a. Bradley JD, Brandt KD, Katz BP: Infectious complications of cyclophosphamide treatment for vasculitis. *Arthritis Rheum* 32:45, 1989.

87. Balow JE, Austin HA III, Tsoko GC, et al: NIH conference. Lupus nephritis. *Ann Intern Med* 106:79, 1987.

87a. Steppat D, Gross WL: Staged-adapted treatment of Wegener's granulomatosis. *Klin Wochensche* 67:666, 1989.

87b. Hoffman GS, Leavitt RY, Fleisher TA, et al: Treatment of Wegener's granulomatosis with intermittent high dose intravenous cyclophosphamide. *Am J Med* 89:403, 1990.

88. Pinching AJ, Rees AJ, Pussell BA, et al: Relapses in Wegener's granulomatosis: The role of infection. *Br Med J* 281:836, 1980.

88a. Sen RP, Walsh TE, Fisher W, Brock N: Pulmonary complications of combination therapy with cytophosphamide and prednisone. *Chest* 99:143, 1991.

89. DeRemee RA: The treatment of Wegener's granulomatosis with trimethoprim/sulfamethoxazole: Illusion or vision? *Arthritis Rheum* 31:1068, 1988.

90. DeRemee RA, McDonald TJ, Weiland LH: Wegener's granulomatosis: Observations on treatment with antimicrobial agents. *Mayo Clin Proc* 60:27, 1985.

90a. Savage CO, Winearls CG, Evans DJ, et al: Microscopic polyarteritis: presentation, pathology and prognosis. *QJ Med* 56:467, 1985.

90b. Savage CO, Winearls CG, Jones S, et al: Prospective study of radioimmunoassay for antibodies for antibodies against neutrophil cytoplasm in diagnosis of systemic vasculitis. *Lancet* 1:1389, 1987.

90c. Jayne DRW, Davies MJ, Fox CJV, et al: Treatment of systemic vasculitis with pooled intravenous immunoglobulin. *Lancet* 337:1137, 1991.

90d. Rossi F, Jayne DRW, Lockwood CM, Kayatchkine MD: Anti-idiotypes against antineutrophil cytoplasmic antigen autoantibodies in normal human polyspecific IgG for therapeutic use and in remission sera of patients with systemic vasculitis. *Clin Exp Immunol* 83:298, 1991.

91. Sigal LH: The neurologic presentation of vasculitis and rheumatologic syndromes. A review. *Medicine (Baltimore)* 66:157, 1987.

92. Moore PM, Cupps TR: Neurological complications of vasculitis. *Ann Neurol* 14:155, 1983.

93. Cohen SB, Hurd ER: Neurological complications of connective tissue and other "collagen vascular" diseases. *Semin Arthritis Rheum* 11.190, 1981.

94. Estes D, Christian CL: The natural history of systemic lupus erythematosus by prospective analysis. *Medicine (Baltimore)* 50:85, 1971.

95. Calabrese LH, Mallek JA: Primary angiitis of the central nervous system. Report of 8 new cases, review of the literature, and proposal for diagnostic criteria. *Medicine (Baltimore)* 67:20, 1987.

96. Reich K, Giansiracusa D, Strongwater S: Neurologic manifestations of giant cell arteritis. *Am J Med,* in press.

97. Katzenstein AL, Carrington CB, Liebow AA: Lymphomatoid granulomatosis: A clinicopathologic study of 152 cases. *Cancer* 43:360, 1979.

98. Sack M, Cassidy JT, Bole GG: Prognostic factors in polyarteritis. *J Rheumatol* 2:411, 1975.

99. Cappiello RA, Espinoza LR, Adelman H, et al: Cholesterol embolism: A pseudovasculitic syndrome. *Semin Arthritis Rheum* 18:240, 1989.

100. Anderson RW: Necrotizing angiitis associated with embolization of cholesterol. *Am J Clin Pathol* 43:65, 1965.

101. Richards AM, Eliot RS, Kanjuh VI, et al: Cholesterol embolism: A multiple system disease masquerading as polyarteritis nodosa. *Am J Cardiol* 15:696, 1965.

102. Carvajal JA, Anderson WR, Weiss L, et al: Atheroembolism: An etiologic factor in renal insufficiency, gastrointestinal hemorrhages, and peripheral vascular diseases. *Arch Intern Med* 119:593, 1967.

103. Snyder HE, Shapiro JL: A correlative study of atheromatous embolism in human beings and experimental animals. *Surgery* 49:195, 1961.

104. Thrulbeck WM, Castleman B: Atheromatous emboli to the kidneys after aortic surgery. *N Engl J Med* 257:442, 1957.

105. Fisher ER, Hellstrom HR, Myers JD: Disseminated atheromatous emboli. *Am J Med* 29:176, 1960.

106. Taylor NS, Gueft B, Lebowich RJ: Atheromatous embolization: A cause of gastric ulcers and small bowel necrosis. *Gastroenterology* 47:97, 1964.

107. Roscher AA, Endlich HL: Atheroembolization. A complication of vascular surgery and-or diagnostic angiography. *Int Surg* 56:82, 1971.

108. Stout C, Hartsuck JM, Howe J, et al: Atheromatous embolization after aortofemoral bypass and aortic ligation. *Arch Pathol* 93:271, 1972.

109. Hertzer NR: Peripheral atheromatous embolization following blunt abdominal trauma. *Surgery* 82:244, 1977.

110. Ramirez G, O'Neill WM, Lambert R, et al: Cholesterol embolization: A complication of angiography. *Arch Intern Med* 138:1430, 1978.

111. Gjesdal K, Orning OM, Smith E: Fatal atheromatous emboli to the kidneys after left-heart catheterisation. *Lancet* 2:405, 1977.

112. Harrington JT, Sommers SC, Kassirer JP: Atheromatous emboli with progressive renal failure. Renal arteriography as the probable inciting factor. *Ann Intern Med* 68:152, 1968.

113. Gaines PA, Cumberland DC, Kennedy A, et al: Cholesterol embolization: A lethal complication of vascular catheterisation. *Lancet* 1:168, 1988.

114. Hendel RC, Cuenoud HF, Giansiracusa DF, et al: Multiple cholesterol emboli syndrome: Bowel infarction after retrograde angiography. *Arch Intern Med* 149:2371, 1989.

114a. Trono R, Sutton C, Hollman J, et al: Multiple myocardial infarctions associated with atheromatous emboli after PTCA of saphenous veing rafts. *Cleveland Clinic Jr of Med* 56:581, 1989.

115. Gore I, Collins DP: Spontaneous atheromatous embolization. Review of the literature and a report of 16 additional cases. *Am J Clin Pathol* 33:416, 1960.

116. Bruns FJ, Segel DP, Adler S: Control of cholesterol embolization by discontinuation of anticoagulant therapy. *Am J Med Sci* 275:105, 1978.

117. Hyman BT, Landas SK, Ashman RF, et al: Warfarin-related purple toes syndrome and cholesterol microembolization. *Am J Med* 82:1233, 1987.

118. Karmody AM, Powers SR, Monaco VJ, et al: "Blue-toe" syndrome: An indication for limb salvage surgery. *Arch Surg* III:1263, 1976.

119. Kempczinski R: Lower extremity arterial emboli from ulcerating atherosclerotic plaques. *JAMA* 241:807, 1979.

120. Kazmier FJ, Sheps SG, Bernatz PE, et al: Livedo reticularis and digital infarcts: A syndrome due to cholesterol emboli arising from atheromatous abdominal aneurysm. *Vasc Dis* 3:12, 1966.

121. Kalter DC, Rufolf A, MacGavran M: Livedo reticularis due to multiple cholesterol emboli. *J Am Acad Dermatol* 13:235, 1985.

122. McGowan JA, Greenberg A: Cholesterol atheroembolic renal disease. *Am J Nephrol* 6:135, 1986.

123. Rosansky SJ, Deschamps EG: Multiple cholesterol emboli syndrome after angiography. *Am J Med Sci* 288:45, 1984.

124. Bloom MG, Winthrop LH, Sarosi GA: Spontaneous cholesterol embolic renal failure. *Minn Med* 55:1009, 1972.

125. Smith MC, Ghose MK, Henry AR: The clinical spectrum of renal cholesterol embolization. *Am J Med* 71:174, 1981.

126. Handler FP: Clinical and pathologic significance of atheromatous embolization with emphasis on etiology of renal hypertension. *Am J Med* 20:366, 1956.

127. Palakos TG, Streeter DPH, Jones D, et al: "Malignant" hypertension resulting from atheromatous embolization predominantly of one kidney. *Am J Med* 57:135, 1974.

128. Harrington D, Amplatz K: Cholesterol embolization and spinal infarction following aortic catheterization. *Am J Radiol* 115:171, 1972.

129. Pfaffenbach DD, Hollenhorst RW: Morbidity and survivorship of patients with embolic cholesterol crystal in the ocular fundus. *Am J Ophthalmol* 75:66, 1973.

130. Sturgill BC, Netsky MG: Cerebral infarction by atheromatous emboli. Report of case and review of literature. *Arch Path (Chicago)* 76:189, 1963.

131. Probstein JG, Joshi RA, Blumenthal HT: Atheromatous embolization: Etiology of acute pancreatitis. *Arch Surg* 75:566, 1957.

132. Anderson NR, Richards AM: Evaluation of lower extremity muscle biopsies in the diagnosis of atheroembolism. *Arch Pathol* 86:535, 1968.

133. Perdue GD Jr, Smith RB III: Atheromatous microemboli. *Ann Surg* 169:954, 1969.

134. Easterbrook JS: Renal and hepatic microaneurysms: Report of a new entity simulating polyarteritis nodosa. *Radiology* 137:629, 1980.

135. Young DK, Burton MF, Herman JH: Multiple cholesterol emboli syndrome simulating systemic necrotizing vasculitis. *J Rheumatol* 13:423, 1986.

136. Asherson RA, Derksen RH, Harris EN, et al: Large vessel occlusion and gangrene in systemic lupus erythematosus and "lupus-like" disease. A report of six cases. *J Rheumatol* 13:740, 1986.

137. Case 33-1974: Case records of the Massachusetts General Hospital: Weekly clinicopathological exercises. *N Engl J Med* 291:406, 1974.

138. Case 50-1977: Case records of the Massachusetts General Hospital: Weekly clinicopathological exercises. *N Engl J Med* 297:1337, 1977.

139. Case 4-1984: Case records of the Massachusetts General Hospital: Weekly clinicopathological exercises. *N Engl J Med* 310:244, 1984.

140. Case 30-1986: Case records of the Massachusetts General Hospital: Weekly clinicopathological exercises. *N Engl J Med* 315:308, 1986.

141. Mehigan JT, Stoney FJ: Lower extremity atheromatous embolization. *Am J Surg* 132:163, 1976.

142. Kinney EL, Nicholas GG, Grallo J, et al: The treatment of severe Raynaud's phenomenon with verapamil. *J Clin Pharmacol* 22:74, 1982.

143. Rodeheffer RJ, Rommer JA, Wigley F, et al: Controlled double-blind trial of nifedipine in the treatment of Raynaud's phenomenon. *N Engl J Med* 308:880, 1983.

144. Darsee JR: Cholesterol embolism: The great masquerader. *South Med J* 72:174, 1979.

145. Kassirer JP: Atheroembolic renal disease. *N Engl J Med* 280:812, 1969.

146. Moldveen-Geronimus M, Merriam JC Jr: Cholesterol embolization: From pathological curiosity to clinical entity. *Circulation* 35:946, 1967.

147. Wagner RB: Peripheral atheroembolism: Confirmation of a clinical concept with a case report and review of the literature. *Surgery* 73:353, 1973.

XVIII. Psychiatric Issues in Intensive Care

Section Editor
Theodore A. Stern

221. Diagnosis and Treatment of Agitation and Delirium in the ICU Patient

George E. Tesar and Theodore A. Stern

An acute change in behavior or mental status in the intensive care unit (ICU) patient requires rapid recognition and treatment [1,2]. The confused patient is often restless and disorganized, and the illusions, hallucinations, and paranoid ideation that accompany confusion can precipitate intense agitation and combativeness. Agitation that is manifest by repeated attempts to get out of bed or pull out intravascular lines, an endotracheal tube, or an intraaortic balloon pump catheter is potentially harmful to the patient. It is also physically and emotionally taxing for nursing staff, who must maintain constant vigilance, rearrange disorganized bedding and equipment, and tolerate physical and verbal abuse from the confused and agitated patient.

The onset of confusion in an ICU patient generally signifies an important change in the patient's medical status that warrants evaluation for systemic and metabolic abnormalities, drug toxicity, withdrawal states, and other reversible factors. Subsequent treatment focuses on the correction of underlying abnormalities, elimination of drug toxicity, and replacement of necessary substances. Frequently, one or more of the factors that precipitate confusion cannot be corrected, or a specific, correctable factor cannot be identified. In these instances, treatment with neuroleptic medication can be instituted to minimize, or possibly reverse, confusion. On occasion, confusion may persist until the offending circumstances (e.g., fever, pneumonia, subarachnoid bleeding, lidocaine infusion) cease or resolve.

Traditionally, the term *ICU psychosis* has been used to designate florid abnormalities of mood and behavior in ICU patients. In our view, the term is outmoded and misleading because it implies a cause and effect relationship between being in an ICU and becoming psychotic. Early theorists drew on clinical and experimental data that suggested a relationship between sleep deprivation and subsequent psychosis [3]. They reasoned that ICU patients became psychotic because they were routinely deprived of sleep and exposed to either sensory deprivation, overload, or monotony. Subsequently, it became clear that other factors, many having no specific relationship to the ICU setting, contribute to neuropsychiatric dysfunction in ICU patients [4,5].

The term *psychosis* does not adequately reflect the range of symptoms seen in confused ICU patients. In a standard psychiatric glossary [6], psychosis is defined as a loss of contact with reality because of a functional (i.e., nonorganic) disturbance in which the sensorium is normal, but thinking is abnormal and associated with abnormal perceptions (e.g., auditory hallucinations) and systematic delusions (i.e., fixed, false beliefs). In fact, mental status changes in ICU patients are usually characterized by an abnormal sensorium, illusions, delusions that are fleeting and disorganized, and all varieties of sensory hallucinations (i.e., olfactory, tactile, visual, and auditory).

A diagnosis of *delirium* more appropriately describes the mental status abnormalities that commonly occur in ICU patients. Although some patients may become psychotic in an ICU, or enter the ICU with a preexisting psychotic condition (e.g., schizophrenia or manic-depressive psychosis), most pa-

tients with mental status changes are delirious because of one or more factors that disrupt the integrity of the central nervous system (CNS).

The purpose of this chapter is to review the evaluation, diagnosis, and treatment of mental status and behavioral abnormalities in ICU patients.

Delirium (Acute Confusional States)

DEFINITION. *Delirium* is a reversible organic mental disorder whose hallmarks are an acute onset of confusion and an altered level of consciousness [7,8]. It has, therefore, also been referred to as an *acute confusional state* [9]. Abnormal consciousness distinguishes delirium from dementia, which is also characterized by confusion, but is associated with a normal level of consciousness. Most cases of delirium, particularly those that develop in the ICU, have an acute onset. Although delirium is usually reversible within a period of days to weeks, some cases progress to irreversible brain failure [7]. The electroencephalogram (EEG) of the delirious patient is characteristically abnormal, suggesting what has been referred to as a state of cerebral insufficiency, or a failure of the normal metabolic processes of the brain [10,11].

INCIDENCE. The frequency of delirium depends on the nature and severity of the patient's illness, the type of treatment involved, the ICU setting, and the diagnostic criteria used to identify delirium. The highest incidence of delirium has been reported in the surgical intensive care unit (SICU), followed by the medical intensive care unit (MICU), the coronary care unit (CCU), and the general medical and surgical wards, respectively [12].

The incidence of delirium after general surgical procedures is less than 0.1 percent [13], although general surgery in the elderly is followed by delirium in 10 to 15 percent of patients [14].

The reported incidence of delirium after cardiac surgery has varied from 13 to 70 percent [15]. This wide range probably reflects inadequate and inconsistent methodologies (i.e., retrospective chart review using varying definitions of delirium) and technical improvements accruing during the 20 years spanned by these studies. A review of postcardiotomy delirium suggests that an average incidence of 32 percent has remained stable over time [16]. In contrast, a prospective study of 59 patients at the Cleveland Clinic found the incidence of delirium after myocardial revascularization to be only 6.8 percent [17].

CLINICAL FEATURES. The delirious patient exhibits a global impairment of cognitive function characterized by abnormal attention and arousal, impaired short-term memory, and disorientation [7,8,9,12]. Typically, levels of consciousness and activity fluctuate throughout the day and achieve peak intensity at night. All types of mood disturbance are seen in delirium; however, the quiet or psychomotorically retarded delirious patient can be mistaken for one with depression. Additionally, there may be abnormalities of perception (e.g., illusions, hallucinations), thought process (e.g., delusions, paranoia), and behavior (e.g., picking at bedsheets and intravenous [IV] tubing) as well as a disturbed sleep-wake cycle with frequent periods of arousal and somnolence throughout the day and night. Cognitive, perceptual, and behavioral dysfunction is often worse at night, undoubtedly giving rise to the popular belief that sleep deprivation is a cause of delirium. In fact, when studied prospectively, delirium has been noted to precede the onset of sleep difficulties in the ICU patient [18].

Florid delirium is easy to detect. The confused, paranoid patient may become combative and act as if the ICU staff are his enemies; this behavior may be reinforced, for example, by mistaking a ceiling light for fire or a shadow for a sinister object. Delirium is less apparent when the patient is quiet and inactive, when a corresponding disturbance of mood (e.g., irritability, depression) is the predominant feature, or when the patient has some awareness of the dysfunction and attempts to conceal it by using defenses of denial, projection, and avoidance [7]. Under these circumstances, a more detailed mental status examination performed at several different times may be necessary. A Mini Mental State Examination (MMSE) score of less than 24 (maximum score 30) reliably detects global cognitive dysfunction [19] but by itself is unable to distinguish delirium from dementia [20]. Trzepacz and colleagues have developed a ten-item clinician-rated scale that reliably distinguishes delirium from both dementia and schizophrenia [20].

ETIOLOGY. Delirium is believed to have an organic basis, although it has not been fully characterized. Romano and Engel's 1944 report [10] of an association between generalized EEG abnormalities and delirium is probably still the most significant pathophysiologic finding in delirium research. Presumably, a derangement of central neurotransmission results in the clinical phenomenology of delirium. It has been suggested that the likelihood of delirium occurring in the ICU patient depends on the number of drugs with anticholinergic properties administered [21]. The susceptibility of elderly patients to delirium may be attributable in part to a relative deficiency of acetylcholine in the aging brain [22]. A preexisting deficit of cholinergic function may be further aggravated by the addition of drugs with anticholinergic properties and result in anticholinergic delirium [22]. These findings suggest that the pathogenesis of delirium depends, at least in part, on a derangement of normal cholinergic transmission.

Numerous organic disturbances have been implicated in the etiology of delirium and can be listed under one of four major categories, according to Lipowski [8]: (1) primary intracranial disease; (2) systemic diseases that secondarily affect the brain; (3) exogenous toxic agents; and (4) withdrawal from substances on which the patient has become dependent (e.g., alcohol and sedative-hypnotic agents). A differential diagnosis of delirium adapted from Ludwig [23] and modified to fit this scheme is listed in Table 221-1. The clinician who evaluates a delirious patient may benefit from reviewing this list, although certain entities (e.g., stroke, shock, drug toxicity, fluid and electrolyte disturbances) occur more frequently than others in the ICU setting. The mnemonic, WWHHHIMP, can assist the clinician in recalling serious or potentially life-threatening causes of delirium (Table 221-2). Finally, Table 221-3 lists drugs commonly used in ICUs that are capable of inducing delirium [1].

Certain procedures and events are commonly associated with delirium. Cardiac surgery, for example, is a well-known precip-

Table 221-1. Differential Diagnosis of Delirium

System/problem	Etiological factors

Primary intracranial disease	Infection
	  HIV encephalopathy
	  Meningitis/encephalitis
	  Neurosyphilis
	Neoplasm
	  Space-occupying lesion
	Seizure
	  Postictal state
	  Complex partial seizure/status
	Vascular
	  Hypertensive encephalopathy
	  Intracranial hemorrhage
	  Vasculitis
	  Stroke
	Miscellaneous
	  Normal pressure hydrocephalus

Systemic diseases that secondarily affect the brain	Cardiopulmonary
	  Cardiac arrest
	  Congestive heart failure
	  Respiratory failure
	  Shock
	Endocrine/metabolic
	  Acid-base disturbance
	  Adrenal dysfunction
	  Fluid/electrolyte imbalance
	  Diabetic ketoacidosis
	  Hypoglycemia
	  Hepatic failure (encephalopathy)
	  Renal failure (uremia)
	  Parathyroid dysfunction
	  Thyroid dysfunction
	  Porphyria
	Infection
	  Sepsis
	  Subacute bacterial endocarditis
	Neoplasm
	  Paraneoplastic syndromes
	Nutritional deficiency
	  Folic acid
	  Niacin (pellagra)
	  Thiamine (Wernicke's encephalopathy, Wernicke-Korsakoff psychosis)
	  Vitamin B_{12} (pernicious anemia)

Exogenous toxic agents	Drugs of abuse
	  Alcohol
	  Amphetamines
	  Cocaine
	  LSD
	  Phencyclidine
	Nonmedicinal
	  Carbon monoxide
	  Heavy metals
	Medications (see Table 187-3)

Drug withdrawal	Alcohol
	Propanediols
	  Chloral hydrate
	  Meprobamate
	Sedative-hypnotic agents
	  Barbiturates
	  Benzodiazepines
	  Narcotics

Source: Adapted from Lipowski ZJ: Delirium in the elderly patient. *N Engl J Med* 320:578, 1989; and Ludwig AM: *Principles of Clinical Psychiatry.* New York, Free Press, 1980.

Table 221-2. Life-Threatening Causes of Delirium (WWHHHIMP)

Wernicke's encephalopathy
Withdrawal from drugs
Hypertensive encephalopathy
Hypoglycemia
Hypoxia
Intracerebral bleed
Meningitis/encephalitis
Poisoning

Source: Adapted from Tesar GE, Stern TA: Evaluation and treatment of agitation in the intensive care unit. *J Intensive Care Med* 1:137, 1986.

Table 221-3. Common Delirium-Inducing Drugs Used in the Intensive Care Unit

Drug group	Agent
Antiarrhythmics	Lidocaine
	Mexiletine
	Procainamide hydrochloride
	Quinidine sulfate
Antibiotics	Penicillin
	Rifampin
Anticholinergics	Atropine sulfate
Antihistamines	Nonselective
	Diphenhydramine hydrochloride
	Promethazine hydrochloride
	H-2 blockers
	Cimetidine
	Ranitidine
Beta-blockers	Propranolol hydrochloride
Narcotic analgesics	Meperidine hydrochloride
	Morphine sulfate
	Pentazocine

Source: Adapted from Tesar GE, Stern TA: Evaluation and treatment of agitation in the intensive care unit. *J Intensive Care Med* 1:137, 1986.

Table 221-4. Factors Contributing to the Development of Delirium After Cardiac Surgery

Time course	Factor
Preoperative	History of myocardial infarction
	Preexisting central nervous system dysfunction
	Psychiatric disorders/factors
	Panic-level anxiety
	Major depression
	Alcohol or drug abuse
	Poor understanding of or reluctance to undergo planned procedure
	Severe physical illness
Intraoperative	Body temperature $\leq$ 28°C
	Complexity of surgical procedure
	Systolic blood pressure $\leq$ 50 – 60 mm Hg
	Total anesthesia time
	Type of oxygenator used in the bypass device (?)
Postoperative	Complications during recovery
	Environment (e.g., sensory overload/deprivation)
	Intraaortic balloon pump (?)
	Medications administered (e.g., excess anticholinergic agents, narcotics, sedative/hypnotics)

Source: Adapted from Tesar GE, Stern TA: Evaluation and treatment of agitation in the intensive care unit. *J Intensive Care Med* 1:137, 1986.

itant of delirium [15,16]. Multiple events occurring in the intervals before, during, and after cardiac surgery have been identified as potential causes of delirium (Table 221-4), although a meta-analysis of studies on delirium associated with cardiac surgery fails to point to an outstanding factor [16]. The hypothetical important contributing factors (see Table 221-4) include the complexity of the surgical procedure (defined by the extent and duration of instrumentation in the intracardiac chambers), a diffuse but transient ischemic brain injury resulting from cardiac surgery [24], and possibly the type of membrane oxygenator used in the bypass device. Recent evidence indicates that significantly fewer patients had angiographic evidence of retinal microemboli after cardiopulmonary bypass using a membrane rather than a bubble oxygenator (56% vs. 100%; p < 0.001) [25]. These studies as well as the reports of delirium after infarction of the territories supplied by the right middle and posterior cerebral arteries [26,27] support the argument that ischemic brain injury accounts for at least some cases of delirium after cardiac surgery.

Drug overdose (OD) is a common cause of delirium in the MICU; agitation may develop during recovery from the acute effects of the OD. Between 1977 and 1981, 5 percent of all admissions to an 18-bed MICU at Massachusetts General Hospital were a direct result of drug OD [28]. The most frequently ingested drugs were alcohol, tricyclic antidepressants (TCAs), benzodiazepines, narcotics, antipsychotics, and barbiturates, in order of decreasing frequency [29].

DIFFERENTIAL DIAGNOSIS. It is important to distinguish delirium from functional psychosis (e.g., schizophrenia), secondary mania, dementia, complex partial seizures, and psychogenic dissociative disorders (e.g., psychogenic fugue or amnesia). The distinctive features of a functional psychotic disorder are a normal sensorium, a history of psychosis, and well-systematized delusions. However, certain psychotic individuals can become so disorganized that they appear delirious, and elderly individuals with functional psychoses and chronic cognitive impairment can also appear to be delirious.

A disturbance of mood is commonly associated with delirium; therefore, affective disorders (e.g., depression, manic-depressive disorder, and secondary mania) may be difficult or impossible to diagnose in the presence of delirium. The presence of mania in an ICU patient always warrants an investigation for an organic or toxic source. Reported causes of secondary mania include medications (e.g., corticosteroids, isoniazid, levodopa, and procarbazine hydrochloride), metabolic disturbance, infection, CNS neoplasm, and right temporal lobe seizures [30,31].

History is also important when differentiating delirium from dementia, because both disorders are characterized by global cognitive dysfunction. In practice, delirium is often superimposed on dementia, which results in further deterioration from the demented patient's cognitive baseline.

Complex partial seizures arising from seizure foci in the limbic system (e.g., the temporal lobes) can produce abnormal psychic and behavioral phenomena that mimic delirium [32]. The failure to make this distinction may lead to use of neuroleptic agents that either fail to treat the underlying disorder or reduce the seizure threshold and result in clinical deterioration.

Although uncommon in the ICU, psychogenic dissociative states can also mimic delirium. Patients with psychogenic amnesia often exhibit globally impaired cognition. However, the deficits are often inconsistent and include the inability to identify oneself (which is usually preserved in patients with delirium or transient global amnesia).

An EEG recording may be helpful in the diagnosis of complicated cases. The EEG is normal in functional psychoses and psychogenic dissociative states. In the presence of delirium, however, the EEG is usually abnormal with diffuse, generalized slowing, the severity of which parallels the intensity of delirium [10,11]. In some cases of mild delirium, the EEG slowing remains within normal limits and is only abnormal relative to fast baseline activity [8,11]. The EEG may also disclose an unexpected seizure focus.

TREATMENT. The treatment of delirium is guided by the following principles: (1) correct metabolic and systemic abnormalities; (2) eliminate drug toxicity; (3) treat withdrawal; and (4) use neuroleptic medication [33].

Correct Metabolic and Systemic Abnormalities. Meticulous examination of the clinical situation and the patient's chart are essential first steps in determining whether specific abnormalities exist so that they can be selectively treated. Treatment of infection, maintenance of a normal perfusion pressure, correction of fluid and electrolyte disturbances, maintenance of normal blood volume, and adequate oxygenation of the blood are essential features of good medical care that will correct or reduce the risk of delirium.

Eliminate Drug Toxicity. When drug toxicity is suspected, elimination or reduction of the offending agent or use of a specific antidote may reverse delirium caused by agents commonly administered to ICU patients (see Table 221-3) [33] (see Section X).

Narcotics and agents with anticholinergic properties probably account for a large portion of drug-induced delirium in the ICU [21,34]. Meperidine toxicity, for example, is probably an underrecognized cause of neuropsychiatric symptoms in ICU patients [34,35]. The CNS-stimulating activity of normeperidine, the long-lasting active metabolite of meperidine, can result in auditory and visual hallucinations, irritability, neuromuscular irritability (tremors, muscle twitching, myoclonus), and generalized seizures. A report by Shochet and Murray emphasizes that meperidine's proconvulsant properties can also induce partial seizures that may be mistaken for a functional (i.e., nonorganic) psychiatric disorder [35].

An antidote such as physostigmine, 1 to 2 mg, may be infused slowly IV on a one-time basis [36] or as a continuous drip [37] to reverse anticholinergic delirium. Naloxone hydrochloride, 0.4 mg subcutaneously or IV, is used to reverse some of the effects of narcotic-induced delirium; repeated doses may be necessary to maintain reversal when long-acting narcotics (e.g., methadone) have been responsible for the delirious state. IV verapamil has been reported to reverse the effects of phencyclidine intoxication [38]. The benzodiazepine antagonist flumazenil has been shown to reverse the effects of benzodiazepine toxicity [39].

A host of other toxins can induce delirium (see chapters in Section X) [40].

Treat Drug Withdrawal. For several reasons, the diagnosis of delirium secondary to drug withdrawal requires a high index of suspicion [1]. First, the emergent nature of many ICU admissions results in sudden discontinuation of the abused drug(s). Second, the ICU patient is often unable to communicate effectively, making it difficult to obtain a history of substance abuse and establish the diagnosis of a withdrawal state. Third, the physical signs of withdrawal (i.e., fever, tremor, and other signs of autonomic arousal) are both nonspecific and commonly present for other reasons. Finally, no laboratory test is available that can confirm the diagnosis of drug withdrawal.

Successful treatment of delirium secondary to drug withdrawal depends on adequate replacement of the same, or a cross-reactive, substance (i.e., one with a similar mechanism of action). Failure to identify the correct substance from which a patient is withdrawing can result in worsening of delirium, seizures, or death as a result of untreated withdrawal (e.g., barbiturate withdrawal) [41]. Although withdrawal-associated delirium resembles other types of delirium, its distinctive features include a greater likelihood of intense agitation and frightening visual hallucinations [42]. Fever, tremulousness, and other manifestations of autonomic arousal should suggest drug withdrawal, but these features may be present for other reasons. The drugs most commonly responsible for withdrawal syndromes include alcohol, sedative-hypnotic agents, and opioids. See Chapter 158 for a complete discussion of treatment of withdrawal syndromes.

Pharmacologic Treatment of Nonspecific Delirium. When a specific cause for delirium cannot be identified or corrected, the administration of a neuroleptic agent such as haloperidol is indicated (see Chap. 209). Haloperidol, a high-potency butyrophenone neuroleptic, is believed to exert its clinical effect through blockade of central dopamine receptor activity like other neuroleptics, although it does not seem to interfere with dopamine-mediated augmentation of renal blood flow [43]. Other neuroleptic agents such as thiothixene, trifluoperazine, or chlorpromazine can be substituted, but haloperidol has an extensive record of safety and efficacy when used in critically ill patients [44–50]. It has trivial effects on cardiovascular and respiratory function [47,48], and unlike most other neuroleptics available in the United States, it can be given intravenously. The Food and Drug Administration (FDA) has not approved use of IV haloperidol for the treatment of delirium or psychosis. Lack of FDA approval should not dissuade one from prescribing a drug approved for other purposes, but physicians are advised to seek approval from the hospital's administration or its formulary committee before using IV haloperidol. It is also recommended that the physician carefully document and inform either the patient, family, or guardian of the indication(s) for its use. Compared with the low-potency neuroleptics (e.g., chlorpromazine, thioridazine), the short-term use of haloperidol is associated with less sedation, less lowering of blood pressure, and fewer anticholinergic effects, but a higher rate of extrapyramidal symptoms (e.g., acute dystonia, akathisia, parkinsonism) [51]. Surprisingly, extrapyramidal symptoms appear to be uncommon when haloperidol is administered intravenously [33,47,48].

The starting dose of haloperidol depends on the patient's hemodynamic stability, integrity of the CNS, and intensity of the accompanying symptoms (e.g., agitation) [2,33,47,48,51]. Older individuals, particularly those with evidence of CNS dysfunction (e.g., dementia, stroke), tend to be less tolerant of haloperidol's side effects, in particular its extrapyramidal effects. The starting dose in this group may be as low as 0.5 mg orally, two or three times per day. A low starting dose and gradual upward titration are also advised in patients with hemodynamic instability. The starting dose of haloperidol in otherwise stable individuals is often 2 to 5 mg orally, three to four times per day, or higher if agitation is intense.

Parenteral administration of haloperidol is indicated when the oral route is not available, when malabsorption is evident, or when a rapid onset of effect is desired. The parenteral dose of haloperidol is approximately half the oral dose [43]. IM administration is effective and assures absorption, but repeated injections may be painful and cause secondary elevation of creatine phosphokinase levels, which can confuse the evaluation of concurrent chest pain.

Observation of haloperidol's effect on the patient should guide the adjustment of dosage and the frequency of administration. In general, a calming effect may be achieved with 2 to 5 mg orally every 4 to 6 hours, adjusting the dosage and frequency of administration according to the patient's mental and behavioral status. The maintenance dose is generally lower than the dose necessary to produce a calming effect. Medication should be maintained as long as the cause or circumstances of delirium persist. Empirically, sudden discontinuation without a taper is generally uneventful. However, gradual reduction reduces the likelihood of a sudden reemergence of delirium and the distant possibility of a withdrawal dyskinesia (i.e., reversible abnormal involuntary movements that resemble those of tardive dyskinesia and develop after sudden discontinuation of a neuroleptic agent).

In the ICU, side effects of haloperidol are usually mild and inconsequential and depend of the presence of other factors (see Chap. 209). In combination with haloperidol, propranolol has been reported to cause complete heart block and hypotension [52].

A recent case report [53] as well as our own experience suggest that prolonged cardiac conduction and *Torsades de pointes* cardiac arrhythmia may occur during haloperidol infusion in some patients. In the report by Metzger and Friedman [53], each of three patients described had a history of chronic alcohol abuse, and all three had cardiac disease and dilated ventricles by echocardiogram. These findings suggest that alcohol-related cardiac disease may have predisposed the patients to the development of haloperidol-associated cardiac arrhythmia. It is recommended that the clinician monitor for factors that might interact with haloperidol to cause cardiac conduction delay and rhythm disturbances (e.g., medications, depletion of magnesium or other electrolytes) and correct these or discontinue IV haloperidol if the QTc increases by more than 25 percent of the baseline value.

Extrapyramidal effects (e.g., acute dystonia, akathisia, parkinsonism) occur with oral and IM haloperidol and are comparatively infrequent with IV use [33,47,48]. Acute dystonia (e.g., laryngeal dystonia) is reversible with administration of benztropine mesylate 1 to 2 mg IV or diphenhydramine 25 to 50 mg IV [51]. A standing dose of either benztropine 1 to 2 mg twice per day or diphenhydramine 25 to 50 mg three to four times per day may be necessary to prevent further episodes. Akathisia, a subjective sense of internal restlessness that can be manifest as motor restlessness, responds best to lowering of neuroleptic dosage, addition of a beta-blocker (e.g., propranolol 10–20 mg three times daily) [54], or addition of a benzodiazepine such as diazepam [55] or lorazepam 0.5 to 1.0 mg, three to four times daily. Older individuals, particularly those with compromised CNS function, are most susceptible to the development of parkinsonian side effects. Reduction of the neuroleptic dosage is often recommended when extrapyramidal symptoms develop. Alternatively, addition of an anticholinergic agent (e.g., benztropine) or conversion of a low-potency neuroleptic (e.g., chlorpromazine) can be considered, but both alternatives introduce the risk of anticholinergic toxicity, to which the elderly are also vulnerable. The possibility of tardive dyskinesia is often mentioned as a reason to avoid use of neuroleptics such as haloperidol; however, there is virtually no risk of this outcome with the short-term use of any neuroleptic.

Agitation

ETIOLOGY. Although delirium is probably the most common cause of agitation in the ICU, many other factors that compromise a patient's ability to tolerate the ICU environment can precipitate agitation. Panic-level anxiety, pain, personality style, and limitations in one's ability to comprehend the nature and demands of intensive care (e.g., sensory, cognitive, or language impairment) are sources of agitation that must be addressed specifically.

Anxiety. Anxiety is a prominent and expected reaction to conditions (e.g., myocardial infarction) that result in ICU admission (see Chap. 222). In CCU patients, Cassem and Hackett [56] found that anxiety was a transient reaction lasting only a few days; most patients became calmer when orientated, educated, and reassured by staff members. However, some patients who are predisposed to panic-level anxiety or claustrophobia may find it difficult to feel comfortable when confined to an ICU. A history of panic attacks or avoidance of circumstances in which the person feels unsafe (e.g., bridges, tunnels, public transportation, church) suggests an anxiety disorder such as panic disorder or agoraphobia [57]. It is important to distinguish such extreme anxiety from paranoia or incipient psychosis, because the respective treatments differ (see following).

The process of weaning from chronic ventilatory support can also generate considerable anxiety (see Chap. 67). Intermittent mandatory ventilation (IMV) may offer an advantage over conventional weaning techniques (e.g., use of the traditional T-tube or trial-and-error) because some patients are reassured and calmed by the presence of the ventilator [58]. Prevention, or at least reduction of anxiety, can be accomplished by attending to six criteria that maximize the likelihood of successful weaning: (1) vital capacity of at least 10 to 15 ml per kilogram body weight; (2) maximal inspiratory force of greater than 25 mm H_2O; (3) oxygen gradient, $P(A-a)O_2^{1.0}$, less than 300 to 350 mm Hg; (4) dead space to tidal volume ratio (V_D/V_T) less than 0.6; (5) cardiovascular stability; and (6) metabolic balance [59]. Failure to fulfill these criteria leads to hypoxia, dyspnea, and subsequent agitation when weaning is attempted.

Fear and panic are the most common causes of a patient's threat or demand to sign out of the ICU [43], although personality factors play a role (see below). Firm but compassionate and reassuring discussion of the situation is indicated. Sometimes this requires the attention of both a psychiatrist and the patient's family. Patients who can be convinced to stay should be medicated with a benzodiazepine (e.g., diazepam or lorazepam) or even a neuroleptic (e.g., haloperidol) if prior benzodiazepine treatment has failed to control mounting anxiety. Those who insist on signing out should be allowed to do so if they demonstrate adequate comprehension of the situation and can satisfactorily weigh the risks and the benefits of their decision. If the patient's judgment is impaired, then she or he should be detained. However, the risk to the patient's health imposed by detention must also be assessed. For example, a patient admitted to the neurosurgical service for clipping of a large cerebral aneurysm was ultimately released from the hospital after he threatened to sign out against medical advice. It was believed that the hemodynamic consequences of combativeness or struggling against physical restraint would produce an unacceptably high risk of aneurysm rupture. In all such instances, careful documentation of the clinical circumstances and the decisions that have been made should be recorded in the patient's chart.

Discomfort. Pain is a source of agitation that may go undetected because of the patient's inability to communicate effectively or because of staff reluctance to provide adequate analgesia. Physicians and nurses sometimes avoid administering sufficient pain medication for fear of promoting addiction [60]. This fear is unwarranted unless the patient has a history of substance abuse or suffers from a chronic pain syndrome.

Akathisia, restlessness that is a side effect of neuroleptic medication, can precipitate agitation. Akathisia is difficult to diagnose because it may be indistinguishable from the restlessness that accompanies delirium, psychosis, or anxiety. Patients often describe this symptom as an experience of internal turmoil or restlessness that makes it difficult to remain inactive.

Personality Factors. Personality is defined in part as a style of coping. Individuals with certain personality types or disorders (e.g., dependent, borderline) cope poorly even under normal circumstances. It is our impression that patients with rigid, compulsive, obsessive, and controlling characteristics have the greatest difficulty coping with being in an ICU. Prolonged or severe illness can also overwhelm normal coping abilities and result in behavioral regression to a more childlike state [61]. Regressed patients are frequently irritable, uncooperative, and hostile, which makes their care more difficult. Sufficient frustration or fear may cause such a patient to sign out of the ICU or to become agitated.

Poor Comprehension or Sensory Impairment. Inability to comprehend fully one's situation because of either a language barrier or intellectual impairment can result in loss of behavioral control. Similarly, patients with hearing or visual impairments are at greater risk of developing auditory and visual hallucinations and may respond to them by becoming agitated. Cognitively impaired (e.g., demented or mentally retarded) patients may become agitated because of an inability to comprehend what is wrong with them, or what is being done to them. These and other patients with CNS dysfunction (e.g., secondary to stroke) are susceptible to further cognitive deterioration because of their vulnerability to CNS insults (e.g., hypoxia, hypoperfusion, or metabolic abnormalities).

When a patient's agitation fails to respond to the measures described above, it may be necessary to resort to the use of mechanical restraint, higher doses of neuroleptic medication, alternative or additional tranquilizing medication, and in extreme situations, intubation, sedation, and paralysis of the patient. Some of the measures to be discussed are controversial and at times have been considered to be alarming; however, they have been found to be useful and safe.

USE OF MECHANICAL RESTRAINT. Intense or explosive agitation must be dealt with expeditiously to ensure the safety of both the patient and the staff. Sedating medication should be infused as rapidly as possible, but mechanical restraint of the patient is generally necessary until the medication can exert its desired, calming effect. Continuous immobilization may still be required to control bursts of agitation. When necessary, the patient's torso can be restrained with a Posey vest and the limbs with gauze strips (e.g., Kerlex) or leather restraints. At times, restraints only intensify the patient's agitation, and some staff members may object to their use. A number of reports attest to the adverse effects of mechanical restraint, including strangulation, brachial plexus injury from vest restraints, increased agitation, and complications of immobilization [62]. Prevention of these adverse effects necessitates continuous observation of the patient. Ultimately, the potentially serious, but generally preventable, consequences of mechanical restraint must be balanced against the risks of uncontrolled agitation in a setting where virtual immobilization of the patient may be required.

PHARMACOLOGIC MANAGEMENT OF AGITATION. No single pharmacologic method has proved to be best for the control of intense agitation. Each agent has characteristics that

suggest its usefulness, and adverse effects associated with each technique are generally infrequent and easily managed in the ICU. Invariably, even the best efforts sometimes fail to control extreme agitation, and intubation, sedation, and paralysis of some patients may be required.

The treatment of choice depends on the cause of agitation. The principles used to evaluate and treat delirium (i.e., correction of systemic and metabolic factors, elimination of drug toxicity, treatment of withdrawal, and use of neuroleptic medication) also apply to the management of agitation. Because delirium is probably the most frequent cause of agitation in ICUs, neuroleptic medication is almost always the pharmacologic treatment of choice. The agitated patient who is psychotic will also benefit from treatment with neuroleptic medication. However, in some instances, agitation is a result of discomfort caused by hypoxia, akathisia, uncontrolled pain, panic-level anxiety, or an inability to comprehend the situation. Identification and correction of the source of discomfort, improved analgesia, or treatment with a high-potency benzodiazepine may be indicated in many of these circumstances.

The pharmacologic methods used to control agitation include (1) IV haloperidol alone, (2) a combination of IV haloperidol and a benzodiazepine, (3) other neuroleptics, (4) a benzodiazepine alone, (5) a narcotic, and (6) intubation, sedation, and infusion of a nondepolarizing muscle relaxant.

IV Haloperidol. When standard doses of haloperidol fail to control agitation, systematic escalation of the dosage has often proved successful [33,47–50,63–66]. IV, rather than oral or IM, administration of haloperidol is preferred for the reasons discussed above and because of the need for frequent dosing. IV injection requires that the IV line be flushed first with saline, because haloperidol can precipitate with both heparin and phenytoin [43]. The rate of infusion is not critical, but should be extended over 5 minutes when the patient is hypotensive. The mean distribution time of IV haloperidol in normal volunteers is 11 minutes and may be longer in critically ill patients [67]. After a steady state has been achieved, the elimination half-life is approximately 24 hours, or longer in patients with hepatic insufficiency [67] (see Chap. 209).

When a given dose of IV haloperidol fails to calm the agitated patient, repeated infusion of the same dose is often not successful. If a calming effect has not occurred within 15 to 20 minutes of the last infusion, doubling the previous dose has proved more effective. For example, if there is no calming effect evident within 20 minutes of a 5-mg bolus of IV haloperidol, the next dose should be 10 mg; if 10 mg is unsuccessful, the next dose should be 20 mg, and so on. If the patient becomes calm, repeat the last dose at the next dosing. The dosing interval is determined by the duration of calm; intense agitation may require hourly dosing. Once the patient is calm and a regular dose of medication and a dosing interval have been determined, the amount of each bolus may be reduced; however, in practice, it is often necessary to continue the same amount of IV haloperidol to maintain a state of behavioral calm. Although the infusion of amounts greater than 50 mg is rarely necessary, an individual bolus of 150 mg, and as much as 1200 mg per day, of IV haloperidol has been required to control severe agitation [63,64].

Continuous infusion of IV haloperidol has been used safely and effectively to control intense agitation [65,66]. In the three cases reported, continuous infusion proved to be superior to the bolus method of haloperidol administration, and in two of three cases, the hourly doses of haloperidol required were less using IV infusion rather than boluses of haloperidol [66]. Consistent with the experience of others [68], no extrapyramidal effects were reported. The IV solution can be prepared by injecting 20 mg of haloperidol into a 100 cc bag of D$_5$W or normal saline.

The use of IV haloperidol in critically ill patients has been associated with fewer extrapyramidal effects than when administered by oral or IM routes [33,47,48]. However, studies in normal controls [69] and in psychotic patients [70] do not show fewer effects, suggesting that medically ill patients may be protected by the often concurrent administration of benzodiazepines and beta-blockers, or that psychotic psychiatric patients are more susceptible to extrapyramidal effects of neuroleptics. In a prospective, double-blind study, Menza and colleagues [68] showed that the incidence of extrapyramidal effects is lower in patients receiving IV haloperidol along with a benzodiazepine than in patients treated with IV haloperidol alone.

It has been argued that neuroleptic-induced akathisia accounts for the high doses of haloperidol used to treat agitated patients in the ICU [71]. In our experience, although akathisia may occur, it probably does not contribute significantly to the high doses of haloperidol used. Once agitation has been controlled by haloperidol, most patients report feeling calm, and there is no evidence of the restlessness typical of akathisia. The escalation to higher doses has generally been preceded not only by increasing agitation, but also by a deterioration of mental status, which resolves after the dosage of haloperidol is increased. Finally, akathisia has not been evident immediately after discontinuation of high-dose haloperidol, an unlikely finding if akathisia had been present during haloperidol administration.

Cardiac conduction intervals should be monitored during high-dose haloperidol therapy, given the potential for prolongation of the QTc and development of *Torsades de pointes* cardiac arrhythmia [53].

Combined Use of IV Haloperidol and a Benzodiazepine.
Use of a benzodiazepine in addition to haloperidol often promotes further calming. Lorazepam has been used more often than other benzodiazepines for this purpose. When compared with diazepam, lorazepam has fewer effects on cardiopulmonary function, a shorter elimination half-life, and an absence of active metabolites [51,72,73]. Lorazepam can also be given with relative safety to patients with hepatic dysfunction because the metabolic step by which it is inactivated, i.e., conjugation with glucuronic acid, is relatively preserved in such patients [51] (see Chap. 209).

Several lines of evidence support the combined use of haloperidol and lorazepam for the treatment of agitation [74,75,76]. In a study of psychiatric patients, the addition of lorazepam to usual doses of haloperidol resulted in a statistically significant reduction of the mean neuroleptic dosage administered over a 6-month period [74]. In critically ill cancer patients who were delirious and agitated, Adams [75] found that doses of IV haloperidol higher than 10 mg seemed to confer no extra advantage. Rather, alternating comparatively high doses of lorazepam with lower doses of haloperidol produced a superior calming effect. Adams and colleagues recommended administering hourly boluses of no more than 10 mg of IV haloperidol alternating with IV lorazepam in doses as high as 350 mg per day, or a mean of 15 mg per hour [76]. Maintaining a lower dose of haloperidol also reduces the theoretical possibility of neuroleptic malignant syndrome [77].

Diazepam or midazolam (see below) rather than lorazepam should be used in combination with haloperidol, particularly when agitation is explosive and rapid control is desired. When administered IV, diazepam has a more rapid onset of both its initial and peak effects than lorazepam (Table 221-5). Its tendency to reduce systolic blood pressure is of little clinical significance, but it may cause significant respiratory depression

[78,79,80]. Case reports [79,80] suggest considerable interindividual variation in susceptibility to this effect, necessitating slow, monitored administration. Respiratory depression and obtundation can also occur unexpectedly after repeated infusions of diazepam as a result of the gradual accumulation of its active metabolite, nordiazepam (t$_{1/2}$ = 60–100 hr).

Other Neuroleptics.
If IV haloperidol alone or in combination with a benzodiazepine has not been effective, it may help to switch to a more sedating neuroleptic, such as droperidol or chlorpromazine. Droperidol, a butyrophenone neuroleptic similar to haloperidol, is less potent and more likely to produce sedation and hypotension than haloperidol. In one study of agitated emergency room patients, droperidol achieved more rapid control of acute agitation than an equivalent dose of haloperidol [81]. Chlorpromazine, an aliphatic phenothiazine neuroleptic, can cause severe orthostatic hypotension and its quinidinelike properties can increase the likelihood of cardiac arrhythmias; it is therefore not the neuroleptic of choice in the ICU setting. However, a retrospective survey documented the safe and effective use of this agent in medical settings, suggesting that it be considered as an alternative when standard treatments of agitation have failed [82]. Oral or IM administration of chlorpromazine is advised, because the risk of serious side effects is greater with IV administration.

Benzodiazepines.
Successful control of psychotic agitation has been achieved with exclusive use of a benzodiazepine [83]. Although neuroleptic medication is thought to be specific for the treatment of delirium and psychosis, attendant agitation may be controlled effectively by use of a benzodiazepine. For example, manic psychosis and agitation have been reported to respond well to clonazepam [84]. A benzodiazepine may also be the treatment of choice when panic and phobic anxiety account for agitated behavior. High-potency benzodiazepines such as alprazolam [85] and clonazepam [86] effectively control panic attacks. However, neither agent is available for parenteral use, and lorazepam (which can be given by oral, IM, and IV routes) is a suitable alternative for the treatment of panic when the oral route is unavailable.

Midazolam, a water-soluble imidazolebenzodiazepine with a rapid onset of action, a short elimination half-life (1–4 hr), and a potency twice that of diazepam, has been used successfully for the management of agitation in both psychiatric and medical settings [87,88]. In one report [87], three acutely agitated, psychotic patients in an emergency psychiatric facility were rapidly sedated with IM injections of midazolam (2.5–3 mg). A calming effect occurred within 6 to 8 minutes, and the patients slept for 25 to 90 minutes. When aroused, they were more cooperative and no longer agitated.

The continuous infusion of midazolam has been used effectively for sedation in the ICU (see Chap. 209). Shapiro and associates [88] studied its effects in six patients aged 22 to 77 years. All patients were either uncooperative or thrashing, and several had pulled out endotracheal, chest, or nasogastric tubes. During the 48-hour interval before starting the midazolam infusion, the six patients had received varying doses and types of IV sedation; morphine, 14 to 123 mg (n = 5); diazepam, 12.5 to 106 mg (n = 4); lorazepam, 8 to 25 mg (n = 4); and haloperidol, 8 to 21 mg (n = 3). Patients received a loading dose of 25 μg/kg/min followed by an infusion of 0.4 μg/kg/min adjusted to achieve an adequate level of sedation. Successful control of agitation was achieved was achieved with a mean loading dose of 17.4 mg (range, 8–32) and a mean infusion rate varying over the 48-hour period of infusion from 0.67 to 6.8 μg/kg/min (range, 0.1–0.4 to 2.5–20.3). All patients were intubated and were monitored with arterial catheters and stan-

Table 221-5. Pharmacology of Drugs Used to Treat Agitation

Drug	Route	Onset (min)	Peak effect (min)	Active metabolites	Starting dose
NEUROLEPTIC					
Haloperidol	IV[a], IM PO	5–20 30–60	15–45 120–240	Insignificant	*Degree of agitation* Mild: 0.5–2.0 mg Moderate: 5.0–10.0 mg Severe: ≥ 10.0 mg
Droperidol	IV, IM	3–10	15–45	Insignificant	2.5–10 mg 25 mg
Chlorpromazine	IM,IV[b]	5–40	10–30		
BENZODIAZEPINE					
Diazepam	IV PO	2–5 10–60	5–30 30–180	Nordiazepam[c]	2–5 mg
Lorazepam	IV, IM SL PO	2–20 2–20 20–60	60–120 20–60 20–120	None	1–2 mg 0.5–1 mg 0.5–1 mg
Midazolam	IM, IV	1–2	30–40	1- and 4-hydroxy-midazolam	0.05–0.15 mg/kg
NARCOTIC					
Morphine sulfate	IM, IV	1–2	20	None	4–10 mg
PARALYTIC					
Metocurine iodide	IV	1–4	2–10		0.2–0.4 mg/kg
Pancurium bromide	IV	½–1	5		0.04–0.1 mg/kg

[a] Intravenous haloperidol is not approved for routine use by the Food and Drug Administration. Permission for its use should be requested from the hospital's formulary.
[b] Intravenous administration of chlorpromazine is more likely to cause cardiovascular disturbance (e.g., hypotension) than intramuscular administration.
[c] Nordiazepam (desmethyldiazepam) is the active metabolite of diazepam). Its half-life is 60–100 hours.
IV = intravenous; IM = intramuscular; PO = oral; SL = sublingual.
Source: Adapted from Tesar GE, Stern TA: Rapid tranquilization of the agitated intensive care unit patient. *J Intensive Care Med* 3:195, 1988.

dard electrocardiography. There were no episodes of cardiovascular or respiratory depression attributable to midazolam.

A midazolam infusion has also been used successfully to control florid delirium tremens in a 25-year-old man [89]. Over a 5-day period, the patient received 2850 mg of midazolam as a constant infusion without evidence of respiratory depression.

Like any benzodiazepine, midazolam can cause respiratory depression if large doses are given. However, the margin of safety is wide with doses of 100 to 150 μg per kilogram necessary to produce clinically significant respiratory depression [90]. Elderly and debilitated patients, especially those with chronic obstructive pulmonary disease (COPD) or hepatic insufficiency, are at particular risk of developing apnea or respiratory arrest. The concurrent administration of opiates potentiates the respiratory depressant effects of midazolam.

Prolonged infusion of midazolam should be followed by a gradual tapering of dosage. Sudden discontinuation has been reported to precipitate a syndrome of benzodiazepine withdrawal [91,92].

In addition to causing respiratory depression, benzodiazepine treatment has the potential for inducing delirium.

Narcotics. Morphine sulfate is used in ICU patients for the dual purposes of pain control and sedation [93]. Parenteral administration is associated with a prompt onset of action that lasts 4 to 5 hours [94]. Mild to moderate agitation, particularly when it is secondary to pain, responds well to morphine. However, other agents are recommended for control of more severe agitation, because high doses of morphine alone or in combination with other CNS depressants may cause respiratory depression and also induce or aggravate delirium.

Nondepolarizing Muscle Relaxants. Intubation, sedation, and paralysis should be reserved for cases of agitation that have not responded successfully to the treatments discussed above. Intubation may result in a higher rate of pulmonary complications, and pharmacologic paralysis increases the risk of traction injuries that can occur in the course of repositioning or moving the patient.

Metocurine iodide or pancuronium bromide can be used to paralyze the patient. The former agent is often preferred because it produces less autonomic instability [95]. Pancuronium bromide has a tendency to increase heart rate, blood pressure, and cardiac output as a result of both its antimuscarinic activity and its ability to release and block the reuptake of norepinephrine [95]. Tricyclic antidepressants share these properties with pancuronium bromide, which may account for the higher incidence of cardiac arrhythmias observed with the combined use of these agents [96]. Infusion of metocurine iodide may produce mild hypotension and a compensatory tachycardia that corresponds to a rate-dependent release of histamine [96].

Liberal use of morphine sulfate is indicated to ensure the tranquility of the paralyzed, but otherwise conscious, patient. Staff members should speak in a professional and compassionate manner in the presence of the patient; although the patient may appear unconscious, she or he may be capable of normal hearing and comprehension.

Conclusion

Agitation is a medical emergency that threatens the well-being of the ICU patient and staff. Delirium, or confusion, frequently heralds agitation, and if treated promptly, may avert potentially serious consequences. A systematic approach to the evaluation of delirium will disclose its cause(s), in many instances permitting specific treatment. When a cause cannot be discovered or corrected, treatment with a neuroleptic agent such as haloperidol should be instituted. In some instances agitation is either so sudden, explosive, or intense that both mechanical restraints and the infusion of rapidly acting sedating agents are required. There is no single best treatment for the control of intense agitation, and the selection of a particular agent or technique depends on careful assessment and monitoring of the clinical circumstances. IV haloperidol has been used successfully to control intense agitation, but benzodiazepines used alone or in combination with haloperidol may offer certain advantages. The use of nondepolarizing muscle relaxants is generally withheld until these treatments have failed.

References

1. Tesar GE, Stern TA: Evaluation and treatment of agitation in the intensive care unit. *J Intensive Care Med* 1:137, 1986.
2. Tesar GE, Stern TA: Rapid tranquilization of the agitated intensive care unit patient. *J Intensive Care Med* 3:195, 1988.
3. Nahum LH: Madness in the recovery room from open-heart surgery, or "They kept waking me up" (editorial). *Con Med* 29:771, 1965.
4. Kornfeld DS, Zimberg S, Malm JR: Psychiatric complications of open-heart surgery. *N Engl J Med* 273:287, 1965.
5. Heller SS, Frank KA, Malm JR, et al: Psychiatric complications of open-heart surgery: A re-examination. *N Engl J Med* 283:1015, 1970.
6. Subcommittee of the Joint Commission of Public Affairs: *A Psychiatric Glossary of the American Psychiatric Association.* Boston, Little, Brown, 1980.
7. Lipowski ZJ: Delirium, clouding of consciousness and confusion. *J Nerv Ment Dis* 145:227, 1967.
8. Lipowski ZJ: Delirium in the elderly patient. *N Engl J Med* 320:578, 1989.
9. Lipowski ZJ: Delirium (acute confusional states). *JAMA* 258:1789, 1988.
10. Romano J, Engel GL: Studies of delirium. I. Electroencephalographic data. *Arch Neurol Psychiatry* 51:356, 1944.
11. Engel GL, Romano J: Delirium, a syndrome of cerebral insufficiency. *J Chronic Dis* 9:260, 1959.
12. Lipowski ZJ: *Delirium: Acute Brain Failure in Man.* Springfield, IL, Charles C Thomas, 1980.
13. Surman OS, Hackett TP, Silverberg EL, et al: Usefulness of psychiatric intervention in patients undergoing cardiac surgery. *Arch Gen Psychiatry* 30:830, 1974.
14. Seymour G: *Medical Assessment of the Elderly Surgical Patient.* Rockville, MD, Aspen Systems, 1986.
15. Dubin WR, Field HL, Gastfriend DR: Postcardiotomy delirium: A critical review. *J Thorac Cardiovasc Surg* 77:586, 1979.
16. Smith LW, Dimsdale JE: Postcardiotomy delirium: Conclusions after 25 years? *Am J Psychiatry* 146:452, 1989.
17. Calabrese JR, Skwerer RG, Gulledge AD: Incidence of postoperative delirium following myocardial revascularization. *Cleve Clin J Med* 54:29, 1987.
18. Harrell RG, Othmer LE: Postcardiotomy confusion and sleep loss. *J Clin Psychiatry* 48:445, 1987.
19. Folstein M, Folstein S, McHugh O: "Mini-mental state": A practical method for grading the cognitive state of patients for the clinician. *J Psychiat Res* 12:189, 1975.
20. Trzepacz PT, Baker RW, Greenhouse J: A symptom rating scale for delirium. *Psychiatry Res* 23:89, 1988.
21. Tune LE, Holland A, Folstein MF, et al: Association of postoperative delirium with raised serum levels of anticholinergic drugs. *Lancet* 2:651, 1981.
22. Sunderland T, Tariot PN, Cohen RM, et al: Anticholinergic sensitivity in patients with dementia of the Alzheimer type and age-matched controls: A dose-response study. *Arch Gen Psychiatry* 44:418, 1987.
23. Ludwig AM: *Principles of Clinical Psychiatry.* New York, Free Press, 1980, p 234.
24. Henriksen L: Evidence suggestive of diffuse brain damage following cardiac operations. *Lancet* 1:816, 1984.
25. Blauth CI, Smith PL, Arnold JV, et al: Influence of oxygenator type on the incidence and extent of microembolic retinal ischemia during cardiopulmonary bypass: Assessment of digital image analysis (abstract). Presented at the Annual Meeting of the American Association for Thoracic Surgery, Boston, MA, May 8, 1989.
26. Mori E, Yamadori A: Acute confusional state and acute agitated delirium: Occurrence after infarction in the right middle cerebral artery territory. *Arch Neurol* 44:1139, 1987.
27. Devinsky O, Bear D, Volpe BT: Confusional states following posterior cerebral artery infarction. *Arch Neurol* 45:160, 1988.
28. Thibault GE, Mulley AG, Barnett GO, et al: Medical intensive care: Indications, interventions, and outcomes. *N Engl J Med* 302:938, 1980.
29. Stern TA, Mulley AG, Thibault GE: Life-threatening drug overdose. *JAMA* 251:1983, 1984.
30. Krauthammer C, Klerman GL: Secondary mania: Manic syndromes associated with antecedent physical illness or drugs. *Arch Gen Psychiatry* 35:1333, 1978.
31. Larson EW, Richelson E: Organic causes of mania. *Mayo Clin Proc* 63:906, 1988.
32. Murray GB: Confusion, delirium, and dementia. In Hackett TP, Cassem HN (eds): *Massachusetts General Hospital Handbook of General Hospital Psychiatry.* 2nd ed. Littleton, MA, PSG Publishing, 1987, p 84.
33. Cassem NH: Critical care psychiatry, in Shoemaker WC, Thompson WL, Holbrook PR (eds): *Textbook of Critical Care.* Philadelphia, WB Saunders, 1984, p 981.
34. Stern TA: Neuropsychiatric effects of narcotic analgesia. *J Intensive Care Med* 3:237, 1988.
35. Shochet RB, Murray GB: Neuropsychiatric toxicity of meperidine. *J Intensive Care Med* 3:246, 1988.
36. Granacher RP, Baldessarini RJ: Physostigmine. *Arch Gen Psychiatry* 32:375, 1975.
37. Stern TA: Continuous infusion of physostigmine. *J Clin Psychiatry* 44:463, 1983.
38. Montgomery PT, Mueller ME: Treatment of PCP intoxication with verapamil (letter). *Am J Psychiatry* 142:882, 1985.
39. Hofer P, Scollo-Lavizzari G: Benzodiazepine antagonist RO 15-1788 in self-poisoning: Diagnostic and therapeutic use. *Arch Intern Med* 145:633, 1985.
40. Haddad LM, Winchester JF (eds): *Clinical Management of Poisoning and Drug Overdose.* Philadelphia, WB Saunders, 1983.
41. Bernstein JG: Psychotropic drug prescribing, in Hackett TP, Cassem NH (eds): *Massachusetts General Hospital Handbook of General Hospital Psychiatry.* 2nd ed. Littleton, MA, PSG Publishing, 1987, p 49.
42. Khantzian EJ, McKenna GJ: Acute toxic and withdrawal reactions associated with drug use and abuse. *Ann Intern Med* 90:361, 1979.
43. Cassem NH, Hackett TP: The setting of intensive care, in Hackett TP, Cassem NH (eds): *Massachusetts General Hospital Handbook of General Hospital Psychiatry.* 2nd ed. Littleton, MA, PSG Publishing, 1987, p 353.
44. Pratt IT: Twilight sleep after infarction. *Br Med J* 3:475, 1971.
45. Cameron OG: Safe use of haloperidol in a patient with cardiac dysrhythmia. *Am J Psychiatry* 135:1244, 1978.
46. Donlon PT, Hopkin J, Schaffer CB, et al: Cardiovascular safety of rapid treatment with intramuscular haloperidol. *Am J Psychiatry* 136:233, 1979.
47. Sos J, Cassem NH: The intravenous use of haloperidol for acute delirium in intensive care settings. Read before the International Symposium: Psychopathological and neurological dysfunctions following open-heart surgery. Hamburg, Germany, 1978.
48. Sos J, Cassem NH: Managing postoperative agitation. *Drug Therapy* 10:103, 1980.
49. Settle EC, Ayd FJ: Haloperidol: A quarter century of experience. *J Clin Psychiatry* 44:440, 1983.

50. Tesar GE, Murray GB, Cassem NH: Use of high-dose intravenous haloperidol in agitated cardiac patients. *J Clin Psychopharmacol* 5:344, 1985.

51. Thompson TL, Thompson WL: Treating postoperative delirium. *Drug Therapy* 13:30, 1983.

52. Alexander HE, McCarty K, Giffen MB: Hypotension and cardiopulmonary arrest associated with concurrent haloperidol and propranolol therapy. *JAMA* 252:87, 1984.

53. Metzger E, Friedman R: Prolongation of the corrected QT and torsades de pointes cardiac arrhythmia associated with intravenous haloperidol in the medically ill. *J Clin Psychopharmacol* 13:128, 1993.

54. Lipinski JF, Zubenko G, Cohen BM, et al: Propranolol in the treatment of neuroleptic-induced akathisia. *Am J Psychiatry* 141:412, 1984.

55. Donlon P: The therapeutic use of diazepam for akathisia. *Psychosomatics* 14:222, 1973.

56. Cassem NH, Hackett TP: Psychiatric consultation in a coronary care unit. *Ann Intern Med* 75:9, 1971.

57. *Diagnostic and Statistical Manual of the American Psychiatric Association, 4th Ed.* Revised. Washington, DC, American Psychiatric Association Press, 1994.

58. Irwin RS, Demers RR: Mechanical ventilation, in Rippe JM, Irwin RS, Alpert JS, et al (eds): *Intensive Care Medicine.* Boston, Little, Brown, 1985, p 462.

59. Feeley TW: Problems in weaning patients from ventilators. *Resident and Staff Physician* 22:291, 1976.

60. Marks RM, Sachar EJ: Undertreatment of medical inpatients with narcotic analgesics. *Ann Intern Med* 78:173, 1973.

61. Weisman AD: Coping with illness, in Hackett TP, Cassem NH (eds): *Massachusetts General Hospital Handbook of General Hospital Psychiatry.* 2nd ed. Littleton, MA, PSG Publishing, 1987, p 297.

62. Francis J: Using restraints in the elderly because of fear of litigation (letter). *N Engl J Med* 320:870, 1989.

63. Stern TA: The management of depression and anxiety following myocardial infarction. *Mt Sinai Med J (NY)* 52:623, 1985.

64. Sanders K, Murray GB, Cassem NH: High-dose intravenous haloperidol for agitated delirium in a cardiac patient on intra-aortic balloon (letter). *J Clin Psychopharmacol* 11:146, 1991.

65. Fernandez F, Holmes VF, Adams F, et al: Treatment of severe, refractory agitation with a haloperidol drip. *J Clin Psychiatry* 49:239, 1988.

66. Dixon D, Craven J: Continuous infusion of haloperidol (letter). *Am J Psychiatry* 150:673, 1993.

67. Forsman A, Ohman R: Pharmacokinetic studies of haloperidol in man. *Curr Ther Res* 20:314, 1976.

68. Menza MA, Murray GB, Holmes VF, et al: Decreased extrapyramidal symptoms with intravenous haloperidol. *J Clin Psychiatry* 48:278, 1987.

69. Magliozzi JR, Gillespie H, Lombrozo L, et al: Mood alteration following oral and intravenous haloperidol and relationship to drug concentration in normal subjects. *J Clin Pharmacol* 25:285, 1985.

70. Moller H-J, Kissling W, Land C, et al: Efficacy and side effects of haloperidol in psychotic patients: Oral versus intravenous administration. *Am J Psychiatry* 139:1571, 1982.

71. Weiden P, Shaw E, Bruun R, et al: High-dose intravenous haloperidol in agitated cardiac patients (letter). *J Clin Psychopharmacol* 6:375, 1986.

72. Rao S, Sherbaniuk RW, Prasad K, et al: Cardiopulmonary effects of diazepam. *Clin Pharmacol Ther* 14:182, 1972.

73. Paulsen BA, Becker LD, Way WL: The effects of intravenous lorazepam alone and with meperidine on ventilation in man. *Acta Anaesthesiol Scand* 27:400, 1983.

74. Salzman C, Green AI, Rodriguez-Villa F, et al: Benzodiazepines combined with neuroleptics for management of severe disruptive behavior. *Psychosomatics* 27(suppl):17, 1986.

75. Adams F: Neuropsychiatric evaluation and treatment of delirium in the critically ill cancer patient. *Cancer Bull* 36:156, 1984.

76. Adams F, Fernandez F, Andersson BS: Emergency pharmacotherapy of delirium in the critically ill cancer patient. *Psychosomatics* 27(suppl):33, 1986.

77. Tesar GE: Neuroleptic malignant syndrome: An update. *Probl Crit Care* 2:149, 1988.

78. Dalen JE, Evans GL, Bands JS, et al: The haemodynamics and respiratory effects of diazepam. *Anesthesiology* 30:259, 1969.

79. Hall SC, Ovassapian A: Apnea after intravenous diazepam therapy. *JAMA* 238:1052, 1977.

80. Del Vecchio PJ: Apnea after intravenous diazepam administration. *JAMA* 239:7, 1978.

81. Resnick M, Burton BT: Droperidol vs. haloperidol in the initial management of acutely agitated patients. *J Clin Psychiatry* 45:298, 1984.

82. Muskin PR, Mellman LA, Kornfeld DS: A "new" drug for treating agitation and psychosis in the general hospital: Chlorpromazine. *Gen Hosp Psychiatry* 8:404, 1986.

83. Cohen BM, Lipinski JF: Treatment of acute psychosis with non-neuroleptic agents. *Psychosomatics* 27(suppl):7, 1986.

84. Sachs GS, Rosenbaum JF, Jones L: Adjunctive clonazepam for maintenance treatment of bipolar affective disorder. *J Clin Psychopharmacol* 10:42, 1990.

85. Ballenger JC, Burrows GD, DuPont RL, et al: Alprazolam in panic disorder and agoraphobia. Results from a multicenter trial. I. Efficacy in short-term treatment. *Arch Gen Psychiatry* 45:413, 1988.

86. Tesar GE, Rosenbaum JF, Pollack MH, et al: Double-blind, placebo-controlled comparison of clonazepam and alprazolam for panic disorder. *J Clin Psychiatry* 52:69, 1991.

87. Mendoza R, Djenderedjian AH, Adams J, et al: Midazolam in acute psychotic patients with hyperarousal. *J Clin Psychiatry* 48:291, 1987.

88. Shapiro JM, Westphal BA, White PF, et al: Midazolam infusion for sedation in the intensive care unit. *Anesthesiology* 64:394, 1986.

89. Lineaweaver WC, Anderson K, Hing DN: Massive doses of midazolam infusion for delirium tremens without respiratory depression. *Crit Care Med* 16:294, 1988.

90. Crippen DW: The role of sedation in the ICU patient with pain and agitation. *Crit Care Clin* 6:369, 1990.

91. Finley PR, Nolan PE: Precipitation of benzodiazepine withdrawal following sudden discontinuation of midazolam. *DICP* 23:151, 1989.

92. Mets B, Horsell A, Linton DM: Midazolam-induced benzodiazepine withdrawal syndrome. *Anaesthesia* 46:28, 1991.

93. Todres D: The role of morphine in acute myocardial infarction. *Am Heart J* 81:566, 1971.

94. Harvey SC: Hypnotics and sedatives: The barbiturates, in Goodman LS, Gilman A (eds): *The Pharmacological Basis of Therapeutics.* 5th ed. New York, Macmillan, 1975, p 102.

95. Miller RD, Savarese JJ: Pharmacology of muscle relaxants, in Miller RD (ed): *Anesthesia,* vol 2, 2nd ed. New York, Churchill Livingstone, 1986, p 889.

96. Edwards RP, Miller RD, Roizen MF, et al: Cardiac responses to imipramine and pancuronium during anesthesia with halothane or enflurane. *Anesthesiology* 50:421, 1979.

222. Recognition and Treatment of Anxiety in the ICU Patient

Mark H. Pollack, Lawrence A. Labbate, and Theodore A. Stern

Anxiety in the critical care setting may be expected as a transient response to the stress of hospitalization; however, excessive or pathologic anxiety has a negative impact on patient morbidity, mortality, and compliance with treatment. It should be diagnosed when present and treated in a timely fashion.

Although the precise nature and prevalence of anxiety in the medical setting are difficult to determine, anxiety disorders are common. It has been reported that anxiety disorders have a prevalence of 6 to 10 percent in primary care settings [1], 10 to 14 percent in cardiology practices [2], and 5 to 20 percent among medical inpatients [3]. Most studies in this field lack uniform instruments, study a heterogeneous patient population, have no control groups, and attempt to study an emotion (anxiety) that is transient and changeable [4]. However, clinical experience suggests an increased prevalence of anxiety in critical care settings. Patients hospitalized in the intensive care unit (ICU) encounter internal and external dangers: fear of death, separation from loved ones and familiar surroundings, loss of control, intimacy with strangers, sleep loss, and frequent procedures that are painful or restrict mobility (e.g., placement of an intraaortic balloon pump). Patients experience anxiety about their illness and their capacity to work and maintain social and family relationships in the future.

Anxiety is a common reason for psychiatric consultation in the ICU; Cassem and Hackett [5] noted that it was the most common reason for consultation during the first 2 days after admission to the coronary care unit (CCU).

Requests for psychiatric consultations from surgical intensive care units (SICUs) and respiratory intensive care units (RICUs) frequently relate to management of anxiety in patients who are attempting to wean from the ventilator. Sixty percent of patients undergoing coronary artery bypass graft (CABG) surgery experience significant postoperative anxiety [6]. Anxiety and depression have been estimated to occur in 65 to 85 percent of patients hospitalized after myocardial infarction (MI) [7,8].

When Cassem and Hackett [5] documented a pattern of psychological responses to MI, anxiety was the most common reason for psychiatric consultation. The fear of death or an increase in cardiopulmonary symptoms often led to anxiety. Mortality was found to be three times lower in the group referred for psychiatric consultation than the group not seen by a psychiatrist. Although a direct correlation in this study was not made between the psychiatric intervention (e.g., prescription of anxiolytics, use of clarification, environmental manipulation, support) and reduced mortality, the evidence suggested that increased anxiety may have been associated with increased morbidity and mortality.

Anxiety is associated with arousal of the sympathetic nervous system and an increase in cardiac output [9]. Stress and anxiety associated with acute MI are often accompanied by increased plasma levels of catecholamines, free fatty acids, and cortisol [10]. These elevated levels may be associated with potentially lethal complications associated with MI, including ventricular arrhythmias, cardiac failure, and cardiogenic shock [11]. Administration of diazepam reduces the elevated urinary excretion of catecholamines and free fatty acids with a concomitant decrease in the incidence of ventricular arrhythmias [12–15]. Elevation of catecholamines causes an increase in heart rate, peripheral resistance, blood pressure, cardiac contractility and cardiac output, and a decreased threshold for ventricular fibrillation (VF) [16]. Stress also has been associated with silent ischemia and disturbances in regional myocardial perfusion in angina patients [17] and has been associated with sudden death in patients with ischemic heart disease.

Because anxiety is common and has a clinical impact on patients in the ICU, clinicians should maintain a high index of suspicion for the presence of anxiety. The timely and effective treatment of anxiety should improve patient compliance and comfort, and reduce morbidity and mortality associated with critical illness.

Definition of Anxiety

Anxiety and fear can be clinically indistinguishable; however, their causes are different. Fear is the sense of dread and foreboding that may occur in response to an external threatening event (e.g., being attacked). "Anxiety is the same distressing experience of apprehension and foreboding as fear except that it derives from an unknown internal stimulus, inappropriate or excessive to the reality of the external stimulus or concerned with a future one" [18].

SYMPTOMS. Anxiety may be manifested by physical, affective, behavioral, or cognitive symptoms. The physical signs and symptoms of anxiety are generally those associated with autonomic arousal (e.g., tachycardia, tachypnea, diaphoresis, and lightheadedness). The diagnosis of anxiety should always be considered in the presence of autonomic hyperactivity. Many physical symptoms of anxiety are also manifestations of critical illness; attention to the characteristics of anxiety is often necessary to minimize diagnostic confusion. The affective component of anxiety ranges from mild edginess to terror and panic. The behavioral consequences of anxiety include the avoidance of distressing situations, noncompliance with procedures, or flight from the hospital. The cognitive aspects include worry, apprehension, and thoughts about emotional or bodily damage.

Though anxiety and fear in the ICU are ubiquitous, nonspecific symptoms of anxiety may lead to underdiagnosis of pathologic anxiety, to incorrect attribution of other physical causes, or to its dismissal as being either insignificant or appropriate to the setting. Pathologic anxiety warrants further evaluation and can be distinguished from "normal" anxiety by four criteria: (1) autonomy, (2) intensity, (3) duration, and (4) behavior [18]. *Autonomy* refers to distress that has a minimal basis in environmental stimuli (i.e., "it has a life of its own"). *Intensity* refers to the level of discomfort and severity of symptoms. *Duration* refers to the persistence of symptoms, and *behavior* refers to the effect of anxiety on coping and normal function. Pathologic anxiety is defined as anxiety that is autonomous, persistent, and causes a level of distress beyond the patient's capacity to bear it, and results in impaired function or abnormal behavior (e.g., avoidance or withdrawal).

ETIOLOGY. The biologic underpinnings for the genesis and propagation of anxiety and fear involve at least two major central nervous system (CNS) mechanisms. Panic attacks appear to be generated by central noradrenergic mechanisms, particularly those emanating from the locus ceruleus, a small retropontine nucleus that is the major source of the brain's noradrenergic innervation [19]. Increased locus ceruleus firing elicits anxious responses in animals and humans; these responses are blocked by agents (e.g., alprazolam and tricyclic antidepressants) that decrease locus ceruleus firing [20].

Limbic system structures, especially the septohippocampal areas, appear to mediate vigilance and generalized anxiety [21]. These structures contain high concentrations of benzodiazepine receptors, which appear to modulate arousal, anxiety, and behavioral inhibition by binding the inhibitory neurotransmitter gamma aminobutyric acid (GABA) [22]. The locus ceruleus and limbic system areas are interconnected and likely serve to modulate the level of anxiety. In addition, other neurotransmitter systems (including the serotonin system and a variety of peptides) appear important in the central regulation of anxiety [23]. Positron emission tomography (PET) scanning suggests limbic activation during panic [24].

DIFFERENTIAL DIAGNOSIS. The diagnostic approach to the anxious patient in the ICU involves consideration of at least three potentially overlapping areas. The clinician needs to assess whether the anxiety is secondary to an organic factor (i.e., a medical illness or its treatment), a primary psychiatric syndrome (e.g., panic disorder or depression), or a reaction by the individual to his or her clinical situation, which is in large part based upon his or her coping style and the meaning of the illness to the patient.

The assessment of the anxious patient can be a diagnostic challenge. The distinction between anxiety as a symptom and as a syndrome may be blurred in the ICU, where situational anxiety or fear, primary anxiety disorders, and anxiety symptoms from organic causes may coincide.

Organic Causes of Anxiety

The list of medical causes of anxiety symptoms is extensive; an exhaustive review of each medical cause of anxiety is beyond the scope of this chapter. However, the following guidelines will help direct an efficient, yet thorough, evaluation of anxiety in the medically ill.

A patient's known medical illness, its complications, and its treatment should be suspected as causes of anxiety. For example, hypoxia, hyperventilation, and sympathomimetic bronchodilators may all contribute to anxiety in a patient with chronic obstructive pulmonary disease. Risk factors such as a family history of a disorder thought to be anxiety related (e.g., hyperthyroidism) may provide important information to guide further assessment.

The quality of anxiety symptoms related to organic factors may differ from symptoms secondary to a primary anxiety disorder. Starkman and colleagues [25] compared the anxiety symptoms of 17 patients with pheochromocytoma with those of 52 patients with primary anxiety disorders. Most of the patients with pheochromocytoma had a significant lack of psychological, as opposed to physical, symptoms of anxiety; most did not meet criteria for panic disorder or generalized anxiety disorder, and none developed phobic symptoms. Harper and Roth [26] compared patients with primary anxiety disorders with those with anxiety secondary to temporal lobe epilepsy (TLE). Patients with primary anxiety disorders were more likely to have had an emotional trauma at the onset of anxiety, daily symptoms, and a gradual resolution of symptoms after an attack, and they were less likely to have either loss of speech or a change in the level of consciousness when anxious.

The presence of an organic cause is suggested by anxiety that occurs in the absence of a psychologically charged situation, or in conjunction with discrete physical events (e.g., a run of supraventricular tachycardia or vasopressor administration). Diagnostic evaluation directed toward the organ system most closely related to the anxiety symptoms may yield the most information.

The differential between an organic anxiety syndrome and a primary anxiety disorder may be clarified by systematic consideration of the following six factors that suggest the presence of an organic cause: (1) onset of anxiety symptoms after the age of 35 years; (2) lack of personal or family history of an anxiety disorder; (3) lack of childhood history of significant anxiety, phobias, or separation anxiety; (4) absence of a significant life event generating or exacerbating the anxiety symptoms; (5) lack of avoidance behavior; and (6) poor responses to standard anti-panic agents (i.e., antidepressants, benzodiazepines) [18].

Particular scrutiny should be directed toward conditions (e.g., arrhythmias, hyperthyroidism) and medications (e.g., excessive caffeine intake, intoxication or withdrawal phenomenon from sedative-hypnotics, alcohol, or other drugs of abuse) that are commonly associated with anxiety.

Intoxication or withdrawal phenomena are often overlooked as potential causes of anxiety symptoms (see Chap. 158). Drug- or alcohol-related phenomena should be considered in cases involving motor vehicle or other accidents, violence, and trauma. The initial workup should include toxicologic screening for drugs of abuse. The emergence of anxiety symptoms within 48 to 72 hours after admission raises the suspicion of withdrawal from alcohol or other drugs (e.g., sedative-hypnotics, opiates). Patients should be examined for stigmata of drug abuse (e.g., needle [track] marks) that may have been overlooked during the initial effort to stabilize a patient.

Complex partial seizures secondary to limbic system irritability may cause anxiety symptoms. Patients may present with episodic anxiety or panic associated with a variety of physical symptoms including chest pain, tachyarrhythmias, syncope, abdominal distress, changes in level of consciousness, staring spells, as well as hallucinations (auditory, olfactory, gustatory, or visual), micropsia, macropsia, and abnormal motor movements (e.g., twitching of extremities). Complex partial seizures may be manifest solely by psychosensory phenomena. The diagnosis of complex partial seizures is clinical and can be supported by, but does not require, abnormal electroencephalographic findings. Patients at risk for developing complex partial seizures often have a history of seizures or head trauma, or take centrally active agents that lower the seizure threshold (e.g., neuroleptics, antidepressants, or alcohol). Carbamazepine is often used for the maintenance treatment of patients with complex partial seizures. During a seizure, administration of intravenous (IV) lorazepam typically resolves abnormal psychosensory phenomena and alterations in consciousness.

Primary Psychiatric Disorders

Patients with a number of primary psychiatric disorders may present with anxiety in the ICU. Usually, a history of psychiatric illness precedes the patient's entry into the ICU and is exacerbated by the acute medical or surgical condition. For some, however, the onset of symptoms associated with a psychiatric disorder may be provoked by the stress of medical illness and hospitalization.

ANXIETY DISORDERS. According to the *Diagnostic and Statistical Manual* (DSM-IV) of the American Psychiatric Association [27], anxiety disorders include panic disorder with and without agoraphobia, generalized anxiety disorder, simple phobia, social phobia, posttraumatic stress disorder, and obsessive-compulsive disorder.

Panic Disorder. Panic disorder is a syndrome characterized by recurrent panic attacks (i.e., discrete episodes of intense anxiety associated with at least four other symptoms of autonomic arousal and anxiety). Attacks generally come on quickly and last from a few minutes to a few hours. The initial attack is usually spontaneous; over time, patients often associate the occurrence of panic attacks with certain situations, such as those from which escape may be difficult, embarrassing (e.g., being in a crowd or in a CT scanner), or where help is not readily available. Patients may avoid feared situations and restrict the scope of their daily activity, or grow to depend on companions. Between panic attacks patients may be apprehensive and suffer anxiety in anticipation of the next attack. Panic disorder usually begins in the third decade of life and becomes chronic with periods of remission and relapse. Panic disorder is usually detected in women, though this may reflect the propensity of men to self-medicate anxiety symptoms with alcohol or other drugs and their reluctance to accept a psychological diagnosis. Risk factors for panic disorder include separation anxiety disorder in childhood, a loss of social supports, and a change in interpersonal relationships [28,29]. Many patients develop the disorder during a medical illness.

Making the diagnosis of panic disorder in the ICU is important for a number of reasons. Patients with panic attacks frequently present to an emergency room for emergent evaluation by a cardiologist or neurologist. The symptoms of panic are on occasion of sufficient intensity that a CCU admission is required to rule out MI. As a result of the physician's failure to recognize the symptoms of panic disorder, patients may undergo painful, expensive, and potentially dangerous diagnostic procedures and continue to suffer significant pain and disability from chest pain. Panic disorder has been found in 40 to 60 percent of patients with chest pain and normal coronary angiograms [30,31]. In one series, panic exacerbated symptoms in patients with preexisting medical conditions and led to more frequent hospitalizations; treatment of the panic disorder reversed this trend [32]. Of patients with chronic asthma, those with high levels of anxiety had more hospitalizations than those with normal levels of anxiety [33].

For some panic patients, the dramatic nature of physical complaints dominates the presentation, especially in patients who do not report feeling anxious. For these patients, "masked panic" is marked by paroxysmal physical symptoms in the absence of affective, behavioral, or cognitive symptoms of panic; this masking obscures the diagnosis and results in continued morbidity [18]. Some patients experience limited-symptom attacks with only one or two panic symptoms (e.g., lightheadedness or tachycardia). Not uncommonly, these symptoms are erroneously attributed to medical illness.

CASE. A 35-year-old man was admitted to the CCU after an episode of chest pain, tachycardia, dyspnea, diaphoresis, and lightheadedness that lasted 20 minutes. The electrocardiogram (ECG) in the emergency room showed nonspecific ST-T wave changes, and the patient was admitted to "rule out MI." The patient reported a history of multiple emergency room and CCU admissions over the past year after similar episodes of chest pain. The patient had received trials of nifedipine, numerous beta-blockers, as well as p.r.n. sublingual nitroglycerin, without relief of symptoms. Results of a stress test and Holter monitor had been unremarkable during a previous workup. Because the patient was becoming increasingly anxious of a return of symptoms, and had severely curtailed his work and social activity, more invasive testing (an angiogram) was considered. However, before the test a psychiatric consultation was obtained. The following features were noted: (1) the episodes were paroxysmal and were superimposed on lower-grade persistent symptoms; (2) diazepam diminished but did not eliminate his symptoms; (3) the symptoms occurred more frequently in crowds or when driving; (4) the symptoms began after a job change; (5) the patient noted his symptoms were relieved by alcohol; and (6) his mother was "very anxious" and was often unable to leave the house for extended periods.

When treated with clonazepam he became completely asymptomatic within 4 weeks. He remained asymptomatic for the next 3 years while taking clonazepam and was able to return to his previous level of function.

Although the man described above presented with cardiac symptoms, a panic disorder with limited-symptom attacks should have been diagnosed. Failure to recognize the anxiety syndrome led to unnecessary hospitalizations and significant patient morbidity. Treatment of the panic disorder resulted in dramatic relief of symptoms. Features consistent with panic disorder not initially recognized were intense paroxysmal and persistent low grade symptoms, an onset with a major life event, avoidant behavior consistent with agoraphobia, partial relief with benzodiazepines and alcohol, and a family history of significant anxiety.

Generalized Anxiety Disorder. Patients with generalized anxiety disorder suffer chronic worry about two or more life circumstances (e.g., finances, or danger to loved ones) in excess of what is reasonable for longer than 6 months [27]. These patients are often called "nervous" or "worriers" by family or friends. Their anxiety is accompanied by a number of somatic symptoms associated with motor tension and autonomic hyperactivity (e.g., sweating, tachycardia, hyperventilation, tremulousness, dizziness). Although the disorder may be differentiated from panic disorder by the persistent, rather than episodic, nature of symptoms, careful questioning often shows that patients with generalized anxiety disorder experience panic attacks as well [34,35]. Many patients with generalized anxiety disorders in the medical setting manifest anxiety in addition to the symptoms of other psychiatric disorders (e.g., panic disorder, depression, or alcohol abuse) [36].

Simple Phobia. Patients with simple phobias are afraid of circumscribed situations or objects (e.g., heights, closed spaces, animals, or the sight of blood) [27]. Exposure to the feared stimulus results in intense anxiety and avoidance that interferes with the patient's life. Some patients are so afraid of needles or blood that compliance with procedures in the ICU is nearly impossible. Acute treatment with benzodiazepines may decrease the patient's anxiety to the point where he agrees to treatment. However, the only consistently effective treatment for simple phobias is behavioral therapy, a technique that involves exposure and desensitization to the feared object or situation [37].

Social Phobia. Social phobia is diagnosed when the patient perceives he or she will be the object of public scrutiny and fears he or she will behave in a way that will be humiliating or embarrassing [27]. This perception leads to persistent fear and avoidance, or endurance with intense distress. Circumscribed situations may be feared (e.g., speaking before a group [i.e., "performance anxiety"], writing or eating in the presence of others, or urinating in public lavatories); some patients experience more global difficulties in which most social interactions are difficult. Patients with social phobias may have intense anxiety in the ICU because they are under intense scrutiny by others. Long-term treatments include antidepressants, beta-blockers, or behavioral therapy. Some reports support the clinical efficacy of high-potency benzodiazepines (e.g., clonazepam [38] and alprazolam [39]) for the treatment of social phobia; when immediate intervention is necessary in the ICU, use of these agents is the treatment of choice.

Posttraumatic Stress Disorder. Patients with posttraumatic stress disorder (PTSD) have experienced a catastrophic event that would be clearly distressing to anyone (e.g., having faced a serious threat to one's life; having one's home suddenly destroyed; or having witnessed a serious accident or act of violence) [27]. Afflicted patients frequently reexperience the traumatic event. They have recurrent dreams or suddenly act or feel like the event is recurring (i.e., a flashback). Individuals with PTSD frequently avoid situations that remind them of the event and may become numb, irritable, hypervigilant, and experience difficulty with sleep or concentration. Although much attention has been directed toward PTSD in combat veterans, PTSD can occur in civilians who suffer life-threatening accidents or who have survived natural disasters. Antidepressants [40], clonidine [41], and psychotherapy have demonstrated some efficacy in the long-term treatment of PTSD patients. The emergence of PTSD should be anticipated in patients who have suffered serious trauma; treatment is aimed at symptomatic relief (e.g., hypnotics for sleep, rapid eye movement [REM] sleep-suppressants for nightmares, and benzodiazepines for anxiety).

Obsessive-Compulsive Disorder. Patients with obsessive-compulsive disorder (OCD) suffer from recurrent, intrusive, unwanted thoughts, i.e., obsessions (e.g., the fear of hurting a loved one, or the fear of contamination), or compulsive behaviors or rituals (e.g., repetitive handwashing, or checking a door multiple times to make sure it is locked) [27]. The obsessions and compulsions are distressing, time consuming (i.e., they may take more than 1 hour per day), and interfere with the patient's normal function. In the ICU, the OCD patient may suffer a marked increase in anxiety if physical disability or unit routine makes it impossible for him or her to perform compulsive rituals. Behavioral therapy aimed at reducing the patient's obsessive thoughts and compulsive behavior may be helpful; benzodiazepine therapy may be necessary to control overwhelming anxiety.

AFFECTIVE ILLNESS. Patients with panic disorder are often depressed: 60 to 90 percent of panic disorder patients develop a major depression sometime in their life [42], and 21 percent of patients with major depression have either a past or current history of panic disorder [43]. Goldberg [44] reported that two

thirds of mentally ill patients in primary care clinics had symptoms of both anxiety and depression. Thus, any patient who presents with anxiety symptoms in the medical setting should be evaluated for the presence of depression. Panic disorder carries a risk for suicidal behavior independent of depression [45]. However, the presence of suicidal ideation, especially when accompanied by psychomotor retardation, persistent dysphoria, early morning awakening, and hopelessness, is more likely to be a consequence of depression than panic. Unfortunately, it is common for physicians to prescribe a benzodiazepine for anxiety and avoid the use of an antidepressant to treat depression. Overlapping anxiety and depressive syndromes can often both be treated with a single antidepressant medication. Antidepressants and certain structured forms of psychotherapy are of proved efficacy for the treatment of depression. Alprazolam, a high-potency benzodiazepine with putative antidepressant properties [46], may be useful in the treatment of patients with mixed anxiety and depressive symptoms in the ICU because of its efficacy and lack of cardiovascular side effects. Clinically, its antidepressant efficacy is limited to mildly depressed patients.

ALCOHOL AND SUBSTANCE ABUSE. Abuse of alcohol and other substances may lead to symptoms associated with anxiety in the ICU. Acute discontinuation of these medications (e.g., alcohol, opiates, barbiturates, and benzodiazepines) can result in potentially dangerous withdrawal reactions that may be heralded by anxiety and signs of autonomic arousal (e.g., tachycardia, tachypnea, and sweating). Patients may consider use of these agents to be trivial, and may neglect to reveal their use of them. Symptoms of alcohol withdrawal typically become manifest 24 to 48 hours after the last ingestion, but can be delayed more than a week when partial treatment has been initiated (see Chap. 158). Recent use of alcohol or other substances may be overlooked while stabilizing the acutely ill patient; the development of anxiety 1 to 2 days after admission may be erroneously attributed to situational stressors or other factors.

The use of stimulants (e.g., cocaine) or other agents (e.g., marijuana or phencyclidine) may be directly associated with anxiety, but goes unidentified because of the patient's reluctance to reveal their use of these illicit substances.

Finally, patients with panic disorder, generalized anxiety, and social phobia may be treating their symptoms with alcohol or sedative agents [47]. Although these substances may be acutely anxiolytic, precipitous drops in blood levels may exacerbate anxiety; recurrent withdrawal may "kindle" the autonomic nervous system and trigger or exacerbate panic or anxiety [48].

SCHIZOPHRENIA. Schizophrenia is a disorder characterized by the presence of hallucinations, delusions, disordered and often bizarre thinking, and social withdrawal. Patients with schizophrenia may manifest severe anxiety and lose touch with reality in the ICU. Conversely, severely anxious patients may have a reduced level of function and manifest social withdrawal that resembles schizophrenia. Differentiation is usually made on the basis of the characteristic symptoms and history. Schizophrenic patients can be managed by using neuroleptics (i.e., antipsychotic medication), minimizing stimulation, and using benzodiazepines judiciously to control anxiety. Akathisia (a side effect of neuroleptics characterized by motor restlessness, anxiety, tension, and an inability to remain still) is in some patients confused with worsening psychosis and treated with increased doses of neuroleptics. This further exacerbates the problem. Akathisia can be managed by decreasing or discontinuing the neuroleptic, and using beta-blockers, benzodiazepines, or anticholinergic agents.

SOMATOFORM DISORDERS. Anxiety can be the great imitator of medical illness because of symptoms related to autonomic arousal [18]. Anxious patients may focus on somatic symptoms (e.g., chest pain or epigastric distress) and make repeated visits to their physician, or "doctor shop" in search for a medical explanation for their symptoms. Many are characterized as hypochondriacs or crocks and receive benzodiazepines or reassurance, but not adequate or definitive treatment. Failure to make the diagnosis of an anxiety disorder may result in the patient's continuing to "make the rounds" in an attempt to discover "what's really wrong with me," while exposing the patient to costly and sometimes dangerous diagnostic and therapeutic procedures.

Katon reported [32,49] that 89 percent of panic disorder patients referred for psychiatric consultation by primary care physicians initially presented with somatic complaints, most commonly cardiac, gastrointestinal, and neurologic. Clancy and Noyes [50] documented the high rate of medical testing and specialty consultations by cardiologists, neurologists, and gastroenterologists for panic disorder patients in medical clinics. Many of these patients focused on physical complaints and denied affective or cognitive symptoms to avoid the stigma of psychiatric illness. Sheehan noted that 70 percent of panic disorder patients had been to at least 10 medical practitioners without receiving either a diagnosis of panic disorder or specific treatment [51]. Many met criteria for somatization disorder and focused on the somatic symptoms of the untreated panic disorder. In addition, panic disorder may exacerbate symptoms of asthma, angina, or diabetes, which then become the focus of attention of both the patient and the physician. In the ICU, cardiac symptoms in panic patients may cause continued suffering, inefficient use of medical personnel, and inappropriate use of costly and potentially dangerous diagnostic and therapeutic technology. Bass and Wade noted that 61 percent of 99 patients with chest pain and insignificant coronary disease (as determined by angiography) had psychiatric morbidity, in comparison with 23 percent of those with significant coronary disease [52]. Anxiety neurosis was the most common psychiatric diagnosis in those with insignificant disease. Katon et al [30] found that 43 percent of patients with chest pain and clean coronary arteries had panic disorder, whereas only 5 percent of those with significant disease had panic disorder. Beitman et al reported that 58 percent of patients with atypical chest pain and no coronary disease by ECG, treadmill, or angiogram [31] had panic disorder. Patients with negative cardiac workups were generally younger and more likely to be female. Forty percent of primary care patients with panic disorder present with chest pain [49]. Recognition and treatment of panic disorder in these patients may eliminate the necessity of angiograms in an otherwise low-risk group (i.e., younger, female patients). Many panic disorder patients exhibit high degrees of somatization and hypochondriasis. However, somatic preoccupation declines markedly with effective panic disorder treatment [53].

The essential features of somatoform disorders are the presence of physical symptoms that suggest a physical disorder, and an absence of demonstrable organic findings or etiology [27]. The patient's symptoms are presumed to be secondary to a psychological disturbance.

Hypochondriasis. Hypochondriasis is characterized by a preoccupation with the fear of being ill and a belief that one is ill based on the patient's unwarranted interpretation of physical signs and symptoms [27]. Appropriate evaluation does not support the diagnosis of a physical disorder and cannot account for the patient's symptoms. The patient's fear or belief persists despite intensive workups and assurance. Frequently, these patients pursue further medical evaluation and treatment.

Somatization Disorder. Patients meeting criteria for somatization disorder have a history of chronic physical complaints and a belief that they are sickly, which begins before the age of 30 years [27]. At least 13 symptoms, involving a number of different organ systems (e.g., gastrointestinal, cardiopulmonary, and genitourinary), must be present that are not accounted for by organic pathology, do not occur only during a panic attack, and have caused the patient to take prescription medication, see a doctor, or alter his or her life-style.

Factitious Disorders. Factitious disorders are characterized by the voluntary production, or feigning, of physical or psychological symptoms in the absence of clear-cut secondary gain [27]. Patients with factitious disorders are also said to have Munchausen's syndrome, or cardiopathica fantastica, when cardiac symptoms dominate the presentation. The disorder is presumably rare and can be difficult to detect when present. Patients with this diagnosis may receive elaborate workups and procedures, including surgery, on the basis of their feigned symptoms. These patients are presumed to be gratifying a psychological need by their aberrant behavior and often present with elaborate and detailed histories, a lack of family and social supports, reports of extensive travel and multiple hospitalizations, and personality disorder characterized by hostility, masochism, and poor impulse control [54].

Common Scenarios of Anxiety in the ICU

FAILURE TO COPE. Patients deal with the stress of hospitalization with a variety of coping strategies. They may rationalize or attempt to reassure themselves (e.g., "The doctors know what they are doing," or "This is the best hospital in the city") and minimize ("It's just heartburn"), have faith in religion, and make use of family support.

However, even for those without a history of anxiety, coping strategies may be overwhelmed in the ICU, and patients may experience anxiety, fear, and feelings of vulnerability. This may happen for a variety of reasons. Some patients may regress in the face of an acute threat, whereas others have difficulty acting passively while accepting nurturance and help. Anxiety often increases if the illness is sudden, if family or social supports are unavailable, if they feel alone, or if an illness or injury has a particularly onerous meaning for them (e.g., loss of potency in its broadest sense, or identification with a sick relative). When coping strategies fail, the patient may become anxious, unable to sleep, needy, noncompliant, and filled with physical complaints. Such a patient can become difficult to manage.

CASE. A 46-year-old man, 3 days after an acute MI, disrupted the CCU routine. He became angry at and sarcastic with caregivers, and was alternately anxious, withdrawn, and entitled. Until then his medical course had been relatively uncomplicated.

He was an active, driven man who built and managed his own successful business. Two critical issues emerged during the psychiatrist's interview. First, the patient was concerned that having an MI meant that he would be unable to continue having sexual relations and playing sports, two areas of his life that were important to him. Second, his son had reassured him at the time of his admission, "Don't worry, I'll take care of everything at the shop." This reassurance was paradoxically unsettling to the patient, who feared losing control; he feared he would no longer be essential to the business.

Two interventions decreased the patient's anxiety. He was provided with detailed information about the course of cardiac rehabilitation and his expected return to satisfactory sexual and athletic function. His condition was explained to his son. From then on, his son apprised him of the situation at work so that he could feel involved and in control.

This case demonstrates that previously well-adapted individuals can become overwhelmed and extremely anxious in the face of serious illness. Though the prescription of anxiolytic medication may have lowered the patient's level of anxiety, recognition of the reasons for the loss of coping ability allowed for appropriate therapy. Anxiety, though understandable in the presence of severe illness, may be triggered or exacerbated by potentially remediable factors. Attention to these issues may enhance patient comfort and compliance and may decrease concern about physical symptoms.

INTERFERENCE WITH EVALUATION OR TREATMENT.
Anxiety can interfere with evaluation or treatment. Patients who fear a painful diagnostic or therapeutic procedure, who catastrophize about physical symptoms or diagnostic tests (e.g., "They're looking for cancer"), or who deny a potentially serious condition may be uncooperative with its evaluation.

CASE. A 54-year-old married woman with a 60 pack-year history of cigarette smoking presented with the acute onset of chest pain and dyspnea. In obvious distress, she adamantly refused a chest x-ray. Though initially refusing explanation, she eventually admitted that she was afraid that an x-ray would show lung cancer. She noted that her sister had died of lung cancer after a long wasting illness, painful surgery, and chemotherapy. She feared a similar lesion.

The patient and her husband were given explicit information about the differential diagnosis (including malignancy and the treatment options for the different possibilities). The husband was very supportive, and the patient eventually agreed to the x-ray, which showed a pneumothorax that was successfully managed.

Interventions to reduce patient anxiety should be guided by an understanding of what the illness or procedure means to the patient. Situational anxiety and the fear of serious illness can be managed with clarification, education, support, behavioral strategies (e.g., relaxation techniques), and the short-term use of benzodiazepines.

Patients with a serious illness may have a worse outcome because of anxiety. In one group of survivors of MI, 95 percent had increased tension and anxiety. Psychological impairment, including anxiety, was the most common reason that some post-MI patients failed to return to work [55]. For the post-MI patient, worry about further heart damage with certain activities (e.g., exercise or sexual relations) impairs rehabilitation and return to independent function. Post-MI patients often benefit from intensive education about their abilities and limitations, supportive or more intensive psychotherapy, behavioral techniques, and pharmacologic care (e.g., anxiolytic or antidepressant medication). Timely diagnosis and treatment of anxiety help to improve patient outcome; for instance, preliminary evidence exists that survival of cancer patients may be affected by changes in the immune system caused by the psychological and emotional state of the patient [56].

Special Situations in the Critical Care Setting

PATIENTS WITH MYOCARDIAL INFARCTION. Hackett and Cassem reported that the mean time between the onset of chest pain and arrival in the hospital was nearly 4 hours [57]. Unfortunately, most deaths of acute MI occur during the first 4 hours secondary to arrhythmias, pump failure, or some combination of both [58]. Therefore, any delay in seeking medical attention (which can be a manifestation of the patient's denial of the implications of the chest pain, or a means to control anxiety) can lead to greater morbidity and mortality. Education of patients and relatives about cardiac symptoms may help overcome denial and extended delays before seeking help.

The MI patient in the ICU is already anxious because of the fear of death and disability and is made uncomfortable by chest pain and monitoring devices. Patients may be overwhelmed by the rapid pace of activity. Clinical staff should maintain a sense of calm, and proffer brief, simple explanations about the situation to the patient and family to decrease the anxiety that surrounds the CCU admission [59]. Stern and colleagues have documented the relative undertreatment of anxiety in the ICU/CCU [60]. Thirty-four percent of a series of suspected or documented MI patients had no benzodiazepines prescribed for them during their ICU/CCU stay. More than a quarter of patients had benzodiazepines prescribed on a prn basis, and in only 16 percent of these patients were benzodiazepines actually administered. Many patients remained anxious. The undermedication of anxiety was attributed to caregivers' failure to inquire about unreported anxiety, the erroneous assumption that "patients who do not request to be sedated are not anxious," and misplaced fears of drug dependency and sedation. The results of the study suggested that management of anxiety in the critical care setting would be improved by wider use of benzodiazepines on a fixed-dosage schedule.

Delirium, manifested by disorientation, clouded consciousness, hallucinations, incoherence, agitation, and confusion, may develop at any point in the CCU stay. The onset of delirium may occur in a bimodal distribution, that is, early during the admission in the setting of cardiogenic shock and high-dose antiarrhythmic therapy, and after a number of days in the unit [59]. Delirium may be misdiagnosed as anxiety; however, the anxious patient does not become disoriented or hallucinate. The management of delirium is predicated on specific treatment of the underlying cause whenever possible; until then, treatment with neuroleptics is helpful.

Disruptive behavior may emerge any number of days into the hospitalization. It can often be understood as the interaction between the clinical situation and the patient's characteristic way of responding to stress. Management strategies should reflect the specific difficulties encountered by different personality types [61]. For example, the paranoid personality may experience any invasive procedure as an attack and respond with mistrust and anger, engendering a similar reaction in caregivers. Paranoid patients are best managed from a dispassionate distance in which the patient's concerns are acknowledged, and simple, direct explanations and information are provided.

PATIENTS WITH VENTRICULAR TACHYARRHYTHMIAS. Patients with recurrent ventricular ectopic activity (VEA) may experience acute and chronic anxiety, vigilance, resistance to being sedated, and fear of sleep [59]. VEA may be precipitated by stress [62,63]; a reduction in anxiety may raise the threshold to developing ventricular fibrillation (VF). Patients with malignant tachyarrhythmias who undergo electrophysiologic studies in the catheterization laboratory commonly experience significant anxiety. Treatment of the anxiety may be accomplished with anxiolytic medication (typically benzodiazepines) and support.

PATIENTS UNDERGOING CARDIAC SURGERY. Anxiety is often prominent in preoperative cardiac patients. It can be minimized by patient education and enlisting the support of family members [64,65]. Delirium occurs in roughly one fourth of patients in the postoperative period after coronary artery bypass grafting (CABG) or cardiac transplant [59] and should be managed by maximizing all physiologic parameters and by using high-potency neuroleptics, such as haloperidol [66].

PATIENTS WHOSE ANXIETY INTERFERES WITH WEANING FROM THE RESPIRATOR. Weaning patients from prolonged ventilatory support may engender a significant degree of anxiety. Weaning by trial and error may increase a patient's anxiety by forcing him or her to breathe during gradually prolonged periods of unassisted ventilation [66]. The continued presence of the ventilator during intermittent mandatory ventilation may provide psychological support for the patient [67]. Relaxation techniques and hypnosis may distract the patient during weaning [68]; however, anxiety may increase to the point of panic, increasing the work of breathing, and making weaning more difficult. Although benzodiazepines can be used to control anxiety, they may depress respiratory effort and should be used cautiously. A high-potency neuroleptic such as haloperidol can be used if nonpharmacologic anxiety-reduction efforts are unsuccessful, especially if the patient is manifesting extreme anxiety. Haloperidol does not significantly depress respiratory effort and can be given in doses of 2 to 5 mg orally per day during the weaning period or 2 to 10 mg IV every 30 minutes to control acute agitation.

If the patient is agitated or extremely anxious, physiologic abnormalities must be assessed and treated before initiation of anxiolytic therapy. Unsuccessful weaning may result in hypercapnia or hypoxia and increased anxiety and agitation. Emotional arousal may result in further metabolic imbalance and a decline in physiologic parameters. Thus, the successful discontinuation of respiratory support often requires the treatment of associated anxiety as well as correction of any physiologic abnormalities (see Chap. 67).

Treatment

The treatment of anxiety in the ICU involves correction of underlying organic factors, use of medication, appropriate reassurance, and education. A combination of treatments is often necessary (Table 228-1).

BENZODIAZEPINES. Benzodiazepines are generally considered the mainstays of anxiolytic pharmacotherapy in the ICU because of their relative safety and rapid therapeutic effects. Drug selection is determined by the clinical situation, the presence of panic attacks, and the pharmacokinetic properties of the agents.

Pharmacokinetics. Drug characteristics determine rapidity of effect onset and offset, degree of accumulation with multiple dose administration, and risk of drug discontinuation. The phar-

Table 222-1. Treatment of Anxiety in the ICU

PHARMACOLOGIC INTERVENTIONS
  Benzodiazepines
  Neuroleptics

NONPHARMACOLOGIC INTERVENTIONS
  Education
  Support
  Behavioral techniques
    Hypnosis
    Relaxation techniques
    Imagery
  Cognitive therapy
  Family therapy
  Cardiac rehabilitation

macologic properties of the commonly used benzodiazepines are noted in Chapter 209.

Drug Selection. The clinician selects an agent to maximize desired effects in a particular clinical situation. A rapid-onset drug such as diazepam may offer more immediate relief, whereas a slower-onset drug (e.g., oxazepam) may minimize initial sedation or spaciness. Shorter-acting drugs may allow more rapid clearing of effects and prevent excessive drug accumulation with attendant confusion or irritability, whereas longer-acting drugs may minimize interdose rebound anxiety and posttreatment rebound.

Patients with impaired hepatic function (e.g., the elderly) should receive agents that have shorter half-lives and fewer active metabolites (e.g., lorazepam or oxazepam) to minimize drug accumulation. The longer-acting agents require oxidative liver processes. Patients with hepatic impairment are likely to accumulate high levels. Short-acting agents require only glucuronide conjugation by the liver; thus, even in patients with liver failure, the half-lives of these agents are not significantly increased. Elderly patients metabolize drugs more slowly; long-acting agents are best avoided to minimize accumulation. Dosages in the elderly should be roughly half those used in younger patients.

For many patients, it is reasonable to initiate treatment with a shorter-acting, easily metabolized agent such as lorazepam (e.g., 1 mg tid–qid). It is usually best to prescribe the medication on a fixed-dose schedule, so the patient does not become more anxious about having to request it or negotiate for it. The dose can be held if the patient refuses it or is overmedicated, or the dose can be increased if the patient's anxiety is inadequately controlled. Patients for whom autonomic lability may be a hazard, such as post-MI patients, should routinely receive benzodiazepines even when they do not appear anxious.

The high-potency benzodiazepines (e.g., alprazolam and clonazepam) have particular antipanic efficacy and are effective for generalized anxiety. Initiation of treatment with the shorter-acting agent alprazolam may be preferable in the ICU because it permits more rapid clearing of effects and minimizes drug accumulation, whereas use of the longer-acting clonazepam may be preferable as a maintenance agent to minimize interdose rebound [69]. Dosing is initiated with 0.25 to 0.5 mg three times per day for alprazolam and 0.25 to 0.5 mg per day to twice a day for clonazepam.

Routes of Administration. Parenteral routes of administration may be necessary when immediate relief of anxiety is required or when the patient is unable to take medications by mouth. Although parenteral forms of diazepam and chlordiazepoxide are available, intramuscular (IM) absorption of these agents is erratic and oral or intravenous (IV) administration is recommended. It is not uncommon for alcoholic patients admitted to the ICU to be unable to take oral medication, and to receive IM chlordiazepoxide to prevent alcohol withdrawal. Because it is poorly absorbed intramuscularly, patients may become increasingly anxious and agitated and develop delirium tremens (DTs). IV diazepam is used routinely as a preanesthetic agent because of its almost immediate onset of sedative effect [70]. IV administration of diazepam is associated with a generally insignificant decrease in systolic blood pressure. However, respiratory depression can occur during IV administration, particularly in patients with compromised pulmonary function [71,72]. The occurrence of apnea after IV administration of diazepam underscores the need for slow administration, titrated against clinical effect [73,74]. Accumulation of the active metabolite nordiazepam ($t\frac{1}{2}$ 100–200 hr) may result in prolonged sedation and clouding of consciousness [70]. Lorazepam is also available parenterally and is well absorbed intramuscularly and sublingually. It has a brief half-life and no active metabolites, and can be used in the elderly and in those with hepatic dysfunction [75].

Midazolam (Versed) is a rapidly active, parenterally administered, high-potency benzodiazepine. It is administered intramuscularly for preoperative sedation and intravenously for conscious sedation before short diagnostic or endoscopic procedures (e.g., bronchoscopy or angiography) and to induce general anesthesia [76]. The onset of sedation is 15 minutes after IM injection and 3 to 5 minutes after IV administration. Many patients have no recall for procedures performed after midazolam administration. It is an effective anxiolytic medication with a rapid onset of effect, no active metabolites, and relatively brief duration of action. However, midazolam may depress respiration and has been associated with apnea and respiratory or cardiac arrest leading to death. Hypotension may occur in patients also receiving a narcotic. IV administration to induce conscious sedation should be initiated with 1 mg and should not exceed 2.5 mg. Midazolam should not be administered as a bolus; doses should be administered over at least 2 minutes, with an additional 2 minutes elapsing to evaluate the sedative effects. A recent study demonstrated that patients may safely self-administer low-dose intravenous midazolam to reduce postoperative anxiety [77]; reduction of anxiety in this setting may reduce postoperative pain [78].

Reversal of Benzodiazepine Effects: Flumazenil. Reversal of benzodiazepine-induced sedation may be required in the ICU for neurologic evaluation, weaning from a ventilator, or treatment of drug overdose. Flumazenil, a potent competitive inhibitor of the benzodiazepine receptor [79], reverses the sedation and motor effects of benzodiazepines [80]. In healthy volunteers 0.1 mg/kg of IV flumazenil reversed apnea and sleep induced by midazolam [81], and it was reported to safely and rapidly reverse midazolam sedation in ICU patients [82]. Flumazenil attains peak levels and effect within 5 minutes after parenteral administration and has a half-life of 55 minutes [83]. It is metabolized by the liver and lacks active metabolites. The duration of flumazenil's effects depends on the dose, potency, and half-life of the benzodiazepine agonist. Repeated doses are required for drugs with long half-lives such as diazepam. It is well tolerated with no relevant agonist effects at low doses, although it may have proconvulsant effects at high doses [84]. Flumazenil specifically reverses the effects of benzodiazepines without affecting other centrally acting drugs, such as opiates. For patients in coma, continued unconsciousness after flumazenil administration suggests nonbenzodiazepine drug intoxication or another cause.

NEUROLEPTICS. When fear and anxiety become severe and the patient is unable to reason or becomes transiently psychotic, then a neuroleptic agent will likely be more effective than a benzodiazepine. The high-potency neuroleptic haloperidol, 2 to 10 mg by mouth or by the parenteral route of administration, is commonly used for this purpose.

NONPHARMACOLOGIC INTERVENTIONS. Appropriate reassurance and explanation can also be an important part of the management of the anxious patient [85]. Patients in the critical care setting experience an understandable fear of death and disability; the clinician should attempt to discern whether any of the patient's fear derives from misconceptions about the clinical situation. For example, many patients assume that their illness will be identical to that of a relative who suffered, or that their diagnosis of cancer or heart failure is an automatic death sentence. Education about the illness and the treatment may be very reassuring to the patient. Positive aspects of the treatment plan, such as the expected gradual increase in level of activity for post-MI patients, should be discussed. For patients with a poor prognosis, the treatment plan should be discussed in a calm, straightforward manner. The patient's fears should be explored and misconceptions clarified, so that a more therapeutic relationship can be established between the patient and clinician. Valid reassurances, such as ensuring that adequate medication will be provided for pain control, should be made; false reassurances undermine the patient's trust in the physician and damage the physician's credibility. Maintaining a calm presence often soothes patients, family, and staff. Relaxation training, hypnosis, and cognitive therapy strategies may also help reduce anxiety in some patients.

Conclusions

The recognition and treatment of anxiety are important components of the management of the ICU patient. Timely and effective intervention will enhance patient comfort and compliance and may have a salutary effect on outcome.

References

1. Rice RL: Symptom patterns of the hyperventilation syndrome. *Am J Med Sci* 8:691, 1951.
2. Wood P: DaCosta's syndrome (or effort syndrome). *Br Med J* 1:767, 1941.
3. Strain JJ, Leisowitz MR, Klein DF: Anxiety and panic attacks in the medically ill. *Psychiatric Clin North Am* 4:333, 1981.
4. Rodin G, Voshart K: Depression in the medically ill: An overview. *Am J Psychiatry* 143:696, 1986.
5. Cassem NH, Hackett TP: Psychiatric consultation in a coronary care unit. *Ann Intern Med* 75:9, 1971.
6. Freeman AM, Fleece L, Folks DG, et al: Alprazolam treatment of postcoronary bypass anxiety. *J Clin Psychopharmacol* 6:39, 1986.
7. Cay E, Vettner N, Philip A, et al: Psychological status during recovery from an acute heart attack. *J Psychosom Res* 16:422, 1972.
8. Stern MJ, Pascale L, McLoone JB: Psychological adaptation following an acute myocardial infarction. *J Chron Dis* 29:513, 1976.
9. Hickman JB, Cargill WH, Golden A: Cardiovascular reactions to emotional stimulus effect on cardiac output, $A\text{-}V\text{-}O_2$ difference, arterial pressure, and peripheral resistance. *J Clin Invest* 27:290, 1948.
10. Vettner NJ, Strange RC, Adams W, et al: Initial metabolic and hormonal response to acute myocardial infarction. *Lancet* 1:284, 1974.
11. Jewitt DE, Mercer CJ, Reid D, et al: Free nor-adrenaline excretion

in relation to the development of cardiac arrhythmias and heart failure in patients with acute myocardial infarction. *Lancet* 1:635, 1969.

12. Melsom M, Andreassen P, Melsom H, et al: Diazepam in acute myocardial infarction: Clinical effects on catecholamines, free fatty acids and cortisol. *Br Heart J* 38:804, 1976.

13. Muenster JJ, Rosenberg MS, Carleton RA, et al: Comparison between diazepam and sodium thiopental during DC countershock. *JAMA* 199:758, 1967.

14. Papp C: New look at arrhythmias. *Br Heart J* 31:267, 1969.

15. Van Loon GR: Ventricular arrhythmias treated by diazepam. *Can Med Assoc J* 98:785, 1968.

16. Lown B: Sudden cardiac death—1978. *Circulation* 60:1593, 1979.

17. Shea MJ, Deanfiel JE, Wilson R, et al: Transient ischemia in angina pectoris: Frequent silent events with everyday activities. *Am J Cardiol* 56(9):E34, 1985.

18. Rosenbaum JF, Pollack MH: Anxiety, in Hackett TP, Cassem NH (eds): *The Massachusetts General Handbook of General Hospital Psychiatry.* 2nd ed. Littleton, MA, PSG Publishing, 1987, p 154.

19. Charney DS, Redmond DE Jr: Neurobiological mechanisms in human anxiety: Evidence supporting noradrenergic hyperactivity. *Neuropharmacology* 22:1531, 1983.

20. Charney DS, Heninger GR: Noradrenergic function and the mechanism of action of antianxiety treatment. *Arch Gen Psychiatry* 42:458, 1985.

21. Gray JA: Issues in the neuropsychology of anxiety, in Tuma AH, Maser JD (eds): *Anxiety and the Anxiety Disorders.* Hillsdale, NJ, L Erlbaum, 1985, p 5.

22. Tallman JF, Gallager DW: The GABA-ergic system: A locus of benzodiazepine action. *Annu Rev Neurosci* 8:21, 1985.

23. Weiss SR, Uhde TW: Animal models of anxiety, in Ballenger J (ed): *Neurobiology of Panic Disorder.* New York, Alan R. Liss, Inc., 1990, p 3.

24. Reiman EM, Raichle ME, Robins E, et al: The application of positron emission tomography to the study of panic disorder. *Am J Psychiatry* 143:469, 1986.

25. Starkman MN, Zelnick TC, Nesse RM, et al: A study of anxiety in patients with pheochromocytoma. *Arch Intern Med* 145:248, 1985.

26. Harper M, Roth M: Temporal lobe epilepsy and the phobic-anxiety depersonalization syndrome. *Compr Psychiatry* 3:129, 1962.

27. American Psychiatric Association. *Diagnostic and Statistical Manual of Mental Disorders.* 4th ed. Washington, D.C., American Psychiatric Association, 1994.

28. Gittelman R, Klein DF: The relationship between separation anxiety and panic and agoraphobic disorders. *Psychopathology* 17(1):56, 1984.

29. Roy-Byrne PP, Geraci M, Uhde T: Life events and the onset of panic disorder. *Am J Psychiatry* 143:1424, 1986.

30. Katon W, Hall ML, Russo J, et al: Chest pain: Relationship of psychiatric illness to coronary arteriographic results. *Am J Med* 84:1, 1988.

31. Beitman BD, Basha I, Flaker G, et al: Atypical or nonanginal chest pain: Panic disorder or coronary artery disease. *Arch Intern Med* 147:1548, 1987.

32. Katon W: Panic disorder and somatization: Review of 55 cases. *Am J Med* 77:101, 1984.

33. Dirks JF, Schraa JC, Brown E, et al: Psycho-maintenance in asthma: Hospitalization rates and financial impact. *Br J Med Psychol* 53:349, 1980.

34. Barlow DH, Blanchard EB, Vermilyea JA, et al: Generalized anxiety and generalized anxiety disorder: Description and reconceptualization. *Am J Psychiatry* 143:40, 1986.

35. Katon W, Vitaliano PP, Anderson K, et al: Panic disorder: Residual symptoms after the acute attacks abate. *Compr Psychiatry* 28:151, 1987.

36. Breslau N, Davis GC: DSM-III generalized anxiety disorder: An empirical investigation of more stringent criteria. *Psychiatry Res* 14:231, 1985.

37. Roy-Byrne PP, Katon W: An update on treatment of the anxiety disorders. *Hospital and Community Psychiatry* 38:835, 1987.

38. Munjack D: Clonazepam for the treatment of social phobia. *J Clin Psychiatry* 51(5 suppl):35, 1990.

39. Lydiard RB, Laraia M, Howell E, et al: Alprazolam in the treatment of social phobia. *J Clin Psychiatry* 49:17, 1988.

40. Bleich A, Siegel B, Garb R, et al: Post-traumatic stress disorder

following combat exposure: Clinical features and psychopharmacologic treatment. *Br J Psychiatry* 149:365, 1986.

41. Kolb LC, Burris BC, Griffiths S: Propranolol and clonidine in post-traumatic stress disorders of war, in Vander Kolk BA (ed): *Post-traumatic Stress Disorder: Psychological and Biological Sequelae.* Washington, D.C., American Psychiatric Press, 1984.

42. National Institute of Mental Health: *Panic Disorder in the Medical Setting,* by Katon W. DMMS Pub. No. (ADM)89-1629. Washington, D.C., U.S. Govt. Printing Office, 1989.

43. Leckman JF, Merikangas KP, Pauls DL, et al: Anxiety disorders and depression: Contradictions between family study data and DSM-III convention. *Am J Psychiatry* 140:880, 1983.

44. Goldberg D: Detection and assessment of emotional disorders in a primary care setting. *Int J Mental Health* 8:30, 1979.

45. Weissman MM, Klerman GL, Markowitz JS, et al: Suicidal ideation and suicide attempts in panic disorder and attacks. *N Engl J Med* 321:1209, 1989.

46. Feighner JP, Aden GC, Fabre LS, et al: Comparison of alprazolam, imipramine and placebo in the treatment of depression. *JAMA* 249:3057, 1983.

47. Quitkin FM, Rifkin A, Kaplan J, et al: Phobic anxiety syndrome complicated by drug dependence and addiction: A treatable form of drug abuse. *Arch Gen Psychiatry* 27:159, 1972.

48. Post RM, Uhde TW, Putnam FW: Kindling and carbamazine in affective illness. *J Nerv Ment Dis* 170:717, 1984.

49. Katon W, Vitaliano P, Russo J, et al: Panic disorder: Epidemiology in primary care. *J Fam Pract* 23:233, 1986.

50. Clancy J, Noyes R: Anxiety neurosis: A disease for the medical model. *Psychosomatics* 17:90, 1976.

51. Sheehan DV, Ballenger J, Jacobsen E: Treatment of endogenous anxiety with phobic, hysterical and hypochondriacal symptoms. *Arch Gen Psychiatry* 37:51, 1980.

52. Bass C, Wade C, Gardner WN, et al: Unexplained breathlessness and psychiatric morbidity in patients with normal and abnormal coronary arteries. *Lancet* 1:605, 1983.

53. Pilowsky I, Spence ND: *Manual for the Illness Behavior Questionnaire (IBQ),* 2nd ed. Adelaide, South Australia, University of Adelaide, Department of Psychiatry, 1983.

54. Stern TA: Munchausen's syndrome revisited. *Psychosomatics* 21:329, 1980.

55. Wishnie HA, Hackett TP, Cassem NH: Psychological hazards of convalescence following myocardial infarction. *JAMA* 215:1292, 1971.

56. Greer S, Morris T, Pettingale KW: Psychological response to breast cancer: Effect on outcome. *Lancet* 2:785, 1979.

57. Hackett TP, Cassem NH: Factors contributing to delay in responding to the signs and symptoms of acute myocardial infarction. *Am J Cardiol* 24:651, 1969.

58. Wallace WA, Yu PN: Sudden death and the prehospital phase of acute myocardial infarction. *Annu Rev Med* 26:1, 1975.

59. Stern TA, Tesar GE: Anxiety and the cardiovascular system. *Mt. Sinai J Med* 55:230, 1988.

60. Stern TA, Caplan RA, Cassem NH: Use of benzodiazepines in a coronary care unit. *Psychosomatics* 28:19, 1987.

61. Geringer ES, Stern TA: Coping with medical illness: The impact of personality types. *Psychosomatics* 27:251, 1986.

62. Lown B, Verrier RL: Neural activity and ventricular fibrillation. *N Engl J Med* 295:1165, 1976.

63. Reich P, deSilva RA, Lown B, et al: Acute psychological disturbances preceding life-threatening ventricular arrhythmias. *JAMA* 246:233, 1981.

64. Abram HS: Adaptation to open heart surgery: A psychiatric study of response to the threat of death. *Am J Psychiatry* 122:659, 1965.

65. Kornfeld DS, Zimberg S, Malm JR: Psychiatric complications of open-heart surgery. *N Engl J Med* 273:287, 1965.

66. Tesar GE, Stern TA: Evaluation and treatment of agitation in the intensive care unit. *Intensive Care Med* 1:137, 1986.

67. Irwin RS, Demers RR: Mechanical ventilation, in Rippe JM, Irwin RS, Alpert JS, et al (eds): *Intensive Care Medicine.* Boston, Little, Brown, 1985, p 462.

68. Cassem NH, Hackett TP: The setting of intensive care, in Hackett TP, Cassem NH (eds): *Massachusetts General Handbook of General Hospital Psychiatry.* 2nd ed. Littleton, MA, PSG Publishing Co., 1987.

69. Herman JB, Rosenbaum JF, Brotman AW: The alprazolam to clon-

azepam switch for the treatment of panic disorder. *J Clin Psychopharmacol* 7:175, 1987.

70. Baldessarini RJ: *Chemotherapy in Psychiatry*. Cambridge, MA, Harvard University Press, 1985.

71. Rao S, Sherbaniuk RW, Prasad K, et al: Cardiopulmonary effects of diazepam. *Clin Pharmacol Ther* 14:182, 1972.

72. Dalen JE, Evans GL, Bands JS, et al: The haemodynamics and respiratory effects of diazepam. *Anesthesiology* 30:259, 1969.

73. Hall SC, Ovassapian A: Apnea after intravenous diazepam therapy. *JAMA* 238:1052, 1977.

74. Del Vecchio PJ: Apnea after intravenous diazepam administration. *JAMA* 239:7, 1978.

75. Tesar GE, Stern TA: Rapid tranquilization of the agitated intensive care unit patient. *J Intensive Care Med* 3:195, 1988.

76. *Physician's Desk Reference 1*. 44th ed. Oradell, NJ, Medical Economics Company, 1990.

77. Egan KJ, Ready LB, Nessley M, et al: Self-administration of midazolam for postoperative anxiety: A double blind study. *Pain* 49:283, 1992.

78. Scott LE, Clum GA: Preoperative predictors of postoperative pain. *Pain* 15:283, 1983.

79. Hunkeler W, Mohler H, Pieri L, et al: Selective antagonists of benzodiazepines. *Nature* 290:514, 1981.

80. O'Boyle C, Lambe R, Darragh A, et al: Ro 15-1788 antagonizes the effects of diazepam in man without affecting bioavailability. *Br J Anesthesia* 55:349, 1983.

81. Amrein R, Hetzel W: Pharmacology of drugs frequently used in ICUs: Midazolam and flumazenil. *Intensive Care Medicine* 17S:1, 1991.

82. Pepperman ML: Double blind study of the reversal of midazolam induced sedation in the ICU with flumazenil: Effect on weaning from ventilation. *Anesthesia and Intensive Care* 18:38, 1990.

83. Roncan G, Zeigler WH, Guenter TW: Pharmacology of the new benzodiazepine antagonist Ro-15-1788 following intravenous and oral administration. *Br J Clin Pharmacol* 22:421, 1986.

84. Scollo-Lavizzari G: The clinical anti-convulsant effects of flumazenil, a benzodiazepine antagonist. *Eur J Anesthesia* (Suppl)2:129, 1988.

85. Geringer ES, Stern TA: Anxiety and depression in critically ill patients. *Probl Crit Care* 2:35, 1988.

223. Recognition and Treatment of Depression in the ICU

Edith S. Geringer and
Theodore A. Stern

Intense emotions are evoked routinely in intensive care units (ICUs), where life and death decisions occur daily. In the ICU, depression occurs as (1) a psychological reaction to an acute medical illness, (2) a manifestation of a primary affective disorder detected at the time of medical evaluation, (3) a mood disorder associated with specific organic pathology, or (4) a result of the confusing overlap of somatic symptoms of depression and symptoms of medical illness. In this chapter we focus on the evaluation and treatment of depression in critical care units: what depression looks like; what looks like depression, but is something else; and how and when to treat depression.

The term *depression* is often used to describe clinical signs and symptoms ranging from transient feelings of discouragement, disappointment, sadness, grief, or despondency to a disorder with neurovegetative symptoms (i.e., major depressive disorder) that may involve psychotic features (e.g., hallucinations and delusions). In this chapter, the term *depression* refers to major depressive disorder, which is defined in the *Diagnostic and Statistical Manual*, Fourth Edition, Revised (DSM-IV) [1] as a syndrome that affects neurovegetative functions (e.g., sleep, appetite, concentration) as well as mood.

Some observers may wonder why it is important to attend to a patient's mood in the ICU when vital organs such as the heart, lungs, liver, kidneys, or brain are not working and when survival is not assured. Moreover, many physicians believe it is appropriate to be depressed in the ICU because severe illness devastates and disrupts a person's life. However, we believe that it is always important to treat depression vigorously. In fact, compelling evidence suggests that untreated depression

decreases survival in general, and increases morbidity and mortality from cardiac conditions.

Overview of the Somatic Effects of Depression

Studies have reported that patients with untreated major depression and untreated bipolar disorder are 6 to 7 times more likely to die than those in the general population [2–4]. Interestingly, in one of these studies, cardiac disease accounted for 40 percent of the deaths in patients with affective illness. Although the possibility has been raised that the higher death rates found in psychiatric populations are attributable to a higher prevalence of medical illnesses [5], more recent data suggest that untreated depression is associated with increased cardiac mortality [6]. Studies have also shown that patients who undergo cardiac surgery are more likely to die in the perioperative phase if they were diagnosed preoperatively as having depression [7,8]. A possible mechanism for increased cardiac deaths may come from the finding that depressed patients have increased cardiac beat-to-beat variability [9]. This has been associated with higher mortality from cardiac sources in other populations [10]. Some have proposed that decreased parasympathetic tone might have accounted for some of the increased mortality among individuals with depression [9].

Besides affecting cardiac function, depression also has effects on other systems. It is well documented that a subgroup of patients with depression have altered hypothalamic-pituitary-adrenal axis functions. Most notably, some people with depression seem to have an increased number and frequency of afternoon and evening secretory bursts of cortisol, an increased plasma cortisol, an early escape of cortisol suppression to dexamethasone, and increased plasma and central nervous system (CNS) metabolites of norepinephrine [11–14]. Major depression is also associated with relative insulin resistance and blunted growth hormone response to insulin-induced hypoglycemia [15] (which can change insulin requirements during an acute depressive phase) and with orthostatic hypotension even before the administration of tricyclic antidepressants (TCAs), implying that major depression is, or involves, a disorder of autonomic function [16].

Changes in the immune system, specifically a decreased response to mitogens of T and B cells [17], have also been associated with major depression. Depression shortens rapid eye movement (REM) latency during sleep [18] and decreases the ventilatory response to carbon dioxide [19]. These findings suggest that untreated depression has profound effects on cardiac and endocrine functions and on the CNS.

Diagnostic Criteria of Depression

Important questions for the clinician who works in the ICU are: "What is depression?" and "What does a patient suffering from depression look like in the ICU?" To qualify for a diagnosis of major depression, a patient must have a sustained period of depressed or hopeless mood for a period of at least 2 weeks, in association with at least four of the following eight neurovegetative symptoms: (1) a change in sleep patterns, (2) a decrease in interests or drives, (3) a sense of guilt or a preoccupation of thought, (4) a decrease in energy (e.g., a patient may think that it is too difficult to get up and walk across the room), (5) a decrease in concentration ability (e.g., not being able to read a newspaper article all the way through or follow a television show), (6) a change in appetite (either an increase or decrease), (7) a change in psychomotor activity (either decreased [psychomotor retardation] or increased [psychomotor agitation]), and (8) suicidal ideation (e.g., with an active plan to commit suicide or the passive wish to be taken by God) or thoughts of death. The mnemonic, SIG: E CAPS (the Latin, *SIG:*, referring to what is said on the label of a prescription, *E*, for energy, *CAPS*, for capsules) is a very helpful guide to remember these eight neurovegetative symptoms (Table 223-1). Each symptom should be asked about specifically. If a patient has suicidal thoughts, he or she should be asked whether there is a specific plan. The physician then assesses the likelihood of a suicidal action. If an active plan for suicide exists, psychiatric consultation is mandatory (see Chap. 224 for details on suicide evaluation).

Table 223-1. Mnemonic for the Eight Neurovegetative Symptoms of Depression (SIG: E CAPS)

*S*leep (decreased or increased)
*I*nterest (decreased)
*G*uilt (or preoccupation of thought)
*E*nergy (decreased)
*C*oncentration (decreased)
*A*ppetite (decreased or increased)
*P*sychomotor (retardation or agitation)
*S*uicidal ideation (or thoughts of death)

The manifestations of depression are varied. The mnemonic "ABCs of depression" refers to the affective, behavioral, and cognitive aspects of depression (Table 223-2). For example, affective symptoms may involve hopelessness, a "blue mood," or lack of interest in daily activities. Anger or tears may also be evident. Behavioral symptoms include apathy, anorexia, impulsivity, or noncompliance with medical regimens. Cognitive symptoms include confusion, impaired ability to concentrate, and guilty ruminations. Individuals can also demonstrate frontal lobe dysfunction from major depression, with a decreased ability to sequence information properly and to think abstractly. Controversy exists about whether it is more useful to rely on the affective and cognitive symptoms of depression than on the behavioral symptoms in patients with medical illness because medical illnesses themselves may affect some behavioral symptoms of depression (e.g., energy and appetite) [20].

Risk Factors for Depression

Major depression is twice as common in women as in men and is more frequent in those with family histories or personal histories of major depression or alcohol or substance abuse [21,22]. Therefore, psychiatric history should be investigated. Major depression is also quite common among medical outpatients and among those with chronic illness (Table 223-3) [23-27].

Particular conflicts and character types may be more likely to produce depression [28]. Depression appears more frequently in patients with oral (clinging, demanding, and attention-seeking); obsessive (orderly, dull, likable, and anxious); narcissistic (self-involved, controlling, angry, and perfectionist); hysterical (dramatic, vivid, seductive, and overinvolved); and masochistic personality types than it does with schizoidal or paranoid personality types. For a more complete discussion of this subject see Chapter 225.

Diagnosing Depression in the Critically Ill: Special Considerations

PATIENTS UNABLE TO SPEAK. It may be particularly difficult to diagnose depression in patients on ventilators or with aphasias. However, much can be learned about patients even when they are mute. It is important to watch their expressions, read their lips, watch their hand gestures, or have them write or point to a letter board to communicate. Changes on the ever-present vital sign monitor screens surrounding most ICU patients can signify intense affect. An individual who averts his or her eyes may be demoralized, discouraged, or depressed (some individuals have a lifelong habit of avoiding direct interpersonal contact). Methods of assessing depression in sensorily compromised patients are summarized in Table 223-4.

If someone on a ventilator has slow, sighing respirations, depression may be more likely than respiratory insufficiency. Assessment should include inquiry about other reportable neurovegetative symptoms (e.g., guilt or suicidal ideation). Neurovegetative symptoms (e.g., related to appetite, concentration, and energy) may be difficult (but not meaningless) to evaluate in the patient on a ventilator. Does the patient respond to the mention of a favorite hobby or grandchild with smiles or with tears? Is the patient's affect labile or consistent with the content of the discussion? Emotional lability is not usually an indicator

Table 223-2. ABCs of Depression: Affective, Behavioral, and Cognitive Symptoms of Depression

Affective symptoms	Behavioral symptoms	Cognitive symptoms
Depressed mood	Insomnia	Guilty ruminations
Hopelessness	Anorexia	Decreased concentration
Crying	Apathy	Suicidal ideation
Blunted affect	Increased sleep	Confusion
Sadness	Increased appetite	Pseudodementia
"Blue" mood	Decreased energy	Thoughts of death
Feeling empty	Psychomotor agitation	
Irritability	Psychomotor retardation	
Anger	Noncompliance	
"No pep"	Suicidal gesture	
"Short fuse"	Impulsivity	
"Don't care"	Poor eye contact	
"Not myself"	Increased or intractable pain	
Decreased interest		

of major depression, but it can suggest frontal lobe dysfunction. Other clues of underlying depression are physical complaints that seem to outweigh the apparent medical problem (e.g., constant complaints of pain that fails to respond to treatment).

One simple screening test that can be used is human figure drawing. The patient is asked to draw one picture of a person and another of what they think is wrong with them (Fig. 223-1). Typically, drawings by depressed patients convey their sense of dejection or hopelessness, or a disordered understanding of their dilemma. If the patient can neither write nor speak, one can probe for affect by telling a joke and observing the reaction. Some particularly angry individuals may act in a controlled fashion. Show them a fist and ask "What would you do if you had one of these?" The patient may say "Well, I wouldn't hit my wife" even though his wife had not been mentioned during the interview. Such an exchange can indicate hidden anger toward his wife.

PATIENTS WITH LIFE-THREATENING ILLNESS. Although depression may be an understandable reaction to a serious medical condition, it is not a normal or appropriate condition. Unfortunately, when a patient has been devastated by illness or injury (e.g., sustaining the loss of a limb, a stroke, or the loss of autonomy associated with a dependence on technology), caregivers can erroneously assume that depression is an appropriate reaction. For example, myocardial infarction (MI) has been described as causing injured self-esteem and depression [29]. Precipitants for depression include the loss of a meaningful

Table 223-3. Epidemiology of Depression

	Lifetime prevalence	Point prevalence
GENERAL POPULATION		
Major depression	5–12% (men)	2–3% (men)
	9–26% (women)	5–9% (women)
MEDICAL POPULATIONS		
Depressive symptoms		
Medical outpatients	?	12–36%
Medical inpatients	?	11–32%
Diabetics	24%	?
Hemodialysis patients	?	18%
Major depression		
Medical outpatients	6%	6%
Crohn's disease	36%	?
Diabetics	33%	14%
Hemodialysis patients	?	7%

object [30], the loss of self-esteem [31], the loss of rewarding situations [32], and the loss of the sense of control and power [33]. An awareness of psychosocial precipitants can contribute to the design of therapeutic interventions; however, the presence of a precipitating event does not preclude the use of biologic therapies.

REACTIVATION OF OLD PSYCHOLOGICAL ISSUES. Another stimulus for depression may be the reactivation of unresolved grief. A patient whose father died of MI and who never grieved the death (because expressions of sadness were not permissible in the home) may become flooded with memories of his father's death while he himself is hospitalized in a coronary care unit (CCU) with chest pain. Depression may result from reactivation of psychological conflict. For example, a patient with a history of multiple childhood hospitalizations for the treatment of asthma who is hospitalized as an adult with severe chronic obstructive pulmonary disease (COPD) may become depressed because of the reactivation of the fear of death and loss of autonomy present during his childhood illness.

DEPRESSION CAUSED BY ORGANIC FACTORS. Various medications and medical illnesses can cause organic (i.e., nonpsychological) affective disorders (Table 223-5). The medical causes of depressive symptoms should be assessed, and

Table 223-4. Methods of Assessing Depression in Sensorily Compromised Patients

1. Facilitate communication
   Watch facial expressions
   Write questions
   Have patients write answers
   Use letter board
2. Observe whether facial expressions are consistent with content of discussion
3. Observe rate of changeability of affect
4. Ask about and observe neurovegetative symptoms of depression
5. Ask about known sources of the patient's enjoyment (e.g., favorite hobby, grandchildren, sports) and observe whether patient can take pleasure in these things
6. Tell a joke or a funny story and observe reaction
7. Ask patient to draw a picture of himself and what's wrong, then assess pictures for a sense of demoralization or hopelessness
8. Make a fist and ask patient "What would you do if you had one of these?" if you think a patient is angry or depressed; assess emotions in response

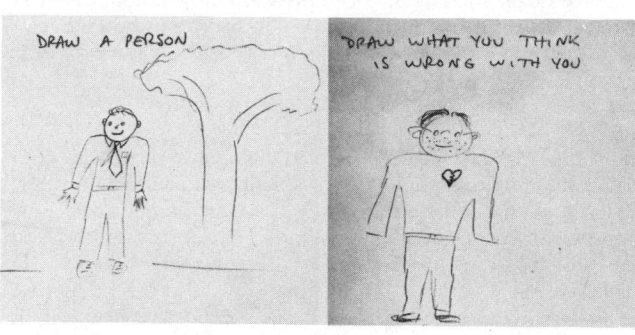

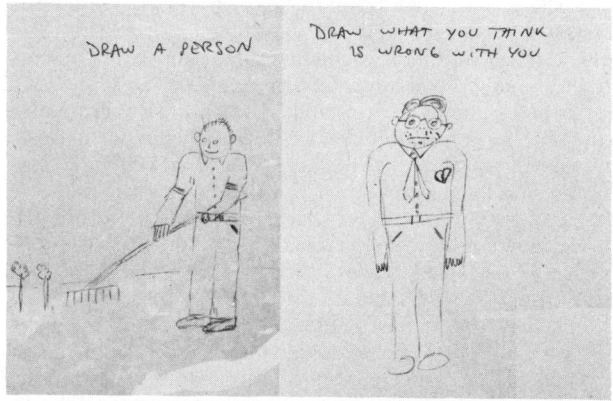

Fig. 223-1. *Above:* Drawings by a 40-year-old man two days after myocardial infarction. *Below:* Drawings by the same 40-year-old man 12 days after the infarction. (From Stern TA: The management of depression and anxiety following myocardial infarction. *Mt Sinai J Med* 52:623, 1985.)

specific treatment of any abnormality should be maximized, if possible. Endocrine disorders (especially hypothyroidism, Cushing's disease, and parathyroid disturbances), neurologic disorders (e.g., post-stroke states), and human immunodeficiency virus (HIV) infections are frequently accompanied by depression.

Depression can occur in the first 6 months after a cerebral vascular accident (CVA) in up to 60 percent of those with left hemispheric lesions and 15 percent of those with right hemispheric lesions [34]. Severity of depression correlates with the lesion's proximity to the left frontal pole or the right parietal region, rather than the degree of functional impairment produced by the CVA. These depressions can persist for 6 to 9 months if left untreated.

HIV infection is becoming an increasingly common cause of depression in critically ill patients. Depression may be the first manifestation of an HIV infection, as well as the first manifestation of an endocrinopathy or a carcinoma [29]. Thyroid function tests and a thorough laboratory screen, including assessment of electrolytes, calcium, magnesium, B₁₂, folate, and VDRL, are useful when ruling out organic causes of depression.

The agents most often responsible for causing depression in the CCU are antihypertensives, beta-blockers, antiarrhythmics, antihistamines (e.g., cimetidine and ranitidine), and steroids (Table 223-6). If a drug regimen or dosage appears to be temporally related to the patient's depression, try to lower the medication dose or eliminate the medication entirely. Some medications may cause depression only after several weeks or even months of continuous use. If the medication cannot be stopped without serious risk to the patient, the depression should be treated.

Table 223-5. Medical Conditions Associated with Depressive Symptoms

CARDIOVASCULAR
  Cardiac tumors
  Congestive heart failure
  Hypertensive encephalopathy
COLLAGEN VASCULAR
  Polyarteritis nodosa
  Systemic lupus erythematosus
ENDOCRINE
  Diabetes
  Hyperadrenalism
  Hypoadrenalism
  Hyperparathyroidism
  Hypoparathyroidism
  Hyperthyroidism
  Hypothyroidism
INFECTION
  Hepatitis
  HIV
  Mononucleosis
  Postinfluenza
METABOLIC
  Acid–base problems
  Hypokalemia
  Hypernatremia
  Hyponatremia
  Renal failure
NEOPLASMS
  Carcinoid
  Pancreatic carcinoma
NEUROLOGIC
  Brain tumor
  Multiple sclerosis
  Parkinson's (especially with on/off phenomenon)
  Temporal lobe epilepsy
  Stroke (CVA)
  Subcortical dementia
VITAMIN DEFICIENCY
  Vitamin B₁₂
  Wernicke's encephalopathy

Differential Diagnosis for Depression in the ICU

CASE EXAMPLE I. A 32-year-old woman was admitted to the ICU after a TCA overdose. When she awoke from coma, the psychiatrist tried to find out what led to the overdose. He considered the following possibilities:

1. She suffered from a *major depression,* was feeling hopeless or lonely, and decided to act on her suicidal ideation, hoping that she would not survive.

2. She overdosed after ending a relationship with a lover. Although some depressive features (e.g., unhappiness, loneliness) were present, there was no concomitant sleep disturbance or concentration difficulty, and the dysphoria had not lasted for a period of 2 weeks. She would have met criteria for an *adjustment disorder with depressed mood,* but not for major depression.

3. She was a diabetic with neuropathy, retinopathy, and nephropathy and an *organic mental disorder* from several frontal strokes. Although irritable or angry, she impulsively ingested too much of her medicine, or merely forgot how much medicine she had taken. In this case, neither major depression nor an acute reaction to a loss caused the overdose.

Table 223-6. Drugs Associated with Depressive Symptoms

Acyclovir (especially at high doses)
Alcohol
Amphetamine-like drugs (withdrawal)
    Phenylpropanolamine, phenmetrazine, fenfluramine
Anabolic steroids
    Methandrostenolone, methyltestosterone
Anticonvulsants (at high doses or plasma levels)
    Carbamazepine, phenytoin, primidone
Antihypertensives
    Reserpine, methyldopa, thiazides, clonidine, hydralazine
Asparaginase
Baclofen
Barbiturates
Benzodiazepines
    Triazolam, alprazolam, clonazepam, clorazepate, diazepam, loraze-
    pam
Beta-blockers
    Atenolol, betaxolol, propranolol, timolol
Bromides
Bromocriptine
Carbon monoxide
Cocaine (withdrawal)
Contraceptives (oral)
Corticosteroids
Cycloserine
Dapsone
Digitalis (at high doses or in elderly patients)
Diltiazem
Disopyramide
Ethionamide
Halothane (postoperatively)
Heavy metals
H$_2$ receptor antagonists
    Cimetidine, ranitidine
Interferon-A
Isoniazid
Isotretinoin
Levodopa (especially in the elderly)
Mefloquine
Metoclopramide
Metrizamide
Metronidazole
Nalidixic acid
Narcotics
    Morphine, meperidine, methadone, pentazocine, propoxyphene
Nifedipine
Nonsteroidal antiinflammatory drugs
Norfloxacin
Phenylephrine
Prazosin
Procaine derivatives
    Pen G procaine, lidocaine, procainamide
Thyroid hormones
Trimethoprim–sulfamethoxazole

Source: Adapted from Klerman G: Depression in the medically ill. *Psychiatr Clin North Am* 4:301, 1981, with permission.

4. She had a *character disorder* replete with anger, emotional lability, and impulsivity. Like many character-disordered individuals, she had an inability to tolerate unpredictability. Constructive criticism at work led her to reach impulsively for her bottle of pills and overdose. She wished to die, to forget, to numb herself, to avoid feelings, to sleep, or to punish the person who caused her some discomfort. When she awakened from her overdose she would probably not be at risk for taking another overdose because the impulse to harm herself had been discharged.

These possibilities highlight a few of the diagnoses associated with overdose, such as major depression, adjustment disorder with depressed mood, organic mental disorder, and character disorder; the stimulus may be anger, confusion, a sense of loss, or impulsivity.

CASE EXAMPLE 2. An 83-year-old diabetic woman with congestive heart failure (CHF) was hospitalized to rule out MI. She denied feeling depressed, but was apathetic and showed new cognitive problems. Making a diagnosis of depression involved assessing the following factors.

Depression in elderly patients may be difficult to diagnose because many elderly people will not readily talk about their mood. This patient may be more likely to let you know that she has lost her energy than talk about feeling depressed, sad, or blue. Sometimes neurovegetative symptoms can be elicited only after taking a careful history of an elderly patient's usual interests and hobbies. For instance, she may tell you that she did not start her garden this year as she usually did, or an elderly man may tell you that he is not as interested in watching baseball games on television.

She may also show the *pseudodementia of depression,* that is, a cognitive decline that appears to be consistent with a diagnosis of dementia, but in fact is a result of impaired concentration and frontal lobe abnormalities that occur with depression. It is important that elderly patients with depression not be prematurely diagnosed as having an irreversible dementia. If dementia is suspected, one should search for supporting evidence such as the presence of abnormal frontal lobe reflexes, perseverative thinking, and impairment of orientation, calculation, memory, and general fund of knowledge. Although pseudodementia associated with depression may result in a lower mini-mental state examination score, extremely low scores on the mini-mental state examination are more consistent with an organic etiology such as delirium or dementia [35].

Depression may also be hidden in chronic pain patients [36]. In these patients, it is all too easy to assume that depression is a normal reaction to the pain, and leave the depression untreated.

In the ICU, depression may occur at different times in different patients. Table 223-7 shows the most common reasons for psychiatric consultations in various ICUs at the Massachusetts General Hospital. Depression is the second most common reason for consultation in the CCU and surgical intensive care unit (SICU), but it is the most common reason for consultation in the respiratory intensive care unit (RICU). Depression is more likely to be the reason for psychiatric consultation from the second to fourth day in the CCU (anxiety and denial are the stimulus for consultation on the first 2 days in the CCU).

Table 223-7. Common Reasons for Psychiatric Consultation in the Coronary Care Unit (CCU), Surgical Intensive Care Unit (SICU), and Respiratory Intensive Care Unit (RICU)

CCU	SICU	RICU
Anxiety	Delirium	Depression
Depression	Depression	Anxiety weaning
Management of behavior (signing out, dependency)	Anxiety weaning from respirator	from respirator
		Management of behavior
Hostility		
Delirium/psychosis		

Adapted from Cassem NH, Hackett TP: The setting of intensive care, in Hackett TP, Cassem NH (eds) *Massachusetts General Hospital Handbook of General Hospital Psychiatry,* 2nd ed. Littleton, MA, PSG Publishing, 1987, with permission.

Treatment of Depression

Patients who meet the criteria for major depression are usually treated with somatic therapy, alone or in combination with psychotherapy. In critical care units, somatic therapies are the most widely used treatments for depression. Somatic therapies include pharmacotherapy and electroconvulsive therapy (ECT). Pharmacotherapy may also be used in critical care units for patients who show adjustment disorder with depressed mood, particularly when these patients have some neurovegetative symptoms. A patient who is not eating or sleeping and who lacks the energy to participate in his rehabilitation may be helped considerably by pharmacotherapy for depression.

Each type of pharmacotherapy has its own indications and contraindications, but some general rules are available when selecting an antidepressant medication. The most common rule is to choose a medication with a side-effect profile that best fits the patient's symptoms. For instance, a patient who is having trouble sleeping will benefit from a sedating antidepressant. Conversely, a patient who has severe psychomotor retardation may benefit from a more stimulating antidepressant. Different antidepressants have different side-effect profiles. The polycyclic antidepressants, as well as the newer generation of selective serotonin reuptake inhibitors (SSRIs), take approximately 4 to 6 weeks until full antidepressant effects are noted. Obviously, in critical care units, quicker effects are generally needed. Stimulants and ECT work more quickly, usually within a week. Lithium carbonate is used to stabilize mood (both highs and lows). Monoamine oxidase inhibitors (MAOIs) are often used to treat atypical depressions and may also take several weeks to reach their full effectiveness; their use is rarely associated with cardiac conduction difficulties. Patients with depression may also manifest considerable anxiety and may be helped by the use of an anxiolytic (e.g., a benzodiazepine) while awaiting response to an antidepressant. Psychotically depressed patients who manifest delusions or hallucinations may need antipsychotic medication (e.g., haloperidol) for control of symptoms.

When using polycyclic antidepressants patients should be monitored closely for signs of orthostatic hypotension, cardiac conduction effects, and anticholinergic effects. Although the full antidepressant effects of medication may take 4 to 6 weeks, changes in sleep and appetite may be noted within the first week of treatment. The patient should be treated with full antidepressant doses of medication for 12 to 18 months after depressive symptoms resolve. In some cases, obtaining blood levels of TCAs can be quite useful. Blood levels help to determine why a patient has had an atypical response to a typical oral dose, to assess the adequacy of a medication trial, and to help establish the severity of overdose.

POLYCYCLIC ANTIDEPRESSANTS. The polycyclic antidepressants include the TCAs, which are familiar to most physicians. TCAs are so named because of their three-ring structure. Although SSRI antidepressants are now prescribed more frequently than TCAs, we will consider the TCAs in detail because of their numerous side effects and toxicity. Some newer or atypical antidepressants have different structures, but act in similar fashion to the tricyclics; therefore, they will be considered in this section. Polycyclic antidepressants and their sedative, anticholinergic, and orthostatic hypotension-producing potencies are listed in Table 223-8. Polycyclics are thought to work by blocking reuptake of norepinephrine or serotonin at presynaptic sites [37]. Although they are used relatively rarely in CCUs [38], they may be used fairly frequently in other critical care units.

Polycyclic antidepressants are lipophilic and are inactivated in the liver through oxidation and aromatic hydroxylation of the tricyclic nucleus and demethylation of the side chain [39,40]. They are then conjugated with glucuronic acid. There are limited data on the use of tricyclics in patients with liver disease. As a general rule, patients with liver disease should be treated with lower doses of TCAs. Because trazodone is mainly excreted unchanged in the urine, it may be the best choice in patients with liver disease [41].

Because tricyclics are metabolized in the liver, renal failure has little effect on them. However, some antacids used to treat renal failure may interfere with the absorption of antidepressants [42]. Changes in the volume of distribution seen in renal failure may also lead to an increased portion of unbound drug in the plasma, leading to increased metabolism and decreased active drug [43]. Assessment of TCA plasma levels may be very difficult when a patient has renal failure.

Cardiovascular Effects. TCAs affect cardiac conduction, orthostatic hypotension, and cardiac rhythm. These effects are summarized in Table 223-9.

CONDUCTION EFFECTS. Early case reports showed that TCAs were associated with sudden cardiac death and life-threatening arrhythmias [44,45]. For this reason it was thought that TCAs could cause grave conduction abnormalities. However, it has been discovered that TCAs have type I or quinidinelike antiarrhythmic properties [46]. They cause a decrease in automaticity; a decrease in conduction velocity; a decrease in conduction through the His-Purkinje system (specifically, the H-V interval); a prolonged effective refractory period; and prolonged PR, QRS, and QTc durations [47–50]. TCAs also decrease premature ventricular contractions (PVCs) [51–54].

Specific polycyclics may affect conduction differently. Conduction delays through the H-V interval have been demonstrated for imipramine at normal therapeutic levels [48]. This prolongation is dose dependent within individuals, but shows marked intraindividual variation. For nortriptyline, there is no effect on the PR or QRS interval with plasma levels of 50 to 100 ng per milliliter [47]. However, in one study, one of every eight patients with plasma levels of 100 to 200 ng per milliliter showed H-V conduction delay, and four of four patients with plasma levels greater than 200 ng per milliliter showed prolongation of the PR and QRS intervals. Although doxepin had been reported to have less effect on conduction than nortriptyline [55], repeated studies have shown that doxepin causes the same cardiac conduction delays as other TCAs when used at equivalent plasma levels [48].

The use of TCAs in patients with preexisting conduction delays is more complex. There is a higher risk of second-degree or third-degree heart block when TCAs are used in patients with bundle branch blocks. In one study of 41 patients, 11 with first-degree A-V block and 30 with a bundle branch block, neither imipramine nor nortriptyline at therapeutic levels caused complications in patients with first-degree A-V block [56]. However, of the 24 patients with a bundle branch block who achieved therapeutic TCA levels, 9 percent developed 2:1 A-V block or a widened QRS complex. This was compared with 0.7 percent of a control population without cardiac disease. (Interestingly, the one patient without preexisting cardiac disease who developed 2:1 A-V block was later found by electrophysiologic studies to have a conduction abnormality). Also of note is the fact that eight out of 38 patients (21%) with conduction abnormalities in the study had to discontinue the medication secondary to severe orthostatic hypotension. This was not seen in the group without conduction abnormalities.

The risk of unforeseen cardiac complications can be averted or reduced by a routine diagnostic electrocardiogram (ECG) before TCA therapy followed by a 24-hour Holter monitor if conduction abnormality is apparent. Some have suggested that

Table 223-8. Comparative Metabolic, Anticholinergic, Sedative, Orthostatic Hypotensive, Cardiac Arrhythmogenic, Convulsive, and Drug Interaction Properties of Antidepressants

Drug	Metabolism	Anticholinergic	Sedation	Orthostatic hypotension	Cardiac arrhythmia	Seizure Risk	Miscellaneous	Target dose (mg/day)	Drug interactions
TRICYCLICS	Liver								Antacids decrease absorption; block uptake of antihypertensive
Imipramine	Liver	++	++	+++	Yes	Increased		≥200	
Amitriptyline	Liver	+++	+++	+++	Yes	Increased	Most anticholinergic	≥150	
Desipramine	Liver	+	++	++	Yes	Increased		≥150	
Nortriptyline	Liver	++	++	+	Yes	Increased	Least orthostatic hypotension	≥100	
Doxepin	Liver	++	+++	++	Yes	Increased	Safest in cardiac disease	≥200	
Protriptyline	Liver	+++	+	++	Yes	Increased		≥30	
OTHERS									
Amoxapine	Liver	+	++	+	Yes	Increased	Risk of tardive dyskinesia	≥200	
Maprotiline	Liver	+	+++	+	Yes	High risk	Difficult to treat overdose	≥150	
Trazodone	Liver	0	+++	++	Yes	Increased	Lowest anticholinergic, priapism	≥150	Digitalis toxicity
Fluoxetine	Liver	+	+	+	Rare	?	Insomnia, $t^{1/2}$ = 2–3 days	≥20	Increased levels of TCAs
Sertraline	Liver	0	0	0	Rare	?	Nausea and vomiting	50–200	Risk serotonin syndrome with MAOI and/or L-tryptophan
Paroxetine	Liver	+	+	0	Rare	?		≥20	
Bupropion	Liver	+	0	+	Rare	Increased	Risk of tardive dyskinesia	≥200	
Alprazolam	Liver	0	++	0	Rare	No	Primarily anxiolytic	Up to 4 mg	
MAOIs	Liver	0	+	+++	Rare	?	Changes ischemia to silent ischemia	45–90	Htn crisis with tyramine or sympathomimetics; avoid meperidine
Lithium	Renal	0	0	0	Rare	?Increased	ECG looks like hypokalemia	Blood level 0.5–1.0 mEq/L	Lithium levels increased by drugs that block sodium resorption
Stimulants	Renal	0	0	0	Rare		Can increase excretion by acidifying urine	5–20	

Key: + = low; + + = moderate; + + + = high.

Table 223-9. The Use of TCAs in Patients with Cardiovascular Disease

Cardiac status	Comments	TCA of choice (based on available data)	Cardiac status	Comments	TCA of choice (based on available data)
Bundle branch block (preexisting)	1. Caution advised 2. All TCAs prolong HV interval 3. Pretreatment ECG recommended in patients >50 years 4. Hospitalization/telemetric monitoring suggested at outset of treatment 5. Maintain lowest effective plasma level	Nortriptyline Doxepin (?)	Left ventricular dysfunction (congestive heart failure)	1. Impairment of contractility is uncommon 2. CHF is very rare; it may occur secondary to heart rate increases from anticholinergic effects	All TCAs
			Essential hypertension	Avoid use of alpha-blockers (clonidine, guanethidine, prazosin) because of drug interaction and decreased effect of antihypertensive agents	All TCAs
Ventricular arrhythmias	1. TCAs possess type I (quinidine-like) effects 2. PVCs may improve on TCAs 3. Antiarrhythmic dosage may require a decrease 4. Holter monitor suggested	Imipramine Desipramine	Recent acute myocardial infarction	Delay use of TCAs for several weeks because of hypotension, tachycardia, and systemic effects	
			Sick sinus syndrome	TCAs contraindicated because of potential for further sinus and AV block	None
Orthostatic hypotension	1. All TCAs can produce further orthostatic changes and can be predicted to some degree by predrug orthostatic changes 2. Effect can occur independent of plasma levels 3. Symptoms may be minimal despite significant fall in blood pressure 4. Symptoms may decrease over time	Nortriptyline	AV block (2° or 3°)	TCAs contraindicated because of potential for further block	None
			Atrial fibrillation	Avoid TCAs unless concurrently treated with digoxin (analogous to use of quinidine in patients with atrial fibrillation)	None
			Prolonged QTC	Use with caution because of risk of sudden death when QTC > 440 msec	Nortriptyline Doxepine (?)
Coronary artery disease	1. Angina or infarction may occur due to tachycardia (anticholinergic effects) and fall in perfusion pressure (orthostasis) 2. Highly anticholinergic agents should be avoided because of potential to increase heart rate	Imipramine Desipramine Nortriptyline	Concomitant treatment with other agents that may adversely affect conduction system (e.g., neuroleptics, antiarrhythmics)	Caution advised because of synergistic effects with TCAs; doses may need to be decreased	Nortriptyline Doxepin (?)

Key: CHF = congestive heart failure; HV = His-ventricular; PVCs = premature ventricular contractions; TCA = tricyclic antidepressant.
Source: Dec GW, Stern TA: *J Intensive Care Med* 5:69, 1990, by permission of Blackwell Scientific Publications, Inc.

nortriptyline at an oral dose that gives a plasma level less than 100 ng per milliliter is safer for patients with conduction anomalies [57]. It is also important to be careful of any additive effects for patients already on type I antiarrhythmics.

ORTHOSTATIC HYPOTENSION. Orthostatic hypotension from TCAs is the most serious and frequent cardiovascular side effect in medically healthy patients [58]. The percentage of patients needing to stop TCAs because of orthostatic hypotension has ranged from 8 to 20 percent in literature reports [45,59–62]. Orthostatic hypotension can lead to falls, fractures, or heart attacks. In one study using imipramine at therapeutic levels, the average fall in systolic pressure was 26 mm Hg on standing [60] and was independent of age, preexisting heart disease, or plasma level of imipramine. Orthostatic hypotension also occurred at subtherapeutic plasma levels, implying that reduction of dose will not necessarily avert orthostatic hypotension. Others have found that orthostatic hypotension was more severe in patients older than 60 years of age [61]. Glassman and co-workers, however, have argued that orthostatic hypotension is not age related, but rather that the risks of orthostasis (e.g., falls) are much greater for the elderly than for younger people.

Nortriptyline is the TCA with the lowest risk of orthostatic hypotension [63,64,65].

For patients with CHF, orthostatic hypotension is a more serious problem. Glassman and colleagues found severe orthostatic hypotension in 50 percent of a group of patients with CHF (mean ejection fraction, 38%) treated with imipramine [66]. In one group, 6 of 15 patients had associated falls; in another, 8 of 19 patients on imipramine had falls associated with orthostatic hypotension. In contrast, nortriptyline appears to cause much less orthostatic hypotension in this group. Roose and associates found that orthostatic hypotension occurred in 1 of 21 patients (4.8%) receiving nortriptyline [67]. Nineteen of these patients had trials of imipramine before, and 8 of the 19 had severe orthostatic hypotension with associated falls. Roose and co-workers also have found that orthostatic hypotension is more common in patients with both CHF and conduction abnormalities [56]. Although the mechanism of orthostatic hypotension is unclear, it may include peripheral alpha-adrenergic blockade or stimulation of central alpha-adrenergic receptors [68].

In general, increased risk of orthostatic hypotension is associated with (1) pretreatment orthostatic hypotension greater than 15 mm Hg, (2) conduction abnormalities, (3) CHF, (4) autonomic neuropathies, and (5) concomitant use of antihypertensives. Treatments include educating the patient to get up slowly; getting inpatients out of bed; tilting the head of the bed up; ensuring adequate hydration; using TED stockings; adding salt to the diet (if not clinically contraindicated); using mineralocorticoids (fludrocortisone); and using caffeine, sympathomimetics, indomethacin, clonidine, or metoclopromide.

CONTRACTILITY. Early studies using systolic time intervals found that imipramine and nortriptyline lowered ejection fractions [69,70,71]. It was later discovered that the systolic time intervals were increased by the lengthened QRS time interval caused by TCAs [67]. More recently, the effect of TCAs on contractility has been studied with the use of radionuclide angiography. Several studies have shown that imipramine, doxepin, and nortriptyline do not affect ejection fractions at rest or during exercise (pretreatment ejection fractions 33–45%) [66,67,72]. Nortriptyline also has no effect on the end systolic volume index, end diastolic volume index, stroke volume index, or cardiac index. In clinical practice, CHF may be worsened with TCA use because the anticholinergic symptom of dry mouth may lead some patients to drink more, resulting in a fluid overload.

ARRHYTHMIAS. As noted before, TCAs have a type I antiarrhythmic effect. Imipramine is a potent premature ventricular contraction (PVC) suppressor in arrhythmic patients with and without depression [51]. This has also been shown for nortriptyline [54].

TCA USE POST-MI. Because of the aforementioned effects on cardiac conduction, rhythm, and orthostatic hypotension, polycyclics are not recommended in the acute post-MI phase. Polycyclics have been used less than 6 weeks after acute MIs with success and without adverse sequelae. In these cases, serial ECG monitoring is warranted, as is close attention to blood pressure, heart rate, and recurrence of ischemia. In severely depressed post-MI patients, the use of ECT has been suggested [57,73]. There are no studies describing the treatment of depression in the acute post-MI period.

Anticholinergic Effects. Anticholinergic symptoms usually consist of increased heart rate, dry mouth, constipation, urinary retention, mydriasis, blurred vision, and confusional states. Relative anticholinergic potencies of TCAs are shown in Table 223-8.

One of the more significant anticholinergic effects is an increase in heart rate. This is mediated through decreased vagal tone and may also be affected by the neuronal catecholamine reuptake blockade and by an increase in plasma catecholamines that occurs with orthostatic hypotension [58]. Most studies have been done on imipramine and desipramine and have shown a modest increase in heart rate in the first few weeks of treatment with decreases in subsequent weeks [51,64]. Although this is normally a trivial increase in heart rate (approximately seven beats per minute), it may be more significant in medically ill patients [51]. Sinus tachycardia can exacerbate angina, MI, or CHF. Increased heart rate is more likely when the pretreatment heart rate is slower [51,64]. Many patients, however, are protected because they are already taking beta-blockers. Increased heart rate is not correlated with TCA blood level, but occurs less with monocyclic antidepressants or with TCAs with lower anticholinergic potencies.

Sedation. Sedation correlates with the antihistaminic potencies of TCAs [29]. When choosing an antidepressant, it is useful to select a more sedating TCA for patients with prominent insomnia or agitation. Often, however, sedative potency correlates with increased potential for weight gain. In general, tertiary amines are more sedating than are secondary amines.

Drug Interactions. TCAs block the effects of many antihypertensives. This is particularly true of adrenergic blocking agents such as guanethidine, clonidine, and reserpine, thereby potentially exacerbating hypertension [57]. Alternatively, if a patient stops taking a TCA while still taking an antihypertensive agent, one may notice hypotension. Loss of blood pressure control may occur because of central TCA interactions with reserpine, alpha-methyldopa, and clonidine [74].

TCAs also interact with antiarrhythmics and anticholinergics. TCAs are additive with both of these groups, particularly with type I antiarrhythmics [48]. TCAs may also potentiate the pressor effects of sympathomimetics (epinephrine and norepinephrine) by blocking the reuptake of these pressors, leading to hypertensive crises [74]. TCAs also have been reported to decrease the hepatic metabolism (i.e., raise plasma levels) of oral anticoagulants [75]. TCAs do not interact with digitalis, but trazodone, an atypical agent, has been reported to increase digoxin toxicity [76]. Concomitant administration of TCAs and propranolol may lead to increased orthostasis. Use of anticonvulsants may lower TCA levels by increasing their metabolism. TCAs may also lower seizure threshold and make anticonvulsants less efficacious.

TCA Overdose. For hypotension associated with TCA overdose, volume expansion and alkalinization with sodium bicarbonate will help to maintain blood pressure. If these fail, vasopressors are useful. Pressors (such as phenylephrine or norepinephrine) with predominant alpha-adrenergic effects are most useful with TCA overdoses [57]. Conduction disturbances and ventricular arrhythmias should be aggressively treated with serum alkalinization and phenytoin.

Ventricular fibrillation and ventricular tachycardia are usually preceded by sinus tachycardia, QRS prolongation, and PVCs. For this reason, aggressive treatment of ectopy is indicated. Although phenytoin loading is useful, serum alkalinization and lidocaine are also part of the initial treatment of ventricular arrhythmias. It is important to note that severe cardiac complications do not necessarily imply a poor prognosis. There is a case report of full recovery from TCA overdose after 5 hours of external cardiac massage in a patient who was healthy before overdose [77]. The treatment of TCA overdose is summarized in Table 223-10. See also Chapter 140.

SELECTIVE SEROTONIN REUPTAKE INHIBITORS. The selective serotonin reuptake inhibitors (SSRIs) are a class of polycyclic antidepressants that cause a potent and selective blockade of serotonin reuptake. The most widely used drug in this class is fluoxetine. Paroxetine and sertraline are also SSRIs, as are fluvoxamine and venlafaxine. These drugs have polycyclic structures and are quite heterogeneous. They are far less anticholinergic, antihistaminic, and alpha-adrenergic than TCAs and therefore are associated with far fewer side effects. They also have fewer effects on cardiac activity and do not commonly cause orthostatic hypotension.

Pharmacokinetics. SSRIs are well absorbed from the gastrointestinal tract, and absorption is generally unaffected by food and antacids [78]. They have a large volume of distribution and are highly protein bound. They are extensively metabolized in the liver, where they are oxidized, methylated, and conjugated. The elimination half-lives of fluvoxamine, sertraline, and paroxetine are all about 1 day (although sertraline has a mildly

Table 223-10. Tricyclic Overdosage: Treatment Recommendations

Symptom/sign	Treatment
Convulsions	Diazepam, 0.1 mg/kg intravenously (IV) per dose as neded Alkalinization Phenytoin, 15 mg/kg IV over 30 min
Coma	Airway support
Hypotension	Crystalloid infusion Alkalinization Vasopressors: norepinephrine preferred Inotropic agents: dobutamine preferred
Ventricular arrhythmias[a]	Alkalinization Lidocaine Phenytoin, 15 mg/kg IV over 30 min
Prolonged QRS ($\geq$0.10 sec)	Alkalinization Phenytoin, 15 mg/kg IV over 30 min
Bradyarrhythmia/ heart block[b]	Isoproterenol Pacemaker

[a]Cardioversion should be considered for any hemodynamically compromising arrhythmia. *Torsades de pointes* ventricular tachycardia may respond only to overdrive pacing or isoproterenol infusion. Quinidine, procainamide, and disopyramide are contraindicated for any tricyclic overdose.
[b] Mobitz II second-degree or third-degree heart block.
Source: Frommer DA, Kulig RW, Marx JA, et al: *JAMA* 257(5):525, 1987, with permission.

active metabolite with a half-life of 66 hours). This allows once-daily dosing. Venlafaxine has a half-life of 3 to 4 hours and must be given 2 or 3 times daily. Fluoxetine has a half-life of 2 to 3 days and a highly active metabolite (norfluoxetine) with a mean half-life of 6.1 days. Fluoxetine takes a much longer time to reach steady state and, more importantly for drug overdoses, can take weeks to months to be fully cleared. Elimination half-lives are also dose dependent, i.e., higher doses and lengthier usage are associated with higher plasma levels and longer half-lives. SSRIs show wide intraindividual variation in pharmacokinetics and as yet do not have a clearly established dose-response curve.

Paroxetine, sertraline, and fluoxetine are unaffected by renal problems. Sertraline has been used at full doses in a small number of patients with serious liver disease without difficulties. Fluoxetine has higher plasma levels and a longer half-life in patients with liver disease; therefore, the dose should be reduced by at least 50 percent in these patients. Venlafaxine clearance is decreased by both renal and hepatic disease. In the elderly, fluoxetine and venlafaxine do not have altered pharmacokinetics. In contrast, paroxetine and sertraline have increased plasma levels and slower clearance.

Side Effects. Fluoxetine can cause tremulousness, agitation, irritability, anorexia, and gastrointestinal distress. In some patients there is marked insomnia, even though fluoxetine is usually taken in the morning to reduce the risk of insomnia. However, some patients become sedated by fluoxetine. Fluoxetine venlafaxine, and paroxetine can also raise the level of hepatically metabolized medications. Fluoxetine has been reported to cause the syndrome of antidiuretic hormone secretion (SIADH), serum sickness, and anorgasmia [79,80,81]. Extrapyramidal symptoms and lithium toxicity have been seen when fluoxetine is used in combination with lithium [82]. Fluoxetine has also been reported to increase suicidal preoccupation [83], but this appears to occur only in a very small percentage of patients taking fluoxetine.

Fluoxetine has been available much longer than paroxetine, venlafaxine, fluvoxamine, and sertraline in the United States.

Consequently, there is a larger literature on reported side effects. Paroxetine and sertraline can cause nausea, vomiting, and diarrhea [84]. They appear to be less activating than fluoxetine. Sertraline does not interact with a wide range of medications, including diazepam, digoxin, haloperidol, amobarbital, oxazepam, and ethanol.

Cardiovascular Effects. None of the SSRIs, except venlafaxine, cause clinically significant changes in heart rate, blood pressure, or ECGs [85,86]. Fluoxetine has been reported to raise TCA levels and may increase conduction delays when used in combination with TCAs [87]. There have been several case reports of bradycardia and syncope with fluoxetine use, and it is estimated that this may occur in 1 to 2 percent of all patients using fluoxetine [88,89]. There have also been case reports of fluoxetine-induced atrial fibrillation, atrial flutter, and A-V block [90]. Venlafaxine can cause dose-dependent 10 to 15 mm Hg increases in diastolic blood pressure.

Drug Overdose/Interactions. The SSRIs have a high margin of safety if taken alone in drug overdose. Fluoxetine can significantly increase TCA cardiac toxicity in combined overdoses. SSRIs in combination with monoamine oxidase inhibitors (MAOIs) or l-tryptophan can cause the serotonin syndrome, a potentially fatal syndrome of serotonergic hyperstimulation. Symptoms of the serotonin syndrome include mental status changes, agitation, diarrhea, myoclonus, hypertension, hyperthermia, hyperreflexia, diaphoresis, tremor, shivering, and seizures [91]. The syndrome can be mild or severe. Treatment is supportive and includes clonazepam for myoclonus and nifedipine for hypertension. It has been reported when SSRIs were taken concomitantly with MAOIs and when there was an insufficient washout period between use of the drugs. Current wisdom suggests a wait of at least five weeks (five half-lives) before starting an MAOI after discontinuation of fluoxetine and at least 2 weeks before starting an SSRI after MAOI therapy is stopped.

ATYPICAL ANTIDEPRESSANTS. Although most of the newer antidepressants have profiles similar to the TCAs, a few words about them are in order. Maprotiline is a tetracyclic antidepressant. It has a cardiac and anticholinergic profile much like that of desipramine [92]. It can also cause orthostatic hypotension and conduction delays at therapeutic doses [93]. In particular, it seems to be associated with a greater risk of seizure than other antidepressants [94]. Overdoses are especially difficult to treat. Maprotiline in overdose has been associated with unusually high cardiac toxicity because of its prolonged half-life.

Trazodone is another atypical antidepressant. It is a triazolopyridine derivative. It has much less intense anticholinergic effects than the polycyclic antidepressants and a more benign cardiac profile than many TCAs [95,96,97]. However, trazodone can cause conduction delays in patients with underlying heart disease [98]. Therefore, an ECG should be checked if there is a history of arrhythmia. It is unclear whether trazodone causes excessive ventricular ectopy. Although early reports noted increased ectopy, a double-blind study comparing trazodone with placebo showed that 40 percent of the placebo-treated patients showed PVCs compared with 38 percent of those patients treated with trazodone [99]. Trazodone does cause significant orthostatic hypotension, although this may decrease 4 to 6 hours after the medication is ingested [100]. It rarely causes a decrease in heart rate or a change in ventricular ejection fraction if patients have a normal myocardium. Trazodone does not possess any antiarrhythmic properties, and overdoses have been reported to be relatively safe [58]. It also causes anorgasmia and has been associated with serious priapism [101]. It is safer than other polycyclic antidepressants for use in patients with liver disease. Nefazadone is a recently released antidepressant closely related to trazodone in structure, with less propensity to cause orthostasis and priapism.

Amoxapine is a newer TCA that works by blocking dopamine reuptake. Because of this, it can cause extrapyramidal symptoms and carries with it a risk of tardive dyskinesia after long-term use. It has also been reported to cause atrial arrhythmias and conduction delays [102]. Although amoxapine has been reported to have minimal cardiac toxicity in overdose, it has caused severe renal failure [103].

Another atypical antidepressant is bupropion, a monocyclic ketone. Like amoxapine, bupropion blocks dopamine reuptake. It is also a partial agonist of serotonin and therefore causes functional serotonin blockade. It has minimal anticholinergic effects and carries with it a low risk of cardiac toxicity, but is associated with an increased risk of seizure. It has not been shown to cause changes in heart rate, blood pressure, cardiac conduction, or left ventricular ejection fraction in patients with mild CHF [104]. Bupropion can cause the serotonin syndrome if used with MAOIs.

MONOAMINE OXIDASE INHIBITORS.

Monoamine oxidase inhibitors (MAOIs) have been used for the treatment of depression since the 1950s. The original MAOIs were derivatives of hydrazine. Of the currently available MAOIs, phenelzine and isocarboxazide are hydrazine derivatives, and tranylcypromine is a nonhydrazine derivative. MAOIs work by blocking the oxidative deamination of biogenic amines such as norepinephrine and serotonin. They are metabolized by acetylation in the liver. Some patients may be slow acetylators and have higher blood levels of these drugs. MAOIs have few direct cardiac effects. In the 1960s, it was found that they reduced the symptoms of angina without changing the ischemic process. In other words, they may convert ischemia into silent ischemia [58]. They also cause a statistically significant but clinically insignificant decrease in heart rate and QTc interval and no change in cardiac conduction (except for one case report of the onset of flutter/fibrillation and syncope with tranylcypromine) [105,106].

The most common and serious cardiovascular side effect of MAOIs is profound orthostatic hypotension. Estimates of the frequency of orthostatic hypotension have ranged from 11 to 47 percent of patients treated with MAOIs [107,108]. The onset of orthostatic hypotension may occur as long as four weeks into MAOI therapy [109]. It is unclear at this time whether different MAOIs have different orthostatic potencies, and at least one study has shown orthostatic hypotension to be dose related [110].

MAOIs may cause profound hypertensive crises when patients taking MAOIs also take sympathomimetic medications or ingest foods containing tyramine. Because tyramine is usually inactivated by MAO, it is thought to act as a false neurotransmitter for norepinephrine and to replace norepinephrine in presynaptic granules, leading to a hypertensive crisis from release of norepinephrine. Patients taking MAOIs must be cautioned to avoid tyramine-containing foods, e.g., aged cheeses, pickled foods, yeast extracts, and other aged foods. Hypertensive crises are also caused by the ingestion of sympathomimetic medications, such as reserpine, guanethidine, pseudephedrine, or ephedrine. The indirect sympathomimetic amines that work through the storage of norepinephrine and dopamine and depend on MAO for metabolism are more likely to produce a hypertensive crisis. Hypertensive crises have been treated with

IV phentolamine, and more recently with sublingual diltiazem or sublingual or oral nifedipine [58]. The incidence of hypertensive crises when sympathomimetics are used with MAOIs is not known. It has been estimated that tyramine causes hypertensive reactions in up to 8 percent of patients on MAOIs [107].

MAOIs and alpha-methyldopa used in combination may cause CNS excitation [111]. MAOIs and hydralazine may lead to hypotension, as may thiazides and MAOIs [112,113]. Narcotics, particularly meperidine, may lead to hypertensive crises and elevated blood levels of meperidine [114]. The use of beta-blockers with MAOIs may lead to unopposed alpha-adrenergic activity and also cause severe hypertension [115]. MAOIs may also interfere with the metabolism of liver-metabolized drugs and raise the levels of many other medications, including oral anticoagulants and benzodiazepines. MAOIs themselves may also produce liver damage in rare instances because of the hydrazine-related structure. MAOIs in conjunction with SSRIs can cause the serotonin syndrome of serotonergic hyperstimulation.

Effects of overdose include agitation, hallucinations, hyperreflexia, and convulsions [116] (see Chap. 149). Both hypertension and hypotension have also been reported. Hypertension should be treated as previously described, with supportive treatment for temperature and respiration, as well as for fluid and electrolyte balance. Because MAOIs produce an irreversible deactivation of MAO, the enzyme is not available until it reconstitutes. This may take up to 2 weeks and may result in late complications of an overdose.

In addition to orthostatic hypotension, less toxic side effects may include excessive stimulation and weight gain. Some patients report difficulty falling asleep and others an increase in myoclonus, particularly at night. Other effects include peripheral edema, anorgasmia, and erectile dysfunction [116]. In general, MAOIs are not useful in ICUs because of their potential interactions with pressors and because their effects are manifest in the body for up to 14 days. They can, however, be used in patients with serious cardiac abnormalities because of their less serious cardiac side effects.

PSYCHOSTIMULANTS.

Psychostimulants have been used to treat depressive symptoms since their development in the 1930s, but they fell into disrepute when they became drugs of abuse in the 1950s and 1960s. There have been numerous reports on the use of stimulants in the treatment of depressed patients, particularly apathetic and geriatric patients [117–124]. In recent years, there has been a renewed interest in the use of psychostimulants in depressed patients who are medically ill and cannot tolerate other treatments for depression (e.g., TCAs and MAOIs) [125]. In a 1987 review of the literature on stimulants for the treatment of depression, Chiarello and Cole stated that the evidence supports judicious use of psychostimulants in some subgroups of patients with depression [126].

The psychostimulants most commonly used are dextroamphetamine and methylphenidate. Both appear to work through the direct neuronal release of dopamine and norepinephrine. Dextroamphetamine also appears to block catecholamine reuptake and has a weak MAOI effect. Both psychostimulants are predominantly excreted by the kidneys, although dextroamphetamine also undergoes a complex biotransformation. Renal excretion of these psychostimulants is enhanced when urine is acidified [126].

Stimulants usually increase motor behavior, increase arousal, and decrease appetite; however, in patients who are anorexic because of depression, appetite will be paradoxically increased. Stimulant effects in the treatment of depression are rapid and are usually evident in the first 2 days of treatment. In a review of 66 patients hospitalized on medical/surgical wards at Massachusetts General Hospital, 93 percent achieved maximum benefit within 2 days of stimulant use [123]. Stimulants do not show any anticholinergic effects or any effects on orthostatic hypotension. They can increase heart rate and can cause coronary spasm, cardiac arrhythmias, or hypertension. However, these effects are rare (even with preexisting cardiac abnormalities) at the low doses usually used for the treatment of depression (5–20 mg/day) [127]. In fact, stimulants have been safely and effectively used in patients with prolonged hospitalizations, patients dependent on respirators, patients with CHF, and postcardiac surgery patients [123]. Contraindications to stimulant use include significant hypertension, pregnancy, seizures, delirium, psychosis, or angina as well as concurrent use of alphamethyldopa (which becomes a sympathoamine when metabolized), MAOIs, or bronchodilators [116].

At Massachusetts General Hospital, psychostimulants are often the first agent used to treat depression in critically ill patients. Patients are started on 2.5 or 5 mg of methylphenidate or dextroamphetamine in the morning. The dose is increased by 5 mg per day until a therapeutic effect is detected or until a maximum daily dose of 20 mg has been reached. Heart rate and blood pressure are closely monitored. Our experience with the use of stimulants in an ICU has been encouraging, and stimulants have been one of the most benign and effective treatments for depression. Stimulants have shown little potential for abuse when used to treat patients with depression. Stimulants are usually given for at least 1 to 2 weeks after the full remission of depressive symptoms. In most cases, after stimulants have been stopped, depression does not recur [29].

Stimulants taken in overdose may cause seizures, coma, hallucinations, paranoia, hypertension, hyperthermia, cardiac arrhythmia, angina, and circulatory collapse. The major treatment for overdose is to acidify the urine and to use supportive measures for all other abnormalities (see Chap. 156). Neuroleptics (e.g., chlorpromazine) have been suggested for the treatment of CNS symptoms, although their alpha-blocking action effects can decrease blood pressure [116].

LITHIUM CARBONATE. Lithium carbonate is a salt that has been used as a mood stabilizer and as an adjunctive agent for numerous other conditions. Lithium-treated patients in critical care units are typically on lithium at the time of their admission to the ICU. It is not entirely clear how lithium works to treat mood instability, but it appears to have some effect on biological membranes. Lithium is almost entirely excreted by the kidney. Therefore, a decrease in renal function will increase the amount of lithium retained in the body. Lithium clearance in the kidney is analogous to that of sodium, i.e., of the 20 percent of glomerular filtrate absorbed, 80 percent of the lithium is resorbed in the proximal tubule. Sodium and lithium, in fact, will replace each other in the kidney; an increase in sodium in the diet will decrease lithium resorbed and vice versa. Therefore, it is important to be mindful of dietary changes involving sodium when treating a person on lithium.

Lithium should be used with caution in patients who have renal failure. In the patient with renal failure, a single dose will typically maintain a blood level until the next dialysis. Lithium also has been reported to be nephrotoxic. Toxic lithium levels in animals cause acute renal toxicity; case reports of acute nephrotoxicity in humans have been published [128]. More commonly, chronic lithium use causes polyuria and a decrease in urine concentrating ability [129,130]. This is believed to be secondary to a decrease in tubular responsiveness to antidiuretic hormone (ADH) [131].

Lithium has several important drug interactions. Thiazide diuretics, which block sodium resorption in the distal tubule, cause increased lithium resorption in the proximal tubule and an increase in the lithium blood level. The same result will occur with potassium-sparing diuretics such as spironolactone, triamterene, and amiloride. Loop diuretics (furosemide and ethacrynic acid) usually have no effect on lithium resorption. Carbonic anhydrase inhibitors and xanthine diuretics will usually increase lithium excretion and lower the lithium plasma level. Some nonsteroidal antiinflammatory drugs may decrease renal prostaglandin and decrease lithium excretion. This does not appear to happen with aspirin or ibuprofen [132].

Lithium causes ECG changes (i.e., flat or inverted T waves and U waves) that look like hypokalemia. This will occur in 20 to 30 percent of patients on lithium carbonate, but is not associated with decreased potassium [133]. ECG changes also occur more commonly in patients older than 60 years of age, and in these patients it is reasonable to monitor the ECG. ECG changes may appear only after a patient has been on medication for more than a year [43]. There have also been case reports of sinoatrial arrest, problems of A-V conduction interference, decreased premature atrial contractions and supraventricular arrhythmias, and increased PVCs and ventricular arrhythmias on lithium [74,134,135,136]. A particularly ominous combination has been that of lithium, bronchodilators, and a history of cardiovascular disease in patients older than 70 years of age. In one study, sudden death was reported in 11 of 100 patients with this combination [137]. This combination should be avoided whenever possible.

Lithium levels are usually monitored by plasma levels, with toxic levels generally being above 1.5 mEq per liter. Acute signs of toxicity include confusion, hyperreflexia, tremor, vomiting, diarrhea, cardiac arrhythmia, ataxia, coma, and convulsions (see Chap. 147). Treatment for overdose is usually supportive unless levels are very high or neurotoxicity develops; there is no known specific antidote for lithium. In milder cases of toxicity, increased renal excretion of lithium may be obtained with nonosmotic diuresis and with IV sodium bicarbonate. In cases of severe toxicity, dialysis is warranted.

ALPRAZOLAM. Alprazolam is a triazolobenzodiazepine. Although it is primarily used as an anxiolytic, several studies have shown that it has antidepressant efficacy when compared with TCAs and placebo [138,139,140]. Alprazolam can be quite useful in ICUs because it has a benign cardiac profile. It primarily acts on the CNS to produce sedation, to decrease anxiety, and to relax muscles. Alprazolam, like all benzodiazepines, is primarily metabolized in the liver through the hepatic microsomal enzyme system. Its metabolism is decreased in the elderly, in the very young, and in those with liver disease. Alprazolam use may result in respiratory depression in the elderly and in those with COPD. Delirium from its use is rare.

Relative contraindications to alprazolam use include liver disease, COPD, and delirium. Like TCAs, alprazolam may take 3 to 4 weeks to show a full antidepressant effect; however, its anxiolytic effects are prompt.

In overdose, alprazolam may cause respiratory depression, confusion, CNS depression, coma, and death. However, like most benzodiazepines, it is relatively safe in overdose. Treatment of alprazolam overdose involves supportive measures.

ELECTROCONVULSIVE THERAPY. Electroconvulsive therapy (ECT) is an effective treatment that may be used in cases of severe or delusional depression, or when more conventional therapies cannot be used (e.g., in patients who are unable to tolerate TCAs). There have been case reports of exaggerated increases in blood pressure, circulatory collapse, MI, and arrhythmias during and after ECT [141–144]. Others have reported S-T depressions and repolarization abnormalities [145,146]. In one series of patients (including 24% who had preexisting heart disease), ECT was found to have no effect on serum cardiac enzymes and ECGs [147]. In another study of patients given ECT (of whom 70% had a history of heart disease), 28 percent had cardiovascular complications [148]. Because of these inconsistencies, we conclude that ECT should be used only in patients with serious underlying heart disease when depression is life threatening. ECT may be used safely in other ICU patients who cannot tolerate antidepressant medication.

Psychological Management of Depression in the ICU

Although pharmacologic treatments are the mainstay of treatment for depression in the ICU, psychological treatments can also be important. Patients often benefit from information, clarification, reassurance, and support. Psychological intervention (i.e., talking therapy) is most useful in cases of adjustment disorder with depressed mood, often as an adjunct to pharmacologic intervention.

When patients come to an ICU, they are often terrified about the outcome of the illness that brings them there. They frequently believe that the illness, no matter how well controlled in the ICU, will continue to be life threatening after discharge. Some patients believe that their illness will necessitate a radical change in lifestyle. For example, many cardiac patients secretly believe that having had a MI means that they will never be able to have sex again. One way to help patients with such concerns is to ask specific questions about how they believe their illness will affect daily life in the future. In this way, one will hear the patient's specific fears and be able to educate the patient about the real effects of the illness. Another example is the patient who is physically weak after a heart attack and thinks he is a cardiac cripple. He fails to understand that his physical weakness is the result of muscle wasting from prolonged bed rest. Education often reassures patients.

Another way of helping patients cope with depression in an ICU involves learning about a patient's premorbid activities. Because patients in the ICU feel stripped of their identity and are demoralized, showing interest in who they are and what is important to them can remind them that they are respected and have a life outside the hospital. Families can also be helped by encouraging realistic expectations and by offering support.

On occasion, depressed ICU patients cause staff to become depressed. The patients may be whining, angry, or intensely sad. Even though caregivers know that patients may need to talk to someone, they may dread seeing the patient. Aversion can be reduced by frequent communication among staff members. Not uncommonly, when it becomes clear that other caregivers are similarly affected, the burden of guilt that leads staff to avoid depressed patients may be lifted. Aversion can also be reduced if aggressive treatment of depression is initiated.

Demoralization of staff can occur when treating depressed patients, especially when patients are not doing well. Sometimes, when a patient's depression is overwhelming, staff begin to believe that the patient is better off dead than suffering from illness. In an interesting study, Leibenluft found that when psychiatric consultation was obtained for suicidal patients with terminal illnesses, many of them were diagnosed as being significantly depressed [149]. Treatment of depression was quite useful in improving the morale of many of these patients.

IMPACT OF DEPRESSION ON COMPETENCY. Depression may complicate the assessment of competency. Competency evaluations are frequently requested when a patient wishes to leave the hospital against medical advice or refuses treatment. Although some patients have the capacity to refuse treatment based on clear and rational thinking, other patients will refuse treatment based on feelings of depression, demoralization, or hopelessness. Depression in such cases makes patients incompetent or lacking in capacity to make sound medical decisions. Depression should be treated before resolution of questions about competency. This interplay between depression, acute behavior problems, character pathology, and staff response is discussed in detail in Chapter 225.

Conclusion

Treatment of depression in ICUs is multifaceted and difficult. Nevertheless, aggressive treatment of depression in the ICU can drastically improve a patient's sense of well-being and change a demoralized, hopeless patient into an active participant in treatment. In this chapter, we have outlined the recognition, differential diagnosis, and treatment of depression in ICUs. We strongly advocate that depression be treated as a serious illness. Although depression is sometimes understandable, it is never appropriate.

References

1. American Psychiatric Association: *Diagnostic and Statistical Manual of Mental Disorders, Fourth Edition, Revised.* Washington, DC, American Psychiatric Association, 1994.
2. Malzberg B: Mortality among patients with involution melancholia. *Am J Psychiatry* 93:1231, 1937.
3. Tsuang MT, Woolson RF: Mortality in patients with schizophrenia, mania, depression and surgical conditions: A comparison with general population mortality. *Br J Psychiatry* 130:162, 1986.
4. Weeke A, Vaeth M: Excess mortality of bipolar and unipolar manic-depressive patients. *J Affective Disord* 11:227, 1986.
5. Winokur G, Black DW: Psychiatric and medical diagnoses as risk factors for mortality in psychiatric patients: A case-control study. *Am J Psychiatry* 144:208, 1987.
6. Avery D, Winokur G: Mortality in depressed patients treated with electroconvulsive therapy and antidepressants. *Arch Gen Psychiatry* 33:1029, 1976.
7. Kimball CP: Psychological responses to the experience of open heart surgery: I. *Am J Psychiatry* 126:348, 1969.
8. Tufo HM, Ostfeld AM: A prospective study of open-heart surgery. Abstract. *Psychosom Med* 30:552, 1968.
9. Roose SP, Glassman AH, Dalack GW: Depression, heart disease, and tricyclic antidepressants. *J Clin Psychiatry* 50:7(suppl):12, 1989.
10. Kleiger RE, Miller JP, Bigger JT Jr, et al: Decreased heart rate variability and its association with increased mortality after acute myocardial infarction. *Am J Cardiol* 59:256, 1987.
11. Sachar E, Asnis G, Halbreich U, et al: Recent studies in the neuroendocrinology of major depressive disorders. *Psychiatr Clin North Am* 3:313, 1980.
12. Rubin R, Poland R, Lesser I, et al: Neuroendocrine aspects of primary endogenous depression: Cortisol secretory dynamics in patients and matched controls. *Arch Gen Psychiatry* 44:328, 1987.
13. Carroll B, Feinberg M, Greden J, et al: A specific laboratory test for the diagnosis of melancholia. *Arch Gen Psychiatry* 38:15, 1981.
14. Schildkraut J, Schatzberg A, Mooney J, et al: Depressive disorders and the emerging field of psychiatric chemistry, in Grinspoon L (ed): *Psychiatry Update.* Washington, DC, American Psychiatric Press, 1983.

15. Ettigi P, Brown G: Psychoneuroendocrinology of affective disorder: An overview. *Am J Psychiatry* 134:493, 1977.
16. Giardina EGV, Johnson LL, Vita J, et al: Effect of imipramine and nortriptyline on left ventricular function and blood pressure in patients treated for arrhythmias. *Am Heart J* 109:992, 1985.
17. Calabrese JR, Kling MA, Gold PW: Alterations in immunocompetence during stress, bereavement and depression: Focus on neuroendocrine regulation. *Am J Psychiatry* 144(9):1123, 1987.
18. Kupfer DJ, Foster FG: Interval between onset of sleep and rapid eye movement sleep as an indication of depression. *Lancet* 2:684, 1972.
19. Jellinek MS, Goldenheim PD, Jenike MA: The impact of grief on ventilatory control. *Am J Psychiatry* 142:121, 1985.
20. Cavanaugh SVA: Diagnosing depression in the hospitalized patient with chronic medical illness. *J Clin Psychiatry* 45:13, 1984.
21. Weissman MM, Boyd JH: The epidemiology of affective disorders: Rates and risk factors, in Grinspoon L (ed): *Psychiatry Update*. Washington, DC, American Psychiatric Press, 1983, p 406.
22. Weissman M, Klerman G: Sex differences and the epidemiology of depression. *Arch Gen Psychiatry* 34:98, 1977.
23. Rodin G, Voshart K: Depression in the medically ill: An overview. *Am J Psychiatry* 143(3):696, 1986.
24. Heizer J, Chammas S, Norland C, et al: A study of the association between Crohn's disease and psychiatric illness. *Gastroenterology* 86:324, 1984.
25. Hoeper F, Nycz G, Cleary P, et al: Estimated prevalence of RDC mental disorder in primary medical care. *Int J Ment Health* 8:6, 1979.
26. Schulberg H, Saul M, McClelland M, et al: Assessing depression in primary medical and psychiatric practices. *Arch Gen Psychiatry* 42:1164, 1985.
27. Lustman PJ, Griffith LS, Clouse RE, et al: Psychiatric illness in diabetes mellitus: Relationship to symptoms and glucose control. *J Nerv Ment Dis* 174:736, 1986.
28. Geringer ES, Stern TA: Coping with medical illness: The impact of personality types. *Psychosomatics* 27:251, 1986.
29. Cassem NH: Depression, in Hackett TP, Cassem NH (eds): *Massachusetts General Hospital Handbook of General Hospital Psychiatry*, 2nd ed. Littleton, MA, PSG Publishing, 1987.
30. Freud S: *Studies on Hysteria*. New York, Basic Books, 1957.
31. Bibring E: The mechanism of depression, in Greenacre P (ed): *Affective Disorders*. New York, International Universities Press, 1953.
32. Fordyce W: *Behavioral Methods for Control of Chronic Pain and Illness*. St. Louis, C.V. Mosby, 1976.
33. Seligman M: Learned helplessness. *Annu Rev Med* 67:695, 1972.
34. Robinson RG, Lipsey JR, Price TR: Diagnosis and clinical management of post-stroke depression. *Psychosomatics* 26:769, 1985.
35. Folstein MF, Folstein SE, McHugh PR: "Mini-Mental State": A practical method for grading the cognitive state of patients for the clinician. *J Psychiatric Res* 12:189, 1975.
36. Blumer D, Heilbronn M: Chronic pain as a variant of depressive disease: The pain prone disorder. *J Nerv Ment Dis* 170:381, 1982.
37. Hollister LE: Tricyclic antidepressants (2 parts). *N Engl J Med* 299:1106, 1978.
38. Cassem NH, Hackett TP: Psychiatric consultation in a coronary care unit. *Ann Intern Med* 75:9, 1971.
39. VanBrunt N: The clinical utility of tricyclic antidepressant blood levels: A review of the literature. *Ther Drug Monitor* 5:1, 1983.
40. Biggs JT: Clinical pharmacology and toxicology of antidepressants. *Hosp Pract* 13:79, 1978.
41. Secor JW, Schenker S: Drug metabolism in patients with liver disease. *Adv Int Med* 32:379, 1987.
42. Harvey SC: Hypnotics and sedatives, in Goodman GA, Goodman LS, Gilman A (eds): *The Pharmacological Basis of Therapeutics*. 6th ed. New York, Macmillan, 1980.
43. Spar JE: Organic mental syndromes, in American Psychiatric Association Task Force on Treatment of Psychiatric Disorders (eds): *Treatments of Psychiatric Disorders*. Washington, DC, American Psychiatric Association, 1989.
44. Williams RB Jr, Sherter C: Cardiac complications of tricyclic antidepressant therapy. *Ann Intern Med* 74:395, 1971.
45. Kantor SJ, Glassman AH, Bigger JT Jr, et al: The cardiac effects of therapeutic plasma concentrations of imipramine. *Am J Psychiatry* 135:534, 1978.
46. Muir WW, Strauch SM, Schaal SF: Effects of tricyclic antidepressant drugs on the electrophysiological properties of dog Purkinje fibers. *J Cardiovasc Pharmacol* 4:82, 1982.
47. Vohra J, Burrows GD, Hunt D, et al: The effect of toxic and therapeutic doses of tricyclic antidepressant drugs on intracardiac conduction. *Eur J Cardiol* 3:219, 1975.
48. Glassman AH, Bigger JT, Jr: Cardiovascular effects of therapeutic doses of tricyclic antidepressants: An overview. *Arch Gen Psychiatry* 38:815, 1981.
49. Weld FM, Bigger JT Jr: Electrophysiological effects of imipramine on bovine cardiac Purkinje and ventricular muscle fibers. *Circ Res* 46:167, 1980.
50. Rawling DA, Fozzard HA: Effects of imipramine on cellular electrophysiological properties of cardiac Purkinje fibers. *J Pharmacol Exp Ther* 209:371, 1979.
51. Giardina EG, Bigger JT Jr, Glassman AH, et al: The electrocardiographic and antiarrhythmic effects of imipramine hydrochloride at therapeutic plasma concentrations. *Circulation* 60:1045, 1979.
52. Bigger JT Jr, Giardina EGV, Perel JM, et al: Cardiac antiarrhythmic effect of imipramine hydrochloride. *N Engl J Med* 296:206, 1977.
53. Giardina EGV, Bigger JT Jr: Antiarrhythmic effect of imipramine hydrochloride in patients with ventricular premature complexes without psychological depression. *Am J Cardiol* 50:172, 1982.
54. Giardina EGV, Barnard T, Johnson LL, et al: The antiarrhythmic effect of nortriptyline in cardiac patients with ventricular premature depolarizations. *J Am Coll Cardiol* 7:1363, 1986.
55. Burrows GD, Vohra J, Dumovic P, et al: TCA drugs and cardiac conduction. *Prog Neuropsychopharmacol* 1:329, 1977.
56. Roose SP, Glassman AH, Giardina EGV, et al: Tricyclic antidepressants in depressed patients with cardiac conduction disease. *Arch Gen Psychiatry* 44:273, 1987.
57. Dec WG, Stern TA: Tricyclic antidepressants in the ICU patient. *J Intensive Care Med* 5:69, 1990.
58. Jefferson JW: Cardiovascular effects and toxicity of anxiolytics and antidepressants. *J Clin Psychiatry* 50(10):368, 1989.
59. Glassman AH, Roose SP: Cardiovascular effects of tricyclic antidepressants. *Psychiatric Ann* 17:340, 1987.
60. Glassman AH, Bigger JT Jr, Giardina EGV, et al: Clinical characteristics of imipramine-induced orthostatic hypotension. *Lancet* 1:468, 1979.
61. Mueller OF, Goodman N, Bellet S: The hypotensive effect of imipramine hydrochloride in patients with cardiovascular disease. *Clin Pharmacol Ther* 2:300, 1961.
62. Nelson JC, Jatlow PI, Bock J, et al: Major adverse reactions during desipramine treatment: Relationship to plasma drug concentrations, concomitant antipsychotic treatment, and patient characteristics. *Arch Gen Psychiatry* 39:1055, 1982.
63. Freyschuss U, Sjoqvist F, Tuck D, et al: Circulatory effects in man of nortriptyline, a tricyclic antidepressant drug. *Pharmacol Clin* 2:68, 1970.
64. Vohra J, Burrows GD, Sloman G: Assessment of cardiovascular side effects of therapeutic doses of tricyclic antidepressant drugs. *Aust N Z J Med* 5:7, 1975.
65. Roose SP, Glassman AH, Siris SG, et al: Comparison of imipramine- and nortriptyline-induced orthostatic hypotension: A meaningful difference. *J Clin Psychopharmacol* 1(5):316, 1981.
66. Glassman AH, Johnson LL, Giardina EGV, et al: The use of imipramine in depressed patients with congestive heart failure. *JAMA* 250:1997, 1983.
67. Roose SP, Glassman AH, Giardina EGV, et al: Nortriptyline in depressed patients with left ventricular impairment. *JAMA* 256:3253, 1986.
68. O'Prichard DC, Greenberg DA, Sheehan PP, et al: Tricyclic antidepressants: Therapeutic properties and affinity for alpha-adrenergic receptor binding sites in the brain. *Science* 199:197, 1978.
69. Burckhardt D, Raeder A, Muller V, et al: Cardiovascular effects of tricyclic and tetracyclic antidepressants. *JAMA* 239:213, 1978.
70. Taylor DJ, Braithwaite RA: Cardiac effects of tricyclic antidepressant medication: A preliminary study of nortriptyline. *Br Heart J* 40:1005, 1978.
71. Raeder EA, Burckhardt D, Neubauer H, et al: Long-term triand tetracyclic antidepressants, myocardial contractility, and cardiac rhythm. *Br Med J* 2:666, 1978.
72. Veith RC, Raskind MA, Caldwell JH, et al: Cardiovascular effects

of tricyclic antidepressants in depressed patients with chronic heart disease. *N Engl J Med* 306:954, 1982.

73. Pitts F: Medical psychology of ECT, in Abrams R, Essman WB (eds): *Electroconvulsive Therapy: Biological Foundations and Clinical Applications.* New York, SP Medical and Scientific Books, 1982.

74. Risch SC, Groom GP, Janowsky D: The effects of psychotropic drugs on the cardiovascular system. *J Clin Psychiatry* 43(sec 2):16, 1982.

75. Vessell ES, Passananti T, Green FE: Impairment of drug metabolism in man by allopurinol and nortriptyline. *N Engl J Med* 283:1484, 1970.

76. Rauch PK, Jenike MA: Digoxin toxicity possibly precipitated by trazodone. *Psychosomatics* 25:334, 1984.

77. Orr DA, Bramble MG: Tricyclic antidepressant poisoning and prolonged external cardiac massage during asystole. *Br Med J* 283:1107, 1981.

78. DeVane CL: Pharmacokinetics of the selective serotonin reuptake inhibitors. *J Clin Psychiatry* 54[suppl]:13, 1992.

79. Hwang AS, Magraw RM: Syndrome of inappropriate secretion of antidiuretic hormone due to fluoxetine. (Letter.) *Am J Psychiatry* 146:399, 1989.

80. Miller LG, Bowman RC, Mann D, et al: A case of fluoxetine induced serum sickness. *Am J Psychiatry* 146:1616, 1989.

81. Kline MD: Fluoxetine and anorgasmia. (Letter.) *Am J Psychiatry* 146:804, 1989.

82. Salama AA, Shafey M: A case of severe lithium toxicity by combined fluoxetine and lithium carbonate (Letter). *Am J Psychiatry* 146:278, 1989.

83. Teicher MH, Glod C, Cole JO: Emergence of intense suicidal preoccupation during fluoxetine treatment. *Am J Psychiatry* 147:207, 1990.

84. Rickels K, Schweizer E: Clinical overview of serotonin reuptake inhibitors. *J Clin Psychiatry* 51[Suppl B]:9, 1990

85. Fisch C: Effect of fluoxetine on the electrocardiogram. *J Clin Psychiatry* 46(3, sec 2):42, 1985.

86. Tulloch IF, Johnson AM: The pharmacologic profile of paroxetine: A new selective serotonin reuptake inhibitor. *J Clin Psychiatry* 53[Suppl]:7, 1992.

87. Aranow RB, Hudson JI, Pope HG, et al: Elevated antidepressant plasma levels after addition of fluoxetine. *Am J Psychiatry* 146:911, 1989.

88. Ellison JM, Milofsky JE, Ely E: Fluoxetine-induced bradycardia and syncope in two patients [see comments]. *J Clin Psychiatry* 51:385, 1990.

89. Feder R: Bradycardia and syncope induced by fluoxetine [Letter; comment]. *J Clin Psychiatry* 52:139, 1991.

90. Buff DD, Brenner R, Kirtane SS, et al: Dysrhythmia associated with fluoxetine treatment in an elderly patient with cardiac disease. *J Clin Psychiatry* 52:174, 1991.

91. Feighner JP, Boyer WF, Tyler DL, et al: Adverse consequences of fluoxetine-MAOI combination therapy. *J Clin Psychiatry* 51:222, 1990.

92. Cassem NH: Cardiovascular effects of antidepressants. *J Clin Psychiatry* 43(11, Sec 2):22, 1982.

93. Edwards JG, Goldie A: Mianserin, maprotiline, and intracardiac conduction. *Br J Pharmacol* 15(suppl):249s, 1983.

94. Ramrize AL: Seizures associated with maprotiline. *Am J Psychiatry* 140:509, 1983.

95. Richelson E: Antimuscarinic and other receptor-blocking properties of antidepressants. *Mayo Clin Proc* 58:40, 1983.

96. Burgess CD, Hames TK, George CF: The electrocardiographic and anticholinergic effects of trazodone and imipramine in man. *Eur J Clin Pharmacol* 23:417, 1982.

97. Hayes RL, Gerner RH, Fairbanks L, et al: ECG findings in geriatric depressives given trazodone, placebo, or imipramine. *J Clin Psychiatry* 44:180, 1983.

98. Rausch JL, Pavlinac DM, Newman PE: Complete heart block following a single dose of trazodone. *Am J Psychiatry* 141:1472, 1984.

99. Lippmann SB: Trazodone cardiac effects. *Int Drug Ther Newsletter* 20:29, 1985.

100. Glassman AH: The newer antidepressant drugs and their cardiovascular effects. *Psychopharmacol Bull* 20:272, 1984.

101. Jami NN, Wise TN, Kass E, et al: Trazadone and anorgasmia. (Letter.) *Am J Psychiatry* 145:896, 1988.

102. Pi EH, Simpson GM: New antidepressants: A review. *Hosp Formul* 20:580, 1985.

103. Pumariega AJ, Muller B, Rivers-Bulkeley N: Acute renal failure secondary to amoxapine overdose. *JAMA* 248:1092, 1982.

104. Wenger TL, Stern WC: The cardiovascular profile of bupropion. *J Clin Psychiatry* 44(5, sec 2):176, 1983.

105. Goldman LS, Alexander RC, Luchins DJ: Monoamine oxidase inhibitors and tricyclic antidepressants: Comparison of their cardiovascular effects. *J Clin Psychiatry* 47:225, 1986.

106. Gorelick DA, Marder SR, Sack D, et al: Atrial flutter/fibrillation associated with tranylcypromine treatment. *J Clin Psychopharmacol* 1:402, 1981.

107. Rabkin JG, Quitkin FM, McGrath P, et al: Adverse reactions to monoamine oxidase inhibitors: II. Treatment correlates and clinical management. *J Clin Psychopharmacol* 5:2, 1985.

108. Robinson DS, Nies A, Ravaris CL, et al: Clinical pharmacology of phenelzine. *Arch Gen Psychiatry* 35:629, 1978.

109. Kronig MH, Roose SP, Walsh BT, et al: Blood pressure effects of phenelzine. *J Clin Psychopharmacol* 3:307, 1983.

110. Mallinger AG, Edwards DJ, Himmelhoch JM, et al: Pharmacokinetics of tranylcypromine in patients who are depressed: Relationship to cardiovascular effects. *Clin Pharmacol Ther* 40:444, 1986.

111. Stockley IH: Monoamine oxidase inhibitors, part 2: Interactions with antihypertensive agents, hypoglycemics, CNS depressants, narcotics, and antiparkinsonian agents. *Pharm J* 211:95, 1973.

112. Gaultieri CT, Powell SF: Psychoactive drug interactions. *J Clin Psychiatry* 39:720, 1978.

113. Moser M: Experience with isocarboxazid. *JAMA* 176:276, 1961.

114. Eade NR, Penton KW: The effect of phenelzine and tranylcypromine on the degradation of meperidine. *J Pharmacol Exp Ther* 173:31, 1970.

115. Frieden J: Propranolol as an antiarrhythmic agent. *Am Heart J* 75:283, 1967.

116. Baldessarini RJ: Drugs and the treatment of psychiatric disorders, in Goodman GA, Goodman LS, Gilman A (eds): *The Pharmacological Basis of Therapeutics.* 6th ed. New York, Macmillan, 1980.

117. Wheatley D: Amphetamines in general practice: Their use in depression and anxiety. *Semin Psychiatry* 1:163, 1969.

118. Myerson A: The effect of benzedrine sulfate on mood and fatigue in normal and neurotic persons. *Arch Neurol Psychiatry* 36:816, 1936.

119. Silberman EK, Reus VI, Jimerson DC, et al: Heterogeneity of amphetamine response in depressed patients. *Am J Psychiatry* 138:1302, 1981.

120. Kerenyi AB, Koranyi EK, Sawer-Foner GJ: Depressive states and drugs: III. Use of methylphenidate (Ritalin) in open psychiatric settings and in office practice. *Can Med Assoc J* 83:1249, 1960.

121. Kaplitz SE: Withdrawn, apathetic geriatric patients responsive to methylphenidate. *J Am Geriatr Soc* 23:271, 1975.

122. Kaufmann M, Murray G, Cassem N: Use of psychostimulants in medically ill depressed patients. *Psychosomatics* 23:817, 1982.

123. Woods SW, Tesar GE, Murray GB, et al: Psychostimulant treatment of depressive disorders secondary to medical illness. *J Clin Psychiatry* 47:12, 1986.

124. Katon W, Raskind M: Treatment of depression in the medically ill elderly with methylphenidate. *Am J Psychiatry* 137:963, 1980.

125. Rosenberg PB, Ahmed I, Hurwitz S: Methylphenidate in depressed medically ill patients. *J Clin Psychiatry* 52:263, 1991.

126. Chiarello RJ, Cole JO: The use of psychostimulants in general psychiatry: A reconsideration. *Arch Gen Psychiatry* 44:286, 1987.

127. Askinazi C, Weintraub RJ, Karamouz N: Elderly depressed females as a possible subgroup of patients responsive to methylphenidate. *J Clin Psychiatry* 47:467, 1986.

128. Jefferson JW, Greist JH: Lithium and the kidney, in Davis JM, Greenblatt D (eds): *Psychopharmacology Update: New and Neglected Areas.* New York, Grune & Stratton, 1979.

129. Jefferson JW, Greist JH, Ackerman DL: *Lithium Encyclopedia for Clinical Practice.* Madison, WS, Lithium Information Center, 1983.

130. Wallin L, Alling C, Aurell M: Impairment of renal function in patients on long-term lithium treatment. *Clin Nephrol* 18:23, 1982.

131. Reisberg B, Gershon S: Side effects associated with lithium therapy. *Arch Gen Psychiatry* 36:879, 1979.

132. Ragheb M, Buchanan D, Frolich JC: Interaction of indomethacin

and ibuprofen with lithium in manic patients under a steady-state lithium level. *J Clin Psychiatry* 41:397, 1980.

133. Mitchell JE, Mackenzie TB: Cardiac effects of lithium therapy in man: A review. *J Clin Psychiatry* 43:47, 1982.

134. Schou M: Electrocardiographic changes during treatment with lithium and with drugs of the imipramine-type. *Acta Psychiatr Scand* [Suppl] 169:258, 1963.

135. Roose SP, Nurnberger JI, Dunner DL, et al: Cardiac sinus node dysfunction during lithium treatment. *Am J Psychiatry* 136:804, 1979.

136. Hagman A, Arnman K, Ryden L: Syncope caused by lithium treatment. Report of two cases and a prospective investigation of the prevalence of lithium-induced sinus node dysfunction. *Acta Med Scand* 205:467, 1979.

137. Lyman GH, Williams CC, Dinwoodie WR, et al: Sudden death in cancer patients receiving lithium. *J Clin Oncol* 2:1270, 1984.

138. Fawcett J, Edwards JH, Krautz HM, et al: Alprazolam: An antidepressant? Alprazolam, desipramine, and an alprazolam-desipramine combination in the treatment of adult depressed outpatients. *J Clin Psychopharmacol* 7:295, 1987.

139. Rickels K, Chung HR, Csanalosi IB, et al: Alprazolam, diazepam, imipramine, and placebo in outpatients with major depression. *Arch Gen Psychiatry* 44:862, 1987.

140. Feighner JP, Aden GC, Fabre LF, et al: Comparison of alprazolam, imipramine and placebo in the treatment of depression. *JAMA* 249:3057, 1983.

141. Brody JI, Bellet S: The use of electric shock therapy in patients with cardiovascular disease. *Am J Med Sci* 233:40, 1957.

142. Alexander SP, Gahagan LH: Deaths following electrotherapy. *JAMA* 161:577, 1956.

143. Sisler GC, Wilt JC: Immediate coronary thrombosis following electric convulsive therapy. *Am J Psychiatry* 110:354, 1953.

144. Lewis WH, Richardson JD, Gahagan LH: Cardiovascular disturbances and their management in modified electrotherapy for psychiatric illness. *N Engl J Med* 252:1016, 1955.

145. McKenna G, Engle R, Brooks H, et al: Cardiac arrhythmias during electroshock therapy: Significance, prevention, and treatment. *Am J Psychiatry* 127:530, 1970.

146. Green R, Woods A: Effects of modified ECT on the electrocardiogram. *Br Med J* 1:1503, 1955.

147. Dec GW, Stern TA, Welch C: The effects of electroconvulsive therapy on serial electrocardiograms and serum cardiac enzyme values: A prospective study of depressed hospitalized inpatients. *JAMA* 253:2525, 1985.

148. Gerring JP, Shields HM: The identification and management of patients with a high risk for cardiac arrhythmias during modified ECT. *J Clin Psychiatry* 43:140, 1982.

149. Leibenluft E, Goldberg RL: The suicidal, terminally ill patient with depression. *Psychosomatics* 29(4):379, 1988.

224. *Suicide*

John L. Shuster and Theodore A. Stern

Attempted suicide is one of the most common noncardiac causes for admission to intensive care units (ICUs) [1]. The care of patients who have attempted suicide and of those critically ill individuals who develop suicidal ideation (caused by major psychiatric disorders, or by despair over their medical illness) is an important part of intensive care medicine [2,3]. The keys to proper treatment are recognition of the problem, informed and careful evaluation, and avoidance of common pitfalls.

Suicide is the tenth leading cause of death in the United States [4], accounting for an estimated 25,000 deaths each year [4]. Approximately one of every nine suicide attempts results in death [5].

Drug ingestion is the most common method of attempted suicide, accounting for 1 to 2 percent of all emergency room visits [5] and for approximately 5 percent of all ICU admissions [1]. Survivors of other means of attempted suicide (e.g., gunshot, jumping from a height, hanging, self-mutilation, and self-immolation) commonly sustain injuries that necessitate intensive care.

The Evaluation of Suicidal Risk

Unfortunately, there are no reliable, easily administered tests for suicidal risk; evaluation is based on clinical judgment. The evaluator needs a detailed understanding of the patient's situation to assess the current risk of suicide. Consideration should also be given to the risk of suicide in the near future. Elements of suicide evaluation are outlined in Table 224-1.

Obviously, survivors of attempted suicide need evaluation. Anyone who complains of suicidal thoughts or urges during ICU admission should always be evaluated, even in the absence of attempted suicide. Evaluation should be considered for those patients whose self-destructive actions suggest that they may have acted with suicidal intent [2,3]. If the diagnosis of suicidal ideation or behavior is not considered, it will not be made.

The approach to the suicidal patient should be calm and uncritical. All suicide attempts should be taken seriously, even those that seem overtly manipulative. Effort should be made to establish rapport with the patient before formal examination begins. It is helpful for the interviewer to introduce himself or herself and to create some degree of privacy in the interview setting. Offers of assistance and actions that maximize the patient's physical comfort during the interview (e.g., providing a drink of water or changing the position of the bed) foster an atmosphere of concern. Empathic connection with the evaluator allows the suicidal patient, who is often angry, frightened, and confused, to trust the examiner and to supply a full and accurate history. Suicidal individuals are usually ambivalent about their wish to die, and even brief contact with a concerned person can be lifesaving.

Evaluation of suicidal potential is an emergency procedure. Failure to assess suicidal potential when it has been suspected is a potentially catastrophic error in patient care. Balanced against the patient's desire for privacy and the maintenance of confidentiality in the doctor-patient relationship is the physician's need for a full and accurate history. All information that can be obtained (e.g., collateral information from family and friends of the patient) should be obtained during the assessment of suicidal risk. This is crucial because patients are often

Table 224-1. Assessment of Suicidal Risk

Take a calm, noncritical approach.
Take suicide attempts seriously.
Establish rapport with the patient.
Obtain collateral history, if available.
Perform a mental status examination and assess:
    General appearance
    Interactive style
    Level of consciousness
    Speech
    Thought content
    Thought process
    Mood
    Cognitive function
    Insight and judgment
Search for the presence of risk factors.
Evaluate suicidal ideation.
    Presence of suicidal thoughts
    Suicide plan
    Suicidal intent
    A wish to die
    Future orientation
    A specific reason to commit suicide now
    A theme of anger, loss, hopelessness, or desperation
If suicide has been attempted, assess:
    The risk-rescue ratio
    The perceived lethality of the attempt
    Any changes in precipitating circumstances
    The degree of impulsivity present

unaware of or are hesitant to share information relevant to their care. Although efforts should always be made to maintain confidentiality and to develop an alliance with the patient, the life-and-death circumstances of suicide evaluation obviate most concerns about obtaining formal consent from the patient before speaking with those familiar with pertinent history.

The evaluation itself consists of several elements: a formal mental status examination, elaboration of suicidal thoughts and behaviors, and assessment of the presence of risk factors for suicide. Mental status examination [6] includes observation of the patient's appearance, style of interaction, speech, and level of consciousness. Mood, cognitive function, insight, judgment, and the content and process of thought should all be examined. Particular attention should be paid to a search for the signs of major affective disorders, psychotic disorders, or cognitive dysfunction, all of which can impair judgment or impulse control.

The patient should be directly questioned about suicidal thoughts. Contrary to common belief, asking about suicide does not plant the thought in the mind of the nonsuicidal patient. Furthermore, many depressed patients with suicidal ideation are often relieved when they are given the opportunity to tell someone of their distress. Questions about suicidal thoughts should be posed tactfully and may be introduced gradually when obtaining the history of illness or when asking about the presence of depressive symptoms. The question "Has it ever seemed like things just aren't worth it?" may lead to the more direct question "Have you gotten so depressed that you've considered killing yourself?" Such inquiries can lead to a more thorough exploration of suicidal ideation and intent. These questions should be asked in a kind but matter-of-fact manner, without apology, as one might do in any routine examination.

If the patient answers "yes" to such questions, more details (about ideas, wishes, and motives regarding suicide) should be obtained. Elaboration of the suicide plan, if the patient has one, is very important. Has a method been chosen? How detailed is the plan? Are the means available? How lethal is the chosen method? The patient should also be questioned about the pres-

ence of a wish or intent to die. The degree to which an individual wants to die can be elicited in part by asking about future plans: "What do you see yourself doing 5 years from now?" or "What things are you still looking forward to doing or seeing?" It is crucial to determine why the patient has become suicidal at this particular time; this should lead to an examination of precipitants and current life events. The reasons for suicide (e.g., anger, loss, hopelessness, desperation) should also be explored in the context of these life events. Social supports available to the patient and prohibitions (including cultural or religious prohibitions) to suicide should also be considered.

When interviewing survivors of a suicide attempt, additional information should be obtained. Assessment should be made of the true danger of the attempt and the chances of rescue or discovery (i.e., the risk-rescue ratio) [7]. It is important to determine how deadly the patient perceived the attempt to be. Did the patient think he or she would die? Was the patient disappointed to have survived? Evaluators should try to find out which (if any) of the precipitating circumstances have changed. If little or nothing has changed since the suicide attempt, the risk of another attempt is high. Patients who make calculated, premeditated suicide attempts are at higher risk for a repeat attempt than are those who have made impulsive attempts (e.g., in a fit of anger, to get attention, to seek revenge against someone, or while intoxicated); an effort should be made to assess the degree of impulsivity associated with an attempt.

Finally, the suicide evaluation should be guided by knowledge of the risk factors for suicide [4,8,9,10]. These risk factors are not infallible predictors of suicidal behavior. They should be placed in the context of a comprehensive clinical evaluation. Risk factors should serve only as guides for clinicians in trying to determine the likelihood of subsequent suicidal behavior. Risk factors for suicide are summarized in Table 224-2.

The most important risk factor for suicide is the presence of psychiatric illness. Major depression accounts for about 50 percent of completed suicides [8]; approximately 15 percent of patients with major depressive illness eventually die by suicide [4]. The features of depression as described in the *Diagnostic and Statistical Manual of Mental Disorders, Fourth Edition, Revised* (DSM-IV) [11] are depressed mood, disturbed sleep (usually decreased sleep and early morning awakening, but on occasion increased amounts of sleep), decreased interest or anhedonia, feelings of guilt or worthlessness, loss of energy, decreased ability to concentrate, disturbed appetite (usually weight loss, but on occasion weight gain), abnormal psycho-

Table 224-2. Risk Factors for Suicide

Major psychiatric illness
    Depression
    Alcohol or substance abuse
    Psychosis
    Character disorder
    Panic disorder/panic attacks
History of suicide attempts
Family history of suicide
Social factors
    Marital status (never married, widowed, divorced)
    Unemployment
    Social isolation, living alone
    Higher education
Age (advanced age, adolescence)
Sex (male)
Race (white)
Chronic or terminal illness
Organic brain syndromes

motor activity (i.e., agitation or psychomotor retardation), and recurrent thoughts of death or suicidal ideation. Severely depressed patients are not difficult to diagnose. They are obviously sad and slow to respond; they appear extremely weak or ill; and they feel hopeless. Depression occurs on a continuum ranging from severe depression to "having the blues." Some cases of severe depression are complicated by psychotic thoughts (including somatic delusions or hallucinations), thus compounding their suicidal risk. For a more complete discussion of the recognition and treatment of depressed patients in the ICU see Chapter 223.

Alcoholism and substance abuse account for another 25 percent of completed suicides [4,12]. Intoxication impairs judgment and impulse control and may thus facilitate suicide attempts of depressed patients. Furthermore, long-term use of drugs such as alcohol, sedatives, and stimulants has adverse effects on mood (i.e., they may induce a depressive state). Most suicidal, intoxicated patients will no longer be suicidal when the effects of the intoxicant (or intoxicants) wear off. These individuals should be detained, should have their safety assured, and should be reevaluated when they are sober.

Psychotic illnesses (schizophrenia, mania, psychotic depression) account for 10 percent of completed suicides [4]. Paranoia and guardedness may interfere with patient cooperation during the suicide evaluation. Paranoid individuals may better tolerate a diagnostic interview if the examiner adopts a relaxed, non-threatening stance and avoids prolonged direct eye contact or sudden, unexpected moves. Disorders of thought and faulty reality testing can interfere with judgment. Patients with hallucinations that instruct or command them to harm themselves are at particular risk and should almost always be hospitalized.

Patients with character disorders account for about 5 percent of completed suicides [4] and a significantly higher percentage of suicide attempts. Personality disorders characterized by impulsivity (e.g., borderline personality disorder) [11] predispose patients to suicidal gestures or attempts. Such patients are likely to make high-risk attempts if they are not taken seriously. It must be remembered that even the most manipulative of suicide gestures can be fatal if the patient miscalculates the lethal dose or misjudges the reactions or plans of others who were expected to intervene. For example, some patients overdose on acetaminophen as a suicide gesture, not understanding the potential danger associated with this over-the-counter medicine. Chapter 225 deals with personality disorders in greater detail.

Patients with panic disorder (or who have panic attacks without meeting full criteria for the disorder) have been shown to have a risk of suicidal ideation and suicide attempts approximately three times greater than a group with other psychiatric diagnoses and approximately 18 times greater than persons without a psychiatric diagnosis [13]. In this study, about 20 percent of those with panic disorder had a previous history of suicide attempts [13].

A history of suicide attempts is an important risk factor. Fifty percent of patients who successfully complete suicide [8] and more than 50 percent of those who take near-fatal overdoses [14] have made previous attempts. One study has shown that 6 percent of patients who have taken a near-fatal drug overdose died by suicide after 10 months of follow-up [14]. Other studies of serious suicide attempts show mortality rates of up to 8 percent at 5 years [15,16]. Family history of suicide also conveys a greater risk, because it provides a behavioral model for resolution of life stresses [8].

Social factors affect the risk of suicide. Patients who have never married are at highest risk, followed by widowed patients, separated and divorced patients, and married patients without children. Those the least at risk are married patients with children [3,10,17]. Unemployment is a risk factor [8], as is living alone or having recently lost a loved one [8]. Higher education, especially in the medical profession, is associated with an increased risk of suicide [8].

Increasing age is correlated with an increased suicidal risk; rates of suicide generally increase steadily with advancing age, although there may be a plateau in suicide rates in females near age 60 [3]. Mood disorders, particularly depression, continue to be important risk factors for attempted suicide in the elderly. In one recent study, 80 percent of geriatric patients attempting suicide had a major depressive syndrome [18]. There is also evidence of recent and substantial increases in the suicide rate among adolescents [19,20].

Male sex is a risk factor: boys and men are two to three times more likely to complete suicide, despite the fact that girls and women are three to four times more likely to attempt suicide [3]. This is probably related to the tendency for boys and men to choose more lethal means (e.g., using a gun or jumping from a height).

Whites are more likely to kill themselves than nonwhites, although among all races American Indians are at the highest risk for suicide.

Chronic or terminal illness and chronic pain also increase suicide risk, especially when the patient feels hopeless [10,21,22]. Patients with cardiorespiratory illnesses [22] and cancer [23] may have an increased suicidal risk. A survey of 3478 renal dialysis patients indicated a suicide rate more than 400 times that of the general population [21]. Recent data suggest that HIV-infected individuals are also at substantially increased risk of suicide, with a suicide rate ranging from 16.3 to 66.1 times that seen in the general population [24,25]. Finally, the presence of an organic brain syndrome elevates the risk of self-harm (ranging from injury to suicide). Confused and delirious patients may be physically agitated, unable to protect themselves from danger, or unable to resist their own destructive impulses.

The nature of suicidal behavior among general hospital patients deserves some mention. Impulsive and unexpected suicide attempts by medical and surgical inpatients were studied over a 7-year period [10]. Reich and Kelly found that all 17 cases reviewed exhibited increasing anger, agitation, a sudden mood swing, or an acute psychotic episode before the attempt. Almost all the attempts were related to disruption in the relationship with caregivers. Fifteen of the 17 patients suffered from mental disorders; patients with personality disorders commonly attempted suicide after the validity of their presenting complaints had been challenged. (Incidentally, none of these attempts occurred in an ICU.)

Treatment of Suicidal Patients

Successful treatment of suicidal individuals requires that their safety be assured. Most suicides are preventable. With treatment of the underlying problems and with passage of time, most suicidal ideation resolves. Patient safety must be maintained until the imminent risk of suicide is past. The ICU can be a difficult place to ensure safety in alert, actively suicidal patients. The suicidal patient should not be left unattended, and access to potential means of self-injury (e.g., glass bottles, scissors, and open windows) should be eliminated. Depending on the size, strength, impulsivity, and intent of the suicidal patient, safety can be assured by one-to-one staff supervision, or by mechanical (wrist and ankle) or chemical (sedation) restraint. If the patient is too strong, impulsive, or agitated to be safely managed with one-to-one supervision, or if staff are unavailable to monitor the patient constantly (as is usually the case in ICU settings), mechanical restraints should be applied. Conservative care is warranted, and restraint should be used when any question of patient safety remains.

Suicide evaluations are complicated and difficult to perform. Multiple factors must be considered (as detailed in the section on evaluation). The evaluator should always err on the side of patient safety. If uncertain as to the proper decision, safety measures should be maintained until psychiatric consultation or transfer to a psychiatric facility can be arranged.

Thorough documentation of the thought process behind the decision to institute or discontinue suicide precautions should be provided for the medical record. It is difficult, if not impossible, to do this in a brief note. As long as decisions regarding suicidal patients are made thoughtfully, considering the elements outlined above and keeping the patient's best interest in mind, there should be little danger of liability. As previously stated, a conservative approach is warranted. It would be much easier to defend a physician against charges of battery brought by a patient who had been restrained against his or her will than it would be to defend a physician against charges of negligence after injury or death after inadequate protection of a patient from known self-destructive urges [2].

Options for disposition after the ICU stay range from discharge home to involuntary admission to a locked psychiatric unit. Once the problems necessitating ICU or general hospital admission are resolved, disposition can be considered. If a patient is judged to be at low risk for suicide, has social supports, and is considered reliable enough to comply with follow-up treatment, a simple discharge with outpatient psychiatric care can be arranged. If the clinician cannot be reasonably certain that the patient will remain safe, psychiatric hospitalization should be arranged. Voluntary admission is ideal, because patient cooperation maximizes the chances for successful treatment. If the patient is unable to control suicidal impulses or urges, or is thought to be at high risk for a repeated suicide attempt, admission to an open psychiatric unit is not appropriate, and a locked facility should be found. If a patient at high risk for suicide refuses voluntary hospitalization, he or she should be sent involuntarily to a locked psychiatric unit for his or her own safety.

Common Problems in Suicide Evaluation

Suicidal patients can be difficult to evaluate. Severe depression, intoxication, serious injury, medical complications, as well as anger, confusion, or shame can hamper patient cooperation. Such impediments to examination can make a challenging task impossible. This section offers a few hints for the management of difficult suicidal patients.

Intoxicated or organically impaired patients cannot be reliably evaluated. If they are intoxicated, they should be allowed to sober up before completing the evaluation. However, useful information can often be obtained while the individual is intoxicated and when the individual is awakening from a stuporous state. At these times, even though cognition may be impaired, psychological defenses may be overridden by the intoxicating agent and the real reasons behind a suicide attempt and the depth of suicidal ideation may be detected.

Efforts should be made to define and treat organic mental disturbances. Angry or threatening patients should be evaluated in the presence of others (preferably hospital security officers).

Restraints should be applied as indicated to assure patient safety (or staff safety if the risk of assault is high). Occasionally, suicidal patients refuse to answer evaluation questions in spite of efforts to establish rapport. A calm but firm statement such as, "I'd like to figure out how to be of help, but I can't do that without some information from you" is useful. Safety measures should not be discontinued until the evaluation has been completed, and uncooperative patients should be informed of this policy. Patients who are potentially suicidal should not be allowed to sign out against medical advice, and competency to make informed decisions should be carefully considered if suicidal patients refuse medical treatments.

A frequent issue during the assessment of suicidal patients is the need for restraint. Patients often complain, "I want these restraints off, and I refuse to cooperate until they are removed." Such statements should be met by an attempt to enlist the patient's cooperation toward this goal, followed by a calm reminder of the importance of the evaluation. "We both agree that the restraints should come off if you don't need them. I am very concerned about your safety, and I need you to answer some questions before I can decide if it's safe to remove the restraints." Patients should not be allowed to talk their way out of appropriate safety measures until a full suicide assessment has been performed.

The evaluator's feelings and reactions to the patient are an additional source of difficulty in the assessment of suicide risk. Also known as countertransference [26], these feelings must be recognized and kept from inappropriately affecting decisions about the patient. Staff can feel anger toward the suicidal patient for a variety of reasons. They may feel that the patient has done something stupid or careless, or that the patient has caused suffering for those who care for him. Anger can lead to a wish to punish the patient by such actions as initiating an inappropriate transfer to a psychiatric facility for a low-risk patient or inappropriately discharging a high-risk patient. Physician denial of a patient's emotional problems (and suicidality) could jeopardize the patient's evaluation and the commencement of life-saving treatment. Depressive symptoms can be contagious; suicidal patients can elicit depressed and hopeless feelings in the ICU staff, impeding proper evaluation and treatment.

Overidentification with patients is common when patients and examiners share personality characteristics. Dangers of overidentification arise when the evaluator's thought "I would never commit suicide" becomes translated into "This patient would never commit suicide." Such thinking interferes with thorough and objective evaluation. An overidentified examiner may try to talk the patient out of his or her suicidality. This may be ineffective and may be perceived by the patient as a painful lack of empathy and understanding, paradoxically increasing the risk of suicide. Suicidal evaluations of "very important patients" (VIPs) are also especially difficult. Staff must be careful not to discharge a suicidal VIP inappropriately as a special favor or to hospitalize a patient unnecessarily for fear of adverse publicity. VIPs should be evaluated for suicide in a fashion similar to that for the non-VIP. Consultation with more experienced clinicians is often very useful in such instances.

The prediction of suicidal risk is exceedingly difficult. Because there are no questionnaires or instruments that accurately predict the risk of future suicide, clinical assessment and judgment remain our best resources. The relatively low base incidence of suicide (about 12:100,000 persons annually) [4] and the fluctuating nature of suicidal ideation guarantee statistically unreliable prediction of suicide [27,28,29]. A multiple logistic regression model using several of the risk factors mentioned above failed to identify any of the 46 patients who committed suicide over a 14-year period from a group of 1906 persons with affective disorders [30]. The only reasonably reliable data regarding suicide assessment pertain to the assessment of risk of suicide in the present and in the near future. Some investigators believe that any suicide assessment is valid for only 24 to 48 hours after examination [31]. Still, there is no reason to abandon suicide evaluation. High-risk patients can be identified and directed toward providers of appropriate care. Causes of suicide are largely treatable. In fact, a concerned and empathic approach during suicide evaluation may well be lifesaving.

Summary

Attempted suicide is one of the most common reasons for admission to an ICU. After injuries and medical complications are treated, psychological evaluation and assessment of suicidal risk should quickly follow. Evaluation consists of full mental status examination; detailed exploration of the suicidal symptoms, ideation, or attempt; and consideration of risk factors. Maintenance of patient safety is crucial, and all necessary steps should be taken to ensure it. A conservative approach is indicated to guarantee patient safety. Suicide evaluations are difficult and are commonly complicated by poor patient cooperation and the evaluator's own feelings toward or about the patient. The suicide evaluation is essentially an informed, carefully considered, clinical judgment. It has little long-term statistical predictive reliability, but is an important and valuable intervention. Proper treatment of causes of suicidal intent can be lifesaving, and the problem must be recognized and understood before appropriate treatment can be instituted.

References

1. Thibault GE, Mulley AG, Barnett GO, et al: Medical intensive care: Indications, interventions, and outcomes. *N Engl J Med* 302:938, 1980.
2. Hackett TP, Stern TA: Suicide and other disruptive states, in Hackett TP, Cassem NH (eds): *Massachusetts General Hospital Handbook of General Hospital Psychiatry.* Littleton, MA, PSG Publishing, 1987.
3. Hyman SE: The suicidal patient, in Hyman SE (ed): *Manual of Psychiatric Emergencies.* 2nd ed. Boston, Little, Brown, 1988.
4. Miles CP: Conditions predisposing to suicide: A review. *J Nerv Ment Dis* 164:231, 1977.
5. O'Brien JP: Increase in suicide attempts by drug ingestion: The Boston experience; 1964-1974. *Arch Gen Psychiatry* 34:1165, 1977.
6. Hyman SE: The emergency psychiatric evaluation, including the mental status examination, in Hyman SE (ed): *Manual of Psychiatric Emergencies.* 2nd ed. Boston, Little, Brown, 1988.
7. Weisman AD, Worden JW: Risk-rescue rating in suicide assessment. *Arch Gen Psychiatry* 26:553, 1972.
8. Roy A: Risk factors for suicide in psychiatric patients. *Arch Gen Psychiatry* 39:1089, 1982.
9. Barraclough B, Bunch J, Nelson B, et al: A hundred cases of suicide: Clinical aspects. *Br J Psychiatry* 125:355, 1974.
10. Reich P, Kelly MJ: Suicide attempts by hospitalized medical and surgical patients. *N Engl J Med* 294:298, 1976.
11. American Psychiatric Association: *Diagnostic and Statistical Manual of Mental Disorders, Fourth Edition, Revised.* Washington, DC, American Psychiatric Association, 1994.
12. Frances RJ, Franklin J, Flavin, DK: Suicide and alcoholism. *Am J Drug Alcohol Abuse* 13: 327, 1987.
13. Weissman MM, Klerman GL, Markowitz JS, et al: Suicidal ideation and suicide attempts in panic disorder and attacks. *N Engl J Med* 321:1209, 1989.
14. Stern TA, Mulley AG, Thibault GE: Life-threatening drug overdose: Precipitants and prognosis. *JAMA* 251:1983, 1984.
15. Motto JA: Suicide attempts: A longitudinal view. *Arch Gen Psychiatry* 13:516, 1965.
16. Rosen DH: The serious suicide attempt: Five-year follow-up study of 886 patients. *JAMA* 235:2105, 1976.
17. Smith JC, Mercy JA, Conn JM: Marital status and the risk of suicide. *Am J Public Health* 78:78, 1988.
18. Lyness JM, Conwell Y, Nelson JC: Suicide attempts in elderly psychiatric inpatients. *J Am Geriatr Soc* 40:320, 1992.
19. Holinger CP: Adolescent suicide: An epidemiological study of recent trends. *Am J Psychiatry* 135:754, 1978.
20. Hellon CP, Solomon MI: Suicide and age in Alberta, Canada, 1951-1977: The changing profile. *Arch Gen Psychiatry* 37:505, 1980.
21. Abram HS, Moore GL, Westervelt FB: Suicidal behavior in chronic dialysis patients. *Am J Psychiatry* 127:1199, 1971.
22. Farberow NL, McKelligott JW, Cohen S, et al: Suicide among patients with cardiorespiratory illness. *JAMA* 195:422, 1966.
23. Farberow NL, Schneidman ES, Leonard CV: Suicide among general medical and surgical hospital patients with malignant neoplasms. *Med Bull Veterans Adm* 9:1, 1963.
24. Marzuk PM, Tierny H, Tardiff K, et al: Increased risk of suicide in persons with AIDS. *JAMA* 259:1333, 1988.
25. Plott RT, Benton SD, Winslade WJ: Suicide of AIDS patients in Texas: A preliminary report. *Tex Med* 85:40, 1989.
26. Maltsberger JT, Buie DH: Countertransference hate in the treatment of suicidal patients. *Arch Gen Psychiatry* 30:625, 1974.
27. Pokorny AD: Prediction of suicide in psychiatric patients. *Arch Gen Psychiatry* 40:249, 1983.
28. Murphy G: On suicide prediction and prevention. *Arch Gen Psychiatry* 40:343, 1983.
29. MacKinnon D, Farberow N: An assessment of the utility of suicide prediction. *Suicide Life Threat Behav* 6:86, 1975.
30. Goldstein RB, Black DW, Nasrallah A, et al: The prediction of suicide: Sensitivity, specificity, and predictive value of a multivariate model applied to suicide among 1906 patients with affective disorders. *Arch Gen Psychiatry* 48:418, 1991.
31. Rethinking approaches to prevention of suicide. *Clin Psychiatry News* 18:1, Jan. 1990.

225. Problematic Behaviors of Patients, Family, and Staff in the ICU

Carol A. Wool, Edith S. Geringer, and Theodore A. Stern

Intensive care units (ICUs) monitor and control life function with exacting detail, but treatment is not always smooth despite sophisticated knowledge and state-of-the-art equipment. Behavioral problems can thwart the normal flow of care for the critically ill patient. Some behavioral problems result from normal reactions to critical illness, others from personality or psychiatric problems predating the illness. When the patient is extremely ill and incapacitated, behavioral problems of family members can further complicate medical care. Interactions between staff, family, and patient can add even more difficulties.

Determinants of Behavior

ENVIRONMENT. ICU monitors, noise, lack of privacy, and paucity of windows, as well as the necessary medical procedures, have a pronounced impact on patients and families. Kornfeld [1] wrote about and studied ICUs when they were only about a decade old. He observed that sleep and sensory deprivation cause abnormal mental status in patients after major cardiac surgery. Keep and co-workers [2] studied patients in two different ICUs. One had no windows; the other had translucent glass that admitted light. They found that the incidence of hallucinations and delusions doubled in the absence of windows. Many authors [3–6] have noted the need to acknowledge that the ICU setting is in and of itself disturbing. With prudent efforts to humanize the physical setting, anxiety can be minimized.

EMOTIONAL RESPONSES TO CRITICAL ILLNESS. Each of us has an idiosyncratic emotional response to critical illness, but there are some common responses [7,8,9]. Anxiety, denial, and depression are common occurrences. Levenson and colleagues [8] studied denial in coronary care unit (CCU) patients with unstable angina and found that denial was correlated with favorable outcomes. They compared 14 "deniers" with 12 "non-deniers." There were no differences between the groups in social or demographic characteristics, history, risk factors, disease, or treatment. The deniers needed less time to stabilize in the ICU, suggesting that there may be no virtue in emphasizing bad news in a zealous attempt to disclose the whole truth [10]. Thomas and associates [11] found that when patients were given a chance to speak about their fears and feelings, they displayed anxiety more often than denial.

Conversely Krantz [12] equated myocardial infarction (MI) to a crisis and suggested that staff help patients use cognitive appraisal processes to reduce reactions to stress. Crises are more manageable if they are predictable, if the patient understands them, and if the patient feels in control. Others have extended this observation to the family of the patient. Fredrickson [13] showed that anxiety was contagious between family

and patient. Doer and Jones [14] showed that anxiety decreased markedly when the family was given a pamphlet describing ICU equipment and what they could expect to occur in the ICU. Families without this input displayed a marked increase in anxiety over the course of the illness. If the family can be made more aware of what is happening and can have a place to voice concerns [13,15,16,17], the patient benefits. An approach tailored to the individual case must balance the need of some patients to deny their medical status and the need of most families for concrete information and a sense of control.

Stress can influence all behavior. Normal adults may respond to critical illness by regressing to behaviors or beliefs that were appropriate and necessary for a dependent child. In fact, some regression is adaptive, because critically ill patients have their most basic needs met by others and must allow staff to feed, wash, and minister to them. Dependency becomes a problem when helplessness and passivity impede the work of the ICU staff. People with histories of abuse or with psychiatric disorders may respond to medically dependent positions with aggressive and obstructive behavior. For example, an individual with a history of sexual abuse might respond to invasive procedures, to being pinned down by monitors and tubes, or to receiving care when only partially conscious as a flashback to past abuse and respond with terror, panic, or even psychosis.

Psychiatric factors can profoundly alter the behavior of a patient. Depression, anxiety, and delirium can be treated effectively. The identification and treatment of these are covered at length in Chapters 221 to 223. It is crucial to include these treatable disorders in the differential diagnosis when considering behavioral problems (see Fig. 225-1). In addition, it is helpful to note that early experiences with caregivers can influence a patient's response to the ICU staff [18]. As noted above, a history of sexual or physical abuse will certainly be a hindrance. Patients in a physical crisis may at times transfer early negative experiences to the current situation.

PERSONALITY TYPES AND COPING STYLES. Each patient brings a unique personality and coping style to a crisis. Initially these factors might not be evident because of the extreme nature of the illness. During hospitalization, the individual's personality may interfere with progress. Bibring and Kahana [19] delineated seven personality types: oral-dependent, overly orderly or obsessive, overly anxious or histrionic, long-suffering or masochistic, isolated or schizoidal, guarded or paranoid, and superior or narcissistic (Tables 225-1 and 225-2). These personality types are variants of normal personality styles; each reacts to medical illness with a characteristic response. Under the stress of illness, the Bibring and Kahana personality types may show impairments characteristic of the *Diagnostic and Statistical Manual, Fourth Edition, Revised* [20] (DSM-IV) personality disorders. The relationship between each type and their clinical manifestations has been more fully described [21].

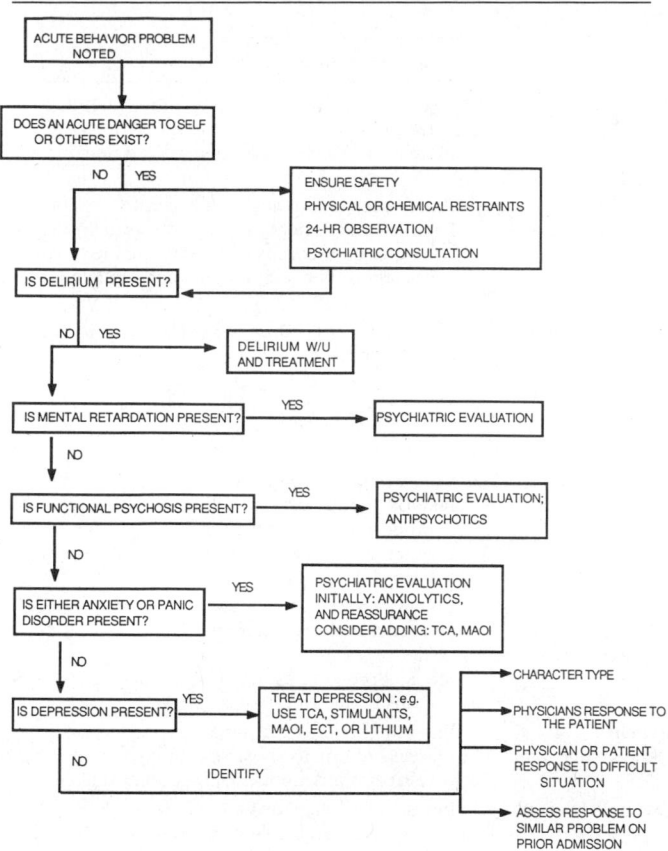

Fig. 225-1. Differential diagnostic schema for behavioral problems in the ICU.

Three common and difficult personality styles are the oral-dependent, the histrionic, and the obsessive. We discuss each with suggestions for management.

The Oral-Dependent or Borderline Personality. The oral-dependent personality type is impulsive, fears being alone, expects boundless care, and experiences illness as a threat of abandonment. The closest DSM-IV personality disorder is the borderline personality disorder. Borderline personality disorder is characterized by impulsivity, chaotic relationships, and an intense fear of being alone. In addition, the diagnostic criteria include unstable identity, recurrent suicidal threats, gestures or physically self-damaging behavior, chronic feelings of emptiness, and inappropriate displays of intense anger.

The strongest clue that a patient's problematic behaviors are caused by an underlying borderline personality disorder is the divisiveness that these patients create within the staff. Formerly friendly staff members can find themselves on opposite sides of an intense disagreement about the true nature and appropriate management of the patient, with both sides convinced that they are right. This occurs because patients with borderline personalities have an ability to present different sides of themselves to different staff members, and each picture appears entirely convincing. Unfortunately, impulsivity, intense fear of being engulfed, and fear of being alone lead these patients to change their behavior from moment to moment to maintain each and every relationship at the appropriate emotional distance. Because of this, it is crucial for staff members to acknowledge their disparate feelings in group meetings, if possible.

Appropriate limits should be set, and actions should be taken by the staff as a cohesive group. Staff can ameliorate difficult behavior by expressing a willingness to care for each patient as completely as possible. There are, of course, practical limits to care, and these must be communicated to the patient. The staff must agree on the limits, and they must present these limits as a unified front. Limits should be clearly explained, and should be adhered to, when possible. In this way the patient gets the care he or she needs consistently and safely (Tables 225-3 and 225-4).

The Obsessive Character. The obsessive patient pays excessive attention to order and detail and keeps emotions in check. Illness is experienced as punishment for letting things get out of control. It threatens the ability to stay in control. For example, an obsessive computer programmer, admitted to the CCU to rule out MI, was frightened by his surroundings. He was at first unable to ask questions lest the staff see his distress. As his anxiety increased, he questioned each new medical intervention intensely, became paralyzed by anxiety, and was unable to agree to any procedure.

For obsessive patients, staff should use a scientific, medical approach and give enough information so that patients can control their anxiety. If the patient is not yet paralyzed by indecision, it is helpful to encourage active participation in decisions (e.g., about exercise or diet) to help the patient feel a sense of control. Patients are also less anxious if given concrete ways to monitor their progress, for example, by encouraging a diabetic to keep a graph of blood glucose levels.

The Histrionic Character. A person with an overly anxious or histrionic character style tends to be very trusting, to personalize many things, and often to eroticize relationships with others. Anxiety is dealt with by denial or avoidance. These patients tend to dramatize everything. Their behaviors can be understood as a manifestation of insecurity and terror. Illness is experienced as a punishment for childhood wishes, and the person is left feeling defective, fearing loss of femininity or virility, and panicked that mutilation by the illness and possibly by the cure is ahead. For instance, a histrionic woman just removed from the ventilator may insist on having her hair washed and wearing makeup. Or, a histrionic man in the CCU may insist on showing the female staff members how virile he is by flirting and talking incessantly about his football-playing days or his success in business. Such a patient is trying desperately to bring the staff close to allay his fears and to prove his attractiveness and manliness.

If staff members find themselves being more disclosing of themselves, using first names, or talking about events or people in their personal lives, they should be alert to the fact that the patient may have a psychiatric problem. It helps to identify clearly the seductive attempts as inappropriate, while acknowledging the underlying distress. All the while, staff members have to maintain an appropriate professional distance, and state firm, nonpunitive limits. They also need to appreciate the patient's attractiveness and courage to offer reassurance against anxiety, and to provide opportunities for discussion of underlying fear. Specific consultation with psychiatric staff can be helpful.

Family Problems and Solutions

Studies show that the anxiety of the family is often conveyed to the patient with detrimental effect. Frederickson [13] studied

Table 225-1. Characteristics and Response to Illness of Seven Personality Types

Personality type	Leading traits	Response to stress or illness
Dependent	Craves special attention Urgently demands services Naively expects total care at all times Constantly seeks reassurance that others care	Fears total abandonment and subsequent help-lessness Increased anxiety leads to increased demands
Overly Orderly/Obsessive	Excessive attention to order and detail Ambiguity, unknowns, surprises increase anxiety Keeps tight reign on expression of emotion, pain, and fear	Illness seen as threat to self-control Double-bind: inner control prevents acknowledgment of confusion, hence unable to ask questions, hence ambiguity and anxiety increase
Dramatic/Histrionic	Trusting person, often forms sexualized relationships Deals with anxiety by denying, avoiding, repressing, or "forgetting" Dramatic presentations May have phobias	Illness experienced as an attack on femininity or masculinity
Long-Suffering/Martyr-Like/Masochistic	History of repeated suffering Steadfast and self-sacrificing Feel that they are unappreciated	Illness experienced as deserved punishment May be "good" patient if illness feels like yet another burden to shoulder May have increased noncompliance if suffering not acknowledged
Paranoid/Guarded	Wary, suspicious Hypersensitive to slights, real or imagined Can be quarrelsome when feeling persecuted	Illness perceived as an assault from the outside Feel unconsciously betrayed by himself for being ill Medical procedures may lead to increased suspicions and fear of being harmed
Superior Feelings/Narcissistic	Difficulty asking for or accepting help Must appear strong, competent, knowledgeable Fears dependence on others	Illness experienced as attack on perfection Increase efforts to show strength (excessive exercise) and independence (sign out AMA)
Aloof/Schizoid	Distant, unsociable, uninvolved with daily events Lives and works with minimum contact with others required. This protects against expected disappointments.	Illness forces closeness Can feel intolerable since protection against expected rejection has been removed Leads to more aloofness and withdrawal Illness is experienced as an intrusion

Adapted from Kahana RJ, Bibring GL: Personality types in medical management, in Zinberg NE (ed): *Psychiatry and Medical Practice in a General Hospital.* New York. International Universities Press, 1965, pp 108–123, with permission.

anxiety transmission in a CCU. He found that there was a very powerful anxiety contagion between family and CCU patient. He also found that such anxiety could be decreased by effective communication between family and staff. Halm [15] offered support groups to family members during a surgical intensive care unit (SICU) stay. Even though most family members attended only one group meeting, anxiety was significantly reduced. A variety of paradigms related to the families' impact on the response to illness have been described [22]. Many times a family meeting can elucidate some of these paradigms, but, if the situation is complex, the team might want to consult with a psychiatric consultant or family therapist.

Individuals in any family can bring their own problems to the ICU setting. Adult children who have depended on an elderly parent for their entire life might find it exceedingly difficult to limit care even when the situation is hopeless and further intervention will only prolong the suffering of the patient. A sibling who has long been estranged from the patient may arrive and insist on heroic care to assuage guilt over the long absence. Wasserman [23] studied the relatives' responses to patients who had attempted suicide. He found that a family request for "do not resuscitate" (DNR) orders sometimes reflected an angry response to the patient, which he termed passive euthanasia. In each of these situations staff members have to be ever cognizant of their duty as advocates for the patient.

Communication is always of critical importance. Ashworth [24] described how staff-patient and staff-visitor communication

is a major component of good CCU care. Obier and Haywood [25] described how therapeutic communication can reassure, instill hope, and alleviate stress. They encouraged staff members to help patients ventilate feelings, to be aware of the effect of an illness on a patient's self-esteem, to limit withdrawal, to support healthy denial, and to give information. Speedling [26] showed how early contact between staff, patient, and family has repercussions on the CCU stay as well as on rehabilitation goals and success. When families were excluded from the medical team's sphere of action, they in turn excluded themselves from active participation in the care of their family member. This was true whether the patient was spouse, sibling, or child. One study found that family difficulties created by the patient's illness significantly contributed to overall anxiety of the patient [27]. For example, when the patient was the primary caretaker of young children, the absence from home would greatly increase the stress in the entire family.

Staff Problems and Solutions

Working in the ICU is very difficult. Caring for critically ill patients, attending to the needs of patient and family, and delivering bad news all take their toll [28] (see Chap. 226 on Staff Stress). In addition, working for awhile in an ICU setting may

Table 225-2. Suggested Staff Management of Patients Based on Personality Type

Personality type	Suggested management
Dependent	Express willingness to care for patient as completely as possible
	Set limits, give thoughtful explanations of limits
	Make small concessions when possible
Overly Orderly/Obsessive	Use scientific medical approach; give enough information
	Help patient establish intellectual control over anxiety
	Allow patient to participate in decisions of care and management (e.g., monitoring diet, exercise)
Dramatic/Histrionic	Appreciate attractiveness, physical prowess and courage
	Give general reassurance (not detailed) if anxiety high
	Provide opportunities to discuss fears
Long Suffering/Masochistic	Appreciate difficulties being endured
	Do not attempt to comfort or assuage
	Present treatment as task that will help others
Paranoid/Guarded	Keep patient thoroughly informed of diagnostic and treatment strategies
	Listen to complaints and appreciate how hard things are to endure in light of illness and hospitalization
Superior Feelings/Narcissistic	Make patient an active partner in proceedings
	Acknowledge strengths
	Expect omissions in history (illness = weakness) and hence question extensively in important areas
Aloof/Schizoid	Accept and respect unsociability and insulation
	Continue interested, caring, and nonintrusive stance

Adapted from Kahana RJ, Bibring GL: Personality types in medical management, in Zinberg NE (ed): *Psychiatry and Medical Practice in a General Hospital.* New York. International Universities Press, 1965, pp 108–123, with permission.

desensitize us to the stresses experienced by patients and family members. Cochron and Ganong [4] caution us to keep an open mind concerning what the actual stress is for a patient. They compared the ratings of nurses and patients when asked about stress. There was a disparity between the two views. Nurses named "being tied down by tubes and not being in control of oneself" as the most stressful experiences for patients. Patients, in contrast, listed being thirsty and not being able to sleep as most stressful. They agreed about the high stress caused by having tubes in the nose and mouth and by being in pain. The nurses uniformly rated all experiences as more stressful than did the patients, and the nurses tended to rate psychological experiences as more stressful, while patients rated physical experiences as more stressful. This shows that, although tenure in an ICU can bring greater skill, it can also enure us to things that are the most troubling to a first-time visitor or patient.

Table 225-3. Examples of Limits

1. Offer medications on fixed-dose schedules with clearly indicated times of administration.
2. Define and adhere to rules (e.g., if and when cigarette smoking is allowed).
3. Specify a time and the amount of time that will be spent assisting patients with routine functions (e.g., baths and getting out of bed).

Table 225-4. Principles of Establishing Limits

1. Have a clear idea of one's own limits before approaching the patient.
2. Explanation of limits should be delivered in a clear, calm, and concise manner.
3. Limits must be presented as coming from the team, not an individual staff member. All staff should be apprised of the plan.
4. Consequences for overstepping limits should be determined at the time of limit setting; these should be explained clearly to the patient.
5. Decide in advance what, if any, areas are negotiable.

Eisendrath and Dunkle [29] have written about psychological problems encountered by ICU staff. They described stressful demands of the physical environment. The social unit may be organized along the lines of a family system with the medical director as father, head nurse as mother, and house and nursing staff as children, giving rise to both supports and stressors. The psychological environment of a unit may include the expectation of producing cures with consequent disappointment when deaths occur. This can be alleviated if staff members believe they are easing a dying patient's suffering rather than failing to find a cure. Other psychological pitfalls include depression, guilt, personality conflicts with patients, the inevitable pain of dealing with dying patients, and rescue fantasies that interfere with a staff member's ability to stop heroic treatment. They recommend staff meetings that attend to psychological issues and encourage the use of humor.

The staff must also be ever vigilant about the perceived similarities that may decrease necessary professional distance between themselves, the patient, and significant others.

CASE EXAMPLE 1. Ms. G was the 35-year-old married daughter of a man with end-stage cardiac disease. She was an only child, and her mother had died 3 years before. Her father's cardiologist was also an only child, and his one surviving parent was dying of lung cancer. His heart went out to Ms. G. He greatly extended himself to her by visiting at home, answering her worried calls no matter when, and spending a good deal of time comforting her. Eventually an intimate relationship developed that ended abruptly when the physician panicked about the liaison. The woman was left feeling hurt and abandoned with the double loss of her father and her lover.

Many doctors and nurses entered medicine because of compassion for the suffering of others and the desire to ameliorate pain. The physician in the above example might have been particularly vulnerable because he suffered losses, which allowed him to overidentify with the patient's daughter. Although his feelings are understandable, his actions overstepped professional bounds. Ethical treatment has distinct limits that often cannot be crossed without harm to others.

Great stress occurs when staff members must inform patients

and families about the intractability of illness. Waller and colleagues [30] discuss this as the "Cassandra Prophesy Phenomenon." In one instance the staff of a pediatric ICU was delivering an honest evaluation of poor prognosis to the parents of a critically ill child. The parents met such news with hostile denial and suspicion. This frustrated the staff and caused a breakdown of the harmonious working relationship between staff and family. To make sure that staff and family work together, physicians and nurses must communicate their medical opinions while explicitly stating their intentions to continue to do everything possible for their patients.

At times the staff is sure that further treatment will only prolong suffering, and there is no hope of improving the patient's condition. This might occur while the family still denies the intractability of the disease and adamantly refuses to allow DNR orders to be written (see Chap. 228). Cassem [31] thoughtfully discusses how one might approach such conflict. He delineates three guiding principles: (1) *primum non nocere* (first, do no harm); (2) the will of the patient, not the family, is the supreme

law; and (3) medical treatment is justified by the benefit it brings to the patient. If the staff has carefully considered all this, explained it to the patient and family, and still meets conflict, a consultation is in order. In some hospitals a committee of physicians and nurses is available to mediate.

Acute Behaviors

Often in the heat of ICU work, behavioral problems arise before staff have had an opportunity to fully appreciate the source. Table 225-5 connects such manifestations with potential etiologies, responses, and management.

The following vignettes illustrate three of the most disruptive behaviors: frightening behavior, helpless behavior, and noncompliant behavior.

Table 225-5. Problematic Acute Behaviors in the ICU and Their Manifestations, Etiology, Staff Response, and Management

Behavior	Manifestations	Etiology	Response	Management
Frightening	Screaming	Pain	Fear	Limit setting
	Crying	Psychosis	Aggression	Restraints
	Threatening	Terror	Avoidance	Sedatives
	Homicidal ideation	Character	Guilt	Antipsychotics
	Litigiousness	Delirium		Narcotics
		Anxiety		
Self-destructive	Drug abuse	Character	Anger	Team communication
	Secret smoking	Psychosis	Repulsion	Limits
	Pulling lines	Anxiety	Sadism	Restraints
	Burning self	Depression	Helplessness	Sedatives
	Cutting self	Delirium	Resignation	Recognition of guilt
	Suicidal actions	Mania	Witholding	
		Substance abuse	Omnipotence	
Inappropriate	Bizarreness	Psychosis	Avoidance	Antipsychotics
	Seductiveness	Paranoia	Fear	Team communication
	Flirtatiousness	Narcissism	Anger	Restraints
	Craziness	Hysteria	Guilt	Limits
		Organic		Sedatives
				Keeping appropriate distance
Helpless	Confusion	Character	Avoidance	Antidepressants
	Childishness	Futile condition	Annoyance	Reassurance
	Inconsolable crying	Depression	Rescue fantasies	Support
	Depression	Family conflict	Helplessness	Exploration of feelings
	Infantile behavior	Culture	Anger	Family meeting
	Whining		Guilt	Enhancement of self-esteem
	Wimpiness			Encourage independence
Noncompliant	Secret smoking	Character	Fury	Paradoxical approaches
	Stealing	Depression	Collusion	Antidepressants
	Lying	Sociopathy	Sadism	Strict limits
	Saying "Yes . . .	Psychosis	Denial	Determine if incompetent; if so,
	but"	Dementia	Annoyance	find guardian
	Leaving AMA	Retardation	Revenge	Limits
	Spitting up pills	Schizoid style	Avoidance	Recognize own limits
	Rudeness	Anxiety		Psychiatric evaluation
	Withdrawal	Mania		
	Refusing procedures	Substance abuse		
	Thwarting	Malingering		
Obnoxious	Insulting	Character	Anger	Limits
	Devaluing	Anxiety	Sadism	Team communication
	Whining	Family conflict	Intrusion	Treat anxiety
	Anger	Culture	Confusion	Treat depression
	Malingering	Psychosis	Guilt	
	Smugness	Delirium	"Yes'em"	
	Self-righteousness			

Key: Table should read down, not across each column.

CASE 1. Mr. A, a 43-year-old large, muscular man, sustained multiple fractures in a motorcycle accident. He had remained quiet until 6 hours after his admission. Then he opened his eyes and began to stir. His nurse, who had been nearby checking his cardiac monitor, suddenly heard an explosive bellow. She turned to see Mr. A trying to pull out his Foley catheter and jump out of bed while screaming obscenities.

Frightening behavior (e.g., being physically threatening, verbally abusive, emotionally intense, or psychotic) is aberrant and inappropriate to the context of ICU care. If the patient or the staff is in danger, swift action must be taken to protect the patient and those around him or her. Physical restraint and later chemical restraint (e.g., benzodiazepines, barbiturates, neuroleptics, narcotics, or paralytic agents) should be used when necessary. Coincident with these emergency measures, assessment of the etiology of the patient's behavior should begin. Delirium, especially its life-threatening causes, needs to be ruled out (see Chap. 221 for further details). Frightening and inappropriate behavior is often related to frontal lobe injuries.

Infrequently, patients may appear to be delirious from dissociative states or a hysterical psychosis [32] when the stress is great and the patient's usual coping mechanisms have failed. In these states there is no waxing or waning of arousal or attention. Psychiatric consultation can determine if these diagnoses are correct and offer immediate assistance to bolster the patient's coping repertoire and to obviate the need for such dissociation. Reassurance, support, encouragement, simplified explanation of the medical situation, and a compassionate, authoritative approach are often useful.

Frightening behavior may also be a manifestation of confusion secondary to mental retardation, dementia, language barriers, fear, or impairment of sight or hearing. A passive, trusting, compliant patient may lash out in a manner antithetical to his character if he or she suddenly feels panicked. Fear and panic may go unnoticed before an outburst, especially when the medical situation is life-threatening and when no old chart is available to provide information. In this case, simple explanations, along with calm, confident assurances, will be of service. Family members and friends can help the staff understand what will help the patient. Anxiolytics or neuroleptics can also be helpful.

CASE 2. Mr. M, a wiry, 62-year-old postal clerk, was in the CCU awaiting bypass surgery. He was constantly vigilant; his eyes darted from side to side. He jumped at any new sound or sudden movement. He answered questions only in a whisper, after looking around to see who was in earshot. Although he began his answers by responding to the questions at hand, he often paused and continued on some unrelated topic; the connection between sentences was hard for others to follow. His questions were unending, his fears legion. Staff felt hopeless about ever being able to reassure him and started to avoid his room as much as possible. After a few days he confided to a nurse that his brain had been altered by the electromagnetic waves emitted by the cardiac monitor.

Psychotic patients can become dangerous when responding to delusions or hallucinations. A paranoid patient may believe that the nurses are plotting against him and try to defend himself by attacking the staff. Alternatively, a patient with psychosis may hear the voice of Satan telling him or her to jump out the window. Psychosis can be caused by an underlying psychiatric condition (e.g., schizophrenia), but even if there is a history of psychosis, an acute psychosis in the ICU can be caused by organic factors (e.g., delirium), and this should be ruled out. Psychosis may develop as an acute emotional reaction to life-threatening illness or in response to exacerbation of a premorbid psychiatric illness.

Psychosis should be treated with neuroleptics. (See Chap. 221 for details.) A psychotic patient who is not acutely dangerous, but who at baseline is delusional or hallucinating, should be continued on his psychiatric medications and talked with in a clear, simple, and calm manner. Psychiatric consultation should also be requested.

HELPLESS BEHAVIOR. Ms. C, a 36-year-old divorced accountant with type I diabetes, was known in her community as a tireless organizer and as one who was devoted to helping others in need. Forty hours before admission she began to vomit uncontrollably. She was admitted to the ICU, where her ketoacidotic state was successfully treated, leaving her with a clear mental status and no frontal release signs. While awaiting transfer out of the ICU she began whining and did not seem able to perform basic activities of daily living. She often let her johnny slip and appeared unkempt. Once staff ran to answer her call-buzzer and found her lying in vomitus, even though a basin was beside her by the bed. After a while, staff moved more slowly to answer her insistent calls, and several nurses angrily stated that she could take care of herself.

A helpless patient can call others to the rescue. Paradoxically, as in the above case, these efforts often increase childish, infantile behavior. The individual becomes more passive, regressed, inconsolable, or depressed. The staff begins to feel they are dealing with someone with bottomless need who soaks up care like a sponge and is always hungry for more. Staff may resent the patient and ultimately provide less than usual care for the patient because of resentment and avoidance.

To change the situation, staff can indicate that circumscribed attempts at self-care are expected, while articulating their confidence in the patient's ability to do for himself or herself. Helplessness can also be a symptom of depression, and this should be actively treated, if present (see Chap. 223 for details of diagnosis and treatment).

Staff responses to helpless behavior may include annoyance, avoidance, and anger. When staff are overextended and exhausted, it is understandable that whining, wimpy behavior will be galling and infuriating. Stepping back and trying to see the behavior in the context of the individual's suffering can be helpful. Awareness of the physician's own reactions to these patients can help avoid frustration. It is a difficult balance to manage care without taking over responsibilities that the helpless patient needs to perform himself or herself with supportive encouragement. An outside consultant can provide perspective in such cases. Staff meetings to ventilate feelings and to share strategies are also useful.

ICU staff may be affected by feelings of helplessness. This occurs when, for example, we care for an aged individual with multiple organ system failure who makes us feel like plate balancers in the carnival. As soon as nine of the ten plates are spinning, the tenth inevitably begins to wobble uncontrollably. The situation is worse if the individual is irascible and difficult to care for. Self-induced illness that is refractory to care often generates feelings of helplessness or anger. We often treat the consequences of ethanol consumption, cigarette smoking, obesity, or self-inflicted wounds, and we know that before too long the person will return, needing our attention for similarly induced injuries. A long-term perspective that looks for behavioral changes over years rather than months can help to decrease the sense of futility. There is also the patient whose condition deteriorates despite the success of all our procedures. Stubbornly, the patient succumbs even though the operation went well, the bypass is patent, and all the laboratory tests have been brought within normal limits. Here it is helpful to recognize that ICU intervention is still very limited in what it can realistically hope to accomplish, despite its very intense, all encompassing internal frame of reference.

We should be mindful of a family's response to the helplessness of the patient, or their feelings of helplessness in response to critical illness. This can be especially difficult if the patient was always the strong, reliable family member who helped others. Fear, disorientation, and anger are natural responses to the situation. Some members of the family may become particularly difficult to deal with and even become angry after being given thorough explanations and abundant attention. The input of a psychiatrist or family therapist can help.

NONCOMPLIANT BEHAVIOR. Ms. D, an obese 46-year-old woman who chain-smoked, was admitted to the CCU to rule out an MI. She was quite angry about the restrictions placed on her. More than once the staff had to tell her to refrain from smoking in her room. She complained of pains in her stomach that moved to her throat. Patiently the staff evaluated the pains, explained diagnostic tests and procedures, and discussed their clinical impressions with her. No explanation was satisfactory. Her agitation grew. She told the nurse she did not trust the doctors and thought they might be experimenting on her. She doubted that the other staff knew what they were doing. In an attempt to allay her fears, further explanations were offered. The resident responsible for her care tried to enlist the help of her 20-year-old son, but he was as wary as his mother. Hours later she insisted on being unhooked from the monitors and leaving the hospital.

Noncompliant behaviors include smoking, spitting up pills, lying, obsequiously agreeing to treatment only to add a countervailing "but" that negates the agreement, and refusing medications or diagnostic evaluations. The anger and frustration that these behaviors evoke can precipitate sadism, collusion, or denial on the part of the staff. Noncompliance can stem from character pathology, depression, psychosis, dementia, or mental retardation. A consultation with a psychiatrist can differentiate among these and suggest appropriate treatment or management for each.

In the case example, the consultant approached the patient and her son to hear their complaints. Only after they had a chance to tell him of their unhappiness in excruciating detail was he able to find the source of the problem. It happened that Ms. D's mother had died of stomach cancer that had gone undiagnosed for several years. She believed her symptoms replicated those of her mother. She could not believe any explanation that did not include stomach cancer. After learning this, the medical team was able to address her fear directly and discuss the difference between her symptoms and those of cancer. After thorough discussions about this, she was able to calm down for the rest of her hospital stay.

Noncompliant Behavior of Family. Mr. R, a well-known trial lawyer, collapsed one day in court. He was brought to the hospital, where over the next 3 days a team of doctors became involved in his case. His wife came immediately to the hospital and was there day and night. She tried repeatedly to meet with her husband's doctors, but in the flurry of activity she was totally excluded. She only received information from her husband. She was at first worried and confused. As days passed and she remained in the dark, she became angry. She wondered if he was receiving good care and planted doubt in his mind. Finally, after intense pressure on her part, her husband threatened to sign out against medical advice (AMA) to seek better care elsewhere.

The ICU staff, realizing their error in not including the patient's wife, immediately met with her. They listened to her complaints without becoming defensive. After hearing her out, they were able to provide concrete information about her husband's condition and progress and specifically answer her questions. They included her in subsequent meetings with her husband. This allayed her fears, and she became an active positive force in her husband's recovery, not the adversary she had been.

The ultimate act of noncompliance is signing out AMA. One study has shown that patients signing out AMA tend to be young men with substance abuse or other psychiatric histories [33], although such behavior is not limited to these populations. Timely attention to anger or anxiety on the part of patient or family and psychiatric consultation can decrease the occurrence of signing out AMA. Many studies [14,25–28] have shown that ICU staff need to attend to families as well as patients to ensure good care. Meijs [16] suggested a treatment plan to relieve family anxiety. This plan includes the family's need for information, the need to be with the patient and be helpful, the need to ventilate feelings, and the need to have their own basic needs (e.g., appropriate accommodations, hospital resources) met.

Conclusion

Physicians confront behaviors in the ICU that may be dangerous, annoying, and frustrating. These are especially difficult for staff focusing on medical and surgical issues. The time-honored approach to these psychiatric problems is to establish patient/staff safety, to diagnose the problem, and to review treatment options. Keeping the concerns of patient, family, and staff in perspective allows for rational management and an end to disruptive behavior.

References

1. Kornfeld DS: Psychiatric view of the intensive care unit. *Br Med J* 1:108, 1969.
2. Keep P, James J, Inman M: Windows in the intensive therapy unit. *Anesthesia* 35:257, 1980.
3. Cox MK: Any nurse can prevent dehumanization by the CCU experience. *Aviat Space Environ Med* 48(6):568, 1977.
4. Cochran J, Ganong LH: A comparison of nurses' and patients' perceptions of intensive care unit stressors. *J Adv Nurs* 14:1038, 1989.
5. Robinson CA, Thorne SE: Understanding disruptive behaviors in the critical care setting. *Crit Care Nurse* 9(4):82, 1989.
6. Rumpler CH, Seigerman C: A behavior modification approach to dealing with violent behavior in an intensive care unit. *Perspect Psychiatr Care* 16:206, 1978.
7. Geiger WJ: Behavioral perspectives in coronary care. *J Fam Pract* 43(2):245, 1975.
8. Levenson JL, Kay R, Monteferrante J: Denial predicts favorable outcome in unstable angina pectoris. *Psychosom Med* 46(1):25, 1984.
9. Weller DJ, Miller PM: Emotional reactions of patient, family and staff in acute-care period of spinal cord injury: part I & II. *Soc Work Health Care* 2(4):369, 1977.
10. Sulman J, Verhaeghe G: Myocardial infarction patients in the acute care hospital: A conceptual framework for social work intervention. *Soc Work Health Care* 11(1):1, 1986.
11. Thomas SA, Sappington E, Gross HS, et al: Denial in coronary care patients. *Heart & Lung* 12(1):74, 1983

12. Krantz DS: Cognitive processes and recovery from heart attack: A review and theoretical analysis. *J Human Stress* 6(3):27, 1980.

13. Frederickson K: Anxiety transmission in the patient with myocardial infarction. *Heart & Lung* 18(6):617, 1989.

14. Doer BC, Jones JW: Effect of family preparation on the state anxiety level of the CCU patient. *Nurs Res* 28(5):315, 1979.

15. Halm MA: Effects of support groups on anxiety of family members during critical illness. *Heart Lung* 19(1):62, 1990.

16. Meijs CA: Care of the family of the ICU patient. *Crit Care Nurse* 9(8):42, 1989.

17. Chartier L, Coutu-Wakulczyk G: Families in ICU: Their needs and anxiety level. *Intensive Care Nurs* 5(1):11, 1989.

18. Strain JJ: Psychological reactions to acute medical illness and critical care. *Crit Care Med* 6(1):39, 1978.

19. Bibring GL, Kahana RJ: *Lectures in Medical Psychology: An Introduction to the Care of Patients*. New York, International Universities Press, 1968.

20. American Psychiatric Association: *Diagnostic and Statistical Manual of Mental Disorders, Fourth Edition, Revised*. Washington, DC, American Psychiatric Association, 1994.

21. Geringer ES, Stern TA: Coping with medical illness: The impact of personality types. *Psychosomatics* 27:251, 1986.

22. Rolland JS: Family illness paradigms: Evolution and significance. *Family Systems Med* 5(4):482, 1987.

23. Wasserman D: Passive euthanasia in response to attempted suicide: One form of aggressiveness by relatives. *Acta Psychiatr Scand* 79:460, 1989.

24. Ashworth PM: Staff-patient communication in coronary care units. *J Adv Nurs* 9(1):35, 1984.

25. Obier K, Haywood LJ: Enhancing therapeutic communication with acutely ill patients. *Heart Lung* 2(1):49, 1973.

26. Speedling EJ: Social structure and social behavior in an intensive care unit: Patient-family perspectives. *Social Work Health Care* 6(2):1, 1980.

27. Hickey M: What are the needs of families of critically ill patients? *Focus Crit Care* 12(1):41, 1985.

28. Williams CC, Rice DG: The intensive care unit: Social work intervention with the families of critically ill patients. *Soc Work Health Care* 2(4):391, 1977.

29. Eisendrath SJ, Dunkle J: Psychological issues in intensive care unit staff. *Heart Lung* 8(4):751, 1979.

30. Waller DA, Todres ID, Cassem NH, et al: Coping with poor prognosis in the pediatric intensive care unit: The Cassandra prophecy. *Am J Dis Child*. 133(11):1121, 1979.

31. Cassem NH: Treatment decisions in irreversible illness, in Hackett TP, Cassem NH (eds): *Massachusetts General Handbook of General Psychiatry*. 2nd ed. Littleton, MA, PSG Publishing, 1987.

32. Hackett TP, Cassem NH, Wishnie HA: The coronary care unit: An appraisal of its psychological hazards. *N Engl J Med* 279:1365, 1968.

33. Holden P, Vogtsberger KN, Mohl PC, et al: Patients who leave the hospital against medical advice: The role of the psychiatric consultant. *Psychosomatics* 29:379, 1988.

226. Recognition and Management of Staff Stress in the ICU

Junius J. Gonzales and
Theodore A. Stern

Intensive-care settings reveal humanity at its best and at its worst. This is as true for the staff as it is for the patients. We who serve in intensive-care settings in a true sense risk our own lives in these settings—our feelings, our self-esteem, our self-respect. By risking these daily we grow; by avoiding the risk we must face the dehumanization of ourselves or of our patients [1].

Cassem and Hackett's statement eloquently captures one of the underlying dangers of intensive care work. Intensive care units (ICUs) have developed rapidly since the 1960s, providing technologically advanced and highly specialized care. Daily and nightly, the staff of the ICU is confronted by questions, challenges, and dilemmas that are driven by unprecedented clinical scenarios.

The structural and functional complexity of an ICU has been well described [2,3,4]. With the growth of intensive care medicine as a discipline, researchers in medical ethics and medical economics have actively tried to understand the impact of intensive care on hospitals, physicians, patients, and society. Some have wondered whether the glamour of the technology has promoted overgrowth of ICUs. However, today these units are often filled to capacity and are an important source of income for hospitals [2]. No one can deny that ICU medicine is more complex today than ever. There are more patients with severe and chronic illness. Ethical questions are more complicated. Technology is ever more advanced and intricate. Moreover, a recent 6-hour public television film documentary heightened the awareness of the general public by showing the day-to-day activities and interactions among doctors, nurses, and patients in an ICU.

For patients and their families who are unfamiliar with the ICU environment and made vulnerable by life-threatening illness, a stay in the ICU can be a physically and psychologically traumatic experience. A range of psychological responses to being a patient or to having a loved one in the ICU has already been described [5,6]. These responses include heightened anxiety, fear, depression, and feelings of grief, which can at times be extreme. The overriding emotion felt by many patients and their families is a fear of disability or death; this is understandable given that 20 to 25 percent of patients admitted to an ICU never leave the hospital [6]. These concerns and fears, as well as environmental disturbances (e.g., noise, congestion, a lack of privacy, and unexpected frenzy) interfere with patient care.

Strain and Grossman [7] have described five conditions or qualities that help patients to adapt to serious illness: (1) the ability to regress in the service of recovery (that is, to cooperate with the physician's recommendations); (2) the ability to maintain defenses against the stresses of critical illness; (3) ready access to personal feelings and fantasies and the ability to communicate personal needs; (4) a basic trust in medical caregivers;

and (5) having the services of an empathic and flexible critical care team.

Working in an ICU affects staff members. Because of technological advances, increased demands placed on caretakers, nursing shortages, and more complicated ethical issues associated with ICU care, the psychological pressures on ICU staff should be addressed. Staff may not be as prepared to handle their own emotional reactions as well as the technical and clinical aspects of intensive care. Today more than ever, ICU staff "face the dehumanization" of themselves and their patients, as Cassem and Hackett warned, if they do not pay attention to their feelings and coping ability.

This chapter briefly reviews general definitions of stress and burnout, discusses common causes of stress for physicians and nurses who work in ICUs, discusses the symptoms of stress and burnout, and discusses the management of staff stress in the ICU.

The Concepts of Stress and Burnout

The concept and definitions of stress have interested and, at times, perplexed investigators. This has resulted in a massive literature on stress [8,9]. Various definitions for stress have been offered that relied on principles derived from cognitive theory and from measurements of physiologic and biochemical (e.g., endocrine) parameters. Selye, a pioneer in stress research, described the general adaptation syndrome or biologic stress syndrome. He defined stress as "the nonspecific (that is, common) result of any demand upon the body, be the effect mental or somatic" [10]. Selye divided stress into *eustress*, "the pleasant stress of fulfillment," and *distress* that has "harmful consequences of damaging stress." Work in an intensive care setting involves both kinds of stress. When intensive care work provides more distress than eustress, burnout is an expected outcome.

Burnout, like stress, is a term that has been conceptualized and defined in many different ways. It has been viewed as a behavioral or psychological condition as well as a process or syndrome [11,12,13]. Burnout is probably the culmination of a sustained and intense response to negative stress; the signs and symptoms of burnout are usually reactions to negative stress.

Very little has been written about burnout in residency training (as compared with the stress associated with ICU nursing). A smoldering or waxing-waning form of burnout may exist as the "house officer stress syndrome" [14]. Civetta, in his 1981 presidential address to the Society of Critical Care Medicine, said:

It is also evident that fewer physicians select careers as full-time intensivists. Though there are fewer than 100 critical care fellowships available in the United States, not all positions are filled. It is also disheartening to note that in contrast to other medical specialties, intensivists tend to practice full-time intensive-care for relatively few years. . . . There are few physicians still practicing full-time bedside—not administrative—intensive care after 10 years in the field. Perhaps "burnout" should be applied to physicians as well [15].

The term *burnout* had its origin in the service fields and was popularized in the late 1970s. It was applied to all professions and organizations (e.g., health professionals, pilots, prison guards, welfare workers, and air-traffic controllers) and generated some interesting and useful schemes for its recognition and management. Most definitions rely on signs and symptoms,

Table 226-1. Definitions of Burnout

A syndrome of emotional exhaustion, depersonalization, and reduced personal accomplishment that can occur among individuals who do "people work" of some kind.

A progressive loss of idealism, energy, and purpose experienced by people in the helping professions as a result of the conditions of their work.

A state of physical, emotional, and mental exhaustion marked by physical depletion and chronic fatigue, feelings of helplessness and hopelessness, and the development of a negative self-concept and negative attitudes toward work, life, and other people.

A syndrome of inappropriate attitudes toward clients and self, often associated with uncomfortable physical and emotional symptoms.

A state of exhaustion, irritability, and fatigue that markedly decreases the worker's effectiveness and capability.

A process in which a professional's attitudes and behavior change in negative ways in response to job strain.

A condition produced by working too hard for too long in a high-pressure environment.

A debilitating psychological condition resulting from work-related frustrations, which results in lower employee productivity and morale.

Source: Adapted from Maslach C: Understanding burnout: Definitional issues in analyzing a complex phenomenon, in Paine WS (ed): *Job Stress and Burnout.* Beverly Hills, Sage Publications, 1982, p 29.

but burnout seems to affect all spheres of existence (intrapsychic or subjective, interpersonal or social, and professional) (Table 226-1) [16]. Burnout is manifest by physical, emotional, attitudinal, cognitive, behavioral, and social changes (Table 226-2) and is probably not related solely to occupational stress. Most authors agree that burnout is a process that can vary in intensity and duration. However, it usually begins slowly and has a somewhat insidious nature [17]. Even if an individual's experience of burnout does not initially reach consciousness, it may affect others, adding another source of stress to the system. Denial and other defense mechanisms may be employed to help cope with feelings of distress. Among the saddest aspects of burnout in ICU personnel are the loss of motivation for creative involvement [18] and the belief that the ability to help people is gone [12].

What are the personal, social, and professional costs of burnout? Feelings of despair, hopelessness, or depression can develop, relationships can become disrupted, and the ability to work can be affected. When this occurs, patient care suffers. At some hospitals, job dissatisfaction and burnout have led to increases in staff turnover and to severe staff shortages, which may limit the number of ICU beds available for patient admissions.

Who is at risk for burnout? Several authors have stated that individuals involved in human services work are probably at the highest risk for burnout because their work is emotionally draining [12,13], in part because patients often have psychological, physical, or economic needs that are not quickly resolved with simple or discrete interventions. Individuals who choose to work in ICUs tend to be idealistic, committed, and driven; these very attributes may make them particularly susceptible to burnout. Little research has been done to determine which personality characteristics predispose an individual to burnout. Until definitive studies can be conducted, it seems reasonable to assume that burnout is an individual experience that should be assessed and managed according to the individual's needs. However, attention should be paid to the impact of job-related stressors and their ramifications.

Table 226-2. Indicators of Burnout

HEALTH INDICATORS

Fatigue and chronic exhaustion, headaches, sleep problems, ulcers, gastrointestinal problems, flare-ups of preexisting medical problems, muscle pain, missed menstrual periods

EXCESSIVE BEHAVIOR INDICATORS

Increased consumption of caffeine, alcohol, tobacco, over-the-counter medications, psychoactive prescription drugs, illicit drugs, high risk-taking behavior (e.g., auto accidents, falls, accident-proneness, gambling), increased propensity for violent and aggressive behavior, over- and undereating, hyperactivity

EMOTIONAL ADJUSTMENT INDICATORS

Emotional distancing, paranoia, depression, decreased emotional control, martyrdom, fear of "going crazy," increased time daydreaming, feelings of being "trapped," nervous tics, undefined fears, difficulty concentrating, increased anger, increased tension, intellectualization

RELATIONSHIP INDICATORS

Isolation from or overbonding with staff, responding to patients in mechanical manner, increased isolation from patients, increased expressions of anger or mistrust, increased interpersonal conflicts with other staff, increased problems with marital or other relationships outside of work, social isolation (e.g., overinvolvement with patients, using patients to meet personal and social needs)

ATTITUDE INDICATORS

Grandiosity; boredom; cynicism; sick humor aimed at patients; distrust of management, supervisors, or peers; air of righteousness; hypercritical attitude toward peers or institution; expressions of hopelessness, powerlessness, meaninglessness

Source: Adapted from Carroll JFX, White WL: Theory building; Integrating individual and environmental factors within an ecological framework, in Paine WS (ed): *Job Stress and Burnout*. Beverly Hills, Sage Publications, 1982, p 41.

Stresses and Their Consequences on Medical Training and Practice

Descriptive literature both from within the medical profession and from outside the profession (e.g., sociology) on stress in medical training and practice is abundant. Some of this literature has been controversial, and much of it (with respect to the training and creation of programs to prevent physician impairment) has been ignored [19–23]. Undeniably, medicine today is more complicated than it was in the 1960s, when ICUs were first created. ICU physicians often struggle to keep up with advances in technology, to remain fiscally solvent, and to survive an ever-increasing bureaucratic barrage.

The most dramatic changes and proposals for reform in medical training (with its attendant stress) followed a grand jury investigation into the death of Libby Zion in 1984. Several articles in a 1988 issue of the *New England Journal of Medicine* reviewed both the case and its implications [24–27]. One author wrote:

In fact, despite changes designed to improve conditions for residents, job stress has grown. . . . There are several reasons for this increased stress. One is the intensification of inpatient medicine. The average patient today is sicker, and more aggressive interventions are employed routinely. . . . Looking to the future, these trends will bring a progressive increase in the overall stress of residency training [25].

Colford and McPhee [20] recently reviewed the stresses of residency training in their aptly titled article, "The Ravelled Sleeve of Care." They discussed stresses common to young

professionals, as well as stresses in residency, and compared them with stresses felt by older practicing physicians. Their list of stresses was divided into those related to the nature of residency, those related to the educational structure of residency, those related to being a female resident, and those related to perceptions about work. Among the most potent stressors were sleep deprivation, information overload, long work hours, and confrontation of chronic or deadly disease (such as AIDS). Other undeniable stresses outside of residency and patient care (e.g., financial debt, personal relationships, and anxiety about malpractice) were thought to be inextricably linked to the training experience. Several of the stresses listed are particularly evident in the ICU (Table 226-3).

Butterfield [21] reviewed the literature on stress during residency from 1980 to 1988 and found similar sources of stress on residents. She concluded that anger was a prominent affect in training (although the implications of this anger on patient care had not been studied), that the body of sleep deprivation research was inconclusive, and that stress in residency was complicated by other factors. She suspected that social support was an important variable for successful coping and stress reduction, and encouraged more active research in this area.

Complex ethical issues face all physicians today but tend to arise more frequently in the ICU setting. Winkenwerder [4] speculated that competing forces interfere with the ability of the resident to make ethical decisions and engender a great deal of stress: the resident's personal values or judgments, conflicts within the team or with the attending physician's decisions, the resident's ability to provide continuing care in conflict situations, and the expectation of the occupational hierarchy. He discussed the strength of decision making by groups, offered recommendations that can be applied in ICU settings, and warned:

One effect of the compromises that result from conflicting judgment and values is a personal cost to caretakers. The experience of interns is most illustrative . . . nothing was more painful during this year than to realize the decision had been made . . . to "flog" a hopeless patient and that they would be the ones doing the flogging . . . similar anxiety when they perceived the actions of the team or attending physician to be under-treatment of salvageable patients.

Table 226-3. Common Stresses for ICU Staff

Physician stressors	Nurse stressors
Being sleep deprived	Having an excessive workload (high patient-nurse ratio)
Having long on-duty assignments	Having too little time to deal with patients' or their families' emotional needs
Providing high-technology care	
Dealing with death	Dealing with death
Dealing with chronically/severely ill patients	Dealing with the unnecessary prolongation of life
Feeling a responsibility to patients' families	Providing high-technology care
Having limited training in ethics	Having unpredictable schedules
Being exposed to contagious and/or deadly diseases (e.g., AIDS)	Being subjected to environmental disturbances (e.g., noise)
	Having administrative conflicts
Performing complex or invasive procedural tasks	Feeling powerless or insecure
Being overloaded with information	
Having a large financial debt	
Anxiety about malpractice	

Finally, McCue [23] reported on stresses that "are an intrinsic part of medical practice," and continue after training is completed:

... working with intensely emotional aspects of life governed by strong cultural codes for behavior, e.g., suffering, fear, sexuality, and death; inadequate training for fundamental professional tasks, e.g., handling "problem" patients; and, demands from society or patients that cannot be reasonably met, e.g., the need for certainty when current medical knowledge allows only approximation [23].

These stresses are strongly felt in ICUs.

What are the consequences of stress associated with medical training and practice? Many articles have tried to assess whether physicians have higher than normal rates of psychological, interpersonal, and professional dysfunction. Small [14] described a "house officer stress syndrome" with seven features: (1) episodic cognitive impairment, (2) chronic anger, (3) pervasive cynicism, (4) family discord, (5) depression, (6) suicidal ideation and suicide, and (7) substance abuse. He believed that the first four were ubiquitous in all house officers at one time or another. Colford and McPhee's review [20] reported that alcohol and drug abuse was a significant problem among 7 to 10 percent of physicians. They also found studies verifying the stress in physicians' relationships, psychological problems (e.g., anxiety and depression), and professional dissatisfaction.

The impaired physician is usually a physician with a substance abuse problem. A 1986 study examined psychoactive drug use in physicians and medical students and reported two important findings: (1) those with drug dependence typically started using drugs for recreational purposes and (2) recreational drugs were not limited to alcohol and marijuana [28]. Morse's review [29] cited a high risk (nearly ten times that of the general population) for narcotic addiction in physicians. Morse noted that impairment in physicians is an important problem that has prompted all 50 state medical societies to develop assistance programs and has led the American Medical Association to make a policy on the ethical responsibilities of all physicians to help impaired colleagues [29].

Colford and McPhee's [20] review confirmed that anxiety and depression exist in house officers, but that these affects tended to diminish over time. Smith, Denny, and Witzke's national survey [30] tried to assess the cumulative effects of emotional impairment in trainees over a 5-year period. They surveyed internal medicine program directors and found that more than half of 274 programs granted at least one resident a leave of absence because of emotional impairment. One percent of residents were affected, and the incidence of leaves was greatest during the first postgraduate year. Thirty-one percent of program directors thought that the emotional impairment was attributable to job-related stress; 45 percent of the impaired residents had no prior evidence of emotional problems. Another important internal psychological stressor in medicine was termed *patient-generated dysphoria* by Herzog, Wyshak, and Stern [31]. They measured dysphoria (involving anger, sadness, anxiety, helplessness, and stress) precipitated by different patient qualities or conditions. The four conditions most frequently cited by residents were typically seen in intensive care settings: patients who were dying, patients who had made repeated suicide attempts, patients who were undergoing cardiac arrest, and patients with burns. The dysphoria, if left unacknowledged or unattended, appears to have negative effects on patient care.

Some [20,32] reported that stress affects professional functioning as measured by levels of job dissatisfaction, leaves of absence, errors in medical care, cynicism, loss of compassion, and inappropriate underconfidence or overconfidence in care providers. Probably the most important consequence of this stress in the ICU is a compromise in patient care. Usually errors by individuals can be picked up or covered for by co-workers. However, Jellinek [33] noted that the recognition of team discord can often be difficult. Because such discord is a source of added stress to the team, it needs to be confronted. If it is not, additional problems may arise. Early signs of team discord include "disagreements about a trivial difference in approach to a patient's care," "academically oriented discussions that have a negative tone," "disparaging looks between team members," and a "decreased willingness to help or 'cover' " [33]. Some signs of more severe team problems include scapegoating, apparent depression in several members of the team, orders that change from day to day depending on which person was on call, and serious patient care errors as a result of negligence.

Thus far there has only been one study of burnout in physicians. Lemkau and colleagues [34] studied 67 family practice residents in four different programs by administering a burnout inventory, two personality inventories, and a general demographic questionnaire. They detected a moderate level of burnout that did not vary with demographic or situational factors. In addition, they found two significant correlations: residents who had high levels of emotional exhaustion had lower levels of satisfaction with their support systems; and "the more extroverted, intuitive, feeling, and perceptive individuals reported lower burnout" [34]. The authors concluded that personality factors may be important variables in causing burnout and that burnout may be linked to more serious emotional disturbances.

Stress and Burnout Among ICU Nurses

Shortly after the development of ICUs, articles began to appear in the literature on the stresses experienced by nurses while working in the ICU. Unlike the literature on physician stress, which includes little or no research on stress or burnout from the ICU experience, there have been a number of studies that specifically examine ICU nursing stress and burnout. One reason for this difference may be that studies of physician stress focus on resident physicians who work relatively few (e.g., two to three rotations), comparatively short (e.g., 4 to 6 weeks at a time) stretches in ICUs, whereas the ICU is a permanent job setting for nurses. Although many of the stresses experienced by physicians are also experienced by nurses, nurses also face other stresses [35] (see Table 226-3). A 1981 study by Gray-Toft and Anderson [36] surveyed nurses on five different units for levels of stress, job satisfaction, trait anxiety, and job turnover. They found three general sources of stress: death, excessive workload, and dealing with emotional needs of patients and families. The top five stressors they uncovered were: (1) a lack of opportunity to share experiences and feelings with other staff on the unit, (2) the death of a patient, (3) insufficient time to provide emotional support to a patient, (4) inadequate preparation to help with the emotional needs of a patient, and (5) uncertainty regarding the operation and function of specialized equipment. They also found a correlation between high trait anxiety and high stress levels and wondered whether personality factors were an important determinant of stress. In addition, they noted correlations between high stress levels and job dissatisfaction and job turnover. Differentiation between results from different units yielded two other potentially important factors in the study of nursing stress: qualities of specific units, and personality types attracted to certain kinds of units.

Cassem and Hackett's 1972 study [37] of cardiac intensive care nurses showed that workload, type of work, and dealing with families were among the top stresses. They described common dilemmas encountered in ICU work [1]: the "competition-cooperation dilemma with its inter-squad conflicts"; the "death watch dilemma" and its potential for interfering with performance; scapegoating; and dealing with death (particularly unexpected deaths).

A 1981 literature review [38] listed other stresses experienced by ICU nurses: technology, environmental disturbances (e.g., noise), administrative conflict, and personal feelings (e.g., insecurity and helplessness). Stehle [38] concluded that despite the use of different research tools in different studies, ICUs were not more stressful than other areas of the hospital.

Are stresses for ICU nurses different from stresses for non-ICU nurses? Gray-Toft and Anderson [36] did not find a significant difference in stress levels between the ICU nurses and general hospital nurses they studied. In fact, they found that ICU nurses had among the lowest levels of trait anxiety. Vincent and Coleman [39] studied sources, levels, and perceptions of stress in ICU and non-ICU nurses. They found no difference in the perceived levels of stress (both groups were deemed to have moderate amounts of stress) or the rank-ordering of major stresses. For these nurses, the top stresses were management of the unit (ranked first by ICU nurses, ranked second by non-ICU nurses) and the nature of direct patient care (ranked third for both groups of nurses). ICU nurses more frequently reported feeling stressed by changing shifts or schedules, by patients not needing ICU care, by the unnecessary prolongation of life, and by working outside the unit. The non-ICU nurses reported a twofold higher frequency of stress when faced with emergencies.

Keane and colleagues' study [40] also determined that ICU nurses did not report higher burnout than non-ICU nurses, were not more negative or dissatisfied with their work, and did not have higher levels of powerlessness. However, "hardiness" variables (feeling alienated from work, feeling alienated from oneself, and being aware of a powerless and external locus of control) did correlate significantly with burnout scores.

Finally, Cronin-Stubbs and Rooks [41] recently investigated stress and burnout in nearly 300 ICU and non-ICU nurses. They found that personal life factors were correlated to burnout. There was no difference in levels of stress between ICU and non-ICU nurses. When factor analysis was performed, the occupational stress experienced in an ICU did not contribute to burnout. Because only 35 percent of the variance in burnout levels was explicable by their study measurements, they recommended investigating other variables (e.g., social and occupational supports, personality traits) that might yield information to facilitate useful interventions. One unique example is the application of computer technology to help ICU staff document and monitor psychological stressors [42].

Management of Staff Stress and Burnout in the ICU

Without a doubt, the ICU is a workplace fraught with a multitude of stresses, which can take a toll on the staff. We have described the common sources of stress and burnout experienced by both physicians and nurses. Most would also agree that how one copes with these stresses is affected by personality factors and social supports. Nearly every article on stress and burnout strongly urges intervention. Unfortunately, although there are descriptive reports on intervention, outcome studies are lacking; stress reduction is the standard solution. However, because stress and burnout are complex phenomena, a huge

number of possible interventions exist; each intervention depends on each identifiable cause. Often the problem is not considered until the first casualty occurs. Preventive strategies are needed. This section describes some ways to handle staff stress and burnout, both tried and untried, to minimize the negative impact on staff, patients, families, and friends.

Because stress occurs on various levels (individual, interpersonal, and organizational), interventions should be made on each of these levels. Just as the stresses are intertwined, so are the interventions. We have noted that personal characteristics (e.g., inadequate coping skills, competitiveness, denial of personal needs) may predispose an individual to succumb to distress. Regulation of stress may be promoted by establishment of goals, better management of time (both in and out of the ICU), relaxation, exercise, and development of the ability to say "no" [43]. To decrease stress and to function better, a nurse or physician may need to seek individual supervision, training, or psychiatric help. Resistance to obtaining individual help is a common problem and is aggravated by fear of being stigmatized, shame about weakness, and constraints imposed by time and finances. Stoudemire and Rhoads [44] described how difficult it is for physicians to receive medical treatment; physicians often try to diagnose and treat themselves and have difficulty assuming the patient role. When they do go for treatment, they are often treated like "very important persons" (VIPs) and, as a consequence, fail to receive the care they need. These difficulties are often fueled by denial, not just by the physician-patient, but by his or her family, colleagues, and other caregivers as well. This may also be true for nurses.

Borenstein [45] reported an interesting and unique program at UCLA that provided full outpatient psychiatric services at no or low cost for house staff. The services were operated autonomously and confidentially off-campus. This model is exemplary and would help to prevent unmanageable stress. Glick and Borus [46] described marital and family therapy for physicians and their loved ones when individual therapy was impossible or refused. Without question, a reduction of marital or family discord will help physicians feel better and function more efficiently.

The interpersonal management of stress with groups and workshops has been reported for both nurses and physicians [1,47–51]. As early as 1975, Cassem and Hackett [1] described having weekly meetings, as well as impromptu group meetings, to examine staff reactions to crises. They recommended that the group leader be familiar with the unit and that the meeting place should be easily accessible to ICU staff. They concluded that these meetings could successfully resolve conflict as well as provide a forum for sharing feelings, experiences, and knowledge. Simon and Whitely [47] described a consultation conference for medical ICU nurses, led by a liaison psychiatrist; this conference successfully evolved into a corrective working group. McCue and Sachs [51] described the effectiveness of a stress management workshop for medical and pediatric residents; it cost little, was positively received, and demonstrated significant short-term improvement in stress and burnout scores.

Weiner and colleagues [49] compared and contrasted a successful support group for ICU nurses with two unsuccessful groups. The two groups failed (as determined by nurses' responses to questionnaires) because the groups were not personally helpful or well attended. The authors concluded that success of support groups is enhanced if there is a need for such a group as communicated by the nurses; if the group leader has positively interacted with them before; if the group is structured; if it quickly suppresses expression of intense negative emotions; and if the problems discussed are intrapersonal or interpersonal (as opposed to problems of the workplace [e.g., noise] or problems with the administration [e.g., scheduling]).

Stern and colleagues at the Massachusetts General Hospital wrote about a group intervention for medical ICU housestaff called Autognosis (self-knowledge or countertransference) Rounds [50]. These weekly 1-hour rounds have been financially and administratively supported by the Department of Medicine for the past 17 years, and are based on the following four goals: (1) to identify subjective reactions to clinical situations; (2) to learn to use personal emotions in clinical practice; (3) to learn to minimize disruptive effects of these reactions in clinical situations; and (4) to share reactions and learn that some reactions are common. Group discussion reduces the feelings of isolation that frequently cause additional stress.

These rounds are distinct from psychotherapy and use various techniques such as humor, fantasy, and a likeability scale to rate the patients, to "create an accepting, protected atmosphere where participants feel free to concentrate on and discuss their reactions to patients, and to provide examples of self-awareness." Stern also introduced the "Red Book" for the ICU (a journal, now 15 years old, kept in the ICU conference room) where house staff can enter any writing (e.g., jokes, philosophical musings, and frank emotions), usually related to the experience of working in a stressful ICU. The longevity of Autognosis Rounds and the Red Book is testimony to their value and effectiveness.

Interventions at the workplace can be extremely helpful and range from making environmental manipulations (e.g., noise reduction [52], improvements in scheduling, placement of a coffee machine in a quiet staff room) to providing financial assistance for further training. It has been noted that there should be a "single responsible physician who is in actual, not nominal, charge" [53]; the presence of this kind of consistent and continuous leader can reduce staff stress.

Koran and colleagues [54] described the use of a questionnaire, the Work Environment Scale (WES), to assess perceptions of the extant and ideal burn unit. This grew out of a support group meeting for the staff led by a liaison psychiatrist. The WES had ten dimensions grouped into three large sections: a relationship section (which rated peer cohesion, involvement, and supervisor support); a goal-orientation section (which assessed autonomy, work pressure, and task orientation); and a system maintenance/change section (which evaluated physical comfort, regulations for control, and clarity of rules and expectations). The WES results were used as a pretext for the group meetings as well as for other interventions (e.g., administrative meetings, conflict resolutions, didactic sessions) by unit staff and the liaison psychiatrist, all of which resulted in improved postintervention WES scores and discrete changes (e.g., schedule changes and regular meetings with attending physicians). The entire staff reported better morale as well as an improved quality of patient care.

This study touched on organizational aspects of the workplace that may produce stress—from the unit itself to administrative policies—and have complex causes such as poor leadership, inadequate supervision, lack of an open communicating atmosphere, and insufficient orientation and education. Certainly many of the proposed methods to decrease residency training stress are at the program, department, or hospital level, which are at times far away from the actual stress or experience [20,22].

Both the nursing and medical literature clearly indicates that significant stress and burnout exist. The cost of ICU staff burnout can be severe. Early identification of dysfunction is paramount, and the system (ICU directors, hospital administrators, and department heads) should be prepared to deal with this problem. There are many organizational approaches to managing ICU stress, involving adequate staffing, sharing the burden of decision making, having an ongoing review of policy and procedures, enacting stress management programs, and promoting education [43]. Perhaps flexibility and support are the main ingredients for the successful management of ICU stress and burnout. Prevention can be achieved through frequent and comprehensive evaluations of each staff member's experience. For example, even though a house officer may rotate through the ICU for only 4 weeks, a reciprocal feedback meeting at the halfway point may help to eradicate potential and unnecessary stress, while it improves satisfaction and performance.

Conclusion

The ICU can be a stressful place to work. Human suffering and death are constants, and uncertainty can sometimes be intolerable. However, ICU work can be tremendously rewarding. The recognition and management of staff stress in the ICU is imperative. Staff stress and burnout, if not attended to, can take a serious and sometimes permanent personal and professional toll. Astute and caring recognition and management of staff stress in the ICU is a way to move "beyond technology" [15]:

We must accentuate the positive qualities of human capabilities that are beyond technological advancement. . . . A smile, a touch, confidence, and security are still beyond our programming capabilities . . . we must focus upon our distinct human qualities of insight and caring. In this way, the popular view that intensive care is a depersonalizing environment can be replaced by the recognition that human beings are caring for human beings [15].

References

1. Cassem NH, Hackett TP: Stress on the nurse and therapist in the intensive-care unit and the coronary-care unit. *Heart Lung* 4:252, 1975.
2. Bryan-Brown C: Pathway to the present: A personal view of critical care, in Civetta JM, Taylor RW, Kirby RR (eds): *Critical Care*. Philadelphia, JB Lippincott, 1988.
3. Fein IA, Strosberg MA (eds): *Managing the Critical Care Unit*. Rockville, Aspen Publishers, 1987.
4. Winkenwerder W: Ethical dilemmas for house staff physicians. *JAMA* 254:3454, 1984.
5. Wallace-Barnhill G: Psychological problems for patients, families, and health professionals, in Shoemaker WC, Ayres S, Grenbik A, et al (eds): *Textbook of Critical Care*. Philadelphia, WB Saunders, 1989.
6. Daley L: The perceived immediate needs of families with relatives in the intensive care setting. *Heart Lung* 13:231, 1984.
7. Strain JJ, Grossman S: *Psychological Care of the Medically Ill: A Primer in Liaison Psychiatry*. New York, Appleton Crofts, 1975.
8. Goldberger L, Breznitz S (eds): *Handbook of Stress*. New York, The Free Press, 1982.
9. Breznitz S (ed): *The Denial of Stress*. New York, International Universities Press, 1982.
10. Selye H: History and present status of the stress concept, in Goldberger L, Breznitz S (eds): *Handbook of Stress*. New York, The Free Press, 1982, p 7.
11. Paine WS (ed): *Job Stress and Burnout*. Beverly Hills, Sage Publications, 1982.
12. Pines AM, Aronson E, Kafry D: *Burnout: From Tedium to Personal Growth*. New York, The Free Press, 1981.
13. Potter BA: *Beating Job Burnout*. San Francisco, Harbor Publishing, 1980.

14. Small GW: House officer stress syndrome. *Psychosomatics* 22:860, 1981.
15. Civetta JM: Beyond technology: Intensive care in the 1980s. *Crit Care Med* 9:763, 1981.
16. Maslach C: Understanding burnout: Definitional issues in analyzing a complex phenomenon, in Paine WS (ed): *Job Stress and Burnout.* Beverly Hills, Sage Publications, 1982, p 29.
17. Carroll JFX, White WL: Theory building: Integrating individual and environmental factors within an ecological framework, in Paine WS (ed): *Job Stress and Burnout.* Beverly Hills, Sage Publications, 1982, p 41.
18. Marshall RE, Kasman C: Burnout in the neonatal intensive care unit. *Pediatrics* 65:1161, 1980.
19. McCue JD: The distress of internship. *N Engl J Med* 312:449, 1985.
20. Colford JM, McPhee SJ: The ravelled sleeve of care: Managing the stresses of residency training. *JAMA* 261:889, 1989.
21. Butterfield PS: The stress of residency: A review of the literature. *Arch Intern Med* 148:1428, 1988.
22. Resident Services Committee, Association of Program Directors in Internal Medicine: Stress and impairment during residency training: Strategies for reduction, identification, and management. *Ann Intern Med* 108:154, 1988.
23. McCue JD: The effects of stress on physicians and their medical practice. *N Engl J Med* 306:458, 1982.
24. Asch DA, Parker RM: The Libby Zion case: One step forward or two steps backward? *N Engl J Med* 318:771, 1988.
25. McCall TB: The impact of long working hours on resident physicians. *N Engl J Med* 318:775, 1988.
26. Levinsky NG: Compounding the error. *N Engl J Med* 318:778, 1988.
27. Glickman RM: House-staff training: The need for careful reform. *N Engl J Med* 318:780, 1988.
28. McAuliffe WE, Rohman M, Santangelo S, et al: Psychoactive drug use among practicing physicians and medical students. *N Engl J Med* 315:805, 1986.
29. Morse G: The impaired physician. *Massachusetts Med* Sept/Oct:39, 1986.
30. Smith JW, Denny WF, Witzke DB: Emotional impairment in internal medicine housestaff. *JAMA* 255:1155, 1986.
31. Herzog DB, Wyshak G, Stern TA: Patient-generated dysphoria in house officers. *J Med Educ* 59:869, 1984.
32. Linn LS, Yager J, Cope D, et al: Health status, job satisfaction, job stress, and life satisfaction among academic and clinical faculty. *JAMA* 254:2775, 1985.
33. Jellinek MS: Recognition and management of discord within house staff teams. *JAMA* 256:754, 1986.
34. Lemkau JP, Purdy RR, Rafferty JP, et al: Correlates of burnout among family practice residents. *J Med Educ* 63:682, 1988.
35. Lewis, DJ, Robinson, JA: ICU nurses' coping measures: Response to work-related stressors. *Crit Care Nurs* 12:18, 1992.
36. Gray-Toft P, Anderson JG: Stress among hospital nursing staff: Its causes and effects. *Soc Sci Med* 15A:639, 1981.
37. Cassem NH, Hackett TP: Sources of tension for the CCU nurse. *Am J Nurs* 72:1426, 1972.
38. Stehle JL: Critical care nursing stress: The findings revisited. *Nurs Res* 30:182, 1981.
39. Vincent P, Coleman WF: Comparison of major stressors perceived by ICU and non-ICU nurses. *Crit Care Nurs* 6:64, 1985.
40. Keane A, Ducette J, Adler D: Stress in ICU and non-ICU nurses. *Nurs Res* 34:231, 1985.
41. Cronin-Stubbs D, Rooks C: The stress, social support, and burnout of critical care nurses: The results of research. *Heart Lung* 14:31, 1985.
42. Malacrida R, Bomio D, Matathia R, et al: Comupter-aided self-observation psychological stressors in an ICU. *Int J Clin Monit Comput* 8:201, 1991.
43. Fein SL: Burnout in nursing: Prevention and management, in Fein IA, Strosberg MA (eds): *Managing the Critical Care Unit.* Rockville, Aspen Publishers, 1987, p 96.
44. Stoudemire A, Rhoads JM: When the doctor needs a doctor: Special considerations for the physician-patient. *Ann Intern Med* 98:654, 1983.
45. Borenstein DB: Should physician training centers offer formal psychiatric assistance to house officers? A report on the major findings of a prototype program. *Am J Psychiatry* 142:1053, 1985.
46. Glick ID, Borus JF: Marital and family therapy for troubled physicians and their families. *JAMA* 251:1855, 1984.
47. Simon NM, Whitely S: Psychiatric consultation with MICU nurses: The consultation conference as working group. *Heart Lung* 6:497, 1977.
48. Siegal B, Donnelly JC: Enriching personal and professional development: The experience of a support group for interns. *J Med Educ* 53:908, 1978.
49. Weiner MF, Caldwell T, Tyson J: Stresses and coping in ICU nursing: Why support groups fail. *Gen Hosp Psychiatry* 5:179, 1983.
50. Stern TA, Prager LM, Cremens MC: Autognosis rounds for medical housestaff. *Psychosomatics* 34:1, 1993.
51. McCue JD, Sachs CL: A stress management workshop improves residents' coping skills. *Arch Intern Med* 151:2273, 1991.
52. Topf M, Dillon E: Noise-induced stress as a predictor of burnout in critical care nurses. *Heart Lung* 17:567, 1988.
53. Waisbren BA: *Critical Care Manual: A Systems Approach Method.* New Hyde Park, Medical Examination Publishing Company, 1985.
54. Koran LM, Moos RH, Moos B, et al: Changing hospital work environments: An example of a burn unit. *Gen Hosp Psychiatry* 5:707, 1983.

227. Neuropsychiatric Aspects of Cancer and AIDS in the ICU

Donna B. Greenberg and
Alexandra Beckett

Care for patients with cancer and with acquired immunodeficiency syndrome (AIDS) often requires judicious use of critical care units. More than three-fourths of patients admitted to a university tertiary cancer center, with either a hematologic cancer or a solid tumor, spent less than 3 months at home before dying [1]. The mortality associated with an intensive care unit (ICU) admission for cancer has been reported to be 70 to 80 percent. Therefore, the use of the ICU for patients with cancer with poor prognosis requires careful thought.

Although some cancers are curable, AIDS resembles a chronic and relapsing cancer with an uncertain but progressively deteriorating course, punctuated by bouts of infection, neutropenia, and other blood dyscrasias. Infections and other life-threatening emergencies are treated aggressively as long as the physician and patient believe that the underlying illness can be controlled sufficiently to maintain a reasonable quality of life. In cancer as well as in AIDS, neurologic compromise is not uncommon, and medical judgments about quality of life and appropriate care require an understanding of which aspects of neuropsychiatric function can be reversed or managed.

There is little controversy about the decision to deliver aggressive medical therapy for a life-threatening illness if potential exists for full reversibility or if the illness occurs in an otherwise healthy individual. The decision to pursue aggressive medical therapy in an individual with a fatal illness that may temporarily improve may be more difficult. Because recurrent infections and marrow failure dominate episodes of critical illness in cancer patients, critical care is most frequently required for sepsis or bleeding. Initially, critical care for patients with AIDS was most often employed for the management of acute respiratory failure attributable to *Pneumocystis carinii* pneumonia (PCP). Now more patients with AIDS are surviving for longer periods; the median survival of homosexual and bisexual men after diagnosis of PCP went from as little as 10.5 months in 1984 to 18 months in 1987 [2,3]. Some individuals have lived more than 5 years after diagnosis. Given the rapidly changing nature and availability of treatments for AIDS, the course of illness is unpredictable. In general, a catastrophic initial presentation of AIDS warrants aggressive treatment. Decisions about how much intensive care individuals with advanced disease should receive are based on our understanding of the prognosis and on the wishes of the patient.

The principles of care that have been applied to cancer patients may be applied to AIDS and other incurable illnesses. The medical judgment of the treating physician, his or her knowledge of illness, and his or her knowledge of the patient's wishes can direct decisions about critical care [4,5]. The goals are to restore health when possible and to relieve suffering. Although the patient's wishes remain most important, at times the patient's judgment may be compromised by intractable pain, treatable depression, or incapacity to assess the risks and benefits of specific procedures. Emergencies are even more likely to be complicated by inadequate information about the patient's wishes. Respect for the patient involves paying attention to the patient's mental status and level of comfort. Delirium, anxiety, depression, or pain should be treated vigorously (see Chaps. 221 to 223). With that in mind, we have devoted this chapter to the neuropsychiatric complications of cancer and AIDS.

Psychiatric Complications of Cancer

PRESENTATIONS OF ANXIETY

Claustrophobia. Restraint by machines and intravenous (IV) lines or confinement in the closed space of the magnetic resonance imaging (MRI) machine arouses panic in those with a history of claustrophobia. Antiphobic agents like lorazepam, alprazolam, or clonazepam are helpful to the patient. Behavioral therapy techniques, relaxation techniques, or hypnosis can also limit anxiety.

Phobia Related to Previous Chemotherapy. Patients who have received anticancer drugs that have provoked vomiting may, after a number of treatments, become conditioned to avoid this aversive experience. The conditioned syndrome is most obvious when patients vomit before receiving the toxic

drug. However, even before they vomit, patients become increasingly anxious at the thought of chemotherapy, the approaching treatment, or the hospital floor. The dread of treatment, or panic associated with the location of treatment, sometimes leads patients to leave the hospital before receiving the scheduled medication. This syndrome is alleviated by use of behavioral therapy or with benzodiazepines administered as anticipatory anxiety begins [6,7]. These treatments for phobias do not replace the standard antiemetic medications used with emetic chemotherapy.

Panic Disorder. Patients with an underlying co-morbid panic disorder, a condition with a 6-month prevalence in the general population of 0.6 to 1.0 percent [8], are likely to develop anticipatory anxiety and experience autonomous panic attacks in the hospital. Episodes of panic often coexist with a diagnosis of major depression. Treatment with high-potency benzodiazepines alleviates symptoms rapidly, whereas a positive response to antidepressants may take several weeks. When both major depression and panic disorder are present, antidepressants should be started as soon as possible because in the long run they may treat both conditions.

Complex Partial Seizures. Complex partial seizures are manifest by psychic phenomena, autonomic changes, or unusual sensory experiences and not by the syncope and tonic-clonic motor activity associated with generalized seizures [9]. Generalized seizures are common among cancer patients because of the high frequency of physiologic insults to the brain by tumor, infection, or drug treatments. Complex partial seizures are more common than generalized seizures and are more difficult to diagnose. The diagnosis is facilitated when classical automatisms of psychomotor seizures (e.g., masticating movements of the lips and jaw) are noted or when the episodes are preceded by an aura, particularly olfactory hallucination (e.g., the smell of burning rubber). Other clues are episodic changes in mental status, visual illusions, loud ringing or buzzing sounds, micropsia, macropsia, bitter taste, or facial numbness [10].

In the critical care unit, autonomic changes may be more easily documented. They include flushing, high blood pressure, salivation, lacrimation, hiccoughs, and shivers. Visceral auras include a rising sensation in the epigastrium, general body heat or cold, nausea, or thirst. Tachycardia, bradycardia, sinoatrial arrest, and paroxysmal atrial tachycardia may also occur [11]. Stereotyped behaviors, rhythmic tremors, incontinence, or the tendency to sleep after an episode may be visible clinical signs.

Anxiety is the most common affect experienced by patients with complex partial seizures (e.g., caused by brain metastases, skull metastases impinging on the brain, carcinomatous meningitis, or use of intrathecal medications). Complex partial seizures must be considered in the differential diagnosis when any episodic change (especially panic attacks or episodic paranoia) in mental status occurs. Patients may experience depersonalization, derealization (the perception that the world is not real), or an unusual sense of familiarity (déjà vu). Rarely, patients have the delusion of being dead or the belief that a time for their death is already appointed [12]. These phenomena may be treated with anticonvulsants, particularly carbamazepine or parenteral lorazepam. However, paranoid and psychotic phenomena usually require antipsychotic medications. Although the electroencephalogram (EEG) may show anterior temporal lobe spikes or sharp waves, a normal EEG does not rule out the diagnosis of complex partial seizures [13].

Akathisia. Akathisia is an internal sense of restlessness that is often relieved by walking. Both the patient and doctor may misdiagnose akathisia as anxiety. This condition occurs as a side effect of neuroleptic medications (e.g., phenothiazines, butyrophenones, and metoclopramide) used commonly for nausea, anxiety, or agitation in cancer patients. Other extrapyramidal symptoms (e.g., dystonias and parkinsonian syndromes) associated with use of these drugs may respond to anticholinergic agents, but akathisia is not as easily treated. Use of diphenhydramine, benzodiazepines, or propranolol may bring some relief [14]. Usually the offending agent can be changed or eliminated. Akathisia may not recur with use of a lower dose or with a different agent, even if it has dopamine-antagonist effects.

MAJOR DEPRESSIVE DISORDER. Among oncology patients, the prevalence of major depressive disorder, 5 to 7 percent, is slightly greater than its prevalence in the general population. Perhaps one-fifth of cancer patients have an adjustment disorder with depressed mood [15,16,17]. Acknowledgment of serious illness is often painful. However, for many patients the acute distress that follows the initial diagnosis abates as they become preoccupied with the rigors of treatment. Those with a history of depression [17], other social and interpersonal problems, and more symptoms of illness are at higher risk for development of depression. Patients with pain are at a higher risk for depression, and the presence of depression exacerbates the experience of the pain [18]. Adenocarcinoma of the pancreas is one particular tumor type that has been associated with a greater risk of dysphoria [19].

SUICIDE. For the oncologist, suicide of a patient is rare. Patients often discuss the possibility of suicide when the threat of complete loss of control has been provoked by critical illness. Patients may fear uncontrolled pain, deformity, or abandonment. Clinical depression is the primary risk factor for suicide. Epidemiologic studies show slightly higher rates for suicide in patients with cancer than in the general population [20,21,22]. Physicians can alleviate some fears by reinforcement of their commitment to continue care and alleviate suffering. Intervention requires maximization of the patient's sense of control, involvement of supportive family or friends, and provision of aggressive pharmacologic treatment of major depressive disorder.

MANIA. Mania is an uncommon side effect of cancer or its treatment. It involves a period of abnormal, expansive, euphoric, or irritable mood, associated with insomnia, increased talkativeness, subjectively racing thoughts, distractibility, psychomotor agitation, and increased goal-directed activity. The most common reason for mania to occur in the context of cancer treatment is as a complication of high-dose steroids [23]. Tumors or strokes only rarely present with mania [24]. Some patients with cancer may have primary manic-depressive illness, which requires treatment with major tranquilizers or lithium.

DELIRIUM. Delirium in cancer patients may result when cancer impinges on the central nervous system (CNS), or from metabolic abnormalities related to the tumor, from anticancer drugs, and from drugs, especially narcotics, used for treatment of symptoms [25]. Delirium caused by cancer may be associated with brain metastases, carcinomatous meningitis, hypercalcemia, or hyponatremia attributable to the syndrome of inappropriate antidiuretic hormone (SIADH). Hyperviscosity is a consideration with lymphomas that produce paraproteins [26].

NEUROPSYCHIATRIC SIDE EFFECTS OF ANTICANCER AGENTS. High-dose corticosteroids may lead to insomnia, agitation, labile mood, depression, or a mixed-manic paranoid psychosis [23]. Cessation of steroids is associated with withdrawal symptoms of muscle aches and emotional let-down. Although withdrawal symptoms of muscle aches and fatigue may be immediate, the dysphoric or psychotic effects of treatment may not abate immediately with cessation of steroids. Insomnia and agitation may be treated with benzodiazepines or neuroleptics. Psychosis must be treated aggressively with antipsychotic medications. For the depressive syndrome, which closely resembles primary major depressive disorder, use of antidepressants is appropriate. Lithium has been used prophylactically to prevent recurrent mania resulting from use of steroids [27].

Other hormones are used primarily in the treatment of patients with breast cancer. Tamoxifen may exacerbate menopausal symptoms (e.g., hot flashes, sleep disorder, irritability). However, it is usually well tolerated. In patients with bone metastases, initial responses may be associated with a flare of bone pain or hypercalcemia. Initial treatment with aminoglutethimide is associated with malaise and fatigue.

Procarbazine causes somnolence, psychosis, and delirium, which occurs as the drug is initiated and resolves rapidly when it is stopped. If taken with alcohol, procarbazine has a disulfiram-like effect, which may provoke flushing, throbbing headache, nausea, vomiting, hypotension, dizziness, seizures, or cardiopulmonary compromise. Although it inhibits monoamine oxidase, the effect is weak [28]. Procarbazine delays the metabolism of barbiturates and phenothiazines.

L-asparaginase, a drug for acute lymphocytic leukemia, causes somnolence, lethargy, and delirium [29]. Change in mental status occurs as the drug is given and resolves when the drug is stopped. These side effects do not seem to be dose-related.

Cytosine arabinoside [30] and 5-fluorouracil (5-FU) [31] have caused delirium and cerebellar syndromes. The neurotoxicity of cytosine arabinoside is related to age and dose.

Methotrexate [32] has caused a transient delirium 10 to 13 days after treatment. Neurotoxicity is more common with higher dose or intrathecal regimens.

Vincristine [33] can cause seizures, SIADH, dysphoria, and lethargy in addition to neuromyopathy and paresthesias. These side effects are related to dose.

Ifosfamide [34] can cause lethargy, seizures, and cerebellar signs; the patient may appear to be intoxicated with alcohol. Catatonia and complex partial seizure status have also been reported [35,36]. Risk for neurotoxicity is related to renal impairment. Like cyclophosphamide and vincristine, it can cause SIADH.

Taxol rarely causes encephalopathy, but it often causes fatigue [37].

Suramin causes gradual onset of a slowly reversible syndrome of malaise, fatigue, and lethargy, first apparent in the third month of therapy [38].

Interferon [39] initially causes a flulike syndrome with fever, myalgias, and malaise. At higher doses, fatigue, difficulty with concentration, psychomotor retardation, and general disinterest have occurred. In those receiving chronic treatment, syndromes of irritability and short temper, as well as syndromes of depression, tearfulness, and hopelessness, have been reported.

Interleukin-2 (IL-2) [40], which has been used with lymphocyte-activated killer (LAK) cells, can also cause delirium and paranoia. Change in mental status is most apt to occur at the end of the course of IL-2 alone, or several days after the onset of combined treatment. Other factors, such as hypoxia or sepsis, may contribute to the changes. The syndrome resolves when the treatment is stopped.

Table 227-1 summarizes the neuropsychiatric side effects of drugs commonly used in the treatment of cancer and AIDS.

Psychiatric Complications of AIDS

A variety of conditions adversely affect neuropsychiatric function in human immunodeficiency (HIV)-infected persons. These include the neurotropic effects of HIV itself, metabolic derangements related to systemic illness, opportunistic malignant and infectious processes, anemia and hypoxemia, and toxicity from chemotherapeutic agents used to treat the primary infection and its complications.

In HIV-infected individuals who manifest a change in mental status, an organic cause must be assumed until proven otherwise. It may be useful to consider the direct effects of HIV on the nervous system as primary and those resulting from opportunistic illnesses and their complications as secondary. Mental status changes that result directly from HIV infection are most often insidious in onset; a sudden change in mental state is likely to have a secondary cause.

Many of the causes of neuropsychiatric dysfunction in HIV-positive individuals are treatable. Individuals in whom there is preexisting HIV-related encephalopathy, even of relatively minor clinical significance, may be particularly vulnerable to the neurologic challenge of a declining hematocrit, impaired oxygenation, or the administration of a drug such as pentamidine, with its attendant CNS effects.

The most common psychiatric diagnoses in HIV-infected patients are adjustment disorder, major depression, and organic mental disorder. In addition, the incidence of substance abuse/dependency disorders is quite high. Because of the high prevalence of organic brain disease in this population, any syndrome that presents primarily as a psychiatric disorder merits a search for an organic cause. For example, mania in an HIV-infected patient may be attributable to an intracranial process such as infection or tumor or may represent an adverse effect of azidothymidine (AZT) or dideoxyinosine (DDI). The evaluation of a psychiatric disorder in an HIV-infected patient is guided by clinical presentation and may include neuroradiologic studies, examination of cerebrospinal fluid (CSF), EEG, and neuropsychological testing. Table 227-2 enumerates a variety of CNS illnesses that occur in HIV-infected individuals.

PRIMARY HIV SYNDROMES

Primary Infection Syndrome. Primary infection syndrome is an acute, mononucleosislike illness occurring within days to weeks of presumed exposure to HIV; seroconversion follows some weeks later. The time from exposure to onset of illness ranges from as short as 6 days [2] to as long as 6 weeks [3]. In Ho and associates' series, seroconversion occurred 8 to 12 weeks after presumed exposure [41].

Primary infection syndrome is sudden in onset and is associated with fevers, sweats, rigors, malaise, lethargy, anorexia, nausea, myalgia, arthralgia, sore throat, and diarrhea. Headaches may be severe and may be accompanied by stiff neck, photophobia, and obtundation, consistent with a diagnosis of meningitis. Examination often shows lymphadenopathy, splenomegaly, and a truncal maculopapular eruption.

Results of a laboratory evaluation may be normal. Abnormalities, when present, include elevated serum transaminases, lymphopenia, thrombocytopenia, and elevated erythrocyte sedimentation rate. Results of CSF examination, when abnor-

Table 227-1. Neuropsychiatric Side Effects of Drugs Used in Cancer and AIDS

Drug	Comments
HORMONES	
Tamoxifen	Exacerbation of menopausal symptoms
Aminoglutethimide	Lethargy in first month
Fluoxymestrone	Irritability
Corticosteroids	Insomnia, lability, depression, psychosis, and mania are dose related
ANTICANCER AGENTS	
Procarbazine	Somnolence, psychosis, and delirium coincide with treatment
L-Asparaginase	Somnolence, lethargy, and delirium common
Cytosine arabinoside	Delirium and cerebellar signs are related to dose and age
5-Fluorouracil	Delirium and cerebellar signs are uncommon
Methotrexate	Transient delirium—uncommon; white matter injury—may be delayed
Vincristine	Dysphoria, lethargy, seizures
Ifosfamide	Lethargy, seizures, dysarthria; more common with renal impairment
Taxol	Rarely causes encephalopathy, often causes fatigue, associated with toxic sensory neuropathy
Suramin	Causes gradual onset of a slowly reversible syndrome of malaise, fatigue, and lethargy, first apparent in third month of therapy, associated toxic sensory neuropathy
Interferon	Initial flu syndrome, encephalopathy (dose related), organic affective and cognitive disorders with chronic use
Interleukin-2	Delirium common
Cisplatin	Consider low magnesium; postural hypotension
Etoposide	Postural hypotension
ANTIVIRAL AGENTS (USED IN AIDS)	
Azidothymidine, Zidovudine (AZT)	Agitation, mania, mental confusion, headaches, somnolence
Dideoxyinosine (DDI)	Mania
Ganciclovir	Mania
ANTIBIOTICS (COMMONLY USED IN AIDS)	
Pentamidine	Hypoglycemia, hypotension, confusion
Dapsone	Agitation, hallucinations
Amphotericin	Headache, disorientation, lethargy, agitation, nausea
Metronidazole	Dizziness, confusion, and delirium; seizures when administered intravenously
ANTICHOLINERGICS	
Antidepressants, low-potency antipsychotics, certain antihistamines, and anti-parkinsonian drugs	*CNS*: confusion, delirium, disorientation, agitation, visual and auditory hallucinations, anxiety, motor restlessness, seizures, myoclonic jerks, and choreoathetoid movements. *Peripheral*: decreased bowel motility, constipation, urinary retention, anhidrosis, mydriasis, dry mouth, cycloplegia, increased body temperature, motor incoordination, flushing, and tachycardia

Table 227-2. Causes of Mental Status Change in the Presence of HIV Infection

Primary HIV syndromes	Primary infection syndrome Aseptic meningitis HIV encephalopathy
Toxic/metabolic	Drug side effects: e.g., AZT, pentamidine, dapsone, alpha-interferon Electrolyte imbalance: hyponatremia, hyperkalemia
Hypoxia	Anemia Pulmonary disease
Neoplasms	Primary or metastatic lymphoma Rarely, metastatic Kaposi's sarcoma
Opportunistic viral infections	Cytomegalovirus (CMV) Herpes simplex virus types I and II Herpes varicella zxoster virus Papovavirus (PML) Adenovirus type 2
Opportunistic nonviral infections	*Toxoplasma gondii* *Cryptococcus neoformans* *Candida albicans* *Aspergillus fumigatus* *Coccidioides immitis* Mucormycosis *Histoplasma capsulatum* *Mycobacterium tuberculosis, Mycobacterium avium intracellularis* *Listeria monocytogenes* *Nocardia asteroides* *Treponema pallidum*
Cerebrovascular disorders	Infarction Hemorrhage Vasculitis
Complex partial seizures	

mal, show mild pleocytosis of 20 to 300 monocytes and an elevated protein.

The illness is self-limited, with resolution over 3 days to 3 weeks. HIV antibodies, absent before illness, are detected within weeks after resolution of the acute disease. The occurrence of such an illness in an individual with known or high risk of exposure to HIV should raise the question of primary infection syndrome [42].

Aseptic Meningitis. Aseptic meningitis due to HIV has a clinical course as described above. It may recur during the course of HIV infection.

HIV Encephalopathy

CLINICAL FEATURES. HIV encephalopathy is a syndrome involving affective, behavioral, cognitive, and motor abnormalities. The clinical findings are often subtle and insidious in onset. Forgetfulness and loss of concentration are the most frequent early symptoms [43]. Patients may complain of confusion, mental slowing, and difficulty with attention. Lapses of attention may be manifested as an inability to read a book, follow a television program, or sustain a conversation. Short-term memory deficits may result in difficulty with adherence to medication regimens and appointment times. Patients may have trouble dividing their attention, doing tasks that were formerly automatic, or planning future activities (making a meal, taking a trip).

Patients may be depressed and have neurovegetative signs such as anorexia, sleep disturbance, or loss of energy. Persons familiar with the patient may notice apathy, social withdrawal, or irritability. Agitation and anxiety can be incapacitating at times. The subtle cognitive and affective complaints that often characterize early HIV encephalopathy closely parallel those of major depression. HIV encephalopathy occasionally presents in a dramatic fashion with acute agitated psychosis, hallucinations, paranoid ideation, or mania [44]. It is often distinguished from purely psychiatric (i.e., nonorganic) syndromes by the presence of focal neurologic deficits or unambiguous evidence of cognitive deterioration.

Motor impairments, when present, include weakness (particularly of the lower extremities) and difficulty with fine motor coordination. There is often dysarthria, tremor, and physical slowing [45]. Patients may notice difficulty walking or climbing stairs, a deterioration in handwriting, or a slight slurring of speech. Nearly 50 percent of patients with HIV encephalopathy complain of motor dysfunction [46]. It is conceivable that these motor deficits result from concomitant vacuolar myelopathy or peripheral neuropathy and not solely from cerebral involvement.

The course of HIV encephalopathy is highly variable. Some individuals remain only minimally symptomatic and can compensate for cognitive problems by keeping written records, using a pocket calendar, or making out daily medication sheets, whereas other patients are dependent on others for activities of daily living. Occasionally, one sees a precipitous decline; severe dementia may occur in a matter of weeks. When HIV encephalopathy becomes severe enough to interfere with occupational or social activities, it is an AIDS-defining illness [47], known as HIV-1 associated dementia complex [48].

LABORATORY FINDINGS. If there are no opportunistic infections or malignancies, the computed tomography (CT) scan of the head in HIV encephalopathy may be normal or may demonstrate diffuse cerebral atrophy. In advanced HIV encephalopathy, the scan often shows a widening of the frontal horns or bilateral low density of the adjacent white matter [49]. Magnetic resonance imaging is more sensitive than CT because of its superior capacity to distinguish white matter disease [50,51]. MRI findings in HIV encephalopathy include cerebral atrophy and ventricular enlargement. In addition, MRI may demonstrate hemispheric white matter abnormalities such as patchy or diffusely increased signal on the T2-weighted image.

CSF abnormalities may occur in individuals with and without clinical findings of encephalopathy. However, the incidence of abnormal findings (WBC > 5/cubic millimeter; total protein > 40 mg/dl; IgG% > 6.1 mg/dl; IgG index > 0.7; oligoclonal bands > 2; HIV culture positive; and HIV p24 antigen present) is greater in symptomatic individuals [52].

TREATMENT. Treatments for HIV encephalopathy include antiretroviral therapy with AZT, DDI, or another antiretroviral agent and palliation of symptoms with psychotropic medications. AZT has been reported to improve clinical status, motor function, nerve conduction velocity, memory and general cognitive ability, the subjective sense of well-being, and the positron emission tomography (PET) scan in persons with HIV encephalopathy [53,54]. There are insufficient data regarding the efficacy of antiretrovirals other than AZT for the treatment of HIV-related neurocognitive deficits; however, other retroviral agents are generally recommended for the AZT-intolerant patient.

PSYCHOSTIMULANTS. Methylphenidate, 5 to 60 mg per day, and dextroamphetamine, 5 to 45 mg per day, provide significant relief of symptoms for a number of patients. Improvement has been shown in neuropsychological test performance and self-esteem, and greater self-sufficiency has been demonstrated in cognitively impaired AIDS-related complex (ARC) and AIDS patients treated with psychostimulants [55]. Few treatment-related side effects have been reported. However, dextroamphetamine may unmask or aggravate abnormal involuntary movements [56].

A trial of antidepressants may be useful to treat depressive symptoms. Because these patients are sensitive to the anticholinergic side effects of these agents, low doses must be used. Bupropion, maprotiline, desipramine, imipramine, nortriptyline, trazodone, fluoxetine, and the newer selective serotonin reuptake inhibitors (sertraline, paroxetine) have all been used successfully according to anecdotal reports. Studies of imipramine and fluoxetine have demonstrated their efficacy in the pharmacologic treatment of major depression in HIV-infected patients [57].

Antipsychotics may be useful in treating agitation, confusion, and hallucinations. Caution is warranted because these agents also have anticholinergic side effects and have the potential to cause extrapyramidal symptoms (EPS). EPS are 2.4 times more common in neurocognitively impaired HIV-infected patients receiving neuroleptics than in controls [58]. The same holds true for use of some antiemetic agents, including prochlorperazine and droperidol. The higher potency antipsychotics are more likely to produce EPS. Again, using low doses is the rule. Anecdotal experience suggests that molindone is a useful agent because of its favorable side effect profile.

OTHER PSYCHIATRIC AND NEUROPSYCHIATRIC SYNDROMES

Delirium. HIV encephalopathy often has a chronic, deteriorating course, which may be punctuated by periods of significantly worse mental functioning secondary to delirium. The incidence of delirium increases with the duration of illness and is higher in patients with opportunistic infections. Delirium is characterized by cognitive dysfunction, difficulty with concentration and attention, and an altered or fluctuating level of consciousness. It may be erroneously diagnosed as depression or another psychiatric disorder. It is usually acute in onset, multifactorial in origin, and in HIV-infected patients, it may not resolve completely. The management of delirium involves treating the underlying cause, orienting the individual, and using neuroleptics (see Chap. 221 for further details on the treatment of delirium). In treating the delirious HIV-infected patient, it is important to bear in mind the special considerations regarding neuroleptics in this population (see HIV Encephalopathy, Treatment).

Anxiety. Anxiety is a common problem in AIDS patients. It may be a symptom of an underlying medical problem, or it may be primarily psychological. Common medical causes of anxiety in this population include hypoxia, anemia, hypoglycemia, complex partial seizure, and drug toxicity.

Nonmedical causes of anxiety are myriad in these patients. They range from concerns about the illness and its prognosis to worries about social isolation and financial difficulties. Uncertainty about the course of the disease is an ever-present issue, and for some patients it is a constant source of anxiety. Pharmacotherapy may be useful for acute anxiety, especially in the hospital; individual and group psychotherapy are often extremely beneficial to help patients develop coping skills.

ANEMIA AND HYPOXEMIA. Patients with HIV infection are particularly prone to anemia. This may ensue from the HIV infection itself, from marrow invasion by opportunistic infections and malignancies, or as a side effect of medications (e.g., antibiotics and AZT). Hypoxia may occur in patients with compromised pulmonary function. The most common pulmonary disease causing hypoxia in the HIV-infected host is PCP.

HYPOGLYCEMIA. Pentamidine may be used intravenously in the treatment of PCP and is also employed in the aerosolized form for prophylaxis. In either form, this drug may cause hypoglycemia.

COMPLEX PARTIAL SEIZURES. Although the incidence of complex partial seizures in patients with AIDS in unknown, there is evidence that HIV-infected persons are at risk for seizures of all types [59]. Seizures in these patients can be attributed to a mass lesion (e.g., toxoplasmosis, lymphoma) in about one third of cases; in another third they are attributed to HIV encephalopathy; and in the remainder the cause is unknown. Because anxiety is commonly associated with complex partial seizures, the occurrence of episodic anxiety, particularly in association with subtle motor signs, should raise the possibility of complex partial seizures (see Complex Partial Seizures, under Psychiatric Complications of Cancer).

AKATHISIA. AIDS patients may be exposed to the same agents that cause akathisia in cancer patients: phenothiazines, butyrophenones, and metoclopramide. (See Akathisia, under Psychiatric Complications of Cancer.)

CLAUSTROPHOBIA. As with oncology patients, the medical evaluation of persons with HIV infection and AIDS may require CT or MRI scans, which may precipitate panic in those with claustrophobia. Confinement secondary to IV lines and other equipment may also arouse severe anxiety. As in cancer patients, pharmacotherapy with antipanic agents (e.g., alprazolam, lorazepam, and clonazepam), relaxation, or hypnosis may prove effective.

Depression. Although the incidence of major depression in hospitalized AIDS patients has been estimated to be between 4.5 percent and 15 percent [60], depressive mood as a feature of adjustment disorder is more common. Dilley and associates [61] reported a diagnosis of adjustment disorder with depressed mood in 7 of 13 hospitalized AIDS patients for whom psychiatric consultation was sought. Depression is also a potential drug side effect of AZT and alpha-interferon. It is impossible to label a depressive syndrome in such individuals as either functional or organic. The symptoms often have roots in both the functional and organic realms. Depression in HIV-infected patients warrants aggressive psychiatric intervention, and should not be assumed to be a reaction to, or a normal outcome of, the diagnosis. Guidelines for pharmacotherapy are outlined above (earlier in this chapter in the discussion of treatment of HIV encephalopathy, and in Chap. 221 on depression in the ICU).

Suicide. The incidence of completed suicide in AIDS patients is a subject of much debate. Suicidal ideation is common, and as with cancer patients, arises in the context of physical deterioration (e.g., with facial Kaposi's sarcoma and wasting as well as with progression of the disease in general) and loss of control. Contributing factors include uncertainty of disease course, threat of neurologic deterioration, social isolation, financial destitution, and homelessness. Populations at highest risk for AIDS are already disenfranchised from society at large, and often their meager connections may be completely ruptured by the onset of this disease. The stigma of the diagnosis is so powerful that even patients whose HIV infection is not related to lifestyle (transfusion recipients, hemophiliacs) take great pains to conceal their illness from others.

Rundell and colleagues discovered an astounding increase in suicidal ideation, suicide attempts, and completed suicides in military personnel who become seropositive [62]. Factors associated with an increased likelihood of suicide attempt include multiple psychosocial stressors, social isolation, substance abuse, physical or serologic evidence of disease progression, loss of effectiveness of the defense mechanism of denial, and the perception of being the victim of events beyond personal control. According to Marzuk and associates, the suicide rate in persons with AIDS is up to 66 times greater than that of the general population and 36 times that of individuals of the same gender and age [63]. The true incidence of completed suicides in the population of symptomatic HIV-infected persons may be obscured by the low rate of postmortem examination.

Physicians and other caretakers may be troubled by patients' decisions to discontinue potentially life-prolonging therapies (e.g., antiretroviral therapy, PCP prophylaxis) or their refusal to undergo medical evaluation for new signs and symptoms of disease. Medical personnel may view such decisions as suicidal. In all circumstances where suicidal ideation is a question, treatable psychiatric disorders such as major depression must be aggressively sought out and treated. In some suicidal patients there is no underlying depressive disorder (see Chap. 223). As with cancer patients, the patient's sense of control should be maximized and psychosocial supports mobilized as much as possible.

Mania. Mania is more common in AIDS patients than in cancer patients. There are numerous potential causes of mania in this population. Intracranial disease, including HIV encephalopathy, mass lesions (e.g., toxoplasmosis, lymphoma), meningitis and encephalitis (e.g., cryptococcal and other meningitides, viral encephalitides), and drug toxicities are frequent causes. Drugs with the potential to cause mania commonly used in this population include AZT, DDI, ganciclovir, dapsone, and corticosteroids. Mania caused by medications has been successfully prevented and treated with use of lithium carbonate.

Neuropsychiatric Side Effects of Medications Used in HIV-Infected Patients. AZT (azidothymidine, zidovudine) has a variety of potential adverse effects on CNS function. These include mental clouding, depression, irritability, headache, and mania. As mentioned, individuals who develop mania while taking AZT may be rechallenged with the drug after initiation of lithium prophylaxis. A recent case report cites DDI-related mania in two HIV-infected patients [64].

For neuropsychiatric side effects of interferon, see Neuropsychiatric Side Effects of Anticancer Agents earlier in this chapter.

Pentamidine, used in the treatment and prophylaxis of PCP, may produce hypoglycemia or hypotension of sufficient severity to interfere with mentation.

Amphotericin, used in the treatment of cryptococcal infections and intractable candidiasis, is associated with headache, disorientation, lethargy, agitation, and nausea.

Metronidazole, an antimicrobial and antiprotozoal medication, may cause dizziness, confusion, and delirium. Used intravenously, it is a convulsant. These side effects are dose related. When combined with alcohol, it has a disulfiramlike effect (see Neuropsychiatric Side Effects of Anticancer Agents).

Corticosteroids may be used during treatment for PCP, for certain intracranial processes, and in the treatment of adrenal failure. For side effects, see Neuropsychiatric Side Effects of Anticancer Agents.

Because HIV-infected patients seem to be particularly sensitive to anticholinergic side effects of a variety of medications, low doses of anticholinergic medications are advised. These side effects include CNS manifestations such as confusion, delirium, disorientation, agitation, visual and auditory hallucinations, anxiety, motor restlessness, and seizures as well as myoclonic jerks and choreoathetoid movements. Peripheral manifestations of anticholinergic toxicity include decreased bowel motility, constipation, urinary retention, anhidrosis, mydriasis, dry mouth, cycloplegia, increased body temperature, motor incoordination, flushing, and tachycardia [65].

Drugs with high anticholinergic potential include certain antidepressants (e.g., amitriptyline, imipramine, and doxepin); certain low-potency antipsychotics (e.g., chlorpromazine and thioridazine); certain antihistamines (e.g., dimenhydrinate, diphenhydramine, hydroxyzine, promethazine, scopolamine, and trimethobenzamide); and anti-parkinsonian drugs.

Summary

Good medical care in cancer and AIDS requires a sound knowledge of the illness, its complications, and its available therapies. Critical care decisions are best made when the physician and patient have a working relationship and when the patient's wishes regarding interventions have been discussed before the acute crisis. Though psychiatric and neuropsychiatric complications are common, many are treatable and even reversible.

References

1. Schapira DV, Studnicki J, Bradham DD, et al: Intensive care, survival, and expense of treating critically ill cancer patients. *JAMA* 269:783, 1993.
2. Lemp GF, Payne SF, Neal D, et al: Survival trends for patients with AIDS. *JAMA* 263:402, 1990.
3. Harris JE: Improved short-term survival of AIDS patients initially diagnosed with *Pneumocystis carinii* pneumonia, 1984 through 1987. *JAMA* 263:397, 1990.
4. Cassem EH: Appropriate treatment limits in advanced cancer, in Billings JA (ed): *Outpatient Management of Advanced Cancer.* Philadelphia, JB Lippincott, 1985.
5. Weisman AD: *On Dying and Denying.* New York, Behavioral Publications, 1972, p 36.
6. Morrow GR, Morrell C: Behavioral treatment for the anticipatory nausea and vomiting induced by cancer chemotherapy. *N Engl J Med* 307:1476, 1982.
7. Greenberg DB, Surman OS, Clarke J, et al: Alprazolam for phobic nausea and vomiting related to cancer chemotherapy. *Cancer Treat Rep* 71:549, 1987.
8. Weissman MM: The epidemiology of panic disorder and agoraphobia, in Frances AJ, Hales RE (eds): *Review of Psychiatry.* Washington, DC, American Psychiatric Press, 1988, vol 7, p 54.
9. Gastaut H: Clinical and electroencephalographical classification of epileptic seizures. *Epilepsia* 11:145, 1971.
10. Theodore WH, Porter RJ, Penry JK: Complex partial seizures: Clinical characteristics and differential diagnosis. *Neurology* 33:1115, 1983.
11. Marshall DW, Westmoreland BF, Sharbrough FW: Ictal tachycardia during temporal lobe seizures. *Mayo Clin Proc* 58:443, 1983.
12. Greenberg DB, Hochberg FH, Murray GB: The theme of death in complex partial seizures. *Am J Psychiatry* 41:1587, 1984.
13. Mesulam M: *Principles of Behavioral Neurology.* Philadelphia, FA Davis, 1985, p 290.
14. Lipinski JF, Zubenko GS, Cohen BM, et al: Propranolol in the treatment of neuroleptic-induced akathisia. *Am J Psychiatry* 141:412, 1990.
15. Derogatis LR, Morrow GR, Fetting J, et al: The prevalence of psychiatric disorders among cancer patients. *JAMA* 249:751, 1983.
16. Lansky SB, List MA, Herrman CA, et al: Absence of major depressive disorder in female cancer patients. *J Clin Oncol* 3:1553, 1985.
17. Weisman AD: *Coping with Cancer.* New York, McGraw-Hill, 1979.
18. Spiegel D, Bloom J: Pain in metastatic breast cancer. *Cancer* 52:341, 1983.
19. Holland JC, Korzun AH, Tross S, et al: Comparative psychological disturbance in patients with pancreatic and gastric cancer. *Am J Psychiatry* 143:982, 1986.
20. Louhivuori KA, Hakama M: Risk of suicide among cancer patients. *Am J Epidemiol* 109:59, 1979.

21. Brown JH, Henteleff P, Barakat S, et al: Is it normal for terminally ill patients to desire death? *Am J Psychiatry* 143:208, 1986.

22. Fos BJ, Stanek EJ, Boyd SC, et al: Suicide rates among cancer patients in Connecticut. *J Chronic Dis* 35:85, 1982.

23. Ling MHM, Perry PJ, Tsuang MT: Side effects of corticosteroid therapy: Psychiatric aspects. *Arch Gen Psychiatry* 38:471, 1985.

24. Greenberg DB, Brown GL: Mania resulting from brain stem tumor. *J Nerv Ment Dis* 173:434, 1985.

25. Silberfarb PM: Chemotherapy and cognitive defects in cancer patients. *Annu Rev Med* 34:35, 1983.

26. Crawford J, Cox EB, Cohen HJ: Evaluation of hyperviscosity in monoclonal gammopathies. *Am J Med* 79:13, 1985.

27. Falk WE, Poskanzer DC: Lithium prophylaxis of corticotropin-induced psychosis. *JAMA* 241:1011, 1979.

28. DeVita VT, Hahn MA, Oliverio VT: Monoamine oxidase inhibition by a new carcinostatic agent, N-isopropyl-a-(2-methylhydrazino)-p-toluamide. *Proc Soc Exp Biol Med* 118:561, 1965.

29. Holland J, Fasanello S, Ohnuma T: Psychiatric symptoms associated with L-asparaginase administration. *J Psychiatr Res* 10:105, 1974.

30. Lazarus M, Herzig RH, Herzig GP, et al: Central nervous system toxicity of high-dose systemic cytosine arabinoside. *Cancer* 48:2577, 1981.

31. Moore DH, Fowler WC, Crumpler LS: 5-Fluorouracil neurotoxicity. *Gynecol Oncol* 36:152, 1990.

32. Walker RW, Allen JC, Rosen G, et al: Transient cerebral dysfunction secondary to high-dose methotrexate. *J Clin Oncol* 4:1845, 1986.

33. Silberfarb PM, Holland JCB, Anbar D: Psychological response of patients receiving two drug regimens for lung carcinoma. *Am J Psychiatry* 140:110, 1983.

34. Zalupski M, Baker LH: Ifosfamide. *JNCI* 80L:556, 1988.

35. Pallotta MG, Valasco A, Sadler A: Ifosfamide extrapyramidal neurotoxicity. *Cancer* 70:2743, 1992.

36. Gilliam F, Simonian N, Chiappa K: Complex partial status epilepticus associated with ifosfamide infusion. *Epilepsia* (supp 33):3, 1992.

37. McGuire WP, Rowinsky EK, Rosenshein NB, et al: Taxol: A unique antineoplastic agent with significant activity in advanced ovarian epithelial neoplasms. *Ann Intern Med* 111:273, 1989.

38. Eisenberger MA, Reyno LM, Jodrell DI, et al: Suramin, an active drug for prostate cancer: Interim observations in a phase I trial. *JNCI* 85:611, 1993.

39. Renault PF, Hoofnagle JH, Park Y: Psychiatric complications of long-term interferon alpha therapy. *Arch Intern Med* 147:1577, 1987.

40. Denicoff KD, Rubinow DR, Papa MZ, et al: The neuropsychiatric effects of treatment with interleukin-2 and lymphokine-activated killer cells. *Ann Intern Med* 107:293, 1987.

41. Ho DD, Sarngadharan MG, Resnick L, et al: Primary human T-lymphotropic virus type III infection. *Ann Intern Med* 103(6 pt 1):880, 1985.

42. Cooper DA, Gold J, MacLean P, et al: Acute AIDS retrovirus infection: Definition of a clinical illness associated with seroconversion. *Lancet* 1:537, 1985.

43. Navia BA, Jordan BD, Price RW: The AIDS dementia complex: I. Clinical features. *Ann Neurol* 19:517, 1986.

44. Beckett A, Summergrad P, Manschreck T, et al: Symptomatic HIV infection of the CNS in a patient with clinical evidence of immune deficiency. *Am J Psychiatry* 144:1342, 1987.

45. Brew BJ, Sidtis JJ, Rosenblum M, et al: AIDS dementia complex. *J R Coll Physicians Lond* 3(3):140, 1988.

46. Gabuzda DH, Hirsch MS: Neurologic manifestations of infection with human immunodeficiency virus: Clinical features and pathogenesis. *Ann Intern Med* 107:383, 1987.

47. Centers for Disease Control: Revision of the CDC surveillance case definition for acquired immunodeficiency syndrome. *MMWR* 36(15), August 14, 1987.

48. Janssen R, Cornblath DR, Epstein LG, et al: Nomenclature and research case definitions for neurological manifestations of human immunodeficiency virus type-1 (HIV-1) infection: Report of a working group of the American Academy of Neurology Task Force. *Neurology* 41(5): 1991.

49. Levy RM, Rosenblum S, Perrett LV: Neuroradiologic findings in AIDS: A review of 200 cases. *Am J Radiol* 147:977, 1986.

50. Jarvick JG, Hesselink JR, Kennedy C, et al: Acquired immunodeficiency syndrome: Magnetic resonance patterns of brain involvement with pathologic correlation. *Arch Neurol* 45:731, 1988.

51. Post MJD, Sheldon JJ, Hensley GT, et al: Central nervous system disease in acquired immunodeficiency syndrome: Prospective correlation using CT, MR imaging, and pathologic studies. *Radiology* 158:141, 1986.

52. Hollander H, Levy J: Neurologic abnormalities and human immunodeficiency virus recovery from cerebrospinal fluid. *Ann Intern Med* 106:692, 1987.

53. Yarchoan R, Berg G, Brouwers P, et al: Response of human-immunodeficiency-virus-associated neurologic disease to 3'-azido-3'-deoxythymidine. *Lancet* 1:132, 1987.

54. Schmitt FA, Bigley JW, McKinnis R, et al: Neuropsychological outcome of zidovudine (AZT) treatment of patients with AIDS and AIDS-related complex. *N Engl J Med* 319:1573, 1988.

55. Fernandez F, Adams F, Levy JK, et al: Cognitive impairment due to AIDS-related complex and its response to psychostimulants. *Psychosomatics* 29:38, 1988.

56. Fernandez F, Levy JK, Galizzi H: Response of HIV-related depression to psychostimulants: Case reports. *Hosp Commun Psychiatry* 39:628, 1988.

57. Hintz S, Kuck J, Peterkin JJ, et al: Depression in the context of human immunodeficiency virus infection: Implications for treatment. *J Clin Psychiatry* 51:497, 1990.

58. Hriso E, Kuhn T, Masdeu JC, et al: Extrapyramidal symptoms due to dopamine-blocking agents in patients with AIDS encephalopathy. *Am J Psychiatry* 148:1558, 1991.

59. Holtzman DM, Kaku DA, So YT: New-onset seizures associated with human immunodeficiency virus infection: Causation and clinical features in 100 cases. *Am J Med* 87:173, 1989.

60. Buhrich N, Cooper DA: Requests for psychiatric consultation concerning 22 patients with AIDS and ARC. *Aust N Z J Med* 21:346, 1987.

61. Dilley JW, Ochitill HN, Perl M, et al: Findings in psychiatric consultation with patients with acquired immunodeficiency syndrome. *Am J Psychiatry* 142:82, 1985.

62. Rundell JR, Kyle KM, Brown GR, et al: Risk factors for suicide attempts in a human immunodeficiency virus screening program. *Psychosomatics* 33:24, 1992.

63. Marzuk PM, Tierney H, Tardiff K, et al: Increased risk of suicide in persons with AIDS. *JAMA* 259:1333, 1988.

64. Orth JP, Ollivier B, Vinti H, et al: Occurrence of acute mania in two AIDS patients during dideoxyinosine treatment at a dose of 750 mg/24h. *Int Conf AIDS 1991,* Jun 16-21;7(1):189 (abstr no. M.B.2031).

65. Bassuk EL, Schoonover SC, Gelenberg AJ (eds): *The Practitioner's Guide to Psychoactive Drugs.* 2nd ed. New York, Plenum Medical Book Company, 1983, p 142.

XIX. Moral, Ethical, Legal, and Public Policy Issues in the Intensive Care Unit

Section Editor
Daniel Teres

228. An Ethical and Legal Analysis of Problems in Critical Care Medicine

John J. Paris and Frank E. Reardon

In one of the first and most significant studies of the public policy implications of intensive care delivery, Knaus and colleagues [1] at George Washington University Medical Center identified two principal roles for intensive care: "life support of organ system failure in critically ill patients or close monitoring of stable non-critically ill patients in case the need for life support suddenly occurs" (p. 562). From their study they determined there is little evidence that the widespread use of such services has resulted in improved survival or quality of life for a substantial portion of the patients presently admitted to such intensive care units (ICUs). In fact, they concluded that approximately 25 percent of the total ICU therapy is used for patients who either have little need for unique ICU services or are too acutely and chronically ill to benefit from them.

Their study confirmed the findings of others who have examined the indications and outcomes of intensive care medicine [2–5], pointing to the need for more vigorous standards for ICU admission and discharge. Such an attempt was made at Memorial Sloan-Kettering Cancer Center, where it was early recognized that many of the patients being admitted to the ICU were surviving their acute episodes only to die shortly thereafter from their underlying cancer. Rather than subject these patients (and their families) to the trauma of spending their final days in an ICU, the medical staff adopted a policy of formally classifying all hospital patients according to the underlying prognosis of their disease. As Turnbull and associates reported [6], those patients whose short-term prognosis was poor and for whom no definitive therapy existed were not considered candidates for transfer to the ICU regardless of the acute problems that might develop.

To limit the inappropriate institution of other invasive "life-saving" therapy, similar classifications were developed for patients suffering from advanced cystic fibrosis [7], severe burns [8], and nontraumatic coma [9]. In addition, work began on establishing quantitative predictive models such as the Acute Physiology and Chronic Health Evaluation (APACHE) scale developed by Knaus and colleagues as an objective measure of the severity of illness of ICU patients [10]. By design, however, the APACHE I and II scales [11] are more appropriate for predicting outcomes for populations of ICU patients, rather than for individuals. That task, at least in the initial stages, remains notoriously uncertain [12] and varied [13].

Knaus' [14] recent data indicated that of 571 acutely ill ventilated patients admitted to the intensive care units of 12 hospitals, 48 percent could be identified on admission to be at a 75 percent or greater risk of hospital death; by day 4 of ICU treatment, estimates for hospital mortality increased to 97 percent. Of those predicted to die, a single 56-year-old patient who had severe long-standing multiple organ system failure with an episode of septic shock survived. Such survivals, even though extremely rare, lead to a reluctance by clinicians to withdraw or withhold intensive care from those too ill to benefit [15].

To overcome the statistical character of the predictive index, Chung [16] proposed the development of a dynamic rather than a static model, one that would identify individual patients who would not survive the course of their illness. Although it remains impossible to predict those acutely ill ICU patients who

will survive, Chung established that focusing on changes in homeostasis will allow the observer to identify accurately that subset of ICU patients who will not survive. With his predictive index, 40 percent of the nonsurvivors can readily be identified.

The remarkable growth of the hospice movement from one program in 1974 to over 1600 programs today [17] is another phenomenon in the attempt to limit inappropriate care of the critically ill. Many of these programs, however, are still in the fledgling stage and are available to only a small fraction of the nation's terminally ill patients. Most critically and terminally ill patients continue to be cared for in institutions in which aggressive intervention and treatment of acute episodes is the norm.

There are many reasons for this general practice of maximal response to crises in the seriously ill patient. Several of them have been identified by Angell [18]: (1) The current fee for service reimbursement schedule, which rewards physicians preferentially for performing tests and procedures; (2) the ever-present spectre of malpractice; and (3) the American propensity to believe that every problem has a solution, often a technical one. This last factor leads to the familiar request of patients and families to "do everything possible," which is all too often translated into what Thurow [19] perceptively characterized as using every experimental technique on the outside chance that one of the procedures just might work.

This process, which Fuchs labeled "the technological imperative" [20], when combined with the other forces now operative in our society, has produced a health care system in crisis. The cost of care has risen beyond our ability or at least our willingness to pay for it. Among the measures to control and limit the rising costs, and thereby curb the demands for "rationing" of health care, Angell [18] suggested that we reexamine the proposition that in health care, as in other commodities, more is better. She insisted that, far from being beneficial, much of the medical care now provided in this country is unnecessary. Much medical care is of no demonstrated value to those who receive it, and some is positively harmful. She cited among the unnecessary items the aggressive treatment of terminally ill patients for whom treatment other than palliative care is no longer appropriate.

In an essay, Moore [21] condemned "desperate measures for desperately ill patients desperately hopeless from the outset." Moore's insight is more readily adopted by European than American physicians. European physicians understand that the ICU is designed for patients with acute reversible diseases and those at risk for developing complications, for example, after extensive surgery. As a result, they have "a policy of admitting only those patients who have a reasonable chance of recovery to a meaningful life and deny ICU admissions to terminally ill patients" [22]. ICU use is confined to those who are expected to recover from acute episodes; it is not used as a high tech hospice.

As Ramsey [23] noted, it is imperative to distinguish between treatments that will benefit the patient and those that are useless and false remedies. For the patient who has truly entered the dying process, comfort and company, not further and futile attempts at treatment, are the appropriate care. Ramsey's comment forces us into the difficult but nonetheless important distinctions of medical ethics, distinctions whose origin can be traced back to the earliest formulations of the Hippocratic corpus.

There we find the antidote to the notion that the physician's duty is to do everything possible to prolong life. As Admundsen's [24] historical analysis established:

The treatise entitled *The Art* in the Hippocratic Corpus defines medicine as having three roles: doing away with the sufferings of the sick, lessening the violence of their diseases, and refusing to treat those who are overmastered by their diseases, realizing that in such cases medicine is powerless. (pp. 23–24)

The best contemporary restatement of the standards for appropriate care of the sick is found in the report of the President's Commission for the Study of Ethical Problems in Medicine and Biomedical and Behavioral Research [25]. That report, which was formulated by ethicists, physicians, lawyers, theologians, and academics, has had enormous impact on hospital policies, regulatory directives, court opinions, and the direction of medicine. Many of the topics in the report responded to the concerns, fears, and worries of physicians, nurses, and patients, particularly those in the highly sophisticated setting of an ICU. The Commission approached its task primarily from the perspective of ethics, the traditions of medicine, and issues of human choice. Only secondarily did the Commission turn to the more narrow and necessarily limited perspective of law for its contributions to the development of standards and formation of public policy. The result is a balanced, sensitive, humane, and strikingly sensible approach to complex, difficult ethical dilemmas, an approach that is helpful to practitioners and patients alike.

Several of the issues reviewed by the Commission are of particular interest to those involved with intensive care medicine: "do not resuscitate" (DNR) orders, brain death, living wills, and decision-making for the incompetent patient.

Do Not Resuscitate Orders

AMA GUIDELINES. After nearly a decade of turmoil concerning do not resuscitate orders, the Ethical and Judicial Council of the American Medical Association has issued a policy statement designed to provide guidance for physicians and hospitals on that topic [26]. As the accompanying *JAMA* editorial by Bernard Lo [27] indicates, the Council's guidance is ambiguous, somewhat convoluted, and certain to evoke hostility from some physicians. The ambiguity and confusion are engendered in part by the Council's efforts to find a compromise between those who support complete patient autonomy [28,29] and those who insist that physician determination [30–33] of potential effectiveness should govern whether to attempt cardiopulmonary resuscitation (CPR).

In its search for a middle course, the Council rejected Blackhall's [34] proposal that futility be defined as survival to discharge. Instead, it defines futility as that which cannot restore heartbeat or, if it can, fails to achieve the expressed goals of the informed patient or the patient's family. The Council's approach thus sides with those who favor patient or family determination on whether to attempt CPR.

The outer reaches of that approach are found in a New York statute enacted on the recommendation of the New York State Task Force on Life and the Law [35] that requires physicians to obtain the informed consent of a competent patient or the family of a decisionally incapable patient before they may legally write a DNR order. The only exception for direct involvement of a competent patient is the assessment by both the attending physician and a second independent physician that the patient would suffer "immediate and severe" harm from the discussion, e.g., the very posing of the question would prove so threatening to the patient as to trigger an immediate cardiac arrest or would prove so unsettling to a patient with severe paranoia, depression, or suicidal tendencies that it might drive the patient to self-inflicted harm (p. 26).

When asked at a medical meeting if this policy meant that a physician would be required to undertake what was believed to be a futile attempt at cardio-resuscitation if requested to do so by a competent patient [or presumably by the family of a decisionally incapable terminally ill patient], the then New York Health Commissioner, Dr. David Axelrod, replied: "There is a right to CPR so I think the patient has to get it." "But," he continued, "that's pretty rare. How often does that happen?" The response from the assembled physicians: "Often," "Everyday," "All the time." [36]

Historical Development of Do Not Resuscitate Orders. In formulating cardiopulmonary or do not resuscitate policies, ethics committees and the hospitals they serve are aware of these conflicting views and the sometimes unreasonable expectations and demands of dying patients and their families. Nurses, physicians, and families regularly find themselves at odds over the topic; yet until recently, the subject was left unaddressed and unresolved. Assistance in designing policies as well as understanding the context for the AMA Guidelines can be found in the historical background of the present debate.

With the development of resuscitation techniques in the 1960s came the need for reflection and guidance on their effectiveness and appropriate usage. These were first provided in the landmark 1974 American Medical Association Report on Standards for Cardiopulmonary Resuscitation [37] which set standards and initiated a massive and highly effective CPR training program. The Report declared:

The purpose of cardiopulmonary resuscitation is the prevention of sudden, unexpected death. Cardiopulmonary resuscitation is not indicated in certain situations, such as in cases of terminal irreversible illness where death is not unexpected or where prolonged cardiac arrest dictates the futility of resuscitation efforts. Resuscitation in these circumstances may represent a positive violation of an individual's right to die with dignity. (p. 864)

That thoughtful and carefully formulated statement has been all but forgotten as paramedics, nurses, and physicians trained in the new lifesaving techniques respond to "code blues" with "crash carts" and portable defibrillators like firefighters answering an alarm. In the words of Dr. Mitchell Rabkin, President of Boston's Beth Israel Hospital, "When the bell rings, you run!"

That response pattern soon led to attempted resuscitations for virtually all in-hospital deaths regardless of individual medical history and prognosis. As Lampton and Winship [38] reported, "Many medical staffs adopted universal, hospital-wide policies stating that CPR would be instituted on all patients experiencing sudden and unexpected cardiopulmonary arrest" (p. 260). And they observed that "ultimately, it appears that many persons view CPR as a mandatory activity for all patients dying in a hospital." In an insightful and humane essay, Steven Spenser [39] noted that tendency has evolved into a fixed policy of attempting to overcome the death of all patients unless the physician has written a specific "no-code" order. Consequently, physicians find themselves in the position of having to write a negative, inhibiting order to protect their terminally ill patients from unwanted and unwarranted intrusions into their dying.

A further complication in this litigation-conscious era is that physicians are now looking to the courts and the legal profession for guidance and protection on the proper treatment of the dying patient. They are also asking families to share the burden of responsibility for such decisions to a degree that Spenser observed would have been unthinkable a few years ago.

How we got ourselves into this predicament, and possible resolutions of it, was the subject of a 2-year study by the President's Commission. Dr. Mitchell Rabkin provided the most complete explanation to the Commission. Rabkin testified that before his institution's well-known 1976 "Orders Not to Resuscitate" directive [40] was in effect, "a significant percentage of patients who died received cardiopulmonary resuscitation upon their *quietus* even though it was acknowledged that the resuscitation efforts for many would be useless" (p. 367). In his words, "The emergency code was called, and all of the troops—cardiologists, anesthetists, nurses, respiratory therapists, and others—responded in full" (p. 367).

The folly of that policy was epitomized for Rabkin when he encountered a nurse weeping in the corridor outside her patient's room. The patient, an octogenarian with widespread terminal cancer, had just stopped breathing, and a staff member called the code. A horde of professionals was applying intravenous medication and electrical current to stimulate the heart, and the anesthetist was ventilating the patient through an endotracheal tube just inserted—all to no avail, of course. "Why can't they just let him die in peace?" wept the nurse. The answer was straightforward and alluded to in the 1976 Beth Israel directive [40]:

Both as a standard of medical care and a statement of philosophy, it is the general policy of hospitals to act affirmatively to preserve the life of all patients, including persons who suffer from irreversibly terminal illness. It is essential that all hospital staff understand this policy and act accordingly (p. 364).

That pro-life policy, good in itself, was so rigidly interpreted that a DNR order could be entered only after (1) it was determined that the patient was irreversibly and irreparably ill and death was imminent (within 2 weeks); (2) an ad hoc committee of senior physicians and nurses concurred in that evaluation; and (3) the informed choice of the competent patient (or the family of an incompetent patient) was given. If, in the judgment of the responsible physician, the patient would be unable to cope psychologically with the consent stipulation, no order could be written. Here a misplaced emphasis on patient autonomy and informed consent pressured the dying patient into the trauma of a code versus no-code choice as a final discretionary decision.

Several years' experience with those stringent stipulations and the increasing realization that these ill-considered resuscitation efforts in no way represent an affirmative act to preserve life led the medical staff to rewrite the DNR policy. In addition to the hospital's own experiences, a Massachusetts appellate court had ruled that DNR decision-making should rest with the physician acting in accordance with the standards of good medical practice and the wishes of the patient or the patient's family [41].

That ruling led numerous Massachusetts hospitals to establish formal DNR policies or to reconsider existing procedures. The 1981 Beth Israel Hospital guidelines omit the attempt to define the candidates for DNR orders; they leave that determination to the judgment of the attending physician. The 1981 policy specifies the process by which such possibilities are to be considered and orders written. It also eliminates the need for a bureaucratic ad hoc committee and substitutes the notification of the chief of service that such an order has been given.

Then, in a dramatic shift from the previous emphasis on individual autonomy and "informed consent," the new guidelines state:

If, in the opinion of the attending physician, the competent patient might be harmed by a full discussion of whether resuscitation would be appropriate in the event of an arrest, the competent patient should be spared the discussion; therefore if the physician and the Chief of Service deem a DNR order appropriate and the family members are in agreement that the discussion might harm the patient and that resuscitation is not appropriate, a DNR order may be entered by the physician [42].

This new policy, which recognizes the difference between an automaton and an autonomous patient, conforms to Spenser's [35] insight that explanations of DNR orders to dying patients "are thoughtless to the point of being cruel except for the extremely unlikely case where the patient himself inquires" (p. 139).

Rabkin et al. [40] reported that the new Beth Israel policy allowed more open discussion among caregivers on the appropriateness of orders not to resuscitate a given patient. Concomitantly, slow codes and partial codes [39] (e.g., "Walk, don't run," "Page but don't stat page," and "Do not intubate if a code is called") have declined. Not only do partial orders such as these place unwarranted burdens on the hospital staff, but they are in Goldenring's [40] explicit phrasing, "an ethical fraud" (p. 1058).

Under the 1981 guidelines a code will be called and answered as a well-considered affirmative act to benefit the patient. As such, when a code is issued, the staff can respond knowing that they will not be deliberately imposing a final, useless indignity on the end of life.

Guidelines for Resuscitation Decisions

In its report, the President's Commission [25] devoted an entire chapter to resuscitation decisions for hospitalized patients. The Commission noted that, among the general hospital population where virtually all deaths were attended by resuscitation efforts, only 3 percent of the attempts were successful. Further, 1 in 20 patients who survived resuscitation sustained severe brain damage, and about 1 in 4 had some serious and permanent injury. Consequently, the Commission concluded that the reflex resuscitation efforts presently attempted in hospitals are frequently a misguided adventure that injures the patient and violates personal control over his or her life.

In response the Commission called for a reevaluation of resuscitation practices by hospitals, health care providers, and especially treatment areas (e.g., ICUs and cardiac care units) where many patients are at risk for cardiac arrest and where CPR frequently is attempted automatically without appropriate prior deliberation.

In the advanced technical setting of an acute care hospital, the physician-patient-family relationship has been expanded to include health teams, rotating residents, triple shifts of nurses, and many other allied health professionals. Decisions that were once commonly agreed upon and easily effected directly by the physician now involve a large, diverse, and frequently unknown cadre of caregivers, hence the emerging need for explicit policies and guidelines for procedures, including for DNR orders.

Prior deliberation in such cases would (1) enable the patient's rights and decisions regarding self-determination to be respected, (2) guarantee that medical interventions serve the patient's best interest, (3) allow adequate evaluation of resource allocation and equity considerations, and (4) reduce nurse-physician-family misunderstandings on resuscitation practices.

To protect both the patient and caregivers, hospital policies should require appropriate communication with the patient (or the family) about the resuscitation decision. If a DNR order is deemed appropriate, that order should be written in the patient's chart, along with the rationale and supporting documentation.

There is an ongoing dispute over the extent to which the competent patient should or must be involved in the decision to write a DNR order [45]. Clearly, if the patient expresses an explicit desire for or against resuscitation, and the patient's comprehension of the medical situation is not questionable, that decision should be honored. The difficulty arises from the fact that most seriously ill patients have not directly expressed any opinion on the subject. Further, many of these patients are unwilling to make a decision [46]. How then should the decision-making process be approached? In its 1976 directive, and its 1991 update, Beth Israel Hospital followed the standard that has now been adopted by the Commission: The focus is on patient autonomy and informed consent, which means that patients must make their preferences known. The New York Task Force on Life and the Law went even further in its recommendation, since adopted as law in that state, that competent patients must provide informed consent for a DNR order unless, in the physician's judgment, the very seeking of the consent would lead to immediate cardiac arrest or suicide.

That pressure, particularly on a dying patient—one already overwhelmed with a deteriorating physical condition and attendant fears—strikes us as misplaced and inappropriate. Nor is the threat of such a mandate and its negative impact on decision-makers lessened by a footnoted reminder that "other caregiving professionals, religious advisors, or family members are in a good or better position to discuss the issue and convey the information (as is the attending physician)" [25] (p. 240, n. 38). Undue and misplaced pressure on the dying patient is not allayed by changing the bearer of the message.

Although Miles and co-workers [47] rightly place the question of resuscitation within the context of the patient's total medical care and prognosis, their insistence on a frank but not overly technical discussion of resuscitation with the patient might well exacerbate the patient's plight. Among the nontechnical factors they believe the patient should understand is that "resuscitation may be followed by the need for life support including intratracheal tube, tracheotomy, respiratory ventilator assistance, arterial lines and monitoring, and continuous intravenous medication, all for an indeterminate period" (p. 660).

Such an approach to CPR decision-making might be modified if compared with the 1974 and 1980 standards for CPR issued by the National Conference of the American Heart Association and with Siegler's [48] reminder that "the principal ethical grounds for making a decision not to resuscitate a patient should be the sound medical judgment that the patient's death from the primary disease is imminent and that further treatment for the primary disease is futile" (p. 28).

THE FUTILITY DEBATE. The futility of attempting CPR in certain cases is documented in a study of Bedell and colleagues [49] that reveals a 98 to 100 percent mortality rate in patients with metastatic disease, acute strokes, sepsis, renal failure, and pneumonia. The same statistics apply to those for whom resuscitation took longer than 30 minutes. The physician, aware of the outcome data and the futility of intervention in such cases,

has a professional obligation to provide care consonant with medical reality. In such cases, Blackhall [34] believes, "the issue of patient autonomy is irrelevant." When they arise, he believes that the physician could write DNR orders on the chart with the following type of documentation: "This patient has a condition for which CPR has been shown not to be effective. In case of cardiopulmonary arrest, CPR should not be performed" (p. 1284).

Tomlinson and Brody [50] distinguish three rationales for DNR orders: no medical benefit; poor quality of life after CPR; and poor quality of life before CPR. They adopt Blackhall's position that "Physicians have no obligation to provide, and patients and families no right to demand, medical treatment that is of no demonstrable benefit" (p. 43). In such cases, they too believe, the patient or family's desire for CPR is irrelevant. The decision is entirely within the physician's technical expertise. The physician's duty is to communicate with the family and explain that the patient's physical condition is such that no intervention will reverse the dying process and, hence, none will be attempted. The most physicians should do when CPR is believed futile is to communicate that information to the patient or family so that they will understand the decision the physician has made.

It is only when the patient declines CPR because of present or anticipated quality of life factors that the patient's values or desires determine the decision. If the present or anticipated quality of life of the patient is such that CPR is not desired by the patient, then the patient's values or desires are of import. In such cases it is personal values, not physician preferences, that prevail.

Murphy and colleagues [51] apply similar thinking to the issue of resuscitation in the elderly. Their data show resuscitation is successful in only 3.8 percent of the cases and never for arrests of elderly patients that are unwitnessed or occur outside the hospital. It is likewise unavailing even in witnessed hospital events in elderly patients with nonventricular arrhythmias.

The same proves true for cardiac arrests in the first 72 hours of life in very low birthweight babies. In a study by Lantos and colleagues [52] at the University of Chicago, none of the 38 babies who received CPR in the first 3 days of life survived. They concluded that in such instances CPR is an "innovative" or "non-validated" therapy. As such, it need not be provided or, if offered, should be presented to the family as an experimental procedure.

Similar outcomes are found by Applebaum and colleagues with regard to CPR initiated in elderly nursing home patients; by Gray, for out of hospital resuscitation efforts in which heartbeat had not been restored in the field; by Blackhall for acutely sick patients in county hospitals; and by McIntyre and independently by Laudoy and colleagues for chronically ill patients in intensive care units.

One additional insight into DNR practice is found in a study by Wachter and colleagues [53] of the discrepancy in the use of DNR orders by disease. Despite similar prognoses by clinicians, physicians are far more willing to write DNR orders for patients with lung cancer and AIDS than those with equally untreatable cirrhosis or severe congestive heart failure. In their study, 52 percent of terminally ill AIDS patients and 47 percent of those with lung cancer had DNR orders, while only 16 percent of those with cirrhosis and 4 percent of those with congestive heart failure and coronary artery disease received a DNR order. The differences persist even after adjustment for severity of illness and similarity of prognosis.

These studies establish that the focus on the process of patient involvement rather than the purpose and restricted effectiveness of CPR is a misplaced emphasis, one that will not affect the outcome of resuscitation efforts appreciably. The misplaced concern with patient autonomy and consent distracts and distorts the attention as well as the actions of patients, families, and caregivers. For most of the dying patients, the issue is purely a technical assessment: Given the patient's physiologic status, the data indicate CPR will be futile.

DO NOT RESUSCITATE POLICYMAKING.

Given that reality, present hospital policies of "full codes" on all patients on whom a DNR order is not written might be mistaken. In those cases where the responding team has no knowledge of the patient, it is imperative to institute a full code. But in many of the codes, the responding residents are fully aware of the terminal status of the patient and the reluctance of the family or the attending physician to authorize a DNR order. The response team is then expected to participate in a charade or an exercise in futility. Neither is good medicine.

In response to such situations, the Tufts-New England Medical Center Hospitals have adopted the following policy [54]. If there is no written DNR order: (1) It is the responsibility of the nursing staff to call a "Code 99" and to initiate CPR; (2) It is the responsibility of all appropriate staff and hospital personnel to respond as quickly as possible to such a "Code 99" when called; and (3) It is the responsibility of the physician(s) responding to a "Code 99" to determine what efforts are medically appropriate to treat the patient who has arrested. This responsibility includes continuing or discontinuing CPR when, in the judgment of the physician(s), aggressive treatment would be medically inappropriate.

The American Heart Association's 1992 Guidelines on Cardiopulmonary Resuscitation and Emerging Cardiac Care [55] also take this position. In addition to withholding CPR when there is a "No CPR order" [The Guidelines prefer that phrase to DNR], the 1992 Guidelines state that resuscitation efforts "should be withheld . . . when, in the judgment of the physician, such efforts cannot restore or sustain cardiopulmonary function; or when widely accepted scientific data indicate that there is no likelihood of survival" (p. 2286).

An even more far-reaching response to the "futility" issue is found in Beth Israel's 1991 Guidelines for Withholding, Withdrawing or Limiting Life-Sustaining Treatment [56]. This updated policy makes a critical distinction between a "Do Not Resuscitate Order," which is based on the patient or surrogate's choice as to whether to attempt resuscitation in the event of a cardiac arrest, and a situation in which a "CPR Not Indicated" order is appropriate. The latter occurs when "a *medical evaluation* of the patient has led to the conclusion that resuscitation efforts would be futile—such efforts would not be expected to restore cardiac or respiratory function or the patient is dying and resuscitative efforts will not benefit the patient" (p. 2). In such situations, the policy follows Blackhall's admonition that patient or (more likely) surrogate authorization is "irrelevant." Consent to withhold CPR is neither sought nor required in such instances since to provide it would be both medically futile and "an unwarranted abuse of the patient."

The Beth Israel policy adopts Tomlinson and Brody's [50] advice that the physician should inform the family that nothing more can be done in the way of resuscitative efforts. This is done to apprise them of the situation; it is not seeking their permission or their approbation. As the Beth Israel policy puts it, "There is no option which benefits the patient; the patient must therefore be allowed to expire in peace" (p. 2). Beth Israel's 1991 Guidelines, which adopt as hospital policy the fact that in some cases CPR will not work, are the first in the nation to incorporate the outcome data of the multiple studies done on the efficacy of CPR. These Guidelines recognize that in certain classes of identifiable patients, CPR is not effective and therefore will not be offered to patients or families as a moral option.

Here it is important to keep in mind Ingelfinger's admonition that "a physician who merely spreads an array of vendibles in front of the patient (or family) and then says, 'Go ahead and choose, it's your life,' is guilty of shirking his duty, if not malpractice" [57] (p. 1509). The physician certainly should explain the patient's condition to the family and the realistic options available. However, Ingelfinger reminded us that it is the physician's responsibility to recommend a specific course of action instead of merely asking the family to choose among them. In addition, the physician is not asking the family to substitute its judgment for that of the patient, but is, rather, asking them to reflect the patient's own value choice as close as humanly possible.

A frustrating situation may arise if, in the physician's judgment, there is no further treatment that can benefit the irreversibly dying patient, yet the family, through ignorance, misunderstanding, fear, or guilt demands that "everything possible" be done. Conversely, the problem may be insistence by the family on a No CPR order for a patient whom the physician believes has a good opportunity of recovery.

In these situations, an intrainstitutional consultation or ethics committee should assess the case. Perhaps a simple airing of the issues or the benefit of consultation will dispel the disagreement. Sometimes a change of physician may be in order. Alternatively, the review committee may decide to petition a court to appoint a legal guardian to protect the patient's interests.

Another problem that frequently arises in major hospital settings is the elderly dying patient who has outlived all family and friends. Rather than unreflectively resuscitating all such patients or overusing the complex and somewhat costly role of legal guardian, decisions against resuscitation might continue to be made as they customarily have been—by the attending physician with the concurrence of a disinterested physician, staff consensus, or an institutionally designated patient advocate. These decisions are well within the scope of common medical practice and should not be elevated to the role of moral dilemma or judicial problem. Decisions that are more complex or uncertain might, of course, demand more formal institutional review or legal guardianship. Here, as in almost all of its recommendations, the Commission is firm in its stance that rarely, if ever, is decision-making about life-sustaining care improved by resort to courts.

In fact, with regard to these questions the only court ever to address itself to the issue ruled that "The question [DNR] is not one for judicial decision, but one for the attending physician, in keeping with the highest traditions of his profession." It is, in the court's words, "a question peculiarly within the competence of the medical profession of what measures are appropriate to ease the imminent passing of an irreversibly, terminally ill patient in light of the patient's history and condition and the wishes of her family" [41] (p. 135).

The possibility that the highly invasive, costly, and often violent resuscitation procedures available in acute care settings might not be appropriate to a particular patient should be considered as a positive and prospective part of the delivery of high-quality medical care. Such decisions should not be made arbitrarily, hastily, or casually, nor should they depend on the personal fears or predilections of the individual physician. Rather, they should reflect a careful consideration of the particular patient's medical condition, prognosis, and values.

Further, the writing of a DNR order does not diminish the

physician's continuing responsibility to provide active medical care to the patient. As the Minnesota Medical Society's Guidelines make clear: "DNR orders are compatible with maximal therapeutic care. The patient may be receiving vigorous support in all other therapeutic modalities and yet justifiably be considered a proper subject for the DNR order" [58] (pp. 499–500).

DO NOT RESUSCITATE ORDERS IN THE OPERATING ROOM.
One small and as yet uncharted issue involving DNR policy is the question of the continuance of a do not resuscitate order for patients who go to the operating room for surgery. The question arises most commonly when a terminally ill patient wants to forgo resuscitation and yet needs amelioration or palliation of symptoms such as insertion of intravenous catheters, a feeding gastrostomy, a tracheostomy wound debridement, or a resection. The problem, as Walker [59] notes, is that deaths in the operating room are generally perceived as a bad outcome that invites professional scrutiny, criticism, and even censure. They also raise the ever-lurking specter of malpractice. For these reasons physicians, though willing to accept "natural" death, are loath to allow a death for which they feel personally responsible [60].

To honor a DNR order in the OR would mean that the surgeons or anesthesiologists not only must restrict their response to a potentially reversible situation, they must stand by idly while their patient dies. Further, Peterson [61] explains that from the surgeon's perspective, "Resuscitation and mechanical ventilation take on an entirely new meaning in the context of an operation" (p. 281). Most arrests in that setting result not from the disease process, but from the administration of anesthetics or from surgical events [62].

These events, as Franklin and Rothenberg [63] note, "are often, but not always, reversible" (p. 182). They argue that since hypotension and/or hypoventilation may not be a sign of incipient death, "it may not be the patient's intent to have intubation, vasopressors, and other maneuvers withheld in this situation." Their response, as is that of Peterson, is to suspend the DNR order during surgery. The overwhelming majority (81%) of accredited residency programs in anesthiology that responded to Franklin and Rothenberg's questionnaire on that issue agree with the policy of automatically suspending DNR orders during anesthesia and surgery. While such a policy might minimize uncertainty regarding the initiation of life support in the OR, the question remains, does it always serve the best interest of the patient? Walker [59] gives two reasons why patients might want to retain their DNR orders during surgery. The first is to avoid the risk of surviving resuscitation only to be left in a worse condition. If that were to occur, the surgery would prove not palliative but injurious. The second is the prospect of death under anesthesia as a peaceful exit. From the dying patient's perspective, if death occurs while under anesthesia, then so much the better.

Two persuasive arguments are presented as to why surgeons and anesthiologists, despite their interest in avoiding operative deaths, should accept the patient's willingness to undergo the risk of intraoperative cardiac arrest and death. One is that otherwise the patient's pain and suffering are not alleviated and the second is that the alternative is to force the patient to undergo morally optional invasive procedures. Such an action not only violates the patient's autonomy, it forces the patient to accept unwanted resuscitation as the price of palliation. While some patients might willingly accede to temporary suspension of a DNR order and others would be willing to risk a few days on a ventilator or even the possibility of being reduced to a comatose state, there are others who would want the assurance

that should they arrest, no resuscitation would be attempted. Here, as in all of medicine, the goal should be the appropriate response to the patient's medical condition, prognosis and, within that context, the patient's values.

DNR orders, which have been described in some detail because of the practical impact they have in an ICU setting, are but one part of the issues about treatment. Two other issues—brain death and living wills—raise troublesome legal and political implications that are out of proportion to the moral consensus on the topics.

BRAIN DEATH.
Despite the opposition of radical right-to-life forces and of a small but influential group of Orthodox Jews [64,65,66] who share their belief that only destruction of the brain can be entertained as a possible definition of death, there is no longer any doubt as to what are the medically accepted standards. The "Guidelines for the Determination of Death," a landmark document summarizing currently accepted medical practices, was published in 1981 [67].

Signed by the nation's leading authorities in neurology, neurosurgery, critical care, and legal medicine, the document represents "a consensus that is truly a remarkable achievement, [one] of which the medical profession can be proud" [68] (p. 2194). That document endorsed the Uniform Determination of Death Act. To date, some 38 states, excluding such major medical areas as Massachusetts, New York, and Minnesota, have adopted brain-death statutes.

The one remaining moral dilemma that some physicians continue to perceive is the need for family permission to remove the respirator from brain-dead patients. A classic statement of that problem is seen in the case of a 4-year-old girl who was brain-dead as the result of meningitis. The physicians approached her parents, informed them of the girl's diagnosis, told them that her condition was hopeless, and recommended the removal of the extraordinary life-support system. Given that moral choice, the parents opted for continued treatment. They did so in the hope of a "miracle." The hospital, fearful of opposing the parents' wishes and unwilling to face the adverse publicity of a court proceeding to override the parents' decision, kept the child in the pediatric ICU until several months later, when she succumbed to kidney failure.

As William Curran, Professor of Legal Medicine at Harvard Medical School and member of the original Harvard ad hoc committee on brain death [69], had repeatedly emphasized the determination of brain death is a technical medical issue, one which does not involve patient consent or family approval. Once the medical staff has made a well-informed determination of brain death, the patient is dead. The only moral issue remaining is the proper disposition of the corpse.

Not only is there no need to ask family permission to remove the respirator, to do so is highly inappropriate: It gives a purported moral choice where, in fact, none exists. Furthermore, to do so, as happened with the meningitis victim, opens the family to unnecessary feelings of ambivalence, anxiety, and guilt, feelings that may result in moral paralysis or a steadfast denial of death. Those emotions, in turn, may result in a decision to continue medical intervention in the hope of a miracle.

An approach more attuned to the reality of the situation would have been to inform the meningitis victim's family of her condition: "She is dead. The motions you see in her body are only the result of air being forced into her lungs by the ventilator."

After allowing the family time to adjust to that reality, the physician should inquire about the family's willingness to donate the organs. If the response is negative, the physician should present the family with the available options: "You may go in and see her before we remove the respirator or you may choose to wait until after it has been removed."

The physician should avoid using the phrase "brain-dead." Dead is dead. Modification of that reality tends to lead to confusion and false hopes on the part of both health care providers and families. As the study by Younger and colleagues [70] reveals, physicians and other health care professionals involved in determining "brain death" and seeking organ procurement have confused and self-contradictory understandings of the concept. Only 38 percent of those surveyed could correctly identify and apply the whole brain-death criterion. If, as proved true, some of the professionals' explanations of brain death suggested they really believed the patient was alive, 40 percent of them rejected any brain-oriented concept of death whatsoever, and the majority (58%) did not use a coherent concept of death consistently, it is clear that the term conveys ambiguity and confusion about its meaning and implications. Consequently, the phrase should be avoided.

Informing the family that the patient who meets the whole brain-death criterion is "dead" avoids the sense that the family is being asked to sign a "death warrant." It also saves them from the possible guilt of thinking they did not do everything possible to save the patient's life.

An alternative approach used by Pitts [71] might be even better. Following the Harvard ad hoc directive that the decision and the responsibility for declaring death and turning off the respirator belongs to the physician, Pitts informs the family that the clinical evidence suggests the patient is brain-dead. He then explains that several tests, including one for apnea, will be done to confirm that diagnosis. The family is asked if it wants to see the patient before these tests are done. After the family has gone, the tests, the last of which is for apnea, are performed. In that controlled situation when the respirator is removed, if the patient is unable to breathe, death is pronounced. The physician then informs the family that the evidence was correct: The patient is dead. There is no question of removing a respirator; none is in use.

Organ Retrieval

Because of the way in which health care professionals now handle brain-death cases, the potential for organ retrieval is often lost. The Centers for Disease Control has estimated that no more than 15 percent of the 20,000 persons who might serve as organ donors actually do so [72]. That fact, coupled with the rapid advances being made in transplantation techniques and the effectiveness of the powerful new immunosuppressive drugs such as cyclosporine, is creating a large gap between the supply and demand for organs.

Nationwide it is estimated that 10,000 people are being maintained on dialysis while awaiting kidney transplant, yet in 1988 only 7096 cadaveric and 1816 living donor transplants were performed [73]. Similar shortages of hearts and livers are marked by the now familiar televised pleas of family and friends to help save the life of a loved one by locating a potential donor. In an attempt to overcome these perennial shortages, Caplan [74] identified the problem as being not a limitation of potential donors or even the willingness of families to consent to donation, but rather the reluctance of physicians and other health care providers to undertake the emotionally charged task of asking the families of the newly dead for the organs. This is particularly true in the case of the young trauma victim in which

death itself comes as a shock to the family. This reticence is compounded when physicians and administrators fear adverse legal and financial consequences from their involvement with organ procurement.

Since the major factors hindering the efficacy of organ procurement from cadaver donors are physician- or hospital-based, Caplan has proposed legislation that would require hospitals in brain-death cases to ask family members to donate the organs of the newly deceased. To assure the family and the public that the determination of death was being made independently of the desire for organs, the request for organs would be made by someone other than the patient's physician or the transplant team.

A policy of "required request," which mandates a request for organ and tissue donation from families of potential donors, is required by state and federal legislation, as well as by new hospital accreditation standards [75]. Though no reliable data yet exist on the actual number of persons who could have donated an organ, preliminary investigations reveal that donations of corneas, skin, bone, and dural tissues are up 200 to 300 percent and organ donations have increased 10 to 20 percent in many states [76].

Despite required request laws, there continues to be an enormous shortfall of harvestable organs [77]. This shortage of desperately needed organs raises anew the question of why the restricted source of vital organs: the dead donor. Why ought we not take organs from the anencephalic, condemned prisoners, the irreversibly comatose, and even the imminently dying? When forced with the Hobson choice between the certain death of two (or more) individuals as opposed to the death of one, why shouldn't the law allow us to take the organs of the dying individual and provide life to others who will surely die without a transplant? The most promising candidate for "dying donor" was the anencephalic infant.

No recent proposal has generated more commentary and produced fewer positive results than that of harvesting organs for transplantation from that class of patients. With the successful transplantation of the heart of a Canadian-born anencephalic into an infant suffering from hypoplastic left heart at Loma Linda Medical Center in 1987 [78], Michael Harrison's [79] proposal that anencephalics be used as ready sources of transplant organs for infants seemed about to be realized. With the prevalence of 0.3 per 1000 births of whom 67 percent are stillborn, the approximately 3756 live-born anencephalic infants each year could serve as potential organ sources [80].

Recognizing that at present the only legitimate source of organs is the brain-dead, Joyce Peabody and colleagues [81] at Loma Linda designed protocols that provide intensive care and respirator support to anencephalics to determine if brain death with intact organs could be achieved. Within the 7-day limitation they imposed on the protocol only 2 of 12 anencephalics met brain-death criteria. Though in one instance there were harvestable organs, no suitable recipients could be identified. The conclusion of that study was that it is not feasible, within the restrictions of current law, to procure solid organs for transplantation from anencephalic infants.

The debate over the use of anencephalics as sources of organs did provide clarification on several ethical issues. It forced a sharper understanding of brain death. Once it was understood that the anencephalic was not brain-dead, but was "brain absent" and dying, we were faced with the issue: Should we consider nonconscious terminally ill patients as potential organ banks? Some commentators tried to finesse the issue by declaring a neocortical standard to be used for "death" [82,83]. That philosophical view equates personhood with consciousness or cognitive functions and argues that in the absence of these qualities there is no person; there is death. The President's Commission considered and rejected that standard as too radical a departure from our understanding of death [84]. The Commission's "deliberately conservative" approach recognized only a new diagnostic measure of death, not a new concept of death.

Other commentators would treat some live births as nonpersons. Loma Linda's Dr. Leonard Bailey, for example, describes the anencephalic as "a nonperson human derivative, a resource we should be able to capitalize on" [85]. Jay Friedman likewise believes that "the anencephalic may be viewed as a biologically functioning entity that is somewhat less than a person" [86]. Once dismissed as a subset of humanity that does not qualify as a person, the anencephalic is viewed as similar to an early developing fetus—an entity with no rights.

Friedman proposed that the various state legislatures (and presumably state courts) should not be prevented from choosing, by majority fiat, a theory that seems most correct to its members (p. 959). That thesis would fit the demands of the parents of Theresa Ann, the Florida child born with anencephaly who petitioned the state courts to declare their child dead so that they could donate her organs. The Florida Supreme Court unanimously rejected that request [87]. It declared that an anencephalic is a person who is not dead, but dying. The question then confronting us is, "Do we want to kill such a person so that others might live?"

The settled law on that issue is found in the unanimous en banc decision of the District of Columbia Court of Appeals in the 1990 case of In re A. C. [88], in which the District's highest court ruled that one could not force a dying pregnant woman to undergo a Cesarean delivery in order to save the fetus. In the court's words, "It matters not what the quality of a patient's life may be; the right of bodily integrity is not extinguished simply because someone is ill or even at death's door" [88]. Pressure to change the settled state of the law continues. Proposals have been made by transplant teams to retrieve cadaveric kidneys from donors whose organs would otherwise be lost because brain-death criteria have not been fulfilled prior to asystole. The donors would be "patients between the ages of 6 and 50 years who have terminal brain damage and for whom next-of-kin consent for organ donation has been obtained" (Teres, personal communication, 1993). Rather than brain death, this proposal would accept as organ donors those suffering "terminal brain injury," which is defined to include "trauma, intracerebral hemorrhage and primary brain tumor." For these classes of patients, once the family grants permission for organ donation, the intensivist would begin a terminal wean. Once asystole is achieved, death is declared and cardiopulmonary resuscitation with intubation and oxygenation is instituted. The femoral vessels are cannulated and systematic heparinization and other organ-saving drugs are induced.

Why wait until asystole is achieved to begin the process? Why not put the vascular catheters in before the patient dies? And how do you restrict the class of donors to those with "terminal brain injury from an irreversible cause of damage?" Why not extend the category to include those in a persistent vegetative state, or those dying of chronic obstructive pulmonary disease (COPD) or irreversible heart disease? Lest these extensions seem far-fetched we need but look at the experience of Dr. Joyce Peabody, the Director of the Loma Linda anencephaly project, who reports that Loma Linda was inundated with calls from "well respected physicians with excellent credentials" with referrals of infants with less severe anomalies for organ donation, such as babies born with an abnormal amount of fluid around the brain or those born without kidneys but with a normal brain. In all, over 20 referrals of babies with conditions entirely different from anencephaly and, more im-

portantly, of babies who did not have a clearly fatal condition had been made to the program. From her experience with a protocol to expand the class of potential organ donors Peabody concludes, "The slippery slope is real and there are significant dangers in extending the criteria for organ donation to include the dying as well as the dead" [89].

Advance Directives

A problem more common in the ICU than brain death or organ donation is what to do with the critically ill patient who is unable to make personal preferences known because of physical condition, age, or medication. The well-documented legal history of informed consent makes clear that the primary responsibility of care-givers in this area is to ascertain as much as possible what the individual, if competent, would choose [90,91]. The decision should reflect the individual's preferences, choices, and values as closely as possible.

That decision can be made, of course, by learning the patient's values and discovering what the patient would have done for others in similar situations. The clearest and most convincing evidence would be the individual's direct testimony on the extent and duration of medical treatment. Ideally, the attending physician would explore and learn this over the course of the illness. Unfortunately, such conversations are rare.

What leads to such a breakdown in communication in an area as vital as life-death decisions? The limited empirical studies of the topic indicate a widespread belief on the part of both patients and physicians that the other party has the responsibility to initiate the conversation. A study by La Puma shows that physicians and providers view advance directives as a patient rather than a professional or institutional responsibility [92]. Further support for that finding comes from a national study of hospitals with policies on advance directives that shows only 4 percent asked their patients whether they had advance directives; 96 percent of the institutions assumed that those who had such directives would inform the hospital [93].

Patients have just the opposite expectation. Emanuel's study of advanced directives reveals that the most frequently cited barrier to their use was patients' expectations that the physician should take the initiative in raising the topic [94]. That study found that while 93 percent of the outpatients and 89 percent of the general public who were surveyed wanted a document specifying future care, only 7 percent had one and only 5 percent had ever had a discussion on the topic with their physicians.

The Patient Self-Determination Act of 1990 (PSDA) [95], which Congress passed as part of the Omnibus Budget Reconciliation Act, is designed, in part, to break that stalemate. The law, which took effect on December 1, 1991, requires all hospitals, nursing facilities, hospices, home health care services, and health maintenance organizations that receive Medicare or Medicaid to inform their adult patients on admission or enrollment of their right to make decisions regarding their medical care and of their right under applicable state law to write a living will or durable power of attorney.

The Act also requires as a condition for Medicare or Medicaid funding that these institutions do the following:

1. Document in the patient's medical record whether the individual has executed an advance directive
2. Follow the directives in compliance with state laws
3. Educate both their own staffs and the general community concerning advanced directives

HISTORICAL BACKGROUND. The PSDA does not create any new rights or privileges for patients. It grants no new rights to citizens. The PSDA merely requires health care providers to inform patients of their existing rights to refuse unwanted medical treatment. As the United States Supreme Court noted in its recent Cruzan opinion, that common-law right is constitutionally protected as part of our basic fundamental "liberty interests" [96]. As an earlier Supreme Court had put it: "No right is held more sacred, or is more carefully guarded by the common law, than the right of every individual to the possession and control of his person, free from all restraint or interference of others, unless by clear and unquestionable authority of law" [97].

The medical implications of a person's right of autonomy were first articulated in 1914 by Justice Benjamin Cardozo, then of the New York Court of Appeals, when he wrote in his now landmark Schloendorff opinion: "Every human being of adult years and sound mind has a right to determine what shall be done with his own body; and a surgeon who performs an operation without his patient's consent commits an assault, for which he is liable in damages" [98]. Schloendorff, which forms the basis for the doctrine of informed consent, made clear, as Cruzan was to reiterate seventy-five years later, that the competent patient has a right to decline any and all medical interventions including those that might be potentially life-prolonging.

Difficulties arise when the question of patient autonomy is applied to noncompetent patients. How do we determine what medical treatment, if any, the unconscious Karen Ann Quinlan or Nancy Cruzan would want? The problem in answering this question is exacerbated by technological advances that have greatly increased medicine's ability to preserve and prolong life. Procedures that once were only dreams have become reality—artificial means to replace failed lungs, hearts, and kidneys are now commonplace. Like all human artifacts, however, sophisticated techniques can be abused: The very means used to preserve life may transform it into a sublethal extension of monitoring machines and sustaining apparatus. Life can become a hellish nightmare from which there is seemingly no exit.

LIVING WILLS. A way around the problem of protecting the rights and dignity of the incompetent patient was proposed in 1969 by Louis Kutner, who described a document, which he termed a "living will," in which a now competent adult could put in writing directions for future medical care to be used by his health care provider should he become incapacitated and unable to communicate his wishes [99].

By 1995, some 47 states and the District of Columbia had enacted such statutes. Though differing widely in detail, all of those statutes grant immunity to physicians and health care providers who follow the patient's expressed wishes [100]. George Annas has noted that most of those statutes suffer from four major shortcomings: (1) They are applicable only to those who are "terminally ill"; (2) They limit the types of treatment that can be refused to "artificial" or "extraordinary" therapies; (3) They make no provisions for the person to designate another person to make the decision on his or her behalf and set criteria for such decisions; and 4) They do not provide for a penalty in the event that health care providers fail to honor these documents [101].

The American Medical Association's Committee on Medico-Legal Problems has also evaluated these statements and found significant drawbacks [102]. First and most important, no matter how carefully drafted, no legislation can provide guidance for unanticipated circumstances. If drafted in general language to cover a broad range of circumstances, the law may be too vague, abstract, or ambiguous to apply to specific situations.

The ambiguity and vagueness of language and the need for physicians to make decisions based on an interpretation of a document, rather than on a discussion with someone acting on behalf of the patient, can result in decisions contrary to what a patient would want. This can be seen in New York's Wirth case [103]. Tom Wirth, a person with AIDS, had signed a living will stating that should he become incapable of making his own decisions and should his condition be "irreversible," he would not want "extraordinary" measures taken to extend his life. When Mr. Wirth developed a brain infection from toxoplasmosis, his physician, over the strenuous objections of Mr. Wirth's companion, continued to treat Mr. Wirth because, in the physician's judgment, "toxoplasmosis is potentially reversible." The court upheld the physician's position.

Mr. Wirth, despite intensive treatment, eventually succumbed to the infection. The appointment of the companion as health care proxy would have obviated the difficulties found in Mr. Wirth's blunt, unnuanced written statement. The appointment of an identifiable person, especially one who knows the person and his or her values, assures that the decision will be clinically situated, attuned to changing conditions, and in the hands of someone the patient knows and whose judgment the patient trusts.

DURABLE POWERS OF ATTORNEY. The static nature of a living will has led to proposals to replace what one commentator labels "a bloodless document" with a flesh and blood person who could speak for the patient [104]. This can be done effectively by assigning a "durable power of attorney" to a designated person who would speak for the individual should that individual become incapacitated. The terminology used for the document that identifies the surrogate, proxy, or agent (the terms are used interchangeably in the literature)—the *durable power of attorney*—is confusing and misleading. The instrument, though developed from probate law, has nothing to do with lawyers. One does not need a lawyer to draft a durable power of attorney, nor need the surrogate, proxy, or agent named therein be an attorney.

Any competent adult can write a statement naming any other competent adult—spouse, parent, child, sibling, companion, or friend—as his or her proxy for health care decisions. To prevent potential abuses or conflicts of interest, it is best that except for relatives, direct health care providers not be named as agents. (Many statutes, in fact, exclude such providers from being named as health care proxies.) Once designated in a written, witnessed document, the proxy has the same health care decision-making power the patient would have had were he or she able to make decisions.

The actual statement need not be complex, nor need it be drafted by an attorney. One can simply write in plain prose what he or she wants done in such circumstances. If the person wishes a prewritten form, the best and most readily available is Bok's "Directions for My Care" [105] (pp. 368–369) (Table 228-1).

Patients with Inadequate Decision-Making Capacity

Although it is relatively easy to make medical decisions for those who have provided clear directives for their care, the overwhelming majority of patients with impaired decision-mak-

Table 228-1. Sample Durable Power of Attorney

I wish to live a full and long life, but not at all costs. If my death is near and cannot be avoided, and if I have lost the ability to interact with others and have no reasonable chance of regaining this ability, or if my suffering is intense and irreversible, I do not want to have my life prolonged. I would then ask not to be subjected to surgery or resuscitation. Nor would I then wish to have life support from mechanical ventilators, intensive care services, or other life prolonging procedures, including the administration of antibiotics, blood products, or artificially provided nutrition and fluids. I would wish, rather, to have care which gives comfort and support, which facilitates my interaction with others to the extent that this is possible, and which brings peace.

In order to carry out these instructions and to interpret them, I authorize _____ to accept, plan and refuse treatment on my behalf in cooperation with my attending physicians and health personnel. This person knows how I value the experience of living, weigh incompetence, suffering and dying. Should it be impossible to reach this person, I authorize _____ to make such choices for me. I have discussed these desires concerning terminal care with them, and I trust their judgment on my behalf. In addition, I have discussed with them the following specific instructions regarding my care:

Signature_____

Address_____

Date_____

Name of proxy_____

Address of proxy_____

Telephone number of proxy_____

Name of substitute_____

Address of substitute_____

Telephone number of substitute_____

Date_____

Witnessed_____

Signed_____

and by_____

ing capacity will not have done so. They present the greatest dilemmas to health care providers. The first of those dilemmas is how to determine that the patient has become so incapacitated that he or she is no longer a competent decision-maker.

When confronted with this situation, many physicians' initial impulse is to call for psychiatric consultation or seek a court order to declare the patient incompetent [106]. In most cases, neither approach is appropriate. As the President's Commission emphatically noted, " 'Decision making incapacity' is not a medical or a psychiatric diagnostic category; it rests on a judgment of the type an informed layperson might make—that the patient lacks sufficient ability to understand a situation and to make a choice in light of that understanding" [25] (p. 123). More specifically, the physician would want to ascertain that the patient understands his or her condition, the treatment options (including nontreatment), and the consequences of each option, and is able to make a reasoned choice among them. This choice need not be what the physician would consider reasonable, rational, or medically appropriate. The patient's decision

need only reflect a reasoned choice among the options. As the Massachusetts Appeals Court stated in Lane v. Candura—a case involving an admittedly confused 78-year-old woman's refusal to have her gangrenous leg amputated—what must be determined is whether the "areas of forgetfulness and confusion cause or relate in any way to impairment of her ability to understand that in rejecting the treatment she is, in effect, choosing death over life" [107].

Once it has been determined that the patient lacks adequate decision-making capacity, the need for a surrogate or proxy arises. Generally, the surrogate should be a family member or a friend who knows the patient's interests and values—and can address them. Ideally, the surrogate would know the patient's actual desires and could address them directly. Even if the patient had never made any specific statements on treatment decisions, the proxy might legitimately be able to infer from the patient's known values and beliefs what he or she would want in such a situation and thereby preserve the subjective and idiosyncratic values of the individual. In the event that no prior discussion of the issues has occurred and the surrogate is unable to assess what the incompetent individual would have chosen, then he or she must use a "best interests" test, which examines the patient's welfare and well-being. The President's Commission spelled out several factors that should be considered in such a determination, factors that the California Court of Appeals in the Barber v. Superior Court [108] case adopted as normative: "relief of suffering, the preservation or restoration of functioning; the quality as well as the extent of life sustained . . . and the impact of a decision on the incapacitated patient's loved ones." The caveat is that the "quality of life and impact on family should be viewed exclusively from the perspective of the patient" (p. 1021).

One attempt to ensure that the process has produced an objective, disinterested, and publicly accountable decision is to take the issue to court [109–112]. That route, however, is terribly costly, cumbersome, traumatic, and uncertain. The personal predilections of judges, the highly diverse formulations of the law, and the fact that judges are poorly equipped for, and not fond of, handling such issues makes that route fraught with potential peril for patients, physicians, hospitals, and society [113,114].

Furthermore, even court approbation will not protect a hospital and physicians from explosive societal repercussions. This is illustrated by the Bloomington Baby Doe case, in which a family physician's decision not to treat a Down's syndrome infant with an esophageal fistula was approved by three courts, including the Indiana Supreme Court. Those repercussions, in the form of the highly restrictive and counterproductive original Baby Doe regulations with their hot line, anonymous tipsters, and "flying Doe squads," proved we need a better way to resolve these problems than inflexible bureaucratic regulations [115].

Decision-Making Process

Whatever the process, good decision-making must consider three factors: the physician, the patient, and the community. Although we have long since surpassed the era of the paternalistic physician and the passive patient [116], the physician continues to have a primary role and responsibility. The physician must make the diagnosis, provide the prognosis, and, after forming a professional judgment on the range of options, make a recommendation. Here, once again, we are reminded of Ingelfinger's [57] admonition that a physician who merely presents options to an uncounseled patient and expects a decision is guilty of, at least, shirking duties and, at most, malpractice.

Given the recommendation, the patient or proxy must then address the subjective values that will determine whether the proposal offers a proportionate benefit. Here the entire range of factors, such as cost, burden, pain, anticipated outcome, dislocation, family structure, and personal plans comes into play. The patient or the person acting on behalf of the patient must plumb these and then choose.

Although the combination of patient-family choice is generally final, a third factor—society—must be considered. With the change in attitude from the strong paternalism of "the doctor knows best" to the elevation of autonomy into a near absolute, individuals sometimes forget that their actions and decisions have implications for, and impact on, others. Consequently, society, for the protection of individuals and the common good, places constraints and limits, both positive and negative, on individual rights [117].

Several examples of those constraints have emerged as ethical problems in health care delivery. A reflection on their resolution provides an insight into how we perceive ourselves as a people. For example, from the Johns Hopkins case [118] to the Bloomington Baby Doe dispute, many persons believe that parents should have the right to deny lifesaving corrective surgery to a Down's syndrome infant because a retarded child would prove a burden on the family [119,120]. Now, however, a strong consensus has emerged in our society that such an infant may not be denied the necessary surgery simply because of its mental handicap [121,122]. Likewise, though parents may have a right to decline blood transfusions based on religious convictions, they have no right to impose those beliefs on their immature minor children [123].

An example of the restriction on one's right to positive claims would be the denial of a family request to have a rapidly deteriorating critically ill patient remain in or moved to the ICU to satisfy their demand that "everything possible be done" [124–127]. Use of that facility must rest on the medical staff's professional assessment of the usefulness of the ICU to the patient and the comparative merit of others' claims for that scarce resource [128]. To hold otherwise would transform the physician from a professional charged with making informed and sometimes difficult judgments into one who simply strives to fulfill family demands no matter how misplaced or misguided.

Perhaps the most succinct statement of the physician's professional role is found in a discussion on termination of treatment decisions in the Vatican's 1980 Declaration on Euthanasia [129]:

For such a decision to be made, account will have to be taken of the reasonable wishes of the patient and the patient's family, as also of the advice of the doctors who are especially competent in the matter. The latter may in particular judge that the investment in instruments and personnel is disproportionate to the results foreseen; they may also judge that the techniques applied impose on the patient strain or suffering out of proportion with the benefits which he or she may gain from such techniques (p. 306).

Here an institution highly protective of the sanctity of life is indicating not only that there are limits to the burdens an individual must undergo to preserve life, but that there are limits that can and ought to be set by physicians concerning what may legitimately be offered to, or demanded for, such patients.

RESPONSIBILITY FOR THE DECISION. It is clear that the judgments concerning burden and benefit to the patient are value judgments, moral choices. They are judgments in which, all things considered, the continuance of life is either called for

or not worthwhile to the patient. Such judgments are the onerous prerogative of those who are primarily responsible for the welfare of the incompetent patient—the family or other surrogate. When the surrogate exercises this prerogative in a way that is questionably no longer in the best interests of the patient, especially by allowing the patient with a good prognosis to go untreated, society has the duty to intervene. That intervention can take many forms, such as legislation, criminal prosecution, or neglect hearings. The purpose of such proceedings is to guarantee that the primary decision-maker acts responsibly in a manner that should be able to sustain public scrutiny. The public accountability and review, which guarantees that the values of the society are respected and adhered to, can be invoked short of judicial intervention.

One approach to achieving that goal is found in the report, *Deciding to Forego Life-Sustaining Treatment* [25]. In the opinion of the President's Commission, "routine judicial oversight [of medical decision-making] is neither necessary or appropriate" (p. 160). The remoteness from the clinical situation and the inability to keep pace with the ongoing fluctuations in the patient's condition, particularly in an intensive care setting, are strong arguments in support of that thesis. The Commission favors having the surrogate's decision in difficult cases reviewed by an in-place, broadly based, multidisciplinary hospital bioethics committee, which would be familiar with both the medical setting and community standards. That consultative body, which would have the ongoing charge of establishing standards of treatment and issuing guidelines for the institution, would provide a framework for impartial but sensitive review of hard choices [130,131,132]. It would also guarantee that the interests of the patient were being considered without the formality and intensely adversarial character of a court proceeding, or worse, the pervasive fear and distrust generated by anonymous tipsters in the ICU.

If, after all this, irreconcilable disagreement still persists, the President's Commission recommends referral to the courts for the appointment of a legal guardian who would be empowered to evaluate the options and make a decision "in the best interest" of the patient. The decision, of course, would be subject to judicial scrutiny as a last resort. Such an approach ensures that the decision-maker has received the most reliable information available, that the decision is within the range of acceptable options, and that those uncomfortable with it have had an opportunity to discuss their reservations with a concerned and disinterested representative of the public. It also insulates the agonizing and often tragic choices from the glare of publicity, the distortion of public posturing, and the costly and tangled involvement of court proceedings.

The implementation of bioethics committees as mediating institutions was greatly enhanced in January 1984, when the Department of Health and Human Services, in response to the criticism of its revised, proposed Infant Doe Regulations [133], adopted the suggestion of the American Academy of Pediatrics [134]: The resolution of treatment-issue decisions for seriously ill newborns should be made in each hospital by a multidisciplinary Infant Care Review Committee [121].

Institutionally based, clinically sensitive, multidisciplinary bodies can educate physicians, staff, and patients on difficult ethical issues. These bodies can also establish institutional policies and guidelines on treatment decisions, and they have proved valuable for consultation on new or particularly difficult cases. Such benefits have led to the widespread use of institutionally based bodies for discussing ethics [135–139].

SUBSTANTIVE GUIDELINES. The procedural aspects of good decision-making assure that patient autonomy, physician responsibility, and societal values are considered. They do not produce the decision; they do not guarantee its character. Further, the range of ethically acceptable options, the complexity of individual cases, and the variable situation of institutions and specific patients preclude prepackaged solutions to ethical dilemmas.

Nonetheless, there are some agreed-upon norms and guidelines that are helpful in resolving difficult ethical questions. The most practical and readily available source for the clinician is Jonsen's *Clinical Ethics* [140], a superb short text in which an ethicist, a physician, and an attorney set out some of the more common principles and illustrate them with brief case studies. That text could well join the *Physician's Desk Reference* as standard equipment in every ICU. Interestingly, the best summary of the ethical norms is found not in discursive philosophical texts but in the major court opinions issued since Quinlan. Four of these, Superintendent of Belchertown State School v. Saikewicz [141], Barber v. Superior Court [108], In the matter of Claire Conroy [142], and Cruzan [96] illustrate the emerging consensus of law and ethics on the appropriate care that is due an incompetent, terminally ill, or irreversibly comatose patient.

In Saikewicz, the Massachusetts Supreme Judicial Court ruled that the court could determine that a 67-year-old, profoundly retarded (IQ of 10), institutionalized man with acute myelogenous leukemia would, if competent, opt for nontreatment. The argument was that the administration of chemotherapy, which for the nonretarded patient might be endured in the hope of a remission, would inexplicably change the character of Joseph Saikewicz's life from a peaceful routine into a bewildering nightmare of pain, fear, and physical restraint. As such, it would surely constitute "extraordinary" treatment. If the patient had no obligation to undergo such treatment, neither had the physician any moral obligation to provide it nor the judge to order it.

In forming this opinion, the Supreme Judicial Court gave judicial support to the distinction between ordinary and extraordinary means: "We should not use *extraordinary* means of prolonging life or its semblance when, after careful consideration . . . it becomes apparent that there is no hope of recovery for the patient" [143]. Further, the court concurred with Quinlan in adopting the thesis of both Ramsey [23] and Kubler-Ross [144] that the distinction between "curing the ill and comforting and easing the dying" can be and ought to be elucidated. It accepted the thesis that physicians ought not to treat the hopeless and the dying as though they are curable. In the court's view, they should recognize that the dying need comfort more than treatment. These positions, buttressed by recent developments in the law on informed consent and respect for the right of privacy, were the basis for the court's authorization of the withholding of chemotherapy for Saikewicz.

In an interesting turn, the court reversed the thesis that the value of life is lessened or cheapened by a decision to refuse treatment. It ruled that the value of life is diminished by the failure to allow a competent human being the right of choice and the right of privacy, that is, the right to be left alone.

The more difficult problem is the attribution of these rights to the incompetent. There are those who argue strenuously that the state must always provide treatment for the incompetent or risk devaluing their dignity and worth. The Supreme Judicial Court rejected that proposition, and in a precedent-shattering contribution to the developing trend in the law ruled that "the principles of equality and respect for all individuals require that a choice exist for incompetents as well as competents. To do otherwise would be to treat wards of the state as a person of lesser status or dignity than others" [141] (p. 424).

Having recognized the right of an incompetent to refuse life-prolonging treatment, the court was faced with the awesome task in a case of first impression of framing an adequate rationale to explain how that right may be exercised. It did so with an interesting yoking of the long-standing legal doctrine of substituted judgment with a Rawlsian reconstruction of the mental world of a "rational" incompetent.

Substituted judgment, a doctrine first articulated in English law over 150 years ago, deals with the authorization of gifts from the estate of incompetents [140]. The English court reasoned this could be done by "donning the mental mantle of the incompetent" (p. 878), that is, what we might reasonably conclude the individual would do if he or she could understand the situation.

That theory of respect for the integrity and autonomy of all persons finds renewed vigor in John Rawls' highly influential *A Theory of Justice* [146], in which he writes that maintaining the integrity of the person means that we act towards him "as we have reason to believe he would choose for himself if he were capable of reasoning and deciding rationally" (p. 14). This does not mean that we can impute preferences that the patient never held. But as is true in the case of Saikewicz where no preferences have been made, the task is to ask how the patient would act if he or she could perceive the present situation.

Applying the substituted judgment theory to Saikewicz, the Supreme Judicial Court concluded that the probate court, the guardian *ad litem,* the physicians, and the staff operated in the best interests of Joseph Saikewicz (i.e., they chose what appeared to be the least detrimental alternative available). That choice, they argued, is what Saikewicz would have chosen if he were capable of doing so.

The California Court of Appeals in Barber refined and developed the ethical standards found in Saikewicz. Reflecting on the moral propriety of the physicians who honored the family request to remove the intravenous feeding tube from the irreversibly comatose Clarence Herbert, the court confronted a host of medical-ethical questions: Is the physician bound by the Hippocratic oath to do everything possible to save life? When, if ever, is it appropriate to stop treatment? What is the difference between killing or letting die, acts of omission or commission, withholding or withdrawing treatment? How does one distinguish ordinary from extraordinary means? Is not use of an intravenous tube ordinary? Who decides for the incompetent patient? Must there be a legal guardian? Is a court order necessary?

In the course of its 25-page opinion, the California Court of Appeals addressed all of these issues. In doing so, it adopted as normative nearly all of the recommendations as to what constitutes appropriate care of the terminally ill or irreversibly comatose patient that were proposed in the President's Commission report, *Deciding to Forego Life-Sustaining Treatment.*

Here, for the first time, a court equated the stopping of intravenous feeding with the removal of a respirator or any other medical intervention [147,148,149]. Each intervention, it declared, is a medical treatment and is to be used only if it benefits the patient. If the intervention merely sustains biologic function, it is not a treatment but a useless and futile gesture, one which the physician need not continue. As the court phrased it, "there is no duty to continue [life-sustaining machinery] once it has become futile in the opinion of qualified medical personnel" (p. 1024) [108].

The court discarded the traditional "ordinary-extraordinary" language in favor of the increasingly common usage of "proportionate-disproportionate" "benefit-burden" to the patient. That approach shifts the emphasis from the technique used to the condition of the patient. In the court's words:

Thus, even if a proposed course of treatment might be extremely painful or intrusive, it would still be proportionate treatment if the prognosis was for complete cure or significant improvement in the patient's condition. On the other hand, a treatment course which is only minimally painful or intrusive may nonetheless be considered disproportionate to the potential benefits if the prognosis is virtually hopeless for any significant improvement in condition (p. 1024).

Finally, bringing to completion a trend in the law that was first articulated in Quinlan, the court noted that in the case of incompetents, the surrogate, if unable to ascertain the patient's actual choices, should be guided by the patient's best interests. These, as previously noted, would include factors such as relief from suffering, the preservation or restoration of functioning, the quality as well as the extent of the life sustained, and the impact of the decision on the family.

In words that it is hoped will sweep away much of the fear and misapprehensions of physicians in such cases, the court held that, without evidence of malevolence, the family is the proper surrogate for the incompetent patient. Further, there is no need for the surrogate to seek prior judicial approval before a decision to withdraw treatment can be made. Such judicial involvement, the court concluded, is not only unnecessary, but may be unwise.

The New Jersey Supreme Court in In the Matter of Claire Conroy [142] further refined the standards articulated in Barber on the withholding or withdrawing of medical treatments, including nutrition and fluids, from incompetent seriously ill patients who, even with treatment, will probably die within approximately 1 year.

After observing that there was no doubt that if competent, an individual in Ms. Conroy's condition would have the right to have a nasogastric tube withdrawn, the New Jersey Supreme Court declared the same right should be accorded to the incompetent. It then articulated three tests to guide the substitute decision-maker. The first test—*subjective standard*—would apply if the patient had previously communicated her wishes by a written living will, an oral directive, or a durable power of attorney.

The other two tests—limited-objective and purely objective—are "best interests" tests to be used if there had been no prior directives from the patient. Here the New Jersey court wished to avoid the naive pretense that it could discern the mind-set of the now incompetent patient or worse, the position of the New York Court of Appeals in O'Connor, which precluded any humane cessation of treatment for persons who had never expressed their desires about life-sustaining treatment, and who are now suffering a prolonged and painful death.

The limited-objective test would allow the termination of treatment for someone in Claire Conroy's situation if there were some trustworthy evidence such as life-style, attitudes, and values that the patient would not want treatment or feeding continued because "it would involve too heavy a burden of unavoidable pain and suffering."

Even in the absence of any reliable evidence, or indeed of any evidence at all, treatment may be withheld or withdrawn if the purely objective test is satisfied. Under this standard "the net burdens of the patient's life with treatment" would "clearly and markedly outweigh the benefits derived from life." This would be true if the patient were suffering from such severe pain that the administration of life-sustaining treatment or feeding would be inhumane. Here the court cautioned that it expressly denied authority under this third test to remove life support from any patient on a "quality of life" basis other than extreme pain or on the ground that the patient's "value to society" was negligible.

In a commentary on this case, Curran [150] observes that the importance of this decision "on the medical obligation to the dying cannot be overstated." Here, for the first time in American jurisprudence, a supreme court had approved the removal of nutrition and hydration as well as other forms of life support and had reinforced the legitimacy of allowing surrogates who, in good faith and without a conflict of interest, determine that the patient's best interests will not be served by prolonging a painful, hopeless existence.

The broad sweep of Conroy reflects one state's approach to treatment decisions for the now incompetent patients. As the U.S. Supreme Court's landmark 1990 opinion in Cruzan v. Director Missouri Department of Health [96] makes clear, individual states can set their own evidentiary standards with regard to treatment decisions for incompetent patients. In its first ruling on the sometimes controversial right-to-die area, the Court stated that though a competent person would have a constitutionally protected right to refuse potentially lifesaving medical treatment, including artificially provided nutrition and hydration, the U.S. Constitution does not prohibit a state from requiring clear and convincing evidence of a now incompetent patient's prior wishes with regard to withdrawal of life-sustaining treatment before such treatment can be terminated.

Since such evidence was found to be lacking in the case of Nancy Cruzan, the Supreme Court upheld the ruling of the Missouri Supreme Court that no surrogate, including her parents, could make the decision to terminate her medical treatment. Since the Cruzans could not meet the evidentiary standard set by Missouri, Nancy Cruzan was to continue to receive artificially provided nutrition and fluids at the state facility where she had been cared for in a persistent vegetative state for some eight years. Despite this untoward outcome for Ms. Cruzan, the Supreme Court's opinion ought not be read overly broadly. The ruling did not consign all incompetent patients who had not made their treatment preferences known to a regimen of unlimited treatment. The ruling says only that there is no constitutional prohibition forbidding states from setting procedural guidelines and evidentiary standards for surrogate decision-makers. The Supreme Court itself set no standards nor did it require the states to establish specific guidelines to control proxy medical decision-making.

POSITIVE ASPECTS OF THE CRUZAN OPINION. The Supreme Court's opinion in Cruzan has provided several positive outcomes in the complex area of law and medicine. It recognized "the principle that a competent person has a constitutionally protected liberty interest in refusing unwanted medical treatment." It also resolved the nearly decade old debate over whether artificially provided nutrition and fluids are medical treatments: they are. Further, it concluded that these treatments should be assessed and evaluated on the same standard as any other medical intervention: on the basis of the patient's subjective assessment of benefits and burdens.

The opinion also gave legal recognition to advance directives. It indicated that the prior expressed wishes of a now incompetent patient are to be accorded the same constitutional protection given to the competent patient's wishes. This assures that even in the absence of specific statutes recognizing their status, written advance directives, the so-called living wills, are to be honored as explicit instructions of the patient. Justice O'Connor's concurrence signaled that a majority of the justices would also afford the same constitutional status to the decisions of a designated proxy or "health care agent." By signing a durable power of attorney, a competent individual could be assured that the same protection given to his or her directions will be accorded to the choices of the person designated to make his or her health care decisions.

The Court also recognized that incompetent persons have and retain constitutional rights with regard to refusing medical treatment. Though all of the justices agree that the state can establish procedural safeguards to protect the "rights" of the incompetent person, they were divided on the level of evidence the state may require as to what the incompetent would want. A majority found that Missouri's requirement of "clear and convincing" evidence of the patient's expressed wishes with regard to the withdrawal of life-sustaining medical treatment did not violate the constitutional rights of the patient.

PRACTICAL IMPLICATIONS FOR PHYSICIANS AND HOSPITALS. The Cruzan opinion does not impose any new standards on the practice of medicine. It recognized that states may establish procedural guidelines for treatment decisions for incompetent patients. And it upheld Missouri's right to demand clear and convincing evidence of the patient's expressed wishes before treatment can be terminated.

Other states are free to set their own standards. New York, like Missouri, requires clear and convincing evidence. Massachusetts uses "substituted judgment." Other states, including California, that have addressed the issue of withholding or withdrawing medical treatment from incompetent patients have allowed caring families or close friends to determine "the best interest" of the patient.

Most states have never addressed the question of medical treatment for incompetents. In those states the traditional practice of physician-family assessment of physical findings and known values or best interest are used to determine what should be done. Nothing in the Cruzan opinion changes the way those decisions are to be made.

In all states—except Missouri and New York—physicians may, at the direction of a caring family, legally withhold or withdraw life-sustaining medical treatments including artificially provided nutrition and fluids from a terminally ill or irreversibly comatose patient.

PHYSICIAN-ASSISTED SUICIDE AND ACTIVE EUTHANASIA. The Hippocratic tradition of western medicine, which has prevailed for 2500 years, had as one of its foundations the proscription against killing. In the oath itself there were prohibitions against abortion and euthanasia. As Pellegrino [151] observes, that tradition, enriched over the years with equally forceful religious prohibitions against killing, stood unchallenged until the 1960s when anti-authoritarianism led to the emergence of competing moral principles.

Recent referenda proposals in the state of Washington and California, authorizing physician-assisted suicide and active euthanasia, though defeated, are manifestations of that shift. In Washington state, for the first time anywhere in the world, voters were asked to approve what its proponents labeled "a new medical service": authorization for physicians actively to assist a terminally ill patient to die. Washington's Initiative 119, which was sponsored by the Hemlock Society, was circulated with the official ballot title, "Shall adult patients who are in a medically terminal condition be permitted to request and receive from a physician aid-in-dying?" Beneath that innocuously worded heading was the reality that "aid-in-dying" meant "aid in the form of a medical service, provided in person by a physician, that will end the life of a conscious and mentally qualified patient in a dignified, painless, and humane manner, when requested voluntarily by the patient through a written directive . . . at the time the medical service is to be provided."

Albert Jonsen, a medical ethicist at the University of Washington Medical School, noted that this was not just a simple amendment to earlier living-will legislation; it represented a radical change in medical practice [152]. For the first time since the Hippocratic tradition established prohibitions against physicians directly taking the lives of their patients, physicians would be authorized to kill dying patients. Jonsen, who is no alarmist, wrote in *Commonweal* just prior to the vote: "The state of Washington is on the edge of a moral cataclysm." Public opinion polls suggested that he was right. A Louis Harris poll indicated that 67 percent of the voters in the state approved of the proposal. A more nuanced poll conducted by the Harvard School of Public Health [153] revealed that 64 percent of Americans favor physician-assisted suicide and euthanasia for terminally ill patients who request it. Of adults under thirty-five, 79 percent supported the idea.

The debate over euthanasia is not new. Only the emphasis has shifted. In a thoughtful and thorough survey of the euthanasia movement, Humphry and Wickett [154] trace the issue from classical Athens, where magistrates kept a supply of poison for anyone who wished to die ("If your existence is hateful to you, die; if you are overwhelmed by fate, drink the hemlock"), through to the rise of Christianity, in which suicide was denounced as violation of God's will.

In the United States, the euthanasia movement gained prominence in the late 1930s with the founding of the Euthanasia Society of America. It had as its agenda "the belief that, with adequate safeguards, it should be made legal to allow incurable sufferers to choose immediate death rather than await it in agony" [155]. In the 1970s and 80s, the movement took two directions, each of which is represented in the current debate and which culminated in the Patient Self-Determination Act and Proposition 119. Legislation recognizing living wills and health care proxies and the court battles over the "right to die" were the vehicles used to protect individuals from unwanted medical treatment. At the same time, such groups as EXIT in England and it American counterpart, the Hemlock Society, pressed for active euthanasia. In 1979, a Scottish EXIT group published the first guide or "suicide recipe book." It gave detailed descriptions of how to end one's life. Derek Humphry soon followed with his guide on "self-deliverance," *Let Me Die Before I Wake*.

Support for physician-assisted suicide remained limited to fringe groups until the publication in 1989 in the *New England Journal of Medicine* of an article in which ten out of twelve physicians from the leading medical centers of the United States went beyond their earlier support for termination of unwanted medical treatment to endorse physician-assisted suicide. In an article entitled "The Physician's Responsibility Toward Hopelessly Ill Patients," these physicians wrote: "All but two of us . . . believe that it is not immoral for a physician to assist in the rational suicide of a terminally ill patient." The group, somewhat surprisingly, stopped short of a similar endorsement of active euthanasia. The reasoning is illuminating: "The social climate in this country is very litigious, and the likelihood of prosecution if a case of euthanasia were discovered is fairly high—much higher than the likelihood of prosecution after a suicide in which the physician has assisted" [156].

That report by distinguished clinicians from the most reputable institutions in the country followed by just one year the publication in *JAMA* of "It's All Over, Debbie" [157], an anonymous account of a gynecology resident's decision to inject a young cancer patient with a lethal dose of morphine. That action, done at 3:00 A.M. by a physician who had no prior knowledge of the patient on the basis of her request, "Let's get this over with," provoked a storm of outrage. Willard Gayland and three of his physician colleagues, in a bluntly worded essay entitled "Doctors Must Not Kill" [158], expressed their horror at what had been done and their incomprehension at *JAMA*'s having published the account. Their incredulity was expressed by their question: "What in the world is going on?" For them, the anonymous author of the "Debbie" essay broke the law, breached medical protocol, and violated the most deeply held and hallowed canon of medical ethics: Doctors must not kill. As they put it, "Generations of physicians and commentators on medical ethics had held fast to the distinction between ceasing useless treatments (or allowing to die) and active, willful taking of life." Since the time of Hippocrates until as recently as a 1989 statement of the Judicial Council of the American Medical Association, Western medicine has regarded the killing of patients, even on request, as a profound violation of the deepest meaning of the medical vocation.

Leon Kass undertook to explain the reasons for this prohibition in a probing essay in *The Public Interest* [159]. There he argued that the basis for the shift in attitude, which has already led to some 5000 cases of active euthanasia or assisted suicide per year in the Netherlands, is an overemphasis on freedom and personal autonomy, expressed in the view that each person has a right to control his or her body and life, including the end of it. In this view, physicians are bound to acquiesce not only to demands for termination of treatment, but also to intentional killing through poison, because the right to choose—freedom—must be respected even more than life itself. The second reason advanced for killing patients is not a concern for choice but the assessment by the patient or others that the patient's life is no longer deemed worth living. It is not autonomy but the miserable or pitiable condition of the body or mind that warrants, in Kass's words, "doing the patient in."

Kass's arguments against those positions constitute a commentary on the now classic essay written in the Minnesota Law Review [160] by Yale Kamisar some thirty years earlier. Kamisar asked: Are not the risks and mistakes in authorizing medically assisted voluntary euthanasia too great and, more importantly, the possible radiations from the proposed change too overwhelming? How is one to establish that the patient's choice is "voluntary"? Will we not sweep up, in the process, some who are not really tired of life, but think others are tired of them? And how much freedom of choice does one really have if a person does not want to die, but feels he or she should not live on because to do so, when there looms the legal alternative of euthanasia, is to be selfish or cowardly?

These realistic problems pale in comparison to the potential difficulties engendered in a society grown indifferent to the taking of life. That indifference would be compounded if the very segment of society committed to saving life were commissioned to destroy it. Once the euthanizing of a patient or two becomes but part of a routine day's work, the brutalization process so vividly described in Leo Alexander's classic essay on "Medical Science Under Dictatorship" [161], which recounts the experience of Nazi Germany, becomes an all too real possibility. And once begun, who sets the limits on "a life not worth living," and how are the limits set?

That such fears are not far-fetched is seen in the actions of Dr. Jack Kevorkian, the Michigan pathologist who in fifteen instances, before the Michigan legislature enacted a statute prohibiting assisted suicide, had used his self-designed "suicide machine" to assist non-dying individuals end their lives [162,163]. The first of those, Janet Adkins, was a functioning, lucid woman who feared that the debilitating consequences of the early onset of Alzheimer's disease would render her unable to end her life when she chose to. The next two were a 43-year-old woman with multiple sclerosis and a 58-year-old woman with a severe, but treatable, pelvic inflammation. Kevorkian's crude device, the primitive surroundings in which the assisted suicides occurred, and his intransigent attitude offended many. It also led to the Michigan Medical Society summarily revoking his medical license. No such penalty has been attached to the actions of Dr. Timothy Quill, a Rochester, New York physician, who reported in the *New England Journal of Medicine* [164] how he had given instructions and provided adequate supplies of barbiturates so that Diane, a patient he had known and treated for years who was dying of cervical cancer, could and did end her life. Unlike the outcry over the publication of "It's All Over, Debbie" and the negative reaction to Dr. Kevorkian, the response to Dr. Quill's participation in a patient's suicide was mostly approval [165]. Typical was the response of a physician who wrote: "Dr. Quill provided his patient with exactly what was lacking in the more notorious cases involving Dr. Jack Kevorkian and the anonymous author of 'It's All Over, Debbie,' comprehensive medical care, with deep concern for the patient's well being and respect for her choices."

Was the shift in response to these cases of euthanasia or physician-assisted suicide limited to the "mode of disposal"? Is aesthetic sensitivity the only barrier to euthanasia? Is our objection that guns and knives and crude homemade "killing machines" used in the back of rusted out vans or backwoods cabins are messy or offend our sense of propriety? Do we object to suicide or euthanasia "only if," in Jo Roman's phrase, "[the victim] looks disgusting and not just dead?" And what of Roman's proposal in *Exit House* [166] that we should make suicide available to all over eighteen who request it? Derek Humphry's best selling *Final Exit* [167] likewise makes no distinction as to who can partake in suicide. With his latest self-help text, all that is required is a desirous individual and a ready source of the lethal potion.

CRITIQUE OF THE CASE FOR EUTHANASIA. Singer and Siegler [168], Kass [169], and Callahan [170] use essentially the same public policy arguments that Kamisar employed in opposition to euthanasia. A special supplement of *Commonweal* devoted to euthanasia [169] contains an essay by Daniel Callahan that succinctly states those public policy arguments. Callahan writes that the fear of dying is frequently surpassed today by the even more powerful fear of being forced to endure destructive pain, or to live out a life of unrelieved, pointless suffering. The movement to legalize euthanasia and assisted suicide is a strong and, as he puts it, "historically inevitable response to that fear" [170]. He traces that response, as do Kass and Kamisar, in part to the failure of modern medicine to reassure us that it can manage our dying with dignity and comfort and to the fact that the intense individualism of our culture leads to the demand that we must be in control, that we be masters of our fate. We resent and reject any kind of dependencies as incompatible with human dignity.

In the face of this powerful, almost relentless, dynamic, Callahan asks how we can regain and retain control. He admits that "for many the answer seems obvious and unavoidable, that of active euthanasia and assisted suicide" [170]. As he put it, "We should not deceive ourselves into thinking of euthanasia or assisted suicide as merely personal acts, just a slight extension of the already-established right to control our bodies and to have medical treatment terminated . . . [Proposition 119] is a radical move into an entirely different realm of morality: that of the killing of one person by another" [170]. As such, it would change the traditional role of the physician from healer to terminator. It would require intrusive regulation and oversight into the most private aspect of life, namely dying. It would also add substantially to the range of permissible killing in our society.

The most notable public policy implication is the potential for abuse in the authorization of "private killings," i.e., those in which the agreement of one person to kill another "is ratified by the persons themselves, but not by public authorities" [170]. How do we control, regulate, or even oversee these killings? What assurance is there or can there be that the limitations enacted in the legislation will be strictly adhered to? The suffering of the person to be killed is, as Callahan notes, "subjective, unmeasurable by, and intangible to an outside observer."

If freedom and suffering are to be the norms of euthanasia, there is no logical way in the future (1) to deny euthanasia to anyone who requests it for whatever reason, terminal illness or not, or (2) to deny it to the suffering incompetent, even if they do not request it. The legal safeguards and procedures we specify to prevent that from happening are, as it were, written in smoke—difficult to discern and easily dissipated. Such barriers cannot provide protection over time.

The problem lies in the flawed logic of the moral premise of euthanasia: our right to self-determination and our claim upon the mercy of others, especially physicians, to end our suffering. Consider self-determination, Callahan suggests. If, as it is proposed, the competent adult has a right to euthanasia for the relief of suffering, is it not a restriction on self-determination to limit euthanasia to those who are terminally ill or profoundly pained? "How," he inquires, "can self-determination have any limits?" As for relief of suffering, why should relief be confined to competent patients? Isn't the suffering of the incompetent as great, if not greater? Doesn't it demand as much concern? Further, if the physician who acts to kill the patient does so in the belief that a life marked by some form of suffering is not worth living, how can the physician deny the same relief to a person who cannot request it, or who requests it but whose competence is in doubt?

Our duty to relieve suffering, Callahan notes, cannot justify the introduction of new evils into society. The risk of doing that is simply too great. It is too great because it would take a disproportionate social change to bring it about, one with implications that extend far beyond the sick and dying. It is too great because in Callahan's powerful words, the history of the twentieth century should demonstrate that "killing is a contagious disease, not easy to stop once unleashed in society" [170].

The fear that restrictions on active euthanasia, once unleashed, could not be restrained is borne out from studies of euthanasia as practiced in the Netherlands. Though technically illegal, active euthanasia is tolerated in the Netherlands where physicians end the lives of their patients under certain specified conditions: The patient's consent must be free, conscious, explicit, and persistent; patient and physician must agree that suffering is intolerable; other measures for relief must have been exhausted; a second physician must concur; these facts must be recorded and the action must be reported to the state prosecutor [171–174].

That actual practice in the Netherlands deviates widely from the agreed-upon constraints is documented in two recent studies. Carlos F. Gomez reports that most acts of euthanasia in the Netherlands go unreported and uninvestigated by public authorities [175]. In his own survey of 26 cases of active euthanasia, only 15 percent had been reported to the prosecutor's office. Despite Proposition 119's assurance of codification into law, Gomez correctly notes that, had it passed, there would be no greater regulation of the private killings in the state of Washington than there is in the Netherlands. If, in instances of euthanasia, the official cause of death is listed as "respiratory arrest," and the massive overdose of narcotics that lead to that arrest is not even mentioned, then cases of physician killing would blend imperceptibly into the larger background of death from natural causes. Under such practice identification and oversight of euthanasia would prove impossible.

Though exact numbers are difficult to ascertain, a survey which was commissioned by the Dutch government and chaired by the attorney general of the Dutch Supreme Court indicates that "1.8% of deaths in the Netherlands are the result of physician assisted suicide." However, Van der Maas sees it

differently [176]. More revealing is the finding that 54 percent of physicians interviewed had participated in at least one case of active euthanasia and another 34 percent stated that, though they had not done so, they would be prepared to do so if asked. Of the 12 percent who said they would not participate in such an action, more than half said they would refer patients requesting euthanasia to a colleague with a more permissive attitude. In other words, the official Dutch study found that an overwhelming majority of physicians in the Netherlands see euthanasia, under certain circumstances, as an accepted element of medical practice. The circumstances mentioned in the study were "loss of dignity, pain, unworthy dying, being dependent on others, or tiredness of life." In only 10 of 107 cases was pain the only reason.

While most of the cases of euthanasia involved explicit patient requests, the attorney general's survey found that 0.8 percent of the deaths occurred without the patient's request. In these cases, it occurred "after consultation with the family, nurses, or one or more colleagues." The authors found that in the Netherlands there are over 25,000 patients each year who seek assurance from their physician that they will assist them if life becomes unbearable. Each year about 9000 explicit requests are made, of which less than one-third are agreed to by physicians.

The Dutch apologists for the practice suggest that euthanasia accounts for 2 to 3 percent, at most, of all deaths in the Netherlands. In a country with a published mortality rate of 120,000, this would imply from 2400 to 3600 cases of euthanasia per year. In the United States, with a rate of approximately two million deaths a year, this would translate into some 40,000 to 60,000 people killed each year by their physician. That not all of these would be voluntary is seen in Gomez's finding that, while most of the cases he studied fit the criteria established by the courts and the Dutch medical profession, in four out of the twenty-six cases he investigated it was clear that the patient was incapable of giving consent, or it was doubtful that consent could have been obtained properly. He reports that in none of these cases was the public prosecutor notified.

The Dutch experience shows that to construct the argument for euthanasia in terms of autonomy is to misconstrue the reality of what happens to those who cannot be truly autonomous. If this is true in a nation with universal health care coverage, how much greater the danger in a society in which 37 percent of the population is uninsured and concern for rising costs dominates the health care agenda? And how much greater in a system in which there are no safeguards built into the legislation to protect the vulnerable? The practice of euthanasia, at least as envisioned in the Washington and California referenda proposals, would place patients, particularly the most vulnerable of patients, at intolerable risk. Those proposals contained no special requirements for the physicians who would administer lethal injections. There was no requirement for determining the mental state or competency of the patient. There was no waiting period required, no notification of family, no minimum residency, and no notification of euthanasia to public authorities.

The demand for active euthanasia is, in part, a response to the fear of being trapped in a technologically sophisticated, seemingly uncaring world of medicine. Unrestrained freedom to end one's life or to have it ended by a physician ought not to be the only response to that fear; nor is such a response without grave social implications. That legitimate fear does not call for state-sanctioned suicide or euthanasia; it calls for a rejection of the mindset that insists we utilize any intervention capable of sustaining life—indifferent to the pain, suffering, and burden to the individual whose life, or dying, is being prolonged.

Conclusion

The high-technology medicine available today not only provides near miraculous benefits for some patients, but also creates challenging and troublesome ethical and legal dilemmas for patients, families, and practitioners. Fortunately, we have begun the process of moral reflection and analysis necessary to meet these challenges. The task before us now is to continue this reflection so that we might come to understand, as others have tried since the time of Hippocrates, the appropriate duties and limits of medicine.

References

1. Knaus W, Draper E, Wagner DP: The use of intensive care: New research initiatives and their implications for national health policy. *Milbank Mem Fund Q* 61:561, 1983.
2. Schroeder SA, Showstack JA, Roberts HE: Frequency and clinical description of high-cost patients in 17 acute-care hospitals. *N Engl J Med* 300:1306, 1979.
3. Thibault GE, Mulley AG, Barnett GO: Medical intensive care: Indications, interventions, and outcome. *N Engl J Med* 302:938, 1980.
4. Zook CJ, Moore FD: High-cost users of medical care. *N Engl J Med* 302:996, 1980.
5. Teres D, Brown RB, Lemeshow S: Predicting mortality of intensive care patients: The importance of coma. *Crit Care Med* 10:65, 1982.
6. Turnbull AD, Goldiner P, Silverman D, et al: The role of an intensive care unit in a cancer center. *Cancer* 37:82, 1976.
7. Davis PB, di Sant'Angnese PA: Assisted ventilation for patients with cystic fibrosis. *JAMA* 239:1851, 1978.
8. Imbus SH, Zawacki BE: Autonomy for burned patients when survival is unprecedented. *N Engl J Med* 297:308, 1977.
9. Levy DE, Bates D, Cardonna JJ, et al: Prognosis in non-traumatic coma. *Ann Intern Med* 94:293, 1981.
10. Knaus WA, Zimmerman JE, Wagner DP, et al: APACHE: Acute physiology and chronic health evaluation: A physiologically based classification system. *Crit Care Med* 9:591, 1981.
11. Knaus WA, Draper EA, Wagner DP, et al: A severity of disease classification system. *Crit Care Med* 13:818, 1985.
12. Rodman GH, Etlint T, Civetta JM, et al: How accurate is clinical judgment? *Crit Care Med* 6:127, 1978.
13. Pearlman RA, Inui TS, Carter WB: Variability in physician bioethical decision-making: A case study of euthanasia. *Ann Intern Med* 97:420, 1982.
14. Knaus WA: Prognosis with mechanical ventilation: The influence of disease, severity of disease, age, and chronic health status on survival from an acute illness. *Am Rev Respir Dis* 140:S8, 1989.
15. Editorial: Intensive care audit. *Lancet* 1:1, 1985.
16. Chung RW: Individual outcome prediction models for intensive care patients. *Lancet* ii:143, 1989.
17. Seale CF: What happens in hospice: A review of research evidence. *Soc Sci Med* 28:551, 1989.
18. Angell M: Cost containment and the physician. *JAMA* 254:1203, 1985.
19. Thurow L: Medicine versus economics. *N Engl J Med* 313:611, 1985.
20. Fuchs VR: Who shall live?, in *Health, Economics and Social Choice*. New York, Basic Books, 1974.
21. Moore FD: The desperate case: CARE (costs, applicability, research, ethics). *JAMA* 261:1483, 1989.
22. Vincent JL, Parquier JN, Preiser JC, et al: Terminal events in the intensive care unit: Review of 258 fatal cases in one year. *Crit Care Med* 17:530, 1989.
23. Ramsey P: *The Patient as Person*. New Haven, Yale University Press, 1970.
24. Admundsen D: The physicians' obligation to prolong life: A medical duty without classical roots. *Hastings Cent Rep* 8:23, 1978.
25. President's Commission for the Study of Ethical Problems in Medicine and Biomedical and Behavioral Research: Deciding to forego life-sustaining treatment. Washington, DC, U.S. Government Printing Office, 1983.
26. Council on Ethical and Judicial Affairs, American Medical Association: Guidelines for the appropriate use of do-not resuscitate orders. *JAMA* 265:1868, 1991.
27. Lo B: Unanswered questions about DNR orders. *JAMA* 265:1874, 1991.
28. Wolfe SM: Near death: In the moment of decision. *N Engl J Med* 322:208, 1990.
29. Shurin S, Pasternak RC: Decision making in "near death" (letter). *N Engl J Med* 322:1604, 1990.
30. Hachler JC, Hiller FC: Family consent to orders not to resuscitate: Reconsidering hospital policy. *JAMA* 264:1281, 1990.
31. Lantos JD, Singer PA, Walker RM: The illusion of futility in clinical practice. *Am J Med* 87:81, 1989.
32. Tomlinson T, Browdy H: Futility and the ethics of resuscitation. *JAMA* 264:1276, 1990.
33. Younger SJ: Who defines futility? *JAMA* 260:2094, 1988.
34. Blackhall L: Must we always use CPR? *N Engl J Med* 317:1281, 1987.
35. The New York State Task Force on Life and the Law: Do not resuscitate orders: The proposed legislation and report. New York, 1986.
36. Rosenthal E: New rules for saving the dying are being misused, doctors say. *New York Times* B20, October 4, 1990.
37. National Conference Steering Committee: Standards for cardiopulmonary resuscitation (CPR) and emergency cardiac care (ECC). *JAMA* 227:837, 864, 1974.
38. Lampton LM, Winship DH: The no-code blue issue: Missouri is not Massachusetts. *Mo Med* 76:259, 1979.
39. Spenser SS: Code or no code: A non-legal opinion. *N Engl J Med* 300:138, 1979.
40. Rabkin MT, Gillerman G, Rice NR: Orders not to resuscitate. *N Engl J Med* 295:364, 1976.
41. *In re Dinnerstein*, 380 N.E.2d 134 (Mass. App. 1978).
42. Beth Israel Hospital: Guidelines: Orders not to resuscitate. Boston, March 5, 1981.
43. Fowler MD: Slow code, partial code, limited code. *Heart Lung* 18:533, 1989.
44. Goldenring J: Code or no code decisions. Correspondence. *N Engl J Med* 300:1058, 1979.
45. Hashimoto DM: A structural analysis of the physician-patient relationship in no-code decision making. *Yale Law Journal* 93:362, 1983.
46. Schade GS, Muslin H: Do not resuscitate discussions with patients. *J Med Ethics* 15:186, 1989.
47. Miles SH, Cranford R, Schulty AL: The do-not resuscitate order in a teaching hospital. *Ann Intern Med* 96:660, 1982.
48. Siegler M: Does everything include CPR? *Hastings Cent Rep* 12:28, 1982.
49. Bedell SE, Delbanco TL, Cook EF, et al: Survival after cardiopulmonary resuscitation in the hospital. *N Engl J Med* 309:569, 1983.
50. Tomlinson T, Brody H: Ethics and communication in do-not-resuscitate orders. *N Engl J Med* 318:43, 1988.
51. Murphy DJ, Murray AM, Robinson BE, et al: Outcomes of cardiopulmonary resuscitation in the elderly. *Ann Intern Med* 111:119, 1989.
52. Lantos JD, Miles SH, Silverstein MD, et al: Survival after cardiopulmonary resuscitation in babies of very low birthweight: Is CPR futile therapy? *N Engl J Med* 318:91, 1988.
53. Wachter RM, Luce JM, Hearst NH, et al: Decisions about resuscitation: Inequities among patients with different diseases but similar prognoses. *Ann Intern Med* 111:525, 1989.
54. Grossman JH: Do not resuscitate (DNR) orders: Revised. New England Medical Center Hospitals, September 1989.
55. The Emergency Cardiac Care Committee, subcommittees American Heart Association: Guidelines on cardiopulmonary resuscitation and emergency cardiac care: Ethical considerations in resuscitation. *JAMA* 268:2282, 1992.
56. Guidelines for withholding, withdrawing or limiting life-sustaining treatment including resuscitation. Boston, Beth Israel Hospital, 1991.

57. Ingelfinger F: Arrogance. *N Engl J Med* 303:1507, 1980.
58. Minnesota Medical Association: Do not resuscitate (DNR) guidelines, in President's Commission for the Study of Ethical Problems in Medicine and Biomedical and Behavioral Research: *Deciding to Forego Life-Sustaining Treatment.* Washington, DC, U.S. Government Printing Office, 1983, p 499.
59. Walker RM: DNR in the OR: Resuscitation as an operative risk. *JAMA* 266:2407, 1991.
60. Cohen CB, Cohen PJ: Do-not-resuscitate orders in the operating room. *N Engl J Med* 325:1879, 1991.
61. Peterson LM: Advance directives, proxies, and the practice of surgery. *Am J Surg* 163:277, 1992.
62. Truog RD: Do-not-resuscitate orders during anesthesia and surgery. *Anesthesiology* 74:606, 1991.
63. Franklin CM, Rothenberg DM: Do-not-resuscitate orders in the presurgical patient. *J Clin Anesth* 4:181, 1992.
64. Committee for Pro-Life Activities, National Conference of Catholic Bishops: *Definition of Death Legislation,* resource paper. Washington, DC, April 1983.
65. Byrne PA, O'Reilly S, Quay PM: Brain death: An opposing viewpoint. *JAMA* 242:1985, 1979.
66. Rosner F, Bleich JD: *Jewish Bioethics.* New York, Hebrew Publishing, 1979.
67. Guidelines for the determination of death. *JAMA* 246:2184, 1981.
68. Barclay WR: Editorial: Guidelines for the determination of death. *JAMA* 246:2194, 1981.
69. Harvard Medical School: Ad hoc committee to examine the definition of brain death report: A definition of irreversible coma. *JAMA* 205:337, 1968.
70. Younger SJ, Landefeldt CS, Coulton CJ: "Brain death" and organ retrieval: A cross-sectional survey of knowledge and concepts among health professionals. *JAMA* 261:2205, 1989.
71. Pitts LH: *Maintenance of a Cadaver Donor for Multiple Organ Procurement.* Presented at the National Institutes of Health Conference, Washington, DC, Jan. 21, 1984.
72. Kotata G: Organ shortage clouds new transplant era. *Science* 221:32, 1983.
73. U.S. Renal Data System: U.S.R.D.S. 1989 annual data report: Counts of renal transplants by year of transplantation and donor type. H. 1, 1989.
74. Caplan A: Ethical and policy issues in the procurement of cadaver organs for transplantation. *N Engl J Med* 311:981, 1984.
75. Martyn S, Wright R, Clark L: Required request for organ donation: Moral, clinical, and legal problems. *Hastings Cent Rep* 18:27, 1988.
76. Caplan AL: Professional arrogance and public misunderstanding. *Hastings Cent Rep* 18:35, 1988.
77. Evans RW, Crieus DE, Ashen NL: The potential supply of organ donors: An assessment of the efficacy of organ procurement effort in the United States. *JAMA* 267:239, 1992.
78. Annas G: From Canada with love: Anencephalic newborns as organ donors? *Hastings Cent Rep* 17:36, 1987.
79. Harrison MR: Organ procurement for children: The anencephalic fetus as donor. *Lancet* 2:1383, 1986.
80. Medical Task Force on Anencephaly: The infant with anencephaly. *N Engl J Med* 322:664, 1990.
81. Peabody JL, Emery JR, Ashwal S: Experience with anencephalic infants as prospective organ donors. *N Engl J Med* 321:391, 1989.
82. Buchanan A: The limits of proxy decision making for incompetents. *UCLA Law Review* 386:403, 1981.
83. Kluge S: The euthanasia of radically defective neonates: Some statutory considerations. *Dalhousie Law Journal* 6:229, 1980.
84. President's Commission for the Study of Ethical Problems in Medicine and Biomedical and Behavioral Research: Defining death: A report on the medical, legal and ethical issues in the determination of death. Washington, DC, U.S. Government Printing Office, 1981.
85. Friedman JA: Taking the camel by the horse: The anencephalic as a source for pediatric organ transplants. *Columbia Law Review* 90:917, 1990.
86. Goldsmith A: Anencephalic organ donor program suspended: Loma Linda report expected to detail findings. *JAMA* 260:1671, 1988.
87. *In re T.A.C.P.,* 609 SO.2d 588(1992).
88. *In re A.C.,* 573 A.2d 1235 (D.C.Cir., 1990).
89. Peabody JL: Reflections on the Loma Linda University experience. *Clin Ethics Rep* 6:1, 1992.
90. Katz J: *The Silent World of Doctor and Patient.* New York, Free Press, 1984.
91. Applebaum PS, Lidz CW, Meisel A: *Informed Consent: Legal Theory and Clinical Practice.* New York, Oxford University Press, 1987.
92. La Puma J, Orentlicher D, Moss RJ: Advanced directives on admission: Clinical implications and analysis of the Patient Self-Determination Act of 1990. *JAMA* 66:402, 1991.
93. Finucaue TE, Schumway JM, Powers RL, et al: Planning with elderly patients for contingencies of severe illness. *J Intern Med* 3:322, 1988.
94. Emanuel LL, Barry MJ, Stockle JD, et al: Advanced directives for medical care: A case for greater use. *N Engl J Med* 324:889, 1991.
95. 42 U.S.C. 1395 §§(a)(1) et seq. (as amended Nov. 1990).
96. *Cruzan v. Director Missouri Dept. of Health,* 110 S. Ct. 2841 (1990).
97. *Union Pacific R. Co. v. Bostford,* 141 U.S. 250 (1891).
98. *Schloendorff v. Society of New York Hospitals,* 105 N.E. 92 (N.Y. 1914).
99. Kutner L: Due process of euthanasia: The living will proposal. *Indiana Law Journal* 44:539, 1969.
100. Silverman HJ, Vinicky JK, Gasner MR: Advance directives: Implications for critical care. *Crit Care Med* 20:1029, 1992.
101. Annas G: The health care proxy and the living will. *N Engl J Med* 324:1210, 1991.
102. Report of the Board of Trustees of the American Medical Association: *Living Wills, Durable Powers of Attorney, and Durable Powers of Attorney for Health Care.* Chicago, American Medical Association, 1989.
103. Rosenthal E: Filling the gap where a living will won't do. *New York Times,* April 4, 1991.
104. Alper PR: A living will is a bloodless document. *Wall Street Journal* January 11, 1991, p 15.
105. Bok S: Directions for my care. *N Engl J Med* 295:367, 1976.
106. Perk M, Shelp EE: Psychiatric consultation making moral dilemmas in medicine. *N Engl J Med* 307:618, 1982.
107. *Lane v. Candura,* 576 N.E.2d 1232 (Mass. 1978).
108. *Barber v. Superior Court,* 195 Cal. 484 (1983).
109. Baron CH: Medical paternalism and the rule of law: A reply to Dr. Relman. *Am J Law Med* 4:337, 1979.
110. Rhoden N: Litigating life and death. *Harvard Law Review* 102:375, 1988.
111. Johnson SH: From medicalization to legalization to politicization: O'Connor, Cruzan and refusal of treatment in the 1990s. *Conn Law Review* 21:685, 1989.
112. Gindes D: Judicial postponement of death recognition: The tragic case of Mary O'Connor. *Am J Law Med* 15:301, 1989.
113. Paris JJ: Court intervention and the diminution of patients' rights: The case of Brother Joseph Fox. *N Engl J Med* 303:876, 1980.
114. Rothenberg LS: The empty search for an imprimatur, or Delphic oracles are in short supply. *Law Med Health Care* 20:115, 1982.
115. Committee on the Legal and Ethical Aspects of Health Care for Children: Comments and recommendations on the "Infant Doe" proposed regulations. *Law Med Health Care* 11:203, 1983.
116. Collins J: Should doctors tell the truth? *Harpers* 155:320, 1927.
117. Callahan D: Shattuck Lecture: Contemporary biomedical ethics. *N Engl J Med* 302:1228, 1980.
118. Gustafson J: Mongolism, parental desires and the right to life. *Perspect Biol Med* 524:429, 1973.
119. Shaw A, Randolph JG, Manard B: Ethical issues in pediatric surgery: A national survey of pediatricians and pediatric surgeons. *Pediatrics* 60:588, 1977.
120. Todres ID, Krane D, Howell MC, et al: Pediatricians' attitudes affecting decision making in defective newborns. *Pediatrics* 60:197, 1977.
121. Office of the Secretary, Department of Health and Human Services: Nondiscrimination on the basis of handicap: Procedures and guidelines relating to health care for handicapped infants. *Federal Register* 49:1622, 1984.
122. Kopelman LM, Irons TG, Kopelman AE: Neonatologists judge the "Baby Doe" regulations. *N Engl J Med* 318:677, 1988.
123. *In re E.G.,* a Minor, 113Ill.2d 98; 549 N.E.2d 322 (1989).

124. Callahan D: Allocating health care resources. *Hastings Cent Rep* 18:14, 1988.
125. Regan M: Health care rationing: A problem in ethics and policy. *J Health Polit Policy Law* 14:627, 1989.
126. Callahan D: *What Kind of a Life: The Limits of Medical Progress.* New York, Simon & Schuster, 1990.
127. Zussman R: *Intensive Care: Medical Ethics and the Medical Profession.* Chicago, University of Chicago, 1992.
128. Schwartz WB, Aaron HJ: Rationing health care: Lessons from Britain. *N Engl J Med* 310:52, 1983.
129. Sacred congregation for the doctrine of the faith: Declaration on euthanasia: Vatican City, 1980, in President's Commission for the Study of Ethical Problems in Medicine and Biomedical and Behavioral Research: *Deciding to Forego Life-Sustaining Treatment.* Washington, DC, U.S. Government Printing Office, 1983, app C, pp 300–307.
130. Ruark JE, Raffin TA, the Stanford University Medical Center Committee on Ethics: Initiating and withdrawing life support. *N Engl J Med* 318:25, 1988.
131. Smedira N, Evans BH, Grais LS, et al: Withholding and withdrawal of life-support from the critically ill. *N Engl J Med* 322:309, 1990.
132. Luce J: Ethical principles in critical care. *JAMA* 263:696, 1990.
133. Office of the Secretary, Department of Health and Human Services: Nondiscrimination on the basis of handicap. *Federal Register* 48:846, 1983.
134. Committee on Bioethics, American Academy of Pediatrics: Treatment of critically ill newborns. *Pediatrics* 72:556, 1983.
135. Cranford RE, Doudera AE (eds): *Institutional Ethics Committees and Health Care Decision Making.* Ann Arbor, MI, Health Administration Press, 1984.
136. Ross JW, Bayley C, Michael V, et al: *Handbook for Hospital Ethics Committees.* Chicago, American Hospital Publishing, 1986.
137. Brennan TA: Ethics committees' decisions to live and decisions to limit care. *JAMA* 260:803, 1988.
138. Wolf SM: Toward a theory of process. *Law Med Health Care* 20:278, 1992.
139. Cohen CB: Avoiding "cloudcuckooland" in ethics committee case review. *Law Med Heath Care* 20:294, 1992.
140. Jonsen AR, Siegler M, Winslade WJ: *Clinical Ethics.* New York, Macmillan, 1982.
141. *Superintendent of Belchertown State School v. Saikewicz,* 370 N.E.2d 417 (1977).
142. *In the matter of Claire Conroy,* 98 N.J. 321; 486 A.2d 1209 (1985) New Jersey Supreme Court.
143. Paris JJ: Withholding of life-supporting treatment from the mentally incompetent. *Linacre Q* 8:237, 1978.
144. Kubler-Ross E: *On Death and Dying.* New York, Macmillan, 1969.
145. *Ex parte Whitebread in re Hinde, a lunatic. English Reporter* 35:878, 1816.
146. Rawls J: *A Theory of Justice.* Cambridge, MA, Harvard University Press, 1971.
147. Lynn J, Childress JF: Must patients always be given food and water? *Hastings Cent Rep* 13:17, 1983.
148. Paris JJ, Fletcher AB: Infant Doe regulations and the absolute requirement to use nourishment and fluids for the dying infant. *Law Med Health Care* 11:210, 1984.
149. Paris JJ, Reardon FE: Court responses to withholding or withdrawing artificial nutrition and fluids. *JAMA* 253:2243, 1985.
150. Curran WJ: Defining appropriate medical care: Providing nutrients and hydration for the dying. *N Engl J Med* 313:940, 1985.
151. Pellegrino ED: The metamorphosis of medical ethics: A 30 year retrospective. *JAMA* 269:1158, 1993.
152. Jonsen AR: What is at stake? *Commonweal* 118:466, 1991.
153. Knox RA: Poll: Americans favor mercy killing. *Boston Globe* 3 Nov. 1991, A1.
154. Humphry D, Wickett A: *The Right to Die: Understanding Euthanasia.* New York, Harper & Row, 1986.
155. Humphry D, Wickett A: *The Right to Die: Understanding Euthanasia.* New York, Harper and Row, 1986, p. 14.
156. Wanzer SH, Federman DD, Edelstein SJ, et al: The physician's responsibility toward hopelessly ill patients: A second look. *N Engl J Med* 320:844, 1984.
157. Anonymous: It's All Over, Debbie. *JAMA* 259:272, 1988.
158. Gayland W, Kass LR, Pellegrino ED, et al: Doctors must not kill. *JAMA* 259:2139, 1988.
159. Kass LR: Neither for love nor money: Why doctors must not kill. *The Public Interest* 94:24, 1989.
160. Kamisar Y: Some non-religious views against proposed mercy killing legislation. *Minnesota Law Review* 42:1042, 1958.
161. Alexander L: Medical science under dictatorship. *N Engl J Med* 214:39, 1949.
162. Wilkerson I: Opponents weigh action against doctor who aided suicides. *New York Times* p. 1., 1991.
163. Annas G: Killing machines. *Hastings Cent Rep* 33, 1991.
164. Quill T: Death and dignity: A case of individualized decision making. *N Engl J Med* 324:691, 1991.
165. Correspondence: Death and dignity: The case of Diane. *N Engl J Med* 325:658, 1991.
166. Roman J: *Exit House.* New York, Seaview, 1980.
167. Humphry D: *Final Exit.* Eugene, OR, Hemlock Society, 1991.
168. Singer PA, Siegler M: Legalized active euthanasia: An aesculapin tragedy. *Am Coll Surg Bull* 74:6, 1989.
169. Euthanasia: Washington State Initiative 119. *Commonweal* 118 (suppl), 1991. (See esp. Jonsen AR: Initiative 119: What is at stake?, p 466; Gomez CF: Euthanasia: Consider the Dutch, p 469; Kass LR: Why doctors must not kill, p 472; Callahan D: Aid-in-dying: The social dimensions, p 476.)
170. Callahan D: Aid-in-dying. The social dimensions. *Commonweal* 118(suppl), 1991 p 476.
171. de Wachter MAM: Active euthanasia in the Netherlands. *JAMA* 262:3316, 1989.
172. Ten Have Henk AMJ: Euthanasia in the Netherlands: The legal context and the cases. *Hospital Ethics Committee Forum* 1:412, 1989.
173. Fenigsen R: Euthanasia in the Netherlands. *Issues Law Med* 6:229, 1990.
174. Fenigsen R: A case against Dutch euthanasia. *Hastings Cent Rep* 22. (Special Supplement, January/February, 1989).
175. Gomez CF: *Regulating Death: Euthanasia and the Case of the Netherlands.* New York, Free Press, 1991.
176. Van der Maas PJ, et al: Euthanasia and other medical decisions concerning the end of life. *Lancet* 338:669, 1991.

229. Public Policymaking for Intensive Care Units

Martin A. Strosberg and Daniel Teres

An examination of a medical specialty society's official literature—newsletters, editorials, special mailings to the membership—will find its leadership calling for "increased involvement in the political process." This involvement may take the form of "engaging the public policymakers in dialogue" or "making the case in Washington" for changes in reimbursement rates, peer review mechanisms, research funding, etc. Almost all specialty societies desire to bring their particular issues and problems to the attention of public policymakers, especially as health care reform moves to the top of the domestic agenda. The Society of Critical Care Medicine (SCCM) is typical in this regard. But there are other specialty organizations with an interest in critical care such as the American Anesthesia Society, subsection on critical care; American College of Chest Physicians; American Thoracic Society; American Trauma Society; American College of Surgeons; American College of Physicians, section on critical care. This chapter will examine the process by which the problems and concerns of critical care are brought to the political arena and placed on the national agenda.

Why focus on specialty organizations and societies? There are certainly many other organizations interested in critical care, e.g., other professional medical and nursing groups, hospitals, government and other third-party payers. We focus on these organizations because they are the interest groups concerned with the widest array of public proposals related to intensive care units (ICUs). An examination of how interest groups act in the political arena will help demonstrate the process of public policymaking, the central purpose of this chapter.

The concept of "agenda" and the agenda-setting process is crucial to our understanding of public policymaking. Political scientist John W. Kingdon describes agenda-setting in his book *Agendas, Alternatives, and Public Policies*. A governmental agenda is the "list of subjects or problems to which governmental officials, and people outside government closely associated with these officials, are paying some serious attention at any given time" [1]. Governmental officials in the health policy arena include relevant congressional committee and subcommittee members and their staffs, high-ranking administrators in the Department of Health and Human Services and in particular in the Health Care Financing Administration (HCFA), the staff of the Office of Management and Budget (OMB), and key members of the White House.

According to Kingdon, certain conditions must be present for an issue to receive a spot on the health policy agenda. Three processes—problem recognition, policy proposal generation, and the unfolding of political events—must converge at the right time and the right place for an issue to receive a spot on the agenda and then move forward into legislative or executive action. At certain times, there are opportunities or "policy windows" when these three processes or "streams," which often operate independently from one another, meet. At this time, one of the alternative proposals is chosen and action is taken in the form of legislation or regulation. As will be argued, the absence of these conditions in the past has impeded many issues important to critical care from receiving a spot on the national agenda.

Problem Recognition

At the time of this writing, we cannot predict how President Clinton's national health care reform proposal will unfold as it wends its way through the legislative process. But we have long known the rhetorical goals of our national health policy. Congressman Willis Gradison explains the inherent dilemma of these goals:

Certainly, the three most important [goals] are to control costs, provide access to health care, and ensure the quality of health care. Of course, today the three goals seem to be cost containment, cost containment, and cost containment. This creates conflict because, at some point, insistence on any one of these goals impinges on the other two and tradeoffs must be made [2].

No one would argue that for some time the central problem on the national health care agenda has been escalating health care costs. Although cost escalation certainly has the attention of policymakers, it is also true that lawmakers have been frustrated in their attempt to enact a comprehensive legislative solution. They have been unable to solve the political puzzle inherent in the tradeoffs among the three goals. Nevertheless, the cost containment bandwagon rolls along in the form of incremental changes made to the reimbursement system. Undoubtedly there is an impact of cost containment on access and quality. One of the tasks facing the leaders of the critical care community is to articulate the consequences of this impact. In terms of agenda-setting, critical care leaders must formulate the problem in such a way so as to get the attention of public policymakers.

The most common way to define a policy problem is to measure it. Chances are that most articles discussing public policy problems contain the word *increasingly* in the first paragraph, if not the first sentence. Discussions of policy problems begin by showing that things are changing, that is, getting worse. And, of course, numbers are preeminently useful in measuring change [3].

In Kingdon's agenda-setting process, indicators, especially numbers, are an important way to recognize problems:

Fairly often, problems come to the attention of government decision makers, not through some sort of political pressure or perceptual sleight of hand, but because some more or less systematic indicator simply shows that there is a problem out there. Such indicators abound in the political world because both governmental and non-governmental agencies routinely monitor various activities and events: highway deaths, disease rates, immunization levels, consumer prices, commuter and intercity ridership, costs of entitlement programs, infant mortality rates, and many others [1].

Trauma is an example rich in indicators. Numbers of injuries and deaths are collected routinely. When these numbers are considered in relation to the lifesaving potential of regionalized trauma systems (a policy proposal), estimates of preventable deaths and injuries can be calculated. "Preventable deaths" is indeed a salient political fact because it clearly indicates deficiencies in the way we do things. Measuring the problem creates pressure to do something about it [3]. Policies are needed to overcome these deficiencies—to close the gap between what is and what should or could be, that is, the "optimal" [4]. Furthermore, in times of proposed budget cutbacks, the consequences of the cuts in terms of added deaths and injuries can be quantified and counterarguments can be made.

In terms of setting agendas, it makes good political sense to improve continually the collection and analysis of data that indicate problems, and to elevate the consideration of those data to highly visible political arenas. It is also helpful if an official method of "counting" the problem exists, for this means that there is an official definition of the problem. For example, in 1987, Congress directed the National Highway Traffic Safety Administration and the Centers for Disease Control to collect and analyze trauma data, monitor the progress of trauma programs, and "report to Congress." The 1989 *Report* includes not only the number of injuries and deaths, but also the direct costs of medical services and the indirect costs of lost productivity due to premature death and short- and long-term disability [5]. A very compelling cost-benefit argument can therefore be made for the policy proposal of a regionalized trauma system, whose benefits in savings from averted premature death and disability compare favorably to the costs of establishing a trauma system.

Embedded in the policy prescription (proposal/solution) of the regionalized trauma system is really a set of programmatic initiatives. These include research and development, demonstration and training, and capacity-building programs. The logic and sequence of these initiatives are followed by most "single disease" coalitions typically composed of lay-groups organized by state chapters to raise funds and lobby on behalf of a particular "dreaded disease," specialty societies (academic- and practitioner-based), graduate medical education credentialing and accrediting associations, and funding organizations, particular institutes of divisions of the NIH, and congressional subcommittees and their staffs [6]. Those groups associated with trauma and emergency medical services have followed a similar path. There have been, for example, predictable calls for the establishment of a National Institute of Trauma since trauma accounts for more years of life lost than cancer and heart disease combined, and yet receives fewer research dollars [7]. Demonstration, training, and capacity-building also follow conventional programmatic lines, as manifested in the Highway Safety Act of 1966 (P.L. 89-564), the Emergency Medical Services System Act of 1973 (P.L. 93-154), and the Trauma Care Systems Planning and Development Act (P.L. 101-590) enacted in 1990.

In contradistinction to the EMS-trauma side of the critical care continuum, it will be argued here that, although indicators of intensive care unit costs are securely established and actively monitored, indicators of benefits are not. In the face of increasing demands and diminished capacity (caused in part by the nursing shortage and resource cutbacks), the first question that we would like policymakers to ask is to what extent are we actually denying, delaying, or otherwise reducing the benefits of intensive care, with what consequences for access and quality? Are things (e.g., preventable deaths) getting worse over time? The inability to decisively answer these questions seriously impedes consideration of ICU resource allocation and other issues on the public policy agenda. This topic will be taken up again at the end of the chapter.

Although ICU cost accounting is primitive, it is possible to estimate and monitor the rising cost of intensive care [8]. The U.S. Office of Technology Assessment estimates that one day in the ICU costs three to four times as much as one day on a regular floor. Fifteen to twenty percent of a hospital's budget is devoted to intensive care [9]. Viewed against the larger backdrop of the increasing percentage of the gross national product devoted to health care, ICU costs are closely identified as a major contributor to the overall problem of cost escalation.

Unfortunately, the benefit side of the picture is missing [10]. Is society getting improved quality for our increasing expenditure? The conventional wisdom is that it is not, i.e., society is not receiving an adequate marginal return on its $60 billion investment in terms of number of lives saved, longevity, and quality of life. There are better places to invest the resources. The most popular representation of this tradeoff is the equation "More money spent on prenatal care = less money spent on neonatal ICU care."

We do not know the extent to which the conventional wisdom is true. According to the NIH Consensus Development Conference of 1983, there are many areas of uncertainty concerning the ability of intensive care to reverse life-threatening conditions [11]. Under the banner of "do everything that might help," questionable procedures may have been incorporated into standard ICU practice. The ongoing debate over the value of Swan-Ganz catheterization points out the difficulty in arriving at a consensus on the effectiveness of many procedures [12,13].

Problems may be recognized through awareness of differences in performance among various health care systems. However, cross-national studies often raise more questions than they answer. Zimmerman et al. conducted a study comparing a small set of hospitals in New Zealand with a group from the United States [14]. Approximately 1.5 percent of hospital beds in New Zealand are allocated to intensive care compared to the approximately 6 percent in the United States. With the same proportion of low-risk monitoring patients and with similar technologic capabilities and quality, physicians in both countries claimed they admitted only those elderly patients who could benefit from the ICU and rejected those who were "too sick to benefit." Knaus concludes, in an editorial comment on the study, "Considering the dramatic differences in utilization, both approaches cannot be correct. Either the American physicians were incredibly extravagant in their use of intensive care or many patients [in New Zealand] were routinely denied life-saving services" [15].

Clearly, for comparative indicators to be useful in problem recognition, there must be risk-benefit and outcomes research to identify those patient groupings for whom ICU intervention is worthwhile. Fortunately, the pressing need for this research is accepted by government as well as professional leaders [16]. We will return to this topic later in the chapter. But it should be abundantly clear that it will be difficult to sell the idea of expanding ICU capacity as a solution to any of the aspects of the cost-escalation, access, or quality of care problems.

Solutions: Policy Proposal Generation

As mentioned previously, and it cannot be overemphasized, problem recognition and policy proposal generation constitute two streams that often flow independently of one another. Whereas it is unlikely that the unique problems of critical care (tradeoffs in access and quality) will be recognized by public policymakers preoccupied with cost escalation, there is greater potential for gaining a spot on the national agenda if somehow the two streams can be joined. To show why this is the case, consider the conventional understanding of the sequence of events leading to the development of public policies: *The rec-*

ognition of a problem generates a search for a solution to the problem. However, an equally likely scenario, according to the Kingdon model is: Solutions (policy proposals) search for problems to attach themselves to. Kingdon points to the pivotal role of the "policy entrepreneur" in creating and taking advantage of opportunities to promote change by hooking solutions to problems and proposals to political momentum [1]. A typical operating mode of policy entrepreneurs is to advocate solutions and look for current problems to which to attach their pet solutions. Policy entrepreneurs originate in interest groups, research organizations, think tanks, universities, and government itself.

In the case of interest groups, it has been argued that the solutions advocated usually advance the well-being of the group. The official goals of professional associations, including specialty societies, are the advancement of science and technology, the improvement of quality of care, the alleviation of pain and suffering, and the furthering of the public interest. However, political economist Paul Feldstein advances a different perspective—the "self-interest paradigm." When lobbying in the public arena, professional associations and specialty societies are interest groups acting according to their self-interest. Specifically, according to Feldstein, they favor legislation and regulation that maximizes income. This is frequently translated into calls for increased autonomy and control over practice, and consequent increased demand for services [17]. In fact, a major service that specialty societies provide their members is to establish and protect the unique reimbursement rates for "recognized" specialists (i.e., members certified by an authoritative body).

THE SOCIETY OF CRITICAL CARE MEDICINE. The SCCM has in fact been drafting proposals that mesh with policymakers' emerging understanding of the cost-escalation problem. In 1992, the SCCM published a booklet entitled "Critical Care in the United States: Coordinating Intensive Care Resources for Positive and Cost-Effective Patient Outcomes." The booklet, with an American flag on the cover (known as the "flag book"), is meant for consumption in the Washington political arena. It clearly stakes out the claims for critical care medicine, "The immediate availability of the qualified critical care physician (QCCP), who provides a coordinated and collaborative approach to care for gravely ill patients, results in strongly improved outcomes at reduced cost" [18].

The booklet gives an example of how this improved outcome at reduced cost might be achieved by illustrating the fate of an ICU patient under two different scenarios. In the first, the patient receives multiple consultations from a cardiologist, pulmonologist, nephrologist, and infectious disease specialist. They are replaced in the second scenario by a single QCCP who, as team leader, coordinates care to achieve a better outcome, shorter length of stay, and fewer external consults and charges.

Needless to say, the claims of critical care medicine are not uncontroversial nor universally accepted. Many single-organ specialists feel that patients are better served by subspecialty consultation rather than by "generalist" intensivists [19]. The struggle to get these claims accepted is the struggle to gain legitimacy within the specialty system of organized medicine. Those seeking acceptance and legitimacy can help their cause by showing how the QCCP addresses the overriding problem of cost escalation.

INTEREST GROUP POWER. In the context of agenda-setting, power may be conceptualized as "the ability to define public problems and place them on governmental agendas for action, to define the terms of debate, limit the alternatives to be considered, and supply the criteria by which they will be evaluated [20].

Specialty recognition is an important variable in explaining the extent of power. Most specialties aspire to reach board certification status—a state that brings economic advantage along with control over technology, working conditions, and "turf." Faced with resistance from rival groups, many budding specialties do not make it. To say the least, the process of specialization is not well understood by politicians, administrators, or the general public, but its influence both on public policymaking and the organization of the U.S. health care system is very important. Specialty societies, parent, and umbrella organizations, through interlocking directorates, dominate the credentialing system which in turn influences accreditation of graduate medical education programs, establishment and certification of new specialties and subspecialties, and the distribution and practice patterns of specialists. Also impacted are the policies, procedures, and organizational structure of the hospital: specification of physician qualifications; staff privileges and responsibilities; technology requirements for quality of care; organizational differentiation into departments, divisions, and sections; referral patterns; the cost of services; and incomes of practitioners — in short many of the essential characteristics of the U.S. health care system.

By 1985, critical care medicine's orbit was finally fixed in the U.S. specialty system: Critical care, as a subspecialty of other primary specialties, has achieved satellite as opposed to planetary status. The model of a broad-based intensivist trained by a multidisciplinary faculty with a common certifying exam has not been achieved. Civetta, a prominent leader of critical care medicine, bemoans this fate:

I believe that one of the saddest developments of the past few years has been the fragmentation of this initial multi-disciplinary commitment. This fragmentation has occurred not within the SCCM; rather, as the primary disciplines have tried to develop isolated critical care subsections, both the professional and personal advantages of the multi-disciplinary interactions were lost that transcended all single disciplines of medicine and other allied health care professions. Our founding fathers were correct in recognizing that this multi-disciplinary characteristic was one of the strengths of the SCCM and we should foster that aim, especially in the face of the popularity of "separatism" today [21].

Opportunities for Policy Entrepreneurs

What are some of the important questions, the answers to which should be of interest to both public policymakers and the critical care community? Presented below are some of these questions, most of which are a subset of larger issues concerning cost containment, quality of care, improvement of the scientific basis of medical practice, and patient autonomy. There are many customers and potential customers for the answers to these questions.

CUSTOMERS, QUESTIONS, CONCERNS. The NIH Consensus Development Conference on Critical Care brought together members of the clinical community to synthesize what was known about the effectiveness of critical care as a distinct technology, to review methods of defining ahead of time which patients would benefit from ICU care, and to outline the major clinical, bioethical, and legal issues that must be addressed.

Clinicians constitute a natural constituency for defining, measuring, and improving performance of ICUs. The scientific and clinical communities are interested in basic and clinical research intended to discover new treatments and establish their effectiveness. But there are other groups who have their own concerns and definitions of ICU performance. In particular these groups include health care plan sponsors/payers, hospital managers, patients, and government/society.

Plan Sponsors/Payers, Including Government and Business. Can they determine the risks, costs, and benefits of ICU interventions and use this information to contain costs and assure quality? Can they identify hospitals with high-quality, low-cost ICUs and steer the patients to these hospitals in the context of managed care? How should effective ICU management activities be supported through the reimbursement system?

Hospital Managers. How can managers provide high-quality, low-cost critical care? What are the organizational characteristics of high-performance ICUs? How can they improve risk-adjusted length of stay (throughput) to optimize reimbursement and to utilize the ICU consistent with the strategic objectives of the hospital? Can they compete under "managed competition"?

Patients. How can ICU staff communicate to patients objective information about the risks and benefits of critical care so that individual patients have an opportunity to place their own values on those risks and benefits? How can patients insure that decision-making will reflect their values? Can the insurance contract provide a vehicle for structuring the decision-making process? If not, what can?

Society/Government. How can society collectively value the risks and benefits of critical care and structure and resource allocation decision-making process?

Pressed by third-party payers, managers, patient advocates, and government, public policymakers will pay increasing attention to these questions. However, they remain as questions or problems unless they can be linked to feasible solutions or policy proposals. Below are some opportunities for creating a linkage:

1. *Outcomes research, appropriateness criteria, practice guidelines.* Outcomes research, now championed by the well-established federal Agency for Health Care Policy and Research (AHCPR), has the support of the major medical associations, specialty societies, and by Congress. The creation of this agency is actually a prime illustration of the agenda-setting process and the role of the policy entrepreneur, in particular Dr. John Wennberg [22]. Many years ago, Wennberg pioneered what has become known as "small-area variation analysis." Wennberg, who can best be described as a medical care epidemiologist, discovered significant variations in medical care utilization among populations in small, geographically distinct towns in New England as well as in large cities such as Boston and New Haven. While he discerned great variation in utilization, there was little difference in outcomes but large differences in expenditures. In searching for an explanation for this variation, Wennberg considered, among other factors, the fact that many medical interventions have been adopted without being well-tested.

Wennberg offered small-area variation analysis—research to find the sources of variation—as a solution to the cost-escalation problem. He reasoned that if there is significant variation among populations in their utilization of medical resources and there is no discernible difference in outcome, why should third-party payers, including government, pay for the expensive practice pattern [23]?

This logic, compelling to both the private and public sectors,

helped spawn a major research endeavor. This research encompasses a variety of approaches including the RAND/UCLA "appropriateness method," which relies on panels of experts to determine when benefits outweigh risks for certain procedures [24]. Outcomes research, appropriateness criteria, and practice guidelines, aimed at finding and implementing the most cost-effective practice patterns, have become a central plank in an overall cost-containment strategy. There is an important role for specialty societies to play in advancing these efforts.

Wide variation in the use of intensive care has long been noted in international comparisons. In response, the critical care community has long advocated outcomes research to identify which patients could best benefit from ICU intervention. The 1983 NIH Consensus Development Conference included a plea for outcomes research. While the majority of the participants at the Conference were clinicians, there is now opportunity to add more constituencies and customers for this research. Third-party payers and business leaders will be active supporters and consumers of this research.

2. *Management roles for intensivists.* While the SCCM and other groups claim that the QCCP and qualified nurses provide the most cost-effective way of managing the individual patient, it can also be argued that a QCCP can best provide the leadership for managing the resources of the intensive care unit. In effect, there is an opportunity to promote the managerial role of intensivists, and in particular the ICU medical director, as a cost-containment strategy. The SCCM, in its "Guidelines for the Definition of an Intensivist and the Practice of Critical Care Medicine," already stakes out the claims for the role of the QCCP in the management of the unit:

The intensivist participates actively in daily unit management activities necessary for the efficient, timely, and consistent delivery of ICU services to the patients of the hospital. These activities include but are not limited to: (a) triage and bed allocation, discharge planning; (b) supervision of the application of unit policies; (c) participation in ongoing quality improvement activities including supervision of data collection; (d) interaction with other departments as necessary to facilitate the smooth operation of the ICU. To provide these services, the intensivist must be physically present in the unit or hospital and free from competing obligations such as operating room or office responsibilities [25].

For the purchasers of health care, the question becomes how to identify high-quality, high-performance, and cost-effective ICUs. The trend toward managed care will generate new ways to understand, analyze, monitor, and control costs. With this information, sponsors, third-party payers, or those choosing on behalf of patients can steer patients to those hospitals with cost-effective units. On the other hand, managers of hospitals and multi-institutional systems may seek ways to improve their performance and compete in the market for physicians, patients, or groups of patients. They will have to recognize and act on the knowledge that different "customers" will have different definitions of performance.

Research is under way to identify the organizational characteristics of high-performance ICUs. Shortell et al. identify the organizational characteristics associated with patient outcomes measured in terms of risk-adjusted mortality and functional status, patient/family satisfaction, and efficiency (risk-adjusted length of stay) [26]. Rapoport and colleagues have a developed a system for assessing ICU performance taking into account both economic and clinical dimensions while adjusting for severity of illness [27].

In terms of influencing public policy, the immediate challenge is to change those reimbursement practices that currently do not adequately compensate intensivists for spending time in managerial activities so as to free the intensivist from "competing obligations" in the operating room and the office.

3. *Resource allocation decision-making methodologies for individuals*. Outcomes research is intended to produce information on the risks and benefits of certain procedures expressed in terms of probabilities or of appropriateness categories (e.g., appropriate, inappropriate, uncertain about appropriateness). Wennberg and others point out that even where an objective determination of probabilities can be made, clinicians and patients may vary among themselves and with each other on the weight or value to be placed on those probabilities, thus leading to different treatment choices.

Value judgments abound in the ICU. ICU care is capable of prolonging life but it is also capable of prolonging the dying process. It is often a thin line that separates these poles and where one draws that line is very much a value judgment. To some, staying in the ICU on a ventilator for a month or more hoping for a 2 percent chance of recovery may be entirely worth the effort. To others it may not be.

Wennberg suggests that if patients' preferences were incorporated into decision-making, the demand for invasive, high-technology medicine would be reduced, especially with regard to care near the end of life, where patients might prefer less rather than more care [28]. Most practice guidelines, however, do not recognize a legitimate role for the patient in the decision-making process, a situation that Wennberg and others think should be rectified. However, it is extremely difficult to systematically structure a decision-process that facilitates a discussion of the risk-benefit probabilities and an articulation of patient preferences. David Eddy, in a series of articles in *JAMA*, explains the methodological challenges and suggests some solutions [29].

Most proposals for incorporating patient preferences into treatment decision-making, however, are narrowly construed and leave out an important economic dimension. Consider the case of Mrs. Helga Wanglie, a ventilator-dependent and permanently unconscious 86-year-old woman whose 15-month stay in a Minneapolis ICU cost $700,000. The hospital doctors wanted to remove her from the ICU and ventilator, not because they thought it was costing too much, but because they believed that continued care was futile. The family wanted her to remain. The courts sided with the family. Ultimately Mrs. Wanglie died in the ICU, but she left a legacy of questions. Whose admission was denied or delayed because Mrs. Wanglie was occupying a bed? Whose insurance premiums became unaffordable because of the $700,000 addition to the budget of the HMO to which Mrs. Wanglie belonged [30]?

Michael Rie proposes using the market to sort out these questions by bringing an economic dimension to the way patients exercise their preferences. Presumably, in a market system, there would not be universal entitlement to unlimited consumption of ICU services. As Rie argues, in a system designed to maximize consumer choice, a buyer should be able to purchase insurance coverage that is linked to a certain level of benefit (services), not unlike automobile and homeowners insurance coverage [31]. For example, some may not wish to purchase coverage guaranteeing access to marginally beneficial therapies and, therefore, they would not be entitled to them. (Presumably the money they save from cheaper insurance premiums would be spent on endeavors more worthwhile to them). Others (e.g., Mrs. Wanglie) may wish to purchase extra coverage even for what many would consider marginally beneficial or futile services. Government may provide a basic level of coverage for the indigent and uninsured. But clearly, a multitiered system is a natural outgrowth of a consumer-choice system. How will insurance policies reflect consumer preferences? Rie, a policy entrepreneur in his own right (see Chapter 230) offers a sample policy:

This policy will limit payment for futile care as defined by a prognostic probability of death of 95% or greater for seven days. Premiums are negotiable depending on the "P" value of uncertainty of the scoring index that the subscriber elects to purchase [32].

Needless to say, the methodology and the rationale are not well-accepted. What is needed is a methodology for effectuating consumer choice, i.e., linking insurance to a desired level of ICU coverage/benefit. Can the task be performed by current prognostic tools and prediction models? Can they be made sufficiently accurate? In spite of considerable research, the questions remain.

RESOURCE-ALLOCATION DECISION-MAKING. The previous section discussed the issue of structuring a decision-making process that would incorporate patient preferences and values, given an objective determination of risks and benefits. The same issue is germane to the society at large. The question for society is how to define the minimally acceptable benefit package that will be offered either in a multitiered, market-driven system as proposed by Dr. Rie and others, or in a single-tiered system like Canada's. How should society collectively determine what preferences and values to place on risks and benefits? In creating this benefit package, society will no doubt decide not to include all the beneficial services that individuals might prefer. This difference between the beneficial care that is offered and that which is preferred is care that is rationed.

Up until recently, rationing was not an issue on the national agenda. There has been no nexus between clinical decision-making at the bedside and our political institutions. "Politicians make choices in ways that will minimize and, if possible, eliminate any public perception that they are rationing care or diminishing its quality." Representative Willis Gradison of the House Ways and Means Subcommittee on Health made this assessment at a 1986 Brookings conference on rationing health care for the critically ill [2]. Only 5 years later, at another Brookings conference, policymakers, analysts, and health care providers met to consider a proposal that would place politicians and public institutions squarely at the center of an explicit rationing plan: The Oregon Medicaid initiative [33].

Before examining the Oregon Plan and its explicit rationing plan, let's examine another type of rationing. A headline in the *New York Times* proclaimed, "Crowding Causes Agonizing Crisis in Intensive Care: As Hopeless Patients Fill Units, Hospitals Adopt Makeshift Settings or Turn People Away" [34]. In spite of media attention, the conditions of decreased access and quality described in the headline cannot be easily transformed into a well-recognized problem for the national agenda. Nor is there an obvious solution. The Oregon Plan may change this.

WHEN IS RATIONING A PROBLEM? In the face of scarce resources, rationing may result in diminished performance. However, it is difficult to operationalize this result for the ICU. To understand this difficulty, consider an electric power company. When there is insufficient power to meet peak demand, the company may "brown out" or ration power to particular areas. Clearly, this is less than ideal performance. Everyone can recognize the rationing of power when the air conditioner goes off. But how does one recognize the negative effects of ICU rationing? Clearly, admitting behavior and treatment decision-making when the ICU is full will be different than when the unit is not. But to what extent is performance diminished? Some studies show no difference in outcome in terms of increased mortality or other adverse impacts [35,36].

In unraveling this puzzle, we have already acknowledged the uncertainty surrounding the values that patients and clinicians place on the risks and benefits of ICU intervention. And frequently missing is an objective determination of those risks and benefits. In triage, the inability to define precisely the likelihood of benefit from a particular treatment for a patient means there is an array of possible alternatives for patient admission and discharge. One study suggests that when independently evaluating the same patients, different intensivists often arrive at different estimates of the potential for discharge [37].

Recognizing the irreducible uncertainty surrounding the facts and values of triage decision-making, we raise the following three points:

1. Perhaps beneficial services are not really being denied; perhaps there is enough slack in the system to absorb safely everyone who can benefit from intensive care. Proponents of this position subscribe to the "rubber band" theory of intensive care delivery. During peak demand, resource capacity can be "stretched" by using the emergency room, postanesthesia care unit, and other holding areas.

From a societal perspective, if resource allocation could be improved, there would be plenty of room for this rubber band to expand. In fact, one prominent spokesperson for the critical care profession, Max Harry Weil, states unequivocally that we are not faced with a scarcity of resources, but rather the inappropriate use of existing resources [38].

2. Perhaps the operative definition of *beneficial* varies, according to the extent of resource scarcity, to mask the emotional consequences of denying services. Clearly, there is some psychological mechanism at work in this "sliding-scale" definition. In their study of the British National Health Service, Aaron and Schwartz discuss the tendency of physicians to redefine standards of care gradually so that they can "avoid the painful realization that they are doing less than the best for the patient" [39].

Just where the balance is struck between prolonging life and prolonging the dying process may depend on the availability of resources. Given clinical uncertainty, there is ample room for maneuvering the sliding-scale definition of benefit.

3. Perhaps the right phenomena are not being measured. Frequently missing from evaluations of rationing during bed shortage is an analysis of those patients outside the ICU, on the floors and in other hospitals, who are potential candidates and may in fact be harmed while waiting to be admitted to the ICU. Data must be collected on patients both inside and outside the ICU.

Alternatively, perhaps we don't want to measure the right things. Although, as Kapp and Lo contend [40], the legal risk of discontinuing futile treatments and nonbeneficial services is greatly exaggerated, it may be very real if beneficial or marginally beneficial treatments are denied, delayed, or diminished. Marginally beneficial treatments are defined as those that provide a slight but real contribution (physical or psychological) to the welfare of all or most patients, or that make a moderately valuable contribution to the welfare of some but not most patients (with no certain foreknowledge of which patients are in the minority that would benefit) [41].

As Morreim argues, there is little flexibility in the legal system to allow the physician to be both the fiduciary agent of the patient and the rationer of marginally beneficial services [42]. Resource and fiscal constraints do not provide physicians with a malpractice defense when the community standard of care is lowered. In a contingency fee environment, lawsuits related to rationing can be expected [43]. Given malpractice fears coupled

with the monitoring activities of the Joint Commission on the Accreditation of Healthcare Organizations (JCAHO) and internal and external peer review committees, it is understandable why there is little systematic documentation of cases of denied, delayed, or diminished benefit.

Is there a crisis in critical care? Apparently, the crisis of denying "truly" beneficial care is being averted. Our discussion raises three possible explanations: (1) There is in fact enough "stretch" capacity to absorb everyone safely, especially if services that are not beneficial or consented to are eliminated; (2) We have conveniently redefined "truly" beneficial service and consequent ICU performance to match available resources; (3) Because of inability and/or unwillingness (based on fear of legal risk or negative publicity), we have failed to measure decreases in ICU performance. No doubt all three factors are combined in U.S. hospitals. Practically speaking, there are no data on case mix, outcomes, and management structures to assess and compare the magnitude of factors among hospitals or even within a single hospital. Nevertheless, it can be argued that critical care delivery capacity cannot be stretched indefinitely. Conceptually, there must be some breaking point to the rubber band, especially given the shortage of staffed beds. Shoemaker et al. graphically describe one such breaking point in an inner-city emergency room [44]. The question is, how many breaking points go unrecognized because of the incentives not to recognize them implicit in factors two and three. With some notable exceptions (Teres [45] and Marshall et al. [46]), this question is not usually addressed.

At least conceptually, the idea of a breaking point focuses attention on the role of the ICU medical director as gatekeeper, a role compatible with JCAHO and Critical Care Society guidelines [47,48]. In weighing competing claims of patients to the communal resources of the ICU, issues of comparative entitlement, fairness (for example, whether patients with similar prognoses but different or even the same diseases have equal access), and accountability are also drawn painfully into focus.

This brings us to the second requirement for bringing an issue to the public policy agenda and then into legislative or executive action. In addition to problem recognition, there must be a policy proposal—a politically feasible solution. The solution to scarce resources and comparative entitlement is to allocate resources rationally, i.e., there must be an explicit mechanism to ration. And yet society is stymied in creating an explicit rationing mechanism. As we have seen:

1. From a legal perspective, malpractice law expects physicians to deliver the same standard of care with the same resources to all patients; tight budgets and scarce resources do not let physicians off the hook.

2. From an ethical perspective, there is nothing in the Hippocratic tradition that allows physicians to be society's resource allocators.

Politicians have not been eager to enter the fray. But now, in a major watershed in public policy, the state of Oregon has adopted a plan that makes politicians and public institutions responsible for an explicit health care rationing plan. What has been done in Oregon is to forge a change of accountability from clinical decision-making at the bedside directly to the Oregon legislature. This chain of accountability will enable the ICU community to: (1) fully recognize the problems of resource scarcity, differential access, and comparative entitlement, and not sweep it under rug, and (2) embrace a rational solution.

In a nutshell, the Oregon Plan expands Medicaid and private insurance to large numbers of people who currently have no health insurance, but at the price of explicitly deciding not to cover some medical procedures generally accepted as beneficial but of low priority. To accomplish this, a publicly appointed Oregon Health Services Commission has created a rank-ordered list of 709 paired medical conditions and treatments prioritized by clinical effectiveness and social importance. The priority list was submitted to the state legislature which, through its allocation of funds to the Medicaid budget, has determined how many of the services on the list can be funded. Those that are too far down on the list are not provided in the basic medical package, even though they might be beneficial services. In July 1991, the legislature allocated funds that covered services down to 587 on the list of 709.

A description of the methodology for the ranking is beyond the scope of this paper and there have been various "generations" of techniques and approaches. However, a perhaps oversimplified formula for calculating the rank of a particular treatment is: *the probability of successful outcome* × *quality of life* × *length of life divided by cost*. Some may recognize this formula as Englehardt and Rie's ICU Entitlement Index [49]. The denominator of the index's formula, cost, enters the Oregon ranking system as the total amount of money that the Oregon legislature decides to allocate, thus determining how far down on the list services can be funded.

At the bottom of the list are aggressive treatments for extremely small infants and aggressive medical treatments for end-stage cancer and end-stage AIDS. Many intensivists would point out that the "vertical" ranking of 709 conditions/treatments lacks a "horizontal" dimension. They would argue that probability rankings should be incorporated into each of the 709 condition/treatments to take into consideration the potential of ICU intervention. As probabilities of survival get worse over time, there would be cutoffs or thresholds for hospice or lower cost options.

In the Oregon Plan, treatments for conditions at the bottom of the list would be deemed marginally beneficial or medically futile. However, some would argue that futility and questions of marginal benefit are individual value judgments (e.g., Mrs. Wanglie). In the Oregon Plan the individual value judgment is replaced by a community value judgment made though the political process.

The Oregon Plan would create a "liability shield" by protecting providers against malpractice and professional disciplinary action when not providing those services that are not in the basic health care package. What this means is that providers can legally have a divided standard of care—a major departure from malpractice law. The state legislature assumes explicit responsibility for the standard of care for the Medicaid population, i.e., it has created the minimum (basic) benefit package.

Rationing is not uncontroversial. Yet most would agree, whether the result of conscious policy choice or not, health care in America is already being rationed for both the uninsured and the Medicaid population. In times of budgetary pressure, instead of raising taxes, state governments typically respond by reducing Medicaid reimbursement to providers who will be less likely to treat Medicaid patients or to drop coverage to a portion of poor persons already on the Medicaid rolls. Such responses ultimately ration care to anonymous people, and government avoids confronting individuals. In making up the shortfall, hospitals are squeezed, trauma services are cut, ICU nurses are overworked and they quit, and the conditions described in the *New York Times* headline take place. Thus, government is implicitly rationing health care resources. Doctors and nurses at the bedside join the ranks of the harassed street-level bureaucrats, including inner-city school teachers, social workers, police officers, and lower court judges, dispensing vital, often life-sustaining services, to an involuntary clientele, yet having inadequate resources, inappropriate performance measures,

contradictory performance expectations, and with great discretion to make life and death decisions [50]. Society has not given them legally or politically defensible allocation rules. But Oregon would.

In Oregon, the debate shifts from whom to cover (often made covertly) to what to cover, based on the degree to which health services improve health status. If revenues fall short, lawmakers cannot, as they usually do, arbitrarily cut people from the Medicaid rolls, or arbitrarily cut what is paid to medical providers. Their only options are to raise more money or to reduce the service level. If the citizens do not like the level of services (e.g., the 587 cut point), all they have to do is to tell their legislators to put more funds into the Medicaid budget. The Oregon Plan and its methodology for the public construction of the basic benefit package empower the citizenry.

In summary, we have argued that the critical care community has not been able to engage the political system with regard to the problems of access, comparative entitlement, and rationing. It has been frustrated in this attempt to articulate its problems and to craft a feasible policy proposal. The Oregon Plan offers a potential resolution to this dilemma by providing an explicit and publicly accountable resource allocation method. In this context, the critical care community can begin to openly articulate its problems of the tradeoffs among cost, access, and quality.

Because Medicaid is a federal/state partnership, Oregon needs a federal waiver from Congress or HCFA in order to modify the current Medicaid requirements in order to implement its plan. The Bush administration denied the request for a waiver. In March 1993, the Clinton administration granted the waiver. At the time of this writing, it is not at all certain that the experiment will be successful. But regardless of the ultimate fate of the plan, many of the ideas embedded in efforts at explicit rationing will resurface, recombine, and enter the policy proposal (solution) stream in the future.

Conclusion: The Policy Window

In space shots, the window presents the opportunity for a launch. The target planets are in proper alignment, but will not stay that way for long. . . Similarly, windows open in policy systems. These policy windows, the opportunities for action on given initiatives, present themselves and stay open for only short periods. If the participants cannot or do not take advantage of the opportunities, they must bide their time until the next opportunity comes along (p. 174) [1].

Typically, policy windows open when new national administrations with new priorities take control. The Clinton administration has staked its reputation on its commitment and ability to reform the health care system. The last time a policy window opened this wide was during the landslide election of President Johnson, which led to the passage of Medicare and Medicaid.

Policy windows provide opportunities for joining the policy proposal stream and the problem recognition stream. Now there is an excellent opportunity for policy entrepreneurs in the critical care community to link their proposals (ranging from QCCP-led coordinated care to regionalized trauma systems) to the problems swimming in the larger political stream.

References

1. Kingdon JW: *Agendas, Alternatives and Public Policies*. Boston, Little, Brown, 1988.

2. Gradison WD: Federal policy and intensive care, in Strosberg MA, Fein IA, Carroll JD (eds): *Rationing of Medical Care for the Critically Ill*. Washington DC, Brookings Institution, 1989, p 37.

3. Stone DA: *Policy, Paradox and Political Reason*. Glenview IL, Scott, Foresman, 1988.

4. Hospital and Prehospital Resources for Optimal Care of the Injured Patient and Appendices A through J. Chicago, American College of Surgeons, 1987.

5. Centers for Disease Control: Cost of injury: United States: A report to Congress, 1989. *JAMA* 262:2803, 1989.

6. Rettig RA: The policy debate on patient care financing for victims of end-stage renal disease. *Law and Contemporary Problems* 40:196, 1976.

7. Trunkey DD: Trauma. *Scientific American* 249:28, 1983.

8. Wagner DP, Wineland TD, Knaus WA: The hidden costs of treating severely ill patients: Changes and resource consumption in an intensive care unit. *Health Care Fin Rev* 5:81, 1983.

9. Berenson RA: Intensive care units (ICUs): Clinical outcomes, costs and decisionmaking OTA-HCS-28. Office of Technology Assessment, Washington, DC, U.S. Government Printing Office, 1984.

10. Birnbaum ML: Cost-containment in critical care. *Crit Care Med* 14:1068, 1986.

11. National Institutes of Health: Consensus development conference statement on critical care medicine, in Parrillo JE, Ayres SM (eds): *Major Issues in Critical Care Medicine*. Baltimore, Williams & Wilkins, 1987, p 277.

12. Robbin ED: The cult of the Swan-Ganz catheter. *Ann Intern Med* 103:445, 1985.

13. Weil MH: Alternatives to rationing, in Strosberg MA, Fein IA, Carroll JD (eds): *Rationing of Medical Care for the Critically Ill*. Washington DC, Brookings Institution, 1989, p 17.

14. Zimmerman JE, Knaus WA, Judson TA, et al: Patient selection for intensive care: A comparison of New Zealand and United States hospitals. *Crit Care Med* 16:318, 1988.

15. Knaus WA: Too sick and old for intensive care. *Br J Hosp Med* 37:381, 1987.

16. Roper WL, Winkenwerder W, Hackbarth GM, et al: Effectiveness in health care: An initiative to evaluate and improve medical practice. *N Engl J Med* 319:1197, 1988.

17. Feldstein P: *The Politics of Health Legislation: An Economic Perspective*. Ann Arbor, MI, Health Administration Press, 1988.

18. *Critical Care in the United States: Coordinating Intensive Care Resources for Positive and Cost-Effective Patient Outcomes*. Anaheim, CA, Society of Critical Care Medicine, 1992, p iii.

19. Kelley M: Critical care medicine: A new specialty? *N Engl J Med* 318:1613, 1988.

20. Johnson WC: *Public Administration: Policy, Politics, and Practices*, Guilford CT, Dishkin Publishing, 1992, p 154.

21. Civetta JM: Critical care: How should we evaluate our progress. *Crit Care Med* 20:1714, 1992.

22. Gray BH: The legislative battle over health services research. *Health Aff*, 1992.

23. Wennberg JE, McPherson K, Caper P: Will payment based on diagnosis related groups control hospital costs? *N Engl J Med* 311:295, 1984.

24. Leape IL, Hilborne LH, Park RE, et al: The appropriateness of the use of coronary bypass graft surgery in New York State. *JAMA* 269:753, 1993.

25. *Guidelines Committee: Guidelines for the Definition of an Intensivist and the Practice of Critical Care Medicine*. Anaheim, CA, Society of Critical Care Medicine, 1991.

26. Shortell SM, Zimmerman JE, Gillies RR et al: Continuously improving patient care: Practical lessons and an assessment tool from the National ICU study. *Quality Rev Bull* May: 150, 1992.

27. Rapoport J, Teres D, Lemeshow S, et al: A method for assessing the clinical performance and cost effectiveness of intensive care units. (Forthcoming)

28. Wennberg JE: Outcomes research, cost containment and the fear of health care rationing. *N Engl J Med* 323:1202, 1990.

29. Eddy D: Anatomy of a decision. *JAMA* 263:441, 1990.

30. Rie MA: The limits of a wish. *Hastings Cent Rep* 21:24, 1991.

31. Rie MA: Professional ethics and political power, in Strosberg MA, Fein IA, Carroll JD (eds): *Rationing of Medical Care for the Critically Ill*. Washington, DC, Brookings Institution, 1989, p 82.

32. Rie MA: The bioethics and structure of managed critical care: Explicit limitation of individual entitlement and provider autonomy. Somers Memorial Lecture, Portland, Oregon, April 4, 1991.

33. Strosberg MA, Wiener JM, Baker R, et al (eds): *Rationing America's Medical Care: The Oregon Plan and Beyond*. Washington DC, Brookings Institution, 1992.

34. Rosenthal E: Crowding causes agonizing crisis in critical care. *New York Times* Aug 22, 1989, p C1.

35. Singer DE, Carr PL, Mulley AG, et al: Rationing intensive care: Physician response to a resource shortage. *N Engl J Med* 309:1155, 1983.

36. Strauss JH, LoGerfo JP, Yeltzie JA, et al: Rationing of intensive care: An everyday occurrence. *JAMA* 255:1143, 1986.

37. Shear L, Steingrub J, Teres D, et al: ICU patient triage ranking: A flawed practice? (abstract). *Crit Care Med* 16:409, 1988.

38. Weil MH: Alternatives to rationing, in Strosberg MA, Fein IA, Carroll JD (eds): *Rationing of Medical Care for the Critically Ill*. Washington DC, Brookings Institution, 1989, p 17.

39. Aaron HJ, Schwartz WE: *The Painful Prescription*. Washington DC, Brookings Institution, 1984.

40. Kapp MB, Lo B: Legal perceptions and medical decision making. *Milbank Mem Q* 64(suppl 2):163, 1986.

41. Bayer R, Callahan D, Fletcher J, et al: The care of the terminally ill: Morality and economics. *N Engl J Med* 309:1490, 1983.

42. Morreim EH: Cost constraints as a malpractice defense. *Hastings Cent Rep* 16:5, 1986.

43. Igelhart JK: From research to rationing: A conversation with William B. Schwartz. *Health Aff* 13:57, 1985.

44. Shoemaker W, James CB, Fleming AW, et al: Defacto rationing of emergency medical services, in Strosberg MA, Wiener JM, Baker R et al (eds): *Rationing America's Medical Care: The Oregon Plan and Beyond*. Washington, DC, Brookings Institution, 1992.

45. Teres D: Civilian triage in the intensive care unit: The ritual of the last bed. *Crit Care Med* 21:598, 1993.

46. Marshall MF, Schwenzer KJ, Orsina M, et al: The influence of political power, medical provincialism and economic incentives on the rationing of surgical intensive care unit beds. *Crit Care Med* 20:387, 1992.

47. *Accreditation Manual for Hospitals 1989*. Chicago, Joint Commission on the Accreditation of Healthcare Organizations, 1988, p 252.

48. Society of Critical Care Medicine Task Force on Guidelines: Recommendations for intensive care unit admissions and discharge criteria. *Crit Care Med* 16:807, 1988.

49. Englehardt HT, Rie MA: Intensive care units, scarce resources and conflicting principles of justice. *JAMA* 255:1143, 1986.

50. Lipsky M: *Street-level Bureaucracy: Dilemmas of the Individual in Public Services*. New York, Russell Sage Foundation, 1980.

230. Health Care Reform and Cost Containment*

Michael A. Rie

"There is nothing more difficult to take in hand, more perilous to conduct or more uncertain in its success, than to take the lead in the introduction of a new order of things. Because the innovator has for enemies all those who have done well under the old conditions and lukewarm defenders in those who may do well under the new . . ."

Machiavelli

Introduction

In Chapter 229, Strosberg and Teres present a general introduction to public policymaking for intensive care units. Though they are quick to point out the rhetorical goals of national health policy, it is worth reemphasizing that the stated principles of the American health care ideology are (1) individual liberty, (2) cost containment, (3) quality care, and (4) universal access to care for all. When President Clinton put forth his legislative proposal for health care reform in 1993, he began with a series of goals that by their very articulation are unattainable. These are summarized as follows: (1) Access to health care for all citizens; (2) Access to the best of health care for all citizens; (3) Freedom of choice of hospitals, physicians, therapies, and an infinite quest for immortality by all those seeking critical care or other health services; and (4) Cost containment and the maintenance of health care costs at a stable level that does not threaten the viability of the national economy.

This chapter begins with the assumption that the American health care ideology is a contemporary public illusion of government, the public, and the collective of health care providers that obstructs critical care medicine from the articulation of its role in serving critically ill patients. It is a large burden on medicine generally and critical care medicine in particular because it forces us to reexamine the societally destructive elements of the Hippocratic Oath and its tradition in medicine [1].

Everything in medical care that might benefit a patient is a new phenomenon that emerged after World War II and the inception of health insurance. Amundsen has chronicled the Hippocratic tradition and corpus and points to the Hippocratic tradition teaching physicians "not to treat those that are overmastered by their disease."

Critical care medicine, perhaps more than any other area of medicine, must confront the basic tension between the use of high technology and the cost of care. The costs of care are increasing faster than the capacity of our society to fund them. We are asked to be the guardians of society's resources and the gatekeepers of technology. We are implored to be "efficient" in our use of resources. Costs, which are escalating at a rate that exceeds the growth of the economy, are the driving force for cost containment. Irrespective of government pronounce-

ments in the United States, "managed care" [2–5] proposals for the larger health policy reform are already in place because of initiatives in the private health sector.

The large macroeconomic policymakers either advocate global budget constraints or discuss health care as an atypical commodity that does not lend itself to a market distribution requiring government regulatory activity. This chapter offers a series of reflections aimed at creating appreciation of health insurance moral packages for retailing in the private economy. In the rationing policy power game, those who can find ways to bring moral economic harmony to the average community will prevail over vague and unpredictable macroeconomic monetary rationing strategies.

Managed care is an organizational structure, which employs primary care physicians as gatekeepers to limit access of patients to specialists who tend to employ high technology interventions. Despite the extensive discussion of managed care as a strategy to limit costs, there has been no discussion to date defining "managed critical care." Though much is written about the organization and management of critical care units as summarized in Chapter 236, and in the chapter on cost containment by Birnbaum in the second edition of this book [6], there is no evidence that such strategies have in any way affected the overall growth rate of costs for critical care services in the United States or other occidental countries. Indeed, even in the single payer Canadian system, the rate of growth of costs and of hospital costs continues to increase at the same rate as occurs in the United States.

The major cost problem of critical care medicine is that it is successful in meeting the short-term goal of physiologic stabilization in a population of aging humans with increasingly complex medical problems and the continued creation of new and successful strategies for dealing with them. Data are lacking to prove the extent to which critical care medicine is beneficial. Nevertheless, its withdrawal can be shown to augment morbidity and mortality. These are the morally meaningful research tasks of our new health research.

Every year, new drugs are added to the critical care formulary and new therapeutic strategies become available. Therefore, the universe of potential therapies that may be of benefit to patients increases as the volume of services and their intensity increase. To contain costs in critical care medicine, we will have to examine and make fundamental moral priority decisions to the basic law of economics which states:

Total Costs = Volume of Services × Unit Costs

As the list of "potentially beneficial services" grows, the unit cost per ICU patient may increase, decrease, or remain unchanged as a function of the intensity (frequency) with which new modalities become part of our daily ICU practice [7].

The cost of providing ICU services is also a function of the desires of citizens to fight disease, strive for immortality, and deny the concept of futility. The principle of autonomy (presently unbounded by public policy) must be addressed by any proposals to contain costs in critical care medicine. This requires policy pronouncements that announce in advance limi-

* The Health Policy Proposal in this chapter was originally presented at the Sommers Memorial Lecture, April 4, 1991, Oregon Health Sciences University. A broader legal/health policy focus appears as "The Oregon ICU: Multitiered Monetarized Morality in Health Insurance Law" [52].

tations on the individual's entitlement to consume resources. This also requires legislative relief from lawsuits alleging that a person is being deprived of their life because a particular service, which has been deemed either experimental or not fundable by an insurance plan, is ruled by a court of law to be the only mechanism of salvation for a particular individual with a life-threatening problem at a given moment [8]. Providers also will need legal relief from accusations that they are participating in murder, assisted suicide, or euthanasia. Confounding these emotion-laden moral issues are pluralist and religious moral values in the greater society that advocate the inviolability of the human life, but make no financial provision for the resources that should be expended for individuals who require large quantities of critical care services with little prospect of return to a physiologically independent functional existence.

We also must confront the public perception that health care providers have a vested interest in their own economic welfare, social status, and well-being. There is the American "open ICU," where physicians are the marketing instruments for a hospital in bringing their patients to the hospital, caring for their patients, and commandeering intensive care resources for them without regard to other patients, and "closed ICU," very common in European hospitals where an intensive care team may function both as resource allocator and primary care-giver and decision-maker for the individual patient. However, in both there are a series of sociologic, economic, power, and turf issues that are better characterized as the enlightened self-interest of providers than a specific morality designed to marshal scarce resources to the care of sick people. Much is ascribed to the ethos and ethical integrity of physicians, but there are few objective data looking at different financial incentives to indicate that physicians in either type of system are able to function without regard to their personal well-being. For example, Levinsky [9] has eloquently documented the inability of the U.S. government to create payments for the use of erythropoietin for uremic anemia; excess payments lead to excess usage and insufficient payments lead to excess anemia. There is no perfect financial incentive. All systems that deal with finance and reimbursement to providers have skewed results depending on the nature of the economic incentive.

In this chapter, I shall examine the necessary moral, financial, legal, and administrative factors that must be fused together in the creation of a democratically derived, horizontally integrated health plan that directs:

1. The allocation of resources to individual patients via a system of entitlement limitations under previously agreed limits;
2. A system of checks and balances to assure that the patient-doctor relationship is preserved;
3. Credible systems of gatekeeping that are administratively, financially, and legally separate from the attempts of individual physicians to garner societal resources for the care of their individual patients and their personal financial gain;
4. The expeditious administrative decision-making in the real-time circumstances of critical care units that will carry the force of law while assuring procedural fairness;
5. A system whereby minority moral views may be recognized in a pluralist society while assigning financial accountability to those who hold such views for the allocation of such resource.

The Political Morality of Health Insurance

The literature of bioethics in critical care medicine is full of lofty principles including autonomy, informed consent, beneficence, nonmaleficence, and justice [10]. Luce and Wachter state simply, "Medical ethics is a set of moral principles or values that govern the behavior of physicians and other health care professionals" [11,12]. But neither the conventional bioethics literature nor sophisticated critical care commentators like Luce and Wachter address forthrightly the need to prioritize some ethical principles above others. When addressing resource allocation, Luce and Wachter sidestep the moral quandary for public policy by suggesting a "relaxed moral rule" for physicians that would permit the selection of a level of probability or a reasonable chance. It would remove from the moral vocabulary of medicine "do everything" and substitute "do as much as is reasonable." But the problem of deciding what is reasonable requires the ability to create moral authority in resource allocation policy, which is a policy decision above the level of gatekeeper physician or fiduciary physician. Justinian (533 A.D.) stated, "Justice is the constant and perpetual desire to give everyone his due."

The framers of the American Declaration of Independence and the Constitution of 1789 faced the same quandary. They wanted a limited democracy, feared the dictatorship of a central state authority, desired local control of their personal lives and deaths (federalism), and thought that liberty, equality, prosperity, and justice for all were the ethical principles of their society. But, as they did not know how the people would relatively value these principles in future generations, they did not rank them in a hierarchy of authority. Conflict on constitutional matters between private parties or private parties and the government was to be resolved by the judiciary.

The purpose of this digression into political philosophy is essential to an understanding of resource-allocation policy and the finite resource issues confronting critical care medicine. To effect reform, contain costs, delineate the private and public ownership of money, and secure a moral policy for allocation of critical care while maximizing individual human freedom, we must focus on creating a morality for health insurance and health law as it pertains to critical care.

In 1989, Dr. John Kitzhaber, an emergency room physician and president of the Oregon senate, was able to guide the Oregon Health Plan to legislative enactment. The fundamental tenets underlying the Oregon Plan are detailed in Table 230-1. While some background has been given on the Oregon Plan in Chapter 229, the internal details remain poorly articulated in the lay press [13]. This is the first governmental legislation in the history of western civilization to face directly the hypocrisy of the American health care ideology. Oregon is the first to face explicitly the moral issue of creating an affordable basic package of health care benefits. Limiting benefits is necessary to increase access to some level of health care for citizens who have no health insurance because of the inability of the market system to solve limited entitlements to health care for the disenfranchised. Though there are complex political issues involved in the federal/state relationships in the United States, the Oregon Plan has attracted great attention in Europe and other countries where there is already universal national health care, because it allows those resource-limited societies to seek democratic solutions to the problem of defining the limits of entitlement of individuals and of defining what is a basic package of health care benefits in health insurance. These political issues are not the subject of this chapter. Rather, this chapter concerns itself with the moral fundamentals that underlie such a health insurance system and its direct application to critical care medicine.

In such a system, and within the universe of public policy, critical care medicine fits at the level that is described as "Mesoallocation Policy" [14]. Mesoallocation is an area of health policy between macroallocation and individual (micro) allocation. In macroallocation, one is deciding fundamental issues such as the percentage of funds that should go to critical care or primary care. Microallocation, on the other hand, is that specific set of duties that would be in the domain of the medical director of an intensive care unit. As the intensive care unit director is not the creator of health insurance policy, and health insurance policy resides at the level of a health insurance plan or program, that level is described in this chapter as being one between the management of an intensive care unit and the larger health policy of macroallocation. For example, although Oregon has created a system in which trauma care may be a covered benefit while metastatic carcinomatosis to the liver or brain is not (for therapy as opposed to comfort), it remains unstated in the Oregon Plan how much intensive care will be accorded an individual with a Glasgow Coma Score of 4. Does such a patient have unlimited coma benefit management services, or will there be some process in which critical care medicine will extend diagnostic and therapeutic evaluation and then withdraw care by specific public policy pronouncement? Dr. Kitzhaber acknowledges that the Oregon Plan holds no mesoallocatory structure [15]. It thus remains both a political and a moral policy problem for critical care in the evolutionary implementation of this new program.

Public and Private Morality

In the Oregon Plan, there have been intense intellectual and political discussions about the propriety of limiting resources to poor people when it does not occur for the middle class or the rich [16,17]. Oregon rejected the morality of Congress as expressed in the Medicaid legislation of 1966 and sought to extend some level of health care to people of unfortunate economic circumstances. As John Kitzhaber so eloquently stated, "We reject the morality of rationing people and choose to ration services." Oregon is committed to a basic minimum decent standard of care for the poor and grounds its system on an egalitarianism of altruism and not one of strict resource distribution equality, which Engelhardt has identified as an egalitarianism of envy [18]. Oregon permits the private ownership of money and the ability of those of more fortunate economic means to either buy more health care or to enter into contracts to freely limit their entitlements to receive critical care in private health insurance plans not subsidized directly by the government. This chapter addresses the latter circumstance and provides a moral framework in health policy that can direct the flow of economic resources, the necessary legal safeguards for individual rights of patients, and litigation relief in explicit health rationing policy for health care providers and institutions. For critical care medicine to participate in this activity will require an agonizing reexamination of its own internal economic moral conflicts. These conflicts will need to be resolved if critical care medicine is to exercise an authoritative moral voice in fashioning health policy.

All governments avoid hard decisions when it comes to limiting care for individual citizens in their countries [6,19,20]. In addition to the problem of health care budgets, there is the problem of what we have previously defined as the moral responses to the natural and social lotteries of life in health care generally and critical care specifically [21]. To the extent that wealth is not evenly distributed in society, there are always problems with how to transfer economic resources from the haves to the have nots [22]. Central to any high-technology health care system is the realization that wealth and resources are produced through the economy of services and industry.

The personal greed of individuals and the desires of corporations to grow and create corporate wealth serve the needs of the society, provide the basis for public taxation, and provide the capacity to care for the medically indigent.

Critical Care Medical and Nursing Organizations

It is not only governments and the public that subscribe to the American health care ideology but medical and nursing organizations as well. In Chapter 229, the focus on medical associations as special interest groups in the world of politics and government is a polite way to sidestep the inherent conflict of interest that all physicians face when they speak to the issue of public policy. As noted by Starr [23], there always has been an inherent bias of physicians to treat patients more rather than less in a fee-for-service payment system. When the patient is not directly the payer, the sense of social responsibility to the resource generator (health insurance premium payers and tax payers) decreases. As the patient assumes greater responsibility for the payment of services rendered, the patient may scrutinize medical bills more closely and physicians will be more attentive to the needs of the "patient/customer" [24]. Fee-for-service is an economic and moral free ride for fiduciary physicians and they are rewarded more for doing more. Whether physicians acknowledge this moral economic reality or not, governments, the public, and health insurers do. The managed care revolution proposes to economically induce hospitals, doctors, and all components of medical care (drugs and technology) to come under the concept of global budgeting. At some point in a global budget system of limited means, one must be prepared for declining standards of care, managerial health insurance plan fraud, administrative domination of physicians, and other system capacity overloads. The United States has two to three times the number of intensive care unit beds (per total hospital beds) as European countries; thus it is necessary to gain objective international data comparing "value purchase" by American critical care units and their European counterparts. The proof of impaired value purchase or excess preventable mortality and morbidity is likely to have quicker political repercussions in Europe where declining quality of care and outcomes due to more centralized resource limitations are felt swiftly. For example, Schnepel and Stopfkuchen [25,26] openly declare that major German pediatric referral intensive care units have experienced decreased nurse-patient staffing ratios in response to governmental budgetary cutbacks. While these authors do not cite absolute outcome decrements from such care, the need to measure them is clear. American hospitals tend to close ICU beds with staffing shortages and decrease access because of the fear of litigation from lowering the standards of care [27].

In Figure 230-1, Shabot et al. [28] studied a group of 5500 abdominal surgery patients at a California medical center with a previously reported group of 3687 comparable patients in France. SAPS I scoring methodology was employed. The suggestion was made that patients in France have statistically higher ICU mortalities than their California counterparts. Although these results may reflect the older French surgical practice of repeated operative intervention for intraabdominal debridement, such comparisons by international collaboration in the critical care community are likely to provide a better index of how insurance system incentives and disincentives affect outcomes in critically ill patients.

Rapoport et al. [29] presented a new standardized methodology for plotting clinical outcomes and resource consumption.

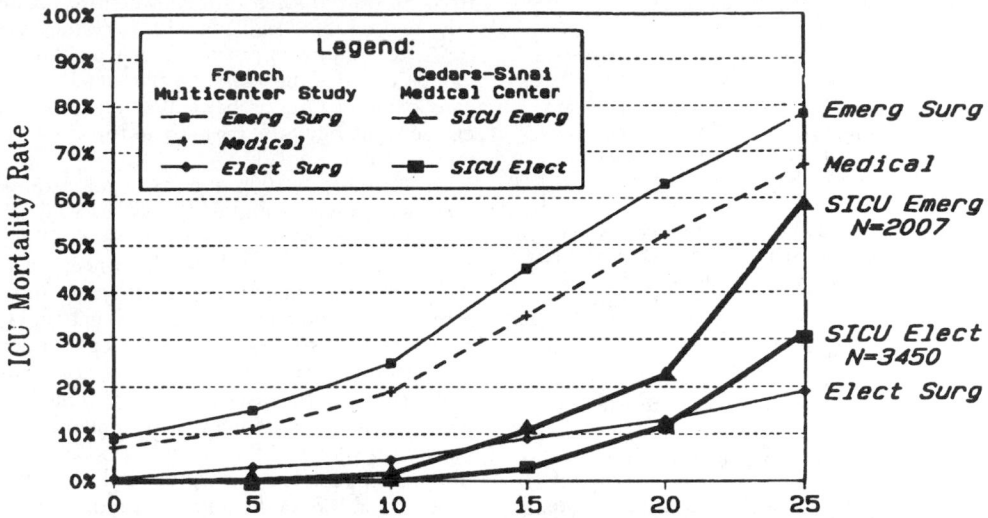

Fig. 230-1. Severity-adjusted survival comparison of American and French ICU outcomes for abdominal surgery. The x-axis represents SAPS I scores. The differences are statistically significant at p = 0.02 for scores of 10 and 15 points and p = 0.005 for scores of 20 points [28] SICU = Surgical Intensive Care Unit.

They showed that hospitals can be measured and compared against one another and that variations exist. The use of such methods in international comparative studies is likely to show still larger variations and the effects of differing national (implicit) resource rationing programs on critical care unit outputs and productivity.

In both America and Europe, physicians learn to network and "game their systems" in response to various incentives. In the only published study analyzing ICU triage at a major American university hospital, Marshall et al. [30] documented that patient acuity was not the prime determinant of ICU admission and triage. Rather, cases with greater institutional reimbursement capability (e.g., cardiothoracic surgery) were preferentially admitted over sicker and more acutely ill general surgical cases. The critical care physicians and nurses were overwhelmed by larger hospital politics beyond their control. It would appear that the profit motive thrives in at least one American university hospital and its surgical staff.

When we examine the behavior of medical organizations such as the Society of Critical Care Medicine (SCCM), we observe further moral confusion regarding the definition of the intensivist and the SCCM's view on the triage of critically ill patients [31,32]. The SCCM defines critical care medicine as encompassing both individual patient advocacy (like that of a primary care fiduciary trust physician) and the function of resource allocation. In the triage consensus statement, the SCCM states, "Conflicts of interest between the health care provider's role as gatekeeper and patient advocate may occur and should be anticipated." The document does not describe what administrative authority and responsibility in health payments and law should obtain in these circumstances. Furthermore, the SCCM offers a legal disclaimer to the statement and refers the reader to "competent legal counsel."

The American Association of Critical Care Nurses (AACCN) does not have a code of ethics and subscribes to the code of ethics of the American Nurses Association [33]. Plank three of the nursing code states "The nurse acts to safeguard the client and the public when health care and safety are effected by an incompetent unethical or illegal practice of any person." This position is silent on the conflict of interest for a nurse required by law or de facto public policy to provide care that might objectively have been documented to provide an increased morbidity or mortality to the individual patient. Though ICU nurses are usually salaried employees of a hospital, it is unstated how an American nurse should divide his or her allegiance, and that of the profession, to societal versus individual health care objectives.

This moral confusion is the same, whether one examines an "open ICU" with ICU critical care consultants and primary admitting physicians and surgeons or a "closed ICU" where the management of the ICU and fiduciary care of critically ill patients is carried out by the same physicians. In either model, conflicting duties to patients and the "power sociologic turf" of the hospital are likely to instill loss of confidence by the public in the critical care enterprise as resources are reduced and patient demands increase.

If there is a legitimate basis for moral confusion in the critical care community because of our cultural immersion in the American health care ideology, the same cannot be said for individuals and organizations representing the primary ICU admitting specialties such as surgery (especially trauma surgery). Vassar and Holcroft [34] provide an example of a specialty of medicine that is attempting to exempt itself from prognostic scoring systems. Despite large quantities of data validating the APACHE III, SAPS II, and MPM II scoring systems for ICU prognosis, trauma specialists argue that these systems are not operative for their patients. There is open hostility to the perceived threat on surgical autonomy that precludes intellectual reason and scientific honesty in the reporting of data [35,36]. Despite the large number of publications showing the validity of these scoring systems, the surgical literature contains continuing negative evaluation. It remains to be seen whether surgery will choose to participate in the creation of explicit resource allocation policies or continue to function at its periphery.

Oregonian Health Policy

For definitional purposes, this chapter takes Oregonian health policy to encompass those pure elements listed in Table 230-

Table 230-1. Fundamentals of a Pure Oregonian Health Care Policy

When resources are insufficient, allocate resources not patients.

In secular pluralist democracies moral authority is acquired in limited measures by negotiation between providers and consumers to prospectively prioritize the creation of a list of health insurance benefits. These policies define the macroeconomic moral response to the natural and social lotteries of life [18].

Health policy that lacks moral prioritization of beneficial care when resources are insufficient mandates declining standards of care with measurable increases in the morbidity and mortality of patient populations.

In limited democracies the creation of universal access to health care in a population of unequal personal wealth requires transfer payments to the poor to be limited by the extent to which the majority of citizens consent to the taxation of their personally created wealth.

People and businesses create wealth. Governments requisition wealth.

The historical liberal maxim that moral conflict requires moral neutrality while resources are consumed by fiat is abandoned [49].

Respect for religious and moral diversity of patients requires public toleration of these expressions of health care desires and their financial support and accountability from private sources of wealth.

Futile medical care is not a disability under the Americans with Disabilities Act. Futility is a publicly derived, morally content definition of unfortunate human circumstances defining the finitude of human life and the limits of our communal resources.

Resource allocation in critical care medicine fuses responsibility and authority in a contractually limited, medically directed managerial structure. Fiduciary trust relationships between doctor and patient are preserved but limited in the extent of resources those relationships may requisition from the limited resources of a basic health insurance plan.

All politics are local, and health insurance morality that fuses responsibility and authority to ration is regionally created. Federalism and the Constitution of 1789 are alive and well in American politics and law.

Oregon morally prioritizes liberty, equality, access, and prosperity in health care. The Constitution of 1789 was silent on this subject.

Resource allocation policy limits individual entitlement claims in the tort system of law by legislation.

Unequal health care is officially acknowledged and the basic package of care is guaranteed to all while the freedom to own and use private wealth to buy more health care is preserved in Oregonian health systems.

The best of care for all is not attainable. The moral dimensions of medical prognostic probability and clinical impression must be monetarized in individual entitlement allocations at the mesoallocatory policy level.

1. These were the original elements of the Oregon Basic Health Services Act passed into law in 1989. Political accommodations to the detractors of the plan and the federal government's participation required the state of Oregon to make several concessions to the federal government in August and October 1992. Many of these attack the Plan's basis, which was the creation of a publicly derived morality to guide macroeconomic resource allocation. Though almost all of the lay media and medical commentators [37] concentrated on the fact that the Plan addressed those patients whose care was economically supported by the public funds of the state, the political structure of the Medicaid program is such that less than half of total public Medicaid economic outlays go to the care of poor women and children while the majority of funds (by congressional mandate)

have subsidized long-term chronic care for the Medicare, elderly, and disabled citizens who become "medically indigent" [38]. The arguments put forward against the Oregon Plan are violent because the Plan directly attacks the American health care ideology. Oregon has called to political, moral, and financial accountability the moral bankruptcy of a system of entitlements without subsidy.

On February 1, 1994, the Medicaid resource allocation program was implemented in Oregon as well as the less publicly known portion of the legislation, Senate Bill 935 [13]. Oregon passed legislation that follows the concept of an employer mandate to provide health insurance for large and small businesses. Although the effective date of this mandate has been pushed back into the late 1990s, it is now legal under Oregon law for managed care plans in the private sector to undertake contractual relations with providers and subscribers that allow for explicit limitation of individual patient care within the benefit package. As long as the benefit package at least equals that in the public Medicaid sector, the legal protections that apply to providers in the Medicaid program of Oregon will also obtain for them in the private health insurance sector. This philosophy of law and health insurance relies heavily on the theory of contracts replacing the theory of unstated human rights in health insurance [39,40]. The nature of the economic relationships in the law is eloquently detailed by Morreim [41,42,43].

The following moral policy proposal replaces the American health care ideology with Oregonian democratic morality. We previously developed this framework in 1986 [21]. In that publication, we laid out the general moral theory for hypothetical contractors possessed of rationality who desired to create a definition of intensive care unit entitlement to benefits based on an Intensive Care Unit Entitlement Index. That index states:

$$ICU\text{--}EI = PQL/C$$

In this index, P indicates the probability of a successful outcome for a specific condition. Q defines the quality of the successful outcome. L defines the length of life remaining. C defines the costs required to achieve therapeutic success. In that publication, we highlighted several clinical examples. We described a range from absolute entitlement within an insurance system, through entitlement leading to subsequent nonentitlement because of a decline in prognosis and potential clinical outcome, to absolute nonentitlement because of inability to benefit from the resource allocation. In 1986, the science of predicting ICU outcome was in its infancy and the computerized software to carry out rapid database acquisition was yet to be developed. In the intervening years, the predictive models have improved sufficiently so that it may now be reasonable to perform mortality probability estimates for individual patients (with significant caveats) that are highlighted in Chapter 231.

It is assumed that any group of individuals wishing to voluntarily enter into the creation of a morally meaningful health insurance contract would have full access to the science of prognostic scoring and be aware of its limitations. It also is assumed that the contract negotiators would have full access to the nature of clinical imprecision and clinical fallibility when physicians are left to their own devices in the practice of medicine. They would have full knowledge of the variability of practice styles, costs, and outcomes.

Since 1986, the SCCM has made fundamental changes in the definition of the ethical integrity of critical care medicine as a medical discipline. In 1994 [32], SCCM published its Consensus Statement on the Triage of Critically Ill Patients. The consensus statement is precedent-setting because it is the first in occidental medicine to specifically call for the limitation of autonomy entitlements and rights of consumption of patients when resources are scarce in a civilian health care setting. The statement strongly supports prognostic scoring instruments as a method for making triage prioritization policy. The consensus statement is offered as an informal guideline to critical care practitioners and suggests (but does not justify) that the locus of policymaking resides within a hospital. Finally, the consensus statement lists a series of categories that do not merit ICU admission. These include (1) patients who competently decline intensive care or request that invasive therapy be withheld, (2) patients declared brain-dead who are not organ donors, and (3) patients in a persistent vegetative or permanently unconscious state. The statement further specifies that moral pluralism in the society may result in situations where individuals holding religious or moral convictions may legitimately have a basis favoring the provision of such treatments of the conditions, but that the costs of such care should not be borne by the general society and the provision of such services should not foreclose the treatment of other patients who would benefit from critical care. The latter is likely to be of great public policy importance because it acknowledges moral diversity, permits the private ownership of money, and respects the free exercise of religion in health care, but it does not burden the majority and their financial obligations to a system of health care that is only desired by the minority. For the first time, a medical organization supports financial accountability for moral diversity and provides the last element so necessary for the creation of an integrated and monetarized critical care resource allocation system.

HEALTH POLICY FRAMEWORK FOR THE 1990s. Shortell and Reinhardt [44] suggest that the evolution of health policy in the 1990s should consider the following seven elements: (1) There is an interdependency that relates to the creation of incremental policy; (2) Health policy should be patient-centered; (3) Health policy should articulate the balance between communitarian values in health insurance vs. individual wishes and expressions of autonomy; (4) Health policy should promote explicit clinical management systems; (5) Health policy should promote fiscal and clinical accountability; (6) The policy should have flexibility to encourage innovation in accountability criteria and provider incentives; and (7) The policy should anticipate implementation issues, midcourse corrections, and input for those directly affected.

What exactly do we know about explicit resource allocation in critical care? The answer to this question is absolutely nothing. We have a *status quo ante* of health financing, conflicting case law, uncertain rights to nebulous insurance benefits in morally empty insurance policies, and the existence of an advancing science of prognosis research that is not being applied to individual clinical entitlement limitations. In addition, we have a series of sophisticated reflections on ethics in critical care medicine and we have evolved a comprehensive system of ethics committees that act as public sounding boards and dispute resolution loci for resolving disputes in American hospitals. However, when patients object to the removal of therapy on ground of futility or nonmedical grounds, they are still able to bring litigation against hospitals and physicians [45]. Accordingly, ethics committees can be obstructed from carrying out any authoritative role with regard to resource allocation.

MORAL AUTHORITY DEVELOPS IN INSURANCE CONTRACTS. The basic construction of the horizontally integrated Oregonian ICU is illustrated in Figure 230-2. In this figure, we begin with the premise that moral authority in health insurance

Administrative Scheme For Provider Reimbursement Eligibility

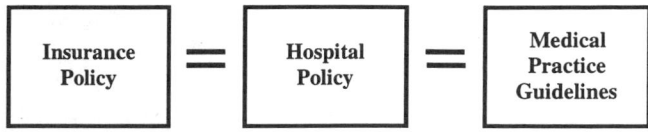

Fig. 230-2. Schematic principle for horizontally integrated critical care resource allocation policy based on the morality of reimbursement criteria. Moral authority is created in the health plan. Institutions and individual providers elect to participate in the morality as expressed in "bylaw symmetry" with the health plan moral limits on individual care and the gatekeeping principle.

is acquired at the time the insurance policy is created. The insurance policy is created and continuously recreated by an ongoing conversation among subscribers, providers, and payers. However, unlike conventional insurance, the insurance laws of the jurisdiction are rewritten to require that subscriber representatives and provider representatives be part of the creation of the health insurance policy. In this system, the benefit manager of a corporation or business is prohibited from having exclusive control of information to employees. Employees in such a system are not eligible for health insurance until such time as they have had full access and understanding of the benefit package at the time they enter employment. Responsible policy requires individual responsibility. Governmental paternalism in policy creation has failed to address rational decisions. On the other side of the equation, the same issues apply to hospitals and to physicians who would admit patients to an ICU.

In this system, neither hospitals nor physicians may qualify as recipients of health insurance payments unless they subscribe to the contractual obligations within the insurance policy. For primary physicians, it will not be possible to be both a primary physician and also an allocator of resources or critical care consultant. The term primary physician in this chapter does not necessarily mean the fields of general medicine, such as family medicine, pediatrics, internal medicine, and obstetrics and gynecology, but instead refers to those physicians, including surgeons, cardiologists, pulmonologists, and oncologists, who will be the principal fiduciary trust physicians within the meaning of the doctor/patient relationship.

In Figure 230-3, the moral insurance and schematic administrative policy organization is further clarified. The health plan creates and directly funds a committee that is identified as the Humanism and Technology Usage Committee. The committee is composed of representatives from the hospital corporation, the medical staff of primary physicians, critical care consultants, and payers and patient subscribers. This is a legally constituted "watch dog process committee" that is specifically created and permitted under the insurance laws of the jurisdiction. Attached to this committee are a group of certified Qualified Critical Care Practitioners (QCCP) in the relevant areas of medicine. These physicians and nurses are direct employees of the health care plan. Although they work as integrated members of the hospital and must possess medical and nursing licensure, the health plan prohibits economic or administrative control of these individ-

Moral Insurance and Administrative Policy

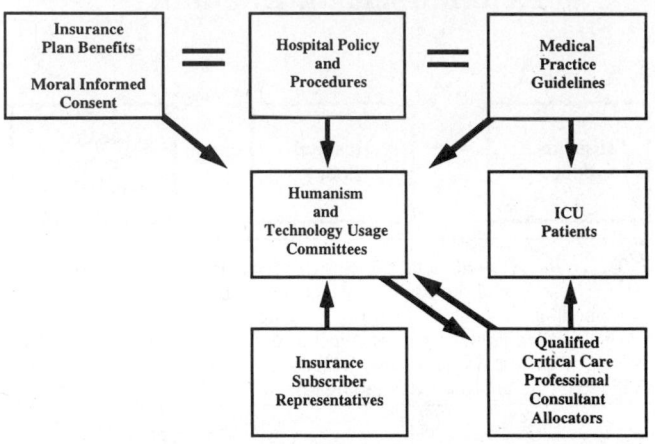

Fig. 230-3. Health plan morality in Figure 230-2 employs the Humanism and Technology Usage Committee to function on-site in the hospital as a combined source of economic authority and the resource allocation oversight function of the critical care consultant gatekeeper.

uals by the hospital and the medical staff as a contingency of hospital and medical staff physician participation in the health plan. These individuals are salaried and are prohibited from fee-for-service medical or nursing practice in this ICU system. These individuals may not rotate to primary care medical status, but must remain as critical care consultants and resource allocation gatekeepers during the entirety of their clinical experience in the applicable hospital. It is expected that these individuals will primarily direct and manage the efficient integrated "case-managed" practice of critical care for critically ill patients. Primary care physicians shall have active participation in the care of their patients in intensive care units, but final authority for questionable usage of technology or usage not sanctioned by the health plan will be under the control of the critical care consultant gatekeeper.

To promote predictable and measurable clinical performance on the part of both primary medical practitioners and critical care consultants, some form of prognostic scoring instrument will be required for health plan participation of providers and the costs of maintaining the surveillance and audit functions will be borne directly by the health insurance plan and not by the providers.

It is expected that there will be wide latitude in the day-to-day practice of medicine for both practitioners and critical care consultants consistent with the unpredictable nature of medical practice. The comprehensive management of critical care patients will have several elements including the choice and number of specialty consultants and the comprehensive attention to the personal needs and desires of patients. The quality and quantity of cognitive service and communication with patients and families will be evaluated by objective scoring systems for their performance. Financial remuneration of both primary care givers and critical care consultants will have a definable component related to customer satisfaction. The terms of these arrangements will be stated within the health insurance plans as arranged by the creators and contractors of the plan.

Closed ICUs in this system will be considered an arrangement that leads to a conflict of economic interest and will be prohib-

ited from the malpractice tort exemption statute for the jurisdiction as described below.

THE HUMANISM AND TECHNOLOGY USAGE COMMITTEE. The critical care consultant gatekeeper is an agent of the committee and reports to the committee and its administrative structure. Should the gatekeeper have irreconcilable conflicts with the committee, there would be a secondary level for conflict resolution within the main body of the health insurance plan. If at any time the gatekeeper believes there to be a breach of the contract conditions on the part of the health plan regarding the resource allocation policy to individual patients, he or she would be free to directly notify the insurance authorities without prejudice. The sensitive and vulnerable status of the gatekeeper position will have specific protections in statute.

The Humanism and Technology Usage Committee (HTUC) is a medico-legally binding decision-making body expressly recognized under the laws of the jurisdiction. It has the economic authority to dispense or deny funds to the hospital and its medical staff. It also serves as the locus for appeals by patients for care rendered in the intensive care unit. It is the locus for denials of individual care occasioned by the entitlement limitation process described below.

The original contract for the health plan describes the appellate process guarantees to patient subscribers. It provides patients and providers with a specifically defined process for resolving grievances from all sides (see Appellate Process). The rights and process are spelled out in the health plan. Under the laws of the jurisdiction, the patient is required to go through the appellate process and the appellate process will be binding on resource allocation by the health plan. The only exception to this rule will be evidence of a sufficient nature to a court of law indicating that there was a breach of the due process provisions in the health insurance contract. Should such an appeal be made to a court of law and that appeal determined to be without merit, then the costs of all medical care between the time that such appeal was made and the final disposition of the matter will be ascribed to the patient. In the alternate circumstance where a court of law determines that a violation of the due process provisions of the contract occurred, the plan will be liable for the costs incurred from the time of appeal until judicial determination was made and the plan shall be assessable for a multiple of those costs as a punitive damage payable directly to the patient.

SAMPLE POLICY. The following is a sample policy of an explicit entitlement limitation defined in the health contract:

This policy limits payments for futile critical care. For the purposes of this contract futile care is defined by the signatories to be a prognostic prediction of death of 95 percent probability after 7 days of ICU care. It is recognized that patients may wish to have more or less degrees of probability attached to the determination of this finding. Accordingly, this contract offers a series of probability tolerances to the certitude of the ultimate diagnosis of futility. The basic package of ICU benefits in this health plan carries a probability variance of x percent. Should you decide as a purchaser of this health plan that you would like to have a higher level of certainty attached to these outcomes, you may elect these degrees of probability as expressed in the premium surcharge table defined by our actuaries in the Appendix of this health insurance policy. These option packages are available annually at the renewal of the contract and may not be changed during a covered benefit year.

MALPRACTICE LAWS AND PROVISIONS. The health insurance laws of the jurisdiction where this contract would be written would be similar to those encompassed under Section 10 of Senate Bill 27 in the original Oregon Basic Health Services Act of 1989. In the Oregon Basic Health Services Act, there is a section prohibiting citizens from bringing malpractice actions in court against health care providers for failing to provide that level of service that was deemed un-fundable by the legislature in the Medicaid benefit package. The Oregon legislature further granted that the tort exemption would apply to health insurance plans under the employer mandate sections of the law. Thus, an Oregonian managed health care plan would contain such exemptions provided they met the minimal basic benefits of the Medicaid program in that state. For purposes of this integrated health insurance morality proposal, the nature of such legislation would apply and a bifurcated standard of care would exist in which providers will still be held to the standard of medical expertise and judgment that exist under the conventional tort law while the standard of resource utilization under the health plan would exempt actions in tort for following the contractually agreed to health plan [41,42,43].

EQUITY IN LIMITATION.

Many critical care professionals look at the issue of triage as a situational activity that occurs when there is an acute shortage of beds and an excess of patients seeking access to the beds. This behavior is likely to lead to unpredictable outcomes for individual patients with regard to their entitlement within a health insurance plan. It is likely that legislatures and courts would look upon situational triage as an unpredictable discrimination in the care of individuals given that some individuals might be forced to leave an intensive care unit on a day when there is busy surgery but not at other times when the hospital census is light. A standard of predictability of decision-making is imposed on the health plan, and situational triage of and by itself is prohibited within this basic benefit health policy.

The abolition of situational triage will be argued to be a destructive event by the prior institutionalization and practices of critical care providers. But that is what it means to function in a resource-limited world. The policy must remain coherent and credible not only in the eyes of providers, but in the eyes of patient subscribers who purchase their health insurance in advance to protect themselves against the perils of the natural and social lotteries of life. If people want situational triage and it is important to them, then the health insurance market, being competitive and freely constituted, will make arrangements for it to exist. Thus, people can have additional "rider provisions" to their health insurance that may be acquired at the time the health insurance is purchased. A la carte health insurance choice also has a positive social benefit to the least well off class of society. To the extent that more people elect to pay additional premiums out of their own personal after-tax dollars, additional tax revenue is created that could be targeted for use to increase benefits to the poor. What we are doing in these circumstances is providing monetarization of morally contentful human values that can be traded in a competitive market system of health insurance. If one wants a single payer system, then it will be necessary to replicate those unique features of a market rationing system, which are (1) resource generation, (2) demand limitation, and (3) value prioritization.

The abolition of situational triage is also necessary to maintain the predictable nature of justice for critical care outcomes and the specific sanctioning of these rationing systems by both the legislative and judicial branches of government. This system of moral judgment-making is one in which the power of contract law takes precedence over tort law [44,45]. If providers of health care claim to be professionally encumbered by the extent to which tort law has dominated, controlled, and distorted the

distribution of health care benefits to their patients, then they will take up and champion the creation of appropriate health insurance contracts for their patients to facilitate appropriate allocation of resources in a morally contentful public manner.

PROBABILITIES OF OUTCOME.

The science of outcomes prediction and objective validated scoring systems in critical care is detailed in Chapter 231. This chapter does not propose to discuss the limitations of these technologies but simply to state that they exist and their degrees of uncertainty are now quantifiable and publicly recognized. We should acknowledge that there is moral confusion when it comes to the termination of care for patients residing in an ICU. Those who oppose the imposition of these external constraints to physicians' autonomy point to the degrees of imprecision that exist in these systems and the degree to which that imprecision may be inferior, equal, or superior to that of the individual practitioner's clinical judgment. Clinical judgment plays a very important role in validating external systems and no claims are made against it. However, in a system where clinical judgments exercised by individual clinicians are publicly perceived to be in a moral conflict of interest with the allocation of resources, it is necessary for the public welfare to establish a system of independent calibration and validation of those judgments so as to have an economic system for the swift daily and implementable flow of resources for all patients covered in the health insurance program. It has been our failure to face this latter point both inside and outside of the medical enterprise that is the cause of rampant cost escalation. As this policy is specifically designed to achieve cost containment in a balance with individual liberty and wealth transfer in a democracy, it is necessary to impose such a system on ourselves as providers and to take a leadership position in a subject of which the public is largely ignorant. From the policy perspective, the advantage of terminating situational triage is that it clearly delineates how an individual health care plan (via finance of entitlement) has chosen to prioritize the elements of liberty, cost, quality of care, and access to care for all who are within the health insurance plan. As health insurance plans will have to compete against each other for market share, the more precisely these matters can be delineated with honesty in health insurance, the more likely it is that people will have confidence in the plans [46]. Health plans will suffer a loss of public image if they sell duplicitous ICU benefits or waste subscriber premiums because of failure to characterize the benefits that will not be realized until the time people need ICU care. These health plans also will experience "contract malpractice" legal suits against them.

On the other hand, the health plan that delivers exactly what it says it will deliver is one that can command public esteem. As unaccustomed as physicians and health providers are to a consumer evaluation standard, that is what it means to be in a commercial enterprise. Conversely, it means that there will be significantly different financial packages for intensive care medicine that will vary in the benefits they offer with regard to resource allocation. If statistical changes can be found for morbidity and mortality from one type of plan to another, it will be an indirect market study of which segments of critical care are truly beneficial and which ones are discretionary. The greatest problem still remains that there has never been a proper technology assessment of the true benefits to be derived from critical care medicine for large numbers of patients [6].

UNCERTAINTY AND THE COST OF STATISTICAL CERTITUDE.

Clinical medicine is not a precise science due to the biologic variability of patients. In the best of diagnostic systems in medicine, there is a degree of statistical imprecision and error. Primary physicians, critical care physicians and nurses, and patients and families all cling to the American health care ideology especially when their individual care is at hand. Accordingly, there will be no resolution to the cost problem in critical care until we accept reasonable probability estimates of failure and avoid the desire to seek miracles and the 1 in 1,000,000 or 1 in 10,000 chance of success for an individual patient. When a patient resides in an intensive care unit and the probability of mortality is estimated to be 95 percent or greater at the end of one week, as suggested in the sample policy, there always will be a statistical measure of imprecision around that value. But the value itself chosen by plan negotiators to be the standard for resource limitation is neither a medical decision nor a strictly financial one. Rather it is the creation of a morality that will determine the degree of imprecision that we as a society, or we as a series of contractors in a health insurance plan, can afford in what will subsequently be our own personal medical care. Of course, at the time we are well and healthy and create the health insurance we won't know whether we will ever require critical care or that category of critical care. However, that is what it means to create a cost-contained, morality of the insurance package within a community of individuals attempting to insure themselves against the perils of the natural and social lotteries of life. The notion that there must be absolute certainty before care is withdrawn, as is so commonly heard every day in the intensive care units of the United States, is simply a cultural delusion that has been adopted by health care providers and citizens at large as they have absorbed and internalized the American health care ideology. If they wish to continue this ideology, they should have no compunction about further diminishing their access to the other commodities besides medical care that would make their lives worthwhile. As the cost of health care grows to 20, 30, or 40 percent of the gross national product of the country, people should anticipate that there will be less higher education, less capacity to own one's own home, or to afford such amenities as vacations, clothing, or expensive textbooks of critical care medicine.

Though the latter may appear somewhat harsh on first impression, the younger generation of researchers will soon be making new analyses of the cost of seeking certitude of death prediction. They will measure the actuarial costs for varying probabilities of error for individual patient predictions. As it will take a given quantum of resources to decide that there is objective evidence of mortality at the 95 percent probability and that the variation of certainty around that will be a given confidence interval, the research is likely to show that it may cost a large multiple of that figure to decrease the confidence interval. It has been the failure of the senior generation of physicians to confront this openly and to share prognoses openly with patients and their families that now are the source of legal suits against physicians for failing to give fatal prognosis information to patients and their families [47]. This is in keeping with the code of ethics for the medical industrial complex [24,46].

These are the foundations for the role of health services research in providing the necessary information to place a monetary value on the cost of probability of fatal outcomes. Even in this system, there always will be a small degree of error. There will be an occasional patient who might have lived had the resources been allocated, but who was denied those resources in the health insurance product. This has been called the technologic imperative applied to the principle of rescue so dominant in the medical culture in the latter twentieth century. But a morally structured cost-containment strategy must encompass a way to create the limits to these expenditures and to lower the relative priority of these expenditures in comparison with other expenditures that are now conceived by the health insurance plan to hold a higher moral and economic priority. As these packages of health insurance would be freely negotiated during periods of health, one would create the quantifiable definitions of unfortunate vs. unfair outcomes. For those who find such limits to be morally objectionable either on personal or religious grounds, it will be necessary for governments and health insurers to sanction the concept of fiscal accountability for moral diversity outlined in the SCCM Triage Consensus Statement [32]. The consensus statement clearly delineates that autonomy is not the master but the servant of communal morality in this setting. This is likely to cause major confrontation in the greater political process and will require a maturation on the part of the American people to realize that individual freedom of patients and their physicians is immoral unless it is circumscribed by the larger morality of the community in which the individual patients and physicians reside.

PATIENT AND PHYSICIAN APPELLATE PROCESS. Limiting situational triage will permit resolution of conflicts in the care of individual patients in the ICU. A health plan offering managed critical care services within the definition of the laws of the jurisdiction in which the health plan operates will require a publicly promulgated list of entitlement screens identifying cutoffs that form the basis for the limits for entitlement to care in an ICU. When we describe these matters in health insurance plans, we are talking about reimbursement only. Should hospitals, physicians, and patients elect to undertake care beyond the limits of the health insurance plan, that would be a matter for them to negotiate privately. It is assumed that the private use of money would allow for black market purchases of such care unless the power of the state was directed at the repression and prohibition of the use of private money to purchase such services. But democracies rarely exercise that power, and when they attempt to exercise it, a black market arises anyway. Examples of this have been abundantly documented in the former Soviet Union where a rich black market with hard western currency developed during the dissolution of the system [48]. Similarly, a black market developed in Alberta, Canada and the Canadian Medicare System generally in 1994 as a consequence of economic decline and public indebtedness. This has resulted in the institution of copayments and the limitation of benefits and hospital resources by government edict as opposed to public negotiation. Canada is able to do this and avoid dissolving its national health care system (as occurred in New Zealand) because a black market exists just south of its border. Though Canadian physicians are prohibited by law from offering private services in a black market, they are still at liberty to refer patients for consultation to American colleagues. It is the American economy that enriches itself by free enterprise, when economic moral repression is practiced north of the American border. The extent to which Canadians opt for cross-border health care is a Canadian plebiscite creating market economics in Canadian health care. Health care may become one of the unintended commodities within the North American Free Trade Agreement of 1993. The beauty of free market transfers is that they establish in money and wealth that which is morally important to a free people. It is therefore necessary to allow for private money and a free market to define the moral adequacy of a governmental health package.

To confront the emotionally charged appeals of patients and their primary physicians, the health insurance plan must be robustly constructed within the meaning of contract law, recognized by legislative authority, and be subject to the sanctions of the judicial system. In this proposal it will be noted in Figure 230-3 that the central source of economic moral authority in this horizontally integrated health care system is the HTUC. This is a conceptually new version of a medico-legally binding ethics committee organized to function within a hospital but under the purview of a health insurance plan. This is necessary to eliminate the division of responsibility and authority between insurers and providers in the American economy. This method assures that there will be legal accountability of the health plan as an integrated portion of a health provider system. This would occur, for example, in a large health maintenance organization (HMO) that owns hospitals and has medical and other providers working as its employees. The large HMOs of the United States have been particularly resistant to this conceptual formulation for fear that they would be accused of primarily looking after their own profits. As previously stated, no system of financial incentives is morally adequate to deal with the entire spectrum of individual health care issues and therefore the following structure is proposed.

A committee is formed by the creation of the health insurance plan and has active participation and voting rights by the hospital corporation and those fiduciary trust physicians who will have primary responsibility for the care of patients when they are admitted to critical care units. To assure that physicians and hospitals will be active and equal participants and not dominate the situation, they agree by economic and legal contract to function within the moral limits of health care benefits assigned to subscribers of the health plan as a condition for their initiation and continued participation in the health plan. Patients and subscribers will have an active role in the creation of the health plan. The health plan would be permitted to have legislatively created tort exemptions as described below unless employers originally sponsoring the health insurance plan had documented an insufficient level of employee participation in the creation of the plan and the ongoing assessment of the benefits and restrictions to individual care benefits within the health plan. Employee organizations or labor components of industries would have an active seat on the HTUC. The HTUC would have two levels of function. The first level would be the creation of health insurance limitations during the contracting process for critical care benefits. A subcomponent of the HTUC would be the oversight committee that would exist for critical care units in a specified hospital. It should be noted that we are dealing only with large hospitals and large critical care components that would meet the criteria for a managed critical care services plan. The need for comprehensive case management and the division of tasks between primary fiduciary physicians and QCCPs as consultant gatekeepers will preclude easy implementation in smaller hospitals. This chapter does not address the issue of efficiency or inefficiency of critical care operations in smaller hospitals. However, there is already documentation of inefficiency of high-technology usage in small hospitals relative to the cost of technology and it is unlikely that people in small communities will continue to possess the freedom to squander large health insurance plan resources for that kind of care. A system of regionalization of critical care is already widely acknowledged to be necessary and is actively supported as a matter of health policy by critical care medical organizations like the SCCM.

The HTUC is a formal structure with a mission, a budget, and contractually defined authority to carry out the individual entitlement limitations of the health care contract. It is a medico-legally binding ethics committee sanctioned in law and health insurance. If a hospital wishes to use this structure to deal with individual ethical issues that do not directly confront resource allocation, the hospital may elect to contract with the health plan to have this function carried out by the HTUC.

QCCPs with specialty certification credentials from any of the existing specialty boards within the American Board of Medical Specialties will be qualified to function as critical care consultants in this system. They will be consultants and case managers only for the care of the critically ill. They are prohibited from being primary, fiduciary trust, admitting physicians and the advocates of patients and their rights of consumption within the health plan. To assure that there is no moral economic conflict, these physicians may not become part of the admitting physician component of the hospital medical staff for patients who would require or could reasonably be anticipated to require critical care services. The contractual mechanism of the health plan, the hospital corporation, and the hospital medical staff component would define the limits of abuse for this privilege and detail the grounds for termination of the critical care physician from health insurance plan employment.

Primary fiduciary trust physicians who would act as the advocates of their patients would be entitled to freely and robustly advocate for the individual circumstances of their patients in a dialogue with the critical care consultant and members of the managed critical care services team. Prior to becoming a recompensable, qualified, admitting physician for patients in this critical care system, the primary fiduciary trust physician will have read and understood the moral economic limits to health benefits that would likely become implementable in the specialties in which he or she works. While some of these limits would obtain directly for issues related to prognostic scoring, it is anticipated that others would relate to the reasonableness of undertaking medical or surgical high-technology strategies prior to admission to an ICU that would subsequently make ICU care and physiologic support necessary. In this chapter we look only at this initial conceptualization of prognostic scoring in defining the moral limits of individual entitlement of patients to consume resources and the autonomy prerogatives of their physician advocates to request such services and requisition them from a health insurance plan.

From time to time, a patient will be identified (through computerized entitlement limitation resource consumption screens) whose limit has been exceeded. At such point, automatic notice of this circumstance would be communicated formally to the primary physician advocate and the patient or the legally documented surrogate. An appropriate period of time (within defined limits) for independent personal response of the patient and the physician advocate would then be permitted. There would be no discretion on the part of the critical care physician consultant gatekeeper as to what the screens would be, as they already would have been decided in the health insurance plan policy. The authority of the critical care gatekeeper is circumscribed in terms of notification of entitlement limitation excess by the rules of the health plan. He or she functions and reports to the HTUC exclusively for all matters that have to do with resource allocation regarding the entitlement limitations in health insurance. As the original model (given as an example only) already contains the definition of medical futility, it will be difficult for individual patients or physicians to make appeals that would have standing in the health insurance plan. The appellate process is designed to assure that all of the necessary information gathered by the critical care gatekeeper and the HTUC is factually correct. When that discovery process has been exhausted, a decision will be made (usually by the critical care gatekeeper) and, if contested, then by the HTUC.

In this system, the committee's decision is final after the individual discovery appellate process has been concluded and all funding for critical care will be terminated. However, for those patients who do not die or are not anticipated to die with the removal of active critical care therapy, the health plan will pay for and assure that the necessary services for critical care hospice services or intermediate care will be fully funded by the health plan. Once a patient enters that category, comfort measures and supportive care will be provided as will counseling and other necessary humanistic supports, and will be supervised by the HTUC. Physicians attempting to reestablish active therapeutic treatment in such patients may not do so without obtaining grounds for such that would be acceptable to the HTUC. Any unilateral decisions taken by primary, fiduciary trust physicians with or without the active or passive permission of the hospital will put the patient, physician, and hospital at financial risk.

If termination of entitlement and triage out of the intensive care unit is carried out under the purview of this policy and is contested after the discovery appellate process has run its course, then a formal hearing before the HTUC will occur and minutes of the proceedings will be kept. The final review will be an impartial review of the gatekeeper's report to the committee with the patient's surrogate and primary attending physician invited to attend. Under such circumstances, we are working under the legal doctrine of contract law. It was specifically noted that as a condition of entering the health insurance plan, both the patient and the physician were fully informed and knew the policies and procedures that would be applied should patients come for care in an intensive care unit. Any notions of ignorance or not understanding these matters will not be acceptable in a court of law because there will be rigid standards required to acquire the health insurance and to enter into the plan either as a patient or as a provider in the original instance. Courts would likely rule in favor of the health plans because the necessary legislative authority would have defined the policy requirements demanded by the judiciary [51].

To allow health plans to function across several jurisdictions, or in large interstate health care enterprises, federal legislation will have been created that will prohibit civil litigation in either state or federal courts against any physician or nurse for adhering to the triage policies created by the contract process for acquiring moral authority in health insurance. Medical negligence suits will continue to exist but will be limited by the absolute resource standard of availability [41,42,43] in Section 10 of Senate Bill 27 of the Oregon Basic Health Services Act of 1989. The fact that a person would die more swiftly than they would have by the continued administration of high-technology care is not a necessary and sufficient grounds legally for seeking recompense and would be recognized as a morally unfortunate but not unfair circumstance within the health insurance system.

It will be noted from Figure 230-3 that physician practice guidelines are mentioned, as opposed to physicians, while hospital policies and procedures are mentioned in contradistinction to a hospital corporation. The reason for this formulation in this conceptual health insurance plan is that there must be latitude accorded to both institutions and to individual providers in the creation of these policies so that they may freely advocate for patients in appellate processes. It is anticipated that as such a system enters implementation within the Oregon Plan, several midcourse corrections in hospital policies and practice guidelines, as well as the entitlement limitations within the health plan, will be made by virtue of economically mandated dialogue between the parties most affected by these issues. This is entirely appropriate as the nature of political and economic conflict is best resolved within the health insurance plan.

Patients like Helga Wanglie [50], who hold specific religious or moral views concerning the sanctity of life in the vegetative state or other "minority moralities," could elect to buy "right to life premium surcharge insurance" when they enter the insurance plan. All systems that choose to forbid a behavior on moral grounds are in trouble. They indicate a lack of tolerance for the freedom of people to hold religious and moral views within a pluralist society. As the American society openly supports the free exercise of religion, we should respect those who hold religious views as they would affect the allocation of health care resources. But when those views require the use of resources that would act to limit the care of others in a resource-constrained society, then the health plan must specifically acknowledge that they must pay to consume such resources.

Unique Cultural, Political, and Economic Obstacles

THE AMERICANS WITH DISABILITIES ACT. The Americans with Disabilities Act (ADA) was employed in 1992 by Secretary of Health and Human Services, Dr. Louis Sullivan, to challenge the Oregon Plan as one that discriminates against disabled citizens. It can be argued that even contractually negotiated definitions of futility violate the ADA because it may be interpreted that permanent coma or other critical illnesses are disabilities. Implementation of the resource allocation policy prepared here will require an amendment to the ADA that specifically exempts publicly or contractually defined futility. If Congress is asked for these exemptions and fails to act, then an argument can be made that Congress is not seriously committed to cost-containment strategies demanded by consumers and providers.

FEDERAL/STATE PAYMENT OBSTACLES. As the health care system will be under increasing competitive pressures, the ability of the federal and state governments to continue to cost-shift underfunded care will become increasingly problematic. This will lead either to further deterioration of the care of Medicare patients or the desire of very efficiently managed care networks to chose not to participate in the Medicare program. The most successful of competitors might be able to contract with enough nongovernmental subscribers to remain viable. Similarly, private providers might see the wisdom of joining plans where the federal cost-shifting can be avoided. Either payments would have to be increased for federally insured subjects or benefits packages would need to be curtailed. Intense friction would likely occur among older Americans, the government, and younger Americans. The younger generation already is subsidizing a large quantity of critical care for the elderly; the elderly are disproportionate consumers of end-of-life critical care. The competitive system in the free market is likely to further drive and accentuate generational competition for resources. The increasing efficiency of critical care medicine occasioned by managed critical care for private nongovernmental programs is likely to further drive the generational disparities that already exist in the country and highlight them in public policy. The larger economic shifts and transformations that will be occasioned by the creation of managed critical care will have to be studied carefully from the earliest dates of inception.

RELIGION AND THEOLOGY. The organized religions will not be silent in this process. Organized religion will have to deal with the impact of a secular pluralist morality. The question that will face all religions is the same, "What does it mean to die as a faithful Catholic, Baptist, Jew, Buddhist, or Confucian in a secular pluralist ICU?"

Enterprise Liability

To guarantee that the insurer is faithful to the subscribers and the providers, the Congress should consider passage of the "National Accountable Health Plan Joint Tort-Feasor Act." (This act would apply to Medicare beneficiaries in state-supervised managed care plans.) This act should include the resource allocation provisions and exemptions for critical care gatekeepers from legal challenges arising from denials of care (provided within the policies and procedures of the process).

Cost Containment and Entitlement Limitation

Some of the most difficult moral problems involving the definition of futility are not encompassed by current scoring systems such as APACHE III or MPM II. As Teres points out in Chapter 231, the highest cost ICU patients includes patients who do not die within a few days but linger for long periods in the ICU. Often the predicted mortality in such patients is not very high. Rather, mortality is probable because of the underlying disease process. Some patients with multiple-organ system failure fall into this category; these patients manifest a high probability of dying only when organ dysfunction become prominent by inspection of routinely available physiologic data.

ICUs that resuscitate patients to predefined end points may lower mortality probability scores. The reason this chapter has emphasized scoring systems is that they are objective, dispassionate, nonprejudicial forms of measurement. Thus, these systems can serve as an analytic tool to inspire public confidence. In the initial implementation of a policy as revolutionary as the one advocated in this chapter, it will be necessary to show the public that critical care medicine is about delivering appropriate medical care to people beyond the issues of personal wealth, greed, and self-interest.

The Oregon Plan is designed to bring the relevant parties in a health care system and a limited democracy closer together in terms of their economic legal relationships so as to arrive at morally meaningful resource allocation decisions. In this way, government may write laws that facilitate the communication of competing entities and differing agendas in a world of free market health care. As the free market system creates efficiencies, the same efficiencies may then accrue to those patients in the publicly financed health system without prejudice to governmentally imposed morality while fairer payments would be required of government to subsidize the care of Medicare and Medicaid recipients. If we expect those in the private sector to ration resources among themselves, then it must be that those under government systems should expect no more. In the Oregon system, the original proposal was in the public sector. However, the private sector seems to be gaining the momentum that will drive moral changes in managed care health insurance policies. As we have previously stated, "The market gains its moral authority from the consent of its participants. It is the result of many individual acts of mutual respect and forbearance. Moreover, in an era when secularism is rampant and plurality of moral viewpoints pronounced, the market offers a

vantage point from which peaceable moral strangers can cooperate in common ventures. The market is one of the driving forces of freedom and tolerance in the post modern world" [24].

Preserving Standards of Medical Care

The risk of budget-constrained systems is the decline in the standards of care with documentable increases in morbidity and mortality. Accordingly, a suitable control mechanism to fuse responsibility and authority for the control of moral standards of resource distribution is needed. Rather than command and control being exercised at the level of central government, legislation becomes permissive to allow resources to be allocated through negotiations among providers, purchasers, and subscribers. But even in this construction there will be the risk of declining standards of care and emasculation of high-technology medicine, as detailed by Levinsky [9]. To avoid the bureaucratic creation of "national circles of blame" as described by Levinsky, we need to establish systems as recommended in this chapter. Free speech of critical care professionals may be one of the last safety valves for the care of critically ill people as they will be among the few to be knowledgeable; to document increased morbidity, mortality, and declining standards of care for the patients in critical care units. Primary physicians also will be aware of these issues and may participate in the education of the public regarding these matters, as they will no longer have any economic conflict of interest with a prejudice to provide more rather than less care in violation of the publicly articulated morality. Such checks and balances systems are at the core of limited democracies and were the basis for the creation of the U.S. Constitution.

Conclusion

This chapter has provided a moral analysis of economic transfers in a free market health insurance society. Though the principles could be applied in a government-run, centrally financed health care system, the policy does not describe how governments could, as a practical matter, acquire moral authority. The strength of the Oregon Plan is that smaller communities may be free to impose high-technology medicine limits on themselves by the creation of a secular pluralist morality. In the belief that peaceful negotiation is better than the use of force, alternate proposals for centrally created governmental systems like the Clinton Health Plan will have to show that they can deliver moral content in health resource allocations by methods other than separating responsibility and authority for health care resource allocations while secretly redistributing wealth from the haves to the have nots of a capitalist democracy.

References

1. Amundsen DW: The physician's obligation to prolong life: A medical duty without classical roots. *Hastings Cent Rep* 8:4:23, 1978.
2. Enthoven AC: The history and principles of managed competition. *Health Aff* 12(suppl):24, 1993.

3. Aaron HJ, Schwartz WB: Managed competition: Little cost containment without budget limits. *Health Aff* 12(suppl):204, 1993.
4. Schwartz WB, Mendelson DN: Why managed care cannot contain hospital costs without rationing. *Health Aff* 11:100, 1992.
5. Fielding JE, Rice T: Can managed competition solve problems of market failure? *Health Aff* 12(suppl):216, 1993.
6. Birnbaum ML: Cost containment in critical care, in Rippe JM, Irwin RS, Alpert JS, et al (eds): *Intensive Care Medicine.* 2nd ed. Boston, Little, Brown, 1991, p 1977.
7. Aaron HI, Schwartz WB: *The Painful Prescription: Rationing Hospital Care.* Brookings Institution, Washington, DC, 1984.
8. Meyer M, Mure A: Not my health care. *Newsweek,* January 10, 1994, p 36.
9. Levinsky NG: The organization of medical care: Lessons from the Medicare end stage renal disease program. *N Engl J Med* 329:1395, 1993.
10. Beauchamp TL, Childress JF: *Principles of Biomedical Ethics,* 4th ed. New York, Oxford University Press, 1994.
11. Luce JM, Wachter RM: The ethical appropriateness of using prognostic scoring systems in clinical management. *Crit Care Clin* 10:229, 1994.
12. Luce JM: Ethical principles in critical care. *JAMA* 263:696, 1990.
13. Oregon Health Services Commission: A Report to the Governor and Legislature Entitled: *Prioritization of Health Services.* Salem, OR, 1991.
14. Lohr KN, Yordy K, Harrison PF: Health care systems: Lessons from international comparisons. *Health Aff* 11:239, 1992.
15. Kitzhaber J: Personal communication.
16. Rosenbaum S: Poor women, poor children, poor policy: The Oregon Medicaid experiment, in Strosberg MA, Wiener JM, Baker R, et al (eds): *Rationing America's Medical Care: The Oregon Plan and Beyond.* Brookings Institution, Washington, DC, 1992, p 21.
17. Ferguson T: Oregon's clue to Clinton's entitlement act, *Wall Street Journal* July 28, 1992.
18. Engelhardt HT: *The Foundation of Bioethics.* 2nd ed. New York, Oxford University Press, 1995.
19. Russel LB: Some of the tough decisions required by a national health plan. *Science* 24:892, 1989.
20. Gradison WD: Federal policy and intensive care, in Strosberg MA, Fein IA, Carroll JD (eds): *Rationing of Medical Care for the Critically Ill.* Washington, DC, Brookings Institution, 1989, p 37.
21. Engelhardt HT, Rie MA: Intensive care units, scarce resources, and conflicting principles of justice. *JAMA* 253:1159, 1986.
22. Brody B: Health care for haves and have nots: Toward a just basis of distribution, in Shelp EE (ed): *Justice and Health Care.* Dordrecht, Holland, D. Reidel, 1981, p 151.
23. Starr P: *The Social Transformation of American Medicine.* New York, Basic Books, 1982.
24. Engelhardt HT, Rie MA: Selling virtue: Ethics as a profit maximizing strategy in health care delivery. *J Health Soc Policy* 4:27, 1992.
25. Schnepel R, Stopfkuchen H: Collaboration between nurses and physicians in Europe. *Crit Care Med* 21(suppl):S388, 1993.
26. Stopfkuchen H: Impact of national health system financing on quality of care in intensive care unit: The German experience. *Crit Care Med* 21(suppl):S406, 1993.
27. *Von Stetina vs. Florida Medical Center,* 436 So. 2d 1022 (Fla. 1983), 10 Fla. L. Weekly 286 (Fla., May 24, 1985).
28. Shabot MM, Bjerke HS, LoBue M, et al: Quality assurance and utilization assessment: The major by products of an ICU clinical information system, in *Proceeding of the XV Symposium on Computer Applications in Medicine, American Medical Informatics Association,* Bethesda, MD, SCAMC, 1992, p 554.
29. Rapoport J, Teres D, Lemeshow S, et al: A method of assessing the clinical performance and cost effectiveness of intensive care units. *Crit Care Med* 22:1385, 1994.
30. Marshall MF, Schwenzer KJ, Orsina M, et al: Influence of political power medical provincialism and economic incentives on the rationing of surgical intensive care unit beds. *Crit Care Med* 20:387, 1992.
31. Guidelines Committee of the SCCM: Guidelines for the definition of an intensivist and the practice of critical care medicine. *Crit Care Med* 20:540, 1992.
32. Ethics Committee of the SCCM: Consensus statement on the triage of critically ill patients. *JAMA* 271:1200, 1994.
33. *Code for Nurses with Interpretative Statements.* Washington, DC, American Nurses Association, 1985.
34. Vassar MJ, Holcroft JW: The case against the use of the APACHE system to predict intensive care unit outcome in trauma patients. *Crit Care Clin* 10:117, 1994.
35. Teres D: Comment on the case against using the APACHE system to predict ICU outcome in trauma patients. *Crit Care Clin* 10:127, 1994.
36. Watts CW, Knaus WA: Comment on the case against using the APACHE system to predict ICU outcome in trauma patients. *Crit Care Clin* 10:129, 1994.
37. Steinbrook R, Lo B: The Oregon Medicaid demonstration project: Will it provide adequate medical care? *N Engl J Med* 326:340, 1992.
38. Rie MA, Engelhardt HT: The Oregon Medicaid controversy. *N Engl J Med* 327:643, 1992.
39. Havighurst C: Altering the applicable standard of care. *Law and Contemporary Problems* 49:265, 1986.
40. Havighurst C: The changing locus of decision making in the health care sector. *J Health Polit Policy Law* 11:697, 1986.
41. Morreim EH: *Balancing Act: The New Medical Ethics of Medicine's New Economics.* Boston, Kluwer Academic Publishers, 1991.
42. Morreim EH: Justice and health care rationing: Lessons from Oregon, in Strosberg MA, Wiener JM, Baker R, et al (eds): *Rationing America's Medical Care: The Oregon Plan and Beyond.* Washington, DC, Brookings Institution, 1991, p 159.
43. Morreim EH: Stratified scarcity: Redefining the standard of care. *Law Med Health Care* 17:356, 1989.
44. Shortell SM, Reinhardt UE: *Improving Health Policy and Management: Nine Critical Research Issues for the 1990's.* Ann Arbor, MI, Health Administration Press, 1992.
45. Greenhouse L: Court order to treat baby prompts a debate on ethics. *New York Times,* February 20, 1994, p 12.
46. Engelhardt HT, Rie MA: Morality for the medical industrial complex: A code of ethics for the mass marketing of health care. *N Engl J Med* 319:1086, 1988.
47. Annas G: Informed consent, cancer and truth in prognosis. *N Engl J Med* 330:223, 1994.
48. Feshbach M: Health in the USSR: Organization, trends and ethics, in Sass HM, Massey RU (eds): *Health Care Systems,* Dordrecht, Holland, D. Reidel, 1988.
49. Emanuel EJ: *The Ends of Human Life: Medical Ethics in a Liberal Polity.* Cambridge, MA, Harvard University Press, 1991.
50. Rie MA: Helga Wanglie's ventilator. *Hastings Cent Rep* 21:24, 1991.
51. National Center for State Courts: *Guidelines for State Court Decision Making in Life Sustaining Medical Treatment Cases.* St. Paul, MN, West Publishing, 1993.
52. Rie MA: Oregonian ICU: Multitiered monetarized morality in health insurance law. *J Law Med Ethics* 23:149, 1995.

231. Severity-of-Illness Modeling and Potential Applications

Daniel Teres and Stanley Lemeshow

"Uncertainty Is Not Chaos"

In 1983 the National Institutes of Health held a Consensus Development Conference to discuss issues related to the practice of critical care medicine. One panel stated that when the capacity of ICUs is strained and ICU resources are limited, priorities should be given to patients with a "reasonable prospect of significant recovery . . . from acutely life-threatening disease or injury" [1]. The panel also concluded that an important evaluation function would be to look at "efficacy of intensive care with respect to mortality and morbidity."

Since that time, considerable advances have been made in the refinement and application of severity-of-illness models to describe patients admitted to ICUs. These models can provide a method for risk stratification for important clinical research trials and for making quality of care comparisons among ICUs with a similar case mix [2].

Because of advanced computer software development and availability and access to large ICU databases, ICU severity models are now commonly utilized. In many institutions, the scores/probabilities can be provided on-line. While there has been elevation of bedside discussion of prognosis of ICU patients with families and on teaching rounds, it is still unclear (and even controversial) how a score or probability estimate of hospital mortality should be applied to an individual patient.

In this chapter we review important severity-of-illness scoring systems and prognostic models and discuss their potential uses and limitations. Some possible applications to certain types of patients and a methodology for evaluating cost-effectiveness also are discussed.

Severity-of-Illness Scoring Systems

The various severity scores for critical care patients have been substantially updated in the past few years. The new versions of these scores are based on much larger databases and have used better statistical methods for development, validation, and field testing. Appropriate methods for measuring discrimination and calibration are now widely used and logistic regression has become the dominant method for converting a score to a probability, scaling physiologic variables, and selecting and weighting clinical variables. Although some critics have raised concerns about the use of severity scores (even for important subgroups of patients), the use of severity scores has achieved a wide level of acceptance, particularly for auditing clinical practice and outcomes within the ICU of an individual hospital and for risk stratification for large-scale clinical trials that include ICU patients. For the latter application, severity scores can be used as an enrollment criterion, a controlling factor for subgroup analysis, a descriptive variable, or an integral component of the analytic technique.

In order to rigorously develop and assess a model, a large database must be available. A separate database using different patients must be employed for validation and field testing. Variables should be clearly defined and reliable. The model should reflect accurately the mortality experience of the patient sample as assessed by objective criteria. The criteria for assessing the reliability of a model are well established and include discrimination, using the area under the receiver/operator curve, and calibration, using formal goodness-of-fit testing [3]. Models should contain a minimum number of variables to reduce the burden of data collection and the potential for error. There should be minimal reliance on ICU treatment variables, laboratory tests, and radiologic examinations.

The common endpoint for the general ICU severity models is vital status at hospital discharge. There also has been preliminary research on ICU models with different endpoints including functional outcome, longer term mortality, efficiency, ICU length of stay, and cost [4].

There also has been a proliferation of general severity scoring systems or case-mix adjustors for hospital-wide patients including a computerized severity index, a cumulative index rating scale, a multiattribute utility model, the use of diagnostic related groups (DRGs), and a medical illness severity grouping system [5–9]. There also are models for subgroups of ICU patients or treatments: ventilator score, trauma scores, therapeutic intervention scoring system, (invasive) critical care scoring system, the clinical sickness score, organ system failure, and septic shock score [10]. Many of these models are based on intuitive selection of variables or are based on small samples on highly selected patients. None of these systems has achieved widespread recognition as being a scientifically derived model. They may serve a variety of clinical, reimbursement, or managerial purposes, but they are not truly validated severity-of-illness models.

The primary models for discussion in this chapter are the general purpose ICU systems: APACHE, MPM, and SAPS.

APACHE II. The Acute Physiology and Chronic Health Evaluation II (APACHE) score is the most widely studied severity illness model. It has been used most often without conversion to a probability of hospital mortality, which requires a logistic regression equation based on the principal precipitating diagnosis [11], and it is widely utilized as a descriptor in clinical studies, both in and out of the ICU setting.

The physiology scoring approach has been criticized by some general surgeons and traumatologists, because physiology scores can be "modified" or "normalized" while a patient is in the operating room or trauma room in the emergency department [12,13,14]. Aggressive stabilization of a patient may mask extreme deviations from the normal values for key physiological parameters that would be present without such clinical intervention [15]. Furthermore, in ICUs where continuous or frequent monitoring and laboratory tests are performed, equivalent patients might have higher scores when compared to an ICU with a clinical practice of intermittent monitoring or a conservative approach to laboratory testing. Cerra et al. have pointed out that APACHE II does not work well in immediate postoperative surgical patients who develop multiorgan failure syndrome [16], and Vassar and Holcroft have reported poor calibration for APACHE II in a large group of trauma patients [17].

Many studies have looked at small groups of unusual ICU patients and have shown that APACHE does not work in these groups of patients. Such results are not surprising since severity methods were developed on large groups of heterogeneous ICU patients which contained only a small number of such unusual patients. Examples include AIDS patients in the ICU [18,19] and patients with metastatic breast cancer [20]. It would be unlikely for a general severity model to provide a reasonable estimate of the hospital mortality of such unusual subgroups of ICU patients. Other studies reporting that APACHE works in subgroups of patients have not utilized sophisticated testing [21,22,23].

Some authors have tried to extrapolate the APACHE ICU physiology scoring system approach to use in patients outside the ICU. For example, Clavien et al. examined the relationship between outcome and APACHE score in patients undergoing cholecystectomy, even though few of these patients were candidates for ICU admission [24]. Others have attempted to use APACHE as a means for case-mix adjustment [25,26] or as a preoperative monitor [27]. Some investigators have argued that the Glasgow Coma Scale (GCS) can replace the physiologic parameters necessary for one of the scoring systems, since neurologic status is such an important determinant of outcome. Thus, in a study of 604 cardiac arrest patients in Finland, GCS alone accounted for a large proportion of the predictive value of APACHE II [28]. Similar studies have been done for stroke and head trauma victims [29,30,31]. Attempts have been made to determine whether APACHE works in cardiac surgery and and coronary care patients [32,33]. In our opinion, results from such studies are inconclusive, because the calibration of the APACHE system in these patients was not fully evaluated. Observing that the proportion of patients who die increases as the score increases does not provide sufficient evidence to say that a model is appropriately calibrated for that group of patients.

International comparisons have been published, which compare mortality data from single ICUs in New Zealand and Hong Kong with the data collected more than 10 years ago in the original APACHE II ICUs [34,35]. These studies are difficult to interpret since the ICUs are not representative, the time periods are different, and APACHE II may no longer be calibrated appropriately for U.S. hospitals, let alone those in New Zealand or Hong Kong. A more detailed study utilized a greater number of hospitals in Japan but did not resolve the issue of poor calibration [36].

It is important to recognize that in order to convert the APACHE score to an estimate of the probability of hospital mortality (prognosis), it is necessary to collect information on the worst values of the APACHE variables during the first 24 hours in the ICU and then use a logistic regression equation to convert the score to a probability. The first 24-hour period of ICU stay is the only time interval that has been validated for making the mathematical link between physiology score and probability of survival. While scores have been proposed at time points other than the first 24 hours as a risk stratifier for descriptive purposes in clinical trials and in describing therapeutic interventions, it has not been established that such scores are meaningful. Nevertheless, in comparing patients undergoing two techniques for draining an intraabdominal abscess, a physiology score is a reasonable way to characterize the two groups [37,38]. Physiology scores also have been shown to be useful in describing patients with acute pancreatitis, presumably during the initial period of hemodynamic instability [39,40].

Is A Single Specific Diagnosis Necessary? In order to convert the APACHE II physiology score to a probability, it is necessary to identify a single, primary precipitating diagnosis from a list of 49 possible conditions. While physicians may prefer that a severity model be based on a single, specific diagnosis, condition, or procedure, such an approach may be problematic. First of all, the APACHE system, which requires that a single diagnosis be specified, has not been shown to be superior to the general models that do not require specific diagnosis [41]. Some diagnoses are poorly defined, even after 24 hours in the ICU. Pneumonia is one example; even with localized lung lavage and protected brush cultures using a bronchoscopy, it is still difficult to diagnose pneumonia [42,43]. It is similarly difficult to diagnose sepsis and pulmonary embolism within the first 24 hours of ICU admission (see Table 231-1). There also are problems of establishing an unambiguous diagnosis for surgical problems during the first day of ICU admission. How should one classify a victim of head trauma if there was a concussion but no computed tomography (CT) evidence of cerebral edema by CT? How would a postoperative trauma patient with a spinal injury be listed: non-head injury multi-trauma or neurologic surgery (Table 231-2)?

Despite the controversies and critiques, the APACHE II system provides a simple, inexpensive way to describe ICU patients and to characterize different patient groups based on a physiology score.

APACHE III. APACHE III follows a pattern similar to the one used in APACHE II [44]. The major components are acute physiology points, chronic health points, and age points collected during the first 24 hours after ICU admission. The APACHE

Table 231-1. Selected Nonoperative Major Disease Categories in Apache II System

Respiratory
    Aspiration pneumonia
    Respiratory neoplasm (including larynx, trachea)
    Respiratory arrest
    Pulmonary edema (noncardiogenic)
    Bacterial/viral pneumonia
    Chronic obstructive pulmonary disease
    Pulmonary embolism
    Mechanical airway obstruction
    Asthma
    Other respiratory diseases
Sepsis
    Sepsis (other than urinary tract)
    Sepsis of urinary tract origin
Trauma
    Head trauma (with/without multiple trauma)
    Multiple trauma (excluding head trauma)

Table 231-2. Selected Operative Major Disease Category

Neurologic
    Intracerebral hemorrhage
    Subdural/epidural hematoma
    Subarachnoid hemorrhage
    Laminectomy/other spinal cord surgery
    Cardiotomy for neoplasm
    Other neurologic diseases
Trauma
    Head trauma (with/without multiple trauma)
    Multiple trauma (excluding head trauma)

score ranges from 0 to 299 points for any patient, with a maximum of 252 points being awarded for physiology variables, up to 23 points for chronic health, and up to 24 points for age. As in the previous versions of APACHE, all variables are assessed as the "worst value in the 24-hour period." There is decreased emphasis on the score except within a specific diagnostic category [44].

Conversion of the score to a probability of hospital mortality is accomplished using a logistic regression equation requiring the specification of one of 79 specific diagnostic categories, as well as one of 9 patient locations (Table 231-3). The score will have a different associated probability of hospital mortality for patients in two different disease categories and for patients in the same disease category but admitted from two different locations. The APACHE III system is proprietary and the statistical weights to convert a score to a probability have not been made public. As a result, performance of the APACHE III system has not been tested independently. The same is true for the statistical equations that convert the score to an estimated length of ICU stay.

It has been suggested that daily physiology scores within diagnostic categories can provide useful information for dynamic modeling and for looking at the change in probability of mortality over time [45]. Again, independent confirmation within specific diagnostic groups has not been performed.

The APACHE III system is more complex than APACHE II. A much larger database has been accumulated with APACHE III through a proprietary network, but it is unclear whether the additional data collection and resulting costs represent a significant improvement over the APACHE II system.

SAPS II. The Simplified Acute Physiology Score follows a similar pattern to the APACHE system but places emphasis on keeping the approach simple. The system is widely used throughout Europe. The SAPS II system has been improved and refined over the original SAPS by having the physiologic variables weighted using logistic regression techniques [46]. The score ranges from 0 to 182 points with up to 120 points for physiologic variables, up to 36 points for chronic health variables, up to 18 points for age, and up to 8 points for type of

Table 231-3. Group Variables in the Apache III System

Physiology
  17 terms
Chronic Health
  AIDS
  Cirrhosis
  Lymphoma
  Hepatic failure
  Metastatic cancer
  Immunosuppression
  Leukemia/multiple myeloma
Surgical status
  Elective
  Emergency
Patient origin
  Direct admission
  Floor
  Other ICU
  Step-down unit
  Transfers from other hospitals
  Emergency room
  Operating room
  Recovery room
  ICU readmission

Table 231-4. Variables in the SAPS II System

Physiology
  Heart rate
  Systolic blood pressure
  Body temperature
  WBC
  Bilirubin
  PaO_2/FIO_2 (if mechanical ventilation or continuous positive airway pressure)
  Urine output
  Blood urea
  Serum K
  Serum Na
  Serum HCO_3
  Glasgow Coma Scale
Chronic health
  AIDS
  Metastatic malignancy
  Hematologic malignancy
Other
  Age
  Type of admission

admission (emergency surgical, scheduled surgical, or nonsurgical) (Table 231-4). There was an initial attempt to maintain SAPS as a "pure" physiology approach, but the model did not calibrate until three chronic conditions were included.

SAPS II provides an algorithm for converting a score to a probability of hospital mortality. All that is necessary at the bedside is to locate the SAPS II score on the horizontal axis of the graph and then match the corresponding probability of hospital mortality on the vertical axis (Fig. 231-1). For bedside availability, this method eliminates the need for expensive computer equipment and specialized software and maintains the

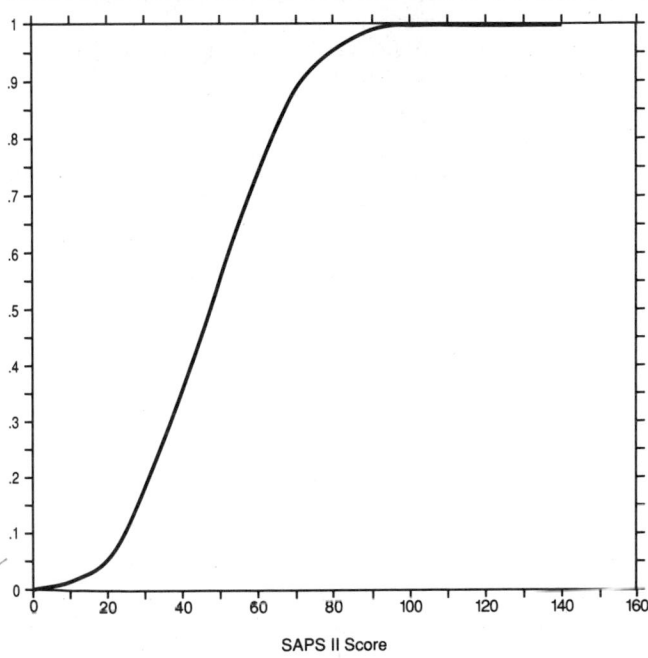

Fig. 231-1. Graph for Converting the SAPS II Score to a Probability of Hospital Mortality

SAPS II Score

overall concept of a simple approach. Obviously, data need to be stored on computers for clinical trials and aggregate group analyses. The calibration and discrimination ability of SAPS II are comparable to the more complex APACHE physiology approach.

MORTALITY PROBABILITY MODEL (MPM II). MPM II was developed on a large database of 19,124 patients from 137 hospitals [47]. The methodology used the statistical technique of multiple logistic regression to identify, as well as to weight, the clinical variables [48,49]. This system is not primarily physiologic and no score is involved. The MPM system is a series of models available at ICU presentation, as well as at 24, 48, and 72 hours [50]. The 24-hour model should be used in comparison with probabilities estimated with APACHE II and APACHE III as well as with SAPS II for patients who are still present in the ICU after 24 hours.

The unique component of MPM is a model, validated on an independent cohort of ICU patients, that is available at the time of ICU presentation. Table 231-5 presents the variables necessary to calculate the probability of mortality at ICU presentation, including diagnostic, condition, prior treatment, and physiologic variables; there is no requirement for a single primary precipitating diagnosis in order to calculate the probability. An ICU presentation model should provide an ideal tool for evaluating ICU quality performance and for stratifying patients prior to randomization in clinical trials before differential ICU treatment patterns have had an opportunity to alter physiology. MPM should be less influenced by treatments started in the emergency room or the postanesthesia care unit than more physiology-based systems.

The MPM 24 is designed for patients still in the ICU at 24 hours. Only eight new variables are collected at the time and are used in conjunction with age, type of admission, cirrhosis, metastatic cancer, and intracranial mass effect. The same variables, but with a different statistical constant value for each time period, comprise the models for calculation of probabilities at 48 and 72 hours. Table 231-6 lists the variables in the MPM 24-hour model.

Is One of the Severity Models Superior to the Others? In a European–North American comparison of ICU severity models by Castella et al., APACHE II, SAPS II, and MPM II were

Table 231-5. Variables for MPM at Admission

Physiology
  Coma or deep stupor
  Systolic blood pressure ≤ 90 mm Hg
  Mechanical ventilation at admission
  CPR prior to admission
  Heart rate ≥ 150 beats/min
Chronic diagnoses
  Metastatic neoplasm
  Cirrhosis
  Chronic renal failure, no acute exacerbation
Acute diagnoses
  Acute renal failure, with or without chronic history
  Intracranial mass effect
  Gastrointestinal bleed
  Cardiac dysrhythmia
  Cerebrovascular disease
Other
  Admission not for elective surgery
  Age (10-year odds ratio)

Table 231-6. Variables for MPM at 24 Hours

Age
Admission diagnosis/condition
  Metastatic neoplasm
  Cirrhosis
  Intracranial mass effect
  Admission not for elective surgery
New measurements
  Coma or deep stupor *at* 24 hours
  Urine output < 150 ml in 8-hr period
  Mechanical ventilation
  Creatinine > 2.0 mg/dl
  Continuous IV vasoactive drug therapy
  Prothrombin time > 3 sec above standard
  Confirmed infection
  $PO_2 < 60$ mm Hg

each computed on a common cohort of patients [51]. These authors also compared APACHE II and APACHE III scores, but the APACHE III probabilities could not be calculated. One important conclusion of this study was that the new systems are an improvement over their older counterparts. The original versions of SAPS and MPM no longer calibrated well enough to be useful today. APACHE II also failed to calibrate well in the large data set. Despite differences in approach, such as need for a specific diagnosis in APACHE II, all three systems could be used with considerable reliability and none was superior to the others. SAPS II is accurate and very easy to use. MPM at 24 hours showed the best fit of the systems analyzed. APACHE II is acceptably simple and has been used most widely in clinical studies. MPM is the only probability that can be calculated at ICU presentation.

Application to Individual Patients

CLINICAL PROGNOSIS VERSUS OBJECTIVELY DERIVED PROBABILITY. There is a natural tendency for physicians to be opposed to the on-line application of severity models for individual patients. Alternatively, a model employing only a small number of variables does not use enough of the extensive information available to the clinician at the bedside. The clinical situation is dynamic over minutes to hours. Each clinical factor has a wide range of possibilities and interactions. A clinical infection may not seem evident at first in the emergency department, but then a second look at the abdominal roentgenogram showing free air may indicate that a major crisis is in progress. These dynamic events and clinical responses seem far removed from the data entered into a "static" model.

There is also a wide range of physiologic responses to resuscitation and therapy. There are ill-defined psychological factors such as "will to live." There also appear to be important clinical factors that are not included in models, such as iatrogenic complications. Several studies caution against using severity models for individual patients, noting occasional wide discrepancies between observed and predicted outcomes [52,53]. Based on probabilistic theory, it should be expected that an occasional patient with a very high severity of illness will survive and one with a very low severity of illness will die.

Advantages of a Parsimonious Model. For obvious reasons, it is impossible to collect data on every clinically interesting variable. It is useful to have a parsimonious model for ease of data collection and for reproducibility. The end product of the combined clinical and statistical effort of model building is to find multivariate relationships that relate to hospital mortality.

It is our experience that some important variables cannot be included because of problems with definition. We already have discussed the example of pneumonia or the clinical variables associated with a pneumonialike picture. Nevertheless, it is intuitively apparent that pneumonia should be an important variable in estimating the hospital probability of mortality for large groups of patients. It is unfortunate that "pneumonia" is ill-defined. However, this term does not appear in the MPM or SAPS systems.

There are concerns regarding the definition for other variables presumed to be more objective. For example, acute renal failure would seem to be a clear, unambiguous, clinical term when a patient presents with shock, oliguria, and granular casts in the urinary sediment. The picture should be considered self-evident and, with fairly simple tests, there should be broad agreement that such a patient has acute renal failure. Severe prerenal failure also would seem to be a clear condition that could be defined in prospect. There are so many patients with mild prerenal failure that it should be an easy decision by a data collector to check "No" for the acute renal failure term. There should be few patients who fall into a gray zone of moderately severe prerenal failure. Consequently, there should be minimal opportunity to overscore a patient.

Interpreting a Probability.
Providing a prognosis to a patient and family is an obligation assumed by the medical team. Such estimates have been provided for many years before "objective" severity models became available. For many conditions, the ranges are broad. For elective, high-risk surgery, the 30-day operative mortality is more narrow.

What is initially disconcerting about severity models is that a single number is presented as the probability estimate. In some ways, it makes the severity output seem like an exact science. In the early history of severity models, there frequently was a reference to a 50-percent cut point or an optimal cut point. Below the cut point (a low score or low probability of dying), the patient was "predicted to live," but limitations of these artificial cut points have been recognized [3]. Presenting probabilities by these artificial cut points was an oversimplification of a probability. Physicians, however, are generally quite comfortable with a probability estimate and appreciate the richness and limitations of such a term. It is important to recognize that the physician or medical team must interpret the probability for the patient or family. It is part of the process of formulating a prognosis. Assuming that all of the variables and rules are properly followed and defined, then the proper interpretation of the "objective" probability is that among a large group of patients with similar findings and the same covariate pattern, it has been shown that X percent of patients will live and (1-X) percent of patients will die.

Such an approach provides valuable information that can be viewed from many perspectives. One component of the discussion between the physician and the patient/family is an explanation of the clinical and physiologic factors that contribute to the probability estimate. A physician can describe the level of confidence in including or excluding the factors used in the calculation. The physician also can describe additional clinical factors that could serve to modify or clinically adjust the calculated probability.

Ideally, probabilities could be presented with a confidence interval surrounding the estimated probability. Such intervals might be useful in helping to avoid oversimplification of the output of the model, particularly by nonphysicians. A common misinterpretation is that a patient with a low probability of dying does not need to be admitted to the ICU while a patient with a high probability of dying should either not be treated in the first place or should not be treated in the ICU for an extended time period. It should be understood or explained that a low calculated probability in a given patient is predicated on the data obtained by studying similar patients who were treated in an ICU. Issues related to patients with a high probability are much more complex.

CAN SEVERITY MODELS BE APPLIED TO INDIVIDUAL PATIENTS?

Patient Requiring Monitoring.
Despite all of these concerns, there may be broad categories where direct application of a severity model to an individual patient may be justifiable and reasonable. The first category applies to patients requiring only monitoring. There are no data and no controlled clinical trials regarding denying admission to the ICU for these types of patients but, surely, their duration of stay could be defined or constrained, especially if one of the severity models were combined with the therapeutic intervention score (TISS), which measures therapeutic effort [54]. A low physiology score, a low risk of dying, and low therapy define a patient's requiring only monitoring [55].

Prolonged, Stable Respiratory Failure.
Severity models also might apply to another category of patients, namely those with chronic respiratory failure requiring a prolonged stay in an ICU. In these patients, the second category would be long-stay patients with chronic respiratory failure. The factors that started the acute illness and the intervening multiorgan dysfunction have resolved leaving the patient with single-system (i.e., pulmonary) failure, requiring chronic mechanical respiratory support. In some of these patients, the daily APACHE or SAPS score remains low, indicating physiologic stability. It has been suggested that these patients may be candidates for an alternative (less costly) treatment setting [56]. It is not established what the best or safest setting would be for these potentially salvageable patients, but they certainly do not require the intensity and constant multidimensional attention and monitoring of an ICU.

Futility Based on Unstable Physiology.
The third category wherein severity scoring on a case-by-case basis may be valuable is more controversial. These are patients who have a steadily increasing degree of physiologic instability. At the extreme end of the spectrum, it is possible to define such patients as reaching a futile situation based on physiologic criteria. In these cases, it should not be necessary to need an hourly or daily APACHE or SAPS score to determine when to stop therapy. The clinical situation should be obvious and if the patient is young, has acute trauma, massive bleeding, or uncontrolled septic shock, it may not be possible or emotionally feasible to stop therapy. If the deranged physiology cannot be reversed and the injury cannot be corrected, then the situation is hopeless. Also at the extreme end of the spectrum are patients with severe head injury who are physiologically unstable. In these patients, a score is not necessary to limit therapy, since the goal often is to try to achieve physiological stability to permit organ donation after declaration of brain death.

For most patients with a more slowly rising physiology score, the accuracy of models is not sufficient to define when to stop care. The science of converting a score to a probability after the first 24 hours is not well established. These patients are truly in a gray zone; many will have care limited or stopped for ethical reasons rather than based on a daily physiology score [57]. In fact, severity models are a poor way to define futility, since many patients with do not resuscitate orders or other limitations of care have already reached that determination by the time the scores have plateaued [58]. Even patients with three or more organs in severe dysfunction or failure for more than 3 days are no longer considered to be in the futile category.

Dynamic Modeling. In order to better apply severity models to individual patients, there will have to be further advances in dynamic modeling [59]. So far, the promise has been far greater than the reality. Perhaps with larger databases, there will be a better opportunity to develop and validate different approaches to this complex problem as it relates to heterogeneous patients with multiple, interacting, comorbid conditions and treatments. Issues related to quality of care, do not resuscitate orders, and patient-mix differences will need better clarification.

Approaches for dynamic modeling have included using the same physiologic variables and weights on a daily basis, looking for changes in the thresholds in the daily scores, and evaluating for iatrogenic complications that impact on mortality [60]. Another approach, requiring a large data collection effort, is to evaluate new and old variables collected at each appropriate time interval and redevelop a model by using logistic regression techniques. An alternative approach may use common variables, but would alter the statistical weights by a method called customization or recalibration.

PROBLEMS ASSOCIATED WITH SPECIAL SUBGROUPS.
All of the currently popular severity models are built on a broad base of heterogeneous medical and surgical patients from a large number of participating multipurpose ICUs. In reality, however, ICUs often are highly specialized. It is, therefore, not surprising that general models may not perform well within subgroups of patients concentrated in special ICUs, even though the models were intended for such patients.

For example, available models may not work well in a highly specialized cancer hospital. Even though cancer patients are common in the general ICU setting and in the databases underlying existing models, these patients are often admitted for a wide range of problems including postoperative monitoring or medical complications. The models validate in an acceptable fashion across the broad range of conditions, but not for the small number of patients with complications related to bone marrow transplantation and/or complications related to therapy of complex advanced hematologic malignancies. Such patients form only a small number of patients in the overall medical/surgical ICU population, but are concentrated in ICUs in specialized cancer centers.

A similar problem occurs for patients for whom the general severity models were not developed. These include burn patients, liver transplant patients, and patients with complications related to AIDS.

What can be done about these special subgroups? The first is to test the general models using formal goodness-of-fit methods to determine whether the model over- or underpredicts across the spectrum of probability ranges. It may be possible to customize or recalibrate for these specialized groups of patients. As long as comparisons are made among similar types of patients, it may be possible that quality testing can be performed. Another approach may be to develop modified models that build on physiologic terms (APACHE/SAPS) and conditions (MPM) but add unique variables related specifically to aspects of the particular subgroup of patients in question.

Cardiac Surgery. New York State developed an outcome prediction model for patients that utilized logistic regression techniques and incorporated special aspects related to myocardial function and intraoperative course [61]. Such a model has been utilized to provide severity-adjusted cardiac surgery mortality rates, so that hospitals and cardiac surgeons can be compared.

Septic Shock. Because of clinical trials of adjuvant therapy of sepsis with expensive new pharmaceuticals, there has been close scrutiny of severity models by the FDA and clinical researchers. The original HA1A study published in the respected peer review journal, *The New England Journal of Medicine,* met high standards for clinical design, but the drug was ultimately not approved by the FDA [62]. One of the subsequent criticisms, seemingly harsh, was that the APACHE score was not identical in the treatment and placebo groups and did not explain important univariate subgroup differences regarding acute respiratory distress syndrome (ARDS) and coagulopathy [63]. The critics suggested that the score should have been converted to a probability or risk of death. It may well be that a probability is a better way to risk-stratify treatment groups; however, the time of sepsis/septic shock did not necessarily correspond to 24 hours after ICU admission. In fact, some of these patients were never in an ICU; others were enrolled in the clinical trial much later than the first 24 hours of their ICU course. For these reasons and also because sepsis may be considered a relatively homogeneous diagnostic subgroup, a physiology score may make more sense than a calculated risk of death. Another approach would be to use specialized severity models developed specifically for septic shock [64]. Before being widely accepted, such models will need to meet very high standards of discrimination and calibration.

THE ROLE OF CALIBRATION.
If a model is to be used in discussions with families about prognosis, it is essential that the model be tested for calibration at the clinical site. The same can be said regarding the use of a model for enrolling patients in a clinical trial. It must be ensured that there is correspondence between observed and expected outcomes across the spectrum of probabilities. The principle is similar to calibrating a blood pressure monitor, both electronically and manometrically, prior to using it to correct for any drift in the readings, especially over time and in different clinical settings. It is not enough to simply say that the pressure is high or rising. If the nurse charts that the blood pressure has gone from 110 to 150 mm Hg systolic, there may be no immediate clinical response. If the nurse notices a problem with the transducer, then recalibrates the monitor and says that the actual blood pressure has gone from 130 to 190 mm Hg, there would obviously be an immediately different clinical response. The same principle of calibration holds for severity models [3].

Quality of Care Comparisons

The main application of severity models is outcome comparisons especially among similar institutions. The three adult systems (APACHE, MPM, and SAPS) plus the pediatric PRISM system have been developed on large databases and have been widely tested. By collecting the appropriate variables on a large number of consecutive ICU patients and then following the patients to determine their vital status at the end of hospitalization, it is possible to calculate the observed-to-expected mortality rate. Since these calculations may be highly politically charged, any "mandated" quality assurance program must have an open and honest feedback loop in order to be successful. Such outcome-oriented quality assessment studies are already commonly employed for internal audits and are increasingly being utilized through confidential database comparisons. However, an externally mandated state or JCAHO outcome study would need to be designed more carefully.

The ideal way to conduct these studies is to use trained ICU or quality assurance nurses as data collectors. It may not be necessary or even beneficial for continuous monitoring (because of the ultimate reduction in the quality of the data collection over time). The ideal time frame is unclear but three months may be satisfactory. Alternatively, data collection can be based on a number of consecutive cases. Using the latter approach, the data collection interval would be shorter in a busy ICU and longer in a smaller unit or one with a low census. The analysis should also evaluate observed-to-expected mortality rates within low, middle, and high severity strata among similar ICU/hospital organizations [65]. And third-party payers may have different requirements from the JCAHO. Ideally, data collectors should undergo a standardized training program on interpreting the definition of the variables and other aspects related to accuracy and reliability of data collection and entry.

LACK OF IMPORTANCE OF CALIBRATION. When used for quality assurance, rather than to make decisions regarding individual patients, failure of calibration (i.e., observed-to-expected mortality rates that are statistically different from the reference group) is the focus. If a model calibrates perfectly in every ICU, then no differences would be identified among ICUs and hospitals. For quality comparisons, the important judgment is whether the ICU is performing better or worse than the reference group; calibration is not necessary.

OBSERVED-TO-EXPECTED MORTALITY RATES. It is important to recognize that if an ICU that has a higher observed-to-expected mortality rate (i.e., more observed deaths than expected, or "excessive deaths"), it does not automatically mean that a quality of care issue has been identified. Interpretation of "excess" mortality must be done with great caution [66]. In the real world, there may be concerns about interpretation of clinical variables. Local practice patterns regarding stabilization of patients in a postanesthesia care unit or in an emergency room or the frequency of laboratory tests may have profound effects on the scores and probabilities generated by physiology-based models. An apparent "excess" mortality for a particular ICU may reflect the occasional need to admit terminal patients from the emergency department or the operating room.

The most important concern regarding the use of outcome models for quality assurance, however, relates to the broader issues of patient mix and selection bias. As noted above, many subtle factors may interact and affect how models perform on selected subgroups of patients. Sample size alone may not compensate for these case-mix factors. There may be important psychosocial or cultural aspects of care that underlie deviations from the predicted mortality rate. For example, consider two patients with bacterial pneumonia and respiratory failure, one being treated in a suburban ICU, the other receiving care in an inner city ICU. Although there may be differences in quality of care in either direction, it is likely that the patient who is employed, fully insured, and blessed with a supportive family will have a better outcome than the patient who is poorly motivated, has no supportive family, is poorly nourished, and has unidentified comorbid conditions that are not scored in chronic health evaluations or identified among the conditions in the MPM system.

Problems identified in ICU quality of care outcome studies,

although focused on the ICU, also may be a bellweather of hospital-wide issues, rather than problems in just the ICU. Excess mortality may occur because patients are discharged from the ICU too early due to bed shortages or sent to acute care wards equipped to handle only sick (but not critically ill) patients. Outcomes from an ICU in such a hospital would be very different from those an ICU that had a "seamless" transfer to a well-organized regular floor or intermediate care unit.

Therefore, since ICUs may be so different, it may not be fair to compare all ICUs against a single reference standard. It may be more appropriate to compare ICUs/hospitals with similar size, geography, patient-mix factors, and organizational and teaching patterns. Although there is no uniform way to distinguish these ICU and hospital characteristics, the goal is achievable with expanding databases. Using a standard deviation or confidence interval also would be preferable to the simple rank order.

Defining a High-Performance Intensive Care Unit

CLINICAL PERFORMANCE INDEX. Rapoport et al. [67] have defined two methodologies for evaluating observed-to-expected mortality rates. The first relates to converting the ICU/hospital mortality rate to a clinical performance index using the standard deviation of all of the hospitals being compared. The formula is the following: the given hospital value minus the mean of all hospitals divided by the standard deviation. Hospitals that are one standard deviation above or below the mean are easily identified (Fig. 231-2). This approach identifies high and low outliers and avoids minor differences. With straight rank ordering, there may be exaggeration of the findings by hospitals, oversight agencies, and the media. In one comparison of outcomes from intensive care at major medical centers, there was a statistically significant difference only for the topmost and bottommost ICUs [68].

The other approach uses a confidence interval around the

Fig. 231-2. High Clinical Performance

HIGH CLINICAL PERFORMANCE

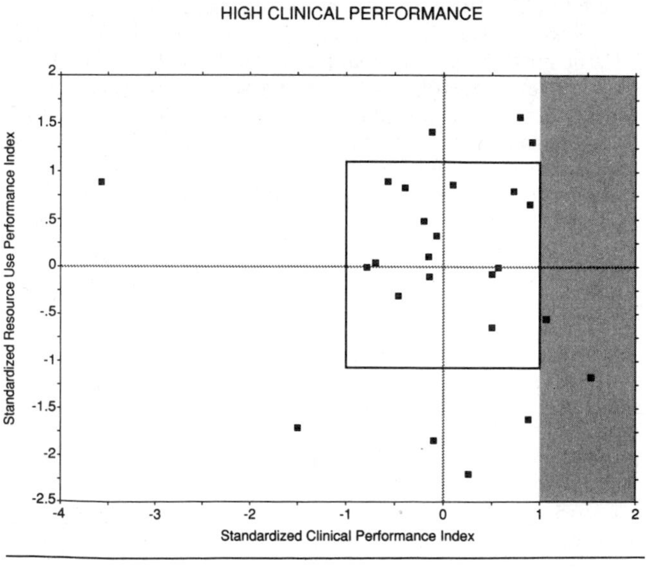

mean value and is particularly useful when relatively small sample sizes are involved. If the confidence interval includes the mean value for the group being compared, then there may not be a statistically significant difference even though the given hospital has an observed-to-expected mortality above or below the mean.

STANDARDIZED RESOURCE PERFORMANCE INDEX. It is possible to create a crude resource index based on length of stay in the ICU and on general wards after the ICU stay. By relating clinical performance to resource use, it is possible to evaluate hospitals on a cost-effectiveness basis [67,69]. The resource index can be created by assigning different units to ICU and floor care. The weighted hospital stay index is related to severity of illness so that a regression analysis is necessary to provide an estimate of predicted resource use. This approach also can be converted to a standardized index to identify ICUs/ hospitals with high or low resource consumption.

Future research in this area will improve this type of index and will need to incorporate factors such as intensity of ICU care, computer acquisition costs, and staffing by nurses and other personnel. Length of ICU stay is obviously one key factor affecting resource utilization, but other factors may be important as well. One preliminary approach is to look at the difference in nurse staff during the patient's last few days in the ICU compared to the next day or so after the patient leaves ICU care. In some ICUs, nursing care is reduced from 1:1 (i.e., one nurse for one patient), then 1:2, and, ultimately, 1:3 in the latter part of the stay. If patients are transferred to an intermediate unit, then nurse staffing may change in a gradual fashion to 1:4. In contrast, other ICUs keep the nurse patient ratio at 1:1 throughout the ICU stay, particularly for intubated patients. After extubation, patients are transferred to a general floor with a nurse:patient ratio as low as 1:10, especially if ICU beds are limited and there is no intermediate care capacity. Since nursing and other personnel comprise such a large proportion of cost, a resource measure index that can capture ICU, intermediate, and general ward nursing and labor costs would be a promising index and more useful than looking at just hospital charges or a crude weighted measure based on length of stay.

COST-EFFECTIVENESS. By cross-tabulating clinical performance versus resource consumption, it is possible to classify ICUs/hospitals into four quadrants (see Figs. 231-2 to 231-4). By using different endpoints, it is possible to identify some ICUs that have excellent clinical performance regardless of cost (see Fig. 231-2) and others that have good clinical performance and low resource consumption (see Fig. 231-3).

Both of these types of ICUs would be exhibiting high performance standards, but there may be very different clinical practice patterns between these two groups of ICUs/hospitals. An important research goal is to identify and analyze the differences between these two types of high-performance units.

Other approaches to regulating ICU practice could be to establish national practice guidelines by convening panels of experts, but there are recognized problems with these panels. Since randomized trials in intensive care are usually considered unethical, it may be more practical, realistic, and productive to analyze actual high-performance units and find out what they are doing right.

Focusing on the left side of the graph, one can identify low-performance ICUs. Clearly, one approach to health care reform places an emphasis on much lower cost ICUs (see Fig. 231-4).

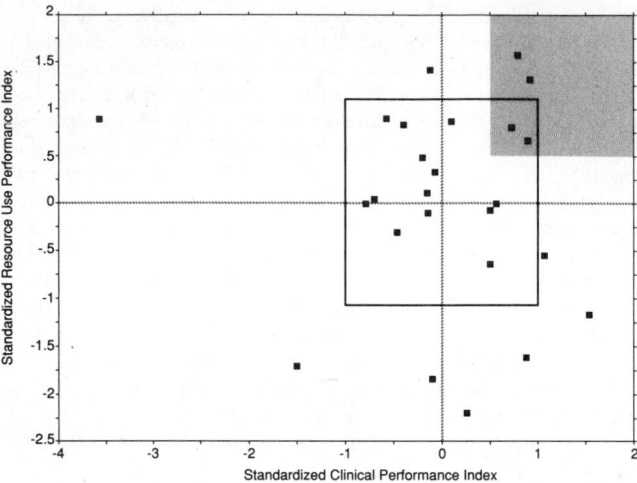

HIGH CLINICAL PERFORMANCE; LOW COST

Fig. 231-3. High Clinical Performance; Low Cost

How Should Severity Models Be Used at the Bedside?

There are ways to use severity models besides the ideal or idealistic approach with a tightly controlled, confidential, quality assessment program described previously. Should the systems be freely available at the bedside for use on teaching rounds or as an adjunct in discussions with families? Should there be a formal severity measure and calculation documented for each individual patient as part of the clinical medical record? Should there be a formal mandate to collect severity measures as part of a uniform national database? Should hospitals be encouraged to participate in more private commercial database ventures to provide more rapid turnaround and feedback and to maintain confidentiality? What are the public's expectations and rights-to-know regarding severity adjusted mortality rates?

PROPOSAL: TECHNOLOGY ASSESSMENT. An interesting and intriguing proposal would be to consider severity models as new technology and therefore subject them to scrutiny under the guidelines for technology assessment. There would be several reasons for considering such a proposal as a clinical trial. First, the cost of computers, software, and data collectors may be considerable. Even with open systems, there is the in-house cost of tracking the data. With systematic data collection on a routine basis, who will collect the information either on admission or daily? How much data should be collected? Nurses, attendants, and residents are all very busy and may not be concerned with filling out additional data forms accurately. Even laboratory values as part of a physiology score need corroboration. Can the models be misused, and what are the possible consequences?

This last question is highlighted by results from a recent clinical trial, which presented an estimated probability of mortality based on the Glasgow Coma Scale in a neurosurgical unit [70]. Compared to the control period of observation prior to presenting the estimated probability, there was no difference

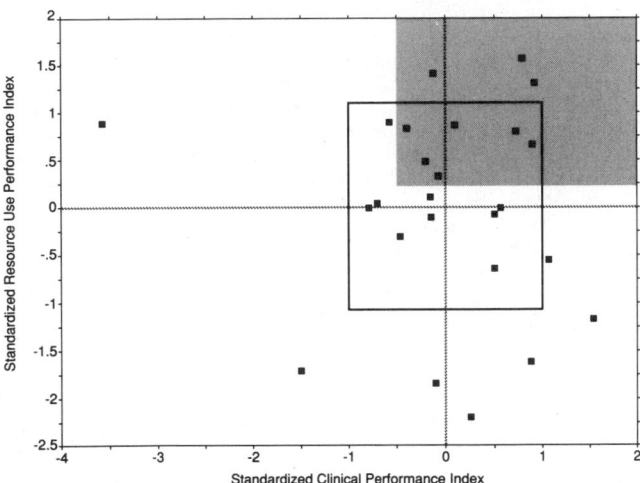

Fig. 231-4. Lowest Cost; Acceptable Quality

in mortality outcome. Nevertheless, during the study period, resources were shifted away from patients with a high likelihood of dying.

The same complex issues relate to presenting at the bedside an estimate of the length of ICU stay. Although not enough research has been done on length-of-stay estimates for individual patients, it is theoretically possible to provide an ICU length-of-stay estimate with a confidence interval 24 hours after the patient is admitted to the ICU. Such an approach might be considered as onerous as DRG report cards, but the information could be a contribution to cost containment.

Summary

ICU severity models have achieved widespread acceptance for providing a reasonable estimate of hospital mortality for groups of heterogeneous ICU patients. The statistical basis for these models is now well established. Application of this methodology for comparing the outcome of similar types of ICUs is gaining acceptance and should help to identify high-performance ICUs. There is now much less uncertainty regarding the hospital outcome of many subgroups of ICU patients. With the availability of larger databases, there will be further progress on application of these scores to individual patients, specialized models for important subgroups of patients, and dynamic modeling over time.

References

1. Parillo JE, Ayres SM: NIH consensus development conference statement on critical care medicine, in *Major Issues in Critical Care Medicine.* Baltimore, Waverly Press, 1984, p 279.
2. Schuster DP: Predicting outcome after ICU admission: The art and science of assessing risk. *Chest* 102:1861, 1992.
3. Lemeshow S, LeGall JR: Update on ICU severity models. (submitted)
4. Wesson DE, Williams JI, Spece LJ, et al: Functional outcome in pediatric trauma. *J Trauma* 29:589, 1989.
5. Sinclair JR, Magee PT, Gould TH, et al: A comparison of APACHE II and a clinical sickness score: A study of 97 consecutive admissions to a district general hospital intensive care unit. *Anaesthesia* 46:442, 1991.
6. Gross PA, Beyt BE, Decker MD, et al: Description of case-mix adjusters by the severity of illness working group of the Society of Hospital Epidemiologists of America (SHEA). *Infect Control Hosp Epidemiol* 9:309, 1988.
7. Selker HP, Griffith JL, D'Agostino RB: A time-insensitive predictive instrument for acute myocardial infarction mortality: A multicenter study. *Med Care* 29:1196, 1991.
8. Brewster AC, Karlin BG, Hyde LA, et al: MEDISGRPS: A clinically based approach to classifying hospital patients at admission. *Inquiry* 12:377, 1985.
9. Horn SD, Horn RA: The computerized severity index: A new tool for case-mix management. *J Med Syst* 10:73, 1986.
10. Yeung HC, Lu MW, Martinez EG, et al: Critical care scoring system: New concept based on hemodynamic data. *Crit Care Med* 18:1347, 1990.
11. Knaus WA, Draper EA, Wagner DP, et al: APACHE II: A severity of disease classification system. *Crit Care Med* 13:818, 1985.
12. Civetta JM: The clinical limitations of ICU scoring systems. *Probl Critical Care* 3:681, 1989.
13. Civetta JM: "New and improved" scoring systems. *Crit Care Med* 18:1487, 1990.
14. McAnena OJ, Moore FA, Moore EE, et al: Invalidation of the APACHE II scoring system for patients with acute trauma. *J Trauma* 33:504, 1992.
15. Teres D, Lemeshow S: Why severity models should be used with caution. *Crit Care Clin* 1994.
16. Cerra FB, Negro F, Abrams J: APACHE II score does not predict multiple organ failure or mortality in postoperative surgical patients. *Arch Surg* 125: 519, 1990.
17. Vassar MJ, Holcroft JW: The case against using the APACHE system to predict ICU outcomes in trauma patients. *Crit Care Clin* 1994.
18. Chu DY: Predicting survival in AIDS patients with respiratory failure: Application of the APACHE II scoring system. *Crit Care Clin* 9:89, 1993.
19. Benson CA, Spear J, Hines D, et al: Combined APACHE II score and serum lactate dehydrogenase as predictors of in-hospital mortality caused by first episode *Pneumocystis carinii* pneumonia in patients with acquired immunodeficiency syndrome. *Am Rev Respir Dis* 144:319, 1991.
20. Headley J, Theriault R, Smith TL: Independent validation of APACHE II severity of illness score for predicting mortality in patients with breast cancer admitted to the intensive care unit. *Cancer* 70:497, 1992.
21. Schein M, D'Egidio A: APACHE II scoring in surgical upper gastro-intestinal emergencies. *Dig Dis* 3:156, 1991.
22. Dart R, Patel B, Perez-Alard J, et al: Prognosis of oncology patients receiving intensive care using the APACHE II scoring system. *Md Med J* 40:273, 1993.
23. Giangiuliani G, Gui D, Bonatti P, et al: APACHE II in surgical lung carcinoma patients. *Chest* 98:627, 1990.
24. Clavien PA, Sanabria JR, Mentha G, et al: Recent results of elective open cholecystectomy in a North American and European center: Comparison of complications and risk factors. *Ann Surg* 216:618, 1992.
25. Thomas JW, Ashcraft ML: Measuring severity of illness: Six severity systems and their ability to explain cost variations. *Inquiry* 28:39, 1991.
26. McMahon LF Jr, Hayward RA, Bernard AM, et al: APACHE II: A new severity of illness adjuster for inpatient medical care. *Med Care* 30:445, 1992.
27. Gagner M, Franco D, Cons C, et al: Analysis of morbidity and mortality rates in right hepatectomy with the preoperative APACHE II score. *Surgery* 110:156, 1991.
28. Niskanen M, Karl A, Nikki P, et al: Acute physiology and chronic health evaluation (APACHE II) and Glasgow coma scores as predictors of outcome from intensive care after cardiac arrest. *Crit Care Med* 10:1465, 1991.

29. Weingarten S, Bolus R, Riedinger MS, et al: The principle of parsimony: Glasgow Coma Scale score predicts the mortality as well as the APACHE II score for stroke patients. *Stroke* 21:1280, 1990.

30. Rhee, KK, Baxt WG, Mackenzie JR, et al: APACHE II scoring in the injured patient. *Crit Care Med* 18:827, 1990.

31. Rocca B, Martin C, Viviand X, et al: Comparison of four severity scores in patients with head trauma. *J Trauma* 29:299, 1989.

32. Moreau R, Soupison T, Vauquelin P, et al: Comparison of two simplified severity scores (SAPS and APACHE II) for patients with acute myocardial infarction. *Crit Care Med* 17:409, 1989.

33. Turner J, Mudalier YM, Chang RW, et al: Acute physiology and chronic health evaluation (APACHE II) scoring in a cardiothoracic intensive care unit. *Crit Care Med* 19:1266, 1991.

34. Zimmerman JE, Knaus WA, Judson JA, et al: Patient selection for intensive care: A comparison of New Zealand and United States hospitals. *Crit Care Med* 16:318, 1988.

35. Oh TE, Hutchinson R, Short S, et al: Verification of the acute physiology and chronic health evaluation scoring system in a Hong Kong intensive care unit. *Crit Care Med* 21:698, 1993.

36. Sirio CA, Tajimi K, Tase C, et al: An initial comparison of intensive care in Japan and the United States. *Crit Care Med* 20:1207, 1992.

37. Levison MA, Zeigler D: Correlation of APACHE II score, drainage technique in outcome in postoperative intra-abdominal abscess. *Surg Gynecol Obstet* 172:89, 1991.

38. Ivatury RR, Nallathambi M, Rao PM, et al: Open management of the septic abdomen: Therapeutic and prognostic considerations based on APACHE II. *Crit Care Med* 17:511, 1989.

39. Wilson C, Heath DI, Imrie CW: Prediction of outcome in acute pancreatitis: A comparative study of APACHE II, clinical assessment and multiple factor scoring systems. *Br J Surg* 77:1260, 1990.

40. Larvin M, McMahon MJ: APACHE II score for assessment and monitoring of acute pancreatitis. *Lancet* 2:201, 1989.

41. Lemeshow S, Teres D, Avrunin JS, et al: A comparison of models to predict mortality of intensive care patients. *Crit Care Med* 15:715, 1987.

42. Scheld WM, Mandell GL: Nosocomial pneumonia: Pathogenesis and recent advances in diagnosis and therapy. *Rev Infect Dis* 13:S743, 1991.

43. Thorpe JE, Baughman RP, Farme PT, et al: Bronchoalveolar lavage for diagnosing acute bacterial pneumonia. *J Infect Dis* 155:855, 1987.

44. Knaus WA, Wagner DP, Draper EA, et al: The APACHE III prognostic system: Risk prediction of hospital mortality for critically ill hospitalized adults. *Chest* 100:1619, 1991.

45. Knaus WA, Wagner DP, Zimmerman JE, et al: Variations in mortality and length of stay in intensive care units. *Ann Intern Med* 118:753, 1993.

46. Le Gall JR, Lemeshow S, Saulnier F: SAPS II.

47. Lemeshow S, Teres D, Klar J, et al: MPM II: Mortality probability models based on 19124 patients. *JAMA* 1993.

48. Lemeshow S, Teres D. Pastides H, et al: A method for predicting survival and mortality of ICU patients using objectively derived weights. *Crit Care Med* 13:519, 1985.

49. Teres D, Lemeshow S, Avrunin JS: A validation of the mortality prediction model for ICU patients. *Crit Care Med* 15:208, 1987.

50. Lemeshow S, Klar J, Teres D, et al: ICU severity models at 48 and 72 hours. (Forthcoming)

51. Castella C, et al: Comparison of ICU severity models in the North American-European Study. (Forthcoming)

52. Castella C, Gilabet J, Torner F: Mortality prediction models in intensive care: Acute physiology and chronic health evaluation II and mortality prediction model compared. *Crit Care Med* 19:191, 1991.

53. Schafer JH, Maurer A, Jochimsen F, et al: Outcome prediction models on admission in a medical intensive care unit: Do they predict individual outcome? *Crit Care Med* 18:1111, 1990.

54. Teres D, Steingrub JS: Can intermediate care substitute for intensive care? *Crit Care Med* 15:280, 1987.

55. Teres D: Using severity-of-illness scores and probabilities to clinically categorize ICU patients: Pulmonary and critical care update. *Chest* 7:2, 1992.

56. Watts CM, Knaus WA: The case for using objective scoring systems to predict ICU outcome. *Crit Care Clin* 1994.

57. Teres D: Trends from the United States with end of life decisions in the intensive care unit. *Intensive Care Med* 19:316, 1993.

58. Smedira NG, Evans BH, Grais LS, et al: Withholding and withdrawal of life support from the critically ill. *N Engl J Med* 322:309, 1990.

59. Lemeshow S, Teres D, Avrunin, et al: Refining ICU outcome prediction by using changing probabilities of mortality. *Crit Care Med* 16:470, 1988.

60. Chang RWS, Jacobs S, Lee B: Predicting outcome among intensive care unit patients using computerized trend analysis of daily APACHE II scores corrected for organ system failure. *Intensive Care Med* 14:558, 1988.

61. Hannan EL, Kiburn H, O'Donnell JF, et al: Adult open heart surgery in New York State. *JAMA* 264:2768, 1990.

62. Ziegler EJ, Fisher CJ, Sprung CL, et al: Treatment of gram-negative bacteremia and septic shock with HA-1A human monoclonal antibody against endotoxin. *N Engl J Med* 324:429, 1991.

63. Warren HS, Danner RL, Munford RS: Anti-endotoxin monoclonal antibodies. *N Engl J Med* 326:1153, 1992.

64. Bone RC: Sepsis, the sepsis syndrome, multi-organ failure: A plea for comparable definitions. *Ann Intern Med* 114:332, 1991.

65. Teres D, Lemeshow S: Using severity measures to describe high performance ICUs. *Crit Care Clin* 1994.

66. Kassirer JP: The quality of care and the quality of measuring it. *N Engl J Med* 329:1263, 1993.

67. Rapoport J, Teres D, Lemeshow S, et al: A method for assessing the clinical performance and cost effectiveness of intensive care units. *Crit Care Med.*

68. Knaus WA, Draper EA, Wagner DP, et al: An evaluation of outcome from intensive care in major medical centers. *Ann Intern Med* 104:410, 1986.

69. Rapoport J, Teres D, Lemeshow S, et al: Explaining variability of cost using a severity of illness measure for ICU patients. *Med Care* 338, 1990.

70. Murry LS, Teasdale GM, Murray GD, et al: Does prediction of outcome alter patient management? *Lancet* 341:1487, 1993.

232. The Special Care Unit Committee

Daniel Teres and Sandra L. Turner

Introduction

Health care reform, by definition, mandates change: how services are delivered, how costs are controlled, how care is accessed, and finally, how quality outcomes are defined. To that end, it is imperative that critical care physicians and nurse managers assume a leadership role in the development of their critical care quality management programs. Only through direct involvement in the identification of meaningful indicators, interpretation and correlation of relevant data, and determination of critical care quality outcomes can the critical care leadership be in a position to set the standards that define quality critical care services [1,2]. To accomplish this, a well-structured quality management program must be established. This program should focus on the appropriateness, efficiency, and effectiveness of services rendered, establish benchmarks against comparable data over time, and continuously strive to improve processes. Development of such a program requires commitment, focus, understanding of total quality management (TQM) principles, collaboration, and leadership.

In this chapter, we review the necessary steps in the development, organization, and implementation of a critical care quality management program, and discuss the strengths and limitations of various elements of that program.

Organization

The Joint Commission on Accreditation of Healthcare Organizations (JCAHO) mandates that the activities of a multipurpose special care unit be coordinated by a multidisciplinary committee of the medical staff (JCAHO Standard SP 2.2) [3]. Ideally, the committee is recognized in the medical staff bylaws, and is identified as an "action body," which is afforded all the rights and responsibilities associated with this position. The organization of such a committee may vary tremendously depending on the size and complexity of the hospital. Typically, membership is made up of the physician director and nurse manager of each of the special care units (MICU, SICU, CCU, CSICU, PICU, NICU, PACU), the medical director of quality management, the nursing director(s) of the critical care units, and the chief of the critical care division, who also acts as chair of the committee. Although the emergency room is not designated as a special care unit, it makes sense to have representation from the emergency medicine department's quality improvement program.

In some settings, it may not be appropriate to have a critical care physician as the overall coordinator. Oversight by a more neutral individual may have some advantages if that person has a commitment to develop a quality improvement program and the leadership skills to provide followthrough. It is important to ensure that the most capable individual is selected to chair the committee.

In full-service hospitals, it may appear that combining pediatric and adult special care units would be especially cumbersome, since the problems in neonatal, perinatal, and pediatric units may be quite dissimilar from those encountered in coronary care and adult intensive care units. Furthermore, physicians and nurses in the pediatric units do not have a daily working relationship with those in the adult units. Nevertheless, issues related to admission and discharge polices, development of collaborative indicators, and interpersonal conflicts are similar in both pediatric and adult units.

There is an additional problem of coordination in major tertiary centers, where there are multiple organ- and department-specific special care units. In community hospitals, medical, surgical, and anesthesia subspecialists are likely to be comfortable working together to develop and use a quality improvement program. In major university academic centers, there are well developed departmental structures in place that make an interdepartmental committee important but also more problematic. There is the additional problem of sheer size in trying to coordinate multiple specialty intensive care units. In such a setting, a small overall coordinating group would fulfill the JCAHO requirement but would lose the impact of peer pressure that pertains when unit medical directors present their quality improvement findings before other unit medical directors. Another advantage of a true multipurpose special care unit committee is the ability to evaluate movement of patients through the hospital, for example from the emergency room to the medical ICU, to the operating room to the post-anesthesia care unit, to the surgical intensive care unit and to a surgical intermediate care (step-down) unit. An evaluation of each site, as well as the transfers between sites, can identify systematic problems, gaps in communication, and issues related to the care of individual patients.

Nonvoting members, who may provide support for this committee, include the department of quality improvement coordinators assigned to the critical care areas, the administrative director of medical records and quality management, and the manager of medical staff services. Invited guests often include the special care unit quality improvement nurses who participate with the unit's leadership in the presentation of unit reports.

The committee must meet at least quarterly, but should meet monthly; the workload requires it. Each leadership team provides regularly scheduled reports to the committee for review and recommendations. Elements of the formal presentation include, but are not limited to, these reports:

Summary of departmental mortality reviews, with specific details on egregious cases
Focused audit results
Summary of morbidity and sentinel events, again with focus on egregious cases
Status of collaborative indicator results, with trend analyses
Status of outstanding issues
Status of Nursing Studies, with trend analyses

In all cases, the reports mirror the information presented to the respective departmental quality improvement committees. The departmental quality improvement committee, however, reviews data on a case-by-case basis; the special care unit committee reviews data specific to the special care units in the aggregate, focusing on *multidisciplinary* trends and patterns.

Horizontal/Vertical Reporting Structure

The physician directors of the special care units are also reporting members of their respective departmental quality improvement committees. This insures that a horizontal communication link exists on an ongoing basis between the clinical departments and the special care unit committee. A horizontal communication link with the nursing quality review board is similarly accomplished through the joint reporting of collaborative indicators to the special care unit committee and the nursing quality review board by the special care unit quality improvement nurse representative. Finally, the special care unit committee chair strives to keep appropriate hospital and medical staff committees apprised of pertinent issues and recommendations identified by the committee while, at the same time, seeking guidance and support as necessary.

There are three potential problems with the horizontal reporting structure. First, in most medical staff bylaws, the duly authorized responsibility for quality improvement fits into a departmental structure along with its support mechanisms. Aside from the application of TQM principles, it is unclear how to reduce parallel or duplicate activities and there is the potential for a strong special care unit quality program to conflict or disagree with the departmental assessment. The usual quality improvement structure is ill-equipped to handle these divisive issues. The special care unit committee should not compete with the departmental mechanism, but, rather, should primarily abstract from their findings for trend analyses. On the other hand, the special care units should continue to identify issues and ask for broad consensus on significant concerns, such as interdepartmental credentialing.

Second, the traditional approach for evaluating and handling quality of care concerns is through a case-by-case review within the departmental quality improvement committee. This method of case review plus secondary evaluation is often tedious, time consuming, excessively deliberative, and too limited in focus. Since each department has somewhat different guidelines and rituals, evaluating a case or sentinel event that crosses individual department boundaries can be troublesome and difficult to resolve even at the level of the departmental chairs. The philosophy that "dirty laundry" should be exposed only *within* the walls of the department is not easily discarded. Thus, interdepartmental case review or policy resolution does not fit into an easily accepted mold or format. The special care unit committee, by definition, straddles these territorial landmines. Although there are many common areas for collaboration and consensus-building, there also are limitations that can be divisive.

The third concern with a horizontal reporting structure relates to the ability to "close the loop." It is sometimes difficult to bring an issue to resolution when the "power bases" are perceived as equal. Fortunately, the move to TQM will diminish this kind of thinking.

There should exist a vertical reporting structure that mandates quarterly and annual reporting of the activities of the special care unit committee to the hospital-wide medical quality improvement committee (MQIC). The MQIC reports its findings to the executive committee of the medical staff and the professional affairs committee of the board of trustees. In this manner, there is an opportunity to have the activities, issues, and concerns of the special care unit committee communicated (and documented) at the highest levels of the organization (Figs. 232-1 and 232-2). Of course, there may be some issues that should be handled on an ad hoc basis, through a special select committee. Other issues may be handled best primarily through

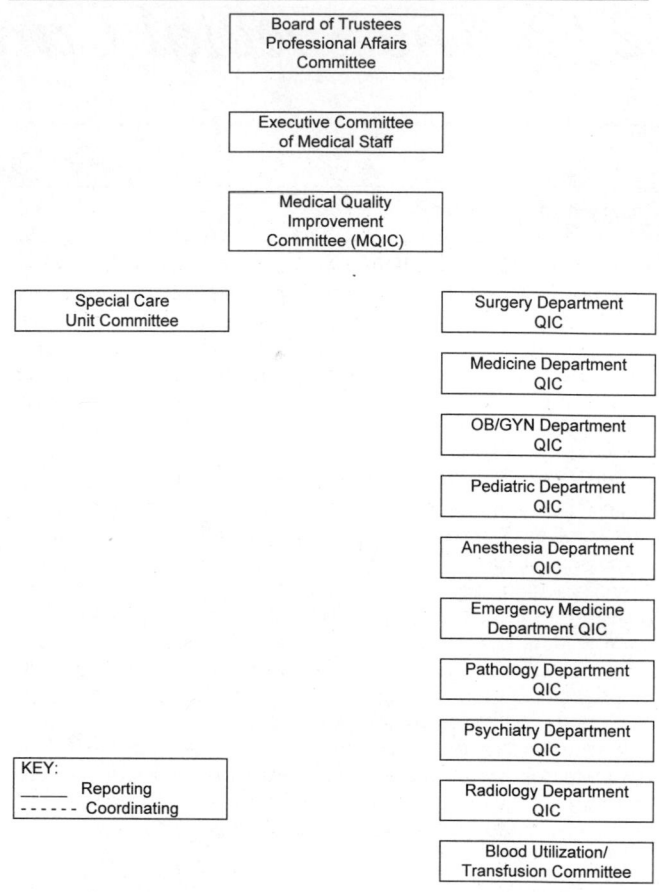

Fig. 232-1. Special Care Unit Committee Organizational Chart

departmental structures. Cases related to a substandard clinical practice pattern of an individual physician must be handled with full adherence to medical staff bylaws and with full attention paid to due process and fairness. At the same time, the process must seek to protect patients. Other issues (e.g., personality conflicts, charges of physical or sexual harassment, conflicts in care, abandonment, stress-related behavior problems, failure to respond to telephone and beeper pages during major patient changes and emergencies, drug-related and other disabilities) must be handled with great care, ensuring full investigation (following departmental or hospital procedures) and strict confidentiality.

The Mission Statement and Committee Responsibilities

The development of an effective, focused, well structured special care unit committee is not an accidental event. It requires vision and preparation and begins when the committee members reach consensus on the mission statement. Briefly, the mission of the special care unit committee should be to oversee the quality of care that each patient receives upon transfer *into*, *within*, and *out* of those areas organized as special care units. Inherent in this concept are the following responsibilities of the committee:

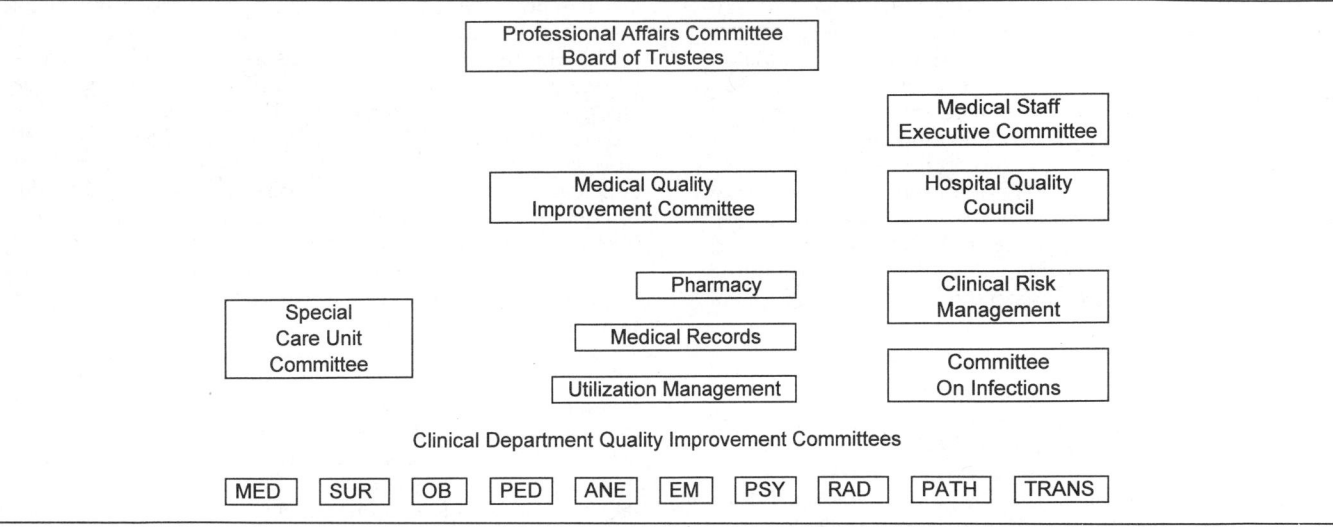

Fig. 232-2. Medical Staff Quality Improvement Reporting Structure

1. To develop, monitor, and evaluate the collaborative indicators that focus on components of care offered by the team of professionals operating within and between units
2. To monitor and evaluate patient management issues and identify patterns and trends relevant to all aspects of patient care
3. To review and approve select policies and procedures associated with the operating of the special care units
4. To assure open and effective horizontal and vertical communication between and among the special care units and within the organization
5. To act on recommendations of the committee to effect positive change

Clearly the work of the committee is much more complex and burdensome than one might first imagine. It is no small task to coordinate the eclectic needs and concerns of varied, multipurpose special care unit managers and directors, focus members on common issues, and provide sufficient time to discuss problems thoroughly, report findings, and make recommendations. Committee meetings must be well planned and well executed. Committee minutes must be prepared thoughtfully so as to provide a trackable record of pertinent discussion points, conclusions, recommendations, actions, evaluations, and follow-up [4,5].

The Joint Commission on Accreditation of Healthcare Organizations Standards

Compliance with the JCAHO standards relevant to special care units is a significant component of the work of the special care unit committee. The committee members must stay current in their knowledge of quality improvement standards for special care units and medical staff. The members must work within the committee structure to assure complete and accurate application of these standards. In particular, the committee members must address themselves to these standards, which historically have proven troublesome. At the same time, the members must assume a leadership role in the implementation of the latest standards. At a minimum, all members of the committee should be able to answer "yes" to the following questions:

Is there a process for implementing new techniques and procedures?
Are the responsibilities of the medical director clearly delineated?
Do medical staff and nursing staff coverage meet the special care needs of the patients?
Are staff appropriately educated/trained to supervise/care for special care unit patients and is that capability routinely assessed and documented?
Is there appropriate orientation for new employees/staff/trainees?
Are there effective written criteria for admission to, discharge from, triage within, and transfer out of the special care units?
Are there clearly delineated privileges for those physicians functioning within the special care units?
Have standards been established that determine when the services of a qualified specialist (consultant) are required?
Is there documentation of age-appropriate care?
Are all policies and procedures reviewed and updated on an annual basis?
Are committee members satisfied with the safety management program for the special care units?
Is there an ongoing planned and systematic process for monitoring, evaluating, and improving care?
Is the quality improvement process fully documented, reflecting identification of patterns and trends, actions taken, and conclusions reached, with documentation of the rationale for those conclusions? [4-8]

If the committee members are not current in their thinking and consistent in their answers regarding these questions, then the committee is not meeting its basic responsibilities.

While the special care unit committee strives to assure compliance with the standards of the JCAHO, it also must insure compliance with its own organizational policies and procedures. At the same time, the committee must also address the ever-evolving guidelines of appropriate specialty medical and nursing societies [9,10]. This issue has become so complex that the American Medical Association has developed and disseminated a "Directory of Practice Parameters" to provide information on approximately 1500 practice guidelines [11]. Additionally, the American Hospital Association also has produced a guidebook to help hospitals understand and use practice guidelines [12]. Requiring regularly scheduled updates regarding the application of current standards and proposed guidelines to be a standing agenda item will go far to ensure that standards are current and consistently followed. Without this self-imposed structure, the likelihood of successfully completing an unannounced survey is questionable. More important, without regular updates, the ability to consistently provide the highest quality care will be jeopardized.

Policies and Procedures

Rewriting policies and procedures in a uniform fashion for several or multiple special care units is a daunting task. It is likely that some units will have sketchy, limited, or even outdated policies and procedures. For instance, it would be surprising for a post-anesthesia care unit to have a statement about triage that is as well developed as the one for the adult multipurpose ICU. When policies are reviewed side-by-side, there may be obvious contradictory statements. In these situations, the special care unit committee must take responsibility. The special care unit committee should review admission, discharge, triage, and transfer policies to ensure clarity and consistency among units. In addition, there may be well thought out policies in one unit, such as methods for resolving conflicts or ensuring appropriate consultation, which could be incorporated into other units.

The JCAHO requirement for annual review of policies increasingly focuses on more quantitative criteria and priorities for admission to the critical care unit. For patients with myocardial infarction (MI), this could mean a hierarchy of priorities for admission as follows: anterior MI > non-Q wave inferior MI > atypical chest pain and no ECG changes (Table 232-1). It also could mean that there is a similar hierarchy in the emergency department and coronary care unit for administering thrombolysis in a timely and safe manner.

For situations when high census exceeds physical space and/or qualified nursing, the responsibilities and authority for triage must be clearly delineated. This is also an opportunity to review

actual or potential areas of cooperation. If the CCU has available beds, they should be able to accept a surgical patient from the PACU who has chest pain and nonspecific ECG changes when the surgical ICU is at capacity. The ultimate authority for discharge and triage usually rests with the unit medical director or the chair of the special care unit committee. It is too often the case that the charge nurse identifies the impending excess patient load, and then initiates telephone calls to various attending physicians to see if it is all right to transfer a particular patient. It is inappropriate to have the medical director function only when the system is in complete gridlock. It is likewise unacceptable if the medical director or designee is unavailable at night to resolve conflicts or be active in triage [13]. Bed utilization should be governed by medical benefit and medical suitability, not by pressure or power [14]. Indeed, failure to provide elementary triage has been the basis for a hospital malpractice suit [15]. Inappropriate triage raises concerns about subtle aspects of discrimination against classes of patients or those with certain types of diseases. Among patients with similarly poor risk of long-term mortality, patients with advanced cirrhosis are more likely to have a do not resuscitate order than are patients with end-stage congestive heart failure with very low ejection fraction. There are also hospital and physician politics that can overrule the authority of the ICU triage officers [16] (Table 232-2).

IDENTIFICATION OF INDICATORS. The identification and development of clinical indicators is perhaps the single most important undertaking of the special care unit committee. Without meaningful indicators, the committee will drift aimlessly from meeting to meeting, failing to recognize potential problematic issues, failing to make timely interventions, and most significantly, failing to weave together the necessary elements for successful pattern analysis and resolution. As a result, the committee's ability to progress effectively and expeditiously to resolve issues of quality will be severely impaired.

There are several components of the process that are worth noting. First, the indicators should relate to important aspects of care especially when an opportunity for improvement clearly exists. For instance, the occasional sentinel event (development of a bed sore in a coronary care unit patient) does not merit consideration as an indicator when one reflects on the greater importance of other aspects of coronary care, such as pain management or the effectiveness and safety of thrombolytic administration. On the other hand, other sentinel events, such as the inadvertent extubation of a patient receiving a continuous infusion of a neuromuscular blocking drug or a pulmonary

Table 232-1. Examples of CCU Admission Criteria

Level I:
1. Strongly suspected acute myocardial infarction with no other severe life-shortening conditions
    A. Chest pain consistent with cardiac origin of > 20 minutes duration
    B. S–T elevation or depression > 1.0 mV in 2 or more contiguous ECG leads
2. Ventricular arrhythmias, bradycardia (HR < 40) requiring titrated IV antiarrhythmic therapy or electric cardioversion
3. Neurologically intact postcardiac arrest patients
Level II:
1. Strongly suspected myocardial infarction in the presence of other known severe life-shortening conditions
2. Unstable angina
Level III:
1. Selected postcardiac surgical patients
2. Postoperative surgical patients, vascular or other "clean" cases as ICU overflow

Table 232-2. Examples of ICU Triage Criteria

Patients who fail to respond to intensive care therapy and who are considered unsalvageable. (Evidence of discussion with the family must be included in the medical record.)

Patients who meet criteria for brain death will remain in the Intensive Care Unit pending organ procurement or discontinuation of mechanical ventilation.

If full criteria for brain death are not met, the patient may be triaged out of the ICU to a general unit where mechanical ventilation may or may not be continued.

In periods of high census (ICU/Hospital) the triage of patients into and out of the ICU will be determined by the triage officer. Elective admissions will be suspended. All surgical cases previously booked and in progress will be evaluated by the triage officer (with the medical director of the operating room).

artery rupture from a pulmonary artery catheter being inserted by an unsupervised intern, should trigger an investigation, review of policies, and even a collaborative indicator study.

Second, it should be recognized that there will be wide diversity regarding important issues from different units. Thus, issues will be different in a neonatal unit (retinopathy of prematurity) as compared to a neurosurgical unit (eye care for comatose patients). Generally speaking, an indicator should be followed for twelve consecutive months unless or until the indicator no longer provides meaningful data. When presented to an audience of special care unit directors and quality improvement personnel, the validity and significance of the indicator, the threshold, and the interpretation of the quality of the data will be challenged regularly. Still, this open format is advantageous and should be viewed as such by a JCAHO surveyor.

Third, the indicators should be *collaborative:* The definition specifically relates to the physician and the nurse. The Society of Critical Care Medicine (SCCM) and the American Association of Critical Care Nurses (AACCN) have issued a joint statement on the coequal status of the unit's medical and nursing leadership [17]. Collaborative indicators are a real test of this policy. What happens if the physician chooses to define the indicator, then expects the nurses to collect and to analyze the data? At the least, the physician should participate in the analysis and both nurse and physician should present the findings. If other special care unit presenters have forged a truly collaborative program it will become evident at the formal presentation. It is also important that the indicator contain some component that is nursing oriented. An evaluation of postoperative bleeding in cardiac surgery patients, while interesting and important, does not contain many nurse-related issues.

It is unclear who should be primarily involved in data collection. Generally speaking, study participation (and outcome analysis) is most effective when both the medical and nursing staff are interested in researching a particular issue. The data forms cannot be overly complex: responses that require a "yes" or "no" answer work best. (Yes/No answers take less time, and lend themselves to clarity of thought in collection, entry, and analysis of data.) It is also important to consider the costs associated with data collection. It could be expensive to have the quality improvement nurses collect all of the components of the data set, if timeliness of access and follow-up are an issue. (A more detailed discussion of the issues involved in quality of the data is presented in Chapter 231.)

To make the indicator program *surveyable*, there should be a final step of analysis of each indicator. Results should be plotted based on quarterly findings. A report including conclusions, recommendations, actions, and continuing follow-up/evaluation should be documented in the committee minutes.

The JCAHO defines a clinical indicator as a "quantitative measure that can be used as a guide to monitor and evaluate the quality of important patient care and support service activities" [18]. It is worth remembering that indicators by and of themselves do not directly measure quality. Rather, indicators are actually performance "screens" designed to flush out situations worthy of further study. The more time and effort that is spent in the effective utilization and refinement of clinical indicators, the more meaningful, and measurable, are the data collected. For an excellent reference on the development, testing, and application of clinical indicators, please refer to the JCAHO's *Primer on Clinical Indicator Development and Application* [19].

An indicator by itself has limited applicability. For an indicator to be truly useful, it must be monitored, plotted, and analyzed quarterly, and whenever possible, applied as a benchmark for comparison against past results for the same indicator

within the institution, other institutions, and established national standards of practice. With increasing availability of national databases being promoted, more useful benchmarking may be achievable.

Indicators that are rate-based are particularly useful for making the shift from a focus on individual cases to a focus on patterns of care. Using statistical process control theory and run rules, the committee can readily identify meaningful variations from the norm, and quickly focus attention to significant issues. Such a shift is in keeping with the move to TQM and away from the negative implications of the individual case review. With the burgeoning of interest in the measurement of outcomes there is an increasing number of tested and reliable indicators available for use. As part of its Agenda for Change, the JCAHO has already developed several Beta indicators that are currently being implemented and may become mandatory JCAHO standards by 1996 [20].

In addition, numerous state hospital associations, health care organizations, medical and nursing societies, and health service researchers are also focusing on the development of practice guidelines, critical pathways, and outcome indicators that will ultimately be used to measure and compare performance among institutions, and against established standards [20,21,22]. With all this activity, it is prudent for the special care unit committee to research what is already developed, determine what is applicable to their own needs and interests, and then capitalize on reasonable opportunities to utilize established indicators whenever possible. Benchmarking against raw data, however, is not enough; the committee also must focus on the *processes* that lead to improvements, and be fully prepared to respond to the variances in the data through an objective and clearly defined program of analysis. Examples of indicators commonly in use may be found on Table 232-2.

One common indicator is unplanned readmission to the ICU. On the surface this would seem like a logical collaborative indicator. Did the patient meet medical and nursing criteria for transfer during the first admission? Did the patient return because of a new complication or because of an extension of a previously identified problem? Was the initial admission elective or emergency? Was the readmission within 48 hours or much later? There are different concerns when an indicator becomes a mandatory benchmark. Consider an ICU that has a high threshold for admitting high risk postoperative patients for monitoring. If a patient at that institution develops congestive heart failure (CHF) while on a "regular" unit and is then transferred to ICU, the patient will be recorded as having had a single ICU admission. In another hospital, the policy may be to admit such patients for overnight monitoring in the ICU. If a patient at this second hospital is admitted to the ICU, transferred

Table 232-3. Example of Indicator Studies

Severity-adjusted hospital mortality of pediatric ICU patients (PRISM)

Severity-adjusted hospital mortality of MICU/SICU patients

Unanticipated complication resulting in measurable clinical sequelae

Readmission to ICU within 48 hours

Unplanned special care transfer

Unplanned return to OR from ICU

Self-extubation

Timing and complications of thrombolytic therapy for patients with myocardial infarct

Adequacy of sedation for patients on neuromuscular blocking drugs

Indication for placing pulmonary artery catheters in PACU

to the ward, and readmitted to the ICU on day two after mobilizing postoperative "third space" fluid developing CHF, the case will be recorded as a readmission. The ICU will be "charged" with a higher rate of readmission, when, in reality, the problem was delay by the floor team in identifying CHF and treating it more promptly.

It is possible to have a very low readmission rate by keeping ICU patients longer, but such a policy would imply poor use of ICU resources. A very high readmission rate might reflect a high ICU census, excess triage, or limited intermediate or step-down capability. The point to remember is that in analyzing and reporting benchmark data, a thorough understanding of the *processes* involved is critical.

Hotline Program

In an effort to expand the methods of reporting quality of care issues, and, at the same time, to create an environment conducive to TQM, the authors initiated a high-intensity quality improvement referral and resource program. This pilot program was designed with two objectives in mind: (1) Provide a highly visible mechanism for rapid identification of issues; and (2) Provide an opportunity at the bedside for staff participation and education, relevant to quality improvement initiatives. This trial program became known as the ICU Quality Improvement "Hotline Program." The goals of the Hotline Program were to define the scope of issues in a given special care unit, distinguish quality improvement issues from other issues, and distinguish hospital system issues from patient management issues. This program was the first major initiative of our hospital's newly formed special care unit committee.

The methodology for achieving the above objectives was specific. Each of the special care areas participated in an intensive 1-week program, which included a preplanning session, a 3-day on-site assessment, and a summary session. First the quality improvement coordinator met with the physician director and nurse manager of each unit to review the Hotline Program. For the next 3 days, the quality improvement coordinator was available in the special care unit to act as a resource for the staff, share in the identification of issues, and aid in the determination of processes for resolution. At the same time, the chair of the special care unit committee visited the area, engaging staff at all levels in focused discussions regarding unit issues. A dedicated Hotline page number was established to ensure ongoing prioritization of unit issues and staff needs beyond the 3 days. This high-profile interface, combined with a strong commitment from the unit's medical and nursing leadership to address all identified issues, were key elements leading to the ultimate success of the program.

The impetus for the Hotline Program came from members of the special care unit committee, who expressed concerns about underreporting of issues. Committee members concluded that existing reporting mechanisms were unknown or confusing to some staff; there was an element of distrust among staff with regard to the reporting structures; the reporting of issues was not considered a priority of the staff; and there was skepticism among staff that the reporting of issues actually led to resolution of issues. With unanimous support from the committee members, a proposal for the initiation of the Hotline Program, as developed by the department of quality improvement, was approved.

Given the concerns expressed by the committee, it was clear that for the proposal to be a success, it would require significant preparation and follow through. Failure to satisfactorily address any one of the identified individual patient care concerns could lead to the failure of the entire program. A critical first step was the selection of the first special care unit to participate in the program. The criteria for selection were the following: evidence that the unit physician director and nurse manager considered the program to have high priority; commitment from the unit leadership to correct identified problems; and finally, a genuine enthusiasm for the project by the unit's leadership. Selection of the appropriate quality improvement coordinator for each unit was also critical. It required an individual knowledgeable in TQM concepts and in critical care, and who also possessed excellent interpersonal skills and teaching abilities.

Once the unit and coordinator were matched, the preplanning session was scheduled. At this time, the physician director and nurse manager were fully briefed on the role of management, the role of the coordinator, and the goals and strategies of the program. On the first of the 3 interface days, time was scheduled for the quality improvement coordinator to meet with the special care unit staff. At this point, instruction was given on the concepts of TQM. It was emphasized that TQM was not a punitive process (pitting staff against management); rather, the focus was on continuous quality improvement with a patient care perspective. The various reporting mechanisms, the confidentiality policy, and the process of follow-up were reviewed. Emphasis was placed on the importance of the involvement of staff in order to accomplish any meaningful change. It also was emphasized that all perceived issues were worthy of review.

At the completion of each unit interface, the quality improvement coordinator produced a summary of all identified issues for review by the unit manager, the unit medical director, and the chair of the special care unit committee. From this review, it was expected that an action plan would be developed. It was planned that the chair of the special care unit committee would meet with the vice president and administrative director for each particular area. Because of the positive energy generated by this process, there was a strong commitment to correct all identified issues.

In a period of 4 months, eight specific special care units completed this process. More than 90 patient care and system issues were identified. While the majority of issues were systematic issues, the range of issues was staggering. Multiple "hidden" issues surfaced. "Hidden" issues were defined as those that had been long tolerated and had come to be accepted as the norm. These hidden issues had led to a situation of "learned helplessness." We learned it was imperative that a tracking system be established to assure that no issue was overlooked. Issues were tracked monthly and were reported and monitored through the special care unit committee, the medical quality improvement committee, and, ultimately, the board of trustees.

Through the combined efforts of the quality assessment department and the special care unit leadership, 90 percent of the issues identified have been resolved. The remaining 10 percent continue to be addressed and are in various stages of resolution. No issue has been lost to follow-up.

In addition to meeting the original goals and objectives of the Hotline Program, multiple secondary gains also have been realized. A renewed spirit of collaboration has been achieved through the sharing of issues and concerns at the special care unit committee meetings. Attendance and participation at these meetings have been significantly strengthened and a greater willingness to bring issues to the table has been identified. The "commitment to correct" by unit and hospital leadership has better positioned staff to move from a quality improvement focus to a total quality management focus. The interface between and among the special care units, including emergency services, also has been strengthened. Finally, a number of prospective indicators have been identified.

As the cycle of tracking, reporting, and bringing to closure identified primary and secondary issue continues, staff and leadership alike are becoming more proficient (and more comfortable) in working together to identify and resolve issues in the true TQM tradition. What began as an attempt to simply identify issues has evolved into a broad-based educational experience in the process and implementation of a TQM program. As a result, the outcome is a more methodological and comprehensive approach to problem solving that focuses on improved patient care.

Analysis of Quality Assessment Hotline Items

The issues uncovered through the Hotline Program were as varied as they were numerous. Identified concerns reflected an array of issues, such as addressograph/printer repair delays, unacceptable turnaround times for "stat" reports, inappropriate removal of name tags, lack of appropriate beds, and sentinel patient care problems (Table 232-4). As issues were identified and corrective actions were taken, events were categorized as either systemic or patient-focused issues; then the issues were tracked over time. Trend analyses revealed that the majority of the issues were systemic issues, related to the *process* of care. Results of the trend analyses identified nine "hard to resolve" issues, which affected most, if not all, special care units (Table 232-5).

As a result of this process, multiple initiatives have been undertaken. The Hospital Quality Council authorized two organization-wide TQM Projects, which specifically addressed concerns identified by the special care unit committee. A proposal for a progressive care ICU was developed and approved. A revised and expanded policy regarding placement of ventilator-dependent patients was established. Resolution of transport problems became a reality with the establishment of a Transport Task Force. Remaining issues continue to be addressed through the activities of the special care unit committee and its subcommittees or have become nonissues through coincident parallel initiatives.

The importance of addressing these issues goes beyond the obvious. Through the Hotline Program, the committee was able

Table 232-4. Examples of Hotline Issues

Environmental safety issues:
    Equipment/unit alarm limitations
    Pediatric furniture safety concerns
Practice issues:
    Sentinel events
    Lack of policy/procedure compliance
    Over/under utilization of services
Equipment limitations:
    Availability
    Functionality
In-hospital transfer issues:
    Delays
    Service coordination issues
    Communication failures

Table 232-5. Hard to Resolve Issues

Placement of stable ventilator patients
Fluctuating SCU bed capacity
Role of attending, consult, intensivist
Delays (e.g., reports, consults, equipment)
Communication failures
Triage: high census
Transfer problems (out of hospital)
Monitoring of MD privileges
Conflicts with consultants: M.D.: M.D./R.N.: M.D.
Communication problems with patient movement to another unit

to clearly *focus* its energies to achieve meaningful outcomes in a timely and effective manner. As a result, the committee has achieved a new level of recognition within the organization and within its own membership. The momentum generated from this approach has done much to empower the committee membership, and the behaviors associated with the phenomenon of "learned helplessness" are minimal.

Trend Analysis: Administrative Action

During the lively discussion that ensues from a substantive report, there exists the possibility that a situation will be unmasked which may require prompt administrative action by the committee. At times it is obvious to the presenter that corrective action should be taken. However, there may be issues presented that require a more global administrative action, especially if the standard approach has not worked. For example, if the issue is that cardiac surgery patients are being transported directly to the cardiac surgery unit without proper labeling of vasoactive infusions, then the problem goes beyond the purview of the cardiac special care unit. This issue involves the pharmacy, the operating room, the anesthesia department, and the cardiac surgery division—areas not directly under the jurisdiction of the special care unit. One mechanism to address this issue is for the special care unit committee to deliver an administrative directive or ultimatum. Although it may be unclear whether the special care unit committee chair has the authority to make such a directive, the various components of the hospital will probably respond promptly and positively.

The special care unit committee has another responsibility: to collate all of the studies and reports into comprehensive trend analyses. This task is difficult to perform. One concern is whether results of the collaborative indicators and morbidity/mortality reviews are perceived as a concrete way of complying with JCAHO standards in order to meet survey requirements. Another issue is the ability to effectively evaluate "real" quality improvement. One approach would be to ask "What are the real problems?"; "What are the weaknesses?"; and "Where is there opportunity for improvement?" Many of these issues are inherent in the running of a complex medical system such as a special care unit. There are special problems in teaching hospitals with various levels of house staff who are overwhelmed with the physical and emotional stresses of working in an ICU [23]. In addition, communication is complicated by the need to coordinate the care among multiple providers, including the primary attending physician, the persons who provide the concurrent titrated medical care (i.e., the intensivists, house officers, physician assistants, and nurse practitioners), the multiple consultants who provide advice, and the bedside nurses. In many settings, the attending tries to coordinate care by telephone. In some units, consultants can write orders relevant to their subspecialty without any comprehensive coordination.

The problems are magnified when a patient moves to another unit where many of the members of the team change. Another complicating factor is that various medical groups read different literature, have different biases, and remember different anecdotes. Some practitioners rely on the "last" case remembered or read little literature and seem stuck in a practice pattern learned when they did their training. It is hoped that the movement toward practice guidelines, evidence-based medicine, comparative databases, and more formal decision-analysis techniques will help critical care units reach consensus on acceptable versus outlier patterns of care. Board certified intensive care specialists are crucial to provide overall coordination on a concurrent care, rather than consultative, basis. The identification and understanding of what constitutes a high-performance critical care unit by lower observed-to-expected mortality, by lower observed-to-expected resource consumption, and a collaborative management style will help support the direction of the special care unit committee [24].

Conclusion

The purposes of this chapter have been to focus the special care unit leadership on the roles and responsibilities of the special care unit committee, to offer a plan of action to assess the current function and purpose of the committee, and to provide guidance in determining the committee's future direction. Clearly there is no one model that will meet the needs and interests of every special care unit committee. It is hoped that the authors have provided the fabric necessary to construct a workable structure. It is left to the committee members to ensure the fit, function, and durability of their committee.

With health care reform on the horizon and the JCAHO Agenda for Change continuing to develop, this truly is an exciting (and perilous) time in health care. Never before have so many divergent groups been so clearly focused on the issues related to the cost and quality of health care. At the same time, never has it been more critical for administrators and clinicians to collaborate, to define, and to quantify meaningful indicators of quality *on which they can agree*. The shift in focus to outcome measurement, while laudable, brings with it a plethora of new concerns. Will national data sources that provide an opportunity to benchmark against comparable institutions continue to protect the confidentiality of individual hospitals? How do we ensure data obtained from nationally established indicators are accurately and fairly interpreted? Will the indicators, in fact, be valid and reliable? With the overwhelming onslaught of practice parameters and clinical indicators in development, how do we effectively assimilate that which is most meaningful to our particular institution? Which software product will best support the institution's needs for data entry and analysis? Needless to say, the effectiveness and strength of the special care unit committee in addressing these issues is linked directly to the committee's understanding of, and commitment to, TQM. The more familiar and current the committee is in its thinking, the more critical and accurate will be the membership in its ongoing assessment of health care reform initiatives. Most important, the credibility of the assessments and recommendations set forth by the special care unit committee will have a

direct bearing on the strength of its voice in the future within the institution, within its specialty societies, and within the nation.

References

1. Cerra FB: Health care reform: The role of coordinated critical care. *Crit Care Med* 21:457, 1993.
2. Merry MD: Physician leadership for the 21st century. *Quality Management in Health Care* 1:31, 1993.
3. *1993 Accreditation Manual for Hospitals.* Vol. I, Oakbrook Terrace, IL. Joint Commission on Accreditation of Healthcare Organizations, 1993.
4. Goodwin ST: *CRAF Minutes Format.* Humana 1993.
5. *1993 Accreditation Manual for Hospitals.* Vol. II, Oakbrook Terrace, IL, Joint Commission on Accreditation of Healthcare Organizations, 1993.
6. Gardiner, WC: Documenting JCAHO standards in assigning nursing staff. *JHQ* 14:50, 1992.
7. Luce, JM: Improving the quality and utilization of critical care. *QRB* 17:42, 1992.
8. Jones L, Strandness DE: Integrating research activities, practice changes, and monitoring and evaluation: A model for academic health centers. *QRB* 17:229, 1991.
9. Guidelines Committee, Society of Critical Care Medicine: Guidelines for granting privileges for the performance of procedures in critically ill patients. *Crit Care Med* 21:292, 1993.
10. International Task Force on Safety in the Intensive Care Unit: International standards for safety in the intensive care unit. *Crit Care Med* 21:453, 1993.
11. *Directory of Practice Parameters, Titles, Sources, and Update.* Chicago, American Medical Association, 1993.
12. *Clinical Practice Guidelines.* Chicago, American Hospital Association, 1992.
13. Strosberg MA, Teres D, Fein IA, et al: Nursing perception of the availability of the intensive care unit medical director for triage and conflict resolution. *Heart Lung* 19:452, 1990.
14. Teres D: Civilian triage in the ICU: The ritual of the last bed. *Crit Care Med* 21:598, 1993.
15. *Von Stetina v. Florida Medical Center,* 436 So. 2d 1022 (Fla. 1993), 10 Fla. L. Weekly 286 (Fla., May 24, 1985)
16. Marshall MF, Schwenzer KJ, Orsina M, et al: The influence of political power, medical provincialism and economic incentives on the rationing of surgical intensive care unit beds. *Crit Care Med* 20:387, 1992.
17. *Collaborative Practice Model: The Organization of Human Resources in Critical Care Units.* Newport Beach, CA, American Association of Critical Care Nurses, 1982.
18. Joint Commission on Accreditation of Healthcare Organizations: *QRB* 15:57, 1989.
19. *Primer on Clinical Indicator Development and Application.* Oakbrook Terrace, IL, Joint Commission on Accreditation of Healthcare Organizations, 1990.
20. *The Quality Agenda: 1993 Update.* Vol. 4, Washington DC, AMHS Institute, 1993.
21. Hudson T: Clinical quality initiatives: The search for meaningful—and accurate—measures. *Hospitals* 66:26, 1992.
22. Lemeshow S, Teres D, Klar J, et al: Mortality probability models based on 19124 ICU patients. *JAMA* 1993.
23. Zussman R: *Intensive Care: Medical Ethics and the Medical Profession.* Chicago, University of Chicago Press, 1992.
24. Teres D, Lemeshow S: Using severity measures to describe high performance intensive care units. *Crit Care Clin* 9:543, 1993.

Suggested Readings

The Quality Agenda: 1993 Update. Vol. 4, Washington DC, AMHS Institute, 1993.

Batalden PB: Building knowledge for quality improvement in health care: An introductory glossary. *JQA* 1991.

Berwick DM: Peer review and quality management: Are they compatible? *QRB* 16:246, 1990.

Blumenthal D: Total quality management and physicians' clinical decisions. *JAMA* 269:2775, 1993.

Burns L, et al: The use of continuous quality improvement methods in the development and dissemination of medical practice guidelines. *QRB* 18:434, 1992.

Cerra FB: Health care reform: The role of coordinated critical care. *Critical Care in Health Care Reform* 21:457, 1993.

Coffey RJ, et al: An introduction to critical paths. *Quality Management in Health Care* 1:45, 1992.

Coleman RL: The use of decision analysis in quality assessment. *QRB* 15:383, 1989.

Davis JW, et al: An analysis of errors causing morbidity and mortality in a trauma system: A guide for quality improvement. *J Trauma* 32:660, 1992.

Friedmann P, Selbovitz L: Continuous quality improvement and physician training. *Quality Management in Health Care* 1:13, 1992.

Goodwin ST: *CRAF Minutes Format, A Learner's Guide.* Humana, 1992.

Groeger JS, et al: Descriptive analysis of critical care units in the United States: Patient characteristics and intensive care unit utilization. *Crit Care Med* 21:279, 1993.

Guidelines Committee, Society of Critical Care Medicine: Guidelines for granting privileges for the performance of procedures in critically ill patients. *Crit Care Med* 21:292, 1993.

Hudson T: Clinical quality initiatives: The search for meaningful—and accurate—measures. *Hospitals* 66:26, 1992.

Iezzoni LI: Using severity information for quality assessment: A review of three cases by five severity measures. *QRB* 15:367, 1989.

International Task Force on Safety in the Intensive Care Unit: International standards for safety in the intensive care unit. *Crit Care Med* 21:453, 1993.

Accreditation Manual for Hospitals. Vols. 1 & 11, Oakbrook Terrace, IL, Joint Commission on Accreditation of Healthcare Organizations, 1993.

Joint Commission on Accreditation of Healthcare Organizations: Characteristics of clinical indicators. *QRB* 15:57, 1989.

How to Prepare for a Survey: Special Care Units. Oakbrook Terrace, IL, Joint Commission on Accreditation of Healthcare Organizations, 1992.

Primer on Clinical Development and Application. Oakbrook Terrace, IL, Joint Commission on Accreditation of Healthcare Organizations, 1990.

Jones L, Strandness DE: Integrating research activities, practice changes and monitoring and evaluation: A model for academic health centers. *QRB* 17:229, 1991.

Kasper J, Plume S, O'Connor G: A methodology for QI in the coronary artery bypass grafting procedure involving comparative process analysis. *QRB* 18:129, 1992.

Keeler E, et al: Hospital characteristics and quality of care. *JAMA* 254: 1990.

Kelly J, Kellie SE: Appropriateness of medical care. *Arch Pathol Lab Med* 114:197, 1990.

Kibbe DC, Scovill RP: Computer software for health care CQI. *Quality Management in Health Care* 1:50, 1993.

Kruse JA, Thill-Baharozian MC, Carlson RW: Comparison of clinical assessment with APACHE II for predicting mortality risk in patients admitted to a medical intensive care unit. *JAMA* 260:1739, 1988.

Latini EE, Foote W: Obtaining consistent quality patient care for the trauma patient by using a critical pathway. *Nurs Q* 15:51, 1992.

Luce JM: Improving the quality and utilization of critical care. *QRB* 17:42, 1991.

Merry M: Physician leadership for the 21st century. *Quality Management in Health Care* 1:31, 1993.

Morris L, Fachet K: Incorporating critical care monitoring tools in your QA program. *Crit Care Nurse* 12:87, 1992.

Nadzam DM: Infection control indicators in critical care settings. *Heart Lung* 21:477, 1992.

Osler T, Horne L: Quality assurance in the surgical intensive care unit. *Surg Clin North Am* 71:887, 1991.

Plsek PE: Tutorial: Introduction to control charts. *Quality Management in Health Care* 1:65, 1992.

Plsek PE: Tutorial: Management and planning tools of TQM. *Quality Management in Health Care* 1:59, 1993.

Plsek PE: Tutorial: Quality improvement project models. *Quality Management in Health Care* 1:69, 1993.

Pollak MM, Ruttiman UE, Getson PR: The pediatric risk of mortality (PRISM) score. *Crit Care Med* 16:1110, 1988.

Pollak MM, et al: Improved outcomes from tertiary center pediatric intensive care: A statewide comparison of tertiary and nontertiary care facilities. *Cent Care Med* 19:150, 1991.

Shortell S, et al: Continuously improving patient care: Practical lessons and an assessment tool from the national ICU study. *QRB* 18:150, 1992.

Sivak E, Perez-Trepichio A: Quality assessment in the medical intensive care unit: Evolution of a data model. *Cleve Clin J Med* 57:273, 1990.

Sivak E, Perez-Trepichio A: Quality assessment in the medical intensive care unit: Continued evolution of a data model. *Cleve Clin J Med* 7:42, 1992.

Sue D: Development of an ICU patient care monitoring and evaluation system in a teaching hospital. *QRB* 17:97, 1991.

Teres D, Avrunin JS, Lemeshow S: Severity of illness modeling, in Rippe J (ed): *Intensive Care Medicine.* 2nd ed. Boston, Little, Brown, 1991.

Wakefield D, Wakefield B: Overcoming the barriers to implementation of TQM/CQI in hospitals: Myths and realities. *QRB* 19:83, 1993.

Weingarten S, Ellrodt AG: The case for intensive dissemination: Adoption of practice guidelines in the coronary care unit. *QRB* 18:449, 1992.

Weingarten S, Agocs L, Tankel N, et al: Reducing lengths of stay for patients hospitalized with chest pain using medical practice guidelines and opinion leaders. *Am J Cardiol* 71:259, 1993.

Wisner DH: History and current status of scoring systems for critical care. *Arch Surg* 127:352, 1992.

233. Beyond Technology: Caring for the Critically Ill Patient

Connie A. Jastremski

The 1990s have brought a myriad of challenges for health care. There will be unprecedented changes as the industry seeks the answers to questions of access to care, quality of care, costs, and ethics. Restructuring to meet patient care needs is the greatest challenge facing hospitals and nursing today.

In addition to the overwhelming cry for health care reform, there is a special concern for critical care practitioners. Predictions made in 1988 show that by the year 2000 the number of critical care beds in the United States will increase from 90,000 to 111,000 [1]. Occupancy rates in critical care units are averaging 84 percent, which is well above the total hospital occupancy rates. In July 1988, the American Association of Critical Care Nurses (AACCN) published the Primary Analysis of the Supply and Requirements for Critical Care. This report estimated that by 1990 between 300,000 and 365,000 full-time critical care nursing positions will be required, with a predicated shortage of 170,000 nurses available [2]. It has been stated by many that unless we do something radically different in the methods of delivering care, the gap between the demand and supply will be an even greater crisis in the future.

The Current Health Care System

In the early 1960s "intensive care" was established. Growth has been unrestrained since then. Associated with this evolution, the relative degree of utilization of resources for the delivery of these services has been increasing at a rate substantially greater than that for the health care system as a whole. Today, the provision of critical care services consumes 15-20 percent ($20-30 billion) of the health care dollars directed toward hospital care [3].

Health care reform, whatever form it will take, has three major goals. The first is to ensure that there is access to needed health care for all. A second goal is to control spending on health care. The final goal is to eliminate unnecessary components of the health care system. Under health care reform, the successful health care organization will be consumer-driven, outcome-focused, and flexible.

Planning for the Future

A number of trends will affect health care delivery and utilization of critical care services. The number and proportion of the elderly in the population will increase rapidly by the year 2012. The population will shift to the southern and western regions of the country and from the densely populated central cities and older suburbs to less populated suburbs and rural areas [4].

Broad social trends have been initiated that will affect requirements for future health care services. People are choosing life-styles with an improved quality of life. Decreases in smoking and alcohol ingestion are reflections of the new health ideal.

Economic growth is being driven by the changing labor force,

capital expenditures, and shift to a service-based economy. Continued economic growth will be necessary to devote significant resources to the provision of health services.

Although health care reform has only begun, health services are undergoing massive changes. The patterns for organizing and delivering health services are being reviewed, revised, and in some cases, replaced [5]. Similarly, the financial arrangements for the delivery of care and the staffing configurations for providing services are being modified or restructured. These transitions will affect the practice patterns of all health professionals and will require new and innovative structures and policies to meet the needs of those seeking health care. One such strategy is redesigning the way in which health care is delivered in hospitals.

Redesigning Patient Care Delivery

The delivery of critical care is expensive. But such service is worth the cost, at least to the practitioners of critical care. As demands for highly specialized critical care services continue to increase, less money will be available to support such services. Many institutions have already begun to examine the current delivery system and have actually experimented with different approaches to care for patients while managing both quality and cost. The common theme which emerges as these innovative systems are examined is that care can be more efficient. Many new models for the delivery of care are being studied and can be used effectively in critical care.

Work redesign is a multidisciplinary approach to restructuring patient care delivery. Useful redesign models link people and technology in ways that optimize the contributions of both [6]. Critical care is resource intensive, in terms of both people and technology. Looking at work redesign in critical care can only benefit the care delivery system.

PRIMARY NURSING REVISITED. Primary nursing is a philosophy of care started in the 1970s. This philosophy places the responsibility and authority into the hands of nurses with 24-hour accountability for the quality of care administered to a given group of patients. Primary nursing is a model that allows for meaningful relationships between nurses and patients. These relationships, and the communication that develops, can ultimately reduce fragmentation of care, enhance collaboration with the medical staff, increase the trust of patients, and reduce length of stay [7]. Primary nursing provides comprehensive and continuous patient care from admission to discharge, using the same registered nurse to coordinate, deliver, and evaluate the care. It implies a philosophy of nursing that places the patient in the center of the focus for the nurse.

There are advantages to using primary nursing as a delivery model. Under this model, the continuity and consistency of patient care are improved, and there is better communication and collaboration with the physicians caring for the patients. In critical care, these advantages are important to ensure quality patient care. Although most patients are in the critical care unit for only a short time, the primary nurse can be a valuable collaborator with the medical staff and a link between the physician and the family.

A recent study reported from Cedars-Sinai Medical Center examined the cost of primary nursing and the relationship of primary nursing to job satisfaction, performance, personnel costs, nursing hours per patient per day, and patient length of stay. Although the nursing unit studied was a 24-bed medical/surgical unit, the results are probably applicable to most critical care units. This study demonstrated that after introduction of primary nursing, job satisfaction improved and there was no turnover of staff during the 10-month study and only a 1 percent sick leave. Nursing hours per patient per day decreased and the average length of stay for patients in the unit decreased. Subjectively, physicians, nurses, and patients all reported an increased satisfaction [7].

CASE MANAGEMENT. The concept of case management is the step beyond primary nursing. Case management, with its foundations in managed care, is a clinical system for the strategic management of cost and quality outcomes [8]. The goals of case management include the following:

The achievement of expected or standardized patient outcomes

Early discharge of patients or discharge within appropriate lengths of stay

Appropriate or reduced utilization of resources

Collaborative practice and coordination and continuity of care

Improved professional development and personal satisfaction on the job

Encouragement of contributions by all care providers to the achievement of improved patient outcomes

To accomplish the stated goals, there should be an interlocking of managed care and case management.

At the core of managed care are critical paths that are based on standards of care for a case type [8]. These paths are shorthand versions of the case management plan. Both of these tools are developed by the multidisciplinary team caring for the patient in the critical care unit. Ongoing evaluation of the care described in the critical path is done and variances from the expected outcomes are documented and analyzed for resolution. Through variance analysis, quality of care is improved. Achievement of expected outcomes using the critical path as a map is a measure of success.

Translating this model for use in critical care can be accomplished easily. Case management can encompass the patient's entire stay while managed care can focus on care delivery in only one area of care, i.e., the ICU. The multidisciplinary team in the critical care unit can develop the appropriate critical path with expected outcomes. This delivery system relies on the collaboration of the entire health care team to be successful. Most units using this model use registered nurse case managers to oversee the achievement of outcomes for a specific patient population.

The case management/managed care delivery system is an effective way to deliver care. The identification of a nurse case manager, working in collaboration with a primary physician, enhances the accountability for patient outcomes. Patient outcomes can be achieved within appropriate time frames when the patient care goals are well defined.

Other benefits of case management in critical care include appropriate or decreased resource utilization, increased conti-

nuity of care, and increased professional development. Efficient and effective management of time, personnel, and resources results in achievement of timely outcomes. To date, managed care/case management has not been shown to impact the costs per patient or hours of care per patient day. Nevertheless, costs are lowered because of decreased length of stay (at least one day per case type) and decreased resource utilization per case [8]. One final benefit is that the model can be applied to outpatients and inpatients equally well. Thus, this approach links all of the arenas of care, including the ICU.

THE PROFESSIONALLY ADVANCED CARE TEAM. Confronted with the imperatives for increased patient care services and the reduction of available professional nurses, the Robert Wood Johnson University Hospital in New Jersey began the process of work redesign in 1987. The project resulted in the creation of the Professionally Advanced Care Team (ProAct) model. The following are the model's four key distinguishing features [10]:

1. Delineation of two distinct professional nursing roles, the primary nurse and the clinical care manager (CCM).
2. Creation of the CCM position combining high-quality clinical management with aggressive business management.
3. Supervised utilization of assistive personnel in the delivery of direct nursing care.
4. Expansion of clinical and nonclinical support services at the unit level to relieve nursing staff of inappropriate tasks and improve the quality of service experienced by the patient.

The model strengthens the bedside relationships between the critical care nurse and the patient by clearly defining the professional nursing roles, expanding support services, and redesigning the environment by decentralizing systems to the bedside [10].

The professional roles of the nurse in the ProAct model speak to two different scopes of practice. The CCM position brings case management into the critical care unit. The CCM is responsible for a caseload of patients in the ICU and uses multidisciplinary clinical care protocols to ensure that the expected patient outcomes are achieved. The CCM initiates the protocols in collaboration with the medical staff and then assesses the patient's progress through the critical care stay. The CCM plans and facilitates patient transfers and coordinates complex diagnostic testing schedules for critically ill patients. The activities of the CCM relieve the primary nurse of the usual interferences that ordinarily take the nurse away from the bedside.

The primary nurses provide the necessary bedside care in this model. They are afforded every opportunity to have input into clinical decisions regarding the patient through collaboration with the CCM and primary physician.

Clinical care managers are salaried in this model;. They work five days a week and participate in an on-call schedule to provide 24-hour, 7-day-a-week coverage [10]. Because of their unique scheduling, the CCMs contribute continuity to the management of patient care.

In addition to the two roles for the professional nurses, the ProAct model utilizes unlicensed support personnel to assist with direct patient care. Using AACCN's position paper on delegation of nursing and nonnursing activities in critical care, the model does not allow for the delegation of nursing activities that "comprise the core of the nursing process and require specialized knowledge, judgment and skill, such as initial patient assessment or intervention" [11].

The model utilizes two different support personnel: the critical care technician (CCT) and the support service host. The CCT is a versatile position designed to perform a variety of tasks delegated by the critical care nurse. The core of the CCT's job is task-oriented and performed on a predictable basis. These tasks include, but are not limited to, taking vital signs, testing stool for occult blood, performing finger sticks for glucose determination, performing 12-lead EKGs, and initiating CPR.

The support service host is also known as a "unit assistant." All hotel functions are managed by these providers including stocking supplies, cleaning and maintaining equipment, and delivering dietary trays. These individuals also perform the duties generally associated with the "unit clerk" or "secretary" role.

A pharmacy technician has been added as a third assistant role [10]. The pharmacy technician in the unit assumes responsibility for preparing all medications, setting up intravenous solutions and tubing, and stocking medications. The nurse is responsible for administering the medications. The presence of the support services host and the pharmacy technician permits the nurse to remain at the bedside providing direct care. It is critical that the primary nurse develop a trusting relationship with the nonlicensed staff.

In the ProAct model, restructuring the delivery system in the critical care units includes redesigning the environment. Several centralized systems have been decentralized to each critical care unit. The goal is to maximize and enhance the primary nurses' direct interactions with the patient and optimize outcomes [10]. The key aspects of environmental restructuring are a bedside supply system, a bedside pharmaceutical system, and a bedside telephone system. With everything the nurse needs at the bedside, the nurse can work more efficiently.

Evaluation of the ProAct model needs to be completed. It appears to have the potential to produce positive financial outcomes through cost avoidance and revenue enhancement [10]. Bed utilization will be maximized and revenues enhanced as a result of increased patient throughput. It is also believed that the model will enhance collaboration between nurses and physicians in critical care.

NURSE EXTENDERS IN CRITICAL CARE. A nurse extender is defined as an individual working as a technical assistant to an experienced RN [12]. The defining characteristic of this model is that each nurse extender (practice partner) works under the auspices of a registered nurse. There are many models of nurse extenders in practice today. Some use the nurse extender as a unit assistant or support service host as was described above. Others use the critical care technician concept to implement the role of nurse extender.

In 1988 Marie Manthey called the nurse extender a "partner in practice" [12]. In her model, the registered nurse and the extender work in a practice partnership; they work as one. This pairing of individuals may allow a 2-patient assignment in the critical care unit to be a safe situation. In contrast, were the nurse to work alone with the same 2 patients, the assignment might be unsafe. The partner is an extender of the nurse much like a physician's assistant is an extender of the physician [13].

The partnership model can be implemented effectively in a critical care unit. Some systems currently using such a model have utilized licensed practical nurses in the extender role. This pairing of RN and LPN has met with mixed success. Other potential partners in the critical care unit may be nursing students, medical students, certified hospital nursing assistants, and paramedics.

This redesign contains some of the elements of the ProAct model, but it is not as extensive a change in the pattern of delivery. It requires a willingness on the nurse's part to delegate some patient care tasks, as well as a willingness to supervise another individual's activities and accept the liabilities associated with that role. It is important to choose the right individual as the nurse extender and to create successful partnerships.

This delivery system has the potential for creating a safe work environment. It also can increase the job satisfaction of the critical care nurse partner while assuring quality patient care.

In addition to assessing the need for nurse extenders in critical care, one study has demonstrated the effectiveness of utilizing physician's assistants (PAs) in critical care. With changes in funding for graduate medical education and a shift to primary care physician preparation, critical care units may soon experience a physician shortage. The study done in an 8-bed medical intensive care unit in Michigan demonstrated that PAs could be utilized effectively in critical care. Appropriate selection and training were the key elements leading to the success of the PAs in the study.

The Future

Creating change is difficult anytime, but particularly if the need to change is being driven primarily from an outside source. There are many models available for redesigning the delivery of critical care. The medical director and nursing director of the unit should take the lead in determining if a change is necessary. As stated in the joint AACN/SCCM position statement on collaborative practice, the responsibility and accountability for effective functioning of the critical care unit must be vested in the physician and nurse directors who are on an equal decision-making level.

The first step in the redesign process is to assess the unit's current level of functioning, and its strengths and areas for improvement. Deciding the outcomes that a redesign would accomplish early will assist in choosing the best model to achieve these outcomes. The directors must also determine the level of administrative support for redesign. Many of these models will require some investment of money. The final component of assessment is to determine the driving and constraining forces for change. Ultimately, these forces will shape the redesign model chosen.

Implementation of the new care delivery system should follow a complete preparation period, which includes getting the medical, nursing, administrative, and support staffs to a thorough understanding of the new delivery system. Involving all of the groups who will ultimately be affected by such a change makes for a smoother transition. An evaluation of the new system should be planned with the key outcomes to be achieved serving as the framework for the evaluation. Following the evaluation, modifications to the new delivery model may be necessary.

Each critical care unit is unique. Determining the delivery system that will work the best and achieve the desired outcomes for the change will require preparation and commitment by the directors of the unit and all affected by the change.

Summary

No one has a crystal ball regarding the future for health care. Critical care services will continue to be demanded, but how they will be delivered remains a question. As providers of critical care, it is our responsibility to assure that these services will be available in the future. In addition, it is our responsibility to create a delivery system that will provide cost-effective, efficient, quality care to the critically ill. In order to create the new system a thorough assessment of the current critical care delivery in this country is necessary. Successful cost-effective ICUs should be defined and studied. Pilot units utilizing different delivery systems should be compared for cost, efficiency and quality. Only in that way can the critical care community as a whole develop the best model for care delivery. The future is ours to create. This chapter has explored some of the new models of care delivery being tested. In order to be proactive rather than reactive towards health care reform, it is wise to examine the care delivery systems in use and determine their applicability in our current practice settings.

References

1. Searle LD: Implications of the nursing shortage. *Heart Lung* 17:219, 1990.
2. *Summary Analysis of Critical Care Nurse Supply and Requirements.* Newport Beach, CA, American Association of Critical Care Nurses, 1988.
3. Birnbaum ML: Cost containment in critical care. *Crit Care Med* 14:1068, 1986.
4. *Long-range Goals for the Profession.* Kansas City, American Nurses Association, 1986.
5. Steel JE: Designing the future. *J Neurosci Nurs* 19:321, 1987.
6. Madden MJ, Lawrenz E: Work redesign, in Mayer GG, Madden MJ, Lawrenz E (eds): *Patient Care Delivery Models.* Gaithersburg, MD, Aspen, 1990.
7. Burnes-Bolton L, Davivier MA, Vosburgh MM, et al: A cost containment model of primary nurses at Cedars-Sinai Medical Center, in Mayer GG, Madden MJ, Lawrenz E (eds): *Patient Care Delivery Models.* Gaithersburg, MD, Aspen, 1990.
8. Zander K: Managed care and nursing case management, in Mayer GG, Madden MJ, Lawrenz E (eds): *Patient Care Delivery Models.* Gaithersburg, MD, Aspen, 1990.
9. Barnsteiner JH, Mohan A, Milberger P: Implementing managed care in a pediatric setting, in Katz R (ed): *Care Delivery Systems: AACN Clinical Issues in Critical Care Nursing.* Philadelphia, JB Lippincott, 1992, p 777.
10. Ritter J, Tonges MC: Work redesign in high intensity environments: ProAct for critical care. *J Nurs Adm* 21:26, 1991.
11. *Delegation of Nursing and Non-nursing Activities in Critical Care: A Framework for Decision Making.* Laguna Niguel, CA, American Association of Critical Care Nurses, 1990.
12. Manthey M: Primary practice partners: A nurse extender system. *Nurs Mgt* 19:11, 1988.
13. Manthey M: Practice partnerships: The newest concept in care delivery. *J Nurs Adm* 19:33, 1989.
14. Dubaybo BA, Samson MK, Carlson RW: The role of physician-assistants in critical care units. *Chest* 99:89, 1991.
15. *Collaborative Practice Model: The Organization of Human Resources in Critical Care Units.* Newport Beach, CA, American Association of Critical Care Nurses, 1982.

234. Rural Critical Care

Michael S. Jastremski

Introduction

The provision of critical care in the rural community hospital health care delivery system may be used as a model to describe the process for providing critical care services in any primary care-focused community hospital. The practice of critical care in a community hospital, be it a farm community in upstate New York or an inner-city neighborhood in Detroit, is considerably different from the practice of critical care medicine in a tertiary care facility. Differences in human and technologic resources determine the patient types that may be cared for effectively in the different levels of hospitals and should form the foundation for a regionalized system of hospital categorization and patient flow. Community primary care hospitals, which will be called rural hospitals for the rest of this chapter, are currently the site of delivery of critical care services for a large number of patients [1]. It is the author's opinion that appropriate and effective critical care can be delivered in this setting with proper planning and appropriate patient selection. This chapter describes a process that will optimize the delivery of critical care in a rural setting through analysis and enhancement of internal resources and their integration into a coordinated, regionalized system of critical care delivery.

The Process for Excellence

The elements of the process for achieving excellence in rural critical care are summarized in Table 234-1. The initiation of this process must begin with a commitment by the administrative, medical, and nursing leadership of the hospital to critically analyze existing practices and to support those changes that will lead to improved outcomes for patients. A committed hospital leadership is necessary to begin the process, provide the resources necessary for system analysis, inform and "sell" the affected members of the hospital staff about practice changes, and provide the resources to implement changes in practice. It is very difficult to accomplish meaningful changes in the delivery of critical care without enthusiastic commitment from the hospital's leadership.

The actual analysis, planning, and implementation process should be coordinated by a multidisciplinary team. This team should include, at a minimum, representatives from administration, nursing, and the medical staff. Respiratory therapy, pharmacy, nutrition, and other elements, such as the emergency medical services system (EMS) when transfer issues are discussed, may be part of the multidisciplinary team for the entire process or may be involved on an ad hoc basis when their

Table 234-1. Rural Critical Care: The Process for Excellence

Institutional commitment
Multidisciplinary team
Needs assessment
   Practice profile
   Resource inventory
Mission statement
Resource enhancement
Collaborative practice
Practice policies and procedures
Education
Continuous quality improvement
Integration into a regional system

expertise is required. The membership of this multidisciplinary team should not be limited to institutional leaders. In fact, it is my belief that the success of such a process requires involvement by the staff nurses and staff physicians who routinely provide critical care in the institution. These individuals who are regularly at the bedside often have the best insights into existing processes and opportunities for improving the care of patients. The chairperson of the multidisciplinary team needs to be committed to the process, actively involved in the bedside practice of critical care at the institution, and have good interpersonal and communication skills. An outside consultant, skilled in critical care management, may be useful for getting the process started, organizing and instructing the multidisciplinary team, and providing an outside unbiased critical assessment of the institution's strengths and weaknesses in its current critical care practices.

The first task for the multidisciplinary team is the completion of a needs assessment of the institution's current and projected future practice profile and an inventory of the institution's critical care resources. This assessment should start by looking at what critical care services the institution currently provides, and how they are provided in terms of people and technologic resources. If possible, the institution's performance should be benchmarked against published outcome data, such as exists for coronary artery bypass grafting and abdominal aortic aneurysm resection [2]. Unfortunately, at present published benchmarks are unavailable for much of the critically ill patient population. If all the required data are available, a scoring system such as the APACHE or MPM may be used to give a broad overview of the institution's present performance in terms of survival [3]. These scores, however, do not provide information about morbidity, quality of life, or cost effectiveness of the critical care delivered in an institution.

The assessment process requires that the multidisciplinary team take a hard and careful look at the institution's current and proposed critical care practice profile. The team needs to decide what is realistic for the institution, and use this assessment as the basis for an institutional critical care mission statement, which should define the institution's role in critical care delivery. This, in turn, will determine what resources the institution must provide to accomplish this mission.

The Society of Critical Care Medicine (SCCM) has developed guidelines for the categorization of critical care units, linking the complexity of care provided and the resources required [4]. These guidelines, although not confirmed by any prospective outcome-based study, represent a consensus of the country's experts, and can be used as a starting point as the multidisciplinary team inventories existing resources and attempts to match them to the practice of critical care at the institution.

A comparison of the institution's resources with the list of resources necessary to fulfill the institution's critical care mission will determine the need for resource enhancement. This comparison might identify needs for additional staff such as 24-hour respiratory therapy support in the ICU or additional nursing positions to meet an increase in patient acuity. Enhancement of personnel resources will require development of a recruitment and retention strategy in conjunction with the hospital's personnel department. Resource enhancement may require capital expenditures to purchase new technology or to redesign and refurbish existing facilities. This will require coordination with biomedical engineering, hospital purchasing, and design and construction entities. It is also possible this process may identify resources that can be eliminated, e.g., an institution might decide that the existing data do not support the provision of pediatric critical care in a community hospital, and thus make a decision to transfer all such cases to a tertiary care hospital. This might allow the institution to eliminate some equipment, such as infant ventilators. This decision also would impact on staff orientation and continuing education, and perhaps on staffing patterns.

There is evidence from the American Association of Critical Care Nurses (AACCN) and a study by Knaus et al that the organizational characteristics and work environment of an intensive care unit influence both patient outcome and staff satisfaction [5,6]. The organizational and management model that seems to best provide such a structure and workplace environment has been termed collaborative practice [7]. Collaborative practice is a management strategy for critical care units that vests responsibility and accountability for the functioning of the critical care unit in a nurse/physician codirector team. The members of this team have equal decision-making authority and accountability. The success of collaborative practice comes with the diffusion of mutual respect and cooperation displayed by the unit codirectors throughout the unit's staff. The medical care-givers of all descriptions become equal partners both in their management of individual patients and in the organizational structure of the ICU. The six main components of collaborative practice are (1) unit codirectors, (2) a collaborative practice committee, (3) the primary nurse and primary physician approach to patient care, (4) individual clinical decision making, (5) the integrated medical record, and (6) collaborative continuous quality improvement. The glue that holds collaborative practice together is collegiality and open, friendly communication. The multidisciplinary planning committee responsible for the mission statement and needs assessment may evolve naturally into the ongoing collaborative practice committee (see Chap. 233).

An early task of the collaborative practice committee should be the development of practice policies and procedures. There is an increasing perception that outcome is improved when standardized approaches to various problems in critically ill patients are adopted [8]. Also, organized preplanned practice approaches may be necessary to achieve guidelines that carry the weight of standards of care. For example, the latest American Heart Association guidelines for emergency cardiac care indicate that thrombolytic therapy should be administered to eligible patients within 30 to 60 minutes of their initial presentation at the emergency department [9]. This time limit is difficult to meet consistently without the existence of preestablished medical and nursing protocols. The impending evolution in our health care delivery system will reward and select systems that are effective in terms of both patient outcome and cost. Standardized practice policies are one way to achieve this goal. Such policies are being developed by a variety of governmental and private entities, and may become the benchmarks against which hospitals and individual physicians are measured.

Unfortunately practice policy development is not easy. The process is time-consuming and expensive, and is often hindered by the paucity of valid outcome studies. In a hospital, different physicians and nurses may have different approaches to the same problems. I recently visited a small suburban hospital that had ten different sets of admission orders for patients with acute myocardial infarction entering the coronary care unit; the standardized orders were for each of the ten physicians on the hospital's staff. This created confusion for the nursing staff, particularly in those areas where the orders were in direct conflict with those of other physicians. The lack of a standardized protocol also led to inconsistent patient care, more frequent nursing errors, and probably adversely affected outcome, although the hospital did not have a continuous quality improvement program in place to prove or disprove that hypothesis.

The collaborative practice committee can begin the process of developing practice policies by picking common, simple, and straightforward problems that are routinely treated in the institution. Two examples are acute myocardial infarction and acute exacerbation of chronic obstructive pulmonary disease. The committee should gather information about the various existing practice approaches used in the institution, and review published guidelines and current data regarding diagnostic and treatment modalities. This information should be used as the basis for a standardized set of medical and nursing protocols for the management of patients with that particular problem. These may be separate medical and nursing protocols or may be integrated into a unified critical pathway. The data from published guidelines and studies of the disease process should serve as a template for developing institutional policies. It can be expected that there will be resistance from individual physicians and nurses, who will be reluctant to change. If possible, these individuals should be identified and involved in the process early, in order to facilitate acceptance of the changes. If consensus cannot be reached, then it is possible to activate the uniform practice policies on a subset of the patients, and compare outcomes between the uniform practice policy and the individualized approaches. Such comparisons should examine mortality, morbidity (including subtle details like medication errors), and cost. Hard data can be used as a lever to change the practice pattern of holdouts and continually improve the standardized practice policies.

The educational activities of the critical care unit need to focus on initial orientation and continuing education. The initial orientation should be based on the unit's mission statement and practice profile. The unit's practice policies and procedures should be integrated into the initial orientation. The initial orientation should be competency-based, and should be flexible enough to address variations in educational background, experience, and individual learning. Credentialing and delineation of privileges should be integrated into the orientation process.

Cross-training is one way to maximize use of personnel, reduce costs, and provide flexibility at times of peak load. For example, critical care nurses may be trained to provide respiratory therapy services during the night shift, thus eliminating the need for an in-house respiratory therapist at night in a low-volume ICU. Cross-training of emergency department and critical care nurses can provide peak load flexibility in these two areas with variable and unpredictable needs for personnel.

Continuous quality improvement is the process by which an entity, be it a widget manufacturer or a critical care unit, analyzes and assesses its activities in an ongoing fashion to identify changes in practices and processes that can produce incremental improvements in both output and processes [10]. The responsibility for continuous quality improvement in critical care

units ultimately rests with the medical director. However, the continuous quality improvement process works best if it involves all the individuals who are directly or indirectly involved in the delivery of care at the bedside. Thus, the unit-based collaborative practice committee is the entity best suited to carry out continuous quality improvement, since it contains representatives of all the involved disciplines (see Chapter 232).

Integration into a Regional System

Regionalization produces an organized, hierarchical system for health care delivery to ensure that each patient is treated in the facility that has the optimal resources necessary for the patient's health care needs [11]. Since a rural critical care service can anticipate that it will be responsible for patients whose needs exceed its capabilities, it behooves rural critical care services to lobby for and be involved in regionalized care systems to increase the ready availability of transfer destinations for complex patients. Regionalization improves outcome for perinatal patients, burn victims, trauma victims, pediatric patients, and some adult patients with acute critical illnesses [12–15]. However, it is important to ensure that only patients who will benefit from tertiary care are transferred. The optimal utilization of rural critical care services should maximize availability of resources at referral centers, and minimize the inconvenience and risks to patients and families of transfer to distant hospitals. Further research is needed concerning the design, implementation, and outcome of regionalized adult critical care systems. Particular emphasis should be placed on developing triage criteria for matching patients to medical resources.

Regionalization is a complex process that requires a considerable degree of planning, education, and effort. Key steps in the regionalization process include the following: (1) Identification of a lead agency and planning committee; (2) Development of categorization criteria for facilities and patients; (3) Creation of an inventory of existing resources; (4) Designation of facilities; (5) Development of treatment, triage, and transfer protocols; (6) System implementation; and (7) Ongoing evaluation of the system by the continuous quality improvement process. By developing formalized linkages with regional tertiary care centers, rural critical care facilities should expect to receive services, such as administrative consultation, education, telephone consultation for management of patients, an efficient referral system, access to a transport team, and feedback regarding patient outcomes.

The rural facility can benefit from borrowing management expertise and policies and procedures from the tertiary care hospital. For example, an infectious disease specialist from the tertiary hospital might provide infection control guidelines for the rural critical care unit.

The tertiary care centers can play a valuable role in the educational process of the rural facilities. In addition to providing traditional lectures, our group also provides on-site physician/ nurse rounds at rural facilities, focused clerkships for both physicians and nurses at the tertiary care facility, and access to critical care nursing orientation courses at the tertiary care hospital.

It may be beneficial for the rural hospital, the tertiary care hospital, the patients, and their families to have a mechanism for transferring patients back to the rural facility when tertiary care is no longer needed. This may occur during the recovery and rehabilitation phase of the illness or during the dying process of hopelessly ill patients. Unfortunately, at present there are

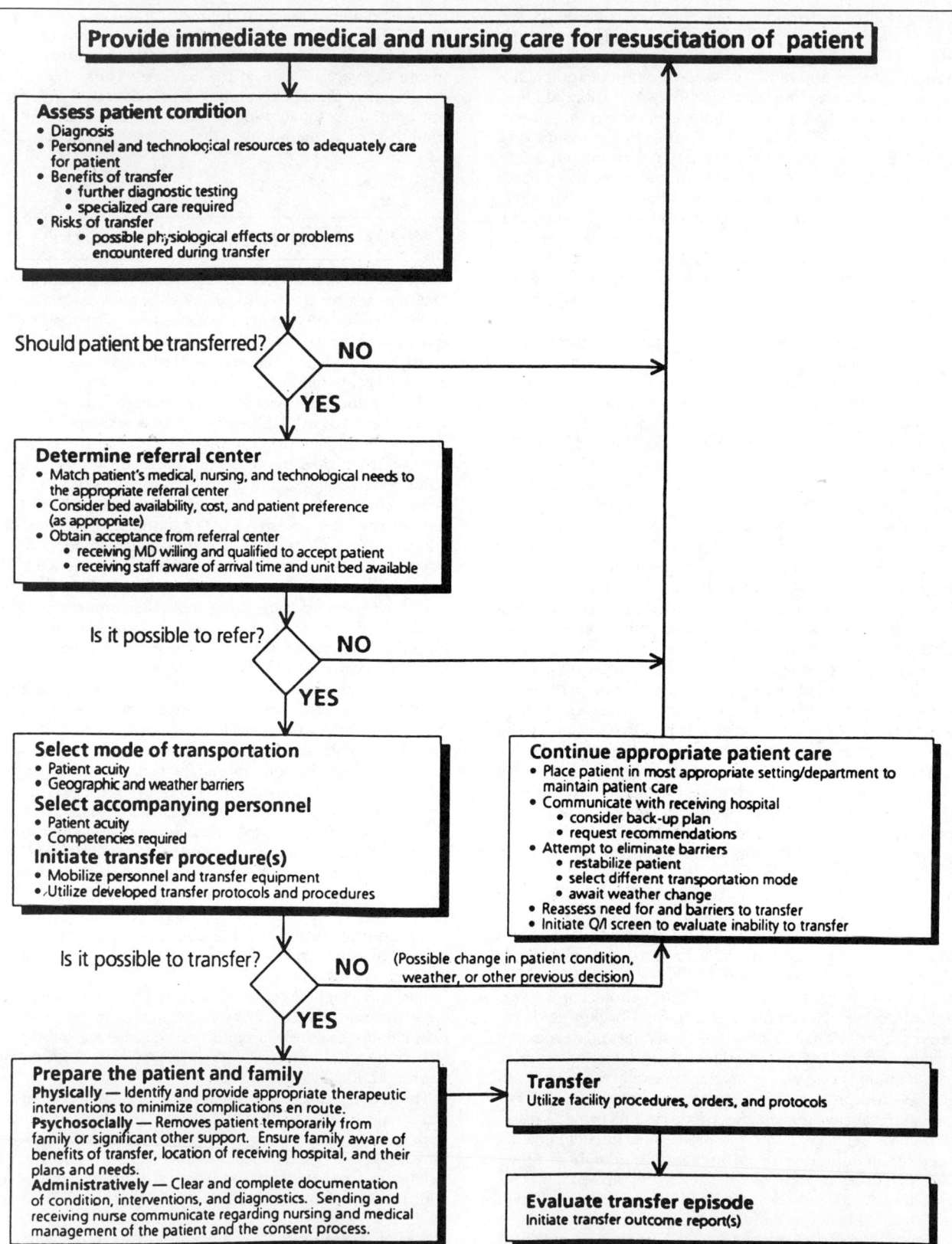

Fig. 234-1. Interfacility transfer algorithm. (From Guidelines Committee, American College of CCM, Transfer Guidelines Task Force of SCCM and AACN: Guidelines for the transfer of critically ill patients. *Crit Care Med* 21:934, 1993. With permission.)

third-party payer regulations that are a disincentive to such back-transfers.

Patient Transfer

The rural critical care facility will need to transfer critically ill patients to tertiary care facilities. Organized transport teams utilizing appropriate personnel and equipment can safely transport critically ill patients long distances. A regionalized critical care system should provide a specialized transport team with access to both air and ground ambulances.

A transport team will not always be available and rural facilities occasionally will have to transfer patients using locally available resources. The algorithm shown in Figure 234-1 summarizes the transfer process [16]. A timely and effective transfer will be most likely if a preconceived plan is in place. The monograph *Guidelines for the Transfer of Critically Ill Patients,* available from the AACCN, is a valuable resource to aid rural critical care facilities in developing contingency plans for transporting critically ill patients [17]. There are federal regulations governing the transfer process that carry serious penalties for noncompliance. In brief, patients must receive timely medical evaluation and stabilization before being transferred and must give informed consent to the transfer [18].

Summary

The process for excellence in rural critical care begins with a commitment by the institution's leadership to analyze and strengthen the critical care delivery process of the institution. This is best carried out by a multidisciplinary team coordinated by the key disciplines of medicine and nursing in an atmosphere of collegiality and equality. The team begins with an assessment that identifies existing and projected critical care practices and inventories existing and needed resources. This self-assessment should lead to a mission statement for the institution's critical care practice. It may be necessary to enhance technologic and/or personnel resources to fulfill this mission. An organizational and management structure should be fostered that will allow collaborative practice and continuous quality improvement. Finally, the rural hospital needs to become a partner in an integrated regionalized critical care system that will ensure timely identification and transfer of those patients whose needs exceed the rural hospital's capabilities.

References

1. Groeger JS, Strosberg M, Halpern N, et al: Descriptive analysis of critical care units in the United States. *Crit Care Med* 20:846, 1992.
2. Hannan EL, O'Donnell JF, Kilburn H, et al: Investigation of the relationship between volume and mortality for surgical procedures performed in New York State Hospitals. *JAMA* 262:503, 1989.
3. Seneff MG, Knaus WA: Predicting patient outcome from intensive care: A guide to APACHE, MPM, SAPS, PRISM and other prognostic scoring systems. *J Intensive Care Med* 5:333, 1990.
4. Task Force on Guidelines, Society of Critical Care Medicine: Guidelines for categorization of services for the critically ill patients. *Crit Care Med* 19:279, 1991.
5. Mitchell P, Armstrong S, Simpson T, et al: 1989 AACN Demonstration project. Profile of excellence in critical care nursing. *Heart Lung* 18:219, 1990.
6. Knaus WA, Draper EA, Wagner DP, et al: An evaluation of outcome from intensive care in major medical centers. *Ann Intern Med* 104:410, 1986.
7. *Collaborative Practice Model: The Organization of Human Resources in Critical Care Units.* Newport Beach, CA, American Association of Critical Care Nurses, 1982.
8. Cohen IL: Establishing and justifying specialized teams in intensive care units for nutrition, ventilation management, and palliative care, in Fein IA (ed): *Critical Care Clinics: Critical Care Unit Management.* Philadelphia, WB Saunders, 1993.
9. American Heart Association Emergency Cardiac Care Committee: Guidelines for cardiopulmonary resuscitation and emergency cardiac care. *JAMA* 268:2171, 1992.
10. Booth FV: ABCs of quality assurance, in Fein IA (ed): *Critical Care Clinics: Critical Care Unit Management.* Philadelphia, WB Saunders, 1993.
11. Jastremski MS: Regionalization and categorization of critical care services, in Fein IA (ed): *Critical Care Clinics: Critical Care Unit Management.* Philadelphia, WB Saunders, 1993.
12. Gortmaker S, Sobol A, Clark C, et al: The survival of very low birth weight infants by level of hospital of birth: A population study of perinatal systems in four states. *Am J Obstet Gynecol* 152:517, 1985.
13. Cales RH: Trauma mortality in Orange County: The effect of implementation of a regional trauma system. *Ann Emerg Med* 13:1, 1984.
14. Pollack MM, Alexander SR, Clarke N, et al: Improved outcomes from tertiary center pediatric intensive care: A statewide comparison of tertiary and nontertiary care facilities. *Crit Care Med* 19:150, 1991.
15. Maerki SC, Luft HS, Hunt SS: Selecting categories of patients for regionalization: Implications of the relationship between volume and outcome. *Med Care* 24:148, 1986.
16. Guidelines Committee, American College of Critical Care Medicine and Transfer Guidelines Task Force Society of Critical Care and American Association of Critical Care Nurses: Guidelines for the transfer of critically ill patients. *Crit Care Med* 21:931, 1993.
17. Transfer Guidelines Task Force of American Association of Critical Care Nurses and Guidelines Committee, American College of Critical Care Medicine: *Guidelines for the Transfer of Critically Ill Patients.* Aliso Viejo, CA, American Association of Critical Care Nurses, 1993.
18. Frew SA: Patient transfers: How to comply with the law. Dallas, American College of Emergency Physicians, 1990.

235. Risk and Information Management

John A. Dawson and
Frank V. McL Booth

Introduction

For the past decade, growing concerns on the part of the public as well as health professionals have led to marked attention to overall quality of care. Although implicit in the concept of professionalism, self-regulation through physician peers is no longer regarded as sufficient by legislative bodies. This has occurred in part because of the erosion in trust previously accorded physicians, and also as a result of the increased commercialization of health care. Consequently, insurance carriers, government, and consumers are reorienting themselves to expect documentation of service received for money spent. As a result, verifiable programs demonstrating ability to provide and improve quality of care for both institutions and individual physicians are now a de facto standard.

In recent years, largely as a result of adapting techniques developed for industry, the emphasis has shifted slightly. It is no longer sufficient to monitor the quality of care and correct deficiencies; it is now necessary to improve the base level of service available. There is increasing demand for meeting specific standards or "benchmarks," which as of yet remain to be developed. The administrative-clinical interface that has formed to meet such demands has undergone several evolutionary cycles and has been given such titles as Quality Care (QC), Quality Assurance (QA), Quality Improvement (QI), Continuous Quality Improvement (CQI), and Re-Engineering. The base goal remains unchanged: Show ability to provide service at a level that follows advances in medicine at a reasonable pace and price while minimizing error and providing correction for individual or institutional aberrations. In the future, to this will be added " . . . [for individual or institutional aberrations] *from the national norm*"[1]. A further outcome of the competitive marketplace in which medicine is practiced is a requirement for malpractice avoidance. Over the past two decades, the field of risk management has blossomed, encompassing hospital safety, injury prevention, and compliance with malpractice insurance and state regulatory requirements. The desired outcome is to reduce financial loss while improving care.

Central to both quality assessment and risk management are the local, state, and federal regulatory bodies that suggest or set policy. Voluntary compliance with standards is certified through independent organizations such as the Joint Commission on Accreditation of Healthcare Organizations (JCAHO). This particular organization's certification is meant to attest that a hospital "[can] provide quality health care" [2]. As is well recognized by most workers in the field, the ideal is hard to meet. It is debatable whether certification signifies quality of care or simply the ability to meet the requirements of the JCAHO surveyors. The approach of a JCAHO review often results in a flurry of activity and hasty adjustment of documentation under the guise of continuous quality improvement. From the individual physician's point of view, this is more often than not regarded as tedious chart review with few obvious results. From the point of the administrator dealing with physicians, such review is believed to be "peer review with teeth" [3]. Neither outlook is very helpful as the intent is not to force a one-shot "witch hunt" but to stimulate long-term programs that become part of ongoing quality endeavors.

Within most institutions, funding now exists to provide focused studies of specific procedures and treatments permitting establishment of physician-specific profiles, identification of problems, remedial education, and enhanced patient care. What is still lacking is universal acceptance of the need to broaden the sphere of attention from individual problem to overall systematic improvement. This concept, often referred to as total quality management (TQM), may be recognized as that which physicians have always attempted via professionalism. If one focuses on the overall process of delivery of health care, maintaining a program of continuous quality improvement is simplified. Confounding variables do exist, however, and overall awareness of regulatory agencies and regulations is suggested, as other entities outside of JCAHO are taking increasing amounts of quality improvement time. These include the Consolidated Omnibus Reconciliation Act, Health Care Financing Administration, Occupational Safety and Health Administration, Clinical Laboratory Improvement Act, and State Departments of Public Health. As this discussion is intended as a framework, it will not specifically address these entities. Neither will it attempt to address the specific problems of the institution as a whole, which must adapt cohesive methods to provide quality care.

Quality improvement in the special care unit (SCU) may be viewed as a microcosm of quality improvement within a hospital. In practice, the JCAHO is the driving force. The JCAHO extracted and expanded on its general requirements within the manual of accreditation for hospitals in a specific section on special care units by 1990 [4]. Some important components of this document are paraphrased below as a basis for discussion (Table 235-1). To these requirements were added the need for a continuous quality improvement education program in 1992. Maintaining of accreditation is now dependent on the implementation of such programs.

It is helpful to define some terms at this juncture, many of which are used interchangeably, adding to the confusion. Quality assurance as applied to either industry or SCUs traditionally has involved the concept of inspection of the steps leading to a product. When product failures were noted, then more inspection steps were added. In industry, up to 50 percent of some plants' workers are employed in inspecting some aspect of the product [5]. In nationalized health systems, such as exist in Great Britain, parallels may be found (for example in the 2.5:1 ratio of administrators to physicians). This is expensive and does little to improve the product. In fact, overall quality may be low as long as the product functions. In the case of hospitals, the products range from improving a patient's status to delivery of ancillary services or provision of jobs and education in the community.

Quality circles (QC), a transplant from Japanese culture, involve employees conversant with a "process," i.e., the steps needed to produce a particular product. This idea was conceived as part of an overall plan for quality and is used successfully when the employees are empowered to change a process. In the U.S. health care industry, incorporation of QCs has often failed. This is due to inadequate training in the techniques required, lack of empowerment, and failure of management to act on employee recommendations. Although currently popular as a means of enhancing communication, as W. Edwards Deming, one of the world's foremost authorities on industrial quality improvement, points out QCs are often a

Table 235-1. JCAHO Required Components of Quality Assurance

A. A clear vertical reporting line for quality assurance activities must be established.
B. The clinical and administration staff must monitor both appropriateness and outcome of care.
C. A written plan must be present.
D. A quality assurance-risk management linkage must exist.
E. Responsibility must be clearly defined.
F. Oversight and review of policies must be documented.
G. Appropriate credentialing shall be required.

"smoke screen"—a way for management to "pretend to be doing something about a problem" [6].

Statistical quality control (SQC) is the basis for the methods Deming used to turn Japanese production around. This involves the application of statistics to help analyze overall processes. The basic premise is that proper design of the model can produce a shortcut method of analysis at crucial steps.

Total quality control (TQC) is J. M. Juran's answer to Deming's teachings. Juran expanded statistical technique into a company-wide philosophy of quality. The methods previously available only at a technical level are used by everyone involved, from the executive to the floor cleaner. The ideal is that everyone in an organization is responsible for quality [7].

Continuous quality improvement is based on the objective of not just meeting a standard but of refining the techniques used to do so and the product itself, one of the foremost goals of forward-thinking health care practitioners. This can be a short-sighted technique, if the specific product does not need or is no longer amenable to improvement. An example of this is offering an excellently executed but unneeded service such as ultrasound ablation of gallstones. By employing this idea in an environment where employees and managers are trained in its techniques, and where management has ceded some degree of authority to those involved in a specific part of the process, the fundamentals for TQM are present.

Total Quality Management Theory

The industrial expression of the philosophy of continuous improvement is an adaptation of techniques utilized by Japanese industry over the past 20 years. It is based on collaborating teams of cross-functional members who examine and improve the processes used in production in a continual feedback cycle. The avowed ideals are production of a quality product in a cost-effective manner. This is achieved through teamwork and results in customer and employee satisfaction and loyalty.

The basic tenets had been developed by a diverse group of efficiency and production experts who fostered production techniques for industry in the United States in the 1930s. After initial success, the techniques were allowed to atrophy at home but were exported to Japan [8]. Paradoxically, the benefit of TQM and the advice of these American consultants has now been enthusiastically and rapidly embraced by manufacturing, health, and financial industries in the United States. What has not been well recognized is that the inherent disparity between cultures may play a large part in success of the technique. A great deal of ideology was added by the Japanese during their learning cycle and may not be easily adapted to Western culture [9].

Nonetheless, the basic ideas of those such as Deming [10] are applicable and should be examined and incorporated into future planning. A framework should include:

1. The primary focus is accepted as coordination of efforts across clinical, administrative, and ancillary care divisions, in order to provide for customer needs and satisfaction. Those responsible should remain cognizant of and moderate expectations. The customer should be recognized as *any* user of the system, e.g., patients, physicians, nurses, families, housekeepers, and orderlies.
2. Processes affecting delivery of care are examined and broken down into a manageable flowchart (see Information Management). Each step in the process is then examined and corrections needed are identified and implemented prior to their becoming problems.
3. A team involved in delivery of product or service is assembled. Each member may (and usually does) belong to several different teams. Necessary improvement is communicated and open discussion and problem solving are instituted by vesting decision-making authority at the team level. Employee involvement enhances satisfaction and cooperation. Ideas are recognized and implemented earlier.
4. Effect is judged on the basis of measurement. Many processes lend themselves to some form of objective measurement of success.
5. Graphics in the form of specific charts of a simple nature, such as Bar or Fishbone (see Information Management), serve to focus attention on vital factors. Training is provided in interpretation and construction. Control charting is used to identify variation and allow measurement.

This broad schema does not comply with the standards such as "Deming's Fourteen Points." The literature is replete with restatements of the principles and should be reviewed for completeness.

As an illustration, a flowchart of delivery of triple lumen catheters to an SCU can be helpful in providing a wide range of information. For example, the overall process is working well. Nurses and physicians are satisfied that availability and delivery is good. The inability to purchase a preferred brand has been accepted by a dissenting physician, when a cost reduction is achieved without an increase in patient discomfort or rate of infection over 3 months. Reexamination by Central Supply one month later reveals a 20 percent variation in usage to the SCU.

The team reassembles and reviews flowcharts and finds no obvious changes. Nursing remarks that the residents are using more catheters as a result of failure to insert after multiple attempts. Under "People" on the flowchart, residents have been forgotten. This instigates direct intervention by attendings with no change in technique required and uneventful insertion by several senior physicians. Observation of the resident staff reveals poor technique in dilator use resulting in catheter damage.

A hands-on training session reduces catheter wastage. The quest to reduce morbidity during insertion by house staff of central venous pressure (CVP) lines shows a decrease in wastage, definable on a percentage basis over a 6-month period, after introducing a written training program. Wastage decreases by a further statistical increment, following implementation of a multimedia technique. The fact that objective and measurable improvement in care is engineered over one year's time is of greater significance than if a particular doctor had been thought to have had bad outcomes and was given individual training. Overall, improvement was achieved for all "customers" in a delivered service above previous baselines. (Purchasing costs came into line, Central Supply returned to previous stocking and delivery levels, nurses spent less time assisting, residents spent less time inserting, physicians were more comfortable with care delivered, and the ultimate goal—patient care—was enhanced.) After a period of time, the cycle is repeated with the aim of maximizing improvement.

The reader may feel this is a laborious and time-consuming process. It is not intended that everything fall into place immediately; rather, it is intended that the basics be implemented and the process begun. Clearly, alternate methods for rapid correction of error will need to be retained (or developed) and utilized where immediate patient detriment cannot be predicted and avoided. The primary clash between industrial and clinical quality improvement is just this. While a defective product may be recycled and examined as a learning experience, it is desirable to minimize this event in the SCU. The "Code Team's" technique may be enhanced, but the team cannot be disbanded on the assumption that care will always be so good that "variation" will be held to minimal levels. It should be noted that the industrial definition for quality is often listed as the absence of variation [11]. Equating this with doing no harm and relieving pain and suffering will not be undertaken by the author. It can be seen, though, that this concept may be applied to approaching standards of care.

Experienced proponents of TQM feel that the "ten-minute mentality" of industry in the United States (i.e., reliance on the quick fix) will doom the technique. It also has been pointed out that traditional job flux and lack of long-term commitment of executive staff are further impediments [12]. To clinical managers, however, the need for immediate action coupled with long-range planning has always been second nature. It is probable that as theory and practice collide, changes in the concept will occur. The overall goals should remain the same: to satisfy or improve the health care of patients in an effective manner while meeting the needs of staff.

Accordingly, outlines for the implementation of a TQM system, while maintaining the current practices of basic QA, may be examined. The need to comply with JCAHO mandates will not change, but this organization clearly recognizes the above-mentioned difficulties and allows health care organizations "a greater latitude to identify and organize their own priorities." This is intended to occur in a manner that permits "establish(ment) and use (of) their own processes" [13]. It should be noted that within the original framework of "The Agenda for Change" and continuing through phase-in plans seeking compliance by 1994, sufficient time has been allowed for some form of functional CQI scheme to have been developed by individual institutions [14].

Practice vs. Theory

REPORTING. Single-discipline critical care quality assurance activities usually are reported directly to the involved department. This may, for example, include surgical, medical, or anesthesiologic quality assurance committees. These committees report through appropriate intermediate levels to the governing body of the hospital. JCAHO guidelines for any special care unit (surgical, multidisciplinary, medical, burn, cardiac, cardiovascular, neonatal, respiratory, and chronic dialysis units are included; post-anesthesia units are excluded) require reporting via an SCU committee of the hospital's medical staff. A multidisciplinary unit must report to a committee of similar disciplines. Additionally, the unit director must sit on or chair this body. Recent revisions require the functional integration of a unit's designated managerial level nursing staff. This integrated

approach assures coherent activity on the part of all departments and early identification of problems. The intermediate levels of reporting may consist of a clinical care evaluation committee, hospital-wide quality assurance committee, or a physician-peer medical quality assurance committee. TQM can be introduced at any of these levels by incorporating executive level staff on the committee. This should be linked to opening meetings to work teams that have been assigned specific portions of a process to examine. The composition of such teams may have a core group, but the ability to incorporate personnel with specific expertise should be recognized. The establishment of a fixed reporting schedule forcing reexamination of overall processes is the key. At some level it is important to allow specifically charged work groups the ability to effect change. These additions allow for prompt identification and correction of problems. The processes that previously went through many committees often meeting months apart are shortened. Still, change can still come slowly with this technique.

MONITORING. Monitoring, the heart of current quality assurance programs, encompasses a wide range of activities. The main direction of quality assurance within the critical care unit is concerned with monitoring of care. Though most hospitals have a QA division, often the chores of monitoring fall on busy clinical staff. TQM delegates these tasks to a larger number of employees. Still, in either a TQM or classic QA schema, immense amounts of information need to be processed.

INDICATORS. Indicators have been in use for some time. This technique is encumbered by the relatively small number of indicators that can be followed. In addition, it is relatively static, the indicator being retracked or dropped at the end of a cycle. As a training tool it is a useful first step and may also help to identify where the "system" or organization as a whole needs to focus attention.

A quality indicator is a variable that is tracked on an ongoing basis. Results are regularly reported, and deviations from the norm are investigated. From time to time, a specific indicator is subjected to a focused audit. When this information is prospectively gathered, carefully analyzed, and promptly acted on, it is the single most powerful tool presently available to the ICU manager to assure the delivery of high-quality care. A list of special care unit quality indicators should be drawn up covering all aspects of patient care. Monitoring should be initiated on each ICU admission and data compiled and entered on discharge (or weekly, for long-stay patients). An example of a data entry form is given in Figure 235-1. Armed with such information, patterns of practice and care can be identified and, where deficient, rectified. The precise list of quality indicators that are to be monitored should be formulated to meet the specific needs of the unit. Certain elements will be common to all lists, such as deaths, emergency readmissions, infections, and complications (Table 235-2). While seemingly obsolete in a true TQM system, indicators serve the function of substituting for the benchmarks against which industrial products are gauged. It is apparent that to fully realize the benefits of TQM, health care will need to develop real standards [15].

REVIEW OF COMPLIANCE. In industry, quality cannot be achieved by the disassembly of products after they have been constructed. This is also true with the delivery of health care. Quality must be built-in from the beginning. Policies and procedures must be well thought out, clearly documented, known

THE BUFFALO GENERAL HOSPITAL
a health care system
48 Hr. REPORT FORM
QUALITY ASSURANCE EVALUATION
OF THE INTENSIVE CARE STAY

PATIENT CARE—WITHIN SICU

1. _____ Stopcock(s) uncovered-SICU
2. _____ Noncompliance with IV care and maintenance
3. _____ Patient without ID band
4. _____ Decubitus Ulcer
5. _____ Line placement/function
6. _____ Accidental Extubation (incident report)
7. _____ Reintubation
8. _____ Unauthorized ventilator change
9. _____ Emergency resp. equip. not at bedside
10. _____ Accidental discontinuation of lines (incident report)
11. _____ Transcription error (incident report)
12. _____ Tubes are resting on floor (including electrical cords)
13. _____ New paresis
14. _____ ECG changes
15. _____ Hypothermia (<34.5)
16. _____ Nonavailability of blood warmer within 15 min of request
17. _____ Monitor malfunction (incident report)
18. _____ Equipment not available
        Specify _____

PATIENT ADMITTED WITH:

1. _____ Stopcock uncovered
2. _____ Noncompliance with IV care and maintenance
3. _____ Patient without ID band
4. _____ NGT not in proper position.
5. _____ NGT not taped as per policy
6. _____ ET tube not taped per policy
7. _____ Noncompliance with pace maker policy
8. _____ Autotransfusion bottle not dated/timed

INTERDEPARTMENTAL

1. _____ Meds not in drawer
2. _____ Stat lab results not received within 1 hr of sending time sent _____
3. _____ Waiting time for x-ray >1 hr time of day _____
4. _____ H.O. did not return call within 15 min. House Officer _____
5. _____ SICU not notified of admission.
6. _____ Waiting time for transfer >1.5 hours
7. _____ Return to OR
8. _____ CPR
9. _____ Death

Fig. 235-1. This form, which is individualized to meet the specific needs of the unit using it, has a number of blank fields at the end of the form. These are used when doing focused audits to enable the form to function as a routine or focused information-gathering tool.

to all, and followed. Knowledge of and compliance with policies and procedures must be continually monitored and reinforced. Evidence of this must be documented and made part of the ongoing quality assurance process. Medical informatics can be employed by this stage. Some ideas are presented below in the section on Information Systems.

FOCUSED AUDITS. Focused audits are a required component of quality assurance. In practice, audits are usually conducted retrospectively; however, the information obtained is more reliable when gathered concurrently. The movement today is toward concurrent rather than retrospective review. As this activity is required by the JCAHO, it is recommended that the unit manager direct a considerable effort to tackling a clearly identified clinical or educational issue or policy. A focused audit

must contain all the steps listed in Table 235-3. The last step of "closing the loop" is often omitted, which makes the previous effort largely futile. The re-audit is the key element in demonstrating management effectiveness. Germane information must be shared as an aid to the educational process. Examples of focused studies are presented in Table 235-4. It is a short but elusive step from the use of indicators and focused audits to the ongoing process of refining CQI.

RED FLAG REVIEW. This aspect of many current QA programs is changing. Some events are considered red flags that automatically raise questions about the quality of care. Such events often trigger an automatic review. Examples include unexpected deaths or unplanned reintubations (within 24 hours). The former is a product quality lapse unique to medicine. The latter, theoretically, should be minimized by adaptation of TQM. These occurrences always should be reviewed. This is another area where quality assurance overlaps risk management. An appropriate risk management program will monitor such occurrences. When not otherwise monitored, morbid-

Table 235-2. Examples of Critical Care Bedside Indicators*

1. Aspiration pneumonitis
   a. Occurred prior to critical care admission
   b. Occurred in critical care (vomitus observed)
2. Cardiac arrest; CPR perfomed in the unit
3. Reintubation within 24 hours
4. Decubitus ulcers
5. Readmission to critical care within 48 hours after transfer
6. Pneumothorax after central line placement

* Developed and reviewed by critical care physicians and nurses.

Table 235-3. Elements of Focused Study or Audit

1. State the problem.
2. The problem should not be a trivial issue.
3. The problem should be physician-specific.
4. Collect the data.
5. Analyze date.
6. Identify deficiencies.
7. Outline education-policy steps to remedy the deficiency.
8. Schedule a re-audit after a suitable interval to demonstrate correction of the problem.

Table 235-4. Examples of Focused Studies

1. Comparison of indications and complications of Swan-Ganz catheter in medical ICU versus surgical ICU.
2. ICU complications after carotid artery surgery (physician-specific).
3. Mortality outcome study: observed-to-expected hospital mortality using Mortality Prediction Model.
4. Evaluation of fluid status in official ICU x-ray report compared to interpretation by "expert radiologist."
5. Review of individual problem patients.
   a. Identified by critical care quality assurance
   b. Reviewed by quality assurance department
   c. Cases generated from emergency room, postanesthesia care unit, medical floor, operating room
6. Identification of ongoing significant and difficult to resolve ICU problems.
   a. Delay in initial antibiotic therapy for severe infections
   b. Poor documentation of fluid balance in ICU
   c. Laboratory discrepancies in the ICU
   d. Back-up resident support when ICU is busy

ity and mortality conferences of the parent department or special care service may be a suitable forum. Efforts should be made to avoid assignment of blame. The emphasis should be on learning and identifying errors in technique or judgment to avoid the same errors in the future. Minutes of these conferences must be kept pursuant to peer review protective statutes (from the point of view of risk management, such minutes should be confidential). Where appropriate, conclusions should be stated. Case summaries should not be duplicated and distributed to participants. Rather transparencies should be made for use with an overhead projector.

SUPPORT SERVICES. The special care unit cannot exist in isolation. A wide range of support services, often outside the direct control or influence of the unit's management, is necessary for the unit to perform at an optimal level. Formal interaction with support services must be part of the quality assurance process. Joint standards of performance should be established. Compliance with these standards should be evaluated regularly. It is helpful to identify a specific staff member with responsibility for such liaison who can improve lines of communication and become familiar with the support service's point of view. Such policies have found expression as collaborative practice committees involving nurses, physicians, respiratory therapists, biomedical engineers, pharmacists, and dieticians. Minutes of the collaborative practice committee should be forwarded to the division team's management for support and action. Continuing these techniques on a smaller scale and with increasing frequency permits a smooth transition into basic TQM.

The above 7 areas meld in a TQM model. The amount of training is minimal and worth the cost [16]. Depending on the skill level of those on a team, further training may be required in analysis of outcomes. The physician or nurse manager for an SCU may need further training.

COMMUNICATING THE RESULTS. The process of quality assurance produces a large quantity of information. Taken together, the various components create an effective and ongoing quality assurance process. The first component demonstrates the results of the information-gathering process along a time line. The second component consists of quality assurance deliberations and conclusions, which usually take the form of revised policies and procedures or simple practice advisories. Feedback of such information to nurses, physicians, and ancillary staff in a timely manner may be regarded as the most important step in the entire quality assurance program (both as an educational tool and to foster appropriate insight into the quality assurance process). Within a TQM model, this is both goal and starting line. Continual review and revision form the basis of the technique. The major difference here is at the level of the second component. Instead of depending on a lengthy process to afford the revised policy or technique, the structured work group itself initiates the correction.

The industrial-medical comparison fails here on occasion due to the legal interface and requisites of risk management. In those cases where individual personal contact is required as a result of inappropriate practice or conduct, confidential documentation of such meetings and any disciplinary action is imperative. Within a conjoint TQM-risk management structure, it will be necessary to incorporate those capable of effecting physician-level discipline on an ad hoc basis. At present, departmental chairs or executive committees serve this function.

THE WRITTEN PLAN. As in all aspects of management, methods, goals, objectives, scope, and organization should be documented. Interim plans need not be elaborate documents. The most useful plan is an executive summary of the process and should rarely exceed one or two pages in length. Special care units are areas of multidisciplinary collaborative practice. Therefore, the overall quality improvement plan and underlying process also should be multidisciplinary and collaborative. Although the basic plan may not be elaborate, the information gathered, analyzed, and charted can be overwhelming. This has been done for years without the use of clinical information systems, but a properly designed database can ease the burden of work. If extended into TQM framework, documentation mostly consists of graphics and text. Collection, creation, review, and maintenance of this material are best automated.

REVIEW OF POLICY. Traditionally, there has been an ongoing and timely review of policies and procedures, such as admission, rules and regulations, triage, and brain death. If continued, this review must be documented. The usual approach is to review a fixed number of existing policies during each meeting of the special care committee and to review the entire set of policies over the course of the clinical year. This can be time- or paper-consuming. Each member of the special care unit committee is assigned several policies to review. They are given ample notice of when presentation is due. The list of policies and procedures up for review at the succeeding meeting should be circulated prior to the meeting, but the policies themselves (unless substantive changes are planned) are kept on file in the office, and are available for members to read before the meeting if they wish to do so.

At the meeting, the policies for reapproval or revision are presented by the individuals previously nominated by the committee. Completing the preparatory work prior to the meeting, if documented, constitutes evidence of appropriate quality assurance activity. JCAHO inspectors will likely examine special care committee minutes for evidence of such activity. Certainly, continuous QI can aid in making these often stagnant tomes into useful implements for improving care.

RESPONSIBILITY. Section SP 2.1 of the 1993 Accreditation Manual for Hospitals specifies that each special care unit be directed by a physician of the active medical staff who has received special training, acquired experience, and demonstrated competence in a specialty related to care provided in the unit. Many hospitals take this as a requirement for certification in critical care medicine. This director is meant to be responsible for implementing policies established by the medical staff for the operation of the unit. Still, the overall activities of such a unit are also required to be guided by a committee of the medical staff including the unit director, nursing supervisor, and appropriate ancillary personnel. A review of the JCAHO standards manual reveals that many aspects of care previously thought to be the domain of "others" are in fact becoming, at least in part, the responsibility of all SCU employees. This is obviously the intent of the JCAHO and meshes well with the TQM theory that every member of the organization is responsible for quality. Unfortunately, this is occasionally translated by upper level management into working more hours. Such an administrative approach is *not* appropriate. Most SCU employees are already working at their educational, emotional, or physical limits and TQM advocates reducing these burdens, not increasing them. If this, however, is perceived to be the case, it is likely that the organization is suffering from lack of adaptation of the fundamental principles or lack of upper management training. In some cases, of course, it is not remediable and either the technique will fail or the impediment will be removed.

FUTURE PLANNING. Although controversy exists concerning who is best positioned to evaluate quality care [17], the evaluation of performance of quality improvement is still largely the province of the JCAHO. Accreditation suggests that an organization provide quality health care; it does not assure that an organization continues to provide quality health care. Recognizing this fact, the JCAHO, in 1987, initiated the "Agenda for Change" [18]. The goal of this program is to develop an outcome-oriented monitoring and evaluation process to assist health care organizations in improving quality of care. The effect or mechanism for such an agenda includes the use of severity-adjusted measurements of clinical indicators, ongoing data reporting, and periodic surveys instead of triannual site visits. Additionally, measures of organizational effectiveness in resolving problems regarding quality of care are incorporated. From the individual physician's or unit manager's perspective, the use of clinical indicators (in a program of ongoing monitoring and evaluation) became JCAHO's essential mechanism in evaluating a health care organization's effectiveness in delivering quality care. Although normative standards for clinical indicators do not yet exist, demonstration projects and prospective studies continue [19].

Clinical indicators are, themselves, not direct measures of quality, but when well chosen they represent a measurable dimension of the quality or appropriateness of an important aspect of care. Reintubation following elective extubation within 24 hours, or readmission to the unit within 48 hours following elective discharge are examples of simple clinical indicators. They allow the collection of measurable data for care processes, complications, or outcomes. Comparisons can then be made with external standards of occurrence rates or sentinel events. This allows the collection of measurable data for care processes, complications, or outcomes. The clinical indicator was designed to be used as an objective pointer leading to in-depth professional peer review. Clinical indicators are, therefore, flags for potentially substandard care or outcome. It remains to be seen whether they can be adapted appropriately for true TQM use. Although the JCAHO's primary thrust is investigation of the organization's response to the highlighted

problem, the unit director can certainly still employ such indicators in an effective, transitional continuous quality assurance program. This will include determining specific physician and ancillary performance profiles, identification or risk factors, and trends toward or away from desired goals. Simply rearranging current indicators into groupings such as process (e.g., catheter complication, medication error) or structure (e.g., triage management, admission protocols) is a satisfactory first step [20]. Including outcome (e.g., actual vs. predicted death, patient satisfaction scales) should be considered a simple second step that aims at eventual reorganization of QA to QI, and QI to CQI.

The JCAHO's agenda for change foresaw a positive feedback system in which clinical and methodologic data from various institutions were collated within a national JCAHO database, analyzed, and presented to individual hospitals. This would, of course, permit interinstitutional comparisons and allow individual hospitals to assess themselves on a measurable scale. At present, the responsibility for overall improvement of patient care and resolution of clinical difficulties resides with the health care organization and not the regulatory body.

To conform with the agenda for change, a ten-step process was suggested [21].

1. Assign responsibility to a designated chairperson for overall departmental review. This director would be expected to delegate responsibility for specific reviews to departmental members.
2. Delineate the scope of care. This is essentially the inventory of what the department does and what aspects of care should be monitored and evaluated. A special care unit, unless it is itself within an individual department, may expect itself to reside within such an inventory. For example, under department of surgery, the SICU may be expected to provide services for the critically ill, perioperative trauma, and specialty service patients.
3. Identify important aspects of care, that is, those that are felt to be high risk, high volume, and/or prone to problems. The evaluation process is expected to focus on those activities with the greatest impact on patient care.
4. Identify indicators. The indicator is a measurable variable related to structure process or outcome of care (previously described).
   a. Sentinel events. A major adverse outcome occurring rarely, requiring immediate review, for example, death following a tracheotomy.
   b. Comparative rate. Events that are statistically predicted to occur during treatment but exceed a threshold rate.
5. Establish thresholds for more detailed evaluation (comparative rate). This is the level at which evaluation of care is flagged for review (generally arranged around a 1 to 100% scale).
6. Collect and organize data. Commonly, this is performed by the hospital's quality assurance data collection personnel. Initial data reduction and comparison with thresholds is performed within this area. Specific cases that are outliers within each individual indicator are then compiled and presented to the appropriate peer review committee.
7. Evaluate care. Individual staff members, identified quality assurance committees within the department, or an institute-wide peer review committee is required to evaluate the care provided and determine overall satisfaction with care. Eventually, it was expected that this review would focus on trends and performance patterns.
8. Take action to solve problems. Following identification of a problem or dissatisfaction of care, an action plan is formulated and implemented at the appropriate departmental

level in an attempt to resolve the problem, improve care, or provide education.

9. Assess actions and document improvement. The outcome of Step 8 is assessed and documented and any necessary recorrections applied before proceeding again to Step 9. *This is the basis for CQI.*

10. Communicate. The appropriate findings should be transmitted to the identified physician or group within the institute.

Items 5, 6 and 7 reflect the current state-of-the-art, though in many institutes 8, 9, and 10 are employed successfully. Some units or institutes have transcended the norm and have incorporated TQM [22]. Still, as a consequence of retrospective review, most studies are set up as an ongoing indicator. Sentinel event indicators are more difficult to program as immediate investigation of the event is required. Doing so, of course, requires increased staffing and time commitments from physicians.

The entire process has in some cases been streamlined, reducing staffing and decreasing physician review time by instituting a program of concurrent review. Instead of calling for discharged patients' charts for indicator data and presenting physician reviewers with de facto retrospective chart review studies, real-time intervention is possible. For example, a unit-based, as opposed to office-bound, quality assurance nurse performs daily chart review of in-house patients. Specific charts are peer reviewed as required, and appropriate corrective and reporting actions taken at the time of discovery. This allows the quality improvement process to immediately affect care of the patients under review. Thus, risk management is incorporated into quality assurance nursing activities, patients benefit (if problems are averted), and the review itself is more pertinent because actual events are more accurately evaluated at the time when participants' memories are fresh. Less skirting of the issues and more immediate patient and physician impact are additionally augmented by an overall quality assurance process. Such programs are already in place in several institutions (and have proved both more effective and pleasant from the reviewers' and reviewed participants' points of view [23].

Concurrent review has the advantage of immediacy but lends itself to excessive rationalization. Retrospective review has one important advantage in that it allows accumulation of data, which is harder for an involved participant to rationalize away. Combining concurrent review with an appropriate database management system and establishing individual health care worker profiles may be the next solution. The goal will be to allow the process to evolve and function as designed, resulting in a quality improvement rather than a quality assessment program. For this reason, it is likely that some form of TQM, irrespective of the acronym or contraction used to represent it, will be employed. As Deming avows, "I'm not interested in stamping out fires—I'm creating a system of profound knowledge that will still be good a century from now." That this is not bravura may be seen from history. The basic techniques (e.g., flowcharting) that have turned around Japanese production and service industries have performed well for 40 years. Moreover, these techniques are the same ones used by American industry to achieve dominance in the 1930s. They were later discarded, but now are again recognized as necessary [24].

Problems

Many problems exist with regard to implementing an SCU TQM system. The sheer volume of work involved is often the greatest stumbling block to any quality program. Fortunately, forced compliance has resulted in increased funding by hospital administrations for quality activities. Still, a large bulk of the work will be found to be "voluntary" on the part of the physician and nonphysician members of the critical care team. Making indicators as specific as possible, choosing those that are easily computer coded into Diagnosis Related Groups (DRG), and providing appropriate training to the initial data reviewers will assure reduction in data bulk and allow timely review. Of course, unless methodology is adapted to reduce the amount of work, dissatisfaction will occur. TQM theory proposes that as members are added, the work burden is reduced. When beneficial outcome is then seen to occur on a timely basis, compliance increases as does satisfaction. In theory this is fine. In operation, it remains to be seen if it will work for particular hospitals. In some cases, the system is too cumbersome and fails [25]. In others, lack of willingness by the executives to delegate or heed unsolicited advice causes failure. As the entrenched paradigm for hospital management in the United States is "From the top down," this sometimes proves to be an insurmountable hurdle. Lack of training is also a formidable impediment. Anyone contemplating TQM should consider, at a minimum, studying the standard texts on the subject and attending a purpose-designed seminar. As always, this should be followed by simulation and practice.

Deming holds management in such poor regard that he has stated, "Export anything to a friendly country except American management" [26]. He describes seven "diseases" that "afflict" American managers: Lack of constancy of purpose; emphasis on short-term profits; evaluation of performance (the annual review); excessive mobility; running the company on accounting alone; excess medical costs, and excess fees for litigation. Those interested are advised to study the rationale behind these errors [27].The last—legal costs—is the province of risk management. One obstacle TQM proponents cite is reliance on QA departments. Downsizing overgrown QA departments (with redistribution of funding) is a popular stratagem. Financially it appeals to management and is intrinsically satisfying to those who have felt burdened by the occasionally unreasonable demands of such services [28].

Interference from outside committees or additional work imposed by outside interests often creates major problems. It is useful for departments to share as many indicators as possible (e.g., both medical and surgical departments could effectively examine an indicator such as cardiac arrest within a unit).

RELUCTANCE TO PARTICIPATE. Reluctance to participate in review may come about either as a result of the tedium involved in reviewing a peer's case or of the responsibility of identifying deviation from the norm due to fear of legal reprisals. QI committee members have been successfully sued, usually for specious reasons [29]. In some cases, liability insurance or indemnification agreements may help protect individual members. Additionally, strict adherence to guidelines and maintenance of accurate but confidential minutes are imperative. It is assumed that any member of a peer review committee will base his or her decisions upon fact and accepted standards of practice as opposed to financial or emotional considerations. With a shift to solving the system problem, and away from apportioning blame, this reluctance may abate. The fears of those who have a purported conflict of interest or constraint of trade are also allayed. In those states where permitted, it may be possible to utilize Continuing Medical Education credit for participation in QI activities as a carrot to induce those who have strayed to reenter the fold.

Risk Management

As alluded to briefly in the preceding sections, risk management is intimately entwined with the quality assurance process. From the point of view of a risk manager, of course, CQI is usually seen as a component of liability control. Within the critical care unit, however, the two major components of risk management control—loss prevention and liability—may be effectively viewed as further components of the overall quality process. Loss prevention, that is, loss of money, consists of a safety program for hospital employees as well as patients. Education and training, an inspection program, fire safety, disaster planning, and incident reporting are the essential components of loss prevention [30].

The quality tie-in with an inspection program has been previously discussed. Of great importance are education, training, and incident reporting. These tie together in that identification of specific incidents or occurrences within a unit are promptly reported. The goal is not just reducing claims, but also identifying problems and providing in-service training. Additionally, as new products are introduced into the highly technical environment, misuse by both staff and patients can be reduced by appropriate education. These components also can help to reduce the feeling of fingerpointing when an incident report is made, by explaining to the staff the purposes for which it is being used.

LIABILITY CONTROL. Liability control deals with the management of claims, insurance programs, patient relations, legal affairs, and, again, quality assurance. The extent of an institute's exposure mandates that legal affairs, claims management, and insurance must be coordinated with a competent risk manager. Actual risk control is directly the responsibility of the critical care physician, as are patient relations. The first line of defense is the point of contact with the patient and family. Patient relations are paramount in liability control; a well-informed family that is encouraged to participate in the decision-making process is less inclined to sue. The salient points are to educate the family in the various aspects of the disease, teach the family what to expect while their loved one is in the critical care unit, provide frequent, frank updates on the patient's condition, and maintain a consistent approach from all the staff involved. For awake and competent patients, similar disclosures are important [31].

RISK CONTROL. Risk control involves several components (Table 235-5). The early components come under the auspices of the critical care physician (or manager or nurse). When an occurrence detrimental to either patient or staff occurs, the first step is to acknowledge the occurrence. Attempting to cover up, obfuscate, or alter records usually results in greater risk. An investigation should be directed toward the degree of injury, any negligence involved, and the standard of care rendered at the time. Following the investigation, a review of the situation with the involved parties, analysis of the outcome, and consultation with risk management, the responsible party, and, potentially, the patient and family may be required. Then, a recommendation is usually made by risk management with the collaboration of all involved employees. In the best of cases, no action is required. In other cases, reduction of liability through offering free services, absorbing costs, or paying damages may be required.

Following any occurrence, ongoing monitors should be employed to determine what effect, if any, this single incident has

Table 235-5. Risk Control Scheme

A. Occurrence
B. Acknowledgment of item A
C. Investigation regarding
   1. Injury sustained
   2. Negligence
   3. Standard of care rendered
D. Assessment-evaluation
E. Recommendations
   1. Communicate with patient
   2. Cost absorption
   3. No action
   4. Prepare for litigation
F. Await patient-family response

had and what the corrections applied (if any) have accomplished. The ultimate goal is to avoid recurrence. The actual aspects of risk financing are beyond the scope of this chapter; however, several other factors involved under risk control are important to the critical care physician.

Documentation standards, credentialing procedure, in-service training, and protocols are central to loss avoidance. Although controversy exists as to the necessity for protocol order sets, such orders may improve delivery of care. Objections to protocolized care can be lessened if protocols are treated as a process to be continuously refined. In this instance, they become the basic "flowchart" component of TQM. Education in such protocols or algorithms may be accomplished by placing them on a database. They may be retrieved for emergent review or perused at leisure. Protocols are amenable to improvement by those affected over many shifts.

DOCUMENTATION. Documentation cannot be overemphasized. In the case of a major disaster, such as important equipment failure or inadvertent extubation leading to death, documentation typically has several components:

1. The minutes of the initial board of inquiry. This ad hoc committee with representation by nursing and physician administration, risk management, hospital administration, the patient's attending physician, and those directly involved in the incident must convene in a timely fashion.
2. The correspondence that arises out of the above deliberations.
3. Conclusions and recommended action. This last item is the most important from the point of view of the accreditors (e.g., JCAHO, state boards). Typical actions under this heading include:
   a. Information placed in the files of individuals involved.
   b. Evidence of interaction with individuals involved such as counseling, reprimand, or other disciplinary action, or a statement that no such action was considered appropriate.
   c. Any new policies or procedures that may have been developed in the light of what had been learned.
   d. Evidence that such new policies and procedures are known to those affected by them.

For the purposes of an ongoing QI program, examining and improving the process that led to the disaster, followed by periodic review of the process, even in the absence of further lapse, is appropriate.

CREDENTIALING. Individuals practicing in critical care must be credentialed to do so. This will often be the responsibility of a hospital department, such as surgery, medicine, or anesthesia. However, the director of the specific unit, perhaps in conjunction with the special care committee, will bear much of the responsibility for setting precise guidelines. In some states, notably in the Northeast, those with responsibility for residency training programs may additionally be required to monitor the number and quality of ICU procedures. Skills such as central line insertions or bronchoscopies performed by trainees need appropriate supervision. The nursing management of more complex technologies, such as extracorporeal membrane oxygenation or intra-arterial balloon pulsation, or even the measurement of cardiac output by thermal dilution must be appropriately verified, documented, and reverified at regular intervals. A major source of help in this area in large institutions is the nursing education department. In smaller hospitals, most of this activity falls on the nursing director and associates.

In situations where trainees rotate through several different institutions, it must be demonstrated that the trainees received adequate orientation to the workings of the unit. This may be conveniently accomplished by mailing a manual to incoming nurses or residents 3 or 4 weeks before starting the rotation. When the trainees actually start, signed statements are collected from the trainees stating that they have read the material contained therein. A number of important institutional policies are distributed along with the manual, such as the patient bill of rights and any required request law (relating to the requesting of tissue after death of the patient). It will be recognized that not everyone who signs will have read every line, but it serves a purpose in conveying a sense of how seriously these matters are taken. With a well-designed information management system, even this problem may be minimized (see below).

WHERE QUALITY ASSURANCE AND RISK MANAGEMENT DIVERGE. It is obvious that despite the great deal of overlap between quality assurance and risk management, there is one area in which the two diverge markedly. Quality improvement centers about standards of care, deviation from standard practice, and ultimate delivery of level of care to patients with the goal of further improving patient care and without an assignment of guilt. An aspect of risk management is that it may specifically attempt to identify patterns of practice that may result in risk (successful law suit for negligence). Simplistically, this may be regarded as unfair. It is, however, a requisite of reporting required by many state boards and is an intrinsically logical program for hospitals to develop. There are four elements required to prove negligence (Table 235-6). A review of them suggests that an appropriate Continuous Quality Improvement program in which the physician or other clinician participates will obviate or minimize the possibility of all of these elements occurring unless there is, in fact, actual negligence or incompetence. In that event, the institution must act to protect the patient and itself. To do otherwise would be unethical. By monitoring the performance of providers, a functional quality improvement program can potentially identify risk and effect prophylaxis.

Championing the Cause

Why should physicians be interested in promulgating TQM? The basic reasons are that those aspects of quality which have always concerned physicians are widely embraced by this discipline; achieving quality is a process which does not end at "good enough"; continuing education improves skills; refining technique improves outcome; and what may not be verbalized but is nonetheless known—the final outcome is dependent upon the efforts of many. To this, TQM adds the proposal that poor quality allowed to persist is a managerial fault. It may also be noted that the work generated by typical QA activities cuts deeply into time commitments and the tedium is not rewarded by marked improvement. With a TQM model, thought and analysis will become the favored process as opposed to chart review, second-guessing, and arguing. A final incentive is the trend away from apportioning blame (often at great professional risk) and toward defining methods for improvement.

Some aspects of TQM are best taught by physicians who as a rule have the greatest degree of scientific training in the hospital setting. (See, for example, Control Charting.) Overall, the process can be emotionally rewarding while permitting the continued existence of financial status quo.

Rationalizations aside, the best reason for promulgating a functional QI scheme (and preferably CQI at the minimum) is the simple fact that we are required to participate. If this is not done on a voluntary basis, the ability to lead and direct will be diminished. Quality in the SCU may then be defined by those least qualified to do so.

Information Management

Many methods may be employed to manage the influx of data that accompanies CQI. Traditional pen-in-hand techniques coupled with chart review are tedious. The use of basic computer technology is urged. For those inclined to continue established QA or CQI, some degree of automation is still valuable. Not only is collation of data improved, but so are interpretation and compliance. The ability to analyze or interpret is enhanced through preprogrammed algorithms that produce flow, pareto, bar, and other charts. Automation permits culling useless information based on reformatted templates. Compliance is enhanced by eliminating redundant work and providing useful information.

Attempting to read and understand the process whereby care was delivered is hard enough for a single patient. Trying to apply it for a multitude of patients is overwhelming. By sharing information in a database, everyone's jobs are enhanced. This idea may be extended to linking terminals throughout the hospital so that charts are available to several people at once, and even more redundancy is eliminated. This of course describes the basic Medical Informatics database now in use in many hospitals.

To expand into institute-wide process control, some form of wide or distributed area network linked to a central system is required. Intuitively, this type of system can be seen to lend itself to the ideals of TQM; work groups may be formed, linked, and altered rapidly. Overall processes may be examined by tracking throughout the institute. Communications via e-mail

Table 235-6. Elements to Prove Negligence

1. The provider (nurse or physician) owed a duty to the patient.
2. The provider failed to meet that duty.
3. The patient sustained damages as a result.
4. The direct cause of the damages was the failure of the provider to meet the accepted duty.

enhance rapid communication and many statistical and graphic analysis components are available to provide modeling of processes. On an institute-wide basis, process control and TQM are expensive and difficult to implement, yet elegant.

Most current medical database systems were designed without attention to future needs, JCAHO mandates, or, most importantly, the ability for local staff to modify basic function to suit their specific needs. Even the major suppliers of software attempt to utilize the same basic interface for each hospital when each instead requires personalization. This can be done retrospectively, but it results in inadequacies and can take years. For the SCU it is possible to purchase integrated monitoring/PC local area network systems that allow elegant clinical information consolidation while at the same time permitting rapid on-site programming for CQI purposes. Regrettably, at an average cost of $30,000 per bed, these systems are beyond the grasp of many units. The idea of beginning the TQM process in the SCU while building in nonobsolescence and allowing expansion into the hospital-wide system makes a great deal of sense. Providing that some basic components are in place, it is possible to begin the transition to TQM while satisfying clinical needs.

BASICS. Choose a "single platform" operating with the same basic system (MacIntosh, DOS, WINDOWS, or OS-2). It is possible to mix platforms, but it results in increased software and hardware costs. Utilize a Local Area Network (LAN). This step will allow overall reduction in software costs as a single license will supply all users. It also assures uniformity of software and data transfer. At the same time, the network reduces costs for peripheral devices as they may be shared. Most important, users will become accustomed to data sharing. The network should be chosen so that it can eventually be connected to the hospital-wide system. A professional consultant with proven abilities will conserve funds in the long run.

ENHANCEMENTS. A workstation or stand-alone computer in a quiet area equipped with multi-media capability is useful. This equipment allows retrieval of CD-ROM stored data at rapid speed. The CD-ROM may contain text (e.g., a collection of journals to which one subscribes) or graphics (e.g., Medical Clip Art). In addition, the computer holds an analog-to-digital, digital-to-analog board with an audio amplifier. Using CD-ROM or disk-based software, the computer now allows high resolution user-machine interaction in both video and audio. A simulation may show a lifelike patient undergoing CPR with full audio. The board allows text-to-speech conversion, (e.g., highlight a word and the machine pronounces it) or speech-to-text (speak and it is recorded). The utility of simulation training is obvious.

A fax/modem/voice mail board should be added. This low-cost option allows one phone line to answer for many individuals, store messages for them for retrieval, or page them automatically. The fax may be used to send a message worldwide, or to receive a fax in the ICU using a single multipurpose machine (the computer). The modem permits linkage to remote services (e.g., bulletin boards, a library) or to a remote computer. The latter allows retrieval of data, or even use of the system from remote locations.

A scanner allows graphics or text (signatures, photos, clinical records, letters) to be entered in digitized form and stored or embedded in the records. The device functions as a front end for entering printed material without needing to retype it. The utility for input of diverse medical information is immense.

Wireless LAN devices are available. A palm or laptop PC may be carried while still transmitting and receiving to and from the LAN. Thus, one machine might replace several, and those areas traditionally barred to computers (clinical walking rounds) would be opened.

DESIGNATE A NETWORK MANAGER. This person can be trained in specific and basic database programming, enabling local problem-solving and programming changes. Educational costs are generally insignificant when compared to returns (see Clinical Operations). Discuss with the users—physician, clerk, nurse—what *they* need from the system and try to comply with reasonable requests. This induces these key personnel to use the system and enter data. Charge an individual (usually the network manager) with maintaining data integrity and security.

CLINICAL OPERATIONS. The simplest form of system should be a local area network personal computer-based system. By beginning to provide information that the staff wants, a basic "buy in" is obtained. Such a system may be provided with an easy-to-use database program, a word processor, basic E-mail, and connection options for on-site or remote library services. At one hospital, the current system supplies all the above as well as clinical modules that train nurses and residents and provide information on drugs, treatment protocols, and scheduling. As an example of how such a system might be put to use consider the following. Intermountain Health Care, Inc. lowered the rate of postoperative wound infections from 1.8 percent to 0.9 percent over one year, and over a further period of time down to 0.4 percent. This was through the simple expedient of noting that many patients scheduled to receive prophylactic perioperative antibiotics often did not receive them. The deficit was corrected by using the bedside computer to request dose administration two hours prior to operation. In addition to improving care, the cost of treating infection was reduced [32].

ADMINISTRATIVE SYSTEMS. Once the basic clinical system is in place and being used, it may be expanded to meet clinical demands. This can include linkages to equipment for real-time data collection from monitors and the addition of software. Connection to the larger hospital network might be considered at this point. Choose a true database management system that will allow either consultant programmers or local programmers to construct easily modified storage and analysis programs for your specific needs. It is important to choose a system that will be able to utilize data from earlier systems and minicomputers (SQL), and to share data across platforms (APPLE/IBM). Data availability is the single most important aspect of information systems. Such programs allow data to be entered and retrieved for manipulation as the need arises. These data can be analyzed directly or through statistical methods or charts. It is useful to have software with the ability to produce a fishbone chart (Fig. 235-2), a flowchart (Fig. 235-3), a pareto chart (Fig. 235-4), or a run chart (Fig. 235-5). Histograms and scattergraphs are usually simple frequency weighting and x-y plots familiar to most health care practitioners.

It is easy to see that these techniques are not overly arduous. However, rapidly creating a readable chart and then manipulating the data on a "what if" basis are aided by computer. Furthermore, the use of basic computing tools reduces the need for extensive statistical analyses. An increased level of knowledge is required for the use of control charts if statistical quality control is required. Relatively simple statistical programs may be used to produce such graphics, which are useful as Deming

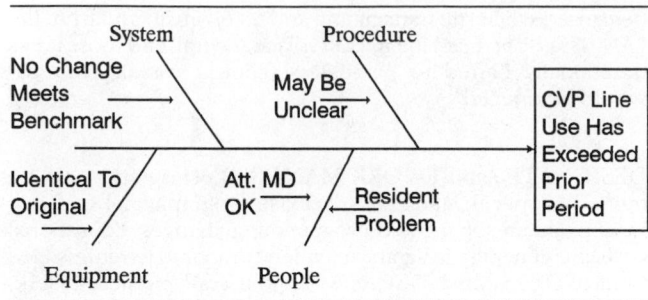

Fig. 235-2. Fishbone (Cause and Effect or Ishikawa) Chart. The chart resembles the backbone of a fish and for medical purposes is often given four major branches: Procedures, People, Equipment, System. A problem is identified (e.g., through an indicator, incident report, or perceived need) and used as the head of the fish. Presentation of data in this form induces discussion, focuses issues, points to need for data collection, and expands level of understanding.

maintains, "to stop people from chasing down causes" [33]. For industrial purposes, measured data are input. For the service industries, the number of perturbations from a desired outcome are counted and used as input. Averages and ranges are used to delineate variability.

BENCHMARKS. The use of benchmarks, i.e., comparing results to a standard and attempting to emulate the standard, can be aided through the use of information systems. The primary problem for most SCUs is that there are no national standards at present. While systems such as APACHE and MPM are undergoing extensive refinement toward outcome prediction, neither defines specific standards of care. However, attempts to do so are being made. Inter Study of Jackson Hole, Wyoming, is inputting treatment and outcome data in a long-term attempt to see how similar patients respond to varying treatment [34]. JCAHO also has proposed collating data in order to provide objective standards of care based on outcome. Although the task is daunting on a national basis due to the vast variation in

Fig. 235-3. Flow Chart. Usually used in reverse, by constructing a chart of how a process should work, then one of how it does work. The resulting discrepancies help clarify areas of misunderstanding while often pointing out areas for change.

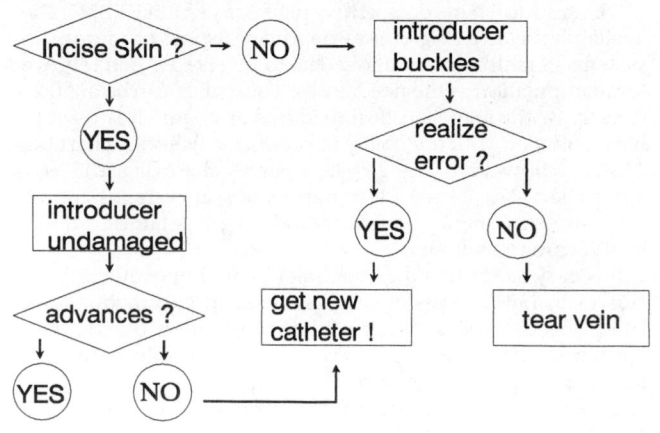

 # Of Events Over Six Months

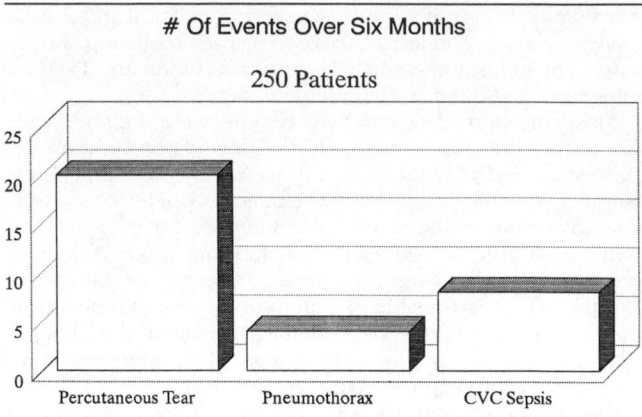

Fig. 235-4. Pareto Chart. This is a technique used to sift vital facts from the total field and prioritize issues. Most often the chart is presented in simple unstacked bar form. A visualization of weight or importance of the information is then available.

treatment and means of reporting, this is not the case in individual hospitals. Here databases may be compiled comparing outcome versus technique (or physician).

Two caveats apply. First, some measure of acuity must be chosen, and these are not particularly specific even though touted loudly. Second, a sufficient number of techniques (or physicians) must be employed. The lone intensivist practicing one form of ventilator weaning is not likely to produce significant data. Over time a significant database exists to make meaningful predictions and create standard profiles.

MODELING. Using the computer to artificially emulate a process and run variations has been used successfully in laboratory research. On an industrial basis, it is a standard methodology. For basic needs in an SCU, some things may be successfully modeled, such as predicting bed needs based on seasonal variation or linking staffing to census and acuity. Clinical improvements may occur if modeling is used for educational purposes. Training is a major focus of TQM, and training by computer is relatively easy to accomplish.

Fig. 235-5. Run Chart. This refers to a basic line chart used to identify trends. As may be seen it is a useful tool for grasping how change occurs over time.

SCU ADMISSIONS

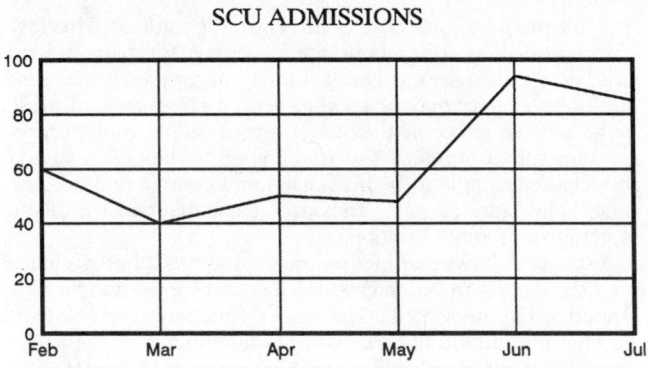

GETTING THE WORD IN AND OUT. Studies show that many workers are reluctant to voice an opinion [35]. Requesting that practitioners read a protocol or policy change results in poor compliance and poor understanding. Both may be aided by an information system. For example, access to a stored resident rotation schedule may be sought after by the residents. On occasion, access may be blocked by a request for specific information or the need to read a protocol and then correctly answer several questions. If access denial is kept to one time in four, these systems work. Many variations on this theme have been used to induce compliance. On a simpler level, eliminating paper forms can be beneficial. If all incident reports, bed transfers, narcotic requests, and the like are electronically inputted, collection of data needed for CQI is enhanced. The user benefits from more rapid input, a permanent record, automatic calculation of needed formulas, and automatic transmission to pharmacy. CQI benefits from assured input and, if properly designed, the ability to track utilization of materials.

The latest variation on this theme is the "help desk." This is the information system analog of applying TQM to an incident reporting system; it can be done without a computer. For example, a system may be established where any SCU problems, real or imagined, may be phoned in by an interested party. Rapid confidential turnaround is assured and the system can be helpful in identifying and correcting many local SCU and system-wide problems. The problem with this technique is that it is labor intensive, costly, and generally tapers off after initial use resulting in cost inefficiency. One solution is to operate this line on a short-term rotating basis. This software provides a link to a database using neural network techniques. Many questions can be answered in an automated format (no concurrent human operator), the details and pathways having been previously entered. The system generates trouble reports and alarm situations may be defined. Specific problems are interpreted by the system and routed to the designated expert or team. As the system operates 24 hours a day, all shifts are included and contribute to input and receive the benefit of seeing more rapid turnaround and ease of reporting. While not obvious to those unfamiliar with "neural networks" or knowlegebases, the ability of the software to switch between report tracking and problem solving is its power. The input from many sources is used to recognize statistically valid patterns often too subtle for real-time identification. This information is then used in combination with inference-forming software and programmed decision trees to mimic human decision-making—without emotion [36].

COMMERCIAL SOLUTIONS. For many SCUs, the use of local skill will be sufficient to produce an effective system. For most institutions this will be the only practical remedy, as commitments involving computer type, mainframe tie-in, and patient care information systems already exist. For those unencumbered with these limits, and a need for improved monitoring, there are several alternatives. A number of commercial hardware-software combinations are on the market and contain proven solutions to combined TQM and SCU patient information needs. The Motorola solution marketed by EMTECH appears to be a reliable system made so in part by the company's commitment to interface the system and provide ongoing training. This is often an added expense or not provided by other vendors. Hewlett Packard's CAREVUE 9000 is also being employed as a tool for quality assurance. Be sure to perform a thorough analysis among contenders in the various areas due to rapid changes in technology.

For those with decreased requirements, there are entry level systems. Though based on a single desktop computer and of-

fering none of the advantages of the monitor-computer LANs, these systems provide a basic yet potent means of tracking trends and performing most TQM functions for moderate size SCUs. The simplicity of these systems permits easy integration into the work routine [37]. Some systems (e.g., MITCCH—Management Information For Critical Care In Hospitals) are supplied as integrated software-hardware combinations or work across multiple platforms eliminating setup problems [38].

Often ignored are those products not considered specific to CQI/TQM. In fact, a large amount of commercial software ranging from simple database programs to graphics programs capable of organization and flowcharting is available. A perusal of any software catalog will reveal project scheduling, form generating, protocol writing, and other applications which may be immediately usable for QI purposes. Stand-alone SCU equipment may come accompanied by specific TQM software. These programs often satisfy regulations for maintaining laboratory certification [39]. Not to be ignored are other programs having nothing to do with QI. These may be useful in an overall strategy that induces users to add information to the system in exchange for receiving useful data. A program that calculates derived hemodynamics may provide entry of data usable for a specific indicator while also reducing resident or nursing workload. Programs that make life easier or save time promote use of the system and familiarity through hands-on learning. A solid decade into desktop use, most SCU managers are unaware of the extent of programs available. Common perception is that word processing, spreadsheets, and customized database programs are the only useful tools. Several hours in the library perusing software reviews will show otherwise.

BRAINSTORMING. This is a conventional technique in many areas of management. Programs are available that enhance this method through the use of a personal computer. Input of the process is accepted and the system generates idea associations that are relevant to the situation. The interplay between team members with diverse ideas and the enhancement provided by digital speed results in more rapid generation of solutions, often along unanticipated lines [40]. This concept is of course adaptable to the LAN. The concept of computer-linked work groups has gained acceptance and is used very successfully in industry. "Groupware," the software for this purpose, allows immediate linkage and file sharing. The software supports idea-generation, consensus-building, alternatives-evaluation, decision-making, and organization. The ability to collaborate from any location improves interaction between workers [41].

PROBLEMS. Deming has grasped the fundamental flaw that many information specialists never perceive: The computer may serve as a repository of data that are never used. A plan must exist for its use, and training is required [42]. Redundancy must be built in to allow for either paper backup or immediate recruitment of a functional computer if a workstation goes "down." Within an ICU environment, fluid-proof keypads and uninterruptable power supplies are mandatory.

DATA INTEGRITY AND SECURITY. By law, an original copy of any patient record must be maintained. All clinical data must be stored with adequate physical protection. This includes actual assault on, or theft of, the media. For magnetic media, a physical backup (using paper, magnetic, or optical media) stored in a separate geographic location is the norm; the manager of the system is responsible for this. The manager also must assure confidentiality. In the case of an LAN in the ICU, the manager may be the unit director [43].

A further legal problem exists with respect to risk management. If any portion of the medical record that would normally require a legal signature (e.g., chart notes) is stored, a means of verifying this is required. For many hospitals, this has meant issuing a code that becomes the "electronic signature." The clinician is exhorted not to divulge this code and it must be changed frequently. The National Institute of Standards and Technology has developed a digital signature methodology. This is composed of a digital signature standard and algorithm [44]. It is suggested that this technique or a similar one be utilized to assure veracity in the case of legal inquiry.

Conclusion

It is clear that the JCAHO wants an identified critical care unit manager to be responsible for assuring overall quality of care. The risk associated with such activities is minimal. When the director or staff become providers of care, however, the financial risk is very real. Accordingly, delegating setup and oversight responsibility for quality improvement and risk management to functionaries is unwise. Enlisting the aid of the staff involved in the actual process, however, epitomizes wisdom. Those with a vested interest in quality are more likely to maintain it. The added incentives of improving quality through collaboration, education, and the opportunity to influence technology acquisition may actually make active participation by the critical care personnel if not pleasurable, at least emotionally rewarding.

Another incentive to improving quality is the thought that, as in industry, salary and employment may soon be linked to quality. This idea is coming to fruition with the Clinton administration's attempt to tap the public sentiment with proposals for health care reform. Those who fail to provide quality care may be out of business.

References

1. An annotated bibliography: Total quality management. *Healthcare Information Management* 6:18, 1992.
2. The Joint Commission on Accreditation of Healthcare Organizations: Examples of monitoring and evaluation in special care units. 1988.
3. Willis RV: Malpractice memo: The perils of professional housecleaning: A legal cross fire. *Surg Rounds* 107, 1987.
4. *Accreditation Manual for Hospitals: Special Care Units (SP):* Chicago, Joint Commission for Accreditation of Healthcare Organizations, 1990, 251–267.
5. Walton M: *The Deming Management Method.* NY, Perigee Books, 1986.
6. Deming WE: *Out of the Crisis.* Cambridge, MA, MIT Center for Advanced Engineering Study, 1986.
7. Juran JM: *Juran's Quality Control Handbook.* 4th ed. New York, McGraw-Hill, 1988.
8. Walton M: *The Deming Management Method.* NY, Perigee Books, 1986.
9. Ishihara S: *The Japan That Can Say No.* NY, Simon & Schuster, 1993.
10. Berwick DM: TQM: Redefining doctoring. *Internist* 34:8, 1993.
11. Juran JM: *Juran's Quality Control Handbook.* 4th ed. New York, McGraw-Hill, 1988.
12. Walton M: *The Deming Management Method.* 4th ed. New York, McGraw-Hill, 1988.
13. *Accreditation Manual for Hospitals: Special Care Units (SP).* Chicago, Joint Commission for the Accreditation of Healthcare Organizations, 1993.
14. *Accreditation Manual for Hospitals: Special Care Units (SP).* Chicago, Joint Commission for the Accreditation of Healthcare Organizations, 1989.
15. Rayworth JF: Total quality management: Involving staff in the search for perfection. *Health Manpower Management* 19:25, 1993.
16. Grignol KA, Jordan S, Tobin R: Improved quality management of central lines demonstrates cost savings. *QRG Advisor* 8:4, 1993.
17. Pinkley DS: Joint Commission, New York battle over evaluations. *American Medical News,* Feb. 24, 1989, p 3.
18. Agenda for change: News from the Joint Commission. 3:1, 1989.
19. Teres D, Lemeshow S: Using severity measures to describe high performance intensive care units. *Crit Care Clin* 9:543, 1993.
20. Dawson JA: Admission, discharge & triage. *Crit Care Clin* 9:555, 1993.
21. Lehmann R: Joint Commission Forum: Forum on clinical indicator development: A discussion of the use and development of indicators. *QRB* 15:223, 1989.
22. Ballinger WF, Hepner JO: Total quality management and continuous quality improvement: An introduction for surgeons. *Surgery* 113:250, 1993.
23. Mahlen KA: Achieving superior performance through process improvement. *Healthcare Financial Management* 47:45, 1993.
24. Hawk AB, Miyamura JB: Quality improvement: How does it differ from quality assurance? *Hawaii Med J* 52:34, 1993.
25. Barrett MJ: Is your organization ready for total quality management? *Am J Med Qual* 7:106, 1992.
26. Walton M: *The Deming Management Method.* New York, Perigee Books, 1986.
27. Thompson TV: Implementing total quality management in health care: How do we get there from here? *J Healthcare Qual* 15:6, 1993.
28. Booth FV: *Quality assurance and computer applications in ICU's.* Presented at the Society of Critical Care Medicine annual meeting, New Orleans, 1989.
29. *Patrick vs. Burget,* 108 S. Ct. 1658 (1988).
30. Kraus GP: *Health Care Risk Management.* National Health Publishing-Rand Communications, 1986.
31. Louden TL: Customer perception counts in quality assurance. *Hospitals* 84, 1989.
32. Green C, et al: *The Quality Imperative.* New York, McGraw-Hill, 1994.
33. Walton M: *The Deming Management Method.* New York, Perigee Books, 1986.
34. Walton M: *The Deming Management Method.* New York, Perigee Books, 1986.
35. National Institute of Business Management: *Mastering Decision Making.* New York, Berkeley, 1991.
36. Wallace P: Help desk software. *Info World* 16:3, 1994.
37. *Acubase.* Seattle, Clinical Information Systems, 1993.
38. Oates PB: *Managing Critical Care Units* course manual. Orlando, 12th Managing Critical Care Units, Critical Care Education Foundation, 1994.
39. Impact 5.0 Data Management System, Lowell, MA, Instrumentation Laboratories, 1993.
40. Ball M: Aspects of CPRs (computerized patient record) and organizational redesign. *Healthcare Informatics* 10:28, 1993.
41. Dawson J: Computerized database management in critical care medicine: The problems of data retrieval, in Fein IA, Strosberg MA (eds): *Managing the Critical Care Unit,* Rockville, MD, Aspen, 1987, pp 198–221.
42. Walton M: *The Deming Management Method.* New York, Perigee Books, 1986.
43. Miller D: Caught with your LAN down: Security issues in an age of networks. *Healthcare Informatics* 10:56, 1993.
44. Schneier B: Digital signatures. *BYTE* 18:309, 1993.

236. Organization and Management of Critical Care Units

I. Alan Fein

The art of management is a complex concatenation of disciplines and methodologies, the significance of which is becoming increasingly evident as the health care industry contends with increasing demands and declining resources. Critical care represents a disproportionate fraction of hospital budgets frequently consuming as much as 20 percent of expenses for as little as 5 percent of total beds. The demand for cost-effective, high-quality medicine is perhaps most acute in the critical care setting, because the very nature of these already high-profile units invites ever closer scrutiny. Historically, the focus of medicine has been on the management of the critically ill patient. Now the forces of regulation, competition, advancing technology, finance and reimbursement, and demographics demand that medicine focus on the management of the critical care unit as well. The challenge for critical care unit directors is to manage their units in a manner that effectively meets the needs of patients, society, and the health care delivery community as well.

Organizational Development

Modern critical care units, having developed in fits and starts from 19th century postoperative recovery rooms, are still evolving in terms of organizational structure. From 1863, when Florence Nightingale noted that many hospitals in Great Britain had a small room adjacent to the operating theater, until the 1940s when centralized recovery rooms gained initial recognition, the impetus for critical care units seems to have been largely in response to widespread civilian and military nursing shortages. Then, as now, change came on the heels of practical necessity, rather than as the result of deliberate, scholarly planning.

Concentrating critically ill or still anesthetized postoperative patients into a single room proved to be a singularly efficient use of an increasingly limited resource. It was years, however, before the practice became commonplace. Despite the manpower shortages during World War II, and despite studies demonstrating that organizing patients, equipment, and personnel into specialized areas reduced postoperative complications and morbidity [1], recovery rooms were still a rarity in America in 1949 [2]. It seemed that the lessons of the 1942 Coconut Grove fire in Boston, which demonstrated the value of intensive care units, were taken to heart primarily by the military and the nursing profession. It was not until the polio epidemics of 1949–1950 and 1953 in Denmark, and 1955 in New England, that general intensive care units began to appear for patients other than those recovering from surgery. The increasing use of mechanical ventilators demanded that a specialized environment be created to accommodate the labor-intensive care associated with the management of patients with respiratory failure.

The political and economic fronts were also conducive to the development of intensive care units. The Hill-Burton Act of 1946 reimbursed hospitals for construction of new facilities, and the postwar mood of the nation was jubilant and expansive. Scientific research and development became national priorities in the 1950s, spurred by events such as the United States–Soviet rivalry in space and the polio epidemics. Much of the basic science research being done to put a person on the moon resulted in developments applicable to other fields such as medicine. The monitoring systems to be used in intensive care units benefited to a large degree from this work.

In the early 1960s, coronary care units established in Toronto, Kansas City, and Philadelphia hospitals demonstrated efficacy in reducing mortality and morbidity in patients with acute myocardial infarctions [3]. These results were extrapolated to encourage the development of general intensive care units. The Medicare and Medicaid acts, by reimbursing hospitals for the high-technology care of the elderly and indigent, respectively, made the construction of intensive care units financially attractive. During this time, there were also significant changes in the medical-legal climate in the United States. There was an increased litigiousness and awareness of malpractice, especially pronounced in metropolitan areas. The newly developed intensive care unit became a resource that physicians could use to demonstrate to families that "everything was being done" for their loved one, the ultimate posture in defensive medicine.

In the 1980s, it became clear that health care was no longer an unlimited resource. Critical care units, consuming a disproportionately large share of the health care dollar, came under increasingly close scrutiny. The management and organization of ICUs, previously left entirely in the hands of nursing, were now being examined by the occasional physician [4]. In an editorial entitled "Enter: The Era of Management," Teres hinted at the managerial roles that critical care physicians would soon have to undertake [5]. Knaus and associates suggested that there was a positive relationship between the level of organization and outcome, when data were analyzed after adjusting for severity of illness [6]. As the issues of quality assurance, utilization management, and resource allocation became increasingly important, the critical care unit came to be viewed as a scarce resource whose efficient management was necessitated from both patient care and financial perspectives. Furthermore, it became obvious that well-managed units should not only provide better patient care, but also provide a better working environment for both the physician and nursing staffs. This can be a critical factor in dealing with the nursing shortages still afflicting many intensive care units throughout the United States.

A more recent evolutionary advance in the development of critical care units has been the recognition of critical care as a valid specialty by the medical profession, a step which the nursing profession had taken previously, albeit via a different pathway. The standards of nursing care for the critically ill are just now being complemented by medical standards of care, with physicians beginning to assume more direct responsibility for the overall management of critical care units. Many decisions and responsibilities that had inappropriately defaulted to nursing (such as resource allocation) are now being assumed by joint physician-nurse teams. Indeed, as physicians begin to enter the management arena, their role demands definition. This can be problematic as there has been little uniformity in the organizational structures of intensive care units. Worse yet is the paucity of information regarding how units are managed or how patients fare in them.

In a scathing critique of intensive care patient management, Robin called for an analysis of current critical care practices in 1983, presaging the 1990's drive for outcomes assessment. He wrote:

The purpose of patient management is to optimize the possibility of happy and productive lives for patients. Much of ICU management, like much of modern medicine, may function tangentially to this main purpose. Physicians do harm as well as good. It is important to recognize this, not for the purpose of *mea culpa,* but so that the harm can be detected and minimized. The actual balance between good and harm has not been established in ICUs. Many patients admitted are irreversibly ill and some would benefit maximally by not being admitted to an ICU. Some patients are clearly salvaged by ICU admission; others are clearly harmed. The relative distribution of these patients is important to establish in guiding our approach to ICUs generally. . . . Our training programs should stress humility, careful recognition of our limitations, and approaches based on what not to do, as well as what to do. . . . Much of modern medicine would benefit from a critical examination. Critical care medicine, as an infant discipline, would benefit particularly [7].

Robin went on to call for a national registry for collecting outcome data of critically ill patients and for the development of "investigational ICUs on a national basis" to conduct prospective studies. The critical examination that Robin demanded is now getting underway in fits and starts. Initial findings suggest a remarkable diversity in structures, care, outcomes, and utilization. While no national registry exists, the Society for Critical Care Medicine (SCCM) has conducted point-in-time surveys, collecting patient characteristics and utilization data on 40 percent of the nation's ICUs, finding significant variations in the type, size, and utilization of units [8]. Knaus and colleagues, studying 42 ICUs in 40 hospitals in depth, found mortality rates varying from 6.4 percent to 40 percent, with 90 percent of the variation due to patient characteristics at the time of admission. Mean lengths of stay also varied significantly, from 3.3 to 7.3 days, with less of the variation accounted for by patient characteristics [9]. Studying the patients in the medical ICUs of a single university hospital, Oye and Bellamy found markedly skewed distributions of resource utilization, with many patients admitted only for either monitoring or for futile treatment [10]. A recent report by Rapoport and colleagues found that even when corrected for severity of illness, patients admitted to an ICU by a managed care group had significantly lower (30–40%) charges and lengths of stay than did traditionally insured patients, in spite of comparable survival statistics [11]. Of note, both groups utilized the same hospital-based intensivists and house officers. Most disturbing, especially in an era of scarce and declining resources, is the study of the utilization and rationing of beds in a surgical intensive care unit conducted by Marshall and colleagues. They found that in situations where surgical ICU beds were unavailable, but other ICU beds were available, decisions about admissions and discharges were not always made based solely on the patient's best interest. They concluded that in many instances, ". . . political power, medical provincialism, and income maximization overrode medical suitability in the provision of critical care services" [12]. One can only conclude that in some cases Robin was correct and that careful analysis of health care delivery practices in the ICU is essential.

Categorization and Standards

The declining pool of resources, both financial and personnel, for health care mandates an organized approach. The problems are especially acute in the critical care arena and organization must be approached at both the hospital and regional levels. The drive for quality assurance, cost containment, and optimization of resource use makes the reassessment and restructuring of current health care delivery systems inevitable.

The need to avoid redundancy has been well recognized. Before Diagnosis-Related Groups (DRGs) were introduced, excess beds and resources resulted in overutilization, possibly inappropriate care, and unnecessary expenditures. In the prospective payment era, the pathway is different but the bottom line is often the same: excessive beds and facilities result in underutilization, loss of skills, and excessive costs. The SCCM recently recommended the categorization of critical care units, with an eye towards regionalization and interhospital cooperation. The ideal situation consists of tertiary care centers surrounded and supported by concentric secondary and primary care hospitals, with patients admitted to hospitals according to their level of injury or disease. This vertical integration demands a high level of cooperation, if political obstacles are to be overcome. A major problem is reimbursement. The current DRG system assumes that there is a normal distribution of patients to each institution. The tools for assessing case-mix and severity of illness under DRGs are generally inadequate when applied to the population of critically ill patients; tertiary care centers can suffer significant financial consequences as a result. Changes must be enacted in the state and federal reimbursement programs to encourage efforts toward regionalization.

The SCCM has suggested two levels of care, with Level I representing optimal care for the most critically ill patients. Level I critical care units should be able to provide a wide range of continuous, sophisticated, tertiary level services, including not only state-of-the-art equipment but the services of specially trained physicians and nurses as well. Level IC units represent this high level of clinical care, while Level IA units have an additional commitment to education and research in the field of critical care nursing and medicine. Level II hospitals are generally smaller institutions with limited resources. While these institutions can provide high-quality care for patients with single organ failure, caring for the desperately ill patient with multisystem failure can be problematic. Therefore, Level II institutions should have comprehensive transfer protocols and agreements with Level I hospitals to assure continuous and optimal care of patients. Table 236-1 attempts to differentiate and establish standards for critical care units. This represents the work of the SCCM's Task Force on Guidelines and is presented here for discussion purposes only.

The specific details of unit organization within the framework of Table 236-1 are problematic. There is little, if any, consensus or uniformity regarding the organization of units apart from that established by the nursing profession. For example, many major tertiary critical care units, which are covered at night by upper level residents, or intermittently by fellows, or by lower level residents with senior resident backup would not be recognized as Level I by this categorization scheme. Many of these units have a large critical care faculty, who are available within 30 minutes and are active in critical care education and research.

Another controversial area is the requirement that primary attending physicians be certified in critical care medicine. What other boards or training would be considered as equivalent qualifications? Why exclude the patient's primary attending physician? One consensus approach would be to have concurrent care provided by a physician with critical care or equivalent credentials. Regardless of specialty, the primary attending physician must be actively involved in the patient's general management; the era of the cursory hospital visit is long past.

It is hard to adequately define the role(s) of the physician director. Collaborative practice, a laudable goal of both the

Table 236-1. Definition of Hospital Resources*

		Level		
		IC	IA	II
I.	Medical Staff Organization			
	A. A distinct medical staff critical care organizational entity (department, division, section or service) exists.	E	E	E
	1. Privileges (both cognitive and procedural) for members of the critical care team are approved by the medical staff credentials committee based on previous training and experience as defined by the medical staff.	E	E	E
	2. A section of the medical staff bylaws spells out the regulations governing the implementation of these conditions.	E	E	E
	3. Budgetary activities relating to unit function, quality assurance, and utilization review are conducted as joint medical/nursing/administrative endeavors.	E	E	E
	4. A critical are representative sits on the medical staff executive committee.	E	E	D
	B. The team is organized and led by an intensivist with time, expertise in, and significant commitment to the care of the critically ill patient.	E	E	D
	C. Each patient's management is directed by an attending-level physician who			
	1. Is privileged by the medical staff to have case management responsibility for critically ill patients.	E	E	E
	2. Is board certified in critical care medicine or has equivalent qualifications.	E	E	D
	3. Sees the patient as often as required by acuity but at least twice daily.	E	E	E
	Note: This physician may be either the patient's attending physician or a consultant designated as the case management physician.			
	D. The medical staff has a Bioethical Committee.	E	E	E
II.	Unit Organization			
	A. A unit director is appointed.	E	E	E
	The unit director is			
	1. A physician who, on the basis of training, interests, type of practice, and time availability can give clinical, administrative, and educational direction to the ICU.	E	E	E
	2. A physician who is board certified in his/her specialty.	E	E	E
	3. Regularly involved in the care of patients in the unit.	E	E	E
	4. Manager of the administrative aspects of the unit, including formation of policies and procedures, enforcement of unit policies, and the education of unit staff.	E	E	E
	5. Responsible for assuring the quality, safety, and appropriateness of care in the ICU.	E	E	E
	6. Certified in critical care medicine or has equivalent qualifications in compliance with the medical staff credentialing process.	E	E	D
	7. Available (or can provide an *equally qualified* alternate) to the unit 24 hr/day, 7 days/wk for both clinical and administrative matters.	E	E	E
	8. Knowledgeable about the development of critical care medicine and participates in national and local societies.	E	E	D
	9. A participant in continuing education programs in the field of critical care medicine.	E	E	E
	10. An advisor and participant in the development of and cooperates with the critical care organization in the community as a whole.	E	E	E
	11. A participant in the education of unit staff, other physicians, house staff, and medical staff as indicated.	E	E	E
	12. A participant in scholarly activity (case reports, clinical, and/or basic research).	E	E	O
	13. An advisor and participant in the review of the appropriate utilization of ICU resources in the hospital.	E	E	E
	B. A nurse manager is appointed to establish clear lines of authority and responsibility for delivery of quality nursing care and for safety and appropriateness of nursing care.			
	The nurse manager is			
	1. An RN with a BSN degree.	E	E	D
	2. Certified as CCRN (critical care nurse) *or* certified in nursing administration.	E	E	D
	3. An experienced ICU nurse having			
	a. At least 3 yrs' experience working in a critical care unit, *and*	E	E	E
	b. Previous management experience	E	E	E
	4. Prepared to participate in the education of			
	a. Unit staff	E	E	E
	b. House staff and fellows	D	E	D
	5. A participant in ongoing continuing education	E	E	E
	6. Prepared to cooperate with scholarly activity (e.g., presentations, clinical research)	D	E	O
III.	Physician Availability			
	A. 24-hr inhouse coverage:			
	1. Physician who can manage emergencies and is not also covering the emergency department, and is certified in ACLS[a]	E	E	E
	2. Critical care physician with case management credentials fully dedicated to the critical care unit to provide titrated medical care[b]	E	E	O
	3. Physician with emergency medicine credentials on duty in the emergency department	E	E	D
	B. On call and available within 30 min			
	1. General surgeon	E	E	E
	2. Neurosurgeon	E	E	O
	3. Cardiovascular surgeon	E	E	O
	4. Obstetric-gynecologic surgeon	E	E	O
	5. Urologic surgeon	E	E	O
	6. Thoracic surgeon	E	E	O
	7. Vascular surgeon	E	E	O
	8. Anesthesiologist	E	E	E
	9. Cardiologist	E	E	D
	10. Pulmonary internist	E	E	D

Table 236-1. (continued)

	Level		
	IC	IA	II
11. Gastroenterologist	E	E	O
12. Hematologist	E	E	O
13. Infectious disease internist	E	E	D
14. Nephrologist	E	E	D
15. Neuroradiologist	D	D	O
16. Pathologist	E	E	D
17. Radiologist	E	E	E
18. Traumatologist (required only if designated trauma center)	E	E	E
19. Neurologist	E	E	D
20. Orthopedic surgeon	E	E	D
IV. Nursing Availability	E	E	D
A. Nursing ratio based on acuity	E	E	E
1. Minimum 1:3 RN/patient ratio with ability to increase to 1:2, 1:1, or 2:1 if acuity demands	—	—	O
2. Minimum 1:2 RN/patient ratio with ability to increase to 1:1 or 2:1 if acuity demands	E	E	D
B. Oriented to the unit before assuming responsibility for patient care	E	E	E
C. Must participate in continuing education activities	E	E	E
V. Respiratory Therapy			
A. A respiratory therapist is available to the unit at all times. Ideal levels of staffing are based on acuity, utilizing objective measures whenever possible.	E	E	E
B. A respiratory therapist is fully dedicated to the ICU.	E	E	D
VI. Services Provided in Unit			
An ICU has the capability of providing basic monitoring and patient support. In order to do so, an ICU is prepared to provide			
A. Continuous monitoring of ECG (with high/low alarms) in all patients	E	E	E
B. Continuous arterial monitoring (invasive and noninvasive)	E	E	E
C. CVP monitoring	E	E	E
D. Equipment to maintain the airway, including laryngoscope, endotracheal tubes	E	E	E
E. Equipment to ventilate, including Ambu bags, ventilators, oxygen, and compressed air	E	E	E
F. Emergency resuscitative equipment	E	E	E
G. Equipment to support hemodynamics, including infusion pumps, blood warmer, pressure bags, blood filters	E	E	E
H. Transport monitor	E	E	E
I. Beds with removable headboard and adjustable position	E	E	E
J. Adequate lighting for bedside procedures	E	E	E
K. Suction	E	E	E
L. Hypo-, hyperthermia blanket	E	E	E
M. Scale	E	E	E
N. Temporary pacemaker	E	E	E
O. Temperature monitoring device	E	E	E
P. Pulmonary artery pressure monitoring	E	E	E
Q. Cardiac output monitoring	E	E	E
R. Continuous inspired oxygen monitoring capability for all ventilators	E	E	E
S. Hemodialysis	E	E	O
T. Peritoneal dialysis	E	E	D
U. Capnography	E	E	D
V. Transcutaneous oxygen monitoring or pulse oximetry for all patients receiving supplemental oxygen	E	E	E
W. Access to CT scanner, cardiac catheterization lab, nuclear medicine testing[c]	E	E	O
X. Fiberoptic and rigid bronchoscopy	E	E	D
Y. Fluoroscopy capability in unit or readily available in radiology	E	E	O
Z. Intracranial pressure monitoring	E	E	O
AA. Extracorporeal membrane oxygen	O	O	O
BB. Left heart assist devices	O	O	O
CC. Hyperbaric chamber	D	D	O
DD Computerized data management systems	D	D	O
EE. Intra-aortic balloon assist device	E	E	O
FF. Magnetic resonance imaging	D	D	O
VII. Support Services			
A. 24-hr availability			
1. Clinical laboratory services			
a. Standard analysis of blood, urine, body fluids	E	E	E
b. Blood typing and cross matching	E	E	E
c. Coagulation studies	E	E	E
d. Blood banking services		E	E
e. Blood gas determination	E	E	E
f. Determination of Na, K, Cl, CO_2, blood glucose, BUN, creatinine	E	E	E
g. Microbiology	E	E	E
h. Toxicology and alcohol screens	E	E	D
2. Portable radiographic equipment	E	E	E
3. Pharmacy	E	E	E

Table 236-1. (continued)

			Level		
			IC	IA	II
	4.	Housekeeping	E	E	E
	5.	Central supply or equivalent	E	E	E
	6.	Biomedical technician	E	E	E
	7.	12-lead ECG recording	E	E	E
	8.	Unit clerk or equivalent	E	E	E
B.		During routine working day			
	1.	Physical/occupational therapy	E	E	E
	2.	Psychiatrist/psychologist	E	E	E
	3.	Clergy	E	E	E
	4.	Social workers	E	E	E
	5.	Noninvasive cardiac investigation lab (echocardiogram/Holter monitoring)	E	E	D
VIII.	Transport Policies				
A.		Interhospital transport is a responsibility shared by Level I and II units.			
	1.	Transfer agreements are in place and specify which patients shall be transferred from Level II to Level I.	E	E	E
	2.	A transport team qualified in life-support techniques exists and is available continuously.	E	E	E
B.		A policy for intrahospital transport exists specifying who accompanies a patient being transported within the hospital and what monitoring/equipment is constantly available.	E	E	E
IX.	Education in Critical Care				
A.		Continuing education activities in critical care provided by hospital for			
	1.	Staff physicians	E	E	O
	2.	Community physicians	D	E	O
	3.	Nurses	E	E	O
	4.	Allied health personnel	E	E	O
B.		Formal training programs in			
	1.	General surgery	D	E	O
	2.	Internal medicine	D	E	O
	3.	Anesthesia	D	E	O
	4.	Nursing	D	D	O
	5.	Respiratory therapy	D	D	O
X.	Critical Care Research Program		D	E	O

E, essential; D, desirable; O, optional.

[a]This requirement may be fulfilled by senior residents, house officers, or physician assistants (or equivalent) capable of handling emergent situations. When residents are used to fulfill this responsibility, an attending physician must be on call and available within 30 min.

[b]This requirement may be fulfilled by critical care fellows. When fellows are used to fulfill this responsibility, an intensivist must be on call and available within 30 min.

[c]If not available in-house, transfer agreements exist with institutions that have this capability.

*From Bekes C, Bayly RW, Branson RD, et al: SCCM Guidelines: Recommendations for Categorization of Services for the Critically Ill Patient, *Concern,* Summer 1990, pp 38–48.

AMA and ANA for many years, has proven equally difficult to implement even though its principles are widely accepted. Most, if not all, critical care units are held hostage to local hospital politics and history.

The medical sociologist Anselm Strauss and his colleagues suggest that the workings of a unit are the result of a "negotiated order," whereby sets of implicit or tacit understandings, agreements, and informal contracts among the professionals, nonprofessionals, and patients, arrived at through negotiation over time, govern relationships [13]. This model suggests the unit is a locale where personnel "are enmeshed in a complex negotiative process in order both to accomplish their individual purposes and to work—in an established division of labor—toward clearly as well as vaguely phrased institutional objectives" [14]. Clarification of objectives and roles, untangling lines of authority and responsibility, and full understanding of the organizational order are the *sine qua non* of effective management and leadership.

Organizational Structures

As intensive care units have evolved organizationally in response to economic, political, human resource, and, occasion-

ally, medical demands, several common models have become apparent:

1. Open unit with no physician director
2. Open unit with a part-time physician director
   a. Nonsalaried volunteer staff physician as director
   b. Paid part-time staff physician director
3. Open unit with a full-time physician director and open medical staff
4. Open unit with a full-time physician director and full-time medical staff
5. Semiclosed unit with a full-time physician director and full-time medical staff
6. Closed unit with a full-time physician director and full-time medical staff
7. Full-time medical staff in models 4, 5, and 6 above may be either:
   a. Direct employees of the hospital, or
   b. Employees of a corporation that contracts with the hospital for management of the critical care unit(s), or
   c. Members of a faculty practice plan.

The terms used in the above outline are defined as follows:

1. *Open unit.* All qualified attending physicians may admit and care for patients in the unit. Triage decisions fall to the unit

director only when there is a bed or staffing shortage. Director and/or associates consult on patients only when requested.

2. *Semiclosed unit.* Director and/or associates(s) must review and approve all admissions, taking into consideration appropriateness of care and staffing levels. All final decisions regarding admission, discharge, and triage rest with the physician director(s). Physician director may consult on all patients, do so only when requested, or consult only in the case of an emergency situation.

3. *Closed unit.* Director and/or associates are responsible for all admissions and discharges. When patients are admitted to the unit, they are formally turned over to the unit team for care. The physician director and associates assume primary responsibility for patient care for the duration, and work collaboratively with the admitting physician.

There is a slowly growing body of evidence suggesting that the organizational structure, degree of communication, and type of physician staffing can affect patient outcomes in critical care units [6,15,16,17]. Until recently, the majority of critical care units in the United States functioned with either no physician director or a part-time director. Often the physician director was a titular position, a member of the medical community who would volunteer his or her time to serve on a committee in order to satisfy regulatory requirements. A recent survey of some 200 critical care unit nursing directors from throughout the United States attending a management conference revealed that only a small number worked in units without a physician director. Nevertheless, many of those who worked in units with a physician director felt that their directors acted in name only, and that many decision-making responsibilities, such as triage, conflict resolution, and bed allocation, unfairly defaulted to them [18].

Some experts argue that a closed unit staffed by full-time intensivists is the most efficient and cost-effective model for managing a critical care unit in large hospitals. Even in small to moderate-size hospitals, full-time intensivists may provide a level of care and service to the community that justifies their cost. Given the increasing sophistication of the physiologic monitoring modalities in use and the labor-intensive nature of critical care, the ongoing presence of a consistent individual or group well versed in state-of-the-art science would seem to be a *sine qua non* of ideal ICU care. While there are many physicians capable of caring for the most seriously ill patient, availability is a quintessential attribute of the intensivist. The ability to respond immediately to changes in patients' conditions, to assess and reassess throughout the day, and to provide a high degree of continuity of care are difficult to achieve when physicians are sequestered in the operating room or in the office with outpatients. Even brief delays can have catastrophic consequences for the critically ill. Finally, private primary practitioners would be freed of the labor-intensive, time-demanding care the critically ill require and have more time for their floor and outpatient practices without losing control of the patients.

Critical care unit directors are routinely charged with the responsibilities of cost containment and quality assurance. Identifying problem areas is a simple task compared with that of rectifying them. Practice patterns of physicians are notoriously difficult to alter. Nursing and administrative policies are also hard to change. While the unit director can ultimately effect change through his or her activities as an educator, timely and effective progress can be achieved only when the director is granted authority appropriate to given responsibilities. This generally implies significant authority over allocation of beds, triage, admissions, and discharges. Appropriate authority also implies the ability to intervene, if not directly manage, all patients in the unit. From a purely managerial perspective, the

most effective situation is one in which there are relatively few physicians involved in the direct care of patients, and where lines of communication, responsibility, authority, availability, and especially accountability are clear and unambiguous. A closed unit with full-time intensivists providing the primary care for all patients, working collaboratively with the admitting physicians, consultants, and nursing staffs comes closest to filling this goal. Although commonplace in Europe and Australia, this model is uncommon in the United States.

There are potential disadvantages to closed units. Unit-based intensivists do not have preexisting relationships with patients and their families, and do not have the details and nuances of patients' medical histories that primary physicians would have. While continuity of care may be improved when patients are in the critical care unit, there is a distinct disruption when patients are transferred in or out. Closed units may alienate referring physicians, resulting, at worst, in decreased admissions (downstream rationing?) and a possibly hostile environment, or, at best, in decreased involvement by physicians in the critical care unit. The latter may lead to decreased scrutiny of medical practices in the unit, complacency on the part of the full-time intensivists, and the loss of valuable medical input from primary medical and surgical practitioners and medical subspecialists. Closed unit directors also may find that when a patient is ready to be transferred to the floor, the primary attending physician may no longer be interested in resuming care of that patient. This leaves the intensivist in the uneasy role of either caring for the patient on the floor or finding a new primary physician. The former situation can lead to a sizable ward and outpatient practice, which will undermine the intensivist's ability and time commitment in the ICU, and possibly compromise his or her reputation in the medical community. The latter situation of finding a new physician disrupts the continuity of care and can generally be awkward for all involved. Furthermore, there may be an erosion of support and commitment for the unit by the medical community at large unless physicians are made to understand and feel that it is indeed a valuable resource for all. Regardless of the organizational structure, there are many reasons why the intensivist should try to keep the primary physician as involved and informed as is possible. As with any large organization, the medical-hospital community is not immune to politicization; perceptions are often more important than is substance. The art of public relations may be as important to the director of a closed as an open unit.

The organizational structures of critical care units have evolved out of, or have been superimposed on, preexisting structures. Establishing a new organizational structure must be done within the framework of the existing order of the institution. Effecting significant change in the politically negotiated order of hospitals is even more difficult to achieve than in the practice patterns of physicians. Frequently, change occurs as a consequence of litigation, state or federal regulation, or financial constraints. A thorough understanding of the political dynamics of the institution and the health care environment in which it exists is required and will have a significant impact on the eventual structure of the unit [19].

A compelling case for team or triad management has been made by Teres and associates [20]. This involves developing an organizational structure that identifies and brings together individuals from administration, nursing, and medicine, clearly identifying their roles to achieve common and mutually beneficial goals. Conflicts among nurses, physicians, and administrators are initially inevitable given their diverse educations, backgrounds, and orientations; however, conflicts are equally likely to arise among medical specialties such as surgery, anesthesia, medicine, cardiology, and pulmonary medicine. The multidisciplinary nature of critical care demands coalition building. It is imperative that differences among specialists be recognized, that each learns the language of the others, understands one another's concerns, and begins the process of cross-cultural team building. When an atmosphere of understanding, communication, and commonalty of purpose exists, then team-building efforts can proceed to the staff level, and true participative decision-making will ensue [21,22].

Achieving this ideal state is far easier said than done. It is certainly possible to design an organizational structure for any hospital unit, and through executive decree attempt to incorporate it into the hospital order. One can draw an organizational chart, formally designate managers, and delineate reporting relationships. This can be facilitated through the use of many devices, such as collaborative practice committees, participatory management, and outside consultants, but there is no guarantee of success in an environment as politically fragmented as most hospitals. The most likely route will be, as Strosberg suggests, through intense coalition formation and bargaining [19]. The probability of success will rest on the ability of the institution to clarify its goals, and of the appointed unit director to understand the negotiated order of the hospital and work within it. Ultimately, success will depend on skilled politicians working to overcome traditional rigidities, historical "baggage," and issues of "turf."

The Medical Director

The Joint Commission on Accreditation of Healthcare Organizations (JCAHO) currently mandates that special care units be directed by a "physician member of the active medical staff who has received special training, acquired experience, and demonstrated competence in a specialty related to the care provided in the unit" [23]. The JCAHO goes on to enumerate the general responsibilities of the physician director in broad terms, without specifying how to implement those activities. The nursing profession has developed the role of the critical care nurse manager over the years. These individuals have been, directly or indirectly, responsible for on-the-job training of many of today's physician intensivists and unit directors. The role of a physician director in a collaboratively managed critical care unit will depend on the relationship between the physician and nurse managers and the environment involved (e.g., trauma unit, surgical, medical, or coronary care unit, community or teaching hospital). Nonetheless, there is a core commonalty to the physician director's job description that applies regardless of the particular situation. A partial listing of a medical director's activities and responsibilities might be as follows:

1. Coordinator of patient care
2. Continuous quality improvement (CQI)
   a. Critical care unit CQI committee and programs
   b. Representation on hospital-wide QA committee
   c. ICU-divisional-departmental morbidity/mortality review and conferences
3. Risk management
4. Safety net for patient care
   a. When attending physician is unavailable
   b. For emergency situations
5. Teacher
   a. Nursing, respiratory therapists, and laboratory staff
   b. Medical students and house staff
   c. Medical-surgical-anesthesia attending staff
6. Medical consultant, both formal and informal

7. Resource on medical ethics and medical-legal issues
   a. Institutional ethics committee
   b. Family conferences
8. Policy maker-policy enforcer
   a. Critical care services/policy committee
   b. Utilization review
9. Critical care cost containment-review-finance
10. Epidemiology and infection control
11. Resource utilization (includes triage)
12. Research
13. Patient advocate
14. Staff advocate
15. Conflict resolution
   a. Physician vs. physician
   b. Physician vs. nurse
   c. Nurse vs. nurse
   d. Staff vs. administration
16. ICU physician-nurse team building
17. Equipment acquisition-assessment-bioengineering
18. Computers-MIS applications
19. Critical care unit design expert
20. Healthcare policy-regulation resource
21. Interhospital relations and regional planning
22. Social services resource
23. Liaison with:
   a. Hospital administration
   b. Physician staff
   c. Nursing staff and administration
   d. Respiratory therapy staff
   e. Pharmacy
   f. Laboratory
   g. Radiology
   h. Physical therapy
   i. Departments of medicine, surgery, anesthesia
   j. Clergy-pastoral care department

Each of these roles, activities, and responsibilities is deserving of extensive exposition and discussion, a task far beyond the scope of this chapter.

The physician director, whether full- or part-time, is jointly responsible, with the nurse manager, for the smooth running of the unit and optimizing patient care. The concept of optimal care, however, is problematic because there are no well-defined standards of care for the critically ill. The diversity of care, expectations, and utilization of critical care units is remarkably wide and, as yet, uncharted. Until there are such standards, optimal care will be defined by local community standards and within the limitations of medical-nursing resources, and financial and organizational constraints.

While all physicians are trained in patient care and management, none are trained in unit care and management. The formal educations provided by medical or nursing schools do little to prepare for the skills necessary to manage the diverse personnel, financial, legal, and regulatory problems that arise daily in critical care units. The on-the-job-training that has constituted the education of current and past unit directors may no longer be adequate to meet the demands of today, and certainly not those of tomorrow.

The current medical-legal-economic climate demands that critical care units be operated at peak efficiency, optimizing quality and resource utilization while minimizing costs and risks. The issue for many unit directors is how to achieve these goals within the politically negotiated order of their institutions. This problem is compounded by the fact that, unlike other, more established specialties, there are no performance standards that are widely accepted for the care of the critically ill. There are, in fact, no well-accepted standards for resource utilization or quality assurance for critical care units. This is especially problematic, in that industrial quality control techniques, such as those developed by W. Edwards Deming [24] and Joseph M. Juran [25], are now being brought to bear on the medical arena. The potential benefits of these techniques are significant for the health care delivery system, but the potential for abuse and misapplication is also substantial. The key element central to these processes is the definition of "quality" [26]. While acceptable complication and mortality rates have been described for most surgical procedures and the management of most discrete diseases, this has not been the case for critically ill patients and critical care units. Severity of illness tools and mortality probability models such as MPM II [27], APACHE III [28], or SAPS II [29] may eventually prove to be useful in defining quality of care and appropriateness of resource utilization for the critically ill. As Berwick has written:

The unabashed rise in health care costs is bringing health services research into center stage as an applied science to help guide health care managers, purchasers, and regulators... [We] must pursue at least four intellectual agendas: the study of efficacy (knowing what works), the study of appropriateness (using what works), the study of the execution of care (doing well what works), and the study of the purposes of care (the values that underlie action). The responsibility for the financing and conduct of the research agendas varies with the level of aggregation of data and effort needed for each topic. All four topics must be pursued effectively if health care quality is to be successfully defined, measured, and protected [30].

These agendas are most pressing for the directors of critical care units for at least two reasons: first, as mentioned above, less is known about this diverse population of multisystem involvement patients than other subgroups in medicine; and second, the demands are more intense because this population consumes a disproportionately large share of financial and personnel resources. In fact, the primary responsibilities of a critical care unit manager or director can be condensed to a three-prong mission:

1. Maintain bed availability and accessibility;
2. Maximize cost effectiveness; and
3. Assure optimal quality care for all patients.

Achieving these goals can be difficult for several reasons. First is the lack of a meaningful national database describing the critical care populations and their care. The currently available studies by the SCCM and others are inherently biased in that they are voluntary databases or registries. Meaningful analysis must be representative of all intensive care unit patients. Berwick's four agendas must be carried out in order to provide the standards, knowledge base, and framework that will be required for unit directors to work toward these goals. The key element will be the ability to recognize well-managed, high-performance critical care units. Indeed, an immediate goal for research is to define objective parameters that can measure performance and quality of care.

Second, there are inherent conflicts of interest for physicians within the aforementioned three goals. Can the physician director adequately fill the role of patient advocate while he or she is attempting to contain costs and allocate beds, and, at the same time, bill for procedures? The ethicist Robert Veatch has examined the role of physicians as managers and cost-containment agents. He warns that clinicians may need to replace the Hippocratic Oath with a sign that says; "Warning, all ye who enter here: I will generally work for your interest but in the case of marginally beneficial, expensive care, I will abandon you in order to serve society as [its] cost-containment agent" [31].

Health care reform in the United States is driven largely by the need to contain costs. As the legislators and the free market rework health care delivery systems, most probably within a managed care or managed competition framework, the future impact on intensivists and critical care is not yet clear. The current emphasis on primary care and the possibility of capitation as a payment scheme may phase out "expensive" specialists such as intensivists. On the other hand, in integrated systems with global budgeting, intensivists may indeed be cost-effective and could well flourish as a specialty. In such systems, hospital-based intensivists who manage to reduce lengths of stay for their patients could easily justify the costs of their positions without posing an economic threat to the primary care physicians in the community [32]. Indeed, by relieving primary practitioners of the high-risk, labor-intensive work that critically ill patients demand, they may well be viewed as assets to physicians whose practices are office-based or who are in the operating room for much of the time.

Ethical dilemmas present the critical care unit manager with as many problems as do any of the other issues mentioned above. Indeed, the ICU is often the ethical crucible for medicine, constantly testing traditions, beliefs, and principles. In an editorial aptly titled "Everything that *Should* Be Done—Not Everything that *Can* Be Done," Schuster underscores Berwick's call to assess the values that underlie our actions, especially among the critically ill [33]. Dealing with the issues of futile care, triage, withholding and withdrawing treatment, and other ethical quandaries discussed elsewhere in this volume, is part of the daily routine in the intensive care unit. Critical care unit directors must be proactive and provide a leadership role in assuring the just, appropriate, and rational allocation of services, regardless of how difficult many of those decisions may be. As Zimmerman and colleagues concluded following an extensive national study of ICU performance, critical care will ". . . continue to be costly and the ethical issues surrounding the use of ICU resources will continue to grow. ICUs will need to become organizationally and managerially competent in order to deal with these challenges" [34]. The role of the physician director of a critical care unit obviously needs to be explored on many levels and clarified to avoid conflicts and misunderstandings. The challenge for the immediate future is to develop managerial structures and processes based on hard information, and to forge multidisciplinary coalitions for the collaborative practice of critical care medicine.

References

1. Dunn FE, Shupp MG: The recovery room: A wartime economy. *Am J Nurs* 43:279, 1943.
2. Charbon HGA, Livingston HM: Planning a recovery room for adequate postoperative care. *Hospitals* 23:35, 1949.
3. Hilberman M: The evolution of intensive care units. *Crit Care Med* 3:159, 1975.
4. Fein IA, Strosberg MS (ed): *Managing the Critical Care Unit.* Rockville, MD, Aspen, 1987.
5. Teres D: Enter: The era of management. *Crit Care Med* 13:137, 1985.
6. Knaus WA, Draper EA, Wagner DP, et al: An evaluation of outcome from intensive care in major medical centers. *Ann Intern Med* 104:410, 1986.
7. Robin ED: A critical look at critical care. *Crit Care Med* 11:144, 1983.
8. Groeger JS, Guntupalli KK, Strosberg M, et al: Descriptive analysis of critical care units in the United States: Patient characteristics and intensive care unit utilization. *Crit Care Med* 21:279, 1993.
9. Knaus WA, Wagner WP, Zimmerman JE, Draper EA: Variations in mortality and length of stay in intensive care units. *Ann Intern Med* 118:753, 1993.

10. Oye RK, Bellamy PE: Patterns of resource consumption in medical intensive care. *Chest* 99:685, 1991.
11. Rapoport J, Gehlbach S, Lemeshow S, et al: Resource consumption among intensive care patients: Managed care vs. traditional insurance. *Arch Intern Med* 152:2207, 1992.
12. Marshall MF, Schwenzer KJ, Orsina M, et al: Influence of political power, medical provincialism, and economic incentives on the rationing of surgical intensive care beds. *Crit Care Med* 20:387, 1992.
13. Strauss A, Fagerhaugh S, Suczek B, et al: *Social Organization of Medical Work*. Chicago, University of Chicago, 1985.
14. Strauss A, Schatzman L, et al: The hospital and its negotiated order, in Friedson E (ed): *The Hospital in Modern Society*. New York, Free Press of Glencoe, 1963.
15. Teres D, Brown RB, Lemeshow S, et al: A comparison of mortality and charges in two differently staffed intensive care units. *Inquiry* 20:282, 1983.
16. Reynolds HN, Haupt MT, Thill-Baharozian MC: Impact of critical care physician staffing on patients with septic shock in a university hospital medical intensive care unit. *JAMA* 260:3446, 1988.
17. Brown JJ, Sullivan G: Effect on ICU mortality of a full-time critical care specialist. *Chest* 96:127, 1989.
18. Strosberg MA, Teres D, Fein IA, et al: Nursing perception of the availability of the intensive care unit director for triage and conflict resolution. *Heart Lung* 19:452, 1990.
19. Strosberg MA: The critical care unit: In search of management and excellence, in Fein IA, Strosberg MA (eds): *Managing the Critical Care Unit*. Rockville, MD, Aspen, 1987.
20. Teres D, Chandler RE, Riddle MM: Critical care unit administration: The management team approach, in Fein IA, Strosberg MA (eds): *Managing the Critical Care Unit*. Rockville, MD, Aspen, 1987.
21. Shortell SM: Theory Z: Implications and relevance for health care management. *HCM Rev* 7:7, 1982.
22. Kuhn R: Nurse and physician collaboration: How to strengthen the team. *Heart Lung* 14:18, 1985.
23. *Accreditation Manual for Hospitals: Special Care Units*. Chicago, Joint Commission of the Accreditation of Healthcare Organizations, 1992.
24. Deming WE: *Quality, Productivity and Competitive Position*. Cambridge, MA, MIT Center for Advanced Engineering Study, 1982.
25. Juran JM: *Managerial Breakthrough*. New York, McGraw-Hill, 1964.
26. Berwick DM: Toward an applied technology for quality measurement in health care. *Med Decis Making* 8:253, 1988.
27. Lemeshow S, Teres D, Klar J, et al: Mortality probability models (MPM II) based on an international cohort of intensive care patients. *JAMA* 270:2478, 1993.
28. Knaus WA, Wagner DP, Draper EA, et al: The APACHE III prognostic system: Risk prediction of hospital mortality for critically ill hospitalized adults. *Chest* 100:1619, 1991.
29. LeGall JR, Lemeshow S, Saulnier F: A new simplified acute physiology score (SAPS II) based on a European/North American multicenter study. *JAMA* 270:2957, 1993.
30. Berwick DM: Health services research and quality of care: Assignments for the 1990s. *Med Care* 27:763, 1989.
31. Veatch RM: DRGs and the ethical reallocation of resources. *Hastings Cent Rep* 83, 1986.
32. Fein IA, Sander B, Cohen IL, et al: Critical care physician billing, unit utilization, and efficiency: Reassessing the financial base of critical care. *Crit Care Med* 21(suppl):S220, 1993.
33. Schuster DP: Everything that should be done—not everything that can be done. *Am Rev Respir Dis* 145:508, 1992.
34. Zimmerman JE, Shortell SM, Rousseau DM, et al: Improving intensive care: Observations based on organizational case studies in nine units: A prospective, multicenter study. *Crit Care Med* 21:1443, 1993.

Appendix

Section Editor
Frederick J. Curley

Calculations Commonly Used in Critical Care

Frederick J. Curley

Table of Contents

Abbreviations Used in the Appendix

A	Alveolar	atm	Atmosphere
D	Dead	BSA	Body surface area
E	Expiration	cap	Capillary
I	Inspiration	cr	Creatinine
P	Pressure	dyn	Dynamic
$\dot{Q}$	Net liquid flow	is	Interstitium
R	Respiratory quotient	st	Static
T	Tidal	ICP	Intracranial pressure
V	Volume	a	Arterial
Δ	Change	d	Distribution
η	Viscosity	l	Length
π	Oncotic pressure	r	Radius
σ	Permeability	t	Time
		$\bar{v}$	Mixed venous

Fahrenheit and Celsius Temperature Conversions

°C	°F
45	113.0
44	111.2
43	109.4
42	107.6
41	105.8
40	104.0
39	.102.2
38	100.4
37	98.6
36	96.8
35	95.0
34	93.2
33	91.4
32	89.6
31	87.8
30	86.0
29	84.2
28	82.4
27	80.6
26	78.8
25	77.0
24	75.2
23	73.4
22	71.6
21	69.8
20	68.0

Hemodynamic Calculations

MEAN BLOOD PRESSURE (mm Hg)

$= \overline{BP}$

$$= \frac{Systolic\ BP + (2 \times Diastolic\ BP)}{3}$$

$= Diastolic\ BP + 1/3\ (Systolic\ BP - Diastolic\ BP)$

Normal values: 85–95 mm Hg

THE FICK EQUATION FOR CARDIAC INDEX (L/min/m^2)

$= CI$

$$= \frac{CO}{BSA}$$

$$= \frac{Oxygen\ consumption}{Arterial\ O_2\ content - Venous\ O_2\ content}$$

$$= \frac{10 \times \dot{V}O_2(\text{ml/min/m}^2)}{Hgb\ (\text{gm/dl}) \times 1.39 \times (Arterial\ \%\ saturation - Venous\ \%\ saturation)}$$

Normal values: 2.5–4.2 L/min/m^2

STROKE INDEX (ml/beat/m^2)

$$= \frac{CI\ (\text{L/min/m}^2) \times 1000}{Heart\ rate\ (\text{beats/min})}$$

Normal values: 33–47 ml/beat/m^2

SYSTEMIC VASCULAR RESISTANCE (dyne-sec-cm^{-5})

$= SVR$

$$= \frac{80 \times (arterial\ \overline{BP} - right\ atrial\ \overline{BP})}{CO\ (\text{L/min})}$$

Normal values: 770–1500 dyne-sec-cm^{-5}

PULMONARY VASCULAR RESISTANCE (dyne-sec-cm^{-5})

$= PVR$

$$= \frac{80 \times (Pulmonary\ artery\ \overline{BP} - Pulmonary\ capillary\ wedge\ pressure)}{CO\ (\text{L/min})}$$

Normal values: 20–120 dyne-sec-cm^{-5}

TOTAL PULMONARY RESISTANCE (dyne-sec-cm^{-5})

$= TPR$

$$= \frac{80 \times Pulmonary\ artery\ \overline{BP}}{CO\ (\text{L/min})}$$

CAPILLARY FLUID FILTRATION

$= \dot{Q}_f$

$= k(P_{cap} - P_{is}) - k\sigma(\pi_{cap} - \pi_{is})$

Nutritional Calculations

BODY MASS INDEX

$= BMI$

$$= \frac{Weight\ (\text{kg})}{(Height\ (\text{cm}))^2}$$

CALORIC CONTENT OF FOODS

Foodtype	Kcal/gm	
Carbohydrate	3.4	*Range 3.4–4.1*
Protein	4.0	*Range 3.3–4.7*
Fat	9.1	*Range 9.1–9.5*

RESPIRATORY QUOTIENT

$$= \frac{CO_2\ production\ (\text{ml/min})}{O_2\ consumption\ (\text{ml/min})}$$

$$= \frac{\dot{V}CO_2}{\dot{V}O_2}$$

RELATIONSHIP OF FUEL BURNED TO RESPIRATORY QUOTIENT

Fuel	*R*
Ketones	<0.6
Fat	0.7
Carbohydrate	1.0
Lipogenesis	>1.0

NITROGEN BALANCE

$= Nitrogen\ consumed - Nitrogen\ excreted$

$$= \frac{Protein\ calories\ (\text{kcal/day})}{25} - Urine\ nitrogen\ (\text{gm/day}) - 5\ (\text{gm/day})$$

HARRIS-BENEDICT EQUATION OF RESTING ENERGY EXPENDITURE (kcal/day)

Males $= 66 + (13.7 \times Weight\ [\text{kg}]) + (5 \times Height\ [\text{cm}]) - (6.8 \times Age)$

Females $= 655 + (9.6 \times Weight\ [\text{kg}]) + (1.8 \times Height\ [\text{cm}]) - (4.7 \times Age)$

WEIR EQUATION (MODIFIED) OF ENERGY EXPENDITURE (kcal/day)

$= (3.94 \times \dot{V}O_2\ [\text{ml/min}]) + (1.11 \times \dot{V}CO_2\ [\text{ml/min}])$

Pulmonary Calculations

TIDAL VOLUME

$= V_T$

$= Dead\ space\ +\ Alveolar\ space$

$= V_D + V_A$

ALVEOLAR GAS EQUATION

$$P_{A}O_2 = P_{I}O_2 - \frac{PaCO_2}{R}$$

$$= F_{I}O_2\ (P_{atm} - P_{H_2O}) - \frac{PaCO_2}{R}$$

$$= 150 - \frac{PaCO_2}{R}\ (room\ air,\ sea\ level)$$

ALVEOLAR ARTERIOLAR GRADIENT

$= A - a\ gradient$

$= P_{A}O_2 - PaO_2$

Normal values (upright): $2.5 + (0.21 \times age)$

MINUTE VENTILATION (L/min)

$= \dot{V}_E$

$$= k\ \frac{\dot{V}CO_2}{PaCO_2}$$

$$= \frac{0.863 \times \dot{V}CO_2\ (ml/min)}{PaCO_2\ (1 - V_D/V_T)}$$

Normal values: 4–6 L/min

BOHR EQUATION OF DEAD SPACE

$$V_D/V_T = \frac{PACO_2 - P_{E}CO_2}{PACO_2}$$

Normal values: 0.2–0.3

PHYSIOLOGIC DEAD SPACE

$$V_D/V_T = \frac{PaCO_2 - P_{E}CO_2}{PaCO_2}$$

Normal values: 0.2–0.3

OXYGEN DISSOLVED IN BLOOD (ml/dl)

$= D_{O_2}$

$= 0.003\ (ml\ O_2/dl) \times PaO_2\ (mm\ Hg)$

OXYGEN CAPACITY OF HEMOGLOBIN (ml O_2/dl)

$= 1.39\ (ml\ O_2) \times Hgb\ (gm/dl)$

Normal values: 17–24 ml/dl

OXYGEN CONTENT OF THE BLOOD (ml/dl)

$= C_{O_2}$

$= D_{O_2} + (1.39 \times Hgb\ [gm/dl] \times [\%\ Hgb\ saturated\ with\ O_2])$

$= D_{O_2} + (1.39 \times Hgb\ [gm/dl] \times S_{O_2})$

Normal values: 17.5–23.5 ml/dl)

PERCENTAGE OF SATURATION OF HEMOGLOBIN WITH OXYGEN

$= S_{O_2}$

$$= 100 \times \frac{C_{O_2} - D_{O_2}}{1.39 \times Hgb\ (gm/dl)}$$

Normal values: >95%

PHYSIOLOGIC SHUNT

$= \dot{Q}_S/\dot{Q}_T$

$$= \frac{C_{cap}O_2 - C_{O_2}}{C_{cap}O_2 - C_{v}O_2}$$

$$= \frac{1.39 \times Hgb\ (gm/dl) + 0.003 \times PaO_2 - CaO_2}{1.39 \times Hgb\ (gm/dl) + 0.003 \times PaO_2 - C\bar{v}O_2}$$

Normal values: <5%

COMPLIANCE

$= \Delta V/\Delta P\ (ml/cm\ H_2O)$

On Mechanical Ventilation

$$Static\ compliance = C_{st} = \frac{V_T}{P_{plateau} - P_{end\ exp}}$$

$$Dynamic\ effective\ complicance = C_{dyn} = \frac{V_T}{P_{peak} - P_{end\ exp}}$$

During Spontaneous Breathing

$$Compliance\ of\ the\ lung = C_L = \frac{V_T}{P_{alveolus} - P_{pleura}}$$

$$Compliance\ of\ the\ chest\ wall = CW_{cw} = \frac{V_T}{P_{pleura} - P_{atm}}$$

$$Compliance\ of\ the\ respiratory\ system = C_{rs} = \frac{V_T}{P_{alveolus} - P_{atm}}$$

Normal values: C_{st} >60 ml/cm H_2O; C_{dyn} >60 ml/cm H_2O
C_L >200 ml/cm H_2O; C_{rs} >100 ml/cm H_2O

RESISTANCE—OHM'S LAW

$= \Delta P/flow = \Delta P/\dot{Q}$

normal values: airway resistance of the lung at functional residual capacity (FRC) = 2 cm H_2O/L/sec

WORK OF BREATHING

$$W_{Thorax} = \int_{t_1}^{t_2} (P_{aw} - P_{atm})\dot{V}dt$$

$$W_{Lung} = \int_{t_1}^{t_2} (P_{aw} - P_{es})\dot{V}dt$$

$$W_{Chest\ wall} = \int_{t_1}^{t_2} (P_{es} - P_{atm})\dot{V}dt$$

Normal values: W_{thorax} = 0.5 kg-M/min

LAPLACE'S LAW OF SURFACE TENSION OF A SPHERE

$P = 2T/r$

POISEUILLE'S LAW OF LAMINAR FLOW

$$\dot{V} = \frac{P\pi r^4}{8\eta l}$$

Electrolyte and Renal Calculations

ANION GAP

$$= [Na^+] - [Cl^-] - [HCO_3^-]$$

Normal values: 9–13 mEq/L

CALCULATED SERUM OSMOLALITY

$$= 2[Na^+] + \frac{[Glucose]}{18} + \frac{[BUN]}{2.8}$$

Normal values: 275–290 mOsm/kg

OSMOLAR GAP

$$= \text{Serum osmolality measured} - \text{Serum osmolality calculated}$$

Normal values: 0–5 mOsm/kg

PH AND K$^+$

$[K^+]$ *increases 0.6 mEq/L for each 0.1 decrease in pH*

$[K^+]$ *decreases 0.6 mEq/L for each 0.1 increase in pH*

NA$^+$ AND GLUCOSE

$[Na^+]$ *decreases 1 mEq/L for each 62 mg/dl increase in [glucose]*

CA$^+$ AND ALBUMIN

$[Ca^+]$ *decreases 0.8 mg/dl for each 1.0 gm/dl decrease in albumin*

GLOMERULAR FILTRATION RATE = GFR

$$\text{Measured} = \text{creatinine clearance} = \frac{U_{Creat}V}{P_{Creat}}$$

$$= \frac{[Creatinine]_{urine}\ (gm/dl) \times \dfrac{Urine\ volume\ (ml/day)}{1440\ (min/day)}}{[Creatinine]_{plasma}\ (mg/dl)}$$

$$\text{Estimated for males} = \frac{(140 - Age) \times (Lean\ body\ weight\ [kg])}{P_{Creat} \times 72}$$

$$\text{Estimated for females} = 0.85 \times Male\ estimate$$

Normal values: 74–160 ml/min

WATER DEFICIT IN HYPERNATREMIA (L)

$$= 0.6 \times (Body\ weight\ [kg]) \times \left(\frac{[Na^+]}{140} - 1\right)$$

WATER EXCESS IN HYPONATREMIA (L)

$$= 0.6 \times (Body\ weight\ [kg]) \times \left(1 - \frac{[Na^+]}{140}\right)$$

FRACTIONAL EXCRETION OF SODIUM

$$= F_E Na$$

$$= \frac{Excreted\ Na^+}{Filtered\ Na^+} \times 100$$

$$= \frac{U_{Na+} \times V}{GFR} \times [Na^+] \times 100$$

$$= \frac{U_{Na+}/[Na^+]}{U_{Creat}/[Creat]}$$

Acid-Base Formulas

HENDERSON-HASSELBALCH EQUATION

$$pH = pK + \log\frac{[HCO_3^-]}{0.03 \times PaCO_2}$$

HENDERSON'S EQUATION FOR CONCENTRATION OF H$^+$

$$[H^+]\ (nM/L) = 24 \times \frac{PaCO_2}{[HCO_3^-]}$$

METABOLIC ACIDOSIS

Bicarbonate deficit (mEq/L) $= 0.5 \times (body\ weight\ [kg]) \times (24 - [HCO_3^-])$

Expected $PCO_2 = 1.5 \times [HCO_3^-] + 8 \pm 2$

METABOLIC ALKALOSIS

Bicarbonate excess $= 0.4 \times (Body\ weight\ [kg]) \times ([HCO_3^-] - 24)$

RESPIRATORY ACIDOSIS

Acute: $\dfrac{\Delta H^+}{\Delta PaCO_2} = 0.8$

Chronic: $\dfrac{\Delta H^+}{\Delta PaCO_2} = 0.3$

Neurologic Calculations

GLASCOW COMA SCALE (3–15)

= *Eyes* (1–4) + *Motor* (1–6) + *Verbal* (1–5)

Normal value: 15

Table A-1. Specific Components of the Glasgow Coma Scale

Eye opening	
Spontaneous	4
To speech	3
To pain	2
Nil	1
Motor response	
Obeys commands	6
Localizes	5
Withdraws	4
Exhibits abnormal flexion	3
Exhibits abnormal extension	2
Nil	1
Verbal response	
Oriented	5
Confused, conversant	4
Uses inappropriate words	3
Uses incomprehensible sounds	2
Nil	1

CEREBRAL PERFUSION PRESSURE (mm Hg)

= $\overline{BP}$ − ICP

Body Surface Area Formula and Nomogram

BODY SURFACE AREA (BSA)

= (*height* [cm])$^{0.718}$ × (*weight* [kg])$^{0.427}$ × 74.49

Fig. A-1. Nomogram for calculation of body surface area (BSA) in square meters by height and weight.

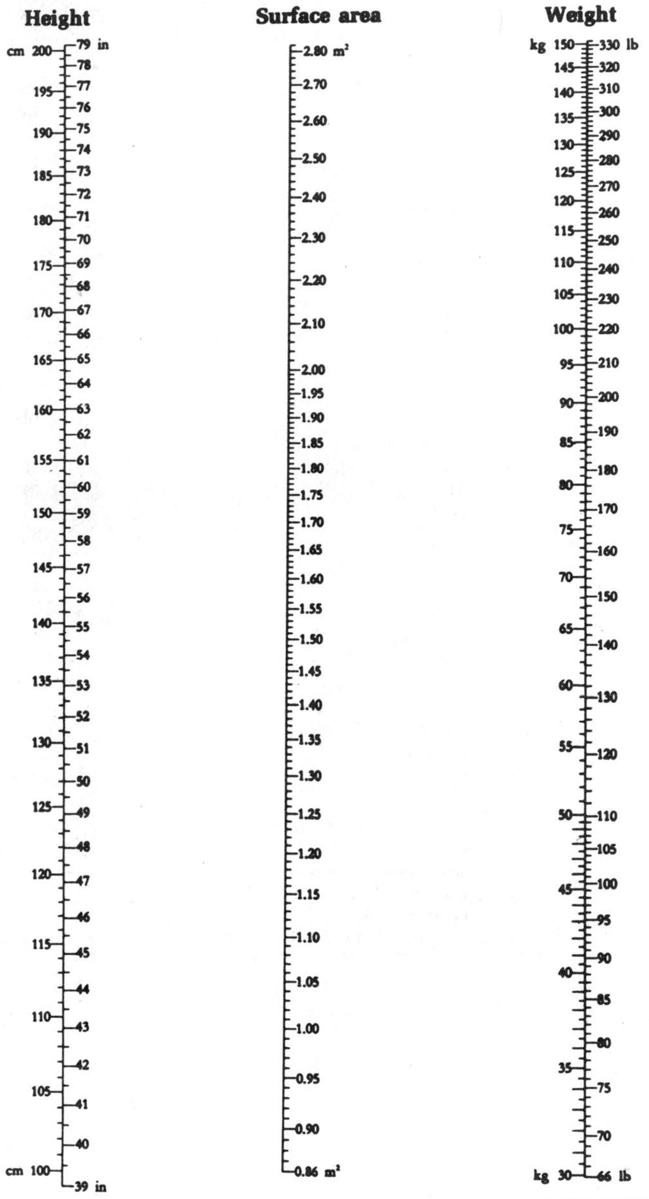

Calculation of Drug Dosage in Renal Failure

The following table summarizes approximate dosage adjustments for drugs commonly used in the ICU. Changes are indicated either as a percentage of the usual dose or as an increase in the usual interval of administration, indicated in hours. Whenever possible, the drug dosage should be adjusted with the aid of serum drug levels.

Table A-2 is not intended to be comprehensive, and more accurate adjustments may become available after the time of publication. For more information, the reader is referred to Chapter 176.

Table A-2. Approximate Drug Dosage Adjustments for Drugs Used in the ICU

Drug	GFR >50 ml/min	GFR 10–50 ml/min	GFR <10 ml/min
Vasoactive drugs			
Captopril/enalapril	100%	75%	50%
Digoxin	24 hr	36 hr	48 hr
Disopyramide	8 hr	12–24 hr	24–40 hr
Methyldopa	8 hr	8–12 hr	12–24 hr
Nadolol	100%	50%	25%
Procainamide	4 hr	6–12 hr	8–24 hr
H2 blockers			
Cimetidine/Ranitidine	100%	75%	50%
Sedatives/anesthetics			
Butorphanol	100%	75%	50%
Meperidine	100%	75%	50%
Phenobarbital	8 hr	8 hr	12–16 hr
Antibiotics			
Amikacin	12 hr	12–18 hr	24–48 hr
Ampicillin/amoxicillin	6 hr	6–12 hr	12–16 hr
Aztreonam	100%	50–75%	25%
Cefazolin	8 hr	12 hr	24–28 hr
Cefotaxime	8 hr	8–12 hr	24 hr
Cefotetan	100%	50%	25%
Cefoxitin	8 hr	8–12 hr	12–24 hr
Ceftazidime	8–12 hr	24–48 hr	48–72 hr
Cefuroxime	45–100%	10–45%	5–10%
Cephalothin	6 hr	6–8 hr	12 hr
Ciprofloxacin	12 hr	12–24 hr	24 hr
Gentamicin	8–12 hr	12 hr	24–48 hr
Imipenem	100%	50%	25%
Mezlocillin/piperacillin	4–6 hr	6–8 hr	8 hr
Penicillin G	100%	75%	25–50%
Ticarcillin	8–12 hr	12–24 hr	24–48 hr
Tobramycin	8–12 hr	12 hr	24–48 hr
Trimethoprim/sulfamethoxazole	12 hr	18 hr	24 hr
Vancomycin	24–72 hr	72–240 hr	240 hr

GFR = glomerular filtration rate.
Modified in part from Bennett WM, Aronoff GR, Golper TA, et al: *Drug Prescribing in Renal Failure.* American College of Chest Physicians, 1987.
*See Chapter 177 for more detailed information on dosing aminoglycosides.

Pharmacologic Calculations

DRUG CLEARANCE

$$= V_d \times K_{el}$$

DRUG HALF-LIFE

$$= t^{1/2}$$

$$= \frac{0.693}{K_{el}}$$

DRUG ELIMINATION CONSTANT

$$= K_{el}$$

$$= \frac{\ln\left(\frac{[Peak]}{[Trough]}\right)}{t_{peak} - t_{trough}}$$

DRUG LOADING DOSE

$$= V_d \times [Target\ peak]$$

DRUG DOSING INTERVAL

$$= \frac{-1}{K_{el}} \times \ln\left(\frac{[Desired\ trough]}{[Desired\ peak]}\right) + Infusion\ time\ (hr)$$

Fig. A-2. Calculation of Apache II Score. From Knaus WA, Draper EA, Wagner DP, et al: APACHE II: A severity of disease classification system. *Crit Care Med* 13:818, 1985. With permission.

THE APACHE II SEVERITY OF DISEASE CLASSIFICATION SYSTEM

PHYSIOLOGIC VARIABLE	HIGH ABNORMAL RANGE					LOW ABNORMAL RANGE			
	+4	+3	+2	+1	0	+1	+2	+3	+4
TEMPERATURE — rectal (°C)	≥41°	39°-40.9°		38.5°-38.9°	36°-38.4°	34°-35.9°	32°-33.9°	30°-31.9°	≤29.9°
MEAN ARTERIAL PRESSURE — mm Hg	≥160	130-159	110-129		70-109		50-69		≤49
HEART RATE (ventricular response)	≥180	140-179	110-139		70-109		55-69	40-54	≤39
RESPIRATORY RATE — (non-ventilated or ventilated)	≥50	35-49		25-34	12-24	10-11	6-9		≤5
OXYGENATION: A-aDO₂ or PaO₂ (mm Hg) a. FIO₂ ≥0.5 record A-aDO₂	≥500	350-499	200-349		<200				
b. FIO₂ <0.5 record only PaO₂					PO₂ >70	PO₂ 61-70		PO₂ 55-60	PO₂ <55
ARTERIAL pH	≥7.7	7.6-7.69		7.5-7.59	7.33-7.49		7.25-7.32	7.15-7.24	<7.15
SERUM SODIUM (mMol/L)	≥180	160-179	155-159	150-154	130-149		120-129	111-119	≤110
SERUM POTASSIUM (mMol/L)	≥7	6-6.9		5.5-5.9	3.5-5.4	3-3.4	2.5-2.9		<2.5
SERUM CREATININE (mg/100 ml) (Double point score for acute renal failure)	≥3.5	2-3.4	1.5-1.9		0.6-1.4		<0.6		
HEMATOCRIT (%)	≥60		50-59.9	46-49.9	30-45.9		20-29.9		<20
WHITE BLOOD COUNT (total/mm3) (in 1,000s)	≥40		20-39.9	15-19.9	3-14.9		1-2.9		<1
GLASGOW COMA SCORE (GCS): Score = 15 minus actual GCS									
[A] Total ACUTE PHYSIOLOGY SCORE (APS): Sum of the 12 individual variable points									
Serum HCO₃ (venous-mMol/L) [Not preferred, use if no ABGs]	≥52	41-51.9		32-40.9	22-31.9		18-21.9	15-17.9	<15

[B] AGE POINTS:
Assign points to age as follows:

AGE(yrs)	Points
≤44	0
45-54	2
55-64	3
65-74	5
≥75	6

[C] CHRONIC HEALTH POINTS
If the patient has a history of severe organ system insufficiency or is immuno-compromised assign points as follows:
a. for nonoperative or emergency postoperative patients — 5 points
or
b. for elective postoperative patients — 2 points

DEFINITIONS
Organ Insufficiency or immuno-compromised state must have been evident prior to this hospital admission and conform to the following criteria:

LIVER: Biopsy proven cirrhosis and documented portal hypertension; episodes of past upper GI bleeding attributed to portal hypertension; or prior episodes of hepatic failure/encephalopathy/coma.

CARDIOVASCULAR: New York Heart Association Class IV.

RESPIRATORY: Chronic restrictive, obstructive, or vascular disease resulting in severe exercise restriction, i.e., unable to climb stairs or perform household duties; or documented chronic hypoxia, hypercapnia, secondary polycythemia, severe pulmonary hypertension (>40mmHg), or respirator dependency.

RENAL: Receiving chronic dialysis.

IMMUNO-COMPROMISED: The patient has received therapy that suppresses resistance to infection, e.g., immuno-suppression, chemotherapy, radiation, long term or recent high dose steroids, or has a disease that is sufficiently advanced to suppress resistance to infection, e.g., leukemia, lymphoma, AIDS.

APACHE II SCORE
Sum of [A] + [B] + [C]

[A] APS points _____

[B] Age points _____

[C] Chronic Health points _____

Total APACHE II _____

Normal Values of Expiratory Peak Flow

There is a wide variability in peak expiratory flows due to individual differences. Values also vary slightly depending on the peak flow meter used.

Table A-3. Normal Values of Expiratory Peak Flow for Males

Age (Yr)	Height				
	60 Inches	65 Inches	70 Inches	75 Inches	80 Inches
20	554	602	649	693	740
25	543	590	636	679	725
30	532	577	622	664	710
35	521	565	609	651	695
40	509	552	596	636	680
45	498	540	583	622	665
50	486	527	569	607	649
55	475	515	556	593	634
60	463	502	542	578	618
65	452	490	529	564	603
70	440	477	515	550	587

Table A-4. Normal Values of Expiratory Peak Flow for Females

Age (Yr)	Height				
	55 Inches	60 Inches	65 Inches	70 Inches	75 Inches
20	390	423	460	496	529
25	385	418	454	490	523
30	380	413	448	483	516
35	375	408	442	476	509
40	370	402	436	470	502
45	365	397	430	464	495
50	360	391	424	457	488
55	355	386	418	451	482
60	350	380	412	445	475
65	345	375	406	439	468
70	340	369	400	432	461

From Leiner GC, et al: Expiratory peak flow. Standards for normal subjects. Use as a clinical test of ventilatory function. *Am Rev Respir Dis* 86:644, 1963. With permission.

Chapter 219 Tables

Nancy Y. N. Liu, David F. Giansiracusa,
and Steven L. Strongwater

Table 219A-1. The 1982 Revised Criteria for the Classification of Systemic Lupus Erythematosus (American Rheumatism Association [ARA], 1982)

1. *Butterfly Rash.* Fixed erythema, flat or raised, over the malar eminences, tending to spare the nasolabial folds.
2. *Discoid Lupus.* Erythematous raised patches with adherent keratotic sealing and follicular plugging; atrophic scarring may occur in older lesions.
3. *Photosensitivity.* Skin rash as a result of unusual reaction to sunlight, by patient history or physician observation.
4. *Oral Ulcers.* Oral or nasopharyngeal ulceration, usually painless, observed by a physician.
5. *Arthritis.* Nonerosive arthritis involving one or more peripheral joints, characterized by tenderness, swelling, or effusion.
6. *Serositis*
   a. Pleuritis—convincing history of pleuritic pain or rub heard by a physician or evidence of pleural effusion, or
   b. Pericarditis—documented by ECG or rub or evidence of pericardial effusion.
7. *Renal Disorder*
   a. Persistent proteinuria greater than 0.5 gm per day or greater than 3 + if quantitation not performed, or
   b. Cellular casts—may be red cell, hemoglobin, granular, tubular, or mixed.
8. *Neurologic Disorder*
   a. Seizures—in the absence of offending drugs or known metabolic derangements, e.g., uremia, ketoacidosis, or electrolyte imbalance, or
   b. Psychosis in the absence of offending drugs.
9. *Hematologic Disorder*
   a. Hemolytic anemia—with reticulocytosis, or
   b. *Leukopenia*—less than 4000/mm³ total on two or more occasions, or
   c. *Lymphopenia*—less than 1500/mm³ on two or more occasions, or
   d. Thrombocytopenia—less than 100,000/mm³ in the absence of offending drugs.
10. *Immunologic Disorder*
    a. Positive LE cell preparation, or
    b. Anti-DNA—presence of antibody to native DNA in abnormal titer, or
    c. Anti-Sm—presence of antibody to SM nuclear antigen, or
    d. False positive STS known to be positive for at least six months and confirmed by TPI or FTA tests.
11. *Antinuclear Antibody.* An abnormal titer of antinuclear antibody by immunofluorescence or an equivalent assay at any point in time and in the absence of drugs known to be associated with "drug-induced lupus" syndrome.

The revised classification is based on 11 criteria. For the purpose of identifying patients in clinical studies, a person shall be said to have systemic lupus erythematosus if any four or more of the 11 criteria are present, serially or simultaneously, during any interval of observation.

Source: From Tan EM, Cohen AS, Fries JF, et al: The 1982 revised criteria for the classification of systemic lupus erythematosus. *Arthritis Rheum* 25:1271, 1982.

Table 219A-2. Lupus Glomerular Nephritis: Summary of Clinical Features and Course

	Focal proliferative (FPGN)	Diffuse proliferative (DPGN)	Membranous (MGN)	Mesangial (MesGN)
Onset	Onset during first year, SLE in about half	Onset during first year, SLE in the majority	Onset during first year, SLE in half	Perhaps characteristic of all SLE from onset
Clinical manifestations	Proteinuria in all, hematuria often; nephrotic syndrome rare; occasional mild renal insufficiency; hypertension absent	Proteinuria and hematuria in all; nephrotic syndrome at onset in over half, eventually in almost all; renal insufficiency at onset in most, occasionally severe; hypertension common	Proteinuria in all at onset with rare exceptions; nephrotic syndrome at onset in four-fifths; microscopic hematuria in half; occasional hypertension and minimal renal insufficiency at onset	No clinical features of renal disease in some; minimal proteinuria and/or hematuria in others; occasional mild renal insufficiency; hypertension absent
Transition	Transitions to DPGN or MGN may occur	Transition to MesGN (with some glomerular sclerosis) or MGN may occur in association with remission	Rare transition to DPGN	Development of nephrotic syndrome with transition to DPGN or MGN may occur
Progression	Renal insufficiency does not develop	Progression to death within 2 years in half of the unremitted; death due to uremia or active SLE often with infection; no progressive renal insufficiency during remission	Slowly progressive renal insufficiency during persistent nephrotic syndrome	No progression unless transition occurs; subsequent course then determined by the form of lupus nephritis that develops
Mortality/pathology	5-year mortality <10%; focal mild proliferative IgG and C3 in mesangium and along GBM	5-year mortality <25%; cell proliferation; crescents; lumpy-bumpy immunoglobulin (Ig) and complement (C) along GBM—subendothelial	5-year mortality <25%; thick GBM; granular Ig and C on GBM (epithelial side)	Ig and C in mesangium

Source: From Schur PH: Clinical Features of SLE, in Kelly WN, Harris ED, Ruddy S, Sledge CB (eds): *Textbook of Rheumatology.* Philadelphia, WB Saunders, 1989, p 1113, with permission.

Table 219A-3. Neuropsychiatric Manifestations of Systemic Lupus

NONFOCAL CEREBRAL DYSFUNCTION (35–60%)

Organic brain disease
  Psychosis
  Affective disorders
  Neurosis

SEIZURES (15–35%)

  Grand mal
  Petit mal
  Temporal lobe
  Focal

FOCAL DEFICITS (10–35%)

  Strokes
  Transverse myelitis
  Cranial neuropathies
  Visual deficits
  Optic neuritis
  Retinal infarction
  Nystagmus
  Ophthalmoplegias
  Ptosis
  Sensorineural hearing loss, tinnitus, vertigo
  Trigeminal neuralgia
  Facial palsy (unilateral or bilateral)

PERIPHERAL NEUROPATHIES (10–15%)

  Stocking glove
  Guillain-Barré syndrome
  Mononeuritis multiplex

MOVEMENT DISORDERS (<5%)

  Athetosis
  Chorea
  Hemiballismus
  Parkinson-like
  Cerebellar infarction

OTHER

  Headache (frequent)
  Aseptic meningitis
  Multiple sclerosis-like
  Eaton-Lambert syndrome
  Myasthenia gravis
  Infection

Source: From McCune WJ, Golbus J: Neuropsychiatric lupus. *Rheum Dis Clin North Am* 14:150, 1988, with permission.

Table 219A-4. Classification of Polymyositis and Dermatomyositis

1. Idiopathic polymyositis
2. Idiopathic dermatomyositis
3. Myositis with features of other connective tissue diseases (overlap group)
4. Idiopathic myositis of childhood
5. Myositis associated with malignancy
6. Miscellaneous
   Inclusion body myositis
   Eosinophilic myositis
   Localized nodular myositis
   Proliferative myositis
   Infectious myositis

Table 219A-5. Drugs Implicated in Human Muscle Disease

PROXIMAL MYOPATHIES WITH ELEVATED MUSCLE ENZYMES

Clofibrate
ε-Aminocaproic acid
Emetine
Heroin
Alcohol
Vincristine
Colchicine
D-Penicillamine
Cocaine
L-Tryptophan

POSSIBLY ASSOCIATED WITH PROXIMAL MYOPATHY

Isoetharine
Danazol
Cimetidine
Metolazone
Bumetanide
Lithium

PROXIMAL MYOPATHY DUE TO HYPOKALEMIA

Diuretics
Purgatives (bulemia)
Liquorice
Carbenoxolone
Amphotericin B

RHABDOMYOLYSIS

Heroin
Amphetamines
Alcohol
Lovastatin

SUBACUTE PAINLESS PROXIMAL MYOPATHY

Chloroquine
Hydroxychloroquine
Corticosteroids
Alcohol

FOCAL MYOPATHY*

Meperidine
Pentazocine
?Opiates

MYASTHENIC SYNDROME

Aminoglycosides
Polymyxin B
Tetracycline
Succinylcholine
C-Penicillamine
Propranolol
Practolol
?Other beta-blockers
Phenytoin
Chlorpromazine
Procainamide
Trimethadione

MALIGNANT HYPERPYREXIA

Suxamethonium
Halothane
Diethyl ether
Cyclopropane
Chloroform
Methoxyflurane
Ketamine
Enflurane
Psychotropics

*Drugs given intramuscularly.

Table 219A-6. Infectious Causes of Myositis

BACTERIAL

Staphylococcus aureus (pyomyositis)
Streptococcus pyogenes; post *S. pneumoniae* infection
Clostridium perfringens

VIRAL

Influenza
Coxsackievirus A and B (particularly B5)
Echovirus 9
Adenovirus 2, 21
Human immunodeficiency virus

PARASITIC

Trichinosis
Toxocariasis
Cysticercosis
Toxoplasmosis
Amebiasis
Sarcosporidiosis
Echinococcosis
Trypanosomiasis
Actinomycosis

Table 219A-7. Immunologic Disorders Reported in Association With Polymyositis and Dermatomyositis

Connective tissue syndromes	Other immunologic disorders
Eosinophilic fasciitis	Agammaglobulinemia
Psoriasis	Amyloidosis
Rheumatoid arthritis	Celiac diseases
Sarcoidosis	Complement (C2) deficiency
Scleroderma	Diffuse interstitial pulmonary fibrosis
Sjögren's syndrome	
Systemic lupus erythematosus	Acquired immunodeficiency syndrome
Vasculitis (polyarteritis nodosa)	IgA deficiency
	Malignancies
	Myasthenia gravis

Table 219A-8. Pathogenic Organisms in Bronchopneumonia Complicating Polymyositis and Dermatomyositis

Pseudomonas aeruginosa
Cryptococcus neoformans
Staphylococcus aureus
Nocardia asteroides
Candida albicans
Mucormycosis
Pneumocystis carinii
Hemophilus influenzae
Streptococcus pyogenes
Streptococcus pneumoniae
Aerobacter aerogenes

Table 219A-9. Cardiac Manifestations in Polymyositis and Dermatomyositis

Myocarditis
Pericarditis
Congestive cardiomyopathy
Hyperdynamic syndrome
Mitral insufficiency; mitral valve prolapse
Conduction disturbances
    Complete heart block (His bundle and/or its branches)
    Atrioventricular or intraventricular delays
Arrhythmias
    Atrial fibrillation
    Supraventricular tachyarrhythmias
    Ventricular tachycardia
Other
    Axis shifts
    Repolarization abnormalities

Source: Strongwater SL, Annesley T, Schnitzer TJ: Myocardial involvement in polymgositis. *J Rheumatol* 10:459, 1983.

Index

Index